Brief Contents

FOCUS ON
ADULT HEALTH
Medical-Surgical Nursing

SECOND EDITION

FOCUS ON
ADULT HEALTH
Medical-Surgical Nursing

SECOND EDITION

Linda Honan, RN, PhD, CNS-BC, ANEF, FAAN

Professor
Yale University School of Nursing
New Haven, Connecticut

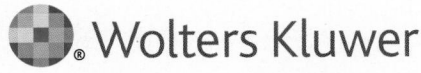

. Wolters Kluwer

Philadelphia • Baltimore • New York • London
Buenos Aires • Hong Kong • Sydney • Tokyo

Vice President and Publisher: Julie K. Stegman
Executive Editor: Kelley Squazzo
Director of Product Development: Jennifer K. Forestieri
Senior Development Editor: Helen Kogut and Michael Kerns
Editorial Coordinator: John Larkin
Senior Marketing Manager: Katie Schlesinger
Editorial Assistant: Leo Gray
Design Coordinator: Holly McLaughlin
Art Director, Illustration: Jennifer Clements
Production Project Manager: Marian Bellus
Manufacturing Coordinator: Karin Duffield
Prepress Vendor: Aptara, Inc.

2nd Edition

9 8 7 6 5 4 3 2 1

Printed in China

Library of Congress Cataloging-in-Publication Data

ISBN-13: 978-1-4963-4928-6
ISBN-10: 1-4963-4928-8
Cataloging-in-Publication data available on request from the Publisher.

LWW.com

For Ryan and Katie

Contributors

Deborah S. Adelman, PhD, RN, NE-BC
Professor
Graduate Nursing Programs
School of Nursing
Kaplan University
Chicago, Illinois
Chapter 56, Nursing Management: Emergencies and Disasters

Laura Kierol Andrews, PhD, APRN, ACNP-BC
Associate Professor
Yale University School of Nursing
New Haven, Connecticut
And
Senior Acute Care Nurse Practitioner
Critical Care Medicine
Hospital of Central Connecticut at New Britain General
New Britain, Connecticut
Chapter 10, Nursing Management: Patients with Chest and Lower Respiratory Tract Disorders

Donna M. Avanecean, RN, FNP-BC, CNRN, DNPc
Nurse Practitioner
Yale New Haven Hospital
New Haven, Connecticut
Chapter 43, Nursing Assessment: Neurologic Function

Mei Bai, RN, PhD
Post-Doctoral Associate
Yale University School of Medicine
New Haven, Connecticut
Chapter 3, Chronic Illness and End-of-Life Care

Lisa M. Barbarotta, MSN, AOCNS, APRN-BC
Program Manager
Oncology Nursing Education & Practice
Smilow Cancer Hospital at Yale-New Haven
New Haven, Connecticut
Chapter 6, Cancer Care
Chapter 19, Nursing Assessment: Hematologic Function
Chapter 20, Nursing Management: Patient with Hematologic Disorders

Mary E. Bartlett, DNP, APRN, FNP-BC, AAHIVS
Family Nurse Practitioner and HIV Specialist
Assistant Professor
Linfield Good Samaritan School of Nursing
Portland, Oregon
Chapter 36, Nursing Assessment: Immune Function
Chapter 37, Nursing Management: Patients with Immunodeficiency, HIV Infection, and AIDS

Cynthia Bautista, PhD, RN, CNRN, SCRN, CCNS, ACNS-BC, FNCS
Associate Professor
Marion Peckham Egan School of Nursing and
    Health Studies
Fairfield University
Fairfield, Connecticut
Chapter 46, Nursing Management: Patients with Neurologic Disorders

Dawn K. Beland, RN, MSN, CCRN-K, ACNS-BC, CNRN, SCRN
Stroke Center Coordinator
Hartford Hospital
Hartford, Connecticut
Chapter 43, Nursing Assessment: Neurologic Function

Lynn S. Bickley, MD, FACP
Clinical Professor of Internal Medicine School of Medicine
University of New Mexico
Albuquerque, New Mexico
Chapter 48, Nursing Assessment: Sensorineural Function

Carolynn Spera Bruno, PhD, APRN, CNS, FNP-C
Clinical Assistant Professor of Nursing
New York University
Rory Meyers College of Nursing
New York, New York
Chapter 49, Nursing Management: Patients with Eye and Vision Disorders
Chapter 50, Nursing Management: Patients with Hearing and Balance Disorders

Nicole C. Colline, RN, MSN, APRN-BC
Clinical Faculty
Yale University School of Nursing
New Haven, Connecticut
And
Nurse Practitioner & Clinical Manager
MedNow Family Walk-In & Industrial Medical Center
Stratford, Connecticut
Chapter 38, Nursing Management: Patients with Allergic Disorders

Jessica Shank Coviello, DNP, APRN, ANP-BC
Associate Professor/Onco-cardiology Nurse Practitioner
Doctor of Nursing Practice Program
Yale University School of Nursing and Smilow Cancer
    Hospital at Yale-New Haven
New Haven, Connecticut
Chapter 15, Nursing Management: Patients with Complications from Heart Disease

Linda S. Dune, RN, PhD, CNL
Program Director
College of Nursing and Public Health at South University
Austin, Texas
Chapter 48, Nursing Assessment: Sensorineural Function

Christa Palancia Esposito, DNP(c), MS, BSN, CNM
Certified Nurse Midwife
Women's Healthcare of Trumbull
Trumbull, Connecticut
Chapter 35, Nursing Management: Patients with Sexually Transmitted Infections

Deborah Bain Fahs
Assistant Professor
Yale University School of Nursing
New Haven, Connecticut
And
Family Nurse Practitioner
Yale Health Center, New Haven, Connecticut
Chapter 21, Nursing Assessment: Digestive, Gastrointestinal, and Metabolic Function
Chapter 26, Nursing Assessment: Renal and Urinary Tract Function

Geriann B. Gallagher, DNP, APRN, MAOM, LicAc
Orthopedic Nurse Practitioner, Acupuncturist
Uconn Health
Storrs, Connecticut
And
Clinical Instructor
Yale University School of Nursing
New Haven, Connecticut
Chapter 40, Nursing Assessment: Musculoskeletal Function
Chapter 41, Nursing Management: Patients with Musculoskeletal Disorders

Kelly S. Grimshaw, DNP(c), RN, MSN, APRN, CCRN, CCTN
Service Line Educator, Transplant
Yale New Haven Hospital
New Haven, Connecticut
And
Member, Board of Directors
Médecins Sans Frontières—USA
New York, New York
Chapter 1, The Nurse's Role in Adult Health Nursing
Chapter 55, Nursing Management: Critical Care

Margaret Campbell Haggerty, APRN, AE-C
Pulmonary Nurse Practitioner
Former Director, Pulmonary Rehabilitation
Norwalk Hospital
Norwalk, Connecticut
Chapter 11, Nursing Management of Patients Diagnosed with Chronic Obstructive Pulmonary Disease and Asthma

Linda Honan, RN, PhD, CNS-BC, ANEF, FAAN
Professor
Yale University School of Nursing
New Haven, Connecticut
Chapter 4, Fluid and Electrolyte and Acid–Base Imbalances
Chapter 7, Pain Management
Chapter 8, Nursing Assessment: Respiratory Function
Chapter 42, Nursing Management: Patients with Musculoskeletal Trauma
Chapter 54, Nursing Management: Shock and Multisystem Failure

Tara Driesen Jennings, MSN, ANP-BC
Adjunct Faculty
Simmons College
And
Nurse Practitioner
Department of Neurology
Massachusetts General Hospital
Boston, Massachusetts
Chapter 45, Nursing Management: Patients with Neurologic Trauma

Jill S. Keller, RN, MSN, FNP-BC, AOCNP
Nurse Practitioner—Oncology
Bridgeport Hospital
Bridgeport, Connecticut
Chapter 44, Nursing Management: Patients with Oncologic Disorders of the Brain and Spinal Cord

Honore Kotler, RN, MSN, ACNP, PhD(c)
Lead Nurse Practitioner
Comprehensive Transplant Center
Cedars Sinai Medical Center
Los Angeles, California
Chapter 25, Nursing Management: Patients with Hepatic and Biliary Disorders

Zachary R. Krom, RN, MSN, CCRN
Education Program Coordinator
Critical Care Services
Cedars-Sinai Medical Center
Los Angeles, California
Chapter 22, Nursing Management: Patients with Oral
and Esophageal Disorders and Patients Receiving
Gastrointestinal Intubation, Enteral, and Parenteral
Nutrition

Jacqueline Laird, BSN, RN, CNML
Nurse Manager
Connecticut Burn Center & Center for Wound Healing and
 Hyperbaric Medicine
Yale-New Haven Health System
Bridgeport Hospital
Bridgeport, Connecticut
Chapter 53, Nursing Management: Patients with
Burn Injury

Michelle J. Lajiness, BSN, MS, FNP-BC
Nurse Practitioner—Urology
Detroit Medical Center
Detroit, Michigan
Chapter 26, Nursing Assessment: Renal and Urinary
Tract Function

James Mark Lazenby, RN, APRN, PhD, FAAN
Associate Professor of Nursing
Divinity Core Faculty
Council on Middle East Studies
Yale University School of Nursing
And
Advanced Oncology Certified Nurse Practitioner
Smilow Cancer Hospital at Yale-New Haven
New Haven, Connecticut
Chapter 3, Chronic Illness and End-of-Life Care

Rosalina Madrid, MSN, RN-C, CHPN, FNP-BC
Nurse Practitioner, Pain Medicine
Inpatient Pain Service
Department of Nursing
Department of Anesthesiology
Cedars-Sinai Medical Center
Los Angeles, California
Chapter 7, Pain Management

Gayge J. Maggio, MSN, FNP-BC, AAHIVS
Street Medicine Program Supervisor—Breaking Ground
Primary Care Provider
Janian Medical Care, P.C.
And
Medical Provider
Callen-Lorde Community Health Center
New York, New York
Chapter 29, Nursing Assessment: Endocrine Function

Andrea Rothman Mann, RN, MSN, CNE
Program Director
Aria Health School of Nursing
Trevose, Pennsylvania
Chapter 13, Nursing Management: Patients with
Hypertension
Chapter 27, Nursing Management: Patients with
Renal Disorders

**Philip R. Martinez, Jr., EdD, MSN, APRN-BC,
CCRN-CMC**
GEPN Program Director & Full-Time Lecturer
 in Nursing
Yale University School of Nursing
New Haven, Connecticut
And
Advanced Practice Registered Nurse
Department of Pulmonary and Critical Care
 Medicine
Middlesex Hospital
Middletown, Connecticut
Chapter 4, Fluid and Electrolyte and Acid–Base
Imbalances
Chapter 24, Nursing Management: Patients with
Intestinal and Rectal Disorders
Chapter 54, Nursing Management: Shock and
Multisystem Failure

**Jeanine L. May, MSN, MPH, APRN,
ACNP-BC**
Nurse Practitioner
Yale Center for Clinical Investigation
Yale School of Medicine
New Haven, Connecticut
Chapter 16, Nursing Management: Patients with
Structural, Inflammatory and Infectious Cardiac
Disorders

Ruth McCorkle, RN, PhD, FAAN
Florence Wald Professor of Nursing
Yale University School of Nursing
New Haven, Connecticut
Chapter 3, Chronic Illness and End-of-Life
Care

Jennifer L. Mosher, MSN, WHNP-BC, CUNP
Women's Health Nurse Practitioner
Mercy Health Bladder Clinic
Muskegon, Michigan
Chapter 32, Nursing Assessment: Female and Male
Reproductive Function

Karin V. Nyström, MSN, APRN, FAHA
Stroke Program Manager and Nurse Practitioner
Department of Neurology
Yale-New Haven Hospital
New Haven, Connecticut
Chapter 47, Nursing Management: Patients with
Cerebrovascular Disorders

Janet A. Parkosewich, RN, DNSc, FAHA
Nurse Researcher
Yale-New Haven Hospital
New Haven, Connecticut
Chapter 12, Nursing Assessment: Cardiovascular and
Circulatory Function

**Mary G. Pierson, MSN, APRN, ACNS-BC,
CNML**
Assistant Patient Services Manager
HVC and Thoracic Surgery Step-Down Unit
Yale-New Haven Hospital
New Haven, Connecticut
Chapter 14, Nursing Management: Patients with
Coronary Vascular Disorders

Linda Alessie Podolak, DNP, RN, ACNS-BC
Director
Bridgeport Hospital School of Nursing
Bridgeport, Connecticut
Chapter 39, Nursing Management: Patients with
Rheumatic Disorders

**Vanessa Pomarico-Denino, EdD(c), MSN, APRN,
FNP-BC, FAANP**
Nurse Practitioner
Northeast Medical Group
Hamden, Connecticut
And
Senior Lecturer
Fitzgerald Health Education Associates (FHEA)
Andover, Massachusetts
Chapter 33, Nursing Management: Patients with
Breast and Female Reproductive Disorders

Joann Preece, MSN, RN, CAPA
Professional Development Specialist
Surgical Services
Middlesex Hospital
Middletown Connecticut
And
Adjunct Faculty
Quinnipiac University
Hamden, Connecticut
And
Part Time Faculty
Chamberlain College of Nursing
Chicago, Illinois
Chapter 5, Perioperative Nursing

Jancee Pust-Marcone, MS, RN, CCRN
Program Director—Post Baccalaureate Nurse Residency &
    VA Academy
VA Connecticut Healthcare System
West Haven, Connecticut
And
Part-Time Faculty—Clinical
School of Nursing at Quinnipiac University
Hamden, Connecticut
Chapter 9, Nursing Management: Patients with Upper
Respiratory Tract Disorders
Chapter 23, Nursing Management: Patients with
Gastric and Duodenal Disorders

**Susanne A. Quallich, PhD, ANP-BC, NP-C, CUNP,
FANNP**
Andrology Nurse Practitioner
Division of Andrology and Urologic Health
Department of Urology
Michigan Medicine
University of Michigan Health System
Ann Arbor, Michigan
Chapter 28, Nursing Management: Patients with
Urinary Disorders
Chapter 32, Nursing Assessment: Female and Male
Reproductive Function
Chapter 34, Nursing Management: Patients with Male
Reproductive Disorders

Susan Seiboldt, RN, MSN, CNE
Assistant Professor of Nursing
Carl Sandburg College
Galesburg, Illinois
Unit Case Studies and Related Answers
NCLEX-Style Review Questions,
Chapters 18, 36, 43, 47, 52

Mary Sieggreen, MSN, NP, APRN-BC, CVN
Nurse Practitioner, Vascular Surgery
DMC Harper University Hospital
Detroit, Michigan
Chapter 18, Nursing Management: Patients with
Vascular Disorders and Problems of Peripheral
Circulation

Elaine Siow, RN, MSN, PhD
Professional Consultant
The Nethersole School of Nursing
The Chinese University of Hong Kong
Hong Kong
Chapter 31, Nursing Management: Patients with
Endocrine Disorders

**Edith Caroline Smith, DNP, CNM, WHNP-BC,
AGN-BC**
Former Director, High Risk and Cancer Genetics Program
Pink Lotus Breast Center
Beverly Hills, California
Chapter 33, Nursing Management: Patients with
Breast and Female Reproductive Disorders

Peter G. Szilagyi, MD, MPH
Professor of Pediatrics and Executive Vice-Chair
  Department of Pediatrics
University of California at Los Angeles (UCLA)
Los Angeles, California
Chapter 48, Nursing Assessment: Sensorineural
Function

Kathryn W. Tierney, MSN, APRN-BC, FNP
Division of Endocrinology
Middlesex Multispeciality Group
Middlesex Hospital
Middletown, Connecticut
Chapter 30, Nursing Management: Diabetes Mellitus

Commander Patina S. Walton-Battle, DNP, APRN, FNP-C, RN-BC, CWCN-AP, CFCN
Commissioned Corps Public Health Services
Health Services Administrator
Advanced Practice Registered Nurse
Federal Bureau of Prisons National Wound Care Team
Edgefield, South Carolina
Chapter 51, Nursing Assessment: Integumentary
Function
Chapter 52, Nursing Management: Patients with
Dermatologic Problems

Carol Ann Wetmore, RN, MSN
Assistant Clinical Professor
University of Connecticut
Storrs, Connecticut
Chapter 2, Health Education and Health
Promotion

Catherine G. Winkler, PhD, MPH, APRN-BC
Nurse Practitioner
Western Connecticut Medical Group
Danbury, Connecticut
And
Adjunct Faculty
Marion Peckham Egan School of Nursing and Health
  Studies
Fairfield University
Fairfield, Connecticut
Chapter 17, Nursing Management: Patients with
Arrhythmias and Conduction Problems

Reviewers

Joyce Brasfield Adams, EdS
Instructor
Hinds Community College
Jackson, Mississippi

Hannah M. Anderson, MSN, RN-BC
Associate Professor and Nursing Program Coordinator
Thomas Nelson Community College
Hampton, Virginia

Sheri L. Banovic, MSN, RN, FNP-BC
Associate Professor and Nursing Program Coordinator
Lewis and Clark Community College
Godfrey, Illinois

Wanda G. Barlow, MSN, RN, FNP
Nursing Instructor
Winston-Salem State University
Winston-Salem, North Carolina

Joyce Basham, MN, CNS
Nursing Instructor
Midlands Technical College
Columbia, South Carolina

Mary Bergmann, MSN, RN
Professor
San Antonio College
San Antonio, Texas

Roberta Bernardini, MSN, BSN
Professor
Tidewater Community College
Portsmouth, Virginia

Sabrina T. Beroz, MSN, RN
Professor
Montgomery College
Takoma Park, Maryland

Jason Berry, MSN, BSN
Nursing Instructor
Winston-Salem State University
Winston-Salem, North Carolina

Sophia Beydoun, MSN, RN
Nursing Faculty
Henry Ford Community College
Dearborn, Michigan

Deborah A. Beyer, MSN, RN
Assistant Professor
Miami University
Hamilton, Ohio

Carol Blakeman, MSN, ARNP
Professor
College of Central Florida
Ocala, Florida

Jill E. Bobb, RN, BSN
Program Administrator of Nursing
Edison State Community College
Piqua, Ohio

Joy Borrero, MSN, RN, APRN
Instructor
Suffolk County Community College in Brentwood
Brentwood, New York

Cynthia A. Bowman, MSN, RNC, CNE
Nursing Instructor
Penn State
Altoona, Pennsylvania

Rebecca Bowman, MSN, BSN
Professor of Nursing
Florida State College at Jacksonville
Jacksonville, Florida

Angie Brindowski, MSN, BSN, RN
Clinical Assistant Professor
Carroll University
Waukesha, Wisconsin

Victoria Brioso-Ang, MSN, RN, CNE
Associate Professor
Sentara College of Health Sciences
Chespeake, Virginia

Michele Bunning, MSN, RN
Associate Professor
Good Samaritan College of Nursing & Health Science
Cincinnati, Ohio

Schvon Bussey, MSN, FNP
Instructor
Albany Technical College
Albany, Georgia

Darlene M. Cantu, MSN, RNC
Assistant Professor
San Antonio College
San Antonio, Texas

Theresa Capriotti, DO, MSN, RN, CRNP
Clinical Associate Professor
Villanova University
Villanova, Pennsylvania

Cecelia Carew, MA, RN-BC, CNE, CCRN, CPAN, CEN, LNC
Associate Professor
Department of Nursing
Bronx Community College
Bronx, New York

Kristine Carey, MSN, RN
Nursing Faculty
Normandale Community College
Bloomington, Minnesota

Arica Carter
Instructor
Atlanta Technical College
Atlanta, Georgia

Mary Rose Chasler, MSN, RN
Associate Professor of Nursing
Jamestown Community College
Jamestown, New York

Fran Cherkis, DHSc, RN, CNE
Instructor
Farmingdale State College
Farmingdale, New York

Maria J. Colón, MSN, RN
Faculty Professor
Inter American University of Puerto Rico---Metropolitan
    Campus
San Juan, Puerto Rico

Ruth S. Conner, PhD(c), RN, FNP-BC
Instructor
Medical University of South Carolina
Charleston, South Carolina

Patricia Dale Cork, MS, BSN, RN
Assistant Director
Riverside School of Professional Nursing and Riverside
    School of Practical Nursing
Newport News, Virginia

Theresa Delahoyde, EdD, RN
Dean of Nursing and Associate Professor of Nursing
BryanLGH College of Health Sciences
Lincoln, Nebraska

Fernande E. Deno, MSN, RN
Instructor
Anoka Ramsey Community College
Coon Rapids, Minnesota

Larinda Dixon, EdD, MS, RN
Professor of Nursing
College of DuPage
Matteson, Illinois

Sarah J. Doty, MSN, BSN, BSW
Instructor and Student Health
Southeast Missouri Hospital College of Nursing and
    Health Sciences
Cape Girardeau, Missouri

Linda K. Dunaway, MSN, RN, SANE
Professor
Maysville Community and Technical College
Maysville, Kentucky

David Dunham, DHEd, MSN, RN
Instructor
Hawaii Pacific University
Honolulu, Hawaii

Shelba Durston, MSN, RN, CCRN, SAFE
Instructor
San Joaquin Delta College
Stockton, California

Carrin Dvorak, MSN, RN, CNE
Assistant Professor of Nursing
Cuyahoga Community College
Cleveland, Ohio

Ellen Elder, MSN, RN
Instructor
Georgia Southwestern State University
Americus, Georgia

Jennifer Ellis, DNP, MSN, RN
Instructor
University of Cincinnati Blue Ash College
Blue Ash, Ohio

Susan Estes, MSN, BSN
Clinical Associate Professor
Georgia Baptist College of Nursing of Mercer University
Atlanta, Georgia

Stacey Estridge, MN, RN
Nursing Faculty
Midlands Technical College
Columbia, South Carolina

Patricia Ferrell, BSN, RN
Nursing Instructor
San Jacinto College North
Houston, Texas

Julie A. Fisher, PhD, MSN, BSN, RNC
Professor of Nursing
Wesley College
Dover, Delaware

Rebecca Flynn, MSN, ARNP, CPNP
Assistant Professor of Nursing
Mercy College of Health Sciences
Des Moines, Iowa

Kristi France, MS, BSN, RN
National Director of Product Development–Nursing &
  Allied Health
Lincoln Educational Services
West Orange, New Jersey

Margie Francisco, EdD, MSN, RN
Instructor
Illinois Valley Community College
Oglesby, Illinois

Connie P. Gazmen, MS, RN, OCN
Instructor and Program Director of Adult Health Clinical
  Nurse Specialist Program
School of Nursing and Dental Hygiene
University of Hawaii at Manoa
Honolulu, Hawaii

Christy Gee, MSN, RN, FNP-BC
Doctoral Student
South College
Asheville, North Carolina

Gwendolyn Greene, MSN/ED, BSN, RN
Nursing Instructor
Midlands Technical College
Columbia, South Carolina

Karla Hall, MSN, RN
Assistant Professor
Mercy College of Health Sciences
Des Moines, Iowa

Janet R. Hamilton, MSN, RN
Allied Health Department Chair
And
Assistant Professor
Lamar State College
Port Arthur, Texas

Janice Hancock, MS, BS, RN
Faculty
North Hennepin Community College
Brooklyn Park, Minnesota

Carol Ann Hanna, PhD, BC, RN
Faculty
Delaware County Community College
Media, Pennsylvania

Elaine C. Hannigan, MSN, RN
Continuing Lecturer
Purdue University
West Lafayette, Indiana

Karla Hanson, MSN, RN
Instructor
College of Nursing at South Dakota State University
Brookings, South Dakota

Lisa Harding, MSN, RN, CEN
Associate Professor
Bakersfield College
Bakersfield, California

Janice Hausauer, MSN, FNP, APRN-BC
Instructor
Montana State University in Bozeman
Bozeman, Montana

Celia G. Hay, PhD, RN
Chair of Nursing Department
LaGrange College
LaGrange, Georgia

Lori Hendrickx, EdD, RN, CCRN
Associate Professor
College of Nursing at South Dakota State University
Brookings, South Dakota

Janet Hertlzer, MSN, FNP-BC
Instructor
Marian University
Indianapolis, Indiana

Barbara A. Hoglund, EdD, MSN, RN, FNP-BC
Associate Professor of Nursing
Bethel University
St. Paul, Minnesota

Nina J. Hollifield, MS, RN
Assistant Professor
College of Southern Idaho
Twin Falls, Ohio

Barbie Hoover, MSN, RN
Instructor
School of Health Sciences
School of Nursing
Pennsylvania College of Technology
Williamsport, Pennsylvania

Laura J. Hope, MSN, RN, CDE
Nursing Faculty
Florence-Darlington Technical College
Florence, South Carolina

Catherine Howell, MSN, RN
Professor of Nursing Education
San Diego City College
San Diego, California

Claudette Jacobs, DNP, MS, BSN, RN-BC
Instructor of Nursing
Howard Community College
Columbia, Maryland

Uletha M. Jones, MSN, CCRN
Nursing Faculty
Pensacola State College
Pensacola, Florida

Melanie M. Jorgenson, BSN, RN
Nursing Instructor
North Seattle Community College
Seattle, Washington

Denise Pruskowski Kavanagh, MSN, RN
Professor
La Salle University
Philadelphia, Pennsylvania

Katie Kay, MSN
Faculty Manager
Chamberlain College of Nursing
Chicago, Illinois

Penny Kessler, DNP, RN
Clinical Assistant Professor
School of Nursing
University of Minnesota
Minneapolis, Minnesota

Jonni K. Pielin Kircher, MSN, RN, CSN
Assistant Professor of Nursing
Westmoreland County Community College
Youngwood, Pennsylvania

Andrea Knesek, DNP, MSN, RN, BC
Nursing Faculty
Macomb Community College
Clinton Township, Michigan

Stephen D. Krau, PhD, RN, CNE
Associate Professor
School of Nursing
Vanderbilt University Medical Center
Nashville, Tennessee

Donna Kubesh, PhD, MS, RN
Associate Professor
Luther College
Decorah, Iowa

Karen Kulhanek, MEd, BSN, RN
Nursing Professor
Kellogg Community College
Battle Creek, Michigan

Marjorie J. Kurt, MSN, RN
Clinical Professor
Indiana University School of Nursing
Indianapolis, Indiana

Jill J. Lambert, MSN, RN, GNP/CNS
Associate Professor
Charity School of Nursing
Delgado Community College
New Orleans, Louisiana

Marci L. Langenkamp, MS, BSN, RN (AD)
Assistant Professor of Nursing
Edison Community College
Piqua, Ohio

Ronnette C. Langhorne, MS, RN
Assistant Professor
Thomas Nelson Community College
Hampton, Virginia

Kelly T. Lawson, MSN, RN
Instructor of Nursing
Francis Marion University
Florence, South Carolina

Kathy Leach, PhD, RN
Adjunct Assistant Professor
St. Louis University
St. Louis, Missouri

Heidi Loucks, MS, RN, CNE
Nurse Educator
Casper College
Casper, Wyoming

Lynn Lowery, MSN, RN, FCN, CCHC, CDE
Associate Professor
Charity School of Nursing
Delgado Community College
New Orleans, Louisiana

Jennifer Lunny, MSN, RN
Assistant Professor of Nursing
Broward College
Coconut Creek, Florida

Elisa Mangosing-Lemmon, MSN, BSN, RN, CMSRN
Nursing Instructor
Riverside School of Health Careers
School of Professional Nursing
Newport News, Virginia

Patricia Ann Martin, MSN, RN, FNP-BC, CNE
Associate Professor
West Kentucky Community and Technical College
Paducah, Kentucky

Ellen McAcoy, MA, RN, CNE
Associate Professor
Hillsborough Community College
Tampa, Florida

Connie McFadden, MSN, RN, CNE
Assistant Professor
The Christ College of Nursing and Health Sciences
Cincinnati, Ohio

Barbara McGraw, MSN, RN, CNE
Nursing Instructor and Curriculum Coordinator
Central Community College
Grand Island, Nebraska

Anthony McGuire, PhD, RN, CCRN, ACNP-BC
Nursing School Lecturer
California State—Long Beach
Long Beach, California

Mary McKay, DNP, ARNP, CNE
Associate Clinical Professor
University of Miami
Coral Gables, Florida

Mary Elizabeth McKenna-Dailey, APRN-BC
Professor and Nurse Education/Family Nurse Practitioner
North Shore Community College
Danvers, Massachusetts

Heather M. McKnight, MSN, RN
Assistant Professor
Texarkana College
Texarkana, Texas

Kathleen McNeese, MN, RN, CNS
Tenured Faculty
Glendale Community College
Glendale, California

Susan McReynolds, MS, RN, CNE
Instructor
Blessing-Rieman College of Nursing
Quincy, Illinois

Dona Molyneaux, PhD, MSN, BSN, RN, ONC
Associate Professor
Gwynedd Mercy University
Gwynedd Valley, Pennsylvania

Cynthia Moore, MSN, RN, PLNC
Nursing Faculty
Minnesota State Community and Technical College
Detroit Lakes, Minnesota

Mary Moseley, EdD, MN, BSN
Professor
Northern Virginia Community College
Springfield, Virginia

Ann Motycka, MSN, RN, CNE
Instructor
Ivy Tech State College, Southwest
Evansville, Indiana

Cindy Neely, MSN, RN
Campus Clinical Lab Coordinator and Professor of Nursing
Oklahoma City Community College
Oklahoma City, Oklahoma

Susan E. Nelson, MSN, RN, WCC, CLNC
Regional Nursing Department Chair
Ivy Tech Community College
Anderson, Indiana

Kathy Newton, MSN, BSN, RN
Nurse Educator
Kellogg Community College
Battle Creek, Michigan

Lynn Noell, MSN, RN
Associate Professor
Department of Nursing Education
Joliet Junior College
Joliet, Illinois

Karen Noss, MSN, RN, OCN
Associate Professor
Luzerne County Community College
Nanticoke, Pennsylvania

Annette Oberhaus, MSN, RN
Clinical Teaching Assistant
Northwest State Community College
Archbold, Ohio

Crystal O'Connell-Schauerte, MSCN, BSCN
Coordinator and Professor
Algonquin College
Ottawa, Ontario

Patricia Brown O'Hara, PhD, RN
Associate Professor of Nursing
Gwynedd Mercy University
Gwynedd Valley, Pennsylvania

Catherine J. Pagel, MSN, RN
Assistant Professor of Nursing
Mercy College of Health Sciences
Des Moines, Iowa

Karen Parker
Professor and Clinical Coordinator
Lorain County Community College
Elyria, Ohio

LaVinda Pearson, PhD, RN, CRRN, CNE
Instructor
St. Catherine University
St. Paul, Minnesota

Michelle M. Pelter, PhD, RN
Assistant Professor
Orvis School of Nursing
University of Nevada
Reno, Nevada

Catherine Pence, MSN, RN
Associate Professor
Northern Kentucky University
Highland Heights, Kentucky

Sherily Pereia, PhD, MSN, RNA
Instructor
Medical Sciences Campus and School of Nursing
University of Puerto Rico
San Juan, Puerto Rico

Norma Jean Peters, MSN
Nursing Instructor
Madison College—Reedsburg
Reedsburg, Wisconsin

Vicki Plagenz, MSN, RN
Assistant Professor
Montana State University Northern
Lewistown, Montana

Julia R. Popp, MSN, RN
Professor of Nursing
Owens Community College
Toldeo, Ohio

Dale Powis, MSN, RN
Professor
Community College of Rhode Island
Warwick, Rhode Island

Kathleen Puri, MSN, RN
Associate Professor
Chattanooga State Community College
Chattanooga, Tennessee

Loretta G. Quigley, MS, RN
Associate Dean
St. Joseph's College of Nursing
Syracuse, New York

Sharon Rappold, MSN, RN, BC
Instructor
Wharton County Junior College
Wharton, Texas

Lucille Rayford, MSN
Adjunct Faculty
California State University—Dominguez Hill
Carson, California

Emily Reece, PhD, MSN, RN
Nursing Professor
El Centro College
Dallas, Texas

Gwendolyn E. Richardson, RN, ACNS-BC
Instructor of Nursing
Midlands Technical College
Columbia, South Carolina

Jennifer Robinson, MSN
Instructor of Nursing
Washington Health System
Atlanta, Georgia

Noelle Rohatinsky, PhD, MN, BSN, RN
Assistant Professor
University of Saskatchewan
Saskatoon, Saskatchewan

Tami Rogers, DVM, MSN, CNE
Lead Nursing Professor, Adult Health
Keiser University
Orlando, Florida

Martha Kathryn Findley Roper, MSN, RN
Nursing Instructor
Wallace State Community College
Hanceville, Alabama

Kathleen S. Rose, MSN, BSN, RN
Associate Professor of Nursing
Coordinator for LPN and Paramedic to RN
    Transition Programs
Chattanooga State Community College
Chattanooga, Tennessee

Kristin E. Sandau, PhD, RN
Associate Professor of Nursing and Staff RN at
    United Hospital
Department of Nursing
Bethel University
St. Paul, Minnesota

Joanne Serembus, EdD, RN, CNE, CCRN
Associate Clinical Professor
College of Nursing and Health Professions
Drexel University
Philadelphia, Pennsylvania

Kathy Sheats, MSN, RN
Associate Professor
University of the Virgin Islands
Kingshill, United States Virgin Islands

Leslee H. Shepard, EdD, MSN, RN, CMSRN
Assistant Professor of Nursing
Winston-Salem State University
Winston-Salem, North Carolina

Margaret Sherer, MS, RN, CEN, CNE
Nursing Faculty
Portland Community College
Portland, Oregon

Mandy M. Sheriff, MSN, RN
Instructor
Western Illinois University
School of Nursing
Macomb, Illinois

Karin Sherill, MSN, RN, CNE
Faculty Nursing Educator and Simulation Coordinator
Maricopa Nursing at Mesa Community College
Mesa, Arizona

Louise A. Shirk, MSN
Instructor, Medical-Surgical Nursing
Midlands Technical College
Columbia, South Carolina

Michelle Sink, MSN, RN
Professor of Nursing
Florida State College at Jacksonville
Jacksonville, Florida

Julie Skrabel, MSN, RN
Assistant Professor
Bryan LGH College of Health Sciences
Lincoln, Nebraska

June R. Soto, MEd, RN, APRN
Assistant Professor of Nursing
Borough of Manhattan Community College
New York, New York

Lisa Sparacino, PhD, MS, RN, CCRN
Instructor
New York Institute of Technology
New York, New York

Denise Spohler, MSN, RN
Professor of Nursing
Owens Community College
Toledo, Ohio

Jodie Steblay, MSN
Instructor
Hibbing Community College
Hibbing, Minnesota

Mary Stedman, EdD, RN
Instructor
Farmingdale State College
Farmingdale, New York

Nancy Steffen, MSN, RN
Nursing Instructor
Century College
White Bear, Minnesota

Elizabeth Zion Stratton, MS, RN
Assistant Professor of Nursing
Monroe Community College
Rochester, New York

Megan Talbot, DNP, MSN, BSN, RN, CNE
Instructor
Merritt College-Oakland
Oakland, California

Stephanie B. Turner, EdD, MSN, RN
Nursing Instructor
Wallace State Community College
Hanceville, Alabama

Patricia Voelpel, EdD
Clinical Assistant Professor
Stony Brook University
Stony Brook, New York

Timothy J. Voytilla, MSN, ARNP
Nursing Program Director
Keiser University–Tampa Campus
Tampa, Florida

Gerry Walker, DHEd, MSN, RN
Nursing Program Chair and Assistant Professor of Nursing
Park University
Parkville, Missouri

Terri L. Walker, MSN, RN
Assistant Nursing Program Director and Team
    Leader NPIV
Oklahoma City Community College
Oklahoma City, Oklahoma

Kathleen Warner, MSN, RN
Assistant Professor of Nursing
Viterbo University
La Crosse, Wisconsin

Cynthia L. Williams, MS, RN, CMSRN
Professor of Nursing
Oklahoma City Community College
Oklahoma City, Oklahoma

Cheryl Winter, MSN, RN, FNP-BC
Associate Professor of Nursing
Erma Byrd Higher Education Center
Bluefield State College
Beaver, West Virginia

Christine Wood, MSN, RN
Nursing Professor
Des Moines Area Community College
Ankeny, Iowa

Mary E. Wright, MSN, RN, BSN, PHN
Professor of Nursing Medical Surgical
Mount San Jacinto College
Menifee, California
MiraCosta College
Oceanside, California

Regina L. Wright, MSN, RN
Assistant Professor of Nursing
Neumann University
Aston, Pennsylvania

Jamie Zwicky, MSN-Ed, RN
Faculty
Bryant and Stratton College
Waukesha, Wisconsin

Preface

I have researched the experience of becoming a nurse and have discovered what you already know—that learning nursing is more difficult than you anticipated. I have also taught educators of nursing and can tell you that they too discover that teaching basic nursing is more difficult than anticipated. Thus, the idea for this book was to meet the needs of both students and teachers. I began this journey with a thoughtful analysis of what core content, values, and skills should form the foundation of medical-surgical nursing, and that is how this book was built. No, this book will not provide all answers to questions related to internal medical and surgical care; rather it focuses on what is essential. That said, it is not a cursory viewpoint but one that will give depth and breadth to essential content. You, the reader, will be the judge of our success.

Additionally, I wanted expert clinicians to write this book. Nurses who continue to live in the real world of clinical practice and have strong opinions about essential nursing knowing have informed this book with their wisdom.

I also know that often seeing the weight and thickness of medical-surgical texts scares you to the point that you never crack the binding. Thus, we have aimed to distill the essential and place the rest online. As an example, although we rigorously researched current references, we have placed them online for you, if needed, rather than add to the pages in this text. I am hoping for cracked binding, dog-eared pages, multicolored highlights, and notes in the margins of this book. They will stand as evidence of our success.

FEATURES

We have designed some special features to help engage you, the reader, and assist you in your understanding of the content and the nurse's role in caring for patients.

Guidelines for Nursing Care provide steps and rationales for important procedures.

Focused Assessment boxes summarize important assessment criteria and significant findings related to a particular disorder.

Risk Factors provide a bulleted list of risk factors for a particular disorder, drawing attention to factors that can impair health.

Patient Education summarizes patient teaching, home care, and discharge planning.

Health Promotion reviews important points the nurse should discuss with the patient to prevent common health problems from developing.

Gerontologic Considerations highlight information that pertains specifically to the care of older adults who comprise the fastest-growing segment of our population.

Laboratory and Diagnostic Tests tables list common lab tests for particular disorders along with normal values, critical values, and nursing implications.

Nursing Research: Bridging the Gap to Evidence-Based Practice demonstrates the nursing implications of important research.

Focus on Pathophysiology highlights and describes important pathophysiologic processes.

Nutrition Alert highlights nutritional considerations for particular disorders.

NURSING ALERTS offer brief tips or highlight red-flag warnings for clinical practice.

DRUG ALERTS highlight key nursing considerations and drug safety information.

Pathophysiology Alerts highlight key pathophysiology concerns.

Unfolding Patient Stories feature patients from Wolters Kluwer's *vSim for Nursing*.

PEDAGOGICAL FEATURES

The following features will help you focus your attention on important content and relate it to the challenges of nursing and patient care.

Unit Case Study Each unit opens with a short case study and related questions to help prepare you for the content to be presented and to engage your critical thinking skills. Answers to the unit case studies appear at the end of the book so that you can instantly check your knowledge of the subject.

Learning Objectives appear at the beginning of each chapter to help guide and focus you on the important content in the chapter.

Critical Thinking Exercises appear at the end of each chapter and use situation-based questions to aid you in applying the knowledge you have gained.

NCLEX-Style Review Questions test your comprehension and application of the content. Answers to these review questions are available on the Instructor's Resource DVD-ROM and the Instructor's Resources on the Point.

References and Selected Readings can be found on the Point in addition to a large array of resources that will aid your comprehension and expand your knowledge of the subject matter.

Glossary appears at the end of the book to assist you in understanding key terminology.

COMPREHENSIVE LEARNING PACKAGE

A carefully designed ancillary package is available to students who purchase the book and to faculty who adopt the book to further facilitate teaching and learning. A wide variety of multimedia tools are readily available and are just a click away on the Web site that accompanies the text. Visit http://thepoint.lww.com/Honan2e.

Resources for Students

Find the following resources on

- E-book
- NCLEX-Style Student Review Questions
- Animations

- Video clips
- Audio glossary
- Journal articles
- Learning objectives
- Breath sounds
- Internet resources
- References from the book
- Plan of Nursing Care for selected chapters
- And more!

Resources for Instructors

Instructor resources are available online at http://thepoint.lww.com/Honan2e.

In addition to all of the student assets, instructor resources include the following items:

- Test Generator Questions
- PowerPoint Presentations
- Image Bank
- Pre-lecture Quizzes
- Guided Lecture Notes
- Topics for Discussion and Suggested Answers
- Assignments and Suggested Answers
- Case Studies and Suggested Answers
- Syllabus
- E-book
- Answers to NCLEX-Style Chapter Review Questions from the book
- QSEN Competency KSAs Mapped to *Focus on Adult Health: Medical-Surgical Nursing*

Linda Honan, RN, PhD, CNS-BC, ANEF, FAAN

Acknowledgments

I must acknowledge and thank the following people who helped clear cobwebs in my understanding. They include Walter Zawalich, my GEPN soul mate who always came through with answers to my pathophysiology questions; Lisa B. Meland, my pharmacology guru who answered questions from standard dosages to interactions, and everything in between; and, finally, my anatomy sages William Stewart and Shanta Kapadia for all their support. To all the nursing staff on 6-4 at Yale New Haven Hospital and all the GEPNs who have honed my skills as a nurse and educator for over a quarter of a century. I am in your debt. To Helen Kogut and Stephanie Kelly who edited this edition with care. Finally, my thanks to all the clinician colleagues who wrote chapters about their day-to-day practice so that this book is grounded in the real world of clinical.

Contents

Basics of Adult Health Nursing

A 70-year-old patient diagnosed with hypertension is being seen in the health clinic. When gathering information on the patient, the nurse notes a definite problem with medication compliance. The patient states, "I just forget to take the medication. It's no big deal!" His current BP is 170/90. His history notes that he has had previous TIAs and a stroke. He also has visual and hearing deficits.

- What areas of health education would be important to emphasize for this patient?
- Discuss variables that could effect this patient's medication compliance.
- What teaching strategies could be incorporated into the plan of care for this 70-year-old patient?

The Nurse's Role in Adult Health Nursing

Kelly S. Grimshaw

Learning Objectives

After reading this chapter, you will be able to:
1. Define nursing.
2. Understand nursing's role in the health care industry and society.
3. Describe the practitioner, leadership, and research roles of nursing.
4. Describe nursing care delivery models.
5. Describe factors causing significant changes in the health care delivery system and their impact on the health care field and the nursing profession.

THE NURSING PROFESSION AND THE HEALTH CARE INDUSTRY

To obtain a foundation for examining the role of the nurse and delivery of nursing care, it is necessary to understand the nursing profession, health care consumers, and the health care delivery system, including their interactions and the forces acting upon them.

Nursing Defined

Since Florence Nightingale wrote (1859) that the goal of nursing was "to put the patient in the best condition for nature to act upon him," nursing leaders have described nursing as both an art and a science. In the 20th century, Virginia Henderson (1966) defined nursing as the professional that "[assists] the individual, sick or well, in the performance of those activities contributing to health or its recovery (or to peaceful death) that he would perform unaided if he had the necessary strength, will, or knowledge. This is done in such a way as to help him gain independence as rapidly as possible." The American Nurses Association (ANA), which is the professional organization representing the interests of the nation's 3.4 million registered nurses (RNs) highlighted the evolving nature of this definition by delineating essential features of professional nursing in its Social Policy Statement (ANA, 2010):

- Provision of a caring relationship that facilitates health and healing
- Attention to the range of human experiences and responses to health and illness within the physical and social environments

- Integration of assessment data with knowledge gained from an appreciation of the patient or the group
- Application of scientific knowledge to the processes of diagnosis and treatment through the use of judgment and critical thinking
- Advancement of professional nursing knowledge through scholarly inquiry
- Influence on social and public policy to promote social justice
- Assurance of safe, quality, and evidence-based practice.

The Health Care Industry

Since Philadelphia Hospital first opened its doors in 1753 with the help of private donations, health care has grown into an industry consuming 17.9% of our gross domestic product spending (World Health Organization [WHO], 2015). Today there are almost 5,700 hospitals registered in the United States with the American Hospital Association (AHA), totaling more than 35.4 million annual admissions and an annual expenditure of $859.4 billion (Fast Facts on US Hospitals, 2015). The health care industry is now comprised of public and private organizations and individuals who provide preventative, diagnostic, and therapeutic services (Health Care Industry, 2015). It also includes research and development groups, professional associations and societies, medical equipment and pharmaceutical manufacturers, regulatory bodies, and health insurance companies. These groups encompass all goods and services designed to maintain and promote health for individuals and populations.

Nursing's Role in the Health Care Industry

There are roughly 150 million adults in the US workforce, of whom approximately 3.4 million are RNs (National Center

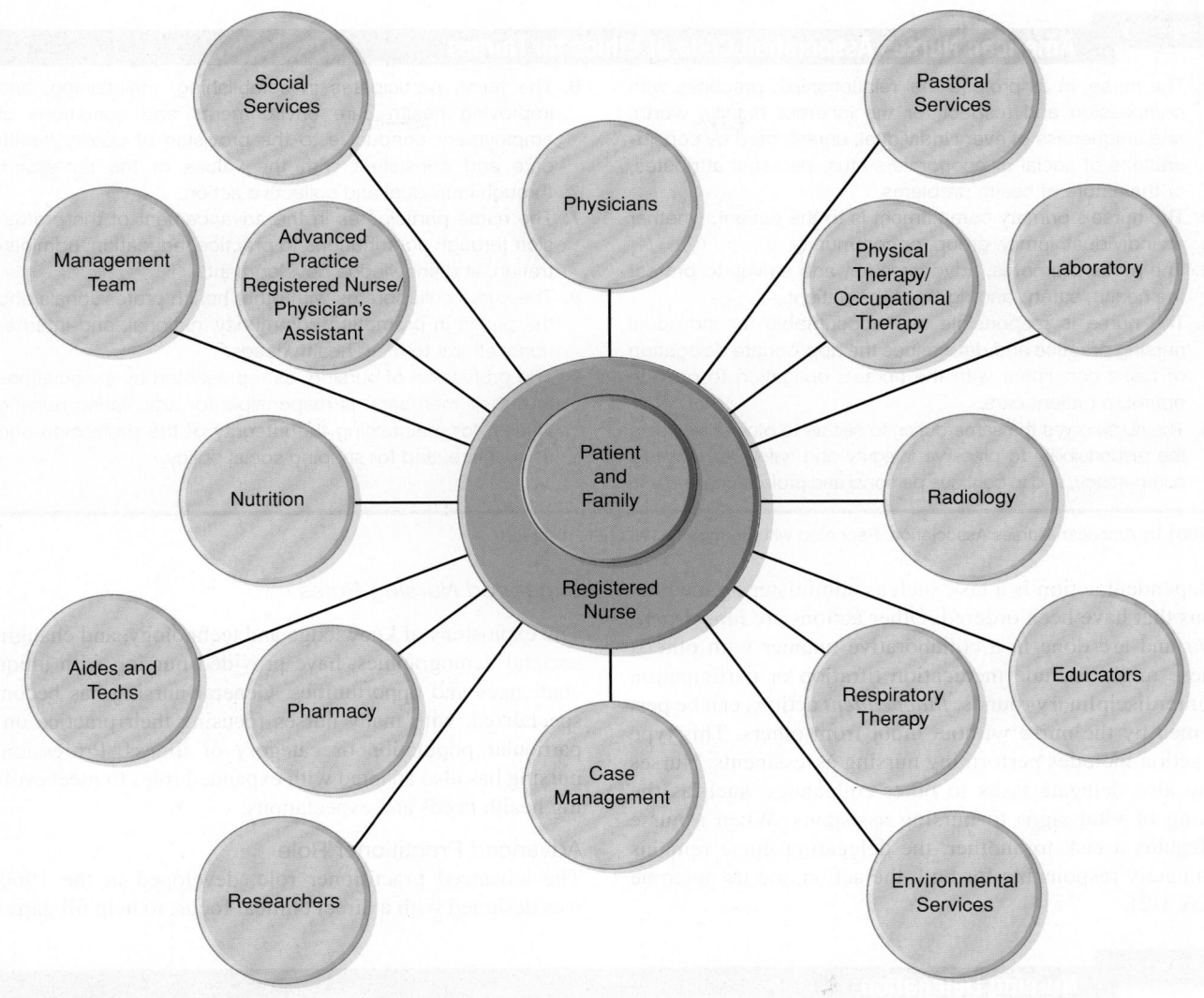

FIGURE 1-1 The Team Player.

for Health Workforce Analysis, 2013; ANA, 2015). Nurses comprise the largest professional group in the health care industry. Each individual nurse is placed in the unique position of standing with the patient and the patient's family at the center of the health care industry. Clinical nurses are at the bedside to act as a care provider and liaison to other health care workers in an effort to provide and coordinate this care (Fig. 1-1).

General Professional Nursing

Each individual nurse has the responsibility to carry out his or her role as described in the Social Policy Statement (ANA, 2010) and to comply with the Code for Nurses (ANA, 2015) and the Nurse Practice Act of the state in which he or she practices. These documents support the definition of nursing and the claim that nurses must be actively involved in

the decision-making process regarding ethical concerns surrounding health care and human responses.

The Code of Ethics (Box 1-1), established by the ANA, consists of ethical standards, each with its own interpretive statements. The interpretive statements provide guidance in addressing nursing responsibilities and ethical decision making.

The role of nurses is specified by individual state boards of nursing and is termed *scope of practice*. Scope of practice is used to delineate actions that are legally permitted for a particular profession, based on specific educational qualifications. It behooves nurses to know and understand their scope of practice, as well as those of other professions with which they interact during patient care. Some actions are described as *dependent*, meaning that a specific action depends upon an order from a medical doctor (MD) or licensed independent practitioner (LIP). An example of

---

BOX 1-1   American Nurses Association Code of Ethics for Nurses

1. The nurse, in all professional relationships, practices with compassion and respect for the inherent dignity, worth, and uniqueness of every individual, unrestricted by considerations of social or economic status, personal attributes, or the nature of health problems.
2. The nurse's primary commitment is to the patient, whether an individual, family, group, or community.
3. The nurse promotes, advocates for, and strives to protect the health, safety, and rights of the patient.
4. The nurse is responsible and accountable for individual nursing practice and determines the appropriate delegation of tasks consistent with the nurse's obligation to provide optimum patient care.
5. The nurse owes the same duties to self as to others, including the responsibility to preserve integrity and safety, to maintain competence, and to continue personal and professional growth.

6. The nurse participates in establishing, maintaining, and improving health care environments and conditions of employment conducive to the provision of quality health care and consistent with the values of the profession through individual and collective action.
7. The nurse participates in the advancement of the profession through contributions to practice, education, administration, and knowledge development.
8. The nurse collaborates with other health professionals and the public in promoting community, national, and international efforts to meet health needs.
9. The profession of nursing, as represented by associations and their members, is responsible for articulating nursing values, for maintaining the integrity of the profession and its practice, and for shaping social policy.

a dependent action is a task such as administering medications that have been ordered. Other actions are *interdependent* and are done in a collaborative manner with others. These might include medication titration or participation in interdisciplinary rounds. *Independent* actions can be performed by the nurse without input from others. This type of action includes performing nursing assessments. Nurses may also delegate tasks to other colleagues, such as the taking of vital signs to nursing assistants. When a nurse delegates a task to another, the delegating nurse remains ultimately responsible for both the action and its outcome (Box 1-2).

Expanded Nursing Roles

The explosions of knowledge and technology, and changing societal demographics, have provided nursing with unique challenges and opportunities. General nursing has become specialized, with many nurses focusing their practice on a particular population or category of illness. Professional nursing has also adapted with expanded roles to meet evolving health needs and expectations.

Advanced Practitioner Role

The advanced practitioner role, developed in the 1960s, was designed with a direct clinical focus, to help fill gaps in

---

BOX 1-2   Nursing Delegation

Who?

The RN
To the LPN or Nursing Assistant or other (e.g., Transport Aide)

What?

Gives authority to a competent individual to perform a selected nursing task
Each task falls within the Nursing Scope of Practice, but can be done by another

Where?

On the nursing unit

When?

When the nurse requires
When the person performing the task has been trained and is deemed competent
When the patient is stable, without unexpected changes in condition

Why?

To achieve a desired patient outcome
To efficiently and effectively make use of personal, financial, and material resources
To efficiently and effectively deliver patient care

How?

Assess the patient need(s), the task(s) required, and the ability of another to perform the task(s)
Delegate the task with clear directions as to priority, timing, and communicating the outcome
Monitor the process of task performance and its completion
Evaluate the patient outcome

Examples of Tasks that Can Be Delegated

Vital signs
Assisting patient out of bed to a chair or to the bathroom
Assisting patient with activities of daily living
Feeding a patient
Phlebotomy

the health care delivery system by providing care to those in geographically and socially underserved areas. These advanced practice RNs who are educated and regulated by state boards of nursing, are present in all specialties. They include, among others, nurse practitioners (NPs), certified nurse–midwives (CNMs), and certified registered nurse anesthetists (CRNA). These and similar advanced practice roles have helped distribute health care services at a decreased cost. The advanced practice role has also provided the nurse with an avenue of personal and professional development. With advanced practice roles has come a continuing effort by professional nursing organizations to yet again define nursing. The nursing profession is coming closer to a single definition of advanced practice with the APRN Consensus Model as explained by Kleinpell and Hudspeth (2013). The model advocates practice to the full extent of licensure, which is defined by the population and health needs of the individuals, not by practice setting. It also states that national standards of preparatory education and completion of ongoing competencies reflect these needs.

More specifically, nurses who function in these roles provide direct care to patients through independent practice, practice within a health care agency, or collaboration with a physician. Advanced practice nurses are credentialed by the American Nurses Credentialing Center (ANCC) or by a specialty's national certification body, such as the Council on Certification for Nurse Anesthetists. Advanced practice professionals have the ability to diagnose disease; order, perform, and interpret diagnostic tests; and prescribe medications.

 Concept Mastery Alert

Underserved populations in geographically remote areas prompted the development of the advanced practitioner role (which first emerged in the 1960s), not government intervention.

Leadership Roles

Nursing has many avenues of practice, and the leadership role is inherent in all of them. Leadership is essentially the art of providing vision, knowledge, and inspiration, and leading change toward a common goal, which in nursing is holistic quality patient care. Leadership involves those actions that all nurses execute when they assume responsibility for the actions of others directed toward determining and achieving patient care goals. Staff nurses work in settings in which they demonstrate leadership as they are held accountable for the nursing care delivered by unlicensed assistive personnel (UAPs), who work under their direct supervision. Beyond the role of direct caregiver, there are a number of leadership roles.

Nurse executives are charged with developing a vision or strategy of a particular institution and ensuring that the

processes required to reach this vision are in place. An example of this may be setting the goal of achieving Magnet status within the Magnet Recognition Program®, in which a hospital is accredited by the ANCC for meeting certain criteria that attract and retain high-functioning nursing staff in order to obtain improved patient outcomes. Nurse Managers are charged with applying the Magnet strategy on the unit level, and they act as translators for putting strategy into actual practice. This may mean scheduling staff to facilitate participation in educational programs or in an institutional activity outside normal job limits, such as community health fairs. Other areas of focus include team coordination, financial responsibilities, policy implementation, staff development, and monitoring of quality of care.

Clinical Nurse Leaders (CNLs), Clinical Nurse Specialists (CNSs), and Clinical Nurse Educators (CNEs) have different advanced degrees, and each role continues to change and develop. These leaders work on improving patient care outcomes in overlapping and complementary ways. According to Moore (2013), CNLs work at the point of care to help nurses improve knowledge, clinical judgment and compliance with evidence-based standards of care. Moore reports that the CNL role has helped institute changes involving improvement in patient care outcomes, patient satisfaction, and decreased length of stay. CNSs are advanced practice nurses whose focus involves advanced assessment skills for assistance to patients, families, and nurses as well as work in the wider system. Harwood (2013) describes their role as "…working across the system to align scientific evidence, necessary resources, provider groups, and organizational policies and practices for improved clinical outcomes." CNEs work within a specific facility or specialty with a focus on nursing education as it relates to orientation, professional development, regulatory requirements, and quality improvement.

The Patient Safety Nurse is one of the newer roles with a focus on prevention of patient and employee harm. They work with all health care disciplines to trend issues that may cause or actually have caused patient harm. This is done in an effort to implement safer practices that, in turn, will prevent future harm. Their role was developed by the health care industry as part of an effort to transform patient care in the wake of two seminal works from the Institute of Medicine (IOM) highlighting preventable harm to our patients: To Err Is Human: Building a Safer Health System (Kohn, Corrigan, & Donaldson, 1999) and Crossing the Quality Chasm: A New Health System for the 21st Century (Kohn, Corrigan, & Donaldson, 2001).

Nurse Researchers

Like other disciplines, nursing strives for scholarship, to obtain new information and advance the art and science of the profession. This would not be possible without nurse researchers. Researchers are prepared at the doctoral level, obtaining degrees such as a doctor of philosophy (PhD) or doctor of nursing science (DNSc), in order to work in academic or research-intensive settings. The goal of nurse researchers is to establish the effectiveness of nursing interventions and nursing care and to further evidence-based practice. Evidence is researched and evaluated to formulate guidelines to be used in clinical practice. This evidence, in turn, is evaluated by the nurse in clinical practice, who is often in the best position to participate in data collection and facilitate the study through communication with the patient, family, and other health care professionals. The nurse directly involved in patient care is also ideally suited to identify nursing problems and important issues that can serve as a basis for research.

THE PATIENT: CONSUMER OF NURSING AND HEALTH CARE

The central figure in health care services is the patient. The term *patient* is derived from a Latin verb meaning "to suffer." It has traditionally been used to describe those who are recipients of care. Patients' needs vary, depending on their roles (as a member of a family, as a member of a particular community), associated circumstances, and past experiences, as well as the problem or problems for which they sought health care. Among the nurse's important functions in health care delivery is obtaining an understanding of the patient's situation and identifying his or her immediate needs, in order to address them.

Certain needs are basic to all people. Noted psychologist Abraham H. Maslow (1954) developed a theory describing basic human needs and how these needs build upon one another to achieve physical, social, and spiritual health and well-being. This model is now known as Maslow's *hierarchy of needs* (Fig. 1-2). Maslow ranked human needs as

physiologic needs, safety and security, sense of belonging and affection, esteem and self-respect, and self-actualization. This last level—self-actualization—refers to fulfilling one's individual potential and includes the desire to know and understand, as well as aesthetics. Once a basic or essential need is met, people usually experience a need on the next level. Depending on an individual's certain situation (e.g., minor vs. major illness or injury), he or she may move among levels. Lower-level needs always remain, but a person's ability to pursue higher-level needs generally indicates movement toward improved health and well-being. This hierarchy provides a useful framework that can be applied to the patient when assessing strengths, limitations, and needs as a consumer of nursing and health care.

The patient who seeks care for a health issue is also an individual person, a member of a family, and a citizen of the community. The ultimate goal of care is to return the patient to the various roles that he or she holds in life. Many patients, as consumers of health care, have become more knowledgeable about health care options and are assuming a collaborative approach with the nurse and the health care system.

Consumers of nursing and health care are as varied as their numbers are large. There are countless differences in demographics, personalities, and abilities that must be understood, so that the patient can participate in his or her own health care decisions. A basic tenet of nursing is to determine the consumers' needs and wants, in order to guide them through their health care experience.

HEALTH, WELLNESS, AND HEALTH PROMOTION

The health care system of the United States, which traditionally has been disease oriented, is placing increasing emphasis on health and health promotion. Many nurses who would formerly have been involved in the care of acutely ill patients are engaged in health promotion and illness prevention. Further, there is a movement toward outpatient care for both acute and chronic conditions.

Health

How health is perceived depends on how health is defined. The WHO, in the preamble to its constitution, defines health as a "state of complete physical, mental, and social well-being and not merely the absence of disease and infirmity" (WHO, 1948). Although this definition of health does not allow for any variation in degrees of wellness or illness, the concept of a health–illness continuum allows for a greater range in describing a person's health status. By viewing health and illness on a continuum, it is possible to consider a person as being neither completely healthy nor completely ill. Instead, a person's state of health is ever-changing and has the potential to range from high-level wellness

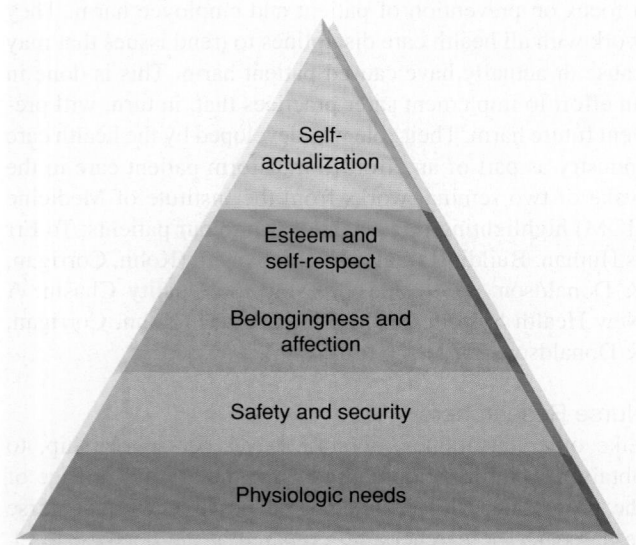

FIGURE 1-2 Maslow's hierarchy of needs.

Self-actualization

Esteem and self-respect

Belongingness and affection

Safety and security

Physiologic needs

to extremely poor health and imminent death. Use of the health–illness continuum makes it possible to view a person as simultaneously possessing degrees of both health and illness.

The limitations of the WHO definition of health are clear in relation to chronic illness and disability. Chronically ill people do not meet the standards of health as established by the WHO definition. However, when viewed from the perspective of the health–illness continuum, people with a chronic illness or disability may be viewed as having the potential to attain a high level of wellness, if they are successful in meeting their health potential within the limits of their chronic illness or disability. Refer to Chapter 3 for details on chronic illnesses.

Wellness

Wellness has been thought of as being equivalent to health. One model of wellness (Hewner, 2014) focuses on various aspects of life that lead to health: emotional, environmental, financial, intellectual, occupational, physical, social, and spiritual.

With this in mind, it is the goal of health care providers to promote positive changes that are directed toward health and well-being. Wellness has a subjective aspect, and the nurse must understand the importance of recognizing and responding to patient individuality and diversity in health care.

Health Promotion

Today, increasing emphasis is placed on health, health promotion, wellness, and self-care. Health is seen as resulting from a lifestyle oriented toward wellness. The result has been the evolution of a wide range of health promotion strategies, including screening, genetic testing, lifetime health monitoring, environmental and mental health programs, risk reduction, and nutrition and health education.

A growing interest in self-care skills is evidenced by the large number of health-related publications, Internet sites, conferences, and workshops designed for the lay public. These programs are designed to promote self-care education, often emphasizing health promotion and disease prevention. As people become increasingly knowledgeable about their health, they often take more interest in and responsibility for their health and well-being.

Special efforts need to be made by health care professionals to determine which organizations, websites, and other venues are providing peer-reviewed and up-to-date information, to ensure people's ability to obtain accurate information concerning health-promoting behaviors. Health-related information and sources of health promotion, whether received from health care professionals, through self-help groups, or from publications, is intended to reach and motivate members of various cultural and socioeconomic groups about lifestyle and health practices.

MODELS OF NURSING CARE

Nursing has evolved from the hospital or home care of the individual during illness to caring for individuals, communities, and populations across the health care continuum in an ever-growing number of ambulatory and inpatient settings. Shortened hospital stays, combined with economic constraints, an aging population, and a greater number of individuals with chronic disease, have necessitated changes in models of nursing care to those best suited to a particular population or setting. Nursing models, such as team nursing, in which nursing staff performed different functions such as medication administration or dressing changes, and primary nursing, in which one nurse provided all assessments and assistance for an individual throughout his or her health care visit, have changed.

Patient- and Family-Centered Care

Patient- and family-centered care can best be described as a model in which the patient and family are cared for by an interdisciplinary group of health care professionals. Active participation of the patient and family and their collaboration in informed decision-making is included.

In their efforts to improve health care quality and safety, hospital leaders today increasingly realize the importance of including a perspective too long missing from the health care equation: the perspective of patients and families. The experience of care, as perceived by the patient and family, is a key factor in health care quality and safety. Bringing the perspectives of patients and families directly into the planning, delivery, and evaluation of health care, and thereby improving its quality and safety, is what patient- and family-centered care is all about. Studies increasingly show that when health care administrators, providers, and patients and families work in partnership, the quality and safety of health care rise, costs decrease, and provider and patient satisfaction increase.

This model appears adaptable to the many facilities through which a person may move during the period of care.

Collaborative Practice

The patient- and family-centered model is a collaborative model and should be a primary goal for nursing. The nursing profession recognizes that it does not practice in a vacuum, and acknowledges the need for participation by the patient and family. With the greater focus on patient safety and improved outcomes at a lower cost, nursing continues to recognize the importance of interaction and communication with other professionals, support staff, and patients and their families in an effort known as *collaborative practice*. Nurses, physicians, and ancillary health personnel perform their particular functions but share in the responsibility of making clinical decisions. The importance of interdisciplinary rounding and collaborative decision-making cannot be underestimated in terms of its ability to provide improved patient care while fostering team cohesion. This is a venture that promotes shared participation, responsibility, and accountability in a health care environment that is striving to meet the complex health care needs of the public.

Care across the Continuum

Regulatory requirements and their financial implications dictate the need for health care organizations to provide the consumer with services of increased value; better health outcomes at a lower price. In order for this to happen, patient- and family-centered care provided by interdisciplinary collaboration needs to happen across the health care continuum. This means that clinicians are aware of the care plan whether in the inpatient or outpatient setting. Hewner (2014) describes the role of nurses in coordinating patient care across providers and settings. Coordinators focus on a group of patients; addressing complex chronic diseases, improving outcomes while reducing hospitalizations and other medical expenses.

INFLUENCES ON HEALTH CARE DELIVERY

Scientific and technologic advances throughout the 20th and into the 21st century have led to social, political, and economic changes. These profound changes have forced the health care industry in general, and nursing practice in particular, to adapt.

Population Demographics

There have been many significant shifts in the demographics of the United States. First of these includes the US Census Bureau (2015) estimation of population increase from 319 million in 2014 to 417 million by the year 2060.

Immigration and Diversity

The United States has been home to an increasingly culturally diverse population, as growing numbers of people from different national backgrounds enter the country.

Again, US Census Bureau (2015) projections indicate that by 2060, one out of every five people will be from a different country, and three out of every fifty people will identify as belonging to two or more races.

As the cultural composition of the population changes, it is increasingly important to address cultural considerations in the delivery of health care. Patients from diverse sociocultural groups not only bring various health care beliefs, values, and practices to the health care setting, but also they have a variety of risk factors for some disease conditions and unique reactions to treatment. These factors significantly affect an individual's responses to health

care problems or illnesses, to caregivers, and to the care itself. Unless these factors are understood and respected by health care providers, the care delivered may be ineffective, and health care outcomes may be negatively affected. In addition, the profession of nursing has set as a goal parity between the nursing workforce and the population of the United States. Thus, a priority is encouraging and fostering the education of ethnic minority groups in health care professions. If achieved, one day a balance will be struck between the health care professional staff and the actual population it serves.

Acknowledging and adapting to the cultural needs of patients and significant others are important components of nursing care. In addition, facilitating access to culturally appropriate health care is critical if nursing care is to be holistic. Culturally competent nursing care is a dynamic process that requires comprehensive knowledge of culture-specific information and an awareness of and sensitivity to the effect that culture has on the care situation. Exploring one's own cultural beliefs and how they might differ from the beliefs of the patient being cared for is a first step toward becoming culturally competent. Specific areas to be considered when providing care include the amount of space and distance needed to feel comfortable, the amount of eye contact, attitudes related to time, the use of touch, observance of civil and religious holidays, and the cultural meanings associated with food. Because the nurse–patient interaction is the focal point of nursing, nurses should consider their own cultural orientation when conducting assessments of patients and patients' families and friends. The guidelines in Box 1-3 may prove useful

---

BOX 1-3   Culturally Appropriate Care

- Know your own cultural attitudes, values, beliefs, and practices.
- Regardless of good intentions, everyone has cultural "baggage" that ultimately results in ethnocentrism.
- Maintain a broad, open attitude. Expect the unexpected. Enjoy surprises.
- Avoid seeing all people as alike; that is, avoid cultural stereotypes, such as "all Chinese like rice" or "all Italians eat spaghetti."
- Try to understand the reasons for any behavior by discussing commonalities and differences.
- If a patient has said or done something that you do not understand, ask for clarification. Be a good listener. Most patients will respond positively to questions that arise from a genuine concern for and interest in them.
- If at all possible, speak the patient's language (even simple greetings and social courtesies are appreciated). Avoid feigning an accent or using words that are ordinarily not part of your vocabulary.
- Be yourself. There is no right or wrong way to learn about cultural diversity.

BOX 1-4   Overcoming Language Barriers

- Greet the patient using the last or complete name. Avoid being too casual or familiar. Point to yourself and say your name. Smile.
- Proceed in an unhurried manner. Pay attention to any effort by the patient or family to communicate.
- Speak in a low, moderate voice. Avoid talking loudly. Remember that there is a tendency to raise the volume and pitch of your voice when the listener appears not to understand. The listener may perceive that you are shouting and/or angry.
- Organize your thoughts. Repeat and summarize frequently. Use audiovisual aids when feasible.
- Use short, simple sentence structure and speak in the active voice.
- Use simple words, such as "pain" rather than "discomfort." Avoid medical jargon, idioms, and slang. Avoid using contractions, such as *don't, can't, won't.*
- Use nouns repeatedly instead of pronouns. *Example*: Do not say: "He has been taking his medicine, hasn't he?" Do say: "Does Juan take medicine?"
- Pantomime words (use gestures) and simple actions while verbalizing them.
- Give instructions in the proper sequence. *Example*: Do not say: "Before you rinse the bottle, sterilize it." Do say: "First, wash the bottle. Second, rinse the bottle."
- Discuss one topic at a time, and avoid giving too much information in a single conversation. Avoid using conjunctions. *Example*: Do not say: "Are you cold and in pain?" Do say (while pantomiming/gesturing): "Are you cold?" "Are you in pain?"
- Talk directly to the patient, rather than to the person who accompanied him or her.
- Validate whether the person understands by having him or her repeat instructions, demonstrate the procedure, or act out the meaning.
- Use any words you know in the person's language. This indicates that you are aware of and respect the patient's primary means of communicating.
- Try a third language. Many Indo-Chinese speak French. Europeans often know three or four languages. Try Latin words or phrases, if you are familiar with the language.
- Be aware of culturally based gender and age differences and diverse socioeconomic, educational, and tribal/regional differences when choosing an interpreter.
- Obtain phrase books from a library or bookstore, make or purchase flash cards, contact hospitals for a list of interpreters, and use both formal and informal networking to locate a suitable interpreter. Although they are costly, some telecommunication companies provide translation services.

to nurses wishing to provide culturally appropriate care. Box 1-4 provides suggestions on overcoming language barriers.

Aging Population

The increase in lifespan experienced in the United States over the last century has resulted in a tripling of the number of elderly citizens, most of whom are women. The elderly population in the United States has increased significantly and will continue to grow in future years with one in four over the age of 65 years (2015). In addition, people 85 years of age and older will continue to increase in numbers. The health care needs of older adults are often chronic in nature, with intermittent exacerbations or acute episodes. This makes their care more complex and demands significant human, material, and financial investment by the health care industry.

Changing Patterns of Disease

The past century has seen a dramatic shift in disease patterns. This is generally considered to be a move from the predominance of infectious disease to that of chronic illness and injury. Perusal of literature and popular media leads us to ask about the impact of major issues on our health: population growth, aging, urbanization, immigration, environmental challenges, and increasing costs of

mitigating their effects. The good news is that innovation continues and science and technology is giving us ever new ways of preventing, treating, and or living with illness and injury.

Advances in Technology

Advances in technology have occurred with greater frequency during the past several decades than in all other periods of civilization. Sophisticated devices have revolutionized how disease is prevented, how patients are diagnosed and treated, and even how communication to and about patients is conducted. Advanced technology has provided access to faster, less invasive, and less painful testing and procedures. In fact, many tests and procedures that once required a hospital stay are performed routinely on an outpatient basis. A disorder that once may have required an operation for diagnosis many times can be diagnosed via computed tomography (CT) or magnetic resonance imaging (MRI). Computers are also significantly changing workflow, as medical records become completely electronic, resulting in improved communication among caregivers, efficient documentation, and ease of medical investigation and research.

Public Safety

The US health care system is based on public trust. This translates to people's confidence that the care they will receive in a hospital or other health care setting will meet legal and social standards. Thus, this large and diverse system is charged with the protection and maintenance of these standards when providing a safe work environment for employees and a healing environment for clients and patients.

Regulatory Bodies

To ensure that minimum standards are maintained, governing and oversight bodies regulate the health care system. Agencies involved in oversight include those in the following discussion.

Occupational Safety and Health Administration

Under the Occupational Safety and Health Act of 1970, employers are responsible for providing a safe and healthy workplace for their employees. The role of the Occupational Safety and Health Administration (OSHA) is to promote the safety and health of working people by setting and enforcing standards; providing training, outreach, and education; establishing partnerships; and encouraging continual process improvement in workplace safety and health.

The Joint Commission

The Joint Commission is a private, nonprofit organization whose mission is to "continuously improve the safety and quality of care provided to the public through the provision of health care accreditation and related services that support performance improvement in health care organizations" (Joint Commission, 2009). At present, the Joint Commission accredits approximately 89% of the nation's hospitals (Joint Commission, 2015).

Patient Protection and Affordable Care Act of 2010

The Patient Protection and Affordable Care Act (PPACA) of 2010 (2015) was designed to improve the health of the population at reduced per capita cost. This is to be accomplished by increasing the number of people with health insurance, improving the insurance policies and reimbursing facilities (hospitals, etc.) based on the quality of care. While relatively new and unstudied, the act has been the target of numerous legal and political challenges. This act is likely to remain a part of the health care landscape impacting both the public and private sectors of health care for the foreseeable future.

Centers for Medicare and Medicaid Services

The Centers for Medicare and Medicaid Services (CMS) is the federal agency that manages Medicare, which is the health insurance program for people over 65 years of age, people under age 65 with certain disabilities, and those with end-stage kidney disease (ESKD). The CMS also manages Medicaid, which is a state-administered program for low-income individuals and families who fit into an eligibility group recognized by federal and state law. In addition, the CMS manages the children's health insurance program (CHIP), which provides coverage for millions of uninsured children.

The CMS exists to ensure effective up-to-date health care coverage and to promote quality care for beneficiaries.

Department of Public Health

Each state has its own Department of Public Health (DPH) with its own mission.

They all are generally charged with the protection of the health and well-being of the state's population and environment. The State Board of Nursing falls within this department and serves to regulate the practice of nursing and the licensing of individual nurses.

Professional Societies and Associations

Associations and societies have a specific focus. They help ensure basic standards as well as promote and recognize advanced knowledge and expertise.

The ANA is the only full-service professional organization representing the nation's more than 3.4 million RNs through its 54 constituent member associations. The ANA advances the nursing profession by fostering high standards of nursing practice, promoting the rights of nurses in the workplace, projecting a positive and realistic view of nursing, and lobbying Congress and regulatory agencies on health care issues affecting nurses and the public.

Hospitals and Institutions

In the 1980s, hospitals and other health care agencies implemented programs designed to measure the quality of care they provided. These programs, known as *quality assurance* (QA) or *quality improvement* (QI), were required to be in place for reimbursement for services and for accreditation by the Joint Commission on Accreditation of Healthcare Organizations (JCAHO; now known simply as the Joint Commission). They sought to establish and maintain accountability to society on the part of the health professions by meeting minimum criteria for the quality, appropriateness, and cost of health services.

In the early 1990s, *continuous quality improvement* (CQI) was identified as a more effective mechanism for improving the quality of health care. Unlike QA, which focuses on individual incidents or errors and minimum expectations, CQI focuses on the processes used to provide care, with the aim of improving quality by assessing and improving those interrelated processes that most affect patient care outcomes and patient satisfaction. CQI involves analyzing, understanding, and improving clinical, financial, and operational processes. Problems that occur as more than isolated events are subject to examination, and all issues that may affect patient outcome are studied. Nurses directly involved in the delivery of care are engaged in analyzing data and refining the processes used in CQI. Their knowledge of the processes and conditions that affect patient care is critical in designing changes to improve the quality of the care provided and ensuring that this care meets or exceeds Joint Commission standards.

Individual Employees

Every individual accepts responsibility for his or her position. For nurses, this entails:

- Maintaining licensure
- Maintaining health requirements, such as annual tuberculosis screening
- Maintaining annual competencies, such as those established by corporate compliance
- Participating in continuing education and certification activities
- Participating in hospital committee and quality review activities
- Providing safe and current care to patients and families.

Economics

The belief that comprehensive, quality health care should be provided for all citizens prompted government concern about rising health care costs and wide variations in charges among providers. In 1983, the US Congress passed significant health legislation termed *prospective payment system* for hospital inpatient services. The federal government was no longer able to afford to reimburse hospitals for patient care that was delivered without any defined limits on costs. Therefore, a *prospective payment system* was approved for hospital inpatient services. Based on diagnosis-related groups (DRGs), prospective payment sets the rates of reimbursement for hospital services for Medicare patients.

Hospitals receive payment at a fixed rate for patients with diagnoses that fall into a specific DRG. A fixed payment has been predetermined for more than 470 possible diagnostic categories, covering the majority of medical diagnoses of patients admitted to the hospital. Hospitals receive the same payment for every patient with a given diagnosis or who falls within a given DRG. If the cost of the patient's care is lower than the payment, the hospital makes a profit; if the cost is higher, the hospital incurs a loss. As a result, hospitals are placing greater emphasis on reducing costs, monitoring utilization of services, and limiting length of patient stay.

There is also the renewed focus on overhauling the nation's health care system in an effort to control its ever-increasing cost. As of this writing, attempts at health care reform are under way although the results and effects remain far from certain. Any future changes most likely will prove to have profound effects on regulatory agencies, health care organizations, individual practitioners, and patients.

Nurses in hospitals now care for patients who are older and sicker and require more nursing services. Nurses in the community are caring for patients who have been discharged earlier and need high-technology acute care services as well as long-term care. The importance of effective discharge planning, along with utilization review and quality improvement, cannot be overstated. Nurses in acute care settings must work with other health care team members to maintain quality care while facing pressures to discharge patients earlier and decrease costs.

CHAPTER REVIEW

Critical Thinking Exercises

1. The roles of nurses continue to develop and change. What avenues of continued education are available to the new nurse in order to adapt to these changing roles?

2. What responsibilities do individual nurses have regarding their participation in monitoring and evaluating patient safety and the quality of care they provide?

3. What other influences on the health care delivery system are not necessarily discussed in this chapter?

NCLEX-Style Review Questions

1. Under the Occupational Safety and Health Act (OSHA) of 1970, employers are responsible for providing a safe and healthy workplace for their employees. Which of the following would be inconsistent with the role of OSHA?
   a. Financial assistance
   b. Outreach
   c. Education
   d. Establishing partnerships

2. Nursing has evolved from the hospital or home care of the individual during illness to caring for individuals, communities, and populations across the health care continuum. Which of the following necessitated changes in models of nursing care?
   a. Fewer individuals with chronic disease
   b. Increased aging population
   c. Fewer inpatient settings
   d. Lengthened hospital stays

3. Which of the following entities is charged with the protection of health and well-being of the state's population and environment?
   a. Joint Commission
   b. Occupational Health and Safety Administration
   c. Department of Public Health
   d. Centers of Medicare and Medicaid Services

4. Based on DRGs, prospective payment sets the rates of reimbursement for hospital services for Medicare patients. Which of the following is an accurate statement regarding the use of DRGs?
   a. If the cost of the patient's care is lower than the payment, the hospital takes a loss.
   b. If the cost of the patient's care is higher than the payment, the hospital takes a loss.
   c. Hospitals receive various payments for every patient with a given diagnosis.
   d. If the cost of the patient's care is higher than the payment, the hospital makes a profit.

Try these additional resources, available at **http://thepoint.lww.com/Honan2e**, to enhance your learning and understanding of this chapter:
- NCLEX-Style Student Review Questions
- Journal Articles

5. Nurses should consider their own cultural orientation when interacting with patients. Which of the following is a technique that can be used to overcome a language barrier when interacting with a patient?
   a. Talk loudly so that the patient will understand.
   b. Give the patient a substantial amount of information.
   c. Give instructions in proper sequence.
   d. Talk directly to the person that accompanied the patient.

REFERENCES AND SELECTED READINGS

References and selected readings associated with this chapter can be found on the website that accompanies the book. Visit **http://thepoint.lww.com/Honan2e** to access the references and other additional resources associated with this chapter.

Health Education and Health Promotion

Carol Ann Wetmore

Learning Objectives

After reading this chapter, you will be able to:

1. Describe the purposes and significance of health education.
2. Describe the concept of adherence to a therapeutic regimen.
3. Identify variables influencing a person's adherence to a therapeutic regimen.
4. Describe strategies that facilitate adults' learning abilities.
5. Describe the relationship of health education to the nursing process.
6. Develop a teaching plan for a patient.
7. Define health promotion and discuss the role of the nurse related to it.

HEALTH EDUCATION

Teaching, as a function of nursing, is included in all state nurse practice acts and in the *Scope and Standards of Clinical Nursing Practice* of the American Nurses Association (2015, p. 65). **Health education** is an independent function of nursing practice and is a primary nursing responsibility. All nursing care is directed toward promoting, maintaining, and restoring health; preventing illness; and helping people adapt to the residual effects of illness. Many of these nursing activities are accomplished through health education or patient teaching. Nurses who serve as teachers are challenged to focus on the educational needs of communities, as well as on specific patient and family educational needs. Health education is important to nursing care because it affects the abilities of people and families to perform important self-care activities.

Every contact an individual nurse has with a health care consumer, whether or not that person is ill, should be considered an opportunity for health teaching. Although people have a right to decide whether or not to learn, nurses have the responsibility to present information that motivates people to recognize the need to learn. Therefore, nurses must use opportunities in all health care settings to promote **wellness**. Educational environments may include homes, hospitals, community health centers, schools, places of business, service agencies, shelters, and consumer action or support groups.

Trends in Health Education

Much of the core of health education today is focused on increasing patient involvement and accountability for individual care and treatment plans. Health education programs are often designed as patient safety initiatives and are geared toward encouraging increased communication between patients and care providers. The effect of improved communication between patients and providers is multifaceted and includes improved patient outcomes, patient safety, and patient perception of quality. The Joint Commission has found consistently that adverse events are caused by breakdowns in communication among caregivers and between caregivers and patients (The Joint Commission, 2016). Therefore, there has been much collaboration to develop processes that encourage improved communication.

The Agency for Healthcare Research and Quality (AHRQ) continues to be a leader in helping both providers and patients to not only understand how important communication is but also develop tools and programs to improve those skills (e.g., evidence-based strategy that hospitals can implement to improve communication and quality [2013, p. 4]). Also AHRQ has built on the foundation of the program, *Questions Are the Answer.* The website offers 10 questions all patients should ask and a "Question Builder" tool to create a list of questions specific to the purpose of the visit—checkup, talking about a problem or health condition, getting a prescription, or discussing a medical test or surgery

(AHRQ, 2012). Whatever the reason for your patient's visit, he or she should be prepared. Even the popular press reveals a number of articles encouraging the public to be active and engaged with their care and providers. One blogger developed the acronym, HEALING, to help patients remember their responsibilities:

- Health summary
- Expert—become an expert yourself
- Accept support
- Look for a second opinion
- Involve yourself
- No—speak up if something does not seem right
- Give thanks to outstanding medical providers (Zeppieri-Caruana, 2016).

Purpose of Health Education

The goal of patient and family education is to improve patient outcomes. For purposes of this discussion, family shall be considered to be the person(s) who plays a significant role in the patient's life. This may include person(s) not legally related to the patient. Effective health education lays a solid foundation for individual and community wellness. Teaching is an integral tool that all nurses use to assist patients and families in developing effective health behaviors and in altering lifestyle patterns that predispose people to health risks.

People with chronic illnesses and disabilities are among those most in need of health education. As the lifespan of the population increases, the number of people with such illnesses also increases. People with chronic illness need health care information to participate actively in and assume responsibility for much of their own care. Health education can help change a patient's behavior favorably, increase the ability to cope with and manage health, and improve understanding of the options, risks, and benefits of care, treatment, and services. It can also prevent crisis situations and reduce the potential for rehospitalization resulting from inadequate information about self-care. The goal of health education is to teach people to live life to its healthiest—that is, to strive toward achieving their maximum health potential.

In addition to the public's right to and desire for health education, patient education is also a strategy for promoting self-care at home and in the community, reducing health care costs by preventing illness, avoiding expensive medical treatments, decreasing lengths of hospital stays, and facilitating earlier discharge.

Adherence to the Therapeutic Regimen

One of the goals of patient education is to encourage people to adhere to their **therapeutic regimen**. **Adherence** to treatment usually requires that a person make one or more lifestyle changes to carry out specific activities that promote and maintain health. Common examples of behaviors facilitating

health include taking prescribed medications, maintaining a healthy diet, increasing daily activities and exercise, self-monitoring for signs and symptoms of illness, practicing specific hygiene measures, seeking recommended health evaluations and screenings, and performing other therapeutic and preventive measures.

Many people do not adhere to their prescribed regimens; rates of adherence are generally low, especially when the regimens are complex or of long duration. Nonadherence to prescribed therapy has been the subject of many studies; a wide range of variables appears to influence the degree of adherence, including the following:

- Inadequate cognitive, psychomotor, or language skills
- Personal values, beliefs, misconceptions, and attitudes coupled with their associated anxiety, depression, and/or fear
- Distrust if loss of control occurs in the decision-making process
- Difficulty in adopting recommended changes
- Insufficient social support or outright sabotage by that support
- Poor self-concept or self-efficacy

Nurses' success with promoting adherence can be improved by creating a collaborative relationship that addresses patient's priorities, circumstances, and goals. Motivational Interviewing (MI) is a collaborative conversational technique intended to strengthen a patient's motivation to change. It has been shown to be effective in addressing many different lifestyle problems as well as in chronic disease management, and many disease prevention guidelines promote use of motivational interviewing. There are four basic principles that are the basis of MI—show empathy, support self-efficacy, roll with resistance, and develop discrepancy. The communication skills often employed include: (1) asking open-ended questions rather than instructing the patient on what they should do, (2) affirming, (3) reflecting, (4) summarizing, and (5) providing individualized information and advice with the patient's permission (Miller & Rollnick, 2013).

Health Literacy and Willingness to Learn

Before initiating a teaching–learning program, it is important to assess the person's physical and emotional readiness to learn, as well as his or her ability to learn what is being taught. This information then becomes the basis for establishing goals that can motivate the person. Involving learners in establishing mutually acceptable goals serves the purpose of encouraging active involvement in the learning process and shared responsibility for learning.

Health literacy is the degree to which an individual has the capacity to obtain, communicate, process, and understand basic health information and services to make appropriate health decisions. Low literacy has been linked to poor health outcomes such as higher rates of hospitalization and

Gerontologic Considerations

Elderly people frequently have one or more chronic illnesses that are managed with numerous medications and complicated by periodic acute episodes. Elderly people also may have other problems that affect adherence to therapeutic regimens, such as increased sensitivity to medications and their side effects, difficulty in adjusting to change and stress, financial constraints, forgetfulness, inadequate support systems, lifetime habits of self-treatment with over-the-counter medications, visual and hearing impairments, and mobility limitations. An important predictor of patient adherence to a therapeutic regimen is concordance of the patient's and providers' perception of their health.

Changes in cognition with age may include slowed mental functioning; decreased short-term memory, abstract thinking, and concentration; and slowed reaction time. Often these changes are accentuated by the health problems that cause the elderly person to seek health care in the first place. Effective teaching strategies include a slow-paced presentation of small amounts of material at a time; frequent repetition of information; and the use of reinforcement techniques, such as audiovisual and written materials and repeated practice sessions. Distracting stimuli should be minimized as much as possible in the teaching environment.

Sensory changes associated with aging also affect teaching and learning. Teaching strategies to accommodate decreased visual acuity include large-print and easy-to-read materials printed on nonglare paper. To maximize hearing, teachers must speak distinctly with a normal or lowered pitch, facing the person so that speech reading can occur as needed. Visual cues often help to reinforce verbal teaching.

Family members should be involved in teaching sessions when possible. They provide another source for reinforcement of material and can help the elderly person recall instructions later. Also family members can provide valuable assessment information about the person's living situation and related learning needs.

When nurses, families, and other involved health care professionals work collaboratively to facilitate the elderly person's learning, chances of success are maximized. Successful learning for the elderly should result in improved self-care management skills, enhanced self-esteem, confidence, and a willingness to learn in the future. Above all, health care professionals must work together to provide continuous, coordinated care; otherwise, the efforts of one health care professional may be negated by those of another.

less frequent use of preventive services (Cajita, Cajita, & Han, 2016). Nearly nine out of ten adults may lack the skills needed to manage their own health and prevent disease. Considering the complexity of medication regimens (dosing, timing, calculations), informed consent, and technology (peak flow meters, glucose monitoring devices, etc.), it is important for the nurse to have insight into how health literacy impacts the patients' well-being. Current evidence shows that nurses overestimate their patients' health literacy consistently and, therefore, may be unaware of creating difficulties for their patients by not providing adequate information or assuming the patient knows more than he or she does (Dickens, Lambert, Cromwell, & Piano, 2013). There are two methods that can be used to quickly assess a patient's health literacy. The *Newest Vital Sign* tests literacy skills for both numbers and words in both English and Spanish and takes approximately 3 minutes to administer ("NVS," n.d.). An alternative health literacy assessment tool is the *Single Item Literacy Screener* (SILS). The SILS is a single question intended to identify adults in need of help with printed health material. The SILS asks, "How often do you need to have someone help you when you read instructions, pamphlets, or other written material from your doctor or pharmacy?" Possible responses are 1—Never, 2—Rarely, 3—Sometimes, 4—Often, and 5—Always. Scores greater than 2 are considered positive, indicating some difficulty with reading printed health-related material (Brice et al., 2014; Morris, MacLean, Chew, & Littenberg, 2006).

Boxes 2-1 and 2-2 provide guidance for patient education in the geriatric population.

NURSING PROCESS
Patient Teaching

The steps of the nursing process—assessment, diagnosis, planning, implementation, and evaluation—are used when constructing a teaching plan to meet people's teaching and learning needs (Box 2-3).

ASSESSMENT

Assessment in the teaching–learning process is directed toward the systematic collection of data about the person's learning needs and style and readiness to learn, as well as the family's learning needs. Box 2-4 discusses the Stages of Change model in relation to teaching and behavior change.

LEARNING READINESS

One of the most significant factors influencing learning is a person's **learning readiness.** This is a crucial step in the assessment process. If patients are not ready to learn, change, or alter their behavior, education can be fruitless. For adults, readiness is based on culture, attitude, personal values, physical and emotional status, and past experiences in learning. Experiential readiness to learn refers to past experiences that may influence a person's ability to learn. Previous educational experiences and life experiences in general are significant determinants of

(continued on page 17)

BOX 2-2   10 Tips for Educating Elderly Patients (HCPro, 2013)

Consider the following tips for teaching elderly patients:

1. Maintain a positive and patient attitude. Treat the older person as intelligent and capable of learning.
2. Take a few minutes to talk and problem-solve before starting to teach. Ask the patient about experience in a given area. Find out what's worked or what hasn't worked in the past.
3. Identify significant cultural or social factors that may affect the teaching–learning process.
4. Include the patient in setting learning goals. Keep the material relevant to the learner's needs.
5. Identify and try to accommodate any disability that may affect the learning process. For example, for patients with visual impairment, encourage the use of glasses (if appropriate), and investigate special learning tools, such as large-print material.
6. Slow the pace of instruction and gear teaching to the patient's rate of absorption. Stop teaching if the patient appears tired or stressed.
7. Break each topic into small parts. Repeat sessions when necessary. Give pertinent, positive feedback.
8. Ask the patient to talk through the procedure before trying it. Provide opportunities for practice sessions and repeat demonstrations. Include role playing, discussion, and problem-solving.
9. Avoid tests or challenges—these can create too much stress and impede learning.
10. Assess responses carefully to make sure the information was understood correctly. Gear the frequency and duration of your teaching to match your patient's learning ability and need to know.

Invite family caregivers to be part of the teaching process. At teaching sessions, you can further assess family dynamics. If one of your goals is to promote patient independence, make sure family members understand that their role is to support the patient, not to take over for the patient. And vice versa, if your goal is to teach the family members—make sure that they understand that it will become their sole responsibility to provide this service for the patient for as long as the need remains. Encourage family caregivers to review and reinforce frequently what the patient is learning.

BOX 2-3   Patient Education

A Nursing Process Guide to Patient Education

Assessment

1. Assess the person's readiness for health education.
   A. What are the person's health beliefs and behaviors?
   B. What physical and psychosocial adaptations does the person need to make?
   C. Is the learner ready to learn?
   D. Is the person able to learn these behaviors?
   E. What additional information about the person is needed (such as availability of resources and tools)?
   F. Are there any variables (e.g., hearing or visual impairment, cognitive issues, and literacy issues) that will affect the choice of teaching strategy or approach?
   G. What are the person's expectations?
   H. What does the person want to learn?
2. Organize, analyze, synthesize, and summarize the collected data.

Planning and Goals

1. Specify the learning goals established by teacher and learner together.
2. Identify teaching strategies appropriate for goal attainment.
3. Establish expected outcomes.
4. Develop the written teaching plan.
   A. Include diagnoses, goals, teaching strategies, and expected outcomes.
   B. Put the information to be taught in logical sequence.
   C. Write down the key points.
   D. Select appropriate teaching aids.
   E. Keep the plan current and flexible to meet the person's changing learning needs.
5. Involve the learner, family or significant others, nursing team members, and other health care team members in all aspects of planning.

Implementation

1. Put the teaching plan into action.
2. Use language the person can understand.
3. Use appropriate teaching aids and provide Internet resources if appropriate.
4. Use the same equipment that the person will use after discharge.
5. Encourage the person to participate actively in learning.
6. Record the learner's responses to the teaching actions.
7. Provide feedback.

Evaluation

1. Collect objective data.
   A. Observe the person.
   B. Ask questions to determine whether the person understands.
   C. Use rating scales, checklists, anecdotal notes, and written tests when appropriate.
2. Compare the person's behavioral responses with the expected outcomes. Determine the extent to which the goals were achieved.
3. Include the person, family or significant others, nursing team members, and other health care team members in the evaluation.
4. Identify alterations that need to be made in the teaching plan.
5. Make referrals to appropriate sources or agencies for reinforcement of learning after discharge.
6. Continue all steps of the teaching process: assessment, diagnosis, planning, implementation, and evaluation.

BOX 2-4   Stages of Change

An approach to health teaching is the use of the transtheoretical model to conceptualize the process of intentional behavior change. This model considers decisional balance (weighing the pros and cons of the proposed behavioral change), self-efficacy (confidence in one's ability to change), and the relationship between stage of change and behavior (Prochaska & Prochaska, 2014). The model considers educational interventions that are not "one size fits all" but rather individualized interventions based upon a patient's current stage of readiness to learn or motivational readiness. At any given time, less than 20% of a population at risk is prepared to take action and make changes, thus this model helps nurses determine teaching interventions for the whole population, not just those prepared to change. Transtheoretical model-based measures have been developed for smoking, alcohol use, sun exposure, and exercise, to name a few. The model is not linear but expects that patients will move between stages until successful behavioral changes are established. The nurse considers the patient's current stage when planning educational needs.

- Precontemplation (the patient is not considering any change in behavior in the next 6 months)
- Contemplation (the patient has serious consideration of change, but it is sometime in the future)
- Preparation (the patient has taken initial behavioral steps toward change and intends to make changes in the next 30 days)
- Action (concrete activities that lead to the desired change have been made for less than 6 months)
- Maintenance (active efforts to sustain the changes made for more than 6 months)

The expectation would be for the patient in the precontemplation stage to disagree with suggestions that a change in behavior is needed. The patient would not be expected to exert effort toward making changes in the "risk" behavior. At this stage, the nurse would offer suggestions and material for the patient to consider the need for behavior change and encourage the patient to consider behavioral changes in the future. On the other hand, the nurse may expect an individual in the action stage to endorse the need for change and engage in specific behaviors that would lead to behavioral change. Engagement in educational activities would be expected at this stage.

---

a person's approach to learning. People with little or no formal education may not be able to understand the instructional materials presented. People who have had difficulty learning in the past may be hesitant to try again. Many behaviors required for reaching maximum health potential require knowledge, physical skills, and positive attitudes. In their absence, learning may be very difficult and very slow. For example, a person who does not understand the basics of normal nutrition may not be able to understand the restrictions of a specific diet. A person who does not view the desired learning as personally meaningful may reject teaching efforts. A person who is not future-oriented may be unable to appreciate many aspects of preventive health teaching. Experiential readiness is closely related to emotional readiness, because motivation tends to be stimulated by an appreciation for the need to learn and by those learning tasks that are familiar, interesting, and meaningful.

A practical way of assessing the patient's learning readiness is to ask how they view their health-related problem and what actions do they see that can be taken. Other open-ended questions that might be asked include, "What changes would you like to make now?" and "Are there any problems that prevent you from learning right now?" Research continues to find that these questions are best asked early in a meeting with a patient. In addition, asking "Do you have any other concerns?" as opposed to "Do you have any other questions?" will illicit more information (Robinson, Tate, & Heritage, 2015, Section 4.1).

DETECTING COMMUNICATION ISSUES

Lack of communication skills is one of the most significant barriers to patient education. This can include both a patient's reading and computer skills. Patients who struggle with written material may appear disinterested in learning rather than admitting that they may not understand. Watch a patient's eyes while he is "reading"; the eyes should move left to right as he examines a document. Using computerized resources to support learning with inexperienced users requires careful assessment and planning. Computer-based education will work best and make the most efficient use of time when it is matched to the skill level of the patient.

Improved health outcomes are achieved when culturally competent nurses acknowledge the patient's culture care values and preferred care practices, and incorporate them into their patient's plan of care. Cultural competence is a recognized standard of care in *Holistic Nursing: Scope and Standards of Practice* (AHNA/ANA, 2007). Completing a cultural assessment will allow the nurse to adapt information and delivery to a patient's cultural beliefs and preferences (Box 2-5). An individual's culture can affect his or her viewpoint in many ways, such as the meaning of a diagnosis, the expectation of reporting symptoms, how much information is desired, how death and dying will be managed, gender roles, family participation, and decision making. Culturally competent communication skills play an important role in your success in influencing your patients' health.

There are a number of cultural mores and rules that a nurse can learn and follow:

- Understand nonverbal behavior (e.g., the cultural meaning of touch, eye contact)
- Allow time to build a relationship and establish a rapport:
  - exchange information
  - greet and respond in culturally appropriate ways

(continued on page 18)

BOX 2-5   Cultural Assessment Components to Consider When Formulating a Teaching Plan

When formulating a teaching plan, consider the patient's beliefs about:

- Body size, shape, boundaries, and functions
- Beauty and strength
- Value of the mind or brain
- Nature and function of blood
- Diet and nutrition
- Communication

- Gender
- Family and social support
- Physical health and illness
- Mental health and illness
- Age-related changes
- Pain
- Medicine, herbs, and talismans
- Spirituality or religion

- smile and be genuine
- pay attention to children
- listen carefully, don't interrupt or put words in one's mouth
- value stories
- Notice eye contact and body language
- Reach out to the appropriate family member
- Check for understanding and ask questions
- Avoid jargon and stereotyping
- Do not impose your personal values, morals, or beliefs on to your patients

One very important key is to learn to laugh at yourself and listen to lessons brought to you by humor (Margalit et al., 2013, pp. 56–57). A balance is necessary; it is important to avoid overemphasizing cultural-specific beliefs so as not to reinforce stereotypes.

Language barriers, once identified, must be addressed. The Joint Commission developed patient-centered communication standards that detail hospital staff's obligation to respect patients' right to and need for effective communication, including the provision of interpreter and translation services when needed (The Joint Commission, 2010). Hospitals are required to provide professional language services to every patient with limited English proficiency (LEP) and tailor written materials to the patient's age, language, and ability to understand (Rorie, 2015). Interpreters must be competent and trained as medical interpreters. Using family members or even untrained support staff as interpreters raises quality, ethical, and possible legal issues. Family members, including children, may incorporate bias into their interpretations; patient confidentiality is compromised; issues about sharing sensitive, private matters with family or friends are an additional issue; and concern over the withholding of bad news or information should also be considered. Often interpreter services are delivered via the telephone, or remote video-phone; however, it does not have applicability for all patients (e.g., for patients who are deaf, where eye contact and nonverbal gestures are essential). Box 2-6 discusses using interpreter services effectively.

DIAGNOSIS

Diagnoses related to health education may include:

- Effective therapeutic regimen management
- Ineffective therapeutic regimen management
- Ineffective family therapeutic regimen management

- Health-seeking behaviors
- Ineffective health maintenance
- Readiness for enhanced management of therapeutic regimen
- Deficient knowledge
- Readiness for enhanced knowledge

PLANNING

Once assessment data are collected, the planning component of the teaching–learning process is established in accordance with the steps of the nursing process:

1. Specify the immediate, intermediate, and long-term goals of learning.
2. Identify specific teaching strategies appropriate for attaining goals.
3. Specify the expected outcomes.
4. Document the goals, teaching strategies, and expected outcomes of the teaching plan.

Developing the plan and goals of teaching should be a joint effort by the nurse and the patient and family members. Consideration must be given to the urgency of the patient's learning needs; the most critical needs should receive the highest priority.

After the learning priorities have been established, it is important to identify the immediate and long-term goals and the teaching strategies appropriate for attaining those goals. A partnership between patients and providers, based on both shared decision making and two-way communication, will develop your patient's skills and confidence needed to self-manage his or her health and prevent chronic disease progression (Gittner, 2015, p. 277). Learning begins with the establishment of goals that are appropriate to the situation and realistic in terms of the patient's ability and desire to achieve them. Involving the patient and family in establishing goals and in planning teaching strategies promotes their cooperation in implementing the teaching plan.

Expected outcomes of teaching strategies can be stated in terms of behaviors of patients, families, or both. Outcomes should be realistic and measurable, and the critical time periods for attaining them should be identified. The desired outcomes and the critical time periods serve as a basis for evaluating the effectiveness of the teaching strategies.

During the planning phase, the nurse must consider the sequence in which the subject matter is presented in each of

BOX 2-6   Working Effectively Through an Interpreter

Knowing the patient:
- Determine ethnicity and nationality of the patient.
- Determine what language(s) the patient speaks, and preferred language.
- Offer an interpreter to all patients where English is not their first language.
- Determine patient preference for face-to-face or telephone interpreter service.

Preparing for the meeting:
- Ensure a private, quiet environment, with space for all meeting participants.
- Maintain a warm, non-rushed environment where patient and interpreter can raise concerns.
- Meet with the interpreter before the meeting to discuss the goals of the meeting and the process (such as pausing for interpretation); if repeat meetings are required, try to use the same interpreter.
- Explain that interpreters are bound by their code of ethics to treat everything that is said as confidential.

Seating arrangements:
- Ensure that the seating is arranged to facilitate communication. When the meeting involves only a client, interpreter, and a clinician, arrange seating in a triangle formation.
- When interpreting with family, caregivers or more than two people, it is advisable to arrange the seating in a horseshoe or circle formation, with the interpreter seated next to the clinician.
- In a large or group meeting situation, arrange the seating in a circular formation, seat the interpreter next to the clinician and close to the client so they are able to understand the proceedings with minimum disruption to others.
- For telephone interpreting, use a dual handset or hands-free phone, and sit facing your client.

Verbal and nonverbal communication (telephone and face-to-face interpreter):
- Speak directly to the patient, not to the interpreter.
- Maintain eye contact and face your patient.
- Speak more slowly rather than more loudly.
- Keep your sentences or questions brief.
- Pause at the end of each statement to allow the interpreter time to interpret, explaining the need to pause to the client.
- Be aware that the interpreter may sometimes have to clarify a statement or answer with the client, family member, or caregiver.

During the medical interview:
- Assume, and insist, that everything you say, everything the patient says, and everything that family members say is interpreted.
- Do not hold the interpreter responsible for what the patient says or doesn't say. The interpreter is the medium, not the source, of the message.
- If you feel that you are not getting the type of response you were expecting, restate the question or consult with the interpreter to better understand if there is a cultural barrier that is interfering with communication.
- Be aware that many concepts you express have no linguistic or conceptual equivalent in other languages. The interpreter may have to paint word pictures of many terms you use. This may take longer than your original speech.
- Respond to nonverbal cues (e.g., quizzical or frightened look, stiffening of body posture)
- If you need to ask questions that may be extremely personal or sensitive, explain to the patient that doing so is part of your evaluation and reiterate that the information will remain confidential.
- Avoid: highly idiomatic speech, complicated sentence structure, sentence fragments, changing your idea in the middle of a sentence, and asking multiple questions at one time. Also avoid making assumptions or generalizations about your patients or their experiences. Common practices or beliefs in a community may not apply to everyone in that community.
- Encourage the interpreter to ask questions and to alert you about potential cultural misunderstandings that may come up. Respect an interpreter's judgment that a particular question is culturally inappropriate and either rephrase the question or ask the interpreter's help in eliciting the information in a more appropriate way.
- Ask the patients what they believe the problem is, what causes it, and how it would be treated in their country of origin.
- Ask the patient to repeat back important information that you want to make sure is understood.
- Be patient. Providing care across a language barrier takes time. However, the time spent up front will be paid back by good rapport and clear communication that will avoid wasted time and dangerous misunderstandings later in the process.

Adapted from Miletic et al. (2006), p. 18–26; Kaur (2014).

the teaching strategies. Critical information (e.g., blood glucose monitoring for a patient with diabetes) and material that the person or family identifies to be of particular importance will be high priority and, thus, should be presented earlier than other information. An outline is often helpful for arranging the subject matter and for ensuring that all necessary information is included. In addition, appropriate teaching aids to be used in implementing teaching strategies are prepared or selected at this time.

THE LEARNING ENVIRONMENT

Although learning can take place without teachers, most people who are attempting to learn new or altered health behaviors benefit from the services of nurses. The interpersonal interaction between the person and the nurse who is attempting to meet the person's learning needs may be formal or informal, depending on the method and techniques of teaching.

(continued on page 20)

Learning may be optimized by minimizing factors that interfere with the learning process. For example, the room temperature, lighting, noise levels, and other environmental conditions should be appropriate to the learning situation.

TIMING

The time selected for teaching should be suited to the needs of the individual person. Scheduling a teaching session at a time of day when a patient is fatigued, uncomfortable, or anxious about a pending diagnostic or therapeutic procedure, or when visitors are present, is not conducive to learning. However, if the family is to participate in providing care, the sessions should be scheduled when family members are present, so that they can learn any necessary skills or techniques.

TEACHING TECHNIQUES

Teaching techniques and methods enhance learning if they are appropriate to the patient's needs (Table 2-1). Numerous

TABLE 2-1 Teaching People with Disabilities

Type of Disability	Teaching Strategy
Physical, Emotional, or Cognitive Disability	Adapt information to accommodate the person's cognitive, perceptual, and behavioral disabilities. Give clear written and oral information. Highlight significant information for easy reference. Avoid medical terminology.
Hearing Impairment	Use slow, directed, deliberate speech. Use sign language or interpreter services if appropriate. Position yourself so that the person can see your mouth if speech reading. Use telecommunication devices (TTY[a] or TDD[b]) for the hearing impaired. Use written materials and visual aids, such as models and diagrams. Use captioned videos, films, and computer-generated materials. Teach on the side of the "good ear" if unilateral deafness is present.
Visual Impairment	Use optical devices such as a magnifying lens. Use proper lighting and proper contrast of colors on materials and equipment. Use large-print materials. Use Braille materials if appropriate. Convert information to auditory and tactile formats. Obtain audiotapes and talking books. Explain noises associated with procedures, equipment, and treatments. Arrange materials in clockwise pattern.
Learning Disabilities	
Input disability—process of recording information in the brain ("LD," n.d.)	If visual perceptual disorder: • Explain information verbally, repeat, and reinforce frequently. • Use audiotapes. • Encourage learner to verbalize information received. If auditory perceptual disorder: • Speak slowly with as few words as possible, repeat, and reinforce frequently. • Use direct eye contact to focus person on task. • Use demonstration and return demonstration such as modeling, role playing, and hands-on experiences. • Use visual tools, written materials, and computers.
Output disability—communication of information from the brain to other people or translation of the information into action ("LD," n.d.)	Use all senses as appropriate. Use written, audiotape, and computer information. Review information and give time to interact and ask questions. Use hand gestures and motions.
Developmental disability	Base information and teaching on developmental stage, not chronologic age. Use nonverbal cues, gestures, signing, and symbols as needed. Use simple explanations and concrete examples with repetition. Encourage active participation. Demonstrate information and have the person perform return demonstrations.

[a]TTY, a special device that lets people who are deaf, hard of hearing, or speech-impaired use the telephone for communication needs (messages are typed back and forth).
[b]TDD, operates similarly to a TTY but is a much smaller desktop machine.

techniques are available, including lectures, group teaching, and demonstrations, all of which can be enhanced with specially prepared teaching materials.

In general, patients remember information in approximately the following ratios:

- 10% of what they read
- 25% of what they hear
- 45% of what they see
- 65% of what they hear and see
- 70% of what they say and write
- 90% of what they say as they perform a task

The lecture or explanation method of teaching is commonly used but should always be accompanied by discussion. Discussion is important because it affords learners opportunities to express their feelings and concerns, to ask questions, and to receive clarification. Group teaching is appropriate for some people because it allows them not only to receive needed information but also to feel secure as members of a group. People with similar issues or learning needs have the opportunity to identify with each other and gain moral support and encouragement. Interactive group education has shown a significant increase in patient knowledge and better outcomes in terms of chronic disease self-management (Lu et al., 2015). Group visits allow interactions in a more natural setting, and conversations between patients help them feel less isolated and, possibly, less threatened. If group teaching is used, assessment and follow-up are imperative to ensure that each person has gained sufficient knowledge and skills. Demonstration and practice are essential ingredients of a teaching program, especially when the nurse is teaching skills to the patient. It is best to demonstrate the skill and then give the learner ample opportunity for practice. When special equipment is involved, such as syringes, colostomy bags, dialysis equipment, dressings, or suction apparatus, it is important to teach with the same equipment that will be used in the home setting. Learning to perform a skill with one kind of equipment and then having to change to a different kind may lead to confusion, frustration, and mistakes.

A tool such as the plan-do-study-act (PDSA) model is a framework for quality improvement activities. This model, or others like it, is used often by health care organizations to approach performance improvement work in a consistent way. A key finding of research about improving the effectiveness of chronic care models found that using the Plan-Do-Study-Act cycle with patients allowed for faster turnaround of information in formats that patients would use and could be individualized (Varkey et al., 2009, pp. 208–209). The PDSA model is a way to engage patients with their own care and have a role in developing their own plan. In addition, it provides opportunity to create learning collaboratives with other patients and health care providers (Davy et al., 2015). Other steps or tools that can improve success include collaborative agendas or goal setting, in which the patient and the nurse build the agenda together regarding items for discussion. Patients should be engaged to help prioritize items for best time management. A communication/demonstration technique known as *ask–tell–ask–close the loop* can help improve communication and patient understanding:

- *Ask* permission to give information about a topic of importance to the patient.
- *Tell:* Explanations and written materials are most effective when given in response to the patient's expressed agenda and tailored to his ability to understand.
- *Ask* for understanding, and provide additional information or clarification as necessary.
- *Close the loop:* Ask the patient to restate the information as the patient understands it (Goldman et al., 2015)

Teaching aids used to enhance learning include books, pamphlets, pictures, films, slides, audio and video tapes, models, programmed instruction, CD-ROMs, and computer-assisted learning modules. These are made available as needed for home, clinic, or hospital use, and they allow review and reinforcement of content and enhanced visual and auditory learning. Such teaching aids are invaluable when used appropriately and can save a significant amount of personnel time and related cost. However, all such aids should be reviewed before use to ensure that they meet the patient's learning needs. Developing tools as part of a multidisciplinary group also has been shown to yield benefits not only for patients who will use the tools but for the staff involved in creating them. Multidisciplinary teams have been shown to be more productive, have less stress, and have enriched professional experience (Reckery et al., 2015).

Reinforcement and follow-up are important because learning takes time. Allowing ample time to learn, and then reinforcing what is learned, are important teaching strategies; rarely is a single teaching session adequate. Follow-up sessions are imperative to promote the learner's confidence in his or her abilities and to plan for additional teaching sessions. For hospitalized patients who may not be able to transfer what they have learned in the hospital to the home setting, follow-up after discharge is essential to ensure that they have realized the full benefits of a teaching program.

The entire planning phase of the teaching–learning process concludes with the documentation of the teaching plan. This teaching plan communicates information to all members of the nursing and health care team. Documentation enhances the continuity of care for the patient and communication among caregivers. Documentation should include:

- The learner, instructor, and interpreter (if used)
- The patient's need assessment
- Learning objectives and goals
- Information and skills taught
- Teaching methods used
- Teaching materials provided or used
- Patient and family response to teaching
- Evaluation of what the patient learned
- Further learning needs
- Revised goals (if necessary)

(continued on page 22)

IMPLEMENTATION

In the implementation phase of the teaching–learning process, the patient, the family, and other members of the nursing and health care team carry out the activities outlined in the teaching plan. The nurse coordinates these activities.

During the implementation phase of the teaching–learning process and throughout the ongoing assessment of patient responses to the teaching strategies, flexibility is indispensable to support modification of the teaching plan as necessary. Creativity is essential in promoting and sustaining the patient's motivation to learn. Be sure to consider new learning needs that may arise after discharge from the hospital or after home care visits have ended.

Feedback about progress also motivates learning. Such feedback should be presented in the form of positive reinforcement when the learner is successful and in the form of constructive suggestions for improvement when he or she is unsuccessful.

The implementation phase ends when the teaching strategies have been completed and when the patient's responses to the actions have been recorded. This record serves as the basis for evaluating how well the defined goals and expected outcomes have been achieved.

EVALUATION

Evaluation of the teaching–learning process determines how effectively the patient has responded to teaching and to what extent the goals have been achieved. An evaluation must be made to determine what was effective and what needs to be changed or reinforced. It cannot be assumed that patients have learned just because teaching has occurred; learning does not automatically follow teaching. An important part of the evaluation phase addresses the question, "What can be done to improve teaching and enhance learning?" Answers to this question direct the changes to be made in the teaching plan.

A variety of measurement techniques can be used to identify changes in patient behavior as evidence that learning has taken place. These techniques include directly observing the behavior; using rating scales, checklists, or anecdotal notes to document the behavior; and indirectly measuring results using oral questioning and written tests. All direct measurements should be supplemented with indirect measurements whenever possible. Using more than one measuring technique enhances the reliability of the resulting data and decreases the potential for error from a measurement strategy.

In many situations, measurement of actual behavior is the most accurate and appropriate technique. Nurses often perform comparative analyses using patient admission data as the baseline: selected data points observed when nursing care is given and self-care is initiated are compared with the patient's baseline data. In other cases, indirect measurement may be used such as patient satisfaction surveys, attitude surveys, and instruments that evaluate specific health status variables.

However, measurement is only the beginning of evaluation, which must be followed by data interpretation and value judgments about learning and teaching. These aspects of evaluation

should be conducted periodically throughout the teaching–learning program, at its conclusion, and at varying periods after the teaching has ended.

Evaluation of learning after hospitalization is highly desirable because the analysis of teaching outcomes must extend into home care. With shortened lengths of hospital stay and with short-stay and same-day surgical procedures, follow-up evaluation in the home is especially important. Coordination of efforts and sharing of information between hospital- and community-based nursing personnel facilitate postdischarge teaching and home care evaluation.

Evaluation is not the final step in the teaching–learning process, but the beginning of the iterative process of a new patient assessment. The information gathered during evaluation should be used to redirect teaching actions, with the goal of improving the patient's responses and outcomes.

HEALTH PROMOTION

Health teaching and **health promotion** are linked by a common goal—to encourage people to achieve as high a level of wellness as possible so that they can live maximally healthy lives and avoid preventable illnesses. Patients are the primary managers of their health conditions. Nurses are in an ideal position to provide the kind of support that patients need to manage their conditions. Health promotion has become a cornerstone in health policy because of the need to control costs and reduce unnecessary sickness and death.

The US Department of Health and Human Services' Healthy People initiative was designed to establish a program of nationwide health-promotion and disease-prevention goals. The first set of goals established in the publication *Healthy People 2000* focused on disease prevention. *Healthy People 2010* added the priorities of health promotion, health protection, and the use of preventive services. *Healthy People 2020* builds on past achievements, reaffirms the overarching goals from the past decade, and adds: promoting quality of life, healthy behaviors across life stages, eliminating health disparities, and creating social and physical environments that promote good health.

Definition

Health promotion is defined as the process of enabling people to increase control over their health and its determinants, thereby improving their health (World Health Organization [WHO], 2016). The purpose of health promotion is to focus on the person's potential for wellness and to encourage appropriate alterations in personal habits, lifestyle, and environment in ways that reduce risks and enhance health and well-being. Health promotion is an active process; that is, it is not something that can be prescribed or dictated. It is up to each person to decide whether to make changes to promote a higher level of wellness. Only the individual can make these choices.

The concepts of health, wellness, health promotion, and disease prevention have been a topic of extensive discussion in the lay literature and news media, as well as in professional journals. As a result, public demand for health information has increased, and health care professionals and agencies have responded by providing this information. As employers strive to reduce costs associated with absenteeism, health insurance, hospitalization, disability, excessive turnover of personnel, and premature death, the workplace has become an important site for health-promotion programs. The concept of health promotion has evolved because of a changing definition of health and an awareness that wellness exists at many levels of functioning. Health is viewed as a dynamic, ever-changing condition that enables people to function at an optimal potential at any given time. The ideal health status is one in which people are successful in achieving their full potential, regardless of any limitations they might have.

Wellness, as a reflection of health, involves a conscious and deliberate attempt to maximize one's health. Wellness does not just happen; it requires planning and conscious commitment and is the result of adopting lifestyle behaviors for the purpose of attaining one's highest potential for well-being. Wellness is not the same for every person. The person with a chronic illness or disability may still be able to achieve a desirable level of wellness. The key to wellness is to function at the highest potential within the limitations over which there is no control.

Self-Responsibility

Taking responsibility for oneself is the key to successful health promotion. The concept of **self-responsibility** is based on the understanding that the individual controls his or her life. Each person alone must make the choices that determine how healthy his or her lifestyle is. As more people recognize that lifestyle and behavior significantly affect health, they may assume responsibility for avoiding high-risk behaviors such as smoking, alcohol and drug abuse, overeating, driving while intoxicated, risky sexual practices, and other unhealthy habits. Also they may assume responsibility for adopting routines that have been found to have a positive influence on health, such as engaging in regular exercise, wearing seat belts, and eating a healthy diet.

A variety of different techniques has been used to encourage people to accept responsibility for their health, ranging from extensive educational programs to reward systems (see Table 2-2). No one technique has been found to be superior to any other. Instead, self-responsibility for health promotion is very individualized and depends on a person's desires and inner motivations. Health-promotion programs are important tools for encouraging people to assume responsibility for their health and to develop behaviors that improve health.

Unfolding Patient Stories: Vincent Brody • Part 1

Vincent Brody, a 67-year-old male with chronic obstructive pulmonary disease (COPD), is experiencing increased fatigue. He spends most of the day in a recliner chair watching television and smoking 1 to 2 packs per day. His nutritional intake is poor due to shortness of breath. What patient education can the nurse provide to promote self-care behaviors for symptom improvement and a healthier lifestyle? (Vincent Brody's story continues in Chapter 51.)

Care for Vincent and other patients in a realistic virtual environment: **vSim** *for Nursing* (thepoint.lww.com/vSimMedicalSurgical). Practice documenting these patients' care in DocuCare (www.lww.com/DocuCareEHR).

Health Promotion throughout the Lifespan

Health promotion is a concept and a process that extends throughout the lifespan. Studies have shown that the health

---

TABLE **2-2** **Guidelines for Developing Patient Education Materials (The American Academy of Ambulatory Care Nursing Patient Education Special Interest Group [AAACN], n.d.)**

- Use visuals as much as possible (DVDs or printed illustrations) of anatomical features of the specific system that relates to the patient's problem or need
- Choose books, pamphlets, and/or brochures that are written at a third to fifth grade level
- Use short sentences (10 words or less) when developing printed materials
- Write paragraphs with no more than two or three sentences with one key point per paragraph
- Focus efforts on key bullet points of "must know" information
- Use visual terms such as "runny nose" and "redness"
- Explain measurements, e.g., "pain that lasts more than 30 minutes"
- Clearly list when the patient needs to call the health care provider and what phone number to call
- Focus on actions patients should do using familiar words
- Use plain language: Define any terms that are difficult to understand
- Have patient and family members "teach back" the information to you to ensure understanding
- Be aware of language, customs, and values to create a culturally sensitive and effective tool
- Use wide margins and leave white space between sections
- Find an advocate for the person with low literacy who will ensure that the individual understands and follows through with instructions

of a child can be affected either positively or negatively by the health practices of the mother during the prenatal period. Therefore, health promotion starts before birth and extends through childhood, adolescence, adulthood, and old age. At any stage of the lifespan, health promotion includes health screening. Screenings are tests that look for diseases before symptoms are present. In general, screening tests can find diseases early, when they are easier to treat. Some conditions that health care providers commonly screen for include breast cancer and cervical cancer in women, prostate cancer in men, as well as colorectal cancer, diabetes, high blood pressure, high cholesterol, osteoporosis, and obesity. Tests needed depend on age, sex, family history, and whether there are risk factors for certain diseases. The Center for Disease Control and Prevention (CDC) offers a website titled *CDC Prevention Checklist* where the public can obtain specific recommendations based upon age and sex for clinical preventative services (see www.cdc.gov, search: prevention checklist).

Young and Middle-Aged Adults

People of all ages are challenged to find the best way to make health behavior changes. Even when highly motivated, people can find it difficult to achieve and or sustain success. Younger people can be driven by different factors than middle-aged and older adults. Physical activity may be more strongly related to personality traits such as achievement orientation and sensation-seeking than to specific beliefs about the behavior (Sallis, Prochaska, & Taylor, 2000). Young adults also have fewer health problems than their older counterparts and unrealistic optimism about health risks. Therefore, young adults' beliefs about their health status may be less dominant in shaping their responses to health communications than their intrinsic motivations. Young and middle-aged adults can differ in their disposition as to the extent to which people are motivated to approach favorable outcomes or avoid unfavorable outcomes. Updegraff, Brick, Emanuel, Mintzer, and Sherman (2015) found that a gain-framed message promoted more interest in a preventive supplement than a loss-framed message among young people told that they were at low risk. In contrast, a loss-framed message promoted more interest for those told that they were at high risk.

Frequently adults are motivated to change their lifestyles in ways that they believe will enhance their health and wellness. Middle to older adults' beliefs can have a moderating effect because beliefs about susceptibility to health issues become more real with age. Many adults who wish to improve their health turn to health-promotion programs to help them make the desired changes in their lifestyles. Many have responded to programs that focus on topics such as general wellness, smoking avoidance or cessation, exercise, physical conditioning, weight control, conflict resolution, and stress management. Because of the nationwide emphasis on health during the reproductive years, young

adults actively seek programs that address prenatal health, parenting, family planning, and women's health issues.

There is a long, broad list of barriers that prevent or limit individuals from taking up and maintaining healthy behaviors in mid-life. The findings are surprisingly consistent across developed countries. Recurring themes include: lack of time (due to family, household and occupational responsibilities), access issues (to transportation, facilities and resources), financial costs, entrenched attitudes and behaviors, restrictions in the physical environment, low socioeconomic status, and lack of knowledge (Kelly et al., 2016). Likewise, research has identified a number of recurring factors that act as facilitators to healthy behaviors such as a focus on enjoyment of the healthy behavior, doing other healthy behaviors, health benefits, prevention of illness, the potential benefits for healthy aging and well-being as motivation; social support and encouragement; clear, accurate health messages, and integration of behaviors into lifestyle and routine (Kelly et al., 2016). Programs should be geared toward minimizing these barriers while maximizing the facilitators.

Programs that provide health screening, such as those that screen for cancer, high cholesterol, hypertension, diabetes, abdominal aneurysm, and visual and hearing impairments, are quite popular with young and middle-aged adults. Programs that involve health promotion for people with specific chronic illnesses, such as cancer, diabetes, heart disease, and pulmonary disease, are also popular. It is becoming more evident that chronic disease and disability do not preclude health and wellness; rather, positive health attitudes and practices can promote optimal health for people who must live with the limitations imposed by their chronic illnesses and disabilities.

Health-promotion programs can be offered almost anywhere in the community. Common sites include the workplace, local clinics, elementary and high schools, community colleges, recreation centers, churches, and even private homes. Frequently health fairs are held in civic centers and shopping malls. The outreach idea for health-promotion programs has served to meet the needs of many adults who otherwise would not avail themselves of opportunities to strive toward a healthier lifestyle.

Workplace programs usually include employee health screening and counseling, physical fitness, nutritional awareness, work safety, and stress management and stress reduction. Many large businesses provide exercise facilities for their employees and offer their health-promotion programs to retirees. If employers can show cost-containment benefits from such programs, their dollars will be considered well spent, and more businesses will provide health-promotion programs as a benefit of employment.

Older Adults

Health promotion is as important for the elderly as it is for other adults and children. Although their chronic illnesses and disabilities cannot be eliminated, these adults can benefit from activities that help them maintain independence and achieve an optimal level of health. Older adults have different health and social circumstances compared to younger people. Because of these differences, there are other strategies that can be used to help promote healthy behaviors. Motivators for older adults include physical and psychological well-being, maintenance of independent lifestyles, social connections, and enjoyment. Older adults who can self-report excellent or very good health, have no history of hip fracture after age 55, no cardiovascular disease, no depression, and have a BMI <25 are predicted to have greater independence. In addition, older adults who self-report "excellent" or "very good" health are also predicted to have little decline in activities of daily living. Older adults also believe that physical activity can protect cognitive health (Vaughan et al., 2016). Health-promotion materials could include information about healthy actions, nutritional information based on ethnicity and a healthy diet, as well as the frequency, duration, and intensity of physical activity and their effect on health. Box 2-1 provides gerontologic considerations.

Nursing Implications

Nurses have a unique relationship with the American public, topping Gallup's Honesty and Ethics ranking of professions every year but one since they were added to the list in 1999. The exception is 2001, when firefighters were included on the list on a one-time basis, shortly after the September 11 terrorist attacks. (Firefighters earned a record-high 90% honesty and ethics rating in that survey.) With an 85% honesty and ethics rating—tying their high point—nurses have no serious competition atop the Gallup rankings (Gallup, 2016). By virtue of nurses' expertise in health and health care and our long-established credibility with consumers, nurses play a vital role in health promotion. In many instances, nurses have initiated health-promotion and health-screening programs or have participated with other health care personnel in developing and providing wellness services in a variety of settings. As health care professionals, nurses have a responsibility to promote activities that foster well-being, self-actualization, and personal fulfillment. Every interaction with consumers of health care must be viewed as an opportunity to promote positive health attitudes and behaviors.

CHAPTER REVIEW

Critical Thinking Exercises

1. A history of GI disease is an independent risk factor for the development of GI adverse reactions during alendronate therapy. Severe reactions requiring hospitalization have occurred. Alendronate should be used with caution in patients with esophageal and GI disease, including dysphagia, esophagitis, gastritis, gastroesophageal reflux disease (GERD), hiatal hernia, duodenitis, ulcers, or GI perforation. What variables made the clinician prescribe this therapy?

2. A home health nurse is instructing a 55-year-old man with a history of coronary artery disease and systolic heart failure about healthy eating habits. He has recently been widowed. What physiologic and psychosocial variables would be relevant to understanding this patient's needs? How would a teaching plan be constructed to promote adequate nutrition? How would you modify the teaching plan if the patient is visually impaired?

3. A 72-year-old man is informed by an advanced practice nurse about a health fair being held at the local community center across the street from his home. He declines to attend, saying, "I am too old, and it is too late to be concerned about health promotion. The damage to my body has already been done." What resources would you use to identify evidence of the effectiveness of health-promotion activities for the elderly? Discuss the strength of the evidence. Identify the criteria used to evaluate the strength of the evidence. What information would you then include in a discussion with the patient about promoting health in the elderly?

NCLEX-Style Review Questions

1. A nurse is providing discharge teaching for an elderly patient who is fully dressed, watching television, and waiting for family. The nurse sits in a chair facing the patient and shows the patient a handout. The patient squints while reading and periodically looks at the television. The nurse is about to review the information and determine the patient's understanding of the material when the family enters the room. The nurse determines the need for further education due to learning barriers. Which barriers affected the patient's ability to comprehend the information? Select all that apply.
   a. Patient is watching television.
   b. The patient is elderly.
   c. The patient squints while reading.
   d. The family entered the room while teaching.
   e. The patient is fully dressed.

2. The nurse is to provide discharge teaching to a patient with newly diagnosed coronary artery disease. In what order should the following steps be prioritized and completed?
   a. Implement teaching plan.
   b. Collect and analyze data regarding the patient's knowledge of coronary artery disease.
   c. Form nursing diagnoses related to patient teaching.
   d. Reassess patient's knowledge as needed.
   e. Develop teaching plan.
   f. Identify learning needs.
   g. Update and change plan.

3. The nurse is discussing postoperative discharge instructions with an Asian American patient. The patient looks at the floor, smiles, and then nods his head. Using cultural awareness, how should the nurse interpret this behavior?
   a. Acceptance of the instructions
   b. Understanding of the material
   c. A reflection of cultural values
   d. The patient's ability to follow through on the instructions

> Try these additional resources, available at **http://thepoint.lww.com/Honan2e**, to enhance your learning and understanding of this chapter:
> • NCLEX-Style Student Review Questions
> • Journal Articles

4. When constructing a teaching plan, the steps of the nursing process are utilized. In which step are teaching strategies identified?
   a. Assessment
   b. Planning
   c. Implementation
   d. Evaluation

5. Which of the following is an accurate statement with regard to adult learner readiness?
   a. Learning readiness is based solely on past life experiences.
   b. Physical skills play little role in learner readiness.
   c. Experimental readiness is not related to emotional readiness.
   d. Learner readiness is based on culture, attitude, and personal values.

REFERENCES AND SELECTED READINGS

References and selected readings associated with this chapter can be found on the website that accompanies the book. Visit **http://thepoint. lww.com/Honan2e** to access the references and other additional resources associated with this chapter.

Chronic Illness and End-of-Life Care

James Mark Lazenby • Ruth McCorkle • Mei Bai

Learning Objectives

After reading this chapter, you will be able to:

1. Define "chronic illness."
2. Identify factors related to the increasing incidence of chronic diseases.
3. Describe characteristics of chronic illness and its impact on patients.
4. Describe implications of caring for patients with chronic illnesses for nursing practice.
5. Define and compare palliative and hospice care.
6. Describe the principles and components of hospice care.
7. Identify barriers to improving care at the end of life.
8. Identify and describe eight tasks that are essential for nurses to manage at the end of a patient's life.
9. Apply skills for communicating with terminally ill patients and their families.

Chronic diseases account for seven of the ten leading causes of death in the United States, including the four most frequently occurring diseases (heart disease, stroke, cancer, and diabetes) that result from preventable causes (tobacco use, improper diet and physical inactivity, and alcohol use). Chronic illnesses affect people of all ages and ethnic, cultural, and racial groups, although some illnesses occur more frequently in some groups than in others (Ward, Schiller, & Goodman, 2014). Although chronic disease occurs in all socioeconomic groups, people who have low incomes and disadvantaged backgrounds are more likely to report poor health (Blackwell, Lucas, & Clarke, 2014). Factors such as poverty and inadequate health insurance decrease the likelihood that people with chronic illness receive health care and preventative services (Office of Disease Prevention and Health Promotion, 2014).

Many people with chronic illnesses function independently with only minor inconvenience to their everyday lives; others require frequent and close monitoring or placement in long-term care facilities. Certain illnesses require advanced technology for survival, as in the late stages of amyotrophic lateral sclerosis or end-stage kidney disease, or intensive care for periods of weeks or months. People with diseases such as these have been described as chronically critically and progressively ill. Some chronic illnesses have little effect on quality of life, but others have a considerable effect because they can result in progressive

decline. The nurse recognizes that many patients admitted to acute care institutions have pre-existing chronic diseases that must continue to be managed in concert with their acute illnesses.

OVERVIEW OF CHRONICITY

Although each chronic disease has its own specific physiologic characteristics, chronic diseases do share common features. Many chronic diseases, for example, have pain and fatigue as associated symptoms. Usually some degree of physical decline is present in severe or advanced chronic illness, limiting the patient's participation in many activities. Many chronic diseases require therapeutic regimens to keep them under control. Unlike the term "acute," which implies a curable and relatively short course of disease, the term "chronic" describes a long course of disease and illnesses that may be incurable. This often makes managing chronic illnesses difficult for those who must live with them (Schulman-Green, Wagner, & McCorkle, 2015).

People who develop chronic illnesses may react with shock, disbelief, depression, anger, resentment, or a number of other emotions. How people react to and cope with chronic illness is usually similar to how they react to other events in their lives, depending, in part, on their understanding of the illness and their perceptions of its potential impact on their own and their family's lives. Adjustment to chronic illness is affected by various factors:

- Suddenness, extent, and duration of lifestyle changes necessitated by the illness
- Family and individual resources for dealing with stress
- Stages of individual/family life cycle
- Previous experience with illness and crises
- Underlying personality characteristics
- Unresolved anger or grief from the past

Psychological, emotional, and cognitive reactions to chronic illnesses are likely to occur at the onset of the illness and recur if symptoms worsen or reappear after a period of remission. Often symptoms associated with chronic illnesses are unpredictable and may be perceived as crisis events by patients and their families, who must contend with both the uncertainty of the chronic illness and the changes it brings to their lives. These possible effects can guide nursing assessment and interventions for the patient who has a chronic illness.

Definition of Chronic Illnesses

The literature does not support a single uniform definition for chronic disease, recurrent themes include the non–self-limited nature, the association with persistent and recurring health problems, and a duration measured in months and years, not days and weeks (Goodman, Posner, Huang, Parekh, & Koh, 2013). Traditionally, chronic diseases have focused on individual chronic pathologies. Now, however, health initiatives have expanded to include not only chronic disease but also chronic conditions such as functional limitations; anatomic problems that are not manifestations of physical disease but are permanent or long-standing; and a broad spectrum of behavioral health problems, some of which have traditionally not been classified as diseases (Goodman et al., 2013). The specific condition may be a result of illness, genetic factors, or injury; it may be a consequence of illnesses or unhealthy behaviors that began during childhood and young adulthood. Management of chronic illnesses includes learning to live with symptoms and coming to terms with identity changes resulting from having a chronic condition. It also consists of carrying out the lifestyle changes and regimens designed to control symptoms and to prevent complications. Although some people assume what might be called a "sick role" identity, most people with chronic illness wish to be involved in health care decision-making, and perform as active participants in their health care with preferences for their treatment and management of disease (Schulman-Green et al., 2015).

Prevalence and Causes of Chronic Illnesses

Chronic illnesses occur in people of every age group, socio-economic level, and culture. In the United States, as of 2012, about half of all adults—117 million people—had one or more chronic health conditions. One of four adults had two or more chronic health conditions (Table 3-1) (Ward et al.,

TABLE **3-1** Percentage of Adults with Chronic Diseases in the United States (2013)

Chronic Diseases	Adults with the Disease (%)
Arthritis	23.7[a]
Asthma	9.0[a]
Cardiovascular Disease	
Hypercholesterolemia	33.6[a]
Hypertension	29.0[a]
Heart attack (myocardial infarction)	4.4
Angina or coronary artery disease	4.1
Stroke	2.8
Diabetes	8.9[a]
Physical, emotional, or psychological problems that causes limitations in activities	35.9[b]

[a]Age-adjusted prevalence%.
[b]Crude prevalence, data for disability among adults aged ≥65 years old (Year 2012).
Adapted from CDC (2015a, 2015b).

2014). As the incidence of chronic illnesses increases, the costs associated with these illnesses (i.e., hospital costs, equipment, medications, supportive services) also increase. Expenditures for health care for people with chronic illnesses exceed billions of dollars every year, and 86% of all health care spending in 2010 was for people with one or more chronic medical conditions in the United States (Gerteis et al., 2014).

Although some chronic health illnesses cause little or no inconvenience, others are severe enough to cause major activity limitations. When people with activity limitations are unable to meet their needs for health care and personal services, they may be unable to carry out their therapeutic regimens or have their prescriptions filled on time, may miss appointments and office visits with their health care providers, and may be unable to carry out their activities of daily living (ADLs).

Chronic disease is a global issue that affects both rich and poor nations. With the advent and distribution of highly active antiretroviral therapies and other treatments for communicable diseases, and, thus, longer lifespans, the incidence of chronic illness is increasing in developing countries of the Global South, even while they try to cope with new and emerging infectious diseases. In developed Western countries of the Global North, chronic illnesses have become the major cause of health-related problems. The Global North represents the economically developed societies of Europe,

North America, Australia, Israel, South Africa, among others, the Global South represents the economically developing or less-developed countries of Africa, India, China, Brazil, Mexico among others.

Causes of the increasing number of people with chronic illnesses include the following:

- A decrease in mortality from infectious diseases, such as smallpox, diphtheria, and other serious illnesses
- Longer lifespans because of advances in technology and pharmacology, improved nutrition, safer working conditions, and greater access (for some people) to health care
- Improved screening and diagnostic procedures, enabling early detection and treatment of diseases
- Prompt and aggressive management of acute illnesses, such as myocardial infarction and AIDS-related infections
- The tendency to develop chronic illnesses with advancing age
- Lifestyle factors, such as smoking, chronic stress, and sedentary lifestyle, which increase the risk for chronic health problems such as respiratory disease, hypertension, cardiovascular disease, and obesity

Consequences of unhealthy lifestyles include an alarming increase in the incidence of diabetes, hypertension, obesity, and cardiac and chronic respiratory disorders. Physiologic changes in the body often occur before the appearance of symptoms of chronic disease. Therefore, the goal of emphasizing healthy lifestyles early in life is to improve overall health status and slow the development of such disorders.

Characteristics of Chronic Illnesses

Sometimes it is difficult for people who are disease-free to understand the often profound effect of chronic illness on the lives of patients and their families. It is easy for health professionals to focus on the illness itself while overlooking the person who has the disorder. In all illnesses, but even more so with chronic illnesses, the illness cannot be separated from the person. People with chronic illness must contend with it daily. To relate to what people must cope with or to plan effective interventions, nurses must understand what it means to have a chronic illness. Characteristics of chronic illness include the following:

- Managing chronic illness involves more than managing medical problems. Also associated psychological and social problems must be addressed because living for long periods with illness symptoms and disability can threaten identity, bring about role changes, alter body image, and disrupt lifestyles. These changes require continuous adaptation and accommodation, depending on age and situation in life. Each decline in functional ability requires physical, emotional, and social adaptation for patients and their families.
- Chronic illnesses usually involve many different phases over the course of a person's lifetime. There can be acute periods, stable and unstable periods, flare-ups, and remissions. Each phase brings its own set of physical, psychological, and social problems, and each requires its own regimens and types of management. Table 3-2 describes the phases in the trajectory model of chronic illness.
- Keeping chronic illnesses under control requires persistent adherence to therapeutic regimens. Failing to adhere to a treatment plan or to adhere consistently increases the risks of developing complications and accelerating the disease process. However, the realities of daily life, including the impact of culture, values, and socioeconomic factors, affect the degree to which people adhere to a treatment regimen. Managing a chronic illness takes time, requires knowledge and planning, and can be uncomfortable and inconvenient. It is not unusual for patients to stop taking medications or alter dosages because of side effects that are more disturbing or disruptive than symptoms of the illness, or to cut back on regimens they consider overly time-consuming, fatiguing, or costly.
- One chronic disease can lead to the development of other chronic illnesses. Diabetes, for example, can affect many parts of the body and is associated with serious complications, such as heart disease and stroke, blindness, kidney failure, and lower-limb amputation (Centers for Disease Control and Prevention [CDC], 2014). The presence of a chronic illness also contributes to a higher risk of morbidity and mortality in patients admitted to the intensive care unit with acute health illnesses.
- Chronic illness affects the entire family. Family life can be altered dramatically as a result of role reversals, unfilled roles, loss of income, time required to manage the illness, decreases in family socialization activities, and the costs of treatment. Stress and caregiver fatigue are common with severe chronic illnesses, and the entire family rather than just the patient may need care. However, some families are able to master the treatment regimen and changes that accompany chronic illness, as well as make the treatment regimen a routine part of life. Furthermore, they are able to keep the chronic illness from becoming the focal point of family life.
- The day-to-day management of illness is largely the responsibility of people with chronic disorders and their families. As a result, the home, rather than the hospital, is the center of care in chronic illnesses. Hospitals, clinics, physicians' offices, nursing homes, nursing centers, and community agencies (home care services, social services, and disease-specific associations and societies) are considered adjuncts or backup services to daily home management.
- The management of chronic illnesses is a process of discovery. People can be taught how to self-manage their illnesses. However, each person must discover how his or her own body reacts under varying circumstances—for example, what it is like to be hypoglycemic, what

TABLE 3-2 Phases in the Trajectory Model of Chronic Illness

Phase	Description	Focus of Nursing Care
Pre-trajectory	Genetic factors or lifestyle behaviors that place a person or community at risk for a chronic condition	Refer for genetic testing and counseling if indicated; provide education about prevention of modifiable risk factors and behaviors
Trajectory onset	Appearance or onset of noticeable symptoms associated with a chronic disorder; includes period of diagnostic workup and announcement of diagnosis; may be accompanied by uncertainty as patient awaits a diagnosis and begins to discover and cope with implications of diagnosis	Provide clear explanations of diagnostic tests and procedures and reinforce information and explanations given by primary health care provider; provide emotional support to patient and family
Stable	Illness course and symptoms are under control as symptoms, resulting disability and everyday life activities are being managed within limitations of illness; illness management centered in the home	Reinforce positive behaviors and offer ongoing monitoring; provide education about health promotion and encourage participation in health-promoting activities and health screening
Unstable	Characterized by an exacerbation of illness symptoms, development of complications, or reactivation of an illness in remission. Period of inability to keep symptoms under control or reactivation of illness; difficulty in carrying out everyday life activities. May require more diagnostic testing and trial of new treatment regimens or adjustment of current regimen, with care usually taking place at home	Provide guidance and support; reinforce previous teaching
Acute	Severe and unrelieved symptoms or the development of illness complications necessitating hospitalization, bed rest, or interruption of the person's usual activities to bring illness course under control	Provide direct care and emotional support to the patient and family members
Crisis	Critical or life-threatening situation requiring emergency treatment or care and suspension of everyday life activities until the crisis has passed	Provide direct care, collaborate with other health care team members to stabilize patient's condition
Comeback	Gradual recovery after an acute period and learning to live with or to overcome disabilities and return to an acceptable way of life within the limitations imposed by the chronic condition or disability; involves physical healing, limitations stretching through rehabilitative procedures, psychosocial coming-to-terms, and biographical reengagement with adjustments in everyday life activities	Assist in coordination of care; rehabilitative focus may require care from other health care providers; provide positive reinforcement for goals identified and accomplished
Downward	Illness course characterized by rapid or gradual worsening of a condition; physical decline accompanied by increasing disability or difficulty in controlling symptoms; requires biographical adjustment and alterations in everyday life activities with each major downward step	Provide home care and other community-based care to help patient and family adjust to changes and come to terms with these changes; assist patient and family to integrate new treatment and management strategies; encourage identification of end-of-life preferences and planning
Dying	Final days or weeks before death; characterized by gradual or rapid shutting down of body processes, biographical disengagement and closure, and relinquishment of everyday life interests and activities	Provide direct and supportive care to patients and their families through hospice programs

Adapted from Corbin, J. M. (1998). The Corbin and Stauss chronic illness trajectory model: An update. *Scholarly Inquiry for Nursing Practice, 12*(1), 33–41.

activities are likely to bring on angina, and how these or other illnesses can best be prevented and managed.

- Managing chronic illnesses must be a collaborative process that involves many different health care professionals working together with patients and their families to provide the full range of services that often are needed for management at home. Often the medical, social, and psychological aspects of chronic health problems are complex, especially in severe illnesses. The goal is to help patients to self-manage and have ultimate responsibility for their own health.
- The management of chronic illnesses is expensive. Many of the expenses incurred by an individual patient (e.g., costs for hospital stays, diagnostic tests, equipment, medications, and supportive services) may be covered by health insurance and by federal and state agencies. However, the cost increases affect society as a whole as insurance premiums increase to cover these costs. Cost increases at the government level decrease resources that might benefit society. In addition, many out-of-pocket expenses are not reimbursed. Many people with chronic disorders, including the elderly and people who are working, are uninsured, or underinsured, and may be unable to afford the high costs of care often associated with chronic illnesses. Absence from work because of chronic disorders may jeopardize job security and income, and consequently health coverage.
- Chronic illnesses raise difficult ethical issues for patients, health care professionals, and society. Problematic questions include how to establish cost controls, how to allocate scarce resources (e.g., organs for transplantation), and what constitutes quality of life and when life support should be withdrawn.
- Living with chronic illness means living with uncertainty. Although health care providers may be aware of the usual progression of a chronic disease such as Parkinson disease, no one can predict with certainty a person's illness course because of individual variation. Even when a patient is in remission or symptom-free, he or she often fears that the illness will reappear.

Implications of Managing Chronic Illnesses

Chronic illnesses have implications for everyday living and management for people and their families as well as for society at large. Most importantly, individual efforts should be directed at preventing chronic illnesses, because many chronic illnesses or disorders are linked to unhealthy lifestyles or behaviors such as smoking, inactivity, and overeating. Therefore, changes in lifestyle can prevent some chronic disorders, or at least delay onset until a later age. Because most people resist change, bringing about alterations in people's lifestyles is a major challenge for nurses today.

Once a chronic condition has emerged, the focus shifts to managing symptoms, avoiding complications (e.g., eye complications in a person with diabetes), and avoiding the development of other acute illnesses (e.g., pneumonia in a person with chronic obstructive pulmonary disease). Quality of life, often overlooked by health professionals in their approach to people with chronic illnesses, is also important. Health-promoting behaviors, such as exercise, are essential to quality of life, even in people who have chronic illnesses, because regular exercise helps to maintain functional status.

Although coworkers, extended family, and health care professionals are affected by chronic illnesses, the problems of living with chronic illnesses are most acutely experienced by patients and their immediate families. They experience the greatest impact, with lifestyle changes that directly affect quality of life. Nurses provide direct care, especially during acute episodes, but they also provide the teaching and secure the resources and other supports that enable people to integrate their illness into their lives and to have an acceptable quality of life despite the illness. To understand what nursing care is needed, it is important to recognize and appreciate the issues that people with chronic illness and their families contend with and manage, often on a daily basis. The challenges of living with chronic illnesses include the need to accomplish the following:

- Alleviate and manage symptoms
- Psychologically adjust to and physically accommodate disabilities
- Prevent and manage crises and complications
- Carry out regimens as prescribed
- Validate individual self-worth and family functioning
- Manage threats to identity
- Normalize personal and family life as much as possible
- Live with altered time, social isolation, and loneliness
- Establish the networks of support and resources that can enhance quality of life
- Return to a satisfactory way of life after an acute debilitating episode (e.g., another myocardial infarction or stroke) or reactivation of a chronic condition
- Die with dignity and comfort

Many people with chronic illness must face an additional challenge: the need to deal with more than one chronic illness at a time. Multiple illnesses are termed comorbidities. The symptoms or treatment of a second chronic condition may aggravate the first chronic condition. Patients need to be able to deal with their various chronic illnesses separately, as well as in combination. Some Medicare beneficiaries have 5 or more chronic illnesses, see an average of 12 physicians per year, and fill an average of 50 prescriptions per year (Gerteis et al., 2014). Furthermore, the effects of increasing longevity among Americans are likely to increase health care costs in the future.

Even more challenging for many people with chronic illness is the need to hire and oversee caregivers who come into their homes to assist with ADLs and instrumental activities of daily living (IADLs). ADLs and IADLs are the activities that let an individual live independently in a community such as preparing meals, shopping, telephone use, and taking medications correctly. It is difficult for many people to be in a position of hiring, supervising, and, sometimes, firing people who may provide them with intimate physical care. The need to balance the role of recipient of care and oversight of the person providing care may lead to blurring of role boundaries.

The challenges of living with and managing a chronic illness are well known, and people with chronic illnesses often report receiving inadequate care, information, services, and counseling. This provides an opportunity for nurses to be responsible for addressing many of the issues experienced, coordinating care, and serving as an advocate for patients and their families who need additional assistance to manage the patient's illness while maintaining a quality of life that is acceptable to all of them.

Phases of Chronic Illnesses

Chronic illnesses can pass through different phases, as described in Table 3-2. However, this course may be too uncertain to predict with any degree of accuracy. The course of an illness can be thought of as a trajectory that can be managed or shaped over time, to some extent, through proper illness management strategies. It is important to keep in mind that not all phases occur in all patients; some phases do not occur at all, and some phases may recur. Each phase is characterized by different medical and psychosocial issues. For example, the needs of a patient with a stroke who is a good candidate for rehabilitation are very different from those of a patient with terminal cancer. By thinking in terms of phases and individual patients within a phase, nurses can target their care more specifically to each person. Not every chronic condition is necessarily life-threatening, and not every patient passes through each possible phase of a chronic condition in the same order.

Using the trajectory model enables the nurse to put the current situation into the context of what might have happened to the patient in the past—that is, the life factors and understandings that might have contributed to the current state of the illness. In this way, the nurse can more readily address the underlying issues and problems.

NURSING CARE OF PATIENTS WITH CHRONIC ILLNESSES

Nursing care of patients with chronic illnesses is varied and occurs in a variety of settings. Care may be direct or supportive. *Direct care* may be provided in the clinic or health provider's office, the hospital, or the patient's home, depending on the status of the illness. Examples of direct care include assessing the patient's physical status, providing wound care, managing and overseeing medication regimens, and performing other technical tasks. The availability of this

type of nursing care may allow the patient to remain at home and return to a more normal life after an acute episode of illness. *Supportive care* may include ongoing monitoring, teaching, counseling, serving as an advocate for the patient, navigating the system to coordinate care, making referrals, and case-managing. Giving supportive care is just as important as giving technical care. For example, through ongoing monitoring, either in the home or in a clinic, a nurse might detect early signs of impending complications and make a referral (i.e., contact the provider or consult the medical protocol in a clinic) for medical evaluation, thereby preventing a lengthy and costly hospitalization.

Working with people with chronic illness requires not only dealing with the medical aspects of their disorders but also working with the whole person—physically, emotionally, and socially. This holistic approach to care requires nurses to draw on their knowledge and skills, including knowledge from the social sciences and psychology in particular. Although quality of life usually is affected by chronic illness, especially if the illness is severe, patients' perceptions of what constitutes quality of life often drive their management behaviors or affect how they view advice about health care. Nurses and other health care professionals need to recognize this, even though it may be difficult to see patients make unwise choices and decisions about lifestyles and disease management. People have the right to receive care without fearing ridicule or refusal of treatment, even if their behaviors (e.g., smoking, substance abuse, overeating, and failure to follow health care providers' recommendations) may have contributed to their chronic disorder.

Unfolding Patient Stories: Skyler Hansen • Part 1

Skyler Hansen is an 18-year-old male recently diagnosed with type 1 diabetes. He lives with his parents and two younger siblings and is active in high school sports. He now requires insulin injections, glucose monitoring, and a diabetic diet. Examine how the psychological, physical, and teaching needs for managing a new diagnosis can be a great source of stress to the patient and family. How can the nurse enhance their ability to cope with and adapt to diabetes management? (Skyler Hansen's story continues in Chapter 30.)

Care for Skyler and other patients in a realistic virtual environment: *vSim for Nursing* (thepoint.lww.com/vSimMedicalSurgical). Practice documenting these patients' care in DocuCare (thepoint.lww.com/DocuCareEHR).

Skills for Communicating with the Chronically Ill

Nurses need to develop skill and comfort in assessing patients' and families' responses to chronic illness and planning interventions that will support their values and choices throughout the continuum of care. Patients and families need ongoing assistance: telling a patient something once is not teaching, and hearing the patient's words is not the same as active listening. Throughout the course of illness, patients and their families encounter complicated treatment decisions, bad news about disease progression, and recurring emotional responses. In addition to the time of initial diagnosis, lack of response to the treatment course, decisions to continue or withdraw particular interventions, and decisions about hospice care are examples of critical points on the treatment continuum that demand patience, empathy, and honesty from nurses. Discussing sensitive issues such as progressive illness, hopes for survival, and fears associated with death is never easy. However, the art of therapeutic communication can be learned and, like other skills, must be practiced to gain expertise. Similar to other skills, communication should be practiced in a "safe" setting, such as a classroom or clinical skills laboratory with other students or clinicians.

Although communication with each patient and family should be tailored to their particular level of understanding and values concerning disclosure, general guidelines for nurses include the following:

- Deliver and interpret the technical information necessary for making decisions without hiding behind medical terminology.
- Realize that the best time for the patient to talk may be when it is least convenient for you.
- Being fully present during any opportunity for communication is often the most helpful form of communication.
- Allow the patient and family to set the agenda regarding the depth of the conversation.
- Realize that beginning the conversation requires additional opportunities to continue the conversation.

When Patients and Families Receive Bad News

Communicating about a life-threatening diagnosis or about disease progression is best accomplished by the interdisciplinary team in any setting: a physician, advanced practice nurse, nurse, and social worker should be present whenever possible to provide information, facilitate discussion, and address concerns. Most importantly, the presence of the team conveys caring and respect for the patient and family. If the patient wishes to have family present for the discussion, arrangements should be made to have the discussion at a time that is best for everyone. A quiet area with a minimum of disturbances should be used. All clinicians present should turn off beepers, cell phones, and other electronic devices for the duration of the meeting and should allow sufficient time for the patient and family to absorb and respond to the news. Finally, the space in which the meeting takes place should be conducive to seating all participants at eye level.

After the initial discussion of a life-threatening illness or progression of a disease, the patient and family have many questions and may need to be reminded of factual information. Coping with news about a serious diagnosis or poor prognosis is an ongoing process. The nurse should be sensitive to these ongoing needs and may need to repeat previously provided information or simply be present while the patient and family react emotionally. Seriously ill patients and their families need time and support to cope with the changes brought about by changes in the patient's condition and the prospect of impending death. The nurse who is able to sit comfortably with another's suffering, time and time again, without judgment and without the need to solve the patient's and family's problems, provides an intervention that is a gift beyond measure.

THE CHANGING TRAJECTORY OF CHRONIC ILLNESS TO END-OF-LIFE CARE

As individuals become chronically ill, their health shifts between stable and unstable and acute and crisis events. During these periods of health status changes, patients will use increased health care services to regain their balance and recover. There are peaks and valleys to these patterns, and eventually patients reach a point from which they do not rebound, and they become progressively ill, decline, and die. It is during these periods of times when chronically ill patients come in contact with members of the health care team who should evaluate them for palliative and supportive services to enhance their care and improve and sustain their quality of living.

Providing end-of-life care for someone chronically ill is very different from providing it to someone who may have died suddenly from an accident, trauma, disaster, or homicide. When a death is sudden, there is tremendous shock and disbelief by the person's survivors that the person has died. The shock is compounded if the death was thought to be preventable, or if it resulted from a reckless act of irresponsibility, such as from a drunken driving accident. When a person has a chronic disease that progresses with a known trajectory, it gives the patient and family members opportunities to plan and participate in decisions about treatment choices and resources to use to facilitate their quality of life individually and as a family.

Sociocultural Context

Although each person experiences terminal illness uniquely, that illness is also shaped substantially by the social and cultural contexts in which it occurs. In the United States, life-threatening illness, life-sustaining treatment decisions, dying, and death occur in a social environment in which illness is largely considered a foe and battles are either lost or won (Benoliel, 1993). A care–cure dichotomy emerged early on in modern medicine, in which health care providers may view cure as the ultimate goal and care as second best, and only acceptable when cure is no longer possible. In this model of health care, alleviating suffering is not as valued as curing disease, and patients who cannot be cured feel distanced from the health care team, concluding that, when treatment has failed, they too have failed. Patients and families who have internalized the socially constructed meaning of care as second-best to cure may fear that any shift from curative goals in the direction of comfort-focused care will result in no care or lower-quality care, and that the clinicians on whom they have come to rely will abandon them if they withdraw from the battle for cure.

The reduction of patients to their diseases is exemplified in the frequently relayed message in late-stage illness that "nothing more can be done." This all-too-frequently used statement communicates the belief of many clinicians that there is nothing of value to offer patients who are beyond cure. In a care-focused perspective, mind, body, and spirit are inextricable, and treating the body without attending to the mind and spirit is considered inadequate to evoke true healing. The idea of healing as care, along with and beyond cure, implies that healing can take place throughout life and outside the boundaries of contemporary medicine. In this expanded definition, there continue to be opportunities for physical, spiritual, emotional, and social healing, even as body systems begin to fail at the end of life.

Clinicians' attitudes toward the terminally ill and dying remain the greatest barrier to improving care at the end of life. Kübler-Ross illuminated the concerns of the seriously ill and dying in her seminal work, *On Death and Dying,* published in 1969. At that time, it was common for patients to be kept uninformed about life-threatening diagnoses, particularly cancer, and for physicians and nurses to avoid open discussion of death and dying with their patients. Kübler-Ross taught the health care community that having open discussion about life-and-death issues did not harm patients and that the patients, in fact, welcomed such openness. She was openly critical of what she called "a new but depersonalized science in the service of prolonging life rather than diminishing human suffering" (Kübler-Ross, 1969). She taught the health care community that healing could not take place in a conspiracy of silence, and that as clinicians break the silence and enter the patient's world, they too can be enriched by being partners with their patients. Her work revealed that, given adequate time and some help in working through the process, patients could reach a stage of acceptance in which they were neither angry nor depressed about their fate.

Clinicians' reluctance to discuss disease and death openly with patients may stem from their own anxieties about death, as well as misconceptions about what and how much patients want to know about their illnesses. In a seminal study of care of the dying in hospital settings, sociologists Glaser and Strauss (1965) identified that health care professionals in hospital settings avoided direct communication about dying in hopes that the patient would discover it on his or her own.

They identified four "awareness contexts" that described awareness of the patient's status by providers, patients, and family members.

- *Closed awareness,* in which the patient is unaware of his or her terminal state
- *Suspected awareness,* in which the patient suspects what others know and attempts to find out details about his or her condition
- *Mutual pretense,* in which the patient, family, and providers are aware that the patient is dying but all pretend otherwise
- *Open awareness,* in which the patient, family, and providers are aware that the patient is dying and openly acknowledge that reality (Glaser & Strauss, 1965).

The two major reasons they identified that clinicians avoided direct communication with patients about the seriousness of their illness were (1) patients already knew the truth or would ask if they wanted to know, or (2) patients would subsequently lose all hope, give up, or be psychologically harmed by disclosure. Glaser and Strauss' findings were published decades ago, yet their observations remain valid today. Although a growing number of health care providers are becoming comfortable with assessing patients' and families' information needs and disclosing honest information about the seriousness of illness, many still avoid the topic of death in hope that the patient will ask or find out on his or her own. Despite progress on many health care fronts, those who work with dying patients have identified the persistence of a "conspiracy of silence" about dying.

The Importance of Palliative Care in Chronic Illness

As patients decline and treatments become complex, there has been an international recognition of the need to help patients transition from a cure orientation to one of care.

Palliative care and hospice care have been recognized as important bridges between a medical bias in the direction of cure-oriented treatment and the needs of the terminally ill patients and their families for comprehensive care in the final years, months, or weeks of life. This bridge has been built by experts in the field who advocate that palliative care needs to be extended throughout the course of life-threatening illness from the time when the patient is first diagnosed and not limited to end-of-life care (World Health Organization [WHO], 2015).

Palliative care encompasses a wide range of therapeutic interventions that aim to prevent and relieve suffering caused by multiple issues that patients and family caregivers face at any stage during an acute or chronic illness. In providing palliative care to the whole person (Lazenby, 2014), health care providers attend to all domains of the human experience of illness that may be involved: physical, psychological, social, and spiritual. A number of models of care have

FIGURE 3-1 Model of cancer care in which only therapies directed at the disease are considered as part of standard care. From Irwin, S. A., & von Guntun, C. F. (2010). The role of palliative care in cancer care transitions. In J. C. Holland, W. S. Bretibart, P. B. Jacobsen, M. S. Lederberg, M. J. Loscalzo, & R. McCorkle (Eds.). *Psycho-Oncology* (2nd ed., pp. 277–283). New York: Oxford University Press.

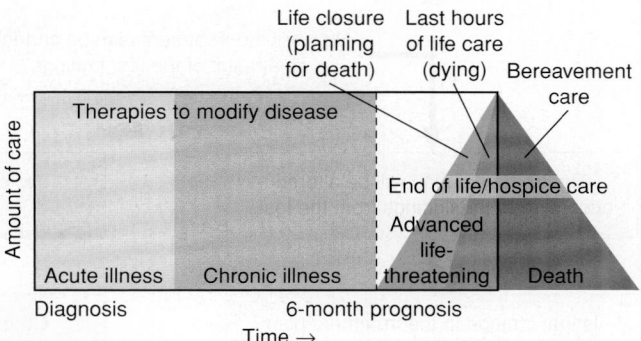

FIGURE 3-3 Model of cancer care in which palliative care begins after efforts directed at the disease end. From Irwin, S. A., & von Guntun, C. F. (2010). The role of palliative care in cancer care transitions. In J. C. Holland, W. S. Bretibart, P. B. Jacobsen, M. S. Lederberg, M. J. Loscalzo, & R. McCorkle (Eds.). *Psycho-Oncology* (2nd ed., pp. 277–283). New York: Oxford University Press.

described the difference in these approaches to treatment. An exclusively "cure-oriented" approach to chronic illness care can be conceptualized in Figure 3-1; here, the treatment is compartmentalized by the type of illness and disease events. In Figure 3-2, the treatment of a disease diminishes over time as treatment becomes less effective. In Figure 3-3, "comfort care" is instituted when the patient with a chronic illness is not responding to the previous treatments and additional symptom management efforts are needed. Figure 3-4 illustrates how palliative care can begin at diagnosis and become integrated throughout the entire course of the chronic illness trajectory for the patient and family caregiver. Ideally, palliative care should precede the time when the provider recognizes that hospice care is needed. When palliative care coexists with disease-oriented treatment, patients and their families benefit from the more comprehensive management of the illness experience.

Goal Setting in Palliative Care

As treatment goals begin to shift in the direction of comfort care over aggressive disease-focused treatment, symptom relief and patient- and family-defined quality of life assume

greater prominence in treatment decision-making. Patients, families, and health care providers all may be accustomed to an almost automatic tendency to pursue exhaustive diagnostic testing to locate and treat the source of patients' illnesses or symptoms. Each decision to withdraw treatment or discontinue diagnostic testing is an extremely emotional one for the patient and family. They may fear that the support from health care providers on whom they have come to rely will be withdrawn along with the treatment.

Throughout the course of the illness, and especially as the patient's functional status and symptoms indicate approaching death, the provider should help the patient and family weigh the benefits of continued diagnostic testing and disease-focused medical treatment against the burdens of those activities. The patient and family may be extremely reluctant to forego monitoring that has become routine throughout the illness (e.g., blood testing, x-rays) but that may contribute little to comfort. Likewise, health care providers from other disciplines may have difficulty discontinuing such diagnostic testing or medical treatment.

FIGURE 3-2 Model of cancer care in which antidisease treatment diminishes over time as it becomes less and less effective. From Irwin, S. A., & von Guntun, C. F. (2010). The role of palliative care in cancer care transitions. In J. C. Holland, W. S. Bretibart, P. B. Jacobsen, M. S. Lederberg, M. J. Loscalzo, & R. McCorkle (Eds.). *Psycho-Oncology* (2nd ed., pp. 277–283). New York: Oxford University Press.

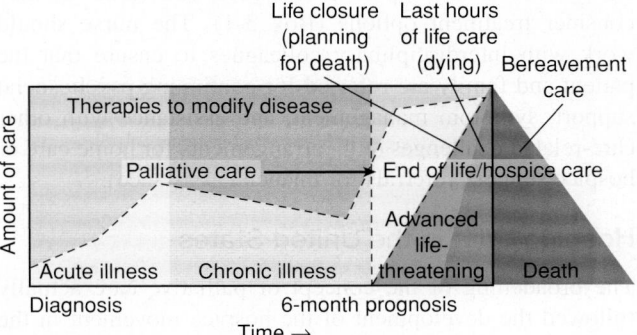

FIGURE 3-4 Model of cancer care in which palliative care begins at diagnosis and is integrated throughout the course of treatment. From Irwin, S. A., & von Guntun, C. F. (2010). The role of palliative care in cancer care transitions. In J. C. Holland, W. S. Bretibart, P. B. Jacobsen, M. S. Lederberg, M. J. Loscalzo, & R. McCorkle (Eds.). *Psycho-Oncology* (2nd ed., pp. 277–283). New York: Oxford University Press.

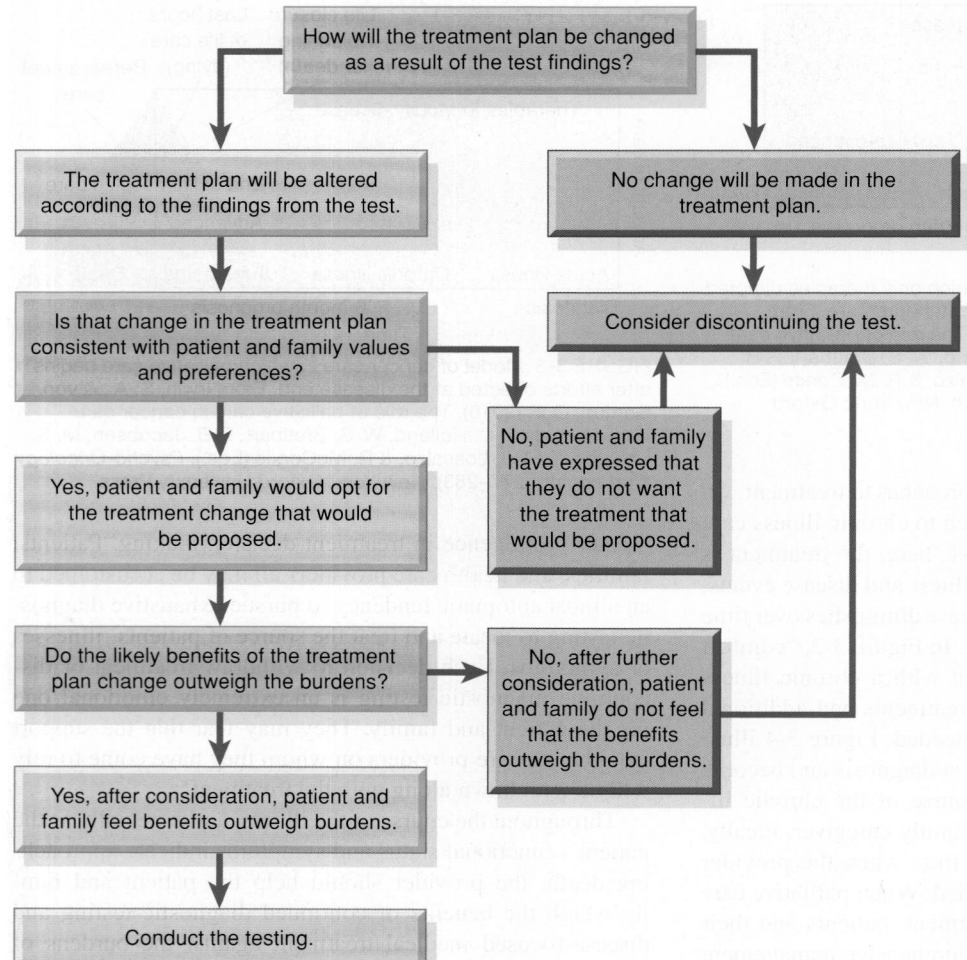

FIGURE 3-5 An algorithm for decision-making about diagnostic testing at the end of life.

Specifically, the nurse should collaborate with other members of the interdisciplinary team to share assessment findings and develop a coordinated plan of care (Fig. 3-5). In addition, the nurse should help the patient and family clarify their goals, expected outcomes, and values as they consider treatment options (Box 3-1). The nurse should work with interdisciplinary colleagues to ensure that the patient and family are referred for continuing psychosocial support, symptom management, and assistance with other care-related challenges (e.g., arrangements for home care or hospice support, referrals for financial assistance).

Hospice Care in the United States

The broadening of the concept of palliative care actually followed the development of the hospice movement in the United States. Hospice care is, in fact, palliative care. The difference is that hospice care is associated with the end of the patient's life, and although it focuses on quality of life, hospice care by necessity usually includes realistic emotional, social, spiritual, and financial preparation for death. The hospice movement in the United States is based on the

BOX 3-1 **Assessing the Patient and Family Perspective: Goal Setting in Palliative Care**

Patient and Family

- **Awareness of diagnosis, illness stage, and prognosis:** "Tell me your understanding of your illness right now."
- **Values:** "Tell me what is most important to you as you are thinking about the treatment options available to you/your loved one."
- **Preferences:** "You've said that being comfortable and pain-free is most important to you right now. Where would you like to receive care (home, hospital, long-term care facility, doctor's office), and how can I help?"
- **Expected/desired outcomes:** "What are your hopes and expectations for this (diagnostic test [e.g., CT scan] or treatment)?"
- **Benefits and burdens:** "Is there a point at which you would say that the testing or treatment is outweighed by the burdens it is causing you (e.g., getting from home to the hospital, pain, nausea, fatigue, interference with other important activities)?"

belief that meaningful living is achievable during terminal illness and that it is best supported in the home, free from technologic interventions that prolong physiologic dying.

The landmark Study to Understand Prognoses and Preferences for Outcomes and Risks of Treatments (SUPPORT Principal Investigators, 1995) documented troubling deficiencies in the care of the dying in hospital settings:

- Many patients received unwanted care at the end of life.
- Clinicians were not aware of patient preferences for life-sustaining treatment, even when preferences were documented in the clinical record.
- Often pain was poorly controlled at the end of life.
- Efforts to enhance communication were ineffective.

Despite more than 40 years of existence in the United States, hospice remains an option for end-of-life care that has not been integrated fully into mainstream health care. Although hospice care is available to people with any life-limiting condition, it has been used primarily by patients with advanced cancer, in which the disease staging and trajectory lend themselves to more reliable prediction about the timing of a person's dying. Many reasons have been suggested to explain the reluctance of providers to refer patients to hospice and the reluctance of patients to accept this form of care. These include the difficulties in making a terminal prognosis and advances in "curative" treatment options in late-stage illness, as well as the values and attitudes of health care providers. The result is that patients who could benefit from the comprehensive, interdisciplinary support offered by hospice programs frequently do not enter hospice care until their final days (or hours) of life.

After hospice care was recognized as a distinct program of services under Medicare in the early 1980s, organizations providing hospice care were able to receive Medicare reimbursement if they could demonstrate that the hospice program met the Medicare "conditions of participation." State Medical Assistance (Medicaid) also provides coverage for hospice care, as do most commercial insurers. Federal reimbursement for hospice care ushered in a new era in hospice, in which program standards developed and published by the federal government codified what had formerly been a grassroots, loosely organized, and somewhat undefined ideal for care at the end of life. In many aspects, Medicare standards have come to largely define hospice philosophy and services.

In most programs, the Medicare definitions for patient eligibility are used to guide all enrollment decisions. According to Medicare, the patient who wishes to use his or her Medicare Hospice Benefit must be certified by a physician as terminally ill, with a life expectancy of 6 months or less if the disease follows its natural course (Box 3-2). Thus, hospice has come to be defined as care provided to terminally ill persons and their families in the last 6 months of the patient's life. Most hospice care is provided at the "routine home care" level and includes the services depicted in Box 3-3. Because of additional Medicare rules concerning

---

BOX 3-2

Eligibility Criteria for Hospice Care

General

- Serious, progressive illness
- Limited life expectancy
- Informed choice of palliative care over cure-focused treatment

Hospice-Specific

- Presence of a family member or other caregiver continuously in the home when the patient is no longer able to safely care for him- or herself (some hospices have created special services within their programs for patients who live alone, but this varies widely)

Medicare and Medicaid Hospice Benefits

- Medicare Part A; Medical assistance eligibility
- Waiver of traditional Medicare/Medicaid benefits for the terminal illness
- Life expectancy of 6 months or less
- Provider certification of terminal illness
- Care must be provided by a Medicare-certified hospice program

Federal rules for hospices require that patients' eligibility be reviewed periodically. There is no limit to the length of time that eligible patients may continue to receive hospice care. Patients who live longer than 6 months under hospice care are not discharged if their physician and the hospice medical director continue to certify that the patient is terminally ill with a life expectancy of 6 months or less, assuming that the disease continues its expected course.

---

completion of all cure-focused medical treatment before the Medicare Hospice Benefit may be accessed, many patients delay enrollment in hospice programs until very close to the end of life. Patients are reassessed for extension of eligibility at regular intervals, and then there is no limit on the amount

---

BOX 3-3

Home Hospice Services Covered Under the Medicare/Medicaid Hospice Benefit Routine Home Care Level

- Nursing care provided by or under the supervision of a registered nurse, available 24 hours a day
- Medical social services
- Physician's services
- Counseling services, including dietary counseling
- Home health aide/homemaker
- Physical/occupational/speech therapists
- Volunteers
- Bereavement follow-up (for up to 13 months after the death of the patient)
- Medical supplies for the palliation of the terminal illness
- Medical equipment for the palliation of the terminal illness
- Medications for the palliation of the terminal illness

of time a patient can spend under hospice care (The National Hospice and Palliative Care Organization [NHPCO], 2015).

NURSING CARE OF TERMINALLY ILL PATIENTS

Nurses can have a significant and lasting effect on the way in which patients live until they die, the manner in which the death occurs, and the enduring memories of that death for the patient's survivors. Knowledge about end-of-life principles of care and patients' and families' unique responses to illness is essential to supporting their unique values and goals (Box 3-4). There is an opportunity to bring research, education, and practice together to change the culture of dying, bringing much needed improvement to care that is relevant across practice settings, age groups, cultural backgrounds, and illnesses.

Factors that Influence Dying

Many factors can directly or indirectly affect how a person dies and what happens to one's body and one's survivors

---

| BOX 3-4 | Nursing Research |

Bridging the Gap to Evidence-Based Practice

The End-of-Life Nursing Education Consortium (ELNEC) project is a national education initiative to improve palliative care in the nursing community and make it readily available and accessible throughout the United States. In the year 2000, the City of Hope and the American Association of Colleges of Nursing (AACN) partnered to develop the ELNEC, with the intent to educate health professionals on how to address the unique needs of the dying and the dying process itself.

The project provides training in palliative care to undergraduate and graduate nursing faculty; CE providers; staff development educators; specialty nurses in pediatrics, oncology, critical care and geriatrics; and other nurses so they can teach this essential information to nursing students and practicing nurses. The project, which began in February 2000, was funded initially by a major grant from The Robert Wood Johnson Foundation (RWJF). Additional funding has been received from the National Cancer (NCI) and Open Society institutes; the Aetna, Archstone, Oncology Nursing, California HealthCare, Milbank, and Cambia Health foundations; and the Department of Veterans Affairs (VA).

The training is comprised of eight modules: an introduction to palliative nursing; pain management; symptom management; ethical issues; cultural and spiritual considerations; communication; loss, grief, and bereavement; and final hours.

The ELNEC curriculum has been translated into many languages, including Spanish, Russian, German, Korean, Japanese, Chinese, Romanian, Armenian, and Chinese.

From Ferrell, Malloy, & Virani (2015); American Association of Colleges of Nursing (AACN, 2015).

---

after death. It is useful for nurses to think of these factors as those that cannot be changed by one's actions and those that can be influenced in some fashion.

Unalterable Factors

Unalterable factors are those that are constant, including the age, gender, and personality of the dying person. Cultural attitudes toward death and dying also cannot be changed and must be taken into account in providing care. Other factors that need to be assessed, and that may affect a person's dying or bereavement, are previous experiences with illness and death, the type of disease of the dying person and its expected course, and the actual cause of death for the bereaved. Death by suicide or from neglected care will affect the family's recovery and grief process negatively compared to a death that is expected. The survivors of people who die suddenly or take their own lives have more emotional and physical problems than do survivors of people with long-term illnesses. In contrast, an expected death provides opportunities for the family to bring closure to their relationships and participate in maintaining the dying person's comfort. Certain diseases are associated, with a trajectory or expected course of dying. Some patients will die very suddenly, and others will have ample time to participate in decisions surrounding their care. The nurse needs to understand the natural course of diseases and the changes that can be expected from treatment regimens in tandem with the responses of those family members left behind.

Changeable Factors

Changeable factors are those that can be influenced by nurses. These factors need ongoing reassessment because they *are* subject to change. These factors include the dying person's previous and current relationship with health care providers, the medical management of the illness, treatment effects, the projected prognosis, the meaning the dying person invests in the experience, and the resources available for support, including the primary caregiver's health and willingness to provide care. The overwhelming majority of patients repeatedly report they prefer to die at home, and if these factors are assessed and the patient's goals are taken into account, dying at home is possible for those patients and families who work together with the nurse and medical staff to accomplish the patient's wishes.

Critical Time Periods of Terminal Care

There are three critical time periods during terminal care: Before death, the death event, and bereavement. In each period, guiding principles can direct nursing care for people who are dying and for their survivors (Institute of Medicine [IOM], 2014). Although a dying person and the survivors progress sequentially through the three time periods of terminal care, unfortunately the same nurse does not care for the patient and family throughout all three phases; therefore, it is essential there is consensus about the critical aspects of care, so that continuity can be provided to the patient and family regardless of who the health care provider is.

Predeath Period

Quint-Benoliel (1967), in her landmark study of the nurse and the dying patient, determined that progressively ill patients need the opportunity for three kinds of experiences that are difficult to achieve in today's society. They need to (1) know what is happening to them and be able to talk about its reality with someone who will listen, (2) be allowed to experience the pain of "feeling bad" instead of having to hide their feelings to protect other people from the pain of their own feelings, and (3) participate in the decisions affecting how they will live their final days and how they will die (Quint, 1967). The primary responsibility of the nurse during the predeath period is to establish a relationship with the dying person. Through this relationship, the nurse should share information with the dying person about what is happening to him or her, as well as the available choices for care. It is important to establish this relationship while the dying person feels well enough to converse with the nurse about his or her goals and wishes as death approaches. It is primarily a time of assessment, not action, in which the nurse gathers data on how the person and family are coping with what is happening to them and how the options available fit within the person's lifestyle and goals for the future. Documentation regarding the person's disease state, responses to treatment, personal goals, and changes in family interactions is essential so that consistent care can be provided over time. As symptoms occur or change, the nurse elicits the meaning of the experience and helps the patient be informed about alternatives in treatment. Specific interventions are planned and evaluated after discussing with the patient the alternatives available, their effects, and long-term consequences.

The Death Event

Many people have misconceptions about how people die and whether dying patients are aware of what is happening to them. Most health care providers have seen people die only in institutional settings and when advanced medical technology had been used to sustain life. The majority of health care providers have not had an opportunity to witness a person dying without medical intervention and in the natural setting of home or another place of preference. Gradually, as the patient becomes more socially and physically dependent on others for assistance, the dying person and the family need increased supervision by providers. The primary purpose in being present as death becomes imminent is to anticipate problems, such as distressing symptoms or family disruptions, before they interfere with the dying person's wishes. The best of plans, well made over a period of months or weeks of preparation, can easily be undermined unintentionally by any member of the health care team or family.

Distressing symptoms that warrant hospitalization generally can be prevented if the nurse and provider are working closely together, and the family has the resources for maintaining the person in the home. Some patients may prefer to be institutionalized because they do not want to be a burden on their family.

If possible, the nurse is present when the patient dies or arranges to be called shortly thereafter, to assist with the preparation of the body and to support the family. If the patient dies in the hospital, the family needs ample time in private to be with the body. The nurse assists the family with answering questions, making telephone calls, and expressing grief. The nurse may assist with helping to clean the patient's room after the death. Some families may want these tasks done for them, and others have a need to do them themselves. Nothing should be removed without the family's permission. Once the death event is over, most nurses need an opportunity to debrief with someone they trust about the experience. It is important for nurses to develop a support network of their own to share their feelings and validate their care with others.

Bereavement

The third critical time period is the time after the death. Most members of the family may need several opportunities to relive the events surrounding the death, and the nurse is in a unique position to listen, having been a part of the experience. Often family and friends do not want to hear the events over and over from each other and frequently send messages that the grieving person should get on with living. Part of the support given in reliving the death experience involves reinforcing the family's sense that they did a good job supporting the dead person's wishes and communicating to the family that everything was done that could be done. The length of time a nurse sees a family for bereavement varies. Usually, at least 3 months are needed to assist with making decisions and disposing of the dead person's belongings as well as to assess the family's coping with the loss. Family members need encouragement not to act impulsively and to think through the consequences of their decisions. The nurse helps the family to discuss options available and to talk not only about the major loss associated with the death but also the consequential losses (e.g., financial, emotional, and social). If a family member needs additional help, the nurse can make a referral to a mental health provider, support group, or primary care provider.

Communicating with the Terminally Ill

To develop a level of comfort and expertise in communicating with seriously and terminally ill patients and their families, nurses and other clinicians should first consider their own experiences with and values concerning illness and death. Reflection, reading, and talking with family members, friends, and colleagues can help nurses examine beliefs about death and dying. Talking with people from different cultural backgrounds can help nurses view personally held beliefs through a different lens and can help nurses become sensitive to death-related beliefs and practices in other cultures. Discussion with nursing and nonnursing colleagues also can be useful; it may reveal the values shared by many health care professionals and identify diversity in the values of patients in their care. Values clarification and personal death awareness exercises can provide a starting point for self-discovery and discussion. Asking a person to share a personal experience of someone who has died and what that experience was like for the person is a place to start.

Ethical Decision-Making in End-of-Life Care

Nurses are responsible for educating patients about the possibilities and probabilities inherent in their illness and their life with the illness, and for supporting them as they conduct life review, values clarification, treatment decision-making, and end-of-life closure. The only way to do this effectively is to try to appreciate and understand the illness from the patient's perspective. It is also important that patients have had an opportunity to identify their preferences for how decisions are made at the end-of-life through legal documents recognized on a federal and state level (Box 3-5).

At the same time, nurses should be both culturally aware and sensitive in their approaches to communication with patients and families about death. Attitudes toward open disclosure about terminal illness vary widely among different cultures, and direct communication with patients about such matters may be viewed as harmful. To provide effective patient- and family-centered care at the end of life, nurses must be willing to set aside their own assumptions and attitudes so that they can discover what type and amount of disclosure is most meaningful to each patient and family within their unique belief systems.

Providing Culturally Sensitive Care at the End of Life

Although death, grief, and mourning are universally accepted aspects of living, one's values, expectations, and practices during serious illness, as death approaches, and after death are culturally bound and expressed. Health care providers may share very similar values concerning end-of-life care or may find that they are inadequately prepared to assess for and implement care plans that support culturally diverse perspectives. Historical mistrust of the health care system and unequal access to even basic medical care may underlie the beliefs and attitudes among ethnically diverse populations. In addition, lack of education or knowledge about end-of-life care treatment options and language barriers influence decisions among many socioeconomically disadvantaged groups.

Much of the formal structure concerning health care decisions in the United States is rooted in the Western notions of autonomy, truth telling, and the acceptability of withdrawing or withholding life-prolonging medical treatment at the end of life. In many cultures, however, interdependence is valued over autonomy, leading to communication styles that favor relinquishment of decision-making to family members or to perceived authority figures, such as physicians. In addition, there is variation in preference regarding the use of life-prolonging medical treatments such as cardiopulmonary resuscitation and artificially provided nutrition and hydration at the end of life; some groups are less likely to agree with withholding or withdrawing such life supports from the patient with a terminal illness.

The nurse's role is to assess the values, preferences, and practices of every patient, regardless of ethnicity, socioeconomic status, or background. The nurse can share knowledge about a patient's and family's cultural beliefs and practices with the health care team and facilitate the adaptation of the care plan to accommodate these practices. For example, a nurse may find that a male patient prefers to have his eldest

---

BOX 3-5 **Methods of Stating End-of-Life Preferences**

Advance directives: Written documents that allow the individual of sound mind to document preferences regarding end-of-life care that should be followed when the signer is terminally ill and unable to communicate his or her wishes verbally. In general, the documents are completed in advance of serious illness but may be completed after a diagnosis of serious illness if the signer is still of sound mind. The most common types are the durable power of attorney for health care and the living will.

Durable power of attorney for health care: A legal document through which the signer appoints and authorizes another individual to make medical decisions on his or her behalf when he or she is no longer able to speak for him- or herself. This is also known as a *health care power of attorney* or a *proxy directive.*

Living will: A type of advance directive in which the individual documents treatment preferences. It provides instructions for care in the event that the signer is terminally ill and not able to communicate his or her wishes directly and often is accompanied by a durable power of attorney for health care. This is also known as a *medical directive* or *treatment directive.*

Information about the advance care planning and state-specific advance directive documents and instructions are available from the website of Caring Connections (http://caringinfo.org). The legality of these documents may vary across states and within institutions, and it is important that people have someone they have spoken to and trust who can advocate for individual preferences if needed.

son make all of his care decisions. Institutional practices and laws governing informed consent are also rooted in the Western notion of autonomous decision-making and informed consent. If a patient wishes to defer decisions to his son, the nurse can work with the team to negotiate informed consent, respecting the patient's right not to participate in decision-making and honoring his family's cultural practices.

The nurse should assess and document the patient's and family's specific beliefs, preferences, and practices regarding end-of-life care, preparation for death, and after-death rituals. The nurse must use judgment and discretion about the timing and setting for eliciting this information. Some patients may wish to have a family member speak for them or may be unable to provide information because of advanced illness. The nurse should give the patient and family a context for the discussion, such as, "It is very important to us to provide care that addresses your needs and the needs of your family. We want to honor and support your wishes, and want you to feel free to tell us how we are doing, and what we could do to better meet your needs. I'd like to ask you some questions; what you tell me will help me to understand and support what is most important to you at this time. You don't need to answer anything that makes you uncomfortable. Is it all right to ask some questions?" The assessment of end-of-life beliefs, preferences, and practices probably should be carried out in short segments over a period of time (e.g., across multiple days of an inpatient hospital stay or in conjunction with multiple patient visits to an outpatient setting). The discomfort of novice nurses with asking questions and discussing this type of sensitive content can be reduced by prior practice in a classroom or clinical skills laboratory, observation of interviews conducted by experienced nurses, and partnering with experienced nurses during the first few assessments.

Symptom Management

Many patients suffer unnecessarily when they do not receive adequate attention for the symptoms accompanying serious illness. Careful evaluation of the patient should include not only the physical problems but also the psychological, social, and spiritual dimensions of the patient's and family's experience of serious illness. This approach contributes to a more comprehensive understanding of how the patient's and family's lives have been affected by illness and leads to nursing care that addresses the needs in every dimension.

Clinical depression should not be accepted as an inevitable consequence of dying, nor should it be confused with sadness and anticipatory grieving, which are normal reactions to the losses associated with impending death. Emotional and spiritual support and control of disturbing physical symptoms are appropriate interventions for situational depression associated with terminal illness. Cancer patients in advanced stages of the disease are especially vulnerable to delirium, depression, suicidal ideation, and severe anxiety. Higher levels of debilitation predict higher levels of pain and

depressive symptoms, and the presence of pain increases the likelihood of developing major psychiatric complications of illness. Patients and their families must be given space and time to experience sadness and to grieve, but patients should not have to endure untreated depression at the end of their lives. An effective combined approach to clinical depression includes relief of physical symptoms, attention to emotional and spiritual distress, and pharmacologic interventions.

Patients approaching the end of life experience many of the same symptoms, regardless of their underlying disease processes. Symptoms in terminal illness may be caused by the disease, either directly (e.g., dyspnea due to chronic obstructive pulmonary disease) or indirectly (e.g., nausea and vomiting related to pressure in the gastric area); by the treatment for the disease; or by a coexisting disorder that is unrelated to the disease. Some of the most frequently encountered symptoms as death approaches include pain, dyspnea, anorexia and cachexia, delirium, and depression (Hinkle & Cheever, 2014). Chapter 7 presents assessment principles for pain that include identifying the effect of the pain on the patient's life, the importance of believing the patient's report of the pain and its effect, and the importance of systematic assessment of pain. Similarly, symptoms such as dyspnea, nausea, weakness, and anxiety should be carefully and systematically assessed and managed. Questions that guide the assessment of symptoms are listed in Box 3-6.

The patient's goals should guide symptom management. Medical interventions may be aimed at treating the

BOX 3-6

Assessing Symptoms Associated with Terminal Illness

Questions to consider:
- When did the symptom start?
- How long has the symptom been present?
- Has the symptom changed in any way?
- Is the symptom intermittent or constant/continuous?
- Are there any other symptoms?

(if symptom is pain specific)
- Does the pain radiate or move anywhere?
- What makes the pain worse or better?
- What has been tried to treat the pain? Has it helped? Are there side effects? What are the scheduled doses?
- What are the patient's goals and expectations regarding pain management for comfort and function? What about those of the family/caregivers?
- How much distress is the pain causing?
- What does the patient think that the pain means (e.g., tumor spread)?
- Who does the patient have for support? Are family members or others available?
- What are cultural, spiritual, or religious concerns about pain?

Adapted from Tickoo, Key, & Breitbart (2015); National Comprehensive Cancer Network (NCCN, 2014).

underlying causes of the symptoms or reducing the impact of symptoms. For example, a medical intervention such as thoracentesis (an invasive procedure in which fluid is drained from the pleural space) may be performed to relieve dyspnea temporarily in a patient with pleural effusion secondary to lung cancer. Pharmacologic and nonpharmacologic methods for symptom management may be used in combination with medical interventions to modify the physiologic causes of symptoms. For example, in addition to having a thoracentesis, many patients find symptoms are reduced by the use of a handheld fan, which has been associated with a reduction in breathlessness (Galbraith, Fagan, Perkins, Lynch, & Booth, 2010). In addition, pharmacologic management with low-dose oral morphine is very effective in relieving dyspnea, and guided relaxation may reduce the anxiety associated with the sensation of breathlessness. As is true with pain, the principles of pharmacologic symptom management call for the use of the smallest dose of the medication to achieve the desired effect, avoidance of polypharmacy, anticipation and management of medical side effects, and creation of a therapeutic regimen that is acceptable to the patient based on his or her goals for maximizing quality of life.

The patient's goals take precedence over the clinicians' goals to relieve all symptoms at all costs. Although clinicians may believe that symptoms must be relieved completely whenever possible, the patient might choose instead to decrease symptoms to a tolerable level rather than to relieve them completely if the side effects of medications are unacceptable to him or her. This often allows the patient to have greater independence, mobility, and alertness, and to devote attention to issues that he or she considers of higher priority and greater importance.

Anticipating and planning interventions for symptoms that have not yet occurred is a cornerstone of end-of-life care. Both patients and family members cope more effectively with new symptoms and exacerbations of existing symptoms when they know what to expect and how to manage it. Hospice programs typically provide "emergency kits" containing ready-to-administer doses of a variety of medications that are useful to treat symptoms in advanced illness. For example, a kit might contain small doses of oral morphine liquid for pain or shortness of breath, a benzodiazepine for restlessness, and an acetaminophen suppository for fever. Family members can be instructed to administer a prescribed dose from the emergency kit, often avoiding prolonged suffering for the patient as well as rehospitalization for symptom management.

Pain Management

Numerous studies have shown that patients with advanced illness, particularly cancer, experience considerable pain. Pain is a significant symptom for many cancer patients throughout their treatment and disease course; it results from both the disease and the modalities used to treat it. Pain and suffering are among the most feared consequences of cancer.

Poorly managed pain affects the psychological, emotional, social, and financial well-being of patients and families.

Patients who are taking an established regimen of analgesics should continue to receive those medications as they approach the end of life. Inability to communicate pain should not be equated with the absence of pain. Although most pain can be managed effectively using the oral route, as the end of life nears, patients may be less able to swallow oral medications due to somnolence or nausea. Patients who have been receiving opioids should continue to receive equianalgesic doses via rectal or sublingual routes. Concentrated morphine solution can be delivered very effectively by the sublingual route because the small liquid volume is well tolerated even if swallowing is not possible. As long as the patient continues to receive opioids, a regimen to combat constipation must be implemented. If the patient cannot swallow laxatives or stool softeners, rectal suppositories or enemas may be necessary.

The nurse should teach the family about continuation of comfort measures as the patient approaches the end of life, how to administer analgesics via alternative routes, and how to assess for pain when the patient cannot verbally report pain intensity. Because the analgesics administered orally or rectally are short-acting, typically scheduled as frequently as every 3 to 4 hours around the clock, there is always a strong possibility that a patient approaching the end of life will die in close proximity to the time of analgesic administration. If the patient is at home, family members administering analgesics should be prepared for this possibility. They need reassurance that they did not "cause" the death of the patient by administering a dose of analgesic medication.

Nutrition and Hydration at the End of Life

Anorexia and cachexia are common problems in the seriously ill. The profound changes in the patient's appearance and the concomitant lack of interest in the socially important rituals of mealtime are particularly disturbing to families. The approach to this problem varies depending on the patient's stage of illness, level of disability associated with the illness, and desires. The anorexia–cachexia syndrome is characterized by disturbances in carbohydrate, protein, and fat metabolism; endocrine dysfunction; and anemia. The syndrome results in severe asthenia (loss of energy).

Although causes of anorexia may be controlled for a period of time, progressive anorexia is an expected and natural part of the dying process. Anorexia may be related to or exacerbated by situational variables (e.g., the ability to have meals with the family vs. eating alone in the "sick room"), progression of the disease, treatment for the disease, or psychological distress. The patient and family should be instructed in strategies to manage the variables associated with anorexia (Table 3-3).

A number of pharmacologic agents are commonly used to stimulate appetite in anorexic patients. Commonly used

TABLE 3-3 Measures for Managing Anorexia

Nursing Interventions	Patient and Family Teaching Tips
Initiate measures to ensure adequate dietary intake without adding stress to the patient at mealtimes.	Reduce the focus on "balanced" meals; offer the same food as often as the patient desires it.
Assess the impact of medications (e.g., chemotherapy, antiretrovirals) or other therapies (radiation therapy, dialysis) that are being used to treat the underlying illness. Administer and monitor effects of prescribed treatment for nausea, vomiting, and delayed gastric emptying.	Increase the nutritional value of meals. For example, add dry milk powder to milk, and use this fortified milk to prepare cream soups, milkshakes, and gravies.
Encourage patient to eat when effects of medications have subsided.	Allow and encourage the patient to eat when hungry, regardless of usual meal times.
Assess and modify environment to eliminate unpleasant odors and other factors that cause nausea, vomiting, and anorexia.	Eliminate or reduce noxious cooking odors, pet odors, or other odors that may precipitate nausea, vomiting, or anorexia.
Remove items that may reduce appetite (soiled tissues, bedpans, emesis basins, clutter).	Keep patient's environment clean, uncluttered, and comfortable.
Assess and manage anxiety and depression to the extent possible.	Make mealtime a shared experience away from the "sick" room whenever possible. Reduce stress at mealtimes. Avoid confrontations about the amount of food consumed. Reduce or eliminate routine weighing of the patient.
Position to enhance gastric emptying.	Encourage patient to eat in a sitting position; elevate the head of the patient's bed. Plan meals (food selection and portion size) that the patient desires.
Assess for constipation and/or intestinal obstruction.	Provide small, frequent meals if they are easier for patient to eat. Ensure that patient and family understand that prevention of constipation is essential, even when the patient's intake is minimal.
Prevent and manage constipation on an ongoing basis, even when the patient's intake is minimal.	Encourage adequate fluid intake, dietary fiber, and use of bowel program to prevent constipation.
Provide frequent mouth care, particularly following nourishment.	Assist the patient to rinse after every meal. Avoid mouthwashes that contain alcohol or glycerine, which dry mucous membranes.
Ensure that dentures fit properly.	Weight loss may cause dentures to loosen and cause irritation. Remove them to inspect the gums and to provide oral care.
Administer and monitor effects of topical and systemic treatment for oropharyngeal pain.	The patient's comfort may be enhanced if medications for pain relief given on an as-needed basis for breakthrough pain are administered before mealtimes.

medications for appetite stimulation include dexamethasone (Decadron), megestrol acetate (Megace), and dronabinol (Marinol). Although several of these agents may result in temporary weight gain, their use is not associated with an increase in lean body mass in the terminally ill patient.

Dexamethasone initially increases appetite and may provide short-term weight gain in some patients. However, therapy may need to be discontinued in patients with a longer life expectancy, because after 3 to 4 weeks, corticosteroids interfere with the synthesis of muscle protein.

Megestrol acetate produces temporary weight gain of primarily fatty tissue, with little effect on protein balance. Because of the time required to see any effect from this agent, therapy should not be initiated if life expectancy is less than 30 days.

Dronabinol is a psychoactive compound found in cannabis that may be helpful in reducing nausea and vomiting, appetite loss, pain, and anxiety, thereby improving food and fluid intake in some patients. However, dronabinol is not as effective as the other agents for appetite stimulation in most patients.

Cachexia

Cachexia refers to severe muscle wasting and weight loss associated with illness. Although anorexia may exacerbate cachexia, it is not the primary cause. Cachexia is associated with changes in metabolism that include hypertriglyceridemia, lipolysis, and accelerated protein turnover, leading to depletion of fat and protein stores. However, the pathophysiology of cachexia in terminal illness is not well understood. In terminal illness, the severity of tissue wasting is greater than would be expected from reduced food intake alone, and typically increasing appetite or food intake does not reverse cachexia in the terminally ill.

Anorexia and cachexia differ from starvation (simple food deprivation) in several important ways. In the case of anorexia and cachexia, appetite is lost early in the process, the body becomes catabolic in a dysfunctional way, and supplementation by gastric feeding (tube feeding) or parenteral nutrition in advanced disease does not replenish lean body mass that has been lost. At one time, it was believed that cancer patients with rapidly growing tumors developed cachexia because the tumor created an excessive nutritional demand and diverted nutrients from the rest of the body. Research links cytokines produced by the body in response to a tumor to a complex inflammatory-immune response present in patients whose tumors have metastasized, leading to anorexia, weight loss, and altered metabolism.

Artificial Nutrition and Hydration

Along with breathing, eating and drinking are essential to survival throughout life. Near the end of life, the body's nutritional needs change, and the desire for food and fluids may diminish. People may no longer be able to use, eliminate, or store nutrients and fluids adequately. For patients with progressive illness, food preparation and mealtimes often become battlegrounds in which well-meaning family members argue, plead, and cajole to encourage ill people to eat. It is not unusual for seriously ill patients to lose their appetites entirely, to develop strong aversions for foods they have enjoyed in the past, or to crave a particular food to the exclusion of all other foods.

Although nutritional supplementation may be an important part of the treatment plan in early or chronic illness, unintended weight loss and dehydration are expected sequelae of progressive illness. As illness progresses, patients, families, and clinicians may believe that, without artificial nutrition and hydration, terminally ill patients will "starve," causing profound suffering and hastened death. However, starvation should not be viewed as the failure to implant tubes for nutritional supplementation or hydration of terminally ill patients with irreversible progression of disease. Studies have demonstrated that terminally ill patients who were hydrated had neither improved biochemical parameters nor improved states of consciousness. Similarly, survival was not increased when terminally ill patients with advanced dementia received enteral feeding. Furthermore, in patients who are close to death, there are beneficial effects to withholding or withdrawing artificial nutrition and hydration, such as decreased complications associated with tube feeding or total parenteral nutrition, which include dislodgement, infection, discomfort, and aspiration (Capasso, Kim, & Perret, 2013).

As the patient approaches the end of life, the family and health care providers should offer the patient what he or she prefers and can tolerate most easily. The nurse should instruct the family how to separate feeding from caring, demonstrating love, and sharing by being with the loved one in other ways. Preoccupation with appetite, feeding, and weight loss diverts energy and time that the patient and family could use in other meaningful activities. Here are tips to promote nutrition for terminally ill patients:

- Offer small portions of favorite foods.
- Do not be overly concerned about a "balanced" diet.
- Cool foods may be better tolerated than hot foods.
- Offer cheese, eggs, peanut butter, mild fish, chicken, or turkey. Meat (especially beef) may taste bitter and unpleasant.
- Add milkshakes, powdered instant drinks, or other liquid supplements.
- Add dry milk powder to milkshakes and cream soups to increase protein and calorie content.
- Place nutritious foods at the bedside (fruit juices, milkshakes in insulated drink containers with straws).
- Schedule meals when family members can be present to provide company and stimulation.
- Avoid arguments at mealtime.
- Help the patient to maintain a schedule of oral care. Rinse the mouth after each meal or snack. Avoid mouthwashes that contain alcohol. Use a soft toothbrush. Treat oral ulcers or lesions. Make sure dentures fit well.
- Treat pain and other symptoms.
- Offer ice chips made from frozen fruit juices.
- Allow the patient to refuse foods and fluids.

Changes in Consciousness and Delirium

Many patients remain alert, arousable, and able to communicate until very close to death. Others sleep for long intervals and awaken only intermittently, with eventual somnolence until death. Delirium refers to concurrent disturbances in level of consciousness, psychomotor behavior, memory, thinking, attention, and sleep–wake cycle. In some patients, a period of agitated delirium precedes death, sometimes causing families to be hopeful that patients who are suddenly active may be getting better. Confusion may be related to underlying, treatable conditions such as medication side effects or interactions, pain or discomfort, hypoxia or dyspnea, or a full bladder or impacted stool. In patients with cancer, confusion may be secondary to brain metastases. Delirium also may be related to metabolic changes, infection, and organ failure.

Patients with delirium may become hypoactive or hyperactive, restless, irritable, and fearful. Sleep deprivation and hallucinations may occur. If treatment of the underlying factors contributing to these symptoms brings no relief, a combination of pharmacologic intervention with neuroleptics or benzodiazepines may be effective in decreasing distressing symptoms. Haloperidol (Haldol) may reduce hallucinations and agitation (Powney, Adams, & Jones, 2012). Benzodiazepines (e.g., lorazepam [Ativan]) can reduce anxiety but do not clear the sensorium and may contribute to worsening cognitive impairment if used alone.

Nursing interventions are aimed at identifying the underlying causes of delirium, acknowledging the family's distress over its occurrence, reassuring family members about what is normal, teaching family members how to interact with and ensure safety for the patient with delirium, and monitoring the effects of medications used to treat severe agitation, paranoia, and fear. Confusion may mask the patient's unmet needs and fears about dying. Spiritual intervention, music therapy, gentle massage, and therapeutic touch may provide some relief. Reduction of environmental stimuli, avoidance of harsh lighting or very dim lighting (which may produce disturbing shadows), presence of familiar faces, and gentle reorientation and reassurance are also helpful.

Dyspnea

Dyspnea is an uncomfortable awareness of breathing or breathlessness that is common in patients approaching the end of life. Dyspnea is a highly subjective symptom that often is not associated with visible signs of distress, such as tachypnea, diaphoresis, or cyanosis. Patients with primary lung tumors, lung metastases, pleural effusion, or obstructive lung disease may experience significant dyspnea. Although the underlying cause of the dyspnea can be identified and treated in some cases, the burdens of additional diagnostic evaluation and treatment aimed at the physiologic problem may outweigh the benefits. The treatment of dyspnea varies depending on the patient's general physical condition and imminence of death. For example, a blood transfusion may provide temporary symptom relief for a patient with anemia earlier in the disease process; however, as the patient approaches the end of life, the benefits are typically short-lived or absent. As with assessment and management of pain, reports of dyspnea by patients must be believed. As is true for physical pain, what dyspnea means to an individual patient may increase his or her suffering. For example, the patient may interpret increasing dyspnea as a sign that death is approaching. For some patients, sensations of breathlessness may invoke frightening images of drowning or suffocation, and the resulting cycle of fear and anxiety may increase the sensation of breathlessness. Therefore, the nurse should conduct a careful assessment of the psychosocial and spiritual components of the dyspnea. Physical assessment parameters include:

- Symptom intensity, distress, and interference with activities (scale of 0 to 10)
- Auscultation of lung sounds
- Assessment of fluid balance
- Measurement of dependent edema (circumference of lower extremities)
- Measurement of abdominal girth
- Temperature
- Skin color
- Sputum quantity and character
- Cough

To determine the intensity of dyspnea and its interference with daily activities, the nurse can ask the patient to report the severity of the dyspnea using a scale of 0 to 10, where 0 is no dyspnea and 10 is the worst imaginable dyspnea. Ongoing objective evidence for the efficacy of the treatment plan is provided by the patient's baseline measurement before treatment and then subsequent measurements taken during exacerbation of the symptom, periodically during treatment, and whenever the treatment plan changes. In addition, physical assessment findings may assist in locating the source of the dyspnea and selecting appropriate nursing interventions to relieve the symptom. The components of the assessment change as the patient's condition changes. Like other symptoms at the end of life, dyspnea can be managed effectively in the absence of assessment and diagnostic data that are standard when a patient's illness or symptom is reversible (i.e., arterial blood gases).

Nursing management of dyspnea at the end of life is directed toward administering medical treatment for the underlying pathology, monitoring the patient's response to treatment, helping the patient and family manage anxiety (which exacerbates dyspnea), altering the perception of the symptom, and conserving energy (Box 3-7). Pharmacologic intervention is aimed at modifying lung physiology and improving performance, as well as in altering the perception of the symptom. Bronchodilators and corticosteroids are examples of medications used to treat underlying obstructive pathology, thereby improving overall lung function. Low doses of opioids are very effective in relieving dyspnea, although the mechanism of relief is not entirely clear. Although dyspnea in terminal illness is typically not associated with diminished blood oxygen saturation, low-flow oxygen often provides psychological comfort to both patients and families, particularly in the home setting.

As previously mentioned, dyspnea may be exacerbated by anxiety, and anxiety may trigger episodes of dyspnea, setting off a respiratory crisis in which the patient and family may panic. For patients receiving care at home, patient and family instruction should include anticipation and management of crisis situations and a clearly communicated emergency plan. The patient and family should be instructed about medication administration, condition changes that should be

---

BOX 3-7 **Palliative Nursing Interventions for Dyspnea**

Decrease Anxiety

- Administer prescribed anxiolytic medications as indicated for anxiety or panic associated with dyspnea.
- Assist with relaxation techniques, guided imagery.
- Provide the patient with a means to call for assistance (call bell/light within reach in a hospital or long-term care facility; handheld bell or other device for home).

Treat Underlying Pathology

- Administer prescribed bronchodilators and corticosteroids (obstructive pathology).
- Administer blood products, erythropoietin as prescribed (typically not beneficial in advanced stages of disease).
- Administer prescribed diuretics and monitor fluid balance.

Alter Perception of Breathlessness

- Administer prescribed oxygen therapy via nasal cannula, if tolerated; masks may not be well tolerated.
- Administer prescribed low-dose opioids via oral route (morphine sulfate is used most commonly).
- Provide air movement in the patient's environment with a portable fan or a cool draft of air as from a handheld fan.

Reduce Respiratory Demand

- Teach the patient and family to implement energy conservation measures.
- Place needed equipment, supplies, and nourishment within reach.
- For home or hospice care, offer a bedside commode, electric bed (with head that elevates).

---

reported to the provider and nurse, and strategies for coping with diminished reserves and increasing symptomatology as the disease progresses. The patient and family need reassurance that the symptom can be managed effectively at home without the need for activation of the emergency medical services or hospitalization, and that a nurse will be available at all times via telephone or to make a visit.

Secretions

If family members have been prepared for the time of death, they are less likely to panic and are better able to be with their loved ones in a meaningful way. Noisy, gurgling breathing or moaning is generally most distressing to family members. In most cases, the sounds of breathing at the end of life are related to oropharyngeal relaxation and diminished awareness. Family members may have difficulty believing that the patient is not in pain or that the patient's breathing could not be improved by suctioning secretions. Patient positioning and family reassurance are the most helpful responses to these symptoms.

When death is imminent, patients may become increasingly somnolent and unable to clear sputum or oral secretions, which may lead to further impairment of breathing from pooled or dried and crusted secretions. Often the sound ("terminal bubbling") and appearance of the secretions are more distressing to family members than is the presence of the secretions to the patient. Family distress over the changes in the patient's condition may be eased by supportive nursing care. Continuation of comfort-focused interventions and reassurance that the patient is not in any distress can do much to ease family concerns. Gentle mouth care with a moistened swab or very soft toothbrush helps maintain the integrity of the patient's mucous membranes. In addition, gentle oral suctioning, positioning to enhance drainage of secretions, and sublingual or transdermal administration of anticholinergic drugs reduces the production of secretions

and provides comfort to the patient and support to the family. Deeper suctioning may cause significant discomfort to the dying patient and is rarely of any benefit, because secretions reaccumulate rapidly. Based on the authors' clinical experience, if anticholinergic drugs are used prophylactic prior to secretions occurring, the drug has an increased chance of being effective. Mercadamte (2014) made a similar suggestion that anticholinergics be used before starting palliative sedation. Refer to Table 3-4 for pharmacologic management of excess oral/respiratory secretions with dying patients.

Palliative Sedation at the End of Life

Effective control of symptoms can be achieved under most conditions, but some patients may experience distressing,

---

TABLE **3-4** **Pharmacologic Management of Excess Oral/Respiratory Secretions When Death is Imminent**

Medication	Dose
Atropine sulfate drops 1%	1 or 2 drops 1% PO/sublingual q4–6h p.r.n. or around the clock (ATC) up to 12 drops/d
Atropine injection	0.4–0.6 mg IV/SC/IM q4–6h p.r.n. or ATC (if PO therapy is ineffective)
Glycopyrrolate (Robinul)	1–2 mg PO/rectal/sublingual TID p.r.n. or ATC (maximum dose 6 mg/d)
Hyoscyamine (Levsin)	0.125–0.25 mg PO/sublingual q4–6h p.r.n. or ATC (maximum dose 1.5 mg/d)
Scopolamine (Transderm Scop)	1–3 patches q3d (maximum dose 3 patches every 72 h)

Reprinted with permission from ExcelleRx, Inc. (2008). *Hospice pharmacia pharmaceutical care tool kit* (9th ed.). Philadelphia, PA: Author.

intractable symptoms. Although **palliative sedation** remains controversial, it is offered in some settings to patients who are close to death or who have symptoms that do not respond to conventional pharmacologic and non-pharmacologic approaches, resulting in unrelieved suffering. Palliative sedation is distinguished from **euthanasia** or physician-assisted suicide in that the intent of palliative sedation is to relieve symptoms, not to hasten death. Palliative sedation is most commonly used when the patient exhibits intractable pain, dyspnea, seizures, or delirium, and it is generally considered appropriate in only the most difficult situations. Before implementing palliative sedation, the health care team should assess for the presence of underlying and treatable causes of suffering, such as depression or spiritual pain. Finally, the patient and family should be informed fully about the use of this treatment and alternatives.

Palliative sedation is accomplished through infusion of sedative drugs such as benzodiazepines to achieve the desired level of sedation to provide relief from the refractory symptoms in the last hours and days of life (Beller, Driel, McGregor, Truong, & Mitchell, 2015). Nurses act as collaborating members of the interdisciplinary health care team, providing emotional support to patients and families, facilitating clarification of values and preferences, and providing comfort-focused physical care. Once sedation has been induced, the nurse should continue to comfort the patient, monitor the physiologic effects of the sedation, support the family during the final hours or days of their loved one's life, and maintain communication within the health care team and between the team and family.

NURSING CARE OF PATIENTS AND FAMILIES IN THE FINAL HOURS OF LIFE

Providing care to patients who are close to death and being present at the time of death can be one of the most rewarding experiences a nurse can have. Patients and their families are understandably fearful of the unknown, and the approach of death may prompt new concerns or cause previous fears or issues to resurface. Family members who have always had difficulty communicating or who are part of families in which there are old resentments and hurts may experience heightened difficulty as their loved ones near death. In contrast, the time at the end of life can also afford opportunities to resolve old hurts and learn new ways of being a family. Regardless of the setting, skilled practitioners can make the dying patient comfortable, make space for their loved ones to remain present when they wish, and can give family members the opportunity to experience growth and healing. Likewise, regardless of setting, the patient and family may be less apprehensive near the time of death if they know what to expect and how to respond.

Expected Physiologic Changes

As death approaches and organ systems begin to fail, observable, expected changes in the body take place. Nursing care measures aimed at patient comfort should be continued: pain medications (administered rectally or sublingually), turning, mouth care, eye care, positioning to facilitate draining of secretions, and measures to protect the skin from urine or feces (if the patient is incontinent) should be continued. The nurse should consult with the provider about discontinuing measures that no longer contribute to patient comfort, such as drawing blood, administering tube feedings, suctioning (in most cases), and invasive monitoring. The nurse should prepare the family for the normal, expected changes that accompany the period immediately preceding death. Although the exact time of death cannot be predicted, it is often possible to identify when the patient is very close to death. Hospice programs frequently provide written information for families so they know what to expect and what to do as death nears (Box 3-8).

Although every death is unique, it is often possible for experienced clinicians to assess that the patient is "actively" or imminently dying and to prepare the family in the final days or hours leading to death. As death nears, the patient may withdraw, sleep for longer intervals, or become somnolent. Family members should be encouraged to be with the patient, to speak and reassure the patient of their presence, to stroke or touch the patient, or to lie alongside the patient (even in the hospital or long-term care facility) if the family members are comfortable with this degree of closeness and can do so without causing discomfort to the patient.

The family may have gone to great lengths to ensure that their loved one will not die alone. However, despite the best intentions and efforts of the family and clinicians, the patient may die at a time when no one is present. In any setting, it is unrealistic for family members to be at the patient's bedside 24 hours a day, and it is not unusual for a patient to die when family members have stepped away from the bedside just briefly. Experienced hospice clinicians have observed and reported that some patients appear to "wait" until family members are away from the bedside to die, perhaps to spare their loved ones the pain of being present at the time of death. Nurses can reassure family members throughout the death vigil by being present intermittently or continuously, modeling behaviors (such as touching and speaking to the patient), providing encouragement in relation to family caregiving, providing reassurance about normal physiologic changes, and encouraging family rest breaks. If a patient dies while family members are away from the bedside, they may express feelings of guilt and profound grief and may need emotional support.

After-Death Care

The time of death is generally preceded by a period of gradual diminishment of bodily functions in which increasing

BOX 3-8 **Patient Education**

Signs of Approaching Death

The person will show less interest in eating and drinking. For many patients, refusal of food is an indication that they are ready to die. Fluid intake may be limited to that which will keep the mouth from feeling too dry.
- What you can do: Offer, but do not force, fluids and medication. Sometimes, pain or other symptoms that have required medication in the past may no longer be present. For most patients, pain medications still will be needed and can be provided by concentrated oral solutions placed under the tongue or by rectal suppository.

Urinary output may decrease in amount and frequency.
- What you can do: No response is needed unless the patient expresses a desire to urinate and cannot. Call the hospice nurse for advice if you are not sure.

As the body weakens, the patient will sleep more and begin to detach from the environment. He or she may refuse your attempts to provide comfort.
- What you can do: Allow your loved one to sleep. You may wish to sit with him or her, play soft music, or hold hands. Your loved one's withdrawal is normal and is not a rejection of your love.

Mental confusion may become apparent as less oxygen is available to supply the brain. The patient may report strange dreams or visions.
- What you can do: As he or she awakens from sleep, remind him or her of the day and time, where he or she is, and who is present. This is best done in a casual, conversational way.

Vision and hearing may become somewhat impaired, and speech may be difficult to understand.
- What you can do: Speak clearly but no more loudly than necessary. Keep the room as light as the patient wishes, even at night. Carry on all conversations as if they can be heard, because hearing may be the last of the senses to cease functioning.
- Many patients are able to talk until minutes before death and are reassured by the exchange of a few words with a loved one.

Secretions may collect in the back of the throat and rattle or gurgle as the patient breathes though the mouth. He or she may try to cough, and his or her mouth may become dry and encrusted with secretions.
- What you can do: If the patient is trying to cough up secretions and is experiencing choking or vomiting, call the hospice nurse for assistance.
- Secretions may drain from the mouth if you place the patient on his or her side and provide support with pillows.

- Cleansing the mouth with moistened mouth swabs will help to relieve the dryness that occurs with mouth breathing.
- Offer water in small amounts to keep the mouth moist. A straw with one finger placed over the end can be used to transfer sips of water to the patient's mouth.

Breathing may become irregular with periods of no breathing (apnea). The patient may be working very hard to breathe and may make a moaning sound with each breath. As the time of death nears, the breathing remains irregular and may become more shallow and mechanical.
- What you can do: Raising the head of the bed may help the patient to breathe more easily. The moaning sound does not mean that the patient is in pain or other distress; it is the sound of air passing over very relaxed vocal cords.

As the oxygen supply to the brain decreases, the patient may become restless. It is not unusual for the patient to pull at the bed linens, to have visual hallucinations, or even to try to get out of bed at this point.
- What you can do: Reassure the patient in a calm voice that you are there. Prevent him or her from falling out of bed. Soft music or a back rub may be soothing.

The patient may feel hot one moment and cold the next as the body loses its ability to control its temperature. As circulation slows, the arms and legs may become cool and bluish. The underside of the body may darken. It may be difficult to feel a pulse at the wrist.
- What you can do: Provide and remove blankets as needed. Avoid using electric blankets, which may cause burns because the patient cannot tell you if he or she is too warm.
- Sponge the patient's head with a cool cloth if this provides comfort.

Loss of bladder and bowel control may occur around the time of death.
- What you can do: Protect the mattress with waterproof padding and change the padding as needed to keep the patient comfortable.

As people approach death, many times they report seeing gardens, libraries, or family or friends who have died. They may ask you to pack their bags and find tickets or a passport. Sometimes they may become insistent and attempt to do these chores themselves. They may try getting out of bed (even if they have been confined to bed for a long time) so that they can "leave."
- What you can do: Reassure the patient that it is all right; he or she can "go" without getting out of bed. Stay close, share stories, and be present.

Used with permission from the Family Home Hospice of the Visiting Nurse Association of Greater Philadelphia.

intervals between respirations, a weakened and irregular pulse, diminishing blood pressure, and skin color changes or mottling may occur. For patients who have received adequate management of symptoms and for families who have received adequate preparation and support, the actual time of death is commonly peaceful and occurs without struggle.

Nurses may or may not be present at the time of a patient's death. In many states, nurses may be authorized to make the pronouncement of death and sign the death certificate. The determination of death is made through a physical examination that includes auscultation for the absence of breathing and heart sounds. Home care or hospice programs in which nurses make the time-of-death visit and pronouncement of death have policies and procedures to guide the nurse's actions during this visit. Immediately on cessation of vital functions, the body begins to change. It becomes dusky or bluish, waxen-appearing, and cool; blood darkens and pools in dependent areas of the body (e.g., the back and sacrum if the body is in a supine position); and urine and stool may be evacuated.

Immediately after death, family members should be allowed and encouraged to spend time with the deceased. Normal responses of family members at the time of death vary widely and range from quiet expressions of grief to overt expressions that include wailing and prostration. The family's desire for privacy during their time with the deceased should be honored. Family members may wish to independently manage or assist with care of the body after death. If the death occurs in a long-term care facility, nurses follow the facility's procedure for preparation of the body and transportation to the facility's morgue. However, the needs of families to remain with the deceased, to wait until other family members arrive before the body is moved, and to perform after-death rituals should be honored. When an expected death occurs in the home setting, the funeral director often transports the body directly to the funeral home or mortuary.

Loss, Grief, and Bereavement

A wide range of feelings and behaviors are normal, adaptive, and healthy reactions to the loss of a loved one. **Grief** refers to the personal feelings that accompany an anticipated or actual loss. **Mourning** refers to individual, family, group, and cultural expressions of grief and associated behaviors. **Bereavement** refers to the period of time during which mourning takes place. Both grief reactions and mourning behaviors change over time as people learn to live with the loss. Although the pain of the loss may be tempered by the passage of time, loss is an ongoing developmental process, and time may never heal the bereaved individual completely. That is, the bereaved do not get over a loss entirely, nor do they return to who they were before the loss. Rather, they develop a new sense of who they are and where they fit in a world that has changed dramatically and permanently without their loved one and that relationship.

Anticipatory Grief and Mourning

Denial, sadness, anger, fear, and anxiety are normal grief reactions in people with life-threatening illness and those close to them. Kübler-Ross (1969) described five common emotional reactions to dying that are applicable to the experience of any loss: denial, anger, bargaining, depression, and acceptance. Kübler-Ross cautioned that not every patient or family member experiences every stage; many patients never reach a stage of acceptance, and patients and families fluctuate on a sometimes daily basis in their emotional responses.

Individual and family coping with the anticipation of death is complicated by the varied and conflicting trajectories that grief and mourning may assume in families. For example, although the patient may be experiencing sadness while contemplating role changes that have been brought about by the illness, the patient's spouse or partner may be expressing or suppressing feelings of anger about the current changes in role and impending loss of the relationship. Others in the family may be engaged in denial (e.g., "Dad will get better; he just needs to eat more"), fear ("Who will take care of us?" or "Will I get sick too?"), or profound sadness and withdrawal. Although each of these behaviors is normal, tension may arise when one or more family members perceive that others are less caring, too emotional, or too detached.

The nurse should assess the characteristics of the family system and intervene in a manner that supports and enhances the cohesion of the family unit. The nurse can encourage family members to talk about their feelings and help them understand what is happening to them in the broader context of anticipatory grief and mourning. Acknowledging and expressing feelings, continuing to interact with the patient in meaningful ways, and planning for the time of death and bereavement are adaptive family behaviors. Professional support provided by grief counselors and social workers, whether in the community, at a local hospital, in the long-term care facility, or associated with a hospice program, can help both the patient and the family sort out and acknowledge feelings and make the end of life as meaningful as possible.

Grief and Mourning After Death

When a loved one dies, the family members enter a new phase of grief and mourning as they begin to accept the loss, feel the pain of permanent separation, and prepare to live a life without the deceased. Even if the loved one died after a long illness, preparatory grief experienced during the terminal illness does not preclude the grief and mourning that follow the death. With a death after a long or difficult illness, family members may experience conflicting feelings of relief that the loved one's suffering has ended, compounded by guilt and grief related to unresolved issues or the circumstances of death. Grief work may be especially difficult if a patient's death was painful, prolonged, accompanied by unwanted interventions, or unattended. Families who had no preparation or support during the period of imminence and death may have a more difficult time finding a place for the painful memories.

Although some family members may experience prolonged or complicated mourning, most grief reactions fall within a "normal" range. The feelings are often profound, but bereaved people eventually reconcile the loss and find a way to reengage with their lives. Grief and mourning are affected by several factors, including individual characteristics, coping skills, and experiences with illness and death; the nature of the relationship to the deceased; factors surrounding the illness and the death; family dynamics; social support; and cultural expectations and norms. Uncomplicated grief and mourning are characterized by emotional feelings of sadness, anger, guilt, and numbness; physical sensations such as hollowness in the stomach and tightness in the chest, weakness, and lack of energy; cognitions that include preoccupation with the loss and a sense of the deceased as still present; and behaviors such as crying, visiting places that are reminders of the deceased, social withdrawal, and restless overactivity.

After-death rituals, including preparation of the body, funeral practices, and burial rituals, are socially and culturally significant ways in which family members begin to accept the reality and finality of death. Preplanning of funerals is becoming increasingly common, and hospice professionals in particular help the family make plans for death, often involving the patient, who may wish to play an active role. Preplanning of the funeral relieves the family of the burden of making decisions in the intensely emotional period after a death.

In general, the period of mourning is an adaptive response to loss during which mourners come to accept the loss as real and permanent, acknowledge and experience the painful emotions that accompany the loss, experience life without the deceased, overcome impediments to adjustment, and find a new way of living in a world without the loved one. Particularly, immediately after the death, mourners begin to recognize the reality and permanence of the loss by talking about the deceased and telling and retelling the story of the illness and death. Societal norms in the United States are frequently at odds with the normal grieving processes of people; time excused from work obligations is typically measured in days, and often mourners are expected to get over the loss quickly and get on with life.

In reality, the work of grief and mourning takes time, and avoiding grief work after the death often leads to long-term adjustment difficulties. Mourning for a loss involves the "undoing" of psychosocial ties that bind mourners to the deceased, personal adaptation to the loss, and learning to live in the world without the deceased. In his classic work, Worden (1991) described four tasks of mourning:

- Acceptance of the reality of the loss
- Working through the pain of grief
- Adjusting to the environment from which the deceased has gone
- Emotional "relocation" of the deceased to move on with life

Although many people complete the work of mourning with the informal support of families and friends, many find that talking with others who have had a similar experience, such as in formal support groups, normalizes the feelings and experiences and provides a framework for learning new skills to cope with the loss and create a new life. Hospitals, hospices, religious organizations, and other community organizations often sponsor bereavement support groups. Groups for parents who have lost a child, children who have lost a parent, widows, widowers, and gay men and lesbians who have lost a life partner are some examples of specialized support groups available in many communities.

Complicated Grief and Mourning

Complicated grief and mourning are characterized by prolonged feelings of sadness and feelings of general worthlessness or hopelessness that persist long after the death, prolonged symptoms that interfere with ADLs (anorexia, insomnia, fatigue, panic), or self-destructive behaviors such as alcohol or substance abuse and suicidal ideation or attempts. Complicated grief and mourning require a referral for a psychiatric assessment and evaluation to determine if pharmacologic and additional psychological interventions are needed. It is important that family members at risk for complicated grief be recognized early so that resources can be identified and mobilized.

COPING WITH DEATH AND DYING: PROFESSIONAL CAREGIVER ISSUES

Whether practicing in the trauma center, intensive care unit or other acute care setting, home care, hospice, long-term care, or the many locations where patients and their families receive ambulatory services, the nurse is closely involved with complex and emotionally laden issues surrounding loss of life. To be most effective and satisfied with the care he or she provides, the nurse should attend to his or her own emotional responses to the losses witnessed every day. Like family members, nurses need opportunities to grieve and express sorrow at the losses experienced and the sadness associated with a person dying before fulfilling one's dreams, leaving children prematurely, or completing one's commitments. Well before the nurse exhibits symptoms of stress or burnout, he or she should acknowledge the difficulty of coping with others' pain on a daily basis and put healthy practices in place that guard against emotional exhaustion. In hospice settings, where death, grief, and loss are expected outcomes of patient care, interdisciplinary colleagues rely on each other for support, using meeting time to express frustration, sadness, anger, and other emotions; to learn coping skills from each other; and to speak about how they were affected by the lives of those patients who have died since the last meeting. In many settings, staff members organize or attend memorial services to support families and other caregivers, who find comfort in joining each other to remember and celebrate the lives of patients. Finally, healthy personal habits, including diet, exercise, stress reduction activities (e.g., dance, yoga, tai chi, meditation), and sleep, help guard against the detrimental effects of stress.

SUMMARY

Chronic illnesses, those that last longer than 3 months, may be caused by injury or disease. Some of these diseases may be the result of genetic factors, while others may be the result of unhealthy lifestyles and behaviors earlier in life. Chronic illness is not merely a disease that has a nonreversible pathology; it is also the slow, progressive decline in normal function that brings with it disability and the need for long-term surveillance. Given its prevalence, chronic illness touches many lives, meaning nurses encounter many people who have been living with the symptoms or disabilities that accompany chronic illness. When they do, nurses will encounter people who are living with uncertainty. Chronic illness waxes and wanes, and with these modulations come a different set of health care regimens and types of management, often placing variable demands on family caregivers. Nurses need to be aware of the phases of the trajectory model of chronic illness, and they need to tailor the care they give to the care demanded, depending on the phase.

As people with chronic illness move in and out of the different phases of the trajectory model of care, and treatments become more complex, focus shifts from cure to care. There has been an international movement to recognize the need to help patients and families transition from cure to care. The goal of this movement is a seamless integration of palliative care into treatment from the beginning—at the time of diagnosis. Palliative care, encompassing a wide range of therapeutic interventions, seeks to prevent and relieve suffering. Because suffering has many and varied sources, nurses who provide palliative care should attend to the whole patient—that is, to the physical, psychological, social, and spiritual domains of human experience. As patients move into the downward phase of chronic illness, they need hospice or hospice-like care. Hospice care includes palliative care, but unlike palliative care, hospice care is associated with the patient's end of life: it helps patients and families prepare for death—emotionally, socially, spiritually, and financially. Nurses who provide end-of-life care have eight tasks: (1) They provide pain and symptom management. (2) With an ease that comes from expertise, they communicate effectively with dying patients and their families. (3) They educate patients and families about end-of-life decision-making and (4) help other professional caregivers to develop a coordinated plan of care that coheres with the wishes of patients and families. (5) They provide care to patients who are close to death, and (6) often, are present at death. (7) After death, they attend to families' loss, grief, and bereavement. (8) Finally, they achieve quality of care at the end of life by providing culturally sensitive care throughout the entire hospice-care experience.

Providing nursing care for patients and families who live with chronic illness is nursing at its fullest and deepest, for from the onset of disease to the end of life, care of the chronically ill centers on the whole person.

CHAPTER REVIEW

Critical Thinking Exercises

1. A 55-year-old married mother of three adult children has been referred for hospice care. During your initial visit to the patient's home, you assess that she is experiencing severe pain in her ribs and pelvis (she reports a score of 8 on a 0–10 pain intensity scale). In addition, she reports that she is unable to sleep. Her provider has prescribed morphine for her pain, but you assess that she has used very few doses of the morphine. Her husband tells you privately that he has discouraged her use of the medicine because it has made her very sleepy and nauseated in the past. The interdisciplinary team is meeting to discuss the patient's treatment plan. What additional assessment data are needed to determine the wishes and expectations of the patient as well as the husband? What are the team's options for intervention? What are the pros and cons of each option?

2. A 28-year-old woman with two children younger than 3 years of age has recently been diagnosed with type 1 diabetes. She is very active in her community and church and states that she cannot fit learning about diabetes, treatments, or blood glucose testing into her busy life. Identify approaches you would use to establish a plan of care with her. Link your teaching to the trajectory onset phase of chronic illness. How would your teaching plan change in the acute and crisis stages of chronic illness?

3. After having a seizure at her law office, a 34-year-old woman, a wife and mother of a 3-year-old son, was diagnosed 2 months ago with an aggressive form of brain cancer. The tumor's growth progresses rapidly. As a result, she experiences uncontrolled seizures, and her cognitive abilities decline. The neuro-oncologist has prognosticated death within a few months. What is one of the primary responsibilities of the nurse in this period of the patient's and family's life? What should the nurse document in the nursing assessment? How should the nurse respond to the patient and family when symptoms, such as seizure and cognitive decline, occur and intensify?

NCLEX-Style Review Questions

1. When educating patients about chronic diseases, such as diabetes, which of the following should the nurse include in the rationale for effective management of the disease? Select all that apply.
   a. An unmanaged chronic disease may lead to the development of other chronic illnesses.
   b. When a patient is admitted to the ICU with a comorbid chronic disease, that patient faces a greater risk of morbidity and mortality.
   c. Although chronic disease affects the entire family system, management of the disease is the patient's sole responsibility.
   d. By managing a chronic disorder early in the disease process, the patient may be able to save him- or herself the high costs associated with the sequelae of unmanaged disease.
   e. Chronic illness management is not influenced by lifestyle changes.

2. A patient is nearing death from metastatic cancer and is receiving hospice care in the home. The home care nurse visits. The patient's family caregiver states that the patient has not eaten well for the last several days and rarely wishes to drink, only sucking on ice now and then. The caregiver thinks that it is cruel to let the dying patient starve to death, or die from dehydration. What would the nurse's best response be?
   a. "I think it is cruel, too. If this were my mother, I would not let her die like that."
   b. "Tell me why you feel that way?"
   c. "It's okay, because this may hasten death and relieve suffering."
   d. "This is what happens when people die."

3. The sounds of breathing, including terminal bubbling, at the time of death may be distressing for families to hear. When the nurse hears these sounds, she should do which of the following? Select all that apply.
   a. Reposition the patient in an attempt to move secretions out of the oropharynx.
   b. Educate the family about what they are hearing and that the sound does not mean that the patient is in any distress.
   c. Suction the patient deeply and often to rid the oropharynx of the build-up of secretions.
   d. Suggest to the provider that now is the time for an anticholinergic drug (such as glycopyrrolate).

4. Chronic illnesses are characterized by which of the following? Select all that apply.
   a. A nonreversible pathology.
   b. A slow, progressive decline in normal physiologic function.
   c. A decreasing prevalence nationally and internationally.
   d. Necessitating long-term surveillance.

5. A dying patient has sudden onset of confusion, waxing and waning consciousness, and loss of orientation, thinking she is at home when she is in the hospital. The nurse recognizes this as _____ and knows that the most appropriate pharmacologic treatment for it includes _____.
   a. Dementia, acetylcholinesterase inhibitor
   b. Delirium, benzodiazepine
   c. Delirium, haloperidol
   d. Dementia, haloperidol

Try these additional resources, available at **http://thepoint.lww.com/Honan2e**, to enhance your learning and understanding of this chapter:
- NCLEX-Style Student Review Questions
- Journal Articles

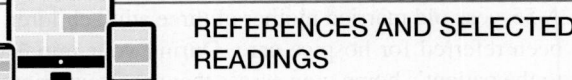

REFERENCES AND SELECTED READINGS

References and selected readings associated with this chapter can be found on the website that accompanies the book. Visit **http://thepoint.lww.com/Honan2e** to access the references and other additional resources associated with this chapter.

Concepts and Challenges in Patient Management

A 45-year-old patient has recently been diagnosed with brain cancer. She will be undergoing surgery, followed by chemotherapy. She is very anxious and has fears about her overall prognosis.

- What psychosocial aspects may be affected by this diagnosis?
- Explain postoperative risks that may occur following surgery.
- Discuss the special needs of a patient undergoing chemotherapy.

Fluid and Electrolyte and Acid–Base Imbalances

Philip R. Martinez, Jr. • Linda Honan

Learning Objectives

After reading this chapter, you will be able to:

1. Differentiate between osmosis, diffusion, filtration, and active transport.
2. Describe the role of kidneys, lungs, and endocrine glands in regulating the body's fluid composition and volume.
3. Identify the effects of aging on fluid and electrolyte regulation.
4. Plan effective care of patients with the following imbalances: hypovolemia, hypervolemia, hyponatremia, hypernatremia, hypokalemia, and hyperkalemia.
5. Describe the cause, clinical manifestations, management, and nursing interventions for the following imbalances: hypocalcemia, hypercalcemia, hypomagnesemia, hypermagnesemia, hypophosphatemia, hyperphosphatemia, hypochloremia, and hyperchloremia.
6. Explain the roles of lungs, kidneys, and chemical buffers in maintaining acid–base balance.
7. Compare metabolic acidosis and alkalosis with regard to causes, clinical manifestations, diagnosis, and management.
8. Compare respiratory acidosis and alkalosis with regard to causes, clinical manifestations, diagnosis, and management.
9. Interpret arterial blood gas measurements.
10. Describe measures used for preventing complications of IV therapy.

Fluid and electrolyte balance is a dynamic process that is crucial for life and **homeostasis**. Potential and actual disorders of fluid and electrolyte balance occur in every setting, with nearly every disorder, and with a variety of changes that affect healthy people as well as those who are ill. The blood's acid–base balance is precisely controlled, and because deviations from the normal pH range of 7.35 to 7.45 can cause severe effects in body function, the nurse needs to competently interpret arterial blood gases (ABGs).

FUNDAMENTAL CONCEPTS

AMOUNT AND COMPOSITION OF BODY FLUIDS

Approximately 60% of the weight of a typical adult consists of fluid (water and electrolytes). Factors that influence the amount of body fluid are age, gender, and body fat. In general, younger people have a higher percentage of body fluid than older people, and men have proportionately more body fluid than women. People who are obese have less fluid than those who are thin because fat cells contain little water.

Body fluid is located in two fluid compartments: the intracellular space (ICS, fluid inside the cells) and the extracellular space (ECS, fluid outside the cells). Approximately two thirds of body fluid is intracellular fluid (ICF) and is located primarily in the skeletal muscle mass; approximately one third is in the extracellular fluid (ECF).

The ECF compartment is further divided into the intravascular, interstitial, and transcellular fluid spaces. The intravascular space (IVS, the fluid within the blood vessels) contains plasma. Plasma is water, along with molecules, electrolytes, and proteins, minus blood cells and platelets. Approximately 3.5 L of the average 6 L of blood volume is made up of plasma, which has a straw-colored appearance. The remaining 2.5 L is made up of erythrocytes (red blood cells [RBC]), leukocytes (white

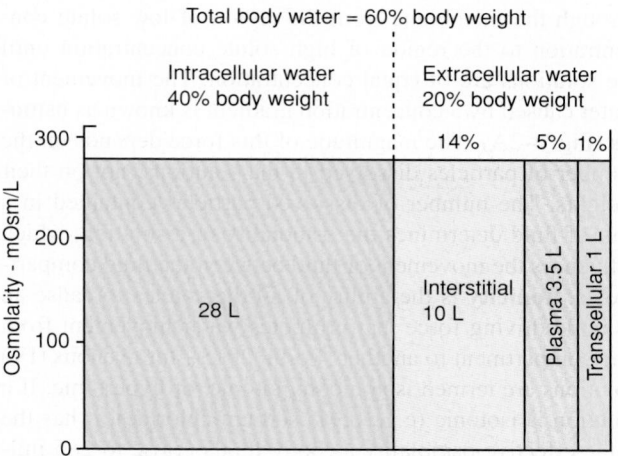

FIGURE 4-1 Approximate size of body compartments in a 70-kg man. (From Porth, C.M., & Matfin, G. (2009). *Pathophysiology: Concepts of altered health status* (8th ed.). Philadelphia, PA: Lippincott Williams & Wilkins.)

blood cells [WBC]), and thrombocytes (platelets). The interstitial space contains the fluid between the cells, tissues, organs, and blood vessels and totals about 10 L in an adult. Lymph fluid is an interstitial fluid. The transcellular space is the smallest division of the ECF compartment and contains approximately 1 L. Examples of transcellular fluids are cerebrospinal, pericardial, synovial, intraocular, pleural, and the peritoneal cavity. Figure 4-1 demonstrates the composition of body compartments.

Body fluid normally shifts between the two major compartments or spaces (ICS and ECS) in an effort to transport gases, nutrients, and wastes while maintaining overall bodily function. Loss of fluid from the body can disrupt this equilibrium. Sometimes fluid is not lost from the body but is unavailable for use by either the ICF or ECF. Loss of ECF into a space that does not contribute to equilibrium between the ICF and the ECF is referred to as an *interstitial fluid shift*, or *third-spacing*.

Nursing Alert

Early evidence of third-space fluid shifting is a decrease in urine output despite adequate fluid intake. Urine output decreases because fluid shifts out of the IVS; the kidneys then receive less blood and attempt to compensate by decreasing urine output. Other signs and symptoms of third-spacing that indicate an intravascular fluid volume deficit (FVD) include increased heart rate, decreased blood pressure, decreased central venous pressure (CVP), edema, increased body weight, and imbalances in fluid intake and output (I&O). Third-space shifts occur in ascites, burns, peritonitis, bowel obstruction, and massive bleeding into a joint or body cavity.

Electrolytes in body fluids are active chemicals (cations that carry positive charges and anions that carry negative charges). The major cations in body fluid are sodium (Na^+), potassium (K^+),

calcium (Ca^{+2}), magnesium (Mg^{+2}), and hydrogen (H^+) ions. The major anions are chloride (Cl^-), bicarbonate (HCO_3^-), phosphate (PO_4^{3-}), sulfate (SO_4^{2-}), and proteinate ions.

These chemicals unite in varying combinations. Therefore, electrolyte concentration in the body is expressed in terms of milliequivalents (mEq) per liter, a measure of chemical activity, rather than in terms of milligrams (mg), a unit of weight. More specifically, a milliequivalent is defined as being equivalent to the electrochemical activity of 1 mg of hydrogen. In a solution, cations and anions are equal in milliequivalents per liter.

Although all body fluid contains equal amounts of cations and anions, the electrolyte concentrations in the ICF are markedly different from those in the ECF, as reflected in Table 4-1. Sodium ions, which are positively charged, far outnumber the other cations in the ECF. Because sodium concentration affects the overall concentration of the ECF, sodium is important in regulating the volume of body fluid. Approximately 90% of the serum osmolality (discussed later) is determined by the serum sodium level. Retention of sodium is associated with fluid retention, and conversely excessive loss of sodium is usually associated with decreased volume of body fluid.

As shown in Table 4-1, the major electrolytes in the ICF are potassium and phosphate. The ECF has a low concentration of

TABLE **4-1** Approximate Major Electrolyte Content in Body Fluid

Electrolytes	mEq/L[a]
Extracellular Fluid (Plasma)	
Cations	
Sodium (Na)	142
Potassium (K)	5
Calcium (Ca^{+2})	5
Magnesium (Mg^{+2})	2
Total cations	154
Anions	
Chloride (Cl^-)	103
Bicarbonate (HCO_3^-)	26
Phosphate (PO_4^{3-})	2
Sulfate (SO_4^{2-})	1
Organic acids	5
Proteinate	17
Total anions	154
Intracellular Fluid	
Cations	
Potassium (K^+)	150
Magnesium (Mg^{+2})	40
Sodium (Na^+)	10
Total cations	200
Anions	
Phosphates and sulfates	150
Bicarbonate (HCO_3^-)	10
Proteinate	40
Total anions	200

[a]Values may vary depending on the method of analysis used.

potassium and can tolerate only small changes in potassium concentrations. Therefore, any condition that causes the release of large stores of intracellular potassium (e.g., trauma to the cells and tissues) can be extremely dangerous.

> **Nursing Alert**
>
> *The nurse understands that the **intracellular** concentration of K^+ is approximately 140 to 150 mEq/L and that the kidneys are primarily responsible for K^+ excretion. The nurse recognizes that hyperkalemia (generally defined as a plasma K^+ of greater than 5.0 mEq/L) is associated with cardiac arrhythmias (discussed in Chapter 17), muscle weakness and acute muscle damage from rhabdomyolysis (discussed in Chapter 42), kidney failure (discussed in Chapter 27), and acidosis (discussed later in this chapter). One of the most common metabolic causes of cardiac arrest is hyperkalemia, which is associated most frequently in patients with kidney failure.*

The body expends a great deal of energy maintaining the high extracellular concentration of sodium and the high intracellular concentration of potassium. It does so by means of cell membrane pumps that exchange sodium and potassium ions.

Normal movement of fluid through the capillary wall into the tissues is dependent on two primary forces (called Starling forces): (1) the capillary hydrostatic pressure generated by cardiac contraction and exerted by plasma fluids on the walls of the blood vessel, and (2) the plasma oncotic (colloid osmotic) pressure, exerted by plasma proteins (primarily by capillary-impermeable albumin). At the arterial end of the capillary bed, fluids are filtered because the hydrostatic pressure exceeds the oncotic pressure; thus, water and electrolytes leave the capillary and enter the interstitial space and/or ICS. Because hydrostatic pressure decreases as blood moves along the capillary bed, the relatively constant plasma oncotic pressure exceeds the hydrostatic pressure at the venous end of the capillary; therefore, fluids now re-enter the capillary. In many capillary beds, the forces favoring filtration slightly exceed those that favor reabsorption. However, excessive interstitial fluid accumulation is prevented since the lymphatic drainage returns this excess fluid to the systemic circulation.

In addition to electrolytes, the ECF transports other substances, such as enzymes and hormones. It also carries blood components, such as RBCs, WBCs, and platelets, throughout the body.

REGULATION OF BODY FLUID COMPARTMENTS

Osmosis and Osmolality

When two different solutions are separated by a membrane that is impermeable to the dissolved substances, fluid shifts through the membrane from the region of low solute concentration to the region of high solute concentration until the solutions are of equal concentration. The movement of water caused by a concentration gradient is known as **osmosis** (Fig. 4-2A). The magnitude of this force depends on the number of particles dissolved in the solutions, not on their weights. The number of dissolved particles contained in a unit of fluid determines the osmolality of a solution, which influences the movement of fluid between the fluid compartments. **Tonicity** is the ability of all the solutes to cause an osmotic driving force that promotes water movement from one compartment to another (Porth, 2015). Intravenous (IV) solutions are termed isotonic, hypotonic, or hypertonic. If a solution is isotonic (e.g., 0.9% sodium chloride), it has the same effective osmolality as body fluids (close to 285 milliosmolal [mOsm]). Sodium, mannitol, glucose, and sorbitol are all effective osmoles (capable of affecting water movement; see later discussion of IV solutions).

> **Nursing Alert**
>
> *It is important to understand osmotic diuresis, which is an increase in urine output caused by the excretion of substances such as glucose, mannitol, or contrast agents in the urine, which exert an osmotic pull on water. For example, because glucose is an osmotic agent (capable of affecting water movement), when glucose is excreted in the urine, it will bring water with it, causing polyuria with resulting FVD.*

Diffusion

Diffusion is the natural tendency of a substance to move from an area of higher concentration to one of lower concentration (see Fig. 4-2B). Examples of diffusion are the exchange of oxygen and carbon dioxide between the pulmonary capillaries and alveoli.

Filtration

Hydrostatic pressure in the capillaries tends to filter fluid out of the intravascular compartment into the interstitial fluid. Movement of water and solutes occurs from an area of high hydrostatic pressure to an area of low hydrostatic pressure. Filtration allows the kidneys to filter 180 L of plasma per day.

Sodium–Potassium Pump

As previously stated, the sodium concentration is greater in the ECF than in the ICF, and, because of this, sodium tends to enter the cell by diffusion. This tendency is offset by the sodium–potassium pump, which is located in the cell membrane and actively moves sodium from the cell into the ECF. Conversely, the high intracellular potassium concentration is maintained by pumping potassium into the cell. By definition,

FIGURE 4-2 **A.** Osmosis: Movement of fluid from an area of lower solute concentration to an area of higher solute concentration with eventual equalization of the solute concentrations. **B.** Diffusion: Movement of solutes from an area of greater concentration to an area of lesser concentration, leading ultimately to equalization of the solute concentrations.

active transport implies that energy must be expended for the movement to occur against a concentration gradient.

ROUTES OF GAINS AND LOSSES

Water and electrolytes are gained in various ways. A healthy person gains fluids by drinking and eating. Fluids may also be provided by the parenteral route (IV or subcutaneously) or by means of an enteral feeding tube in the stomach or intestine.

Kidneys

The usual daily urine volume in the adult is 1.5 L. A general rule is that the output is approximately 0.5 to 1 mL of urine per kilogram of body weight per hour (0.5 to 1 mL/kg/hr) in all age groups, with boundaries of 0.5 to 2 mL/kg/hr.

Skin

Sensible perspiration refers to visible water and electrolyte loss through the skin (sweating). The chief solutes in sweat are sodium, chloride, and potassium. Actual sweat loss can vary from 0 to 1,000 mL or more every hour, depending on the environmental temperature. Continuous water loss by evaporation (approximately 600 mL/day) occurs through the skin as insensible perspiration, a nonvisible form of water loss. Fever greatly increases insensible water loss through the lungs and the skin as does loss of the natural skin barrier (e.g., through major burns). Although sodium content in sweat is low (ranging from approximately 20 to 50 mmol/L), with increased sweat loss, sodium deficit and FVD can occur (Slotki & Skorecki, 2016).

Lungs

The lungs normally eliminate water vapor (insensible loss) at a rate of approximately 400 mL every day. The loss is much greater with increased respiratory rate or depth, or in a dry climate.

Gastrointestinal Tract

The usual loss through the gastrointestinal (GI) tract is only 100 mL daily, even though approximately 8 L of fluid

TABLE **4-2** Average Daily Intake and Output in an Adult

Intake (mL)			
Oral liquids	1,300	Urine	1,500
Water in food	1,000	Stool	100
Water produced by metabolism	300	Insensible	
		Lungs	400
		Skin	600
Total gain[a]	2,600	Total loss[a]	2,600

[a]Approximate volumes.

circulates through the GI system every 24 hours. Because the bulk of fluid is normally reabsorbed in the small intestine, diarrhea and fistulas cause large losses. To illustrate, worldwide, infectious diarrhea is a leading cause of death from hypovolemia (Slotki & Skorecki, 2016). In healthy people, the daily average I&O of water are approximately equal (Table 4-2).

LABORATORY TESTS FOR EVALUATING FLUID STATUS

Osmolality is the concentration of fluid that affects the movement of water between fluid compartments by osmosis. Osmolality measures the solute concentration per kilogram of solvent in blood and urine. It is also a measure of a solution's ability to create osmotic pressure and affect the movement of water. Serum osmolality primarily reflects the concentration of sodium, although blood urea nitrogen (BUN) and glucose also play a major role in determining serum osmolality (Porth, 2015). Urine osmolality is determined by urea, creatinine, and uric acid. When measured with serum osmolality, urine osmolality is the most reliable indicator of the concentrating ability of kidneys. Osmolality is reported as milliosmoles per kilogram of water (mOsm/kg).

Osmolarity, another term that describes the concentration of solutions, is measured in milliosmoles per liter (mOsm/L). The term *osmolality* is used more often in clinical practice. Normal serum osmolality is 275 to 300 mOsm/kg, and normal urine osmolality is 50 to 1,400 mOsm/kg in a random urine test and 300 to 900 mOsm/kg in a 24-hour urine collection (Fischbach & Dunning, 2015).

Nursing Alert
When concerned about renal concentrating ability, a serum and urine osmolality test is obtained at the same time. In general, the normal ratio of urine and serum is 3:1. Higher ratios are seen in concentrated urine, whereas lower ratios are seen with poor concentrating ability.

Factors that increase and decrease serum and urine osmolality are identified in Table 4-3. Serum osmolality may be

TABLE **4-3** Factors Affecting Serum and Urine Osmolality

Fluid	Factors Increasing Osmolality	Factors Decreasing Osmolality
Serum (275–300 mOsm/kg water)	• Severe dehydration • Free water loss • Diabetes insipidus • Hypernatremia • Hyperglycemia • Stroke or head injury • Renal tubular necrosis • Consumption of methanol or ethylene glycol (antifreeze)	• Fluid volume excess • Syndrome of inappropriate antidiuretic hormone (SIADH) • Kidney failure • Diuretic use • Adrenal insufficiency • Hyponatremia • Overhydration • Paraneoplastic syndrome associated with lung cancer
Urine (250–900 mOsm/kg water)	• Fluid volume deficit (FVD) • SIADH • Congestive heart failure • Acidosis	• Fluid volume excess • Diabetes insipidus • Hyponatremia • Pyelonephritis

measured directly through laboratory tests or estimated at the bedside by doubling the serum sodium level or by using the following formula:

$$\text{Plasma osmolality (mOsm/kg)} = 2\,[\text{serum sodium}] + \text{Glucose}/18 + \text{BUN}/2.8$$

The calculated value usually is within 10 mOsm of the measured osmolality.

The specific gravity of urine measures the kidneys' ability to excrete or conserve water. The specific gravity of urine is compared to the weight of distilled water, which has a specific gravity of 1.000. The normal range of urine specific gravity is 1.010 to 1.025. Specific gravity of urine can be measured at the bedside by placing a calibrated hydrometer or urinometer in a cylinder of approximately 20 mL of urine. Specific gravity can also be assessed with a refractometer or dipstick with a reagent for this purpose. Specific gravity varies inversely with urine volume; normally, the larger the volume of urine, the lower the specific gravity.

Nursing Alert
Specific gravity is a less reliable indicator of concentration than urine osmolality because it is influenced by both the number and size of particles in urine; increased glucose or protein in urine can cause a falsely elevated specific gravity. Factors that increase or decrease urine osmolality are the same as those for urine specific gravity.

The laboratory value BUN, part of the basic metabolic panel, is made up of urea, which is an end product of the metabolism of protein (from both muscle and dietary intake) by the liver. The normal BUN is 10 to 20 mg/dL (3.6 to 7.2 μmol/L). The BUN level varies with urine output. Factors that increase BUN include decreased kidney function, GI bleeding, dehydration, increased protein intake, fever, and sepsis. Any condition that increases tissue necrosis and protein catabolism will cause the BUN to rise; a critical value for BUN is when it is over 100 mg/dL (Fischbach & Dunning, 2015). Those factors that decrease BUN include end-stage liver disease, a low-protein diet, starvation, syndrome of inappropriate antidiuretic hormone (SIADH), and any condition that results in expanded fluid volume (e.g., pregnancy).

Creatinine is the end product of muscle metabolism. It is a better indicator of kidney function than BUN because it does not vary with protein intake and metabolic state. The normal serum creatinine is approximately 0.6 to 1.4 mg/dL (53 to 124 mmol/L); however, its concentration depends on lean body mass and varies from person to person. Serum creatinine levels increase when kidney function decreases.

Hematocrit measures the volume percentage of RBC (erythrocytes) in whole blood and normally ranges from 42% to 52% for males and 36% to 48% for females. Conditions that increase the hematocrit value are dehydration and polycythemia, and conditions that decrease hematocrit are overhydration and anemia.

Urine sodium values change with sodium intake and the status of fluid volume: as sodium intake increases, excretion increases; as the circulating fluid volume decreases, sodium is conserved. Normal urine sodium levels range from 40 to 220 mEq every 24 hours (40 to 220 mmol/day). A random specimen usually contains more than 40 mEq/L of sodium. Urine sodium levels are used to assess volume status and are useful in the diagnosis of hyponatremia and acute kidney failure (AKF).

HOMEOSTATIC MECHANISMS

The body is equipped with remarkable homeostatic mechanisms to keep the composition and volume of body fluid within narrow limits of normal. Organs involved in homeostasis include the kidneys, lungs, heart, adrenal glands, parathyroid glands, and pituitary gland.

Kidney Functions

Vital to the regulation of fluid and electrolyte balance, the kidneys normally filter 170 L of plasma every day in the adult, while excreting only 1.5 L of urine. They act both autonomously and in response to blood-borne messengers, such as aldosterone and antidiuretic hormone (ADH) (Porth, 2015). Major functions of the kidneys in maintaining normal fluid balance include the following:

- Regulation of ECF volume and osmolality by selective retention and excretion of body fluids;
- Regulation of electrolyte levels in the ECF by selective retention of needed substances and excretion of unneeded substances;
- Regulation of pH of the ECF by excretion or retention of hydrogen ions and/or bicarbonate ions (HCO_3^-);
- Excretion of metabolic wastes and toxic substances.

Given these functions, it is readily apparent that kidney failure results in multiple fluid and electrolyte abnormalities. Kidney function declines with advanced age, as do muscle mass and daily exogenous creatinine production. Therefore, high-normal and minimally elevated serum creatinine values actually may indicate substantially reduced kidney function in the elderly.

Heart and Blood Vessel Functions

The pumping action of the heart circulates blood through the kidneys under sufficient pressure to allow for urine formation. Failure of this pumping action interferes with renal perfusion and thus with water and electrolyte regulation.

Lung Functions

The lungs are also vital in maintaining homeostasis. Through exhalation, the lungs remove approximately 400 mL of water daily in the normal adult. Abnormal conditions, such as hyperpnea (abnormally deep respiration) or continuous coughing, increase this loss; mechanical ventilation with excessive moisture decreases it. The lungs also play a major role in maintaining acid–base balance. Normal aging results in decreased respiratory function, causing increased difficulty in pH regulation in older adults, especially those with major illness or trauma.

Pituitary Functions

The hypothalamus manufactures ADH, which is stored in the posterior pituitary gland and released as needed. ADH is sometimes called the *water-conserving hormone* because it causes the body to retain water. Functions of ADH include maintaining the osmotic pressure of the cells by controlling the retention or excretion of water by the kidneys and by regulating blood volume (Fig. 4-3).

Adrenal Functions

Aldosterone, a mineralocorticoid secreted by the zona glomerulosa (outer zone) of the adrenal cortex, has a profound effect on fluid balance. Increased secretion of aldosterone causes sodium retention (and, thus, water retention) and potassium loss. Conversely, decreased secretion of aldosterone causes sodium and water loss and potassium retention.

Cortisol, another adrenocortical hormone, has only a fraction of the mineralocorticoid potency of aldosterone.

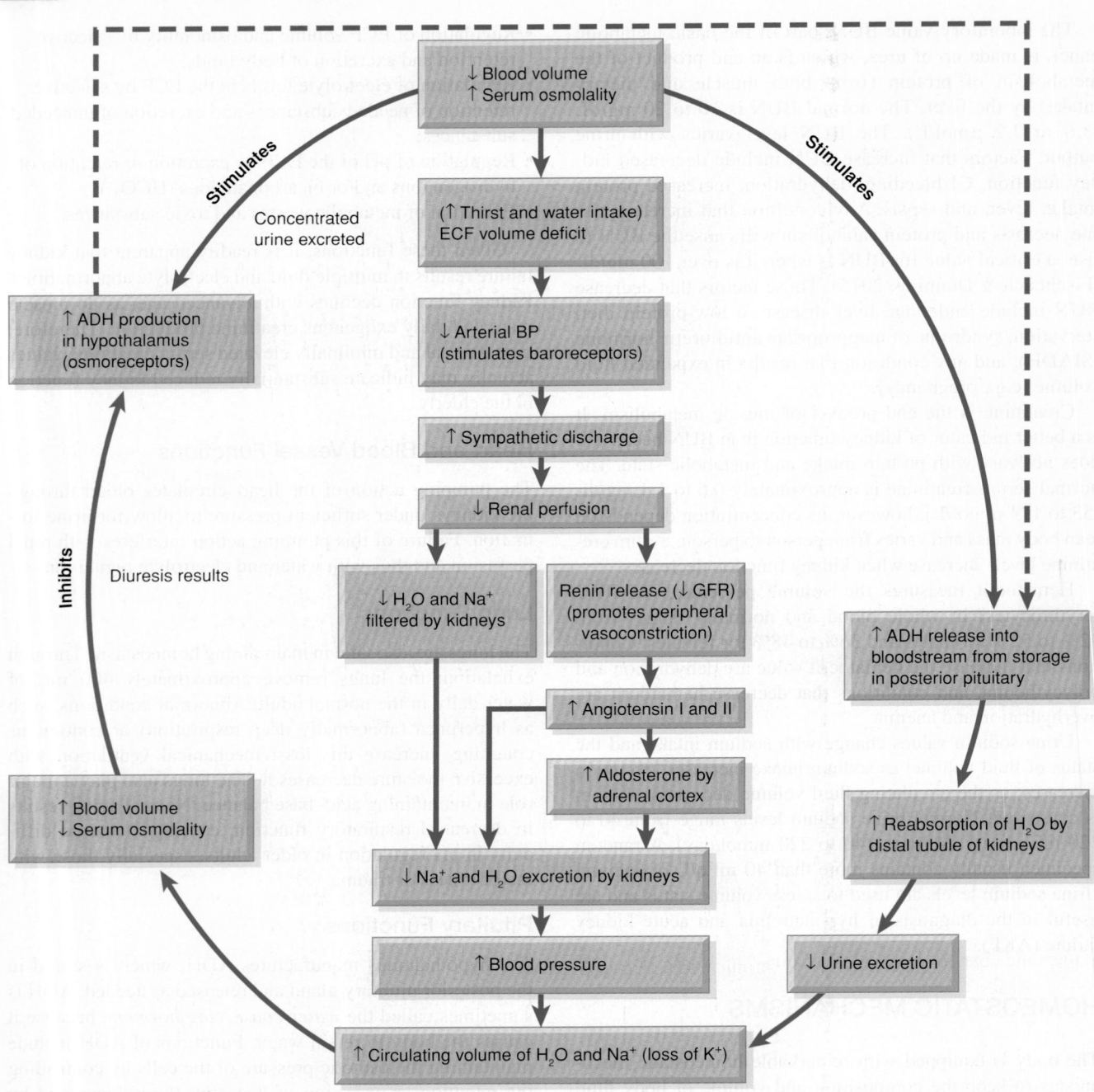

FIGURE 4-3 Fluid regulation cycle.

However, when secreted in large quantities (or administered as corticosteroid therapy), it can also produce sodium and fluid retention.

Parathyroid Functions

The parathyroid glands, embedded in the thyroid gland, regulate calcium and phosphate balance by means of parathyroid hormone (PTH). PTH influences bone resorption (movement of calcium out of bone to the blood), calcium absorption from the intestines, and calcium reabsorption from the renal tubules. A decrease in serum calcium is the primary stimulus for PTH secretions, whereas a rise in serum calcium inhibits secretion.

Other Mechanisms

Changes in the volume of the interstitial compartment within the ECF can occur without affecting body function. However, the vascular compartment cannot tolerate change as readily and must be carefully maintained to ensure that tissues receive adequate nutrients.

Baroreceptors

The baroreceptors are small nerve receptors that detect changes in pressure within blood vessels and transmit this information to the central nervous system (CNS). They are responsible for monitoring the circulating volume, and they regulate sympathetic and parasympathetic neural activity as well as endocrine activities. They are categorized as either low-pressure or high-pressure baroreceptors. Low-pressure baroreceptors are in the cardiac atria, particularly the left atrium. High-pressure baroreceptors are nerve endings in the aortic arch and the carotid sinus, as well as in the afferent arteriole of the juxtaglomerular apparatus of the nephron.

As arterial pressure decreases, baroreceptors transmit fewer impulses from the carotid sinuses and the aortic arch to the vasomotor center. A decrease in impulses stimulates the sympathetic nervous system and inhibits the parasympathetic nervous system. The outcome is an increase in cardiac rate, conduction, and contractility as well as an increase in circulating blood volume. Sympathetic stimulation constricts renal arterioles; this increases the release of aldosterone, decreases glomerular filtration, and increases sodium and water reabsorption and potassium loss (discussed below). Conversely, if high-pressure baroreceptors are stimulated, the outcome is a lowered heart rate and lowered blood vessel resistance.

Renin–Angiotensin–Aldosterone System

Renin is an enzyme that converts angiotensinogen, an inactive substance formed by the liver, into angiotensin I (AI) (Porth, 2015). Renin is released by the juxtaglomerular cells of the kidneys in response to decreased renal perfusion. Angiotensin-converting enzyme (ACE) converts AI to angiotensin II (AII). AII, with its vasoconstrictor properties, increases arterial perfusion pressure and also stimulates thirst. When the sympathetic nervous system is stimulated, aldosterone is released in response to an increased release of renin. Aldosterone is a volume regulator and is also released as serum potassium increases, serum sodium decreases, or adrenocorticotropic hormone (ACTH) increases. The net effect of aldosterone is to increase the reabsorption of sodium, which increases water reabsorption thus increasing plasma volume.

Antidiuretic Hormone and Thirst

ADH and the thirst mechanism play important roles in maintaining sodium concentration and oral intake of fluids. Oral intake is controlled by the thirst center, located in the hypothalamus (Porth, 2015). As serum concentration or osmolality increases or blood volume decreases, neurons in the hypothalamus are stimulated by intracellular dehydration; thirst then occurs, and the person increases his or her intake

of oral fluids. An increase in osmolality of only 1% to 2% is sufficient to stimulate thirst. Water excretion is controlled by ADH, aldosterone, and baroreceptors, as mentioned previously. The presence or absence of ADH is the most significant factor in determining whether the urine that is excreted is concentrated or dilute.

Osmoreceptors

Located on the surface of the hypothalamus, osmoreceptors sense changes in sodium concentration. As the serum osmolality increases, the neurons become dehydrated and quickly generate action potentials resulting in increased release of ADH from the posterior pituitary. The ADH then travels in the blood to the kidneys, where it alters permeability to water, causing increased reabsorption of water and decreased urine output. The retained water dilutes the ECF and returns its concentration to normal. Restoration of normal serum osmolality provides feedback to the osmoreceptors to inhibit further ADH release (see Fig. 4-3).

Release of Atrial Natriuretic Peptide

Atrial natriuretic peptide (ANP), also called *atrial natriuretic factor,* is synthesized, stored, and released by muscle cells of the atria of the heart in response to several factors. ANP secretion is enhanced by increases in atrial pressure, endothelin (a powerful peptide vasoconstrictor of vascular smooth muscle released from damaged endothelial cells in the kidneys or other tissues) and sympathetic stimulation (Porth, 2015). In addition, any condition that results in volume expansion (e.g., pregnancy), hypoxia, or increased cardiac filling pressures (e.g., high sodium intake, heart failure, chronic kidney failure (CKF), atrial tachycardia, or use of vasoconstrictor agents such as epinephrine) increases the release of ANP. The action of ANP is the direct opposite of the renin–angiotensin–aldosterone system (RAAS); ANP decreases blood pressure and volume (Fig. 4-4). The ANP measured in plasma is normally 20 to 77 pg/mL (20 to 77 ng/L). This level increases in paroxysmal atrial tachycardia, hyperthyroidism, subarachnoid hemorrhage, and small cell lung cancer. In congestive heart failure and cirrhosis with ascites, ANP is elevated but not sufficiently to prevent fluid volume excess (FVE). Brain natriuretic peptide (BNP) that is stored primarily in ventricular myocardium and released when ventricular diastolic pressure rises, has actions similar to **ANP**. Normal BNP levels are less than 100 pg/mL. For reasons that are not understood, the renal effects of the natriuretic peptides appear to become dampened with advancing heart failure, leaving the effects of RAS unopposed (Hasenfuss & Mann, 2015).

GERONTOLOGIC CONSIDERATIONS

Normal physiologic changes of aging, including reduced cardiac, kidney, and respiratory function and reserve; and

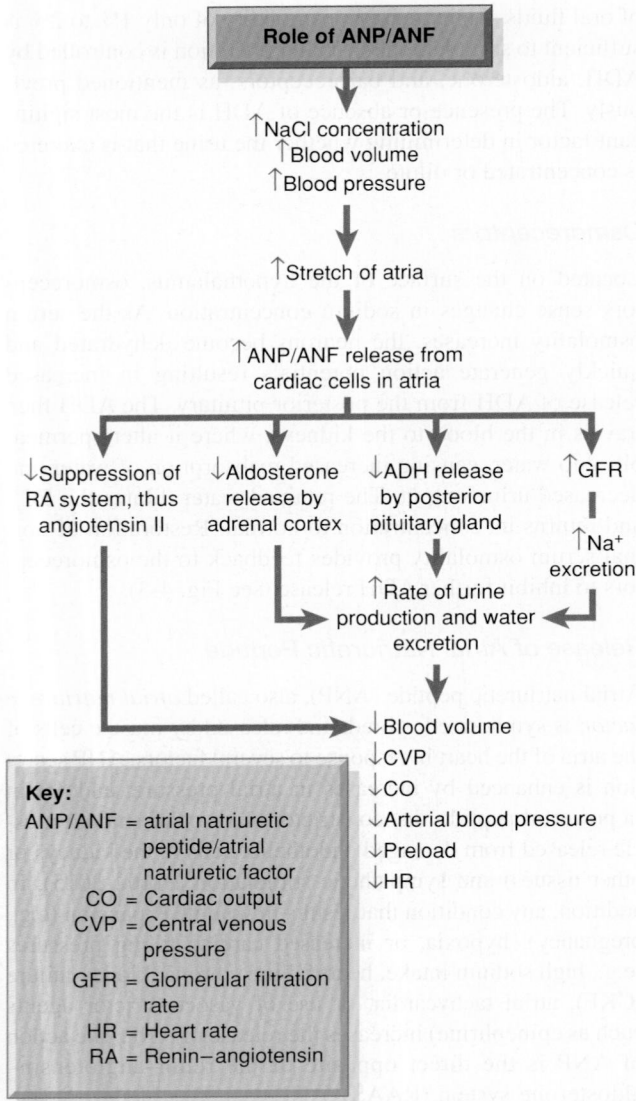

FIGURE 4-4 Role of atrial natriuretic peptide (ANP) in maintenance of fluid balance.

alterations in the ratio of body fluids to muscle mass, may alter the responses of elderly people to fluid and electrolyte changes and acid–base disturbances. In addition, the frequent use of medications in the older adult can affect kidney and cardiac function and fluid balance, thereby increasing the likelihood of fluid and electrolyte disturbances. Routine procedures, such as the vigorous administration of laxatives before GI studies, may produce a serious FVD, necessitating the use of IV fluids to prevent hypotension and other effects of hypovolemia.

Alterations in fluid and electrolyte balance that may produce minor changes in young and middle-aged adults have the potential to produce profound changes in older adults, accompanied by a rapid onset of signs and symptoms. In elderly patients, the clinical manifestations of fluid and electrolyte disturbances may be subtle or atypical. For example, fluid deficit may cause confusion or cognitive impairment in the elderly person, whereas in the young or middle-aged person the first sign commonly is increased thirst. Rapid infusion of an excessive volume of IV fluids may produce fluid overload and cardiac failure in the elderly patient. These reactions are likely to occur more quickly and with the administration of smaller volumes of fluid than in healthy young and middle-aged adults because of the decreased cardiac reserve and reduced kidney function that accompany aging. Dehydration in the elderly is common as a result of decreased reserve capacity of the kidney from the aging process, disease, and use of medications.

Increased sensitivity to fluid and electrolyte changes in elderly patients requires careful assessment, with attention to I&O of fluids from all sources and to changes in daily weight; careful monitoring of side effects and interactions of medications; and prompt reporting and management of disturbances.

FLUID VOLUME DISTURBANCES

Appendix A summarizes the major fluid and electrolyte imbalances that are described in this chapter.

HYPOVOLEMIA

FVD, or hypovolemia, occurs when loss of ECF volume exceeds the intake of fluid. It occurs when water and electrolytes are lost in the same proportion as they exist in normal body fluids, so that the ratio of serum electrolytes to water remains the same. FVD should not be confused with the term *dehydration,* which refers to loss of water alone, with increased serum sodium levels. FVD may occur alone or in combination with other imbalances. Unless other imbalances are present concurrently, serum electrolyte concentrations remain essentially unchanged.

Pathophysiology

FVD results from loss of body fluids and occurs more rapidly when coupled with decreased fluid intake. FVD can develop from inadequate intake alone if the decreased intake is prolonged. The nurse considers NPO status of patients for diagnostic tests, those with difficulty swallowing, nausea, decreased level of consciousness (LOC), or depression when IV fluids are not administered. The elderly are at risk for FVD because of poor oral intake and potential difficulty gaining access to water. Causes of FVD also include abnormal fluid losses, such as those resulting from vomiting, diarrhea, GI suctioning (nasogastric or intestinal tubes, drains [biliary, pancreatic]), fever, and sweating. Additional risk factors include burns, surgery, diabetes insipidus, adrenal insufficiency, osmotic diuresis, hemorrhage, and coma. Third-space fluid shifts, or the movement of fluid from the vascular system to other body spaces (e.g., with edema formation in burns, ascites with liver dysfunction), also cause FVD because although the fluid has not left the body, it is not available in the IVS.

Clinical Manifestations and Assessment

FVD can develop rapidly and can be mild, moderate, or severe, depending on the degree of fluid loss. Important signs include acute weight loss; decreased skin turgor; oliguria (urinary output below 400 mL/day); concentrated urine with a high specific gravity; postural hypotension (a 20 mm Hg decrease in systolic pressure or a 10 mm Hg decrease in diastolic pressure with position change); a weak, rapid heart rate; flattened neck veins; decreased CVP; cool, clammy skin related to peripheral vasoconstriction; a smaller tongue with additional longitudinal furrows; dry oral mucous membranes; delayed capillary refill (greater than 2 seconds); altered sensorium; and thirst. Diagnostic testing includes BUN and its relation to serum creatinine concentration. A volume-depleted patient has a BUN elevated out of proportion to the serum creatinine (ratio greater than 20:1). The BUN can also be elevated because of decreased renal perfusion and function. The cause of abnormal laboratory findings may be determined through the health history and physical findings.

The hematocrit level is greater than normal in dehydration because the RBC become suspended in a decreased plasma volume, which is also known as *hemoconcentration.*

Serum electrolyte changes may also exist. Potassium and sodium levels can be reduced (hypokalemia, hyponatremia) or elevated (hyperkalemia, hypernatremia):

- Hypokalemia occurs with GI and kidney losses;
- Hyperkalemia occurs with adrenal insufficiency;
- Hyponatremia occurs with increased thirst and ADH release;
- Hypernatremia results from increased insensible losses and diabetes insipidus.

Specific gravity of urine is increased in relation to the kidneys' attempt to conserve water and decreased with diabetes insipidus. The range of urine specific gravity will vary with

- the hydration status of the patient (increased with FVD, decreased with FVE),
- the volume of urine (increased with decreased urine output, decreased specific gravity with increased urine output), and
- the number of the particles in the urine (increased with increased particles, decreased with less particles).

A urine specific gravity of 1.005 or less indicates the diluting ability of the kidney, whereas 1.020 or greater indicates concentrating ability of the kidney. For example, a patient with preserved kidney function who is volume depleted will have a specific gravity greater than 1.020 because the patient is able to concentrate his or her urine. However, there are times that the specific gravity is falsely elevated, such as during kidney excretion of radiopaque x-ray contrast (high-molecular-weight substance). Thus, a urine osmolality test is a more exact measurement than specific gravity and may be required when assessment of the concentrating or diluting function of the kidney is needed.

Medical Management

When planning the correction of fluid loss for the patient with FVD, the health care provider considers the usual maintenance requirements of the patient and other factors (e.g., fever) that can influence fluid needs. If the deficit is not severe, the oral route is preferred, provided the patient can drink. However, if fluid losses are acute or severe, the IV route is required. Isotonic electrolyte solutions (e.g., lactated Ringer solution, 0.9% sodium chloride) are frequently used to treat the hypotensive patient with FVD because those solutions expand plasma volume. ICS is essentially sodium free; thus, for every liter of 0.9% sodium chloride administered, 1,000 mL will remain in the ECS, of which approximately 250 mL will remain in the IVS, re-expanding the plasma volume. Because this solution can expand the IVS, patients must be assessed for signs and symptoms of FVE (discussed shortly). As soon as the patient becomes normotensive (normalization of their blood pressure), a hypotonic electrolyte solution (e.g., 0.45% sodium chloride) is often used to provide both electrolytes and water for renal excretion of metabolic wastes. These and additional fluids are discussed later in the chapter.

> **Nursing Alert**
> *The nurse understands that when the patient is hypotensive, restoration of the IVS is imperative. If an isotonic solution such as Dextrose 5% Water (D5W) (primarily water as the sugar is metabolized quickly) was administered, two thirds of the fluid would move to the ICS (approximately 666 mL); recall the discussion earlier when we noted two thirds of the water in the body is intracellular, which will not increase the blood pressure! The remaining 333 mL will be in the ECS, but approximately 75% will move to the interstitial space, leaving only 83 mL in the IVS, which is unlikely to increase the blood pressure significantly. Thus, in emergency situations, a solution such as normal saline (0.9% NaCl) is selected because 75% of the solution will move to the interstitial space, leaving 25% in the circulating blood volume (IVS).*

Accurate and frequent assessments of I&O, weight, vital signs, CVP, LOC, breath sounds, and skin color should be performed to determine when therapy should be slowed to avoid volume overload. The rate of fluid administration is based on the severity of loss and the patient's hemodynamic response to volume replacement.

If the patient with severe FVD is not excreting enough urine and is, therefore, oliguric (less than 400 mL/24 hrs), the health care provider needs to determine whether the depressed function is caused by reduced renal blood flow secondary to FVD (prerenal azotemia or increased nitrogen levels in the blood) or, more seriously, by acute tubular necrosis from prolonged FVD. The test used in this situation is referred to as a *fluid challenge test*. During a fluid challenge test, volumes of fluid are administered at specific rates and intervals while the patient's hemodynamic response to this treatment is monitored (i.e., vital signs, breath sounds, sensorium, CVP, pulmonary capillary wedge pressure values, and urine output).

An example of a typical fluid challenge involves administering 100 to 200 mL of normal saline solution over 15 minutes. The goal is to provide fluids rapidly enough to attain adequate tissue perfusion without compromising the cardiovascular system. The response by a patient with FVD but normal kidney function is increased urine output and an increase in blood pressure and CVP.

Shock can occur when the volume of fluid lost exceeds 25% of the intravascular volume, or when fluid loss is rapid. Shock and its causes and treatment are discussed in detail in Chapters 20 and 54.

Nursing Management

Assessing Fluid Status

To assess for FVD, the nurse monitors and measures fluid I&O at least every 8 hours; depending on the patient's status, the assessment may be done hourly. As FVD develops, body fluid losses exceed fluid intake. This loss may be in the form of excessive urination (polyuria), diarrhea, vomiting, and so on. Later, after FVD progresses, the kidneys attempt to conserve needed body fluids, leading to a urine output of less than 30 mL/hr in an adult. Urine in this instance is concentrated; the specific gravity generally is greater than 1.020, indicating healthy renal conservation of fluid.

Daily body weights are monitored; an acute loss of 1 lb represents a fluid loss of approximately 500 mL, whereas 1 L is approximately 1 kg, or 2.2 lbs.

> **Nursing Alert**
> *The nurse recognizes that the FVD is associated with weight loss; however, if the patient is edematous or third-spacing (e.g., developing ascites), weight gain may be seen despite FVD.*

Vital signs are closely monitored. The nurse observes for a weak, rapid pulse and postural hypotension (i.e., a decrease in systolic pressure exceeding 20 mm Hg when the patient moves from a lying to a sitting position). Skin and tongue turgor is monitored on a regular basis. In a healthy person, pinched skin immediately returns to its normal position when released. This elastic property, referred to as *turgor*, is partially dependent on interstitial fluid volume. In a person with FVD, the skin flattens more slowly after the pinch is released. In a person with severe FVD, the skin may remain elevated for many seconds. Skin turgor is best measured by pinching the skin over the sternum, inner aspects of the thighs, or forehead.

> **Nursing Alert**
> *Skin turgor is a less valid assessment in the elderly patient because the skin has lost some of its elasticity due to the decreased number of papillae and collagen fibers; therefore, other assessment measures become more useful in detecting FVD (e.g., slowness in filling of veins of the hands and feet: veins in hands generally fill within 3 to 5 seconds; if filling takes longer than 5 seconds, consider FVD or hypovolemia). In elderly patients, skin turgor is best tested over the forehead or the sternum because alterations in skin elasticity are less marked in these areas.*

Tongue turgor is not affected by age. In a normal person, the tongue has one longitudinal furrow. In the person with FVD, there are additional longitudinal furrows, and the tongue is smaller because of fluid loss. The degree of oral mucous membrane moisture is also assessed; a dry mouth may indicate either FVD or mouth breathing.

Mental function is eventually affected in severe FVD as a result of decreasing cerebral perfusion. Decreased peripheral perfusion can result in cold extremities. In patients with relatively normal cardiopulmonary function, a low CVP is indicative of hypovolemia. Patients with acute cardiopulmonary decompensation require more extensive hemodynamic monitoring of pressures in both sides of the heart to determine if hypovolemia exists.

Preventing Fluid Volume Deficit

To prevent FVD, the nurse identifies patients at risk and takes measures to minimize fluid losses. The nurse recognizes that patients who are semidependent on another for care (related to sensorium or mobility) are at a higher risk for limited fluid intake. For example, if the patient has diarrhea, diarrhea-control measures should be implemented and replacement fluids administered. These measures may include administering antidiarrheal medications and small volumes of oral fluids at frequent intervals or, if necessary, IV therapy. Given the typical sensible and insensible loss of approximately 2,600 mL per day, if a patient is NPO, the nurse expects that the total daily water requirement for a 70-kg man is about 2,000 mL: This translates to approximately 30 mL/kg/day. However, fluid and electrolyte therapy should be individualized based upon physical examination findings, daily weight, and serum electrolytes.

Nursing Alert
The nurse is aware that when a patient has an increased insensible loss, it is associated with FVD. As an example, when the patient has an elevated temperature between 101°F and 103°F, an increase of 1,000 mL of fluid may be needed; fluid needs also increase in clinical scenarios such as diarrhea, vomiting, and an increased respiratory rate (greater than 35 breaths per minute). In general, insensible loss is calculated as 5 to 10 mL/kg per day (Mount, 2015).

Correcting Fluid Volume Deficit

When administering oral fluids, consideration is given to the patient's likes and dislikes. The type of fluid the patient has lost is also considered, and attempts are made to select fluids most likely to replace the lost electrolytes. If the patient is reluctant to drink because of oral discomfort, the nurse assists with frequent mouth care and provides non-irritating fluids. If nausea is present, antiemetics may be ordered and administered before oral fluid replacement is initiated.

If the patient cannot eat and drink, fluid may need to be administered by an alternative route (enteral or parenteral) until adequate circulating blood volume and renal perfusion are achieved. Isotonic fluids are prescribed to increase ECF volume.

Nursing Alert
When fluid balance is critical, all routes of gain and all routes of loss must be recorded and all volumes compared. Organs of fluid loss include the kidneys, skin, lungs, and GI tract.

HYPERVOLEMIA

FVE, or hypervolemia, refers to an isotonic expansion of the ECF caused by the abnormal retention of water and sodium in approximately the same proportions in which they normally exist in the ECF. It is always secondary to an increase in the total body sodium content, which, in turn, leads to an increase in total body water. Because there is isotonic retention of body substances, the serum sodium concentration remains essentially normal.

Nursing Alert
There are conditions that cause retention of water relative to sodium, such as SIADH. In these situations, hemodilution of the ECF will be reflected by decreased sodium, as well as BUN, and hematocrit. The term used for this situation is hypervolemic (increased volume) hyponatremia (decreased sodium related to dilution).

Pathophysiology

The maintenance of an effective circulating volume—that part of the "extracellular fluid that is in the arterial system and, therefore, effectively perfusing tissues" (Rennke & Denker, 2010)—is essential to sustain blood pressure to ensure organ vitality is monitored and tightly regulated. It may be increased in a number of situations, including fluid overload; excessive water ingestion; iatrogenic overadministration of IV fluids; or the ectopic secretion of ADH. Since the kidneys are responsible for regulating fluid excretion, kidney failure, either acute or chronic, is also associated with FVE. Excessive salt intake or the administration of sodium-containing fluids in a patient with impaired renal regulatory mechanisms may predispose the patient to serious FVE. On the other hand, a decrease in the effective circulating volume results in activation of the RAAS. Consider that since circulation is critical for survival, if the heart pump does not work effectively to generate enough volume for perfusion and function of vital organs, this "underfilling" results in activation of RAAS. This activation of RAAS results in increased circulating ADH or AVP and aldosterone, which increases sodium reabsorption and renal water reabsorption. This occurs in situations where cardiac output is decreased (heart failure) or when the patient suffers from hypovolemia (blood loss), increased capillary permeability (anaphylaxis), or extreme vasodilation (neurogenic shock).

Nursing Alert
The nurse understands that a normal serum sodium is 135 to 145 mEq/L (135 to 145 mmol/L), and that normal saline or 0.9% NaCl has 154 mEq/L of sodium, thus overadministration of normal saline leads to hypernatremia and potential for FVE.

Clinical Manifestations and Assessment

Clinical manifestations of FVE stem from expansion of the ECF and include edema, distended neck veins or jugular vein distention (JVD), and crackles (abnormal lung sounds) in lung fields. Other manifestations include tachycardia; increased blood pressure, pulse pressure, and CVP; increased weight; increased urine output (with normal kidney function); shortness of breath, and/or wheezing.

Laboratory data useful in diagnosing FVE include BUN and hematocrit levels. In FVE, both of these values may be decreased because of plasma dilution, termed *hemodilution*. Other causes of abnormalities in these values include low protein intake and anemia. Azotemia (increased nitrogen levels in the blood) can also occur with FVE when urea and creatinine are not excreted due to decreased perfusion by the kidneys and decreased excretion of wastes. In CKF, both serum osmolality and the sodium level are decreased due to excessive retention of water (inability of the kidneys to excrete the normal 1.5 L/day). The urine sodium level is increased if the kidneys are attempting to excrete excess volume. Chest x-rays may reveal pulmonary congestion. Hypervolemia occurs when aldosterone is chronically stimulated (i.e., cirrhosis, heart failure, and nephrotic syndrome). Therefore, the urine sodium level does not increase in these conditions.

Medical Management

Management of FVE is directed at the causes. If the fluid excess is related to excessive administration of sodium-containing fluids, discontinuing the infusion may be all that is needed. Symptomatic treatment consists of administering diuretics and restricting fluids and sodium.

Pharmacologic Therapy

Diuretics are prescribed when dietary restriction of sodium alone is insufficient to reduce fluid excess, which inhibits the reabsorption of sodium and water by the kidneys. The choice of diuretic is based on the severity of the hypervolemic state, the degree of impairment of kidney function, and the potency of the diuretic. Thiazide diuretics block sodium reabsorption in the distal tubule, where only 5% to 10% of filtered sodium is reabsorbed. Loop diuretics, such as furosemide (Lasix), or bumetanide (Bumex), can cause a greater loss of both sodium and water because they block sodium reabsorption in the ascending limb of the loop of Henle, where 20% to 30% of filtered sodium is normally reabsorbed. Generally, thiazide diuretics, such as hydrochlorothiazide or metolazone (Zaroxolyn), are prescribed for mild to moderate hypervolemia and loop diuretics for severe hypervolemia.

Electrolyte imbalances may result from the effect of the diuretic. Hypokalemia can occur with all diuretics except those that work in the last distal tubule of the nephrons (e.g., spironolactone). Potassium supplements can be prescribed to avoid this complication. Hyperkalemia can occur with diuretics that work in the last distal tubule, especially in patients with decreased kidney function.

Hemodialysis

If kidney function is so severely impaired that pharmacologic agents cannot act efficiently, other modalities are considered to remove sodium and fluid from the body. Hemodialysis or peritoneal dialysis may be used to remove nitrogenous wastes and control potassium and acid–base balance, and to remove sodium and fluid. Continuous renal replacement therapy may also be required. See Chapter 27 for discussion of these treatment modalities.

Nutritional Therapy

Treatment of FVE usually involves dietary restriction of sodium. An average daily diet not restricted in sodium contains 6 to 15 g of salt, whereas low-sodium diets can range from a mild restriction to as little as 250 mg of sodium per day, depending on the patient's needs. A mild sodium-restricted diet allows only light salting of food (about half the usual amount) in cooking and at the table as well as no addition of salt to commercially prepared foods that are already seasoned. Of course, foods high in sodium must be avoided. It is the sodium salt, sodium chloride, rather than sodium itself that contributes to edema. Therefore, patients are instructed to read food labels carefully to determine salt content.

Because about half of ingested sodium is in the form of seasoning, seasoning substitutes can play a major role in decreasing sodium intake. Lemon juice, onions, and garlic are excellent substitute flavorings, although some patients prefer salt substitutes. Most salt substitutes contain potassium and, therefore, must be used cautiously by patients taking potassium-sparing diuretics (e.g., spironolactone, triamterene, amiloride). They should not be used at all in conditions associated with potassium retention, such as advanced kidney disease. Salt substitutes containing ammonium chloride can be harmful to patients with liver damage.

In some communities, the drinking water may contain too much sodium for a sodium-restricted diet. Depending on its source, water may contain as little as 1 mg or more than 1,500 mg per quart. Patients may need to use distilled water if the local water supply is very high in sodium. Bottled water can have a sodium content from 0 to 1,200 mg/L; therefore, if sodium is restricted, the label must be examined carefully for sodium content before purchasing and drinking bottled water. Also, patients on sodium-restricted diets should be cautioned to avoid water softeners that add sodium to water in exchange for other ions, such as calcium.

Nursing Management

Assessing the Patient

To assess for FVE, the nurse measures I&O at regular intervals to identify excessive fluid retention. The patient is weighed daily, and acute weight gain is noted. An acute weight gain of 2.2 lb (1 kg) is equivalent to a gain of approximately 1 L of fluid. The nurse also needs to assess breath sounds at regular intervals in at-risk patients, particularly if parenteral fluids are being administered. The nurse monitors the degree of edema in the most dependent parts of the body, such as the feet and ankles in ambulatory patients and the sacral region in patients confined to bed. The degree of pitting edema is assessed, and the extent of peripheral edema is monitored by measuring the circumference of the extremity or the abdomen (in ascites) with a tape marked in millimeters. In general, edema that is apparent is associated with a minimum of 2.5 L of fluid in the interstitial space, and pitting edema is associated with a gain of 4.5 L (approximately 10 lb) (Longo et al., 2015). Often a history of weight gain will correlate with the edema.

> **Nursing Alert**
> *The etiology of edema—visible or palpable (pitting) tissue swelling produced by the expansion of interstitial fluid volume—is not as simple as it may appear. Edema occurs in response to many factors, including increased venous pressure, as with a deep vein thrombosis (DVT) or venous clot; lymphatic drainage obstruction (often an unwanted side effect of removal of the breast [mastectomy] and underarm lymph tissue); decreased plasma albumin oncotic pressure (seen in malnutrition, nephrotic syndrome, or liver damage); increased capillary leakage (caused by burns, sepsis); local injury (a result of sprains, fractures, surgery); infection (cellulitis), or inadequate valves in the venous system (chronic venous insufficiency) (Nadler & Gonzales, 2016). The nurse must consider a variety of etiologies when assessing edema.*

Preventing Fluid Volume Excess

Specific interventions vary somewhat with the underlying condition and the degree of FVE. However, most patients require sodium-restricted diets in some form, and adherence to the prescribed diet is strongly recommended. Patients are instructed to avoid over-the-counter medications without first checking with a health care provider because these substances may contain sodium. If fluid retention persists despite adherence to a prescribed diet, hidden sources of sodium, such as the water supply or use of water softeners, should be considered.

Correcting Fluid Volume Excess

It is important to detect FVE before the condition becomes critical. Interventions include restricting sodium intake, monitoring parenteral fluid therapy, and administering appropriate medications.

Sodium and fluid restriction should be instituted as indicated. Because most patients with FVE require diuretics, the patient's response to these agents is monitored. The rate of parenteral fluids and the patient's response to these fluids are also closely monitored. If dyspnea or orthopnea is present, the patient is placed in a semi-Fowler position to promote lung expansion. The patient is turned and positioned at regular intervals, and skin is assessed at regular intervals because edematous tissue is fragile and more prone to skin breakdown than normal tissue. Because conditions predisposing to FVE are likely to be chronic, patients are taught to monitor their response to therapy by monitoring their fluid I&O and documenting daily body weight changes.

Teaching Patients about Edema

Because edema is a common manifestation of FVE, patients need to recognize its symptoms and understand its importance. As noted earlier, edema can occur as a result of increased capillary fluid pressure, decreased capillary oncotic pressure, or increased interstitial oncotic pressure, causing expansion of the interstitial fluid compartment (Porth, 2015). Edema can be localized (e.g., in the ankle, as in rheumatoid arthritis) or generalized (as in cardiac and kidney failure). Severe generalized edema is called *anasarca*.

Edema occurs when there is a change in the capillary membrane, increasing the formation of interstitial fluid or decreasing the removal of interstitial fluid. Sodium retention is a frequent cause of the increased ECF volume. Burns and infection are examples of conditions associated with increased interstitial fluid volume. Obstruction to lymphatic outflow, decreased plasma albumin levels, or a decrease in plasma oncotic pressure contributes to increased interstitial fluid volume. The kidneys retain sodium and water when decreased ECF volume occurs as a result of decreased cardiac output from heart failure. A thorough medication history is necessary to identify any medications that could cause edema, such as nonsteroidal anti-inflammatory drugs (NSAIDs), estrogens, corticosteroids, and antihypertensive agents.

Ascites is a form of edema in which fluid accumulates in the peritoneal cavity; it results from nephrotic syndrome, cirrhosis, and some malignant tumors. The patient commonly reports shortness of breath and a sense of pressure because of pressure on the diaphragm.

Edema usually affects dependent areas. It can be seen in the ankles, sacrum, scrotum, or the periorbital region of the face. Pitting edema is so named because a pit forms after a finger is pressed into edematous tissue. In pulmonary edema, the amount of fluid in the pulmonary interstitium and the alveoli increases. Manifestations include shortness of breath, increased respiratory rate, diaphoresis, and crackles and wheezing on auscultation of the lungs. Decreased hematocrit resulting from hemodilution as well as decreased serum sodium and osmolality from retention of fluid may occur with edema. The goal of treatment is to preserve or restore the circulating intravascular fluid volume. In addition to treating the cause, other treatments may include diuretic therapy, restriction of fluids and sodium, elevation of the extremities, application of elastic compression stockings, paracentesis, dialysis, and continuous renal replacement therapy in cases of kidney failure or life-threatening fluid volume overload.

ELECTROLYTE IMBALANCES

Disturbances in electrolyte balances are common in clinical practice and must be corrected for the patient's health and safety.

SODIUM IMBALANCES

Sodium is the most abundant electrolyte in the ECF; its concentration ranges from 135 to 145 mEq/L (135 to 145 mmol/L). Consequently, sodium is the primary determinant of ECF osmolality. Sodium plays a major role in controlling water distribution throughout the body because it does not easily cross the intracellular membrane and because of its abundance and high concentration in the body. Sodium also functions in establishing the electrochemical state necessary for muscle contraction and the transmission of nerve impulses. Sodium is regulated by ADH, thirst, and the RAAS. A loss or gain of sodium is usually accompanied by a loss or gain of water.

The sodium imbalances commonly seen are: sodium deficit (hyponatremia) and sodium excess (hypernatremia).

HYPONATREMIA (SODIUM DEFICIT)

Hyponatremia refers to a serum sodium level that is below normal (less than 135 mEq/L [135 mmol/L]).

Pathophysiology

Plasma sodium concentration represents the ratio of total body sodium to total body water. A decrease in this ratio can occur because of salt loss that is greater than water loss (e.g., diarrhea, diuretics, NG tube suctioning), or there is an excess of water relative to total body sodium (e.g., congestive heart failure, cirrhosis of the liver, excessive water intake without salt, SIADH). Therefore, a hyponatremic state can be superimposed on an existing FVD or FVE.

Sodium may be lost by way of vomiting, diarrhea, fistulas, or prolonged or excessive sweating, or it may be lost as the result of the use of diuretics, particularly in combination with a low-salt diet. A deficiency of aldosterone, as occurs in adrenal insufficiency, also predisposes a patient to sodium deficiency. Potomania, otherwise known as beer potomania, due to the chronic consumption of large amounts of beer (a hypotonic solution) and protein malnutrition, may also cause hyponatremia due to an inability of the kidneys to excrete free water.

In dilutional hyponatremia (water intoxication), the patient's serum sodium level is diluted by an increase in the ratio of water to sodium. Dilutional hyponatremia, therefore, results from an increased ECF volume and a normal or increased total body sodium. Predisposing conditions for this type of hyponatremia include cirrhotic ascites; SIADH; hyperglycemia, which causes increased water to be drawn into the IVS; and increased water intake through the administration of electrolyte-poor parenteral fluids, the use of tap-water enemas, or the irrigation of nasogastric tubes with water instead of normal saline solution. Water may be gained abnormally by the excessive parenteral administration of hypotonic solutions such as dextrose and water solutions, particularly during periods of stress. It may also be gained by compulsive water drinking (psychogenic polydipsia).

> **! Nursing Alert**
> *Psychogenic polydipsia has been linked to a number of psychiatric conditions; however, it can also occur in a variety of individuals, including high endurance athletes, users of 3,4-Methylenedioxymethamphetamine (MDMA, commonly known as ecstasy), and in patients receiving total parenteral nutrition (TPN) or partial parenteral nutrition (PPN) (Gill & McCauley, 2015).*

The basic physiologic disturbances in SIADH are excessive ADH activity, with water retention and dilutional hyponatremia, and inappropriate urinary excretion of sodium in the presence of hyponatremia. SIADH can be the result of either sustained secretion of ADH by the hypothalamus or production of an ADH-like substance from a tumor (aberrant ADH production). Conditions associated with SIADH include oat-cell lung tumors, head injuries, endocrine and pulmonary disorders, physical or psychologic stress, and a variety of medications (e.g., vincristine, phenothiazines, tricyclic antidepressants, and thiazide diuretics). SIADH is discussed in more detail in Chapter 31.

Clinical Manifestations and Assessment

Clinical manifestations of hyponatremia depend on the cause, magnitude, and speed with which the deficit occurs. Patients can present with FVD, as euvolemic (SIADH), or with FVE. With true salt loss, a number of conditions occur, including poor skin turgor, dry mucosa, headache, decreased saliva production, orthostatic blood pressure (decreased with position changes), nausea, and abdominal cramping. With water gain in excess of sodium, clinical manifestations are associated with FVE, such as edema, crackles, ascites, and JVD. Symptoms are primarily neurologic. They are related to osmotic water shift as water from the relatively dilute ECF is pulled into the cell, leading to increased ICF volume, specifically brain cell swelling or cerebral edema (Fig. 4-5). The skull limits the brain's ability to expand, which results in increased intracranial pressure (ICP), the precursor to brain damage. Neurologic changes include altered mental status, headache, lethargy, seizures, and a progressively decreased LOC eventuating in coma. When the serum sodium level decreases to less than 115 mEq/L (115 mmol/L), signs of increasing intracranial pressure may occur, such as lethargy, confusion, muscle twitching, focal weakness, hemiparesis, papilledema, and seizures. In general, patients with an acute decrease in serum sodium levels have more cerebral edema and higher mortality rates than those with more slowly developing hyponatremia. Acute decreases in sodium, developing in less than 48 hours, may be associated with brain herniation and compression of midbrain structures.

Regardless of the cause of hyponatremia, the serum sodium level is less than 135 mEq/L; in SIADH it may be

FIGURE 4-5 Effect of extracellular sodium level on cell size.

as low as 100 mEq/L (100 mmol/L) or even less. Serum osmolality is also decreased, except in azotemia or ingestion of toxins. When hyponatremia is due primarily to sodium loss, the urinary sodium content is less than 20 mEq/L (20 mmol/L), suggesting increased renal reabsorption of sodium secondary to ECF volume depletion, and the specific gravity is low (1.002 to 1.004). However, when hyponatremia is due to SIADH, the urinary sodium content is greater than 20 mEq/L, and the urine specific gravity is usually greater than 1.012. Although the patient with SIADH retains water abnormally and, therefore, gains body weight, there is no peripheral edema; instead, fluid accumulates equally within the three compartments (intracellular, interstitial, and intravascular).

Medical Management

Treatment depends on the cause of the hyponatremia, the amount of time the individual has had hyponatremia, and the presence of signs and symptoms. Hyponatremia is considered acute if it developed within the last 24 hours and chronic if the duration of time since the initiation of hyponatremia is more than 24 hours or unknown. If the etiology is related to sodium and (to a lesser extent) water loss, sodium and water replacement is expected; if the etiology is related to water intoxication, restriction of fluid intake and diuretics are anticipated.

Sodium Replacement

If treatment for hyponatremia is warranted, careful administration of sodium by mouth, nasogastric tube, or a parenteral route may be ordered. For patients who can eat and drink,

sodium is easily replaced because sodium is consumed abundantly in a normal diet. For those who cannot consume sodium, lactated Ringer solution or isotonic saline (0.9% sodium chloride) solution may be prescribed. Serum sodium must not be increased by more than 12 mEq/L in the first 24 hours to avoid neurologic damage due to osmotic demyelination. This condition, termed *central pontine myelinolysis (CPM)*, may occur when the serum sodium concentration is overcorrected (exceeding 140 mEq/L) too rapidly, causing a relatively hypotonic ICS compared to the ECS. This causes water to flow from the ICS to the ECS, causing cell volume collapse. Osmotic demyelination presents as flaccid paralysis, dysarthria (speech that is slurred, slow, and difficult to produce), dysphagia (difficulty in swallowing), and quadriparesis. The usual daily sodium requirement in adults is approximately 100 mEq, provided no abnormal losses occur. Selected water and electrolyte solutions are described later in the chapter.

In SIADH, the administration of hypertonic saline solution alone cannot change the plasma sodium concentration. Excess sodium would be excreted rapidly in highly concentrated urine. With the addition of the diuretic furosemide (Lasix), urine is not concentrated, and isotonic urine is excreted to effect a change in water balance. In patients with SIADH, in whom water restriction is difficult, lithium or demeclocycline can antagonize the osmotic effect of ADH on the medullary collecting tubule.

In patients with severe symptoms of hyponatremia, such as seizures or obtundation, or in patients with acute hyponatremia, administration of hypertonic saline solution may be ordered to stabilize the patient and prevent brain herniation. In this setting, the goal increase of sodium is 4 to 6 mEq/L and a maximum of 8 mEq/L in a 24-hour period; however, these values are often debated. The adage of "go slow" has particular utility in symptomatic hyponatremia.

Water Restriction

In a patient with normal or excess fluid volume, hyponatremia is treated by restricting fluid to a total of 800 mL in 24 hours. This is far safer than sodium administration and is usually effective. However, if neurologic symptoms are present, it may be necessary to administer small volumes of a hypertonic sodium solution, such as 3% sodium chloride. Incorrect use of these fluids is extremely dangerous because 1 L of 3% sodium chloride solution contains 513 mEq of sodium with an osmolality of 1,026! Recall normal serum osmolality is 275 to 300 mOsm/kg. A 3% saline solution is three times higher; thus if administered rapidly, the blood osmolality would increase dramatically. However, because of the blood–brain barrier, the osmolality in the brain would be the same, thus intracellular water would attempt to try to dilute the bloodstream causing CPM (see alert below). If edema exists alone, sodium is restricted; if edema and hyponatremia occur together, both sodium and water are restricted.

Nursing Alert
A 3% saline solution has an osmolality of 1,026 mOsm/kg. A normal serum osmolality varies from approximately 275 to 300 mOsm/kg. Thus, a 3% saline solution is three times more concentrated than normal blood osmolality. Rapid administration would have an adverse impact on the brain. The blood osmolality would increase dramatically. However, because the blood–brain barrier limits capillary sodium but not water permeability, the movement of interstitial and neuronal intracellular water into the capillary may potentially culminate in cerebral shrinkage, osmotic demyelination, and the constellation of clinical symptoms (including paraparesis, dysphagia, and coma) known as CPM. In addition, a solution this concentrated must be administered via a central IV line because it is too concentrated for peripheral veins; it is tolerated when administered in central lines because it is diluted by vena cavae blood.

Nursing Management

The nurse needs to identify patients at risk for hyponatremia so that they can be monitored. Early detection and treatment of this disorder are necessary to prevent serious consequences. For patients at risk, the nurse monitors fluid I&O as well as daily body weight. It is also necessary to note abnormal losses of sodium or gains of water as well as GI manifestations such as anorexia, nausea, vomiting, and abdominal cramping. The nurse must be particularly alert for CNS changes, such as lethargy, confusion, muscle twitching, and seizures. In general, more severe neurologic signs are associated with very low sodium levels that have fallen rapidly because of fluid overloading. Serum sodium is monitored very closely in patients who are at risk for hyponatremia; when indicated, urine sodium and specific gravity are also monitored.

Hyponatremia is a frequently overlooked cause of confusion in elderly patients, who have an increased risk for hyponatremia because of changes in kidney function and subsequent decreased ability to excrete excessive water loads. Administration of medications causing sodium loss or water retention is a predisposing factor.

Correcting Hyponatremia

For a patient who is experiencing abnormal losses of sodium and can consume a general diet, the nurse encourages foods and fluids with a high sodium content. For example, broth made with one beef cube contains approximately 900 mg of sodium; 8 oz of tomato juice contains approximately 700 mg of sodium. The nurse also needs to be familiar with the sodium content of parenteral fluids (see later discussion and Table 4-6 on page 93).

For the patient taking lithium, the nurse observes for lithium toxicity, particularly when sodium is lost by an abnormal route. In such instances, supplemental salt and fluid are administered. Because diuretics promote sodium loss, the patient taking lithium is instructed not to use diuretics without close medical supervision. For all patients on lithium therapy, adequate salt intake should be ensured.

Excess water supplements are avoided in patients receiving isotonic or hypotonic enteral feedings, particularly if abnormal sodium loss occurs or water is being retained abnormally (as in SIADH). Actual fluid needs are determined by evaluating fluid I&O, urine specific gravity, and serum sodium levels.

HYPERNATREMIA (SODIUM EXCESS)

Hypernatremia is a higher-than-normal serum sodium level (exceeding 145 mEq/L [145 mmol/L]).

Pathophysiology

Hypernatremia can be caused by a gain of sodium in excess of water or by a loss of water in excess of sodium. It can occur in the euvolemic patient or in those with FVD or FVE. With a water loss, the patient loses more water than sodium; as a result, the serum sodium concentration increases and the increased concentration pulls fluid out of the cell. This is both an extracellular and an intracellular FVD. In sodium excess, the patient ingests or retains more sodium than water.

A common cause of hypernatremia is fluid deprivation in unconscious patients who cannot perceive, respond to, or communicate their thirst (Soiza, Cumming, Clarke, Wood, Myint, 2014). Most often affected are very old, very young, and cognitively impaired patients. Administration of hypertonic enteral feedings without adequate water supplements leads to hypernatremia, as does watery diarrhea and greatly increased insensible water loss (e.g., hyperventilation, denuding effects of burns).

Diabetes insipidus, a deficiency of ADH or AVP from the posterior pituitary gland, leads to hypernatremia if the patient does not experience, or cannot respond to, thirst or if fluids are excessively restricted. Neurogenic or nephrogenic causes of diabetes insipidus should be considered in the assessment (refer to Chapter 31).

IV administration of hypertonic saline, hypertonic feeding preparations, or excessive use of sodium bicarbonate can also cause hypernatremia.

Clinical Manifestations and Assessment

The clinical manifestations of hypernatremia are primarily neurologic and are the consequence of increased plasma osmolality caused by an increase in plasma sodium concentration. Water moves out of the ICS into the ECS, resulting in cellular dehydration (see Fig. 4-5). Clinically, these changes may be manifested by restlessness and weakness in moderate hypernatremia and by disorientation, delusions, and hallucinations in severe hypernatremia. Dehydration (resulting in hypernatremia) is often overlooked as the primary reason for behavioral changes in elderly patients. If hypernatremia is severe, permanent brain damage can occur (especially in children). Brain damage is apparently due to subarachnoid hemorrhages that result from brain contraction. A primary characteristic of hypernatremia is thirst. Thirst is such a strong defender of serum sodium levels in healthy people that hypernatremia never occurs unless the person is unconscious or does not have access to water. However, ill people may have an impaired thirst mechanism. Other signs include a dry, swollen tongue and sticky mucous membranes. Flushed skin, peripheral and pulmonary edema, postural hypotension, and increased muscle tone and deep tendon reflexes are additional signs and symptoms of hypernatremia. Body temperature may increase mildly, but it returns to normal after the hypernatremia is corrected. In hypernatremia, the serum sodium level exceeds 145 mEq/L (145 mmol/L), and the serum osmolality exceeds 300 mOsm/kg (300 mmol/L). The specific gravity and osmolality of urine are increased as the kidneys attempt to conserve water (provided the water loss is from a route other than the kidneys).

Medical Management

Treatment of hypernatremia consists of a gradual lowering of the serum sodium level by the infusion of a hypotonic electrolyte solution or an isotonic nonsaline solution (e.g., dextrose 5% in water [D$_5$W]). D$_5$W is indicated when water needs to be replaced without sodium. Many clinicians consider a hypotonic sodium solution (e.g., 0.45% NaCl or ½ normal saline) to be safer than D$_5$W because it allows a gradual reduction in the serum sodium level, thereby decreasing the risk of cerebral edema. It is the solution of choice in severe hyperglycemia with hypernatremia. A rapid reduction in the serum sodium level temporarily decreases the plasma osmolality below that of the fluid in the brain tissue, causing dangerous cerebral edema. Diuretics also may be prescribed to treat the sodium gain.

There is no consensus about the exact rate at which serum sodium levels should be reduced. As a general rule, the serum sodium level is reduced at a rate no faster than 0.5 to 1 mEq/L/hr to allow sufficient time for readjustment through diffusion across fluid compartments. Desmopressin acetate (DDAVP), a synthetic ADH, may be prescribed to treat diabetes insipidus if it is the cause of hypernatremia (Grossman & Porth, 2014).

! Nursing Alert
One of the most common causes of hypernatremia is the inadequate intake of free water accompanied by total body sodium depletion, deemed hypovolemic hypernatremia. This may be seen in elderly or severely debilitated individuals who may be unable to ask for or take in water adequately. In this population, restoration of ECF volume with 0.9% normal saline solution may occur prior to correcting the water deficit. Hypovolemic patients with signs of hemodynamic compromise (e.g., tachycardia, hypotension) should receive volume resuscitation initially to restore perfusion prior to administration of hypotonic fluids (to replace free water deficit).

Nursing Management

As in hyponatremia, fluid losses and gains are carefully monitored in patients who are at risk for hypernatremia. The nurse should assess for abnormal losses of water or low water intake and for large gains of sodium as might occur with ingestion of over-the-counter medications that have high sodium content (e.g., Alka-Seltzer). In addition, the nurse obtains a medication history because some prescription medications have high sodium content. The nurse also notes the patient's thirst or elevated body temperature and evaluates it in relation to other clinical signs. The nurse monitors for changes in behavior, such as restlessness, disorientation, and lethargy.

Preventing Hypernatremia

The nurse attempts to prevent hypernatremia by offering fluids at regular intervals, particularly in debilitated patients who may be unable to perceive or respond to thirst. If fluid intake remains inadequate, the nurse consults with the provider to plan an alternative route for intake, either by enteral feedings or by the parenteral route. If enteral feedings are used, sufficient water should be administered to keep the serum sodium and BUN within normal limits. As a rule, the higher the osmolality of the enteral feeding, the greater the need for water supplementation.

For patients with diabetes insipidus, adequate water intake must be ensured. If the patient is alert and has an intact thirst mechanism, merely providing access to water may be sufficient. If the patient has a decreased LOC or other disability interfering with adequate fluid intake, parenteral fluid replacement may be prescribed. This therapy can be anticipated in patients with neurologic disorders, particularly in the early postoperative period.

POTASSIUM IMBALANCES

Potassium is the major intracellular electrolyte; in fact, 98% of the body's potassium is inside the cells. The remaining 2% is in the ECF, and it is this 2% that is important in neuromuscular function. The normal serum potassium concentration ranges from 3.5 to 5.0 mEq/L (3.5 to 5 mmol/L), and even minor variations are significant.

To maintain potassium balance, the renal system must function because 80% of the potassium excreted daily leaves the body by way of the kidneys; the other 20% is lost through the bowel. Intestinal fluid may contain as much as 30 mEq/L of potassium. However, the kidneys are the primary regulators of potassium balance; they accomplish this by adjusting the amount of potassium that is excreted in the urine. Aldosterone also increases the excretion of potassium by the kidney. Because the kidneys do not conserve potassium as well as they conserve sodium, potassium may still be lost in urine in the presence of a potassium deficit. Potassium imbalances are commonly associated with a variety of diseases, injuries, medications (diuretics, laxatives, antibiotics), and special treatments, such as parenteral nutrition and chemotherapy.

HYPOKALEMIA (POTASSIUM DEFICIT)

Hypokalemia (below-normal serum potassium concentration) usually indicates an actual deficit in total potassium stores. However, it may occur in patients with normal potassium stores, such as when alkalosis is present, since it causes a temporary shift of serum potassium into the cells (see later discussion).

Pathophysiology

Hypokalemia (less than 3.5 mEq/L) is a common imbalance. It is associated with conditions that cause an increased output of K^+ (use of diuretics, diarrhea, vomiting, gastric suction, recent ileostomy, intestinal drains, villous adenoma [a tumor of the intestinal tract characterized by excretion of potassium-rich mucus]); decreased intake (NPO, anorexia, vomiting, alcoholism, fasting diets); or redistribution of K^+ (metabolic alkalosis).

The nurse considers clinical conditions that cause increased loss. Approximately 5 to 10 mEq/L K^+ are found in upper GI fluid, whereas 30 to 100 mEq/L are lost with diarrhea. Thus, relatively large amounts of potassium are lost in intestinal fluids.

Potassium-losing diuretics, such as the thiazides, can induce hypokalemia, particularly when administered in large doses to patients with inadequate potassium intake. Other medications that can lead to hypokalemia include corticosteroids, sodium penicillin, carbenicillin, and amphotericin B.

Increased loss is also seen with hyperaldosteronism, which causes reabsorption of sodium and renal excretion of K^+. Primary hyperaldosteronism is seen in patients with adrenal adenomas. Secondary hyperaldosteronism occurs in disorders that activate RAAS to maintain serum sodium concentrations such as cirrhosis, nephrotic syndrome, or heart failure.

Decreased intake occurs in patients who are unable or unwilling to eat a normal diet. This may occur in debilitated elderly people, patients with alcoholism, and patients with anorexia nervosa. In addition to poor intake, people with bulimia frequently suffer increased potassium loss through self-induced vomiting and abuse of laxatives and diuretics.

Redistribution is associated with alterations in acid–base balance or certain medications, such as insulin. In general, a hypokalemia is associated with an alkalosis and, in turn, an alkalosis can cause hypokalemia. The mechanism involves shifts of hydrogen and potassium ions between the ICS and the ECF. For example, hydrogen ions move out of the cells in alkalotic states to help correct the high pH, and potassium ions move in to maintain an electrically neutral state (see later discussion of acid–base balance).

Because insulin promotes the entry of potassium into skeletal muscle and hepatic cells, patients with persistent insulin hypersecretion may experience hypokalemia, which is often the case in patients receiving high-carbohydrate parenteral fluids (as in parenteral nutrition). The nurse anticipates that patients requiring IV insulin are at risk for hypokalemia.

Finally, a magnesium depletion can cause a renal potassium loss and must be corrected or loss of potassium in the urine will continue.

Clinical Manifestations and Assessment

Potassium deficiency can result in widespread derangements in physiologic function. Severe hypokalemia can cause death through cardiac or respiratory arrest. Clinical signs rarely develop before the serum potassium level has decreased to less than 3 mEq/L (3 mmol/L) unless the rate of decline has been rapid. Manifestations of hypokalemia include fatigue, anorexia, nausea, vomiting, muscle weakness, leg cramps, decreased bowel motility, paresthesias (numbness and tingling), arrhythmias, and increased sensitivity to digitalis.

If prolonged, hypokalemia can lead to an inability of the kidneys to concentrate urine, causing dilute urine (resulting in polyuria, nocturia) and excessive thirst. Potassium depletion depresses the release of insulin and results in glucose intolerance. Decreased muscle strength and tendon reflexes can be found on physical assessment.

In hypokalemia, the serum potassium concentration is less than the lower limit of normal. Electrocardiographic (ECG) changes can include flat T waves or inverted T waves or both, suggesting ischemia, and depressed ST segments (Fig. 4-6). An elevated U wave is specific to hypokalemia. Hypokalemia increases sensitivity to digitalis, predisposing the patient to digitalis toxicity at lower digitalis levels.

Medical Management

If hypokalemia cannot be prevented by conventional measures, such as increased intake in the daily diet, it is treated with oral or IV replacement therapy. Potassium loss must be corrected daily; administration of 40 to 80 mEq/day of potassium is adequate in the adult if there are no abnormal losses of potassium.

For patients who are at risk for hypokalemia, a diet containing sufficient potassium should be provided. Dietary intake of potassium in the average adult is 50 to 100 mEq/day. If dietary intake is inadequate for any reason, the provider may prescribe oral or IV potassium

A
Normal ECG

B
Hypokalemia

Moderate   Extreme

C
Hyperkalemia

Moderate   Extreme

FIGURE 4-6 Effect of potassium on the electrocardiogram (ECG). **A.** Normal tracing. **B.** Hypokalemia: Serum potassium level below normal. **Left:** Flattening of the T wave and the appearance of a U wave. **Right:** further flattening with prominent U wave. **C.** Hyperkalemia: Serum potassium level above normal. **Left:** moderate elevation with wide, flat P wave, wide QRS complex, and peaked T wave. **Right:** ECG changes seen with extreme potassium elevation: widening of QRS complex and absence of P wave.

supplements. Many salt substitutes contain 50 to 60 mEq of potassium per teaspoon and may be sufficient to prevent hypokalemia.

If oral administration of potassium is not feasible, the IV route is indicated. The IV route is mandatory for patients with severe hypokalemia (e.g., serum level of less than 2 mEq/L). Although potassium chloride is usually used to correct potassium deficits, potassium acetate or potassium phosphate may be prescribed.

> ***Nursing Alert***
> *Serum potassium levels on average will rise by .1 mEq/L for each 10 mEq of potassium given to a patient.*

Nursing Management

Because hypokalemia can be life-threatening, the nurse needs to monitor for its early presence in patients who are at risk. Fatigue, anorexia, muscle weakness, decreased bowel motility, paresthesias, and arrhythmias are signals that warrant assessing the serum potassium concentration. When available, the ECG may provide useful information. For example, patients receiving digitalis who are at risk for potassium deficiency should be monitored closely for signs of digitalis toxicity, because hypokalemia potentiates the action of digitalis.

Preventing Hypokalemia

Measures are taken to prevent hypokalemia when possible. Prevention may involve encouraging the patient at risk to eat foods rich in potassium (when the diet allows). If the hypokalemia is caused by abuse of laxatives or diuretics, patient education may help alleviate the problem.

> ***Nursing Alert***
> *Sources of potassium include fruit and fruit juices (bananas, melon, citrus fruit, avocado, coconut water), fresh and frozen vegetables, fresh meats, milk, and processed foods.*

Correcting Hypokalemia

Great care should be exercised when administering potassium, particularly in older adults who have lower lean body mass and total body potassium levels and, therefore, lower potassium requirements. In addition, because of the physiologic loss of kidney function with advancing years, potassium may be retained more readily in older than in younger people.

> ***Nursing Alert***
> *Oral potassium supplements can produce small-bowel lesions; therefore, the patient must be assessed for and cautioned about abdominal distention, pain, or GI bleeding.*

Potassium should be administered only after adequate urine flow has been established. A decrease in urine volume to less than 20 mL/hr for 2 consecutive hours is an indication to stop the potassium infusion until the situation is evaluated. Potassium is primarily excreted by the kidneys; therefore, when oliguria occurs, potassium administration can cause the serum potassium concentration to rise dangerously. Each health care facility has its own standard of care for the administration of potassium, which should be consulted; however, the maximum concentration of potassium that should be administered on a medical–surgical unit through a peripheral IV line is 10 mEq/100 mL at a rate no faster than 10 mEq/hr. Concentrations of potassium greater than 20 mEq/100 mL should be administered through a central IV catheter using an infusion pump with the patient monitored by ECG. Caution must be used when selecting the correct premixed solution of IV fluid containing potassium chloride as the concentrations range from 10 to 40 mEq/100 mL. IV bags of 1,000 mL of fluid containing potassium are also available with 20 to 40 mEq/L. IV pumps should always be used with potassium administration. Rapid infusion can cause sudden hyperkalemia and cardiac arrest.

 Nursing Alert
Potassium is never administered by IV push or intramuscularly. IV potassium is available as a premixed solution; the nurse is aware that it must be administered using an infusion pump.

Kidney function should be monitored through BUN and creatinine levels and urine output if the patient is receiving potassium replacements, and the provider should be notified of changes in kidney function to prevent complications.

 Nursing Alert
Potassium supplements are extremely dangerous for patients who have impaired kidney function and thus decreased ability to excrete potassium. Even more dangerous is the IV administration of potassium to such patients because serum levels can rise very quickly. Aged (stored) blood should not be administered to patients with impaired kidney function because the serum potassium concentration of stored blood increases as the storage time increases, a result of deterioration of RBCs. It is possible to exceed the renal tolerance of any patient with rapid IV potassium administration, as well as when large amounts of oral potassium supplements are ingested.

HYPERKALEMIA (POTASSIUM EXCESS)

Hyperkalemia (greater-than-normal serum potassium concentration) seldom occurs in patients with normal kidney function.

Pathophysiology

Like hypokalemia, hyperkalemia is often caused by iatrogenic (treatment-induced) causes. Although hyperkalemia is less common than hypokalemia, it is usually more dangerous because cardiac arrest is more frequently associated with high serum potassium levels.

Pseudohyperkalemia (a variation of hyperkalemia) has a number of causes. The most common causes are the use of a tight tourniquet around an exercising extremity while drawing a blood sample and hemolysis of the sample before analysis. Other causes include marked leukocytosis (WBC count exceeding 200,000) or thrombocytosis (platelet count exceeding 1 million); drawing blood above a site where potassium is infusing; and familial pseudohyperkalemia, in which potassium leaks out of the RBC while the blood is awaiting analysis. Failure to be aware of these causes of pseudohyperkalemia can lead to aggressive treatment of a nonexistent hyperkalemia, resulting in serious lowering of serum potassium levels. Therefore, measurements of grossly elevated levels should be verified by retesting.

Hyperkalemia (K^+ greater than 5 meq/L) is associated with increased intake (salt substitutes, potassium supplements); administration of medications that increase K^+ load such as penicillin-K^+; K^+-sparing diuretics such as spironolactone and ACE inhibitors; or cell injuries such as crushing injuries, burns, trauma, intravascular hemolysis, rhabdomyolysis (see Chapter 42) or chemotherapy, decreased output (renal disease [AKF/CKF], hypoaldosteronism), or redistribution (acidosis).

The major cause of hyperkalemia is decreased renal excretion of potassium and is commonly seen in patients with untreated kidney failure, particularly those in whom potassium levels increase as a result of infection or excessive intake of potassium in food or medications. In addition, patients with hypoaldosteronism or Addison disease are at risk for hyperkalemia because of deficient aldosterone.

Although a high intake of potassium can cause severe hyperkalemia in patients with impaired kidney function, hyperkalemia rarely occurs in people with normal kidney function. However, improper use of potassium supplements predisposes all patients to hyperkalemia, especially if salt substitutes are used. Not all patients receiving potassium-losing diuretics require potassium supplements, and patients receiving potassium-conserving diuretics should not receive supplements.

In **acidosis**, potassium moves out of the cells and into the ECF. This occurs as hydrogen ions enter the cells, a process that buffers the pH of the ECF (see later discussion). An elevated ECF potassium level should be anticipated when extensive tissue trauma has occurred, as in burns, crushing injuries, or severe infections. Similarly, it can occur with lysis of malignant cells after chemotherapy.

Clinical Manifestations and Assessment

The most important consequence of hyperkalemia is its effect on the myocardium. Cardiac effects of elevated serum potassium are usually not significant when the level is less than 7 mEq/L (7 mmol/L), but they are almost always present when the level is 8 mEq/L (8 mmol/L) or greater. As the plasma potassium level rises, disturbances in cardiac conduction occur. The earliest changes, often occurring at a serum potassium level greater than 6 mEq/L (6 mmol/L), are peaked, narrow T waves; ST-segment depression; and a shortened QT interval. If the serum potassium level continues to increase, the PR interval becomes prolonged and is followed by disappearance of the P waves. Finally, there is decomposition and prolongation of the QRS complex (see Fig. 4-6). Ventricular arrhythmias and cardiac arrest may occur at any point in this progression. Severe hyperkalemia causes skeletal muscle weakness and even paralysis, related to a depolarization block in muscle. Similarly, ventricular conduction is slowed. Although hyperkalemia has marked effects on the peripheral nervous system, it has little effect on the CNS. Rapidly ascending muscular weakness leading to flaccid quadriplegia has been reported in patients with very high serum potassium levels. Paralysis of respiratory and speech muscles can also occur. In addition, GI manifestations, such as nausea, intermittent intestinal colic, and diarrhea, may occur in hyperkalemic patients. Serum potassium levels and ECG changes are crucial to the diagnosis of hyperkalemia, as discussed previously. ABG analysis may reveal metabolic acidosis; in many cases, hyperkalemia occurs with acidosis, owing to shifts of hydrogen and potassium ions between the ICS and the ECF. For example, hydrogen ions move into the cells in acidotic states to help correct the low serum pH, and potassium ions move out of the cells in exchange, causing a hyperkalemia.

Medical Management

In nonacute situations, restriction of dietary potassium and potassium-containing medications may suffice. For example, eliminating the use of potassium-containing salt substitutes in a patient who is taking a potassium-conserving diuretic may be all that is needed to deal with mild hyperkalemia.

Prevention of serious hyperkalemia by the administration, either orally or by retention enema, of cation exchange resins (e.g., Kayexalate) may be necessary in patients with renal impairment. Cation exchange resins were once used as the primary agent for physical removal of potassium in the body; they act by binding potassium within the bowel and excreting it within the stool. However, research now suggests that cation exchange resins actually increase the risk of bowel ischemia, and no study to date has clearly stated that cation exchange resins do, in fact, lower the potassium levels. Therefore, this practice has begun to fall out of favor among health care providers. A newer medication, patiromer, which reduces potassium levels by binding to potassium in the GI tract, has been approved by the FDA for use in hyperkalemia (Garimella & Jaber, 2016).

Emergency Pharmacologic Therapy

If serum potassium levels are dangerously elevated, it may be necessary to administer IV calcium gluconate. Within minutes after administration, calcium antagonizes the action of hyperkalemia on the heart. Infusion of calcium does not reduce the serum potassium concentration, but it immediately antagonizes the adverse cardiac conduction abnormalities. Calcium chloride and calcium gluconate are not interchangeable: calcium gluconate contains 4.5 mEq of calcium, and calcium chloride contains 13.6 mEq of calcium; therefore, caution must be used.

Monitoring the blood pressure is essential to detect hypotension, which may result from the rapid IV administration of calcium gluconate. The ECG should be monitored continuously during administration; the appearance of bradycardia is an indication to stop the infusion. The myocardial-protective effects of calcium are transient, lasting about 30 minutes. Extra caution is required if the patient has been "digitalized" (i.e., has received accelerated dosages of a digitalis-based cardiac glycoside to reach a desired serum digitalis level rapidly) because parenteral administration of calcium sensitizes the heart to digitalis and may precipitate digitalis toxicity.

IV administration of sodium bicarbonate may be necessary to alkalinize the plasma and cause a temporary shift of potassium into the cells. Also, sodium bicarbonate furnishes sodium to antagonize the cardiac effects of potassium. Effects of this therapy begin within 30 to 60 minutes and may persist for hours; however, they are temporary.

IV administration of regular insulin and a hypertonic dextrose solution causes a temporary shift of potassium into the cells. Glucose and insulin therapy has an onset of action within 30 minutes and lasts for several hours. Loop diuretics, such as furosemide (Lasix), increase excretion of water by inhibiting sodium, potassium, and chloride reabsorption in the ascending loop of Henle and distal renal tubule.

Beta-2 agonists, such as albuterol (Proventil, Ventolin), can be effective in decreasing potassium; however, large doses are needed to elicit potassium shifting into the cells. The nurse is aware that beta-2 agonists may cause tachycardia and observes cardiac response to treatment, and the provider may consider other options in the patient with ischemic cardiac disease. Administration of these medications is a stopgap measure that only temporarily protects the patient from hyperkalemia. If the hyperkalemic condition is not transient, actual removal of potassium from the body is required; this may be accomplished by using peritoneal dialysis, hemodialysis, or other forms of renal replacement therapy.

Nursing Management

Patients at risk for potassium excess (e.g., those with kidney failure) should be identified so that they can be monitored closely for signs of hyperkalemia. The nurse observes for signs of muscle weakness and arrhythmias. The presence of paresthesias and GI symptoms, such as nausea and intestinal colic, should be monitored for and reported if identified.

Because measurements of elevated serum potassium levels may be erroneous, highly abnormal levels should always be verified by repeating the test. To avoid false reports of hyperkalemia, prolonged use of a tourniquet while drawing the blood sample is avoided, and the patient is cautioned not to exercise the extremity immediately before the blood sample is obtained. The blood sample is delivered to the laboratory as soon as possible because hemolysis of the sample results in a falsely elevated serum potassium level.

Preventing Hyperkalemia

Measures are taken to prevent hyperkalemia in patients at risk, when possible, by encouraging the patient to adhere to the prescribed potassium restriction. Potassium-rich foods to be avoided include many fruits and vegetables, legumes, whole-grain breads, meat, milk, eggs, coffee, tea, and cocoa. Conversely, foods with minimal potassium content include butter, margarine, cranberry juice or sauce, ginger ale, gumdrops or jellybeans, hard candy, root beer, sugar, and honey.

Correcting Hyperkalemia

As previously stated, it is possible to exceed the tolerance for potassium in any person if it is administered rapidly by the IV route. Therefore, great care should be taken to administer and monitor potassium solutions closely, paying attention to the solution's concentration and rate of administration. When potassium is added to parenteral solutions, the potassium is mixed with the fluid by inverting the bottle several times. Potassium chloride should never be added to a hanging bottle because the potassium might be administered as a bolus (potassium chloride is heavy and settles to the bottom of the container).

It is important to caution patients to use salt substitutes sparingly if they are taking other supplementary forms of potassium or potassium-conserving diuretics. Also, potassium-conserving diuretics, potassium supplements, and salt substitutes should not be administered to patients with kidney dysfunction. Most salt substitutes contain approximately 50 to 60 mEq of potassium per teaspoon.

CALCIUM IMBALANCES

More than 99% of the body's calcium is located in the skeletal system, where it provides strength and stability to the skeletal system and serves as a source for extracellular calcium (Grossman & Porth, 2014). Approximately 0.1% to 0.2% of calcium (8.5 to 10.5 mg/dL) circulates in the serum, 40% is bound to plasma proteins (mostly albumin), 10% is complexed or chelated with substances such as phosphorus and sulfate, and approximately 50% is ionized or free to leave the blood stream and participate in cellular function (Grossman & Porth, 2014). Calcium plays a major role in the transmission of nerve impulses, regulation of muscle contraction and relaxation including cardiac muscle, and coagulation pathways; thus, it is important for cardiac conduction,

neuromuscular activity, and blood clotting. Calcium is also instrumental in activating enzymes that stimulate many essential chemical reactions in the body. Because many factors affect calcium regulation, both hypocalcemia and hypercalcemia are relatively common disturbances.

Calcium is absorbed from foods (milk and milk products) in the presence of normal gastric acidity and vitamin D. Calcium is excreted in feces and urine. The serum calcium level is controlled by PTH and calcitonin. As ionized or free serum calcium decreases, the parathyroid glands secrete PTH. This, in turn, increases calcium absorption from the GI tract (mediated by an increase in renal vitamin D synthesis), increases calcium reabsorption from the renal tubule, and releases calcium from the bone. The subsequent increase in calcium ion concentration suppresses PTH secretion. When calcium increases excessively, the thyroid gland secretes calcitonin, the antagonist of PTH. It briefly inhibits calcium reabsorption from bone, encourages calcium salt deposits in the bone matrix, and decreases the serum calcium concentration. In addition, blood phosphate (most phosphorus is present as phosphate) levels have a reciprocal relationship with calcium levels. Increases in blood phosphate result in a fall in free calcium concentrations. PTH secretion is stimulated, and this reduces renal excretion of calcium and increases renal phosphate excretion. These adaptations prevent the potentially damaging effects of calcium phosphate crystal deposition that can form in soft tissues when the normal calcium–phosphorus ratio is disturbed.

> **! Nursing Alert**
> *In conditions such as kidney failure, excess phosphate is not excreted, nor is vitamin D activated, which decreases absorption of calcium. This excess phosphate binds with free calcium, forming an insoluble compound that can be deposited in the heart, lungs, eyes, kidneys, skin, and soft tissues. The subsequent fall in serum calcium increases PTH secretion, which dissolves more calcium from the bone to attempt to maintain a normal serum calcium level. The net effect is the development of hyperparathyroidism and a variety of symptoms (renal osteodystrophy, bone pain, fractures, and bleeding) (see Chapters 27 and 31).*

HYPOCALCEMIA (CALCIUM DEFICIT)

Hypocalcemia (lower-than-normal serum concentration of calcium), or less than 8.5 mg/dL and an ionized calcium of less than 4.6 mg/dL, occurs in a variety of clinical situations (Fischbach & Dunning, 2015).

Pathophysiology

Factors associated with hypocalcemia include inadequate calcium intake, increased calcium loss, malabsorption of calcium, decreases in serum protein levels, and increased binding of calcium. Inadequate intake is associated with chronic alcoholism and malnutrition. Increased calcium loss is associated with pancreatic insufficiency and acute pancreatitis. Inflammation of the pancreas causes the breakdown of proteins and lipids. It is thought that calcium ions combine with the fatty acids released by lipolysis, forming soaps. As a result of this process, hypocalcemia occurs and is common in pancreatitis. It has also been suggested that hypocalcemia might be related to excessive secretion of glucagon from the inflamed pancreas, which results in increased secretion of calcitonin (a hormone that lowers serum calcium). Inadequate secretion of PTH by the parathyroid gland results in hypocalcemia and can be related to hypoparathyroidism or other parathyroid gland disorders, use of certain drugs, surgery of the thyroid gland with inadvertent removal of the parathyroids, radiation injury to the thyroid, and radical neck dissection. This is likely to occur in the first 24 to 48 hours postoperatively.

Medications predisposing the patient to hypocalcemia include aluminum-containing antacids, aminoglycosides, anticonvulsants (phenytoin and phenobarbital), corticosteroids, mithramycin, phosphates, isoniazid, and loop diuretics. Malabsorption of calcium may be seen in severe diarrhea, laxative abuse, decreased exposure to sunlight or conditions that impair vitamin D, high phosphorus level in the intestines, reduced gastric acidity, and kidney failure. In addition, hypoalbuminemia, alkalosis, and massive blood transfusion are associated with hypocalcemia. Recall that approximately 40% of calcium is bound to albumin; thus, a decrease in serum albumin will result in a decrease in total serum calcium, but it does not affect the concentration of the ionized form of calcium that is essential for body function (Fischbach & Dunning, 2015). When the arterial pH increases (alkalosis), more calcium binds to protein. As a result, the ionized portion decreases, thus symptoms of hypocalcemia may occur with alkalosis. Transient hypocalcemia can occur with massive administration of citrated blood (adults who experience massive hemorrhage and shock), because citrate (which is used in blood transfusions to prevent clotting in blood) can combine with ionized calcium and temporarily remove it from the circulation.

Clinical Manifestations and Assessment

If ionized calcium level is normal despite low total calcium levels, patients are generally asymptomatic, whereas large changes in ionized calcium levels lead to a variety of symptoms associated with neuromuscular hyperactivity and cardiovascular effects detailed below. Tetany (the most characteristic manifestation of hypocalcemia) and convulsions are seen when the total calcium level is less than 4.4 mg/dL and/or the ionized calcium is less than 2.0 mg/dL (Fischbach & Dunning, 2015). *Tetany* refers to the entire symptom complex induced by increased neural excitability. These symptoms are caused by spontaneous discharges of both sensory and motor fibers in peripheral nerves. Sensations

FIGURE 4-7 Trousseau sign. Ischemia-induced carpal spasm can occur with hypocalcemia or hypomagnesemia. Occluding the brachial artery with a blood pressure cuff for 3 minutes can produce carpal spasm that mimics the spasm that occurs with hypocalcemia or hypomagnesemia.

of tingling may occur in the tips of the fingers, around the mouth, and, less commonly, in the feet. Spasms of the muscles of the extremities and face may occur. Pain may develop as a result of these spasms.

Trousseau sign (Fig. 4-7) can be elicited by inflating a blood pressure cuff on the upper arm to about 20 mm Hg above systolic pressure; within 2 to 5 minutes, carpal spasm (an adducted thumb, flexed wrist and metacarpophalangeal joints, extended interphalangeal joints with fingers together) occurs as ischemia of the ulnar nerve develops. *Chvostek sign* consists of twitching of muscles supplied by the facial nerve when the nerve is tapped about 2 cm anterior to the earlobe, just below the zygomatic arch.

Seizures occur because hypocalcemia causes irritability of the CNS as well as of the peripheral nerves. Other changes associated with hypocalcemia include mental changes, such as depression, impaired memory, confusion, delirium, and even hallucinations. A prolonged QT interval is seen on the ECG due to prolongation of the ST segment, which predisposes patients to a form of ventricular tachycardia called *torsades de pointes* (see Chapter 17). Respiratory effects with decreasing calcium include dyspnea and laryngospasm (stridor). Signs and symptoms of chronic hypocalcemia include hyperactive bowel sounds, dry and brittle hair and nails, and abnormal clotting. When evaluating serum calcium levels, variables such as the serum albumin level and the arterial pH must be considered. Because abnormalities in serum albumin levels may affect interpretation of the serum calcium level, it may be necessary to calculate the corrected serum calcium if the serum albumin level is abnormal. For every decrease in serum albumin of 1 g/dL below 4 g/dL, the total serum calcium level is underestimated by approximately 0.8 mg/dL. The following is a quick method to calculate the corrected serum calcium level:

Corrected calcium = measured calcium
+ 0.8 (4.0 − measured serum albumin)

An example of the calculations needed to obtain the corrected total serum calcium level is as follows: A patient's reported serum albumin level is 2.5 g/dL; the reported serum calcium level is 10.5 mg/dL. First, the decrease in serum albumin level from normal (i.e., the difference from the normal albumin concentration of 4 g/dL) is calculated: 4 g/dL – 2.5 g/dL = 1.5 g/dL. Next, multiply 0.8 (1.5) = 1.2.

Finally, 1.2 mg/dL is added to 10.5 mg/dL (the reported serum calcium level) to obtain the corrected total serum calcium level: 1.2 mg/dL + 10.5 mg/dL = 11.7 mg/dL.

The ionized calcium level is usually normal in patients with reduced total serum calcium levels and concomitant hypoalbuminemia.

Ideally, the ionized level of calcium should be measured in the laboratory. However, in many laboratories, only the total calcium level is reported; therefore, the concentration of the ionized fraction must be estimated by simultaneous measurement of the serum albumin level or specifically ordered by the provider. In addition, PTH levels and magnesium and phosphorus levels need to be assessed to identify possible causes of decreased calcium.

Medical Management

Acute symptomatic hypocalcemia is life-threatening and requires prompt treatment with IV administration of calcium. Although calcium chloride produces a significantly higher ionized calcium level than calcium gluconate, it is not used as often because it is more irritating to the vasculature and can cause sloughing of tissue if it infiltrates. Administering IV calcium too rapidly can cause cardiac arrest, which may be preceded by bradycardia in patients. IV administration of calcium is particularly dangerous in patients receiving digitalis-derived medications because calcium ions exert an effect similar to that of digitalis and can cause digitalis toxicity, with adverse cardiac effects. Therefore, calcium should be diluted in D_5W and administered via a slow IV infusion using a volumetric infusion pump. The IV site must be observed often for any evidence of infiltration because of the risk of extravasation and resultant cellulitis or necrosis. A 0.9% sodium chloride solution should not be used with calcium because it increases renal calcium loss. Solutions containing phosphates or bicarbonate should not be used with calcium because they cause precipitation when calcium is added. The nurse must clarify with the provider which calcium salt to administer because calcium gluconate yields 4.5 mEq of calcium, and calcium chloride provides 13.6 mEq of calcium. Because calcium can cause postural hypotension, the patient is kept in bed during IV replacement, and blood pressure is monitored.

Vitamin D therapy may be instituted to increase calcium absorption from the GI tract. Aluminum hydroxide, calcium acetate, or calcium carbonate antacids may be prescribed to decrease elevated phosphorus levels before treating hypocalcemia in the patient with CKF. Increasing the dietary intake of calcium to at least 1,000 to 1,200 mg/day in the adult is recommended. Calcium-containing foods include milk products; green, leafy vegetables; canned salmon; sardines; and fresh oysters. Hypomagnesemia can also cause tetany; if the tetany does not respond to IV calcium, then a low magnesium level is considered as a possible cause.

Nursing Management

It is important to observe for hypocalcemia in patients at risk. Seizure precautions are initiated if hypocalcemia is severe. The status of the airway is closely monitored because laryngeal stridor can occur. A tracheotomy tray should be kept at the bedside and a manual resuscitation bag nearby in case of laryngospasm in patients with audible stridor. Safety precautions are taken, as indicated, if confusion is present. Because of the cardiac complications, ECG monitoring should be instituted to detect changes in heart rate and rhythm, especially if the patient is receiving digoxin.

People who have a high risk for osteoporosis are instructed about the need for adequate dietary calcium intake; it is important to teach the patient which foods are rich in calcium. The nurse must also advise the patient to consider calcium supplements if sufficient calcium is not consumed in the diet. Such supplements should be taken in divided doses with meals. In addition, the value of regular weight-bearing exercise in decreasing bone loss should be emphasized, as well as the effect of medications on calcium balance. For example, alcohol and caffeine in high doses inhibit calcium absorption, and moderate cigarette smoking increases urinary calcium excretion. Additional teaching includes discussion of bisphosphonate medications to reduce the rate of bone loss. Teaching also includes strategies to reduce the risk of falls. The patient is also cautioned to avoid the overuse of laxatives and antacids that contain phosphorus because their use decreases calcium absorption.

HYPERCALCEMIA (CALCIUM EXCESS)

Hypercalcemia (excess of calcium in the plasma) is a dangerous imbalance. Hypercalcemic crisis (an acute increase in calcium level) has an extremely high mortality rate if not corrected promptly, often related to cardiac arrest (Grossman & Porth, 2014).

Pathophysiology

Ninety percent of hypercalcemia cases are related to either malignancy or hyperparathyroidism (Thomas & Chung, 2016). Considered an oncologic emergency, hypercalcemia occurs in 20% to 30% of patients with cancer at some point in their disease process (Thomas & Chung, 2016). It is associated with increased osteoclast activity resulting in bone demineralization, direct bone destruction by tumor cells and subsequent release of calcium, and/or tumor-produced factors that affect bone resorption and/or tubular calcium reabsorption. Tumor cells can secrete PTH-related protein, resulting in increased serum calcium. The excessive PTH secretion associated with hyperparathyroidism causes increased release of calcium from the bones and increased intestinal and renal absorption of calcium. Calcifications of soft tissue occur when the calcium–phosphorus product (serum calcium × serum phosphorus) exceeds 70 mg/dL.

Bone mineral is lost during immobilization, and sometimes this causes elevation of total (and especially ionized) calcium in the bloodstream. Symptomatic hypercalcemia from immobilization is rare; when it does occur, it is virtually limited to people with high calcium turnover rates (e.g., adolescents during a growth spurt). Most cases of hypercalcemia secondary to immobility occur after severe or multiple fractures or spinal cord injury.

Thiazide diuretics can cause a slight elevation in serum calcium levels because they potentiate the action of PTH on the kidneys, reducing urinary calcium excretion. A rare condition, called *milk–alkali syndrome,* has occurred in patients with peptic ulcer treated previously for a prolonged period with milk and alkaline antacids, particularly calcium carbonate. Vitamin A and D intoxication, as well as the use of lithium, can cause calcium excess.

Clinical Manifestations and Assessment

As a rule, the symptoms of hypercalcemia are proportional to the degree of elevation of the serum calcium level. Hypercalcemia reduces neuromuscular excitability because it suppresses activity at the myoneural junction. Symptoms such as muscle weakness, incoordination, anorexia, and constipation may be caused by decreased tone in smooth and striated muscle. Cardiovascular effects include hypertension and a shortened QT interval, which can cause increased sensitivity to digitalis and deposition of calcium in heart valves, myocardium, or coronary arteries (Lycans et al., 2016). Cardiac standstill can occur when the serum calcium level is about 18 mg/dL (4.5 mmol/L).

Anorexia, nausea, vomiting, and constipation are common symptoms of hypercalcemia. Abdominal and bone pain may also be present. Abdominal distention and paralytic ileus may complicate severe hypercalcemic crisis. Excessive urination due to disturbed renal tubular function produced by hypercalcemia may occur. In fact, nephrogenic diabetes insipidus can be seen in patients with this disorder (Abbas, Iqbal, Iqbal, Javaid, & Ashraf, 2016). Severe thirst secondary to the polyuria caused by the high solute (calcium) load is expected. Although uncommon, patients with chronic hypercalcemia may develop symptoms similar to those of peptic ulcer because hypercalcemia increases the secretion of acid and pepsin by the stomach.

Confusion, impaired memory, slurred speech, lethargy, acute psychotic behavior, or coma may occur. The more severe symptoms tend to appear when the serum calcium level is approximately 16 mg/dL (4 mmol/L) or higher.

However, some patients become profoundly disturbed with serum calcium levels of only 12 mg/dL (3 mmol/L). These symptoms resolve as serum calcium levels return to normal after treatment.

Hypercalcemic crisis refers to an acute rise in the serum calcium level to 17 mg/dL (4.3 mmol/L) or higher. Severe thirst and polyuria are often present. Other findings may include muscle weakness, intractable nausea, abdominal cramps, obstipation (very severe constipation) or diarrhea, peptic ulcer symptoms, and bone pain. Lethargy, confusion, and coma may also occur. This condition is very dangerous and may result in cardiac arrest.

The double-antibody PTH test may be used to differentiate between primary hyperparathyroidism and malignancy as a cause of hypercalcemia: PTH levels are increased in primary or secondary hyperparathyroidism and suppressed in malignancy. X-rays may reveal the presence of osteoporosis if the patient has hypercalcemia secondary to a malignancy or bone cavitation. A 24-hour urine calcium collection may be ordered; hypercalciuria is defined as calcium excretion of greater than 400 mg/day.

> **Nursing Alert**
> *The mnemonic "bones (bone pain), stones (kidney), groans (pain), and psychic moans (anxiety, psychiatric symptoms)" may be helpful to recall the cascade of symptoms associated with hypercalcemia.*

Medical Management

Therapeutic aims in hypercalcemia include decreasing the serum calcium level and reversing the process causing hypercalcemia. Treating the underlying cause (e.g., chemotherapy for a malignancy, partial parathyroidectomy for hyperparathyroidism) is essential. For example, drugs such as thiazides and Vitamin D compounds, as associated with hypercalcemia, may be discontinued and dietary calcium restricted (Thakker, 2016).

General measures include intravenous fluids to dilute serum calcium and promote its excretion by the kidneys, mobilizing the patient, and restricting intake of fluids and medications that contain calcium. IV administration of 0.9% sodium chloride solution is expected since it temporarily dilutes the serum calcium level and increases urinary calcium excretion by inhibiting tubular reabsorption of calcium. Furosemide (Lasix) is often used in conjunction with administration of a saline solution; in addition to causing diuresis, furosemide increases calcium excretion and is useful in preventing FVE associated with saline administration.

Bisphosphonates are the drugs of choice for hypercalcemia due to secondary hyperparathyroidism. Glucocorticoid therapy is effective when the hypercalcemia is due to diseases such as lymphoma, myeloma, or granulomatous disease. Dialysis using a low or zero calcium dialysate should be considered if these treatments are not effective or if the patient has kidney failure. When the acute management of hypercalcemia has been completed, appropriate treatment for the underlying cause needs to be undertaken. Calcitonin can be used to lower the serum calcium level and is particularly useful for patients with heart disease or kidney failure who cannot tolerate large sodium loads. Calcitonin reduces bone resorption, increases the depositing of calcium and phosphorus in the bones, and increases urinary excretion of calcium and phosphate. Although several forms are available, calcitonin derived from salmon is commonly used. Skin testing for allergy to salmon calcitonin is necessary before the hormone is administered. Systemic allergic reactions are possible because this hormone is a protein; resistance to the medication may develop later because of antibody formation. Calcitonin is administered by intramuscular injection rather than subcutaneously because patients with hypercalcemia have poor perfusion of subcutaneous tissue.

For patients with cancer, treatment is directed at controlling the condition by surgery, chemotherapy, or radiation therapy. Corticosteroids may be used to decrease bone turnover and tubular reabsorption for patients with sarcoidosis, myelomas, lymphomas, and leukemias; patients with solid tumors are less responsive. The bisphosphonates inhibit osteoclast activity and may be used to lower serum calcium levels. Mithramycin, a cytotoxic antibiotic, inhibits bone resorption and thus lowers the serum calcium level. This agent must be used cautiously because it has significant side effects, including thrombocytopenia, nephrotoxicity, rebound hypercalcemia when discontinued, and hepatotoxicity. Finally, hemodialysis or peritoneal dialysis with low calcium levels in dialysis fluid may be considered since both treatments are effective for removing calcium from circulation. In addition, dialysis may be considered for patients with renal insufficiency and congestive heart failure in which saline infusion is not suitable (Ahmad, Kuraganti, & Steenkamp, 2015).

Nursing Management

It is important to monitor for hypercalcemia in patients who are at risk. Interventions such as increasing patient mobility and encouraging fluids can help prevent hypercalcemia, or at least minimize its severity. Fluids containing sodium should be administered unless contraindicated because sodium favors calcium excretion. Patients are encouraged to drink 3 to 4 quarts of fluid daily. Adequate fiber should be provided in the diet to offset the tendency for constipation. Safety precautions are implemented, as necessary, when mental symptoms of hypercalcemia are present. The patient and family are informed that these mental changes are reversible with treatment. Increased calcium potentiates the effects of digitalis; therefore, the patient is assessed for signs and symptoms of digitalis toxicity. Because ECG changes (premature ventricular contractions, paroxysmal atrial tachycardia, and

heart block) can occur, the cardiac rate and rhythm are monitored for any abnormalities.

MAGNESIUM IMBALANCES

Magnesium is the most abundant intracellular cation after potassium. It acts as an activator for many intracellular enzyme systems and plays a role in both carbohydrate and protein metabolism. The normal serum magnesium level is 1.3 to 2.3 mEq/L (1.8 to 3.0 mg/dL; 0.8 to 1.2 mmol/L). Approximately one third of serum magnesium is bound to protein; the remaining two thirds exists as free cations—the active component (Mg^{+2}). Magnesium balance is important in neuromuscular function. Because magnesium acts directly on the myoneural junction, variations in the serum concentration of magnesium affect neuromuscular irritability and contractility. Magnesium produces its sedative effect at the neuromuscular junction, probably by inhibiting the release of the neurotransmitter acetylcholine.

Magnesium exerts effects on the cardiovascular system, acting peripherally to produce vasodilation. Magnesium is thought to have a direct effect on peripheral arteries and arterioles, which results in a decreased total peripheral resistance. IV magnesium may also be helpful in patients with acute asthma by potentially improving both bronchodilation and airflow. Magnesium is predominantly found in bone and soft tissues. It is primarily eliminated by the kidneys.

HYPOMAGNESEMIA (MAGNESIUM DEFICIT)

Hypomagnesemia refers to a below-normal serum magnesium concentration (1.3 to 2.3 mEq/L; 1.8 to 3.0 mg/dL; 0.8 to 1.2 mmol/L). Magnesium is similar to calcium in two aspects: (1) it is the ionized fraction of magnesium that is primarily involved in neuromuscular activity and other physiologic processes, and (2) magnesium levels should be evaluated in combination with albumin levels. Low serum albumin levels decrease total magnesium.

Pathophysiology

Hypomagnesemia is a common yet often overlooked imbalance in acutely and critically ill patients. It may occur with withdrawal from alcohol and administration of tube feedings or parenteral nutrition.

An important route of magnesium loss is the GI tract. Loss of magnesium from the GI tract may occur with nasogastric suction, diarrhea, or fistulas. Because fluid from the lower GI tract has a higher concentration of magnesium (10 to 14 mEq/L) than fluid from the upper tract (1 to 2 mEq/L), losses from diarrhea and intestinal fistulas are more likely to induce magnesium deficit than are those from gastric suction. Although magnesium losses are relatively small in nasogastric suction, hypomagnesemia will occur if losses are prolonged and magnesium is not replaced through IV infusion. Because the distal small bowel is the major site of magnesium absorption, any disruption in small-bowel function, as in intestinal resection or inflammatory bowel disease, can lead to hypomagnesemia.

Alcoholism is currently the most common cause of symptomatic hypomagnesemia in the United States. Hypomagnesemia is particularly troublesome during treatment of alcohol withdrawal. Therefore, the serum magnesium level should be measured routinely in patients undergoing withdrawal from alcohol. The serum magnesium level may be normal on admission but may decrease as a result of metabolic changes, such as the intracellular shift of magnesium associated with IV glucose administration.

During nutritional replacement, the major cellular electrolytes move from the serum to newly synthesized cells. Patients on enteral (feeding that uses the GI tract) or parenteral (delivery of calories and nutrients into a vein, i.e., TPN, PPN) feedings should have magnesium levels measured routinely as serious hypomagnesemia can occur with magnesium-deficient formulas, especially in those who have undergone a period of starvation. Other causes of hypomagnesemia include the administration of aminoglycosides, cyclosporine, cisplatin, diuretics, digitalis, and amphotericin, as well as the rapid administration of citrated blood, especially to patients with kidney or hepatic disease. Magnesium deficiency often occurs in diabetic ketoacidosis, secondary to increased renal excretion during osmotic diuresis and shifting of magnesium into the cells with insulin therapy. Other contributing causes are sepsis, burns, and hypothermia.

Clinical Manifestations and Assessment

Clinical manifestations of hypomagnesemia are largely confined to the neuromuscular system. Some of the effects are due directly to the low serum magnesium level; others are due to secondary changes in potassium and calcium metabolism. Symptoms do not usually occur until the serum magnesium level has dropped to less than 1 mEq/L (0.5 mmol/L).

Among the neuromuscular changes are hyperexcitability with muscle weakness, tremors, and *athetoid movements* (slow, involuntary twisting and writhing). Others include tetany, generalized tonic–clonic or focal seizures, laryngeal stridor, and positive Chvostek and Trousseau signs (see earlier discussion), which occur, in part, because of accompanying hypocalcemia.

Hypomagnesemia may be accompanied by marked alterations in mood. Apathy, depression, apprehension, and extreme agitation have been noted, as well as ataxia, dizziness, insomnia, and confusion. At times, delirium, auditory or visual hallucinations, and frank psychoses may occur.

On laboratory analysis, the serum magnesium level is less than 1.3 mEq/L or 1.8 mg/dL (0.75 mmol/L). Hypomagnesemia is frequently associated with hypokalemia and hypocalcemia. About 25% of magnesium is protein-bound, principally to albumin. A decreased serum albumin level can, therefore, reduce the measured total magnesium concentration. ECG evaluations reflect magnesium, calcium, and potassium deficiencies, tachyarrhythmias, prolonged PR and QT intervals, widening QRS, depression of the ST-segment, flattened T waves, and a prominent U wave. Torsades de pointes is associated with a low magnesium level. Premature ventricular contractions, paroxysmal atrial tachycardia, and heart block may also occur. Digitalis toxicity is associated with low serum magnesium levels. This is important because patients receiving digoxin are also likely to be receiving diuretic therapy, predisposing them to renal loss of magnesium. Urine magnesium levels may be helpful in identifying causes of magnesium depletion and are measured after a loading dose of magnesium sulfate is administered.

Medical Management

Mild magnesium deficiency can be corrected by diet alone. Principal dietary sources of magnesium, which is a component of chlorophyll, are green leafy vegetables, nuts, seeds, legumes, whole grains, and seafood. Magnesium is also plentiful in peanut butter and cocoa.

If necessary, magnesium salts can be administered orally in an oxide or gluconate form to replace continuous excessive losses. Diarrhea is a common complication of excessive ingestion of magnesium. Patients receiving parenteral nutrition require magnesium in the IV solution to prevent hypomagnesemia. Magnesium sulfate must be administered intravenously by an infusion pump typically at a rate of 1 to 2 g over an hour. A bolus dose of magnesium sulfate given too rapidly can produce alterations in cardiac conduction, leading to heart block or asystole. Vital signs must be assessed frequently during magnesium administration to detect changes in cardiac rate or rhythm, hypotension, and respiratory distress. Monitoring urine output is essential before, during, and after magnesium administration; the provider is notified if urine volume decreases to less than 30 mL/hr (Nettina & Lippincott, 2014). Calcium gluconate must be readily available to treat hypocalcemic tetany or hypermagnesemia.

Overt symptoms of hypomagnesemia are treated with parenteral administration of magnesium. Magnesium sulfate is the most commonly used magnesium salt. Serial measurements of serum magnesium levels can be used to regulate the dosage.

Nursing Management

The nurse should be aware of patients who are at risk for hypomagnesemia and observe them for its signs and symptoms. Patients receiving digitalis are monitored closely because a deficit of magnesium can predispose them to digitalis toxicity. If hypomagnesemia is severe, seizure precautions are implemented. Other safety precautions are instituted, as indicated, if confusion is observed.

Because difficulty in swallowing (dysphagia) may occur in magnesium-depleted patients, a swallowing evaluation should be performed before oral medications or foods are offered. Dysphagia is probably related to the athetoid or *choreiform* (rapid, involuntary, and irregular jerking) movements associated with magnesium deficit. To determine neuromuscular irritability, the nurse needs to assess and grade deep tendon reflexes (refer to Chapter 43).

Teaching plays a major role in treating magnesium deficit, particularly that resulting from abuse of diuretic or laxative medications. In such cases, the nurse instructs the patient about the need to consume magnesium-rich foods. For patients experiencing hypomagnesemia from abuse of alcohol, the nurse provides teaching, counseling, support, and possible referral to alcohol abstinence programs or other professional help.

HYPERMAGNESEMIA (MAGNESIUM EXCESS)

Hypermagnesemia is a rare electrolyte abnormality because usually the kidneys are efficient in excreting magnesium. A serum magnesium level can appear falsely elevated if blood specimens are allowed to hemolyze or are drawn from an extremity with a tourniquet that was applied too tightly or for too long a period of time prior to blood draw.

Pathophysiology

By far the most common cause of hypermagnesemia is kidney failure. In fact, most patients with advanced kidney failure have at least a slight elevation in serum magnesium levels. This condition is aggravated when such patients receive magnesium to control seizures or inadvertently take one of the many commercial antacids that contain magnesium salts.

Hypermagnesemia can occur in a patient with untreated diabetic ketoacidosis when catabolism causes the release of cellular magnesium that cannot be excreted because of profound fluid volume depletion and resulting oliguria (less than 400 mL/24 hrs). An excess of magnesium can also result from excessive magnesium administered to treat hypertension of pregnancy or to treat low hypomagnesemia. Increased serum magnesium levels can also occur in adrenocortical insufficiency, Addison disease, or hypothermia. Excessive use of antacids (e.g., Maalox, Riopan, Mylanta); laxatives (Milk of Magnesia); and medications that decrease GI motility, including opioids and anticholinergics, can also increase serum magnesium levels. Decreased elimination of magnesium or its increased absorption due to intestinal hypomotility from any cause can contribute to hypermagnesemia. Lithium intoxication can also cause an increase in serum magnesium levels.

Clinical Manifestations and Assessment

Acute elevation of the serum magnesium level depresses the CNS as well as the peripheral neuromuscular junction. At mildly increased levels, there is a tendency for lowered blood pressure because of peripheral vasodilation. Nausea,

vomiting, weakness, soft tissue calcifications, facial flushing, and sensations of warmth may also occur. At higher magnesium concentrations, lethargy, difficulty speaking (dysarthria), and drowsiness can occur. Deep tendon reflexes are lost, and muscle weakness and paralysis may develop. The respiratory center is depressed when serum magnesium levels exceed 10 mEq/L (5 mmol/L). Coma, atrioventricular heart block, and cardiac arrest can occur when the serum magnesium level is greatly elevated and not treated. High levels of magnesium also result in platelet clumping and delayed thrombin formation. On laboratory analysis, the serum magnesium level is greater than 2.5 mEq/L or 3.0 mg/dL (1.25 mmol/L). Increased potassium and calcium are present concurrently. ECG findings may include a prolonged PR interval, tall T waves, a widened QRS, and a prolonged QT interval, as well as an atrioventricular block.

Medical Management

Hypermagnesemia can be prevented by avoiding the administration of magnesium to patients with kidney failure and by carefully monitoring seriously ill patients who are receiving magnesium salts. In patients with severe hypermagnesemia, all parenteral and oral magnesium salts are discontinued. In emergencies, such as respiratory depression or defective cardiac conduction, ventilatory support and IV calcium gluconate are indicated. In addition, hemodialysis with a magnesium-free dialysate can reduce the serum magnesium to a safe level within hours. Administration of loop diuretics (Lasix) and sodium chloride or lactated Ringer IV solution enhances magnesium excretion in patients with adequate kidney function. IV calcium gluconate antagonizes the cardiovascular and neuromuscular effects of magnesium.

Nursing Management

Patients at risk for hypermagnesemia are identified and assessed. The nurse monitors the vital signs, noting hypotension and shallow respirations, or ECG abnormalities. The nurse also observes for decreased deep tendon reflexes and changes in the LOC. Medications that contain magnesium are not administered to patients with kidney failure or compromised kidney function, and patients with kidney failure are cautioned to check with their health care providers before taking over-the-counter medications. Caution is essential when preparing and administering magnesium-containing fluids parenterally because available parenteral magnesium solutions (e.g., 2 mL ampules, 50 mL vials) differ in concentration.

PHOSPHORUS IMBALANCES

Phosphorus is a critical constituent of all the body's tissues. It is essential to the function of muscle and RBC; the formation of adenosine triphosphate (ATP) and of 2,3-diphosphoglycerate, which facilitates release of oxygen from hemoglobin;

and the maintenance of acid–base balance, as well as to the nervous system and the intermediary metabolism of carbohydrate, protein, and fat. It provides structural support to bones and teeth in the form of phosphate. Phosphorus is the primary anion of the ICF. About 85% of phosphorus is located in bones and teeth, 14% in soft tissue, and less than 1% in the ECF. The normal serum phosphorus level is 2.5 to 4.5 mg/dL (0.8 to 1.45 mmol/L).

HYPOPHOSPHATEMIA (PHOSPHORUS DEFICIT)

Pathophysiology

Hypophosphatemia is a below-normal serum concentration of inorganic phosphorus; it may occur under a variety of circumstances in which total body phosphorus stores are normal. Conversely, phosphorus deficiency is an abnormally low content of phosphorus in lean tissues that may exist in the absence of hypophosphatemia. It can be caused by an intracellular shift of potassium from serum into cells, by increased urinary excretion of potassium, or by decreased intestinal absorption of potassium.

Hypophosphatemia may occur during the administration of calories to patients with severe protein–calorie malnutrition. It is most likely to occur with overzealous intake or administration of simple carbohydrates. This syndrome can be induced in anyone with severe protein–calorie malnutrition, such as patients with anorexia nervosa or alcoholism, or elderly debilitated patients who are unable to eat. Approximately 50% of patients hospitalized due to chronic alcoholism have hypophosphatemia.

Marked hypophosphatemia may develop in malnourished patients who receive parenteral nutrition if the phosphorus loss is not adequately corrected. Other causes of hypophosphatemia include pain, heat stroke, prolonged intense hyperventilation, alcohol withdrawal, poor dietary intake, diabetic ketoacidosis, hepatic encephalopathy, and major thermal burns. Low magnesium levels, low potassium levels, and hyperparathyroidism related to increased urinary losses of phosphorus contribute to hypophosphatemia. Loss of phosphorus through the kidneys also occurs with acute volume expansion, osmotic diuresis, use of carbonic anhydrase inhibitors (acetazolamide [Diamox]), and some malignancies. Respiratory alkalosis can cause a decrease in phosphorus because of an intracellular shift of phosphorus, which often stimulates intracellular glycolysis.

Excess phosphorus binding by antacids containing magnesium, calcium, or albumin may decrease the phosphorus available from the diet to an amount lower than required to maintain serum phosphorus balance. The degree of hypophosphatemia depends on the amount of phosphorus in the diet compared to the dose of antacid. Phosphate loss can occur with chronic diarrhea or through severe potassium restriction. Vitamin D regulates intestinal ion absorption; therefore, a deficiency of vitamin D may cause decreased calcium and phosphate (phosphorus) levels, which may lead to osteomalacia (softened, brittle bones).

Clinical Manifestations and Assessment

A wide range of neurologic symptoms may occur, including irritability, fatigue, apprehension, weakness, numbness, paresthesias, dysarthria, dysphagia, diplopia, confusion, seizures, and coma. Low levels of diphosphoglycerate may reduce the delivery of oxygen to peripheral tissues, resulting in tissue anoxia. Hypoxia then leads to an increase in respiratory rate and respiratory alkalosis, causing phosphorus to move into the cells and potentiating hypophosphatemia. Hemolytic anemia may lead to pale skin and conjunctivae. It is thought that hypophosphatemia may predispose a person to infection due to a decrease in granulocyte function.

Muscle damage may develop as the ATP level in the muscle tissue declines. Clinical manifestations are muscle weakness, which may be subtle or profound and may affect any muscle group, muscle pain, and at times acute rhabdomyolysis (disintegration of striated muscle). Weakness of respiratory muscles may greatly impair ventilation. Hypophosphatemia also may predispose a person to insulin resistance and thus hyperglycemia. Chronic loss of phosphorus can cause bruising and bleeding from platelet dysfunction.

On laboratory analysis, the serum phosphorus level is less than 2.5 mg/dL (0.80 mmol/L) in adults. When reviewing laboratory results, the nurse should keep in mind that glucose or insulin administration causes a slight decrease in the serum phosphorus level. If hypophosphatemia is associated with hyperparathyroidism, the serum PTH levels are increased. Likewise, if etiology of hypophosphatemia is related to increased osteoblastic activity serum alkaline, phosphatase is increased. X-rays may show skeletal changes of osteomalacia or rickets.

Medical Management

Prevention of hypophosphatemia is the goal. In patients at risk for hypophosphatemia, serum phosphate levels should be monitored closely and correction initiated before deficits become severe. Adequate amounts of phosphorus should be added to parenteral solutions, and attention should be paid to the phosphorus levels in enteral feeding solutions.

Severe hypophosphatemia is dangerous and requires prompt attention. Aggressive IV phosphorus correction is usually limited to the patient whose serum phosphorus levels decrease to less than 1 mg/dL (0.3 mmol/L) and whose GI tract is not functioning. Possible dangers of IV administration of phosphorus include tetany from hypocalcemia and calcifications in tissues (blood vessels, heart, lung, kidney, eyes) from hyperphosphatemia. IV preparations of phosphorus are available as sodium or potassium phosphate. The rate of phosphorus administration should not exceed 10 mEq/hr, and the site should be monitored carefully because tissue sloughing and necrosis can occur with infiltration. In less acute situations, oral phosphorus replacement is usually adequate.

Nursing Management

The nurse identifies patients who are at risk for hypophosphatemia and monitors them. Because malnourished patients receiving parenteral nutrition are at risk when calories are introduced too aggressively, preventive measures involve gradually introducing the solution to avoid rapid shifts of phosphorus into the cells.

For patients with documented hypophosphatemia, careful attention is given to preventing infection because hypophosphatemia may alter the granulocytes. In patients requiring correction of phosphorus losses, the nurse frequently monitors serum phosphorus levels and documents and reports early signs of hypophosphatemia (apprehension, confusion, change in LOC). If the patient experiences mild hypophosphatemia, foods such as milk and milk products, organ meats, nuts, fish, poultry, and whole grains should be encouraged. With moderate hypophosphatemia, supplements such as Neutra-Phos capsules (250 mg phosphorus/capsule) or Fleet's Phospho-Soda (815 mg phosphorus/5 mL) may be prescribed.

HYPERPHOSPHATEMIA (PHOSPHORUS EXCESS)

Hyperphosphatemia is a serum phosphorus level that exceeds normal. Various conditions can lead to this imbalance, but the most common is kidney failure. Other causes include increased intake, decreased output, or a shift from the ICS to ECS. Other causes include chemotherapy for neoplastic disease, hypoparathyroidism, metabolic or respiratory acidosis, diabetic ketoacidosis, acute hemolysis, high phosphate intake, profound muscle necrosis, and increased phosphorus absorption. The primary complication of increased phosphorus is metastatic calcification (soft tissue, joints, and arteries), which occurs when the calcium–magnesium product (calcium × magnesium) exceeds 70 mg/dL.

Clinical Manifestations and Assessment

An increased serum phosphorus level causes few symptoms. Symptoms that do occur usually result from decreased calcium levels and soft tissue calcifications. The most important short-term consequence is tetany. Because of the reciprocal relationship between phosphorus and calcium, a high serum phosphate level tends to cause a low serum calcium concentration. Tetany can result, causing tingling sensations in the fingertips and around the mouth. Anorexia, nausea, vomiting, bone and joint pain, muscle weakness, hyperreflexia, and tachycardia may occur.

The major long-term consequence is soft tissue calcification, which occurs mainly in patients with a reduced glomerular filtration rate. High serum levels of inorganic

phosphorus promote precipitation of calcium phosphate in nonosseous sites, decreasing urine output, impairing vision, and producing palpitations.

On laboratory analysis, the serum phosphorus level exceeds 4.5 mg/dL (1.5 mmol/L) in adults. Serum phosphorus levels are normally higher in children presumably because of the high rate of skeletal growth. The serum calcium level is useful also for diagnosing the primary disorder and assessing the effects of treatments. X-ray studies may show skeletal changes with abnormal bone development. PTH levels are decreased in hypoparathyroidism. BUN and creatinine levels are used to assess kidney function. Renal ultrasonography may be indicated as part of the diagnostic assessment for kidney failure; bone studies and coronary calcification studies also provide information about the chronicity and prognosis of kidney failure.

Medical Management

When possible, treatment is directed at the underlying disorder. For example, hyperphosphatemia may be related to volume depletion or respiratory or metabolic acidosis. In kidney failure, elevated PTH production contributes to a high phosphorus level and bone disease. Measures to decrease the serum phosphate level in these patients include vitamin D preparations, such as calcitriol, which is available in both oral and parenteral forms. IV administration of calcitriol does not increase the serum calcium unless its dose is excessive, thus permitting more aggressive treatment of hyperphosphatemia with calcium-binding antacids (calcium carbonate or calcium citrate), phosphate-binding gels or antacids, restriction of dietary phosphate, forced diuresis with a loop diuretic, volume repletion with saline, and dialysis. Surgery may be indicated for removal of large calcium–phosphorus deposits.

Nursing Management

The nurse monitors patients at risk for hyperphosphatemia. If a low-phosphorus diet is prescribed, the patient is instructed to avoid phosphorus-rich foods such as hard cheese, cream, nuts, meats, whole-grain cereals, dried fruits, dried vegetables, kidneys, sardines, sweetbreads, and foods made with milk. When appropriate, the nurse instructs the patient to avoid phosphate-containing substances such as laxatives and enemas. The nurse also teaches the patient to recognize the signs of impending hypocalcemia and to monitor for changes in urine output.

CHLORIDE IMBALANCES

Chloride, the major anion of the ECF, is found more in interstitial and lymph fluid compartments than in blood. Chloride is also contained in gastric and pancreatic juices, sweat, bile, and saliva. The choroid plexus, where cerebrospinal fluid forms in the brain, depends on sodium and chloride to attract water to form the fluid portion of the cerebrospinal fluid. Sodium and chloride in water make up the composition of the ECF and assist in determining osmotic pressure. The serum level of chloride reflects a change in dilution or concentration of the ECF and does so in direct proportion to the sodium concentration. Serum osmolality parallels chloride levels as well. The normal serum chloride level is 97 to 107 mEq/L (97 to 107 mmol/L). Inside the cell, the chloride level is 4 mEq/L.

Plasma bicarbonate has an inverse relationship with chloride. For example, the carbonic anhydrase reaction in RBCs generates both hydrogen and bicarbonate from metabolically produced CO_2. Hydrogen facilitates the dissociation of oxygen from hemoglobin. The intracellular accumulation of bicarbonate is prevented by its movement out of the cell into the plasma. To maintain electrical neutrality, chloride enters the RBC, a response referred to as the *chloride shift*. It is important to note that when the level of one of these three electrolytes (sodium, bicarbonate, or chloride) is disturbed, the other two are also affected. Chloride is important not only in maintaining acid–base balance, but it also mediates the hyperpolarizing effect of many neurotransmitters on the membrane potential. Chloride is primarily obtained from the diet as table salt.

HYPOCHLOREMIA (CHLORIDE DEFICIT)

Chloride control depends on the intake of chloride and the excretion and reabsorption of its ions in the kidneys. Chloride is produced in the stomach, where it combines with hydrogen to form hydrochloric acid. A small amount of chloride is lost in the feces. GI tube drainage and severe vomiting and diarrhea, laxatives, ileostomy, and fistulas are risk factors for hypochloremia. Administration of chloride-deficient formulas, low sodium intake, decreased serum sodium levels, metabolic alkalosis, prolonged therapy with IV dextrose (water intoxication), diuretic therapy, burns, and fever may also cause hypochloremia. As chloride decreases (usually because of volume depletion), sodium and bicarbonate ions are retained by the kidney to balance the loss. Bicarbonate accumulates in the ECF, which raises the pH and leads to hypochloremic metabolic alkalosis.

Clinical Manifestations and Assessment

Because hypochloremia rarely occurs in the absence of other abnormalities, signs and symptoms of hypochloremia are associated with hyponatremia, hypokalemia, and metabolic alkalosis. Metabolic alkalosis is a disorder that results in a high pH and a high serum bicarbonate level as a result of excess alkali intake or loss of hydrogen ions. With compensation, the partial pressure of carbon dioxide in arterial blood ($PaCO_2$) increases to 50 mm Hg. Hyperexcitability of muscles, tetany, hyperactive deep tendon reflexes, weakness, twitching, and muscle cramps may result. Hypokalemia can

cause hypochloremia, resulting in cardiac arrhythmias. In addition, because low chloride levels parallel low sodium levels, a water excess may occur. Hyponatremia can cause seizures and coma.

In addition to the chloride level, sodium and potassium levels are also evaluated because these electrolytes are lost along with chloride. ABG analysis identifies the acid–base imbalance, which is usually metabolic alkalosis. The urine chloride level, which is also measured, decreases in hypochloremia.

Medical Management

Treatment involves correcting the cause of hypochloremia and the contributing electrolyte and acid–base imbalances. Normal saline (0.9% sodium chloride) or half-strength saline (0.45% sodium chloride) solution is administered by IV to replace the chloride. The provider may re-evaluate whether the patient receiving a diuretic (loop, osmotic, or thiazide) should discontinue the medications or change to another diuretic.

Foods high in chloride are provided; these include tomato juice, bananas, dates, eggs, cheese, milk, salty broth, canned vegetables, and processed meats. A patient who drinks free water (water without electrolytes) or bottled water excretes large amounts of chloride; therefore, the patient is instructed to avoid this kind of water. Ammonium chloride, an acidifying agent, may be prescribed to treat metabolic alkalosis; the dosage depends on the patient's weight and serum chloride level. This agent is metabolized by the liver, and its effects last for about 3 days. Its use should be avoided in patients with impaired liver or kidney function.

Nursing Management

The nurse monitors the patient's I&O, ABG values, and serum electrolyte levels as well as LOC and muscle strength and movement. Changes are reported to the provider promptly. Vital signs are monitored, and respiratory assessment is carried out frequently. The nurse teaches the patient about foods with high chloride content.

HYPERCHLOREMIA (CHLORIDE EXCESS)

Hyperchloremia exists when the serum level of chloride exceeds 107 mEq/L (107 mmol/L).

Pathophysiology

Because chloride has an affinity for sodium and an inverse relationship with bicarbonate, hyperchloremia is related to hypernatremia, bicarbonate loss, and metabolic acidosis. Hyperchloremic metabolic acidosis is also known as *normal anion gap acidosis* (see later discussion). It is usually caused by the loss of bicarbonate ions via the kidney or the GI tract with a corresponding increase in chloride ions. Chloride ions in the form of acidifying salts accumulate and acidosis occurs with a decrease in bicarbonate ions. Hyperchloremia results from increased intake either by mouth or by isotonic or hypertonic IV fluid administration (e.g., 9% NaCl has a chloride content of 154 mEq/L. Since normal chloride is 97 to 107 mEq/L, the nurse recognizes that prolonged administration of normal saline can results in hyperchloremic metabolic acidosis (electroneutrality is maintained by a decrease in the serum HCO_3^- [bicarbonate or base] concentration in the presence of a high chloride level, thus a hyperchloremic acidosis ensues). It can also result from decreased chloride excretion as in hyperparathyroidism, hyperaldosteronism, and kidney failure.

Clinical Manifestations and Assessment

The signs and symptoms of hyperchloremia are the same as those of metabolic acidosis, hypervolemia, and hypernatremia and can include tachypnea; weakness; lethargy; deep, rapid respirations; diminished cognitive ability; and hypertension. If untreated, hyperchloremia can lead to a decrease in cardiac output, arrhythmias, and coma. A high chloride level is often accompanied by a high sodium level and fluid retention. Laboratory analysis reveals the serum chloride level of 108 mEq/L (108 mmol/L) or greater, the serum sodium level greater than 145 mEq/L (145 mmol/L), the serum pH less than 7.35, and the serum bicarbonate level less than 22 mEq/L (22 mmol/L).

Medical Management

Correcting the underlying cause of hyperchloremia and restoring electrolyte, fluid, and acid–base balance are essential. Hypotonic IV solutions may be given to restore balance. Lactated Ringer solution may be prescribed to convert lactate to bicarbonate in the liver, which increases the base bicarbonate level and corrects the acidosis. IV sodium bicarbonate may be administered to increase bicarbonate levels, which leads to the renal excretion of chloride ions as bicarbonate and chloride compete to combine with sodium. Diuretics may be administered to eliminate chloride as well. Sodium, chloride, and fluids are restricted.

Nursing Management

Monitoring vital signs, ABG values, and the patient's I&O status is important to assess the patient's status and the effectiveness of treatment. Assessment findings related to respiratory, neurologic, and cardiac systems are documented, and changes are discussed with the provider. The nurse teaches the patient about the diet that should be followed to manage hyperchloremia and maintain adequate hydration.

ACID–BASE DISTURBANCES

Acid–base disturbances are commonly encountered in clinical practice. Identification of the specific acid–base imbalance is important in identifying the underlying cause of the disorder and determining appropriate treatment.

Plasma pH is an indicator of hydrogen ion (H^+) concentration. Homeostatic mechanisms keep pH within a normal range (7.35 to 7.45). These mechanisms consist of buffer systems, the kidneys, and the lungs. The H^+ concentration is extremely important: the greater the concentration, the more acidic the solution and the lower the pH; the lower the H^+ concentration, the more alkaline the solution and the higher the pH. The process causing an acidemia (condition when the blood is acid) is termed either *metabolic* or *respiratory acidosis,* whereas the process causing an alkalemia (condition when the blood is alkaline) is either *metabolic* or *respiratory alkalosis.* Blood pH must be kept within narrow limits because a pH outside the range of 6.8 to 7.8 is incompatible with life.

Buffer systems prevent major changes in the pH of body fluids by removing or releasing H^+; they can act quickly to prevent excessive changes in H^+ concentration. Hydrogen ions are buffered by both intracellular and extracellular buffers. The body's major extracellular buffer system is the bicarbonate–carbonic acid buffer system, which is assessed when ABGs are measured. The sources for bicarbonate (HCO_3^-) are the intestinal lumen, the pancreas, kidney, and, to a lesser extent, diet. The role of the kidneys is to reabsorb filtered bicarbonate and make new bicarbonate. The bicarbonate ion acts as a H^+ ion acceptor and is responsible for buffering 90% of the hydrogen ions in blood. Normally, there are 20 parts of bicarbonate (HCO_3^-) to one part of carbonic acid (H_2CO_3). If this ratio is altered, the pH will change. It is the ratio of HCO_3^- to H_2CO_3 that is important in maintaining pH, not absolute values. Carbon dioxide (CO_2) is regulated by the lungs and, when dissolved in water, becomes carbonic acid ($CO_2 + H_2O = H_2CO_3$). Therefore, when CO_2 is increased, the carbonic acid content is also increased, and vice versa. If either bicarbonate or carbonic acid is increased or decreased so that the 20:1 ratio is no longer maintained, an acid–base imbalance will result. Less important buffer systems in the ECF include the inorganic phosphates and the plasma proteins. Intracellular buffers include proteins, organic and inorganic phosphates, and, in RBC, hemoglobin.

The kidneys regulate the bicarbonate level in the ECF; they can regenerate bicarbonate ions as well as reabsorb them from the renal tubular cells. In respiratory acidosis, the kidneys respond to the increased CO_2 (carbon dioxide) and decreased pH by excreting hydrogen ions and conserving bicarbonate ions to help restore balance. Conversely, in respiratory alkalosis, the kidneys' response to the decreased CO_2 and increased pH is to retain hydrogen ions and excrete bicarbonate ions to help restore balance. However, the renal compensation for imbalances described above is relatively slow (a matter of hours or days).

The lungs, under the control of the pons and the medulla, regulate the CO_2 and, thus, the carbonic acid content of the ECF. They do so by adjusting ventilation in response to the amount of CO_2 in the blood. A rise in the partial pressure of CO_2 in arterial blood ($PaCO_2$) is a powerful stimulant to respiration. Of course, the partial pressure of oxygen in arterial blood (PaO_2) also influences respiration. However, its effect is not as marked as that produced by the $PaCO_2$.

In metabolic acidosis, the respiratory rate increases, causing greater elimination of CO_2 (to reduce the acid load). In contrast, in metabolic alkalosis, the respiratory rate decreases, causing CO_2 to be retained (to increase the acid load). Both mechanisms are an attempt to return the pH to normal, and the respiratory response is instantaneous.

To review, a normal pH is 7.35 to 7.45 and is associated with three conditions: (1) a normal level of acid and base; (2) an abnormal process in which too many bases are produced (alkalosis), and the body counteracts this base load by allowing more acids to accumulate (20 base to 1 acid ratio maintained); (3) an abnormal process in which too many acids are produced, and the body counteracts by allowing more base to accumulate (20 base to 1 acid ratio maintained). The second and third conditions are considered compensation and will be discussed later in the chapter. If the pH is greater than 7.45, an alkalemia (blood is excessively alkaline) exists. If the pH is less than 7.35, an acidemia (blood is excessively acid) exists.

BASE BICARBONATE IMBALANCES

ACUTE AND CHRONIC METABOLIC ACIDOSIS (BASE BICARBONATE DEFICIT)

Metabolic acidosis is a clinical disturbance characterized by a low pH (increased H^+ concentration) and a low plasma bicarbonate concentration (less than 22 mEq/L). It can be produced by a gain of hydrogen ions or a loss of bicarbonate, and it is divided clinically into two forms according to the values of the serum anion gap: high anion gap acidosis and normal anion gap acidosis. The anion gap reflects unmeasured anions (phosphates, sulfates, and proteins) in plasma. Recall cations are positively charged ions (Na^+, K^+, H^+), and anions are negatively charged ions (HCO_3^-, Cl^-). Under normal conditions the ratio of cation to anion is not equal; that is, the Na^+ and K^+ levels are greater than the number of HCO_3^- and Cl^-. In actuality, the ECF is, under normal circumstances, electroneutral, and the sum of cations does equal the sum of anions. However, since not all anions are measured, there is a gap. The anion gap can be calculated by either one of the following equations:

$$(Na^+ + K^+) - (HCO_3^- + Cl^-)$$

or

$$Na^+ - (HCO_3^- + Cl^-)$$

Potassium is often omitted from the equation because of its low level in the plasma; therefore, the second equation is used more often than the first.

The normal value for an anion gap is about 8 to 12 mEq/L (8 to 12 mmol/L) without potassium in the equation. If potassium is included in the equation, the normal value for the anion gap is 12 to 16 mEq/L (12 to 16 mmol/L). An anion gap greater than 16 mEq/L (16 mmol/L) is termed a *high anion gap metabolic acidosis* and results from excessive accumulation of fixed acid. High anion gap occurs in the ketoacidosis of uncontrolled diabetes or starvation, lactic acidosis, the late phase of salicylate poisoning, uremia, and methanol or ethylene glycol toxicity. In each of these situations the excess hydrogen is buffered by HCO_3^-, causing the bicarbonate concentration to fall. This is the reason for the high anion gap.

Normal anion gap acidosis results from the direct loss of bicarbonate, and can occur in diarrhea, lower intestinal fistulas, ureterostomies, diuretic therapy, early renal insufficiency, excessive administration of chloride (recall 0.9% NaCl contains 154 mEq of Cl^- per liter), and the administration of parenteral nutrition without bicarbonate or bicarbonate-producing solutes (e.g., lactate). Pancreatic drains are also associated with the direct loss of bicarbonate. In these situations, the direct loss of HCO_3^- is associated with an increase in plasma chloride, and the anion gap remains normal. This condition is also referred to as *hyperchloremic acidosis.*

Clinical Manifestations and Assessment

Signs and symptoms of metabolic acidosis vary with the severity of the acidosis. They may include headache, lethargy, confusion, sluggishness, increased respiratory rate and depth, nausea, and vomiting. Peripheral vasodilation and decreased cardiac output occur when the pH drops to less than 7. Additional physical assessment findings include decreased blood pressure, arrhythmias, and shock. Chronic metabolic acidosis is usually seen with CKF. The bicarbonate and pH decrease slowly, and the patient is asymptomatic until the bicarbonate is approximately 15 mEq/L or less.

ABG measurements reveal a low bicarbonate level (less than 22 mEq/L) and a low pH (less than 7.35). Hyperkalemia may accompany metabolic acidosis as a result of the shift of potassium out of the cells. Later, as the acidosis is corrected, potassium moves back into the cells and hypokalemia may occur. Hyperventilation decreases the CO_2 level as a compensatory action. As stated previously, calculation of the anion gap is helpful in determining the cause of metabolic acidosis. An ECG detects arrhythmias caused by the associated increased serum potassium.

Medical and Nursing Management

Treatment is directed at correcting the underlying metabolic defect. When the problem results from excessive intake of chloride, treatment is aimed at eliminating the source of the chloride (discontinuation of offending medication). When necessary, in general bicarbonate is administered if the pH is less than 7.1 and the serum bicarbonate level is less than 10 mEq/L. Although hyperkalemia occurs with acidosis, hypokalemia may occur with reversal of the acidosis and subsequent movement of potassium back into the cells. Therefore, the serum potassium level is monitored closely, and hypokalemia is corrected as acidosis is reversed.

In chronic metabolic acidosis, low serum calcium levels are treated before the chronic metabolic acidosis is treated, to avoid tetany resulting from an increase in pH and subsequent decrease in ionized calcium. Alkalizing agents may be administered if the serum bicarbonate level is less than 12 mEq/L. Treatment modalities may also include hemodialysis or peritoneal dialysis.

ACUTE AND CHRONIC METABOLIC ALKALOSIS (BASE BICARBONATE EXCESS)

Metabolic alkalosis is a clinical disturbance characterized by a high pH (decreased H^+ concentration) and a high plasma bicarbonate concentration. It can be produced by a gain of bicarbonate or a loss of H^+.

Pathophysiology

A common cause of metabolic alkalosis is related to volume depletion from vomiting or gastric suction, with loss of hydrogen and chloride ions. The disorder also occurs in pyloric stenosis, in which only gastric fluid is lost. Gastric fluid has an acid pH (usually 1 to 3), and loss of this highly acidic fluid increases the alkalinity of body fluids. Other situations predisposing the patient to metabolic alkalosis include those associated with loss of potassium, such as diuretic therapy that promotes excretion of potassium (e.g., thiazides, furosemide), and excessive adrenocorticoid hormones (as in hyperaldosteronism and Cushing syndrome).

Hypokalemia produces alkalosis in two ways: (1) the kidneys conserve potassium, and, therefore, H^+ excretion increases; and (2) cellular potassium moves out of the cells into the ECF in an attempt to maintain near-normal serum levels (as potassium ions leave the cells, hydrogen ions must enter to maintain electroneutrality). A helpful cue to recall the association of a decreased K^+ to alkalosis is "al-K^+-low-sis" (Diepenbrock, 2015).

Excessive alkali ingestion from antacids containing bicarbonate or from use of sodium bicarbonate during cardiopulmonary resuscitation can also cause metabolic alkalosis.

Chronic metabolic alkalosis can occur with long-term diuretic therapy (thiazides or furosemide), villous adenoma (GI polyp), external drainage of gastric fluids, significant potassium depletion, cystic fibrosis, and the chronic ingestion of milk and calcium carbonate.

Clinical Manifestations and Assessment

Alkalosis is primarily manifested by symptoms related to decreased calcium ionization, such as tingling of the fingers and toes, dizziness, and hypertonic muscles. The ionized fraction of serum calcium decreases in alkalosis as more calcium combines with serum proteins. Because it is the ionized fraction of calcium that influences neuromuscular activity, symptoms of hypocalcemia are often the predominant symptoms of alkalosis. Respirations are depressed as a compensatory action by the lungs. Atrial tachycardia may occur. As the pH increases to greater than 7.6 and hypokalemia develops, ventricular disturbances may occur. Decreased motility and paralytic ileus may also occur.

Symptoms of chronic metabolic alkalosis are the same as for acute metabolic alkalosis, and as potassium decreases, frequent premature ventricular contractions or U waves are seen on the ECG.

Evaluation of ABG reveals a pH greater than 7.45 and a serum bicarbonate concentration greater than 26 mEq/L. The $PaCO_2$ increases as the lungs attempt to compensate for the excess bicarbonate by retaining CO_2. This hypoventilation is more pronounced in semiconscious, unconscious, or debilitated patients than in alert patients. The former may develop marked hypoxemia as a result of hypoventilation. Hypokalemia and hypocalcemia are expected.

Medical and Nursing Management

Treatment of metabolic alkalosis is aimed at correcting the underlying acid–base disorder. Because of volume depletion from GI loss, the patient's fluid I&O must be monitored carefully.

Sufficient chloride must be supplied for the kidney to absorb sodium with chloride (allowing the excretion of excess bicarbonate). Treatment also includes restoring normal fluid volume by administering sodium chloride fluids (because continued volume depletion serves to maintain the alkalosis). In patients with hypokalemia, potassium is administered as KCl to replace both K^+ and Cl^- losses. Carbonic anhydrase inhibitors are useful in treating metabolic alkalosis in patients who cannot tolerate rapid volume expansion (e.g., patients with heart failure).

CARBONIC ACID IMBALANCES

ACUTE AND CHRONIC RESPIRATORY ACIDOSIS (CARBONIC ACID EXCESS)

Respiratory acidosis is a clinical disorder in which the pH is less than 7.35 and the $PaCO_2$ is greater than 45 mm Hg. It may be either acute or chronic.

Pathophysiology

Respiratory acidosis is always due to inadequate excretion of CO_2 with inadequate ventilation, resulting in elevated plasma CO_2 concentrations and, consequently, increased levels of carbonic acid. Any condition that causes hypoventilation is associated with an elevated $PaCO_2$, and usually a decrease in PaO_2. Acute respiratory acidosis occurs in emergency situations, such as aspiration of a foreign object, atelectasis, diaphragmatic paralysis, overdose of sedatives, sleep apnea syndrome, administration of high-flow oxygen to a patient with chronic hypercapnia (excessive CO_2 in the blood), severe pneumonia, and acute respiratory distress syndrome. Respiratory acidosis can also occur in diseases that impair respiratory muscles, such as muscular dystrophy, myasthenia gravis, and Guillain–Barré syndrome.

Mechanical ventilation may be associated with hypercapnia if the rate of effective alveolar ventilation is inadequate (respiratory rate or tidal volume too low).

In addition, some disorders, such as pulmonary edema and pneumothorax, may initially cause hyperventilation, but as respiratory fatigue develops, the CO_2 level will rise and acidosis will develop. Therefore, the nurse cannot assume that a clinical condition will cause a predicted disturbance. Rather, the nurse considers whether the respiratory center is capable of continuing to exhale the respiratory acid.

Clinical Manifestations and Assessment

Clinical signs in acute and chronic respiratory acidosis vary. Sudden hypercapnia (elevated $PaCO_2$) can cause increased pulse and respiratory rate, mental cloudiness, dull headache, or weakness. An elevated $PaCO_2$ causes cerebrovascular vasodilation and increased cerebral blood flow, particularly when it is greater than 60 mm Hg. Ventricular fibrillation may be the first sign of respiratory acidosis in anesthetized patients.

If respiratory acidosis is severe, intracranial pressure may increase, resulting in papilledema and dilated conjunctival blood vessels. Hyperkalemia may result as the hydrogen concentration overwhelms the compensatory mechanisms and H^+ moves into cells, causing a shift of potassium out of the cell.

Chronic respiratory acidosis occurs with pulmonary diseases such as chronic emphysema and bronchitis, obstructive sleep apnea, and obesity. As long as the $PaCO_2$ does not exceed the body's ability to compensate, the patient will be asymptomatic. However, if the $PaCO_2$ increases rapidly, cerebral vasodilation will increase the intracranial pressure, and cyanosis and tachypnea will develop. Patients with chronic obstructive pulmonary disease (COPD) who gradually accumulate CO_2 over a prolonged period (days to months) may not develop symptoms of hypercapnia because compensatory renal changes have had time to occur.

ABG analysis reveals a pH lower than 7.35, a $PaCO_2$ greater than 45 mm Hg, and a variation in the bicarbonate level, depending on the duration of the acute respiratory acidosis. When compensation (renal retention of bicarbonate) has fully occurred, the arterial pH may be within the lower limits of normal. Depending on the cause of respiratory acidosis, other diagnostic measures would include monitoring of serum electrolyte levels, chest x-ray for determining any respiratory disease, and a drug screen if an overdose is suspected. An ECG to identify any cardiac arrhythmias may be indicated.

Medical and Nursing Management

Treatment is directed at treating the cause of the hypoventilation; exact measures vary with the cause of inadequate ventilation. Pharmacologic agents are used as indicated. For example, bronchodilators help reduce bronchial spasm, antibiotics are used for respiratory infections, and thrombolytics or anticoagulants are used for pulmonary emboli.

Pulmonary hygiene measures are initiated, when necessary, to clear the respiratory tract of mucus and purulent drainage. Adequate hydration (2 to 3 L/day) is indicated to keep the mucous membranes moist and thereby facilitate the removal of secretions as long as not contraindicated by cardiac, liver, or kidney disease. Supplemental oxygen is administered as necessary.

> **Nursing Alert**
> *If the $PaCO_2$ is chronically higher than 50 mm Hg, the respiratory center becomes relatively insensitive to CO_2 as a respiratory stimulant, leaving hypoxemia as the major drive for respiration. Oxygen administration may remove the stimulus of hypoxemia, and the patient develops "carbon dioxide narcosis" unless the situation is quickly reversed. Additional reasons for the increased CO_2, beyond oxygen administration, include oxygen administration increases the release of CO_2 from hemoglobin (which would cause the CO_2 to rise), or pulmonary arteriolar vasodilation increases perfusion to poorly ventilated alveoli with O_2 administration, causing a rise in the CO_2 (Effros & Swenson, 2015; Reid & Innes, 2014). While the exact etiology has not been elucidated for carbon dioxide narcosis, it is prudent to administer the amount of oxygen necessary to improve the patient's oxygen saturation to approximately 90%. Typically low flow oxygen (24% or 28% or 1–2 L/min) is administered; however, oxygen administration may need to be above this level. Therefore, the nurse recognizes that failure to achieve appropriate oxygenation is an indication for assisted ventilation.*

Mechanical ventilation may be required to improve pulmonary ventilation. Inappropriate mechanical ventilation (e.g., increased dead space, insufficient rate or volume settings, high fraction of inspired oxygen [FiO_2] with excessive CO_2 production) must be corrected with appropriate changes to the ventilator setting. Proper patient positioning in a semi-Fowler position facilitates expansion of the chest wall.

ACUTE AND CHRONIC RESPIRATORY ALKALOSIS (CARBONIC ACID DEFICIT)

Respiratory alkalosis is a clinical condition in which the arterial pH is greater than 7.45 and the $PaCO_2$ is less than 35 mm Hg. As with respiratory acidosis, acute and chronic conditions can occur.

Pathophysiology

Respiratory alkalosis is always caused by hyperventilation, which causes excessive "blowing off" of CO_2 and, hence, a decrease in the plasma carbonic acid concentration. Causes of respiratory alkalosis can include extreme anxiety, hypoxemia, the early phase of salicylate intoxication (since the medulla is directly stimulated by the drug and the respiratory rate increases), high fever, gram-negative bacteremia, or inappropriate ventilator settings that do not match the patient's requirements. Acute exposure to a high altitude also can result in a hypoxia-induced hyperventilation, which can take several days before the patient is fully adapted.

Chronic respiratory alkalosis results from chronic hypocapnia, and decreased serum bicarbonate levels are the consequence. Chronic hepatic insufficiency and cerebral tumors are predisposing factors.

Clinical Manifestations and Assessment

Clinical signs consist of lightheadedness due to vasoconstriction and decreased cerebral blood flow, inability to concentrate, numbness and tingling from decreased calcium ionization, tinnitus, and, sometimes, loss of consciousness. Recall that cerebral blood flow is significantly decreased by hypocapnia, which is a potent vasoconstrictor; thus many of the clinical manifestations of respiratory alkalosis are related to the CNS and reduced free calcium. Cardiac effects of respiratory alkalosis include tachycardia and ventricular and atrial arrhythmias.

Analysis of ABG reveals an elevated pH (greater than 7.45) as a result of a low $PaCO_2$ (less than 35 mm Hg) and a normal bicarbonate level. (The kidneys cannot alter the bicarbonate level quickly; it will take up to 3 days for compensation to occur). The response of the kidneys will be to reduce hydrogen ion excretion (holding on to acids to maintain the 20:1 relationship) and increase bicarbonate excretion. In the compensated state, the kidneys have had sufficient time to lower the bicarbonate level to a near-normal level. Evaluation of serum electrolytes is indicated to identify a decrease in potassium as hydrogen is pulled out of the cells in exchange for potassium. As the blood pH rises and blood becomes more alkaline, proteins such as albumin become more negatively charged causing a higher affinity for binding with free calcium in the bloodstream. As a result, the ionized portion of calcium decreases, thus symptoms of carpopedal spasms and tetany occur. A toxicology screen should be performed to rule out salicylate intoxication.

Patients with chronic respiratory alkalosis are usually asymptomatic, and the diagnostic evaluation and plan of care are the same as for acute respiratory alkalosis.

Medical and Nursing Management

Treatment depends on the underlying cause of respiratory alkalosis. If the cause is anxiety, the patient is instructed to breathe more slowly to allow CO_2 to accumulate. A sedative may be required to relieve hyperventilation in very anxious patients. Treatment of other causes of respiratory alkalosis is directed at correcting the underlying problem.

MIXED ACID–BASE DISORDERS

Patients can simultaneously experience two or more independent acid–base disorders. A normal pH in the presence of changes in the $PaCO_2$ and plasma HCO_3^- concentration immediately suggests a mixed disorder. The only mixed disorder that cannot occur is a mixed respiratory acidosis and alkalosis because it is impossible to have alveolar hypoventilation and hyperventilation at the same time. An example of a mixed disorder is the simultaneous occurrence of metabolic acidosis and respiratory acidosis during respiratory and cardiac arrest.

Compensation

Generally, the pulmonary and renal systems compensate for each other to return the pH to normal. In a single acid–base disorder, the system not causing the problem will try to compensate by returning the ratio of bicarbonate to carbonic acid to the normal 20:1. The lungs compensate for metabolic disturbances by changing CO_2 excretion. The kidneys compensate for respiratory disturbances by altering bicarbonate retention and H^+ secretion.

In respiratory acidosis, excess hydrogen is excreted in the urine, and bicarbonate is retained. In respiratory alkalosis, the renal excretion of bicarbonate increases, and hydrogen ions are retained. In metabolic acidosis, the compensatory mechanisms increase the ventilation rate; in metabolic alkalosis, the respiratory system compensates by decreasing ventilation to conserve CO_2 and increase the $PaCO_2$. Because the lungs respond to acid–base disorders within minutes, compensation for metabolic imbalances occurs faster than does compensation for respiratory imbalances. Table 4-4 summarizes compensation effects.

Blood Gas Analysis

Blood gas analysis is often used to identify the specific acid–base disturbance and the degree of compensation that has occurred (see Boxes 4-1 and 4-2). The analysis is usually based on an arterial blood sample, but if an arterial sample cannot be obtained, a mixed venous sample may be used. Results of ABG analysis provide information about alveolar ventilation, oxygenation, and acid–base balance. The health history, physical examination, previous blood gas results, and serum electrolytes should always be part of the assessment used to determine the cause of the acid–base disorder. Before obtaining an ABG from the radial artery, the nurse assesses patency of the ulnar artery by performing the Allen test (refer to Chapter 12). Treatment of the underlying condition

TABLE 4-4 Acid–Base Disturbances and Compensation

Disorder	Initial Event	Compensation
Respiratory acidosis	↓ pH, ↑ or normal HCO_3^-, ↑ $PaCO_2$	↑ Renal acid excretion and ↑ serum HCO_3^-
Respiratory alkalosis	↑ pH, ↓ or normal HCO_3^-, ↓ $PaCO_2$	↓ Renal acid excretion and ↓ serum HCO_3^-
Metabolic acidosis	↓ pH, ↓ HCO_3^-, ↓ $PaCO_2$	Hyperventilation with resulting ↓ $PaCO_2$
Metabolic alkalosis	↑ pH, ↑ HCO_3^-, ↑ $PaCO_2$	Hypoventilation with resulting ↑ $PaCO_2$

usually corrects most acid–base disorders. Table 4-5 compares normal ranges of venous and ABG values.

PARENTERAL FLUID THERAPY

When no other route of administration is available, fluids are administered intravenously in hospitals, outpatient diagnostic and surgical settings, clinics, and homes to replace fluids, administer medications, and provide nutrients. Typical indications for giving a fluid bolus include hypotension, low urine output, and inadequate cardiac output for tissue needs (Rewa & Bagshaw, 2015).

Purpose

The choice of an IV solution depends on the purpose of its administration. Generally, IV fluids are administered to achieve one or more of the following goals:

BOX 4-1 Assessing Arterial Blood Gases

The following steps are recommended to evaluate arterial blood gas (ABG) values. They are based on the assumption that the average values are:

pH = 7.4
$PaCO_2$ = 40 mm Hg (normal 35 to 45 mm Hg)
HCO_3^- = 24 mEq/L (normal 22 to 26 mEq/L)

First, note the pH. It can be high, low, or normal, as follows:

pH greater than 7.4 (alkalosis)
pH less than 7.4 (acidosis)
pH equal to 7.4 (normal)

A normal pH may indicate perfectly normal blood gases, *or* it may be an indication of a *compensated* imbalance. A compensated imbalance is one in which the body has been able to correct the pH by either respiratory or metabolic changes (depending on the primary problem). For example, a patient with primary metabolic acidosis starts out with a low bicarbonate level but a normal CO_2 level. Soon afterward, the lungs try to compensate for the imbalance by exhaling large amounts of CO_2 (hyperventilation). As another example, a patient with primary respiratory acidosis starts out with a high CO_2 level; soon afterward, the kidneys attempt to compensate by retaining bicarbonate. If the compensatory mechanism is able to restore the bicarbonate to carbonic acid ratio back to 20:1, full compensation (and thus normal pH) will be achieved.

The next step is to determine the primary cause of the disturbance. This is done by evaluating the $PaCO_2$ and HCO_3^- in relation to the pH.

Example: pH greater than 7.4 (alkalosis)

a. If the $PaCO_2$ is less than 35 mm Hg, the primary disturbance is respiratory alkalosis. (This situation occurs when a patient hyperventilates and "blows off" too much CO_2. Recall that CO_2 dissolved in water becomes carbonic acid, the acid side of the "carbonic acid–bicarbonate buffer system.")

b. If the HCO_3^- is greater than 26 mEq/L, the primary disturbance is metabolic alkalosis. (This situation occurs when the body gains too much bicarbonate, an alkaline substance. Bicarbonate is the basic or alkaline side of the "carbonic acid–bicarbonate buffer system.")

Example: pH less than 7.4 (acidosis)

a. If the $PaCO_2$ is greater than 45 mm Hg, the primary disturbance is respiratory acidosis. (This situation occurs when a patient hypoventilates and thus retains too much CO_2, an acidic substance.)

b. If the HCO_3^- is less than 22 mEq/L, the primary disturbance is metabolic acidosis. (This situation occurs when the body's bicarbonate level drops, either because of direct bicarbonate loss or because of gains of acids such as lactic acid or ketones.)

The next step involves determining if compensation has begun. This is done by looking at the value other than the primary disorder. If it is moving in the same direction as the primary value, compensation is under way. Consider the following gases:

pH	$PaCO_2$	HCO_3^-
(1) 7.2	60 mm Hg	24 mEq/L
(2) 7.4	60 mm Hg	37 mEq/L

The first set (1) indicates acute respiratory acidosis without compensation (the $PaCO_2$ is high, the HCO_3^- is normal). The second set (2) indicates chronic respiratory acidosis. Note that compensation has taken place; that is, the HCO_3^- has elevated to an appropriate level to balance the high $PaCO_2$ and produce a normal pH.

Two distinct acid–base disturbances may occur simultaneously. These can be identified when the pH does not explain one of the changes.

Example: Metabolic and respiratory acidosis

a. pH	7.2 decreased acid
b. $PaCO_2$	52 increased acid
c. HCO_3	13 decreased acid

This is an example of metabolic and respiratory acidosis.

BOX 4-2

Nursing Research

Bridging the Gap to Evidence-Based Practice

Guérin, L., Teboul, J., Persichini, R., Dres, M., Richard, C., & Monnet, X. (2015). Effects of passive leg raising and volume expansion on mean systemic pressure and venous return in shock in humans, *Critical Care*, 19, 411.

Purpose

The aim of this study was to assess how mean systemic pressure and resistance to venous return (RVR) behave during passive leg raising (PLR) in cases of fluid responsiveness and fluid unresponsiveness.

Design

In 30 patients with an acute circulatory failure, in order to estimate the venous return curve, the authors constructed the regression line between pairs of cardiac index (CI) and central venous pressure (CVP). Values were measured during end-inspiratory and end-expiratory ventilatory occlusions performed at two levels of positive end-expiratory pressure. The x-axis intercept was used to estimate the mean systemic pressure and the inverse of the slope to quantify RVR. These measurements were obtained at baseline, during PLR, and after fluid infusion. Patients in whom fluid infusion increased CI by more than 15% were defined as "fluid-responders."

Findings

In fluid-responders (n = 15), CVP and mean systemic pressure significantly increased (from 7 ± 3 to 9 ± 4 mm Hg and from 25 ± 13 to 31 ± 13 mm Hg, respectively) during PLR. The mean systemic pressure -CVP gradient significantly increased by 20% to 30% while RVR did not change significantly during PLR. In fluid-nonresponders, CVP and mean systemic pressure increased significantly, but the mean systemic pressure -CVP gradient did not change significantly during PLR. PLR did not change the intra-abdominal pressure in the whole population (14 ± 6 mm Hg before vs. 13 ± 5 mm Hg during PLR, p = 0.26) and in patients with intra-abdominal hypertension at baseline (17 ± 4 mm Hg before vs. 16 ± 4 mm Hg during PLR, p = 0.14). In the latter group, PLR increased mean systemic pressure from 22 ± 11 to 27 ± 10 mm Hg (p < 0.01) and did not change RVR (5.1 ± 2.6 to 5.2 ± 3 mm Hg/min/m^2/mL, p = 0.71). In fluid-responders, mean systemic pressure, CVP and the mean systemic pressure -CVP gradient significantly increased during fluid infusion while the RVR did not change. In fluid-nonresponders, CVP and mean systemic pressure increased significantly during fluid infusion while the mean systemic pressure -CVP gradient and RVR did not change.

Nursing Implications

Passive leg raising (PLR) significantly increased mean systemic pressure and central venous pressure (CVP), confirming that it represents a powerful preload challenge without modifying resistance to venous return. In acute circulatory failure, PLR is a test that predicts whether cardiac output will increase with volume expansion by transferring a volume of around 300 mL of venous blood from the lower body toward the right side of the heart. There are specific rules: the head of the bed should be 45 degrees to begin. PLR should start from the semi-recumbent since trunk lowering and leg raising should mobilize venous blood from the large splanchnic compartment, thus magnifying the increasing effects of leg elevation on cardiac preload and increasing the test's sensitivity. The nurse should follow institutional protocols on PLR as this represents a potential test that will mimic a fluid challenge but has the advantage of having no fluid infused and being rapidly reversible (by lowering the extremities), thereby avoiding the risks of fluid overload (Monnet & Teboul, 2015).

- To provide water, electrolytes, and/or nutrients to meet daily requirements;
- To replace water and correct electrolyte deficits;
- To administer medications and blood products.

IV solutions contain dextrose or electrolytes mixed in various proportions with water. Pure, electrolyte-free water can never be administered IV because it enters RBCs rapidly and causes them to rupture.

Types of IV Solutions

Crystalloid solutions are often categorized as **isotonic**, **hypotonic**, or **hypertonic**, according to whether their total osmolality is the same as, less than, or greater than that of plasma (see earlier discussion of osmolality). Crystalloid fluids generally contain three basic components: water, electrolytes, and sugar (dextrose).

Electrolyte solutions are considered isotonic if the total electrolyte content (anions + cations) is approximately 310 mEq/L, hypotonic if the total electrolyte content is less than 250 mEq/L, and hypertonic if the total electrolyte content is greater than 375 mEq/L. The nurse must also consider a solution's osmolality, keeping in mind that the osmolality of plasma is approximately 300 mOsm/L (300 mmol/L). For example, a 10% dextrose solution has an osmolality of approximately 505 mOsm/L.

TABLE **4-5** Normal Values for Arterial and Mixed Venous Blood

Parameter	Arterial Blood	Mixed Venous Blood
pH	7.35–7.45	7.33–7.41
PaCO$_2$	35–45 mm Hg	41–51 mm Hg
PaO$_2$[a]	80–100 mm Hg	35–40 mm Hg
HCO$_3^-$	22–26 mEq/L	22–26 mEq/L
Base excess/deficit	±2 mEq/L	±2 mEq/L
Oxygen saturation	over 94%	75%

[a]At altitudes of 3,000 feet and higher, the values for oxygen are decreased.

When administering parenteral fluids, the nurse monitors the patient's response to the fluids, considering the fluid volume, the content of the fluid, and the patient's clinical status. Some fluids may actually initiate an inflammatory process within the body, especially when overused in patients with hemorrhage shock (Horeczko, Green, & Panacek, 2014). Refer to Table 4-6 for various IV solutions.

Nursing Alert

When administering fluids to patients with cardiovascular disease, the nurse assesses for signs of circulatory overload (e.g., cough, dyspnea, puffy eyelids, dependent edema, weight gain in 24 hours). The lungs are auscultated for crackles. Extreme care is taken when administering highly

TABLE 4-6 Selected Water and Electrolyte Solutions

Solution	Comments
Isotonic Solutions 0.9% NaCl (isotonic, also called normal saline [NS]) Na^+ 154 mEq/L Cl^- 154 mEq/L (308 mOsm/L) Also available with varying concentrations of dextrose (the most frequently used is a 5% dextrose concentration)	• An isotonic solution that expands the ECF volume • Used in hypovolemic states, resuscitative efforts, shock, diabetic ketoacidosis, metabolic alkalosis, hypercalcemia, mild Na^+ deficit • Supplies an excess of Na^+ and Cl^-; can cause FVE and hyperchloremic acidosis if used in excessive volumes, particularly in patients with compromised kidney function, heart failure, or edema • Not desirable as a routine maintenance solution as it provides only Na^+ and Cl^- (and these are provided in excessive amounts) • When mixed with 5% dextrose, the resulting solution becomes hypertonic in relation to plasma and, in addition to the above described electrolytes, provides 170 cal/L • Only solution that may be administered with blood products
Lactated Ringer solution Na^+ 130 mEq/L K^+ 4 mEq/L Ca^{+2} 3 mEq/L Cl^- 109 mEq/L Lactate (metabolized to bicarbonate) 28 mEq/L (274 mOsm/L) Also available with varying concentrations of dextrose (the most common is 5% dextrose)	• An isotonic solution that contains multiple electrolytes in roughly the same concentration as found in plasma (note that solution is lacking in Mg^{+2}): provides 9 cal/L • Used in the treatment of hypovolemia, burns, fluid lost as bile or diarrhea, and for acute blood loss replacement • Lactate is rapidly metabolized into HCO_3^- in the body. Lactated Ringer solution should not be used in lactic acidosis because the ability to convert lactate into HCO_3^- is impaired in this disorder • Not to be given with a pH over 7.5 because bicarbonate is formed as lactate breaks down, causing alkalosis • Should not be used in kidney failure (because it contains potassium and can cause hyperkalemia) or in liver disease (due to altered lactate metabolism) • Similar to plasma
5% dextrose in water (D_5W) No electrolytes 50 g of dextrose	• Initially an isotonic solution, once the dextrose is metabolized it becomes a hypotonic solution that supplies 170 cal/L and free water to aid in renal excretion of solutes • Used in treatment of hypernatremia, fluid loss, and dehydration • Should not be used in excessive volumes in the early postoperative period (when antidiuretic hormone secretion is increased due to stress reaction) • Should not be used solely in treatment of FVD because it dilutes plasma electrolyte concentrations • Contraindicated in head injury because it may cause increased intracranial pressure • Should not be used for fluid resuscitation because it can cause hyperglycemia and will not expand the IVS • Should be used with caution in patients with kidney or cardiac disease because of risk of fluid overload • Electrolyte-free solutions may cause peripheral circulatory collapse, anuria in patients with sodium deficiency, and increased body fluid loss • Over time, D_5W without NaCl can cause water intoxication (ICF volume excess [FVE]) because the solution is hypotonic
Hypotonic Solutions 0.45% NaCl (half-strength saline) Na^+ 77 mEq/L Cl^- 77 mEq/L (154 mOsm/L) Also available with varying concentrations of dextrose (the most common is a 5% concentration)	• Provides Na^+, Cl^-, and free water • Free water is desirable to aid the kidneys in elimination of solute • Lacking in electrolytes other than Na^+ and Cl^- • When mixed with 5% dextrose, the solution becomes slightly hypertonic to plasma and, in addition to the above-described electrolytes, provides 170 cal/L • Used to treat hypertonic dehydration, Na^+ and Cl^- depletion, and gastric fluid loss • Not indicated for third-space fluid shifts or increased intracranial pressure • Administer cautiously because it can cause fluid shifts from vascular system into cells, resulting in cardiovascular collapse and increased intracranial pressure.

(continued on page 94)

TABLE **4-6** Selected Water and Electrolyte Solutions (*continued*)

Solution	Comments
Hypertonic Solutions 3% NaCl (hypertonic saline) Na^+ 513 mEq/L Cl^- 513 mEq/L (1,026 mOsm/L)	• Used to increase ECF volume, decrease cellular swelling • Highly hypertonic solution used only in critical situations to treat hyponatremia • Must be administered slowly and cautiously because it can cause intravascular volume overload and pulmonary edema • Supplies no calories • Assists in removing ICF excess
5% NaCl (hypertonic solution) Na^+ 855 mEq/L Cl^- 855 mEq/L (1710 mOsm/L)	• Highly hypertonic solution used to treat symptomatic hyponatremia • Administered slowly and cautiously because it can cause intravascular volume overload and pulmonary edema • Supplies no calories
Colloid Solutions Dextran in NS or 5% D_5W Available in low-molecular-weight (Dextran 40) and high-molecular-weight (Dextran 70) forms	• Colloid solution used as volume/plasma expander for intravascular part of ECF • Affects clotting by coating platelets and decreasing ability to clot • Remains in circulatory system up to 24 hours • Used to treat hypovolemia in early shock to increase pulse pressure, cardiac output, and arterial blood pressure • Improves microcirculation by decreasing RBC aggregation • Contraindicated in hemorrhage, thrombocytopenia, kidney disease, and severe dehydration • Not a substitute for blood or blood products

hypertonic sodium fluids (e.g., 3% or 5% sodium chloride) because these fluids can be lethal if infused carelessly.

Isotonic Fluids

Isotonic fluids have a total osmolality close to that of the ECF and do not cause RBCs to shrink or swell. The composition of these fluids may or may not approximate that of the ECF. Isotonic fluids expand the ECF volume. One liter of isotonic fluid expands the ECF by 1 L; however, it expands the plasma by only 0.25 L because it is a crystalloid fluid and diffuses quickly into the ECF compartment. In patients hospitalized for shock, as much as 20 to 40 mL/kg of isotonic fluid boluses may be required initially to maintain renal perfusion. However, since these fluids expand the IVS, patients with hypertension and heart failure should be monitored carefully for signs of fluid overload.

D_5W

A solution of D_5W has a serum osmolality of 252 mOsm/L. Once administered, the glucose is metabolized rapidly, and this initially isotonic solution then disperses as a hypotonic fluid, one third extracellular and two thirds intracellular. It is essential to consider this action of D_5W, especially if the patient is at risk for ICP. During fluid resuscitation, this solution should not be used because of its limited ability to expand the intravascular volume. Therefore, D_5W is used mainly to supply water and to correct an increased serum osmolality. About 1 L of D_5W provides fewer than 200 kcal and is a minor source of the body's daily caloric requirements.

Normal Saline Solution

Normal saline (0.9% sodium chloride) solution has a total osmolality of 308 mOsm/L. Because the osmolality is contributed entirely by electrolytes, the solution remains within the ECF. For this reason, normal saline solution is often used to correct an extracellular volume deficit. Normal saline contains only sodium and chloride and does not actually simulate the ECF. It is used with administration of blood transfusions and to replace large sodium losses, as in burn injuries. It is not used for heart failure, pulmonary edema, kidney impairment, or sodium retention. Normal saline does not supply calories. Historically, in patients with trauma or penetrating injury, initial treatment consisted of large amounts of isotonic saline administration to maintain a systolic blood pressure greater than 90 mm Hg. Hemorrhage can also begin a process of coagulopathy, acidosis, and hypothermia within the body, necessitating a decision for light versus aggressive parenteral fluid administration (Rewa & Bagshaw, 2015).

Other Isotonic Solutions

Several other solutions contain ions in addition to sodium and chloride and are somewhat similar to the ECF in composition. Lactated Ringer solution contains potassium and calcium in addition to sodium and chloride and can be used to correct dehydration and sodium depletion or to replace GI losses. Lactated Ringer solution contains bicarbonate precursors as well. Lactated Ringer is typically not used in patients with severe acidosis or in advanced liver disease, which can affect lactate metabolism.

Hypotonic Fluids

One purpose of hypotonic solutions is to replace cellular fluid. Another is to provide free water for excretion of body wastes. At times, hypotonic sodium solutions are used to treat hypernatremia and other hyperosmolar conditions. Half-strength saline (0.45% sodium chloride) solution, with an osmolality of 154 mOsm/L, is frequently used. Multiple-electrolyte solutions are also available. Excessive infusions of hypotonic solutions can lead to intravascular fluid depletion by causing a fluid shift from blood vessels to cells, resulting in decreased blood pressure, cellular edema, and cell damage. These solutions exert less osmotic pressure than the ECF.

Hypertonic Fluids

When normal saline solution or lactated Ringer solution contains 5% dextrose, the total osmolality exceeds that of the ECF. However, the dextrose is quickly metabolized, and only the isotonic solution remains. Therefore, any effect on the intracellular compartment is temporary.

Higher concentrations of dextrose, such as 50% dextrose in water, are administered to help meet caloric requirements or to treat hypoglycemia in the NPO patient. These solutions are strongly hypertonic and must be administered into central veins so that they can be diluted by rapid blood flow.

Saline solutions are also available in osmolar concentrations greater than that of the ECF. These solutions draw water from the ICF to the ECF and cause cells to shrink. If administered rapidly or in large quantity, they may cause an extracellular volume excess and precipitate circulatory overload. As a result, these solutions must be administered cautiously and usually only when the serum osmolality has decreased to dangerously low levels. Hypertonic solutions exert an osmotic pressure greater than that of the ECF.

Nursing Alert

Highly hypertonic sodium solutions (3% and 5% sodium chloride) should be administered only in intensive care settings under close observation because only small volumes are needed to elevate the serum sodium concentration. These fluids are administered slowly and in small volumes, and the patient is monitored closely for fluid overload. Frequent checks of the patient's electrolyte panel are warranted. The purpose is to relieve acute manifestations of cerebral edema and to prevent neurologic complications rather than to specifically correct the sodium concentration. Along with the sodium solution, the patient may receive a loop diuretic to prevent ECF volume overload and to increase water excretion.

Other IV Substances

When the patient's GI tract is unable to tolerate food, nutritional requirements are often met using the IV route. Parenteral solutions may include high concentrations of glucose, protein, or fat to meet nutritional requirements (see Chapter 22). The parenteral route may also be used to administer colloids, plasma expanders, and blood products including packed RBCs, fresh frozen plasma, and platelets.

Many medications are also delivered by the IV route, either by infusion or directly into the vein. Because IV medications enter the circulation rapidly, administration by this route is potentially very hazardous. While all medications may produce reactions, IV medications are especially dangerous due to the rapid introduction and absorption within the bloodstream. Astute nursing includes knowledge of the administration rates and recommended dilutions for any medication given.

Nursing Management of the Patient Receiving IV Therapy

The ability to perform venipuncture to gain access to the venous system for administering fluids and medication is an expected nursing skill in many settings. This responsibility includes selecting the appropriate venipuncture site and type of cannula and being proficient in the technique of vein entry. This skill should be mastered by all bedside nurses, and it is up to each individual nurse to seek out the opportunity to learn and practice venipuncture.

Preparing to Administer IV Therapy

Before performing venipuncture, the nurse performs hand hygiene, applies gloves, and informs the patient about the procedure. Next, the nurse selects the most appropriate insertion site and type of cannula for a particular patient. See Box 4-3 for the factors that influence these choices. Some institutions have organized specialized "IV therapy" teams who assist in IV placement and management.

Choosing an IV Site

Veins of the extremities are designated as peripheral locations and are ordinarily the only sites used by nurses. Because they are relatively safe and easy to enter, arm veins are most commonly used (Fig. 4-8). The metacarpal, cephalic, basilic,

---

BOX 4-3   **Factors in Selecting a Venipuncture Site**

The following factors should be considered when selecting a site for venipuncture:
- Condition of the vein
- Type of fluid or medication to be infused
- Duration of therapy
- Patient's age and size
- Whether the patient is right- or left-handed
- Patient's medical history and current health status
- Skill of the person performing the venipuncture

Anterior (palmar) view | Posterior (dorsal) view

Labels: Cephalic vein, Accessory cephalic vein, Perforating vein, Cephalic vein, Intermediate antebrachial vein, Palmar digital veins, Basilic vein, Median cubital vein, Dorsal metacarpal veins, Cephalic vein, Basilic vein, Dorsal venous arch, Dorsal digital veins

FIGURE 4-8 Site selection for peripheral cannulation of veins: anterior (palmar) veins at left, posterior (dorsal) veins at right. (Adapted from Agur, A. M. R., Lee, M. J., & Boileau Grant, M. J. (1999). *Grant's atlas of anatomy* (10th ed.). Philadelphia, PA: Lippincott Williams & Wilkins.)

and median veins and their branches are recommended sites because of their size and ease of access. More distal sites should be used first, with more proximal sites used subsequently. Leg veins should rarely, if ever, be used because of the high risk of thromboembolism. Additional sites to avoid include veins distal to a previous IV infiltration or phlebitic area, sclerosed or thrombosed veins, an arm with an arteriovenous shunt or fistula, and an arm affected by edema, infection, blood clot, or skin breakdown.

> **Nursing Alert**
> *Due to the interruption in the lymphatic system in patients who have had a mastectomy or lymph node removal, blood pressure measurements (both manual and automatic) or IV therapy placement should not occur on the same side. Performing either of these procedures on the affected arm can cause fluid to back up in the arm, and lymphedema (accumulation of lymph fluid) can develop. This is a painful condition that also increases the risk of infection to the patient.*

Central veins commonly used by physicians and trained advanced practice providers include the subclavian and

internal jugular veins. It is possible to gain access to (or cannulate) these larger vessels even when peripheral sites have collapsed, and they allow for the administration of hyperosmolar solutions and vasoconstrictive drugs. However, the potential hazards are much greater and include inadvertent entry into an artery or the pleural space, as well as a higher risk of infection.

Ideally, both arms and hands are carefully inspected before choosing a specific venipuncture site that does not interfere with mobility. For this reason, the antecubital fossa is avoided, except as a last resort. The most distal site of the arm or hand is generally used first so that subsequent IV access sites can be moved progressively upward. Refer back to Box 4-3 for factors to consider in selecting an IV site.

After applying a tourniquet, the nurse palpates and inspects the vein. The tourniquet remains applied for a maximum of 3 minutes before the tension must be released. The vein should feel firm, elastic, engorged, and round—not hard, flat, or bumpy. Because arteries lie close to veins in the antecubital fossa, the vessel should be palpated for arterial pulsation (even with a tourniquet on), and cannulation of pulsating vessels should be avoided.

Using Venipuncture Devices

Cannulas. Most peripheral access devices are cannulas. "Catheter" and "cannula" are terms that are used interchangeably. General guidelines for selecting a cannula include the following:

- Length: 0.75 to 1.25 in long
- Diameter: Narrow diameter of the cannula to occupy minimal space within the vein
- Gauge: 20 to 22 gauge for most IV fluids; a larger gauge for caustic or viscous solutions; 14 to 18 gauge preferred for trauma patients and those undergoing surgery; and blood administration can now safely use as small as a 24-gauge needle (Infusion Nurses Society, 2011).

Cannulas have an obturator inside a tube that is later removed. The main types of cannula devices available are those referred to as winged infusion sets (butterfly) with a steel needle or as over-the-needle catheters with wings; indwelling plastic cannulas that are inserted over a steel needle; and indwelling plastic cannulas that are inserted through a steel needle. Scalp vein or butterfly needles are short steel needles with plastic wing handles. These are easy to insert, but because they are small and nonpliable, infiltration occurs easily. The use of these needles should be limited to obtaining blood specimens and not for IV medications because they increase the risk of vein injury and infiltration.

Plastic cannulas inserted through a hollow needle are usually called *intracatheters*. They are available in long lengths and are well suited for placement in central locations. Because insertion requires threading the cannula through the vein for a relatively long distance, these can be difficult to insert. The most commonly used infusion device is the over-the-needle catheter. A hollow metal stylet is pre-inserted into the catheter and extends through the distal tip of the catheter to allow puncture of the vessel in an effort to guide the catheter as the venipuncture is performed. The vein is punctured and a flashback of blood appears in the closed chamber behind the catheter hub. Once the flash-back has occurred, the catheter is threaded through the stylet into the vein, and then the stylet is removed. All insti-tutions should carry safety over-the-needle catheter designs with retracting stylets to protect health care workers from needlestick injuries.

Many types of cannulas are available for IV therapy. Some of the variations in these cannulas include the thick-ness of the cannula wall (affects rate of flow), the sharpness of the insertion needles (determines needle insertion tech-nique), the softening properties of the cannula (influences the length of time the cannula can remain in place), safety features (minimizes risk of needlestick injuries and blood-borne exposure), and the number of lumens (determines the number of solutions that can be infused simultaneously).

Needleless IV Delivery Systems. The federal Needlestick Safety and Prevention Act, which was signed into law in November 2000, requires needleless systems in an effort to decrease needlestick injuries and exposure to HIV, hepati-tis, and other blood-borne pathogens. These systems have built-in protection against needlestick injuries and provide a safe means of using and disposing of an IV administration set (which consists of tubing, an area for inserting the tubing into the container of IV fluid, and an adapter for connect-ing the tubing to the needle). Numerous companies produce needleless components. IV line connectors allow the simul-taneous infusion of IV medications and other intermittent medications (known as a *piggyback delivery*) without the use of needles. Technology is advancing and moving away from use of the traditional stylet. Many examples of these devices are on the market. Each institution must evaluate products to determine its own needs based on Occupational Safety and Health Administration (OSHA) guidelines and the institu-tion's policies and procedures.

Peripherally Inserted Central Catheter or Peripheral-Midline Catheter Access Lines. Patients who need moderate- to long-term parenteral therapy often receive a peripherally inserted central catheter (PICC or PIC line) or a peripheral-midline catheter. These catheters are also used for patients with limited peripheral access who require IV antibiotics, blood, vasopressors, or parenteral nutrition. For these devices to be used, the median cephalic, basilic, and cephalic veins must be patent and undamaged. Typically insertion of these catheters is performed by specialized nurses who are trained in the use of them as well as in the use of ultrasonography (which is used to visualize the vein to be cannulized).

If these veins are damaged, then central venous access via the subclavian or internal jugular vein, or surgical placement of an implanted port or a vascular access device, must be considered as an alternative. Table 4-7 compares peripher-ally inserted central and peripheral-midline catheters.

The provider prescribes the line and the solution to be infused. Insertion of either catheter requires sterile tech-nique. The size of the catheter lumen chosen is based on the type of solution, the patient's body size, and the vein to be used. The patient's consent is obtained before use of these catheters. Use of the dominant arm is recommended as the site for inserting the cannula into the superior vena cava to ensure adequate arm movement, which encourages blood flow and reduces the risk of dependent edema or emboli formation. Contraindications to arm choice include prior mastectomy, pacemaker placement, hemiparesis, and dialysis shunt. Review each institution's policy regarding PICC lines for further contraindications.

Teaching the Patient

Except in emergency situations, a patient should be pre-pared in advance for an IV infusion. The venipuncture, the expected length of infusion, and activity restrictions are explained. Then, the patient should have an opportunity to ask questions and express concerns. For example, some patients believe that they will die if small bubbles in the tub-ing enter their veins. After acknowledging this fear, the nurse can explain that usually only relatively large volumes of air administered rapidly are dangerous.

Preparing the IV Site

Before preparing the skin, the nurse should ask the patient whether he or she is allergic to latex or iodine, products commonly used in preparing for IV therapy. Excessive hair at the selected site may be removed by clipping to increase the visibility of the veins and to facilitate insertion of the cannula and adherence of dressings to the IV insertion site. Shaving should not be performed due to increased risk of infection.

Because infection can be a major complication of IV therapy, the IV device, the fluid, the container, and the tub-ing must be sterile. The insertion site is scrubbed with a sterile pad soaked in 10% povidone–iodine (Betadine) or chlorhexidine gluconate solution for 30 seconds, work-ing in a circular motion from the center of the area to the periphery and allowing the area to air dry for approximately 2 minutes. The site should not be wiped with 70% alcohol because the alcohol negates the effect of the disinfecting solution. (Alcohol pledgets are used for 30 seconds instead, only if the patient is allergic to iodine.) The nurse must per-form hand hygiene and put on gloves. Gloves (nonsterile, disposable) must be worn during the venipuncture proce-dure because of the likelihood of coming into contact with the patient's blood.

TABLE **4-7** Comparison of Peripherally Inserted Central and Peripheral-Midline Catheters

	Peripherally Inserted Central Catheter (PICC)	Peripheral-Midline Catheter
Indications	Parenteral nutrition; IV fluid replacement; administration of chemotherapy agents, analgesics, and antibiotics; removal of blood specimens	Parenteral nutrition; IV fluid replacement; administration of analgesics and antibiotics (no solution or medications with a pH less than 5 or greater than 9 or osmolarity greater than 500 mOsm/L); removal of blood specimens
Features	Single- and double-lumen catheters available 40–60 cm long; gauge variable (16–24 gauge)	Single- and double-lumen catheters available 7.5–20 cm long; gauge variable (16–24 gauge). Can increase two gauges in size as it softens
Material	Radiopaque, polymer (polyurethane), Silastic materials. Flexible.	Silicone, polyurethane, and their derivatives; available impregnated with heparin to ↓ thrombogenicity (radiopaque or clear, with radiopaque strip)
Insertion sites	Venipuncture performed in the antecubital fossa, above or below it into the basilic, cephalic, or axillary veins of the dominant arm. The median basilic is the ideal insertion site.	Venipuncture performed 1½ in above or below the antecubital fossa through the cephalic, basilic, or median cubital vein.
Catheter placement	The tip of the catheter lies in the superior vena cava. The catheter is placed via the basilic or cephalic vein at the antecubital fossa.	Between the antecubital area and the head of the clavicle (tip in axilla region). The tip terminates in the proximal portion of the extremity below the axilla and proximal to central veins and is advanced 3–10 in
Insertion method	Through-the-needle technique, with or without a guide wire, breakaway needle with introducer or cannula with introducer (peel-away sheath). (A peripherally inserted central catheter can also be used as a midline catheter.)	No separate guide wire or introducer is needed. Stiff catheter is passed using the catheter advancement tab.
	Insertion can be accomplished at the bedside using sterile technique. Arm to be used should be positioned in abduction to 90-degree angle. Consent is required	Insertion can be accomplished at the bedside using sterile technique. Arm to be used should be positioned in abduction to 45-degree angle. Consent is required
	Catheter may stay in place for up to 12 months or as long as required without complications	Catheter may stay in place for 2–4 weeks
Potential complications	Malposition, pneumothorax, hemothorax, hydrothorax, arrhythmias, nerve or tendon damage, respiratory distress, catheter embolism, thrombophlebitis, or catheter occlusion. Compared with centrally placed catheters, venipuncture in the antecubital space reduces risk of insertion complications	Thrombosis, phlebitis, air embolism, infection, vascular perforation, bleeding, catheter transection, occlusion
Contraindications	Dermatitis, cellulitis, burns, high fluid volume infusions, rapid bolus injections, hemodialysis, and venous thrombosis. No clamping of this catheter or splinting of the arm permitted. No blood pressure or tourniquets to be used on extremity where PICC is inserted.	Dermatitis, cellulitis, burns, high fluid volume infusions, rapid bolus injection, hemodialysis, and venous thrombosis. No blood pressure or tourniquet to be used on extremity where midline catheter is placed
Catheter maintenance	Sterile dressing changes according to agency policy and procedures. Generally, dressing is changed every 2–3 days or when wet, soiled, or nonocclusive. Line is flushed every shift with 3 mL normal saline followed by 3 mL of heparin (100 U/mL) per lumen. The nurse follows institutional policy for flushing catheter	Sterile dressing changes according to agency policy and procedures. Generally, dressing is changed every 2–3 days or when wet, soiled, or nonocclusive. Line is flushed after each infusion or every shift with 5–10 mL normal saline followed by 1 mL of heparin (100 U/mL). Catheter must be anchored securely to prevent its dislodgment. The nurse follows institutional policy for flushing catheter

	Peripherally Inserted Central Catheter (PICC)	Peripheral-Midline Catheter
Postplacement	Chest x-ray needed to confirm placement of catheter tip	Chest x-ray to assess placement may be obtained if unable to flush catheter, if no free flow blood return, if difficulty with catheter advancement, or if guide wire is difficult to remove or bent on removal
Assessment	Daily measurement of arm circumference (4 in above insertion site) and length of exposed catheter	Daily measurement of arm circumference (4 in above insertion site) and length of exposed catheter
Removal	Catheter should be removed when no longer indicated for use, if contaminated, or if complications occur	Catheter should be removed when no longer indicated for use, if contaminated, or if complications occur
	Arm is abducted during removal. Patient should be in a dorsal recumbent position with head of bed flat and should perform the Valsalva maneuver while catheter is withdrawn	Arm is abducted during removal
	Pressure is applied on removal with a sterile dressing and antiseptic ointment to site. Dressing is changed every 24 hours until epithelialization occurs	Pressure is applied on removal with a sterile dressing and antiseptic ointment to site. Dressing is changed every 24 hours until epithelialization occurs
Advantages	Reduces cost and avoids repeated venipunctures compared with centrally placed catheters. Decreases incidence of catheter-related infections	Reduces cost and avoids repeated venipunctures compared with centrally placed catheters. Decreases incidence of catheter-related infections

Performing Venipuncture

IV therapy initiation is a specialized nursing skill. Institutional policies and procedures determine whether all nurses must be certified to perform venipuncture. A nurse certified in IV therapy or an IV team can be consulted to assist with initiating IV therapy. Refer to each institution's guidelines on venipuncture for specific policies regarding this skill.

Understanding Factors Affecting Flow

The flow of an IV infusion is governed by the same principles that govern fluid movement in general. Flow is directly proportional to the height on the infusion. Raising the infusion bag may improve sluggish flow. The clamp on IV tubing regulates the flow by changing the tubing diameter. In addition, the flow is faster through large-gauge rather than small-gauge cannulas. Issues such as length of IV tubing and viscosity of the fluid being infused may also affect the flow rate.

Monitoring Flow

Because so many factors influence gravity flow, a solution does not necessarily continue to run at the speed originally set. Therefore, the nurse monitors IV infusions frequently to make sure that the fluid is flowing at the intended rate. The IV container should be marked with tape to indicate at a glance whether the correct amount has infused. The flow rate is calculated when the solution is originally started and

then monitored at least hourly. To calculate the flow rate, the nurse determines the number of drops delivered per milliliter; this varies with equipment and is usually printed on the administration set packaging. In an effort to decrease the amount of medication errors, it has become standard for all intermittent IV infusions to be given with an electronic infusion device.

A variety of electronic infusion devices are available to assist in IV fluid delivery. These devices allow more accurate administration of fluids and medications than is possible with routine gravity-flow setups. A pump is a positive-pressure device that uses pressure to infuse fluid at a pressure of 10 psi; newer models use a pressure of 5 psi. The pressure exerted by the pump overrides vascular resistance (increased tubing length, low height of the IV container).

Volumetric pumps calculate the volume delivered by measuring the volume in a reservoir that is part of the set and is calibrated in milliliters per hour (mL/hr). A controller is an infusion assist device that relies on gravity for infusion; the volume is calibrated in drops (gtt) per minute. A controller uses a drop sensor to monitor the flow. Factors essential for the safe use of pumps include alarms to signify the presence of air in the IV line or an occlusion. The standard for the accurate delivery of fluid or medication via an electronic IV infusion pump is plus or minus 5%. The manufacturer's directions must be read carefully before use of any infusion pump or controller because there are many variations in available models. Use of these devices does not eliminate the need for the nurse to monitor the infusion and the patient frequently; however, it does limit the amount of bedside drug calculations and medication administration errors.

Flushing of a vascular device is performed to ensure patency and to prevent the mixing of incompatible medications or solutions. This procedure should be carried out at established intervals, according to hospital policy and procedure, especially for intermittently used catheters. Most manufacturers and researchers suggest the use of saline for flushing. The volume of the flush solution should be at least twice the volume capacity of the catheter. The catheter should be clamped before the syringe is completely empty and withdrawn to prevent reflux of blood into the lumen, which could cause catheter clotting and infiltration.

Discontinuing an Infusion

The removal of an IV catheter is associated with two possible dangers: bleeding and catheter embolism. To prevent excessive bleeding, a dry, sterile pressure dressing should be held over the site as the catheter is removed. Firm pressure is applied until hemostasis occurs.

If a plastic IV catheter is severed, the patient is at risk for catheter embolism. To detect this complication when the catheter is removed, the nurse compares the expected length of the catheter with its actual length. Plastic catheters should be withdrawn carefully and their length measured to make certain that no fragment has broken off in the vein.

Great care must be exercised when using scissors around the dressing site. If the catheter clearly has been severed, the nurse can attempt to occlude the vein above the site by applying a tourniquet to prevent the catheter from entering the central circulation (until surgical removal is possible). However, as always, it is better to prevent a potentially fatal problem than to deal with it after it has occurred. Fortunately, catheter embolism can be prevented easily by following simple rules:

- Avoid using scissors near the catheter.
- Avoid withdrawing the catheter through the insertion needle.
- Follow the manufacturer's guidelines carefully (e.g., cover the needle point with the bevel shield to prevent severance of the catheter).

Managing Systemic Complications

IV therapy predisposes the patient to numerous hazards, including both local and systemic complications. Systemic complications occur less frequently but are usually more serious than are local complications. They include circulatory overload, air embolism, febrile reaction, and infection.

Overloading the circulatory system with excessive IV fluids causes increased blood pressure and CVP. Signs and symptoms of fluid overload include moist crackles on auscultation of the lungs, edema, weight gain, dyspnea, and respirations that are shallow and have an increased rate.

Possible causes include rapid infusion of an IV solution or hepatic, cardiac, or kidney disease. The risk of fluid overload and subsequent pulmonary edema is especially increased in elderly patients with cardiac disease; this is referred to as *circulatory overload.*

The treatment for circulatory overload is decreasing the IV rate, monitoring vital signs frequently, assessing breath sounds, and placing the patient in a high Fowler position. The provider is contacted immediately. This complication can be avoided by using an infusion pump for infusions and by carefully monitoring all infusions. Complications of circulatory overload include heart failure and pulmonary edema.

The risk of air embolism is rare but ever-present. It is most often associated with cannulation of central veins. Manifestations of air embolism include dyspnea and cyanosis; hypotension; weak, rapid pulse; loss of consciousness; and chest, shoulder, and low back pain. Treatment calls for immediately clamping the cannula and replacing a leaking or open infusion system, placing the patient on the left side in the Trendelenburg position, assessing vital signs and breath sounds, and administering oxygen. Air embolism can be prevented by using a Luer Lock adapter on all lines, filling all tubing completely with solution, and using an air detection alarm on an IV pump. Complications of air embolism include shock and death. The amount of air necessary to induce death in humans is not known; however, the rate of entry is probably as important as the actual volume of air.

Pyrogenic substances in either the infusion solution or the IV administration set can induce a febrile reaction and septicemia. Signs and symptoms include an abrupt temperature elevation shortly after the infusion is started, backache, headache, increased pulse and respiratory rate, nausea and vomiting, diarrhea, chills and shaking, and general malaise. In severe septicemia, vascular collapse and septic shock may occur. Causes of septicemia include contamination of the IV product or a break in aseptic technique, especially in immunocompromised patients. Treatment is symptomatic and includes culturing of the IV cannula, tubing, or solution if it is suspect as well as establishing a new IV site for medication or fluid administration. See Chapter 54 for a discussion of septic shock.

Infection ranges in severity from local involvement of the insertion site to systemic dissemination of organisms through the bloodstream, as in septicemia. Measures to prevent infection are essential at the time the IV line is inserted and throughout the entire infusion. Prevention includes the following:

- Careful hand hygiene before every contact with any part of the infusion system or the patient
- Examining the IV containers for cracks, leaks, or cloudiness; these findings may indicate a contaminated solution
- Using strict aseptic technique
- Firmly anchoring the IV cannula to prevent to-and-fro motion

- Inspecting the IV site daily and replacing a soiled or wet dressing with a dry sterile dressing (antimicrobial agents that should be used for site care may include 2% tincture of iodine, 10% povidone–iodine, alcohol, or chlorhexidine gluconate, used alone or in combination per the institution's policy)
- Disinfecting injection/access ports with antimicrobial solution before use
- Removing the IV cannula at the first sign of local inflammation, contamination, or complication
- Replacing the peripheral IV cannula every 72 hours, or as indicated
- Replacing the IV cannula inserted during emergency conditions (with questionable asepsis) as soon as possible
- Using a 0.2-μm air-eliminating and bacteria/particulate retentive filter with non–lipid-containing solutions that require filtration. The filter can be added to the proximal or distal end of the administration set. If added to the proximal end between the fluid container and the tubing spike, the filter ensures sterility and particulate removal from the infusate container and prevents inadvertent infusion of air. If added to the distal end of the administration set, it filters air particles and contaminants introduced from add-on devices, secondary administration sets, or interruptions to the primary system. The nurse would choose where to place the filter depending on whether the administration set is on a dedicated line.
- Replacing the solution bag and administration set in accordance with agency policy and procedure
- Infusing or discarding medication or solution within 24 hours of its addition to an administration set
- Changing primary and secondary continuous administration sets every 96 hours, or immediately if contamination is suspected (Ling et al., 2016)
- Changing primary administration sets containing lipid-based solutions every 24 hours, or immediately if contamination is suspected (Ling et al., 2016).

Managing Local Complications

Local complications of IV therapy include infiltration and extravasation, phlebitis, thrombophlebitis, hematoma, and clotting of the needle.

Infiltration is the unintentional administration of a non-vesicant solution or medication into surrounding tissue. This can occur when the IV cannula dislodges or perforates the wall of the vein. Infiltration is characterized by edema around the insertion site, leakage of IV fluid from the insertion site, discomfort and coolness in the area of infiltration, and a significant decrease in the flow rate. When the solution is particularly irritating, sloughing of tissue may result. Close monitoring of the insertion site is necessary to detect infiltration before it becomes severe.

Infiltration is usually easily recognized if the insertion area is larger than the same site of the opposite extremity;

however, it is not always so obvious. A common misconception is that a backflow of blood into the tubing proves that the catheter is properly placed within the vein. However, if the catheter tip has pierced the wall of the vessel, IV fluid will seep into tissues as well as flow into the vein. Although blood return occurs, infiltration has occurred as well. A more reliable means of confirming infiltration is to apply a tourniquet above (or proximal to) the infusion site and tighten it enough to restrict venous flow. If the infusion continues to drip despite the venous obstruction, infiltration is present.

As soon as the nurse notes infiltration, the infusion should be stopped, the IV discontinued, and a sterile dressing applied to the site after careful inspection to determine the extent of infiltration. The infiltration of any amount of blood product, irritant, or vesicant is considered the most severe.

The IV infusion should be started in a new site or proximal to the infiltration if the same extremity must be used again. A warm compress may be applied to the site if small volumes of noncaustic solutions have infiltrated over a long period or if the solution was isotonic with a normal pH; the affected extremity should be elevated to promote the absorption of fluid. If the infiltration is recent and the solution was hypertonic or had an increased pH, a cold compress may be applied to the area. Infiltration can be detected and treated early by inspecting the site every hour for redness, pain, edema, coolness at the site, and IV fluid leaking from the IV site. Using the appropriate size and type of cannula for the vein prevents this complication.

Extravasation is similar to infiltration with an inadvertent administration of vesicant or irritant solution or medication into the surrounding tissue. Medications such as dopamine, calcium preparations, and chemotherapeutic agents can cause pain, burning, and redness at the site. Blistering, inflammation, and necrosis of tissues can occur. The extent of tissue damage is determined by the concentration of the medication, the quantity that extravasated, the location of the infusion site, the tissue response, and the duration of the process of extravasation.

The infusion must be stopped and the provider notified promptly. The agency's protocol to treat extravasation is initiated; the protocol may indicate specific treatments, including antidotes specific to the medication that extravasated, and may indicate whether the IV line should remain in place or be removed before treatment. The protocol often specifies infiltration of the infusion site with an antidote prescribed after assessment by the provider, removal of the cannula, and application of warm compresses to sites of extravasation from vinca alkaloids or cold compresses to sites of extravasation from alkylating and antibiotic vesicants (Al-Benna, O'Boyle, & Holley, 2013). The affected extremity should not be used for further cannula placement. Thorough neurovascular assessments of the affected extremity must be performed frequently.

Reviewing the institution's IV policy and procedures, incompatibility charts and checking with the pharmacist before administering any IV medication, whether given peripherally or centrally, is a prudent way to determine incompatibilities and vesicant potential to prevent extravasation. Careful, frequent monitoring of the IV site, avoiding insertion of IV devices in areas of flexion, securing the IV line, and using the smallest catheter possible that accommodates the vein help minimize the incidence and severity of this complication. In addition, when vesicant medication is administered by IV push, it should be given through a side port of an infusing IV solution to dilute the medication and decrease the severity of tissue damage if extravasation occurs.

Signs of phlebitis and infiltration may be assessed using a scale such as the Infusion Nurses Society (INS) infiltration scale (Ray-Barruel, Polit, Murfield, & Rickard, 2014). The scale ranges from 0, or no edema, to 4, which includes pitting edema, moderate to severe pain at the site, or circulatory impairment. Extravasation should always be rated as a grade 4 on the infiltration scale.

Phlebitis is defined as inflammation of a vein, which can be categorized as chemical, mechanical, or bacterial; however, two or more of these types of irritation often occur simultaneously. Chemical phlebitis can be caused by an irritating medication or solution (increased pH or high osmolality of a solution), rapid infusion rates, and medication incompatibilities. Mechanical phlebitis results from long periods of cannulation, catheters in flexed areas, catheter gauges larger than the vein lumen, and poorly secured catheters. Bacterial phlebitis can develop from poor hand hygiene, lack of aseptic technique, failure to check all equipment before use, and failure to recognize early signs and symptoms of phlebitis. Other factors include poor venipuncture technique, catheter in place for a prolonged period, and failure to adequately secure the catheter. Phlebitis is characterized by a reddened, warm area around the insertion site or along the path of the vein, pain or tenderness at the site or along the vein, and swelling. The likelihood of phlebitis increases with the length of time the IV line is in place, the composition of the fluid or medication infused (especially its pH and tonicity), the size and site of the cannula inserted, ineffective filtration, inadequate anchoring of the line, and the introduction of microorganisms at the time of insertion. Treatment consists of discontinuing the IV and restarting it in another site as well as applying a warm, moist compress to the affected site. Phlebitis can be prevented by using aseptic technique during insertion, using the appropriate-size cannula or needle for the vein, considering the composition of fluids and medications when selecting a site, observing the site hourly for any complications, anchoring the cannula or needle well, and changing the IV site according to agency policy and procedures.

Thrombophlebitis refers to the presence of a clot plus inflammation in the vein. It is evidenced by localized pain, redness, warmth, and swelling around the insertion site or along the path of the vein, immobility of the extremity because of discomfort and swelling, sluggish flow rate, fever, malaise, and leukocytosis.

Treatment includes discontinuing the IV infusion; applying a cold compress first, to decrease the flow of blood and increase platelet aggregation, followed by a warm compress; elevating the extremity; and restarting the line in the opposite extremity. If the patient has signs and symptoms of thrombophlebitis, the IV line should not be flushed (although flushing may be indicated in the absence of phlebitis to ensure cannula patency and to prevent mixing of incompatible medications and solutions). The catheter must be removed promptly. In some circumstances, the catheter tip may be sent to the laboratory for culture, and it should be removed and placed in a sterile container prior to sending to the lab. Thrombophlebitis can be prevented by avoiding trauma to the vein at the time the IV is inserted, observing the site every hour, and checking medication additives for compatibility.

A hematoma results when blood leaks into tissues surrounding the IV insertion site. Leakage can result if the opposite vein wall is perforated during venipuncture, the needle slips out of the vein, or insufficient pressure is applied to the site after removal of the needle or cannula. The signs of a hematoma include ecchymosis, immediate swelling at the site, and leakage of blood at the insertion site.

Treatment includes removing the needle or cannula and applying light pressure with a sterile, dry dressing; applying ice for 24 hours to the site to avoid extension of the hematoma; elevating the extremity; assessing the extremity for any circulatory, neurologic, or motor dysfunction; and restarting the line in the other extremity if indicated. A hematoma can be prevented by carefully inserting the needle and by using diligent care with patients who have a bleeding disorder, are taking anticoagulant medication, or have advanced liver disease.

Blood clots may form in the IV line as a result of kinked IV tubing, a very slow infusion rate, an empty IV bag, or failure to flush the IV line after intermittent medication or solution administrations. The signs are decreased flow rate and blood backflow into the IV tubing. If blood clots in the IV line, the infusion must be discontinued and restarted in another site with a new cannula and administration set. The tubing should not be irrigated or milked. Neither the infusion rate nor the solution container should be raised, and the clot should not be aspirated from the tubing. Clotting of the needle or cannula may be prevented by not allowing the IV solution bag to run dry, taping the tubing to prevent kinking and maintain patency, maintaining an adequate flow rate, and flushing the line after intermittent medication or other solution administration. In some cases, a specially trained nurse or provider may inject a thrombolytic agent.

CHAPTER REVIEW

Critical Thinking Exercises

1. A 28-year-old man with a history of diabetes mellitus has an open fracture of the tibia as the result of a motorcycle crash. In the emergency department, his temperature is 103°F. His laboratory test results are as follows: blood glucose, 450 mg/dL; BUN, 35 mg/dL; sodium, 140 mEq/L; potassium, 4.1 mEq/L; pH, 7.1; PCO_2, 10 mm Hg; and HCO_3^-, 12 mEq/L. His urine ketones are 3+. What fluid and electrolyte or acid–base disorders is the patient experiencing? What IV fluids would you anticipate being prescribed? Give the rationale for their use. What treatments would address the patient's fluid and electrolyte or acid–base disorders?

2. A 30-year-old woman comes to the emergency department with nausea, confusion, dehydration, and oliguria. Her mother reports that she has been depressed after losing her job as a bank executive. An empty bottle of aspirin was found in her bathroom sink. Her laboratory values are as follows: pH, 7.35; $PaCO_2$, 16 mm Hg; PaO_2, 98 mm Hg; and HCO_3^-, 15 mEq/L. What acid–base disorder does this patient have? What treatments and relevant nursing actions related to the underlying disorder and its treatment should the nurse anticipate?

3. A 58-year-old woman is vomiting bright red blood. She is hypotensive. Her pulse rate is 108 bpm, and her pulse is weak and thready. Her ABG results are as follows: pH, 7.34; $PaCO_2$, 35 mm Hg; PaO_2, 69 mm Hg; and HCO_3^-, 20 mEq/L. Her hemoglobin is 4 g/dL. How do you interpret the patient's blood gas values? What treatment would you anticipate?

NCLEX-Style Review Questions

1. A nurse is analyzing her patient's ABG values. Which result is inconsistent with the diagnosis of respiratory acidosis?
   a. pH 7.3
   b. $PaCO_2$ 50
   c. Hyperventilation ($PaCO_2$ 25)
   d. Hypoventilation ($PaCO_2$ 60)

2. A patient is diagnosed with SIADH. What disturbance should the nurse be aware of related to this diagnosis?
   a. Excess water loss
   b. Dilutional hyponatremia
   c. Serum sodium level of 148 mg/dL
   d. Decreased urine osmolality

3. A nurse working on a trauma unit is initiating IV fluids for a patient. For what condition would the nurse administer normal saline?
   a. Renal impairment
   b. Pulmonary edema
   c. Burns
   d. Heart failure

4. When entering a patient's room, the nurse notices blood clots in the IV line. What is the most appropriate nursing intervention at this time?
   a. Milk the tubing.
   b. Discontinue the infusion.
   c. Irrigate the tubing and catheter.
   d. Aspirate the clot from the tubing.

5. What does the nurse expect to see on the ECG reading when serum potassium levels rise to greater than 6 mEq/L?
   a. Peaked, widened T waves
   b. ST-segment elevation
   c. Lengthened QT interval
   d. ST-segment depression

Try these additional resources, available at **http://thepoint.lww.com/Honan2e**, to enhance your learning and understanding of this chapter:

• NCLEX-Style Student Review Questions
• Journal Articles

REFERENCES AND SELECTED READINGS

References and selected readings associated with this chapter can be found on the website that accompanies the book. Visit **http://thepoint. lww.com/Honan2e** to access the references and other additional resources associated with this chapter.

Perioperative Nursing

Joann Preece

Learning Objectives

After reading this chapter, you will be able to:

1. Define the three phases of perioperative nursing.
2. Describe a comprehensive preoperative assessment to identify surgical risk factors.
3. Identify legal and ethical considerations related to informed consent.
4. Describe the immediate preoperative preparation, and intraoperative and postoperative management of the surgical patient.
5. Identify the nurse's role in patient safety and regulatory compliance in the perioperative setting.
6. Describe the principles of surgical asepsis.
7. Identify adverse effects of surgery and anesthesia.
8. Describe types of anesthetic approaches and the implications for nursing care in the perioperative setting.
9. Describe perioperative nursing measures that decrease the risk for complications.

Surgery, whether elective or emergent, is a stressful, complex event. The special field known as **perioperative** and perianesthesia nursing includes a wide variety of nursing functions associated with the patient's surgical experience during the perioperative period.

INTRODUCTION

Phases

Perioperative and perianesthesia nursing addresses the nursing roles relevant to the three phases of the surgical experience: preoperative, intraoperative, and postoperative. Each phase begins and ends at a particular point in the sequence of events that constitutes the surgical experience, and each includes a wide range of activities that the nurse performs using the nursing process and based on the standards of practice (American Society of Perianesthesia Nurses [ASPAN], 2015). Box 5-1 represents nursing activities characteristic of the three perioperative phases of care.

Surgical Settings

Today, as a result of advances in surgical techniques and instrumentation, as well as in **anesthesia,** the number of surgeries, imaging studies, and diagnostic tests performed outside of hospitals is growing rapidly. These procedures are primarily moving to **ambulatory surgery centers** (ASCs), which provide outpatient surgical services not requiring an overnight stay, independent diagnostic and testing facilities, and health providers' offices. Innovation in medical technology and surgical techniques, along with preferences of multiple players in the health care system, has driven the migration of care to nonhospital settings. Less invasive surgical techniques and advances in anesthesia have made it possible for more procedures to be performed in outpatient settings, where recovery time is limited. As a result, today, many patients arrive at the hospital on the morning of surgery and go home after recovering from the anesthesia in the postanesthesia care unit (PACU). Often, surgical patients who require hospital stays are trauma patients, acutely ill patients, and/or patients undergoing major surgery.

Although each setting (ambulatory, outpatient, or inpatient) offers its own unique advantages for the delivery of patient care, they all require comprehensive preoperative nursing assessment and nursing interventions, and a sound knowledge of all aspects of perioperative and perianesthesia nursing.

Surgical Classifications

A surgical procedure may be diagnostic (e.g., biopsy, exploratory laparotomy), curative (e.g., excision of a tumor or an inflamed appendix), or reparative (e.g., multiple wound

| BOX 5-1 | **Examples of Nursing Activities in the Perioperative Phases of Care** |

Preoperative Phase

Preadmission Testing

1. Initiates initial preoperative health history and physical assessment
2. Initiates teaching appropriate to patient's needs
3. Involves family in interview
4. Verifies completion of preoperative testing
5. Verifies understanding of surgeon-specific preoperative orders (e.g., bowel preparation, preoperative shower)
6. Discharge planning—assesses patient's need for postoperative transportation and care

Admission to Surgical Center or Unit

1. Verification of patient identification and expected procedure
2. Completes preoperative assessment
3. Assesses patient's status, including nutritional status and baseline level of pain
4. Assesses for risks for postoperative complications
5. Assesses for and manages perioperative nomothermia
6. Reports unexpected findings or any deviations from normal
7. Verifies that operative consent and all appropriate documents have been signed
8. Coordinates patient teaching with other nursing staff and reinforces previous teaching
9. Explains phases in perioperative period and expectations; answers patient's and family's questions
10. Develops a plan of care
11. Removes and secures prosthesis, dentures, glasses, jewelry
12. Ensures interpreter is present if patient requires
13. Encourages patient to void immediately pre-op
14. Establishes IV line
15. Obtains pre-op blood glucose or pregnancy testing as ordered
16. Administers medications if prescribed, reminds patient not to get OOB after premedicated
17. Takes measures to ensure patient's comfort
18. Provides psychological support
19. Communicates patient's emotional status to other appropriate members of the health care team

Intraoperative Phase

Maintenance of Safety

1. Maintains aseptic, controlled environment
2. Effectively manages human resources, equipment, and supplies for individualized patient care
3. Transfers patient to operating room bed or table
4. Safely positions the patient:
   a. Confirms functional alignment and secures patient to operating room table
   b. Initiates pressure ulcer reduction and skin injury processes
   c. Ensures appropriate exposure of surgical site
5. Applies grounding device to patient
6. Ensures that the sponge, needle, and instrument counts are correct
7. Ensures that the final verification (time out) is conducted and documented
8. Completes intraoperative documentation
9. Maintains an environment to support patient's body temperature as per procedural protocol

Psychological Support (Before Induction and when Patient is Conscious)

1. Provides emotional support to patient
2. Stands near or touches patient during procedures and induction
3. Continues to assess patient's emotional status

Postoperative Phase

Transfer of Patient to Postanesthesia Care Unit

1. Communicates intraoperative information:
   a. Identifies patient by name
   b. States type of surgery performed
   c. Identifies type of anesthetic used
   d. Reports patient's response to surgical procedure and anesthesia
   e. Describes intraoperative factors (e.g., insertion of drains or catheters; administration of blood, analgesic agents, or other medications during surgery; occurrence of unexpected events)
   f. Describes physical limitations
   g. Reports patient's preoperative level of consciousness
   h. Communicates necessary equipment needs
   i. Communicates presence of family and/or significant others

Postoperative Assessment Recovery Area

1. Determines patient's immediate response to surgical intervention
2. Integrates data received at transfer of care
3. Monitors patient's physiologic status
4. Assesses patient's pain level and administers appropriate pain relief measures
5. Maintains patient's safety (airway, circulation, prevention of injury)
6. Administers medications, fluid, and blood component therapy, if prescribed
7. Provides oral fluids if prescribed for ambulatory surgery patient
8. Assesses patient's readiness for transfer to in-hospital unit or for discharge home based on institutional policy

Surgical Unit

1. Continues close monitoring of patient's physical and psychological response to surgical intervention
2. Assesses patient's pain level and administers appropriate pain relief measures
3. Provides teaching to patient during immediate recovery period
4. Assists patient in recovery and preparation for discharge home
5. Determines patient's psychological status
6. Assists with discharge planning

Home or Clinic

1. Provides follow-up care during office or clinic visit or by telephone contact
2. Reinforces previous teaching and answers patient's and family's questions about surgery and follow-up care
3. Assesses patient's response to surgery and anesthesia and their effects on body image and function
4. Determines family's perception of surgery and its outcome

TABLE **5-1** Categories of Surgery Based on Urgency

Classification	Indications for Surgery	Examples
I. Emergent—Patient requires immediate attention; disorder may be life-threatening	Without delay	Severe bleeding Bladder or intestinal obstruction Fractured skull Gunshot or stab wounds Extensive burns
II. Urgent—Patient requires prompt attention	Within 24–30 hours	Acute gallbladder infection Kidney or ureteral stones
III. Required—Patient needs to have surgery	Plan within a few weeks or months	Prostatic hyperplasia without bladder obstruction Thyroid disorders Cataracts
IV. Elective—Patient should have surgery	Failure to have surgery not catastrophic	Repair of scars Simple hernia
V. Optional—Decision rests with patient	Personal preference	Cosmetic surgery

repair). It may be reconstructive or cosmetic (e.g., mammoplasty or a facelift) or palliative (e.g., to relieve pain or correct a problem—for instance, a gastrostomy tube may be inserted to compensate for the inability to swallow food). Surgery may also be classified according to the degree of urgency involved (Table 5-1).

Emergency Surgery

Emergency surgeries are unplanned and occur with little time for preparation of the patient or the perioperative team. The unpredictable nature of trauma and emergency surgery poses unique challenges to the nurse throughout the perioperative period. All of the factors that affect patients preparing to undergo surgery apply to these patients, usually in a very condensed time frame. There may be only one preoperative assessment, and it may take place at the same time as resuscitation in the emergency department. For the unconscious patient, informed consent and essential information, such as pertinent past medical history and allergies, need to be obtained from a family member, if one is available. A quick visual survey of the patient is essential to identify all sites of injury if the emergency surgery is due to trauma. The patient, who may have undergone a very frightening experience, may need extra support, including an explanation of the surgery.

Special Populations

Patients Who are Elderly

Advances in nutrition, public health, education, and social services have produced a major change in human longevity in industrialized societies, and elderly patients now account for more than one third of all hospital care days in the United States. Patients 65 years of age and older have surgery at a rate two to three times that of younger patients

and tend to have longer hospital stays (Sieber & Pauldine, 2015). Although the decision to operate lies within the purview of the physician, perioperative nurses should be aware of the surgery's implications. Surgical intervention should be tailored to the patient's symptoms, overall functional and health status, and predicted benefit of the intervention. Important factors that need to be evaluated are (1) disease course versus life expectancy, (2) state of independence, (3) personal motivation, and (4) surgical risk factors versus nonoperative management (Rothrock, 2014).

Preoperative pain assessment and teaching are important in the elderly patient. The older person undergoing surgery may have a combination of chronic illnesses and health issues in addition to the specific one for which surgery is indicated. Elderly people frequently do not report symptoms, perhaps because they fear a serious illness may be diagnosed or because they accept such symptoms as part of the aging process. Subtle clues alert the nurse to underlying problems. A complete pain assessment and review of the patient's medical history will assist with identifying the risk for postoperative complications. Delirium is a common but often undiagnosed complication in the elderly following a major operation.

Health care staff must remember that the hazards of surgery for the aged are proportional to the number and severity of coexisting health problems and the nature and duration of the operative procedure. The underlying principle that guides the preoperative assessment, surgical care, and postoperative care is that the aged patient has less physiologic reserve (the ability of an organ to return to normal after a disturbance in its equilibrium) than does a younger patient. Refer to Table 5-2 for the implications of aging on operative course. The nurse plans interventions based upon the patient's medical history, clinical presentation, and knowledge of the physiologic impact of aging. For example,

TABLE 5-2 GERONTOLOGIC CONSIDERATIONS / Age-Related Changes and Impact on Operative Course

Structural or Functional Change	Impact
Increased incidence of coexisting disease	Higher risks from anesthesia and surgery than younger adult patients
Aging heart and blood vessels	Decreased ability to respond to stress
Reduced cardiac output and limited cardiac reserve	Increased vulnerability to changes in circulating volume and blood oxygen levels; in addition, excessive or rapid administration of IV solutions can cause pulmonary edema.
Decreased ability to compensate for hypoxia	Increased risk of cerebral ischemia, thrombosis, embolism, infarction, and anoxia
Decrease in the percentage of lean body tissue and a steady increase in fatty tissue (from 20 to 90 years of age).	Anesthetic agents that have an affinity for fatty tissue concentrate in body fat and the brain. The elderly patient needs fewer and smaller amounts of anesthetic agents to produce anesthesia and eliminates the anesthetic agent over a longer period of time, compared with a younger patient.
If malnourished or has low plasma protein levels (hypoalbuminemia)	With decreased plasma proteins, more of the anesthetic agent remains free or unbound, resulting in more potent action.
Reduced liver size and potential for reduced kidney function	Decreases the rate at which the liver can inactivate many anesthetic agents, and decreased kidney function slows the elimination of waste products and anesthetics
Impaired ability to increase metabolic rate and impaired thermoregulatory mechanisms	Increased susceptibility to hypothermia
Bone loss (25% in women, 12% in men)	Increased risk of musculoskeletal problems postoperatively
Loss of collagen and muscle; thinning, sagging skin	Increased risk of skin complications
Impaired vision or hearing and reduced tactile sensitivity	Increased potential for communication issues, increased risk of skin complications
Increased tooth loss and periodontal disease, increased incidence of dental devices (dentures, partial plates, crowns)	Increased risk of airway occlusion due to dental device dislodgement

arthritis is common in older people and may affect mobility, making it difficult for the patient to turn from one side to the other or ambulate without discomfort. The elderly patient has less subcutaneous fat, poor skin turgor, and tissue fragility. Aging-related changes in the musculoskeletal system accentuate bony prominences and decrease range of motion. These changes, along with limitations imposed by chronic pain, make positioning one of the most important considerations for this population of surgical patients. Protective measures include adequate padding for tender areas, moving the patient slowly, and protecting bony prominences from prolonged pressure. Precautions are taken when moving an elderly person because of the fragility of skin, and a lightweight cotton blanket is an appropriate cover when an elderly patient is moved to and from the operating room (OR) because of temperature sensitivity.

In addition, many elderly people have experienced personal illnesses and possibly life-threatening illnesses of friends and family. Such experiences may result in fears about the surgery and about the future. By providing an opportunity for the patient to express these fears, the nurse enables the patient to gain some peace of mind.

Because the elderly patient may face greater risks during the perioperative period, the following factors are critical: (1) skillful preoperative assessment and treatment, (2) skillful anesthesia and surgery, and (3) meticulous and competent postoperative and postanesthesia management. In addition, the nurse should incorporate pain management information and pain communication skills when teaching the elderly patient how to obtain greater postoperative pain relief.

Patients Who are Obese

Like age, obesity increases the risk and severity of complications associated with surgery. During surgery, fatty tissues are especially susceptible to infection. In addition, obesity increases technical and mechanical problems related to surgery. Therefore, dehiscence (wound separation) and wound infections are more common. Moreover, the obese patient may be more difficult to care for because of the added weight. The patient tends to have shallow respirations when supine, which increases the risk of hypoventilation and postoperative pulmonary complications. It has been estimated that for each 30 lb of excess weight, about 25 additional miles of blood vessels are needed, and this places increased demands on the heart. Thus, nursing management includes careful assessment of the cardiopulmonary status of obese patients and thorough wound assessments.

Patients with Disabilities

Special considerations for patients with mental or physical disabilities include the need for appropriate assistive devices, modifications in preoperative teaching, and additional assistance with and attention to positioning or transferring. Assistive devices include hearing aids, eyeglasses, braces, prostheses, and other devices. People who are hearing-impaired may need a sign interpreter or some alternative communication system perioperatively. If the patient relies on signing or speech (lip) reading, and his or her eyeglasses or contact lenses are removed or the health care staff wears surgical masks, an alternative method of communication will be needed. These needs must be identified during the preoperative evaluation and clearly communicated to the appropriate personnel. Specific strategies for accommodating the patient's needs must be identified in advance. Ensuring the security of assistive devices is important, because these devices are expensive and can be misplaced easily.

Most patients are directed to move from the stretcher to the OR table and back again. In addition to being unable to see or hear instructions, the patient with a disability may be unable to move without special devices or a great deal of assistance. The patient with a disability that affects body position (e.g., cerebral palsy, post-polio syndrome, and other neuromuscular disorders) may need special positioning during surgery to prevent pain and injury. Moreover, these patients may be unable to sense whether their extremities are positioned incorrectly.

Patients with respiratory problems related to a disability (e.g., multiple sclerosis, muscular dystrophy) may experience pulmonary difficulties unless the problems are made known to the anesthesia provider, who can make adjustments. These factors need to be identified clearly in the preoperative period and communicated to the appropriate personnel.

PREOPERATIVE NURSING

The **preoperative phase** begins when the decision to proceed with surgical intervention is made, and ends with the transfer of the patient onto the OR table. The nursing roles during this phase focus on assessing the patient and

developing a plan of care. This process is performed utilizing diverse modalities. Telephone interviews, face-to-face assessments and computer-aided tools are used to review the physical, psychological, sociocultural, and spiritual needs of the patient. Preadmission units work collaboratively with anesthesia providers to interview and assess the patient to identify potential or actual problems that may occur. The goals of preoperative assessment are to reduce the patient's surgical and anesthetic perioperative morbidity or mortality. Medical history, laboratory values, and diagnostic tests help practitioners evaluate the patient. Preadmission nurses actively participate in pre-op education to prepare the patient and family to take an active role in their experience.

Informed Consent

The surgical experience, except in extreme emergencies, begins after a patient has consented to a recommended surgical procedure. Voluntary and written **informed consent** from the patient is necessary before nonemergent surgery can be performed. The Department of Health and Human Services, Centers for Medicare and Medicaid Services (CMS), believes that a patient or his or her representative (as allowed under state law) has the right to make informed decisions regarding the patient's care. The guidelines further indicate that, for the surgical patient, a properly executed informed consent form for the operation must be in the patient's chart prior to surgery, except in emergencies. The primary purpose of the informed consent process is to ensure that the patient, or the patient's representative, is provided information necessary to enable him or her to evaluate the proposed surgery before agreeing to it (Centers for Medicare and Medicaid Services, 2017; Waisel, 2015). A written consent protects the patient from unsanctioned surgery and protects the surgeon from claims of an unauthorized operation (The Joint Commission, 2016b). It is normally the responsibility of the performing surgeon to obtain the informed surgical consent, which should consist of the following four basic elements:

1. The physician documents that the patient or surrogate has decision-making capacity, which is distinct from the legal concept of competency as determined by courts. Adults are presumed to be legally competent unless declared otherwise by a court (Waisel, 2015, p. 258).
2. The surgeon discloses to the patient details regarding the diagnosis and treatment options sufficiently for the patient to make an informed choice.
3. The patient demonstrates understanding of the disclosed information.
4. The patient freely authorizes a specific treatment plan without undue influence (Waisel, 2015).

Informed consent is necessary in the following circumstances:

- Invasive procedures, such as a surgical incision, a biopsy, a cystoscopy, or paracentesis

- Procedures requiring sedation and/or anesthesia
- A nonsurgical procedure, such as an arteriography, that carries more than slight risk to the patient
- Procedures involving radiation

If the patient has doubts and has not had the opportunity to investigate alternative treatments, a second opinion may be requested. No patient should be urged or coerced to give informed consent. Refusing to undergo a surgical procedure is a person's legal right and privilege.

The consent process can be improved by providing audiovisual materials to supplement discussion, by ensuring that the wording of the consent form is understandable, and by using other strategies and resources as needed to help the patient understand its content. It is required to have the consent available in multiple languages or have a trained medical interpreter available for non–English-speaking patients. In many cases, it is required to have alternative forms of communication (e.g., Braille, large print, sign interpreter) for the elderly and disabled.

Preoperative Health Assessment

Before any surgical treatment is initiated, a health history is obtained, a physical examination is performed during which vital signs are noted, and a database is established for future comparisons. Preoperative blood tests, x-rays, and other diagnostic tests are obtained as needed.

The goal in the preoperative period is for the patient to have as many positive health factors as possible. Many risk factors may lead to complications (Box 5-2). Every attempt is made to stabilize those conditions that otherwise hinder recovery.

Nutritional and Fluid Status

Optimal nutrition is an essential factor in promoting healing and resisting infection and other surgical complications. Assessment of a patient's nutritional status identifies factors that can affect the patient's surgical course, such as obesity, under nutrition, weight loss, malnutrition, deficiencies in specific nutrients, metabolic abnormalities, and the effects of medications on nutrition. Nutritional needs may be determined by measurement of body mass index (BMI) and waist circumference (U.S. Department of Health and Human Services, 2015). A BMI of 18.5 to 24.9 is normal; less than 18.5 is underweight, greater than 25 is overweight, greater than 30 is obese, and 40 and greater is extreme obesity. A waist circumference measurement of greater than 40 in in men and 35 in in women is associated with increased cardiac risk.

If possible, any nutritional deficiency, such as malnutrition, should be corrected before surgery to provide adequate protein for tissue repair. The nutrients needed for wound healing are summarized in Table 5-3. Dehydration, hypovolemia, and electrolyte imbalances can also lead to significant problems in patients with comorbid medical conditions

| BOX 5-2 | **Risk Factors for Surgical Complications** |

- Hypovolemia
- Dehydration or electrolyte imbalance
- Nutritional deficits
- Extremes of age (very young, very old)
- Extremes of weight (emaciation, obesity)
- Infection and sepsis
- Toxic conditions
- Immunologic abnormalities
- Pregnancy (because of diminished maternal physiologic reserve)
- Cerebrovascular disease
- Pulmonary disease:
  - Obstructive disease
  - Restrictive disorder
  - Respiratory infection
- Renal or urinary tract disease:
  - Decreased renal function
  - Urinary tract infection
  - Obstruction
- Cardiovascular disease:
  - Coronary artery disease or previous myocardial infarction
  - Cardiac failure
  - Arrhythmias
  - Hypertension
  - Prosthetic heart valve
  - Thromboembolism
  - Hemorrhagic disorders
- Endocrine dysfunction:
  - Diabetes mellitus
  - Adrenal disorders
  - Thyroid malfunction
- Hepatic disease:
  - Cirrhosis
  - Hepatitis
- Pre-existing mental or physical disability

or in patients who are elderly. The severity of fluid and electrolyte imbalances is often difficult to determine. Mild volume deficits may be treated during surgery; however, additional time may be needed to correct pronounced fluid and electrolyte deficits to promote the best possible preoperative condition.

Drug or Alcohol Use

People who abuse drugs or alcohol frequently deny or attempt to hide it. In such situations, the nurse who is obtaining the patient's health history needs to ask frank questions with patience, care, and a nonjudgmental attitude. Because acutely intoxicated people are at higher risk for potential injury, surgery is postponed if possible. If emergency surgery is required, local, spinal, or regional block anesthesia is used for minor surgery. Otherwise, to prevent vomiting and potential aspiration, a nasogastric tube is inserted before general anesthesia is administered.

TABLE **5-3** Nutrients Important for Wound Healing

Nutrient	Rationale for Increased Need
Protein	To allow collagen deposition and wound healing to occur; clotting factor production; white blood cell (WBC) production and migration; cell-mediated phagocytosis; fibroblast proliferation; granulation tissue formation, neovascularization
Arginine (amino acid)	To provide necessary substrate for collagen synthesis and nitric oxide (crucial for wound healing) at wound site To increase wound strength and collagen deposition To stimulate T-cell response To support a variety of essential reactions of intermediary metabolism
Carbohydrates and fats	To be a primary source of energy in the body and, consequently, in the wound-healing process To meet the demand for increased essential fatty acids needed for cellular function after an injury To spare protein Fibroblast proliferation is sensitive to glucose deficiencies.
Water	To maintain homeostasis
Vitamin C	To support capillary formation, tissue synthesis, and wound healing through collagen formation To allow for antibody formation, WBC production; deficiency is associated with abnormal scar tissue formation
Vitamin B complex	To influence host resistance, indirectly supporting wound healing
Vitamin E	An antioxidant responsible for normal fat metabolism and collagen synthesis
Vitamin A	Increases inflammatory response in wounds, reduces anti-inflammatory effects of corticosteroids on wound healing; is essential for epidermal proliferation, reepithelialization, and epithelium maintenance
Vitamin K	Important for normal blood clotting To help avoid impaired intestinal synthesis associated with the use of antibiotics
Magnesium	Essential cofactor for many enzymes that are involved in the process of protein synthesis and wound repair
Copper	Responsible for collagen cross-linking and erythropoiesis
Zinc	A cofactor for collagen formation, also metabolizes protein, liberates vitamin A from storage in the liver, interacts with platelets in blood clotting, and assists in immune function

The person with a history of chronic alcoholism often suffers from malnutrition and other systemic problems that increase surgical risk. Alcohol withdrawal syndrome or delirium tremens (DTs) may be anticipated between 48 and 72 hours after alcohol withdrawal and is associated with a significant mortality rate when it occurs postoperatively.

 Nursing Alert
The nurse is aware that DTs usually appear within 72 hours of withdrawal and is often preceded by tremulousness, anxiety, and insomnia; progressing to tachycardia, diaphoresis, anorexia, agitation, headache, and gastrointestinal distress. Late symptoms include visual hallucinations, delirium or seizures (Ferri, 2016). Many institutions use the Clinical Institute Withdrawal Assessment-Alcohol (CIWA-A) scale to measure the severity of alcohol withdrawal. The CIWA-A scale consists of 10 symptoms, and treatment is either a fixed-dose regimen or individualized benzodiazepine administration dose.

Respiratory Status

The goal for surgical patients is optimal respiratory function. Because adequate ventilation is potentially compromised during all phases of surgical treatment, surgery is usually postponed if the patient has a respiratory infection. Patients with underlying respiratory disease (e.g., asthma, chronic obstructive pulmonary disease [COPD]) are assessed carefully for current threats to their pulmonary status. Patients should be evaluated for conditions such as respiratory infection and neuromuscular diseases, such as Parkinson disease, which may affect respiratory function.

The use of tobacco is an important risk factor but one that usually cannot be influenced. Even among smokers who have not developed chronic lung disease, smoking is associated with significant changes in lung function. While cessation for 2 days prior to surgery is recommended, a prospective study by Warner, Divertie, & Tinker (1984) revealed that smoking cessation for up to 8 weeks was necessary to reduce the rate of postoperative pulmonary complications. However, the ideal duration of cessation of smoking before surgery remains unclear. What it known is that, within 12 hours of quitting smoking, the patient would experience a decrease in carbon monoxide levels; improved oxygen delivery; lower nicotine levels, which improves vasodilatation; and a decrease in toxic substances that impair wound healing (Stoelting, Hines, & Marschall, 2012).

Cardiovascular Status

The goal in preparing any patient for surgery is to ensure a well-functioning cardiovascular system to meet the oxygen, fluid, and nutritional needs of the perioperative period. If the patient has uncontrolled hypertension, surgery may be postponed until the blood pressure is stabilized. At times, surgical treatment can be modified to meet the cardiac tolerance of the patient. For example, in a patient with obstruction of the descending colon and coronary artery disease, a temporary simple colostomy may be performed rather than a more extensive colon resection that would require a prolonged period of anesthesia.

Hepatic and Kidney Function

The presurgical goal is optimal function of the liver and urinary systems, so that medications, anesthetic agents, body wastes, and toxins are adequately processed and removed from the body.

The liver is important in the biotransformation of anesthetic compounds. Therefore, any disorder of the liver has an effect on how anesthetic agents are metabolized. The limited ability of a failing liver increases the perioperative risks and presents significant challenges. Increased morbidity and mortality is associated with varying degrees of liver insufficiency; thus, it is important to quantify and grade preoperative liver dysfunction using various serum liver function tests (Kaufman & Roccaforte, 2013). Because the kidneys are involved in excreting anesthetic medications and their metabolites, and because acid–base status and metabolism are also important considerations in anesthesia administration, surgery is contraindicated if a patient has acute nephritis, acute kidney injury with oliguria or anuria, or other acute kidney problems. The exception is surgery that is performed as a life-saving measure or that is necessary to improve urinary function, as in the case of an obstructive uropathy.

Endocrine Function

Diabetes is the most common endocrinopathy and has both acute and chronic disease manifestations. Because of this and other factors, patients with diabetes are more likely to require surgery. The majority of patients with diabetes develop disease in more than one body system, thus a thorough assessment of major organ disease (cardiac, renal, peripheral vascular) must be identified and managed carefully during the perioperative period. The patient with diabetes who is undergoing surgery is at risk for hypoglycemia and hyperglycemia. Hypoglycemia may develop during anesthesia or postoperatively from inadequate carbohydrates or excessive administration of insulin. Hyperglycemia, which can increase the risk for surgical wound infection, and fluid and electrolyte loss, may result from the stress of surgery because it triggers increased release of catecholamines. An increase in catecholamines contributes to an elevation in the blood glucose level. Previously, blood sugar was tightly controlled with intensive insulin therapy— this practice is no longer recommended routinely. Surgical patients with type 1 diabetes are also at risk for developing ketoacidosis. Refer to Chapter 30 for details on management of patients with diabetes.

Patients who have received corticosteroids are at risk of adrenal insufficiency. Therefore, the use of corticosteroids for any purpose during the preceding year must be reported to the anesthesia provider and surgeon. The patient is monitored for signs of adrenal insufficiency, which frequently presents with hyponatremia, hypoglycemia, hyperkalemia, and complaints of weakness and fatigue.

Patients with uncontrolled thyroid disorders are at risk for thyrotoxicosis (with hyperthyroid disorders) or respiratory failure (with hypothyroid disorders). Therefore, the patient is assessed for a history of these disorders. Refer to Chapter 31 for further discussion of endocrine disorders.

Immune Function

The nurse determines the presence of allergies. It is especially important to identify and document any sensitivity to medications and past adverse reactions to these agents. The nurse asks the patient to identify any substances that precipitated previous allergic reactions, including medications, herbal supplements, blood transfusions, contrast agents, latex, and food products, and to describe the signs and symptoms produced by these substances. A sample latex allergy screening questionnaire is shown in Figure 5-1.

Immunosuppression is common with corticosteroid therapy, kidney transplantation, radiation therapy, chemotherapy, and disorders affecting the immune system, such as AIDS and leukemia. The mildest symptoms or slightest temperature elevation must be investigated. Because patients who are immunosuppressed are highly susceptible to infection, the health care team should take great care to ensure strict asepsis.

Medication Use

A medication history is obtained from each patient because of the possible effects of medications on the patient's perioperative course, including the possibility of drug interactions. Any medication the patient is using or has used in the past is documented, including the frequency with which the medication is used. Potent medications have an effect on physiologic functions; interactions of such medications with anesthetic agents can cause serious problems, such as arterial hypotension and circulatory collapse.

The potential effects of prior medication therapy are evaluated by the anesthesia provider, who considers the length of time the patient has used the medication, the physical condition

Ask the patient the following questions. Check "Yes" or "No" in the box.	YES	NO
1. Has a doctor ever told you that you are allergic to latex?		
2. Do you have on-the-job exposure to latex?		
3. Were you born with problems involving your spinal cord?		
4. Have you ever had allergies, asthma, hay fever, eczema, or problems with rashes?		
5. Have you ever had respiratory distress, rapid heart rate, or swelling?		
6. Have you ever had swelling, itching, hives, or other symptoms after contact with a balloon?		
7. Have you ever had swelling, itching, hives, or other symptoms after a dental examination or procedure?		
8. Have you ever had swelling, itching, hives, or other symptoms following a vaginal or rectal examination or after contact with a diaphragm or condom?		
9. Have you ever had swelling, itching, hives, or other symptoms during or within 1 hour after wearing rubber gloves?		
10. Have you ever had a rash on your hands that lasted longer than 1 week?		
11. Have you ever had swelling, itching, hives, runny nose, eye irritation, wheezing, or asthma after contact with any latex or rubber product?		
12. Have you ever had swelling, itching, hives, or other symptoms after being examined by someone wearing rubber or latex gloves?		
13. Are you allergic to bananas, avocados, kiwi, or chestnuts?		
14. Have you ever had an unexplained anaphylactic episode?		

Preop RN Signature: _____

Patient Name: _____

Procedure: _____

Scheduled Date / Time: _____

Surgeon: _____

FIGURE 5-1 Example of a latex allergy assessment form. (Courtesy of Inova Fairfax Hospital, Falls Church, Virginia.)

of the patient, and the nature of the proposed surgery. Medications that cause particular concern are listed in Table 5-4.

In addition, many patients take self-prescribed or over-the-counter (OTC) medications. Aspirin is a common OTC medication that inhibits platelet aggregation; therefore, it is prudent to stop aspirin at least 7 to 10 days before surgery if possible, especially for surgeries in which excess bleeding would cause significant complications, such as brain or spinal cord surgeries. Because of the effects of aspirin or other OTC medications and possible interactions with prescribed medications and anesthetic agents, it is important to ask a patient

about their use. The information is noted in the patient's chart and conveyed to the anesthesia provider and surgeon.

The use of herbal medications is widespread among patients; because of their potential effects on coagulation and potentially lethal interactions with other medications, the nurse must ask surgical patients specifically about the use of these agents, document their use, and inform the surgical team and anesthesia provider. Decisions should be made by the surgical team about the discontinuation of herbal medications prior to surgery. Currently, there are no studies demonstrating specific adverse interactions between herbals and anesthetic drugs; however, some have been implicated to be related to pharmacokinetic and pharmacodynamic interactions (Wijeysundera & Sweitzer, 2015).

Psychosocial Factors

All patients have some type of emotional reaction before any surgical procedure, be it obvious or hidden, normal or abnormal. For example, preoperative anxiety may be an anticipatory response to an experience the patient views as a threat to his or her customary role in life, body integrity, or life itself. Psychological distress directly influences body functioning. In addition to providing anticipatory guidance about what the patient will experience during the operative procedure, the nurse provides opportunities for the patient to ask questions, so that concerns can be addressed.

Most patients who are about to undergo surgery have fears, including fear of the unknown, of death, of anesthesia, of pain, or of cancer. Concerns about loss of work time, loss of job, increased responsibilities or burden on family members, and the threat of permanent incapacity further contribute to the emotional strain created by the prospect of surgery. Less obvious concerns may occur because of previous experiences with the health care system and people the patient has known with the same condition.

People express fear in different ways. For example, some patients may repeatedly ask many questions, even though answers were given previously. Others may withdraw, deliberately avoiding communication, perhaps by reading, watching television, or talking about trivialities. Assessing the patient's readiness to learn and determining the best approach to maximize comprehension provides the basis for preoperative patient education. Consequently, the nurse must be empathetic, listen well, and provide information that helps alleviate concerns.

An important outcome of the psychosocial assessment is the determination of the extent and role of the patient's support network. The value and reliability of all available support systems are assessed. Other information, such as usual level of functioning and typical daily activities, may assist in the patient's care and rehabilitation plans.

Spiritual and Cultural Beliefs

Spiritual beliefs play an important role in how people cope with fear and anxiety. Regardless of the patient's religious

TABLE 5-4 Examples of Medications with the Potential to Affect the Surgical Experience

Agent (Generic and Trade Example)	Effect of Interaction with Anesthetics
Corticosteroids Prednisone (Deltasone)	Cardiovascular collapse can occur if discontinued suddenly. Therefore, a bolus of corticosteroid may be administered intravenously immediately before and after surgery.
Diuretics Hydrochlorothiazide (HydroDIURIL)	During anesthesia, may cause excessive respiratory depression resulting from an associated electrolyte imbalance
Phenothiazines Chlorpromazine (Thorazine)	May increase the hypotensive action of anesthetics
Tranquilizers Diazepam (Valium)	May cause anxiety, tension, and even seizures if withdrawn suddenly
Insulin	Interaction between anesthetics and insulin must be considered when a patient with diabetes is undergoing surgery. IV insulin may need to be administered to keep the blood glucose within the normal range.
Antibiotics Erythromycin (Ery-Tab)	When combined with a curariform muscle relaxant, nerve transmission is interrupted and apnea from respiratory paralysis may result.
Anticoagulants Warfarin (Coumadin)	Can increase the risk of bleeding during the intraoperative and postoperative periods; should be discontinued in anticipation of elective surgery. The surgeon will determine how long before the elective surgery the patient should stop taking an anticoagulant, depending on the type of planned procedure and the medical condition of the patient.
Antiseizure Medications	IV administration of medication may be needed to keep the patient seizure-free in the intraoperative and postoperative periods.
Monoamine Oxidase (MAO) Inhibitors Phenelzine sulfate (Nardil)	May increase the hypotensive action of anesthetics
Thyroid Hormone Levothyroxine sodium (Levothroid)	IV administration may be needed during the postoperative period to maintain thyroid levels.

affiliation, spiritual beliefs can be as therapeutic as medication. Every attempt must be made to help the patient obtain the spiritual support that he or she requests. Faith has great sustaining power. Therefore, the beliefs of each patient should be respected and supported. In addition, the nurse needs to communicate and document if the patient declines blood transfusions for religious reasons (Jehovah's Witnesses), as this information needs to be clearly identified in the preoperative period. Some nurses avoid the subject of a clergy visit lest the suggestion alarm the patient. Asking whether the patient's spiritual advisor knows about the impending surgery is a caring, nonthreatening approach.

Showing respect for a patient's cultural values and beliefs facilitates rapport and trust. Some areas of assessment include identifying the ethnic group to which the patient relates and the customs and beliefs the patient holds about illness and health care providers. For example, patients from some cultural groups are unaccustomed to expressing feelings openly. Nurses need to consider this pattern of communication when assessing pain. Nurses should familiarize themselves with these cultural similarities and differences (see Box 1-3 in Chapter 1) and, recently, the Joint Commission has developed standards of cultural competency for health care workers (The Joint Commission, 2016a).

Perhaps the most valuable skill at the nurse's disposal is listening carefully to the patient, especially when obtaining the history. Invaluable information and insights may be gained through effective communication and interviewing skills. An unhurried, understanding, and caring nurse promotes confidence on the part of the patient.

Presence of Genetic Disorders

In the preoperative period, attention needs to be paid to patients with various genetic disorders (listed below) since surgical outcomes may be altered related to complications with anesthesia.

- Malignant hyperthermia (MH) (discussed on page 130)
- Central core disease (CCD), is a genetic disorder that presents in the neonatal period or infancy with muscle

weakness and hypotonia and mild facial weakness. This condition increases the risk of developing MH.
- Duchenne muscular dystrophy and Becker dystrophy are two types of muscular dystrophies associated with risk of developing MH.
- Hyperkalemic periodic paralysis is a genetic disorder that causes episodes of extreme muscle weakness and occasionally hyperkalemia. It is also associated with MH.
- King–Denborough syndrome, a rare genetic disorder associated with musculoskeletal abnormalities, is associated with MH.

Preoperative Nursing Management

Providing Preoperative Teaching

Preoperative education is important for improved patient outcomes. Each patient is taught as an individual, with consideration for any unique concerns or learning needs. Preoperative teaching is initiated as soon as possible, includes different modalities (verbal, written, electronic, return demonstration), and should be tailored to the needs of the patient. It should start in the surgeon's office or at the time of Pre-Admission Testing (PAT), continue until the patient arrives in the OR, and extend to and through discharge.

Timing and Technique

It is best to begin teaching early, when the patient and family may be less anxious and can make adjustments or prepare for the postoperative period more effectively. The ideal timing for preoperative teaching is not on the day of surgery but during the preadmission visit, when diagnostic tests are performed. At this time, the nurse or resource person answers questions and provides important patient teaching. During this visit, the patient can meet and ask questions of the perioperative nurse and health care team members, view audiovisual resources, receive written materials, and be given the telephone number to call as questions arise closer to the date of surgery. Many institutions provide access to websites where patients can view and review written instructions, communicate electronically, and ask questions with caregivers.

Teaching should go beyond descriptions of the procedure and should include explanations of the sensations the patient will experience. For example, telling the patient only that preoperative medication will cause relaxation before the operation is not as effective as also noting that the medication may result in lightheadedness and drowsiness. Knowing what to expect will help the patient anticipate these reactions and, thus, attain a higher degree of relaxation than might otherwise be expected. Knowing ahead of time about the possible need for a ventilator, drainage tubes, or other types of equipment helps decrease anxiety in the postoperative period. In addition, preoperative teaching includes instruction in the breathing and leg exercises used to prevent postoperative complications such as pneumonia and deep vein thrombosis (DVT). These exercises may be performed in the hospital or at home. The nurse should guide the patient through the experience and allow ample time for questions. For some patients, overly detailed descriptions increase anxiety; the nurse should be sensitive to this and provide as much detail as necessary to ensure patient preparation.

Deep Breathing, Coughing, and Incentive Spirometry

One goal of preoperative nursing care is to teach the patient how to promote optimal lung expansion and consequent blood oxygenation after anesthesia. The patient assumes a sitting position to enhance lung expansion. The nurse then demonstrates how to take a deep, slow breath and how to exhale slowly (see Box 11-7 in Chapter 11). After practicing deep breathing several times, the patient is instructed to breathe deeply, exhale through the mouth, take a short breath, and cough deeply (see Box 5-3). The nurse also demonstrates how to use an incentive spirometer, a device that provides measurement and feedback related to breathing effectiveness. In addition to enhancing respiration, these exercises may help the patient relax.

If a thoracic or abdominal incision is anticipated, the nurse demonstrates how to splint the incision to minimize pressure and control pain. The patient should put the palms of both hands together, interlacing the fingers snugly. Placing the hands across the incisional site acts as an effective splint when coughing. In addition, the patient is informed that medications are available to relieve pain and should be taken regularly for pain relief, so that effective deep breathing and coughing exercises can be performed. The goal in promoting coughing is to mobilize secretions, so that they can be removed. Deep breathing before coughing stimulates the cough reflex. If the patient does not cough effectively, atelectasis (collapse of the alveoli), pneumonia, or other lung complications may occur.

Promoting Mobility

The goals of promoting mobility postoperatively are to improve circulation, prevent venous stasis, and promote optimal respiratory function. The nurse explains the rationale for frequent position changes after surgery and then shows the patient how to turn from side to side and how to assume the lateral position without causing pain or disrupting IV lines, drainage tubes, or other equipment. The nurse uses proper body mechanics when turning the patient and instructs the patient to do the same. Whenever the patient is positioned, his or her body needs to be properly aligned.

In addition, some patients require instruction about special positions that are required after surgery (e.g., abduction or elevation of an extremity). The importance of maintaining as much mobility as possible despite restrictions is discussed. Reviewing the process before surgery is helpful, because the patient may be too uncomfortable or drowsy after surgery to absorb new information.

BOX 5-3 **Patient Education**

Preoperative Instructions to Prevent Postoperative Complications

Coughing

1. Lean forward slightly from a sitting position in bed, interlace your fingers together, and place your hands across the incisional site to act as a splint-like support when coughing.

Splinting of chest when coughing

Leg Exercises

1. Lie in a semi-Fowler position and perform the following simple exercises to improve circulation.
2. Bend your knee and raise your foot—hold it a few seconds, then extend the leg and lower it to the bed.

Straighten Flex

Down

Leg exercises

3. Do this five times with one leg, and then repeat with the other leg.
4. Then trace circles with the feet by bending them down, in toward each other, up, and then out.
5. Repeat these movements five times.

Foot exercises

Turning to the Side

1. Turn on your side with the uppermost leg flexed most and supported on a pillow.
2. Grasp the side rail as an aid to maneuver to the side.
3. Practice coughing while on your side.

Getting Out of Bed

1. Turn on your side.
2. Push yourself up with one hand as you swing your legs out of bed.

Exercise of the extremities includes extension and flexion of the knee and hip joints (similar to bicycle riding while lying on the side). The foot is rotated as though tracing the largest possible circle with the great toe (see Box 5-3). The elbow and shoulder are also put through their range of motion. At first, the patient is assisted and reminded to perform these exercises. Later, the patient is encouraged to do them independently. Muscle tone is maintained so that ambulation will be easier.

Pain Management

The nurse is guided by the recommendations of the Joint Commission that the "hospital uses methods to assess pain that are consistent with the patient's age, conditions, and ability to understand" (www.jc.org, 2015). A pain assessment should include differentiation between acute and chronic pain. A pain intensity scale should be introduced and explained to the patient to promote more effective postoperative pain management.

Once a patient answers yes to whether he or she has pain, the nurse should perform a comprehensive pain assessment and select an appropriate pain assessment scale (see Chapter 7).

Patients are informed that medications will be administered to relieve pain and maintain comfort without compromising the cardiopulmonary and neurologic status. Anticipated methods of administration of analgesic agents for inpatients include patient-controlled analgesia (PCA), epidural catheter bolus or infusion, peripheral nerve blockades, or patient-controlled epidural analgesia (PCEA). A patient who is expected to go home likely will receive local anesthetic and oral analgesic agents. These methods are discussed with the patient before surgery, and the patient's interest and willingness to use them are assessed.

Instruction for Patients Undergoing Ambulatory Surgery

Preoperative education for the same-day or ambulatory surgical patient comprises all the material presented above as well as collaborative planning with the patient and family for discharge and follow-up home care. The major difference in outpatient preoperative education is the teaching environment.

Preoperative teaching content may be presented in a group class, on a videotape, at PAT, or by telephone in conjunction with the preoperative interview. In addition to answering questions and describing what to expect, the nurse tells the patient when and where to report, what to bring (insurance card, copayment, and list of medications and allergies), what to leave at home (jewelry, watch, medications, contact lenses), and what to wear (loose-fitting, comfortable clothes; flat shoes). During the final preoperative telephone call, teaching is completed or reinforced as needed, and last-minute instructions are given. The patient is reminded not to eat or drink as directed.

Unfolding Patient Stories: Vernon Watkins • Part 1

Vernon Watkins, a 69-year-old male, came to the emergency department with severe abdominal pain, and a bowel perforation was diagnosed. He is being prepared for surgery. Significant medical history includes controlled hypertension and smoking for 50 years. What preoperative education should the nurse discuss with Mr. Watkins prior to his emergent surgery? (Vernon Watkins' story continues in Chapter 49.)

Care for Vernon and other patients in a realistic virtual environment: *vSim for Nursing* (thepoint.lww.com/vSimMedicalSurgical). Practice documenting these patients' care in (thepoint.lww.com/DocuCareEHR).

Managing Nutrition and Fluids

The major purpose of withholding food and fluid before surgery is to prevent aspiration. Until recently, fluid and food were restricted preoperatively overnight and often longer. However, the American Society of Anesthesiologists (ASA) reviewed this practice and has made new recommendations for people undergoing elective surgery who are otherwise healthy.

The American Society of Anesthesiologists published practice guidelines pertaining to preoperative fasting in non-laboring individuals undergoing elective procedures. The recommended fasting period after consuming clear fluids for all patients is 2 hours. In general, the volume of liquid ingested is less important than the type of liquid ingested (e.g., clear liquids vs. milk products) (Wijeysundera & Sweitzer, 2015, p. 1147).

Preparing the Bowel

Enemas are not commonly prescribed preoperatively unless the patient is undergoing abdominal or pelvic surgery. In this case, a cleansing enema or laxative may be prescribed the evening before surgery and may be repeated the morning of surgery. The goals of this preparation are to allow satisfactory visualization of the surgical site and to prevent trauma to the intestine or contamination of the peritoneum by feces. Unless the condition of the patient presents some contraindication, the toilet or bedside commode, rather than the bedpan, is used for evacuating the enema if the patient is hospitalized during this time. In addition, antibiotics may be prescribed to reduce intestinal flora.

Preparing the Skin

The goal of preoperative skin preparation is to decrease bacteria without injuring the skin. If the surgery is not performed as an emergency, the patient may be instructed to use a soap containing a detergent-germicide to cleanse the skin area for several days before surgery to reduce the number of skin organisms; this preparation may be carried out at home.

In general, hair is not removed preoperatively unless the hair at or around the incision site is likely to interfere with the operation. If hair must be removed, electric clippers are used for safe hair removal immediately before the operation.

Providing Immediate Preoperative Care

The patient changes into a hospital gown that is tied loosely and opens in the back. The patient with long hair may braid it, remove hairpins, and cover the head completely with a disposable bouffant cap.

The mouth is inspected, and dentures or plates are removed. If left in the mouth, these items could easily fall to the back of the throat during induction of anesthesia and cause respiratory obstruction.

Jewelry is not worn to the OR; wedding rings and jewelry of body piercings should be removed to prevent injury (The Association of PeriOperative Registered Nurses [AORN], 2015). If a patient objects to removing a ring, some institutions allow the ring to be securely fastened to the finger with tape. All articles of value, including assistive devices, dentures, glasses, and prosthetic devices, are given to family members or are labeled clearly with the patient's name and stored in a safe and secure place according to the institution's policy.

All patients (except those with urologic disorders) should void immediately before going to the OR to promote continence during low abdominal surgery and to make abdominal organs more accessible. Urinary catheterization is performed in the OR as necessary.

Maintaining the Preoperative Record

Since the release of the World Health Organization's Surgical Safety Checklist in 2008, surgical safety checklists have been used to foster an environment of teamwork and communication while ensuring that staff members consistently adhere to safety standards (Fig. 5-2). The nurse completes the preoperative assessment and plan of care, as well as the portion of the universal protocol/safety checklist that focuses on patient identification, correct documents, and patient understanding of the surgical procedure. The surgical site should be marked by the surgeon during this phase if the surgery involves laterality, and the marking is documented by the admitting nurse. The completed chart (with the preoperative checklist and verification form) accompanies the patient to the OR with the most recent history and physical (within the past 30 days), anesthetic assessment, and surgical consent form attached, along with all laboratory reports and nurses' records per hospital policy. Any unusual last-minute observations that may have a bearing on anesthesia or surgery are noted prominently at the front of the chart. Many institutions document these preoperative requirements electronically. To support this process, institutions are required to ensure that a standard hand-off process is in place to communicate critical and pertinent information to the next caregiver.

Administering Preanesthetic Medication

The rare use of preanesthetic medication is a minimal dose with ambulatory or outpatient surgery. If prescribed, it is usually administered in the preoperative holding area. If a preanesthetic medication is administered, the patient is kept

---

Before induction of anaesthesia →	Before skin incision →	Before patient leaves operating room
(with at least nurse and anaesthetist)	(with nurse, anaesthetist and surgeon)	(with nurse, anaesthetist and surgeon)

Before induction of anaesthesia (with at least nurse and anaesthetist)

Has the patient confirmed his/her identity, site, procedure, and consent?
☐ Yes

Is the site marked?
☐ Yes
☐ Not applicable

Is the anaesthesia machine and medication check complete?
☐ Yes

Is the pulse oximeter on the patient and functioning?
☐ Yes

Does the patient have a:

Known allergy?
☐ No
☐ Yes

Difficult airway or aspiration risk?
☐ No
☐ Yes, and equipment/assistance available

Risk of >500ml blood loss (7ml/kg in children)?
☐ No
☐ Yes, and two IVs/central access and fluids planned

Before skin incision (with nurse, anaesthetist and surgeon)

☐ **Confirm all team members have introduced themselves by name and role.**

☐ **Confirm the patient's name, procedure, and where the incision will be made.**

Has antibiotic prophylaxis been given within the last 60 minutes?
☐ Yes
☐ Not applicable

Anticipated Critical Events

To Surgeon:
☐ What are the critical or non-routine steps?
☐ How long will the case take?
☐ What is the anticipated blood loss?

To Anaesthetist:
☐ Are there any patient-specific concerns?

To Nursing Team:
☐ Has sterility (including indicator results) been confirmed?
☐ Are there equipment issues or any concerns?

Is essential imaging displayed?
☐ Yes
☐ Not applicable

Before patient leaves operating room (with nurse, anaesthetist and surgeon)

Nurse Verbally Confirms:

☐ The name of the procedure

☐ Completion of instrument, sponge and needle counts

☐ Specimen labeling (read specimen labels aloud, including patient name)

☐ Whether there are any equipment problems to be addressed

To Surgeon, Anaesthetist and Nurse:

☐ What are the key concerns for recovery and management of this patient?

This checklist is not intended to be comprehensive. Additions and modifications to fit local practice are encouraged.

FIGURE 5-2 Surgical safety checklist. Based on the WHO Surgical Safety Checklist, http://whqlibdoc.who.int/publications/2009/9789241598590_eng_Checklist.pdf.

in bed with the side rails raised, because the medication can cause lightheadedness or drowsiness. During this time, the nurse observes the patient for any untoward reaction to the medications. The immediate surroundings are kept quiet to promote relaxation.

Nursing Alert
Protecting patients from injury is one of the major roles of the perioperative nurse. Specific nursing interventions to decrease the risk of falling after the premedication is administered are to raise the side rails of the bed, provide the call light if available, and remind the patient that out of bed (OOB) activity is not permitted due to potential medication side effects such as dizziness.

Transporting the Patient to the Presurgical Area

Patient safety in the preoperative area is a priority. Use of a process to verify patient identification, the surgical procedure, and the surgical site is imperative to maximize patient safety. This process should be performed at the time of admission in the presurgical unit and during all hand-offs from caregiver to caregiver. This allows for prompt intervention if any discrepancies are identified.

Attending to Family Needs

Most hospitals and ASCs have a waiting room where family members and significant others can wait while the patient is undergoing surgery. This room may be equipped with comfortable chairs, television, telephones, and facilities for light refreshment. Volunteers may remain with the family, offer them coffee, and keep them informed of the patient's progress. After surgery, the surgeon should meet the family in the waiting room or call the family and discuss the outcome.

The family and significant others should never judge the seriousness of an operation by the length of time the patient is in the OR. A patient may be in surgery much longer than the actual operating time for several reasons:

- Patients are routinely transported well in advance of the actual operating time.
- The anesthesia provider often makes additional preparations that may take 30 to 60 minutes.
- Patient positioning may take up to 45 minutes prior to procedure start time.
- The surgeon may take longer than expected with the preceding case, which delays the start of the next surgical procedure.

After surgery, the patient is taken to the PACU to ensure safe emergence from anesthesia. Family members and significant others waiting to see the patient after surgery should be informed that the patient may have certain equipment or devices (e.g., IV lines, indwelling urinary catheter, nasogastric tube, oxygen lines, monitoring equipment, blood transfusion lines) in place when he or she returns from surgery.

Many hospitals now adopt the model of patient- and family-centered care and allow visitations in the PACU for short periods after the patient is stabilized and made comfortable. In ambulatory surgery and pediatric settings, family members are brought in early in the recovery process and are integral to the preparation for discharge. When the patient returns to the room, the nurse provides explanations regarding the frequent postoperative observations that will be made. However, it is the responsibility of the surgeon, not the nurse, to relay the surgical findings and the prognosis, even when the findings are favorable.

INTRAOPERATIVE NURSING

The **intraoperative phase** begins when the patient is transferred onto the OR table and ends with admission to the PACU. In this phase, the scope of nursing activities includes:

- providing for the patient's safety
- maintaining an aseptic environment
- ensuring proper function of equipment
- providing the surgeon with specific instruments and supplies for the surgical field
- completing appropriate documentation
- providing emotional support during induction of general anesthesia
- assisting in positioning the patient on the OR table using appropriate principles of body alignment
- acting as scrub nurse, circulating nurse, or registered nurse first assistant (RNFA)

The intraoperative experience has undergone many changes that make it safer and less disturbing to patients. However, even with these advances, anesthesia and surgery place the patient at risk for several complications or adverse events. Consciousness or full awareness, mobility, protective biologic functions, and personal control are totally or partially relinquished by the patient when entering the OR. Staff from the departments of anesthesia, nursing, and surgery work collaboratively to implement professional standards of care, to control iatrogenic (adverse condition in a patient resulting from treatment) and individual risks, to prevent complications, and to promote high-quality patient outcomes.

The Surgical Team

The surgical team includes the **circulating nurse** (also known as the **circulator**), scrub person (scrub role), RNFA, surgeon, and anesthesia providers. Table 5-5 summarizes the roles of each member. Every member of the surgical team verifies the patient's name, procedure, and surgical site using objective documentation and data before beginning the surgery, as mandated by the Joint Commission. This is referred to as the "time out" or final pause and must be performed prior to incision, preferably with the patient involved; if patient's surgical site was marked, the mark should be visible.

TABLE 5-5 The Surgical Team

Team Member	Responsibilities
Circulating Nurse (Circulator)	Using the nursing process to develop individualized plans of care Checking and managing the OR conditions (ensuring cleanliness, proper temperature, humidity, lighting, safe function of equipment, and the availability of supplies and materials) Continually assessing the patient for signs of injury and implementing appropriate interventions Verifying consent and ensuring documentation is correct Coordinating the team Monitoring aseptic practices to avoid breaks in technique while coordinating the movement of related personnel (medical, x-ray, and laboratory) Implementing fire safety precautions and accounting for all surgical counts in collaboration with scrub person Ensuring that the second verification of the surgical procedure and site takes place and is documented Managing specimens
Scrub person	Performing a surgical hand scrub Setting up the sterile tables Preparing sutures, ligatures, and special equipment (e.g., laparoscope) Anticipating the instruments and supplies that will be required, such as sponges, drains, and other equipment As the surgical incision is closed, counting all needles, sponges, and instruments with the nurse to be sure they are accounted for and not retained as a foreign body within the patient's body
Registered nurse first assistant (RNFA)	Handling tissue Providing exposure at the operative field Suturing Maintaining hemostasis
Surgeon (he or she is a licensed physician, osteopath, oral surgeon, or podiatrist who is specially trained and qualified)	Performing the surgical procedure Heading the surgical team
Anesthesia Provider—Anesthesiologist (a physician specifically trained in the art and science of anesthesiology) and anesthetist (a qualified health care professional who administers anesthetics; most are certified registered nurse anesthetists [CRNAs])	Assessing the patient before surgery Selecting the anesthesia and administering it Intubating the patient if necessary Managing any technical problems related to the administration of the anesthetic agent Supervising the patient's condition throughout the surgical procedure

The Surgical Environment

The surgical environment is known for its stark appearance and cool temperature. The surgical suite is behind double doors, and access is limited to authorized personnel. To provide the best possible conditions for surgery, the OR is situated in a location that is central to all supporting services (e.g., pathology, x-ray, laboratory). The OR has special air filtration devices to screen out contaminating particles, dust, and pollutants.

Maintaining the Environment

Most of the Joint Commission's 2015 National Patient Safety Goals pertain to the perioperative areas (see Box 5-4). External precautions include adhering to principles of surgical asepsis, and strict control of the OR environment is required, including traffic pattern restrictions. Policies governing this environment address such issues as the health of the staff; the cleanliness of the rooms; the sterility of equipment and surfaces; processes for scrubbing, gowning, and gloving; and OR attire.

BOX 5-4 Primary National Patient Safety Goals for 2015

- Identify patients correctly
- Improve staff communication
- Use medicines safely
- Use alarms safely
- Prevent infection
- Identify patient safety risks
- Prevent mistakes in surgery

From http://www.jointcommission.org/assets/1/6/2015_HAP_NPSG_ER.pdf.

Preventing Surgical Fire

Fire is a risk to both patients and personnel in the operating room due to the three elements of the fire triangle that are necessary for a fire: fuel, oxidizer, and ignition source (AORN, 2015; Norton, Gorgone, & Belanger, 2014). Although rare, the possibility of surgical fires can result in devastating disfigurement, serious injury, and death. Fires can occur at any time in the OR; for example, surgical drapes provide an opportunity for oxygen to concentrate; a stray spark could more easily ignite a fire. To evaluate safety in the facility, electrical hazards, emergency exit clearances, and storage of equipment and anesthetic gases are monitored periodically by official agencies, such as the state department of health and the Joint Commission. All operating room personnel must be familiar with and educated about fire prevention and how to respond in the event that a fire should occur in the operating room. A fire risk assessment should be completed and communicated to the surgical team prior to the start of a procedure (AORN, 2015).

Donning Proper Attire

To help decrease microbes, the surgical area is divided into three zones: the **unrestricted zone**, where street clothes are allowed; the **semirestricted zone**, where attire consists of scrub clothes and caps; and the **restricted zone**, where scrub clothes, shoe covers, caps, and masks are worn. The surgeons and other surgical team members wear additional sterile clothing and protective devices during the operation.

The Association of Perioperative Registered Nurses, formerly known as the Association of Operating Room Nurses (still abbreviated as AORN), recommends specific practices for personnel wearing surgical attire to promote a high level of cleanliness in a particular practice setting (AORN, 2015). Shirts and waist drawstrings should be tucked inside the pants to prevent accidental contact with sterile areas and to contain skin shedding. Wet or soiled garments should be changed.

Masks are worn at all times in the restricted zone of the OR. High-filtration masks decrease the risk of postoperative wound infection by containing and filtering microorganisms from the oropharynx and nasopharynx. Masks should fit tightly, should cover the nose and mouth completely, and should not interfere with breathing, speech, or vision. Masks must be adjusted to prevent venting from the sides. Disposable masks have a filtration efficiency exceeding 95%. Masks are changed between patients and should not be worn outside the surgical department. The mask must be either on or off; it must not be allowed to hang around the neck.

Headgear should cover the hair completely (head and neckline, including beard), so that single strands of hair, bobby pins, clips, and particles of dandruff or dust do not fall on the sterile field.

Shoes should be comfortable and supportive. Shoe covers are worn when it is reasonably anticipated that spills or splashes will occur or if shoes are worn outside of the Operating Room Suite. Shoe covers should be changed when they become wet, torn, or soiled (AORN, 2015).

Barriers such as scrub attire and masks do not entirely protect the patient from microorganisms. Upper respiratory tract infections, sore throats, and skin infections in staff and patients are sources of pathogens and must be reported.

Because artificial fingernails harbor microorganisms and can cause nosocomial infections, a ban on artificial nails by OR personnel is supported by the Centers for Disease Control and Prevention (CDC), AORN, and the Association of Professionals in Infection Control. Short, natural fingernails are encouraged.

Using Environmental Controls

In addition to the protocols described previously, surgical asepsis requires meticulous cleaning and maintenance of the OR environment. Floors and horizontal surfaces are cleaned frequently with detergent, soap, and water or a detergent germicide. Sterilizing equipment is inspected regularly to ensure optimal operation and performance.

All equipment that comes into direct contact with the patient must be sterile. Sterilized linens, drapes, and solutions are used. Instruments are cleaned and sterilized in Central Sterile Services (CSS). Individually wrapped sterile items are used when additional individual items are needed.

Airborne bacteria are a concern. To decrease the amount of bacteria in the air, standard OR ventilation provides 15 air exchanges per hour, at least three of which are fresh air (CDC, 2015). A temperature of 20° to 24°C (68° to 73°F), humidity between 30% and 60%, and positive pressure relative to adjacent areas are maintained. Staff members shed skin scales, resulting in about 1,000 bacteria-carrying particles (or colony-forming units [CFUs]) per cubic foot per minute. With the standard air exchanges, air counts of bacteria are reduced to 50 to 150 CFUs per cubic foot per minute. Unnecessary personnel and physical movement may be restricted to minimize bacteria in the air and achieve an OR infection rate no greater than 3% to 5% in clean, infection-prone surgery.

Some ORs have laminar airflow units. These units provide 400 to 500 air exchanges per hour (CDC, 2015). The goal for a laminar airflow–equipped OR is an infection rate of less than 1%. An OR equipped with this unit is frequently used for total joint replacement or organ transplant surgery. Constant surveillance and conscientious technique in carrying out aseptic practices are necessary to reduce the risk of contamination and infection.

Health Hazards Associated with the Surgical Environment

Safety issues in the OR include exposure to blood and body fluids, latex and adhesive substances, radiation, toxic agents, and laser plumes. Internal monitoring of the OR includes the analysis of surface swipe samples and air samples for infectious and toxic agents. In addition, policies and procedures have been established for minimizing exposure to body fluids and reducing the dangers associated with lasers and radiation.

An additional hazard is the unintentional leaving of an object in a person during a surgical procedure. The risk that foreign objects may be left in a person increases in the following situations: when the procedure is performed on an emergency basis, when there is an unplanned change in the procedure, and when the patient has a high BMI. Many complications can occur from the retention of an object, and the patient is subjected to the risk of an additional surgical procedure.

Exposure to Blood and Body Fluids

OR attire has changed dramatically since the advent of HIV/AIDS. Double-gloving is routine in trauma and other types of surgery where sharp bone fragments are present. Goggles, or a wrap-around face shield, are worn to protect against splashing when the surgical wound is irrigated or when bone drilling is performed. In hospitals where numerous total joint procedures are performed, a complete face shield may be used. This shield provides full-barrier protection from bone fragments and splashes. Ventilation is accomplished through an accompanying hood with a separate air-filtration system.

Latex Allergy

The AORN has recommended standards of care for the patient with latex allergy (AORN, 2015). These recommendations include early identification of patients with latex allergies, preparation of a latex allergy supply cart, and maintenance of latex allergy precautions throughout the perioperative period. Because of the increased number of patients with latex allergies, most products are latex free. For safety, manufacturers and hospital material managers need to take responsibility for identifying the latex content in items used by patients and health care personnel. Additional discussion of latex allergy can be found in Chapter 38.

Laser Risks

The AORN has recommended practices for laser safety. While lasers are in use, warning signs must be posted clearly to alert personnel. Safety precautions are implemented to reduce the possibility of exposing the eyes and skin to laser beams, to prevent inhalation of the laser plume (smoke and particulate matter), and to protect the patient and personnel from fire and electrical hazards. Several types of lasers are available for clinical use; perioperative personnel should be familiar with the unique features, specific operation, and safety measures for each type of laser used in the practice setting.

All personnel wear special protective goggles, specific to the type of laser used in the procedure (ANSI, 2014).

Whether protection is needed to avoid the laser plume and the effects of its inhalation is controversial. Smoke evacuators are used in some procedures to remove the laser plume from the operative field. In recent years, this technology has been used to protect the surgical team from the potential hazards associated with the generalized smoke plume generated by standard electrocautery units.

The Surgical Experience

During the surgical procedure, the patient will need sedation, anesthesia, or some combination of these. In addition, strict surgical asepsis is maintained.

Anesthesia and Sedation

Anesthesia today is very safe, and although anesthesia-related morbidity and mortality is difficult to quantify, more recent studies estimate anesthesia-related death rate in the United States to be less than 1 per 10,000 anesthetics (Barash et al., 2013). When the patient arrives in the OR, the anesthesia provider reassesses the patient's physical condition immediately prior to initiating anesthesia. For the patient, the anesthesia experience consists of having an IV line inserted, if it was not inserted earlier; receiving a sedating agent prior to induction with an anesthetic agent; losing consciousness; being intubated, if indicated; and then receiving a combination of anesthetic agents. Typically, the experience is a smooth one, and the patient has no recall of the events. The main types of anesthesia are general anesthesia, regional anesthesia, moderate sedation, monitored anesthesia care, and local anesthesia.

During surgery, the anesthesia provider monitors the patient's blood pressure, pulse, and respirations as well as the electrocardiogram (ECG), blood oxygen saturation level, tidal volume, blood gas levels, blood pH, alveolar gas concentrations, and body temperature. Monitoring by electroencephalography (measure of brain waves) is sometimes required. Levels of anesthetics in the body also can be determined; a mass spectrometer can provide instant readouts of critical concentration levels on display terminals. This information helps personnel assess the patient's ability to breathe unassisted or the need for mechanical assistance if ventilation is poor and the patient is not breathing well independently. Even with the availability of automatic monitoring equipment, the anesthesia provider and/or nurse must remain in close contact with the patient to observe any significant physiologic changes immediately.

General Anesthesia

Anesthesia is a state of narcosis (severe central nervous system [CNS] depression produced by pharmacologic agents), analgesia, relaxation, and reflex loss. Patients under general anesthesia are not arousable, not even to painful stimuli. They lose the ability to maintain ventilatory function and require assistance in maintaining a patent airway. Cardiovascular function may be impaired as well.

General anesthesia consists of four stages, each associated with specific clinical manifestations (Box 5-5) (Rothrock, 2014).

Stages of General Anesthesia

- *Stage I: Beginning anesthesia.* As the patient breathes in the anesthetic mixture, warmth, dizziness, and a feeling of detachment may be experienced. The patient may have a ringing, roaring, or buzzing in the ears and, although still conscious, may sense an inability to move the extremities easily. During this stage, noises are exaggerated; even low voices or minor sounds seem loud and unreal. For this reason, unnecessary noises and motions are avoided when anesthesia begins.
- *Stage II: Excitement.* The excitement stage, characterized variously by struggling, shouting, talking, singing, laughing, or crying, is often avoided if the anesthetic is administered smoothly and quickly. Because of the possibility of uncontrolled movements of the patient during this stage, the anesthesia provider must always be assisted by someone ready to help restrain the patient. The patient should not be touched except for purposes of restraint, but restraints should not be applied over the operative site.
- *Stage III: Surgical anesthesia.* Surgical anesthesia is reached by continued administration of the anesthetic vapor or gas. The patient is unconscious and lies quietly on the table. With proper administration of the anesthetic, this stage may be maintained for hours in one of several planes, ranging from light (1) to deep (4), depending on the depth of anesthesia needed.
- *Stage IV: Medullary depression.* This stage is reached when too much anesthesia has been administered. Cyanosis develops and, without prompt intervention, death follows rapidly. If this stage develops, the anesthetic is discontinued immediately and respiratory and circulatory support is initiated to prevent death. Stimulants, although rarely used, may be administered; narcotic antagonists can be used if the overdosage is due to opioids.

When opioid agents (narcotics) and neuromuscular blockers (relaxants) are administered, several of the stages are absent. During smooth administration of an anesthetic, there is no sharp division between stages I, II, and III, and there is no stage IV. The patient passes gradually from one stage to another, and it is through close observation of the signs exhibited by the patient that an anesthesia provider controls the situation. The responses of the pupils, the blood pressure, and the respiratory and cardiac rates are among the most reliable guides to the patient's condition.

Anesthetic agents used in general anesthesia are inhaled or administered by IV (Fig. 5-3). Anesthetics produce anesthesia because they are delivered to the brain at a high partial pressure that enables them to cross the blood–brain barrier. Relatively large amounts of anesthetic must be administered during induction and the early maintenance phases because the anesthetic is recirculated and deposited in body tissues. As these sites become saturated, smaller amounts of the anesthetic agent are required to maintain anesthesia because equilibrium or near equilibrium has been achieved among brain, blood, and other tissues.

Any condition that diminishes peripheral blood flow, such as vasoconstriction or shock, may reduce the amount of anesthetic required. Conversely, when peripheral blood flow is unusually high, as in a muscularly active or apprehensive patient, induction is slower, and greater quantities of anesthetic are required because the brain receives a smaller quantity of anesthetic.

Inhaled Administration. Inhalation anesthetics are commonly used for the provision of general **anesthesia**. With the addition of a volatile (readily vaporized) anesthetic to inspired oxygen, a state of unconsciousness and amnesia can be established. When combined with additional medications (e.g., opioids and benzodiazepines), further sedation/hypnosis and amnesia are established. They are considered easy to administer, inexpensive, and reliable in terms of ability to monitor their effects with both clinical signs and end-tidal

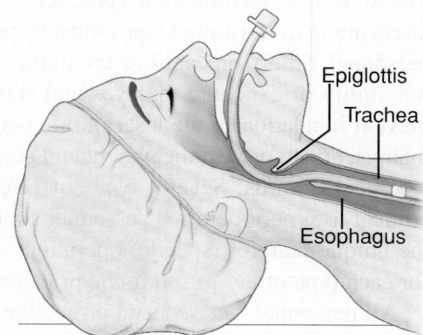

A. Laryngeal Mask Airway (LMA)   **B.** Intranasal intubation   **C.** Oral intubation

FIGURE 5-3 Anesthetic delivery methods: (**A**) laryngeal mask airway (LMA), (**B**) nasal endotracheal catheter (in position with cuff inflated), and (**C**) oral endotracheal intubation (tube is in position with cuff inflated).

concentrations (Perouansky, Pearce, & Hemmings, 2015). In addition, they are important in situations where there is a lack of venous access and anticipated airway difficulty.

Intravenous Administration. General anesthesia can be produced by the IV administration of various substances, such as barbiturates, benzodiazepines, nonbarbiturate hypnotics, dissociative agents, and opioid agents. Table 5-6 lists commonly used IV anesthetic and analgesic agents, including IV medications used as muscle relaxants in the intraoperative period. These medications may be administered to induce (initiate) or maintain anesthesia. Although they are often used in combination with inhalation anesthetics, they may be used alone. They may also be used to produce moderate sedation.

An advantage of IV anesthesia is that the onset of anesthesia is pleasant; there is none of the buzzing, roaring, or dizziness known to follow administration of an inhalation anesthetic. For this reason, induction of anesthesia usually begins with an IV agent and often is preferred by patients who have experienced various methods. The duration of action is brief, and the patient awakens with little nausea or vomiting.

The IV anesthetic agents are nonexplosive, require little equipment, and are easy to administer. The low incidence of postoperative nausea and vomiting (PONV) makes the method useful in eye surgery because in this setting vomiting would increase intraocular pressure and endanger vision in the operated eye. IV anesthesia is useful for short procedures but is used less often for the longer procedures of abdominal surgery. It is not indicated for children, who have small veins, or for those who require intubation because of their susceptibility to respiratory obstruction.

A disadvantage of an IV anesthetic such as thiopental (Pentothal) is its powerful respiratory depressant effect. It must be administered by a skilled anesthesia provider and only when some method of oxygen administration is available immediately in case of difficulty. Sneezing, coughing, and laryngospasm are sometimes noted with its use.

TABLE 5-6 Commonly Used Intravenous Medications

Medication	Common Usage	Advantages	Disadvantages	Comments
Opioid Analgesics				
Morphine sulfate (MS)	Perioperative pain; premedication	Inexpensive; duration of action 4–5 hours; euphoria; good cardiovascular stability	Nausea and vomiting; histamine release; respiratory depression; postural ↓ BP and ↓ SVR	Used intrathecally and epidurally for postoperative pain; elimination half-life 90 minutes
Alfentanil (Alfenta)	Surgical analgesia in ambulatory patients	Duration of action 0.5 hour; used as bolus or infusion		Potency: 750 µg = 10-mg morphine sulfate; elimination half-life 1.6 hours
Fentanyl (Sublimaze)	Surgical analgesia: epidural infusion for postoperative analgesia; add to SAB	Good cardiovascular stability; duration of action 0.5 hour		Most commonly used opioid; potency: 100 µg = 10-mg morphine sulfate; elimination half-life 3.6 hours
Remifentanil (Ultiva)	IV infusion for surgical analgesia; small boluses for brief, intense pain	Easily titratable; metabolized by blood and tissue esterases; very short duration; good cardiovascular stability	New; expensive; requires mixing; may cause muscle rigidity	Potency: 25 µg = 10-mg morphine sulfate; 20–30 times the potency of alfentanil; elimination half-life 3–10 minutes
Sufentanil (Sufenta)	Surgical analgesia	Good cardiovascular stability; duration of action 0.5 hour; prolonged analgesia	Prolonged respiratory depression	Potency: 15 µg = 10-mg morphine sulfate; elimination half-life 2.7 hours
Nondepolarizing Muscle Relaxants—Intermediate Onset and Duration				
Rocuronium (Zemuron)	Intubation; maintenance of relaxation	Rapid onset (dose dependent); elimination via kidney and liver	Vagolytic; may ↑ HR	Duration similar to atracurium and vecuronium
Vecuronium (Norcuron)	Intubation; maintenance of relaxation	No significant cardiovascular or cumulative effects; no histamine release	Requires mixing	Mostly eliminated in bile, some in urine

(continued on page 124)

TABLE 5-6 **Commonly Used Intravenous Medications** (*continued*)

Medication	Common Usage	Advantages	Disadvantages	Comments
Intravenous Anesthetics				
Etomidate (Amidate)	Induction	Good cardiovascular stability; fast, smooth induction and recovery	May cause pain with injection and myotonic movements	May cause adrenal suppression
Diazepam (Valium, Dizac)	Amnesia; hypnotic; preoperative medication	Good sedation	Prolonged duration	Residual effects for 20–90 hours; increased effect with alcohol
Ketamine (Ketalar)	Induction, occasional maintenance (IV or IM)	Short acting; patient maintains airway; good in small children and burn patients	Large doses may cause hallucinations and respiratory depression	Need darkened, quiet room for recovery; often used in trauma cases
Midazolam (Versed)	Hypnotic; anxiolytic; sedation; often used as adjunct to induction	Excellent amnesia; water-soluble (no pain with IV injection); short acting	Slower induction than thiopental	Often used for amnesia with insertion of invasive monitors or regional anesthesia
Propofol (Diprivan)	Induction and maintenance; sedation with regional anesthesia or MAC	Rapid onset; awakening in 4–8 minutes	May cause pain when injected	Short elimination half-life (34–64 minutes)
Sodium methohexital (Brevital)	Induction	Ultrashort-acting barbiturate	May cause hiccups	Can be given rectally
Thiopental sodium (Pentothal)	Induction	Induction	May cause laryngospasm; can be given rectally	Large doses may cause apnea and cardiovascular depression

BP, blood pressure; HR, heart rate; IM, intramuscular; IV, intravenous; MAC, monitored anesthesia care; SAB, subarachnoid block; SVR, stroke volume ratio.

IV neuromuscular blockers (muscle relaxants) block the transmission of nerve impulses at the neuromuscular junction of skeletal muscles. Muscle relaxants are used to relax muscles in abdominal and thoracic surgery, relax eye muscles in certain types of eye surgery, facilitate endotracheal intubation, treat laryngospasm, and assist in mechanical ventilation.

Local Anesthesia

Local anesthesia is used to block nerves in the peripheral nervous system and CNS. Local anesthesia provides anesthesia and analgesia by blocking the transmission of pain sensation along nerve fibers. The degree of blockage depends on both drug concentration and volume.

Local anesthesia can be used alone or in conjunction with other types of anesthesia. Usually it is administered by the surgeon to a specific area of the body by topical application or local infiltration. In most cases, the patient will be monitored by a nurse. To ensure safety and quality of care, the AORN has developed recommended practices for nurses who monitor patients receiving local anesthesia (AORN, 2015). The nurse should also monitor the quantity of medication administered since toxic reactions are dose related (AORN, 2015).

Regional Anesthesia. Regional anesthesia is a form of local anesthesia in which an anesthetic agent is injected around nerves, so that the area supplied by these nerves is anesthetized. The most common techniques are spinal, epidural, and peripheral nerve blocks. Regional anesthesia is an attractive anesthetic option for many types of operative procedures and can provide excellent postoperative pain management in selected patients (Berde & Strichartz, 2015). The effect depends on the type of nerve involved. A local anesthetic blocks motor nerves least readily and sympathetic nerves most readily. An anesthetic cannot be regarded as having worn off until all three systems (motor, sensory, and autonomic) are no longer affected.

The patient receiving regional anesthesia is awake and aware of his or her surroundings unless medications are given to produce mild sedation or to relieve anxiety. The nurse must avoid careless conversation, unnecessary noise, and unpleasant odors; these may be noticed by the patient in the OR and may contribute to a negative response to the surgical experience. A quiet environment is therapeutic. The diagnosis must not be stated aloud if the patient is not to know it at this time.

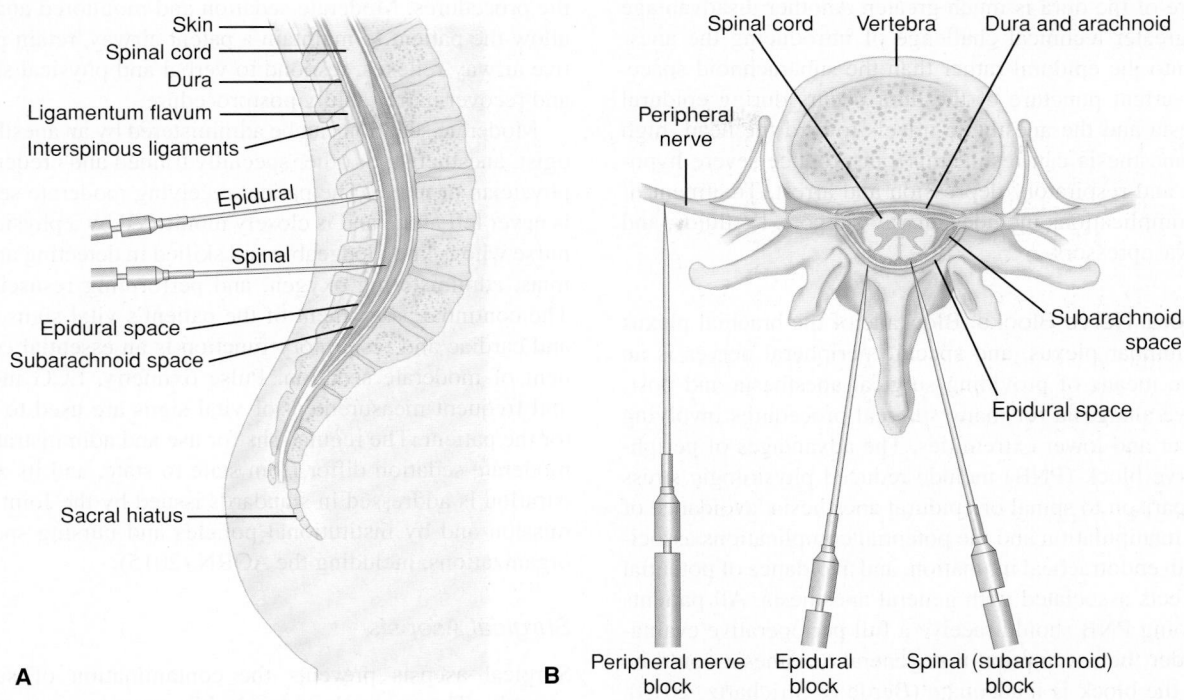

FIGURE 5-4 (**A**) Injection sites for spinal and epidural anesthesia. (**B**) Cross-section of injection sites for peripheral nerve, epidural, and spinal blocks.

Spinal Anesthesia. Spinal anesthesia is an extensive conduction nerve block that is produced when a local anesthetic is introduced into the subarachnoid space at the lumbar level, usually between L4 and L5 (Fig. 5-4). It produces anesthesia of the lower extremities, perineum, and lower abdomen. For the lumbar puncture procedure, the patient usually lies on the side in a knee-to-chest position. Sterile technique is used as a spinal puncture is made and the medication is injected through the needle. As soon as the injection has been made, the patient is positioned on his or her back. If a relatively high level of block is sought, the head and shoulders are lowered.

A few minutes after induction of a spinal anesthetic, anesthesia and paralysis affect the toes and perineum and then gradually the legs and abdomen. If the anesthetic reaches the upper thoracic and cervical spinal cord in high concentrations, a temporary partial or complete respiratory paralysis results. Paralysis of the respiratory muscles is managed by mechanical ventilation until the effects of the anesthetic on the cranial and thoracic nerves have worn off.

Nausea, vomiting, and pain may occur during surgery when spinal anesthesia is used. As a rule, these reactions result from manipulation of various structures, particularly those within the abdominal cavity. The simultaneous IV administration of a weak solution of thiopental and inhalation of nitrous oxide may prevent such reactions.

Headache may be an after-effect of spinal anesthesia. Several factors are related to the incidence of headache: the size of the spinal needle used, the leakage of fluid from the subarachnoid space through the puncture site, and the patient's hydration status. Measures that increase cerebrospinal pressure are helpful in relieving headache. These include maintaining a quiet environment, keeping the patient lying flat, and keeping the patient well hydrated.

In continuous spinal anesthesia, the tip of a plastic catheter remains in the subarachnoid space during the surgical procedure, so that more anesthetic may be injected as needed. This technique allows greater control of the dosage, but there is greater potential for postanesthetic headache because of the large-gauge needle used.

Epidural Anesthesia. Epidural anesthesia, a commonly used conduction block, is achieved by injecting a local anesthetic into the epidural space that surrounds the dura mater of the spinal cord (refer to Fig. 5-4). In contrast, spinal anesthesia involves injection through the dura mater into the subarachnoid space surrounding the spinal cord. Epidural anesthesia blocks sensory, motor, and autonomic functions; it differs from spinal anesthesia by the site of the injection and the amount of anesthetic agent used. Epidural doses are much higher because the epidural anesthetic does not make direct contact with the spinal cord or nerve roots.

Epidural anesthetics, if placed correctly, can cause less hypotension and less hemodynamic changes. However, since the needle used for epidural anesthesia is much larger (17 to 18 gauge) than that used in spinal anesthesia (22 to 24 gauge), the severity of the headache with inadvertent puncture of the dura is much greater. Another disadvantage is the greater technical challenge of introducing the anesthetic into the epidural rather than the subarachnoid space. If inadvertent puncture of the dura occurs during epidural anesthesia and the anesthetic travels toward the head, high spinal anesthesia can result; this can produce severe hypotension and respiratory depression and arrest. Treatment of these complications includes airway support, IV fluids, and use of vasopressors.

Peripheral Nerve Blocks. Blockade of the brachial plexus (arm), lumbar plexus, and specific peripheral nerves is an effective means of providing surgical anesthesia and postoperative analgesia for many surgical procedures involving the upper and lower extremities. The advantages of peripheral nerve block (PNB) include reduced physiologic stress in comparison to spinal or epidural anesthesia, avoidance of airway manipulation and the potential complications associated with endotracheal intubation, and avoidance of potential side effects associated with general anesthesia. All patients undergoing PNB should receive a full perioperative evaluation under the assumption that general anesthesia could be used if the block is inadequate (Berde & Strichartz, 2015). Examples of common local conduction blocks are:

- Brachial plexus block, which produces anesthesia of the arm
- Paravertebral anesthesia, which produces anesthesia of the nerves supplying the chest, abdominal wall, and extremities
- Transsacral (caudal) block, which produces anesthesia of the perineum and, occasionally, the lower abdomen
- Femoral nerve block, which produces anesthesia of the nerves supplying the leg.

Moderate Sedation/Analgesia and Monitored Anesthesia Care

It is important to distinguish between moderate sedation/analgesia and **monitored anesthesia care**. *Moderate sedation/analgesia* is a term used by the ASA in their practice guidelines for sedation and analgesia by nonanesthesiologists. *Monitored anesthesia care* implies the potential for a level of sedation deeper than what provided by sedation/analgesia and is always administered by an anesthesiologist (ASPAN, 2015). **Moderate sedation/analgesia**, previously referred to as *conscious sedation,* and monitored anesthesia are forms of anesthesia that involve the IV administration of sedatives and/or analgesic medications to reduce patient anxiety and control pain during diagnostic or therapeutic procedures. It is being used increasingly for specific short-term surgical procedures in hospitals and ambulatory care centers (Rothrock, 2014). The goal is to depress a patient's level of consciousness (LOC) to a moderate level to enable surgical, diagnostic, or therapeutic procedures to be performed while ensuring the patient's comfort during and cooperation with

the procedures. Moderate sedation and monitored analgesia allow the patient to maintain a patent airway, retain protective airway reflexes, respond to verbal and physical stimuli, and recover more rapidly postprocedure.

Moderate sedation can be administered by an anesthesiologist, anesthetist, or other specially trained and credentialed physician or nurse. The patient receiving moderate sedation is never left alone and is closely monitored by a physician or nurse who is knowledgeable and skilled in detecting arrhythmias, administering oxygen, and performing resuscitation. The continual assessment of the patient's vital signs, LOC, and cardiac and respiratory function is an essential component of moderate sedation. Pulse oximetry, ECG monitor, and frequent measurement of vital signs are used to monitor the patient. The regulations for use and administration of moderate sedation differ from state to state, and its administration is addressed in standards issued by the Joint Commission and by institutional policies and nursing specialty organizations, including the AORN (2015).

Surgical Asepsis

Surgical asepsis prevents the contamination of surgical wounds. The patient's natural skin flora or a previously existing infection may cause postoperative wound infection. Rigorous adherence to the principles of surgical asepsis by OR personnel is basic to preventing surgical site infections (SSIs).

Traditionally, the surgeon, surgical assistants, and nurses prepared themselves by scrubbing their hands and arms with antiseptic soap and water, but this traditional practice is being challenged by research investigating the optimal length of time to scrub and the best preparation to use. Many institutions have now introduced a scrubless process for cleaning the hands prior to surgery. Box 5-6 provides guidelines for maintaining surgical asepsis.

Intraoperative Nursing Management

The major goals for care of the patient during surgery are to reduce his or her anxiety, keep the patient free of perioperative injury related to positioning, avoid threats to safety, maintain patient dignity, and avoid complications associated with operative events.

Reducing Anxiety

The OR environment can seem cold, stark, and frightening to the patient, who may be feeling isolated and apprehensive. Introductions, addressing the patient by name warmly and frequently, verifying details, providing explanations, and encouraging and answering questions convey a sense of professionalism and friendliness that can help the patient feel secure. When discussing what the patient can expect in surgery, the nurse uses basic communication skills, such as touch and eye contact, to reduce anxiety. Attention to

BOX 5-6 Basic Guidelines for Maintaining Surgical Asepsis

All practitioners involved in the intraoperative phase have a responsibility to provide and maintain a safe environment. Adherence to aseptic practice is part of this responsibility. Here are the basic principles of aseptic technique:

- All materials in contact with the surgical wound or used within the sterile field must be sterile. Sterile surfaces or articles may touch other sterile surfaces or articles and remain sterile; contact with unsterile objects at any point renders a sterile area contaminated.
- Gowns of the surgical team are considered sterile in front from the chest to the level of the sterile field. The sleeves are also considered sterile from 2 in above the elbow to the stockinette cuff.
- Sterile drapes are used to create a sterile field. Only the top surface of a draped table is considered sterile. During draping of a table or patient, the sterile drape is held well above the surface to be covered and is positioned from front to back.
- Items are dispensed to a sterile field by methods that preserve the sterility of the items and the integrity of the sterile field. After a sterile package is opened, the edges are considered unsterile. Sterile supplies, including solutions, are delivered to a sterile field or handed to a scrubbed person in such a way that the sterility of the object or fluid remains intact.
- The movements of the surgical team are from sterile to sterile areas and from unsterile to unsterile areas. Scrubbed persons and sterile items contact only sterile areas; circulating nurses and unsterile items contact only unsterile areas.
- Movement around a sterile field must not cause contamination of the field. Sterile areas must be kept in view during movement around the area. At least a 1-foot distance from the sterile field must be maintained to prevent inadvertent contamination.
- Whenever a sterile barrier is breached, the area must be considered contaminated. A tear or puncture of the drape permitting access to an unsterile surface underneath renders the area unsterile. Such a drape must be replaced.
- Every sterile field is constantly monitored and maintained. Items of doubtful sterility are considered unsterile. Sterile fields are prepared as close as possible to the time of use.

physical comfort (warm blankets, position changes) helps the patient feel more comfortable. Telling the patient who else will be present in the OR, how long the procedure is expected to take, and other details helps the patient prepare for the experience and gain a sense of control.

Preventing Intraoperative Positioning Injury

The patient's position on the operating table depends on the surgical procedure to be performed as well as on the patient's physical condition (Fig. 5-5). The potential for transient discomfort or permanent injury is present because many positions are awkward. Hyperextending joints, compressing arteries, or pressing on nerves and bony prominences usually results in discomfort simply because the position must be sustained for a long period of time (Rothrock, 2014). Factors to consider include the following:

- The patient should be in as comfortable a position as possible, whether conscious or unconscious.
- The operative field must be exposed adequately.
- An awkward position, undue pressure on a body part, or use of stirrups or traction should not obstruct the vascular supply.
- Respiration should not be impeded by pressure of arms on the chest or by a gown that constricts the neck or chest.
- Nerves must be protected from undue pressure. Improper positioning of the arms, hands, legs, or feet can cause serious injury or paralysis. Shoulder braces must be well padded to prevent irreparable nerve injury, especially when the Trendelenburg position (head down) is necessary. The postoperative complication of compartment syndrome is associated with intraoperative positioning (AORN, 2015). Refer to Chapter 42 for information related to clinical manifestations of compartment syndrome.

- Precautions for patient safety must be observed, particularly with thin, elderly, or obese patients as well as those with a physical deformity.
- The patient may need light restraint before induction in case of excitement.

The usual position for surgery, called the dorsal recumbent position, is flat on the back. One arm is positioned at the side of the table, with the hand placed palm down; the other is carefully positioned on an arm board to facilitate IV infusion of fluids, blood, or medications. This position is used for most abdominal surgeries except for surgery of the gallbladder or pelvis (see Fig. 5-5A).

The Trendelenburg position usually is used for surgery on the lower abdomen and pelvis to obtain good exposure by displacing the intestines into the upper abdomen. In this position, the head and upper body are lowered. The patient is held in position by padded shoulder braces (see Fig. 5-5B).

The lithotomy position is used for nearly all perineal, rectal, and vaginal surgical procedures (see Fig. 5-5C). The patient is positioned on the back with the legs and thighs flexed. The position is maintained by placing the feet in stirrups.

The Sims' or lateral position is used for renal surgery. The patient is placed on the nonoperative side with an air pillow or beanbag 12.5 to 15 cm (5 to 6 in) thick under the loin, or on a table with a kidney or back lift (see Fig. 5-5D).

Other procedures, such as neurosurgery or abdominothoracic surgery, may require unique positioning and supplemental apparatus, depending on the operative approach.

A. Patient in position on the operating table for a laparotomy. Note the strap above the knees.

B. Patient in Trendelenburg position on operating table. Note padded shoulder braces in place. Be sure that brace does not press on brachial plexus.

C. Patient in lithotomy position. Note that the hips extend over the edge of the table.

D. Patient lies on unaffected side for kidney surgery. Table is spread apart to provide space between the lower ribs and the pelvis. The upper leg is extended; the lower leg is flexed at the knee and hip joints; a pillow is placed between the legs.

FIGURE 5-5 Positions on the operating table. Captions call attention to safety and comfort features. All surgical patients wear caps to cover the hair completely.

Protecting the Patient from Injury

A variety of activities are used to address the diverse patient safety issues that arise in the OR. The nurse protects the patient from injury by providing a safe environment. Verifying information, checking the chart for completeness, and maintaining surgical asepsis and an optimal environment are critical nursing responsibilities. Verifying that all required documentation is completed is one of the first functions of the intraoperative nurse. The patient is identified, and the planned surgical procedure, correct surgical site, and type of anesthesia are verified. It is important to review the patient's record for the following:

- Correct informed surgical consent, with patient's and surgeon's signatures
- Completed records for health history and physical examination

- Results of diagnostic studies
- Allergies (including latex)

In addition to checking that all necessary patient data are complete, the perioperative nurse obtains the necessary equipment specific to the procedure. The need for nonroutine medications, blood components, instruments, and other equipment and supplies is assessed, and the readiness of the room, completeness of physical setup, and completeness of instrument, suture, and dressing setups are determined. Any aspects of the OR environment that may negatively affect the patient are identified. These include physical features, such as room temperature and humidity; electrical hazards; potential contaminants (dust, blood, and discharge on floor or surfaces, uncovered hair, faulty attire of personnel, jewelry worn by personnel); and unnecessary traffic. The circulating nurse also sets up and maintains suction equipment in working order, sets up invasive monitoring equipment, assists with insertion of vascular access and monitoring devices (arterial, Swan-Ganz, central venous pressure, IV lines), and initiates appropriate physical comfort measures for the patient.

Preventing physical injury includes using safety straps and side rails and not leaving the sedated patient unattended. Transferring the patient from the stretcher to the OR table requires safe transferring practices. Other safety measures include properly positioning the grounding pad under the patient to prevent electrical burns and shock, removing excess antiseptic solution from the patient's skin, and promptly and completely draping exposed areas after the sterile field has been created to decrease the risk for hypothermia.

The importance of nursing measures to prevent "never events" in surgery such as prevention of retained foreign objects, wrong site surgery, and pressure ulcers cannot be overemphasized. The Joint Commission and the AORN have developed guidelines that should be implemented in each facility to prevent these from occurring. There are also technologic devices that can support the safe counting of surgical instruments and supplies to prevent retention of foreign objects. The unintended retention of foreign objects (URFOs)—also called retained surgical items (RSIs)—after invasive procedures can cause death, and surviving patients may sustain both physical and emotional harm, depending on the type of object retained and the length of time it is retained (Joint Commission, 2013). The risk of URFOs increases during certain surgical conditions (Box 5-7).

Nursing measures to prevent injury from excessive blood loss include blood conservation using equipment such as a cell-saver (a device for recirculating the patient's own blood cells) and administration of blood products. Few patients undergoing an elective procedure require blood transfusion, but those undergoing higher-risk procedures (such as orthopedic or cardiac surgeries) may require an intraoperative transfusion. The circulating nurse anticipates this need, checks that blood has been cross-matched and held in reserve, and is prepared to support the anesthesia provider with administration when needed.

BOX 5-7   Risk Factors for Unintended Retention of Foreign Objects (URFOs)

- The absence of policies and procedures
- Failure to comply with existing policies and procedures
- Problems with hierarchy and intimidation
- Failure in communication with physicians
- Failure of staff to communicate relevant patient information
- Inadequate or incomplete education of staff

From The Joint Commission, 2016.

Serving as Patient Advocate

Because the patient undergoing general anesthesia or moderate sedation experiences temporary sensory/perceptual alteration or loss, he or she has an increased need for protection and advocacy. Patient advocacy in the OR entails maintaining the patient's physical and emotional comfort, privacy, rights, and dignity. Patients, whether conscious or unconscious, should not be subjected to excess noise, inappropriate conversation, or, most of all, derogatory comments. As surprising as this sounds, banter in the OR occasionally includes jokes about the patient's physical appearance, job, personal history, and so forth. Cases have been reported in which seemingly deeply anesthetized patients recalled the entire surgical experience, including disparaging personal remarks made by OR personnel. As an advocate, the nurse never engages in this conversation and discourages others from doing so. Other advocacy activities include minimizing the clinical, dehumanizing aspects of being a surgical patient by making sure the patient is treated as a person, respecting cultural and spiritual values, providing physical privacy, and maintaining confidentiality.

Monitoring and Managing Potential Complications

It is the responsibility of the surgeon, anesthesia provider, and the circulating nurse to monitor and manage complications. Important nursing functions include being alert to and reporting changes in vital signs and symptoms of nausea and vomiting, anaphylaxis, hypoxia, hypothermia, MH, or disseminated intravascular coagulation (DIC) and assisting with the management of those complications. Each of these complications will be discussed shortly. It is the responsibility of all members of the health care team to maintain asepsis.

Nausea and Vomiting

Nausea and vomiting, or regurgitation, may affect patients during the intraoperative period. If gagging occurs, the patient is turned to the side, the head of the table is lowered, and a basin is provided to collect the vomitus. Suction is used to remove saliva and vomited gastric contents. The advent of new anesthetics has reduced the incidence; however, there is no single way to prevent nausea and vomiting. An interdisciplinary approach involving the surgeon, anesthesia provider, and nurse is best.

In some cases, the anesthesia provider administers antiemetics preoperatively or intraoperatively to counteract possible aspiration. If the patient aspirates vomitus, it will trigger an asthma-like attack with severe bronchial spasms and wheezing. Pneumonitis and pulmonary edema can subsequently develop, leading to extreme hypoxia. Increasing medical attention is being paid to silent regurgitation of gastric contents (not related to preoperative fasting times), which occurs more frequently than previously realized. The volume and acidity of the aspirate determine the extent of damage to the lungs.

Anaphylaxis

Anaphylaxis is an acute life-threatening allergic reaction to a specific antigen or hapten (a small molecule that can cause an immune response when bound to a protein) resulting in urticaria (hives), pruritus (itching), or angioedema (swelling beneath the skin rather than on the surface), and quickly deteriorating to vascular collapse, shock, and respiratory distress. Any time the patient comes into contact with a foreign substance, there is the potential for an anaphylactic reaction. Because medications are the most common cause of anaphylaxis, intraoperative nurses must be aware of the type and method of anesthesia used as well as the specific agents. An anaphylactic reaction can occur in response to many medications, latex, or other substances. Chapter 38 provides additional detail on anaphylaxis.

Hypoxia and Other Respiratory Complications

Inadequate ventilation, occlusion of the airway, inadvertent intubation of the esophagus, and hypoxia are significant potential complications associated with general anesthesia. Many factors can contribute to inadequate ventilation. Respiratory depression caused by anesthetic agents, aspiration of respiratory tract secretions or vomitus, and the patient's position on the operating table can compromise the exchange of gases. Anatomic variation can make the trachea difficult to visualize and result in the artificial airway being inserted into the esophagus rather than into the trachea. In addition to these dangers, asphyxia can occur from foreign bodies in the mouth, spasm of the vocal cords, relaxation of the tongue, or aspiration of vomitus, saliva, or blood. Brain damage from hypoxia occurs within minutes; therefore, vigilant monitoring of the patient's oxygenation status is a primary function of the anesthesia provider and the circulating nurse. Peripheral perfusion is checked frequently, and pulse oximetry values are monitored continuously.

Hypothermia

During anesthesia, the patient's temperature may fall. This condition is called *hypothermia* and is indicated by a core body temperature that is lower than normal (36.6°C [98.0°F] or less). Inadvertent hypothermia may occur as a result of a low temperature in the OR, infusion of cold fluids, inhalation of cold gases, open body wounds or cavities, decreased muscle activity, advanced age, or the pharmaceutical agents used (e.g., vasodilators, phenothiazines, general anesthetics). Also hypothermia may be induced intentionally in selected surgical procedures (e.g., cardiac surgeries requiring cardiopulmonary bypass) to reduce the patient's metabolic rate and energy demands.

Preventing unintentional hypothermia is a major objective. If hypothermia occurs, the goal of intervention is to minimize or reverse the physiologic process. If hypothermia is intentional, the goal is safe return to normal body temperature. Environmental temperature in the OR can be set temporarily at 25° to 26.6°C (78° to 80°F). IV and irrigating fluids are warmed to 37°C (98.6°F). Wet gowns and drapes are removed promptly and replaced with dry materials because wet linens promote heat loss. Whatever methods are used to rewarm the patient, warming must be accomplished gradually, not rapidly. Conscientious monitoring is required for core temperature, urinary output, ECG, blood pressure, arterial blood gas (ABG) levels, and serum electrolyte levels.

 Nursing Alert

Shivering is associated with hypothermia. The nurse is aware that shivering can increase oxygen demand by 300% to 400%, thus supplemental oxygen should be administered, and oxygen saturation monitoring should be continuous.

Malignant Hyperthermia

MH is a rare inherited muscle disorder that is chemically induced by anesthetic agents (Rothrock, 2014). At one time, mortality rates exceeded 80%. Since the introduction of dantrolene sodium in 1979, the development of genetics testing, and early detection and treatment with specific protocols, fatalities have been reduced to approximately less than 10% (Zhou, Bose, Allen, & Pessah, 2015). Identification of patients at risk for MH is imperative. Susceptible people include those with strong and bulky muscles, familial genetic mutations as described earlier, first-degree relatives of persons who have been diagnosed or suspected of MH, and an unexplained death of a family member during surgery that was accompanied by a febrile response.

During anesthesia, potent agents such as inhalation anesthetics (halothane, enflurane) and muscle relaxants (succinylcholine) may trigger the symptoms of MH (refer to Table 5-5 for list of anesthetic agents). Stress and some medications, such as sympathomimetics (epinephrine), theophylline, aminophylline, anticholinergics (atropine), and cardiac glycosides (digitalis), can induce or intensify such a reaction. The pathophysiology is related to a hypermetabolic condition in skeletal muscle cells that involves altered mechanisms of calcium function at the cellular level. This disruption of calcium causes clinical symptoms of hypermetabolism, which, in turn, increases muscle contraction (rigidity). The sustained muscle contraction causes hyperthermia (fever may exceed 110°F) and subsequent damage to the CNS.

The skeletal muscle cells, when depleted of their source of cellular energy (adenosine triphosphate [ATP]), break down and release the muscle cell contents, including myoglobin (a protein released from muscle when injury occurs), creatine phosphokinase (CPK), and potassium into the systemic circulation. The resulting hyperkalemia has a dramatic effect on the heart, causing ventricular arrhythmias. The muscle pigment myoglobin has an affinity for the kidneys, resulting in potential for kidney failure (refer to Chapter 42, Box 42-7 for details). If untreated, cardiac arrest, kidney failure, blood coagulation problems, internal hemorrhage, brain injury, liver failure, and death can result.

The initial symptoms of MH are related to cardiovascular and musculoskeletal activity. Tachycardia (heart rate >150 bpm) is often the earliest sign. In addition to the tachycardia, sympathetic nervous stimulation leads to ventricular arrhythmia, hypotension, decreased cardiac output, oliguria (less than 400 mL), and, later, cardiac arrest. With the abnormal transport of calcium, rigidity or tetanus-like movements occur, often in the jaw. The rise in temperature is actually a late sign that develops rapidly; body temperature can increase 1° to 2°C (2° to 4°F) every 5 minutes (Rothrock, 2014). The core body temperature can reach or exceed 42°C (104°F) in a very short time and must be properly monitored and recorded during surgery. Clinical signs of patients with MH include: hypercarbia (elevated carbon dioxide in blood), sinus tachycardia, rapidly increasing temperature, elevated temperature, masseter muscle spasm, also known as masseter muscle spasm after succinylcholine administration (the muscle covering the side of the jaw nearest the ear, responsible for mastication [chewing]), generalized muscular rigidity, tachypnea (increased respiratory rate), profuse diaphoresis, cola-colored urine, cyanosis, skin mottling, ventricular tachycardia, excessive bleeding, unstable blood pressure, and ventricular fibrillation (Zhou et al., 2015). The entire health team is alert for the presence of any of the aforementioned signs.

Recognizing symptoms early and discontinuing anesthesia promptly are imperative. The immediate response is the discontinuation of the triggering agent and hyperventilation of the patient with 100% oxygen and immediate administration of at least 2.5 mg/kg of dantrolene sodium intravenously (Zhou et al., 2015). Additional incremental doses may be required until the signs of MH are controlled. Because dantrolene is available in 20-mg multidose vials that must be reconstituted with 50 mL of sterile water only, it is expected that at least two nurses will be reconstituting the drug during the crisis. If the patient is hyperthermic, active cooling is initiated with iced saline administration, lavage of the stomach, bladder, rectum, and open body cavities if appropriate with iced saline, use of a hypothermia blanket, and use of ice packs. It is essential to monitor the patient's temperature to assess treatment efficacy and avoidance of hypothermia. Antiarrhythmic medications, such as amiodorone, are expected for management of ventricular arrhythmias; infusion by IV glucose and insulin, as well as calcium chloride, is anticipated for the hyperkalemia. Sodium bicarbonate may be administered to treat the metabolic acidosis based upon ABG analysis. In addition, diuretics may be administered to assist with the clearance of filtered myoglobin into the urine; hourly urine output and color of urine are observed closely (Zhou et al., 2015).

Goals of treatment are to decrease metabolism, reverse metabolic and respiratory acidosis, correct arrhythmias, decrease body temperature, provide oxygen and nutrition to tissues, and correct electrolyte imbalance. The Malignant Hyperthermia Association of the United States (MHAUS)

publishes a treatment protocol that should be posted in the OR and be readily available on an MH cart. Although MH is uncommon, all providers must identify patients at risk, recognize the signs and symptoms, have the appropriate medication and equipment available, and be knowledgeable about the protocol to follow. This preparation may be life-saving for the patient.

Disseminated Intravascular Coagulation

DIC is a dynamic systemic disorder that results in widespread hemorrhage and microthrombosis with ischemia. It can be a side effect of MH or a precursor to the development of MH. The mortality rate can exceed 80%, and clinical manifestations may be bleeding from mucous membranes, venipuncture sites, and the GI and urinary tracts. Bleeding can range from minimal occult internal bleeding to profuse hemorrhage from all orifices. It is important that all providers are alert for the subtle cues of developing DIC. Refer to Chapter 20 for complete details of DIC.

POSTOPERATIVE NURSING

The **postoperative phase** begins when the patient is transferred to the PACU and report is given by the anesthesia provider and circulating nurse to the perianesthesia nurse. The postoperative phase ends when the patient is discharged from all phases of postoperative care. The scope of nursing care in this phase covers a wide range of activities, including maintaining the patient's airway, monitoring vital signs, assessing the effects of the anesthetic agents, assessing the patient for complications, and providing comfort and pain relief. Nursing activities also focus on promoting the patient's recovery and initiating the teaching, follow-up care, and referrals essential for recovery and rehabilitation after discharge.

Nursing Management During Postanesthesia Care

Postanesthesia care in some hospitals and ambulatory surgical centers is divided into two phases. In **phase I PACU**, which is the immediate recovery phase, intensive nursing care is provided. In **phase II PACU**, the patient is prepared for self-care or care in the hospital, an extended-care setting, or discharge. Recliners rather than stretchers or beds are standard in many phase II units. In facilities without separate phases, the patient remains in the PACU and may be discharged home directly from this unit (ASPAN, 2015).

The nursing management objectives for the nurse in the PACU are to provide care until the patient has recovered from the effects of anesthesia (e.g., until resumption of motor and sensory functions), is oriented or returns to baseline cognition, has stable vital signs and adequate pain control, and shows no evidence of hemorrhage or other complications. All PACU nurses have special skills, including strong assessment skills. The PACU nurse provides frequent monitoring (every 15 minutes) of the patient's pulse, ECG, respiratory rate, blood pressure, and pulse oximeter value (blood oxygen level). In some cases, the end-tidal carbon dioxide ($ETCO_2$) level is monitored as well. The patient's airway may become obstructed because of the latent effects of recent anesthesia, and the PACU nurse must be prepared to assist in reintubation and in handling other emergencies that may occur. Nurses in PACUs must also possess excellent patient teaching skills.

Admitting the Patient to the PACU

Transferring the postoperative patient from the OR to the PACU is the responsibility of the anesthesia provider. During transport from the OR to the PACU, the anesthesia provider remains at the head of the stretcher (to maintain the airway), and a surgical team member remains at the opposite end. Transporting the patient involves special consideration of the incision site, potential vascular changes, and exposure. The surgical incision is considered every time the postoperative patient is moved; many wounds are closed under considerable tension, and every effort is made to prevent further strain on the incision. The patient is positioned so that he or she is not lying on or obstructing drains or drainage tubes. Serious orthostatic hypotension may occur when a patient is moved too quickly from one position to another (e.g., from a lithotomy position to a horizontal position or from a lateral to a supine position), so the patient must be moved slowly and carefully. As soon as the patient is placed on the stretcher or bed, the soiled gown is removed and replaced with a dry gown. The patient is covered with lightweight blankets and warmed. Three side rails may be raised to prevent falls.

Assessing the Patient

The cornerstones of nursing care in the PACU are frequent, skilled assessments of the blood oxygen saturation level, pulse rate and regularity, depth and nature of respirations, skin color, LOC, and ability to respond to commands. The nurse performs a baseline assessment and then checks the surgical site for drainage or hemorrhage and makes sure that all drainage tubes and monitoring lines are connected and functioning. The nurse checks any IV fluids or medications currently infusing and verifies dosage and rate.

After the initial assessment, the patient's vital signs and general physical status are assessed at least every 15 minutes. Patency of the airway and respiratory function are always evaluated first, followed by assessment of cardiovascular function, the condition of the surgical site, and function of the CNS. Any surgical procedure has the potential for injury due to disrupted neurovascular integrity resulting from prolonged awkward positioning in the OR, manipulation of tissues, inadvertent severing of nerves, or tight bandages. Any orthopedic surgery or surgery involving the extremities carries a risk of peripheral nerve damage. Vascular surgeries, such as replacing sections of diseased peripheral arteries or inserting an arteriovenous graft, put the patient at risk for thrombus formation at the surgical site and subsequent ischemia of tissues distal to the thrombus. Assessment of *circulation, sensation, and mobility* (CSM) includes having the patient move the hand or foot distal to the surgical site through a full range of motion, assessing all surfaces for intact sensation, and assessing peripheral pulses and capillary refill (Rothrock, 2014). Refer to Table 40-3, Assessing for Peripheral Nerve Function for specific nerve monitoring on page 1180. The nurse must be aware of any pertinent information from the patient's history that may be significant (e.g., patient is deaf or hard of hearing, has a history of seizures, has diabetes, is allergic to certain medications or to latex, etc.).

Maintaining a Patent Airway

The primary objective in the immediate postoperative period is to maintain pulmonary ventilation and, thus, prevent hypoxemia (reduced oxygen in the blood) and hypercapnia (excess carbon dioxide in the blood). Both can occur if the airway is obstructed and ventilation is reduced (hypoventilation). Besides checking the provider's orders for and administering supplemental oxygen, the nurse assesses respiratory rate and depth, ease of respirations, oxygen saturation, and breath sounds.

Patients who have experienced prolonged anesthesia usually are unconscious, with all muscles relaxed. This relaxation extends to the muscles of the pharynx. When the patient lies on his or her back, the lower jaw and the tongue fall backward and the air passages become obstructed (Fig. 5-6). This is called *hypopharyngeal obstruction*.

Nursing Alert
Signs of hypopharyngeal occlusion include choking; noisy and irregular respirations; decreased oxygen saturation; and within minutes, a blue, dusky color (cyanosis) of the skin. Because movement of the thorax and the diaphragm does not necessarily indicate that the patient is breathing, the nurse needs to place the palm of her hand at the patient's nose and mouth to feel the exhaled breath.

The anesthesia provider may leave a hard rubber or plastic airway in the patient's mouth or nares to maintain a patent airway. Such a device should not be removed until signs such as gagging indicate that reflex action is returning. Alternatively, the patient may enter the PACU with an endotracheal tube still in place and may require continued mechanical ventilation. The nurse assists in initiating the use of the ventilator and in the weaning and extubation processes. Some patients, particularly those who have had extensive or lengthy surgical procedures, may be transferred from the OR directly to the intensive care unit (ICU) or from the PACU to the ICU while still intubated and receiving mechanical ventilation.

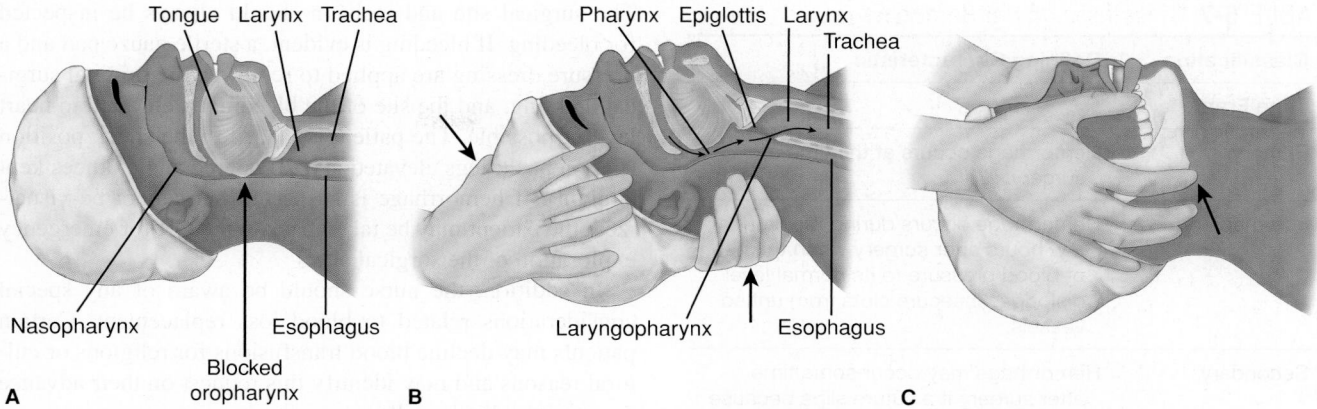

FIGURE 5-6 (**A**) A hypopharyngeal obstruction occurs when neck flexion permits the chin to drop toward the chest; obstruction almost always occurs when the head is in the midposition. (**B**) Tilting the head back to stretch the anterior neck structure lifts the base of the tongue off the posterior pharyngeal wall. The direction of the arrows indicates the pressure of the hands. (**C**) Opening the mouth is necessary to correct valve-like obstruction of the nasal passage during expiration, which occurs in about 30% of unconscious patients. Open the patient's mouth (separate lips and teeth) and move the lower jaw forward, so that the lower teeth are in front of the upper teeth. To regain backward tilt of the neck, lift with both hands at the ascending rami of the mandible.

Respiratory difficulty also can result from excessive secretion of mucus or aspiration of vomitus. Placing the patient on his or her side in the recovery position will allow the fluid to escape from the mouth. The head of the bed is elevated 15 to 30 degrees unless contraindicated, and the patient is closely monitored to maintain the airway as well as to minimize the risk of aspiration. If vomiting occurs, the patient is turned to the side to prevent aspiration, and the vomitus is collected in the emesis basin. Mucus or vomitus obstructing the pharynx or the trachea is suctioned with a pharyngeal suction tip or a nasal catheter introduced into the nasopharynx or oropharynx. Caution is necessary in suctioning the throat of a patient who has had a tonsillectomy or other oral or laryngeal surgery because of risk of bleeding and discomfort.

Maintaining Cardiovascular Stability

To monitor cardiovascular stability, the nurse assesses the patient's mental status; vital signs; cardiac rhythm; skin temperature, color, and moisture; and urine output. Central venous pressure, pulmonary artery pressure, and arterial lines are monitored if the patient's condition requires such assessment. The nurse also assesses the patency of all IV lines. The primary cardiovascular complications seen in the PACU include hypotension and shock, hemorrhage, hypertension, and arrhythmias.

Hypotension and Shock

Hypotension can result from blood loss, hypoventilation, position changes, pooling of blood in the extremities, or side effects of medications and anesthetics. The most common cause is loss of circulating volume through blood and plasma loss. If the amount of blood loss exceeds 500 mL (especially if the loss is rapid), replacement is usually indicated.

Fluid loss is a significant potential problem for surgical patients, owing to their preoperative NPO status, evaporation of fluid intraoperatively, and significant shifting of sodium-rich fluid from the intravascular space to the extracellular space because of inflammatory process, trauma, or infection. The fluid lost from the blood stream sequesters in the tissues or "third spaces," which may be noted by the presence of edema. It is important for the nurse to understand that, although the patient may clinically present with edema (often associated with fluid volume excess), a hypovolemia exists intravascularly that can progress to shock if fluids are not managed adequately. In addition, the nurse considers fluid loss related to evaporation in the OR. For example, it is estimated that, with surgery involving an open abdomen, insensible fluid losses can reach 500 to 1,000 mL/hr (Rothrock, 2014). When evaluating the patient's fluid volume status, the nurse considers fluid loss from the nasogastric tube, urinary output, drains, estimated blood loss (EBL), and evaporation.

Shock, one of the most serious postoperative complications, can result from hypovolemia and decreased intravascular volume. The types of shock are classified as hypovolemic, cardiogenic, neurogenic, anaphylactic, and septic. See Chapter 54 for more information on shock.

Hemorrhage

Hemorrhage is an uncommon yet serious complication of surgery that can result in death. It can present insidiously or emergently at any time in the immediate postoperative period or up to several days after surgery (Table 5-7). When blood loss is extreme, the patient is apprehensive, restless, agitated and thirsty; the skin is cold, moist, and pale. The pulse rate increases, the temperature falls, hypotension is seen with a

TABLE **5-7** **Classifications of Hemorrhage**

Classification	Defining Characteristic
Time Frame	
Primary	Hemorrhage occurs at the time of surgery.
Intermediary	Hemorrhage occurs during the first few hours after surgery when the rise of blood pressure to its normal level dislodges insecure clots from untied vessels.
Secondary	Hemorrhage may occur some time after surgery if a suture slips because a blood vessel was not tied securely, became infected, or was eroded by a drainage tube.
Type of Vessel	
Capillary	Hemorrhage is characterized by a slow, general ooze.
Venous	Darkly colored blood bubbles out quickly.
Arterial	Blood is bright red and appears in spurts with each heartbeat.
Visibility	
Evident	Hemorrhage is on the surface and can be seen.
Concealed	Hemorrhage is in a body cavity and cannot be seen.

narrowed pulse pressure (difference between systolic and diastolic pressure; normal pulse pressure is approximately 40 mm Hg), and respirations are rapid and deep, often of the gasping type spoken of as "air hunger." Capillary refill is prolonged (normal is less than 2 seconds), and there is diminished urine output. If hemorrhage progresses untreated, cardiac output decreases, arterial and venous blood pressure and hemoglobin levels fall rapidly, the lips and the conjunctivae become pale, and the patient grows weaker and obtunded but remains conscious until near death.

Nursing Alert

The term obtunded *comes from the root word,* obtund, *which means "dulled or less sharp" and is used to describe a patient who presents with less than full alertness (altered LOC). Rather than use terms like* stuporous *or* obtunded, *it is beneficial to describe the behavior in detail rather than use a broad term.*

The initial therapeutic measures are to transfusing blood or blood products and determining the cause of hemorrhage.

The surgical site and incision should always be inspected for bleeding. If bleeding is evident, a sterile gauze pad and a pressure dressing are applied to reinforce the original surgical dressing, and the site of the bleeding is elevated to heart level if possible. The patient is placed in the shock position (flat on back; legs elevated at a 20-degree angle; knees kept straight). If hemorrhage is suspected but cannot be visualized, the patient may be taken back to the OR for emergency exploration of the surgical site.

In addition, the nurse should be aware of any special considerations related to blood loss replacement. Certain patients may decline blood transfusions for religious or cultural reasons and may identify this request on their advance directives or living will.

Nursing Alert

*Always wear gloves when handling blood. To prevent warming of the blood, administration should begin within 30 minutes of retrieving the blood. If this is not possible, the blood should be returned to the blood bank. Baseline vital signs are obtained. Normal saline injection (0.9% sodium chloride) is used to initiate a transfusion of red blood cells (RBCs), whole blood, platelets, or leukocytes. Hypotonic or hypertonic solutions are **never used** because hemolysis of the RBCs occurs. No medications or other solutions except 0.9% sodium chloride should be added to or infused simultaneously through the same blood set. Refer to Chapter 20 for more details on blood transfusion.*

Nursing Alert

Hemoglobin levels of 7 to 9 g/dL are generally tolerated by most asymptomatic patients. Symptomatic patients with cardiac, pulmonary, or cerebrovascular disease may require RBC transfusions to achieve higher hemoglobin levels (Rosen, 2015). The nurse understands that the transfusion of 1 unit of packed RBCs should increase the hemoglobin level by 1 g/dL and the hematocrit by 3%.

Hypertension and Arrhythmias

Hypertension is common in the immediate postoperative period secondary to sympathetic nervous system stimulation from pain, hypoxia, or bladder distention. Arrhythmias are associated with electrolyte imbalance, altered respiratory function, pain, hypothermia, stress, and anesthetic agents. Both hypertension and arrhythmias are managed by treating the underlying causes.

Relieving Pain and Anxiety

IV opioid analgesics are administered judiciously and often in the PACU. IV opioids provide immediate pain relief and are short acting, thus minimizing the potential for drug interactions or prolonged respiratory depression while there are anesthetics still active in the patient's system. The PACU nurse monitors the patient's physiologic status, manages pain, and provides psychological support in an effort to relieve the patient's fears and concerns. The nurse checks the medical record for special needs and concerns of the patient. When the patient's condition permits, a close member of the family may visit in the PACU. This often decreases the family's anxiety and makes the patient feel more secure.

Controlling Nausea and Vomiting

Postoperative and postdischarge nausea and vomiting (PONV/PDNV) is one of the most commonly occurring postoperative complications, frequently resulting in prolonged postoperative stay, unanticipated admission, and increased health care costs. Health care providers have yet to reach consensus regarding an evidence-based multidisciplinary, multimodel treatment approach to PONV/PDNV. The nurse should intervene at the patient's first report of nausea to control the problem rather than wait for it to progress to vomiting.

Many medications are available to control nausea and vomiting without oversedating the patient; they are commonly administered during surgery, as well as in the PACU. Medications such as metoclopramide (Reglan), prochlorperazine (Compazine), promethazine (Phenergan), dimenhydrinate (Dramamine), hydroxyzine (Vistaril, Atarax), and scopolamine (Transderm-Scop) are commonly prescribed (Rothrock, 2014). Although it is costly, ondansetron (Zofran) is frequently used as an effective antiemetic with few side effects.

ASPAN has developed a practice guideline for nurses to treat this postoperative complication (ASPAN, 2015). It includes the identification of risk factors (e.g., for adults undergoing general inhaled anesthesia, risks include female gender, being a nonsmoker, history of PONV or motion sickness, and the use of postoperative intravenous opioids (Apfel, 2015). Recommended treatments can range from no prophylaxis treatment to several antiemetic combinations for patients at higher risk (ASPAN, 2014).

Preparing for Discharge from the PACU

A patient remains in the PACU until fully recovered from the anesthetic agent. Indicators of recovery include stable blood pressure, adequate respiratory function, adequate oxygen saturation level compared with baseline, and spontaneous movement or movement on command. Discharge criteria should be developed collaboratively with the anesthesia department using the standards below (ASPAN, 2015):

- Stable vital signs
- Return to baseline LOC
- Uncompromised pulmonary function and adequate airway
- Pulse oximetry readings indicating adequate blood oxygen saturation

- Intake and output
- Nausea and vomiting absent or under control
- Pain level
- Sensory and motor function
- Condition of surgical site

Many hospitals use a scoring system (e.g., Aldrete score) to determine the patient's general condition and readiness for transfer from the PACU. Throughout the recovery period, the patient's physical signs are observed and evaluated by means of a scoring system based on a set of objective criteria (Aldrete & Wright, 1992; Theodora, 2015) that includes consciousness, activity, breathing, pulse oximetry, and circulation. The patient is assessed at regular intervals (e.g., every 15 minutes), and a total score is calculated and recorded on the assessment record. Patients remain in the PACU until their condition improves or they can be transferred safely to an ICU or surgical unit, or discharged (depending on their preoperative baseline score).

The patient is discharged from the phase I PACU by the anesthesia provider to the critical care unit, the medical-surgical unit, the phase II PACU, or home with a responsible family member.

Nursing Management of Direct Discharge Home

To ensure patient safety and recovery, expert patient teaching and discharge planning are necessary when a patient undergoes same-day or ambulatory surgery. Because anesthetics cloud memory for concurrent events, verbal and written instructions should be given to both the patient and the adult who will be accompanying the patient home. Alternative formats (e.g., large print, Braille) of instructions or use of a sign interpreter may be required to ensure patient and family understanding. A translator may be required if the patient and family members do not understand English.

The patient and caregiver (e.g., family member or friend) are informed about expected outcomes and immediate, anticipated postoperative changes. The nurse provides written instructions about wound care, activity and dietary recommendations, medications, and follow-up visits to the surgeon. The patient's caregiver at home is provided with verbal and written instructions about what to look for and about the actions to take if complications occur. Prescriptions and medication reconciliation are given to the patient and/or caregiver. The nurse's or surgeon's telephone number is provided, and the patient and caregiver are encouraged to call with questions and to schedule follow-up appointments.

Nursing Alert
Medication reconciliation is the process of creating the most accurate list possible of all medications a patient is taking—including drug name, dosage, frequency, and route—and comparing that list against the provider's admission, transfer, and/or

discharge orders, with the goal of providing correct medications to the patient at all transition points within the hospital (Institute for Healthcare Improvement [IHI], 2016).

Although recovery time varies depending on the type and extent of surgery and the patient's overall condition, instructions usually advise limited activity for 24 to 48 hours. During this time, the patient should not drive a vehicle, drink alcoholic beverages, or perform tasks that require energy or skill. Fluids may be consumed as desired, and smaller-than-normal amounts may be eaten at mealtime. Patients are cautioned not to make important decisions at this time, because the medications, anesthesia, and surgery may affect their decision-making ability.

Nursing Management of the Hospitalized Postoperative Patient

Given the complexities of patient care treatment and management, multisystem disease, and workplace demands, it is important that the traditional "nurse-to-nurse" patient hand-off now be a comprehensive, thorough, and sophisticated account of patient information focusing on patient safety (AORN, 2015). Hand-off communication must also allow opportunity for questions to be answered. The *SBAR* format is an increasingly popular approach to the standardization of relaying of this crucial information. SBAR is a mnemonic for:

Situation (What is happening at the present time?)
Background (What are the circumstances leading up to this situation?)
Assessment (What do I think the problem is?)
Recommendation (What should we do to correct the problem?) (IHI, 2017).

Whatever approach is used in each institution, it is essential that the method is used by all staff members during all hand-offs across all phases of surgical patient care.

Receiving the Patient in the Clinical Unit

The patient's room is readied by assembling the necessary equipment and supplies: IV pole, drainage receptacle holder, suction equipment, oxygen, emesis basin, tissues, disposable pads, blankets, and postoperative documentation. When the call comes to the unit about the patient's transfer from the PACU, the need for any additional items should be communicated. The PACU nurse reports data about the patient to the receiving nurse. The report includes relevant demographic data, medical diagnosis, procedure performed, type of anesthesia, comorbid conditions, allergies, unexpected intraoperative events, EBL, types and amounts of fluids received, medications administered for pain, types of IV fluids or medications infused, whether the patient has voided, and information that the patient and family have received about the patient's condition. Usually, the surgeon speaks to the family

after surgery and relays the general condition of the patient. The receiving nurse reviews the postoperative orders, admits the patient to the unit, performs an initial assessment, and attends to the patient's immediate needs.

Providing Care for the First 24 Hours After Surgery

During the first 24 hours after surgery, nursing care of the hospitalized patient on the general medical-surgical unit involves continuing to help the patient recover from the effects of anesthesia, frequently assessing the patient's physiologic status, monitoring for complications, managing pain, and implementing measures designed to achieve the long-range goals of independence with self-care, successful management of the therapeutic regimen, discharge to home, and full recovery. In the initial hours after admission to the clinical unit, primary concerns include adequate ventilation, hemodynamic stability, incisional pain, surgical site integrity, nausea and vomiting, neurologic status, and spontaneous voiding. The pulse rate, blood pressure, respiration rate, and oxygen saturation are recorded per institutional policy. Typically, vital signs are recorded frequently until stable and then regularly until the patient is discharged. Frequency of vital sign measurements will depend upon the nature of the operation and the clinical course. Thereafter, vital signs are measured less frequently if they remain stable.

Typically, patients begin to return to their usual state of health several hours after surgery or after waking up the next morning. Although pain may still be intense, many patients feel more alert, less nauseous, and less anxious. They have begun their breathing and leg exercises, and many will have dangled their legs over the edge of the bed, stood, and ambulated a few feet or been assisted out of bed to the chair at least once. Many will have tolerated a light meal and had IV fluids discontinued. The focus of care shifts from intense physiologic management and symptomatic relief of the adverse effects of anesthesia to regaining independence with self-care and preparing for discharge (all discussed in the following nursing process section).

NURSING PROCESS
The Hospitalized Patient Recovering from Surgery

ASSESSMENT

Assessment of the hospitalized postoperative patient includes monitoring vital signs, completing a review of the systems, and observing for potential postoperative complications on arrival of the patient to the clinical unit and at regular intervals thereafter.

Respiratory status is important, because pulmonary complications are among the most frequent and serious problems encountered by the surgical patient. The nurse observes for airway patency, watching for laryngeal edema, which is often heralded by inspiratory stridor. The quality of respirations, including depth, rate, and sound, are assessed regularly. Chest auscultation verifies that breath sounds are normal (or abnormal) bilaterally, and the findings are documented as a baseline for later comparisons. Pulse oximetry is assessed to monitor respiratory status. Often, because of the effects of analgesic and anesthetic medications, respirations are slow. Shallow and rapid respirations may be caused by pain, constricting dressings, gastric dilation, abdominal distention, or obesity. Noisy breathing may be due to obstruction by secretions or the tongue.

The nurse assesses the patient's pain level using a verbal or visual analog scale and assesses the characteristics of the pain. The patient's appearance, pulse, respirations, blood pressure, skin color (adequate or cyanotic), and skin temperature (cold and clammy, warm and moist, or warm and dry) are clues to cardiovascular function. When the patient arrives in the clinical unit, the surgical site is observed for bleeding, type and integrity of dressings, and functioning of all tubes and drains.

The nurse also assesses the patient's mental status and LOC, speech, and orientation, and compares them with the preoperative baseline. Although a change in mental status or postoperative restlessness may be related to anxiety, pain, or medications, it may also be a symptom of oxygen deficit, hypoglycemia, or hemorrhage. These serious causes must be investigated and excluded before other causes are pursued.

General discomfort resulting from lying in one position on the operating table, the surgeon's handling of tissues, the body's reaction to anesthesia, and anxiety are also common causes of restlessness. These discomforts may be relieved by administering the prescribed analgesics, changing the patient's position frequently, and assessing and alleviating the cause of anxiety. Drainage-soaked bandages may cause discomfort. The nurse reinforces or changes the dressing completely, as prescribed by the provider, which may make the patient more comfortable. The bladder is assessed for distention, because urinary retention can also cause restlessness.

DIAGNOSIS

Major nursing diagnoses may include the following:

- Risk for ineffective airway clearance related to depressed respiratory function, pain, and bed rest
- Acute pain related to surgical incision
- Decreased cardiac output related to shock or hemorrhage
- Risk for activity intolerance related to generalized weakness secondary to surgery
- Impaired skin integrity related to surgical incision and drains
- Ineffective thermoregulation related to surgical environment and anesthetic agents
- Risk for imbalanced nutrition, less than body requirements related to decreased intake and increased need for nutrients secondary to surgery
- Risk for constipation related to effects of medications, surgery, dietary change, and immobility
- Impaired urinary elimination related to urinary retention

- Risk for injury related to surgical procedure/positioning or anesthetic agents
- Anxiety related to surgical procedure
- Risk for ineffective self-health management of therapeutic regimen related to wound care, dietary restrictions, activity recommendations, medications, follow-up care, or signs and symptoms of complications

PLANNING

The major goals for the patient include optimal respiratory function, relief of pain, optimal cardiovascular function, increased activity tolerance, unimpaired wound healing, maintenance of body temperature, and maintenance of nutritional balance. Further goals include resumption of usual pattern of bowel and bladder elimination, identification of any perioperative positioning injury, acquisition of sufficient knowledge to manage self-care after discharge, and absence of complications.

NURSING INTERVENTIONS

PROMOTING RESPIRATORY FUNCTION

Increasing age, smoking, COPD, long duration of surgery, and incisional site (chest and upper abdomen), as well as comorbidities, such as heart failure, arrhythmias, diabetes mellitus, and patients with swallowing disorders, are associated with an increased risk for **postoperative** pulmonary **complications**. Respiratory depressive effects of opioid medications, decreased lung expansion secondary to pain, operative position that may have limited maximum respiratory function, impaired mucociliary clearance of secretions, and decreased mobility combine to put the patient at risk for common respiratory complications, particularly atelectasis (alveolar collapse; incomplete expansion of the alveoli), pneumonia, and hypoxemia (Rothrock, 2014). Atelectasis remains a risk for the patient who is not moving well or ambulating, who is not performing deep breathing or coughing out retained secretions, or who is not using an incentive spirometer. Signs and symptoms include decreased breath sounds over the affected area, crackles, and cough. Pneumonia is characterized by chills and fever, tachycardia, and tachypnea. Cough may or may not be present and may or may not be productive. Risk factors for postoperative pneumonia are patients with COPD, impaired cough, and acute bronchitis or lower airway infections.

The types of hypoxemia that can affect postoperative patients are subacute and episodic. Subacute hypoxemia is a constant low level of oxygen saturation, although breathing appears normal. Episodic hypoxemia develops suddenly, and the patient may be at risk for cerebral dysfunction, myocardial ischemia, and cardiac arrest. Risk for hypoxemia is present in patients who have undergone major surgery (particularly thoracic or abdominal), are obese, or have pre-existing pulmonary problems. Hypoxemia can be detected by pulse oximetry, which measures blood oxygen saturation. Factors that may affect the accuracy of pulse oximetry readings include cold extremities, tremors, atrial fibrillation, and acrylic nails. Current research

(continued on page 138)

reveals that different colored nail polish demonstrated altered pulse oximetry readings in healthy subjects (Hakverdioğlu Yönt, Akin Korhan, & Dizer, 2014), thus it seems reasonable that nail polish should be removed prior to SpO_2 (peripheral capillary oxygen saturation) determination to ensure accurate readings.

Preventive measures and timely recognition of signs and symptoms help avert pulmonary complications. Strategies to prevent respiratory complications include use of an incentive spirometer and deep-breathing exercises, and sitting in an upright position that is unrestricted, thus allowing for maximum pulmonary expansion. Mobilization of patients is an important nursing intervention that will assist in maximizing lung expansion and improving circulation, thus facilitating gas exchange while additionally decreasing the risk of DVT (Rothrock, 2014). Crackles indicate static pulmonary secretions that need to be mobilized by coughing retained secretions and deep-breathing exercises. When a mucus plug obstructs one of the bronchi entirely, the pulmonary tissue beyond the plug collapses, and massive atelectasis results. Thus, coughing is also encouraged to dislodge mucus plugs.

 Nursing Alert
It is important to consider that coughing is a forced expiratory maneuver, thus the nurse should encourage the patient to use the incentive spirometer or take deep breaths after coughing to re-expand alveoli. A common recommendation for use of the incentive spirometer is 10 deep breaths every hour while awake.

To clear secretions and prevent pneumonia, the nurse encourages the patient to turn frequently (every 2 hours) and take deep breaths hourly. These pulmonary exercises should begin as soon as the patient arrives on the clinical unit and continue until the patient is discharged. Even if he or she is not fully awake from anesthesia, the patient can be asked to take several deep breaths. This helps expel residual anesthetic agents, mobilize secretions, and prevent alveolar collapse (atelectasis). Careful splinting of abdominal or thoracic incision sites helps the patient overcome the fear that the exertion of coughing might open the incision. Analgesic agents are administered to permit more effective coughing, and oxygen is administered as prescribed to prevent or relieve hypoxia. To encourage lung expansion, the patient is encouraged to yawn or take sustained maximal inspirations to create a negative intrathoracic pressure and expand lung volume to total capacity.

 Nursing Alert
Coughing is contraindicated in patients who have head injuries or who have undergone intracranial surgery (because of the risk for increasing intracranial pressure), as well as in patients who have undergone eye surgery (because of the risk for increasing intraocular pressure) or plastic surgery (because of the risk for increasing tension on delicate tissues).

RELIEVING PAIN

Most patients experience some pain after a surgical procedure. Many factors (motivational, affective, cognitive, and emotional) influence the pain experience. The degree and severity of postoperative pain and the patient's tolerance for pain depend on the incision site, the nature of the surgical procedure, the extent of surgical trauma, the type of anesthetic agent, and how the agent was administered. The Agency for Healthcare Research and Policy reports that the most reliable indicator of the existence and intensity of pain is the patient's self-report. Therefore it is important to complete a thorough preoperative pain evaluation and develop pain goals for the surgical patient. This preparation, which includes information such as what to expect, how the pain will be managed, how to report, and reassurance, can contribute to reducing anxiety and, possibly, the level of postoperative pain experienced. Refer to Chapter 7 for details on patient-controlled analgesia (PCA) and epidural infusions.

For pain that is difficult to control, a subcutaneous pain management system may be used. This is a silicone catheter that is inserted at the site of the affected area. The catheter is attached to a pump that delivers a continuous amount of local anesthetic at a specific amount determined and prescribed by the provider.

Complete absence of pain in the area of the surgical incision may not occur for a few weeks, depending on the site and nature of the surgery, but the intensity of postoperative pain gradually subsides on subsequent days. However, pain control continues to be an important concern for the patient and the nurse. Effective pain management allows the patient to participate in care, perform deep-breathing and leg exercises, and tolerate activity. Poor pain control contributes to postoperative complications and increased length of stay. The nurse continues to assess the pain level, the effectiveness of analgesic agents, and factors that influence pain tolerance (e.g., energy level, stress level, cultural background, meaning of pain to the patient). The nurse explains that taking an analgesic agent before the pain becomes intense is more effective and offers medication to the patient at appropriate intervals rather than waiting for the patient to request it.

Nonpharmacologic pain relief measures, such as imagery, music, relaxation, massage, application of heat or cold (if prescribed), and distraction, are discussed in Chapter 7.

PROMOTING CARDIAC OUTPUT

If signs and symptoms of shock or hemorrhage occur, treatment and nursing care are implemented as described previously in the discussion of care in the PACU.

Although most patients do not hemorrhage or go into shock, changes in circulating volume, the stress of surgery, and the effects of medications and preoperative preparations all affect cardiovascular function. IV fluid replacement is standard for up to 24 hours after surgery or until the patient is stable and tolerating oral fluids. Close monitoring is indicated to detect and correct conditions such as fluid volume deficit, altered tissue perfusion, and decreased cardiac output, all of which can increase the patient's discomfort, place him or her at risk of complications, and prolong the hospital stay. Some patients are at risk of fluid volume excess secondary to existing cardiovascular or renal disease, advanced age, or the release of adrenocorticotropic hormone and antidiuretic hormone as a result of the stress of surgery (Rothrock, 2014). Consequently, fluid replacement must be managed carefully, and intake and output records must be accurate.

Nursing management includes assessing the patency of the IV lines and ensuring that the correct fluids are administered at the prescribed rate. Intake and output, including emesis and output from wound drainage systems, are recorded separately and totaled to determine fluid balance. If the patient has an indwelling urinary catheter, hourly outputs are monitored, and rates of less than 30 mL/hr (0.5–1 mL/kg/hr) are reported; if the patient is voiding, an output of less than 240 mL per 8-hour shift is reported. Levels of electrolytes, hemoglobin, and hematocrit are monitored. Decreased hemoglobin and hematocrit levels can indicate blood loss or dilution of circulating volume by IV fluids. Recall that the fluid changes associated with surgery cause fluid extravasation into the tissues. This "third spaced" fluid usually returns to the intravascular space by postop day (POD) 2 or 3. At this time period, the nurse assesses for evidence of fluid volume excess. If hemodilution is contributing to the decreased hemoglobin and hematocrit levels, the nurse expects that, as the stress response abates and fluids are mobilized and excreted, the hemoglobin and hematocrit will rise.

Venous stasis from dehydration, immobility, and pressure on leg veins during surgery put the patient at risk for DVT. Leg exercises and frequent position changes are initiated early in the postoperative period to stimulate circulation. Patients should avoid positions that compromise venous return, such as raising the bed's knee gatch, placing a pillow under the knees, sitting for long periods, and dangling the legs with pressure at the back of the knees. Venous return is promoted by elastic compression stockings, sequential compression devices (SCDs), and early ambulation. Early ambulation has a significant effect on recovery and the prevention of complications and can begin, in many instances, on the evening of surgery. Postoperative activity orders are checked before the patient is assisted in getting out of bed. Sitting up at the edge of the bed for a few minutes may be all that the patient who has undergone a major surgical procedure can tolerate at first.

ENCOURAGING ACTIVITY

Most surgical patients are encouraged to be out of bed as soon as possible. Early ambulation reduces the incidence of postoperative complications, such as atelectasis, hypostatic pneumonia, GI discomfort, and circulatory problems. Ambulation improves ventilation and reduces the stasis of bronchial secretions in the lungs. It also reduces postoperative abdominal distention by increasing GI tract and abdominal wall tone and stimulating peristalsis. Early ambulation prevents stasis of blood by increasing the rate of circulation in the extremities; as a result, thrombophlebitis or phlebothrombosis occurs less frequently. Often

pain is decreased when early ambulation is possible, and the hospital stay is shorter and less costly, a further advantage to the patient and the hospital.

Despite the advantages of early ambulation, patients may be reluctant to get out of bed on the evening of surgery. Reminding them of the importance of early mobility in preventing complications may help patients overcome their fears. When a patient gets out of bed for the first time, orthostatic hypotension, also called postural hypotension, is a concern. Orthostatic hypotension is an abnormal drop in blood pressure that occurs as the patient changes from a supine to a standing position. It is common after surgery because of changes in circulating blood volume and bed rest. Approximately 500 to 700 mL of blood momentarily shifts to the lower body when changing position to standing from supine, resulting in decreased venous return and arterial pressure. Signs and symptoms include an increase in heart rate of 15 beats per minute (bpm) with a decrease in systolic pressure of 20 mm Hg or a 10 mm Hg decrease in diastolic pressure with position change (typically within 3 minutes). Patients often also complain of weakness, dizziness, leg buckling, and visual blurring. Older adults are at increased risk for orthostatic hypotension secondary to age-related changes in vascular tone. Refer to Chapter 12 for details on assessing for orthostatic hypotension.

To assist the postoperative patient in getting out of bed for the first time after surgery, the nurse:

- Helps the patient move gradually from the lying position to the sitting position by raising the head of the bed, and encourages the patient to splint the incision when applicable. It may be easier for postoperative patients with abdominal incisions to roll on their side first with the head of the bed elevated. Once the patient is on his side, the nurse has the patient move his feet off the side of the bed and push off his elbow into a sitting position.
- Positions the patient completely upright (sitting) and turned, so that both legs are hanging over the edge of the bed. The nurse allows the patient to sit for a few minutes and assesses for dizziness and vital sign changes if indicated. If patient is asymptomatic, the nurse asks the patient to push down with his arms on the mattress and stand up.
- Helps the patient stand beside the bed

After becoming accustomed to the upright position, the patient may start to walk. The nurse should be at the patient's side to give physical support and encouragement. Care must be taken not to tire the patient; the extent of the first few periods of ambulation varies with the type of surgical procedure and the patient's physical condition and age.

Whether or not the patient can ambulate early in the postoperative period, bed exercises are encouraged to improve circulation. Unless contraindicated by the operative event, bed exercises consist of the following:

- Arm exercises (full range of motion, with specific attention to abduction and external rotation of the shoulder)
- Hand and finger exercises

(continued on page 140)

TABLE **5-8** Phases of Wound Healing

Phase	Duration	Events
Inflammatory (also called lag or exudative phase)	1–4 days	Blood clot forms Wound becomes edematous Debris of damaged tissue and blood clot are phagocytosed
Proliferative (also called fibroblastic or connective tissue phase)	5–20 days	Collagen produced Granulation tissue forms Wound tensile strength increases
Maturation (also called differentiation, resorptive, remodeling, or plateau phase)	21 days to months or even years	Fibroblasts leave wound Tensile strength increases Collagen fibers reorganize and tighten to reduce scar size

- Foot exercises to prevent DVT, foot drop, and toe deformities, and to aid in maintaining good circulation
- Leg flexion and leg-lifting exercises to prepare the patient for ambulation
- Abdominal and gluteal contraction exercises

Hampered by pain, dressings, IV lines, or drains, many patients cannot engage in activity without assistance. Prolonged inactivity may lead to pressure ulcers, DVT, atelectasis, constipation, anorexia, and malaise. Helping the patient increase his or her activity level on the first postoperative day is an important nursing function. One way to increase the patient's activity is to have the patient perform as much routine hygiene care as possible. Setting up the patient to bathe with a bedside wash basin or, if possible, assisting the patient to the bathroom to sit in a chair at the sink not only gets the patient moving but also helps restore a sense of self-control and prepares the patient for discharge.

To be discharged safely to home, patients need to be able to ambulate a functional distance (e.g., length of the house or apartment), get in and out of bed unassisted, and be independent with toileting. Patients can be asked to perform as much as they can and then to call for assistance. The patient and the nurse can collaborate on a schedule for progressive activity that includes ambulating in the room and hallway and sitting out of bed in the chair. Assessing the patient's vital signs and oxygen saturation before, during, and after a scheduled activity helps the nurse and patient determine the rate of progression. By providing physical support, the nurse maintains the patient's safety; by communicating a positive attitude about the patient's ability to perform the activity, the nurse promotes the patient's confidence. The nurse should make sure the patient continues to perform bed exercises, wears pneumatic compression or elastic compression stockings when in bed, and rests as needed. If the patient has had orthopedic surgery of the lower extremities or will require a mobility aid (i.e., walker, crutches) at home, a physical therapist may be involved the first time the patient gets out of bed to teach him or her to ambulate safely or to use the mobility aid correctly. If patients are required to climb steps at home, their ability to do so must be assessed before discharge.

PROMOTING WOUND HEALING

Ongoing assessment of the surgical site involves inspection for approximation of wound edges, integrity of sutures or staples, redness, discoloration, warmth, swelling, unusual tenderness, or drainage. The area around the wound should also be inspected for a reaction to tape or trauma from tight bandages.

Principles of Wound Healing

With shorter hospital stays, much of the healing takes place at home, and both the hospital and home care nurse should be informed about the principles of wound healing. Surgical wound healing occurs in three phases: inflammatory, proliferative, and maturation (Table 5-8). Wounds also heal by different mechanisms, depending on the condition of the wound. These mechanisms are first-, second-, and third-intention wound healing (Fig. 5-7) (Rothrock, 2014).

First-Intention Healing. Wounds made aseptically with a minimum of tissue destruction that are properly closed will heal with little tissue reaction by first intention (primary union). When wounds heal by **first-intention healing,** granulation tissue is not visible and scar formation is minimal. Postoperatively, many of these wounds are covered with a dry sterile dressing. If a cyanoacrylate tissue adhesive (LiquiBand®) was used to close the incision without sutures, a dressing is contraindicated.

Second-Intention Healing. Second-intention healing (granulation) occurs in infected wounds (abscess) or in wounds in which the edges have not been approximated. When an abscess is incised, it collapses partly, but the dead and dying cells forming its walls are still being released into the cavity. For this reason, drainage tubes or gauze packing is inserted into the abscess pocket to allow drainage to escape easily. Gradually, the necrotic material disintegrates and escapes, and the abscess cavity fills with a red, soft, sensitive tissue that bleeds easily. This tissue is composed of minute, thin-walled capillaries and buds that later form connective tissue. These buds, called granulations, enlarge until they fill the area left by the destroyed tissue. Healing is complete when skin cells (epithelium) grow over these granulations. This method of repair is called healing

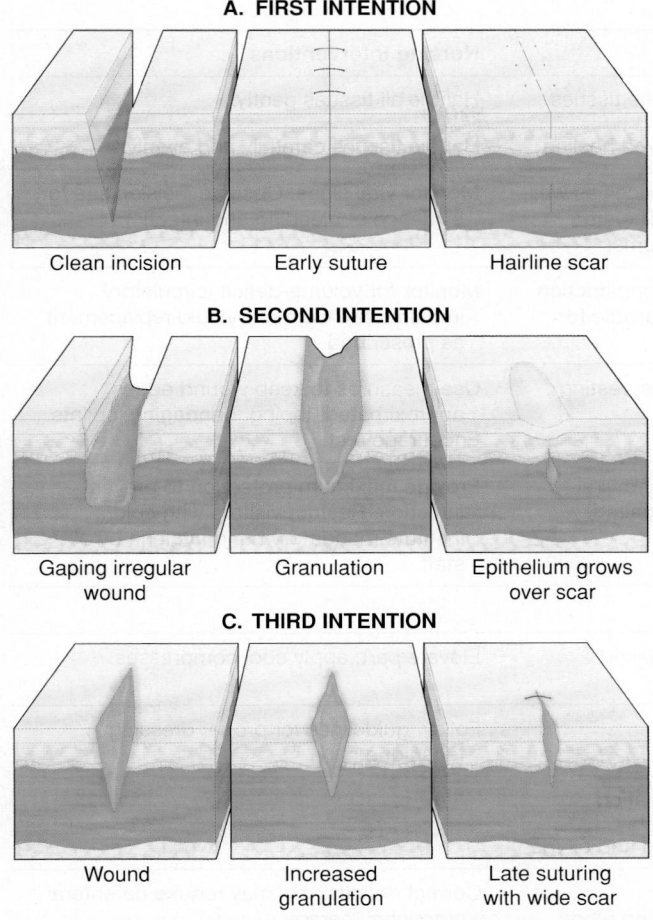

A. FIRST INTENTION

Clean incision   Early suture   Hairline scar

B. SECOND INTENTION

Gaping irregular   Granulation   Epithelium grows
wound   over scar

C. THIRD INTENTION

Wound   Increased   Late suturing
          granulation   with wide scar

FIGURE 5-7 Types of wound healing: first-intention healing, second-intention healing, and third-intention healing.

by granulation, and it takes place whenever pus is formed or when loss of tissue has occurred for any reason. When the postoperative wound is to be allowed to heal by secondary intention, it is usually packed with saline-moistened sterile dressings and covered with a dry sterile dressing.

Third-Intention Healing. **Third-intention healing** (secondary suture) is used for deep wounds that either have not been sutured early or break down and are resutured later, thus bringing together two opposing granulation surfaces. This results in a deeper and wider scar. These wounds are also packed postoperatively with moist gauze and covered with a dry sterile dressing.

Alternatively, wound vacuum-assisted closure (VAC) may be used in the management of open wounds (Fig. 5-8). It applies subatmospheric pressure to the wound surface and consists of a foam dressing, semiocclusive adhesive cover, fluid collection system, and suction pump. The wound VAC, also known as negative pressure therapy, has been shown to speed up the development of granulation tissue. Contraindications include wounds with necrotic tissue; malignancy within the wound; exposed arteries, veins, or vascular grafts; and untreated osteomyelitis (Adams, Heffernan, & Cioffi, 2013). Vacuum dressings, if used, are usually replaced within 24 to 72 hours (Rosen, 2015).

As a wound heals, many factors, such as adequate nutrition, cleanliness, rest, and position determine how quickly healing occurs. Specific nursing assessments and interventions that address these factors and help promote wound healing are presented in Table 5-9. Management of surgical drains and dressings is discussed in more detail below.

(continued on page 143)

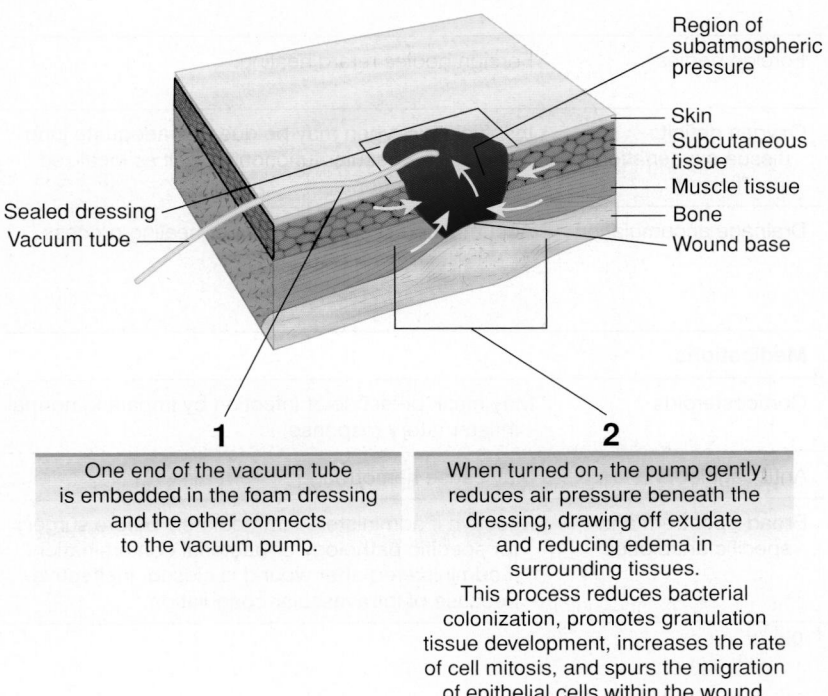

Region of subatmospheric pressure

Skin
Subcutaneous tissue
Muscle tissue
Bone
Wound base

Sealed dressing
Vacuum tube

1
One end of the vacuum tube is embedded in the foam dressing and the other connects to the vacuum pump.

2
When turned on, the pump gently reduces air pressure beneath the dressing, drawing off exudate and reducing edema in surrounding tissues.
This process reduces bacterial colonization, promotes granulation tissue development, increases the rate of cell mitosis, and spurs the migration of epithelial cells within the wound.

FIGURE 5-8 Wound vacuum-assisted closure (VAC).

TABLE 5-9 Factors Affecting Wound Healing

Factors	Rationale	Nursing Interventions
Age of patient	The older the patient, the less resilient the tissues.	Handle all tissues gently.
Handling of tissues	Rough handling causes injury and delayed healing.	Handle tissues carefully and evenly.
Hemorrhage	Accumulation of blood creates dead spaces as well as dead cells that must be removed. The area becomes a growth medium for organisms.	Monitor vital signs. Observe incision site for evidence of bleeding and infection.
Hypovolemia	Insufficient blood volume leads to vasoconstriction and reduced oxygen and nutrients available for wound healing.	Monitor for volume-deficit (circulatory impairment). Correct by fluid replacement as prescribed.
Patient overactivity	Prevents approximation of wound edges; resting favors healing.	Use measures to keep wound edges approximated: taping, bandaging, splints. Encourage rest.
Immunosuppressed state	Patient is more vulnerable to bacterial and viral invasion; defense mechanisms are impaired.	Provide maximum protection to prevent infection. Restrict visitors with colds; institute mandatory hand hygiene by all staff.
Local Factors		
Edema	Reduces blood supply by exerting increased interstitial pressure on vessels	Elevate part; apply cool compresses.
Inadequate dressing technique		Follow guidelines for proper dressing technique.
Too small	Permits bacterial invasion and contamination	
Too tight	Reduces blood supply carrying nutrients and oxygen	
Nutritional deficits	Protein–calorie depletion may occur. Insulin secretion may be inhibited, causing blood glucose to rise.	Correct deficits; this may require parenteral nutritional therapy. Monitor blood glucose levels. Administer vitamin supplements as prescribed.
Foreign bodies	Foreign bodies retard healing.	Keep wounds free of dressing threads and talcum powder from gloves.
Oxygen deficit (tissue oxygenation insufficient)	Insufficient oxygen may be due to inadequate lung and cardiovascular function as well as localized vasoconstriction.	Encourage deep breathing, turning, controlled coughing, and supplemental oxygen as prescribed.
Drainage accumulation	Accumulated secretions hamper healing process.	Monitor closed drainage systems for proper functioning. Institute measures to remove accumulated secretions.
Medications		
Corticosteroids	May mask presence of infection by impairing normal inflammatory response	Be aware of action and effect of medications patient is receiving.
Anticoagulants	May cause hemorrhage	
Broad-spectrum and specific antibiotics	Effective if administered immediately before surgery for specific pathology or bacterial contamination. If administered after wound is closed, ineffective because of intravascular coagulation.	

Factors	Rationale	Nursing Interventions
Systemic Disorders		

Hemorrhagic shock
Acidosis
Hypoxia
Kidney failure
Hepatic disease
Sepsis
Smoking
Immunodeficiency
  diseases;
  chemotherapy;
  radiation
Poor nutrition
Obesity
Diabetes
	These depress cell functions that directly affect
	  wound healing.
		Be familiar with the nature of the specific
		  disorder. Administer prescribed treatment.
		  Cultures may be indicated to determine
		  appropriate antibiotic.

Wound Stressors		

Vomiting
Valsalva maneuver
Heavy coughing
Straining
	Produce tension on wounds, particularly of the torso	Encourage frequent turning and ambulation
		  and administer antiemetic medications
		  as prescribed. Assist patient in splinting
		  incision.

Managing Drains

Wound drains are tubes that exit the peri-incisional area, either into a portable wound suction device (closed) or into the dressings (open). The principle involved is to allow the escape of blood and serous fluids that could otherwise serve as a culture medium for bacteria. In portable wound suction, the use of gentle, constant suction enhances drainage of these fluids and collapses the skin flaps against the underlying tissue, thus removing "dead space." Types of wound drains include the Penrose, Hemovac, and Jackson-Pratt drains (Fig. 5-9). Output from wound drainage systems and all new drainage is recorded. The amount of bloody drainage on the surgical dressing is assessed frequently. Spots of drainage on the dressings are outlined with a pen, and the date and time of the outline are recorded on the dressing, so that increased drainage can be seen easily. A certain amount of bloody drainage in a wound drainage system or on the dressing is expected, but excessive amounts should be reported to the surgeon. Increasing amounts of fresh blood on the dressing should be reported immediately. Some wounds are irrigated heavily before closure in the OR, and open drains exiting the wound may be embedded in the dressings. These wounds may drain large amounts of blood-tinged fluid that saturate the dressing. The dressing can be reinforced with sterile gauze bandages; the time at which they were reinforced should be documented. If drainage continues, the surgeon should be notified, so that the dressing can be changed. Multiple similar drains are numbered or otherwise labeled (e.g., left lower quadrant, left upper quadrant), so that output measurements can be recorded reliably and consistently. Careful positioning and safeguarding that any drains are secure can prevent the dislodgment of nasogastric tubes, chest tubes, and the drains themselves.

(continued on page 144)

FIGURE 5-9 Types of surgical drains: (**A**) Penrose, (**B**) Jackson-Pratt, (**C**) Hemovac.

Changing the Dressing

Although the first postoperative dressing is usually changed by a member of the surgical team, subsequent dressing changes in the immediate postoperative period are usually performed by the nurse. A dressing is applied to a wound for one or more of the following reasons: (1) to provide a proper environment for wound healing; (2) to absorb drainage; (3) to splint or immobilize the wound; (4) to protect the wound and new epithelial tissue from mechanical injury; (5) to protect the wound from bacterial contamination and from soiling by feces, vomitus, and urine; (6) to promote hemostasis, as in a pressure dressing; and (7) to provide mental and physical comfort for the patient.

The patient is told that the dressing is to be changed and that changing the dressing is a simple procedure associated with little discomfort. The dressing change is performed at a suitable time (e.g., not at mealtimes or when visitors are present). Privacy is provided, and the patient is not unduly exposed. The nurse should avoid referring to the incision as a scar, because the term may have negative connotations for the patient. Assurance is given that the incision will shrink as it heals and that the redness will fade.

The nurse carries out hand hygiene before and after the dressing change and wears disposable gloves for the dressing change itself. The tape or adhesive portion of the dressing is removed by pulling it parallel with the skin surface and in the direction of hair growth, rather than at right angles. Nonirritating solvents aid in removing adhesive painlessly and quickly. The old dressing is removed and then deposited in a container designated for disposal of biomedical waste. In accordance with standard precautions, dressings are never touched by ungloved hands because of the danger of transmitting pathogenic organisms.

Nursing Alert

There is a dearth of research regarding the influence of sterile or aseptic versus clean gloves and SSIs related to wound care. Therefore the nurse will perform dressing changes depending upon institutional policy. However, the nurse should consider the patient's immune status and depth of a wound when selecting dressing technique of sterile versus clean technique. In addition, use of gloves does not preclude meticulous hand hygiene (Leonard, 2016).

If the patient is sensitive to adhesive tape, the dressing may be held in place with hypoallergenic tape. Many tapes are porous to permit ventilation and prevent skin maceration. The correct way to apply tape is to place the tape at the center of the dressing and then press the tape down on both sides, applying tension evenly, away from the midline. The incorrect way to apply tape—to fix one end of the tape to the skin and to pull it tight over the dressing—often wrinkles and pulls the skin in the process. The resulting continuous and forceful traction produces a shearing effect, causing the epidermal layer to slip sideways and become separated from the deeper dermal layers.

Some wounds become edematous after having been dressed, causing considerable tension on the tape. If the tape is not flexible, the stretching bandage will also cause a shear injury to the skin. This can result in denuded areas or large blisters and should be avoided. An elastic adhesive bandage (Elastoplast, 3M Microfoam) may be used to hold dressings in place over mobile areas, such as the neck or the extremities, or where pressure is required. Or a tubular band netting (which stretches and holds dressing in place without tape) can be considered.

While changing the dressing, the nurse has an opportunity to teach the patient how to care for the incision and change the dressings at home. The nurse observes for indicators of the patient's readiness to learn, such as looking at the incision, expressing interest, or assisting in the dressing change.

MAINTAINING NORMAL BODY TEMPERATURE

The patient is still at risk for MH and hypothermia in the postoperative period. Efforts are made to identify MH and to treat it early and promptly.

Patients who have been anesthetized are susceptible to chills and drafts. Attention to hypothermia management, begun in the intraoperative period, extends into the postoperative period to prevent significant nitrogen loss and catabolism. Signs of hypothermia are reported to physician member of the surgical team. The room is maintained at a comfortable temperature, and blankets are provided to prevent chilling. Treatment includes oxygen administration, adequate hydration, and proper nutrition. The patient is also monitored for cardiac arrhythmias. The risk of hypothermia is greater in the elderly and in patients who were in the cool OR environment for a prolonged period.

MANAGING GI FUNCTION AND RESUMING NUTRITION

GI discomfort (nausea, vomiting, hiccups) and resumption of oral intake are issues for both the patient 'and the nurse. Nausea and vomiting are common after anesthesia (Rothrock, 2014). They are more common in women, in obese people (fat cells act as reservoirs for the anesthetic), in patients prone to motion sickness, and in patients who have undergone lengthy surgical procedures. Other causes of postoperative vomiting include an accumulation of fluid in the stomach, inflation of the stomach, and the ingestion of food and fluid before peristalsis resumes.

If vomiting is likely because of the nature of surgery, a nasogastric tube is inserted intraoperatively and remains in place throughout the surgery and the immediate postoperative period. A nasogastric tube (NG tube) also may be inserted before surgery if postoperative distention is anticipated. In addition, an NG tube may be inserted if a patient who has food in the stomach requires emergency surgery. Refer to Chapter 22 for further details on NG tubes.

Hiccups, produced by intermittent spasms of the diaphragm secondary to irritation of the phrenic nerve, can occur after surgery. The irritation may be direct, such as from stimulation of the nerve by a distended stomach, subdiaphragmatic abscess, or abdominal distention; indirect, such as from toxemia or uremia that stimulates the nerve; or reflexive, such as irritation from a drainage tube or obstruction of the intestines. Usually, these occurrences are mild, transitory attacks that cease spontaneously. If hiccups persist, they may produce considerable distress and serious effects such as vomiting, exhaustion, and wound dehiscence. The provider may prescribe phenothiazine medications (e.g., Thorazine) for intractable hiccups (Chang & Lu, 2012).

Once nausea and vomiting have subsided and the patient is fully awake and alert with the nurse having documented resumption of bowel sounds, the nurse should offer the patient something to drink or eat. The sooner the patient can tolerate a usual diet, the more quickly normal GI function will resume. Taking food by mouth stimulates digestive juices and promotes gastric function and intestinal peristalsis. The return to normal dietary intake should proceed at a pace set by the patient. Of course, the nature of the surgery and the type of anesthesia directly affect the rate at which normal gastric activity resumes. Liquids are typically the first substances desired and tolerated by the patient after surgery. Water, juice, and tea may be given in increasing amounts. Cool fluids are tolerated more easily than are those that are ice cold or hot. Soft foods (gelatin, custard, milk, and creamed soups) are added gradually after clear fluids have been tolerated. As soon as the patient tolerates soft foods well, solid food may be given.

Assessment and management of GI function are important after surgery because the GI tract is subject to uncomfortable or potentially life-threatening complications. Any postoperative patient may suffer from abdominal distention, resulting from the accumulation of gas in the intestinal tract. Manipulation of the abdominal organs during surgery may produce a loss of normal peristalsis for 24 to 48 hours, depending on the type and extent of surgery. Even though nothing is given by mouth, swallowed air and GI secretions enter the stomach and intestines; if not propelled by peristalsis, they collect in the intestines, producing distention and causing the patient to complain of fullness or pain in the abdomen. Most often, the gas collects in the colon. Abdominal distention is increased further by immobility, anesthetic agents, and the use of opioid medications.

After major abdominal surgery, distention may be avoided by having the patient turn frequently, exercise, and ambulate as early as possible. This also alleviates distention produced by swallowing air, which is common in anxious patients. An NG tube inserted before surgery may remain in place until full peristaltic activity (indicated by the passage of flatus) has resumed. The nurse can determine when peristaltic bowel sounds return by listening to the abdomen with a stethoscope (normal frequency of bowel sounds are 5 to 34 clicks and gurgles per minute). Bowel sounds are documented so that diet progression can occur.

Paralytic ileus (failure of forward movement of bowel contents; when due to paralysis of the intestinal muscles, also termed postoperative adynamic ileus) and intestinal obstruction are potential postoperative complications that occur more frequently in patients undergoing intestinal or abdominal surgery.

PROMOTING BOWEL FUNCTION

Constipation is common after surgery and can range from a minor to a serious complication. Decreased mobility, decreased oral intake, and opioid analgesics contribute to difficulty having a bowel movement. In addition, irritation and trauma to the bowel during surgery may inhibit intestinal movement for several days. The combined effect of early ambulation, improved dietary intake, and a stool softener (if prescribed) promotes bowel elimination. Until the patient reports return of normal bowel function, the nurse should assess the abdomen for distention and the presence and frequency of bowel sounds. If the abdomen is not distended and bowel sounds are normal, and if the patient does not have a bowel movement by the second or third postoperative day, the provider should be notified.

MANAGING VOIDING

Urinary retention after surgery can occur for various reasons. Anesthetics, anticholinergic agents, and opioids interfere with the perception of bladder fullness and the urge to void and inhibit the ability to initiate voiding and completely empty the bladder. Abdominal, pelvic, and hip surgery may increase the likelihood of retention secondary to pain. In addition, some patients find it difficult to use the bedpan or urinal in the recumbent position.

Bladder distention and the urge to void should be assessed at the time of the patient's arrival on the unit and frequently thereafter. The patient is expected to void within 6 to 8 hours after surgery (this includes time spent in the PACU). If the patient has an urge to void and cannot, or if the bladder is distended and no urge is felt or the patient cannot void, a portable ultrasound device (bladder scan) should be performed to assess degree of distention and possible need for urinary catheterization. All methods to encourage the patient to void should be tried (e.g., letting water run, applying heat to the perineum). The bedpan should be warm; a cold bedpan causes discomfort and automatic tightening of muscles (including the urethral sphincter). If the patient cannot void on a bedpan, it may be possible to use a commode rather than resorting to catheterization. Male patients are often permitted to sit up or stand beside the bed to use the urinal, but safeguards should be taken to prevent the patient from falling or fainting due to loss of coordination from medications or orthostatic hypotension. If the patient cannot void in the specified time frame and a bladder scan verifies distention, the patient is catheterized and the catheter is removed after the bladder has emptied. Straight intermittent catheterization is preferred over indwelling catheterization, because the risk of infection is increased with an indwelling catheter.

Even if the patient voids, the bladder may not necessarily be empty. The nurse notes the amount of urine voided and uses the bladder scan to assess residual volume. If more than 100 mL of residual urine is seen on the bladder scanner, it is considered diagnostic of urinary retention. If a bladder scan is not available in your institution, the nurse can palpate the suprapubic area for distention or tenderness after the patient urinates to assess for

(continued on page 146)

residual urine. Intermittent catheterization may be prescribed every 4 to 6 hours until the patient can void spontaneously and the postvoid residual is less than 100 mL.

MAINTAINING A SAFE ENVIRONMENT

During the immediate postoperative period, the patient recovering from anesthesia should have two side rails up, and the bed should be in the low position. The nurse assesses the patient's LOC and orientation and determines whether the patient needs his or her eyeglasses or hearing aid, because impaired vision, inability to hear postoperative instructions, or inability to communicate verbally places the patient at risk for injury. All objects the patient may need should be within reach, especially the call light. Any immediate postoperative orders concerning special positioning, equipment, or interventions should be implemented as soon as possible. The patient is instructed to ask for assistance with any activity. Although restraints are occasionally necessary for the disoriented patient, they should be avoided if at all possible. Agency policy on the use of restraints must be consulted and followed.

PROVIDING EMOTIONAL SUPPORT TO THE PATIENT AND FAMILY

Although patients and families are undoubtedly relieved that surgery is over, anxiety levels may remain high in the immediate postoperative period. Many factors contribute to this anxiety: pain, being in an unfamiliar environment, inability to control one's circumstances or care for oneself, fear of the long-term effects of surgery, fear of complications, fatigue, spiritual distress, altered role responsibilities, ineffective coping, and altered body image are all potential reactions to the surgical experience. The nurse helps the patient and family work through their anxieties by providing reassurance and information and by spending time listening to and addressing their concerns. The nurse describes hospital routines and what to expect in the ensuing hours and days until discharge, and explains the purpose of nursing assessments and interventions. Informing patients when they will be able to drink fluids or eat, when they will be getting out of bed, and when tubes and drains will be removed helps them gain a sense of control and participation in recovery and engages them in the plan of care. Acknowledging family members' concerns and accepting and encouraging their participation in the patient's care assists them in feeling that they are helping their loved one. The nurse can modify the environment to enhance rest and relaxation by providing privacy, reducing noise, adjusting lighting, providing enough seating for family members, and encouraging a supportive atmosphere.

MANAGING POTENTIAL COMPLICATIONS

The RN must be alert for the development of additional postoperative complications that include cardiac complications, DVT and pulmonary embolism (PE), hematoma, wound infection, and/or wound dehiscence and evisceration. The following sections detail each of these complications.

Cardiac Complications

A postoperative cardiac complication is a myocardial ischemia/infarction (MI). The nurse is aware that in the postoperative patient, clinical presentation is often subtle. Perioperative MIs are frequently silent or may present with dyspnea, hypotension, or atypical pain. If suspected, the nurse alerts the surgical team; obtains vital signs and oxygen saturation; performs a cardiac, peripheral vascular, and pulmonary assessment, electrocardiogram; and anticipates laboratory work to assess cardiac biomarkers will be obtained. Refer to Table 14-5 for cardiac laboratory tests on page 446.

As a result of excessive IV fluid administration intraoperatively, the nurse is alert for the development of congestive heart failure (CHF), which can present in the immediate postoperative period, or on POD 2 to 3 when fluid shifting causes increased intravascular volume. Daily weights are an important parameter for judging fluid balance. The nurse is aware that when calculating new gain or loss that 500 mL approximates 1 lb or 1,000 mL approximates 1 kg (2.2 lb). In addition, the nurse observes for jugular vein distention, rales, dyspnea, wheezing, cough, and fatigue. Refer to Chapters 14 and 15 for details of care of the patient with MI and CHF.

Deep Vein Thrombosis and Pulmonary Embolism

DVT and other complications, such as PE, are serious potential complications of surgery (Box 5-8). The stress response that is initiated by surgery inhibits the fibrinolytic system, resulting in blood hypercoagulability. Dehydration, low cardiac output, blood pooling in the extremities, and bed rest add to the risk of thrombosis formation. Although all postoperative patients are at some risk, factors such as a history of thrombosis, malignancy, trauma, obesity, indwelling venous catheters, and hormone use (e.g., estrogen) increase the risk. The first symptom of DVT may be swelling of the involved extremity, often accompanied by a low grade fever. The edema is associated with impaired venous flow. Tenderness, which usually occurs later,

---

BOX 5-8 **Risk Factors for Postoperative Deep Vein Thrombosis**

- Orthopedic patients having hip surgery, knee reconstruction, and other lower extremity surgery
- Urologic patients having transurethral prostatectomy and older patients having urologic surgery
- General surgical patients older than 40 years of age, those who are obese, those with a malignancy, those who have had prior DVT or PE, and those undergoing extensive, complicated surgical procedures
- Gynecologic (and obstetric) patients older than 40 years of age with added risk factors (varicose veins, previous venous thrombosis, infection, malignancy, obesity)
- Neurosurgical patients, similar to other surgical high-risk groups (in patients with stroke, for instance, the risk of DVT in the paralyzed leg is as high as 75%)

TABLE **5-10** Wound Classification and Associated Surgical Site Infection Risk

Surgical Category	Determinants of Category	Expected Risk of Postsurgical Infection (%)
Clean	Nontraumatic site Uninfected site No inflammation No break in aseptic technique No entry into respiratory, alimentary, genitourinary, or oropharyngeal tracts	1–3
Clean-contaminated	Entry into respiratory, alimentary, genitourinary, or oropharyngeal tracts without unusual contamination Appendectomy Minor break in aseptic technique Mechanical drainage	3–7
Contaminated	Open, newly experienced traumatic wounds Gross spillage from GI tract Major break in aseptic technique Entry into genitourinary or biliary tract when urine or bile is infected	7–16
Dirty	Traumatic wound with delayed repair, devitalized tissue, foreign bodies, or fecal contamination Acute inflammation and purulent drainage encountered during procedure	16–29

is produced by inflammation of the vein wall, and firmness may be detected along the involved veins by gently palpating the affected extremity (palpated cord). Refer to Chapter 18 for details on DVT.

Prophylactic treatment for postoperative patients at risk is common practice, until the patient is ambulatory. External pneumatic compression and thigh-high elastic compression stockings can be used alone or in combination with low-dose heparin. The benefits of early ambulation and hourly leg exercises in preventing DVT cannot be overemphasized, and these activities are recommended for all patients, regardless of their risk. It is important to avoid the use of blanket rolls, pillow rolls, or any form of elevation that can constrict vessels under the knees. Even prolonged "dangling" (having the patient sit on the edge of the bed with legs hanging over the side) can be dangerous and is not recommended in susceptible patients because pressure under the knees can impede circulation. Adequate hydration is also encouraged; the patient can be offered juices and water throughout the day to avoid dehydration.

PE from DVT is a postoperative risk for patients owing to immobility, venous stasis, venous trauma, and hypercoagulability. Clinically, symptoms of a PE include sudden onset of shortness of breath, tachypnea, tachycardia, low-grade temperature, chest pain (pleuritic in nature), and apprehension. Patients who have had major orthopedic surgery of a lower extremity, including hip or knee arthroplasty and hip fracture surgeries, as well as major trauma patients, are at high risk for PE. Some form of prophylactic therapy is expected in high-risk patients to reduce the risk of DVT and PE. Refer to Chapter 10 for more details on PE.

Hematoma

At times, concealed bleeding occurs beneath the skin at the surgical site. This hemorrhage usually stops spontaneously but results in clot (hematoma) formation within the wound. If the clot is small, it will be absorbed and need not be treated. If the clot is large, the wound usually bulges somewhat, and healing will be delayed unless the clot is removed. After several sutures are removed by a member of the surgical team, the clot is evacuated and the wound is packed lightly with gauze. Healing occurs usually by granulation, or a secondary closure may be performed.

Infection (Wound Sepsis)

The creation of a surgical wound disrupts the integrity of the skin and its protective function. Exposure of deep body tissues to pathogens in the environment places the patient at risk for infection of the surgical site, a potentially life-threatening complication. SSI increases hospital length of stay, costs of care, risk for further complications, and readmission to a hospital.

Multiple factors place the patient at risk for wound infection. One risk factor relates to the type of wound. Surgical wounds are classified according to the degree of contamination. Table 5-10 defines the terms used to describe surgical wounds and gives the expected rate of wound infection per category. Other risk factors include both patient-related factors and those associated with the surgical procedure. Factors related to the surgical procedure include the method of preoperative skin preparation, surgical attire of the team, method of sterile draping, duration of surgery, antimicrobial prophylaxis, aseptic technique, factors related to surgical technique, drains or foreign material, OR ventilation, length of procedure, and exogenous microorganisms. Efforts to

(continued on page 148)

prevent wound infection are directed at reducing these risks. Current guidelines to prevent SSIs suggest that an appropriate prophylactic antibiotic that is based on current recommendation be administered within 1 hour of surgical incision (2 hours are allowed for the administration of vancomycin and fluoroquinolones) and discontinuation of prophylactic antibiotics within 24 hours after surgery, owing to the link between the development of resistant organisms and excessive use of antibiotics. Discontinuation of the antibiotic is extended to within 48 hours for cardiothoracic procedures for adult patients. The Surgical Care Improvement Project (SCIP) is a national quality partnership of organizations interested in improving surgical care by significantly reducing surgical complications. They provide guidelines for antibiotic therapy throughout the patient's hospitalization (Joint Commission, 2014).

Wound infection may not be evident until at least POD 5. Most patients are discharged before that time, and more than half of wound infections are diagnosed after discharge, highlighting the importance of patient education regarding wound care. Risk factors for wound sepsis include wound contamination, foreign body, faulty suturing technique, devitalized tissue, hematoma, debilitation, dehydration, malnutrition, anemia, advanced age, extreme obesity, shock, length of preoperative hospitalization, duration of surgical procedure, and associated disorders (e.g., diabetes mellitus, immunosuppression). Signs and symptoms of wound infection include increased pulse rate and temperature; an elevated white blood cell count; wound swelling, warmth, tenderness, or discharge; and incisional pain. Local signs may be absent if the infection is deep. Staphylococcus aureus accounts for many postoperative wound infections. Other infections may result from Escherichia coli, Proteus vulgaris, Aerobacter aerogenes, Pseudomonas aeruginosa, and other organisms. Although they are rare, beta-hemolytic streptococcal or clostridial infections can develop rapidly and be deadly. If wound infection due to beta-hemolytic streptococcus or clostridium occurs, strict infection-control practices are needed to prevent the spread of infection to others. Intensive medical and nursing care is essential if the patient is to survive.

When a wound infection is diagnosed in a surgical incision, the surgeon may remove one or more sutures or staples and, using aseptic precautions, separate the wound edges with a pair of blunt scissors or a hemostat, opening the incision to allow for drainage. Another option is for the patient to be referred to interventional radiology for percutaneous drainage. Antimicrobial therapy and a wound care regimen are also initiated.

Wound Dehiscence and Evisceration

Wound **dehiscence** (disruption of surgical incision or wound) and **evisceration** (protrusion of wound contents) are serious surgical complications (Fig. 5-10). Dehiscence and evisceration are especially serious when they involve abdominal incisions or wounds. These complications result from sutures giving way, from infection, or, more frequently, from marked distention or strenuous cough. They may also occur because of increasing

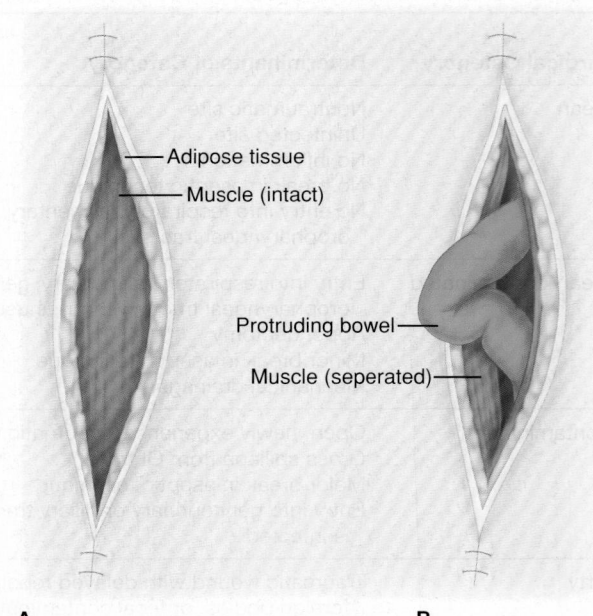

FIGURE 5-10 (**A**) Wound dehiscence; (**B**) wound evisceration.

age; obesity; poor nutritional status (hypoproteinemia, hypoalbuminemia); steroid use or immunosuppression (cancer); or the presence of diabetes, uremia, or sepsis; or pulmonary or cardiovascular disease in patients undergoing abdominal surgery. Local risk factors include inadequate closure, increased intra-abdominal pressure, and deficient wound healing (Chu & Agarwal, 2015).

When the wound edges separate slowly, the intestines may protrude gradually or not at all, and the earliest sign may be a gush of bloody (serosanguineous) peritoneal fluid from the wound. When a wound ruptures suddenly, coils of intestine may push out of the abdomen. The patient may report that "something gave way." The evisceration causes pain and may be associated with vomiting.

An abdominal binder, properly applied, is a prophylactic measure against an evisceration and often is used along with the primary dressing, especially in patients with weak or pendulous abdominal walls or when rupture of a wound has occurred. If evisceration occurs, the nurse aseptically covers the abdominal contents with moist saline dressings to prevent drying of the bowel, notifies the surgical team immediately and assesses the patient's vital signs, including oxygen saturation. The patient remains in bed with knees bent to reduce abdominal muscle tension. The patient should be NPO and an IV established for fluid management. After the patient returns from surgery, review splinting of the abdomen and anticipate the use of an abdominal binder.

PROVIDING DISCHARGE TEACHING

Patients have always required detailed discharge instructions to become proficient in special self-care needs after surgery;

BOX 5-9

Patient Education

Wound Care Instructions

Until Sutures are Removed

1. Keep the wound dry and clean:
   - If there is no dressing, ask your nurse or provider if you can bathe or shower.
   - If a dressing or splint is in place, do not remove it unless it is wet or soiled.
   - If wet or soiled, change dressing yourself if you have been taught to do so; otherwise, call your nurse or provider for guidance.
   - If you have been taught, instruction might be as follows:
     - Cleanse area *gently* with sterile normal saline once or twice daily.
     - Cover with a sterile Telfa pad or gauze square large enough to cover the wound.
     - Apply hypoallergenic tape (Dermicel or paper). Adhesive is not recommended because it is difficult to remove without possible injury to the incisional site.
2. Immediately report any of these signs of infection:
   - Increasing redness, swelling, tenderness, pain, or increased warmth around the wound
   - Red streaks in the skin near the wound
   - Pus or discharge, foul odor
   - Chills or temperature higher than 37.7°C (100°F)
3. If soreness or pain causes discomfort, apply a dry cool pack (containing ice or cold water) or take prescribed acetaminophen tablets (2) every 4–6 hours. Avoid using aspirin

without direction or instruction because bleeding can occur with its use.

4. Swelling after surgery is common. To help reduce swelling, elevate the affected part to the level of the heart:
   - Hand or arm:
     - Sleep: Elevate arm on pillow at side
     - Sitting: Place arm on pillow on adjacent table
     - Standing: Rest affected hand on opposite shoulder; support elbow with unaffected hand
   - Leg or foot:
     - Sitting: Place a pillow on a facing chair; provide support underneath the knee
     - Lying: Place a pillow under affected leg

After Sutures are Removed

Although the wound appears to be healed when sutures are removed, it is still tender and will continue to heal and strengthen for several weeks.

1. Follow recommendations of your provider or nurse regarding extent of activity.
2. Keep the suture line clean; do not rub vigorously; pat dry. Wound edges may look red and may be slightly raised. This is normal.
3. If the site continues to be red, thick, and painful to pressure after 8 weeks, consult the health care provider. (This may be due to excessive collagen formation and should be checked.)

---

however, dramatically reduced hospital lengths of stay during the past decade have greatly increased the amount of information needed while reducing the amount of time in which to provide it. Box 5-9 provides patient education about wound care.

EVALUATION

Expected patient outcomes may include the following:

1. Maintains optimal respiratory function:
   a. Performs deep-breathing exercises
   b. Displays clear breath sounds
   c. Uses incentive spirometer as prescribed
   d. Splints incisional site when coughing to reduce pain
2. Indicates that pain is decreased in intensity or acceptable to patient
3. Increases activity as prescribed:
   a. Alternates periods of rest and activity
   b. Progressively increases ambulation
   c. Resumes normal activities within prescribed time frame
   d. Performs activities related to self-care
4. Wound heals without complication
5. Maintains body temperature within normal limits
6. Resumes oral intake:
   a. Reports absence of nausea and vomiting
   b. Eats at least 75% of usual diet

   c. Is free of abdominal distress and gas pains
   d. Exhibits normal bowel sounds
7. Reports resumption of usual bowel elimination pattern
8. Resumes usual voiding pattern
9. Is free of injury
10. Exhibits decreased anxiety
11. Acquires knowledge and skills necessary to manage therapeutic regimen
12. Experiences no complications

Gerontologic Considerations

Elderly patients recover more slowly, have longer hospital stays, and are at greater risk for the development of postoperative complications. Some of the major threats to recovery include pneumonia, decline in functional ability, exacerbation of comorbid conditions, pressure ulcers, decreased oral intake, GI disturbance, and falls. Expert nursing care can help the older adult avoid these complications or minimize their effects.

Postoperative delirium, characterized by confusion, perceptual and cognitive deficits, altered attention levels, disturbed sleep patterns, and impaired psychomotor skills, is a significant problem for older adults. Causes of delirium

BOX 5-10 **Causes of Postoperative Delirium**

- Acid–base disturbances
- Age greater than 80 years
- Fluid and electrolyte imbalance
- Dehydration
- History of dementia-like symptoms
- Hypoxia
- Hypercarbia
- Infection (urinary tract, wound, respiratory)
- Medications (anticholinergics, benzodiazepines, central nervous system depressants)
- Unrelieved pain
- Blood loss
- Decreased cardiac output
- Cerebral hypoxia
- Heart failure
- Acute myocardial infarction
- Hypothermia or hyperthermia
- Unfamiliar surroundings and sensory deprivation
- Emergent surgery
- Alcohol withdrawal
- Urinary retention
- Fecal impaction
- Polypharmacy
- Presence of multiple diseases
- Sensory impairments
- High stress or anxiety levels

are multifactorial (refer to Box 5-10 for causes of delirium). Skilled and frequent assessment of mental status and of all physiologic factors influencing mental status helps the nurse plan care because delirium may be the initial or only early indicator of infection, fluid and electrolyte imbalance, or deterioration of respiratory or hemodynamic status in the elderly patient.

Recognizing postoperative delirium and identifying and treating its underlying cause are the goals of care. Sometimes postoperative delirium is mistaken for pre-existing dementia or is attributed to age. In addition to monitoring and managing identifiable causes, the nurse implements supportive interventions. Keeping the patient in a well-lit room and close to the nurses' station can help with sensory deprivation. At the same time, distracting and unfamiliar noises should be minimized. Because pain can contribute to postoperative delirium, adequate pain control is essential. The nurse collaborates with the physician or geriatric nurse specialist and the patient to achieve pain relief without oversedation.

The patient is reoriented as often as necessary, and staff should introduce themselves each time they come in contact with the patient. Engaging the patient in conversation and care activities and placing a clock and calendar nearby may improve cognitive function. Physical activity should not be neglected while the patient is confused because physical deterioration can worsen delirium and place the patient at increased risk for other complications. Restraints should be avoided because they also can worsen confusion. If possible, a family member or staff member is asked to stay with the patient instead.

Other problems confronting the elderly postoperative patient, such as pneumonia, altered bowel function, DVT, weakness, and functional decline, often can be prevented by early and progressive ambulation. Ambulation means walking, not just getting out of bed and sitting in a chair. Prolonged sitting positions that promote venous stasis in the lower extremities should be avoided. Assistance with ambulation may be required to keep the patient from bumping into objects and falling. A physical therapy referral may be indicated to promote safe, regular exercise for the older adult.

Urinary incontinence can be prevented by providing easy access to the call bell and the commode and by prompting voiding. Early ambulation and familiarity with the room help the patient to become self-sufficient sooner.

Optimal nutritional status is important for wound healing, return of normal bowel function, and fluid and electrolyte balance. The nurse and patient can consult with the dietitian to plan appealing, high-protein meals that provide sufficient fiber, calories, and vitamins. Nutritional supplements, such as Ensure® or Sustacal, may be recommended. Multivitamins, iron, and vitamin C supplements aid in tissue healing, formation of new RBCs, and overall nutritional status and are commonly prescribed postoperatively.

In addition to monitoring and managing physiologic recovery of the older adult, the nurse identifies and addresses psychosocial needs. The older adult may require much encouragement and support to resume activities, and the pace may be slow. Sensory deficits may require frequent repetition of instructions, and decreased physiologic reserve may necessitate frequent rest periods. The older adult may require extensive discharge planning to coordinate both professional and family care providers, and the nurse, social worker, or nurse case manager may institute the plan for continuing care.

CHAPTER REVIEW

Critical Thinking Exercises

1. An 80-year-old patient with Parkinson disease is scheduled for surgery to replace a fractured hip. Identify the considerations and associated responsibilities of the OR nurse for safe intraoperative care of this patient.

2. A patient develops a temperature of 38°C (100°F) and becomes tachycardic halfway through an abdominal surgery. Five minutes later, the patient's temperature is 42°C (104°F). Describe the protocol you would follow and the medication you would administer for this condition.

3. A male patient is scheduled for major surgery and asks how long before the surgery will he be without food and fluids. What resources would you use to identify the current fasting guidelines? What is the evidence base for the patient's being NPO after midnight as opposed to a 2-hour fast before surgery? Identify the criteria used to evaluate the strength of the evidence for this practice.

NCLEX-Style Review Questions

1. A 70-year-old elderly patient is admitted to the preoperative unit for a liver resection that is scheduled for 6 hours of surgery. What is one of the basic principles that should guide the preoperative nurse's assessment?
   a. Elderly patients do not experience as much preoperative anxiety as younger patients.
   b. The elderly patient has less physiologic reserve than the younger patient.
   c. Elderly patients experience less pain.
   d. Preoperative pain assessment and teaching should occur following the procedure as the elderly patient may not retain the information.

2. A nurse is caring for a postoperative patient who had spinal anesthesia. The patient complains of headache. What action should the nurse take?
   a. Lower the head of the patient's bed.
   b. Keep the patient lying flat, maintain a quiet environment, and keep the patient hydrated.
   c. Encourage the patient to lay on his right side.
   d. Do nothing, as this is a normal response to the spinal anesthesia.

3. When does the postoperative phase begin?
   a. Admission of the patient to the OR
   b. Admission of the patient to the PACU and ending when the patient is discharged to the unit or home
   c. Admission of the patient to the PACU and ending with follow-up evaluation in the clinical setting or home
   d. Admission to the PACU

4. A nurse is caring for a postoperative patient on POD 2. The patient had a large upper abdominal incision. While assessing the patient at the beginning of the shift, the nurse noted decreased breath sounds, crackles, and a mild cough. What is the patient most likely experiencing?
   a. Atelectasis
   b. Pneumonia
   c. Acute bronchitis
   d. Hypoxemia

5. Surgical wound healing occurs in:
   a. Two phases: inflammatory and maturation
   b. Three phases: inflammatory, proliferative, and maturation
   c. First-, second-, and third-intention wound healing
   d. First and proliferative phase

Try these additional resources, available at **http://thepoint.lww.com/Honan2e**, to enhance your learning and understanding of this chapter:
- NCLEX-Style Student Review Questions
- Journal Articles

REFERENCES AND SELECTED READINGS

References and selected readings associated with this chapter can be found on the website that accompanies the book. Visit **http://thepoint. lww.com/Honan2e** to access the references and other additional resources associated with this chapter.

Cancer Care

Lisa M. Barbarotta

Learning Objectives

After reading this chapter, you will be able to:

1. Compare the structure and function of the normal cell and the cancer cell.
2. Differentiate between benign and malignant tumors.
3. Identify agents and factors that have been found to be carcinogenic.
4. Describe the significance of health education and preventive care in decreasing the incidence of cancer.
5. Differentiate among the various types of surgical procedures used in cancer treatment, diagnosis, prophylaxis, and palliation.
6. Describe the roles of surgery, radiation therapy, chemotherapy, targeted agents, and immunotherapy in treating cancer.
7. Describe the special nursing needs of patients receiving chemotherapy and immunotherapy.
8. Describe common nursing diagnoses and collaborative problems of patients with cancer.
9. Describe the concept of hospice in providing care for patients with advanced cancer.
10. Discuss the role of the nurse in assessment and management of common oncologic emergencies.

Cancer is not a single disease with a single cause; rather, it is a highly heterogeneous group of diseases with different causes, manifestations, treatments, and prognoses. Cancer nursing, also called **oncology** nursing, encompasses all age groups and nursing specialties and is carried out in a variety of health care settings, including the home, community, acute care institutions, rehabilitation centers, and hospice. The scope, responsibilities, and goals of oncology nursing are as diverse and complex as those of any nursing specialty. Oncology nurses must be prepared to support patients and families through a wide range of physical, emotional, social, cultural, and spiritual experiences from diagnosis through end of life and survivorship.

EPIDEMIOLOGY OF CANCER

Although cancer affects people of all ages, most cancers occur in people older than 65 years of age. Overall, the incidence of cancer is higher in men than in women and higher in industrialized nations.

In 2016 there were 1.68 million new cancer cases and 595,690 cancer deaths projected in the United States, with cancer being the second leading cause of death (Siegel, Miller, & Jemal, 2016). The most common causes of cancer death include lung and bronchus, prostate, and colorectal cancers in men and lung and bronchus, breast, and colorectal cancer in women (Fig. 6-1) (Siegel et al., 2016). These four cancer types are responsible for 46% of all cancer deaths. Notable trends in the United States include stabilization of the incidence rates for cancer in women and declining rates in men due to decreasing numbers of prostate cancers diagnosed (Siegel et al., 2016).

Over the last 30 years, 5-year survival rates for cancer have increased by 20% in whites and 23% in blacks (Siegel et al., 2016). Progress has been most dramatic for diseases including acute lymphoblastic leukemia (ALL) and chronic myelogenous leukemia (CML) due to the discovery of targeted therapies such as tyrosine kinase inhibitors. Unfortunately, similar advances for lung and pancreatic cancers have been slower to evolve (Siegel et al., 2016).

Cancer incidence and mortality rates vary among racial groups. Black men have the highest overall incidence of cancer and higher mortality rates (Siegel et al., 2016). Higher mortality rates may be a reflection of being diagnosed at an advanced stage of disease. Other factors to account for

Estimated New Cases*

Male	Female
Prostate 180,890 (21%)	Breast 246,660 (29%)
Lung and bronchus 117,920 (14%)	Lung and bronchus 106,470 (13%)
Colon and rectum 70,820 (8%)	Colon and rectum 63,670 (8%)
Urinary bladder 58,950 (7%)	Uterine corpus 60,050 (7%)
Melanoma of the skin 46,870 (6%)	Thyroid 49,350 (6%)
Non-Hodgkin lymphoma 40,170 (5%)	Non-Hodgkin lymphoma 32,410 (4%)
Kidney and renal pelvis 39,650 (5%)	Melanoma of the skin 29,510 (3%)
Oral cavity and pharynx 34,780 (4%)	Leukemia 26,050 (3%)
Leukemia 34,090 (4%)	Pancreas 25,400 (3%)
Liver and intrahepatic bile duct 28,410 (3%)	Kidney and renal pelvis 23,050 (3%)
All sites 841,390 (100%)	*All sites 843,820 (100%)*

Estimated Deaths

Male	Female
Lung and bronchus 85,920 (27%)	Lung and Bronchus 72,160 (26%)
Prostate 26,120 (8%)	Breast 40,450 (14%)
Colon and rectum 26,020 (8%)	Colon and rectum 23,170 (8%)
Pancreas 21,450 (7%)	Pancreas 20,330 (7%)
Liver and intrahepatic bile duct 18,280 (6%)	Ovary 14,240 (5%)
Leukemia 14,130 (4%)	Uterine corpus 10,470 (4%)
Esophagus 12,720 (4%)	Leukemia 10,270 (4%)
Urinary bladder 11,820 (4%)	Liver and intrahepatic bile duct 8,890 (3%)
Non-Hodgkin lymphoma 11,520 (4%)	Non-Hodgkin lymphoma 8,630 (3%)
Brain and other nervous system 9,440 (3%)	Brain and other nervous system 6,610 (2%)
All sites 314,290 (100%)	*All sites 281,400 (100%)*

FIGURE 6-1 Ten Leading Cancer Types for the Estimated New Cancer Cases and Deaths by Sex, United States, 2016. *Excludes basal and squamous cell skin cancers and in situ carcinomas except urinary bladder. Estimates rounded to the nearest 10. Adapted from Siegel, R. L., Miller, K. D., & Ahmedin, J. (2016). Cancer statistics, 2016. *CA: Cancer Journal for Clinicians, 66*, 7–30.

the disparities include differences in risk factor prevalence, increased incidence of poverty, and less access to high-quality health care (Siegel et al., 2016).

Characteristics of Malignant Cells

The primary difference between malignant (cancerous) and benign cells is that malignant cells have abnormal regulation of growth. Cancer cells continue to grow, even at the expense of their host. They demonstrate uncontrolled cell growth that follows no physiologic demand.

Benign and malignant growths are classified and named by tissue of origin. Benign and malignant cells differ in many cellular growth characteristics, including the method and rate of growth, ability to metastasize or spread, general effects, destruction of tissue, and ability to cause death. These differences are summarized in Table 6-1.

Despite their individual differences, all cancer cells share some common cellular characteristics in relation to the cell membrane, special proteins, the nuclei, chromosomal abnormalities, and the rate of mitosis and growth. Characteristics of cancer cells include:

- Pleomorphism: Cells vary in size and shape
- Polymorphism: Nucleus is enlarged and variable in shape
- Chromosomal mutations including translocations, deletions, amplification, and aneuploidy (abnormal number of chromosomes)
- Production of surface enzymes that aid in invasion and metastasis
- Loss of antigens that label the cell as "self"
- Production of new tumor-associated antigens that label the cell as "nonself"
- Increased rate of anaerobic metabolism
- Loss of contact inhibition, which normally halts cell division once cells are in contact with one another
- Defect in cell recognition and adhesion (cancer cells do not recognize and adhere to each other as normal cells do)

TABLE **6-1** Characteristics of Benign and Malignant Neoplasms

Characteristics	Benign Neoplasms	Malignant Neoplasms
Cell characteristics	Well-differentiated cells that resemble cells in the tissue of origin	Cells are undifferentiated, with anaplasia (loss of differentiation of cells) and atypical structure that often bear little resemblance to cells in the tissue of origin
Mode of growth	Grows by expansion without invading the surrounding tissues; usually encapsulated	Grows by invasion, sending out processes that infiltrate the surrounding tissues
Rate of growth	Usually progressive and slow; may come to a standstill or regress	Variable and depends on level of differentiation; the more undifferentiated the cells, the more rapid the rate of growth
Metastasis	Does not spread by metastasis	Gains access to the blood and lymph channels to metastasize to other areas of the body

Grossman, S., & Porth, C. (2014). *Pathophysiology: Concepts of altered health states* (9th ed.). Philadelphia, PA: Lippincott Williams & Wilkins.

- Loss of control of proliferation
- Increased mitotic index: Tumors have a larger number of cells that are in mitosis
- Abnormal lifespan: Cancer cells tend to live longer than do normal cells

Carcinogenesis

Carcinogenesis, the process in which healthy cells become malignant, is a multi-step process involving both environmental exposure to cancer-causing agents (carcinogens) and random errors in replication of DNA that result in genetic mutations over time (Lemoine, 2014). The end result of these mutations is uncontrolled proliferation of abnormal cells.

 Pathophysiology Alert
Although cancer originates from a single mutated cell (monoclonal origin), over time due to subsequent mutations, the tumor cells become heterogeneous in their cellular properties. In addition, cells within different regions of an established tumor may express different genes and different mutations (Harrington, Bristow, Hill, & Tannock, 2013). Understanding the characteristics of the cancer cells assists in developing novel therapies to eliminate it.

The following cellular changes are essential to carcinogenesis:

- loss of sensitivity to growth inhibitory signals
- evasion of apoptosis (programmed cell death)
- limitless replicative potential
- angiogenesis (growth of new blood vessels)
- potential for metastatic/tissue invasion

Cells acquire these properties through genetic and epigenetic alterations (external modifications to DNA that turn genes "on" or "off" but do not change the DNA sequence itself) over time as a result of genomic instability, acquired and inherited mutations, changes in the microenvironment, cell selection, and clonal expansion (Grant, 2013).

Carcinogenesis has been described previously as a three-step process, including tumor initiation, promotion, and progression. *Initiation* involves the interaction between DNA with a reactive chemical species that results in damage. If this damage is not repaired before the next cell division, erroneous DNA replication ensues, resulting in fixed mutations within the genome of individual cells (Grant, 2013). Although initiation is irreversible, not all initiated cells will go on to become a tumor as many of these cells may die by apoptosis. *Promotion* involves the clonal expansion of the initiated cell, in which the initiated cell divides into other cells that now have the same alterations in DNA if not repaired in time (Grant, 2013). Initiated cells may have a selective growth advantage allowing the cells to divide and evade death, resulting in the proliferation and survival of premalignant cells and the formation of benign lesions like polyps. *Progression* is the stage in which benign lesions acquire the ability to proliferate and invade adjacent tissue and establish distant sites of metastasis through the acquisition of additional mutations (Grant, 2013). While this simplistic model has been used over time to understand the multi-step process of carcinogenesis, we now understand that cancer is a complex result of multiple sequential mutations in combination with epigenetic changes and prolonged changes in the cellular microenvironment (Grant, 2013).

Mutations can be either germ-line mutations or somatic mutations. Germ-line mutations occur in the DNA of sperm or egg cells. These are inheritable mutations that can also be passed on to offspring. Somatic mutations are acquired mutations that occur in nongerm cells and cannot be inherited or passed on. However, any cells that result from division of a cell with a somatic mutation will have that same mutation if the mutation is not corrected before the cell is able to divide (Lemoine, 2014). Mutations can involve an alteration in a single base pair (point mutation) as well as deletions, translocations, or insertions of chromosomes or large parts of DNA. The end results of these mutations are highly variable. Some mutations are silent and do not have any clinical implications. Other mutations, especially those that involve deletions of large amounts of DNA, can be more significant as they result in an inability to make essential proteins needed for cell growth (Lemoine, 2014).

The two most common groups of genes that are mutated are proto-oncogenes, which promote cell proliferation, and tumor suppressor genes, which inhibit cell proliferation (Lemoine, 2014). Oncogenes are the end product of a mutated proto-oncogene and stimulate a cell's ability to move through the cell cycle (called a *gain of function mutation*). Mutations in tumor suppressor genes are referred to as *loss of function mutations* because the normal function of suppressing growth is lost (Harrington et al., 2013). Fusion oncogenes are a result of translocations among normal genes; BCR-ABL and PML–RARα (discussed in Chapter 20) are two examples of fusion oncogenes that stimulate abnormal cell growth (Lemoine, 2014).

The p53 gene (*TP53*) is a tumor suppressor gene that is frequently mutated in more than 50% of human cancers (Grant, 2013). This gene determines whether cells will live or die after their DNA is damaged. **Apoptosis** is the innate cellular process of programmed cell death. Alterations in *TP53* may decrease apoptotic signals, thus decreasing the body's ability to kill mutated cells, giving rise to a survival advantage for mutant cell populations. Mutant *TP53* is associated with a poor prognosis and may be used to determine response to treatment.

Pathophysiology Alert

Carcinogenesis is the result of both genetic and epigenetic changes. The term epigenetics refers to heritable, reversible changes in gene expression that do not involve changes to the underlying DNA sequence. Epigenetic changes result in a change in phenotype without a change in genotype. Epigenetics are critical to the process of transcription regulation and gene expression (Miozzo, Vaira, & Sirchia, 2015). Epigenetic changes include alterations in DNA methylation, histone modification, changes in chromatin, and noncoding RNA (ncRNA)-associated gene silencing. These changes may result in overexpression or underexpression of genes (Lemoine, 2014; Harrington et al., 2013; Shao, Khokha, & Hill, 2013; Miozzo et al., 2015).

All cells, both healthy and malignant, proliferate by way of the cell cycle (see Fig. 6-2). The cell cycle time is the time required for one cell to divide and reproduce two identical daughter cells. The cell cycle of any cell has four distinct phases, each with a vital underlying function:

1. G_1 phase: RNA and protein synthesis occur
2. S phase: DNA synthesis occurs

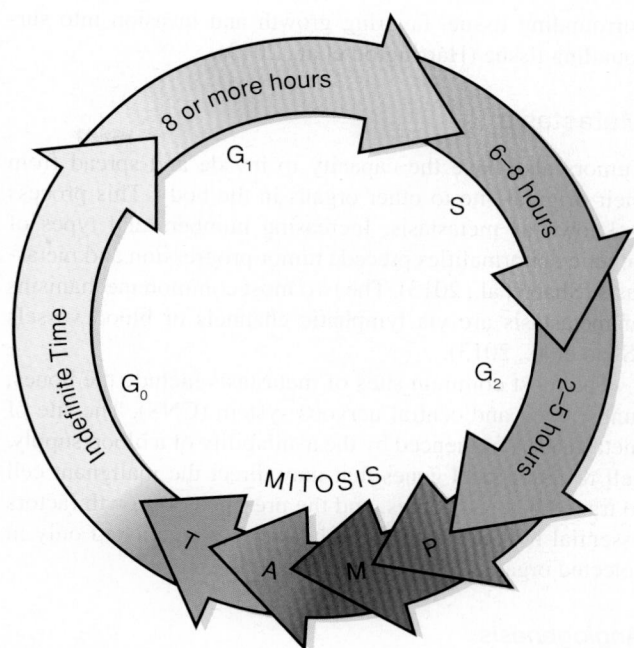

FIGURE 6-2 Phases of the cell cycle extend over the interval between the midpoint of mitosis and the subsequent end point in mitosis in a daughter cell. G_0 is the resting, or dormant, phase of the cell cycle. G_1 is the postmitotic phase during which ribonucleic acid (RNA) and protein syntheses are increased and cell growth occurs. In the S phase, nucleic acids are synthesized and chromosomes are replicated in preparation for cell mitosis. During G_2, RNA and protein synthesis occur as in G_1. P, prophase; M, metaphase; A, anaphase; T, telophase. Redrawn from Porth, C. M. (2002). *Pathophysiology: Concepts of altered health states* (6th ed.). Philadelphia, PA: Lippincott Williams & Wilkins.

3. G_2 phase: Premitotic phase; DNA synthesis is complete, mitotic spindle forms
4. Mitosis: Cell division occurs

The G_0 phase, the resting or dormant phase of cells, can occur after mitosis and during the G_1 phase. In the G_0 phase there are cells that are not actively dividing but have the potential to enter into the cell cycle. Mitosis (cell division) occurs more frequently in malignant cells than in normal cells. As the cells grow and divide, more glucose and oxygen are needed. If glucose and oxygen are unavailable, malignant cells use anaerobic metabolic channels to produce energy, which makes the cells less dependent on the availability of a constant oxygen supply.

Proliferation through the cell cycle is controlled by a balance of positive and negative signals received from inside and outside of the cell (known as *signal-transduction pathway*) (Harrington et al., 2013). A decrease or increase in the cell's ability to respond to a signal may result in increased proliferation.

Thus, cancer development and progression is a result of a series of mutations over time that destabilize the genome and allow for uncontrolled cell growth. This makes the cells further susceptible to mutations and causes alterations in the surrounding tissue, favoring growth and invasion into surrounding tissue (Harrington et al., 2013).

Metastasis

Tumors also have the capacity to invade and spread from their original site to other organs in the body. This process is known as metastasis. Increasing numbers and types of genetic abnormalities precede tumor progression and metastasis (Shao et al., 2013). The two most common mechanisms of metastasis are via lymphatic channels or blood vessels (Shao et al., 2013).

The most common sites of metastasis include the bones, lungs, liver, and central nervous system (CNS). The site of metastasis is influenced by the availability of a blood supply, cell receptors and genes that may direct the malignant cell to travel to specific sites, and the presence of growth factors essential for metastatic growth that may be elicited only in selected organs.

Angiogenesis

Angiogenesis is the process by which a new blood supply is formed, creating an interface between the tumor and the vascular surface of the host (Rak, 2013). Once a tumor reaches a size of 2 mm^3, this blood supply is necessary for continued growth and facilitation of metastasis. The newly formed blood vessels allow inflow of nutrition, oxygen, growth factors, metabolites, hormones, and regulatory molecules to the tumor and also provide an essential route for metastasis. Angiogenesis also allows the export of metastatic cancer cells, proinflammatory, procoagulant, metabolic, and angiogenesis-regulating substances from the tumor to the vascular system and distant sites (Rak, 2013). The process of angiogenesis is mediated by the release of growth factors and key molecules such as vascular endothelial growth factor (VEGF). These proteins rapidly stimulate formation of new blood vessels. Therapies that target VEGF or its receptors are being used effectively to treat many cancers (Rak, 2013).

Lymphatic Spread

The transport of tumor cells through the lymphatic circulation is the most common mechanism of metastasis. Tumor emboli enter the lymph channels by way of the interstitial fluid, which communicates with lymphatic circulation. Malignant cells also may penetrate lymphatic vessels by invasion. After entering the lymphatic circulation, malignant cells either lodge in the lymph nodes or pass between the lymphatic and venous circulations. Tumors arising in areas of the body with rapid and extensive lymphatic circulation are at high risk for metastasis through lymphatic channels. Breast tumors frequently metastasize in this manner through axillary, clavicular, and thoracic lymph channels.

Hematogenous Spread

Hematogenous spread is the dissemination of malignant cells via the bloodstream and is directly related to the vascularity of the tumor. Malignant cells are able to travel through the bloodstream, attach to endothelium and attract fibrin, platelets, and clotting factors to seal themselves from immune system surveillance. The endothelium retracts, allowing the malignant cells to enter the basement membrane and secrete lysosomal enzymes. These enzymes destroy surrounding body tissues and thereby allow implantation.

Etiology

Genetic mutations can result from inherited mutations, acquired mutations due to exposure to chemical- or radiation-induced DNA damage, exposure to viruses, and random errors that may occur during DNA synthesis (Harrington et al., 2013). Recent evidence has demonstrated that the environment can also profoundly influence the epigenome: diet, smoking, and alcohol consumption can negatively impact the gene expression profile (Miozzo et al., 2015).

Other factors implicated in carcinogenesis include viruses and bacteria, physical agents, chemical agents, genetic or familial factors, dietary and life style factors, and hormonal agents.

Viruses and Bacteria

Viruses are thought to incorporate themselves into the genetic structure of cells, thus altering future generations of that cell population—perhaps leading to cancer.

The human papillomavirus (HPV) family includes over 170 different types of viruses that infect the mucosa of the anogenital region (anus and genital), upper-respiratory tract, or the skin. HPV16 is a high-risk type of HPV associated with cervical, anogenital, and oral mucosal cancers (Ghittoni, Accardi, Chiocca, & Tommasino, 2015; Hay & Ganley, 2015).

Chronic viral infection with hepatitis C is associated with an increased risk for hepatocellular carcinoma (Mitchell, Lemon, & McGivern, 2015).

A few bacteria are associated with the development of cancer. An example is *Helicobacter pylori (H pylori)* which is linked with gastric ulcers. Because the inner layer of the stomach can also become inflamed and damaged, *H. pylori* can lead to cancer in the lower part of the stomach and is also associated with some types of stomach lymphoma.

Physical Agents

Physical factors associated with carcinogenesis include exposure to sunlight or radiation. Exposure to ionizing radiation can occur with repeated diagnostic x-ray procedures or with radiation therapy used to treat disease. Fortunately, improved x-ray equipment appropriately minimizes the risk to healthy tissue of extensive radiation exposure. Radiation therapy used in disease treatment and exposure to radioactive materials at nuclear weapon manufacturing sites or nuclear power plants is associated with a higher incidence of leukemias; multiple myeloma; and cancers of the lung, bone, breast, thyroid, and other tissues. Background radiation from the natural decay process produces radon that has also been associated with lung cancer.

Chemical Agents

Chemicals can contribute to the initiation, promotion, and progression stages of carcinogenesis either through their ability to damage DNA directly and produce somatic mutations in cells or as a result of an altered microenvironment that provides initiated cells with a growth advantage via metabolic changes, local vascular changes, and/or the ability to evade apoptosis, terminal differentiation, and contact inhibition (Grant, 2013).

Over one third of cancer-related deaths are associated with tobacco use, including cancers of the lung and bronchus, oral cavity and pharynx, larynx, esophagus, stomach, pancreas, kidney and renal pelvis, urinary bladder, and cervix as well as acute myeloid leukemia (Underwood et al., 2015). Incidence rates for tobacco-related cancers have decreased significantly from 152.9 (per 100,000 persons) in 2005 to 145.8 in 2009 (Underwood et al., 2015). In men, death from lung cancer has been reduced by 38% from 1990 to 2014; rates in women have also declined but not as dramatically (Loeb, 2016). Despite these improvements, tobacco continues to account for a large number of cancers in the United States and worldwide (Underwood et al., 2015; Loeb, 2016.)

Alcohol consumption is strongly linked to the development of cancers of the mouth and pharynx, larynx, esophagus, liver, stomach, gallbladder, colon, breast, and lung. An estimated 4% of all cancers can be attributed to daily alcohol consumption; 30% to 40% of cancers of the oral cavity and pharynx and 20% to 50% of esophageal cancers may be attributed to daily alcohol use (Katzke, Kaaks, & Kuhn, 2015). There is a strong synergistic interaction between alcohol consumption and smoking with regard to cancer risk (Katzke et al., 2015).

Many chemical substances found in the workplace have proved to be carcinogens or co-carcinogens. The extensive list of suspected chemical substances continues to grow and includes aromatic amines and aniline dyes; pesticides and formaldehydes; arsenic, soot, and tars; asbestos; benzene; betel nut and lime; cadmium; chromium compounds; nickel and zinc ores; wood dust; beryllium compounds; and polyvinyl chloride.

Genetics or Familial Factors

Observations over time have shown that cancers cluster in some families. This may be due to genetics, shared environments, cultural or lifestyle factors, or chance alone. Obtaining an accurate family history is essential in guiding referrals to genetic counseling and testing for hereditary cancer syndromes, such as hereditary breast and ovarian cancer syndrome (HBOC) and Lynch syndrome. *BRCA1* and *BRCA2* are the genes associated with hereditary breast and ovarian cancer syndrome, and *MLH1*, *MSH2*, *MSH6*, and *PMS2* are the genes associated with Lynch syndrome. Lynch syndrome, also known as *hereditary nonpolyposis colorectal cancer (HNPCC)*, is an inherited disorder that increases the risk of developing many other types of cancer, particularly colorectal cancer. Patients who test positive for mutations in these genes need more careful follow-up and surveillance for cancer over their lifespan (Estrada, LeGrazie, McKamie, and Montgomery, 2015). In addition, lifestyle changes to minimize cancer risk may be recommended (Mahon, 2015).

Multigene panel testing, also known as *next-generation gene sequencing*, which tests for germline mutations in a number of genes associated with increased cancer risk, has recently become available to patients. Some of these genetic mutations carry a significantly elevated lifetime cancer risk (greater than 50%), whereas others carry less of a risk (Estrada et al., 2015). For example, mutations in the *MSH2* gene are associated with an 80% lifetime risk for developing colorectal cancer and a 70% chance of developing endometrial cancer (Mahon, 2013b). It is essential to identify individuals or families most likely to benefit from testing and ensure pre- and posttest counseling, preferably done by genetics experts (Mahon, 2013a).

Common errors that may result when nongenetics professionals order genetic tests include: the wrong genetic test is ordered, genetic test results are misinterpreted, and inappropriate or inadequate genetic counseling leads to psychosocial distress or other negative outcomes (Mahon, 2013b).

The *BRCA1/2* genes account for approximately 25% of hereditary breast cancer cases. However, additional genes have been discovered that may contribute to hereditary breast cancer risk. Next-generation gene sequencing has the potential to detect these other lower penetrance genes that may be responsible for hereditary breast cancer. One commercially available targeted panel that tests for 17 of these genes is called Breast Next™ (Ambry Genetics Laboratories, n.d.).

Approximately 5% of cancers in adults display a familial predisposition. Key indicators of hereditary risk include:

- younger than usual age at time of diagnosis (e.g., colon cancer before age 50);
- multiple family members in one generation with cancer;
- multiple generations with cancer(s) associated with hereditary risk;
- presence of nonmalignant changes associated with hereditary risk (e.g., Dysplastic nevi);
- presence of rare tumors commonly associated with hereditary risk (e.g., medullary thyroid cancer);
- any pattern of cancers associated with a hereditary cancer syndrome (e.g., Lynch syndrome);
- bilateral cancer in a paired organ (e.g., breast cancer in both breasts);

- multiple synchronous cancers (e.g., colon cancer with more than one tumor in the colon); or
- an individual with more than one primary cancer (Mahon, 2015).

Cancers associated with familial inheritance include retinoblastomas; nephroblastomas (kidney tumor); pheochromocytomas (adrenal medulla tumor); malignant neurofibromatosis (tumors of nerve tissue); and breast, ovarian, colorectal, stomach, prostate, and lung cancers.

Dietary and Lifestyle Factors

After tobacco, obesity, diet, and levels of physical activity are the most important modifiable determinants of cancer risk. Poor diet is linked to 25% of cancers. Obesity contributes to as much as 20% of cancer-related deaths (Mahon, 2015). Obesity is also associated with increased risk for cancer, including renal cell cancer; postmenopausal breast cancer; and cancers of the endometrium, pancreas, colon, and esophagus (adenocarcinomas) (Katzke et al., 2015).

Prospective studies have shown that diets with higher intake of fruits, vegetables, and wholegrain foods, and lower intake of red and processed meats and salt, are related to reduced risks of cancer and death and that a healthy diet can improve overall survival after diagnosis of breast and colorectal cancers. There is evidence that high dietary intake of fruit and vegetables may reduce the risk of cancers of the aerodigestive tract (combined organs and tissues of the respiratory tract and the upper part of the digestive tract [lips, mouth, tongue, nose, throat, vocal cords, and part of the esophagus and windpipe]) and dietary fiber protects against colorectal cancer. Red and processed meats increase the risk of colorectal cancer (Norat et al., 2015).

Dietary substances that appear to increase the risk of cancer include fats, alcohol, salt-cured or smoked meats, and nitrate- and nitrite-containing foods. A high-caloric dietary intake and obesity are associated with an increased cancer risk (Norat et al., 2015).

There is some evidence that exercise, independent of weight, may provide a protective benefit against cancer. A demonstrated inverse association between physical activity and the risk of cancers for which obesity may not be a major risk factor, such as bladder cancer and gastric cancer, may suggest benefits of physical activity beyond preventing obesity (Katzke et al., 2015).

Hormonal Agents

Tumor growth may be promoted by disturbances in hormonal balance, including prolonged exposure to the hormone either by the body's own (endogenous) hormone production or by administration of exogenous hormones. Cancers of the breast and uterus (estrogen dependent) and prostate (androgen dependent) are thought to depend on endogenous hormonal levels for growth.

A lower risk of estrogen and progesterone receptor positive breast cancer is associated with an earlier age at first full-term pregnancy, a higher number of full-term pregnancies, and longer cumulative duration of breast-feeding. Longer duration of breast-feeding is also associated with a decreased risk of hormone receptor negative and HER2 negative (known as *triple negative*) breast cancer (Katzke et al., 2015).

A higher number of full-term pregnancies and longer cumulative lifetime duration of breast-feeding also confer relatively strong protection against ovarian cancer, reducing risk by up to 50% or more (Katzke et al., 2015).

Use of oral contraceptives has been linked to clear reduction in risk of ovarian cancer, with risk reduction of up to 50% depending on duration of use. In addition, oral contraceptive use is associated with up to 40% reductions in risk of endometrial cancer and a more modest (up to around 15%) reduction in risk of colorectal cancer, but a weak (less than 10%) increase in risk of breast cancer (Katzke et al., 2015).

Postmenopausal hormone replacement therapy (HRT), especially combined estrogen-plus-progestin regimens, causes an increase in risk of breast cancer. There is a strong correlation between use of estrogen-only HRT and increased endometrial cancer risk in contrast to the use of combined estrogen-plus-progestin regimens, which may reduce the risk for endometrial cancer (Katzke et al., 2015).

Role of the Immune System

In humans, malignant cells can develop at any time in the life span. However, some evidence indicates that the immune system can detect the development of malignant cells and destroy them before cell growth becomes uncontrolled. When the immune system fails to identify and stop the growth of malignant cells, clinical cancer develops.

An intact immune system has the ability to combat cancer cells in several ways. Usually, the immune system recognizes as foreign certain antigens on the cell membranes of many cancer cells. These antigens, known as *tumor-associated antigens* (also called *tumor cell antigens*), are capable of stimulating both cellular and humoral immune responses.

Along with the macrophages, T lymphocytes are responsible for recognizing tumor-associated antigens. When T lymphocytes, the soldiers of the cellular immune response, recognize tumor antigens, other T lymphocytes that are toxic to the tumor cells are stimulated. These lymphocytes proliferate and are released into the circulation. In addition to possessing cytotoxic (cell-killing) properties, T lymphocytes can stimulate other components of the immune system to rid the body of malignant cells.

A three-phase model has been proposed to describe the role of the immune response during various stages of tumor progression. These stages include elimination, equilibrium, and escape.

During the elimination phase, the immune system recognizes tumor cells and mounts a response against the tumor.

During the equilibrium phase, the immune system and the tumor are in dynamic equilibrium, where the combination of the genomic instability of tumor cells and the pressure exerted by the antitumor immune response results in editing of the tumor cell population. The elimination of certain tumor cells by the immune system results in the selection of less immunogenic tumors. During the escape phase, there are too many tumor cells, which overwhelm the immune system and allow the tumor to evade elimination (Nguyen, Lind, & Ohashi, 2013).

The ability to evade the immune response may be, in part, a result of reduced immunogenicity of tumor cells, such as reduced expression of tumor antigens. However, there are many other mechanisms whereby the tumor can evade the immune system (Nguyen et al., 2013).

The failure of the immune system to respond promptly to the malignant cells allows the tumor to grow too large to be managed by normal immune mechanisms. Newer therapies are attempting to restore or stimulate the immune response to treat cancer (discussed later in chapter).

Patients who are immunocompromised have been shown to have an increased incidence of cancer. Organ transplant recipients who receive immunosuppressive therapy to prevent organ rejection have an increased incidence of lymphoma, Kaposi sarcoma, squamous cell cancer of the skin, and cervical and anogenital cancers. Patients with immunodeficiency diseases, such as AIDS, have an increased incidence of Kaposi sarcoma, lymphoma, and rectal and head and neck cancers.

Treatment with certain types of chemotherapy, including alkylating agents and topoisomerase II inhibitors can increase the risk of developing another malignancy over the course of a lifetime. Autoimmune diseases, such as rheumatoid arthritis and Sjögren syndrome, are associated with increased cancer development. Finally, age-related changes, such as declining organ function, increased incidence of chronic diseases, and diminished immunocompetence, may contribute to an increased incidence of cancer in older people.

PREVENTION

Nurses play a critical role in every level of prevention, including primary prevention, secondary prevention, and tertiary prevention. Primary prevention efforts focus on preventing or delaying onset of cancer. Secondary prevention focuses on the early detection of cancer with the goal of identifying cancer in early stages before symptoms develop. Tertiary prevention includes the management of the disease and prevention of progression to later stages. Nurses must be familiar with current guidelines and recommendations for cancer prevention and screening in order to provide accurate, relevant patient education (Mahon, 2015). A major barrier to adherence to screening standards is lack of a recommendation from a health care provider (Mahon, 2015). Nurses can play a critical role in informing patients about recommended screening tests and provide anticipatory guidance to alleviate any fears patients may have about the tests.

Primary Prevention

As discussed, primary prevention strategies are aimed at preventing or delaying the development of cancer (Mahon, 2015). Nurses play a critical role in educating the community about cancer prevention. Nurses can use their teaching and counseling skills to encourage participation in cancer prevention programs, minimize exposure to known carcinogens, and to adopt healthy lifestyles, including avoiding all forms of tobacco; maintaining a healthy weight; performing regular exercise (150 min/wk); eating a diet rich in fruits and vegetables (at least five servings per day); limiting red meat, high fat, and processed foods; limiting alcohol; using sun protection; getting regular checkups; and being familiar with their own family history and personal cancer risks (Kushi, Doyle, McCullough, 2012; American Cancer Society, 2015). Other primary prevention strategies include immunization against cancer-associated viruses, such as hepatitis and HPV (Mahon, 2015).

For individuals at high risk for cancer, medications or prophylactic surgery may be recommended (Mahon, 2015). Several clinical trials have been conducted to identify medications that may help reduce the incidence of certain types of cancer. For example, a number of studies have demonstrated that daily use of the medication tamoxifen can significantly reduce a woman's lifetime risk of developing breast cancer in high-risk populations (Cuzik et al., 2014).

Secondary Prevention

Nurses must be aware of factors such as race, cultural influences, access to care, provider–patient relationship, level of education, income, and age, which influence the knowledge, attitudes, and beliefs people have about cancer. These factors also may affect the health-promoting behaviors people practice.

Public awareness about health-promoting behaviors can be provided in a variety of ways, including health education and health maintenance programs. Although primary prevention programs may focus on the hazards of tobacco use or the importance of nutrition, secondary prevention programs focus on early detection. Nurses and providers must encourage people to comply with detection efforts as suggested by the American Cancer Society (Table 6-2). Many organizations conduct cancer-screening events that focus on cancers with the highest incidence rates or those that have improved survival rates if diagnosed early, such as breast cancer. These events offer education and examinations, such as mammograms, for minimal or no cost. Often these programs are targeted at people who lack access to health care or cannot afford to participate on their own. In developing these programs, nurses must use strategies that are culturally sensitive to foster participation.

TABLE **6-2** American Cancer Society Recommendations for Early Detection of Cancer in Asymptomatic, Average Risk People

Site	Gender	Age-Specific Evaluation and Frequency
Breast	F	Women ages 40–44 may start annual mammograms if they wish to do so Starting at age 45, mammograms should be done every year, then, Every other year beginning at age 55 Clinical breast examination and self-examination are no longer recommended
Colon/rectum	F/M	Beginning at age 50, one of the following strategies should be used: • Flexible sigmoidoscopy every 5 years*, or • Colonoscopy every 10 years, or • Double-contrast barium enema every 5 years*, or • CT colonography (virtual colonoscopy) every 5 years* • Yearly guaiac-based fecal occult blood test (gFOBT) done via multi-sample take-home test, or • Yearly fecal immunochemical test (FIT) done via multi-sample take-home test, or • Stool DNA test (sDNA) every 3 years* *If test is positive, colonoscopy must be done High-risk patients may be tested on a different schedule.
Prostate	M	Starting at age 50, men should talk to a health care provider about the risks and benefits of testing and then decide about screening. African-American men or those with a father or brother with a history of prostate cancer should have this discussion beginning at age 45. If the decision is made to pursue testing, testing includes a PSA test +/− a digital rectal examination.
Cervix	F	• **Cervical cancer testing should start at age 21.** • **Women between the ages of 21 and 29** should have a Pap test done every 3 years. HPV testing should not be used in this age group unless it's needed after an abnormal Pap test result. • **Women between the ages of 30 and 65** should have a Pap test plus an HPV test (called "cotesting") done every 5 years. This is the preferred approach, but it is also acceptable to have a Pap test alone every 3 years. • **Women over age 65** who have had regular cervical cancer testing in the past 10 years with normal results should not be tested for cervical cancer. Once testing is stopped, it should not be started again. Women with a history of a serious cervical precancer should continue to be tested for at least 20 years after that diagnosis, even if testing goes past age 65. • **A woman who has had her uterus and cervix removed (a total hysterectomy)** for reasons not related to cervical cancer and who has no history of cervical cancer or serious precancer should not be tested. • **All women who have been vaccinated against HPV** should still follow the screening recommendations for their age groups.
Endometrium	F	The American Cancer Society recommends that at the time of menopause, all women should be told about the risks and symptoms of endometrial cancer. Women should report any unexpected vaginal bleeding or spotting to their doctors.
Lung cancer	M/F	For patients: • 55–74 years of age • In good health • Have at least a 30 pack/year smoking history AND are either still smoking or have quit within the last 15 years Screening is done with an annual low-dose CT scan (LDCT) of the chest.
Cancer-related checkups	M/F	For people aged 20 or older who get periodic health examinations, a cancer-related check-up should include health counseling and, depending on a person's age and gender, examinations for cancers of the thyroid, oral cavity, skin, lymph nodes, testes, and ovaries.

Adapted from Oeffinger, K. C., Fontham, E. H., Etzioni, R., et al. (2015); The American Cancer Society Guidelines for the early detection of cancer (2015) available at http://www.cancer.org/healthy/findcancerearly/cancerscreeningguidelines/american-cancer-society-guidelines-for-the-early-detection-of-cancer

DIAGNOSIS

A cancer diagnosis is based on an assessment of physiologic and functional changes and results of the diagnostic evaluation.

Diagnostic Evaluation

The diagnostic evaluation is guided by information obtained through a complete history and physical examination. Knowledge of suspicious symptoms and of the behavior of particular types of cancer assists in determining which diagnostic tests are most appropriate. Patients with suspected cancer undergo extensive testing to (1) determine the presence of a tumor and its extent, (2) identify possible spread (metastasis) of disease or invasion of other body tissues, (3) evaluate the function of involved and uninvolved body systems and organs, and (4) obtain tissue and cells for analysis to assist in the evaluation of tumor type, stage, grade, and molecular and genetic changes.

Patients undergoing extensive testing are usually fearful of the procedures and anxious about the possible test results. The nurse can help relieve the patient's fear and anxiety by explaining the tests to be performed, the sensations likely to be experienced, and the patient's role in the test procedures. The nurse encourages the patient and family to voice their fears about the test results, supports the patient and family throughout the test period, and reinforces and clarifies information conveyed by the primary care provider.

Tumor Staging and Grading

A complete diagnostic evaluation includes identifying the stage and grade of the tumor. This is accomplished before treatment begins to provide baseline data for evaluating outcomes of therapy and to maintain a systematic and consistent approach to ongoing diagnosis and treatment. Treatment options and prognosis are based on stage and grade of disease as well as the molecular and genetic profile.

Staging

Staging determines the size of the tumor and the extent of disease. Several systems exist for classifying the disease stage. The TNM system is frequently used for many solid tumor types. In this system, "T" refers to the extent of the primary tumor, "N" refers to lymph node involvement, and "M" refers to the extent of metastasis (Box 6-1) (Shao et al., 2013). A variety of other staging systems are used to describe the extent of cancers that are not well described by the TNM system, such as CNS cancers, hematologic cancers, and malignant melanoma. Staging systems also provide

---

BOX 6-1	**TNM Classification System**		
T	The extent of the primary tumor	**Regional Lymph Nodes (N)**	
N	The absence or presence and extent of regional lymph node metastasis	Nx	Regional lymph nodes cannot be assessed
M	The absence or presence of distant metastasis	N0	No regional lymph node metastasis
The use of numerical subsets of the TNM components indicates the progressive extent of the malignant disease.		N1, N2, N3	Increasing involvement of regional lymph nodes
		Distant Metastasis (M)	
Primary Tumor (T)		Mx	Distant metastasis cannot be assessed
Tx	Primary tumor cannot be assessed	M0	No distant metastasis
T0	No evidence of primary tumor	M	Distant metastasis
Tis	Carcinoma in situ		
T1, T2, T3, T4	Increasing size and/or local extent of the primary tumor		

From Edge, S., Byrd, D. R., Compton, C. C., Fritz, A. G., Greene, F. L., & Trotti, A. (Eds.). (2010). *AJCC cancer staging manual* (7th ed.). New York: Springer-Verlag.

a convenient shorthand notation that condenses lengthy descriptions into manageable terms for comparisons of treatments and prognoses.

Grading

Grading refers to the classification of the tumor cells. Grading systems seek to define the type of tissue from which the tumor originated and the degree to which the tumor cells retain the functional and histologic characteristics of the tissue of origin. Samples of cells to be used to establish the grade of a tumor may be obtained through cytology (examination of cells from tissue scrapings, body fluids, secretions, or washings), biopsy, or surgical excision.

This information helps the health care team predict the behavior and prognosis of various tumors. The tumor is assigned a numeric value ranging from I to IV (Box 6-2). Grade I tumors, also known as *well-differentiated tumors,* closely resemble the tissue of origin in structure and function. Tumors that do not clearly resemble the tissue of origin in structure or function are described as *poorly differentiated* or *undifferentiated* and are assigned grade IV. These tumors tend to be more aggressive and less responsive to treatment than are well-differentiated tumors.

Genetic Testing: Precision Medicine

Over the last decade there has been a paradigm shift toward a more personalized approach to cancer treatment. Precision medicine, also called *personalized medicine,* is defined by the National Cancer Institute as "a form of medicine that uses information about a person's genes, proteins, and environment to prevent, diagnose, and treat disease" (National Cancer Institute, 2016).

Precision medicine emerged in oncology with the discovery of molecularly targeted agents based on DNA molecular information of the patients' tumors. While traditional chemotherapy destroys rapidly dividing cells by interfering with DNA replication and cell division, molecularly targeted agents alter the function of specific molecular targets in cell signaling, proliferation, apoptosis, angiogenesis, metabolism, migration, or invasion. Some tumor types share the same targetable molecular alterations (e.g., HER2 overexpression in both breast and gastric cancers) (Le Tourneau et al., 2015).

Molecular profiling of key oncogenic factors has allowed many types of cancers to be more carefully classified. For example, a breast tumor is now defined not just by TNM stage and grade but whether the tumor is estrogen and progesterone receptor positive or negative and whether the tumor expresses HER2. These results allow the provider to recommend treatment targeted to the patient's profile (e.g., tamoxifen or arimidex for estrogen-receptor (ER) positive breast cancer and Herceptin, which targets the HER2 receptor in HER2 positive patients) (Harrington et al., 2013). The

BOX 6-2	**Grading**
GX	Grade cannot be assessed
G1	Well differentiated
G2	Moderately differentiated
G3	Poorly differentiated
G4	Undifferentiated

advent of readily available, cost-effective tests that identify targetable molecular alterations in a reasonable timeframe has allowed wide integration into oncology practice (Le Tourneau et al., 2015).

MANAGEMENT

The range of possible treatment goals may include cancer prevention, complete eradication of malignant disease (**cure**), prolonged survival and prevention of progression (**control**), or relief of symptoms associated with the disease (**palliation**).

A number of factors are considered when determining a treatment plan, including the tumor type, stage, and grade; functional or **performance status (PS)** of the patient; comorbidities; and organ function.

PS is one of the most important factors in determining eligibility for treatments, including clinical trials, and predicting prognosis (West & Jin, 2015). There are two widely used scales for PS. The most commonly used is typically referred to as the Zubrod or ECOG (Eastern Cooperative Oncology Group) scale. The ECOG scale uses a range of 0–4 with 0 being independent and 4 being restricted to bed. The other commonly used scale, the Karnofsky scale, ranges from 10 (moribund) to 100 (fully independent) (West & Jin, 2015).

A variety of approaches, including surgery, radiation therapy, chemotherapy, targeted therapy and immunotherapy, may be used at various times throughout treatment. Understanding the principles of each treatment modality and how they interrelate is important in understanding the rationale and goals of treatment.

The health care team, the patient, and the patient's family must have a clear understanding of the treatment options, goals, and potential impact on quality of life. Open communication and support are vital as the patient and family periodically reassess treatment plans and goals when complications of therapy develop or disease progresses.

Surgery

Surgery is used for a variety of different reasons and at different times during the cancer trajectory. Surgery may be the primary method of treatment, or it may be prophylactic, palliative, or reconstructive. Diagnostic surgery is the definitive method for identifying the cellular characteristics of the tumor that influence all treatment decisions.

Diagnostic Surgery

Diagnostic surgery, such as a **biopsy**, must be performed to obtain a tissue sample for analysis of cells suspected to be malignant. In most instances, the biopsy is taken from the actual tumor, but in some situations, it is necessary to biopsy lymph nodes near the suspicious tumor. Many cancers metastasize from the primary site to other areas of the body through the lymphatic circulation. Knowing whether adjacent lymph nodes contain tumor cells is critical to staging the cancer and will impact the need for systemic therapies instead of or in addition to surgery, to combat tumor cells that have gone beyond the primary tumor site.

Surgery as Primary Treatment

When surgery is the primary approach in treating cancer, the goal is to remove the entire tumor or as much as is feasible (a procedure sometimes called *debulking*) and any involved surrounding tissue, including regional lymph nodes.

Two common surgical approaches used for treating primary tumors are local and wide excisions:

- A *local excision* is warranted when the mass is small. It includes removal of the mass and a small margin of normal tissue that is easily accessible.
- *Wide* or *radical excisions* (*en bloc dissections*) include removal of the primary tumor, lymph nodes, adjacent involved structures, and surrounding tissues that may be at high risk for tumor spread. This surgical method can result in disfigurement and altered functioning. However, wide excisions are considered if the tumor can be removed completely and the chances of cure or control are good.

Prophylactic Surgery

Prophylactic surgery involves removing nonvital tissues or organs that are likely to develop cancer. Several factors are considered when providers and patients discuss possible prophylactic surgery; these include family history and genetic predisposition, presence or absence of symptoms, potential risks and benefits, ability to detect cancer at an early stage, and the patient's acceptance of the postoperative outcome.

Colectomy (surgical resection of the colon), mastectomy (removal of breast), and oophorectomy (removal of ovary[ies]) are examples of prophylactic surgeries. Recent developments in the ability to identify genetic markers indicative of a predisposition to develop some types of cancer may play a role in decisions concerning prophylactic surgeries. Several factors are considered when deciding to proceed with a prophylactic mastectomy, including a strong family history of breast cancer; positive results in *BRCA1* or *BRCA2*

testing; an abnormal physical finding on breast examination, such as progressive nodularity and cystic disease; a proven history of breast cancer in the opposite breast; abnormal mammography findings; and abnormal biopsy results.

Because the long-term physiologic and psychological effects are unknown, prophylactic surgery is offered selectively to patients with a thorough discussion of potential risks and benefits with patients and families. Preoperative teaching and counseling, as well as long-term follow-up, are provided.

> **Nursing Alert**
> BRCA1 (breast cancer 1) *and* BRCA2 (breast cancer 2) *are clinical markers associated with the hereditary development of breast and ovarian cancer. Mutations of the BRCA1 and BRCA2 genes account for most inherited breast cancers. Carriers of BRCA1 (a tumor suppressor gene) mutation have an 85% risk for developing breast cancer and a 45% risk for developing ovarian cancer by age 85 (Fischbach & Dunning, 2014). BRCA2 is also a tumor suppressor gene; mutations in this gene are associated with hereditary breast and ovarian cancer syndrome, and often presents as premenopausal breast cancer, ovarian cancer, and/or male breast cancer (Axilbund & Wiley, 2015). Those who test positive for the mutations should be monitored annually or semi-annually. Discussions with providers may include chemoprevention (e.g., tamoxifen), and consideration of prophylactic surgery (Fischbach & Dunning, 2014).*

Palliative Surgery

When cure is not possible, the goals of treatment are to make the patient as comfortable as possible and to improve quality of life as defined by the patient. Palliative surgery is performed in an attempt to relieve complications of cancer, such as ulcerations, obstructions, hemorrhage, pain, and malignant effusions. Honest and informative communication with the patient and family about the risks, benefits, and goals of surgery is essential.

Nursing Management in Cancer Surgery

A multidisciplinary approach to patient care is essential before, during, and after any type of surgery. The effects of surgery on the patient's body image, self-esteem, and functional abilities are addressed. If necessary, a plan for postoperative rehabilitation is made before the surgery is performed.

The nurse must complete a thorough preoperative assessment for factors that may affect the patient undergoing the surgical procedure, including medical history, prior cancer treatments, and any complications associated with those treatments. The nurse targets interventions to minimize the risk of complications (Morgan, 2014). Cardiac risk factors that increase the risk for complications in noncardiac surgery include a history of stroke, heart failure, angina or MI, renal insufficiency, and diabetes (Morgan, 2014). Pre-existing pulmonary disease can increase the risk for postoperative pneumonia and pleural effusions. Patients with cancer may be at increased risk for bleeding (see Chapter 20) and may require additional tests prior to surgery to assess individual bleeding risk. Elective surgery should be delayed until the patient has an absolute neutrophil count of at least 1,000 cells/mm^3 and a platelet count more than 50 platelets/mm^3 (and more than 100 for any neurosurgery) (Morgan, 2014).

Patients who are undergoing surgery for the diagnosis or treatment of cancer are often anxious about the surgical procedure, possible findings, postoperative limitations, changes in normal body functions, and prognosis. The patient and family require time, support, and assistance to deal with the possible changes and outcomes resulting from the surgery.

The nurse provides education and emotional support by assessing the needs of the patient and family and by discussing their fears and coping mechanisms with them. The nurse encourages the patient and family to take an active role in decision-making when possible. If the patient or family asks about the results of diagnostic testing and surgical procedures, the nurse's response is guided by the information the provider has previously conveyed to the patient and family. The patient and family may also ask the nurse to explain and clarify information that the provider initially gave but that they did not grasp because they were anxious at the time. It is important that the nurse communicate frequently with providers and other members of the health care team to be certain that the information provided is consistent.

After surgery, the nurse assesses the patient's responses to the surgery and monitors the patient for possible complications, such as infection, bleeding, thrombophlebitis, wound dehiscence, fluid and electrolyte imbalance, and organ dysfunction. The nurse also provides for the patient's comfort. Postoperative teaching addresses decreasing the risk for complications, including deep vein thrombosis (DVT) and pneumonia, as well as education on wound care, activity, nutrition, and medication information.

Patients undergoing surgery for cancer require general perioperative nursing care, as described in Chapter 5, along with specific care related to age, organ impairment, nutritional deficits, disorders of coagulation, and altered immunity that may increase the risk of postoperative complications. Combining other treatment methods, such as radiation and chemotherapy, with surgery also contributes to postoperative complications, such as infection, impaired wound healing, altered pulmonary or kidney function, and the development of venous thromboembolism (VTE), also known as DVT. Some cancer types result in an increase in circulating procoagulants, which can significantly increase the risk for DVT. Patients with cancer account for 20% of all DVT cases (Morgan, 2014).

Nursing Alert
Approximately 50% of patients with DVT are asymptomatic. The nurse should inquire about an ache or pain in the calf that is aggravated by standing or walking. In addition, it is important to assess for asymmetry of the limbs as slight swelling may be noted as well as erythema and warmth of the involved extremity. Venous distention in the affected limb that persists despite elevation of the extremity may be noted. Patients may also present with low-grade fever and tachycardia.

Plans for discharge, follow-up and home care, and treatment are initiated as early as possible to ensure continuity of care from hospital to home or from a cancer referral center to the patient's local hospital and health care provider. Patients and families are also encouraged to use community resources, such as the American Cancer Society, for support and information.

Radiation Therapy

In **radiation therapy**, ionizing radiation is used to interrupt cellular growth. More than half of patients with cancer receive a form of radiation therapy at some point during treatment. Radiation may be used to cure the cancer, as in head and neck, prostate, lung, and bladder cancers. Radiation therapy may also be used to control malignant disease when a tumor cannot be removed surgically or when local nodal metastasis is present, or it can be used prophylactically to prevent leukemic infiltration to the brain (Iwamoto, Haas, & Gosselin, 2012).

Palliative radiation therapy is used to relieve the symptoms of metastatic disease, especially when the cancer has spread to brain, bone, or soft tissue, or to treat oncologic emergencies, such as superior vena cava syndrome (SVCS) or spinal cord compression.

Two types of ionizing radiation—electromagnetic rays (x-rays and gamma rays) and particles (electrons [beta particles], protons, neutrons, and alpha particles)—can lead to tissue disruption. Radiation disrupts malignant cell proliferation through the alteration in DNA structure. Ionizing radiation breaks the strands of the DNA helix, leading to cell death. Ionizing radiation can also ionize constituents of body fluids, especially water, leading to the formation of free radicals and irreversible DNA damage. If the DNA is incapable of repair, the cell may die immediately, or it may initiate apoptosis (Iwamoto et al., 2012).

Cells are most vulnerable to the disruptive effects of radiation during DNA synthesis and mitosis. Therefore, those body tissues that undergo frequent cell division are most sensitive to radiation therapy. These radiosensitive tissues include bone marrow, lymphatic tissue, epithelium of the GI tract, hair cells, and gonads. Slower-growing tissues and tissues at rest are relatively radioresistant (less sensitive to the effects of radiation). Such tissues include muscle, cartilage, and connective tissues.

A radiosensitive tumor is one that can be destroyed by a dose of radiation that still allows for cell regeneration in the normal tissue. Tumors that are well oxygenated also appear to be more sensitive to radiation (Iwamoto et al., 2012). In theory, therefore, radiation therapy may be enhanced if more oxygen can be delivered to tumors. In addition, if the radiation is delivered when most tumor cells are cycling through the cell cycle, the number of cancer cells destroyed (cell kill) is maximal. Certain chemicals, including chemotherapy and some targeted agents (e.g., EGFR inhibitors) act as radiosensitizers and sensitize more hypoxic (oxygen-poor) tumors to the effects of radiation therapy (Iwamoto et al., 2012).

Radiation Delivery

Radiation is delivered to tumor sites by external or internal methods.

External Radiation

If external radiation therapy is used, one of several delivery methods may be chosen, depending on the depth of the tumor. Kilovoltage therapy devices deliver the maximal radiation dose to superficial lesions, such as lesions of the skin and breast. Conversely, linear accelerators and betatron machines produce higher-energy x-rays and deliver their dosage to deeper structures with less harm to the skin and less scattering of radiation within the body tissues.

Internal Radiation

Internal radiation implantation, or **brachytherapy**, delivers a high dose of radiation to a localized area. The specific radioisotope for implantation is selected on the basis of its half-life, which is the time it takes for half of its radioactivity to decay. This internal radiation can be implanted by means of needles, seeds, beads, or catheters into body cavities (e.g., vagina, abdomen, pleura) or interstitial compartments (e.g., breast). With internal radiation therapy, the farther the tissue is from the radiation source, the lower the radiation exposure. This spares the noncancerous tissue from the radiation dose and toxicity. Brachytherapy may also be administered orally, as with the isotope iodine-131, which is used to treat thyroid carcinomas.

Intracavitary Radiation. Intracavitary radioisotopes are used frequently to treat gynecologic cancers. In these malignancies, the radioisotopes are inserted into applicators specially positioned in the cervix and vagina, after the position is verified by x-ray. These radioisotopes remain in place for a prescribed time period and then are removed. The patient is maintained on bed rest and carefully log-rolled to prevent displacement of the intracavitary delivery device. The head of the bed must not be elevated greater than 15 degrees due to the risk of perforating the uterus with the appliance. An indwelling urinary catheter is inserted to ensure that the bladder remains empty, which minimizes the exposure of the bladder to radiation. Low-residue diets and antidiarrheal agents, such as diphenoxylate (Lomotil), are provided to prevent bowel movements during therapy that might displace the radioisotopes. Pain management is also a priority for these patients as the presence of the appliance can be painful. Patient-controlled analgesia is a common method used for pain management in this population. Patient are also at risk for atelectasis, pressure ulcers, and DVT due to bed rest so preventative measures, including incentive spirometry, a pressure-relieving mattress, sequential compression devices, and prophylactic anticoagulation, are essential to preventing these complications.

Safety. Because patients receiving internal radiation emit radiation while the implant is in place, contacts with the health care team are guided by principles of *time, distance,* and *shielding* to minimize exposure of personnel to radiation. As the amount of *time* with the patient increases, the nurses' exposure to radiation increases. The goal of nursing care for this population is to deliver safe, efficient care that meets the patients' needs in the shortest amount of time; in general, no more than 30 minutes per 8-hour shift. The *principle of distance* means that the closer you are to the patient, the greater the radiation exposure. When not providing direct care (e.g., when talking with the patient), stand at least 6 feet from the patient to minimize exposure. Organize activities outside the room when possible; for example, preparation of meals and medication. *Shielding* refers to the use of a lead shield to buffer the exposure to radiation. Often, the rooms that patients stay in may be lead-lined, or portable lead shields or aprons may be available to minimize exposure.

Other safety precautions used in caring for a patient receiving brachytherapy include assigning the patient to a private room, posting appropriate notices about radiation safety precautions, having staff members wear dosimeter badges (to track cumulative radiation exposure), ensuring that pregnant staff members are not assigned to the patient's care, prohibiting visits by children or pregnant visitors, limiting visits from others to 30 minutes daily, and seeing that visitors maintain a 6-foot distance from the radiation source.

Nurses must be prepared to respond to a radiation emergency. If the radiation implant becomes dislodged, the nurses' first priority is to ensure the safety of the patient. Metal forceps and a lead-lined container should be available in the room. The nurse can use the forceps to pick up the radiation source and place the source into the lead-lined container. Once the source is contained, the radiation safety officer should be contacted immediately. Then the patient, nurse, and room will be monitored for radioactivity using a Geiger counter. The staff exposed should report to their Occupational Health department for an evaluation. Nurses should refer to their institution's radiation safety committee's guidelines for specific measures.

Radiation Dosage

The radiation dosage is dependent on the sensitivity of the target tissues to radiation and on the tumor size. The lethal tumor dose is defined as the dose that will eradicate 95% of the tumor yet preserve normal tissue. With external radiation, the total radiation dose is delivered over several weeks to allow healthy tissue to repair and to achieve greater cell kill by exposing more cells to the radiation as they begin active cell division. Repeated radiation treatments over time (fractionated doses) also allow for the periphery of the tumor to be reoxygenated repeatedly because tumors shrink from the outside inward. This increases the radiosensitivity of the tumor, thereby increasing tumor cell death.

Toxicity

Toxicity of radiation therapy is localized to the region being irradiated. Toxicity may be increased if concomitant chemotherapy is administered. Acute local reactions occur when normal cells in the treatment area are also destroyed and cellular death exceeds cellular regeneration. Altered skin integrity is a common effect and can include **alopecia** (hair loss), erythema, and shedding of skin (desquamation). Re-epithelialization occurs after treatments have been completed; healing can take several weeks.

Alterations in oral mucosa secondary to radiation therapy include **stomatitis**, **xerostomia** (dryness of the mouth), change and loss of taste, and decreased salivation. The entire GI mucosa may be involved, possibly resulting in esophageal irritation with chest pain and dysphagia. Anorexia, nausea, vomiting, and diarrhea may occur if the stomach or colon is in the irradiated field. Symptoms subside and GI re-epithelialization occurs after treatments have been completed; however, it may take several weeks for stomatitis to resolve. Xerostomia and taste changes may never return to normal.

Bone marrow cells proliferate rapidly, and if sites containing bone marrow (e.g., the iliac crest, sternum) are included in the radiation field, anemia, leukopenia (decreased WBCs), and **thrombocytopenia** (a decrease in platelets) may result. The patient is then at increased risk for infection and bleeding until blood cell counts return to normal. Chronic anemia may occur commonly due to the cumulative effects of radiation and may be evidenced by shortness of breath, dizziness, fatigue, decreased oxygen saturation, and decreased activity tolerance.

Acute side effects to radiation therapy can occur within hours to days of receiving the first treatment. Bone marrow suppression, gonadal toxicity, skin changes, salivary changes, and GI side effects, such as nausea, may occur acutely.

Late effects from radiation are seen months to years after therapy even in the absence of acute symptoms. These effects include changes to the pituitary and thyroid glands, lungs, bones, breasts, cartilage, and pancreas (Iwamoto et al., 2012).

Nursing Management in Radiation Therapy

Providing Patient Education

Patients receiving radiation therapy, and their families, often have questions and concerns about its safety. To answer questions and allay fears about the effects of radiation on the tumor and on the patient's normal tissues and organs, the nurse explains the procedure for delivering radiation and describes the equipment, the duration of the procedure (often minutes only), the methods for immobilizing the patient during the procedure, and the sensory experience, including the absence of pain, during the procedure.

If a radioactive implant is used, the nurse informs the patient and family about the restrictions placed on visitors and health care personnel and other radiation precautions. The patient also should understand his or her own role before, during, and after the procedure. Patients with seed implants may be able to return home because the radiation exposure to others is minimal. Information about any precautions, if needed, is provided to the patient and family members to ensure safety. See Chapters 33 and 34 for further discussion of radiation treatment for gynecologic cancers and prostatic cancer, respectively.

Protecting Skin and Oral Mucosa

The nurse regularly assesses the patient's skin, oral mucosa, nutritional status, and general feeling of well-being. As many as 95% of patients receiving radiation experience radiation dermatitis. The nurse must educate the patient on early identification of symptoms and self-care guidelines to minimize further damage (Bauer, Laszewski, & Magnan, 2015).

The skin in the radiation field must be protected from irritation, and the patient is instructed to avoid using ointments, lotions, or powders on the treated area. The patient is instructed to gently cleanse the skin with lukewarm water and a mild, nondeodorant soap using the fingertips or a soft washcloth (no scrubbing) and then gently pat the area dry. If temporary skin markings were applied to facilitate external radiation treatments, warn the patient not to remove the markings. Avoid any perfumed lotion or powder; avoid applying makeup to the treatment field. Emollients such as Aquaphor® may be used as directed by the radiation oncologist to soothe and moisturize irritated skin. However, even approved emollients should not be used up to 4 hours before the treatment time. Lotions and emollients may amplify the effects of the radiation on the skin. Electric razors should be used for shaving, but aftershave products should be avoided. Patients should be instructed to avoid constrictive clothing that may irritate skin. Loose, cotton clothing is usually most comfortable. Other instructions include avoiding sun exposure, wind, extreme temperatures, heating lamps, heating pads, and ice packs to the area being treated—these are all potential sources of thermal injury. Avoid itching skin and avoid applying tape to radiated areas to minimize trauma to the skin (Iwamoto et al., 2012; Bauer et al., 2015).

BOX 6-3 **Patient Education**

Mouth Care for Patients Receiving Head and Neck Radiation Therapy

- Use a bland mouth rinse (such as salt water or baking soda and water) often. Gently swish and gargle with this before and after meals and at bedtime. You may use it more often as needed to soothe a dry or sore mouth. To make the mouth rinse: Mix 1 teaspoon of baking soda with 16 oz of water; or 1 teaspoon of table salt with 16 oz of water.
- Use fluoride preparations daily as instructed by your dentist. Brush your teeth using a soft-bristled toothbrush three to four times a day. Floss your teeth daily.
- Dentures should be left out if they are irritating to the gums or are poorly fitting.
- Avoid alcoholic beverages, tobacco, highly spiced foods, and commercial mouthwashes containing alcohol.

- Once you begin to experience pain or sensitivity in your mouth, avoid foods and drinks that are too hot or too cold. Room temperature is best. Avoid carbonated drinks such as soda or sparkling water.
- Avoid acidic fruits and juices like tomato, orange, lemon, grapefruit, and pineapple. Avoid rough, crunchy foods such as pretzels, nuts, and chips.
- Inspect your mouth daily and report any changes to your nurse or doctor.
- For a dry mouth, drink 8 oz of water or other noncaffeinated beverage every 2 to 3 hours. Keep a cool mist humidifier running, especially at night.
- Moisturize lips frequently with water-based moisturizer.

Gentle oral hygiene is essential to remove debris, prevent irritation, and promote healing (see Box 6-3 for detailed instructions). If systemic symptoms, such as weakness and fatigue, occur, the patient may need assistance with activities of daily living and personal hygiene (see Nursing Process later in the chapter). In addition, the nurse offers reassurance by explaining that these symptoms are a result of the treatment and do not represent deterioration or progression of the disease.

Chemotherapy

In **chemotherapy**, antineoplastic agents are used in an attempt to destroy tumor cells by interfering with cellular functions, including replication. Chemotherapy is used primarily to treat systemic disease rather than localized lesions that are amenable to surgery or radiation. Chemotherapy

may be combined with surgery, radiation therapy, or both to reduce tumor size preoperatively (neoadjuvant), to destroy any remaining tumor cells postoperatively (adjuvant), for conditioning therapy prior to stem cell transplant, or to treat hematologic malignancies, such as lymphoma and leukemia (Polovich, Olsen, & LeFebvre, 2014). The goals of chemotherapy (cure, control, palliation) define the medications to be used and the aggressiveness of the treatment plan. Chemotherapy may also be delivered in the setting of a clinical trial (see Box 6-4).

Cell Kill and the Cell Cycle

Each time a tumor is exposed to a chemotherapeutic agent, a percentage of tumor cells (20% to 99%, depending on dosage) are destroyed. Repeated doses of chemotherapy are necessary over a prolonged period to achieve regression

BOX 6-4 **Investigational Antineoplastic Therapies and Clinical Trials**

Evaluation of the effectiveness and toxic potential of promising new modalities for preventing, diagnosing, and treating cancer is accomplished through clinical trials. Before new therapies are approved for clinical use, they are subjected to rigorous and lengthy evaluations to identify beneficial effects, adverse effects, and safety.
- *Phase I* clinical trials determine optimal dosing, scheduling, toxicity, and pharmacokinetics. The goal is to determine a tolerable dose and schedule for drug administration.
- *Phase II* trials determine effectiveness with specific tumor types and further define toxicities. Phase I and II trials often involve small numbers of patients to help guide decisions about the utility of further research on a given agent. Participants in early trials are often those who have not responded to standard forms of treatment. Since the goals of Phase I and II trials are not focused on efficacy and extending

survival, patients and families must be fully informed about the experimental nature and goal of the trial.
- *Phase III* clinical trials establish the effectiveness of new medications or procedures as compared with conventional approaches.
- *Phase IV* testing further investigates medications in terms of new uses, dosing schedule, and toxicities.

Nurses may assist in the recruitment, eligibility screening, consent, and education processes for patients who participate in clinical trials. In many cases, nurses are instrumental in monitoring and promoting adherence as well as documenting data describing patients' responses and adverse effects. The physical and emotional needs of patients in clinical trials are addressed in much the same way as those of patients who receive standard forms of cancer treatment.

Adapted from Amir, E. & Tannock, 2013.

of the tumor. Eradication of 100% of the tumor is almost impossible. Instead, the goal of treatment is eradication of enough of the tumor so that the remaining tumor cells can be destroyed by the body's immune system.

Cells that are actively dividing within a tumor are the most sensitive to chemotherapeutic agents. Nondividing cells capable of future proliferation (cells in the G_0 phase, see Fig. 6-2) are the least sensitive to antineoplastic medications and, consequently, are potentially dangerous. However, the nondividing cells must also be destroyed to eradicate a cancer. As dividing cells are killed by chemotherapy, nondividing cells are recruited into the cell cycle to divide, in order to replace the dying cells. Repeated cycles of chemotherapy must be used to kill these newly dividing cells.

Chemotherapy drugs are often given in combination (referred to as a *protocol* or *regimen*). The goal of combination chemotherapy is to overcome drug resistance and take advantage of the synergistic effects of some drugs while minimizing toxicity. As described earlier, tumors are heterogeneous so agents with different mechanisms of action are used in combination to increase the number of cells killed; combination approaches also reduce the risk of drug resistance. Considerations for combination chemotherapy include the use of drugs with different mechanisms of action and different side effect profiles (Polovich et al., 2014).

Classification of Chemotherapeutic Agents

Chemotherapeutic agents may be classified by their relationship to the cell cycle. Certain chemotherapeutic agents that are specific to certain phases of the cell cycle are termed *cell cycle–specific agents*. These agents destroy cells that are actively reproducing by means of the cell cycle; most affect cells in the S phase by interfering with DNA and RNA synthesis. Other agents, such as the vinca or plant alkaloids, are specific to the M phase, where they halt mitotic spindle formation. Chemotherapeutic agents that act independently of the cell cycle phases are termed *cell cycle–nonspecific agents*. These agents usually have a prolonged effect on cells, leading to cellular damage or death. Many treatment plans combine cell cycle–specific and cell cycle–nonspecific agents to increase the number of vulnerable tumor cells killed during a treatment period (Polovich et al., 2014).

Chemotherapeutic agents are also classified by chemical group, each with a different mechanism of action. These include the alkylating agents, nitrosoureas, antimetabolites, antitumor antibiotics, plant alkaloids, hormonal agents, and miscellaneous agents. The classification, mechanism of action, common medications, and common side effects of selected antineoplastic agents are listed in Table 6-3.

Administration of Chemotherapeutic Agents

Chemotherapeutic agents may be administered in the hospital, clinic, or home setting by a variety of routes including topical, oral, IV, intramuscular, subcutaneous, arterial, intracavitary, and intrathecal routes. Intrathecal chemotherapy is the administration of medication into the cerebrospinal fluid. This can be accomplished through a lumbar puncture or through the placement of an intraventricular catheter

TABLE 6-3 Selected Antineoplastic Agents

Drug Class and Examples	Mechanism of Action	Cell Cycle Specificity	Most Common Side Effects
Alkylating Agents			
Altretamine, Bendamustine, Busulfan, carboplatin, chlorambucil, cisplatin, cyclophosphamide, dacarbazine, ifosfamide, melphalan, nitrogen mustard, oxaliplatin, temozolomide, thiotepa	Alter DNA structure by misreading DNA code, initiating breaks in the DNA molecule, cross-linking DNA strands	Cell cycle—nonspecific	Bone marrow suppression, nausea, vomiting, cystitis (cyclophosphamide, ifosfamide), stomatitis, alopecia, gonadal suppression, renal toxicity (cisplatin)
Nitrosoureas			
Carmustine (BCNU), lomustine (CCNU), semustine (methyl CCNU), streptozocin	Similar to the alkylating agents; cross the blood–brain barrier	Cell cycle—nonspecific	Delayed and cumulative myelosuppression, especially thrombocytopenia; nausea, vomiting
Topoisomerase I Inhibitors			
Irinotecan, topotecan	Induce breaks in the DNA strand by binding to enzyme topoisomerase I, preventing cells from dividing	Cell cycle—specific (S phase)	Bone marrow suppression, diarrhea, nausea, vomiting, hepatotoxicity

Drug Class and Examples	Mechanism of Action	Cell Cycle Specificity	Most Common Side Effects
Antimetabolites			
5-Azacitidine, capecitabine, cladribine, clofarabine, cytarabine, decitabine, floxuridine, fludarabine, 5-fluorouracil (5-FU), gemcitabine, 6-mercaptopurine, methotrexate, nelarabine, pemetrexed, pralatrexate, 6-thioguanine	Interfere with the biosynthesis of metabolites or nucleic acids necessary for RNA and DNA synthesis	Cell cycle—specific (S phase)	Nausea, vomiting, diarrhea, bone marrow suppression, stomatitis, renal toxicity (methotrexate), hepatotoxicity
Antitumor Antibiotics			
Bleomycin, dactinomycin, daunorubicin, doxorubicin, epirubicin, idarubicin, mitomycin, mitoxantrone, valrubicin	Interfere with DNA synthesis by binding DNA; prevent RNA synthesis	Cell cycle—nonspecific	Bone marrow suppression, nausea, vomiting, alopecia, anorexia, cardiac toxicity (doxorubicin, daunorubicin, idarubicin, mitoxantrone)
Mitotic Spindle Poisons			
Plant alkaloids: etoposide, teniposide, vinblastine, vincristine (VCR), vindesine, vinorelbine *Taxanes:* cabazitaxel, docetaxel, paclitaxel	Arrest metaphase by inhibiting mitotic tubular formation (spindle); inhibit DNA and protein synthesis Arrest metaphase by inhibiting tubulin depolymerization	Cell cycle—specific (M phase) Cell cycle—specific (M phase)	Plant alkaloids: Bone marrow suppression (mild with VCR), neuropathies (VCR), stomatitis Taxanes: Alopecia, bone marrow suppression, bradycardia, hypersensitivity reactions, neuropathy
Hormonal Agents			
Androgens and antiandrogens, estrogens and antiestrogens, progestins and antiprogestins, aromatase inhibitors, luteinizing hormone–releasing hormone analogs, steroids	Bind to hormone receptor sites that alter cellular growth; block binding of estrogens to receptor sites (antiestrogens); inhibit RNA synthesis; suppress aromatase of P450 system, which decreases estrogen level	Cell cycle—nonspecific	Hypercalcemia, increased appetite, masculinization, feminization, sodium and fluid retention, nausea, vomiting, hot flashes, vaginal dryness
Miscellaneous Agents			
Arsenic trioxide, Asparaginase, hydroxyurea, mitotane, procarbazine Romidepsin Vorinostat	Unknown or too complex to categorize Inhibit histone deacytelase	Varies	Anorexia, nausea, vomiting, bone marrow suppression, hepatotoxicity, anaphylaxis, hypotension, altered glucose metabolism

Adapted from Polovich et al. (2014).

with the tip lying in the fourth ventricle of the brain. This route is used to treat or prevent CNS metastasis. The route of administration usually depends on the type of agent; the required dose; and the type, location, and extent of tumor being treated. Guidelines for the administration of chemotherapy have been developed by the Oncology Nursing Society (ONS) (Polovich et al., 2014). The use of oral agents to treat cancer is increasing dramatically. Patient education and consistent monitoring of patient adherence is essential to maximize safety.

Dosage
Dosage of antineoplastic agents is based primarily on the patient's total body surface area, previous response to chemotherapy or radiation therapy, function of major organ systems, and PS.

 Nursing Alert
Because of the high potential for error related to chemotherapy dosing, the standard expectation is that two nurses verify the chemotherapy

doses to ensure accuracy. The Mosteller Equation *for calculation of body surface area is the most commonly used formula in the United States:*

$$\sqrt{\frac{height\ (cm) \times weight\ (kg)}{3600}}$$

Infusion-Related Events

Nurses administering chemotherapy must carefully assess the patient for infusion-related events, such as infusion reactions, hypersensitivity, and extravasation. Specific assessments vary based on the medication being administered (see Table 6-3).

Infusion Reaction. Reactions that occur during or shortly after drug infusion are described as infusion reactions. These reactions may be allergic or nonallergic in nature. Infusion reactions can often be anticipated when administering drugs such as monoclonal antibodies. Most infusion reactions are mild (e.g., chills) and, if recognized and treated promptly, should resolve. Initial management is interruption of the infusion and symptom management with antihistamines, antiemetics, steroids, or anxiolytics. In most cases, the infusion can be reinitiated and completed at a slower rate with careful monitoring (Jakel, Carsten, Braskett, & Carino, 2016).

Hypersensitivity. About 5% to 15% of patients receiving chemotherapy and biotherapy agents experience hypersensitivity reactions (HSRs). The risk of hypersensitivity varies based on the type of agent being administered. Platinum- and taxane-containing agents have the most frequent incidence of HSRs (Tham, Cheng, Tay, Alcasabas, & Shek, 2015). Prompt recognition of the symptoms of HSRs and quick intervention are critical roles of oncology nurses who administer these agents. Common symptoms observed in patients experiencing HSRs range from flushing, rash (urticarial), nausea, vomiting, flushing, back pain, shortness of breath, and anxiety or sense of impending doom to bronchospasm and hemodynamic collapse (Jakel et al., 2016). Response to HSRs includes stopping the infusion as soon as symptoms are observed; monitoring vital signs; maintaining a patent airway; administering oxygen as needed; maintaining a patent IV with running normal saline; administering emergency medications such as antihistamines, epinephrine, bronchodilators, and corticosteroids as ordered; and providing emotional support to the patient. In mild reactions, reinitiation of the infusion at a slower rate may be considered. For patients with more severe reactions, additional considerations are required for retreatment, including premedication with steroids and antihistamines (H_1 and H_2 blockers) and, in some cases, desensitization protocols (Tham et al., 2015).

Extravasation. Special care must be taken whenever IV vesicant agents are administered. **Vesicants** are agents that, if deposited into the subcutaneous tissue (**extravasation**), cause tissue ulceration and necrosis as well as damage to underlying tendons, nerves, and blood vessels. Although the complete mechanism of tissue destruction is unclear, it is known that the pH of many antineoplastic drugs is responsible for the severe inflammatory reaction as well as the ability of some of these drugs (e.g., anthracyclines) to bind to tissue DNA. Sloughing and ulceration of the tissue may be so severe that skin grafting may be necessary. The full extent of tissue damage may take several weeks to become apparent. Some examples of medications classified as vesicants include actinomycin D, dacarbazine, doxorubicin (Adriamycin), epirubicin, nitrogen mustard, mitomycin, vinblastine, vincristine, vinorelbine (Kreidieh, Moukadem, & El Saghir, 2016).

 Nursing Alert
Prior to administration of any anticancer agent, the nurse must be aware of a drug's vesicant potential. If frequent administration of antineoplastic vesicants is anticipated in a patient with poor veins, or if a vesicant agent requires administration over more than 1 hour, a central venous access device (CVAD) must be inserted to promote safety during medication administration. Complications associated with CVAD use include infection and thrombosis. Educating the patient about all risks associated with vesicant chemotherapy administration is critical.

Irritants are drugs that can cause pain or irritation at the extravasation site and burning sensation during administration but do not cause tissue damage. Examples of irritants include bendamustine or carboplatin (Kreidieh et al., 2016).

Exfoliants are drugs that can cause inflammation and peeling or blistering of the skin without tissue necrosis. Examples of exfoliants include Cisplatin, Docetaxel, Liposomal Doxorubicin, Mitoxantrone, Oxaliplatin, and Paclitaxel (Kreidieh et al., 2016).

Patients must understand the importance of prompt reporting of any signs and symptoms of extravasation. Risk factors for extravasation include small and/or fragile veins, lymphedema, obesity, impaired level of consciousness (LOC), history of multiple venipunctures, poor cannula size selection, and poor vein selection. Extravasation can occur as a result of accidental puncturing of the vein or with movement of the cannula itself due to patient activity or a poorly secured catheter. Prolonged peripheral IV infusions of vesicants carry an increased risk of extravasation, and, therefore, vesicant infusions lasting more than 1 hour should be administered through a CVAD (Figs. 6-3 and 6-4).

Strategies to decrease the risk of extravasation include:

- Appropriate training of nurses following the ONS standards
- Selection of appropriate vascular access location, including avoiding veins in the hand, wrist, or antecubital regions
- Avoiding veins that are small and/or fragile
- Avoiding an extremity with lymphedema or recent venipuncture

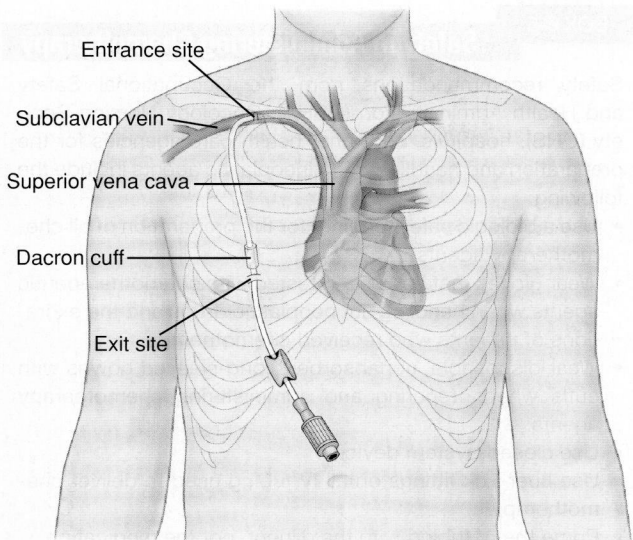

FIGURE 6-3 Central venous access device. The central venous catheter is inserted into the subclavian vein and advanced until its tip lies in the superior vena cava just above the right atrium. The proximal end is then tunneled from the entry site through the subcutaneous tissue of the chest wall and brought out through an exit site on the chest. The Dacron cuff anchors the catheter in place and serves as a barrier to infection.

- Use of the smallest size of cannula in the largest available vein
- Use of a small bore plastic cannula that is 1.2 to 1.5 cm long
- Use of a clear dressing
- Avoiding the use of a butterfly needle

Nursing Alert
Indications of extravasation during administration of vesicant agents include:
- *Absence of blood return from the IV catheter*
- *Resistance to flow of IV fluid*
- *Leaking around the insertion site*
- *Swelling, pain, burning, or redness or blistering at the site, or if using a CVAD, pain in the upper arm, upper back, chest, neck, or jaw*
- *For some drugs (anthracyclines such as doxorubicin), signs and symptoms of extravasation may continue for weeks after drug administration (Kreidieh et al., 2016).*

If any one of the above signs is present, extravasation should be suspected. The medication administration should be stopped immediately. The nurse should attempt to aspirate any residual drug from the IV line. If an antidote is indicated, the nurse should administer it immediately (as ordered). Selection of the neutralizing solution or antidote depends on the extravasated agent.

Dexrazoxane is approved in the setting of anthracycline extravasation with efficacy rates as high as 98% in

FIGURE 6-4 Implanted vascular access device. **(A)** A schematic diagram of an implanted vascular access device used for administration of medications, fluids, blood products, and nutrition. The self-sealing septum permits repeated puncture by Huber needles without damage or leakage. **(B)** Two Huber needles used to enter the implanted vascular port. The 90-degree needle is used to access the port.

preventing tissue damage. Dexrazoxane is administered as a 1- to 2-hour IV infusion for 3 consecutive days. Treatment with dexrazoxane should be initiated within 6 hours of extravasation for best results (Kreidieh et al., 2016).

Examples of neutralizing solutions include sodium thiosulfate, hyaluronidase, and sodium bicarbonate. Hyaluronidase is an enzyme administered as a subcutaneous injection into the extravasation site that degrades hyaluronic acid in tissues and promotes diffusion of the extravasated agent. It is recommended for vinca-alkaloids, etoposide and taxanes extravasation with low levels of evidence supporting its use. Sodium thiosulfate is also administered via subcutaneous injection for nitrogen mustard extravasations (Kreidieh et al., 2016). It is essential for nurses to keep up with the research findings related to extravasation and to apply the evidence to clinical practice.

The involved extremity should be elevated for the first 48 hours. Ice is applied to the site (unless the extravasated vesicant is a vinca-alkaloid in which case warm compresses are used) (four times a day for 20 minutes for the first 48 hours), and the patient is educated to avoid further trauma to the site (including heat, constrictive clothing, sunlight) and to report changes in the skin integrity and appearance of the extravasation site to the provider immediately. A plastic surgery consult should be considered within the first 24 hours (Pluschnig et al., 2014). Recommendations and guidelines for managing vesicant extravasation have been issued by individual medication manufacturers, pharmacies, and the ONS, and they differ for each medication.

Protecting Caregivers

Chemotherapy agents are hazardous and have the potential for carcinogenicity, genotoxicity, teratogenicity, reproductive toxicity, and organ toxicity (Redmond, 2016). Nurses involved in handling chemotherapeutic agents may be exposed to low doses of the agents by direct contact, inhalation, or ingestion. Nurses who handle these agents must receive education on safe handling measures to minimize risks of exposure. Exposure is often accidental and can happen during preparation, transport, administration, waste disposal, and spills (Redmond, 2016). Urinalyses of personnel repeatedly exposed to cytotoxic agents have demonstrated the presence of these agents. Although long-term studies of nurses who handle chemotherapeutic agents have not been conducted, chemotherapeutic agents are associated with secondary formation of cancers and chromosomal abnormalities. In addition, nausea, rashes, alopecia, and hearing loss have been reported in health care personnel who have handled chemotherapeutic agents (CDC, 2015). In an effort to minimize the exposure of health care workers to hazardous substances, the Occupational Safety and Health Administration, ONS, hospitals, and other health care agencies have developed specific precautions for health care providers involved in the preparation and administration of chemotherapy (Box 6-5).

Toxicity

Cells with rapid growth rates (e.g., epithelium, bone marrow, hair follicles, sperm) are most susceptible to the effects of chemotherapy.

GI System

Chemotherapy-induced nausea and vomiting (CINV) is a common and feared side effect of chemotherapy and may persist for as long as 24 to 48 hours after its administration. Delayed nausea and vomiting may persist for several days after chemotherapy. Delayed nausea and vomiting is commonly seen with cisplatin, carboplatin, cyclophosphamide, and doxorubicin (Polovich et al., 2014). Anticipatory nausea

---

BOX 6-5 | **Safety in Administering Chemotherapy**

Safety recommendations from the Occupational Safety and Health Administration (OSHA), Oncology Nursing Society (ONS), hospitals, and other health care agencies for the preparation and handling of antineoplastic agents include the following:

- Use a biologic safety cabinet for the preparation of all chemotherapy agents.
- Wear gloves that have been tested with chemotherapeutic agents when handling antineoplastic drugs and the excretions of patients who received chemotherapy.
- Wear disposable, nonabsorbent long-sleeved gowns with cuffs when preparing and administering chemotherapy agents.
- Use closed-system devices.
- Use Luer-Lok fittings on all IV tubing used to deliver chemotherapy.
- Prime the IV tubing with the diluent, not the medication.
- Work below eye level. Use eye protection if there is a risk of splashing.
- Do not open or crush oral medication.
- Dispose of all equipment used in chemotherapy preparation and administration in appropriate, leak-proof, puncture-proof containers.
- Dispose of all chemotherapy wastes as hazardous materials.

When followed, these precautions greatly minimize the risk of exposure to chemotherapy agents.

---

may be experienced after the first cycle and is caused by classical conditioning; nausea is triggered by taste, odors, sights, thoughts, or anxiety related to a poor initial experience with CINV (Aapro, Jordan, & Fever, 2015). The primary risk factor for CINV is the emetogenic potential of the agents being used (how likely the agents are to cause nausea and vomiting). Patient-specific risk factors include a history of CINV, female sex, under 50 years of age, and history of motion sickness. A history of heavy alcohol use is associated with decreased risk for CINV (Aapro et al., 2015).

The pathophysiology of CINV is not fully understood and is the result of a complex interplay of many different factors. A vagal-dependent pathway is considered a primary mechanism for CINV. A number of important neurotransmitter receptors, including 5-HT3 (palonosetron), NK-1 (aprepitant), and cholecystokinin-1, are located on the terminal ends of the vagal afferents. These receptors lie in close proximity to the enterochromaffin cells located in the gastrointestinal mucosa of the proximal small intestine, which contains a number of local mediators, such as serotonin, substance P, and cholecystokinin. When patients are treated with cytotoxic drugs that damage the enterochromaffin cells, serotonin is released, activating vagal afferent neurons through interaction with the 5-HT3 receptors. The activation of vagal afferent neurons leads to an emetic response mediated through the chemoreceptor trigger zone within the area postrema (medullary structure in the brain that controls vomiting) (Aapro et al., 2015).

The goal of antiemetics is to prevent CINV. Antiemetic regimens are tailored based on the emetogenicity of the regimen (Polovich et al., 2014). Newer antiemetics have been developed that target 5-HT3 and NK-1 and a combination medication, NEPA, which combines a highly selective NK1RA (netupitant) and the 5-HT3RA (palonosetron) (Jordan, Jahn, & Aapro, 2015). For patients with a high risk of nausea and vomiting who are receiving regimens, a combination of a 5-HT3 antagonist, an NK1 antagonist, and a corticosteroid are given prior to initiation of treatment. NK1 antagonists and long-acting 5-HT3 antagonists are particularly useful in prevention of delayed nausea and vomiting. Patients should also have medication at home for as-needed use for breakthrough nausea and vomiting; options for breakthrough CINV include prochlorperazine, metoclopramide, olanzapine, lorazepam, dronabinol, and ondansetron (for patients who have not received the long-acting medication palonosetron) (Polovich et al., 2014; Jordan et al., 2015). For anticipatory CINV, benzodiazepines are most effective. Nonpharmacologic interventions, such as relaxation, can also be helpful in this setting (Polovich et al., 2014).

Hematopoietic System

Most chemotherapeutic agents cause **myelosuppression** (depression of bone marrow function), resulting in decreased production of blood cells. Myelosuppression decreases the number of WBCs (leukopenia), red blood cells (RBCs) (anemia), and platelets (thrombocytopenia) and increases the risk of infection and bleeding. Depression of these cells is a common reason for decreasing the dose of the chemotherapeutic agents. Monitoring blood cell counts frequently is essential because it allows strategies to be implemented to protect patients from infection and injury.

Other agents, called colony-stimulating factors (granulocyte colony-stimulating factor [G-CSF], granulocyte-macrophage colony-stimulating factor [GM-CSF], and erythropoietin [EPO]), can be administered after chemotherapy. G-CSF and GM-CSF stimulate the bone marrow to produce WBCs, including neutrophils, at an accelerated rate, thus decreasing the duration of **neutropenia**. GCSF decreases the episodes of infection and reduce the need for antibiotics, allowing for timelier cycling of chemotherapy with less need for dose reductions.

Erythropoietin-stimulating agents (ESAs) stimulate RBC production, thus decreasing the symptoms of chronic anemia and reducing the need for blood transfusions. Recent evidence has demonstrated that the use of ESAs in certain malignancies, including head and neck, nonsmall cell lung, lymphoid, cervical, and breast cancers, has resulted in decreased survival rates. Based on this data, the use of ESAs is not recommended in those diseases when the goal is cure (Polovich et al., 2014). Other studies have demonstrated an increase in cardiac events, including cerebrovascular events and myocardial infarction, when hemoglobin (Hgb) targets of greater than 12 mg/dL were used. Specific guidelines are now available to improve the safety of ESA administration, including holding ESAs for Hgb levels greater than 10 mg/dL, assessing the hemoglobin (Hgb) and hematocrit (Hct) prior to each ESA dose, and discontinuing ESA use in patients who do not achieve a significant benefit within the first 8 weeks of administration.

Reproductive System

Ovarian and testicular function can be affected by chemotherapeutic agents, resulting in possible sterility. Abnormal ovulation, early menopause, or permanent sterility may occur. In men, temporary or permanent azoospermia (absence of spermatozoa) may develop. Reproductive cells may be damaged during treatment, resulting in chromosomal abnormalities in offspring. Banking of sperm is recommended for males of reproductive age before treatments are initiated. Sperm banking requires daily sperm collections for 2 to 3 days in order to collect a sufficient sample. Women should be counseled regarding options for fertility preservation prior to initiating treatment. Embryo cryopreservation is the most well-established method for fertility preservation. Oocyte cryopreservation and cryopreservation of ovarian tissue are considered investigational. Fertility preservation options for women require more time (2 to 6 weeks) and may result in cancer treatment delays, which may impact overall outcomes (Polovich et al., 2014).

Prior to initiating treatment, patients and their partners need to be informed about potential changes in reproductive and sexual function resulting from chemotherapy. They are advised to use reliable methods of birth control while receiving chemotherapy and not to assume that sterility has resulted.

Nursing Management in Chemotherapy

Nurses play an important role in assessing and managing many of the problems experienced by patients undergoing chemotherapy. Chemotherapeutic agents have systemic effects on normal cells as well as malignant ones, which means that these problems are often widespread, affecting many body systems. Nurses must recognize the potential side effects specific to the drug or drug(s) that the patient is receiving and target assessments based on expected side effects. Common side effects seen with chemotherapy include myelosuppression, alopecia, nausea and vomiting, anorexia, and fatigue. The nursing care specific to these side effects is discussed in the nursing process section on page 181.

Targeted Therapies

Recent advances in the fields of molecular biology, biochemistry, immunology, and genetics have led to an improved understanding of cancer development. Traditional therapies such as chemotherapy and radiation are nonspecific, affecting all rapidly dividing cells. As a result, both healthy and malignant cells are subject to harmful systemic effects of treatment. **Targeted therapies** seek to minimize the negative effects on healthy tissues by disrupting specific cancer cell functions, such as malignant transformation, communication pathways (also called *cell signaling* or *signal transduction*), processes for growth and metastasis, as well as genetic coding. Targeted therapies can be divided into two categories: those with an extracellular target, such as receptors on the surface of the cells (e.g., Monoclonal antibodies or mAbs) and those with an intracellular target (e.g., Tyrosine kinase inhibitors).

Monoclonal antibodies (mAbs) have a specific target that may be unique to the tumor cell or may target proteins that support tumor growth. Monoclonal antibodies may inhibit the binding of growth factors to receptors on the cell surface, which shuts down the subsequent steps necessary for tumor cell division. Monoclonal antibodies also can act directly on the tumor cell to induce death. In addition, mAbs are involved in stimulating antibody-dependent cellular cytotoxicity (ADCC) in which the antibody binds to tumor cell antigen, NK cells recognize the antibody-covered cell, stimulating cytotoxic proteins to be released to destroy the tumor cell (Polovich et al., 2014). Monoclonal antibodies can be conjugated or unconjugated. Unconjugated mAbs kill tumor cells from the direct action of the antibody on the target (e.g., Rituximab, which targets C20; Trastuzumab, which targets HER2; Cetuximab, which targets EGFR). Conjugated mAbs are antibodies attached to antitumor agents (radioisotopes, chemotherapy drugs, toxins). The mAb attaches to its target and releases the antitumor agent into the cell, stimulating cell death (e.g., brentuximab vedotin). Infusion reactions are common with mAbs and require careful monitoring (see section on infusion related events) (Polovich et al., 2014).

Drugs that target intercellular pathways include tyrosine kinase inhibitors, which target the tyrosine kinase receptor and inhibit cell signaling. Examples of tyrosine kinase targets include BCR-ABL, mTOR, and BRAF. Growth factors and growth factor receptors are also targets; examples of growth factors include EGFR and VEGF (Polovich et al., 2014). Many of the drugs targeting these kinases and growth factors are taken orally, and adherence is critical to response. See Tables 6-4 and 6-5 for examples of targeted therapies and approved cytokines.

Immunotherapy

As discussed earlier, the immune system is critical in preventing, controlling, and eliminating cancer. Malignancy develops as a result of multiple mechanisms of immune failure or suppression. Immune therapies, including cytokines, vaccines, and checkpoint inhibitors, were developed in an attempt to restore or stimulate the body's own immune response to treat the cancer.

Cytokines, including interferon (IFN) alpha and interleukin-2 (IL-2), have been in use for many years in the treatment of melanoma. They both have significant side effects, which have limited widespread use. Eight percent of patients treated with IFN experience fever and fatigue. Psychiatric side effects are also common, including depression (45%) with rare reports of suicide. GI side effects include diarrhea, nausea, and anorexia. High-dose IL-2 is associated with capillary leak syndrome leading to hypotension, which may require vasopressor support. Flu-like symptoms are also seen. These patients require expert nursing care and vigilant monitoring (Weber, Yang, Atkins, & Disis, 2015).

Vaccines are used to stimulate the immune system to kill malignant cells. Vaccines are also used to prevent cancer-causing infections (hepatitis, HPV) (Polovich et al., 2014). Sipuleucel-T (Provenge®) is an FDA-approved vaccine for the treatment of advanced prostate cancer. Side effects, including chills, fever, and fatigue, are common in the first 24 hours (Weber et al., 2015).

Three checkpoint inhibitor antibodies are approved for use in the United States, and a number of others are in development: ipilimumab, which blocks CTLA-4; and pembrolizumab and nivolumab, which block PD-1 (Weber et al., 2015). CTLA-4 is a negative regulator of the immune response. Blockade of CTLA-4 using anti CTLA4 antibody, such as ipilimumab, results in T-cell stimulation. PD-1 is a negative regulator of T-cell activity and dampens the immune response when it interacts with PD-L1 and PD-L2. When PD-1 is blocked, signaling pathways necessary for cell growth are inhibited; PD-1 also inhibits effector T-cell activity, so when PD-1 is blocked, effector T cells are able to function (Postow, Callahan, & Wolchok, 2015).

Ipilimumab, a CTLA-4 inhibitor, has demonstrated significant improvements in survival in patients with advanced melanoma (with 18% of patients alive after 2 years compared to 5% in the control group) (Postow et al., 2015). Both nivolumab and pembrolizumab have shown durable response rates in advanced melanoma, renal cell carcinoma, and nonsmall cell lung cancer (Postow et al., 2015). This group of drugs has a unique side effect profile requiring expert care and management. Immune-related adverse events (irAEs) are a result of immune system stimulation and resemble autoimmune disorders, including colitis, pneumonitis, hypophysitis (endocrinopathies), hepatitis, and skin rashes. Skin-related side effects often occur first. Colitis is seen after 4 to 6 weeks; and hepatitis and endocrinopathies occur later, as late as 12 to 24 weeks into treatment (Weber et al., 2015). Prompt initiation of steroids is essential to avoid severe, life-threatening autoimmune effects.

Nursing Management in Immunotherapy

Patients receiving immunotherapy require careful monitoring and thorough patient education regarding reportable side effects and self-care. The nurse should be familiar with each agent given and its potential effects. Adverse effects, including flu-like symptoms such as fever, chills, myalgia,

TABLE **6-4** Selected Food and Drug Administration—Approved Targeted Therapies

Monoclonal Antibody	Indication	Target	Selected Side Effects
Alemtuzumab (Campath)	Chronic lymphocytic leukemia	CD52, a marker on cell membrane of lymphocytes, monocytes, and macrophages	Infusion reactions; fever; chills; rash; hives; itching; decreased WBC, platelet, and RBC counts
Bevacizumab (Avastin)	Metastatic colorectal cancer	Vascular endothelial growth factor	Arterial and venous thrombosis, hypertension, hemorrhage, GI perforation, proteinuria, congestive heart failure
Cetuximab (Erbitux)	Metastatic colorectal cancer	Epidermal growth factor	Infusion reactions, fever, chills, rash, hives, itching, acne-like rash, lung inflammation, kidney failure, diarrhea, nausea, abdominal pain, vomiting
Gemtuzumab ozogamicin (Mylotarg)	Acute leukemia	CD33, a marker on cell membrane of leukemic cells	Infusion reactions; fever; chills; weakness; headache; tachycardia; hemorrhage; local skin reaction; rash; stomatitis; decreased platelet, WBC, and RBC counts; increased liver function tests
Ibritumomab-tiuxetan (Zevalin; anti-CD20 B cells)	Non-Hodgkin lymphoma	CD20, a marker on cell membrane of lymphocytes	Decreased platelets, WBC, and RBC counts; weakness; fever; chills
Ofatumumab (anti-CD20 B cells)	Non-Hodgkin lymphoma	CD20, a marker cell membrane of lymphocytes	Infusion reactions, neutropenia, thrombocytopenia, hepatitis B reactivation, intestinal obstruction
Panitumumab (anti-EGFR antibody)	EGFR + metastatic colorectal cancer	Binds to EGFR receptor	Acneform rash, paronychia, dry skin, fissures, fatigue, low magnesium, infusion reactions
Pertuzumab	HER2 + metastatic breast cancer	Targets extracellular domain for HER2	Cardiomyopathy, infusion reactions, peripheral edema, alopecia, rash, diarrhea, myelosuppression
Rituximab (Rituxan; anti-CD20, B cells)	Non-Hodgkin lymphoma	CD20, a marker on cell membrane of lymphocytes	Infusion reactions, fever, chills, back pain, night sweats, infection
Tositumomab (Bexxar; anti-CD20, B cells)	Non-Hodgkin lymphoma	CD20, a marker on cell membrane of lymphocytes	Infusion reactions, fever chills, rash, hives, itching, anemia, thrombocytopenia, decreased WBC count
Trastuzumab (Herceptin)	Breast cancer	HER2, a growth factor protein on cell membrane	Infusion reactions, hypotension, fever, chills, heart failure
Small Molecule Inhibitors	Indication	Target	Selected Side Effects
Axitinib	Advanced renal cell carcinoma	Inhibits VEGF	Hypertension, DVT/PE, bleeding, hypothyroidism, GI perforation, proteinuria, elevated LFTs
Bortezomib	Myeloma	Inhibits proteasome 26S	Peripheral neuropathy, hypotension, nausea, vomiting, diarrhea, constipation, fatigue, myelosuppression, reactivation of herpesvirus
Bosutinib	CML	Inhibits BCR-ABL	Diarrhea, nausea, vomiting, abdominal pain, myelosuppression, LFT elevation, rash, headache

(continued on page 176)

TABLE **6-4** Selected Food and Drug Administration—Approved Targeted Therapies (*continued*)

Small Molecule Inhibitors	Indication	Target	Selected Side Effects
Cabozantinib	Metastatic medullary thyroid cancer	Tyrosine kinase inhibitor	GI perforation, bleeding, DVT/PE, wound complications, hypertension, proteinuria, mucositis, abdominal pain, nausea vomiting, taste changes, myelosuppression
Carfilzomib	Myeloma	Inhibits proteasome 20S	CHF, MI, dyspnea, infusion reactions, myelosuppression, LFT elevation, renal toxicity, fatigue, peripheral edema, peripheral neuropathy, reactivation of herpesvirus
Crizotinib	ALK + NSCLC	Inhibits multiple kinases including ALK	LFT abnormalities, QT prolongation, pneumonitis, nausea, diarrhea, vomiting, edema, anorexia, fatigue, dyspnea, neutropenia
Dasatinib	CML	Inhibits BCR-ABL	Myelosuppression, fluid retention, pleural effusion, diarrhea, nausea, vomiting, bleeding, pulmonary hypertension
Erlotinib	NSCLC	Inhibits tyrosine kinase interfering with EGFR	Rash, diarrhea, anorexia, fatigue, dyspnea, GI bleeding, kidney and liver toxicity, MI, CVA, eye problems
Everolimus	ER + HER2neg breast cancer; metastatic neuroendocrine tumors; renal cell carcinoma	FKBP12 and mTOR	Pneumonitis, infections, mucositis, kidney failure, diarrhea, nausea, vomiting, fatigue, taste changes, headache, cough, dyspnea, myelosuppression, hyperglycemia
Imatinib	CML	BCR-ABL	Nausea, vomiting, myalgias, fluid retention, myelosuppression, hypothyroidism, rash
Lapatinib	Advanced HER2+ breast cancer	EGFR and HER2	Diarrhea, palmar-plantar erythrodysesthesia (hand-foot syndrome), nausea, vomiting, rash, fatigue, QT prolongation, cardiomyopathy, liver and lung toxicity
Nilotinib	CML	BCR ABL	Rash, headache, fatigue, nausea, vomiting, diarrhea, constipation, myelosuppression, liver toxicity, QT prolongation, lipase elevation
Pazopanib	Advanced renal cell carcinoma	VEGF	Liver toxicity, cardiomyopathy, DVT/PE, GI perforation, hypertension, hypothyroidism, proteinuria, infection, myelosuppression, low magnesium and phosphorous, headache, myalgias
Regorafenib	Metastatic colorectal cancer; locally advanced or unresectable gastrointestinal stromal tumors (GIST)	Inhibits multiple kinases	Liver toxicity, bleeding, skin reactions, hypertension, poor wound healing, asthenia, fatigue, anorexia, diarrhea, mucositis, infection, myelosuppression, low calcium/potassium/sodium/phosphorous, proteinuria
Ruxolitinib	Myelofibrosis	JAK1 and JAK2	Myelosuppression, infection

Small Molecule Inhibitors	Indication	Target	Selected Side Effects
Sorafenib	Unresectable hepatocellular carcinoma and advanced renal cell cancer	Multikinase inhibitor	Palmar plantar erythrodysesthesia (hand-foot syndrome) is erythema, edema, numbness, and desquamation (skin sloughing or peeling) on palms of the hands and soles of the feet (and, occasionally elsewhere), rash, hypertension, MI, mucositis, dyspepsia, elevated lipase, diarrhea, nausea, vomiting, loss of appetite, QT prolongation, low phosphorous, myelosuppression
Sunitinib	GIST Advanced renal cell carcinoma Unresectable pancreatic neuroendocrine tumors	Tyrosine kinase inhibition	Myelosuppression, liver toxicity, decreased LVEF, hypothyroidism, diarrhea, constipation, nausea, vomiting, stomatitis, skin changes, fatigue, hypertension, QT prolongation, impaired wound healing, DVT/PE
Temsirolimus	Advanced renal cell carcinoma	FKBP12, mTOR inhibition	Rash; asthenia; mucositis; nausea; anorexia; myelosuppression; elevated blood sugar, lipids, and cholesterol; elevations in creatinine; low phosphorous; LFT abnormalities; infections
Vandetanib	Unresectable, locally advanced or metastatic medullary thyroid cancer	VEGFR and EGFR inhibition	Skin changes, photosensitivity, QT prolongation, pneumonitis, ischemic cardiovascular events, diarrhea, hypothyroidism, hypertension, fatigue, nausea, anorexia, headache
Vemurafenib	Unresectable melanoma or melanoma with BRAF mutation	BRAF inhibition	Hypersensitivity, skin reactions, QT prolongation, liver toxicity, photosensitivity, eye changes, alopecia, itching, nausea, fatigue, headache, diarrhea
Vismodegib	Metastatic basal cell carcinoma	Hedghog pathway inhibitor	Alopecia, taste changes, weight loss, fatigue, anorexia, nausea, vomiting, arthralgias
Zivaflibercept	Metastatic colorectal carcinoma	VEGF	Bleeding, impaired wound healing, GI perforation, hypertension, arterial thrombolic events, CVA, angina, proteinuria, nephrotic syndrome, myelosuppression, anorexia, diarrhea, fatigue, elevated LFTS

Adapted from Polovich et al. (2014).

nausea, and vomiting, as seen with IFN therapy, may not be life threatening. However, the nurse must be aware of the impact of these side effects on the patient's quality of life and should implement supportive care measures, such as NSAIDs for flu-like symptoms and antiemetics for nausea and vomiting to relieve symptoms. Other life-threatening adverse effects (e.g., capillary leak syndrome, pulmonary edema, hypotension) may occur with IL-2 therapy, requiring aggressive fluid resuscitation and, at times, vasopressors

(refer to Chapter 54 for details on managing shock). The nurse must work closely with providers to assess and manage potential toxicities of immunotherapy. The specific nursing care required will depend on the agent being administered.

The nurse teaches patients self-care and assists in providing for continuing care. Some cytokines, such as IFN, EPO, and G-CSF, can be administered by the patient or family members at home. As needed, the nurse teaches the

TABLE **6-5** Selected Side Effects of Food and Drug Administration—Approved Cytokines

Agent Cytokines	Selected Side Effects
Interferon alfa	Flu-like symptoms (fever, chills, weakness, muscle and joint pain, headaches); fatigue; anorexia; mental status changes; depression; irritability; insomnia; rash; pruritus; irritation at the injection site; decreased WBC, RBC, and platelet counts; abnormal liver function values
Interleukin-2	Flu-like symptoms (fever, chills, weakness, muscle and joint pain, headaches); fatigue, anorexia, nausea, vomiting, diarrhea, capillary leak syndrome, edema and fluid retention, hypotension, tachycardia, skin rash, erythema, desquamation
Filgrastim (granulocyte growth factor)	Bone pain, malaise, fever, fatigue, headache, skin rash
Sargramostim (granulocyte-macrophage growth factor)	Allergic/anaphylactic reaction with first dose, bone pain, fever, fatigue, headache, weakness, chills, skin rash, infection
Epoetin alfa (erythrocyte growth factor)	Fever, fatigue, weakness, diarrhea, dizziness, edema, shortness of breath
Oprelvekin (platelet growth factor)	Edema, fever, headache, rash, chills, bone pain, fatigue, nausea, vomiting, abdominal pain, constipation, rhinitis, cough, arrhythmia, skin discoloration, bleeding

Adapted from Polovich et al. (2014).

patient and family how to administer these agents through subcutaneous injections. The nurse also provides instructions about side effects and helps the patient and family identify strategies to manage many of the common side effects of cytokine therapy, such as fatigue, anorexia, and flu-like symptoms.

Patients being treated with checkpoint inhibitor therapies must be monitored carefully over long periods of time for autoimmune-related adverse effects; monitoring should include complete blood counts, liver function tests (LFTs) and metabolic panels, and thyroid function tests. For fatigue and nonspecific syndromes, cortisol should be checked to rule out adrenal insufficiency; and in men, testosterone should be checked as it may be low as a result of pituitary suppression (Weber et al., 2015). Hypothyroidism is also seen and replacement with thyroid hormone may be necessary. Patients must be counseled to report any signs of diarrhea, bloody stool, or abdominal pain promptly as colitis can be life threatening if untreated. Corticosteroids are the primary treatment, and patients may have to be on steroids for prolonged periods; the nurse should provide education on short- and long-term effects of steroids and the importance of taking steroids with food to minimize stomach upset.

Referral for home care may be indicated to monitor the patient's responses to treatment and to continue to reinforce patient and family teaching. During home visits, the nurse assesses the patient's and family members' technique in administering medications. The nurse collaborates with providers, third-party payers, and pharmaceutical companies to help the patient obtain reimbursement for home administration of these therapies. The nurse also reminds the patient about the importance of keeping follow-up appointments with providers and assesses the patient's need for changes in care.

Hematopoietic Stem Cell Transplantation (HSCT)

Many malignancies exhibit a dose-related response to chemotherapy; by increasing the dose of chemotherapy, the number of malignant cells destroyed is increased. The dose of chemotherapy that is delivered is limited by the toxicity, specifically myelosuppression. The use of bone marrow or stem cells from either the patient (autologous) or from a donor (allogeneic) allows the bone marrow to be "rescued" from the toxic effects of the chemotherapy, therefore allowing higher doses of chemotherapy to be delivered safely (Niess, 2013).

The process of obtaining donor cells has evolved over the years. Traditionally, donor cells were obtained by harvesting large amounts of bone marrow tissue under general anesthesia in the operating room. Currently, a process referred to as *peripheral blood stem cell transplantation* (PBSCT) has gained widespread use. This method of collection uses apheresis methods to collect donor peripheral blood stem cells (PBSCs) for reinfusion. This is a safer and more cost-effective means of collection, rather than the traditional harvesting of marrow.

Types of Stem Cell Transplantation (SCT)

Types of SCT are based on the source of donor cells and include:

- Autologous (from patient)
- Allogeneic (from a donor other than the patient); either a related donor (i.e., family member) or a matched unrelated donor (national bone marrow registry, cord blood registry)
- Syngeneic (from an identical twin)

Autologous hematopoietic SCT, or HSCT, is considered for patients with hematologic malignancies requiring treatment with myeloablative doses of chemotherapy (doses high enough to obliterate marrow function) to achieve cure or prolong survival. Malignancies most commonly treated with autologous transplant include myeloma and lymphoma (Niess, 2013). In autologous transplant, cells are collected from the patient and preserved for reinfusion at a later date. Then the patient is treated with myeloablative chemotherapy and, in some cases, total body irradiation to eradicate any remaining tumor (Polovich et al., 2014). Stem cells are reinfused to "rescue" the marrow from the toxic effects of treatment (Niess, 2013). Until engraftment (repopulation of the marrow with healthy cells) occurs in the bone marrow, there is a high risk of infection, sepsis, and bleeding. Acute toxicities from chemotherapy and radiation therapy may be severe, including mucositis (inflammation and ulceration of the mucous membranes lining the digestive tract), diarrhea, poor appetite, and myelosuppression. No immunosuppressant medications are necessary after autologous bone marrow transplant because the patient does not receive foreign cells. A disadvantage of autologous transplantation is the risk that viable tumor cells may remain despite high-dose chemotherapy.

Allogeneic stem cell transplant is used primarily for disease of the bone marrow, including acute leukemia and aplastic anemia, and depends on the availability of a human leukocyte antigen–matched donor. A patient with one sibling has a 25% chance of having a matched-sibling donor (Niess, 2013). Prior to transplant, patients and potential donors undergo a thorough clinical assessment to evaluate eligibility (Niess, 2013).

Allogeneic HSCT involves either myeloablative (high-dose) or nonmyeloablative (reduced-intensity) chemotherapy. In myeloablative allogeneic HSCT, the recipient must undergo high doses of chemotherapy and, in some cases, total body irradiation to destroy all existing bone marrow and residual malignant disease. The harvested donor marrow or PBSCs are infused intravenously, similar to a blood transfusion, into the recipient. The infused cells travel to the bone marrow, where the cells mature and proliferate. When the new bone marrow becomes functional, producing RBCs, WBCs, and platelets, engraftment is considered complete (2 to 4 weeks). An advantage of allogeneic HSCT is that the transplanted cells are immunologically intolerant of a patient's malignancy. The donor's healthy immune system is able to recognize the patient's malignancy as foreign and kill any remaining tumor cells. This is referred to as the **graft-versus-tumor effect**. However, patients can also experience graft versus host disease (GVHD) as a result of the donor's immune system (T cells) recognizing the recipient's tissues as foreign.

In nonmyeloablative allogeneic HSCT, the chemotherapy doses are lower and are aimed at suppressing the recipient's immune system to allow engraftment of donor bone marrow or PBSCs. The lower doses of chemotherapy create less organ toxicity and, thus, can be offered to older patients or those with underlying organ dysfunction, for whom high-dose chemotherapy would be prohibitive. Once the transplanted donor cells begin to grow and reproduce, a process referred to as *engraftment*, a graft-versus-disease effect results in which the donor's healthy immune system keeps the patient's cancer cells from growing.

Before engraftment, patients are at high risk for infection, sepsis, and bleeding. Side effects of the high-dose chemotherapy and total body irradiation can be acute and chronic. Acute side effects include alopecia, hemorrhagic cystitis (inflammation of the bladder), nausea, vomiting, diarrhea, and severe stomatitis. Chronic side effects include sterility, pulmonary dysfunction, cardiac dysfunction, cataracts, and liver disease (McAdams & Burgunder, 2013).

To prevent **GVHD**, patients receive immunosuppressant drugs, such as cyclosporine (Neoral), tacrolimus (FK 506, Prograf), or sirolimus (Rappamune). In allogeneic transplant recipients, GVHD occurs when the T lymphocytes proliferating from the transplanted donor marrow or PBSCs become activated and mount an immune response against the recipient's tissues (skin, GI tract, liver). T lymphocytes respond in this manner because they view the recipient's tissue as "foreign," immunologically different from what they recognize as "self" in the donor. GVHD may occur acutely (within the first 100 days) or chronically (after 100 days) (Mitchell, 2013).

The first 100 days after allogeneic HSCT are crucial for patients; the immune system and blood-making capacity (hematopoiesis) must recover sufficiently to prevent infection and hemorrhage. Most acute side effects, such as nausea, vomiting, and mucositis, also resolve in the initial 100 days after transplantation. In addition to acute GVHD, patients are also at risk for hepatic venous occlusive disease (VOD) or hepatic sinusoidal obstruction syndrome (HSOS), a vascular injury to the liver caused by high-dose chemotherapy (McAdams & Burgunder, 2013). Incidence of VOD is as high as 30% (Anderson-Rietz & Clancy, 2013). VOD can lead to acute liver failure and death and presents as painful hepatomegaly (enlarged liver), elevated bilirubin levels, ascites, and weight gain in the absence of other causes. Coagulopathy and acute kidney failure can also accompany VOD. Onset is within the first 20 days posttransplant. There are no standard treatments for VOD; defibrotide has shown promise with response rates of 30% to 60%. Ursodiol has shown some efficacy in the preventative setting and is initiated prior to transplant in some institutions. Fortunately, 70% of patients have resolution of VOD without intervention. Supportive care includes maintaining fluid balance through strict monitoring of I/O and twice-daily weights, pain management, monitoring for signs of bleeding and administering blood products as ordered, and ensuring patient safety (Anderson-Rietz & Clancy, 2013).

Syngeneic transplants use an identical twin as the donor. Syngeneic transplants result in less incidence of GVHD and graft rejection; however, there is also less graft-versus-tumor effect to fight the malignancy. For this reason, even when an identical twin is available for marrow donation, another matched sibling or even an unrelated donor may be the most suitable option to combat an aggressive malignancy (Niess, 2013).

Nursing Management in Stem Cell Transplantation

Providing Care During Treatment

Skilled nursing care is required during all phases of transplant. In the pretransplant phase, the nurse educates the patient about what to expect, pretransplant testing, and finding a donor. When the patient is admitted for high-dose chemotherapy with or without total body irradiation, the nurse educates the patient about expected side effects, expected onset and recovery, and critical self-care measures to decrease the risk of infection. The acute toxicities of nausea, vomiting, diarrhea, mucositis, myelosuppression, and hemorrhagic cystitis require close monitoring and constant attention by the nurse.

Nursing management during the bone marrow or stem cell infusions consists of monitoring the patient's vital signs and blood oxygen saturation; assessing for adverse effects, such as fever, chills, shortness of breath, chest pain, cutaneous reactions (hives), nausea, vomiting, hypotension or hypertension, tachycardia, anxiety, and taste changes; and providing ongoing support and patient teaching.

Throughout the period of bone marrow aplasia (inability to create new cells) until engraftment of the new marrow occurs, the patient is at high risk for death from sepsis and bleeding. The patient requires support with blood products and hematopoietic growth factors. Potential infections may be bacterial, viral, fungal, or protozoan in origin. Renal complications may arise from the nephrotoxic chemotherapy agents used in the conditioning regimen or those used to treat infection (amphotericin B, aminoglycosides). Tumor lysis syndrome (Box 6-6) is an uncommon occurrence with conditioning as most patients do not have a large disease burden at the time of transplant. Acute tubular necrosis is a risk following conditioning therapy.

GVHD requires skillful nursing assessment to detect early effects on the skin, liver, and GI tract, including red maculopapular rash commonly found on the palms of the hands and soles of the feet, elevated LFTs, weight gain, jaundice, right upper quadrant pain, diffuse abdominal pain, early satiety, and diarrhea. Diarrhea resulting from GVHD may be of large volume; therefore, all stools must be measured and monitored for the presence of blood. VOD resulting from the conditioning regimens used in HSCT can result in fluid retention, jaundice, abdominal pain, ascites, tender and enlarged liver, and encephalopathy. Pulmonary complications, such as pulmonary edema, interstitial pneumonia, and other pneumonias, often complicate the recovery after transplant. Immunosuppressive agents, including cyclosporine, tacrolimus, and rapamycin, require close monitoring of blood levels and kidney function; doses

---

> **BOX 6-6** **Focus on Pathophysiology**
>
> **Tumor Lysis Syndrome**
>
> Malignant cells contain higher intracellular levels of potassium, phosphorous, and nucleic acids than do healthy cells. As the malignant cells are killed by chemotherapy, biotherapy, or corticosteroids, the intracellular contents are released into the bloodstream, leading to hyperkalemia, hyperphosphatemia, and hyperuricemia. The elevation in phosphorous results in an inverse decline in calcium levels. The crystallization of phosphates and uric acid salts in the kidneys can result in acute kidney injury, evidenced by an increase in serum creatinine and acidemia. The treatment plan includes aggressive hydration, administration of medications that block uric acid accumulation (such as Allopurinol) and medications that break uric acid down into a soluble substance that can be excreted through the urine (Rasburicase®), and control of electrolyte disturbances (Porth, 2015). Nursing considerations include strict monitoring of urine output and intake, monitoring of weight changes, and assessment of signs and symptoms of electrolyte disturbances.

are adjusted based on blood levels. Patients also require education about timing of medication around blood draws and meals, as well as the potential for drug–drug interactions (Mitchell, 2013).

Providing Posttransplantation Care

Ongoing nursing assessment and coordination of care in follow-up visits is essential to detect and manage late effects of therapy after HSCT, which occur 100 days or more after the procedure. Late effects include infections (e.g., varicella zoster infection), restrictive pulmonary abnormalities, and recurrent pneumonias. Sterility may result. Chronic GVHD involves the skin, liver, intestine, esophagus, eyes, lungs, joints, and oral and vaginal mucosa. Cataracts may also develop after total body irradiation.

Psychosocial assessments by nursing staff must be ongoing. In addition to the stressors affecting patients at each phase of the transplantation experience, marrow donors and family members also have psychosocial needs that must be addressed.

NURSING PROCESS
The Patient with Cancer

Nurses play a critical role in monitoring for changes over time; identifying problems and alterations in quality of life; and collaborating with patients, families, and members of the multidisciplinary team to optimize patient care. The nursing approach to the most common problems in patients with cancer will be discussed here. A plan of nursing care for a patient with cancer is available online at http://thepoint.lww.com/Honan2e.

ASSESSMENT

Individuals with cancer may experience a range of side effects with varying severity depending on the cancer type, tumor stage, and treatment modalities being used. Assessment of common problems is presented with related interventions below.

DIAGNOSIS

Appropriate nursing diagnoses of the patient with cancer may include:

- Impaired oral mucous membranes
- Impaired skin integrity
- Nausea
- Pain, acute
- Pain, chronic
- Imbalanced nutrition: Less than body requirements
- Fatigue
- Activity intolerance
- Risk for infection
- Risk for bleeding
- Disturbed body image

Based on the assessment data, potential complications include the following:

- Infection and sepsis
- Hemorrhage
- SVCS
- Spinal cord compression
- Hypercalcemia
- Pericardial effusion
- Disseminated intravascular coagulation (DIC)
- Syndrome of inappropriate secretion of antidiuretic hormone (SIADH)
- Tumor lysis syndrome

See Table 6-6 for more information on oncologic emergencies.

PLANNING

The major goals for the patient may include relief of fatigue, absence of complications, management of stomatitis, maintenance of nutrition, body image, relief of pain, and effective progression through the grieving process.

NURSING INTERVENTIONS

PREVENTING/MINIMIZING FATIGUE

Cancer-related fatigue is an unusual, distressing, persistent, subjective sense of physical, cognitive, or emotional tiredness related to cancer or cancer treatment and not proportional to recent activity but interfering with usual activity (National Comprehensive Cancer Network [NCCN], 2016a). Fatigue is a prevalent symptom that most patients experience at some point along their cancer experience. Fatigue is a subjective symptom that must be assessed in a systematic way, similarly to pain, relying on the patient's self-report. The nurse should ask the patient to describe the severity of the fatigue. The patient can use a scale of 0 to 10, with 0 being no fatigue and 10 being severe fatigue, or patients can simply state none, mild, moderate, or severe. The nurse should also assess the onset of fatigue as well as aggravating and alleviating factors, including physiologic and psychological stressors that can contribute to fatigue, such as pain, nausea, dyspnea, constipation, fear, and anxiety. The nurse assesses for feelings of weariness, weakness, lack of energy, inability to carry out necessary and valued daily functions, lack of motivation, and inability to concentrate. The patient may become less verbal and may appear pale, with relaxed facial musculature. The nurse helps the patient and family understand that fatigue is an expected side effect of cancer and cancer treatment. Fatigue may be exacerbated by the stress of coping with cancer. It does not always signify that the cancer is advancing or that the treatment is failing.

Nursing strategies are implemented to minimize fatigue or to help the patient cope with existing fatigue. Educational interventions and cognitive behavioral therapies, including providing anticipatory guidance that fatigue is an expected side effect of cancer treatment, have been shown to reduce the severity of cancer-related fatigue (NCCN, 2016a). Helping the patient identify sources of fatigue aids in selecting appropriate and individualized interventions.

Ways to conserve energy are developed to help the patient plan daily activities. Alternating periods of rest and activity are beneficial. Strong evidence exists to support that regular exercise may decrease fatigue and facilitate coping, whereas lack of physical activity and "too much rest" can actually contribute to deconditioning and associated fatigue (Mitchell et al., 2014; NCCN, 2016a). Yoga has also shown to improve cancer-related fatigue (NCCN, 2016a; Sprod et al., 2015). The nurse assists in educating the patient on local resources for exercise and yoga. The nurse also counsels on sleep hygiene, including not staying in bed if the patient is not sleeping; going to bed only when sleepy and at the same time every night; using the bed only for sleep and sexual activity; avoiding daytime napping or, if needed, limiting naps to 30 minutes; avoiding caffeine, nicotine, and alcohol after noon; and using a relaxing routine within 2 hours of going to bed, such as a warm bath or shower, reading, or listening to music (NCCN, 2016a).

The patient is encouraged to maintain as normal a lifestyle as possible by continuing with activities that he or she values and enjoys. Prioritizing necessary and valued activities can help the patient plan for each day. The patient and family are encouraged to plan to reallocate responsibilities, such as attending to childcare, cleaning, and preparing meals. Patients who are employed full-time may need to reduce the number of hours worked each day or week. The nurse helps the patient and family cope with these changing roles and responsibilities. The nurse also addresses factors that contribute to fatigue, such as poor nutrition, pain, nausea, and depression, and implements pharmacologic and nonpharmacologic strategies to manage these symptoms. The nurse provides nutrition

(continued on page 187)

TABLE **6-6** Oncologic Emergencies: Manifestations and Management

Emergency	Diagnostic Approaches and Clinical Manifestations	Medical and Nursing Management
Superior Vena Cava Syndrome (SVCS) Compression or invasion of the superior vena cava by tumor, enlarged lymph nodes, or intraluminal thrombus that obstructs venous circulation, or drainage of the head, neck, arms, and thorax. Compression of the SVC restricts venous return, decreasing cardiac output. Typically SVCS is associated with bronchogenic cancer but can be associated with other cancers such as lymphoma. Internal occlusion can precipitate SVCS if a central vein catheter becomes occluded. If untreated, SVCS may lead to cerebral anoxia (due to cerebral edema), laryngeal edema, bronchial obstruction, and death.	*Diagnostic* Diagnosis is confirmed by • Clinical findings • Chest CT with contrast is preferred test (Shelton, 2013) • CXR • MRI • Biopsy to obtain tissue diagnosis to determine cause is important in initiating treatment. *Clinical* Gradually or suddenly impaired venous drainage giving rise to: • Progressive dyspnea (most common symptom), cough, hoarseness, chest pain, and facial swelling, cyanosis, plethora (redness) of the face, complaints of difficulty buttoning shirt collars • Engorged and distended jugular, temporal, and arm veins • Dilated thoracic vessels causing prominent venous patterns on the chest wall Blood pressure that is falsely elevated in the upper extremities and low in the lower extremities Tachycardia Late signs: Increased intracranial pressure, associated visual disturbances, headache, dizziness, syncope and altered mental status, irritability, lethargy (Shelton, 2013)	*Medical* • The goal is control or cure of the underlying malignancy or cause by: • Radiation therapy to shrink tumor size, relieving symptoms • Chemotherapy for chemosensitive cancers (e.g., lymphoma, small cell lung cancer) or when the mediastinum has been irradiated to maximum tolerance • Anticoagulant or thrombolytic therapy for intraluminal thrombosis • Stent placement to restore blood flow • Supportive measures such as oxygen therapy, bronchodilators, corticosteroids, diuretics, and anxiolytics (Shelton, 2013) *Nursing* • Identify patients at risk for SVCS. • Monitor and report clinical manifestations of SVCS. • Monitor vital signs as well as cardiopulmonary and neurologic status. • Facilitate breathing by positioning the patient properly. Assist the patient to maintain an upright position (elevated 45 degrees). This helps to promote comfort and reduce anxiety; it also reduces intracranial pressure. • Remove rings and restrictive clothing. Assist patient with ADLs to minimize energy expenditures. Monitor the patient's fluid volume status: Assess weights and I/Os regularly. Ensure that the patient avoids the Valsalva maneuver, which may worsen symptoms, by providing cough suppressants and stool softeners as needed.
Spinal Cord Compression (SCC) Occurs when a malignant disease or a pathologically collapsed vertebrae compresses or displaces the thecal sac that contains the spinal cord, leading to neurologic impairment. The prognosis depends on the severity and rapidity of onset with median of 6 months survival from time of SCC diagnosis. Presenting signs and symptoms depend on the location of compression. 20% of patients present with SCC. About 60% of compressions occur at the thoracic level, 30% in the lumbosacral level, and 10% in the cervical region. Metastatic cancers (breast, lung, kidney, prostate, myeloma, lymphoma) and related bone erosion are associated with spinal cord compression (Pi et al., 2016)	*Diagnostic* • MRI (preferred test), myelogram, spinal cord x-rays, bone scans, and CT scan • Imaging should include the entire thecal sac as there may be multiple sites of disease involvement (Pi et al., 2016). *Clinical* • Percussion tenderness at the level of compression • Abnormal reflexes • Sensory (40–90%) and motor (60–85%) abnormalities • Local or radicular back or neck pain along the dermatomal areas innervated by the affected nerve root (e.g., thoracic radicular pain extends in a band around the chest or abdomen) • Pain exacerbated by movement, supine recumbent position, coughing, sneezing, or the Valsalva maneuver	*Medical* • Radiation therapy is the initial treatment of choice for those with a radiosensitive tumor type who are not surgical candidates; radiation will reduce tumor size to halt progression. • Corticosteroid therapy at time of presentation to decrease inflammation and swelling at the compression site • Surgery if: patient is medically able to undergo surgical decompression and fixation, direct compression in setting of intraspinal bony fragments unlikely to respond to radiation, an unstable spine where direct fixation and stabilization is the only way to preserve ambulation, impending sphincter dysfunction, lack of response to initial radiation therapy, paraplegia in less than 48 hours, unknown primary tumor type (Pi et al., 2016). • Chemotherapy or hormonal therapy as adjuvant to radiation therapy • *Note:* Despite treatment, patients with poor neurologic function before treatment are less likely to regain complete motor and sensory function; less than 30% of patients who have

Emergency	Diagnostic Approaches and Clinical Manifestations	Medical and Nursing Management
	• Back pain is the most common (83–95%) and often the first symptom preceding other symptoms by as much as 2 months. • Neurologic dysfunction, and related motor and sensory deficits (numbness, tingling, feelings of coldness in the affected area, inability to detect vibration, loss of positional sense) • Motor loss ranging from subtle weakness to flaccid paralysis • Bladder and/or bowel dysfunction depending on level of compression (above S2, overflow incontinence; from S3 to S5, flaccid sphincter tone and bowel incontinence). These tend to be late symptoms and match degree of weakness. (Pi et al., 2016)	lost the ability to walk before radiation was started regain the ability to ambulate. Pain management is a priority. ***Nursing*** • Perform ongoing assessment of neurologic status, including motor and sensory function to identify existing and progressing dysfunction (Kaplan, 2013c). • Control pain with pharmacologic and nonpharmacologic measures. • Prevent complications of immobility resulting from pain and decreased function (e.g., skin breakdown, urinary stasis, thrombophlebitis, decreased clearance of pulmonary secretions). • Maintain muscle tone by assisting with range-of-motion exercises in collaboration with physical and occupational therapists. • Institute intermittent urinary catheterization and bowel training programs for patients with bladder or bowel dysfunction. • Maintain safety by assisting the patient with ADLs and ambulation.
Hypercalcemia In patients with cancer, hypercalcemia is a potentially life-threatening metabolic abnormality resulting when the calcium released from the bones exceeds the amount that the kidneys have the ability to excrete or the bones can reabsorb. It may be the result of: • Bone destruction by tumor cells and subsequent release of calcium • Production of prostaglandins and osteoclast-activating factors, which stimulate bone breakdown and calcium release • Tumors that produce parathyroid-like substances that promote calcium release • Overproduction of vitamin D analogues (calcitriol), seen most commonly in hematologic malignancies (Pi et al., 2016) • Most commonly seen in breast cancer, lung cancer, and myeloma (Pi et al., 2016)	***Diagnostic*** Serum calcium level exceeding 11 mg/dL (2.74 mmol/L) Moderate hypercalcemia: 12–14 mg/dL Severe hypercalcemia: greater than 14 mg/dL (Pi et al., 2016) ***Clinical*** Early signs: Fatigue, weakness, lethargy, irritability, cognitive changes, personality changes, confusion, decreased level of responsiveness, hyporeflexia, nausea, vomiting, constipation, anorexia, polyuria (excessive urination), polydipsia (excessive thirst), nocturia, dehydration. Late signs: ataxia, stupor, seizures, coma, arrhythmias, ileus, kidney failure, heart block, cardiac arrest	***Medical*** See Chapters 4 and 31. ***Nursing*** • Identify patients at risk for hypercalcemia and assess for signs and symptoms of hypercalcemia. • Educate patient and family on prevention, including hydration and ambulation/weight-bearing activity. • Teach at-risk patients to recognize and report signs and symptoms of hypercalcemia promptly. • Ensure that patients consume (PO or IV) a total of 3 L of fluid daily unless contraindicated by existing kidney or cardiac disease. • Monitor I/O and daily weight. • Explain the use of dietary and pharmacologic interventions, such as stool softeners and laxatives for constipation. • Discuss antiemetic therapy if nausea and vomiting occur. • Advise patients to maintain nutritional intake without restricting normal calcium intake. • Implement safety measures, including fall and seizure precautions. Promote mobilization by assisting with ambulation and providing active resistive exercises for patients on bed rest; emphasize the importance of mobility in preventing demineralization and breakdown of bones. (Kaplan, 2013b)

(continued on page 184)

TABLE 6-6 Oncologic Emergencies: Manifestations and Management (*continued*)

Emergency	Diagnostic Approaches and Clinical Manifestations	Medical and Nursing Management
Pericardial Effusion and Cardiac Tamponade Cardiac tamponade is an accumulation of fluid in the pericardial space. The fluid compresses the heart and thereby impedes expansion of the ventricles, limiting cardiac filling during diastole. As ventricular volume and cardiac output fall, the heart pump fails, and circulatory collapse develops. With gradual onset, fluid accumulates slowly, and the outer layer of the pericardial space stretches to compensate for rising pressure. Large amounts of fluid accumulate before symptoms of heart failure occur. With rapid onset, pressures rise too quickly for the pericardial space to compensate. Malignancies, particularly from adjacent thoracic tumors (lung, breast, lymphoma), and side effects of cancer treatment are the most common causes of cardiac tamponade. High doses of radiation to fields involving the heart also have been implicated in pericardial fibrosis, pericarditis, and resultant cardiac tamponade. Untreated pericardial effusion and cardiac tamponade lead to circulatory collapse and cardiac arrest (Turner Story, 2013.) Tamponade is associated with late-stage disease and carries a high mortality rate (Turner Story, 2013).	**Diagnostic** • Electrocardiography (ECG) • Echocardiogram is preferred imaging test (Turner Story, 2013) • In small effusion, chest x-rays show small amounts of fluid in the pericardium; in large effusions, x-ray films disclose "water-bottle" heart (obliteration of vessel contour and cardiac chambers) • CT scans help diagnose pleural effusions and evaluate effect of treatment **Clinical** • Fatigue, dyspnea, orthopnea, nonproductive cough, dull or diffuse chest pain • Neck vein distention during inspiration (Kussmaul sign) • Pulsus paradoxus (systolic blood pressure decrease exceeding 10 mm Hg during inspiration; pulse gets stronger on expiration) • Distant heart sounds, rubs and gallops, cardiac dullness • Shifted Point of Maximal Impulse (PMI) • Compensatory tachycardia (heart beats faster to compensate for decreased cardiac output) • Increased venous and vascular pressures • Narrow pulse pressure (the difference between systolic and diastolic blood pressure) • Shortness of breath and tachypnea • Weakness, chest pain, orthopnea, anxiety, diaphoresis, lethargy, and altered consciousness from decreased cerebral perfusion • Low voltage QRS on EKG; electrical alternans	**Medical** • Pericardiocentesis (the aspiration or withdrawal of pericardial fluid by a large-bore needle inserted into the pericardial space). In malignant effusions, pericardiocentesis provides only temporary relief; fluid usually reaccumulates. Windows or openings in the pericardium can be created surgically as a palliative measure to drain fluid into the pleural space. Catheters may also be placed in the pericardial space, and sclerosing agents (such as doxycycline, talc, bleomycin) are injected to prevent fluid from reaccumulating. • Radiation therapy; antineoplastic agents. In mild effusions, prednisone and diuretic medications may be used. **Nursing** • Monitor vital signs, oxygen saturation, cardiac and respiratory examination frequently. • Assess for pulsus paradoxus. • Monitor ECG tracings. • Assess heart and lung sounds, neck vein filling, level of consciousness, respiratory status, and skin color and temperature. • Monitor and record intake and output. • Review laboratory findings (e.g., arterial blood gas and electrolyte levels). • Elevate the head of the patient's bed to ease breathing. • Minimize patient's physical activity to reduce oxygen requirements; administer supplemental oxygen as prescribed. • Provide frequent oral hygiene. • Reposition and encourage the patient to cough, use pursed-lip breathing, and take deep breaths. Assist patient with ADLs to conserve energy. Maintain oxygen saturation greater than 92%. Administer analgesics and anxiolytics as ordered. Assist patients with relaxation techniques (Turner Story, 2013.)
Disseminated Intravascular Coagulation (DIC, also called consumption coagulopathy) Complex disorder of coagulation and fibrinolysis (destruction of clots), which results in thrombosis and bleeding. DIC is most commonly associated with hematologic cancers (leukemia); cancer of prostate, GI tract, and lungs; chemotherapy (methotrexate, prednisone, ʟ-asparaginase, vincristine, and 6-mercaptopurine); and disease processes such as sepsis, hepatic failure, and anaphylaxis.	**Diagnostic** • Prolonged prothrombin time (PT or protime) • Prolonged international normalized ratio (INR) • Prolonged partial thromboplastin time (PTT) • Prolonged thrombin time (TT) • Decreased fibrinogen level • Decreased platelet level • Decrease in clotting factors • Decreased hemoglobin • Decreased hematocrit • Elevated fibrin split products (or fibrin degradation products) • Elevated D-dimer test • Positive protamine sulfate precipitation test (thrombin activation test)	**Medical** The underlying cause of DIC must be treated. • Chemotherapy, biologic response modifier therapy, radiation therapy, or surgery is used to treat the underlying cancer. • Antibiotic therapy is used for sepsis. • Anticoagulants, such as heparin or antithrombin III, decrease the stimulation of the coagulation pathways. Anticoagulants must be used with caution in patients who have experienced or are at risk for bleeding.

Emergency	Diagnostic Approaches and Clinical Manifestations	Medical and Nursing Management
Blood clots form when normal coagulation mechanisms are triggered. Once activated, the clotting cascade continues to consume clotting factors and platelets faster than the body can replace them, which can result in bleeding. Clots are deposited in the microvasculature, placing the patient at great risk for impaired circulation, tissue hypoxia, and necrosis. In addition, fibrinolysis occurs, breaking down clots and increasing the circulating levels of anticoagulant substances, thereby placing the patient at risk for hemorrhage.	**Clinical** *Chronic DIC:* Characterized by diffuse thrombosis or subacute bleeding. Few or no observable symptoms or easy bruising, prolonged bleeding from venipuncture and injection sites, bleeding of the gums, and slow GI bleeding *Acute DIC:* life-threatening hemorrhage and infarction; clinical symptoms of this syndrome are varied and depend on the organ system involved in thrombus and infarction or bleeding episodes. Bleeding can occur anywhere.	• Transfusions of fresh-frozen plasma (containing clotting factors) or cryoprecipitate (containing fibrinogen), packed RBCs, and platelets may be used as replacement therapy in patients with evidence of bleeding. • Although controversial, antifibrinolytic agents such as aminocaproic acid (Amicar), which is associated with increased thrombus formation, may be used (Kaplan, 2013a). **Nursing** • Monitor vital signs. • Measure and document intake and output. • Assess skin color and temperature; lung, heart, and bowel sounds; level of consciousness; headache; visual disturbances; chest pain; decreased urine output; and abdominal tenderness. • Inspect all body orifices, tube insertion sites, incisions, and bodily excretions for bleeding. • Review laboratory test results. • Minimize physical activity to decrease injury risks and oxygen requirements. • Prevent bleeding; apply pressure to all venipuncture sites, and avoid nonessential invasive procedures; avoid the use of tourniquets; provide electric rather than straight-edged razors; avoid tape on the skin and advise gentle but adequate oral hygiene with use of a soft toothbrush or toothette. • Assist the patient to turn, cough, and take deep breaths every 2 hours. • Reorient the patient, if needed; maintain a safe environment; and provide appropriate patient education and supportive measures.
Syndrome of Inappropriate Secretion of Antidiuretic Hormone (SIADH) SIADH is a result of the failure in the negative feedback mechanism that normally regulates the release of antidiuretic hormone (ADH). Some malignancies, such as small-cell lung cancer, inappropriately release antidiuretic hormone (ADH). The excessive release of ADH produced by tumor cells or by the abnormal stimulation of the hypothalamic–pituitary network leads to uncontrolled water reabsorption. The most common cause of SIADH is cancer, especially small cell cancer of the lung. Medications, including antineoplastics—vincristine, vinblastine, cisplatin, and cyclophosphamide—and morphine also stimulate ADH secretion (see Chapters 4 and 31 for details on SIADH).	**Diagnostic** • Decreased serum sodium level • Decreased serum osmolality • Increased urine osmolality • Increased urinary sodium level • Increased urine-specific gravity • Decreased blood urea nitrogen (BUN), creatinine, and serum albumin levels secondary to dilution • Abnormal water load test results **Clinical** *Mild SIADH:* serum sodium 125–134 mEq/L *Signs and symptoms include:* increased thirst, anorexia, nausea, fatigue, weakness, headache *Moderate SIADH:* Serum sodium levels between 115 and 124 mEq/L (120 mmol/L) *Signs and symptoms include:* personality changes, irritability, nausea, anorexia, vomiting, weight gain, oliguria, fatigue, muscular pain (myalgia), headache, lethargy, and confusion	**Medical** The underlying cause of SIADH must be treated in order to effectively treat SIADH. Discontinue the offending medication. Fluid intake limited to 500–1,000 mL/day to increase the serum sodium level. If water restriction alone is not effective in correcting or controlling serum sodium levels, demeclocycline is often prescribed to inhibit ADH secretion and promote water excretion. If neurologic symptoms are severe, parenteral sodium replacement and diuretic therapy are indicated. Electrolyte levels are monitored carefully to detect secondary magnesium, potassium, and calcium imbalances. After the symptoms of SIADH are controlled, the underlying cancer is treated. If water excess continues despite treatment, pharmacologic intervention may be indicated. Hypertonic (3%) saline may be administered for a short time (1–3 hours) in an intensive care setting with frequent (q2h) serum sodium levels (Lahoti et al., 2016) The goal is to increase the serum sodium level slowly. Increasing the serum sodium level too quickly can cause intracellular dehydration,

(continued on page 186)

TABLE **6-6** Oncologic Emergencies: Manifestations and Management (*continued*)

Emergency	Diagnostic Approaches and Clinical Manifestations	Medical and Nursing Management
	Severe SIADH: Serum sodium levels less than 115 mEq/L *Signs and symptoms include:* seizure, abnormal reflexes, delirium, ataxia, papilledema, coma, and death. Number and severity of symptoms depends on the rate of onset; the faster the onset of SIADH, the more symptomatic the patient may be. Signs and symptoms of fluid volume overload, including edema, are rare.	which may result in serious neurologic impairment. *Nursing* Early identification of at-risk patients is essential to promote early intervention. • Maintain intake and output measurements; assess urine-specific gravity. • Assess level of consciousness, lung and heart sounds, vital signs, daily weight; also assess for nausea, vomiting, anorexia, edema, fatigue, and lethargy. • Monitor laboratory test results, including serum electrolyte levels, osmolality, and BUN, creatinine, and urinary sodium levels. • Minimize the patient's activity; provide appropriate oral hygiene; maintain environmental safety; and restrict fluid intake if necessary. • Maintain safety: implement fall and seizure precautions for sodium levels below 120 mEq/L.
Tumor Lysis Syndrome (TLS) TLS is a rapidly developing oncologic emergency that results from the rapid release of intracellular contents as a result of radiation- or chemotherapy-induced cell destruction of large or rapidly growing cancers, such as leukemia, lymphoma, and small cell lung cancer. Cancer cells have an abnormally high amount of potassium, phosphate, and nucleic acids. The release of these intracellular contents from the tumor cells leads to electrolyte imbalances—hyperkalemia, hypocalcemia, hyperphosphatemia, and hyperuricemia—because the kidneys can no longer excrete large volumes of the released intracellular metabolites. These metabolic abnormalities may result in life-threatening arrhythmias, seizures, and kidney failure.	*Diagnostic* Electrolyte imbalances identified by laboratory test results, including: Uric acid greater than 8 mg/dL Phosphorus greater than 4.5 mg/dL Potassium greater than 5.5 mEq/L Calcium less than 7 mg/dL (Pi et al., 2015) *Clinical* Clinical manifestations depend on the extent of metabolic abnormalities. • Neurologic: fatigue, weakness, memory loss, altered mental status, muscle cramps, irritability, paresthesias (numbness and tingling), tetany seizures • Cardiac: hypotension, peaked T waves, flattened P waves, widened QRS waves, ST depression, dysrhythmias, cardiac arrest • GI: anorexia, nausea, vomiting, abdominal cramps, diarrhea • Renal: flank pain, oliguria, anuria, kidney failure, hematuria, acidic urine pH	*Medical* Prevention, early detection, and prompt management are critical in decreasing morbidity and mortality. • To prevent kidney failure and restore electrolyte balance, aggressive hydration (one to two times the daily maintenance requirement) is initiated 48 hours before the initiation of cytotoxic therapy to increase urine volume and eliminate uric acid and electrolytes. Alkalinization of urine is no longer recommended due to lack of clear benefit (Pi et al., 2015). • Following aggressive hydration, diuretic therapy may be used to increase electrolyte excretion (potassium, uric acid). • Allopurinol therapy should be started prior to the initiation of chemotherapy to inhibit the conversion of nucleic acids to uric acid (Pi et al., 2015). Rasburicase therapy may be initiated as prophylaxis or treatment of hyperuricemia. Rasburicase converts uric acid into allantoin, which is a substance that is soluble in urine. • Administration of a cation-exchange resin, such as sodium polystyrene sulfonate (Kayexalate) to treat hyperkalemia by binding and eliminating potassium through the bowel. (Refer to Chapter 4 for treatment of hyperkalemia.) • Administration of hypertonic dextrose and regular insulin temporarily shifts potassium into cells and lowers serum potassium levels. • Administration of phosphate-binding gels, such as aluminum hydroxide, treats hyperphosphatemia by promoting phosphate excretion in the feces. • Hemodialysis is performed when patients have persistently elevated electrolytes with worsening kidney function or in patients with symptomatic electrolyte imbalances or fluid volume overload from TLS management.

Emergency	Diagnostic Approaches and Clinical Manifestations	Medical and Nursing Management
		Nursing • Identify at-risk patients. • Institute essential preventive measures as described above. • Assess patient for signs and symptoms of electrolyte imbalances. • Monitor serum electrolyte and uric acid levels. • Assess for evidence of fluid volume overload secondary to aggressive hydration by monitoring I/O and daily weights. • Instruct patients to report symptoms indicating electrolyte disturbances.

counseling to patients who are not eating enough calories or protein. Small, frequent meals require less energy for digestion. The nurse monitors the patient for deficiencies in serum hemoglobin and hematocrit and administers blood products or ESAs as prescribed. In addition, the nurse monitors the patient for alterations in oxygenation and electrolyte balances. Physical therapy and assistive devices are beneficial for patients with impaired mobility. Studies have evaluated the use of psychostimulants, such as methylphenidate and modafinil, for the treatment of fatigue with mixed results; more data are needed before these interventions can be recommended safely (NCCN, 2016a).

MONITORING AND MANAGING INFECTION AND SEPSIS

Monitoring for Infection. For patients in all stages of cancer, the nurse assesses risk factors for infection and observes for clinical signs and symptoms, as infection is the leading cause of death in cancer patients. The nurse monitors laboratory studies to detect early changes in WBC counts. Common sites of infection, such as the oropharynx, skin, perianal area, urinary tract, GI tract, and respiratory tract, are assessed frequently. The typical signs of infection (swelling, redness, drainage, and pain) may not occur in immunosuppressed patients because of a diminished local inflammatory response. Fever or localized tenderness may be the only sign of infection. The nurse also monitors the patient for sepsis, particularly if invasive catheters or venous access devices are in place.

WBC function is often impaired in patients with cancer. There are two types of WBCs: granulocytes (neutrophils, eosinophils, basophils) and agranulocytes (lymphocytes, monocytes, macrophages). The neutrophils, totaling 60% to 70% of the body's total WBCs, play a major role in combating infection by engulfing and destroying microorganisms in a process called *phagocytosis*. Both the total WBC count and the number of neutrophils are important in determining the patient's ability to fight infection. A decrease in circulating WBCs is referred to as *leukopenia*. *Granulocytopenia* or *neutropenia* is a decrease in neutrophils (see Chapters 19 and 20).

A differential WBC count identifies the relative numbers of WBCs and permits tabulation of the absolute neutrophil count (ANC). The ANC includes the number of polymorphonuclear neutrophils (mature neutrophils, reported as "polys," PMNs, or "segs") and immature forms of neutrophils (reported as bands, metamyelocytes, and "stabs"). The ANC is calculated by the following formula:

$$\text{Total WBC} \times [\%\text{segs} + \%\text{bands}]$$

For example, if the total WBC count is 6,000 cells/mm³, with segmented neutrophils 25% and bands 25%, the ANC is 3,000 cells/mm³. That is $6,000 \times [0.25 + 0.25] = 6,000 \times 0.5 = 3,000$.

Neutropenia, an abnormally low ANC, is associated with an increased risk for infection. The risk for infection rises as the ANC decreases and persists. An ANC less than 500 cells/mm³ reflects a severe risk of infection. **Nadir** is the lowest ANC after myelosuppressive chemotherapy or radiation therapy. Therapies that suppress bone marrow function are called *myelosuppressive.* Therapies that severely suppress bone marrow function are called *myeloablative.* The nadir is reached, on average, 7 to 10 days following chemotherapy treatment and takes an additional 7 to 14 days to recover. The patient is at increased risk for infection throughout the duration of neutropenia.

Gram-positive bacteria (*Streptococcus* and *Staphylococcus* species) and gram-negative organisms (*Escherichia coli, Klebsiella pneumoniae,* and *Pseudomonas aeruginosa*) are the most frequently isolated causes of infection. Fungal organisms, such as *Candida albicans,* also contribute to the incidence of serious infection. Viral infections in immunocompromised patients are caused most commonly by herpes viruses and respiratory viruses.

Nursing Alert
Normal WBC levels in adults are 4.5 to 10.5 × 10³ cells/mm³ or 4,500 to 10,500 cells/mm³. For African-American adults, normal levels are 3,200 to 10,000 cells/mm³. A WBC level (count) below 500 or above 30,000 is a critical value.

(continued on page 188)

Managing Patients with Febrile Neutropenia. A fever in a patient with neutropenia is considered an emergency due to the high mortality rate associated with sepsis in neutropenic patients. Hospitalized patients who are neutropenic and become febrile are assessed immediately for infection. Cultures of blood, sputum, urine, stool, catheter, or wounds are obtained. In addition, a chest x-ray is often included to assess for pulmonary infections. If a patient is at home and develops neutropenic fever, the patient is instructed to notify their health care provider and seek medical attention immediately.

> **Nursing Alert**
> *Fever is often the only sign of infection in immunocompromised patients. Although fever may be related to a variety of noninfectious conditions, including the underlying cancer, any temperature of 38.3°C (100.9°F) or higher or a sustained temperature of 38.0°C (100.4°F) for 1 hour is reported and addressed promptly (NCCN, 2016b).*

Empiric antibiotics are initiated to treat infections immediately after cultures are obtained. The term *empiric antibiotics* refer to the use of broad-spectrum antibiotics used to treat infection before a definitive organism is identified. Often, Gram stains are ordered along with cultures to assist providers in identifying the most appropriate antibiotic. Empiric antibiotics have been employed due to the high incidence of mortality associated with untreated infection in neutropenic patients. Broad-spectrum antibiotic coverage or empiric therapy most often includes a combination of medications to defend the body against the major pathogenic organisms (both gram-positive and gram-negative). It is important for the nurse to administer these medications promptly, immediately after two sets of blood cultures are obtained, according to the prescribed schedule, to achieve adequate blood levels of the medications (NCCN, 2016b).

Minimizing the Risk of Infection in Neutropenic Patients. Strict asepsis is essential when handling IV lines, catheters, and other invasive equipment. Patients are advised to minimize contact with anyone who might be sick and to avoid crowds. Patients with profound immunosuppression, such as allogeneic HSCT recipients or patients with acute leukemia, should be placed in single rooms where the air is filtered. To reduce the risk of foodborne illnesses, patients are educated to avoid raw meat, eggs, or fish; deli meats; unroasted raw nuts or nuts in the shell; miso products; raw grain products; unpasteurized milk products; and soft cheese, cheese with uncooked vegetables, or cheese with mold. Fruits and vegetables must be washed well, eliminating soft fruits such as berries that are difficult to wash.

Hand hygiene and appropriate general hygiene are critical to reduce exposure to potentially harmful bacteria and to eliminate environmental contaminants. Invasive procedures, such as injections, vaginal or rectal examinations, rectal temperatures, and surgery, are avoided. The patient is encouraged to cough and to perform deep-breathing exercises frequently to prevent atelectasis and other respiratory problems. Prophylactic antimicrobial therapy may be used for patients who are expected to be profoundly immunosuppressed and at risk for certain infections, such as patients undergoing autologous or allogeneic stem cell transplant and patients with acute leukemia. The nurse teaches the patient and family to recognize signs and symptoms of infection that should be reported, performs effective hand hygiene, uses antipyretics, maintains skin integrity, and administers hematopoietic growth factors when indicated.

MONITORING AND MANAGING BLEEDING AND HEMORRHAGE

The nurse assesses the patient with cancer for factors that may contribute to bleeding. Bleeding may result from a reduction in the quantity or quality of platelets, a decrease in clotting factors, or from DIC (see Chapter 20 for details on DIC). Treatment-related factors include bone marrow suppression from radiation, chemotherapy, and other medications that interfere with coagulation and platelet functioning, such as aspirin and other nonsteroidal anti-inflammatory medications, dipyridamole, heparin, or warfarin (Coumadin).

Thrombocytopenia often results from bone marrow depression after certain types of chemotherapy and radiation therapy. Tumor infiltration of the bone marrow can also impair the normal production of platelets. In some cases, platelet destruction is associated with an enlarged spleen (hypersplenism) and abnormal antibody function, which occur with leukemia and lymphoma. Chapter 19 details thrombocytopenia. Refer to Box 19-2 for thrombocytopenia precautions.

 Concept Mastery Alert

> A nurse can best detect early signs and symptoms of thrombocytopenia by closely observing the client's skin for petechiae and bruising.

The nurse administers platelet transfusions as ordered and monitors for signs of transfusion reaction, including fever, chills, urticaria, and shortness of breath. In limited circumstances, the nurse may administer Interluekin (IL)-11 (Oprelvekin), which has been approved by the U.S. Food and Drug Administration (FDA) to prevent severe thrombocytopenia and to reduce the need for platelet transfusions after myelosuppressive chemotherapy in patients with nonmyeloid malignancies. In some instances, the nurse teaches the patient or family members to administer IL-11 in the home (Wyeth, 2013).

When a hospitalized patient experiences bleeding, the nurse monitors blood pressure and pulse and respiratory rates every 15 to 30 minutes. Serum hemoglobin and hematocrit are monitored carefully for changes indicating blood loss. The nurse tests all urine, stool, and emesis for occult blood. Neurologic assessments are performed to detect changes in orientation and behavior. Headaches reported by the patient or abnormal neurologic findings must be reported to the provider immediately as even subtle signs may indicate an intracranial hemorrhage. The nurse administers fluids and blood products as prescribed to replace any losses.

> **Nursing Alert**
> *One unit of platelets is approximately 50 to 70 mL; in general, four to six units are pooled for a platelet transfusion and infused according to the patient's tolerance. The platelet transfusion is anticipated to increase the platelet count 5,000 to 10,000/µL per unit.*

ASSESSING AND MANAGING STOMATITIS

Mucositis is a common side effect of radiation and some types of chemotherapy that may lead to inflammation and ulceration of any portion of the GI tract from the oral cavity throughout the alimentary canal. One form of mucositis, stomatitis, is an inflammatory response of the oral tissues that is characterized by mild redness (erythema) and edema or, if severe, by painful ulcerations, bleeding, and secondary infection. Stomatitis commonly develops 5 to 14 days after patients receive myelosuppressive chemotherapeutic agents and often coincides with the WBC nadir. As many as 40% of patients receiving standard-dose chemotherapy experience some degree of stomatitis during treatment, and up to 100% of patients receiving high-dose chemotherapy or combination therapy with radiation and chemotherapy for treatment of head and neck cancers may experience stomatitis (Eilers et al., 2014).

As a result of normal everyday wear and tear, the epithelial cells that line the oral cavity undergo rapid turnover and slough off routinely. Until recently, stomatitis was thought to occur because chemotherapy and radiation interfered with this process. Mucositis is now understood as a complex process involving inflammation, tissue damage, cell death, cytokine release, and microbes in the oral cavity (Eilers et al., 2014). Poor oral hygiene, existing dental disease, use of other medications that dry mucous membranes, advanced age, smoking, previous cancer treatment, diminished kidney function, and impaired nutritional status all contribute to morbidity associated with stomatitis. Radiation-induced xerostomia (dry mouth) associated with decreased function of the salivary glands may contribute to stomatitis in patients who have received radiation to the head and neck.

Myelosuppression (bone marrow depression), resulting from underlying disease or its treatment, predisposes the patient to oral bleeding and infection. Severe pain associated with ulcerated oral tissues can significantly interfere with nutritional intake, speech, and a willingness to maintain oral hygiene. Severe stomatitis may cause or prolong hospitalizations. In addition, stomatitis may lead to interruptions in chemotherapy and radiation administration or decreases in the intended dosing until the inflammation subsides. Further, it may significantly reduce the patient's quality of life.

Nurses must perform routine oral assessments in patients at risk for developing stomatitis and in patients with established stomatitis. Standardized oral assessment guides exist to facilitate objective descriptions of the oral mucosa (Eilers et al., 2014). The assessment should include the color and moisture of the lips and oral mucosa; presence of ulcerations; presence of edema of the lips, buccal mucosa, or tongue; and quantity and quality of saliva. The nurse also assesses the level of pain that the patient experiences secondary to stomatitis, alterations in the patient's ability to talk or sleep, and nutritional intake (Polovich et al., 2014).

Although multiple studies on stomatitis have been published, the optimal prevention and treatment approaches have not been identified. Future studies will focus on addressing the cascade of inflammatory events and release of chemical substances that leads to the cellular and tissue destruction underlying stomatitis. Routine, good oral hygiene, including brushing, flossing, and rinsing, is necessary to minimize the risk of oral complications associated with cancer therapies. Soft-bristled toothbrushes and nonabrasive toothpaste prevent or reduce trauma to the oral mucosa. Oral swabs with sponge-like applicators may be used in place of a toothbrush for painful oral tissues. Flossing may be performed unless it causes pain or bleeding. Oral rinses with saline solution or tap water after meals and at bedtime may be necessary for patients who cannot tolerate tooth brushing. Products that irritate oral tissues or impair healing, such as alcohol-based mouth rinses, are avoided. Foods that are difficult to chew or that are hot or spicy are avoided to minimize further trauma. The patient's lips are lubricated to keep them from becoming dry and cracked. Topical anti-inflammatory and anesthetic agents may be prescribed to promote healing and minimize discomfort. Products that coat or protect oral mucosa are used to promote comfort and prevent further trauma. Patients who experience severe pain and discomfort with stomatitis require systemic analgesics.

Adequate fluid and food intake is encouraged. In some instances, parenteral hydration and nutrition are necessary. Topical or systemic antifungal and antibiotic medications are prescribed to treat local or systemic infections.

Cryotherapy (sucking on ice chips) has demonstrated a reduction in pain incidence and severity in patients being treated with drugs with a short half-life (e.g., bolus 5-fluorouracil, melphalan) (Eilers et al., 2014). Low-level laser therapy has also demonstrated a reduction in prevalence, severity, pain, and duration of mucositis (Eilers et al., 2014; Polovich et al., 2014).

Palifermin, a synthetic form of human keratinocyte growth factor, is an IV medication approved in 2005 by the FDA for treatment of mucositis in patients with hematologic malignancies who are undergoing high-dose chemotherapy or total body radiation prior to HCST. Palifermin appears to promote more rapid replacement of cells in the mouth and GI tract, decreasing the incidence and duration of severe mucositis. It has not yet been tested in other patients with cancer. Careful timing of administration and monitoring are essential for maximum effectiveness and to detect adverse effects (Eilers et al., 2014; Polovich et al., 2014).

(continued on page 190)

CARING FOR PATIENTS WITH NAUSEA AND VOMITING

Nausea is an unpleasant sensation experienced in the back of the throat, epigastrium, or stomach that may result in vomiting. Nausea is one of the most feared side effects of cancer treatment. The potential causes of nausea are numerous, and nurses should not assume that nausea is due to chemotherapy; all potential causes must be considered. Causes of nausea include primary or metastatic tumor involving the CNS; gastroparesis (slowed gastric emptying); obstruction in the GI tract; infection; hypercalcemia; kidney or liver dysfunction; hyponatremia; and side effects of medications including chemotherapy, morphine, and antibiotics. Risk factors for treatment-induced nausea include younger age, female sex, and a history of treatment-induced nausea and vomiting.

Nausea is a subjective phenomenon analogous to pain. Nausea is best assessed by eliciting the patient's self-report. The following components should be assessed: timing of nausea in relation to treatment, perceived meaning of nausea to the patient, onset, frequency, associated symptoms, precipitating and alleviating factors, and previous experiences with nausea. Physical assessment should include signs of sweating, tachycardia, dizziness, pallor, excessive salivation, weakness, gastric distention, abdominal tenderness, and evaluation of bowel sounds. Laboratory values including electrolytes and kidney function should be monitored.

The prevention of chemotherapy-induced nausea and vomiting is a priority (see earlier discussion). For nausea and vomiting unrelated to chemotherapy, medications including serotonin receptor antagonists (e.g., ondansetron), dopamine receptor antagonists (e.g., metoclopramide), phenothiazines (e.g., prochlorperazine), corticosteroids (e.g., dexamethasone), and cannabinoids (e.g., dronabinol) can be used. Antiemetics should be administered around the clock with breakthrough doses as needed. Nonpharmacologic interventions that have proven to be effective in decreasing nausea include relaxation, guided imagery, acupressure, acupuncture, deep breathing, and eliminating odors. Patients should be instructed to avoid reclining within the first 30 minutes after eating. Dietary interventions include eating small, frequent meals and eating bland, chilled foods.

MAINTAINING SKIN INTEGRITY

The nurse assesses the patient with cancer for any skin problems. Maintaining integrity of skin and tissue poses a problem for patients with cancer because of the effects of chemotherapy, radiation therapy, surgery, and invasive procedures carried out for diagnosis and therapy. Targeted therapies are associated with cutaneous toxicity, including skin and nail changes (Shi, Levy, & Choi, 2016). Nail changes can include loss of all or a portion of the nail, transverse ridges across the nail plate (Beau lines), and hyperpigmentation (Polovich et al., 2014). The EGFR inhibitors commonly cause skin rash appearing as acneform eruptions or a papulopustular rash (Polovich et al., 2014). The rash can cause itching and discomfort. Up to 30% of patients experience an infection due to alteration in skin integrity.

Treatment of EGFR inhibitor rash includes topical steroids and oral antibiotics (Shi et al., 2016).

As part of the assessment, the nurse identifies which of these predisposing factors is present and assesses the patient for risk factors, including treatment type, nutritional deficits, bowel and bladder incontinence, immobility, immunosuppression, multiple skin folds, and changes related to aging. The nurse notes the presence of skin lesions, ulcers, rashes, or ulcerations secondary to the tumor or the effects of treatment.

Some of the most frequently encountered disturbances of tissue integrity, in addition to stomatitis, include skin and tissue reactions to radiation therapy, alopecia, and metastatic skin lesions. Patients with skin and tissue reactions to radiation therapy require careful skin care to prevent further skin irritation, drying, and damage. The skin over the affected area is handled gently; avoiding rubbing and use of hot or cold water, soaps, powders, lotions, and cosmetics. Patients may avoid tissue injury by wearing loose-fitting, cotton clothes and avoiding clothes that constrict, irritate, or rub the affected area. If blistering occurs, care is taken not to disrupt the blisters, thus reducing the risk of introducing bacteria. Moisture- and vapor-permeable dressings, such as hydrocolloids and hydrogels, are helpful in promoting healing and reducing pain. Aseptic wound care is indicated to minimize the risk for infection and sepsis. Topical antibiotics, such as 1% silver sulfadiazine cream (Silvadene), may be prescribed for use on areas of moist desquamation (painful, red, moist skin). As many cancer treatments cause photosensitivity, patients must be counseled on sun protection and use of sunscreen (Polovich et al., 2014).

Helping Patients Cope with Alopecia. The nurse notes the presence of alopecia (hair loss), which is another form of tissue disruption common in patients with cancer who receive radiation therapy or chemotherapy. In addition, the nurse assesses the psychological impact of this side effect on the patient and family.

The temporary or permanent thinning or complete loss of hair is a potential adverse effect of various radiation therapies and chemotherapeutic agents. The extent of alopecia depends on the type, dose, and duration of therapy. Combination chemotherapy is more likely to cause complete hair loss than monotherapy. These treatments cause alopecia by damaging stem cells and hair follicles. As a result, the hair is brittle and may fall out or break off at the surface of the scalp. Hair loss may be patchy or total, involve scalp hair and body hair, although loss of body hair is less frequent (Dua, Heiland, Kracen, & Deshields, 2017). Hair loss usually begins 2 to 3 weeks after the initiation of treatment; regrowth begins within 8 weeks after the last treatment and may take up to 6 months for complete regrowth. Some patients who undergo radiation to the head may sustain permanent hair loss. Many health care providers view hair loss as a minor problem when compared with the potentially life-threatening consequences of cancer. However, for many patients, hair loss is a major assault on body image, resulting in depression, anxiety, anger, rejection, and isolation. To patients and families, hair loss can serve as a constant reminder of the challenges cancer places on coping abilities, interpersonal relationships, and sexuality.

Scalp cooling or scalp hypothermia has been studied with mixed results. It is not recommended for patients with hematologic malignancies and should be used in the context of clinical trials in patients with solid tumors (Polovich et al., 2014). Topical minoxidil has demonstrated decreased severity and duration of alopecia but does not prevent it entirely (Polovich et al., 2014).

The nurse provides information about alopecia and supports the patient and family in coping with changes in body image. The patient is advised to use shampoos without detergents, menthol, salicylic acid, alcohol, or heavy perfume to minimize damage; avoiding hair color, perms and bleach, hot rollers or excessive heat, or aggressive hair brushing or combing (Polovich et al., 2014). The patient is encouraged to acquire a wig or hairpiece before hair loss occurs, so that the replacement matches the patient's own hair. Use of attractive scarves and hats may make the patient feel less conspicuous. The nurse can refer the patient to supportive programs, such as "Look Good, Feel Better," offered by the American Cancer Society. The scalp should be protected from cold and sun with hats, scarves, wigs, and sunscreen; eye protection (sunglasses) is also important, especially if eyelashes are lost (Polovich et al., 2014). Knowledge that hair usually begins to regrow after therapy is completed may comfort some patients, although patients must be prepared that the color and texture of the new hair may be different.

IMPROVING NUTRITIONAL STATUS

Assessment of the patient's nutritional status is an important nursing role. Impaired nutritional status may contribute to disease progression, decreased survival, immune incompetence, increased incidence of infection, delayed tissue repair, diminished functional ability, decreased capacity to continue antineoplastic therapy, increased length of hospital stay, and impaired psychosocial functioning. Altered nutritional status, weight loss, and cachexia (muscle wasting, emaciation) are complex states and may be secondary to decreased protein and caloric intake, metabolic or mechanical effects of the cancer, systemic disease, side effects of the treatment, or the patient's emotional status.

The nursing assessment of nutritional status includes monitoring the patient's weight and caloric intake consistently. Other information obtained by assessment includes diet history, any episodes of anorexia, changes in appetite, situations and foods that aggravate or relieve anorexia, and medication history. Difficulty in chewing or swallowing is identified, and the presence of nausea, vomiting, or diarrhea is noted. The patient should also be asked about the ability to prepare and obtain food to assist in identifying the need for additional resources.

Clinical and laboratory data useful in assessing nutritional status include anthropometric measurements (triceps skin fold and middle-upper arm circumference), serum protein levels (albumin, prealbumin, and transferrin), serum electrolytes, lymphocyte count, hemoglobin levels, hematocrit, urinary creatinine levels, and serum iron levels.

> **Nursing Alert**
> *A normal serum albumin is 3.5 to 5.2 g/dL or 35 to 52 g/L and gives the clinician a quick assessment of protein stores. In a seminal study by Seltzer et al. (1979), a sixfold increase in mortality was seen with an albumin level of less than 35 g/L, while additional studies associate serum albumin levels of less than 30 g/L with significant morbidity and mortality regardless of patient age and diagnosis (Jellinge, Henriksen, Hallas, & Brabrand, 2014). However, since albumin is degraded over 14 to 21 days, it is not a good measure for assessing recent nutritional deficits. Prealbumin has a half-life of 2 days and, therefore, is a better measure of response to dietary treatments. The normal reference range for prealbumin in males is 19 to 37 mg/dL, and in females, 17 to 31 mg/dL.*

Understanding Cancer-Related Causes of Malnutrition. Most patients with cancer experience some weight loss during their illness. Anorexia, malabsorption, and cachexia are examples of nutritional problems that commonly occur in patients with cancer; special attention is needed to prevent weight loss and promote nutrition.

Anorexia. Anorexia is defined as an involuntary loss of appetite. Among the many causes of anorexia in patients with cancer is alterations in taste, manifested by increased salty, sour, and metallic taste sensations, and altered responses to sweet and bitter flavors. These changes lead to decreased appetite, decreased nutritional intake, and protein–calorie malnutrition. Taste alterations may result from mineral (e.g., zinc) deficiencies, increases in circulating amino acids and cellular metabolites, or the administration of chemotherapeutic agents. Patients undergoing radiation therapy to the head and neck may experience "mouth blindness" (MacCarthy-Leventhal, 1959) which is a severe impairment of taste. Alterations in the sense of smell also alter taste; this is a common experience of patients with head and neck cancers.

Anorexia may occur because people feel full after eating only a small amount of food. This is referred to as *early satiety.* This sense of fullness occurs secondary to a decrease in digestive enzymes, abnormalities in the metabolism of glucose and triglycerides, and prolonged stimulation of gastric volume receptors, which convey the feeling of being full. Psychological distress (e.g., fear, pain, depression, and isolation) throughout illness may also have a negative impact on appetite. Patients may develop an aversion to food because of nausea and vomiting after treatment.

Cachexia. Cachexia is common in patients with cancer with prevalence ranging from 40% at cancer diagnosis to 70% to 80% in advanced phases of the disease (Alexander, Goldberg, & Korc-Grodzicki, 2016). It is a multifactorial syndrome marked by loss of skeletal muscle mass without loss of fat mass that cannot be entirely reversed by nutritional support alone (Penet

(continued on page 192)

& Bhujwalla, 2015). Cachexia is defined as a weight loss of 10% body weight or more within 6 months, a BMI below 20, and any weight loss greater than 2% (Penet & Bhujwalla, 2015; Polovich et al., 2014). Cachexia is characterized by negative protein and energy balance as a result of decreased food intake and abnormal metabolism (Polovich et al., 2014). Cachexia often leads to a decline in functional status, quality of life, and decreased tolerance to treatment. Progressive cachexia suggests a poor prognosis and accounts for 20% of all cancer deaths (Penet & Bhujwalla, 2015). Treatment includes nutritional support and counseling and treatment of the underlying malignancy.

Promoting Nutrition. Whenever possible, every effort is used to maintain adequate nutrition through the oral route. Referral to a registered dietitian is essential as this has been shown to improve calorie intake (Polovich et al., 2014). High calorie/high protein supplements should be encouraged. Food should be prepared in ways that make it appealing. Unpleasant smells are avoided. Family members are included in the plan of care to encourage adequate food intake. The patient's preferences, as well as physiologic and metabolic requirements, are considered when selecting foods. Small, frequent meals are provided with supplements between meals. Patients often tolerate larger amounts of food earlier in the day rather than later, so meals can be planned accordingly. To avoid early satiety, the patient should avoid drinking fluids while eating. Oral hygiene before mealtime often makes meals more pleasant. It is important to assess and manage pain, nausea, and other symptoms that may interfere with nutrition. Medications, such as corticosteroids, dronabinol, and progestational agents such as megestrol acetate, have been used successfully as appetite stimulants (Alexander et al., 2016). Prokinetic agents, such as metoclopramide, are used to increase gastric emptying in patients with early satiety and delayed gastric emptying.

If adequate nutrition cannot be maintained by oral intake, nutritional support via the enteral route may be necessary. Short-term nutritional supplementation may be provided through a nasogastric tube. However, if nutritional support is needed for longer than several weeks, a gastrostomy or jejunostomy tube may be inserted. The patient and family are taught to administer enteral nutrition in the home.

If malabsorption is a problem, enzyme and vitamin replacement may be instituted. Additional strategies include changing the feeding schedule, using simple diets, and relieving diarrhea. If malabsorption is severe, parenteral nutrition may be necessary. Parenteral nutrition can be administered in several ways: by a long-term venous access device (e.g., right atrial catheter), by an implanted venous port, or by a peripherally inserted central catheter (PICC) (Fig. 6-5). The nurse teaches the patient and family to care for venous access devices and to administer parenteral nutrition when appropriate. Home care nurses may assist with or supervise parenteral nutrition administration in the home.

Interventions to reduce cachexia usually do not prolong survival or improve nutritional status significantly. Optimal management of other symptoms that may be contributing, such as

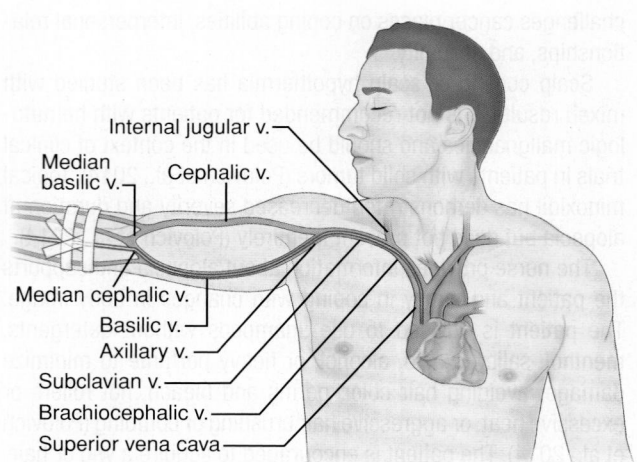

Internal jugular v.
Median basilic v.
Cephalic v.
Median cephalic v.
Basilic v.
Axillary v.
Subclavian v.
Brachiocephalic v.
Superior vena cava

FIGURE 6-5 A peripherally inserted central catheter (PICC) is advanced through the cephalic or basilic vein to the axillary, subclavian, or brachiocephalic vein or the superior vena cava.

depression, anxiety, nausea or xerostomia, is critical to promoting improved nutritional intake. Further study is needed to assess the effects of nutritional intervention on disease status and the patient's quality of life. Before invasive nutritional strategies are instituted, the nurse should assess the patient carefully and discuss goals of care and options with the patient and family.

RELIEVING PAIN

The nurse assesses the patient with cancer for the source and site of pain. In cancer, pain and discomfort may be related to underlying disease, pressure exerted by the tumor, diagnostic procedures, or the cancer treatment itself. As in any other situation involving pain, cancer pain is affected by both physical and psychosocial influences. A comprehensive pain assessment is completed including onset, duration, location, quality or characteristics, quantity, aggravating and alleviating factors, associated symptoms, and the treatments that the patient has used to relieve pain.

The nurse also assesses those factors that increase the patient's perception of pain, such as fear and apprehension, fatigue, anger, and social isolation. Pain assessment scales (see Chapter 7) are useful for assessing the patient's pain before pain-relieving interventions are instituted and for evaluating the effectiveness of these interventions.

Various pharmacologic and nonpharmacologic options are available for managing cancer pain. No reasonable approaches, even those that may be invasive, should be overlooked because of a poor or terminal prognosis. The nurse helps the patient and family take an active role in managing pain. The nurse provides education and support to correct fears and misconceptions about opioid use. Inadequate pain control leads to suffering, anxiety, fear, immobility, isolation, and depression. The goal, regardless of the patient's disease status, is to maximize quality of life and optimize functional ability by adequately managing pain. Refer to Chapter 7 for details on managing cancer pain.

IMPROVING BODY IMAGE

The nurse identifies potential threats to the patient's body image and assesses the patient's ability to cope with the many assaults to body image that he or she experiences throughout the course of disease and treatment. Entry into the health care system is often accompanied by depersonalization. Threats to self-concept are enormous as the patient faces the realization of illness, disfigurement, possible disability, and possible death. To accommodate treatments or because of the disease, many patients with cancer are forced to alter their lifestyles. Priorities and values change when body image is threatened. Disfiguring surgery, hair loss, cachexia, skin changes, altered communication patterns, and sexual dysfunction are some of the devastating results of cancer and its treatment that threaten the patient's self-esteem and body image.

A positive approach is essential when caring for patients with altered body image. To help the patient retain control and positive self-esteem, it is important to encourage independence and continued participation in self-care and decision-making. The patient is assisted to assume those tasks and participate in those activities that are personally of most value. Any negative feelings that the patient has or threats to body image should be identified and discussed. The nurse serves as a listener and counselor to both the patient and the family. Referral to a support group can provide the patient with additional assistance in coping with the changes resulting from cancer or its treatment. In many cases, cosmetologists can provide ideas about hair or wig styling, makeup, and the use of scarves and other head coverings to help with body image concerns.

Patients who experience alterations in sexuality and sexual function are encouraged to discuss concerns openly with the health care team and with their partners. Alternative forms of sexual expression are explored with patients and their partners to promote positive self-worth and acceptance. Nurses who identify serious physiologic, psychological, or communication difficulties related to sexuality or sexual function are in a key position to help patients and partners seek further counseling if necessary.

TEACHING PATIENTS SELF-CARE

Many patients with cancer return home from acute-care facilities to receive treatment in the home or outpatient area. The shift from the acute-care setting also shifts the responsibility for care to the patient and family. As a result, family members and friends must assume increased involvement in patient care, which requires teaching that enables them to provide quality care. Teaching initially focuses on providing information needed by the patient and family to address the most immediate care needs likely to be encountered at home.

Side effects of treatments and changes in the patient's status that should be reported are reviewed verbally and reinforced with written information. Strategies to deal with side effects of treatment are discussed with the patient and family. Other learning needs are identified based on the priorities conveyed by the patient and family as well as on the complexity of care provided in the home.

Technologic advancements allow home administration of chemotherapy, parenteral nutrition, blood products, parenteral antibiotics, and parenteral analgesics as well as management of symptoms and care of vascular access devices. Although home care nurses provide care and support for patients receiving this advanced technical care, patients and families need instruction and ongoing support that allow them to feel comfortable and proficient in managing these treatments at home. Follow-up visits and telephone calls from the nurse are often reassuring and increase the patient's and family's comfort in dealing with complex and new aspects of care. Continued contact facilitates evaluation of the patient's progress and assessment of the ongoing needs of the patient and family.

CONTINUING CARE

Referral for home care is often indicated for patients with cancer. The responsibilities of the home care nurse include assessing the home environment, suggesting modifications in the home or in care to help the patient and family address the patient's physical needs, providing physical care, and assessing the psychological and emotional impact of the illness on the patient and family.

Assessing changes in the patient's physical status and reporting relevant changes to the provider help ensure that appropriate and timely modifications in therapy are made. The home care nurse also assesses the adequacy of pain management and the effectiveness of other strategies to prevent or manage the side effects of treatment modalities.

It is necessary to assess the patient's and family's understanding of the treatment plan and management strategies and to reinforce previous teaching. The nurse often facilitates coordination of patient care by maintaining close communication with all involved health care providers. The nurse may make referrals and coordinate available community resources (e.g., local office of the American Cancer Society, home aides, church groups, parish nurses, support groups) to assist patients and caregivers.

EVALUATION

Nurses play an important role in evaluating the expected outcomes for patients with cancer. To maximize beneficial outcomes and intervene in the presence of potential complications, evaluation of the patient's and family's needs are assessed because cancer affects not only the patient but also the family members. In addition, with the shift away from inpatient care, many families are caring for patients at home and should be considered members of the health care team. The nurse can refer the patient and family to a variety of support groups sponsored by the American Cancer Society or available community resources. The nurse also collaborates with a variety of providers (e.g., physical and occupational therapists, wound and ostomy nurses, nutritionists, pharmacists, social workers,

(continued on page 194)

psychologists, and clergy or spiritual advisors) to help identify appropriate interventions that support the goal of regaining the highest level of function and independence possible for the patient.

Expected patient outcomes may include the following:
1. Maintains integrity of oral mucous membranes
2. Maintains adequate tissue integrity
3. Maintains adequate nutritional status
4. Achieves relief of pain and discomfort
5. Demonstrates increased activity tolerance and decreased fatigue
6. Exhibits improved body image and self-esteem
7. Progresses through the grieving process
8. Experiences no complications, such as infection, or sepsis, and no episodes of bleeding or hemorrhage

GERONTOLOGIC CONSIDERATIONS

As a result of an increased life expectancy and an increased risk of cancer with age, nurses are providing cancer-related care for growing numbers of elderly patients. More than half of all cancers occur in people older than 65 years of age, and 70% of all cancer deaths with prostate, bladder, colon, uterine, pancreatic, gastric, rectal and lung carcinomas accounting for the majority of cases (Suhag, Sunita, Sarin, & Singh, 2015). Nursing care of this population addresses special needs, including physical, psychosocial, and financial concerns.

Oncology nurses working with the elderly population must understand the normal physiologic changes that occur with aging. These changes include decreased skin elasticity; decreased skeletal mass, structure, and strength; decreased organ function and structure; impaired immune system mechanisms; alterations in neurologic and sensory functions; and altered drug absorption, distribution, metabolism, and elimination. These changes ultimately influence the ability of elderly patients to tolerate cancer treatment. In addition, many elderly patients have other chronic diseases and associated treatments that may limit tolerance to cancer treatments. Polypharmacy is common in the elderly and the growing number of drug–drug interactions with newer anti-cancer therapies must be considered carefully (Thompson & Dale, 2015). Treatment decisions should not be based on age alone; a thorough consideration of the patient's performance status and comorbidities is essential in decision making (Suhag et al., 2015).

Potential chemotherapy-related toxicities, such as renal impairment, myelosuppression, fatigue, and cardiomyopathy, may increase as a result of declining organ function and diminished physiologic reserves. The recovery of normal tissues after radiation therapy may be delayed, and older patients may experience more severe adverse effects, such as mucositis, nausea and vomiting, and myelosuppression. Because of decreased tissue-healing capacity and declining

pulmonary and cardiovascular functioning, older patients are slower to recover from surgery. Elderly patients are also at increased risk for complications such as atelectasis, pneumonia, and wound infections.

Access to cancer care for elderly patients may be limited by discriminatory or fatalistic attitudes of health care providers, caregivers, and patients themselves. Issues such as the gradual loss of supportive resources, declining health or loss of a spouse, and unavailability of relatives or friends may result in limited access to care and unmet needs for assistance with activities of daily living. In addition, the economic impact of health care may be difficult for those living on fixed incomes.

Nurses must be aware of the special needs of the aging population. Nurses carefully monitor elderly patients receiving cancer treatments for signs and symptoms of adverse effects. In addition, elderly patients are instructed to report all symptoms to their provider. It is not uncommon for elderly patients to delay reporting symptoms, attributing them to "old age." Many elderly people do not want to report illness for fear of losing their independence or financial security. Sensory losses (e.g., hearing and visual losses) and memory deficits are considered when planning patient education because they may affect the patient's ability to process and retain information. In such cases, the nurse acts as a patient advocate, encouraging independence and identifying resources, such as home care, for support when indicated. Often elderly patients see a number of different doctors and subspecialists; coordination of care becomes critical (Suhag et al., 2015).

END-OF-LIFE CONSIDERATIONS

The needs of patients with terminal illnesses are best met by a comprehensive multidisciplinary program that focuses on quality of life, palliation of symptoms, and provision of psychosocial and spiritual support for patients and families when cure and control of the disease are no longer possible. The concept of hospice, which originated in Great Britain, best addresses these needs. Most important, the focus of care is on the family, not just the patient. Hospice care can be provided in several settings: free-standing, hospital-based, and community- or home-based settings. Research has demonstrated that use of palliative care teams can improve patient care and reduce costs at the end of life (Gebauer, 2015; Nekhlyudov, Levit, Hurria, & Ganz, 2014).

Hospice care is often delivered through coordination of services provided by hospitals and the community. Although physicians, social workers, clergy, dietitians, pharmacists, physical therapists, and volunteers are involved in patient care, nurses are most often the coordinators of hospice activities. It is essential that home care and hospice nurses possess advanced skills in communication, assessing and managing pain, nutrition, dyspnea, bowel dysfunction, and skin impairments.

In addition, hospice programs facilitate clear communication among family members and health care providers. Most patients and families are informed of the prognosis and are encouraged to participate in decisions regarding pursuing or terminating cancer treatment. Through collaboration with other support disciplines, the nurse helps the patient and family cope with changes in role identity, family structure, grief, and loss. Hospice nurses are actively involved in bereavement counseling. In many instances, family support for survivors continues for approximately 1 year.

CHAPTER REVIEW

Critical Thinking Exercises

1. Your patient has been receiving high doses of chemotherapy to treat leukemia. She reports that she wants to stop the chemotherapy because of the oral ulcerations and pain that have developed since she started on the chemotherapy. What would be your response to her? What evidence-based nursing interventions would you implement to relieve the ulcers and her pain? What is the evidence for the interventions that you identified? How strong is that evidence, and what criteria did you use to assess the strength of that evidence?

2. A 74-year-old patient with prostate cancer and metastasis to the bone is to begin a continuous subcutaneous infusion of analgesia through an ambulatory infusion pump to relieve his severe pain. The patient's wife is afraid that he will become addicted, and his adult children state that his pain remains unrelieved. As a home care nurse, what assessments would be of highest priority to you during your initial visit to this patient? What nursing interventions and teaching would be indicated in this situation? How would you modify your interventions if the patient is receiving fentanyl by transdermal patch and still reporting severe pain?

3. Your 68-year-old patient with lung cancer has been admitted for emergent radiation therapy for the diagnosis of SVCS. Describe the underlying pathology that can lead to the signs and symptoms of SVCS. What patient monitoring will be essential during this patient's course of care? Describe the medical and nursing management strategies that will be used for this patient.

NCLEX-Style Review Questions

1. In assessing the neutropenic patient's understanding of discharge education, which patient statement indicates that the nurse needs to provide further education?
   a. "I should stay away from crowds and people who are sick."
   b. "I should wash my hands carefully after using the bathroom and before eating meals."
   c. "If I have a fever or chills, I should take acetaminophen immediately and recheck my temperature an hour later."
   d. "My WBC count should recover about 14 days after my treatment is completed."

2. A nurse is caring for a patient receiving brachytherapy for cervical cancer. Which of the following statements regarding the nursing care of this patient is true? Select all that apply.
   a. The patient must be maintained on bed rest.
   b. The head of the bed must be elevated more than 30 degrees to decrease the risk of aspiration.
   c. Pain management is a priority.
   d. The patient will have an indwelling urinary catheter.

3. A patient is receiving external beam radiation therapy for head and neck cancer. The patient reports moderate pain to the tongue and buccal mucosa that is interfering with his ability to eat, sleep, and speak. Which of the following interventions would you recommended for this patient? Select all that apply.
   a. Take pain medication 30 minutes before meals.
   b. Avoid acidic, spicy, and sharp foods such as chips.
   c. Keep dentures out when not eating to promote healing.
   d. Rinse the oral mucosa regularly with an alcohol-based solution.

4. A nurse is creating a public health intervention that targets teenagers at risk for skin cancer secondary to sun and tanning bed exposure. Which of the following is an example of primary prevention?
   a. Establishing a van that travels to high schools to perform skin assessments
   b. Establishing a clinic based in the school nurse's office that performs screening examinations for skin cancer
   c. Developing an educational intervention to teach skin self-assessment
   d. Developing a television commercial, to be aired on the music television network, educating teens on the risks of sun exposure

5. A nurse is caring for a patient with newly diagnosed leukemia who is receiving chemotherapy for the first time. Twenty-four hours after the first dose of chemotherapy, the patient experiences decreased urine output, an abnormal heart rate, and lethargy. Which of the following laboratory results would help support the nurse's suspicion for tumor lysis syndrome?
   a. Serum calcium 13.0 mg/dL, potassium 3.5 mEq/L, magnesium 2.0 mg/dL
   b. Potassium 2.0 mEq/L, phosphorous 3.0 mg/dL, calcium 6.0 mg/dL
   c. Uric acid 4.0 mg/dL, creatinine 3.0
   d. Uric acid 10.0 mg/dL, potassium 5.5 mEq/L, phosphorous 5.0 mg/dL

Try these additional resources, available at **http://thepoint.lww.com/Honan2e**, to enhance your learning and understanding of this chapter:
- NCLEX-Style Student Review Questions
- Journal Articles

REFERENCES AND SELECTED READINGS

References and selected readings associated with this chapter can be found on the website that accompanies the book. Visit **http://thepoint. lww.com/Honan2e** to access the references and other additional resources associated with this chapter.

Pain Management

Linda Honan • Rosalina Madrid

Learning Objectives

After reading this chapter, you will be able to:

1. Compare characteristics of acute pain, chronic (persistent) pain, and cancer pain.
2. Describe the effects of acute and chronic pain.
3. Describe the pathophysiology of pain.
4. Describe factors that can alter the response to pain.
5. Demonstrate appropriate use of pain measurement instruments.
6. Explain the nursing role in multidisciplinary pain management.
7. Identify nonpharmacologic pain relief interventions for selected groups of patients.
8. Develop a plan to prevent and treat the adverse effects of analgesic agents.
9. Use the nursing process as a framework for the care of patients with pain.

Pain has been defined as an unpleasant sensory and emotional experience associated with actual or potential tissue damage (Merskey & Bogduk, 1994). It is the most common reason for seeking health care (Cohen & Raja, 2016). It is associated with many disorders, diagnostic tests, and treatments. It disables, distresses more people than any single disease, varies widely in intensity, and spares no age group. Because nurses spend more time with patients in pain than other health care providers, nurses need to understand the pathophysiology of pain, the physiologic and psychological consequences of acute and chronic (persistent) pain, and the methods used to treat pain. Nurses encounter patients in pain in a variety of settings, including acute care, outpatient, and long-term care settings, as well as in the home. Therefore, they must have the knowledge and skills to assess pain, implement pain relief strategies, and evaluate the effectiveness of these strategies, regardless of setting.

TYPES OF PAIN

Pain is categorized according to its duration, location, and etiology. In general, three basic categories of pain are recognized: acute pain, chronic (persistent, nonmalignant) pain, and cancer-related pain.

Acute Pain

Usually of recent onset and commonly associated with a specific injury, trauma, or painful medical procedures, acute pain indicates that damage or injury has occurred. Pain is significant in that it draws attention to a threat and teaches people to avoid similar potentially painful situations. Thus, pain is both a sensation and a warning signal. If no lasting damage occurs and no systemic disease exists, acute pain usually decreases as healing occurs or as the underlying cause is treated. Acute pain can be an isolated one-time incident or recur at regular intervals, such as menstrual cramping, or sporadically, as with angina or migraine headaches. If untreated, acute pain may lead to chronic pain.

Chronic Pain

Chronic pain is a persistent or intermittent pain that lingers beyond the expected healing time (generally over 3 months). It is associated with a variety of degenerative or traumatic conditions, such as arthritis, degenerative disk disease, and intervertebral disk herniation, but often a specific cause or injury for the chronic pain may not be found. It may have a poorly defined onset, and it is often difficult to treat because the cause or origin may be unclear. Although acute pain may be a useful signal that something is wrong, chronic or persistent pain may become a patient's primary disorder with symptoms of refractory pain, functional and psychological impairment, and disability (Dinakar, 2016). Medical-surgical nurses care for patients with chronic pain when these patients are admitted to the hospital for management or when they develop other new etiologies.

Cancer-Related Pain

Pain associated with cancer may be acute or chronic. Pain resulting from cancer is so ubiquitous that when cancer patients are asked about the most feared consequences of cancer, pain is reported most frequently. Approximately one third of cancer patients who receive active therapy, and 60% to 90% of patients with advanced disease, experience moderate to severe pain (LeBlanc & Abernethy, 2015). Pain in patients with cancer can be directly associated with the cancer (e.g., bony infiltration with tumor cells or nerve compression), a result of cancer treatment (e.g., surgery or radiation), or unrelated to the cancer (e.g., trauma). However, most pain associated with cancer is a direct result of tumor involvement. Although the pain may be acute, it is characterized more frequently as chronic. As in other situations involving pain, the experience of cancer pain is influenced by both physical and psychosocial factors.

Cancer can cause pain in various ways. Pain may be associated with various cancer treatments. Acute pain is linked with trauma from surgery. Occasionally, chronic pain syndromes, such as postsurgical neuropathies (pain related to nerve tissue injury), occur. Some chemotherapeutic agents cause tissue necrosis, peripheral neuropathies, and stomatitis—all potential sources of pain—whereas radiation therapy can cause pain secondary to skin or organ inflammation.

For some patients with advanced cancer, pain that continues to increase over time may be a sign that the tumor growth has progressed and that death is near. It is vital for the nurse to recognize the progression of symptoms correlating with the disease process so as to provide physical and emotional support to both the patient and loved ones. As patients anticipate the pain and their anxiety increases, pain perception heightens, producing fear and further pain. Chronic cancer pain, then, can be best described as a cycle progressing from pain to anxiety to fear and back to pain.

EFFECTS OF PAIN

Regardless of its nature, pattern, or cause, pain that is inadequately treated has harmful effects beyond the suffering it causes.

Effects of Acute Pain

Unrelieved acute pain can affect the pulmonary, cardiovascular, GI, endocrine, and immune systems. The stress response (neuroendocrine response to stress) that occurs with trauma also occurs with severe pain. The widespread endocrine, immunologic, and inflammatory changes that occur with stress can have significant negative effects. This is particularly harmful in patients whose health is already compromised by age, illness, or injury.

The stress response generally consists of increased metabolic rate and cardiac output, impaired insulin response, increased production of cortisol, and increased retention of fluids. Box 7-1 discusses the physiologic impact of acute pain. The stress response may increase the risk of physiologic disorders (e.g., myocardial infarction, pulmonary infection, thromboembolism, prolonged paralytic ileus). Patients with severe pain and associated stress may be unable to take deep breaths and may experience increased fatigue and decreased mobility. Although these effects may be tolerated by young, healthy people, they may hamper recovery in elderly, debilitated, or critically ill people. Effective pain relief may result in faster recovery and improved outcomes.

Effects of Chronic Pain

Like acute pain, chronic pain also has adverse effects. Suppression of the immune function associated with chronic pain may promote tumor growth. In addition, chronic pain often results in anger, depression, anxiety, fatigue, and disability.

BOX 7-1	**Physiologic Response to Acute Pain**	
Endocrine and metabolic response	Activation of sympathetic nervous system and an increase in glucagon secretion, which causes hyperglycemia, increased lipolysis (fat breakdown), accelerated protein breakdown, and nitrogen loss.	
	The stress response presents as hypertension, tachycardia, arrhythmias, myocardial ischemia, protein catabolism, immune system suppression, and impaired renal excretory function.	
Pulmonary function	Decreased phrenic nerve activity and diaphragmatic dysfunction manifested as a decrease in functional residual capacity and a decrease in tidal volume.	
GI motility	Decreased gastric motility, especially in the colon. The stomach and small intestines recover within 12–24 hours after abdominal surgery; however, the colon is inhibited for at least 48–72 hours.	
Cardiovascular	Increased sympathetic tone, which causes an increase in heart rate and blood pressure as well as redistribution of blood to and within various organs. The redistribution predisposes patients to myocardial ischemia in the presence of coronary artery disease and may induce arrhythmias.	
Immune system	Decreased responsiveness to antigens, delayed hypersensitivity, natural killer cell activity, and antibody response.	

Adapted from Peeters-Asdourian, C., & Akhouri, V. (2004). Acute pain management in the adult. In C. Warfield & Z. Bajwa (Eds.), *Principles and practices of pain management* (2nd ed.). New York: McGraw-Hill.

Patients may be unable to continue the activities and inter-personal relationships that they had engaged in before the pain began, with resultant impact on their quality of life. Disabilities may range from curtailing participation in physical activities to being unable to take care of personal needs, such as dressing or eating. Regardless of how patients cope with persistent pain, disability can result if the pain persists for an extended period.

Nurses should understand the effects of chronic pain on patients and families and should be knowledgeable about pain relief strategies and appropriate resources to assist effectively with pain management. Chronic pain that has become refractory to conventional treatment modalities can predispose a patient to take large quantities of opioid medications. Health care providers face the challenge of uncontrolled pain despite continued opioid dose increases. In some cases, patients can become hyperalgesic or have opioid-induced hyperalgesia (OIH), which is defined as the state of nociceptive sensitization caused by long-term exposure to opioids. A patient will report more pain or uncontrolled pain despite an increase in opioid dose. It may be hard for the patient to understand that reducing opioids in the state of hyperalgesia will help with the reduction of pain. The general health care provider can seek referral to available pain resources, such as a consult from an existing pain service or an evaluation by a certified pain nurse specialist.

Effects of Cancer Pain

As noted above, cancer pain may have aspects that are both acute and chronic. In addition, patients with cancer often have multiple causes of pain (e.g., direct tumor involvement, tumor invasion of the nerve and hollow viscera) involving multiple sites (bone pain, pain from chemotherapy, radiation, surgery). There can be significant changes in the patient's personality (mood disturbances, anxiety, and depression), lifestyle (lack of confidence in ability to control pain limits actions, decreased social interactions), and functional ability. Given the multidimensional aspects of cancer pain, it follows that a multidimensional plan is needed to manage the challenging aspects of cancer pain effectively.

PATHOPHYSIOLOGY OF PAIN

The processing of noxious stimuli and the resulting perception of pain involve the peripheral nervous system and central nervous system (CNS). Various nerve mechanisms and structures are involved in the transmission of pain to and from the brain, including nociceptors, or pain receptors, and chemical mediators. **Nociceptors** are free nerve endings found in the skin. These receptors are preferentially sensitive to intense, potentially damaging mechanical, thermal, or chemical stimuli. Although the skin contains the highest density of nociceptors, they also are found in joints, connective tissues,

blood vessels, periosteum, skeletal muscle, fascia, tendons, most visceral organs, and the corneas, and have the potential to respond to painful stimuli. When stimulated, nociceptors send signals to local blood vessels, mast cells, hair follicles, and sweat glands, often resulting in clinical findings associated with pain, such as vasomotor, autonomic, and visceral effects.

The nociceptors transmit information about the noxious, distressing, or damaging stimuli to neurons located in the spinal cord or brainstem, and this sensory information is integrated in the thalamus along with higher brain structures generating protective somatic and autonomic reflexes, endocrine actions, emotional responses, learning and memory about the event, and cortical awareness of pain (Westlund, 2014, p. 87).

Peripheral Nervous System Response

A number of **algogenic** (pain-causing) substances that enhance the sensitivity of nociceptors are released into the extracellular tissue as a result of tissue damage. Histamine, bradykinin, acetylcholine, serotonin (5-HT), calcitonin gene-related peptide (CGRP), and substance P are chemicals that increase the transmission of pain (Barrett, Barman, Boitano, & Brooks, 2016). The injured tissue releases bradykinin and prostaglandins that sensitize or activate nociceptors, which, in turn, release substance P. Substance P acts on mast cells to release histamine and CGRP, which dilates the blood vessels, resulting in edema and an inflammatory process. Serotonin (5-HT) is released from platelets and activates nociceptors. **Prostaglandins** are chemical substances that are believed to increase the sensitivity of pain receptors by enhancing the pain-provoking effect of bradykinin. It is interesting to note that aspirin and other nonsteroidal anti-inflammatory drugs (NSAIDs) block the enzyme needed for prostaglandin synthesis, resulting in pain control. At the peripheral nervous system level, two main types of fibers are involved in **nociception** (the neurologic transmission of pain impulses). The larger, myelinated A delta fibers transmit the initial pain sensation rapidly, at a rate of 12 to 34 m/sec, to the brain (acute pain, or "fast pain"). This type of pain frequently is associated with mechanical or thermal stimuli. The smaller, unmyelinated C fibers transmit impulses at a rate of 0.5 to 2 m/sec (Barrett et al., 2016). This is called "second pain" or "slow-wave pain" due to delayed onset and longer duration. It has dull, aching, diffuse, or burning qualities, which last longer than the initial fast pain. Chronic pain is believed to be associated with C-fiber stimulation.

If there is repeated C-fiber stimulation, there is a heightened response in spinal cord neurons, causing the person to perceive more pain. For this reason, it is important to treat patients with analgesic agents when they first feel pain. Patients require less medication and experience more effective pain relief if analgesia is administered before they become sensitized to the pain.

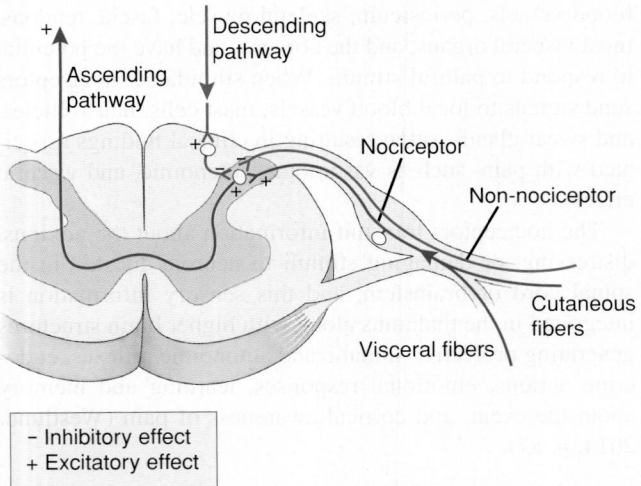

- Inhibitory effect
+ Excitatory effect

FIGURE 7-1 A schematic representation of aspects of nociceptive system.

Central Nervous System Response

For pain to be consciously perceived, neurons in the ascending system must be activated. Activation occurs as a result of input from the nociceptors. After tissue injury occurs, nociception continues and relays the impulses to the dorsal horn of the spinal cord. Upon entering the spinal cord at the dorsal horn, the pain impulse crosses the spinal cord and passes upward to the brain by the anterolateral pathway to the thalamus. Then the pain signals are transmitted to other areas of the brain and sensory cortex where the conscious experience or perception of pain occurs. Figure 7-1 illustrates pain transmission.

Chemicals that reduce or inhibit the transmission or perception of pain include **endorphins**, **enkephalins**, and **dynorphins** (Porth, 2015). These chemical, morphine-like neurotransmitters are endogenous (produced by the body) and reduce nociceptive transmission.

Just as the ascending system relays signal up to the brain for interpretation, the descending control system is considered inhibitory. It is always somewhat active, and it prevents continuous transmission of painful stimuli, partly through the action of the endorphins. Cognitive processes may stimulate endorphin production in the descending control system. The effectiveness of this system is illustrated by the effects of distraction. The distractions of visitors or a favorite television show may increase activity in the descending control system. Therefore, patients who have visitors or who are engaged in a television program may not report pain because activation of the descending control system results in less noxious or painful information being transmitted to consciousness. In addition, tactile stimulation can modulate pain through a complex process of tactile information being transmitted by large and small fibers throughout the CNS (Porth, 2015).

The neuromatrix theory of pain proposed by Melzack (2001) provides a conceptual framework to examine chronic pain. It proposes in response to injury, inflammation, disease, or chronic stress, the body–self neuromatrix activates perceptual, homeostatic, and behavioral responses. Endocrine, autonomic, immune, and opioid systems contribute to this interactive cognitive interpretation of pain. The pain experience is distinctive to each individual, shaped by sensory, psychosocial, and genetic factors, and modulated by various sensory inputs from the environment and by cognitive events, such as psychological stress (Stanos, Tyburski, & Harden, 2016). Thus, pain occurs in response to a widely distributed neural network in the brain (sensory, affective, and cognitive dimensions) rather than only to the sensory input of injury, inflammation, or pathology.

> **Nursing Alert**
> *Large internal organs (viscera) have a low density of nociceptors; as a result, typically visceral pain is poorly localized, nauseating, and frequently associated with diaphoresis and autonomic symptoms. Typically, pain originating in these large, internal organs results from intense stimulation of multipurpose receptors that respond to inflammation, stretching, ischemia, dilation, and spasm of the internal organs. An intense response in these fibers can cause severe pain.*

FACTORS INFLUENCING PAIN RESPONSE

Several factors, including past experiences with pain, anxiety, culture, age, gender, genetics, and expectations about pain relief, influence a person's experience of pain. These factors may increase or decrease perception of pain, increase or decrease tolerance for pain, and affect responses to pain.

Past Experience

The way a person responds to pain is a result of many separate painful events during a lifetime. The nurse understands that a patient's pain history may provide vital information on how a person has been able to either positively cope and manage their pain as well as what has hindered their physical and emotional well-being. This information will shape the patient's current expectation of pain and or pain management. If pain is relieved promptly and adequately, the person may be less fearful of future pain and better able to tolerate it.

Anxiety and Depression

Although it is commonly believed that anxiety increases pain, this is not necessarily true (see Box 7-2 for common misconceptions about pain). However, anxiety that is associated with pain may increase the patient's perception of pain. For example, the patient who was treated 2 years ago for breast cancer and who now has hip pain may fear that the

Common Concerns and Misconceptions About Pain and Analgesia

Misconception	Evidence
Patients with chronic pain have a higher tolerance to pain.	Patients with chronic pain have a decreased tolerance to pain associated with decreased endorphins, the effect of neurotransmitters, and physiologic responses. In patients with chronic pain, signals for pain and muscle spasm continue to be transmitted by the nervous system.
Chronic pain is due to psychological disturbance.	When unable to find a physiologic reason for pain, providers often attribute chronic pain to a psychological issue and, in addition, have demonstrated more positive responses to patients when pathology is found.
Chronic pain is caused by stress, and if the stress is relieved, pain abates.	Coping with chronic pain can be stressful which can lead to suffering and depression.
Patients will exaggerate their pain in order to receive increased compensation payments.	No evidence exists that patients report increased pain when seeking compensation or litigation.
Patients in chronic pain demonstrate manipulative behavior.	It is rare for patients with chronic pain to misrepresent their symptoms. Rather, some patients may seek out a variety of providers to obtain relief.
Depression causes chronic pain.	There is a corollary between chronic pain and depression; however, it is more likely that the stress of managing the chronic pain leads to depression.
People get addicted to pain medicine easily.	Research suggests a negligible risk of addiction when patients are prescribed opioids for pain. Misconceptions are related to a lack of knowledge of tolerance, physical dependence, and addiction.
Often patients are noncompliant and to blame for their physical symptoms.	Evidence shows that patients with chronic pain are generally compliant, and, if not, the reasons are attributed to treatment side effects or lack of treatment response.

From Shaw, S., & Lee, A. (2009). Student nurses' misconceptions of adults with chronic nonmalignant pain. *American Society for Pain Management Nursing, 11*(1), 2–14.

pain indicates metastasis. In this case, the patient's anxiety may result in increased pain. However, anxiety that is unrelated to the pain (e.g., anxiety about who is taking care of the pets while the patient is in the hospital) may distract the patient and may actually decrease the perception of pain.

Just as anxiety is associated with pain because of concerns and fears about an underlying disease, depression is associated with chronic pain and unrelieved cancer pain. In cases of chronic pain, the incidence of depression is increased with variable rates of 5% to 87% (Stanos et al., 2016) and often is associated with major life changes caused by the limiting effects of persistent pain.

Culture

Beliefs about pain and how to respond to it differ from one culture to the next. Early in childhood, people learn from those around them what responses to pain are acceptable or unacceptable. For example, a child may learn that a sports injury is not expected to hurt as much as a comparable injury caused by a motor vehicle crash. The child also learns what stimuli are expected to be painful and what behavioral responses are acceptable.

Cultural factors must be taken into account to manage pain effectively. Factors that help explain differences in a cultural group include age, gender, education level, and income. In addition, the degree to which patients identify with a culture influences the extent to which they will adopt

new health behaviors or rely on traditional health beliefs and practices. A wide range of behaviors may be seen in response to pain, ranging from moaning and complaining about pain and describing pain as "unbearable" to behaving in a quiet, stoic manner rather than expressing the pain verbally. The nurse must respond to the person's perception of pain and assess the person's behavior taking into consideration cultural influences. The nurse who recognizes cultural differences has insight into the impact of pain on the patient and is more accurate in assessing pain and in planning appropriate treatments to relieve pain.

The main issues to consider when caring for patients of a different culture are:

- What does the illness mean to the patient?
- Are there culturally based stigmas related to this illness or pain?
- What is the role of the family in health care decisions?
- Are traditional pain relief remedies used?
- What is the role of stoicism in the patient's culture?
- Are there culturally determined ways of expressing and communicating pain?
- Does the patient have any fears about the pain?
- Has the patient seen or does the patient want to see a traditional healer?

The nurse should avoid stereotyping the patient by culture and should provide individualized care rather than

TABLE 7-1   GERONTOLOGIC CONSIDERATIONS / For Pain Management

Physiologic Changes Influencing Pain Response	Pain Management Interventions
• Higher incidence of chronic illnesses • Increased use of prescription and OTC medications • Sensitivity to medications and increased risk for drug toxicity • Changes in medication absorption and metabolism due to decreased function of the liver, kidney, and GI system • Altered distribution of medications due to changes in body weight, protein stores, and distribution of body fluid • Slowed metabolism of medications • Higher blood levels of medications • Susceptibility to depression of both the nervous and the respiratory systems; hypoxia and hypercarbia can worsen workload on the heart, resulting in myocardial ischemia • Decreased binding of meperidine by plasma proteins, with possible result of twice the levels found in younger patients	• Obtain a careful medication history to identify potential drug interactions. • Administer analgesic agents, keeping a balance between minimal side effects and effective pain relief. • Consider possible need for slightly smaller initial dose of analgesic medication than prescribed for younger patients. • Patient may need prolonged dosing interval for subsequent doses. • Nurse may not administer meperidine because its active neurotoxic metabolite, normeperidine, is more likely to accumulate and cause CNS excitation and seizures. • Refer to clinical practice guidelines for managing persistent pain as needed. • Perform frequent assessments and evaluation of patient responses to pain interventions.

OTC, over the counter.

assuming that a patient of a specific culture will exhibit more or less pain. In addition to avoiding stereotyping, health care providers should individualize the amount of medications or therapy according to the information provided by the patient. The nurse should recognize that stereotypes exist and become sensitive to how they negatively affect care; refer to Box 7-2 for common misconceptions.

Age

Age-related changes that impact the assessment and management of pain include physiologic changes in the peripheral and CNS, kidneys, and liver function. Aging brings about a reduction of endorphin and serotonin receptors (Stewart, Schofield, Gooberman-Hill, Mehta, & Reid, 2014). In addition, the speed of processing nociceptive stimuli via A delta and C fiber function decreases, which may result in reduction in reaction time and a susceptibility to injury (Stewart et al., 2014). Kidney and liver function may decrease with aging, and, as a result, if medications are cleared by the kidney or liver, then increased half-lives are seen. Thus to avoid the risk of toxicity, dosages and/or frequency modifications may be necessary for medications. The nurse also recognizes that total body water decreases with aging (approximately 50% vs. 60% for adults), and total body fat generally increases, which translates into higher peak plasma concentrations for water-soluble drugs and prolonged half-lives for lipid-soluble drugs (Stewart et al., 2014, p. 467). Finally, the nurse considers the impact of high rates of polypharmacy among older adults, when administering medications.

Unrelieved pain contributes to the problem of depression as well as poor sleep quality, social relationships, performance of activities of daily living, and symptom management in older adults (Stewart et al., 2014). Older adults deal with pain according to their lifestyle, personality, and cultural background, as do younger adults. Many elderly people are afraid of the side effects related to pain medications, such as

constipation, as a result, do not report that they are in pain or ask for medication to relieve pain. Others fail to seek care because they fear that the pain may indicate serious illness or that pain relief will be associated with a loss of independence. Nurses are aware that confusion in the elderly may be a result of untreated and unrelieved pain. In some cases, postoperative confusion clears once the pain is relieved. Pain assessment and the adequate treatment of pain in the elderly should not only be based on the patient's report of pain but age related changes and their implication to treatment. Table 7-1 provides gerontologic considerations related to pain management.

Gender

Women and African Americans are more likely to report pain than are men and whites, respectively; however, because of the highly individualized nature of pain, a "one size fits all" treatment plan for pain is ineffective and potentially harmful (Cohen & Raja, 2016).

PAIN ASSESSMENT

The role of primary health care providers is to assess and relieve pain by administering medications and other treatments. Nurses collaborate with other health care professionals while administering most pain relief interventions, evaluating their effectiveness, and serving as patient advocates when the intervention is ineffective. In addition, nurses serve as educators to patients and families, teaching them to manage the pain relief regimen themselves when appropriate.

The definition of pain forwarded by the International Association for the Study of Pain identified at the beginning of this chapter encompasses the multidimensional nature of pain. An early broad definition of pain by McCaffery is, "whatever the person says it is, existing whenever the experiencing person says it does" (McCaffery & Pasero, 1999, p. 5). This definition emphasizes the highly subjective nature of pain and pain management. Patients are the best authority on the existence of pain. Therefore, validation of the existence of pain is based on the patient's report that it exists.

Pain assessment is one core element of patient care that requires ongoing surveillance. Self-report of pain intensity and distress should be used whenever possible. Regular assessment and documentation of pain assessment help monitor the efficacy of analgesic modalities.

Although it is important to believe patients who report pain, it is equally important to be alert to patients who deny pain in situations where pain would be expected. A nurse who suspects pain in a patient who denies it should explore with the patient the reason for suspecting pain, such as discussing the fact that the disorder or procedure is painful for most people or pointing out that the patient grimaces when moving or avoids movement. It also may be helpful to explore why the patient may be denying pain. Some people deny pain because they fear the treatment that may result if they report or admit pain. Others deny pain for fear of becoming addicted to **opioids** (previously referred to as narcotics) if these medications are prescribed. The American Pain Foundation developed the Pain Care Bill of Rights, which addresses the importance of pain management (Box 7-3).

The highly subjective nature of pain means that pain assessment and management present challenges for all clinicians. The report of pain is a social transaction; that is, the assessment and management of pain will require the establishment of rapport and trust with the person in pain. In assessing a patient with pain, the nurse reviews the patient's description of the pain and other factors that may influence

pain (e.g., previous experience, anxiety, age) as well as the patient's response to pain relief strategies. Documentation of the pain level as rated on a pain scale becomes part of the patient's medical record, as does the record of the pain relief obtained from interventions.

Pain assessment includes determining what level of pain relief the acutely ill patient believes is needed to recover quickly or improve function, or what level of relief the chronically or terminally ill patient requires to maintain comfort. Part of a thorough pain assessment is understanding the patient's expectations and misconceptions about pain, which may include the notion that pain is a normal experience, that pain builds character, that pain medication side effects are worse than the pain, and the fear of becoming addicted to opioids. People who understand that pain relief not only contributes to comfort but also hastens recovery are more likely to request or self-administer treatment appropriately.

Nursing Alert
Previously, pain assessment had been referred to as "the fifth vital sign" to emphasize its significance in data collection and to increase the awareness among health care professionals of the importance of the relationship between pain and health. However, research reveals that the routine measurement of pain as the fifth vital sign did not increase the quality of pain management (Alexander, Kruszewski, & Webster, 2012). Since pain is subjective and not an objective sign that can be measured, it is important for nurses to recognize that routine documentation of pain intensity (i.e., rating of 0 to 10), while important to care, is limited in its singular ability to improve the quality of pain management. The intent of this chapter is to present the scope of pain assessment and interventions available for the RN. In addition, it is important for nurses to know that pain assessment and management are mandated by The Joint Commission (2016).

Characteristics of Pain

The factors to consider in a complete pain assessment are the intensity, timing, location, quality, and personal meaning of pain; aggravating and alleviating factors; and pain behaviors. Pain assessment begins by careful patient observation, noting overall posture and presence or absence of overt pain behaviors. In addition, it is essential to ask the patient to describe the specifics of the pain. The words used to describe the pain may point toward the cause. For example, the classic description of chest pain that results from a myocardial infarction includes pressure or squeezing on the chest. A detailed history should follow the initial description of pain.

Intensity

The intensity of pain ranges from none to mild discomfort to excruciating. There is no correlation between reported

---

BOX 7-3 Pain Care Bill of Rights

Although not always required by law, these are the rights you should expect and, if necessary, demand, for your pain care.
As a person with pain, you have the right to:

- Have your report of pain taken seriously and be treated with dignity and respect by doctors, nurses, pharmacists, and other health care professionals.
- Have your pain thoroughly assessed and promptly treated.
- Be informed by your health care provider about what may be causing the pain, possible treatments, and the benefits, risks, and cost of each.
- Participate actively in decisions about how to manage your pain.
- Have your pain reassessed regularly and your treatment adjusted if your pain has not been eased.
- Be referred to a pain specialist if your pain persists.
- Get clear and prompt answers to your questions, take time to make decisions, and refuse a particular type of treatment if you choose.

Courtesy of the American Pain Foundation, 201 N. Charles Street, Suite 710, Baltimore, Maryland, 21201, www.painfoundation.org

intensity and the stimulus that produced it. The reported intensity is influenced by the person's **pain threshold** and **pain tolerance**. Pain threshold is the smallest stimulus for which a person reports pain, and pain tolerance is the maximum amount of pain a person can tolerate. To understand variations, the nurse can ask about the present pain intensity as well as the least and the worst pain intensity. Various scales and surveys are helpful to patients trying to describe pain intensity; see the later discussion of Instruments for Assessing the Perception of Pain on page 205.

Timing

Sometimes the cause of pain can be determined when its temporal aspects are known. Therefore, the nurse inquires about the onset and duration of pain, the relationship between time and intensity (e.g., at what time is the pain worst), and changes in rhythmic patterns. The patient is asked if the pain began suddenly or increased gradually. Sudden pain that rapidly reaches maximum intensity is indicative of tissue rupture; thus immediate assessment and intervention is necessary. Pain from chronic ischemia gradually increases and becomes intense over a longer time. The chronic (or persistent) pain of arthritis illustrates the usefulness of determining the relationship between time and intensity because people with arthritis usually report that pain is worse in the morning.

Location

The location of pain is best determined by having the patient point to the area of the body involved. Some general assessment forms include drawings of human figures, on which the patient is asked to shade in the area involved. This is especially helpful if the pain radiates (**referred pain**). The

shaded figures are helpful in determining the effectiveness of treatment or change in the location of pain over time.

Nursing Alert
Patients with irritation of a visceral organ frequently complain of pain that is referred—that is, pain is sensed not at that site but a distance away. A factor associated with this finding is that the structure developed from the same embryonic segment or dermatome. Thus, since the heart and the arm have the same segmental origin, chest pain may be referred to the arm, and since the testicle migrated from where the kidney and ureter also developed, ureter distension may cause testicular pain. In addition, irritation under the diaphragm may be referred to the shoulder. Common sites of pain referral assist the clinician in considering sources for the patient's complaints. See Figure 7-2.

Quality

The nurse asks the patient to describe the pain without offering clues. For example, the nurse asks the patient to describe what the pain feels like. The nurse must give the patient sufficient time to describe the pain and then record all words in the answer. If the patient cannot describe the quality of the pain, the nurse can suggest words such as burning, aching, throbbing, or stabbing. It is important to document the exact words used by the patient to describe the pain and which words were suggested by the nurse conducting the assessment.

Personal Meaning

Pain means different things to different people; as a result, patients experience pain differently. The meaning of the

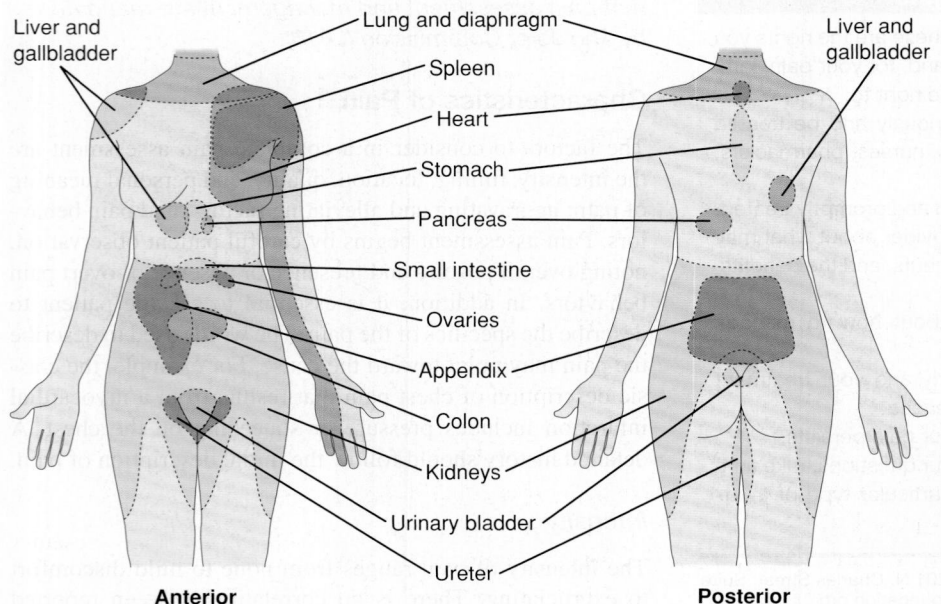

Liver and gallbladder — Lung and diaphragm — Spleen — Heart — Stomach — Pancreas — Small intestine — Ovaries — Appendix — Colon — Kidneys — Urinary bladder — Ureter

Liver and gallbladder

Anterior **Posterior**

FIGURE 7-2 Referred pain. Certain visceral organs can refer pain to specific cutaneous areas. If all special tests are negative yet the individual continues to feel pain at a specific site, it may be referred pain. (From Marcia K Anderson, Foundations of Athletic Training.)

pain experience helps the clinician understand how the patient is affected and assists in planning treatment. It is important to ask how the pain impacts the person's daily life. Some people with pain can continue to work or study, whereas others may be disabled by their pain, which may affect family finances. For some patients, the recurrence of pain may mean worsening of disease, such as the spread of cancer.

Aggravating and Alleviating Factors

The nurse asks the patient what, if anything, makes the pain worse and what makes it better, and asks specifically about the relationship between activity and pain. This helps detect factors associated with pain. For example, in a patient with advanced metastatic cancer, pain with coughing may signal spinal cord compression. The nurse also ascertains whether environmental factors influence pain because they may be modified more easily than other factors. For example, making the room warmer may aid in patient relaxation, which may decrease the person's pain. Finally, the nurse asks the patient whether the pain is influenced by or affects the quality of sleep or anxiety. Both can significantly influence pain intensity and the quality of life.

Knowledge of alleviating factors assists the nurse in developing a treatment plan. Therefore, it is important to ask about the patient's use of medications (prescribed and over-the-counter [OTC]), including amount and frequency. In addition, the nurse asks if herbal remedies, nonpharmacologic interventions, or alternative therapies have been used with success. This information assists the nurse in determining teaching needs.

Pain Behaviors

When experiencing pain, people express pain through many different behaviors. Nonverbal and behavioral expressions of pain can be useful indicators of the quality or intensity of pain. A patient may grimace, cry, rub the affected area, guard the affected area, or immobilize it. Others may moan, groan, grunt, or sigh. Not all patients exhibit the same behaviors, and different meanings may be associated with the same behavior.

Sometimes, in nonverbal patients, pain behaviors are used as a proxy to assess pain. It is unwise to make judgments and formulate treatment plans based on behaviors that may or may not indicate pain. In unconscious patients, pain should be assumed to be present and treated. All patients have a right to adequate pain management.

Physiologic responses to acute pain, such as tachycardia, hypertension, tachypnea, pallor, diaphoresis, mydriasis (pupillary dilatation), hypervigilance, and increased muscle tone, are related to stimulation of the autonomic nervous system. These responses are short-lived as the body adapts to the stress. These physiologic signs could be the result of a change in the patient's condition, such as the onset of

hypovolemia. Use of physiologic signs to indicate pain is unreliable. Although it is important to observe for any and all pain behaviors, the absence of these behaviors does not indicate an absence of pain.

Instruments for Assessing the Perception of Pain

Only the patient can describe and assess the individual pain experience accurately. Therefore, a number of pain assessment tools have been developed to assist in the assessment of the patient's perception of pain. Such tools may be used to document the need for intervention, to evaluate the effectiveness of the intervention, and to identify the need for alternative or additional interventions if the initial intervention is ineffective in relieving the pain. For a pain assessment tool to be useful, it must require little effort on the part of the patient, be easy to understand and use, be easily scored, and be sensitive to small changes in the characteristic being measured. Figure 7-3 shows a pain assessment pathway that can be used at the time of assessment to direct clinical decisions for pain management.

> **Nursing Alert**
> *Pain scores represent an important component of pain management; however, other assessments can add data to your assessment and may include consideration of functional ability, psychological and emotional functioning, satisfaction ratings with their current treatment, and inquiring about any adverse treatment effects.*

Visual Analogue Scales

Visual analogue scales (VAS) are useful in assessing the intensity of pain (Fig. 7-4). One version of the scale includes a horizontal 10-cm line, with anchors (ends) indicating the extremes of pain. The patient is asked to place a mark indicating where the current pain lies on the line. The left anchor usually represents "none" or "no pain," whereas the right anchor usually represents "severe" or "worst possible pain." To score the results, a ruler is placed along the line, and the distance the patient marked from the left or low end is measured and reported in millimeters or centimeters.

Some patients (e.g., children, elderly patients, visually or cognitively impaired patients) may find it difficult to use an unmarked VAS. In those circumstances, ordinal scales, such as a simple descriptive pain intensity scale or a 0-to-10 numeric pain intensity scale, may be used.

Faces Pain Scale—Revised

The revised faces pain scale uses six facial expressions that range from contented to obvious distress (Fig. 7-5). The patient is asked to point to the face that most closely resembles the experienced pain intensity.

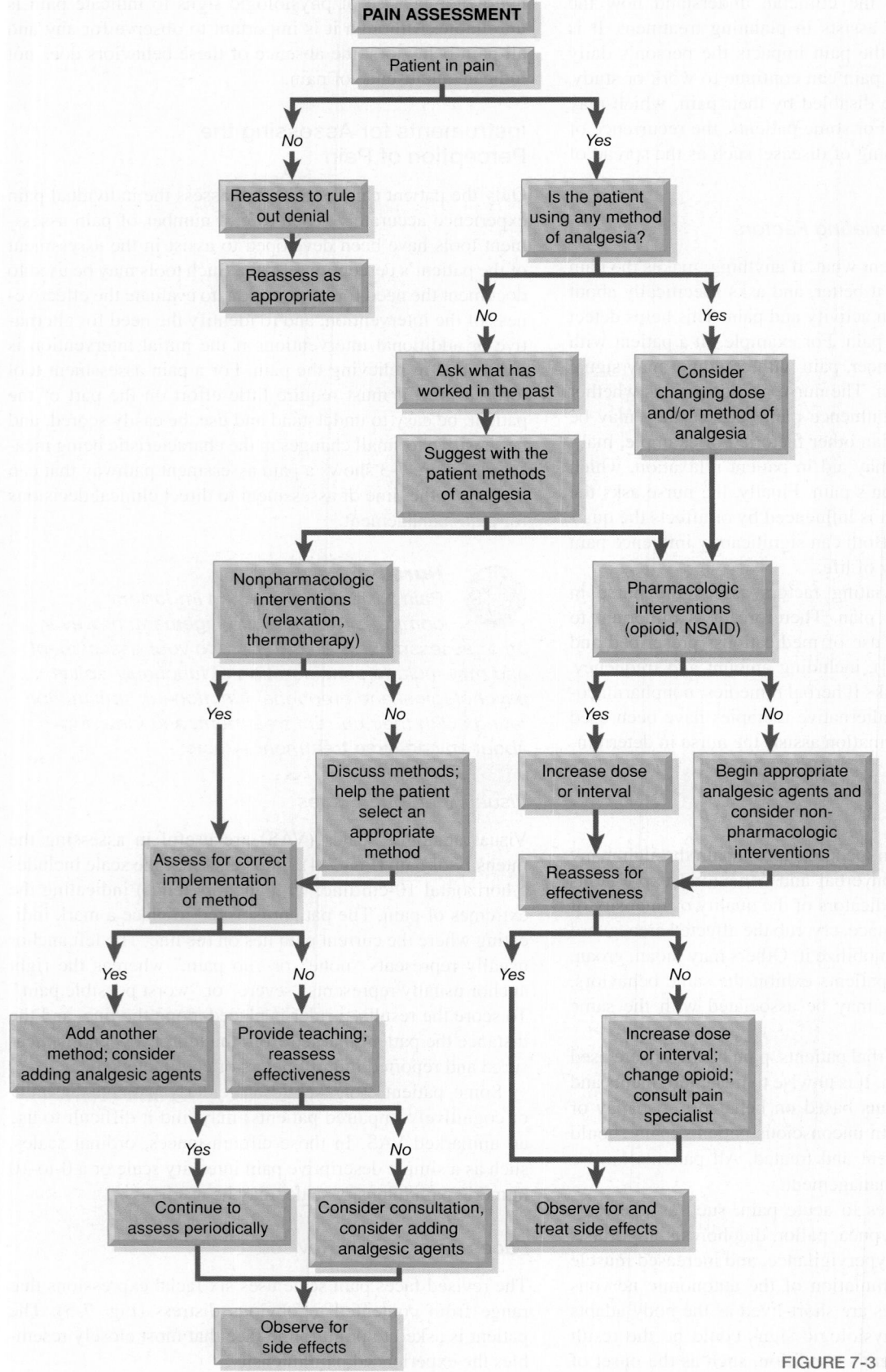

FIGURE 7-3 Pain assessment pathway.

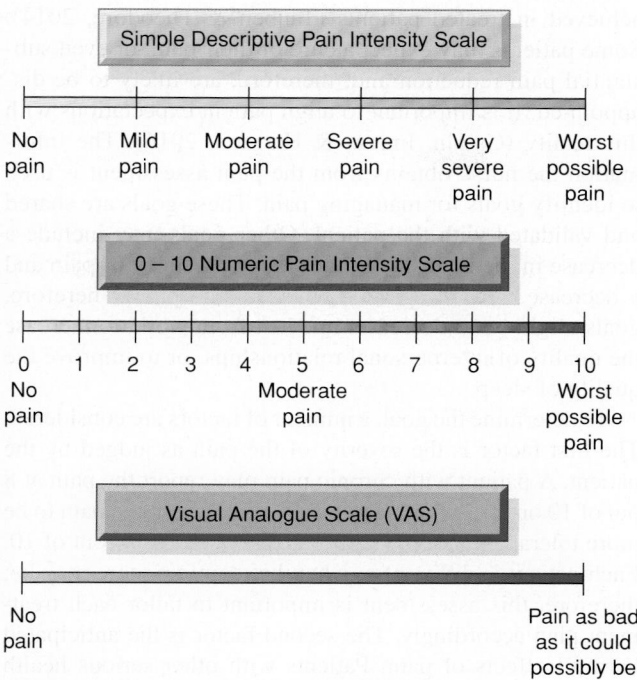

FIGURE 7-4 Examples of pain intensity scales.

and explain "pain that is a 5 or 6" is pain that can interrupt focus or concentration. This means the patient has difficulty reading a book or watching TV because the pain can be disruptive intermittently. Pain that is higher than "7 or 8" may cause the patient to think or focus only on pain. A "pain that is a 9 or 10" can mean the patient cannot even think clearly or do anything because the pain is the worst pain imaginable. The patient's numerical rating is documented and used to assess the effectiveness of pain relief interventions.

If a particular patient does not speak English or cannot clearly communicate information needed to manage pain, an interpreter/translator and/or caregivers familiar with the person's method of communication should be consulted and a method established for pain assessment. Often, a chart can be constructed with English words on one side and the foreign language on the other. Then the patient can point to the corresponding word to tell the nurse about the pain.

When people with pain are cared for at home by family caregivers or home care nurses, a pain scale may help assess the effectiveness of the interventions if the scale is used before and after the interventions are implemented. Scales that address the location and pattern of pain may be useful in identifying new sources or sites of pain in patients who are chronically or terminally ill and in monitoring changes in the patient's level of pain. For example, a home care nurse who sees a patient only at intervals may benefit from consulting the patient's or family's written record of pain scores to evaluate how effective the pain management strategies have been over time.

Guidelines for Using Pain Assessment Scales

Using a written scale to assess pain may not be possible if a person is seriously ill, is in severe pain, or has just returned from surgery. In these cases, the nurse can ask the patient, "On a scale of 0–10, 0 being no pain and 10 being the worse pain that you can ever imagine, how bad is your pain?" For patients who have difficulty with a 0 to 10 scale, a 0 to 5 scale may be tried. Whichever scale is used, it should be used consistently. Most patients usually can respond without difficulty. Ideally, the nurse teaches the patient how to use the pain scale before the pain occurs (e.g., before surgery). The nurse can integrate function into the pain scale

Guidelines for Assessing Pain in Patients with Disabilities

Alternative forms of communication may be necessary for people with sensory impairments or other disabilities.

- For people who are blind and who know how to read Braille, pain assessment instruments can be obtained in

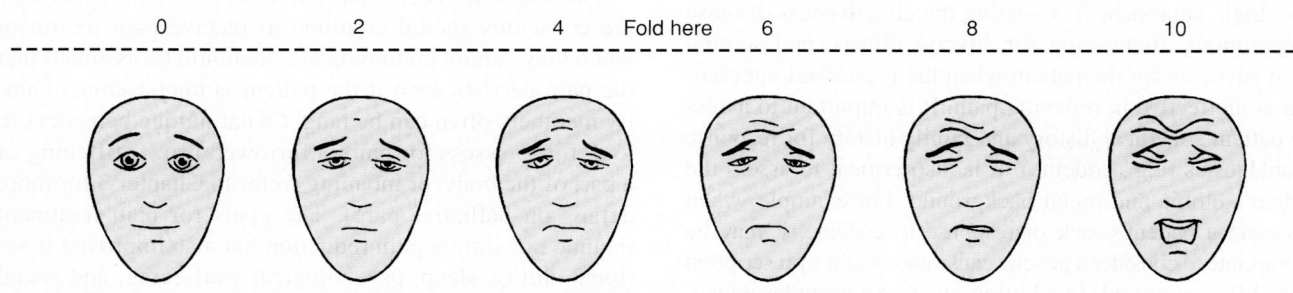

FIGURE 7-5 Faces Pain Scale—Revised. This pain scale is especially suited for helping children describe pain. Instructions for using this scale follow: "These faces show how much something can hurt. This face (*point to left-most face*) shows *no pain*. The faces show more and more pain (*point to each from left to right*) up to this one (*point to right-most face*). It shows *very much pain*. Point to the face that shows how much you hurt (right now)." Score the chosen face 0, 2, 4, 6, 8, or 10, counting left to right, so 0 = no pain and 10 = very much pain. Do not use words like "happy" or "sad." This scale is intended to measure how children feel inside, not how their face looks. (From *The pediatric pain sourcebook*. Used with permission of the International Association for the Study of Pain and the Pain Research Unit, Sydney Children's Hospital, Randwick NSW 2031, Australia.)

Braille. In addition, computer software is available that allows written documents to be scanned and converted into Braille. If these programs are not available, agencies that provide services for people who are blind may be able to assist in developing Braille versions.

- For people who are deaf or hard of hearing, outside interpreters (i.e., not family members) should be used. Other useful communication strategies may include sign language, written notes, or pictures. When writing notes on a "magic slate" or making written notes, it is necessary to make every effort to guard the patient's privacy and confidentiality.
- For people with disabilities that result in communication impairment, computer-generated speech may be useful.

> ### Nursing Alert
> *For people with cognitive impairment, a triangulated approach may be useful, which includes self-report, caregiver report, and direct observation. For acute pain, behaviors that are suggestive of pain may include sympathetic nerve stimulation (increased heart rate, dilated pupils, diaphoresis, hypertension), grimacing, frowning, changes in sleep patterns and nutritional intake, vocalizations (noisy respirations, moaning), changes in mental status (confusion, irritability), guarding, bracing, and behavioral changes (aggressive, disruptive, social withdrawal) (Stewart et al., 2014). The nurse is aware that chronic pain is usually not associated with autonomic activation that causes the vital sign changes noted above.*

THE NURSE'S ROLE IN PAIN MANAGEMENT

The nurse helps relieve pain by administering pain-relieving interventions (including both pharmacologic and nonpharmacologic approaches), assessing the effectiveness of those interventions, monitoring for adverse effects, and serving as an advocate for the patient when the prescribed intervention is ineffective in relieving pain. It is important to assess the patient's medical history and family history for response to analgesics (e.g., codeine). It is also critical to assess the patient's ethnic and racial background. For example, when assessing a patient's lack of response to codeine, it may be appropriate to consider a genetic cause and obtain a prescription for a different opioid. In addition, the nurse provides education to the patient and family to enable them to manage the prescribed intervention themselves when appropriate.

Identifying Goals for Pain Management

Pain is a common reason most people seek care, but the literature indicates a pain reduction of only 30% is typically

achieved in treated patients (Tauben & Theodore, 2014). Some patients may expect a cure of their pain, or even substantial pain reduction and, therefore, are likely to be disappointed. It is important to align patient expectations with this reality (Calpin, Imran, & Harmon, 2016). The information the nurse obtains from the pain assessment is used to identify goals for managing pain. These goals are shared and validated with the patient. Other goals may include a decrease in the intensity, duration, or frequency of pain and a decrease in the negative effects of the pain. Therefore, goals might be to decrease time lost from work, to increase the quality of interpersonal relationships, or to improve the quality of sleep.

To determine the goal, a number of factors are considered. The first factor is the severity of the pain as judged by the patient. A patient with chronic pain may report the pain at 8 out of 10 on a daily basis; the patient may want the pain to be more tolerable and strive for a comfort score of 5 out of 10. Each patient is different in what that comfort score may be; therefore, this assessment is important to tailor each treatment plan accordingly. The second factor is the anticipated harmful effects of pain. Patients with other serious health issues are at much greater risk for harmful effects of pain than are young, healthy patients (e.g., elderly patients with unrelieved pain who have contributing comorbidities and are on chronic pain-relieving medications may be at higher risk for falls). The third factor is the anticipated duration of the pain. In patients with pain from a disease such as cancer, the pain may be prolonged, possibly for the remainder of the patient's life. Therefore, interventions will be needed for some time and should not detract from the patient's quality of life. In the acute stages of illness, the patient may be unable to participate actively in relief measures, but when the patient has sufficient mental and physical energy, the patient may learn self-management techniques to relieve the pain. Therefore, as the patient progresses through the stages of recovery, increased patient use of self-management of pain relief measures may be a goal.

Patients who receive palliative care for pain when they are conscious should continue to receive pain treatment when they cannot communicate. It should be assumed that the pain persists even if the patient is unconscious. Family members often can be taught what unique behaviors to look for to assess for pain: a furrowed brow, stiffening of a part of the body, or moaning (refer to Chapter 3 for more details on palliative care). The goals for pain treatment include not simply pain reduction but also improved functional ability, sleep, psychological well-being, and social interaction.

Providing Patient Education

Patient education is extremely important since the patient or family may be responsible for managing the pain at home and preventing or managing side effects. Teaching about pain and strategies to relieve it may reduce the threat of the pain and, thus, the pain itself, in the absence of other relief measures and may enhance the effectiveness of the pain relief measures used.

The nurse also provides information by explaining how pain can be controlled. For example, the patient should be informed that pain should be reported in the early stages. When the patient waits too long to report pain, **sensitization** may occur, and the pain may become so intense that it is difficult to relieve. Sensitization results from a heightened nervous system response after exposure to a noxious (pain) stimulus. This results in an increased and prolonged pain experience. When health care providers assess and treat pain before it becomes severe, sensitization is diminished or avoided, and less medication is needed.

Providing Physical Care

Patients in pain may be unable to participate in the usual activities of daily living or to perform usual self-care and may need assistance to carry out these activities. Usually patients are more comfortable when physical and self-care needs have been met and efforts have been made to ensure the patient is in as comfortable a position as possible. A fresh gown and change of bed linens, along with efforts to make the person feel refreshed (e.g., brushing teeth, combing hair), often increase the level of comfort and improve the effectiveness of the pain relief measures.

In acute, long-term, and home settings, the nurse who provides physical care to patients also has the opportunity to perform complete assessments and to identify problems that may contribute to the patient's discomfort and pain. Appropriate and gentle physical touch during care may be reassuring and comforting. If transdermal treatments such as fentanyl (an opioid analgesic) patches or IV or epidural catheters are used, the skin around the patch or catheter should be assessed for integrity during physical care.

Managing Anxiety Related to Pain

Anxiety may affect the patient's response to pain. A patient who anticipates pain may become increasingly anxious. Anticipatory guidance about the nature of the impending painful experience and the ways to reduce pain often decreases anxiety. Pain relief measures should be used **before** pain becomes severe. It is important to explain to all patients that pain relief or control is more successful if such measures begin before the pain becomes unbearable. Administering medications early before an expected painful procedure or activity will lessen pain more effectively and allow the patient to meet goals of care. A patient who experiences nausea after pain medication may feel compelled to pass on subsequent pain medication dosing, causing anxiety and pain to build. Premedicating with antiemetics or other medications is recommended to mitigate the side effects of the pain medications. The nurse is aware that, often, people who experience pain use previously learned strategies; therefore, it is important to teach the patient about measures to relieve pain. This nursing action may lessen the threat of pain and give the patient a sense of control. The patient's anxiety may be reduced by explanations that point out the degree of pain relief that can be expected from each measure. For example, a patient who is informed that an intervention may not eliminate pain completely is less likely to become anxious when a certain amount of pain persists. A positive nurse–patient relationship characterized by trust is essential. Acknowledging to the patient, "I know that you have pain," often has positive impact on the patient's psychological state. Occasionally, patients who fear that no one believes their pain feel relieved to know that the nurse believes that the pain exists.

A patient who is anxious about pain may be less tolerant of the pain, which, in turn, may increase anxiety levels. To prevent the pain and anxiety from escalating, the anxiety-producing cycle must be interrupted. A patient who suffers from an anxiety disorder that is not under control will have an effect on pain perception. Pain intensity is heightened, and the response to pain may cause more undue stress.

PAIN MANAGEMENT STRATEGIES

Reducing pain to a "tolerable or comfort" level is considered the goal of pain management. Looking further, even patients who have described pain relief as adequate often report disturbed sleep and marked distress because of pain. In view of the harmful effects of pain and inadequate pain management, the goal of the nurse is that of relieving pain. Pain management strategies include both pharmacologic and nonpharmacologic approaches. These approaches are selected on the basis of the requirements and goals of particular patients.

> **Nursing Alert**
> *Analgesic medications are appropriate when patients are in pain. These agents are not considered a last resort to be used only when other pain relief measures fail. Any intervention is most successful if it is initiated before pain sensitization occurs, and usually the greatest success is achieved if several interventions are applied simultaneously. Nonpharmacologic interventions include efforts to create a quiet environment, comfort measures (e.g., back rub, change of position, use of heat or cold compresses), use of relaxation exercises (e.g., focused breathing, visualization, guided imagery), and diversional or distraction activities (Murr & Doenges, 2016).*

Pharmacologic Interventions

Pharmacologic management of pain is accomplished in collaboration and communication with health care providers, patients, and, often, families. A physician, nurse practitioner, or physician assistant prescribes specific medications for pain or may insert an IV line for administration of analgesic medications. Alternatively, an anesthesiologist or nurse anesthetist may insert an epidural catheter for administration of such analgesic agents. However, it is the nurse who maintains the analgesia, assesses its effectiveness, and reports whether the intervention is ineffective or produces side effects.

There are three general categories of analgesic agents: opioids, NSAIDs, and adjuvants. These agents work by different mechanisms. Adjunctive agents, such as antidepressant and antiseizure medications, local anesthetics, topical agents, baclofen, and NMDA receptor antagonists also may be used.

Opioid Analgesic Agents

The goal of administering opioids is to relieve pain and improve quality of life; therefore, the route of administration, dose, and frequency of administration are determined on an individual basis. Factors that are considered in determining the route, dose, and frequency of medication include the characteristics of the pain (e.g., its expected duration and severity), the overall status of the patient (e.g., NPO status), the patient's response to analgesic medications, and the patient's report of pain. Opioids can be administered by various routes—oral, IV, subcutaneous, intraspinal, intranasal, buccal mucosa, rectal, and transdermal. Although the oral route is usually preferred for opioid administration, oral opioids must be given frequently enough to be effective. Opioid analgesic agents given orally may provide a more consistent serum level than those given intravenously.

> **Nursing Alert**
> *The nurse recognizes that the route of administration determines response time to the medication. Intravenous (IV) medications are the most direct route, and responses are expected in the shortest time frame. The nurse also recognizes that when intramuscular (IM) or subcutaneous (SC) routes are selected, there will be variable responses depending on blood flow to the extremity.*

If the patient is expected to require opioid analgesic agents at home, the clinician should consider the ability of the patient and family to administer opioids as prescribed at the planning stages and should take steps to ensure that the required medications will be available to the patient. Many pharmacies, especially those in smaller rural areas or inner cities, may be reluctant to stock large amounts of opioids. Therefore, arrangements must be made ahead of time for obtaining these prescription medications.

Side Effects

With the administration of opioids by any route, side effects must be considered and anticipated. Clinicians who take steps to minimize the side effects increase the likelihood that the patient will receive adequate pain relief without interrupting therapy to treat the effects.

Respiratory Depression and Sedation. Respiratory depression is the most serious adverse effect of opioid analgesic agents administered intravenously, subcutaneously, or by an epidural route. However, respiratory depression is relatively rare because doses administered through these routes are small, and tolerance to respiratory depressant effects increases if the dose is increased slowly. The risk of respiratory depression increases with age and with the concomitant use of other opioids or other CNS depressants.

A patient who receives opioids by any route must be assessed frequently for changes in respiratory status (see Box 7-6). Specific notable changes are shallow respirations, decreasing respiratory rate, hypercarbia (increased carbon dioxide in blood), and decreasing oxygen saturation. Sedation, which may occur with any method of opioid administration, is likely to occur when opioid doses are increased. However, patients often develop tolerance so that, in time, they are no longer sedated by the dose that had caused sedation initially. Increasing the time between doses or reducing the dose temporarily, as prescribed, usually prevents deep sedation from occurring. The institution of a continuous pulse oximetry and or end tidal CO_2 monitoring may be initiated by the nurse for closer monitoring for patients at risk for respiratory depression. Patients at risk for sedation must be monitored closely for changes in respiratory status. Patients are also at risk for problems associated with sedation and immobility. The nurse must initiate strategies to prevent problems, such as skin breakdown.

Nausea and Vomiting. Nausea and vomiting frequently occur with opioid use. Usually these effects can occur immediately or hours after initial administration. Patients, especially postoperative patients, may not think to tell the nurse that they are nauseated, particularly if the nausea is mild. However, a patient receiving opioids should be assessed for nausea and vomiting, which may be triggered by a position change and may be prevented by having the patient change positions slowly. Adequate hydration and the administration of antiemetic agents may also decrease the incidence of nausea. Opioid-induced nausea and vomiting often subside within a few days.

Constipation. Constipation, a common side effect of opioid use, may become so severe that the patient is forced to choose between relief of pain and relief of constipation. This situation can occur in patients after surgery and in patients receiving large doses of opioids to treat cancer-related pain. Preventing constipation must be a high priority in all patients receiving opioids, and an effective bowel program is needed. Whenever a patient receives opioids, a bowel regimen should begin at the same time. Tolerance to this side effect does not occur; rather, constipation persists even with long-term use of opioids.

Several strategies may help prevent and treat opioid-related constipation. Mild laxatives and a high intake of fluid and fiber may be effective in managing mild constipation. Unless contraindicated, a mild laxative and a stool softener should be administered on a regular schedule. However, continued severe constipation often requires the use of a stimulating cathartic agent, such as senna derivatives (Senokot™) or bisacodyl (Dulcolax™). Additional laxatives used include suppositories, enemas, and lactulose, along with diet modification and increased intake of fluid and fiber (Leonard & Baker, 2015). Three medications are approved specifically for opioid-induced constipation: naloxegol, lubiprostone, and methylnaltrexone. The newest medication, naloxegol, is pegylated naloxone (narcan) molecule with mu-opioid antagonist activity and is effective in countering the gastric peristaltic effects of morphine without a significant effect on analgesia (Leonard & Baker, 2015). However, it is classified as a Schedule II drug under the Controlled Substance Act because of its structural relationship to noroxymorphone, thus it remains to be seen if the increased cost and increased provider visits will limit its use.

Pruritus and Urinary Retention. When asked about drug allergies, patients with previous hospital experience (especially for surgery) may report that they are "allergic" to morphine. This report should be investigated thoroughly. Commonly, this allergy is described as itching only. Pruritus (itching) is a frequent side effect of opioids administered by any route, but it is not an allergic reaction. It can be relieved by administering prescribed antihistamines. Epidural or continuous intravenous administration of opioids also may cause urinary retention. The patient should be monitored and may require urinary catheterization. A weight-based low-dose naloxone infusion may be prescribed to relieve problems of nausea, vomiting, itching, urinary retention, and ileus in patients who are receiving continuous opioids for the relief of acute postoperative pain.

Endocrine Deficiencies. The nurse understands that chronic use of opioids is associated with decreased testosterone levels, leading to hypogonadism, sexual dysfunction, infertility, and accelerated osteoporosis (exact mechanism for osteopenia and osteoporosis is not known). Opioid-induced hypogonadism is treatable with appropriate hormone replacement therapy. Screening should be considered for osteoporosis for patients on chronic opioid medication. Refer to Chapter 41 for details on osteoporosis.

Inadequate Pain Relief
One factor commonly associated with ineffective pain relief is an inadequate dose of opioids. This is most likely to occur when the caregiver underestimates the patient's pain or fails to consider differences in absorption and action after a change in the route of administration. Consequently, the patient receives doses that are too small to be effective and, possibly, too infrequent to relieve pain. For example, if opioid delivery is changed from the IV route to the oral route, the oral dose must be approximately three times greater than that given parenterally to provide relief. Because of differences in absorption of orally administered opioids among individuals, patients must be assessed carefully to ensure that the pain is relieved.

Table 7-2 lists opioids and dosages that are equivalent to morphine; Table 7-3 is an equianalgesic table that providers may use when changing routes of administration (e.g., from IV to oral medications in preparation for patient discharge). These tables serve only as a guide; the doses listed are not necessarily the most appropriate doses for all patients. However, the tables do give clinicians some idea of equivalency.

After administering the first dose of an opioid, the nurse should perform a complete pain assessment to determine the efficacy of that dose. The time, date, patient's pain rating (scale of 0 to 10), analgesic agent, other pain relief measures, side effects, and patient activity are recorded. If the pain has not decreased in 30 minutes (sooner if an IV route is used) and the patient is reasonably alert and has a satisfactory respiratory status, blood pressure, and pulse rate, then some change in analgesia is indicated. In general, calculate the equianalgesic dose of the new opioid, and then reduce the dose by 50% to avoid potential cross-tolerance (Therapeutic Research Center [TRC], 2012). Cross-tolerance is a phenomenon that occurs when a patient who is tolerant to the effects of a certain pharmaceutical agent also develops a tolerance to another agent. From here, the dose can be adjusted to each individual response. Although extended-release agents come in the same dosage form and contain the same drug, they are not considered therapeutically equivalent because they use different release mechanisms. Patients who need to change brands should be monitored carefully both for overdose and for inadequate pain relief.

Because of the fear of promoting addiction or causing respiratory depression, health care providers tend to prescribe and administer inadequate dosages of opioid agents to treat acute pain or persistent pain, particularly in patients who are terminally ill. Long-term use of opioids can lead to dependence and addiction (Slover, Zieg, & Clopton, 2015). In the past decade there has been a dramatic increase in opioid prescriptions, which is associated with increased abuse, overdose, and accidental deaths. In primary care settings, prevalence of opioid abuse ranged from 0.6% to 8%. In pain clinic settings, prevalence of addiction ranged from 2% to 14% (Chou et al., 2015). Currently, there is a general agreement that opioids are overprescribed; that education regarding management of acute and chronic pain by health care providers is essential; and that efforts must be made to balance between treating patients in pain and mitigating abuse, overdoses, and related deaths (Atkinson, Schatman, & Fudin, 2014).

Genetic factors play a role in the varied responses to NSAIDs and opioids seen in patients. There appears to be

TABLE 7-2 Selected Opioid Analgesic Agents Commonly Used for Moderate and Severe Pain in Adults

| Name | Starting Dose (milligrams) | | Comments | Precautions and Contraindications |
	Moderate Pain	Severe Pain		
Morphine	—	30–60 (oral) 10 (parenteral)	Agonist at specific opioid receptors in the CNS to produce analgesia, euphoria, and sedation	Use with caution, especially in elderly patients, very ill patients, and those with respiratory impairment. Major risks include respiratory depression, apnea, circulatory depression, and respiratory arrest, shock, and cardiac arrest. Obtain history of hypersensitivity to opioids. Monitor patient closely. If prescribed in correct dose, oral preparations are effective in treating moderate and severe pain.
Codeine	15–30 (oral)	60 (oral) up to 360/24 hr	Agonist at specific opioid receptors in the CNS to produce analgesia, euphoria, and sedation. Is also an antitussive. 10% of people lack the enzyme needed to make codeine active. Codeine may cause more nausea and constipation per unit of analgesia than other mu-agonist opioids.	Many preparations of codeine and the other opioids in this table are combinations with nonopioid analgesics. Caution must be used in patients with impaired ventilation, bronchial asthma, increased intracranial pressure, or impaired liver function and in elderly and very ill patients.
Oxycodone (OxyContin™)	5 (oral)	10–20 (oral)	Agonist at specific opioid receptors in the CNS to produce analgesia, euphoria, and sedation	Caution must be used in patients with impaired ventilation, bronchial asthma, increased intracranial pressure, or impaired liver function and in elderly and very ill patients.
Meperidine (Demerol™)	50 (oral)	300 (oral) 75 (parenteral)	Agonist at specific opioid receptors in the CNS to produce analgesia, euphoria, and sedation. Shorter acting than morphine. Meperidine is biotransformed to normeperidine, a toxic metabolite.	Normeperidine, a toxic metabolite of meperidine, accumulates with repetitive dosing, causing CNS excitation. High risk for seizures. No longer recommended for the management of pain due to its transformation to a toxic metabolite and poor analgesic properties. Used in the presence of postoperative shivering. Avoided in patients with impaired kidney function who are receiving MAO inhibitors. Is irritating to tissues with repeated intramuscular injections. Should not be used for more than 1 or 2 days.
Hydrocodone (Vicodin™)	5–10 (oral)	—	—	Most preparations are combined with nonopioid analgesics.
Tramadol (Ultram™)	50–100 (oral)	—	Unique mechanism; analgesia results from the synergy of two mechanisms. Maximum dose is 400 mg/day.	Most common side effects are dizziness, nausea, constipation, and somnolence. Lowers seizure threshold.

CNS, central nervous system; MAO, monoamine oxidase.
Adapted from American Pain Society. (2008). *Principles of analgesic use in the treatment of acute pain and chronic cancer pain* (6th ed.). Skokie, I. L., and Karch, A. M. (2013). *Focus on nursing pharmacology*. Philadelphia, PA: Lippincott Williams & Wilkins.

TABLE 7-3 Approximate Dose Equivalents for Opioid Analgesics[a]

Drug	Oral Dose (mg)	Parenteral Dose[b]
Morphine[c]	30	10 mg
Codeine[d]	200	100–120 mg
Fentanyl[e,f]	NA	100 µg or 0.1 mg
Hydrocodone (Vicodin)	30–45	NA
Hydromorphone (Dilaudid)[c]	7.5	1.5 mg
Levorphanol	4	1 mg
Methadone[g,h]	The conversion ratio of methadone is variable. Please refer to specific conversion tables based upon single opioid or multiple opioid regimens.	
Oxycodone (OxyContin)[d]	20	Only available orally (tablet and liquid), not available parenterally
Oxymorphone (Opana, Opana ER, and OpanaIV[c])	10	1 mg
Buprenorphine	NA	0.4 mg

IV, IV; NA, not available.

[a]Published tables vary in the suggested doses that are equianalgesic to morphine. Many of these doses are based on clinical consensus rather than well-controlled trials. Clinical response is the criterion that must be applied for each patient; titration to clinical response is necessary. Because there is not complete cross-tolerance among these drugs, usually it is necessary to use a lower-than-equianalgesic dose when changing drugs and reiterate according to response.

[b]Parenteral dosing includes IV and subcutaneous administration. Onset and duration may vary slightly between these routes; however, doses remain approximately equal. The intramuscular route is not recommended because of variability in uptake of the drug and painful injection.

[c]Caution: For morphine, hydromorphone, and oxymorphone, rectal administration is an alternate route for patients unable to take oral medications. Equianalgesic doses may differ from oral to parenteral doses because of pharmacokinetic differences. Note: A short-acting opioid normally should be used for initial therapy of moderate to severe pain.

[d]Caution: Doses of aspirin and acetaminophen in combination opioid/NSAID preparations must be adjusted to the patient's body weight.

[e]Transdermal fentanyl is an alternative. Transdermal fentanyl dosage is not calculated as equianalgesic to a single morphine dosage but is calculated based on a 24-hour opioid dose. See package insert for dosing calculations. Transdermal fentanyl should not be used in opioid-naïve patients.

[f]Transmucosal and buccal fentanyl are also available and indicated for breakthrough pain, although they are not bioequivalent. Titration of either should be conducted gradually; neither should be used in opioid-naïve patients.

[g]Caution: Methadone is much more potent than indicated in older published literature.
Potency varies and is not linear—it is noted to be between two and ten times as potent as morphine—depending on opiate history. When morphine at lower doses (e.g., 30–60 mg/d orally) is switched to methadone, the potency may be three to five times; when switched from high doses (e.g., more than 300 mg/d orally), the potency may be 12 times or even higher.

[h]Caution: The oral-to-IV dose ratio of methadone is not well established. The IV route is used very seldom except in cancer centers with a pain service that is familiar with parenteral methadone. IV use of methadone is associated with QTc wave prolongation.

a higher incidence of poor drug metabolism among Caucasians and Asian Americans compared with African Americans. The most **extensively** studied genetic variation related to pain in humans is in the metabolism of codeine. Drug metabolism involves genetically controlled enzyme activity for absorption, distribution, inactivation, and excretion. In studies of both experimental and clinical pain, multiple polymorphisms (DNA proteins with variant alleles) result both in poor metabolism and poor analgesic efficacy, leading to changes in drug absorption, distribution, and elimination (Edmondson, 2017).

 Nursing Alert
Conversion tables available for the transdermal systems should be used only to establish the initial dose of the transdermal fentanyl or buprenorphine when patients switch from oral morphine to the transdermal route of delivery (and not vice versa). If these tables are used inappropriately to determine the dosages of oral morphine for patients who have been receiving transdermal fentanyl or buprenorphine, many patients will not achieve satisfactory analgesia and will require an increase in their opioid dose to treat breakthrough pain.

Nursing Alert
If the conversion table or equation is used incorrectly to calculate a morphine dose, there is a risk of overdose. If a patient requires a change from transdermal fentanyl or buprenorphine back to oral or IV morphine (as in the case of surgery), the patch should be removed and IV morphine administered on an as-needed basis. Before a new patch is applied, the patient should be checked carefully for any older, forgotten patches, which should be removed and discarded. Patches should be replaced every 72 hours.

Opioid Use with Selected Conditions and Medications

A number of factors may influence the safety and effectiveness of opioid administration. Opioid analgesic agents are primarily metabolized by the liver and excreted by the kidney. Therefore, metabolism and excretion of analgesic medications are impaired in patients with liver or kidney disease, increasing the risk of cumulative or toxic effects.

Patients with untreated hypothyroidism are more susceptible to the analgesic effects and side effects of opioids. In contrast, patients with hyperthyroidism may require larger doses for pain relief. Patients with a decreased respiratory reserve from disease or aging may be more susceptible to the depressant effects of opioids and must be monitored carefully for respiratory depression.

Patients who are dehydrated are at increased risk for the hypotensive effects of opioids. Patients who become hypotensive after the administration of an opioid should be kept recumbent and rehydrated unless fluids are contraindicated. Patients who are dehydrated also are more likely to experience nausea and vomiting with opioid use. Rehydration usually relieves these symptoms.

Patients receiving certain other medications, such as monoamine oxidase (MAO) inhibitors, phenothiazines, or tricyclic antidepressants, may have an exaggerated response to the depressant effects of opioids. Patients taking these medications should receive small doses of opioids and must be monitored closely. Continued pain in these patients indicates that a therapeutic level of the analgesic has not been achieved. Patients must be monitored for sedation even if an analgesic effect has not been obtained.

Tolerance and Addiction
There is no maximum safe dosage of opioids, nor is there any easily identifiable therapeutic serum level. Both the maximal safe dosage and the therapeutic serum level are relative and individual.

Tolerance (the need for increasing doses of opioids to achieve the same therapeutic effect) develops in almost all patients taking opioids for extended periods. Patients requiring opioids over a long term, especially cancer patients, need increasing dosages to relieve pain, although after the first few weeks of therapy, the progressively increasing dosages will no longer be required and the patient can be placed on maintenance dosages. Patients who become tolerant to the analgesic effects of large doses of morphine may obtain pain relief by changing to a different opioid. Symptoms of physical dependence may occur when the opioids are discontinued; dependence often occurs with opioid tolerance and does not indicate an addiction. It is an expected physiologic response that will occur in all people exposed to continuous opioid administration (Slover et al., 2015).

Nursing Alert
Although patients may need increasing levels of opioids, they are not addicted. Physical tolerance usually occurs in the absence of addiction. Tolerance to opioids is common and becomes a problem primarily in terms of delivering or administering the medication.

Addiction is a behavioral pattern of substance use characterized by a compulsion to take the substance (drug or alcohol) primarily to experience its psychic effects. Fear that patients will become addicted or dependent on opioids has contributed to inadequate treatment of pain. This fear is commonly expressed by health care providers as well as patients and results from lack of knowledge about the risk of addiction. Current research suggests that patients with a history of other substance abuse are at higher risk for opioid addiction. About 4% of patients treated for trauma had problems with opiates but showed other indications of addictive

behavior that correlated with their increased use (Slover et al., 2015, p. 462). Therefore, patients and health care providers should be discouraged from withholding opioid analgesics for patients in acute pain because of concerns about addiction.

Currently, over 20 million people in the United States are dealing with substance abuse disorders; thus, it is likely that nurses in acute care will encounter patients with a history of addiction seeking care for acute or chronic pain (SAMHSA, 2016). When caring for people with a known history of addiction, nurses should consider that each individual person has the right to be treated for pain. The use of multimodal analgesia is treatment strategy useful for the treatment of pain in patients with a history of addiction; the use of NSAIDs or acetaminophen, gabapentin, or duloxetine regional blocks and local infiltration of anesthetics also should be considered (Slover et al., 2015). If opioids are necessary, the use of long-acting agents is suggested, with collaboration of a multidisciplinary team (Garimella & Cellini, 2013). If prescribed, the opioids should be tapered slowly to prevent withdrawal symptoms; the use of a mutually agreeable pain contract should be considered (Garimella & Cellini, 2013). The use of complementary therapies is also suggested and is described later in the chapter.

Nursing Alert
Patients admitted to the hospital suffering from an acute illness who have a history of substance abuse and are currently on methadone maintenance treatment (MMT) should have their methadone dose continued or an equivalent opioid given to prevent craving. Also the patient's methadone treatment facility should be consulted. Additional opioids can be prescribed on an as-needed basis if indicated while applying the same monitoring guidelines for potential opioid-induced side effects. Patients can also be taking sublingual buprenorphine for the treatment of both pain and opioid use disorder (Salsitz, 2016).

Nursing Alert
Patients may be monitored during opioid therapy with urine toxicology studies. They should be informed to avoid eating poppy seeds, which can make a urine drug screen (UDS) positive for opiates, depending on where the threshold for opioid screening is set.

NSAIDs

NSAIDs are thought to decrease pain by inhibiting cyclo-oxygenase (COX), the enzyme involved in the production of prostaglandin (which is believed to increase the sensitivity of pain receptors) from traumatized or inflamed tissues. There are two types of COX: COX-1 and COX-2.

COX-1 mediates prostaglandin formation involved in the maintenance of physiologic functions, such as platelet aggregation, which prevents ischemia and promotes mucosal integrity. Inhibition of COX-1 may result in gastric ulceration, bleeding, and kidney damage.

COX-2 mediates prostaglandin formation that results in symptoms of pain, inflammation, and fever. Therefore, inhibition of COX-2 is desirable. Celecoxib (Celebrex™) is an example of a COX-2 inhibitor. There is evidence of increased cardiovascular risk associated with COX-2 inhibitors. Ibuprofen (Advil™, Motrin™), another NSAID, blocks both COX-1 and COX-2. It is effective in relieving mild to moderate pain and has a low incidence of adverse effects. Aspirin, the oldest NSAID, also blocks COX-1 as well as COX-2; however, because it causes frequent and severe side effects, aspirin is used infrequently to treat significant acute or persistent pain.

NSAIDs are very helpful in treating arthritic diseases and may be especially powerful in treating cancer-related bone pain. They have been combined effectively with opioids to treat postoperative and other severe pain. The use of NSAIDs in combination with opioids relieves pain more effectively than the use of opioids alone. In such cases, patients may obtain pain relief with decreased doses of opioids and with fewer side effects. A regimen of a fixed-dose, time-contingent NSAID (e.g., every 6 hours) and a separately administered fluctuating dose of opioid may be effective in managing moderate to severe cancer pain. In more severe pain, the opioid dose is also fixed, with an additional fluctuating dose as needed for **breakthrough pain** (a sudden increase in pain despite the administration of pain-relieving medications). Most patients tolerate NSAIDs well. However, those with impaired kidney function may require a smaller dose and must be monitored closely for side effects. Patients taking NSAIDs bruise easily because the agents have some anticoagulant effect. Furthermore, NSAIDs may displace other medications, such as warfarin (Coumadin™), from serum proteins and increase their effects. Thus, high doses or prolonged use can irritate the stomach and, in some cases, result in gastric ulcers and GI bleeding as well. For this reason, the use of NSAIDs is dependent on the individual patient's risk factors. If administered, monitoring for GI bleeding is indicated, and gastroprotective agents should be considered to prevent this complication (Ralston & McInnes, 2014).

Drug Alert!

Cardiovascular risks of NSAIDs: NSAIDs, especially COX-2 inhibitors, should be avoided or used with caution in patients with a cardiac history. The use of COX-2 inhibitors may decrease prostacyclin levels, which may lead to increased thrombotic risk (Dinakar, 2016). In addition, NSAIDs may exacerbate hypertension and heart failure as well as impair kidney function.

Local Anesthetic Agents

Local anesthetics work by blocking nerve conduction when applied directly to the nerve fibers. They can be applied directly to the site of injury (e.g., a topical anesthetic spray for sunburn) or directly to nerve fibers by injection or at the time of surgery. Also they can be administered through an epidural catheter (see later discussion of Intraspinal and Epidural Administration).

Local anesthetic agents have been successful in reducing the pain associated with thoracic or upper abdominal surgery when injected by the surgeon intercostally. Local anesthetic agents are rapidly absorbed into the bloodstream, resulting in decreased availability at the surgical or injury site and an increased anesthetic level in the blood, increasing the risk of toxicity. Therefore, a vasoconstrictive agent (e.g., epinephrine or phenylephrine) is added to the anesthetic agent to decrease its systemic absorption and maintain its concentration at the surgical or injury site.

A topical anesthetic agent known as *eutectic mixture* (emulsion of local anesthetics), or EMLA cream, has been effective in preventing the pain associated with invasive procedures, such as lumbar puncture or the insertion of IV lines. To be effective, EMLA must be applied to the site 60 minutes before the procedure.

A lidocaine 5% patch acts locally by targeting damaged nerves responsible for discharging pain impulses and is approved for limited use. The lidocaine 5% patch provides sufficient medication for anesthetic effect but not enough to cause total sensory block in the area of application so it has a wide margin of safety. The recommended dose is one to three patches at a time applied over the affected area for 12 hours daily.

Topical NSAIDs also have been beneficial in randomized controlled studies for patients with rheumatologic disorders and have demonstrated comparable efficacy for regional pain conditions but with fewer adverse effects than systemic NSAIDs (Cohen & Raja, 2016).

Antidepressant and Antiseizure Medications

Pain of neurologic origin (e.g., causalgia [intense burning pain and sensitivity to the slightest vibration or touch]), tumor impingement on a nerve, postherpetic neuralgia) is difficult to treat and, in general, is not responsive to opioid therapy. If these pain syndromes are accompanied by dysesthesia (burning or cutting pain), then they may be responsive to tricyclic antidepressants or antiseizure agents. When indicated, tricyclic antidepressant agents, such as amitriptyline (Elavil™) or imipramine (Tofranil™), are prescribed in doses considerably smaller than those generally used for depression. Since antidepressants have the FDA warnings of worsening mood and suicidal ideations, patients should be informed about side effects before beginning this treatment (Dinakar, 2016). Patients also need to know that a therapeutic effect may not occur until they have taken the medication for 4 weeks. Antiseizure medications, such as phenytoin (Dilantin™) or carbamazepine (Tegretol™), may be used in doses lower than those prescribed for seizure disorders. They may be beneficial in patients with neuropathic pain who do not respond to antidepressants; however, they also have the FDA warnings of mood changes, worsening depression, and suicidal ideation, predominantly in adolescents and young adults (Dinakar, 2016, p. 725). Because a variety of medications can be tried, nurses should be familiar with the possible side effects of each and should teach patients and families how to recognize these effects.

Approaches to Using Analgesic Agents

The nurse obtains the patient's medication history (e.g., current, usual, or recent use of prescription or OTC medications or herbal agents), along with a history of health disorders and allergies. Certain medications or conditions may affect the analgesic medication's effectiveness or its metabolism and excretion. Table 7-4 lists adverse interactions of herbal substances or foods with analgesics. Before administering analgesic agents, the nurse should assess the patient's pain status, including the intensity of current pain, changes in pain intensity after the previous dose of medication, and side effects of the medication. Medications are most effective when the dose and interval between doses are individualized to meet the needs of a particular patient.

Balanced Analgesia

Pharmacologic interventions are most effective when a multimodal, or balanced, analgesia approach is used. Multimodal analgesia combines two or more analgesic agents or techniques that act by different mechanisms to provide analgesia with better pain relief and less opioid side effects. Using two or three types of agents simultaneously can maximize pain relief while minimizing the potentially toxic effects of any one agent (Manworren, 2015). When one agent is used alone, it usually must be used in a higher dose to be effective.

Treating Cancer Pain

Different kinds of pain are treated with different medications. Multimodal analgesia is the use of opioids, nonopioid analgesics, and adjuvant agents together to maximize the efficacy and minimize side effects from one analgesic (mainly opioids) (Grisenko, Khelemsky, & Urman, 2014). The World Health Organization advocates a three-step approach to treat cancer pain (Fig. 7-6). Analgesics are administered based on the patient's level of pain. Nonopioid analgesics (e.g., acetaminophen) are used for mild pain; weak opioid analgesics (e.g., codeine) are used for moderate pain; and strong opioid analgesics (e.g., morphine) are used for severe pain. Also adjuvant medications are administered to enhance the effectiveness of analgesics. Examples of adjuvant medications include antidepressants, antiseizure agents, antispasmodics,

FIGURE 7-6 Adapted from the World Health Organization three-step ladder approach to relieving cancer pain. Various opioid (narcotic) and nonopioid medications may be combined with other medications to control pain.

local anesthetics, radiopharmaceuticals (radioactive agents that may be used to treat painful bone tumors), and corticosteroids. A cancer pain algorithm, developed as a set of analgesic guiding principles, is given in Figure 7-7.

Preventing and reducing pain help to decrease anxiety and break the pain cycle. This can be accomplished best by administering analgesics on a regularly scheduled basis as prescribed (the preventive, preferred approach to pain management), with additional analgesics administered for breakthrough pain as needed and as prescribed.

Preventive Approach

With the preventive approach, analgesic agents are administered at set intervals so that the medication acts before the pain becomes severe and before the serum opioid level decreases to a subtherapeutic level. For example, a patient takes prescribed morphine or a prescribed NSAID (e.g., ibuprofen) every 4–6 hours rather than waiting until the pain is severe. If the pain is likely to occur around the clock or for a substantial portion of a 24-hour period, a regular around-the-clock schedule of administering analgesia may be indicated. Even if the analgesic is prescribed *pro re nata* (PRN), or "as needed," it can be administered on a preventive basis before the patient is in severe pain as long as the prescribed interval between doses is observed. The preventive approach reduces the peaks and troughs in the serum level and provides more pain relief with fewer adverse effects.

Smaller doses of medication are needed with the preventive approach because the pain does not escalate to a level of severe intensity. Therefore, a preventive approach may

TABLE **7-4** Adverse Interactions of Herbal Substances or Food with Analgesics

Analgesic	Herb, Supplement, or Food	Potential Interaction
NSAID	Bilberry fruit (*Vacciniummyrtillus*)	Potential for increased bleeding if taken with anticoagulants and other antiplatelet drugs; use cautiously if taking medicinal quantities
	Chondroitin	Do not take with anticoagulants; may potentiate bleeding
	German or Hungarian chamomile (*Matricariarecutita*)	Anticoagulants may potentiate effect; use cautiously together
	Dong quai (*Angelica sinensis*)	May increase bleeding time if used with warfarin and other anticoagulant drugs
	Fenugreek (*Trigonellafoenum-graecum*)	May potentiate effects of anticoagulants
	Feverfew (*Tanacetumparthenium*)	May increase bleeding; use cautiously with anticoagulants
	Garlic (*Allium sativum*)	May increase bleeding; use cautiously with anticoagulants
	Ginger (*Zingiberofficinale*)	May increase bleeding; use cautiously with anticoagulants
	Melatonin (N-acetyl-5-methoxytryptamine)	NSAIDs and antidepressants may deplete melatonin
	Pau D'arco (*Tabebuiaimpetiginosa, T. ipe*)	May potentiate effects of anticoagulants; avoid concurrent use
	Red clover (*Trifoliumpratense*)	May increase bleeding; use cautiously with anticoagulants and antiplatelet agents
	Turmeric (*Curcuma longa*)	Avoid using large doses with anticoagulants and NSAIDs; possible additive effect for bleeding
	Willow (*Salix* spp.)	Use cautiously with NSAIDs; may increase likelihood of GI irritation and bleeding due to tannins.
Ibuprofen	St. John wort (*Hypericumperforatum*)	Mean residence time of ibuprofen may be reduced with concurrent use of St. John wort.
Acetaminophen	Watercress	May inhibit the oxidative pathway of acetaminophen metabolism.
Aspirin	Ginkgo (*Ginkgo biloba*)	May increase bleeding tendencies; patients taking aspirin should avoid concurrent use of ginkgo biloba.
	Dan shen (*Salvia miltiorrhiza*)	Avoid concurrent use with sedatives, warfarin, and aspirin.
Opioids (sedatives)	Kava-kava (*Piper methysticum*)	May potentiate action of alcohol, tranquilizers (barbiturates), and antidepressants; may increase sedative effect of anesthetics
	Sarsaparilla (*Smilax* spp.)	May increase elimination of sedatives
	Valerian (*Valeriana officinalis*)	May intensify effects of sedatives
Alfentanil, fentanyl, sufentanil	Grapefruit	Inhibits CYP3A4 and P-glycoprotein; if used in combination with drugs that are metabolized through 3A4 or via P-glycoprotein, may increase in concentration leading to potential adverse effects
	St. John wort (*Hypericumperforatum*)	May increase or decrease cyclic P-450 activity; may affect medications that are metabolized by this pathway

From Drug interactions facts™: Herbal supplements and food. (2008). St. Louis, MO: Wolters Kluwer Health/Facts and Comparisons; Kuhn, M., & Winston, D. (2008). *Herbal therapy & supplements: A scientific and traditional approach*. Philadelphia, PA: Wolters Kluwer Health/Lippincott Williams & Wilkins.

result in the administration of less medication over a 24-hour period, helping prevent tolerance to analgesic agents and decreasing the severity of side effects (e.g., sedation, constipation). Better pain control can be achieved with a preventive approach, reducing the amount of time patients are in pain.

In using the preventive approach, the nurse assesses the patient for sedation before administering the next dose. It is not safe to medicate the patient with opioids repeatedly if the patient is sedated or not in pain.

Individualized Dosage
The dosage and the interval between doses should be based on the patient's requirements rather than on an inflexible standard or routine. As noted earlier, metabolism and absorption of medications are highly variable. Therefore, a certain dose of an opioid medication given at specified intervals may be effective for one patient but ineffective for another.

As in the preventive approach discussed above, the nurse does not wait for the patient to complain of pain and then

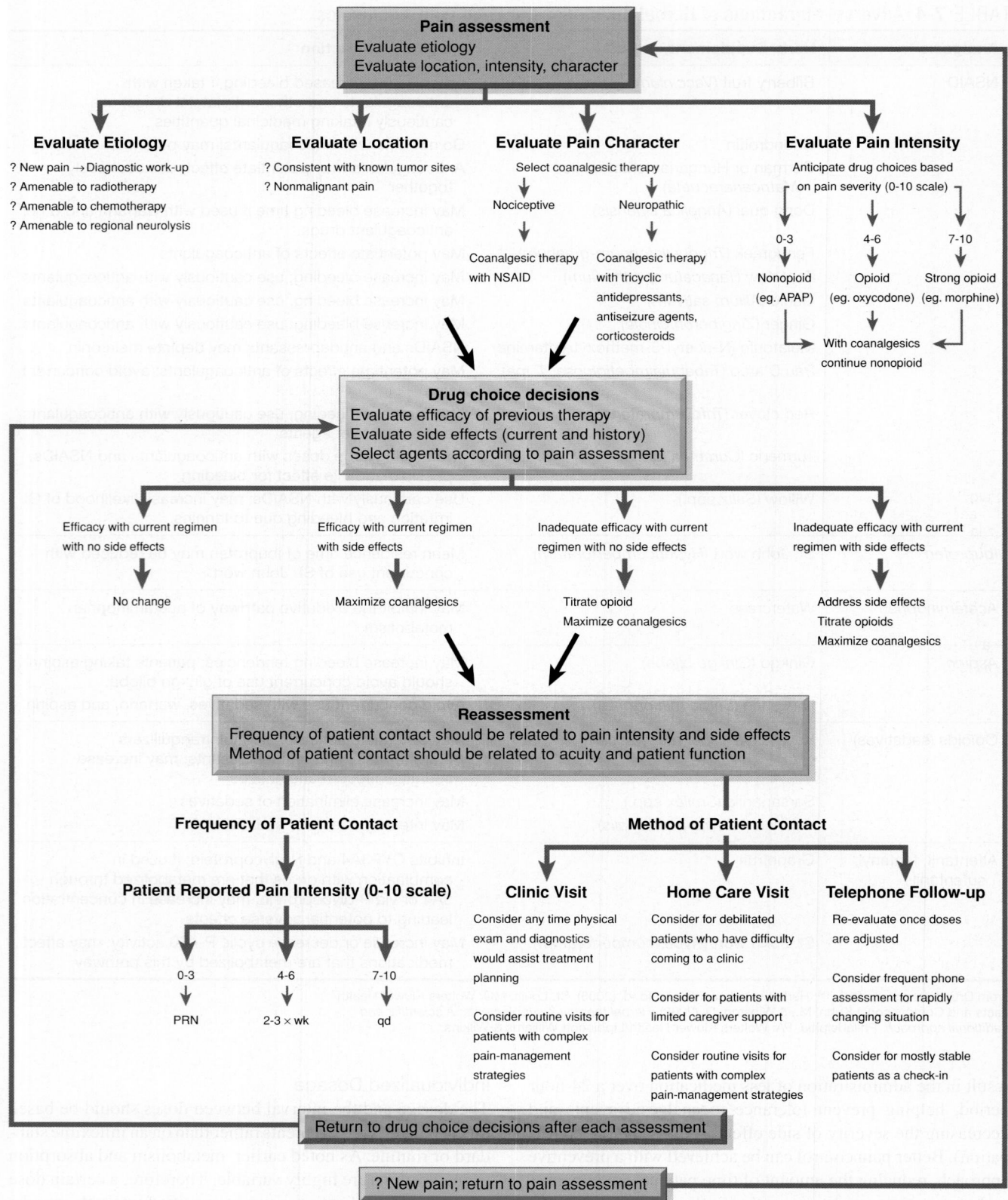

FIGURE 7-7 The cancer pain algorithm (highest-level view) is a decision-tree model for pain treatment that was developed as an interpretation of the AHCPR Guideline for Cancer Pain, 1994. (Reproduced with permission from DuPen, A. R., DuPen, S., Hansberry, J., et al. (2000). An educational implementation of a cancer pain algorithm for ambulatory care. *Pain Management Nursing*, *1*(4), 118.)

FIGURE 7-8 Relationship of mode of delivery of analgesia to serum analgesic level. *Top:* Intramuscular (IM) and IV patient-controlled analgesia (PCA). *Bottom:* Transdermal (TD) and transmucosal (•) delivery.

TD = Transdermal
• = Transmucosal

administer analgesia. To receive pain relief from an opioid analgesic, the serum level of that opioid must be maintained at a minimum therapeutic level (Fig. 7-8). The lower the serum opioid level, the more difficult it is to achieve the therapeutic level with the next dose. If pain is reported to be continuous, then a long-acting or around-the-clock administration of an opioid needs to be considered.

Routes of Administration

The route selected for administration of an analgesic agent (Table 7-5) depends on the condition of the individual patient and the desired effect of the medication. Analgesic agents can be administered by parenteral, oral, rectal, transdermal (skin patch), transmucosal, intraspinal, or epidural routes. Each method of administration has advantages and disadvantages. The route chosen should be based on patient need. Box 7-4 discusses the safe use of transdermal fentanyl administration.

Patient-Controlled Analgesia

Used to manage postoperative pain as well as persistent pain in hospitals or home settings, **patient-controlled analgesia** (PCA) allows patients to control the administration of their own medication within predetermined safety limits.

The PCA pump permits the patient to self-administer a predetermined amount of medication safely and to administer extra medication (demand doses) with episodes of increased pain or painful activities. A PCA pump is electronically controlled by a timing device. A patient experiencing pain can administer small amounts of medication directly into the IV,

subcutaneously, or into the epidural catheter by pressing a button. The pump then delivers a preset amount of medication.

The PCA pump also can be programmed to deliver a constant, background infusion of medication (or basal rate) and still allow the patient to administer additional bolus doses as needed. The nurse also can administer clinician doses, which typically are higher doses than the demand dose. The timer can be programmed to prevent additional doses from being administered until a specified time period has elapsed (lockout time) and until the first dose has had time to exert its maximal effect. Even if the patient pushes the button multiple times in rapid succession, no additional doses are released. If another dose is required at the end of the delay period, the button must be pushed again for the dose to be delivered. Patients who are controlling their own opioid administration usually become sedated and stop pushing the button before any significant respiratory depression occurs. Nevertheless, assessment of respiratory status remains a major nursing role.

Pain should be brought under control before a PCA is started with the use of intravenous pain medication. Then, after control is achieved, the pump is programmed to deliver small doses of medication at a time. If a patient with severe pain has a low serum level of opioid analgesic, it is difficult to regain control with the small doses available by pump. The patient is instructed not to wait until the pain is severe before pushing the button to obtain a bolus dose. Since the patient can maintain a near-constant level of medication, the periods of severe pain and sedation that occur with the traditional PRN regimen are avoided. If PCA is to be used in the patient's home, the patient and family are taught about the operation of

TABLE 7-5 **Administration Routes for Analgesics**

Route	Patient Factors	Advantages	Disadvantages
IV	Can be used if patient has had nothing by mouth. Side effects are nausea, vomiting.	Rapid, reliable effect, helps make patient feel more comfortable; may be administered by push or slow push (e.g., over a 5- to 10-minute period); may be administered by continuous infusion with a pump. Continuous infusion provides a steady level of analgesia over 24-hour period.	Short duration; careful calculation of dosage needed. Possible respiratory depression
Intramuscular	Can be used if patient has had nothing by mouth. Side effects are nausea, vomiting.	Limited to emergency setting where no IV access can be obtained or patient preference	Slower entry into bloodstream; slow metabolism. Absorption depends on site selected and amount of body fat.
Subcutaneous	Use if patient is in severe pain or had limited IV sites. Use for home pain management	Effective, convenient	Limited to small volume that can be administered at one time into the subcutaneous tissue
Oral	Preferred over parenteral administration if patient can take medication by mouth	Easy, noninvasive, not painful. Severe pain can be relieved with oral opioids if dose is high enough. Gradual dose increase provides additional pain relief without producing respiratory depression or sedation	Increased doses needed as the disease progresses; tolerance may develop to the medication. Change from parenteral to oral route requires equianalgesic dosing to avoid withdrawal reaction and recurrence of pain
Rectal	Use if patient is unable to take medications by any other route. Side effects include bleeding problems.	Prolonged duration of action	Onset of action unclear; delayed absorption compared with other routes of administration
Transdermal	Use for home pain management or hospice care in patients currently taking oral sustained-release opioid.	Consistent opioid serum level; slightly less constipation than oral opioids; less costly than parenteral route	Delay in effect while the dermal layer is saturated. Increased absorption in febrile patients. Require short-acting opioids for breakthrough pain; more expensive than sustained-release opioids
Transmucosal	Use in patients on sustained-release opioid who experience breakthrough pain.	Rapid onset of action nasal sprays allows analgesia to be achieved within 5–10 minutes; significant decreases in pain intensity; high patient satisfaction.	This route promotes rapid absorption and high bioavailability as a result of a highly vascularized oral mucosa entering systemic circulation directly and bypassing the GI tract and first-pass effect in the liver.

the pump as well as about the side effects of the medication and strategies to manage them.

Nursing Alert
Family members are cautioned not to push the button for a patient, especially if the patient is asleep, because this overrides some of the safety features of the PCA system.

Intrathecal and Epidural Administration
Infusion of opioids or local anesthetic agents into the intrathecal space or epidural space has been used for effective control of pain in postoperative patients and those with chronic pain unrelieved by other methods. A catheter is inserted into the epidural space at the thoracic or lumbar level for administration of opioid or anesthetic agents (Fig. 7-9). With intrathecal administration, medications infuse

Safe Use of Transdermal Fentanyl

The U.S. Food and Drug Administration issued a public health advisory in 2009 about the use of fentanyl skin patches and warned patients and health care providers about the need for the patches to be used as intended. The advisory also included precautions about safe storage and disposal of fentanyl skin patches:

- Fentanyl skin patches are very strong opioids and always should be prescribed at the lowest dose needed for pain relief. They should be used only for patients with chronic pain that is not well controlled with shorter-acting opioids.
- Patients should be cautioned that a sudden and possibly dangerous rise in the level of fentanyl in their blood can occur with use of alcohol or other medications that affect brain function, an increase in body temperature or exposure to heat, or use of other medicines that affect the metabolism of fentanyl.
- Patients should be informed about signs and symptoms of fentanyl overdose (i.e., shallow or difficult breathing; fatigue, extreme sleepiness, or sedation; inability to think, talk, or walk normally; and feeling faint, dizzy, or confused).

A

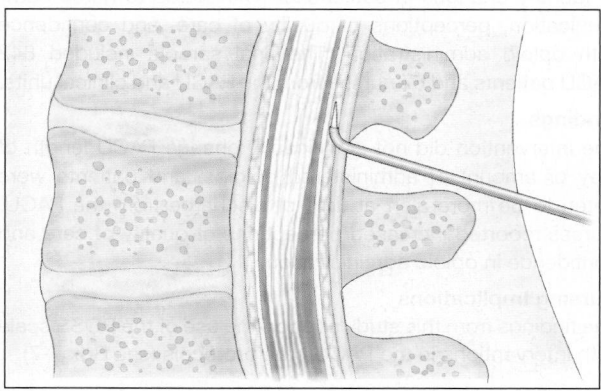

B

FIGURE 7-9 Placement of intraspinal catheters for administration of analgesic medications: (**A**) intrathecal route; (**B**) epidural route.

directly into the subarachnoid space and cerebrospinal fluid, which surrounds the spinal cord. With epidural administration, medication is deposited in the epidural space of the spinal canal and diffuses into the subarachnoid space. It is believed that pain relief from intrathecal administration of opioids is based on the existence of opioid receptors in the spinal cord.

An epidural anesthetic agent can be administered continuously in low doses, intermittently on a schedule, or on demand as the patient requires it, and it is often combined with the epidural administration of opioids. Typically, an opioid and local anesthetic (0.5% bupivacaine) administered at induction of anesthesia results in good postoperative analgesia for up to 24 hours (Garimella & Cellini, 2013, p. 192). Morphine is the intrathecal drug most commonly used for pain relief. Research reveals no difference in length of hospital stay and adverse events when comparing PCA versus continuous epidural analgesia (CEA) in patients undergoing abdominal surgery; however, patients achieved better pain control in the first 72 postoperative hours with CEA (Garimella & Cellini, 2013). In addition, epidural analgesia for thoracic surgery provides superior pain control, less sedation, and better pulmonary function than parenteral opiates (Hernandez & Sherwood, 2017, p. 381).

For patients who have persistent, severe pain that fails to respond to other treatments or for those who obtain pain relief only with the risk of serious side effects, medication administered by a long-term intrathecal or epidural catheter may be effective.

Nursing Alert
Epidural catheters inserted for pain control are usually managed by nurses. Baseline information necessary to provide safe and effective pain control includes the level or site of catheter insertion, the medications (e.g., local anesthetic agents, opioids) that have been administered, and the medications anticipated in the future. The infusion rate is increased with caution when anesthetic agents are combined with opioids. Sensory deficits can occur, and patients must be assessed frequently. An infusion with a lower concentration of anesthetic agent allows for administration of a greater concentration of opioid with a lower risk of sensory deficits.

Adverse effects associated with intrathecal administration include spinal headache resulting from loss of spinal fluid when the dura is punctured. The dura must be punctured with the intrathecal route, and dural puncture may occur inadvertently with the epidural route. If dural puncture occurs inadvertently, spinal fluid seeps out of the spinal canal. Headache resulting from spinal fluid loss may be delayed. Therefore, the nurse needs to assess regularly for headache after either type of catheter is placed. If headache develops, the patient should remain flat in bed and should

Pasero Opioid-Induced Sedation Scale (POSS)

S = Sleep, easy to arouse
Acceptable; no action necessary; may increase opioid dose if needed

1 = Awake and alert
Acceptable; no action necessary; may increase opioid dose if needed

2 = Slightly drowsy, easily aroused
Acceptable; no action necessary; may increase opioid dose if needed

3 = Frequently drowsy, arousable, drifts off to sleep during conversation
Unacceptable; monitor respiratory status and sedation level closely until sedation level is stable at less than 3 and respiratory status is satisfactory; decrease opioid dose 25% to 50% or notify prescriber or anesthesiologist for orders; consider administering a nonsedating, opioid-sparing nonopioid, such as acetaminophen or an NSAID, if not contraindicated.

4 = Somnolent, minimal or no response to verbal and physical stimulation
Unacceptable; stop opioid; consider administering naloxone; notify prescriber or anesthesiologist; monitor respiratory status and sedation level closely until sedation level is stable at less than 3 and respiratory status is satisfactory.

Pasero Opioid-Induced Sedation Scale (POSS). Copyright 1994, Chris Pasero. Used with permission.

be given large amounts of fluids (provided the medical condition allows), caffeinated drinks and the provider should be notified. An epidural blood patch may be performed to reduce leakage of spinal fluid (typically if the headache does not resolve within 36 hours) (Barr, 2015).

Respiratory depression generally peaks 6 to 12 hours after epidural opioids are administered, but it can occur earlier or up to 24 hours after the first injection. It is important for the nurse to monitor the patient closely during the postoperative period with particular attention to sedation and oxygen saturation. Depending on the lipophilicity (affinity for body fat) of the opioid injected, the time frame for respiratory depression can be short or long. Morphine is hydrophilic (it has an affinity to water), and the time for peak effect is longer than that of fentanyl, which is lipophilic. The nurse must assess and record respiratory status and sedation levels using a sedation scale according to agency policy. The health care provider will need to be notified if the patient has a sedation scale of less than 3 on the Pasero Opioid-Induced Sedation Scale (POSS) (Kobelt, Burke, & Renker, 2014). The POSS evaluates the patient's level of consciousness since sedation precedes respiratory depression (Boxes 7-5 and 7-6 [research brief]). The patient should be easily aroused if slightly drowsy, and should be able to remain awake during conversation. Opioid antagonist agents such as naloxone must be available for IV use if respiratory depression occurs (see Box 7-7).

Cardiovascular effects (hypotension) may result from relaxation of the vasculature in the lower extremities.

Nursing Research

Bridging the Gap to Evidence-Based Practice

Kobelt, P., Burke, K., & Renker, P. (2014). Evaluation of a standardized sedation assessment for opioid administration in the postanesthesia care unit. *Pain Management Nursing, 3*(15), 672–681.

Purpose

The impact of opioid-related sedation progressing to respiratory depression in the Post Anesthesia Care Unit (PACU) can be extensive; however, there is a paucity of research on the subject of standardized assessment tools to prevent adverse events. The purposes of this study were: (1) to measure the efficacy of a standardized method of assessing sedation and administering opioids for pain management via the Pasero Opioid-Induced Sedation Scale (POSS) with interventions in the PACU; (2) to increase PACU nurses' confidence in assessing sedation associated with opioid administration for pain management and in the quality of care provided in their clinical area; and (3) to facilitate communications between PACU and postoperative clinical unit nurses during patient handoffs regarding safe opioid administration.

Design

A quasi-experimental design was used to evaluate the POSS protocol. Two PACUs and six nursing units receiving

postsurgical patients in a Midwestern inner-city hospital served as the setting for this research. Medical records were surveyed for outcome data to evaluate the efficacy of the care protocol in two patient cohorts before and after implementation of the POSS protocol. Nurses completed a written survey to identify changes in satisfaction with nurse-to-nurse communication, perceptions of quality of care, and confidence with opioid administration. The final sample included 842 PACU patients and 67 nurses from the PACU and clinical units.

Findings

The intervention did not significantly change PACU length of stay or amount of administered opioids, and patients were noted to be more alert at time of discharge from the PACU. Nurses reported increased perceptions of quality of care and confidence in opioid administration.

Nursing Implications

The findings from this study support the use of the POSS scale with interventions in the PACU care protocols (see Box 7-7).

BOX 7-7

BOX 7-7 Opioid Analgesic Orders: General Considerations for the Nurse

A. Opioid analgesic orders or a hospital protocol should include the expectation that a nurse will hold the opioid dose if a patient is sedated excessively. The nurse documents the rationale for holding the dose. The nurse also recognizes that a fall in oxygen saturation can represent a critical level of respiratory depression and the need for immediate intervention to prevent life-threatening hypoxemia.

B. In the event of oversedation or life-threatening respiratory depression, the hospital protocol should include that naloxone should be available for the nurse. In general, 0.1–0.4 mg of naloxone and 9 mL of normal saline are mixed in a syringe, and this dilute solution is administered very slowly (e.g.,

1 mL or 0.04 mg over 1 minute) while observing the patient's response (titrate to effect). Patients should be monitored after being recovered with naloxone because the patient can fall back into unresponsiveness as the half-life of naloxone is only about 30 minutes before wearing off.

C. The nurse is aware that naloxone is administered incrementally in order to improve respiratory function but not reverse all analgesia, to avoid recurrence of severe pain.

D. When naloxone is administered in excessive doses, excitement, blood pressure liability, pulmonary edema, ventricular tachycardia and fibrillation, and seizures may be caused in postoperative patients (Vallerand, Sanoski, & Deglin, 2017).

Adapted from Pasero, C., Portenoy, R. K., McCaffery M. (1999). Opioid analgesics. In *Pain: Clinical manual* (2nd ed.). St. Louis, MO: Mosby, p. 267; American Pain Society (APS). (2003). *Principles of analgesic use in the treatment of acute pain and chronic cancer pain* (5th ed.), Glenview, IL: American Pain Society.

However, bradycardia, may occur with placement of a high thoracic epidural affecting the cardiac accelerator nerves. Therefore, the nurse should assess frequently for decreases in blood pressure, pulse rate, and urine output.

Urinary retention and pruritus may develop, and the health care provider may prescribe intravenous infusion of low-dose naloxone to combat these effects. The nurse administers doses that are small enough to reverse the side effects of the opioids without reversing the analgesic effects. Diphenhydramine or low-dose intravenous infusion of naloxone also may be used to relieve opioid-related pruritus.

Precautions must be taken to avoid infection at the catheter site and catheter displacement. The epidural catheter insertion site should be inspected routinely for any signs of infection or drainage. Only medications without preservatives should be administered into the subarachnoid or epidural space because of the potential neurotoxic effects of preservatives.

Nursing Alert

Because of the risk of an epidural hematoma, a general consensus exists that the epidural catheter should not be removed earlier than 12 hours after the last dose of low–molecular-weight heparin (LMWH), and LMWH should not be restarted earlier than 2 hours after catheter removal. The nurse is aware that symptoms of an epidural hematoma include back pain, sensory and motor dysfunction of the lower limbs, and bladder and bowel abnormalities (Hernandez & Sherwood, 2017).

Placebo Effect

A **placebo effect** occurs when a person responds to the medication or other treatment because of an expectation that the treatment will work rather than because it actually

does so. The American Society for Pain Management Nurses contends that placebos (tablets or injections with no active ingredients) should not be used to assess or manage pain in any patient, regardless of age or diagnosis (Arnstein, Broglio, Wuhrman, & Kean, 2011). Furthermore, the group recommends that all health care institutions have policies in place prohibiting the use of placebos for this purpose. Educational programs should be conducted to educate nurses and other health care providers about effective pain management, and ethics committees should assist in developing and disseminating these policies.

Nonpharmacologic Interventions

Analgesic medication is the most powerful tool for pain relief that is available, but it is not the only one. Nonpharmacologic nursing interventions can assist in pain relief, usually with low risk to the patient. Although such measures are not a substitute for medication, they may be all that is necessary or appropriate to relieve episodes of pain lasting only seconds or minutes. In instances of severe pain that lasts for hours or days, combining nonpharmacologic interventions with medications may be the most effective way to relieve pain.

Cutaneous Stimulation and Massage

Massage, which is generalized cutaneous stimulation of the body, often concentrates on the back and shoulders. A massage does not specifically stimulate the nonpain receptors in the same receptor field as the pain receptors, but it may have an impact through the descending control system (see previous discussion). Although the exact mechanism of massage therapy is not known, it is purported to improve local circulation, tone of supportive musculature, joint flexibility, and decrease inflammation (Perlman, 2016). Massage also promotes comfort, improves function, produces muscle relaxation and relieves stress (Perlman, 2016). It has demonstrated potential benefit for neck pain, low back pain, constipation, high blood pressure, lymphedema, stress, depression, and osteoarthritis (Perlman, 2016).

Thermal Therapies

Ice and heat therapies may be effective pain relief strategies in some circumstances; however, their effectiveness and mechanisms of action need further study. Proponents believe that ice and heat stimulate the nonpain receptors in the same receptor field as the injury. Both ice and heat therapy must be applied carefully and monitored closely to avoid injuring the skin. Neither therapy should be applied to areas with impaired circulation or used in patients with impaired sensation.

For greatest effect, ice should be placed on the injury site immediately after injury or surgery. Ice therapy after joint surgery can significantly reduce the amount of analgesic medication required. Ice therapy also may relieve pain if applied later. Care must be taken to assess the skin before treatment and to protect the skin from direct application of the ice. Ice should be applied to an area for no longer than 15 to 20 minutes at a time and should be avoided in patients with compromised circulation (Arthritis Foundation, 2015). Prolonged applications of ice may result in frostbite or nerve injury.

Application of heat increases blood flow to an area and contributes to pain reduction by speeding healing. Both dry and moist heat may provide some analgesia, but their mechanisms of action are not well understood.

 Nursing Alert
Heat should not be applied to a painful area that is the site of acute, untreated infection (e.g., mastitis, tooth abscess) because it may cause increased pain with increased blood flow to the site.

Transcutaneous Electrical Nerve Stimulation

Transcutaneous electrical nerve stimulation (TENS) uses a battery-operated unit with electrodes applied to the skin to produce a tingling, vibrating, or buzzing sensation in the area of pain. It has been used in both acute and chronic pain relief and is thought to decrease pain by stimulating the nonpain receptors in the same area as the fibers that transmit the pain. Research studies have demonstrated that low-frequency high-intensity TENS has inhibitory effects on pain perception (Treede, 2016). The mechanism of action of TENS is related to the gate control theory of pain, which was proposed in 1965 and held that the perception of pain can be inhibited by activation of nerves that do not transmit pain signals, thus interrupting the nociceptors signals. This theory explains the effectiveness of cutaneous stimulation when applied in the same area as an injury. Although much has been learned about the complexity of spinal circuitry, the gate control theory model predicted the efficacy of TENS.

Distraction

Distraction helps relieve both acute and chronic pain (Slover et al., 2015; Schreiber et al., 2014). Distraction, which involves focusing the patient's attention on something other than the pain, may be the mechanism responsible for other effective cognitive techniques. Distraction is thought to reduce the perception of pain by stimulating the descending control system, resulting in fewer painful stimuli being transmitted to the brain. The effectiveness of distraction depends on the patient's ability to receive and create sensory input other than pain. Distraction techniques may range from simple activities, such as watching television or listening to music, to highly complex physical and mental exercises. Pain relief generally increases in direct proportion to the patient's active participation, the number of sensory modalities used, and interest in the stimuli. Therefore, the stimulation of sight, sound, and touch is likely to be more effective in reducing pain than is the stimulation of only a single sense.

Visits from family and friends are effective in relieving pain. Watching an action-packed movie on a large screen with "surround sound" through headphones may be effective (provided the patient finds it acceptable). Others may benefit from games and activities (e.g., chess, crossword puzzles) that require concentration. Not all patients obtain pain relief with distraction, especially those in severe pain. Severe pain may prevent patients from concentrating well enough to participate in complex physical or mental activities.

Relaxation Techniques/Meditation

Skeletal muscle relaxation is believed to reduce pain by relaxing tense muscles that contribute to the pain. A simple relaxation technique consists of abdominal breathing at a slow, rhythmic rate. The patient may close both eyes and breathe slowly and comfortably. A constant rhythm can be maintained by counting silently and slowly with each inhalation ("in, two, three") and exhalation ("out, two, three"). When teaching this technique, the nurse may count out loud with the patient at first. Slow, rhythmic breathing may also be used as a distraction technique. Relaxation techniques, as well as other noninvasive pain relief measures, may require practice before the patient becomes skilled in using them. Patients who already know a relaxation technique may need to be reminded to use it to reduce or prevent increased pain. Almost all people with persistent pain can benefit from some method of relaxation. Meditation has demonstrated impact on lowering of blood pressure and heart rate, increased cerebral blood flow, and decreased levels of hormones associated with stress (Perlman, 2016). Regular relaxation periods may help combat the fatigue and muscle tension that occur with and increase chronic pain.

Guided Imagery

Guided imagery is using one's imagination in a special way to achieve a specific positive effect. Guided imagery for relaxation and pain relief may consist of combining slow, rhythmic breathing with a mental image of relaxation and comfort. The nurse instructs the patient to close the eyes and breathe slowly in and out. With each slowly exhaled breath, the patient imagines muscle tension and discomfort being breathed out, carrying away pain and tension and leaving behind a relaxed and comfortable body. With each inhaled breath, the patient imagines healing energy flowing to the area of discomfort.

If guided imagery is to be effective, it requires a considerable amount of time to explain the technique and time for the patient to practice it. Usually, the patient is asked to practice guided imagery for approximately 5 minutes, three times per day. Several days of practice may be needed before the intensity of pain is reduced. Many patients begin to experience the relaxing effects of guided imagery the first time they try it. Pain relief can continue for hours after the imagery is used. Patients should be informed that guided imagery may work only for some people. Guided imagery should be used only in combination with all other forms of treatment that have demonstrated effectiveness.

Hypnosis

Hypnosis, which has been effective in relieving pain or decreasing the amount of analgesic agents required in patients with acute and chronic pain, may promote pain relief in particularly difficult situations (e.g., burns). The mechanism by which hypnosis acts is unclear. Its effectiveness depends on the hypnotic susceptibility of the individual (Jensen & Patterson, 2014). In some cases, hypnosis may be effective in the first session, with effectiveness increasing in additional sessions. In other cases, hypnosis does not work at all. Usually, hypnosis must be induced by specially skilled people (a psychologist or a nurse with specialized training in hypnosis). Some patients may learn to perform self-hypnosis.

Music Therapy

Music therapy is an inexpensive and effective therapy for the reduction of pain and anxiety in some patient populations. Research has shown that it reduces postoperative pain, fatigue, anxiety, and cumulative opioid consumption (Sin & Chow, 2015). Music therapy was also found to decrease pain in persons with chronic pain (Stanos, Tyburski, & Harden, 2016). More research needs to be done to determine the mechanism by which music exerts its positive effect on pain relief.

Acupuncture

The insertion of the needles is intended to stimulate or improve the balance of the flow of "life energy" or *qi* (pronounced chi), whereas a blockage of flow or imbalance of *qi* is associated with patient complaints or disease. Although very different from a Western medical view of pathophysiology, acupuncture has been shown to have various

physiologic effects on the body, including stimulation of endorphins (Perlman, 2016). Research suggests that acupuncture may be beneficial for pain associated with fibromyalgia, headache, and chronic pain and has been used with varied conditions such as stroke, analgesia during childbirth, and infertility treatment. In addition, stimulation of the acupuncture point at the wrist is potentially effective in reducing postoperative nausea and vomiting (Perlman, 2016).

Movement Therapy

Restoring balance to the body by using physical movement, such as yoga, and tai chi have gained in popularity and have had positive health benefits in patients with low back pain and back-related disabilities. In addition, often tai chi can be practiced even by patients with heart disease or arthritis as well as patients who are at risk of falling (Perlman, 2016).

Alternative Therapies

The National Institutes of Health has established the National Council for Complementary and Alternative Medicine (CAM) to examine the effectiveness of complementary and alternative therapies. The new field of integrative medicine allows for a combination of mainstream medicine and alternative therapies that enhance effectiveness and safety for patients seeking CAM therapies for pain and other disorders. The use of CAM has increased in the United States, and patients with cancer or rheumatologic conditions use CAM at a higher rate than the general population. For example, a study noted that 75% of cancer patients surveyed had used at least one CAM modality, compared to usage in 38% of the general population (Perlman, 2016).

When caring for patients who are using or considering using untested therapies, it is imperative for the nurse not to diminish the patient's hope. This must be weighed against the nurse's responsibility to protect the patient from costly and potentially harmful and dangerous therapies that the patient is not in a position to evaluate scientifically. The nurse encourages the patient to assess the effectiveness of the therapy, continually using standard pain assessment techniques. All use of alternative and complementary therapies needs to be discussed with the patient's health care provider.

Neurologic and Neurosurgical Approaches to Pain Management

In some situations, especially with long-term and severe intractable pain, usual pharmacologic and nonpharmacologic methods of pain relief are ineffective. In those situations, neurologic and neurosurgical approaches to pain management may be considered. *Intractable pain* refers to pain that cannot be relieved satisfactorily by the usual approaches, including medications. Such pain often is the result of malignancy (especially of the cervix, bladder, prostate, and lower bowel), but it may occur in other conditions, such as postherpetic neuralgia, trigeminal neuralgia, spinal cord arachnoiditis, and uncontrollable ischemia and other forms of tissue destruction.

Neurologic and neurosurgical methods available for pain relief include: (1) stimulation procedures (intermittent electrical stimulation of a tract or center to inhibit the transmission of pain impulses), (2) administration of intraspinal opioids (see previous discussion), and (3) interruption of the tracts conducting the pain impulse from the periphery to cerebral integration centers. Stimulation of nerves with minute amounts of electricity is used if other pharmacologic and nonpharmacologic treatments fail to provide adequate relief. These treatments are reversible. If they need to be discontinued, the nervous system continues to function. However, methods that involve interruption of the tracts are destructive or ablative procedures. They are used only after other methods of pain relief have failed because their effects are permanent.

Stimulation Procedures

Electrical stimulation, or neuromodulation, is a method of suppressing pain by applying controlled low-voltage electrical pulses to the different parts of the nervous system. Electrical stimulation is thought to relieve pain by blocking painful stimuli. This pain-modulating technique is administered by many modes. TENS (discussed earlier) and dorsal spinal cord stimulation are the most common types of electrical stimulation used. There are also brain-stimulating techniques in which electrodes are implanted in the periventricular area of the posterior third ventricle, allowing the patient to stimulate this area to produce analgesia.

Spinal cord stimulation is a technique used for the relief of persistent, intractable pain, ischemic pain, spinal stenosis pain, pain from angina, and other neuropathic pain syndromes. A surgically implanted device allows the patient to apply pulsed electrical stimulation to the dorsal aspect of the spinal cord to block pain impulses (the largest accumulation of afferent fibers is found in the dorsal column of the spinal cord (Al-Kaisy et al., 2014). The dorsal column stimulation unit consists of a radiofrequency stimulation transmitter, a transmitter antenna, a radiofrequency receiver, and a stimulation electrode. The battery-powered transmitter and antenna are worn externally; the receiver and electrode are implanted. A laminectomy is performed above the highest level of pain input, and the electrode is placed in the epidural space over the posterior column of the spinal cord. The placement of the stimulating systems varies. A subcutaneous pocket is created over the clavicular area or at some other site for placement of the receiver. The two are connected through a subcutaneous tunnel. As implantable devices carry higher risks than conservative nonoperative approaches, this treatment is generally reserved for patients who have exhausted more conservative options (Eli, Konrad, & Neimat, 2015).

Deep brain stimulation is performed in patients with special pain problems if there is no response to the usual techniques of pain control. Under local anesthesia, electrodes are introduced through a burr hole in the skull and inserted into a selected site in the brain, depending on the location or type of pain. After the effectiveness of stimulation is confirmed, the implanted electrode is connected to a radiofrequency device or pulse-generator system operated by external telemetry. It is used in patients with neuropathic pain that may be caused by damage or injury from a stroke, chronic cluster headaches, brain or spinal cord injuries, or Parkinson disease.

Interruption of Pain Pathways

Pain-conducting fibers can be interrupted at any point from their origin to the cerebral cortex. In doing so, some part of the nervous system is destroyed, resulting in varying amounts of neurologic deficit and incapacity. For example, a spinal ablation procedure of the dorsal root, which selectively destroys neurons located in the posterolateral spinal cord where sensory fibers enter into the spinal cord, may be used in neuropathic pain, phantom limb pain, and traumatic brachial and lumbosacral plexus avulsion injuries. Studies report 60% of patients demonstrated good pain relief with an average follow-up of 71 months (Eli et al., 2015). Destructive procedures used to interrupt the transmission of pain also include cordotomy, myelotomy, and rhizotomy. A cordotomy is destruction of the lateral spinothalamic tract (which carries pain signals) in the anterolateral part of the spinal cord and is used for intractable unilateral cancer pain (Eli et al., 2015). A percutaneous technique can be used for this procedure, which limits risks. A myelotomy is a neuroablation treatment used for patients with intractable oncologic visceral pain in the abdomen or pelvis. A rhizotomy is an ablative procedures of the sensory and pain fibers of the trigeminal nerve either centrally or peripherally to provide pain relief. These procedures are offered if it is thought that the procedure will result in an improved quality of life. The use of other methods to interrupt pain transmission is reserved for a patient with intractable pain where medical therapy has been exhausted.

Unfolding Patient Stories: Stan Checketts • Part 1

Stan Checketts, a 52-year-old male, is in the emergency department with severe abdominal pain. The provider has ordered buprenorphine 0.3 mg IV push for pain. Explain the assessments performed by the nurse prior to, during, and following the administration of the medication. Also consider nonpharmacologic interventions the nurse can incorporate to assist with his pain relief. (Stan Checketts' story continues in Chapter 24.)

Care for Stan and other patients in a realistic virtual environment: **vSim** *for Nursing* (thepoint.lww.com/vSimMedicalSurgical). Practice documenting these patients' care in DocuCare (thepoint.lww.com/DocuCareEHR).

BOX 7-8

Expected Patient Outcomes for the Patient with Pain

Relief of pain, evidenced when the patient rates pain at a lower intensity:
- On a scale of 0–10 after intervention.
- For longer periods.

Correct administration of prescribed analgesic medications, evidenced when the patient or family:
- States correct dose of medication.
- Administers correct dose using correct procedure.
- Identifies side effects of medication.
- Describes actions taken to prevent or correct side effects.

Use of nonpharmacologic pain strategies as recommended, evidenced when the patient:
- Reports practice of nonpharmacologic strategies.
- Describes expected outcomes of nonpharmacologic strategies.

Minimal effects of pain and minimal side effects of interventions, evidenced when the patient:
- Participates in activities important to recovery (e.g., drinking fluids, coughing, ambulating).
- Participates in activities important to self and to family (e.g., family activities, interpersonal relationships, parenting, social interaction, recreation, work).
- Reports adequate sleep and absence of fatigue and constipation.

EVALUATING PAIN MANAGEMENT STRATEGIES

An important aspect of caring for patients in pain is reassessing the pain after the intervention has been implemented. The measure's effectiveness is based on the patient's assessment of pain, as reflected in pain assessment tools. If the intervention was ineffective, the nurse should consider other measures. If these are ineffective, pain relief goals need to be reassessed in collaboration with the primary care provider and or interdisciplinary team. The nurse serves as the patient's advocate in obtaining additional pain relief.

After interventions have had a chance to work, the nurse asks the patient to rate the intensity of pain. The nurse repeats this assessment at appropriate intervals after the intervention and compares the result with the previous rating. These assessments indicate the effectiveness of the pain relief measures and provide a basis for continuing or modifying the plan of care. A plan of nursing care for a patient with pain is available at http://thepoint.lww.com/Honan2e. Expected patient outcomes are given in Box 7-8.

CHAPTER REVIEW

Critical Thinking Exercises

1. A 35-year-old man who is a recovering heroin addict is admitted to the hospital for an emergency appendectomy. During surgery, the appendix ruptures, and the patient remains hospitalized for several days for IV antibiotics. He tells the nurse that he has been "clean" for the past 3 months. He complains of pain (7 on a 0 to 10 scale) and refuses to use the patient-controlled analgesia that is prescribed for him. He states, "I don't want to get hooked again." Describe how you would address pain relief in this patient, and give the rationale for your actions. Who would you consult to help with this patient's pain management?

2. A 48-year-old woman has severe chronic pain associated with cancer metastasis to the bone. She is reluctant to take opioids because she wants to remain alert to enjoy being around her family. Furthermore, she is concerned about having opioids around the house because of the presence of young children in the home. Identify pharmacologic alternatives and nonpharmacologic interventions that might be appropriate. Identify the evidence base and the strength of the evidence for the use of the nonpharmacologic interventions.

NCLEX-Style Review Questions

1. The nurse is managing an epidural catheter for a patient diagnosed with cancer. The patient has developed a spinal headache. Which intervention should be completed at this time?
   a. Increase the dosage of anesthetic.
   b. Place in semi-Fowler position.
   c. Continue to monitor the patient.
   d. Initiate administration of prescribed fluids.

2. The nurse is caring for an 80-year-old patient following right hip surgery. When administering pain medication to this patient, what is important for the nurse to remember?
   a. Elderly patients have a faster metabolism than their younger counterparts.
   b. Elderly patients have an increased risk for drug toxicity.
   c. Elderly patients have a lower incidence of chronic illness.
   d. Elderly patients infrequently use OTC medications.

3. A patient has a pancreatic tumor and history of alcoholism. The patient receives morphine 2 mg subcutaneously every 3 to 4 hours for treatment of pain associated with the tumor. After 2 days of receiving this dose every 4 hours, the patient tells the nurse that the medication is needed more frequently to control the pain. What is the nurse's best response to this situation?
   a. The patient is becoming addicted to the morphine, and the medication should be administered less frequently than every 4 hours.
   b. A tolerance to the morphine is developing, and the patient should receive the drug every 3 hours.
   c. Administering the morphine every 3 hours will increase the patient's physical dependence on the drug.
   d. Physical dependence should be avoided at all costs, and the drug should continue to be administered every 4 hours.

4. A patient who had abdominal surgery 5 days ago complains of sharp, throbbing abdominal pain that ranks 8 on a scale of 0 (no pain) to 10 (worst pain). The patient's pain rating has averaged at a 3/10 for the first 5 days postoperatively on epidural administration of hydromorphone. However, narcotic administration via epidural catheter was discontinued earlier this morning. Which of the following would be the nurse's first action?
   a. Obtain an order to restart the epidural narcotic administration.
   b. Assess the patient to rule out possible complications secondary to surgery.
   c. Check the patient's chart to determine what additional pain medications can be administered.
   d. Explain to the patient that his pain should not be this severe 5 days postoperatively.

5. What instruction should the nurse stress when teaching the preoperative patient about correct use of the PCA device?
   a. Push the button when you feel the pain beginning rather than waiting until the pain is at its worst.
   b. Push the button every 15 minutes whether you feel pain at that time or not.
   c. Instruct your family or visitors to press the button for you when you are sleeping.
   d. Try to go as long as you possibly can before you press the button.

Try these additional resources, available at **http://thepoint.lww.com/Honan2e**, to enhance your learning and understanding of this chapter:
- NCLEX-Style Student Review Questions
- Journal Articles

REFERENCES AND SELECTED READINGS

References and selected readings associated with this chapter can be found on the website that accompanies the book. Visit **http://thepoint. lww.com/Honan2e** to access the references and other additional resources associated with this chapter.

Problems Related to Gas Exchange and Respiratory Function

A 43-year-old patient diagnosed with laryngeal cancer will undergo a total laryngectomy. He is very anxious about how he will deal with his care at home. How can the nurse address his fears?

- Discuss potential complications that may arise following a total laryngectomy.
- Discuss areas to be included in teaching the patient self-care.
- Discuss area support groups for laryngectomy patients.

Nursing Assessment: Respiratory Function

Linda Honan

Learning Objectives

After reading this chapter, you will be able to:

1. Describe the structures and functions of the upper and lower respiratory tracts.
2. Define ventilation, perfusion, diffusion, and shunting.
3. Explain the use of inspection, palpation, percussion, and auscultation for respiratory assessment.
4. Discriminate between normal and abnormal breath sounds.
5. Use assessment parameters appropriate for determining the characteristics and severity of the major symptoms of respiratory dysfunction.
6. Identify the nursing implications of the various procedures used for diagnostic evaluation of respiratory function.

Disorders of the respiratory system are commonly encountered by nurses in every setting from the community to the intensive care unit. Expert assessment skills must be developed and used when caring for patients with acute and chronic respiratory problems. In addition, an understanding of respiratory function and the significance of abnormal diagnostic test results is essential.

ANATOMIC AND PHYSIOLOGIC OVERVIEW

The respiratory system is composed of the upper and lower respiratory tracts, blood vessels, thoracic cage (spine, ribs, and sternum) and respiratory muscles, chiefly the diaphragm (Fig. 8-1). Respiration requires concert of **ventilation** (movement of air from the atmosphere to the alveoli [the functional unit of the lung]), **diffusion** (exchange of oxygen [O_2] and carbon dioxide [CO_2] at the alveolar–capillary membrane), and perfusion (blood flow). In addition, innervations of the respiratory system are controlled by the neurologic system (medulla, pons, spinal nerves), muscular system (diaphragm, intercostal muscles), and chemical regulation.

Anatomy of the Upper Respiratory Tract

Upper airway structures consist of the nose, sinuses and nasal passages, pharynx, tonsils and adenoids, and larynx, which warm, humidify, and filter atmospheric air.

Nose

The anterior nares (nostrils) are the external openings of the nasal cavities. The internal portion of the nose is divided into two by a narrow vertical divider, the *septum*, which is richly supplied with sensory nerves and blood vessels. Each nasal cavity is divided into three passageways by the projection of the turbinates (also called conchae), which are highly sensitive. The middle passageway, or meatus, lies under the middle turbinate and contains the ostia (openings) of three of the paranasal sinuses (discussed below) that drain into this area. The nasal cavities are lined with highly vascular ciliated mucous membranes (nasal mucosa). Mucus, secreted continuously by goblet cells, covers the surface of the nasal mucosa and is moved back to the nasopharynx by the action of the **cilia** (fine hairs).

 Nursing Alert
The nurse considers that prolonged obstruction of the ostia (as with a nasotracheal tube or nasogastric [NG] tube) is associated with sinusitis (Bennett, Dolan, & Blaser, 2014). Patients with endotracheal intubation are also at risk for nosocomial sinusitis because of pooling of nasopharyngeal secretions.

Paranasal Sinuses

The paranasal sinuses include four pairs of bony cavities or air spaces that drain into the nasal cavity and lighten the

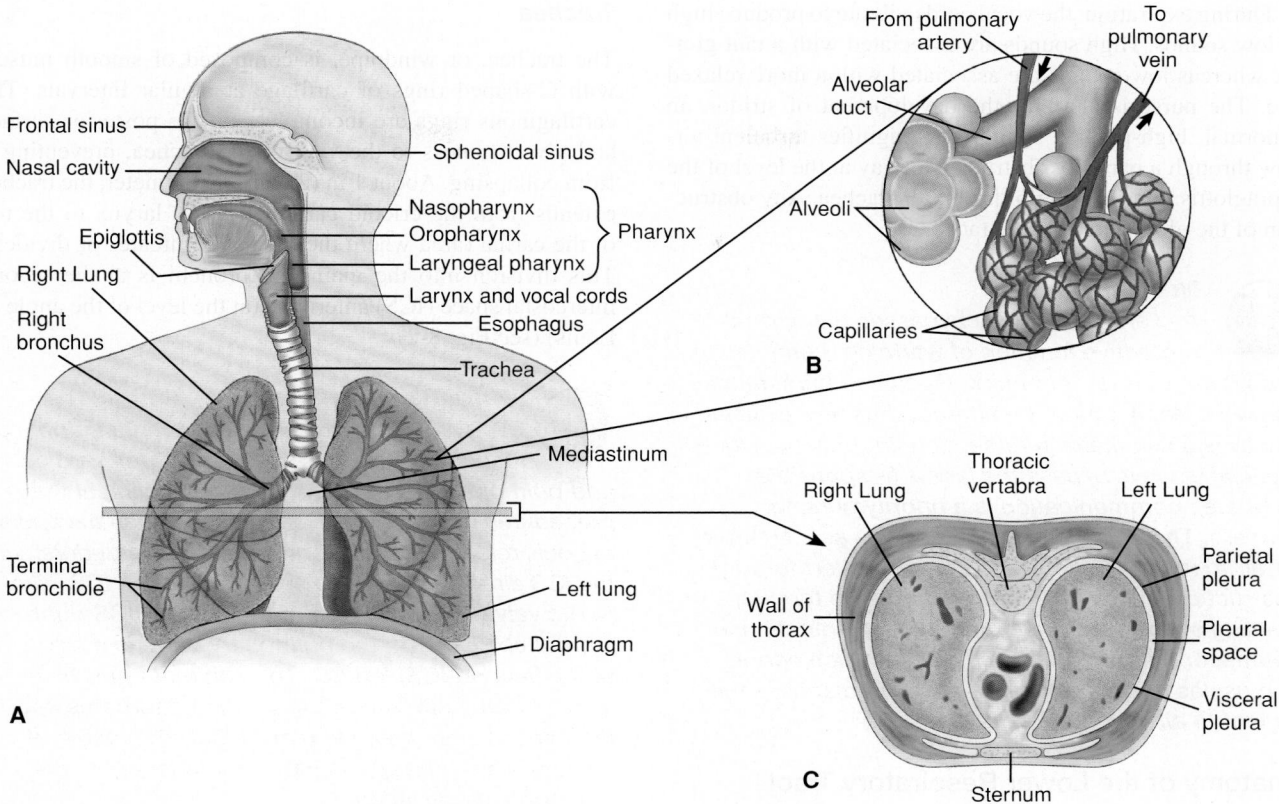

FIGURE 8-1 The respiratory system. **A.** Upper respiratory structures and the structures of the thorax. **B.** Alveoli. **C.** A horizontal cross-section of the lungs.

weight of the skull. The sinuses are named by their location: frontal (above the eyebrows), ethmoidal (between the eyes and behind the nose), sphenoidal (behind the ethmoid sinuses), and maxillary (located on the cheeks below the eyes). They serve as a resonating chamber in speech and are a common site of infection.

Pharynx, Tonsils, and Adenoids

The pharynx, or throat, is a tube-like structure that connects the nasal and oral cavities to the larynx and is a passageway for the respiratory and digestive tracts. It is divided into three regions: nasal, oral, and laryngeal. The nasopharynx is located posterior to the nose and above the soft palate. The adenoids, or pharyngeal tonsils, are located in the roof of the nasopharynx. Air entering reaches the nasopharynx, where it contacts sensitive nerves. Some of these nerves detect odors; others provoke sneezing to expel irritating dust. The eustachian tubes are also located here, they connect the middle ear to the nasopharynx and function to drain mucus and equalize pressures. The oropharynx houses the faucial, or palatine, tonsils. The tonsils, the adenoids, and other lymphoid tissue encircle the throat. These structures are important links in the chain of lymph nodes guarding the body from invasion by organisms entering the nose and the throat. The laryngopharynx extends from the hyoid bone to the cricoid cartilage.

Larynx

The larynx, or voice organ, connects the pharynx and the trachea. The major function of the larynx is vocalization. It also protects the lower airway from foreign substances and facilitates coughing. It is frequently referred to as the voice box and consists of the following:

- *Epiglottis:* A valve flap of cartilage (lid-like structure) that covers the entrance to the larynx during swallowing; it is essential to prevent aspiration (inhalation of food or fluid into the lungs)
- *Glottis:* The opening between the vocal cords in the larynx
- *Thyroid cartilage:* The largest of the cartilage structures; it can be felt anteriorly as the "Adam's apple"
- *Cricoid cartilage:* The only complete cartilaginous ring in the larynx (located below the thyroid cartilage)
- *Arytenoid cartilages:* Used in vocal cord movement with the thyroid cartilage
- *Vocal cords:* Ligaments controlled by muscular movements that produce sounds; located in the lumen of the larynx

During expiration, the vocal cords vibrate to produce high or low sounds. High sounds are associated with a taut glottis, whereas low sounds are associated with a more relaxed one. The nurse is alert for the development of stridor, an abnormal, high-pitched sound, as it signifies turbulent airflow through a partially obstructed airway at the level of the supraglottis, glottis, subglottis, and/or trachea. Any obstruction of the glottis area can be fatal.

> **Nursing Alert**
> *Any artificial airway bypasses the normal protective function of warming, humidifying, and filtering the air. Although, O_2 can be humidified and warmed, it cannot be filtered, thus any artificial airway is a risk factor for infection. In addition, since artificial airways bypass the larynx (responsible for voice), communication is a priority nursing concern. The upper airway also serves as a conduit for air to reach the lungs. The nurse is alert for any obstruction—such as a foreign body; the tongue; swelling secondary to allergic reaction, infection, or trauma; or neurologic impairment in which nerves or muscles may be impaired—that predisposes the patient to airway obstruction.*

Anatomy of the Lower Respiratory Tract

The lower respiratory tract consists of the trachea, right and left mainstem bronchi, secondary bronchi, bronchioles, and lungs, and can be further subdivided into the conducting airways and the acinus, where the respiratory bronchioles and alveoli (functional unit of the lung) are located.

Trachea

The trachea, or windpipe, is composed of smooth muscle with C-shaped rings of cartilage at regular intervals. The cartilaginous rings are incomplete on the posterior surface and give firmness to the wall of the trachea, preventing it from collapsing. About 1 in (2.5 cm) in diameter, the trachea extends from the cricoid cartilage of the larynx to the top of the carina (area where the trachea bifurcates or divides). This division into the mainstem bronchi is at the second intercostal space (ICS) anteriorly (at the level of the angle of Louis) (see Fig. 8-2).

> **Nursing Alert**
> *The angle of Louis is a significant anatomical landmark that has implications for cardiac and pulmonary assessment as well as clinical procedures (i.e., EKG lead placement). Since the angle of Louis relates to the second rib, the nurse understands the ICS directly **below** this rib is the second ICS. The aortic valve is auscultated at the second ICS right sternal border (SB); the pulmonary valve is heard at the second ICS, left SB. The angle of Louis is also anatomically where the trachea bifurcates into the left and right mainstem bronchus. The angle of Louis is also referred to as the sternal angle or the manubriosternal junction.*

Lungs

The lungs are paired elastic structures enclosed in the thoracic cage, which is an airtight chamber with distensible

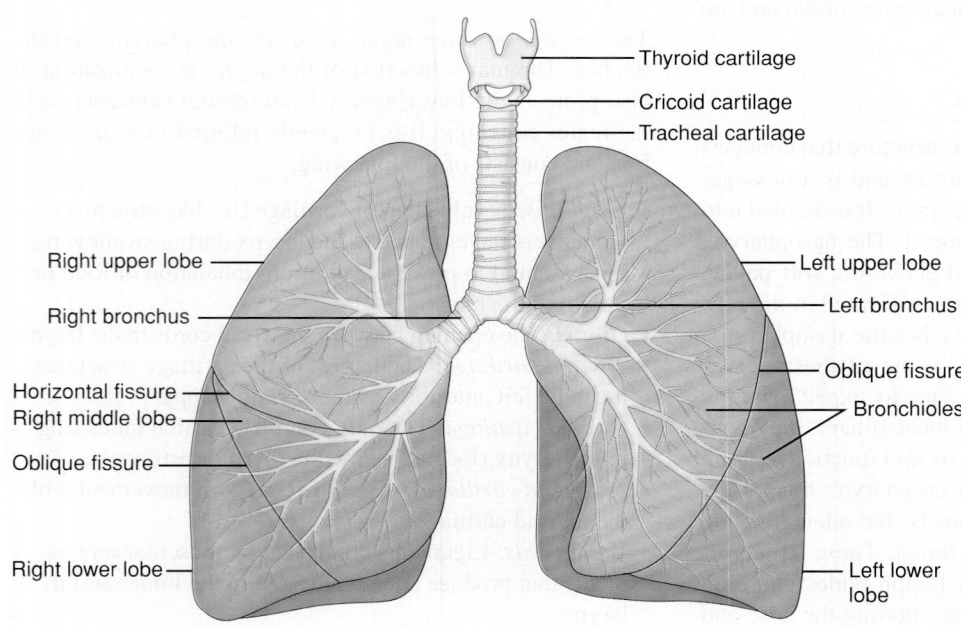

Thyroid cartilage
Cricoid cartilage
Tracheal cartilage

Right upper lobe
Right bronchus

Horizontal fissure
Right middle lobe
Oblique fissure

Right lower lobe

Left upper lobe
Left bronchus

Oblique fissure
Bronchioles

Left lower lobe

FIGURE 8-2 Anterior view of the lungs. The lungs consist of five lobes. The right lung has three lobes (upper, middle, lower); the left has two (upper and lower). The lobes are further subdivided by fissures. The bronchial tree, another lung structure, inflates with air to fill the lobes.

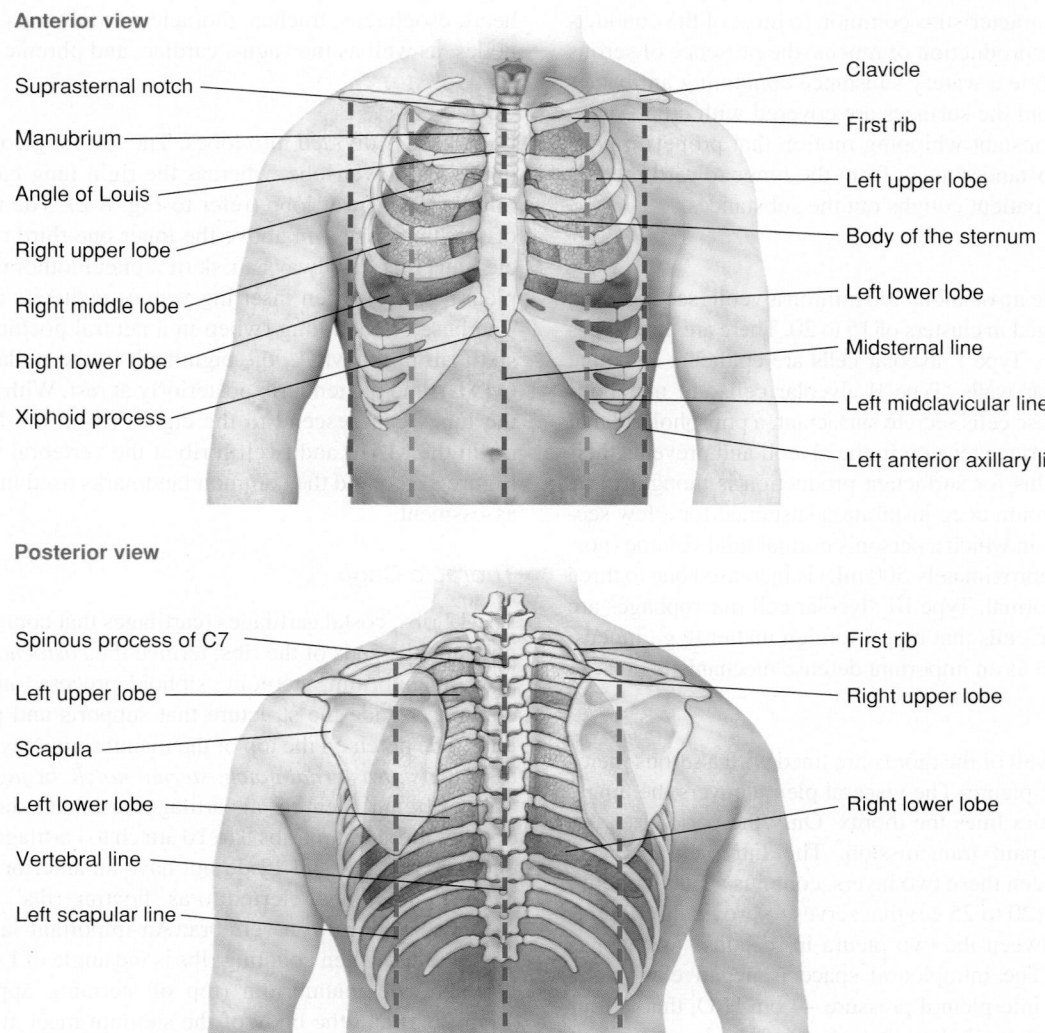

Anterior view

- Suprasternal notch
- Manubrium
- Angle of Louis
- Right upper lobe
- Right middle lobe
- Right lower lobe
- Xiphoid process

- Clavicle
- First rib
- Left upper lobe
- Body of the sternum
- Left lower lobe
- Midsternal line
- Left midclavicular line
- Left anterior axillary line

Posterior view

- Spinous process of C7
- Left upper lobe
- Scapula
- Left lower lobe
- Vertebral line
- Left scapular line

- First rib
- Right upper lobe
- Right lower lobe

FIGURE 8-3 Landmarks in respiratory assessment.

walls (Fig. 8-3). They are divided into lobes by fissures. The lungs are separated into upper and lower lobes by the oblique or major fissures that begin at T3 posteriorly and terminate at the sixth rib in the midclavicular line (MCL) bilaterally. To find T3, the nurse asks the patient to flex the neck forward; the most protruding spinous process is C7. The nurse palpates below this process from here to T1, T2, and T3. An additional horizontal fissure produces the middle lobe of the right lung. It begins anteriorly at approximately the fourth rib at the right SB and extends to the fifth rib in the midaxillary line. It is essential for nurses to understand that the right middle lobe can be auscultated only anteriorally (see later discussion and Box 8-7 on page 248).

Bronchi and Bronchioles

The bronchi begin at the carina. The right main bronchus, which provides air to the right lung, is wider, shorter (about 2.5 cm long), and more vertical in direction than the left main bronchus, which supplies the left lung. Because of the

anatomical structure, aspiration of material tends to occur in the right lung. The mainstem bronchi divide into five lobar bronchi: three in the right lung and two in the left lung, to correspond with each respective lobe of the lung. The lobar bronchi enter the lung at the hilum (a fissure or opening) along with blood vessels, nerves, and lymphatics. The lobar bronchi branch into segmental bronchi (10 on the right and 8 on the left). They are the structures identified when choosing the most effective postural drainage position for a given patient. The segmental bronchi further subdivide until they branch into bronchioles. Bronchioles have no cartilage in their walls, thus patency depends entirely on the elastic recoil of the surrounding smooth muscle and on the alveolar pressure. The terminal bronchioles then become respiratory bronchioles that have actual alveolar sacs imbedded in their walls, so that gas exchange can occur. Up until this point, the exchange of O_2 and CO_2 has not occurred, thus it is termed *anatomical dead space* and is calculated to be 150 mL.

There are characteristics common to most of the conducting airways: the production of mucus, the presence of serous glands that secrete a watery substance containing antibacterial enzymes, and the surfaces are covered with cilia. These cilia create a constant whipping motion that propels mucus and foreign substances away from the lungs toward the larynx, where the patient coughs out the substances.

Alveoli

The lung is made up of about 300 million alveoli (see Fig. 8-1), which are arranged in clusters of 15 to 20. There are three types of alveolar cells. Type I alveolar cells are epithelial cells that form the alveolar walls. Type II alveolar cells are metabolically active. These cells secrete surfactant, a phospholipid that decreases the surface tension in the alveoli and prevents their collapse. Stimulus for surfactant production is thought to be related to maximum deep inspiration sustained for a few seconds or sighing, in which a person's normal tidal volume (normal breath of approximately 500 mL) is increased one to three times what is normal. Type III alveolar cell macrophages are large phagocytic cells that ingest foreign matter (e.g., mucus, bacteria) and act as an important defense mechanism.

Pleura

The lungs and wall of the thorax are lined with a serous membrane called the pleura. The visceral pleura covers the lungs; the parietal pleura lines the thorax. Only the parietal pleura has fibers for pain transmission. The intrapleural space, which lies between these two layers, contains a small amount of pleural fluid (20 to 25 cc) that serves to provide a frictionless surface between the two pleura in response to changes in respiration. The intrapleural space is negative with the average resting interpleural pressure –4 cm H_2O, that is four centimeters of water, below that of atmospheric pressure at rest, and remains so during inspiration and expiration. Refer to Table 8-1 for pleural pressures.

Mediastinum

The mediastinum is in the middle of the thorax, between the pleural sacs. It contains the great vessels of the heart, the

TABLE 8-1 Pressures: Atmospheric, Intrapulmonary, and Intrapleural

Pressure	At Rest	Inspiratory	Expiratory
Atmospheric	760	760	760
Intrapulmonary	760	757	763
Intrapleural	756	750	756

Atmospheric pressure remains constant at 760 mm Hg. For air to enter the lungs, the pressure within the airways and alveoli (intrapulmonary pressure) must become less than atmospheric so that the air can be pulled in. This is accomplished in inspiration because of the action of the diaphragm and the external intercostal muscles. At expiration, the intrapulmonary pressure is now higher than atmospheric pressure and air escapes from the lungs. The intrapleural pressure (pressure within the pleural cavity) fluctuates with inspiration and expiration but always remain negative.

heart, esophagus, trachea, thoracic duct, thymus, and lymph nodes, as well as the vagus, cardiac, and phrenic nerves.

Lobes

Each lung is divided into lobes. The left lung consists of an upper and lower lobe, whereas the right lung has an upper, middle, and lower lobe (refer to Fig. 8-2). The upper lobes of the lungs rise 1 in above the inner one third of the clavicle, thus there is always a risk of a pneumothorax (air in the pleural space) when inserting venous catheters in the neck. The base of each lung (when in a neutral position) is at the sixth rib in the MCL, the eighth rib in the midaxillary line (MAL), and the tenth rib posteriorly at rest. With inspiration, the lungs can descend to the eighth rib in the MCL, tenth rib in the MAL, and twelfth rib at the vertebral border. Use Figure 8-3 to find the common landmarks used in respiratory assessment.

Thoracic Cage

The 12 ribs, costal cartilages (cartilages that connect the sternum and the ends of the ribs; termed the *costochondral junction*), manubrium, sternum, xiphoid process, and vertebral column provide the structure that supports and protects the lung. The notch on the top of the manubrium may be referred to as the *suprasternal notch, sternal notch,* or *jugular notch.* Seven ribs and their costal cartilages articulate directly to the body of the sternum, ribs 8 to 10 attach to cartilage of the seventh rib. Ribs 11 and 12 do not have an anterior attachment and are sometimes referred to as 'floating ribs'. Posteriorly, each rib attaches to a vertebra. An important landmark for nurses to use when counting ribs is the angle of Louis, which is where the manubrium (top of sternum, approximately 4 cm long) and the body of the sternum meet at the second rib. This area is also termed the manubriosternal junction and can be palpable as a transverse ridge in most patients. The second costal cartilages articulate with the sternum here at the angle of Louis; the ICS below the angle is the second ICS.

It is important to recognize that any disorder to the bony structure of the thorax affects the ability of the lungs to function. The costal angle (lower parts of the anterior rib cage near the xiphoid process) normally is about 90 degrees.

Respiratory Muscles

Ventilation requires movement of the walls of the thoracic cage and of its floor, the *diaphragm.* The diaphragm is a dome-shaped muscle that, when contracted (during inspiration), pulls the lungs in a downward and forward direction; the abdomen appears to enlarge because the abdominal contents are being compressed by the diaphragm. With inspiration, the diaphragmatic pull elongates the chest cavity, and the external intercostal muscles (located between and along the lower borders of the ribs) contract to raise the ribs, which expands the anteroposterior (AP) diameter. The effect of these movements is to decrease the intrapulmonary pressure

(pressure within the lung) to less than atmospheric pressure, which causes air to rush into the lung (see Table 8-1). With expiration, the diaphragm and intercostals recoil, which increases the intrapulmonary pressure over atmospheric pressure so that gases are expelled from the lung. While inspiration is an active process, expiration is passive. In respiratory diseases, such as chronic obstructive pulmonary disease (COPD), the act of breathing becomes work requiring energy.

Additional accessory muscles of inspiration, including the scalene (elevates the first two ribs), sternocleidomastoid (raise the sternum), and the alae nasi (faring of nostrils), which may be called upon to assist with inspiration when exercising, while the abdominal and internal intercostal muscles may be used to increase expiration.

> **Nursing Alert**
> The diaphragm is innervated by the phrenic nerve, which exits the spinal column at the level of C3 to C5. Any fracture at or above this level will cause respiratory paralysis.

Neuroanatomy Related to Respiration

The rhythm of breathing is controlled by the medulla oblongata and pons. In addition, central chemoreceptors located in the medulla respond to changes in PCO_2 and pH levels in the cerebrospinal fluid and alter the depth and then the rate of ventilation to correct an imbalance. In addition, peripheral chemoreceptors are located in the aortic arch and the carotid arteries that respond first to changes in PaO_2 (less than 60 mm Hg) and then to $PaCO_2$ and pH by altering the depth and rate of respiration (Porth, 2015). These chemoreceptors no longer respond to $PaCO_2$ or pH in patients with COPD because of the persistently high levels of $PaCO_2$ that exist with this disorder, thus the primary drive to breathe comes from a low O_2 level rather than a high CO_2 level. If O_2 is administered at a high enough rate to raise the PaO_2 to normal, there is a risk of obliterating the hypoxic drive. Therefore low-flow O_2 is administered to a patient with COPD while the nurse carefully assesses for complications.

A final reflex to consider is the Hering–Breuer reflex that prevents overinflation of the lung. It is activated by stretch receptors located within the smooth muscle of large and small airways that inhibit further inspiration. Tidal volumes increased to approximately three times normal (greater than approximately 1,500 mL) are generally required to elicit this reflex in conscious, normally breathing adults (Hall, 2016a).

Function of the Respiratory System

The cells of the body require O_2. Certain vital tissues, such as the brain and the heart, cannot survive for long without a continuous supply. However, as a result of oxidation in the body tissues, CO_2 is produced and must be removed from the cells to prevent the buildup of acid waste products. The respiratory system performs this life-sustaining function of gas exchange.

Respiration

The process of **respiration** requires gas exchange both in the lungs, termed *external or pulmonary respiration,* and, ultimately, in the tissues, termed *internal or cellular respiration.* External respiration requires three processes: (1) *ventilation,* the act of breathing (inspiration and expiration); (2) *perfusion,* blood flow to the alveoli, so that gases can be exchanged; and (3) *diffusion,* movement of gases from a higher area of concentration to a lower area across the alveolar–capillary membrane. Systemic veins carry venous blood richer in CO_2 and poorer in O_2 than the systemic arteries to the pulmonary circulation. The O_2 concentration in blood within the capillaries of the lungs is lower than in the alveoli. Because of this concentration gradient, O_2 diffuses from the alveoli to the blood. Carbon dioxide, which has a higher concentration in the blood than in the alveoli, diffuses from the blood into the alveoli. The end result is O_2-rich blood leaving the pulmonary veins (the only veins other than the umbilical vein to carry oxygenated blood) to systemic circulation. Internal respiration refers to the process by which O_2 is supplied to, and CO_2 is removed from, the body cells by way of the circulating blood. Cells are in close contact with capillaries, the thin walls of which permit easy passage or exchange of O_2 and CO_2. Oxygen diffuses from the capillaries through the capillary walls to the interstitial fluid. At this point, O_2 diffuses through the membrane of tissue cells, where it is used by mitochondria for cellular respiration. The movement of CO_2 occurs by diffusion in the opposite direction—from cell to blood. These processes are critical for survival.

Ventilation

During inspiration, air flows from the environment into the trachea, bronchi, bronchioles, and alveoli. During expiration, alveolar gas travels the same route in reverse.

Physical factors that govern air flow in and out of the lungs are collectively referred to as the *mechanics of ventilation* and include air pressure variances, resistance to air flow (the narrower the airway, the greater the resistance to flow), and lung compliance (the dispensability of the lung, or how well the lung stretches).

Airway Resistance

Resistance is determined chiefly by the radius or size of the airway through which the air is flowing. Any process that changes the bronchial diameter or width affects airway resistance and alters the rate of air flow for a given pressure gradient during respiration (Box 8-1). With increased resistance, greater-than-normal respiratory effort is required to achieve normal levels of ventilation.

Compliance

Compliance is a measure of the elasticity, expandability, and distensibility of the lungs and thoracic structures. Consider an elastic band: When it is stretched, it easily returns to its normal shape; so too should the lungs. Factors that determine lung compliance are the surface tension of the alveoli (normally low with the presence of surfactant) and the connective tissue (i.e., collagen and elastin) of the lungs.

Compliance is normal (1.0 L/cm H_2O) if the lungs and thorax easily stretch and distend when pressure is applied. High or increased compliance occurs if the lungs have lost their elasticity (cannot return to normal state) and the thorax is overdistended (i.e., in emphysema). Low or decreased compliance occurs if the lungs and thorax are "stiff" (difficult to stretch). Conditions associated with decreased compliance include pneumothorax, hemothorax, pleural effusion, pulmonary edema, atelectasis, pulmonary fibrosis, and acute respiratory distress syndrome (ARDS), all of which are discussed in later chapters in this unit.

Lung Volumes and Capacities

Lung function, which reflects the mechanics of ventilation, is viewed in terms of lung volumes and lung capacities. These terms are described in Table 8-2 and illustrated in Figure 8-4. Three common measurements that the medical-surgical nurse should understand are tidal volume, minute ventilation, and vital capacity. The volume of each breath is referred to as the *tidal volume* and can be measured by a bedside spirometer. If the patient is breathing through an endotracheal tube or tracheostomy, the spirometer is attached directly to it, and the exhaled volume is obtained from the reading on the gauge. In other patients, the spirometer is attached to a face mask or a mouthpiece positioned so that it is airtight, and the exhaled volume is measured.

The tidal volume may vary from breath to breath. To ensure that the measurement is reliable, it is important to measure the volumes of several breaths and to note the range of tidal volumes, together with the average tidal volume. But measurements like respiratory rates and tidal volume alone are unreliable indicators of adequate ventilation because both can vary widely from breath to breath. However, together the tidal volume and respiratory rate are important because the minute ventilation is useful in detecting respiratory failure.

FIGURE 8-4 Spirometry recordings of respiratory volumes (*left*) and diagram of lung capacities (*right*). The tidal volume (TV, *yellow*) is the amount of air inhaled and exhaled during normal breathing; the inspiratory reserve volume (IRV, *pink*) is the maximal amount of air in excess of the tidal volume that can be forcefully inhaled; the maximal expiratory reserve (ERV, *blue*) is the maximal amount of air that can be exhaled in excess of tidal volume; and the residual volume (RV, *green*) is the air that continues to remain in the lung after maximal expiratory effort. The functional residual capacity (FRC) is the sum of the ERV and the RV. The vital capacity is the sum of IRV, TV, and ERV. (From Porth, C. M. (2015). *Essentials of pathophysiology* (4th ed.). Philadelphia, PA: Lippincott Williams & Wilkins.)

TABLE 8-2 Lung Volumes and Lung Capacities

Term	Symbol	Description	Normal Value[a]	Significance
Lung Volumes				
Tidal volume	VT or TV	The volume of air inhaled and exhaled with each breath	500 mL or 5–10 mL/kg	The tidal volume may not vary, even with severe disease.
Inspiratory reserve volume	IRV	The maximum volume of air that can be inhaled after a normal inhalation	3,100 mL	Inspiratory reserve volume is decreased in obstructive lung disorders.
Expiratory reserve volume	ERV	The maximum volume of air that can be exhaled forcibly after a normal exhalation	1,200 mL	Expiratory reserve volume is decreased with restrictive conditions, such as obesity, ascites, or pregnancy.
Residual volume	RV	The volume of air remaining in the lungs after a maximum exhalation	1,200 mL	Residual volume may be increased with obstructive disease.
Lung Capacities				
Vital capacity	VC	The maximum volume of air exhaled from the point of maximum inspiration VC = TV + IRV + ERV	4,800 mL	A decrease in vital capacity may be found in neuromuscular disease, generalized fatigue, atelectasis, pulmonary edema, and COPD.
Inspiratory capacity	IC	The maximum volume of air inhaled after normal expiration IC = TV + IRV	3,600 mL	A decrease in inspiratory capacity may indicate restrictive disease; may also be decreased in obesity.
Functional residual capacity	FRC	The volume of air remaining in the lungs after a normal expiration FRV = ERV + RV	2,400 mL	Functional residual capacity may be increased with COPD and decreased in ARDS.
Total lung capacity	TLC	The volume of air in the lungs after a maximum inspiration TLC = TV + IRV + ERV + RV	6,000 mL	Total lung capacity may be decreased with restrictive disease (atelectasis, pneumonia) and increased in COPD.

[a]Values for healthy men; women are 20–25% less.
ARDS, acute respiratory distress syndrome; COPD, chronic obstructed pulmonary disease.

Minute ventilation is the volume of air expired per minute. It is equal to the product of the tidal volume in liters multiplied by the respiratory rate or frequency. In practice, the minute ventilation is not calculated but is measured directly using a spirometer. Minute ventilation may be decreased by a variety of conditions that result in hypoventilation. When the minute ventilation falls, alveolar ventilation in the lungs also decreases, and the $PaCO_2$ increases.

Forced vital capacity requires having the patient take in a maximal breath and exhale fully and forcefully. Most patients can exhale at least 80% of their vital capacity in 1 second (forced expiratory volume in 1 second, or FEV_1) and almost all of it in 3 seconds (FEV_3). A reduction in FEV_1 (ability to get the air OUT of the lung) suggests abnormal pulmonary air flow. If the patient's FEV_1 and forced vital capacity are reduced proportionately, maximal lung expansion is restricted in some way. If the reduction in FEV_1 greatly exceeds the reduction in forced vital capacity, the patient may have some degree of airway obstruction. Often forced vital capacity is reduced in COPD because of air trapping, and a decreased FEV is a valuable clue to the severity of the expiratory airway obstruction.

Thus, pulmonary function tests (PFTs) can aid in diagnosing restrictive or obstructive pulmonary disorders. Restrictive disorders are ones that make the lungs stiff; they decrease the total volume of air the lungs can hold. This is typically due to a decrease in the elasticity of the lungs or the inability of the chest wall to expand during inhalation. Examples of restrictive lung diseases are asbestosis, sarcoidosis, and pulmonary fibrosis. Obstructive disorders cause a narrowing or blockage in exhaled airflow and are commonly associated with COPD (discussed in Chapter 11).

Diffusion and Perfusion

Diffusion is the process by which O_2 and CO_2 are exchanged at the air–blood interface. The alveolar–capillary membrane is ideal for diffusion because of its thinness and large surface area. In the normal, healthy adult, O_2 and CO_2 travel across the alveolar–capillary membrane without difficulty as a result of differences in gas concentrations in the alveoli and capillaries.

Pulmonary perfusion is the actual blood flow through the pulmonary circulation. The blood is pumped into the lungs by the right ventricle (RV) through the pulmonary artery. The pulmonary artery divides into the right and left branches to supply both lungs. These two branches divide further to supply all parts of each lung. Normally, about 2% of the blood pumped by the RV does not perfuse the alveolar capillaries. This "shunted" blood drains into the left side of the heart without participating in alveolar gas exchange.

The pulmonary circulation is considered a low-pressure system because the systolic blood pressure in the pulmonary artery is 20 to 30 mm Hg and the diastolic pressure is 8 to 15 mm Hg. Because of these low pressures, the pulmonary vasculature normally can vary its capacity to accommodate the blood flow it receives. However, pulmonary blood flow is also not consistent. Regardless of body position, the lower (dependent) areas of the lung receive greater blood flow than upper (nondependent) areas (Butterworth, Mackey, & Wasnick, 2013). When a person is in an upright position, the pulmonary artery pressure is not great enough to supply blood to the apex of the lung against the force of gravity. Thus, when a person is upright, the lung may be considered to be divided into three sections: an upper part with poor blood supply, a lower part with maximal blood supply, and a section between the two with an intermediate supply of blood. When a person lying down turns to one side, more blood passes to the dependent lung. Thus, the nurse should consider that the dependent lung, regardless of position, is better perfused.

Perfusion is also influenced by alveolar pressure. The pulmonary capillaries are sandwiched between adjacent alveoli. If the alveolar pressure is sufficiently high, the capillaries are squeezed. Depending on the pressure, some capillaries completely collapse, whereas others only narrow.

Pulmonary artery pressure, gravity, and alveolar pressure determine the patterns of perfusion. In lung disease, these factors vary, and the perfusion of the lung may become very abnormal.

Ventilation and Perfusion Balance and Imbalance

Ventilation is the flow of gas in and out of the lungs (normally at a rate of 4 L/min), and perfusion is the filling of the pulmonary capillaries with blood (normally at a rate of 5 L/min). Thus, the alveolar (ventilation) to capillary (perfusion) ratio is 4:5 or 0.8. Adequate gas exchange depends on an adequate ventilation–perfusion ($\dot{V}/\dot{Q}$) ratio.

$\dot{V}/\dot{Q}$ imbalance occurs as a result of inadequate ventilation, inadequate perfusion, or both. There are four possible $\dot{V}/\dot{Q}$ states in the lung: normal $\dot{V}/\dot{Q}$ ratio, low $\dot{V}/\dot{Q}$ ratio (shunt), high $\dot{V}/\dot{Q}$ ratio (dead space), and absence of ventilation and perfusion (silent unit) (Box 8-2).

Shunting is the term used to describe conditions in which ventilation is impaired and perfusion is adequate. Normal shunting is about 2%; severe **hypoxia** results when the amount of shunting exceeds 20%. This can occur secondary to airway obstruction from a variety of causes (mucus plug, atelectasis, infective process, tumor), where blood is bypassing the alveoli without gas exchange. Adequate ventilation but impaired perfusion (as in pulmonary emboli, which is a blood clot in pulmonary vessels) is termed *increased dead space*. In this situation, the alveolus has inadequate perfusion, and gas exchange does not occur. Both conditions result in **hypoxia** (low levels of cellular O_2). Supplemental O_2 is of use in conditions causing an increase in dead space, as long as the impaired perfusion is not massive; supplemental O_2 may not improve **hypoxemia** in shunting, however, as the O_2 does not come in contact with alveoli (areas of diffusion).

Physiology Alert

The nurse understands that with low O_2 saturation (especially when it falls below 70% of normal, i.e., below 73 mm Hg PO_2), the adjacent blood vessels constrict, with resulting increased vascular resistance. The lower the O_2 level, the higher the pulmonary vasoconstriction, which, in turn, causes strain on the RV. Recall the RV must push blood through this increased resistance, leading to RV strain. This effect is opposite *to the effect observed in systemic vessels, which dilate rather than constrict in response to low O_2 levels. Although not completely understood, it is thought low O_2 concentration may stimulate the release of vasoconstrictor substances or decrease release of a vasodilator, such as nitric oxide, from the lung tissue (Hall, 2016b).*

Concept Mastery Alert

When ventilation exceeds perfusion (exhibited by a pulmonary embolus), a dead space exists. A low ventilation–perfusion ratio (shunting) exists when ventilation is impaired and perfusion is adequate.

Gas Exchange

The air we breathe is a gaseous mixture consisting mainly of nitrogen (78.62%) and O_2 (20.84%), with traces of CO_2 (0.04%), water vapor (0.05%), helium, and argon.

Oxygen and CO_2 are transported simultaneously, dissolved in blood, or combined with some of the elements of blood. Oxygen is carried in the blood in two forms: first, as physically dissolved O_2 in the plasma, and second, in combination with the hemoglobin of the red blood cells. Each 100 mL of normal arterial blood carries 0.3 mL of O_2 physically dissolved in the plasma and 20 mL of O_2 in

BOX 8-2
Understanding Ventilation and Perfusion

Normal Ventilation and Perfusion

When ventilation and perfusion ($\dot{V}/\dot{Q}$) are matched, unoxygenated blood from the venous system returns to the right side of the heart through the pulmonary arteries to the lung, carrying carbon dioxide (CO_2). The arteries branch into alveolar capillaries. Gas exchange takes place in the alveolar capillaries. Normal ventilation is 4 L/min, and perfusion is normally at a rate of 5 L/min. Thus, the alveolar (ventilation) to capillary (perfusion) ratio is 4:5 or 0.8.

From pulmonary artery
To pulmonary vein
Alveolus
Normal capillary

Ventilation and Perfusion Mismatch

Conditions that may produce a $\dot{V}/\dot{Q}$ mismatch include the following:

1. Shunting (reduced ventilation to a lung unit) causes unoxygenated blood to move from the right side of the heart to the left side and into systemic circulation; it may result from obstruction of the distal airways, such as with pneumonia, atelectasis, tumor, or a mucus plug. When the $\dot{V}/\dot{Q}$ ratio is low, pulmonary circulation is adequate, but not enough oxygen (O_2) is available to the alveoli for normal diffusion. To illustrate, assume the ventilation is now 2 L/min versus a perfusion of 5 L/min. The ratio is now 2:5 or reduced to 0.4. A portion of the blood flowing through the pulmonary vessels doesn't become oxygenated.

Ventilation blockage
From pulmonary artery
To pulmonary vein
Alveolus

2. Dead-space ventilation (reduced perfusion to a lung unit) occurs when alveoli do not have adequate blood supply for gas exchange to occur, such as with pulmonary emboli (PE) and pulmonary infarction. When the $\dot{V}/\dot{Q}$ ratio is high, as shown here, ventilation is normal, but alveolar perfusion is reduced or absent. Note the narrowed capillary, indicating poor perfusion. This commonly occurs from a perfusion defect, such as PE, or a disorder that decreases cardiac output (cardiogenic shock). In this situation, assume the ventilation is normal at 4 L/min but perfusion is reduced to 3 L/min; thus, the ratio is 4:3 or increased to 1.3.

From pulmonary artery
To pulmonary vein
Perfusion blockage
Alveolus
Narrowed capillary

3. A silent unit (a combination of shunting and dead-space ventilation) occurs when little or no ventilation and perfusion are present, such as in acute respiratory distress syndrome.

The silent unit indicates an absence of ventilation and perfusion to the lung area.

Ventilation blockage
From pulmonary artery
To pulmonary vein
Perfusion blockage
Alveolus

Key to the figures: Blue, blood with CO_2; red, blood rich in O_2; purple, blood with CO_2 and O_2.
Adapted from *Hemodynamic monitoring made incredibly visual.* (2011). Philadelphia, PA: Lippincott Williams & Wilkins.

combination with hemoglobin. Thus, much more O_2 is normally transported in combination with hemoglobin (approximately 98%) than is physically dissolved in the blood (2%) (Porth, 2015). Hemoglobin is essential to supply sufficient O_2 to meet tissue demands. Figure 8-5 demonstrates differences in O_2 and CO_2 in venous, arterial, alveolus, and atmosphere.

Nursing Alert

Hemoglobin rapidly combines reversibly with O_2 (half-time of 0.01 second or less); that is, it allows O_2 to be released quickly to the tissues to satisfy metabolic needs. Some hemoglobin exists in forms such as methemoglobin (commonly seen in drug reaction) or is combined with carbon monoxide

Abbreviation
A = alveolar
a = arterial
$\bar{v}$ = venous
P = partial pressure
O_2 = oxygen
CO_2 = carbon dioxide
N_2 = nitrogen
H_2O = water vapor

PO_2 158 mm Hg
PCO_2 0.3 mm Hg

Air into the lungs

PAO_2 100 mm Hg
$PACO_2$ 40 mm Hg
PAH_2O 47 mm Hg
PAN_2 573 mm Hg

Air in the alveolus

CO_2 O_2

$P\bar{v}O_2$ 40 mm Hg
$P\bar{v}CO_2$ 46 mm Hg

PaO_2 97 mm Hg
$PaCO_2$ 40 mm Hg

CO_2 Pulmonary O_2
Capillary

Venous system blood
(Desaturated)

Arterial system blood
(Oxygenated)

FIGURE 8-5 Changes occur in the partial pressure of gases during respiration. These values vary as a result of the exchange of O_2 and CO_2 as well as the changes that occur in their partial pressures as venous blood flows through the lungs.

(as in smoke inhalation), in which case the hemoglobin cannot bind O_2, resulting in tissue hypoxia and lactic acidosis. Thus, the nurse is aware that O_2 delivery to tissues is dependent upon hemoglobin, O_2 content, and cardiac output. While a healthy heart generally can increase cardiac output to compensate for diseased lungs or a low hemoglobin level, a diseased heart may be unable to. It is important for the nurse to consider that a combination of poor oxygenation, low hemoglobin level, and low cardiac output may be rapidly fatal.

Gerontologic Considerations

A gradual decline in respiratory function begins in early to middle adulthood and affects the structure and function of the respiratory system. With aging (age 40 years and above), changes occur in the alveoli that reduce the surface area available for the exchange of O_2 and CO_2. At approximately 50 years of age, the alveoli begin to lose elasticity. A decrease in vital capacity occurs with loss of chest wall mobility, which restricts the tidal flow of air. The amount of respiratory dead space increases with age. These changes result in a decreased diffusion capacity for O_2 with increasing age, producing lower O_2 levels in the arterial circulation. Also, there is degeneration of the bronchial epithelium and mucous glands, which increases the susceptibility to infections (Swartz, 2014a,b). Gerontologic changes in the respiratory system are summarized in Table 8-3.

ASSESSMENT OF THE RESPIRATORY SYSTEM

Health History

The health history focuses on the physical and functional problems of the patient and the effects of these problems on the patient, including his or her ability to carry out activities of daily living (ADLs).

Common Complaints

Common signs and symptoms of respiratory disease are **dyspnea** (shortness of breath [SOB]), cough, sputum production, chest pain, wheezing, clubbing of the fingers, **hemoptysis** (coughing up blood), and cyanosis. These clinical manifestations are related to the duration and severity of the disease. In addition to identifying the chief reason why the patient is seeking health care, the nurse tries to determine when the health problem or symptom started, how long it has lasted, if it was relieved at any time, and how relief was obtained. The nurse obtains information about precipitating factors, duration, severity, and any associated factors or symptoms.

Dyspnea

Dyspnea is the subjective experience of "shortness of breath" (Swartz, 2014b). Dyspnea (difficult or labored breathing, breathlessness, SOB) is a symptom common in life-threatening conditions such as pulmonary

TABLE 8-3 Age-Related Changes in the Respiratory System

Component	Structural Changes	Functional Changes	History and Physical Findings
Defense mechanisms (respiratory and nonrespiratory)	↓ Number of cilia and ↓ mucus; ↓ thirst response ↓ Cough and gag reflex Loss of surface area of the capillary membrane Lack of a uniform or consistent ventilation and/or blood flow	↓ Protection against foreign particles; may have less moisture within the mucous membranes of the upper and lower respiratory tracts ↓ Protection against aspiration ↓ Antibody response to antigens ↓ Response to hypoxia and hypercapnia (chemoreceptors)	Thickened mucus, cough reflex may be reduced ↑ Infection rate History of respiratory infections, COPD, pneumonia Risk factors: smoking, environmental exposure, TB exposure
Lung	↓ Size of airway ↑ Diameter of alveolar ducts ↑ Collagen of alveolar walls ↑ Thickness of alveolar membranes ↓ Elasticity of alveolar sacs	↑ Airway resistance ↑ Pulmonary compliance ↓ Expiratory flow rate ↓ Oxygen diffusion capacity ↑ Dead space Premature closure of airways ↑ Air trapping ↑ Expiratory flow rates Ventilation–perfusion mismatch ↓ Exercise capacity ↑ Anteroposterior (AP) diameter	Unchanged total lung capacity (TLC) ↑ Residual volume (RV) ↓ Inspiratory reserve volume (IRV) ↓ Expiratory reserve volume (ERV) ↓ Forced vital capacity (FVC) and vital capacity (VC) ↑ Functional residual capacity (FRC) ↓ PaO_2 ↑ CO_2
Chest wall and muscles	Calcification of intercostal cartilages Arthritis of costovertebral joints ↓ Continuity of diaphragm ↓ Muscle mass Muscle atrophy	↑ Rigidity and stiffness of thoracic cage ↓ Respiratory muscle strength ↑ Work of breathing ↓ Capacity for exercise ↓ Peripheral chemosensitivity ↑ Risk for inspiratory muscle fatigue	Barrel chest ↑ AP diameter Shortness of breath ↑ Abdominal and diaphragmatic breathing ↓ Maximum expiratory flow rates
Skeletal changes	↑ dorsal curve of the thoracic spine Osteoclastic activity is greater than osteoblastic activity.	↑AP/lateral chest diameter Enlargement of the cancellous bone spaces and a thinning of the trabeculae	Kyphosis; loss of height; ↑ AP/lateral chest diameter; skeletal changes also contribute to a decrease in vital capacity ↑ Risk of osteoporosis

↑, increased; ↓, decreased.

embolism (PE), pulmonary edema, acute airway obstruction from anaphylaxis or foreign bodies, pneumothorax, pneumonia, myocardial infarction, or cardiac tamponade. Chronic dyspnea (longer than 4 weeks in duration) is associated with COPD, asthma, interstitial lung disease, heart failure, cardiomyopathy, gastroesophageal reflux disease (GERD), or other respiratory diseases (Braithwaite & Perina, 2014; Kraft, 2016; Peters, 2013). It may also be associated with neurologic or neuromuscular disorders (i.e., myasthenia gravis, Guillain–Barré syndrome, muscular dystrophy), renal (failure, acidosis), hepatic (ascites), endocrine (hyperthyroidism), and hematologic (anemia, hemoglobinopathy) diseases that affect respiratory function or physical deconditioning. Dyspnea can also occur after physical exercise in people without disease (Porth, 2015). It is also a symptom at the end of life, associated with anxiety, depression, and fear in patients and helplessness in caregivers (Blinderman & Billings, 2015). If the patient is experiencing severe dyspnea, the nurse may need to modify or abbreviate the questions asked and the timing of the health history to avoid increasing the patient's breathlessness and anxiety.

Clinical Significance. In general, acute diseases of the lungs produce a more severe grade of dyspnea than do chronic diseases. Sudden dyspnea in a healthy person may indicate pneumothorax (air in the pleural space), acute respiratory obstruction, or ARDS. In immobilized patients, sudden dyspnea may denote PE. *Orthopnea* (inability to breathe unless sitting or standing) may be found in patients with heart disease and occasionally in patients with COPD; dyspnea with an expiratory **wheeze** occurs with COPD. Noisy breathing may result from a narrowing of the airway or localized obstruction of a major bronchus by a tumor or foreign body. The presence of both inspiratory and expiratory wheezing usually signifies asthma if the patient does not have heart failure. Since dyspnea can occur with a variety of disorders, a thorough health history is essential.

The circumstance that produces the dyspnea must be determined; it is important to ask the patient the following questions:

- How much exertion triggers SOB?
- Is there an associated cough?
- Is the SOB related to other symptoms?
- Was the onset of SOB sudden or gradual?
- At what time of day or night does the SOB occur?
- Is the SOB worse when the patient is flat in bed?
- Does the SOB occur at rest? With exercise? Running? Climbing stairs?
- Is the SOB worse while walking? If so, when walking how far? How fast?
- How many level blocks can you walk without becoming short of breath?
- How many level blocks could you walk 6 months ago?
- What makes the SOB worse? What relieves it?

Other issues that are important in the assessment of dyspnea include the following: the patient's rating of the intensity of breathlessness, the effort required to breathe, and the severity of the breathlessness or dyspnea. Patients use a variety of terms and phrases to describe breathlessness, such as "can't get enough air," "hard to breath," "feeling tight," and the nurse needs to clarify what terms are most familiar to the patient and what these terms mean. Several scales are available to assess the severity of dyspnea, including visual analog scales similar to pain scales, where one side denotes no dyspnea and the extreme is maximal dyspnea. These scales can be used to assess changes in the severity of dyspnea over time (Porth, 2015). Box 8-3 illustrates one such scale.

Relief Measures. The management of dyspnea is aimed at identifying and correcting its cause. Relief of the symptom sometimes is achieved by placing the patient at rest with the head elevated (high Fowler position), encouraging

the patient to lean forward with arms and upper body supported on a table (orthopneic position), and using pursed-lip breathing (i.e., breathing in through the mouth and exhaling slowly through pursed lips to facilitate exhalation of air). Using a handheld fan (blowing air across the nose and mouth) has demonstrated success in reducing the sensation of breathlessness (Booth, Chin, & Spathis, 2015), and, in some cases, administering O_2 may help (Box 8-4). Strategies that enable patients with chronic or persistent dyspnea to decrease or prevent breathlessness and to cope with it can lead to improved quality of life (Moriyama, Takeshita, Haruta, Hattori, & Ezenwaka, 2015). Medical and nursing intervention may include use of opioids (Blinderman & Billings, 2015), O_2 administration in patients with hypoxemia (low O_2 saturation), pulmonary rehabilitation programs (Kiongera & Houde, 2015), or treatment specific to the cause of the dyspnea (i.e., proton-pump inhibitors [PPIs] for GERD, or angiotensin-converting enzyme [ACE] inhibitor or an angiotensin II receptor blocker [ARB], and a beta blocker for heart failure [HF]). See Chapter 11 for interventions for COPD.

Cough

Although cough is a reflex that protects the lungs from the accumulation of secretions or the inhalation of foreign bodies, it can also be a symptom of a number of disorders of the pulmonary system, or it can be suppressed in other disorders. It is the most common reason for seeking heath care in the United States (Kraft, 2016).

Involuntary coughing can be initiated by a variety of nerve receptors in the oropharynx, larynx, and tracheobronchial tree that can be stimulated by irritation (airborne irritants such as smoke, smog, perfume, powders, or dust), excess secretions, or a foreign body. These signals are transmitted to the vagus nerve and to the cough center (medulla).

A persistent and frequent cough can be exhausting and have significant impact on the patient's lifestyle and sense of well-being. Coughs can be significant enough to cause incontinence, vomiting, rib fractures, pain, and syncope. They may indicate serious pulmonary disease, but they may be caused by a variety of other problems, including cardiac disease, medications (e.g., amiodarone, ACE inhibitors), smoking, postnasal drip, pertussis, and GERD (Kraft, 2016).

It is important to consider that the cough reflex may be impaired by weakness or paralysis of the respiratory or abdominal muscles. Risk factors include prolonged inactivity, surgery, the presence of an NG tube (may prevent closure of the glottis), or depressed function of the medullary centers in the brain (e.g., anesthesia, drugs that depress the cough center, brain disorders) predisposing the patient to pulmonary problems (Porth, 2015).

Clinical Significance. To help determine the cause of the cough, the nurse needs the patient to describe the characteristics of the cough. A dry, irritative cough is a feature of

> **BOX 8-3** **Grading Dyspnea**
>
> To assess **dyspnea** as objectively as possible, ask your patient to briefly describe how various activities affect his breathing. Then document his response using this grading system:
> - *Grade 0:* Not troubled by breathlessness except with strenuous exercise
> - *Grade 1:* Troubled by shortness of breath when hurrying on a level path or walking up a slight hill
> - *Grade 2:* Walks more slowly on a level path because of breathlessness than do people of the same age or has to stop to breathe when walking on a level path at his own pace
> - *Grade 3:* Stops to breathe after walking about 100 yards (91 m) on a level path
> - *Grade 4:* Too breathless to leave the house or breathless when dressing or undressing

BOX 8-4

Nursing Research

Bridging the Gap to Evidence-Based Practice

Incentive spirometry (IS) for prevention of postoperative pulmonary complications in upper abdominal surgery

Nascimento, P., Módolo, N., Andrade, S., Guimarães, M., Braz, L., & Dib, R. (2014). *The Cochrane Database of Systemic Reviews*. 2:CD006058. Doi: 10.1002/14651858.CD006058.pub3.

Purpose

Since upper abdominal surgical procedures are associated with a high risk of postoperative pulmonary complications, the authors assessed the effect of incentive spirometry compared to no therapy or physiotherapy, including coughing and deep breathing, on all-cause postoperative pulmonary complications and mortality in adult patients admitted to a hospital for upper abdominal surgery.

Design

Meta-analysis of 12 studies was originally proposed, however this was decreased to 8 studies because of problems with the methodologic quality of the included studies. A total of 1,160 participants are reported below.

Findings

Four trials (152 patients) compared the effects of IS with no respiratory treatment. No statistically significant difference between the participants receiving IS and those who had no respiratory treatment for clinical complications (relative risk [RR] 0.59, 95% confidence interval [CI] 0.30 to 1.18). Two trials (194 patients) compared incentive spirometry with deep breathing exercises (DBE). No statistically significant differences between the participants receiving IS and those receiving DBE in the meta-analysis for respiratory failure (RR 0.67, 95% CI 0.04 to 10.50). Two trials (946 patients) compared IS with other chest physiotherapy. No statistically significant differences between the participants receiving IS and those receiving physiotherapy in the risk of developing a pulmonary condition or the type of complication. There was no evidence that IS is effective in the prevention of pulmonary complications.

Nursing Implications

It is important for nurses to be aware of current research findings. In this study, the evidence suggests there is a lack of effectiveness of incentive spirometry for prevention of postoperative pulmonary complications in patients after upper abdominal surgery. However, this review underlines the urgent need to conduct well-designed trials in this field. It seems prudent that for patients who are at risk for pulmonary complications, nurses should continue to educate patients regarding the use of IS, encourage them to use it hourly, and consider the minimal cost and noninvasive nature of IS therapy. Finally, nurses should participate in research studies that evaluate the efficacy of IS in well-designed studies.

---

an upper respiratory tract infection of viral origin, or a side effect of ACE inhibitor therapy. Laryngotracheitis causes an irritative, high-pitched cough. Tracheal lesions produce a brassy cough. Pertussis has a characteristic long, strident inspiratory noise (a whoop) before the cough. A hacking cough may be suggestive of pneumonia. A severe or changing cough may indicate bronchogenic carcinoma. Pleuritic chest pain that accompanies coughing may indicate pleural or chest wall (musculoskeletal) involvement.

The time of coughing is also noted. Coughing at night may herald the onset of left-sided heart failure or bronchial asthma. A cough in the morning with sputum production may indicate bronchitis. A cough that worsens when the patient is supine suggests postnasal drip (sinusitis) or reflux (spill-over of gastric contents into the larynx). Coughing after food intake may indicate aspiration of material into the tracheobronchial tree. A cough of recent onset is usually from a viral or upper respiratory tract infection. Duration is also a factor; a cough is considered acute if present for less than 3 weeks, persistent if between 3 and 8 weeks, and chronic if greater than 8 weeks.

! Nursing Alert

Coughs are not localized only to a pulmonary problem. For example, chronic cough is the only symptom in 75% of patients with GERD.

Eight common conditions associated with 98% of cases of chronic cough are: postnasal drip; asthma; GERD; chronic bronchitis; eosinophilic bronchitis, bronchiectasis; use of ACE inhibitors, and postinfectious cough (Kraft, 2016).

Relief Measures. Treatment depends on the cause of the cough. Treatment may include cautious use of cough suppressants because, while they may relieve the cough, they do not address the etiology of the cough. Other treatments are antihistamines, decongestants, or nasal corticosteroids if the etiology of the cough is postnasal drip; or H_2-blockers or PPIs when cough is associated with GERD. If the cough is a result of irritation, smoking cessation strategies are indicated. Drinking warm beverages may relieve cough caused by throat irritation.

Sputum Production

A patient who coughs long enough almost invariably produces sputum. Sputum production is the reaction of the lungs to any constantly recurring irritant. It also may be associated with a nasal discharge. The amount of sputum a person produces daily varies widely with mean values of 200 mL to over 500 mL (Santini, Cavallesco, & Grossi, 2015). Sputum production is unnoticed and sputum is swallowed, thus any complaint of sputum needs to be investigated. To help quantify the amount of sputum production, patients are asked to describe the volume of sputum production in terms of teaspoon (~5 mL) to cupful (~240 mL); however, this is difficult to calculate because of how much sputum may have been swallowed by the patient.

Clinical Significance. The nature of the sputum is indicative of the causal condition. A profuse amount of purulent sputum (thick and yellow or green) is a common sign of bacterial infection, lung abscess, or bronchiectasis. A small amount of purulent sputum is associated with acute bronchitis, pneumonia during resolution, small tuberculous cavities, or lung abscess. Sputum that looks like currant jelly is associated with *Klebsiella pneumoniae* or *Streptococcus pneumoniae*. Purulent rust-colored sputum suggests *pneumococcal pneumonia*. Thin, mucoid sputum frequently results from viral bronchitis. A gradual increase of sputum over time may indicate the presence of chronic bronchitis or bronchiectasis. Pink-tinged mucoid sputum suggests a lung tumor. Expectorated blood-stained sputum tends to be a complaint of patients with bronchogenic carcinoma, PE, and TB (Raftery, Lim, & Ostor, 2014). Profuse, frothy, white or pink material, often welling up into the throat, may indicate pulmonary edema. Foul-smelling sputum and bad breath point to the presence of a lung abscess, bronchiectasis, or an infection caused by anaerobic organisms (LeBlond, Brown, Suneja, & Szot, 2015b). A musty odor may indicate pseudomonas infection (Alspach, 2013).

Relief Measures. If the sputum is too thick for the patient to expectorate, it is necessary to decrease the sputum's viscosity by increasing its water content through adequate hydration (drinking water) and inhalation of aerosolized solutions, which may be delivered by any type of nebulizer.

Smoking is contraindicated with excessive sputum production because it interferes with ciliary action, increases bronchial secretions, causes inflammation and hyperplasia of the mucous membranes, and reduces production of surfactant. When a person stops smoking, sputum volume decreases and resistance to bronchial infections increases.

The patient's appetite may decrease because of the odor of the sputum or the taste it leaves in the mouth. The nurse encourages adequate oral hygiene and wise selection of food, measures that stimulate the appetite. Citrus juices at the beginning of the meal may increase palatability, because these juices cleanse the palate of the sputum taste.

Hemoptysis

Hemoptysis is a symptom of both pulmonary and cardiac disorders. The onset of hemoptysis is usually sudden, and it may be intermittent or continuous. Signs, which vary from blood-stained sputum to a large sudden hemorrhage, always merit investigation. Frank bloody sputum (obvious, visible presence of blood) may indicate a pulmonary emboli, bronchogenic carcinoma, or erosion of a bronchial artery

by cavitary tuberculosis, whereas blood-stained sputum (streaks of blood) may indicate inflammation in the nose, nasopharynx, gums, larynx, or bronchi, or airway trauma from severe coughing (Kraft, 2016). The amount of blood produced is not always proportional to the seriousness of the cause. If the oropharynx is colonized with *Serratia marcescens*, a red-pigment–producing aerobic gram-negative rod, the sputum can also be red and be confused with hemoptysis (Kraft, p. 589).

 Nursing Alert
Blood from the lung is usually bright red, frothy, and mixed with sputum. Initial symptoms include a tickling sensation in the throat, a salty taste, a burning or bubbling sensation in the chest, and perhaps chest pain, in which case the patient tends to splint the bleeding side. The term hemoptysis is reserved for the coughing up of blood arising from a pulmonary hemorrhage. This blood has an alkaline pH (greater than 7.0). If the hemorrhage is in the stomach, the blood is vomited (hematemesis) rather than coughed up. Blood that has been in contact with gastric juice is sometimes so dark that it is referred to as "coffee grounds." This blood generally has an acid pH.

Chest Pain

Chest pain or discomfort may be associated with pulmonary or cardiac disease. Chest pain associated with pulmonary conditions may be sharp, stabbing, and intermittent, or it may be dull, aching, and persistent. The pain usually is felt on the side where the pathologic process is located, but it may be referred elsewhere—for example, to the neck, back, or abdomen.

Clinical Significance. Chest pain may occur with pneumonia, PE with lung infarction, and pleurisy. It also may be a late symptom of bronchogenic carcinoma. In carcinoma, the pain may be dull and persistent because the cancer has invaded the chest wall, mediastinum, or spine.

Lung disease does not always cause thoracic pain because the lungs and the visceral pleura lack sensory nerves and are insensitive to pain stimuli. However, the parietal pleura has a rich supply of sensory nerves that are stimulated by inflammation and stretching of the membrane. Pleuritic pain from irritation of the parietal pleura is sharp and seems to "catch" on inspiration; patients often describe it as "like the stabbing of a knife." The nurse assesses the quality, intensity, and radiation of pain and identifies and explores precipitating factors and their relationship to the patient's position. In addition, it is important to assess the relationship of pain to the inspiratory and expiratory phases of respiration.

Relief Measures. Analgesic medications may be effective in relieving chest pain, but care must be taken not to depress the respiratory center or a productive cough, if present. Non-steroidal anti-inflammatory drugs (NSAIDs) achieve this goal and, therefore, are used for pleuritic pain. A regional anesthetic block may be performed to relieve extreme pain. Patients may be more comfortable when they lie on the affected side because this splints the chest wall, limits expansion and contraction of the lung, and reduces the friction between the injured or diseased pleura on that side. Pain associated with cough may be reduced manually by splinting the rib cage.

Wheezing

Wheezing is often the major finding in a patient with bronchoconstriction or airway narrowing. It is heard with or without a stethoscope, depending on its location. Wheezing is a high-pitched, musical sound heard mainly on expiration; however, it may be heard on both inspiration and expiration. Wheezing is associated with a variety of clinical conditions other than asthma. The nurse needs to assess for all possible etiologies (discussed later in this chapter). Oral or inhalant bronchodilator medications reverse wheezing in most instances.

 Nursing Alert
If a patient has severe bronchospasm, there may be an absence of wheezing or gas movement. Thus a "quiet" chest is a "scary" chest.

Patient and Family History

The nurse also assesses for risk factors and genetics factors that may contribute to the patient's lung condition (Boxes 8-5 and 8-6).

Social History

The nurse inquires about current or past smoking and calculates pack/year history. This is calculated by the number of packs smoked per day times the number of years the patient has smoked. Thus, 2 packs per day times 20 years equals a 40 pack/year history.

The impact of signs and symptoms on the patient's ability to perform ADLs and to participate in usual work and family activities is assessed. Questions related to sleep–rest patterns should include asking about nocturnal dyspnea (waking up

---

BOX 8-5
Risk Factors for Respiratory Disease

- Smoking (the single most important contributor to lung disease)
- Exposure to secondhand smoke
- Personal or family history of lung disease
- Genetic makeup
- Allergens and environmental pollutants
- Recreational and occupational exposure

BOX 8-6
Risk Factors for Hypoventilation

- Limited neurologic impulses transmitted from the brain to the respiratory muscles, as in spinal cord trauma, cerebrovascular accidents, tumors, myasthenia gravis, Guillain–Barré syndrome, polio, and drug overdose
- Depressed respiratory centers in the medulla, as with anesthesia, sedation, and drug overdose
- Limited thoracic movement (kyphoscoliosis), limited lung movement (pleural effusion, pneumothorax), or reduced functional lung tissue (chronic pulmonary diseases, severe pulmonary edema)

---

with SOB) or orthopnea as well as quantifying the number of pillows used at night. In addition, psychosocial factors that may affect the patient are explored. These factors include anxiety, role changes, family relationships, financial problems, employment status, and the strategies the patient uses to cope with them. It is also important to ask questions concerning immunizations, medications, exposure to environmental hazards, use of O_2, hospitalizations, and medical and surgical history.

Many respiratory diseases are chronic and progressively debilitating and disabling. Therefore, ongoing assessment of the patient's physical abilities, psychosocial supports, and quality of life is needed to plan appropriate interventions. It is important that the patient with a respiratory disorder understand the condition and be familiar with necessary self-care interventions. The nurse evaluates these factors over time and provides education as needed.

Physical Assessment

Complete respiratory assessment includes assessment of the integument and upper and lower respiratory structures. The nurse also observes the work of breathing (e.g., nasal flaring, mouth breathing, use of accessory muscles, splinting, etc.).

Assessment of the Integumentary System

Respiratory conditions may have skin and nail manifestations.

Inspection of Color

Cyanosis, a bluish coloring of the skin, is a very late indicator of hypoxia. The presence or absence of cyanosis is determined by the amount of unoxygenated hemoglobin in the blood. Cyanosis appears when there is at least 5 g/dL of unoxygenated hemoglobin (normal hemoglobin is approximately 15 g/dL). Thus, a full one third of the hemoglobin is deoxygenated before cyanosis is observed. In addition, a patient with anemia rarely manifests cyanosis, and a patient with polycythemia may appear cyanotic even if adequately oxygenated. Thus, cyanosis is *not* a reliable sign of hypoxia.

Assessment of cyanosis is affected by room lighting, the patient's skin color, and the distance of the blood vessels from the surface of the skin. Central cyanosis (tongue and lips), often associated with clubbing of the fingers and toes, indicates inadequate oxygenation of blood, whereas peripheral cyanosis (nailbeds) results from vasoconstriction or diminished peripheral blood flow in the distal extremities from a variety of causes and does not necessarily indicate a central systemic problem. In addition, the two may coexist. In people of color, the nurse assesses for central cyanosis by examining for dull, dark color in the buccal mucosa (inside of the cheek) and hard palate (roof of the mouth).

Inspection for Clubbing of the Fingers

Clubbing of the fingers is found in patients with chronic hypoxic conditions, chronic lung and pleural infections, or malignancies of the lung and pleural. It is also associated with cyanotic congenital heart disease, infective endocarditis, and cirrhosis (Tosti, 2016). It is painless, usually bilateral, and may be reversed if the causative factor is removed (Usatine, Smith, Chumley, & Mayeaux, 2013). This finding may be manifested initially as sponginess of the nail bed and loss of the nail bed angle, resulting in a bulbous enlargement of the distal segments of the fingers and toes (see Chapter 51, Box 51-4).

Assessment of Upper Respiratory Structures

For a routine examination of the upper airway, only a simple light source, such as a penlight, is necessary.

Inspection and Palpation of Nose and Sinuses

The nurse inspects the external nose for lesions, asymmetry, or inflammation and then asks the patient to tilt the head backward. Gently pushing the tip of the nose upward, the nurse examines the internal structures of the nose, inspecting the mucosa and septum for color, swelling, exudate, or bleeding. The nasal mucosa is normally redder than the oral mucosa. It may appear swollen and hyperemic if the patient has a common cold, but in allergic rhinitis, the mucosa appears pale and swollen. Most people have a slight degree of septal deviation, but actual displacement of the cartilage into either the right or left side of the nose may produce nasal obstruction. Such deviation usually causes no symptoms. Observation of nasal flaring and mouth breathing suggests respiratory distress. Next, the nurse may palpate the frontal and maxillary sinuses for tenderness, which suggests inflammation. Using the thumbs, gentle pressure is applied in an upward fashion at the supraorbital ridges (frontal sinuses) and in the cheek area adjacent to the nose (maxillary sinuses) (Fig. 8-6).

Inspection of Pharynx and Mouth

The mouth and pharynx are assessed by asking the patient to open the mouth wide and take a deep breath. Usually, this flattens the posterior tongue and briefly allows a full view of the anterior and posterior pillars, tonsils, uvula, and posterior pharynx (Fig. 8-7). These structures are inspected for color, symmetry, and evidence of exudate, ulceration,

FIGURE 8-6 Technique for palpating the frontal sinuses at left and the maxillary sinuses at right.

or enlargement. If a tongue blade is needed to depress the tongue to visualize the pharynx, it is pressed firmly down on the midpoint of the arched tongue to avoid a gagging reflex (Bickley, 2017).

Palpation of the Trachea

The position and mobility of the trachea are noted by placing the thumb and index finger of one hand on either side of the trachea just above the sternal notch. The trachea is highly sensitive, and palpating too firmly may trigger a coughing or gagging response. The trachea is normally in the midline as it enters the thoracic inlet behind the sternum, but it may be deviated by masses in the neck or mediastinum. The trachea may deviate away from a life-threatening tension

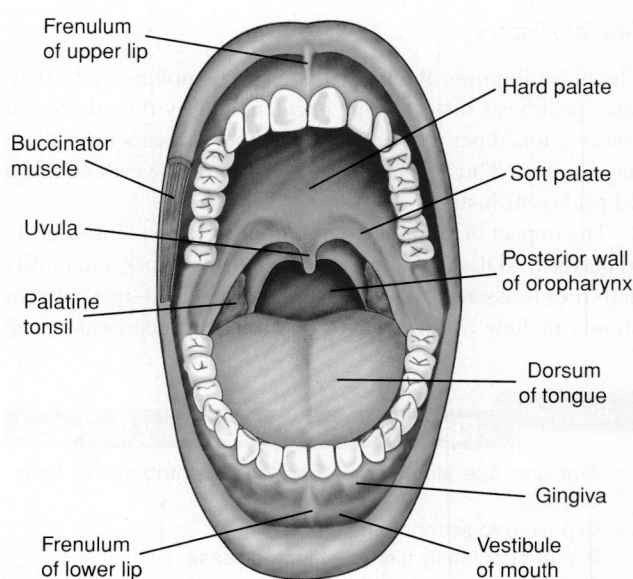

FIGURE 8-7 The pharynx and other oral structures—pillars, tonsils, uvula, hard and soft palates, posterior pharynx, and tongue—are easily seen when the mouth is open.

pneumothorax, and toward an atelectasis or fibrosis of the lung (Mootz & Matuschak, 2015).

Physical Assessment of the Lower Respiratory Structures and Breathing

Lower respiratory assessment consists of four areas: inspection, palpation, percussion, and auscultation. The patient should be positioned upright, if possible, to assess the posterior thorax and lungs, and supine to assess the anterior chest and lung with chest exposed.

Thoracic Inspection

The nurse observes the skin over the thorax for color and turgor and for evidence of loss of subcutaneous tissue. In recording or reporting the findings, anatomic landmarks are used as points of reference (Box 8-7). Normally, there is symmetry in chest movement. It is important to note asymmetry, if present. In thin people, it is quite normal to note a slight retraction of the ICSs during quiet breathing. Bulging of the ICSs during expiration implies obstruction of expiratory airflow, as in emphysema. Marked retraction on inspiration, particularly if asymmetric, implies blockage of a branch of the respiratory tree. Asymmetric bulging of the ICSs, on one side or the other, is created by an increase in pressure within the hemithorax. This may be a result of air trapped under pressure within the pleural cavity, where it is not normally present (pneumothorax), or the pressure of fluid within the pleural space (pleural effusion).

> **! Nursing Alert**
> *Frequently, patients with COPD are found to have cachexia and muscle dysfunction. These patients should be screened for malnutrition*

and referred to a nutrition practitioner when there is diminished nutritional intake or weight loss (Seres, 2015).

Chest Configuration. Normally, the ratio of the AP diameter to the lateral diameter is 1:2. However, four main deformities of the chest are associated with respiratory disease that alter this relationship: barrel chest, funnel chest (pectus excavatum), pigeon chest (pectus carinatum), and kyphoscoliosis (see Fig. 8-8).

Barrel chest occurs as a result of lung hyperinflation, as in emphysema. There is an increase in the AP diameter of the thorax so that it approximates a 1:1 ratio. In a patient with emphysema, note the costal angle will also be greater than 90 degrees.

Funnel chest or pectus excavatum is a common developmental deformity where there is a depression in the lower portion of the sternum, so that the sternum appears "bowl-like," and the ratio may be less than 1:2. It may be symmetrical or asymmetrical to the midline of the sternum. Refer to a pediatric resource for further details. Most patients are asymptomatic but may have mild restriction on PFTs (Tzelepis & Dennis McCool, 2015) and decreased thoracic volume with aging; thus, medical-surgical nurses should assess these patients' pulmonary function thoroughly and encourage the use of the incentive spirometer (IS).

Pectus carinatum is also a congenital structural abnormality in which the sternum is displaced anteriorly, increasing the AP diameter. For some patients, this deformity is associated with a rigid chest wall in which the AP diameter is almost fixed in full inspiration. In these patients, respiratory efforts are less efficient, and use of IS should be encouraged.

A *kyphoscoliosis* is characterized by elevation of the scapula and a corresponding S-shaped spine. This deformity

(A)   **(B)**

Anteriorly
displaced sternum

Depressed
costal cartilages

(C)

FIGURE 8-8 Deformities of the thoracic wall. **(A)** Funnel chest (pectus excavatum); **(B)** Barrel chest; **(C)** Pigeon chest (pectus carinatum).

BOX 8-7 **Locating Thoracic Landmarks**

With respect to the thorax, location is defined both horizontally and vertically. With respect to the lungs, location is defined by lobe.

Horizontal Reference Points

Horizontally, thoracic locations are identified according to their proximity to the rib or the intercostal space under the examiner's fingers. On the anterior surface, identification of a specific rib is facilitated by first locating the angle of Louis. This is where the manubrium joins the body of the sternum in the midline. The second rib joins the sternum at this prominent landmark.

Other ribs may be identified by counting down from the second rib. The intercostal spaces are referred to in terms of the rib immediately above the intercostal space; for example, the fifth intercostal space is directly below the fifth rib.

Locating ribs on the posterior surface of the thorax is more difficult. The first step is to identify the spinous process. This is accomplished by finding the seventh cervical vertebra (*vertebra prominens*), which is the most prominent spinous process. When the neck is slightly flexed, the seventh cervical spinous process stands out. Other vertebrae are then identified by counting downward.

Vertical Reference Points

Several imaginary lines are used as vertical referents or landmarks to identify the location of thoracic findings. The *midsternal line* passes through the center of the sternum. The *midclavicular line* is an imaginary line that descends from the middle of the clavicle. The *point of maximal impulse* of the heart normally lies medial to this line on the left thorax.

When the arm is abducted from the body at 90 degrees, imaginary vertical lines may be drawn from the anterior axillary fold, from the middle of the axilla, and from the posterior axillary fold. These lines are called, respectively, the *anterior axillary line,* the *midaxillary line,* and the *posterior axillary line.* A line drawn vertically through the superior and inferior poles of the scapula is called the *scapular line,* and a line drawn down the center of the vertebral column is called the *vertebral line.* Using these landmarks, for example, the nurse communicates findings by referring to an area of dullness extending from the vertebral to the scapular line between the seventh and tenth ribs on the right.

Lobes of the Lungs

The lobes of the lung may be mapped on the surface of the chest wall in the following manner. The fissure that divides the right and left lung into upper and lower lobes posteriorly is termed the oblique fissure. It begins at T3 (spinous process) and obliquely to sixth rib in the midclavicular line (MCL) bilaterally. The right lung is further divided anteriorly by the horizontal fissure, which runs close to the fourth rib at the sternal border (SB) to the fifth rib in the midaxillary line (MAL). There is no presentation of the right middle lobe on the posterior surface of the chest.

Anterior thorax

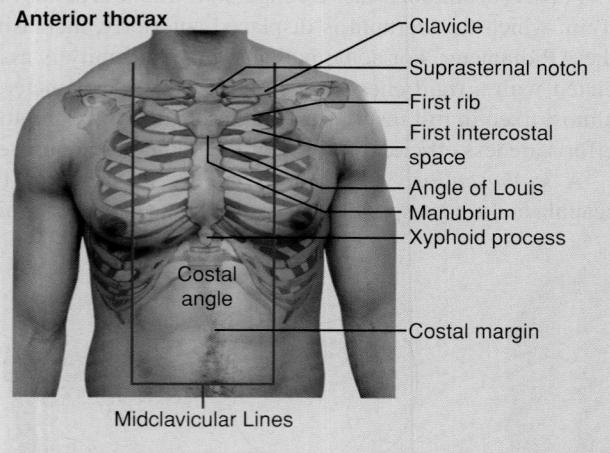

- Clavicle
- Suprasternal notch
- First rib
- First intercostal space
- Angle of Louis
- Manubrium
- Xyphoid process
- Costal angle
- Costal margin

Midclavicular Lines

Posterior thorax

- C7
- T1
- Scapula
- Spinous process
- T12

Midscapular lines

Anterior view of lungs

- Midsternal line
- Midclavicular line
- Right upper lobe
- Right middle lobe
- Right lower lobe
- Left upper lobe
- Left lower lobe

Lateral view of lungs

- Midaxillary line
- Anterior axillary line
- Right upper lobe
- Right middle lobe
- Right lower lobe
- Posterior axillary line

limits lung expansion within the thorax. It may occur with osteoporosis and other skeletal disorders that affect the thorax.

In addition, the nurse notes the presence of paradoxical chest movements known as a *flail chest*, which occurs with multiple ipsilateral (same side) rib fractures. In this condition, asymmetrical chest movements are observed; during inspiration, the unstable chest wall collapses inward and then bulges outward with expiration. It is associated with respiratory distress and crepitus (see later discussion). The nurse is aware that early intubation and ventilatory assistance in patients with flail chest reduce mortality compared with delaying intubation until the onset of respiratory failure (Jones, Nelson, & Ma, 2016).

Breathing Patterns and Respiratory Rates. Observing the rate and depth of respiration is a simple but important aspect of assessment. The normal adult who is resting comfortably takes 12 to 20 breaths per minute. Except for occasional sighs, respirations are regular in depth and rhythm. This normal pattern is described as *eupnea.*

Certain patterns of respiration are characteristic of specific disease states. Respiratory rhythms and their deviation from normal are important observations that the nurse reports and documents. The rates and depths of various patterns of respiration are presented in Table 8-4.

![Nursing Alert icon] ***Nursing Alert***
One should not rely on only visual inspection of the rate and depth of a patient's respiratory excursions to determine the adequacy of ventilation. Respiratory excursions may appear normal or exaggerated due to an increased work of breathing, but actually the patient may be moving only enough air to ventilate the dead space. If there is any question regarding adequacy of ventilation, auscultation or pulse oximetry (or both) should be used for additional assessment of respiratory status.

Thoracic Palpation

The nurse palpates the thorax for tenderness, masses, lesions, respiratory excursion, vocal fremitus, and crepitus.

Respiratory Excursion. Respiratory excursion is an estimation of thoracic range and expansion and may disclose significant information about thoracic movement during breathing. The patient is instructed to inhale deeply while the movement of the nurse's thumbs is observed (placed along the costal margin on the anterior chest wall) during inspiration and expiration. This movement is normally symmetric.

Posterior assessment is performed by placing the thumbs adjacent to the spinal column at the level of the tenth rib (Fig. 8-9). The hands lightly grasp the lateral rib cage. Sliding

FIGURE 8-9 Method for assessing posterior respiratory excursion. Place both hands posteriorly at the level of T9 or T10. Slide hands medially to pinch a small amount of skin between your thumbs. Observe for symmetry as the patient exhales fully following a deep inspiration.

the thumbs medially about 2.5 cm (1 in) raises a small skinfold between the thumbs. The patient is instructed to take a full inspiration and to exhale fully. The nurse observes for normal flattening of the skinfold and feels the symmetric movement of the thorax.

Asymmetric excursion may be due to a problem in the underlying chest wall, pleura, or lung; causes include pain (fractured ribs, trauma, splinting secondary to pleurisy or incisional pain), fibrosis, consolidation (lobar pneumonia), pleural effusion, or unilateral bronchial obstruction (Bickley, 2013). Equal but diminished expansion is seen in neurologic disease and emphysema.

Tactile Fremitus. The detection of palpable sound vibration transmitted to the chest wall as the patient speaks is called *tactile fremitus.* Normal fremitus is widely varied. It is influenced by thickness of the chest wall, especially with an increase in subcutaneous tissue associated with obesity, and pitch (lower-pitched sounds travel better and produce greater vibration of the chest wall). Fremitus is most pronounced in the second ICS lateral to the sternum and medial to the scapula, the level of the bronchus. Therefore, it is most palpable in the upper thorax, anteriorly and posteriorly.

The patient is asked to repeat "99" or "1, 2, 3" as the nurse's hands move down the patient's thorax comparing vibrations from similar areas (Fig. 8-10). Some clinicians test for fremitus using both hands simultaneously to compare the two sides, whereas others prefer a systematic survey

TABLE 8-4 Rates and Depths of Respiration

	Definition
Eupnea	Normal, breathing at 12–20 breaths/min
Bradypnea	Slower than normal rate (<10 breaths/min), with normal depth and regular rhythm; associated with increased intracranial pressure, brain injury, CNS depressants (e.g., opiates, benzodiazepines, barbiturates, alcohol), and drug overdose
Tachypnea	Rapid, shallow breathing >24 breaths/min; commonly seen in patients with a number of causes including metabolic acidosis, septicemia, severe pain, and rib fracture
Hypoventilation	Decreased depth of breathing; associated with decreased medullary respiratory center drive, weakness of the respiratory muscles from a variety of neurologic disorders (e.g., myasthenia gravis, amyotrophic lateral sclerosis, Guillain–Barré)
Hyperventilation	Increased rate and depth of breathing (called *Kussmaul respiration* if caused by diabetic ketoacidosis); associated with severe acidosis of diabetic or renal origin and hypoxemia
Apnea	Period of cessation of breathing. Time duration varies; apnea may occur briefly during other breathing disorders, such as with sleep apnea. Life-threatening if sustained.
Cheyne–Stokes	Regular cycle in which the rate and depth of breathing increase and then decrease until apnea (usually about 20 seconds) occurs. It may be seen during the sleep of normal children and the aged, also associated with heart failure and damage to the respiratory center (drug-induced, tumor, trauma).
Biot respiration	Periods of normal breathing (3–4 breaths) followed by a varying period of apnea (usually 10–60 seconds). Uncommon, but associated with some central nervous system disorders, meningitis.

of the chest wall with one hand. The vibrations are detected with the palmar surfaces of the fingers and hands, or the ulnar aspect of the extended hands, on the thorax. Bony areas are not tested.

Air does not conduct sound well, but a solid substance such as a tumor, or fluid that increases the density of the lung,

such as occurs in pneumonia, does. Therefore, an increase in solid tissue of the normally air-filled lung enhances fremitus, and an increase in air of the lung impedes sound. Patients with emphysema, which results in trapping of air, exhibit almost no tactile fremitus. A patient with consolidation of a lobe of the lung from pneumonia has increased tactile

FIGURE 8-10 The palpation sequence for tactile fremitus.

fremitus over that lobe. Air in the pleural space does not conduct sound; thus, a pneumothorax will have absent fremitus (Bickley, 2013). In the case of pleural effusion, decreased fremitus is noted at the effusion; however, the lung above the effusion may reveal increased fremitus as the fluid has increased the density of the lung.

Crepitus. Crepitus or subcutaneous emphysema is indicated by the presence of air bubbles in the subcutaneous tissues or underlying muscle; upon palpation, the sensation of bubbles under the fingers can be felt and, occasionally, crackling can be heard. Crepitus is not painful. The gas bubbles move with palpation. It is associated with pneumothorax, trauma (e.g., fractured rib piercing the lung), surgical wounds, or gas gangrene.

Thoracic Percussion

Percussion sets the chest wall and underlying structures in motion, producing audible and tactile vibrations. It helps to determine whether underlying tissues are filled with air, fluid, or solid material and is used to estimate diaphragmatic excursion. If possible, the patient is positioned in a sitting position with the head flexed forward and the arms crossed in front of the chest touching the patient's shoulders, which exposes more lung area for assessment by separating the scapulae widely. The nurse maintains a position to the side of the patient in order to comfortably and firmly hyperextend the middle finger of the nondominant hand (pleximeter finger) in the ICSs, being careful to avoid contact with any other finger on the chest wall as sound will be dampened. Bony structures (scapulae or ribs) are not percussed. While the middle finger is positioned firmly against the chest wall

in the ICS, the middle finger of the opposite hand strikes the pleximeter finger in a quick and sharp manner. The striking finger aims for the distal interphalangeal joint (below the nail and above the distal joint). The term to describe the sound heard over a normal lung is resonant. Normally dullness is heard over bone, thus if this sound is noted over lung tissue, it is associated with consolidation, such as from pneumonia or a tumor. Hyperresonant sounds, which are louder and lower-pitched sounds, are associated with COPD or pneumothorax. It takes practice to develop comfort striking the finger with a quick, sharp but relaxed wrist motion and training to distinguish dullness, resonance, and hyperresonance (Bickley, 2013). The sound will penetrate only 5 to 7 cm, thus any density below this depth will not be discovered. The nurse proceeds down the posterior thorax, percussing symmetric areas at intervals of 5 to 6 cm (2 to 2.5 in) (Fig. 8-11). Dullness over the lung occurs when air-filled lung tissue is replaced by fluid or solid tissue.

Diaphragmatic Excursion. The normal resonance of the lung stops at the diaphragm. The position of the diaphragm is different during inspiration and expiration. Initially, the nurse determines the change from resonance (normal lung) to dullness (structures below the diaphragm) during normal breathing. Posteriorly, the lung normally ends at the tenth ICS with quiet respiration, and the diaphragm is generally two interspaces below this level. The point on the midscapular line at which the percussion changes from resonance to dullness is marked with a pen. An additional area medial or lateral to this area should be assessed to confirm the change to dullness. Then the patient is instructed to inhale fully and hold it while the nurse again percusses downward from the

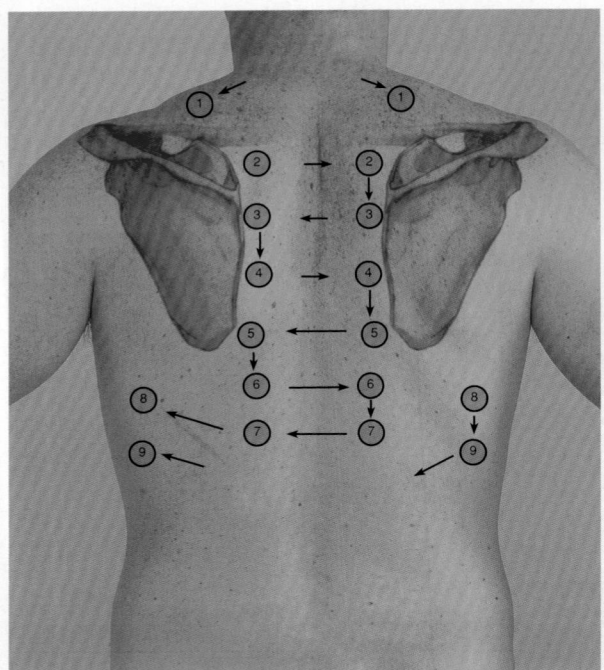

FIGURE 8-11 Percussion of the posterior thorax. With the patient in a sitting position, symmetric areas of the lungs are percussed at 5-cm intervals. This progression starts at the apex of each lung and concludes with percussion of each lateral chest wall.

marked area to the new level of dullness of the diaphragm. With deep inspiration, the diaphragm descends. This point is also marked. The distance between the two markings indicates the range of motion of the diaphragm. The new position for the transition between resonance and dullness is 5 to 6 cm lower in healthy adults as their diaphragms descend with deeper breaths (LeBlond et al., 2015a). Decreased diaphragmatic excursion may occur with pleural effusion, a paralyzed hemidiaphragm, and emphysema.

Thoracic Auscultation

Auscultation is useful in assessing the flow of air through the bronchial tree and in evaluating the presence of fluid or solid obstruction in the lung. The nurse auscultates for normal breath sounds, adventitious sounds, and voice sounds.

Examination includes auscultation of the anterior, posterior, and lateral thorax and is performed as follows. The nurse places the diaphragm of the stethoscope firmly against the chest wall as the patient breathes slowly and deeply through the mouth. Corresponding areas of the chest are auscultated in a systematic fashion from the apices to the bases and along MALs. The sequence of auscultation and the positioning of the patient are similar to those used for percussion. Often it is necessary to listen to two full inspirations and expirations at each anatomic location for valid interpretation of the sound heard. Repeated deep breaths may result in symptoms of hyperventilation (e.g., light-headedness); this is avoided by having the patient rest and breathe normally periodically during the examination.

Breath Sounds. The diaphragm of the stethoscope is used to assess for lung sounds. Normal breath sounds are distinguished by their location over a specific area of the lung and are identified as bronchial (tubular), which may possibly be heard over the manubrium; bronchovesicular, which are heard at the first and second ICS, at approximately the angle of Louis anteriorly and between the scapula posteriorly; and vesicular (dominant sound over the remaining lung) breath sounds. In bronchial breath sounds, the inspiration phase is shorter than expiration; in bronchovesicular sounds, inspiration and expiration phases are equal; and with vesicular sounds, inspiration is longer than expiration.

The location, quality, and intensity of breath sounds are determined during auscultation. As the nurse moves down the chest wall, the sounds decrease. When airflow is decreased by fluid (pleural effusion) or tissue (obesity), breath sounds may be diminished or absent. For example, the breath sounds of the patient with emphysema are faint or often completely inaudible. Bronchial and bronchovesicular sounds that are audible anywhere except over the main bronchus in the lungs signify pathology, usually indicating consolidation in the lung (e.g., pneumonia). This finding requires further evaluation.

Adventitious Sounds. An abnormal condition that affects the bronchial tree and alveoli may produce adventitious (additional or abnormal) sounds that are superimposed over usual breath sounds. Adventitious sounds are divided into two categories: discrete, noncontinuous sounds (**crackles**), and continuous musical sounds (wheezes) (Table 8-5). The duration of the sound is the important distinction to make in identifying the sound as noncontinuous or continuous.

Crackles (formerly referred to as *rales*) are discrete, noncontinuous sounds that result from delayed reopening of deflated airways. Crackles may or may not be cleared by coughing. They reflect underlying inflammation or congestion and often are present in such conditions as pneumonia, bronchitis, heart failure, bronchiectasis, atelectasis, and pulmonary fibrosis. Usually crackles are heard on inspiration, but they also may be heard on expiration.

Pleural friction rubs are specific examples of crackles. Friction rubs result from inflammation of the pleural surfaces that induces a crackling, grating sound usually heard in inspiration and expiration (late in inspiration and early in expiration) (Grippi, Senior, & Callen, 2015). The sound can be enhanced by applying pressure to the chest wall with the diaphragm of the stethoscope. Pleural fluid can accumulate in the pleural space because of transudation of fluid from the pleural and pulmonary vessels (increased venous hydrostatic pressure, decreased oncotic pressure, capillary leak), increased production of pleural fluid (inflamed pleura or pleural neoplasm), decreased pleural absorption of fluid (lymphatic obstruction, systemic venous hypertension), or by bleeding into the pleural space (LeBlond, Brown, Suneja, & Szot, 2015b). Pleural fluid dampens vibrations from the

TABLE 8-5 Abnormal (Adventitious) Breath Sounds

Breath Sound	Description	Etiology
Crackles		
Crackles in general	Soft, high-pitched, discontinuous popping sounds that occur during inspiration; sounds like several hairs rubbing together between the thumb and index finger	Secondary to fluid in the airways or alveoli or to opening of collapsed alveoli; When present in patients without lung disease, crackles (formerly termed rales) are specific for heart failure.
Coarse crackles	Discontinuous popping sounds heard in early inspiration; harsh, louder, lower-pitched moist sound originating in the large bronchi	Associated with obstructive pulmonary disease, asthma
Fine crackles	Discontinuous popping sounds heard in late inspiration; originates in the alveoli	Associated with interstitial pneumonia, restrictive pulmonary disease (e.g., fibrosis), atelectasis, congestive heart failure (CHF). In CHF, crackles may be heard widely over both lung fields (typically beginning at the bases) and may be accompanied by expiratory wheezing (cardiac asthma). Fine crackles in early inspiration are associated with bronchitis or pneumonia.
Wheezes		
Wheezes in general	Usually heard on expiration but may be heard on inspiration or both phases	Associated with turbulent airflow and small airway vibration in which there is partial obstruction, commonly seen with COPD, asthma, and bronchitis
Rhonchi	Deep, low-pitched rumbling sounds heard primarily during expiration; caused by air moving through narrowed tracheobronchial passages	Secretions within the larger airways that clear or change significantly after an effective cough; heard in a wide variety of pathologies, any of which cause increased secretions (e.g., cystic fibrosis, pneumonia, bronchitis or emphysema)
Stridor	Loud, rough, continuous, high-pitched sound that is pronounced during inspiration; it indicates proximal airway obstruction.	Turbulent air flowing through a narrowed trachea or larynx; loudest over the trachea. Commonly a medical emergency that needs to be recognized early. Diagnoses include epiglottitis, vocal cord dysfunction, croup, and airway edema (which could be secondary to trauma or an allergic reaction)
Friction Rubs		
Pleural friction rub	Harsh, crackling sound, like two pieces of leather being rubbed together. Heard during inspiration alone or during both inspiration and expiration. May subside when patient holds breath. Coughing will not clear sound. Auscultate in the region where patient complains of pleuritic pain.	Secondary to inflammation and loss of lubricating pleural fluid

bronchotrachea so vocal fremitus, breath sounds, and whispered and spoken voice are decreased (see below), and dullness is noted on percussion in the area of fluid accumulation.

Rhonchi are low-pitched gurgling sounds produced by secretions within the larger airways. They clear or change significantly after an effective cough.

Wheezes are associated with bronchial wall oscillation and changes in airway diameter. Although usually heard on expiration, wheezes may be heard on inspiration, or both phases. They are commonly heard in patients with asthma, chronic bronchitis, or bronchiectasis. *Stridor*, a high-pitched, harsh inspiratory wheeze associated with partial obstruction

of the larynx or trachea, demands immediate attention (Bickley, 2013).

Voice Sounds. The sound heard through the stethoscope as the patient speaks is known as *vocal resonance*. The vibrations produced in the larynx are transmitted to the chest wall as they pass through the bronchi and alveolar tissue. During the process, the sounds are diminished in intensity and altered so that syllables are not distinguishable. Voice sounds are usually assessed by having the patient repeat "99" or "eee" while the nurse listens with the stethoscope in corresponding areas of the chest, from the apices to the bases.

TABLE **8-6** Assessment Findings in Common Respiratory Disorders

Disorder	Tactile Fremitus	Percussion	Auscultation
Consolidation (e.g., pneumonia)	Increased	Dull	Bronchial breath sounds, crackles, bronchophony, egophony, whispered pectoriloquy
Bronchitis	Normal	Resonant	Normal to decreased breath sounds, wheezes
Emphysema	Decreased	Hyperresonant	Decreased intensity of breath sounds, usually with prolonged expiration
Asthma (severe attack)	Normal to decreased	Resonant	Wheezes
Pulmonary edema	Normal	Resonant	Crackles at lung bases, possibly wheezes
Pleural effusion	Absent	Dull	Decreased to absent breath sounds, bronchial breath sounds and bronchophony, egophony, and whispered pectoriloquy above the effusion over the area of compressed lung
Pneumothorax	Decreased	Hyperresonant	Absent breath sounds
Atelectasis	Absent	Dull (if large)	Decreased to absent breath sounds, fine crackles

Bronchophony describes vocal resonance that is more intense and clearer than normal. *Egophony* describes voice sounds that are distorted. It is best appreciated by having the patient repeat the letter E. The distortion produced by consolidation transforms the sound into a clearly heard "A" rather than "E." Bronchophony and egophony have precisely the same significance as bronchial breathing with an increase in tactile fremitus. When an abnormality is detected, it should be confirmed using more than one assessment method. A change in tactile fremitus is more subtle and can be missed, but bronchial breathing and bronchophony can be noted loudly and clearly.

Whispered pectoriloquy is a very subtle finding, which is heard only in the presence of rather dense consolidation of the lungs. Transmission of the high-frequency components of sound is so enhanced by the consolidated tissue that even whispered words are heard, a circumstance not noted in normal physiology. The significance is the same as that of bronchophony (Bickley, 2013).

The physical findings for the most common respiratory diseases are summarized in Table 8-6.

Diagnostic Evaluation

A wide range of diagnostic studies, described in the following sections, may be performed to aid in diagnosing or monitoring patients with a variety of respiratory conditions.

Pulmonary Function Tests

PFTs are used routinely in patients with chronic respiratory disorders. These tests are performed to assess respiratory function and to determine the extent of dysfunction. PFTs are useful in screening patients for major surgery, monitoring the course of a patient with an established respiratory disease, and assessing the response to therapy. They are useful as screening tests in potentially hazardous industries, such as coal mining and those that involve exposure to asbestos and other noxious fumes, dusts, or gases.

PFTs generally are performed by a technician using a spirometer that has a volume-collecting device attached to a recorder that demonstrates volume and time simultaneously. A number of tests are carried out because no single measurement provides a complete picture of pulmonary function.

PFT results are interpreted on the basis of the degree of deviation from normal, taking into consideration the patient's height, weight, age, and gender. Because there is a wide range of normal values, PFTs may not detect early localized changes.

Patients with respiratory disorders may be taught how to measure their peak flow rate (which reflects maximal expiratory flow) at home using a spirometer to monitor progress of therapy, assess effect of alteration of medications, and use as a guide for when to notify the health care provider.

Arterial Blood Gas Studies

Measurements of blood pH and of arterial O_2 and CO_2 tensions are obtained when managing patients with respiratory problems and adjusting O_2 therapy as needed. The arterial O_2 tension (PaO_2) indicates the degree of oxygenation of the blood, and the arterial CO_2 tension ($PaCO_2$) indicates the adequacy of alveolar ventilation (i.e., how effectively CO_2 is exhaled from the body). Arterial blood gas (ABG) studies aid in assessing the ability of the lungs to provide adequate O_2 and remove CO_2 as well as the ability of the kidneys to reabsorb or excrete bicarbonate ions to maintain normal body pH. ABG levels are obtained through an arterial puncture at the radial, brachial, or femoral artery or through an indwelling arterial catheter. Before obtaining an ABG from the radial artery, it is necessary to test the patency of the ulnar artery by performing the Allen test (refer to Chapter 12 for details).

Pulse Oximetry

Pulse oximetry is a noninvasive method of continuously monitoring the O_2 saturation of hemoglobin (SaO_2). When O_2 saturation is measured with pulse oximetry, it is referred to as SpO_2. Although pulse oximetry does not replace ABG measurement, it is an effective tool to monitor for subtle or sudden changes in O_2 saturation as this measurement is available in real time.

A probe or sensor is attached to a well-perfused fingertip (Fig. 8-12), forehead, earlobe, or bridge of the nose. The sensor detects changes in O_2 saturation levels by monitoring light signals generated by the oximeter and reflected by blood pulsing through the tissue at the probe. Normal SpO_2 values are 95% to 100%. Values of less than 90% imply inadequate oxygenation, and further evaluation is needed. SpO_2 values obtained by pulse oximetry are unreliable in cardiac arrest and shock (decreased pulsatile force of blood), if dyes (i.e., methylene blue) or vasoconstrictor medications have been used or if the patient has severe anemia or a high carbon monoxide level (smoke inhalation and carbon monoxide poisoning). Furthermore, they are not reliable detectors of hypoventilation or rising CO_2 which leads to respiratory acidosis.

End Tidal CO₂

End-tidal CO_2 ($ETCO_2$) is a continuous recording of the concentration of CO_2 at the end of expiration. An $ETCO_2$ monitor may be a separate monitor or part of the patient's bedside hemodynamic monitoring system. Because end-tidal gas is primarily alveolar gas and is virtually identical to $PaCO_2$ (arterial partial pressure of CO_2), $ETCO_2$ is used clinically as an estimate of $PaCO_2$. In addition, it is used to (1) ensure that airway adjuncts (such as endotracheal tubes) are placed correctly in the trachea (and not in the esophagus) of a mechanically ventilated patient, (2) assess the effectiveness of interventions related to mechanical ventilation, neuromuscular blockade used with mechanical ventilation, and changing body positioning, and (3) assess the adequacy of chest compressions during cardiopulmonary resuscitation. Normally, $ETCO_2$ is 2 to 5 mm Hg lower than arterial CO_2 pressure so the typical range is 30 to 40 mm Hg versus 35 to 45 mm Hg for arterial CO_2. An early sign of malignant hyperthermia is a rapidly rising $ETCO_2$ especially if it is unresponsive to hyperventilation (refer to Chapter 5). The nurse should notify the provider of an increase or decrease in readings of 10% (Walsh, 2015).

Sputum Studies

Sputum is obtained for analysis to identify pathogenic organisms and to determine whether malignant cells are present. It also may be used to assess for hypersensitivity states (in

FIGURE 8-12 Measuring blood oxygenation with pulse oximetry reduces the need for invasive procedures, such as drawing blood for analysis of O_2 levels. **A.** Self-contained digital fingertip pulse oximeter, which incorporates the sensor and display into one unit. **B.** Table top model with sensor attached. Memory permits tracking heart rate and O_2 saturation over time.

which there is an increase in eosinophils). In general, sputum cultures are used in diagnosis, for drug sensitivity testing, and to guide treatment.

Expectoration is the usual method for collecting a sputum specimen. The patient is instructed to clear the nose and throat and rinse the mouth to decrease contamination of the sputum. After taking a few deep breaths, the patient coughs forcefully on exhalation (rather than spits), using the diaphragm, and expectorates into a sterile container. An early morning specimen is best for collection; 2 to 3 mL is generally a sufficient amount (Fischbach & Dunning, 2015).

If the sputum cannot be raised spontaneously, respiratory therapy personnel may assist the patient in obtaining an "aerosol-induced" specimen with an ultrasonic nebulizer until a strong cough reflex is initiated. The specimen is labeled as being aerosol induced. Other methods of collecting sputum specimens include chest physiotherapy, nasotracheal or tracheal suctioning, and bronchoscopy.

 Nursing Alert
A sputum specimen is sealed in a sterile container and placed in a leak-proof biohazard bag. The specimen is sent as soon as possible to the laboratory after being labeled properly. Usually sputum specimens are not refrigerated. Allowing the specimen to stand for several hours in a warm room results in the overgrowth of contaminant organisms and may make it difficult to identify the pathogenic organisms (especially Mycobacterium tuberculosis).

Imaging Studies

Imaging studies, including x-rays, computed tomography (CT), magnetic resonance imaging (MRI), contrast studies, and radioisotope diagnostic scans may be part of any diagnostic workup, ranging from a determination of the extent of infection in sinusitis to tumor growth in cancer.

Chest X-Ray
Normal pulmonary tissue is radiolucent; therefore, densities produced by fluid, tumors, foreign bodies, and other pathologic conditions can be detected by x-ray examination. The routine chest x-ray consists of two views—the posteroanterior projection and the lateral projection. Usually chest x-rays are taken after full inspiration (a deep breath) because the lungs are best visualized when they are well aerated. Also, the diaphragm is at its lowest level, and the largest expanse of lung is visible.

Computed Tomography
CT is an imaging method in which the lungs are scanned in successive layers by a narrow-beam x-ray. The images produced provide a cross-sectional view of the chest. CT can distinguish fine tissue density. They may be used to define pulmonary nodules and small tumors adjacent to pleural surfaces that are not visible on routine chest x-rays as well as to demonstrate mediastinal abnormalities and hilar adenopathy, which are difficult to visualize with other techniques. Contrast agents are useful when evaluating the mediastinum and its contents. Computed tomography pulmonary angiography (CTPA), which is the injection of contrast media directly into a vein or artery via a needle and/or catheter, has become the standard imaging technique for diagnosing PE (Solaiman & Bartholomew, 2013).

Magnetic Resonance Imaging
MRI is similar to CT except that with MRI, magnetic fields and radiofrequency signals are used instead of a narrow-beam x-ray. MRI yields a much more detailed diagnostic image than CT. MRI is used to characterize pulmonary nodules, to help stage bronchogenic carcinoma (assessment of chest wall invasion), and to evaluate inflammatory activity in interstitial lung disease, acute PE, and chronic thrombolytic pulmonary hypertension.

Positron Emission Tomography
Positron emission tomography (PET) imaging involves the combined use of positron-emitting radionuclides and emission CT. PET generates high-resolution images of body function and metabolism, thus PET provides physiologic, anatomic, and biochemical data. PET images include glucose metabolism, O_2 utilization, blood flow, and tissue perfusion. Clinical PET is useful for aiding in diagnosis of many disease states, primarily in oncology, neurology, and cardiology.

 Nursing Alert
Nurses must assess patient allergy to iodine contrast media before diagnostic studies; the nurse asks about iodine-containing substances (e.g., seafood, cabbage, kale, raw leafy vegetables, turnips, iodized salt) and documents findings in the patient record. The risk for subsequent reactions increases three to four times after the first reaction; however, subsequent reactions will not necessarily be more severe than the first (Fischbach & Dunning, 2015).

Fluoroscopic Studies
Fluoroscopy is used to assist with invasive procedures, such as a chest needle biopsy or transbronchial biopsy, that are performed to identify lesions. It also may be used to study the movement of the chest wall, mediastinum, heart, and diaphragm; to detect diaphragm paralysis; and to locate lung masses.

Pulmonary Angiography
Pulmonary angiography remains the reference standard for which most studies are compared in the diagnosis of PE despite these factors: (1) it is not universally available, (2) it is invasive, and (3) it is costly (Solaiman & Bartholomew, 2013). It involves the rapid injection of a radiopaque agent into the vasculature of the lungs for radiographic study of the pulmonary vessels. It is not without complications; morbidity of 5% and mortality of 0.5% were reported (Solaiman & Bartholomew, 2013). Due to introduction of CTPA, pulmonary angiography is used infrequently.

Radioisotope Diagnostic Procedures (Lung Scans)
Several types of lung scans—ventilation/perfusion (V/Q) scan, gallium scan, and PET—are used to assess normal lung functioning, pulmonary vascular supply, and gas exchange.

A V/Q lung scan is performed by injecting a radioactive agent into a peripheral vein and then obtaining a scan of the chest to detect radiation. The isotope particles pass through the right side of the heart and are distributed into the lungs in proportion to the regional blood flow, making it possible to trace and measure blood perfusion through the lung. This procedure is used clinically to measure the integrity of the pulmonary vessels relative to blood flow and to evaluate blood flow abnormalities, as seen in pulmonary emboli. The imaging time is 20 to 40 minutes, during which the patient lies under the camera with a mask fitted over the nose and mouth. This is followed by the ventilation component of the scan. The patient takes a deep breath of a mixture of O_2 and radioactive gas, which diffuses throughout the lungs. A scan is performed to detect ventilation abnormalities in patients who have regional differences in ventilation. Ventilation without perfusion is seen with pulmonary emboli. V/Q scanning has been replaced by CTPA and currently is considered a second-line modality in the diagnosis of PE. However, V/Q scan remains a valuable tool in the diagnosis of acute PE in patients with a normal chest x-ray or patients who cannot undergo CTPA (contrast allergy, renal insufficiency, or pregnancy) (Solaiman & Bartholomew, 2013).

A gallium scan is a radioisotope lung scan used to detect inflammatory conditions, abscesses, adhesions, and the presence, location, and size of tumors. It is used to stage bronchogenic cancer and document tumor regression after chemotherapy or radiation. Gallium is injected intravenously, and scans are taken at intervals (e.g., 6, 24, and 48 hours) to evaluate gallium uptake by the pulmonary tissues. Although gallium is radioactive, the risk of radiation exposure is lower than x-ray or CT scan.

Endoscopic Procedures

Bronchoscopy

Bronchoscopy is the direct inspection and examination of the larynx, trachea, and bronchi for diagnosis of infectious, inflammatory, and malignant disease of the chest through a flexible or rigid fiberoptic bronchoscope (Fig. 8-13).

Therapeutic bronchoscopy is used to (1) remove foreign bodies from the tracheobronchial tree, (2) perform difficult endotracheal intubations, (3) remove secretions obstructing the tracheobronchial tree when the patient cannot clear them, (4) diagnose lung infection, inflammation, and interstitial diseases, (5) destroy and excise lesions, (6) place endobronchial radiation therapy (brachytherapy) and laser therapy of obstructive airway lesions, (7) stent obstructing endobronchial lesions, and (8) dilate stenotic airways.

Possible complications of bronchoscopy include a reaction to the local anesthetic, infection, aspiration, bronchospasm, **hypoxemia** (low blood O_2 level), pneumothorax, bleeding, and perforation.

Before the procedure, a signed consent form is obtained from the patient. Food and fluids are withheld for 8 hours before the test to reduce the risk of aspiration when the

Fiberoptic bronchoscopy

Rigid bronchoscopy

FIGURE 8-13 Endoscopic bronchoscopy permits visualization of bronchial structures. The bronchoscope is advanced into bronchial structures orally. Bronchoscopy permits the provider not only to diagnose but also to treat various lung problems.

cough reflex is blocked by anesthesia. The nurse explains the procedure to the patient to reduce fear and decrease anxiety and administers preoperative medications if required.

The patient must remove dentures and other oral prostheses. Usually the examination is performed under local anesthesia or moderate sedation. A topical anesthetic such as lidocaine (Xylocaine) may be sprayed on the pharynx or dropped on the epiglottis and vocal cords and into the trachea to suppress the cough reflex and minimize discomfort. Sedatives or opioids are administered intravenously as prescribed to provide moderate sedation. Resuscitative and suctioning equipment should be available.

After the procedure, it is important that the patient takes nothing by mouth until the cough reflex returns, because the preoperative sedation and local anesthesia impair the protective laryngeal reflex and swallowing for several hours. The patient is instructed to spit out saliva rather than swallow it until the gag reflex returns. Once the patient demonstrates a cough reflex, the nurse may offer ice chips and, eventually, fluids. The nurse also monitors the patient's respiratory status and observes for hypoxia, hypotension, tachycardia, arrhythmias, hemoptysis, subcutaneous air or crepitus, stridor, or dyspnea. Any abnormality is reported promptly. The patient is not discharged from the recovery area until adequate cough reflex and respiratory status are present. The nurse instructs the patient and family caregivers to report any SOB or bleeding immediately.

Nursing Alert
Anesthesia can temporarily impair the pharyngeal reflex (ninth, tenth, CN), which

is responsible for the gag reflex and swallowing; to prevent aspiration, before refeeding the patient, the nurse must reassess return of this reflex (refer to Chapter 43 for details on assessment).

Thoracentesis

A thoracentesis (aspiration of fluid or air from the pleural space) is performed on patients with various clinical problems. As a diagnostic or therapeutic procedure, thoracentesis may be used for removal of fluid and air from the pleural cavity, aspiration of pleural fluid for analysis, pleural biopsy, or instillation of medication into the pleural space. Care of the patient undergoing thoracentesis is discussed in Box 8-8 on pages 258–259. A needle biopsy of the pleura may be performed at the same time. Studies of pleural fluid include: gram stain culture and sensitivity, acid-fast staining and culture, differential cell count, cytology, pH, specific gravity, total protein, and lactic dehydrogenase.

BOX 8-8

GUIDELINES FOR NURSING CARE

Assisting the Patient Undergoing Thoracentesis

Equipment

- Thoracentesis tray
- Local anesthetic
- Sterile gloves

- Sterile collection bottles
- Germicide solution

Implementation

ACTIONS	RATIONALE
1. Ascertain in advance that a chest x-ray and ultrasound (if available) has been ordered and completed and the consent form has been signed. The nurse also anticipates that coagulation studies are evaluated and any coagulopathy corrected before the procedure.	1. Posteroanterior and lateral decubitus chest x-ray films are obtained before the procedure and ultrasound if available to determine optimal site for thoracentesis When thoracentesis is performed under ultrasound guidance, it has a lower rate of complications than when it is performed without ultrasound guidance, including a decrease in post-procedure pneumothorax, less accidental organ puncture, and improved site selection. If fluid is loculated (isolated in a pocket of pleural fluid), ultrasound scans are performed to help select the best site for needle aspiration. Correction of coagulopathy may be necessary to decrease the bleeding risk with this procedure.
2. Assess the patient for allergy to the local anesthetic to be used.	2. If the patient is allergic to the anesthetic prescribed initially, then assessment findings provide an opportunity to use a safer anesthetic.
3. Administer sedation if prescribed.	3. Sedation enables the patient to cooperate with the procedure and promotes relaxation.
4. Inform the patient about the nature of the procedure and: a. The importance of remaining immobile b. Pressure sensations to be experienced c. That minimal discomfort is anticipated after the procedure	4. An explanation helps to orient the patient to the procedure, provides anticipatory guidance, and provides an opportunity to ask questions and verbalize anxiety.
5. Position the patient comfortably with adequate supports. If possible, place the patient upright or in one of the following positions: a. Sitting on the edge of the bed with the feet supported and arms and head on a padded over-the-bed table b. Straddling a chair with arms and head resting on the back of the chair c. Lying on the unaffected side with the head of the bed elevated 30–45 degrees if unable to assume a sitting position	5. The upright position facilitates the removal of fluid that usually localizes at the base of the thorax. A position of comfort helps the patient to relax.
6. Support and reassure the patient during the procedure: a. Prepare the patient for the cold sensation of skin germicide solution and for a pressure sensation from infiltration of local anesthetic agent. b. Encourage the patient to refrain from coughing.	6. Sudden and unexpected movement, such as coughing, by the patient can traumatize the visceral pleura and lung.

CHAPTER 8 NURSING ASSESSMENT: RESPIRATORY FUNCTION **259**

ACTIONS	RATIONALE

7. Expose the entire chest. The site for aspiration is visualized by chest x-ray and percussion. If fluid is in the pleural cavity, the thoracentesis site is determined by the chest x-ray, ultrasound scanning, and physical findings, with attention to the site of maximal dullness on percussion.

7. If air is in the pleural cavity, the thoracentesis site is usually in the second or third intercostal space in the midclavicular line because air rises in the thorax.

8. The procedure is performed under aseptic conditions. After the skin is cleansed, the provider uses a small-caliber needle to inject a local anesthetic slowly into the intercostal space.

8. An intradermal wheal is raised slowly; rapid injection causes pain. The parietal pleura is very sensitive and should be well-infiltrated with anesthetic before the physician passes the thoracentesis needle through it.

9. The provider advances the thoracentesis needle with the syringe attached. When the pleural space is reached, suction may be applied with the syringe:

9. Use of thoracentesis needle allows proper insertion:

   a. A 20-mL syringe with a three-way stopcock is attached to the needle (one end of the adapter is attached to the needle and the other to the tubing leading to a receptacle that receives the fluid being aspirated).

   a. When a large quantity of fluid is withdrawn, a three-way stopcock serves to keep air from entering the pleural cavity.

   b. If a considerable quantity of fluid is removed, the needle is held in place on the chest wall with a small hemostat.

   b. The hemostat steadies the needle on the chest wall. Sudden pleuritic chest pain or shoulder pain may indicate that the needle point is irritating the visceral or the diaphragmatic pleura.

   c. The nurse should anticipate that no more than 1 L will be removed from the chest. Amounts greater than 1 to 1.5 L can result in re-expansion pulmonary edema (Longo et al., 2013).

   c. To prevent re-expansion pulmonary edema.

10. After the needle is withdrawn, pressure is applied over the puncture site and a small, airtight, sterile dressing is fixed in place.

10. Pressure helps to stop bleeding, and the airtight dressing protects the site and prevents air from entering the pleural cavity.

11. Advise the patient that he or she will be on bed rest and a chest x-ray will be obtained after thoracentesis.

11. A chest x-ray verifies that there is no pneumothorax.

12. Record the total amount of fluid withdrawn from the procedure and document the nature of the fluid, its color, and its viscosity. If indicated, prepare samples of fluid for laboratory evaluation. A specimen container with formalin may be needed for a pleural biopsy.

12. The fluid may be clear, serous, bloody, purulent, etc.

13. Monitor the patient at intervals for increasing respiratory rate; increased dyspnea, asymmetry in respiratory movement; faintness; vertigo; tightness in chest; uncontrollable cough; blood-tinged, frothy mucus; a rapid pulse; and signs of hypoxemia.

13. Pneumothorax, tension pneumothorax, subcutaneous emphysema, and pyrogenic infection are complications of a thoracentesis. Pulmonary edema or cardiac distress can occur after a sudden shift in mediastinal contents when large amounts of fluid are aspirated.

Pleural effusion

CHAPTER REVIEW

Critical Thinking Exercises

1. A man with a long history of smoking (60 pack/year) is scheduled for surgery to remove a nonfunctioning kidney. In preparation for surgery, he is scheduled for PFTs, which he refuses to have because he says his breathing has nothing to do with his kidney problem or his scheduled kidney surgery. How would you respond to his statement? What impact does his 60 pack/year history of cigarette smoking have on your preoperative, intraoperative, and postoperative assessment?

2. When obtaining a health history from a 55-year-old patient who is seeking health care because of a persistent cough and extreme fatigue, you note that she is able to speak only in short sentences before having to stop to catch her breath. What specific information about signs and symptoms would you obtain during the health history? How would you modify your physical examination based on your observations? What initial laboratory tests would you anticipate will be ordered for this patient?

NCLEX-Style Review Questions

1. Before an ABG is drawn from the patient's radial artery, what test should be performed?
   a. Doppler flow test
   b. Allen test
   c. Babinski test
   d. Ankle Brachial Index (ABI)

2. A patient has a chronic cough with thick sputum. He undergoes a bronchoscopy for diagnostic purposes. Following the bronchoscopy, which action by the nurse is most appropriate?
   a. Encourage fluid intake to promote elimination of contrast media.
   b. Monitor hemoglobin and hematocrit to evaluate blood loss.
   c. Check vital signs every 15 minutes for 4 hours.
   d. Keep NPO until the gag reflex returns.

3. A patient is admitted to the ICU after falling from a roof and sustaining fractures of the first three ribs on the right side. The patient is dyspneic, and crepitus (subcutaneous emphysema) can be palpated. Auscultation reveals decreased breath sounds on the right. The chest x-ray reveals a pneumothorax. Upon percussion, what does the nurse expect to hear?
   a. Dullness on the right
   b. Resonance on the right
   c. Tympany on the right
   d. Hyperresonance on the right

4. The finding of normal breath sounds on the right chest and diminished, distant breath sounds on the left chest of a newly intubated patient is probably due to which of the following?
   a. A left pneumothorax
   b. A right hemothorax
   c. Intubation of the right mainstem bronchus
   d. A malfunctioning mechanical ventilator

5. A patient presents to the emergency room with pulmonary edema. The nurse expects to hear what adventitious sound?
   a. Decreased breath sounds
   b. Inspiratory and expiratory wheezing
   c. Crackles
   d. Friction rub

Try these additional resources, available at **http://thepoint.lww.com/Honan2e**, to enhance your learning and understanding of this chapter:
- NCLEX-Style Student Review Questions
- Journal Articles

REFERENCES AND SELECTED READINGS

References and selected readings associated with this chapter can be found on the website that accompanies the book. Visit **http://thepoint.lww.com/Honan2e** to access the references and other additional resources associated with this chapter.

Nursing Management: Patients with Upper Respiratory Tract Disorders

Jancee Pust-Marcone

Learning Objectives

After reading this chapter, you will be able to:

1. Compare and contrast the upper respiratory tract infections with regard to cause, incidence, clinical manifestations, management, and the significance of preventive health care.
2. Use the nursing process as a framework for care of patients with upper airway infection.
3. Describe the nursing management of the patient with obstructive sleep apnea.
4. Describe the nursing management for patients receiving continuous positive-pressure (CPAP) or bi-level (BiPAP) breathing.
5. Describe nursing management of the patient with epistaxis.
6. Describe nursing management of patients undergoing laryngectomy.
7. Describe the nursing care for a patient with an endotracheal tube or a tracheostomy.
8. Demonstrate the procedure of tracheal suctioning.

Many upper airway disorders are relatively minor, and their effects are limited to mild and temporary discomfort for the patient. Others may be acute, severe, and life-threatening and may require permanent alterations in breathing and speaking. The nurse must have expert assessment skills, an understanding of the wide variety of disorders that may affect the upper airway, and an awareness of the impact of these alterations on patients.

UPPER AIRWAY INFECTIONS

Upper airway infections, also known as upper respiratory tract infections (URIs), are the most common cause of illness, and affect most people on occasion. There are many causative organisms, and people are susceptible throughout their lives.

Some infections are acute, with symptoms that last several days, while others are chronic, with symptoms that last a long time or recur. Patients with these conditions seldom require hospitalization. URIs affect the nasal cavity; ethmoidal air cells; and frontal, maxillary, and sphenoid sinuses (see Fig. 9-1), as well as the larynx and trachea. About 90% of upper respiratory disorders stem from a viral infection

of the upper respiratory passages and subsequent mucous membrane inflammation.

RHINITIS

Rhinitis is a group of disorders characterized by inflammation and irritation of the mucous membranes of the nose as well as ocular symptoms. Rhinitis may be acute or chronic, nonallergic or allergic (see Chapter 38 for information about allergic rhinitis).

Viral rhinitis is the most frequent viral infection in the general population and is referred to as the "common cold." It affects between 10% and 30% of adults and 40% of children (Borish, 2016).

Pathophysiology

Nonallergic rhinitis may be caused by a variety of factors, including environmental factors such as changes in temperature or humidity, odors, or foods; infection; age; systemic disease; illegal drugs (e.g., cocaine); over-the-counter (OTC) and prescribed nasal decongestants; and the presence of a foreign body.

The most common cause of nonallergic rhinitis is the common cold. Colds are believed to be caused by as many as

FIGURE 9-1 Sinuses are air-filled cavities in your head. This image details the: sphenoid sinuses; frontal sinuses; ethmoid sinuses. (From Anatomical Chart Company.)

200 different viruses. Rhinoviruses are the most likely causative organisms and are believed to cause more than 40% of colds. Other viruses implicated in the common cold include coronavirus, adenovirus, respiratory syncytial virus (RSV), influenza virus, and parainfluenza virus. Each virus may have multiple strains. Because of this diversity of causes, development of a vaccine is almost impossible. Immunity after recovery is variable and depends on many factors, including a person's natural host resistance and the specific virus that caused the cold. Drug-induced rhinitis is associated with use of antihypertensive agents, oral contraceptives, and chronic use of nasal decongestants. Other causes of rhinitis are identified in Table 9-1. Figure 9-2 shows the pathologic processes involved in rhinitis and sinusitis.

Risk Factors

Colds are highly contagious because virus is shed for about 2 days before the symptoms appear and during the first part of the symptomatic phase. Adults in the United States average two to four colds each year mostly between September and May (American Lung Association, 2015). Adult women are more susceptible than adult men. Viral rhinitis can occur at any time of the year, but three time periods account for the epidemics in the United States: in September, just after the opening of school; in late January; and toward the end of April. Contrary to popular belief, cold temperatures and exposure to cold, rainy weather do not increase the incidence or severity of the common cold.

Clinical Manifestations and Assessment

The signs and symptoms of nonallergic rhinitis include **rhinorrhea** (excessive nasal drainage, runny nose); nasal

TABLE **9-1** Causes of Rhinitis

Category	Causes
Allergic	Seasonal (pollens) Perennial (dust/mold)
Vasomotor	Idiopathic Abuse of nasal decongestants (rhinitis medicamentosa) Drugs (reserpine, prazosin, cocaine abuse) Psychological stimulation (anger, sexual arousal) Irritants (smoke, air pollution, exhaust fumes, cocaine)
Mechanical	Tumor Deviated septum Crusting Hypertrophied turbinates Foreign body Cerebrospinal fluid leak
Chronic inflammatory	Polyps (in cystic fibrosis) Sarcoidosis Wegener granulomatosis Midline granuloma
Infectious	Acute viral infection Acute or chronic sinusitis Rare nasal infections (syphilis, tuberculosis)
Hormonal	Pregnancy Hypothyroidism Use of oral contraceptives Hypothyroidism

Adapted from Carr, M. M. Differential diagnosis of rhinitis. Retrieved from http//icarus.med.utoronto.ca/carr/manual/ddxrhinitis.html.

congestion; nasal discharge (purulent with bacterial rhinitis); sneezing; and pruritus of the nose, roof of the mouth, throat, eyes, and ears (Borish, 2016). Headache may occur particularly if sinusitis is also present. In addition to the above symptoms, viral rhinitis may present with sore throat, general malaise, low-grade fever, chills, and muscle aches. As the illness progresses, cough usually appears. In some people, the virus exacerbates **herpes simplex**, commonly called a "cold sore."

The symptoms of viral rhinitis may last from 1 to 2 weeks.

Medical and Nursing Management

Management consists of symptomatic therapy. Medication therapy for allergic and nonallergic rhinitis focuses on symptom relief. The choice of medications depends on the symptoms, adverse reactions, adherence factors, risk of drug interactions, and cost to the patient. Acetaminophen or nonsteroidal anti-inflammatory agents (NSAIDs), such as aspirin or ibuprofen, relieve the aches, pains, and fever.

A Rhinitis

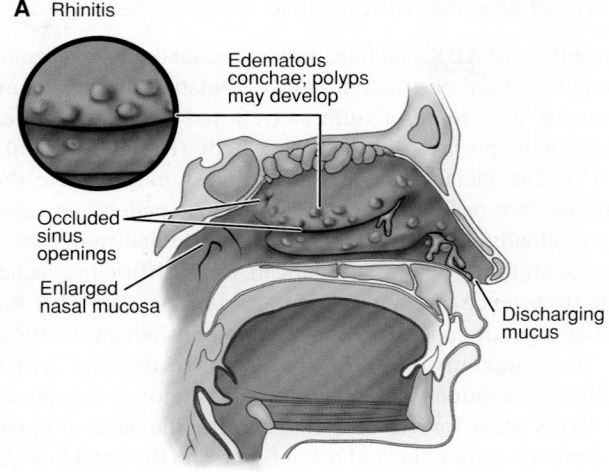

Edematous
conchae; polyps
may develop

Occluded
sinus
openings

Enlarged
nasal mucosa

Discharging
mucus

B Rhinosinusitis

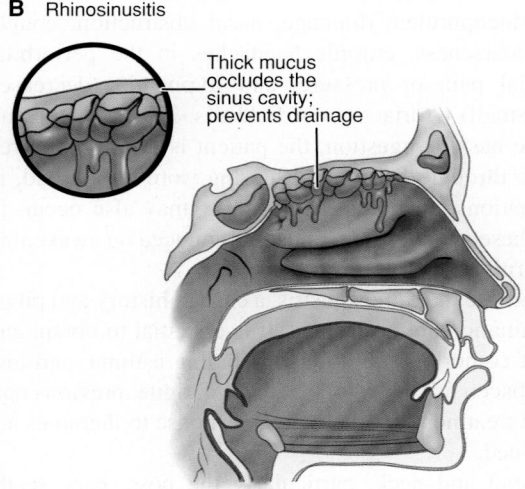

Thick mucus
occludes the
sinus cavity;
prevents drainage

FIGURE 9-2 Pathophysiologic processes in rhinitis and rhinosinusitis. Although pathophysiologic processes are similar in rhinitis and sinusitis, they affect different structures. In rhinitis (**A**), the mucous membranes lining the nasal passages become inflamed, congested, and edematous. The swollen nasal conchae block the sinus openings, and mucus is discharged from the nostrils. Rhinosinusitis (**B**) is also marked by inflammation and congestion, with thickened mucous secretions filling the sinus cavities and occluding the openings.

The four major categories of medications used to manage cold symptoms are antihistamines, decongestants, antitussives, and expectorants. Antihistamines remain the most common treatment and are administered for sneezing, nasal congestion, pruritus, and rhinorrhea. The most common adverse effects of antihistamines are sedation, dry mouth, GI upset, and cardiac arrhythmias. Antihistamines have been show to aggravate certain conditions and should be used with caution in patients with asthma, urinary retention, hypertension, open-angle glaucoma, and prostatic hypertrophy. Topical nasal decongestants should be used with caution. Topical therapy delivers medication directly to the nasal mucosa, but

its overuse can produce *rhinitis medicamentosa* (an increase in the severity or duration of rhinitis that results from prolonged use of decongestant nasal spray) or rebound rhinitis (Borish, 2016). Oral decongestant agents may be used for congestive nasal obstruction. Use of saline nasal spray can act as a mild decongestant and can liquefy mucus to prevent crusting. Expectorants are available without a prescription and are used to promote removal of secretions. Several antiviral medications are available by prescription. Antimicrobial agents (antibiotics) should not be used because they do not affect the virus or reduce the incidence of bacterial complications, and they have been implicated in development of organisms resistant to therapy.

Herbal medicines (e.g., echinacea, zinc lozenges, zinc nasal spray) are used frequently to treat the common cold; however, evidence regarding their effectiveness in shortening the symptomatic phase is questionable (American Lung Association, 2015). The inhalation of steam or heated, humidified air has been a mainstay of home remedies for common cold sufferers, but the value of this therapy has not been demonstrated.

If symptoms suggest a bacterial infection, an antimicrobial agent will be used. Other treatment measures include adequate fluid intake, adequate rest, prevention of chilling, and warm saltwater gargles to soothe the sore throat. Patients with nasal septal deformities or nasal polyps may be referred to an ear, nose, and throat (ENT) specialist.

RHINOSINUSITIS

Rhinosinusitis, formerly called *sinusitis*, is an inflammatory process involving the paranasal sinuses and nasal cavity (Rosenfeld et al., 2015). The clinical practice guideline for adult rhinosinusitis released by the American Academy of Otolaryngology–Head and Neck Surgery Foundation recommends use of the term *rhinosinusitis* because sinusitis is almost always accompanied by inflammation of the nasal mucosa (Peters et al., 2014; Rosenfeld et al., 2015). Rhinosinusitis affects 1 in 8 Americans, about 31 million people in the United States, and accounts for billions of dollars in direct health care costs (Peters et al., 2014; Rosenfeld et al., 2015). Uncomplicated rhinosinusitis does not extend beyond the paranasal sinuses and nasal cavity. Rhinosinusitis is classified by duration of symptoms as acute (less than 4 weeks), subacute (4 to 12 weeks), and chronic (more than 12 weeks) with or without acute exacerbations (Peters et al., 2014; Rosenfeld et al., 2015). Rhinosinusitis can be further classified as an **acute bacterial rhinosinusitis** (ABRS) or **acute viral rhinosinusitis** (AVRS) (Rosenfeld et al., 2015). Recurrent acute rhinosinusitis is characterized by three or more acute episodes of ABRS per year without symptoms of rhinosinusitis between episodes (Peters et al., 2014; Rosenfeld et al., 2015). Chronic rhinosinusitis (CRS) is defined as an inflammation of the nose and the paranasal sinuses characterized by two or more symptoms, one of which should be either nasal blockage or discharge, and/or facial pain and/or reduced smell. CRS affects 2% to 16% of the U.S. population (Halawi, Smith, & Chandra, 2013). It occurs more often in women than men and accounts for almost 20 million visits to providers' offices annually. In about 29% to 36% of patients, CRS is accompanied by nasal polyps.

Pathophysiology

Acute rhinosinusitis usually follows a viral URI or cold, such as an unresolved viral or bacterial infection, or an exacerbation of allergic rhinitis. Nasal congestion, caused by inflammation, edema, and transudation of fluid secondary to URI, leads to obstruction of the sinus cavities (see Fig. 9-2). This provides an excellent medium for bacterial growth.

CRS occurs with episodes of prolonged inflammation and with repeated or inadequate treatment of acute infections. Irreversible damage to the mucosa may occur, and symptoms last for longer than 3 months.

Bacterial organisms account for more than 60% of the cases of acute rhinosinusitis. *Streptococcus pneumoniae, Haemophilus influenzae,* and, less commonly, *Staphylococcus aureus* and *Moraxella catarrhalis* (Papadakis, McPhee, & Rabow, 2015; Rosenfeld et al., 2015) are implicated. Other organisms that are occasionally isolated include *Chlamydia pneumoniae, Streptococcus pyogenes,* viruses, and fungi (*Aspergillus fumigatus*). Immunodeficiency should be considered in patients with CRS or acute recurrent rhinosinusitis. Acute fulminant/invasive sinusitis is a life-threatening illness and is commonly attributed to *Aspergillus.*

Risk Factors

Some people are more prone to rhinosinusitis because of chronic inflammation of the nasal passages due to exposure to environmental hazards such as paint, sawdust, and chemicals. If sinus drainage is obstructed by a deviated septum or by hypertrophied turbinates, spurs, or nasal polyps or tumors, sinus infection may persist as a smoldering (persistent) secondary infection or progress to an acute suppurative process (causing purulent discharge). Other conditions that can block the normal flow of sinus secretions include abnormal structures of the nose, enlarged adenoids, diving and swimming, tooth infection, trauma to the nose, tumors, and the pressure of foreign objects. Immunocompromised patients are at increased risk for the development of fungal sinusitis. Fungal sinusitis in immunocompromised patients can be divided into three categories: (1) fungus ball, (2) chronic erosive (noninvasive) sinusitis, and (3) allergic fungal sinusitis. *A. fumigatus* is the most common organism associated with fungal sinusitis. The fungus ball is usually a brown or greenish-black material with the consistency of peanut butter or cottage cheese.

Clinical Manifestations and Assessment

Symptoms of ABRS include purulent nasal drainage accompanied by nasal obstruction or a combination of facial pain, pressure, or a sense of fullness (referred to collectively as facial pain–pressure–fullness), or both (Rosenfeld et al., 2015). The facial pain–pressure–fullness may involve the anterior face or the periorbital region. The patient may also report cloudy or colored nasal discharge, congestion, blockage, or stuffiness, as well as a localized or diffuse headache. The occurrence of symptoms for 10 days or more after the initial onset of upper respiratory symptoms indicates ABRS.

The symptoms of AVRS are similar to those of ABRS with the exceptions of the duration of symptoms. Symptoms of AVRS occur for less than 10 days after the onset of upper respiratory symptoms and do not worsen (Rosenfeld et al., 2015).

Clinical manifestations of CRS are similar to ABRS and include mucopurulent drainage, nasal obstruction, cough, chronic hoarseness, chronic headaches in the periorbital area, facial pain or pressure, and **hyposmia** (decreased sense of smell) (Adriaensen & Fokkens, 2013). As a result of chronic nasal congestion, the patient is usually required to breathe through the mouth. Snoring, sore throat, and, in some situations, adenoidal hypertrophy may also occur. In general, these symptoms are most pronounced on awakening in the morning.

To diagnose the rhinosinusitis, a careful history and physical examination are performed. It is essential to obtain any history of comorbid conditions, including asthma, and history of tobacco use. A history of fever, fatigue, previous episodes and treatments, and previous response to therapies are also obtained.

The head and neck, particularly the nose, ears, teeth, sinuses, pharynx, and chest, are examined. The physical assessment includes examination of the external nose for evidence of anatomical abnormality. Nasal mucous membranes are assessed for erythema, pallor, atrophy, edema, crusting, discharge, polyps, erosions, and septal perforations or deviations. There may be tenderness to palpation over the infected sinus area.

Diagnostic imaging (x-ray, computed tomography [CT], magnetic resonance imaging [MRI]) is not recommended for the diagnosis of acute rhinosinusitis if the patient meets clinical diagnostic criteria (Adriaensen & Fokkens, 2013; Rosenfeld et al., 2015). Diagnostic testing may be required to rule out other local or systemic disorders, such as tumor, fistula, and allergy for the patient with CRS. Nasal endoscopy may be indicated to rule out underlying diseases, tumors, and sinus mycetomas (fungus balls).

Medical and Nursing Management

Treatment of acute and chronic rhinosinusitis depends on the cause. The goals of treatment of acute rhinosinusitis are to treat the infection, shrink the nasal mucosa, and relieve pain.

General measures include adequate hydration, steam inhalation for 20 to 30 minutes three times per day if possible, saline irrigation (Adriaensen & Fokkens, 2013), and saline nose drops. Patients are instructed to sleep with the head of the bed elevated and to avoid exposure to cigarette smoke and fumes. Patients are cautioned to avoid caffeine and alcohol, which can lead to dehydration.

Treatment of acute and chronic rhinosinusitis typically involves nasal saline lavage and decongestants. Decongestants or nasal saline spray can improve patency of the ostiomeatal unit (area where the frontal and maxillary sinuses normally drain into the nasal cavity) and improve drainage of the sinuses. Topical decongestants are used only in adults and should not be used for longer than 3 or 4 days. Oral decongestants must be used cautiously in patients with hypertension. OTC antihistamines and prescription antihistamines are used if an allergic component is suspected. Heated mist and saline irrigation also may be effective for opening blocked passages. If the patient continues to have symptoms after 7 to 10 days, the sinuses may need to be irrigated (Prokopakis, Vlastos, Pan, & Ferguson, 2013).

Observation without the use of antibiotics is an option for some patients with uncomplicated ABRS (mild pain, temperature of less than 38.3°C [101°F]). Follow-up is essential. Studies suggest that most patients will improve spontaneously, and antibiotics should be reserved for those with prolonged symptoms (Rosenfeld et al., 2015). When ABRS is confirmed, antibiotic therapy is prescribed. The recommended first-line drug for both children and adults is amoxicillin-clavulanate. Doxycycline may be used as an alternative for patients who cannot tolerate amoxicillin-clavulanate. For patients with a penicillin allergy, doxycycline or a respiratory fluoroquinolone such as levofloxacin or moxifloxacin is recommended (Murr, 2016; Teeters, Boles, Ethier, Jenkins, & Curtis, 2013). Prescribed medications may be required for a period of 3 to 4 weeks for CRS and recurrent acute rhinosinusitis.

For patients with concomitant asthma, leukotriene inhibitors may be used. Leukotriene inhibitors block the binding of *leukotrienes,* which are inflammatory mediators. If allergies are a possible cause of CRS, oral antihistamines or nasal corticosteroids may be prescribed (Borish, 2016; Adriaensen & Fokkens, 2013). The use of intranasal inhalations has been associated with a significant improvement of symptoms of CRS and a reduction in nasal bacteria (Dunn, Dion, & McMains, 2013; Huang & Govindaraj, 2013; Rosenfeld et al., 2015). Intranasal corticosteroids have been shown to produce complete or marked improvement in acute symptoms of CRS, with or without the presence of nasal polyps (Manes & Batra, 2013; Rosenfeld et al., 2015).

If standard medical therapy fails to treat CRS and symptoms persist, endoscopic sinus surgery (ESS) may be indicated to correct structural deformities that obstruct the ostia (openings) of the sinuses (Borish, 2016; Settipane, Peters, & Chandra, 2013). Patients undergoing ESS report a reduction of symptoms including headache, nasal obstruction, fatigue, body pains, and hyposmia (Settipane et al., 2013). Excising and cauterizing nasal polyps, correcting a deviated septum, incising and draining the sinuses, aerating the sinuses, and removing tumors are some of the specific procedures performed. If sinusitis is caused by a fungal infection, surgery is required to excise both the fungus ball and necrotic tissue and drain the sinuses. Antimicrobial agents are administered before and after surgery. Some patients with severe chronic sinusitis obtain relief only by relocating to a dry climate.

Complications

If untreated, acute rhinosinusitis may lead to severe complications. Local complications include osteomyelitis and mucocele (cyst of the paranasal sinuses). Osteomyelitis requires prolonged antibiotic therapy and, at times, removal of necrotic bone. Intracranial complications are rare but include cavernous sinus thrombosis, meningitis, brain abscess, ischemic brain infarction, and severe orbital cellulites (Papadakis et al., 2015; Ocampo & Grammer, 2013). Complications of CRS, although uncommon, include severe orbital cellulitis, subperiosteal abscess, cavernous sinus thrombosis, meningitis, encephalitis, and ischemic infarction. CRS can also lead to intracranial infection.

PHARYNGITIS

Acute **pharyngitis** is a sudden inflammation of the pharynx involving the back portion of the tongue, soft palate, and tonsils. Chronic pharyngitis is a persistent inflammation of the pharynx.

Pathophysiology

Most cases of acute pharyngitis are caused by viral infection. Responsible viruses include the adenovirus, influenza virus, Epstein–Barr virus, and herpes simplex virus. Bacterial organisms account for the remainder of the cases. Ten percent of adults with pharyngitis have group A beta-hemolytic streptococcus, more commonly known as group A streptococcus (GAS), streptococcal pharyngitis or "strep throat". Other bacterial organisms found in acute pharyngitis include *Mycoplasma pneumoniae, Neisseria gonorrhoeae,* and *H. influenzae* type B.

Risk Factors

Acute pharyngitis is more common in patients less than 25 years of age (usually between 5 and 15 years). Chronic pharyngitis is common in adults who work or live in dusty surroundings, use their voice to excess, suffer from chronic cough, or habitually use alcohol and tobacco.

Clinical Manifestations and Assessment

The signs and symptoms of acute pharyngitis include a fiery-red pharyngeal membrane and tonsils, lymphoid follicles

FIGURE 9-3 Pharyngitis, inflammation without exudate. **A.** Redness and vascularity of the pillars and uvula are mild to moderate. **B.** Redness is diffuse and intense. Each patient would probably complain of a sore throat. (From Bickley, L. S., & Szilagyi, P. G. (2013). *Bates' guide to physical examination and history taking* (9th ed.). Philadelphia, PA: Lippincott Williams & Wilkins.)

that are swollen and flecked with white-purple exudate, enlarged and tender cervical lymph nodes, and no cough (Fig. 9-3). Creamy exudates may be present in the tonsillar pillars. A fever greater than 100.4°F (38°C), malaise, and sore throat also may be present. Patients with GAS pharyngitis may exhibit vomiting, anorexia, and a scarlatina-form rash with urticaria known as *scarlet fever.*

Patients with chronic pharyngitis complain of a constant sense of irritation or fullness in the throat, mucus that collects in the throat and can be expelled by coughing, and difficulty swallowing. A sore throat that is worse with swallowing in the absence of pharyngitis suggests the possibility of thyroiditis and should be referred for evaluation.

Accurate diagnosis of pharyngitis is essential to determine the causative organism and to initiate treatment early. Rapid antigen detection testing (RADT) strep test and strep culture (sometimes referred to as STCX) should be used and require proper collection technique because improper collection reduces the accuracy of the test (Borchardt, 2013).

Medical and Nursing Management

Viral pharyngitis is treated with supportive measures. Antibiotics will have no effect on the organism.

If a bacterial cause is suggested or demonstrated, penicillin is usually the treatment of choice in the treatment of acute pharyngitis (Spinks, Glasziou, & Del Mar, 2013). Nasal congestion may be relieved by short-term use of nasal sprays or medications containing ephedrine sulfate or phenylephrine hydrochloride. For a patient with a history of allergy, one of the antihistamine decongestant medications is prescribed orally every 4 to 6 hours. Aspirin or acetaminophen is recommended for its anti-inflammatory and analgesic properties.

Treatment of chronic pharyngitis is based on relieving symptoms, avoiding exposure to irritants, and correcting any upper respiratory, pulmonary, or cardiac condition that might cause a chronic cough. For adults with chronic pharyngitis, tonsillectomy is an effective option.

Complications

Uncomplicated viral infections usually subside promptly, within 3 to 10 days after the onset. However, pharyngitis caused by more virulent bacteria, such as GAS, is a more severe illness. If left untreated, the complications can be severe and life-threatening. Complications include rhinosinusitis, otitis media, peritonsillar abscess, mastoiditis, and cervical adenitis. In rare cases, the infection may lead to bacteremia, pneumonia, meningitis, rheumatic fever, rheumatic heart disease or glomerulonephritis. Acute poststreptococcal glomerulonephritis (APSGN) is a complication that follows roughly 10 days after the onset of streptococcal infection and results in temporary kidney failure. APSGN is characterized by the rapid onset of gross hematuria, edema (leading to respiratory distress and pulmonary edema), and hypertension, and is usually preceded by an episode of group A streptococcal (GAS) pharyngitis or pyoderma (skin infection with pustules) (Borchardt, 2013).

LARYNGITIS

Laryngitis is inflammation of the larynx.

Pathophysiology

Laryngitis often occurs as a result of voice abuse or exposure to dust, chemicals, smoke, and other pollutants, or as part of a URI. It also may be caused by infection involving the vocal cords. Laryngitis is also associated with gastroesophageal reflux.

Laryngitis is very often caused by the same pathogens that cause the common cold and pharyngitis: a virus. Laryngitis is often associated with allergic rhinitis or pharyngitis. The onset of infection may be associated with exposure to sudden temperature changes, dietary deficiencies, malnutrition, or an immunosuppressed state. Viral laryngitis is common in the winter and is easily transmitted to others.

Clinical Manifestations and Assessment

Signs of acute laryngitis include hoarseness or **aphonia** (complete loss of voice) and severe cough. Other signs of acute laryngitis include sudden onset aggravated by cold dry wind. The throat feels worse in the morning and improves when the patient is indoors in a warmer climate. At times, the patient presents with a dry cough and a dry, sore throat that worsens in the evening hours. If allergies are present, the uvula will be visibly edematous. Many patients also complain of a "tickle" in the throat that is made worse by cold air or cold liquids. Chronic laryngitis is marked by persistent hoarseness.

Medical and Nursing Management

Management of acute or chronic laryngitis includes resting the voice, avoiding irritants (including smoking), getting enough rest drinking additional fluids, and inhaling cool steam or an aerosol. Decongestants should be avoided due to their drying effects. In addition, alcohol and caffeine should be avoided because of their diuretic effects (Fort, 2016). The majority of patients recover with conservative treatment; however, laryngitis tends to be more severe in elderly patients and may be complicated by pneumonia.

If laryngitis is part of a more extensive respiratory infection caused by a bacterial organism, or if it is severe, appropriate antibacterial therapy is instituted. For chronic laryngitis, the use of topical corticosteroids may be given by inhalation. These preparations have few systemic or long-lasting effects and may reduce local inflammatory reactions. Treatment for reflux laryngitis typically involves use of proton pump inhibitors given once daily.

NURSING PROCESS
The Patient with Upper Airway Infection

ASSESSMENT

A health history may reveal signs and symptoms of headache, sore throat, pain around the eyes and on either side of the nose, difficulty in swallowing, cough, hoarseness, fever, stuffiness, and generalized discomfort and fatigue. Determining when the symptoms began, what precipitated them, what (if anything) relieves them, and what aggravates them is part of the assessment. Inspection may reveal swelling, lesions, or asymmetry of the nose, as well as bleeding or discharge. The nurse inspects the nasal mucosa for abnormal findings such as increased redness, swelling, exudate, and nasal polyps, which may develop in chronic rhinitis. The mucosa of the nasal turbinates may also be swollen (boggy) and pale, bluish-gray. The nurse palpates the frontal and maxillary sinuses for tenderness, which suggests inflammation, and then inspects the throat by having the patient open the mouth wide and take a deep breath. The tonsils and pharynx are inspected for abnormal findings such as redness, asymmetry, or evidence of drainage, ulceration, or enlargement. The nurse also palpates the trachea to determine the midline position in the neck and to detect any masses or deformities. The neck lymph nodes are palpated for enlargement and tenderness.

DIAGNOSIS

Appropriate nursing diagnoses may include:

- Ineffective airway clearance related to excessive mucus production secondary to retained secretions and inflammation.
- Acute pain related to upper airway irritation secondary to an infection.
- Impaired verbal communication related to physiologic changes and upper airway irritation secondary to infection, swelling, hoarseness, or loss of speech.
- Deficient fluid volume related to decreased fluid intake and increased fluid loss secondary to diaphoresis associated with a fever.
- Deficient knowledge regarding prevention of URIs, treatment regimen, surgical procedure, or postoperative care.

PLANNING

The major goals for the patient may include maintenance of a patent airway, relief of pain, maintenance of effective means of communication, normal hydration, knowledge of how to prevent upper airway infections, and absence of complications.

NURSING INTERVENTIONS

MAINTAINING A PATENT AIRWAY

An accumulation of secretions can block the airway in patients with URI. As a result, changes in the respiratory pattern occur, and the work of breathing increases to compensate for the blockage. The nurse can implement several measures to loosen thick secretions or to keep the secretions moist so that they can be expectorated easily. Increasing fluid intake helps thin the mucus. Use of room vaporizers or steam inhalation also loosens secretions and reduces inflammation of the mucous membranes. To enhance drainage from the sinuses, the nurse instructs the patient about the best position to assume; this depends on the location of the infection or inflammation.

PROMOTING COMFORT

URIs usually produce localized discomfort. The nurse encourages the patient to take analgesics as prescribed. Other helpful measures include topical anesthetic agents for symptomatic relief of herpes simplex blisters and sore throats, hot packs to relieve the congestion of rhinosinusitis and promote drainage, and warm-water gargles or irrigations to relieve the pain of a sore throat. The benefits of this treatment depend on the degree of heat that is applied. The nurse encourages rest to relieve the generalized discomfort and fever that accompany many upper URIs.

PROMOTING COMMUNICATION

URIs may result in hoarseness or loss of speech. The nurse instructs the patient to refrain from speaking as much as possible. Additional strain on the vocal cords may delay full return of

(continued on page 268)

the voice. The nurse encourages the patient and family to use alternative forms of communication, such as a memo pad.

ENCOURAGING FLUID INTAKE

In URIs, the work of breathing and the respiratory rate increase as inflammation and secretions develop. This may increase insensible fluid loss. Fever further increases the metabolic rate, diaphoresis, and fluid loss. Sore throat, malaise, and fever may interfere with a patient's willingness to eat and drink. The nurse provides a list of easily ingested foods to increase caloric intake during the acute phase of illness. These include soups, pudding, yogurt, cottage cheese, high-protein drinks, and popsicles. The nurse encourages the patient to drink 2 to 3 L of fluid per day during the acute stage of airway infection, unless contraindicated, to thin the secretions and promote drainage. Liquids (hot or cold) may be soothing, depending on the disorder. In severe situations, IV fluids may be needed.

PREVENTING INFECTION

Prevention of most URIs is difficult because of the many potential causes. But because most URIs are transmitted by hand-to-hand contact, the nurse teaches the patient and family techniques to minimize the spread of infection to others, including frequent handwashing. The nurse advises the patient to avoid exposure to people who are at risk for serious illness including elderly adults, immunosuppressed people, and those with chronic health problems. The nurse may advise elderly patients and those at increased risk from a respiratory infection to consider an annual influenza and pneumococcal vaccine as recommended by the primary care provider (PCP). A follow-up appointment with the PCP may be indicated for patients with compromised health status to ensure that the respiratory infection has resolved.

MONITORING AND MANAGING POTENTIAL COMPLICATIONS

Because most patients with URIs are managed at home, patients and their families must be instructed to monitor for signs and symptoms and to seek immediate medical care if the patient's condition does not improve or if the patient's physical status appears to be worsening. Symptoms that require further attention include persistent or high fever, increasing shortness of breath, confusion, and increasing weakness and malaise. Potential complications include sepsis, meningitis or brain abscess, and peritonsillar abscess, otitis media, or rhinosinusitis.

Sepsis and meningitis may occur in patients with compromised immune status or in those with an overwhelming bacterial infection. The nurse explains to the patient that fever, severe headache, and **nuchal rigidity** (stiffness of the neck/inability to bend the neck) are signs of potential complications. The patient with sepsis requires expert care to treat the infection, stabilize vital signs, and prevent or treat septicemia and shock. Deterioration of the patient's condition necessitates intensive care

measures (e.g., hemodynamic monitoring and administration of vasoactive medications, IV fluids, nutritional support, corticosteroids) to monitor the patient's status and to support the patient's vital signs. High doses of antibiotics may be administered to treat the causative organism. The nurse's role is to monitor the patient's vital signs, hemodynamic status, and laboratory values; administer needed treatment; alleviate the patient's physical discomfort; and provide explanations, teaching, and emotional support to the patient and family. Refer to Chapter 54 for management of septic shock.

The patient and family are instructed about the signs and symptoms of otitis media and rhinosinusitis (periorbital edema, severe facial pain on palpation) and about the importance of follow-up with the PCP to ensure adequate evaluation and treatment of these conditions.

Potential for airway compromise is possible in severe pharyngitis. Symptoms that require provider referral include dyspnea, drooling, inability to swallow, and inability to fully open the mouth. The skin should be examined for possible rash because acute pharyngitis may precede some other communicable diseases (e.g., rubella). For the patient with laryngitis, the signs and symptoms that require contacting the health care provider include loss of voice with sore throat that makes swallowing saliva difficult, hemoptysis, and noisy respirations.

EVALUATION

Expected outcomes include:

1. Maintains a patent airway by managing secretions:
   a. Reports decreased congestion.
   b. Assumes best position to facilitate drainage of secretions.
   c. Uses self-care measures appropriately and consistently to manage secretions during the acute phase of illness.
2. Reports relief of pain and discomfort using pain intensity scale:
   a. Uses comfort measures: Analgesics, hot packs, gargles, rest.
   b. Demonstrates adequate oral hygiene.
   c. Free of pain in ears, sinuses, and throat.
3. Demonstrates ability to communicate needs, wants, level of comfort.
4. Maintains adequate fluid and nutrition intake.
5. Utilizes strategies to prevent upper airway infections:
   a. Demonstrates hand hygiene technique.
   b. Identifies the value of the influenza and pneumococcal vaccines.
6. Absence of complications:
   a. No signs of sepsis: Fever, hypotension, deterioration of cognitive status.
   b. Vital signs and hemodynamic status normal.
   c. No evidence of neurologic involvement.
   d. No signs of development of brain abscess.
   e. Resolution of URI without development of otitis media or rhinosinusitis.

OBSTRUCTION AND TRAUMA OF THE UPPER RESPIRATORY AIRWAY

OBSTRUCTION DURING SLEEP

Obstructive sleep apnea syndrome (OSA) is a disorder characterized by recurrent episodes of upper airway obstruction and a reduction in ventilation. It is defined as cessation of breathing (**apnea**) during sleep, usually caused by repetitive upper airway obstruction. It interferes with the person's ability to obtain adequate rest and, ultimately, can affect memory, learning, and decision-making (Carlucci, Smith, & Corbridge, 2013). As many as 18 million Americans suffer from sleep apnea (Jordan, McSharry, & Malhotra, 2014).

Various definitions of OSA—also referred to as obstructive sleep apnea/hypopnea syndrome (OSAHS) or upper respiratory resistance syndrome (UARS)—exist, leading to overestimation of the prevalence of this syndrome.

Pathophysiology

OSA is a disorder characterized by recurrent episodes of upper airway obstruction, causing a reduction in ventilation followed by frequent arousals and periodic oxyhemoglobin desaturations during sleep (Jordan et al., 2014). OSA is defined as the presence of at least five obstructive events (apneas and hypopneas [slow or shallow breathing]) per hour during sleep (Jordan et al., 2014; Paiva & Attarian, 2014). Repetitive apneic events result in hypoxia and hypercapnia, which trigger a sympathetic response (increased heart rate and increased tone and contractility of smooth muscle). An obstruction may be caused by mechanical factors such as a reduced diameter of the upper airway or dynamic changes in the upper airway during sleep.

Patients with OSA have a higher prevalence of hypertension and an increased risk of myocardial infarction, stroke, and death (Basner, 2016; Jordan et al., 2014). Patients with underlying cardiovascular disease may find the nocturnal **hypoxemia** may predispose them to arrhythmias. Patients who have a diagnosis of heart failure and who have untreated OSA are at increased risk of death (Pavia & Attarian, 2014; Jordan et al., 2014). OSA can also increase insulin resistance and other metabolic changes that can increase the risk of vascular disease (Drager, Togeiro, Polotsky, & Lorenzi-Filho, 2013). OSA is more prevalent in people with coronary artery disease, congestive heart failure, metabolic syndrome, and type 2 diabetes, suggesting that screening for OSA is indicated in patients with these pathologies (Carlucci et al., 2013).

Risk Factors

Sleep apnea is more prevalent in men, especially those who are older and overweight (Jordan et al., 2014). However, postmenopausal and obese women are at increased risk of developing OSA as well (Basner, 2016). The major risk factor for OSA is obesity around the neck that narrows and compresses the upper airway. The elderly have a higher prevalence of OSA (Jordan et al., 2014). Other associated factors include alteration in the upper airway, such as structural changes (e.g., tonsillar hypertrophy, abnormal posterior positioning of one or both jaws, excessive fat deposits in the lateral walls of the pharynx, and craniofacial structural abnormalities) that contribute to the collapsibility of the airway and increase the risk of sleep apnea (Pavia & Attarian, 2014).

Clinical Manifestations and Assessment

OSA is characterized by frequent and loud snoring with breathing cessation for 10 seconds or longer, for at least five episodes per hour, followed by awakening abruptly with a loud snort as the blood oxygen level drops. Classic signs and symptoms of OSA are presented in Box 9-1. Symptoms typically progress with increases in weight and aging as well as during the transition to menopause (Jordan et al., 2014).

Several screening tools/questionnaires are available to assess the frequency and severity of symptoms (Jordan et al., 2014). The diagnosis of sleep apnea is based on clinical symptoms plus polysomnographic findings (sleep study). This overnight sleep study measures multiple physiologic signals related to sleep (electroencephalogram [EEG], electrocardiogram [ECG], and airflow), in order to gauge oxyhemoglobin saturation, brain activity, eye movement, thoracic muscle activity, body position, respiratory rate, heart rate, cardiac arrhythmias, chest impedance, and airflow (Jordan et al., 2014).

Medical Management

Treatments are varied but include weight loss and avoidance of alcohol and hypnotic medications initially (Papadakis et al., 2015; Pavia & Attarian, 2014). Weight loss reduces the

---

BOX 9-1   Focused Assessment

Obstructive Sleep Apnea (OSA)

Be alert for the following signs and symptoms:
- Excessive daytime sleepiness
- Frequent nocturnal awakening
- Insomnia
- Loud snoring
- Morning headaches
- Intellectual deterioration
- Personality changes, irritability
- Impotence
- Systemic hypertension
- Arrhythmias
- Pulmonary hypertension, cor pulmonale
- Polycythemia
- Enuresis

number of apneas and hypopneas per hour of total sleep time as measured by the apnea–hypopnea index (AHI) (Carlucci et al., 2013; Baby, Aronow, & Chandy, 2013). Oral appliances designed to reposition the mandible or tongue may be useful in select patients. These devices are not very beneficial in the elderly patient as full dentition is required (Baby et al., 2013; Jordan et al., 2014).

Noninvasive Positive-Pressure Ventilation

In more severe cases of OSA involving hypoxemia with severe carbon dioxide retention (hypercapnia), the treatment includes continuous positive airway pressure (CPAP) or bilevel positive airway pressure (BiPAP) therapy with supplemental oxygen (Carlucci et al., 2013). Patients are considered candidates for noninvasive ventilation if they have acute or chronic respiratory failure, acute pulmonary edema, chronic obstructive pulmonary disease (COPD), chronic heart failure, or OSA. The device also may be used at home to improve tissue oxygenation and to rest the respiratory muscles while the patient sleeps at night.

CPAP provides positive pressure to the airways throughout the respiratory cycle, preventing collapse (Basner, 2016; Baby et al., 2013; Jordan et al., 2014). A CPAP delivery system is comprised of an air pump that is connected to a nasal, oral, or combined mask by a flexible tube. The air pump extracts external filtered air to deliver the pressurized airflow that can be adjusted (Basner, 2016; Baby et al., 2013). The leak-proof mask keeps the alveoli open, thereby preventing respiratory failure. CPAP is the most effective treatment for OSA because the positive pressure acts as a splint, keeping the upper airway and trachea open during sleep. To use CPAP, the patient must be breathing independently (Baby et al., 2013; Carlucci et al., 2013).

BiPAP ventilation offers independent control of inspiratory and expiratory pressures while providing pressure-support ventilation. It delivers two levels of positive airway pressure via a nasal or oral mask, nasal pillow, or mouthpiece with a tight seal and a portable ventilator. Each inspiration can be initiated either by the patient or by the machine (programmed backup rate). The backup rate ensures that the patient will receive a set number of breaths per minute. BiPAP is most often used for patients who require ventilatory assistance at night, such as those with severe COPD or sleep apnea. Tolerance is variable; BiPAP usually is most successful with highly motivated patients (Baby et al., 2013).

Problems with CPAP or BiPAP therapy are common. Commonly reported adverse effects of CPAP include skin irritations, pain, rash, or breakdown at the mask contact points (usually the bridge of the nose). Dryness or irritation of the nasal and pharyngeal membranes, nasal congestion, and eye irritation from leakage from the mask are also reported (Basner, 2016; Baby et al., 2013; Hu, Yu, & Tsao, 2013). Gastrointestinal bloating secondary to air swallowing is another common side effect (Basner, 2016). Proper fitting of the mask should allow for therapy to continue. Although these treatments are effective in managing OSA, patient compliance with treatment continues to be a major concern (Carlucci et al., 2013). Nursing research on the factors (physical, psychological, and social) influencing the use and nonuse of CPAP therapy is described in Box 9-2.

Surgical Management

Surgical procedures (e.g., tonsillectomy or **uvulopalato-pharyngoplasty** [termed UPPP, the surgical resection of pharyngeal soft tissue and uvula]) may be performed to correct the obstruction should the airway be in jeopardy or the patient has been unsuccessful with CPAP therapy. Effective in about 50% of patients, UPPP is more effective in eliminating snoring than in eliminating apnea (Baby et al., 2013). UPPP has been shown to reduce the AHI by 50% (Pavia & Attarian, 2014). Nasal septoplasty may be performed for anatomic nasal septal deformities. Tracheostomy relieves upper airway obstruction but has many adverse effects, including speech difficulties and increased risk of infections. These procedures, as well as other maxillofacial surgeries, are reserved for patients with life-threatening arrhythmias or severe disabilities who have not responded to conventional therapy (Baby et al., 2013; Papadakis et al., 2015).

Pharmacologic Therapy

Although medications are not generally recommended for OSA, modafinil (Provigil) has been shown to reduce daytime sleepiness (Jordan et al., 2014). Protriptyline (Triptil), Theophylline (Aminophylline), and estrogen therapy are not recommended for treating OSA (Baby et al., 2013). Patients must understand that medications are not a substitute for CPAP or BiPAP therapy. Administration of low-flow nasal oxygen at night can help relieve hypoxemia in some patients but has little effect on the frequency or severity of apnea. Further study on the effectiveness of pharmacologic therapy is needed.

Nursing Management

The patient with OSA may not recognize the potential consequences of the disorder. The nurse explains the disorder and relates symptoms (daytime sleepiness, morning headaches, heartburn, insomnia, snoring) to the underlying disorder. The nurse also instructs the patient and family about treatments, including weight loss, avoiding alcohol and sedative medications, and the correct and safe use of prescribed therapies such as CPAP, BiPAP, and oxygen therapy.

EPISTAXIS (NOSEBLEED)

Epistaxis, a hemorrhage from the nose, is caused by the rupture of tiny, distended vessels in the mucous membrane of any area of the nose. Most commonly, the site is the anterior septum, where three major blood vessels enter the nasal

BOX 9-2   **Nursing Research**

Bridging the Gap to Evidence-Based Practice

Is Inconsistent Pretreatment Bedtime Related to CPAP Non-adherence?

Sawyer, A. M., King, T. S., Sawyer, D. A., & Rizzo, A. (2014). *Research in Nursing & Health*, 37(6), 504–511.

Purpose

Continuous positive airway pressure (CPAP) is the treatment of choice for patients with obstructive sleep apnea (OSA). Lack of adherence to continuous positive airway pressure therapy (CPAP) is a well-recognized limitation to the effectiveness of treatment of OSA. Patterns of CPAP use are established early in the treatment period, generally during the first week of home therapy. These patterns have been shown to be consistent with long-term CPAP outcomes. It is important to determine predictors of CPAP nonadherence prior to treatment initiation to minimize noncompliance. Multiple factors have been examined as related to CPAP compliance, including patient characteristics, titration method, sleep quality, disease and symptom severity, and psychological and psychosocial factors. Some important insights into CPAP adherence have emerged, but challenges still surround CPAP nonadherence.

Design

In a prospective longitudinal study conducted at two clinical sleep centers in the United States, the authors examined whether inconsistent self-reported bedtime before initiation of CPAP treatment, operationalized as bedtime variability, was (1) different among those adherent (more than 4 hours a night) and nonadherent to CPAP treatment at 1 week and 1 month; and/or (2) related to 1-week and 1-month CPAP use when other variables were accounted for. Participants were recruited from those referred to the sleep centers for CPAP titration polysomnogram (PSG). Patients who responded to an invitation to participate in the study were contacted and screened. Inclusion criteria for the study were (1) newly diagnosed OSA with AHI of at least five events/hour on in-laboratory PSG; (2) referral to CPAP titration PSG; and (3) able to speak and read English. Exclusion criteria were (1) supplemental oxygen or bilevel positive airway pressure required during titration PSG; (2) newly diagnosed psychiatric disorder within 6 months; and (3) medical contraindications to using CPAP for treatment of OSA. A total of 102 patients were enrolled with a final complete data collection from 79 patients.

Data collection included an 18-item, self-reported demographic questionnaire; a diagnostic PSG; and a 1-week sleep diary completed after PSG but before CPAP titration PSG. Participants completed the diary by recording date; day of the week; whether it was a work day, vacation day, and/or weekend day; time to bed; and time of terminal awakening. The independent variable, pretreatment bedtime variability (inconsistency in time of going to bed to initiate sleep), was derived from sleep diary recordings. Objective CPAP use data were collected from the internal microprocessor on standard CPAP devices after 1 month of home CPAP treatment. The CPAP use data were hours per night at effective pressure for at least 20 minutes. Nonadherence was defined as less than 4 hours per night of CPAP use.

Findings

The study sample (N = 79) were predominantly white non-Hispanic, college-educated, obese, and employed full-time, with slightly more males than females. Most (68%) had been referred. The majority had severe OSA. Participants' CPAP use averaged 4.6 hours per night (SD 2.5) at 1 week, with 27 participants (34.2%) below the minimal adherence level of 4 hours per night. The sample averaged 4.3 hours per night (SD 2.4) of CPAP at 1 month, with 31 (39.2%) below the 4-hour minimum for adherence. Hours of CPAP use per night were significantly different between CPAP adherents and nonadherents at both time points. There were no differences between 1-month CPAP adherents and nonadherents on any baseline characteristic except marital status.

Mean pretreatment bedtime variability was 63.1 minutes (SD 38.04; median 55.93, IQR 38.17). Pretreatment bedtime variability was not statistically different between CPAP adherents and nonadherents at 1 week and did not predict CPAP nonadherence at 1 week. The 31 participants who were nonadherent at 1 month had significantly greater variability in pretreatment bedtime. Men who were nonadherent to CPAP had greater bedtime variability than did adherent men; while for female participants, the difference in bedtime variability between nonadherent and adherents was not statistically significant. Educational level was examined as potential modifiers for the effect of bedtime variability. Lower educational levels were associated with an increased bedtime variability and CPAP nonadherence.

These results suggest that pretreatment bedtime variability, or inconsistency in time of going to bed to initiate sleep, is an important and modifiable predictor of 1-month CPAP nonadherence, especially among men and those with little completed education. More than 75 minutes of bedtime variability conferred significantly more statistical risk for CPAP nonadherence than having less than 75 minutes of bedtime variability. These findings provide preliminary evidence to support the inclusion of sleep schedule stabilization, or minimizing bedtime inconsistency, in future interventions aimed at reducing CPAP nonadherence.

Nursing Implications

Strategies for patient education, assessment, and management of therapies to treat disorders of sleep related to OSA can be strengthened as the variables leading to adherence or nonadherence to CPAP therapy are studied and reported in the literature. Incorporating knowledge and behavioral changes, including incorporating scheduled repetitive behaviors around bedtime, can lead to increase in adherence to CPAP treatment.

Risk Factors for Epistaxis

- Local infections/inflammation (vestibulitis, rhinitis, rhinosinusitis, sinusitis, nasal polyps)
- Systemic infections (scarlet fever, malaria)
- Drying of nasal mucous membranes (cold, dry environment); overuse of decongestant nasal sprays
- Structural deformities (deviated septum, chronic perforations)
- Nasal inhalation of illicit drugs (e.g., cocaine), irritants
- Trauma (digital trauma as in picking the nose; blunt trauma; fracture; forceful nose-blowing)
- Nasal or facial surgery
- Arteriosclerosis
- Hypertension
- Tumor (sinus or nasopharynx)
- Coagulopathy (thrombocytopenia, hemophilia, von Willebrand disease)
- Drugs: Use of aspirin, nonsteroidal anti-inflammatory drugs (NSAIDs), warfarin
- Liver disease
- Osler–Weber–Rendu (hereditary hemorrhagic telangiectasia)
- Foreign bodies in the nasal cavity

cavity. Several risk factors may be associated with epistaxis and are described in Box 9-3.

Medical Management

Management of epistaxis depends on its cause and the location of the bleeding site. Initial treatment includes applying direct pressure. The patient sits upright with the head tilted forward to prevent swallowing and aspiration of blood and is directed to pinch the soft outer portion of the nose against the midline septum for 5 or 10 minutes continuously. If this measure is unsuccessful, the nose must be examined using good illumination and suction to determine the site of bleeding (Murr, 2016). Cotton applicators soaked in a vasoconstricting solution (i.e., epinephrine, ephedrine, cocaine) may be inserted into the nose to reduce the blood flow. Visible bleeding sites may be cauterized with silver nitrate or electrocautery (high-frequency electrical current). A supplemental patch of Surgicel or Gelfoam may be used (Papadakis et al., 2015). If the origin of the bleeding cannot be identified, the nose may be packed with gauze impregnated with petroleum jelly or antibiotic ointment. The packing may remain in place for 48 hours or up to 5 or 6 days if necessary to control bleeding. Antibiotics may be prescribed because of the risk of iatrogenic sinusitis and toxic shock syndrome.

Nursing Management

The nurse monitors the patient's vital signs, assists in the control of bleeding, and provides tissues and an emesis basin to allow the patient to expectorate any excess blood. The nurse continuously assesses the patient's airway and breathing, as well as vital signs. On rare occasions, a patient with significant hemorrhage requires IV infusions of crystalloid solutions (normal saline) as well as cardiac and pulse oximetry monitoring.

Once the bleeding is controlled, the nurse instructs the patient to avoid vigorous exercise for several days and to avoid hot or spicy foods and tobacco, as they may cause vasodilation and an increased risk of rebleeding. Discharge teaching includes reviewing ways to prevent epistaxis: avoiding forceful nose-blowing, straining, high altitudes, and nasal trauma. Adequate humidification may prevent drying of the nasal passages. The nurse instructs the patient how to apply direct pressure to the nose in case of a recurrent nosebleed. If recurrent bleeding cannot be stopped, the patient is instructed to seek additional medical attention.

NASAL OBSTRUCTION

The passage of air through the nostrils is frequently obstructed by a deviation of the nasal septum, hypertrophy of the turbinate bones, or the presence of nasal polyps. Chronic nasal congestion forces the patient to breathe through the mouth, producing dryness of the oral mucosa and other problems including persistent dry, cracked lips. Patients with chronic nasal congestion often suffer from sleep deprivation due to difficulty maintaining an adequate airway while lying flat during sleep.

Medical Management

The treatment of nasal obstruction requires the removal of the obstruction, followed by measures to treat chronic infection. Measures to reduce or alleviate nasal obstruction include nonsurgical as well as surgical techniques. Commonly used medications include nasal corticosteroids. Treatment with nasal corticosteroids for 1 to 3 months is beneficial in treatment of small polyps, avoiding surgical intervention. Additional medications may include antibiotics for the treatment of underlying infection or antihistamines for management of allergies. Hypertrophied turbinates may be treated by applying an astringent agent to shrink them. A more aggressive approach in treating nasal obstruction caused by turbinate hypertrophy involves surgical reduction of the hypertrophy, a procedure known as functional rhinoplasty.

Nursing Management

Most of these surgical procedures are performed on an outpatient basis. Postoperatively, the nurse elevates the head of the bed to promote drainage and to alleviate discomfort from edema. Frequent oral hygiene is encouraged to overcome dryness caused by breathing through the mouth. Before discharge, the patient is instructed to avoid blowing the nose with force during the postoperative recovery period. The patient is also instructed about the signs and symptoms of bleeding and infection and when to contact the provider.

FRACTURES OF THE NOSE

Nasal fracture is the most common fracture involving the face. Fractures of the nose usually result from a direct assault. Nasal fractures may affect the ascending process of the maxilla and the septum. The torn mucous membrane results in a nosebleed. In a series of complications, the patient could ultimately experience a hematoma, infection, abscess, and a vascular/septic necrosis. However, as a rule, serious consequences usually do not occur.

Clinical Manifestations and Assessment

The signs and symptoms of a nasal fracture are pain, bleeding from the nose externally and internally into the pharynx, swelling of the soft tissues adjacent to the nose, periorbital ecchymosis, nasal obstruction, and deformity. The patient's nose may have an asymmetric appearance that may not be obvious until the edema subsides.

The nose is examined internally to rule out the possibility that the injury may be complicated by a fracture of the nasal septum and a submucosal septal hematoma (Papadakis et al., 2015). Clear fluid draining from either nostril suggests a fracture of the cribriform plate with leakage of cerebrospinal fluid (CSF). Because CSF contains glucose, it can readily be differentiated from nasal mucus by means of a dipstick. Refer to Chapter 45 for details of CSF leaks.

Nursing Alert
If CSF is suspected, the patient is instructed not to cough or blow the nose. If the patient has to sneeze, do so with an open mouth. The head of bed should be elevated, and nothing should be inserted into the nares. The primary concern of CSF rhinorrhea (leakage of CSF via the nares) is the complication of meningitis.

Careful inspection or palpation discloses any deviations of the bone or disruptions of the nasal cartilages. An x-ray may reveal displacement of the fractured bones and may help rule out extension of the fracture into the skull.

Medical Management

Any bleeding is controlled with the use of packing. For the patient who has sustained traumatic force to break the nose or any facial bone, the possibility of a cervical spine fracture must be considered. If suspected, stabilize the cervical spine and log roll the patient if turning is required. Uncomplicated nasal fractures may be treated initially with analgesic agents, use of ice to reduce swelling, and ENT follow-up.

Treatment of nasal fractures is aimed at restoring nasal function and returning the aesthetic appearance of the nose to baseline. Reduction of the fracture is performed as soon as possible. If edema is too severe to reduce the fraction immediately, reduction is performed within 3 to 7 days. Fractures that heal but are misaligned may require surgical intervention, such as rhinoplasty, to reshape the external appearance of the nose. In patients who develop a septal hematoma, the provider will drain the hematoma through a small incision. Antibiotic coverage is expected after septal hematoma evacuation. A septal hematoma that is not drained can lead to permanent deformity of the nose.

Nursing Management

Immediately after the fracture, the nurse applies ice and encourages the patient to keep the head elevated. The nurse instructs the patient to apply ice packs to the nose for 20 minutes, four times each day, to decrease swelling. The packing inserted to stop the bleeding may be uncomfortable and unpleasant, and obstruction of the nasal passages by the packing forces the patient to breathe through the mouth. This, in turn, causes the oral mucous membranes to become dry. Mouth rinses help to moisten the mucous membranes and to reduce the odor and taste of dried blood in the oropharynx and nasopharynx. Use of analgesic agents, such as acetaminophen, is preferred initially over NSAIDs, such as ibuprofen or naproxen, in the first 2 days to avoid increasing the risk of bleeding. The nurse reminds the patient to avoid sports activities, especially contact sports, for 6 weeks.

LARYNGEAL OBSTRUCTION

Obstruction of the larynx caused by edema is a serious, often fatal, condition. The larynx contains a narrow space between the vocal cords (glottis), through which air must pass. Swelling of the laryngeal mucous membranes may close off the opening tightly, leading to life-threatening hypoxia or suffocation.

Pathophysiology

Edema of the glottis occurs rarely in patients with acute laryngitis, occasionally in patients with urticaria, and more frequently in patients with severe inflammation of the throat, as in scarlet fever. It is an occasional but usually preventable cause of death in severe anaphylaxis (angioedema). Hereditary angioedema (HAE) is also characterized by episodes of life-threatening laryngeal edema. Laryngeal edema in people with HAE can occur at any age, although young adults are at greatest risk. Laryngospasm, a severe form of airway obstruction, may be triggered by mechanical stimulation of the larynx or by cord irritation due to aspiration of oral secretions, blood, or vomitus (Lavery & Craig, 2014).

Risk Factors

Risk factors for laryngeal obstruction are provided in Box 9-4. Foreign bodies frequently are aspirated into the pharynx, the larynx, or the trachea.

BOX 9-4
Risk Factors for Laryngeal Obstruction

- History of allergies that may result in anaphylaxis
- Inhalation/ingestion of foreign body (balloon fragments, chewing gum, drug packets)
- Heavy alcohol consumption or tobacco use (causing a tumor)
- Family history of airway problems (suggests angioedema)
- Use of ACE inhibitors
- Recent throat pain or fever (suggests infectious process)
- History of surgery or previous tracheostomy (suggests possible subglottic stenosis)

Clinical Manifestations and Assessment

The foreign objects obstruct the air passages and cause difficulty in breathing, hoarseness, and stridor, which may lead to asphyxia; and later, the obstructing objects may be drawn farther down, entering the bronchi or a bronchial branch and causing symptoms of irritation, such as a croupy cough, expectoration of blood or mucus, or labored breathing. The patient may demonstrate lowered oxygen saturation; however, normal oxygen saturation should not be interpreted as a sign that the obstruction is not significant. Use of accessory muscles to maximize airflow may occur and is often manifested by retractions in the neck or abdomen during inspirations. Patients who demonstrate these symptoms may need ventilatory support (i.e., mechanical ventilation or positive-pressure ventilation).

A thorough history can be very useful to the health care team in diagnosing and treating the patient with a laryngeal obstruction. The nurse obtains a history from the patient or family about alcohol or tobacco consumption, current medications, family history of airway problems, recent infections, pain or fever, dental pain or poor dentition, and any previous surgeries or trauma. Emergency measures to secure the patient's airway should not be delayed to obtain a history or perform tests. The patient's clinical presentation and x-ray findings confirm the diagnosis of laryngeal obstruction.

Medical and Nursing Management

Medical management is based on the initial evaluation of the patient and the need to ensure a patent airway. If the airway is obstructed by a foreign body and signs of asphyxia are apparent, immediate treatment is necessary. Frequently, if the foreign body has lodged in the pharynx and can be visualized, the finger can dislodge it. If the obstruction is in the larynx or the trachea, the clinician or other rescuer tries the subdiaphragmatic abdominal thrust (Heimlich) maneuver. If all efforts are unsuccessful, an immediate tracheotomy is necessary. If the obstruction is caused by edema resulting from an allergic reaction, treatment may include administration of subcutaneous epinephrine and a corticosteroid (see Chapter 38). Continuous pulse oximetry is essential. Box 9-5 describes nursing management of an upper airway obstruction.

CANCER OF THE LARYNX

Cancer of the larynx is a malignant tumor in and around the larynx (voice box). Squamous cell carcinoma is the most common form of cancer of the larynx (95%). Approximately 55% of patients with laryngeal cancer present with involved lymph nodes at the time of diagnosis (DeVita, Lawrence, & Rosenberg, 2014).

Carcinogens associated with laryngeal cancer include tobacco (smoke, smokeless) and alcohol and their combined effects. Occupational or environmental exposure to asbestos, wood dust, coal dust, steel dust, cement dust, tar products, leather, formaldehyde, and iron compounds and fumes have also been implicated. Other contributing factors include straining the voice, chronic laryngitis, nutritional deficiencies (riboflavin), family predisposition, and a weakened immune system.

Metastatic disease from the true vocal cords is very rare because they are devoid of lymph nodes. The prognosis for patients who have small laryngeal cancers without evidence of spread to the lymph nodes is about 75% to 95%. Recurrence occurs usually within the first 2 to 3 years after diagnosis. The presence of disease after 5 years is very often secondary to a new primary malignancy.

Risk Factors

Cancer of the larynx occurs more frequently in men than in women, and it is most common in people between the ages of 60 and 70 years (American Cancer Society, 2015). The incidence of laryngeal cancer continues to decline, but the incidence in women versus men continues to increase. The disease is also about 50% more common among African Americans than among Caucasian Americans.

Clinical Manifestations and Assessment

Hoarseness of more than 2 weeks' duration occurs in the patient with cancer in the glottic area because the tumor impedes the action of the vocal cords during speech. The voice may sound harsh, raspy, and lower in pitch. Affected voice sounds are not early signs of subglottic or supraglottic cancer. The patient may complain of a persistent cough or sore throat and pain and burning in the throat, especially when consuming hot liquids or citrus juices. A lump may be felt in the neck. Later symptoms include **dysphagia**, dyspnea (difficulty breathing), unilateral nasal obstruction or discharge, persistent hoarseness, persistent ulceration, and foul breath. Cervical lymph adenopathy, unintentional weight loss, a general debilitated state, and pain radiating to the ear may occur with metastasis.

An initial assessment includes a complete history and physical examination of the head and neck. An indirect laryngoscopy, using a flexible endoscope, is initially performed by the otolaryngologist to visually evaluate the pharynx, larynx, and possible tumor. Mobility of the vocal cords

BOX 9-5
Management of Upper Airway Obstruction

Adequate ventilation is dependent on free movement of air through the upper and lower airways. Maintaining a patent (open) airway is achieved through meticulous airway management, whether in an emergency situation, such as airway obstruction, or in long-term management, as in caring for a patient with an endotracheal or a tracheostomy tube. The patient with an altered level of consciousness from any cause is at risk for upper airway obstruction because of loss of the protective reflexes (cough and swallowing) and loss of the tone of the pharyngeal muscles, which causes the tongue to fall back and block the airway.

The nurse makes rapid observations to assess for signs and symptoms of upper airway obstruction: assessing the patient's level of consciousness (LOC), inspecting the chest for movement and use or retraction of accessory muscles, and noting skin color and any obvious signs of deformity or obstruction of the airway (trauma, food, teeth, tongue, vomitus). The nurse should palpate the trachea for midline location and look for any specific areas of tenderness, fracture, or subcutaneous emphysema (crepitus). Auscultation is performed to assess for audible air movement, stridor (inspiratory crowing sound), or wheezing (high-pitched musical sound) that may be present over the lower trachea and bilaterally in all lobes. As soon as an upper airway obstruction is identified, the nurse takes the following emergency measures:

Clearing the Airway

- Hyperextend the patient's neck by placing one hand on the forehead and placing the fingers of the other hand underneath the jaw and lifting upward and forward. This action pulls the tongue away from the back of the pharynx. **Note that this position is used only if the cervical spine is free of injury**. Assess the patient by observing the chest and listening and feeling for the movement of air.

- Use a cross-finger technique to open the mouth and observe for obvious obstructions, such as secretions, blood clots, or food particles.
- If no passage of air is detected, apply five quick sharp abdominal thrusts just below the xiphoid process to expel

the obstruction. Repeat this procedure until the obstruction is expelled.

- After the obstruction is expelled, roll the patient as a unit onto the side for recovery.
- When the obstruction is relieved, if the patient can breathe spontaneously but not cough, swallow, or gag, insert an oral or nasopharyngeal airway.

Bag and Mask Resuscitation

- Use a resuscitation bag and mask if assisted ventilation is required.
- Apply the mask to the patient's face and create a seal by pressing the thumb of the nondominant hand on the bridge of the nose and the index finger on the chin. Using the rest of the fingers on that hand, pull on the chin and the angle of the mandible to maintain the head in extension. Use the dominant hand to inflate the lungs by squeezing the bag to its full volume.

is assessed; if normal movement is limited, the growth may affect muscle, other tissue, and even the airway. The neck and the thyroid gland are palpated for enlarged lymph nodes or thyroid gland.

Diagnostic procedures that may be utilized include endoscopy, optical imaging, and CT scans. A direct laryngoscopic examination performed under local or general anesthesia may be required to evaluate all areas of the larynx. Direct visualization and palpation of the vocal folds may yield a more accurate diagnosis.

CT and MRI are used to assess regional adenopathy and soft tissue and to help stage and determine the extent of a tumor. MRI is also helpful in posttreatment follow-up to detect a recurrence. Positron emission tomography (PET) scanning may also be used to detect recurrence of a laryngeal tumor after treatment.

Medical Management

The goals of treatment of laryngeal cancer include cure; preservation of safe, effective swallowing; preservation of useful voice; and avoidance of permanent tracheostomy (Papadakis et al., 2015). Treatment options include surgery, radiation therapy, and chemotherapy. The prognosis depends on a variety of factors: tumor stage, the patient's gender and age, and pathologic features of the tumor, including the grade and depth of infiltration. The treatment plan also depends on whether this is an initial diagnosis or a recurrence.

Surgery and radiation therapy are both effective methods in the early stages of cancer of the larynx. Chemotherapy traditionally has been used for recurrence or metastatic disease. It has also been used more recently in conjunction with radiation therapy, to avoid a total laryngectomy, or preoperatively, to shrink a tumor before surgery.

Surgical Management

Surgical management depends largely on the stage of the disease. Complete removal of the larynx (total **laryngectomy**) can provide the desired cure, but it also leaves the patient with significant loss of the natural voice and the need to breathe through a stoma created in the lower neck. The stoma is a permanent opening into the trachea. Several different procedures are available that can offer voice-sparing results while achieving a positive cure rate for the patient who has an early laryngeal carcinoma. These procedures include vocal cord stripping and cordectomy. Vocal cord stripping involves removal of the mucosa of the edge of the cord using an operating microscope. It is used to treat dysplasia, hyperkeratosis, and leukoplakia and is often the curative treatment for this classification of lesions. A cordectomy is an excision of the vocal cord performed via transoral laser and is used for confined lesions involving the middle third of the vocal cord. The probability of poor voice quality is related to the extent of tissue removed.

These partial resections are increasingly common surgical procedures, using total laryngectomy as salvage therapy for recurrences (Tomeh & Holsinger, 2014; Lewis, 2012). Several different types of laryngectomy are considered for patients with more extensive involvement. These include partial laryngectomy, supraglottic laryngectomy, hemilaryngectomy, or total laryngectomy.

- *Partial laryngectomy* (laryngofissure–thyrotomy): A portion of the larynx is removed, along with one vocal cord and the tumor; all other structures remain. The airway remains intact, and the patient is expected to have no difficulty swallowing. The voice quality may change, or the patient may sound hoarse. It is associated with a high cure rate.
- *Supraglottic laryngectomy:* A voice-sparing operation; the hyoid bone, glottis, and false cords are removed. The true vocal cords, cricoid cartilage, and trachea remain intact. A tracheostomy is left in place until the glottic airway is established. Postoperative irradiation may be indicated. The quality of the voice may change.
- *Hemilaryngectomy:* The thyroid cartilage of the larynx is split in the midline of the neck, and the portion of the vocal cord (one true cord and one false cord) is removed with the tumor. Some change may occur in the voice quality. The voice may be rough, raspy, and hoarse and have limited projection. The airway and swallowing remain intact.
- *Total laryngectomy:* A complete removal of the larynx, including the hyoid bone, epiglottis, cricoid cartilage, and two or three rings of the trachea. The tongue, pharyngeal walls, and trachea are preserved. This procedure is performed for advanced laryngeal cancer and results in permanent loss of the voice and a change in the airway.

Surgery for laryngeal cancer is more difficult when the lesion involves the midline structures or both vocal cords. With or without neck dissection, a total laryngectomy requires a permanent tracheal stoma (Fig. 9-4) because the larynx that provides the protective sphincter is no longer present. The tracheal stoma prevents the aspiration of food and fluid into the lower respiratory tract. The patient will have no voice but will have normal swallowing. A total laryngectomy changes the manner in which airflow is used for breathing and speaking, as depicted in Figure 9-5. Patients who have this procedure require alternatives to normal speech.

Complications that may occur include a salivary leak, wound infection from the development of a pharyngocutaneous fistula, stomal stenosis, and dysphagia secondary to pharyngeal and cervical esophageal stricture. Advances in surgical techniques for treating laryngeal cancer may minimize the cosmetic and functional deficits previously seen with total laryngectomy. Some microlaryngeal surgery can be performed endoscopically. Many patients who have undergone a total laryngectomy report a good quality of life overall (Singer et al., 2013).

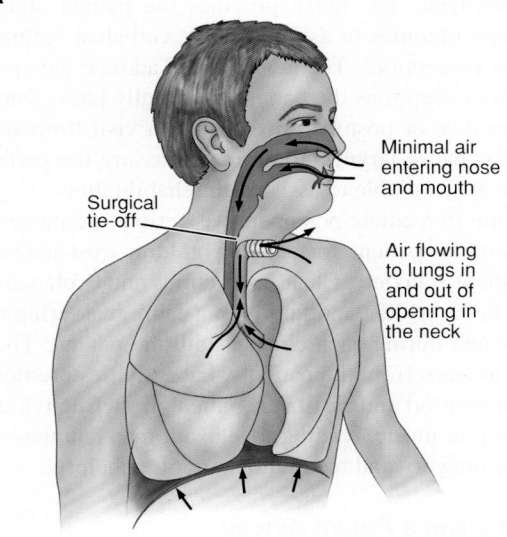

FIGURE 9-4 Total laryngectomy produces a change in airflow for breathing and speaking. **A.** Normal airflow. **B.** Airflow after total laryngectomy.

FIGURE 9-5 Schematic representation of tracheoesophageal puncture speech (TEP). Air travels from the lung through a puncture in the posterior wall of the trachea into the esophagus and out the mouth. A voice prosthesis is fitted over the puncture site.

Radiation Therapy

The goal of radiation therapy is to eradicate the cancer and preserve the function of the larynx. The decision to use radiation therapy is based on several factors, including the staging of the tumor and the patient's overall health status, lifestyle (including occupation), and personal preference. Early-stage vocal cord tumors are treated initially with irradiation. One of the benefits of radiation therapy is that patients retain a near-normal voice. A few develop chondritis (inflammation of the cartilage) or stenosis; a small number may require laryngectomy later. Radiation therapy may also be used preoperatively to reduce the tumor size. Radiation therapy is combined with surgery in advanced laryngeal cancer as adjunctive therapy to surgery or chemotherapy and as a palliative measure.

Advances in research and treatment of these tumors with surgery, chemotherapy, and radiation therapy have improved outcomes and decreased incidence of posttreatment morbidities (DeVita et al., 2014). Complications from radiation therapy are a result of external radiation to the head and neck area, which may also include the parotid gland, which is responsible for mucus production. Symptoms may include acute mucositis, ulceration of the mucous membranes, pain, **xerostomia** (dry mouth), loss of taste, dysphasia, fatigue, and skin reactions. Complications occurring later may include laryngeal necrosis, edema, and fibrosis.

Speech Therapy

The patient who undergoes a laryngectomy faces potentially complex and frustrating communication problems. These are related to alterations in communication methods, perceived voice quality, and perceptions of quality of life related to communication, disfigurement, and socialization. To minimize anxiety and frustration for the patient and family, the nurse discusses the loss or alteration of speech with the patient and family before surgery, and the speech therapist conducts a preoperative evaluation. The nurse discusses with the patient and family those methods of communication that will be available in the immediate postoperative period. These include writing, lip speaking, and communication or word boards. A system of communication is established with the patient, family, nurse, and provider, and is implemented consistently after surgery.

In addition, a long-term postoperative communication plan for **alaryngeal communication** is developed. The three most common techniques of alaryngeal communication are esophageal speech, artificial larynx (electrolarynx), and tracheoesophageal puncture.

With esophageal speech, patients compress air into the esophagus and expel it, setting off a vibration of the pharyngeal esophageal segment. The technique can be taught once the patient begins oral feedings after surgery. The patient learns to belch and use this action to transform simple explosions of air from the esophagus to sound for speech purposes. The speech therapist continues to work with the patient to make speech intelligible. The success rate is low.

With the electrolarynx, a battery-powered apparatus projects sound into the oral cavity. When the mouth forms words (articulation), the sounds from the electrolarynx become audible words. The voice that is produced sounds mechanical, and some words may be difficult to understand. The advantage is that the patient is able to communicate with relative ease while working to become proficient at either esophageal or tracheoesophageal puncture speech.

With tracheoesophageal puncture, a valve is placed in the tracheal stoma to divert air into the esophagus and out the mouth. Once the puncture is surgically created and has healed, a voice prosthesis (Blom-Singer) is fitted over the puncture site. A speech therapist teaches the patient how to produce sounds. Moving the tongue and lips to form the sound into words produces speech. To prevent airway obstruction, the prosthesis is removed and cleaned when mucus builds up (see Fig. 9-5). This method most resembles normal speech and is easily learned.

The success of these various approaches to preserve or restore speech varies. In studies that evaluated the effectiveness of these methods, the electrolarynx was used more often than the other methods of speaking, and tracheoesophageal speech was preferred over esophageal speech (DeVita et al., 2014; Pereira da Silva, Feliciano, Vaz Freitas, Esteves, & Almeida E Sousa, 2015; Vilaseca et al., 2013).

> **⚠ Nursing Alert**
> *The ability to speak intelligibly after total laryngectomy increases with time and speech rehabilitation, although it has been reported that some patients are never able to speak intelligibly—if at all— following surgery (Singer et al., 2013).*

Nursing Management

Teaching the Patient Preoperatively

The nurse reinforces information related to diagnosis and treatment options given to the patient and family by the provider and clarifies any misconceptions. Informational materials (written and audiovisual) about the surgery are given to the patient and family for review and reinforcement. If a complete laryngectomy is planned, the patient must understand that the natural voice will be lost but that special training can provide a means for communicating. The patient needs to know that temporarily communication will be possible by writing or by using a special communication board. The patient's ability to sing, laugh, and whistle will be lost.

The nurse reviews equipment and treatments for postoperative care with the patient and family, teaches important coughing and deep-breathing exercises, and assists the patient to perform return demonstrations. The nurse clarifies the patient's role in the postoperative and rehabilitation periods.

Reducing Anxiety and Depression

Patients undergoing surgery for laryngeal cancer may have many fears. These fears may relate to the diagnosis of cancer and the possibility of permanent loss of the voice and disfigurement. The nurse provides the patient and family with opportunities to ask questions, verbalize feelings, and discuss perceptions. The nurse should address any questions and misconceptions the patient and family have. During the preoperative or postoperative period, a visit from someone who has had a laryngectomy may reassure the patient that people are available to assist with rehabilitation.

In the immediate postoperative period, the nurse spends time with the patient, focusing on building trust and reducing the patient's anxiety. Clear instructions and explanations are given to the patient and family in a calm, reassuring manner before and during each contact with the patient. The nurse seeks to learn from the patient what activities promote feelings of comfort and assists the patient in such activities (e.g., listening to music, reading). Relaxation techniques, such as guided imagery and meditation, are often helpful.

Maintaining a Patent Airway

The nurse promotes a patent airway by positioning the patient in the semi-Fowler or Fowler position after recovery from anesthesia. This position decreases surgical edema and promotes lung expansion. Observing the patient for restlessness, labored breathing, apprehension, and increased pulse rate helps to identify possible respiratory or circulatory problems. The nurse assesses the patient's lung sounds and reports changes that may indicate impending complications. Medications that depress respiration, particularly opioids, should be used cautiously. Adequate use of analgesic medications is essential for pain relief, as postoperative pain can result in shallow breathing and an ineffective cough. The nurse encourages the patient to turn, cough, and take deep breaths. If needed, suctioning may be performed to remove secretions, but the nurse must avoid disruption of suture lines. The nurse also encourages and assists the patient with early ambulation to prevent atelectasis, pneumonia, and deep vein thrombosis. Pulse oximetry is used to monitor the patient's oxygen saturation level.

If a total laryngectomy was performed, a laryngectomy tube may not be used; in others, it is used temporarily; and in many, it is used permanently. The laryngectomy tube, which is shorter than a tracheostomy tube but has a larger diameter, is the patient's only airway. The care of this tube is the same as for a tracheostomy tube (see discussion later in the chapter). If a tracheostomy tube without an inner cannula is used, humidification and suctioning of this tube are essential to prevent formation of mucous plugs.

Frequently, the patient coughs up large amounts of mucus through this opening. Because air passes directly into the trachea without being warmed and moistened by the upper respiratory mucosa, the tracheobronchial tree compensates by secreting excessive amounts of mucus. The patient will have frequent coughing episodes and may develop a brassy-sounding, mucus-producing cough. The nurse reassures the patient that these problems will diminish in time, as the tracheobronchial mucosa adapts to the altered physiology.

After the patient coughs, the tracheostomy opening must be wiped clean and clear of mucus. A simple gauze dressing, washcloth, or even paper towel (because of its size and absorbency) worn below the tracheostomy may serve as a barrier to protect the clothing from the copious mucus that the patient may expel initially.

One of the most important factors in decreasing cough, mucus production, and crusting around the stoma is adequate humidification of the environment. Mechanical humidifiers and aerosol generators (nebulizers) increase the humidity and are important for the patient's comfort. The laryngectomy tube may be removed when the stoma is well healed, within 3 to 6 weeks after surgery. The nurse teaches the patient how to clean and change the tube and remove secretions.

Wound drains, inserted during surgery, may be in place to assist in removal of fluid and air from the surgical site. Suction also may be used, but cautiously, to avoid trauma to the surgical site and incision. The nurse observes, measures, and records drainage. When drainage is less than 30 mL/day for 2 consecutive days, a member of the surgical team usually removes the drains.

Promoting Alternative Communication Methods

Establishing an effective means of communication is the primary goal in the rehabilitation of the patient with a laryngectomy. To understand and anticipate the patient's postoperative needs, the nurse works with the patient, speech therapist, and family to encourage use of alternative communication methods. These means of communication are established preoperatively and must be used consistently by all personnel who come in contact with the patient. The patient is unable to use an intercom system. A call bell or hand bell must be placed within easy reach of the patient. A reusable writing board often is used for communication so the nurse documents which hand the patient uses for writing so that the opposite arm can be used for IV infusions. To ensure the patient's privacy, the nurse discards any old notes used for communication. If the patient cannot write, a picture–word–phrase board or hand signals can be used. Writing everything or communicating through gestures can be very time-consuming and frustrating. The patient must be given adequate time to communicate his or her needs. The patient may become impatient and angry when not understood.

Promoting Adequate Nutrition and Hydration

Postoperatively, the patient may not be permitted to eat or drink for several days. Alternative sources of nutrition and hydration include IV fluids, enteral feedings through a nasogastric or gastrostomy tube, and parenteral nutrition.

When the patient is ready to start oral feedings, a speech therapist or radiologist may conduct a swallow study to evaluate the patient's risk for aspiration. Once the patient is cleared for oral feedings, the nurse explains that thick liquids will be used first because they are easy to swallow. Different swallowing maneuvers are attempted with various food consistencies. Once the patient is cleared for food intake, the nurse stays with the patient during initial oral feedings and keeps a suction setup at the bedside for needed suctioning. The nurse observes the patient for any difficulty swallowing, particularly when eating resumes, and reports its occurrence to the provider.

The nurse instructs the patient to avoid sweet foods, which increase salivation and suppress the appetite. Solid foods are introduced as tolerated. The patient is instructed to rinse the mouth with warm water or mouthwash after oral feedings and to brush the teeth frequently.

Because taste and smell are so closely related, taste sensations are altered for a while after surgery because inhaled air passes directly into the trachea, bypassing the nose and the olfactory end organs. Over time, the patient usually accommodates to this change and olfactory sensation adapts, often with return of interest in eating. The patient's weight and laboratory data are monitored to ensure that nutritional and fluid intake are adequate. Skin turgor and vital signs are assessed for signs of decreased fluid volume.

Promoting Positive Body Image and Self-Esteem

Disfiguring surgery and an altered communication pattern are a threat to a patient's body image and self-esteem. The reaction of family members and friends is a major concern for the patient. The nurse encourages the patient to express feelings about the changes brought about by surgery, particularly feelings related to fear, anger, depression, and isolation. Encouraging use of previous effective coping strategies may be helpful. Referral to a support group, such as the International Association of Laryngectomees (IAL) and I Can Cope (the American Cancer Society), may help the patient and family deal with the changes in their lives. In addition to its work through support groups, the IAL encourages an exchange of ideas and methods for teaching and learning alaryngeal methods of communication.

Promoting Self-Care

A positive approach is important when caring for the patient and includes promotion of self-care activities. The patient and family should begin participating in self-care activities as soon as possible. The nurse assesses the patient's readiness for decision-making and encourages the patient to participate actively in performing care. The nurse needs to support the patient and the family, especially when explaining the tubes, dressings, and drains that are in place postoperatively.

Monitoring and Managing Potential Complications

The potential complications after laryngectomy include respiratory distress and hypoxia, hemorrhage, infection, wound breakdown, aspiration, and tracheostomal stenosis.

Respiratory Distress and Hypoxia

The nurse monitors the patient for signs and symptoms of respiratory distress and hypoxia, particularly restlessness, irritation, agitation, confusion, tachypnea, use of accessory muscles, and decreased oxygen saturation on pulse oximetry (SpO_2). Any change in respiratory status requires immediate intervention. Hypoxia may cause restlessness and an initial rise in blood pressure; this is followed by hypotension and somnolence. Cyanosis is a late sign of hypoxia. Obstruction needs to be ruled out immediately by suctioning and by having the patient cough and breathe deeply. Hypoxia and airway obstruction, if not immediately treated, are life-threatening.

Other nursing measures include repositioning of the patient to ensure an open airway and administering oxygen as prescribed. Oxygen should be used with caution in patients with chronic obstructive pulmonary disease.

> **Nursing Alert**
> *Adequate oxygenation is important in the management of hypoxia and should never be withheld. Key in the care of patients with COPD on supplemental oxygen is monitoring and assessment, with the goal of achieving and maintaining an oxygen saturation of greater than or equal to 90%. Pulse oximetry is helpful in assessing response to therapy. The nurse considers patency of the airway, protective reflexes, inspired oxygen concentration, and respiratory drive when assessing adequacy of the airway.*

The nurse should always be prepared for possible intubation and mechanical ventilation. The nurse must be knowledgeable about the hospital's emergency code protocols and skilled in use of emergency equipment. The nurse must remain with the patient at all times during respiratory distress. The emergency call bell and telephone should be used to initiate a code, call for further assistance, and summon the provider immediately if nursing measures do not improve the patient's respiratory status.

> **Nursing Alert**
> *After a total laryngectomy, it is advisable to have a properly sized replacement laryngectomy tube and an appropriately sized replacement cuffed tracheostomy tube at the bedside should the treatment of the patient's respiratory distress require placement on a mechanical ventilator. If the patient suffers a respiratory arrest, the nurse is aware that the naso/oro pharynx is now distinct from the tracheal bronchial tree, meaning the patient CAN NOT be intubated orally. The airway must be managed via a laryngectomy tube or tracheostomy tube, allowing for rescue breathing via mouth-to-neck or bag-valve mask with supplemental oxygen delivery.*

Hemorrhage

Bleeding from the drains at the surgical site or with tracheal suctioning may signal the occurrence of hemorrhage. The nurse promptly notifies the surgeon of any active bleeding from the surgical site, drains, and trachea. Rupture of the carotid artery is especially dangerous. Should this occur, the nurse must apply direct pressure over the artery, summon assistance, and provide emotional support to the patient until the vessel is ligated. The nurse monitors vital signs for increased pulse rate, decreased blood pressure, and rapid deep respirations, as well as restlessness and delayed capillary refill. Cold, clammy, pale skin may indicate active bleeding. IV fluids and blood components may be administered and other measures implemented to prevent or treat hemorrhagic shock.

Infection

The nurse monitors the patient for signs of postoperative infection. These include an increase in temperature and pulse, a change in the type of wound drainage, and increased areas of redness or tenderness at the surgical site. Other signs include purulent drainage, odor, and increased wound drainage. The nurse monitors the patient's white blood cell (WBC) count. An elevation in WBCs (leukocytosis) may indicate the body's effort to combat infection. In elderly patients, infection can be present without an increase in the patient's WBC count. WBCs will be suppressed in the patient with decreased immune function (e.g., patients with HIV infection or those receiving chemotherapy or radiation therapy); this predisposes the patient to a severe infection and sepsis. Antimicrobial (antibiotic) medications must be administered as scheduled. All suspicious drainage is cultured, and the patient may be placed in isolation as indicated. The nurse reports any significant change in the patient's status to the surgeon.

Wound Breakdown

Wound breakdown caused by infection, poor wound healing, development of a fistula, radiation therapy, or tumor growth can create a life-threatening emergency. The carotid artery, which is close to the stoma, may rupture from erosion if the wound does not heal properly. The nurse observes the stoma area for wound breakdown, hematoma, and bleeding and reports this to the surgeon. If wound breakdown occurs, the patient must be monitored carefully and identified as being at high risk for carotid hemorrhage.

Aspiration

The patient who has undergone a laryngectomy is at risk for aspiration and aspiration pneumonia due to depressed cough, the sedating effects of anesthetic and analgesic medications, alteration in the airway, impaired swallowing, and the administration of tube feedings. The nurse assesses for the presence of nausea and administers antiemetic medications as prescribed. The nurse keeps a suction setup available in the hospital and instructs the family to do so at home for use if needed. Patients receiving tube feedings are positioned with the head of the bed at 30 degrees or higher during feedings and for 30 to 45 minutes after tube feedings. For patients with a nasogastric or gastrostomy tube, the placement of the tube must be checked before each feeding. High residual volumes may indicate delayed gastric emptying and can lead to reflux and aspiration. Risks for aspiration include a low level of consciousness, heavy sedation, low head-of-bed elevation, and vomiting. Gastric residual volumes (GRVs) have not been shown to be correlated with pneumonia, regurgitation, or aspiration (McClave et al., 2016). The American Society of Parenteral and Enteral Nutrition and the Society of Critical Care Medicine continue to suggest that GRVs of 250 to 500 mL appear to be tolerated and do not increase the risk of regurgitation, aspiration, or pneumonia (McClave et al., 2016). Because individual procedures vary widely and uncertainty exists regarding the assessment and treatment for high residual volumes, it is important to follow institutional procedures (McClave et al., 2016). Residual volumes from the small bowel are usually less than 10 mL; however, limited research is available to suggest a volume that might contribute to aspiration risk. If intestinal residual volumes are similar to GRVs, the nurse should be suspicious for dislocation of the distal portion of the intestinal tube upward into the stomach (Preiser et al., 2015). Refer to Chapter 22 for details of gastric and intestinal feedings.

Tracheostomal Stenosis

Tracheostomal stenosis is an abnormal narrowing of the trachea or the tracheostomy stoma. Infection at the stoma site, excessive traction on the tracheostomy tube by the connecting tubing, and persistent high tracheostomy cuff pressure are risk factors for tracheostomal stenosis. Cuff pressures should be below 25 cm H_2O (18 mm Hg) (Morris, Whitmer, & McIntosh, 2013). The incidence of this condition varies widely and is often preventable. The nurse assesses the patient's stoma for signs and symptoms of infection and immediately reports any evidence of this to the provider. Tracheostomy care is performed routinely. The nurse assesses the connecting tubing (e.g., ventilation tubing) and secures the tubing to avoid excessive traction on the patient's tracheostomy. The nurse ensures that, for the patient who is breathing independently (without ventilator), the tracheostomy cuff is deflated (for a patient with a cuffed tube).

Nursing Alert
An inflated tracheostomy cuff will not prevent aspiration. The decision to administer medications or food in a patient with a tracheostomy should be made as a team, which should include a formal swallowing evaluation and consideration of the patient's medical and psychological status (Morris et al., 2013).

Teaching Patients Self-Care

In preparing the patient to go home, the nurse assesses the patient's readiness to learn and the level of knowledge about self-care management. The patient will need to learn a variety of self-care behaviors, including tracheostomy and stoma care (described later in the chapter), wound care, and oral hygiene. The nurse also instructs the patient about the need for adequate dietary intake, safe hygiene, and recreational activities.

Special precautions are needed in the shower to prevent water from entering the stoma. Wearing a loose-fitting plastic bib over the tracheostomy or simply holding a hand over the opening is effective. Swimming is not recommended because a person with a laryngectomy can drown without submerging his or her face. Hair sprays, loose hair, and powder should not get near the stoma, because they can block or irritate the trachea and possibly cause infection.

The nurse teaches the patient and caregiver the signs and symptoms of infection and identifies indications that require contacting the provider after discharge. The nurse teaches the patient and family to wash their hands before and after caring for the tracheostomy, to use tissue to remove mucus, and to dispose of soiled dressings and equipment properly. If the patient's surgery included cervical lymph node dissection, the nurse teaches the patient exercises for strengthening the shoulder and neck muscles.

Recreation and exercise are important for the patient's well-being and quality of life, and all but very strenuous exercise can be enjoyed safely. Avoidance of strenuous exercise and fatigue is important because the patient will have more difficulty speaking when tired, which can be discouraging. Additional safety points to address include the need for the patient to wear or carry medical identification—such as a bracelet or card—to alert medical personnel to the special requirements for resuscitation should this need arise. If resuscitation is needed, direct mouth-to-stoma ventilation should be performed. For home emergency situations, prerecorded emergency messages for police, the fire department, or other rescue services can be kept near the phone to be used quickly.

The nurse instructs and encourages the patient to perform oral care on a regular basis to prevent halitosis and infection. Brushing the teeth or dentures and rinsing the mouth several times a day will assist in maintaining proper oral hygiene. If the patient is receiving radiation therapy, synthetic saliva may be required because of decreased saliva production. The nurse instructs the patient to drink water or sugar-free liquids throughout the day and to use a humidifier at home.

It is important that the person who has had a laryngectomy have regular physical examinations and seek advice concerning any problems related to recovery and rehabilitation. The patient is also reminded to participate in health promotion activities and health screening as well as about the importance of keeping scheduled appointments with the provider, speech therapist, and other health care providers.

ARTIFICIAL AIRWAYS

The patient with an airway disorder such as a laryngeal obstruction or cancer may require the use of a temporary or, in some cases, a permanent artificial airway. Two types of artificial airways that may be used include an endotracheal tube (ETT) or a tracheostomy tube. General recommendations are to favor a tracheostomy tube rather than ETT if the patient will be intubated for 21 days or greater, and to favor the ETT over a tracheostomy if support will be required for 10 days or less (Morris et al., 2013). To provide for adequate ventilation, mechanical ventilation may be required to ensure adequate oxygenation.

ETT and tracheostomy tubes have several disadvantages. The tubes cause discomfort, the cough reflex is depressed because closure of the glottis is hindered, and secretions tend to become thicker because the warming and humidifying effect of the upper respiratory tract has been bypassed. The swallowing reflexes are depressed because of prolonged disuse and the mechanical trauma produced by the endotracheal or tracheostomy tube, thus increasing the risk of aspiration. In addition, ulceration and stricture of the larynx or trachea may develop. Of great concern to the patient is the inability to talk and to communicate needs.

ENDOTRACHEAL INTUBATION

Endotracheal intubation is a temporary means of providing an airway for patients who cannot maintain an adequate airway on their own (e.g., comatose patients, patients with upper airway obstruction), for patients needing mechanical ventilation, and for suctioning secretions from the pulmonary tree.

FIGURE 9-6 Endotracheal tube in place. The tube has been inserted using the oral route. The cuff has been inflated to maintain the tube's position and to minimize the risk of aspiration.

 Nursing Alert
For any patient with an artificial airway, a self-inflating bag-valve mask device or Ambu bag must be at the bedside as well as suction catheters and suctions source.

Endotracheal intubation involves passing an ETT through the mouth or nose into the trachea (Fig. 9-6) with the aid of a laryngoscope or illuminated glidescope by specifically trained personnel. It is the method of choice in emergency care. Once the tube is inserted, a cuff is inflated to prevent air from leaking around the outer part of the tube, to minimize the possibility of subsequent aspiration, and to prevent movement of the tube.

The nurse should be aware that complications could occur from pressure exerted by the cuff on the wall of the trachea. Low cuff pressure can increase the risk for aspiration pneumonia. High cuff pressure can cause tracheal bleeding, ischemia, and pressure necrosis. Routine deflation of the cuff is not recommended because of the increased risk for aspiration and hypoxia. The cuff must be deflated before the ETT is removed. Tracheobronchial secretions are suctioned through the tube (see description in Tracheostomy section). Warmed, humidified oxygen should always be introduced through the tube, whether the patient is breathing spontaneously or is receiving ventilatory support. Endotracheal intubation should be used until a time when it is prudent to consider a tracheostomy to decrease oropharyngeal irritation and trauma to the tracheal lining, to reduce the incidence of vocal cord paralysis (secondary to laryngeal nerve damage), and to decrease the work of breathing.

Unintentional or premature removal of the tube is a potentially life-threatening complication of endotracheal intubation that is a frequent problem in intensive care units and occurs mainly during nursing care or by the patient.

TRACHEOSTOMY

A **tracheotomy** is a surgical procedure in which an opening is made into the trachea. The indwelling tube inserted into the trachea is called a **tracheostomy tube**. A tracheostomy may be either temporary or permanent.

A tracheostomy is used to bypass an upper airway obstruction, to allow removal of tracheobronchial secretions, to permit the long-term use of mechanical ventilation, to prevent aspiration of oral or gastric secretions in the unconscious or paralyzed patient (by closing off the trachea from the esophagus), and to replace an ETT. Many disease processes and emergency conditions make a tracheostomy necessary, including total laryngectomy.

Procedure

A surgical opening is made between the second and third tracheal rings. After the trachea is exposed, an obturator guides insertion of the cuffed tracheostomy tube by creating a pathway for the tracheostomy tube. The obturator is removed immediately after the tracheostomy tube is in place. This procedure can be done in the Operating Room or is increasingly being done percutaneously as a bedside procedure in the ICU (Morris et al., 2013). A spare tracheostomy tube (cuffed) and the obturator should be available in the room in case of accidental dislodgement of the tracheostomy tube. The cuff is inflated to occlude the space between the tracheal walls and the tube, to permit effective mechanical ventilation, and to decrease the risk of aspiration. The tracheostomy tube is held in place by twill tape or a cloth neckband with velcro band fasteners placed around the patient's neck.

Usually a square of sterile gauze is placed between the tube and the skin to absorb drainage and reduce the risk for infection (Morris et al., 2013). The nurse should refer to institutional protocols regarding tracheostomy management.

Tube Types

Types of tracheostomy tubes include (Fig. 9-7):

- *Cuffed tracheostomy tube*: This is required when placing a patient on a ventilator because the balloon prevents air from being diverted out to the upper airway (Fig. 9-7A).
- *Fenestrated tube*: This tube allows some air flow up to the larynx, which allows for vocalization (Fig. 9-7B).
- *Uncuffed (cuffless) tube*: This tube does not permit ventilator management but will allow talking if the airway is not edematous and the patient covers or "buttons" the end of the tube. This allows air to flow from the nose and mouth past the larynx and vocalization (Fig. 9-7C).

 Nursing Alert
In an emergency, if an Ambu bag or ventilator was used on a cuffless tube, then the nurse needs to understand that air will follow the path of least resistance, out the nose and mouth rather than into the lungs. Therefore, any patient who has a cuffless tracheostomy must have the exact size tracheostomy tube at the bedside with a cuff. In an

FIGURE 9-7 Tracheostomy tubes. **A.** Cuffed tracheostomy tube; used for patients on mechanical ventilation. **B.** Cuffed fenestrated tube; allows the patient to talk. **C.** Uncuffed tracheostomy tube; not used for adult patients on mechanical ventilation; often used for permanent tracheostomy patients who are not ventilator dependent.

Preventing Complications Associated with Endotracheal and Tracheostomy Tubes

- Administer adequate warmed humidity.
- Maintain cuff pressure at appropriate level.
- Suction as needed per assessment findings.
- Maintain skin integrity. Change tape and dressing as needed or per protocol.
- Auscultate lung sounds.
- Monitor for signs and symptoms of infection, including temperature and white blood cell count.
- Administer prescribed oxygen and monitor oxygen saturation.
- Monitor for cyanosis.
- Maintain adequate hydration of the patient.
- Use sterile technique when suctioning and performing tracheostomy care.

emergency, the provider will change the cuffless tube to a cuffed tube and inflate the balloon, allowing for ventilation with an Ambu bag or ventilator.

Complications

Complications may occur early or late in the course of tracheostomy tube management. Early complications include bleeding, pneumothorax, air embolism, aspiration, subcutaneous or mediastinal emphysema, recurrent laryngeal nerve damage, and posterior tracheal wall penetration. Long-term complications include airway obstruction from accumulation of secretions or protrusion of the cuff over the opening of the tube, infection, rupture of the innominate artery, dysphagia, tracheoesophageal fistula, tracheal dilation, and tracheal ischemia and necrosis. Tracheal stenosis may develop after the tube is removed. Box 9-6 provides information about preventing complications.

Nursing Management

The patient with an artificial airway requires continuous monitoring and assessment. The airway must be kept patent by proper suctioning of secretions. After the vital signs are stable, the patient is placed in a semi-Fowler position to facilitate ventilation, promote drainage, minimize edema, and prevent strain on the suture lines. Analgesia and sedative agents must be administered with caution because of the risk of suppressing the cough reflex.

Major objectives of nursing care are to alleviate the patient's apprehension, provide an effective means of communication, and prevent infection. The nurse keeps paper and pencil or a reusable writing board and the call light within the patient's reach at all times to ensure a means of communication. The care of the patient with a tracheostomy tube is summarized in Box 9-7.

For the patient with a tracheostomy tube, a Passy-Muir Valve (PMV) allows the patient to speak. The devise is a positive-closure, one-way speaking valve. The PMV opens upon inspiration to allow the patient to inspire through the tracheostomy tube and then closes after inspiration, redirecting the exhaled air around the tube, through the vocal cords, and out of the mouth. The tracheostomy cuff must be deflated completely before the PMV is placed.

GUIDELINES FOR NURSING CARE

Providing Care for a Patient with a Tracheostomy Tube

Equipment

- Sterile gloves
- Goggles, mask, or face shield
- Sterile cotton-tipped applicators
- Disposable inner cannula, size for patient
- Sterile dressing
- Twill tape or commercially prepared tracheostomy holder
- Normal saline solution or sterile water

Implementation

ACTIONS	RATIONALE
1. Gather the needed equipment.	1. Everything needed to care for a tracheostomy should be readily on hand for the most effective care.
2. Provide patient and family instruction on the key points for tracheostomy care; inspect the tracheostomy dressing for moisture or drainage.	2. The tracheostomy dressing is changed as needed to keep the skin clean and dry. To prevent potential breakdown, moist or soiled dressings should not remain on the skin.
3. Perform hand hygiene.	3. Hand hygiene reduces bacteria on hands.
4. Explain procedure to patient and family.	4. A patient with a tracheostomy is apprehensive and requires ongoing assurance and support.
5. Put on clean gloves; remove and discard the soiled dressing in an appropriate container. Discard gloves.	5. Observing body substance isolation reduces cross-contamination from soiled dressings. Having necessary supplies and equipment readily available allows the procedure to be completed efficiently.

ACTIONS	RATIONALE
6. Prepare sterile supplies, including normal saline solution or sterile water, cotton-tipped applicators, dressing, and tape.	6. Sterile equipment minimizes transmission of surface flora to the sterile respiratory tract.
7. Put on sterile gloves. (Some providers approve clean technique for long-term tracheostomy patients in the home.)	7. Clean technique may be used in the home because of decreased exposure to potential pathogens.
8. Cleanse the wound and the plate of the tracheostomy tube with sterile cotton-tipped applicators moistened with sterile saline solution.	8. Rinsing prevents retention of residue.
9. Soak inner cannula in peroxide or sterile saline; rinse with saline solution; inspect to be sure all dried secretions have been removed. Dry and reinsert inner cannula or replace with a new disposable inner cannula.	9. Soaking loosens and removes secretions from the inner lumen of the tracheostomy tube. Retained secretions could harbor bacteria, leading to infection. Some plastic tracheostomy tubes may be damaged by using peroxide.
10. Place clean twill tape in position to secure the tracheostomy tube by inserting one end of the tape through the side opening of the outer cannula. Take the tape around the back of the patient's neck and thread it through the opposite opening of the outer cannula. Bring both ends around, so that they meet on one side of the neck. Tighten the tape until only two fingers can be inserted comfortably under it. Secure with a knot. **For a new tracheostomy, two people should assist with tape changes.** Remove soiled twill tape after the new tape is in place. In place of twill tape, a commercially prepared tracheostomy tube holder may be used.	10. This taping technique provides a double thickness of tape around the neck, which is needed because the tracheostomy tube can be dislodged by movement or by a forceful cough if left unsecured. However, it cannot be so tight that it causes constriction of the jugular vein. Therefore, changing ties should always be a two-person task. A dislodged tracheostomy tube is difficult to reinsert, and respiratory distress may occur. Dislodgement of a new tracheostomy is a medical emergency.
11. Remove old tapes and discard in a waste container after the new tape is in place.	11. Tapes with old secretions may harbor bacteria.
12. Although some long-term tracheostomies with healed stomas may not require a dressing, other tracheostomies do. Use a sterile tracheostomy dressing, fitting it securely under the twill tape and flange of tracheostomy tube, so that the incision is covered, as shown below. A sterile pre-cut "drain" sponge may be available also.	12. Healed tracheostomies with minimal secretions do not need a dressing. Dressings that will shred are not used around a tracheostomy because of the risk that pieces of material, lint, or thread may get into the tube and eventually into the trachea, causing obstruction or abscess formation.
13. Dispose of all used equipment in waste receptacle, remove and discard gloves, and perform hand hygiene.	13. Disposing of all used equipment, cleaning agents, and gloves prevents the spread of contaminants/bacteria. Performing hand hygiene prevents the spread of infection.

A   B   C

(**A**) The cuff of the tracheostomy tube fits smoothly and snugly in the trachea in a way that promotes circulation but seals off the escape of secretions and air surrounding the tube. (**B**) For a dressing change, a specially designed drain sponge or a 4 × 4-in gauze pad may be folded (cutting would promote shredding, placing the patient at risk for aspiration) around the tracheostomy tube and (**C**) stabilized by slipping the neck tape ties through the neck plate slots of the tracheostomy tube. The ties may be fastened to the side of the neck to eliminate the discomfort of lying on the knot.

Suctioning the Tracheal Tube (Tracheostomy or Endotracheal Tube)

When a tracheostomy or ETT is in place, it is necessary to suction the patient's secretions because of the decreased effectiveness of the cough mechanism. Tracheal suctioning is performed when adventitious breath sounds are detected or whenever secretions are obviously present. Unnecessary suctioning can initiate bronchospasm and cause mechanical trauma to the tracheal mucosa.

All equipment that comes into direct contact with the patient's lower airway must be sterile to prevent pulmonary and systemic infections. The procedure for suctioning a tracheostomy is presented in Box 9-8. Recent research analysis suggests using minimally invasive endotracheal

suctioning, in which the suction catheter is inserted to the length of the ETT or tracheostomy tube only. The suction catheter is inserted to the carina and then retracted 1 to 2 cm before suctioning is performed; an alternative option is to measure the length of the suction catheter estimated by measuring an identical ETT (Maggiore et al., 2013; Morris et al., 2013; Schrieber, 2015). However, deep suctioning may be necessary in patients with large amounts of secretions in the lower airways, since minimally invasive suctioning removes secretions from central airways only. Deep suctioning may lead to episodes of bradycardia. As research data are analyzed, best practice related to suctioning practices will be established.

In mechanically ventilated patients, an inline suction catheter may be used to allow rapid suction when needed

---

BOX 9-8

GUIDELINES FOR NURSING CARE

Performing Tracheal Suction

Equipment

- Suction catheters, may be available in a commercially prepared kit
- Gloves (sterile and nonsterile), mask, and goggles. Additional PPE as required.

- Basin for sterile normal saline solution for irrigation
- Manual resuscitation bag with supplemental oxygen
- Portable or wall suction unit with tubing

Implementation

ACTIONS	RATIONALE
1. Explain the procedure to the patient before beginning and offer reassurance during suctioning. Unless contraindicated, elevate the head of the patient's bed; semi-Fowler position is preferred.	1. Patients are apprehensive and require ongoing assurance and support. Elevation of bed maximizes diaphragmatic excursion.
2. Perform hand hygiene. Put on nonsterile gloves, goggles, gown, and mask.	2. Hand hygiene reduces transmission of microorganisms and body secretions; donning PPE follows standard precautions.
3. Secure the end of the suction tubing to the suction device. Place the open end within reach in preparation for connecting to the suction catheter. Turn on suction source (pressure should not exceed 150 mm Hg).	3. High vacuum pressures are associated with mucosal injury.
4. To perform open-suction technique: Open-suction catheter kit on a clean surface, using the inside of the wrapping as a sterile field. Suction catheter should be less than half of the internal lumen of the endotracheal tube or tracheostomy.	4. If the catheter is too small, it will not adequately remove secretions, and if it is too large, it will obstruct airflow around the catheter during insertion. To calculate the catheter size needed, note the interior diameter (ID) of the tracheostomy tube, divide by two, and then multiply by three to obtain the French size. For example, a size 8 tracheostomy tube would accommodate a 12-French suction catheter.
Set up a sterile solution container. Fill basin with approximately 100 mL of sterile normal saline or water. Be careful not to touch the inside of the container. Don sterile gloves.	This maintains sterility and follows standard precautions.
Pick up suction catheter; avoid touching nonsterile surfaces. With the nondominant hand, pick up the connecting tubing. Secure the suction catheter to the suction tubing.	This maintains catheter security. The dominant hand should not come in contact with the connecting tubing. Wrapping the sterile catheter around the sterile dominant hand helps to prevent inadvertent contamination of the catheter.

ACTIONS	RATIONALE
Check equipment for proper functioning by suctioning a small amount of sterile saline solution from the container. To perform closed-suction technique: Connect the suction tubing to the closed system suction port, according to the manufacturer's guidelines. The sterile suction catheter is in a clear plastic sleeve (see illustration). This system allows the patient to remain connected to the ventilator during suctioning.	Ensures equipment function.

A   B

T-piece

Suction catheter

Catheter sleeve

Closed airway suction system. **(A)** Closed tracheal suction system. **(B)** Closed system connected by a T-piece to the endotracheal tube and ventilator.

5. Follow institution guidelines related to hyperoxygenating the patient's lungs before suctioning. In general, for the nonventilator-dependent patient, humidified oxygen via a tracheostomy mask is placed over the tracheostomy for several deep breaths before suctioning, or if on a ventilator, preoxygenate the patient with 100% oxygen for at least 30 seconds prior to and after suctioning. OR Increase the baseline faction of inspired oxygen (FIO$_2$) level on the mechanical ventilator. Disconnect the ventilator or gas delivery tubing from the end of the endotracheal or tracheostomy tube, attach the manual resuscitation bag (MRB) to the tube with the nondominant hand, and administer five to six breaths. Attach a PEEP valve to the MRB for patients on more than 5 cm H$_2$O PEEP (refer to Chapter 55). Verify 100% oxygen delivery capabilities of MRB.	5. Routine use of hyperinflation is not recommended due to the risk of barotrauma (damage to the lung from rapid or excessive pressure changes) from large volumes, high peak pressures, and patient discomfort. Hyperoxygenation with 100% oxygen is used to prevent a decrease in arterial oxygen levels during the suctioning procedures. Press the suction hyperoxygenation button on the ventilator with the nondominant hand. Using this added valve increases the amount of air left in the lungs at the end of exhalation, increasing functional residual capacity.

(continued on page 288)

BOX 9-8   GUIDELINES FOR NURSING CARE (*continued*)

Performing Tracheal Suction (*continued*)

ACTIONS	RATIONALE
6. With the suction off, gently and quickly insert the catheter with the dominant hand into the artificial airway to the extent of the tracheostomy or ETT (not to pass beyond the tip of the tubes), which can be measured. Other researchers suggest passing the catheter to the carina (strong cough reflex or where resistance is felt), then pull back 1–2 cm before suctioning is performed; this is termed *minimally invasive suctioning*. Deeper suctioning may be necessary in patients with large amounts of secretions in the lower airways since minimally invasive suctioning removes secretions from central airways only.	6. Suction should be applied only as needed to remove secretions and for as short a time as possible to minimize decreases in arterial oxygen levels.
7. Place the nondominant thumb over the control vent of the suction catheter and apply continuous or intermittent suction. Rotate the catheter 360 degrees between the dominant thumb and forefinger as you withdraw the catheter in the sterile catheter sleeve (closed-suction technique) or out of the open airway (open-suction technique). The suctioning procedure should take no more than 15 seconds, waiting at least 1 minute between suctioning events.	7. Tracheal damage from suctioning is similar with intermittent or continuous suction. Decreases in arterial oxygen levels during suctioning can be kept to a minimum with brief suction periods.
8. After suctioning, hyperoxgenate the patient for at least 1 minute as described earlier. Inflate the patient's lungs for several breaths. Assess oxygen saturation and evidence of bradycardia and arrhythmias (particularly if deep suctioning was required).	8. Arterial oxygen desaturation and cardiopulmonary complications increase with each successive pass.
9. Repeat steps until the airway is clear.	
10. Rinse catheter by suctioning a few milliliters of sterile saline solution from the basin between suction attempts.	10. Removes the buildup of secretions in the connecting tubing and/or the inline suction catheter.
11. When the lower airway has been adequately cleared of secretions, suction the nasal or oropharyngeal cavity.	11. Prevents contamination of the lower airways with upper airway organisms.
12. Rinse suction tubing.	12. Removes contaminates from tubing
13. Discard catheter, gloves, and basin appropriately. If using the open-suction technique, wrap the catheter around the dominant hand. Pull glove off inside out. Catheter remains in the glove. Pull other glove off in the same manner. Discard both gloves, and turn off suction device.	13. Reduces transmission of microorganisms. Solutions and catheters that come in direct contact with the lower airways during suctioning must be kept sterile to decrease the risk of nosocomial pneumonia.
14. Perform hand hygiene.	

and to minimize cross-contamination by airborne pathogens. An inline suction device allows the patient to be suctioned without being disconnected from the ventilator circuit.

Nursing Alert

Evidence-based research reveals that the routine instillation of normal saline prior to endotracheal suctioning increases the risk of infections and patient discomfort, and therefore is not recommended. Research indicates no evidence to support the claims of improving secretion clearance (Caparros & Forbes, 2015; Dawson, 2014).

Managing the Cuff

For the patient being supported with a mechanical ventilator, the cuff on the endotracheal or tracheostomy tube must be inflated. The pressure within the cuff should be the lowest possible pressure that allows delivery of adequate tidal volumes. Cuff pressure must be monitored at least every 8 hours by attaching a handheld pressure gauge to the pilot balloon of the tube or by using the minimal leak volume or minimal occlusion volume technique. Usually the pressure is maintained at less than 25 cm H_2O to prevent injury; when cuff pressure exceeds capillary perfusion pressure, necrosis of the tracheal wall, ischemia and stenosis can occur.

CHAPTER REVIEW

Critical Thinking Exercises

1. A 55-year-old woman is brought to the emergency department by her husband, who tells you that her nose has been bleeding for more than 3 hours. The patient reports that she takes one aspirin a day (325 mg), has a history of atrial fibrillation, and takes medication for hypertension. What immediate action would you take to care for this patient? What are the risk factors for epistaxis in this patient? What medical treatment would you anticipate for her? What nursing measures would you provide for this patient? How would you modify your discharge instructions if the patient lived alone? What strategies would you recommend to the patient and her husband to stop a nosebleed if it occurs again at home? What is the evidence for your recommendations? How will you determine the strength of the evidence on which your recommendations are based?

2. You are caring for a 78-year-old patient on a medical-surgical nursing unit. He has recently been diagnosed with cancer of the larynx and is scheduled for a total laryngectomy in the morning. What patient education is needed before this patient's surgery? Discuss nursing management of the patient's airway in the immediate postoperative period. What critical elements would you include in teaching the patient how to care for his tracheostomy? What community resources would you provide or arrange for this patient once he is discharged? What modifications in teaching and care would be necessary if this man had one-sided weakness secondary to an earlier stroke?

3. A 65-year-old man is referred for home care after a total laryngectomy performed to treat cancer of the larynx. As the home health nurse, you are responsible for providing continued patient education regarding tracheostomy care and gastric tube feedings. The overall plan is for the patient to begin oral feedings; however, both the patient and his wife believe that he is not ready to begin to eat. What are your priorities in terms of assessment of this patient? What are your recommendations to the patient regarding fear, anxiety, communication, and nutrition? What additional medical and support services will the patient need to assist him in his recovery? How would your care differ if this patient lived alone?

NCLEX-Style Review Questions

1. The nurse is providing preoperative teaching for the patient who is to undergo a total laryngectomy. Which nursing intervention is most important?
   a. Having the patient restrict food and fluids
   b. Teaching the care required for the tracheostomy tube
   c. Assessing the patient's ability to communicate postoperatively
   d. Demonstrating cough and deep-breathing exercises

2. A patient who has just had a total laryngectomy for cancer is being discharged. Which statement indicates the patient needs further teaching on care of the tracheostomy?
   a. "I must avoid getting any objects in the stoma."
   b. "I can take a shower when I get home."
   c. "I can learn to speak with an electric larynx."
   d. "I need to clean around the stoma every day."

3. Which statement indicates further teaching is required for the patient diagnosed with obstructive sleep apnea (OSA)?
   a. "The CPAP machine will help me be more awake during the day."
   b. "If I exercise and lose weight, I may not need to use CPAP."
   c. "I will use the CPAP machine only when I really need to sleep well."
   d. "The CPAP helps to keep my airway open when I sleep."

4. The nurse assesses the patient with acute pharyngitis for what signs and symptoms that indicate a complication of GAS pharyngitis?
   a. Pain and spasm of the lower leg muscles
   b. Gross hematuria, edema, and hypertension
   c. Reduced visual fields, blurred vision
   d. Insomnia, heartburn, and abdominal distension

5. A patient will be going home with a tracheal stoma. What information does the nurse include in the discharge teaching for this patient?
   a. Water sports are permitted.
   b. Wear a medical identification bracelet.
   c. Mouth-to-mouth ventilation should be performed in an emergency.
   d. Fifteen minutes of strenuous exercise will improve overall strength.

Try these additional resources, available at **http://thepoint.lww.com/Honan2e**, to enhance your learning and understanding of this chapter:

- NCLEX-Style Student Review Questions
- Journal Articles

REFERENCES AND SELECTED READINGS

References and selected readings associated with this chapter can be found on the website that accompanies the book. Visit **http://thepoint.lww.com/Honan2e** to access the references and other additional resources associated with this chapter.

Nursing Management: Patients with Chest and Lower Respiratory Tract Disorders

Laura Kierol Andrews

Learning Objectives

After reading this chapter, you will be able to:

1. Identify patients at risk for atelectasis and describe nursing interventions related to its prevention and management.
2. Compare the various pulmonary infections with regard to causes, clinical manifestations, nursing management, complications, and prevention.
3. Use the nursing process as a framework for care of the patient with pneumonia.
4. Describe the nursing management for patients receiving oxygen therapy, mini-nebulizer therapy, incentive spirometry, chest physiotherapy, and breathing retraining.
5. Relate pleurisy, pleural effusion, and empyema to pulmonary infection.
6. Relate the therapeutic management techniques of acute respiratory distress syndrome (ARDS) to the underlying pathophysiology of the syndrome.
7. Describe risk factors and measures appropriate for prevention and management of pulmonary embolism (PE).
8. Describe risk factors for the development of occupational lung disease.
9. Discuss the modes of therapy and related nursing management for patients with lung cancer.
10. Describe the complications of chest trauma and their clinical manifestations and nursing management.
11. Describe nursing measures to prevent aspiration.
12. Explain the principles of chest drainage and the nursing responsibilities related to the care of the patient with a chest drainage system.

It is common for patients in medical and surgical areas to have lower respiratory tract conditions. The care of these patients requires judicious assessment and management skills as these conditions are often serious and life-threatening and have a significant impact on activities of daily living and quality of life.

ATELECTASIS

Atelectasis is the collapse of alveoli, leading to the loss of lung volume. It is classified by its cause (absorptive, obstructive, or compressive) and can affect subsegmental, segmental, lobar, or whole lung areas. The diagnosis of atelectasis is based on both clinical and radiologic findings.

Pathophysiology

Absorptive atelectasis occurs by surfactant inactivation or when less than normal levels of inhaled nitrogen (*nitrogen wash-out*) are present in the alveoli. The most common condition that causes an inactivation of surfactant is acute respiratory distress syndrome (ARDS), in which pulmonary edema fluid dilutes and/or reduces surfactant production. The loss of surfactant causes a reduction in alveoli surface tension and leads to their collapse. Nitrogen wash-out is a condition that occurs when high levels of inhaled oxygen (FiO_2 greater than 60%) lessen the amount of nitrogen gas needed to stent open alveoli. In addition, the use of some general anesthetics can cause an absorptive atelectasis.

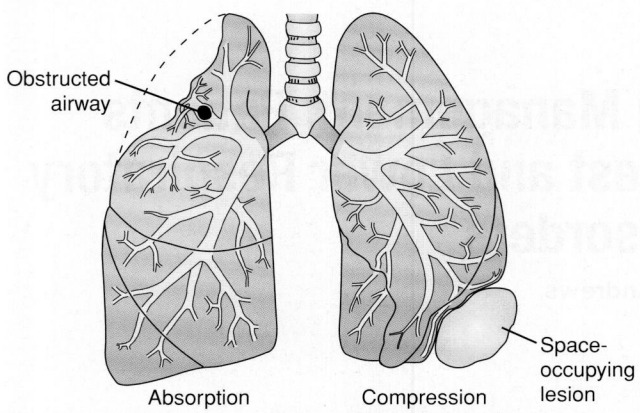

FIGURE 10-1 Atelectasis caused by airway obstruction and absorption of air from the involved lung area (*left*) and by compression of the lung tissue (*right*). (From Grossman, S., & Porth, C. M. (2014). *Pathophysiology: Concepts of altered health states* (9th ed.). Philadelphia, PA: Lippincott Williams & Wilkins.)

Compressive atelectasis occurs as a result of external forces compressing pleural and/or lung tissues. Common causes of this type of atelectasis are pleural effusions, lung tumors, pneumothoraces (air in the pleural space), hemothoraces (blood in the pleural space), and abdominal distention.

Obstructive atelectasis occurs when there is a mechanical obstruction of airways (secretions, mucous plugs, airway tumors, peribronchial lymph node enlargement, foreign bodies) or from low-tidal-volume breathing (which results in hypoventilation of alveoli and then absorption of alveolar gases), causing lung tissue collapse (Fig. 10-1).

Each type of atelectasis can cause a mismatching of lung ventilation in relation to perfusion that results in deoxygenated blood reaching systemic circulation and lowering oxygen supply to tissues. The most common cause of atelectasis is the obstruction of airways by secretions, mucus, foreign bodies, bronchial tumors, and oxygen toxicity.

Risk Factors

Postoperative patients, especially those who undergo abdominal and/or thoracic procedures, are at risk to develop atelectasis due to anesthetic- and/or narcotic-induced hypoventilation, incisional pain, abdominal distention, and immobility, all of which impair the ability to breathe deeply (expand lung volume) and cough (expel secretions). Additional risk factors for developing atelectasis include chronic lung disease, morbid obesity, tobacco use, anesthesia time greater than 4 hours, prior cerebrovascular accident (CVA), lung cancer, pleural effusions, and nasogastric tube placement.

Clinical Manifestations and Assessment

Signs and symptoms include dyspnea, cough, leukocytosis, diminished breath sounds, and sputum production. Fever is often cited as a clinical sign of atelectasis, but there is no correlation between the severity of atelectasis on chest radiology and the presence of fever. However, atelectasis should be suspected in postoperative patients with low-grade temperature (O'Donnell, 2016). Physical examination findings relate to the severity of collapse. For a small atelectatic area, findings include crackles, decreased breath sounds, and decreased tactile fremitus over the affected lung area(s). For a large atelectatic area, findings include tracheal deviation toward the atelectatic area, decreased fremitus, bronchial breath sounds, egophony (secondary to lobar or lung collapse), and asymmetry of the chest.

If obstruction by an airway tumor or foreign body is the cause, wheezing and stridor can occur. Patients with acute atelectasis or atelectasis involving large areas, such as segments, lobes, or whole lung areas, can develop significant respiratory distress manifested by dyspnea, tachycardia, tachypnea, anxiety, restlessness, pleural pain, and hypoxemia. They may also have paroxysmal breathing, retractions, and use of accessory muscles. Chronic atelectasis has manifestations similar to those of acute atelectasis, and chronic patients are at risk of developing a postobstructive pneumonia.

Atelectasis is diagnosed by radiologic studies such as chest x-ray, computed tomography (CT) scanning, or ultrasound. Radiologic findings of atelectasis may reveal opacity or patchy infiltrates underlying the affected tissue. Larger areas of collapse can reveal shifting of the heart border, hilar vessels, and hemidiaphragm toward the affected sections. Ultrasound can detect several lung pathologies, is portable, and does not expose patients to radiation (Dietrich et al., 2015).

Hypoxemia can be detected by arterial blood gas (ABG) analysis, which shows a decreased PaO_2 and oxygen saturation. Noninvasive pulse oximetry (POX) can be used to detect hypoxemia (SpO_2 less than 90%), but ABGs are the gold standard.

Medical and Nursing Management

The prevention of atelectasis is the primary management goal in at-risk patients (Box 10-1). Patients need to be educated and able to perform maneuvers that can improve ventilation and remove secretions. Immobile patients should be turned frequently, and all patients should be ambulated as soon as possible to improve lung expansion and mobilization of secretions. Lung volume expansion maneuvers, such as controlled deep breathing, coughing exercises, and use of incentive spirometry (IS), should be initiated early in the postoperative period. Patients who have asthma, chronic obstructive pulmonary disease (COPD), lung cancer, and thoracic or abdominal surgeries are at very high risk for developing atelectasis. These patients require additional interventions to prevent atelectasis. The use of aerosolized (nebulized) bronchodilators and/or mucolytics, followed by chest physiotherapy (CPT) (chest percussion and postural drainage), may be instituted.

BOX 10-1
Health Promotion

Preventing Atelectasis

- Change patient's position frequently, especially from supine to upright position, to promote ventilation and prevent secretions from accumulating.
- Encourage early mobilization from bed to chair, followed by early ambulation.
- Encourage appropriate deep breathing and coughing to mobilize secretions and prevent them from accumulating.
- Teach/reinforce appropriate technique for incentive spirometry.
- Administer prescribed opioids and sedatives judiciously to prevent respiratory depression.
- Perform postural drainage and chest percussion, if indicated.
- Institute suctioning to remove tracheobronchial secretions, if indicated.

BOX 10-2
Patient Education

Using an Incentive Spirometer

The inhalation of air, in a slow and controlled manner, helps inflate the lungs. The marker within the spirometer will measure the depth of each breath.

- Assume an upright position if possible (sitting or semi-Fowler's).
- Breathe using your diaphragm.
- Place mouthpiece firmly in the mouth, to breathe in **deeply and slowly**, holding each breath in for 3–4 seconds and exhaling slowly.
- Repeat 6–10 times per session.
- Use spirometer every hour while awake (keep it within reach).
- Try coughing, with splinting of incision, after each use.

Incentive Spirometry

Incentive spirometry (IS) is a method of deep breathing that provides visual feedback to encourage the patient to inhale slowly and deeply via a handheld spirometer. This prevents or reduces atelectasis by stimulating alveolar cells to secrete surfactant, which decreases the surface tension in the alveoli and improves inspiratory muscle performance. The use of IS is discussed in Box 10-2.

> ### Nursing Alert
> *Surfactant, which decreases the surface tension in the alveoli, thus reducing their risk of collapse, needs to be replaced continuously. One stimulus for replacement is maximum deep inhalation that is sustained for a few seconds. Adults sigh or deep breath at one and a half to two times their normal tidal volume (~500 mL) six to eight times every hour. Any etiology that results in monotonous hypoventilation will lead to atelectasis. IS encourages the patient to sigh or deep breath. The IS is typically graduated to 1.5 L and allows the user to see the depth of their breath by the rise of the three balls inside. Coughing is a forced expiratory maneuver that can "squeeze" alveoli. If coughing is needed to expel secretions, the nurse should follow the coughing maneuvers with the use of IS to re-expand the alveoli and encourage surfactant replacement. Assisting a patient to splint incisions will help improve the efficacy of coughing.*

Nebulizer Therapy

Nebulizer therapy dispenses aerosolized medications to a patient's lungs via handheld or face mask devices. The medication is inhaled with a flow of compressed air or oxygen, producing a visible mist. The patient breaths through the mouth, taking slow, deep breaths, and then holds the breath for a few seconds. The patient is encouraged to cough during the treatment, which assists in increasing intrathoracic pressure and promoting secretion expectoration. Antibiotics, bronchodilators, and mucolytic medications can be nebulized.

Chest Physiotherapy

Chest physiotherapy (CPT), with or without nebulizer medications, also can be used to prevent or treat atelectasis, bronchial obstructions, and pneumonias. CPT includes **postural drainage**, **chest percussion**, vibration, and breathing retraining. The goals of CPT are to remove bronchial secretions, improve ventilation, and increase the efficiency of the respiratory muscles. In addition, teaching the patient effective coughing technique is an important part of CPT.

Postural drainage uses specific positions that allow gravity to aid in the removal of pulmonary secretions. Patients who lie supine will have secretions accumulate in the posterior lung sections, whereas upright patients will pool secretions in their lower lobes. By having the patient change positions (Fig. 10-2), secretions can drain from the affected bronchioles into the bronchi and trachea and then be removed by coughing or suctioning. Postural drainage is usually performed two to four times daily, prior to meals (to prevent nausea, vomiting, or aspiration) and at bedtime. Prescribed nebulizer therapy should be given prior to postural drainage to dilate the bronchioles, reduce bronchospasm, and thin secretions. The patient is instructed to remain in each position for 10 to 15 minutes, inhaling slowly through the nose and exhaling slowly through pursed lips. If the patient cannot tolerate a position, the nurse modifies it for comfort. When changing positions, the patient should be instructed to deep breath and cough out secretions, or the nurse may have to suction if the patient is unable to cough.

Lower lobes, anterior basal segments

Upper lobes, anterior segments

Lower lobes, lateral basal segments

Upper lobes, apical segments

Lower lobes, superior segments

Upper lobes, posterior segments

FIGURE 10-2   Positions used in lung drainage.

FIGURE 10-3 Percussion and vibration. **A.** Proper hand position for vibration. **B.** Proper technique for vibration. The wrists and elbows remain stiff; the vibrating motion is produced by the shoulder muscles. **C.** Proper hand position for percussion.

Chest percussion and vibration can be used in each position to loosen secretions (Fig. 10-3). Percussion is performed by the nurse or respiratory therapist by rapidly "clapping" their cupped hands over the affected lung lobe. This is done for 1 to 2 minutes in each postural area. Commercial percussion vests and beds are also available for use. Vibration is performed either manually or with a mechanical device. The nurse places his or her hands over the affected area and rapidly contracts the arms and shoulders while the patient exhales. This maneuver is done for 5 to 10 breaths over each lung area.

Other Treatments

If the cause of atelectasis is bronchial obstruction from secretions, the secretions must be removed by forceful coughing or suctioning to allow air to reenter that portion of the lung. Mucolytic agents such as acetylcysteine (Mucomyst) or dornase alfa (Pulmozyme) can be added to loosen and thin tenacious mucus. If intensive pulmonary toilet maneuvers and nebulizers fail to remove the obstructive mucus, a bronchoscopy can be performed. A bronchoscopy can also be used to remove foreign bodies from airways. Patients with airways tumors also may undergo biopsy for diagnostic purposes, cryotherapy (cold therapy), or laser therapy via bronchoscopy. Additional therapies for these patients include airway stents or radiation and chemotherapy.

If the cause of atelectasis is compression of lung tissue, the goal is to decrease or remove the compression. Large pleural effusions that collapse lung tissue can be removed by **thoracentesis** (removal of fluid by needle aspiration) or chest tube insertion (thoracostomy). A **hemothorax** or **pneumothorax** usually is treated by inserting a chest tube to drain the blood or air that is collapsing the lung. No matter what the cause of atelectasis, in patients with significant hypoxemia, intubation and mechanical ventilation with

positive end-expiratory pressure (PEEP) may be necessary to provide adequate ventilation and oxygenation.

Complications

Usually mild atelectasis can be managed with lung expansion maneuvers, CPT, and mobilization of the patient, but in some cases patients can develop severe hypoxia, respiratory distress, or pneumonia. Mortality is highest in patients who require intubation and mechanical intubation, especially for more than 48 hours. Complications also can occur from treatments used to treat atelectasis, such as bronchoscopy, thoracentesis, and thoracostomy, all of which place the patient at risk for infection, bleeding, and pneumothorax.

RESPIRATORY INFECTIONS

PNEUMONIA

Pneumonia is the infection of the lower respiratory tract caused by a variety of microorganisms, including bacteria, viruses, fungi, protozoa, and parasites. Pneumonia is common, affecting 1% of the population. Pneumonia causes more than 1.25 million hospitalizations annually and is associated with considerable mortality and morbidity (Mandell et al., 2007; Musher, 2016). It is the most common infectious cause of death and the eighth leading cause of death in the United States (Centers for Disease Control and Prevention [CDC], 2016c).

Classifications

Pneumonia may be classified in a wide variety of ways, including by its microbiologic cause, host condition, and host setting. Currently, the most common classifications for pneumonia are community-acquired pneumonia (CAP), hospital-acquired (**nosocomial**) pneumonia (HAP), ventilator-associated pneumonia (VAP), health care–associated pneumonia (HCAP), and pneumonia in an immunocompromised patient.

Community-Acquired Pneumonia

CAP occurs either in the community-dwelling person or within the first 48 hours after hospitalization or institutionalization. Most cases of CAP occur in the winter and early spring months, and prevalence rates are higher in men and in African Americans. Each year approximately 12% to 57% of CAP patients require hospitalization; these patients have a mortality rate of 1% to 36% (Lee et al., 2014; McLaughlin, Johnson, Kagan, & Baer, 2015). The need for hospitalization for CAP depends on the severity of the pneumonia, which is assessed by factors such as

- altered mental status,
- azotemia (higher than normal blood levels of urea or other nitrogen-containing compounds),
- respiratory rate greater than or equal to 30 breaths per minute (BPM),
- low blood pressure (BP) (systolic BP less than 90 or diastolic BP less than 60),
- tachycardia (HR greater than 125 bpm),
- high fever (temperature greater than 104°F) or afebrile,
- age of 65 years or older, arterial pH <7.35, and
- poor oxygenation (PaO_2 less than 70 mm Hg if less than 50 years old, PaO_2 less than 60 mm Hg if over 50 years old), or an inability to reliably take medications (Ferri, 2016; Musher, 2016).

In addition, people of advanced age with at least one comorbid disorder are at higher risk for needing hospitalization (Lee et al., 2014). The most common causative microbe of CAP is the gram-positive *Streptococcus pneumoniae* (pneumococcus); however, that causative agent is identified definitively in less than 30% of CAP cases. Other causative agents are *Haemophilus influenzae, Staphylococcus aureus, Legionella* spp., and viruses.

Hospital-Acquired and Ventilator-Associated Pneumonia

HAP is defined as the onset of pneumonia symptoms more than 48 hours after admission in patients who had no evidence of infection at the time of hospitalization. HAP is the second most common nosocomial infection but carries the highest mortality rate (33% to 50%). VAP is a type of HAP that is associated with **endotracheal intubation** and mechanical ventilation; it is defined as pneumonia that develops in patients who have been receiving mechanical ventilation for at least 48 hours (Montravers, Harpan, & Guivarch, 2016). It is reported that HAP accounts for 25% of intensive care unit infections and causes increased length of stay, leading to greater costs of care (Musher, 2016). VAP carries a

mortality rate of 20% to 50%, and can be even higher when lung infection is caused by high-risk pathogens (Chastre & Luyt, 2016).

HAP occurs when at least one of three conditions exists: host defenses are impaired, microorganisms reach the lower respiratory tract (usually by microaspiration of oropharyngeal microorganisms), or a highly virulent organism is present. Certain factors may predispose patients to HAP because of impaired host defenses (e.g., severe acute or chronic illness), a variety of comorbid conditions, supine positioning, aspiration, altered mental status, malnutrition, prolonged hospitalization, hypotension, and metabolic disorders. Hospitalized patients are also exposed to potential bacteria from other sources (e.g., transmission of pathogens from health care workers' hands, respiratory devices, and water reservoirs that are contaminated). Numerous intervention-related factors also may play a role in the development of HAP (e.g., therapeutic agents that cause central nervous system [CNS] depression with hypoventilation, endotracheal intubation, or inappropriate use of antibiotics). Alterations in the gastric pH due to illness and medications can disrupt the stomach lining, exposing patients to enteric bacteria. The mortality of HAP is related to the virulence of the organisms, their resistance to antibiotics, and the patient's underlying condition. The common organisms responsible for HAP and VAP include gram-negative bacilli and gram-positive cocci. Gram-negative organisms include *Pseudomonas aeruginosa, Escherichia coli, Klebsiella pneumoniae, Acinetobacter* spp., *Serratia* spp., *Stenotrophomonas maltophilia,* and *H. influenzae.* Gram-positive organisms include *S. aureus* (MSSA and MRSA) and *Streptococcus pneumoniae.* Viruses or fungi are less common causative agents, except in the immunocompromised patient.

Health Care–Associated Pneumonia

HCAP occurs in nonhospitalized patients who have had extensive health care contact, as defined as one of the following: resident of a nursing home or other type of long-term care facility, acute care hospitalization for 2 or more days within the last 90 days, intravenous antibiotic therapy, wound care, or chemotherapy, or attended a hospital or hemodialysis clinic within the last 30 days (Barbier, Andremont, Wolff, & Bouadma, 2013; Sopena, Hera, Casas, et al., 2014). Causative microorganisms are similar to those listed for HAP and VAP.

Pneumonia in the Immunocompromised Hosts

Pneumonia in the immunocompromised hosts includes *Pneumocystis* pneumonia (PCP), fungal pneumonias, and *Mycobacterium tuberculosis.* Pneumonia in the immunocompromised hosts occurs with use of corticosteroids or other immunosuppressive agents, chemotherapy, nutritional depletion, use of broad-spectrum antimicrobial agents, acquired immune deficiency syndrome (AIDS), genetic immune disorders, and long-term life-support technology (mechanical ventilation). In addition, increasing numbers of patients with impaired defenses develop HAP from gram-negative bacilli, which poses difficulty in providing coverage. In addition, the combination of an immunocompromised patient and some gram-negative bacilli impacts the incidence of mortality.

Pneumonia in immunocompromised hosts may be caused by the organisms also observed in CAP or HAP. PCP is rarely observed in immunocompetent hosts and is often an initial AIDS-defining complication. Whether patients are immunocompromised or immunocompetent, the clinical presentation of pneumonia is similar, but PCP has a subtle onset, with progressive dyspnea, fever, and a nonproductive cough. Refer to Chapter 37 for more information about PCP and HIV.

Pathophysiology

Pneumonia can arise from several vectors: from normal flora present in patients whose resistance has been altered; aspiration of flora present in the nasopharynx or oropharynx; the inhalation of airborne microorganisms from other persons (sneezing, coughing, or talking); contaminated water sources or respiratory equipment; or blood-borne organisms that enter the pulmonary circulation (hematogenous spread) and become trapped in the pulmonary capillary beds.

Normal host defenses (cough, ciliary clearance, and alveolar macrophages) and intact upper airway defense mechanisms usually prevent potentially infectious particles from reaching the sterile lower respiratory tract.

Once the microorganisms reach the lower airways and alveoli, their presence activates an inflammatory response that begins with the migration of white blood cells (WBCs) (mainly neutrophils), plasma fluid, and immune complexes into the alveoli, filling the normally air-filled spaces with exudative liquids and cellular debris. This causes alveolar edema and lung tissue consolidation. Additional damage can occur when some microorganisms release toxins that further damage respiratory cells. Alveolar and bronchial tissues become swollen and infiltrated with WBCs, causing **consolidation** of lung tissue that can be seen on x-ray. The damage caused by toxins and inflammatory mediators and immune complexes interferes with the diffusion of oxygen and carbon dioxide, leading to clinical manifestations of the pneumonia. A mismatch between ventilation and perfusion occurs in the affected area of the lung, and poorly oxygenated blood returns from the pulmonary vasculature to the heart, resulting in arterial hypoxemia.

Risk Factors

Risk factors for pneumonia are summarized in Box 10-3. Patients with comorbid diseases such as COPD, heart failure, diabetes, and chronic liver or kidney disease have higher mortality rates than do those without comorbid diseases.

BOX 10-3 | **Risk Factors for Pneumonia**

Community-Acquired Pneumonia (CAP)
- Smoking
- Alcohol abuse
- Pre-existing hypoxemia
- Acidosis
- Toxic inhalations
- Pulmonary edema
- Altered mental status (e.g., seizure, CVA)
- Presence of comorbid conditions, including chronic respiratory (COPD, asthma) and cardiovascular diseases (HF), cerebrovascular disease, Parkinson disease, epilepsy, dementia, dysphagia, HIV, or chronic kidney or liver disease
- Malnutrition; underweight
- Immunosuppressive therapies
- Poor dental hygiene
- Age older than 65 years
- Intravenous drug abuse
- Regular contact with children
- 10 or more people living in a household
- Previous episodes of pneumonia
- Working and environmental conditions (contact with dust and sudden changes of temperature)

Hospital-Acquired Pneumonia (HAP) and Ventilator-Associated Pneumonia (VAP)
- Debilitation
- Malnutrition
- Altered mental status
- Previous exposure to antibiotics (within the last 90 days)
- Hospital stays of 5 days or longer
- High rates of antibiotic resistance (hospital or unit-specific)
- Immunosuppressive therapies or diseases
- Prolonged (greater than 48 hours) intubation or a tracheostomy
- Male gender

Health Care–Acquired Pneumonia (HCAP)
- Hospitalization for 2 or more days in the last 3 months
- Chronic dialysis within the last month
- Home wound care within 30 days
- Recent home IV therapy (antibiotic, chemotherapy)
- Resident of a skilled nursing or extended-care facility
- Family member with drug-resistant microorganism

Clinical Manifestations and Assessment

Pneumonia varies in its signs and symptoms depending on the causal organism and the presence of underlying disease; however, it is not possible to diagnose a specific type of pneumonia by clinical manifestations alone. The classic clinical manifestations of pneumonia are fever, cough (productive or nonproductive), dyspnea, and leukocytosis (elevated WBCs). Patients can also present with rigors (shaking chills), pleuritic chest pain, tachypnea, use of accessory muscles, tachycardia, fatigue, and anorexia. Some patients initially exhibit an upper respiratory tract infection (nasal congestion, sore throat), and the onset of symptoms of pneumonia is gradual and nonspecific. Then the predominant symptoms may be headache, low-grade fever, pleuritic pain, myalgia (muscle pain), rash, and pharyngitis.

Physical examinations findings may reveal bronchial breath sounds over consolidated lung areas, crackles, increased tactile fremitus (vocal vibration detected on palpation), percussion dullness, egophony, and whispered pectoriloquy (whispered sounds are easily auscultated through the chest wall). These changes occur because sound is transmitted better through solid or dense tissue (consolidation) than through normal air-filled tissue. **Purulent** sputum or slight changes in respiratory symptoms may be the only sign of pneumonia in patients with COPD. It may be difficult to determine whether an increase in symptoms is an exacerbation or an infectious process.

The diagnosis of pneumonia is made by history (particularly of a recent respiratory tract infection), physical examination, chest x-ray, blood culture (bloodstream invasion, called *bacteremia*, occurs frequently), sputum examination (Gram stain and culture), and rapid bacterial antigen testing of urine or oropharyngeal swabs. A urine test may be ordered when pneumococcal pneumonia is suspected since the enzyme-linked immunosorbent assay (ELISA) can detect pneumococcal cell wall or capsular polysaccharide in the urine of 60% to 80% of patients with bacteremic pneumococcal pneumonia (Musher, 2016). In addition, a urinary antigen test can be obtained to assess for *Legionella pneumophila* if suspected.

The sputum sample is obtained by having patients do the following: (1) rinse the mouth with water to minimize contamination by normal oral flora, (2) breathe deeply several times, (3) cough deeply, and (4) expectorate the raised sputum into a sterile container. The best time to collect the sputum culture is in the morning because the sputum is more concentrated and less likely to be contaminated with saliva and nasopharyngeal secretions. More invasive procedures may be used to collect sputum specimens (nasotracheal or orotracheal suctioning or bronchioalveolar lavage via bronchoscopy).

> ### ! Nursing Alert
> *Since timely initiation of antibiotic treatment is important, the nurse understands that a STAT sputum Gram stain may be obtained. The Gram stain will inform the provider whether the organisms are gram-positive (thick cell walls) or gram-negative (thin cell walls). Since results are available rapidly, the provider can prescribe an antibiotic with efficacy to the identified bacteria (positive, negative) and fungi (yeasts, molds), but not viruses. Thus the nurse understands the difference between empiric coverage and culture documented. Culture documented will name the specific organism and antibiotics that are sensitive or resistant to the specified organism.*

Chest x-ray findings associated with pneumonia vary depending upon microbial causes, but a new pulmonary infiltrate or consolidation is often seen within 48 hours of onset of symptoms. Infiltrates can involve segments or lobes, or be multilobar.

Unfolding Patient Stories: Kenneth Bronson • Part 1

Kenneth Bronson, a 27-year-old male, has a history of fatigue, high fever, and a productive cough for a week and arrives in the emergency department with difficulty breathing. A chest x-ray reveals a right lower lobe pneumonia. What are the clinical manifestations and assessment findings associated with a right lower lobe pneumonia that the nurse should investigate when evaluating the patient? (Kenneth Bronson's case continues in Chapter 17.)

Care for Kenneth and other patients in a realistic virtual environment: **vSim** *for Nursing* (thepoint.lww.com/vSimMedicalSurgical). Practice documenting these patients' care in (thepoint.lww.com/DocuCareEHR).

Medical and Nursing Management

Pharmacologic Therapy

The treatment of pneumonia includes administration of the appropriate antibiotic. The choice of antibiotic is determined by the classification of pneumonia (i.e., CAP vs. HAP), results of Gram stains, culture sensitivities, antigen testing, and patient's comorbid conditions. Initial treatment for CAP is empiric unless sputum culture and sensitivity results are available. Empiric therapy for non-CAP is usually initiated with a broad-spectrum IV antibiotic and may be monotherapy or combination therapy. The choice of antibiotics is based on assessment of risk of multidrug resistance (MDR) pathogens and early versus late onset of HAP or VAP symptoms (Table 10-1). Once the microbacterial cultures and sensitivities are available, therapy should be narrowed to avoid emergence of drug-resistant pathogens. Box 10-4 depicts the risk factors for developing MDR pathogens.

Prompt administration of antibiotics in patients is a key treatment measure. If specific pathogens responsible for the pneumonia are identified, more specific, less broad-spectrum agents should be used. The recommended duration of treatment for CAP is a minimum of 5 days. Patients should be afebrile for at least 2 days before antibiotics are discontinued. Patients with nosocomial pneumonias are treated for 7 to 10 days, as long as the patient is showing signs of clinical improvement. Emerging data are demonstrating that shorter durations of antibiotic use are producing good clinical

TABLE **10-1**   Empiric Antibiotic Therapy for Hospital-Acquired, Ventilator-Associated, or Health Care–Acquired Pneumonia

Type	Drugs
Early onset (less than 5 days), with no risk factors for multi drug-resistant pathogens	Ampicillin-sulbactam OR Ceftriaxone OR Levofloxacin, moxifloxacin, or ciprofloxacin OR ertapenem
Late onset (5 days or more) or risk factors for multidrug-resistant pathogens	Cefepime or ceftazidime OR Imipenem or meropenem OR Piperacillin-tazobactam AND Ciprofloxacin or levofloxacin OR amikacin, gentamicin or tobramycin AND Linezolid or vancomycin (MRSA)

Data from American Thoracic Society & Infectious Disease Society of America. (2005). Guidelines for management of adults with hospital-acquired ventilator associated, and healthcare-associated pneumonia. *American Journal of Respiratory and Critical Care Medicine, 171,* 388–416; Musher, D. (2016). Overview of pneumonia. In L. Goldman & A. Schafter (Eds.), *Goldman-Cecil medicine* (25th ed.). New York: Elsevier, Saunders.

responses and fewer emergences of MDR pathogens (Montravers, Harpan, & Guivarch, 2016).

Antibiotics are ineffective in viral pneumonia, and their use may be associated with adverse effects (superinfections, MDR pathogens). Patients who develop pneumonia or who are at risk for influenza can be treated with antiviral agents. The CDC (2015b, 2016c) recommends initiating antiviral therapy for persons with suspected/confirmed influenza who are severely ill or hospitalized, or are at risk for complications.

Oxygen Inhalation Therapy

Oxygen inhalation therapy is the administration of oxygen at a concentration greater that that found in the environmental atmosphere. At sea level, the concentration of oxygen in room air is 21% and has a relative humidity of 50% under normal circumstances; the lungs contribute about 250 mL of H_2O per day to maximally saturate inspired air. The goal of using oxygen therapy is to prevent or correct tissue hypoxia,

---

BOX 10-4

Risk Factors for the Development of Multidrug-Resistant Pathogens

- Antibiotic use in preceding 90 days
- Current hospitalization 5 days or longer
- Immunocompromised (by disease or therapies)
- Increased frequency of drug resistance in the community or hospital unit
- Presence of risk factors for HCAP

---

which is decreased oxygen supply to the tissues (Box 10-5). Hypoxia is often confused with hypoxemia. Hypoxemia is a decrease in the arterial oxygen content or arterial oxygen tension (partial pressure of oxygen, PaO_2) and is measured by ABG or POX. Hypoxemia is defined as a PaO_2 level of less than 60 mm Hg and/or a POX level of less than 90%. When administering oxygen to a patient, a nurse must keep in mind that oxygen transport to the tissues is dependent not only on the arterial oxygen content but also on cardiac output, hemoglobin concentration, and metabolic requirements.

Indications for Oxygen Therapy

The use of oxygen to *treat* patients with hypoxia is based on clinical indicators such as subjective information (dyspnea, chest pain), ABG analysis, POX, and physical examination findings. A change in respiratory rate or pattern (bradypnea, tachypnea, Cheyne–Stokes breathing), change in mental status (agitation, anxiety, disorientation, confusion, lethargy, coma), change in BP, change in heart rate (bradycardia or tachycardia), development of arrhythmias, cyanosis (late sign), diaphoresis, or cool extremities are signs of hypoxia. The development of these signs and symptoms depends on how suddenly the hypoxia develops. Acute onset tends to show signs of neurologic and cardiovascular impairment, while with chronic onset, patients complain of fatigue, drowsiness, dyspnea on exertion (DOE), and inattentiveness.

The administration of oxygen to *prevent* hypoxemia in high-risk patients who do not have clinical indicators of hypoxia is common in hospitals. High-risk patients are those who are at risk of rapidly developing hypoxemia or who will not tolerate even mild hypoxemia. Patients with pneumonia,

Types of Hypoxia

Hypoxia can occur from either severe pulmonary disease (inadequate oxygen supply) or from extrapulmonary disease (inadequate oxygen delivery) affecting gas exchange at the cellular level. The four general types of hypoxia are hypoxemic hypoxia, circulatory hypoxia, anemic hypoxia, and histotoxic hypoxia.

Hypoxemic Hypoxia

Hypoxemic hypoxia is a decreased oxygen level in the blood resulting in decreased oxygen diffusion into the tissues. It may be caused by hypoventilation, high altitudes, ventilation–perfusion mismatch (as in pulmonary embolism), shunts in which the alveoli are collapsed and cannot provide oxygen to the blood (commonly caused by atelectasis), and pulmonary diffusion defects. It is corrected by increasing alveolar ventilation or providing supplemental oxygen.

Circulatory Hypoxia

Circulatory hypoxia results from inadequate capillary circulation. It may be caused by decreased cardiac output, local

vascular obstruction, low-flow states such as shock, or cardiac arrest. Although tissue partial pressure of oxygen (PO_2) is reduced, arterial oxygen (PaO_2) remains normal. Circulatory hypoxia is corrected by identifying and treating the underlying cause.

Anemic Hypoxia

Anemic hypoxia is a result of decreased effective hemoglobin concentration, which causes a decrease in the oxygen-carrying capacity of the blood. It is rarely accompanied by hypoxemia. Carbon monoxide poisoning, because it reduces the oxygen-carrying capacity of hemoglobin, produces similar effects but is not strictly anemic hypoxia because hemoglobin levels may be normal.

Histotoxic Hypoxia

Histotoxic hypoxia occurs when a toxic substance, such as cyanide, interferes with the ability of tissues to use available oxygen.

PE, suspected myocardial injury or infarction, and head trauma or injury are just a few examples.

Methods of Oxygen Administration

Oxygen is dispensed from a cylinder or a piped-in system, and a flow meter regulates the flow of oxygen in liters per minute. When oxygen is used at flow rates greater than or equal to 4 L/min, it should be moistened by passing it through a humidification system to prevent it from drying the mucous membranes of the respiratory tract (Tokarczyk, Greenberg, & Vender, 2013). A variety of oxygen delivery systems is available (Table 10-2). Each system and oxygen flow rate is designed to provide a specific **fraction of inspired oxygen** (FiO_2) or percentage of oxygen. The appropriate form of oxygen therapy is best determined by ABG levels, which indicate the patient's oxygenation status, and/or POX.

Oxygen delivery systems are classified as low-flow or high-flow delivery systems. Low-flow systems contribute partially to the inspired gas the patient breathes, which means that the patient breathes some room air along with the oxygen. These systems do not provide a constant or known concentration of inspired oxygen. The amount of inspired oxygen changes as the patient's breathing changes. Examples of low-flow systems include nasal cannula, simple mask, partial-rebreather, and nonrebreather masks. In contrast, high-flow systems provide the total amount of inspired air. A specific percentage of oxygen is delivered independent of the patient's breathing. High-flow systems are indicated for patients who require a constant and precise amount of oxygen. Examples of such systems include transtracheal catheters, Venturi masks, aerosol masks, tracheostomy collars, and face tents.

 Concept Mastery Alert

For patients fitted with partial rebreathing masks, the masks should always be filled, whether the patient is inhaling or exhaling.

A nasal cannula is used when the patient requires a low to medium concentration of oxygen for which precise accuracy is not essential. This method is relatively simple and allows the patient to move about in bed, talk, cough, and eat without interrupting oxygen flow. Flow rates in excess of 6 to 8 L/min may lead to swallowing of air or may cause irritation and drying of the nasal and pharyngeal mucosa. When oxygen is administered via cannula, the percentage of oxygen reaching the lungs varies with the depth and rate of respirations, particularly if the nasal mucosa is swollen or if the patient is a mouth breather.

 Nursing Alert
The nurse is aware that patients with nasal cannula often develop irritation and erythema on their ears and cheeks due to pressure of the cannula tubing. Gauze or protective devices that pad the pressure points may be used around the cheeks and ears during prolonged use.

Oxygen masks come in several forms (Fig. 10-4). Each is used for different purposes. *Simple masks* are used to administer low to moderate concentrations of oxygen. The body of the mask itself gathers and stores oxygen between breaths. The patient exhales directly through openings or ports in the body of the mask. If oxygen flow ceases, the patient

TABLE **10-2** Oxygen Administration Devices

Device	Suggested Flow Rate (L/min)	O₂ Percentage Setting	Advantages	Disadvantages
Low-Flow Systems				
Cannula	1–2 3–5 6	23–30 30–40 42	Lightweight, comfortable, inexpensive, continuous use with meals and activity	Nasal mucosal drying, variable FiO₂
Oropharyngeal catheter	1–6	23–42	Inexpensive, does not require a tracheostomy	Nasal mucosa irritation; catheter should be changed frequently to alternate nostril
Mask, simple	6–8	40–60	Simple to use, inexpensive	Poor fitting, variable FiO₂, must remove to eat
Mask, partial rebreather	8–11	50–75	Moderate O₂ concentration	Warm, poorly fitting, must remove to eat
Mask, nonrebreather	12	80–100	High O₂ concentration	Poorly fitting
High-Flow Systems				
Transtracheal catheter	¼–4	60–100	More comfortable, concealed by clothing, less oxygen liters per minute needed than nasal cannula	Requires frequent and regular cleaning, requires surgical intervention
Mask, Venturi	4–6	24, 26, 28	Provides low levels of supplemental O₂	Must remove to eat
	6–8	30, 35, 40, 50	Precise FiO₂, additional humidity available	
Mask, aerosol	8–10	30–100	Good humidity, accurate FiO₂	Uncomfortable for some
Tracheostomy collar	8–10	30–100	Good humidity, comfortable, fairly accurate FiO₂	
Face tent	8–10	30–100	Good humidity, fairly accurate FiO₂	Bulky and cumbersome
Oxygen-Conserving Devices				
Pulse dose (or demand)	10–40 mL/breath		Deliver O₂ only on inspiration, conserve 50–75% of O₂ used	Must carefully evaluate function individually

can draw air in through these openings around the mask edges. Although widely used, these masks cannot be used for controlled oxygen concentrations and must be adjusted for proper fit. They should not press too tightly against the skin because this can cause a sense of claustrophobia as well as skin breakdown; adjustable elastic bands are provided to ensure comfort and security.

Partial-rebreathing masks have a reservoir bag that *must remain inflated during both inspiration and expiration*. The nurse adjusts the oxygen flow to ensure that the bag does not collapse during inhalation. A high concentration of oxygen can be delivered because both the mask and the bag serve as reservoirs for oxygen. Oxygen enters the mask through small-bore tubing that connects at the junction of the mask and bag. As the patient inhales, gas is drawn from the mask, from the bag, and potentially from room air through the exhalation ports. As the patient exhales, the first third of the exhalation fills the reservoir bag. This is mainly dead space and does not participate in gas exchange in the lungs.

Therefore, it has a high oxygen concentration. The remainder of the exhaled gas is vented through the exhalation ports. The actual percentage of oxygen delivered is influenced by the patient's ventilatory pattern.

Nonrebreathing masks are similar in design to partial-rebreathing masks except that they have additional valves. A one-way valve located between the reservoir bag and the base of the mask allows gas from the reservoir bag to enter the mask on inhalation but prevents gas in the mask from flowing back into the reservoir bag during exhalation. One-way valves located at the exhalation ports prevent room air from entering the mask during inhalation. They also allow the patient's exhaled gases to exit the mask on exhalation. As with the partial-rebreathing mask, *it is important to adjust the oxygen flow so that the reservoir bag does not completely collapse on inspiration*. In theory, if the nonrebreathing mask fits the patient snugly, and both side exhalation ports have one-way valves, it is possible for the patient to receive 100% oxygen, making the nonrebreathing mask a high-flow

FIGURE 10-4 Types of oxygen masks used to deliver varying concentrations of oxygen. **A.** Venturi mask. **B.** Nonrebreather. **C.** Partial rebreather.

oxygen system. However, because it is difficult to get an exact fit from the mask on every patient, and some nonrebreathing masks have only one one-way exhalation valve, it is almost impossible to ensure 100% oxygen delivery, thus making it a low-flow oxygen system.

The *Venturi mask* is the most reliable and accurate method for delivering precise concentrations of oxygen through non-invasive means. The mask is constructed in a way that allows a constant flow of room air blended with a fixed flow of oxygen. It is used primarily for patients with COPD because it can accurately provide appropriate levels of supplemental oxygen, thus avoiding the risk of suppressing the hypoxic drive (refer to Chapter 11 for further details).

 Nursing Alert
The nurse is aware that patients with severe COPD characteristically have a chronically elevated $PaCO_2$, a normal pH, an elevated HCO_3, and a PaO_2 level that usually is less than 60 mm Hg. As a result, the chemoreceptors in the aortic and carotid bodies are desensitized to the ventilatory stimulation from an increased $PaCO_2$ level but instead remain sensitive to PaO_2. Thus the goal of oxygen therapy is to raise the oxygen level to the patient's chronic baseline level (or a POX of 88% to 92%), not above it.

The Venturi mask uses the Bernoulli principle of air entrainment (trapping the air like a vacuum), which provides a high air flow with controlled oxygen enrichment. For each liter of oxygen that passes through a jet orifice, a fixed proportion of room air is entrained. A precise volume of oxygen can be delivered by varying the size of the jet orifice and adjusting the flow of oxygen. Excess gas leaves the mask through the two exhalation ports, carrying with it the exhaled carbon dioxide. This method allows a constant oxygen concentration to be inhaled regardless of the depth or rate of respiration.

The mask should fit snugly enough to prevent oxygen from flowing into the patient's eyes. The nurse checks the patient's skin for irritation. It is necessary to remove the mask so that the patient can eat, drink, and take medications, at which time supplemental oxygen is provided through a nasal cannula.

The nurse must understand how to convert percentage of oxygen with a mask to liters per minute for a nasal cannula (Box 10-6).

The *transtracheal oxygen catheter* is inserted directly into the trachea and is indicated for patients with chronic oxygen therapy needs. These catheters are more comfortable, less dependent on breathing patterns, and less obvious than other

---

BOX 10-6

Approximate FiO_2 of Nasal Cannula Flow Rates

Each liter (L) of flow is approximately an addition of 4% FiO_2
- 1 L/min = 24% FiO_2
- 2 L/min = 28% FiO_2
- 3 L/min = 32% FiO_2
- 4 L/min = 36% FiO_2
- 5 L/min = 40% FiO_2
- 6 L/min = 44% FiO_2

Tokrczyk et al. (2013).

oxygen delivery methods. Because no oxygen is lost into the surrounding environment, the patient achieves adequate oxygenation at lower rates, making this method less expensive and more efficient.

Other oxygen devices include *aerosol masks, tracheostomy collars,* and *face tents,* all of which are used with aerosol devices (nebulizers) that can be adjusted for oxygen concentrations from 27% to 100% (0.27 to 1.00). If the gas mixture flow falls below patient demand, room air is pulled in, diluting the concentration. The aerosol mist delivered by the nebulizer must be available for the patient during the entire inspiratory phase. The nurse notifies the respiratory therapist if the nebulizer is not functioning properly.

Hyperbaric oxygen therapy is the administration of oxygen at pressures greater than 1 atmosphere. As a result, the amount of oxygen dissolved in plasma is increased, which increases oxygen levels in the tissues. During therapy, the patient is placed in a small (single patient use) or large (multiple patient use) cylindrical chamber. Hyperbaric oxygen therapy is used to treat conditions such as air embolism, carbon monoxide poisoning, gangrene, tissue necrosis, and hemorrhage. Potential side effects include ear trauma, CNS disorders, and oxygen toxicity.

Complications

Oxygen, like other medications, should be administered with caution and a careful assessment of patient response. A high concentration of oxygen is contraindicated in the patient with COPD because it may worsen alveolar ventilation by decreasing the patient's ventilatory drive, leading to further respiratory decompensation.

When oxygen is metabolized, it produces free radicals that can cause cellular damage. This side effect of oxygen therapy is called *oxygen toxicity.* Although healthy lungs may be able to tolerate FiO_2 levels of less than 60%, when lungs are damaged FiO_2 over 50% may result in a toxic alveolar O_2 concentration and absorptive atelectasis (Tokrczyk et al., 2013). Toxic levels of oxygen are reached when FiO_2 levels are greater than 50% for longer than 48 hours (Marino, 2014). Signs and symptoms of oxygen toxicity include chest pain, paresthesias, dyspnea, restlessness, fatigue, malaise, progressive respiratory distress, atelectasis, pulmonary infiltrates, and fibrosis. The prevention of oxygen toxicity is achieved by using the lowest level of oxygen needed clinically. If a patient remains hypoxemic on toxic levels of oxygen, additional measures should be instituted, such as intubation and mechanical ventilation.

Oxygen supports combustion; therefore, its use is a fire hazard. No smoking or open flames should be allowed near oxygen use. In addition, the risk of cross-contamination of oxygen supplies (mask, tubing, cannulas) should be addressed and equipment changed per infection control policy.

Supportive Care

Supportive care for pneumonia includes hydration to combat insensible fluid losses from fever and tachypnea. Antipyretics

may be used to treat headache, aches, and fever. Warm, moist inhalations are helpful in relieving bronchial irritation.

Additional therapies must be considered for the hospitalized pneumonia patient. Nutritional assessment and support, deep vein thrombosis prophylaxis, nebulized bronchodilators or mucolytics, and comfort care measures should be individualized for each patient.

Gerontologic Considerations

Pneumonia in elderly patients may occur as a primary diagnosis or as a complication of a chronic disease process. Pulmonary infections in older people frequently are difficult to treat and result in a higher mortality rate than in younger people. General deterioration, weakness, abdominal symptoms, incontinence, anorexia, confusion, tachycardia, and tachypnea may signal the onset of pneumonia. The diagnosis of pneumonia may be missed because the classic symptoms of cough, chest pain, and sputum production may be absent or masked in elderly patients. Fever as a symptom can be missed as well because 30% to 40% of older patients are afebrile. Also, the presence of some signs may be misleading. Abnormal breath sounds, for example, may be caused by atelectasis that occurs as a result of decreased mobility, decreased lung volumes, or other respiratory function changes. It may be necessary to obtain chest x-rays to differentiate chronic heart failure, which is often seen in the elderly, from pneumonia as the cause of clinical signs and symptoms.

Supportive treatment includes hydration (with caution and with frequent assessment because of the risk of fluid overload in the elderly), supplemental oxygen therapy, and assistance with deep breathing, coughing, frequent position changes, and early ambulation. All of these are particularly important in the care of elderly patients with pneumonia. To reduce or prevent serious complications of pneumonia in the elderly, vaccination against pneumococcal and influenza infections is recommended.

Prevention

Pneumococcal disease is more prevalent (three- to fivefold higher) in African-American adults as compared with Caucasians. Pneumococcal vaccination has been demonstrated to prevent pneumonia in otherwise healthy populations by 90%. The vaccine provides specific prevention against pneumococcal pneumonia and other infections caused by *S. pneumoniae* (otitis media, other upper respiratory tract infections). Vaccines should be avoided during the first trimester of pregnancy (CDC, 2016d).

To reduce or prevent serious complications of CAP in high-risk groups, vaccination against pneumococcal infection is advised for persons 2 to 64 years of age with chronic illnesses, those who are immunocompromised or are asplenic (spleen is removed), and for all those 65 years or older. Also smokers or those with asthma between the ages of 19 and 64 should get vaccinated. If vaccine was given prior to age 65, it should be repeated once after 5 years (CDC, 2016d).

NURSING PROCESS
The Patient with Pneumonia

ASSESSMENT

Nursing assessment is critical in detecting pneumonia. Patients with fever, chills, dyspnea, and cough should alert the nurse to the possibility of pneumonia. Respiratory assessment further identifies the clinical manifestations of pneumonia: pleuritic-type pain, fatigue, tachypnea, use of accessory muscles for breathing, tachycardia, coughing, and purulent sputum. The nurse monitors the patient for the following:

- Changes in temperature and pulse
- Amount, odor, consistency, and color of secretions
- Frequency and severity of cough
- Degree of tachypnea or shortness of breath
- Pulse oximetry
- Changes in physical assessment findings (primarily assessed by inspecting and auscultating the chest)
- Changes in the chest x-ray findings
- Changes in WBCs; leukocytosis is seen in *S. pneumoniae, H. influenzae*, and gram-negative bacilli whereas leukopenia may be seen with pneumococcal or gram-negative bacillary pneumonia (Torres, Menendez, & Wunderink, 2016).

In addition, it is important to assess patients, especially elderly patients, for unusual behavior, altered mental status, dehydration, excessive fatigue, and concomitant heart failure.

DIAGNOSIS

Appropriate nursing diagnoses may include:

- Ineffective airway clearance related to copious tracheobronchial secretions
- Impaired gas exchange
- Activity intolerance related to impaired respiratory function
- Risk for deficient fluid volume related to fever, a rapid respiratory rate, and sepsis
- Imbalanced nutrition: less than body requirements
- Deficient knowledge about the treatment regimen and preventive health measures

Collaborative problems or potential complications that may occur include the following:

- Continuing symptoms after initiation of therapy
- Shock
- Respiratory failure
- Atelectasis
- Pleural effusion
- Confusion
- Superinfection

PLANNING

The major goals may include improved airway patency, rest to conserve energy, maintenance of proper fluid volume, maintenance of adequate nutrition, an understanding of the treatment protocol and preventive measures, and absence of complications.

NURSING INTERVENTIONS

IMPROVING AIRWAY PATENCY

Removing secretions is important because retained secretions interfere with gas exchange and may slow recovery. The nurse encourages hydration (2 to 3 L/day) because adequate hydration thins and loosens pulmonary secretions. Hydration must be achieved more slowly and with careful monitoring in patients with pre-existing conditions, such as heart failure. Humidification may be used to loosen secretions and improve ventilation. A high-humidity face mask (using either compressed air or oxygen) delivers warm, humidified air to the tracheobronchial tree and helps to liquefy secretion. Coughing can be initiated either voluntarily or by reflex. Lung expansion maneuvers, such as deep breathing with an incentive spirometer, may induce a cough. A directed cough may be necessary to improve airway patency. The nurse encourages the patient to perform an effective, directed cough, which includes correct positioning, a deep inspiratory maneuver, glottic closure, contraction of the expiratory muscles against the closed glottis, sudden glottic opening, and an explosive expiration.

> ### ⚠ Nursing Alert
> *In general, the dependent lung is associated with improved perfusion. If the goal is to match ventilation with perfusion, the "good lung down" is a position that will facilitate this. However, any position for a prolonged period of time is associated with stagnation of secretions and pressure on the dependent lung, increasing the risk of atelectasis in the dependent lung. Therefore, the nurse turns the patient at regular intervals. The nurse is aware that when the affected lung is positioned dependently, the oxygen saturation should be assessed to note the impact of this position on oxygen level. In addition, the nurse is aware that in the case of unilateral (one lung) pulmonary hemorrhage or pulmonary abscess, "good lung down" is contraindicated to prevent blood or infected material from draining into the good lung.*

CPT is important in loosening and mobilizing secretions. Indications for CPT include sputum retention not responsive to spontaneous or directed cough, a history of pulmonary problems previously treated with CPT, continued evidence of retained secretions (decreased or abnormal breath sounds, change in vital signs), abnormal chest x-ray findings consistent with atelectasis or infiltrates, and deterioration in oxygenation.

The nurse may consult the respiratory therapy department for volume-expansion protocols and secretion-management protocols that help direct the respiratory care of the patient and match the patient's needs with appropriate treatment schedules.

After each position change, the nurse encourages the patient to breathe deeply and cough. If the patient is too weak to cough effectively, the nurse may need to remove the mucus by nasotracheal suctioning. It may take time for secretions to mobilize and move into the central airways for expectoration. Therefore, it is important for the nurse to monitor the patient for cough and sputum production after the completion of CPT.

The nurse also administers and titrates oxygen therapy as prescribed or via protocols. The effectiveness of oxygen therapy is monitored by improvement in clinical signs and symptoms, patient comfort, and adequate oxygenation values as measured by POX or ABG analysis.

PROMOTING REST AND CONSERVING ENERGY

The nurse encourages the debilitated patient to rest and avoid overexertion and possible exacerbation of symptoms. The patient should assume a comfortable position to promote rest and breathing (e.g., semi-Fowler position) and should change positions frequently to enhance secretion clearance as well as ventilation and perfusion in the lungs. It is important to instruct outpatients not to overexert themselves and to engage in only moderate activity during the initial phases of treatment.

PROMOTING FLUID INTAKE

The respiratory rate of patients with pneumonia increases because of the increased workload imposed by labored breathing and fever. An increased respiratory rate leads to an increase in insensible fluid loss during exhalation and can lead to dehydration. Therefore, it is important to encourage increased fluid intake (at least 2 L/day), unless contraindicated.

MAINTAINING NUTRITION

Many patients with shortness of breath and fatigue have a decreased appetite and consume only fluids. Fluids with electrolytes and protein-supplementation drinks can be prescribed to patients. In addition, IV fluids and nutrients may be administered if necessary.

PROMOTING PATIENTS' KNOWLEDGE

The patient and family are instructed about the cause of pneumonia, management of symptoms of pneumonia, signs and symptoms that should be reported to the health care provider or nurse, and the need for follow-up. The patient also needs information about factors (both patient risk factors and external factors) that may have contributed to development of pneumonia and strategies to promote recovery and prevent recurrence. If the patient is hospitalized, he or she is instructed about the purpose and importance of management strategies that have been implemented and about the importance of adhering to them during and after the hospital stay. Explanations should be given in simple and clear language that the patient can understand. If possible, written instructions and information should be provided, with alternative formats available for patients with hearing or vision loss, if necessary. Because of the severity of symptoms, the patient may require that instructions and explanations be repeated several times.

MONITORING AND MANAGING POTENTIAL COMPLICATIONS

Continuing Symptoms after Initiation of Therapy. The patient is observed for response to antibiotic therapy; patients usually begin to respond to treatment within 24 to 48 hours after antibiotic therapy is initiated. If the patient started taking antibiotics before evaluation by culture and sensitivity of the causative organisms, antibiotics may need to be changed once the results are available. The patient is monitored for changes in physical status (deterioration of condition or resolution of symptoms) and for persistent or recurrent fever, which may be a result of medication allergy (signaled possibly by a rash); medication resistance or slow response (greater than 48 hours) of the susceptible organism to therapy; superinfection; pleural effusion; or pneumonia caused by an unusual organism, such as *P. jiroveci* or *Aspergillus fumigatus.* Failure of the pneumonia to resolve or persistence of symptoms despite improvement on the chest x-ray raises the suspicion of other underlying disorders, such as lung cancer. As previously described, lung cancers may invade or compress airways, causing an obstructive atelectasis that may lead to pneumonia.

In addition to monitoring for continuing symptoms of pneumonia, the nurse also monitors for other complications, such as shock and multisystem failure and atelectasis, which may develop during the first few days of antibiotic treatment.

Shock and Respiratory Failure. Severe complications of pneumonia include sepsis and septic shock as well as respiratory failure. These complications are encountered primarily in patients who have received nonspecific, inadequate, or delayed treatment in combination with particularly virulent pathogens. These complications are also encountered when the infecting organism is resistant to therapy, when a comorbid disease complicates the pneumonia, or when the patient is immunocompromised.

Severe sepsis is defined as a systemic inflammatory response related to an infection such as pneumonia, with dysfunction or failure of one or more organs (e.g., renal insufficiency, ARDS, or disseminated intravascular coagulation). *Septic shock* occurs when severe sepsis is accompanied by hypotension that is refractory to the infusion of IV fluids. Severe sepsis and septic shock can lead to multiorgan dysfunction and carry a high mortality rate.

If the patient is seriously ill, aggressive therapy may include hemodynamic and ventilator support to combat peripheral vascular collapse, maintain arterial blood pressure, and provide adequate oxygenation. A vasopressor agent may be administered by continuous IV infusion and at a rate adjusted in accordance with the blood pressure response. Corticosteroids may be

(continued on page 306)

administered parenterally to combat shock and toxicity in patients who are extremely ill with pneumonia and at apparent risk for death from the infection, or who have adrenal insufficiency. However, whether corticosteroids are beneficial in patients with pneumonia remains uncertain (Musher, 2016). Patients may require endotracheal intubation and mechanical ventilation. Heart failure, cardiac arrhythmias, pericarditis, and myocarditis also are complications of pneumonia that may lead to shock.

The nurse assesses for signs and symptoms of shock and respiratory failure by evaluating the patient's vital signs, POX values, and hemodynamic monitoring parameters. The nurse reports signs of deteriorating patient status and assists in administering IV fluids and medications prescribed to combat shock. Intubation and mechanical ventilation may be required if respiratory failure occurs.

Atelectasis and Pleural Effusion. Atelectasis (from obstruction of a bronchus or small airways by accumulated secretions) may occur at any stage of acute pneumonia. Parapneumonic **pleural effusions** occur in at least 40% of bacterial pneumonias. A parapneumonic effusion is any pleural effusion associated with bacterial pneumonia, lung abscess, or bronchiectasis. After the pleural effusion is detected on a chest x-ray or CT scan, a thoracentesis may be performed to remove the fluid. The fluid is sent to the laboratory for analysis. There are three stages of parapneumonic pleural effusions based on pathogenesis: uncomplicated, complicated, and empyema. An **empyema** occurs when thick, purulent fluid accumulates within the **pleural space**, often with fibrin development and a loculated (walled-off) area where the infection is located (see later discussion). A chest tube may be inserted to treat pleural infection by establishing proper drainage of the empyema. Sterilization of the empyema cavity usually requires 4 to 6 weeks of antibiotics, but sometimes surgical management is required.

The patient is assessed for atelectasis, and preventive measures are initiated to prevent its development. If pleural effusion develops and thoracentesis is performed to remove fluid, the nurse assists in the procedure and explains it to the patient. After thoracentesis, the nurse monitors the patient for pneumothorax or recurrence of pleural effusion. If a chest tube needs to be inserted, the nurse monitors the patient's respiratory status and assesses functioning of the chest drainage system (see later discussion).

Superinfection. Superinfections may occur with the administration of any antibiotic but are more common with the use of high-dose, broad-spectrum, and multiple antibiotics. Superinfections are the overgrowth of endogenous flora. Common superinfections are oral yeast (thrush) and vaginal candidiasis, and *Clostridium difficile* colitis (pseudomembranous colitis). The patient is monitored for manifestations of superinfection (i.e., white coating of tongue or oral mucosa, vaginal discharge, and diarrhea). These signs are reported, and the nurse assists in implementing therapy to treat superinfection.

Confusion. A patient with pneumonia is assessed for confusion and other more subtle changes in cognitive status. Confusion and changes in cognitive status resulting from pneumonia are poor prognostic signs. Confusion may be related to hypoxemia, fever, dehydration, sleep deprivation, or developing sepsis. Also the patient's underlying comorbid conditions may play a part in the development of confusion. Addressing the underlying factors and ensuring patient safety are important nursing interventions.

PROMOTING HEALTH

The nurse encourages the patient to stop smoking. Smoking inhibits tracheobronchial ciliary action, which is the first line of defense of the lower respiratory tract. Smoking also irritates the mucous cells of the bronchi and inhibits the function of alveolar macrophage (scavenger) cells. The patient is instructed to avoid stress, fatigue, sudden changes in temperature, and excessive alcohol intake, all of which lower resistance to pneumonia. The nurse reviews with the patient the principles of adequate nutrition and rest because one episode of pneumonia may make a patient susceptible to recurring respiratory tract infections.

EVALUATION

Expected patient outcomes may include the following:
1. Demonstrates improved airway patency, as evidenced by adequate oxygenation by POX or ABG analysis, normal temperature, normal breath sounds, and effective coughing
2. Rests and conserves energy by limiting activities and remaining in bed while symptomatic and then slowly increasing activities
3. Maintains adequate hydration, as evidenced by an adequate fluid intake and urine output as well as normal skin turgor
4. Consumes adequate dietary intake, as evidenced by maintenance or increase in body weight without excess fluid gain
5. States explanation for management strategies
6. Complies with management strategies
7. Exhibits no complications:
   - Exhibits acceptable vital signs, POX, and ABG measurements
   - Reports productive cough that diminishes over time
   - Has absence of signs or symptoms of shock, respiratory failure, or pleural effusion
   - Remains oriented and aware of surroundings
   - Maintains or increases weight
   - Complies with treatment protocol and prevention strategies

PULMONARY TUBERCULOSIS

Tuberculosis (TB) is an infectious disease that primarily affects the lung parenchyma. The primary infectious agent, *M. tuberculosis*, is an acid-fast aerobic bacilli that grows slowly and is sensitive to heat and ultraviolet light. It is a resistant bacterium that can persist in calcified and necrotic lesions and remain able to reinitiate growth.

TB is a worldwide public health problem, and mortality and morbidity rates continue to rise. *M. tuberculosis* infects an estimated one third of the world's population and remains the leading cause of death from infectious disease in the world, although cases in the United States have declined slightly. TB is closely associated with poverty, malnutrition, overcrowding, substandard housing, and inadequate health care (American Thoracic Society, Centers for Disease Control and Prevention, Infectious Disease Society of America [ATS, CDC, & IDSA], 2003; CDC, 2014b, 2014c).

Pathophysiology

TB spreads from person to person by airborne transmission. An infected person releases droplet nuclei (usually particles 1 to 5 μm in diameter) through talking, coughing, sneezing, laughing, or singing. Larger droplets settle; smaller droplets remain suspended in the air and are inhaled. Several factors determine the transmission of *M. tuberculosis* and include characteristics of the source case, exposed person, and the exposure; and the virulence of the *M. tuberculosis* strain. Box 10-7 depicts risk factors for tuberculosis.

BOX 10-7
Risk Factors for Tuberculosis (TB)

- Being born in foreign countries with high prevalence of TB
- Being medically underserved and/or with low income. Populations include:
  - Homeless
  - Impoverished
  - Minorities, particularly children under age of 15 years and people between 15 and 44 years
  - Those living in overcrowded, substandard housing
- Being a resident or employee of correction centers, homeless shelters, long-term care facilities
- Being a health care worker caring for high-risk patients
- Being a health care worker performing high-risk activities:
  - Administration of aerosolized medications
  - Sputum-induction procedures, including suctioning and coughing procedures
  - Bronchoscopy
  - Intubations
- Unprotected exposure to TB patients
- Advanced age
- Traveling abroad to work in endemic areas (Southeastern Asia, Africa, Latin America, Caribbean)
- Infants and children exposed to high-risk patients
- Substance abuse (IV/injection drug users and alcoholics)
- Immunocompromise:
  - Human immunodeficiency virus (HIV) infections
  - Malignancies: Head, neck, lung, hematologic
  - Long-term corticosteroid use
  - Immunosuppressive drug therapies
  - Organ transplantation
- Comorbidities:
  - Malnutrition
  - Diabetes
  - Silicosis
  - Chronic kidney disease
  - Gastric or intestinal bypass surgery

TB begins when a susceptible person inhales mycobacteria and the bacteria are transmitted through the airways to the alveoli, where macrophages ingest the bacilli. If the bacilli escape the antimicrobial activities of the macrophages, an infection begins. This stage, called *primary TB*, usually is clinically silent and is due to the chronic inflammatory response that the bacterium provokes. The bacilli may be transported via the lymph system and bloodstream to other parts of the body (kidneys, bones, cerebral cortex) and other areas of the lungs (upper lobes). The spreading of TB via lymphatics and blood is called *miliary TB*. The body's immune system responds by initiating an inflammatory reaction. Phagocytes (neutrophils and macrophages) engulf many of the bacteria, and TB-specific lymphocytes destroy the bacilli along with normal tissue. This tissue reaction results in the accumulation of exudate in the alveoli, causing bronchopneumonia. The initial infection usually occurs 2 to 10 weeks after exposure.

Granulomas, new tissue masses of live and dead bacilli, are surrounded by macrophages, which form a protective wall. Then they are transformed to a fibrous tissue mass, the central portion of which is called a Ghon tubercle. The material (bacteria and macrophages) becomes necrotic, forming a cheesy mass. This mass may become calcified and form a collagenous scar. At this point, the bacteria become dormant, and there is no further progression of active disease.

After initial exposure and infection, active disease may develop because of a compromised or inadequate immune system response. Active disease also may occur with reinfection and activation of dormant bacteria. In this case, the Ghon tubercle ulcerates, releasing the cheesy material into the bronchi. Then the bacteria become airborne, resulting in further spread of the disease. The ulcerated tubercle heals and forms scar tissue. This causes the infected lung to become more inflamed, resulting in further development of bronchopneumonia and tubercle formation.

Unless the process is arrested, it spreads slowly downward to the hilum of the lungs and later extends to adjacent lobes. The process may be prolonged and is characterized by long remissions when the disease is arrested, followed by periods of renewed activity. Approximately 10% of people who are initially infected develop active disease. Some people develop reactivation TB. This type of TB results from a breakdown of the host defenses. It most commonly occurs in the lungs, usually in the apical (upper) or posterior segments of the upper lobes or the superior segments of the lower lobes.

Clinical Manifestations and Assessment

The signs and symptoms of pulmonary TB are insidious. Most patients have a low-grade fever, cough, night sweats, fatigue, and weight loss. Initially the cough is nonproductive but progresses to be mucopurulent. Dyspnea, chest pain, and **hemoptysis** (bloody sputum) occur as the disease progresses. Both the systemic and the pulmonary symptoms are

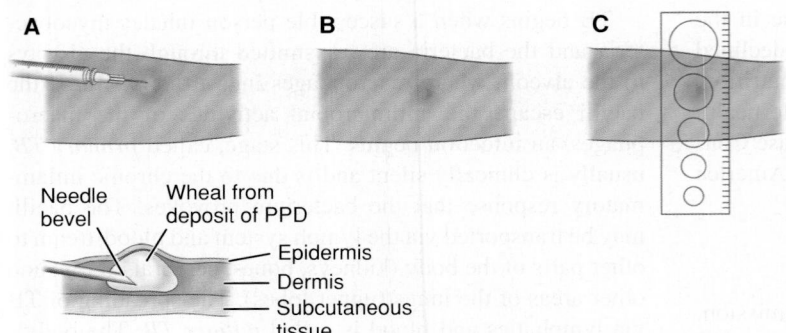

Needle bevel
Wheal from deposit of PPD
Epidermis
Dermis
Subcutaneous tissue

FIGURE 10-5 The Mantoux test for tuberculosis. **A.** Correct technique for inserting the needle involves depositing the purified protein derivative (PPD) intradermally with the needle bevel facing upward. **B.** The reaction to the Mantoux test usually consists of a *wheal,* a hive-like, firm welt. **C.** To determine the extent of the reaction, the wheal is measured using a commercially prepared gauge. Interpretation of the Mantoux test is discussed on this page.

chronic and may have been present for weeks to months. Elderly patients usually present with less pronounced symptoms than do younger patients. Extrapulmonary disease occurs in up to 16% of cases in the United States. In patients with AIDS, extrapulmonary disease is more prevalent and is manifested by neurologic deficits, bone pain, meningitis symptoms (stiff neck, headache, fever, confusion, and seizures), and urinary tract symptoms (dysuria).

A complete history, physical examination, tuberculin skin test, chest x-ray, AFB smear, and sputum culture are used to diagnose TB. If the patient is infected with TB, the chest x-ray usually reveals lesions in the upper lobes, and the AFB smear contains mycobacteria.

Tuberculin Skin Test

The Mantoux test is used to determine whether a person has been infected with the TB bacillus. The Mantoux test is a standardized procedure and should be performed only by those trained in its administration and reading (Fig. 10-5). Tubercle bacillus extract (tuberculin), purified protein derivative (PPD), is injected into the intradermal layer of the inner aspect of the forearm, approximately 4 in below the elbow. Intermediate-strength PPD, in a tuberculin syringe with a 0.5-in 26- or 27-gauge needle, is used. The needle, with the bevel facing up, is inserted beneath the skin. Then, 0.1 mL of PPD is injected, creating an elevation in the skin, a *wheal* or *bleb*. The site, antigen name, strength, lot number, date, and time of the test are recorded. The test result is read 48 to 72 hours after injection. Tests read after 72 hours tend to underestimate the true size of **induration** (hardening).

A reaction occurs when an induration at the injection site is present. After the area is inspected for induration, it is lightly palpated across the injection site, from the area of normal skin to the margins of the induration. The diameter of the induration (not erythema) is measured in millimeters at its widest part, and the size of the induration is documented. Erythema without induration is not considered significant. The size of the induration determines the significance of the reaction. A reaction of 0 to 4 mm is considered not significant; a reaction of 5 mm or greater may be significant in people who are considered to be at risk. An induration of 10 mm or greater is usually considered significant in people

who have normal or mildly impaired immunity. A significant reaction indicates past exposure to *M. tuberculosis* or vaccination with Bacille Calmette–Guérin (BCG) vaccine. The BCG vaccine is used in Europe and Latin America but not routinely in the United States.

> **Nursing Alert**
> *Ambiguity exists in interpretation of the tuberculin skin test (TST) when patients were vaccinated with BCG; however, data reveal that the BCG administered once at birth has little effect on the TST beyond the first year, and by year 10, only 1% of positive TSTs can be attributed to previous BCG administration (Ellner, 2016, p. 2035).*

A reaction of 5 mm or greater is defined as positive in patients who are HIV positive or have HIV risk factors and are of unknown HIV status; in those who are close contacts of someone with active TB; and in those who have chest x-ray results consistent with TB. HIV-positive patients are at risk for developing cutaneous anergy from impaired cellular immunity and may have a false-negative reaction to PPD skin testing. These patients may undergo Mantoux-method skin testing with mumps and candida antigens to assess for anergy. A positive test result is an induration of 5 mm or greater, meaning the patient has relatively intact cell-mediated immunity and can mount a reaction to PPD testing (Chapter 37 details anergy further).

A significant (positive) reaction does not necessarily mean that active disease is present in the body. More than 90% of people who are tuberculin-significant reactors do not develop clinical TB. However, all significant reactors are candidates for active TB. In addition, a nonsignificant (negative) skin test does not exclude TB infection or disease because patients who are immunosuppressed cannot develop an immune response that is adequate to produce a positive skin test.

TB Blood Testing

There are two FDA-approved blood tests for the detection of TB by interferon-gamma release assay, the QuantiFERON-TB Gold and the T-spot. A positive test indicates that the person has been infected with TB and further testing is needed to determine latency versus active disease. These blood tests are recommended when a person has received the BCG vaccine or when it is impractical to return for a second visit to read a TST (CDC, 2014b).

Classification

Data from the history, physical examination, TB test, chest x-ray, and microbiologic studies are used to classify TB into one of five classes. A classification scheme provides public health officials with a systematic way to monitor epidemiology and treatment of the disease (ATS & CDC, 2000; WHO, 2014):

- Class 0: No exposure; no infection
- Class 1: Exposure; no evidence of infection
- Class 2: Latent infection; no disease (e.g., positive PPD reaction but no clinical evidence of active TB)
- Class 3: Disease; clinically active
- Class 4: Disease; not clinically active
- Class 5: Suspected disease; diagnosis pending

Gerontologic Considerations

TB may have atypical manifestations in elderly patients, whose symptoms may include unusual behavior and altered mental status, fever, anorexia, and weight loss. In many elderly patients, the tuberculin skin test produces no reaction (loss of immunologic memory) or delayed reactivity for up to 1 week (recall phenomenon). A second skin test is performed in 1 to 2 weeks.

Medical and Nursing Management

Pharmacologic Therapy

Pulmonary TB is treated primarily with antituberculosis agents, as either active disease treatment or prophylactic treatment for persons exposed and at risk for developing the disease. A prolonged treatment duration is necessary to ensure eradication of the organisms and to prevent relapse. The continuing (since the 1950s) and increasing resistance of *M. tuberculosis* to TB medications is a worldwide concern and challenge in TB therapy. Several types of drug resistance must be considered when planning effective therapy:

- *Primary drug resistance:* Resistance to one of the first-line antituberculosis agents in people who have not had previous treatment
- *Secondary or acquired drug resistance:* Resistance to one or more antituberculosis agents in patients undergoing therapy
- *MDR:* Resistance to two agents, isoniazid (INH) and rifampin. The populations at greatest risk for MDR are those who are HIV positive, institutionalized, or homeless.

The increasing prevalence of drug resistance points out the need to begin TB treatment with three or more medications to ensure completion of therapy and to develop and evaluate new anti-TB medications.

Treatment Regimens

In current TB therapy, four first-line medications are used: INH, rifampin, pyrazinamide, and ethambutol. Combination medications, such as INH and rifampin (Rifamate) or INH, pyrazinamide, and rifampin (Rifater), and other medications administered twice a week (e.g., rifapentine) are available to help improve patient adherence. Capreomycin, ethionamide, para-aminosalicylate sodium, and cycloserine are second-line medications. Additional potentially effective medications include other aminoglycosides, quinolones, rifabutin, clofazimine, and combinations of medications (ATS, CDC, & IDSA, 2003).

Recommended treatment guidelines for newly diagnosed cases of presumably drug-susceptible active pulmonary TB have two parts: an initial treatment phase and a continuation phase. The initial phase consists of multiple medications (INH, rifampin, pyrazinamide, and ethambutol) and multiple dosing regimen choices of these four medications. This initial intensive treatment regimen is administered for 8 weeks and has 4 dosing options that range from daily to 2 or 5 times per week. Once susceptibilities of the TB to INH, rifampin, and pyrazinamide are confirmed, ethambutol can be discontinued (Horsburgh, Barry, & Lange, 2015). The continuation phase of treatment, which includes INH and rifampin or INH and rifapentine, lasts for an additional 18 or 31 weeks. The 18-week period is used for the large majority of patients. The 31-week period is recommended for patients with cavitary pulmonary TB whose sputum culture after the initial 2 months of treatment is positive; those whose initial phase of treatment did not include pyrazinamide (PZA); and those being treated once weekly with INH and rifapentine whose sputum culture is positive at the end of the initial phase of treatment. In general, people are considered noninfectious after 2 to 3 weeks of continuous medication therapy. Usually vitamin B (pyridoxine) is administered with INH to prevent INH-associated peripheral neuropathy. The total number of doses taken, not simply the duration of treatment, more accurately determines whether a course of therapy has been completed (Ellner, 2016).

Several types of drug-resistant TB have emerged over the last two decades. Multidrug resistant and extensively drug resistant TB are identified by sputum culture and sensitivity, but it may take weeks for results to be available. Nucleic acid testing (GeneXpert MTB/RIF and MTBDRplus) can provide results in a few days (Theron et al., 2014; Steingart et al., 2014). Treatment for resistant TB requires additional antimicrobial agents (up to six) and for a longer duration (Horsburgh et al., 2015; Wilson & Tsukayama, 2016).

INH also may be used as a prophylactic (preventive) measure for people who are at risk for significant disease, including:

- Household family members of patients with active disease
- Patients with HIV infection who have a PPD test reaction with 5 mm of induration or greater

- Patients with fibrotic lesions suggestive of old TB detected on a chest x-ray and a PPD reaction with 5 mm of induration or greater
- Patients whose current PPD test results show a change from former test results, suggesting recent exposure to TB and possible infection (skin test converters)
- Users of IV/injection drugs who have PPD test results with 10 mm of induration or greater
- Patients with high-risk comorbid conditions and a PPD result with 10 mm of induration or greater

Other candidates for preventive INH therapy are those 35 years or younger who have PPD test results with 10 mm of induration or more and one of the following criteria:

- Foreign-born individuals from countries with a high prevalence of TB
- High-risk, medically underserved populations
- Institutionalized patients

Prophylactic INH treatment involves taking daily doses for 6 to 12 months. Liver enzymes, blood urea nitrogen (BUN), and creatinine levels are monitored monthly to detect changes in liver and kidney function. Sputum culture results are monitored for AFB to evaluate the effectiveness of treatment and the patient's adherence to the treatment regimen.

Side Effects of Medication Therapy

It is important to assess medication side effects, because often they are a reason why patients fail to adhere to the prescribed medication regimen. Efforts are made to reduce the side effects and to motivate the patient to take the medications as prescribed.

The nurse instructs the patient to take the medication either on an empty stomach or at least 1 hour before meals because food interferes with medication absorption (although taking medications on an empty stomach frequently results in gastrointestinal upset). Patients taking INH should avoid foods that contain tyramine and histamine (tuna, aged cheese, red wine, soy sauce, yeast extracts) because eating them while taking INH may result in headache, flushing, hypotension, lightheadedness, palpitations, and diaphoresis.

In addition, rifampin can increase the metabolism of certain other medications, making them less effective. These medications include beta-blockers, oral anticoagulants such as warfarin, digoxin, quinidine, corticosteroids, oral hypoglycemic agents, oral contraceptives, theophylline, and verapamil. This issue should be discussed with the prescriber and pharmacist so that medication dosages can be adjusted accordingly. The nurse informs the patient that rifampin may discolor contact lenses and that the patient may want to wear eyeglasses during treatment. The nurse monitors for other side effects of anti-TB medications, including hepatitis, neurologic changes (hearing loss, neuritis, visual changes, neuropathy), and rash. Renal and hepatic function tests as well as sputum AFB results are monitored closely. The nurse

carefully monitors vital signs and observes for spikes in temperature or changes in the patient's clinical status. Changes in the patient's respiratory status are reported to the primary health care provider. The nurse instructs the patient about the risk of drug resistance if the medication regimen is not followed strictly and continuously.

The strict adherence to complex medication regimens is an important area of education of the TB patient. Drugs must be taken exactly as prescribed, and noncompliance can lead to continued infection and drug resistance. Directly observed therapy (DOT) can be implemented to ensure that patients are compliant with medications regimens. In DOT, a trained health care provider administers each dose of anti-TB medication. DOT can be prescribed by a health care provider such as a physician, nurse practitioner, or a local board of health.

Patient Teaching

The care of TB patients involves education related to halting the spread of the infection and its complex drug regimens. Patients should be instructed to cover their mouth and nose when they cough or sneeze, dispose of facial tissues in plastic bags, and wear a mask when in public until sputum samples are documented as free of AFB.

Patients in hospital settings will be placed on airborne precautions, including staying in a negative-pressure room that vents air to the outside, and staff must wear fitted filtration masks (N95 or high-efficiency particulate air respirators) when in the room. Health care providers who have the potential to be in contact with TB patients must be fit tested at least yearly and when their weight changes or if they have respiratory disorders such as asthma. Also patients must wear surgical masks when outside of the negative-pressure rooms.

Malnutrition may be a consequence of the patient's lifestyle, lack of knowledge about adequate nutrition and its role in health maintenance, lack of resources, fatigue, or lack of appetite because of coughing and mucus production and medication side effects. To counter the effects of these factors, the nurse collaborates with the dietitian, provider, social worker, family, and patient to identify strategies to ensure an adequate nutritional intake and the availability of nutritious food. Identifying facilities (e.g., shelters, soup kitchens, Meals on Wheels) that provide meals in the patient's neighborhood may increase the likelihood that the patient with limited resources and energy will have access to a more nutritious intake. High-calorie nutritional supplements may be suggested as a strategy for increasing dietary intake using food products normally found in the home. Purchasing food supplements may be beyond the patient's budget, but dietitians can help develop recipes to increase caloric intake despite minimal resources.

PULMONARY EDEMA

Pulmonary edema is defined as abnormal accumulation of fluid within the lung tissue, the alveolar space, or both.

Acute pulmonary edema, often called "flash" pulmonary edema, is a severe, life-threatening condition. Classification of pulmonary edema is based on its causative origin: cardiogenic or noncardiogenic. Noncardiogenic pulmonary edema includes ARDS, neurogenic, re-expansion, and negative-pressure pulmonary edema. ARDS will be discussed later in this chapter, and cardiogenic pulmonary edema is discussed in Chapter 15.

Pathophysiology

In each type of pulmonary edema, capillary fluid leaks or is forced by high capillary hydrostatic pressure into alveolar spaces. The edematous alveoli are unable to participate in gas exchange, causing intrapulmonary shunting of blood and hypoxemia. The pathophysiology of cardiogenic pulmonary edema is discussed in Chapter 15. The most common form of noncardiogenic pulmonary is ARDS, a form of acute lung injury (ALI) in which a precipitating injury (direct or indirect) to the lung triggers a systemic inflammatory response that causes pulmonary capillaries to leak fluid into the alveoli. Neurogenic pulmonary edema can occur after epileptic seizures or injuries to the head, brain, or spine. It is theorized to occur as the result of the massive surge of central sympathetic output, which increases blood flow to pulmonary vasculature. The vasoconstriction causes elevations in hydrostatic pressure, which results in extravasation of fluid into the pulmonary interstitium. Re-expansion pulmonary edema may result from a rapid reinflation of the lung after removal of air from a pneumothorax or evacuation of fluid from a large pleural effusion or hemothorax. This rapid negative-pressure change within the lungs causes capillary fluid to be pulled into the alveolar spaces. This is similar to negative-pressure pulmonary edema, in which an obstruction in the trachea or large bronchi causes a person to attempt to forcefully inhale against a closed glottis or airway. This pulls fluid into the alveolar spaces. Common causes of this type of edema are choking, angioedema, and manual strangulation.

Clinical Manifestations and Assessment

Increasing respiratory distress, characterized by dyspnea, air hunger, and hypoxemia is present. Usually patients are very anxious and often agitated. As the fluid leaks into the alveoli and mixes with air, a foam or froth is formed (more common in cardiogenic edema). The patient coughs up (or the nurse suctions out) these foamy, frothy, and often blood-tinged or pink secretions. The patient experiences acute respiratory distress and may become confused or stuporous.

Auscultation reveals crackles in the lung bases (especially in the dependent lung areas) that rapidly progress toward the apices of the lungs. These crackles are caused by the movement of air through the alveolar fluid. Also patients may present with wheezing. The chest x-ray reveals increased bilateral interstitial markings, often in a patchy appearance, with or without cardiomegaly. The patient may have tachycardia. Pulse oximetry values begin to fall, and ABG analysis demonstrates worsening hypoxemia.

Medical Management

Management focuses on correcting the underlying disorder. If the pulmonary edema is cardiac in origin, then improvement in left ventricular function is the goal (see Chapter 15). Oxygen is administered to correct the hypoxemia; in some circumstances, intubation and mechanical ventilation are necessary. Noncardiogenic pulmonary edema treatment is aimed at treating the underlying cause of the ALI (i.e., infection), removing obstructions causing negative-pressure edema, and providing supportive care such as oxygen, mechanical ventilation, and judicious IV fluids.

Nursing Management

Nursing management includes assisting with administration of oxygen and intubation and mechanical ventilation if respiratory failure occurs. The nurse also administers medications (e.g., morphine, vasodilators, inotropic medications, diuretics, and pre- and afterload agents) as prescribed, and monitors the patient's responses.

PLEURAL CONDITIONS

Pleural conditions are disorders that involve the membranes covering the lungs (visceral pleura) and the surface of the chest wall (parietal pleura) or disorders affecting the pleural space. The most common pleural conditions are pleurisy, pleural effusions, and empyemas.

PLEURISY

Pathophysiology

Pleurisy (pleuritis) refers to inflammation of both layers of the pleurae (parietal and visceral). Pleurisy may develop in conjunction with pneumonia or an upper respiratory tract infection, TB, or collagen diseases; after trauma to the chest, pulmonary infarction, or PE; in patients with primary or metastatic cancer; and after **thoracotomy**. The parietal pleura has nerve endings; the visceral pleura does not. When the inflamed pleural membranes rub together during respiration (intensified on inspiration), the result is severe, sharp, knifelike pain.

Clinical Manifestations and Assessment

The key characteristic of pleuritic pain is its relationship to respiratory movement: Taking a deep breath, coughing, or sneezing worsens the pain. Pleuritic pain is limited in distribution rather than diffuse; it usually occurs only on one side. The pain may become minimal or absent when the breath is held, leading to rapid shallow breathing. It may be localized or may radiate to the shoulder or abdomen. Later, as pleural fluid accumulates, the pain decreases. A pleural friction rub may be heard on auscultation.

Medical and Nursing Management

The objectives of treatment are to discover the underlying condition causing the pleurisy and to relieve the pain. As the underlying disease (e.g., pneumonia, infection) is treated, the pleuritic inflammation usually resolves. At the same time, it is necessary to monitor for signs and symptoms of pleural effusion, such as shortness of breath, pain (typically sharp and worsens with inspiration), assumption of a position that decreases pain, decreased chest wall excursion, dullness to percussion in the area of the effusion, along with diminished breath sounds and absent tactile fremitus.

Prescribed analgesics and topical applications of heat or cold provide symptomatic relief. Nonsteroidal anti-inflammatory agents (NSAIDs) may provide pain relief while allowing the patient to take deep breaths and cough more effectively. If the pain is severe, a narcotic or an intercostal nerve block may be required.

PLEURAL EFFUSION AND EMPYEMA

Pleural effusion, a collection of fluid in the pleural space, is rarely a primary disease process but usually occurs secondary to other diseases (Fig. 10-6). Normally, the pleural space contains a small amount of fluid (20 to 25 cc), which acts as a lubricant that allows the pleural surfaces to move without friction. Pleural effusion may be a complication of heart failure, TB, pneumonia, pulmonary infections (particularly viral infections), nephrotic syndrome, connective tissue disease, pulmonary embolus, and neoplastic tumors. In addition, abdominal processes such as pancreatitis or cirrhosis

with ascites can cause pleural effusions. The most common malignancies associated with a pleural effusion are bronchogenic carcinoma and breast cancer. An empyema is an accumulation of thick, purulent fluid (pus) within the pleural space and is a type of pleural effusion.

Pathophysiology

In certain disorders, fluid may accumulate in the pleural space to a point at which it becomes clinically evident. This almost always has pathologic significance. A pleural effusion can be composed of a relatively clear fluid or it can be bloody or purulent. An effusion of clear fluid may be a transudate or an exudate. A transudate (filtrate of plasma that moves across intact capillary walls) occurs when factors influencing the formation and reabsorption of pleural fluid are altered, usually by imbalances in hydrostatic or oncotic pressures. The finding of a transudative effusion generally implies that the pleural membranes are not diseased. A transudative effusion most commonly results from heart failure or volume resuscitation causing volume overload. An exudate (extravasation of fluid into tissues or a cavity) usually results from inflammation by bacterial products or tumors involving the pleural surfaces. Empyemas are exudative pleural effusions by definition.

Most empyemas occur as complications of bacterial pneumonia or lung abscess, with streptococcus pneumonia being the most common causative microbe. They also result from penetrating chest trauma, hematogenous infection of the pleural space, nonbacterial infections, and iatrogenic causes (after thoracic surgery or thoracentesis). At first, the pleural fluid is thin, with a low leukocyte count, but it frequently progresses to a fibropurulent stage and, finally, to a stage at which it encloses the lung within a thick exudative membrane ("peel"). A chest x-ray, CT scan, or ultrasound determines whether fluid is free flowing or loculated (fixed pocket).

Clinical Manifestations and Assessment

Usually, the clinical manifestations are caused by the underlying disease. Pneumonia causes fever, chills, and pleuritic chest pain, whereas a malignant effusion may result in dyspnea, difficulty lying flat, and coughing. The severity of symptoms is determined by the size of the effusion, the speed of its formation, whether it is a transudate or exudate, and the underlying lung disease. A large pleural effusion causes dyspnea. A small to moderate pleural effusion usually causes minimal or no dyspnea. Patients with empyemas tend to be acutely ill, with more severe inflammatory symptoms (fever, chills, pain, cough, dyspnea, and tachycardia).

Assessment of the area of the pleural effusion reveals decreased or absent breath sounds, decreased fremitus, and a dull, flat sound on percussion. In the case of an extremely large or rapidly accumulating pleural effusion, the assessment reveals a patient in acute respiratory distress. The

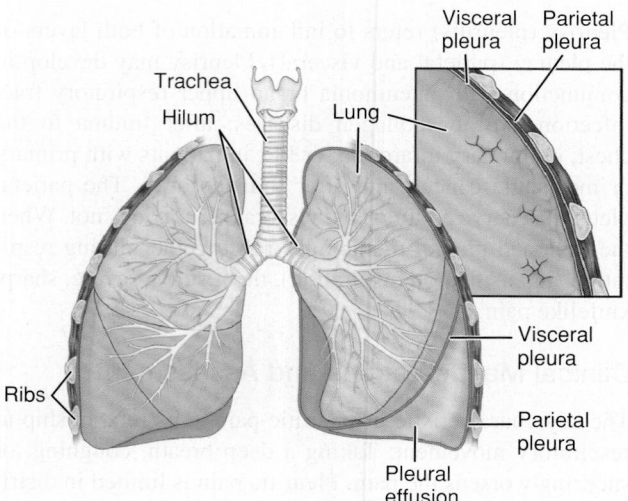

FIGURE 10-6 In pleural effusion, an abnormal volume of fluid collects in the pleural space, causing pain and shortness of breath. Pleural effusion is usually secondary to other disease processes.

patient may have tracheal deviation away from the affected side, hypoxemia (SpO_2 less than 90%), hypotension, and tachycardia.

Physical examination, chest x-ray, chest CT, ultrasound, and thoracentesis confirm the presence of fluid. In some instances, a lateral decubitus x-ray is obtained. For this x-ray, the patient lies on the unaffected side in a side-lying position. A pleural effusion can be diagnosed because this position allows for the "layering out" of the fluid, and an air-fluid line is visible.

Pleural fluid is analyzed by bacterial culture, Gram stain, AFB stain (for TB), red blood cell and WBC counts and differential, chemistry studies (glucose, amylase, lactic dehydrogenase, protein), cytologic analysis for malignant cells, and pH. A pleural biopsy also may be performed as a diagnostic tool.

Medical Management

The objectives of treatment are to discover the underlying cause of the pleural effusion; to prevent reaccumulation of fluid; and to relieve discomfort, dyspnea, and respiratory compromise. Specific treatment is directed at the underlying cause (e.g., heart failure, pneumonia, cirrhosis). If the pleural fluid is an exudate, more extensive diagnostic procedures are performed to determine the cause. Treatment for the primary cause is then instituted.

Thoracentesis is performed to remove fluid, to obtain a specimen for analysis, and to relieve dyspnea and respiratory compromise. Thoracentesis may be performed under ultrasound guidance or blindly. Depending on the size of the pleural effusion, the patient may be treated by removing the fluid during the thoracentesis procedure or by inserting a chest tube connected to a water-seal drainage system or suction to evacuate the pleural space and re-expand the lung. If the empyema is loculated, fibrinolytic agents, such as tissue plasminogen activator (TPA) and DNase, can be instilled via a chest tube to dissolve fibrinous septations and improve drainage (Rahman et al., 2011; Hedley et al., 2013; Mccool, 2016). Often surgical management via thoracotomy or video-assisted thoracoscopic surgery (VATS) with lung decortication is required for patients with acute respiratory compromise, sepsis, or hemodynamic instability. Decortication is the surgical removal of fibrous tissue in the pleural space; this procedure is called a *pleural peel.*

However, if the underlying cause is a malignancy, the effusion tends to recur within a few days or weeks. Repeated thoracenteses result in pain, depletion of protein and electrolytes, and sometimes pneumothorax. Once the pleural space is drained adequately, a chemical pleurodesis may be performed to obliterate the pleural space and prevent reaccumulation of fluid. Pleurodesis may be performed using either a VATS or a chest tube. A chemically irritating agent (e.g., talc, bleomycin, doxycycline) is instilled into the pleural space. With the chest tube approach, after the agent is instilled, the chest tube is clamped for 60 to 90 minutes, and the patient is assisted to assume various positions to promote uniform distribution of the agent and to maximize its contact with the pleural surfaces. The tube is unclamped as prescribed, and chest drainage may be continued several days longer to prevent reaccumulation of fluid and to promote the formation of adhesions between the visceral and parietal pleurae.

Other treatments for malignant pleural effusions include repeated needle thoracentesis, tube thoracostomy, chemical pleurodesis, surgical pleurectomy and decortication, pleuroperitoneal shunt, and tunneled pleural catheters (TPCs). Pleuracotomy involves the insertion of a small catheter attached to a drainage bottle for outpatient management (PleurX catheter [Denver Biomedical]), or implantation of a pleuroperitoneal shunt. A pleuroperitoneal shunt consists of two catheters connected by a pump chamber containing two one-way valves. Fluid moves from the pleural space to the pump chamber and then to the peritoneal cavity. The patient manually pumps on the reservoir daily to move fluid from the pleural space to the peritoneal space. Because pleuroperitoneal shunts have a median length of patency of 2.5 months due to clotting of the shunt (25% of the time), risk of shunt infection, and need for manual operation, pleuroperitoneal shunts have largely been replaced with TPCs (Thomas & Musani, 2013). The TPC catheter is a soft silicone tube inserted percutaneously as an outpatient, allowing the patient to return home with minimum sedation and less time spent in the hospital. Patients manage their catheter drainage in their home.

Nursing Management

The nurse's role in the care of patients with a pleural effusion or empyema includes implementing the medical regimen. The nurse prepares and positions the patient for thoracentesis and offers support throughout the procedure. The nurse is responsible for making sure the thoracentesis fluid amount is recorded and sent for appropriate laboratory testing. If a chest tube drainage and water-seal system is used, the nurse is responsible for monitoring the system's function and recording the amount of drainage at prescribed intervals. Nursing care related to the underlying cause of the pleural effusion is specific to the underlying condition. Pain management is a priority, and premedication for the procedure with a narcotic analgesic and antianxiety drug should be considered. If the patient is undergoing TPA/DNase or pleurodesis, the patient requires frequent turning and movement to facilitate adequate spreading of the agents over the pleural surface. Treatment of pleurisy pain is similar to the care of patients with chest tubes because the patient has considerable pain on inspiration. The nurse offers suggestions to enhance comfort, such as turning frequently onto the affected side to splint the chest wall and reduce the stretching of the pleurae. The nurse also teaches the patient to use the hands or a pillow to splint the rib cage while coughing.

Administration and assessment of the effects of narcotics or NSAIDs is necessary.

ACUTE RESPIRATORY FAILURE

Acute respiratory failure (ARF) is a sudden and life-threatening deterioration of the gas exchange function of the lung. It exists when the exchange of oxygen for carbon dioxide in the lungs cannot keep up with the rate of oxygen consumption and carbon dioxide production by the cells of the body. ARF is classified as hypoxemic (decrease in arterial oxygen tension [PaO$_2$] to less than 50 mm Hg on room air) and or hypercapnic (increase in arterial carbon dioxide tension [PaCO$_2$] to greater than 50 mm Hg with an arterial pH of less than 7.35).

It is important to distinguish between ARF and chronic respiratory failure. Chronic respiratory failure is defined as deterioration in the gas exchange function of the lung that has developed insidiously or has persisted for a long period. The absence of acute symptoms and the presence of a chronic respiratory acidosis (elevated PaCO$_2$ and bicarbonate, and hypoxemia) suggest the chronicity of the respiratory failure. Two causes of chronic respiratory failure are COPD (discussed in Chapter 11) and neuromuscular diseases (discussed in Chapter 46). Patients with these disorders develop a tolerance to the gradually worsening hypoxemia and hypercapnia. However, patients with chronic respiratory failure can develop ARF. For example, a patient with COPD may develop an exacerbation or infection that causes additional deterioration of gas exchange. The principles of management of acute versus chronic respiratory failure are different; the following discussion is limited to ARF.

Pathophysiology

In ARF, the ventilation or perfusion mechanisms in the lung are impaired. Impaired respiratory system mechanisms leading to ARF include:

- *Alveolar hypoventilation,* which is the inability to deliver oxygen to the alveoli and remove CO$_2$ from the alveoli, may be due to a variety of causes including obesity, chest wall deformities, neuromuscular disorders, CNS depression, or COPD.
- *Diffusion abnormalities* are related to problems with gas transfer across the alveolar–capillary membrane, which may be due to increased resistance, increased thickness of the alveolar–capillary membrane, or any pathology that impacts the alveolar epithelium, the capillary endothelium, or the interstitial space between them.
- *Ventilation–perfusion mismatching.* Alveolar ventilation brings oxygen to the lung and removes the alveolar CO$_2$ (ventilation), while blood brings CO$_2$ to the alveoli and takes up the O$_2$ from the alveoli (perfusion). Thus, the O$_2$ and CO$_2$ levels are determined by the matching of ventilation with perfusion.

- *Shunting* occurs when perfusion is adequate to the lung but ventilation is impaired, thus deoxygenated blood continues to the left side of the heart. (Conditions associated with this include right-to-left shunts with cardiac abnormalities such as septal defects, or pulmonary diseases such as pneumonia, ARDS, or pulmonary edema, in which the alveoli are affected and unable to be ventilated.)
- *Increased physiologic dead space,* which describes situations in which ventilation of the lung is adequate but perfusion is impaired, as with pulmonary emboli. This mismatch also results in impaired gas exchange.

Common causes of ARF can be classified into four categories: decreased respiratory drive, dysfunction of the chest wall, dysfunction of the lung parenchyma, and other causes.

Decreased Respiratory Drive

Decreased respiratory drive may occur with severe brain injury with increased intracranial pressure, lesions or trauma of the brainstem (multiple sclerosis, tumor, or herniation), use of sedative medications, and metabolic disorders such as severe hypothyroidism. These disorders impair the response of chemoreceptors in the brain to normal respiratory stimulation.

Dysfunction of the Chest Wall

The impulses arise in the respiratory center and travel through nerves that extend from the brainstem down the spinal cord to receptors in the muscles of respiration. Any disease or disorder of the nerves, spinal cord, muscles, or neuromuscular junction involved in respiration seriously affects ventilation and may ultimately lead to ARF. These include musculoskeletal disorders (muscular dystrophy, polymyositis, chest wall trauma), neuromuscular junction disorders (myasthenia gravis, poliomyelitis), some peripheral nerve disorders, and spinal cord disorders (amyotrophic lateral sclerosis, Guillain–Barré syndrome, and cervical spinal cord injuries). Chest wall trauma, such a flail chest, can cause instability of the thorax and impair ventilation.

 Nursing Alert
With cervical spinal injuries, the rigid cervical collar is left in place until the provider confirms stability of the C spine. The nurse is aware that motor innervations to the diaphragm are from the phrenic nerve at the C3–C5 level, thus any fracture in the area risks respiratory paralysis.

Dysfunction of Lung Parenchyma

Pleural effusion, hemothorax, pneumothorax, and airway obstruction are conditions that interfere with ventilation by preventing expansion of the lung. These conditions, which may cause respiratory failure, usually are produced by an underlying lung disease, pleural disease, or trauma and injury. Other diseases and conditions of lung parenchyma that lead to ARF include pneumonia, pulmonary contusions, status asthmaticus, atelectasis, PE, exacerbation of COPD, ARDS, and pulmonary edema.

Other Causes

In the postoperative period, especially after major thoracic or abdominal surgery, inadequate ventilation and respiratory failure may occur because of several factors. During this period, for example, ARF may be caused by the effects of anesthetic agents, analgesics, and sedatives, which may depress respiration (as described earlier) or enhance the effects of opioids and lead to hypoventilation. Pain may interfere with deep breathing and coughing.

Clinical Manifestations and Assessment

Early signs are those associated with impaired oxygenation and may include restlessness, fatigue, headache, dyspnea, air hunger, mild tachycardia and tachypnea, and increased BP. As the hypoxia progresses, more obvious signs may be present, including confusion, lethargy, tachycardia, tachypnea, **central cyanosis**, diaphoresis, and finally respiratory arrest. Physical findings are those of acute respiratory distress, including use of accessory muscles, decreased breath sounds if the patient cannot adequately ventilate, and other findings related specifically to the underlying disease process and cause of ARF.

Medical Management

The objectives of treatment are to correct the underlying cause and to restore adequate gas exchange in the lungs. Supplemental oxygen administration is used to improve hypoxemia. If narcotics are thought to be the cause of hypoventilation, reversal agents, such as naloxone (for opiates) or flumazenil (for benzodiazepines) can be administered. Mechanical ventilation may be required to maintain adequate ventilation and oxygenation while the underlying cause is corrected.

Nursing Management

Nursing management of patients with ARF includes assisting with intubation and maintaining mechanical ventilation. Usually patients are managed in the ICU. The nurse assesses the patient's respiratory status by monitoring the level of responsiveness, ABG levels, POX, and vital signs. In addition, the nurse assesses the entire respiratory system and implements strategies (e.g., turning schedule, mouth care, skin care, range-of-motion exercises for the extremities) to prevent complications. The nurse also assesses the patient's understanding of the management strategies that are used and initiates some form of communication to enable the patient to express concerns and needs to the health care team.

Finally, the nurse addresses the problems that led to the ARF. As the patient's status improves, the nurse assesses the patient's knowledge of the underlying disorder and provides teaching as appropriate to address the disorder.

ACUTE RESPIRATORY DISTRESS SYNDROME

Acute respiratory distress syndrome (ARDS) (previously called adult respiratory distress syndrome) is a severe form of **acute lung injury** that affects over 200,000 persons each year. This clinical syndrome is characterized by a sudden and progressive pulmonary edema, increasing bilateral infiltrates on chest x-ray, hypoxemia refractory to supplemental oxygen, and reduced lung compliance. These signs occur in the absence of left-sided heart failure. Patients with ARDS usually require mechanical ventilation with a higher-than-normal airway pressure. ARDS has been associated with a mortality rate as high as 50% to 60%. The major cause of death in ARDS is multisystem organ failure.

Pathophysiology

ARDS occurs as a result of an inflammatory trigger that initiates the release of cellular and chemical mediators, causing diffuse epithelial cell injury to the alveolar capillary membrane. This leads to leakage of protein-rich fluid and blood cells into the alveolar interstitial spaces and alterations in the capillary bed.

Severe ventilation–perfusion mismatching occurs in ARDS. Alveoli collapse because of the inflammatory infiltrate, blood, fluid, and surfactant dysfunction. Small airways are narrowed because of interstitial fluid and bronchial obstruction. Lung compliance becomes markedly decreased (stiff lungs), and the result is a characteristic decrease in functional residual capacity (FRC) and severe hypoxemia. The blood returning to the lung for gas exchange is pumped through the nonventilated, nonfunctioning areas of the lung, causing shunting. This means that blood is interfacing with nonfunctioning alveoli, and gas exchange is markedly impaired, resulting in severe, refractory hypoxemia. Figure 10-7 shows the sequence of pathophysiologic events leading to ARDS.

Risk Factors

A wide range of factors are associated with the development of ARDS, including direct injury to the lungs (e.g., smoke inhalation, near drowning) or indirect insult to the lungs (e.g., septic shock, massive fluid resuscitation) (see Box 10-8 for risk factors). Transfusion-related acute lung injury (TRALI) and transfusion-associated circulatory overload (TACO) are two forms of ALI that result from transfusion of blood products. TRALI is an immune reaction that causes an increase in pulmonary vascular permeability, and TACO causes an

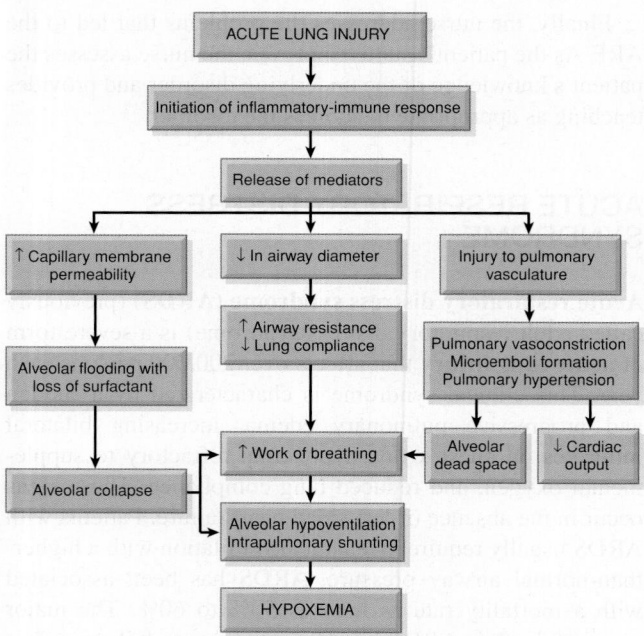

FIGURE 10-7 Pathogenesis of acute respiratory distress syndrome (ARDS).

increase in hydrostatic pressure, both causing pulmonary edema.

Clinical Manifestations and Assessment

Clinically, the acute phase of ARDS is marked by a rapid onset of severe dyspnea that usually occurs 12 to 48 hours after the initiating event. A characteristic feature is arterial

---

BOX 10-8
Risk Factors for Acute Respiratory Distress Syndrome (ARDS)

- Systemic sepsis (40%)
- Aspiration: near-drowning, aspiration of gastric contents (more than 30% of cases)
- Trauma (more than 20% of cases)
- Multiple transfusions, blood products
- Drugs (overdose of morphine, methadone, heroin; reaction to nitrofurantoin)
- Hematologic disorders (e.g., disseminated intravascular coagulopathy, massive transfusions, cardiopulmonary bypass)
- Noxious inhalation (high concentrations of oxygen; chlorine gas)
- Postresuscitation
- Localized infection
- Metabolic disorders (pancreatitis, uremia)
- Shock
- Major surgery
- Fat or air embolism

Adapted from Ferri (2016).

---

hypoxemia that does not respond to supplemental oxygen. On chest x-ray, the findings are similar to those seen with cardiogenic pulmonary edema and appear as bilateral, patchy infiltrates that quickly worsen. On chest CT, bilateral, patchy infiltrates with consolidation are usually more pronounced in the dependent (posterior) lung areas. The ALI then progresses to fibrosing alveolitis with persistent, severe hypoxemia. The patient also has increased alveolar dead space (ventilation to nonperfused alveoli) and decreased pulmonary compliance ("stiff lungs," which are difficult to ventilate). Clinically, the patient is thought to be in the recovery phase if the hypoxemia begins to resolve, the chest x-ray improves, and the lungs become more compliant.

Intercostal retractions and crackles, as the fluid begins to leak into the alveolar interstitial space, are evident on physical examination. ABGs are analyzed to assess the severity of hypoxemia. A diagnosis of ARDS may be made based on the following criteria: a history of systemic or pulmonary risk factors, acute onset of respiratory distress, bilateral pulmonary infiltrates, clinical absence of left-sided heart failure, and a ratio of PaO_2 to fraction of inspired oxygen (FiO_2) of less than 300 mm Hg (severe refractory hypoxemia). The normal ratio of PaO_2 to FiO_2 is over 300 mm Hg. Severity of ARDS is measured by calculation of PaO_2/FiO_2 ratio. A ratio of 200 to 300 is mild, 100 to 199 is moderate, and less than 100 is severe (Matthay & Slutsky, 2016).

> **Nursing Alert**
> A quick calculation the nurse can perform to assess the patient's pulmonary status is the ratio of the patient's arterial oxygen level (PaO_2), obtained from ABGs and the amount of oxygen inspired (FiO_2). This is also known as the P/F ratio. If the patient's PaO_2 is 75 mm Hg on 45% FiO_2, then the nurse converts the FiO_2 to a percentage. Thus an FiO_2 of 45% become 0.45. The simple calculation is 75/0.45, which equals a P/F ratio of 167, suggesting a moderate ARDS. To illustrate a patient with normal pulmonary function, an ABG may reveal a PaO_2 of 100 mm Hg on room air (FiO_2 of 21%); therefore the patient's PF ratio would be 100/0.21 = 476.

Medical Management

The primary focus in the management of ARDS includes identification and treatment of the underlying causative condition. Aggressive, supportive care must be provided to compensate for the severe respiratory dysfunction. This supportive therapy almost always includes intubation and mechanical ventilation. In addition, circulatory support, adequate fluid volume, and nutritional support are important. Supplemental oxygen is used as the patient begins the initial spiral of hypoxemia. As the hypoxemia progresses, intubation and mechanical ventilation are instituted. The concentration of oxygen and ventilator settings and modes are determined by the patient's status. This is monitored by ABG analysis, POX, and bedside pulmonary compliance testing.

Positive End-Expiratory Pressure

PEEP is a critical part of the treatment of ARDS. Use of PEEP helps increase FRC and reverse alveolar collapse by keeping the alveoli open, resulting in improved arterial oxygenation and a reduction in the severity of the ventilation–perfusion imbalance. Also the use of PEEP can allow for the use of lower, safer FiO_2 levels (60% or less FiO_2). The goal is a PaO_2 of greater than 60 mm Hg or an oxygen saturation level of greater than 90% at the lowest possible FiO_2. Evidence suggests that ARDS should be managed with a low tidal volume (6 cc/kg of ideal body weight), pressure-limited approach (plateau pressure of 30 mm Hg or less) with low or moderately high PEEP. Although the optimal level of PEEP has not been established, higher levels of PEEP may be beneficial for moderate to severe ARDS (Matthay & Slutsky, 2016).

The use of positive-pressure ventilation (as opposed to normal negative-pressure breathing) increases intrathoracic pressure and causes a decrease in preload to the heart. This drop in preload can result in decreased cardiac output and hypotension. Systemic hypotension also may occur in ARDS as a result of hypovolemia secondary to leakage of fluid into the interstitial spaces. Hypovolemia must be treated carefully without causing further fluid overload. IV crystalloid or colloid solutions are administered with careful monitoring of pulmonary status. Inotropic (e.g., dobutamine) or vasopressor agents (e.g., norepinephrine, dopamine, and epinephrine) may be required. Central venous catheters and, occasionally, pulmonary artery pressure catheters may be used to monitor the patient's fluid status and the severe and progressive pulmonary hypertension sometimes observed in ARDS. Arterial catheterization is required as patients with ARDS need frequent blood gas analysis.

Pharmacologic Therapy

Numerous pharmacologic treatments are under investigation to stop the cascade of events leading to ARDS; however, the mainstay of treatment is related to improving oxygenation and preventing complications. Thus prophylaxis for prevention of DVT and stress ulcer is common.

ARDS patients often require IV sedation and pain medication to combat anxiety and agitation from hypoxemia and intubation. In extreme cases, patients may require chemical paralysis with neuromuscular blockers in order to adequately ventilate and oxygenate them.

Nutritional Therapy

Adequate nutritional support is vital in the treatment of ARDS. Patients with ARDS require 20 to 25 kcal/kg/day to meet caloric requirements. Enteral feeding is the first consideration; however, parenteral nutrition also may be required (McClave et al., 2016).

Nursing Management

General Measures

A patient with ARDS is critically ill and requires close monitoring in the intensive care unit. Many different respiratory modalities can be used in this situation (oxygen administration, nebulizer therapy, CPT, endotracheal intubation or tracheostomy, mechanical ventilation, suctioning, bronchoscopy). Frequent assessment of the patient's status is necessary to evaluate the effectiveness of treatment.

In addition to implementing the medical plan of care, the nurse considers other patient needs. Positioning is important. The nurse turns the patient frequently to improve ventilation and perfusion in the lungs and enhance secretion drainage. However, the nurse must monitor the patient closely for deterioration in oxygenation with changes in position. Oxygenation in patients with ARDS is sometimes improved in the prone position, and data indicate this position reduces mortality in patients with moderate to severe ARDS (initial P/F less than 150 mm Hg) (Matthay & Slutsky, 2016). This position may be evaluated for improvement in oxygenation and used in special circumstances. Devices and specialty beds are available to assist the nurse in placing the patient in a prone position.

The patient can be extremely anxious and agitated because of the increasing hypoxemia, dyspnea, and intubation. The nurse explains all procedures and provides care in a calm, reassuring manner. It is important to reduce the patient's anxiety, because anxiety increases oxygen expenditure by preventing rest. Rest is essential to limit oxygen consumption and reduce oxygen needs.

Ventilator Considerations

If the patient is intubated and receiving mechanical ventilation with PEEP, several considerations must be addressed. PEEP is an unnatural pattern of breathing that feels strange to patients. The patients may be anxious and "fight" the ventilator. It is important for the nurse to assess for problems with ventilation that may be causing the anxiety reaction: tube blockage by kinking or retained secretions, other acute respiratory problems (e.g., pneumothorax, pain), a sudden decrease in the oxygen level, the level of dyspnea, or ventilator malfunction. In most cases, sedation may be required to decrease the patient's oxygen consumption, allow the ventilator to provide full support of ventilation, and decrease the patient's anxiety. Sedatives that may be used are lorazepam, midazolam, dexmedetomidine, and propofol. Judicious use of sedatives is necessary to prevent or reduce ICU delirium.

If satisfactory oxygen levels cannot be maintained despite the use of sedatives, neuromuscular blocking agents, such as pancuronium, vecuronium, atracurium, or rocuronium, may be administered to paralyze the patient. These agents paralyze skeletal muscles, including respiratory muscles, leading to respiratory arrest if the patient is not intubated and on adequate ventilator settings. With paralysis, the patient appears to be unconscious, loses motor function, and cannot breathe, talk, or blink independently. However, the patient retains sensation and is awake and able to hear. Paralytic agents should be used only by personnel who are trained in airway and ventilator management. The nurse must reassure the patient that the paralysis is a result of the medication and is temporary. Paralysis should be used for the shortest possible time and never without adequate sedation and pain management.

Use of paralytic agents has many dangers and side effects. The nurse must be sure the patient does not become disconnected from the ventilator because respiratory muscles are paralyzed and the patient will be apneic. Consequently, the nurse ensures that the patient is closely monitored, and all ventilator and patient alarms must be on at all times. Eye care is important as well, because the patient cannot blink, thus increasing the risk of corneal abrasions. Neuromuscular blockers predispose the patient to deep venous thrombosis (DVT), muscle atrophy, and skin breakdown; therefore, passive range-of-motion exercises and skin assessment are important nursing actions.

 Nursing Alert
If a patient is on concurrent administration of aminoglycosides and/or steroids, this increases the chance of the chemically paralyzed patient developing critical illness polyneuropathy. This is a severe form of muscle atrophy and deconditioning that can occur within 24 hours; it requires intensive physical therapy to correct, increases the patient's risks of developing complications, and prolongs hospital lengths of stay.

The patient may have discomfort or pain but cannot communicate these sensations. Signs of pain, such as tachycardia, diaphoresis, and hypertension, must be assessed for and treated. Analgesia **must** be administered concurrently with neuromuscular blocking agents. The nurse must anticipate the patient's needs regarding pain and comfort. The nurse checks the patient's position to ensure it is comfortable and in normal body alignment.

The nurse talks to, and not about, the patient while in the patient's presence; remember the patient is awake and able to hear. In addition, it is important for the nurse to describe the purpose and effects of the paralytic agents to the patient's family. If family members are unaware that these agents have been administered, they may become distressed by the change in the patient's status.

PULMONARY ARTERIAL HYPERTENSION

Pulmonary circulation is a low-pressure system intended to accommodate high blood flow from the right ventricle. The pulmonary vasculature is compliant and thin walled in order to facilitate gas exchange. The normal mean pulmonary pressure is 12 to 15 mm Hg with the capacity to dilate and constrict as needed. Pulmonary arterial hypertension (PAH) exists when the mean pulmonary artery pressure exceeds 25 mm Hg at rest or 30 mm Hg with activities. Unlike systemic BP, these pressures cannot be measured indirectly; instead, they must be measured via right-sided heart catheterization with a pulmonary artery catheter or estimated with an echocardiogram. In the absence of these measurements, clinical recognition becomes the only indicator for the presence of pulmonary hypertension; however, PAH is a condition that is not clinically evident until late in its progression.

There are two types of PAH: idiopathic PAH (formerly known as primary) and secondary PAH due to a known cause. Idiopathic PAH is a very uncommon disease. It occurs most often in women 20 to 40 years of age, either sporadically or in patients with a family history, and is usually fatal within 5 years of diagnosis. There are several possible causes, but the exact cause is unknown (Papadakis, McPhee, & Rabow, 2016).

In contrast, secondary PAH due to a known cause is more common and results from existing cardiac (left ventricular failure, mitral stenosis) or pulmonary disease (emphysema, pulmonary fibrosis, or thromboembolism). The prognosis depends on the severity of the underlying disorder and the changes in the pulmonary vascular bed. A common cause of PAH is pulmonary artery constriction due to chronic hypoxemia and hypercapnia from COPD (Box 10-9) (Papadakis et al., 2016). Conditions such as collagen vascular disease, congenital heart disease, portal hypertension, and HIV infection increase the risk for PAH in susceptible patients.

Pathophysiology

In patients with PAH, the pulmonary vasculature is injured, which leads to endothelial and smooth muscle thickening and hypertrophy, leading to noncompliant and narrowed vessels.

BOX 10-9 **Causes of Pulmonary Arterial Hypertension (PAH)**

- Collagen vascular diseases
- Congenital systemic-to-pulmonary shunts
- Portal hypertension
- Altered immune mechanisms (HIV infection)
- Diseases associated with significant venous or capillary involvement
- Chronic thrombotic or embolic disease
- Pulmonary venous hypertension
- Pulmonary vasoconstriction due to hypoxemia
- Chronic obstructive pulmonary disease (COPD), interstitial lung disease, sleep-disordered breathing
- Miscellaneous causes: Sarcoidosis, histiocytosis, compression of pulmonary vessels

Normally, the pulmonary vascular bed can handle the blood volume delivered by the right ventricle. It has a low resistance to blood flow and compensates for increased blood volume by dilation of the vessels in the pulmonary circulation. However, if the pulmonary vascular bed is destroyed or obstructed, the ability to handle whatever flow or volume of blood it receives is impaired, and the increased blood flow then increases the pulmonary artery pressure. As the pulmonary arterial pressure increases, the pulmonary vascular resistance also increases. This increased workload affects right ventricular function. The myocardium ultimately cannot meet the increasing demands imposed on it, leading to right ventricular hypertrophy (enlargement and dilation) and failure (cor pulmonale).

Clinical Manifestations and Assessment

Dyspnea, the main symptom of both types of PAH, occurs at first with exertion and eventually at rest. Other signs and symptoms include chest pain, weakness, fatigue, syncope, occasional hemoptysis, and signs of right-sided heart failure (peripheral edema, ascites, distended neck veins, hepatomegaly, crackles, heart murmur, splitting of second heart sound).

Diagnosis of idiopathic PAH is made by exclusion of secondary causes such as COPD, pulmonary emboli (PE), HIV, and cardiac disease. Several tests are used to determine whether there is a known cause for the pulmonary hypertension. Complete diagnostic evaluation includes a history, physical examination, chest x-ray, pulmonary function studies, electrocardiogram (ECG), echocardiogram, ventilation–perfusion scan ($\dot{V}/\dot{Q}$ scan), CT or magnetic resonance (MR) angiography, sleep studies, autoantibody tests (to identify diseases of collagen vascular origin), HIV tests, liver function testing, hypercoagulation studies, and cardiac catheterization. Pulmonary function studies may be normal or show a slight decrease in vital capacity and lung compliance with a mild decrease in the diffusing capacity. The PaO_2 also is decreased (hypoxemia). Complete blood count is usually normal but may show polycythemia (hematocrit of more than 54% in males or 51% in females). The ECG reveals right atrial enlargement (and tall peaked P waves in inferior leads), right axis deviation, right ventricular hypertrophy (tall R waves in V_2 and tall R waves in V_5); and ST-segment depression, T-wave inversion, or both in V_{1-4}. An echocardiogram can assess the progression of the disease and rule out other conditions with similar signs and symptoms. A $\dot{V}/\dot{Q}$ scan or pulmonary CT or MR angiography detects defects in pulmonary vasculature, such as pulmonary emboli. Cardiac catheterization of the right side of the heart reveals elevated pulmonary arterial pressure and determines whether there is a vasoactive component to the pulmonary hypertension. Acute vasodilator testing can be performed with the right heart catheterization to determine if there is a reduction in mean pulmonary artery pressure when a short-acting vasodilator (adenosine, epoprostenol, or inhaled nitric oxide) is administered. A

positive response is a decrease in mean PAP of more than 10 mm Hg to a value of less than 40 mm Hg, with increased or unchanged cardiac output (Ferri, 2016). Fewer than 10% of patients are responsive in idiopathic PAH, but these patients benefit from calcium-channel blockers.

Medical Management

The goal of treatment is to manage the underlying condition related to PAH of known cause. Hypoxemia, at rest or during exertion, should be treated with supplemental oxygen. Appropriate oxygen therapy can reverse the vasoconstrictive effect and reduce the pulmonary hypertension. Pharmacologic agents such as diuretics, digoxin, anticoagulant therapy (increased incidence of clots in pulmonary system), and calcium-channel blockers (nifedipine, diltiazem) (if they responded to the vasodilator testing described above) may be prescribed. Because calcium-channel blockers are effective in only a small percentage of patients, other treatment options, including prostacyclin, which acts as a potent vasodilator of pulmonary arteries and inhibitor of platelet aggregation, are often necessary (Ferri, 2016).

Vasodilating agents can be used to improve exercise tolerance and hemodynamic function as well as extend survival. Epoprostenol is given by continuous infusion, treprostinil by subcutaneous injection, bosentan and sildenafil by mouth, and iloprost by inhalation. Current therapies are not curative, have considerable side effects, and are often quite expensive. Lung or heart–lung transplantation is reserved for patients who have advanced disease despite maximal medical therapy (Hill, Cawley, & Heggen-Peay, 2016; Papadakis et al., 2016).

Nursing Management

The major nursing goal is to identify patients at high risk for PAH, such as those with COPD, pulmonary emboli, congenital heart disease, and mitral valve disease. The nurse also must be alert for signs and symptoms of deterioration such as worsening dyspnea, hypoxemia, and right ventricular failure. Oxygen therapy is administered as ordered, and the patient and family are instructed about the use of home oxygen supplementation. In patients treated with prostacyclin (i.e., epoprostenol or treprostinil), education about the need for central venous access (epoprostenol), or subcutaneous infusion (treprostinil) is discussed. In addition, the nurse reviews proper administration and dosing of the medication, usual side effects such as pain at the injection site, and potential severe side effects of hypotension, flushing of skin, bradycardia, and headache associated with IV administration. Emotional and psychosocial aspects of this disease must be addressed.

PULMONARY EMBOLISM

Pulmonary embolism (PE) refers to the obstruction of the pulmonary artery or one of its branches by a thrombus (or

BOX 10-10

Risk Factors for Thromboembolism

BOX 10-10

- Acute medical illness (CVA, acute MI, heart failure, neuromuscular diseases)
- Major surgery (abdominal, orthopedic, gynecologic, urologic, neurosurgical, oncologic)
- Trauma (multisystem trauma, spinal cord injury or fracture, hip or pelvic fractures)
- Cancer (localized or metastatic) receiving chemotherapy or radiation therapy
- History of thromboembolism
- Obesity
- Immobility for more than 2 days
- Age older than 40 years
- Hypercoagulable conditions
- Prolonged mechanical ventilation
- Neuromuscular paralytic use
- Central venous catheters
- Severe sepsis
- Heparin-induced thrombocytopenia (HIT)

thrombi) that originates somewhere in the venous system or right side of the heart. Hospitalized patients are at a high risk for PE; it is estimated that more than 900,000 people suffer from DVT/PE, and almost 100,000 deaths are attributed to PE annually (CDC, 2015c). It is the third leading cause of death in hospitalized patients, often not diagnosed until autopsy. PE is a common disorder and often is associated with trauma, arrhythmia (atrial fibrillation), surgery (orthopedic, major abdominal, pelvic, gynecologic), pregnancy, heart failure, malignancies, age greater than 50 years, hypercoagulable states, and prolonged immobility. It also may occur in apparently healthy people. Risk factors for thromboembolism are identified in Box 10-10.

Pathophysiology

Most commonly, PE is due to a blood clot or thrombus. However, there are other types of emboli: air, fat, amniotic fluid, tumor cells, intravenously injected particulates, and septic (from bacterial invasion of the thrombus). Although most thrombi originate in the deep veins of the legs, other sites include the pelvic veins and the right atrium of the heart. Venous thrombosis can result from slowing of blood flow (stasis) secondary to damage to the blood vessel wall (particularly the endothelial lining) or changes in the blood coagulation mechanism. In atrial fibrillation, blood stagnates in the fibrillating atria, and stagnant blood forms clots. These clots can travel into the pulmonary circulation.

When a thrombus completely or partially obstructs a pulmonary artery or its branches, the alveolar dead space is increased. Alveolar dead space is an area that is ventilated but receives little or no blood flow. Therefore, gas exchange is impaired or absent in this area. In addition, various vasoactive substances are released from the clot and surrounding area, and these cause regional blood vessels and bronchioles to constrict. The reflex bronchoconstriction and vasoconstriction causes impaired gas exchange and the loss of alveolar surfactant, which results in atelectasis and hypoxemia. The hemodynamic consequences are increased pulmonary vascular resistance and pulmonary artery pressures, which put a strain on the right ventricle. When the work requirements of the right ventricle exceed its capacity, right ventricular failure occurs, leading to a decrease in cardiac output followed by a decrease in systemic blood pressure and the development of shock.

Clinical Manifestations and Assessment

Symptoms depend on the size of the thrombus and the area of the pulmonary artery occluded by the thrombus. Acute onset of dyspnea is the most frequent symptom, followed by pleuritic chest pain, cough, hemoptysis, and palpitations. The most common signs found on physical assessment are tachypnea, crackles, tachycardia, and presence of an S_4 heart sound and split S_2. Deep venous thrombosis (DVT) is closely associated with development of PE. Typically, these patients report sudden onset of pain and/or swelling and warmth of the proximal or distal extremity, skin discoloration (red or dusky blue in color), and superficial vein distention.

Shock can develop with massive PEs ("saddle" embolisms) or in patients with pre-existing heart failure. Pronounced dyspnea, sudden substernal pain, rapid and weak pulse, hypotension, syncope, and sudden death can occur. Multiple small emboli can lodge in the terminal pulmonary arterioles, producing multiple small infarctions of the lungs. A pulmonary infarction causes necrosis of an area of the lung. The clinical picture may mimic that of bronchopneumonia or heart failure. In atypical instances, PE causes few signs and symptoms, whereas in other instances it mimics various other cardiopulmonary disorders.

Death from PE commonly occurs within hours of the onset of symptoms; therefore, early recognition and diagnosis are priorities. Because the symptoms of PE can vary from mild to severe, a diagnostic workup is performed to rule out other diseases. The initial diagnostic workup includes chest x-ray, ECG, peripheral vascular studies (duplex ultrasound, venogram), ABG analysis, and D-dimer.

The chest x-ray is most helpful in excluding other possible causes such as pneumonia, COPD, and pulmonary edema due to heart failure. ABG analysis may show hypoxemia and hypocapnia (from tachypnea); however, ABG measurements may be normal even in the presence of PE. The classic ECG pattern associated with PE, although rare, is S_1, Q_3, T_3, meaning a deep S wave in lead I, a Q wave in lead III and an inverted T wave in lead III. More common ECG findings are sinus tachycardia, PR-interval depression, and nonspecific T-wave changes. Peripheral vascular studies used to diagnose a DVT may include impedance plethysmography, Doppler ultrasonography, or venography. If a DVT is present with the associated signs and symptoms of PE, the patient is treated for both. The D-dimer assay is used to evaluate patients with possible PE. Emergency departments in particular have used this as a rapid, cost-effective test. D-dimer is a product of fibrin degradation and occurs as a result of fibrin lysis. D-dimer is used only to rule out a PE; as a negative result, it has a 95% predictive ability, meaning 95% of patients with PE have an elevated D-dimer. If the D-dimer is negative, the diagnosis of PE is excluded, whereas a positive test generally prompts a computed tomographic pulmonary angiography (CTPA) (Weitz, 2016), or spiral CT. For most patients with suspected PE, CTPA is the first-choice diagnostic imaging modality because it is sensitive and specific for the diagnosis of PE (Thompson, 2016).

Nursing Alert
The nurse understands that there is a higher rate of false-positive D-dimers in patients with acute illness, those over 50 years, pregnant women, and those with kidney disease (Thompson, 2016).

If a facility does not have access to a spiral CT scanner or CTPA, a $\dot{V}/\dot{Q}$ scan is ordered. The $\dot{V}/\dot{Q}$ scan was once the second choice for diagnosis of a PE (with pulmonary angiogram [discussed below] considered the best diagnostic procedure). It is minimally invasive, involving the administration of a radioactive agent (both IV and inhaled). This scan evaluates different regions of the lung (upper, middle, lower) and allows comparisons of the percentage of ventilation and perfusion in each area. This test has a high sensitivity but can be more cumbersome than a CT scan and is not as accurate as a pulmonary angiogram. Patients who have an underlying lung disease, such as COPD or pneumonia, often have inconclusive $\dot{V}/\dot{Q}$ scan results; also patients who are mechanically ventilated cannot undergo this test.

Contrast angiogram CT scan has gained popularity for use in the diagnosis of PE. Limitations to the use of CT scanning are that patients must be cooperative and able to have IV contrast (no contrast allergies, normal renal function), and it is less sensitive than a pulmonary angiogram. Pulmonary angiography allows for the visualization of the pulmonary vasculature under fluoroscopy with IV contrast. It requires interventional radiologists to perform the test with specific equipment and personnel that may not be available in many hospitals, and the test is costly.

Prevention

For patients at risk for PE, the most effective approach for prevention is to prevent DVT. General preventive measures include active leg exercises to avoid venous stasis, early ambulation, and use of elastic compression or intermittent pneumatic compression stockings.

Prophylactic anticoagulation therapy is prescribed based on assessment of a patient's risk level. Table 10-3 illustrates the risk stratification and recommended prophylaxis. Anticoagulant therapy may be prescribed for patients who are older than 40 years of age, whose hemostasis is adequate, and who are undergoing major abdominal or thoracic surgery. Low doses of heparin may be administered before surgery to reduce the risk of postoperative DVT and PE. Heparin should be administered subcutaneously 2 hours before surgery and continued every 8 to 12 hours until the patient is discharged. Low-dose heparin is thought to enhance the activity of antithrombin III, a major plasma inhibitor of clotting factor X. This regimen is not recommended for patients with an active thrombotic process or for those undergoing major orthopedic surgery, open prostatectomy, or surgery on the eye or brain. Low–molecular-weight heparins (e.g., enoxaparin [Lovenox], dalteparin [Fragmin], fondaparinux [Arixtra]) are additional therapies. They have a longer half-life, enhanced subcutaneous absorption, a reduced incidence of thrombocytopenia, and reduced interaction with platelets, compared with unfractionated heparin (Kearon et al., 2016).

Often sequential compression devices (SCDs) are used to prevent venous stasis through compression and relaxation of the calf muscles, similar to the effect of muscle contraction. SCDs have been proved to effectively reduce the risk of DVT and have been shown to be an effective primary therapy for patients who are unable to receive anticoagulation therapy, but a combination of pharmacologic agents with SCDs is more effective (Kakkos et al., 2011). Several types of SCDs, using foot, calf, and thigh-high compression as well as graduated, asymmetric, and circumferential compression, are available. There is little evidence favoring any particular type of compression. Graduated compression involves the sequential movement of air in the sleeve up the leg, followed by relaxation of the sleeve. The advantage of this therapy is the extended duration of compression compared with standard inflation. Asymmetric compression involves inflating only the area on the back of the leg or foot, whereas, circumferential compression involves even compression of the entire leg. Assessment of the patient's skin is an important nursing function when SCDs are in use.

Medical Management

Because PE is often a medical emergency, emergency management is of primary concern. After emergency measures have been initiated and the patient is stabilized, the treatment goal is to dissolve (lyse) the existing emboli and prevent new ones from forming. Treatment may include a variety of modalities:

- General measures to improve respiratory and vascular status
- Anticoagulation therapy
- Thrombolytic therapy
- Surgical intervention

TABLE 10-3 Recommended Deep Vein Thrombosis Prophylaxis

Risk Level	Recommended Prophylaxis
Low risk:	Early mobilization mechanical aid (intermittent pneumatic compression devices) until ambulatory (>300 feet/day)
Minor surgery + age under 40 years and no additional DVT risk factors	Mechanical aid (intermittent pneumatic compression devices) until ambulatory
Moderate risk: Major surgery + age over 40 years and no additional DVT risk factors	Mechanical aid (intermittent pneumatic) until ambulatory >300 feet per day OR Heparin: 5,000 units SC q12h (start 2 hours prior to surgery) or Enoxaparin) 40 mg. SC daily or Dalteparin 2,500 units SC daily
High risk: Major surgery + Age over 40 years and/or other DVT risk factors	Mechanical aid (intermittent pneumatic compression or graded compression stockings) AND Heparin 5,000 units SC q8h (start 2 hours prior to surgery) or Enoxaparin 40 mg SC daily or Dalteparin 5,000 units SC daily
Hip arthroplasty	Enoxaparin 30 mg SC q 12 hours × 10–14 days Fondaparinux 2.5 mg SC daily × 10–14 days Dabigatran 220 mg PO daily × 28–35 days Warfarin (INR 2.0–3.0) for 14–21 days
Knee arthroplasty	Enoxaparin 30 mg SC q 12 hours × 10–14 days Apixaban 2.5 mg PO BID × 12 days Edoxaban 30 mg PO daily × 11–14 days Rivaroxaban 10 mg PO daily × 12 days Warfarin (target INR 2.0–3.0) for 14–21 days

Emergency Management

Massive PE is a life-threatening emergency. The immediate objective is to stabilize the cardiopulmonary system. A sudden increase in pulmonary resistance increases the work of the right ventricle, which can cause acute right-sided heart failure with cardiogenic shock. Emergency management consists of the following actions:

- Oxygen is administered immediately to relieve hypoxemia, respiratory distress, and central cyanosis.
- Intravenous infusion lines are inserted to establish routes for medications or fluids that will be needed.
- A perfusion scan, hemodynamic measurements, and ABG determinations are performed. CT angiogram or pulmonary angiography may be performed.
- An echocardiogram can be done at the bedside to assess right ventricular function.
- Hypotension is treated with IV fluid resuscitation, vasopressors (dopamine, norepinephrine, epinephrine) or inotropic support (dobutamine).
- The ECG is monitored continuously for arrhythmias and right ventricular failure, which may occur suddenly.
- Digitalis glycosides, IV diuretics, and antiarrhythmic agents are administered when appropriate.
- Blood is drawn for serum electrolytes, complete blood count, and coagulation studies (PT, international normalized ratio [INR], partial thromboplastin time [PTT], D-dimer).

- If clinical assessment and ABG analysis indicate the need, the patient is intubated and placed on a mechanical ventilator.
- If the patient has suffered massive embolism and is hypotensive, an indwelling urinary catheter is inserted to monitor urinary output.
- Small doses of IV morphine or sedatives are administered to relieve patient anxiety, to alleviate chest discomfort, to improve tolerance of the endotracheal tube, and to ease adaptation to the mechanical ventilator.
- IV thrombolytic agents (tissue plasminogen activator [Alteplase, Reteplase]) may be used in patients who are hemodynamically unstable (hypotension, ECG strain patterns or echocardiographic evidence of right ventricular strain or failure) to lyse the clot(s).
- Initiation of low–molecular-weight heparins (SC route) or IV heparin should be considered.

Pharmacologic Therapy

Anticoagulation Therapy

Anticoagulant therapy (unfractionated or low–molecular-weight heparins) is traditionally the primary method for managing acute DVT and PE. Heparin is used to prevent recurrence of emboli but has no effect on emboli that are already present. Heparin is generally recommended for all patients who have been diagnosed with PE and should be administered by continuous intravenous infusion and dosed using weight-based nomograms. In general, a therapeutic heparin dose is administered as a one-time 80 units/kg bolus, and then a continuous IV infusion (18 units/kg/hr) is started to maintain the PTT at 1.5 to 2.5 times the normal level (Weitz, 2016). Rapid achievement and maintenance of a therapeutic PTT are important to reduce the risk for recurrent PE. In addition to examining the PTT, a complete blood count is monitored, generally a minimum of two to three times per week due to the risk for bleeding and heparin-induced thrombocytopenia (HIT), discussed in Chapter 14 (Weitz, 2016). Enoxaparin, a low–molecular-weight heparin, is administered subcutaneously at 1 mg/kg every 12 hours. This should be reserved for hemodynamically stable patients in order to ensure that the drug is being absorbed into the vasculature. Enoxaparin has an advantage over heparin as its levels do not need to be monitored and IV access is not an issue (Marino, 2014).

Therapy may be changed to an oral regimen, such as warfarin, as soon as the patient is able to take oral medications. Heparin must be continued until the INR is within a therapeutic range, typically 2.0 to 3 (Weitz, 2016). Once the patient starts an oral regimen, it is important that he or she continues to take the same brand of warfarin because the bioavailability may vary greatly among brands.

High doses of subcutaneous low–molecular-weight heparin or heparinoids may also be used to maintain a therapeutic PTT while oral anticoagulation therapy is being adjusted. Lepirudin (Refludan) and argatroban are alternatives for patients in whom heparin or heparinoids are contraindicated (e.g., patients with HIT). These agents are direct thrombin inhibitors; therefore, they require less frequent monitoring and dose adjustment. Both medications have contraindications and side effects that the nurse must be aware of before administration. Heparins, lepirudin, and argatroban are all contraindicated in patients with overt major bleeding and in patients who are hypersensitive to these agents or at high risk for bleeding (e.g., recent CVA), anomaly of vessels or organs, recent major surgery, recent puncture of large vessels, or organ biopsy. Major side effects are bleeding anywhere in the body and anaphylactic reaction resulting in shock or death. Other side effects include fever, abnormal liver function, and allergic skin reaction. Patients must continue to take some form of anticoagulation for at least 3 to 6 months after the embolic event.

Novel oral anticoagulants such as apixaban and rivaroxaban (factor Xa inhibitors) are now approved for the initial treatment of DVT and PE. Dabigatran (direct thrombin inhibitor) and edoxaban (factor Xa inhibitor) are approved for treatment or DVT and PE after initial therapy with parenteral anticoagulation is used (Meyer, Vieillard-Baron, & Planquette, 2016). These agents have the advantage of not requiring monitoring of INR or PTT levels, but renal function must be assessed during therapy (refer to Chapter 18 for more details on DVT).

Thrombolytic Therapy

Thrombolytic therapy (urokinase, streptokinase, alteplase, anistreplase, reteplase) also may be used in treating PE, particularly for patients who are severely compromised (e.g., those who are hypotensive, RV dysfunction, patent foramen ovale, large or saddle embolism, or have significant hypoxemia despite oxygen supplementation). Thrombolytic therapy dissolves the thrombi or emboli more quickly and restores more normal hemodynamic functioning of the pulmonary circulation, thereby reducing pulmonary hypertension and improving perfusion, oxygenation, and cardiac output. However, bleeding is a significant side effect. Absolute contraindications to thrombolytic therapy include history of hemorrhagic CVA, active intracranial neoplasm, recent brain or spinal surgery (less than 2 months), and internal bleeding within the last 6 months. Relative contraindications for thrombolytic therapy are bleeding tendency, uncontrolled hypertension (SBP greater than 200 or DBP greater than 100), nonhemorrhagic CVA within 2 months, surgery in the last 10 days, or thrombocytopenia of less than 100,000 platelets per mm^3.

Before thrombolytic therapy is started, INR, PTT, hematocrit, and platelet counts are obtained. Heparin is stopped prior to administration of a thrombolytic agent. During therapy, all but essential invasive procedures are avoided because of potential bleeding. If necessary, packed red cells, cryoprecipitate, or frozen plasma is administered to replace blood loss and reverse the bleeding tendency. After the thrombolytic infusion is completed (which varies in duration according to the agent used and the condition being treated), anticoagulant therapy is initiated.

Surgical Management

A surgical embolectomy is rarely performed but may be indicated if the patient has a massive PE or hemodynamic instability and must have the clot removed to help reduce right-sided heart failure, or if there are contraindications to thrombolytic therapy. This invasive procedure involves removal of the actual clot and must be performed by a cardiovascular surgical team with the patient on cardiopulmonary bypass. The procedure has a high intraoperative mortality rate and has typical postoperative complications.

Venous catheter embolectomy via rheolytic (injection of pressured saline or TPA) or rotating blades can be used to break up clots in the pulmonary vasculature. These catheters are placed via the femoral vein, threaded through the right heart, and up to the clot. An inferior vena cava (IVC) filter is usually inserted at the time of surgery to protect against a recurrence.

IVC filters are mesh-like devices used to trap thrombi from the pelvic and lower extremities to prevent them from traveling to the lungs. The IVC filters can be either permanent or retrievable. Recent research reveals that the filters

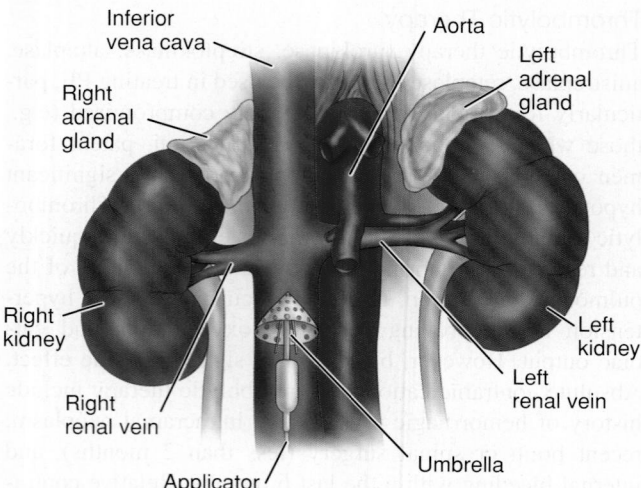

FIGURE 10-8 An umbrella filter is in place in the inferior vena cava to prevent pulmonary embolism. The filter (compressed within an applicator catheter) is inserted through an incision in the right internal jugular vein. The applicator is withdrawn when the filter fixes itself to the wall of the inferior vena cava after ejection from the applicator.

do not have prolonged survival, in part because permanent filters can be associated with complications such as IVC occlusion because of clots, and recurrent DVT. Alternatively retrievable filters have recently been noted for problems of device migration or thrombosis in up to 10% of patients. Thus the insertion of IVC filters generally is restricted to patients who have high risk for recurrent PE and an absolute contraindication for anticoagulation, experience significant bleeding while on anticoagulation, or have recurrent PE despite adequate treatment. The IVC filters (e.g., Greenfield filter) are inserted via the femoral or internal jugular vein (Fig. 10-8). This filter is advanced into the IVC, where it is opened.

Nursing Management

Minimizing the Risk of Pulmonary Embolism

A key role of the nurse is to identify the patient at high risk for PE and to minimize the risk of PE in all patients. The nurse must have a high degree of suspicion for PE in all patients but particularly in those with conditions predisposed to a slowing of venous return.

Preventing Thrombus Formation

Preventing thrombus formation is a major nursing responsibility. The nurse encourages ambulation and active and passive leg exercises to prevent venous stasis in patients who are prescribed bed rest. The nurse instructs the patient to move the legs in a "pumping" exercise so that the leg muscles can help increase venous flow. The nurse also advises the patient not to sit or lie in bed for prolonged periods, not to cross the legs, and not to wear constrictive clothing. Legs should not be dangled or feet placed in a dependent position while the patient sits on the edge of the bed; instead, feet should rest on the floor or on a chair. In addition, IV catheters (for parenteral therapy or measurements of central venous pressure) should not be left in place for prolonged periods.

Assessing Potential for Pulmonary Embolism

All patients are evaluated for risk factors for thrombus formation and PE. The nurse does a careful assessment of the patient's health history, family history, and medication record. On a daily basis, the patient is asked about pain or discomfort in the extremities. In addition, the extremities are evaluated for unilateral leg warmth, redness, and inflammation.

Monitoring Thrombolytic Therapy

The nurse is responsible for monitoring thrombolytic and anticoagulant therapy. Thrombolytic therapy (streptokinase, urokinase, tissue plasminogen activator) causes lysis of deep vein thrombi and pulmonary emboli, which helps dissolve the clots. During thrombolytic infusion, while the patient remains on bed rest, vital signs are assessed every 15 minutes for 2 hours, then every 2 hours for 4 hours, and invasive procedures are avoided. PTT testing should be performed every 6 hours after thrombolytics are started.

 Nursing Alert
The activated PTT (APTT) is a more sensitive test than the PTT for the monitoring of heparin therapy. A normal APTT is 21 to 35 seconds. The goal of heparin therapy is to extend the APTT to 2 or 2.5 the normal level. The nurse is aware that when the APTT is over 70 seconds, the risk for spontaneously bleeding increases. Many institutions have protocols for increasing or decreasing the heparin dosage depending on the APTT. The nurse follows hospital protocol but anticipates that if the APTT is over 90 seconds to stop the anticoagulant for 1 hour and restart as mandated by protocol, typically at a lower rate per hour. In general, heparin infusion should be restarted (without a bolus) when PTT is less than 60 seconds. If no protocols are available, the nurse contacts the provider immediately with APTTs of greater than 90 seconds.

The INR was developed as a consistent way of monitoring prothrombin times, which are used for monitoring Coumadin therapy. A normal INR is about 1. The goal of Coumadin therapy is to extend the INR to 2 to 3, depending on the reason the patient is anticoagulated. The higher the number, the longer the blood takes to clot. A patient with atrial fibrillation may have a goal INR of 2.5, whereas a patient with a mechanical heart valve may have a maximum goal of an INR of 3.5. Any INR over 3.6 is a critical value that necessitates notification of the patient's provider. With an elevated APTT and/or INR, the nurse observes the patient for hematuria, hematemesis, melena, petechiae, unusual bruising, and any evidence of bleeding (hypotension, tachycardia, dyspnea, etc.) (Fischbach & Dunning, 2014; Smithburger, Campbell, & Kane-Gill, 2013).

Managing Pain

Chest pain, if present, is usually pleuritic rather than cardiac in origin. A semi-Fowler position provides a more comfortable position for breathing. It is important to continue to turn patients frequently and reposition them to improve the **ventilation–perfusion ratio** in the lung. The nurse administers opioid analgesics as prescribed for severe pain.

Managing Oxygen Therapy

It is important to ensure that the patient understands the need for continuous oxygen therapy. The nurse assesses the patient frequently for signs of hypoxemia and monitors the POX values to evaluate the effectiveness of the oxygen therapy. Deep breathing and IS are indicated for all patients to minimize or prevent atelectasis and improve ventilation. Nebulizer therapy or percussion and postural drainage may be used for management of secretions.

Relieving Anxiety

The nurse encourages the stabilized patient to talk about any fears or concerns related to this frightening episode, answers the patient's and family's questions concisely and accurately, explains the therapy, and describes how to recognize untoward effects early.

Monitoring for Complications

When caring for a patient who has had PE, the nurse must be alert for the potential complication of cardiogenic shock or right ventricular failure subsequent to the effect of PE on the cardiovascular system.

Providing Postoperative Care

The nurse measures the patient's pulmonary arterial pressure or central venous pressure (CVP), and urinary output. The nurse also assesses the insertion site of the arterial catheter for hematoma formation and infection. It is important to maintain the BP at a level that supports perfusion of vital organs. To prevent peripheral venous stasis and edema of the lower extremities, the nurse encourages isometric exercises, use of elastic compression stockings or SCDs, and walking when the patient is permitted out of bed. Sitting is discouraged, because hip flexion compresses the large veins in the legs.

Nursing Alert
The nurse is aware that a mean arterial pressure (MAP) of 65 mm Hg is recommended to maintain adequate tissue perfusion.

OCCUPATIONAL LUNG DISEASES

Diseases of the lungs occur in numerous occupations as a result of exposure to several different types of agents. Examples include mineral dusts (asbestos, silica, coal), metal dusts, biologic dusts (spores, mycelia, bird droppings), manufactured fibers (glass or ceramic fibers), and toxic fumes (nitrogen dioxide, sulfur dioxide, chlorine, ammonia). One category of occupational lung disease that causes chronic fibrotic lung disease is pneumoconiosis, which is caused by the inhalation of inert, inorganic, or silicate dusts. The effects of inhaling these materials depend on the composition of the substance, its concentration, its ability to initiate an immune response, its irritating properties, the duration of exposure, and the individual's response or susceptibility to the irritant. The most common types of pneumoconiosis are coal worker's pneumoconiosis, silicosis, and **asbestosis**. Smoking may compound the problem and may increase the risk of lung cancers in people exposed to the mineral asbestos and other potential carcinogens. Many people with early pneumoconiosis are asymptomatic, but advanced disease often is accompanied by disability and premature death. Between 1996 and 2005, pneumoconiosis was cited as the cause of death of 9,646 people in the United States (CDC, 2014a).

Silicosis is a chronic fibrotic pulmonary disease caused by inhalation of silica dust (silicon dioxide). Exposure to silica and silicates occurs in almost all mining, quarrying, and tunneling operations. Glass manufacturing, stonecutting, manufacturing of abrasives and pottery, and foundry work are other occupations with exposure hazards. Finely ground silica, such as that found in soaps, polishes, and filters, is extremely dangerous (Papadakis, McPhee, & Rabow, 2016).

Asbestosis is a disease characterized by diffuse nodular interstitial fibrosis from the inhalation of asbestos dust. Current laws restrict the use of asbestos, but many industries used it in the past. Therefore, exposure occurred, and may still occur, in people in numerous occupations, including asbestos mining and manufacturing, shipbuilding, demolition of structures containing asbestos, and roofing. Materials such as shingles, cement, vinyl asbestos tile, fireproof paint and clothing, brake linings, and filters all contained asbestos at one time, and many of these materials are still in existence. Chronic exposure may also occur by washing clothes that have been in contact with asbestos. Additional diseases related to asbestos exposure include lung cancer, mesothelioma, and asbestos-related pleural effusion (Papadakis, McPhee, & Rabow, 2016).

Coal worker's pneumoconiosis ("black lung disease") includes a variety of respiratory diseases found in coal workers who have inhaled coal dust over the years. Coal miners are exposed to dusts that are mixtures of coal, kaolin, mica, and silica (Papadakis, McPhee, & Rabow, 2016).

Pathophysiology

The pathophysiology of each type of pneumoconiosis (any chronic lung disease caused by the inhalation of particles) begins with the inhalation and deposition of industrial dusts or particles in the lungs. In silicosis, the inhaled silica particles form nodular lesions throughout the lungs. With the passage of time and further exposure, the nodules enlarge and coalesce. Dense masses form in the upper portion of the lungs, resulting in the loss of pulmonary volume. **Restrictive lung disease** (disease of the lungs that limits their ability to expand fully) and obstructive lung disease from secondary emphysema result. Cavities can form as a result of superimposed TB. Exposure of 15 to 20 years is usually required before the onset of the disease and shortness of breath occurs. Fibrotic destruction of pulmonary tissue can lead to emphysema, pulmonary hypertension, and cor pulmonale (right ventricular failure).

In asbestosis, inhaled asbestos fibers enter the alveoli, where they are surrounded by fibrous tissue. The fibrous tissue eventually obliterates the alveoli. Fibrous changes also affect the pleura, which thickens and develops plaque. The result of these physiologic changes is a restrictive lung disease, with a decrease in lung volume, diminished exchange of oxygen and carbon dioxide, and hypoxemia.

When coal dust is deposited in the alveoli and respiratory bronchioles, macrophages engulf the particles (by phagocytosis) and transport them to the terminal bronchioles, where they are removed by mucociliary action. In time, the clearance mechanisms cannot handle the excessive dust load, and the macrophages aggregate in the respiratory bronchioles and alveoli. Fibroblasts appear and a network of reticulin (similar in composition to collagen) is laid down surrounding the dust-laden macrophages. The bronchioles and the alveoli become clogged with coal dust, dying macrophages, and fibroblasts. This leads to the formation of the coal macule, the primary lesion of the disorder. Macules appear as blackish dots on the lungs. Fibrotic lesions develop and, as the macules enlarge, the weakening bronchioles dilate, with subsequent development of localized emphysema. The disease begins in the upper lobes of the lungs but may progress to the lower lobes.

Clinical Manifestations and Assessment

Patients with acute silicosis present with dyspnea, fever, cough, and weight loss, and progression of the disease is rapid. Symptoms are more severe in patients whose disease is complicated by progressive massive fibrosis. More commonly, this disease is a chronic problem with a long latency period. In patients with asbestosis, the onset of the disease is insidious, and patients have progressive dyspnea, persistent, dry cough, mild to moderate chest pain, anorexia, weight loss, and malaise. Early physical findings include bibasilar fine, end-inspiratory crackles, and, in more advanced cases, clubbing of the fingers. Patients with coal miner's disease usually present with a chronic cough and sputum production, similar to the signs encountered in chronic bronchitis. As the disease progresses, patients develop dyspnea and cough up large amounts of sputum with varying amounts of black fluid (melanoptysis), particularly if they are smokers.

As each of these diseases progresses, worsening dyspnea and hypoxemia occur. Eventually, patients develop respiratory failure and cor pulmonale. A high proportion of workers who have been exposed to asbestos dust, especially those who smoke or have a history of smoking, die of lung cancer. Malignant mesothelioma, a rare cancer of the pleura or peritoneum that is strongly associated with asbestos exposure, may also occur.

Medical Management

The medical treatment for these specific pneumoconioses is limited to supportive care, as the fibrotic process is irreversible. Oxygen therapy, diuretics, inhaled beta-adrenergic agonists, anticholinergics, and bronchodilator therapy can be used to maximize pulmonary and cardiac function and preserve activity tolerance. It is imperative that patients avoid any additional environmental exposures and stop smoking. There is a higher incidence of TB in patients with silicosis; therefore, they should have a tuberculin skin test and chest radiograph. Preventing this disease is key because there is no effective treatment. Instead, treatment focuses on early diagnosis and management of complications.

CHEST TUMORS

Tumors of the lung may be benign or malignant. A malignant chest tumor can be primary, arising within the lung, chest wall, or mediastinum, or it can be a metastasis from a primary tumor site elsewhere in the body. Metastatic lung tumors occur frequently because the bloodstream transports cancer cells from primary cancers elsewhere in the body to the lungs.

LUNG CANCER (BRONCHOGENIC CARCINOMA)

Lung cancer is the leading cancer killer among men and women in the United States. In 2012, 210,828 people in the United States were diagnosed with lung cancer. That same year, 157,423 people died of the disease (CDC, 2016b). There has been a statistically significant decrease in the incidence of lung cancer in both men and women (except American Indian, Alaska Native, and Asian/Pacific Islander women) in the years between 2002 and 2011 (CDC, 2016b). In approximately 70% of patients with lung cancer, the disease has spread to regional lymphatics and other sites by the time of diagnosis. As a result, the long-term survival rate is low.

Pathophysiology

Eighty percent of lung cancer in women and 90% in men are caused by cigarette smoking, with the remainder being attributed to other carcinogens, including radon gas and occupational and environmental agents (CDC, 2015b).

Classification and Staging

For purposes of staging and treatment, most lung cancers are classified into one of two major categories: small cell lung cancer (25% of lung cancers) and nonsmall cell lung cancer (75% of lung cancers) (Table 10-4). In nonsmall cell lung carcinoma (NSCLC), the cell types include squamous cell carcinoma (20% to 30%), large cell carcinoma (10%), and adenocarcinoma (30% to 40%), including bronchoalveolar carcinoma. Most small cell carcinomas arise in the major bronchi and spread by infiltration along the bronchial wall.

In addition to classification according to cell type, lung cancers are staged. The stage of the tumor refers to the size of the tumor, its location, whether lymph nodes are involved, and whether the cancer has metastasized, referred to as the TNM ("T" refers to the extent of the primary tumor, "N" refers to lymph node involvement, and "M" refers to the extent of metastasis) (Goldstraw, Chansky, Crowley, et al., 2015). NSCLC is staged as I to IV. Stage I is the earliest stage and has the highest cure rates, whereas stage IV designates metastatic spread. Small cell lung cancers are classified as limited or extensive. Diagnostic tools and further information on staging were described in Chapter 6.

Risk Factors

Various factors have been associated with the development of lung cancer (Box 10-11). Other factors that have been associated with lung cancer include genetic predisposition and underlying respiratory diseases, such as COPD and TB.

Clinical Manifestations and Assessment

Often, lung cancer develops insidiously and is asymptomatic until late in its course. The signs and symptoms depend on the location and size of the tumor, the degree of obstruction, and

TABLE 10-4 Lung Cancer Types and Characteristics

Tumor Classification	Growth Rate	Clinical Manifestations	Treatment	Metastasis
Nonsmall Cell Lung Cancer (NSCLC)				
Squamous cell	Slow	Cough, hemoptysis, pneumonia, atelectasis, chest pain (late sign), unexplained weight loss	Surgical resection, adjunctive chemotherapy	Late: Brain, liver, bones, adrenals
Adenocarcinoma	Moderate	Dyspnea, pleuritic chest pain, pleural effusions, unexplained weight loss	Surgical resection, adjunctive chemotherapy	Early: Liver, brain, bones, kidneys, adrenals
Large cell (undifferentiated)	Rapid	Chest wall pain, cough, sputum production, hemoptysis, pleural effusion, pneumonia, unexplained weight loss	Surgical resection	Early: Brain, liver, bones, adrenals
Small Cell Lung Cancer (SCLC)				
Oat cell and intermediate cell type	Very rapid	Cough, unexplained weight loss, dyspnea, airway obstruction, hilar mass on x-ray, pneumonia, paraneoplastic syndromes (SIADH, hypercalcemia, Cushing's, myopathies)	Chemotherapy, Radiation therapy	Early: Liver, bone, bone marrow, brain, adrenals

SIADH, syndrome of inappropriate antidiuretic hormone secretion.

the existence of metastases to regional or distant sites. The most frequent symptom of lung cancer is cough or change in a chronic cough. The cough starts as a dry, persistent cough, without sputum production. When obstruction of airways occurs, the cough may become productive due to infection.

Dyspnea occurs in many patients. Hemoptysis or blood-tinged sputum may be expectorated. Chest or shoulder pain may indicate chest wall or pleural involvement by a tumor. Pain also is a late manifestation and may be related to metastasis to the bone.

In some patients, a recurring fever is an early symptom in response to a persistent infection in an area distal to the tumor. In fact, cancer of the lung should be suspected in people with repeated unresolved upper respiratory tract infections. If the tumor spreads to adjacent structures and regional lymph nodes, the patient may present with chest pain and tightness, hoarseness (involving the recurrent laryngeal nerve), dysphagia, head and neck edema, and symptoms of pleural or pericardial effusion. The most common sites of metastases are lymph nodes, bone, brain, contralateral lung, adrenal glands, and liver. Nonspecific symptoms of weakness, anorexia, and weight loss also may be present.

If pulmonary symptoms occur in smokers, cancer of the lung should always be considered. A chest x-ray is performed to search for pulmonary densities, pulmonary nodules, atelectasis, and infection. CT scans of the chest are used to identify small nodules not easily visualized on the chest x-ray and also to examine areas for lymphadenopathy.

Fiberoptic bronchoscopy provides a detailed study of the tracheobronchial tree and allows for brushings, washings, and biopsies of suspicious areas. For peripheral lesions not amenable to bronchoscopic biopsy, a transthoracic **fine-needle aspiration** may be performed under CT guidance to aspirate cells from a suspicious area. In some circumstances, an endoscopy with esophageal ultrasound may be used to obtain a transesophageal biopsy of enlarged subcarinal (below the carina) lymph nodes that are not easily accessible by other means.

A variety of scans may be used to assess for metastasis of the cancer. These may include bone scans, abdominal scans,

positron emission tomography (PET) scans, and liver ultrasound. CT of the brain, magnetic resonance imaging (MRI), and other neurologic diagnostic procedures are used to detect CNS metastases. Mediastinoscopy or mediastinotomy may be used to obtain biopsy samples from lymph nodes in the mediastinum.

If surgery is a potential treatment, the patient is evaluated to determine whether the tumor is resectable and whether the patient can tolerate the physiologic impairment resulting from such surgery. Pulmonary function tests, ABG analysis, $\dot{V}/\dot{Q}$ scans, and exercise testing may all be used as part of the preoperative assessment.

Medical Management

The objective of management is to provide a cure, if possible. Treatment depends on the cell type, the stage of the disease, and the patient's physiologic status (particularly cardiac and pulmonary status). In general, treatment may involve surgery, radiation therapy, or chemotherapy—or a combination of these. Newer and more specific therapies to modulate the immune system (gene therapy, therapy with defined tumor antigens) are under study.

Surgical Management

Surgical resection is the preferred method of treating patients with localized nonsmall cell tumors, no evidence of metastatic spread, and adequate cardiopulmonary function. The cure rate of surgical resection depends on the type and stage of the cancer. Surgery is primarily used for NSCLCs because small cell cancer of the lung grows rapidly and metastasizes early and extensively. Lesions of many patients with bronchogenic cancer are inoperable at the time of diagnosis.

Several different types of lung resection may be performed. The most common surgical procedure for a small, apparently curable tumor of the lung is lobectomy (removal of a lobe of the lung). In some cases, an entire lung may be removed (pneumonectomy).

Radiation Therapy

Radiation therapy (XRT) may offer cure in a small percentage of patients. It is useful in controlling neoplasms that cannot be surgically resected but are responsive to radiation. Irradiation also may be used to reduce the size of a tumor, to make an inoperable tumor operable, or to relieve the pressure of the tumor on vital structures. It can reduce symptoms of spinal cord metastasis and superior vena caval compression. Also, XRT is used to treat metastases to the brain. Radiation therapy may help relieve cough, chest pain, dyspnea, hemoptysis, and bone and liver pain. Relief of symptoms may last from a few weeks to many months and is important in improving the quality of the remaining period of life. Radiofrequency ablation and cryoablation are two types of nonsurgical therapies that have been used to treat lung tumors.

Chemotherapy

Chemotherapy is used to alter tumor growth patterns, to treat distant metastases or small cell cancer of the lung, and as an adjunct to surgery or radiation therapy. Chemotherapy may provide relief, especially of pain, but it does not usually cure the disease or prolong life to any great degree. Chemotherapy is also accompanied by side effects. It is valuable in reducing pressure symptoms of lung cancer and in treating brain, spinal cord, and pericardial metastases.

The choice of agent depends on the growth of the tumor cell and the specific phase of the cell cycle that the medication affects. In combination with surgery, chemotherapy may be administered before surgery (neoadjuvant therapy) or after surgery (adjuvant therapy). Combinations of two or more medications may be more beneficial than single-dose regimens.

Palliative Therapy

Palliative therapy may include radiation therapy or chemotherapy to shrink the tumor to provide pain relief, a variety of bronchoscopic interventions to open a narrowed bronchus or airway, and pain management and other comfort measures. Evaluation and referral for hospice care are important in planning for comfortable and dignified end-of-life care for the patient and family.

Treatment-Related Complications

A variety of complications may occur as a result of treatment for lung cancer. Surgical resection may result in respiratory failure, particularly if the cardiopulmonary system is compromised before surgery. Surgical complications and prolonged mechanical ventilation are potential outcomes. Radiation therapy may result in diminished cardiopulmonary function and other complications, such as pulmonary fibrosis, pericarditis, myelitis, and cor pulmonale. Chemotherapy, particularly in combination with radiation therapy, can cause pneumonitis. Pulmonary and systemic toxicity is a potential side effect of chemotherapy.

Nursing Management

Nursing care of patients with lung cancer is similar to that for other patients with cancer and addresses the physiologic and psychological needs of the patient. The physiologic problems are primarily due to the respiratory manifestations of the disease. Nursing care includes strategies to ensure relief of pain and discomfort and to prevent complications.

Managing Symptoms

The nurse instructs the patient and family about the potential side effects of the specific treatment and strategies to manage them. Strategies for managing such symptoms as dyspnea, fatigue, nausea and vomiting, anorexia, and fatigue help the patient and family cope with therapeutic measures. See Chapter 6.

Relieving Breathing Problems

Airway clearance techniques are key to maintaining airway patency through the removal of excess secretions. This may be accomplished through deep-breathing exercises, CPT, directed cough, suctioning, and, in some instances, bronchoscopy. Bronchodilator medications may be prescribed to promote bronchial dilation. As the tumor enlarges or spreads, it may compress a bronchus or involve a large area of lung tissue, resulting in an impaired breathing pattern and poor gas exchange. At some stage of the disease, supplemental oxygen will probably be necessary.

Nursing measures focus on decreasing dyspnea by encouraging the patient to assume positions that promote lung expansion and to perform breathing exercises for lung expansion and relaxation. Patient education about energy conservation and airway clearance techniques is also necessary. Many of the techniques used in pulmonary rehabilitation can be applied to patients with lung cancer. Depending on the severity of disease and the patient's wishes, a referral to a pulmonary rehabilitation program may be helpful in managing respiratory symptoms.

Providing Psychological Support

Another important part of the nursing care of patients with lung cancer is provision of psychological support and identification of potential resources for the patient and family. Refer to Chapter 6.

Gerontologic Considerations

At the time of diagnosis of lung cancer, most patients are older than 65 years of age and have stage III or IV disease (CDC, 2016b). Although age is not a significant prognostic factor for overall survival and response to treatment for either NSCLC or small cell lung cancer, older patients have specific needs. Depending on the comorbidities and functional status of elderly patients, chemotherapy agents, doses, and cycles may need to be adjusted to maintain quality of life. Issues that must be considered in the care of elderly patients with lung cancer include functional status, comorbid conditions, nutritional status, cognition, concomitant medications, and psychological and social support.

TUMORS OF THE MEDIASTINUM

Tumors of the mediastinum include neurogenic tumors, tumors of the thymus, lymphomas, germ cell tumors, cysts, and mesenchymal tumors. These tumors may be malignant or benign. They are usually described in relation to location: anterior, middle, or posterior masses or tumors.

Clinical Manifestations and Assessment

Nearly all symptoms of mediastinal tumors result from the pressure of the mass against important intrathoracic organs.

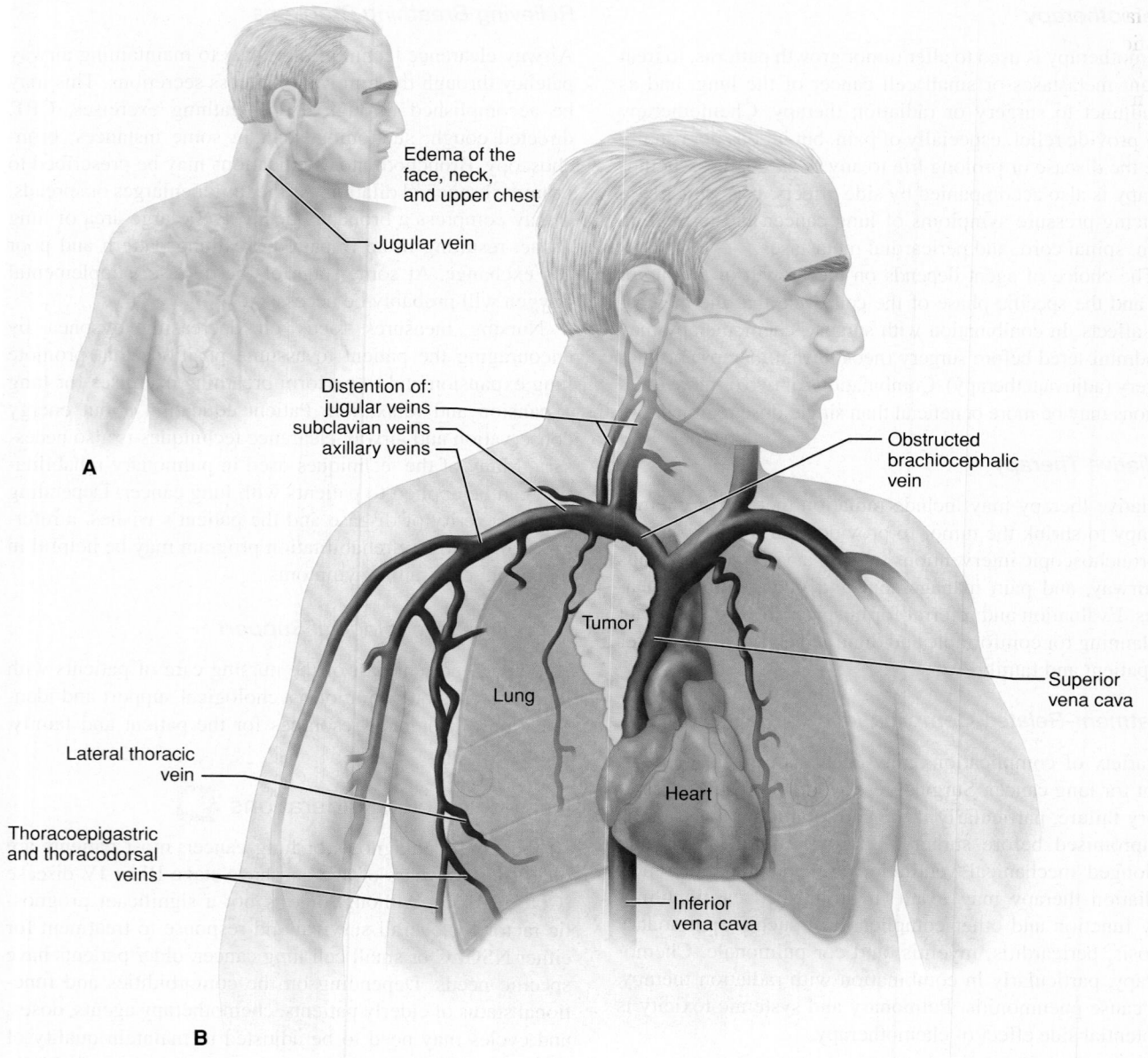

FIGURE 10-9 Clinical signs of the superior vena cava syndrome. (**A**) shows facial edema, plethora, jugular venous distention, and prominent superficial vessels in the neck and upper chest. (**B**) depicts the vascular anatomy and collateral vessel formation in a patient with superior vena cava syndrome. (DeVita, V. T., Jr., Lawrence, T. S., & Rosenberg, S. A. *DeVita, Hellman, and Rosenberg's cancer, principles and practice of oncology: Review* (10th ed.). Philadelphia, PA: Wolters Kluwer. (2016). Used with permission.)

Symptoms may include cough, wheezing, dyspnea, anterior chest or neck pain, bulging of the chest wall, heart palpitations, angina, other circulatory disturbances, central cyanosis, superior vena cava syndrome (i.e., swelling of the face, neck, and upper extremities; Fig. 10-9), marked distention of the veins of the neck and the chest wall (evidence of the obstruction of large veins of the mediastinum by extravascular compression or intravascular invasion), and dysphagia and weight loss from pressure or invasion into the esophagus.

Most often, chest x-rays are used to diagnose mediastinal tumors and cysts. CT is the standard diagnostic test for assessment of the mediastinum and surrounding structures. MRI, as well as PET, may be used in some circumstances.

Medical and Nursing Management

If the tumor is malignant and has infiltrated the surrounding tissue and complete surgical removal is not feasible, radiation therapy, chemotherapy, or both are used.

Many mediastinal tumors are benign and operable. The location of the tumor (anterior, middle, or posterior compartment) in the mediastinum dictates the type of incision. The common incision used is a median sternotomy; however, a thoracotomy may be used, depending on the location of the tumor. Additional approaches include a bilateral anterior thoracotomy (clamshell incision) and video-assisted thoracoscopic surgery (VATS). The care is the same as for any patient undergoing thoracic surgery. Major complications include hemorrhage, injury to the phrenic or laryngeal nerve, and infection.

CHEST TRAUMA

Major chest trauma may occur alone or in combination with multiple other injuries. Chest trauma is classified as either blunt or penetrating. Blunt chest trauma results from rapid deceleration injury (e.g., motor vehicle accident [MVA], falls) or direct injury (abuse, crushing, and explosions). Penetrating trauma occurs when a foreign object penetrates the chest wall (stabbing, gunshot wounds, and shrapnel).

BLUNT TRAUMA AND PENETRATING TRAUMA

Blunt thoracic injures are responsible for 53% of trauma deaths (Davis et al., 2014). It is often difficult to identify the extent of the damage because the symptoms may be occult and vague.

Pathophysiology

The most common causes of blunt chest trauma are MVAs (trauma from steering wheel, seat belt), falls, and bicycle crashes (trauma from handlebars) (Fair et al., 2015). Mechanisms of blunt chest trauma include acceleration (moving object hitting the chest or patient being thrown into an object), deceleration (sudden decrease in rate of speed or velocity, such as an MVA), shearing (stretching forces to areas of the chest causing tears, ruptures, or dissections), and compression (direct blow to the chest, such as a crush injury or explosion). Injuries to the chest are often life-threatening and result in one or more of the following pathologic states:

- Hypoxemia from disruption of the airway; injury to the lung parenchyma, rib cage, and respiratory musculature; massive hemorrhage; collapsed lung; pulmonary contusion and pneumothorax
- Hypovolemia from massive fluid loss from the great vessels, cardiac rupture, or hemothorax
- Cardiac failure from cardiac tamponade, cardiac contusion, or increased intrathoracic pressure

These pathologic states frequently result in impaired ventilation and perfusion leading to ARF, hypovolemic shock, and death.

Gunshot and stab wounds are the most common causes of penetrating chest trauma. These wounds are classified according to their velocity. In general, stab wounds are considered low-velocity trauma because the weapon destroys a small area around the wound. The appearance of the external wound may be very deceptive because pneumothorax, hemothorax, lung contusion, and cardiac tamponade, along with severe and continuing hemorrhage, can occur from any small wound, even one caused by a small-diameter instrument such as an ice pick.

Gunshot wounds may be classified as low-, medium-, or high-velocity. The factors that determine the velocity and resulting extent of damage include the distance from which the gun was fired, the caliber of the gun, and the construction and size of the bullet. A bullet can cause damage at the site of penetration and along its pathway, and a gunshot wound to the chest can produce a variety of pathophysiologic changes. The bullet may ricochet off bony structures and damage the chest organs and great vessels or can travel into the abdomen. If the diaphragm is involved in a gunshot wound or a stab wound, injury to the chest cavity must be considered.

Clinical Manifestations and Assessment

Time is critical in treating chest trauma. Therefore, it is essential to assess the patient immediately to determine the following:

- Time elapsed since injury occurred
- Mechanism of injury
- Level of responsiveness
- Specific injuries
- Estimated blood loss
- Recent drug or alcohol use
- Prehospital treatment

Initial assessment of thoracic injuries includes assessment for airway obstruction, **tension pneumothorax**, open pneumothorax, massive hemothorax, flail chest, and cardiac tamponade and rupture. These injuries are life-threatening and require immediate treatment. Secondary assessment includes assessment for simple pneumothorax, hemothorax, pulmonary contusion, traumatic aortic rupture, tracheobronchial disruption, sternal fracture, esophageal perforation, traumatic diaphragmatic injury, and penetrating wounds to the mediastinum. Although listed as secondary, these injuries may be life-threatening as well (Davis et al., 2014; Fair et al., 2015; Sarkar, Brunsvold, Cherry-Bukoweic, et al., 2011).

The rapid assessment of thoracic injuries involves the use of the Advanced Trauma Life Support (ATLS) algorithm of "**C**irculation, **A**irway, **B**reathing, **D**isability (neurologic), and **E**xposure/Environmental control":

- *Circulation:* The vital signs and skin color are assessed for signs of shock.
- *Airway:* Assessment includes noting the rate and depth of breathing and observing for abnormalities such as

stridor, cyanosis, nasal flaring, use of accessory muscles, drooling, and overt trauma to the face, mouth, or neck.

- *Breathing:* The chest is assessed for symmetric movement, symmetry of breath sounds, open chest wounds, entrance or exit wounds, impaled objects, distended neck veins, and paradoxical chest wall motion. The thorax is palpated for tenderness and crepitus (subcutaneous emphysema), and the position of the trachea is also assessed. In addition, the chest wall is assessed for bruising, petechiae, lacerations, and burns.
- *Disability:* Assess the patient's level of consciousness and note if concurrent head or spinal cord injuries are present.
- *Exposure/Environmental:* Assess for exposure injuries such as hypothermia or hyperthermia.

The initial diagnostic workup includes a chest x-ray, CT scan, complete blood count, clotting studies, type and cross-match, electrolytes, oxygen saturation, ABG analysis, and ECG. The patient is completely undressed to avoid missing additional injuries that may complicate care. Many patients with injuries involving the chest have associated head and abdominal injuries that require attention. Ongoing assessment is essential to monitor the patient's response to treatment and to detect early signs of clinical deterioration.

Medical Management

The medical management of penetrating and blunt chest trauma are similar. The objective of immediate management is to restore and maintain cardiopulmonary function. After an adequate airway is ensured and ventilation is established, examination for shock and intrathoracic and intra-abdominal injuries is necessary. There is a high risk for associated intra-abdominal injuries with stab wounds below the level of the fifth anterior intercostal space.

The diagnostic workup includes a chest x-ray, chemistry profile, ABG analysis, POX, and ECG. The patient's blood is typed and cross-matched in case blood transfusion is required. After the status of the peripheral pulses is assessed, a large-bore IV line is inserted. An indwelling catheter is inserted to monitor urinary output. A nasogastric tube is inserted and connected to low suction to prevent aspiration, minimize leakage of abdominal contents, and decompress the gastrointestinal tract.

Shock is treated simultaneously with colloid solutions, crystalloids, or blood, as indicated by the patient's condition. Diagnostic procedures are carried out as dictated by the needs of the patient (e.g., CT scans of chest or abdomen, flat plate x-ray of the abdomen, abdominal ultrasound to check for bleeding).

A chest tube is inserted into the pleural space in most patients with penetrating wounds of the chest to achieve rapid and continuing re-expansion of the lungs, especially in wounds above the fifth intercostal space (nipple line). The insertion of the chest tube frequently results in a complete evacuation of the blood and air. The chest tube also allows early recognition of continuing intrathoracic bleeding, which would make surgical exploration necessary. If the patient has a penetrating wound of the heart or great vessels, the esophagus, or the tracheobronchial tree, surgical intervention is required.

Patients with penetrating chest wound usually require exploratory surgery. In extreme cases, an emergency thoracotomy may be performed in the trauma room to access bleeding from large vessels such as the aorta, pulmonary artery, or heart.

Chest Tubes

Chest tubes may be inserted to drain fluid or air from any of the three compartments of the thorax (the right and left pleural spaces and the mediastinum). The pleural space, located between the visceral and parietal pleura, normally contains 25 mL or less of fluid, which helps lubricate the visceral and parietal pleura. Surgical incision of the chest wall almost always causes some degree of pneumothorax (air accumulating in the pleural space) or hemothorax (buildup of serous fluid or blood in the pleural space). Air and fluid collect in the pleural space, restricting lung expansion and reducing gas exchange. Placement of a chest tube in the pleural space restores the normal negative intrathoracic pressure needed for lung re-expansion after surgery or trauma.

The mediastinal space is an extrapleural space that lies between the right and left thoracic cavities and contains the large blood vessels, heart, mainstem bronchus, and thymus gland. If fluid accumulates here, the heart can become compressed and stop beating, causing death. Mediastinal chest tubes can be inserted either anteriorly or posteriorly to the heart to drain blood after surgery.

Catheters

There are two types of chest tubes: small-bore and large-bore catheters. Small-bore catheters (7 to 12 Fr) have a one-way valve apparatus to prevent air from moving back into the patient. They can be inserted through a small skin incision. Large-bore catheters, which range in size up to 40 Fr, are usually connected to a **chest drainage system** (Fig. 10-10) to collect any pleural fluid and monitor for air leaks. After the chest tube is positioned, it is sutured to the skin and connected to a drainage apparatus to remove the residual air and fluid from the pleural or mediastinal space. This results in the re-expansion of remaining lung tissue.

Chest Drainage Systems

Chest drainage systems have a suction source, a collection chamber for pleural drainage, and a mechanism to prevent air from re-entering the chest with inhalation. Various types of chest drainage systems are available for use in removal of air and fluid from the pleural space and re-expansion of the lungs. Chest drainage systems come with either wet (water seal) or dry suction control. In wet suction systems,

FIGURE 10-10 Chest drainage systems. **A.** The Atrium Ocean is an example of a water-seal chest drain system composed of a drainage chamber and water-seal chamber. The suction control is determined by the height of the water column in that chamber (usually 20 cm). *A*, suction control chamber; *B*, water-seal chamber; *C*, air leak zone; *D*, collection chamber. **B.** The Atrium Oasis is an example of a dry suction water-seal system that uses a mechanical regulator for vacuum control, a water-seal chamber, and a drainage chamber. *A*, dry suction regulator; *B*, water-seal chamber; *C*, air leak monitor; *D*, collection chamber; *E*, suction monitor bellows. (Art redrawn with permission from Atrium Medical Corporation, Hudson, New Hampshire.)

the amount of suction is determined by the amount of water instilled in the suction chamber. Wet systems use a water seal to prevent air from moving back into the chest on inspiration. Dry systems use a one-way valve and may have a suction control dial in place of the water. Both systems can operate by gravity drainage, without a suction source (Fig. 10-10; Box 10-12).

Water-Seal Systems

The traditional water-seal system (or wet suction) for chest drainage has three chambers: a collection chamber, a water-seal chamber, and a wet suction control chamber. The collection chamber acts as a reservoir for fluid draining from the chest tube. It is graduated to permit easy measurement of drainage. Suction may be added to create negative pressure and promote drainage of fluid and removal of air. The

suction control chamber regulates the amount of negative pressure applied to the chest. The amount of suction is determined by the water level. It is usually set at 20 cm H_2O; adding more fluid results in more suction. After the suction is turned on, bubbling appears in the suction chamber. A positive-pressure valve is located at the top of the suction chamber that automatically opens with increases in positive pressure within the system. Air is automatically released through a positive-pressure relief valve if the suction tubing is inadvertently clamped or kinked.

The water-seal chamber has a one-way valve or water seal that prevents air from moving back into the chest when the patient inhales. There is an increase in the water level with inspiration and a return to the baseline level during exhalation; this is referred to as *tidaling*. If bubbling is present, either intermittent or continuous, an air leak is present

BOX 10-12

GUIDELINES FOR NURSING CARE

Managing Chest Drainage Systems

Equipment

- Chest drainage system
- Dressings
- Sterile water

- Tape
- Marker

ACTION	RATIONALE

ACTION

1. If using a chest drainage system with a water seal, fill the water-seal chamber with sterile water to the level specified by the manufacturer.

2. When using suction in chest drainage systems with a water seal, fill the suction control chamber with sterile water to the 20 cm level or as prescribed. In systems without a water seal, set the regulator dial at the appropriate suction level.

Pleur-evac system.

3. Attach the drainage catheter exiting the thoracic cavity to the tubing coming from the collection chamber. Tape securely with adhesive tape.

4. If suction is used, connect the suction control chamber tubing to the suction unit. If using a wet suction system, turn on the suction unit and increase pressure until slow but steady bubbling appears in the suction control chamber. If using a chest drainage system with a dry suction control chamber, turn the regulator dial to 20 cm H_2O.

5. Mark the drainage from the collection chamber with tape on the outside of the drainage unit. Mark hourly/daily increments (date and time) at the drainage level.

RATIONALE

1. Water-seal drainage allows air and fluid to escape into a drainage chamber. The water acts as a seal and keeps the air from being drawn back into the pleural space.

2. The water level regulator dial setting determines the degree of suction applied.

3. In chest drainage units, the system is closed.

4. With a wet suction system, the degree of suction is determined by the amount of water in the suction control chamber and is not dependent on the rate of bubbling or the pressure gauge setting on the suction unit.
   With a dry suction control chamber, the regulator dial replaces the water.

5. This marking shows the amount of fluid loss and how fast fluid is collecting in the drainage chamber. It serves as a basis for determining the need for blood replacement, if the fluid is blood. Visibly bloody drainage will appear in the chamber in the immediate postoperative period but should gradually become serous. If the patient is bleeding as heavily as 100 mL every 15 minutes, check the drainage every few minutes. A reoperation or autotransfusion may be needed. Drainage of 200 mL/hr is usually associated with bleeding complications. The transfusion of blood collected in the drainage chamber must be reinfused within 4–6 hours. Usually, however, drainage decreases progressively in the first 24 hours.

ACTION	RATIONALE
6. Ensure that the drainage tubing does not kink, loop, or interfere with the patient's movements.	6. Kinking, looping, or pressure on the drainage tubing can produce back pressure, which may force fluid back into the pleural space or impede its drainage.
7. Encourage the patient to assume a comfortable position with good body alignment. With the lateral position, make sure that the patient's body does not compress the tubing. The patient should be turned and repositioned every 1.5 to 2 hours. Provide adequate analgesia.	7. Frequent position changes promote drainage, and good body alignment helps prevent postural deformities and contractures. Proper positioning also helps breathing and promotes better air exchange. Analgesics may be needed to promote comfort.
8. Assist the patient with range-of-motion exercises for the affected arm and shoulder several times daily. Provide adequate analgesia.	8. Exercise helps to prevent ankyloses (abnormal stiffening and immobility of a joint) of the shoulder and to reduce postoperative pain and discomfort. Analgesics may be needed to relieve pain.
9. If the drainage is bloody, gently drain the tubing in the direction of the drainage chamber. Gentle "milking" may be warranted if allowed according to institutional policy in cases of active bleeding to prevent obstruction in the tubing. If "gentle milking" is allowed, ***do not compress the tubing completely***. In general, the prevention of dependent loops, laying of the tubing horizontally across the bed that then drops vertically into the chest drainage system is sufficient for fluid drainage.	9. Gentle "milking" may prevent the tubing from becoming obstructed by clots and fibrin. Constant attention to maintaining the patency of the tube facilitates prompt expansion of the lung and minimizes complications. However, compressing the tubing may cause high negative pressure in the pleural space and lung entrapment, thus routine "milking" is discouraged.
10. Make sure there is fluctuation ("tidaling") of the fluid level in the water-seal chamber (in wet systems), or check the air leak indicator for leaks (in dry systems with a one-way valve). *Note:* Fluid fluctuations in the water-seal chamber or air leak indicator area will stop when: • The lung has re-expanded • The tubing is obstructed by blood clots, fibrin, or kinks • A loop of tubing hangs below the rest of the tubing • Suction motor or wall suction is not working properly	10. Fluctuation of the water level in the water seal shows effective connection between the pleural cavity and the drainage chamber and indicates that the drainage system remains patent. Fluctuation is also a gauge of intrapleural pressure in systems with a water seal (wet and dry, but not with the one-way valve).
11. With a dry system, assess for the presence of the indicator (bellows or float device) when setting the regulator dial to the desired level of suction.	11. An air leak indicator shows changes in intrathoracic pressure in dry systems with a one-way valve. Bubbles will appear if a leak is present. The air leak indicator takes the place of fluid fluctuations in the water-seal chamber. The indicator shows that the vacuum is adequate to maintain the desired level of suction.
12. Observe for air leaks in the drainage system; they are indicated by constant bubbling in the water-seal chamber, or by the air leak indicator in dry systems with a one-way valve. Also assess the chest tube system for correctable external leaks. Notify the provider immediately of excessive bubbling in the water-seal chamber not due to external leaks.	12. Leaking and trapping of air in the pleural space can result in tension pneumothorax.
13. When turning down the dry suction, depress the manual high-negativity vent, and assess for a rise in the water level of the water-seal chamber.	13. A rise in the water level of the water-seal chamber indicates high negative pressure in the system that could lead to increased intrathoracic pressure.
14. Observe and immediately report rapid and shallow breathing, cyanosis, pressure in the chest, subcutaneous emphysema, symptoms of hemorrhage, or significant changes in vital signs.	14. Many clinical conditions can cause these signs and symptoms, including tension pneumothorax, mediastinal shift, hemorrhage, severe incisional pain, pulmonary embolus, and cardiac tamponade. Surgical intervention may be necessary.
15. Encourage the patient to breathe deeply and cough at frequent intervals. Provide adequate analgesia. If needed, request an order for patient-controlled analgesia. Also teach the patient how to perform incentive spirometry.	15. Deep breathing and coughing help to raise the intrapleural pressure, which promotes drainage of accumulated fluid in the pleural space. Deep breathing and coughing also promote removal of secretions from the tracheobronchial tree, which, in turn, promotes lung expansion and prevents atelectasis (alveolar collapse).

(continued on page 336)

BOX 10-12

GUIDELINES FOR NURSING CARE (*continued*)

Managing Chest Drainage Systems (*continued*)

ACTION	RATIONALE
16. If the patient is lying on a stretcher and must be transported to another area, place the drainage system below the chest level. If the tubing disconnects, cut off the contaminated tips of the chest tube and tubing, insert a sterile connector in the cut ends, and reattach to the drainage system. Do *not* clamp the chest tube during transport.	16. The drainage apparatus must be kept at a level lower than the patient's chest to prevent fluid from flowing backward into the pleural space. Clamping can result in a tension pneumothorax.
17. When assisting in the chest tube's removal, instruct the patient to perform a gentle Valsalva maneuver or to breathe quietly. Then the chest tube is clamped and removed quickly. Simultaneously, a small bandage is applied and made airtight with petrolatum gauze covered by a 4 × 4-inch gauze pad and thoroughly covered and sealed with nonporous tape.	17. The chest tube is removed as directed when the lung is re-expanded (usually within 24 hours to several days), depending on the cause of the pneumothorax. During tube removal, the chief priorities are preventing air from entering the pleural cavity as the tube is withdrawn and preventing infection.

within the system or the patient. The nurse must investigate the system for loose connections. Bubbling and tidaling do not occur when the tube is placed in the mediastinal space; however, fluid may pulsate with the patient's heartbeat. If the chest tube is connected to gravity drainage only, suction is not used. Two-chamber chest drainage systems (water-seal chamber and collection chamber) are available for use with patients who need only gravity drainage.

The water level in the water-seal chamber reflects the negative pressure present in the intrathoracic cavity. A rise in the water level of the water-seal chamber indicates negative pressure in the pleural or mediastinal space. Excessive negative pressure can cause trauma to tissue. Most chest drainage systems have an automatic means to prevent excessive negative pressure. By pressing and holding a manual high-negativity vent (usually located on the top of the chest drainage system) until the water level in the water-seal chamber returns to the 2-cm mark, excessive negative pressure is avoided, thus preventing damage to tissue.

Dry Suction Water-Seal Systems

Dry suction water-seal systems, also referred to as dry suction, have a collection chamber for drainage, a water-seal chamber, and a dry suction control chamber. The water-seal chamber is filled with water to the 2 cm level. Bubbling in this area can indicate an air leak. The dry suction control chamber contains a regulator dial that regulates vacuum to the chest drain. Water is not needed for suction in these systems. Without the bubbling in the suction chamber, the system is quieter. However, if the container is knocked over, the water seal may be lost.

Once the tube is connected to the suction source, the regulator dial allows the desired level of suction to be dialed in; the suction is increased until an indicator appears. The indicator has the same function as the bubbling in the traditional water-seal system; that is, it indicates that the vacuum is

adequate to maintain the desired level of suction. Some drainage systems use a bellows (a chamber that can be expanded or contracted) or an orange-colored float device as an indicator of when the suction control regulator is set.

When the water in the water seal rises above the 2 cm level, intrathoracic pressure increases. Dry suction water-seal systems have a manual high-negativity vent located on top of the drain. The manual high-negativity vent is pressed until the indicator appears (either a float device or bellows) and the water level in the water seal returns to the desired level, indicating that the intrathoracic pressure is decreased.

Dry Suction Systems with a One-Way Valve

A third type of chest drainage system is dry suction with a one-way mechanical valve. This system has a collection chamber, a one-way mechanical valve, and a dry suction control chamber. The valve permits air and fluid to leave the chest but prevents their movement back into the pleural space. This model lacks a water-seal chamber and therefore can be set up quickly in emergency situations, and the dry control drain still works even if it is knocked over. This makes the dry suction systems useful for the patient who is ambulating or being transported. However, without the water-seal chamber, there is no way to tell by inspection whether the pressure in the chest has changed, even though an air leak indicator is present so that the system can be checked. If an air leak is suspected, 30 mL of water is injected into the air leak indicator or the container is tipped so that fluid enters the air leak detection chamber. Bubbles will appear if a leak is present.

If the chest tube has been inserted to re-expand a lung after pneumothorax, or if very little fluid drainage is expected, a one-way valve (Heimlich valve) may be connected to the chest tube (Fig. 10-11). This valve may be attached to a collection bag or covered with a sterile dressing if no drainage is expected.

FIGURE 10-11 One-way (Heimlich) valve, a disposable, single-use chest drainage system with 30-mL collection volume. Used when minimal volume of chest drainage is expected.

STERNAL AND RIB FRACTURES

Sternal fractures are most common in MVAs, caused by a direct blow to the sternum via the steering wheel. Rib fractures are the most common type of chest trauma, occurring in more than 62% of patients admitted with blunt chest injury (Sharma et al., 2008). Most rib fractures are benign and are treated conservatively. Fractures of the first three ribs are rare but can result in a high mortality rate because they are associated with laceration of the subclavian artery or vein. The fifth through ninth ribs are the most common sites of fractures. Fractures of the lower ribs are associated with injury to the spleen and liver, which may be lacerated by fragmented sections of the rib.

Clinical Manifestations and Assessment

Patients with sternal fractures have anterior chest pain, overlying tenderness, ecchymosis, crepitus, swelling, and possible chest wall deformity. For patients with rib fractures, clinical manifestations are similar: severe pain, point tenderness, and muscle spasm over the area of the fracture that is aggravated by coughing, deep breathing, and movement. The area around the fracture may be bruised. To reduce the pain, the patient splints the chest by breathing in a shallow manner and avoids sighs, deep breaths, coughing, and movement. This reluctance to move or breathe deeply results in diminished ventilation, atelectasis (collapse of unaerated alveoli), pneumonitis, and hypoxemia. Respiratory insufficiency and failure can be the outcomes of such a cycle.

The patient must be evaluated closely for underlying cardiac or abdominal injuries. A crackling, grating sound in the thorax (subcutaneous crepitus) may be detected with auscultation or palpation. The diagnostic workup may include a chest x-ray, rib films of a specific area, ECG, continuous POX, and ABG analysis.

Medical and Nursing Management

Medical management is directed toward relieving pain, avoiding excessive activity, and treating any associated injuries. Surgical fixation is rarely necessary unless fragments are grossly displaced and pose a potential for further injury.

The goals of treatment for rib fractures are to control pain and to detect and treat the injury. Narcotics are most often used to relieve pain and to allow deep breathing and coughing. Care must be taken to avoid oversedation and suppression of respiratory drive. Alternative strategies to relieve pain include an intercostal nerve block and ice over the fracture site. A chest binder may be used as supportive treatment to provide stability to the chest wall and may decrease pain. The patient is instructed to apply the binder snugly enough to provide support but not so tight as to impair respiratory excursion. Usually the pain abates in 5 to 7 days, and discomfort can be relieved with epidural analgesia, patient-controlled analgesia, or nonopioid analgesia (NSAIDs). Most rib fractures heal in 3 to 6 weeks.

FLAIL CHEST

Flail chest is frequently a complication of blunt chest trauma from a steering wheel injury. It usually occurs when three or more adjacent ribs (multiple contiguous ribs) are fractured at two or more sites, resulting in free-floating rib segments. It may also result as a combination fracture of ribs and costal cartilages or sternum (Fig. 10-12). As a result, the chest wall loses stability, causing respiratory impairment and usually severe respiratory distress. In addition, due to the force needed to break ribs or the sternum, often an underlying pulmonary or cardiac contusion is present.

Pathophysiology

During inspiration, as the chest expands, the detached part of the rib segment (flail segment) moves in a paradoxical manner (pendelluft movement) in that it is pulled inward during inspiration, reducing the amount of air that can be drawn into the lungs. On expiration, because the intrathoracic pressure exceeds atmospheric pressure, the flail segment bulges outward, impairing the patient's ability to exhale. The mediastinum then shifts back to the affected side. This paradoxical action results in increased dead space, a reduction in alveolar ventilation, and decreased compliance. Retained airway secretions and atelectasis frequently accompany flail chest. The patient has hypoxemia, and if

A. Inspiration

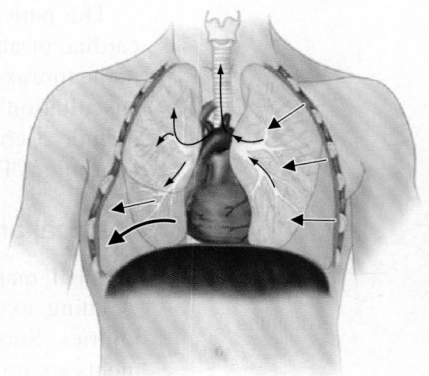

B. Expiration

FIGURE 10-12 Flail chest is caused by a free-floating segment of rib cage resulting from multiple rib fractures. **A.** Paradoxical movement on inspiration occurs when the flail rib segment is sucked inward and the mediastinal structures shift to the unaffected side. The amount of air drawn into the affected lung is reduced. **B.** On expiration, the flail segment bulges outward, and the mediastinal structures shift back to the affected side.

gas exchange is greatly compromised, respiratory acidosis develops as a result of carbon dioxide retention. Hypotension, inadequate tissue perfusion, and metabolic acidosis often follow as the paradoxical motion of the mediastinum decreases cardiac output.

Medical and Nursing Management

As with rib fracture, treatment of flail chest is usually supportive. Management includes providing ventilatory support, clearing secretions from the lungs, and controlling pain. Specific management depends on the degree of respiratory dysfunction. If only a small segment of the chest is involved, the objectives are to clear the airway through positioning, coughing, deep breathing, and suctioning to aid in the expansion of the lung, and to relieve pain by intercostal nerve blocks, high thoracic epidural blocks, or cautious use of IV opioids.

For mild to moderate flail chest injuries, the underlying pulmonary contusion is treated by monitoring fluid intake and appropriate fluid replacement while relieving chest pain. Pulmonary physiotherapy focusing on lung volume expansion includes deep breathing exercises, IS, and nebulized bronchodilators and mucolytics.

For severe flail chest injuries, endotracheal intubation and mechanical ventilation are required to provide internal pneumatic stabilization of the flail chest and to correct abnormalities in gas exchange. This helps treat the underlying pulmonary contusion, serves to stabilize the thoracic cage to allow the fractures to heal, and improves alveolar ventilation and intrathoracic volume by decreasing the work of breathing. In rare circumstances, surgery may be required to more quickly stabilize the flail segment.

Regardless of the type of treatment, the patient is carefully monitored by serial chest x-rays, ABG analysis, POX, and bedside pulmonary function monitoring. Pain management is key to successful treatment. Patient-controlled analgesia, intercostal nerve blocks, epidural analgesia, and intrapleural administration of opioids may be used to relieve or manage thoracic pain.

PULMONARY CONTUSION

Pulmonary contusion is a common thoracic injury and is frequently associated with blunt trauma. It is defined as damage to the lung tissues resulting in hemorrhage and localized edema (i.e., bruised lung). Pulmonary contusion represents a spectrum of lung injury characterized by the development of infiltrates and various degrees of respiratory dysfunction and sometimes respiratory failure. A contusion is sustained in up to 64% of patients who experience blunt force trauma (Hammer et al., 2016). Pulmonary contusion may not be evident initially on examination but develops in the posttraumatic period; it may involve a small portion of one lung, a massive section of a lung, one entire lung, or both lungs.

Pathophysiology

The primary pathologic defect is an abnormal accumulation of fluid in the interstitial and intra-alveolar spaces. It is thought that injury to the lung parenchyma and its capillary network results in a leakage of serum protein and plasma. The leaking serum protein exerts an osmotic pressure that enhances loss of fluid from the capillaries. Blood, edema, and cellular debris (from cellular response to injury) enter the lung and accumulate in the bronchioles and alveoli, where they interfere with gas exchange. The patient has hypoxemia and carbon dioxide retention. Occasionally, a contused lung occurs on the other side of the point of body impact; this is called a *contrecoup contusion*.

Clinical Manifestations and Assessment

The clinical manifestations of pulmonary contusions can vary based on the severity of bruising and parenchymal involvement. The most common signs and symptoms are crackles, decreased breath sounds, or bronchial breath sounds in peripheral lung areas, dyspnea, tachypnea, tachycardia, chest pain, blood-tinged secretions, hypoxemia, and respiratory acidosis. Patients with moderate pulmonary contusions often have a constant, but ineffective cough and cannot clear their secretions. Patients with severe pulmonary contusion have the signs and symptoms of ARDS; these may include hypoxemia, dyspnea, agitation, combativeness, and productive cough with frothy, bloody secretions.

The efficiency of gas exchange is determined by POX and ABG measurements. Pulse oximetry is also used to measure oxygen saturation continuously. The initial chest x-ray may show no changes; changes may not appear for 1 or 2 days after the injury and appear as pulmonary infiltrates on chest x-ray.

Medical and Nursing Management

Treatment priorities include maintaining the airway, providing adequate oxygenation, and controlling pain. In mild pulmonary contusion, judicious hydration via IV fluids and oral intake is important to mobilize secretions. However, fluid intake must be monitored closely to avoid hypervolemia, which can worsen the contusion. Volume expansion techniques, postural drainage, physiotherapy including coughing, and endotracheal suctioning are used to remove the secretions. Pain is managed by intercostal nerve blocks or by opioids via patient-controlled analgesia or other methods. Usually supplemental oxygen is given by mask or cannula for hypoxemia (saturation less than 90%).

In patients with moderate pulmonary contusions, bronchoscopy may be required to remove secretions. Intubation and mechanical ventilation with PEEP may also be necessary to maintain the pressure and keep the lungs inflated. In patients with severe contusion, who may develop respiratory failure, aggressive treatment with endotracheal intubation and ventilatory support, diuretics, and fluid restriction may be necessary.

Antimicrobial medications may be prescribed for the treatment of pulmonary infection. This is a common complication of pulmonary contusion because the fluid and blood that extravasates into the alveolar and interstitial spaces serve as an excellent culture medium.

CARDIAC TAMPONADE

Cardiac tamponade is compression of the heart resulting from fluid or blood within the pericardial sac. It usually is caused by blunt or penetrating trauma to the chest. A penetrating wound of the heart is associated with a high mortality rate. Cardiac tamponade also may follow diagnostic cardiac catheterization, angiographic procedures, and pacemaker insertion, which can produce perforations of the heart and great vessels. Pericardial effusion with fluid compressing the heart also may develop from metastases to the pericardium from malignant tumors of the breast, lung, or mediastinum and may occur with lymphomas and leukemias, renal failure, TB, and high-dose radiation to the chest. Cardiac tamponade is discussed in detail in Chapter 15.

PNEUMOTHORAX

Pneumothorax occurs when the parietal or visceral pleura are punctured and the pleural space is exposed to positive atmospheric pressure. Normally, the pressure in the pleural space is negative or subatmospheric; this negative pressure is required to maintain lung inflation. When either pleura is breached, air enters the pleural space, and the lung or a portion of it collapses.

Types of Pneumothorax

Types of pneumothorax include simple, traumatic, and tension pneumothorax (Fig. 10-13).

Simple Pneumothorax

A simple, or spontaneous, pneumothorax most commonly occurs as air enters the pleural space through the rupture of a bleb or a bronchopleural fistula. A spontaneous pneumothorax may occur in an apparently healthy person (most commonly in young men) in the absence of trauma due to rupture of an air-filled bleb, or blister, on the surface of the lung, allowing air from the airways to enter the pleural cavity. It may also be associated with bullous lung diseases such as emphysema or pulmonary fibrosis.

Traumatic Pneumothorax

A traumatic pneumothorax occurs when air escapes from a laceration in the lung itself and enters the pleural space or enters the pleural space through a wound in the chest wall. It may result from blunt trauma, penetrating chest or abdominal trauma, or diaphragmatic tears. Traumatic pneumothorax may occur during invasive thoracic procedures (i.e., thoracentesis, **transbronchial** lung biopsy, insertion of a subclavian line) in which the pleura is punctured inadvertently or with barotrauma from mechanical ventilation. A traumatic pneumothorax resulting from major trauma to the chest is often accompanied by a hemothorax (collection of blood in the pleural space resulting from torn intercostal vessels, lacerations of the great vessels, or lacerations of the lungs). Often both blood and air are found in the chest cavity (hemopneumothorax) after major trauma.

Open pneumothorax is one form of traumatic pneumothorax. It occurs when a wound in the chest wall is large enough to allow air to pass freely in and out of the thoracic cavity with each attempted respiration. Because the rush of air through the wound in the chest wall produces a sucking sound, such injuries are termed *sucking chest wounds.*

Tension Pneumothorax

A tension pneumothorax occurs when air is drawn into the pleural space from a lacerated lung or through a small opening or wound in the chest wall. It may be a complication of other types of pneumothorax. In contrast to open pneumothorax, the air that enters the chest cavity with each inspiration is trapped; it cannot be expelled during expiration through the air passages or the opening in the chest wall. In effect, a one-way valve or ball valve mechanism occurs, where air

FIGURE 10-13 Open and tension pneumothorax.

enters the pleural space but cannot escape. With each breath, tension (positive pressure) is increased within the affected pleural space. This causes the lung to collapse and the heart, the great vessels, and the trachea to shift toward the unaffected side of the chest (mediastinal shift). Both respiration and circulatory function are compromised because of the increased intrathoracic pressure, which decreases venous return to the heart, causing decreased cardiac output and impairment of peripheral circulation. In extreme cases, cardiac arrest can occur.

Clinical Manifestations

The signs and symptoms associated with pneumothorax depend on its size and cause. Usually pain is sudden and may be pleuritic. The patient may have only minimal respiratory distress with slight chest discomfort and tachypnea with a small simple or uncomplicated pneumothorax. If the pneumothorax is large and the lung collapses totally, acute respiratory distress occurs. The patient is anxious, has dyspnea and air hunger, has increased use of the accessory muscles, and may develop severe hypoxemia. In assessing the chest for any type of pneumothorax, the nurse assesses tracheal alignment, expansion of the chest, and breath sounds, and percusses the chest. In a simple pneumothorax, the trachea is midline, expansion of the chest is decreased, breath sounds may be diminished, and percussion of the chest may reveal normal sounds or hyperresonance depending on the size of the pneumothorax. The nurse assesses the affected lung for crepitus or subcutaneous emphysema and notes the extent of it in the patient's record.

In a tension pneumothorax, the trachea may shift away from the affected side, chest expansion may be decreased or fixed in a hyperexpansion state, breath sounds are diminished or absent, and percussion to the affected side is hyperresonant. The clinical picture is one of air hunger, agitation, increasing hypoxemia, central cyanosis, hypotension, and tachycardia.

Medical and Nursing Management

Medical management of pneumothorax depends on its cause and severity. The goal of treatment is to evacuate the air or blood from the pleural space. A thoracostomy tube (chest tube) is used to evacuate any accumulated air or fluid. A small, simple pneumothorax is treated with a small chest tube (20 Fr, or 10–12 Fr pigtail catheter) inserted at the second intercostal space, at the midclavicular line. Larger pneumothoraxes, especially if there is fluid or blood present, are managed with larger-sized tubes (32–36 Fr) that are placed in the fourth or fifth intercostal space at the midaxillary line. The tube is directed posteriorly to drain the fluid and air. Once the chest tube or tubes are inserted and suction is applied (usually to –20 mm Hg suction), effective decompression of the pleural cavity (drainage of blood or air) occurs.

The severity of open pneumothorax depends on the amount and rate of thoracic bleeding and the amount of air in the pleural space. The pleural cavity can be decompressed by needle aspiration (thoracentesis) or by chest tube drainage of the blood or air. Then the lung is able to re-expand and resume the function of gas exchange. As a rule of thumb, the chest wall is opened surgically (thoracotomy) if more than 1,500 mL of blood is aspirated initially by thoracentesis (or is the initial chest tube output) or if chest tube output continues at greater than 200 mL/hr. The urgency with which the blood must be removed is determined by the degree of respiratory compromise. An emergency thoracotomy may also be performed in the emergency department if a cardiovascular injury secondary to penetrating trauma is suspected. The patient with a possible tension pneumothorax should be given a high concentration of supplemental oxygen immediately to treat the hypoxemia, and POX should be used to monitor oxygen saturation.

In an emergency situation, a tension pneumothorax can be decompressed or quickly converted to a simple pneumothorax by inserting a large-bore needle (14-gauge) at the second intercostal space, midclavicular line on the affected side. This relieves the pressure and vents the positive pressure to the external environment. A chest tube is then inserted and connected to suction to remove the remaining air and fluid, reestablish the negative pressure, and re-expand the lung. If the lung re-expands and air leakage from the lung parenchyma stops, further drainage may be unnecessary. If a prolonged air leak continues despite chest tube drainage to underwater seal, surgery may be necessary to close the leak. A plan of nursing care for the patient after thoracotomy is available online at http://thepoint.lww.com/Honan2e.

SUBCUTANEOUS EMPHYSEMA

No matter what kind of chest trauma a patient has, when the lung or the air passages are injured, air may enter the tissue planes and pass for some distance under the skin (e.g., neck, chest). The tissues give a crackling sensation when palpated, and the subcutaneous air produces an alarming appearance as the face, neck, body, and scrotum become misshapen by subcutaneous air. Fortunately, subcutaneous emphysema in and of itself usually is not a serious complication. The subcutaneous air is absorbed spontaneously if the underlying air leak is treated or stops spontaneously. In severe cases, in which there is widespread subcutaneous emphysema, a tracheostomy is indicated if airway patency is threatened.

ASPIRATION

Aspiration of stomach contents into the lungs is a serious complication that can cause pneumonia and result in the clinical picture of tachycardia, dyspnea, hypoxemia, hypertension, hypotension, and, finally, death. It can occur when the protective airway reflexes are decreased or absent due to a variety of factors.

Pathophysiology

The primary factors responsible for death and complications after aspiration of gastric contents are the volume and character of the aspirated gastric contents. For example, a small, localized aspiration from regurgitation can cause pneumonia and acute respiratory distress; a massive aspiration is usually fatal. Factors that increase the risk of aspiration are discussed in Box 10-13.

A full stomach contains food particles. If these are aspirated, the problem then becomes one of mechanical blockage of the airways and secondary infection or chemical pneumonitis. During periods of fasting, the stomach contains acidic gastric juice, which, if aspirated, can be very destructive to the alveoli and capillaries. Fecal contamination (more likely seen in intestinal obstruction) increases the likelihood of death because the endotoxins produced by intestinal organisms may be absorbed systemically, or the thick proteinaceous material found in the intestinal contents may obstruct the airway, leading to atelectasis and secondary bacterial invasion.

Aspiration pneumonitis may develop from aspiration of gastric contents, which can also cause a chemical burn of the tracheobronchial tree and pulmonary parenchyma.

BOX 10-13 **Risk Factors for Aspiration**

- Altered level of consciousness (cerebrovascular accident, head trauma, intracranial mass/tumor, drug overdose, alcohol intoxication, seizures, oversedation)
- Neurologic disorders (Parkinson disease, myasthenia gravis, multiple sclerosis, amyotrophic lateral sclerosis)
- Dysphagia (esophageal stricture, diverticula or neoplasm, tracheoesophageal fistula, cardiac sphincter incompetence, achalasia [lack of the lower esophageal sphincter to relax, preventing food from passing into the stomach])
- Altered airway or oropharyngeal anatomy (head and neck malignancy, surgery and/or radiation therapy to head and neck)
- Disruption via mechanical instruments (endotracheal intubation, tracheostomy, naso-/orogastric tube [any size], bronchoscopy, laryngoscopy, upper GI endoscopy)
- Recumbent position
- Protracted vomiting
- Nasogastric feeding
- Gastric outlet obstruction

An ensuing inflammatory response occurs. This results in the destruction of alveolar–capillary endothelial cells, with a consequent outpouring of protein-rich fluids into the interstitial and intra-alveolar spaces. As a result, surfactant is lost, which, in turn, causes the airways to close and the alveoli to collapse. Finally, the impaired exchange of oxygen and carbon dioxide causes respiratory failure.

Aspiration pneumonia develops after inhalation of colonized oropharyngeal material. The pathologic process involves an acute inflammatory response to bacteria and bacterial products. Most commonly, the bacteriologic findings include gram-positive cocci, gram-negative rods, and, occasionally, anaerobic bacteria.

Prevention

Prevention is the primary goal when caring for patients at risk for aspiration. Examples of risk factors for aspiration include decreased level of consciousness, supine positioning, presence of a nasogastric tube, tracheal intubation and mechanical ventilation, and advanced age (Christiani, 2016). Evidence confirms that one of the main preventive measures for aspiration is placing at-risk patients in a semirecumbent position (elevation of the head of the bed to a 30- to 45-degree angle) (American Association of Critical Care Nurses [AACN], 2016).

Compensating for Absent Reflexes

Aspiration may occur if the patient cannot adequately coordinate protective glottic, laryngeal, and cough reflexes. This hazard is increased if the patient has a distended abdomen, is supine, has the upper extremities immobilized by IV infusions or hand restraints, receives local anesthetics to the oropharyngeal or laryngeal area for diagnostic procedures, has been sedated, or has had long-term intubation.

When vomiting, people can normally protect their airway by sitting up or turning on the side and coordinating breathing, coughing, gag, and glottic reflexes. If these reflexes are active, an oral airway should not be inserted. If an airway is in place, it should be pulled out the moment the patient gags so as not to stimulate the pharyngeal gag reflex and promote vomiting and aspiration. Suctioning of oral secretions with a catheter should be performed with minimal pharyngeal stimulation.

In addition, using the smallest effective level of sedation is prudent in patients at risk for aspiration.

Assessing Feeding Tube Placement

When a patient is intubated, aspiration may occur even with a nasogastric tube in place and may result in nosocomial pneumonia. Assessment of nasogastric tube placement is key to the prevention of aspiration. The best method for determining tube placement is via an x-ray taken immediately after an enteral feeding tube is placed and prior to beginning feeds. Nurses should mark the place where the tube exits the nares or lips and note this in the patient's chart. This marking should be assessed whenever medication is administered via the tube or at least every 4 hours. Other methods of tube confirmation have been studied, such as observation of the aspirate color, testing of its pH or glucose content, and auscultation over the stomach for an air bolus. None of these methods has been shown to accurately assess the placement of the tube (AACN, 2016). A combination of methods is recommended: assessment of the patient's tolerance to medication and feeding administration (noting abdominal distention and complaints of abdominal pain, observing for passage of flatus and stool) as well as measurement of tube length, while assessing the pH measurement of aspirate remains an area where further research is warranted. It is important for the nurse to understand that where research is ongoing, he or she should follow institutional procedures. Refer to the AACN Prevention of Aspiration Practice Alert (with AACN Levels of Evidence and complete reference list).

Patients who receive continuous or timed-interval tube feedings must be positioned properly. Patients receiving continuous infusions are given small volumes under low pressure in an upright position, which helps prevent aspiration. Patients receiving tube feedings at timed intervals are maintained in an upright or semirecumbent position (elevation of the head of the bed to a 30- to 45-degree angle) during the feeding and for a minimum of 30 minutes afterward to allow the stomach to empty partially. Because there is controversy over the assessment of gastric residual volume (GRV) since research does not demonstrate prevention of early detection of feeding intolerance or aspiration (McClave et al., 2016), the nurse should follow institutional procedures related to GRV. Tube feedings must be given only when it is certain that the feeding tube is positioned correctly in the stomach or in the small bowel. Many patients today receive enteral feeding directly into the small intestine through a small-bore flexible feeding tube or surgically implanted tube. Feedings are given slowly and are regulated by a feeding pump (refer to Chapter 22 for more details). The nurse should be aware that the results of routine chest and abdominal x-ray will report tube location.

CHAPTER REVIEW

Critical Thinking Exercises

1. You are caring for an 82-year-old woman who was recently transferred to the hospital from a nursing home with the diagnosis of presumed health care–associated pneumonia. She has a gastrostomy feeding tube in place and is lethargic, dehydrated, and confused. What strategies would you initiate to prevent aspiration? What nursing care interventions would you use to assess for aspiration? What is the evidence base for the interventions that you consider? How will you evaluate the strength of the evidence? What suggestions might you have regarding appropriate devices for long-term enteral feeding in this patient once she is discharged back to the nursing home?

2. On a surgical unit, you are caring for a 42-year-old woman who underwent a total abdominal hysterectomy and bilateral salpingo-oophorectomy and has developed a postoperative DVT that resulted in a PE. She is a smoker and is taking multiple medications. She was stable when you started your shift, but she has become increasingly anxious with some shortness of breath in the past hour. What are potential risk factors you might observe or identify in this patient? What assessment strategies would you use to evaluate changes in her respiratory status? What decision process would you use to determine when the provider should be contacted?

3. You are caring for a patient who experienced blunt chest trauma in an MVA. A chest tube has been inserted to treat a simple pneumothorax and hemothorax. The chest drainage system has drained 400 mL of light red fluid during the first 6 hours after insertion. The patient has become increasingly short of breath during the past hour. You note that there is no longer an air leak noted in the water-seal chamber. What physical assessment skills and strategies would you use to determine potential changes in the patient's respiratory condition? What are potential causes of this increasing shortness of breath? What would you do to prepare for an emergency situation in this patient?

4. On a surgical unit, you are caring for a 62-year-old man who has undergone right upper lobectomy for lung cancer. The patient has COPD and has continued to smoke despite the diagnoses of COPD and lung cancer. What strategies would you use to prevent or minimize pulmonary complications in this patient? What are the methods you might use to assess the patient's progress from a respiratory standpoint? What strategies would you consider to encourage the patient to stop smoking? What is the evidence base for the strategies that you consider? How will you evaluate the strength of the evidence?

NCLEX-Style Review Questions

1. The nurse is caring for a client diagnosed with ARDS. In evaluating the use of PEEP, what outcome would the nurse expect to find?
   a. Increased ventilation–perfusion mismatch
   b. Increased FRC
   c. Decreased intrathoracic pressure
   d. Decreased FRC

2. A nurse working on a general medical-surgical floor is discussing the clinical manifestations of pulmonary arterial hypertension (PAH) with a recent nursing graduate. What is the main symptom of PAH that the nurse would explain?
   a. Chest pain
   b. Fatigue
   c. Dyspnea
   d. Hemoptysis

3. A patient is receiving thrombolytic therapy for treatment of a pulmonary emboli. For what side effect should the nurse must monitor the patient?
   a. Chest pain
   b. Rash
   c. Hyperthermia
   d. Bleeding

4. A nurse is caring for a patient diagnosed with lung cancer who has a chest tube. The chest tube has continuous bubbling in the water-seal chamber. What does the nurse understand that this indicates?
   a. Tidaling
   b. The tube in the mediastinum
   c. A properly functioning system
   d. An air leak in the system

5. The nurse is assessing a patient with a blunt chest trauma due to an MVA. What finding would be indicative of a flail chest?
   a. Hypertension
   b. Metabolic alkalosis
   c. Paradoxical chest movement
   d. Respiratory alkalosis

Try these additional resources, available at **http://thepoint.lww.com/Honan2e**, to enhance your learning and understanding of this chapter:

- NCLEX-Style Student Review Questions
- Journal Articles

REFERENCES AND SELECTED READINGS

References and selected readings associated with this chapter can be found on the website that accompanies the book. Visit **http://thepoint. lww.com/Honan2e** to access the references and other additional resources associated with this chapter.

Nursing Management of Patients Diagnosed with Chronic Obstructive Pulmonary Disease and Asthma

Margaret Campbell Haggerty

Learning Objectives

After reading this chapter, you will be able to:

1. Describe the pathophysiology of chronic obstructive pulmonary disease (COPD).
2. Discuss the major risk factors for developing COPD and interventions used to minimize or prevent these risk factors.
3. Use the nursing process as a framework for care of patients with COPD.
4. Develop a teaching plan for patients with COPD.
5. Describe the pathophysiology of asthma.
6. Discuss the medications used in asthma management.
7. Describe asthma self-management strategies.

Chronic obstructive pulmonary disease (COPD) and asthma are the most common chronic pulmonary disorders. Nurses working with patients with these chronic pulmonary diseases care for them across the spectrum of care, from outpatient and home care to emergency, inpatient, and critical care and, finally, in the hospice setting. Patients with COPD and asthma need care from nurses who not only have astute assessment and clinical management skills but who also understand how these disorders can affect quality of life. In addition, the nurse's knowledge of palliative and end-of-life care is important for affected patients. Patient and family teaching is an important nursing intervention to enhance self-management in patients with any chronic pulmonary disorder.

COPD

Chronic obstructive pulmonary disease (COPD) is a disease state characterized by chronic airflow limitation that is not fully reversible. The airflow limitation in COPD is usually progressive and is associated with an inflammatory response of the lungs (GOLD, 2015).

An estimated 13.7 million Americans have the diagnosis of COPD. The actual incidence of COPD is thought to be much higher as many cases are undiagnosed. COPD is the fourth leading cause of death in the United States; more women than men die from COPD. In addition, COPD is a major cause of morbidity and accounts for an annual cost estimated to be nearly $50 billion, including health care expenditures, mortality costs, lost work days, and other indirect costs (Ford et al., 2013; COPD Fast Stats, 2015).

Pathophysiology

The pathologic changes that characterize COPD are complex and include changes to the airways, lung parenchyma, and pulmonary vasculature (GOLD, 2015). Increased levels of proinflammatory cytokines that result in small airway injury, an imbalance between mediators that promote inflammation and those that protect lung tissue and increased airway hyperresponsiveness, are among the pathophysiologic changes that occur (Hoepers, Menezes, & Frode, 2015). Inflammation and narrowing of peripheral airways lead to a loss of pulmonary function, specifically FEV_1 (forced expired volume in one second). Destruction of the lung parenchyma results in emphysematous changes and contributes to airflow limitation and impaired gas exchange.

FIGURE 11-1 Changes in the alveolar structure in centrilobular and panlobular emphysema. In panlobular emphysema, the bronchioles, alveolar ducts, and alveoli are destroyed, and the airspaces within the lobule are enlarged. On centrilobular emphysema, the pathologic changes occur in the lobule, whereas the peripheral portions of the acinus are preserved.

> ### Nursing Alert
> *Normally, 80% or more of the expiratory volume can be expelled in 1 second. Obstructive lung disease is defined as a postbronchodilator FEV₁/FVC (forced expired volume in one second as a ratio of forced vital capacity [volume of lungs from full inspiration to forced maximal expiration that is expressed as a percentage of the predicted normal for a person]) ratio of less than 70%. The patient demonstrates a degree of reversibility if the pulmonary function values improve significantly (more than 12%) after administration of the bronchodilator. Usually patients who demonstrate complete reversibility to normal values are diagnosed with asthma. Patients who demonstrate some*

reversibility that does not reach normal values may be diagnosed with COPD with some reversible component or an overlap of COPD and asthma.

Emphysema is a pathologic term that describes an abnormal enlargement of the airspaces beyond the terminal bronchioles with destruction of the walls of the alveoli (parenchymal destruction) (Fig. 11-1). **Chronic bronchitis**, a disease of the airways, is defined as the presence of cough and sputum production for at least 3 months in each of 2 consecutive years. Chronic mucus hypersecretion has been implicated as a cause of lung function decline, exacerbations, and infections. Thickening of the epithelium, smooth muscle hypertrophy, and airway inflammation are implicated in remodeling of the airways (Fig. 11-2). Emphysema and chronic bronchitis may exist in patients with normal lung function and in patients with COPD (GOLD, 2015).

In the later stages of COPD, gas exchange is often impaired. As the alveolar walls continue to break down, the pulmonary capillary bed is reduced in size. Resistance to pulmonary blood flow is increased, forcing the right ventricle to maintain a higher and a higher pressure in the pulmonary artery. Chronic hypoxemia (low oxygen) increases pulmonary artery pressures and can lead to pulmonary hypertension. This higher pressure in the pulmonary artery results in right ventricular hypertrophy. Ultimately, cor pulmonale, or right ventricular failure, can occur. In addition, decreased carbon dioxide elimination results in increased carbon dioxide tension in arterial blood (hypercapnia) and leads to respiratory acidosis and chronic respiratory failure. In acute illness, worsening hypercapnia can lead to acute respiratory failure. COPD is considered a systemic disease and may affect skeletal muscle as well as the functioning of the cardiovascular, neurologic, psychiatric, and endocrine systems.

Risk Factors

The risk factors for the development for COPD are outlined in Box 11-1. The most important risk factor is tobacco

FIGURE 11-2 Pathophysiology of chronic bronchitis as compared to a normal bronchus. The bronchus in chronic bronchitis is narrowed and has impaired air flow due to multiple mechanisms: inflammation, excess mucus production, and potential smooth muscle constriction (bronchospasm).

BOX 11-1
Known Risk Factors for Chronic Obstructive Pulmonary Disease

- Tobacco smoke (cigarette, pipe, cigar, water pipe, marijuana)
- Environmental tobacco smoke
- Genetic factors, e.g., severe inherited alpha-1 antitrypsin deficiency
- Exposure to particles: organic and inorganic dusts, open fires from wood, animal dung, crop residue, and coal
- Biomass cooking in poorly ventilated areas

Possible Risk Factors
- Poverty
- Asthma/bronchial hyperreactivity
- Chronic bronchitis/mucus hypersecretion
- Severe respiratory infections in childhood

smoking (cigarettes, pipe, cigar, water pipe, marijuana). Environmental tobacco smoke (ETS), also known as secondhand smoke, is also a risk factor for the development of COPD. The effects of cigarette smoke are complex and lead to the development of COPD in approximately 15% to 20% of smokers. Many experts now think the incidence may be as high as 30% to 50% in smokers (GOLD, 2015). Tobacco smoke irritates the airways and, in susceptible individuals, results in mucus hypersecretion and airway inflammation.

Fetuses exposed to maternal smoking in utero have impaired lung development and may go on to develop COPD later in life. Biomass (open fire) cooking and heating in poorly ventilated areas is a major risk factor for the development of COPD in third world nations. Other factors that put people at risk for COPD include prolonged and intense exposure to occupational dusts and chemicals, a history or respiratory infections as a child, and outdoor air pollution. (GOLD, 2015).

A host risk factor for COPD is a deficiency of an enzyme inhibitor that protects the lung parenchyma from injury: alpha$_1$-antitrypsin. **Alpha$_1$-antitrypsin deficiency** affects approximately 1 in every 3,000 Americans and accounts for approximately 80,000 to 100,000 cases of COPD (Izaguiree, 2014). Genetically susceptible people are more sensitive to environmental factors (e.g., smoking, air pollution, infectious agents, allergens) and have a higher risk of developing chronic obstructive symptoms. Not all smokers get COPD, but it does occur more frequently in families. Studies to identify other genetic factors that may be associated with COPD are as yet inconclusive (GOLD, 2015).

Clinical Manifestations and Assessment

COPD is characterized by three primary symptoms: dyspnea, chronic cough, and sputum production. Dyspnea is defined as an awareness of uncomfortable breathing that may vary in intensity. It often starts as mild and is noticed only with vigorous activities, such as stair-climbing and playing sports. As the disease progresses, dyspnea may become severe and often interferes with the person's activities of daily living. In more severe cases of COPD, dyspnea can occur at rest. Chronic cough and sputum production often precede the development of airflow limitation by many years. In early stage disease, the person may note an early morning cough productive of a small to moderate amount of white to clear sputum. During exacerbations, an increase in the amount and viscosity of sputum may occur, and the sputum may change color.

COPD is diagnosed based on history, physical examination, and pulmonary function testing. A positive history of progressive dyspnea and/or a productive cough in a cigarette smoker leads to a suspicion of COPD. Smoking history is usually expressed as "pack/years": the number of packs smoked per day times the number of years of smoking. A person who has smoked an average of 2 packs per day for 20 years has a smoking history of 40 pack/years.

Physical examination findings may be near normal in those with beginning and sometimes moderate disease. Findings consistent with more advanced COPD may include signs of hyperinflation: an increased anterior to posterior diameter of the chest, referred to as "barrel chest"; bilateral intercostal retractions at the posterior axillary line; horizontal fixation of the ribs in the inspiratory position; and hyperresonance to percussion, particularly in thin individuals. Breath sounds may be diminished; prolonged exhalation (bronchovesicular breath sounds) is usually heard throughout the chest; often adventitious sounds (coarse crackles and wheezes) are heard when the patient has increased secretions or bronchial hyperreactivity as well as during an exacerbation.

Pulmonary function studies are used to help confirm the diagnosis, determine disease severity, and monitor disease progression. **Spirometry** is used to evaluate airflow obstruction. Spirometry results are expressed as an absolute value and as a percentage of the predicted value using appropriate normal values for gender, race, age, weight, and height. With obstruction, the patient has difficulty exhaling or cannot forcibly exhale air from the lungs, reducing the **FEV$_1$**. Obstructive lung disease is defined as a postbronchodilator FEV$_1$/FVC ratio of less than 70%. The lower the FEV$_1$, the more severe the disease process.

Bronchodilator reversibility testing may be performed to rule out asthma and to guide initial treatment. Spirometry is first obtained; the patient is given an inhaled bronchodilator and spirometry is repeated. The patient demonstrates a degree of reversibility if the pulmonary function values improve significantly (more than 12%) after administration of the bronchodilator. Usually patients who demonstrate complete reversibility to normal values are diagnosed with asthma. Patients who demonstrate some reversibility that does not reach normal values may be diagnosed with COPD with some reversible component or an overlap of COPD and asthma. Patients who do not show a significant response to a bronchodilator test still may be given a trial of broncho-dilator treatment to determine if it helps relieve symptoms. Additional tests of pulmonary function include total lung capacity (TLC) and diffusion capacity. These tests are used to diagnose coexisting restrictive disease, in which the lung is restricted from filling to its normal capacity of air, and to help predict the contribution of emphysematous changes in the diagnosis.

Arterial blood gas (ABG) measurements may be obtained to assess baseline oxygenation and gas exchange and are especially important in advanced COPD. In addition, a chest x-ray may be obtained to establish the patient's base-line and to exclude alternative diagnoses. A chest x-ray is seldom diagnostic in COPD unless obvious bullous disease or severe hyperinflation is present. Chest x-rays are more commonly used in exacerbations to determine if the patient has an infiltrate or a concomitant lung mass. A computed tomography (CT) scan is not routinely obtained in the diag-nosis of COPD, but a high-resolution CT scan may help in the differential diagnosis or to evaluate patients for surgical procedures such as bullectomy or lung-volume reduction surgery (LVRS). Screening for alpha$_1$-antitrypsin deficiency is usually recommended for symptomatic patients younger than 45 years and for those with a strong family history of COPD.

Different methods are used to classify COPD by stages depending on severity. The updated GOLD guidelines include lung function measurement and exacerbation history to stage patients. Staging is used to determine prognosis, guide therapy, and to develop research protocols. In mild disease, the patient may be asymptomatic. As lung function (FEV$_1$/FVC%) declines, symptoms start to appear. The more severe the decline in lung function is, the more severe the COPD. When the FEV$_1$ is less than 50% predicted, COPD is classified as severe. Other factors that determine progno-sis include history cigarette smoking in terms of pack/years, continued cigarette smoking, passive smoking exposure, age, rate of decline of FEV$_1$, hypoxemia, pulmonary artery pressure, resting heart rate, weight loss, number of exacerba-tions, and reversibility of airflow obstruction. Staging sever-ity serves as a guideline to treatment protocols, but variation occurs depending on the patient characteristics, comorbid conditions, and response to interventions.

The differential diagnosis of COPD includes: asthma, heart failure, bronchiectasis (abnormal widening of the bronchi or their branches, causing a risk of infection), tuber-culosis, lung cancer, and bronchiolitis (inflammation of the bronchioles). These conditions may also coexist with COPD, and as many as 66% of patients have one comorbid-ity. Cardiac disease, peripheral atherosclerosis, stroke, dia-betes mellitus, arthritis, malignancy, anxiety, and depression are common comorbid conditions. Phenotypes or overlap syndromes that are heterogeneous and usually disease man-ifestations are worse than when each disease is considered separately. Recent reports include COPD linked to asthma,

---

BOX 11-2 | **COPD, Common Co-existing Disorders with Overlap of Clinical Presentation**

- COPD/Asthma overlap syndrome (ACOS) (Papaiwannou et al., 2014)
- Combined pulmonary fibrosis and emphysema syndrome (Portillo & Morera, 2012)
- Sleep-disordered breathing and COPD: the overlap syn-drome (Owens & Malhota, 2012)
- Bronchiectasis phenotype (Martinez-Garcia et al., 2015)

---

obstructive sleep apnea, pulmonary fibrosis, bronchiectasis, and heart failure (see Box 11-2).

Medical Management

The goals of medical therapy are to stabilize, manage, and monitor the disease; reduce symptoms; assess and reduce exacerbation risk and rate; promote maximal functional ability; prevent premature disability; assist the individual to adapt to the handicap caused by the disorder and limit adverse prognosis as the disease progresses. The management of the patient depends on the severity of the COPD. In early-stage disease, clinical strategies are aimed at maximizing pulmo-nary function, keeping the patient active, preventing exac-erbations, and engaging the patient in self-management. In progressive stages, more intensive therapies are added. In very late-stage disease, palliative care should be considered (see Fig. 11-3).

Stabilizing Disease Progression

Smoking cessation slows the accelerated decline in lung function and the progression of COPD (GOLD, 2015). Fac-tors associated with continued smoking vary among patients and may include the strength of the nicotine addiction,

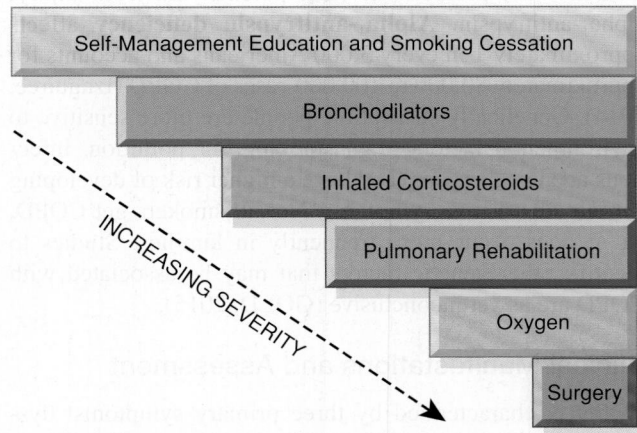

FIGURE 11-3 Treatment options for COPD. (Redrawn from *Breath-ing better with a COPD diagnosis,* U.S. Department of Health and Human Services, NIH publication No. 07-5841.)

continued exposure to smoking-associated stimuli (at work or in social settings), stress, depression, and habit.

Because multiple factors are associated with continued smoking, successful cessation often requires multiple strategies. Health care providers should promote cessation by explaining the risks of smoking and personalizing the "at-risk" message to the patient. Encouraging the patient to set a definite "quit date" is associated with more successful smoking cessation. Brief counseling may work for many smokers; referral to a smoking cessation program may be helpful for those unable to quit on their own. Follow-up from the nurse within a few days after the established "quit date" is associated with an increased rate of success; the nurse can review progress and address any problems with the patient. Continued reinforcement with telephone calls or clinic visits is also beneficial. Relapses should be analyzed, and the patient and health care provider should jointly identify possible solutions to prevent future backsliding.

Pharmacotherapy increases long-term smoking abstinence rates when used in conjunction with smoking cessation counseling. Nicotine replacement (gum, inhaler, nasal spray, transferal patch, sublingual tablet, or lozenges) may be used as a single agent or in combination with other pharmacologic agents. Antidepressants such as bupropion SR (Zyban®, Wellbutrin®) and nortriptyline also have been shown to increase long-term quit rates. Bupropion is particularly useful in those concerned with weight gain during smoking abstinence as it may result in weight loss.

 Drug Alert!
Bupropion is contraindicated in patients with a history of seizures as it may lower the seizure threshold.

Varenicline (Chantix®) reduces nicotine withdrawal symptoms and has been associated with increased quit rates. Electronic cigarettes, or "e-cigarettes, produced by a variety of manufactures are usually battery-operated devices that vaporize a mist of nicotine to the user. They have been used by some smokers when trying to quit. The Federal Drug Administration (FDA) has limited authority to regulate e-cigarettes as long as they are marketed as therapeutic. Concerns over unregulated additives that are potentially toxic and conflicting reports about efficacy exist. In addition, e-cigarettes may promote tobacco smoking in previous non-smokers. A position statement issued by the multinational Forum of International Respiratory Societies (Schraufnagel et al., 2014) recommends banning or more closely regulating these products until more safety information becomes available.

Smoking cessation can begin in a variety of health care settings: outpatient clinics, pulmonary rehabilitation, community health programs, and hospitals as well as in the home. Regardless of the setting, nurses have the opportunity to teach patients about the risks of smoking and the benefits of smoking cessation. Various materials, resources, and programs developed by several organizations (e.g., Agency for Healthcare Research and Quality, U.S. Public Health Service, CDC, National Cancer Institute, American Lung Association, American Thoracic Society, American Cancer Society) are available to assist with this effort. Online programs may be useful to some smokers. One such program is "the ex" plan, which can be found at BecomeAnEX.org. Box 11-3 outlines a smoking cessation approach that incorporates the current concepts in a concise outline.

Pharmacologic Therapy

Pharmacologic agents are an important part of the treatment of COPD and fall into several categories.

Bronchodilators

Bronchodilators relieve bronchospasm, reduce airway obstruction, and aid in secretion clearance. The most frequently used classes of bronchodilators include sympathomimetics, also called beta adrenergic (both short and long acting); anticholinergics, also called muscarinic antagonists (both short and long term), or a combination of the two agents. Methylxanthines, for example, theophylline-like medications, are used less frequently than in the past but may still be useful for some patients. The methylxanthines that are currently available have a narrow therapeutic range and have serious side effects. They are often used as a third-line agent when other bronchodilators don't completely control symptoms.

Bronchodilators are usually delivered by the inhaled route (metered dose inhalers, dry powder inhalers [DPIs], or by nebulization). Oral forms of bronchodilators are rarely given because of side effects. Long-acting sympathomimetics (also known as **LABAs** or long-acting beta adrenergics) and anticholinergic bronchodilators (also known as **LAMAs** or long-acting muscarinic antagonists) are considered maintenance medications and are usually administered on a regular basis. Short-acting sympathomimetics (also known as **SABAs** or short-acting beta adrenergics) are most often used on an as-needed basis to help with dyspnea and secretion clearance. SABAs may be used prophylactically, before the patient participates in dyspnea-producing activity such as eating or walking. Short-acting muscarinic antagonists (**SAMAs**) are sometimes used for quick relief.

Corticosteroids

Inhaled and systemic corticosteroids (oral or intravenous) may also be used in COPD. Systemic steroids are usually reserved for acute exacerbations and for those with severe symptoms that do not respond adequately to bronchodilators. Long-term treatment with oral corticosteroids is associated with an increased incidence of side effects, some of which are serious (hyperglycemia, osteoporosis). Inhaled corticosteroids may be used alone by inhaler devices or in

BOX 11-3

Health Promotion

Quitting Smoking: Help for the Smoker

Cigarette smoking has long been known to damage the heart, lungs, and other organs of the body. Cancer, problems with circulation, and premature wrinkling are among its other effects. Cigar, pipe, and marijuana smoke are also known to be harmful. Smoking is the single most preventable cause of premature death and disability. Quitting smoking increases your chance of living a longer, healthier life. Here are some tips for helping you quit.

- *Determine your readiness to quit: how motivated are you?*
  - Have you set a date to quit? A willingness to set a quit-date within 2 weeks indicates good motivation for quitting.
  - Can you list your reasons for wanting to quit? Health, saving money, feeling control over your habits, smelling better, and setting an example for others are some reasons for quitting. Make your reasons for quitting personal.
  - What obstacles do you anticipate?
  - Have you prepared for quitting?
    - Throw away all smoking-related materials: cigarettes, ashtrays, lighters
    - Make a plan for dealing with smoking urges
- *Develop an action plan.*
  - For immediate urges to smoke: practice the "4 Ds"
    - *Delay*: the urge to smoke will lessen in 3 minutes whether or not you have a cigarette

- *Deep breathe*: take several deep breaths when the urge strikes to help take the edge off
- *Drink water*: it helps to clear out the nicotine faster
- *Do something else*: distraction helps you ignore the urges to smoke
- Change your Thinking: remind yourself that you are choosing to become a nonsmoker and that it takes active work to do so
- Reward Yourself for Not Smoking: set aside the money you would have spent on cigarettes and buy yourself something as a reward
- *Discuss the need for nicotine replacement or other medications.*
  - Many smokers are much more successful in quitting with the assistance of medications like Zyban™, Chantix™, and/or one of the nicotine replacement products (patch, gum, inhaler, nasal spray, or lozenge). Discuss this with your health care provider.
- *Don't give up if you have a slip or relapse.*
  - Many people need several tries at quitting before they are successful. Keep at it, and you will be successful.
- *Seek help if trying to quit on your own hasn't worked.*
  - Find a local stop smoking program in your area. Your PCP, local hospital, visiting nurse, or Lung Association may know of a local program.

Adapted from the Norwalk Hospital Patient Education Guidelines.

combination with LABAs and/or LAMAs. Patients should be instructed to rinse and gargle after using inhaled steroid preparations to decrease the risk of oral thrush. An association between inhaled corticosteroids and pneumonia has been shown. Most clinicians reserve their use for those with more severe disease.

Medication regimens used to manage the symptoms of COPD are based on disease, symptom severity, and risk for exacerbation. For mild COPD, a short-acting bronchodilator is usually prescribed for symptom relief. For moderate to severe COPD, a short-acting bronchodilator along with regular treatment with a LABA, a LABA/steroid combination, and/or LAMA may be used. For severe or very severe COPD, medication therapy includes regular treatment with one or more bronchodilators and may include a methylxanthine and inhaled or systemic corticosteroids (GOLD, 2015).

A **metered-dose inhaler** (MDI) is a pressurized device that contains an aerosolized suspension of medication. A measured amount of medication is released with each activation of the canister. Patients must be instructed on the correct use of inhalers. With correct technique, 15% to 20% of the dose of medication is inhaled into the lung. Proper technique is important to ensure adequate deposition into the

airways. Common mistakes made by patients using MDIs include having difficulty coordinating actuation with inhalation, breathing in too quickly, and not breath-holding after inhalation.

A spacer (holding chamber) may also be used for patients who have difficulty coordinating activation of the MDI with inspiration. They are particularly useful for MDI steroids as less medication is deposited in the oropharynx, decreasing inhaled steroid side effects. Spacers come in several designs, but all are attached to the MDI and have a mouthpiece on the opposite end. Once the canister is activated, the aerosol particles stay suspended in the chamber for several seconds, allowing the patient to inhale after actuating the inhaler. Box 11-4 outlines the important steps for using a metered dose inhaler and spacer correctly. Patients need periodic review of correct inhaler technique to increase optimal therapeutic effect. DPIs include a variety of medications and devices. Specific package insert information is available on the use of these inhalers from the manufacturer. The most common medications administered by metered dose or DPIs used for both COPD and asthma are shown in Table 11-1. Nebulized medications (aerosolization of medication via a jet nebulizer and an air compressor) may also be effective

BOX 11-4

Patient Education

Using Inhalers Correctly

Many medicines taken for breathing are given by the inhaled method. Inhaled medicine goes directly to the lungs. But you need to learn to use inhalers correctly. With perfect technique, you get about 15–20% of the medication in your lungs. So, **good** technique is very important.

Correct Technique for Using Inhalers

- Remove the cap from mouthpiece of inhaler.
- Shake your inhaler for 5–6 seconds.
- Place the mouthpiece of the inhaler in your mouth with your tongue and teeth out of the way.
- As you depress the inhaler take a deep breath with your mouth wide open. Inhale for 5–6 seconds if you can. *Slow is the way to go.* The more slowly you breathe in, the deeper the medicine gets.
- At the end of the deep breath, hold your breath for at least 3–10 seconds.
- Exhale through pursed lips.
- If more than one puff is prescribed, repeat the above steps.
- After your last puff, rinse your mouth with mouthwash or water to help prevent dryness. If you are using inhaled steroids, rinse, gargle, and spit out the water or mouthwash.
- Rinse the mouthpiece thoroughly with warm water at least once a day. Let it air dry before assembling and storing it.

Other points: Do not use your inhaler more often than your health care provider recommends. An occasional extra puff or treatment of your quick-acting bronchodilator is ok, but, if you find yourself using your inhaler more frequently than usual, that may be a sign that you're getting ill and need to contact your provider.

Other inhaled medicines, e.g., those obtained without a prescription, should not be used unless approved by your Primary Care Provider (PCP). You can have serious side effects by mixing certain medications.

Spacer Devices

Spacer devices are used with inhalers when:
- You have a hard time using your inhaler correctly
- When the taste of the propellant in the inhaler is disturbing
- When you are using inhaled steroids and have problems with yeast infections in your mouth

The technique for using an inhaler with a spacer:
- Take the cap off the inhaler and the spacer
- Place the inhaler mouthpiece in the end of the spacer
- Shake your inhaler for 5–6 seconds
- Place the spacer mouthpiece in your mouth
- Depress the inhaler into the spacer
- Inhale slowly—over 5–6 seconds
- Hold your breath for about 10 seconds
- Repeat for the steps for each puff of medication

---

in patients who cannot use an MDI properly or who prefer this method of administration. Several formulations of medications are available for nebulization: SABAs used alone or in combination with anticholinergics, LABAs, and some corticosteroids. Patients need to learn proper technique for administration by nebulizers. Disinfection of the medication cup needs to be performed on a regular basis to avoid bacterial growth and inhalation by the patient.

Other Medications

Influenza and pneumococcal vaccinations reduce the incidence of pneumonia, hospitalizations for cardiac conditions, and deaths in the general elderly population. Patients should receive a yearly influenza vaccine. The CDC currently recommends the two-step pneumococcal vaccine (PCV13/Prevnar 13® and 12 months later PPSV23/Pneumovax23®) for patients with COPD. A one-time booster of pertussis (TDAP-tetanus, diphtheria, and pertussis), is also recommended (CDC, 2016).

Roflumilast (Daliresp®) is a phosphodiesterase-4 inhibitor that suppresses inflammatory activity in the lungs and is associated with decreased COPD exacerbations and hospitalizations. Side effects, including severe nausea, weight loss, mood disturbances, and suicidal ideation, may limit its usefulness in some patients.

Other pharmacologic treatments that may be used in COPD include alpha1-antitrypsin augmentation therapy for those with a diagnosed deficiency, antibiotic agents for acute infection, and mucolytic agents for help with secretion clearance. Cough suppressants are usually reserved for nighttime use when cough interferes with sleep. In very severe COPD, narcotics and other agents may be administered to relieve uncontrolled dyspnea (Schwartzstein, 2015).

Pharmacologic treatment of COPD poses many challenges for patients. Multiple drugs and drug classes are included in treatment regimens, and many drugs go by multiple names. In addition, multiple delivery methods, poly-pharmacy particularly with other comorbid conditions, expense, and side effects can add to poor adherence. Patients often confuse the concepts of maintenance medications and "quick-relief" medications and may not use them correctly. Repeated patient education is important.

Exacerbations and Complications

Exacerbations of COPD are defined as "an acute event characterized by a worsening of the patient's symptoms that is beyond normal day-to-day variations and leads to a change in medications" (GOLD, 2015). Exacerbations of COPD are associated with worsening prognosis and an accelerated decline in pulmonary function. Signs and symptoms may

TABLE 11-1 Common Inhaled Medications Used in COPD and Asthma

Medication Class	Generic Name (Trade Name®)	
Short-acting beta-adrenergic (SABA) aka beta2 agonist	**albuterol solution for nebs** *(comes in three strengths)* **albuterol sulfate HFA** *ProAir®* *Proventil®* *Ventolin®* **levalbuterol HFA** *Xopenex®*	• Used "as-needed for quick relief" or may be on a timed basis • MDIs generally given as two puffs as needed or four times a day • May or may not need a spacer with MDI for good technique • MDIs now come with a dose counter • ProAir also available in RespiClick™ device
Short-acting muscarinic antagonist (SAMA) aka short-acting anticholinergic	**ipratropium HFA** *Atrovent®*	• Used as a timed medication or as alternative for "quick relief" • Generally given as two puffs four times a day (up to 12 puffs in 24 hours)
SAMA/SABA combination	**ipratropium/albuterol** *Combivent®* *Duoneb® for nebs*	• May be used as first-line therapy or quick relief • Combivent generally administered four times a day by Respimat® device
Long-acting muscarinic antagonist (LAMA) aka LA anticholinergic	**tiotropium** *Spiriva HandiHaler®* **aclidinium** *Tudorza Pressair®* **umeclidinium** *Incruse Ellipta®*	• First-line therapy for moderate to severe disease • Tiotropium given once a day; aclidinium given twice a day • Tiotropium approved for reducing COPD exacerbations • Tiotropium also available in Respimat™ device • Each medication comes with its own delivery device
Long-acting beta adrenergic (LABA) aka LA beta2 agonist	**arformoterol tartrate solution** *Brovana® for nebs* **salmeterol DPI** *Serevent®* **formoterol DPI** *Foradil®* *Perforomist® for nebs* **indacaterol** *Arcapta Neohaler®*	• Used in moderate to severe COPD often in combination with corticosteroids • Each medication comes with its own delivery device • Not for acute symptoms • Salmeterol and formoterol both one puff twice a day, indacaterol once daily • This class not used as monotherapy in asthma
Combinations of long-acting: LAMA/LABA	**umeclidinium/vilanterol** *Anoro Ellipta®* **tiotropium/olodaterol** *Stiolto*	• Used for moderate to severe COPD • Given one puff once daily • Stiolto is given two actuations once a day by Respimat®
Inhaled glucocorticosteroids (ICS)	**ciclesonide HFA** *Alvesco®* **mometasone** *Asmanex Twisthaler®* **fluticasone HFA** *Flovent®* **budesonide DPI** *Pulmicort Flexhaler®* **beclomethasone** *QVAR HFA®*	• Generally used in persistent asthma/later stages of COPD • Patients need to rinse out their mouths to prevent oral thrush • Spacers are also useful to help prevent thrush • All devices have counters except for QVAR • All come in two strengths except for Flovent, which comes in three • Are maintenance or controller medications in both asthma and COPD, not to be used as needed • Most are given twice a day, strength varies based on patient's severity of illness and history of recent exacerbation
Combinations of long acting: LABA/ Corticosteroid combination	**fluticasone/salmeterol** *Advair HFA® (steroid comes in three strengths), two puffs twice a day, Advair Discus® one puff twice a day* **budesonide/formoterol** *Symbicort HFA® (steroid comes in two strengths), two puffs twice a day* **mometasone/formoterol** *Dulera® (comes in two strengths), two puffs twice a day* **fluticasone/vilanterol** *Breo Ellipta® (one strength), one puff once a day*	• Used in moderate to severe COPD and asthma • Patients need to rinse out their mouths to prevent oral thrush • Each drug has its own delivery device and technique • Breo Elipta given once daily, others every 12 hours

HFA, hydrofluoroalkane used as propellant; **DPI,** dry powder inhaler.

include increased dyspnea, increased sputum production and purulence, respiratory failure, changes in mental status, or worsening blood gas abnormalities. The primary causes of acute exacerbations include infection (bacterial and viral), heart failure, and response to pollutants and allergens. Severe exacerbations requiring hospitalization are associated with an increase in mortality.

Prevention of exacerbations is associated with preservation of pulmonary function and a decrease in hospitalizations. Smoking cessation, influenza and pneumococcal vaccines, inhaled drugs (LABAs, LAMAs with or without corticosteroids), and phosphodiesterase inhibitors (Daliresp®) have been associated with a prolonged time between exacerbations (GOLD, 2015).

During an exacerbation, optimization of bronchodilator medications, inhaled or systemic corticosteroids, antibiotic agents, oxygen therapy, and intensive respiratory interventions may also be used. Early treatment with antibiotics in patients needing hospitalization for an acute exacerbation may result in improved outcomes.

Indications for hospitalization for an acute exacerbation of COPD include: severe COPD, marked increase in intensity of symptoms that does not respond adequately to initial therapy, inadequate home support, confusion or lethargy, respiratory muscle fatigue, paradoxical chest wall movement, peripheral edema, worsening or new onset of central cyanosis, persistent or worsening hypoxemia, and the need for noninvasive or invasive assisted mechanical ventilation (GOLD, 2015). The risk of death from an exacerbation of COPD is closely related to the development of respiratory acidosis, the presence of significant comorbidities, and the need for noninvasive or invasive positive-pressure ventilatory support (Stoller, 2015).

Respiratory insufficiency and failure are major life-threatening complications of COPD. The acuity of the onset and the severity of respiratory failure depend on baseline pulmonary function, pulse oximetry or ABG values, comorbid conditions, and the severity of other complications of COPD. Respiratory insufficiency and failure may be chronic (with severe COPD) or acute (with a severe exacerbation or pneumonia in a patient with severe COPD). Acute respiratory insufficiency and failure may necessitate ventilatory support until the underlying cause, such as infection, can be treated. Management of the patient requiring ventilatory support is discussed in Chapter 55.

Other complications of COPD include pneumonia, atelectasis, pneumothorax, and pulmonary arterial hypertension. Pulmonary hypertension is more common in patients with hypoxemia and severe disease and is associated with decreased survival. The diagnosis of pulmonary hypertension associated with COPD is suspected in patients complaining of dyspnea and fatigue that appear to be disproportionate to pulmonary function abnormalities. Enlargement of the central pulmonary arteries on chest radiograph, echocardiography suggestive of right ventricular enlargement and elevated plasma brain natriuretic peptide (BNP) may be present.

Pneumothorax is a less common complication of COPD but can be life-threatening in patients who have minimal pulmonary reserve. Patients with severe emphysematous changes can develop large bullae, which may rupture and cause a pneumothorax. Development of a pneumothorax may be spontaneous or related to an activity such as severe coughing or large intrathoracic pressure changes. Signs and symptoms of a pneumothorax include: sudden chest pain that is sharp and abrupt, a significant and sudden increase in severe shortness of breath, asymmetry of chest movement, unilateral retractions, hyperresonance on percussion, crepitus (cracking sensation when touching affected area), bilateral differences in breath sounds, and/or oxygen desaturation. Pneumothorax in a patient with underlying lung disease is a medical emergency. Rapid response teams or emergency services should be initiated.

Medical management of pulmonary hypertension associated with COPD includes stabilization of the underlying lung disease, administration of long-term supplemental oxygen and diuretics. During acute episodes, treatment may include positive-pressure ventilation.

Pathophysiology Alert
Brain Natriuretic Peptide (BNP) is secreted from the overdistended cardiac chambers. High BNP levels (greater than 100 pg/mL) indicate abnormal ventricular function or symptomatic heart failure. BNP levels are useful for diagnosing heart failure.

The clinical and economic impact of frequent readmissions has prompted an examination of factors that contribute to frequent hospitalizations. Patients with comorbidities, a history of prior exacerbations, individual patient and caregiver factors, and lack of integration of inpatient and outpatient care are suggested as possible contributing factors. Integrated care and other programs to reduce readmission rates have met with varying degrees of success (Crisafulli, Ortega, & Torres, 2015; Coughlin, Liang, & Parthasarathy, 2015).

Oxygen Therapy

Oxygen therapy may be administered during an acute exacerbation, as long-term continuous therapy for chronic hypoxemia, and during exercise and sleep for selected patients. The goal of oxygen therapy is to maintain tissue oxygenation and decrease the work of the cardiopulmonary system. Oxygen is generally administered to acutely ill COPD patients when their room air oxygen saturation is less than 90% or if they are showing signs of increased cardiopulmonary work: increased shortness of breath, tachypnea, tachycardia, or elevated blood pressure. Oxygen is administered to maintain an oxygen saturation of greater than or equal to 90%.

A small subset of COPD patients with chronic hypercapnia (elevated $PaCO_2$ levels) may be at some risk for respiratory failure should they receive too high an oxygen concentration. Concern persists that such patients would lose their "drive to breathe," also called "hypoxic drive." Over-concern may lead patients to receive too little oxygen and result in hypoxemia. While hypercapnic patients are at increased risk for respiratory failure, the risk is related to the severity of their COPD. Adequate oxygenation is as important in their management and should never be withheld. Key in the care of patients with COPD on supplemental oxygen is monitoring and assessment. Pulse oximetry is helpful in assessing response to therapy. ABGs are needed to assess $PaCO_2$ levels. Adequate oxygenation of patients (keeping the oxygen saturation *at or above* 90%) is important to prevent vital organ damage while monitoring for any possible complications of oxygen supplementation. Alternate delivery devices such as venturi-masks or ventilatory support (noninvasive by mask or by intubation) may be necessary during acute exacerbations to ensure adequate gas exchange (Stoller, 2015).

 Concept Mastery Alert

For patients with advanced COPD, a venturi-mask is needed to promote adequate gas exchange.

Two seminal landmark studies showed the value of long-term supplemental oxygen in patients who are chronically hypoxemic (Nocturnal Oxygen Therapy Trial Group, 1980; British Medical Research Working Party, 1981). Long-term oxygen therapy (worn more than 15 hours per day) was associated with increased survival, improved quality of life, a modest reduction in pulmonary arterial pressure, and decreased dyspnea. Long-term oxygen therapy is usually introduced in severe COPD. Indications generally include: a PaO_2 of 55 mm Hg or less or an oxygen saturation of 88% or less. Evidence of tissue hypoxia and organ damage such as pulmonary hypertension, secondary polycythemia, edema from right-sided heart failure, or impaired mental status indicates a need for long-term oxygen therapy. For patients with exercise-induced hypoxemia, oxygen supplementation during exercise may improve performance. Patients who are hypoxemic while awake are likely to be so during sleep. Therefore, nighttime oxygen therapy is recommended as well; the prescription for oxygen therapy is for continuous, 24-hour use. Intermittent oxygen therapy is indicated for patients who desaturate only during exercise or sleep. Oxygen may also be prescribed in patients who become hypoxemic at high-altitude situations, for example, air travel and high-altitude environments. Specialized studies done in a pulmonary function laboratory can determine which patients may need oxygen at high altitude.

Home oxygen is usually supplied by several different methods: by oxygen concentrators, compressed gas cylinders, liquid oxygen, or some combination of these. Newer concentrator/compressors allow appropriate patients to fill their own gas cylinders. Demand portable oxygen systems (liquid and gas systems) and small portable oxygen concentrators have allowed many patients to have more freedom and time away from their stationary systems. Patients need to be evaluated with the chosen system to ensure adequate oxygen saturation.

Surgical Treatments

Bullae are enlarged airspaces that do not contribute to ventilation but occupy space in the thorax. Bullae may compress areas of healthier lung and impair gas exchange. If they are limited in number, bullae may be surgically excised. A bullectomy (surgical excision of the bullae) may help reduce dyspnea and improve lung function. It can be performed thoracoscopically (with a video-assisted thoracoscope) or via a limited thoracotomy incision.

LVRS is an option for a subset of patients with severe emphysema. Patients with predominately upper lobe disease benefit the most. LVRS involves the removal of a portion of the diseased lung parenchyma. Successful LVRS results in reduced hyperinflation and improvement in the elastic recoil and diaphragmatic mechanics. LVRS is not curative but may decrease dyspnea, improve lung function, and improve the patient's overall quality of life. Careful selection of patients for LVRS is essential to decrease morbidity and mortality. The National Emphysema Treatment Trial found that the addition of LVRS to optimal medical management and rehabilitation led to overall improvement in exercise tolerance and survival in a subgroup of patients with predominantly upper lobe disease (GOLD, 2015).

Lung transplantation is an alternative surgical treatment for end-stage COPD. It has been shown to improve quality of life and functional capacity in a selected group of patients with COPD (GOLD, 2015). Single-lung transplantation may be considered for patients with end-stage emphysema who have an FEV_1 of less than 25% of the predicted and who have complications such as pulmonary hypertension, marked hypoxemia, and hypercapnia. Specific criteria exist for referral for lung transplantation. Patients are prioritized based on the severity of their disease, age, and prognosis. Limited organ availability is a concern and may limit transplantation as an option. Patients who have had a lung transplant need special care when hospitalized. Transplanted patients are on multiple medications to prevent organ rejection and are at markedly increased risk for infection. Coordinating care with the transplant center should be made when patients require hospitalization.

Pulmonary Rehabilitation

Pulmonary rehabilitation for patients with COPD is well established and widely accepted as a means to alleviate symptoms and optimize functional status. It is now considered part of the recommended treatment for symptomatic COPD. The primary goals of rehabilitation are to reduce symptoms, improve quality of life, and increase

BOX 11-5 **Nursing Research**

Bridging the Gap to Evidence-Based Practice

Effectiveness of a partnership-based self-management program for patients with mild and moderate chronic obstructive pulmonary disease: A pragmatic randomized controlled trial

Jonsdottir, H., Amundadottir, O., Gudmundsson, G., ...Stefansdottir, I. (2015). *Journal of Advanced Nursing, 71*(11), 2634–2648.

Purpose

The purpose of this study was to evaluate the effectiveness of a 6-month, partnership-based self-management program for patients with mild and moderate chronic obstructive pulmonary disease (COPD).

Design

This was a pragmatic randomized control trial where patients aged 45–65 years, with mild and moderate COPD were invited with a family member to participate in a 6-month, partnership-based self-management program consisting of: (a) three to four conversations between nurse and patient-family member; (b) 6 months of smoking cessation; and (c) interdisciplinary team-patient-family member group meeting. The control group ($n = 52$) received usual care. The experimental group consisted of 48 participants ($n = 48$). Data were collected at months 0, 6, and 12. The trial lasted from June 2009 to March 2013.

Findings

Patients with mild and moderate COPD who participated in the partnership-based self-management program perceived less intrusiveness of the disease and its treatment than patients in the control group. Patients in the experimental group did not have better health-related quality of life, less anxiety or depression, increased physical activity, fewer exacerbations, or better smoking status than patients in the control group. Patients in both groups found participation in the research useful and important.

Nursing Implications

A concerted effort needs to be put into developing a comprehensive, long-term self-management program that takes account for that which is of concern to young people with COPD in its early stages and their families regarding life with the disease, into which an effective smoking cessation treatment is incorporated. Action needs to be taken to reach out to young people with COPD in its early stages, who might not realize that they have the disease nor comprehend the likely consequences of their own smoking. These actions should include not only development and use of health care but recruitment into research programs as well. Smoking cessation treatment for young people with COPD in its early stages warrants further developments. Family involvement was complicated for participants and is thus an area for further exploration.

participation in everyday activities (Nici & ZuWallack, 2012; GOLD, 2015). Pulmonary rehabilitation services are multidisciplinary and include assessment, education, physical reconditioning, skills training, and psychological support (refer to Box 11-5). Patients are taught methods to alleviate symptoms through breathing exercises and learning how to pace activities. Physical conditioning through endurance and strength training is an essential component of rehabilitation. Energy conservation skills are used to improve functional status and decrease dyspnea and fatigue. Nutritional counseling and medication education are other important components of rehabilitation.

The demonstrated benefits of pulmonary rehabilitation include: improvement in symptoms and exercise tolerance, improved quality of life, and a reduction in hospitalizations. Selection of a program depends on the patient's physical, functional, and psychosocial status; insurance coverage; geographic location; and preference. Patients with moderate to severe lung disease may benefit the most from pulmonary rehabilitation. Patients with very severe disease may also benefit.

Nursing Management

Nurses play a key role in the care of the patient with COPD. In an office setting, nurses may assist in the assessment of patients suspected of having COPD or help manage patients with known COPD, teach techniques for managing the common problems associated with living with COPD, and review the use of prescribed medications. In acute care settings, nursing care focuses on assessing patients for problems with dyspnea, gas exchange, and secretion clearance. In addition, nurses assess for and help manage respiratory failure, administer medications and treatments to support the cardiopulmonary system, assist the patient to recover from an acute exacerbation, and help prepare patients for discharge. Nursing care in extended-care facilities and home care focuses on helping patients maintain disease stability, improve functional capacity, and learn self-management strategies. Nursing care of patients with very severe and end-stage disease focuses on palliative measures aimed at symptom relief and helping the patient and family cope with limited prognosis.

In addition, nurses may identify potential candidates for pulmonary rehabilitation and reinforce the material learned in the rehabilitation program. Not all patients have access to a formal rehabilitation program. Nurses can teach patients and families rehabilitation concepts as well as facilitate specific services: respiratory therapy for equipment and oxygenation needs, physical therapy for exercise and breathing retraining, occupational therapy for conserving energy during activities of daily living, psychosocial therapy, and nutritional counseling. Numerous educational materials are available to assist nurses in teaching patients with COPD.

Potential resources include those of organizations such as the American Lung Association, the American Association of Cardiovascular and Pulmonary Rehabilitation, the American Thoracic Society, the American College of Chest Physicians, and the American Association for Respiratory Care. Online information is also available through these organizations (see resource list at the end of the chapter).

Assessing the Patient

Assessment includes obtaining information about current symptoms as well as previous disease manifestations. In addition to the questions obtained in a basic health history, key questions should focus around the main symptoms of patients with COPD: shortness of breath (dyspnea), cough, and sputum production. Patients with moderate to severe COPD may always have some symptoms. It is helpful to ask patients how their current symptoms compare to their usual amount of shortness of breath, cough, and sputum. When quantifying dyspnea, it can be helpful to use a numerical scale based on 0 to 10, with 0 being no shortness of breath and 10 being the worst. For example, if the patient's usual rating of shortness of breath is a 4 and is now a 7, a significant change has occurred. A change in sputum color, quantity or thickness is also significant. Additional symptoms of a change in condition may include increased fatigue and a decreased ability to perform one's usual activities.

Other assessment questions may include: the presence of other medical problems (cardiovascular, diabetes, stroke, history of pneumonia, cancer), allergies, history of smoking in pack/years, current smoking, a history of past exacerbations and pulmonary hospitalizations including a history of intubations, a description of how the patient spends a usual day, sleep quality and amount, problems with mood (anxiety and/or depression), and what self-care measures the patient is currently using.

Physical examination should focus on observing the patient's breathing pattern and body position. Accessory muscle use, shoulder elevation, and the tripod position (leaning forward with the arms braced on the knees) are associated with increased respiratory distress. A change in respiratory rate is also a significant examination finding. A normal resting respiratory rate is 8 to 16 breaths per minute (a respiratory rate of 20 is considered the upper limit of normal by some sources). Many patients with COPD will have respiratory rates of 20 to 24 at baseline. When the respiratory rate is greater than the patient's baseline, it may signal an acute problem. It is helpful to ask patients if they are aware of their increased respiratory rate. They may relate this to a recent exacerbation of symptoms. Assessment of breath sounds should include: quality (good aeration or diminished), the presence of adventitious sounds (crackles or wheezes), and whether the adventitious sounds clear with cough. Patient assessment is aided by a review of laboratory data, including pulmonary function tests, tests of oxygenation, and radiologic studies.

TABLE 11-2 Common Problems Associated with COPD

- Continued smoking
- Dyspnea
- Impaired gas exchange
- Cough and ineffective airway clearance
- Fatigue
- Decreased exercise tolerance
- Decreased functional capacity
- Deficient knowledge of self-care strategies to be performed at home
- Anxiety
- Depression
- Limited prognosis in severe disease
- Potential complications:
  - Respiratory insufficiency or failure
  - Pulmonary infection and pneumonia
  - Pulmonary hypertension
  - Cor pulmonale (right-sided heart failure)

A systematic assessment of the patient helps the nurse determine if the patient is stable, becoming acutely ill and needs medical intervention, or becoming more severely ill and needs emergency medical attention.

Common Problems

COPD is a chronic illness and by its definition is not curable. Several common problems of COPD are amenable to treatment and nursing interventions. Table 11-2 lists the most common problems associated with a diagnosis of COPD. The nursing goals for patients are compatible with other members of the health care team and may include: smoking cessation, improved dyspnea, improved gas exchange, more effective airway clearance, increased exercise tolerance, maintaining ideal body weight, increased self-management, improved coping ability, adherence to the therapeutic program including medications and oxygen, home care, and absence of complications.

Nursing Interventions

Smoking
Although many patients believe that smoking cessation is futile, continued smoking does increase the rate of lung function decline and disabling symptoms. Even brief counseling by nurses and other health professional about the hazards of smoking can be beneficial. Hospitalized smokers may present a "teachable moment." Relating the cause of the hospitalization to smoking behavior personalizes the message to the patient. Administering and teaching patients about pharmacologic agents that increase the likelihood of a successful quit attempt is an additional nursing intervention. Refer to Box 11-3 on page 350 for helping smokers to quit.

Chronic Dyspnea
Chronic dyspnea is one of the most common problems of patients with moderate to severe COPD. Dyspnea or shortness

of breath is an uncomfortable awareness of breathing that is often described by patients as an inability to get enough air into the lungs. Acute dyspnea occurs during an exacerbation, with increased activity, from anxiety and panic, and because of acute coexisting medical conditions (e.g., anemia, heart failure, pneumonia). Chronic dyspnea is different from acute dyspnea in that the patient may exhibit no visible signs of distress. Analogous to pain, dyspnea occurs "when the patient says it does" and feels like "the patient says it does."

The management of dyspnea focuses on assessing the underlying causes and administering therapies to reduce the symptoms. Nursing management includes administering bronchodilators to increase airway patency, assisting acutely ill patients with activities of daily living to decrease the work of breathing, administering oxygen therapy when hypoxemia contributes to dyspnea, and teaching strategies for relieving increased shortness of breath and for limiting future episodes.

Ineffective breathing patterns and shortness of breath are partially due to the ineffective respiratory mechanics of the chest wall, lungs, and diaphragm; airway obstruction; the metabolic cost of breathing; and stress. Breathing retraining may help improve breathing patterns. Pursed-lip breathing helps slow exhalation and is thought to prevent the collapse of the small airways, effectively allowing more air to be exhaled and decreasing hyperinflation. A simple explanation to patients is that pursed-lip breathing makes "more room to breathe." It may promote relaxation and reduce feelings of panic, allowing patients to gain control of their breathing. Box 11-6 provides a patient handout and method of helping patients deal with an acute episode of their chronic dyspnea.

An additional patient teaching strategy is to advise the use of a small handheld fan and let the air flow on the cheek. Patients frequently report that cool and moving air reduces their sensation of dyspnea. Relaxation techniques such as progressive muscle relaxation may also be useful.

Diaphragmatic breathing has long been taught to patients with COPD. However, the technique is difficult to learn by most patients, and its benefits are limited. Patients with milder disease and those with voice or woodwind musical training may feel the technique to be beneficial, but those with more severe disease may find diaphragm breathing too difficult to do. Inspiratory muscle training (IMT) involves having the patient train against a resistive load. Several commercial devices are available for use. Training may be of benefit in some patients, but it is not currently recommended as standard care (GOLD, 2015).

Limiting future episodes of shortness of breath include exercise training to improve endurance, teaching patients how to pace their activities with their breathing, and helping patients anticipate dyspnea-producing activities and plan how they will keep their dyspnea at a manageable level. For example, if a patient is short of breath when climbing stairs, climbing more slowly and only during exhalation may help keep dyspnea at a manageable level. A simple teaching strategy is "pause-breathe in, exhale, and climb one to two steps."

In very severe COPD, simple tasks may cause severe dyspnea that is not adequately responsive to medications and breathing techniques. The administration of opioids may be needed to keep dyspnea under control. Patients and families need to be taught how to use opioids effectively. Concerns over physical dependence, addiction, and respiratory

---

BOX 11-6 **Patient Education**

Managing an Acute Episode of Shortness of Breath

(Use this method to control your breathing when you become more short of breath from over exertion or anxiety and to help you avoid panic)

Step One: Position *(find the most comfortable position to allow the air to move in and out of your lungs)*

- Leaning forward with your back straight
- Leaning over a table with your arms resting on the table
- Placing pillows under your arms and keeping them supported and relaxed

Step Two: Breathing *(begin to control your breathing)*

- Breathe out through pursed or slightly puckered lips
- Breathe in through your mouth if you are very short of breath
- It may help to puff your cheeks out as you breathe out
- Breathe out longer and longer each breath until it starts to feel more comfortable
- As your breathing gets more comfortable, breathe in through your nose and out through pursed lips

Step 3: Relaxation *(once your breathing starts to slow down)*

- Relax your neck and shoulders
- Allow your arms to become limp
- Close your eyes if that helps you to relax

Additional Points

- When your breathing is in control, resume your previous activity but at a slower pace.
- It may help to use your "quick-relief" medication in addition to pursed-lip breathing.
- Breathe out for the hardest part of the exertion.
  Example: While climbing stairs, breathe in while standing still; breathe out while climbing one or more steps. Pause again to breathe in; breathe out while you climb.
- Practice **position, breathing, and relaxation** when you are not short of breath to help you avoid panic.
- **If your shortness of breath continues or gets worse, call your primary care provider.**

depression need to be addressed, but opioids should not be withheld in very severe patients for whom palliative care is the goal. Noninvasive positive-pressure ventilation (NPPV) also has been used for the treating dyspnea in patients with severe COPD.

Impaired Gas Exchange

Patients with more severe disease and those experiencing an exacerbation are at increased risk for hypoxemia, oxygen desaturation, and hypercapnia. Nursing care includes monitoring the patient for hypoxemia by oximetry and ABG measurements and administering supplemental oxygen. As mentioned under Medical Management, over-concern about hypercapnia should never result in under treating the patient. Adequate oxygenation (keeping the oxygen saturation *at or above* 90%) is important to protect vital organ function.

Patients requiring oxygen therapy need to be taught the importance of adhering to the oxygen prescription. Patients often think they can tell when they need oxygen by their symptoms. The presence or absence of dyspnea is unreliable in detecting the need for supplemental oxygen. Many hypoxemic patients do not feel dyspnea. In addition, many patients who are dyspneic do not have significant hypoxemia or oxygen desaturation.

The pulmonary arteries respond to hypoxemia by constricting, causing increased pressure to occur. Pulmonary hypertension and right ventricular hypertrophy and failure may occur as a result of chronic, untreated hypoxemia. Chronic hypoxemia affects the function of other vital organs. Cognitive impairment is greater in hypoxemic patients. Long-term oxygen is

the prescribed treatment. Teaching patients who need home oxygen should include an explanation of supplemental oxygen's effect on improved cardiac and cognitive function as well as improved prognosis. The teaching plan should include the number of hours per day to wear oxygen, the dose of oxygen (usually give as number of liters per minute), and special instructions for using oxygen for sleep and exercise. Home care companies supplying oxygen to patients usually employ respiratory therapists and/or nurses. Home care professionals help patients use their oxygen more effectively, identify special equipment needs, troubleshoot equipment, and explore the use of oxygen for work and travel.

Cough and Ineffective Airway Clearance

Patients with mucus hypersecretion or a comorbidity of bronchiectasis as well as those experiencing an acute exacerbation may have increased sputum quantity and viscosity. In addition, many patients are too weak or fatigued to clear secretions effectively.

Diminishing the quantity and viscosity of sputum can help clear the airways and improve pulmonary ventilation and gas exchange. Pulmonary irritants should be eliminated or reduced, particularly cigarette smoking, secondhand smoke, aerosol cleaning and household products, cooking that produces fumes, and powders used when bathing patients. Nursing interventions include instruction in directed or controlled coughing and drinking enough fluid to prevent dehydration. Box 11-7 can be used to teach patients effective coughing and how to deal with uncontrolled coughing spasms.

BOX 11-7   Patient Education

Controlled Cough

An effective cough moves secretions (also called sputum, phlegm, or mucus) out of the smaller airways of the lungs. An effective cough should use just enough effort to remove secretions but not so much as to cause pain, coughing spasms, or exhaustion.

One Coughing Technique

*   Sit up leaning slightly forward with your back straight and your head tilted down.
*   Take 2 slow deep breaths and exhale through pursed lips.
*   Take another deep breath in, and hold your breath for 2–3 seconds.
*   Open your mouth so that your lips are slightly parted. Cough, cough, cough from your stomach without breathing in (coughing the air out of your lungs with little coughs).
*   If coughing from the stomach is too hard, try: huff, huff, huffing the air out.
*   Finish exhaling through pursed lips.
*   Breathe in slowly through your nose, and exhale through pursed lips, 2–3 times. Then try clearing your throat or coughing the secretions out of your mouth.

*   Repeat, if necessary.
*   Check your sputum for color, quantity, and consistency.

If you don't cough out any sputum after 2–3 controlled coughs, wait 15–20 minutes and try again. Avoid continuous coughs to minimize your risk of injury or fatigue. Try using your inhaled bronchodilator before coughing to make it easier to get results.

Controlling Coughing Spasms

If you go into a coughing spasm:

*   Take several short sniffs of air in through your nose to help cut down on the irritation.
*   Avoid a inhaling quickly through your mouth as it may make you cough more; breathe out through pursed lips and relax your shoulders.

It may take a few breaths to control the coughing spasm so be patient and keep trying.

Once you get the cough under control and after resting a few minutes, try the controlled cough.

Some patients require more intense secretion-clearance techniques. Chest physiotherapy with postural drainage and/or mechanical percussion and vibration, the use of positive expiratory pressure devices (PEP therapy), and suctioning may be needed for patients who are unable to cough sputum out effectively. Patients receiving one or more of these more intense techniques need to be monitored for their response to treatment. Very frail patients may experience too much fatigue, pain, or dyspnea. Respiratory therapists are often consulted when these more intense forms of secretion clearance are needed.

Decreased Exercise Tolerance

Patients with advanced COPD experience progressive intolerance and disability during activity and exercise. Exacerbations and hospitalizations add to decreased activity, muscle weakness, and fatigue. Interventions used during acute exacerbations may weaken the patient further, for example, systemic corticosteroids are associated with myopathy (muscle weakness), particularly in the leg muscles.

Nursing interventions focus on therapies to help the patient recover from the effects of an acute exacerbation, maintain or regain independence in ambulation and performing activities of daily living, and improve stamina and strength. Early mobilization in patients experiencing an acute exacerbation, including those in intensive care, is associated with improvements in exercise tolerance and may help patients recover more quickly. Box 11-8 provides a simple handout to use with patients.

Interventions preparing the patient for discharge or when working with outpatients may include teaching alternating high-energy with low-energy activities throughout the day to better manage energy expenditure. The patient may benefit from exercise training to strengthen the muscles of the upper and lower extremities and to improve exercise tolerance and endurance. Use of walking aids may be recommended to improve activity levels, balance, and ambulation. Pulmonary rehabilitation staff, occupational therapists, and physical therapists can be consulted to assist patients with improving exercise tolerance and self-care.

Nutrition

Patients with COPD may have a number of issues related to nutrition. Some individuals become underweight and have difficulty consuming enough calories to meet their body's metabolic requirements. Others may be normal weight but have decreased muscle mass. Some may be overweight because of increased fat mass or increased fluid retention. Overweight patients may need the help of nutrition education by a dietician to help them lose weight safely. Exercise should be encouraged to help them increase muscle mass.

Hospitalized patients may have difficulty eating because the act of eating may cause increased dyspnea. Oral nutritional supplements are useful for increasing body weight and respiratory function. Weight gain in underweight patients results in improved exercise capacity and quality of life. However, some patients negate the effectiveness of the supplements by using them as meal substitutes.

Therapy is aimed at assessing the nutritional status of the patient, treating the underlying cause, and stabilizing weight and body composition. Nursing interventions include:

- timing bronchodilator therapy before meals
- assisting severely dyspneic patients during meal times to minimize energy spent eating

---

BOX 11-8   **Patient Education**

Exercises to Do in Bed or in a Chair When You Are in the Hospital or Recovering from Being Sick

Deep Breathing

Every hour you are awake, take **10 slow, deep breaths.** Exhale through pursed lips.

If you get tired after five breaths, rest a minute or two and do the second set of five.

Moving in Bed

Roll from side to side in the bed at least every hour. This helps your breathing, circulation, and skin.

Leg Work to Keep Your Muscles from Getting Too Weak

Ankle Pumps: Flex your ankles and point your toes toward your head, and then point your toes down.

Quad Sets: Tighten your knee and press it into the bed or chair for a count of 5.

Buttocks Squeeze: Squeeze your buttocks together for a count of 5.

Leg Lifts: Bend your knee and bring your leg up toward your chest. Lower your knee slowly back down on the bed. You can also try lifting your leg up and down slowly with your knee in the straight position.

Arm Work

Raise your arms above your head as you breathe in, and then lower them back down to your sides as you breathe out.

Additional Points

- *Remember to breathe as you do the exercises.* Avoid holding your breath.
- Try doing five of each arm or leg exercise every 2–3 hours.
- *As soon as you can, get out of bed to a chair.* Get up several times a day for short periods to improve your stamina and avoid too much fatigue.
- *Take short walks.* Walk with your nurse if you feel unsure of your balance.
- Wear your oxygen for activity if your provider prescribes it.

- teaching patients to eat small, frequent meals to help them avoid becoming too full
- encouraging choices of calorie-rich foods; and providing patients with oral supplements
- referring patients to dieticians
- encouraging progressive periods of exercise aimed at increased muscle mass

Enhancing Self-Care Strategies

Self-management strategies are aimed at involving the patient in the decision-making process and goal formation. It is important for patients to participate in setting and accepting realistic short-term and long-term goals. If COPD is mild or moderate, the goals may be to increase exercise tolerance and prevent further loss of pulmonary function. In severe disease, the goals are to preserve current pulmonary function, increase activity tolerance, and relieve symptoms as much as possible. In very severe disease, the goals may shift to relief of severe dyspnea and preparing for a peaceful death. As severity increases, goals and expectations may change.

Examples of patient goals compatible with the concept of self-care include: learning to balance diminished exercise tolerance with the desire to maintain participation in important activities; recognizing the effect that environmental factors have on breathing, and dealing with respiratory irritants; preventing and recognizing the signs and symptoms of exacerbations and complications; learning how to handle an exacerbation and/or complication; managing a complex medical regimen that includes medication, exercise, oxygen, nutrition, and other medical conditions; and deciding on the course of treatment in very severe disease.

Interventions that help patients plan participation in favorite activities with less shortness of breath can be very helpful. For example, attendance at a special event such as a wedding or graduation may be very tiring for patients with more severe disease, yet they still may wish to participate. Strategies to minimize stress and shortness of breath may include: using quick-relief medications prior to the event; planning to attend part of the event such as only the ceremony or reception to minimize fatigue; using an assistive device during the event; and maintaining prescribed medications, oxygen, and exercise program to maximize physical health. Helping patients delineate and decide on possible strategies may allow participation and enhance self-efficacy.

Many patients with COPD are sensitive to changes in air quality, fluctuations in temperature and humidity, and respiratory irritants in the environment. Nursing interventions include teaching patients to check local weather conditions and air alerts for extremes of temperature, humidity, and poor air quality. Teaching patients to create "transitions zones" when they go from one extreme temperature to another can be useful. For example, during hot, humid weather, patients can be taught to turn the air-conditioning off in the car and crack the window to allow the outside air to gradually mix with the inside air. The more gradual transition to hotter, more humid air may make breathing easier for many patients.

Prevention and early recognition of exacerbations of COPD are important self-care measures for patients to learn. Preventative measures include: handwashing to minimize the transmission of infectious agents, avoiding or minimizing contact with sick individuals, and receiving immunizations against influenza and pneumococcal pneumonia. Patients should be taught to report signs of infection, including increased dyspnea as well as fever or change in sputum color, character, consistency, or amount. Any marked worsening of symptoms (chest tightness, dyspnea, and fatigue) also suggests infection and should be reported by patients to their PCP. Viral infections may make patients more susceptible to more serious bacterial infections.

Nursing Alert
High fevers of 102°F or greater accompanied by shaking chills are signs of a more serious infection such as pneumonia. Patients should be instructed to go to the nearest emergency room as soon as possible.

Patients with more severe disease often have significant variation in daily symptoms and may have difficulty determining if they are becoming acutely ill. A change in normal routines, increased activity, family events, increased stress; and fatigue are some of the causes of "bad-breathing days." A knowledge of the patient's past response to "bad-breathing" days can help guide patient teaching. For example, a patient with moderate disease may note a slight increase in sputum volume, no change in sputum color, a slight increase in usual dyspnea (from a 4 out of 10 to a 5) and denies fever or chills. This patient had one exacerbation in the last 2 years that responded to outpatient treatment with bronchodilators and antibiotics. Instruction might include using prescribed quick-relief medication (usually a SABA), using pursed-lip breathing and cough techniques, monitoring for increased symptoms, and contacting the primary care provider should symptoms worsen or persist. Conversely, a patient with similar symptoms but a history of requiring more intensive intervention such as systemic corticosteroids, antibiotics, emergency room visits, or hospitalizations may be instructed to contact their provider more quickly.

Respiratory Failure

Patients with severe and very severe COPD and those with hypercapnia are at increased risk for acute respiratory failure. Nursing interventions of hospitalized patients include frequent monitoring for signs and symptoms of impending respiratory failure, more intensive treatments aimed at clearing the airways, and frequent communication and coordination of care with other members of the health care team, for example, internists, hospitalists, pulmonologists, and respiratory therapists.

 Nursing Alert
Signs of impending respiratory failure and need for intensive care:

- *Severe dyspnea not responding to treatment*
- *Tachypnea alternating with bradypnea (slow respiratory rate below 8 breaths per minute) and apnea as fatigue ensues*
- *Hyperventilation that may deteriorate to rapid and shallow breathing*
- *Anxiety*
- *Change in mental status*
- *Worsening hypoxemia that is unresponsive to oxygen therapy*
- *Worsening hypercapnia*
- *Evidence of respiratory muscle fatigue: increased use of accessory muscles paroxysmal respiratory movement (inward movement of abdomen on inspiration) (GOLD, 2015)*

Patients who show signs and symptoms of impending acute respiratory failure must be monitored more closely until transfer to an intensive care can be accomplished. Additional interventions include providing adequate oxygenation, administration of medications to maximize bronchodilatation, and keeping the patient awake until more intensive therapy can be initiated. NPPV may be initiated. Patients not responding to NPPV may require intubation and invasive ventilatory support. Chapter 55 covers these therapies in more detail. Patients transferred to a medical unit following an acute episode of respiratory failure require the same close monitoring to avoid another episode.

Enhancing Individual Coping Strategies

COPD and its progression promote a cycle of physical, social, and psychological consequences, all of which are interrelated. Depression may occur in as many as 30% to 50% of patients with significant disease. Nursing interventions include: assessing patients for anxiety and depression, promoting interventions to maximize physical functioning and psychological and emotional stability, and social support. After the initial assessment of the patient, the nurse may provide referrals to psychiatric and social services, pulmonary rehabilitation, pastoral care, and home care.

 Nursing Alert
Anxiety may be a sign of worsening respiratory status and impending respiratory failure. Anxiety should not be attributed to psychological causes until the patient is assessed: vital signs, tests of oxygenation, mental status changes. Anxiolytics are generally contraindicated in patients with impending acute respiratory failure. Certain medications, in particular high-dose systemic corticosteroids, also can make patients feel extremely anxious and should be considered as a possible cause.

Any factor that interferes with normal breathing may induce anxiety, depression, and changes in behavior. Fatigue is a major symptom in many patients with COPD. Restricted activity, reversal of family roles due to loss of employment, the frustration of having to work to breathe, and the realization that the disease is prolonged and unrelenting may cause the patient to become angry, depressed, and demanding. Sexual function may be compromised, which also diminishes self-esteem. Nursing interventions include discussions with patients and families about the chronic nature of lung disease, support as roles change and spouses or significant others assume responsibilities once managed by the patient, and palliative and hospice care when patients near end-stage disease. Patients with severe anxiety and depression may need a referral to a mental health specialist. Many areas have support groups for patients with chronic lung disease that are usually administered by local pulmonary rehabilitation programs or local chapters of the American Lung Association. Participation in support groups may help many patients discuss common problems with professionals and patients with similar issues.

Continuing Care

Nursing interventions include assessment for and referral to community resources when hospitalized patients are nearing discharge. Nurses caring for outpatients with COPD may also identify community care needs as patients become more disabled. Referral to an inpatient pulmonary rehabilitation program or extended-care facility may be needed for patients who have had prolonged hospital stays and are severely disabled. Home care through a nursing agency may be appropriate for many patients. Home visits provide a more accurate assessment of the patient's daily life, physical and psychological status, and adherence to the prescribed regimen. Home care visits by physical and occupational therapists may help the patient gain endurance and strength enough to attend an outpatient pulmonary rehabilitation program.

As patients become more severely ill, medical therapy may not adequately relieve symptoms. Discussions about prognosis and end of life are difficult for many patients, families, and professionals. Fears of suffering, a desire to stay alive as long as possible, and depression are some of the factors that may interfere with discussions about the end of life. Areas identified as being of major importance for patients with end-stage COPD include adequate symptom management (particularly avoiding severe, uncontrolled dyspnea); psychological, emotional, and spiritual needs; and privacy and dignity. Assurances that patients and families will not be abandoned as the disease progresses and every effort to help the patient avoid suffering are important parts of caring.

Advanced care planning includes discussing patients' wishes should the need for more invasive procedures arise such as intubation, acute and long-term mechanical ventilation, feeding tubes, and placement of a tracheostomy tube. Nursing interventions include participation in these discussions with patients and families and providing support to them as they struggle with decision-making. Chapter 3 presents a more thorough discussion of end-of-life care.

ASTHMA

Asthma is a common disease of the airways that is complex and characterized by recurring and variable symptoms, airflow obstruction, and bronchial hyperresponsiveness. Inflammation is the key underlying feature and leads to recurrent episodes of asthma symptoms: cough, chest tightness, wheeze, and dyspnea. Symptoms occurrence and severity may vary over time.

An estimated 18.7 million American adults (8%) have asthma. Asthma accounts for 14.2 million outpatient visits, 1.8 million emergency room visits, approximately 439,000 hospitalizations, and 3,630 deaths per year (COPD Fast Stats, 2015).

The U.S. National Heart Lung and Blood Institute Expert Panel Guidelines (first produced in 1997 and updated in 2002 and 2007) provide evidence-based information to assist in the diagnosis and management of patients with asthma. A portion of the guidelines "Quick Reference for Asthma Care" was updated in 2011. Multinational guidelines known as the Global Strategy for Asthma Management and Prevention (GINA) were updated in 2015.

Recent research has led to the description of asthma "phenotypes." Common phenotypes include: allergic asthma, nonallergic asthma, late-onset asthma, asthma with fixed airflow limitation, and asthma with obesity (GINA, 2015).

Atopy, the genetic predisposition for the development of an IgE-mediated response to allergens, is the most common identifiable predisposing factor for asthma. Chronic exposure to airway allergens may sensitize IgE antibodies and the cells of the airway. Common allergens can be seasonal (grass, tree, and weed pollens) or perennial (e.g., mold, dust, roaches, animal dander). Atopy may also occur in the absence of asthma.

A variety of nonallergen triggers may also cause asthma symptoms and exacerbation. Most people with asthma are sensitive to a variety of triggers, both allergens and nonallergens. Asthma may vary in an individual person at different points in time. The dose and response to environmental exposures, activities engaged in, the particular asthma control measures used, the frequency of exacerbations, and other factors all influence the disease course in a given individual.

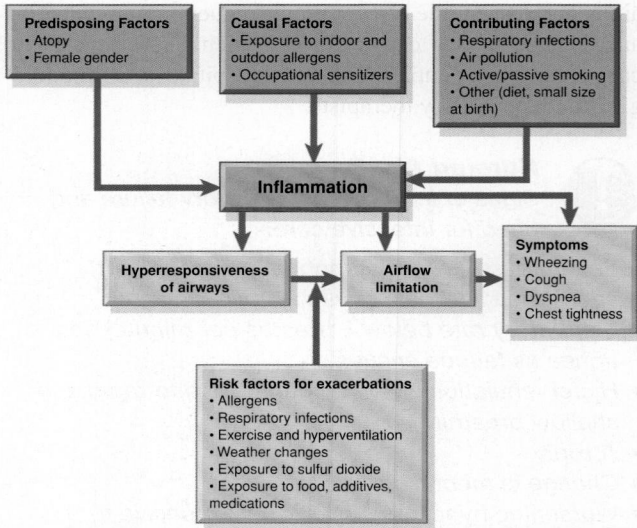

FIGURE 11-4 Pathophysiology of asthma. (Adapted from material developed for the Global Initiative for Asthma (GINA). Retrieved from http:www.ginasthma.org)

Pathophysiology

The underlying pathology in asthma is reversible and diffuse airway inflammation. Acute inflammation leads to airflow limitation and changes in the airways. Bronchoconstriction, the contraction of the smooth muscle of the airways, occurs in response to a variety of allergens and irritants. The airways become hyperresponsive (respond to stimuli in an exaggerated manner). Airway edema (swelling of the membranes that line the airways) becomes more progressive as asthma severity increases. Mucus hypersecretion and mucus plugs can occur. The airways of some asthmatics may undergo "remodeling," which includes persistent changes in airway structure, the development of sub-basement fibrosis, injury to the cells lining the airways, and hypertrophy of airway smooth muscle. Advanced changes in the airways lead to airway narrowing and potentially irreversible airflow limitation. Figure 11-4 depicts some of the pathophysiologic features of asthma.

Many cells and cellular elements play a role in the inflammation of asthma. Mast cells, neutrophils, eosinophils, and lymphocytes are implicated. Mast cells, when activated, release several chemicals called mediators which include: histamine, bradykinin, prostaglandins, and leukotrienes. These mediators perpetuate the inflammatory response and cause increased blood flow, vasoconstriction, fluid leak into the airways, attraction of white blood cells to the area, and bronchoconstriction (Porth, 2015). Regulation of these chemicals is the aim of much of the current research regarding pharmacologic therapy for asthma.

Clinical Manifestations and Assessment

Asthma is diagnosed based on history, physical examination, and spirometry. Symptoms often occur at night or early in

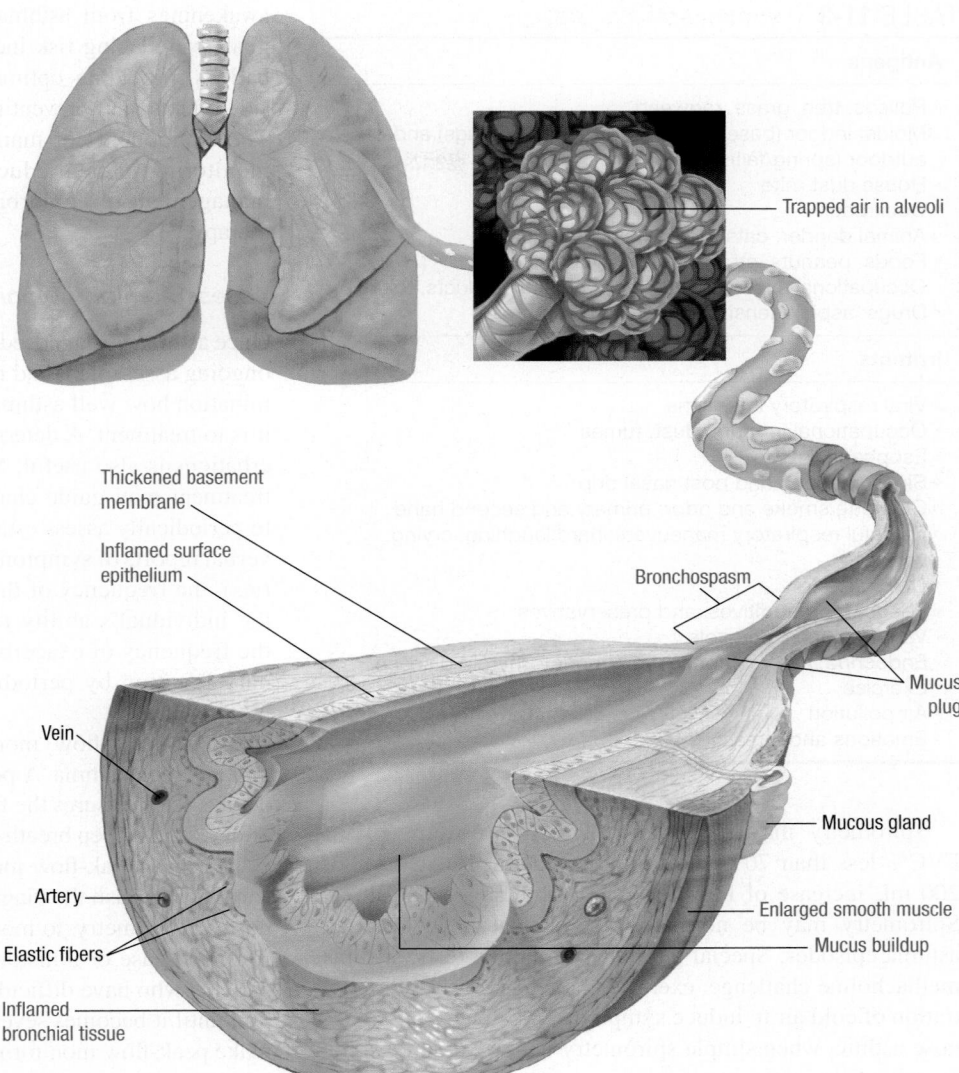

Trapped air in alveoli

Thickened basement
membrane

Inflamed surface
epithelium

Bronchospasm

Mucus
plug

Vein

Mucous gland

Artery

Enlarged smooth muscle

Elastic fibers

Mucus buildup

Inflamed
bronchial tissue

FIGURE 11-5 In asthma, inflammation and smooth muscle spasms severely constrict the airways. Released histamine stimulates the mucous membranes to secrete excessive mucus, further narrowing the bronchial lumen. On inhalation, the narrowed bronchial lumen can still expand slightly, allowing air to reach the alveoli. On exhalation, increased intrathoracic pressure may close the bronchial lumen. Mucus fills the lung bases, inhibiting alveolar ventilation. (Figure courtesy of the Anatomical Chart Company.)

the morning and may awaken patients. Asthma symptoms may occur suddenly or develop over several hours or days. Asthma is categorized according to symptoms and objective measures of airflow obstruction (Fig. 11-5).

A complete family, environmental, and occupational history helps establish the diagnosis. A history of cough, especially at night, recurrent wheeze, chest tightness, and/or difficulty breathing may indicate the presence of asthma. A report of symptoms that occur or worsen with exercise, exposure to allergens, irritants, occupational irritants, weather changes, stress, menstrual cycles, or strong expression of emotions such as hard laughing or crying increase the suspicion. Table 11-3 lists common allergens and irritants that may trigger an asthma episode. Cough, with or without mucus production may be the only symptom reported by some patients. Exercise-induced asthma is common and is defined as symptoms occurring during or soon after stopping exercise. Occupational asthma is worse

on work days and improved on days off. Many patients develop chronic asthma after years of exposure to an occupational trigger and may have persistent asthma even when not working.

Physical examination findings may reveal generalized wheezing initially heard during expiration. In between asthma episodes, physical examination findings may be normal.

Nursing Alert
The occurrence of a severe, continuous reaction is referred to as status asthmaticus and is considered life-threatening. In more severe episodes, diaphoresis, wheezing heard on inspiration, tachycardia, and a widened pulse pressure may occur along with hypoxemia. When airflow rates are very low, the "quiet chest" with minimal air movement may signal impending respiratory failure (Porth, 2015).

TABLE 11-3 Common Asthma Triggers

Antigens

- Pollens: tree, grass, ragweed
- Molds: indoor (basements, bathrooms, wet rugs) and/or outdoor (spring/fall)
- House dust mite
- Cockroach
- Animal dander: cats, dogs, guinea pigs, birds
- Foods: peanuts, strawberries, shellfish
- Occupational exposures: animals, baking products, toluene
- Drugs: aspirin sensitivity

Irritants

- Viral respiratory infections
- Occupational irritants: dust, fumes
- Esophageal reflux
- Sinus infection and post nasal drip
- Cigarette smoke and odor: primary and second hand
- Forceful respiratory maneuvers: hard laughing, crying, yelling
- Cold, dry air
- Foods, food additives, and preservatives
- Vapors, gases, aerosols
- Endocrine factors: menses, pregnancy, thyroid disease
- Exercise
- Air pollution
- Emotions and stress

Spirometry may reveal an obstructive pattern (FEV_1/FVC% less than 70%). Reversibility, defined as a 12% or 200 mL increase of FEV_1, FVC, or both suggests asthma. Spirometry may be normal if the patient is in between asthma episodes. Special pulmonary function tests, such as methacholine challenge, exercise challenge, or the administration of cold air to induce symptoms, may be used to diagnose asthma when simple spirometry is normal and asthma is suspected.

Other laboratory tests that are done less often may include: blood tests to detect elevated levels of eosinophils and immunoglobulin E, chest x-rays to exclude alternative diagnoses, and blood gases when patients experience symptoms of a severe exacerbation. The most common differential diagnoses in adults include: vocal cord dysfunction, foreign-body obstruction, congestive heart failure, pulmonary embolism, cough secondary to drugs, for example, angiotensin-converting enzyme (ACE) inhibitors, benign or malignant tumors obstructing airways, eosinophilic pneumonia, and COPD. In addition to being part of the differential diagnosis, COPD and asthma can coexist (GINA, 2015).

Medical Management

The overall goals of management are to reduce impairment and reduce the risk of adverse outcomes. Reducing impairment includes: freedom from symptoms, minimal need of inhaled short-acting beta agonist (SABA) to two or fewer times a week, fewer than two nights a month of nocturnal awakenings from asthma, and satisfaction with care. The goals of reducing risk include: preventing recurrent exacerbations, providing optimal pharmacotherapy with minimal side effects, and preventing loss of function (Fanta, 2015a). The components of management include assessment and monitoring, patient education, environmental control and management of comorbid conditions, and pharmacologic therapy.

Assessment and Monitoring

Once asthma is diagnosed and disease severity is determined, ongoing assessment and monitoring which includes a determination how well asthma is controlled and how responsive it is to treatment. A determination of potential risk for exacerbations is also useful. Monitoring adverse reactions from treatment may guide changes in treatment. Measures used to periodically assess established asthma include: written or verbal reports of symptoms and symptom relief (asthma diaries), the frequency of the use of quick-relief medications, the individual's ability to participate in normal activities, the frequency of exacerbations, and monitoring of pulmonary function by periodic spirometry or home peak-flow monitoring.

Home peak-flow monitoring may be useful in some patients with asthma. A peak flow meter is a small handheld device that measures the fastest flow the patient can generate after taking a deep breath in and blowing out as hard and fast as possible. Peak-flow monitoring is used for different reasons: to establish the diagnosis in symptomatic patients with normal spirometry, to monitor disease in patients with more severe disease or a history of frequent exacerbations, or in patients who have difficulty perceiving an asthma exacerbation until it becomes severe. Proper technique is essential to make peak-flow monitoring useful (see Box 11-9). Once the baseline or personal best peak flow is determined, changes in peak flow can be used to determine the need to adjust medication protocols. Written asthma action plans based

BOX 11-9 Patient Teaching

How to Use a Peak Flow Meter

- Stand or sit up straight.
- Put the marker on the peak-flow meter at zero.
- Take a full, deep breath in.
- Place the meter in your mouth with your tongue and teeth out of the way and seal your lips around the meter.
- Blow out as hard and fast as possible.
- Repeat the procedure two more times.
- Write down the highest reading.

Use your peak-flow meter at the same time of day for 2 weeks to establish your "personal best." Work with your PCP, nurse, or asthma educator to help you use your peak-flow numbers to help you control your asthma better and help you decide when to call your provider or go to the emergency room.

on fluctuations in peak flow and/or symptoms are useful for many patients.

Newer form of assessment may include analysis of expectorated sputum for eosinophilia and exhaled nitric oxide (NO). NO exhaled in breath is a method used to measure airway inflammation and provides a tool to assess airways disease, including asthma. These two techniques are not yet widely used (Fanta, 2015).

Patient Education

Asthma is a chronic illness and requires lifelong management by patients and clinicians to achieve the goals of therapy. The concept of partnership is one in which the clinician and patient work together to establish mutually agreed upon goals and treatments. Patients need to learn and manage multiple areas, for example, identification and management of triggers, monitoring for early warning signs of an acute episode, and taking prescribed medications correctly. Comorbid conditions, side effects, financial issues, living conditions, different beliefs about asthma, and other factors may influence the patient's adherence to the asthma management plan. Involving the patient in the decision-making process may increase adherence and positively affect outcomes.

Exacerbations and Complications

An asthma exacerbation is an acute or sub-acute episode of worsening shortness of breath, cough, wheeze, and/or chest tightness. Asthma exacerbations are classified by the severity of symptoms, the response to treatment, and peak-flow measurements. The standard classifications are: mild, moderate, severe, and life-threatening. Mild exacerbations are usually treated by the patient at home. Moderate exacerbations usually require an office visit or close contact with the patient's health care provider. Severe exacerbations usually result in an emergency room visit followed by possible admission to the hospital. Very severe episodes require emergency room visits and probable admission to the hospital or intensive care.

> **Nursing Alert**
> *Patients at high risk for asthma death need to seek medical care early during an exacerbation. Risk factors that place the patient at high risk include: a history of a previous severe exacerbation requiring intensive care and/or intubation, two or more hospitalizations or more than three emergency room visits in the past year, using more than two canisters of a SABA per month, difficulty perceiving worsening asthma, low socioeconomic status/inner city residence, illicit drug use, severe psychiatric illness, and major comorbid conditions.*

Complications of asthma may include worsening disease, status asthmaticus, and respiratory failure. Airway obstruction, particularly during acute asthmatic episodes, often results in hypoxemia, requiring the administration of oxygen and the monitoring of pulse oximetry and ABGs. Antibiotics are rarely needed but may be used for concomitant pneumonia or bacterial sinusitis.

Status asthmaticus is a severe asthma episode that is refractory to initial therapy. It is a medical emergency. Patients report rapid progressive chest tightness, wheezing, dry cough, and shortness of breath. Status asthmaticus may occur following a viral respiratory infection, exposure to a trigger, or following exercise in a cold environment. Infection, anxiety, nebulizer abuse, nonadherence to controller medications, dehydration, increased adrenergic blockage, and nonspecific irritants may contribute to these episodes. It may also occur with little or no warning and can progress rapidly to severe obstruction.

Patients in *status asthmaticus* are monitored closely in the emergency room or intensive care unit. Oxygen, adequate hydration, frequent or continuous nebulization of SABAs, ipratropium, theophylline, and systemic corticosteroids are frequently used to manage *status asthmaticus*. Other treatments that have been tried include intravenous magnesium sulfate, inhaled heliox (a mixture of oxygen and helium that is seven times lighter than air), and inhaled leukotriene modifiers. These latter three treatments have not been well tested in patients with status asthmaticus and are not routinely used (Saadeh, 2017). Intubation and mechanical ventilation may be needed when patients do not respond to initial treatment (Saadeh, 2017).

Pharmacologic Therapy

The pharmacologic management of asthma involves a stepwise approach (see Fig. 11-6). Medication prescriptions are based on the severity and control of asthma symptoms. Quick-relief medications are used for the immediate treatment of asthma symptoms; long-acting medications are used to achieve and maintain control of persistent asthma. The lowest dose of medications to achieve control is recommended. When patients are stable for 3 months, a decrease in medications may be tried (Expert Panel 3 Report, Quick Reference Guide 2011). The major inhaled medications used for asthma are listed in Table 11-1 on page 352. The pharmacologic management of asthma includes many medications that are used in COPD. The stepwise approach is somewhat different from COPD and is illustrated in Figure 11-6.

For patients with mild intermittent disease, a SABA administered by MDI may be all that is needed. Control of persistent asthma is accomplished primarily with regular use of anti-inflammatory medications. Inhaled corticosteroids are the treatment of choice. The dose of inhaled corticosteroids is adjusted based on patient symptoms and asthma control. A spacer should be used with inhaled corticosteroids; patients should gargle and spit out water after administration to prevent thrush, a troublesome complication

Stepwise Approach for Pharmacologic Management of Asthma

Intermittent Asthma

Persistent Asthma: Daily Medication
Consult with asthma specialist if step 4 care or higher is required.
Consider consultation at step 3.

Step up if needed
(first, check adherence, environmental control, and comorbid conditions)

Assess control

Step down if possible

(and asthma is well controlled at least 3 months)

Step 1

Preferred:
SABA PRN

Step 2

Preferred:
Low-dose ICS

Alternative:
Cromolyn, LTRA, nedocromil, or theophylline

Step 3

Preferred:
Low-dose ICS + LABA
OR
Medium-dose ICS

Alternative:
Low-dose ICS + either LTRA, theophylline, or zileuton

Step 4

Preferred:
Medium-dose ICS + LABA

Alternative:
Medium-dose ICS + either LTRA, theophylline, or zileuton

Step 5

Preferred:
High-dose ICS + LABA

AND

Consider omalizumab for patients who have allergies

Step 6

Preferred:
High-dose ICS + LABA + oral corticosteroid

AND

Consider omalizumab for patients who have allergies

Each step: Patient education, environmental control, and management of comorbidities.
Steps 2–4: Consider subcutaneous allergen immunotherapy for patients who have allergic asthma (see notes).

Quick-Relief Medication for All Patients
- SABA as needed for symptoms. Intensity of treatment depends on severity of symptoms: up to 3 treatments at 20-minute intervals as needed. Short course of oral systemic corticosteroids may be needed.
- Use of SABA >2 days a week for symptom relief (not prevention of EIB) generally indicates inadequate control and the need to step up treatment.

Key: Alphabetical order is used when more than one treatment option is listed within either preferred or alternative therapy. EIB, exercise-induced bronchospasm; ICS, inhaled corticosteroid; LABA, inhaled long-acting beta$_2$-agonist; LTRA, leukotriene receptor antagonist; SABA, inhaled short-acting beta$_2$-agonist

Notes:

- The stepwise approach is meant to assist, not replace, the clinical decision making required to meet individual patient needs.

- If alternative treatment is used and response is inadequate, discontinue it and use the preferred treatment before stepping up.

- Zileuton is a less desirable alternative due to limited studies as adjunctive therapy and the need to monitor liver function. Theophylline requires monitoring of serum concentration levels.

- In step 6, before oral systemic corticosteroids are introduced, a trial of high-dose ICS + LABA + either LTRA, theophylline, or zileuton may be considered, although this approach has not been studied in clinical trials.

- Steps 1, 2, and 3 preferred therapies are based on evidence A; step 3 alternative therapy is based on evidence A for LTRA, evidence B for theophylline, and evidence D for zileuton. Step 4 preferred therapy is based on evidence B, and alternative therapy is based on evidence B for LTRA and theophylline and evidence D for zileuton. Step 5 preferred therapy is based on evidence B. Step 6 preferred therapy is based on (EPR—2 1997) and evidence B for omalizumab.

- Immunotherapy for steps 2–4 is based on evidence B for house-dust mites, animal danders, and pollens; evidence is weak or lacking for molds and cockroaches. Evidence is strongest for immunotherapy with single allergens. The role of allergy in asthma is greater in children than in adults.

- Clinicians who administer immunotherapy or omalizumab should be prepared and equipped to identify and treat anaphylaxis that may occur.

FIGURE 11-6 Stepwise approach for managing asthma in youths 12 years of age and older and adults. Evidence A: Quality of evidence is high (further research is very unlikely to change confidence in the estimate of effect); Evidence B: Moderate (further research is likely to have an important impact on confidence in the estimate of effect and may change the estimate); Evidence D: Very low: Estimate of effect is very uncertain. (Credit: Redrawn from Expert Panel 3 Report. (2007). Guidelines for the diagnosis and management of asthma (p. 343). NIH Publication Number 08–5846. National Asthma Education and Prevention Program. Summary Report. Bethesda, MD. U.S. Department of Health and Human Services, National Heart, Lung and Blood Institute.)

associated with the use of inhaled corticosteroids. Inhaled corticosteroids may be used alone or in combination with LABAs.

Drug Alert!
A black box warning has been issued for a LABA for patients with asthma. One large clinical trial found an increase in asthma deaths and exacerbations in patient using a LABA. The current guidelines recommend using LABAs only in combination with inhaled corticosteroids (FDA Drug Safety Communication, 2010).

Leukotriene modifiers (inhibitors), or antileukotrienes, are a class of medications that include montelukast (Singulair®), zafirlukast (Accolate®), and zileuton (Zyflo®). Leukotriene inhibitors act either by interfering with leukotriene synthesis or by blocking the receptors where leukotrienes exert their action. They may provide an alternative to inhaled corticosteroids for mild persistent asthma, or they may be added to a regimen of inhaled corticosteroids in more severe asthma to improve control. Careful monitoring of liver function is recommended for patients taking zileuton.

Cromolyn sodium and nedocromil, also known as cromoglycates, stabilize mast cells. They are used primarily for mild persistent asthma as an alternative medication in patients not tolerating inhaled corticosteroids or as a preventive treatment for exercise asthma.

Omalizumab (anti-IgE) is used as an additional therapy for patients with severe, persistent asthma who have sensitivity to specific allergens, for example, cats, dogs, and cockroaches. Omalizumab is administered intravenously. Because of the potential for serious allergic reactions during administration, careful monitoring and possible treatment for anaphylaxis is required.

Nursing Alert
It is important for the nurse to recognize an anaphylactic reaction and initiate prompt emergency interventions. Signs and symptoms include: urticaria (hives), angioedema, bronchoconstriction, cough, stridor, cardiac arrhythmias, hypotension, and GI symptoms of nausea, vomiting, and diarrhea. Assessment of the patient's airway and cardiovascular status is essential. Supplemental oxygen therapy is administered, and endotracheal intubation may be required to provide sufficient oxygenation.

Other occasionally useful medications include methylxanthines and anticholinergics. Methylxanthines, sustained-release theophylline medications, are mild to moderate bronchodilators. They are mainly used as an adjunct when long-term controllers fail to achieve relieve of nighttime symptoms. Methylxanthines have a narrow therapeutic range

that necessitates monitoring of the serum theophylline level. The anticholinergic, ipratropium, may be used as an alternative quick-relief medication when the patient cannot tolerate SABAs.

Oral corticosteroids are used to gain quick control of asthma and during acute exacerbations. Patients with severe persistent asthma that is not adequately controlled may need long-term oral corticosteroids.

Environmental Control and Management of Triggers and Comorbid Conditions

Reducing exposure to asthma triggers may reduce asthma symptoms, inflammation, and the need for higher doses of medications. Skin testing is useful in some patients to identify specific allergens and in patients who may be candidates for immunotherapy. Effective allergen and trigger avoidance may be complicated when the patient's asthma is triggered by multiple allergens and irritants. Ongoing education and prioritizing the contribution of specific triggers in individuals may be needed. When patients have many triggers, specific trigger management may need to be designed to stress the management of the most troublesome triggers first and manage less troublesome triggers later. For example, if a patient has a severe reaction to cockroach antigen and less of a reaction to dust mites, initial efforts should be directed at cockroach control.

Drug Alert!
Patients with persistent asthma, nasal polyps, and sensitivity to aspirin or nonsteroidal anti-inflammatory drugs (NSAIDs) need to avoid using these drugs because of the risk of severe or even fatal reactions.

Asthma management is complicated by comorbid conditions, particularly COPD, allergic bronchopulmonary aspergillosis (aspergillosis, commonly found in soil, is a fungi to which patients with asthma or cystic fibrosis may have an allergic or hypersensitive reaction), gastroesophageal reflux disease (GERD), obesity, obstructive sleep apnea, rhinitis, sinusitis, stress, and depression. Adequately treating these conditions may improve the control of asthma. Most patients with comorbid conditions should be referred to a pulmonary or asthma specialist.

Nursing Management

Nursing care of patients with asthma depends on the setting the nurse works in and on the severity of the patient's disease. Patients may be treated successfully as outpatients if asthma symptoms are relatively mild or may require hospitalization and intensive care if symptoms are acute and severe. Asthma episodes may be frightening to patients and families. Reassurance and a calm approach are important aspects of care.

Nursing assessment includes taking a history of the patient's symptoms, self-care measures used, sequence of the current asthma episode, and response to medication and treatments used. A history of allergic reactions to medications, current prescription and nonprescription medications (including complementary and alternative therapy [CAM]), recent exposure to allergens and triggers, previous hospitalizations, emergency room visits, intensive care unit admissions, intubations for asthma, and the patient's perception of asthma severity are additional elements to include in a nursing assessment. Physical examination is similar to that used with COPD. Peak-flow measurements and pulse oximetry are additional assessment measures.

Nursing interventions for patients admitted for an asthma exacerbation include administering medications and treatments as prescribed, monitoring patients' response, preparing patients for discharge, and educating patients about treatment, medication administration, identification and management of asthma triggers, prevention and treatment of future exacerbations, and medical follow-up.

The main focus of nursing management of patients in *status asthmaticus* is to actively assess the patient's airway and the response to treatment. Nursing care includes: frequent monitoring of the patient's vital signs, oxygen saturation, and cardiac rhythm until status asthmaticus is under control; assessing for signs of dehydration and managing fluid intake; administering systemic corticosteroids, bronchodilators, and other medications as ordered (often given as continuous therapy); assisting patients with daily activity to help them conserve energy; and providing a quiet environment that is free of respiratory irritants including flowers, perfumes, powders, or odors of cleaning agents. The administration of heliox and magnesium sulfate are additional interventions that may be used and require close monitoring.

Patients in *status asthmaticus* who are not responding adequately to treatment and patients with severe comorbidities may need to be transferred to intensive care. Intubation and mechanical ventilation may also be needed. Frequent communication and consultation with physicians, respiratory therapists, and rapid response teams is important in any patient hospitalized for asthma. Discharge criteria include an FEV_1 or peak flow *measurement of* 70% or higher predicted (good response) or a *measurement of* 50% to 70% predicted in some patients (moderate response), a sustained response to bronchodilator treatment, no or mild distress, and the absence of hypoxemia. Patients being discharged from an emergency room or hospital may benefit from referral to an asthma clinic, asthma or pulmonary specialist, and/or visiting nurse agency. Home visits may be particularly useful for patients with recurrent exacerbations and emergency room visits. The home visit may give a more accurate picture of the individual's allergens and triggers.

Patient Teaching

Patient teaching is a critical component of the nursing care of patients with asthma. Complex treatment regimens, including multiple and different types of inhalers, monitoring of asthma control, antiallergy therapy, therapy for comorbid conditions, identification of early warning signs, and recognition and avoidance of triggers are essential for long-term control. Patient education may include: the nature of asthma as a chronic inflammatory disease, the definition of inflammation and bronchoconstriction, the goals of asthma control, the purpose and action of each medication (quick-relief medications and controllers), triggers to avoid and how to do so, proper inhalation technique, performance and recording of peak flow, implementation of an action plan designed with their health care provider, and recognition of the signs and symptoms indicating the need for prompt medical assistance.

An assortment of excellent educational materials is available from the NHLBI and other sources. The choice of educational materials used should be based on the patient's diagnosis, causative factors, educational and reading level, and cultural background. Selected references and websites for professionals and patients can be found on the website that accompanies the book. Visit http://thepoint.lww.com/Honan2e to access the references and other additional resources associated with this chapter.

Unfolding Patient Stories: Jennifer Hoffman • Part 1

Jennifer Hoffman is 33 years old and was diagnosed with asthma in childhood. She has come to the clinic multiple times over the last 2 months complaining of continued symptoms. Her asthma action plan was adjusted by her primary provider last month. What measures can the nurse take to determine areas needing education reinforcement? How can the nurse ensure that Jennifer is accurately following the prescribed asthma regimen and monitoring medication effectiveness? (Jennifer Hoffman's story continues in Chapter 38.)

Care for Jennifer and other patients in a realistic virtual environment: *vSim for Nursing* (thepoint.lww.com/vSimMedicalSurgical). Practice documenting these patients' care in (thepoint.lww.com/DocuCareEHR).

CHAPTER REVIEW

Critical Thinking Exercises

1. A 74-year-old man with severe COPD has been admitted with an acute exacerbation. He is extremely anxious and short of breath. He is unable to lie flat in bed and is on supplemental oxygen at 2 L/min. What tests or examinations might be appropriate to assess the severity of the patient's respiratory symptoms and his oxygenation status? What other nursing measures would you institute for this patient?

2. A 69-year-old woman with COPD reports that she has been using continuous oxygen for the past 5 years. She reports that she doesn't always use her oxygen as prescribed, only when she "feels she needs it." What should you teach her about oxygen?

3. As a nurse in an outpatient asthma clinic in a tertiary care medical center, you see a 35-year-old woman with asthma. When you inquire about symptom management and medication history, she reports that she uses an inhaler a few times a day when her breathing gets "really bad." She notes wheeze and cough several times a day. The inhaler she has with her is albuterol. She wakes up 3 times a week with asthma symptoms. In her medical record, you note that use of a combination LABA/corticosteroid to be taken twice a day has been repeatedly prescribed for her, but she reports that she does not use it very often. Describe the assessment method you would use to evaluate her asthma symptoms and severity. Describe teaching techniques you might use to assess the patient's knowledge of her medications, and provide education about the action of her controller and quick-relief medications, frequency of use, and correct administration. What methods would you use to monitor use of her medications and reinforce teaching?

4. As a nurse in your hospital's community outreach clinic, you are responsible for providing group education and counseling to patients with newly diagnosed asthma. What areas would you address regarding triggers for asthma? How might you have patients assess or change their home and work environments? What resources might you suggest?

NCLEX-Style Questions

1. During morning rounds on a medical floor, the nurse assesses a patient admitted the previous evening with an exacerbation of COPD. The patient is complaining of increased dyspnea. He is sitting on the side of the bed with his arms braced against his knees. His respiratory rate was 20 on admission and is now 28. His breath sounds are diminished with coarse crackles heard throughout. His oxygen saturation is 93% on 2 L/min of supplemental oxygen. The nurse would perform which of the following (Select all that apply) *except:*
   a. Administer albuterol using a spacer that has been ordered "as needed"
   b. Switch the patient's oxygen to a venturi-mask at 32%
   c. Instruct the patient to begin pursed-lip breathing
   d. Instruct the patient in controlled cough

2. The following day the patient's symptoms are improving. He is less dyspneic and able to walk to the bathroom with minimal assistance. In preparing for discharge, a home oxygen assessment is ordered. The patient's room air oxygen saturation is 88% at rest and 86% with exertion. Oxygen administered by nasal cannula at 2 L/min raises the oxygen saturation to 94% at rest and 92% when walking. Home oxygen is ordered as 2 L/min 24 hours a day. Teaching about home oxygen would include:
   a. Oxygen improves cardiac and cognitive function and improves prognosis
   b. Oxygen needs to be worn only when the patient is short of breath
   c. Oxygen improves cardiac and cognitive function but does not improve prognosis
   d. Home oxygen is dangerous and will explode

3. A 62-year-old woman is being seen at the health care provider's office for an initial evaluation of her symptoms of shortness of breath, cough, and sputum production. Her spirometry reveals an FEV_1 of 65% predicted. Her FVC is 90%. Her FEV_1/FVC is 60%. She has been given a diagnosis of COPD. She reports a smoking history of 35 years. She now smokes 10 cigarettes a day. She has tried to quit several times and was able to stay quit for 1 week a few years ago. She is concerned about weight gain if she quits smoking. The provider gave her a prescription for bupropion and nicotine nasal spray. The nurse is asked to review an approach to smoking cessation. What should be included in the teaching plan (Select all that apply) *except:*
   a. Bupropion and nicotine replacement can assist in the quitting process
   b. Successful smoking cessation includes multiple approaches
   c. Dealing with the habit of smoking is important to success
   d. Quitting smoking once COPD is diagnosed has no effect on prognosis

4. A hospital conducts an outpatient clinic for patients with asthma. The nurse working in the clinic is responsible for teaching patients about their medications. Which is true about inhaled medications?
   a. All inhalers must be given with a spacer device
   b. Inhaled corticosteroids are used on an as-needed basis for quick relief
   c. LABAs (long-acting beta adrenergics) can be used as monotherapy to control asthma
   d. LABAs and inhaled corticosteroids are used as controllers in the management of asthma

5. A 45-year-old woman with a diagnosis of asthma comes to the emergency room with worsening symptoms of cough and wheeze. She has been using her albuterol inhaler every 3 hours for the past 2 days. She denies allergies to medications, foods, and the environment. She has no other major medical problems and has never been a smoker. She is recovering from a viral respiratory infection. Her respiratory rate is 28; she is sitting upright on the stretcher. Her breath sounds are markedly diminished. Her room air oxygen saturation is 89%. The nurse should take the following next step:
   a. Administer oxygen to keep her oxygen saturation at 90–92% or above
   b. Recommend discharge with follow-up to her primary care provider (PCP)
   c. Administer inhaled corticosteroids
   d. Review asthma triggers and early warning signs

Try these additional resources, available at **http://thepoint.lww.com/Honan2e**, to enhance your learning and understanding of this chapter:
- NCLEX-Style Student Review Questions
- Journal Articles

REFERENCES AND SELECTED READINGS

References and selected readings associated with this chapter can be found on the website that accompanies the book. Visit **http://thepoint. lww.com/Honan2e** to access the references and other additional resources associated with this chapter.

Problems Related to Cardiovascular and Circulatory Function

The nurse is caring for an obese 60-year-old patient who smokes two packs of cigarettes a day. He is being seen in the cardiology clinic for evaluation and treatment of hypertension. His current blood pressure is 180/90. He has congestive heart failure and is currently nonadherent with his medication regimen and has not followed up with a doctor for 3 years.

- Discuss current and potential problems of the patient's nonadherence.
- What areas of teaching would be important to emphasize with this patient?
- Discuss target organs that may be affected by the patient's nonadherence with prescribed medications.

Nursing Assessment: Cardiovascular and Circulatory Function

Janet A. Parkosewich

Learning Objectives

After reading this chapter, you will be able to:

1. Describe the relationship between the anatomic structures and physiologic function of the heart and peripheral circulation.
2. Discuss the significance of the health history and physical assessment to the diagnosis of cardiovascular disorders.
3. Discuss the clinical indications, patient preparation, and other related nursing implications for common tests and procedures used to assess cardiovascular and circulatory function.
4. Compare the various methods of hemodynamic monitoring (e.g., central venous pressure, pulmonary artery pressure, and arterial pressure monitoring) with regard to indications for use, potential complications, and nursing responsibilities.

Cardiovascular disease (CVD) refers to diseases involving the heart and blood vessels. CVD affects more than 85.6 million Americans and claims the life of 1 person every 37 seconds (American Heart Association [AHA], 2016). Given the prevalence of CVD, nurses practicing in most settings will be assessing and managing patients with one or more disorders associated with the heart or blood vessels. An understanding of the structure and function of the cardiovascular system in health and disease is essential to the development of cardiovascular assessment skills.

ANATOMIC AND PHYSIOLOGIC OVERVIEW

The unique function of the cardiovascular system is to circulate blood through a network of blood vessels (arteries, capillaries, and veins) via two interdependent circulatory systems called the *pulmonary circulatory system* (right heart) and *systemic circulatory system* (left heart) (Fig. 12-1). The *lymphatic system* complements the function of the circulatory system by draining excessive interstitial fluid from the tissues and returning it into the bloodstream via the internal jugular and subclavian veins.

Anatomy and Physiology of the Vascular System

The vascular system is composed of blood vessels that circulate blood throughout the body and back to the heart. There are several types of blood vessels, including arteries, arterioles, capillaries, venules, and veins.

Arteries and Arterioles

Arteries are thick-walled structures that transport blood containing oxygen and nutrients from the heart to the tissues of the body. The aorta, the largest artery, has a diameter of approximately 25 mm (1 in) in the average-sized adult. It has numerous branches that continue to divide into progressively smaller arteries, eventually reaching 4 mm in diameter. Once these vessels diminish to approximately 30 µm in diameter, they become *arterioles,* which are embedded within the tissues.

The walls of the arteries and arterioles are composed of the *intima,* a thin, smooth endothelial cell layer; the *media,* the middle layer of smooth muscles and elastic fibers; and the *adventitia,* a protective layer of connective tissue that anchors these vessels to surrounding structures. The media is well developed in the arteries, whereas in smaller arteries and arterioles there is much less elastic tissue.

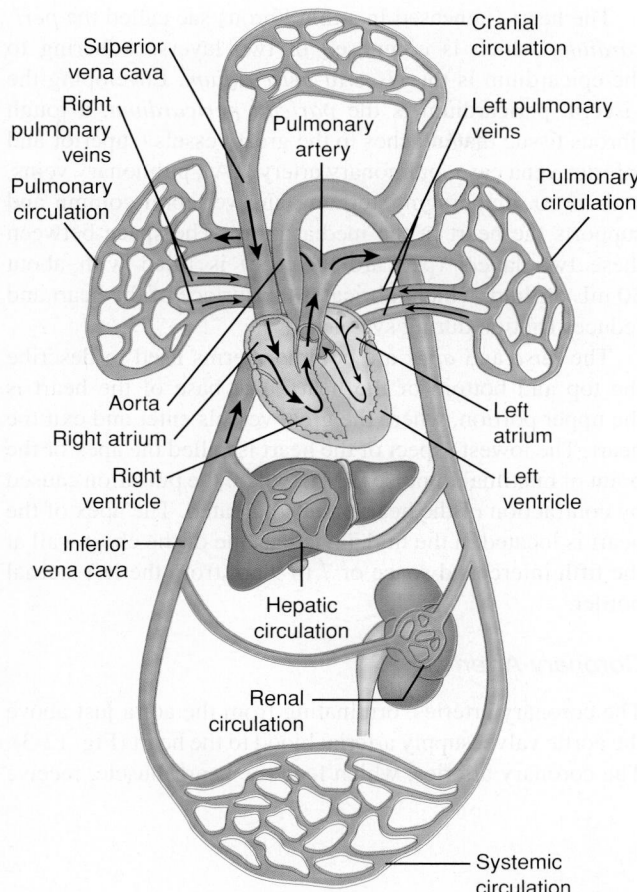

Superior vena cava
Right pulmonary veins
Pulmonary circulation
Cranial circulation
Pulmonary artery
Left pulmonary veins
Pulmonary circulation
Aorta
Right atrium
Right ventricle
Left atrium
Left ventricle
Inferior vena cava
Hepatic circulation
Renal circulation
Systemic circulation

FIGURE 12-1 Pulmonary and systemic circulation. Oxygen-rich blood from the pulmonary circulation is pumped from the left side of the heart into the aorta and the systemic arteries to the capillaries, where the exchange of nutrients and waste products takes place. The deoxygenated blood returns to the right side of the heart by way of the systemic veins and is pumped into the pulmonary circulation. *Arrows* represent the direction of blood flow through the great vessels and chambers of the heart. The blue shading represents venous blood and the red shading represents arterial blood.

Capillaries

Capillaries are narrow vessels (5 to 10 μm) formed by a single layer of endothelial cells that permit continuous movement of fluid and exchange of oxygen and nutrients to the cells and removal of carbon dioxide and other metabolic wastes. The amount of oxygen extracted differs by tissue type. For example, the heart has large metabolic requirements, extracting approximately 70% to 80% of the oxygen delivered, whereas other organs extract about 25%.

Capillary membrane permeability and hydrostatic and osmotic pressures are the primary controls for the amount and direction of fluid filtering across the capillary membrane into the interstitium (space around the cells). Under normal conditions, capillary permeability remains constant. Hydrostatic pressure is generated by the blood pressure

(BP), whereas osmotic pressure is created by plasma proteins (primarily albumin). The hydrostatic pressure, which is higher on the arterial side of the capillaries, tends to drive fluid out of the capillaries and into the interstitium. Interstitial fluid is reabsorbed into the capillaries on the venous side of the capillary bed, as the osmotic force predominates over hydrostatic pressure at this location. The excess interstitial fluid that is not reabsorbed into the venous end of the capillary enters the lymphatic system. These processes— filtration, reabsorption, and lymph formation—aid in maintaining tissue fluid volume and removing tissue waste and debris.

Tissue *edema*, an accumulation of excessive interstitial fluid, occurs for a variety of reasons including: abnormal conditions that obstruct lymph drainage, increased capillary membrane permeability, significantly elevated venous pressure, or decreased osmotic force generated by the plasma proteins.

Venules and Veins

The venous system has venules and veins, which are responsible for returning blood to the heart after cellular exchange of oxygen, nutrients, and metabolic waste products. The return of blood to the heart begins as capillaries merge to form thin-walled vessels called *venules* that merge to form larger vessels or veins. The veins contain approximately 75% of total blood volume. Compared with arteries, veins have three thin, less muscular layers. Thus, veins readily distend, permitting large volumes of blood to accumulate in these blood vessels under low pressure. Transport of venous blood back to the right side of the heart is facilitated by the pumping action of the skeletal muscles and the presence of one-way valves, which prevent backward blood flow and enhance the pumping action of skeletal muscles.

Circulatory Needs of Tissues

The amount of arterial blood flow needed to meet the demand for oxygen and other substances is determined by the rate of tissue metabolism, the availability of oxygen, and the function of the tissues. The central nervous system, circulating hormones, and certain chemicals are primarily responsible for regulating blood flow. When metabolic requirements increase (e.g., due to physical activity, local heat application, fever, or infection) blood vessels dilate (vasodilatation) to increase blood flow to the tissues. Vasodilatation and resultant lowering of BP is caused by relaxation of the blood vessel smooth muscles. This develops when potent substances, such as nitric oxide, prostacyclin, histamine, bradykinin, and prostaglandin, enter the circulation.

Blood vessels constrict (vasoconstriction) to reduce blood flow when metabolic demands are low (e.g., due to rest, local cold application, and cooling of the body). Vasoconstriction is due to contraction of the smooth muscles of the arteries, arterioles, and veins. This action causes narrowing of the lumen of the blood vessels and an elevation in BP. It is stimulated by the release of norepinephrine from the sympathetic nervous system, epinephrine from the adrenal medulla, and angiotensin II. Angiotensin II is the end result of a series of interactions beginning with renin (synthesized by the kidney) and angiotensinogen, a circulating serum protein produced by the liver, which forms angiotensin I. An enzyme (angiotensin-converting enzyme) secreted by the pulmonary vasculature converts angiotensin I into angiotensin II.

Anatomy and Physiology of the Heart

The heart is a hollow, muscular organ located in the center of the thorax, where it occupies the space between the lungs (mediastinum) and rests on the diaphragm. It weighs approximately 300 g (10.6 oz) and is about the size of a clenched fist, although size varies based on age, gender, body stature, physical condition, and presence of CVD.

The walls of the heart are made up of three layers (Fig. 12-2). The inner layer, or *endocardium*, consists of endothelial tissue and lines the inside of the heart and valves. The middle layer, or myocardium, forms an interconnected network of muscle fibers, which encircles the heart in a figure-of-eight pattern. During myocardial contraction, this configuration facilitates a twisting and compressive movement beginning from the top to the bottom of the heart. The exterior layer of the heart is called the *epicardium.*

The heart is encased in a thin fibrous sac called the *pericardium*, which is composed of two layers. Adhering to the epicardium is the *visceral pericardium*. Enveloping the visceral pericardium is the *parietal pericardium*, a tough fibrous tissue that attaches to the great vessels (superior and inferior vena cava, pulmonary artery [PA], pulmonary veins, and aorta), diaphragm, sternum, and vertebral column and supports the heart in the mediastinum. The space between these two layers (pericardial space) is filled with about 30 mL of fluid, which lubricates the surface of the heart and reduces friction during systole.

The *base* and *apex* are common terms used to describe the top and bottom of the heart. The base of the heart is the upper portion, where the great vessels enter and exit the heart. The lowest aspect of the heart is called the apex or the point of maximal impulse (PMI), where the pulsation caused by contraction of the heart can be palpated. The apex of the heart is located in the midclavicular line of the chest wall at the fifth intercostal space or 7 to 9 cm from the left sternal border.

Coronary Arteries

The coronary arteries, originating from the aorta just above the aortic valve, supply arterial blood to the heart (Fig. 12-3). The coronary arteries, which feed the heart muscle, receive

Superior vena cava
Right pulmonary artery
Interatrial septum
Pulmonary veins
Pulmonic valve
Right atrium
Tricuspid valve
Inferior vena cava
Right ventricle
Papillary muscle

Aortic arch
Left pulmonary artery
Descending aorta
Pulmonary veins
Left atrium
Aortic valve
Mitral valve
Left ventricle
Chordae tendinae
Papillary muscle

Interventricular septum
Endocardium
Myocardium
Epicardium
Pericardial space

Visceral pericardium
Parietal pericardium

→ Unoxygenated blood
→ Oxygenated blood

FIGURE 12-2 Anatomy of the heart. *Arrows* represent blood flow through the chambers of the heart.

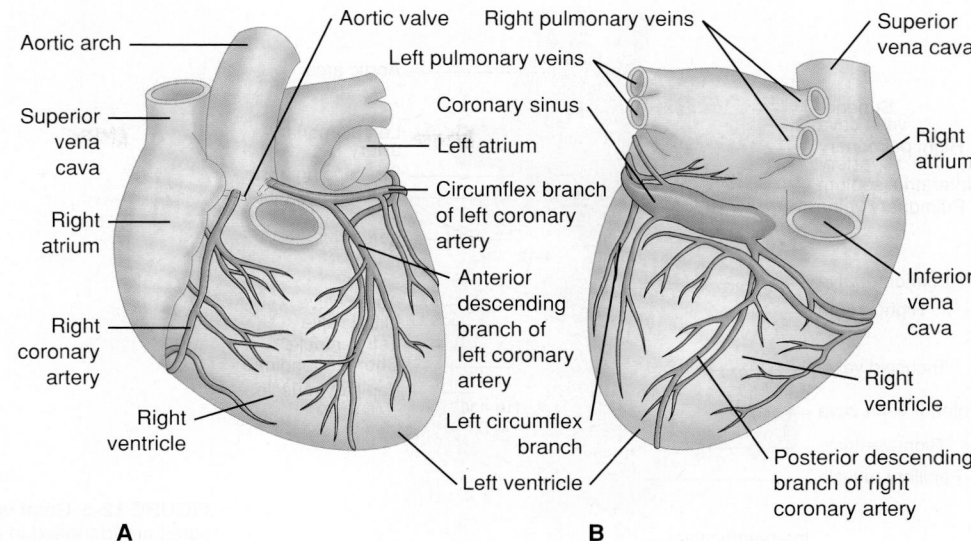

FIGURE 12-3 The coronary arteries supply the heart muscle with oxygenated blood, adjusting the flow according to metabolic needs. (**A**) Anterior view and (**B**) posterior view of the heart.

most of the blood during diastole, when the aortic valve closes. The left coronary, often referred to as the *left main coronary artery,* bifurcates into the left anterior descending artery that supplies the anterior wall of the heart and the *circumflex artery* that circles to the left side feeding the lateral wall of the heart.

The right side of the heart is supplied by the right coronary artery, which progresses around to the bottom or inferior wall of the left ventricle. The right coronary artery branches into the posterior descending artery, which supplies the posterior wall of the left ventricle. Superficial to the coronary arteries are the coronary veins. Venous blood from these veins returns to the heart primarily through the coronary sinus, which is located in the posterior wall of the right atrium.

Heart Chambers, Valves, and Great Vessels

The right and left sides of the heart each have an upper chamber, or atrium, that collects blood and a larger lower pumping chamber, called a *ventricle* (see Fig. 12-2). Blood flows into the right atrium from the superior and inferior vena cava, passes through the tricuspid valve to the right ventricle. The right ventricle pumps the blood in need of oxygenation across the pulmonary valve into the PA. The PA is the only artery carrying deoxygenated blood (other than the umbilical arteries in the fetus). Oxygenated blood returns to the left atrium via the pulmonary veins. The left atrium contracts, and blood flows through the mitral valve to the left ventricle. The left ventricle pumps the blood through the aortic valve into systemic circulation. Thus, two sets of valves are located within the right and left heart that provide one-way blood flow through these chambers. Valves separating the atria from the ventricles are termed *atrioventricular (AV) valves,* whereas valves located between the right and

left ventricles and their respective great vessels (PA and aorta) are called *semilunar valves.*

Cardiac Conduction System

The cardiac conduction system is composed of specialized cells that are capable of spontaneously initiating an electrical impulse (automaticity), responding to an electrical impulse (excitability), and propagating these impulses from one cell to another (conductivity) (Fig. 12-4). The **sinoatrial (SA) node**, the primary pacemaker of the heart, initiates electrical impulses at an inherent rate of 60 to 100 beats per minute (bpm). These impulses move across the atria via internodal pathways causing the atria to contract and then move onto the AV node. At the AV node, a slight delay occurs, which synchronizes atrial and ventricular activity and permits adequate time for the ventricles to fill. If the SA node fails in

FIGURE 12-4 Cardiac conduction system. AV, atrioventricular; SA, sinoatrial.

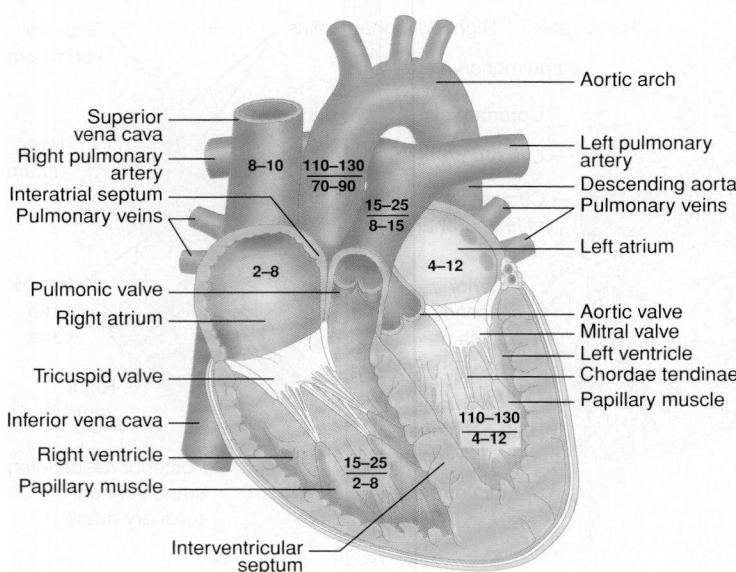

FIGURE 12-5 Great vessel and chamber pressures. Pressures are identified in mm Hg as mean pressure or systolic over diastolic pressure.

its pacemaker role, the AV node is capable of assuming this function by discharging electrical impulses at an inherent rate of 40 to 60 bpm. Impulses are then conducted to the ventricles via the bundle of His, to the right bundle branch (located in the right ventricle) and left bundle branches (located in the left ventricle), and finally to the Purkinje fibers, the point at which the ventricles are stimulated to contract (ventricular systole). The conduction tissue in the ventricles has an inherent rate of 30 to 40 bpm, which will assume the pacemaker role should the SA and AV nodes fail to provide electrical impulses.

At the cellular level, the electrical activity of the heart is due to the exchange of electrically charged particles, called *ions*, across channels located in the cellular membranes. These channels regulate the movement and speed of ions, specifically sodium and potassium. When the cell is in its resting or polarized state, sodium is the primary extracellular ion, whereas potassium is the primary intracellular ion. This difference in ion concentration causes the inside of the cell to have a negative charge, compared with the positive charge on the outside. A reversal of these charges occurs during electrical stimulation of the myocardial cells, as sodium ions move into the cell and potassium ions exit. This exchange of ions characterizes the period known as **depolarization**, which is followed rapidly by the contraction of the stimulated myocardium. Once depolarization is complete, the exchange of ions reverts back to its polarized state. This period is known as **repolarization**. It is analogous to a rest period that allows the myocardial cells to prepare for the next depolarization and subsequent contraction.

Cardiac Hemodynamics

Cardiac hemodynamics describes the pumping forces or pressure required by the heart to maintain blood flow throughout the cardiovascular system. An important determinant of blood flow is the principle that fluid flows from a region of higher pressure to one of lower pressure. The pressures responsible for blood flow are generated during systole and diastole. Figure 12-5 identifies the pressures in the great vessels and heart chambers during systole and diastole.

Cardiac Cycle

The cardiac cycle is the term used to describe the events that occur in the heart from the beginning of one heartbeat to the beginning of the subsequent one. Therefore, the number of cardiac cycles completed in a minute is dependent on the heart rate. Each cardiac cycle has three major sequential events, which include **diastole**, atrial **systole**, and ventricular systole. Diastole is the period in which the atria and ventricles are in a relaxed state, allowing the ventricles to fill with blood. Systole refers to the period of myocardial contraction.

Deoxygenated blood (venous blood) from the tissues enters the pulmonary circulation by flowing into the right atrium via the superior vena cava (head, neck, and upper extremities), inferior vena cava (trunk and lower extremities), and coronary sinus (heart). On the left side of the heart, oxygenated blood from the pulmonary circulation returns to the left atrium via the pulmonary veins. During diastole, the pressure in the ventricles is reduced, allowing the AV valves (tricuspid valve in the right heart and mitral valve in the left heart) to open. Blood flows freely from both atria into the ventricles. At the end of diastole, the atria contract (atrial systole), forcing the remaining blood into the ventricles. Atrial systole, better known as the "atrial kick," is an important event because it augments ventricular blood volume by 15% to 25%.

Nursing Alert
Loss of the atrial kick decreases cardiac output, leading to the development of symptoms in the patient such as dizziness, lightheadedness, syncope, decreased activity tolerance, and hypotension. Atrial fibrillation is an arrhythmia that is known to be associated with the loss of the atrial kick. Loss of coordinated atrial contraction into the ventricle will decrease the left ventricular preload and significantly lower cardiac output.

During ventricular systole, rising pressure in the ventricles closes the AV valves and forces the semilunar valves (pulmonic valve in the right side of the heart and aortic valve in the left side of the heart) to open. Additional structures attached to the AV valves (chordae tendineae and papillary muscles) keep the valve leaflets closed, thereby preventing regurgitation of blood into the atria. This function permits the one-way flow of blood from the right ventricle into the PA and into the lungs for oxygenation (pulmonary circulation) and from the left ventricle into the aorta and out into the remainder of the body via the systemic circulation.

Cardiac Output

Cardiac output refers to the amount of blood pumped by each ventricle in liters per minute (L/min). In an adult at rest, the cardiac output is about 4 to 6 L/min but varies greatly depending on the metabolic needs of the body.

Cardiac output is a function of the **stroke volume** and the heart rate. Stroke volume is the amount of blood ejected with each heartbeat. The average resting stroke volume is about 70 mL. Each time the heart beats, only a fraction of the blood present in the ventricles is ejected, which is referred to as the **ejection fraction** (EF). The EF of the left ventricle (normally 50% to 70%) is commonly assessed because it is an important noninvasive measure of myocardial contractility: the EF is lower in conditions that depress myocardial contractility (e.g., myocardial infarction [MI] and heart failure [HF]).

Effect of Heart Rate on Cardiac Output. Cardiac output meets the metabolic demands of the tissues, in part, by changes in heart rate. For example, the heart rate increases during periods of high oxygen demand, such as physical activity, and returns to baseline heart rate at rest. Changes in heart rate are accomplished by inhibition or stimulation of the SA node, through the parasympathetic and sympathetic divisions of the autonomic nervous system. The parasympathetic impulses, which travel to the SA node via the vagus nerve, slow the heart rate, whereas sympathetic innervations via beta$_1$ receptor sites increase heart rate.

Heart rate is also stimulated by an increased level of circulating catecholamines (secreted by the adrenal gland) and by excess thyroid hormone, which produces a catecholamine-like effect.

In addition, heart rate is affected by central nervous system and baroreceptor activity. **Baroreceptors**, located in the aortic arch and the right and left internal carotid arteries (at the point of bifurcation from the common carotid arteries), are sensitive to changes in BP. During elevations in BP (**hypertension**), these cells increase their rate of discharge, transmitting impulses to the medulla. This initiates parasympathetic activity and inhibits sympathetic response, lowering the heart rate and the BP. In contrast, low BP (hypotension) exerts less baroreceptor stimulation, decreasing the parasympathetic action on the SA node and allowing for enhanced sympathetic activity. The resultant vasoconstriction and increased heart rate elevate the BP.

Effect of Stroke Volume on Cardiac Output. Stroke volume is a major determinant of cardiac output and is influenced by three interdependent factors: preload, afterload, and contractility.

Preload refers to the pressure generated in the ventricles at the end of diastole and the resultant stretching of the muscle fibers. A direct relationship exists between end-diastolic blood volume and the degree of stretch. As the volume of blood increases, the degree of stretch increases, resulting in stronger contraction and a greater stroke volume. This relationship, called the Frank-Starling (or Starling) law of the heart, is maintained until the physiologic limit of the muscle is reached.

Preload is decreased by a reduction in the volume of blood returning to the ventricles. Vasodilatation and loss of fluid volume from bleeding, diuresis, vomiting, or excessive diaphoresis reduce preload. Preload is increased by increasing the return of circulating blood volume to the ventricles. Controlling the loss of blood or body fluids and replacing fluids (i.e., blood transfusions and intravenous [IV] fluid administration) are examples of ways to increase preload.

Afterload, the amount of resistance to ejection of blood from the ventricle, is the second determinant of stroke volume. The right side of the heart collects venous blood, which has a very low pressure and is met with little resistance as blood is ejected into the pulmonary vascular system, better known as **pulmonary vascular resistance (PVR)**. On the other hand, the left side of the heart requires significantly higher pressures to overcome resistance created by the arteries in the systemic circulation. This resistance is called **systemic vascular resistance (SVR)**.

An inverse relationship exists between afterload and stroke volume. For example, afterload is increased by arterial vasoconstriction, which leads to decreased stroke volume. The opposite is true with arterial vasodilation, a situation that reduces afterload and improves stroke volume.

Nursing Alert
Preload reflects the volume of blood returning to the right and left ventricles at the end of diastole. Central venous pressure (CVP)

monitoring measures right heart preload, whereas, PA monitoring measures left ventricular preload.

Afterload is directly affected by arterial vascular tone. Afterload is increased as SVR increases due to vasoconstriction of the aorta and arteries. The opposite affect occurs with arterial vasodilatation. SVR greater than 1,200 dynes implies vasoconstriction, whereas SVR less than 900 dynes implies vasodilation.

Contractility refers to the force generated by the contracting myocardium under any given condition. Contractility is enhanced by circulating catecholamines, sympathetic neuronal activity, and certain medications (e.g., digoxin [Lanoxin], IV dopamine [Intropin], or dobutamine [Dobutrex]). Increased contractility results in increased stroke volume. Contractility is depressed by hypoxemia, acidosis, and certain medications (e.g., beta-adrenergic blocking medications).

Anatomy and Physiology of the Lymphatic System

The lymphatic system and the cardiovascular system are closely linked. The lymphatic system is formed by lymph, lymph vessels, and lymph nodes. This system collects interstitial fluid, called lymph, and returns it to the cardiovascular system, thus helping to maintain preload. The lymphatic system plays an important role in the immune system as well by producing lymphocytes (a white blood cell [WBC]), which defend the body against disease.

Lymph is a fluid similar to plasma that contains plasma proteins, lymphocytes, and other factors. It is formed by the filtration of interstitial fluid into the lymph vessels. Lymph vessels are a complex network of thin-walled vessels that resemble veins with a few exceptions: lymph vessels have thinner walls, have more valves, and contain lymph nodes. Lymph readily filters into these vessels because they are very permeable and are not pressurized.

As lymph circulates through these vessels, it passes through one or more lymph nodes before it is returned to the venous blood via openings in the right or left subclavian vein. Lymph nodes, small bean-shaped structures, filter lymph and provide an environment for lymphocytes to perform their immune function after exposure to foreign antigens, such as bacteria or viruses. Lymph nodes are located in clusters primarily in the neck, axilla, and groin.

The lymphatic vessels converge into two main structures: the thoracic duct and the right lymphatic duct. The lymphatic vessels rely on one-way valves, arterial pulsations, and contraction of the lymphatic walls and adjacent skeletal muscle to propel lymph toward the venous drainage points in the subclavian veins.

Gerontologic Considerations

As people age, myocardial muscle mass shrinks (atrophy) and its walls thicken (hypertrophy). The aging process also results in decreased elasticity and widening of the aorta, calcification and stiffening of the blood vessels, thickening and increased rigidity of the cardiac valves, and increased connective tissue in the cardiac conduction system. These changes lead to decreased cardiac output and impaired blood flow to the tissues. As a result, the aging heart has limited ability to respond to increased demands for oxygen and nutrients caused by physical or emotional stress and disease states. These age-associated changes place the elderly at risk for the development of serious symptoms, including fatigue, shortness of breath, angina, palpitations, leg pain, dizziness, or syncope. Age-related changes of the cardiovascular system are summarized in Table 12-1.

Gender Considerations

The heart of a woman is smaller and weighs less, compared with the heart of a man. Coronary arteries of the female heart are smaller and thus occlude from **atherosclerosis** more easily and make procedures such as cardiac catheterization and percutaneous coronary interventions technically more difficult, with a higher incidence of postprocedural complications. In addition, the resting heart rate, stroke volume, and EF of a woman's heart are higher than those of a man's heart. The first onset of coronary artery disease (CAD) in women is almost a decade later than in their male counterparts. These gender differences in disease presentation are attributed to the premenopausal protection of circulating estrogen.

ASSESSMENT OF THE CARDIOVASCULAR SYSTEM

The frequency and extent of the nursing assessment of the cardiovascular system are based on several factors, including the severity of the patient's symptoms, the presence of risk factors, the practice setting, and the purpose of the assessment. Although the key components of the cardiovascular assessment remain the same, the assessment priorities vary according to the needs of the patient. For example, an emergency department nurse caring for a patient who is admitted with symptoms associated with acute coronary syndrome (ACS—a term used for any condition brought on by a sudden blockage of blood flow to the heart) performs a rapid and focused assessment because treatment of ACS is time-dependent.

Health History

Nurses practicing in settings where patients with CVD are seen must be expert at recognizing cardiac symptoms as well as expediting timely and, oftentimes, lifesaving care. Likewise, patients must be able to recognize when they are experiencing these symptoms and know how to manage them. All too often, patients fail to appreciate the significance of new or worsening cardiac symptoms. This problem results

TABLE 12-1 GERONTOLOGIC CONSIDERATIONS / Age-Related Changes in the Cardiovascular System

Cardiovascular System Component	Structural Changes	Functional Changes	History and Physical Examination Findings
Ventricular myocardium	Loss of muscle mass Hypertrophy	Stiff, noncompliant ventricles Decrease in cardiac output	Fatigue, ↓ exercise tolerance HF or arrhythmia signs/symptoms PMI palpated lateral to midclavicular line Auscultation reveals S_4
Valves	Calcification of AV valves	Turbulent blood flow across valves	Murmurs and thrills
Conduction system	Deposits of connective tissue	↓ SA node rate and ↓ speed of conduction	Bradycardia Heart block
Sympathetic nervous system	↓ response to beta-adrenergic stimulation	↓ HR and contractility "in" response "to" exercise ↑ time for HR to return to baseline	Fatigue and ↓ exercise tolerance
Aorta and arteries	Calcification and stiffening of the blood vessels ↓ Elasticity and widening of aorta	Left ventricular hypertrophy	Progressive ↑ systolic BP; ↑ diastolic BP Widening pulse pressure
Baroreceptor response	↓ Baroceptor sensitivity to episodes of hypertension and hypotension	Baroreceptors fail to regulate HR and vascular tone, causing a slow response to postural changes	Postural hypotension, dizziness, or syncope when sitting or standing up

AV, atrioventricular; BP, blood pressure; HF, heart failure; HR, heart rate; PMI, point of maximal impulse; SA, sinoatrial; ↓, decreased; ↑, increased.

in prolonged delays in seeking treatment. Major barriers to seeking prompt lifesaving care include lack of knowledge about personal risk and symptoms of heart disease, attributing symptoms to a benign source, denying symptom significance, and feeling embarrassed about having symptoms (Gillis, Arslanian-Engoren, & Struble, 2014). Box 12-1 discusses results of a study testing the effect of an educational intervention on Latinas' knowledge of CVD risk factors and prevention strategies.

Common Complaints

Common CVD signs and symptoms, with related medical diagnoses in parentheses, are covered in the section below.

- Chest pain or discomfort (ACS that includes unstable angina and acute MI, arrhythmias, valvular heart disease)
- Pain or discomfort in other areas of upper body, including one or both arms, back, neck, jaw, or stomach (ACS)
- Dizziness, syncope, or changes in level of consciousness (ACS, cardiogenic shock, cerebrovascular disorders, arrhythmias, hypotension, postural hypotension, vasovagal episode)
- **Intermittent claudication** or rest pain in lower extremities, especially at night (peripheral arterial disease [PAD])

- Palpitations or tachycardia (ACS, caffeine or other stimulants, electrolyte imbalances, HF, stress, valvular heart disease, ventricular aneurysm)
- Peripheral edema (HF, PAD), weight gain (HF), or ascites and abdominal distension due to enlarged liver and spleen (HF)
- Shortness of breath or dyspnea, with or without chest pain (ACS, cardiogenic shock, HF, pulmonary edema, valvular heart disease)
- Unusual fatigue characterized by feeling more tired or fatigued than usual (early warning symptom of ACS, HF, valvular heart disease)

Chest Pain

Chest pain and chest discomfort are common symptoms caused by a number of cardiac and noncardiac problems. Table 12-2 identifies the characteristics of common causes of chest pain. To differentiate among these causes of pain, the nurse asks the patient to identify the quantity (0 = no pain to 10 = worst pain), location, and quality of pain. It is important to identify the events that precipitated symptom onset, the duration of the symptom, measures that aggravate or relieve the symptom, and associated signs and symptoms, such as diaphoresis or nausea. The nurse should keep the

---

BOX 12-1 Nursing Research

Bridging the Gap to Evidence-Based Practice

What does the current evidence reveal about the effect of an educational intervention on immigrant Latinas' knowledge of cardiovascular risk factors and prevention strategies?

Koniak-Griffin, D., & Brecht, M. L. (2015). Awareness of cardiovascular disease and preventive behaviors among overweight immigrant Latinas. *Journal of Cardiovascular Nursing, 30*(5), 447–455.

Purpose

Almost one third of Latino women die from all forms of cardiovascular disease (CVD), including heart disease and stroke, making it the leading cause of death in this population. It is alarming to note that disparities in Latino women's awareness and knowledge about CVD risk factors and prevention strategies exist despite efforts made by the American Heart Association, the National Alliance for Hispanic Health, the Office of Women's Health, and other community outreach programs. The purpose of this study was to evaluate the effect of a lifestyle behavior intervention (LSBI) on awareness and knowledge of CVD risk factors and prevention strategies in overweight, Spanish-speaking, immigrant Latinas.

Design

This randomized controlled trial was conducted in two communities of Los Angeles, California. Eligible participants were Spanish and/or English-speaking Latina, between the ages of 35 and 64 years, and had a body mass index (BMI) of 25 or greater. Exclusion criteria included impaired physical mobility, type 1 diabetes, uncontrolled hypertension, or history of a heart attack or stroke. A health clearance was required for those with type 2 diabetes or hypertension controlled by diet and/or oral medications prior to enrollment. The women were randomly assigned to an experimental group and received a 6-month LSBI (2 months of group education on CVD prevention followed by 4 months of individual teaching and coaching) or a control group in which women received 6 months of safety and disaster preparedness education. The LSBI curriculum was based upon Su Corazón, Su Vida/Your Heart, Your Life, a National Heart Lung and Blood program designed specifically for use with Latinos. The intervention group was facilitated by promotora, specially trained lay health advisors. CVD knowledge was examined using an 11-item true-or-false test. Dietary habits were determined using a 27-item survey with a Likert scale response that had been used extensively in previous projects. The study was approved by the institutional review board of the University of California, Los Angeles.

Findings

The results of a preliminary analysis of data from 90 women in the intervention group were reported in this publication. These women had a mean age of 42.6 years, were obese (BMI, mean, 32.5 ± 5.2) and the majority was of Mexican descent (83%). This group of low income women had low acculturation and educational attainment with 51.7% having completed eighth grade or less.

There was a statistically significant improvement in total CVD knowledge scores and in nine of the 11 items postintervention, controlling for age and education. Almost all of the women postintervention knew that overweight women face increased risk for heart disease and diabetes (97.8%), eating smaller portions of a variety of foods lower in fat and calories is the healthiest way to lose weight (96.67%), physical activity can lower a woman's risk for heart disease (95.6%), and high blood pressure is a heart disease risk factor that you can do something about (94.4%). Although the item regarding heart disease as the leading cause of death in women improved significantly, eight women answered incorrectly despite the intensive education. Another concern was related to the fact that 87.8% of the women failed to recognize that women may have heart attack symptoms that are different from those in men. There were no significant correlations between CVD knowledge scores and overall dietary habits score, demographic characteristics (age, education, acculturation, and years living in the United States), BMI, or physical activity.

Nursing Implications

More than a decade of public education campaigns aimed at enhancing women's CVD awareness have not reached all women. Latino women with lower acculturation and socioeconomic status may benefit most from local community-based LSBI lead by promotora. Knowledge alone is not associated with lifestyle behaviors including heart-healthy nutrition and physical activity. Latino women at high risk for CVD may benefit from ongoing support to translate new knowledge into lifestyle changes. The results of this study illustrate the need for continued testing of interventions designed to effect CVD risk reduction over the lifespan.

---

following points in mind when assessing patients with chest pain or discomfort:

- The severity and duration of chest pain or discomfort does not predict the seriousness of its cause. For example, a patient experiencing esophageal spasm may rate chest pain as a "10/10," whereas, a patient experiencing an acute MI may report only mild to moderate chest pressure.
- More than one cardiac condition may occur simultaneously. During an acute MI, patients may report chest pain from myocardial **ischemia** (inadequate oxygen supply to the tissues), shortness of breath from HF, and palpitations from arrhythmias. Both HF and arrhythmias are complications of acute MI.

Symptoms of Acute Coronary Syndrome

Nurses must take complaints of patients with cardiac symptoms seriously until the cause is determined. Because CAD is so prevalent, all patients reporting new or worsening cardiac symptoms, particularly those at risk for CAD or who have a history of CAD, should be evaluated initially for ACS.

TABLE **12-2** Characteristics of Cardiac and Noncardiac Causes of Chest Pain

Location	Character	Duration	Precipitating Events and Aggravating Factors	Alleviating Factors
Angina pectoris Acute coronary syndrome (ACS) (unstable angina, myocardial infarction [MI]) Usual distribution of pain with myocardial ischemia Jaw Epigastrium Right side Back Less common sites of pain with myocardial ischemia	Angina: Uncomfortable pressure, squeezing, or fullness in substernal chest area Can radiate across chest to the medial aspect of one or both arms and hands, jaw, shoulders, upper back, or epigastrium Radiation to arms and hands, described as numbness, tingling, or aching ACS: Same as angina pectoris Pain or discomfort ranges from mild to severe Associated with shortness of breath, diaphoresis, palpitations, unusual fatigue, and nausea or vomiting	Angina: 5–15 minutes ACS: 15 min or more	Angina: Physical exertion, emotional upset, eating large meal, or exposure to extremes in temperature ACS: Emotional upset or unusual physical exertion occurring within 24 hours of symptom onset Can occur at rest or while asleep	Angina: Rest, nitroglycerin, oxygen ACS: Morphine, reperfusion of coronary artery with thrombolytic agent or percutaneous coronary intervention
Pericarditis	Sharp, severe substernal or epigastric pain Can radiate to neck, arms, and back Associated symptoms include fever, malaise, dyspnea, cough, nausea, dizziness, and palpitations	Intermittent	Sudden onset Pain increases with inspiration, swallowing, coughing, and rotation of trunk	Sitting upright, analgesia, anti-inflammatory medications
Pulmonary disorders (pneumonia, pulmonary embolism)	Sharp, severe substernal or epigastric pain arising from inferior portion of pleura (referred to as pleuritic pain). Patient may be able to localize the pain	30 minutes or more	Follows an infectious or noninfectious process (MI, cardiac surgery, cancer, immune disorders, uremia) Pleuritic pain increases with inspiration, coughing, movement, and supine positioning Occurs in conjunction with community-acquired or nosocomial lung infections (pneumonia) or deep vein thrombosis (pulmonary embolism)	Treatment of underlying cause

(continued on page 382)

TABLE **12-2** **Characteristics of Cardiac and Noncardiac Causes of Chest Pain** (*continued*)

Location	Character	Duration	Precipitating Events and Aggravating Factors	Alleviating Factors
Esophageal disorders (hiatal hernia, reflux esophagitis or spasm)	Substernal pain described as sharp, burning, or heavy. Often mimics angina. Can radiate to neck, arm, or shoulders	5–60 minutes	Recumbency, cold liquids, exercise	Food or antacid
Anxiety and panic disorders	Pain described as stabbing to dull ache. Associated with diaphoresis, palpitations, shortness of breath, tingling of hands or mouth, feeling of unreality, or fear of losing control	Peaks in 10 minutes	Can occur at any time, including during sleep. Can be associated with a specific trigger	Removal of stimulus, relaxation, medications to treat anxiety or underlying disorder
Musculoskeletal disorders (costochondritis)	Sharp or stabbing pain localized in anterior chest. Most often unilateral. Can radiate across chest to epigastrium or back	Hours to days	Most often follows respiratory tract infection with significant coughing, vigorous exercise, or posttrauma. Some cases are idiopathic. Exacerbated by deep inspiration, coughing, sneezing, and movement of upper torso or arms	Rest, ice, or heat. Analgesic or anti-inflammatory medications
Dissecting aorta	Severe, persistent tearing pain in anterior chest/back. Radiates to shoulders, epigastrium or abdomen. Associated with diaphoresis and tachycardia	Sudden onset	Hypertension, blunt chest trauma, or cocaine use	Medical or surgical interventions

There are several distinct characteristics of ACS symptoms that need to be kept in mind during assessment:

- The majority of patients with ACS experience prodromal symptoms sometimes a month or more prior to developing this acute event. Prodromal symptoms include unusual fatigue, shortness of breath, sleep disturbances, anxiety, or fleeting chest discomfort (aching, pressure) that comes and goes. Because these symptoms are less severe than what is experienced during ACS, patients often attribute them to a benign problem, such as stress, and fail to seek medical care. Nurses should include a question regarding presence of prodromal symptoms when assessing patients with cardiac symptoms.
- Approximately 50% of men and women with ACS experience chest symptoms, whereas the remainder may develop a variety of symptoms such as upper back, shoulder, arm, or neck pain; epigastric burning; or shortness of breath. There are many misconceptions that men and women have about their cardiac risk factors and signs and symptoms of heart disease.
- During the onset of ACS, people experience a group of at least four or more symptoms that can include chest discomfort or pain; upper back, shoulder, arm, or neck pain; epigastric burning or indigestion; shortness of breath; unusual fatigue; and diaphoresis. The combination of symptoms can vary from person to person (Gillis, Arslanian-Engoren, & Struble, 2014).
- Neuropathies in elderly patients and those with diabetes may prevent these patients from experiencing pain or discomfort associated with myocardial ischemia. Instead, they may report unusual fatigue or shortness of breath. In some patients, ACS may be asymptomatic, which is referred to as *silent ischemia*.
- A 12-lead electrocardiogram (ECG) and serum laboratory analysis of cardiac biomarkers are necessary to determine if the patient with ACS symptoms is experiencing unstable angina or acute MI.

History

Epidemiologic studies show that certain conditions or behaviors (i.e., risk factors) are associated with a greater incidence of CAD, cerebrovascular disease, and PAD (AHA, 2016). The nurse might ask some of the following questions:

- How is your health? Have you noticed any changes from last year? From 5 years ago?
- Do you have a cardiologist or primary health care provider? How often do you go for checkups?
- What are your risk factors for heart disease? What do you do to reduce these risk factors? Box 12-2 lists risk factors for CVD and treatment goals.

Patients who lack understanding of their risk factors and diagnosis may be less motivated to make lifestyle changes or manage their cardiac disease effectively. On the other hand,

---

BOX 12-2

Risk Factors for Cardiovascular Diseases (CVD)

Nonmodifiable Risk Factors

- Older age
- Male gender
- Heredity, including race

Modifiable Risk Factors and Treatment Goals[a]

- Hyperlipidemia (LDL less than 100 mg/dL and preferably less than 70 mg/dL if CAD present; LDL less than 160 mg/dL if one or more risk factors or 130 mg/dL if two or more risk factors; HDL greater than 40 mg/dL and triglycerides less than 150 mg/dL)
- Hypertension (less than 140/90 mm Hg; less than 130/80 if diabetes or chronic renal disease present)
- Cigarette smoking (complete cessation, no secondhand tobacco exposure)
- Diabetes mellitus (fasting serum glucose less than 110 mg/dL and hemoglobin A_{1c} less than 7%)
- Obesity and overweight (BMI 18.5–24.9 kg/m^2; waist circumference: male 40 in or less, female 35 in or less)
- Physical inactivity (30–60 minutes moderate intensity aerobic activity 5 days or more)

[a]American Heart Association; recommended goals are given in parentheses.

---

patients who have this awareness and believe that they have the power to modify their risk factors may be more likely to engage in prevention measures. Once patients' risk factors are identified, the nurse determines if patients have a plan for making necessary lifestyle changes and if assistance is needed to support these changes.

Family History

The nurse inquires about a history of cardiac disease in the patient's family, including:

- A history of sudden death in family members of all ages with or without symptoms or known CAD
- A family member with a biochemical or neuromuscular condition (e.g., hemochromatosis [excessive iron retention in the body] or muscular dystrophy)
- DNA mutation or other genetic testing that was performed on any family member

Cardiovascular disorders associated with genetic abnormalities include familial hypercholesterolemia, hypertrophic cardiomyopathy, long QT syndrome, hereditary hemochromatosis, and elevated homocysteine levels (discussed later in this chapter).

Social History

Medications

Nurses collaborate with other health care providers to obtain a complete list of the patient's medications, including dose and frequency. Vitamins, herbals, and over-the-counter medications are included on this list. During this aspect of the health assessment, the nurse solicits answers to the following questions to ensure that patients are taking their medications safely and effectively:

- Is the patient independent in taking medications?
- Are the medications taken as prescribed?
- Does the patient know what side effects to report to the prescriber?
- Does the patient understand why the medication regimen is important?
- Are doses ever forgotten or skipped, or does the patient ever decide to stop taking a medication?
- An aspirin a day is a common nonprescription medication that improves patient outcomes after an acute MI. However, if patients are not aware of this benefit, they may be inclined to stop taking aspirin if they think it is a trivial medication. A careful medication history often uncovers common medication errors and causes for nonadherence to the medication regimen.

Nutrition and Metabolism

Dietary modifications, exercise, weight loss, and careful monitoring are important strategies for managing three major cardiovascular risk factors: hyperlipidemia, hypertension, and diabetes mellitus. Diets that are restricted in sodium, fat, cholesterol, and/or calories are commonly prescribed. The nurse obtains the following information:

- How often the patient self-monitors BP, blood glucose, and weight as appropriate to the medical diagnoses
- The patient's knowledge regarding target goals for each of the risk factors, and any problems achieving or maintaining these goals
- What the patient normally eats and drinks in a typical day, and any food preferences (including cultural or ethnic preferences)
- Eating habits (canned or commercially prepared foods versus fresh foods, restaurant cooking versus home cooking, assessing for high-sodium foods, dietary intake of fats)
- Who shops for groceries and prepares meals

Elimination

Typical bowel and bladder habits need to be identified. Nocturia (awakening at night to urinate) is common in patients with HF. Fluid collected in the dependent tissues (extremities) during the day redistributes into the circulatory system once the patient is recumbent at night. The increased circulatory volume is excreted by the kidneys (increased urine production).

When straining during defecation, the patient bears down (the Valsalva maneuver), which momentarily increases pressure on the baroreceptors. This triggers a vagal response, causing the heart rate to slow, which may lead to syncope in some patients. Straining during urination can produce the same response.

Because many cardiac medications can cause GI side effects or bleeding, the nurse asks about bloating, diarrhea, constipation, stomach upset, heartburn, loss of appetite, nausea, and vomiting. Patients taking platelet-inhibiting medications such as aspirin and clopidogrel (Plavix); platelet aggregation inhibitors such as abciximab (ReoPro), eptifibatide (Integrilin), and tirofiban (Aggrastat); and IV anticoagulants such as low–molecular-weight heparin (i.e., dalteparin [Fragmin], enoxaparin [Lovenox]), heparin, or oral anticoagulants (i.e., warfarin [Coumadin] rivaroxaban [Xarelto] or apixaban [Eliquis]) are screened for bloody urine (hematuria) or stools (red, black, or tarry), epistaxis (nosebleed), or unusual bruising.

Activity and Exercise

Changes in patients' activity tolerance may be gradual and go unnoticed. The nurse determines if there are recent changes by comparing the patient's current activity level with that performed in the past 6 to 12 months. New symptoms or a change in the usual symptoms during activity is a significant finding. Activity-induced angina or shortness of breath (SOB) may indicate CAD, which requires medical attention. Arterial insufficiency is suspected if the patient experiences intermittent claudication, described as a lower extremity muscular, cramping pain that occurs with activity and is relieved by rest. Angina and intermittent claudication occur when there is tissue ischemia or inadequate arterial blood supply, in the setting of increased demand (e.g., exercise, stress, or anemia). As the tissues are forced to function without adequate nutrients and oxygen, muscle metabolites and lactic acid are produced. Pain is experienced as the metabolites aggravate the nerve endings of the surrounding tissue. **Rest pain** is a persistent pain in the anterior portion of the foot at rest that can worsen at night and indicates significant arterial insufficiency and a critical state of ischemia.

Fatigue, associated with a low left ventricular EF (less than 40%) and certain medications (e.g., beta-adrenergic blocking agents), can result in activity intolerance. Patients with fatigue may benefit from having their medications adjusted and learning energy-conservation techniques.

Additional areas to explore include the presence of architectural barriers in the home (stairs, multilevel home), the patient's involvement in cardiac rehabilitation, and the patient's typical exercise pattern, including intensity, frequency, and duration.

Sleep and Rest

Clues to worsening cardiac disease, especially HF, can be revealed by sleep-related events. Determining where the patient sleeps or rests and any recent changes in sleep habits is important. Worsening HF is characterized by pulmonary congestion resulting in dyspnea at rest or when lying down. *Orthopnea* is the term used to indicate the need to sit upright or stand to avoid dyspnea. Thus, patients with worsening HF will report that they sleep upright in a chair instead of in bed; increase the number of pillows used; awaken from sleep with sudden onset of dyspnea, often associated with coughing and wheezing, called *paroxysmal nocturnal dyspnea* (PND); or awaken with angina (nocturnal angina). PND occurs at night and is caused by the reabsorption of fluid from dependent areas of the body (arms and legs) back into the circulatory system within hours of lying in bed. This sudden fluid shift increases preload and places too great a demand on the heart of patients with HF, causing sudden pulmonary congestion.

There is mounting evidence pointing to the cardiac consequences associated with sleep-disordered breathing (SDB). SDB is an abnormal respiratory pattern due to intermittent episodes of upper airway obstruction causing apnea and hypopnea (shallow respirations) during sleep. These abnormal sleep events cause intermittent hypoxemia, sympathetic nervous system activation, and increased intrathoracic pressure that puts mechanical stress on the heart and large artery walls. Untreated SDB has been linked to CAD, hypertension, HF, and arrhythmias. SDB is treated by the use of continuous positive airway pressure (CPAP) and mandibular advancement devices (MAD). These devices maintain an open airway during sleep, preventing hypoxemia and resulting abnormal elevations in BP. The cardinal signs of SBD are loud, disruptive snoring and apnea lasting 10 seconds or more. Obesity and large neck circumference are two important risk factors for SDB (Ayas, Owens, & Kheirandish-Gozal, 2015).

During the health history, the nurse assesses for SDB by asking high-risk patients if they snore loudly, have frequent bouts of awakening from sleep, waking with a headache, or experience severe daytime sleepiness (hypersomnolence). For patients with a diagnosis of SDB, the nurse determines if the patient has been prescribed a CPAP or MAD and the frequency of its use. Patients who are being admitted to the hospital or going for an ambulatory surgical procedure should be instructed to bring their sleep aid devices with them.

Cognition and Perception

Evaluating cognitive ability helps determine whether the patient has the capacity to manage safe and effective self-care independently. Is the patient's short-term memory intact? Is there any history of dementia? Is there evidence of depression or anxiety? Can the patient read? Can the patient read English? What is the patient's reading level? What is the patient's preferred learning style? What information does the patient perceive as important? Providing the patient with written information can be a valuable part of patient education but only if the patient can read and comprehend the information.

Related assessments include possible hearing or visual impairments. If vision is impaired, patients with HF may not be able to weigh themselves independently or keep records of weight, BP, pulse, or other data requested by the health care team.

Self-Perception and Self-Concept

Self-perception and self-concept are related to the cognitive and emotional processes that people use to formulate their beliefs and feelings about themselves. It is important for the nurse to understand patients' beliefs and feelings about their health as these concepts are key determinants of patients' adherence to new medical regimens and lifestyle changes (e.g., smoking cessation, weight reduction, exercise), which are necessary for effective self-management after an acute cardiac event. Patients who have misperceptions about the health consequences of their cardiac illness are at risk for nonadherence to their treatment plan. Responses of patients to the following questions will guide the nurse in planning interventions to assure that patients are prepared to manage their illness and that adequate services are in place to support the patient's recovery and self-management needs.

- What is your cardiac problem, and what do you think has contributed to this problem?
- What consequences do you think this illness will have on your current lifestyle (leisure and physical activities, work, role in the family and social relationships)?
- How much of an influence do you think you have on controlling this illness?

Sexuality and Reproduction

A common problem for patients with cardiac diseases is a decrease in frequency of and satisfaction with sexual activity. These changes are associated with inadequate information, depression, and fear of having a cardiac event (e.g., AMI, sudden death) or development of bothersome symptoms (e.g., chest discomfort, shortness of breath, palpitations). In men, impotence may develop as a side effect of cardiac medications (e.g., beta-blockers); some men will stop taking their medication as a result. Other medications may be substituted so patients should be encouraged to discuss this problem with their health care providers.

Patients and their partners may not have adequate information about the physical demands related to sexual activity and ways in which these demands can be modified. The physiologic demands are greatest during orgasm, reaching 5 or 6 metabolic equivalents (METs), which is equivalent to walking 3 to 4 miles per hour on a treadmill. The METs expended before and after orgasm are considerably less, at 3.7 METs. Sharing this information may make the patient and his or her partner more comfortable about resuming sexual activity (Steinke et al., 2013).

A reproductive history is necessary for women of childbearing age, particularly those with seriously compromised cardiac function. These women may be advised by their health care providers not to become pregnant. The reproductive history includes information about previous pregnancies, plans for future pregnancies, oral contraceptive use (especially in women older than 35 years of age who smoke), menopausal status, and use of hormone therapy.

Coping and Stress Tolerance

Anxiety, depression, and stress are known to influence both the development of and recovery from CAD and HF. High levels of anxiety are associated with an increased incidence of CAD and in-hospital complications after MI. Patients with a diagnosis of an acute MI and depression have an increased risk of rehospitalization and death, more frequent angina, more physical limitations, and poorer quality of life, compared with people without depression. Although the association between depression and CAD is not completely understood, it is postulated that both biologic factors (e.g., platelet abnormalities, inflammatory responses) and lifestyle factors contribute to the development of CAD. People who are depressed are known to be less motivated to adhere to the recommended lifestyle changes and medical regimens necessary to prevent future cardiac events. Patients with CVD should be assessed for depression by asking them if they are feeling sad or blue, if they have lost interest in things they usually enjoy, or have thoughts about death or suicide. Other indications of depression include feelings of worthlessness or guilt, problems falling asleep or staying asleep, having difficulty concentrating, restlessness, and recent changes in appetite or weight (Havranek et al., 2015; Lichtman et al., 2014).

Stress initiates a variety of physiologic responses, including increased levels of catecholamines and cortisol, and has been strongly linked to cardiovascular events. Therefore, patients need to be assessed for sources of stress, previous coping styles and effectiveness, and perception of their current mood and coping ability. Consultation with a psychiatric advanced practice nurse, psychologist, psychiatrist, or social worker is indicated for anxious or depressed patients or those patients having difficulty coping with their cardiac illness.

Roles and Relationships

Patients with CVD are being managed with complex medical regimens and sophisticated technology, such as implantable cardioverter defibrillators and left ventricular assist devices. Hospital stays for cardiac disorders have shortened, and many invasive diagnostic cardiac procedures, such as cardiac catheterization, are being performed in the ambulatory setting. Therefore, social support is often necessary to facilitate patient's self-management of cardiac illnesses. Patients with lower levels of social support have been shown to have an increased risk for cardiac-related mortality and stroke, compared with others having higher levels of support (Havranek et al., 2015).

To assess patients' role in the family and their relationships, both components of social support, the nurse asks the patient: With whom do you live? Who is your primary caregiver at home? Who helps you manage your health? The nurse also assesses for any significant effects that the cardiac illness has had on the patient's role in the family. Are there adequate finances and health insurance? The answers to these questions help the nurse determine if consultation with social services or others is necessary to tailor the plan of care to meet the patient's self-care needs.

Physical Assessment

During the physical assessment, the nurse is evaluating the cardiovascular system for any deviations from normal with regard to the following (examples of abnormalities are in parentheses):

- The heart as a pump (reduced pulse pressure, gallop sounds, murmurs, displaced PMI)
- Atrial and ventricular filling volumes and pressures (elevated jugular venous distension [JVD], peripheral edema, ascites, crackles, postural changes in BP)
- Cardiac output (reduced pulse pressure, hypotension, tachycardia, reduced urine output, or level of consciousness)
- Compensatory mechanisms (peripheral vasoconstriction, tachycardia)

Assessment of General Appearance and Cognition

The nurse notes signs of distress, which may include pain or discomfort, SOB, or anxiety.

The patient's height and weight are measured to calculate body mass index (BMI) (weight in kilograms/square of the height in meters), as well as the waist circumference. These measures are used to determine if obesity (BMI greater than 30 kg/m^2) and abdominal fat (males, waist circumference greater than 40 in; and females, waist circumference greater than 35 in) are placing the patient at risk for CAD.

To assess cognition, the nurse evaluates the patient's level of consciousness (alert, lethargic, stuporous, comatose) and mental status (oriented to person, place, time; coherence). Changes in level of consciousness and mental status may be attributed to inadequate perfusion of the brain from a compromised cardiac output or thromboembolic event (stroke).

Inspection and Palpation of the Skin

The signs and symptoms of an acute obstruction of arterial blood flow in the extremities are referred to as the six Ps, which are pain, pallor, pulselessness, paresthesia, poikilothermia (coldness), and paralysis. Additional changes resulting from a chronically reduced supply of oxygen and nutrients to the skin include hair loss, brittle nails, dry or scaling skin, atrophy, skin color changes, and ulcerations. Table 12-3 summarizes common skin findings in patients with CVD.

The nurse assesses capillary refill time, which indicates the adequacy of arterial perfusion to the extremities. To perform this test, the nurse compresses the nail bed briefly to occlude perfusion (nail bed blanches). Then, the nurse releases pressure and determines the time it takes to restore perfusion. Normally, reperfusion occurs within 2 seconds, as evidenced by the return of color to the nail bed. Prolonged capillary refill time indicates compromised arterial perfusion, a problem associated with cardiogenic shock and HF.

TABLE 12-3 Common Skin Findings Associated with Cardiovascular Diseases

Findings	Associated Causes and Conditions
Clubbing of the fingers or toes (thickening of the skin under the fingers or toes)	Chronic hemoglobin desaturation most often due to congenital heart disease, advanced pulmonary diseases and lung cancer; also associated with malignancies and inflammatory bowel disease
Cool/cold skin and diaphoresis	Low cardiac output (e.g., cardiogenic shock, AMI) causing sympathetic nervous system stimulation with resultant vasoconstriction
Cold, pain, pallor of the fingertips or toes	Intermittent arteriolar vasoconstriction (Raynaud disease). Skin may change in color from white, to blue and red accompanied by numbness, tingling, and burning pain.
Cyanosis, central (a bluish tinge observed in the lips, tongue, and buccal mucosa)	Serious cardiac disorders (pulmonary edema, cardiogenic shock, congenital heart disease) as venous blood passes through the pulmonary circulation without being oxygenated.
Cyanosis, peripheral (a bluish tinge, most often of the nails and extremities)	Peripheral vasoconstriction, allowing more time for the hemoglobin molecules to become desaturated. It can be caused by exposure to cold environment, anxiety, or ↓ cardiac output.
Ecchymosis or bruising (a purplish-blue color fading to green, yellow, or brown)	Blood leaking outside of the blood vessels. Excessive bruising is a risk for patients on anticoagulants or platelet-inhibiting medications; coagulopathies, trauma.
Edema, lower extremities (collection of fluid in the interstitial spaces of the tissues)	HF and vascular problems (PAD, chronic venous insufficiency, DVT, thrombophlebitis)
Hematoma (localized collection of clotted blood in the tissue)	Bleeding after catheter removal/tissue injury in patients on anticoagulant/antithrombotic agents.
Pallor (↓ skin color in fingernails, lips, oral mucosa and lower extremities)	Anemia or ↓ arterial perfusion. Suspect PAD if feet develop pallor after elevating legs 60° from a supine position.
Rubor (A reddish-blue discoloration of the legs, seen within 20 seconds to 2 minutes after placing the patient in a dependent position)	Filling of dilated capillaries with deoxygenated blood, indicative of PAD.
Ulcers, feet and ankles (Superficial, irregular ulcers at medial malleolus. Red to yellow granulation tissue). (Painful, deep, round ulcers on feet or from exposure to pressure. Pale to black wound base)	Rupture of small skin capillaries from chronic venous insufficiency. Prolonged ischemia to tissues due to PAD. Can lead to gangrene.
Thinning of skin around a pacemaker or an implantable cardioverter defibrillator	Erosion of the device through the skin.
Xanthelasma (yellowish, raised plaques observed along nasal portion of eyelids)	Elevated cholesterol levels (hypercholesterolemia)

AMI, acute myocardial infarction; DVT, deep vein thrombosis; HF, heart failure; PAD, peripheral arterial disease.
Adapted from Bickley, 2013.

Peripheral edema, fluid accumulation in dependent areas of the body (feet, legs, and sacrum in the bedridden patient) is a common finding in patients with CVD. The nurse assesses the patient for pitting edema (a depression over an area of pressure) by using the thumb to place firm pressure over the dorsum of each foot, behind each medial malleolus, and over the shins or sacral area for 5 seconds. The depression created by this pressure is graded as absent or as present on a scale from slight (1+) to very marked (4+). Scales exist to measure the degree of pitting edema that rely on a clinician's judgment of depth of edema or time the indentation remains after release of pressure. It is important that clinicians use a consistent scale in order to ensure reliable clinical measurements and management.

Peripheral edema is observed in patients with HF and peripheral vascular diseases, such as deep vein thrombosis or chronic venous insufficiency.

Assessment of Blood Pressure

Systemic arterial BP is the pressure exerted on the walls of the arteries during ventricular systole and diastole. It is affected by factors such as cardiac output; distention of the arteries; and the volume, velocity, and viscosity of the blood.

The ideal BP is 120/80 mm Hg. A BP of 140/90 mm Hg or greater is defined as *hypertension,* whereas a BP of less than 90/60 mm Hg is called *hypotension.*

During the first encounter with a new patient, BP measurements should be obtained in both arms. There may be a 5 to 10 mm Hg difference in pressure between extremities. A BP difference greater than 10 mm Hg may be indicative of arterial obstruction (on the limb with lower pressure) or aortic dissection and requires further evaluation. See Chapter 13 for more information on BP.

Pulse Pressure

Pulse pressure is the difference between the systolic and the diastolic pressures, which normally is 30 to 40 mm Hg. It indicates how well the body is maintaining cardiac output.

Nursing Alert
A pulse pressure of less than 30 mm Hg signifies a serious reduction in cardiac output and requires further evaluation.

Postural Blood Pressure Changes

Postural (orthostatic) hypotension is a significant decrease in BP with a change in body position from supine to sitting/standing or from sitting to standing. It may be accompanied by dizziness, lightheadedness, or syncope.

The most common cause of postural hypotension in patients with CVD is due to a reduction in preload from over-diuresis, dehydration, or use of medications that cause vasodilatation (nitrates and antihypertensive agents). The following recommendations are important when assessing the patient for postural changes in BP:

- The patient is positioned supine for 10 minutes before obtaining the initial BP and heart rate.
- After obtaining supine measurements, the patient is positioned on the side of the bed with feet dangling, then, if appropriate, with the patient standing at the side of the bed.
- Wait 1 to 3 minutes after each position change before obtaining the BP and heart rate.
- Return the patient to a supine position if dizziness or lightheadedness is reported after the patient sits or stands.
- Record heart rate and BP in each position and any symptoms that accompany the postural change.

Normal postural responses that occur when a person moves from a lying to a sitting or standing position include (1) a heart rate increase of 5 to 20 bpm above the resting rate (to offset reduced stroke volume and maintain cardiac output); (2) a decrease of 10 mm Hg or less in systolic pressure; and (3) a slight increase of 5 mm Hg in diastolic pressure. An increase in heart rate of 15 bpm with either a 20 mm Hg decrease in systolic pressure or a 10 mm Hg decrease in diastolic pressure within 3 minutes are abnormal findings and require further evaluation to determine etiology (Bickley, 2013; LeBlond, Brown, Suneja, & Szot, 2015).

Palpation of Arterial Pulses

The examination of arterial pulses involves assessment of the pulse rate, rhythm, and quality.

Pulse Rate

The normal pulse rate varies from a low of 50 bpm in healthy, athletic young adults to rates well in excess of 100 bpm after exercise or during times of excitement. Anxiety frequently raises the pulse rate during the physical examination. If the rate is higher than expected, the nurse should reassess the pulse at the end of the physical examination when the patient may be more relaxed. A heart rate less than 60 is termed bradycardia, whereas a heart rate greater than 100 is termed tachycardia.

Pulse Rhythm

The rhythm of the pulse is normally regular; although slight irregularities in rhythm can occur due to changes in vagal tone during the respiratory cycle (pulse rate accelerates with inspiration and slows with expiration). This phenomenon, called *sinus arrhythmia,* normally occurs in children and young adults.

During the initial cardiac examination, or if the pulse rhythm is irregular, the nurse assesses pulse rate for a *pulse deficit,* defined as the difference between the apical (apex of the heart, apical impulse is visible in 20% of normal people) and the peripheral pulse rates (Leblond et al., 2015). The pulse deficit is ascertained by simultaneously auscultating the apical pulse and palpating the radial pulse for 1 minute. The nurse should anticipate finding a pulse deficit in patients with arrhythmias, especially atrial fibrillation, atrial flutter, and ventricular arrhythmias. Some of the ventricular systoles generated by these arrhythmias may be much weaker than others; therefore, they are heard during auscultation but do not produce a palpable pulse.

Pulse Quality

The pulse quality or amplitude is indicative of the BP in the artery and is used to assess peripheral arterial circulation. The right and left temporal, common carotid, brachial, radial, and lower extremity arteries are palpated, one side at a time, and compared for symmetry in quality. Light palpation is essential as firm finger pressure can obliterate the temporal, dorsalis pedis, and posterior tibial arteries.

The quality of each of the pulses is reported by using descriptors (absent, diminished, normal, or bounding) or the following 0-to-4 scale:

0: Pulse not palpable or absent
+1: Weak, thready pulse; difficult to palpate; obliterated with pressure
+2: Diminished pulse; cannot be obliterated
+3: Easy to palpate, full pulse; cannot be obliterated
+4: Strong, bounding pulse; may be abnormal

When documenting the pulse quality, specify the artery location and scale range (e.g., "left radial +3/+4"). Other pulse scales exist; the nurse uses the institution's scale to ensure consistent clinical measurements and management.

Inspection of Jugular Venous Pulsations

Right-sided heart function can be estimated by observing the pulsations of the jugular veins of the neck, which reflects the CVP (right ventricular end-diastolic pressure or right ventricular preload). If internal jugular vein pulsations are difficult to visualize, the external jugular veins are used because they are more superficial and visible right above the clavicles, adjacent to the sternocleidomastoid muscles. In the supine position, the patient's external jugular veins are quite visible but disappear as the head is elevated greater than 30 degrees. The nurse assesses the right internal jugular vein rather than the left because it is anatomically straighter.

Obvious distention of the veins with the patient's head elevated 45 to 90 degrees indicates an abnormal increase in the CVP. This occurs with right-sided HF, cardiac tamponade (see Chapter 15), less commonly with obstruction of blood flow in the superior vena cava, and rarely with acute massive pulmonary embolism.

Inspection and Palpation of the Heart

The heart is examined by inspection, palpation, and auscultation of the precordium or anterior chest wall that covers the heart and lower thorax. A systematic approach is used to examine the precordium in the following areas (see Fig. 12-6).

1. *Aortic area:* Second intercostal space to the right of the sternum. To determine the correct intercostal space, the nurse first finds the angle of Louis by locating the bony ridge at the junction of the body of the sternum and the manubrium. From this angle, the second intercostal space is located by sliding one finger to the right of the

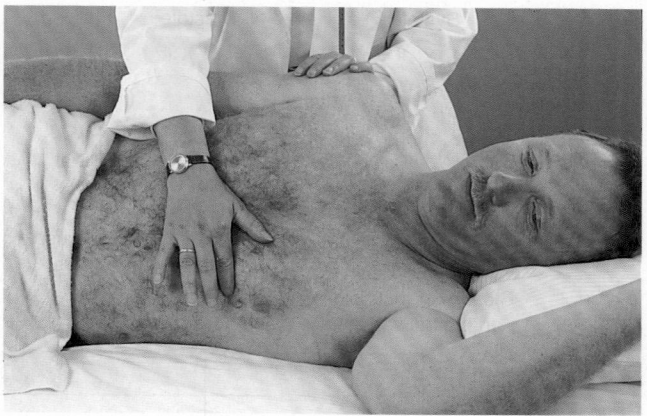

FIGURE 12-7 Locating and palpating the apical impulse, also called the point of maximal impulse (PMI), in the left lateral position. The apical pulse is normally located at the fifth intercostal space to the left of the sternum at the midclavicular line. The nurse locates the impulse with the palm of the hand and palpates with the fingerpads. (© B. Proud.)

sternum. Subsequent intercostal spaces are located from this reference point by palpating down the rib cage.
2. *Pulmonic area:* Second intercostal space, left sternal border (LSB)
3. *Erb's point:* Third intercostal space, LSB
4. *Tricuspid area:* Fourth and fifth intercostal spaces, LSB
5. *Mitral (apical area):* Left fifth intercostal space at the midclavicular line (MCL)

For most of the examination, the patient lies supine with the head of the bed slightly elevated. A right-handed examiner stands at the right side of the patient; a left-handed examiner at the left side.

Each area of the precordium is inspected for abnormal pulsations. A subtle pulsation located over the apical area, called the **apical impulse** or PMI, is a normal finding observed in young patients and adults who have thin chest walls. The nurse uses the palm of the hand to locate the apical impulse initially and the fingerpads to assess its size and quality. Palpation of the apical impulse may be facilitated by placing the patient in the left lateral position as this position brings the heart into closer contact with the chest wall (see Fig. 12-7).

Normally, the apical impulse is palpable in only one intercostal space and is no larger than 2 cm in diameter. Feeling the impulse in two or more adjacent intercostal spaces indicates left ventricular enlargement. A vibration or purring sensation felt over any of the precordial areas indicates abnormal, turbulent blood flow. It is best detected by using the palm of the hand. This vibration is called a *thrill*, which is associated with a loud murmur. Depending on the location of the thrill, it may be indicative of serious valvular heart disease or a defect (abnormal opening) in the septum of the atria or ventricles. Thrills that are palpated over blood vessels are associated with significant obstruction of a large artery, such as the carotid artery.

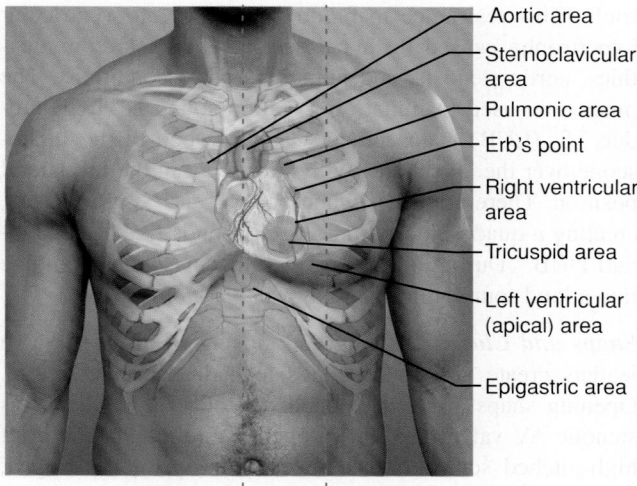

Aortic area
Sternoclavicular area
Pulmonic area
Erb's point
Right ventricular area
Tricuspid area
Left ventricular (apical) area
Epigastric area

Midsternum Midclavicular line

FIGURE 12-6 Areas of the precordium to be assessed when evaluating heart function.

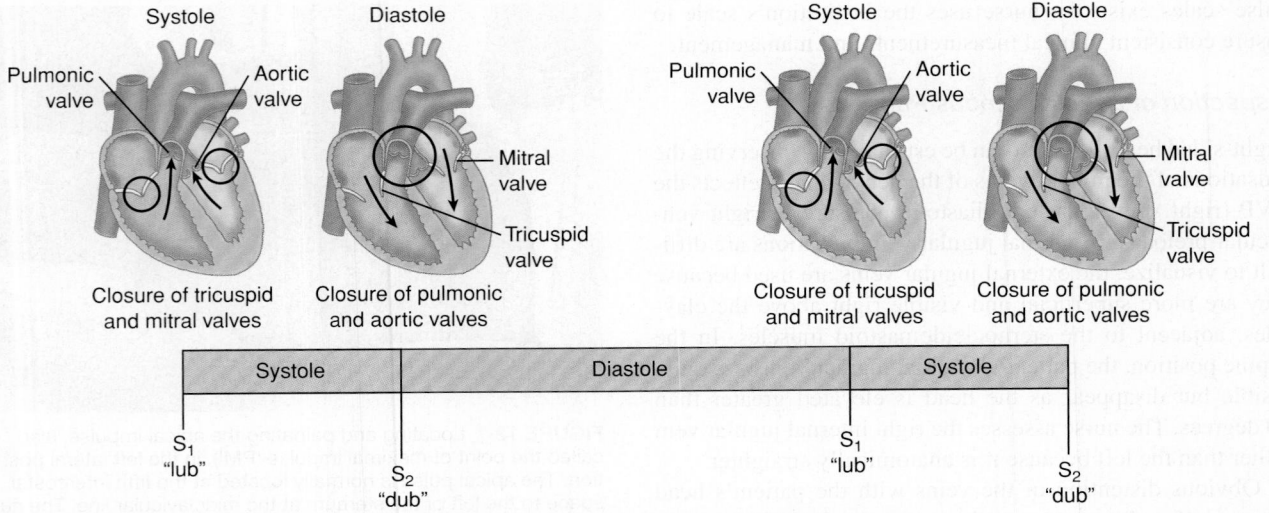

FIGURE 12-8 Normal heart sounds. The first heart sound (S_1) is produced by closure of the mitral and tricuspid valves ("lub"). The second heart sound (S_2) is produced by closure of the aortic and pulmonic valves ("dub"). *Arrows* represent the direction of blood flow during systole and diastole.

Auscultation of the Heart

A stethoscope is used to auscultate each of the locations identified in Figure 12-6, to assess heart rate and rhythm, and to evaluate heart sounds. The apical area is auscultated for 1 minute to determine the apical pulse rate and the regularity of the heartbeat.

Heart Sounds
Normal Heart Sounds. Normal heart sounds, referred to as S_1 and S_2, are produced by closure of the AV valves and the semilunar valves, respectively. The period between S_1 and S_2 corresponds with ventricular systole (Fig. 12-8). When the heart rate is within the normal range, diastole (period between S_2 and S_1) is twice as long as systole. However, as the heart rate increases, diastole shortens.

S_1—First Heart Sound. Tricuspid and mitral valve closure creates the first heart sound (S_1). The word "lub" is used to replicate its sound. S_1 is usually heard the loudest at the apical area (5th ICS left MCL). S_1 is easily identifiable and serves as the point of reference for the remainder of the cardiac cycle. If you are having difficulty determining S_1 from S_2, palpate the pulse, which will cue you into the S_1.

S_2—Second Heart Sound. Closure of the pulmonic and aortic valves produces the second heart sound (S_2), commonly referred to as the "dub" sound. S_2 is heard the loudest over the aortic (2nd ICS, RSB) and pulmonic areas (2nd ICS LSB).

Abnormal Heart Sounds. Abnormal sounds develop during systole or diastole when structural or functional heart problems are present. High-pitched heart sounds are heard best with the diaphragm of the stethoscope (e.g., aortic, pulmonic, tricuspid and mitral valve closure, and regurgitant murmurs),

whereas low-pitched sounds (e.g., gallop rhythms or mitral stenosis) are better heard with the bell.

S_3—Third Heart Sound. An S_3 is an abnormal sound heard early in diastole as blood flows from the atrium into a noncompliant ventricle. It is heard immediately after S_2. "Lub-dub-DUB" is used to imitate the abnormal sound of a beating heart when an S_3 (DUB) is present. It represents a normal finding in children and young adults, up to 35 or 40 years of age. In these cases it is called a *physiologic S_3* (Fig. 12-9). In adults, S_3 is a significant finding, suggesting HF. It is heard best by using the bell of the stethoscope with the patient in the left lateral position.

S_4—Fourth Heart Sound. S_4 occurs late in diastole (see Fig. 12-9). S_4, heard just before S_1, is generated during atrial contraction as blood forcefully enters a noncompliant ventricle. This resistance to blood flow is due to ventricular hypertrophy caused by hypertension, CAD, cardiomyopathies, aortic stenosis, and numerous other conditions. The mnemonic used to imitate this gallop sound is "LUB-lub-dub." S_4 (LUB) is auscultated using the bell of the stethoscope over the apical area with the patient in the left lateral position. There are times when both S_3 and S_4 are present, creating a quadruple rhythm, which sounds like "LUB lub-dub DUB." During a tachycardia, all four sounds combine into a loud sound, referred to as a *summation gallop.*

Snaps and Clicks. Opening and closing of diseased valve leaflets create abnormal sounds, called snaps and clicks. Opening snaps are high-pitched diastolic sounds heard as stenotic AV valves are forced open. Systolic clicks, a brief high-pitched sound, are heard early in systole as ridged, calcified semilunar valves are forced open during ventricular contraction. These sounds are the loudest in the areas directly over the diseased valve.

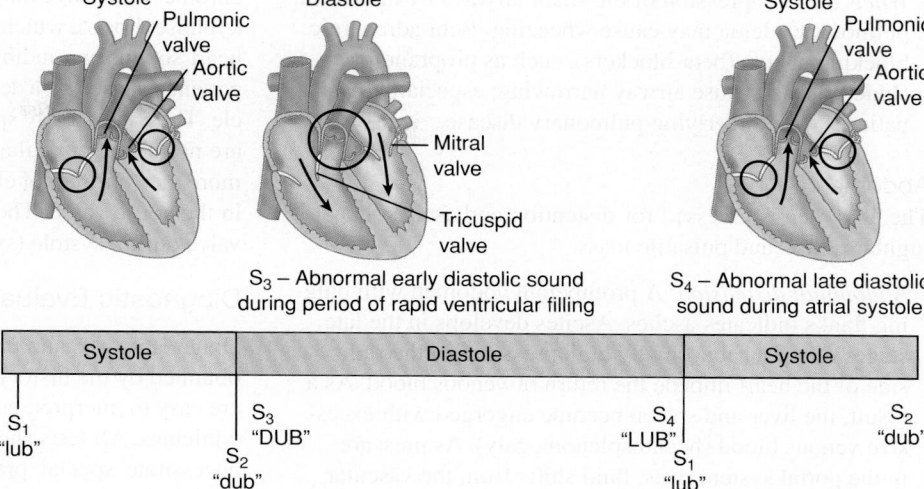

FIGURE 12-9 Gallop sounds. An S_3 ("DUB") is an abnormal sound heard early in diastole, immediately following S_2 (closure of the semilunar valves). This sound is generated very early in diastole as blood flowing into the right or left ventricle is met with resistance. S_4 ("LUB") is an abnormal sound created during atrial systole as blood flowing into the right or left ventricle is met with resistance. *Arrows* show the direction of blood flow.

Murmurs. These are a result of turbulent blood flow across rigid, calcified valves; leaky valves that allow backward blood flow (regurgitation); defects (abnormal openings) in the septum, aorta, or PA; or abnormally high velocity of blood flow through a normal structure (e.g., with fever, pregnancy, hyperthyroidism). Murmurs are described by several characteristics (see Box 12-3) that are used to determine the cause and clinical significance.

BOX 12-3 Characteristics of Heart Murmurs

The following characteristics provide information needed to determine the cause and clinical significance of heart murmurs.

Location: Pinpoints where the murmur is heard the loudest to identify the involved underlying structures (see Fig. 12-6)

Timing: Describes when the murmur is heard (systole, diastole, or both)

Intensity: A grading system is used to describe the intensity or loudness of a murmur:

Grade 1: Very faint and difficult for the inexperienced clinician to hear

Grade 2: Quiet, but readily perceived by the experienced clinician

Grade 3: Easily heard, no palpable thrill

Grade 4: Loud and may be associated with a thrill (a thrill feels like a purring cat under the area)

Grade 5: Very loud; heard when stethoscope is partially off the chest; associated with a thrill

Grade 6: Extremely loud; detected with the stethoscope off the chest; associated with a thrill

Pitch: Describes the sound frequency, ranging from high to medium to low

Quality: Describes the sound that the murmur resembles (rumbling, blowing, whistling)

Radiation: Identifies if the sound of the murmur is transmitted to other precordial areas

---

Friction Rub. A harsh, grating sound that can be heard in both systole and diastole is called a friction rub. It is caused by abrasion of the inflamed pericardial surfaces from pericarditis. A pericardial friction rub can be heard best using the diaphragm of the stethoscope, with the patient sitting up and leaning forward.

Auscultative Procedure

During auscultation, the patient remains supine. Using the diaphragm of the stethoscope, the nurse auscultates the precordium to identify S_1 and S_2 and then listens for abnormal systolic or diastolic sounds. Repositioning the patient into the left lateral position may facilitate detection of S_3, S_4, and murmurs. Positioning the patient sitting and leaning forward will facilitate detection of the high-pitched diastolic murmur of aortic regurgitation. Ask the patient to exhale and hold their breath as you listen. The characteristics of abnormal findings are documented by identifying the location, timing, intensity, pitch, quality, and presence of radiation (see Box 12-3).

Evaluation of Other Systems

Lungs

The details of the respiratory assessment are described in Chapter 8. Abnormal findings exhibited by patients with CVD include the following:

- *Hemoptysis:* Pink, frothy sputum indicative of acute pulmonary edema.
- *Cough:* A dry, hacking cough from irritation of small airways from pulmonary congestion associated with HF.
- *Crackles:* Typically, first noted at the bases (due to the effect of gravity on fluid accumulation and decreased ventilation of basilar tissue). Crackles may progress to all portions of the lung fields as a result of worsening HF or atelectasis associated with bed rest; splinting from ischemic pain; or the effects of analgesics, sedatives, or anesthetic agents.

- *Wheezes:* Compression of the small airways by interstitial pulmonary edema may cause wheezing. Beta-adrenergic blocking agents (beta-blockers), such as propranolol (Inderal), may cause airway narrowing, especially in patients with underlying pulmonary disease.

Abdomen

The abdomen is assessed for distention and ascites, hepato-jugular reflux, and pulsatile mass.

- *Abdominal distension:* A protuberant abdomen with bulging flanks indicates ascites. Ascites develops in the late stages of HF as abnormally high pressures in the right side of the heart impede the return of venous blood. As a result, the liver and spleen become engorged with excessive venous blood (hepatosplenomegaly). As pressure in the portal system rises, fluid shifts from the vascular bed into the abdominal cavity. Ascitic fluid, found in the dependent or lowest points in the abdomen, will shift with position changes.
- *Hepatojugular reflux:* This test is performed when right ventricular or biventricular HF is suspected. The patient is positioned so that the jugular venous pulse is visible in the lower part of the neck. While observing the jugular venous pulse, firm pressure is applied over the right upper quadrant of the abdomen for at least 5 seconds (see Chapter 15 for further details). An increase of 1 cm or more in jugular venous pressure is indicative of a positive hepatojugular reflux. This positive test aids in confirming the diagnosis of HF.
- *Pulsatile mass:* The most important diagnostic indication of an abdominal aortic **aneurysm** (a localized dilation formed at a weak point in the arterial wall) is a pulsatile mass in the middle and upper abdomen. About 80% of aneurysms that are 5 cm or larger can be palpated. A systolic **bruit** (abnormal sound associated with turbulent blood flow in an artery) may be heard over the mass.

Gerontologic Considerations

Peripheral pulses of elderly patients are readily palpable because of decreased elasticity of the arteries and a loss of adjacent connective tissue. In older patients, symptoms of PAD may be more pronounced than in younger patients. Intermittent claudication may occur after walking only a few blocks or after walking up a slight incline. Prolonged pressure exerted on areas of the toes or feet further compromises arterial perfusion, which can lead to ulceration, infection, and gangrene.

Isolated systolic hypertension, associated with significant cardiovascular morbidity and mortality, is a common finding in the elderly. There is a higher risk for postural hypotension in the elderly, reflecting a decrease in the sensitivity of the postural reflexes and must be considered prior to prescribing new cardiovascular medications.

It may be difficult to palpate the PMI or detect audible heart sounds due to changes in the shape of the chest (e.g.,

chronic obstructive lung disease) and spinal deformities (e.g., kyphoscoliosis), which worsen with the aging process. When heart sounds are audible, an S_4 is detectable in most elderly patients, caused by a decrease in compliance of the left ventricle. The S_2 is usually split, meaning that the semilunar valves are not closing simultaneously. Murmurs are also audible in more than one half of elderly patients due to sclerotic changes in the aortic valve. These murmurs are heard over the aortic valve during systole (systolic ejection murmur).

Diagnostic Evaluation

Diagnostic tests and procedures are used to confirm the data obtained by the history and physical assessment. Some tests are easy to interpret, but others must be interpreted by expert clinicians. All tests should be explained to the patient. Some necessitate special preparation before they are performed and special monitoring by the nurse after the procedure.

Laboratory Tests

Laboratory tests may be performed for the following reasons:

- To assist in identifying the cause of cardiovascular signs and symptoms
- To identify abnormalities in the blood that affect the prognosis of a patient with CVD
- To assess the degree of inflammation
- To screen for risk factors associated with CAD
- To determine baseline values before initiating therapeutic interventions
- To ensure that therapeutic levels of medications (e.g., antiarrhythmic agents and warfarin) are maintained
- To assess the effects of medications (e.g., the effects of diuretics on serum potassium levels)

Because different laboratories use various types of equipment and methods of measurements, normal test values may vary depending on the laboratory and the health care institution.

Cardiac Biomarker Analysis

Plasma levels of cardiac biomarkers are used to diagnose acute MI in conjunction with the history, physical examination, and ECG. These substances leak into the bloodstream after injured myocardial cells rupture their cell membranes. Biomarkers have a specific timeline for when they first rise, peak, and then return to normal. This timeline helps the clinician decide which test to order, based on the timing of patient's symptom onset.

- *Creatine kinase (CK)/CK-MB:* CK is released from three types of damaged tissue (myocardium, skeletal muscle, brain). CK-MB is the cardiac-specific isoenzyme that rises within 4 to 8 hours after myocardial injury, peaks in 12 to 24 hours, and returns to normal within 3 to 4 days.
- *Myoglobin:* This heme protein transports oxygen. Its small molecular structure allows it to be released rapidly

from damaged myocardial tissue and accounts for its early rise. Myoglobin is not used alone to diagnose MI because elevations can also occur in patients with renal or musculoskeletal disease. However, negative results are helpful in ruling out acute MI. Myoglobin rises within 1 to 3 hours of tissue injury, peaks in 4 to 12 hours, and returns to normal in 24 hours.

• *Troponin T and I:* These heme proteins regulate the contractile function of the myocardium. After myocardial injury, these biomarkers rise early (within 3 to 4 hours), peak in 4 to 24 hours, and remain elevated for 1 to 3 weeks. These early and prolonged elevations make very early diagnosis of acute MI possible and allow for late diagnosis in patients who have delayed seeking care for several days after the onset of acute MI symptoms.

Blood Chemistry, Hematology, and Coagulation Studies

Table 12-4 provides information about common serum laboratory tests and the implications for patients with CVD.

Lipid Profile. The lipid profile helps evaluate a person's risk for developing atherosclerosis or to diagnose a specific lipoprotein abnormality. Cholesterol and triglycerides are transported in the blood by combining with protein molecules to form lipoproteins. The lipoproteins are referred to as low-density lipoproteins (LDL) and high-density lipoproteins (HDL). The risk of CAD increases as the ratio of LDL to HDL or the ratio of total cholesterol (LDL + HDL) to HDL increases. The blood specimen for the lipid profile should be obtained after a 12-hour fast.

Cholesterol Levels. Cholesterol is a lipid required for hormone synthesis and cell membrane formation. Cholesterol comes from the diet (animal products) and the liver, where cholesterol is synthesized. Elevated cholesterol levels increase the risk of atherosclerosis. Factors that contribute to variations in cholesterol levels include age, gender, diet, exercise patterns, genetics, menopause, tobacco use, and stress levels. Normal level is less than 200 mg/dL.

LDL is the primary transporter of cholesterol and triglycerides into the cell. One harmful effect of LDL is the

TABLE 12-4 Common Serum Laboratory Tests and Implications for Patients with Cardiovascular Disease (CVD)

Laboratory Test/Reference Range	Implications
Blood Chemistries	
Sodium (Na⁺) 135–145 mEq/L	*Hyponatremia:* ↓ Na levels can be due to thiazide diuretics or from fluid excess, as seen in HF. *Hypernatremia:* ↑ Na levels indicate fluid deficits and can result from ↓ water intake or hypovolemia.
Potassium (K⁺) 3.5–5 mEq/L	*Hypokalemia:* ↓ K levels often due to use of K-excreting diuretics, which can cause ventricular tachycardia and fibrillation and predispose digitalis toxicity in patients taking digoxin. *Hyperkalemia:* ↑ K levels due to ↑ intake of foods high in K or overuse of K supplements; ↓ renal excretion of K; use of K-sparing diuretics (e.g., spironolactone); or use of angiotensin-converting enzyme inhibitors (ACE inhibitors). Can cause heart block, asystole, and ventricular arrhythmias.
Calcium (Ca⁺⁺) 8.5–10.2 mg/dL	Necessary for blood coagulability, neuromuscular activity, and automaticity of the sinoatrial and atrioventricular nodes. *Hypocalcemia:* ↓ calcium levels slow nodal function and impair myocardial contractility. Latter effect ↑ risk of HF. *Hypercalcemia:* ↑ Ca levels are associated with use of thiazide diuretics that ↓ renal excretion of Ca. Hypercalcemia potentiates digitalis toxicity, causes ↑ myocardial contractility, and ↑ risk of heart block and ventricular fibrillation.
Magnesium (Mg⁺⁺) 1.3–2.3 mEq/L	Needed to absorb Ca, maintain K stores, metabolize adenosine triphosphate, synthesize protein and carbohydrate, and maintain muscular contraction. *Hypomagnesemia:* ↓ Mg levels are due to enhanced renal excretion of Mg from diuretic or digitalis therapy. ↓ Mg levels predispose patients to atrial or ventricular tachycardias. *Hypermagnesemia:* ↑ magnesium levels are caused by use of cathartics or antacids containing Mg. ↑ Mg levels depress myocardial contractility and excitability heart block or asystole.
Blood urea nitrogen (BUN) 10–20 mg/dL Creatinine Males: 0.9–1.4 mg/dL Females: 0.8–1.3 mg/dL	End products of protein metabolism excreted by the kidneys. Renal impairment is detected by an ↑ in BUN and creatinine. A normal creatinine level and an ↑ BUN detect an intravascular fluid volume deficit, bleeding, or increased protein intake.

(continued on page 394)

TABLE 12-4 **Common Serum Laboratory Tests and Implications for Patients with Cardiovascular Disease (CVD)** (*continued*)

Laboratory Test/Reference Range	Implications
Glucose (fasting): 65–110 mg/dL	↑ Glucose levels result from stress as endogenous epinephrine is mobilized to convert of liver glycogen to glucose.
Glycosylated hemoglobin (HbA$_{1c}$) 2.2–4.8%	Monitored in people with diabetes, as it reflects blood glucose levels over 2–3 months. Goal: hemoglobin A$_{1c}$ less than 7%.
Coagulation Studies	
Activated partial thromboplastin time (aPTT) 23–32 seconds	It is used to monitor patient's response to unfractionated heparin. Heparin dose is adjusted to maintain a therapeutic range of 1.5–2.5 times baseline values. aPTT is a more sensitive version of partial thromboplastin time (PTT) used to monitor heparin therapy.
Prothrombin time (PT) 12–15 seconds	Measures the activity of five factors in the blood clotting pathway (prothrombin, fibrinogen, factors V, VII, X). Used to monitor patients on warfarin therapy. Therapeutic range is 1.5–2 times normal.
International Normalized Ratio (INR)	Standardized method for monitoring prothrombin levels in patients receiving warfarin therapy. Therapeutic range 2–3.5, depending upon diagnosis.
Hematologic Studies	
Complete blood count (CBC)	Identifies the total number of white and red blood cells and platelets, and measures hemoglobin and hematocrit.
White blood cell count (WBC) 4,500–11,000/mm^3	WBC counts are monitored in immunocompromised patients (e.g., post-heart transplant) or those at risk for infection (e.g., after invasive procedures or surgery).
Red Blood Cells (RBC) Normal range men: 4.32–5.72 million cells/mm^3; non-pregnant women 3.90–5.03 million cells/mm^3	RBCs, also called erythrocytes, are primarily composed of hemoglobin needed for oxygen transport from the lungs to the tissues.
Hematocrit Male: 40–50% Female: 38–47% Hemoglobin Male: 13.5–18 g/100 mL Female: 12–16 g/100 mL	Represents the percentage of red blood cells found in 100 mL of whole blood. The red blood cells contain hemoglobin, which transports oxygen to the cells. Low hemoglobin and hematocrit levels can cause more frequent angina episodes or acute MI in patients with cardiovascular diseases.
Platelets 150,000–400,000/mm^3	Initiate thrombus formation by clumping together at sites of vessel wall injury. Monitor for thrombocytopenia if aspirin, clopidogrel (Plavix), eptifibatide (Integrilin), or tirofiban (Aggrastat) is prescribed.

Refer to Table 14-5 for cardiac biomarkers.

deposition of these substances into the walls of arteries. Normal level is less than 160 mg/dL. Elevated LDL levels are associated with a greater incidence of CAD. In people with known CAD or diabetes, the LDL goal is less than 70 mg/dL.

HDL has a protective action by transporting cholesterol away from the arterial wall to the liver for excretion. Normal level for men is 35 to 70 mg/dL, for women, 35 to 85 mg/dL. Higher HDL levels are known to lower CAD risk; therefore, an HDL level over 40 mg/dL is desirable in patients with known CAD. Factors associated with lowering HDL levels are smoking, diabetes, obesity, and physical inactivity.

Triglycerides. Triglycerides, composed of free fatty acids and glycerol, are stored in the adipose tissue and are a source

of energy. Normal level is less than 150 mg/dL. Triglyceride levels increase after meals and are affected by stress. Diabetes, alcohol use, and obesity can elevate triglyceride levels. Triglyceride levels have a direct correlation with LDL and an inverse one with HDL.

Brain (B-Type) Natriuretic Peptide. Brain (B-type) natriuretic peptide (BNP), secreted from the ventricles, is a neurohormone that responds to volume overload in the heart by acting as a diuretic and vasodilator. BNP levels are useful for the prompt diagnosis of HF. A BNP level of 100 to 300 pg/mL indicates HF is present, and increasingly higher values are correlated with greater severity of HF.

C-Reactive Protein. C-Reactive protein (CRP) is protein produced by the liver in response to systemic inflammation. Inflammation is thought to play a role in the development and progression of atherosclerosis. High levels of CRP (3.0 mg/dL) are used as an adjunct to other tests to predict CAD risk.

Homocysteine. Homocysteine, an amino acid, can damage the endothelial lining of arteries and promote thrombus formation. Elevated levels are linked to the development of atherosclerosis and an increased risk for CAD, stroke, and peripheral vascular disease. Elevated homocysteine levels are associated with genetic factors and a diet low in folic acid, vitamin B_6, and vitamin B_{12}. A 12-hour fast is necessary prior to obtaining the blood sample. Test results are interpreted as normal (5 to 15 µmol/L), moderate (16 to 30 µmol/L), intermediate (31 to 100 µmol/L), and severe (more than 100 µmol/L).

Electrocardiogram

The ECG is a graphic recording of the electrical activity of the heart. The ECG is obtained by placing disposable electrodes in standard positions on the skin of the chest wall and extremities. The standard 12-lead ECG records electrical impulses of the heart on special graph paper from 12 different reference points referred to as *leads*. It is used to diagnose arrhythmias, conduction abnormalities, enlarged heart chambers, and myocardial ischemia or infarction.

The ECG is observed continuously by placing the patient on a bedside (hardwire) monitor or **telemetry** (battery-operated transmitting device worn by the patient), both of which transmit to a central bank of monitors. The telemetry system is wireless and allows patients to be monitored while ambulating. These forms of monitoring have graded visual and audible alarms that sound when an arrhythmia is detected. However, many of the alarms can be false alarms, caused by artifact that mimics an arrhythmia. Muscular activity, patient movement, electrical interference, or equipment malfunction are common causes of artifact. Nurses dealing with excessive alarms may become desensitized to these sounds and develop alarm fatigue. Alarm fatigue delays the nurse's response time or results in missed alarms. Alarm fatigue has serious consequences as undetected arrhythmias have led to serious adverse events, including death of patients (Honan et al., 2015).

Several nursing interventions facilitate acquisition of accurate data, reduce risk of alarm fatigue, and ensure patient safety when using various forms of cardiac monitoring (Hannibal, 2014; Sendelbach & Funk, 2013; Sendelbach & Jepsen, 2013). Key to the elimination of artifact is using proper skin preparation before applying electrodes and changing the electrode every 24 hours. Continuous ECG monitoring is discussed in Chapter 17.

Patients requiring ECG monitoring need to be informed of the purpose of the monitoring and cautioned that it does not detect symptoms such as dyspnea or chest pain. Therefore, patients need to be advised to report symptoms to the nurse whenever they occur.

Stress Testing

Stress testing is used to evaluate the response of the cardiovascular system to increased demands for oxygen and nutrients. It is used to determine the (1) presence of atherosclerosis in the arteries of the heart and lower extremities, (2) functional capacity of the heart after an MI or heart surgery, and (3) effectiveness of the medical regimen. The stress test is usually combined with a radionuclide imaging technique or echocardiogram to examine myocardial function during exercise and at rest.

Procedure

During an exercise stress test, the patient walks on a treadmill (most common) or pedals a stationary bicycle. Exercise intensity progresses according to established protocols in which the speed and grade of the treadmill are increased every few minutes. If the patient is unable to exercise, a pharmacologic stress test is performed. Patients undergoing a pharmacologic stress test with radionuclide imaging will receive an infusion of a vasodilating agent (dipyridamole [Persantine], adenosine [Adenocard], or regadenoson [Lexiscan]) to mimic the physiologic effects of exercise. If echocardiography is used, the patient receives an infusion of dobutamine, a synthetic sympathomimetic agent to increase the metabolic demands of the heart.

Throughout the test, the patient is assessed for signs and symptoms of myocardial or leg ischemia (claudication) by monitoring the ECG, BP, physical appearance, perceived exertion, and symptoms, including chest pain, dyspnea, dizziness, leg cramping, and fatigue. The stress test is said to be "positive" if evidence of myocardial ischemia is detected by changes in the patient's ECG or claudication is validated by a decrease in ankle pressure. A positive stress test is an indication for additional testing.

Nursing Interventions

Patients are instructed to fast for 4 hours before the test, avoiding tobacco, caffeine, and other stimulants. Medications may be taken with sips of water. Clothes and rubber-soled shoes suitable for exercising should be worn. The nurse describes the monitoring equipment, symptoms to report, and reviews the exercise protocol and the need for the patient to put forth his or her best efforts to complete the test. If vasodilating agents are used, patients are informed that they may have transient flushing or nausea. If the stress test is to be combined with imaging techniques, information related to these techniques is also reviewed. After the test, patients are monitored for 10 to 15 minutes or until stable, and then patients may resume their usual activities.

Radionuclide Imaging

Radionuclide imaging studies involve the use of radioisotopes to evaluate coronary artery perfusion noninvasively, to detect myocardial ischemia and infarction, and to assess left ventricular function. Radioisotopes are atoms in an unstable form that give off small amounts of energy in the form of gamma rays as they decay. When radioisotopes are injected into the bloodstream, the energy emitted can be detected by a gamma scintillation camera positioned over the body. These radioisotopes are called tracers.

Myocardial Perfusion Imaging

Myocardial perfusion imaging is performed using two types of techniques—single-photon emission computed tomography (SPECT) or positron emission tomography (PET). It is commonly performed after an acute MI to determine if arterial perfusion to the heart is compromised during activity and to evaluate the extent of myocardial damage. It is also used to evaluate if myocardial ischemia from CAD is the cause of chest pain or other CAD-related symptoms.

These imaging techniques are performed in combination with stress testing to compare images obtained when the heart is resting to images of the heart in a stressed state resulting from exercise or medications. An area of the myocardium that shows no perfusion or reduced perfusion is said to have a "defect" present. Comparing resting images with images taken after the stress test help differentiate ischemic myocardium from infarct-related myocardium. A defect that does not change in size before and after stress is called a fixed defect. Fixed defects indicate that there is no perfusion in that area of the myocardium, which is the case after an MI. Defects that appear or that get larger after the stress test images are taken indicate reduced perfusion to that area of the heart. Because the defect disappears with rest, it is called a reversible defect. Reversible defects constitute positive stress test findings. Typically, cardiac catheterization is recommended after a positive test result to determine the severity of obstructions to blood flow caused by CAD.

SPECT is a painless, noninvasive procedure that involves the injection of one of three commercially available tracers (technetium [Tc]-99m sestamibi, Tc-99m-tetrofosmin, or thallium-201). During SPECT, patients are positioned supine on the table with their arms over their heads. The gamma camera circles around the chest area converting the signals from the traces into pictures of the heart. The procedure takes approximately 30 minutes. The second scan is repeated following the exercise or pharmacologic stress test.

During PET, tracers are administered by injection; one compound is used to determine blood flow in the myocardium, and another determines the metabolic function. The PET camera provides detailed three-dimensional images of the distributed compounds. The viability of the myocardium is determined by comparing the extent of glucose metabolism in the myocardium to the degree of blood flow. For example, ischemic but viable tissue will show decreased blood flow and elevated metabolism. For a patient with this finding, revascularization through surgery or percutaneous coronary interventions will probably be indicated to improve heart function. Restrictions of food intake before the test vary among institutions, but because PET evaluates glucose metabolism, the patient's blood glucose level should be within the normal range before testing.

The patient undergoing nuclear imaging techniques with stress testing should be prepared for the type of stressor to be used (exercise or drug) and the type of imaging technique (SPECT or PET). The patient may be concerned about receiving a radioactive substance and needs to be reassured that these tracers are safe—the radiation exposure is similar to that of other diagnostic x-ray studies. No postprocedure radiation precautions are necessary.

Test of Ventricular Function and Wall Motion

Equilibrium radionuclide angiocardiography (ERNA), also known as multiple-gated acquisition (MUGA) scanning, is a noninvasive technique that uses a conventional scintillation camera interfaced with a computer to record images of the heart during several hundred heartbeats. The computer processes the data and allows for sequential images of the functioning heart. These images are analyzed to evaluate left ventricular function, wall motion, and EF. This scanning procedure can be used to assess for differences in left ventricular function during rest and exercise. The patient is reassured that there is no radiation danger and is instructed to remain motionless during the scan.

Echocardiography

Traditional Echocardiography

Echocardiography, a noninvasive ultrasound test, is used to examine cardiac structures and function.

Procedure. A handheld transducer generates high-frequency sound waves through the chest wall into the heart and records the return signals for display on an oscilloscope and recording on a videotape. An ECG is recorded simultaneously to assist with interpreting the echocardiogram. Two-dimensional or cross-sectional echocardiography, an enhancement of this technique, creates a sophisticated, spatially correct image of the heart. Other techniques, such as Doppler and color flow imaging echocardiography, show the direction and velocity of the blood flow through the heart.

Nursing Interventions. The nurse prepares the patient for the test by explaining that it is a painless procedure and that the transducer emits sound waves as it is moved across the surface of the chest wall. Gel applied to the skin helps transmit the sound waves. Periodically, the patient is asked to turn onto the left side or hold a breath. The test takes about 30 to 45 minutes.

Transesophageal Echocardiography

Procedure. Transesophageal echocardiography (TEE) involves threading a small transducer through the mouth and into the esophagus. This technique provides clearer images than other ultrasound methods because ultrasound waves are passed through less dense tissue. It is an important diagnostic tool for determining if atrial or ventricular thrombi are present in patients with HF, valvular heart disease, and arrhythmias.

A topical anesthetic and moderate sedation are used during a TEE because of the discomfort associated with the positioning of the transducer. Once the patient is sedated, the transducer is inserted into the mouth and the patient is asked to swallow several times until it is positioned in the esophagus.

Complications are uncommon during TEE, but if they do occur they are serious. These complications are caused by sedation and impaired swallowing resulting from the topical anesthesia (respiratory depression and aspiration) and by insertion and manipulation of the transducer into the esophagus and stomach (vasovagal response or esophageal perforation). The patient must be assessed before TEE for a history of dysphagia or radiation therapy to the chest, which increases the risk of complications.

Nursing Interventions. Prior to the test, the nurse provides preprocedure education and ensures that patients have a clear understanding of what the test entails and why it is being performed. Patients are instructed not to eat or drink anything for 6 hours before the study; that an IV will be inserted to administer medications, including a sedative to keep the patient comfortable; and after the removal of dentures, a topical anesthetic agent is used to numb the throat. After the procedure, the nurse informs patients that they will remain in bed with the head of the bed elevated to 45 degrees and will be offered something to drink as soon as they are recovered from the sedation and swallow, cough, and gag reflexes have returned. Patients are reminded that a sore throat may be present for the next 24 hours. They are to report the presence of a persistent sore throat, shortness of breath, or difficulty swallowing. If the procedure is performed in an outpatient setting, patients must have someone transport them home.

The nurse follows the organization's moderate sedation policy. During the test, the nurse provides emotional support and monitors the patient's comfort level, level of consciousness, BP, ECG, respiration, and oxygen saturation (SpO_2). Liquids and food are withheld until patients are fully alert and the effect of the topical anesthetic agent is reversed; swallowing reflexes may be diminished for several hours. Once the patient begins taking liquids, the patient should be assessed for dysphagia (difficulty swallowing).

Cardiac Catheterization

This invasive diagnostic procedure uses fluoroscopy (an imaging technique that visualizes the heart on an x-ray screen) to guide catheter placement into the heart and to view chambers and coronary arteries. This procedure is usually performed in the outpatient setting, unless the condition of the patient is serious enough to require hospitalization, such as HF or acute MI.

Cardiac catheterization is the gold standard for diagnosing CAD and quantifying the extent of coronary artery obstruction (reported as percentage). Cardiac catheterization is also used to diagnose pulmonary hypertension and valvular heart disease. Results of this procedure are used to determine if revascularization procedures (percutaneous coronary intervention or coronary artery bypass surgery) or valve replacement/repair are indicated.

In preparation for the procedure, patients have blood tests performed to evaluate metabolic function (electrolytes and glucose) and renal function (blood urea nitrogen and creatinine level). Baseline coagulation studies (activated thromboplastin time, international normalized ratio, and prothrombin time) are obtained to guide dosing of anticoagulation during the procedure. Because bleeding and hematoma formation are procedure risks, a complete blood cell count (hematocrit, hemoglobin, platelets) is necessary to establish baseline values. Later these results are compared with postprocedure results to monitor for blood loss. Patients who are managed on warfarin (Coumadin) are informed to discontinue the medication 3 days before the procedure, and the INR is assessed preprocedure. An INR of less than 1.8 is recommended to minimize bleeding, and an INR less than 2.2 is considered acceptable if the radial artery is used (Davidson & Bonow, 2015, p. 366). For patients with diabetes, metformin is discontinued the day before any diagnostic testing because of the potential development of lactic acidosis; normal renal function should be confirmed before the medication is restarted after the procedure.

Patients are NPO for at least 6 hours, and an IV is established for sedation, fluids, heparin, and other medications. BP and multiple ECG leads are monitored to observe for hemodynamic instability and arrhythmias, and pulse oximetry is used to monitor respiratory status. Prior to the procedure, patients having experienced a reaction to contrast agents are premedicated with antihistamines and steroids. Contrast agents can induce contrast-induced nephropathy (CIN), a form of acute kidney failure in patients who have diabetes, HF, renal insufficiency or renal disease, hypotension, dehydration, or are older aged. Patients at risk for CIN receive pre- and postprocedure preventive strategies. IV hydration increases vascular volume and facilitates removal of contrast from the kidneys. Administration of sodium bicarbonate and the antioxidant acetylcysteine (Mucomyst), both urine-alkalizing agents, aid in protecting the renal tubules from an acidic environment (Jorgensen, 2013). Advise the patient that he or she may feel warm and have a metallic taste and/or a burning sensation for a few seconds behind the eyes or in the jaw, teeth, tongue, or lips during injection of contrast medium (Daniels, 2014). In addition, an important role of the nurse is to prepare the patient and family for the cardiac catheterization. Box 12-4 outlines the information that should be reviewed prior to the procedure.

Patient Education

Preparing for a Cardiac Catheterization

Goal: To assure adequate preparation for the procedure
- Ask patients about any concerns or fears they have about the procedure.
- Remind patients to fast for 8 to 12 hours before the procedure.
- Understand the procedure involves lying on a hard table for about an hour.
- Assure patient that medications will be given to maintain comfort.
- Tell patients they may experience palpitations due to extra heartbeats that can occur as the catheter is advanced through the heart. Flushing and a sensation similar to the need to void may occur after injection of the contrast agent, which subsides in 1 minute or less.

Procedure

Right-Heart Catheterization. Right-heart catheterization is performed to evaluate pressures and oxygen saturations in the chambers of the right side of the heart and the function of the tricuspid and pulmonary valves. It involves the passage of a catheter from an antecubital, internal jugular, subclavian, or femoral vein into the right atrium, right ventricle, and PA. Complications, although rare, include arrhythmias, infection, and perforation of the septum or chamber wall.

Left-Heart Catheterization. Left-heart catheterization is performed to evaluate the patency of the coronary arteries and the function of the left ventricle and the mitral and aortic valves. It is performed by the insertion of a catheter into the radial or femoral artery that is advanced into the aorta, left ventricle, and coronary arteries. If the radial artery approach is selected, the Allen test is performed to assess arterial perfusion of the hand (discussed later in this chapter). The radial artery approach is associated with reduction in major bleeding, access-related complications, mortality, and major adverse cardiac events (Mahla, Mahla, Choudhary, & Nahata, 2015; Ruiz-Rodriguez, Asfour, Lolay, Ziada, & Abdel-Latif, 2016). Rare complications include arrhythmias, acute MI, perforation of the heart or great vessels, and systemic embolization.

Angiography. Angiography involves the injection of a contrast agent into the vascular system to visualize the heart and blood vessels. *Coronary angiography* is produced through the injection of the contrast agent into the coronary arteries to determine patency. An *aortogram* is produced through the injection of the contrast agent to highlight the aorta and its major arteries.

Arterial Hemostasis. Once the arterial catheter is removed, either manual pressure, mechanical compression devices, percutaneously deployed vascular closure devices, or external patches are used to achieve hemostasis. Major benefits of the vascular closure devices include immediate hemostasis and a shorter time on bed rest. Rare complications associated with these devices include bleeding around the closure device, infection, and arterial obstruction.

Nursing Interventions

After cardiac catheterization, the nurse:

- Assesses the catheter access site frequently for bleeding or hematoma formation. If hematoma develops, notify the provider and apply direct pressure with gloved hand for 15 minutes (Daniels, 2014).
- Assesses for arrhythmias using cardiac monitoring or by assessing the apical and peripheral pulses for a pulse deficit. A vagal response, causing bradycardia and hypotension, can be triggered by discomfort from manual pressure used to obtain hemostasis as the arterial or venous catheter is removed. It is reversed by promptly elevating the lower extremities above heart level, infusing IV fluid, and administering IV atropine to treat the bradycardia, as prescribed.
- Maintains the patient on bed rest after the procedure until hemostasis of the involved blood vessels is achieved, which is based upon variables such as catheter insertion site, size of the catheter used, anticoagulation status of the patient, and other patient variables (e.g., advanced age, obesity, bleeding disorder). Variations exist in time on bedrest and range from 2 to 8 hours. If manual or mechanical pressure was used, bed rest is maintained for up to 6 hours with the affected leg straight and the head elevated to 30 degrees. For comfort, the patient may be turned from side to side with the affected extremity straight. If a percutaneous closure device or patch was deployed, the nurse reviews local nursing care standards and anticipates that the patient will have fewer activity restrictions. Analgesic medication is administered for discomfort.
- Instructs the patient to report chest pain and bleeding or sudden discomfort from the catheter insertion sites immediately.
- Assesses for contrast agent–induced renal failure by monitoring for an increase in creatinine levels. IV hydration is used to flush the contrast agent from the urinary tract; accurate intake and output are recorded.
- Assesses peripheral perfusion of the involved limb, including peripheral pulses, capillary refill, and neurovascular status per institution policy until discharge, as embolization is infrequent but can cause limb or end-organ ischemia.
- Ensures patient safety by instructing the patient to ask for help when getting out of bed the first time. The patient is assessed for bleeding from the catheter access site and for orthostatic hypotension.
- Provides patients with additional instructions at time of discharge (see Box 12-5).

BOX 12-5 **Patient Education**

Self-Management After Cardiac Catheterization

Goal: To assure that patients have information they need to reduce the risk of postprocedure complications and to understand their treatment plan.

- For the next 24 hours, do not bend at the waist, strain, or lift heavy objects.
- If the radial artery was used, avoid sleeping on the affected arm for 24 hours and refrain from repetitive movement of the affected extremity for 24–48 hours.
- Avoid tub baths, but shower as desired.
- Ask your provider about when you may resume your usual activities.

- Call your provider if you have any bleeding, swelling, new bruising, or pain from your procedure puncture site, or a temperature of 101.5°F (38.6°C) or more.
- Talk with your provider about getting assistance with lifestyle changes to reduce your risk for future heart problems. If test results show that you have coronary artery disease, ask your provider to refer you to a local cardiac rehabilitation program.
- Your provider may prescribe new medications. If you suspect that any of these are causing side effects, call your provider immediately. Do not stop taking any medications before talking to your provider.

Hemodynamic Monitoring

Hemodynamic monitoring continuously assesses the cardiovascular function of critically ill patients. It requires a special catheter and pressure monitoring system composed of a continuous flushing device to maintain catheter patency, a transducer to convert the pressure coming from the artery or heart chamber into an electrical signal, and a monitor, which displays the pressure waveform on a bedside oscilloscope.

Procedure

Central Venous Pressure Monitoring. CVP is measured by positioning a catheter in the vena cava (superior or inferior) or right atrium. It reflects right ventricle preload because pressure in the vena cava, right atrium, and right ventricle are all equal at the end of diastole. Normal CVP is 2 to 8 mm Hg. A CVP of greater than 8 mm Hg indicates hypervolemia (excessive fluid circulating in the body) or right-sided HF. On the contrary, a CVP of less than 2 mm Hg indicates a reduction in preload or hypovolemia. Complications of CVP monitoring are infection, pneumothorax, and air embolism.

Pulmonary Artery Pressure Monitoring. PA pressure monitoring involves the use of a balloon-tipped catheter that is inserted through a large vein (subclavian, jugular, or femoral) and connected to the pressure monitoring system (see Fig. 12-10). The catheter is threaded through the right side of the heart into the PA. It is used in critically ill patients to measure the cardiac output and right atrial, PA systolic and diastolic, and pulmonary capillary wedge pressures (see Fig. 12-5, for normal pressures).

The PA diastolic and PA wedge pressures are used most often because they reflect left ventricular preload. These readings are possible because, at the end of diastole, when the ventricle is completely filled and the mitral valve is open, there is equalization of pressure within all left heart chambers and vessels (left ventricle and atrium, pulmonary veins and arteries). The PA diastolic and PA wedge pressures

are used to diagnose the etiology of shock and evaluate the response of the patient's cardiovascular system to medical interventions.

The pulmonary capillary wedge pressure is obtained by inflating the balloon tip that causes the catheter to float out into a smaller branch of the PA. This is an occlusive maneuver; therefore, the measurement must be taken immediately, the balloon deflated, and the waveform assessed to ensure that the catheter returned to its normal position in the PA.

Complications of PA pressure monitoring include infection, PA rupture, pulmonary thromboembolism, pulmonary infarction, arrhythmias, and air embolism.

Intra-arterial BP Monitoring. Intra-arterial BP monitoring is used to obtain continuous systolic, diastolic, and mean arterial pressure (MAP) readings and blood samples. MAP is used to reflect the perfusion pressure to major organs. During one cardiac cycle, the heart spends two thirds of the time in diastole, compared with systole. The formula for calculating MAP is: $\text{MAP} = (2 \times \text{diastolic}) + \text{systolic}/3$. The cardiac monitor automatically makes the calculation, or if the BP is taken by cuff pressure, it can be calculated manually. Major organs require an MAP of 65 mm Hg (normal range is 70 to 110 mm Hg).

The Allen test is used to assess for adequate perfusion of the hand via the ulnar artery prior to cannulating the radial artery for pressure monitoring. The Allen test is performed by compressing the radial and ulnar arteries simultaneously and asking the patient to make a fist, which causes the hand to blanch. After the patient opens the fist, the nurse releases the pressure on the ulnar artery while maintaining pressure on the radial artery. The patient's hand will turn pink within 3 to 5 seconds if the ulnar artery is patent (Bickley, 2013). If other arteries are selected for cannulation, a Doppler ultrasound is used to assess perfusion to the involved limb.

Complications associated with arterial monitoring include arterial obstruction with distal ischemia, hemorrhage, air embolism, arteriospasm, and infection.

FIGURE 12-10 Pulmonary artery (PA) catheter and pressure monitoring systems. **(A)** Bedside monitor that connects with cables to **(B)** the pressure monitoring systems (includes IV solution in a pressure bag, IV tubing, and two transducers with stopcocks and flush devices). This system connects to **(C)** the proximal infusion port that opens in the right atria and is used to infuse fluids or medications and monitor central venous pressures and **(D)** the distal infusion port. This port opens in the PA and is used to monitor PA pressures. **(E)** The thermistor connector is attached to the bedside cardiac monitor to obtain cardiac output. **(F)** An air filled-syringe is attached to the balloon inflation valve during catheter insertion and measurement of PA wedge pressure. **(G)** PA catheter positioned in the PA. Note the sterile sleeve over the PA catheter. The PA catheter is threaded through the sheath until it reaches the desired position in the PA. The side port on the sheath is used to infuse medications or fluids. ECG, electrocardiogram; RA, right atrium.

Nursing Interventions

Nurses receive comprehensive training prior to using hemodynamic monitoring technologies. The following guidelines are used to ensure safe and effective care:

• The insertion site is prepared following local hospital policy, which includes clipping excessive hair, cleansing with an antiseptic solution, and using a local anesthetic.

• CVP and PA catheters are used for infusing IV fluids and drugs as well as drawing blood specimens.
• The nurse assures that the system is set up and maintained properly. The pressure monitoring system must be kept patent, free of air bubbles, and calibrated to atmospheric pressure (referred to as the zero reference point).

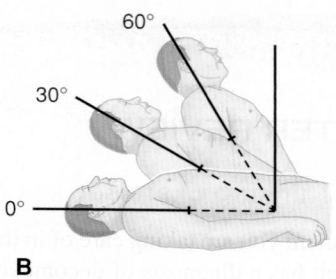

FIGURE 12-11 **A.** The phlebostatic axis is the reference point for the atrium when the patient is in supine position. It is the intersection of two lines on the left chest wall: (1) the midaxillary line drawn between the anterior and posterior surfaces of the chest and (2) the line drawn through the fourth intercostal space. Its location is identified with a skin marker. The stopcock of the transducer used in hemodynamic monitoring is "leveled" at this mark prior to obtaining pressure measurements. **B.** Measurements can be taken with the head of the bed (HOB) elevated to 60 degrees. Note the phlebostatic axis changes as the HOB is elevated, so that the stopcock and the transducer must be repositioned after each position change.

- Before the pressure measurements are obtained, the nurse positions the stopcock of the transducer at the phlebostatic axis. Figure 12-11 describes landmarks to use to locate the phlebostatic axis.
- The pressure monitoring system and catheter insertion site dressing are changed according to hospital policy. In general, the dressing is kept dry and air occlusive. Dressing changes are performed using sterile technique.
- CVP and PA catheter placement is confirmed by chest x-ray.
- The nurse monitors the patient for complications associated with the various forms of hemodynamic monitoring and reports findings immediately.

Doppler Ultrasound Flow Studies

Doppler ultrasound studies are most often used to detect obstruction of blood flow to the extremities or head due to a thrombus and determine if atherosclerosis is present in the lower extremities in patients with intermittent claudication. This technology uses a handheld device, called a *transducer,* which sends and receives sound waves that "echo" or bounce off blood cells. The transducer is placed in contact with the skin over the blood vessel being examined. Normally, the transducer detects rhythmic changes in the sound waves that are generated as blood cells flow through patent blood vessels. Obstruction to blood flow is evidenced by no change in sound waves.

Standard Doppler ultrasound studies are combined with computer technology to provide additional information about blood flow. Duplex Doppler ultrasound provides a picture of the blood vessel and a graph describing the speed and direction of blood flow, and color Doppler ultrasound produces colors to visualize these dimensions of blood flow.

When the nurse has difficulty finding a pulse, the continuous wave Doppler, a portable device, can be used. This device is used to hear, rather than feel the pulse. Box 12-6 describes how to use the continuous wave Doppler to evaluate pulses in the lower extremities.

The continuous wave Doppler is also used to obtain systolic BPs in the extremities to calculate the **ankle-brachial index (ABI)**. This ratio compares the ankle to arm systolic BPs and is an indicator of perfusion to the lower extremities. The ABI for each lower extremity is calculated by selecting the higher of the two ankle systolic pressures (obtained from both the posterior tibial and dorsalis pedis arteries) and dividing it by the higher of the right and left brachial systolic pressures. The ankle systolic pressure is normally the same or slightly higher than the brachial systolic pressure, resulting in an ABI of 1 to 1.1. As PAD progresses, the systolic BP in the ankle of the affected extremity decreases. An ABI of 0.8 to 0.99 indicates mild PAD, 0.5 to 0.79 moderate PAD (claudication present), and less than 0.5 severe PAD (pain at rest).

- Example: The patient's right brachial systolic pressure is 160 mm Hg; the right posterior tibial systolic pressure is 80 mm Hg.

$$80/160 = 0.5 \text{ ABI}$$

BOX 12-6	**Evaluating Lower Extremity Pulse Using a Continuous Wave Doppler**

The patient is placed in supine position with the head of the bed elevated to 20–30 degrees; the legs are externally rotated to permit adequate access to the medial malleolus. Acoustic gel is applied to the skin to permit uniform transmission of the ultrasound wave (do not use electrocardiogram gel). The tip of the Doppler transducer is positioned at a 45- to 60-degree angle over the expected location of the artery and angled slowly to identify arterial blood flow. Avoid using excessive pressure as diseased arteries can collapse if too much pressure is applied over the artery.

CHAPTER REVIEW

Critical Thinking Exercises

1. The patient you are taking care of in the cardiac intensive care unit has a diagnosis of decompensated heart failure and is having a pulmonary artery catheter inserted to help guide medical therapy. Describe the process you will use to obtain pulmonary artery systolic, diastolic, and wedge pressure measurements. Discuss the correlation between pulmonary artery pressure measurements and the patient's symptoms and physical assessment findings. What is your role in assuring that the pulmonary catheter is properly maintained and that the patient is free from catheter-related complications?

2. You are admitting a 65-year-old woman with rapid atrial fibrillation who will be undergoing a number of tests and treatment for this arrhythmia. She has an order for telemetry, and a transesophageal echocardiography (TEE) is planned for later today. What nursing interventions will you perform to minimize false ECG alarms? How will you prepare the patient for ECG monitoring? Why is it important for the patient to undergo a TEE? How will you describe this procedure to the patient? What is your role in managing the patient when she returns from having the TEE?

3. You are considering taking a position in an emergency department and plan to observe the triage nurse on the evening shift. You want to prepare for this experience by familiarizing yourself with the common types of patients who present with cardiovascular-related complaints. Name five common cardiovascular diseases and signs and symptoms associated with these disorders. What additional information do you need to consider when quickly assessing patients for a potentially life-threatening illness? Describe how you will focus your physical assessment on the cardiovascular system.

NCLEX-Style Review Questions

1. The nurse is performing a cardiac examination of a patient who has HF. When auscultating over the apical area, the nurse hears an extra sound between S_1 and S_2. This sound may be caused by:
   a. S_3, indicating worsening HF
   b. S_4, indicating the sound of blood moving into a noncompliant left ventricle
   c. A diastolic murmur, suggesting aortic regurgitation
   d. A systolic murmur, indicating a mitral valve regurgitation

2. After which of the following diagnostic tests will the patient need to remain on bedrest for 2 to 6 hours?
   a. Exercise stress test
   b. Cardiac catheterization
   c. Myocardial perfusion imaging
   d. Traditional echocardiography

3. A man was just admitted after experiencing chest pain and shortness of breath. Blood tests were sent while he was in the emergency department, and the nurse is evaluating the results. An elevation in which one of the following blood tests indicates that he is having an acute myocardial infarction?
   a. Troponin
   b. Cholesterol
   c. Brain natriuretic peptide (BNP)
   d. C-reactive protein (CRP)

4. A 45-year-old woman who has a history of diabetes, hypertension, and cigarette smoking walks into the emergency room with shortness of breath, indigestion, and diaphoresis. She should be evaluated immediately for:
   a. Community-acquired pneumonia
   b. Acute coronary syndrome
   c. Pulmonary embolus
   d. Aortic dissection

5. Which of the following signs or symptoms are indications for performing an ankle-brachial index (ABI)?
   a. Irregular, superficial ulcer along the medial malleolus
   b. 4+ pitting edema to lower extremities
   c. Intermittent claudication
   d. Pulse deficit greater than 20 mm Hg

Try these additional resources, available at **http://thepoint.lww.com/Honan2e**, to enhance your learning and understanding of this chapter:

- NCLEX-Style Student Review Questions
- Journal Articles

REFERENCES AND SELECTED READINGS

References and selected readings associated with this chapter can be found on the website that accompanies the book. Visit **http://thepoint. lww.com/Honan2e** to access the references and other additional resources associated with this chapter.

Nursing Management: Patients with Hypertension

Andrea Rothman Mann

Learning Objectives

After reading this chapter, you will be able to:

1. Compare and contrast the continuum of normotension, prehypertension, hypertension, and hypertensive crisis.
2. Assess for risk factors for primary and secondary hypertension.
3. Correlate pathophysiology of hypertension to complications in target organs.
4. Identify nursing management of patients with prehypertension and hypertension, including lifestyle changes and pharmacologic therapy.
5. Summarize management of the patient experiencing hypertensive crisis.
6. Incorporate current evidence when caring for the client with prehypertension and hypertension.

Currently, **about 78 million** American adults in the United States have hypertension; that amounts to almost one in three people over 18 years of age. In addition, hypertension affects 1 billion individuals worldwide (NIH, 2013; CDC, 2015). Another one **in three American adults** has **prehypertension**—blood pressure higher than the normal 120/80 or lower but not yet in the high blood pressure range. Hypertension is the most common condition causing visits to a health care provider (Krader, 2014). Diagnosis of hypertension may be missed easily as it is asymptomatic and must be measured to be detected; hence the term "silent killer" (Bostock-Cox, 2013). About one in five adults is unaware of having high blood pressure (CDC, 2015). Undiagnosed, untreated, or undertreated hypertension may lead to target organ damage causing myocardial infarction (MI), kidney damage or failure, cerebrovascular accident (CVA), or hypertensive retinopathy.

High blood pressure was a primary or contributing cause of death for more than 360,000 Americans in 2013—that's nearly 1,000 deaths each day. High blood pressure costs the nation $46 billion each year. This total includes the cost of health care services, medications to treat high blood pressure, and missed days of work (CDC, 2015).

Almost 91% of adults aged 18 years and older had their blood pressure measured within the preceding 2 years and could state their blood pressure. The target of Healthy People 2020 is to increase this awareness to 92.6%, for a 2% improvement nationwide. Over the past decade, blood pressure control increased by 55% among adults aged 18 years and above, up from 48.9% in the data from 2009 to 2012.

Yet, of individuals treated for hypertension, approximately 50% do not achieve adequate blood pressure (BP) control (ODPHP, 2014; CDC, 2015).

Nursing Alert
Every 10 years, the U.S. Department of Health and Human Services (HHS) provides scientific insights and lessons from the decade, along with new knowledge from current data, trends, and innovations. Healthy People 2020 reflects assessments of major risks to health and wellness, changing public priorities, and emerging issues related to national preparedness and prevention.

HYPERTENSION

The Joint National Committee on Prevention, Detection, Evaluation and Treatment of High BP (**JNC7**) of the National Institute of Health (2003) defines a BP of less than 120/80 mm Hg diastolic as normal, BP of 120 to 139/80 to 89 mm Hg as **prehypertension**, and a BP of 140/90 mm Hg or higher as hypertension. The JNC8 of 2014 did not focus on or change classifications but rather introduced evidence-based age and pharmacologic treatment options.

The JNC8 defined diagnosis for hypertension based on those under 60 years of age and those over 60 years of age (Weber, 2014). In addition, JNC8 addressed evidence-based thresholds for initiating pharmacologic therapy (James et al.,

TABLE 13-1 Classification of Blood Pressure (BP) for Adults Age 18 and Older[a]

BP Classification[a]	Systolic BP (mm Hg)		Diastolic BP (mm Hg)
Normal	Less than 120	and	Less than 80
Prehypertension	120–139	or	or 80–89
Stage 1 hypertension	140–159	or	90–99
Stage 2 hypertension	160 or higher	or	100 or higher
Hypertensive crisis	Greater than 180		Greater than 120

[a]Based on the average of two or more properly measured, seated readings taken on each of two or more office visits. From the Seventh Report of the Joint National Committee on Prevention, Detection, Evaluation, and Treatment of High BP. (2003). *Hypertension*, 42(6), 1206–1252; Ferri, 2018.

2013) and concluded hypertensive persons ages 30 through 59 years without diabetes or chronic kidney disease (CKD) should receive treatment when the BP is greater than 140/90. The panel based the recommendation of maintaining BP of less than 140/90 mm Hg for individuals 59 years of age or less on expert opinion. Treatment threshold for diagnosis of hypertension in those age 60 or older without diabetes or CKD is considered a blood pressure reading above 150/90. All individuals who have diabetes and/or CKD should receive treatment to keep the BP below 140/90 (James et al., 2013). While this may seem like the standards for diagnosis and treatment for hypertension have been relaxed, Weber (2014) points out that evidence-based recommendations need not be applied rigidly. The blood pressure targets and therapies should be based on patient response to treatment and practitioner judgment regardless of age. Further evidence is needed to clarify treatment for patients up to 80 years of age.

Hypertension is further classified as stage 1 or 2 depending on its severity (Table 13-1). Stage 1 hypertension occurs when the systolic pressure is 140 to 159 mm Hg or greater and/or the diastolic pressure is 90 to 99 mm Hg or greater. Stage 2 hypertension occurs when the systolic pressure is 160 mm Hg or higher, or the diastolic pressure is 100 mm Hg or higher. Severe hypertension is demonstrated with the systolic BP greater than or equals to 180 mm Hg or the diastolic BP *greater than or equals to* 110 mm Hg (O'Connell, 2014). If the systolic and diastolic pressures are in separate categories, the higher classification is used. The term *resistant hypertension* is used to define patients whose conventional blood pressure remains uncontrolled by three classes of antihypertensive agents, including a diuretic (Franklin et al., 2013). The terms *refractory* and *resistant* are used interchangeably (Ferri, 2018).

Classifying hypertension on a continuum as opposed to a single value promotes an understanding that elevation in BP from prehypertension through stages 1 and 2 is associated with increasing morbidity and mortality. This health risk rises with elevations of either the systolic or diastolic pressure. Diagnosis of hypertension should be based on the average of two or more accurate BP measurements taken during two or more contacts with a health care provider (D'Amico & Barbenit, 2016).

Blood pressure should be measured accurately in both arms, using the higher reading. The nurse should palpate the brachial pulse prior to measurement and use the correct cuff size. The patient should be seated for at least 5 minutes; smoking and eating should be avoided for 30 minutes. In addition, the arm should be at heart level.

 Nursing Alert
*As this book is ready to print, the American College of Cardiology and the American Heart Association recommended new guidelines for the definition of **elevated** blood pressure (Systolic 120 to 129 mm Hg and diastolic <80 mm Hg); and **Hypertension** (Stage 1 is defined as Systolic 130 to 139 mm Hg or diastolic 80 to 89 mm Hg), and Stage 2 is a Systolic at least 140 mm Hg or diastolic at least 90 mm Hg). While evidence can seem conflicting at this point, it is continually evolving. Awareness of current literature is essential to providing evidenced based care, and since science is continually evolving, nurses must commit to continuous lifelong learning. Current emphasis supports non-pharmacologic interventions, in addition to pharmacologic therapy individualized by the provider.*

Pathophysiology

BP is the product of cardiac output (CO) multiplied by peripheral vascular resistance (PVR). CO is the volume of blood being pumped by the heart per minute and is the product of the heart rate (HR) multiplied by the stroke volume (SV), which is the amount of blood pumped out from the ventricles per beat. PVR is related to the diameter of the blood vessel and the viscosity of the blood. The thicker the blood or smaller the radius of the blood vessel, the higher the resistance. Conversely, the larger the diameter of the vessel or thinner the blood, the lower the PVR (Grossman & Porth, 2014). For hypertension to develop, there must be a change in one or more factors affecting PVR or CO (Fig. 13-1). In addition, there must also be a problem with the body's control systems that monitor or regulate pressure. Management of hypertension aims to decrease peripheral resistance or blood volume, or the strength, force, and rate of myocardial contraction.

Circadian variations in blood pressure occur. Blood pressure tends to be highest shortly after awakening and then

FIGURE 13-1 Factors involved in control of BP. (Adapted from Kaplan, N. M., Lieberman, E., & Neal, W. (2014). *Kaplan's clinical hypertension* (11th ed.). Philadelphia, PA: Lippincott Williams & Wilkins.)

decreases throughout the day, reaching the lowest point between 2 AM and 5 AM. Individuals who reflect this pattern are known as dippers; those who reflect a pattern of a flattened 24-hour blood pressure profile are referred to as nondippers. Nondippers may be at higher risk for cardiovascular and kidney disease; however, additional research is needed to determine optimal therapy (Grossman & Porth, 2014).

Of patients with hypertension, 90% to 95% have **primary hypertension**; that is, high BP from an unidentified cause (Felicilda-Reynaldo & Kenneally, 2015; Grossman & Porth, 2014). This type of hypertension has also been called *essential* or *idiopathic* hypertension. The remainder of this group have **secondary hypertension**, which is high BP related to an identified cause. These causes include narrowing of the renal arteries or renal artery stenosis, kidney disease, hyperaldosteronism (mineralocorticoid hypertension), medications, pregnancy, and coarctation of the aorta (Grossman & Porth, 2014).

White-coat hypertension and *masked hypertension* are two additional types of hypertension with emerging concern for complications (AHA, 2016a). The patient with white-coat hypertension has normal ambulatory BP readings but elevated pressures (greater than 140/90) in a health care office or clinic. Those identified as having white-coat hypertension should have follow-up with ambulatory home blood pressure monitoring to determine if the situation is, indeed, isolated. Ambulatory monitoring will also determine if masked hypertension exists (discussed below) and if systolic hypertension is present; in addition, it will help to prevent overdiagnosis and treatment, which may cause unnecessary side effects (ACP, 2012; AHA, 2014b; Franklin et al., 2013). Additional studies of individuals with white-coat hypertension demonstrated an increased risk of developing systolic hypertension; 37% developed a diagnosis of hypertension in 2.5 years (Franklin et al., 2013). It is important that these clients receive active follow-up and lifestyle counseling (Sivén, Niiranen, Kantola, & Jula, 2016). Additional evidence suggests that elevations in blood pressure without tachycardia or complaints of pain, can be predictive of developing hypertension later in life (Shiber-Ofer, Shohat, & Grossman, 2015; Grossman & Porth, 2014).

Masked hypertension presents as normal pressure readings in provider settings but elevated BPs at home or work. Masked hypertension is known to be a precursor of sustained hypertension. The prevalence of masked hypertension is known to be as high as 70% in African Americans, a rate significantly higher than the approximately 10% reported in the general population (O'Riordan, 2011). In addition, as many as 10% to 40% of patients who are normotensive by conventional clinic measurement are hypertensive by ambulatory blood pressure monitoring (ABPM) (Kaplan & Townsend, 2016). Masked hypertension may be related to daily stressors at work, smoking or alcohol use, oral contraceptive use, and sedentary habits. The nurse should also suspect masked hypertension in men, those with diabetes or kidney disease, and those with transiently elevated BPs. In addition, masked hypertension may appear in those with nighttime blood pressure elevation using ABPM, those with normal/high-normal daytime ABPM of 130 to 135/80 to 85 mm Hg, and those with obstructive sleep apnea and autonomic dysfunction (Franklin et al., 2013). Those with masked hypertension have an increased prevalence of metabolic risk factors, left ventricular hypertrophy, and carotid plaque, demonstrating the impact of hypertension on organ function. Among baseline-masked hypertensives, hypertension progressed after 5 years to sustained hypertension in approximately one third of patients; about one out of five remained masked. This demonstrates individuals with masked hypertension may be at particular risk for cardiovascular disease because of delays in diagnosis and treatment (Trudel, Milot, & Brisson, 2013).

When the at-risk individual is identified, the nurse advocates for the use of home BP monitoring to confirm the diagnosis and monitor treatment. Engaging the patient in the process of self-care results in improved outcomes.

Risk Factors

Although no precise cause can be identified for most cases of hypertension, it is understood that hypertension is a multifactorial condition. Associated factors for essential hypertension include heredity, obesity, sleep apnea, advancing age, renal changes, and ethnicity/race. Possible factors include diabetes, type A personality, smoking, sedentary lifestyle, and hypothyroidism (Bellestas & Caico, 2014; Weber, 2014). A diet high in sodium and low in potassium may contribute to hypertension especially in those who are sodium sensitive (CDC, 2015). About 5% of individuals have sodium sensitivity that can affect their BP.

Factors contributing to hypertension may include increased sympathetic nervous system activity and increased renal reabsorption of sodium, chloride, and water. Other contributors to hypertension include increased activity of the renin–angiotensin–aldosterone system, causing expansion of extracellular fluid volume and increased SVR, or dysfunction of the vascular endothelium. Resistance to insulin may be a common factor linking hypertension, type 2 diabetes mellitus, hypertriglyceridemia, obesity, and glucose intolerance (Grossman & Porth, 2014).

The prevalence of hypertension increases with aging. A rise in systolic pressure continues throughout life; while diastolic pressure rises until approximately 50 years old, it tends to level off over the next decade, and may remain the same or fall later in life. About 65% of Americans aged 60 or older have hypertension. Those who are normotensive at age 55 have a 90% lifetime risk for developing hypertension. Men and women are equally likely to develop hypertension during their lifetimes. Before age 45, men are more likely to have hypertension than women. When women reach menopause, loss of hormonal protection occurs, at which time the risk for hypertension rises. After age 64, hypertension is more likely to affect women.

Men younger than 55 are more likely to have uncontrolled hypertension than women; after age 65, women are more likely to have uncontrolled high blood pressure (HBP) (NIH, 2015a; Davis, 2015). Black males, Mexican-American males, and younger adults ages 20 to 39 have a higher likelihood of uncontrolled blood pressure (Davis, 2015).

While hypertension can affect anyone, it is more common in African-American adults than in Caucasian adults. African Americans have an earlier onset, higher prevalence, and a greater rate of stage 2 hypertension, leading to higher incidences of nonfatal stroke, death from heart disease, and end-stage kidney disease. In addition, African Americans are less likely than Caucasians to achieve target control levels with treatment. This increases when the African-American individual is male, overweight or obese, physically inactive, smokes, and/or has diabetes. Hypertension risks vary among different groups of Hispanic-American adults. For instance, Puerto Rican-American adults have higher rates of HBP-related death than all other Hispanic groups and Caucasians. However, Cuban Americans have lower rates of HBP-related deaths than Caucasians (NIH, 2015a).

Systolic hypertension is the most common form of hypertension and is a major risk factor for cardiovascular disease. As the "baby boomer" generation ages, its incidence is expected to increase (Grossman & Porth, 2014).

Obesity is one of the common risk factors for the development of hypertension. A rise in childhood obesity forewarns of increasing numbers of hypertensive adults (Bellestas & Caico, 2014; NIH, 2015a). Hypertension, a risk factor for atherosclerotic heart disease, often coexists with **dyslipidemia** (see Chapter 14), diabetes mellitus (see Chapter 30), and a sedentary lifestyle. Metabolic syndrome or syndrome X occurs when three of the following symptoms are present simultaneously: BP elevation greater than 130/85, insulin resistance, dyslipidemia, and/or abdominal obesity. Metabolic syndrome places the patient at risk for cardiovascular disease and diabetes (AHA, 2014b). The risk for cardiovascular disease doubles with each increment of 20/10 mm Hg above 115/75 mm Hg.

Oral contraceptive use causes a small increase in systolic and diastolic BP, which, when accompanied by smoking and obesity, results in hypertension three times more often than in those without these risk factors. Cigarette smoking does not cause high BP; however, if a person with hypertension smokes, his or her risk of dying from heart disease or related disorders increases significantly (Grossman & Porth, 2014).

 Nursing Alert
Use of oral contraceptive is probably the most common cause of secondary hypertension in women. Question female clients regarding medication use (Grossman & Porth, 2014).

Gerontologic Considerations

The number of people in the United States over 65 years of age is expected to reach 75 million by the year 2040. People over 85 years of age are the fastest growing subset of the US population (Chaudhry, Chavez, Gasowski, Grodzicki, & Messerli, 2012).

The prevalence of hypertension increases with aging; half of individuals aged 60 to 69 and 75% of individuals over age 70 are affected (Grossman & Porth, 2014). Aging causes structural and functional changes in the heart and blood vessels, including atherosclerosis and decreased elasticity of the major blood vessels. Because of increased wall stiffness, the arteries are less able to buffer the pressure created as blood is ejected from the left ventricle and unable to store the energy to exert diastolic pressure. The elderly also are more likely to suffer from the complications of hypertension and are more likely to have uncontrolled disease (Egan, 2016). Isolated systolic hypertension with widened pulse pressure is more common in older adults. This is associated with cardiovascular and cerebrovascular morbidity and mortality, as well as dementia (Grossman & Porth, 2014).

Compared with younger patients with similar blood pressure, elderly hypertensive patients have lower CO, higher peripheral resistance, wider pulse pressure, lower intravascular volume, and lower renal blood flow. These age-related pathophysiologic differences must be considered when treating hypertension in the elderly.

The average elderly American is on more than six medications, putting them at risk for polypharmacy. Not all medications are for high blood pressure, but many interact with antihypertensive medications, such as NSAIDs used for arthritis, which can raise blood pressure. Therefore, the drug regimen of an elderly patient with hypertension should be reviewed carefully at every visit.

An orthostatic decline in blood pressure accompanies advanced age and contributes to an inevitable adverse effect with some antihypertensive drugs (refer to Chapter 12 for details on assessing for orthostatic hypotension). Accordingly, systolic blood pressure lower than 130 and diastolic blood pressure lower than 70 mm Hg are best avoided in octogenarians. An initial goal of less than 140/90 mm Hg is reasonable in elderly patients, and an achieved systolic blood pressure of 140 to 145 mm Hg is acceptable in octogenarians (Chaudhry et al., 2012).

Nursing Alert
When hypertension is treated initially, the nurse monitors the blood pressure to evaluate response to the treatment. It is important to recognize that if the mean BP is lowered more than 40% in the initial 24 hours, then symptoms of cerebral hypoperfusion may occur (Ferri, 2018).

Restricting sodium intake has been shown to lower blood pressure more in older adults than in younger adults. In the DASH trial, systolic blood pressure decreased by 8.1 mm Hg with sodium restriction in hypertensive patients aged 55 to 76 years, compared with 4.8 mm Hg for adults aged 23 to 41 years. Thiazide diuretics should be used with caution in the elderly because of the risk of hyponatremia and volume depletion.

Nursing Alert
Pulse pressure is the difference between the systolic and diastolic pressure; normally, it is approximately 40 mm Hg. As an example, 120/80 equals a pulse pressure of 40 mm Hg. A widened pulse pressure, over 50 mm Hg, is associated with increasing intracranial pressure, atherosclerosis, aortic insufficiency, and fever. It is detected with routine BP measurement. Elevated systolic pressure is a key indicator for the development of coronary heart disease (Franklin & Wong, 2013).

To reduce the cardiovascular and cerebrovascular risks, older adults should begin treatment with lifestyle modifications. If medications are needed to achieve the BP goal, the starting dose should be half that used in younger patients and increased slowly. Many practitioners advocate for "start low and go slow" with medication regimens in the geriatric population. Compliance may be more difficult for the elderly when memory impairment exists or due to the

expense of treatment plans. The nurse should ensure that the patient understands the regimen and can see and read instructions, open the medication container, and get the prescription refilled. Family or caregivers should be included in the teaching program so that they can assist with the regimen as necessary, encourage adherence to the treatment plan, and know when and whom to call for questions or problems.

Nursing Alert
The elderly are more sensitive to volume depletion caused by diuretics and to sympathetic inhibition caused by adrenergic antagonists. Teach patients to change positions slowly when moving from a lying or sitting position to a standing position and to use supportive devices, such as handrails and walkers, to prevent falls that could result from dizziness.

Clinical Manifestations and Assessment

Proper technique for assessment of BP is essential. The nurse should ensure proper BP measurement technique is being used (see Box 13-1) and that manometers used are calibrated. The nurse should select a cuff with a length of about 80% of the arm circumference and a width of about 40% of the arm circumference (D'Amico & Barbenito, 2016). To avoid undermeasurement of the SBP with **auscultatory gap**, the nurse should inflate the cuff to palpate the brachial artery until the pulse is obliterated, deflate the cuff, add 30 mm Hg to the palpated pressure, and then auscultate the BP and record results (D'Amico & Barbenito, 2016).

Automated or semiautomated blood pressure measurement devices are usually less accurate than are trained observers using the auscultatory method. It is recommended their use be limited to when frequency and less accurate methods of blood pressure assessment are needed. Providers should auscultate blood pressure (as described previously) to diagnose and/or evaluate the management of hypertension (Grossman & Porth, 2014).

Nursing Alert
Normally, the BP should vary by no more than 5 mm Hg between arms. If there is a difference, record both initially. Later, record the higher number. A difference of 10 mm Hg or more between the patient's arms may indicate thoracic outlet syndrome or arterial obstruction on the side with the lower value.

Pathophysiology Alert
Thoracic outlet syndrome is a condition where upper extremity symptoms are believed to result from neurovascular compression at the thoracic outlet. Compression may occur in three anatomical structures—arteries, veins, and nerves (Ferri, 2016b). If arterial compression is present, the

BOX 13-1

GUIDELINES FOR NURSING CARE

Measuring BP

Assessment is based on the average of at least two readings. (If two readings differ by more than 5 mm Hg, additional readings are taken and an average reading is calculated from the results.)

Equipment

- Recently calibrated aneroid manometer, or validated electronic device
- Cuff
- Stethoscope

Implementation

NURSING ACTION	RATIONALE
1. Instruct the patient to: • Avoid smoking cigarettes or ingesting nicotine, exercising, or drinking caffeine for 30 minutes before BP is measured. • Sit quietly for 5 minutes before the measurement. • Sit comfortably with the forearm supported at heart level on a firm surface, palm up, both feet firmly on the ground, back supported; avoid talking while the measurement is being taken. The selected arm should be bare to the shoulder, and if the garment sleeve is raised, it should be loose so blood flow is not impinged.	1. Listening carefully helps ensure an accurate measurement is taken. Stimuli such as food, alcohol, caffeine, nicotine, and exercise within 30 minutes before blood pressure measurement may affect the reading. Crossing legs, talking, and doing mental tasks while the BP is measured increase blood pressure.
2. Select the size of the cuff based upon the size of the patient. (The cuff size should have a bladder width of at least 40% of limb circumference and length at least 80% of limb circumference.) The average adult cuff is 12–14 cm wide and 30 cm long.	2. Using a cuff that is too small will give a higher BP measurement, and using a cuff that is too large results in a lower BP measurement compared to one taken with a properly sized cuff.
3. Wrap the cuff firmly around the arm (half the distance between the acromion [bony process on the shoulder blade] and the olecranon [elbow] is used to determine the midpoint of the arm). Center the cuff bladder approximately 2 cm (~1 in) above the elbow crease, with the midline of the bladder directly over the brachial artery. One finger should fit between the cuff and the patient's arm.	3. Proper setup is required for accurate reading. If the cuff is too loose, a falsely high reading occurs and vice versa.
4. Position the patient's arm at the level of the heart, preferably by resting the arm on a firm surface such as the examination table.	4. Positioning the arm above heart level will give a falsely low reading; a reading when the patient's arm is below heart level will be falsely elevated.
5. Palpate the systolic pressure before auscultating, using the radial or brachial artery (inflate the cuff until the pulse disappears; then deflate the cuff and note the pressure at which the pulse reappears. This is the systolic pressure by palpation).	5. This technique prevents the risks of overinflation, undue patient discomfort, and/or underestimation of systolic blood pressure. It also helps to detect the presence of an auscultatory gap more readily; an auscultatory gap is present when there is intermittent disappearance of the initial Korotkoff sounds after their first appearance (associated with older patients with hypertension), leading to underestimation of systolic blood pressure.
6. Ask the patient to sit quietly while the BP is measured.	6. BP can increase when the patient is engaged in conversation.
7. The nurse positions himself/herself so that the manometer is at the eye level. Tighten the thumbscrew of the pressure bulb and rapidly inflate the cuff to 30 mm Hg above the palpated systolic pressure. Slowly loosen the thumbscrew to deflate the cuff of the sphygmomanometer, releasing the pressure at 2 mm Hg per second. Listen carefully. Note the pressure at which the first sound is auscultated. This is the systolic reading. Continue to listen to the Korotkoff sounds. Determine the pressure when the pulsations disappear completely, this is the diastolic reading.	7. Misalignment between the eye and the mercury meniscus or aneroid manometer may cause the meniscus to be read as higher or lower than the actual position. Listening carefully ensures an accurate measurement.

NURSING ACTION	RATIONALE
8. Initially, record BP results of both arms and take subsequent measurements from the arm with the higher BP.	8. A difference of 10–15 mm Hg may indicate arterial obstruction on the side with the lower value.
9. Record the site where the BP was measured and the position of the patient (e.g., right arm).	9. This is especially important when assessing for orthostatic changes.
10. Inform the patient of his or her BP value and what it means. Emphasize the need for periodic reassessment, and encourage patients who measure BP at home to keep a written record of readings.	10. This engages the patient in the teaching process and correlates diet and medication adherence with BP.

Adapted from D'Amico & Barbenito, 2016.

involved extremity will be cool with a weak or absent pulse. A decrease in blood pressure (on the involved limb) greater than 20 mm Hg compared with the opposite arm is sometimes noted.

Because there are typically no symptoms of hypertension, physical examination may be unremarkable, other than elevated BP. Rarely patients may report early morning headaches, dull aching headache throughout the day, visual disturbances, orthostatic hypertension or hypotension; fatigue and proteinuria may be found on assessment (Bellestas & Caico, 2014). Many symptoms are associated with target or end-organ damage. The nurse should question the patient asking about anginal pain; shortness of breath; alterations in speech, vision, or balance; epistaxis (nosebleeds); headaches; dizziness; or nocturia. Further assessment includes asking about personal, social, or financial factors, or unacceptable pharmaceutical side effects that may interfere with the patients' ability to adhere to the medication regimen.

Hypertension may be asymptomatic and remain so for many years; however, when signs and symptoms appear, vascular damage related to the organs served by the involved vessels has occurred (Bellestas & Caico, 2014). Coronary artery disease with angina or MI is a common consequence of hypertension. Left ventricular hypertrophy occurs in response to the increased workload placed on the ventricle as it contracts against higher systemic pressure. When heart damage is extensive, heart failure follows; 90% of the time, hypertension precedes congestive heart failure (Aschenbrenner & Venable, 2012). Pathologic changes in the kidneys, indicated by microalbuminuria, increased blood urea nitrogen (BUN) and serum creatinine levels, and nocturia result. Cerebrovascular involvement may lead to stroke or transient ischemic attack, manifested by alterations in vision or speech, dizziness, weakness, a sudden fall, or hemiplegia. Occasionally, retinal changes such as hemorrhages, exudates (fluid accumulation), arteriolar narrowing, and cotton-wool spots (small infarctions) occur. In severe hypertension, papilledema (swelling of the optic disc) may be seen. A risk factor assessment is needed to classify and guide the treatment of the hypertensive individual at risk for cardiovascular damage. Risk factors and cardiovascular problems related to hypertension are presented in Box 13-2.

Routine laboratory tests evaluate for end-organ damage. These include urinalysis, evaluation for microalbuminuria or proteinuria, blood chemistry (i.e., analysis of sodium, potassium, BUN and creatinine, fasting glucose, and total and high-density lipoprotein [HDL] cholesterol levels), and a 12-lead electrocardiogram (ECG). Left ventricular hypertrophy can be assessed by echocardiography. Additional studies, including creatinine clearance, renin level, urine tests, and 24-hour urine protein, may be performed. The eyes should be assessed for hypertensive retinopathy (Bellestas & Caico, 2014).

BOX 13-2

Risk Factors for Cardiovascular Problems in Hypertensive Patients

Major Risk Factors (in Addition to Hypertension)

- Smoking
- Dyslipidemia (elevated LDL [or total] cholesterol and/or low HDL cholesterol)[a]
- Diabetes mellitus[b]
- Impaired renal function (GFR less than 60 mL/min and/or microalbuminuria)
- Obesity (body mass index [BMI] of 30 kg/m^2 or higher)[c]
- Physical inactivity
- Age (over 55 years for men, 65 years for women)
- Alcohol use
- Family history of cardiovascular disease (in female relative under 65 years or male relative under 55 years)

Target Organ Damage or Clinical Cardiovascular Disease

- Heart disease (left ventricular hypertrophy, angina, or previous myocardial infarction, previous coronary revascularization, heart failure)
- Stroke (cerebrovascular accident, brain attack) or TIA
- Chronic kidney disease
- Peripheral arterial disease
- Retinopathy

Grossman & Porth, 2014.

[a]These risk factors plus hypertension, elevated triglyceride levels, and abdominal obesity are components of the metabolic syndrome.
[b]These risk factors plus hypertension, elevated triglyceride levels, and abdominal obesity are components of the metabolic syndrome.
[c]These risk factors plus hypertension and elevated triglyceride levels are components of the metabolic syndrome.

Medical and Nursing Management

The treatment goal for most individuals under 60 years of age with hypertension, regardless of complicating conditions, is a BP of less than 140/90 mm Hg. The aim for individuals with prehypertension and no complicating conditions is to lower BP to normal. To prevent or delay progression to hypertension, JNC7 urges health care providers to encourage people with BPs in the prehypertension category to begin lifestyle modifications, such as dietary changes and exercise (see below). JNC8 recommends that people over the age of 60 begin pharmacologic treatment when the blood pressure is greater than 150/90; lifestyle changes should also be emphasized. Health care providers should monitor these patients every 1 to 3 months until their BP goal is reached and then every 3 to 6 months thereafter. While JNC7 recommended those with diabetes or CKD attain a target pressure of less than 130/80 mm Hg, current JNC8 guidelines call for similar treatment goals for all hypertensive populations, maintaining blood pressure less than 140/90 (Krader, 2014).

The management of hypertension is summarized in the treatment algorithm issued by JNC8 (Fig. 13-2). The

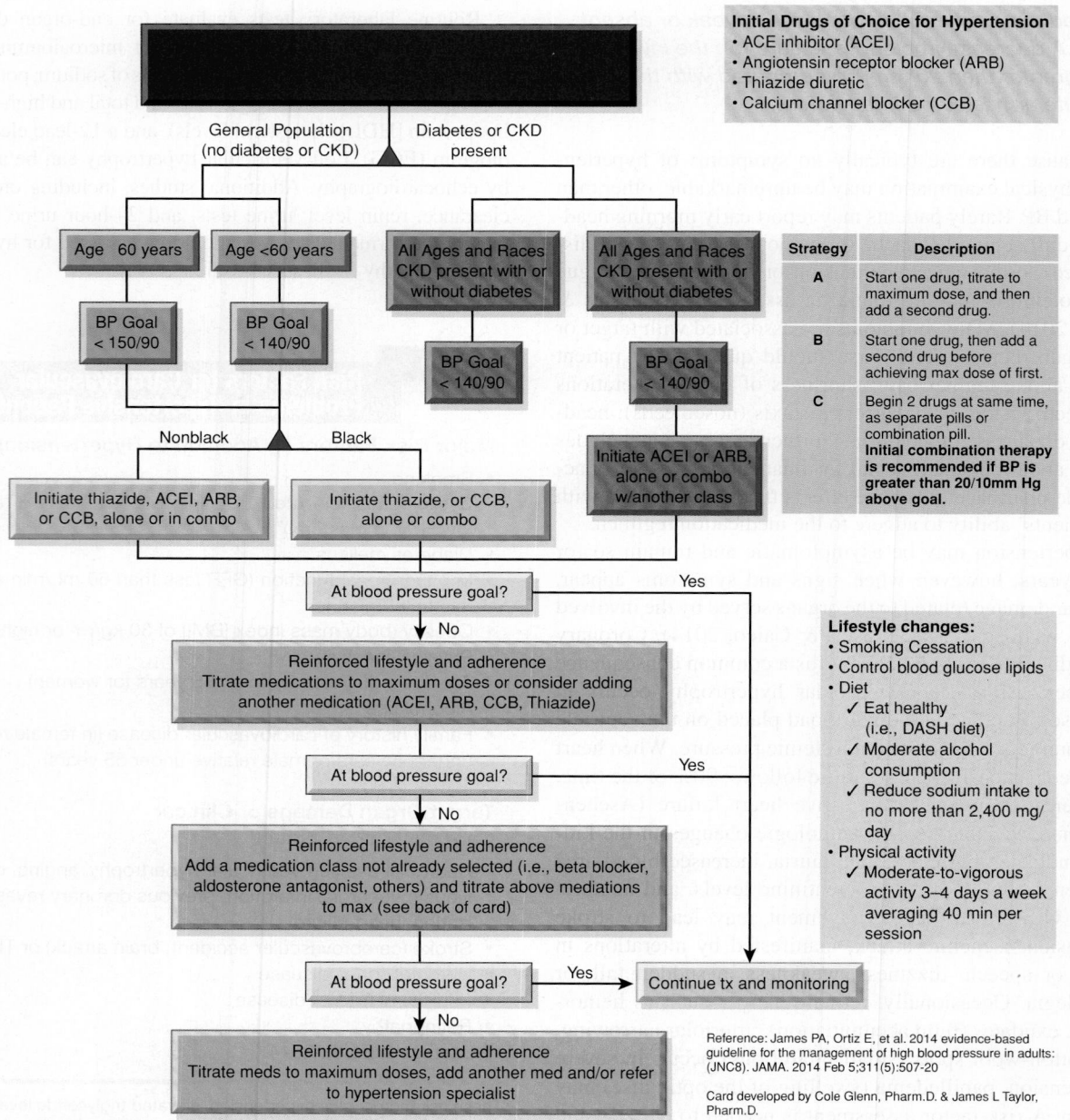

FIGURE 13-2 Algorithm of hypertension treatment. Treatment begins with lifestyle modifications and continues with various medication regimens. ACEI, angiotensin-converting enzyme inhibitor; ALDO ANT, aldosterone antagonist; ARB, angiotensin receptor blocker; BB, beta blocker; CCB, calcium-channel blocker; THIAZ, thiazide diuretic. (From the Eighth Report of the Joint National Committee on Prevention, Detection, Evaluation, and Treatment of High BP (JNC8).)

Compelling indications	
Indication	**Treatment Choice**
Heart failure	ACEI/ARB + BB + diuretic + spironolactone
Post-MI/Clinical CAD	ACEI/ARB AND BB
CAD	ACEI, BB, diuretic, CCB
Diabetes	ACEI/ARB, CCB, diuretic
CKD	ACEI/ARB
Recurrent stroke prevention	ACEI, diuretic
Pregnancy	labetolol (first line), nifedipine, methyldopa

Hypertension treatment

Beta-1 Selective Beta-blockers – possibly safer in patients with COPD, asthma, diabetes, and peripheral vascular disease:
- metoprolol
- bisoprolol
- betaxolol
- acebutolol

Drug Class	Sample Dose Ranges	Comments
Diuretics	HCTZ 12.5–50mg, chlorthalidone 12.5–25mg, indapamide 1.25–2.5mg triamterene 100mg *K+ sparing* – spironolactone 25–50mg, amiloride 5–10mg, triamterene 100mg furosemide 20-80mg twice daily, torsemide 10–40mg	Monitor for hypokalemia Most side effects (SE) are metabolic in nature Most effective when combined w/ ACEI Stronger clinical evidence w/chlorthalidone Spironolactone - gynecomastia and hyperkalemia Loop diuretics may be needed when GFR <40mL/min
ACEI/ARM	*ACEI:* lisinopril, benazapril, fosinopril and quinapril 10–40mg, ramipril 5–10mg, trandolapril 2–8mg *ARB:* candesartan 8–32mg, valsartan 80–320mg, losartan 50–100mg, olmesartan 20-40mg, telmisartan 20–80mg	SE: Cough (ACEI only), angioedema (more with ACEI), hyperkalemia Losartan lowers uric acid levels; candesartan may prevent migraine headaches
Beta-blockers	metoprolol succinate 50–100mg and tartrate 50-100mg twice daily, nebivolol 5–10mg, propranolol 40–120mg twice daily, carvedilol 6.25–25mg twice daily, bisoprolol 5–10mg, labetalol 100–300mg twice daily	Not first line agents – reserve for post-MI/CHF Cause fatigue and decreased heart rate Adversely affect glucose; mask hypoglycemic awareness
Calcium channel blockers	*Dihydropyridines:* amlodipine 5–10mg, nifedipine ER 30–90mg, *Non-dihydropyridines:* diltiazem ER 180–360 mg, verapamil 80–120mg 3 times daily or ER 240–480mg	Cause edema; dihydropyridines may be safely combined w/ B-blocker Non-dihydropyridines reduce heart rate and proteinuria
Vasodilators	hydralazine 25–100mg twice daily, minoxidil 5–10mg terazosin 1–5mg, doxazosin 1–4mg given at bedtime	Hydralazine and minoxidil may cause reflex tachycardia and fluid retention – usually require diuretic + B-blocker Alpha-blockers may cause orthostatic hypotension
Centrally-acting agents	clonidine 0.1–0.2mg twice daily, methyldopa 250–500mg twice daily guanfacine 1–3mg	Clonidine available in weekly patch formulation for resistant hypertension

FIGURE 13-2 *(Continued)*

clinician uses the treatment algorithm, risk factor assessment data, and the patient's BP category to choose treatment plans for the patient.

The nurse encourages self-management, which may include self BP monitoring, and education to initiate and maintain lifestyle changes. It is important to assess the patient's beliefs about hypertension (Box 13-3). Self-management and education empowers patients to ask questions and voice concerns. These individuals are less likely to be hospitalized, have fewer emergency department and unscheduled medical visits, and have fewer days off from work.

The nurse should routinely ask whether patients take herbal supplements or over-the-counter (OTC) medications that may increase BP. These include caffeine and ephedra, which are stimulants; licorice, which has an aldosterone-like effect; and oral contraceptives, acetaminophen and NSAIDs, which may lead to fluid retention. In addition, certain agents have been touted as BP-lowering agents, such as coenzyme Q10, garlic, vitamin C, and L-arginine. Patients should be cautioned that nutritional supplements are not regulated in the same manner as pharmaceuticals, and all products used should be reported to the health care provider (FDA, 2016).

Lifestyle Changes

Table 13-2 summarizes recommended lifestyle modifications. Research findings demonstrate that weight loss, reduced alcohol and sodium intake, and regular physical activity for 30 minutes on most days are effective lifestyle adaptations to reduce BP (Grossman & Porth, 2014). Counsel the client that smoking cessation will decrease the risk for heart disease. Treatment of sleep apnea, underlying thyroid disorders, and management of blood glucose are also recommended (Harvard Letter, 2015). The nurse should emphasize the concept of lifelong BP control and adherence to treatment rather than cure and absolute compliance.

Every patient with hypertension should be offered information regarding lifestyle modifications to reduce blood pressure (O'Connell, 2014). Specific information regarding diet, exercise, avoidance of salt/sodium intake and alcohol as well as smoking cessation should be included. Adhering to the American Heart Association's DASH approach (Dietary Approaches to Stop Hypertension) helps decrease BP and lower lipid levels, reducing the risk of cardiovascular diseases (NIH, 2015b). Refer to Table 13-3 for details on DASH diet.

DASH is low in saturated and trans fats as well as rich in potassium, calcium, magnesium, fiber, and protein. Further,

BOX 13-3 **Nursing Research**

Bridging the Gap to Evidence-Based Practice

Using Culturally Sensitive Education to Improve Adherence With Anti-Hypertension Regimen.

Gross, B., Anderson, E., Busby, S., Frith, K., & Panco, C. (2013). Using culturally sensitive education to improve adherence with anti-hypertension regimen. *Journal of Cultural Diversity, 20*(2), 75–79.

Purpose
The purpose of the project was to assess the outcomes of culturally sensitive education programs for African Americans on antihypertensive treatment regimens.

Design
A culturally sensitive, evidence-based education program was designed to promote adherence to an antihypertensive regimen among African-American patients receiving care at a nonprofit ambulatory walk-in clinic. Thirty-five clinic patients with elevated BP were enrolled initially. The theory of Planned Behavior was used to assess for an association among beliefs, attitudes, social influences and perceived ability to perform the expected behavior. Baseline literacy was assessed using the Newest Vital Sign literary assessment tool. Patients were asked to maintain a medication diary to determine if outcomes were met.

Findings
Economic factors impact adherence to the prescribed diet and exercise, as well as ability to purchase healthy food choices. Eighty percent of the participants were women ages 29–70 years of age. Several patients desired to eat healthfully but expressed concern their families and friends would not eat food prepared with unfamiliar food choices. Participants made statements such as, "I had to stop eating in restaurants with my friends because they made fun of me when I ordered salads instead of fried and seasoned food." In addition, eating healthfully required participants to travel several miles to a full-service supermarket.

Some patients who were nonadherent to the medical regimen felt home remedies such as "a little cold water on my forehead" could help get blood pressure down. Others stated they took the medication only when they "felt bad."

Of the 10 patients who completed the program, all stated their knowledge of hypertension treatment had increased. Only one maintained the medication diary; the others forgot to bring it to the clinic but stated they followed the regimen. Lifestyle changes such as eating healthier, maintaining a record of weight, smoking cessation, and beginning a safe exercise program were agreed to; however the elderly did not agree to the exercise program due the fear of crime. The 10 patients who completed the program had blood pressure readings within normal limits at the end of the project.

Nursing Implications
Barriers to treatment included friends and families who did not encourage participants to change their diets. Culturally, hypertension may be seen as an episodic, rather than chronic, condition by this group. Fear of being robbed while walking around the neighborhood, even in broad daylight, and lack of financial resources to join a gym or fitness club were reported. Walking in the mall was also difficult as the mall was several miles from home and participants had no transportation. Natural remedies are passed down by family members, and lack of trust of health care providers can impact adherence with prescription medications.

African-American's attitudes regarding health and illness have been influenced by their culture and are often passed on to future generations. Nurses should be conscious of the importance of culture and treatment and ensure the treatment is congruent with the patient's cultural background, income, and religious practices. The authors conclude education programs should be offered in churches and community centers. Churches in the African-American community serve as spiritual as well as social and cultural gathering sites. Education programs that support both spiritual and social support will promote healthy lifestyle modification.

---

the DASH approach emphasizes vegetables, fruits, and fat-free or low-fat dairy products. It includes whole grains, fish, poultry, beans, seeds, nuts, and vegetable oils and limits sodium, sweets, sugary beverages, and red meats, which not only lowers blood pressure but also prevents cardiovascular disease (NIH, 2015c).

The average daily sodium intake for Americans age 2 years and older is 3,400 mg (CDC, 2016). Consistent with the DASH approach, the target sodium intake should be 2,300 to 2,400 mg daily (1 teaspoon). Those who already have hypertension, diabetes, or CKD as well as African-American individuals and adults aged 51 and over should reduce sodium intake further, to 1,500 mg of sodium daily (Oza & Garcellano, 2015). When salt intake is reduced, blood pressure begins decreasing within weeks (CDC, 2016). About 5% of patients have sodium-sensitive hypertension and should be very cautious with sodium intake, especially the elderly.

A diet high in fruits and vegetables is associated with lower systolic and diastolic blood pressure. Maintaining or attaining normal weight is advised. Obesity may increase the risk of hypertension through overactivation of the sympathetic nervous system, activation of renin–angiotensin–aldosterone system, sodium retention, and increased HR. Increased inflammatory markers such as C-reactive protein, leads to endothelial dysfunction and abnormal lipid levels. The impaired production of nitric oxide, a potent vasodilator, impairs vasodilation and causes an increased resting blood pressure (O'Connell, 2014). Regular exercise is associated with lower blood pressure regardless of body mass index (BMI). Exercise may improve inflammatory markers and cause an increase in endothelial nitric oxide synthase, a potent vasodilator.

Exercise and lifestyle changes should include the importance of achieving a waist circumference of less than 40 inches for a man and less than 35 inches for a woman and a BMI

TABLE 13-2 Lifestyle Modifications to Prevent and Manage Hypertension[a]

Modification	Recommendation	Goal of SBP[b] Reduction (Range)[c]
Weight reduction	Maintain normal body weight (body mass index 18.5–24.9 kg/m²).	5–20 mm Hg/10 kg
Adopt DASH (Dietary Approaches to Stop Hypertension) eating plan	Consume a diet rich in fruits, vegetables, fiber, potassium, and low-fat dairy products, and reduce consumption of animal protein, fat, and saturated fat.	8–14 mm Hg
Dietary sodium reduction	Reduce dietary sodium intake to 2.4-g sodium or 6-g sodium chloride per day.	2–8 mm Hg
Physical activity	Engage in regular aerobic physical activity such as 30 minutes of brisk walking 3–5 days per week	4–9 mm Hg
Moderation of alcohol consumption	Limit consumption to no more than two drinks (e.g., 24-oz beer, 10-oz wine, or 3-oz 80-proof whiskey) per day in most men and to no more than one drink per day in women and lighter-weight people.	2–4 mm Hg

[a]For overall cardiovascular risk reduction, stop smoking.
[b]SBP, Systolic BP.
[c]The effects of implementing these modifications are dose- and time-dependent and could be greater for some individuals.
From the Seventh Report of the Joint National Committee on Prevention, Detection, Evaluation, and Treatment of High BP. (2003). *Hypertension, 42*(6), 1206–1252.

between 18.5 and 24.9 kg/m². For patients not meeting that goal, modification involves caloric restriction and increased physical activity. A weight loss of only 10 lb may result in a 5 to 20 mm Hg reduction in SBP, offering tangible results to the patient. The nurse encourages the patient to formulate a plan for weight loss, consulting a dietician or using support groups if necessary. The bariatric patient may benefit from surgical intervention. Mobile health technology (Fitbit, pedometer, etc.) may assist the patient in increasing his physical activity.

TABLE 13-3 The DASH (Dietary Approaches to Stop Hypertension) Diet

Food Group	Number of Servings Per Day
Grains and grain products	6–8
Vegetables	4 or 5
Fruits	4 or 5
Low-fat or fat-free dairy foods	2 or 3
Meat, fish, and poultry	6 or fewer
Nuts, seeds, and dry beans	4 or 5 weekly
Sodium	2,300 mg/day (1,500 mg if over 51 years of age)
Fats and oils	2–3
Sweets and added sugars	5 or less weekly

The diet is based on 2,000 calories per day.
Retrieved from http://www.nhlbi.nih.gov/health/health-topics/topics/dash/followdash. Last updated June 2014.

Specific information should be provided on reading labels for foods that contain less than 400 mg of sodium per serving and for reducing the intake of table salt to 1 teaspoon (2.3 to 2.4 g of sodium) daily. Most sodium intake comes from packaged, processed, and restaurant foods and, therefore, is in the product at the time of purchase. Teach the patient that it takes 2 to 3 months for the taste buds to adapt to changes in salt intake to encourage perseverance (Dudek, 2014). Recognizing that hypertension is a common cause of morbidity and mortality of cardiovascular disease, the American Public Health Association has published a resolution that food manufacturers and restaurants reduce sodium in the food supply by 50% over the next decade (Jackson, King, Zhao, & Cogswell, 2016) (apha.org, 2014).

 Nursing Alert
Reducing table salt to about 1 teaspoon per day, or 2.3 to 2.4 g of sodium, can reduce systolic BP by 2 to 8 mm Hg.

While moderate alcohol consumption has shown to lower blood pressure, those who do not drink alcohol already should not start for the purpose of lowering blood pressure (Oza & Garcellano, 2015). Limiting one's daily alcohol intake to 24 oz of beer, 10 oz of wine, or 3 oz of whiskey for men, and half that for women, is recommended (AHA, 2016a). Smoking cessation is encouraged in all hypertensive patients because it can significantly increase the progression of renal insufficiency as measured by the serum creatinine concentration, which rose from 1.5 to 1.9 mg/dL in a study conducted over 35 months (Kaplan, 2016). There has been some concern regarding the impact of nicotine replacement therapy (NRT) on blood pressure in patients with hypertension; a recent study conducted with patients with hypertension, CAD, and/or MI revealed no significant clinical change in blood pressure or HR during the use of NRT and/or bupropion (Zevin & Pacheco, 2016). Based on these data, nurses may advocate for behavioral therapies and/or pharmacotherapies for those interested in quitting smoking.

Alternate Therapies

Complementary and alternative medicine therapies and mind–body interventions are potentially effective in reducing BP. Relaxation, meditation, guided imagery, hypnosis, biofeedback, yoga, and Tai Chi are some examples of these therapies. Yoga has been shown to have beneficial effects on the cardiovascular system. Physical activity and exercise has been demonstrated to reduce morbidity and mortality for coronary heart disease, hypertension, obesity, diabetes, and osteoporosis as well as have a positive effect on the patient's psychological well-being (Lo, Yeh, Chang, Sung, & Smith, 2012; Oza & Garcellano, 2015).

Blood Pressure Monitoring

The nurse must ensure that follow-up is provided for any person identified as having an elevated BP level. Each person should be given a written record of his or her BP at the screening. The American Heart Association and the National Heart, Lung, and Blood Institute provide printed and electronic patient education materials (see reference resources web addresses). Reductions in BP are greater when patients are partners and participate in self-management; some options include diaries and technology-based applications (smartphone products, web-based self-monitoring programs).

Pharmacologic Therapy

The nurse collaborates with the patient to support adherence to the medication regimen. Studies have shown consistently that 20% to 30% of medication prescriptions are never filled and that, on average, 50% of medications for chronic disease are not taken as prescribed (AHRQ, 2012). In addition, patients with limited income as well as those who do not have health insurance are at high risk for not purchasing their medication after receiving a prescription (Adams & Urban, 2016). Motivation for adherence to the prescribed regimen improves when patients have positive experiences with and trust in the clinician. Empathy and culturally sensitive education build trust and is a potent motivator to achieve better outcomes with medication adherence and lifestyle changes (Gross, Anderson, Busby, Frith, & Panco, 2013). Cene et al. (2013) identified African-American men with depressive symptoms, psychosocial stressors, and substance abuse as a population at high risk for nonadherence to treatment. Screening for such symptoms should be undertaken when nonadherence is noted along with referral to appropriate resources (Cene et al., 2013).

Evidence-based guidelines for management of hypertension from JNC8 suggests the general population aged over 60 years initiates pharmacologic therapy to lower BP when systolic BP is over 150 mm Hg or diastolic BP is over 90 mm Hg (James et al., 2013; Felicilda-Reynaldo & Kenneally, 2015). While exact target range for B/P control vary for subgroups such as the elderly or those with kidney disease, current evidence suggests more intensive control of B/P is warranted because of the association between higher BP and increased CVD risk. Most recent guidelines recommend a systolic pressure of 130 mm Hg is the upper limit of normal at all ages (ACC/AHA, 2017). In the general population, including those with diabetes but excluding all African Americans, initial antihypertensive treatment should include a thiazide-like diuretic, calcium-channel blocker (CCB), angiotensin-converting enzyme inhibitor (ACEI), or angiotensin-receptor blocker (ARB). In the general African American population, including those with diabetes, initial antihypertensive treatment should include a thiazide-type diuretic or CCB. In the population aged 18 or older, regardless of race or presence of diabetes, those who have CKD as well as initial or added antihypertensive treatment should include an ACEI or ARB to improve kidney outcome.

The main objective of hypertension treatment is to attain and maintain goal BP. If the goal is not attained within 1 month of treatment, increasing the dose of the first drug or adding a second drug from one of the classes was recommended (thiazide-type diuretic, CCB, ACEI, or ARB). The advantage of adding a medication, rather than increasing the dose of the first medication, is that side effects may be avoided. Most patients requiring pharmacologic intervention need two medications for effective treatment as hypertension is caused by multiple factors.

Blood pressure should be assessed and the treatment adjusted until the goal is reached. If the goal is not met with two medications, a third drug is added and titrated; note that an ACEI and ARB are not recommended for use at the same time. A third drug from another class may be added as needed (Krader, 2014).

There is a recommendation against use of beta-blockers for the initial treatment of hypertension (Krader, 2014), since evidence suggested a higher rate of cardiovascular death, MI, or stroke when compared to use of an ARB. The following are not recommended as first-line therapy: dual alpha$_1$- + beta-blocking agents (e.g., carvedilol), vasodilating beta-blockers (e.g., nebivolol), central alpha$_2$-adrenergic agonists (e.g., clonidine), direct vasodilators (e.g., hydralazine), aldosterone receptor antagonists (e.g., spironolactone), adrenergic neuronal depleting agents (e.g., reserpine), and loop diuretics (e.g., furosemide) (James, 2014).

Thiazide diuretics are useful in the elderly and in patients with osteoporosis because they decrease bone breakdown and preserve bone integrity. ACEIs or angiotensin receptor blockers (ARBs) protect and preserve kidney function and protect the vascular endothelium (Felicilda-Reynaldo & Kenneally, 2015). CCBs, such as amlodipine, exert their major effect on blood vessels and are recommended for the treatment of hypertension, while medications that affect HR, such as diltiazem, are better suited to rhythm control.

 Drug Alert!
The JNC8 recommends initial therapy with thiazide diuretics and CCBs for African-American individuals. They provide the greatest blood pressure reduction in this population (Adams & Urban, 2016).

 Drug Alert!
Use of NSAIDs with ACEIs and ARBs may decrease antihypertensive effects due to prostaglandin inhibition and fluid retention.

 Drug Alert!
Maximum antihypertensive effect from thiazide diuretics used for hypertension is delayed and does not occur for 3 to 4 weeks. Inform patients of this information to decrease risk of nonadherence to therapy (Felicilda-Reynaldo & Kenneally, 2015).

 Drug Alert!
ACEIs exert their therapeutic effect within 1 hour of administration, and the risk for severe hypotension is increased during the first 5 hours. To prevent first-dose hypotension and the risk for falls, the patient should be in a supine position for the first dose and have blood pressure assessed (Felicilda-Reynaldo & Kenneally, 2015).

 Drug Alert!
Observe patients receiving ACEIs for the first time for angioedema, a dangerous adverse effect. Symptoms include difficulty breathing or swelling in the face, neck, or tongue (Felicilda-Reynaldo & Kenneally, 2015).

When the BP is at goal for at least 1 year, gradual reduction of the types and doses of medication is indicated. To promote persistence (adherence), clinicians try to prescribe the simplest treatment schedule possible, ideally one or two pills daily. The nurse needs to emphasize and support both pharmacologic and nonpharmacologic strategies; contracting, goal-setting, counseling, referral to support groups, and use of web-based technology are some of the strategies used. If a patient who is diagnosed with resistant hypertension fails to reach goal BP when adhering to a three-drug regimen that includes a diuretic and the patient has multiple drug intolerances or contraindications, a referral to a hypertension specialist is indicated (Ferri, 2016a). Obstructive sleep apnea has been recognized as one of the most common risk factors for resistant hypertension (Oza & Garcellano, 2015).

Table 13-4 describes the pharmacologic agents that are recommended for the treatment of hypertension.

The nurse should include education when medication for other risk factors is combined with antihypertensive therapy. For example, a statin to lower cholesterol is prescribed if the patient has a cardiovascular disease risk or has target organ damage. The nurse teaches the patient that high cholesterol does not directly increase BP but can increase vascular damage leading to cardiovascular complication (Harvard Health Letter, 2015). Low-dose aspirin therapy may be indicated once BP is controlled to limit cardiovascular complications. There is evidence that depression is associated with poor adherence to medication regimens and that posttraumatic stress disorder (PTSD) is associated with hypertension, thus directing the nurse to develop further psychosocial interventions and reinforce collaborative pharmacologic interventions (Kibler, Joshi, & Ma, 2008).

The nurse provides written information about the expected effects and side effects of antihypertensive medications, warning the patient not to stop medications abruptly because **rebound hypertension** may occur. As always, the patient should be encouraged to provide honest feedback to the health care provider to achieve optimum BP control. Patients should be cautioned to avoid OTC medications, especially nasal decongestants containing vasoconstrictors, which can further elevate BP.

Medication compliance increases when patients actively participate in self-care, including self-monitoring of BP, diet, and exercise—possibly because patients receive immediate feedback and have a greater sense of control. Evidence demonstrates that compliance further increases when the provider takes time in counseling, takes into account cultural perspectives on causes and treatment of hypertension, and avoids viewing the patient as responsible for treatment failures.

Complications

Prolonged BP elevation damages blood vessels, particularly in target organs such as the heart, kidneys, brain, and eyes. The consequences of prolonged, uncontrolled hypertension are MI, heart failure, left ventricular hypertrophy, kidney failure, stroke, and impaired vision. An acute elevation in BP associated with end-organ damage is termed *hypertensive emergency*.

HYPERTENSIVE CRISES

Hypertensive crisis is defined as a diastolic BP of higher than 180/120 mm Hg. Approximately 1% of individuals with hypertension will have a hypertensive crisis at some point. Hypertensive crises occur when hypertension is untreated or has been poorly controlled as well as in those who have discontinued their medications. These crises are more common in men, older adults, and African Americans

TABLE **13-4** Medication Therapy for Hypertension

Medication	Major Action	Considerations
Diuretics (Thiazide and Thiazide-Like, Loop, Potassium-Sparing)		
Hydrochlorothiazide and metolazone, furosemide, spironolactone	Decreases blood volume, renal blood flow, and cardiac output Natriuresis, negative sodium balance Directly affects vascular smooth muscle	Side effects: Dry mouth, thirst, nausea, weakness, drowsiness, postural hypotension Considerations: Monitor for signs of sodium, potassium, and magnesium imbalance.
Central Alpha$_2$-Agonists and Other Centrally Acting Drugs—No Longer Recommended as First-Line Treatment		
Clonidine, methyldopa	Impairs synthesis and reuptake of norepinephrine Displaces norepinephrine from storage sites Stimulates central alpha$_2$-adrenergic receptors	Side effects: Hypotension, postural hypotension, bradycardia, dizziness, drowsiness, dry mouth, depression, nasal congestion, rebound hypertension, impotence
Beta Blockers—No Longer Recommended as First-Line Treatment in Any Subgroup (Krader, 2014)		
Atenolol, propranolol, metoprolol, nadolol, timolol	Blocks beta adrenergic receptors of sympathetic nervous system causing vasodilation, decreased cardiac output and heart rate	Side effects: Hypotension, bradycardia, congestive heart failure, fatigue, depression, weakness, impotence, rebound hypertension, hypoglycemia Contraindications: Asthma, COPD
Alpha$_1$ Blockers—No Longer Recommended as First-Line Treatment in Any Subgroup (Krader, 2014)		
Doxazosin, prazosin hydrochloride, terazosin	Peripherally acting vasodilator	Side effects: Vomiting and diarrhea, urinary frequency, and tachycardia if not controlled with beta blocker, drowsiness
Combined Alpha and Beta Blockers—No Longer Recommended as First-Line Treatment in Any Subgroup (Krader, 2014)		
Carvedilol, labetalol hydrochloride	Blocks alpha- and beta-adrenergic receptors; causes peripheral dilation and decreases peripheral vascular resistance	Side effects: Orthostatic hypotension, tachycardia or bradycardia Contraindications: Asthma and COPD
Vasodilators		
Fenoldopam mesylate	Stimulates dopamine and alpha$_2$-adrenergic receptors	Side effects: Headache, flushing, hypotension, sweating
Hydralazine	Decreases peripheral resistance; concurrently elevates cardiac output; acts directly on smooth muscle of blood vessels	Side effects: Headache, tachycardia, flushing, and dyspnea, lupus erythematosus–like syndrome
Minoxidil	Direct-acting arterial vasodilator	Side effects: Hirsutism, dizziness, headache, nausea, edema, tachycardia, profound hypotension, thiocyanate toxicity
Sodium nitroprusside	Peripheral vasodilation by relaxation of smooth muscle	Side effects: Hypotension, tachycardia, flushing, headache
Angiotensin-Converting Enzyme (ACE$_1$) Inhibitors		
Captopril, enalaprilat/enalapril, fosinopril, lisinopril, quinapril, ramipril	Inhibits conversion of angiotensin I to angiotensin II; reduces peripheral resistance	Side effects: Hypotension, tachycardia, hyperkalemia, azotemia, angioedema (rare but life threatening) Contraindications: Pregnancy

Medication	Major Action	Considerations
Angiotensin II Receptor Blockers (ARBs)		
Candesartan irbesartan, losartan olmesartan, telmisartan, valsartan	Blocks the effects of angiotensin II at the receptor; reduces peripheral resistance	Side effects: Hypotension, hyperkalemia Contraindications: Pregnancy
Calcium-Channel Blockers		
Nondihydropyridines Diltiazem, verapamil **Dihydropyridines** Amlodipine, felodipine, isradipine, nifedipine	Inhibits calcium ion influx; reduces cardiac afterload, workload	Do not discontinue suddenly. Side effects: Hypotension, bradycardia, CHF dizziness, edema Contraindications: Sick sinus syndrome, heart blocks
Direct renin inhibitor (DRI)	Not considered first-line agent for treatment	
Aliskiren		Side effect, diarrhea, cough, flulike symptoms, and rash. DRI aliskiren can injure or be fatal to the developing fetus.

COPD, chronic obstructive pulmonary disease; CHF, congestive heart failure; DRI, direct renin inhibitor.

(Adams & Urban, 2016). Other causes of hypertensive crises include head injury, pheochromocytoma (a tumor of the adrenal medulla that causes excess secretion of catecholamines), food–drug interactions (such as tyramine combined with a monamine oxidase [MAO] inhibitors), eclampsia or preeclampsia, substance abuse (e.g., cocaine intoxication), and kidney disease (Adams & Urban, 2016).

Once the crisis has been managed, the nurse strategizes with the patient and provider to take control of his or her BP and prevent recurrence. There are two classes of hypertensive crisis that require immediate intervention: hypertensive emergency and hypertensive urgency (Adams & Urban, 2016).

A **hypertensive emergency** is a situation in which diastolic BP is greater than 120 mm Hg and must be lowered quickly to halt or prevent damage to the target organs (Adams & Urban, 2016; Grossman & Porth, 2014). Conditions associated with hypertensive emergency include eclampsia or preeclampsia, MI, dissecting aortic aneurysm, intracranial hemorrhage, and hyperthyroidism or thyroid storm. In hypertensive emergencies, patients present with severe elevations in blood pressure, accompanied by rapidly progressive target organ dysfunction, such as myocardial or cerebral ischemia or infarction, pulmonary edema, or kidney failure (Victor, 2016). Patient complaints include headaches, confusion, blurred vision, nausea and vomiting, seizures, pulmonary edema, oliguria, and hypertensive retinopathy (Victor, 2016, p. 394). The therapeutic goals are a controlled, gradual reduction of the BP by 10% in the first hour and by an additional 15% during the next 3 to 12 hours to a blood pressure of no less than 160/110 mm Hg (Victor, 2016). Additional gradual reductions are made over the next 48 hours until blood pressure normalizes. It is important not to become overeager and lower the BP too quickly (cerebral

hypoperfusion may occur if the mean BP is lowered more than 40% in the initial 24 hours); because of hypoperfusion to the brain, heart, kidneys, and retina an MI or CVA could result (Ferri, 2016a). The exceptions include aortic dissection and postoperative bleeding from vascular suture lines, in which a more rapid normalization of blood pressure is required (Victor, 2016). A patient experiencing hypertensive emergency most likely will receive care in the intensive care unit with BP measured every 5 minutes while unstable. The nurse evaluates the patient for a precipitous drop in BP, which requires immediate action to restore BP and perfusion to normal levels.

Hypertensive urgency describes a situation in which BP is severely elevated, but there is no evidence of impending or progressive target organ damage (Adams & Urban, 2016). Elevated BPs associated with severe headache, epistaxis, or anxiety are classified as urgencies. Reducing blood pressure can be accomplished by increasing the dose of the patient's current medications or by adding a second medication. Oral medications with rapid onset of action may be used, including clonidine (Catapres), captopril (Capoten), or labetalol (Trandate). This can be accomplished by keeping the patient in the emergency department for several hours, followed by outpatient assessment within 1 to 3 days (Adams & Urban, 2016).

Pharmacologic Management of Hypertensive Crises

The medications of choice in hypertensive emergencies are best managed with continuous IV infusion of a short-acting titratable antihypertensive agent. The nurse avoids the sublingual and IM routes as their absorption and dynamics are unpredictable. Medications may include clevidipine hydrochloride, fenoldopam mesylate, enalaprilat, esmolol, hydralazine, nicardipine, or sodium nitroprusside, which have immediate, short-lived actions. Nitroprusside should be used cautiously due to thiocyanate toxicity, erratic responses, and risk for severe hypotension (Adams & Urban, 2016). For more information about these medications, see Table 13-4.

Oral doses of fast-acting agents such as clonidine or labetalol are recommended for the treatment of hypertensive urgencies (see Table 13-4).

Drug Alert!
ACEIs and ARBs block aldosterone and may cause hyperkalemia when used with potassium-sparing diuretics or salt substitutes that contain potassium. The nurse should monitor the potassium level and teach the patient to avoid salt substitutes.

The nurse follows up with teaching about a hypertensive crisis and encourages the patient to take charge of managing hypertension.

CHAPTER REVIEW

Critical Thinking Exercises

1. A 72-year-old man arrives in the emergency department with a laceration of his right forearm from a minor gardening injury, which will require suturing. The patient's BP on his left arm is 184/96 and his heart rate is 82 and regular. You express concern to the patient that his BP is high. He shrugs and tells you, "The top number is always elevated, but it's nothing to worry about." Based on current evidence, what teaching should the nurse provide regarding untreated hypertension? What other information do you plan to gather from this patient? What plan of action might you initiate?

2. You are volunteering at a church-sponsored BP screening offered after Sunday services, in tandem with a fund-raising buffet breakfast. The pastor approaches you and notes that the breakfast buffet contains a variety of egg dishes, hash browns, sausage patties, bacon, and pastries. He asks you what effects, if any, this food may have on his parishioners' BPs. What effect might this type of diet have on the parishioners' BPs today? Discuss the evidence that supports specific dietary strategies aimed at preventing and treating hypertension and its complications. Include the DASH approach.

NCLEX-Style Review Questions

1. The nurse is reviewing the vital signs of a patient admitted with cellulitis whose BP is 136/86. Which of the following should the nurse teach the patient about this BP reading?
   a. "Your BP is in the normal range, you don't need to worry."
   b. "This BP shows prehypertension; try to cut down on sodium and see your health care provider."
   c. "I will notify the provider of your BP; a BP of 136/86 indicates you have hypertension."

   d. "You are at risk for organ damage; this BP indicates a hypertensive urgency."

2. During routine screening, the nurse notes a BP of 172/96. The patient states, "I feel fine—what's the big deal?" Which of the following indicates the best response by the nurse?
   a. "As long as you are feeling well and you are under 60 years old, there is no need to worry."
   b. "Untreated high BP may result in kidney failure, heart attack, or stroke."
   c. "This BP elevation indicates you have not been compliant with your medication."
   d. "Have you had any unusual nosebleeds or headaches lately?"

3. A patient is admitted with angina and hypertensive crisis. On admission, the BP is 240/120. The nurse recognizes which of the following is consistent with current BP management strategies?
   a. In 2 hours, the target BP is 140/90.
   b. In 1 hour, the patient's target BP should be 180/90.
   c. Lowering the BP too quickly may lead to rebound hypertension.
   d. The nurse should anticipate using oral medications for hypertensive crisis.

4. The nurse is teaching a patient about BP self-monitoring. What direction should be included in the plan of care?
   a. You may sit or stand when taking your BP.
   b. Do not eat or drink for at least 2 hours before measuring your BP.
   c. Make sure the cuff is loose enough to avoid squeezing your arm too tightly.
   d. Keep your arm at heart level and avoid talking during BP measurement.

5. A nurse is completing medication teaching for a patient diagnosed with hypertension. What directive is important to include in the plan to prevent rebound hypertension?
   a. Caution the client about the use of OTC vitamins.
   b. Inform the client that beta blockers can cause sexual dysfunction.
   c. Avoid abruptly stopping antihypertensive medication.
   d. Teach the patient/client to arise slowly.

Try these additional resources, available at **http://thepoint.lww.com/Honan2e**, to enhance your learning and understanding of this chapter:
- NCLEX-Style Student Review Questions
- Journal Articles

REFERENCES AND SELECTED READINGS

References and selected readings associated with this chapter can be found on the website that accompanies the book. Visit **http://thepoint. lww.com/Honan2e** to access the references and other additional resources associated with this chapter.

Nursing Management: Patients with Coronary Vascular Disorders

Mary G. Pierson

Learning Objectives

After reading this chapter, you will be able to:

1. Summarize the pathophysiology, risk factors, clinical manifestations, and treatment of coronary atherosclerosis.
2. Summarize the pathophysiology, clinical manifestations, and treatment of angina pectoris.
3. Describe percutaneous coronary intervention (PCI) and coronary artery revascularization procedures.
4. Explain the nursing care of a patient who has had a PCI procedure for treatment of coronary artery disease.
5. Describe the nursing care of a patient who has undergone cardiac surgery.
6. Summarize the pathophysiology, clinical manifestations, and treatment of myocardial infarction.

Cardiovascular disease (CVD) is the leading cause of death in the United States and globally, and accounts for more than 17.3 million deaths per year, a number that is expected to increase to more than 23.6 million by 2030 (Mozaffarian et al., 2016). About one of every three deaths in America and 31% of all deaths globally can be attributed to CVD, affecting all segments of the population. Coronary artery disease (CAD) is the most prevalent type of CVD in adults. For this reason, it is important for nurses to become familiar with various manifestations of coronary artery conditions and methods for assessing, preventing, and treating these disorders medically and surgically.

CORONARY ATHEROSCLEROSIS

The most common cause of CVD in the United States is **atherosclerosis**, an abnormal accumulation of lipid or fatty substances and fibrous tissue in the lining of arterial blood vessel walls. These substances create blockages and narrow the coronary vessels in a way that reduces blood flow to the myocardium. It is now known that atherosclerosis involves a repetitious inflammatory response to injury to the artery wall and subsequent alteration in the structural and biochemical properties of the arterial walls.

Pathophysiology

Atherosclerosis begins as fatty streaks of lipids that are deposited in the intima of the arterial wall. These lesions commonly begin early in life, perhaps even in childhood. Not all fatty streaks develop into more advanced lesions later. Genetics and environmental factors influence the progression of these lesions. The continued development of atherosclerosis involves an inflammatory response, which begins with injury to the vascular endothelium. The injury may be initiated by smoking, hypertension (HTN), and other factors. The presence of inflammation has multiple effects on the arterial wall, including the attraction of inflammatory cells (including macrophages or monocytes, white blood cells [WBCs]) (Swirski & Nahrendorf, 2013). The macrophages infiltrate the injured vascular endothelium and ingest lipids, which turns them into what are called "foam cells." These foam cells are present in all stages of atherosclerotic plaque formation (Porth, 2015). Activated macrophages also release biochemical substances that can further damage the endothelium, attracting platelets and initiating clotting.

Smooth muscle cells within the vessel wall subsequently proliferate and form a fibrous cap over a center that is filled with lipid and inflammatory infiltrate. These deposits, called **atheromas** or plaques, protrude into the lumen of the vessel, narrowing it and obstructing blood flow (Fig. 14-1). If the

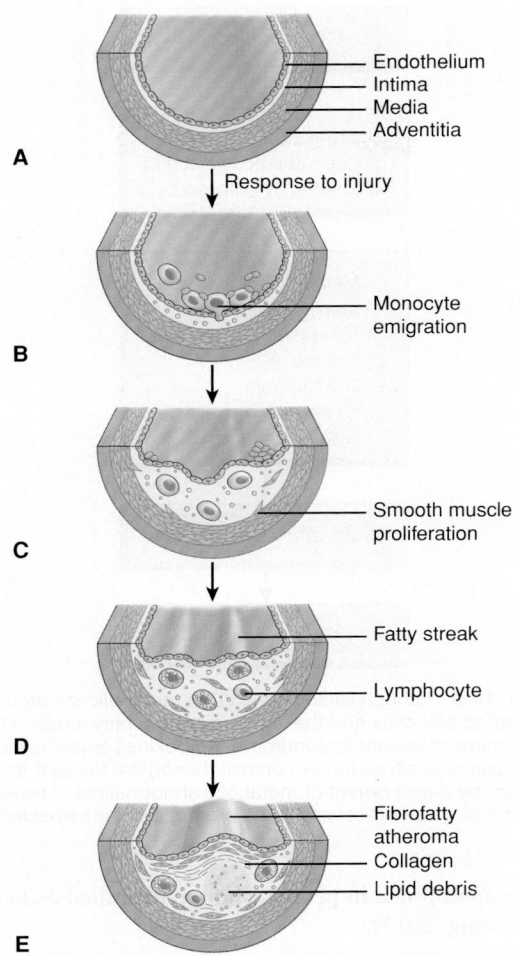

FIGURE 14-1 Atherosclerosis begins as monocytes and lipids enter the intima of an injured vessel (**A, B**). Smooth muscle cells proliferate within the vessel wall (**C**) contributing to the development of fatty accumulations and atheroma (**D**). As the plaque enlarges, the vessel narrows and blood flow decreases (**E**). The plaque may rupture and a thrombus might form, obstructing blood flow.

fibrous cap of the plaque is thick and the lipid pool remains relatively stable, it can resist the stress from blood flow and vessel movement. If the cap is thin and inflammation is ongoing, the lipid core may grow, causing it to rupture, and this ruptured plaque is a focus for thrombus formation. Then the thrombus may obstruct blood flow, leading to sudden cardiac death or an acute **myocardial infarction (MI)**, which is the death of a portion of the heart muscle. Thus, atherosclerosis can produce narrowing of the lumen of a blood vessel, sudden obstruction of a blood vessel due to plaque rupture, and weakening of a blood vessel, resulting in aneurysm formation or emboli formation because of direct damage to the endothelium.

The anatomic structure of the coronary arteries makes them particularly susceptible to the mechanisms of atherosclerosis. There are three major coronary arteries and they have multiple branches; atherosclerotic lesions most often form where the vessels branch (Fig. 14-2). Although heart disease is most often caused by atherosclerosis of the coronary arteries, other phenomena may also decrease blood flow to the heart. Examples include vasospasm (sudden constriction or narrowing) of a coronary artery, myocardial trauma from internal or external forces, structural disease, congenital anomalies, decreased oxygen supply (e.g., from acute blood loss, anemia, or low blood pressure), and increased oxygen demand (e.g., from rapid heart rate, thyrotoxicosis, or use of cocaine).

Risk Factors

Epidemiologic studies point to several factors that increase the probability that CAD will develop in a person. Some risk factors are uncontrollable, including:

- Age (men over 45 years old, women over 55 years old)
- Gender (in people less than 55 years of age, men are at a greater risk; after 55 years of age, men and women have

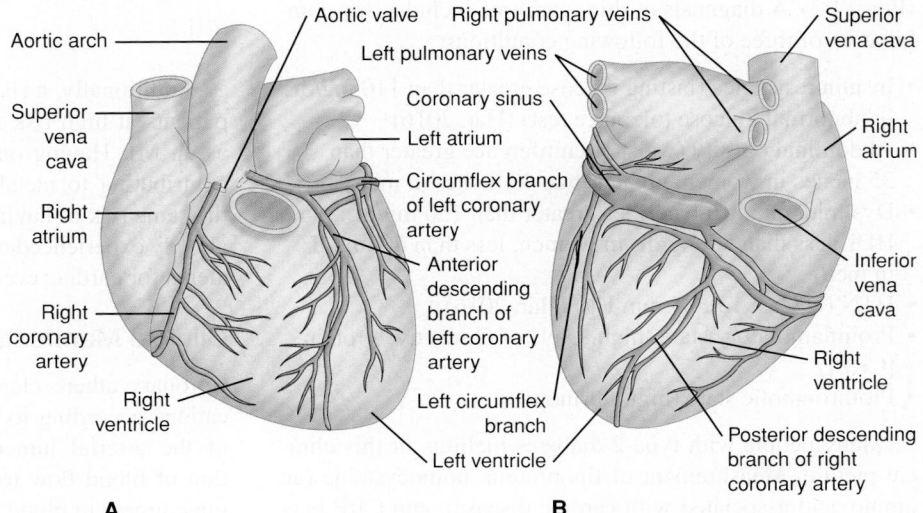

FIGURE 14-2 The coronary arteries supply the heart muscle with oxygenated blood, adjusting the flow according to metabolic needs: (**A**) anterior view and (**B**) posterior view of heart.

the same risk; or women under 55 years of age who have premature menopause without estrogen replacement therapy)
- Race (African Americans, Mexican Americans, Native Americans, and some Asian Americans demonstrate increased risk)
- Family history of first-degree relative with premature diagnosis of heart disease

Known modifiable risk factors include diabetes and pre-diabetes, HTN, smoking, obesity, physical inactivity, high blood cholesterol, unhealthy diet, and stress (National Heart, Lung, and Blood Institute [NHLBI], 2016).

Risk factors identified more recently include sleep apnea, metabolic syndrome (discussed below), increased body mass index (BMI), chronic kidney disease, chronic infections (Hui, Leung, & Padwal, 2015), nonalcoholic fatty liver disease (NAFLD) (Targher & Byrne, 2013), and influenza; additional risk factors may include conditions thought to be proinflammatory (e.g., rheumatoid arthritis) (Udel et al., 2013; Wilson, 2016).

> ### Nursing Alert
> *Obesity (BMI of 35% or higher) in and of itself is associated with all-cause mortality regardless of level of physical activity. Questions exist regarding whether obesity itself is a risk factor for CAD or cardiovascular events, or if it is the relationship of obesity to glucose intolerance, insulin resistance, HTN, physical inactivity, and dyslipidemia that increases risk. Given the significant risk that diabetes, HTN, and hyperlipidemia impose on coronary disease, nurses need to make efforts toward increasing awareness of the crucial role that these disorders have on cardiovascular mortality and morbidity.*

A cluster of metabolic abnormalities now known as **metabolic syndrome** is known to be a major risk factor for CAD (Fig. 14-3). A diagnosis of this syndrome includes any combination of three of the following conditions:

- Insulin resistance (fasting glucose greater than 110 mg/dL or abnormal glucose tolerance test) (Har, 2016)
- Abdominal obesity (waist circumference greater than 35 inches in women, greater than 40 inches in men)
- Dyslipidemia (triglycerides greater than 150 mg/dL; HDL less than 50 mg/dL in women, less than 40 mg/dL in men)
- HTN (at least 130/85 mm Hg) (Har, 2016)
- Proinflammatory state (high levels of C-reactive protein [CRP])
- Prothrombotic state (high fibrinogen)

Many people with type-2 diabetes mellitus fit this clinical picture. Measurement of lipoprotein, homocysteine (an amino acid associated with cardiac disease), and CRP may

FIGURE 14-3 Pathophysiology of CVD in metabolic syndrome. Both central adiposity and the immune system play a role in the development of metabolic syndrome. Adipokines (such as leptin) and cytokines (such as tumor necrosis factor) are thought to contribute to the development of metabolic abnormalities. The eventual effect of these processes is the promotion of atherosclerosis.

also be appropriate in people who are identified as being at risk (Koenig, 2013).

> ### Nursing Alert
> *CRP is a protein that is released in the blood during inflammatory states. The high-sensitivity CRP (hs-CRP) may be useful in assessing the risk of a cardiac event (Yousuf et al., 2013). A normal level is less than 0.1 mg/dL or less than 1 mg/L (Kaptoge, Di Angelantonio, & Pennells, 2012; Koenig, 2013).*

Additionally, a risk equivalent is a condition that places patients at high risk for experiencing a cardiac event, such as an MI. Having one or more of the conditions listed as contributing to metabolic syndrome may place patients at the same risk of having a cardiac event as someone who has already experienced one (Lackland et al., 2012). Risk equivalents for cardiac events are detailed in Box 14-1.

Clinical Manifestations and Assessment

Coronary atherosclerosis produces symptoms and complications according to the location and degree of narrowing of the arterial lumen, thrombus formation, and obstruction of blood flow to the myocardium (Libby, 2013). This impediment to blood flow is usually progressive, causing an

BOX 14-1

Coronary Artery Disease Risk Equivalents

Individuals at highest risk for a cardiac event within 10 years are those with known existing coronary artery disease (CAD) who have experienced a cardiac event, and those without a known history of cardiac event but have any one or more of the following diseases, which are called CAD risk equivalents (Lackland et al., 2012). Risk equivalents are essentially disease processes that involve atherosclerotic disease.

- Diabetes
- Peripheral arterial disease
- Abdominal aortic aneurysm
- Carotid artery disease
- Chronic kidney disease (CKD)
- Large vessel atherosclerotic ischemic stroke

inadequate blood supply that deprives the cardiac muscle cells of oxygen needed for their survival. The condition is known as **ischemia**. **Angina pectoris** refers to chest pain that is brought about by myocardial ischemia. If the decrease in blood supply is significant enough, of long enough duration, or both, death of myocardial cells, or MI, may result. Over time, irreversibly damaged myocardium undergoes degeneration and is replaced by scar tissue, causing various degrees of myocardial dysfunction. Significant myocardial damage may result in persistently low cardiac output (CO), and if the heart cannot support the body's needs for oxygenated blood, the result is heart failure. Myocardial hypoxia due to CAD may also lead to lethal cardiac rhythm disturbances that may result in sudden cardiac death.

Nursing Alert

Classic signs and symptoms of myocardial ischemia include acute onset of chest pain (often described as crushing pain, usually substernal but may be in other areas of the chest, jaw, back, or arms), shortness of breath (SOB) (dyspnea [particularly in the elderly]), extreme fatigue, diaphoresis, and nausea and vomiting. The pain of an MI may be differentiated from angina by persistence of the pain despite rest and nitroglycerine. Women often complain of atypical chest pain and nonspecific signs and symptoms.

In the elderly, sometimes there will not be a classic presentation of symptoms (referred to as "silent" ischemia), making recognition and diagnosis a clinical challenge. Elderly patients should be encouraged to recognize their chest pain–like symptom (anginal equivalent), for example, weakness, as an indication that they should rest or take prescribed medications and contact their provider with concerns. Pharmacologic stress testing may be used to diagnose CAD in elderly patients or those who have a limited ability

to exercise because of other conditions (e.g., peripheral vascular disease, arthritis, degenerative disk disease, physical disability, foot problems).

Prevention and Medical and Nursing Management

Controlling cholesterol, treating hyperlipidemia, and managing HTN and diabetes mellitus are discussed here; additional medical and nursing management is discussed under angina.

Controlling Cholesterol Abnormalities

The association of a high blood cholesterol level with CAD is well established. The metabolism of fats is an important contributor to the development of CAD. Fats, which are insoluble in water, are encased in water-soluble lipoproteins that allow them to be transported within the circulatory system. The various lipoproteins are categorized by their protein content, which is measured in density. The density increases when more protein is present. Four elements of fat metabolism—total cholesterol, LDL, HDL, and triglycerides—affect the development of heart disease. Cholesterol is processed by the GI tract into lipoprotein globules called *chylomicrons*. These are reprocessed by the liver as lipoproteins (Fig. 14-4). This is a physiologic process necessary for the formation of lipoprotein-based cell membranes and other important metabolic processes. When an excess of LDL is produced, LDL particles adhere to vulnerable points in the arterial endothelium. Here, macrophages ingest them, leading to the formation of foam cells and the beginning of plaque formation.

All adults 20 years of age or older should have a fasting lipid profile (total cholesterol, LDL, HDL, and triglyceride) performed at least once every 5 years and more often if the profile is abnormal. Patients younger than 20 years of age with known family history of hyperlipidemia and/or vascular disease should probably be tested earlier. Patients who have had an acute event (e.g., MI), a **percutaneous coronary intervention (PCI)**, or a **coronary artery bypass graft (CABG)** require assessment of the LDL cholesterol level within a few months of the event or procedure because LDL levels may be low immediately after the acute event or procedure. Subsequently, lipids should be monitored regularly until the desired level is achieved.

LDL exerts a harmful effect on the coronary vasculature because the small LDL particles can be transported easily into the vessel lining. In contrast, HDL promotes the use of total cholesterol by transporting LDL to the liver, where it is biodegraded and then excreted. The level of HDL should exceed 40 mg/dL and ideally should be more than 60 mg/dL. A high HDL level is a strong negative risk factor for heart disease (i.e., it protects against disease). In 2013, the guidelines for the treatment of high blood cholesterol levels were updated by the American College of Cardiology and the American Heart Association (ACC-AHA) Task Force on Practice Guidelines. The current guidelines represent a

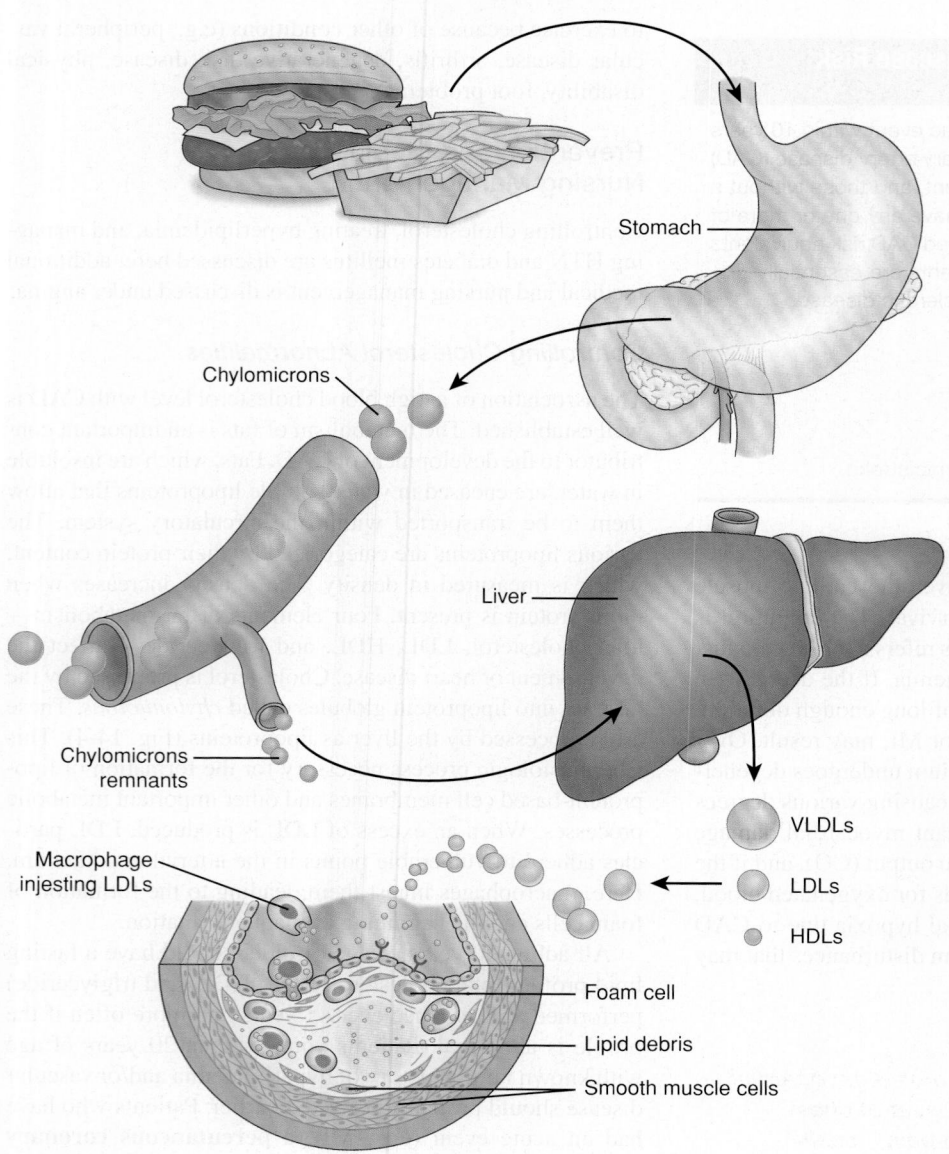

Stomach

Chylomicrons

Liver

Chylomicrons remnants

Macrophage injesting LDLs

VLDLs

LDLs

HDLs

Foam cell

Lipid debris

Smooth muscle cells

FIGURE 14-4 Lipoproteins and the development of atherosclerosis. As dietary cholesterol and saturated fat are processed by the GI tract, chylomicrons enter the blood. They are broken down into chylomicron remnants in the capillaries. The liver processes them into lipoproteins. When these are released into the circulation, excess low-density lipoproteins (LDLs) adhere to receptors on the intimal wall. Macrophages also ingest LDLs and transport them into the vessel wall, beginning the process of plaque formation. HDLs, high-density lipoproteins; VLDL, very-low-density lipoprotein.

substantial change from previous recommendations, which promoted specific lipid-level goals for patients that were dependent on the patient's level of risk. Patients now fall into a group dependent upon risk, their factors, and history rather than on their LDL level. The groups who would benefit from statin therapy (cholesterol lowering medications) are those:

1. With clinically evident atherosclerotic CVD
2. With primary low-density lipoprotein (LDL) cholesterol levels of at least 190 mg/dL
3. With type-1 or type-2 diabetes (ages 40 to 75 years) and an LDL cholesterol level of 70 mg/dL or higher, without clinically evident atherosclerotic CVD
4. Without clinically evident atherosclerotic CVD or diabetes with an LDL cholesterol level range of 70 to 189 mg/dL and an estimated 10-year risk of

atherosclerotic CVD of at least 7.5% (Note: A downloadable spreadsheet enabling estimation of 10-year and lifetime risk for atherosclerotic CVD and a web-based calculator are available at http://my.americanheart.org/cvriskcalculator and http://www.cardiosource.org/science-and-quality/practice-guidelines-and-quality-standards/2013-prevention-guideline-tools.aspx).

In these patient groups, high-intensity statin therapy (designed to reduce LDL cholesterol levels by as much as 50% or more) is generally recommended; it is believed that the benefit outweighs the risk. Research has demonstrated that primary prevention with statins reduces total mortality as well as nonfatal atherosclerotic cardiovascular events (see Table 14-1 for commonly prescribed medications affecting lipoprotein metabolism).

TABLE **14-1** Medications Affecting Lipoprotein Metabolism

Medication	Lipid/Lipoprotein Effects	Side Effects	Contraindications
HMG-CoA Reductase Inhibitors (Statins)			
Lovastatin (Mevacor®) Pravastatin (Pravachol®) Simvastatin (Zocor®) Fluvastatin (Lescol®) Atorvastatin (Lipitor®)[a] Rosuvastatin (Crestor®)[a] Pitavastatin (Livalo®)	LDL ↓ 18–55% HDL ↑ 5–15% TG ↓ 7–30%	Myopathy, myalgias, increased liver enzyme levels, ↑ blood sugar	**Absolute:** Active liver disease, pregnancy, lactation **Relative:** Drug–drug interactions can increase the risk of adverse events—refer to pharmacist.
Nicotinic Acid			
Niacin (Niacor®, Niaspan®) Immediate-release nicotinic acid Extended-release nicotinic acid Sustained-release nicotinic acid	LDL ↓ 5–25% HDL ↑ 15–35% TG ↓ 20–50%	Flushing, hyperglycemia, hyperuricemia (or gout), upper GI distress, hepatotoxicity	**Absolute:** Chronic liver disease, severe gout **Relative:** Diabetes, hyperuricemia, peptic ulcer disease
Fibric Acids			
Fenofibrate (TriCor®, Trilipix®, Lipofen®, Fenoglide®, Antara®, Lofibra®) Gemfibrozil (Lopid®) Fenofibric acid (Fibricor®)	LDL ↓ 5–20% (may be increased in patients with high TG) HDL ↑ 10–20% TG ↓ 20–50%	Dyspepsia, rash, pruritis, gallstones, myopathy, unexplained non-CHD deaths	**Absolute:** Severe kidney disease, severe liver disease
Bile Acid Sequestrants			
Cholestyramine (LoCholest®, Questran®, Prevalite®) Colesevelam (WelChol®) Colestipol HCl (Colestid®)	LDL ↓ 15–30% TG no change or increase	GI distress, constipation, vitamin K deficiency, Decreased uptake of fat-soluble vitamins, drug interactions (binds to other drugs and prevents absorption)	**Absolute:** dysbetalipoproteinemia, TG > 400 mg/dL, bowel obstruction, TG induced pancreatitis **Relative:** TG > 200 mg/dL
Omega-3 Fatty Acids *eicosapentaenoic acid/ docosahexaenoic acid (EPA/DHA)*	TG ↓ 25–30% LDL ↑ 5–10% (with dose of 4 g/day)	Flushing, elevated liver enzymes, bleeding risk eructation, and gastric irritation (taste perversion, dyspepsia) and allergic reactions (fish); When used in amounts greater than 3 g/day, EPA is POSSIBLY UNSAFE, and can thin the blood and increase the risk for bleeding.	**Absolute:** hypersensitivity to any component of this medication Use caution if hypersensitivity to fish/shellfish, bleeding risk, active liver disease
PCSK9 INHIBITOR Evolocumab (Repatha®) Alirocumab (Praluent®) (self-injected under the skin with a prefilled, single-use SureClick® Autoinjector)	↓ LDL 58–71%	Allergic reaction; flu-like symptoms; back pain; redness, pain, or bruising at the injection site	**Absolute:** hypersensitivity reaction to evolocumab
Cholesterol Absorption Inhibitor Ezetimibe (Zetia®)	↓ LDL (~18%), ↑ HDL 1–4%, ↓ TG 5–10%	Allergic reaction, arthralgia, diarrhea, back pain, stomach or abdominal pain, fever, sore throat	Allergy to ezetimibe; active liver disease

Note: Statin therapy are considered first line agents; the other agents listed below are generally reserved for patients with tolerability issues or hypertriglyceridemia.
HMG-CoA, 3-hydroxy-3-methylglutaryl coenzyme A; LDL, low-density lipoprotein; HDL, high-density lipoprotein; TG, triglycerides; ↓, decrease; ↑, increase; CHD, coronary heart disease.
[a]Atorvastatin (Lipitor) and Rosuvastatin (Crestor) are both "High-Intensity Statins", High-Intensity Statins daily dose lowers LDL-C by approx ≥50% and are the most commonly prescribed (Foley et al., 2017).

Moderate-intensity statin therapy (aims for a reduction of 30% to less than 50% in LDL cholesterol levels) is recommended for patients who cannot tolerate high-intensity treatment or patients with diabetes and a 10-year risk of atherosclerotic CVD of less than 7.5%. People receiving statin therapy should be monitored for muscle and hepatic injury and for new-onset diabetes.

Serum cholesterol and LDL levels often can also be influenced by diet and physical activity. Depending on the patient's LDL level and risk of CAD, medication to treat hyperlipidemia may also be prescribed. Medication should be used in conjunction with a heart-healthy diet and an exercise program (Keaney, Curfman, & Jarcho, 2014). Refer to Table 14-1.

Treating Hyperlipidemia

Lipid-lowering medications can reduce CAD mortality in patients with elevated lipid levels and in at-risk patients with normal lipid levels. Patients with elevated cholesterol levels should be monitored for adherence to the therapeutic plan, the effect of cholesterol-lowering medications, and the development of side effects. Lipid levels are obtained and adjustments made to the diet and medication every 6 weeks until the lipid goal or maximum dose is achieved and then every 6 months thereafter (Morris, Ballantyne, Birtcher, Dunn, & Urbina, 2014). Lifestyle changes need to be incorporated into any treatment regimen and include:

- Dietary measures include a heart-healthy diet (monitor and treat hyperlipidemia if dietary control is not enough).
  - Increase physical activity;150 minutes of moderate exercise weekly (i.e., brisk walking) or about 75 minutes of vigorous exercise weekly (i.e., running) (Ridker, Libby, & Buring, 2015)
- Smoking cessation (people who stop smoking reduce their risk of heart disease 30% to 50% within the first year, and the risk continues to decline thereafter)
- Stress management
- HTN management
- Diabetes management

Managing Hypertension

The risk of CVD increases as blood pressure increases. Elevated blood pressure may result in increased stiffness of the vessel walls, leading to vessel injury and a resulting inflammatory response within the intima. Inflammatory mediators then lead to the release of growth-promoting factors that cause vessel hypertrophy and hyperresponsiveness. These changes result in acceleration and aggravation of atherosclerosis. HTN also increases the work of the left ventricle, which must pump harder to eject blood into the arteries. Over time, the increased workload causes the heart to enlarge and thicken and may, eventually, lead to cardiac failure.

Early detection of high blood pressure and adherence to a therapeutic regimen can prevent the serious consequences associated with untreated elevated blood pressure. HTN is discussed in detail in Chapter 13.

Controlling Diabetes Mellitus

The relationship between diabetes mellitus and heart disease has been confirmed. Patients with diabetes are two to four times more likely than nondiabetic patients to experience development of CVD (Ferri, 2016). And diabetes is considered equivalent to existing CAD as a risk factor for a secondary cardiac event (Lackland et al., 2012). For 50% to 75% of patients with diabetes, CVD is identified as the cause of death (Grossman & Porth, 2014).

Hyperglycemia fosters dyslipidemia, increased platelet aggregation, and altered red blood cell function, which can lead to thrombus formation. Effective treatment with appropriate anti-hyperglycemic agents and diet has shown improvement in endothelial function and improved endothelial-dependent dilation (Strain & Smith, 2016). Thus, control of diabetes is essential in preventing or modulating the development of CAD. Diabetes is discussed in detail in Chapter 30.

Unfolding Patient Stories: Carl Shapiro • Part 1

Carl Shapiro, who has a family history of atherosclerotic CVD, is diagnosed with HTN and hyperlipidemia during a routine visit to his primary provider. He is overweight, smokes a half pack of cigarettes per day, and describes his job as stressful. What questions can the nurse ask Carl Shapiro to help develop a plan for patient education? What topics are important for the nurse to address, and how can the information be presented? (Carl Shapiro's story continues in Chapter 56.)

Care for Carl and other patients in a realistic virtual environment: ***vSim*** *for Nursing* (thepoint.lww.com/vSimMedicalSurgical). Practice documenting these patients' care in (thepoint.lww.com/DocuCareEHR).

ANGINA PECTORIS

Angina pectoris is a clinical syndrome usually characterized by episodes or paroxysms of pain, pressure, or discomfort in the chest, jaw, shoulder, back, or arm that is caused by myocardial ischemia (Ferri, 2016). The cause is insufficient coronary blood flow (usually caused by atherosclerotic disease), resulting in a decreased oxygen supply when there is increased myocardial demand for oxygen in response to physical exertion or emotional stress. In other words, the demand for oxygen exceeds the supply. The severity of angina is based on the precipitating activity and its effect on activities of daily living. Types of angina are listed in Box 14-2.

Pathophysiology

Angina is usually caused by atherosclerotic disease. Almost invariably, angina is associated with a significant obstruction

Types of Angina

- *Stable angina:* Predictable and consistent pain that occurs on exertion and is relieved by rest
- *Unstable angina* (also called preinfarction angina or crescendo angina): Symptoms occur more frequently and last longer than in stable angina. The threshold for pain is lower, and pain may occur at rest.
- *Intractable or refractory angina:* Severe incapacitating chest pain
- *Variant angina* (also called **Prinzmetal's angina**): Pain at rest with reversible ST-segment elevation; thought to be caused by coronary artery vasospasm
- *Silent ischemia:* Objective evidence of ischemia (such as electrocardiogram changes with a stress test), but patient reports no symptoms

of a major coronary artery. Normally, the myocardium extracts a large amount of oxygen from the coronary circulation to meet its continuous demands. When there is an increase in demand, flow through the coronary arteries needs to be increased. When there is blockage in a coronary artery, flow cannot be increased, and ischemia results. Because angina is a symptom of coronary atherosclerosis, the risk factors are the same.

Clinical Manifestations and Assessment

Ischemia of the heart muscle may produce pain or other symptoms, varying in severity from mild indigestion to a choking or heavy sensation in the upper chest that ranges from discomfort to agonizing pain accompanied by severe apprehension and a feeling of impending death. Typically, the pain or discomfort is poorly localized and may radiate to the neck, jaw, shoulders, and inner aspects of the upper arms, usually the left arm. The patient often feels tightness or a heavy, choking, or strangling sensation that has a vise-like, insistent quality. The patient with diabetes mellitus may not have severe pain with angina because diabetic neuropathy can dull the perception of pain. A woman may have different symptoms than a man, because coronary disease in women tends to be more diffuse and affects long segments of the artery rather than discrete segments. Table 14-2 discusses anginal pain.

The nurse is alert for complaints of unusual fatigue; weakness or numbness in the arms, wrists, and hands; SOB; pallor; diaphoresis; anxiety; dizziness or lightheadedness; and nausea and vomiting that may accompany the pain (called *associated signs and symptoms*). Angina may subside with rest or nitroglycerin. In many patients, anginal symptoms follow a stable, predictable pattern.

The diagnosis of angina begins with the patient's history related to the clinical manifestations of ischemia. A 12-lead electrocardiogram (ECG) and blood laboratory biomarker values help in making the diagnosis. The patient may undergo an exercise or pharmacologic stress test in which the heart is monitored by ECG, echocardiogram, or both. The patient may also be referred for a nuclear scan or invasive procedure (e.g., cardiac catheterization, coronary artery angiography).

Medical Management

The objectives of the medical management of CAD and angina are to decrease the oxygen demand of the myocardium and to increase the oxygen supply. Medically, these objectives are met through pharmacologic therapy and control of risk factors. Alternatively, reperfusion procedures

TABLE 14-2 Assessing Angina

Acronym	Factors About Pain That Need To Be Assessed	Assessment Questions
P	Position/Location Provocation/Palliation	"Where is the pain? Can you point to it?" "What were you doing when the pain began?" "What makes it worse?" "What makes it better?"
Q	Quality Quantity	"How would you describe the pain?" "Is it like any pain you had before?" "Has the pain been constant?"
R	Radiation	"Can you feel the pain anywhere else?"
S	Severity Symptoms	"How would you rate the pain on a 0–10 scale, with 0 being no pain and 10 being the most amount of pain?" (or use visual analog scale or adjective rating scale) "Did you notice any other symptoms with the pain?" (such as nausea, vomiting, diaphoresis)
T	Timing	"How long ago did the pain start?"

Adapted from Bickley, L. S. (2013). *Bates' guide to physical examination and history taking* (11th ed.). Philadelphia, PA: Lippincott Williams & Wilkins.

may be used to restore the blood supply to the myocardium. These include PCI procedures (e.g., percutaneous transluminal coronary angioplasty [PTCA] with intracoronary stent placement, atherectomy) and CABG. PCI is currently the preferred method of treatment for patients with simple coronary artery lesions (Iqbal, Serruys, & Taggert, 2013).

Pharmacologic Therapy

Several types of drugs are used to treat coronary vascular disease:

- *Positive inotrope:* A medication that increases myocardial contractility (force of contraction)
- *Negative inotrope:* A medication that decreases myocardial contractility
- *Positive chronotrope:* A medication that increases heart rate
- *Negative chronotrope:* A medication that decreases heart rate

Nitrates

Nitrates remain the mainstay for treatment of coronary ischemia. A vasoactive agent (Nitroglycerin, Nitrostat, Nitrol, Nitro-Bid, Nitro-paste) is administered to reduce myocardial oxygen consumption, which decreases ischemia and relieves pain. Nitroglycerin dilates primarily the veins and, in higher doses, also the arteries. Dilation of the veins causes venous pooling of blood throughout the body. As a result, less blood returns to the heart, and filling pressure (preload) is reduced. If the patient is hypovolemic (does not have adequate circulating blood volume), the decrease in filling pressure can cause a significant decrease in CO and blood pressure; thus it is important for the nurse to monitor the patient's response to nitrates. Nitrates also relax the systemic arteriolar bed and increase oxygen supply, bringing about a more favorable balance between supply and demand.

Nursing Alert
The nurse must evaluate for hypotension before administering nitrates. Once hypotension is excluded, a sublingual nitroglycerin tablet is administered. Vital signs are monitored while evaluating for resolution of symptoms since even small doses can produce sudden hypotension and bradycardia. Usually this reaction can be reversed with intravenous atropine (Mega & Morrow, 2015).

When nitroglycerin is administered sublingually (SL), the patient's response is assessed (relief of chest pain and effect on blood pressure and heart rate). If the chest pain is unchanged or is lessened but still present, nitroglycerin SL administration is repeated up to a total of three doses. Each time, blood pressure, heart rate, and the ST segment (if the patient is on a monitor with ST-segment monitoring capability) are assessed. If the pain is significant and continues after

these interventions, the patient is evaluated further for acute MI and further intervention is necessary.

Nursing Alert
As with any medication, the nurse should always check the expiration dates on the bottle of nitroglycerin tablets.

Most patients with angina pectoris must self-administer nitroglycerin on an as-needed basis. A key nursing role in such cases is educating patients about the medication and how to take it (Box 14-3). SL nitroglycerin comes in tablet and spray forms.

Beta-Adrenergic Blocking Agents

Beta-blockers such as metoprolol (Lopressor, Toprol) and atenolol (Tenormin) reduce myocardial oxygen consumption by blocking beta-adrenergic sympathetic stimulation to the heart. The result is a reduction in heart rate, slowed conduction of impulses through the conduction system, decreased blood pressure, and reduced myocardial **contractility** (negative chronotrope and negative inotrope) to balance the myocardial oxygen needs (demands) and the amount of oxygen available (supply). This helps control chest pain and delays

---

BOX 14-3	**Patient Education**

Self-Administration of Nitroglycerin

- Instruct the patient to make sure the mouth is moist, the tongue is still, and saliva is not swallowed until the nitroglycerin tablet dissolves. Place the tablet under the tongue or between the cheek and gum, and let it dissolve.
- Advise the patient to carry the medication at all times as a precaution. However, because nitroglycerin is very unstable, it should be carried securely in its original container (e.g., capped, dark, glass bottle); tablets should never be removed and stored in metal or plastic pillboxes.
- Explain that nitroglycerin is volatile and is inactivated by heat, moisture, air, light, and time. Instruct the patient to renew the nitroglycerin supply every 6 months.
- Inform the patient that the medication should be taken in anticipation of any activity that may produce pain. Because nitroglycerin increases tolerance for exercise and stress when taken prophylactically (i.e., before angina-producing activity, such as exercise, stair-climbing, or sexual intercourse), it is best taken before pain develops.
- Recommend that the patient note how long it takes for the nitroglycerin to relieve the discomfort. Advise the patient that if pain persists after taking three sublingual tablets at 5-minute intervals, emergency medical services should be called.
- Discuss possible side effects of nitroglycerin, including flushing, throbbing headache, hypotension, and tachycardia.
- Advise the patient to sit down for a few minutes when taking nitroglycerin to avoid hypotension and syncope.

the onset of ischemia during work or exercise. Beta-blockers reduce the incidence of recurrent angina, infarction, and cardiac mortality. Patients taking beta-blockers are cautioned not to stop taking them abruptly because angina may worsen and MI may develop.

Calcium-Channel Blocking Agents

Calcium-channel blockers (calcium ion antagonists such as Norvasc, Cardizem) have a variety of effects. These agents decrease sinoatrial node automaticity and atrioventricular node conduction, resulting in a slower heart rate and a decrease in the strength of the heart muscle contraction (negative inotropic and negative chronotropic effects). These effects decrease the workload of the heart. Calcium-channel blockers also relax the blood vessels, causing a decrease in blood pressure and an increase in coronary artery perfusion. Calcium-channel blockers increase myocardial oxygen supply by dilating the smooth muscle wall of the coronary arterioles; they decrease myocardial oxygen demand by reducing systemic arterial pressure and the workload of the left ventricle. They may be prescribed to prevent and treat vasospasm (as in variant angina).

The calcium-channel blockers most commonly used are amlodipine (Norvasc) and diltiazem (Cardizem, Tiazac).

Antiplatelet and Anticoagulant Medications

Antiplatelet medications are administered to prevent platelet aggregation and subsequent thrombosis, which impedes blood flow. The patient receiving anticoagulation therapy should be monitored for signs and symptoms of external and internal bleeding, such as low blood pressure, increased heart rate, and decreased serum hemoglobin and hematocrit. The patient should be placed on bleeding precautions, which include:

- Applying pressure to the site of any needle puncture for a longer time than usual
- Avoiding intramuscular (IM) injections
- Avoiding tissue injury and bruising from trauma or use of constrictive devices (e.g., continuous use of an automatic blood pressure cuff)

Examples of antiplatelet and anticoagulant medications include aspirin, clopidogrel, heparin, and glycoprotein and IIb/IIIa inhibitors.

Aspirin prevents platelet activation and reduces the incidence of MI and death in patients with CAD.

Clopidogrel (Plavix) or ticlopidine (Ticlid) is given to patients who are allergic to aspirin or is given in addition to aspirin in patients at high risk for MI. Unlike aspirin, these medications take a few days to achieve their antiplatelet effect. They also may cause GI upset.

IV unfractionated heparin (UFH) prevents the formation of new blood clots. Treating patients with unstable angina with heparin reduces the occurrence of MI. A decrease in platelet count or evidence of thrombosis may indicate a serious complication called *heparin-induced thrombocytopenia* (HIT), an antibody-mediated reaction to heparin that may result in thrombosis. Patients who have received heparin within the past 3 months and those who have been receiving UFH for 5 to 15 days are at high risk for HIT.

> **Nursing Alert**
> *HIT is a complication of anticoagulation with UFH or low–molecular-weight heparin (LMWH). It is an immune-mediated disorder in which antibodies form against the heparin-platelet factor 4 complex. The antibody complex attaches to the platelet, causing its aggregation. The reticuloendothelial system destroys activated platelets, thus resulting in decreased platelet counts. Frequently, procoagulants are also generated, resulting in thrombosis. A complication of HIT is heparin-associated thrombocytopenia and thrombosis (HITT). In the presence of unexplained thrombocytopenia, or venous or arterial thrombosis associated with thrombocytopenia, HIT should be considered. Discontinuation of heparin as soon as diagnosis is suspected is warranted (Lee & Arepally, 2013).*

IV administration of glycoprotein (*GP*) *IIb/IIIa agents* (abciximab [ReoPro], tirofiban [Aggrastat], and eptifibatide [Integrilin]) is indicated for hospitalized patients with unstable angina and as adjunct therapy for PCI. These agents prevent platelet aggregation by blocking the GPIIb/IIIa receptors on the platelets, preventing adhesion of fibrinogen and other factors that cross-link platelets to each other and thereby would normally allow platelets to form a thrombus (clot). As with heparin, bleeding is the major side effect, and bleeding precautions should be initiated.

Oxygen Administration

Oxygen therapy is usually initiated at the onset of chest pain in an attempt to increase the amount of oxygen delivered to the myocardium and to decrease pain. Blood oxygen saturation is monitored by pulse oximetry; the normal oxygen saturation (SpO_2) level is greater than 95%.

Percutaneous Coronary Interventions

PCIs to treat angina and CAD most commonly include balloon angioplasty with intracoronary stent implantation. The patient in whom an acute MI is suspected may be referred for an immediate intervention, in which case the occluded coronary artery is opened and reperfusion to the area that had been deprived of oxygen is re-established. The duration of oxygen deprivation is directly related to the number of cells that die; therefore, the time from the patient's arrival in the emergency department to the time PCI is performed is critical and should be less than 60 minutes (time is muscle!). This is frequently referred to as *door-to-balloon time*,

"*DTB*," or "*time to device*." A cardiac catheterization laboratory and staff must be available 24 hours a day, 7 days a week if an emergent PCI is to be performed within this short time.

> **Nursing Alert**
> *It is imperative that an accurate assessment of a patient's peripheral vascular system is documented preprocedurally. This data will be used to evaluate postoperative vascular status. The assessment should include extremities color, sensation, temperature, capillary refill, and peripheral perfusion using the grading scale common to the nurse's institution. The affected extremity is assessed every 15 minutes for the first hour and then according to hospital protocol.*

Diagnostic Cardiac Catheterization and Percutaneous Coronary Intervention

A cardiac catheterization is a diagnostic procedure carried out in the cardiac catheterization laboratory where a vascular catheter is inserted in an artery (mostly radial or femoral) and threaded through your blood vessels to your heart; dye that is seen on fluoroscopy (x-ray) is then injected, and the structures of the heart and the patency of the coronary arteries are visualized. Coronary vessels with blockages are definitively identified, and often during the same procedure, are opened by a PCI. During PCI, the vascular catheter that is balloon-tipped is used to open blocked coronary arteries. Most often a stent is then deployed to maintain patency of the artery. PCI is used in patients with angina and as an intervention for acute MI. Catheter-based interventions can also be used to open blocked CABGs.

PCI is used more often now than ever before; it is the fifth most common procedure carried out yearly in the United States (Mullin, 2014). Hollow catheters called *sheaths* are inserted usually via the radial or femoral artery and occasionally the brachial artery. Catheters are then threaded through the sheaths, up through the aorta, and into the coronary arteries. Angiography is performed using injected radiopaque contrast agents (commonly called *dye*) to identify the location and extent of the blockage. A balloon-tipped dilation catheter is passed through the sheath and positioned over the lesion. The physician determines the catheter position by examining markers on the balloon that can be seen with fluoroscopy. When the catheter is positioned properly, the balloon is inflated with high pressure for several seconds and then deflated. The pressure compresses and possibly "cracks" the atheroma (Fig. 14-5). The media and adventitia of the coronary artery are also stretched. The appropriate stent is then put into place to keep the artery open (see Fig. 14-6).

> **Nursing Alert**
> *It is critical that an "Allen's test" is assessed pre-intervention to ensure ulnar arterial flow*

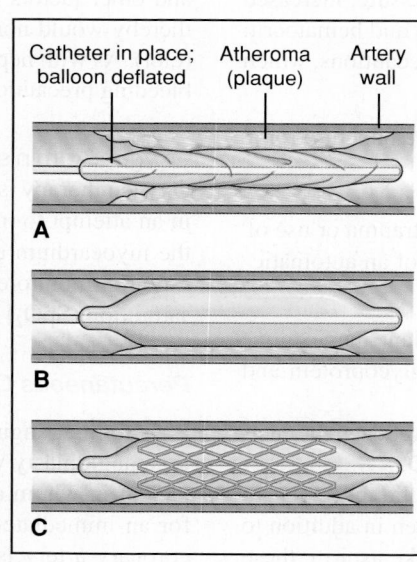

Catheter in place; balloon deflated — Atheroma (plaque) — Artery wall

A

B

C

FIGURE 14-5 Percutaneous coronary intervention. **A.** A balloon-tipped catheter is passed into the affected coronary artery and placed across the area of the atheroma (plaque). **B.** The balloon is then rapidly inflated and deflated with controlled pressure. **C.** A stent is placed to maintain patency of the artery, and the balloon is removed.

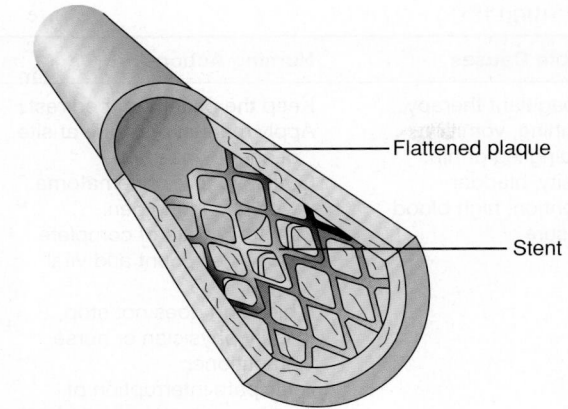

FIGURE 14-6 Vascular stent.

to the hand since adequacy will permit a radial artery approach for a PCI procedure (refer to Chapter 12). The radial approach provides direct access to the ascending aorta and allows for immediate mobilization following PCI.

Several inflations and several balloon sizes may be required to achieve the goal, usually defined as an improvement in blood flow and a residual stenosis of less than 20%. Other measures of the success of a PCI are an increase in the artery's lumen, a difference of less than 20 mm Hg in blood pressure from one side of the lesion to the other, and no clinically obvious arterial trauma. Because the blood supply to the coronary artery decreases while the balloon is inflated, the patient may complain of chest pain and the ECG may display significant ST-segment changes. Intracoronary stents are usually positioned in the intima of the vessel to maintain patency after the balloon is withdrawn. PCI procedures have a success rate of greater than 95%; the only exception is a chronic total coronary (100%) obstruction of the lumen, where the ability to negotiate a guidewire through the blockage is only about 50% to 90% (and varies substantially with the operator's expertise) (Teirstein & Lytle, 2016). Refer to Table 14-3 for complications after PCI.

Coronary Artery Stent

After PCI, the area that has been treated may potentially close off partially or completely, a process called *restenosis*. The intima of the coronary artery has been injured and responds by initiating an acute inflammatory process. This process may include release of mediators that lead to vasoconstriction, clotting, and scar tissue formation. A coronary artery stent is placed to overcome these risks. Restenosis happens in 10% to 50% of patients with PCI after balloon angioplasty *without* stenting, usually within 6 months (Teirstein & Lytle, 2016). A **stent** is a metal mesh that provides structural support to a vessel at risk of acute closure. Either bare metal or "drug eluting" stents are used; there are guidelines in place to aid in determining which the cardiologist should choose.

Stents have been shown to improve long-term outcomes of PCI (Grossman & Porth, 2014). The stent is positioned over the angioplasty balloon. When the balloon is inflated, the mesh expands and presses against the vessel wall, holding the artery open. The balloon is withdrawn, but the stent is left permanently in place within the artery; eventually endothelium covers the stent, and it is incorporated into the vessel wall. Because of the risk of thrombus formation in the stent, the patient receives antiplatelet medications (examples are clopidogrel [Plavix] and aspirin). These medications are routinely continued for at least 3 to 6 months to decrease the risk of thrombus formation.

Complications that can occur during a PCI procedure include dissection, perforation, abrupt closure, or vasospasm of the coronary artery; acute MI; acute arrhythmias (e.g., ventricular tachycardia); and cardiac arrest. These may require emergency surgical treatment. Complications after the procedure may include abrupt closure of the coronary artery and vascular complications, such as bleeding at the insertion site, retroperitoneal bleeding, hematoma, pseudoaneurysm, arteriovenous fistula, or arterial thrombosis and distal embolization, as well as acute kidney failure. Risk factors for the aforementioned complications include older age, female gender, larger vascular sheath size, low BMI, renal insufficiency, and degree of anticoagulation during the procedure (Mauri & Bhatt, 2015).

Nursing Alert

Severe kidney failure is associated with post-PCI procedural mortality and is directly related to the extent of the patient's baseline kidney disease (Mauri & Bhatt, 2016). Patients admitted with mild kidney dysfunction are at a higher risk for kidney failure and more adverse cardiac events (MACE) after PCI; therefore, monitoring of urinary output and renal function tests is particularly critical in this patient population. There is a 20% higher risk for death at 1 year following PCI than in those with preserved renal function (Mauri & Bhatt, 2016). The risk for nephropathy is dependent on the dose of contrast dye used and level of hydration. Ensuring adequate intravenous hydration surrounding the procedure can help protect against renal compromise.

Postprocedure Care

Patient care is similar to that for a cardiac catheterization. Many patients are admitted to the hospital the day of the PCI and discharged the next day; increasingly selected patients are treated as outpatients and released 6 to 12 hours after the procedure without an overnight stay (Teirstein & Lytle, 2016). When the PCI is performed emergently to relieve acute coronary syndrome (ACS), the patient will usually go to a critical care unit to be monitored closely for a slightly longer period of time. During the PCI, patients receive IV heparin and are monitored for signs of bleeding. Patients

TABLE 14-3 Complications After Percutaneous Coronary Intervention (PCI)

Complication	Signs and Symptoms	Possible Causes	Nursing Actions
Bleeding or hematoma	Expanding mass surrounding puncture site; hard lump or bluish tinge at sheath insertion site	Anticoagulant therapy, coughing, vomiting, bending leg or hip, obesity, bladder distention, high blood pressure	Keep the patient on bed rest. Apply manual pressure at site of sheath insertion. Outline extent of hematoma with a marking pen. Monitor results of complete blood cell count and vital signs. If bleeding does not stop, notify physician or nurse practitioner. Anticipate interruption of anticoagulant and antiplatelet therapies. Blood transfusion may be indicated.
Lost or weakened pulse distal to sheath insertion site	Extremity cool, cyanotic, pale, or painful	Arterial thrombus or embolus	Assess peripheral circulation by comparing bilateral pulses; note temperature, capillary refill, sensation, and movement, as well as color of the affected extremity. Notify physician or nurse practitioner. Anticipate surgery and anticoagulation or thrombolytic therapy.
Pseudoaneurysm and arteriovenous fistula; if they rupture, sudden massive swelling and severe pain will be seen.	A large painful pulsatile mass felt or bruit heard near sheath insertion site	Vessel trauma during procedure	Notify physician or nurse practitioner. Anticipate ultrasound-guided compression. If the pseudoaneurysm is small (less than 2 cm), it may be observed and monitored clinically. Assess circulation, sensation, and motility of involved extremity. Prepare patient for surgery to close fistula if indicated.
Retroperitoneal bleeding (blood collecting in the retroperitoneal space may not produce obvious swelling or skin color changes)	Back or flank pain Unexplained hypotension Tachycardia Restlessness and agitation Decreased hemoglobin/hematocrit Cullen sign (bluish to purplish periumbilical discoloration) and Grey Turner sign (flank discoloration) may be noted with retroperitoneal bleed (see Fig. 27-10 on page 843).	Arterial tear causing bleeding into flank area	Notify physician or nurse practitioner immediately. Stop any anticoagulation medication. Anticipate need for IV fluids and/or administration of blood.
Acute kidney failure	Decreased urine output, elevated blood urea nitrogen (BUN), creatinine	Nephrotoxic contrast agent	Provide hydration to promote excretion of contrast material. Monitor urine output. Monitor BUN and creatinine. Administer renal protective agents (e.g., acetylcysteine [Mucomyst] before and after procedure as prescribed.

Complication	Signs and Symptoms	Possible Causes	Nursing Actions
Allergic reaction	Urticaria, hives, sneezing, and bronchospasm	Allergic reaction to dye is higher in patients allergic to penicillin or shellfish and in those with known prior reaction to contrast material.	Anticipate administering prednisone, antihistamines, and H$_2$ blockers before the coronary procedure for patients with known prior reaction to contrast material or shellfish. If anaphylaxis occurs, the nurse anticipates administering epinephrine and IV saline for hydration.
Cardiac tamponade	Tachypnea, tachycardia, hypotension, jugular venous distention, and muffled heart sounds; cool extremities from hypoperfusion in some patients	Most common cause is perforation due to rupture of a coronary artery.	Anticipate a pericardiocentesis in patients with compromised hemodynamic status.
Chest pain/acute ischemic event/spasm	Complaints of chest pain	Benign stent sensation, acute stent thrombosis, abrupt vessel closure, transient coronary spasms, side branch occlusion, and distal embolization of debris	Notify the provider when patient complains of chest pain. Monitor vital signs, O$_2$ sat, and lung and cardiac sounds. Assess peripheral perfusion. Monitor electrocardiogram (ECG). Perform serial tests for cardiac markers. Measure troponin. Obtain a 12-lead ECG with any episodes of chest pain.

Adapted from Gomes, B. B. (2015). Care of the patient undergoing radial approach heart catheterization: Implications for medical-surgical nurses. *Medsurg Nursing, 24*(3), 173–176; Mullin, M. (2014). Transradial approach versus transfemoral approach for coronary angiography and coronary angioplasty. *Critical Care Nursing Quarterly, 37*(2), 159–169.

may also receive a GPIIb/IIIa agent (e.g., eptifibatide [Integrilin]) for several hours following the PCI to prevent platelet aggregation and thrombus formation in the coronary artery and stent. Hemostasis at the access site is achieved, and sheaths may be removed at the end of the procedure by using a vascular closure device (e.g., Angio-Seal, VasoSeal) or a device that sutures the vessels. Hemostasis after sheath removal may also be achieved by direct manual pressure, a mechanical compression device (e.g., C-shaped clamp), or a pneumatic compression device (e.g., FemoStop® or TR band®).

Occasionally, the patient may return to the nursing unit with the femoral or brachial vascular access sheaths in place. This may happen if there is a planned trip back to the catheterization lab or if the activated clotting time (ACT) is too high to remove the sheath safely. The sheaths are removed when blood studies (e.g., ACT) indicate that the heparin is no longer active and the clotting time is within an acceptable range. This usually takes a few hours, depending on the amount of heparin given during the procedure. As long as a sheath is in place, the patient must remain in bed and avoid bending the affected limb. The head of bed (HOB) is not elevated beyond 30 degrees if there is a femoral sheath in place. After the sheath removal, the patient maintains bed rest for 3 to 6 hours according to the hospital's policy. Sheath removal and the application of pressure on the vessel insertion site may cause the heart rate to slow and the blood pressure to decrease (vasovagal response). An IV bolus of atropine is usually given to treat this response. If the radial approach was used, the patient will have fewer restrictions on mobility but should not bend or put pressure on the affected area; the nurse should follow institutional policy for specific restrictions. Refer to Box 14-4 for care of patient after radial artery approach.

Some patients with unstable lesions and at high risk for abrupt vessel closure are restarted on heparin after sheath removal, or they receive an IV infusion of a GPIIb/IIIa inhibitor. These patients are monitored more closely and may recover more slowly.

Nursing Alert

Post PCI, IV fluids may be administered to promote excretion of the contrast medium. The nurse is alert for signs of fluid volume excess

BOX 14-4

Nursing Care After Cardiac Cath/PCI via Radial Approach

Assessment

- Monitor vital signs (including pulse oximetry*), neurovascular checks**, site and limb assessment per policy and/or provider's order (expect Q15 minutes x4, Q30 minutes x4, Q1 hour x4, and then Q4 hours or routine).
- Observe site for any bleeding, ecchymosis or hematoma. Observe appearance of skin under and around the compression device (i.e., TR band®).
- Avoid use of affected arm for blood pressure and blood draws for 24 hours.
- After a diagnostic cardiac catheterization, the TR band® is likely to remain in place for a minimum of 1 hour (follow provider's order).
- After an interventional procedure (angioplasty with stent placement) the TR band® is likely to remain in place for a minimum of 2 hours (follow provider's order).

*The Pulse oximetry probe should be on either the thumb or index finger of the affected hand because impaired radial artery circulation will be revealed in these digits.

**Neurovascular checks include color, temperature, sensation (presence or absence of numbness and tingling), pulses (radial and ulnar of the affected limb), and capillary refill.

Activity

- The patient may be out of bed with assistance (per provider's order) while the radial artery compression device is in place. Typically there is no restriction on head of bed elevation; the affected arm is kept straight and no pressure is applied to the limb. An ace wrap or an arm board can be applied to prevent wrist flexing. As noted above, avoid blood pressures and blood draws from the procedural arm for 24 hours.
- When removing the Radial compression device, the nurse should position the patient either in a bed or stretcher or in a chair that allows for elevation of legs in the event of a vagal response (drop in blood pressure and/or heart rate).

Reportable to the Provider

- Changes in sensation or pain in affected extremity, hematoma, bleeding, ecchymosis, blistering of the skin, appearance of mottling, absence of radial or ulnar pulse
- Any variance of the patient's vital signs

Patient and Family Education

- Report any symptoms of pain, numbness, or tingling in the affected extremity, as well as redness or streaking, swelling, and discharge from the site.
- For 24 hours after procedure, minimize manipulation of the affected wrist (no flexing), including no weight-bearing on wrist when rising from bed/chair. Elevating the affected arm and applying ice will promote comfort and decrease swelling.
- Do not drive.
- Remove occlusive dressing after 24 hours and leave open to air. If minor oozing occurs, apply dressing for 12 more hours; the site may be washed with mild soap and water. Avoid excess moisture to the access site, especially submerging the hand in water. and flexing the wrist for 72 hours after procedure.
- If bleeding should occur: sit down and hold pressure at the site for 10 minutes. If bleeding stops, sit with the wrist straight for 2 hours and notify the provider. If bleeding does not stop after 10 minutes or a large amount of bleeding is noted, call 911 and lie down. DO NOT drive yourself to the hospital.
- Avoid heavy lifting (over 5 lbs.).
- Do not operate heavy equipment.
- Avoid excessive wrist movement.
- Avoid vigorous exercise using arm.
- Plan for a follow-up appointment within 1 to 2 weeks; use the call-back number with 24-hour service if needed.

Adapted from Gomes, B. B. (2015). Care of the patient undergoing radial approach heart catheterization: Implications for medical-surgical nurses. *Medsurg Nursing, 24*(3), 173–176; Mullin, M. (2014). Transradial approach versus transfemoral approach for coronary angiography and coronary angioplasty. *Critical Care Nursing Quarterly, 37*(2), 159–169.

that may include complaints of SOB at rest or with exertion, orthopnea, paroxysmal nocturnal dyspnea, cough, development or increased crackles in the lungs, S_3 gallop, jugular vein distention (JVD), and pulsus alternans (characterized by alternating strong and weak peripheral pulses). Changes in vital signs will vary depending on whether CO is increased (HTN) or reduced (hypotension).

After hemostasis is achieved, a pressure dressing is applied to the site. Patients resume self-care and ambulate unassisted within a few hours of the procedure. The duration of immobilization depends on the size and location of the sheath inserted, the amount of anticoagulant administered, the method of hemostasis, the patient's underlying condition, and the physician's preference. On the day after the procedure, the site is inspected and the dressing replaced with an adhesive bandage. The nurse teaches the patient to monitor the site for bleeding or development of a hard mass indicative of hematoma. On discharge, heavy lifting is discouraged for several days if the femoral artery was used, and intense aerobic exercise is typically discouraged for 2 to 4 weeks (especially after stent implantation). There is usually no driving for 24 hours (Teirstein & Lytle, 2016).

Surgical Procedures: Coronary Artery Revascularization

Advances in diagnostics, medical management, and surgical and anesthesia techniques, as well as the care provided in critical care and surgical units, home care, and rehabilitation programs, have continued to make surgery a viable treatment option for patients with CAD. CABG has been done for nearly 50 years now, with techniques ever evolving and improving. CABG is a surgical procedure in which a blood vessel is grafted to the occluded coronary artery so that blood can flow beyond the occlusion; it is also called a bypass graft.

Major indications for CABG include:

- Alleviation of angina that cannot be controlled with medication or PCI
- Treatment of multivessel CAD and complicated lesions
- Prevention and treatment of MI, arrhythmias, or heart failure
- Treatment for complications from an unsuccessful PCI

The recommendation for CABG is determined by a number of factors, including the number of diseased coronary vessels, the location complexity of the lesions (blockages), the degree of left ventricular dysfunction, the presence of comorbidities, the patient's symptoms, and any previous treatment. CABG surgery remains the standard of care for patients with complex CAD, although technological advancements in both PCI and in CABG surgery make it difficult to compare these interventions historically. Cardiologists and cardiac surgeons work together to determine the most appropriate treatment for an individual patient (Iqbal et al., 2013).

For a patient to be considered for CABG, the coronary arteries to be bypassed must have approximately a 70% occlusion (60% if in the left main coronary artery). If significant blockage is not present, the flow through the artery will compete with the flow through the bypass, and circulation to the ischemic area of myocardium may not be improved. It is also necessary that the artery be patent beyond the area of blockage or the flow through the bypass will be impeded.

Vessels commonly used for CABG are the greater saphenous vein, followed by the lesser saphenous vein (other veins may also be used) as well as the internal thoracic arteries (Fig. 14-7). If a vein is be used, it is removed from its original location and grafted to the ascending aorta and to the coronary artery distal to the lesion. The saphenous veins are used in emergency CABG procedures because they can be obtained quickly by one surgeon while another performs the chest surgery. A common adverse effect of vein removal is edema in the extremity from which the vein was taken. The degree of edema varies and usually diminishes over time. Within 5 to 10 years, atherosclerotic changes often develop in saphenous vein grafts.

The right and left internal mammary arteries and, less frequently, the radial arteries are also used for CABG. Arterial grafts are preferred to venous grafts because they do not develop atherosclerotic changes as quickly and remain patent longer. The surgeon leaves the proximal end of the mammary artery intact and detaches the distal end of the artery

FIGURE 14-7 The greater and lesser saphenous veins are commonly used in bypass graft procedures.

from the chest wall. This end of the artery is then grafted to the coronary artery distal to the occlusion. The internal mammary arteries may not be long enough to use for multiple bypasses. Because of this, many CABG procedures are performed with a combination of venous (reversed segments of veins [reversed because of venous valves]) and arterial grafts.

After CABG, as many as 63% to 89% of patients develop pleural effusions (fluid collection within the pleural space) in the immediate postoperative period (Heffner, 2016), which is associated with a variety of etiologies, including accumulation of pleural fluid because of congestive heart failure, surgical tissue trauma, hemorrhage from harvesting of the IMA, postoperative atelectasis and diaphragmatic dysfunction, or chylothorax (lymphatic fluid in the pleural space) because of unintended thoracic duct injury during the operative event. Signs and symptoms vary based upon the etiology; however, the nurse is alert for dyspnea, cough, orthopnea (SOB when lying flat), splinting, dullness to percussion, decreased breath sounds, and decreased respiratory excursion on the affected side (for further details, refer to Chapter 10).

Coronary Artery Bypass Graft Surgery

Traditional Technique. The traditional CABG procedure is performed with the patient under general anesthesia. The surgeon makes a median sternotomy incision and connects the patient to the cardiopulmonary bypass (CPB) machine (discussed below). Next, a blood vessel from another part of the patient's body (e.g., saphenous vein, left internal mammary artery) is grafted distal to the coronary artery lesion, bypassing the obstruction (Fig. 14-8). Then CPB is discontinued,

FIGURE 14-8 Coronary artery bypass grafts. One or more procedures may be performed using various veins and arteries. **A.** Left internal mammary artery, used frequently because of its functional longevity. **B.** Saphenous vein, also used as bypass graft.

isotonic crystalloid solution (usually 5% dextrose in lactated Ringer's solution). Venous blood removed from the body by the cannula is filtered, oxygenated, cooled or warmed by the machine, and then returned to the body. The cannula used to return the oxygenated blood is usually inserted in the ascending aorta, or it may be inserted in the femoral artery. The heart is stopped by the injection of cardioplegia solution, which is high in potassium, into the coronary arteries. The patient receives heparin to prevent clotting and thrombus formation in the bypass circuit when blood comes in contact with the foreign surfaces of the tubing. At the end of the procedure, when the patient is disconnected from the bypass machine, protamine sulfate is administered to reverse the effects of heparin.

During the procedure, hypothermia is maintained, usually 28° to 32°C (82.4° to 89.6°F). The blood is cooled during CPB and returned to the body. The cooled blood slows the body's basal metabolic rate, thereby decreasing the demand for oxygen. Cooled blood usually has a higher viscosity, but the crystalloid solution used to prime the bypass tubing dilutes the blood. When the surgical procedure is completed, the blood is rewarmed as it passes through the CPB circuit. Urine output, arterial blood gases (ABGs), electrolytes, and coagulation studies are monitored to assess the patient's status during CPB.

chest tubes and epicardial pacing wires are placed, and the incision is closed. Next, the patient is admitted to a critical care unit and typically stays for about 24 hours before being transferred to the step-down unit.

Many cardiac surgical procedures are possible because of CPB (i.e., extracorporeal circulation) (Fig. 14-9). The procedure mechanically circulates and oxygenates blood for the body while bypassing the heart and lungs. CPB maintains perfusion to body organs and tissues, and allows the surgeon to complete the anastomoses in a motionless, bloodless surgical field.

CPB is accomplished by placing a cannula in the right atrium, vena cava, or femoral vein to withdraw blood from the body. The cannula is connected to tubing filled with an

Alternate Technique. Another type of CABG procedure often done today is the "off pump" CABG or "OPCAB." The potential benefits of OPCAB include a decrease in the incidence of stroke and other neurologic complications, reduced blood usage, less kidney failure, and fewer cardiac rhythm disturbances. Also done today is the "MIDCAB," or minimally invasive coronary artery bypass surgery. The MIDCAB is performed on a beating heart via a thoracotomy incision and is only suitable for certain lesions that are located in the

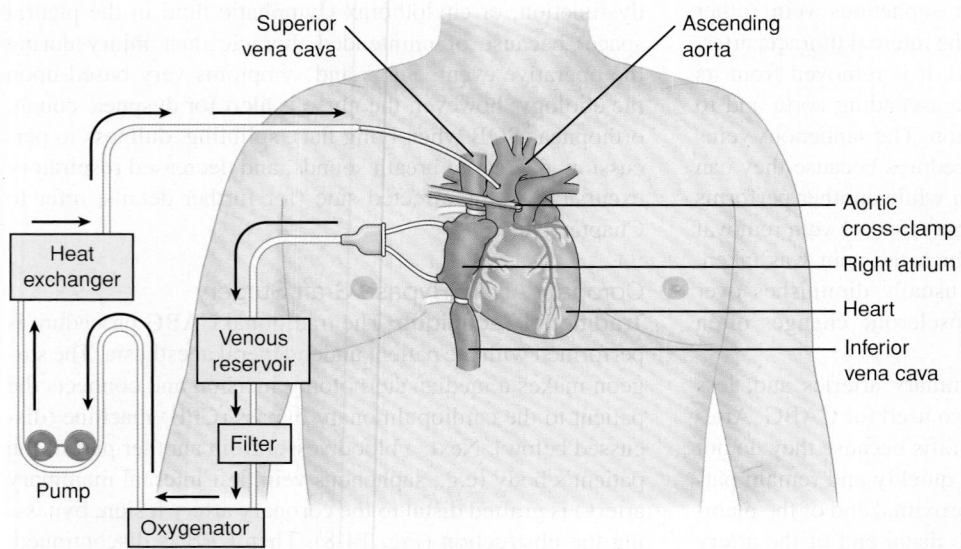

FIGURE 14-9 The cardiopulmonary bypass (CPB) system, in which cannulas are placed through the right atrium into the superior and inferior vena cavae to divert blood from the body and into the bypass system. The pump system creates a vacuum, pulling blood into the venous reservoir. The blood is cleared of air bubbles, clots, and particulates by the filter and then is passed through the oxygenator, releasing carbon dioxide and obtaining oxygen. Next, the blood is pulled to the pump and pushed out to the heat exchanger, where its temperature is regulated. Then the blood is returned to the body via the ascending aorta.

arteries on the anterior portions of the heart. Patients undergoing any type of CABG surgery will go to the intensive care unit for approximately 24 hours, and then transfer to the step-down unit. The average overall hospital stay for CABG surgery is anticipated at 5 days.

Complications of Coronary Artery Bypass Graft

CABG may result in complications such as MI, arrhythmias, hemorrhage, and kidney dysfunction. Table 14-4 presents an

overview of the potential complications in the postoperative cardiac surgical patient. Although most patients improve symptomatically following surgery, CABG is not a cure for CAD, and angina, exercise intolerance, or other symptoms experienced before CABG may recur. Medications required before surgery may need to be continued. Lifestyle modifications recommended before surgery remain important to treat the underlying CAD and for the continued viability of the newly implanted grafts.

TABLE 14-4 Potential Complications of Cardiac Surgery

Complication	Description	Assessment and Management
Cardiac Complications **Decreased Cardiac Output**		
Hypovolemia (most common cause of decreased cardiac output after cardiac surgery)	• Net loss of blood and intravascular volume • Surgical hypothermia (as the reduced body temperature rises after surgery, blood vessels dilate and more volume is needed to fill the vessels). • IV fluid loss to the interstitial spaces because surgery and anesthesia make capillary beds more permeable. • Increased heart rate, arterial hypotension, low pulmonary artery wedge pressure (PAWP), and low central venous pressures (CVP) often are seen.	• Fluid replacement may be prescribed. Replacement fluids include: Colloid (albumin, heta-starch), packed red blood cells, or crystalloid solution (normal saline, lactated Ringer's solution).
Persistent bleeding	• Cardiopulmonary bypass may cause platelet dysfunction, and hypothermia alters clotting mechanisms. • Surgical trauma causing tissues and blood vessels to ooze bloody drainage. • Intraoperative anticoagulant (heparin) therapy • Postoperative coagulopathy may also result from liver dysfunction and depletion of clotting components.	• Accurate measurement of wound bleeding and chest tube blood is essential. Bloody drainage should not exceed 200 mL/hr for the first 4 to 6 hours. Drainage should decrease and stop within a few days, while progressing from sanguineous to seros anguineous and serous drainage. • Protamine sulfate may be administered to neutralize unfractionated heparin; vitamin K and blood products may be used to treat hematologic deficiencies. • If bleeding persists, the patient may return to the operating room.
Cardiac tamponade	• Fluid and clots accumulate in the pericardial sac, which compresses the heart, preventing blood from filling the ventricles. • Signs and symptoms include arterial hypotension, tachycardia, muffled heart sounds, decreasing urine output, and ↑ CVP. Additional signs and symptoms: arterial pressure waveform demonstrating a pulsus paradoxus (decrease of more than 10 mm Hg during inspiration) and decreased chest tube drainage (suggesting that the drainage is trapped or clotted in the mediastinum).	• The chest drainage system is checked to eliminate possible kinks or obstructions in the tubing. • Patency of the tubing in the chest drainage system must be maintained, the nurse can facilitate movement of the fluid by adjusting the position of the tubing therefore helping with forward flow. • Chest x-ray may show a widening mediastinum. • Emergency medical management is required; may include pericardiocentesis or return to surgery.
Fluid overload	• High PAWP, CVP, and pulmonary artery diastolic pressures, as well as crackles indicate fluid overload.	• Diuretics are prescribed and the rate of IV fluid administration is reduced. • Alternative treatments include continuous renal replacement therapy and dialysis.
Hypothermia	• Low body temperature leads to vasoconstriction, shivering, and arterial hypertension.	• Patient is rewarmed gradually after surgery, decreasing vasoconstriction.

(continued on page 438)

TABLE **14-4** Potential Complications of Cardiac Surgery (*continued*)

Complication	Description	Assessment and Management
Hypertension	• Results from postoperative vasoconstriction. It may stretch suture lines and cause postoperative bleeding. The condition may be transient.	• Vasodilators (nitroglycerin [Tridil], nitroprusside [Nipride, Nitropress]) may be used to treat hypertension. Administer cautiously to avoid hypotension.
Tachyarrhythmias	• Increased heart rate is common with perioperative volume changes. Uncontrolled atrial fibrillation commonly occurs during the first few days postoperatively.	• If a tachyarrhythmia is the primary problem, the heart rhythm is assessed and medications (e.g., adenosine [Adenocard, Adenoscan], amiodarone [Cordarone], digoxin [Lanoxin], diltiazem [Cardizem], esmolol [Brevibloc], lidocaine [Xylocaine], procainamide [Pronestyl]), may be prescribed. Patients may be prescribed antiarrhythmics before coronary artery bypass graft (CABG) to minimize the risk of postoperative tachyarrhythmias. • Carotid massage may be performed by a provider to assist with diagnosing or treating the arrhythmia. • Cardioversion and defibrillation are alternatives for symptomatic tachyarrhythmias. • For patients who cannot attain normal sinus rhythm, an alternate goal may be to establish a stable rhythm that produces a sufficient cardiac output.
Bradycardias	• Decreased heart rate	• Many postoperative patients will have temporary pacer wires that can be attached to a pulse generator (pacemaker) to stimulate the heart to beat faster. Less commonly, atropine, epinephrine, or isoproterenol may be used to increase heart rate.
Cardiac failure (decreased cardiac output)	• Myocardial contractility may be decreased perioperatively.	• The nurse observes for and reports falling mean arterial pressure; rising PAWP, pulmonary artery diastolic pressure, and CVP; increasing tachycardia; restlessness and agitation; peripheral cyanosis; venous distention; labored respirations; and edema. • Medical management includes diuretics, digoxin, and IV inotropic agents.
MI (may occur intraoperatively or postoperatively)	• Portion of the cardiac muscle dies; therefore, contractility decreases. Impaired ventricular wall motion further decreases cardiac output. Symptoms may be masked by the postoperative surgical discomfort or the anesthesia–analgesia regimen.	• Careful assessment to determine the type of pain the patient is experiencing; myocardial infarction (MI) suspected if the mean blood pressure is low with normal preload. • Serial electrocardiograms (ECGs) and cardiac biomarkers assist in making the diagnosis (alterations may be due to the surgical intervention). Analgesics are prescribed in small amounts while the patient's blood pressure and respiratory rate are monitored (because vasodilation secondary to analgesics or decreasing pain may occur and compound the hypotension). • Activity progression depends on the patient's activity tolerance.
Pulmonary Complications		
Impaired gas exchange	• During and after anesthesia, patients require mechanical assistance to breathe. • Potential exists for postoperative atelectasis. • Anesthetic agents stimulate production of mucus, and chest incision pain may decrease the effectiveness of ventilation.	• Pulmonary complications are often detected during assessment of breath sounds, oxygen saturation levels, arterial blood gases, and when monitoring peak pressure and exhaled tidal volumes on the ventilator. • Extended periods of mechanical ventilation may be required while complications are treated.

Complication	Description	Assessment and Management
Fluid Volume Complications		
Hemorrhage	• Untoward and excessive bleeding may be life-threatening.	• Serial hemoglobin, hematocrit, and coagulation studies are performed to guide therapy. • Administration of fluids, colloids, and blood products: packed red blood cells, fresh frozen plasma, platelet concentrate. • Administration of aprotinin (Trasylol) perioperatively to reduce blood transfusion needs. • Administration of desmopressin acetate (DDAVP) to enhance platelet function.
Neurologic Complications		
Neurologic changes; stroke	• Inability to follow simple commands within 6 hours of recovery from anesthetic; different capabilities on right or left side of body	• Neurologically, most patients begin to recover from anesthesia in the operating room. • Patients who are elderly or who have kidney or hepatic failure may take longer to recover. • Patient should be evaluated for stroke when neurologic changes are evident.
Kidney Failure and Electrolyte Imbalance		
Kidney failure	• Usually acute and resolves within 3 months but may become chronic and require ongoing dialysis	• May respond to diuretics or may require continuous renal replacement therapy (CRRT) or dialysis
Acute kidney Injury	• Often results from hypoperfusion of the kidneys or from injury to the renal tubules by nephrotoxic medications	• Fluids, electrolytes, BUN, creatinine, and urine output are monitored frequently. Follow your medical center's protocol for postprocedure hydration
Electrolyte imbalance	• Postoperative imbalances in potassium, magnesium, sodium, calcium, and blood glucose are related to surgical losses, metabolic changes, and the administration of medications and IV fluids.	• Monitor electrolytes and basic metabolic studies frequently. • Implement treatment to correct electrolyte imbalance promptly
Other Complications		
Hepatic failure	• Most common in patients with cirrhosis, hepatitis, or prolonged right-sided heart failure	• Use of medications metabolized by the liver must be minimized. • Bilirubin, albumin, and amylase levels are monitored, and nutritional support must be provided.
Infection	• Surgery and anesthesia alter the patient's immune system. Many invasive devices are used to monitor and support the patient's recovery and may serve as a source of infection.	• The following must be monitored to detect signs of possible infection: body temperature, white blood cell (WBC) counts and differential counts, incision and puncture sites, cardiac output and systemic vascular resistance, urine (clarity, color, and odor), bilateral breath sounds, sputum (color, odor, amount), as well as nasogastric secretions. • Antibiotic therapy may be expanded or modified as necessary. • Invasive devices must be discontinued as soon as they are no longer required. Institutional protocols for maintaining and replacing invasive lines and devices must be followed to minimize the patient's risk for infection.

Note: The patient may require interventions for more than one complication at a time. Collaboration among nurses, physicians, pharmacists, respiratory therapists, and dietitians is necessary to achieve the desired patient outcomes.

NURSING PROCESS
The Postoperative Cardiac Surgery Patient

Initial postoperative care focuses on achieving or maintaining hemodynamic stability and recovery from general anesthesia. Care will be provided in the PACU or intensive care unit, with the patient transferred to the step-down or progressive care unit usually within 24 hours. Care focuses on the monitoring of cardiopulmonary status, pain management, wound care, progressive activity, and nutrition. Education about medications and risk factor modification is emphasized. Discharge from the hospital may occur 3 to 5 days after CABG in patients without complications.

The immediate postoperative period for the patient who has undergone cardiac surgery presents many challenges to the health care team. Specific information about the surgical procedure and important factors about postoperative management are communicated by the surgical team and anesthesia personnel to the critical care nurse, who then assumes responsibility for the patient's care. A plan of nursing care for the patient after cardiac surgery is available online at http://thepoint.lww.com/Honan2e.

ASSESSMENT

In the critical care environment, a complete assessment of all systems is performed hourly for at least 12 hours to determine the postoperative status of the patient compared with the preoperative baseline and to identify anticipated changes since surgery. The following parameters are assessed:

- *Neurologic status:* Level of responsiveness, pupil size and reaction to light, reflexes, facial symmetry, movement and strength of upper and lower extremities
- *Cardiac/hemodynamic status:* Heart rate and rhythm, heart sounds, pacemaker status, arterial blood pressure, central venous pressure (CVP), pulmonary artery pressure, pulmonary artery wedge pressure (PAWP), waveforms from the invasive blood pressure lines, cardiac output (CO) or index, systemic and pulmonary vascular resistance, pulmonary artery oxygen saturation (SvO_2), and bleeding (from mediastinal chest tubes). Refer to Chapter 55 for a detailed description of hemodynamic monitoring.
- *Respiratory status:* Chest movement, breath sounds, ventilator settings, respiratory rate, peak inspiratory pressure, arterial oxygen saturation (SaO_2), percutaneous oxygen saturation (SpO_2), end-tidal CO_2, ABGs
- *Peripheral vascular status:* Peripheral pulses; color of skin, nail beds, mucosa, lips, and earlobes; skin temperature; edema; condition of dressings and invasive lines
- *Kidney function:* Urinary output; urine-specific gravity and osmolality may be assessed, serum blood urea nitrogen (BUN) and creatinine
- *Fluid and electrolyte status:* Intake, output from all drainage tubes, all CO parameters, mucous membranes, skin turgor, presence of edema, and analysis of laboratory values including electrolytes, calcium, and magnesium
- *Pain:* Nature, type, location, and duration (incisional pain must be differentiated from anginal pain); apprehension; response to analgesics

Assessment also includes observing all equipment and tubes to determine whether they are functioning properly (Fig. 14-10).

As the patient regains consciousness and progresses through the postoperative period, the nurse also assesses indicators of psychological and emotional status. The patient may exhibit behavior that reflects denial or depression or may experience postcardiotomy delirium. Characteristic signs of delirium include transient perceptual illusions, visual and auditory hallucinations, disorientation, and paranoid delusions.

DIAGNOSIS

Appropriate nursing diagnoses of the patient recovering from cardiac surgery may include:

- Decreased CO/tissue perfusion
- Fluid volume and electrolyte imbalance
- Impaired gas exchange
- Impaired cerebral circulation
- Pain

PLANNING

The goal after CABG surgery is to maintain hemodynamic stability, adequate gas exchange, fluid volume balance, and cerebral perfusion. As the patient progresses toward hospital discharge, patient education and activity progression must be included in the plan of care.

NURSING INTERVENTIONS

RESTORING CARDIAC OUTPUT

To evaluate the patient's cardiac status, the nurse primarily determines the effectiveness of the CO through clinical observations and routine measurements: serial readings of blood pressure, heart rate, CVP, arterial pressure, and pulmonary artery pressures.

Kidney function is related to cardiac function as blood pressure and heart rate drive glomerular filtration; therefore, urinary output is measured and recorded. Urine output of less than 30 mL/hr or 0.5 mL/kg/hr may indicate a decrease in CO. Body tissues depend on adequate CO to provide a continuous supply of oxygenated blood to meet the changing demands of the organs and body systems. Because the buccal mucosa, nail beds, lips, and earlobes are sites with rich capillary beds, they should be observed for cyanosis or duskiness as possible signs of reduced CO. The nurse notes distention of the neck veins along with an elevated CVP, signaling right-sided heart failure. Generally, if cardiac output has decreased, the skin becomes cool, moist, and cyanotic or mottled.

Arrhythmias may develop when perfusion of the heart is poor. Common arrhythmias encountered during the

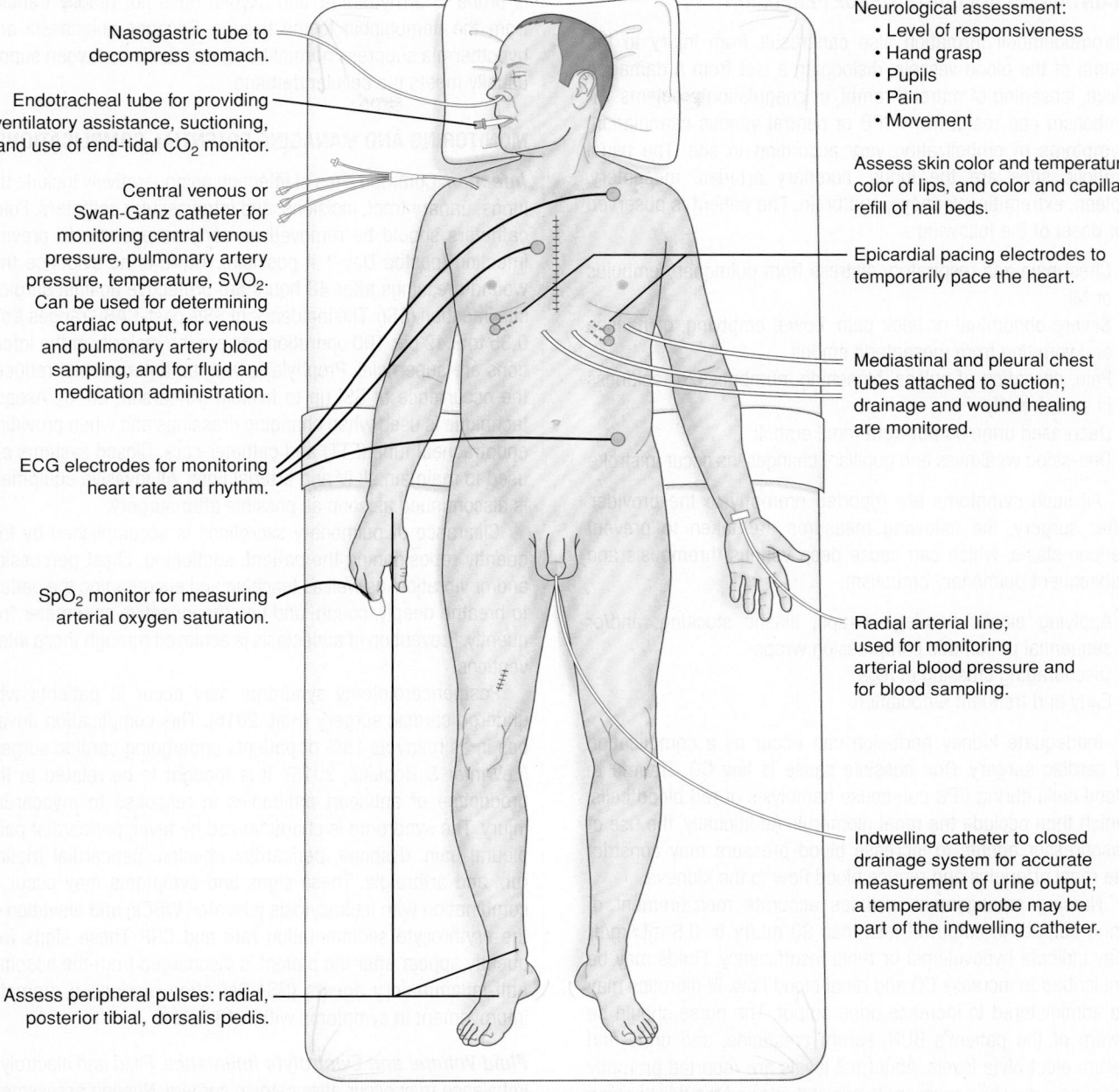

Nasogastric tube to decompress stomach.

Endotracheal tube for providing ventilatory assistance, suctioning, and use of end-tidal CO_2 monitor.

Central venous or Swan-Ganz catheter for monitoring central venous pressure, pulmonary artery pressure, temperature, SVO_2. Can be used for determining cardiac output, for venous and pulmonary artery blood sampling, and for fluid and medication administration.

ECG electrodes for monitoring heart rate and rhythm.

SpO_2 monitor for measuring arterial oxygen saturation.

Assess peripheral pulses: radial, posterior tibial, dorsalis pedis.

Neurological assessment:
• Level of responsiveness
• Hand grasp
• Pupils
• Pain
• Movement

Assess skin color and temperature, color of lips, and color and capillary refill of nail beds.

Epicardial pacing electrodes to temporarily pace the heart.

Mediastinal and pleural chest tubes attached to suction; drainage and wound healing are monitored.

Radial arterial line; used for monitoring arterial blood pressure and for blood sampling.

Indwelling catheter to closed drainage system for accurate measurement of urine output; a temperature probe may be part of the indwelling catheter.

FIGURE 14-10 Postoperative care of the cardiac surgical patient requires the nurse to be proficient in interpreting hemodynamics, correlating physical assessments with laboratory results, sequencing interventions, and evaluating progress toward desired outcomes.

postoperative period are atrial fibrillation (Afib), bradycardias, tachycardias, and ectopic beats. Afib is one of the most frequently encountered arrhythmias of CABG, occurring in up to 40% of patients, typically within 2 to 3 days (Morrow & Boden, 2015). Afib increases the risk of clot formation and embolization (two- to threefold increase in incidence of postoperative stroke); therefore, patients at risk for this arrhythmia may be prescribed prophylactic beta-blocking agents (Morrow & Boden, 2015). Risk factors for developing postoperative Afib are older, hypertensive, previous Afib, and heart

failure. Epicardial pacing wires are typically placed during the surgery, and the nurse and provider work collaboratively if pacing is needed postoperatively to stabilize a rhythm. Continuous observation of the cardiac monitor for arrhythmias is essential.

Any indications of decreased CO are reported promptly to the provider. These assessment data and results of diagnostic tests are used to determine the cause of the problem. After a diagnosis has been made, the provider and the nurse work together to restore CO and prevent further complications.

(continued on page 442)

MAINTAINING ADEQUATE TISSUE PERFUSION

Thromboemboli formation also can result from injury to the intima of the blood vessels, dislodging a clot from a damaged valve, loosening of mural thrombi, or coagulation problems. Air embolism can result from CPB or central venous cannulation. Symptoms of embolization vary according to site. The usual embolic sites are the lungs, coronary arteries, mesentery, spleen, extremities, kidneys, and brain. The patient is observed for onset of the following:

- Chest pain and respiratory distress from pulmonary embolus or MI
- Severe abdominal or back pain, bowel emptying, or nausea and vomiting from mesenteric emboli
- Pain, cessation of pulses, blanching, numbness, or coldness in an extremity
- Decreased urine output from renal emboli
- One-sided weakness and pupillary changes, as occur in stroke

All such symptoms are reported promptly to the provider. After surgery, the following measures are taken to prevent venous stasis, which can cause deep venous thrombosis and subsequent pulmonary embolism:

- Applying elastic bandage wraps, elastic stocking, and/or sequential pneumatic compression wraps
- Discouraging crossing of legs
- Early and frequent ambulation

Inadequate kidney perfusion can occur as a complication of cardiac surgery. One possible cause is low CO. Trauma to blood cells during CPB can cause hemolysis of red blood cells, which then occlude the renal glomeruli. Additionally, the use of vasopressor agents to increase blood pressure may constrict the renal arterioles and reduce blood flow to the kidneys.

Nursing management includes accurate measurement of urine output. An output of less than 30 mL/hr or 0.5 mL/kg/hr may indicate hypovolemia or renal insufficiency. Fluids may be prescribed to increase CO and renal blood flow. IV diuretics may be administered to increase urine output. The nurse should be aware of the patient's BUN, serum creatinine, and urine and serum electrolyte levels. Abnormal levels are reported promptly because it may be necessary to adjust fluids and the dose or type of medication administered. If efforts to maintain kidney perfusion are ineffective, the patient may require continuous renal replacement therapy (CRRT) or dialysis (refer to Chapter 27).

MAINTAINING NORMAL BODY TEMPERATURE

Patients are usually hypothermic when admitted to the critical care unit following the cardiac surgical procedure if their surgery was done using CPB. The patient must be warmed to a normal temperature gradually. This is accomplished partially by the patient's own basal metabolic processes and often with the assistance of warmed ventilator air, warm air via a warming system, blankets, or heat lamps. While the patient is hypothermic, the clotting process is less efficient, the heart is prone to arrhythmias, and oxygen does not readily transfer from the hemoglobin to the tissues. Because anesthesia and hypothermia suppress normal basal metabolism, oxygen supply usually meets the cellular demand.

MONITORING AND MANAGING POTENTIAL COMPLICATIONS

Infection. Common sites of infection postoperatively include the lungs, urinary tract, incisions, and intravascular catheters. Foley catheters should be removed as early as possible to prevent infection (postop Day 1 if possible). There is no evidence that wound dressings after 48 hours are protective against surgical site infection (SSI). The incidence of SSIs post-CABG ranges from 0.35 to 8.49 per 100 operations where the majority of the infections are superficial. Prophylaxis with an antimicrobial reduces the occurrence of SSI up to fivefold (Anderson, 2016). Aseptic technique is used when changing dressings and when providing endotracheal tube (ETT) and catheter care. Closed systems are used to maintain all IV and arterial lines. All invasive equipment is discontinued as soon as possible after surgery.

Clearance of pulmonary secretions is accomplished by frequently repositioning the patient, suctioning, chest percussion and/or vibration, as well as teaching and encouraging the patient to breathe deeply, cough, and use the incentive spirometer frequently. Prevention of atelectasis is achieved through these interventions.

Postpericardiotomy syndrome may occur in patients who undergo cardiac surgery (Hoit, 2016). This complication develops in as many as 15% of patients undergoing cardiac surgery (LeWinter & Hopkins, 2015). It is thought to be related to the production of antiheart antibodies in response to myocardial injury. The syndrome is characterized by fever, pericardial pain, pleural pain, dyspnea, pericardial effusion, pericardial friction rub, and arthralgia. These signs and symptoms may occur in combination with leukocytosis (elevated WBCs) and elevation of the erythrocyte sedimentation rate and CRP. These signs frequently appear after the patient is discharged from the hospital. Anti-inflammatory agents (NSAIDs) often produce a dramatic improvement in symptoms within 48 hours.

Fluid Volume and Electrolyte Imbalance. Fluid and electrolyte imbalance may occur after cardiac surgery. Nursing assessment includes monitoring of intake and output, weight, hemodynamic parameters, hematocrit levels, distention of neck veins, edema, breath sounds, and electrolyte levels. Changes in serum electrolytes are reported promptly so that treatment can be instituted. Especially important are high or low levels of potassium, magnesium, sodium, and calcium. Elevated blood glucose levels are common in the postoperative period. Administration of insulin may be required in patients both with and without diabetes to achieve the glycemic control necessary for promoting wound healing.

Impaired Gas Exchange. Impaired gas exchange is another possible complication after cardiac surgery. All body tissues require an adequate supply of oxygen for survival. To achieve this after surgery, an ETT with ventilator assistance will be needed initially postop (for an average of about 6 hours). The assisted ventilation is continued until the patient's blood gas measurements are acceptable and the patient demonstrates the ability to breathe independently. To ensure adequate gas exchange, the nurse assesses and maintains the patency of the ETT. The patient is suctioned when necessary. Because a patent airway is essential for oxygen and carbon dioxide exchange, the ETT must be secured to prevent it from slipping into the right mainstem bronchus or accidental dislodgment. The patient is weaned from the ventilator and extubated as soon as possible, usually within 6 hours of CABG. Physical assessment and ABG results guide the process. Before being extubated, the patient should have cough and gag reflexes and stable vital signs; be able to lift the head off the bed or give firm hand grasps; have adequate vital capacity, negative inspiratory force, and minute volume appropriate for body size; and have acceptable ABG levels while breathing without the assistance of the ventilator. Refer to Chapter 55 for additional information related to ventilators and weaning.

During this time, the nurse assists with the weaning process and eventually with the removal of the ETT. Deep breathing and coughing are encouraged at least every 1 to 2 hours after extubation to open the alveolar sacs and provide for increased ventilation as well as to clear secretions (preventing atelectasis).

The patient is assessed continuously for signs of impaired gas exchange: restlessness, anxiety, cyanosis of mucous membranes and peripheral tissues, and tachycardia. Breath sounds are assessed frequently, as well as ABGs, oxygen saturation, and end-tidal CO_2. Following extubation, aggressive pulmonary interventions, such as turning, coughing of secretions, using incentive spirometer, and deep breathing, are necessary to prevent atelectasis and pneumonia.

When the patient's condition stabilizes, body position is changed every 1 to 2 hours. Frequent changes of patient position provide for optimal pulmonary ventilation and perfusion by allowing the lungs to expand more fully.

Impaired Cerebral Circulation. Brain function depends on a continuous supply of oxygenated blood. The brain does not have the capacity to store oxygen and must rely on adequate continuous perfusion by the heart. Hypoperfusion or microemboli may produce central nervous system injury after cardiac surgery.

It is important to observe the patient for any symptoms of hypoxia: restlessness, headache, confusion, dyspnea, hypotension, and cyanosis. An assessment of the patient's neurologic status includes level of consciousness (LOC), response to verbal commands and painful stimuli, pupil size and reaction to light, facial symmetry, movement of the extremities, and hand grip strength. Any indication of a change in status is immediately reported to the provider and documented in the medical record.

MINIMIZING SENSORY-PERCEPTION IMBALANCE

Some patients exhibit abnormal behaviors that occur with varying intensity and duration. In the early years of cardiac surgery, this phenomenon occurred more frequently than it does today. Advances in surgical techniques and in the delivery of anesthetic

agents have significantly decreased the incidence of postoperative delirium. However, incident rates of 3% to 32% of delirium after cardiac surgery are seen in those with pre-existing organic mental disorders (e.g., stroke, dementia), significant prior alcohol consumption, advanced age, or intracranial cerebral artery disease (McGarvey, Cheung, & Stecker, 2016). In those without the aforementioned risk factors, the nurse should consider etiologies of anxiety, sleep deprivation, increased sensory input, medications, and physiologic problems such as hypoxemia. Delirium may appear after a 2- to 5-day stay in an intensive care environment and is associated with increased morbidity and mortality, including postoperative complications of respiratory insufficiency and sternal instability, prolonged length of stay, increased need for skilled nursing facility placement, and reduced cognitive and functional recovery, making early recognition and response crucial. Treatment of postoperative delirium requires an assessment for the etiology and correction of potentially reversible causes (McGarvey et al., 2016).

Careful explanations of all procedures and of the need for cooperation help keep the patient oriented throughout the postoperative course. Continuity of care is desirable; a familiar face and a nursing staff with a consistent approach help the patient feel safe. The patient's family should be welcomed at the bedside. Some patients have difficulty learning and retaining information after cardiac surgery. Many patients have difficulties in cognitive function after cardiac surgery, a phenomenon that does not occur after other types of major surgery. The patient may experience recent memory loss, short attention span, difficulty with simple math, poor handwriting, and visual disturbances. Patients with these difficulties often become frustrated when they try to resume normal activities and learn how to care for themselves at home. The patient and family are reassured that the difficulty usually resolves gradually and most patients will return to their preoperative baseline by 3 to 12 months after surgery (McGarvey et al., 2016). A well-designed plan of nursing care can assist the nursing team in coordinating their efforts for the emotional well-being of the patient.

RELIEVING PAIN

Deep pain may not be felt in the peri-incisional area but may occur in a broader, more diffuse area. Patients who have had cardiac surgery experience pain caused by the interruption of intercostal nerves along the incision route and irritation of the pleura by the chest catheters. Incisional pain may also be experienced from peripheral vein or artery graft harvest sites. IV and oral NSAIDs decrease the amount of opioids required for pain relief and increase patient comfort. Patients report the most pain during coughing, turning, and moving. Physical support of the incision with a folded bath blanket or small pillow during deep breathing and coughing helps to minimize pain (often referred to as "splinting"). Then the patient should be able to participate in respiratory exercises and increase self-care progressively. Patient comfort improves after removal of the chest tubes. The patient is observed for any adverse effects of opioids,

(continued on page 444)

which may include respiratory depression, hypotension, ileus, or urinary retention. If serious side effects occur, an opioid antagonist (e.g., naloxone [Narcan]) may be used.

EVALUATION

Expected patient outcomes may include:

- Maintains adequate CO
- Maintains adequate gas exchange
- Maintains fluid and electrolyte balance
- Experiences decreased symptoms of sensory-perception disturbances
- Experiences relief of pain
- Maintains adequate tissue perfusion
- Maintains normal body temperature
- Incisions are well healed
- Performs self-care activities
- Engages in follow-up care with health care providers and cardiac rehabilitation services
- Adheres to recommendations for diet and lifestyle changes to maintain optimal future health
- Exhibits no complications

MYOCARDIAL INFARCTION (MI)

Coronary occlusion, heart attack, and **MI** are terms used synonymously, but the preferred term is **MI**.

Pathophysiology

In an MI, an area of the myocardium is permanently destroyed. MI is usually caused by reduced blood flow in a coronary artery due to rupture of an atherosclerotic plaque and subsequent occlusion of the artery by a thrombus. In unstable angina, the plaque ruptures, but the artery is not completely occluded. Because unstable angina and acute MI are considered to be the same process but occurring at different points along a continuum, the term **acute coronary syndrome (ACS)** may be used in lieu of these diagnoses. Other causes of MI include vasospasm (sudden constriction or narrowing) of a coronary artery, decreased oxygen supply (e.g., from acute blood loss, anemia, or low blood pressure), and increased demand for oxygen (e.g., from a rapid heart rate, thyrotoxicosis, or ingestion of cocaine). In each case, a profound imbalance exists between myocardial oxygen supply and demand.

The area of infarction develops over minutes to hours. As the cells are deprived of oxygen, ischemia develops, cellular injury occurs, and the lack of oxygen results in infarction, or the death of cells. The expression "time is muscle" reflects the urgency of appropriate treatment to improve patient outcomes. Each year in the United States, more than 1,500,000 people die from acute MIs; it is the most common cause of death in those over 40 years (Ferri, 2016). Half of those who die never reach a hospital.

Various descriptions are used to further identify an MI: the type of MI (ST-segment elevation, non–ST-segment elevation), the location of the injury to the ventricular wall (anterior, inferior, posterior, or lateral wall), the point in time within the process of infarction (acute, evolving, or old), and the extent of the damage to the myocardium caused by the MI (partial or full thickness). Partial infarcts are associated with severely narrow coronary arteries and present as non–ST-segment elevation, while full-thickness infarcts commonly occur with obstruction of a single coronary artery and present as ST elevation on ECG readings (Porth, 2015).

The ECG usually identifies the type and location, and other ECG indicators such as a Q wave and patient history identify the timing. Regardless of the location of the infarction of cardiac muscle, the goal of medical therapy is to prevent or minimize myocardial tissue death and to prevent complications.

Risk Factors

Risk factors for MI are the same as those described for atherosclerosis and angina.

Clinical Manifestations and Assessment

Chest pain that occurs suddenly and continues despite rest and medication is the presenting symptom in most patients with an MI. Although patients with diabetic neuropathy may not experience chest pain, a high degree of suspicion must be maintained for an MI in diabetic patients admitted with associated symptoms of dyspnea, syncope, fatigue, diaphoresis, or lightheadedness. Up to 30% of patients with ST elevation myocardial infarction (STEMI) have prodromal (early nonspecific) symptoms. Box 14-5 discusses assessment parameters. In many cases, the signs and symptoms of MI cannot be distinguished from those of unstable angina. The diagnosis of MI is generally based on the presenting symptoms, physical findings, ECG, and laboratory test results (e.g., serial cardiac biomarker values). The prognosis depends on the severity of coronary artery obstruction and the extent of myocardial damage.

Nursing Alert
Women often present with symptoms different from those seen in men; in fact, 50% of women with an MI do not complain of chest pain (Chesler, Ho, & Ramkissoon, 2014). Therefore, a high level of suspicion is associated with vague complaints such as fatigue, shoulder blade discomfort, and/or SOB (Chesler et al., 2014).

Patient History

The patient history has two parts: the description of the presenting symptom(s) (e.g., pain) and the history of previous illnesses and family history of heart disease. The patient's risk factors for heart disease should also be evaluated.

Focused Assessment

Acute Myocardial Infarction (MI) or Acute Coronary Syndrome (ACS)

Be alert for the following signs and symptoms:

Cardiovascular

- Chest pain or discomfort, palpitations
- S_3, S_4, and new onset of a murmur
- Increased jugular venous distention (may be seen if the MI has caused heart failure)
- Elevated blood pressure (because of sympathetic stimulation) or decreased blood pressure (because of decreased contractility, impending cardiogenic shock, or medications)
- Pulse deficit, indicating atrial fibrillation
- In addition to ST-segment and T-wave changes, tachycardia, bradycardia, or arrhythmias on electrocardiogram (ECG)

Respiratory

- Shortness of breath, dyspnea, tachypnea, and crackles if MI has caused pulmonary congestion
- Pulmonary edema

Gastrointestinal

- Nausea and vomiting

Genitourinary

- Decreased urinary output (may indicate cardiogenic shock)

Skin

- Cool, clammy, diaphoretic, and pale appearance (due to sympathetic stimulation, may indicate cardiogenic shock)

Neurologic

- Anxiety, restlessness, and lightheadedness (may indicate increased sympathetic stimulation or a decrease in contractility and cerebral oxygenation or cardiogenic shock)

Psychological

- Fear with feeling of impending doom
- Denial

Electrocardiogram

The ECG provides information that assists in diagnosing acute MI. It should be obtained within 10 minutes from the time a patient reports pain or arrives in the emergency department. By monitoring serial ECG changes over time, the location, evolution, and resolution of an MI can be identified and monitored. The ECG changes that occur with an MI are seen in the leads that view the involved surface of the heart. The extent of ischemia and resultant injury through the various layers of the heart determine the type of ECG changes seen. The classic ECG changes are T-wave inversion, ST-segment elevation, and development of an abnormal Q wave (Fig. 14-11). The first ECG signs of an acute MI occur as a result of myocardial ischemia and injury. As the area becomes ischemic, myocardial repolarization is delayed, causing the T wave (representing ventricular depolarization) to invert. The ischemic region may remain depolarized while adjacent areas of the myocardium return to the resting state. As ischemia progresses to injury, the T wave becomes enlarged and symmetric. Myocardial injury also causes ST-segment changes. The ST segment may rise at least 1 mm above the isoelectric line (area between the T wave and the next P wave is used as the reference for the isoelectric line), or there may be non–ST-segment elevation. Remember that there may be a combination of ischemia, injury, and infarction occurring simultaneously, thus resulting in mixed ECG patterns.

Nursing Alert
Because lethal arrhythmias can appear suddenly in patients with MIs (most deaths with STEMI occur within the first hour of its onset and usually result from ventricular fibrillation [Mega

& Morrow, 2015]), all patients should have bedside monitoring of the ECG and intravenous access!

The beginning of the ST segment is usually identified by a change in the thickness or angle of the terminal portion of

Endocardium Myocardium Epicardium

FIGURE 14-11 Effects of ischemia, injury, and infarction on an electrocardiogram (ECG) recording. Ischemia causes inversion of the T wave because of altered repolarization. Cardiac muscle injury causes elevation of the ST segment and tall, symmetrical T waves. Later, Q waves develop because of the absence of depolarization current from the necrotic tissue and opposing currents from other parts of the heart.

FIGURE 14-12 Using the electrocardiogram (ECG) to diagnose acute myocardial infarction (MI). (ST-segment elevation is measured 0.06 to 0.08 seconds after the J point. An elevation of more than 1 mm in contiguous leads is indicative of acute MI.)

the QRS complex and is called the *J point* (Fig. 14-12). The J point is the end of ventricular depolarization (QRS) and the beginning of the ventricular repolarization (ST segment) and is identified by a change from an essentially vertical angle (QRS) to a more horizontal angle (ST segment). This J point is normally on the baseline, and elevation in the ST segment in two contiguous leads is a key diagnostic indicator for MI. The nurse assesses for ST elevation, as it relates to the isoelectric line, at a point 0.08 seconds past the J point.

The appearance of abnormal Q waves is another indication of MI. A Q wave is a negative deflection that signals the beginning of ventricular depolarization; however, abnormal Q waves represent myocardial necrosis and can develop within 1 to 3 days of an MI. A pathological Q wave is identified by an abnormal depth and duration of the Q wave or the appearance of "new" Q waves not previously seen in ECG tracings. The pathological Q wave, therefore, reflects the conduction from other parts of the heart because of necrotic tissue. An abnormal Q wave is 0.04 seconds or longer, 25% of the R-wave depth (provided the R wave exceeds a depth of 5 mm), or did not exist before the event. An acute MI may also cause a significant decrease in the height of the R wave. During an

acute MI, injury and ischemic changes are usually present. An abnormal Q wave may be present without ST-segment and T-wave changes, which indicates an old, not acute, MI. For some patients, there are no persistent ECG changes, and the MI is diagnosed by blood levels of cardiac biomarkers.

Using the above information, patients are diagnosed with one of the following forms of ACS:

- *Unstable angina:* The patient has clinical manifestations of coronary ischemia, but ECG or cardiac biomarkers show no evidence of acute MI.
- *STEMI:* The patient has ECG evidence of acute MI with characteristic changes in two contiguous leads on a 12-lead ECG. In this type of MI, significant damage to the myocardium occurs.
- *Non-STEMI:* The patient has elevated cardiac biomarkers but no definite ECG evidence of acute MI.

During recovery from an MI, the ST segment often is the first ECG indicator to return to normal (in 1 to 6 weeks). The T wave becomes large and symmetric for 24 hours, and it then inverts within 1 to 3 days for 1 to 2 weeks. Q-wave alterations are usually permanent. An old ST-segment elevation MI is usually indicated by an abnormal Q wave or decreased height of the R wave without ST-segment and T-wave changes.

Echocardiogram

The echocardiogram is used to evaluate ventricular function. It may be used to assist in diagnosing an MI, especially when the ECG is nondiagnostic. The echocardiogram can detect hypokinetic and akinetic wall motion, can determine the ejection fraction, and can also assess valvular function.

Laboratory Tests

Laboratory tests called *cardiac biomarkers* are used to diagnose an MI (Table 14-5). Newer laboratory tests with faster results, and thus producing earlier diagnosis, include troponin analysis. These tests are based on the release of cellular contents into the circulation when myocardial cells die.

Creatine Kinase and Its Isoenzymes
Creatinine kinase–myocardial band (CK-MB) is the cardiac-specific isoenzyme; CK-MB is found mainly in cardiac

TABLE 14-5 Biomarkers of Acute Myocardial Infarction

Serum Test	Earliest Increase (hours)	Test Running Time (minutes)	Peak (hours)	Return to Normal
Total creatinine kinase (CK)	3–6	30–60	24–36	3 days
CK-MB:isoenzyme	4–8	30–60	12–24	3–4 days
Mass assay	2–3	30–60	10–18	3–4 days
Myoglobin	1–3	30–60	4–12	12 hours
Troponin T or I	3–4	30–60	4–24	1–3 weeks

cells and, therefore, increases only when there has been damage to these cells. Elevated CK-MB assessed by mass assay is an indicator of acute MI; its level begins to increase within a few hours and peaks within 24 hours of an MI. A normal CK-MB is 0 to 3 ng/mL or 1 to 3 µg/L. If the patient has cardiac complaints and negative CK-MB for more than 48 hours, then etiologies for the symptoms outside of an MI will be assessed.

Myoglobin

Myoglobin is a hemeprotein that helps transport oxygen. Like CK-MB enzyme, myoglobin is found in cardiac and skeletal muscle. A normal level is 5 to 70 ng/mL or 5 to 70 µg/L. The myoglobin level starts to increase within 1 to 3 hours and peaks within 12 hours after the onset of symptoms. An increase in myoglobin is not very specific in indicating an acute cardiac event; however, negative results are an excellent parameter for ruling out an acute MI.

Troponin

Troponin, a protein found in the myocardium, regulates the myocardial contractile process. There are three isomers of troponin: C, I, and T. Troponin C binds calcium to activate muscle contraction, while troponins I and T are specific for cardiac muscle, and are currently recognized as reliable and critical biomarkers of myocardial injury. A normal troponin I level is less than 0.5 ng/mL. An increase in the level of troponin in the serum can be detected within a few hours during acute MI. It remains elevated for a long period, often as long as 3 weeks, and it, therefore, can be used to detect recent myocardial damage.

Nursing Alert
Troponin I levels of greater than 1.5 ng/mL or greater than 1.5 µg/L are critical.

Medical Management

The goals of medical management are to minimize myocardial damage, preserve myocardial function, and prevent complications. These goals are facilitated by the use of guidelines developed by the American College of Cardiology and American Heart Association (Box 14-6). They may be achieved by reperfusing the area with the emergency PCI or use of thrombolytic medications in a medical center not capable of doing a PCI. Minimizing myocardial damage is also accomplished by reducing myocardial oxygen demand and increasing oxygen supply with medications, oxygen administration, and bed rest. The resolution of pain and ECG changes indicate that demand and supply are in equilibrium; they may also indicate reperfusion. Visualization of blood flow through an open vessel in the catheterization laboratory is evidence of reperfusion.

Pharmacologic Therapy

The patient with suspected MI is given aspirin, nitroglycerin, morphine, a beta-blocker, and other medications as indicated,

---

BOX 14-6

Medical Treatment Guidelines for Acute Myocardial Infarction

Use rapid transit to the hospital.
Obtain 12-lead electrocardiogram (ECG) to be read within 10 minutes.
Obtain laboratory blood specimens of cardiac biomarkers, including troponin.
Obtain other diagnostics to clarify the diagnosis.
Begin routine medical interventions:
- Supplemental oxygen
- Nitroglycerin
- Morphine
- Aspirin 162 to 325 mg
- Beta-blocker
- Angiotensin-converting enzyme inhibitor or angiotensin-receptor blocker within 24 hours

Evaluate for indications for reperfusion therapy:
- Percutaneous coronary intervention
- Thrombolytic therapy

Continue therapy as indicated:
- IV heparin or low–molecular-weight heparin
- Clopidogrel (Plavix) or antiplatelet-like agent
- Glycoprotein IIb/IIIa inhibitor

---

while the diagnosis is being confirmed. Patients should receive a beta-blocker initially, throughout the hospitalization, and upon discharge. Also on discharge, there needs to be documentation that the patient was discharged on a statin, an **angiotensin-converting enzyme (ACE)** inhibitor or an **angiotensin-receptor blocking agent (ARB)**, and aspirin. These are "quality indicators" for ACS treatment and are now publicly reported measures. Remember **SAAB:** *s*tatin, *a*ce or arb, *a*spirin, *b*eta-blocker. If any of these are not prescribed, clear documentation as to why not must be provided.

Thrombolytics

In non–PCI-capable hospitals, initial assessment of patients should include evaluation of the contraindications to administration of a thrombolytic agent. The purpose of **thrombolytics** is to dissolve and lyse the thrombus in a coronary artery (thrombolysis), allowing blood to flow through the coronary artery again (reperfusion), minimizing the size of the infarction, and preserving ventricular function. Hospitals monitor their ability to administer these medications **within 30 minutes** from the time the patient arrives in the emergency department. This is called *door-to-needle time* or "*time to needle*." The thrombolytic agents used most often are alteplase (t-PA, Activase) and reteplase (r-PA, TNKase). Box 14-7 discusses administration of and contraindications for thrombolytic therapy.

Analgesics

The analgesic of choice for acute MI is morphine sulfate administered in IV boluses to reduce pain and anxiety. It

BOX 14-7

Administration of Thrombolytic Therapy

Indications

- No PCI-capable center available in the next 120 minutes (O'Gara et al., 2013)
- Chest pain for longer than 20 minutes, unrelieved by nitroglycerin
- ST-segment elevation in at least two leads that face the same area of the heart
- Less than 6 hours from onset of pain

Absolute Contraindications

- Active bleeding (excluding menses)
- Known bleeding disorder
- History of hemorrhagic stroke
- History of intracranial vessel malformation
- Known malignant intracranial neoplasm
- Ischemic stroke within 3 months (except acute ischemic stroke within 4.5 hours)
- Recent major surgery or trauma
- Uncontrolled hypertension
- Suspected aortic dissection
- Pregnancy

Nursing Considerations

- Minimize the number of times the patient's skin is punctured.
- Avoid intramuscular injections.
- Draw blood for laboratory tests when starting the IV line.
- Start IV lines before thrombolytic therapy; designate one line to use for blood draws.
- Avoid continual use of noninvasive blood pressure cuff.
- Monitor for acute arrhythmias and hypotension.
- Monitor for reperfusion; resolution of angina or acute ST-segment changes on the EKG.
- Check for signs and symptoms of bleeding: decrease in hematocrit and hemoglobin values, decrease in blood pressure, increase in heart rate, oozing or bulging at sites of invasive procedure, back pain, muscle weakness, changes in level of consciousness, complaints of headache.
- Treat major bleeding by discontinuing thrombolytic therapy and any anticoagulants; apply direct pressure and notify the provider immediately.
- Treat minor bleeding by applying direct pressure if accessible and appropriate; continue to monitor for bleeding.

Note: If possible, a patient should always be transferred to a hospital with PCI capability within 2 hours.
O'Gara, P. T., Kushner, F. G., Ascheim, D. D., et al. (2013). ACCF/AHA guideline for the management of ST-elevation myocardial infarction: A report of the American College of Cardiology Foundation/American Heart Association Task Force on Practice Guidelines. *Journal of the American College of Cardiology*, *61*, e78.

reduces preload and afterload (peripheral arterial and venous dilation), which decreases the workload of the heart. Morphine also relaxes bronchioles to enhance oxygenation. The cardiovascular response to morphine is monitored carefully, particularly the blood pressure, which can decrease, and the respiratory rate, which can be depressed. Because morphine decreases the sensation of pain, ST-segment monitoring may be a better indicator of subsequent ischemia than assessment of pain.

 Nursing Alert
Maintaining the patient in a supine position and elevating the lower extremities if blood pressure falls can minimize hypotension following the administration of nitroglycerin and morphine. Such positioning is undesirable in patients with pulmonary edema, but morphine rarely produces hypotension in these circumstances (Mega & Morrow, 2015).

Angiotensin-Converting Enzyme Inhibitors

ACE inhibitors prevent the conversion of angiotensin I to angiotensin II. In the absence of angiotensin II, the blood pressure decreases and the kidneys excrete sodium and fluid (diuresis), decreasing the oxygen demand of the heart. Use of ACE inhibitors in patients after MI decreases mortality rates and prevents remodeling of myocardial cells, which is associated with the onset of heart failure. It is important to ensure that the patient is not hypotensive, hyponatremic, hypovolemic, or hyperkalemic before administering ACE inhibitors. Blood pressure; urine output; and levels of serum sodium, potassium, and creatinine need to be monitored closely. An ARB can be used in lieu of an ACE inhibitor.

 Nursing Alert
The nurse remembers the mnemonic MONA when treating potential MI patients: morphine, oxygen, nitrates, and aspirin.

Reperfusion Procedures

Reperfusion procedures may be used to restore the blood supply to the myocardium. These include PCI procedures (e.g., intracoronary stents, atherectomy), and CABG. See discussion under "angina pectoris" section for detailed descriptions.

Cardiac Rehabilitation

After the MI patient is free of symptoms, an active rehabilitation program is initiated. Cardiac rehabilitation is a program that targets risk reduction by means of education, individual and group support, and physical activity. Most insurance programs, including Medicare, cover the cost of cardiac rehabilitation. The nurse needs to encourage the patient and ensure that referral from the hospital for outpatient cardiac rehabilitation is accomplished.

Cardiac rehabilitation is categorized in three phases. Phase I begins with the diagnosis of atherosclerosis, which may occur when the patient is admitted to the hospital for ACS (e.g., unstable angina or acute MI). It includes any postprocedural activity that occurs during the hospitalization. Phase I consists of low-level activities and initial education for the patient and family.

Phase II occurs after the patient has been discharged. It usually lasts for 4 to 6 weeks but may extend to 6 months. This outpatient program consists of supervised, often ECG-monitored, exercise training that is individualized based on the results of an exercise stress test.

Phase III focuses on maintaining cardiovascular stability and long-term conditioning. The patient is usually self-directed during this phase and does not require a supervised program, although it may be offered. The goals of each phase build on the accomplishments of the previous phase. Health promotion is discussed in Box 14-8.

Nursing Management

Relieving Pain and Other Signs and Symptoms of Ischemia

Balancing myocardial oxygen supply with demand (e.g., as evidenced by the relief of chest pain) is the top priority in the care of the patient with an acute MI. Although medication therapy is required to accomplish this goal, nursing interventions are also important.

The recommended treatment for acute MI is reperfusion with thrombolytic therapy (*time to needle*) or emergent PCI (*time to device*) for patients who present to the health care facility immediately and who have no major contraindications. These therapies are important because, in addition to relieving symptoms, they aid in minimizing or avoiding permanent injury to the myocardium. With or without reperfusion, administration of aspirin, an IV beta-blocker, and nitroglycerin is indicated. Use of a GPIIb/IIIa agent or heparin may also be indicated. Aspirin (300 mg) should be administered unless already given (e.g., by emergency services or home treatment) or contraindicated (known allergy). A previous history of gastritis or indigestion is not a contraindication to the use of aspirin in ACS (Kelly, 2015). Since the goal is rapid therapeutic aspirin level in the blood, the

---

Health Promotion

Promoting Health After Myocardial Infarction and Other Acute Coronary Syndromes

To extend and improve the quality of life, a patient who has had an MI must learn to adjust his or her lifestyle to promote heart-healthy living. With this in mind, the nurse and patient develop a program to help the patient achieve desired outcomes.

Changing Lifestyle During Convalescence and Healing

Adaptation to an MI is an ongoing process and usually requires some modification of lifestyle. Some specific modifications include:

- Avoiding any activity that produces chest pain, extreme dyspnea, or undue fatigue
- Avoiding extremes of heat and cold and walking against the wind
- Losing weight, if indicated
- Stopping smoking and use of tobacco; avoiding secondhand smoke
- Using personal strengths to support lifestyle changes
- Developing heart-healthy eating patterns, including avoiding large meals and hurrying while eating
- Modifying meals to align with the Therapeutic Lifestyle Changes (TLC) or the Dietary Approaches to Stopping Hypertension (DASH) diet
- Adhering to medical regimen, especially in taking medications
- Following recommendations that ensure blood pressure and blood glucose are in control
- Pursuing activities that relieve and reduce stress

Adopting an Activity Program

Additionally, the patient needs to undertake an orderly program of increasing activity and exercise for long-term rehabilitation as follows:

- Engaging in a regimen of physical conditioning with a gradual increase in activity duration and then a gradual increase in activity intensity
- Walking daily, increasing distance and time as prescribed
- Monitoring pulse rate during physical activity until the maximum level of activity is attained
- Avoiding activities that tense the muscles: isometric exercise, weight-lifting, any activity that requires sudden bursts of energy
- Avoiding physical exercise immediately after a meal
- Alternating activity with rest periods (some fatigue is normal and expected during convalescence)
- Participating in a daily program of exercise that develops into a program of regular exercise for a lifetime

Managing Symptoms

The patient must learn to recognize and take appropriate action for possible recurrences of symptoms as follows:

- Call 911 if chest pressure or pain (or anginal equivalent) is not relieved in 15 minutes by nitroglycerin.
- Contact the provider if any of the following occur: shortness of breath, fainting, slow or rapid heartbeat, swelling of feet and ankles.

patient should chew the tablet to promote buccal absorption rather than absorption through the gastric mucosa (Mega & Morrow, 2015). The nurse administers morphine to relieve pain and anxiety and to promote vasodilation, reducing preload and afterload.

 Nursing Alert
Bleeding complications are most common after thrombolytic therapy, and intracranial hemorrhage is the most serious complication (frequency is generally less than 1%); therefore, any change in the LOC, cranial nerve changes, motor weakness, etc. is reported immediately to the provider.

Oxygen should be administered along with medication therapy to assist with relief of symptoms. Administration of oxygen, even in low doses, raises the circulating level of oxygen to reduce pain associated with low levels of myocardial oxygen. The route of administration, usually by nasal cannula, and the oxygen flow rate are documented. A flow rate of 2 to 4 L/min is usually adequate to maintain oxygen saturation levels of 96% to 100% if no other disease is present.

Vital signs are assessed frequently as long as the patient is experiencing pain and other signs or symptoms of acute ischemia. Physical rest in bed with the backrest elevated (semi-Fowler's position) helps decrease chest discomfort and dyspnea. Elevation of the head and torso is beneficial for the following reasons:

- Tidal volume improves because of reduced pressure from abdominal contents on the diaphragm and better lung expansion and gas exchange.
- Drainage of the upper lung lobes improves.
- Venous return to the heart (preload) decreases, reducing the work of the heart.

Nursing Alert
HOB elevation is beneficial for patients with cardiac disease; however, if the patient becomes hypotensive, the patient may be placed in the supine position with legs elevated to increase venous return.

Improving Respiratory Function

Regular and careful assessment of respiratory function can help the nurse detect early signs of pulmonary complications. Scrupulous attention to fluid volume status prevents overloading the heart and lungs.

Promoting Adequate Tissue Perfusion

Limiting the patient to bed or chair rest during the initial phase of treatment is particularly helpful in reducing myocardial oxygen consumption. This limitation should remain until the patient is pain-free and hemodynamically stable. Checking skin temperature and peripheral pulses frequently is important in monitoring tissue perfusion. Pulse oximetry should be in use, and efforts toward minimizing myocardial oxygen consumption should be in place. Maintaining the patient at rest both physically and emotionally by providing a quiet atmosphere and mild anxiolytic medications may be considered in some cases.

Reducing Anxiety

Alleviating anxiety and decreasing fear are important nursing functions that reduce the sympathetic stress response. Decreased sympathetic stimulation decreases the workload of the heart, which may relieve pain and other signs and symptoms of ischemia.

Monitoring and Managing Potential Complications

Complications that can occur after acute MI are caused by the damage that occurs to the myocardium and to the conduction system as a result of the reduced coronary blood flow. Because these complications can be life-threatening, close monitoring for and early identification of their signs and symptoms are critical. Refer to Chapter 54 for details of cardiogenic shock.

The nurse closely monitors and reports changes in cardiac rate/rhythm, heart and lung sounds, blood pressure, pain, respiratory status, urinary output, skin color/temperature, LOC, ECG changes, and laboratory values. Also, stool softeners should be considered to prevent constipation and straining. The nurse institutes emergency measures when necessary.

CHAPTER REVIEW

Critical Thinking Exercises

1. You are working in a cardiology office and you receive a phone call from a patient who had an MI 2 years ago. She reports that she is experiencing some SOB and mild back pain. What evidence base is there to suggest that symptoms of an MI may be different for women than men? Discuss the strength of this evidence and its significance in determining assessment criteria to be used for women and men. What questions would you ask this patient?

What would you instruct her to do? Provide rationale for your instructions.

2. You are taking over the care of a patient who returned from the catheterization laboratory 2 hours ago following a successful PCI. He was reported to be stable on bed rest, with no bleeding from the right femoral site. The patient appears very pale and complains of right flank pain. Identify the key parameters that need to be assessed. Describe the actions you would take and state why.

3. You are caring for a patient who has been hospitalized awaiting CABG surgery. As you deliver his morning medications, he states that he is feeling "pressure" in the lower sternal area, but he thinks it is just "nerves." What questions would you ask and what would you assess? What would your next actions be?

NCLEX-Style Review Questions

1. A patient arrives in the emergency room complaining of nausea, diaphoresis, SOB, and squeezing substernal chest pain that radiates to the left shoulder and jaw. The nurse should perform which interventions?
   a. Complete admission registration, alert the catheter laboratory team, establish an IV access, and record all vital signs
   b. Alert the catheter laboratory team, administer oxygen, obtain blood work, and notify the health care provider
   c. Establish an IV, give sublingual nitroglycerin as ordered, insert a Foley catheter, and alert the catheter laboratory team
   d. Administer oxygen, apply a cardiac monitor, record patient's vital signs, and give sublingual nitroglycerin as ordered

2. What does the nurse recognize as an absolute contraindication for thrombolytic therapy?
   a. Active bleeding
   b. Current anticoagulant therapy
   c. Over age 75
   d. Severe hepatic disease

3. The nurse is caring for a nonsmoking female patient with the diagnosis of coronary atherosclerosis who has been admitted to the hospital with angina. The patient states that she never experiences chest pain going down her arm or in the middle of her chest. The nurse is not surprised at this statement and explains to the patient that:
   a. Women who have ischemia are usually totally asymptomatic.
   b. Women have been found to have more atypical symptoms such as dyspnea, nausea, and weakness.
   c. Chest pain occurs only with strenuous exercise.
   d. Cigarette smoking is usually the contributing factor to chest pain.

4. Two hours after cardiac catheterization that was accessed via the right femoral artery route, an adult client complains of numbness and pain in the right foot. What action should the nurse take first?
   a. Call the provider immediately.
   b. Check the client's peripheral pulses (pedal/posterior tibial).
   c. Take the client's blood pressure.
   d. Recognize that this is an expected response and reassess the patient in 1 hour.

5. A 54-year-old man comes to triage complaining of severe, left-sided, pressure-like chest pain and left arm numbness. The pain began 2 hours ago and is unrelieved by rest. The patient is anxious, diaphoretic, and complaining of nausea. Cardiac monitoring is begun, and oxygen is given at 2 L/min. An intermittent infusion device (IID) is in place, and vital signs are as follows: BP of 128/68 mm Hg; pulse, 76 beats/min; respirations easy and regular at 20 breaths/min. ECG reveals normal sinus rhythm with occasional unifocal premature ventricular contractions (PVCs).
   The nurse suspects an MI based on an elevation in the which lab study?
   a. CK-MB and LDH
   b. LDH and troponin I
   c. CK-MB and troponin I
   d. Troponin I and SGPT

REFERENCES AND SELECTED READINGS

References and selected readings associated with this chapter can be found on the website that accompanies the book. Visit **http://thepoint. lww.com/Honan2e** to access the references and other additional resources associated with this chapter.

Nursing Management: Patients with Complications from Heart Disease

Jessica Shank Coviello

Learning Objectives

After reading this chapter, you will be able to:

1. Compare and contrast diastolic and systolic heart failure (HF), including pathophysiology and clinical manifestations.
2. Describe the management of patients with HF.
3. Develop a teaching plan for patients with HF.
4. Describe the assessment and management of patients with pulmonary edema.
5. Describe the management of patients with cardiogenic shock.
6. Describe the management of patients with pericardial effusion.
7. Describe emergency management of patients with cardiac arrest.

Today, patients with heart disease can be assisted to live longer and achieve a higher quality of life than they could even a decade ago. Through advances in diagnostic procedures that allow earlier and more accurate diagnoses, treatment can begin well before significant debilitation occurs. Newer treatments, technologies, and pharmacotherapies are being developed rapidly. However, heart disease remains a chronic condition, and complications may develop. This chapter presents the complications most often resulting from heart diseases and the treatments provided by the health care team for these complications.

HEART FAILURE

Heart failure (HF) is the inability of the heart to pump sufficient blood to meet the needs of the tissues for oxygen and nutrients. In the past, HF was often referred to as **congestive heart failure** (CHF), because many patients experience pulmonary or peripheral congestion. Currently HF is recognized as a clinical syndrome characterized by signs and symptoms of fluid overload or of inadequate tissue perfusion. Fluid overload and decreased tissue perfusion result when the heart cannot generate a cardiac output (CO) sufficient to meet the body's demands (see Chapter 12 for a review of cardiac hemodynamics). The term *heart failure* indicates myocardial disease in which there is a problem with contraction of the heart

(systolic dysfunction) or filling of the heart (diastolic dysfunction) that may or may not cause pulmonary or systemic congestion. Some cases of HF are reversible, depending on the cause. Most often, HF is a progressive, lifelong diagnosis that is managed with lifestyle changes and medications to prevent acute congestive episodes.

CHRONIC HEART FAILURE

As with coronary artery disease (CAD), the incidence of chronic heart failure increases with age. The nature of chronic heart failure can be either systolic or diastolic with systolic failure the most common at 60% (Hobbs & Boyle, 2014). In the United States, the lifetime risk of developing HF is 20% for those *age* 40 years and older. Currently, over 5.7 million people *age 20 years or older* in the United States have HF, and 650,000 new cases are diagnosed each year (Muzaffarian et al., 2015). Although HF can affect people of all ages, the incidence increases from approximately 20 per 1000 individuals 65 to 69 years of age to more than 80 per 1000 among those age 85 years or older. HF is the most common reason for hospitalization of people older than 65 years of age and the second most common reason for visits to a health care provider. The rate of hospital readmission remains staggeringly high. The economic burden caused by HF is estimated to rise from $30.7 billion in 2012 to $69.7 billion in 2030 (Muzaffarian et al., 2015).

The increase in the incidence of HF reflects the increased number of elderly people and improvements in treatment of cardiac diseases, resulting in increased survival rates. Many hospitalizations could be prevented by appropriate outpatient care. Prevention and early intervention to arrest the progression of HF are major health initiatives in the United States.

Types and Classification

There are two types of HF, which are identified by assessment of left ventricular functioning, usually by echocardiogram. The more common type is an alteration in ventricular contraction called **systolic heart failure**, which is characterized by a weakened heart muscle. The less common alteration is **diastolic heart failure**, which is characterized by a stiff and noncompliant heart muscle, making it difficult for the ventricle to fill. An assessment of the **ejection fraction (EF)** is performed to assist in determining the type of HF. EF, an indication of the volume of blood ejected with each contraction, is calculated by subtracting the amount of blood at the end of systole from the amount at the end of diastole and calculating the percentage of blood that is ejected. A normal EF is 50% to 70% of the ventricular volume; the ventricle does not empty completely between contractions. The EF is normal in diastolic HF but severely reduced in systolic HF.

Pathophysiology Alert
In diastolic heart failure there is a normal EF; therefore, a normal EF does not mean or equate to normal CO. A normal EF is not a reliable gauge of normal CO. The nurse is aware that a low CO is the fundamental pathophysiologic abnormality of all HF.

Although a low EF is a hallmark of HF, the severity of HF is frequently classified according to the patient's symptoms. In 2008, the American College of Cardiology and the American Heart Association (Schocken et al.) developed a classification system for HF that incorporates a patient's clinical status and pathophysiology of the disease in its classification. Stages of HF (A–D) were defined for use in understanding and managing the progression of HF, including risk factors for HF and primary prevention strategies; the stage classifications continue to be used today. Additionally, Figure 15-1 considers the natural history and progressive nature of HF. Treatment guidelines have been developed for each stage.

Pathophysiology

HF results from a variety of cardiovascular (CV) conditions (including chronic hypertension [HTN], CAD, valvular disease, congenital heart defects, and arrhythmias) as well as from conditions such as diabetes mellitus, fever, infection, thyrotoxicosis, iron overload, hypoxia, anemia, and pulmonary embolus (Mann, Zipes, Libby, & Bonow, 2014). These conditions can result in decreased contraction (systole), decreased filling (diastole), or both. Significant myocardial dysfunction most often occurs before the patient experiences signs and symptoms of HF, such as shortness of breath, edema, or fatigue.

As HF develops, the body activates neurohormonal compensatory mechanisms. These mechanisms represent the body's attempt to cope with the HF and are responsible for the signs and symptoms that eventually develop. Understanding these mechanisms is important because the treatment of HF is aimed at relieving them (Fig. 15-2).

Systolic HF results in a decrease in the volume of blood being ejected from the ventricle. The decreased ventricular stretch is sensed by baroreceptors (sensors in blood vessels that respond to perfusion pressure of blood flow) in the aortic and carotid bodies (Mann et al., 2014). The sympathetic nervous system is stimulated to release epinephrine and norepinephrine. The purpose of this initial response is to increase heart rate and **contractility** and support the failing myocardium, but the continued response has multiple negative effects. Sympathetic stimulation causes vasoconstriction of the skin, gastrointestinal tract, and kidneys. A decrease in renal perfusion due to low CO and vasoconstriction then causes the release of renin by the kidney. Renin promotes the formation of angiotensin I, a benign, inactive substance. Angiotensin-converting enzyme (ACE) in the lumen of pulmonary blood vessels converts angiotensin I to angiotensin II, a potent vasoconstrictor, which then increases the blood pressure and **afterload** (see alert below). Angiotensin II also stimulates the release of aldosterone from the adrenal cortex, resulting in retention of sodium and fluid, excretion of potassium (K^+) by the renal tubules, and stimulation of the thirst center. This leads to the fluid volume overload commonly seen in HF. Angiotensin, aldosterone, and other neurohormones (e.g., endothelin, prostacyclin) lead to an increase in **preload** (see alert below) and afterload, which increases stress on the ventricular wall, causing an increase in the workload of the heart. Additionally, the combination of medication treatments for HF coupled with the release of aldosterone predisposes patients with HF to hypokalemia. A counter-regulatory mechanism is attempted through the release of natriuretic peptides. Atrial natriuretic peptide (ANP) and B-type natriuretic peptide (BNP) are released from the over distended cardiac chambers (Fig. 15-3). These substances promote vasodilation and diuresis. However, their effect is usually not strong enough to overcome the negative effects of the other mechanisms.

Nursing Alert
Preload should be considered as the stretching of the cardiac muscle prior to contraction. Ventricular preload is determined by the volume of blood in the ventricle prior to the onset of systole and is a function of both venous return and end-systolic volume of the chamber. For example, when venous return or volume of blood entering the heart is

At Risk for Heart Failure

Stage A
At high risk for HF but without structural heart disease or symptoms of HF

Stage B
Structural heart disease but without signs or symptoms of HF

Heart Failure

Stage C
Structural heart disease with prior or current symptoms of HF

Stage D
Refractory HF requiring specialized interventions

e.g., **Patients with:**
•hypertension
•atherosclerotic disease
•diabetes
•obesity
•metabolic syndrome
or
Patients
•using cardiotoxins
•with FHx CM

Structural heart disease

e.g., **Patients with:**
•previous MI
•LV remodeling including LVH and low EF
•asymptomatic valvular disease

Development of symptoms of HF

e.g., **Patients with:**
•known structural heart disease
and
•shortness of breath and fatigue, reduced exercise tolerance

Refractory symptoms of HF at rest

e.g., **Patients** who have marked symptoms at rest despite maximal medical therapy (e.g., those who are recurrently hospitalized or cannot be safely discharged from the hospital without specialized interventions.)

Therapy
Goals
•Treat hypertension
•Encourage smoking cessation
•Treat lipid disorders
•Encourage regular exercise
•Discourage alcohol intake, illicit drug use
•Control metabolic syndrome
Drugs
•ACEI or ARB in appropriate patients for vascular disease or diabetes

Therapy
Goals
•All measures under stage A
Drugs
•ACEI or ARB in appropriate patients
•Beta blockers in appropriate patients
Devices in selected patients
•Implantable defibrillators

Therapy
Goals
•All measures under stages A and B
•Dietary salt restriction
Drugs for routine use
•Diuretics for fluid retention
•ACEI
•Beta blockers
Drugs in selected patients
•Aldosterone antagonist
•ARBs
•Digitalis
•Hydralazine/nitrates
Devices in selected patients
•Biventricular pacing
•Implantable defibrillators

Therapy
Goals
•Appropriate measures under stages A, B, C
•Decision re: appropriate level of care
Options
•Compassionate end-of-life care/hospice
•Extraordinary measures
 •heart transplant
 •chronic inotropes
 •permanent mechanical support
 •experimental surgery or drugs

© 2009, American Heart Association, Inc.

FIGURE 15-1 Stages in the development of heart failure. ACEI, angiotensin-converting enzyme inhibitor; ARB, angiotensin receptor blocker; EF, ejection fraction; FHx CM, family history of cardiomyopathy; LV, left ventricle; LVH, left ventricular hypertrophy; MI, myocardial infarction. (From American Heart Association (AHA). (2009). *Circulation*, *119*, 1977–2016. Reprinted with permission.)

increased, preload increases. In contrast, if there is a loss of blood due to hemorrhage, less blood returns to the atria and this leads to decreased ventricular filling and reduced preload. Regardless of the chamber (atria or ventricle), preload is related to the volume just prior to contraction. Afterload should be considered as resistance to flow (the pressure gradient that the ventricles must overcome to pump blood out the ventricles to either the lungs or systemic circulation).

As the heart's workload increases, contractility of the myocardial muscle fibers decreases. Decreased contractility results in an increase in end-diastolic blood volume (preload) in the ventricle, stretching the myocardial muscle fibers and

increasing the size of the ventricle (ventricular dilation). The increased size of the ventricle further increases the stress on the ventricular wall, adding to the workload of the heart. One way the heart compensates for the increased workload is to increase the thickness of the heart muscle (ventricular hypertrophy). However, hypertrophy results in an abnormal proliferation of myocardial cells, a process known as *ventricular remodeling*. Under the influence of neurohormones (e.g., angiotensin II), large myocardial cells are produced that are dysfunctional and die early, leaving the other normal myocardial cells to struggle to maintain CO (Mann et al., 2014). The heart does not pump sufficient blood to the body, which causes the body to stimulate the heart to work harder; the heart cannot respond, and failure becomes worse. This

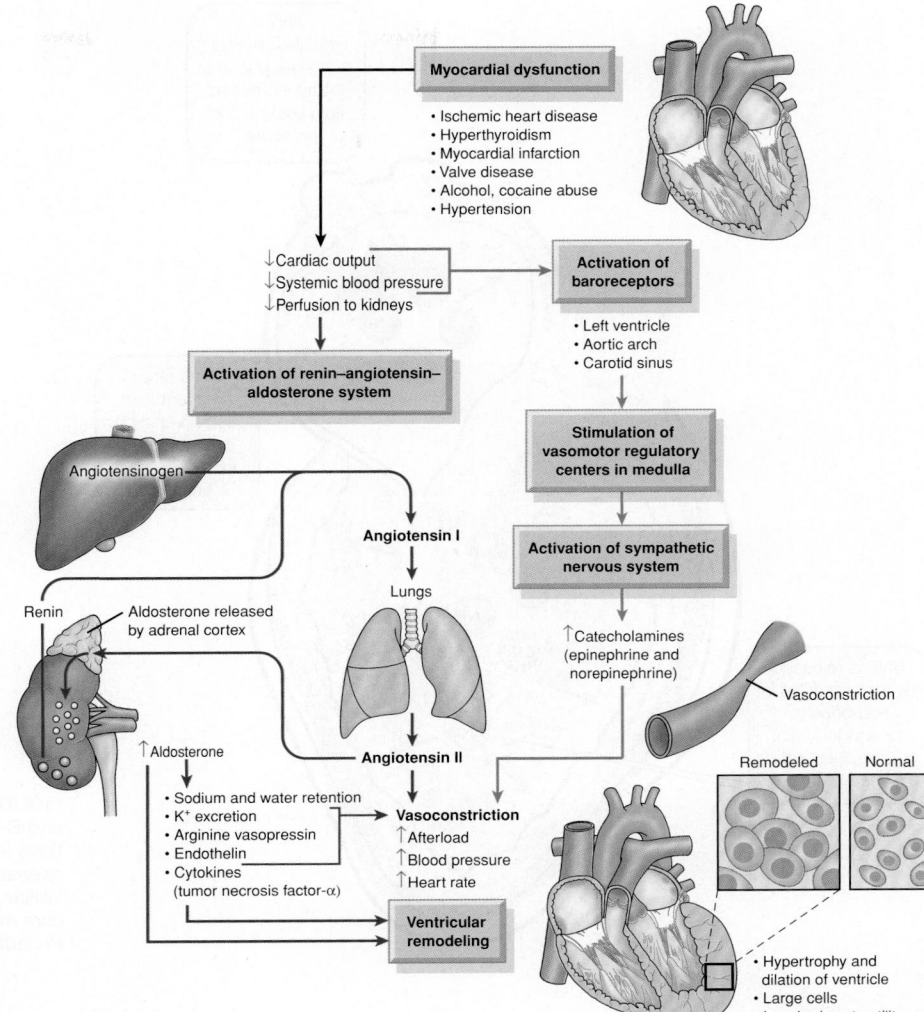

FIGURE 15-2 The pathophysiology of heart failure. A decrease in cardiac output activates multiple neurohormonal mechanisms that ultimately result in the signs and symptoms of HF.

cycle repeats itself, thus contributing to an ongoing process of further cardiac decline.

Diastolic HF develops because of continued increased workload on the heart, which responds by increasing the number and size of myocardial cells (i.e., ventricular hypertrophy and altered cellular functioning). These responses cause resistance to ventricular filling, which increases ventricular filling pressures despite a normal or reduced blood volume. Less blood in the ventricles causes decreased CO. The low CO and high ventricular filling pressures can cause the same neurohormonal responses as described for systolic HF. Table 15-1 provides a comparison of systolic and diastolic HF (Van Wacher & Edelmann, 2014).

Additionally, HF may present as right sided versus left sided (Table 15-2).

Risk Factors

There are important risk factors for HF that can be modified before actual structural heart disease occurs. Early

identification and treatment of these risk factors, or comorbidities may prevent or decrease the occurrence of the onset of HF. Risk factors that are asymptomatic for HF are included in stage A HF.

An example of such an HF risk factor is HTN. HTN is a risk for both men and women, but it is more profound in women. In fact, it is the primary etiology of HF in women. The incidence of HF increases as blood pressure increases, duration increases, and the patient's age increases. Long-term treatment of HTN reduces the risk by 50% (Yancy et al., 2013). It has been estimated that the lifetime risk of HTN in the United States is more than 75%. It is, therefore, an important risk factor to treat early, and patients should be encouraged to maintain their blood pressure below 140/90 mm Hg consistently (Yancy et al., 2013).

Those with diabetes mellitus or metabolic syndrome are at greater risk of HF. Remember metabolic syndrome is confirmed in patients who have any three of the following: abdominal obesity, elevated triglyceride levels (over 150 mg/dL), decreased high-density lipoprotein (HDL) (<40 mg/dL for men, <50 mg/dL for women) HTN, and elevated fasting

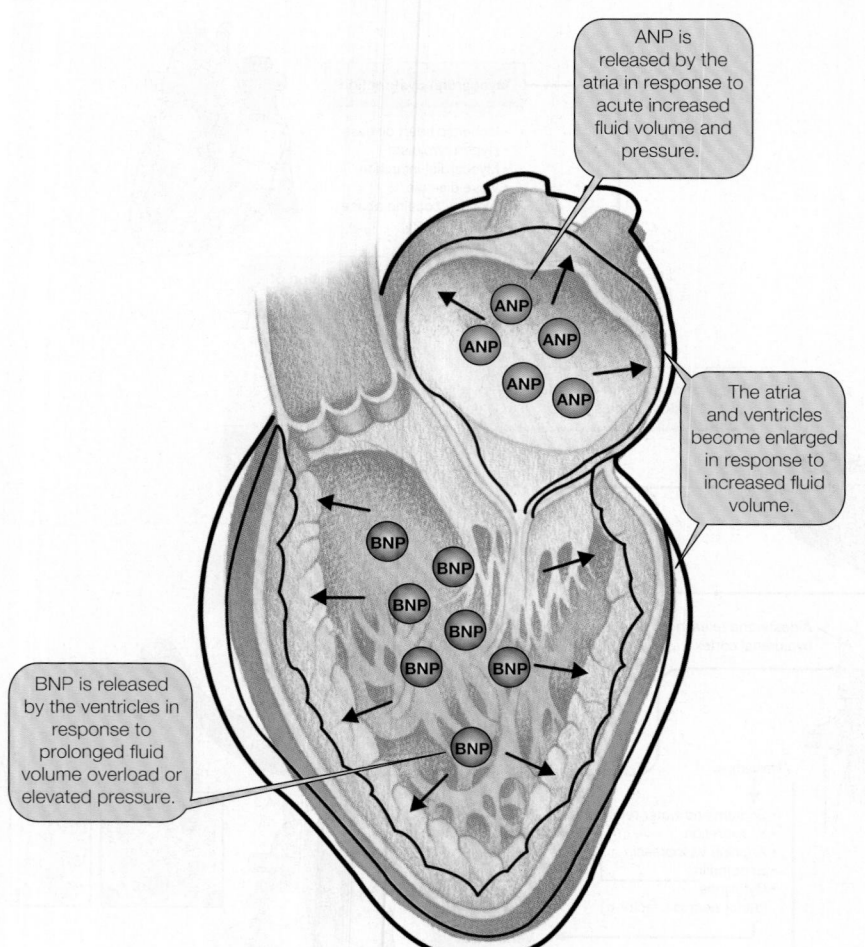

FIGURE 15-3 A-type natriuretic peptide (ANP) and B-type natriuretic peptide (BNP). Disruptions in intravascular fluid balance trigger the release of ANP and BNP. (From Lippincott Williams & Wilkins. (2010). *Cardiovascular care made incredibly visual* (2nd ed., p. 50). Philadelphia, PA: Lippincott Williams & Wilkins.)

glucose. These comorbidities also negatively affect outcomes for those with HF (Yancy et al., 2013).

Finally, those diagnosed with atherosclerotic disease (CAD, stroke, or peripheral vascular disease) are likely to develop HF without adequate control of CV risk. It is important to note that the primary cause of HF in men is CAD (Schocken et al., 2008; Yancy et al., 2013; Goff et al., 2013; Katz, 2015; van Deursen et al., 2014a).

TABLE 15-1 Comparison of Systolic and Diastolic Heart Failure

	Systolic Failure	Diastolic Failure
Pathophysiology	• Impaired ventricular pumping of blood during systole • Characterized by reduced stroke volume, incomplete ventricular emptying, cardiac dilation, and elevated left ventricular diastolic pressure • Reduced cardiac output evokes compensatory neurohormonal responses that increase heart rate, sodium and water retention, and vasoconstriction	• Impaired ventricular relaxation filling during diastole • Characterized by a stiffened left ventricle that cannot relax and fill sufficiently at normal diastolic pressure • The result is either decreased left ventricular end-diastolic volume (leading to decreased cardiac output) or a compensatory rise in left ventricular filling pressure, which can lead to pulmonary venous hypertension
Causes/etiology	Usually caused by ischemic or idiopathic dilated cardiomyopathy, when the left ventricle cannot adequately contract or squeeze out its contents, so that preload increases and stroke volume decreases	Usually caused by hypertensive, hypertrophic, or restrictive cardiomyopathy

TABLE 15-2 Symptom Comparison of Left- Versus Right-Sided Heart Failure

	Left-Sided HF	Right-Sided HF
Pathophysiology	• Pulmonary congestion from impaired left ventricle (LV) function • LV cannot pump blood out of the ventricle effectively into the aorta and the systemic circulation • Pulmonary venous blood volume and pressure increase, forcing fluid from the pulmonary capillaries into the pulmonary tissues and alveoli, causing pulmonary interstitial edema and impaired gas exchange	• Right ventricle pump failure leading to congestion in the peripheral tissues and the viscera • Right side of the heart cannot eject blood and cannot accommodate all the blood that normally returns to it from the venous circulation • Increased venous pressure leads to jugular vein distension (JVD) and increased hydrostatic pressure throughout the venous system. Normal central venous pressure (CVP) is 2–8 mm Hg. A CVP greater than 8 mm Hg associated with hypervolemia (excessive fluid circulating in the body) or right-sided HF

Clinical Manifestations and Assessment

Systolic and diastolic HF share similar clinical findings. Overt signs of HF include resting dyspnea, cyanosis, and cachexia (physical wasting), resulting from long-standing heart disease. A baseline height and weight should be documented on admission and weight rechecked each morning. Obtaining daily weights and tracking trends in weight, along with an accurate intake and output log, provide an easy and accurate way to monitor fluid balance. Fluid balance is an important surveillance strategy in controlling HF symptoms.

Nursing Alert
Daily weights should be at the same time, on the same scale, and with the patient wearing the same clothes for accuracy. The nurse is aware that when calculating new gain or loss that 500 mL approximates 1 lb, or 1000 mL approximates 1 kg (2.2 lb).

A thorough CV assessment is performed, which includes blood pressure measurement in both sitting and standing positions in order to detect orthostatic hypotension.

Tachycardia (heart rate over 120 bpm) may signal worsening HF. When the heart rate is rapid, the stroke volume (SV) decreases because the ventricle has less time to fill. This, in turn, produces increased pressure in the atria and, eventually, in the pulmonary vascular bed. A weak, thready pulse and *pulsus alternans* (pulse is regular but force of amplitude varies with alternating beats from large to small) are signs of decreased left ventricular function.

Left ventricular hypertrophy (LVH) may displace the apical pulse left and downward from its normal location at the fifth intercostal space, medial to the midclavicular line. Right-sided HF may present with an elevation in jugular venous pressure greater than 4 cm above the sternal angle. This is an estimate, not a precise measurement, of central venous pressure.

An S_3 heart sound is a sign that the heart is beginning to fail and that increased blood volume is filling the ventricle with each beat. Other sounds may include mitral and tricuspid regurgitation murmurs. The nurse may detect an S_4 sound if the patient has increased resistance to ventricular filling because of increased stiffness of the ventricular myocardium.

The nurse assesses the lungs. Crackles (formerly called rales) are discrete, discontinuous crackling sounds heard at the end of inspiration. They are produced by the sudden delayed reopening of edematous small airways and alveoli and are not cleared with coughing. It is recommended that the nurse begins auscultation at the base of the lungs to detect crackles in HF patients and notes the extent. Typically crackles start at the lung bases and are heard progressively higher in the lungs as HF worsens. Wheezing may also be heard in some patients. The rate and depth of respirations are also documented. Dullness to percussion may indicate pleural effusions due to HF.

The nurse assesses dependent parts of the patient's body for perfusion and edema. With significant decreases in SV, there is a decrease in perfusion to the periphery, causing the skin to feel cool and to appear pale or cyanotic. If the patient is sitting upright, the feet and lower legs are examined for edema; if the patient is supine in bed, the sacrum and back are also assessed for edema. Fingers and hands may also become edematous. The nurse notes the location and extent of the edema and assesses for evidence of pitting edema (refer to Chapter 12).

Hepatomegaly, hepatojugular reflux, and ascites can occur with venous congestion due to right-sided HF. Recall with right-sided HF, there is accumulation of fluid in the systemic venous circulation. To assess for hepatojugular reflux, the patient is positioned in bed so that the nurse can observe the blood column of the jugular veins above the clavicle. The patient is asked to breathe normally while manual pressure is applied over the right upper quadrant of the abdomen for at least 5 seconds (Kusumoto Heart Disease, 2013). If the top of the jugular venous column in the neck rises and persists as long as the abdominal pressure is continued, it is considered positive hepatojugular reflux, which indicates that the right ventricle cannot accommodate the additional volume of displaced blood; when the right ventricle cannot accommodate this additional volume,

BOX 15-1
Focus on Assessment

Left-Sided Versus Right-Sided Heart Failure

Be alert for the following signs and symptoms:

Left-Sided HF
- Dyspnea, orthopnea, PND
- Cough
- Pulmonary crackles (rales)
- Decrease O_2 saturation levels
- S_3 ventricular gallop
- Oliguria, if kidney perfusion is diminished (Note: Nocturia may occur when perfusion improves with sleeping due to improved perfusion at rest.)
- Decreased perfusion to other systemic organs (advanced failure):
  - Sluggish GI motility
  - Dizziness, lightheadedness, confusion, restlessness
  - Anxiety
  - Skin cool and clammy
  - Decrease in EF
  - Tachycardia and/or weak/thready pulse
  - Fatigue or activity intolerance

Right-Sided HF
- Lower extremity dependent edema (dependent edema is swelling that follows the position of the body):
  - Legs and feet
  - May progress to thighs, external genitalia, lower trunk, abdomen, and sacral edema (in a bed-bound patient)
  - Pitting edema (indentations in the skin remain even after slight compression with the fingertips)
- Hepatomegaly (enlargement of the liver)
- Ascites (accumulation of fluid in the peritoneal cavity)
- Anorexia and nausea
- Weight gain due to retention of fluid
- Weakness/fatigue from reduced CO and impaired cognition
- Decreased perfusion to other systemic organs (advanced failure)

an increase in jugular venous pressure is seen. A positive hepatojugular reflux is associated with right HF and constrictive pericarditis.

Sensorium and level of consciousness must be evaluated. As the volume of blood ejected by the heart decreases, so does the amount of oxygen transported to the brain. Patients may complain of dizziness or lightheadedness. Box 15-1 compares and contrasts assessment findings in left- and right-sided HF.

Diagnostic evaluation includes:

- A chest x-ray can determine the presence and extent of cardiac enlargement or pulmonary congestion and can help identify pulmonary disease. Cardiomegaly indicates systolic dysfunction; a normal heart size suggests diastolic dysfunction.

- A 12-lead electrocardiogram (ECG) determines the presence of cardiac arrhythmias, LVH, and previous or current myocardial infarction (MI). If the patient has left ventricular dysfunction, the ECG usually indicates a left ventricular electrical abnormality specific to ventricular dilation or hypertrophy.

- A two-dimensional (2D) echocardiogram with Doppler flow study is a noninvasive test to look for structural cardiac abnormalities and to measure EF. An EF of less than 40% indicates systolic dysfunction; an EF of greater than 40% with signs and symptoms of HF and impaired ventricular relaxation indicates diastolic dysfunction.

- Although the 2D echocardiogram remains the more common approach to assessing left ventricular function, three-dimensional (3D) echocardiogram with strain (−20% plus or minus 2 SD) measurements is quickly replacing the 2D mode due to greater accuracy (Jasilyte et al., 2013; Yingchoncharoen, Agarwal, Popvic, & Marwick, 2013).

- Cardiac magnetic resonance testing is now considered the gold standard for assessing cardiac function. It is a more expensive test than both the 2D and 3D with strain and can be found only in large or regional medical facilities (Manolis, Chamodraka, & Zacharopoulou, 2015).

- Laboratory tests that may help diagnose HF include complete blood cell count, electrolyte levels (including calcium and magnesium), blood urea nitrogen, creatinine, serum glucose, serum albumin, liver function tests, thyroid-stimulating hormone, urinalysis, and BNP levels. High BNP levels (greater than 100 pg/mL) indicate abnormal ventricular function or symptomatic HF.

- A right-sided heart catheterization also can be performed to determine the heart's preload pressures and pulmonary pressures to determine the degree of HF and the need for further intervention. A patient with angina who is a candidate for coronary revascularization may undergo a full cardiac catheterization with coronary arteriography.

Medical Management

Treatment begins with prevention. Identifying patients at risk is the first step in the care and treatment of HF.

The overall goals of management of HF are to relieve patient symptoms, improve functional status and quality of life, and extend survival. Treatment is based on the type, severity, and cause of HF. Specific objectives include the following:

- Eliminate or reduce any etiologic contributory factors, especially those that may be reversible (e.g., atrial fibrillation, excessive alcohol ingestion, uncontrolled HTN).
- Reduce the workload on the heart by reducing afterload and preload.
- Optimize all therapeutic regimens.
- Prevent exacerbations of HF.

Treatment options vary according to the severity of the patient's condition (see Fig. 15-1).

Lifestyle Changes

Managing the patient with HF includes providing general education and counseling to the patient and family. It is important that the patient and family understand the nature of HF and the importance of their participation in the treatment regimen. Lifestyle recommendations include restriction of dietary sodium; avoidance of excessive fluid intake, alcohol, and smoking; weight reduction when indicated; and regular exercise. The patient must know how to recognize signs and symptoms that need to be reported to the health care professional such as weight gain, increasing shortness of breath, fatigue, and edema.

Pharmacologic Therapy

Several medications (Table 15-3) are prescribed routinely for systolic HF, including ACE inhibitors, beta blockers,

TABLE 15-3 Pharmacologic Treatment of Heart Failure

Drug Class	Pharmacokinetics	Indications and Nursing Implications
Diuretics	Diuretics prompt the kidneys to excrete sodium, chloride, and water, reducing fluid volume. They are a preload reducer.	• Diuretics should never be used alone to treat HF because they don't prevent further myocardial damage. • Loop diuretics such as furosemide, bumetanide, and torsemide, are the preferred first-line diuretics because of their efficacy in patients with and without kidney impairment. • Low-dose spironolactone may be added to a patient's regimen if he or she has recent or recurrent symptoms at rest despite therapy with angiotensin-converting enzyme (ACE) inhibitors, beta blockers, digoxin, and diuretics.
Inotropes	Inotropes affect the force of myocardial contraction. Positive inotropes increase force of myocardial contraction and also increase workload of heart and oxygen demand. Negative inotropes decrease force of myocardial contraction and decrease workload of heart and oxygen demand.	• Digoxin increases the heart's ability to contract and improves HF symptoms and exercise tolerance in patients with mild to moderate HF. • Major adverse reactions to positive inotropes include arrhythmias; gastrointestinal problems, such as anorexia; and neurologic symptoms, such as confusion (Adams et al., 2014). • IV-positive inotropes, such as dobutamine, dopamine, and milrinone, can also be used for long-term support (e.g., patients awaiting cardiac transplant) via a tunneled central venous catheter or peripherally inserted central catheter.
ACE inhibitors	ACE inhibitors, such as captopril and enalapril, block the conversion of angiotensin I to angiotensin II, a vasoconstrictor that can raise blood pressure. These drugs alleviate HF symptoms by causing vasodilation and decreasing myocardial workload. They are preload and afterload reducers that provide renal protection.	• The most common adverse reaction to ACE inhibitors is a dry cough. Other adverse reactions include hypotension, worsening kidney function, and potassium retention.
Angiotensin-II receptor blockers	Angiotensin-II receptor antagonists selectively block the binding of angiotensin II to specific tissue receptors in vascular smooth muscle and the adrenal glands. Overall effects include: blocking the vasoconstricting effect of the renin–angiotensin system; blocking aldosterone release, leading to a reduction in sodium and water retention; they have little effect on potassium. They are preload and afterload reducers.	• Patients who cannot take ACE inhibitors may be prescribed angiotensin receptor blockers instead. This therapy reduces the effects of sodium and water retention, vasoconstriction, and myocardial remodeling.
Aldosterone receptor antagonists	Aldosterone receptor antagonists, such as eplerenone, block aldosterone from binding to receptors in the kidneys. This allows the kidneys to eliminate excess sodium and water. They are a preload reducer.	• Aldosterone receptor antagonists are similar to ACE inhibitors for nursing implications. Evidence suggests patients may not exhibit the side effect of a cough as they do with ACE inhibitors.

(continued on page 460)

TABLE **15-3** Pharmacologic Treatment of Heart Failure (*continued*)

Drug Class	Pharmacokinetics	Indications and Nursing Implications
Beta blockers	Beta-adrenergic blockers, such as bisoprolol, metoprolol, and carvedilol, block the effects of catecholamines, resulting in reduction of heart rate, decreased peripheral vasoconstriction and decreased myocardial demand. Beta blockers can interfere with the passage of air into the lungs. However, selective beta blockers avoid this problem. They are a negative inotrope.	• Long-term therapy reduces HF symptoms and improves the patient's functional status.
Nesiritide	Nesiritide (Natrecor) is a preparation of human B-type natriuretic peptide (BNP) that mimics the action of endogenous BNP, causing diuresis and vasodilation, reduced BP, and improved cardiac output. It is a preload and afterload reducer.	• It is given via the IV route only. **The use of nesiritide has come into question recently with outcomes similar to those of diuretics (van Deursen et al., 2014b).**
Vasodilators/nitrates	Vasodilators/nitrates are used for arterial and venous smooth muscle relaxation. They are preload and afterload reducers.	• The combination of hydralazine and nitrates is recommended to improve outcomes for patients self-described as African American (Khazanie et al., 2016) with moderate–severe HF symptoms who are on optimal ACE inhibitors, beta blockers, and diuretics.

diuretics, and digoxin. Medications for diastolic failure depend on the underlying condition, such as HTN or valvular dysfunction.

Additional Therapies

Additional therapy and surgical treatment are described in Table 15-4. Box 15-2 discusses the psychological impact of these therapies.

Nursing Management

Despite advances in medical and surgical approaches to HF, mortality remains high. Nurses can make a major difference in promoting positive outcomes. Caring for patients with HF requires a collaborative, interdisciplinary team approach. Nurses play a pivotal role in the care and ongoing teaching of this patient population (Danna, Garbee, & Kensler, 2014).

Assessing the Patient

The nursing assessment for the patient with HF focuses on observing for effectiveness of therapy and for the patient's ability to understand and implement self-management strategies. Signs and symptoms of pulmonary and systemic fluid overload are recorded and reported immediately so that adjustments can be made in therapy. The nurse also explores the patient's emotional response to the diagnosis of HF, a chronic and often progressive condition.

The health history focuses on the signs and symptoms of HF, such as shortness of breath, **dyspnea on exertion (DOE)**, (shortness of breath that occurs with exertion), and cough. Sleep disturbances, particularly sleep suddenly interrupted by shortness of breath termed *paroxysmal nocturnal dyspnea* (PND), may be reported. The nurse also asks about the number of pillows needed for sleep (an indication of **orthopnea**—shortness of breath while lying flat), edema, abdominal symptoms, altered mental status, activities of daily living, daily weight, and the activities that cause fatigue. The nurse explores the patient's understanding of HF, self-management strategies, and the desire to adhere to those strategies. The nurse helps patients identify the impact the illness has had on their quality of life and successful coping skills that they have used. Often family and significant others are included in these discussions.

Monitoring Intake and Output

If the patient is hospitalized, the nurse measures output carefully to establish a baseline against which to assess the effectiveness of diuretic therapy. Intake and output records are rigorously maintained. It is important to know whether the patient has ingested more fluid than he or she has excreted (positive fluid balance), which then is correlated with a gain in weight. The patient must be monitored for **oliguria** (diminished urine output, less than 400 mL/24 hours) or anuria (urine output less than 100 mL/24 hours).

The patient is weighed daily in the hospital or at home, at the same time of day, with the same type of clothing, and on the same scale. If there is a significant change in weight (i.e., 2 to 3 lb increase in a day or 5 lb increase in a week), the patient is instructed to notify his or her provider or to adjust the medications (e.g., increase the diuretic dose) per the provider's directions.

TABLE **15-4** Modalities for Treatment of Heart Failure

Modality	Indications	Description/Procedure
Ultrafiltration (UF)	Eases symptoms for patients in decompensated HF and can help some patients to respond again to conventional drug therapy; it is a low-volume extracorporeal process that removes fluid from the intravascular compartment. Recent studies show inconsistent findings on the benefit of UF vs. standard diuretic therapy (Mehra, 2015; Marenzi, Kazory, & Agostoni, 2015).	• Uses a mechanical pump and a hemofilter to remove a specified amount of fluid with each treatment, alleviating the patient's symptoms. • Treatment time varies depending on patient needs. • During treatment, the intravascular fluid volume remains stable, since fluid shifts from the interstitial space to replace fluid lost in treatment, which reduces edema and third-spacing. Typically, patients do not become hypotensive or hypovolemic with this treatment (Klein, 2014).
Cardiac resynchronization therapy (CRT)	In the patient with HF who does not improve with standard therapy, CRT may be beneficial. CRT involves the use of a biventricular pacemaker to treat electrical conduction defects. Left bundle branch block is a feature of delayed conduction that is frequently seen in patients with HF that results in dyssynchronous conduction and contraction of the right and left ventricles, which can further decrease EF (Yancy et al., 2013).	• Use of a pacing device with leads placed in the right atrium, right ventricle, and left ventricular can synchronize the contractions of the right and left ventricles. This intervention has been shown to improve cardiac output, optimize myocardial energy consumption, reduce mitral regurgitation, and slow the ventricular remodeling process. For selected patients, this results in fewer symptoms and increased functional status (Yancy et al., 2013; Krishnamoorthy & Felker, 2014). For patients who require CRT and an implantable cardiac defibrillator (ICD), combination devices are available.
Implantable cardiac defibrillators (ICDs)	Patients with HF are at high risk for arrhythmias. In patients with life-threatening arrhythmias, placement of an ICD can prevent sudden cardiac death and extend survival.	• ICDs can provide a range of therapies that include cardioversion, defibrillation, and pacing. A lead or leads are placed in the appropriate chamber's endocardium and attached to a generator box that can be implanted in the right or left side of the chest, under the clavicle. • Wearable cardioverter defibrillators have recently been used as a bridge to implantable defibrillators (Chung, 2014).
Ventricular access devices/destination therapy	Patients with end-stage HF may require a ventricular assist device (VAD) for greater support for the failing ventricle(s). A VAD can reduce myocardial ischemia and workload, limit permanent cardiac damage, and restore adequate organ perfusion. Indications for use include: as a bridge to myocardial recovery in acute ventricular failure (e.g., shock, acute MI, etc.), as a bridge to heart transplantation in chronic ventricular failure, and for permanent therapy for end-stage chronic HF. VADs are also known as *destination therapy*.	• VADs are mechanical blood pumps that work by augmenting or replacing the function of either the left or right ventricle. • There are currently four FDA-approved devices that are used as bridges to transplantation in adults. One of the four is also approved for use as destination therapy or as long-term mechanical support of the heart. The devises may be pulsatile or continuous flow (nonpulsatile) (Sunagawa et al., 2017). • All shares a common problem with infectious complications, risk for thromboembolic complications, and possibility of mechanical failure common to any machine.
Heart transplant	For some patients with end-stage HF, cardiac transplantation is the only option for long-term survival. Some of these patients require mechanical circulatory assistance with an implanted ventricular assist device as a bridge therapy to cardiac transplantation. Research continues toward perfection of a totally implantable artificial heart that may be used as an alternative to transplantation.	• Heart transplantation involves replacing a person's diseased heart with a donor heart. This is an option for advanced HF patients when all other therapies have failed (Ammirate et al., 2014).

BOX 15-2   Nursing Research

Bridging the Gap to Evidence-Based Practice

What are the evidence-based approaches and key factors associated with successful outcomes in teaching patients with heart failure?

Rasmusson, K., Flattery, M., Baas, L. S. (2015). American Association of Heart Failure Nurses position paper on educating patients with heart failure. *Heart & Lung, 44*(2), 173–177.

Purpose

To provide supporting evidence associated with successful educational approaches for patients with heart failure.

Design

This is a position paper. Position papers represent a policy or opinion of a panel of experts representing an organization (e.g., American Heart Association). They are based on a synthesis and analysis of the literature and expert testimony.

Nursing Implications

The nurse's approach to teaching self-care measures to heart failure patients should be guideline directed and evidence based. It should include:

- Early instruction reinforced through the hospital stay and at discharge (Andrikopoulou, Abbate, & Whellan, 2014)
- Assessment of patient's health literacy, educational preferences, and knowledge of heart failure tailored to the patient's needs, including preferred language and learning style (visual, verbal, and/or multimedia)

- Sixty minutes of heart failure education, which has demonstrated a reduction in 30-day readmission (Koelling, Johnson, Cody, & Aaronson, 2005)
- Teach-back methods (White, Garbez, Carroll, Brinker, & Howie-Esquivel, 2013)
- Family and caregivers (Agren, Evangelista, Hjelm, & Stromber, 2012; Hwang, Fleischmann, Howie-Esquivel, Stotts, & Dracup, 2011; Kurylo, Elliot, & Deviro, 2004)
- Evidence-based and novel teaching techniques to enhance knowledge as well as build skills and confidence (Yancy et al., 2013; Lindenfeld et al., 2010)
- Clarification with patient of who will be providing posthospitalization management and then communication of the plan to that provider in order to coordinate care, reduce polypharmacy, and reduce readmissions
- Assessment of learning after discharge through telephone follow-up and repeating information at each outpatient visit (Andrikopoulou et al., 2014)
- Assessment of patient's adherence with self-care monitoring at each outpatient visit and addressing factors that limit adherence
- Community-based classes, groups, or other creative programming

ACUTE HEART FAILURE AND PULMONARY EDEMA

Pulmonary edema is the abnormal accumulation of fluid in the lungs. The fluid may accumulate in the interstitial spaces and in the alveoli. Pulmonary edema can be categorized into two subsets depending on the etiology: cardiogenic and noncardiogenic (Sovari, 2014; Givertz et al., 2014).

Pathophysiology

Cardiogenic pulmonary edema is an acute event that results from HF. It can occur acutely, such as with MI, or it can occur as an exacerbation of chronic HF. Myocardial scarring as a result of ischemia can limit the dispensability of the ventricle and render it vulnerable to a sudden increase in workload. With increased resistance to left ventricular filling, blood backs up into the pulmonary circulation. The patient quickly develops pulmonary edema, sometimes called *flash pulmonary edema,* from the blood volume overload in the lungs. Pulmonary edema can also be caused by noncardiac disorders, such as kidney failure, liver failure, and oncologic conditions that cause the body to retain fluid. The pathophysiology is similar to that seen in HF, in that the left ventricle cannot handle the volume overload, and blood volume and pressure build up in the left atrium. The rapid increase in atrial pressure results in an acute increase in pulmonary

venous pressure, which produces an increase in hydrostatic pressure that forces fluid out of the pulmonary capillaries into the interstitial spaces and alveoli.

Impaired lymphatic drainage also contributes to the accumulation of fluid in the lung tissues. The fluid within the alveoli mixes with air, creating "bubbles" that are expelled from the mouth and nose, producing the classic symptom of pulmonary edema: frothy sputum; alveoli are flooded with fluid from the capillaries, producing thin secretions containing air bubbles that frequently are colored with hemoglobin (LeBlond, Brown, Suneja, & Szot, 2015). Because of the fluid within the alveoli, air cannot enter, and gas exchange is impaired. The result is hypoxemia, which is often severe. The onset may be preceded by premonitory symptoms of pulmonary congestion, but it also may develop quickly in the patient with a ventricle that has little reserve to meet increased oxygen needs.

Clinical Manifestations and Assessment

As a result of decreased cerebral oxygenation, the patient becomes increasingly restless and anxious. Clinical manifestations include a sudden onset of breathlessness, sense of suffocation, cough that produces a large amount of frothy sputum (that may be blood tinged), cold and moist skin, cyanotic (bluish) nail beds, a weak and rapid pulse, pulmonary crackles (rales), expiratory wheezing, and distended neck veins.

Additionally oxygen demand increases, yet oxygen saturation is significantly decreased. The patient, nearly suffocated by the blood-tinged, frothy fluid filling the alveoli, is literally drowning in secretions. The situation demands immediate action.

Medical and Nursing Management

Although the etiology of pulmonary edema may vary, management of symptoms follows the similar clinical management plan for treating acute decompensated HF (oxygen, diuretics, pharmacologic preload [volume] and afterload [resistance to flow] reduction, and, possibly, hemodynamic monitoring). Additional therapies may include early rescue with noninvasive mask ventilation and bronchodilator therapy with select beta$_2$ agonist medications like albuterol (Lazzari et al., 2016).

CARDIOGENIC SHOCK

Cardiogenic shock occurs when decreased CO leads to inadequate tissue perfusion and initiation of the shock syndrome. Cardiogenic shock may occur following MI, when a large area of myocardium becomes ischemic, necrotic, and hypokinetic (slow or diminished muscle motion). It also can occur as a result of end-stage HF, cardiac tamponade, pulmonary embolism (PE), cardiomyopathy, and arrhythmias. Cardiogenic shock is a life-threatening condition with a high mortality rate.

Pathophysiology

The signs and symptoms of cardiogenic shock reflect the circular nature of the pathophysiology of HF. The degree of shock is proportional to the extent of left ventricular dysfunction. The heart muscle loses its contractile power, resulting in a marked reduction in SV and CO. The decreased CO, in turn, reduces arterial blood pressure and tissue perfusion in the vital organs (heart, brain, lung, kidneys). Flow to the coronary arteries is reduced, resulting in decreased oxygen supply to the myocardium, which increases ischemia and further reduces the heart's ability to pump. Inadequate emptying of the ventricle also leads to increased pulmonary pressures, pulmonary congestion, and pulmonary edema, exacerbating the hypoxia, causing ischemia of vital organs, and setting a vicious cycle in motion.

Clinical Manifestations and Assessment

The classic signs of cardiogenic shock are those of tissue hypoperfusion and result from HF and the overall shock state. They include cerebral hypoxia (restlessness, confusion, agitation), low blood pressure, rapid and weak pulse, cold and clammy skin, tachypnea with respiratory crackles, and decreased urinary output. Initially, arterial blood gas

(ABG) analysis may show respiratory alkalosis related to the tachypnea. Arrhythmias are common and result from myocardial ischemia.

The patient with cardiogenic shock is managed in an intensive care unit. A pulmonary artery catheter may be inserted to measure CO and other hemodynamic parameters that are used to assess the severity of the problem and to guide patient management. The pulmonary artery wedge pressure (indirect estimate of left atrial pressure or left ventricular preload) is elevated and the CO is decreased as the left ventricle loses its ability to pump. The systemic vascular resistance is elevated because of the sympathetic nervous system stimulation that occurs as a compensatory response to the decrease in blood pressure. The decreased blood flow to the kidneys causes a hormonal response (i.e., activation of the renin–angiotensin–aldosterone system) that causes fluid retention and further vasoconstriction. Increases in HR, circulating volume, and vasoconstriction occur to maintain circulation to the brain, heart, kidneys, and lungs but at a cost: an increase in the workload of the heart.

The reduction in blood volume delivered to the tissues results in an increase in the amount of oxygen extracted from the blood that is delivered to the tissues (to try to meet the cellular demand for oxygen). The increased systemic oxygen extraction results in decreased venous (mixed and central) oxygen saturation. When the cellular oxygen needs cannot be met, anaerobic metabolism and buildup of lactic acid occur. As a result, ABGs would reveal metabolic acidosis. Continuous central venous oximetry and measurement of blood lactic acid levels may help assess the severity of the shock as well as the effectiveness of treatment. Refer to Chapter 55 for further discussion on lactic acid levels.

Continued cellular hypoperfusion eventually results in organ failure. The patient becomes unresponsive, severe hypotension ensues, and the patient develops shallow respirations and cold, cyanotic or mottled skin. Laboratory tests results indicate organ dysfunction.

Medical Management

The most important approach to treating cardiogenic shock is to correct the underlying problem, reduce any further demand on the heart, improve oxygenation, and restore tissue perfusion. For example, if the ventricular failure is the result of an acute MI, emergency percutaneous coronary intervention may be indicated. Major arrhythmias are corrected because they may have caused or contributed to the shock. If the patient has hypervolemia, diuresis is indicated. Diuretics, vasodilators, and mechanical therapies, such as continuous renal replacement therapy, have been used to reduce the circulating blood volume. If hypovolemia (low intravascular volume) is suspected or detected through hemodynamic pressure readings, the patient is given IV volume expanders (e.g., normal saline solution, lactated Ringer solution, albumin) to increase the amount of circulating fluid. The patient is placed on strict bed rest to conserve energy. If the patient has hypoxemia, as detected by pulse oximetry or ABG analysis, oxygen administration is increased, often under positive pressure when regular flow is insufficient to meet tissue demands. Intubation and sedation may be necessary to maintain oxygenation. The settings for mechanical ventilation are adjusted according to the patient's oxygenation status and the need for conserving energy. Ventilator management is discussed in Chapter 55.

PERICARDIAL EFFUSION AND CARDIAC TAMPONADE

Pericardial effusion (accumulation of fluid in the pericardial sac) may accompany pericarditis, advanced HF, metastatic carcinoma, chemotherapy, cardiac surgery, or trauma.

Pathophysiology

Normally, the pericardial sac contains less than 50 mL of fluid, which is needed to decrease friction for the beating heart. An increase in pericardial fluid raises the pressure within the pericardial sac and compresses the heart. This has the following effects:

• Increased right ventricular end-diastolic pressure (RVEDP) and left ventricular end-diastolic pressure (LVEDP)
• Decreased venous return
• Inability of the ventricles to distend and fill adequately

Pericardial fluid may accumulate slowly without causing noticeable symptoms until a large amount accumulates. However, a rapidly developing effusion can stretch the pericardium to its maximum size and, because of increased pericardial pressure, venous return to the heart is obstructed and the amount of blood pumped out with each contraction is reduced, which decreases CO. The result is cardiac tamponade (e.g., compression of the heart).

Clinical Manifestations and Assessment

The patient may report a feeling of fullness within the chest or may have substantial or ill-defined pain. The feeling of pressure in the chest may result from stretching of the pericardial sac. Because of increased pressure within the pericardium, venous pressure tends to increase, as evidenced by engorged neck veins during inspiration. This rise in venous pressure and vein distension during inspiration is known as Kussmaul sign (Mansoor & Karlapuclir, 2015). If hemodynamic pressures are monitored, the nurse will note equivalent diastolic pressures in all chambers, so that right and left atrial pressures, RVEDP, LVEDP, and pulmonary artery diastolic pressures become equal or nearly equal (a difference of less than 3 to 5 mm Hg) (Imazio, 2014). Other signs include dyspnea, cough, and labile or low blood pressure.

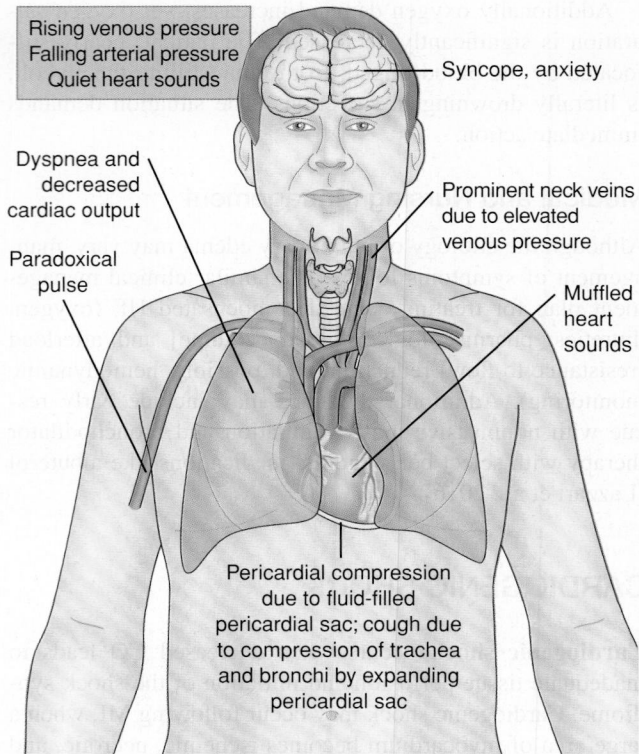

FIGURE 15-4 Assessment findings in cardiac tamponade resulting from pericardial effusion include feelings of faintness, shortness of breath, and anxiety from decreased cardiac output; cough from pressure created in the trachea from swelling of the pericardial sac; distended neck veins from rising venous pressure; Kussmaul sign; paradoxical pulse; and muffled or distant heart sounds.

Systolic blood pressure that is markedly lower during inhalation is called **pulsus paradoxus**. The difference in systolic pressure between the point that is heard during exhalation and the point that is heard during inhalation is measured. Pulsus paradoxus exceeding 10 mm Hg is abnormal. A pericardial friction rub may be heard. The cardinal signs of cardiac tamponade are falling systolic blood pressure, narrowing pulse pressure (difference between the systolic and diastolic pressure, should normally be above 40 mm Hg), rising venous pressure (increased JVD) during inspiration, and distant (muffled) heart sounds (Fig. 15-4). If untreated, shock and death can result.

A chest x-ray shows a large pericardial effusion. An echocardiogram is performed to confirm the diagnosis.

Medical and Nursing Management

Pericardiocentesis

If cardiac function becomes seriously impaired as a result of pericardial effusion, **pericardiocentesis** (puncture of the pericardial sac to aspirate pericardial fluid) is performed to remove fluid from the pericardial sac (Fig. 15-5). The major goal of this procedure is to prevent cardiac tamponade, which restricts normal heart filling and contraction.

Parietal layer of
pericardial sac

Visceral layer (epicardium)

Myocardium

Pericardial
fluid

RA

LA

V₁ lead

Syringe

To ECG

RL   LL

FIGURE 15-5 Pericardiocentesis. (From Lippincott Williams & Wilkins. (2010). *Cardiovascular care made incredibly visual* (2nd ed., p. 231). Philadelphia, PA: Lippincott Williams & Wilkins.)

During the procedure, vital signs, oxygen saturation, ECG and, if applicable, hemodynamic pressures are measured. Emergency resuscitation equipment should be readily available. The head of the bed is elevated to 45 to 60 degrees, placing the heart in proximity to the chest wall so that the needle can be inserted into the pericardial sac more easily. If a peripheral IV line is not already in place, one is inserted, and a slow IV infusion is started in case it becomes necessary to administer emergency medications or blood products.

The pericardial aspiration needle is attached to a 50-mL syringe by a three-way stopcock. Several possible sites are used for pericardial aspiration. Typically, ultrasound imaging is used to guide placement of the needle into the pericardial space. The needle is advanced slowly until it has entered the pericardium and fluid is obtained.

A resulting decrease in central venous pressure and an associated increase in blood pressure after withdrawal of pericardial fluid indicate that the cardiac tamponade has been relieved. The patient almost always feels immediate relief. If there is a substantial amount of pericardial fluid, a small catheter may be left in place to drain recurrent accumulation of blood or fluid. Pericardial fluid is sent to the laboratory for examination for tumor cells, bacterial culture, chemical and serologic analysis, and differential blood cell count.

Complications of pericardiocentesis include ventricular or coronary artery puncture, arrhythmias, pleural laceration, gastric puncture, and myocardial trauma. After pericardiocentesis, the patient's heart rhythm, blood pressure, venous pressure, and heart sounds are monitored to detect possible recurrence of cardiac tamponade. If it recurs, repeated aspiration is necessary. Cardiac tamponade may require surgical treatment by open pericardial drainage called a pericardiotomy.

Pericardiotomy

Recurrent pericardial effusions, usually associated with neoplastic disease, may be treated by a **pericardiotomy** (pericardial window). Under general anesthesia, a portion of the pericardium is excised to permit the pericardial fluid to drain continuously into the mediastinum and is reabsorbed via lymphatics (Imazio, 2014). The nursing care is the same as that for other cardiac surgery (see Chapter 14).

CARDIAC ARREST

Cardiac arrest occurs when the heart ceases to produce an effective pulse and circulate blood.

Pathophysiology

Cardiac arrest may be caused by a cardiac electrical event such as ventricular fibrillation, progressive profound bradycardia, or when there is no heart rhythm at all (asystole). Cardiac arrest may follow respiratory arrest; it may also occur when electrical activity is present but there is ineffective cardiac contraction or circulating volume, which is called **pulseless electrical activity (PEA)**. PEA can be caused by hypovolemia (e.g., with excessive bleeding), hypoxia, hypothermia, hyperkalemia, massive PE, MI, and medication overdose (e.g., beta blockers, calcium-channel blockers).

Clinical Manifestations and Assessment

In cardiac arrest, consciousness, pulse, and blood pressure are lost immediately. Ineffective respiratory gasping may occur. The pupils of the eyes begin dilating within 45 seconds. Seizures may or may not occur.

The risk of irreversible brain damage and death increases with every minute from the time that circulation ceases. The interval varies with the age and underlying condition of the patient. During this period, the diagnosis of cardiac arrest must be made, and measures must be taken immediately to restore circulation.

Emergency Management: Cardiopulmonary Resuscitation

Cardiopulmonary resuscitation (CPR) provides blood flow to vital organs until effective circulation can be reestablished. Once loss of consciousness has been established, the resuscitation priority for the adult in most cases is placing a phone call to activate the code team or the emergency medical system (EMS). The "A-B-Cs" (airway, breathing, and circulation) of CPR were replaced with a new standard from the American Heart Association in 2010 and continued in 2015. "C-A-B" (compression, airway, and breathing) is the new sequence for CPR in basic life support (Box 15-3). Compressions are performed first. Exceptions to this include near-drowning and respiratory arrest situations for which 2 minutes of conventional CPR (A-B-C) with rescue breathing should be performed before activating the EMS (Hazinski, 2010, 2015).

Resuscitation of adults consists of the following steps:

1. Establish unresponsiveness: no breathing or no normal breathing (gasping). Activate EMS and get defibrillator or automatic external defibrillator (AED).

BOX 15-3   Performing One-Person CPR

1. Establish unresponsiveness by asking, "Are you okay?" Tap or gently shake the patient along with recognition of no breathing or no normal breathing (i.e., only gasping).
2. After initiating the emergency response team or calling for a defibrillator when a patient is unresponsive, position the patient supine on a hard surface.

Unless a definite pulse is felt, initiate chest compressions.

3. Place one hand on top of the other on the lower half of the sternum between the nipples, with elbows locked. Compress the chest 2 in (or one third the depth of the chest) at a rate of 100–120 compressions per minute, keeping your hands on the chest. Allow equal time for compressions and full chest recoil. Continue for 30 compressions, then give 2 ventilations and resume compressions quickly for 5 cycles (2 minutes) before rechecking the pulse.

2. Check pulse at carotid artery for no more than 10 seconds.
3. Perform chest compressions to a depth of at least 2 in for 30 times allowing for chest recoil after each compression.
4. Airway/breathing: Open airway, give 2 quick breathes followed by 30 compressions.
5. Defibrillation: Shock with standard defibrillator or AED for ventricular tachycardia and ventricular fibrillation.

If the patient is already being monitored or is immediately placed on the monitor using the multifunction pads or the quick-look paddles (found on most defibrillators) and the ECG shows ventricular tachycardia or ventricular fibrillation, immediate defibrillation rather than CPR is the treatment of choice (Boggust, 2016). Survival from pulseless ventricular tachycardia or ventricular fibrillation is inversely related to the time interval between its onset and termination. Optimization occurs with CPR and advanced cardiac life support, including defibrillation and drug therapy, if they are provided at the earliest opportunity (Ornato, 2016). If the patient has not been defibrillated within 10 minutes, the chance of survival is close to zero. Refer to Chapter 17 for more details on defibrillation.

Recent research on CPR performed in the field for persons in out-of-hospital cardiac arrest by bystanders supports eliminating mouth to mouth or rescue breathing and using "hands-only" cardiac compression only. No differences in patient survival were seen when bystanders received emergency dispatcher instructions for compression-only versus compression-plus rescue breathing CPR (Myerburg & Castellanos, 2015).

CHAPTER REVIEW

Critical Thinking Exercises

1. Compare the pathophysiology of systolic and diastolic failure.

2. Describe the effect of ACE inhibitors and angiotensin receptor blockers on the renin–angiotensin–aldosterone system (RAAS) and its therapeutic effect for HF.

NCLEX-Style Review Questions

1. Which outcome best demonstrates the effectiveness of treatment for a patient with right ventricular failure?
   a. Clear breath sounds
   b. Oxygen saturation greater than 96%
   c. Moist mucous membranes
   d. Central venous pressure of 4 mm Hg

2. The nurse is caring for a patient with right ventricular failure. What symptom will the patient most likely exhibit?
   a. Crackles on auscultation
   b. Jugular vein distention
   c. Pulmonary edema
   d. Normal CVP

3. A patient with CHF is being discharged home. What instruction will the nurse likely give this patient to assess fluid balance?
   a. Monitor blood pressure
   b. Assess radial pulses
   c. Monitor weight daily
   d. Monitor bowel movements

4. What condition includes the classic signs and symptoms of jugular vein distention, muffled heart sounds, and decreasing systolic pressure?
   a. HF
   b. Pericardial tamponade
   c. Pulmonary edema
   d. Cardiogenic shock

5. What medication is commonly used to treat cardiogenic shock related to hypervolemia?
   a. Diuretics
   b. Beta blockers
   c. Vasoconstrictors
   d. Inotropes

Try these additional resources, available at **http://thepoint.lww.com/Honan2e**, to enhance your learning and understanding of this chapter:
- NCLEX-Style Student Review Questions
- Journal Articles

REFERENCES AND SELECTED READINGS

References and selected readings associated with this chapter can be found on the website that accompanies the book. Visit **http://thepoint.lww.com/Honan2e** to access the references and other additional resources associated with this chapter.

Nursing Management: Patients with Structural, Inflammatory and Infectious Cardiac Disorders

Jeanine L. May

Learning Objectives

After reading this chapter, you will be able to:

1. Define valvular disorders of the heart and describe the pathophysiology, clinical manifestations, and management of patients with mitral and aortic regurgitation and/or stenosis.

2. Describe types of cardiac valve repair and replacement procedures used to treat valvular problems and the care needed by patients who undergo these procedures.

3. Describe the pathophysiology, clinical manifestations, and management of patients with the intracardiac septal defects.

4. Describe the pathophysiology, clinical manifestations, and management of patients with cardiomyopathy.

5. Describe the pathophysiology, clinical manifestations, and management of patients with infections of the heart.

6. Describe the rationale for prophylactic antibiotic therapy for patients with valvular heart disease, rheumatic heart disease, and infective endocarditis.

Structural disorders of the heart present many challenges for the patient, family, and health care team. Dysfunctional heart valves, intracardiac septal defects, cardiomyopathies, and inflammatory and infectious diseases of the heart muscle alter cardiac output (CO) and interfere with the heart's ability to pump blood sufficiently to meet the body's demand for oxygen. Nursing care for patients with these disorders requires an understanding of cardiac anatomy; structure and physiology (function) of heart valves, pericardium, myocardium, and endocardium; as well as knowledge of the causes and management of each disorder. Noninvasive and invasive treatments include options such as medication management, supportive care, valve repair or replacement, septal repair, mechanical circulatory assist devices, and cardiac transplantation. Nurses play an integral role in the care of patients with structural, infectious, and inflammatory cardiac conditions.

VALVULAR DISEASE

Properly functioning heart valves allow blood to flow in one direction through the heart and vasculature. Acquired valvular heart disease is a chronic, progressive disorder that develops slowly, although it can occur acutely in certain conditions. Compensatory mechanisms can maintain equilibrium for an extended period of time, and it may be years before the disease progresses, the patient becomes symptomatic, and require treatment. Common causes include degenerative disease, rheumatic heart disease, and infective endocarditis (inflammation of the inner lining of the heart, the endocardium).

Progression of valvular heart disease can result in heart failure, arrhythmias, stroke, and sudden death. Interventions for the management and treatment of acquired valvular heart disease are aimed at preventing the sequelae of atrial fibrillation (AF), thromboembolism, pulmonary artery hypertension, and heart failure, and significant advances in treatment and outcomes have been made in the past several decades. This is primarily due to the development of management guidelines, improvements in noninvasive monitoring of cardiac function, advancements in valvular reconstruction procedures, and improved prosthetic valves.

A detailed review of normal cardiac valvular anatomy is found in Chapter 12 and shown in Figure 16-1. When heart valves do not close or open properly, blood flow is affected.

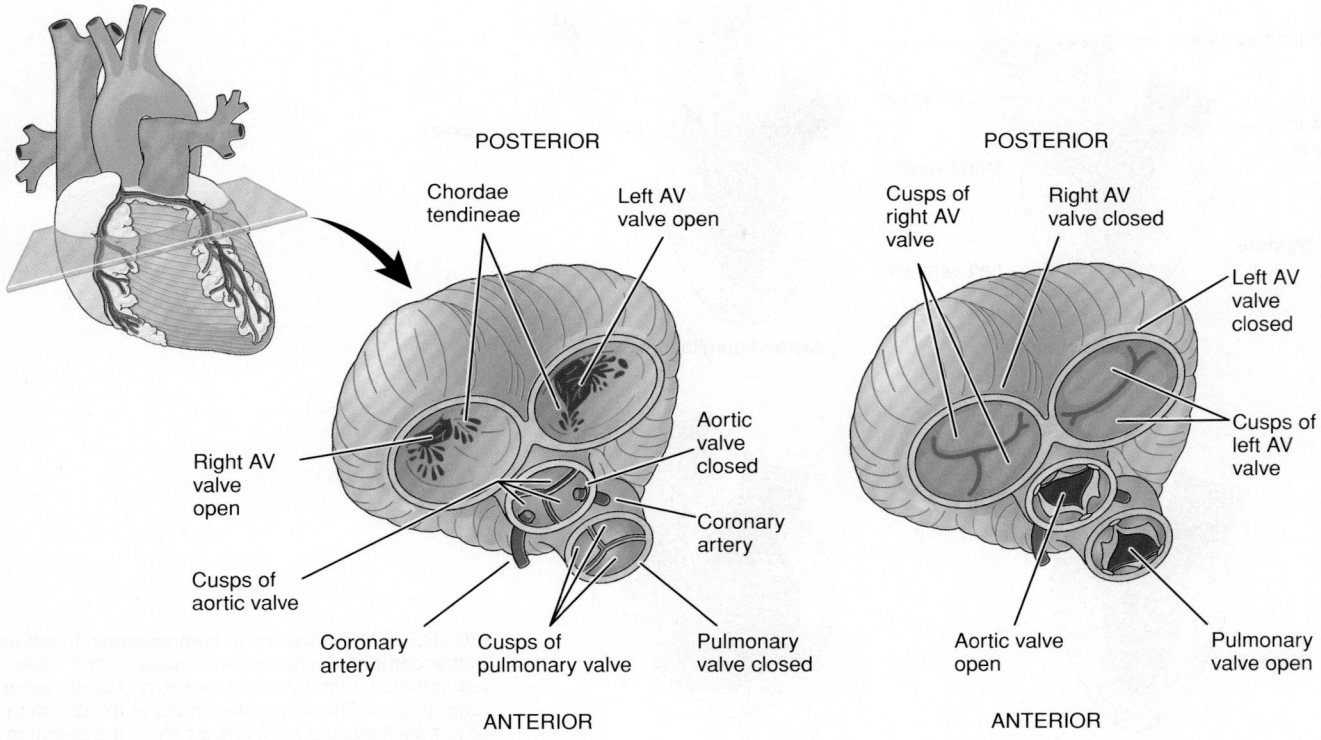

A Ventricular relaxation (diastole)

B Ventricular contraction (systole)

FIGURE 16-1 Heart valves (superior view from anterior, atria removed). Valves keep blood flowing in a forward direction through the heart. **A.** When the heart is relaxed (diastole), the AV valves are open and blood flows freely from the atria to the ventricles. The pulmonary and aortic valves are closed. **B.** When the ventricles contract (systole), the AV valves close and blood pumped out of the ventricles opens the pulmonary and aortic valves. ZOOMING IN How many cusps does the right AV valve have? The left? Answer the right AV valve has three cusp (Tricuspid valve) versus two on the left or mitral valve.

The turbulent flow of blood through a heart valve opening results in a murmur, as described in Table 16-1. Characteristic **stenosis** occurs when the opening of the valve is narrowed, valve leaflets fail to open properly and the forward flow of blood through the valve is reduced, as shown in Figure 16-2A. The increase in resistance results in turbulent blood flow. The volume of blood in the chamber increases and the heart is forced to work harder to eject blood through the narrowed valve, resulting in increased afterload and eventually, decreased CO. Refer to Figure 16-3 for pathophysiology of heart failure related to valvular heart disease.

Regurgitation, or valvular insufficiency, occurs when valves do not close completely and blood flows backward through the valve, as shown in Figure 16-2. If the aortic valve is affected, blood will flow backward into the left ventricle (LV) during diastole, and if the mitral valve is affected,

TABLE 16-1 Heart Murmurs

Murmur	Timing	Description	Auscultation Site
Mitral Stenosis	Diastole (S2)	Low-pitched, rumbling, decrescendo	Apex
Mitral Regurgitation	Systole (S1)	High-pitched, loud, rumbling	Apex
Aortic Stenosis	Midsystolic (S1)	Loud, crescendo-decrescendo	2nd ICS right sternal border; may radiate into the neck
Aortic Regurgitation	Early Diastole (S2)	High-pitched blowing sound, decrescendo	Left sternal border, at the 3rd ICS

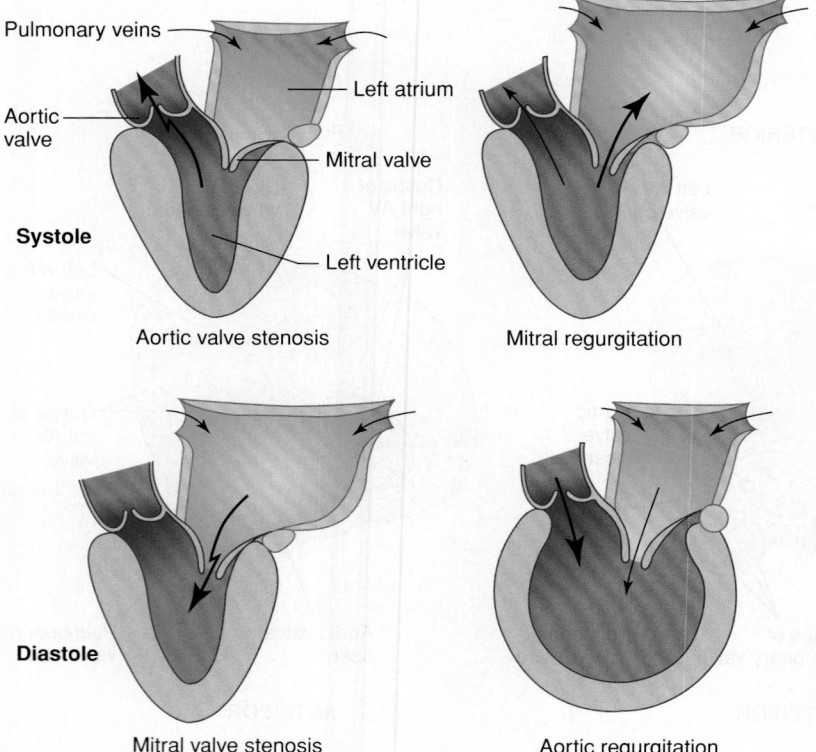

FIGURE 16-2 Alterations in hemodynamic function that accompany aortic valve stenosis, mitral valve regurgitation, mitral valve stenosis, and aortic valve regurgitation. The *thin arrows* indicate the direction of normal flow, and *thick arrows* show the direction of abnormal flow.

FIGURE 16-3 Pathophysiology: Left-sided heart failure as a result of aortic and mitral valvular heart disease and the development of right ventricular failure.

blood will flow back into the left atrium (LA) during systole. Preload is increased. Mitral valve **prolapse** (MVP) occurs when the **mitral valve** does not close properly and the valve leaflets balloon back into the LA during systole. An understanding of the structure and function of heart valves, pathophysiology, as shown in Figures 16-2 and 16-3, and the causes and management of valvular disorders is necessary in order to provide appropriate nursing care for patients with valvular heart disease. Valvular disorders may require surgical repair or replacement of the valve to correct the problem, depending on the severity of symptoms.

Pulmonic and **tricuspid valve** disorders also occur, although with less frequency and usually with fewer symptoms and complications. Tricuspid regurgitation usually occurs with mitral stenosis because of the increased volume and pressure load on the right side of the heart but also can result from infective endocarditis. Tricuspid valve repair is done only if there is severe regurgitation. Tricuspid valve replacement is uncommon. Multivalvular disease is possible: regurgitation and stenosis may occur at the same time in the same or different valves, or one disease may occur in two or more valves.

Nursing Alert
Stenosis is a pressure problem, and regurgitation is a volume problem. Blood volume and pressures are increased behind the affected valve and reduced in front of the affected valve.

MITRAL STENOSIS

In mitral stenosis (MS), the valve opening is narrowed, and blood flow from the LA into the LV is slowed during diastole. MS is slow and progressive. Symptoms may take decades to appear. Over time, heart failure will develop.

Pathophysiology

Normally, the mitral valve opening is 4 to 6 cm², but over time as fibrous tissue replaces normal valve tissue, the leaflets begin to thicken and fuse. In cases of marked stenosis, the opening narrows to the width of 1 cm² or less. Left atrial pressure increases because of the resistance caused by slowed blood flow into the LV through the narrowed orifice. The LA dilates and hypertrophies because of the increased blood volume. Sluggish atrial blood flow can lead to clot formation and thromboembolism. Because there is no functional valve to protect the pulmonary veins from the backward flow of blood from the atrium, pulmonary venous pressure rises and circulation becomes congested. As a result, the right ventricle (RV) must contract against an abnormally high pulmonary pressure. Pulmonary hypertension increases the work of the RV, and the RV and right atrium become enlarged. Eventually, this results in right-sided heart failure.

Risk Factors

Most often MS is caused by rheumatic fever (RF) or endocarditis, which gradually causes the mitral valve leaflets to thicken and can result in leaflet fusion. Typically MS occurs 20 to 40 years after RF, and symptoms do not develop for another 10 years. Although rheumatic disease is rare in developed countries, MS is still prevalent in developing nations where RF is common (Carabello, 2016). Radiation therapy to the chest area also can result in MS. It is more common in women than in men. Rarely, it can result from a congenital defect.

Clinical Manifestations and Assessment

Although patients with MS can remain asymptomatic, symptoms usually develop when the pressure in the LA becomes greater than that of the LV, after the valve opening is reduced by one third to one half its usual size. Dyspnea on exertion (DOE) results from pulmonary congestion. Patients become progressively fatigued as a result of low CO. Palpitations, chest pain, and paroxysmal nocturnal dyspnea (PND) can occur. As the LA becomes more distended, palpitations, premature beats, AF, and paroxysmal atrial tachycardia may occur. AF is common in people with symptomatic MS, and AF increases the risk of developing a stroke. Dyspnea at rest is likely with severe MS. Other symptoms include cough, sometimes with hemoptysis from ruptured pulmonary veins, hoarseness from the dilated atrium impinging on the left recurrent laryngeal nerve, palpitations, orthopnea, and recurrent respiratory infections. Later, symptoms of right heart failure, including peripheral edema and ascites, occur.

A loud S1 and an opening snap can be heard because of the elevated left atrial pressure. The opening snap is a high-pitched sound heard in early diastole (S2) by the opening of a stenotic valve. The murmur is caused by turbulent blood flow through the abnormally tight valve opening from the LA into the LV. Due to the increased blood volume and pressure, the atrium dilates and becomes electrically unstable, leading to atrial arrhythmias. The pulse can be irregular because of AF. Echocardiography is the most sensitive and specific noninvasive method to diagnose MS and is used to evaluate valve morphology and to measure cardiac pressures. Cardiac catheterization is not indicated unless clinical findings and echo results are discordant.

MITRAL VALVE PROLAPSE

In MVP, a portion of one or both mitral valve leaflets bulge back into the LA during systole, usually with little or no mitral regurgitation (MR). Rarely, the leaflet stretches to the point where the valve does not remain closed during systole and then blood flows from the LV back into the LA.

Pathophysiology

Myxomatous degeneration (pathologic weakening of connective tissue) can cause one or both of the valve leaflets to become enlarged and floppy, causing them to billow into the LA during systole. Over time, as the leaflets prolapse, they can stretch to a degree where the leaflet edges do not fully coapt, or close, resulting in MR.

Risk Factors

Female gender and family history are associated with MVP. It often occurs in people with Marfan syndrome, a connective tissue disorder.

Clinical Manifestations and Assessment

MVP is commonly asymptomatic. However, over time, fatigue, dyspnea, palpitations, and chest pain may develop. Atypical chest pain is not related to activity and may be caused by abnormal stress placed on the chordae tendineae and papillary muscles. Shortness of breath (SOB) is not correlated with activity levels or pulmonary function.

Cardiac auscultation may reveal a mitral midsystolic click. This is a sign that a valve leaflet is ballooning into the LA. A late systolic murmur may be heard if progressive valve leaflet stretching and regurgitation have occurred. Echocardiography is used to diagnose and monitor the progression of MVP.

MITRAL REGURGITATION

MR, also termed *mitral insufficiency,* is the backward flow of blood from the LV into the LA during systole because the valve fails to close completely. Disease processes, including

MVP, that alter valve leaflets, mitral annulus, chordae tendineae, and the papillary muscle may result in MR.

Pathophysiology

When the mitral valve leaflets thicken, fibrose, and contract, they cannot close completely. With each heartbeat, blood is forced backward into the LA during systole. Regurgitation of blood into the LA causes left atrial pressure to rise. The LA stretches to accommodate the increased volume, and left atrial dilation occurs. During diastole, regurgitant blood from the LV increases volume load in the LA. With chronic MR, hemodynamic changes occur slowly. Over time, compensatory left ventricular dilation and hypertrophy occur to maintain a normal CO. Eventually this leads to left ventricular failure. The backward flow of blood from the LV reduces blood volume flowing into the atrium from the lungs, and pulmonary venous pressure increases. Pulmonary congestion results, elevating pulmonary artery pressure; this adds further strain on the RV, causing enlargement and right ventricular failure.

Risk Factors

MR is more common in older adults and can result over time from normal aging. Having MVP or mitral valve stenosis can lead to the development of chronic primary MR, although most people with MVP never develop severe regurgitation. Rheumatic heart disease can result in a thick, rigid mitral valve that does not open and close completely, leading to MR.

Clinical Manifestations and Assessment

Patients with chronic MR can remain asymptomatic for years; symptoms develop gradually. As the LV becomes progressively impaired and CO diminishes, fatigue, tachycardia, and weakness can occur. As left atrial pressure increases, orthopnea, DOE, and PND result from pulmonary congestion. Palpitations are related to a hyperdynamic LV and/or AF. Peripheral edema and ascites occur when the RV fails. Acute MR (discussed shortly) manifests as severe left-sided heart failure. Patients may report a sudden inability to breathe accompanied by chest pain.

Physical examination may reveal a hyperdynamic point of maximal impulse, displaced leftward and downward because of the hypertrophied LV. A holosystolic (pansystolic) murmur is heard as a high-pitched, blowing sound at the apex; radiation to the axilla is possible. An S3 may be present because of increased, rapid blood flow into the ventricle during diastole.

Chest x-ray may reveal left ventricular and left atrial enlargement. An echocardiogram provides information regarding left ventricular size and function, left atrial size, and pulmonary artery pressures as well as the anatomy of the valve. Also, echocardiography is used to monitor the severity and progression of MR. Cardiac catheterization may be used if there is a discrepancy between clinical and noninvasive findings to determine the severity of MR.

ACUTE MITRAL REGURGITATION

Acute MR occurs abruptly, when papillary muscle rupture occurs as a complication of myocardial infarction (MI) or if infective endocarditis or trauma leads to rupture of the chordae tendineae. This is a cardiac emergency because of the sudden and severe hemodynamic compromise. It is almost always symptomatic.

Pathophysiology

An acute MI can damage the ventricular wall and disrupt the attachment of the papillary muscle or the chordae tendineae, resulting in acute MR. Without a normally functioning valve to direct the flow of blood forward, a large amount of blood from the LV flows backward into the LA. This compromises forward flow of blood and CO is diminished, which can lead to cardiogenic shock. Compensatory mechanisms lead to an increase in systemic vascular resistance (SVR), which can worsen regurgitation. At the same time, additional blood flows back into the LA causes an increase in left atrial pressure and forces blood back into the pulmonary circulation.

Clinical Manifestations and Assessment

Signs of left- and right-sided heart failure are seen in acute MR: severe SOB, pallor, tachycardia, crackles, and hypotension, as well as peripheral edema, jugular venous distention (JVD), and ascites. Poor tissue perfusion is common as is acute pulmonary decompensation.

Rapid assessment with an echocardiogram is necessary to establish a diagnosis. Often the LA and ventricle are normal in size, and systolic function can be hyperdynamic or normal; also a flail leaflet may be seen.

AORTIC STENOSIS

Aortic stenosis (AS) is narrowing of the valve opening between the LV and the aorta, resulting in obstruction of blood flow across the valve.

Pathophysiology

Progressive narrowing of the valve orifice develops gradually over several years to several decades, increasing afterload. Because the narrowing occurs slowly, the LV is able to adapt by contracting more slowly and stronger than normal, forcibly squeezing the blood through the smaller opening. Normal blood volume in the LV is maintained for a while, but, eventually, left ventricular pressure increases, causing the ventricular wall to hypertrophy to maintain CO. Diastolic dysfunction leads to increased work of the heart, which results in left ventricular failure. This results in elevated left atrial pressure, pulmonary congestion, and, ultimately, heart failure.

Risk Factors

The buildup of calcium deposits on heart valves is the most common cause of AS. As calcification progresses, valve leaflets become more rigid and outflow from the LV becomes obstructed. Acquired AS is common in those over 70 years of age, particularly in males. Besides degeneration of the valve, rheumatic heart disease also can lead to AS. Having a congenital malformation, such as a bicuspid aortic valve, is another risk factor.

Clinical Manifestations and Assessment

Since it develops slowly, and the LV is able to compensate, AS can be asymptomatic for decades. Exertional dyspnea or decreased exercise tolerance can be early signs. The triad of symptoms associated with AS includes angina due to LV hypertrophy and diminished coronary blood flow; dyspnea due to increased pulmonary venous pressure from LV failure; and syncope, usually with exertion, due to a reduction in cerebral blood flow that occurs when vasodilation leads to a decrease in arterial pressure in the setting of fixed CO. With AS, the heart rate will increase in an attempt to increase CO, but CO does not improve. Symptomatic AS has a poor prognosis if untreated.

Nursing Alert
Patients with AS have SAD symptoms: syncope, angina, and dyspnea.

On physical examination, a thrill, or a vibration, may be felt. The vibration is caused by turbulent blood flow across the narrowed valve orifice. A loud, systolic ejection murmur may be heard over the aortic area (second intercostal space, right sternal border) and may radiate into the neck. This is caused by blood flowing through the narrowed opening of the stenotic valve. The patient should be instructed to lean forward during auscultation, especially upon exhalation, to accentuate the murmur. An S4 gallop may be heard.

Echocardiography is used to diagnose and monitor the progression of AS and will demonstrate calcification of the valve or decreased mobility of valve cusps, as well as size and function of LV. Cardiac catheterization can measure the severity of AS when noninvasive testing is inconclusive.

AORTIC REGURGITATION

AR, also referred to as aortic insufficiency, is the backward flow of blood into the LV from the aorta during diastole. This occurs when the valve leaflets do not close completely.

Pathophysiology

When the aortic valve is incompetent, blood from the aorta returns to the LV during diastole in addition to the blood normally delivered by the LA. The LV dilates in an attempt to accommodate blood volume overload, causing hypertrophy.

Dilatation and hypertrophy allow the LV to expel more blood with above-normal force, increasing afterload and, as a result, systolic blood pressure, while maintaining a normal ejection fraction (EF). The arteries attempt to compensate for the higher pressures by reflex vasodilation; the peripheral arterioles relax, reducing peripheral resistance and diastolic blood pressure. Although compensatory mechanisms allow patients to remain asymptomatic for some time despite pressure and volume overload, when left ventricular dysfunction develops, symptoms appear.

Risk Factors

Calcific valve disease and bicuspid aortic valve are the most common risk factors for AR. Because they affect the valve leaflets, rheumatic heart disease and infective endocarditis can cause AR. Disorders affecting the aortic root, such as Marfan syndrome and dissecting aortic aneurysms, can lead to AR, as can chronic hypertension (Nishimura et al., 2014a, 2014b; Otto & Bonow, 2015).

Clinical Manifestations and Assessment

AR is asymptomatic for years, but as the disease progresses, symptoms related to increased stroke volume become apparent. Palpitations, particularly when lying down, and visible neck vein pulsations are a result of the increased force and volume of the blood ejected from the hypertrophied LV. Later symptoms, including dyspnea, fatigue, angina, orthopnea, and pulmonary congestion, signify decreased cardiac reserve and LV failure.

Pulse pressure, the difference between systolic and diastolic pressures, widens, resulting in high systolic and low diastolic blood pressure. Another characteristic sign of AR is the water-hammer pulse, in which the pulse has a rapid upstroke and collapses. Systolic blood pressure in the lower extremities is higher than in the upper extremities. A decrescendo diastolic murmur is heard as a high-pitched blowing sound at the 3rd or (4th) intercostal space (ICS) at the left sternal border with the patient sitting up and leaning forward. If the AR is severe, the murmur may be holodiastolic (throughout the S2) and radiate widely along the left sternal border.

Diagnosis is confirmed by echocardiography; valve morphology, degree of LV hypertrophy, and functional capacity are determined. Cardiac catheterization is not necessary in most patients with AR. Patients with symptoms usually have echocardiograms every 4 to 6 months, and those without symptoms have annual echocardiograms. Exercise stress testing will assess functional capacity and symptom response.

MEDICAL AND NURSING MANAGEMENT OF VALVULAR DISORDERS

Patients with any of the valvular diseases discussed thus far in the chapter share some commonalities in medical and nursing management of their varying conditions.

No treatment is required for asymptomatic patients with valvular pathology. The goal of medical therapy is not curative; it is symptom relief. Definitive therapy for a valvular problem is mechanical restoration of valve function. Management is guided by findings on the echocardiogram and is aimed at the specific valvular problem, i.e., decreasing regurgitant volume, improving CO, and reducing pulmonary congestion. Beta-blockers (BBs) and calcium channel blockers (CCBs) may be used for rate control, to treat palpitations, for chest discomfort, and for anxiety, and are particularly useful when there is concomitant coronary artery disease. Less commonly, digoxin is given to increase contractility and slow rapid rates to allow for improved ventricular filling. Antiarrhythmics and electrical cardioversion are utilized to restore sinus rhythm, and anticoagulation is indicated if AF is persistent. Diuretics, vasodilators, and sodium restriction may be used to reduce preload and pulmonary congestion. Because patients with severe AS are dependent on preload to maintain CO, diuretics should be used with caution. Angiotensin-converting enzyme inhibitors (ACE-Is) are prescribed to reduce preload, afterload, and hypertension by causing vasodilation. ACE-Is are commonly prescribed for patients with concomitant hypertension but may be avoided in patients with AS because the vasodilation reduces pressure distal to the obstruction without increasing CO and may cause syncope. Afterload reduction may be managed with angiotensin blockers (ARBs), nitrates, or hydralazine. In acute cases of decompensation, intravenous nitroprusside is the vasodilator used most commonly for afterload reduction, but nitrates should be used with great caution with AS because their use can result in reduced CO.

Nursing Alert
Venous dilation that results from nitroglycerin decreases blood return to the heart, thus decreasing CO and increasing the risk of syncope and decreased coronary artery blood flow. The nurse teaches the patient about the importance of attempting to relieve chest pain with rest before taking nitroglycerin and to anticipate the potential adverse effects (orthostatic hypotension and syncope).

Nursing Alert
Although diuretics and nitrates are used to treat decompensated heart failure in patients with incompetent valves, the nurse understands that caution must be taken if diuretics or nitrates are ordered for a patient with AS. The risk associated with these medications is that preload will be critically reduced and/or systemic arterial blood pressure (with administration of diuretics and nitrates). The treatment for symptomatic AS is valve replacement.

Valvular problems increase the patient's risk of developing bacterial endocarditis. Thrombi may occur on the valve

leaflets and, if they embolize, transient ischemic attacks (TIAs) can occur. Daily aspirin is recommended for people who have had documented TIA, even when they are in sinus rhythm. Elimination of caffeine and alcohol may control or reduce symptoms, and the nurse encourages the patient to read labels on over-the-counter products, such as cough medicine, because these products may contain alcohol, caffeine, ephedrine, and epinephrine, which may produce arrhythmias and other symptoms. Symptoms may appear or worsen when the heart rate increases, such as during exercise, and also may be triggered by pregnancy or other stress on the body, such as a pulmonary infection. Strenuous activity is avoided since it increases workload of the heart.

Treatment of arrhythmias, heart failure, or other complications is described in Chapters 15 and 17. If symptoms develop on optimal medical therapy, then surgical repair with valvuloplasty or valve replacement should be considered before ventricular dysfunction worsens. Intra-aortic balloon counterpulsation may be considered as it aids afterload reduction until surgery is performed; however, it is contraindicated in AR because it increases regurgitation.

Assessing Valvular Heart Disorders

Heart and lung sounds are auscultated and peripheral pulses palpated. The nurse assesses the patient with valvular heart disease for signs and symptoms of heart failure, arrhythmias, and other symptoms such as dizziness, syncope, weakness, or chest pain. The nurse teaches the patient about the diagnosis, the progressive nature of valvular disease, and treatment, and also teaches the patient to report new symptoms or changes in symptoms to the health care provider. Treatment is not required until the patient becomes symptomatic. Management should include cardiovascular risk reduction of hyperlipidemia, hypertension, tobacco use, physical inactivity, and weight. Patients should be monitored for signs of activity intolerance, including excessive fatigue, palpitations, diaphoresis, pallor, dyspnea, and tachycardia, and should be instructed to rest if symptoms occur.

Nursing Alert
Evaluating the patient's response to physical activity is important because a decrease in activity tolerance may indicate deterioration in cardiac function, not overexertion. This occurs when the heart can no longer increase CO sufficiently to meet the oxygen demands associated with exercise.

VALVE REPAIR AND REPLACEMENT PROCEDURES

Most patients with valvular heart disease are managed medically until symptoms become unmanageable or the ventricles begin to fail. However, medication cannot cure valve disease. If the condition worsens, or if medication fails to control symptoms, a percutaneous intervention or surgery is

FIGURE 16-4 Balloon valvuloplasty: Cross section of heart illustrating the guide wire and dilation catheter placed through an atrial transseptal puncture and across the mitral valve. The guide wire is extended out from the aortic valve into the aorta for catheter support.

indicated to repair or replace diseased heart valves. Percutaneous balloon valvotomy is a nonsurgical procedure used to increase the opening of a stenotic (narrowed) valve, typically performed in the cardiac catheterization laboratory. Although the balloon valvotomy is available for AS, research reveals it is relatively ineffective in improving aortic flow and has a mortality rate postprocedure that is similar to that in untreated patients. Thus, balloon aortic valvotomy generally has been abandoned but may be used when immediate temporary relief is required (Carabello, 2016). For a percutaneous balloon mitral valvotomy, a guide wire is advanced percutaneously from the femoral vein to the right atrium, through a puncture in the septum to the mitral valve, as shown in Figure 16-4. A balloon catheter is placed over the guide wire and positioned

so that the balloon tip is directly inside the narrowed valve. The balloon is inflated and deflated several times to widen the valve opening. During the procedure, an echocardiogram may be done to determine the mobility of the valve leaflets and function of the valve. The procedure is contraindicated for patients with heavily calcified valves, left atrial thrombus, or moderate to severe coexisting MR. Patients may have some MR after the procedure. Other potential complications include left-to-right atrial shunts through an atrial septal defect caused by the procedure and emboli from dislodged left atrial thrombus.

Concept Mastery Alert

Commissurotomy is the splitting or separating of fused cardiac valve leaflets. Valvuloplasty is a general term for repairing a stenosed or regurgitant cardiac valve by commissurotomy, annuloplasty (repair of a cardiac valve's outer ring), leaflet repair, or chordoplasty.

The decision to proceed with a transcatheter versus surgical approach and valve repair or replacement should be made after a detailed discussion between the patient and medical team, and the discussion should include the patient's preferences, risks of anticoagulant therapy, and the possible need for and risk of a repeat surgery (Nishimura et al., 2014a, 2014b).

Regurgitation can be treated surgically by **annuloplasty** (repair of a cardiac valve's outer ring) (see Fig. 16-5), valve **leaflet** repair (see Fig. 16-6), and **chordoplasty** (repair of the tendinous fibers that connect the edges of the atrioventricular valve leaflets to the papillary muscles). Mitral annuloplasty narrows the diameter of the valve's orifice to treat valvular regurgitation. An annuloplasty ring prosthesis is sutured to the annulus and leaflets, creating an annulus of the desired size, as shown in Figure 16-5.

Leaflet repair, as shown in Figure 16-5, includes removal of excess leaflet tissue and the repair of leaflet damage from stretching or tearing by using pericardial or synthetic patches.

For example, mitral valve leaflets are often repaired by chordoplasty. Stretched chordae tendineae can be shortened,

FIGURE 16-5 Annuloplasty ring insertion. **A.** Mitral valve regurgitation; leaflets do not close. **B.** Insertion of an annuloplasty ring. **C.** Completed valvuloplasty; leaflets close.

FIGURE 16-6 Valve leaflet resection and repair with a ring annuloplasty. **A.** Mitral valve regurgitation; the section indicated by dashed lines is excised. **B.** Approximation of edges and suturing. **C.** Completed valvuloplasty, leaflet repair, and annuloplasty ring.

lengthened, or replaced with synthetic chordae. Torn chordae can be reattached to the leaflet. Generally valvular repair is preferred over valve replacement since it avoids the risks associated with cardiopulmonary bypass, anticoagulation for artificial mechanical valve, and lessens pain and recovery time.

Surgery is too risky for some patients. A minimally invasive treatment option, called the MitraClip, was recently approved by the FDA to treat high-risk patients with MR. A small clip is attached to the leaky mitral valve, allowing it to close more completely (https://mitraclip.com/can_the_mitraclip_procedure_help_me; accessed September 17, 2016). This transcatheter mitral valve repair (TMVr) procedure may be used in people with severe degenerative MR who are not candidates for surgery. Patients who are older, symptomatic, and very high risk or not surgical candidates may benefit from a minimally invasive procedure. A transcatheter aortic valve replacement (TAVR) also can be performed for aortic valve pathology. A collapsible artificial valve is inserted into the stenotic aortic valve through a catheter that is inserted either into the femoral artery (transcatheter) or through a small incision in the chest wall allowing insertion through the LV (transapical). Then the replacement valve is positioned in the damaged valve, and, as it expands, it pushes the damaged valve leaflets aside and becomes the functional valve. Rarely, percutaneous aortic balloon valvuloplasty is used as a bridge to valve replacement surgery in an unstable patient. Aortic balloon valvuloplasty is performed by introducing a

balloon catheter across the aortic valve and into the LV. As the balloon is inflated, the calcified leaflets are cracked and split open and the valve ring is stretched. Potential complications include AR, emboli, ventricular perforation, rupture of the aortic valve annulus, ventricular arrhythmias, mitral valve damage, and bleeding from the catheter insertion sites.

Surgical procedures include an open commissurotomy (splitting or separating fused cardiac valve leaflets), which is performed to increase the size of the specific valve orifice when the valve is not calcified. Although some valves can be repaired by commissurotomy, most require replacement because of significant calcification or regurgitation.

Surgical valve replacement is the definitive treatment for symptomatic AS. However, surgical valve replacement for MS is indicated when the valvular problem is not amenable to a percutaneous procedure, percutaneous valvotomy failed, or when there is another indication for surgery, such as coronary artery disease, aortic valve disease, or concomitant mitral or tricuspid regurgitation (Nishimura et al., 2014a, 2014b).

Valvuloplasty, the repair of a cardiac valve, can be done percutaneously or surgically. Percutaneous balloon dilatation of stenotic valves is an appropriate alternative to surgical valve replacement or repair in some patients with valvular heart disease. In general, patients do not require continuous anticoagulation when they undergo valvuloplasty.

When surgical **valve replacement** is indicated, a decision must be made to use either a mechanical or a bioprosthetic (tissue, biologic) valve. Figure 16-7 shows a prosthetic valve

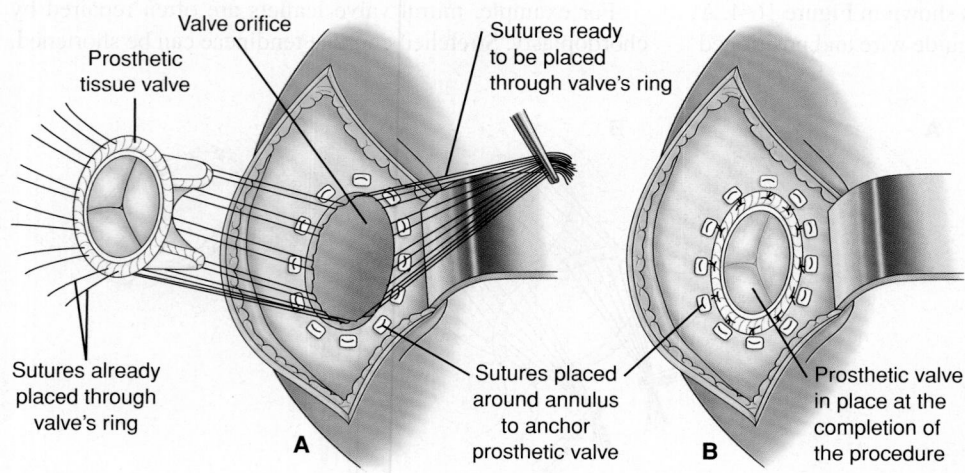

FIGURE 16-7 Valve replacement. **A.** The native valve is trimmed, and the prosthetic valve is sutured in place. **B.** Once all sutures are placed through the ring, the surgeon slides the prosthetic valve down the sutures and into the natural orifice. The sutures are then tied off and trimmed.

FIGURE 16-8 Common mechanical and tissue valve replacements. Different types of prosthetic heart valves. **A.** Bileaflet mechanical valve (St. Jude's); this is the most commonly used prosthetic valve, which consists of two semicircular leaflets that pivot on hinges. The leaflets swing partially open and are designed to close so that an acceptable amount of regurgitant blood flow is permitted. **B.** Monoleaflet, tilting disk mechanical valve (Medtronic Hall). **C.** Caged ball valve (Starr-Edwards); this valve was discontinued in 2007; however, you may care for patients who had this valve implanted. **D.** Stented porcine bioprosthesis (Medtronic Mosaic). **E.** Stented pericardial bioprosthesis (Carpentier-Edwards Magna). **F.** Stentless porcine bioprosthesis (Medtronic Freestyle). **G.** Percutaneous bioprosthesis expanded over a balloon (Edwards Sapien). **H.** Self-expandable percutaneous bioprosthesis (CoreValve).

replacement surgery. Consideration must be given to durability, risk of thrombosis, survival rates, and technical issues.

Types of Valve Prostheses

Two types of valve prostheses are available: mechanical and bioprosthetic (tissue, biological) and are depicted in Figure 16-8. The advantage of a mechanical valve is durability. The major disadvantage is the need for anticoagulation. Bioprosthetic valves have the advantage that they do not require anticoagulation; however, they are less durable. Age, lifestyle, medical history, and valve location are factors that determine whether a mechanical or biologic valve is used.

Mechanical Valves

Three major types of mechanical valves exist: (a) bi-leaflet valve, (b) tilting disk, and (c) caged-ball. The bi-leaflet valve, manufactured by St. Jude, CarboMedics, and On-X, and the single-tilting disc valve (e.g., Medtronic Hall) are used today; the caged-ball valve (Starr-Edwards) is no longer used because of the higher risk of thromboembolism associated with it.

The age and life expectancy of the patient determine the need for durability of a bioprosthetic valve. Mechanical valves are more durable than bioprosthetic valves and may be more likely to be used in a younger patient. However, patients with mechanical valves require lifelong anticoagu-lation due to the risk of thromboembolism and valve thrombosis, and with this comes the additional risk of bleeding complications.

Bioprosthetic Valves

Bioprosthetic valves are less durable than mechanical valves because of the structural degeneration that occurs over time. This can lead to the need for reoperation. Generally, older patients have shorter anticipated survival, so the risk of reoperation is less than it would be for a younger person. Because long-term anticoagulation generally is not recommended for bioprosthetic valves after the first 3 months of implantation, these valves are used when anticoagulation is contraindicated or should be avoided, such as in women of childbearing age, patients who are noncompliant with medications and follow-up, patients with a history of bleeding disorders, and others who cannot tolerate long-term anticoagulation. The major disadvantage of tissue valves is that they lack longevity.

Types of bioprosthetic valves include **homograft** (preserved human cadaver), pericardial, and **xenograft** (bovine, porcine, or equine). Generally homografts are used for the treatment of valve endocarditis. Newer tissue valves demonstrate improved hemodynamics compared with older models. Refer to Figure 16-8 for additional images of bioprosthetic valves.

Nursing Management: Valvuloplasty and Replacement

Before surgery, compensatory mechanisms allowed the heart to adjust gradually to the valvular pathology; surgery abruptly "corrects" blood flow through the heart. Complications unique to valve replacement are related to the sudden changes in intracardiac blood pressures. With valve replacement for a stenotic valve, blood flow through the heart is improved. Symptoms of the backward heart failure resolve in hours to days. With valve replacement for a regurgitant valve, it may take months for the chamber into which blood had been regurgitating to achieve its optimal postoperative function. Signs and symptoms of heart failure resolve as heart function improves.

Patients with percutaneous valvuloplasty procedures must be assessed for signs and symptoms of emboli and heart failure. Postprocedure care is the same as for patients having percutaneous coronary intervention and is discussed in Chapter 14.

Patient care following valve repair or replacement is similar to that of a patient recovering from coronary artery bypass surgery and is discussed in Chapter 14. In the immediate postoperative phase, attention is given to hemodynamic stabilization: augmenting preload, reducing afterload, and enhancing contractility, recognizing that the heart is adjusting to improved function. Patients are at risk for postoperative complications, including thromboembolism, bleeding, infective endocarditis, arrhythmias, structural deterioration (bioprosthetic valves), and hemolytic anemia.

Thromboembolism is the most common complication of prosthetic valves and can lead to hemodynamic compromise by occluding the valve orifice. Long-term anticoagulation with warfarin, a vitamin K antagonist, is indicated after mechanical valve replacement. Heparin is used as a "bridge" until an acceptable level of anticoagulation is achieved with warfarin. Frequently low-dose aspirin is used with warfarin. Newer oral anticoagulants, such as dabigatran, rivaroxaban, and apixaban, are not used (Nishimura et al., 2014a, 2014b).

The risk of thromboembolism is lower in patients with bioprosthetic valves. Usually low-dose (75 to 100 mg daily) aspirin is recommended. For patients with additional thrombotic risk factors, such as concurrent AF, anticoagulation with warfarin generally is prescribed for 3 months postoperatively. The nurse educates the patient about long-term anticoagulant therapy, including the risks associated with it as well as the need for frequent follow-up appointments and blood laboratory studies. Patients receiving warfarin will have individualized target international normalized ratios (INRs), typically between 2 and 3.5 seconds, and will vary based upon the type of valve.

Prosthetic valve endocarditis occurs more often with tissue valves. It can occur early, within the first 60 days after surgery, or later. Signs include fever, heart failure, embolic events, and new murmur. In general, for a patient with a prosthetic heart valve, if the temperature is higher than 100°F, endocarditis must be excluded by blood culture; whereas for fever with signs of sepsis, broad-spectrum antibiotics must be begun while awaiting culture results (Carabello, 2016). Hemolytic anemia results from the destruction of red blood cells by the movement of the prosthetic valve disk or caged ball.

Conduction disturbances and atrial arrhythmias occur frequently following valve surgery, likely due to circulating catecholamines, myocardial inflammation, and electrolyte imbalances. Digoxin, BBs, and CCBs may be used for the treatment of arrhythmias.

The nurse provides teaching about all prescribed medications: Patients with prosthetic valves require education to prevent infective endocarditis with antibiotic prophylaxis. The American Heart Association (AHA) recommends antibiotic prophylaxis for dental procedures that involve manipulation of gingival tissue, the periapical region of teeth, or perforation of the oral mucosa, not for routine cleaning (Nishimura et al., 2014a, 2014b).

INTRACARDIAC SEPTAL DEFECTS AND REPAIR

The atrial or ventricular septum may have an abnormal opening between the right and left sides of the heart, causing oxygenated blood to be shunted from the left side of the heart, which is under greater pressure, to the right. A small septal defect will be asymptomatic and have minimal effect on heart function, but larger ones may require repair to prevent problems related to excess blood volume in the right side of the heart. Over time, a large defect can cause pulmonary congestion, which can cause elevated right heart pressure; eventually this may cause right heart failure and pulmonary hypertension.

Most large septal defects are repaired during infancy or childhood to prevent later problems. A patent foramen ovale (PFO) is a small atrial septal wall defect (ASD) that may not be detected in an adult until the patient presents with symptoms of a TIA or a stroke. Normally thrombi are filtered out of the blood by the lungs. With an ASD, however, there is a risk that the clot could bypass the lungs and travel directly to the brain, causing a TIA or stroke. AF is common in patients with ASDs and further increases risk of stroke. Closure of the PFO is usually a percutaneous procedure to implant a device to plug the opening. Often anticoagulation with aspirin is prescribed. Small ventricular septal defects (VSDs) are rarely closed in adults unless there is evidence of endocarditis or if valve function is compromised due to the location of the defect. A stitch or pericardial or synthetic patch is used to close the opening. Atrial septal defect repairs have low morbidity and mortality rates. Patients should be taught the importance of infective endocarditis antibiotic prophylaxis for 6 months after the repair.

CARDIOMYOPATHY

Cardiomyopathies are diseases of the myocardium (heart muscle) characterized by mechanical and electrical dysfunction and structural abnormalities. Cardiomyopathy is *not* the result of another disease or dysfunction of the heart (such as valve disease). Cardiomyopathy results from various etiologies that are most frequently genetic and is characterized by abnormal hypertrophy or dilatation of the ventricles. Other causes include autoimmune disorders, excessive alcohol intake, pregnancy, chemotherapeutic agents, or infection (usually viral). Regardless of cause, cardiomyopathy results in impaired CO. Decreased stroke volume stimulates the sympathetic nervous system and the renin–angiotensin–aldosterone response, resulting in increased SVR and increased sodium and fluid retention, which places an increased workload on the heart. These alterations lead to severe heart failure, lethal arrhythmias, myocardial destruction, and death.

DILATED CARDIOMYOPATHY

Dilated cardiomyopathy (DCM) is the most common cardiomyopathy and is distinguished by significant irreversible dilation of the ventricles and systolic dysfunction without hypertrophy. It is a common cause of heart failure and the major reason for cardiac transplantation. The ventricles have increased systolic and diastolic volumes with decreased left ventricular function. As the LV becomes dilated (enlarged), contractility is impaired and becomes less forceful. The LV is unable to pump blood out of the heart effectively because of impaired contractility, and this often results in heart failure, ventricular arrhythmias, and sudden cardiac death (SCD). DCM occurs more often in men than in women and is generally seen between 20 and 60 years of age. As much as 40% of DCM is thought to be familial (Lakdawal, Winterfield, & Funke, 2013).

Pathophysiology

Microscopic examination of cardiac muscle tissue shows both atrophic and hypertrophic myocardial fibers with diffuse necrosis of myocardial cells and interstitial fibrosis. The result is poor systolic function. Structural changes (ventricular dilation) decrease the amount of blood ejected from the ventricle with systole, increasing the amount of blood remaining in the ventricle after contraction. Then less blood is able to enter the ventricle during diastole, increasing end-diastolic pressure and eventually increasing pulmonary and systemic venous pressures.

Clinical Manifestations and Assessment

Initial presentation is often with heart failure; symptoms of dyspnea, fatigue, weight gain, and volume overload are most common and are progressive. Arrhythmias and SCD frequently occur. Altered valve function, usually regurgitation,

can result from an enlarged stretched ventricle. Poor blood flow through the ventricle also may cause ventricular or atrial thrombi, which can embolize to other locations in the body. A persistent gallop rhythm, JVD, and a holosystolic murmur due to severe MR may be present. An echocardiogram is the preferred diagnostic tool as it can evaluate LV function and size, as well as valvular abnormalities. Cardiac catheterization is important to exclude coronary artery disease.

HYPERTROPHIC CARDIOMYOPATHY

Hypertrophic cardiomyopathy (HCM) is characterized by a hypertrophied, nondilated LV that can lead to obstruction of left ventricular outflow. HCM is an inherited autosomal dominant heart muscle disorder and is one of the most common types of cardiomyopathy, occurring in 1 out of 500 people. It is the most common cause of SCD in young athletes.

Pathophysiology

Cardiac muscle cells normally lay parallel to and end-to-end with each other. However, in HCM, the hypertrophied myofibrils are in disarray, and interstitial fibrosis develops. The heart muscle enlarges and asymmetrically thickens, especially along the septum. The increased thickness of the heart muscle reduces the size of the ventricles, making it more difficult to pump blood. The walls of the ventricle stiffen, and, as a result, the ventricle is less able to relax and fill with blood. The smaller-than-normal ventricular chamber creates a higher velocity flow of blood out of the LV into the aorta. Left ventricular outflow tract obstruction may occur if the mitral valve presses on the septum and blocks blood flow. This causes high systolic pressure in the LV that leads to prolonged ventricular relaxation and diminished CO, resulting in impaired diastolic filling. This decreases the effectiveness of contractions and increases the risk of ventricular arrhythmias.

Clinical Manifestations and Assessment

Clinical presentation varies widely: Many patients with HCM remain asymptomatic or experience only minor symptoms. Others may exhibit dyspnea with exercise or at rest, fatigue, chest pain, palpitations, dizziness, or presyncope and syncope. Some present with ventricular arrhythmias, SCD, or end-stage heart failure requiring cardiac transplantation. AF is common and may result from atrial enlargement. Patients with HCM may have systolic ejection murmurs that become more pronounced when the patient moves from standing to a squatting position. Mitral murmurs occur because of regurgitation. Echocardiography is used to detect HCM; a hypertrophied LV confirms diagnosis when other causes are excluded.

RESTRICTIVE CARDIOMYOPATHY

Restrictive cardiomyopathy (RCM) is characterized by diastolic dysfunction and impaired ventricular filling during diastole. RCM is rare and frequently idiopathic. Other causes of RCM are amyloidosis sarcoidosis and radiation fibrosis. It can occur after a heart transplant. Abnormal myocardial relaxation with interstitial fibrosis and calcifications are the fundamental abnormalities of restrictive cardiomyopathies.

Pathophysiology

Abnormally rigid ventricular walls result in poor ventricular compliance. Stiff ventricular walls lack ventricular stretch, or flexibility, to expand as they fill with blood. Typically, there is normal ventricular wall thickness and the ventricular chambers are not dilated. Systolic function (contractility) is normal or near normal. Atrial enlargement may be present. Impaired diastolic filling occurs because the rigid ventricular walls do not relax and fill with normal blood volume. CO can be increased by an increase in heart rate but, eventually, becomes ineffective due to shortened filling time. As the disease progresses, diastolic heart failure occurs.

Clinical Manifestations and Assessment

Signs and symptoms of RCM are similar to constrictive pericarditis: dyspnea, orthopnea, nonproductive cough, PND, and chest pain. Peripheral edema, fatigue, and hepatomegaly may be present. Echocardiography typically demonstrates normal ventricular dimensions with normal or nearly normal systolic function. With disease progression, edema worsens, and ascites, anasarca, or pulmonary edema may develop. Signs and symptoms of heart failure appear. Often JVD is present on physical examination, and an S3 and S4 can be heard with auscultation.

ARRHYTHMOGENIC RIGHT VENTRICULAR CARDIOMYOPATHY/DYSPLASIA

Arrhythmogenic right ventricular cardiomyopathy/dysplasia (ARVC/D) is an inherited cardiomyopathy, often with an autosomal dominant trait. It is a disease of the RV characterized by ventricular tachycardia and right heart failure; however, it may be seen in the left or both ventricles. Although relatively rare, ARVC/D accounts for up to 20% of cases of SCD primarily in young athletes, making it the second leading cause of SCD after DCM (Romero, Mejia-Lopez, Manrique, & Lucariello, 2013).

Presenting symptoms range from palpitations and syncope to SCD. ARVC/D myocardial electrical instability comprises the main clinical manifestation with ventricular ectopy and ventricular tachycardia. Biventricular or RV failure is less common and observed mainly in patients with long-term disease protected from SCD by implantable cardioverter defibrillator (ICD) implantation.

Pathophysiology

ARVC/D occurs when the RV is progressively infiltrated and replaced with fibrous scar and fatty tissue. Initially, localized areas of the RV are affected, but, as the disease progresses, the entire heart can be affected. Eventually, the RV dilates and develops poor contractility, and arrhythmias occur.

Clinical Manifestations and Assessment

Usually presentation is in early adulthood, with symptoms ranging from palpitations and syncope to supraventricular and ventricular arrhythmias or right-sided heart failure. Ventricular tachycardia originating in the RV (left bundle branch block morphology) is the classic presentation. SCD may be the initial presentation. ARVC/D should be suspected in patients with palpitations, syncope, or ventricular tachycardia originating in the RV or SCD, especially among previously symptom-free athletes. Family history, electrocardiogram (ECG), and a history of arrhythmias can help establish a diagnosis of ARVC/D.

STRESS-INDUCED (TAKOTSUBO) CARDIOMYOPATHY

Stress-induced (Takotsubo) cardiomyopathy is a syndrome of acute, reversible LV dysfunction that is frequently, but not always, precipitated by profound emotional, psychological, or physical distress. Ventricular function fully returns within several days to several months. LV morphology, as seen with echocardiography or ventriculogram, demonstrates apical and midventricular contractile abnormalities (akinesis) with sparing of the base as well as resultant ballooning of the ventricle that is seen with angiography. Stress-induced cardiomyopathy has been identified predominantly in white, postmenopausal women. Noncardiac comorbidities, such as anxiety, chronic pulmonary disease, and thyroid disease, are associated.

Pathophysiology

The pathophysiology of stress-induced cardiomyopathy is not completely understood. Catecholamine release triggered by activation of the sympathetic system during sudden stress is thought to result in stress-induced cardiomyopathy. Very happy events, such as the birth of a grandchild, also can cause Takotsubo cardiomyopathy, and it is thought that happy events may increase activation of the sympathetic and parasympathetic systems, acting similarly to stressful events (Ghadri et al., 2016). There are also cases of stress-induced cardiomyopathy occurring from iatrogenic causes, such as during catecholamine administration for dobutamine stress echocardiography (Lyon et al., 2016).

Clinical Manifestations and Assessment

Clinical presentation of stress-induced cardiomyopathy is similar to that of ST-segment elevation myocardial infarction (STEMI). Acute presentation may be severe and reportedly can include life-threatening arrhythmias, pulmonary edema, heart failure, cardiogenic shock, and SCD (Liang,

Cha, Oh, & Prasad, 2013). Typically, patients present with acute substernal pain and SOB following an emotionally or physically stressful trigger. Palpitations induced from tachycardia or arrhythmia may be present. ST-segment elevation may be present on ECG, and cardiac enzymes may be mildly elevated, although disproportionately low to levels seen with acute MI. Conversely, serum brain natriuretic peptide (BNP) is extremely elevated. The diagnosis of Takotsubo cardiomyopathy should be suspected in postmenopausal women with acute heart failure or cariogenic shock following an emotionally stressful event. Typically, patients are treated as if they are having an acute MI and undergo urgent cardiac catheterization. An absence of significant coronary artery disease with ballooning of the LV seen during ventriculography, with rapid and complete recovery, is the hallmark feature of stress-induced cardiomyopathy. See Table 16-2.

 Nursing Alert
DCM is a floppy heart; HCM is an enlarged, thickened heart; RCM is a stiff, rigid heart; ARVC/D is an arrhythmia-prone heart; and Takotsubo cardiomyopathy is a stressed heart.

MEDICAL AND NURSING MANAGEMENT OF CARDIOMYOPATHY

The echocardiogram is used in the evaluation of cardiomyopathy because it allows assessment of both the structure and function of the ventricles, including valvular abnormalities and EF. A chest x-ray can identify the extent of cardiac enlargement and the presence of pulmonary congestion, an electrocardiogram (ECG) can confirm the presence of arrhythmias, and cardiac catheterization can detect the presence of coronary artery disease. Endomyocardial biopsy may be performed; analysis of myocardial tissue may be used to guide therapy or to establish a precipitating cause, if unknown. Because genetic factors may be involved, detailed and careful family history, should be obtained. Screening of first-degree blood relatives (e.g., parents, siblings, and children) for HCM, DCM, and ARVC/D with echocardiography (echo), and ECG should be considered, as early diagnosis and treatment can prevent or delay significant symptoms and SCD.

Regardless of the type of cardiomyopathy, symptoms are primarily those associated with heart failure. Treatment is supportive and is focused on symptom management. In addition to symptom relief, treatment priorities are prevention of complications, including prevention of lethal arrhythmias to reduce the risk of SCD. Specific treatment for the underlying cause is given if it is known.

Supportive care with standard heart failure therapy, including ACE inhibitors, aldosterone receptor antagonists (ARBs), BB and diuretics, should be administered for all cardiomyopathies. BBs and CCBs reduce catecholamine response and decrease heart rate. ACE inhibitors are prescribed to reduce preload, afterload, and hypertension by causing vasodilation. ARBs reduce afterload by blocking the action of Angiotensin II, resulting in vasodilation, which subsequently decreases preload and helps regulate fluid and electrolyte balance. Diuretics remove excess sodium and fluid to reduce pulmonary congestion. Nitrates and dehydration should be avoided in HCM to maintain CO. Systemic anticoagulation may be needed to prevent thromboembolic events. Because mural thrombi (a thrombus formed on and attached to a diseased patch of endocardium, not on a valve or on one side of a large blood vessel) are also a risk, the patient's neurologic status should be monitored carefully. Often antiarrhythmic medications are initiated to prevent and treat arrhythmias. For stress-induced cardiomyopathy, accurate diagnosis and differentiation from STEMI is critical to avoid unnecessary treatments, such as administration of thrombolytics, which can cause harm to the patient.

Unstable patients may require positive inotropic medications, vasopressors and intra-aortic balloon pumps (IABPs), implantable devices, or surgery. Pacemakers are used to correct conduction abnormalities and control heart rate when tachyarrhythmias or bradyarrythmias are present. Cardiac resynchronization therapy with biventricular pacing can resynchronize the ventricles to improve contractility. ICDs are recommended when there is a high risk for life-threatening arrhythmias, particularly with ARVC/D. IABP (described in Chapter 55), septal myectomy (removal of hypertrophied portion of the septum that is obstructing the flow of blood from the LV to the aorta) or alcohol septal ablation, left ventricular assist devices (VADs), and heart transplantation may be necessary in the most severe cases.

Nursing management of cardiomyopathy includes careful cardiovascular assessment for signs of worsening heart failure, particularly dyspnea, congested lungs, peripheral edema, and the presence of abnormal heart sounds.

 Nursing Alert
The nurse should assess for changes in mentation; pallor; cyanosis; cool, clammy skin; arrhythmias; and a decrease in urine output. These are manifestations of diminished tissue perfusion and suggest reduced CO.

Arrhythmias occur frequently; continuous cardiac monitoring is recommended with personnel and equipment readily available to treat life-threatening arrhythmias. Bed rest is maintained to decrease cardiac workload. Physical activity is increased slowly, and the patient is asked to report symptoms that occur with increasing activity. For stress-induced cardiomyopathy, the nurse must evaluate for the presence of anxiety and guide stress management practices. Encouraging a heart-healthy lifestyle by maintaining a healthy weight and physical activity, smoking cessation, and stress reduction, is integral.

TABLE 16-2 Cardiomyopathies

Type	Description	Etiology	Pathophysiology	Clinical Manifestations
Dilated Cardiomyopathy (DCM)	Significant, irreversible dilation of the ventricles Systolic dysfunction without hypertrophy Increased ventricular systolic and diastolic volumes with decreased left ventricular (LV) function Impaired contractility may result in HF, ventricular arrhythmias, and sudden cardiac death.	As much as 40% of DCM is thought to be familial. It occurs most often in adults 20 to 60 years of age, and men are affected more than women.	Reduced ventricular wall thickness and increased myocardial mass result in poor systolic function. Decreased blood volume ejected from the ventricle during systole increases blood volume remaining in the ventricle after contraction. Then less blood is able to enter the ventricle during diastole, increasing end-diastolic pressure and, eventually, increasing pulmonary and systemic venous pressures. Valvular regurgitation can result from an enlarged stretched ventricle. Poor blood flow through the ventricle may cause ventricular or atrial thrombi, which may embolize to other locations in the body.	Symptoms are progressive and include dyspnea, fatigue, volume overload, weight gain, chest pain due to coronary artery disease or pulmonary embolism, or abdominal discomfort from hepatomegaly. Signs include: holosystolic murmur (heard on S1) due to MR, thromboembolism, ventricular arrhythmias, and sudden cardiac death. HF may be the initial presentation.
	Increased chamber size Thin left ventricular muscle			
Hypertrophic Cardiomyopathy (HCM)	Hypertrophied, nondilated LV leads to obstruction of left ventricular outflow, without cardiac or systemic disease	HCM is an inherited autosomal dominant heart muscle disorder and one of the most common types of cardiomyopathy. It is the most common cause of sudden cardiac death (SCD) in young athletes.	Heart muscle asymmetrically increases in mass, especially along the septum, and increased thickness reduces the size of the ventricular cavities, taking longer to relax after systole. During diastole, ventricular filling is impaired; atrial contraction at the end of diastole becomes critical for filling and systolic contraction. Smaller-than-normal LV cavity creates high-velocity blood flow from the LV into the aorta. Left ventricular outflow tract obstruction causes high systolic pressure in the LV that leads to prolonged ventricular relaxation and diminished cardiac output, resulting in diastolic dysfunction. Systolic function is normal or high, resulting in an above-normal ejection fraction.	Most patients with HCM are asymptomatic, but some present with ventricular arrhythmias, SCD, or other symptoms: syncope, dyspnea, or chest pain. Atrial fibrillation commonly occurs from atrial enlargement. Systolic ejection murmurs (heard on S1) do not radiate to the neck. Mitral murmurs result from regurgitation.
	Decreased chamber size Thickened intraventricular septum			

Type	Description	Etiology	Pathophysiology	Clinical Manifestations
Restrictive Cardiomyopathy (RCM) Stiff ventricular walls	Characterized by diastolic dysfunction that negatively affects or "restricts" the heart's ability to fill with blood Uncommon cardiomyopathy	Frequently idiopathic Associated with amyloidosis and endomyocardial fibrosis (scarring of the heart) Often occurs after a heart transplant	Stiff ventricular walls lack ventricular stretch (flexibility to expand as they fill with blood). This impairs diastolic filling, resulting in diastolic HF. Normal, or slightly increased, ventricular wall thickness and atrial enlargement with normal systolic function are characteristic. Atrioventricular block and symptomatic bradycardia can occur.	Symptoms are similar to constrictive pericarditis: dyspnea, nonproductive cough, chest pain, and exercise intolerance. Signs may include jugular venous distention, edema, ascites, anasarca, pulmonary edema, and an S3 and S4 can be heard with auscultation.
Arrhythmogenic Right Ventricular Cardiomyopathy/ Dysplasia (ARVC/D) Fibrofatty replacement of right ventricular myocardium	Rare but increasingly recognized condition ARVC/D should be suspected in patients with ventricular tachycardia originating in the right ventricle (i.e., left bundle branch block on ECG) or SCD, especially among previously symptom-free athletes.	Familial in more than 50% of patients and usually occurs in early adulthood	ARVC/D occurs when the right ventricle is progressively infiltrated and replaced with fibrous scar and adipose tissue. Initially, only localized areas of the right ventricle are affected, but, as the disease progresses, the entire heart is affected. Eventually, the right ventricle dilates and develops poor contractility, and arrhythmias occur.	Symptoms are consistent with right HF. Supraventricular arrhythmias may occur. Ventricular arrhythmias and SCD may be the initial presentation, and often diagnosis is made postmortem. Family history, ECG, and a history of arrhythmias can help establish a diagnosis of ARVC/D.
Stress-induced (Takotsubo) Cardiomyopathy Akinesis (absence of or decreased movement) with sparing of the base and left ventricular apical ballooning	Syndrome of transient LV dysfunction. Ventricular function fully returns within weeks. LV morphology, seen with echocardiography or ventriculogram, demonstrates apical akinesis (absence of or decreased movement) with sparing of the base and resultant ballooning of the ventricle. It has been identified predominantly in white, postmenopausal women. Noncardiac comorbidities, such as anxiety, chronic pulmonary disease, and thyroid disease are associated.	Precipitated by emotional or physical distress	The pathophysiology of stress-induced cardiomyopathy remains unclear. One theory gaining acceptance is catecholamine excess triggered by activation of the sympathetic system.	Clinical presentation is identical to that of acute ST-segment elevation MI: acute substernal pain and shortness of breath following an emotionally or physically stressful trigger. ST-segment elevation may be present on ECG, and cardiac enzymes may be mildly elevated, disproportionate to levels seen with acute MI. Acute presentation may be severe; arrhythmias, HF, pulmonary edema, and cardiogenic shock have been reported in the absence of significant coronary artery disease. Ballooning of the LV, with rapid and complete recovery, is the hallmark feature.

SURGICAL INTERVENTIONS FOR CARDIOMYOPATHY

When heart failure progresses and medical treatment is no longer effective, surgical intervention, including cardiac transplantation, is considered.

Septal Myectomy and Alcohol Septal Ablation

Septal myectomy generally is used for younger patients with obstructive HCM and severe symptoms refractory to medical management. Removing part of the thickened septum that is bulging into the LV improves blood flow through the heart and out to the body.

Septal ablation is the destruction of the hypertrophied septum caused by injecting alcohol into the artery that supplies blood to that area. Alcohol septal ablation can improve symptoms, but possible complications with this procedure include permanent heart block, which can occur in as many as 10% of the cases and requires implantation of a pacemaker. Generally this is thought to be an acceptable alternative to myectomy when concomitant cardiac surgery is not necessary, coronary anatomy is appropriate, in older patients at risk for operative morbidity, or for those with a strong desire to avoid surgery (Maron & Nishimura, 2014a, 2014b).

Mechanical Circulatory Support

Mechanical circulatory support (MCS) has evolved greatly, and its use has increased dramatically since the late 1960s when a VAD was first used for postcardiotomy shock (McLarty, 2015). MCS has three main functions: (a) reduce or assume the workload of the heart, (b) support systemic circulation, completely or partially, and (c) improve myocardial oxygenation. Patients who cannot be weaned from cardiopulmonary bypass, patients in cardiogenic shock, and patients with refractory heart failure may benefit from short-term (hours to days) MCS for the management of hemodynamically unstable acute, decompensated heart failure while the patient's own heart recovers. Typically, an IABP, described in Chapter 55, or an extracorporeal membrane oxygenator (ECMO) is used to provide support in these cases.

Intra-aortic Balloon Pump Counterpulsation

The IABP decreases the workload of the heart by reducing left ventricular afterload. Additionally, it improves coronary artery blood flow by increasing coronary artery perfusion pressure. The IABP is used pre- and postoperatively in patients with severely compromised left ventricular function, in patients with myocardial ischemia undergoing complex percutaneous coronary interventions, and for patients with complications resulting from acute myocardial infarction,

such as papillary muscle rupture, awaiting surgical repair. Bleeding, limb ischemia, infection, and vascular injury are potential complications of IABP, and monitoring the patient for compromised circulation and hemodynamic instability is a priority for nursing management.

Extracorporeal Membrane Oxygenator

ECMO uses a pump to circulate blood through an oxygenator outside the body to provide both cardiac and respiratory support by artificially removing the carbon dioxide and re-oxygenating red blood cells. The purpose of ECMO is to allow time for intrinsic recovery of the lungs and heart; a standard cardiopulmonary bypass provides support during various types of cardiac surgical procedures.

Increasingly, MCS is used long term (months to years) for the management of advanced heart failure from causes including cardiomyopathy (heart failure is described in detail in Chapter 15). Investigation continues for devices for permanent use (Yancy et al., 2013a, 2013b).

Ventricular Assist Devices

VADs can support a failing heart by generating blood flow to the systemic circulation and unloading the ventricle. Most patients receive a left VAD, but some may receive a biventricular device (BiVAD) or a total artificial heart (TAH). Initially this therapy was used temporarily for patients with difficulty weaning from cardiopulmonary bypass following cardiothoracic surgery, VADs were mainly a bridge to recovery. Nondurable (temporary) support indications include cardiogenic shock, acute myocarditis (discussed shortly), and acute, reversible heart failure. Another nondurable indication is the use of a VAD as a bridge to the decision regarding candidacy for transplantation or to a more permanent VAD when the patient becomes more clinically stable.

Durable or long-term indications include using a VAD as a bridge to transplantation, to sustain life until a donor heart becomes available, or as destination therapy (DT) in patients with end-stage heart failure who are ineligible for transplantation and for whom ventricular recovery is not possible. Increasingly, VADs are being used as DT. See Figure 16-9 for an example of a long-term use of VAD. VAD therapies are also categorized as a bridge to decision (BTD) and a bridge to bridge (BTB). VADs used for a BTD allow time to evaluate whether a transplant or other treatment is most suited to a patient. Similarly, a BTB VAD is used when emergent stabilization is necessary, with a plan to transition to a longer-term device when the patient becomes more clinically stable. Long-term indications include using a VAD as a bridge to transplant (BTT) in patients failing on maximal medical therapy, or for DT in patients with end-stage heart failure who are not transplant candidates.

These devices can have pumps that are outside the body (extracorporeal) or implantable and can be broadly classified as pulsatile volume displacement or continuous flow (axial

FIGURE 16-9 Left ventricular assist device.

flow, centrifugal). Most are surgically inserted via sternotomy, but some short-term use VADs can be inserted percutaneously. First-generation volume-displacement pumps provided good hemodynamic support but were limited by lack of long-term durability, an extensive surgical procedure for insertion, and a large external driveline that was prone to infection. These are rarely implanted today.

Second- and third-generation LVADs are continuous flow pumps and have only one moving part, making them more durable. Because they have smaller drivelines, the risk of infection and surgical trauma is reduced. Second-generation axial flow pumps contain a spinning impeller that generates a continuous, nonpulsatile flow by a rotor spinning around a central shaft and return blood to the aorta at a constant rate. Third-generation centrifugal VADs generate centrifugal force from the spinning cone-shaped rotor, resulting in a nonpulsatile flow of blood and have been designed for long-term use. Compared with earlier LVADs, the third-generation VADs optimize blood flow to reduce the risk of thrombus formation and are smaller in size to facilitate surgical implantation.

Long-term use of VADs has been shown to improve survival in patients with symptomatic late-stage heart failure; however, it is not without adverse events and an impact on quality of life. Some researchers had suggested that potential survival benefit would offset the increased rates of adverse effects (Rose et al., 2001). More recently, researchers have acknowledged that although LVADs pose significant risks,

they have been shown to improve both quantity and quality of life of patients living with Stage D heart failure and have sought to describe and explain patients' preimplantation decision-making and pre- and postimplantation expectations regarding LVADs, as seen in Box 16-1 (Kitko, Hupcey, Birriel, & Alonso, 2016).

Nursing Alert
The nurse understands that there is no palpable pulse or measurable "normal" systolic or diastolic blood pressure in patients with continuous flow LVADs where the majority of blood flow is through the LVAD. The nurse can attempt to palpate the pulse as occasionally some patients may have a weak pulsation. Obtain a traditional manual blood pressure cuff and, using a Doppler, assess the VAD pressure at the brachial artery, often referred to as the MAP (mean arterial pressure, although with LVAD, it is not the traditional MAP). Refer to your health care facility's target VAD pressure (generally 65 to 80 mm Hg, NOT TO EXCEED 90 mm Hg). The nurse auscultates below the heart to hear the hum of the device running. Use level of consciousness, skin color, respiratory rate, and temperature, and assess the system controller for messages. Observe for the cables, being careful not to put undue stress on them. Additionally for patients that will be discharged with a VAD, patient education focuses on contingency plans, including ensuring uninterrupted electrical access, ensuring access to a working telephone for emergencies, and understanding the limitations of battery life (Devore, Mentz, & Patel, 2014).

Total Artificial Hearts

TAHs are designed to replace both ventricles. The SynCardia Temporary Total Artificial Heart has been FDA-approved for use since 2004 as a BTT in patients waiting for a donor heart who have biventricular failure unresponsive to other therapies and who are at imminent risk of death (U.S. Food and Drug Administration website. Syncardia Systems, Inc. CardioWest total artificial heart (TAH): directions for use. http://www.fda.gov/ohrms/dockets/ac/04/briefing/4029b1_final.pdf. Accessed September 3, 2017). More than 1100 patients have been supported by this device, the longest duration being 1374 days before the patient received a donor heart. In December 2014, Syncardia received FDA approval for this device to be tested in a clinical trial evaluating its effectiveness as DT (http://www.syncardia.com/2015-multimedia-releases/fda-approves-the-syncardia-total-artificial-heart-for-destination-therapy-study/itemid-1737.html).

Complications

Complications of VADs and TAHs include infection, ventricular arrhythmias, thrombus, thromboemboli, hemolysis,

Kitko, L. A., Hupcey, J. E., Birriel, B., & Alonso, W. (2016). Patients' decision-making process and expectations of a left ventricular assist device (LVAD) pre- and postimplantation. *Heart and Lung: The Journal of Acute and Critical Care, 45*, 95–99.

BOX 16-1 Nursing Research

Purpose

Five percent to 10% of the nearly 6 million Americans with heart failure have advanced (Stage D) heart failure (HF) with progressive signs and symptoms despite optimal medical, device, and surgical management. Increasing, left ventricular assist devices (LVADs) are being used as a treatment for advanced heart failure. Although LVADs have been shown to improve both the quantity and quality of life in patients living with Stage D HF, they also pose significant risks. Most patients will experience a significant adverse event within 2 years, including malfunctioning pump, infection, bleeding arrhythmias, and stroke. The purpose of this research was to examine patients' preimplantation decision-making and pre- and postimplantation expectations of LVADs.

Design

Thematic analysis of semi-structured, serial interviews of 15 patients with Stage D HF and LVADs was used in this longitudinal, qualitative study to obtain a strong understanding of the decision-making process of patients undergoing LVAD placement and their postimplant expectations.

Findings

"No choice" was the main theme among patients in the preimplantation period. Postimplantation, two themes emerged: "I thought I would be doing better" and "I feel good, but now what." Evidence from preimplantation to postimplantation suggested that patients' perceived expectations of quality-of-life improvement were not met.

Nursing Implications

Faced with rapidly declining health, most patients felt that death, an unacceptable option, was their only alternative to LVAD implantation. Ongoing discussion of treatment goals and all treatment options, including the benefits and risks of each, is critical prior to implantation. In the postimplantation period, patients expected greater improvements in their quality of life. This strongly suggests that postimplantation, ongoing palliative care is necessary as are evidence-based guidelines for discussions of goals of care that include detailed and realistic expectations.

---

hemorrhage, right heart failure, multisystem failure, and mechanical failure of the device. Appropriate anticoagulation to reduce the risk of thrombus formation and thromboembolism, while avoiding the risk of bleeding, is a challenge, and anticoagulation therapy depends on device type, patient history, and platelet responsiveness. Infection is another major complication, particularly with extracorporeal devices as the percutaneous driveline exit site commonly becomes infected. Infection at this site can spread quickly through the entire system causing sepsis, a systemic infection.

Nursing care for patients with mechanical assist devices (MAD) focuses on the assessment of and minimization of complications as well as providing emotional support and education about the mechanical assist device and the underlying cardiac disease. If a durable VAD is being considered, the patient's ability to manage the VAD should be assessed. When assessing the patient with a VAD, it is important to remember that there may not be any palpable pulse because blood flow throughout the cardiac cycle is continuous, not pulsatile. Pulse oximetry may be unmeasurable or unreliable, and obtaining VAD pressure may be difficult or not possible. It is recommended that a Doppler ultrasound be used with a sphygmomanometer to obtain a VAD pressure.

Heart Transplantation

The first human-to-human heart transplant was performed in 1967. Since then, transplant procedures, equipment, and medications continue to improve. In 1983, when cyclosporine became available, transplantation became an option for patients with end-stage heart disease. Cyclosporine is an immunosuppressant that significantly decreases the body's rejection of transplanted organs. The use of tacrolimus, another immunosuppressant drug, and better methods for monitoring rejection have greatly improved survival rate and expanded selection criteria.

There is a critical shortage of donor hearts; in 2014, 2655 cardiac transplants were performed in the United States, and as of July 2015, there were more than 4100 people on the transplant list awaiting a heart (Mozaffarian et al., 2016). For cardiac transplants occurring between 2009 and 2010, the one-year survival rate after cardiac transplantation was more than 90.8% for men and 90.6% for women (Mozaffarian et al., 2016, p. e345). Typical candidates have advanced heart failure, severe symptoms and functional limitations uncontrolled by medical therapy, no other surgical options, and a poor life expectancy from heart disease. As discussed earlier, VADs serve as a "BTT," for patients waiting for a heart transplant.

A multidisciplinary team screens the candidate before recommending the transplantation procedure. A primary factor to be considered is the candidate's prognosis after transplantation. Function of major organ systems (lungs, liver, and kidneys), chronic health conditions, infections, history of other transplantations, psychosocial status, family support, compliance, and current health status are evaluated (Mancini & Naka, 2016).

Transplant candidates cannot have irreversible pulmonary hypertension as this would lead to right ventricular

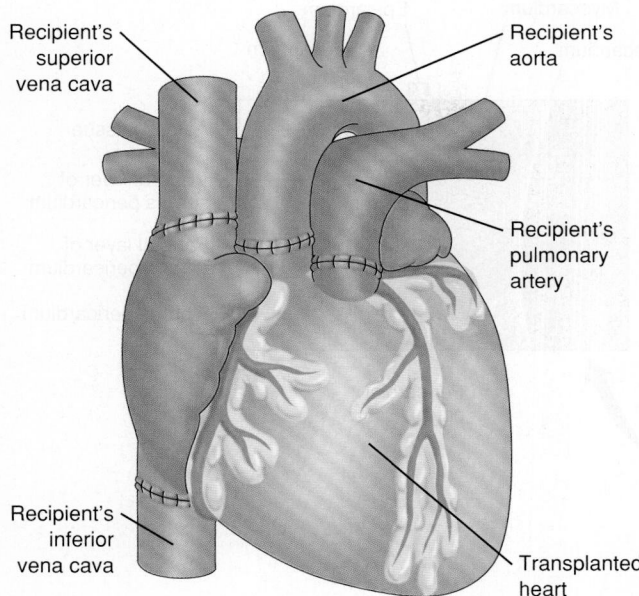

FIGURE 16-10 Orthotopic method of heart transplantation.

failure of the transplanted heart. Other contraindications include malignancy and active infection as both of these can worsen as a result of the antirejection medications.

In addition to having severely compromised physical health, patients also struggle with psychosocial issues. Waiting for a donor heart is stressful for the patient and family. Much unpredictability and uncertainty exist regarding when or whether a donor heart will become available.

Orthotopic Transplantation

Orthotopic transplantation, as depicted in Figure 16-10, is the most common surgical procedure for cardiac transplantation. The recipient's heart is removed, leaving a portion of the recipient's atria with the vena cava and pulmonary veins in place. The donor heart, which usually has been preserved in ice, is prepared for implant by cutting away a small section of the atria that corresponds with the sections of the recipient's heart that were left in place. The donor heart is implanted by suturing the donor atria to the residual atrial tissue of the recipient's heart. After the venous or atrial anastomoses are complete, the recipient's pulmonary artery and aorta are sutured to those of the donor heart.

Rarely (less than 1%), a heterotopic cardiac transplant may be performed because of significant pulmonary hypertension, small donor heart, or expected poor function of the donor heart. In this case, the recipient's heart is left in place and the donor heart is placed next to it and they are joined together.

Postoperative Course

Patients who have had heart transplants constantly balance the risk of rejection with the risk of infection. They must adhere to a complex regimen of diet, medications, activity, follow-up laboratory studies, biopsies of the transplanted heart (to diagnose rejection), and clinic visits. Commonly, patients receive cyclosporine or tacrolimus, azathioprine or mycophenolate mofetil (CellCept), and corticosteroids to minimize rejection.

The transplanted heart is denervated; it has no nerve connections to the recipient's body, and the sympathetic and vagus nerves do not affect the transplanted heart. The resting rate of the transplanted heart is approximately 70 to 90 beats/minute, but it increases gradually if catecholamines are in the circulation. Patients must gradually increase and decrease their exercise (i.e., extended warm-up and cooldown periods), because 20 to 30 minutes may be required to achieve the desired heart rate. Atropine does not increase the heart rate of transplanted hearts.

Rejection is most common in the first 3 to 6 months following transplant, although the risk of infection continues to be a significant risk even after the first year because of the immunosuppressant medications. In addition to rejection and infection, other complications include posttransplant lymphoproliferative disease and the development of allograft vasculopathy or rapidly progressing atherosclerosis in the arteries of the transplanted heart. Osteoporosis frequently occurs as a side effect of the anti-rejection medications and pretransplantation dietary insufficiency and long-term sedentary lifestyle. Immunosuppressants and corticosteroids can cause weight gain, diabetes, dyslipidemia, kidney failure, and disturbances of the central nervous and gastrointestinal systems, and toxicity from immunosuppressants can occur.

Transplant recipients face a number of stressors, including (a) coping with complications such as graft rejection; (b) managing a complex posttransplant regimen consisting of multiple medications; exercise and dietary prescriptions; regular medical follow-up evaluations and laboratory tests; lifestyle restrictions related to smoking, alcohol, and other potentially harmful substances; (c) transitioning from their roles as critically ill or dying patients to roles and lifestyles that are less illness-focused; (d) psychological acceptance of the transplant and the fact that someone else lost their life when the patient regained his or hers; and (e) coping with financial issues, such as the cost of surgery and medications.

INFLAMMATORY DISEASES OF THE HEART

Any of the heart's three layers can become inflamed or affected by a variety of causes including infections (viral, bacterial, fungal), inflammatory disorders (connective tissue disorders, inflammatory bowel disease, drug-induced, postoperative (heart and lung surgeries), or idiopathic (no specific cause can be found). The diseases are named for the layer of the heart most involved in the infectious process:

FIGURE 16-11 The layers of the heart. Layers of the heart and pericardium. This schematic diagram shows the anatomic relationship between the layers of the heart. In the middle mediastinum, the heart and roots of the great vessels are surrounded by the pericardium, which is often covered by highly variable amounts of adipose tissue. The pericardium has two layers: a tough external fibrous layer called the fibrous pericardium and a parietal layer of serous pericardium that lines its inner surface. The parietal layer of the serous pericardium is reflected back at the great vessels entering and leaving the heart as the visceral layer of the serous pericardium or epicardium. The epicardium lines the outer surface of the heart. The pericardial cavity is a space between the visceral and parietal layers of the serous pericardium, and it is lined by the mesothelial cells. Deep within the epicardium is the myocardium, which consists of cardiac muscle. Note the small amount of adipose tissue of the epicardium, which contains the coronary arteries and cardiac veins. The inner layer of the myocardium is called the endocardium, which is lined by the mesothelium with an underlying thin layer of connective tissue.

endocarditis (endocardium), myocarditis (myocardium), and pericarditis (pericardium) (see Fig. 16-11). These diseases may damage heart muscle, valves, or pericardium and impact cardiac function and, indirectly, quality of life. The ideal management for all infectious diseases is prevention.

RHEUMATIC FEVER AND RHEUMATIC HEART DISEASE

Rheumatic fever (RF) is a systemic inflammatory condition that is a complication of Group A beta-hemolytic streptococcal (GAS) pharyngitis, commonly known as strep throat. RF almost always occurs in children or adolescents; however, because suspected strep throat is treated swiftly with antibiotics, RF now occurs rarely in the United States.

Pathophysiology

RF results in damage to connective tissues, especially in the heart, brain, joints, and skin. It is triggered by the body's immune response to GAS bacteria. It is thought that the immune system is unable to distinguish between the invading bacteria and its own host tissues, resulting in inflammation

and tissue damage. Rheumatic heart disease is a condition in which permanent damage to the heart valves occurs from a prior episode of RF.

Clinical Manifestations and Assessment

Symptoms of RF include sore throat, fever, headache, weakness, diaphoresis, nausea, irritability, and swollen glands. Other manifestations result from the inflammatory process in the affected structures. Polyarthritis occurs in 75% of cases, and swollen, tender, painful joints can persist for up to 4 weeks. Erythema marginatum is a nonitchy macular rash on the trunk and proximal extremities that blanches with pressure, is not indurated, and does not scar. It often occurs with subcutaneous nodules: round, firm, painless bumps beneath the skin that usually disappear after 1 to 2 weeks. Patients also may develop chorea, which is characterized by spontaneous, purposeless movements of the trunk and extremities. Typically self-limiting, chorea can last for weeks to months. The existence and extent of cardiac damage may not be apparent during the acute phase of RF but will manifest later in life as rheumatic heart disease.

Rheumatic carditis is inflammation of the pericardium, myocardium, or endocardium, separately or in combination. Rheumatic myocarditis can temporarily weaken the pumping ability of the heart and cause conduction abnormalities. Rheumatic pericarditis occurs during the acute illness and may result in accumulation of fluid in the pericardial sac. Myocardial and pericardial inflammation usually resolves without sequelae, but rheumatic endocardial inflammation often results in permanent adverse effects. Heart valves become swollen, and tiny vegetations or growths develop on the valve leaflets. They can lead to thickening of the leaflets, causing them to shorten and preventing them from closing completely. As a result, blood regurgitates backward through the valve. The most common site of valvular regurgitation is the mitral valve, although any of the heart valves may be affected. Heart murmurs characteristic of valvular regurgitation, stenosis, or both become audible on auscultation. Since most patients with rheumatic heart disease develop mitral insufficiency, a blowing, high-pitched holosystolic murmur is frequently heard. Diastolic murmurs are heard if AR occurs. The myocardium compensates for some time, but as the valvular pathology progresses, compensatory mechanisms fail, and heart failure can develop.

Medical and Nursing Management

Throat cultures are necessary to diagnose the presence of a GAS infection. If group A beta-hemolytic streptococcus (GAS) is identified, aggressive treatment with penicillin for a 10-day course of therapy is prescribed. Clarithromycin or clindamycin may be prescribed for patients who are penicillin-allergic. Aspirin, or other anti-inflammatory medicines, is usually prescribed.

Since no diagnostic studies are specific for rheumatic endocarditis and symptoms may not develop until years after the RF, the Jones criteria help standardize the diagnosis of RF by classifying the signs of RF into major and minor categories. Having two major (e.g., polyarthritis, carditis, subcutaneous nodules, erythema marginata, or chorea) or one major and two minor (e.g., fever, elevated erythrocyte sedimentation rate [ESR] or serum C-reactive protein level) clinical findings with a throat culture indicating recent infection with GAS pharyngitis indicates a high probability of RF. Although the Jones criteria were developed in the 1940s, they have been revised several times. The most recent review by the AHA in 2015 recommended the expanded use of echocardiography to aid in diagnosis, even in the absence of confirmed heart murmur.

After acute RF has resolved, the long-term risks are related to the risk of developing rheumatic heart disease. Long-term antibiotic prophylaxis against group A strep is indicated in cases of known RF or rheumatic heart disease because recurrent RF is associated with worsening rheumatic heart disease. Recommended antibiotic prophylaxis for RF is shown in Box 16-2 (Nishimuri et al., 2014a, 2014b). People who

BOX 16-2	**Duration of Antibiotic Prophylaxis for Rheumatic Fever/Rheumatic Heart Disease**
Rheumatic fever without carditis:	5 years or until age 21 (whichever is longer)
Rheumatic fever with carditis:	10 years or until age 21 (whichever is longer)
Rheumatic fever with valvular heart disease:	10 years or until age 40 (whichever is longer)

have recovered from RF should have annual cardiac evaluations to identify the presence of new heart murmurs, which suggest the presence of rheumatic heart disease. Echocardiograms should be done to determine whether rheumatic valvular disease is developing. When a new murmur is detected in a patient with a systemic infection, endocarditis should be suspected.

Patients who have rheumatic endocarditis with mild valvular dysfunction may require no further treatment. However, there is a risk of recurrent attacks of acute RF; bacterial endocarditis; embolism from vegetations or mural thrombi to the lung, kidney, spleen, brain, or peripheral vessels; and cardiac failure. The nurse monitors the patient for signs and symptoms of valvular disease, heart failure, thromboemboli, and arrhythmias. Rheumatic heart disease may be prevented through early recognition and adequate treatment of oropharyngeal streptococcal infections to prevent RF.

INFECTIVE ENDOCARDITIS

Endocarditis is a serious infection of the endocardium, the membrane that lines the interior chambers of the heart and forms the valves. Certain factors, such as the presence of a prosthetic heart valve, a structural cardiac defect, an implantable device, or a previous episode of endocarditis, account for the majority of infectious endocarditis (IE). Other conditions, such as immunosuppression, neutropenia, malignancy, intravenous drug use (IVDU), and nosocomial hospital exposures, such as the presence of an indwelling central venous catheter, can predispose the patient to IE because they can introduce bacteria into the bloodstream. The risk of exposure to antibiotic-resistant bacteria is greater in the hospital and can result in a more virulent infection.

Pathophysiology

Most IE is caused by staphylococci, followed by streptococci and enterococci bacteria. IE also can be fungal. Systemic infection can result in IE, but pathogens also can enter the bloodstream because of surgical or dental procedures or through direct contamination, such as through an injection by IVDUs. Then the microbes colonize at the site of an abnormality or injury of the endocardium, such as a prolapsed mitral valve or a prosthetic valve site. Inflammation and infection result in endothelial damage; platelets, fibrin, blood cells, and the pathogens cluster as vegetations on the endocardium. The infection may erode through the endocardium into the underlying structures (e.g., valve leaflets), causing tears or deformities of valve leaflets, dehiscence of prosthetic valves, deformity of the chordae tendineae, or paravalvular abscesses. The vegetations are friable and fragments can break off, move through the bloodstream, and cause systemic or pulmonary embolization.

Acute IE has a rapid onset, occurring within days to weeks, and often is accompanied by high fever and chills. Subacute IE occurs gradually and is notable by low-grade fever, malaise, and lethargy, and its course is prolonged. Often, the onset of IE is insidious, and signs and symptoms slowly develop from inflammation, destruction of the heart valves, and embolization of the vegetative growths on the heart.

Risk Factors

Pre-existing heart disease increases the risk of developing IE. A cardiac valve with epithelial damage will attract bacteria to its surface, and this can result in endocardial infection. This injury may be the result of rheumatic heart disease, previous endocarditis, a prosthetic valve, a congenital abnormality such as a bicuspid aortic valve, a structural abnormality such as MVP, or it may be age-related, degenerative valvular changes. Central venous access devices and long-term indwelling catheters, such as those used for hemodialysis, are associated with the hospital-acquired IE. IVDU and body piercing are risk factors for IE (see Box 16-3).

Clinical Manifestations and Assessment

The clinical presentation of IE varies and diagnosis may be difficult, as symptoms are often vague and may include anorexia,

---

BOX 16-3

Risk Factors for Infective Endocarditis

- Acquired valvular dysfunction
- Atrial septal defect (unrepaired or repaired)
- Bicuspid aortic valve
- Body piercing
- Coarctation of the aorta
- Complex cyanotic congenital malformations
- Degenerative valve disease
- History of infective endocarditis
- Indwelling, long-term hemodialysis catheters
- IV drug use
- Mitral regurgitation
- MVP with valvular regurgitation or thickened leaflets
- Nosocomial endocarditis
- Parenteral nutrition lines or IV lines into the right atrium
- Health care exposure
- Patent ductus arteriosus
- Prosthetic cardiac valves
- Ventricular septal defect

---

myalgias, fever, chills, weight loss, back and joint pain, and night sweats. Fever is common, but may be intermittent or absent, especially in patients who are receiving antibiotics or corticosteroids, in the elderly, or in those who have heart failure or kidney failure. A heart murmur may be absent initially but develops in almost all patients. Murmurs that worsen over time are indicative of progressive damage from vegetations or perforation of the valve or chordae tendineae.

In addition to fever and heart murmur, Osler nodes, Janeway lesions, and Roth spots are distinguishing signs of IE, and are the result of microembolization (see Fig. 16-12). Osler nodes are painful, erythematous nodules present on the pads of fingers or toes. Janeway lesions are painless, red or purple macules found on the palms and soles. Roth spots, seen on fundoscopic exam, are oval retinal hemorrhages with pale centers. Splinter hemorrhages may be seen under the fingernails and toenails, and petechiae may appear on the neck, chest, abdomen, conjunctiva, and mucous membranes. Central nervous system manifestations of IE include headache, transient cerebral ischemia, and strokes, which may be caused by emboli to the cerebral arteries. Embolization may be a presenting symptom; it may occur at any time and may involve other organ systems. Cardiomegaly, heart failure, tachycardia, or splenomegaly may occur. Abdominal discomfort, particularly in the left upper quadrant, is suggestive of splenic embolization or infarction. It is notable that because of earlier diagnosis and improved treatment, these classic signs of IE (with the exception of conjunctival hemorrhages and petechiae) are now seen in less than 10% of patients with IE (Murdoch et al., 2009).

Positive blood cultures are highly sensitive for diagnosis; however, negative blood cultures do not definitely rule out infective endocarditis, especially if a patient has received antibiotics or if slow-growing bacteria are present. Three sets of blood cultures should be obtained 24 hours apart before administration of any antimicrobial agents.

The modified Duke Criteria are used to aid in the diagnosis of IE. Major clinical criteria are positive blood cultures and evidence of endocardial involvement. When these are supplemented by minor clinical criteria, such as predisposing cardiac conditions or IVDU, persistent fever without an alternative cause, systemic or pulmonary embolism, Osler nodes, or Roth spots, a diagnosis of IE can be made. A diagnosis of IE is established with two major criteria or one major and three minor criteria, or five minor criteria. A possible diagnosis of IE is made when one major and one minor or three minor criteria are present (Fowler, Bayer, & Baddour, 2016).

Echocardiography can detect the presence of vegetations or abscesses, prosthetic valve dehiscence, new regurgitation, or heart failure, and is recommended for all patients with suspected IE. Other abnormal findings include anemia, elevated white blood cell (WBC) count, elevated sedimentation rate (ESR), and elevated C-reactive protein. Abnormal electrocardiographic (ECG) findings include atrioventricular blocks, bundle branch blocks, and fascicular blocks.

FIGURE 16-12 Common peripheral manifestations of infective endocarditis. Splinter hemorrhages (**A**) are normally seen under the fingernails or toenails. They are usually linear and red for the first 2 to 3 days and brownish thereafter. Osler's nodes (**B**) are tender subcutaneous nodules, often in the pulp of the digits or the thenar eminence (the fleshy prominence at the base of the thumb). **C.** Conjunctival petechiae. Janeway's lesions (**D**) are nontender erythematous, hemorrhagic, or pustular lesions, often on the palms or soles. (From Mylonakis, E. & Calderwood, S. B. (2001). Infective endocarditis in adults. *New England Journal of Medicine, 345,* 1318–1330.)

Medical and Nursing Management

Treatment of IE focuses on eliminating the infection and preventing complications. Treatment with long-term intravenous antibiotic therapy is targeted to the pathogen identified by the blood cultures. It is administered for a significant period, often up to 6 weeks, in doses that produce a high serum concentration to ensure eradication of the infection. Antibiotics are initiated as soon as blood cultures have been obtained. Many patients have peripherally inserted central catheters (PICC) or other long-term IV access. Nursing management of patients with endocarditis includes prevention of the complications of long-term IV therapy. Invasive lines and wounds must be assessed for erythema (redness), tenderness, warmth, swelling, drainage, or other signs of infection. Blood cultures are taken periodically to monitor the effect of therapy, and serum levels of the selected antibiotic are monitored to ensure the serum demonstrates bactericidal activity.

Even if the patient responds to therapy, endocarditis can be destructive to the heart and other organs. Nurses should be alert for complications such as persistent infection, heart failure, kidney failure, or emboli. A new or worsening murmur may indicate dehiscence of a prosthetic valve, rupture of an abscess, or injury to valve leaflets. When IE is complicated by persistent or recurrent infection, heart failure, systemic emboli, neurologic complication, myocardial abscess, or fungal endocarditis, surgery is indicated. Most patients who have prosthetic valve endocarditis require valve replacement. If the patient has undergone surgical treatment, the nurse provides postoperative care and instructions.

The patient should be taught to recognize the symptoms of endocarditis and to seek medical assistance should symptoms recur. The patient and family should be instructed about medications as well as signs and symptoms of infection. The nurse provides the patient and family with emotional support and facilitates coping strategies during the prolonged course

---

BOX 16-4

Indications for Infective Endocarditis Antibiotic Prophylaxis

- Prosthetic heart valve
- Previous infective endocarditis
- Cardiac transplant recipients with a structurally abnormal valve with regurgitation.
- Congenital heart disease with persistent risk of IE:
  - Unrepaired cyanotic congenital abnormalities
    - Completely repaired congenital defects with prosthetic material, during first 6 months after surgery
  - Repaired congenital defects with residual defect adjacent to prosthetic material

Dental Procedures for Which Endocarditis Prophylaxis Is Recommended for High-Risk Patients (see the below list)

All dental procedures that involve manipulation of gingival tissue or the periapical region of teeth or perforation of the oral mucosa *except* the following:
- Routine anesthetic injections through noninfected tissue
- Taking dental radiographs
- Placement of removable prosthodontic or orthodontic appliances
- Adjustment of orthodontic appliances
- Placement of orthodontic brackets
  - Shedding of deciduous teeth and bleeding from trauma to the lips or oral mucosa

Adapted from Baddour, L. M., Freeman, W. K., Suri, R. M., & Wilson, W. R. (2015). Cardiovascular Infections. In *Braunwald's heart disease: A textbook of cardiovascular medicine* (Vol. 64, pp. 1524–1550). Philadelphia, PA: Elsevier Saunders.

---

of the infection and antibiotic treatment. The nurse instructs all patients with IE about the importance of excellent daily dental hygiene and the highest-risk patients about the need for prophylactic before certain dental procedures.

Infectious Endocarditis Prophylaxis

Prevention of IE is important, and antibiotic prophylaxis is recommended prior to dental procedures for only the subset of patients who are at highest risk of adverse outcomes. For patients with a (1) prosthetic cardiac valve, (2) history of infective endocarditis, (3) congenital heart disease with persistent risk of IE, and (4) heart transplantation with valvular disease, antibiotic prophylaxis is warranted for dental procedures that involve manipulation of gingival tissue, the periapical region of teeth, or perforation of the oral mucosa. Antibiotic prophylaxis is not recommended for (1) routine anesthetic injections through noninfected tissue, (2) taking dental radiographs, or (3) placement or adjustment of removable prosthodontic or orthodontic appliances (Nishimura et al., 2014a, 2014b). A summary of indications for infective endocarditis antibiotic prophylaxis is found in Box 16-4.

MYOCARDITIS

Myocarditis is an inflammation of the heart muscle (myocardium), commonly resulting from viral infection. It also may be caused by bacterial infections, immune-mediated mechanisms, and toxic agents. Frequently, the cause is unknown. It can be acute or chronic. Mortality varies with the severity of symptoms. Mild cases with few symptoms may resolve without treatment, while more serious cases result in cardiogenic shock and death.

Pathophysiology

Cardiac muscle inflammation that results in myocyte necrosis (e.g., cardiac cell death) is the hallmark of myocarditis.

Acute myocarditis is characterized by myocyte damage from viral infection, autoimmunity, or other precipitating event. Myocyte antigens and cytokines are released. In the subacute phase (days 4 through 14), T and B lymphocytes infiltrate the myocardium, and the virus is cleared. The immune response continues, and infected myocytes are lysed. Myocyte necrosis results in fibrosis. During the chronic phase, myocyte injury continues and can lead to DCM, left ventricular failure, and ventricular arrhythmias.

Clinical Manifestations and Assessment

Clinical presentation can vary widely; symptoms can range from mild systemic findings of fever, myalgias, fatigue, and dyspnea to ventricular arrhythmias, cardiogenic shock, and DCM. Other signs and symptoms include an S3 gallop, tachycardia, tachypnea, JVD, edema, ECG abnormalities, orthopnea, and palpitations. Fulminant heart failure or SCD can develop quickly.

A minority of patients will have elevated cardiac enzymes and WBC count. ESR will be elevated approximately 60% of the time. Echocardiography is widely used when myocarditis is suspected and may show nonspecific findings or demonstrate impaired heart muscle function or pericardial effusion. Endomyocardial biopsy is used to confirm diagnosis.

Medical and Nursing Management

For patients with myocarditis, supportive care is of primary importance with a goal of maintaining hemodynamic stability and improving symptoms. ACE-Is, ARBs, BBs, and diuretics may be prescribed to treat heart failure symptoms. Self-limiting, mild cases may resolve with bed rest and supplemental oxygen, while more severe cases will require hemodynamic support. Surgical options, such as the placement of a VAD or TAH or heart transplantation, should be considered when there is no improvement in symptoms or hemodynamic status despite maximal medical therapy.

Nursing care of the patient with myocarditis includes an assessment whether the patient's symptoms are improving or worsening. In addition to monitoring vital signs, heart sounds, lung sounds, and peripheral perfusion, the nurse must assess hemodynamic, oxygenation, and fluid status. Nurses should be prepared to use emergency equipment as there is a high risk for life-threatening ventricular arrhythmias. Nurses must also provide emotional support to the patient and family; myocarditis can be particularly stressful due to its variable presentation and course.

PERICARDITIS

Pericarditis is an inflammation of the pericardium, the membranous sac surrounding the heart. The pericardium holds the heart in place, prevents it from over-expanding if blood volume increases, and protects the heart from infection and malignancy (see Figs. 16-11 and 16-13). Pericarditis can be infectious (viral, bacterial, or fungal) or noninfectious. Approximately 80% to 90% of pericarditis is idiopathic and assumed to be caused by viral infection (Imazio, Gaita, & LeWinter, 2015). Causes of the less common, noninfectious pericarditis include acute myocardial infarction, chest trauma or cardiac surgery, autoimmune disorders, medications (e.g., isoniazid, hydralazine), and malignancy. A list of the most frequently occurring causes of pericarditis is provided in Box 16-5.

Pathophysiology

The pericardial sac consists of two layers, the parietal (outer) layer and the visceral (inner) layer that is affixed to the heart. A small amount of fluid (15 to 50 mL) separates the layers. Acute pericarditis develops rapidly, occurring when the pericardial sac becomes inflamed. Pericarditis may lead to an accumulation of fluid in this space, called *pericardial effusion*. This may result in increased pressure on the heart, leading to cardiac tamponade (refer to Chapter 15).

FIGURE 16-13 Tissue changes in pericarditis. Normally, the epicardium and pericardium slide over each other easily because they are lubricated by a small amount of fluid. Thicker material replaces this fluid in pericarditis.

BOX 16-5 Causes of Pericarditis

- Acute myocardial infarction (MI)
- Bacterial infection (e.g., streptococci, staphylococci, meningococci)
- Cancer, particularly metastasis to the heart from lung or breast tumors or lymphoma
- Chest Trauma: chest injury, invasive cardiac procedures, such as implantation of pacemaker or defibrillator (ICD) or cardiac surgery
- Disorders of adjacent structures: dissecting aneurysm, pulmonary disease (e.g., pneumonia)
- Fungal infection (e.g., *Aspergillus, Candida, Histoplasma*)
- Idiopathic
- Medications (e.g., procainamide, hydralyzine, and isoniazid)
- Metabolic disorders, primarily kidney failure and uremia
- Radiation therapy of chest and upper torso, especially for breast cancer, lung cancer, or lymphoma (peak occurrence 5 to 9 months after treatment)

Rheumatic diseases (systemic lupus erythematosus, rheumatoid arthritis, and mixed connective tissue disease)
- Viral infection (e.g., coxsackie, hepatitis B, influenza, mononucleosis, mumps, varicella)

Pericarditis that reappears 4 to 6 weeks after an episode of acute pericarditis is termed *recurrent pericarditis*. In chronic *effusive* pericarditis, fluid slowly accumulates in the pericardial space, between the two layers of the pericardium.

Chronic *constrictive* pericarditis is rare. Frequent or prolonged episodes of pericarditis can lead to thickening and decreased elasticity of the pericardium, and scarring may fuse the visceral and parietal pericardium. This compresses the heart and restricts its ability to fill with blood. Over time, the pericardium may become calcified, further restricting ventricular expansion during diastole. With less filling, the ventricles pump less blood, leading to decreased CO and signs and symptoms of heart failure. Because higher pressure is required to fill the compressed heart, pressure increases in the veins that return blood to the heart. This increased systemic venous pressure will lead to peripheral edema and liver failure.

Clinical Manifestations and Assessment

The clinical presentation of pericarditis can range from minor chest pain to cardiogenic shock. However, the most common symptom is chest pain. Irritation of the pericardium causes pain that is typically persistent, sharp, pleuritic, and retrosternal. Although usually felt in the midchest, it may radiate to the neck, shoulders, or arms, making it difficult to differentiate from chest pain associated with an MI. However, in contrast to myocardial ischemic pain, the discomfort is usually aggravated by deep inspiration, coughing, lying down, or turning. It is characteristically relieved with a forward-leaning or sitting position because that position reduces pressure on the parietal pericardium. Although not heard in all patients with pericarditis, a common finding is a creaky or scratchy friction rub.

> **Nursing Alert**
> *A pericardial friction rub is diagnostic of pericarditis. It has a creaky or scratchy sound and is louder at the end of exhalation. Nurses can assess for the presence of a pericardial friction rub by placing the diaphragm of the stethoscope tightly against the thorax and auscultating the left lower sternal border in the fourth intercostal space, the site where the pericardium comes into contact with the left chest wall. The rub is best heard when the patient is sitting and leaning forward. The friction rub is caused by the inflamed layers of the pericardium rubbing against each other and is often intermittent.*

Other signs may include a mild fever, increased WBC count, anemia, and an elevated ESR or C-reactive protein level. Patients may have a nonproductive cough. Dyspnea unrelated to exertion is typical of pericarditis; SOB occurs as a result of pericardial compression from cardiac tamponade.

A diagnosis of pericarditis can be made if two of the following are present: pleuritic chest pain, pericardial friction rub, 12-lead ECG demonstrating widespread ST elevation without reciprocal changes or T-wave inversion, and pericardial effusion. Echocardiography is done to assess for pericardial effusion or tamponade, but the absence of effusion does not exclude pericarditis.

Medical and Nursing Management

The goals of management are to provide symptom relief and detect signs and symptoms of cardiac tamponade. If the underlying cause is known, it should be treated; however, typically it is not necessary to confirm the etiology as most pericarditis is viral in nature and resolves without sequelae. Nonsteroidal anti-inflammatory medications (NSAIDs) and aspirin constitute first-line treatment. In the past, corticosteroids were commonly prescribed if a pericardial effusion was present or if the patient did not respond to NSAIDs, but more recently, it has been shown that corticosteroids may prolong the course of recovery or can increase the risk of a recurrent pericarditis (Imazio et al., 2015; Snyder, Bepko, & White, 2014). Colchicine is used to treat recurrent pericarditis, and recent research suggests it may be beneficial when added to NSAIDs for initial management of acute pericarditis (Adler, Charron, & Imazio, 2015). In cases of constrictive pericarditis, surgical removal of the pericardium (pericardectomy) may be necessary to provide relief from restrictive inflammation and scarring.

In addition to pain management, patients with acute pericarditis benefit from positioning: sitting upright and leaning forward will relieve pressure on the pericardium. Patients with chest pain often benefit from psychological support, education, and reassurance that the chest pain they are experiencing is not a heart attack.

Complications

Nurses caring for patients with pericarditis must be aware of the potential of serious complications. The two major complications of pericarditis are pericardial effusion, the accumulation of fluid in the pericardial sac, and cardiac tamponade, compression of the heart from excessive fluid buildup (refer to Chapter 15).

NURSING PROCESS
The Patient with Pericarditis

ASSESSMENT

Pain is the primary symptom of the patient with pericarditis, and it is assessed while repositioning the patient. The nurse tries to identify whether the pain is influenced by inspiration or expiration; breath holding; flexion, extension, or rotation of the spine and neck; by movements of the shoulders and arms; and by coughing or swallowing. Recognizing that deep inspiration or coughing intensifies pain may help to differentiate the pain of pericarditis from the pain of MI. To distinguish a pericardial friction rub from a pleural friction rub, the patient is asked to hold his or her breath; a pericardial friction rub will continue. A pericardial friction rub occurs when the pericardial surfaces lose their lubricating fluid because of inflammation. The rub is audible on auscultation and is synchronous with the heartbeat but is often intermittent and does not always occur. The patient's temperature is monitored frequently. Pericarditis may cause an abrupt onset of fever in a patient who has been afebrile.

DIAGNOSIS

Based on the assessment data, a major nursing diagnosis may be:
- Acute pain related to inflammation of the pericardium

PLANNING

The nursing plan focuses on two goals: pain relief and absence of complications.

NURSING INTERVENTIONS

PAIN RELIEF

Relief of pain is achieved by chair rest because sitting upright and leaning forward is the posture that tends to relieve pain. It is important to instruct the patient to restrict activity until the pain subsides. As the chest pain and friction rub abate, activities of daily living may be resumed gradually. If the patient is taking analgesics or colchicine for the pericarditis, his or her responses are monitored and recorded. Patients taking NSAIDs are assessed for gastrointestinal adverse effects. If chest pain and friction rub recur, bed rest or chair rest is resumed.

MONITORING AND MANAGING POTENTIAL COMPLICATIONS

Pericardial Effusion. Fluid that accumulates between the pericardial linings or in the pericardial sac is called *pericardial effusion* (see Chapter 15). The fluid can constrict the myocardium and impair its ability to pump. CO declines with each contraction. Failure to identify and treat this problem can lead to cardiac tamponade and possible sudden death.

Cardiac Tamponade. The first symptoms of cardiac tamponade are often SOB, chest tightness, dizziness, or restlessness. Assessment of blood pressure may reveal a pulsus paradoxus, a decrease of 10 mm Hg or more in the systolic blood pressure during inspiration. Usually, the systolic pressure decreases and the diastolic pressure remains stable; hence, pulse pressure narrows. The patient may have tachycardia, and the ECG voltage may be decreased or the QRS complexes may alternate in height (electrical alternans). Heart sounds may progress from distant to imperceptible. Neck vein distention and other signs of rising central venous pressure develop. These signs occur as the fluid-filled pericardial sac compresses the myocardium. Blood continues to return to the heart from the periphery but cannot flow into the heart to be pumped back into the circulation. The nurse notifies the provider immediately and prepares to assist with diagnostic echocardiography and pericardiocentesis (see Chapter 15). The nurse stays with the patient and continues to assess and record signs and symptoms while intervening to decrease patient anxiety.

EVALUATION

Expected patient outcomes include:
1. Freedom from pain
   a. Performs activities of daily living without pain, fatigue, or SOB
   b. Temperature returns to normal range
   c. Exhibits no pericardial friction rub
2. Absence of complications
   a. Sustains blood pressure in normal range
   b. Has heart sounds that are strong and can be auscultated
   c. No evidence of effusion or tamponade

CHAPTER REVIEW

Critical Thinking Exercises

1. A friend tells you she does not like to take drugs and does not plan to adhere to advice from her health care providers to use antibiotics before routine dental checkups. You know your friend has had a heterograft mitral valve replacement. How would you respond to your friend? On what evidence do you base your response? What is the strength of that evidence?

2. A 19-year-old man with HCM is being discharged from the hospital. He lives alone and states he really needs to get back to the gym to resume his weight training. Based on your knowledge about the developmental tasks of 19-year olds, what do you anticipate his psychosocial needs would be? His family came to the hospital during the first 2 days of his hospital stay, but they live out of town and have returned home. Should they be included in the plan of care? The cardiologist has requested a consult with transplant services. How will this consult be included in the plan of care?

3. A 68-year-old man with AF, who is recovering from an aortic valve replacement for AS and three coronary artery bypass grafts, has been prescribed a BB, an ACE inhibitor, digoxin, and warfarin. The cardiologist advises the patient to continue to carry nitroglycerin spray for treatment of angina, should it occur. What are the teaching and discharge planning needs? As you care for the patient on the third postoperative day, you assess that the patient has short-term memory deficits. What are your plans to achieve discharge as expected on postoperative day 5 to 7?

NCLEX-Style Review Questions

1. Incomplete closure of the mitral valve results in backflow of blood from the:
   a. RV to the right atrium
   b. Right atrium to RV
   c. LV to LA
   d. LA to LV

2. Severe AS is consistent with all of the following *except:*
   a. Pulmonary edema
   b. Increased CO
   c. Right-sided heart failure
   d. Left ventricular hypertrophy

3. The following are symptoms associated with AS:
   a. Angina, syncope, dyspnea
   b. Diastolic murmur, syncope, dyspnea
   c. Syncope, diastolic murmur, angina
   d. Dyspnea, angina, diastolic murmur

4. Which diagnostic test is preferred for evaluation of heart function?
   a. Electrocardiogram
   b. Chest x-ray
   c. Echocardiogram
   d. Cardiac catheterization

5. Management of patients with cardiomyopathy is directed at preventing and treating heart failure. The treatment of heart failure includes (*select all that apply*):
   a. Reducing circulating blood volume
   b. Reducing myocardial oxygen needs
   c. Increasing CO by improving contractility or reducing peripheral resistance
   d. Increasing preload

6. All of the following are indications for a VAD to be used as a bridge to recovery *except:*
   a. Acute myocarditis
   b. Cardiogenic shock following an acute myocardial infarction
   c. End-stage heart failure
   d. Failure to wean from cardiopulmonary bypass following cardiac surgery

7. A patient presents with chest pain. Acute myocardial infarction is excluded and the patient is diagnosed with pericarditis. Which of the following medications would the provider be most likely to prescribe initially? *Select all that apply.*
   a. Acetaminophen (Tylenol)
   b. Ibuprofen (Motrin)
   c. Colchicine
   d. Broad Spectrum Antibiotic
   e. Coumadin (Warfarin)

8. Which of the following describes the best place to auscultate for the presence of a pericardial friction rub?
   a. Left lower sternal border in the fourth intercostal space
   b. Right lower sternal border in the fourth intercostal space
   c. Left lower sternal border in the second intercostal space
   d. Right lower sternal border in the second intercostal space

9. What condition requires IE prophylaxis?
   a. MVP
   b. Rheumatic heart disease
   c. Bicuspid valve disease
   d. Prosthetic valve

Try these additional resources, available at **http://thepoint.lww.com/Honan2e**, to enhance your learning and understanding of this chapter:
• NCLEX-Style Student Review Questions
• Journal Articles

REFERENCES AND SELECTED READINGS

References and selected readings associated with this chapter can be found on the website that accompanies the book. Visit **http://thepoint. lww.com/Honan2e** to access the references and other additional resources associated with this chapter.

Nursing Management: Patients with Arrhythmias and Conduction Problems

Catherine G. Winkler

Arrhythmias (also called *dysrhythmias*) are disorders of the electrical impulse within the heart that cause disturbances of heart rate, heart rhythm, or both. Without a normal rate and regular rhythm, the heart does not perform efficiently as a pump to circulate oxygenated blood. Arrhythmias may initially produce symptoms related to the hemodynamic effect they cause, such as a decrease in cardiac output. Refer to Table 17-1 for signs and symptoms of a decreased cardiac output. In addition to decreasing the cardiac output, some arrhythmias increase the risk of clot formation within the chambers of the heart. Arrhythmias are named according to the site of origin of the impulse (e.g., atria or ventricle) and the mechanism of formation or **conduction** involved (e.g., bradycardia [too slow], tachycardia [too fast], premature [early], etc.). Their presence is confirmed by an electrocardiogram.

THE ELECTROCARDIOGRAM

The electrical impulse that travels through the heart can be viewed by means of an electrocardiogram (ECG). Each phase of the cardiac cycle is reflected by specific waveforms (discussed later in the chapter). The number and placement of the electrodes used depend on the type of ECG needed. The electrodes record waveforms that appear on the paper or monitor and represent the electrical current in relation to the two electrodes (Fig. 17-1). Heart rate and rhythm may be monitored effectively through only two electrodes; however, the use of 10 electrodes (resulting in 12 leads) provides more detailed information and is the basis for understanding other types of electrocardiographic monitoring. The difference between electrodes, wires, and leads is described in Box 17-1.

TABLE 17-1 Signs and Symptoms of Decreased Cardiac Output

System	Signs and Symptoms of Decreased Cardiac Output
Respiratory	Tachypnea, shortness of breath (SOB), orthopnea, dyspnea on exertion (DOE), hypoxemia, crackles on lung auscultation, wheeze, dry or productive cough
Cardiac and peripheral vascular	Edema, jugular vein distention (JVD), displaced point of maximum impulse (PMI), S_3 gallop rhythm, tricuspid and/or mitral regurgitation murmurs, hypotension, decreased mean arterial pressure (MAP), narrow pulse pressure, cool skin and extremities, delayed capillary refill, tachycardia
Renal	Decreased urinary output, oliguria, rising creatinine
Gastrointestinal	Abdominal distention, ascites, liver engorgement, positive abdominojugular reflex
Central nervous	Dizziness, decreased sensorium, syncope, fatigue
Behavioral/ emotional	Anxiety, restlessness

BOX 17-1 Understanding Electrodes, Wires, and Leads

Electrodes

Electrodes are electrical contacts that are placed on the patient's skin. They come in various shapes. Today's electrodes are disposable for single patient use. They all contain conductive gel and a connector for a wire.

Wires

The electrode is connected to a recording device by a set of wires or cables. The wires are color coded, although the coding system is not internationally consistent. For 12-lead ECGs, there are 10 wires, one for each electrode. For continuous monitoring, there may be anywhere from three to five wires. Three- and four-wire systems allow monitoring of limb leads only, whereas five-wire systems allow monitoring of limb leads plus a chest lead. Some wires come preattached to the electrodes and are disposable; others need to be attached to the electrode and are reusable.

Leads

Leads are the images the nurse sees on the paper or monitor. They represent an examination of the heart from a specific viewpoint. The direction of the ECG complex varies depending on which lead is viewed. The direction of the electric current determines how the waveforms appear on paper.

THE 12-LEAD ELECTROCARDIOGRAM

An ECG contains information about the contraction and relaxation of heart chambers. This diagnostic information could change due to various cardiovascular diseases (Dandapat, Sharma, & Tripathy, 2015). The 12-lead ECG is a diagnostic tool that uses 10 electrodes: one placed on each limb and six placed on the chest (precordial). In combination, these 10 electrodes produce 12 different waveforms (or leads). These 12 leads include three bipolar leads (I, II, III) and nine unipolar leads (aVR, aVL, aVF, V_1–V_6). Bipolar leads measure electrical activity traveling between a positive and negative electrode, while unipolar leads record electrical activity from a single reference point. Together, the 12 leads show electrical activity in both a frontal plane and a transverse plane. When viewed together, these two planes provide important diagnostic information beyond heart rate and rhythm, including conduction abnormalities such as bundle branch block (BBB), heart chamber enlargement, localization of ischemia or infarction, and even noncardiac conditions such as electrolyte imbalances caused by hypocalcemia, hyperkalemia, or hypomagnesemia (Hale & Hovey, 2014; Winkler, 2015). Consider taking a picture of a statue from 12 different angles: When merged, a composite picture of the entire statue is achievable, but the viewer is

also capable of analyzing unique details of the picture when selecting to view a specific angle—this is the same principle behind ECG monitoring. The 12-lead ECG produces an image of the heart, whereas particular leads view specific areas of the heart.

Electrode placement for a 12-lead ECG must be accurate and consistent as misplacement can result in altered waveforms, which can lead to an inaccurate diagnosis and treatment. Electrode placement is important in arrhythmia identification and is crucial in identifying changes related to ischemia (decreased blood flow often due to atherosclerosis), infarction (cellular damage or death because of limited blood supply), and many arrhythmias. In addition, electrode placement is important in terms of customization to the patient to ensure that clinically relevant data is obtained through placing electrodes strategically on the patient to capture or view the best clinical ECG data.

The four limb electrodes are placed on the lower legs, near the ankles, and on the arms, near the wrists. The remaining six electrodes are placed across the left side of the chest. Locating the specific anatomical landmark is critical for correct chest electrode placement (Box 17-2). If the patient needs a series of ECGs, consistency of electrode placement is also important. In some cases, the chest electrodes are left in place or the correct location is marked

FIGURE 17-1 Relationship of electrocardiogram (ECG) complex, lead system, and electrical impulse. The heart conducts electrical activity, which the ECG measures and records. The configurations of electrical activity displayed on the ECG vary depending on the lead (or view) of the ECG and on the rhythm of the heart. Therefore, the configuration of a normal rhythm tracing from lead I will differ from the configuration of a normal rhythm tracing from lead II, lead II will differ from lead III, and so on. The same is true for abnormal rhythms and cardiac disorders. To make an accurate assessment of the heart's electrical activity or to identify where, when, and what abnormalities occur, the ECG needs to be evaluated from every lead, not just from lead II. Here the different areas of electrical activity are identified by color. RA, right arm; LA, left arm; SA, sinoatrial; AV, atrioventricular; LL, left leg.

with an indelible pen to ensure the identical placement for follow-up ECGs.

The specific locations for electrode placement are shown in Figure 17-2.

V_1 Right side of the sternum, fourth intercostal space
V_2 Left side of the sternum, fourth intercostal space
V_3 Midway between V_2 and V_4
V_4 Midclavicular line, fifth intercostal space (under the breast in women)
V_5 Left anterior axillary line, same level as V_4
V_6 Left midaxillary line, same level as V_4 (Davies & Scott, 2014)

The precordial (anterior surface over the heart) leads reflect the electrical activity primarily in the left ventricle. In some circumstances, an alternative electrode placement may be required. For example, in patients with suspected right-sided heart damage, right-sided chest leads are required to evaluate the right ventricle (see Fig. 17-2). Electrodes for V_1R (R refers to the right side of the chest) through V_6R are placed in the mirror image of the electrodes on the left side of the chest as detailed here:

V_1R Left side of the sternum, fourth intercostal space
V_2R Right side of the sternum, fourth intercostal space
V_3R Midway between V_2 and V_4

BOX 17-2 Correct Electrode Placement

Too often, arbitrary markings are used to determine rib positions, such as the areola of the breast. Valid ECG monitoring requires counting ribs for correct placement of electrodes. Begin by finding the sternal notch and slowly move your finger down the manubrium, until a rise is noted. Next, move your hand laterally from the rise until you note the rib at the sternal margin; this is the second rib. Underneath this rib is the second intercostal space (ICS). Count down two more ribs to the fourth ICS and place V_1 electrode on right side of sternum and V_2 on left side of sternum. V3 electrode will be placed midway between V_2 and V_4. The V_4 electrode is placed at the fifth ICS at the midclavicular line. The V_5 electrode is placed at the same level of V_4 at the left anterior axillary line, and the V_6 electrode is at same level as V_4 and V_5 at the left midaxillary line. It may be helpful to mark this placement for consistent ECG placements in the future.

V_4R Midclavicular line, fifth intercostal space (under the breast in women)

V_5R Right anterior axillary line, same level as V_4

V_6R Right midaxillary line, same level as V_4

CONTINUOUS MONITORING

Targeted or patient-centric ECG monitoring is best applied when an immediate assessment of the patient can be made to determine the optimal monitoring level. Based on the admission diagnosis and changes in the clinical course during hospitalization, ongoing medical decisions are predicated on the goals of care and specific interventions. Patients are monitored for a variety of reasons: to detect changes in the patient's clinical condition, to diagnose a problem, to assess a response to an intervention, to prevent an undesirable event, and for surveillance before and after cardiac surgery (Winkler, 2015).

The American Heart Association (AHA) practice standards for ECG monitoring in the hospital setting were last published in 2004 by Drew and colleagues and provide direction in deciding which patients are best served by cardiac monitoring during an episode of illness. The practice standards group patients into the following classes:

- Class I: indicated for all patients such as those who have been resuscitated from cardiac arrest
- Class II: possibly indicated, but not essential, which includes patients who are post-acute myocardial infarction (MI) for 24 to 48 hours for ECG monitoring of arrhythmia, ST-segment ischemia, and/or QTc interval, and
- Class III: not indicated because risk is so low for patients such as those who have permanent, rate-controlled atrial fibrillation (AF).

FIGURE 17-2 ECG electrode placement. The standard left precordial leads are V_1—fourth intercostal space, right sternal border; V_2—fourth intercostal space, left sternal border; V_3—diagonally between V_2 and V_4; V_4—fifth intercostal space, left midclavicular line; V_5—same level as V_4, anterior axillary line; V_6 (not illustrated)—same level as V_4 and V_5, midaxillary line. The right precordial leads, placed across the right side of the chest, are the mirror opposite of the left leads. RA, right arm; LA, left arm; RL, right leg; LL, left leg. (Adapted from Molle, E. A., Kronenberger, J., West-Stack, C., & Durham, L. S. (2005). *Lippincott Williams & Wilkins' Pocket Guide to Medical Assisting* (2nd ed.). Philadelphia, PA: Lippincott Williams & Wilkins.)

After a decision is made regarding the class of ECG monitoring and the intensity that is required for the patient, the specific inpatient setting and the timeframe for monitoring are selected. Monitoring is an important diagnostic tool for heart disease and changes in health status. Important clinical decisions are made based on the data, to include medication therapy, device (pacemaker, ICD) adjustments, further diagnostic testing, referral for cardiac consultation, unit transfers, and length of stay (Winkler, 2015).

However, as important as understanding when a patient does require ECG monitoring is recognizing when the patient does not. Unnecessary monitoring increases health care costs, diverts nursing and medical staff from other important work, and may give the patient an incorrect message about his or her cardiac health (i.e., that the patient is more ill than he or she actually is). In addition, the ubiquitous nature of alarms in hospitals has been associated with compromised patient safety to such an extent that the Joint Commission has deemed alarm management a National Patient Safety Goal (2013).

Accordingly, ECG monitoring with human oversight of the patient remains indispensable but needs to be evaluated continuously because the standard of care evolves over time and the aim needs to be to deliver the right "type" and "dose" of cardiac monitoring (Winkler, 2015). Through an understanding of the patient's underlying condition and the pathology, the nurse can select the leads that will supply the most clinically significant information.

ECG monitoring systems vary in sophistication but, in general, can do the following:

- Monitor one limb lead or one limb lead plus one chest lead
- Monitor ST segments (ST-segment depression is a marker of myocardial ischemia; ST-segment elevation provides evidence of an evolving MI)
- Monitor QT segments for prolongation
- Provide graded visual and audible alarms (based on priority, asystole would be highest)
- Provide computerized rhythm monitoring (arrhythmias are interpreted and stored in the memory of the monitoring system)
- Produce a graphical recording
- Interface with the electronic medical record (as applicable)

Continuous monitoring systems have anywhere from three to five electrodes with capability of viewing two to ten leads. Box 17-3 provides helpful hints on how to apply these electrodes. In continuous monitoring, although limb electrodes are still used, they are positioned on the torso as opposed to the lower legs and arms, as in a 12-lead ECG. This allows for greater patient movement and comfort and reduced interference from skeletal muscle artifact. The four disposable electrodes are positioned in specific locations on the patient's chest, and a cable is connected to the monitor or telemetry device in the following arrangement: the right arm (RA) electrode placed on the right upper chest (below the clavicle) and the RA wire (usually white) attached; the left arm (LA) electrode placed on the left upper chest (below the clavicle) and the LA wire (usually black) attached; the left leg (LL) electrode placed on the left torso below the rib cage and on the left side of the abdomen and the LL wire (usually red) attached; the right leg (RL) electrode placed on the right torso and the RL wire (usually green) attached. A maxim used to recall placement is "white on right (snow over grass [green]) and smoke (black) over fire (red)." The color-coding

---

BOX 17-3

Helpful Hits for Applying Electrodes

These guidelines optimize skin adherence and the conduction of electrical currents.

- Have the patient positioned supine with the head of the bed at an angle of 30–40 degrees. This will make it easier to find the intercostal spaces for electrode placement. Provide as much privacy for the patient as possible.
- Débride the skin surface of dead cells with soap and water, and dry well. This decreases skin impedance and increases conductivity.
- Clip (do not shave) hair from around the electrode site if needed.
- If the patient is diaphoretic, apply a small amount of benzoin to the skin or wipe with alcohol, avoiding the area under the center of the electrode. (These are controversial recommendations. Benzoin, like alcohol, may increase the risk of burns if the patient requires cardioversion or defibrillation.)
- Connect the electrodes to the lead wires prior to placing them on the chest; peel the backing off the electrode and make sure the center is moist with electrode gel.
- Locate the landmarks for lead placement and use light, consistent pressure to secure the electrode.
- Change the electrodes every 24–48 hours (or as recommended by the manufacturer), examine the skin for irritation, and apply the electrodes to different locations. This, too, is debatable although evidence suggests that changing the electrodes daily decreases the number of "false alarms" according to the AACN Practice Alert on Alarm Management (Sendelbach & Jepsen, 2013).
- If the patient is sensitive to the electrodes, use hypoallergenic electrodes.

---

of wires is not an international standard. To reduce interference from skeletal muscle when placing electrodes, it is helpful to avoid boney prominences or areas that have significant movement. It is also important to ensure that the electrodes have not expired (expiration date on package) and, if the package has been opened, that the electrodes have not dried out. In addition, the electrodes need to be applied properly to the skin by prepping the skin according to manufacturer's directions and removing excessive chest hair. Expert opinion and research support proper skin preparation to reduce the number of false alarms. Walsh-Irwin and Jurgens (2015) found that electrocardiographic alarms decreased significantly ($p < 0.05$) after proper skin preparation and electrode placement (95% confidence interval). Reducing alarm frequency or the number of false alarms is central to decreasing alarm fatigue and increasing patient safety in the inpatient environment (Walsh-Irwin & Jurgens, 2015).

The signals are transmitted either directly to a bedside monitor (hardwire) or by radio waves from a small transmitter box to a central monitoring station (telemetry).

The most basic monitoring system uses three electrodes to allow monitoring in one of three bipolar limb leads. Leads

TABLE **17-2** Monitoring Recommendations, Vessels, and Recommended Leads

Type of Monitoring	Coronary Vessel Involved	Lead Selection
Arrhythmia monitoring Primary lead	LAD	V_1—intraventricular septum
Arrhythmia monitoring Secondary lead	Left circumflex	V_6—lateral wall
Ischemia monitoring	LAD	V_3—anterior wall V_1, V_2, V_4
Ischemia monitoring	RCA	III—inferior wall II, aVF
Ischemia monitoring	Left circumflex	V_5 and V_6—lateral wall I, aVL—sometimes no change V_1, V_2, or V_3 for reciprocal changes posterior wall
If ischemic footprint unknown	LAD and RCA	V_3 and III—anterior and inferior leads
Demand ischemia	Left circumflex	V_5—lateral wall
QT-interval monitoring	N/A	Monitor in the lead with best defined T wave

LAD, left anterior descending; RCA, right coronary artery.

that can be monitored are lead I (positive electrode on the LA, negative electrode on the RA), lead II (positive electrode on the LL and negative electrode on the RA), and lead III (positive electrode on the LL and negative electrode on the LA). These are useful for heart rate and basic rhythm recognition. They are inadequate for accurately identifying many arrhythmias, especially tachycardias (increased heart rate) with a wide QRS. Bipolar limb lead monitoring systems are often found on portable monitors, defibrillators, and some telemetry ECG devices.

Five-electrode monitoring systems use four electrodes placed as above, in the LA, RA, LL, and RL positions, as well as one chest electrode that can be placed in any one of the precordial locations (V_1–V_6). Monitoring systems with five electrodes permit the nurse to decide which leads will be monitored based on the patient's diagnosis and condition. Five-electrode systems have a display that allows two leads to be monitored simultaneously; typically, the nurse chooses one limb lead and one precordial lead to be viewed. The ability to monitor a limb lead and precordial lead simultaneously is often necessary for accurate identification of many arrhythmias, including arrhythmias with a wide QRS complex (BBBs, ventricular pacemaker rhythms, and wide QRS tachycardias). Two leads commonly used for continuous monitoring are leads II and V_1. Lead II provides the best visualization of atrial depolarization (represented by the P wave) and is preferred for monitoring atrial activity and heart rate. Lead V_1 best records ventricular depolarization and is most helpful when monitoring the patient for tachycardias. The AACN Practice Alert for dysrhythmia monitoring

and the AHA Practice Standards for ECG monitoring recommend V_1 as the preferred lead to monitor for wide QRS complex tachycardia. The next best lead is V_6. Monitoring for ST-segment changes is also important in terms of detecting ischemia. If the patient's history is known, it is best to monitor the patient in a more directed way using the leads that reflect the vessels involved in the ischemic event. Refer to the monitoring recommendations in Table 17-2 when the patient's history is known.

Further, patients who have or are at risk for prolongation of the QT interval should also be monitored. Prolongation of the QT interval can occur because of a genetic predisposition or through acquired abnormalities such as kidney failure, hypokalemia, and acute pancreatitis. However, in the acute care setting, QT prolongation is often due to medications, such as some antibiotics, antipsychotics, antiarrhythmics, and antiemetics (Ferri, 2016a). The QTc is considered prolonged when it is above 0.47 second in males and 0.48 second in females. If the QTc is above 0.50 second in anyone, it can be associated with a higher risk of torsade de pointes (Roden, 2015).

Ambulatory Electrocardiography

Ambulatory ECG is a continuous form of monitoring used in the outpatient setting to identify the etiology of distressing symptoms (pre-syncope, syncope, palpitations) that may be caused by arrhythmias, myocardial ischemia, or pacemaker dysfunction. In addition to monitoring for arrhythmias and evaluation of silent ischemia, ambulatory monitoring is used to evaluate arrhythmia and device therapy as well as prognosis and risk stratification of various cardiac populations. Ambulatory ECG monitoring may also be used in patients who have had a cryptogenic stroke (strokes that cannot be attributable to any specific cause) where paroxysmal AF is suspected (Afzal et al., 2015) or with hypertrophic cardiomyopathy, or in patients with variant angina. The patient wears a portable recording device (i.e., Holter monitor) that is connected to the chest by electrodes and lead wires. The patient keeps a diary while wearing this device, noting the type and time of symptoms or performance of unusual activities. The patient may also wear an event loop monitor or an implantable loop recorder, which are categorized as intermittent recorders and selected when patients have infrequent symptoms. The monitoring period may be as short as 24 to 48 hours or as long as several months.

Transtelephonic Monitoring

Transtelephonic monitoring (TTM), a form of outpatient ECG monitoring, transmits ECG signals via the telephone. Chest electrodes are connected to a transmitter box. To send the ECG, the telephone mouthpiece is placed over the transmitter box, and the ECG is evaluated at another location. This method is used for diagnosing arrhythmias and evaluating permanent cardiac pacemakers. It is a patient-activated recording that can be sent directly over the phone line and captures data when symptoms present during activities of daily living.

Wireless Mobile Cardiac Monitoring Systems

This outpatient monitoring system, mobile cardiac telemetry (MCT), uses a small sensing device worn by the patient; it transmits the ECG signal to a monitor. When an arrhythmia is detected, the system transmits the ECG to a monitoring center via a telephone line or a wireless communication system. This system enhances detection and early treatment of arrhythmias.

INTERPRETING THE ELECTROCARDIOGRAM

ECG waveforms are printed on graph paper that is divided by light and dark vertical and horizontal lines at standard intervals (Fig. 17-3). Time and rate are measured on the horizontal axis of the graph, and amplitude or voltage is measured on the vertical axis. Each small block on the graph paper equals 0.04 second, and five small blocks form a large block, which equals 0.2 second. When an ECG waveform moves toward the top of the paper, it is called a *positive deflection.* When it moves toward the bottom of the paper, it is called a *negative deflection.*

The ECG is composed of waveforms (including the P wave, the QRS complex, the T wave, and possibly a U wave) and of segments or intervals (PR interval, the ST segment, and the QT interval) (see Fig. 17-3).

The **P wave** represents the electrical impulse starting in the sinus node and spreading through the atria (atrial **depolarization** leading to atrial contraction).

The **PR interval** is measured from the beginning of the P wave to the beginning of the QRS complex and represents the time needed for sinus node stimulation, atrial depolarization, and conduction through the AV node before ventricular depolarization. In adults, the normal range for the PR is 0.12 to 0.20 second.

FIGURE 17-3 ECG and commonly measured components. Each small box represents 0.04 second on the horizontal axis and 1 mm or 0.1 millivolt on the vertical axis. The PR interval is measured from the beginning of the P wave to the beginning of the QRS complex; the QRS complex is measured from the beginning of the Q wave to the end of the S wave; the QT interval is measured from the beginning of the Q wave to the end of the T wave; and the TP interval is measured from the end of the T wave to the beginning of the next P wave.

The **QRS complex** represents ventricular depolarization. Not all QRS complexes have all three waveforms. The Q wave is the first negative deflection after the P wave. The R wave is the first positive deflection after the P wave, and the S wave is the first negative deflection after the R wave. The QRS complex is normally less than 0.10 second in duration (2.5 small boxes).

The **T wave** represents ventricular repolarization or electrical recovery. It follows the QRS complex and is usually in the same direction as the QRS complex. Atrial repolarization also occurs but is not visible on the ECG because it occurs at the same time as the QRS.

The **U wave** may or may not be present and is thought to represent repolarization of the Purkinje fibers; it is, however, sometimes seen in patients with hypokalemia (low potassium levels), hypertension, or heart disease. If present, the U wave follows the T wave and is usually smaller than the P wave. If tall, it may be mistaken for an extra P wave.

The **ST segment**, which represents early ventricular repolarization, lasts from the end of the QRS complex to the beginning of the T wave. The beginning of the ST segment is usually identified by a change in the thickness or angle of the terminal portion of the QRS complex and is called the *J point*. The end of the ST segment may be more difficult to identify because it merges into the T wave. The ST segment is analyzed to identify whether it is above or below the **isoelectric line**, which may be, among other signs and symptoms, a sign of cardiac ischemia.

 Nursing Alert
Nurses should note ST-segment changes and obtain a 12-lead ECG because:

- *ST-segment depression is seen with ischemia*
- *ST-segment elevation is seen with injury*
- *Q waves are seen with necrosis and infarction*
- *Patients sometimes have silent myocardial ischemia with no associated symptoms such as chest pain. Often silent ischemia occurs in patients with diabetes. Therefore, ST-segment changes viewed on an ECG may be the only way to know that there is a significant cardiac problem.*

The **QT interval**, which represents the total time for ventricular depolarization and repolarization, is measured from the beginning of the QRS complex to the end of the T wave. The QT interval varies with heart rate, gender, and age. If the QT interval becomes prolonged, the patient may be at risk for a lethal ventricular arrhythmia called *torsade de pointes*. The corrected QT (QTc) is calculated based on heart rate and is a determinant of risk for torsade de pointes arrhythmia. The nurse should measure the QT interval every 8 to 12 hours and calculate the QTc on printouts of rhythm strips from the bedside or telemetry monitor for patients at risk for torsade de pointes. An alternative is to use the cardiac monitoring system QT measurement if your hospital system has it as a feature. As referenced earlier, QTc greater than

0.47 second for males or greater than 0.48 second for females is indicative of increased risk of torsade de pointes, and a QTc of more than 0.50 second is considered dangerously prolonged (Ferri, 2016).

 Nursing Alert
The QT interval (QTc) using the Bazett formula: QT interval divided by the square root of the RR interval. The RR interval is measured from one R wave to the next R wave that comes before the QT interval being measured (Bazett, 1920).

The **PP and RR intervals** are measured from the beginning of one P or R wave to the beginning of the next P or R wave. The PP interval is used to determine atrial rate and rhythm. The RR interval is measured from one QRS complex to the next QRS complex. The RR interval is used to determine ventricular rate and rhythm (Fig. 17-4).

ANALYZING THE ELECTROCARDIOGRAM RHYTHM STRIP

The ECG must be analyzed in a systematic manner to determine the patient's cardiac rhythm and to detect arrhythmias and conduction disorders. If continuous ST-segment monitoring is in use, evidence of myocardial ischemia, injury, and infarction may also be detected.

Box 17-4 is an example of a method that can be used to analyze the patient's rhythm.

Normal **sinus rhythm** occurs when the electrical impulse starts at the sinus node and travels through the normal conduction pathway. Normal sinus rhythm serves as a baseline for comparison in identifying all other arrhythmias. ECG characteristics are as follows:

Rate: 60 to 100 in the adult
Rhythm: Regular
P wave: Normal and consistent shape; always in front of the QRS
PR interval: Consistent interval between 0.12 and 0.20 second
QRS duration: Less than 0.10 second

See Figure 17-5.

ARRHYTHMIAS

As our population grows older, where we now define elder groups who range from youngest old (65 to 74 years of age) to elite old (centenarians), the normative aging processes coupled with high incidences of heart disease and polypharmacy with frequent drug–drug interactions show that arrhythmias will continue to be a growing health care concern requiring monitoring, ongoing assessment, and treatment. Nurses are in

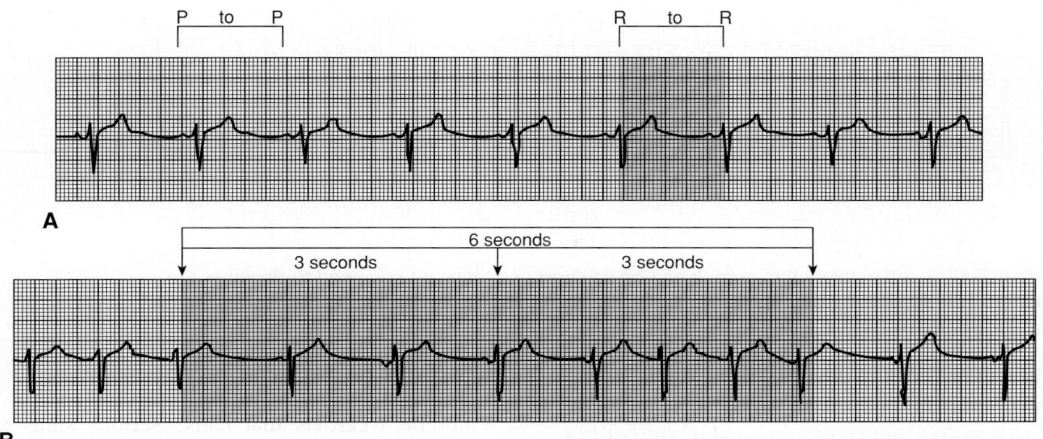

FIGURE 17-4 **A.** Ventricular and atrial heart rate determination with a regular rhythm: 1,500 divided by the number of small boxes between two P waves (atrial rate) or between two R waves (ventricular rate). In this example, there are 25 small boxes between both the R waves and the P waves, so the heart rate is 60 bpm. **B.** Heart rate determination if the rhythm is irregular. There are approximately 7 RR intervals in 6 seconds, so there are about 70 RR intervals in 60 seconds (7 × 10 = 70). The ventricular heart rate is 70 bpm.

BOX 17-4

Interpreting Arrhythmias: Systematic Analysis of the Electrocardiogram

Step 1: Determine the Heart Rate

The heart rate is usually visible on the monitor display or on the printed rhythm strip. However, the monitor will also record "artifact," which may alter the heart rate. The heart rate should always be confirmed by one of the following methods.

Note: the term artifact refers to "noise" that is not related to the heart and produces a "fuzzy" or obscured waveforms. It may be associated with electrical interference by outside sources, poor electrode contact, patient tremors, and malfunction of equipment.

Six-second Method

Locate the 3-second markers along the top or bottom of the ECG paper. Count the number of R waves (ventricular rate) or P waves (atrial rate) occurring between two 3-second markers (thus total time is 6 seconds) and multiply by 10 (thus, 60 seconds or 1 minute).

Large-box Method

Count the number of large boxes between two consecutive R waves (ventricular rate) or P waves (atrial rate) and divide into 300. If, for example, there are four large boxes between two R waves, the heart rate is 300/4, or 75.

Small-box Method

Count the number of small boxes between two consecutive R (ventricular rate) or P waves (atrial rate) waves and divide into 1,500. If, for example, there are 10 small boxes between two R waves, the heart rate is 1500/10, or 150 (see Fig. 17-4).

The normal heart rate is between 60 and 100. The term *bradycardia* is used when the heart rate is below 60, whereas *tachycardia* refers to rates above 100.

Step 2: Determine the Rhythm Regularity

Measure the distance between two consecutive R waves (ventricular regularity) or between two consecutive P waves (atrial regularity). Compare the distance between other RR or PP intervals. If the distance is consistent, the rhythm is regular; if the distance varies, the rhythm is irregular. The normal rhythm is regular.

Step 3: Determine if the Rhythm Originated in the SA Node

Look for a P wave and determine if there is one P wave for every QRS. Determine if the size and shape of the P wave is consistent. The normal rhythm has one P wave for every QRS complex. Because P waves represent the contraction across both atria, irregularities in shape are noted with conduction defect within the atrium, atrial enlargement, or hypertrophy.

Step 4: Evaluate Conduction

Measure the PR interval and the QRS duration. The normal PR interval is between 0.12 (three small boxes) and 0.20 (five small boxes) second. The normal QRS interval is less than 0.10 second (2.5 small boxes). QRS duration of more than 0.10 is termed "wide QRS" and is indicative of abnormal ventricular conduction, such as BBBs or ventricular tachycardia.

Step 5: Evaluate the Appearance of the Rhythm

Look for premature beats or elevated or depressed ST segments. ST elevation/depression is associated with ventricular injury/ischemia.

Step 6: Interpret the Rhythm

Compare the findings to the defining characteristics of specified arrhythmias.

Step 7: If a change is noted from the patient's baseline, evaluate the patient, consider obtaining a 12-lead ECG, and report the change to the provider as appropriate.

FIGURE 17-5 A typical rhythm strip. It can be as short or as long as you need to decipher the rhythm. This particular strip represents a continuous recording of lead II in a patient with normal sinus rhythm, the normal rhythm of the heart.

a unique position to be the ones who first discover the arrhythmia and, later, to educate the patient on the management of this condition to preserve and support a good quality of life.

SINUS NODE ARRHYTHMIAS

SINUS ARRHYTHMIA

Sinus arrhythmia occurs when the sinus node creates an impulse at an irregular rhythm. Sometimes the irregularity is associated with the respiratory cycle. The rate increases with inspiration and decreases with expiration because the SA node fires more quickly with inspiration. Sinus arrhythmia does not cause any significant hemodynamic effect and is not clinically significant. It occurs frequently in the young and decreases in frequency with age.

SINUS BRADYCARDIA

Pathophysiology

Sinus bradycardia occurs when the sinus node creates an impulse at a slower-than-normal rate. The causes include lower metabolic needs (e.g., sleep, athletic training, hypothyroidism), vagal stimulation (e.g., from vomiting, suctioning, severe pain, extreme emotions), medications (e.g., calcium-channel blockers, amiodarone, beta blockers), increased intracranial pressure (ICP), and MI specifically the inferior wall (10% to 15% of patients with inferior MIs develop sinus bradycardia) (Olgin & Zipes, 2015).

Clinical Manifestations and Assessment

Sinus bradycardia often does not cause symptoms though the context or etiology may be important to treat. The patient is assessed to determine the hemodynamic effect, if any, and the possible cause of the arrhythmia.

ECG characteristics are:

Rate: Less than 60 beats per minute (bpm)
Rhythm: Regular
P wave: Present before each QRS and consistent in size and shape
PR interval: Normal
QRS duration: Normal

See Figure 17-6.

Medical and Nursing Management

Only bradycardias that cause serious signs and symptoms (altered mental status, ongoing chest pain, hypotension, or shock) require immediate treatment. Treatment of symptomatic bradycardia includes transcutaneous pacing and atropine. If pacing is unavailable or ineffective, a dopamine or epinephrine infusion may be considered (Neumar et al., 2015). If significant bradycardia is due to medications, the medications should be withheld while their necessity is re-evaluated.

> **Nursing Alert**
> *For new-onset syncope and bradycardia, the nurse asks the patient about recent medications during patient admission history, since medications are the cause of most cases of symptomatic bradycardia. Consider a wide variety of medications, including beta-adrenergic blocking eye drops for the treatment of glaucoma. Recall that if the puncta is not occluded with administration, the medication can drain into tear ducts and be systemically absorbed, resulting in syncope secondary to bradycardia (Miller & Zipes, 2015).*

SINUS TACHYCARDIA

Pathophysiology

Sinus tachycardia occurs when the sinus node creates an impulse at a faster-than-normal rate. Causes may include the following:

- Physiologic or psychological stress (e.g., acute blood loss, anemia, shock, hypervolemia, hypovolemia, heart failure, pain, pulmonary emboli, hypermetabolic states, fever, exercise, anxiety)

FIGURE 17-6 Sinus bradycardia. More than seven large squares separate each beat, and the rate is 40 to 45 beats per minute.

FIGURE 17-7 Sinus tachycardia. Each beat is separated by two and one half large squares for a rate of 120 beats per minute.

- Medications that stimulate the sympathetic response (e.g., catecholamines, aminophylline, atropine, thyroid medications), stimulants (e.g., caffeine, alcohol, nicotine), and illicit drugs (e.g., amphetamines, cocaine, ecstasy)

Clinical Manifestations and Assessment

Sinus tachycardia often does not cause symptoms like bradycardia, the context is important to determine if an intervention is clinically indicated. As the heart rate increases, the diastolic filling time decreases, possibly resulting in reduced cardiac output and associated symptoms (refer to Table 17-1). If the rapid rate persists and the heart can no longer compensate for the decreased ventricular filling, the patient may develop acute pulmonary edema or cardiac ischemia.

ECG characteristics are:

Rate: Greater than 100 bpm
Rhythm: Regular
P wave: Present before each QRS and consistent in size and shape
PR interval: Normal
QRS duration: Normal

See Figure 17-7.

Medical and Nursing Management

Treatment of sinus tachycardia is usually determined by the severity of symptoms and directed at identifying and treating its cause. For example, tachycardia caused by acute blood loss would be treated with intravenous (IV) fluid replacement and blood transfusion. Common causes of sinus tachycardia in hospitalized patients include agitation, hemorrhage, or sepsis; in outpatient settings consider hyperthyroidism, anemia, infection or inflammation, and hypovolemia (Olgin & Zipes, 2015).

ATRIAL ARRHYTHMIAS

PREMATURE ATRIAL COMPLEX

Pathophysiology

A premature atrial complex (PAC) is a single ECG complex that occurs when an electrical impulse starts in the atrium before the next normal impulse of the sinus node. The PAC may be caused by caffeine, alcohol, nicotine, stretched atrial myocardium (e.g., as in hypervolemia), anxiety, hypokalemia (low potassium level), hypermetabolic states (e.g., with pregnancy), hypoxemia, or atrial ischemia, injury, or infarction.

Clinical Manifestations and Assessment

PACs are common ECG findings, often found without cardiac pathology. The patient may report, "My heart skipped a beat"; however, many times the patient is asymptomatic.

ECG characteristics are:

Rate: Depends on the underlying rhythm
Rhythm: Irregular
P wave: Size and shape of the P wave associated with the premature beat is different from sinus node–generated P wave
PR interval: The PR interval of the premature beat is greater than 0.12 second but shorter than the sinus generated PR interval
QRS duration: Normal

See Figure 17-8.

Medical and Nursing Management

If PACs are infrequent, no treatment is necessary since hemodynamic stability is maintained. If they are frequent (more than six per minute), this may be a sign of a worsening condition or the onset of more serious arrhythmias, such as AF, and further work-up may be clinically indicated.

ATRIAL FLUTTER

Pathophysiology

Atrial flutter occurs in the atrium and creates impulses at a rapid but regular atrial rate between 220 and 350 times per minute. Because the atrial rate is faster than the atrioventricular (AV) node can conduct, not all atrial impulses are conducted into the ventricle. This is an important feature of this arrhythmia because if all atrial impulses were conducted to the ventricle, the ventricular rate would also be 220 to 350, which would result in a life-threatening arrhythmia. Causes include coronary artery disease (CAD), hypertension, mitral or tricuspid valve disease, hyperthyroidism or thyrotoxicosis, chronic lung disease, cor pulmonale (right ventricular

FIGURE 17-8 Premature atrial complex (PAC). Normal sinus rhythm with one premature atrial contraction (PAC).

failure), pulmonary emboli, previous extensive atrial ablation, and cardiomyopathy. A clinical relationship between atrial flutter and AF can be appreciated often in the same patient post open heart surgery (Olgin & Zipes, 2015).

Clinical Manifestations and Assessment

Atrial flutter may not cause any symptoms or, instead, may cause serious signs and symptoms, such as fatigue, light-headedness, chest pain, shortness of breath, and low blood pressure. The risk of mural (wall) emboli forming in the atria increases with this arrhythmia because without a strong atrial contraction, stasis of blood occurs; therefore, the nurse remains alert for signs of pulmonary or systemic emboli.

ECG characteristics are:

Rate: Atrial rate ranges between 220 and 350 bpm; ventricular rate usually ranges between 75 and 150 depending on AV node conduction
Rhythm: Usually regular but may be irregular because of a change in the AV conduction
P wave: Flutter waves in a characteristic "sawtooth" pattern
PR interval: Not measurable
QRS duration: Normal

See Figure 17-9.

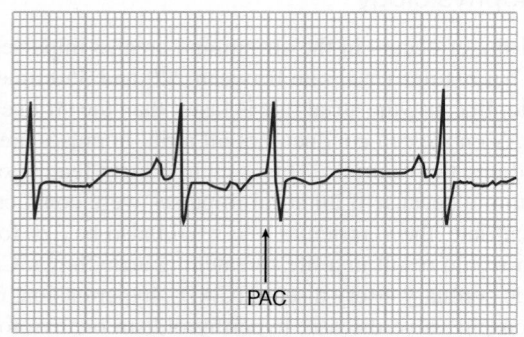

FIGURE 17-9 The classic saw-toothed pattern of atrial flutter.

Medical and Nursing Management

As noted in the 2014 AHA/ACC/HRS Guidelines, the initial treatment for atrial flutter commonly is cardioversion or radiofrequency ablation (discussed later in this chapter) to terminate it and restore NSR (January et al., 2014). If the patient is unstable, urgent electrical **cardioversion** is usually indicated (discussed later in this chapter). For patients who have atrial flutter, antithrombotic therapy is recommended per the same risk profile used for AF (AHA/ACC/HRS, 2014). In addition, flecainide, dofetilide, propafenone, and intravenous ibutilide are useful for pharmacologic cardioversion of AF or atrial flutter, provided there are no contraindications to the selected medication (AHA/ACC/HRS, 2014). Refer to Table 17-3 for medication management of AF.

ATRIAL FIBRILLATION

Pathophysiology

AF should be distinguished from atrial flutter. AF causes rapid, disorganized, and uncoordinated electrical activity within the atria. AF may be transient, starting and stopping suddenly and occurring for a very short time (**paroxysmal**), or it may be persistent, requiring treatment to terminate the rhythm or to control the ventricular rate. Further, AF may be described in terms of duration of episodes, such as long-standing, permanent, or nonvalvular AF. Long-standing persistent AF is continuous or AF lasting longer than 12 months in duration; permanent AF is used when the physician and patient together decide to stop further attempts to restore and maintain NSR. Finally, the term nonvalvular AF is used when AF exists in the absence of rheumatic mitral stenosis, a mechanical or bioprosthetic heart valve, or mitral valve repair (AHA/ACC/HRS, 2014). The erratic atrial contraction promotes formation of thrombi within the atria, increasing the risk for an embolic event such as stroke (brain attack). In fact, patients with AF have a fivefold

TABLE 17-3 Common Medication Dosage for Rate Control of AF

	Intravenous Administration	Usual Oral Maintenance Dose
Beta Blockers		
Metoprolol tartrate	2.5–5.0 mg IV bolus over 2 minutes; up to 3 doses	25–100 mg BID
Metoprolol XL (succinate)	N/A	50–400 mg QD
Atenolol	N/A	25–100 mg QD
Esmolol	500 mcg/kg IV bolus over 1 minute, then 50–300 mcg/kg/min IV	N/A
Propranolol	1 mg IV over 1 minute, up to 3 doses at 2-minute intervals	10–40 mg TID or QID
Nadolol	N/A	10–240 mg QD
Carvedilol	N/A	3.125–25 mg BID
Bisoprolol	N/A	2.5–10 mg QD
Nondihydropyridine Calcium-Channel Antagonists		
Verapamil	0.075–0.15 mg/kg IV bolus over 2 minutes; may give an additional 10.0 mg after 30 minutes if no response, then 0.005 mg/kg/min infusion	180–480 mg QD (ER)
Diltiazem	0.25 mg/kg IV bolus over 2 minutes, then 5–15 mg/hr	120–360 mg QD (ER)
Digitalis Glycosides		
Digoxin	0.25 mg IV with repeat dosing to a maximum of 1.5 mg over 24 hours	0.125–0.25 mg QD
Others		
Amiodarone[a]	300 mg IV over 1 hour, then 10–50 mg/hr over 24 hours	100–200 mg QD

[a]Multiple dosing schemes exist for the use of amiodarone.
AF, atrial fibrillation; BID, twice daily; ER, extended release; IV, intravenous; N/A, not applicable, QD, once daily; QID, 4 times a day; TID, 3 times a day.
January, C. T., Wann, L. S., Alpert, J. S., Calkins, H., Cigarroa, J. E., Cleveland, J. C.,... Yancy, C. W. (2014). 2014 AHA/ACC/HRS Guideline for the Management of Patients With Atrial Fibrillation: Executive Summary. *Circulation*, 130, 2071–2104.

increase in the risk for stroke and a twofold increase in mortality (Morady & Zipes, 2015). AF is usually associated with increasing age, valvular heart disease, CAD, hypertension, heart failure, cardiomyopathy, diabetes, obstructive sleep apnea, obesity, hyperthyroidism, pulmonary disease, chronic lung disease, and surgery (especially open heart surgery). Physiologic stressors, such as hypoxia, infection, and hypoglycemia; as well as the use of caffeine, alcohol, or sympathomimetic drugs; and smoking are also associated with AF. An additional risk factor for AF is psoriasis, which, if severe, triples the risk for AF in patients younger than 50 years (Morady & Zipes, 2015, p. 800). It is important to note that sometimes AF occurs in people without any underlying pathophysiology.

Clinical Manifestations and Assessment

Some people with AF may be asymptomatic. However, there is a rapid ventricular response, which reduces the time for ventricular filling, resulting in a smaller stroke volume. In addition, loss of the atrial contraction (sometimes referred to as *atrial kick*) reduces ventricular filling volume and reduces cardiac output by 25%. This often leads to symptoms of fatigue and malaise. The shorter time in diastole reduces the time available for coronary artery perfusion, thereby increasing the risk for myocardial ischemia. In addition, patients are at risk for the development of heart failure (Morady & Zipes, 2015).

ECG characteristics are:

Rate: Atrial rate is 300 to 400, with a variable ventricular response rate (typically rapid)
Rhythm: Irregular
P wave: No discernible P waves; irregular undulating waves may be seen and are referred to as *fibrillatory waves*
PR interval: Not measurable
QRS duration: Normal

See Figure 17-10.

FIGURE 17-10 Atrial fibrillation with a slow, irregular ventricular rate.

Nursing Alert

The three cornerstones of AF management include rate control, rhythm control, and prevention of thromboembolism.

Medical and Nursing Management

Treatment of AF depends on its cause and duration and the patient's symptoms, age, and comorbidities. Once the pattern, clinical history, and symptoms are established, it is important to then assess for the presence of structural heart disease and identification of any correctable secondary causes, such as sleep apnea or substance abuse. The management of AF includes controlling the ventricular rate and achieving rhythm conversion to sinus rhythm if possible. Cardioversion of AF can be done either by medication or an electrical shock. Direct-current cardioversion is more effective than pharmacologic cardioversion (Knight, 2013). It is important to consider that when AF onset is more recent, then pharmacologic cardioversion will be more effective. However, electrical cardioversion is indicated when a patient with new-onset AF is hemodynamically unstable (Knight, 2013). Shocks are delivered in sync with the QRS wave. Biphasic defibrillators are used more often with less energy required (150 to 200 J) than when using the older, monophasic defibrillators with higher-energy settings. Pharmacologic cardioversion is done with intravenous (IV) ibutilide, procainamide, or amiodarone. For AF episodes shorter than 48 to 72 hours duration, the efficacy of ibutilide is approximately 60% to 70%, whereas amiodarone's efficacy is approximately 40% to 50%, and procainamide's efficacy is 30% to 40% (Morady & Zipes, 2015). Commonly used oral medications include flecainide and propafenone. For ventricular rate control, the medications that are used are beta blockers and calcium-channel antagonists along with Digoxin (reserved for those patients who are sedentary or with systolic HF). For rhythm control after cardioversion, patients will often be placed on dofetilide, amiodarone, or dronedarone (Knight, 2013).

Nursing Alert

For a patient with new-onset AF for over 48 hours, or when the onset is unknown, the nurse is aware that a transesophageal echocardiography (TEE) should be performed before cardioversion to rule out a left atrial thrombus. The rationale behind this is that with cardioversion, if the patient converts to a sinus rhythm, the risk increases for embolization of the clot resulting in a potential

CVA. If no thrombi are present, then cardioversion can be performed safely; however, the patient needs to be educated that 4 weeks of anticoagulation will be maintained after cardioversion to prevent thromboembolism (Morady & Zipes, 2015).

If delayed cardioversion is selected rather than emergent cardioversion, then the patient typically receives 3 weeks of therapeutic anticoagulation (Knight, 2013) to prevent a thrombus and a TEE should be performed prior to cardioversion. Accordingly, all patients with AF, regardless of whether a rhythm or rate control plan is chosen, should be treated with antithrombotic therapy.

If the QRS is wide and the ventricular rhythm is irregular, AF with an accessory pathway, such as Wolff–Parkinson–White syndrome, should be suspected. Medications that block AV conduction (e.g., adenosine [Adenocard], digoxin, diltiazem [Cardizem], and verapamil [Calan]) should be avoided because they may actually cause an increase in ventricular rate given that conduction is via an alternative pathway rather than via the AV node. Expert consultation will be required to determine appropriate treatment.

Antithrombotic therapy prevents thromboembolism, and long-term anticoagulant therapy is prescribed using warfarin, or warfarin alternatives—factor Xa inhibitor (rivaroxaban or apixaban) or direct thrombin inhibitor (dabigatran). These therapies are indicated if the patient with AF is at high risk for stroke using the CHADS 2 scoring system (i.e., over 75 years of age or has hypertension, diabetes, heart failure, or history of stroke). There are no effective reversal agents for these warfarin-alternative agents. If immediate anticoagulation is necessary, the patient may be placed on heparin until the warfarin level is therapeutic (AHA/ACC/HRS, 2014).

Nursing Alert

No therapy, cardiac medications or cardioversion may be used to convert lone AF (also referred to as idiopathic AF [where there is no clear cause for the rhythm]) for patients over 65 years of age without heart disease. If there are no contraindications, anticoagulation therapy may be started without direct treatment of arrhythmia itself. If warfarin is used, the international normalized ratio (INR) should be 2.0 to 3.0 with a target of 2.5. An INR below 2.0 is not effective at preventing strokes. If the patient has a mechanical valve, then the target INR should be 2.5 (Knight, 2013).

Pacemaker implantation or catheter ablation is sometimes indicated for patients who are unresponsive to medications. Catheter ablation is a minimally invasive procedure during which high-frequency radio waves are applied to destroy the tissue at the site of the arrhythmia. Ablation procedures are usually performed in electrophysiology (EP) laboratories and are similar to other types of heart catheterization procedures in that a catheter is used. However, the differences include longer procedure times (approximately 6 to 8 hours) for ablation, the catheter delivers high energy to stop an arrhythmia, and it is indicated for conduction diagnosis and treatment alone—not for diagnosis and treatment of disease in the coronary arteries. During a catheter ablation, long, thin, flexible tubes are placed in the heart via the vascular system. A diagnostic catheter determines where the abnormal tissue that is causing the arrhythmia is located. High-frequency energy is sent into the tissue, creating a lesion or scar. The area is now ablated (destroyed), thus facilitating normal electrical conduction. Cryoballoon ablation is a new procedure that has been effective in preventing paroxysmal AF in patients who were unable to be medically managed with antiarrhythmic medications (Packer et al., 2013). Pulmonary vein isolation using cryoablation can be achieved in most people with shorter procedure times. However, the potential complications of this procedure include phrenic nerve injury or stroke (Packer et al., 2013).

Several approaches are effective in preventing the occurrence of postoperative AF, including preoperative administration of a beta blocker or immediate postoperative administration of IV amiodarone (AHA/ACC/HRS, 2014).

SUPRAVENTRICULAR TACHYCARDIA

Pathophysiology

Supraventricular tachycardia (SVT) is a broad term used to describe tachycardias where the atrial and/or the ventricular rates exceed 100 bpm at rest (Page et al., 2016). The mechanism involves an electrical impulse originating above the ventricles, commonly from tissue at the HIS bundle and above (AV node). The heart rate is increases by an abnormal electrical impulse starting in the atria, and the ventricular rate follows the atrial impulse resulting in this "tachy" arrhythmia. Broadly, SVT includes sinus tachycardia, focal and multifocal atrial tachycardias, junctional tachycardias, AV nodal re-entry tachycardia (AVNRT), and various other accessory pathway-mediated reentrant tachycardias. Technically, AF is an SVT, but it is not grouped this way in the AHA guidelines and was addressed separately. SVTs even without AF included are among the most common arrhythmias that require treatment. Conduction abnormalities may occur because of aberrant conduction, a pre-existing BBB, or an accessory pathway that results in pre-excitation (Page et al., 2015). Further, the presence of AV dissociation (where the ventricular rate is faster than the atrial rate or in other cases where fusion complexes occur that represent the dissociation of supraventricular impulses from ventricular) provides assistance with diagnosis of VT versus SVT. It is sometimes difficult to differentiate between the two without a 12-lead ECG.

Clinical Manifestation

SVTs effect on a patient's quality of life varies; the degree of impact is often affected by the frequency of episodes, the duration, and the timing of the SVT (whether with exercise or also at rest). Symptoms vary depending on the rhythm and the patient, with reports of palpitations, chest pain, shortness of breath, dizziness, and syncope, along with panic and anxiety, which heighten the degree of symptoms and confounds the diagnosis of SVT (Page et al., 2015).

ECG characteristics are:

Rate: over 100 bpm
Rhythm: Regular
P wave: If visible, inverted P waves sometimes seen after the QRS
PR interval: Not measurable
QRS duration: In paroxysmal SVT, the QRS is normal.

See Figure 17-11.

FIGURE 17-11 Supraventricular tachycardia: note rate above 220, abnormal P waves, no beat-to-beat variability.

Medical and Nursing Management

Treatment of atrial SVT depends on its cause and duration and the patient's symptoms, age, and comorbidities. Vagal maneuvers are recommended as a first step to discontinue the rhythm in patients who are hemodynamically stable. Often this intervention does not work or only works in the short term. Medical management in the short term in a patient who is stable with a regular SVT is with adenosine. If the patient becomes hemodynamically unstable, cannot be rate controlled with medication or it is ineffective, the treatment recommendation is synchronized cardioversion. Intravenous beta blockers, IV diltiazem, or IV verapamil (class IIa) can also be used to convert the patient's rhythm to NSR (Page et al., 2015).

For ongoing management, patients are placed on oral beta blockers, diltiazem, or verapamil and taught how to do the vasovagal maneuver. Antiarrhythmic medications do carry the potential for adverse side effects. Therefore, today more often patients are referred for catheter ablation with a high degree of success and low rate of complications (Page et al., 2015).

JUNCTIONAL ARRHYTHMIAS

JUNCTION RHYTHM

Pathophysiology

Junctional rhythm occurs when the AV node, instead of the sinus node, becomes the pacemaker of the heart. When the sinus node slows (e.g., from increased vagal tone) or when the impulse cannot be conducted through the AV node (e.g., because of complete heart block), the AV node automatically discharges an impulse. Junctional escape rhythm may

be caused by acute coronary syndromes; valvular disease; hypoxia; increased parasympathetic tone; or the effects of medication, including digoxin, beta blockers, and calcium-channel blockers.

Clinical Manifestations and Assessment

The patient may be asymptomatic or experience signs and symptoms associated with a decreased cardiac output.

ECG characteristics are:

Rate: 40 to 60 bpm
Rhythm: Regular
P wave: If visible, may be before, during, or after the QRS
PR interval: If a P wave is visible, less than 0.12 second
QRS duration: Normal

See Figure 17-12.

Medical and Nursing Management

If the patient is symptomatic, the treatment is the same as for bradycardia; the patient may be paced (temporary or permanent) or is given IV atropine or epinephrine.

VENTRICULAR ARRHYTHMIAS

ABNORMAL VENTRICULAR CONDUCTION (BBB)

Pathophysiology

If there is a delay or defect in the conduction system within the ventricles (right and left bundle branches), the

FIGURE 17-12 Junctional rhythm note short PR intervals. **A.** A junctional premature beat. The third beat is obviously premature, and there is no P wave preceding the QRS complex. **B.** The third beat is a junctional escape beat, establishing a sustained junctional rhythm. It looks just like a junctional premature beat, but it occurs late, following a prolonged pause, rather than prematurely.

QRS complex will be prolonged or widened (greater than 0.12 second). A BBB may be described as right or left and complete or incomplete. They may occasionally be present in otherwise healthy individuals; however, they may also be caused by ventricular enlargement (ventricular hypertrophy or cardiomyopathy) or anteroseptal myocardial ischemia or infarction. A BBB may be clinically insignificant, though it can be serious when associated with an acute MI.

Medical and Nursing Management

The goal is to treat the underlying cause of the BBB when possible, such as by maximizing medical management of CAD or cardiomyopathy. However, in the presence of an acute MI, BBB may progress to complete heart block, which may require temporary pacing during the acute phase of illness.

PREMATURE VENTRICULAR COMPLEX

Pathophysiology

A premature ventricular complex (PVC) is an impulse that starts in a ventricle and is conducted through the ventricles before the next normal sinus impulse. Premature ventricular contractions can occur in healthy people, especially with intake of caffeine, nicotine, or alcohol. They are also caused by cardiac ischemia or infarction, increased workload on the heart (e.g., exercise, fever, hypervolemia, heart failure, tachycardia), digitalis toxicity, hypoxia, acidosis, or electrolyte imbalances, especially hypokalemia. Prevalence of PVCs increases with age, in males, and with hypokalemia (Olgin & Zipes, 2015). New research suggests that PVCs may be an early marker for the development of heart failure. In a population-based study by Dukes et al. (2015) a higher frequency of PVCs was associated with a decrease in left ventricular ejection fraction (LVEF, which is the amount of blood ejected out of the left ventricle per each ventricular contraction), an increase in incident CHF, and increased mortality. More studies are needed to refine and evaluate efficacy for both preventative therapies and treatment options for PVCs. What is clear is that prevention of PVCs through ablation is possible, thus the future may include PVCs as a modifiable risk factor for HF (Dukes et al., 2015).

Clinical Manifestations and Assessment

The patient may be asymptomatic or complain that their heart "skipped a beat." The effect of a PVC depends on its timing in the cardiac cycle and how much blood was in the ventricles when they contracted. *Bigeminy* is a rhythm in which every other complex is a PVC. In *trigeminy,* every third complex is a PVC, and in *quadrigeminy*, every fourth complex is a PVC. PVCs may present singly or in pairs (often referred to as couplets). Three or more successive PVCs are termed *ventricular tachycardia* (VT) (discussed next).

ECG characteristics are:

Rate: Depends on the underlying rhythm

Rhythm: Regular

P wave: Visibility of P wave depends on the timing of the PVC; may be absent (hidden in the QRS or T wave) or in front of the QRS. If the P wave follows the QRS, the shape of the P wave may be different.

PR interval: If the P wave is in front of the QRS, the PR interval is less than 0.12 second.

QRS duration: Duration of the QRS in a PVC is 0.12 second or longer (wide); shape is bizarre and abnormal.

See Figure 17-13.

FIGURE 17-13 Dangerous forms of premature ventricular contractions (PVCs): **(A)** bigeminy, **(B)** couplets, **(C)** run, **(D)** multifocal, and **(E)** R-on-T phenomenon.

Medical and Nursing Management

Initial treatment is aimed at correcting the cause of the arrhythmia (e.g., treat hypokalemia). Long-term pharmacotherapy for PVCs is not indicated unless the patient is symptomatic. In the absence of disease, PVCs usually are not serious. In the patient with an acute MI or in the context of HF, PVCs may be more frequent and reflect the underlying heart disease or represent an early modifiable risk factor for heart failure.

Unfolding Patient Stories: Kenneth Bronson • Part 2

Recall from Chapter 10 Kenneth Bronson, who came to the emergency department with difficulty breathing after a week of flu-like symptoms, productive cough, and high fever. He was diagnosed with a right lower lobe pneumonia. Sinus tachycardia with occasional unifocal premature ventricular contractions (PVCs) is seen on the cardiac monitor. What are potential causes for the tachycardia and PVCs that the nurse should investigate when considering his age of 27 years, symptoms experienced over the last week, and the clinical manifestations associated with his diagnosis?

Care for Kenneth and other patients in a realistic virtual environment: *vSim for Nursing* (thepoint. lww.com/vSimMedicalSurgical). Practice documenting these patients' care in (thepoint.lww.com/ DocuCareEHR).

VENTRICULAR TACHYCARDIA

Pathophysiology

Ventricular tachycardia is defined as three or more consecutive ventricular beats occurring at a rate exceeding 100 bpm. The causes are similar to those of PVCs. Ultimately, those causes will determine the course of treatment with consideration to the underlying disease; the projected, associated risk; the period of time that the risk exists; and the benefits

and risks as well as tolerance of the planned treatment. VT is usually associated with ACS but can also occur in specific clinical conditions:

- after an MI,
- with inherited primary arrhythmia syndromes, such as long QT syndrome,
- with electrolyte imbalances,
- cardiomyopathies,
- structural heart disease, and
- due to proarrhythmic medications that may precede ventricular fibrillation.

Untreated VT can deteriorate into ventricular fibrillation, a lethal arrhythmia and sudden cardiac death.

Clinical Manifestations and Assessment

The patient can experience a range of symptoms related to decreased cardiac output, such as hypotension or syncope, pulselessness, and unresponsiveness. In contrast, some patients may be initially asymptomatic but usually will decompensate hemodynamically.

ECG characteristics are:

Rate: 100 to 250 bpm
Rhythm: Regular
P wave: Usually not visible; if visible are not associated with the QRS complex (called *dissociation*)
PR interval: None
QRS duration: Greater than 0.12 second

See Figure 17-14.

Medical and Nursing Management

The patient's tolerance for this rapid rhythm depends on the ventricular rate and underlying disease. Several factors together with the ventricular rate and the etiology determine the initial treatment, including the following: identifying the rhythm as monomorphic (having a consistent QRS shape and rate) or polymorphic (having varying QRS shapes and rhythms); determining the existence of a

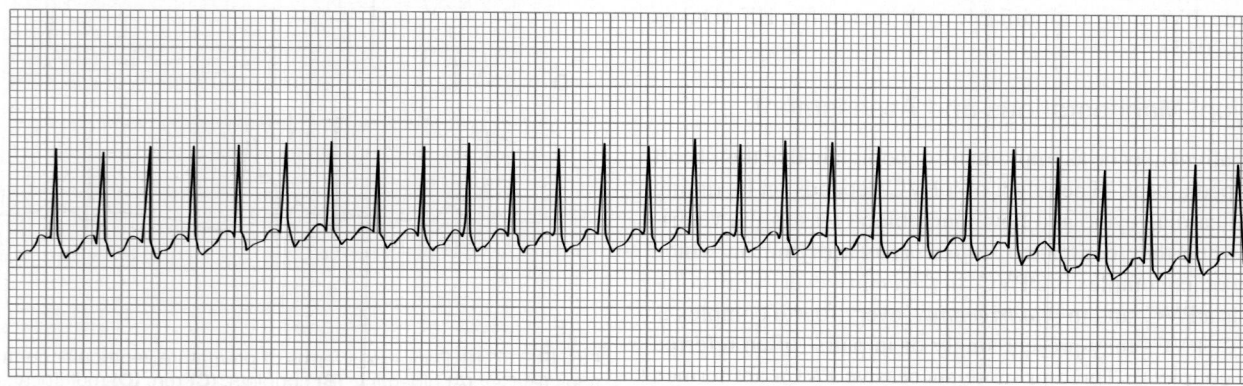

FIGURE 17-14 Ventricular tachycardia: rapid and regular rhythm, wide QRS complex without P waves.

prolonged QT interval before the initiation of VT; and ascertaining the patient's heart function. If the patient is stable, continuing the assessment, especially obtaining a 12-lead ECG, may be the only action necessary.

Vasopressin with epinephrine is no longer administered to patients in cardiac arrest because the evidence does not support it, according to the AHA Guidelines Update (Hazinski et al., 2015). However, per these guidelines, epinephrine alone should be considered to establish a rhythm that can be treated in the event that the initial rhythm is a nonshockable one. Amiodarone administered IV is often the antiarrhythmic medication of choice for a stable patient with VT. Cardioversion is the treatment of choice for monophasic VT in a symptomatic patient. However, many antiarrhythmic drugs other than beta blockers have not been shown to be effective in the treatment of primary ventricular arrhythmia or in sudden cardiac death prevention but may be helpful as an adjunct therapy in management of patients who are arrhythmia prone (Priori et al., 2015). Importantly, AF should be suspected as the cause of a wide, complex tachycardia with an irregular rhythm, and it should be treated appropriately.

Nursing Alert

The nurse observes the patient's response hemodynamically to the VT. Obtain vital signs, auscultate lungs and heart, monitor urine output, and assess the patient's level of consciousness. If a patient demonstrates hypotension, shock, angina, symptoms of congestive heart failure (crackles, decreasing oxygen saturation, SOB [left-sided HF] or edema, jugular vein distention [right-sided HF]), or symptoms of cerebral hypoperfusion, the nurse prepares for cardioversion.

Torsade de pointes (Fig. 17-15) is a polymorphic VT usually preceded by a prolonged QT interval that can be congenital or acquired and is relatively uncommon. Acquired torsades is frequently associated with drug therapy, hypokalemia, or hypomagnesemia (Berul, Seslar, Zimetbaum, & Josephson, 2016). Risk factors for torsade de pointes are described in Box 17-5 which includes some of the

---

BOX 17-5 **Risk Factors for Torsade de Pointes**

1. QT interval prolongation
2. Female gender
   a. Risk increased two- to threefold
3. Electrolyte imbalance
   a. Primarily hypokalemia
4. Structural heart disease
   a. Ischemic heart disease
   b. Cardiomyopathy
5. Pharmacologic factors
   a. Antiarrhythmic medications—most potent QT interval prolonging
      i. Ia Class—quinidine and procainamide
      ii. III Class—dofetilide, ibutilide, sotalol, and amiodarone
         • More than 50 drugs medications are noted to prolong the QT interval
   b. Other medications with ability to prolong QT have been found in almost every other class of therapeutic agent.
6. Congenital
   a. Congenital severe bradycardia (long QT syndrome)
   b. Autosomal-dominant syndromes
   c. Autosomal-recessive cases
7. Other
   a. Intracranial events (e.g., subarachnoid hemorrhage) may be as high as 8% if associated with hypokalemia
   b. Cocaine
   c. Hypothermia
   d. HIV infection

Adapted from Ferri, F. (2016). Torsade de Pointes. In: *Ferri clinical advisor*. Philadelphia, PA: Elsevier Inc.

QT-prolonging medications. Since QT-prolonging agents can be found in all classes of medications, a website has been established for patients and health care professionals (e.g., www.QTdrugs.org). Up-to-date information is provided at this site regarding QT-prolonging medications and drug-to-drug interactions that can also affect the QT interval. Because this rhythm is likely to cause the patient to deteriorate and become pulseless, immediate treatment is usually required. Standard antiarrhythmic agents may be administered with temporary pacing, but treatment will depend on the cause of

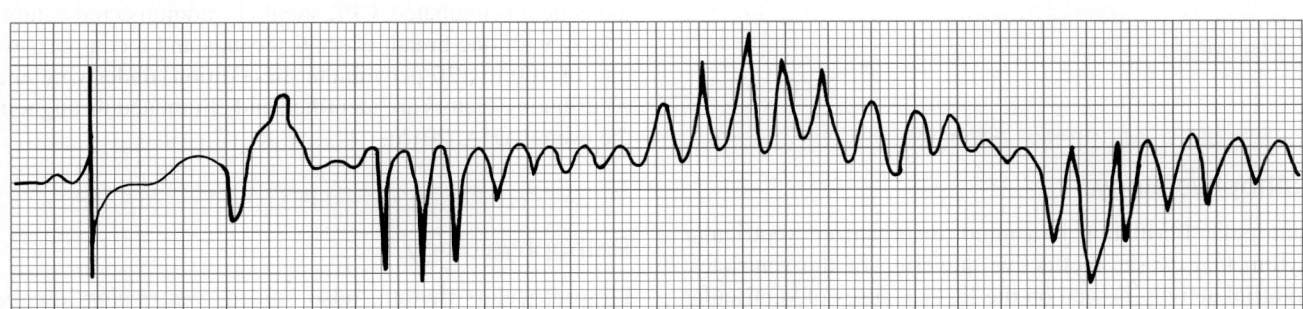

FIGURE 17-15 Torsades de pointes. (From Lippincott. (2005). *Just the Facts: ECG interpretation*. Philadelphia, PA: Lippincott Williams & Wilkins.)

FIGURE 17-16 Coarse ventricular fibrillation: Chaotic electrical activity.

torsades and management should focus on removing the etiology of this arrhythmia. For example, in acquired torsades, intravenous magnesium is the initial treatment of choice followed by temporary ventricular or atrial pacing (Olgin & Zipes, 2015, p. 783). Any type of VT in a patient who is unconscious and without a pulse is treated in the same manner as ventricular fibrillation: immediate **defibrillation** is the action of choice. In addition, it is important in the hospital setting to monitor patients closely, noting those who have a QTc above 500 ms and discontinuing the offending medications.

 Nursing Alert
When caring for a patient experiencing an emergent cardiac arrhythmia, consider the following.

1. *Assess the patient's condition.*
2. *If patient has a loss of respirations, a loss of pulse, a decrease in level of consciousness, or significant change in blood pressure, call a cardiac arrest code. If the patient is alert without a significant change in vital signs, call for a rapid response team (RRT) or alert the provider stat to the patient's change in condition. Speak with the patient as it applies to keep the patient informed and calm.*
3. *While awaiting arrival of the medical team, continue to assess the patient, apply supplemental oxygen, ensure adequate IV access, and bring emergency equipment and a bedside monitor to the patient's bedside.*

VENTRICULAR FIBRILLATION

Pathophysiology

Ventricular fibrillation is a rapid, disorganized ventricular rhythm that causes ineffective quivering of the ventricles. No atrial activity is seen on the ECG. Causes of ventricular fibrillation are the same as for VT; it may also result from untreated or unsuccessfully treated VT.

Clinical Manifestations and Assessment

Clinical manifestations include absence of an audible heartbeat, a palpable pulse, and respirations. Cardiac arrest and death are imminent.

ECG characteristics are:

Rate: Often cannot be determined, but is greater than 220 bpm
Rhythm: Irregular
P wave: Not visible
PR interval: Not visible
QRS duration: Not visible

See Figure 17-16.

Medical and Nursing Management

Treatment of choice is immediate defibrillation if available, immediate cardiopulmonary resuscitation (CPR), and activation of emergency services. After the initial defibrillation, five cycles of CPR, alternating with a rhythm check and defibrillation, are used to convert ventricular fibrillation to an electrical rhythm that produces a pulse. Vasoactive medications (epinephrine) should be administered as soon as possible after the second rhythm check (immediately before or after the second defibrillation). Often antiarrhythmic medications (amiodarone, lidocaine, or possibly magnesium) will be administered though there is lack of evidence to support their routine use after a cardiac arrest (AHA, 2015). Once the patient is intubated, CPR should be administered continuously with one breath every 6 seconds and a compression rate of 100 to 120 per minute. In addition, underlying and contributing factors are identified and eliminated throughout the event (AHA, 2015).

IDIOVENTRICULAR RHYTHM

Pathophysiology

Idioventricular rhythm, also called *ventricular escape rhythm*, occurs when the impulse starts in the conduction system below the AV node. When the sinus node fails to

FIGURE 17-17 Idioventricular rhythm. There are no P waves, the QRS complexes are wide, and the rate is about 75 beats per minute.

create an impulse (e.g., from increased vagal tone) or when the impulse is created but cannot be conducted through the AV node (e.g., due to complete AV block), the Purkinje fibers automatically discharge an impulse.

Clinical Manifestations and Assessment

Idioventricular rhythm commonly causes the patient to lose consciousness and experience other signs and symptoms of reduced cardiac output.

ECG characteristics are:

Rate: 20 to 40; if the rate exceeds 40, the rhythm is known as *accelerated idioventricular rhythm* (AIVR)
Rhythm: Regular
P wave: Not visible
PR interval: Not visible
QRS duration: Duration is 0.12 second or more

See Figure 17-17.

Medical and Nursing Management

If the patient is in cardiac arrest, treatment is the same as for asystole (absence of electrical activity and pulse); if the patient is not in cardiac arrest, treatment is the same as for bradycardia. Interventions include identifying the underlying cause, administering IV atropine and vasopressor medications, and initiating emergency pacing. In some cases, idioventricular rhythm may cause no symptoms of reduced cardiac output.

VENTRICULAR ASYSTOLE

Pathophysiology

Commonly called *flatline*, ventricular asystole is characterized by absent QRS complexes confirmed in two different leads. Asystole is seen in the absence of cardiac electrical activity; because there is no contraction, there is no perfusion.

Clinical Manifestations and Assessment

There is no heartbeat, no palpable pulse, and no respiration. Without immediate treatment, ventricular asystole is fatal.

ECG characteristics are:

Rate: Not measurable
Rhythm: Not measurable
P wave: Usually not visible
PR interval: Not measurable
QRS duration: Absent

See Figure 17-18.

Medical and Nursing Management

Asystole is treated by focusing on high-quality CPR with minimal interruptions and identifying underlying and contributing factors. The guidelines for advanced cardiac life support (AHA, 2015) state that the key to successful treatment is rapid assessment to identify a possible cause, which may be hypoxia, acidosis, severe electrolyte imbalance, drug overdose, hypovolemia, cardiac tamponade, tension pneumothorax, coronary or pulmonary thrombosis, trauma, or hypothermia. Because of the poor prognosis associated with asystole, if the patient does not respond to CPR, medical management, and other interventions aimed at correcting underlying causes, resuscitation efforts are usually ended ("the code is called") unless special circumstances (e.g., hypothermia, transportation to a hospital is required) exist.

PULSELESS ELECTRICAL ACTIVITY

In some situations, the patient may have an organized electrical rhythm visible on the monitor display but is unresponsive, not breathing, and pulseless. This is termed *pulseless electrical activity* (PEA) and is considered a cardiac arrest. The patient should receive immediate CPR and life support.

FIGURE 17-18 Asystole. Always check two different leads to confirm rhythm.

CONDUCTION ABNORMALITIES

AV blocks occur when the conduction of the impulse through the AV nodal area is decreased or stopped. These blocks can be caused by medications (e.g., digitalis, calcium-channel blockers, beta blockers), myocardial ischemia and infarction, valvular disorders, or myocarditis.

The clinical signs and symptoms of a heart block vary with the ventricular rate and the severity of any underlying disease processes. Whereas first-degree AV block rarely causes any hemodynamic effect, the other blocks may result in decreased heart rate, causing a reduction in perfusion to vital organs, such as the brain, heart, kidneys, lungs, and skin. A patient with third-degree AV block caused by digitalis toxicity may be stable; another patient with the same rhythm caused by acute MI may be unstable. Therefore the context and general condition of the patient are factors. Health care providers must always keep in mind the need to treat the patient, not the rhythm. The treatment is based on the hemodynamic effect of the rhythm.

FIRST-DEGREE ATRIOVENTRICULAR BLOCK

First-degree AV block occurs when atrial conduction is delayed through the AV node, resulting in a prolonged PR interval.

Pathophysiology

First-degree block may occur without an underlying pathophysiology or may be the result of medications such as beta blockers, calcium-channel blockers, or digoxin. It can also result from conditions that increase parasympathetic (vagal) tone, such as vomiting or Valsalva maneuver.

Clinical Manifestations and Assessment

The patient is usually asymptomatic.
ECG characteristics are:

Rate: Depends on underlying rhythm
Rhythm: Regular
P wave: Present before each QRS and consistent in size and shape
PR interval: Greater than 0.20 second
QRS duration: Normal

See Figure 17-19.

Medical and Nursing Management

The patient with first-degree AV block is only treated if symptoms related to bradycardia are present. If the AV block is new, the patient should be observed for potential progression to second-degree block.

FIGURE 17-19 First-degree AV block. Note the prolonged PR interval.

SECOND-DEGREE ATRIOVENTRICULAR BLOCK, TYPE I (WENCKEBACH)

Second-degree AV block, type I, occurs when there is a repeating pattern in which all but one of a series of atrial impulses are conducted through the AV node into the ventricles (e.g., every four of five atrial impulses are not conducted). Each atrial impulse takes a longer time for conduction than the one before, until one impulse is fully blocked, thus an increasing PR interval is seen with each successive beat until a P wave is seen without a resulting QRS. Because the AV node is not depolarized by the blocked atrial impulse, the AV node has time to fully repolarize so that the next atrial impulse can be conducted within the shortest amount of time.

Pathophysiology

Second-degree AV block, type I, is caused by a gradual and progressive conduction delay through the AV node. It may be related to increased parasympathetic (vagal) tone, ischemia, or medications that slow conduction, such as beta blockers, calcium-channel blockers, and digoxin.

Clinical Manifestations and Assessment

Signs and symptoms are related to bradycardia and may include chest discomfort, dyspnea, and hypotension.
ECG characteristics are:

Rate: Atrial rate faster than ventricular rate
Rhythm: The atrial rhythm is usually regular; the ventricular rhythm is usually irregular.
P wave: Size and shape normal
PR interval: PR interval becomes longer with each succeeding ECG complex until there is a P wave not followed by a QRS
QRS duration: Normal

See Figure 17-20.

Medical and Nursing Management

If the patient has symptomatic bradycardia, treatment with atropine or transcutaneous pacing is indicated.

FIGURE 17-20 Mobitz type I second-degree AV block (Wenckebach block). The PR intervals become progressively longer until one QRS complex is dropped.

SECOND-DEGREE ATRIOVENTRICULAR BLOCK, TYPE II

Second-degree AV block, type II, occurs when only some of the atrial impulses are conducted through the AV node into the ventricles. The ECG will reveal P waves not followed by a QRS. It is less common but more severe as it can progress to complete third-degree heart block.

Pathophysiology

Conduction is blocked below the AV node. It is caused by ischemia, usually due to blockage of the left coronary artery.

Clinical Manifestations and Assessment

Signs and symptoms are related to bradycardia and may include chest discomfort, dyspnea, and hypotension.

ECG characteristics are:

Rate: Atrial rate 60 to 100 bpm; ventricular rate less than atrial rate

Rhythm: Atrial rhythm is regular (constant PP interval); ventricular rhythm is irregular.

P wave: Normal

PR interval: Constant, no progressive prolongation with conducted beats

QRS duration: Normal or wide depending on the location of the block relative to the AV node

See Figure 17-21.

Medical and Nursing Management

If the patient has symptomatic bradycardia, treatment with atropine or pacing is indicated.

★ = nonconducted P-waves

FIGURE 17-21 Mobitz type II second-degree AV block. On this EKG, each third P wave is not followed by a QRS complex (dropped beat).

FIGURE 17-22 Third-degree AV block. The P waves appear at regular intervals, as do the QRS complexes, but they have nothing to do with one another. The QRS complexes are wide, implying a ventricular origin.

THIRD-DEGREE ATRIOVENTRICULAR BLOCK

Third-degree AV block occurs when no atrial impulse is conducted through the AV node into the ventricles. In third-degree AV block, two separate impulses stimulate the heart: one stimulates the atria, represented by the P wave, and one stimulates the ventricles, represented by the QRS complex, but there is no relationship or synchrony between the atrial and the ventricular contraction. Each is beating at its own inherent rate and independent of each other, thus the cardiac output is affected. P waves may be seen, but the atrial electrical activity is not conducted down into the ventricles. This is called *AV dissociation*.

Pathophysiology

Complete heart block is caused by injury to the conduction system so that there is no conduction between the atria and the ventricles.

Clinical Manifestations and Assessment

Signs and symptoms are related to bradycardia and may include syncope, chest discomfort, angina, dyspnea, and hypotension.

ECG characteristics are:

Rate: Atrial rate 60 to 100 bpm, ventricular rate 20 to 40 bpm
Rhythm: Atrial and ventricular rhythms are both regular but independent of each other.
P wave: Normal, more P waves than QRS complexes
PR interval: Not present; no relationship between the P wave and the R wave
QRS duration: Normal or wide depending on the location of the block relative to the AV node

See Figure 17-22.

Medical and Nursing Management

If the patient has symptomatic bradycardia, treatment with atropine or pacing is indicated.

NURSING PROCESS
The Patient with an Arrhythmia

ASSESSMENT

Major areas of assessment include possible causes of the arrhythmia, contributing factors, the associated risks, and the arrhythmia's effect on the heart's ability to pump an adequate blood volume.

A health history is obtained to identify any previous occurrences of possible decreased cardiac output, such as near-syncope or syncope (fainting), light-headedness, dizziness, fatigue, chest discomfort, shortness of breath, and/or palpitations. Comorbidities or coexisting conditions that could be a possible cause of the arrhythmia (e.g., heart disease, chronic obstructive pulmonary disease, pre-existing thyroid disease or Lyme disease) may also be identified. All medications, prescribed and over-the-counter, are reviewed. Laboratory results are reviewed to assess levels of medications, as well as factors that could contribute to the arrhythmia (e.g., anemia, hypokalemia, hypomagnesemia). A psychosocial assessment is performed to identify the possible effects of the arrhythmia, the patient's perception of the arrhythmia, and whether anxiety is a significant contributing factor.

During physical assessment, the nurse assesses the patient's skin, which may be pale and cool. Signs of fluid retention, such as neck vein distention and crackles and wheezes auscultated in the lungs, may be detected. The presence of peripheral edema is assessed as well as its extent and whether it is pitting or not. The rate and rhythm of apical and peripheral pulses are also assessed, and any pulse deficit (see Chapter 12) is noted. The nurse auscultates for extra heart sounds (especially S_3 and S_4) and for heart murmurs, evaluates blood pressure, and assesses the patient's usual versus current weight.

> **Nursing Alert**
> *Cardiac output is calculated as heart rate (HR) × stroke volume (SV). Stroke volume is the amount of blood ejected by the left ventricle*

with each contraction. If an arrhythmia occurs, the HR and SV can be affected, decreasing the filling times for the ventricle and, ultimately, causing a decreased cardiac output. The nurse is alert for patient complaints of dizziness, syncope, shortness of breath, peripheral edema, weight gain, crackles, fatigue, chest pain, or discomfort.

DIAGNOSIS

Appropriate nursing diagnoses of the patient with an arrhythmia may include:

- Cardiac output, decreased
- Anxiety related to fear of the unknown
- Knowledge deficit regarding the arrhythmia and its treatment

  Potential complications may include the following:

- Cardiac arrest (see Chapter 15)
- Heart failure (see Chapter 15)
- Thromboembolic event, especially with AF (see Chapter 15)

PLANNING

The major goals for the patient would include eliminating or decreasing the occurrence of the arrhythmia, minimizing anxiety, and acquiring knowledge about the arrhythmia and its treatment.

NURSING INTERVENTIONS

MONITORING AND MANAGING THE ARRHYTHMIA

The nurse regularly evaluates the patient's blood pressure, pulse rate and rhythm, rate and depth of respirations, breath sounds, and daily weights. The nurse also asks the patient about episodes of chest pain, syncope, light-headedness, dizziness, or fainting as part of the ongoing assessment as well as frequency of palpitations and overall level of fatigue. If a patient with an arrhythmia is hospitalized, the nurse may obtain a 12-lead ECG, continuously monitor the patient, and analyze rhythm strips to track and trend the arrhythmia. The patient should have vascular access and supplemental oxygen at the bedside.

The nurse assesses and observes for the beneficial and adverse effects of each antiarrhythmic medication. The nurse also manages medication administration carefully so that a constant serum blood level of the medication is maintained.

In addition to medication, the nurse assesses for factors that contribute to the arrhythmia, such as caffeine and stress, and assists the patient in developing a plan to make lifestyle changes that eliminate or reduce these factors.

MINIMIZING ANXIETY

When the patient experiences episodes of arrhythmia, the nurse maintains a calm and reassuring attitude. This assists in reducing anxiety (reducing the sympathetic response) and fosters a trusting relationship with the patient. In addition, the nurse can help the patient develop a system to identify possible causative,

influencing, and alleviating factors (e.g., keeping a diary). The nursing goal is to maximize the patient's control and to make the episode less threatening. In addition, involving family members can also be beneficial for the patient; the family can be involved in providing an educated support system and a plan of action if the patient experiences a hemodynamically unstable rhythm.

TEACHING PATIENTS SELF-CARE

The nurse explains the importance of maintaining therapeutic serum levels of antiarrhythmic medications so that the patient understands why medications should be taken regularly each day. If the patient has a potentially lethal arrhythmia, it is also important to establish with the patient and family a plan of action to take in case of an emergency. Family members should be encouraged to learn CPR as well as how to use an automated external defibrillator (AED). Occasionally patients wear a defibrillator vest to manage arrhythmias in the short term while allowing time to determine if the patient's cardiac output will improve post-MI or while trying to diagnose the cause of a clinically significant arrhythmia. This wearable defibrillator is worn only for a period of a few weeks to months, and then, depending on the patient's progress, the device is discontinued with no further device used or a permanent ICD is placed (discussed shortly) (Figs. 17-23 and 17-24). The patient and family should also be taught about potential effects or presentation of the arrhythmia and the signs and symptoms. This information allows the patient and family to feel more in control and better prepared for possible events.

(continued on page 522)

FIGURE 17-23 The implantable cardioverter defibrillator (ICD) consists of a generator and a sensing/pacing/defibrillating electrode.

FIGURE 17-24 The LifeVest is a wearable defibrillator. Unlike an implantable cardioverter defibrillator (ICD), the LifeVest is worn outside the body rather than implanted in the chest. This device continuously monitors the patient's heart with dry, nonadhesive sensing electrodes to detect life-threatening abnormal heart rhythms. If a life-threatening rhythm is detected, the device alerts the patient prior to delivering a treatment shock, and thus allows a conscious patient to delay the treatment shock. If the patient becomes unconscious, the device releases a Blue™ gel over the therapy electrodes and delivers an electrical shock to restore normal rhythm. Dry, non-adhesive sensing electrodes on this electrode belt continuously monitor patient's heart (**A**). This monitor is worn in a holster around the waist and collects ECG data from the sensing electrodes which can later be sent to a provider via modem (**B**).

CONTINUING CARE

Home care is warranted if the patient has significant comorbidities, socioeconomic issues, or limited self-management skills that could increase the risk for nonadherence to the therapeutic regimen.

EVALUATION

Expected patient outcomes may include:
1. Maintains cardiac output:
   a. Demonstrates heart rate, blood pressure, respiratory rate, and level of consciousness within normal ranges
   b. Demonstrates no or decreased episodes of arrhythmia
2. Experiences reduced anxiety:
   a. Expresses a positive attitude about living with the arrhythmia
   b. Expresses confidence in ability to take appropriate actions in an emergency

3. Expresses understanding of the arrhythmia and its treatment:
   a. Explains the arrhythmia and its effects
   b. Describes the medication regimen and its rationale
   c. Explains the need to maintain a therapeutic serum level of the medication
   d. Describes a plan to eliminate or limit factors that contribute to the arrhythmia
   e. States actions to take in the event of an emergency

ADJUNCTIVE MODALITIES AND MANAGEMENT

Acute arrhythmias may be treated with medications or with electrical therapy (emergency defibrillation, cardioversion, or pacing), or, in many cases, both are used concurrently and sequentially to prevent the occurrence of arrhythmias. Many antiarrhythmic medications are used to treat atrial and ventricular tachyarrhythmias. The choice of medication depends on the specific arrhythmia and its duration, the presence of heart failure and other diseases, and the patient's response to previous treatment. Electrical therapies include cardioversion and defibrillation for acute tachyarrhythmia, and implantable devices (pacemakers for bradycardias and implantable cardioverter defibrillator [ICD] for chronic tachyarrhythmias). These devices are often referred to as cardiovascular implantable electronic devices (CIEDs). Catheter ablation is also available depending on the type of arrhythmia. The nurse is responsible for assessing the patient's understanding of and response to therapy, as well as the patient's self-management abilities.

CARDIOVERSION AND DEFIBRILLATION

Cardioversion and defibrillation are used to treat tachyarrhythmias by delivering an electrical current that depolarizes a critical mass of myocardial cells. When the cells repolarize, the sinus node is usually able to recapture its role as the heart's pacemaker. One major difference between cardioversion and defibrillation is the timing of the delivery of electrical current. In cardioversion, the delivery of the electrical current is synchronized with the patient's intrinsic rhythm; in defibrillation, the delivery of the current is unsynchronized or delivered independent of the patient's intrinsic rhythm.

The electrical current may be delivered externally through the skin with the use of paddles or with electrode pads, or it may be delivered internally as part of open heart surgery. The paddles or pads may be placed on the front of the chest (Fig. 17-25) (standard paddle placement), or one paddle may be placed on the front of the chest and the other connected to an adapter with a long handle and placed under the patient's back (anteroposterior placement) (Fig. 17-26). Whether using pads or paddles, the nurse must observe two

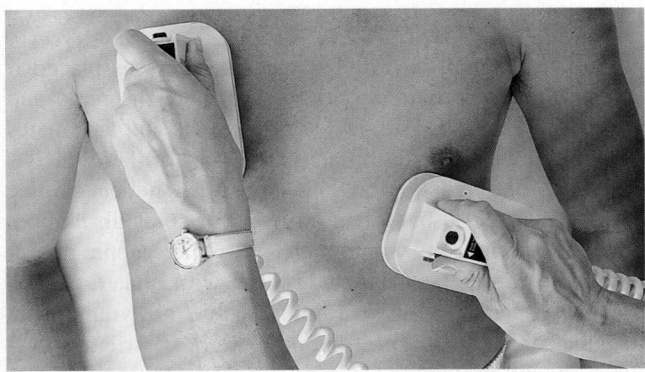

FIGURE 17-25 Standard paddle placement for defibrillation and for pads.

safety measures. First, good contact must be maintained between the pads or paddles and the patient's skin (with a conductive medium in between them) to prevent electrical current from leaking into the air (arcing) when the defibrillator is discharged. Second, no one is to be in contact with the patient or with anything that is touching the patient when the defibrillator is discharged, to minimize the chance that electrical current will be conducted to anyone other than the patient. Box 17-6 lists key points for assisting with cardioversion or defibrillation.

Nursing Alert

Two types of defibrillators are used today for external cardioversion and defibrillation: the older, monophasic sinusoidal waveform and the newer, biphasic truncated waveform. The new biphasic defibrillators use less energy to convert arrhythmias to normal sinus rhythm, which is a benefit. These defibrillators work through automatically adjusting to the patient's transthoracic impedance. The nurse understands that the amount of energy delivered to the heart is inversely related to transthoracic resistance so lowering the resistance helps to deliver optimal current to "shock" the heart. Refer to recommendations in Box 17-6 for further details.

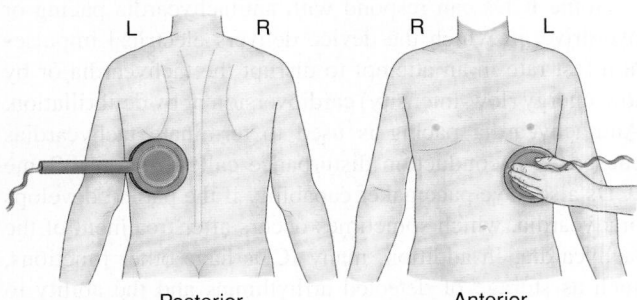

FIGURE 17-26 Anteroposterior paddle placement for defibrillation.

BOX 17-6

Assisting with External Cardioversion or Defibrillation

When assisting with external cardioversion or defibrillation, the nurse should remember these key points:

- Use multifunction conductor pads or paddles with a conducting medium between the paddles and the skin (the conducting medium is available as a sheet, gel, or paste). Do not use gels or pastes with poor electrical conductivity (e.g., ultrasound gel). Conductive electrode gel has been noted to reduce the transthoracic resistance by approximately 30% (Open Anesthesia, 2013).
- Place paddles or pads so that they do not touch the patient's clothing or bed linen and are not near medication patches or direct oxygen flow.
- If using paddles, exert 20–25 lb of pressure to ensure good skin contact. This lowers the transthoracic resistance.
- Before pressing the discharge button, call "Clear!" three times. Ensure that you and everyone else are not touching the patient, bed, or equipment. Perform a final visual check to ensure that you, and everyone else, are clear of the patient and anything touching the patient.
- Record the delivered energy.
- After the event is complete, inspect the skin under the pads or paddles for burns; if any are detected, consult with the physician or a wound care nurse about treatment.
- If cardioverting, ensure that the monitor leads are attached to the patient and that the defibrillator is in the synchronized mode ("sync"). If defibrillating, ensure that the defibrillator is not in the synchronized mode (most machines default to the "not-sync" mode).

Electrical Cardioversion

Electrical cardioversion involves the delivery of a "timed" electrical current to terminate a tachyarrhythmia. In cardioversion, the defibrillator is set to synchronize with the ECG on a cardiac monitor so that the electrical impulse discharges during ventricular depolarization (QRS complex). The synchronization prevents the discharge from occurring during the vulnerable period of repolarization (T wave), which could result in VT or ventricular fibrillation. When the synchronizer is on, no electrical current is delivered if the defibrillator does not discern a QRS complex. Because there may be a short delay until recognition of the QRS, the discharge buttons of an external defibrillator must be held down until the shock has been delivered.

If the cardioversion is elective and the arrhythmia has lasted longer than 48 hours, anticoagulation for a few weeks before cardioversion may be indicated. Digoxin is usually withheld for 48 hours before cardioversion to ensure the resumption of sinus rhythm with normal conduction. The patient is instructed not to eat or drink for at least 4 hours before the procedure. Before cardioversion, the patient receives IV moderate sedation as well as an analgesic medication or anesthesia. The amount of voltage used varies, depending on the defibrillator's technology and the type of arrhythmia.

> ⚠️ **Nursing Alert**
> *When the heart returns to a normal sinus rhythm after cardioversion, the atria beat forcefully. If a clot has formed in the atria, systemic emboli may result, thus anticoagulation is needed if the arrhythmia has lasted over 48 hours. The nurse is alert for systemic signs of embolization, such as sudden onset shortness of breath with pulmonary emboli or neurologic changes (visual, motor, sensory, headache, etc.; refer to Chapter 47) with cerebral emboli.*

Defibrillation

Defibrillation is used in emergency situations as the treatment of choice for ventricular fibrillation and pulseless VT. Defibrillation is not used on patients who are conscious or have a pulse. It has been established that early defibrillation is the major determinant of survival in cardiac arrest and is recommended in the guidelines as the first step when there is access to a defibrillator (AHA, 2015).

The electrical voltage required to defibrillate the heart is usually greater than that required for cardioversion and may cause more myocardial damage. Defibrillators are classified as monophasic or biphasic as discussed in the Alert. Monophasic defibrillators deliver current in only one direction and require increased energy loads; they are rarely used today. Newer biphasic defibrillators deliver the electrical charge to the positive paddle, which then reverses back to the originating paddle. The recommended energy levels for defibrillation vary according to the type of waveform and the manufacturer of the defibrillator. Following defibrillation, CPR is initiated immediately if a rhythm resulted that did not resume perfusion, and other advanced life support treatments are begun. This treatment with continuous CPR, medication administration, and defibrillation continues until a stable rhythm resumes or it is determined that the patient cannot be revived.

Often AEDs are used today by both laypersons and health care providers where the device once attached to the patient interprets the rhythm. Based on an algorithm when the patients' rhythm is determined to be "shockable," the defibrillator will guide the operator's or rescuer's action to discharge a shock. The AEDs are commonly placed in locations where large groups of people meet and/or in remote locations. They are often found in schools, airports, stadiums, on board aircraft, and in hospitals. The assignment of AEDs in the hospital setting makes sense to facilitate early rescue by providers who—although they are clinically oriented—are not necessarily proficient in interpreting arrhythmias due to infrequent occurrences of lethal arrhythmias, such as on a maternal child health unit.

Implantable Cardioverter Defibrillator

Often patients will have ICD/Pacemaker devices placed if they have tachyarrhythmias to manage both the rapid and slow rates. The ICD is a device that detects and terminates life-threatening episodes of tachycardia or fibrillation. ICDs are used for patients who have survived sudden cardiac death syndrome, usually caused by ventricular fibrillation, or have experienced symptomatic VT. Other people at risk of sudden cardiac death include those with dilated cardiomyopathy, hypertrophic cardiomyopathy, arrhythmogenic (capable of inducing an arrhythmia) right ventricular dysfunction, and prolonged QT syndrome. In addition, patients with moderate to severe left ventricular dysfunction, with a low ejection fraction (less than 30%), or with or without nonsustained VT are at high risk for cardiac arrest; therefore, prophylactic implantation may be indicated. ICDs may also be implanted in patients with symptomatic, recurrent, medication-refractory AF.

An ICD consists of a generator and at least one lead that can sense intrinsic electrical activity and deliver an electrical impulse. The device is usually implanted much like a pacemaker (Fig. 17-23). ICDs are designed to respond to two criteria: a rate that exceeds a predetermined level, and a change in the isoelectric line segments. When an arrhythmia occurs, the device automatically charges and delivers the programmed charge through the lead to the heart. ICD surveillance is similar to that of the pacemaker; however, it includes information about the number and frequency of shocks that have been delivered. Each device offers a different delivery sequence, but all are capable of delivering high-energy defibrillation to treat a tachycardia (atrial or ventricular). Antiarrhythmic medication usually is administered with this technology to minimize the occurrence of the tachyarrhythmia and to reduce the frequency of ICD discharge. In patients who have SVT, there is a choice between a single- and dual-chamber ICD dependent on the patient's clinical condition. The dual-chamber algorithm senses and interprets data from the atrium and ventricle to classify the rhythm and treat. However, early nonrandomized and small studies have not shown the dual chamber to be superior to single chamber at this time probably due to atrial sensing malfunctions (Madhavan & Friedman, 2013).

Some ICDs can respond with antitachycardia pacing or overdrive, in which the device delivers electrical impulses at a fast rate in an attempt to disrupt the tachycardia or by low-energy (low-intensity) cardioversion or by defibrillation. Antitachycardia pacing is used to terminate tachycardias caused by a conduction disturbance called *re-entry*. Some ICDs also have pacemaker capability if the patient develops bradycardia, which sometimes occurs after treatment of the tachycardia. In addition, many ICDs have other functions, such as storage of detected arrhythmias and the ability to perform electrophysiologic testing.

! Nursing Alert

Patients who have ICDs must take care when coming into contact with devices that have strong magnetic fields. These devices may interfere with ICD function especially with prolonged exposure.

It is important for the nurse to refer the patient to the AHA website: http://www.heart.org/ to learn more about the potential environmental issues associated with ICDs so that the patient can take the necessary precautions.

The primary complication associated with the ICD is surgery-related infection. A few complications are associated with the technical aspects of the equipment, such as premature battery depletion and dislodged or fractured leads. In original research by Stoier, Preben, and Berg (2013), the findings suggest that patients who receive an ICD as secondary prevention experience an increase in negative emotions to include sadness, disgust, anger, and surprise. Accordingly, the literature also suggests that more research and work need to be done in the area of communication with the patient about the ICD prior to implantation. Patient–provider communication about the ICD has been reported to be unclear with omission of information considered important to the patient, use of medical jargon, and lack of attention to the psychological burden of the device and the impact on patient's quality of life (Hauptman, Chibnall, Guild, & Armbrecht, 2013). Nurses should advocate for patients and their families to ensure that informed consent is achieved before implantation of an ICD.

Support may need to be provided to assist individuals with adjustment to the uncertainty and psychological distress related to ICD delivering a shock. In past research, inappropriate shocks occurred in 13% of ICD patients, usually due to misinterpretation of an SVT (vanRees et al., 2011). However, newer features in modern ICDs (e.g., antitachycardia pacing therapy) coupled with the broad goals of both preventing inappropriate shocks and delivering shocks for symptomatic ventricular arrhythmias are offering advances in providing medical devices safely to such patients (Rickard & Wilkoff, 2016). Patients who have ICDs are clinically monitored, and their devices can be interrogated remotely and in-person to program them to meet the specific clinical indications (Wilcoff et al., 2015).

Deactivation of the ICD at End of Life

When a patient is in the terminal phases of illness, the ICD is no longer an appropriate intervention in the management of clinical care, and thoughtful consideration is required of the deactivation plan. Ideally, the conversation regarding the ICD and the possible need to deactivate it in a terminal illness should be discussed before the device is even implanted in the patient. Guidelines or protocols are needed in the United States to provide both patients and providers with direction for management of this lifesaving device in the context of life-ending disease along with ethical and legal implications. Further, both pacemakers and ICDs should be considered fully as they relate to the end of life to then estimate the potential benefits and harm associated with the device while allowing death with dignity. Pacemakers are not as controversial because in contrast with the ICD, there are no associated painful discharges of shocks to treat an arrhythmia in a patient who is dying. Deactivation of an ICD would not cause the death of a patient; rather this will allow a natural death to occur. Nurses, along with the interdisciplinary team, will need to collaborate to address the ethical challenges associated with withdrawal of life-sustaining treatments, such as the CIEDs (Wiegand, MacMillan, Rogrigues dos Santos, & Bousso, 2015).

PACEMAKER THERAPY

A pacemaker is an electronic device that delivers electrical stimulation to the heart to regulate the heart rate when a patient has a slower-than-normal heart rate or conduction disturbance. They may also be used to control some tachyarrhythmias or to treat advanced heart failure that does not respond to medication. Pacemakers may be temporary or permanent. Temporary pacemakers may be transvenous, transcutaneous, or epicardial.

Pacemaker Design and Types

Pacemakers consist of two components: an electronic pulse generator and pacemaker electrodes, or leads. The generator contains the energy source that determines the rate (measured in bpm) and the strength or output (measured in milliamperes [mA]) of the electrical stimulus delivered to the heart. The generator can be programmed to detect the heart's intrinsic electrical activity and to cause an appropriate response; this component of pacing is called *sensitivity* and is measured in millivolts (mV). Leads can be threaded through a major vein into the right ventricle (endocardial leads), or they can be lightly sutured onto the outside of the heart and brought through the chest wall during open heart surgery (epicardial wires). The endocardial leads may be placed temporarily with catheters through a great vessel (transvenous wires), usually guided by fluoroscopy. The endocardial and epicardial wires are connected to a temporary external generator.

Endocardial leads may also be placed permanently, usually through the external jugular vein, and connected to a permanent generator. The generator is implanted in a subcutaneous pocket created in the pectoral region below the clavicle (Fig. 17-27). The procedure usually takes about 1 hour, and it is performed in a cardiac catheterization or EP laboratory using a local anesthetic. Batteries need replacement after approximately 10 years; and battery replacement is usually performed using a local anesthetic.

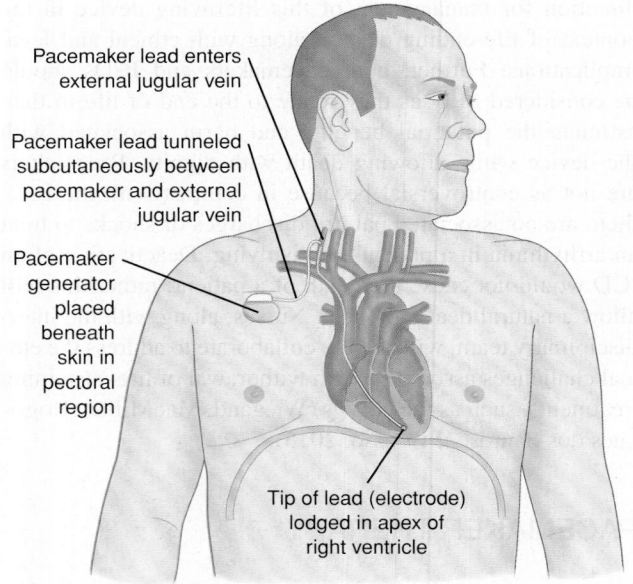

Pacemaker lead enters external jugular vein

Pacemaker lead tunneled subcutaneously between pacemaker and external jugular vein

Pacemaker generator placed beneath skin in pectoral region

Tip of lead (electrode) lodged in apex of right ventricle

FIGURE 17-27 Implanted transvenous pacing lead (with electrode) and pacemaker generator.

FIGURE 17-28 Transcutaneous pacemaker with electrode pads connected to the anterior and posterior chest walls.

If a patient suddenly develops a symptomatic bradycardia, emergency pacing may be started with transcutaneous pacing. Large pacing ECG electrodes (pads) are placed on the patient's chest and back. The electrodes are connected to the temporary pacemaker generator (Fig. 17-28). Because the impulse must travel through the patient's skin and tissue before reaching the heart, transcutaneous pacing can cause significant discomfort and is intended to be used only in emergencies. If the patient is alert, sedation and analgesia may be administered.

When pacing is initiated, the ECG tracing will display a straight vertical line, called a *pacemaker spike,* with each pacemaker impulse. The appropriate ECG complex should immediately follow the pacing spike; therefore, a P wave should follow an atrial pacing spike and a QRS complex should follow a ventricular pacing spike. Because the impulse

starts in a different place than the patient's normal rhythm, the QRS complex or P wave that responds to pacing looks different from the patient's normal ECG complex. *Capture* is a term used to denote that the appropriate complex followed the pacing spike (Fig. 17-29). *Synchronized biventricular pacing,* also called *cardiac resynchronized therapy* (CRT), has been found to modify the intraventricular, interventricular, and atrial-ventricular conduction defects identified with symptomatic moderate to severe (New York Heart Association Functional Class III and IV) left ventricular dysfunction and heart failure. The generator for biventricular pacing has three leads: one for the right atrium; one for the right ventricle, as with most standard pacemaker generators; and one for the left ventricle, usually placed in the left lateral wall. Studies have shown that this therapy improves cardiac function, resulting in decreased heart failure symptoms and an improved quality of life. The American College of Cardiology Foundation and the AHA developed four stages for HF, and it is at the level of stage B that a pacemaker or, in many cases, an ICD is recommended to prevent sudden cardiac death (Chapter 15 reviews the stages for HF).

FIGURE 17-29 Pacing with appropriate sensing (on-demand pacing) in lead V$_1$. *Arrows* denote pacing spike. Asterisk (*) denotes intrinsic (patient's own) beats, therefore no pacing.

Complications of Pacemaker Use

Complications associated with pacemakers relate to their presence within the body and improper functioning. The following complications may arise from a pacemaker:

- Local infection
- Bleeding and hematoma
- Hemothorax
- Ventricular ectopy and tachycardia
- Movement or dislocation of the lead placed
- Phrenic nerve stimulation (hiccuping may be a sign)
- Rarely, cardiac tamponade

In the initial hours after a temporary or permanent pacemaker is inserted, the most common complication is dislodgment of the pacing electrode. Minimizing patient activity can help prevent this complication. If a temporary electrode is in place, the extremity through which the catheter has been advanced is immobilized. With a permanent pacemaker, the patient is instructed initially to restrict activity on the side of the implantation for 2 to 4 weeks (Olshansky & Hayes, 2016).

The ECG is monitored very carefully to detect pacemaker malfunction. Improper pacemaker function, which can arise from failure in one or more components of the pacing system, is outlined in Table 17-4. Pacemaker settings (e.g., rate, energy output [mA], sensitivity [mV], and duration of interval between atrial and ventricular impulses [AV delay]) should be noted in the patient's record.

A patient experiencing pacemaker malfunction may develop bradycardia as well as signs and symptoms of decreased cardiac output. The degree to which these symptoms become apparent depends on the severity of the malfunction, the patient's level of dependency on the pacemaker, and the patient's underlying condition. Pacemaker malfunction is diagnosed by analyzing the ECG and through *interrogation* of the pacemaker's stored bank of activity, performed by trained personnel.

Inhibition of permanent pacemakers or reversion to asynchronous fixed rate pacing can occur with exposure to strong electromagnetic fields (electromagnetic interference [EMI]). However, recent pacemaker technology allows patients to safely use most household electronic appliances and devices (e.g., microwave ovens, electric tools). Objects that contain magnets (e.g., the earpiece of a phone; large stereo speakers; portable media players; magnet therapy products, such as mattresses, jewelry, and wraps) should not be near the generator for longer than a few seconds. Patients are advised to keep digital cellular phones at least 6 to 12 in away from (or on the side opposite of) the pacemaker generator and not to carry them in a shirt pocket.

Pacemaker Surveillance

Pacemaker clinics have been established to monitor patients and to test pulse generators for impending pacemaker battery failure. A computerized device is held over the generator to interrogate it with painless radio signals; it detects the generator's settings, battery status, pacing threshold, sensing function, lead integrity, and other stored information. Several factors, such as lead fracture, muscle inhibition, and insulation disruption, also may be assessed. If indicated,

TABLE 17-4 Assessing Pacemaker Malfunction/Complications

Problem	Possible Cause	Intervention
Failure to pace; the pacemaker fails to deliver the correct number of electrical stimuli per minute	Output failure—oversensing and undersensing Battery failure Loose connection between lead wire and generator Fracture or displacement of pacing lead wire Pulse generator failure Electromagnetic interference (Potential causes of EMI include use of the TENS unit, electroconvulsive therapy, and monopolar electrocautery) Sensitivity setting too high Lead displacement	Replace the pulse generator battery Tighten the connections between pacing lead and pulse generator Replace the lead wire Replace pulse generator unit Remove the source of electromagnetic interference or moderate it if possible. Check with pacemaker manufacturer. Adjust sensitivity setting Adjust lead May require programming adjustment
Failure to capture; the pacemaker does not depolarize the heart	Battery failure Fracture or displacement of pacing lead wire Perforation of the myocardium by the lead wire Scar tissue or edema formation at lead tip Energy output (mA) too low Increase in stimulation threshold due to medication Electrolyte imbalance Myocardial Infarction	Replace battery Reposition patient; Replace the lead wire Surgical repair Replace pacing lead Increase the output (mA) Increase the output (mA) Correct electrolyte imbalances May require programming adjustment

EMI, electromechanical interference; TENS, transcutaneous electrical nerve stimulation; mA, miliamperage.
Neelankavil et al., 2013.

the pacemaker is turned off for a few seconds, using a magnet or a programmer, while the ECG is recorded to assess the patient's underlying cardiac rhythm. Changes may be made in the programming of the pacemaker or ICD prior to surgery or procedures where the device may need to be adjusted. Therefore, it is very important that the perioperative team is made aware of the device that the patient has implanted. In addition, it is important to have a list of manufacturer contacts should there be an emergent need requiring technical support. Transtelephonic transmission of the generator's information is another follow-up method. Special equipment is used to transmit information about the patient's pacemaker over the telephone to a receiving system at a pacemaker clinic. The information is converted into tones; equipment at the clinic converts these tones to an electronic signal and records them on an ECG strip. The pacemaker rate and other data concerning pacemaker function are obtained and evaluated by a cardiologist. This simplifies the diagnosis of a failing generator, reassures the patient, and improves management when the patient is physically remote from pacemaker testing facilities.

ELECTROPHYSIOLOGIC STUDIES

An EP study is a minimally invasive procedure used to evaluate and treat significant arrhythmias. It also is indicated for patients with symptoms that suggest an arrhythmia that has gone undetected and undiagnosed by other methods. An EP study is used to do the following:

- Identify the impulse formation and propagation through the cardiac electrical conduction system
- Assess the function or dysfunction of the SA and AV nodal areas
- Identify the location (called *mapping*) and mechanism of dysrhythmogenic foci
- Assess the effectiveness of antiarrhythmic medications and devices for the patient with an arrhythmia
- Treat certain arrhythmias through the destruction of the causative cells (**ablation**)

An EP procedure is a type of cardiac catheterization that is performed in a specially equipped cardiac catheterization laboratory by an electrophysiologist. One of the main purposes of programmed stimulation is to assess the ability of the area of the myocardium to cause an arrhythmia. If the arrhythmia can be reproduced by programmed stimulation, it is called *inducible*. Once an arrhythmia is induced, a treatment plan is determined and implemented. If, on the follow-up EP study, the tachyarrhythmia cannot be induced, then the treatment is determined to be effective. Different medications may be administered and combined with electrical devices (pacemaker, ICD) to determine the most effective treatment to suppress the arrhythmia.

Patient care, patient teaching, and associated complications of an EP study are the same as those associated with cardiac catheterization (see Chapter 14). The study is usually about 2 hours in length; however, if the electrophysiologist conducts not only a diagnostic procedure but also treatment, the study can take up to 8 hours.

Patients who are to undergo an EP study may be anxious about the procedure and its outcome. Before the procedure, the patient should receive instructions, including its usual duration, the environment where the procedure is performed, and what to expect. Although an EP study is not painful, it does cause discomfort and can be tiring. It may also cause feelings that were experienced when the arrhythmia occurred in the past. In addition, the nurse should prepare the patient for the procedure and what will be expected of him or her (e.g., lying very still during the procedure, reporting symptoms or concerns, etc.).

The patient should also know that the arrhythmia may occur during the procedure. It often stops on its own; if it does not, treatment is given to restore the patient's normal rhythm. The arrhythmia may have to be terminated using cardioversion or defibrillation, but this is performed under more controlled circumstances than if performed in an emergency. Postprocedural care is similar to that for cardiac catheterization.

CARDIAC CONDUCTION SURGERY

Atrial tachycardias and VTs that do not respond to medications and are not suitable for antitachycardia pacing may be treated by methods that include a maze procedure and ablation. The *maze procedure* is an open heart surgical procedure for refractory AF. Sometimes, it is referred to as a Cox procedure or a mini-maze. The surgeon will ablate and/or use small incisions to create nonconducting scar tissue to stop the arrhythmia. This procedure is sometimes done together with an EP procedure or done when a patient is having another surgery such as a CABG or with valve replacement.

Catheter ablation done by radiofrequency destroys specific cells that are the cause or central conduction route of a tachyarrhythmia. It is performed with or after an EP study. Usual indications for ablation are recurrent atrial arrhythmias or VT unresponsive to previous therapy (or for which the therapy produced significant side effects). In addition to the standard catheter radiofrequency ablation, as mentioned earlier in the chapter, cryoablation is a newer type of treatment where the cardiac tissue is frozen, usually in the area of the pulmonary arteries. It often can be done faster since the tissue is frozen in a circle with the end of the catheter all at one time, discontinuing the arrhythmia. This is becoming a safe and effective alternative to radiofrequency ablation.

CHAPTER REVIEW

Critical Thinking Exercises

1. You are caring for a 79-year-old woman who was admitted for control of heart failure 3 days ago. Today, her telemetry monitor alarmed and displayed a new sustained tachycardia with a wide QRS (0.14 second). What are some of the possible causes of this arrhythmia? Identify some of the key factors that would need to be included in your assessment to assist in identification of the arrhythmia. What nursing interventions are needed?

2. You are caring for a 40-year-old man who recently had a pacemaker inserted, with the rate set at 72 bpm. When taking his pulse, you note that his heart rate is 66 bpm. Describe the possible causes of this difference in heart rates and the nursing actions that are needed.

3. The wife of this same patient tells you that her husband has informed her that now he has a pacemaker, they must get rid of their microwave oven and that he can no longer speak on the cell phone. What would you say to the wife? How would you discuss this with the patient? What other education would you provide to this patient and his wife about safety in relation to the pacemaker? What is the evidence base that supports this education? Discuss the strength of the evidence and the criteria used to evaluate the strength of the evidence.

NCLEX-Style Review Questions

1. In interpreting a patient's rhythm strip, the nurse is most concerned with which of the finding?
   a. A PR interval of 0.22 second
   b. Progressively lengthening PR interval
   c. A premature and short PR interval
   d. A PR interval of 0.10 second

2. The nurse is observing the central monitoring station and notes the following rhythm alarms. Which alarm should the nurse respond to first?
   a. Atrial fibrillation rate of 90
   b. First-degree heart block, rate of 80

c. Ventricular tachycardia (monomorphic)
   d. Torsade des pointes (polymorphic)

3. A patient presents to the emergency room in atrial fibrillation. The nurse understands that the treatment plan for this patient will be determined based on which factor?
   a. Whether or not the patient has a "do not resuscitate" prescription
   b. How long the patient has been in atrial fibrillation
   c. The number of episodes of atrial fibrillation the patient has experienced in the past year
   d. The rate of atrial contractions

4. The nurse notes a new wide complex tachycardia on the telemetry monitor. Upon assessing the patient, the nurse finds the patient cannot be aroused and has gasping respirations. The nurse's next action is to:
   a. Call a code
   b. Notify the provider stat
   c. Document the findings in the telemetry record
   d. Defibrillate the patient at 100 J

5. The nurse notes that a patient has a new second-degree type I block (Wenckebach). The patient denies chest pain or other symptoms, and the patient's blood pressure is 90/60. After paging the provider stat, what intervention would the nurse perform first?
   a. Apply oxygen, assess IV access, bring the portable monitor/external pacemaker to the bedside
   b. Administer nitroglycerin as ordered p.r.n. for chest discomfort and obtain a 12-lead ECG
   c. Call for stat labs to be drawn and prepare the patient for surgical pacemaker implantation
   d. Ask the nurse's aide to stay with the patient and monitor the blood pressure every 5 minutes

Try these additional resources, available at **http://thepoint.lww.com/Honan2e,** to enhance your learning and understanding of this chapter:
- NCLEX-Style Student Review Questions
- Journal Articles

REFERENCES AND SELECTED READINGS
References and selected readings associated with this chapter can be found on the website that accompanies the book. Visit **http://thepoint. lww.com/Honan2e** to access the references and other additional resources associated with this chapter.

Nursing Management: Patients with Vascular Disorders and Problems of Peripheral Circulation

Mary Sieggreen

Learning Objectives

After reading this chapter, you will be able to:

1. Identify factors that affect peripheral blood flow and tissue oxygenation.
2. Identify clinical manifestations, management, and prevention of arterial disorders.
3. Describe prevention and management of deep venous thrombosis.
4. Describe medical and nursing management of venous and arterial ulcers.
5. Describe nursing management of lymphedema.

Conditions of the vascular system include arterial disorders, venous disorders, lymphatic disorders, and cellulitis. Nursing management depends on an understanding of the structure and function of the vascular and lymphatic systems.

Intact, patent, and responsive blood vessels are necessary to deliver adequate amounts of oxygen to tissues and to remove metabolic wastes. Reduced blood flow through blood vessels characterizes all peripheral vascular diseases (PVDs). Perfusion is about supply versus demand. If tissue needs are high, even modestly reduced blood flow may be inadequate to maintain tissue integrity. When arterial blood flow decreases, ischemia follows, and tissues become malnourished and, ultimately, die unless blood flow is restored. Thus, the effect of decreased blood flow depends on the extent to which tissue demands exceed the supply of oxygen.

Nurses are in key positions to help patients with vascular disorders learn about the disease and their personal risk factors. Learning to modify the risk factors and manage their disorders may increase the lifespan of patients with vascular disorders.

ARTERIAL DISORDERS

Arteries become damaged or obstructed as a result of atherosclerotic plaque, thromboemboli, chemical or mechanical trauma, infections or inflammatory processes, vasospastic disorders, and congenital malformations. A sudden arterial occlusion causes profound and often irreversible tissue ischemia and tissue death. When arterial occlusions develop gradually, there is less risk of sudden tissue death because **collateral** circulation may develop (the rerouting of blood vessels, in which new blood vessels join to take over some of the circulation of blocked vessels), giving that tissue the opportunity to adapt to gradually decreased blood flow. However, over time, continued decreased perfusion results in ischemia and tissue death (Treat-Jacobson, 2014).

PERIPHERAL ARTERIAL DISEASE

Peripheral artery disease (PAD) refers to any disease process that affects the arteries. Various PADs result in ischemia and produce the signs and symptoms described in Box 18-1. The type and severity of symptoms depend in part on the type, stage, and extent of the disease process and on the speed with which the disorder develops. Arterial insufficiency of the extremities is a common cause of disability. Frequently the legs are affected more than the upper extremities.

Clinical recognition of PAD varies in individuals; it is a slow process that begins in early adulthood and increases with age. PAD is one manifestation of **atherosclerosis**, thus systemic diseases that affect arteries of the brain, heart, kidneys, mesentery, and limbs should be suspected. Over one third of patients with PAD have significant coronary disease, and up to one quarter have carotid artery disease (White, 2016). Patients with PAD have an increased risk of mortality, myocardial infarction (MI), and cerebrovascular disease. Many patients with PAD are not receiving any treatment for their

Focused Assessment

Lower Extremity Peripheral Arterial Disease

Be alert for the following signs and symptoms:

- Structural changes, resulting from chronic lack of oxygen and nutrient delivery to the tissues:
  - Hair loss distal to the occlusion
  - Thick, opaque nails; shiny, dry skin
  - Skeletal muscle atrophy
- Skin color changes:
  - Elevational pallor
  - Dependent rubor (red color when limb dependent from dilated damaged vessels)
- Pulse changes:
  - Pulses diminished or absent below area of stenosis/obstruction-pedal, posterior tibial, popliteal, femoral
  - Cool extremity distal to occlusion
- Sensation changes:
  - Paresthesias
  - Numbness
  - Tingling of extremities
- Ulcers or gangrene (traumatic or spontaneous on onset) located at tips of toes, between toes, over areas of pressure, such as the heel, or areas susceptible to trauma like the shin; defined punched out (circular), necrotic/yellow ulcer base, dry, pale in appearance; usually very painful; poor healing of injuries on the extremities.
- Edema, although frequently absent, may be present and related to dependency

disease because they do not realize they have the condition (Naito et al., 2016).

Pathophysiology

As the lumen narrows and blood flow decreases, ischemia occurs, progressing to infarction in the distal tissues. In PAD, obstructive lesions are predominantly confined to segments of the arterial system extending from the aorta below the renal arteries to the popliteal artery. Distal occlusive disease is frequently seen in patients with diabetes mellitus and in the elderly.

Arteriosclerosis, the most common disease of the arteries, is a diffuse process whereby muscle fibers and endothelial linings of the walls of small arteries and arterioles become thickened. Atherosclerosis involves changes of the intima consisting of accumulation of lipids, calcium, blood components, complex carbohydrates, and fibrous tissue, referred to as *atheromas* or *plaques*. Atherosclerosis causes arterial **stenosis**, obstruction by thrombosis, **aneurysm**, ulceration, and vessel rupture.

Arterial bifurcations are more vulnerable to atherosclerosis than other areas of the arteries (Fig. 18-1). These include the distal abdominal aorta; the common iliac arteries; the orifice of the superficial femoral and *profunda femoris* arteries;

the superficial femoral artery in the adductor canal, which is particularly narrow; and anywhere along the arteries distal to the knee. Gradual narrowing of the arterial lumen stimulates the development of collateral circulation (Fig. 18-2) from pre-existing vessels.

Risk Factors

Risk factors for developing PAD are similar to those for developing coronary artery disease (Eraso et al., 2014) (Box 18-2). The age of onset and disease severity are influenced by the type and number of atherosclerotic risk factors. Risk factors include modifiable (e.g., diet, smoking) and non-modifiable (e.g., race and age) factors. Evidence indicates modification may slow the disease process. Of those that can be modified, tobacco use is one of the most important in atherosclerotic lesion development. Nicotine decreases blood flow, increases heart rate and blood pressure, and increases the risk for clot formation by increasing platelet aggregation. According to research findings (Lu, Mackay, & Pell, 2013), smokers have a three- to fivefold increased risk of developing PAD compared to nonsmokers.

Hyperhomocysteinemia is considered an independent risk factor for atherosclerosis (Brunelli, Fusco, Iosa, Ricciardi, & Traballesi, 2015). Homocysteine is a protein that promotes coagulation. Elevated homocysteine levels are associated with genetic factors and a diet low in folic acid, vitamin B_6, and vitamin B_{12}. Treatment includes intake of vitamins B_6, B_{12}, and folate, which often lowers homocysteine levels (refer to Chapter 12 for more details on homocysteine levels). In addition, since inflammation plays a fundamental role in the development and progression of atherosclerosis, elevated levels of C-reactive protein (CRP) are strongly associated with the development of PAD (White, 2016).

Hypertension also accelerates the rate at which atherosclerotic lesions form in high-pressure vessels and, therefore, is a major PAD risk factor. Patients with diabetes have about seven to fifteen times the amputation rate of those without diabetes. Therefore, tight control of diabetes is important; the risk of developing PAD increases by 28% for every 1% increase in glycosylated hemoglobin (White, 2016). Obesity, stress, and lack of exercise also have been identified as contributing to the disease process.

Clinical Manifestations and Assessment

Most patients with PAD are initially asymptomatic. Studies have demonstrated that for every patient who has symptomatic disease, approximately three to four patients have no symptoms (Eraso et al., 2014).

Approximately 1% to 5% of patients with PAD have **critical limb ischemia** (CLI), with chronic ischemic pain at rest (rest pain), nonhealing, ulcers, or gangrene. A small number of patients with PAD have **acute limb ischemia** (ALI), a sudden decrease in limb perfusion, most commonly caused by

Right common carotid

Vertebral

Right subclavian

Aortic arch

Celiac trunk

Right renal

Superior mesenteric

Internal iliac

Common femoral

Deep femoral

Superficial femoral

Anterior tibial

Posterior tibial

Left common iliac

Popliteal

FIGURE 18-1 Common sites of atherosclerotic obstruction in major arteries.

Anterior cerebral

Middle cerebral

Posterior cerebral

Internal carotid

Anterior spinal

External carotid

Vertebral

Common carotid

Left subclavian

Posterior communicating

Basilar

Aortic arch

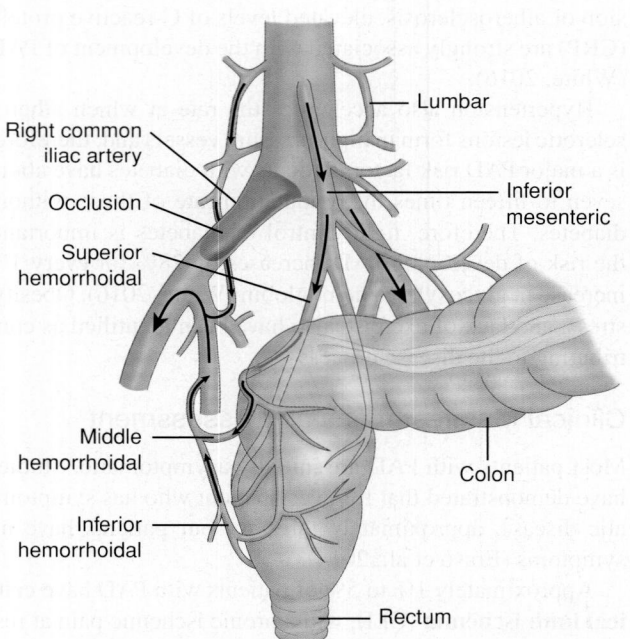

Lumbar

Right common iliac artery

Occlusion

Superior hemorrhoidal

Inferior mesenteric

Middle hemorrhoidal

Colon

Inferior hemorrhoidal

Rectum

FIGURE 18-2 Development of channels for collateral blood flow in response to occlusion of the right common iliac artery and the terminal aortic bifurcation.

either thrombosis or embolism, that produces new or worsening symptoms that may threaten limb viability. Other potential causes of acute arterial occlusion include atherosclerotic stenosis, aneurysm, arterial dissection, arterial embolization, cardiac embolization, trauma (blunt injuries, fractures), tumor compression, graft thrombosis, drug abuse, low cardiac

---

BOX 18-2

Risk Factors for Peripheral Arterial Disease (PAD)

- Family history
- Age (14.5% of adults over 70 years of age have PAD) (White, 2016)
- Obesity
- Smoking
- Pre-existing health conditions:
  - Coronary artery disease
  - Cerebral artery disease
  - Diabetes
  - Hypertension
  - Dyslipidemia
  - Clotting disorders
  - Hyperhomocysteinemia

output, phlegmasia cerulea dolens (massive iliofemoral venous thrombosis), and compartment syndrome. Box 18-3 summarizes clinical manifestations of acute arterial occlusion.

Nursing Alert
In patients with CLI, minor trauma from poorly fitting shoes or carelessly clipped toenails can cause a nonhealing wound or infection that can progress to amputation.

Clinical signs and symptoms resulting from atherosclerosis are manifested in the end organ supplied by arterial blood flow. Patients complain of pain in the fingers or feet or pain in muscle groups with use (not the joints). Walking causes pain in the leg muscles, and upper extremity physical activity causes pain in the arm muscles. A description of pain and its precipitating factors, assessment of skin color and temperature, and peripheral pulse presence and character are important assessment parameters in the diagnosis of arterial disorders.

Pain

The hallmark symptom for PAD in the lower extremity is **intermittent claudication** (Box 18-4). This pain may be

described as aching or cramping in a muscle that occurs with the same degree of exercise or activity and is relieved with rest. Intermittent claudication is caused by the inability of the arterial system to provide adequate blood flow to the tissues in the face of increased demand for nutrients and oxygen during exercise. As the tissues are forced to complete the energy cycle without adequate nutrients and oxygen, muscle metabolites and lactic acid are produced. Pain is experienced as the metabolites aggravate the nerve endings of the surrounding tissue. When the patient stops muscle activity and thereby decreases the metabolic needs of the muscles, the pain subsides. If the patient must sit to relieve lower extremity pain, the pain may be caused by a nerve injury to the back or another noncirculatory etiology. Progression of arterial disease can be monitored by documenting the ambulatory distance before pain is felt. Because the pain is associated with decreased perfusion, it is important to determine that the pain is reproducible from one day to the next on similar terrain.

The location of disease within the arterial system can be determined by the location of claudication symptoms because pain occurs in muscle groups distal to the diseased vessel. Calf pain may accompany reduced blood flow through the superficial femoral or popliteal artery, whereas pain in the hip or buttock may result from reduced blood flow in the abdominal aorta or the common iliac or hypogastric arteries. Persistent pain in the anterior portion of the foot when the patient is resting indicates a severe degree of arterial insufficiency and a critical state of ischemia. Known as **rest pain**, this discomfort is often worse at night and may interfere with sleep. This pain frequently requires the extremity be lowered to a dependent position to improve perfusion to the distal tissues. The dependent position of the lower extremity may cause edema in the leg and foot, thus edema may be associated with PAD. Rest pain is associated with limb-threatening ischemia. Refer to Table 18-1 for information on how to differentiate claudication from other causes.

Upper extremity atherosclerotic stenosis may cause arm fatigue and pain with exercise (forearm claudication) and inability to hold or grasp objects (e.g., painting, combing hair, placing objects on shelves above the head).

Changes in Skin Appearance and Temperature

Inadequate blood flow results in cool and pale extremities. Further reduction of blood flow to the tissues, which occurs when the extremity is elevated, for example, results in an even whiter or more blanched appearance to the skin compared to the contralateral limb. When the extremity is placed in a dependent position after elevation, it becomes a reddish-blue color called **rubor**. This color change suggests severe peripheral arterial damage, in which vessels that cannot constrict remain dilated. *Cyanosis*, a bluish tint of the skin, is manifested when the amount of oxygenated hemoglobin contained in the blood is reduced. Skin color changes

TABLE **18-1** Differentiation of Claudication from Other Disorders in the Lower Extremities

	Intermittent Claudication	Spinal Stenosis	Arthritis	Venous Congestion	Compartment Syndrome
Character	Aching, cramping	Same as claudication or tingling, weakness, clumsiness	Aching	Tightness	Tightness, tense
Location	Dependent on area of obstruction: buttock, hip, thigh, calf, foot	Buttock, hip, thigh	Hip, thigh, knee	Groin, thigh	Dependent on area of high pressure; frequently the tibia, however can occur in foot, thigh, gluteal region
Response to exercise	Yes	Variable	Variable	After walking	Can occur because of inordinate stress or exercise
Response to walking	Reproducible	Variable	Variable	Variable	Excessive exercise
Relief of discomfort	Relief with cessation of muscle activity	Relief with sitting or changing position	Slow relief with avoidance of weight bearing	Slow relief with leg elevation	Unrelieved
Other	Associated with atherosclerosis and decreased pulses	History of back problems	Discomfort at the joints	History of deep vein thrombosis, signs of venous congestion; edema	Seen in athletes May occur with trauma

Adapted from White, C. J. (2016). Atherosclerotic peripheral arterial disease. In L. Goldman, A. I., Schafer Al (Eds.), *Goldman-Cecil Medicine* (25th ed.). Philadelphia, PA: Elsevier, Saunders.

may be more subtle in darkly pigmented individuals. Comparing the contralateral limb is the best way to discern color changes. Capillary refill time (CRT) is frequently used as an assessment of peripheral perfusion. The nurse depresses the nail bed of the finger or toe between his or her fingers until it blanches. After releasing the pressure, the skin color in normal tissue is expected to return in fewer than 2 seconds. However, recent research findings call into question the efficacy of this test in assessing circulatory volume because of poor agreement among observers. The nurse considers this test not as a definitive marker for impaired perfusion but rather as an adjunctive tool to consider when clustering other manifestations of peripheral perfusion.

Additional changes resulting from a chronically reduced nutrient supply include loss of hair; brittle nails; dry, shiny, or scaling skin; atrophy; and ulcerations. Skin and nail changes, ulcers, gangrene, and muscle atrophy may be evident in chronic arterial disease but cannot be relied on for diagnosis of acute arterial insufficiency.

Pulses

Unequal pulses between extremities or the absence of a normally palpable pulse is a sign of PAD. Palpation of pulses (Fig. 18-3) is subjective. Box 18-5 provides tips for palpating pulses. The presence of foot pulses does not exclude the possibility of PAD, and further investigation is required in the presence of leg pain. After exercise, the pulses may not be palpable. This is known as "disappearing pulses," and it is caused by the increased need for blood flow in the working muscle, which the arteries cannot provide. This change in pulses is reproducible and is consistent with the distance the patient walks before experiencing claudication. **Bruits** may be auscultated with a stethoscope just distal to an arterial stenosis, indicating turbulent blood flow that occurs with vessel stenosis (Sieggreen & Walsh, 2014).

Ankle-brachial Index

The presence of PAD is defined as an ankle-brachial index (ABI) of less than 0.90. ABI is calculated as the ratio of the systolic blood pressure in the ankle divided by the higher of the two brachial systolic blood pressures (see Chapter 12).

Sensory changes

Numbness, paresthesias, and motor deficits indicate tissue anoxia. Motor deficits typically progress from distal to proximal; therefore, the nurse assesses initially for weakness of

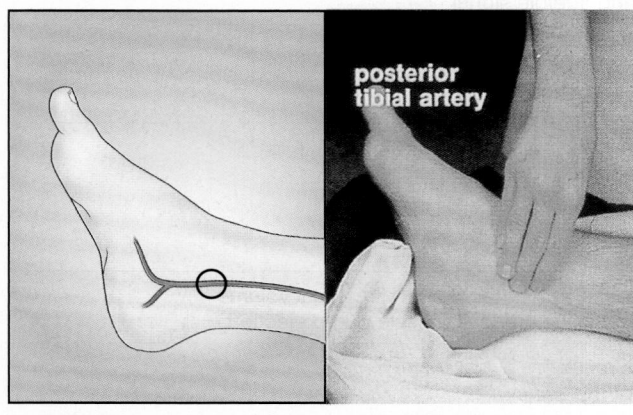

FIGURE 18-3 Assessing peripheral pulses. (*Left*) Popliteal pulse. (*Right*) Dorsalis pedis pulse. (*Bottom*) Posterior tibial pulse.

the foot muscles. In contrast, paresthesia denotes ischemia that threatens limb survival.

Nursing Alert

The nurse is aware that in the event of acute occlusion of arterial circulation, symptoms will include pain, pallor, poikilothermia (coldness), paresthesias, delayed capillary refill, cyanosis, and decreased or absent pulses. With chronic arterial disease, the nurse expects to see hair loss, thickened nails, and smooth and shiny skin.

BOX 18-5   Tips for Palpating Peripheral Pulses

- Use tips of fingers to palpate. To avoid mistaking your own pulse for that of the patient, use light touch and avoid using only the index finger for palpation because this finger has the strongest arterial pulsation of all the fingers. The thumb should not be used for the same reason.
- Palpate bilaterally and simultaneously.
- Compare both sides for symmetry in rate, rhythm, and quality (the nurse should grade according to the institution's/facility's scale).
- Document as present, absent, or bounding (Ex. aneurysm).

Diagnostic Tests

Various noninvasive and invasive tests are performed to diagnose abnormalities that affect the arteries. When pulses cannot be palpated reliably, a handheld continuous wave (CW) Doppler ultrasound device may be used to hear (*insonate*) signals in the vessels (Fig. 18-4). The Doppler emits a signal through the tissues, which is reflected off the moving blood

FIGURE 18-4 Continuous-wave (CW) Doppler ultrasound detects blood flow in peripheral vessels (demonstrated in obtaining ABI).

TABLE 18-2 Noninvasive and Invasive Vascular Tests

Test	Purpose
Doppler Ultrasound Flow Studies	Evaluation of arterial signals Blood pressure measurement in the limbs Assessment of vessel size and compressibility Assessment for presence of thrombus Assessment of valve function
Exercise Testing	Assessment of ankle systolic blood pressure in response to walking on treadmill (normal response is little or no drop in ankle systolic pressure after exercise) Assessment for claudication (a drop in ankle pressure correlates with claudication distance reported by the patient)
Duplex Ultrasonography	Localization of vascular obstruction Evaluation of stenosis Assessment for vascular reflux Provides both image and audible signal
Computed Tomography Angiography (CTA) (spiral or helical CT that provides a series of images in continuous spiral)	Demonstration of cross-sectional images of soft tissue Diagnoses of abdominal aneurysms, graft infections or occlusions, hemorrhage
Magnetic Resonance Angiography (MRA) (standard magnetic resonance imaging [MRI] scanner with software programmed to isolate blood vessels and reassemble images in three dimensions)	Detection of changes, aneurysms, DVT Useful in poor kidney function or contrast agent allergy
Air Plethysmography	Measurement of volume, ejection fraction, and residual volume Quantification of venous reflux and calf muscle pump ejection
Venous Duplex	Assessment of venous reflux Manual compression of the veins
Angiography	Confirmation of occlusive arterial disease when considering interventions Patient may report sensation of warmth during injection and may have immediate or delayed allergic reaction to the iodine in the contrast agent Digital subtraction angiography (DSA) has bony structures removed from the image
Venography	Radiopaque contrast agent injected into the venous system produces an image showing unfilled segment of vein Used to outline vein for thrombolytic therapy Infrequently used (duplex ultrasound is standard for diagnosing venous thrombosis)
Vascular Endoscopy (Angioscopy)	Use of fiber optics to visualize the vessel lumen Used to identify plaque, thrombus, hemorrhage, ulcers Used to remove debris or remove venous valves

cells and returned to the device. Then the filtered output Doppler signal is transmitted to a loudspeaker or headphones, where it can be heard for interpretation. Doppler studies are more useful when combined with the **ankle-brachial index (ABI)**. (Chapter 12 provides detailed discussion of Doppler, ultrasound, and ABI.) The "gold standard" for diagnosis and evaluation of PAD is the invasive digital angiography (White, 2016). Additional diagnostic tools are discussed in Table 18-2.

Medical Management

Medical management is aimed at reducing the patient's risk for life-threatening complications of atherosclerosis; improving walking distance; and salvaging the limb, which includes the use of exercise, pharmacologic treatment, risk factor modification (control of hypertension, hypercholesterolemia, and diabetes, and cessation of smoking), and invasive options. Revascularization is recommended if there is a reasonable likelihood of symptomatic improvement and there has been an inadequate response to pharmacologic or exercise therapy. Invasive methods include surgery and percutaneous endoscopic procedures.

Management of Intermittent Claudication

Treatment goals for patients with intermittent claudication are to relieve symptoms, improve exercise performance, and improve functional abilities. In general, patients with intermittent claudication feel better when on an exercise program. Initial treatment should be focused on a structured exercise program and pharmacotherapy. Patients are advised to "walk into the pain" of claudication, pause until the pain subsides, and continue walking. If this program is combined with weight reduction and tobacco cessation, patients may improve their activity tolerance and experience pain relief without further intervention.

Pharmacologic Therapy

Cilostazol is a phosphodiesterase III inhibitor that is a vasodilator and interferes with platelet aggregation. It is prescribed in combination with an exercise program to improve walking distance (U.S. National Library of Medicine, 2015). Guidelines recommend a 3- to 6-month course of Cilostazol as first-line pharmacotherapy treatment for patients with intermittent claudication (Schirmer & Mosier, 2014).

Antiplatelet agents, such as aspirin or clopidogrel, help prevent the formation of thromboemboli, which can lead to MI and stroke. Aspirin (usually 75 to 325 mg/day) has been shown to reduce the risk of MI, stroke, and death in patients with vascular disease. Clopidogrel is indicated for the prevention of cardiovascular ischemic events in patients with PAD but not for treatment of claudication (Schirmer & Mosier, 2014).

Thrombolysis

A thrombotic stenosis or occlusion may be treated by **thrombolysis**. After catheter insertion into the affected vessel, the thrombolytic agent is injected directly into the thrombus. It will lyse the thrombus (clot). The patient is admitted to a special or critical care unit for continuous monitoring. Vital signs are taken frequently, according to the facility's protocol. The patient is monitored closely for any signs of bleeding, as this is the most common side effect of thrombolytic therapy. The nurse minimizes the number of punctures for IV lines and obtaining blood samples, avoids intramuscular injections, prevents tissue trauma, and applies pressure at least twice as long as usual after any puncture is performed. Patients will have follow-up images to determine treatment effectiveness. Refer to Table 18-2 for discussion of thrombolytic agents.

Nursing Alert
In order to monitor patients post intervention, it is essential that a baseline assessment of the extremity is documented so that the nurse can determine changes in perfusion of the extremity post instrumentation.

Surgical Management

Disabling claudication or risk for amputation is an indication for surgical or percutaneous intervention. Percutaneous, catheter-based endovascular treatments with or without

stenting are seen increasingly over open surgical approaches because of the relative safety, success, and durability of stenting (White, 2016). The initial treatment goals for ALI are to prevent worsening ischemia and thrombus propagation, to manage pain, and to preserve tissue. Anticoagulation is started immediately upon recognizing the acute ischemia. Revascularization or **arterial bypass** is the first-line intervention used in ALI treatment. Vascular surgical procedures are divided into two groups: inflow procedures, which improve blood supply from the aorta into the femoral artery, and outflow procedures, which provide blood supply to vessels below the femoral artery. The type of procedure performed depends on the degree and location of the stenosis or occlusion. When diffuse disease is present, an inflow procedure is performed first. The restoration of arterial flow may be sufficient after this procedure so that other procedures may not be needed. The overall health of the patient and the ability to tolerate a procedure factors into the decision as to what approach is best for each patient. For some patients who are at high risk or in a life-threatening situation, a primary amputation may be the best choice.

Bypass grafts are placed to reroute blood flow around the stenosis or occlusion. Grafts below the knee require the use of native vein (i.e., autologous; the patient's own vein) to ensure patency; however, synthetic grafts may be used for bypass procedures on larger vessels above the knee. Several synthetic materials are available for use as a peripheral bypass graft. Cryopreserved saphenous veins and umbilical veins are also available but usually do not last as long as native veins or synthetic grafts. Graft patency is determined by the graft size, graft type, and location. Great care is taken to prevent graft infection as the graft must be removed if infected. Vein grafts are reversed before creating the graft conduit to prevent the valves from causing an occlusion, or they are left in place (in situ) and the valves are removed with a special instrument (valvulotome).

Doppler evaluation of the graft and the proximal vessels beyond the graft is usually performed for postprocedure vascular patients. Patients may have arterial studies, ABI, and arterial wave form analysis performed in the vascular laboratory after arterial reconstructive procedures and prior to discharge. Disappearance of a pulse or a Doppler signal that was previously present may indicate an occluded graft and requires notification of the surgeon.

Endovascular Intervention

Several percutaneous interventional techniques are available to remove plaque and dilate vessels. **Angioplasty**, also called percutaneous transluminal **balloon angioplasty** (PTA), may be performed with or without a **stent**. Balloons are inserted into the vessels via a catheter and expanded at the stenotic site within the vessel. The expanding balloon cracks the atherosclerotic plaque and opens the vascular lumen. Stents may be inserted to support the vessel wall and maintain patency.

Complications from PTA include hematoma, embolization, dissection of the vessel, bleeding, intimal damage (dissection), and stent migration. The advantage of angioplasty, stents, and **stent-grafts** compared to open surgical procedures is the decreased length of hospital stay required for the treatment and less physical trauma to the patient than open surgical procedures. Often percutaneous catheter procedures are performed in an outpatient setting (White, 2013).

Nursing Management

Providing Postoperative Care

In the postoperative period, the nurse collaborates with the surgeon about the patient's appropriate activity level based on the patient's condition (Chung, Modrall, Ahn, Lavery, & Valentine, 2015). In general, every effort is made to encourage patients to move the involved extremity and be active. The primary objective in the postprocedure period is to maintain adequate circulation. Anticoagulant therapy may be continued after surgery to prevent thrombosis of the graft. Metabolic abnormalities, kidney failure, and **compartment syndrome** are potential complications after arterial occlusions or operations (refer to Chapter 42 for details of compartment syndrome). The nurse assesses for evidence of local complications, such as hemorrhage or thrombosis, by performing neurovascular checks of the limb and systemic complications, by monitoring vital signs, intake and output, physical assessment parameters (e.g., pulmonary, cardiac, PV, GI, mental status), and laboratory data. Any evidence of deterioration is reported to the surgical team immediately (cool; dusky; weakened pulses; delayed capillary refill; decreased sensory/motor function; progressive, unrelieved pain).

Providing Pain Relief

Often narcotics are needed to manage rest pain until circulation can be restored. After interventions, pain management is similar to other postoperative patient care, keeping in mind that the patient may have been taking large doses of narcotics preoperatively and may need more pain medication than expected to relieve symptoms.

Maintaining Tissue Integrity

Poorly perfused tissues are susceptible to damage and infection. When lesions develop, healing may be delayed or inhibited because of the poor blood supply to the area. Infected, nonhealing ulcers of the extremities can be debilitating and may require prolonged, often expensive treatments and run the risk of potential limb loss. Measures to prevent tissue loss and amputation are a high priority. Patients are taught to avoid trauma; wear sturdy, well-fitting shoes or slippers; and use neutral soaps and body lotions. Patients with vascular disease are taught the same precautions that patients with diabetes are taught for foot care (see Chapter 30, Box 30-8). Patients who have an open arterial or venous ulcer are given detailed wound care instructions. Risk factor modification is the most effective intervention for preventing progression of vascular disease (e.g., maintain A1c within target range for patients with diabetes).

Patients and their families are educated on environmental and behavioral risk factors associated with ischemia. For example, excess heat may increase the metabolic rate of the extremities and increase the need for oxygen beyond that provided by the reduced arterial flow through the diseased artery. Cold temperature is associated with vasoconstriction, which decreases perfusion to the extremities. Nicotine from tobacco products causes vasospasm and can dramatically reduce circulation to the extremities. Tobacco smoke also impairs transport and cellular use of oxygen and increases blood viscosity. Patients with arterial insufficiency who use tobacco must be fully informed of the effects of nicotine on circulation and encouraged to stop using tobacco. Secondhand smoke is also harmful to the vascular system.

Emotional upsets cause vasoconstriction by stimulating the sympathetic nervous system. This can be minimized to some degree by avoiding stressful situations or by following a stress-management program. Counseling services or relaxation training may be indicated for people who cannot cope effectively with situational stressors.

Constrictive clothing and accessories are avoided, as are heating pads and hot water bottles. The temperature of bath water should also be evaluated and the overall water temperature in the home decreased to prevent scalding. Tight socks, panty girdles, belts, and shoelaces are discouraged because they may impede arterial circulation to the extremities and promote venous congestion and edema.

 Nursing Alert
Lower extremity elevation is associated with decreased arterial flow, which lessens perfusion to the tissues and increases pain. A dependent position improves flow and decreases pain.

UPPER EXTREMITY ARTERIAL OCCLUSIVE DISEASE

Arterial occlusions from atherosclerosis occur less frequently in the upper extremities than in the legs.

Pathophysiology

Upper extremity arterial symptoms and occlusive disease are more likely to be caused by vasospasm, trauma, or arterial constrictive disorders than by atherosclerosis.

Stenosis may occur at the origin of the subclavian artery proximal to the vertebral artery. Arterial blood flows to the brain via the carotid and the vertebral arteries. If there is diminished flow to the arm from the subclavian artery due to the stenosis, there will be preferential reverse flow down the vertebral artery to the arm when the arm is being used. This is called *subclavian steal syndrome* as the arm is "stealing" blood from the brain.

Clinical Manifestations and Assessment

The patient may complain of arm fatigue and pain when using the arm to paint or comb hair and occasionally may report difficulty when driving. Patients also report dizziness, vertigo, ataxia, syncope, or bilateral visual changes when using the arm.

Assessment findings in the ischemic upper extremity may include coolness and pallor of the affected extremity, decreased capillary refill, a decreased amplitude and delay in radial artery pulse on the affected side, and a difference in arm blood pressures of more than 20 mm Hg (affected limb pressure is lower). Noninvasive studies performed to evaluate for upper extremity arterial occlusions include upper and forearm blood pressure determinations and duplex ultrasound to identify the anatomic location of the lesion and to evaluate the hemodynamics of the blood flow.

Medical and Nursing Management

Surgical bypass or a PTA procedure may be indicated. If the stenosis involves the subclavian artery with siphoning of blood from the intracranial circulation to the arm, a carotid-to-subclavian artery bypass or reimplantation of the subclavian to the carotid artery may be performed.

INFLAMMATORY DISORDERS

Various inflammatory diseases affect the arterial system. Examples of these are Takayasu arteritis, Behçet disease, and giant cell arteritis. The inflammatory response creates granuloma formation and causes vessel destruction. Initial treatment for active vascular inflammatory diseases is high-dose corticosteroids. Revascularization, if indicated, is delayed until the inflammatory process in under control.

RAYNAUD DISEASE AND RAYNAUD PHENOMENON

Primary *Raynaud disease* (primary Raynaud phenomenon or idiopathic Raynaud phenomenon) refers to vasospasm that occurs with cold or stress. Patients with scleroderma or systemic lupus erythematosus may have the same signs and symptoms. This is called *Secondary Raynaud phenomenon.*

Pathophysiology

Raynaud disease is of unknown etiology. While its exact cause is unknown, it may be associated with immunologic disorders. Emotional factors or cold may trigger episodes.

It usually occurs in women between 16 and 40 years of age, and it occurs more frequently in cold climates and during the winter. It may cause skin and muscle atrophy.

The prognosis varies; patients may slowly improve, become progressively worse, or show no change.

Clinical Manifestations and Assessment

The patient's skin becomes cyanotic due to vasospasm, and then vasodilation causes redness (rubor). Numbness, tingling, and burning pain occur. Although typically the fingers are involved, the toes are affected in as many as 40% of patients (Mark, 2015). Typically, the radial, ulnar, and pedal pulses are normal; fingers and toes may be cool between attacks and may perspire excessively.

Medical and Nursing Management

With appropriate patient teaching and lifestyle modifications, the disorder is generally benign and self-limiting. The patient is instructed to avoid the stimuli (e.g., cold, tobacco) that provoke vasoconstriction. Patients are encouraged to dress warmly; wear gloves and mittens; and protect the trunk, head, and feet with warm clothing to prevent cold-induced reflex vasoconstriction. Tobacco use is contraindicated. The patient may be prescribed calcium-channel blockers to relieve symptoms. Digital sympathectomy (interrupting the sympathetic nerves) may help some patients.

> **!** *Nursing Alert*
> *Remember the red, white, and blue of Raynaud's! The intense spasm of the digital arteries produces initial pallor (white), followed over minutes by capillary dilation and filling with deoxygenated venous blood, resulting in cyanosis (blue). On relaxation of the arterial spasm, the circulation improves (warm red digits).*

THROMBOANGIITIS OBLITERANS (BUERGER DISEASE)

Buerger disease is characterized by recurring inflammation of the intermediate and small arteries and vein, resulting in thrombus formation and vessel occlusion. It occurs in both upper and lower extremities. It is differentiated from vessel diseases by microscopic appearance.

Buerger disease is an autoimmune disease. While its etiology is unknown, it is believed to be an autoimmune **vasculitis** (inflammation of a blood vessel). It most often occurs in men between 20 and 35 years of age and is reported in all races. Tobacco use is a causative factor, and continued use interferes with healing. Pain is generally bilateral and symmetric with focal lesions.

Treatment is essentially the same as for atherosclerotic PAD; sympathetic block may dilate vessels and increase

Adventitia

Media

Intima

FIGURE 18-5 Characteristics of arterial aneurysm. (**A**) Normal artery. (**B**) False aneurysm (pseudoaneurysm); actually a pulsating hematoma. The clot and connective tissue are outside the arterial wall. (**C**) True aneurysm. One, two, or all three layers of the artery may be involved. (**D**) Fusiform aneurysm; symmetric, spindle-shaped expansion of entire circumference of involved vessel. (**E**) Saccular aneurysm; a bulbous protrusion of one side of the arterial wall. (**F**) Dissecting aneurysm; this usually is a hematoma that splits the layers of the arterial wall. (**G**) Ruptured aneurysm.

blood flow. Tobacco cessation is mandatory for healing to occur.

ANEURYSMS

An aneurysm is a localized out-pouching, sac, or dilation formed at a weak point in the artery wall (Fig. 18-5). It may be classified by its shape or form. The most common forms of aneurysms are saccular and fusiform. A *saccular aneurysm* projects from one side of the vessel only. If an entire arterial segment becomes dilated, a *fusiform aneurysm* develops. Very small aneurysms due to localized infection are called *mycotic aneurysms. Aortic aneurysms* occur in the abdominal and thoracic aorta and are characterized by disruption and loss of elastic fibers, resulting in degeneration of the medial vessel wall. It is thought to be an inflammatory process.

ABDOMINAL AORTIC ANEURYSM

The cause of abdominal aortic aneurysm (AAA), the most common type of degenerative aneurysm, has historically been attributed to atherosclerotic changes in the aorta. Recently, the pathogenesis of AAAs has been linked to genetic, environmental, hemodynamic, and immunologic factors, with atherosclerosis contributing to the process (Lederle, 2016). Most AAAs are asymptomatic and are found on routine examinations or during a workup for another condition. The U.S. Preventive Services Task Force recommends one-time ultrasound screening for men 65 to 75 years of age who have ever smoked (Guirguis-Blake, Beil, Senger, & Whitlock, 2014). Aneurysms are serious because they can rupture, leading to hemorrhage and death. If the AAA ruptures, mortality rates as high as 80% are seen (Latessa & Aquila, 2014).

Pathophysiology

All aneurysms involve a damaged media layer of the vessel. This may be caused by congenital weakness, trauma,

or disease. The degradation of the medial elastin fibers and collagen (which gives the vessel strength) leads to the weakening and dilation of the aorta and the development of aneurysm. After an aneurysm develops, it tends to enlarge, growing at a rate of 0.3 to 0.4 cm per year on average; however, there is no predictable pattern (Mohler, 2016).

Risk Factors

Risk factors include age (over 50 years of age), male sex, tobacco use, family history, occlusive atherosclerotic disease, and hypertension. Many types of aneurysms have a genetic basis. Patient education includes advising biologic family members to be evaluated for aneurysms.

Clinical Manifestations and Assessment

Not all patients with AAAs have symptoms. Some patients complain that they can feel their heart beating in their abdomen when lying down, or they may say they feel an abdominal mass or abdominal throbbing. If the AAA is associated with thrombus, a major vessel may be occluded, or smaller distal occlusions may result from emboli. Small **cholesterol**, platelet, or fibrin emboli may lodge in the digital arteries, causing cyanosis and mottling of the toes.

Signs of impending aneurysm rupture include severe back or abdominal pain, which may be persistent or intermittent. Abdominal pain is often localized in the middle or lower abdomen to the left of the midline. Low back pain may be present because of pressure of the aneurysm on the lumbar nerves. This is a significant symptom, usually indicating that the aneurysm is expanding rapidly and is about to rupture. Indications of a rupturing AAA include constant, intense back pain; falling blood pressure; and decreasing hematocrit. Rupture into the peritoneal cavity is rapidly fatal, and surgical repair is the only chance for survival. A retroperitoneal rupture of an aneurysm may result in hematomas in the scrotum, perineum, flank, or penis. Cullen sign (bluish to purplish periumbilical discoloration) and Grey Turner sign (flank discoloration) may be noted with retroperitoneal blood from leaking or ruptured AAA (see Fig. 27-10 on page 843). Symptoms of abdominal distention, constipation, or urinary retention may be caused by a hematoma that compresses the bowel or the urinary tract or by impaired blood supply to these organs (Lederle, 2016).

The most important diagnostic indication of an AAA is a pulsatile mass in the abdomen. These aneurysms can be palpated if the patient is not obese. The aorta is slightly left of midline, measures approximately 2 cm, and is palpated a few centimeters above the umbilicus (level of bifurcation to the iliac arteries). The aortic width is measured using both hands by noting the width of the pulsations, not the intensity. A systolic bruit may be heard over the mass. Duplex ultrasonography or computed tomography (CT) is used to determine the size, length, and location of the aneurysm. An aorta that is 3 cm or greater in width is indicative of an AAA.

Medical Management

Screening intervals are proposed based upon the size of the aneurysm. When the aneurysm is small (3.0 to 3.9 cm), ultrasonography is conducted at 3-year intervals, whereas an AAA greater than 4.5 cm is evaluated annually (Lederle, 2016). Some aneurysms remain stable over many years of observation; however, when the AAA exceeds 5.5 cm, elective repair should be considered.

Pharmacologic Therapy

If an aneurysm is stable in size based on serial duplex ultrasound scans, the blood pressure is closely monitored over time. There is an association between increased diastolic blood pressure, size increase, and rupture. Antihypertensive agents, including diuretics, beta blockers, angiotensin-converting enzyme (ACE) inhibitors, angiotensin II receptor antagonists, and calcium-channel blockers, may be prescribed to maintain the patient's blood pressure within acceptable limits.

Surgical Management

An expanding or enlarging AAA is likely to rupture. Surgery is the treatment of choice for AAAs more than 5.5 cm wide or those that are enlarging (Stone & Cronenwett, 2013). An alternative for treating an infrarenal (below the renal arteries) AAA is endovascular grafting, which involves percutaneous transluminal placement and attachment of an aortic graft prosthesis across the aneurysm (Fig. 18-6). This procedure is performed under local or regional anesthesia. Potential complications are similar to those of other endograft procedures (discussed later). It is important to consider that the overall surgical mortality rate associated with a ruptured aneurysm is 75% to 80%; therefore, early intervention is warranted (Latessa & Aquila, 2014). Nursing management after surgery can be found after the discussion of other types of aneurysms (see Nursing Management After Surgical Interventions, p. 543).

FIGURE 18-6 AneuRx Endograft repair of an abdominal aortic aneurysm (Medtronic).

THORACIC AORTIC ANEURYSM

Approximately 85% of all cases of thoracic aortic aneurysm are caused by atherosclerosis. Ascending thoracic aortic aneurysms are often associated with genetic mutations such as Marfan syndrome (Lederle, 2016). They occur most frequently in men between 40 and 70 years of age. The thoracic area is the most common site for a dissecting aneurysm. About one third of patients with thoracic aneurysms die of rupture of the aneurysm.

Clinical Manifestations and Assessment

Symptoms are variable and depend on how rapidly the aneurysm dilates and how the pulsating mass affects surrounding intrathoracic structures. Some patients are asymptomatic. In most cases, pain is the most prominent symptom. The pain is usually constant and of a boring quality, but it may occur only when the person is supine. Other symptoms are dyspnea, the result of pressure of the aneurysm sac against the trachea, a main bronchus, or the lung itself; cough, frequently paroxysmal and with a brassy quality; hoarseness, stridor, or weakness or complete loss of the voice (aphonia), resulting from pressure against the laryngeal nerve; and dysphagia (difficulty in swallowing) due to impingement on the esophagus by the aneurysm (Latessa & Aquila, 2014).

When large veins in the chest are compressed by the aneurysm, the superficial veins of the chest, neck, or arms become dilated; edematous areas on the chest wall and cyanosis are often evident. Pressure against the cervical sympathetic chain can result in unequal pupils. Diagnosis of a thoracic aortic aneurysm is principally made by chest x-ray, transesophageal echocardiography (TEE), and CT.

Medical Management

Aneurysms are sometimes managed medically with risk factor modification, especially blood pressure control, pain management, and close monitoring of symptoms. However, in most cases, an aneurysm is treated by open surgical method or an endovascular procedure. General measures such as controlling blood pressure and correcting risk factors are important. Systolic pressure is maintained at about 100 to 120 mm Hg with antihypertensive medications or a beta blocker. The goal of surgery is to repair the aneurysm and restore vascular continuity with a vascular graft. Intensive monitoring is usually required after an open surgical procedure, and the patient is cared for in the critical care unit. Endovascular graft repair of unruptured thoracic aneurysms decreases postoperative recovery time and decrease complications compared with traditional surgical techniques; however, it has not improved the adjusted 5-year survival rate (Lederle, 2016). These endovascular grafts are inserted into the thoracic aorta via various vascular access routes, including the femoral or iliac artery (Eagleton & Upchurch, 2013).

Postoperatively the immediate concern is blood pressure control and a device-related complication termed an *endoleak* from the endovascular graft. An endoleak is a persistent leaking of blood out of the graft and into the aneurysm sac. Early leaks have the potential to rupture within the first 30 postoperative days (primary endoleaks), but late endoleaks (secondary endoleaks) can occur as late as 7 years after the procedure. An endoleak is screened by CT scanning and duplex ultrasound. The nurse considers that during the operative procedure, necessary vessel clamping can have profound effect on the mesentery circulation (gut), renal circulation (kidneys), and artery of Adamkiewicz (supplies the lower two thirds of the spinal cord). Postoperatively, regardless of type of procedure performed, the patient is assessed for changes in mentation, vision, speech, or motor strength, as well as pain in the abdomen or flank, vomiting, or bloody diarrhea, which may indicate embolization to cerebral, mesentery circulation, or other organs and should be reported to the surgeon immediately. In addition, depending on length of time the aorta was clamped during the surgery, concerns include spinal cord ischemia with resultant paraplegia and renal insufficiency—thus, both kidney function and sensory/motor function are assessed postoperatively. Patients undergoing open surgical procedures go to the intensive care unit and typically are on mechanical ventilation postoperatively. Endovascular procedures may not require intensive care unit monitoring postprocedure.

PERIPHERAL ANEURYSMS

Aneurysms may also arise in the peripheral vessels, most often as a result of atherosclerosis. These may involve the renal artery, femoral artery, or (most frequently) popliteal artery. Between 50% and 60% of popliteal aneurysms are bilateral and may be associated with AAAs.

The aneurysm produces a pulsating mass and disturbs peripheral circulation distal to it. Pain and swelling develop because of pressure on adjacent nerves and veins. Diagnosis is made by duplex ultrasonography and CT to determine the size, length, and extent of the aneurysm. Arteriography may be performed to evaluate the level of proximal and distal involvement.

DISSECTING ANEURYSM

Occasionally, in an aorta diseased by arteriosclerosis, a tear develops in the intima or the media degenerates, resulting in a dissection (a false lumen that communicates with the true lumen) (refer to Fig. 18-5). Dissections may be treated medically or surgically.

Pathophysiology

Arterial dissections are commonly associated with poorly controlled hypertension, blunt force chest trauma, and cocaine use. Dissection is caused by rupture in the intimal layer. A rupture may occur through adventitia or into the lumen through the intima, allowing blood to reenter the main channel, resulting in chronic dissection or occlusion of branches of the aorta.

As the separation progresses, the arteries branching from the involved area of the aorta shear and occlude. The tear occurs most commonly in the region of the aortic arch, with the highest mortality rate associated with ascending aortic dissection, which accounts for about 3,000 deaths per year in the United States (Lederle, 2016). The dissection of the aorta may progress toward the heart, obstructing the orifices of the coronary arteries, producing hemopericardium (effusion of blood into the pericardial sac), or aortic insufficiency, or it may extend distally, occluding the arteries supplying the GI tract, kidneys, spinal cord, and legs.

Clinical Manifestations and Assessment

Onset of symptoms is usually sudden. Severe and persistent pain, described as tearing or ripping, may be reported. The pain is in the anterior chest or back and extends to the shoulders, epigastric area, or abdomen. Aortic dissection may be mistaken for an acute MI, which could confuse the clinical picture and initial treatment. Cardiovascular, neurologic, and GI symptoms are responsible for other clinical manifestations, depending on the location and extent of the dissection. For example, if the dissection extends to the renal arteries, patients can present with acute kidney failure (AKF); with mesentery involvement, abdominal pain and bloody diarrhea may be seen; and lower extremity ischemia can be seen with iliac involvement. The patient may appear pale. Diaphoresis and tachycardia may be detected. Blood pressure may be elevated or markedly different from one arm to the other if dissection involves the orifice of the sub-clavian artery on one side. Because of the variable clinical picture associated with this condition, early diagnosis is difficult.

Nursing Management After Surgical Interventions

Surgical repair of the aorta is performed for dissection, rupture, and aneurysm. General postoperative nursing assessment involves frequent vital signs; recording of intake and output; assessment of oxygen saturation; bilateral comparison of upper arm blood pressures and peripheral pulses; and assessment of motor and sensory function, temperature of extremities, color changes, and capillary refill. The patient who has had an endovascular repair must lie supine according to a protocol. The patient needs to use a bedpan or urinal while on bed rest. The access site (usually the femoral or iliac artery) is assessed when vital signs and pulses are monitored. The nurse assesses for bleeding, pulsation, swelling, pain, and hematoma formation. In addition, the patient is monitored for signs of embolization to the lower extremities; therefore, skin changes of the lumbar area, buttocks, and lower extremity (plantar area of the feet or toes is often affected) are assessed for extremely tender, irregularly shaped, cyanotic areas.

The patient's temperature should be monitored according to a protocol, and any signs of postimplantation syndrome should be reported. Postimplantation syndrome typically begins within 24 hours of stent-graft placement and consists of a spontaneously occurring fever, leukocytosis, and, occasionally, transient thrombocytopenia. The exact etiology is unknown, but the symptoms are thought to be related to the activation of cytokines, which results from thrombosis in the repaired aneurysm that occurs because of the release of coagulation proteins and platelets. These symptoms can be managed with mild analgesics or anti-inflammatory agents, such as acetaminophen or ibuprofen, and usually subside within a week.

Because of the increased risk for hemorrhage, the surgeon is notified of persistent coughing, sneezing, vomiting, or systolic blood pressure greater than 180 mm Hg. Most patients can resume their preprocedure diet and are encouraged to drink fluids. An IV infusion may be continued until the patient can drink normally. Fluids are important to maintain blood flow through the arterial repair site and to assist the kidneys with excreting IV contrast agent and other medications used during the procedure. According to a protocol, after a procedure that involves a catheter in the groin, the patient may be able to roll from side to side and may be able to ambulate with assistance to the bathroom. After the

patient can take adequate fluids orally, the IV infusion may be discontinued and the IV access converted to a saline lock. Postoperative care requires intense monitoring of pulmonary, cardiovascular, renal, and neurologic status. Pulmonary complications include the potential development of acute respiratory distress syndrome (ARDS), particularly if large quantities of blood were required intraoperatively (refer to Chapter 10 for discussion of ARDS). MI and arrhythmias are potential cardiac complications and are discussed in Chapters 14 and 17, respectively. GI complications include a risk for ischemic colitis, and symptoms include bloody diarrhea, abdominal distention, leukocytosis, fever, and abdominal pain. Because AKF is a potential complication, urine output is monitored hourly and laboratory parameters are monitored (blood urea nitrogen [BUN] and creatinine values) for significant changes. Potential injury to the spinal cord with resultant paraplegia requires that the nurse assess the patient's sensory motor function postoperatively. In addition, since it is important that perfusion to the spinal cord be maintained, the nurse frequently assesses blood pressure measurements, and the surgeon is alerted upon evidence of decreasing parameters.

Before discharge, the patient is assisted in developing and implementing a plan to stop using tobacco and to manage pain. The patient may need to be encouraged to make the lifestyle changes necessary to adequately manage a chronic disease, including modifications in diet, activity, and hygiene. The nurse assesses the patient's resources, including family and friends to assist as needed. The nurse ensures that the patient has the knowledge and ability to assess for disease progression and postoperative or postprocedure complications as needed.

VENOUS DISORDERS

Venous blood flow is reduced by a thrombus or **embolus** obstructing a vein, by incompetent venous valves, or by a reduction of the pumping action effectiveness of surrounding muscles. Decreased venous blood flow causes increased venous pressure, which increases capillary hydrostatic pressure, facilitating filtration of fluid out of the capillaries into the interstitial space, with resultant development of tissue edema. Edematous tissue does not receive adequate nutrition from the blood and is more susceptible to breakdown, injury, and infection. Thus, the nurse is aware that edematous tissue is fragile tissue.

VENOUS THROMBOSIS

The terms *venous thrombosis, deep vein thrombosis* (DVT), *thrombophlebitis, venous thromboembolism,* and *phlebothrombosis* do not necessarily reflect identical disease processes, but they are grouped together for clinical purposes.

1. *Stasis of blood:* Caused by immobility (bed rest, long plane/car/train rides, obesity, constrictive devices, paralysis, paresis, recent surgery, varicose veins, pregnancy)
2. *Vessel wall injury:* Caused by trauma (fractures, contusions), central venous catheterization, vascular devices (PICC, central lines, pacemaker wires), IV medications, cancer therapy (hormonal, chemotherapy, or radiotherapy)
3. *Altered coagulation:* Caused by estrogen-containing oral contraception or hormone replacement, cancer (secretes procoagulants), smoking, dehydration, hypercoagulable states, late pregnancy, and the postpartum period

Pathophysiology

The exact cause of venous thrombosis remains unclear. Three factors, known as *Virchow triad* (Box 18-6), are believed to play a significant role in the development of venous thrombosis. Some hypercoagulable states are hereditary. Patients with these states should have a hematology consult.

Upper extremity venous thrombosis is not as common as lower extremity thrombosis. However, it may occur in patients with IV catheters (IV lines or wires from pacemaker leads, chemotherapy ports, dialysis catheters, or parenteral nutrition lines) or in patients with an underlying hypercoagulation disorder. Effort thrombosis is caused by repetitive motion (as in competitive swimmers, tennis players, and construction workers) that irritates the vessel wall, causing inflammation and subsequent thrombosis.

Venous thrombi are aggregates of platelets attached to the vein wall that have a tail-like appendage containing fibrin, white blood cells, and many red blood cells. The thrombus can propagate as successive layers of thrombus form. A propagating venous thrombosis is dangerous because it is often the source of a pulmonary embolism (PE). Thrombus fragmentation can occur spontaneously or in association with an elevated venous pressure, as when a person stands suddenly or engages in muscular activity after prolonged inactivity. After an episode of acute DVT, recanalization of the lumen of the vessel occurs. However, the venous valves remain open and are ineffective. Reverse venous flow contributes to chronic venous insufficiency. Over time, postphlebitic syndrome (Box 18-7) occurs, manifested by skin and tissue changes.

Clinical Manifestations and Assessment

A major problem associated with recognizing DVT is that the signs and symptoms are nonspecific. The exception is *phlegmasia cerulea dolens* (massive iliofemoral venous thrombosis), in which the entire extremity becomes massively swollen, tense, and painful, with arterial ischemia (bluish color) and potential loss of distal pulses. Despite this variability, clinical signs should always be investigated.

Deep venous obstruction is associated with edema of the extremity due to inhibition of venous outflow. The nurse should note any differences in leg circumference bilaterally from thigh to ankle; increase in the surface temperature of the leg, particularly the calf or ankle; and areas of tenderness or superficial thrombosis. Swelling can be measured by obtaining the circumference of the affected extremity at specific levels and comparing one extremity with the other at the same level. Asymmetry of extremities (calf swelling at least 3 cm larger than asymptomatic leg), measured 10 cm below the tibial tuberosity, should alert the nurse to a potential DVT. In addition, the nurse should assess for the presence of a low-grade fever.

Tenderness, which usually occurs later, is produced by inflammation of the vein wall, and firmness may be detected along the involved veins by gently palpating the affected extremity (palpated cord). *Homans sign* (pain in the calf after the foot is sharply dorsiflexed) used to be considered a sign of DVT, but it is not reliable and is not used anymore. Dilation and prominence of the superficial veins may be noted. In some cases, signs and symptoms of a PE are the first indication of DVT.

Superficial vein thrombosis produces pain or tenderness, redness, and warmth in the involved area. Many of these thromboses dissolve spontaneously. This condition can be treated at home with bed rest, limb elevation, analgesics, and anti-inflammatory medication. It should be noted that while nonsteroidal anti-inflammatory drugs (NSAIDs) provide analgesia, they are associated with an increase in venous thromboembolism (VTE), caused by an embolism breaking off and lodging in a smaller vein (Ungprasert, Srivali, Wijarnpreecha, Charoenpong, & Knight, 2015).

Careful assessment is the key in detecting early signs of lower extremity venous disorders. Patients with a history of varicose veins, hypercoagulation, neoplastic disease, cardiovascular disease, or recent major surgery or injury are at high risk. Other patients at high risk include those who are obese, immobile, or elderly, as well as women taking oral contraceptives.

Postphlebitic Syndrome

Postphlebitic syndrome develops as follows:
1. Venous valve injury results in an incompetent valve and reverse venous flow.
2. Fluid, plasma, and red blood cells leak into the interstitial tissue.
3. Edema forms around ankles and/or lower legs.
4. Staining of skin occurs as red blood cells break down, releasing hemosiderin.
5. Subcutaneous tissue becomes firm and fibrotic.
6. Loss of elasticity in the skin and subcutaneous tissue results.
7. Tissue becomes vulnerable to trauma and ulcer formation.

> ### ! Nursing Alert
> *The D-dimer blood assay is a marker of coagulation activity. When a clot lyses, fibrin degradation occurs and a D-dimer is positive. When positive, it is associated with clot breakdown, such as the presence of DVT or PE, but it is also associated with a variety of nonthrombotic disorders, including recent surgery, hemorrhage, trauma, cancer, MI, pneumonia, and sepsis. Thus, D-dimers are frequently elevated due to some systemic illness; however, a negative D-dimer decreases the likelihood of a DVT or PE.*

Prevention

Preventive measures should be instituted for patients at risk for DVT. These might include physical interventions, such as elastic compression stockings, intermittent pneumatic compression devices, and body positioning and exercise. Medications to prevent thrombosis include anticoagulant therapy, such as subcutaneous unfractionated or low–molecular-weight heparin (LMWH). Studies are ongoing as to which prevention method works best with which patient population. Guidelines for intervention are continuously evolving. It is up to the practitioner to keep up with the research findings and to apply the evidence to clinical practice.

Medical Management

The objectives of treatment for DVT are to prevent the thrombus from growing and fragmenting (risking PE) and to prevent recurrent thromboemboli. Interventions to prevent thrombus formation are indicated in patients with thrombophlebitis, recurrent embolus formation, persistent leg edema from heart failure, and in any patients who may require lengthy immobilization.

Pharmacologic Therapy

Heparin
Anticoagulant therapy is effective prophylaxis; however, anticoagulants do not dissolve a thrombus that has already formed.

Unfractionated Heparin. Unfractionated heparin is administered subcutaneously to prevent development of DVT. In the event of a DVT, although heparin can be administered subcutaneously, common practice is to administer heparin via an IV drip to prevent the extension of a thrombus and the development of new thrombi. IV heparin produces an immediate anticoagulant effect, and, therefore, is used when rapid anticoagulant effects are desired. Unfractionated heparin is administered via an infusion pump to carefully control the rate. Dosage is based on the patient's weight, and any possible bleeding tendencies are detected by a pretreatment clotting profile. If renal insufficiency exists, lower doses of heparin are required. Periodic coagulation tests and hematocrit levels are obtained. Heparin is in the effective, or therapeutic, range when the activated partial thromboplastin time (aPTT) is 1.5 to 2.5 times the baseline control. Normal aPTT level is 21 to 35 seconds (Fischbach & Dunning, 2014). If the PTT is greater than 100 seconds, the risk for hemorrhage is significant! Typically, the PTT level is measured 6 hours after therapy is started. The nurse is aware that heparin has a half-life of about 60 minutes; therefore, in an emergency, the heparin is discontinued for a period of at least 1 hour.

Coumadin, an oral anticoagulant, is administered soon after initiating heparin therapy, since Coumadin may require 3 to 5 days to achieve a therapeutic effect. Until a therapeutic international normalized ratio (INR) is achieved, both medications are administered concurrently. Medication dosage is regulated by monitoring the aPTT for heparin, the INR for Coumadin, and the platelet count, to assess for potential complications of heparin therapy (discussed later in this chapter).

Low–Molecular-Weight Heparin. Subcutaneous LMWH is an effective treatment for some cases of DVT. These agents have longer half-lives than unfractionated heparin so doses can be given in one or two subcutaneous injections each day. Doses are adjusted according to patient weight. LMWH prevents the extension of a thrombus and development of new thrombi, and they are associated with fewer bleeding complications and lower risks of heparin-induced thrombocytopenia (HIT) than is unfractionated heparin. Because there are several preparations, the dosing schedule must be based on the product used and the protocol at each institution. Because LMWH is cleared almost entirely by the kidneys, clearance can be variable in patients with renal insufficiency, thus a longer half-life may be expected. The cost of LMWH is higher than that of unfractionated heparin; however, another benefit is that LMWH may be used safely in pregnant women.

Direct Thrombin Inhibitor. Thrombin's role in clot formation is to convert soluble fibrinogen to insoluble fibrin, while stimulating platelet activation; thus direct thrombin inhibitors (DTIs) impede this process. In addition, DTIs have a more predictable anticoagulant effect compared with heparin and do not cause an immune-mediated thrombocytopenia. Three parenteral DTIs are approved for use as anticoagulants in the United States: desirudin, bivalirudin, and argatroban. Currently, there is no specific antidote to reverse the effects of parenteral DTIs. Thus, the nurse observes for evidence of bleeding and reports to the provider any concerns. There is one oral DTI that is available: dabigatran. Currently reversal of dabigatran's anticoagulant effects can be achieved in emergency situations with the use of idarucizumab.

In addition to parenterally administered heparins, oral direct factor Xa inhibitors can be utilized although clinical applications differ. Oral direct factor Xa inhibitors include rivaroxaban, apixaban, and edoxaban. They are at least as effective and safe as warfarin, and their ability to be administered in fixed doses without routine coagulation monitoring

TABLE **18-3** Arterial and Venous Thrombolysis

Indications (Arterial and Venous)	Drug	Advantages (All Drugs in Arterial and Venous Thrombosis)	Disadvantages (All Drugs in Arterial and Venous Thrombosis)
In situ thrombosis of less than 14 days	Alteplase	Clot lysis between 6 and 72 hours Preferred choice for clot removal if no contraindications Avoidance of invasive surgical operations May be repeated if needed.	Limited in DVT lysis by long infusion times and risks of hemorrhagic complications associated with large doses
Nonlife-threatening limb ischemia (arterial)	Reteplase	Superior thrombus penetration	Risk factors for hemorrhagic complications: older age, lower body weight, elevated pulse pressure, uncontrolled hypertension, recent stroke, recent operation, bleeding disorder, congestive heart failure

Please refer to the latest guidelines from the manufacturer for indications, dosages, general warnings and precautions. Currently complications (among others) associated with thrombolysis include: 1. increased risk of bleeding, 2. orolingual angioedema, 3. cholesterol embolism, 4. Reembolization from the lysis.
Alteplase (Activase) (2016). www. Activase.com. South San Francisco, CA: Genentech Inc.; Reteplase (Reteplase) (2015). Chiesi, Cary, NC; Sobieszcyk, P. S. (2013). Acute arterial occlusion. In M. A. Creager, J. A. Beckman, J. Loscalzo (Eds.), *Vascular medicine: A companion to Braunwald's heart disease.* Philadelphia, PA: Elsevier Saunders.

has led to an increase in their use. However, it has yet to be determined if the reduced need for monitoring overrides the increase in cost and absence of an easy antidote when patients have major bleeding as a current concern.

Thrombolytic Therapy

Unlike heparin, thrombolytic (fibrinolytic) therapy lyses and dissolves thrombi. There is an increase in bleeding complications with thrombolytics compared with heparin. Since thrombolytics have not decreased the incidence of postthrombotic syndrome or pulmonary emboli, this therapy is generally reserved for patients with life-threatening limb ischemia as a result of massive thrombosis. If bleeding occurs, the thrombolytic agent is discontinued. See Table 18-3 for thrombolytic therapy.

Oral Anticoagulants

Warfarin is a vitamin K antagonist (VKA) that is frequently used for extended anticoagulant therapy. Routine coagulation monitoring is essential to ensure that a therapeutic response is obtained and maintained over time. Interactions with a range of other medications and various foods with vitamin K can reduce or enhance the anticoagulant effects of warfarin. Warfarin has a narrow therapeutic window, and there is a slow onset of action. Oral

anticoagulants, such as warfarin (Coumadin), are monitored by the INR. Because the full anticoagulant effect of warfarin is delayed for 3 to 5 days, treatment is initially supported with concomitant parenteral anticoagulation with heparin until the warfarin demonstrates anticoagulant effectiveness; then the heparin can be discontinued and the patient maintained on oral Coumadin. A normal INR is approximately 1. The target INR depends on why the person is being anticoagulated. If, for example, anticoagulation is related to atrial fibrillation or DVT, the INR range will be 2 to 3, with a goal of 2.5. Once INR is stable, levels are checked weekly for 2 to 4 weeks, progressing to monthly thereafter. Refer to Table 18-4 for list of therapeutic goals for INR.

Surgical Management

Surgery is necessary for DVT when anticoagulant or thrombolytic therapy is contraindicated, the danger of PE is likely, or the venous drainage is so severely compromised that permanent damage to the extremity is likely. A thrombectomy (removal of the thrombosis) is the procedure of choice. A vena cava filter may be placed at the time of the thrombectomy; this filter traps large emboli and prevents PE (see Chapter 10, Fig. 10-8). Recent research noted that placement of an inferior vena cava (IVC) filter for 3 months did not

TABLE **18-4** Therapeutic Context

	INR	Target
Non–hip surgery	1.5–2.5	2.0
Hip surgery	2.0–3.0	2.5
Primary and secondary prevention of deep vein thrombosis	2.0–3.0	2.5
Prevention of systemic embolism in patients with atrial fibrillation	2.0–3.0	2.5
Recurrent systemic embolism	3.0–4.5	3.5
Prevention of recurrent deep vein thrombosis (two or more episodes)	2.5–4.0	3.0
Cardiac stents	3.0–4.5	3.5
Prevention of arterial thrombosis, including patients with mechanical heart valves	2.5–3.5	3.0

Fischbach, F. T., & Dunning, M. B. (2014). *A manual of laboratory and diagnostic tests* (8th ed.). Philadelphia, PA: Lippincott Williams & Wilkins.

reduce recurrent PE, including fatal PE, in anticoagulated patients who had additional risk factors for recurrent VTE (Mismetti et al., 2015). A vena cava filter may be indicated if there is a contraindication to or complication of anticoagulation therapy (DeHart, 2015, p. 212). The filter does not prevent other thrombi from forming. Balloon angioplasty and stent placement are being used in the iliac veins of patients with acute and chronic venous disease.

Nursing Management

Monitoring Drug Therapy

When the patient is receiving anticoagulant therapy, the nurse frequently monitors the aPTT, prothrombin time (PT), INR, activated coagulation time (ACT), hemoglobin and hematocrit values, platelet count, and fibrinogen level, depending on which medication is being given.

Nurses must watch for potential complications; the principal one is spontaneous bleeding anywhere in the body. Bleeding from the kidneys is detected by microscopic examination of the urine and is often the first sign of excessive dosage. Bruises, nosebleeds, and bleeding gums are also early signs. To promptly reverse the effects of heparin, protamine sulfate may be administered. Risks of protamine administration include bradycardia and hypotension, which can be minimized by slow administration. Protamine sulfate can be used in patients receiving LMWH, but it is less effective with LMWH than with unfractionated heparin. Reversing the anticoagulation effects of warfarin is more difficult, but effective measures may include administration of vitamin K and/or infusion of fresh-frozen plasma or prothrombin concentrate. Oral vitamin K significantly reduces the INR within 24 hours. Low-dose IV vitamin K is also effective.

HIT may be another complication of therapy, which is defined as a sudden decrease in the platelet count by at least 30% of baseline levels in patients receiving heparin.

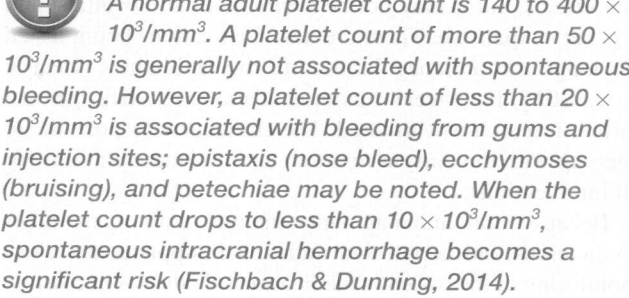

Nursing Alert

A normal adult platelet count is 140 to 400 × 10³/mm³. A platelet count of more than 50 × 10³/mm³ is generally not associated with spontaneous bleeding. However, a platelet count of less than 20 × 10³/mm³ is associated with bleeding from gums and injection sites; epistaxis (nose bleed), ecchymoses (bruising), and petechiae may be noted. When the platelet count drops to less than 10 × 10³/mm³, spontaneous intracranial hemorrhage becomes a significant risk (Fischbach & Dunning, 2014).

Patients at greatest risk for bleeding are those who receive unfractionated heparin for a long period of time (i.e., several days or weeks). Therefore, it is preferable not to anticoagulate patients with unfractionated heparin over the long term. Beginning warfarin concomitantly with heparin can provide a stable INR by day 5 of heparin treatment, at which time the heparin may be discontinued.

The administration of LMWH is less frequently associated with HIT. The thrombocytopenia is thought to result from an autoimmune mechanism that causes destruction of platelets. If the process is not arrested, platelets may aggregate, initiating inappropriate clotting, and thrombosis may occur. This serious complication results in thromboembolic manifestations throughout the body, and the prognosis is extremely guarded.

Prevention of thrombocytopenia depends on regular monitoring of platelet counts. Early signs of complications associated with anticoagulants include a decreasing platelet count, the need for increasing doses of heparin to maintain the therapeutic level, and thromboembolic or hemorrhagic complications, such as skin necrosis at the injection site and at distal sites of thromboses, and skin discoloration consisting of hemorrhagic areas, hematomas, purpura, and blistering. If thrombocytopenia does occur, platelet aggregation studies are conducted, the heparin is discontinued, and alternate anticoagulant therapy is initiated rapidly because the continued prothrombotic state poses an ongoing threat of continuous clot development.

Lepirudin (Refludan) and argatroban are DTIs approved for treatment of HIT. Lepirudin has a half-life of 1.3 hours, is excreted by the kidneys, and can be monitored using the aPTT. An initial IV bolus infusion followed by a continuous infusion with subsequent adjustments to maintain the aPTT between 1.5 and 2.5 times baseline has been recommended. Strict dosage adjustment in kidney failure is required because the clearance of lepirudin is proportional to the patient's creatinine clearance. Argatroban has a half-life of 30 to 45 minutes, is metabolized by the liver, and is unaffected by kidney function. The anticoagulant effect of argatroban is predictable, with low variability between patients, but it is dose-dependent and requires monitoring with either the aPTT or ACT. There is no safe, rapidly acting antidote if the patient develops bleeding complications from DTIs. Recombinant factor VIIa may reverse the anticoagulant effects, but it may not be available in all hospitals, and it is very expensive. There are new medications being tested for long-term anticoagulation, but the Guidelines (Kearon et al., 2016) have weak recommendations for their use and further research is warranted. The clinician is responsible to keep up with the current research and recommendations for all interventions.

Because oral anticoagulants interact with many other medications and herbal and nutritional supplements, close monitoring of the patient's medication schedule is necessary. Many medications and supplements potentiate or inhibit oral anticoagulants; it is always wise to check to see if any medications or supplements the patient is taking are contraindicated with warfarin. In general, 3 months of therapy is expected (Ginsberg, 2016).

Providing Comfort

Elevation of the affected extremity, elastic compression stockings, and analgesics for pain relief are adjuncts to therapy. They help improve circulation and increase comfort.

Warm, moist packs applied to the affected extremity reduce the discomfort associated with DVT, as do mild analgesics prescribed for pain control. When the patient begins to ambulate, elastic compression stockings are used. Walking is better than standing or sitting for long periods. The patient is advised to elevate the legs when not ambulating.

Nursing Alert
Does research show that bed rest or ambulation is best for a patient with a DVT?
Early ambulation has demonstrated the ability to decrease the risk of thrombus extension without increasing the risk of PE (DeHart, 2015). In addition, ventilation/perfusion scanning studies (V/Q scanning) demonstrate no decrease in PE with the use of bed rest, while pain and swelling have been shown to resolve more rapidly with early ambulation (Dehart, 2015, p. 212). However, the use of bed rest versus activity continues as an institutional protocol in many hospitals. The nurse should follow the facility's protocol but be cognizant of the findings described here.

Applying Compression Therapy

Increased venous pressure causes the long-term negative effects of venous disease. Treatment for venous insufficiency is external compression, which counteracts this pressure and protects the tissues from further damage.

Elastic compression stockings are prescribed for patients with chronic venous insufficiency. These stockings exert a sustained, graduated compression over the extremity, compressing the superficial veins, minimizing venous blood pooling, and resulting in increased flow toward the deep veins. They also prevent the sequelae of postphlebitic syndrome (fibrosis, ulceration). Stockings are available in knee-high, thigh-high, or waist-high lengths.

Short stretch elastic wraps may be applied from the toes to the knee in a 50% spiral overlap. These wraps are available in two-, three-, or four-layer systems, which include an inner layer of soft padding. Other types of compression include the Unna boot, which consists of a gauze roll impregnated with glycerin, gelatin, and sometimes zinc oxide or calamine. It is applied without tension in a circular, angular fashion from the base of the toes to the tibial tuberosity with a 50% spiral overlap. This type of compression may remain in place for as long as 1 week. Other manufactured rigid dressings are available to effectively augment the calf muscle pump during ambulation. Patients may find these dressings easier to wear than the Unna boot or a compression stocking.

Intermittent pneumatic compression devices can be used with elastic compression stockings to prevent DVT and to reduce edema. They consist of an electric motor attached to plastic knee-high or thigh-high sleeves, with single-chamber or multiple sequential chamber air bladders. These devices mimic muscle contraction and apply pressure to the veins, increasing blood velocity during bed rest.

Body Positioning and Exercise

When the patient is on bed rest, the feet and lower legs should be elevated periodically above the level of the heart. This position allows the veins to empty rapidly. Active and passive leg exercises, particularly those involving calf muscles, should be performed to increase venous flow. Early ambulation is most effective in preventing venous stasis. Deep-breathing exercises produce increased negative pressure in the thorax, which assists in emptying the large veins. Once ambulatory, the patient is instructed to avoid sitting for more than 2 hours at a time and to perform active and passive leg exercises during long car, train, and plane trips when ambulation is not possible.

VARICOSE VEINS

Varicose veins (varicosities) are abnormally dilated, tortuous, superficial veins caused by incompetent venous valves. They occur more frequently in the lower extremities, the saphenous veins, or the lower trunk, but they can occur elsewhere in the body.

Pathophysiology

Varicose veins may be primary (without involvement of deep veins) or secondary (resulting from obstruction of deep veins). A reflux of venous blood in the veins results in venous stasis. If the superficial veins are affected without deep vein involvement, the patient may be asymptomatic but may be troubled by the appearance of the distended veins.

Risk Factors

Varicose veins are more common in women than men and in people whose occupations require prolonged standing, such as salespeople, hair stylists, teachers, nurses, and ancillary medical personnel, and construction workers. A hereditary weakness of the vein wall may contribute to the development of varicosities, and it commonly occurs in several members of the same family. Varicose veins are rare before puberty. Pregnancy may cause varicosities because of hormonal effects related to venous distensibility, increased pressure by the gravid uterus, and increased blood volume.

Clinical Manifestations and Assessment

Symptoms, if present, may include dull aches, muscle cramps, increased muscle fatigue in the lower legs, ankle edema, and a feeling of heaviness of the legs. Nocturnal cramps are common. When deep venous obstruction results in varicose veins, the patient may develop the signs and symptoms of chronic venous insufficiency: edema, pain, pigmentation changes, and ulcers. Susceptibility to injury and infection is increased.

Diagnostic tests for varicose veins include the duplex scan, which documents the anatomic site of reflux and provides a quantitative measure of the severity of valvular reflux. Air plethysmography measures the changes in venous blood volume. Venography is not routinely performed to evaluate for valvular reflux.

Prevention

The patient should avoid activities that increase venous hypertension, such as wearing constricting clothing, crossing the legs at the thighs, and sitting or standing for long periods. Changing position frequently, elevating the legs when they are tired, and getting up to walk for several minutes of every hour promote circulation. The patient is encouraged to walk 1 or 2 miles each day if there are no contraindications. Walking up the stairs rather than using the elevator or escalator is helpful, and swimming is good exercise. Walking must incorporate the heel–toe step rather than a shuffle to elicit the calf muscle pump effect. Overweight patients should be encouraged to begin a weight-reduction plan.

Surgical Management

Ligation and Stripping

Surgery for varicose veins requires that the deep veins be patent and functional. The saphenous vein is ligated and divided. The vein is ligated high in the groin, where the saphenous vein meets the femoral vein. Pressure and

elevation minimize bleeding during surgery. Vein stripping, which used to be a common surgical procedure, has been replaced by the venous ablation techniques.

Ablation Procedures

Thermal ablation is a nonsurgical approach using thermal energy. Radiofrequency ablation uses an electrical contact inside the vein. As the device is withdrawn, the vein is sealed. Laser ablation uses a laser fiber tip that seals the vein (decompresses it). Topical gel may be used first to numb the skin along the course of the saphenous vein. To protect the surrounding tissue, a series of small punctures are made along the vein, and 100 to 200 mL of dilute lidocaine is delivered to the perivenous space using ultrasound guidance. The goal of this tumescent anesthesia (i.e., anesthesia that causes localized swelling) is to provide analgesia, thermal protection (the cuff of fluid surrounds the veins and accompanying nerves), and extrinsic compression of the vein. The saphenous vein is entered percutaneously near the knee using ultrasound guidance. The device is then activated and withdrawn, sealing the vein. Small bandages and compression stockings are applied after the procedure. The patient is asked not to remove the stockings for at least 48 hours and then to rewrap the legs and wear the compression stockings while ambulatory for a period of time according to a protocol. Patients are ambulatory prior to being discharged from the outpatient facility and have no activity restrictions, except that swimming is discouraged for 3 weeks. NSAIDs, such as ibuprofen or acetaminophen, are used as needed for pain. The patient is informed that bruising along the course of the vein, leg cramps (for a few days), and difficulty straightening the knees (for up to 1.5 weeks) may be experienced post procedure.

Sclerotherapy

Sclerotherapy involves injection of an irritating chemical into a vein to produce localized phlebitis and fibrosis, thereby obliterating the lumen of the vein. This treatment may be performed alone for small varicosities or may follow vein ablation or ligation. Sclerosing is palliative rather than curative. Sclerotherapy is typically performed in an examination or procedure room and does not require any sedation. After the sclerosing agent is injected, elastic compression bandages are applied to the leg and are worn according to a protocol, followed by elastic compression stockings. Walking activities are encouraged to maintain blood flow and to dilute the sclerosing agent within the deep venous system.

Post Procedure Nursing Management

After venous ablation procedures, bed rest is discouraged; the nurse encourages the patient to become ambulatory as soon as sedation has worn off. The patient is instructed to walk according to an individual protocol and to increase walking and activity as tolerated. Elastic compression stockings may be worn continuously or just when awake and upright (depending on the individual care provider's protocol) for 1 to 2 weeks after vein procedures. The nurse assists the patient in performing exercises and moving the legs. The foot of the bed should be elevated. Standing and sitting are discouraged. Jogging and hard-impact exercises are avoided according to individual protocols.

Analgesics are prescribed to help the patient move the affected extremities more comfortably. Dressings are inspected for bleeding, particularly at the groin, where the risk of bleeding is greatest. The nurse is alert for reported sensations of "pins and needles," as sensation is regained. Hypersensitivity to touch in the involved extremity may indicate a temporary or permanent nerve injury resulting from the procedure because the saphenous vein and nerve are close to each other in the leg.

Usually, the patient may shower after the first 24 hours. The patient is instructed to dry the incisions well with a clean towel, using a patting technique, rather than rubbing. Application of skin lotion is avoided until the incisions are completely healed to avoid infection. The patient is instructed to apply sunscreen or zinc oxide to the incision area prior to sun exposure for 6 months; otherwise, hyperpigmentation of the incision, scarring, or both may occur. The nurse may encourage the use of a mild analgesic as prescribed and regular short walking to provide relief.

CHRONIC VENOUS INSUFFICIENCY

Venous insufficiency results from obstruction of the venous valves in the legs and a reflux of blood. Both superficial and deep leg veins can be involved. A prolonged increase in venous pressure causes venous hypertension. Because the walls of veins are thinner and more elastic than arterial walls, they distend readily when venous pressure is elevated consistently. In this state, leaflets of the venous valves are stretched and prevented from closing completely, allowing a backflow or reflux of blood in the veins (Fig. 18-7). Duplex ultrasound confirms the obstruction and identifies incompetent venous valves.

Clinical Manifestations and Assessment

Classic signs of venous disease are edema and increased pigmentation of the skin, termed *hemosiderosis*. Because of the poor venous return, there is extravasation of red blood cells, which break down and deposit hemosiderin (a pigment that gives red blood cells their color), staining the skin a gray-brown. Varicosities and telangiectasias are also commonly noted. The extremity is warm, and pulses are present (assuming there is no concomitant arterial disease) but may be difficult to feel due to the extensive edema.

Postthrombotic syndrome is the long-term result of an incompetent venous system and venous hypertension. Venous obstruction or poor calf muscle pumping, in addition

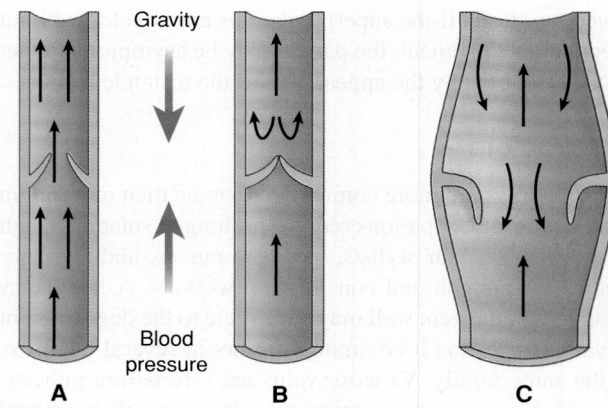

FIGURE 18-7 Competent valves showing blood flow patterns when the valve is open (**A**) and closed (**B**), allowing blood to flow against gravity. (**C**) With faulty or incompetent valves, the blood cannot move toward the heart.

to valvular reflux, also contributes to the development of severe postthrombotic syndrome. It is characterized by chronic edema, altered pigmentation, pain, and stasis dermatitis. This is called *dermatosclerosis*. The patient may notice aching and heaviness less in the morning after rest and elevation and more in the evening. The disorder is longstanding, difficult to treat, and often disabling.

Medical and Nursing Management

Management of the patient with venous insufficiency is directed at reducing venous stasis and preventing ulcers (see additional discussion below). Measures that increase venous blood flow are antigravity activities, such as elevating the leg, and compression of superficial veins with elastic compression stockings.

Elevating the legs decreases edema, promotes venous return, and provides symptomatic relief. The legs should be elevated frequently throughout the day. At night, the patient should sleep with the foot of the bed elevated. Prolonged sitting or standing in one position is detrimental; walking should be encouraged.

VASCULAR ULCERS

Vascular ulcers include arterial ischemic ulcers, venous ulcers, and ulcers on the lymphatic limb (Table 18-5). Treatment is different for each of these ulcers because treatment is based on etiology, which varies for each type of ulcer. Ulcers are not common on lymphatic limbs. When they occur, usually, associated venous disease or trauma to the already compromised tissue is present.

Pathophysiology

Venous ulceration is the most serious complication of chronic venous insufficiency and can be associated with other conditions

TABLE 18-5 Arterial and Venous Ulcer Characteristics

	Arterial	Venous
Location	Distal to arterial stenosis, heels, toes, over bony prominences, metatarsals, malleoli, between toes, trauma points	Around ankle, lower third of leg, more often on medial side
Ulcer base	Dry, pale gray or yellow; may be necrotic	Generally shallow but may be deep. Pink, but may be beefy red with granulation tissue. Ulcer bed usually moist. May have copious drainage
Shape	Border regular and well demarcated	Irregular border
Surrounding tissue	Pale; cooler than other skin areas. In longstanding insufficiency, skin is thin.	Darkened color in gaiter area. Temperature higher than other skin areas. Brawny edema. Skin may be thick and fibrotic (woody). May be oozing and crusted
Edema	Minimal unless leg is dependent often	May be severe
Pain	Claudication. Rest pain; continuous pain worsens with elevation and eases with dependency.	Aching, throbbing, heaviness. Superficial stinging when open to air during dressing changes
Pulses	May be absent or diminished; often disappears with exercise	Usually present with only venous etiology but may be difficult to palpate with edema
ABI	Less than 0.90	Greater than 0.90
Wound treatment	Moist wound healing after revascularization. Monitor for infection. Keep dry gangrene dry.	Compression. Elevation above heart. Absorptive dressings
Operative procedures	Arterial bypass. Angioplasty. Stent placement	Vein ligation/stripping. Valve grafts. Sclerotherapy. Laser or radiofrequency ablation

affecting the circulation of the lower extremities. Cellulitis or dermatitis may complicate the care of chronic venous insufficiency and venous ulcer. Venous ulcers develop as a result of increased venous pressure or external trauma.

Atherosclerosis, the most common cause of peripheral arterial occlusive disease, primarily affects the superficial femoral and popliteal vessels, reducing blood flow to the lower extremities. Ulceration will develop as a result of ischemia.

Clinical Manifestations and Assessment

Venous ulcers occur in the lower part of the extremity, in the area of the medial malleolus of the ankle, called the *gaiter area*. They range from small to large in size, are superficial, irregular in shape, highly exudative, and associated with periulcer hemosiderin staining of the skin. The skin becomes dry, cracked, and pruritic; subcutaneous tissues fibrose and atrophy. The risk for injury and infection of the extremities is increased.

Typically, arterial ulcers are small lesions on the tips of toes or in the web spaces between the toes. Ulcers often occur on the medial side of the hallux or lateral fifth toe and may be caused by a combination of ischemia and pressure.

Arterial insufficiency may result in gangrene of the toe (digital gangrene), which may be precipitated by trauma (Box 18-8) (Sieggreen & Kline, 2016a).

Medical and Nursing Management

Patients with ulcers can be effectively managed by advanced practice nurses or wound-ostomy-continence nurses in collaboration with health care providers. The nurse is aware that all ulcers have the potential to become infected.

Pharmacologic Therapy

All ulcers are colonized with superficial bacteria. Most leg ulcers do not need antibiotics. Antibiotic therapy is prescribed when the ulcer is infected; the specific antibiotic agent is based on culture and sensitivity test results. When indicated, oral or intravenous antibiotics usually are prescribed because topical antibiotics have not proven to be effective for leg ulcers.

Wound Cleansing and Débridement

As a general rule, arterial ulcers are kept dry and necrotic tissue is not débrided until revascularization procedures are performed because of the risk of infection and the likelihood of nonhealing associated with poor peripheral perfusion.

Venous ulcers with necrotic tissue should be débrided. To promote healing, the wound is kept clean of drainage. The wound is cleaned with each dressing change using normal saline solution or a non cytotoxic wound-cleansing agent.

BOX 18-8
Gangrene of the Toe

Gangrene of the toes, resulting from severe arterial ischemia, causes the digits to turn black. Débridement is contraindicated in these instances. Although the toes are gangrenous, this is the dry form of gangrene. Managing dry gangrene is preferable to débriding and creating an open wound that will not heal because of insufficient circulation. A distal amputation requires adequate circulation to heal. Without it, further amputation, such as below the knee or above the knee may be necessary. A higher-level amputation in an elderly person often results in loss of independence and possibly the need for institutional care. Dry gangrene of the toe(s) in an elderly person with poor circulation, who is asymptomatic, is usually left undisturbed. The toes are kept clean and dry until they separate from the viable tissue. Soaking is avoided.

The cleansing agent should be applied to the wound with enough force to wash the surface debris away. If there is necrotic tissue at the base of the venous wound, debridement, or removal of nonviable tissue, may be necessary. Removing the dead tissue is important to promote wound healing. There are several methods of debridement.

- *Surgical debridement:* This is the fastest method and can be performed by a physician, skilled advanced practice nurse, or wound-ostomy-continence nurse in collaboration with the physician.
- *Wet to dry or nonselective debridement:* This method can be accomplished by applying saline-impregnated gauze to the ulcer. When the dressing dries, it is removed, along with the debris adhering to the gauze. Pain management is usually necessary.
- *Enzymatic debridement:* This method involves application of enzyme ointments prescribed to treat the ulcer. The ointment is applied to the lesion but not to normal surrounding skin. Most enzymatic ointments are covered with saline-soaked gauze that has been thoroughly wrung out. Then a dry gauze dressing and a loose bandage are applied. The enzymatic ointment is discontinued when

the necrotic tissue has been débrided, and an appropriate wound dressing is applied.
- *Autolytic debridement:* With this method, an occlusive absorptive dressing, such as a hydrocolloid, is placed over the wound and left in place for a few (3 to 7) days to allow enzymes from the body to liquefy the necrotic tissue and separate it from the viable tissue. The wound is irrigated copiously during dressing changes to cleanse away the necrotic tissue. This type of dressing promotes granulation tissue growth (Sieggreen & Kline, 2016).

Wound Dressings

After the circulatory status has been assessed and determined to be adequate for healing, surgical dressings can be used to promote a moist environment. The simplest method is to use a wound contact material next to the wound bed and cover it with gauze. Other available options that promote the growth of granulation tissue and reepithelialization include the *hydrocolloids*. These materials also provide a barrier for protection because they adhere to the wound bed and surrounding tissue. However, these dressings may not be effective treatment for deep wounds and infected wounds. Patient and family education is necessary before beginning and throughout the wound care program. See Chapter 52 for further information about wound care.

Stimulated Healing

Tissue-engineered human skin equivalent is a skin product cultured from human dermal fibroblasts and keratinocytes used in combination with therapeutic compression. When applied, it seems to react to factors in the wound and may interact with the patient's cells to stimulate the production of growth factors. Application is not difficult, no suturing is involved, and the procedure is painless.

Hyperbaric Oxygenation

Hyperbaric oxygenation (HBO) may be beneficial as an adjunct treatment in patients with diabetes who evidence no signs of wound healing after standard wound treatment. HBO is accomplished by placing the patient into a chamber that increases barometric pressure while the patient is breathing 100% oxygen. The process by which HBO is thought to work involves several factors. The edema in the wound area is decreased because high oxygen tension facilitates vasoconstriction and enhances the ability of leukocytes to phagocytize and kill bacteria. In addition, HBO is thought to increase diffusion of oxygen to the hypoxic wound, thereby enhancing epithelial migration and improving collagen production.

Compression

Leg elevation helps to promote edema reduction. Venous ulcers require external compression. The Unna boot or commercial two- and three-layer compression bandages are available for this treatment. An Unna boot is a gauze dressing impregnated with a paste of glycerin, zinc oxide, and, sometimes, calamine. It is layered on the leg like a cast, from the tips of the toes to just below the knee. Extra padding is used if there is copious wound drainage, and an elastic bandage is placed over the dressing. Once the dressing dries, it becomes rigid. The boot is changed weekly. Its effectiveness depends on healthy calf muscle and the ability to ambulate.

LYMPHATIC DISORDERS

The lymphatic system consists of a set of vessels that start as lymph capillaries, which drain unabsorbed plasma from the interstitial spaces (spaces between the cells). The lymphatic capillaries unite to form the lymph vessels, which pass through the lymph nodes and then empty into progressively larger channels, most of which drain into the thoracic duct that joins the jugular vein on the left side of the neck.

Fluid drained from the interstitial space by the lymphatic system is called *lymph*. Lymph flow depends on the intrinsic contractions of the lymph vessels, the contraction of muscles, respiratory movements, and gravity. The lymphatic vessels of the extremities empty into nodes of the axillae and the groin. Under certain abnormal conditions, the fluid filtered out of the capillaries may greatly exceed the amounts reabsorbed and carried away by the lymphatic vessels. This imbalance can result from a variety of etiologies, including damage to capillary walls and subsequent increased permeability, obstruction of lymphatic drainage, elevation of venous pressure, or decrease in plasma protein osmotic force. Accumulation of excess interstitial fluid that results from these processes is known as lymphedema. In general, the nurse is aware that edema usually represents accumulation of 2.5 to 3 L of interstitial fluid. If the edema is *pitting*—that is, when the nurse presses the thumb into the edematous area for 5 seconds an imprint of the finger is noted—it is estimated that approximately 4.5 kg (10 lb) of fluid has accumulated (Leblond, DeGowin, & Brown, 2015). Refer to Chapter 12 for more details on assessing pitting edema.

Lymphangiography and lymphoscintigraphy are two diagnostic tests to assess lymphatic function. Lymphangiography involves injecting a contrast agent into a lymphatic vessel in each foot (or hand), followed by taking a series of x-rays at the conclusion of the injection, 24 hours later, and periodically thereafter. A diagnosis of lymphedema can be confirmed by the failure to identify subcutaneous lymphatic collection of contrast agent and the persistence of contrast agent in the tissue for days afterward.

Lymphoscintigraphy is a reliable alternative to lymphangiography. A radioactively labeled colloid is injected subcutaneously in the second interdigital space. The extremity is then exercised to facilitate the uptake of the colloid by the lymphatic system, and serial images are obtained at preset intervals.

LYMPHANGITIS AND LYMPHADENITIS

Lymphangitis is an acute inflammation of the lymphatic channels. It arises most commonly from an infection in an extremity. Usually, the infectious organism is a hemolytic streptococcus. The characteristic red streaks that extend up the arm or the leg from an infected wound outline the course of the lymphatic vessels as they drain.

The lymph nodes located along the course of the lymphatic channels also become enlarged, red, and tender (acute lymphadenitis). They can also become necrotic and form an abscess (suppurative lymphadenitis). The nodes involved most often are those in the groin, axilla, or cervical region. Because these infections are nearly always caused by organisms that are sensitive to antibiotics, it is unusual to see abscess formation. Recurrent episodes of lymphangitis are often associated with progressive lymphedema. After acute attacks, and if the edema has subsided, an elastic compression stocking or sleeve should be worn on the affected extremity for several months to prevent long-term edema.

LYMPHEDEMA AND ELEPHANTIASIS

Lymphedema is swelling in the extremities due to an accumulation of lymph from blocked lymphatic vessels.

Pathophysiology

Lymphedemas are classified as primary (congenital malformations) or secondary (acquired obstructions). Tissue swelling occurs in the extremities because of an increased quantity of lymph that results from obstruction of lymphatic vessels. It is especially marked when the extremity is in a dependent position. Initially, the edema is soft and pitting. As the condition progresses, the edema becomes firm, nonpitting, and less responsive to treatment. The most common type is congenital lymphedema (*lymphedema praecox*), which is caused by hypoplasia (underdevelopment) of the lymphatic system of the lower extremity.

The obstruction may be in the lymph nodes and the lymphatic vessels. Sometimes, it is seen in the arm after an axillary node dissection (e.g., for breast cancer) and in the leg in association with varicose veins or chronic thrombophlebitis. In the latter case, the lymphatic obstruction usually is caused by chronic lymphangitis. Lymphatic obstruction caused by a parasite (filaria) is seen frequently in patients in the tropics and is the most common cause of lymphedema worldwide. When chronic swelling is present, there may be frequent bouts of acute infection characterized by high fever and chills and increased residual edema after the inflammation has resolved. These lead to chronic fibrosis, thickening of the subcutaneous tissues, and hypertrophy of the skin. This condition, in which chronic swelling of the extremity recedes only slightly with elevation, is referred to as *elephantiasis*.

Clinical Manifestations and Assessment

The diagnosis of lymphedema is made by clinical evaluation and exclusion of other causes of edema. In the early stages, the tissue is soft and pliable, but in advanced lymphedema, the tissue becomes firm and thick, often with overlapping folds of tissue. Early diagnosis is important to prevent tissue destruction. In the lower extremities the toes are squared, and the skin of the second toe fails to "tent" when pinched (Fife, Sieggreen, & Kline, 2016).

Medical Management

Treatment is focused on reducing the edema and preventing increased edema, infections, and tissue damage. Treatment may consist of comprehensive decongestive therapy provided by a certified lymphedema therapist, use of a pump to reduce the edema, and elastic and nonelastic compression wraps or garments to maintain the edema reduction.

Care must be taken to avoid any break in the skin that would allow bacteria to enter the tissue. Antibiotics are prescribed for infection. Antibiotics used to be prescribed frequently for prophylaxis because chronic infections were common in some individuals. They are very selectively prescribed now because of the increase in antibiotic-resistant infections. Patients need support and must be taught that lymphedema requires lifelong vigilance. The individual needs to learn as much as possible about the condition and how to manage it (Box 18-9). The nurse provides access to resources available, both in the local area and credible references found online. Certified therapists can be located by accessing http://www.lymphnet.org.

Pharmacologic Therapy

As initial therapy, the diuretic furosemide (Lasix) may be prescribed to prevent fluid overload while the extracellular fluid is mobilized. The use of diuretics alone has little benefit because their main action is to limit capillary filtration by decreasing the circulating blood volume. If lymphangitis or cellulitis is present, antibiotic therapy is initiated in addition to the administration of diuretics. Skin care is important to maintain moisture.

Exercise and Compression

Active and passive exercises assist in moving lymphatic fluid into the bloodstream. External compression devices move the fluid proximally from the foot to the hip or from the hand to the axilla. When the patient is ambulatory, and the limb is reduced to an acceptable size, custom-fitted elastic compression stockings or sleeves are worn; those with the highest compression strength, 30–40 mm Hg, may be required. When the leg is affected, continuous bed rest with the leg elevated for a limited time may aid in mobilizing the fluids. Manual lymphatic drainage is a highly specialized massage technique designed to direct or shift the congested lymph through functioning lymphatics that have preserved drainage capacity. Manual lymphatic drainage used in combination with compression bandages, exercises, skin care, pressure gradient sleeves, and, sometimes, pneumatic pumps, depending on the severity and stage of the lymphedema. If the patient is in the hospital and in bed, there may be a reduction of the size of the limb in 24 hours. In this case a compression garment can be placed on to maintain the reduction. If the patient is at home, it is impractical to expect a 24-hour bed rest so the patient may be advised to sit with the legs elevated for 20 minutes three to four times a day. The nurse recognizes there are complications associated with prolonged bed rest, so the plan must be individualized for each person and agreed upon between the patient and the practitioner.

Surgical Management

Surgery is performed if the edema is severe and uncontrolled by medical therapy, if mobility is severely compromised, or if infection persists. One surgical approach involves the excision of the affected subcutaneous tissue and fascia, followed by skin grafting to cover the defect. Copious amounts of lymphatic fluid may make skin grafts nonadherent. Another procedure involves the surgical relocation of superficial lymphatic vessels into the deep lymphatic system by means of a buried dermal flap to provide a conduit for lymphatic drainage. This procedure has had limited success. Surgery is rarely performed in these patients in most hospitals. Patients who would benefit from surgery are referred to specialized centers.

Nursing Management

After surgery, the management of skin grafts and flaps is the same as when these therapies are used for other conditions. Antibiotics are prescribed. Constant elevation of the affected extremity and observation for complications are essential. Complications may include flap necrosis, hematoma or abscess under the flap, and cellulitis. The nurse instructs the patient or caregiver to inspect the dressing daily. Unusual

---

BOX 18-9 | **Patient Education for Lymphedema**

- Keep skin clean and dry.
- Wear compression support garments as prescribed.
- Avoid blood pressure cuffs, needle sticks, injections, or procedures on the affected limb.
- Report new swelling, redness, pain, heat, rash, blisters, or fever to the provider/nurse.
- Avoid tight clothing.
- Check feet with a mirror for sores, rashes, or cracks in the skin.
- Avoid trauma: Pet scratches, insect bites, burns, sports injuries, bruising.
- Clean cuts or insect bites with soap and water and apply antibiotic ointment.
- Elevate the affected limb whenever possible.

drainage or any inflammation around the wound margin suggests infection and should be reported to the surgeon. The patient is informed that there may be a loss of sensation in the skin graft area. The patient is also instructed to avoid the application of heating pads or exposure to sun to prevent burns or trauma to the area. The patient is taught to inspect the skin for evidence of infection.

CELLULITIS

Cellulitis is the most common infection of the skin and subcutaneous tissue that causes limb swelling. Cellulitis can occur as a single isolated event or a series of recurrent events. It is often misdiagnosed, usually as recurrent thrombophlebitis or chronic venous insufficiency. It occurs when an entry point through normal skin barriers allows bacteria to enter. Cellulitis is a frequent complication in tissues with lymphedema. It is also diagnosed in otherwise healthy tissue.

Pathophysiology

Cellulitis occurs when there is an entry point through the normal skin barrier. This allows bacteria to enter the subcutaneous tissue.

Clinical Manifestations and Assessment

The acute onset of swelling, localized redness, and pain is frequently associated with systemic signs of fever, chills, and sweating. The redness may not be uniform and often skips areas. Dimpling in the skin may be seen when the edema surrounds hair follicles. Regional lymph nodes may also be tender and enlarged.

Medical Management

Mild cases of cellulitis can be treated on an outpatient basis with oral antibiotic therapy. If the cellulitis is severe, the patient is treated with IV antibiotics. The key to preventing recurrent episodes of cellulitis lies in adequate antibiotic therapy for the initial event and in identifying the site of bacterial entry. The most commonly overlooked areas are the cracks and fissures that occur in the skin between the toes. Other possible locations are drug-use injection sites, contusions, abrasions, ulcerations, ingrown toenails, and hangnails.

Nursing Management

The patient is instructed to elevate the affected area above heart level and apply warm, moist packs to the site. Patients with sensory and circulatory deficits, such as those caused by diabetes and paralysis, should use caution when applying warm packs because burns may occur; it is advisable to use a thermometer or have a caregiver ensure that the temperature is not more than lukewarm. Education should focus on preventing a recurrent episode. The patient with PVD or diabetes mellitus should receive education or reinforcement about skin and foot care.

CHAPTER REVIEW

Critical Thinking Exercises

1. A 75-year-old male patient has been diagnosed with a stenosis of his external iliac artery and is scheduled for an angiogram with a possible balloon angioplasty and stent placement. What factors should be considered when planning his post procedure and continuing care? If the patient is taking warfarin for atrial fibrillation and has renal insufficiency (creatinine of 1.8 mg/dL) as a complication of diabetes, how would these factors be addressed in the plan of care?

2. A 96-year-old patient presents with a 2-year history of chronic venous ulceration of the left lower extremity, requiring weekly placement of an Unna boot. The patient lives alone, six blocks from any mass transit or shopping area, and no longer drives a vehicle. The patient wants to continue living at his current location. What options and plan of care should be discussed with the patient?

3. One of your patients has been diagnosed with a recurrent DVT of the femoral vein. The patient has been treated previously with unfractionated heparin and developed HIT. Discuss strategies for DVT prophylaxis that you will include in your teaching plan with this patient.

NCLEX-Style Review Questions

1. The nurse is caring for a patient diagnosed with peripheral arterial disease. Based on assessment, which clinical manifestation would be inconsistent with acute arterial occlusion?
   a. Pallor
   b. Paresthesia
   c. Hyperthermia
   d. Poikilothermia

2. A new postsurgical patient has been prescribed unfractionated heparin to prevent DVT. What is a true statement regarding the use of heparin?
   a. Heparin has a half-life of approximately 60 minutes.
   b. Therapeutic PT level is three times the baseline control
   c. Vitamin K interferes with the action of heparin
   d. Heparin is administered by gravity drip

3. The nurse is using a hydrocolloid dressing for a patient who is undergoing autolytic debridement of a necrotic venous ulcer. What is characteristic of this type of debridement?
   a. Accomplished by applying enzymatic ointment to the lesion
   b. Left in place for 3 to 7 days

   c. The fastest method of debridement
   d. Accomplished by applying saline impregnated gauze to the ulcer

4. Which of the following is not a reliable indicator of a possible DVT?
   a. Calf tenderness
   b. Edema of the extremity
   c. Homan sign
   d. Increased circumference of affected extremity

5. Which characteristic is consistent with an arterial ulcer?
   a. Pink or beefy red appearance with granulation tissue
   b. May have severe edema
   c. Darkened color tissue in gaiter area
   d. Pale and cool extremity

Try these additional resources, available at **http://thepoint.lww.com/Honan2e**, to enhance your learning and understanding of this chapter:
- NCLEX-Style Student Review Questions
- Journal Articles

REFERENCES AND SELECTED READINGS

References and selected readings associated with this chapter can be found on the website that accompanies the book. Visit **http://thepoint.lww.com/Honan2e** to access the references and other additional resources associated with this chapter.

Problems Related to Hematologic Function

A 65-year-old woman has been diagnosed with chronic myeloid leukemia (CML). Previously she had been complaining of fatigue. She has lost 10 lb in the last month. She is very apprehensive about starting chemotherapy.

- What is the only curative treatment for CML?
- Discuss the three phases of the disease.
- Discuss important nursing considerations of the patient undergoing treatment for CML (Gleevec).

Nursing Assessment: Hematologic Function

Lisa M. Barbarotta

Learning Objectives

After reading this chapter, you will be able to:

1. Describe the process of hematopoiesis.
2. Describe the processes involved in maintaining hemostasis.
3. Differentiate between normal and abnormal hematologic laboratory values.
4. Describe the pertinent components of nursing assessment based on abnormal hematologic laboratory values.
5. Describe the procedure and patient preparation for a bone marrow biopsy.

Unlike many other body systems, the hematologic system truly encompasses the entire human body. Patients with hematologic disorders often have significant abnormalities in blood tests but few or no symptoms. Therefore, the nurse must have an understanding of the pathophysiology of the patient's condition and the ability to make a thorough assessment that relies heavily on the interpretation of laboratory tests. It is equally important for the nurse to anticipate potential patient needs and to target nursing interventions accordingly. A basic appreciation of blood cells and bone marrow function is critical to the understanding of hematologic diseases.

ANATOMIC AND PHYSIOLOGIC OVERVIEW

The hematologic system consists of the blood and the sites where blood is produced, including the bone marrow and the **reticuloendothelial system** (RES). Blood is a specialized organ that differs from other organs in that it exists in a fluid state. Blood is composed of plasma and various types of cells. **Plasma** is the fluid portion of blood; it is thin and colorless and contains various proteins, such as albumin, globulin, **fibrinogen**, and other factors necessary for clotting, as well as electrolytes, waste products, and nutrients. Approximately 55% of blood volume is plasma, and 45% consists of various cellular components.

Blood

The cellular component of blood consists of three primary cell types (Table 19-1): **erythrocytes (red blood cells [RBCs])**, **leukocytes (white blood cells [WBCs])**, and **thrombocytes (platelets)**. As noted above, these cellular components of blood normally make up approximately 45% of the blood volume. Because most blood cells have a short lifespan, the need for the body to replenish its supply of cells is continuous; this process is termed **hematopoiesis** (the formation and production of blood cells). RBCs generally live for 120 days, WBCs live from days to years depending on the type, and platelets live 7 to 10 days. The primary site for hematopoiesis is the bone marrow. During embryonic development and in other conditions, the liver and spleen may also be involved; production of blood cells outside of the bone marrow is often referred to as **extramedullary hematopoiesis** (Golub, Vieira, & Cumano, 2014).

Under normal conditions, the adult bone marrow produces approximately 175 billion erythrocytes, 70 billion **neutrophils** (a mature type of WBC), and 175 billion platelets each day. When the body needs more blood cells, as in infection (when neutrophils are needed to fight the invading pathogen) or in bleeding (when more RBCs and platelets are needed), the marrow increases its production of the cells required. Thus, under normal conditions, the marrow responds to increased demand and releases adequate numbers of cells into the circulation.

Blood makes up approximately 7% to 10% of the normal body weight and amounts to 5 to 6 L of volume. Blood circulates through the vascular system carrying oxygen and nutrients to the various cells throughout the body to promote cell growth and function. Blood also carries proteins such as hormones, antibodies, and other substances to their sites of action or use. In addition, blood carries waste products

TABLE 19-1 Blood Cells

Cell Type	Major Function
WBC (Leukocyte)	Fights infection
Neutrophil	Essential in preventing or limiting bacterial infection via phagocytosis
Monocyte	Enters tissue as macrophage; highly phagocytic, especially against fungus
Eosinophil	Involved in allergic reactions (neutralizes histamine); digests foreign proteins
Basophil	Contains histamine; integral part of hypersensitivity reactions
Lymphocyte	Integral component of immune system
T lymphocyte	Responsible for cell-mediated immunity; recognizes material as "foreign"
B lymphocyte	Responsible for humoral immunity; many mature into plasma cells to form antibodies
Plasma cell	Secretes immunoglobulin (Ig, antibody); most mature form of B lymphocyte
RBC (Erythrocyte)	Carries hemoglobin to provide oxygen to tissues; average lifespan is 120 days
Platelet (Thrombocyte)	Fragment of megakaryocyte; provides basis for coagulation to occur; maintains hemostasis; average lifespan is 7 days

produced by cellular metabolism to the lungs, skin, liver, and kidneys for elimination.

To prevent blood loss as a result of trauma or injury, an intricate clotting mechanism is activated to seal any leak in the blood vessels. Excessive clotting is equally as dangerous as excessive blood loss because it can obstruct blood flow to vital tissues. To prevent this, the body has a fibrinolytic mechanism that eventually dissolves clots (**thrombi**) formed within blood vessels. The balance between these two systems, clot (**thrombus**) formation and clot dissolution, or **fibrinolysis**, is called **hemostasis**.

Bone Marrow

The bone marrow is the site of hematopoiesis, or blood cell formation (Fig. 19-1). In children, blood formation involves all skeletal bones, but with aging, marrow activity is usually limited to the pelvis, ribs, vertebrae, and sternum.

Marrow, which accounts for up to 4% to 5% of total body weight, consists of islands of cellular components (red marrow) separated by fat (yellow marrow). As the adult ages, the proportion of active marrow is gradually replaced by fat; however, in the healthy person, the fat can again be replaced by active marrow when more blood cell production is required. In adults with disease that causes marrow destruction, fibrosis, or scarring, the liver and spleen can also resume production of blood cells (*extramedullary hematopoiesis*).

The marrow is highly vascular. Within it are primitive cells called **stem cells**, which have the ability to self-replicate, thereby ensuring a continuous supply of stem cells throughout the lifecycle. When stimulated, stem cells can begin a process of **differentiation** into either **myeloid** or **lymphoid** stem cells. Lymphoid stem cells produce either T or B **lymphocytes**, whereas myeloid stem cells differentiate into three broad cell types: erythrocytes, leukocytes, and platelets. Thus, with the exception of lymphocytes, all blood cells are derived from myeloid stem cells. A defect in a myeloid stem cell can cause problems with erythrocyte, leukocyte, and platelet production. Many complex mechanisms are involved in hematopoiesis, many at the molecular level.

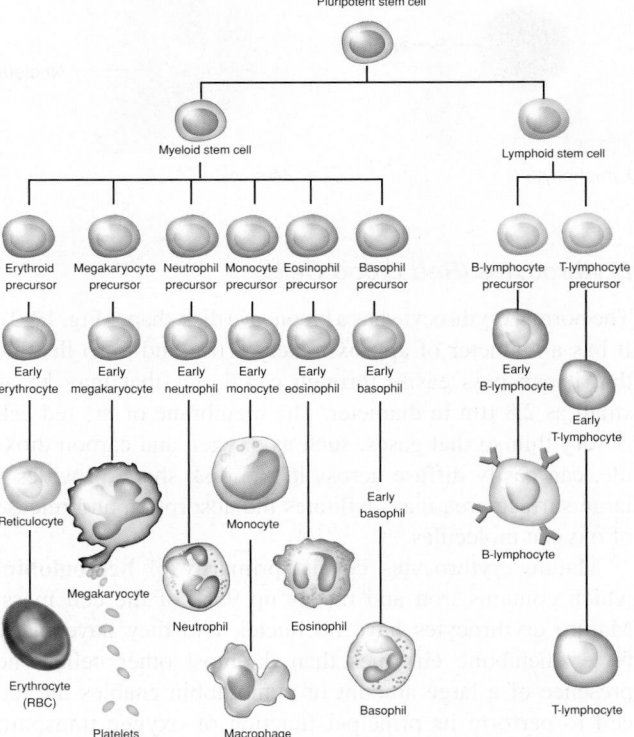

FIGURE 19-1 Hematopoiesis. Uncommitted (pluripotent) stem cells can differentiate into myeloid or lymphoid stem cells. These stem cells then undergo a complex process of differentiation and maturation into normal cells that are released into the circulation. The myeloid stem cell is responsible not only for all nonlymphoid white blood cells (WBCs) but also for the production of red blood cells (RBCs) and platelets. Each step of the differentiation process depends in part on the presence of specific growth factors for each cell type. When the stem cells are dysfunctional, they may respond inadequately to the need for more cells, or they may respond excessively, sometimes uncontrollably, as in leukemia.

Blood smear

Note the clump of platelets

Granulocytes

Neutrophil

Basophil

Eosinophil

Non-granulocytes

Lymphocyte

Monocyte

FIGURE 19-2 Normal types of blood cells. (From Cohen, B. J. (2016). *Memmler's the human body in health and disease* (12th ed.). Philadelphia, PA: Lippincott Williams & Wilkins.)

Erythrocytes (Red Blood Cells)

The normal erythrocyte has a biconcave disk shape (Fig. 19-2). It has a diameter of approximately 8 μm and is so flexible that it can pass easily through capillaries that may be as small as 2.8 μm in diameter. The membrane of the red cell is very thin so that gases, such as oxygen and carbon dioxide, can easily diffuse across it; the disk shape provides a large surface area that facilitates the absorption and release of oxygen molecules.

Mature erythrocytes consist primarily of **hemoglobin**, which contains iron and makes up 95% of the cell mass. Mature erythrocytes have no nuclei, and they have many fewer metabolic enzymes than do most other cells. The presence of a large amount of hemoglobin enables the red cell to perform its principal function of oxygen transport. Occasionally, the marrow releases slightly immature forms of erythrocytes, called **reticulocytes**, into the circulation. An elevation in the reticulocyte count may occur as a normal response to an increased demand for erythrocytes (as in bleeding) or in some disease states.

The oxygen-carrying hemoglobin molecule is made up of four subunits, each containing a heme portion attached to a globin chain. Iron is present in the heme component of the molecule. An important property of heme is its ability to bind to oxygen loosely and reversibly. Oxygen readily binds to hemoglobin in the lungs and is carried as **oxyhemoglobin** in arterial blood. Oxyhemoglobin is a brighter red than hemoglobin that contains lesser amounts of oxygen (reduced hemoglobin), which is why arterial blood is a brighter red than venous blood. The oxygen readily dissociates (detaches) from hemoglobin in the tissues, where the oxygen is needed for cellular metabolism. In venous blood, hemoglobin combines with hydrogen ions produced by cellular metabolism and thus buffers excessive acid. Whole blood normally contains approximately 15 g of hemoglobin per 100 mL of blood.

Erythropoiesis

Erythroblasts arise from the primitive myeloid stem cells in bone marrow. The erythroblast is an immature nucleated cell that accumulates hemoglobin and then gradually loses its nucleus. At this stage, the cell is known as a *reticulocyte*. Further maturation into an erythrocyte entails the loss of the dark-staining material within the cell and slight shrinkage. Then the mature erythrocyte is released into the circulation.

Differentiation of the primitive myeloid stem cell of the marrow into an erythroblast is stimulated by **erythropoietin**, a hormone produced primarily by the kidney. If the kidney detects low levels of oxygen (as would occur in **anemia**, in which fewer red cells are available to bind to oxygen, or with people living at high altitudes), the release of erythropoietin is stimulated. The increase in erythropoietin production then stimulates the marrow to increase production of erythrocytes. The entire process typically takes 5 days.

For normal erythrocyte production, the bone marrow also requires iron, vitamin B_{12}, folic acid, pyridoxine (vitamin B_6), protein, and other factors. A deficiency in any one of these factors during erythropoiesis can result in decreased red cell production and anemia.

Iron Stores and Metabolism. The average daily diet in the United States contains 10 to 15 mg of elemental iron, but only 0.5 to 1 mg of ingested iron is normally absorbed from the small intestine daily. The rate of iron absorption is regulated by the amount of iron already stored in the body and by the rate of erythrocyte production. Additional amounts of iron, up to 2 mg daily, must be absorbed by women of childbearing age to replace that lost during menstruation. Total body iron content in the average adult is approximately 3 to 4 g. The majority of iron stores (2 to 3 g) is carried in hemoglobin. The remainder of iron is stored in hepatocytes and macrophages, with a small portion stored in other proteins (ferroproteins) (Ganz & Nemeth, 2012a, 2012b).

The concentration of iron in blood is normally about 75 to 175 µg/dL (13 to 31 µmol/L) for men and 65 to 165 µg/dL (11 to 29 µmol/L) for women. With iron deficiency, bone marrow iron stores are depleted rapidly; hemoglobin synthesis is depressed, and the erythrocytes produced by the marrow are small and low in hemoglobin. This is known as *microcytic anemia* (characterized by small RBCs). Part of a standard complete blood count (CBC) includes the mean corpuscular volume (MCV), which measures the size of the RBCs. In microcytic anemia, a small (less than 82 µm³) MCV is seen. Causes of microcytic anemia include iron deficiency related to dietary inadequacy, malabsorption, increased iron loss (blood loss), and increased iron requirements (Fischbach & Dunning, 2014, p. 99). In the adult, lack of dietary iron is rarely the sole cause of iron deficiency anemia. Iron deficiency in the adult generally indicates that blood has been lost from the body (e.g., most commonly from bleeding in the GI tract or heavy menstrual flow). The source of iron deficiency should be investigated promptly because iron deficiency in an adult may be a sign of bleeding in the GI tract or colon cancer.

Vitamin B_{12} and Folic Acid Metabolism. Vitamin B_{12} and folic acid are required for the synthesis of DNA in many tissues. Deficiencies of either of these vitamins have a significant impact on erythropoiesis. Both vitamin B_{12} and folic acid are derived from the diet and depend on a functioning intestinal mucosa for absorption. Vitamin B_{12} combines with intrinsic factor produced in the stomach and is absorbed in the distal ileum.

Nursing Alert

It is important for nurses to recall that patients who have had a partial or total gastrectomy may have limited amounts of intrinsic factor, and, therefore, the absorption of vitamin B_{12} may be diminished, leading to anemia. The effects of either decreased absorption or decreased intake of vitamin B_{12} may not be apparent for 2 to 4 years.

Red Blood Cell Destruction

Aged erythrocytes lose their elasticity and become trapped in small blood vessels and the spleen. They are removed from the blood by the reticuloendothelial cells, particularly in the liver and the spleen. As the erythrocytes are destroyed, most of their hemoglobin is recycled. Some hemoglobin also breaks down to form bilirubin and is secreted in the bile. Most of the iron is recycled to form new hemoglobin molecules within the bone marrow; small amounts are lost daily in the feces and urine and monthly in menstrual flow.

Leukocytes (White Blood Cells)

Leukocytes are divided into two general categories: granulocytes and agranulocytes. In normal blood, the total leukocyte count is 5,000 to 10,000 cells per cubic millimeter. Of these, approximately 60% to 70% are granulocytes, and 30% to 40% are lymphocytes. Both of these types of leukocytes protect the body against infection and tissue injury.

Granulocytes

Granulocytes are defined by the presence of granules in the cytoplasm of the cell. Granulocytes are divided into three main subgroups (see Fig. 19-2): eosinophils, basophils, and neutrophils. **Neutrophils** are the most numerous cells of this class. Neutrophils are also called *polymorphonuclear neutrophils* (PMNs, or polys) or *segmented neutrophils* (segs).

The nucleus of the mature neutrophil has multiple lobes (usually two to five), or a "segmented" nucleus. The immature granulocyte has a single-lobed, elongated nucleus and is called a **band cell**. Ordinarily, band cells account for only a small percentage of circulating granulocytes, although their percentage can increase greatly under conditions in which neutrophil demand increases, such as infection. An increased number of band cells is sometimes called **bandemia**. A patient with bandemia should be evaluated thoroughly for infection.

Fully mature neutrophils result from the gradual differentiation of myeloid stem cells, specifically myeloid **blast cells**. The process, called **myelopoiesis**, takes an average of 10 days (see Fig. 19-1). Once the neutrophil is released into the circulation from the marrow, it stays there for only about 6 hours before it migrates into the body tissues to perform its function of **phagocytosis** (ingestion and digestion of bacteria and particles; Fig. 19-3). Here, neutrophils survive no more than 1 to 2 days before they die.

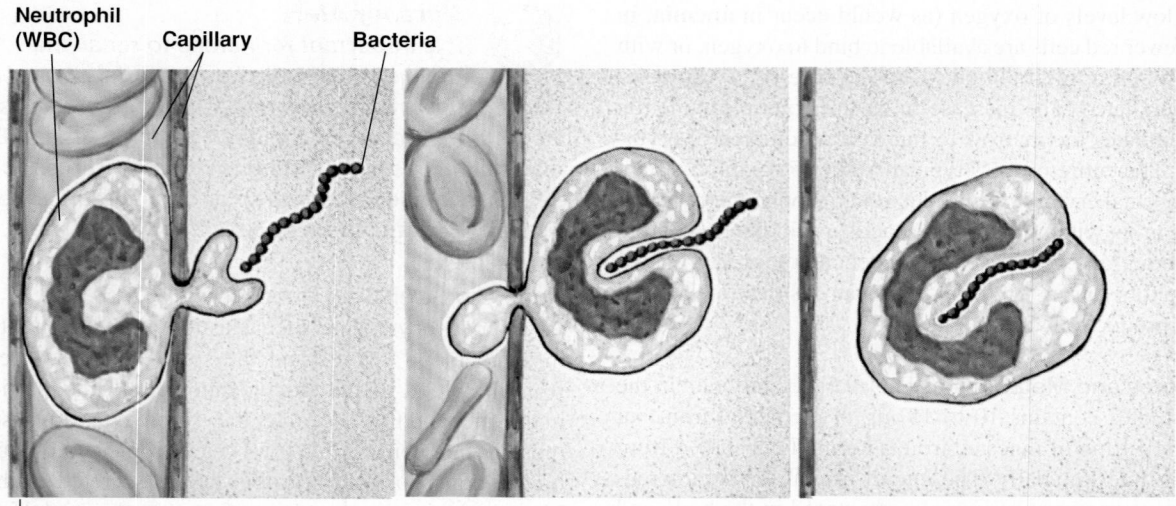

Neutrophil (WBC) **Capillary** **Bacteria**

Endothelial cell

FIGURE 19-3 Phagocytosis. In order for phagocytosis to occur, a foreign body (such as bacteria, parasites, or cellular debris) must adhere to the cell wall of the phagocyte. The phagocyte then extends around the foreign body by projecting out pseudopods, engulfing the foreign body. Once inside the phagocyte, the engulfed material is left in a vacuole, where enzymes within the cell destroy the foreign material.

Eosinophils play a key role in response to parasitic and allergic diseases. The presence of certain microbes (such as parasites) results in the release of the granular contents of the eosinophil, allowing for destruction and phagocytosis of the organism.

Basophils are the least numerous of the circulating leukocytes and have characteristically large, dark-purple granules. The granules contain heparin and histamine and are released in response to exposure to allergens.

The number of circulating granulocytes found in the healthy person is relatively constant. An elevation in the total number of WBCs may indicate infection, trauma, tissue injury, or malignancy (such as leukemia), or it may be a side effect of certain medications, such as corticosteroids. A WBC count that is below normal may be related to viral infections, the result of side effects from medications such as antiviral medications, or may hint of a more serious condition, such as leukemia or myelodysplastic syndrome (MDS).

Agranulocytes

Monocytes and lymphocytes are leukocytes with granule-free cytoplasm—hence the term *agranulocyte* (see Fig. 19-2).

Monocytes

Monocytes (also called *mononuclear leukocytes*) have a single-lobed nucleus. They are the largest of the leukocytes. In normal adult blood, monocytes account for approximately 5% of the total leukocyte count. When released from the marrow, monocytes spend a short time in the circulation (approximately 24 hours) and then enter the body tissues. Within the tissues, the monocytes continue to differentiate

into **macrophages**, which can survive for months. Macrophages are particularly active in the spleen, liver, peritoneum, and alveoli; they remove debris from these areas and phagocytize bacteria within the tissues (see discussion of the Reticuloendothelial System on page 563).

Lymphocytes

Mature lymphocytes are small cells with scanty cytoplasm (see Fig. 19-2). Immature lymphocytes are produced in the marrow from the lymphoid stem cells. A second major source of production is the cortex of the thymus. Cells derived from the thymus are known as T lymphocytes (or T cells); those derived from the marrow can also be T cells but are more commonly B lymphocytes (or B cells). Lymphocytes complete their differentiation and maturation primarily in the lymph nodes and in the lymphoid tissue of the intestine and spleen after exposure to a specific antigen. Mature lymphocytes are the principal cells of the immune system, producing antibodies and identifying other cells and organisms as foreign.

Function of Leukocytes

Granulocytes protect the body from invasion by bacteria and other foreign entities. Neutrophils arrive at a given site within 1 hour after the onset of an inflammatory reaction and initiate phagocytosis, but they are short lived. An influx of monocytes follows; these cells continue their phagocytic activities for long periods as macrophages. This process constitutes a second line of defense for the body against inflammation and infection. Although neutrophils often can work adequately against bacteria without the help of macrophages, macrophages are particularly effective against fungi and viruses.

The primary function of lymphocytes is to produce substances that aid in attacking foreign material. T lymphocytes kill foreign cells directly or release a variety of *lymphokines*, substances that enhance the activity of phagocytic cells. T lymphocytes are responsible for delayed allergic reactions, rejection of foreign tissue (e.g., transplanted organs), and destruction of tumor cells. This process is known as *cellular immunity*. B lymphocytes are capable of differentiating into plasma cells. Plasma cells, in turn, produce antibodies called immunoglobulin (Ig), which are protein molecules that destroy foreign material. This process is known as *humoral immunity*.

Both eosinophils and basophils are active in allergic reactions. For example, a patient with an allergic rash may have an elevated eosinophil count (Fischbach & Dunning, 2014, p. 76). Eosinophils also have a role in the destruction of parasites.

Platelets (Thrombocytes)

Platelets, or thrombocytes, are not technically cells; rather, they are granular fragments of giant cells in the bone marrow, called *megakaryocytes*. Platelet production in the marrow is regulated in part by the hormone thrombopoietin, which stimulates the production and differentiation of megakaryocytes from the myeloid stem cell.

Platelets play an essential role in the control of bleeding (hemostasis). They circulate freely in the blood in an inactive state, where they nurture the endothelium of the blood vessels, maintaining the integrity of the vessel. When vascular injury occurs, platelets collect at the site and are activated. They adhere to the site of injury and to each other, forming a platelet plug that temporarily stops bleeding. Substances released from platelet granules activate coagulation factors in the blood plasma and initiate the formation of a stable clot composed of **fibrin**, a filamentous protein.

Plasma and Plasma Proteins

After cellular elements are removed from blood, the remaining liquid portion is called *plasma*. More than 90% of plasma is water. The remainder consists primarily of plasma proteins, clotting factors (particularly fibrinogen), and small amounts of other substances such as nutrients, enzymes, waste products, and gases. If plasma is allowed to clot, the remaining fluid is called **serum**. Serum has essentially the same composition as plasma, except that fibrinogen and several clotting factors have been removed in the clotting process.

Plasma proteins consist primarily of albumin and the globulins. The globulins can be separated into three main fractions (alpha, beta, and gamma), each of which consists of distinct proteins that have different functions. Important proteins in the alpha and beta fractions are the transport globulins and the clotting factors that are made in the liver. The transport globulins carry various substances in bound form in the circulation. For example, thyroid-binding globulin carries thyroxin, and transferrin carries iron. The clotting factors, including fibrinogen, remain in an inactive form in the blood plasma until activated by the clotting cascade. The gamma globulin fraction refers to the immunoglobulins, or antibodies. These proteins are produced by the well-differentiated lymphocytes and plasma cells. The actual fractionation of the globulins can be measured on a specific laboratory test (serum protein electrophoresis or SPEP).

Albumin is particularly important for the maintenance of fluid balance within the vascular system. Capillary walls are impermeable to albumin, so its presence in the plasma creates an osmotic force that keeps fluid within the vascular space. Albumin, which is produced by the liver, has the capacity to bind to several substances that are transported in plasma (e.g., certain medications, calcium, bilirubin, and some hormones). People with poor liver function may have low concentrations of albumin with a resultant decrease in osmotic pressure and the development of edema.

Reticuloendothelial System

The reticuloendothelial system (RES) (also called the *mononuclear phagocytic system*, or MPS) is a system of phagocytic cells, including monocytes and macrophages. The RES is divided into primary and secondary lymphoid systems. The primary lymphoid system is the site of RES cell production and includes the bone marrow and thymus. The secondary lymphoid system is the site of RES cell function and includes the liver, spleen, and lymph nodes. In the liver, spleen, lymph nodes, and other areas throughout the body, these cells function to recognize foreign cells and trigger an immune response.

The spleen has a number of additional functions, including recycling of iron, pooling of platelets, and blood volume regulation. It also acts as a filter for bacteria. In addition, the spleen is a major source of fetal hematopoiesis. It can resume hematopoiesis later in adulthood if necessary, particularly when marrow function is compromised (e.g., in bone marrow fibrosis, also known as myelofibrosis).

Hemostasis

Hemostasis refers to prevention of blood loss from intact vessels as well as the termination of bleeding when blood vessels are damaged. The prevention of blood loss from intact vessels requires adequate numbers of functional platelets. Platelets nurture the endothelium and thereby maintain the structural integrity of the vessel wall. Two processes are involved in arresting bleeding: primary hemostasis and secondary hemostasis (Fig. 19-4).

In primary hemostasis, the severed blood vessel constricts. Von Willebrand factor (vWf) binds to the collagen exposed on the damaged vessel and creates a binding site for platelets (DeLoughery, 2015b). Acting as the "glue" between platelets and the damaged vessel (Israels, 2015, p. 23), vWf also carries factor VIII to the vessel to assist in fibrin clot formation.

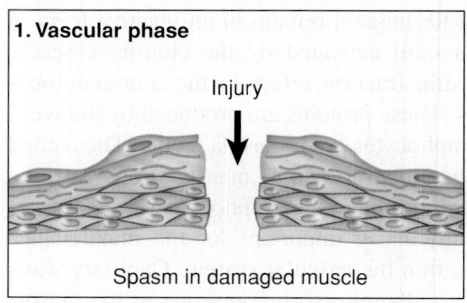

1. Vascular phase

Injury

Spasm in damaged muscle

2. Platelet phase

Platelet aggregation and adhesion

3. Coagulation phase

Intrinsic pathway

Common pathway

Extrinsic pathway

Platelet thromboplastin

Prothrombin

Tissue thromboplastin

Clotting factors VIII, IX, X, XI, XII

Thrombin

Fibrinogen

Clotting factor VII

Ca²⁺

Ca²⁺

Platelet factors

Fibrin

Tissue factors

Plasminogen

Activation of clotting system and clot formation

4. Clot retraction

Contraction of blood clot

5. Clot destruction

Plasmin

Plasmin

Enzymatic destruction of clot

FIGURE 19-4 Hemostasis. When the endothelial surface of a blood vessel is injured, several processes occur. In primary hemostasis, platelets within the circulation are attracted to the exposed layer of collagen at the site of injury. They adhere to the site of injury, releasing factors that stimulate other platelets to aggregate at the site, forming an unstable platelet plug. In secondary hemostasis, based on the type of stimulus, one of two clotting pathways is initiated—the intrinsic or extrinsic pathway—and the clotting factors within that pathway are activated. The end result from either pathway is the conversion of prothrombin to thrombin. Thrombin is necessary for fibrinogen to be converted into fibrin, the stabilizing protein that anchors the fragile platelet plug to the site of injury to prevent further bleeding and permit the injured vessel or site to heal. (Modified from www.irvingcrowley.com/cls/clotting.gif.)

For the coagulation process to be activated correctly, circulating inactive coagulation factors must be converted to active forms. This process occurs on the surface of the aggregated platelets at the site of vessel injury. The end result is the formation of fibrin, which reinforces the platelet plug and anchors it to the injury site. This process is termed *secondary hemostasis*.

The process of blood coagulation is highly complex. It can be activated by the intrinsic or the extrinsic pathway. Both pathways are needed for maintenance of normal hemostasis.

Many factors are involved in the coagulation cascade that forms fibrin. When tissue is injured, the extrinsic pathway is activated by the release of thromboplastin from the tissue. As the result of a series of reactions, prothrombin is converted to **thrombin**, which, in turn, catalyzes the conversion of fibrinogen to fibrin.

Clotting by the intrinsic pathway is activated when the collagen that lines blood vessels is exposed. Clotting factors are activated sequentially until, as with the extrinsic pathway, ultimately fibrin is formed.

As the injured vessel is repaired and again covered with endothelial cells, the fibrin clot is no longer needed. The fibrin is digested via two systems: the plasma fibrinolytic system and the cellular fibrinolytic system. The substance **plasminogen** is required to lyse (break down) the fibrin. Plasminogen, which is present in all body fluids, circulates with fibrinogen and, therefore, is incorporated into the fibrin clot as it forms. When the clot is no longer needed (e.g., after an injured blood vessel has healed), the plasminogen is activated to form plasmin. Plasmin digests the fibrinogen and fibrin. The by-products of clot digestion, called *fibrin degradation products*, are released into the circulation. Through this system, clots are dissolved as tissue is repaired, and the vascular system returns to its normal baseline state.

Gerontologic Considerations

In elderly patients, the bone marrow's ability to respond to the body's need for blood cells (erythrocytes, leukocytes, and platelets) may be decreased. This decreased ability is a result of many factors, including diminished production of the growth factors necessary for hematopoiesis by stromal cells within the marrow or a diminished response to the growth factors (in the case of erythropoietin). In addition, in elderly patients, the bone marrow may be more susceptible to the myelosuppressive effects of medications. As a result of these factors, when an elderly person needs more blood cells (e.g., leukocytes in infection, erythrocytes in anemia), the bone marrow may not be able to increase production of these cells adequately. **Leukopenia** (a decreased number of circulating leukocytes), thrombocytopenia (a decrease in the platelet count), and/or anemia can result.

Anemia is the most common hematologic condition affecting elderly patients; with each successive decade of life, the incidence of anemia increases. Anemia frequently results from iron deficiency (in the case of blood loss) or from a nutritional deficiency, particularly folate or vitamin B_{12} deficiency or protein–calorie malnutrition; it may also result from inflammation, chronic disease such as an underlying malignancy, or alcohol abuse. Management of the disorder varies, depending on the etiology. Therefore, it is important to identify the cause of the anemia rather than to consider it an inevitable consequence of aging. Elderly people with concurrent cardiac or pulmonary problems may not tolerate anemia well, and a prompt, thorough evaluation is always warranted.

ASSESSMENT AND DIAGNOSTIC EVALUATION

Most hematologic diseases reflect a defect in the hematopoietic or hemostatic systems, or in the RES. The defect can be quantitative (e.g., increased or decreased production of cells), qualitative (e.g., the cells that are produced are not functioning normally), or both.

Many hematologic conditions lack symptoms initially. Therefore, an extensive history and laboratory tests are used to determine a diagnosis. For many hematologic conditions, continued monitoring of laboratory results over time is essential to establish trends. Trends help to establish the acuity of the condition and also help to assess the response to interventions.

Hematologic Studies

The most common tests used to assess bone marrow function are the CBC and the peripheral blood smear (PBS). Blood for both the CBC and PBS is typically obtained by venipuncture. The CBC identifies the total number of blood cells (leukocytes, erythrocytes, and platelets) as well as the hemoglobin, **hematocrit** (percentage of blood volume consisting of erythrocytes), and RBC indices (Table 19-2). Because cellular morphology (shape and appearance of the cells) is particularly important in most hematologic disorders, the blood cells involved must be examined. This process is referred to as the *manual examination of the peripheral smear*. In this test, a drop of blood is spread on a glass slide, stained, and examined under a microscope. Visualizing the shape and size of the leukocytes, erythrocytes, and platelets provides useful information in identifying hematologic conditions. Increases or decreases in any one parameter of the CBC may indicate a hematologic disorder and indicate the need for further testing (refer to Chapter 20). However, an abnormal CBC should always be assessed relative to the patient's baseline; up to 5% of the general population may have labs outside of the normal limits in the absence of disease. In addition, people of African descent may have lower Hgb, WBC, neutrophil and platelet counts (Tefferi et al., 2005; Fischbach & Dunning, 2014). Nurses must be familiar with the normal CBC parameters and be aware of potential implications of hematologic alterations.

Nursing Alert
A falsely elevated hematocrit is noted in conditions of fluid volume loss (such as dehydration). Since no single test confirms hemoconcentration, the nurse must assess for signs of fluid deficit, such as weight loss, dry mucous membranes, delayed skin turgor, orthostatic hypotension, decreased pulse pressure (the difference between the systolic and diastolic pressure), decreasing urinary output with elevated urine specific gravity, and vital sign changes (increasing heart rate and decreasing blood pressure as volume is lost). Regardless of the etiology, a hematocrit of greater than 60% is associated with spontaneous clotting (Fischbach & Dunning, 2014, p. 91). Likewise, in times of hemodilution (i.e., fluid gain), a falsely lower hematocrit is noted. The nurse assesses for weight gain, moist mucous membranes, edema, hypertension, crackles in the lung fields, an S_3 gallop over the mitral area, increased urinary output with decreased specific gravity, and distended neck veins. A hematocrit of less than 20% is associated with

TABLE 19-2 Normal Complete Blood Count with Differential

Example: 42-Year-Old Caucasian Man[a]		
Tests	Normal Reference Range	Case Example
WBC	5,000–10,000/µL Absolute neutrophil count >1,800/µL	5,300/µL
Segments	38–71% of total WBC	61%
Bands	0–10% of total	5%
Monocytes	2–15% of total	11%
Basophils	0–1% of total	0%
Eosinophils	0–5% of total	1%
Lymphocytes	20–40% of total	22%
Hemoglobin	Male: 14–18 g/dL Female: 12–16 g/dL	17 g/dL
Hematocrit	Male: 40–52% Female: 37–47%	51%
Red blood cells (RBCs)	Male: $4.5–5.5 \times 10^6/mm^3$ Female: $3.8–5.2 \times 10^6/mm^3$	$5 \times 10^6/mm^3$
RBC distribution width (%)	Male: 11.8–15.6% Female: 11.9–15.5%	12%
Mean corpuscular volume (MCV)	Male: 81–101.4 (fL) Female: 81.1-99.8 (fL)	90 fL
Mean corpuscular hemoglobin (MCH)	28–34 pg/cell	30 pg/cell
Mean corpuscular hemoglobin concentration (MCHC)	32–36 g/dl	32 g/dL
Platelets	$150–400,000/mm^3$	$200,000/mm^3$
Mean Platelet Volume	7.4–10.3 fL	8 fL

[a]People of African ancestry may have lower WBC, neutrophil and platelet counts.
Fischbach and Dunning (2014).

increased risk of cardiac failure and death (Fischbach & Dunning, 2014, p. 91).

Assessing the Patient with Low Hemoglobin and Hematocrit

Patients with mildly to moderately lowered hemoglobin and hematocrit levels may be asymptomatic due to effective compensatory mechanisms. However, a careful history may uncover the following: progressive fatigue, poor activity tolerance, headaches, dizziness, irritability, difficulty sleeping or concentrating, tinnitus, anorexia, dyspnea, palpitations, chest pain, indigestion, abnormal menstruation in females, impotence in males, and loss of libido. On physical examination, pallor is the most common and obvious sign of anemia. Pallor can be most easily assessed in the oral mucous membranes, nail beds, conjunctiva, and creases of the palms. Other findings may include tachypnea, tachycardia and flow murmurs, and hypotension. Tachypnea and tachycardia may be seen with activity. Patients with hemolytic anemia may exhibit jaundice and splenomegaly.

Assessing the Patient with a Low White Blood Cell Count

When assessing a patient with low WBC count, the nurse must examine the WBC differential to see which type of WBC is low. The myeloid and/or lymphoid lines may be low. However, the most critical factors influencing an individual's risk for infection are the severity and duration of neutropenia. Nurses caring for a patient with a low WBC count should calculate the absolute neutrophil count (ANC; Box 19-1). Neutropenia severity is classified using the following guidelines:

- ANC 1,500 to $1,000/mm^3$ indicates mild neutropenia;
- ANC 999 to $500/mm^3$ indicates moderate neutropenia;
- ANC of less than $500/mm^3$ indicates severe neutropenia.

BOX 19-1

Calculating the Absolute Neutrophil Count (ANC)

Normally, the neutrophil count is greater than $2,000/mm^3$. The actual (or absolute) neutrophil count (ANC) is calculated using this formula:

$$\text{Total WBC} \times [\%segs + \%bands] = ANC$$

For example, if the total white blood cell (WBC) count is $3,000/mm^3$ with 72% neutrophils and 3% bands, the ANC would be calculated as follows:

$$3,000 \times [72\% + 3\%] = 2,250/mm^3$$

This result is not indicative of neutropenia because the ANC is greater than $1,000/mm^3$ despite the low total WBC count ($3,000/mm^3$).

Conversely, in the following example, neutropenia is evident despite a normal WBC count ($5500/mm^3$) with 8% neutrophils and 0% bands:

$$5,500 \times [8\% + 0\%] = 440/mm^3$$

Here, the ANC is severely low ($440/mm^3$) despite the normal total WBC count ($5,500/mm^3$).

When evaluating neutropenia, it is important to calculate the ANC and not to rely solely on the total WBCs and percentage of neutrophils alone.

Patients with severe neutropenia are at significantly increased risk for developing opportunistic infections and sepsis. The most common sites of infection in neutropenic patients include the respiratory tract, GI and GU tracts, and the skin (Vioral & Wentley, 2015). Patients with neutropenia must be assessed carefully for the following:

- *Skin*: Check for tenderness, erythema, edema, breaks in skin integrity, moisture, drainage, lesions (especially under breasts, axillae, groin, skin folds, bony prominences, perineum, and perirectum); check all puncture sites (e.g., IV sites) and central venous access device sites for erythema, tenderness, induration, and drainage.
- *Oral mucosa*: Check for moisture, lesions, color (check palate, tongue, buccal mucosa, gums, lips, oropharynx); assess level of pain and taste changes, which may precede objective signs of mucosal damage by 3 to 5 days.
- *Respiratory*: Check for presence of cough, sore throat, tachypnea, pain on inspiration; auscultate breath sounds. Note color, amount, and consistency of sputum.
- *Gastrointestinal*: Check for abdominal discomfort and distention by palpating the abdomen, assess for nausea, change in bowel pattern; auscultate bowel sounds.
- *Genitourinary*: Check for dysuria, urgency, frequency; check urine for color, clarity, and odor.
- *Neurologic*: Ask about headache, neck stiffness, visual disturbances; assess level of consciousness, orientation, and behavior.
- *Temperature*: Check for elevation (greater than 38°C [greater than 100.4°F]).

Often patients with neutropenia are not able to manifest the classic signs of infection, such as pus, because pus is comprised of WBCs. Signs of infection may be subtle; therefore, the presence of fever may be the only sign that the patient has an infection and should be addressed immediately.

Nursing Alert

Agranulocytosis or marked neutropenia and leukopenia place the patient at significant risk for infection. The nurse is aware that handwashing is critical to prevent infection (Bossaer & Cluck, 2013). Strict reverse isolation procedures, such as the use of mask, gown, and gloves to prevent infection, have not been demonstrated to decrease infection rates and are no longer routinely implemented (Vioral & Wentley, 2015). Patients should be cautioned to avoid large crowds and sick contacts. See Chapter 6 for further discussion.

Assessing the Patient at Risk for Bleeding

Assessment of bleeding risk should include a thorough examination of bleeding history, family history, laboratory tests, and a thorough physical examination (Stasi, 2012; Israels, 2015). The strongest predictor of bleeding risk is a history of bleeding (DeLoughery, 2015c). Assessment of bleeding history should include questions about frequency and severity of nosebleeds; bleeding with dental work, both immediate and delayed; bleeding with surgery and need for blood transfusions; bruising; length of menstrual periods, need for iron replacement due to heavy menses, excessive bleeding with childbirth necessitating blood transfusion; blood in stool or urine; and gum bleeding (DeLoughery, 2015c). History of mucocutaneous bleeding may signal inherited or acquired defects in platelet number or function, or von Willebrand disease (vWd) (Israels, 2015). The patient may report easy bruising, bleeding gums, and frequent nosebleeds (DeLoughery, 2015c). In comparison, patients with coagulation factor defects, such as hemophilia, are more likely to experience muscle and joint bleeding (DeLoughery, 2015c). Coagulation problems result in bleeding that is excessive (DeLoughery, 2015c). For example, patients with hemophilia may bleed for several hours after a minor procedure (DeLoughery, 2015).

Family history of bleeding is also important. Hemophilias A (factor VIII deficiency) and B (factor IX deficiency) are inherited and sex linked; family history should include questioning of bleeding in brothers, male cousins, and uncles (DeLoughery, 2015c).

Laboratory Tests to Assess Type of Bleeding Defect

Patients with a bleeding history should have a CBC, peripheral blood smear (PBS), prothrombin time and International Normalized Ratio (PT/INR), partial thromboplastin time (PTT), and assessment of platelet function assay-100 (PFA-100) (DeLoughery, 2015b). Testing for vWd should also be considered if the patient has a low platelet count (Israels, 2015).

A CBC and PBS are performed to assess platelet count, size, and shape. The presence of schistocytes on PBS suggests disseminated intravascular coagulation (DIC) or thrombotic thrombocytopenia purpura (TTP); these must be ruled out as they require prompt intervention. See Chapter 20 for further discussion (Stasi, 2012).

Pseudothrombocytopenia may occur as a result of platelet clumping when collected in Ethylenediaminetetraacetic acid (EDTA); recollecting a sample in a citrate-based anticoagulant will provide an accurate platelet count (Stasi, 2012; Israels, 2015).

Bleeding may be due to a decrease in platelet number or function (Stasi, 2012). A decrease in platelet number does not exclude the possibility of platelet dysfunction. Some of the inherited platelet disorders are marked by both a decrease in platelet number and abnormal function (Israels, 2015). The Platelet Function Assay (PFA)-100 test is a screening tool for primary hemostasis and assesses platelet function (Francis et al., 1999; Fischbach & Dunning, 2014). An abnormal result suggests a problem with platelet function.

Thrombocytopenia severity can be described as follows: excess bleeding that may occur as a result of injury, trauma,

Nursing Interventions for Patients with Thrombocytopenia (Platelet Count Below 50,000/mm³)

Prevent Complications: Implement Bleeding Precautions

- Avoid giving aspirin and aspirin-containing medications or other medications known to inhibit platelet function (NSAIDs), if possible.
- Assess for use of herbal medications, such as **Ginkgo biloba,** which can predispose the patient to bleeding.
- Do not give intramuscular injections.
- Do not insert indwelling catheters.
- Do not use the rectal route for taking temperatures or administering medications.
- Use stool softeners and oral laxatives to prevent constipation.
- Use the smallest possible needles when performing venipuncture.
- Apply pressure to venipuncture sites for 5 minutes or until bleeding has stopped.
- Use only soft-bristled toothbrush for mouth care.
- Do not permit wearing of restrictive clothing; avoid tourniquets or overinflation of blood pressure cuffs.
- Lubricate lips with water-soluble lubricant every 2 hours while patient is awake.
- Avoid suctioning if at all possible; if unavoidable, use only gentle suctioning.
- Discourage vigorous coughing or blowing of the nose.
- Use only electric razor for shaving.
- Pad side rails as needed.
- Prevent falls by ambulating with patient as necessary and keeping the environment safe.
- Teach patient to avoid contact sports and sports with risk for falling or injury (such as biking or roller-blading).
- Teach patient to avoid sexual intercourse (both vaginal and anal) until platelet count is over 50,000/mm³.
- Hematest secretions and excretions for occult blood for early identification of internal bleeding.

Control Bleeding

- Apply direct pressure.
- Use manual pressure with gauze over the source of bleeding.
- For epistaxis, position patient in high Fowler position with body tilted forward and the mouth open so that the blood can be spit out instead of swallowed; apply ice pack to the bridge of the nose and direct pressure to nose.
- Hemostatic agents such as thromboplastin, absorbable gelatin, fibrin sealants, collagen, and alginate can be used for hemostasis at wound sites and central venous access device sites that are bleeding.
- Notify health care provider for prolonged bleeding (e.g., unable to stop within 10 minutes).
- Administer platelets, fresh-frozen plasma, and/or packed red blood cells as prescribed.

Adapted from Doenges (2016).

or surgery, with a platelet count of 50,000 to 100,000/mm³; platelet counts of 20,000/mm³ or less increase the risk for spontaneous bleeding; and platelet counts of 10,000/mm³ or less are associated with serious episodes of spontaneous bleeding, including intracranial hemorrhage. Bleeding precautions are recommended for patients with a platelet count of less than 50,000/mm³. The nursing care and patient education required to safely care for patients with thrombocytopenia are outlined in Box 19-2.

PT measures the time needed for factor VIIa to form a complex with tissue factor and form a clot (DeLoughery, 2015b). Prolongation/elevation of the PT alone often indicates a factor VII deficiency. In the past, PT was used to monitor response to warfarin therapy; however, due to laboratory variations, a more consistent way to monitor response to warfarin is the INR. The INR is a method of standardizing PT times obtained from different labs (DeLoughery, 2015b). INR is calculated by dividing the PT by the control and then applying the International Sensitivity Index, which adjusts the PT for the differing sensitivities of reagents by laboratory (DeLoughery, 2015b). Use of INR has resulted in more accurate monitoring of warfarin use.

Elevation of the PTT may indicate a deficiency in Factor VIII, IX, or XI. Prolongation of both the PT and PTT may indicate a deficiency in factor X, II, or V, or a combination of deficits in these factors (DeLoughery, 2015).

A thorough physical examination can be very useful in determining the source of the hemostatic defect. Abnormalities of the vascular system give rise to local bleeding, usually into the skin. Because platelets are primarily responsible for hemostasis in small vessels, patients with platelet defects develop petechiae (see Fig. 19-5), often in clusters; these are most often seen first on the extremities and then the mucous membranes. With prolonged thrombocytopenia, petechiae may also be seen on the trunk.

Other pertinent assessment findings include ecchymoses or hematomas, conjunctival hemorrhages, bleeding gums, bleeding at puncture sites (venipuncture); hypotension, tachycardia, dizziness, epistaxis (nosebleed); respiratory distress, tachypnea, hemoptysis (coughing of blood); abdominal or back pain, hematemesis (vomiting blood), abdominal distention, rectal bleeding; vaginal or urethral bleeding; and headache, blurred vision, and mental status changes.

Nursing Alert
Because of the risk of spontaneous intracranial bleeding, patients with very severe thrombocytopenia (platelet count below 10,000/mm³) must be monitored closely for subtle changes in mental status, including irritability and restlessness, and educated to report even mild headaches immediately.

FIGURE 19-5 Petechiae of limb and oral cavity. (Laurin Council, M., Sheinbein, D. M., Cornelius, L. A. *The Washington Manual of Dermatology Diagnostics*. Sharon Jensen, Nursing Health Assessment.)

In contrast to platelet defects, coagulation factor defects do not tend to cause superficial bleeding because the primary hemostatic mechanisms are still intact. Instead, bleeding occurs deeper within the body (e.g., subcutaneous or intramuscular hematomas, hemorrhage into joint spaces). Because of this bleeding, the patient may report joint pain.

External bleeding diminishes very slowly when local pressure is applied; it often recurs several hours after pressure is removed. For example, severe bleeding may start several hours after a tooth extraction.

Bone Marrow Aspiration and Biopsy

The bone marrow aspiration and biopsy are indicated to further assess the underlying cause of an abnormal CBC, when additional information is needed to assess the quantity and quality of each type of cell produced within the marrow. Bone marrow aspiration and biopsy are used in the diagnosis and classification of malignancies, benign hematologic disorders, infections, and storage disorders, as well as for assessment of response to treatment (Jackson, Guinigundo, & Waterhouse, 2012; Fischbach & Dunning, 2014; Malempati, Joshi, Lai, Braner, & Tegtmeyer, 2009 [The later reference is a video of a Bone Marrow Aspiration and Biopsy video]).

For example, a patient with an abnormal CBC undergoes a bone marrow biopsy and aspirate with results revealing acute myeloid leukemia. After receiving chemotherapy to treat the leukemia, another bone marrow aspirate and biopsy are done to assess response to treatment; if the treatment was effective, no leukemia cells should be seen in the biopsy or aspirate specimens.

Normal bone marrow is in a semifluid state and can be aspirated through a special hollow core, large-bore needle. In adults, bone marrow is usually aspirated from the posterior iliac crest. The aspirate provides a sample of cells. Aspirate alone may be adequate for evaluating certain conditions, such as anemia. However, in most cases, a biopsy is also performed. Biopsy samples are taken from the posterior iliac crest; occasionally, an anterior iliac approach is required. The sternum can be used to obtain an aspirate but should not

be used to obtain a biopsy because of its proximity to vital organs. A bone marrow biopsy shows the architecture of the bone marrow as well as its degree of cellularity.

The first step in the procedure is obtaining informed consent. Informed consent is obtained by the physician, nurse practitioner, or physician's assistant performing the procedure and includes the reason the procedure is being performed, alternatives, and risks of the procedure. Risks include infection, bleeding, and pain. The risk for bleeding is somewhat increased if the patient's platelet count is low (less than 20/mm³) or if the patient has been taking a medication (e.g., aspirin) that alters platelet function. Rare, serious complications include trauma to nearby structures, such as the gluteal artery, retroperitoneal hematomas, and fractures of the underlying bone. Fortunately these complications are very rare (incidence less than 1% [0.05 to 0.07% in two studies]) (Malempati et al., 2009; Zehnder, 2015).

Most adult patients need no more preparation than a careful explanation of the procedure and the sensations that will be experienced, but for some very anxious patients, administration of an antianxiety agent, such as lorazepam, may be useful. Pediatric patients usually require deeper sedation. Though this procedure is potentially painful, generous local anesthesia and a skilled operator minimize the risk for discomfort.

After informed consent is obtained, the patient is assisted to either a prone or lateral decubitus position. The skin is cleansed using aseptic technique and either a chlorhexidine-based solution or povidone-iodine. A sterile drape is applied; then the skin is numbed using local anesthesia. The periosteum, which contains many nerve endings, is numbed next. The bone itself cannot be numbed. An aspirate needle is inserted with a stylet in place through the numbed skin into the cortical bone through to the marrow; when the needle is felt to go through the outer cortex of bone and into the marrow cavity, the stylet is removed, a syringe is attached, and a small volume (10 to 20 mL) of marrow is aspirated (this is often referred to as the aspirate sample). Patients typically feel a sensation of pressure as the needle is advanced into position. The aspiration of fluid causes a sudden and sharp but brief pain, resulting from the suction exerted as the marrow is aspirated into the syringe; the patient should be warned about this. Taking deep breaths or using relaxation techniques often helps ease the discomfort.

Once the aspirate sample is obtained, the aspirate needle is removed and then a longer hollow core needle with stylet is inserted through the same hole in the skin. A drilling motion is used to advance the needle through the cortical bone; once the needle is anchored into the cortical bone, the stylet is removed and the hollow needle is advanced into the marrow to a depth of 2 to 3 cm (Fischbach & Dunning, 2014; Malempati et al., 2009). Next the needle is turned clockwise and then counterclockwise several times to help loosen the specimen; the needle is carefully removed revealing a solid core specimen of bone and bone marrow inside the hollow needle. A probe is used to gently push the specimen out of the needle and into a specimen container. During the biopsy, the patient may feel pressure but should not feel pain; if the patient experiences pain radiating down the leg, repositioning of the needle may be necessary.

After the marrow sample is obtained, pressure is applied to the site for several minutes. Then the site is covered with a sterile dressing. Most patients have no discomfort after a bone marrow aspiration, but the site of a biopsy may ache for 1 or 2 days. Patients should be instructed not to submerge in a bath for 24 hours, until the site heals. A mild analgesic (e.g., acetaminophen) may be useful. Aspirin-containing analgesics should be avoided because of the increased risk of bleeding.

The nurses' role is to reinforce patient education pre- and postprocedure, provide emotional support during the procedure, assist the operator, and assess for pain and anxiety. The nurse also reviews postprocedure care with the patient,

including keeping the site clean and dry for 24 hours and instructing the patient and family to call if any signs or symptoms of bleeding or infection develop (Fischbach & Dunning, 2014; Malempati et al., 2009).

The bone marrow aspirate and biopsy samples are evaluated by a pathologist who ultimately provides a summary of findings. The aspirate provides information on the cell type, size, shape, and number present in the marrow and also allows for specialized tests, including flow cytometry, cytogenetic studies, and molecular studies to be conducted, all of which help classify the bone marrow disorder. The bone marrow biopsy provides information on the cellularity of the marrow as well as the severity of disease or dysfunction; normal cellularity can be estimated based on the patient's age and subtracting the age from 100. For example, a 30-year-old woman should have a cellularity of 70%. Fewer cells than expected is referred to as hypocellular; more cells than expected is called hypercellular.

Unfolding Patient Stories: Lloyd Bennett • Part 1

Lloyd Bennett is a 76-year-old male who fell while working outdoors. He presents to the emergency department with a hip fracture. What physical assessment and laboratory data can assist the nurse in evaluation for possible internal blood loss from the fracture or indications that the patient is at higher risk of bleeding? (Lloyd Bennett's story continues in Chapter 26.)

Care for Lloyd and other patients in a realistic virtual environment: **vSim** *for Nursing* (thepoint.lww.com/vSimMedicalSurgical). Practice documenting these patients' care in (thepoint.lww.com/DocuCareEHR).

CHAPTER REVIEW

Critical Thinking Exercises

1. You are caring for a patient with acute leukemia and sepsis who has a declining platelet count of 10,000/mm^3. On assessment, you observe oozing blood from the Hickman catheter site, petechiae to the upper and lower extremities, and epistaxis. What are the potential causes of this patient's bleeding? What other laboratory results would you assess? What further assessments would you perform? What nursing interventions would you implement? What medical interventions would you anticipate?

2. You are working in a hematology–oncology clinic. The laboratory reports a critical laboratory result for one of your patients presenting with possible acute leukemia:

the leukocyte count is 1,200/mm^3 with 10% neutrophils. What other laboratory results would be important to review or consider? The patient is also anemic (hemoglobin 8.2 mg/dL), and platelets are 110,000/mm^3. What observations will you include in your assessment of this patient? Determine the extent to which this patient is neutropenic. What medical treatments would you anticipate? How would you educate the patient about neutropenia precautions? What information do you need to obtain about the patient's home setting that will assist you in determining the patient's risk of developing an infection at home? How will you modify this education if the patient has mild dementia? Lives alone? Does not understand or speak English well?

NCLEX-Style Review Questions

1. A nurse is caring for a patient who is 73 years old with a platelet count of 5,000/mm³ resulting from myelodysplastic syndrome. At 10 PM, the patient complains of a headache. What should be the nurse's immediate action to take?
   a. Administer aspirin per p.r.n. order.
   b. Administer acetaminophen per p.r.n. order.
   c. Notify the health care provider.
   d. Administer a nonpharmacologic intervention, such as a cool compress.

2. A patient presents to her primary care provider with a complaint of a "cold that just won't go away." She has a CBC drawn, revealing the following: WBC 4.5: segs 5, bands 0, lymphs 45, eosinophils 5, basophils 5, monocytes 5, blasts 35. What is the patient's absolute neutrophil count?
   a. 500
   b. 250
   c. 225
   d. 2,250

3. What is the priority nursing diagnosis for a client experiencing anemia?
   a. Risk for injury related to poor blood clotting
   b. Fatigue related to decreased cellular oxygenation
   c. Risk of infection related to decreased leukocytes
   d. Imbalanced nutrition; less than body requirements related to anorexia

4. A patient with thrombocytopenia due to chemotherapy develops a nose bleed (epistaxis). What is the nurse's expected response?
   a. Apply ice to the anterior surface of the nose and place the patient in a supine position
   b. Apply pressure to the nares and position the patient in a high Fowler position, leaning slightly forward
   c. Squeeze the nares together firmly and position the patient in prone position with mouth open
   d. Ask the patient to blow the nose vigorously as the nurse applies firm pressure to the nares

5. The nurse recognizes this as the most common hematologic condition associated with aging.
   a. Thrombocytopenia
   b. Leukopenia
   c. Agranulocytosis
   d. Anemia

Try these additional resources, available at **http://thepoint.lww.com/Honan2e**, to enhance your learning and understanding of this chapter:
• NCLEX-Style Student Review Questions
• Journal Articles

REFERENCES AND SELECTED READINGS

References and selected readings associated with this chapter can be found on the website that accompanies the book. Visit **http://thepoint. lww.com/Honan2e** to access the references and other additional resources associated with this chapter.

Nursing Management: Patients with Hematologic Disorders

Lisa M. Barbarotta

Learning Objectives

After reading this chapter, you will be able to:

1. Differentiate between the different types of anemias and compare and contrast the physiologic mechanisms, clinical manifestations, medical management, and nursing interventions for each.
2. Compare the leukemia types in terms of incidence, physiologic alterations, clinical manifestations, management, and prognosis.
3. Discuss physiologic mechanisms, clinical manifestations, medical management and nursing interventions for myelodysplastic syndromes.
4. Discuss nursing management of patients with lymphoma and multiple myeloma.
5. Discuss nursing management of patients with bleeding or thrombotic disorders.
6. Identify therapies for blood disorders, including the nursing implications for the administration of blood components.

Hematologic disorders include both benign and malignant conditions. These disorders can impact every system in the body. Nursing care of these patients requires an understanding of the anatomy and physiology of hematopoiesis and immunology, as well as astute assessment skills.

RED BLOOD CELL DISORDERS

Anemia

Anemia, a condition in which the **hemoglobin** concentration is lower than normal, reflects the presence of fewer than normal **erythrocytes** (red blood cells; RBCs) within the circulation. As a result, the amount of oxygen delivered to body tissues is also diminished. Anemia is not a specific disease state per se but a sign of an underlying disorder. It is by far the most common hematologic condition, affecting one fourth of the world population (Jiminez, Kulnigg-Dabsch, & Gasche, 2015). Anemia is a common occurrence among all age groups, with prevalence increasing with age (Jiminez et al., 2015).

Overview

Anemia, a decrease in the number of red blood cells (RBCs), has a number of different etiologies. The treatment varies based on the cause. The different classifications of anemia, as well as the nursing management of each, will be discussed here.

Classification of Anemias

Anemia can be classified by cellular morphology (shape) or by physiologic process. Morphologic classification is the most common approach and includes the cell size, color, and shape. Changes in the size of the RBC are described as normocytic (normal or average size), macrocytic (larger than normal), or microcytic (smaller than normal). Changes in the color of the RBC are described as **normochromic** (normal in color), hyperchromic (darker cellular contents), or hypochromic (pale or lighter cellular contents) (see Table 20-1). A physiologic approach (see Table 20-2) classifies anemia according to whether the deficiency in erythrocytes is caused by a defect in their production (hypoproliferative anemia), by their destruction (hemolytic anemia), or by their loss (e.g., bleeding) (Fig. 20-1).

In hypoproliferative anemias, the marrow cannot produce adequate numbers of erythrocytes. The reticulocyte count reflects bone marrow production of RBCs. In anemia due to blood loss, a healthy bone marrow compensates for losses and increases RBC production, reflected as an increased reticulocyte count. In hypoproliferative anemias, the bone marrow cannot mount an adequate response to anemia, and this lack of RBC production is reflected as a low reticulocyte count.

Inadequate production of erythrocytes may result from marrow damage due to medications (e.g., chloramphenicol) or chemicals (e.g., benzene) or from a lack of essential

TABLE **20-1** Classification of Anemia by Morphology

Type of Anemia	Morphology	Examples	Laboratory Values Expected
Normocytic (MCV 80–100 fL), normochromic	Cells of normal size with normal Hgb content	Aplastic anemia Acute blood loss Hemolytic anemia Anemia of chronic disease Sickle cell anemia	Normal MCV Normal MCHC ↓ Hgb ↓ Hct
Microcytic (MCV less than 80 fL), hypochromic	Small, reduced amount of Hgb	Iron deficiency anemia Sideroblastic anemia Thalassemia	↓ MCV ↓ MCHC ↓ Hgb ↓ Hct
Macrocytic (MCV greater than 100 fL), normochromic	Large in size, thickness, and volume	Folic acid deficiency Vitamin B_{12} deficiency Alcohol abuse Medications (e.g., hydroxyurea)	↑ MCV Normal MCHC ↓ Hgb ↓ Hct

MCV, mean corpuscular volume; MCHC, mean corpuscular hemoglobin concentration; Hgb, hemoglobin; Hct, hematocrit.

factors (e.g., iron, vitamin B_{12}, folic acid, **erythropoietin**) necessary for erythrocyte formation.

In hemolytic anemias, premature destruction of erythrocytes results in the liberation of hemoglobin from the erythrocytes into the plasma. The increased erythrocyte destruction leads to tissue hypoxia, which, in turn, stimulates erythropoietin production. This increased production is reflected in an increased reticulocyte count as the bone marrow responds to

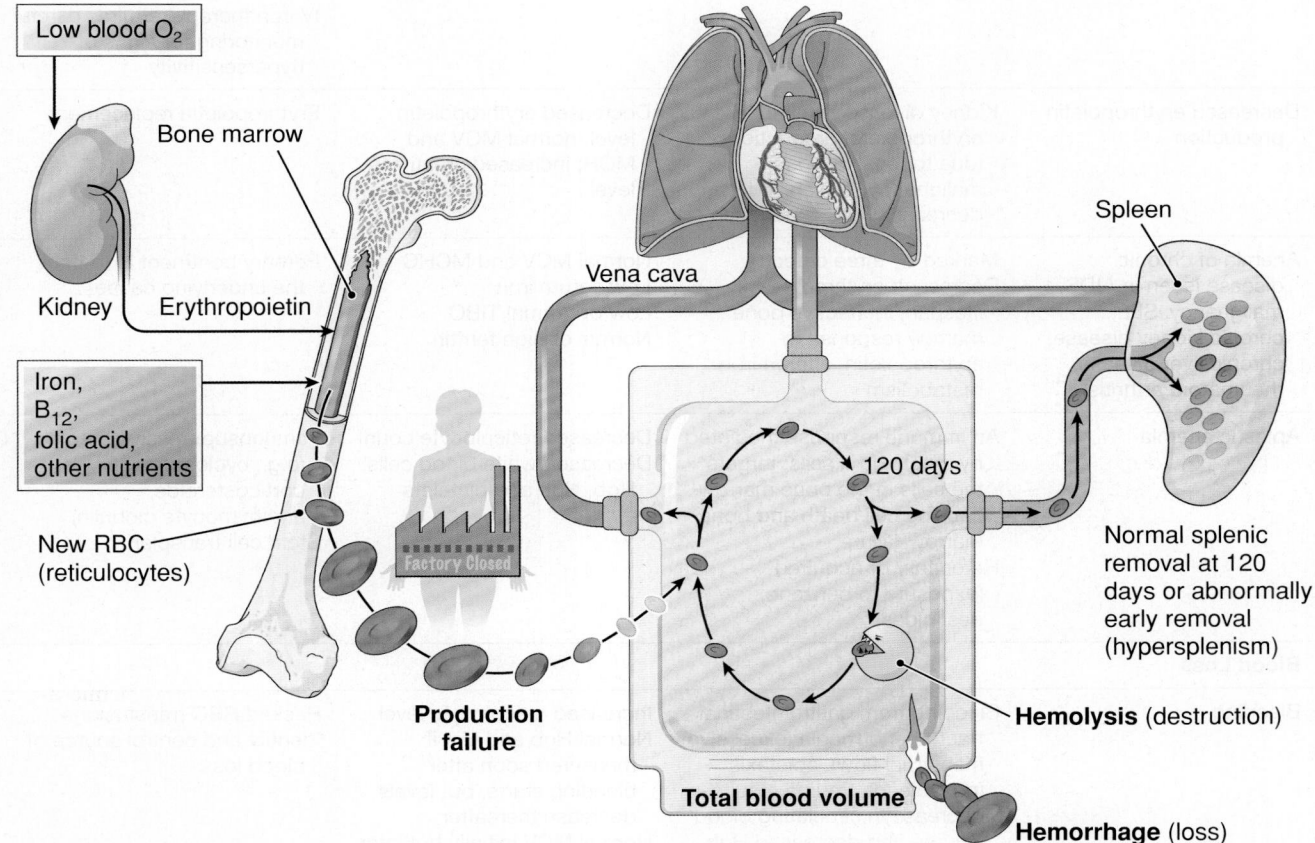

FIGURE 20-1 Production, circulation, and death of red blood cells. Every anemia is caused by at least one of three problems: (1) decreased red cell production, (2) loss of red cells by hemorrhage, or (3) early death (destruction) of RBCs. (From McConnell, T. H. (2007). *The nature of disease pathology for the health professions.* Philadelphia, PA: Lippincott Williams & Wilkins.)

TABLE **20-2** Anemia Classification by Etiology

Type of Anemia	Pathophysiology	Laboratory Findings	Treatment
Hypoproliferative (Decreased Production)			
Pernicious, megaloblastic	Vitamin B_{12} deficiency; lack of intrinsic factor required for B_{12} absorption	Decreased vitamin B_{12} level; increased MCV Elevated methylmalonic acid and homocysteine levels Low reticulocyte count	B_{12} replacement Cyanocobalamin 1,000 µg IM monthly
Folate deficiency	Decreased folic acid intake; impaired absorption; alcohol impairs folate metabolism in the liver, causing a significant depletion in folate reserves Decreases in folate impair DNA synthesis and increase erythroblast cell deaths	Decreased folate levels Increased MCV	Oral folic acid 1–5 mg/day PO
Iron deficiency	Chronic blood loss, failure to recapture iron from recycled RBCs Demands for iron exceed iron intake. Decreased iron intake results in use and depletion of iron stores, resulting in decreased Hgb production	Decreased reticulocytes, iron, ferritin, iron saturation, MCV Increased TIBC	Iron replacement therapy: ferrous sulfate 325 mg PO t.i.d. Parenteral iron therapy reserved for those who cannot take oral replacement due to intolerance, poor enteral absorption, or continued blood loss IV iron therapy requires careful monitoring for signs of hypersensitivity
Decreased erythropoietin production	Kidney disease can impair erythropoietin production (due to renal disease, malignancy), which, in turn, decreases RBC production	Decreased erythropoietin level; normal MCV and MCH; increased creatinine level	Erythropoietin replacement
Anemia of chronic disease (seen in AIDS, malignancy, SLE, chronic kidney disease, chronic liver disease, rheumatoid arthritis)	Marked by three defects: Decreased erythrocyte lifespan, ineffective bone marrow response to erythropoietin, altered iron metabolism	Normal MCV and MCHC Low serum iron Low or normal TIBC Normal or high ferritin	Primary treatment is to treat the underlying cause
Aplastic anemia	An immune response mediated by cytotoxic T cells; targets the cells in the bone marrow, causing cell death and bone marrow failure Hereditary or acquired (exposure to benzene, pesticides)	Decreased reticulocyte count Decreased white blood cells, Hgb, Hct, and platelets	Immunosuppressive therapy (e.g., cyclosporine, corticosteroids, antithymocyte globulin) Stem cell transplant
Blood Loss			
Bleeding	Bleeding from gastrointestinal tract, menorrhagia (excessive menstrual flow), epistaxis (nosebleed), trauma results in decrease in circulating blood volume and decreased Hgb and Hct	Increased reticulocyte level Normal Hgb and Hct if measured soon after bleeding starts, but levels decrease thereafter Normal MCV initially but later decreases Decreased ferritin and iron levels (later)	Packed RBC transfusions Identify and control source of blood loss

Type of Anemia	Pathophysiology	Laboratory Findings	Treatment
Hemolysis (Destruction of RBCs)			
Autoimmune hemolytic anemia Acquired; caused by extrinsic insults such as infection, medications, venom, trauma	Both inherited and acquired forms result in hemolysis within blood vessels and/or lymphoid tissue	Presence of schistocytes Increased spherocyte level Increased reticulocytes	Immunosuppressive therapy (i.e., corticosteroids) Acquired: remove insult, treat underlying disorder
Thalassemias A group of inherited forms of autoimmune hemolytic anemia	Caused by cellular abnormalities of the Hgb structure, marked by an imbalance between the beta chain and alpha chain of Hgb, resulting in RBC membrane damage, ineffective RBC production, and hemolysis	Decreased MCV; fragmented RBCs Increased reticulocyte level	Transfusion therapy with PRBCs Monitor ferritin regularly to assess for iron overload
Sickle cell disease	Inherited disorder in which abnormal hemoglobin (HbS) polymerizes when deoxygenated, creating a semisolid gel that makes an RBC rigid with a distorted shape (sickle cell) that leads to hemolytic anemia, pain (stasis of RBCs in capillaries) and organ failure	Anemia (resulting from chronic hemolysis), reticulocytosis, leukocytosis, and thrombocytosis are common. Elevations of bilirubin and lactate dehydrogenase are also common. Peripheral blood smear may reveal sickle cells	Transfusion therapy with PRBCs Monitor ferritin regularly to assess for iron overload Hydroxyurea

MCV, mean corpuscular volume; MCHC, mean corpuscular hemoglobin concentration; TIBC, total iron binding capacity; Hgb, hemoglobin; Hct, hematocrit; AIDS, acquired immune deficiency syndrome; SLE, systemic lupus erythematosus; RBCs, red blood cells; PRBCs, packed RBCs.

the destruction of erythrocytes. The released hemoglobin is converted in large part to bilirubin; therefore, the bilirubin concentration rises. **Hemolysis** can result from an abnormality within the erythrocyte itself (e.g., sickle cell anemia, glucose-6-phosphate dehydrogenase [G-6-PD] deficiency) or within the plasma (e.g., immune hemolytic anemias), or from direct injury to the erythrocyte within the circulation (e.g., hemolysis caused by mechanical heart valve).

To determine whether the presence of anemia in a given patient is caused by destruction or by inadequate production of erythrocytes, consider the following factors:

- The marrow's ability to respond to decreased erythrocytes (as evidenced by an increased reticulocyte count in the circulating blood)
- The degree to which young erythrocytes (**nucleated RBCs**) proliferate in the bone marrow and the manner in which they mature (as observed on bone marrow biopsy)
- The presence or absence of end products of erythrocyte destruction within the circulation (e.g., increased bilirubin level, decreased haptoglobin [a protein produced by the liver] level)

Clinical Manifestations and Assessment

Aside from the severity of the anemia itself, several factors influence the development of anemia-associated symptoms:

- The rapidity with which the anemia has developed
- The duration of the anemia (i.e., chronicity)
- The metabolic requirements of the patient
- Other concurrent disorders or disabilities (e.g., cardiopulmonary disease)

In general, the more rapidly an anemia develops, the more severe its symptoms. An otherwise healthy person can often tolerate as much as a 50% gradual reduction in hemoglobin without pronounced symptoms or significant incapacity, whereas the rapid loss of as little as 30% may precipitate profound vascular collapse in the same person. A person who has become gradually anemic, with hemoglobin levels between 9 and 11 g/dL, may have few or no symptoms other than mild tachycardia on exertion and fatigue.

People who usually are very active or who have significant demands on their lives (e.g., a single, working mother of small children) are more likely to experience symptoms. Patients with hypothyroidism with decreased oxygen needs may be completely asymptomatic, without tachycardia or increased cardiac output, at a hemoglobin level of 10 g/dL. Similarly, patients with coexistent cardiac, vascular, or pulmonary disease may develop more pronounced symptoms of anemia (e.g., dyspnea, chest pain, muscle pain or cramping) at a higher hemoglobin level than those without these concurrent health problems.

BOX 20-1 **Focused Assessment**

Anemia

Be alert for the following signs and symptoms:
- General:
  - Weakness, fatigue
  - Dizziness
  - Pica (craving unusual items including: ice, starch, or dirt)
- Neurologic:
  - Numbness and tingling (paresthesias), irritability
  - Weakness
  - Headache
  - Poor coordination, confusion
  - Gait disturbances
  - Reflex abnormalities
  - Loss of position (proprioception) and vibration sense
  - Spasticity
  - Roaring, rushing, ringing, or pounding sensation in the ears
- Integumentary:
  - Pallor of the skin and mucous membranes
  - Jaundice (hemolytic anemia)
  - Brittle, ridged, concave nails
  - Impaired wound healing
  - Loss of elasticity
  - Early thinning and graying of hair
  - Dry skin
  - Painful mouth sores
- Beefy red, sore tongue (megaloblastic anemia)
- Smooth and red tongue (iron deficiency anemia)
- Ulcerated corners of the mouth (angular cheilitis)
- Cardiovascular:
  - Palpitations
  - Chest pain
  - Tachycardia
  - Hypotension
  - Peripheral edema
  - Murmurs
- Respiratory:
  - Dyspnea
  - Orthopnea
  - Tachypnea
- Gastrointestinal:
  - Anorexia, nausea, vomiting
  - Dysphagia
  - Abdominal pain
  - Flatulence
  - Diarrhea
  - Hepatomegaly
  - Splenomegaly
- Musculoskeletal:
  - Muscle pain (claudication)

[a]Neurologic signs and symptoms are most commonly seen in pernicious anemia.

The most common signs and symptoms of anemia are discussed in Box 20-1. A careful and thorough assessment is essential in identifying potential complications and targeting nursing interventions.

A variety of hematologic studies are performed to determine the type and cause of the anemia (see Chapter 19 for a detailed overview). In an initial evaluation, the hemoglobin, **hematocrit**, reticulocyte count, and RBC indices, particularly the mean corpuscular volume (MCV) and red cell distribution width (RDW), are particularly useful. Iron studies (**serum** iron level, total iron-binding capacity [TIBC], % saturation, and ferritin), as well as serum vitamin B_{12} and folate levels are also frequently obtained. Other tests include haptoglobin (if hemolysis is suspected) and erythropoietin levels. The remaining complete blood count (CBC) values are useful in determining whether the anemia is an isolated problem or part of another hematologic condition, such as **leukemia** or myelodysplastic syndrome (MDS) (a group of disorders where the bone marrow does not produce enough healthy blood cells). Bone marrow aspiration and biopsy may be performed. In addition, other diagnostic studies, including endoscopy and colonoscopy, may be performed to determine the presence of underlying chronic illness, such as malignancy, or the source of any blood loss, such as polyps or ulcers within the gastrointestinal (GI) tract.

Medical Management

Management of anemia is directed toward correcting or controlling the cause of the anemia; if the anemia is severe, the erythrocytes that are lost or destroyed may be replaced with a transfusion of packed RBCs (PRBCs). The management of the various types of anemia is covered in the discussions that follow.

Nursing Management

Managing Fatigue

The most common symptom and complication of anemia is fatigue. This distressing symptom is too often minimized by health care providers. Fatigue is often the symptom that has the greatest negative impact on a patient's level of functioning and consequent quality of life. Patients often describe the fatigue from anemia as oppressive. Fatigue can interfere with a person's ability to work, both inside and outside the home. It can disrupt relationships with family and friends. Patients often lose interest in hobbies and activities, including sexual activity. The severity of distress from fatigue is often related to a person's responsibilities and life demands as well as the amount of assistance and support received from others.

Other factors that may be contributing to fatigue should also be assessed and managed including pain, emotional distress, sleep disturbances, comorbidities, physical deconditioning, and nutritional deficiencies (NCCN, 2016a).

Nursing interventions can focus on assisting the patient to prioritize activities and to establish a balance between activity and rest that is realistic and feasible from the patient's perspective. Patients with chronic anemia need to maintain some physical activity and exercise to prevent the deconditioning that results from inactivity. Short periods of daily exercise can also decrease the severity of fatigue (Tomlinson, Diorio, Beyene, & Sung, 2014).

Maintaining Adequate Nutrition

Inadequate intake of essential nutrients, such as iron, vitamin B_{12}, and folic acid can cause anemia. The symptoms associated with anemia (e.g., fatigue, anorexia) can, in turn, interfere with maintaining adequate nutrition. A healthy diet should be encouraged. The nurse should inform the patient that alcohol interferes with the utilization of essential nutrients and should advise the patient to avoid alcoholic beverages or to limit intake. Dietary teaching sessions should be individualized and culturally sensitive to food preferences and food preparation. The involvement of family members enhances compliance with dietary recommendations. Dietary supplements (e.g., vitamins, iron, folate, protein) may be prescribed as well depending on the results of testing.

Equally important, the patient and family must understand the underlying cause of the anemia because many forms of anemia are not the result of a nutritional deficiency. In such cases, even an excessive intake of nutritional supplements will not improve the anemia. A potential problem in patients with chronic transfusion requirements occurs with the indiscriminate use of iron supplements. These individuals are at risk for iron overload from their transfusions. The addition of an iron supplement will only increase their iron burden, contributing to risk for end-organ damage.

Maintaining Adequate Perfusion

Patients with acute blood loss or severe hemolysis may have decreased tissue perfusion from decreased blood volume or reduced circulating erythrocytes (decreased hematocrit). Lost volume is replaced with transfusions or IV fluids, based on the symptoms and the laboratory test results. Supplemental oxygen may be necessary, but it is rarely needed on a long-term basis unless there is underlying severe cardiac or pulmonary disease. The nurse monitors the patient's vital signs and pulse oximetry readings closely; other medications, such as antihypertensive agents, may need to be adjusted or withheld.

Complications

General complications of severe anemia include heart failure, paresthesias (abnormal sensation of pricking, tingling, numbness, burning, etc.), and confusion. At any given level of anemia, patients with underlying heart disease are far more likely to have angina or symptoms of heart failure than those without heart disease.

HYPOPROLIFERATIVE ANEMIAS

IRON DEFICIENCY ANEMIA

The development of iron deficiency anemia occurs when the body's iron stores are depleted and there is no iron available for hemoglobin synthesis. The volume of individual iron stores is dependent upon sex, age, rate of growth, and the balance between dietary iron absorption and losses. Iron is stored primarily in the liver, spleen, and bone marrow. The remainder of iron exists as hemoglobin and proteins. Iron deficiency anemia is diagnosed based on the presence of a microcytic anemia, transferrin saturation below 20%, and ferritin below 30 ng/mL (Jiminez et al., 2015).

Iron deficiency anemia is the most common type of anemia in all age groups, and it is the most common anemia in the world. It is particularly prevalent in developing countries, where inadequate iron stores can result from inadequate intake of iron (seen with vegetarian diets) or from blood loss (e.g., from intestinal hookworm). Iron deficiency is also common in the United States. In children, adolescents, and pregnant women, the cause is typically inadequate iron in the diet to keep up with increased growth. However, for most adults with iron deficiency anemia, the cause is blood loss. In fact, in adults, the cause of iron deficiency anemia should be considered to be bleeding until proven otherwise.

The most common cause of iron deficiency anemia in men and postmenopausal women is bleeding (from ulcers, gastritis, inflammatory bowel disease, or GI tumors). The most common cause of iron deficiency anemia in premenopausal women is menorrhagia (excessive menstrual bleeding) and pregnancy with inadequate iron supplementation. Patients with chronic alcoholism often have chronic blood loss from the GI tract, which causes iron loss and eventual anemia. Other causes include iron malabsorption, as is seen after gastrectomy or with celiac disease.

Medical Management

Except in the case of pregnancy, the cause of iron deficiency should be investigated. Anemia may be a sign of a curable GI cancer or of uterine fibroid tumors. Stool specimens should be tested for occult blood and *H. pylori* infection. Blood samples should be sent for celiac serology and antiparietal cell antibodies (to rule out pernicious anemia). In the presence of iron deficiency, patients over 50 years of age, those with a family history of GI disorders, those with GI symptoms, men with Hgb below 13 g/dL or women with Hgb below 10 g/dL should undergo endoscopy and colonoscopy to rule out GI blood loss (Jiminez et al., 2015).

Several oral iron preparations—ferrous sulfate, ferrous succinate, ferrous gluconate, and ferrous fumarate—are available for treating iron deficiency anemia. The oral route of administration is preferred over IV. The recommended daily dose for treatment of iron deficiency is 100 mg/day of elemental iron. Oral preparations are inexpensive and readily available. Ferrous sulfate, fumarate, and gluconate each contain 50 to 65 mg of elemental iron per tablet with recommended dosing of one tab three times/day (Auerbach & Adamson, 2016). Despite the development of a number of orally effective iron-containing compounds, the original salt, ferrous sulfate (325 mg three times daily), remains the most useful. However, some newer oral iron preparations, such as ferrous gluconate (300 mg two or three times daily) or ferrous fumarate (325 mg two or three times daily), may induce fewer GI side effects.

Food can decrease iron absorption by as much as 50% although vitamin C facilitates the absorption of iron. Therefore, oral iron should be taken with a glass of orange juice or a vitamin C tablet on an empty stomach to maximize absorption. However, taking iron on an empty stomach and taking iron with vitamin C can increase GI side effects. GI side effects, including nausea and epigastric discomfort, occur in up to 70% of patients taking oral iron and are dose dependent (Auerbach & Adamson, 2016). Taking iron with meals may decrease nausea and epigastric discomfort but may result in decreased absorption. In addition, calcium supplements can decrease iron absorption; therefore, administration of these two medications should be staggered (Ferri, 2016a).

The hemoglobin level should begin to rise after 1 week of replacement and should increase by 1 to 2 g/dL within 4 to 8 weeks. If hemoglobin levels fail to improve within this time frame, adherence to the regimen should be assessed and IV iron replacement should be considered. If the patient has been adherent to the prescribed regimen, then assess for absorption problems, continued blood loss, concomitant deficiencies (folate, B$_{12}$, copper), and drug interactions. Diet has been implicated when large quantities of phytates from cereals or tannate from teas inhibit iron absorption (Ginder, 2016). In addition, iron absorption is impaired by conditions that affect the duodenum's ability to absorb iron, as in extensive gastric surgery, generalized intestinal malabsorption, and atrophic gastritis; whereas proton pump inhibitors (PPIs) or histamine 2 receptor blockers (H2) do not appear to cause iron deficiency (Ginder, 2016). Iron store repletion takes much longer (goal ferritin greater than 100 ng/mL), so it is important that the patient continue taking the iron for as long as 6 to 12 months (Auerbach & Adamson, 2016).

In some cases, oral iron is poorly absorbed or poorly tolerated, or iron supplementation is needed in large amounts. In these situations, IV administration of iron may be needed. There are currently six available intravenous iron preparations:

- INFeD® (low–molecular-weight [LMWH] iron dextran),
- Ferrlecit® (ferric gluconate),
- Venofer® (iron sucrose),
- Feraheme® (ferumoxytol),
- Monofer® (iron isomaltoside 1,000), and
- Injectafer® (ferric carboxymaltose).

All IV iron preparations carry some risk for hypersensitivity. INFeD® is the only formulation that requires a test dose due to the risk of hypersensitivity. INFed® also allows the delivery of higher doses of iron (1,000 mg) over 1 hour. Ferrlecit® and Venofer® must be given in smaller doses. Feraheme®, Monofer®, and Injectafer® allow higher doses to be given over shorter periods of time (15 minutes). Feraheme® and Injectafer® are available in the United States and Europe; Monofer® is available only in Europe (Auerbach & Macdougall, 2014). In most cases, multiple doses of IV iron replacement are required to replace the patient's iron stores.

Nursing Management

Preventive education is important, because iron deficiency anemia is common in menstruating and pregnant women. Food sources high in iron include organ meats (beef or calf's liver, chicken liver), other red meats, beans (black, pinto, and garbanzo), leafy green vegetables, raisins, and molasses. Taking iron-rich foods with a source of vitamin C (e.g., orange juice) enhances the absorption of iron.

The nurse helps the patient select a healthy diet and refers the patient to a registered dietitian as appropriate. Nutritional counseling can be provided for those whose usual diet is inadequate. Patients with a history of eating fad diets or strict vegetarian diets are counseled that such diets often contain inadequate amounts of absorbable iron. The nurse encourages the patient to continue iron therapy as long as it is prescribed, even if the symptoms of anemia resolve. The nurse helps to assess and manage side effects of oral iron replacement.

Because iron is best absorbed on an empty stomach, the patient is instructed to take the supplement an hour before meals. Iron supplements are usually given in the oral form, typically as ferrous sulfate. Most patients can use the less expensive, more standard forms of ferrous sulfate. Tablets with enteric coating may be absorbed poorly and should be avoided. Many patients have difficulty tolerating iron supplements because of GI side effects (diarrhea, constipation, epigastric discomfort, nausea, and vomiting). Some iron formulations are designed to limit GI side effects by the addition of a stool softener or use of sustained-release formulations to limit nausea or gastritis. Specific patient teaching aids (Box 20-2) can assist patients with the use of iron supplements.

IV supplementation may be used when the patient's iron stores are completely depleted, if the patient has impaired iron absorption, or the patient cannot tolerate oral forms of iron supplementation (see Medical Management). The IV route is preferred for administration of iron dextran. Due to the risk for hypersensitivity reactions with parenteral iron formulations, the patient should be monitored closely during

Patient Education

Taking Oral Iron Supplements

- Take iron on an empty stomach (1 hour before or 2 hours after a meal). Because iron absorption is reduced with food, especially dairy products and antacids, avoid taking iron with these items.
- To prevent gastrointestinal distress, the following schedule may work better if more than one tablet a day is prescribed: Start with only one tablet per day for a few days, then increase to two tablets per day, and then three tablets per day. This method permits the body to adjust gradually to the iron.
- Increase the intake of vitamin C (citrus fruits and juices, strawberries, tomatoes, broccoli), to enhance iron absorption.
- Eat foods high in fiber to minimize problems with constipation.
- Remember that stools will become dark in color.
- To prevent staining the teeth with a liquid preparation, use a straw or place a spoon at the back of the mouth to take the supplement. Rinse the mouth thoroughly afterward.

and shortly after the infusion; vital signs should be monitored carefully per institution guidelines.

ANEMIA IN KIDNEY DISEASE

The degree of anemia in patients with end-stage kidney disease (ESKD) varies greatly, but in general patients do not become significantly anemic until the serum creatinine level exceeds 3 mg/dL.

Pathophysiology

This anemia is caused by both a mild shortening of erythrocyte lifespan and a deficiency of erythropoietin (necessary for **erythropoiesis**). As kidney function decreases, erythropoietin, which is produced by the kidney, also decreases. Because erythropoietin is also produced outside the kidney, some erythropoiesis continues, even in patients whose kidneys have been removed. However, the number of RBCs produced is small and the degree of erythropoiesis is inadequate.

Patients undergoing long-term hemodialysis lose blood into the dialyzer and, therefore, may become iron deficient. Folic acid deficiency develops because this vitamin passes into the dialysate. Therefore, patients who receive hemodialysis and who have anemia should be evaluated for iron and folate deficiency and treated appropriately.

Clinical Manifestations and Assessment

For patients with ESKD, the symptoms of anemia, including fatigue and decreased activity tolerance, are often the most disturbing. If untreated, the hematocrit may fall to between 20% and 30%, although in rare cases it may fall to less than 15%. The erythrocytes appear normal in shape, size, and color on the peripheral smear.

Medical and Nursing Management

The availability of recombinant erythropoietin (also referred to as erythropoiesis stimulating agents or ESAs) (epoetin alfa [Epogen, Procrit]; darbepoetin alfa [Aranesp]) has dramatically altered the management of anemia in ESKD by decreasing the need for RBC transfusion, with its associated risks. Iron stores, including transferrin saturation and ferritin, must be measured prior to starting ESAs, and iron replacement should be initiated in patients with a ferritin of less than 100 ng/mL; adequate iron stores are essential for optimal response to erythropoietin. Erythropoietin, in combination with oral iron supplements, can raise and maintain hematocrit levels to between 33% and 38%. This treatment has been successful with dialysis patients. ESAs carry an increased risk of death and cardiovascular events, including stroke, venous thromboembolism (VTE), and myocardial infarction (MI) when hemoglobin targets exceed 11 g/dL; therefore, the lowest dose required to reduce transfusion requirements is recommended (Aranesp® package insert, Amgen 2015).

Hypertension is also seen in this patient population when the hematocrit rapidly increases to a high level. Therefore, the hemoglobin and blood pressure should be checked frequently when a patient with kidney disease begins erythropoietin therapy. The dose of erythropoietin should be titrated to the goal hemoglobin based on available guidelines (Aranesp® package insert, Amgen 2015). Some patients may require initiation of antihypertensive therapy.

ANEMIA OF CHRONIC DISEASE

The term "anemia of chronic disease" is a misnomer in that only the chronic diseases of inflammation, infection, and malignancy cause this type of anemia. Many chronic inflammatory diseases are associated with a **normochromic**, **normocytic** anemia (i.e., the erythrocytes are normal in color and size). These disorders include rheumatoid arthritis; severe, chronic infections; and many cancers. It is, therefore, imperative that the "chronic disease" be diagnosed when this form of anemia is identified so that it can be managed appropriately.

The anemia is usually mild to moderate and nonprogressive. It develops gradually over 6 to 8 weeks and then stabilizes at a hematocrit seldom less than 25%. The hemoglobin level rarely falls below 9 g/dL, and the bone marrow has normal cellularity with increased stores of iron as the iron is diverted from the serum.

Most of these patients have few symptoms and do not require treatment for the anemia. With successful treatment of the underlying disorder, the bone marrow iron is used to make erythrocytes and the hemoglobin level rises.

MEGALOBLASTIC ANEMIAS

In the anemias caused by deficiencies of either vitamin B_{12} or folic acid, identical bone marrow and peripheral blood changes occur because both vitamins are essential for normal

DNA synthesis. In either anemia, the erythrocytes that are produced are abnormally large and are called *megaloblastic red cells*; therefore, the MCV is elevated. Other cells derived from the **myeloid** stem cell (nonlymphoid leukocytes, platelets) are also abnormal, resulting in low leukocyte and platelet counts in advanced stages of disease. A bone marrow analysis reveals **hyperplasia** (abnormal increase in the number of cells), and the precursor erythroid and myeloid cells are large and bizarre in appearance.

Pathophysiology

Folic Acid Deficiency

Folic acid is stored as compounds referred to as *folates*. The folate stores in the body are much smaller than those of vitamin B_{12}, and they are quickly depleted when the dietary intake of folate is deficient (within 4 months). Folate is found in green leafy vegetables, legumes, egg yolks, fortified foods like cereal, and liver (Lolin, 2014). Folate deficiency occurs in people who rarely eat uncooked vegetables. Alcohol increases folic acid requirements; patients with alcoholism usually have a diet that is deficient in the vitamin. Folic acid requirements are also increased in patients with chronic hemolytic anemias and in women who are pregnant because the need for erythrocyte production is increased in these conditions. Folate is absorbed in the upper small intestine; therefore, some patients with malabsorptive diseases of the small bowel, such as celiac sprue, may not absorb folic acid normally (Lolin, 2014).

Vitamin B_{12} Deficiency

A deficiency of vitamin B_{12} can occur in several ways. Inadequate dietary intake is rare but can develop in strict vegans (who consume no meat or dairy products). Faulty absorption from the GI tract is a more common cause. This occurs in conditions such as Crohn disease, or after ileal resection, bariatric gastric bypass surgery, or gastrectomy. Even if adequate vitamin B_{12} and intrinsic factor are present, a deficiency may occur if disease involving the ileum or pancreas impairs absorption. Another cause is the absence of intrinsic factor, as in pernicious anemia. Intrinsic factor is normally secreted by cells within the gastric mucosa; normally, it binds with the dietary vitamin B_{12} and travels with it to the ileum, where the vitamin is absorbed. Without intrinsic factor, orally consumed vitamin B_{12} cannot be absorbed, and eventually erythrocyte production is diminished. Pernicious anemia, which tends to run in families, is primarily a disorder of adults, particularly the elderly. Pernicious anemia is an autoimmune disorder involving autoantibodies to intrinsic factor and parietal cells resulting in poor absorption of B_{12} (Rojas Hernandez & Oo, 2015). For unknown reasons, patients with pernicious anemia have a higher incidence of gastric cancer, adenocarcinomas, and other cancers compared to the general population (Murphy et al., 2015). Though routine screening

for this population has not yet been recommended, these patients should understand their risks and be educated on reporting any new symptoms promptly to health care providers. It is recommended that patients with newly diagnosed pernicious anemia or any patient with pernicious anemia and GI symptoms undergo screening endoscopy (Evans et al., 2015). The body normally has large stores of vitamin B_{12} so years may pass before the deficiency results in anemia. Because the body compensates so well, the anemia can be severe before the patient becomes symptomatic.

Clinical Manifestations and Assessment

People with vitamin B and/or folic acid deficiency may present with nonspecific symptoms including fatigue, mood changes, memory difficulty, and weakness (Lolin, 2014). Assessment of patients who have or are at risk of megaloblastic anemia includes inspection of the skin and mucous membranes. Mild jaundice may be apparent and is best seen in the sclera without using fluorescent lights. Vitiligo (patchy loss of skin pigmentation) and premature graying of the hair are often seen in patients with pernicious anemia. The tongue is smooth, red, and sore (referred to as glossitis).

Symptoms of folic acid and vitamin B_{12} deficiencies are similar, and the two anemias may coexist. However, the neurologic manifestations of vitamin B_{12} deficiency do not occur with folic acid deficiency, and they persist if vitamin B_{12} is not replaced. Therefore, careful distinction between the two anemias must be made. Serum levels of both vitamins can be measured. In the case of folic acid deficiency, even small amounts of folate increase the serum folate level. Therefore, measuring the amount of folate within the red cell itself (red cell folate) is a more sensitive test in determining true folate deficiency (Lolin, 2014).

Neurologic symptoms are seen in severe vitamin B_{12} deficiency and pernicious anemia and include psychiatric symptoms and peripheral neuropathy (Lolin, 2014). This presentation happens infrequently due to earlier diagnosis.

After the body's stores of vitamin B_{12} are depleted, the patient may begin to show signs and symptoms of the anemia. However, because the onset and progression of the anemia are so gradual, the body can compensate very well until the anemia is severe so that the typical manifestations of anemia (weakness, listlessness, fatigue) may not be apparent initially. The hematologic effects of deficiency are accompanied by effects on other organ systems, particularly the GI tract and nervous system (see Box 20-1). These symptoms are progressive, although the course of illness may be marked by spontaneous partial remissions and exacerbations. Without treatment, patients can die after several years, usually from heart failure secondary to anemia.

Medical Management

Underlying causes for vitamin B_{12} and folate deficiency should be investigated and treated.

Dietary counseling should include discussion on increasing dietary sources of folic acid. Supplemental oral folic acid should be administered at a dosage of 1 to 5 mg daily until recovery (Lolin, 2014). Patients with malabsorption will need to continue folic acid supplements over the long term. Pregnant patients should take folic acid (0.4 to 0.8 mg daily) when planning for pregnancy as well as throughout the course of pregnancy (Antony, 2016).

Vitamin B_{12} deficiency is treated by vitamin B_{12} replacement. Vegetarians can prevent or treat deficiency with oral supplements, vitamins, or fortified soy milk. When the deficiency is due to the more common defect in absorption or the absence of intrinsic factor, replacement by IM injections of vitamin B_{12} is necessary. The replacement schedule includes daily or every other day administration of 1 mg (1,000 μg) of cyanocobalamin IM for 1 week, followed by weekly administration for 1 to 2 months and then monthly through the remainder of the patient's life (Rojas Hernandez & Oo, 2015; Stabler, 2013).

As vitamin B_{12} is replaced, the reticulocyte count rises within 1 week, and in several weeks all the blood counts should improve to normal. The characteristic beefy red, sore tongue feels better and appears less red in several days. However, the neurologic manifestations require more time for recovery; if there is severe neuropathy, the patient may never recover fully. To prevent recurrence of pernicious anemia, vitamin B_{12} therapy must be continued for life.

> **Nursing Alert**
> *Even when the megaloblastic anemia is severe, RBC transfusions may not be used because the patient's body has compensated over time by expanding the total blood volume. Administration of blood transfusions to such patients, particularly those who are elderly or who have cardiac dysfunction, can precipitate pulmonary edema. If transfusions are required, the RBCs should be transfused slowly, with careful attention to signs and symptoms of fluid overload.*

Nursing Management

In the setting of peripheral neuropathy, the nurse needs to pay particular attention to ambulation and should assess the patient's gait and stability as well as the need for assistive devices (e.g., canes, walkers) and for assistance in managing daily activities. Of particular concern is ensuring safety when position sense, coordination, and gait are affected. Physical and occupational therapy referrals may be needed. If sensation is altered, the patient needs to be instructed to avoid excessive heat and cold.

Because mouth and tongue soreness may restrict nutritional intake, the nurse advises the patient to eat small amounts of bland, soft foods frequently and educates the patient on routine mouth care. The nurse also may explain

that other nutritional deficiencies, such as alcohol-induced anemia, can induce neurologic problems.

HEMOLYTIC ANEMIAS

In hemolytic anemias, the erythrocytes have a shortened lifespan; thus, their number in the circulation is reduced. Fewer erythrocytes result in decreased available oxygen, causing hypoxia, which, in turn, stimulates an increase in erythropoietin release from the kidney. The erythropoietin stimulates the bone marrow to compensate by producing new erythrocytes and releasing some of them into the circulation somewhat prematurely as reticulocytes. If the red cell destruction persists, the hemoglobin is broken down excessively; about 80% of the heme is converted to bilirubin, conjugated in the liver, and excreted in the bile.

The mechanism of erythrocyte destruction varies, but all types of hemolytic anemia share certain laboratory features: the reticulocyte count is elevated, the fraction of indirect (unconjugated) bilirubin is increased, and the supply of haptoglobin (a binding protein for free hemoglobin) is depleted as more hemoglobin is released. As a result, the plasma haptoglobin level is low. The severity of anemia will increase if the marrow does not compensate by replacing the hemolyzed erythrocytes (poor response indicated by a decreased reticulocyte count). Causes of hemolytic anemia are discussed in Box 20-3.

THALASSEMIA

The thalassemias are a group of hereditary anemias characterized by **hypochromia** (an abnormal decrease in the hemoglobin content of erythrocytes), extreme **microcytosis** (smaller-than-normal erythrocytes), destruction of blood elements (hemolysis), and variable degrees of anemia due to impaired hemoglobin production and ineffective RBC production (Tubman et al., 2015). The thalassemias occur worldwide, but the highest prevalence is found in people of Mediterranean, African, and Southeast Asian ancestry.

Thalassemias are classified into two major groups according to which hemoglobin chain is diminished: alpha or beta. The alpha thalassemias occur mainly in people from Asia and the Middle East, and the beta thalassemias are most prevalent in people from Mediterranean regions but also occur in those from the Middle East or Asia. The alpha thalassemias are milder than the beta forms and often occur without symptoms; the erythrocytes are extremely microcytic, but the anemia, if present, is mild.

The severity of beta thalassemia varies depending on the extent to which the hemoglobin chains are affected. Patients with mild forms have a microcytosis and mild anemia. If left untreated, severe beta thalassemia (*thalassemia major*, or *Cooley anemia*) can be fatal within the first few years of life. Peripheral blood stem cell transplant (PBSCT) offers a

Causes of Hemolytic Anemias

Inherited Hemolytic Anemia

- Abnormal hemoglobin:
  - Sickle cell anemia
  - Thalassemia
- RBC membrane abnormality:
  - Hereditary spherocytosis
  - Hereditary elliptocytosis
  - Acanthocytosis
  - Stomatocytosis
- Enzyme deficiencies:
  - Glucose-6-phosphate dehydrogenase (G-6-PD) deficiency

Acquired Hemolytic Anemia

- Antibody-related:
  - Iso-antibody/transfusion reaction
  - Autoimmune hemolytic anemia (AIHA)
  - Cold agglutinin disease
- Not antibody-related:
  - RBC membrane defects
  - Paroxysmal nocturnal hemoglobinuria (PNH)
  - Liver disease
  - Uremia
  - Trauma
  - Mechanical heart valve
  - Microangiopathic hemolytic anemia
  - Infection
  - Bacterial
  - Parasitic
  - Disseminated intravascular coagulation (DIC)
  - Toxins
  - Hypersplenism

chance of cure, but when this is not possible, the disease is usually treated with transfusion of PRBCs. Complications related to lifelong transfusions include the development of anti-RBC antibodies, transfusion-associated infections, and iron overload. Transfusional iron overload is the primary cause of death in patients with thalassemia (90% of deaths). In the 1980s, life expectancy was not expected to exceed the third decade of life. However, with improvements in methods to measure iron overload as well as treatments for iron overload, life expectancy has improved (Tubman et al., 2015).

Patient teaching during the reproductive years should include preconception counseling about the risk of thalassemia major.

Treatment of iron overload involves the use of chelating agents. Deferoxamine (given IV or SQ), deferasirox (oral), and deferiprone (oral) are used alone or in combination to treat iron overload. Each medication requires monitoring for toxicity, including bone marrow suppression (deferiprone), liver function abnormalities (deferasirox), annual eye and hearing examinations (due to risk for ocular toxicity and ototoxicity) (all) (Tubman et al., 2015). Side effects of the oral agents

include nausea, vomiting, diarrhea, and abdominal pain and may contribute to interruptions in therapy. Adherence with these agents is essential to response; therefore, nursing education should focus on necessary monitoring parameters and the importance of taking agents as directed.

AUTOIMMUNE HEMOLYTIC ANEMIA

Autoimmune hemolytic anemia (AIHA) results when the patient's own immune system hemolyzes RBCs (Hill, 2015). Hemolysis results from exposure of the erythrocyte to antibodies, which coat the RBCs, resulting in early destruction. In half of the cases, no identifiable cause for AIHA can be found. In the other half, other disorders, including chronic lymphocytic leukemia (CLL), lupus, or some infections, trigger the AIHA (Hill, 2015). Medications can also trigger immune hemolysis.

Pathophysiology

Autoantibodies may develop for many reasons. In many instances, the person's immune system is dysfunctional so that it falsely recognizes its own erythrocytes as foreign and produces antibodies against them. This mechanism is seen in people with CLL. Another mechanism is a deficiency in suppressor lymphocytes, which normally prevent antibody formation against a person's own antigens. Autoantibodies tend to be of the IgG type. The erythrocytes are sequestered in the spleen and destroyed by the **macrophages** outside the blood vessel (extravascular hemolysis).

AIHAs can be classified based on the body temperature involved when the antibodies react with the RBC antigen. Warm-body antibodies bind to erythrocytes most actively in warm conditions (37°C); cold-body antibodies react in cold conditions (0°C). Most AIHAs are the warm-body type. AIHA is associated with other disorders in most cases (e.g., medication exposure, lymphoma, CLL, other malignancy, collagen vascular disease, autoimmune disease, infection). In idiopathic autoimmune hemolytic states, the etiology of autoantibody production is not known. All ages and both genders are equally vulnerable to this form, whereas the incidence of secondary forms is greater in people older than 45 years of age and in females.

Medical Management

Treatment depends on the severity of the anemia, the type of AIHA, and the presence or absence of an underlying disorder. Treatment of the underlying disorder may improve the AIHA (Hill, 2015). Mild, asymptomatic AIHA may not require intervention other than close monitoring over time. Since medications can also trigger immune hemolysis, any possible offending medication should be discontinued immediately.

In warm AIHA, the treatment includes high doses of corticosteroids until hemolysis decreases. Corticosteroids decrease the macrophage's ability to clear the antibody-coated erythrocytes. If the hemoglobin level returns to normal, usually after several weeks, the corticosteroid dose can be lowered or, in some cases, tapered and discontinued. However, corticosteroids rarely produce a lasting remission. In severe cases, blood transfusions may be required. Because the antibodies may react with all possible donor cells, careful blood typing is necessary, and the transfusion should be administered slowly and cautiously.

In the setting of steroid failure, other immunosuppressive medications may be attempted to decrease antibody production. The immunosuppressive agents most frequently used are cyclophosphamide (Cytoxan), which has a more rapid effect but more toxicity, and azathioprine (Imuran), which has a less rapid effect but less toxicity. The monoclonal antibody, Rituximab, has been used with success in 45% to 60% of patients with AIHA, and studies are ongoing to determine the duration of remission following Rituximab therapy (Hill, 2015). The synthetic androgen, danazol, can be useful in some patients, particularly in combination with corticosteroids. The mechanism for this success is unclear. If corticosteroids or immunosuppressive agents are used, the taper must be very gradual to prevent a rebound "hyperimmune" response and exacerbation of the hemolysis.

Immunoglobulin administration is effective in about one third of patients, but the effect is transient and the medication is expensive. Transfusions may be necessary if the anemia is severe; it may be extremely difficult to cross-match samples of available units of PRBCs with that of the patient. Splenectomy (removal of the spleen) removes the major site of erythrocyte destruction; therefore, splenectomy may be performed if medications do not produce a remission.

For patients with cold-antibody hemolytic anemia, no treatment may be required other than to advise the patient to keep warm; relocation to a warm climate may be necessary. Intravenous solutions and blood products that have been refrigerated must have their temperature raised before infusion. Treatment with Rituximab may be considered for severe symptoms or anemia requiring transfusion (Hill, 2015).

Nursing Management

Patients may have great difficulty understanding the pathologic mechanisms underlying the disease and may need repeated explanations in terms they can understand. Patients who have had a splenectomy should be vaccinated against pneumococcal and encapsulated bacteria infections (e.g., Pneumovax) and informed that they are permanently at greater risk for infection. Patients receiving long-term corticosteroid therapy, particularly those with concurrent diabetes or hypertension, need careful monitoring of blood sugar and blood pressure. They must understand the need for adherence to the medication and the importance of never abruptly discontinuing it. A written explanation and a tapering schedule should be provided, and needed adjustments based on hemoglobin levels should be emphasized. Similar teaching should be provided when immunosuppressive agents are

used. Corticosteroid therapy is not without significant risk, and patients need to be monitored closely for complications.

Polycythemia, literally meaning "too many cells in the blood," refers to an increased number of erythrocytes. It is a term used when the hematocrit is elevated (to greater than 55% in males, greater than 50% in females). Polycythemia is classified as either primary or secondary (Porth, 2015). Primary polycythemia, also known as polycythemia Vera (PV) is a malignant condition that will be described later in the chapter; secondary polycythemia is a benign condition, discussed below.

Long-term complications of corticosteroid therapy are presented in Chapter 31 (Table 31-7).

SECONDARY POLYCYTHEMIA

Pathophysiology

Secondary polycythemia is caused by excessive production of erythropoietin. This may occur in response to a reduced amount of oxygen, which acts as a hypoxic stimulus, as in cigarette smoking, obstructive sleep apnea, chronic obstructive pulmonary disease (COPD), or cyanotic heart disease, or in nonpathologic conditions, such as living at a high altitude. It can also result from certain hemoglobinopathies (e.g., hemoglobin Chesapeake), in which the hemoglobin has an abnormally high affinity for oxygen. Secondary polycythemia can also occur from neoplasms (e.g., renal cell carcinoma) that stimulate erythropoietin production.

Medical and Nursing Management

Management of secondary polycythemia may not be necessary; when management is necessary, the goal is to treat the underlying primary conditions. If the cause cannot be corrected (e.g., by treating the renal cell carcinoma or improving pulmonary function), therapeutic phlebotomy may be necessary in symptomatic patients to reduce blood viscosity and volume.

PLATELET DISORDERS

Thrombocythemia

Thrombocythemia is the overproduction of platelets. There are two types with very different etiologies and treatment approaches: primary or essential (a malignant condition described later in the chapter) and secondary (a benign condition discussed here). Refer to Chapter 19 for discussion of bleeding disorders.

SECONDARY THROMBOCYTOSIS

Increased platelet production is the primary mechanism of secondary, or reactive, **thrombocytosis**. The platelet count is above normal, but, in contrast to primary thrombocythemia, an increase to more than 1 million/mm^3 is rare. Platelet function is normal; the platelet survival time is normal or decreased. Consequently, symptoms associated with hemorrhage or thrombosis are rare. Many disorders or conditions can cause a reactive increase in platelets, including infection, chronic inflammatory disorders, iron deficiency, malignant disease, acute hemorrhage, and splenectomy (see later discussion of primary thrombocythemia). Treatment is aimed at the underlying disorder. With successful management, the platelet count usually returns to normal.

THROMBOCYTOPENIA

Thrombocytopenia (low platelet level) can result from various factors: decreased production of platelets within the bone marrow, increased destruction of platelets, or increased consumption of platelets. There are numerous causes of thrombocytopenia, including malignancy, infection, medications, autoimmunity (ITP), and DIC. The primary strategy for managing thrombocytopenia is correction or treatment of the underlying cause or removal of the offending agent.

Clinical Manifestations and Assessment

Bleeding and petechiae usually do not occur with platelet counts greater than 50,000/mm^3, although excessive bleeding can follow surgery or trauma. When the platelet count drops to less than 20,000/mm^3, petechiae can appear, along with spontaneous nasal and gingival bleeding, excessive menstrual bleeding, and excessive bleeding after surgery or dental extractions. When the platelet count is less than 10,000/mm^3, spontaneous, potentially fatal CNS or GI hemorrhage can occur. If the platelets are dysfunctional due to disease (e.g., MDS) or medications (e.g., aspirin), the risk for bleeding may be much greater even when the actual platelet count is not significantly reduced.

A platelet deficiency that results from decreased production (e.g., leukemia, MDS) is diagnosed by examining the bone marrow via aspiration and biopsy. Infections, either viral or bacterial, as well as alcoholism can suppress platelet production. Therefore, laboratory tests should include testing for HIV and hepatitis B and C.

When platelet destruction is the cause of thrombocytopenia, the marrow shows increased megakaryocytes (the cells from which the platelets originate) and normal or even increased platelet production as the body attempts to compensate for the decreased platelets in circulation. Another cause of thrombocytopenia is sequestration. Approximately one third of the circulating platelets are within the spleen, and a greatly enlarged spleen results in increased sequestration of platelets.

Many medications (e.g., sulfa drugs, methotrexate) can either decrease platelet production or shorten their lifespan. Numerous genetic causes of thrombocytopenia have been discovered, including autosomal dominant, autosomal recessive, and X-linked mutations (Abrams, 2016).

An important cause to exclude is *pseudothrombocytopenia*. Here, platelets aggregate and clump in the presence of ethylenediamine tetra-acetic acid (EDTA), the anticoagulant present in the tube used for CBC collection. This clumping accounts for 15% to 30% of instances of isolated thrombocytopenia (Diz-Küçükkaya & López, 2016; Greenberg & Kaled, 2013). A manual examination of the peripheral smear can easily determine platelet clumping as the cause of thrombocytopenia; newer cell counter machines can also detect this.

Medical Management

The management of thrombocytopenia is usually treatment of the underlying cause. If the platelet count is low due to medications, removal of the offending agent may improve the platelet count. Medications strongly associated with thrombocytopenia include antibiotics (quinine, quinidine, penicillin, cephalosporin, vancomycin, trimethoprim-sulfamethoxazole, sulfonamides, and sulfonylureas), cardiovascular medications (digoxin, salicylates, and abciximab), and some miscellaneous agents (Cimetidine, Famotidine, Ranitidine, Valproate, and Interferon) (Abrams, 2016). When the platelet count is predictably lowered as a result of chemotherapy treatment, platelet transfusions may be needed to support the patient and prevent bleeding.

In hospitalized patients with chemotherapy-induced thrombocytopenia, platelets should be transfused to maintain a platelet count of more than 10,000/mm^3 to reduce the risk for spontaneous bleeding (Kaufman et al., 2015). Outpatients may be transfused more liberally (e.g., a platelet count less than 20,000/mm^3) because they may not be able to get daily transfusions due to logistical constraints (e.g., transportation availability). See Table 20-6 for further information on platelet transfusion parameters.

If excessive platelet destruction occurs, transfused platelets are also destroyed, and the platelet count does not increase. The most common cause of excessive platelet destruction is immune thrombocytopenia purpura (ITP) (see the following discussion). In some instances, splenectomy can be a useful therapeutic intervention, but often it is not an option; for example, in patients in whom the spleen is enlarged due to portal hypertension related to cirrhosis, splenectomy may cause more bleeding disorders.

Nursing Management

Nursing interventions for patients with thrombocytopenia are listed in Chapter 19, Box 19-3.

IMMUNE THROMBOCYTOPENIA PURPURA (ITP)

ITP is the most common autoimmune blood disorder, affecting people of all ages, although it is more common among children and young women. Historically, this disorder was referred to as "idiopathic" thrombocytopenia purpura because in many cases the underlying causes were unknown. In recent years, scientists have uncovered a number of etiologies leading to our current understanding of ITP as an autoimmune process, thus leading to the change in terminology from *idiopathic* to *immune* (Abrams, 2016). There are two forms of ITP: acute and chronic. Acute ITP, which occurs predominantly in children, often appears 1 to 6 weeks after a viral illness. This form is self-limited; remission often occurs spontaneously within 6 months. Chronic ITP is often diagnosed by exclusion of other causes of thrombocytopenia.

Pathophysiology

Although the precise cause of ITP remains unknown, the platelet count is decreased by a combination of antibody-mediated platelet destruction and impaired platelet production secondary to antiplatelet antibodies produced by B cells (Neunert, 2013). In addition, there is an inappropriately low rise in serum thrombopoietin, a hormone that stimulates platelet production (Abrams, 2016). Normally, in the presence of a low platelet count, the serum thrombopoietin rises to stimulate platelet production. In ITP, there is a low platelet count and an inappropriately low thrombopoietin level. While antiplatelet antibodies that bind to the platelets can be found in the blood of patients with ITP, testing for these antibodies is not currently recommended due to poor test sensitivity (Neunert, 2013). When the platelets are bound by the antibodies, the RES or tissue macrophage system ingests the platelets, destroying them. The production of autoantibodies may be triggered by medications or infections. Viral infections sometimes precede the disease in children. Occasionally medications, such as sulfa drugs, can induce ITP. Other conditions, such as systemic lupus erythematosus or pregnancy, can also induce ITP.

Clinical Manifestations and Assessment

Many patients have no symptoms, and the low platelet count (often below $20,000/mm^3$; below $5,000/mm^3$ is not uncommon) is an incidental finding. Common physical manifestations are easy bruising, heavy menses, and petechiae on the extremities or trunk. Patients with simple bruising or petechiae, termed "dry purpura," tend to have fewer complications from bleeding than do those with bleeding from mucosal surfaces, such as the GI tract (including the mouth) and pulmonary system (e.g., hemoptysis), termed "wet purpura." Patients with wet purpura have a greater risk of intracranial bleeding than do those with dry purpura.

Severe bleeding is rare in patients with platelet counts exceeding $30,000/mm^3$ (Neunert, 2013). Despite low platelet quantity, the platelets are young and very functional. They adhere to endothelial surfaces and to one another so that spontaneous bleeding does not always occur. Thus, treatment may not be initiated unless bleeding becomes severe

or life-threatening, the platelet count is extremely low (less than $10,000/mm^3$), or in those with risk factors for bleeding, such as uncontrolled hypertension or peptic ulcer disease (Diz-Küçükkaya & López, 2016; Abrams, 2016).

Medical Management

The primary goal of treatment is a "safe" platelet count. Because the risk for bleeding typically does not increase until the platelet count is less than $10,000/mm^3$, a patient whose count exceeds $30,000/mm^3$ to $50,000/mm^3$ may be carefully observed without additional intervention. However, if the count is less than $30,000/mm^3$ or if bleeding occurs, treatment with steroids (prednisone) should be initiated (Abrams, 2016). The goal is to improve the patient's platelet count rather than to cure the disease. The decision to treat should not be made merely on the basis of the patient's platelet count but also on his or her lifestyle and activity level. A person with a sedentary lifestyle can tolerate a low platelet count more safely than one with a more active lifestyle.

ITP patients with severe thrombocytopenia (less than $5,000/\mu L$) and/or those who have internal bleeding should be treated promptly with high doses of pulse corticosteroids and intravenous immunoglobulin IVIG (Abrams, 2016).

Treatment for ITP first focuses on removing any possible inciting agents. If the patient is taking a medication known to cause ITP (e.g., quinine, sulfa-containing medications), then the medication must be stopped immediately.

Traditional first-line therapies often include corticosteroids or corticosteroids in combination with IVIG (Neunert, 2013). A substantial number of adults with newly diagnosed ITP (40% to 60%) achieve and maintain a response to first-line therapy that can last up to 6 months; however, very few maintain this response at 1 year (Cuker, Luning Prak, & Cines, 2015).

Because of the associated side effects, patients cannot take high doses of corticosteroids indefinitely. It is not unusual for the platelet count to drop once the corticosteroid dose is tapered. Some patients can be maintained successfully on low doses of prednisone.

IVIG is also commonly used to treat ITP. The timing of IVIG in the treatment of ITP is controversial as other treatments offer comparable efficacy at a lower cost with less toxicity (Kessler, 2015). IVIG works by binding receptors on the macrophages; the effects are more rapid than daily oral prednisone, and response rates are approximately 80% with effects that are transient, lasting 2 to 4 weeks (Abrams, 2016).

Second-line therapies for patients whose platelet count drops after cessation of steroids include splenectomy, rituximab, and thrombopoietin receptor antagonists (TPO-RAs) (Neunert, 2013; Abrams, 2016).

The spleen is the primary site of platelet destruction and antiplatelet antibody production; removal of the spleen removes the mechanism for platelet destruction (Neunert,

2013). Splenectomy is the only curative therapy for ITP, with studies demonstrating a durable response in 66% to 72% of patients (Mikhael et al., 2009; Neunert, 2013; Abrams, 2016). Approximately half of the remaining patients who do not have normal platelet counts following splenectomy do achieve a partial response that is clinically meaningful (i.e., no bleeding events) (Abrams, 2016). However, even those who do respond initially to splenectomy may have recurrences of severe thrombocytopenia months or years later. Unfortunately, 10% to 15% of patients derive no benefit from splenectomy, and there is no test to predict whether a particular patient will respond to this treatment (Abrams, 2016).

Despite promising rates of success with splenectomy, the availability of newer medications (such as TPO-RAs) has resulted in reluctance from patients and providers to recommend invasive surgery for splenectomy (Neunert, 2013).

Patients who have undergone splenectomy are permanently at risk for sepsis, most commonly caused by pneumococcus or encapsulated bacteria. Though the incidence of sepsis in asplenia is relatively rare, when sepsis does develop in asplenic patients, there is a mortality rate of up to 50% (Rubin & Schaffner, 2014). Prevention of fatal infection depends on comprehensive patient education, vaccination, and early antibiotic initiation in the onset of fever (Rubin & Schaffner, 2014). Prior to splenectomy, these patients should receive pneumococci (Pneumovax), *Haemophilus influenzae* B, influenza virus, and meningococcal vaccines. PCV13 followed by PPSV23 8 weeks later is recommended for the prevention of pneumococcal infection; the series should be completed at least 2 weeks before splenectomy. A second dose of PPSV23 should be repeated in 5 years. Boosters of the meningococcal vaccine must be given every 5 years, and influenza vaccines should be given every year (Rubin & Schaffner, 2014). If an asplenic patient has a fever, antibiotics should be administered immediately. For this reason, asplenic patients are often given prescriptions for antibiotics such as amoxicillin or levofloxacin so that they always have antibiotics on hand.

Rituximab, a monoclonal antibody that targets the CD 20 marker on B cells, has been used successfully to treat ITP following treatment with steroids. Rituxan depletes the B cells that produce platelet-destroying autoantibodies, effectively increasing the platelet count. Although rituximab has not been approved by the U.S. Food and Drug Administration (FDA) for the treatment of ITP, it is widely used in clinical practice. It is well tolerated and has few side effects. Studies have demonstrated a response rate between 28% and 44%; however, when used in combination with dexamethasone, higher response rates have been seen (Abrams, 2016).

The treatment of ITP has changed dramatically with the discovery of drugs that target the point of platelet production. Romiplostim (Nplate®) and Eltrombopag (Promacta®) are thrombopoietin receptor agonists that stimulate platelet production by stimulating proliferation and differentiation of platelet precursors (Cuker, Luning Prak, & Cines, 2015). Romiplostim is administered weekly via subcutaneous injection, and Eltrombopag is a pill given once daily. Both medications have demonstrated efficacy in increasing the platelet count by 70% (Abrams, 2016). These drugs are not currently considered curative, and most patients require continuation of therapy to maintain response (Cuker et al., 2015; Neunert, 2013).

Despite the extremely low platelet count, platelet transfusions are usually avoided. Transfusions tend to be ineffective because the patient's antiplatelet antibodies bind with the transfused platelets, causing them to be destroyed. Platelet counts can actually drop after platelet transfusion. Occasionally, transfusion of platelets may protect against catastrophic bleeding in patients with severe wet purpura.

Nursing Management

Nursing care includes an assessment of the patient's lifestyle to determine the risk of bleeding from activity. Also a careful medication history is obtained, including use of over-the-counter medications, herbs, and nutritional supplements. The nurse must be alert for sulfa-containing medications and others that alter platelet function (e.g., aspirin-based or other nonsteroidal anti-inflammatory drugs [NSAIDs]) (see Box 20-4). The nurse assesses for any history of recent viral illness and for risk factors for hepatitis and HIV. Reports of headache or visual disturbances should be reported to the licensed provider immediately as these symptoms can signal intracranial bleeding. Patients who are admitted to the hospital with wet purpura and low platelet counts should have a neurologic assessment incorporated into their routine vital sign measurements. All intramuscular injections and rectal medications should be avoided, and rectal temperature measurements should not be performed because they can stimulate bleeding.

Patient teaching addresses signs of exacerbation of disease (petechiae, ecchymoses, wet purpura), how to contact appropriate health care personnel, the name and type of medication inducing ITP (if appropriate), current medical treatment (medications, tapering schedule if relevant, side effects), and the frequency of monitoring the platelet count. The patient is instructed to avoid all agents that interfere with platelet function (see Box 20-4). The patient should avoid constipation, as well as the Valsalva maneuver (straining to have a bowel movement). Electric razors should be used for shaving, and soft-bristled toothbrushes should replace stiff-bristled ones. The patient is also counseled to refrain from sexual intercourse when the platelet count is less than 50,000/mm³. Patients who are receiving corticosteroids long term are at risk for complications, including osteoporosis, proximal muscle wasting, cataract formation, and dental caries. Bone mineral density should be monitored, and these patients may benefit from calcium and vitamin D

Medications and Substances that Impair Platelet Function

- Anesthetic agents:
  - Local anesthetics
  - Halothane
- Antibiotics:
  - Beta-lactam antibiotics
  - Penicillins
  - Cephalosporins
  - Nitrofurantoin
  - Sulfonamides
- Anticoagulation agents:
  - Heparin
  - Fibrinolytic agents
- Anti-inflammatory agents (Nonsteroidal):
  - Aspirin
  - Ibuprofen
  - Naproxen
- Antineoplastic agents:
  - Carmustine
  - Daunorubicin
  - Mithramycin
- Cardiovascular drugs:
  - Beta blockers
  - Calcium-channel blockers
  - Isosorbide
  - Nitroglycerine
  - Nitroprusside
  - Quinidine
- Medications that increase platelet cAMP:
  - Dipyridamole
  - Prostacyclin
  - Theophylline

- Food and food additives:
  - Caffeine
  - Chinese black tree fungus
  - Clove
  - Cumin
  - Ethanol
  - Fish oils
  - Garlic
  - Onion extract
  - Turmeric
- Plasma expanders:
  - Dextrans
  - Hydroxyethyl starch
- Psychotropic agents:
  - Tricyclic antidepressants
  - Phenothiazines
- Miscellaneous:
  - Antihistamines
  - Clofibrate
  - Furosemide
  - Heroin
  - Contrast agents
  - Ticlopidine
  - Vitamin E
- Herbal supplements:
  - Feverfew
  - Ginger
  - Gingko
  - Ginseng
  - Kava kava

supplementation and bisphosphonate therapy to prevent significant bone disease.

PLATELET DEFECTS

Quantitative platelet defects are relatively common (thrombocytopenia), but qualitative defects can occur also. With qualitative defects, the number of platelets may be normal, but the platelets do not function normally. See Chapter 19 for an outline of testing for platelet defects.

An important functional platelet disorder is that induced by aspirin. Even small amounts of aspirin reduce normal platelet aggregation, and the prolonged bleeding time lasts for several days after aspirin ingestion. Although this does not cause bleeding in most people, patients with a coagulation disorder (e.g., hemophilia) or thrombocytopenia can have significant bleeding after taking aspirin, particularly if invasive procedures or trauma has occurred.

NSAIDs can also inhibit platelet function, but the effect is not as prolonged as with aspirin (about 5 days vs. 7 to 10 days). Other causes of platelet dysfunction include,

possibly metabolic products affecting platelet function, MDS, multiple myeloma (MM) (due to abnormal proteins interfering with platelet function), cardiopulmonary bypass, and other medications (see Box 20-4).

Clinical Manifestations and Assessment

Bleeding may be mild or severe. The extent is not necessarily correlated with the platelet count or with tests that measure coagulation (prothrombin time [PT], partial thromboplastin time [PTT]). Ecchymoses are common, particularly on the extremities. Patients with platelet dysfunction may be at risk for significant bleeding after trauma or invasive procedures (e.g., biopsy, dental extraction).

Medical Management

If the platelet dysfunction is caused by medication, use of the offending medication should be stopped, if possible, particularly when bleeding occurs or prior to an invasive procedure. If platelet dysfunction is marked, bleeding often can be prevented by transfusion of normal platelets before or during invasive procedures. Aminocaproic acid (EACA, Amicar), an anti-fibrinolytic agent, may be required to prevent significant bleeding after such procedures.

Nursing Management

Patients with significant platelet dysfunction need to be instructed to avoid substances that can diminish platelet function, such as certain over-the-counter medications, herbs, nutritional supplements, and alcohol. They also need to serve as their own advocates and inform their health care providers (including dentists) of the underlying condition before any invasive procedure is performed so that appropriate steps can be initiated to diminish the risk of bleeding. Bleeding precautions should be initiated as appropriate (see Chapter 19, Box 19-2).

BLEEDING DISORDERS

Von Willebrand Disease

Von Willebrand disease (vWD) is the most common inherited bleeding disorder in humans (Taylor, 2015). The disease affects males and females equally. The prevalence of this disease is estimated to be 1% to 2%; thus, it is the most common inherited bleeding disorder (Ferri, 2016b). The disease is a result of deficiency, dysfunction, or absence of von Willebrand Factor (vWF) (Ferri, 2016b). vWF is necessary for factor VIII activity and is essential for platelet adhesion at the site of vascular injury. Although synthesis of factor VIII is normal in vWD, its half-life is shortened; therefore, factor VIII levels are mildly low (15% to 50% of normal).

There are three types of vWD. Type 1, the most common (accounting for 60% to 80% of cases), is a quantitative defect in vWF and is inherited in an autosomal dominant pattern (Taylor, 2015). Type 2 shows variable qualitative defects based on the specific vWF subtype involved (with subtypes 2A, 2B, 2M, and 2N). Type 3 is very rare and is characterized by a severe vWF deficiency as well as by a significant deficiency of factor VIII.

Clinical Manifestations and Assessment

The history should include questions related to bleeding following a procedure, such as a dental procedure; need for blood transfusions following surgery or childbirth; history of heavy menses; and easy bruising (Ferri, 2016b). Patients commonly have mucocutaneous bleeding, including nosebleeds and large bruises (Taylor, 2015). Women may report heavy menses. Bleeding with minor surgery may also be seen. Joint bleeding is uncommon (Taylor, 2015).

Laboratory test results show a normal platelet count but a prolonged bleeding time and a normal or slightly prolonged PTT. These defects are not static, and laboratory test results can vary widely within the same patient over time. As the laboratory values can vary over time so can the history and extent of bleeding. For example, a careful history of prior bleeding may show little problem with postoperative bleeding on one occasion but significant bleeding from a dental extraction at another time. Laboratory tests required to diagnose vWD include the vWF ristocetin cofactor activity, vWF antigen, factor VIII activity, and, for patients with suspected type 2 defects, vWF multimers (Taylor, 2015).

Medical Management

The goal of treatment is to replace the deficient protein (e.g., vWF or factor VIII) at the time of spontaneous bleeding or prior to an invasive procedure to minimize postprocedural bleeding. There are two general strategies to meet this goal. For types 1 and 1A, the first line of treatment is administration of a synthetic form of the hormone vasopressin, called desmopressin (DDAVP). Desmopressin causes the release of vWF stored within the endothelium, resulting in a temporary increase in circulating vWF and factor VIII (Taylor, 2015). Desmopressin can be administered intranasally or intravenously. With major surgery or invasive procedures, IV administration is preferable. DDAVP is contraindicated in patients with unstable coronary artery disease because it can induce platelet aggregation and cause an MI. Side effects include headache, facial flushing, tachycardia, hyponatremia from free water retention, and, rarely, seizures. It is contraindicated in type 2B vWD because of risk of thrombocytopenia and has no efficacy for type 3 vWD (Nichols, 2016).

The second strategy is the administration of replacement products, such as Alphanate SD/HT (Grifols), Humate-P (CSL Behring), and Wilate (Octapharma), which are commercial concentrates of vWF and factor VIII (Nichols, 2016). Administration of these agents shortens bleeding time through normalization of multimer patterns (Taylor, 2015). Replacement continues for several days to ensure correction of the factor VIII deficiency. Treatment should continue for 4 days following minor surgery, and up to 14 days of treatment may be necessary after major surgery. The dosage and frequency of administration depend on factor VIII levels; doses may need regular adjustment based on trough levels. Antibody (inhibitor) formation is usually seen only in patients with type 3 vWD when large amounts of replacement products have been administered.

Other agents may be effective in reducing the bleeding. Aminocaproic acid (EACA, Amicar) is useful in managing mild forms of mucosal bleeding, for example, prior to dental work (Taylor, 2015). Hormonal contraceptives, such as the levonorgestrel-releasing intrauterine device, have demonstrated efficacy in reducing menorrhagia in women with bleeding disorders (Nichols, 2016). Platelet transfusions may be useful when significant bleeding is present.

Nursing Alert
Avoidance of aspirin and other NSAIDs is important nursing education to share with patients who have vWD.

ACQUIRED COAGULATION DISORDERS

The most common causes of acquired coagulation disorders include liver disease, vitamin K deficiency, and disseminated intravascular coagulation (DIC), all of which can result in abnormal bleeding.

LIVER DISEASE

With the exception of factor VIII, most blood coagulation factors are synthesized in the liver. Therefore, liver dysfunction (due to cirrhosis, tumor, or hepatitis; see Chapter 25) can result in diminished amounts of the factors needed to maintain coagulation and hemostasis. Prolongation of the PT, unless it is caused by vitamin K deficiency, may indicate severe liver dysfunction. Although minor bleeding is common (e.g., ecchymoses), these patients are also at risk for significant bleeding, related especially to trauma or surgery. Transfusion of fresh-frozen plasma may be required to replace clotting factors and to prevent or stop bleeding. Patients may also have life-threatening hemorrhage from peptic ulcers or esophageal varices. In these cases, replacement with fresh-frozen plasma, PRBCs, and platelets is usually required.

VITAMIN K DEFICIENCY

The synthesis of many coagulation factors depends on vitamin K. Vitamin K deficiency is common in malnourished patients, and some antibiotics decrease the intestinal flora that produce vitamin K, depleting vitamin K stores. Administration of vitamin K (phytonadione [Mephyton]), either orally or as a subcutaneous injection, can correct the deficiency quickly; adequate synthesis of coagulation factors is reflected by normalization of the PT.

COMPLICATIONS OF ANTICOAGULANT THERAPY

Anticoagulants are used in the treatment or prevention of thrombosis. These agents, particularly warfarin or heparin, can cause bleeding. If the PT or PTT is longer than desired, and bleeding has not occurred, the medication can be stopped or the dose decreased. Vitamin K is administered as an antidote for warfarin toxicity. Protamine sulfate is rarely needed for heparin toxicity because the half-life of heparin is very short. With significant bleeding, fresh-frozen plasma is needed to replace the vitamin K–dependent coagulation factors.

DISSEMINATED INTRAVASCULAR COAGULATION (DIC)

DIC is not a disease but a sign of an underlying condition. DIC may be triggered by sepsis, trauma, cancer, shock, abruptio placentae, toxins, or allergic reactions. The severity of DIC is variable, but it is potentially life-threatening. The mortality rate can exceed 80% of patients who develop severe DIC with ischemic thrombosis and frank hemorrhage. Identification of patients who are at risk for DIC and recognition of the early clinical manifestations of this syndrome can result in earlier medical intervention, which may improve the prognosis. However, the primary prognostic factor is the ability to treat the underlying condition that precipitated DIC.

Pathophysiology

Normal hemostatic mechanisms are altered in DIC so that a massive amount of tiny clots forms in the microcirculation. Initially, the coagulation time is normal. However, as the platelets and clotting factors are consumed to form the microthrombi, coagulation fails. Thus, the paradoxical result of excessive clotting is bleeding. The clinical manifestations of DIC are reflected in the organs, which are affected either by excessive clot formation (with resultant ischemia to all or part of the organ) or by bleeding. The excessive clotting triggers the fibrinolytic system to release fibrin degradation products, which are potent anticoagulants, furthering the bleeding. The bleeding is characterized by consumption of platelets and clotting factors, thus precipitating low platelet and fibrinogen levels (due to the consumption of fibrinogen); prolonged PT, PTT, and **thrombin** time; and elevated fibrin degradation products (**D-dimers**) (see Table 20-3 for an overview of laboratory values commonly found in DIC).

Clinical Manifestations and Assessment

Patients with frank DIC may bleed from mucous membranes, venipuncture sites, and the GI and urinary tracts. The bleeding can range from minimal occult internal bleeding to profuse hemorrhage from all orifices. The patient may also develop organ dysfunction, such as kidney failure and pulmonary and multifocal CNS infarctions, as a result of microthromboses, macrothromboses, or hemorrhages.

During the initial process of DIC, the patient may have no new symptoms, the only manifestation being a progressive decrease in the platelet count. As the thrombosis becomes more extensive, the patient exhibits signs and symptoms of thrombosis in the organs involved. Then, as the clotting factors and platelets are consumed to form these thrombi, bleeding occurs. Initially, the bleeding is subtle, but it can develop into frank hemorrhage. Signs and symptoms, which depend on the organs involved, are listed in Table 20-4.

Medical Management

The most important management factors in DIC are early recognition and treatment of the underlying cause; until the cause is controlled, the DIC will persist (Toh & Alhamdi, 2013). Correcting the secondary effects of tissue ischemia by improving oxygenation, replacing fluids, correcting electrolyte

TABLE **20-3** Laboratory Values Commonly Found in Disseminated Intravascular Coagulation (DIC)[a]

Test	Function Evaluated	Normal Range	Changes in DIC
Platelet count	Platelet number	150,000–450,000/mm^3	↓
Prothrombin time (PT)	Extrinsic pathway	11–12.5 seconds	↑
Partial thromboplastin time (PTT)	Intrinsic pathway	23–35 seconds	↑
Thrombin time (TT)	Clot formation	8–11 seconds	↑
Fibrinogen	Amount available for coagulation	170–340 mg/dL	↓
D-dimer	Local fibrinolysis	0–250 ng/mL	↑
Fibrin degradation products (FDPs) or fibrin split products (FSPs)	Fibrinolysis	0–5 μg/mL	↑
Euglobulin clot lysis	Fibrinolytic activity	2 or more hours	1 hour or less

[a]Because DIC is a dynamic condition, the laboratory values measured will change over time. Therefore, a progressive increase or decrease in a given laboratory value is likely to be more important than the actual value of a test at a single point in time.

imbalances, and administering vasopressor medications is also important.

Blood product support includes platelets, fresh-frozen plasma, and cryoprecipitate (to replace fibrinogen). The decision to transfuse should be based on laboratory trends and the patient's condition. FFP should be given in the presence of bleeding and prolonged PT/PTT; platelets are transfused if the platelet count is less than 50,000/mm^3; cryoprecipitate is considered in patients with a fibrinogen below 1.5 g/L (less than 150 mg/dL) (Toh & Alhamdi, 2013).

TABLE **20-4** Assessing for Thrombosis and Bleeding in Disseminated Intravascular Coagulation (DIC)[a]

System	Signs and Symptoms of Microvascular Thrombosis	Signs and Symptoms of Microvascular and Frank Bleeding
Integumentary system (skin)	↓ Temperature and sensation; ↑ pain; cyanosis in extremities, nose, earlobes; focal ischemia, superficial gangrene	Petechiae, including oral mucosa; bleeding: gums, oozing from wounds, previous injection sites, around catheters (IV or foley); tracheostomies; epistaxis; diffuse ecchymoses; subcutaneous hemorrhage; joint pain
Circulatory system	↓ Pulses; capillary filling time greater than 3 sec	Tachycardia
Respiratory system	Hypoxia (secondary to clot in lung); dyspnea; chest pain with deep inspiration; ↓ breath sounds over areas of large embolism	High-pitched bronchial breath sounds; tachypnea; ↑ consolidation; signs and symptoms of acute respiratory distress syndrome
Gastrointestinal system	Gastric pain; "heartburn"	Hematemesis (heme⊕ NG output) melena (heme⊕ stools → tarry stools → bright-red blood from rectum) retroperitoneal bleeding (abdomen firm and tender to palpation; distended; ↑ abdominal girth; back pain)
Kidney system	↓ Urine output; ↑ creatinine, ↑ blood urea nitrogen	Hematuria
Neurologic system	↓ Alertness and orientation; ↓ pupillary reaction; ↓ response to commands; ↓ strength and movement ability	Anxiety; restlessness; ↓ mentation, altered level of consciousness; headache; visual disturbances; conjunctival hemorrhage

heme⊕, positive for hemoglobin.
[a]Signs of microvascular thrombosis are the result of an inappropriate activation of the coagulation system, causing thrombotic occlusion of small vessels within all body organs. As the clotting factors and platelets are consumed, signs of microvascular bleeding appear. This bleeding can quickly extend into frank hemorrhage. Treatment must be aimed at the disorder underlying the DIC; otherwise, the stimulus for the syndrome will persist.

A controversial treatment strategy is to interrupt thrombosis through the use of heparin infusion. Heparin may inhibit the activation of the coagulation pathway in sepsis, inhibiting microthrombi formation and thereby correcting perfusion of the organs. However, a beneficial effect of heparin on outcomes in patients with DIC has never been demonstrated in controlled trials and may increase the incidence and risk for bleeding in patients with DIC. Heparin is indicated only in patients with clinically evident thromboembolism in a large blood vessel or with evidence of tissue damage secondary to thromboemboli; extreme caution must be used due to the high risk for bleeding (Schafer, 2016). There is a recent trend toward using LMWH due to decreased bleeding risks and predictable half-life (Toh & Alhamdi, 2013).

Another therapy in the treatment of DIC includes recombinant activated protein C (APC; drotrecogin alfa [Xigris®]), which is effective in diminishing inflammatory responses on the surface of the vessels and has anticoagulant properties. APC has been used in the setting of DIC secondary to sepsis; however, the overall survival benefit with these agents in patients with DIC has not been demonstrated (Schafer, 2016). APC is contraindicated in patients with bleeding and increases the risk for bleeding in patients with low platelet counts (less than 30,000/mm^3) or an international normalized ratio (INR) of more than 3.0. Bleeding is common, can occur at any site, and can be significant. Antithrombin (AT) infusions can also be used for their anticoagulant and anti-inflammatory properties. Bleeding can be significant, particularly when administered in association with heparin. Use of AT has yet to demonstrate a survival advantage and needs further study (Toh & Alhamdi, 2013).

Nursing Management

Nurses need to be aware of which patients are at risk of DIC. Sepsis and acute promyelocytic leukemia (APML) are the most common causes of DIC. Patients need to be assessed thoroughly and frequently for signs and symptoms of thrombi and bleeding and monitored for any progression of these signs. Timely recognition of symptoms and prompt reporting to the medical team can help facilitate early intervention and improve outcomes (see Table 20-4).

In addition, the nurse monitors and manages potential complications. Assessment and interventions should target potential sites of end-organ damage (see Table 20-4). As organs are inadequately perfused because of occlusion by microthrombi, organ function diminishes; the kidneys, lungs, brain, and skin are particularly vulnerable, and kidney dysfunction is common. Lack of renal perfusion may result in acute tubular necrosis and kidney failure, sometimes requiring dialysis. Placement of a large-bore dialysis catheter is extremely hazardous for this patient population and should be accompanied by adequate platelet and plasma transfusions. Liver dysfunction is also relatively common, reflected in altered liver function tests, depleted albumin stores, and diminished synthesis of clotting factors. Respiratory function warrants careful monitoring and aggressive measures to diminish alveolar compromise, such as incentive spirometry. Suctioning (if required) should be performed as gently as possible to diminish the risk for additional bleeding. CNS involvement can be manifested as headache, visual changes, and alteration in level of consciousness. A plan of nursing care for the patient with DIC is available online at http://thepoint.lww.com/Honan2e.

THROMBOTIC DISORDERS

Several conditions can alter the balance within the normal hemostatic process and cause excessive thrombosis. Abnormalities that predispose a person to thrombotic events include decreased clotting inhibitors within the circulation (which enhances coagulation), altered liver function (which may decrease production of clotting factors or clearance of activated coagulation factors), lack of fibrinolytic enzymes, and tortuous vessels (which promote platelet aggregation). Thrombosis can be caused by more than one predisposing factor. Several conditions can result from thrombosis, such as myocardial infarction (MI) (see Chapter 14), Cerebral Vascular Accident (CVA) (brain attack or stroke; see Chapter 47), and peripheral arterial occlusion (see Chapter 18). Several inherited or acquired deficiency conditions, including hyperhomocysteinemia, AT III deficiency, protein C deficiency, APC resistance, factor V Leiden, and protein S deficiency, can predispose a patient to repeated episodes of thrombosis; these are referred to as hypercoagulable states or thrombophilia. Table 20-5 lists these disorders, their abnormal laboratory values, and the need for family testing.

Thrombosis requires anticoagulation therapy. The duration of therapy varies with the location and extent of the thrombosis, precipitating events (e.g., trauma, immobilization), and concurrent risk factors (e.g., use of oral contraceptives, tortuous blood vessels, history of thrombotic events). With some conditions, lifelong anticoagulant therapy is necessary. Refer to Chapter 18 for details on anticoagulation.

MALIGNANT HEMATOLOGIC CONDITIONS

Myeloproliferative Neoplasms

Myeloproliferative neoplasms (MPNs) are a group of myeloid malignancies with varying clinical presentation, disease course, treatment, and prognosis. In 2014, the World Health Organization (WHO) convened to revise the classification of MPNs to include: PV, essential thrombocythemia (ET), primary myelofibrosis, chronic myelogenous leukemia (CML), chronic neutrophilic leukemia (CNL), systemic mastocytosis, chronic eosinophilic leukemia, and MPN-unclassifiable (Tefferi & Pardanani, 2015). Here we will focus on the most common MPNs: PV, ET, and CML.

TABLE 20-5 Hypercoagulable States

Disorder	Abnormal Laboratory Value[a]
Inherited Disorders (Family Testing Necessary)	
Hyperhomocysteinemia	Homocysteine ↑ after methionine load
Antithrombin III (AT III) deficiency	AT III ↓
Protein C deficiency	Protein C activity ↓ (must be measured off warfarin [Coumadin])
Activated protein C (APC) resistance	Must be measured off anticoagulant; less than 2× prolongation of PTT when APC added. Patients with APC resistance have a smaller increase in clotting time than normal (i.e., the prolongation of clotting time is less than normal).
Factor V Leiden	Positive
Protein S deficiency	Protein S activity ↓; must be measured off warfarin (Coumadin)
Dysfibrinogenemia	↑ thrombin time; ↑ reptilase time; ↓ functional fibrinogen; often requires special fibrinogen assays
Acquired Disorders (Family Testing Unnecessary)	
Anticardiolipin antibody	Positive
Cancer	Varied, depending on disorder
Lupus anticoagulant	Positive
Hyperhomocysteinemia	Homocysteine ↑ after methionine load
AT III deficiency	AT III ↓
Paroxysmal nocturnal hemoglobinuria	+ Hamm test; acid hemolysis
Myeloproliferative disorders	Varied, depending on disorder
Nephrotic syndrome	Varied, depending on disorder
Cancer chemotherapy	Varied, depending on specific agent

[a]Protein C and protein S are vitamin K–dependent proteins. Warfarin (Coumadin) interferes with the hepatic synthesis of vitamin K–dependent factors, which may decrease levels of protein C or protein S; therefore, protein C and protein S should be measured while the patient is off warfarin.

POLYCYTHEMIA VERA

Polycythemia vera (PV), or primary polycythemia, is a clonal myeloproliferative disorder in which the myeloid stem cells have escaped normal control mechanisms. In most cases, PV is the result of a mutation in the JAK-STAT pathway, which stimulates cell growth (Ferri, 2016c). The bone marrow is hypercellular, and the erythrocyte, leukocyte, and platelet counts in the peripheral blood are elevated. The erythrocyte elevation is predominant; the hematocrit can exceed 60%. This phase can last for an extended period (10 years or longer). Over time, the spleen resumes its embryonic function of hematopoiesis and enlarges. Splenomegaly (enlarged spleen) is a hallmark of PV, present in 75% of patients (Ferri, 2016c). Eventually, the bone marrow may become fibrotic, with a resultant inability to produce as many cells ("burnt out" or spent phase). The disease evolves into myeloid metaplasia with myelofibrosis, MDS, or acute myeloid leukemia (AML) in approximately 10% of patients at 20 years from diagnosis; this form of AML is usually refractory to standard treatments (Tefferi, 2015). The incidence of polycythemia has been estimated at 1 per 100,000 people. The median age at onset is 60 years, occurring most commonly in patients 50 to 75 years of age; men are affected more than women (Ferri, 2016c). Median survival duration is 14 years (Tefferi, 2015).

Pathophysiology

PV is a clonal myeloid disorder driven by mutations in JAK2. According to criteria from WHO proposed in 2015, a diagnosis of PV requires the presence of an elevated Hgb (greater than 16.5 g/dL in men and greater than 16.0 g/dL in women) or evidence of increased RBC mass (over 49% in men; over 48% in women) and the presence of a JAK2 genetic mutation; additional criteria include a hypercellular bone marrow and low serum erythropoietin levels (Tefferi & Barbui, 2015; Passamonti, 2012). More than 95% of patients with PV have mutations in JAK2V617F, and patients with suspected PV should be screened for these mutations. A test that is positive for the mutation supports the diagnosis of PV.

Clinical Manifestations and Assessment

Patients may present with a ruddy complexion (referred to as plethora) and complaints related splenomegaly, including left upper quadrant pain and early satiety. Symptoms result from increased blood volume (headache, dizziness, tinnitus, fatigue, paresthesias, and blurred vision) or from increased blood viscosity (angina, claudication, dyspnea, and thrombophlebitis), particularly if the patient has atherosclerotic blood vessels. For this reason, blood pressure is often elevated. Uric acid may be elevated, resulting in gout and kidney stone formation. Another common and bothersome problem is generalized pruritus, which may be caused by histamine release due to the increased number of basophils. A hallmark feature of PV is severe and painful itching that is triggered by exposure to water (referred to as aquagenic pruritus) (Ferri, 2016c). Erythromelalgia a syndrome of painful burning, warmth, and redness in a localized distal area of the extremities; it most commonly occurs in the fingers and toes and is only partially relieved by cooling.

Patients who present with elevated hemoglobin and hematocrit should be assessed for the presence of PV. Causes of secondary erythrocytosis should not be present (see earlier discussion). Patients typically have a normal oxygen saturation level and splenomegaly on physical examination.

Complications

Patients with PV are at increased risk for thromboses, including: cerebrovascular accident (CVA or stroke), MI, and deep vein thrombosis (DVT); thrombotic complications are the most common cause of death. Risk factors for thrombosis in PV include age over 60 years, a history of vascular events, and smoking (Passamonti, 2012; Ferri, 2016c). Nearly 20% of patients experience arterial or venous thrombosis as their initial symptom (Ferri, 2016c). Bleeding is also a complication in the setting of extremely high platelet counts (exceeding 1.5 million) and associated acquired vWD (Passamonti, 2012; Tefferi, 2015). The bleeding can be significant and can occur in the form of nosebleeds, ulcers, frank GI bleeding, hematuria, and intracranial hemorrhage.

Medical Management

The goals of therapy include preventing thrombosis, palliating disease-associated symptoms, and delaying progression of disease to myelofibrosis or AML (Ferri, 2016c). Treatment strategies to achieve these goals include phlebotomy to reduce the hematocrit, antiplatelet therapy to reduce thrombosis risk, cytoreduction to control the blood counts, and modification of cardiovascular risk factors (Passamonti, 2012).

Phlebotomy is a critical part of therapy to lower the hematocrit and is the only treatment that has demonstrated improved survival; phlebotomy extends the average survival time to 12 years and is recommended in all PV patients (Ferri, 2016c; Tefferi, 2016a). It involves removing enough blood (initially 500 mL once or twice weekly) to diminish the blood viscosity and then intermittently to maintain the hematocrit below 45% in men and 42% in women. Many patients are managed by routine phlebotomy on an intermittent basis.

Additional therapy may be indicated based on the individual risk for thrombosis (high risk vs. low risk). Risk factors include a history of venous or arterial thrombosis, the presence of a JAK2 mutation, and age over 60 years (Tefferi, 2016a; Tefferi, 2016b). Risk factors for high-risk disease include a history of thrombosis or age over 60 years with a JAK2 mutation. Patients with high-risk disease with a history of venous thrombosis are treated with hydroxyurea and systemic anticoagulation; patients with high-risk disease and a history of arterial thrombosis are treated with hydroxyurea and once-daily aspirin (Tefferi, 2016b). High-risk patients with additional cardiovascular risk factors and a history of arterial thrombosis should be advised to take aspirin twice a day; if they are high risk with additional CV risk factors and a history of venous thrombosis, once-daily aspirin may be added to systemic anticoagulation (Tefferi, 2016b). Patients with very low risk (no history of thrombosis, age under 60 years, and no JAK2 mutation) and low-risk disease (no risk of thrombosis, age under 60 years, JAK2 mutation present) may be managed with aspirin alone (Tefferi, 2016b).

Randomized studies have demonstrated the value of low-dose aspirin (40 to 100 mg/day) and should be administered in the absence of contraindications (i.e., history of GI bleeding, hemorrhagic stroke). Aspirin is also effective in alleviating vasomotor symptoms, including painful erythromelalgia (a symptom that affects the extremities causing redness, warmth, and burning pain), headaches, pruritus, lightheadedness, tinnitus, paresthesias, and chest pain (Tefferi, 2015). Aspirin must be used with caution in patients with platelet counts exceeding 1 million/mm^3 given the risks for acquired vWD and associated bleeding risk.

Patients receiving hydroxyurea (Hydrea) appear to have a lower incidence of thrombotic complications than do those treated by phlebotomy alone; this may result from a more effectively controlled platelet count. Patients on hydrea must be counseled on avoiding pregnancy. Other side effects include mouth sores, skin (leg) ulcers, and nail changes (Passamonti, 2012). There is no conclusive data showing that hydrea increases the risk for leukemic transformation (Tefferi, 2014).

For patients unable to tolerate or who are resistant to hydroxyurea, interferon alpha-2b (Intron-A) is also an effective treatment for cytoreduction (Tefferi, 2016b). Interferon alpha is also effective in alleviating the pruritus associated with PV (Passamonti, 2012; Tefferi, 2015) but may be difficult for patients to tolerate because of its frequent side effects (e.g., flu-like syndrome, depression).

Ruxolitinib, an oral JAK1-2 inhibitor that targets the JAK mutation, was recently approved for use in hydroxyurea-resistant or hydroxyurea-intolerant patients (Tefferi, 2016b). Studies have demonstrated that ruxolitinib lowers hematocrit to target goals, reduces spleen size, controls white blood cell (WBC) and platelet counts, and improves patient reported symptoms; however ruxolitinib has yet to demonstrate improvements in survival (Passamonti, 2012; Ferri, 2016c; Tefferi, 2016b).

Aquagenic pruritus is seen in 31% to 69% of patients with PV and can have a negative impact on quality of life (Lelonek & Szepietowski, 2016). It is a challenging symptom to manage. Improvement in pruritus often correlates with improvement in blood counts. Interferon alpha is often most effective in alleviating pruritus when used as treatment for PV. Antihistamines have demonstrated inconsistent efficacy and should not be recommended routinely. Selective serotonin receptor inhibitors have demonstrated efficacy (80%) in a small study of patients with PV (Tefferi et al., 2002; Lelonek & Szepietowski, 2016). Allopurinol (Zyloprim) is used to prevent gout in patients with elevated uric acid concentrations.

Patients with PV who smoke must be counseled on smoking cessation. Other modifiable cardiovascular risk factors, including obesity, hypertension, and diabetes, should also be addressed (Passamonti, 2012).

Nursing Management

The nurse's role is primarily that of educator. Risk factors for thrombotic complications, particularly smoking, obesity, and poorly controlled hypertension, should be assessed, and the patient should be instructed about risk reduction as well as the signs and symptoms of thrombosis. To reduce the likelihood of DVT, activity should be promoted, and crossing the legs and use of restrictive clothing should be avoided. The nurse instructs patients to walk around frequently on long flights. Patients with a history of bleeding are usually advised to avoid aspirin and aspirin-containing medications because these medications alter platelet function. The nurse encourages minimizing alcohol intake to further diminish the risk of bleeding. The patient needs to be instructed to avoid iron supplements, including those within multivitamin supplements, because the iron can further stimulate RBC production. For pruritus, the nurse may recommend bathing in tepid or cool water (hot water can exacerbate the symptom), limiting bathing time to 30 minutes or extending to every other day, and avoiding vigorous toweling-off after bathing. Use of mild soaps, application of emollient lotions, adding colloidal oatmeal treatment to bath water, use of cotton blankets and clothing, and washing sheets, clothing, and undergarments with baby detergent may also decrease pruritus.

ESSENTIAL THROMBOCYTHEMIA

ET (primary thrombocythemia) is a chronic, clonal, MPN. It most commonly occurs in women over 50 years of age and is marked by an overproduction of platelets. Women are 1.5 times more likely to have ET than men. Twenty percent of ET patients are under 40 years of age. Median survival is 20 years (Tefferi & Barbui, 2015).

Pathophysiology

Similar to PV, most cases of ET are driven by acquired mutations in *JAK2* (60% of ET cases); the remainder of patients will have mutations in either *CALR* or *MPL* genes (Tefferi & Barbui, 2015). The criteria proposed in 2015 by WHO for diagnosis of ET include: a platelet count of $450/mm^3$ or higher; a bone marrow biopsy with increased numbers of large, mature megakaryocytes and no significant increase in neutrophil granulopoiesis or erythropoiesis; not meeting WHO criteria for CML, PV, primary myelofibrosis, MDS or

other myeloid neoplasm; and/or presence of a clonal marker (such as *JAK2, MPL,* or *CALR* mutation) (Tefferi & Barbui, 2015).

Clinical Manifestations and Assessment

The diagnosis of ET is made by ruling out secondary causes of thrombocytosis (see earlier discussion). Iron deficiency should be excluded because a reactive increase in the platelet count often accompanies this deficiency. Occult malignancy should be excluded. The CBC shows markedly large and abnormal platelets. CBC, bone marrow aspiration and biopsy, and mutational testing for *JAK2, MPL,* and *CALR* are the cornerstones of diagnostic evaluation for ET (Tefferi & Barbui, 2015).

Many patients with ET are asymptomatic; the illness is diagnosed as the result of finding an elevated platelet count on a CBC. Symptoms, when they do occur, result primarily from hemorrhage or vaso-occlusion in the microvasculature. Symptoms occur most often when the platelet count exceeds 1 million/mm^3. However, symptoms do not always correlate with the extent to which the platelet count is elevated. Thrombosis is common and can be either arterial or venous; the life-threatening complications include large-vessel thrombosis (both arterial and venous), and hemorrhage (Tefferi, 2016b). Common sites of large vessel arterial occlusion include the arteries of the legs, the coronary arteries, and the renal arteries. Vasomotor symptoms are not infrequent complaints and can include visual disturbances, lightheadedness, headaches, palpitations, atypical chest pain, and distal paresthesias (Tefferi, 2016b). Headache is the most common neurologic complication, followed by transient ischemic attacks, dizziness, syncope, and seizures. More common forms of venous thrombosis include DVT and pulmonary embolism; less commonly, stroke and MI occur. Small vessel vaso-occlusive manifestations cause symptoms of erythromelalgia (described earlier).

Because these platelets can be dysfunctional, minor or major hemorrhage can also occur. The GI tract is the most common site of bleeding, followed by the skin, eyes, urinary tract, tooth socket and gums, joints, or brain. Bleeding typically does not occur unless the platelet count exceeds 1 million/mm^3. The spleen may be enlarged but usually not to a clinically significant extent.

No data reliably predict the development of complications. Risk factors for the development of thrombotic complications are age older than 60 years, gender (men are at greater risk than women), smoking, prior thrombotic or bleeding events, and pre-existing cardiac risk factors (obesity, hypertension, hypercholesterolemia, and smoking) (Lai, 2015).

Medical Management

The approach to therapy in ET is similar to PV; the goals are to reduce thrombotic risk and alleviate symptoms (Tefferi

& Pardanani, 2015). The risk for significant thrombotic or hemorrhagic complications may not be increased until the platelet count exceeds 1.5 million/mm^3. A careful assessment of other risk factors, such as history of peripheral vascular disease, history of tobacco use, atherosclerosis, and prior thrombotic events, should be used in making the decision regarding when to initiate therapy.

As in PV, a risk-adapted strategy for ET is recommended with high risk defined as a history of thrombosis or age greater than 60 years with a JAK2 mutation (Tefferi, 2016a). High-risk patients are treated with hydroxyurea and either systemic anticoagulation (history of venous thrombosis) or aspirin (history of arterial thrombosis) (Tefferi, 2016a). Low-risk patients may be treated with aspirin alone.

Aspirin (81 mg/day) is recommended for patients with *JAK2*-mutated ET and also can be used to relieve the neurologic symptoms (e.g., headache), erythromelalgia, and visual symptoms of ET (Tefferi & Pardanani, 2015). As in PV, in the setting of very high platelet counts, acquired vWD can occur; use of aspirin should be avoided unless the Ristocetin Cofactor Activity test is greater than 30% (Lai, 2015; Tefferi & Barbui, 2015).

For patients unable to tolerate or resistant to hydroxyurea, interferon alpha is an option for second-line therapy (Tefferi, 2016). Interferon alpha has been associated with hematologic response rates up to 80% for ET, but its use is limited by side effects, including cytopenias, flu-like symptoms, and fatigue, contributing to discontinuation in up to 20% of patients (Kaplan et al., 2016).

Rarely, the occlusive symptoms of ET are so great that the platelet count must be reduced immediately. When necessary, plateletpheresis (see later discussion) can reduce the amount of circulating platelets but only transiently. The extent to which symptoms and complications (e.g., thromboses) are reduced by pheresis remains unclear.

Nursing Management

Patients with ET need to be instructed about the accompanying risks of hemorrhage and thrombosis. The patient is informed about signs and symptoms of thrombosis, particularly the neurologic manifestations, such as visual changes, numbness, tingling, and weakness as well as chest pain, and extremity swelling, redness, or pain. Risk factors for thrombosis are assessed, and measures to diminish risk factors (particularly cessation of tobacco use and weight management) are encouraged.

Patients receiving aspirin therapy should be informed about the increased risk of bleeding. Patients who are at risk for bleeding should be instructed about medications (e.g., aspirin, NSAIDs) and other substances (e.g., alcohol) that can alter platelet function and, therefore, should be avoided. Patients receiving interferon therapy are taught to self-administer the medication and manage any side effects promptly (primarily fatigue, flu-like symptoms, and depression).

CHRONIC MYELOID LEUKEMIA (CML)

There were an estimated 5,900 new cases of CML in 2013 (ACS, 2013). The incidence of CML increases with age; the median age at diagnosis is 67 years. Thus, the prevalence of CML is predicted to increase because of demographics (aging population), and the acknowledgment that because of highly effective therapies for CML, there will be an increased number of those living with the disease. Prevalence is expected to reach 250,000 in the next 20 years. CML may be seen at any age, but is uncommon in children and adolescents (NCCN, 2016b). CML is slightly more common in men and accounts for 15% to 20% of adult leukemias (Rathore, 2017a).

Pathophysiology

CML is a clonal myeloid MPN marked by the presence of the Philadelphia chromosome; a balanced mutation of chromosomes 9 and 22 (t9;22) resulting in the production of the bcr/abl kinase protein, which is responsible for aberrant cell growth.

CML involves an overproduction of myeloid WBCs. The platelet count may also be elevated. Because there is an uncontrolled proliferation of cells, the marrow expands into the cavities of long bones (e.g., the femur), resulting in bone pain, and myeloid cells may also be produced in the liver and spleen (extramedullary hematopoiesis), resulting in enlargement of these organs that is sometimes painful.

There are three phases of the disease: the chronic phase, where most of the leukocytes produced are mature and retain some ability to function normally; the accelerated phase, in which the numbers of abnormal cells are being produced at a faster rate; and blast crisis, in which the predominant cell type is immature. Most patients are diagnosed in the chronic phase. Untreated CML will progress to advanced phases in 3 to 5 years (NCCN, 2016b). Once the disease transforms to the acute phase (blast crisis), the overall survival rarely exceeds several months.

Clinical Manifestations and Assessment

The clinical picture of CML varies based on the phase of the disease. During the chronic phase, 40% to 50% of patients are asymptomatic, and so the diagnosis may be detected based on abnormal blood work. The most common symptoms include fatigue, night sweats, abdominal pain, early satiety, and weight loss (O'Brien & Jabbour, 2016).

Patients with extremely high leukocyte counts (over 100,000/mm^3) may exhibit signs of leukostasis (the excessive volume of leukocytes slows and inhibits blood flow through the capillaries via increased viscosity) including confusion, vision changes, shortness of breath, or chest pain due to decreased capillary perfusion to the brain, eyes, and lungs. The patient may have an enlarged, tender spleen. The liver may also be enlarged.

Medical Management

Advances in understanding of the pathology of CML at a molecular level have led to dramatic changes in its treatment. The development of drugs that target and inhibit the bcr/abl tyrosine kinase protein (called tyrosine kinase inhibitors or TKIs) have significantly extended survival for patients with CML and have shifted the paradigm of CML management to that of a chronic disease. The 5-year survival rate for patients diagnosed in the chronic phase and treated with TKIs is as high as 90% (Cortes et al., 2016).

Therapy depends on the stage of disease. In the chronic phase, the expected outcome is correction of the chromosomal abnormality (i.e., conversion of the malignant stem cell population back to normal), and the standard therapy is a TKI. TKIs approved for the front-line setting include imatinib, nilotinib, and dasatinib. TKIs approved in the second-line setting include dasatinib, nilotinib, and bosutinib (Bauer, Buchanan, & Ryan, 2016). Initial response to therapy is through monitoring of the CBC with expected normalization of blood counts within the first 4 to 6 weeks of therapy, called a complete hematologic response. Subsequent response to TKI therapy using blood measurement of bcr/abl quantity (molecular testing) is done every 3 months with the goal of reaching major molecular response. Achievement and maintenance of early major molecular response is predictive of longer survival (Cortes, Goldman, & Hughes, 2012). There are established goals for molecular response at set time points, including 3 months, 6 months, 12 months, etc. (NCCN, 2016b). If patients do not meet established milestones, assessment of adherence must be performed as well as resistance testing. There is a blood test to assess for the development of mutational resistance to TKIs. The test will alert the provider if the patient has developed resistance to a particular TKI and will direct the provider to TKIs to which the disease remains sensitive. Adherence to prescribed therapy is essential to response; when adherence falls below 90%, response to therapy declines.

During the initial phase of treatment, if there is significant leukocytosis, the WBC needs to be reduced quickly to minimize complications from leukostasis. This goal can be achieved by using drugs like hydroxyurea in conjunction with initiation of TKI therapy. In the case of an extreme leukocytosis at diagnosis (e.g., leukocyte count greater than 300,000/mm^3), a more emergent treatment may be required. In this instance, *leukapheresis* (in which the patient's blood is removed and separated, with the leukocytes withdrawn, and the remaining blood returned to the patient) can reduce the number of leukocytes temporarily.

The treatment of CML in the accelerated and blast phases is more challenging, as many patients in advanced stages of disease have developed resistance to TKIs. There is no consensus on optimal treatment of patients with advanced CML (Mukherjee & Kalycio, 2016). Options for treatment include second-line TKIs based upon mutation analysis or allogeneic hematopoietic stem cell transplantation (AHSCT) (discussed in Chapter 6) (O'Brien & Jabbour, 2016). Prognosis at time to progression is 7 to 11 months (Mukherjee & Kalycio, 2016).

The accelerated or transformation phase can be insidious or rapid. In the accelerated phase, the patient may complain of bone pain and may report fevers (without any obvious sign of infection), night sweats, and weight loss. Even with treatment, the spleen may continue to enlarge. The patient may become more anemic and thrombocytopenic.

In the acute form of CML (blast crisis), the disease progresses to either Acute lymphocytic leukemia (ALL) or Acute Myeloid Leukemia (AML) blast phase, and treatment is targeted to the specific type. Patients whose disease evolves into a "lymphoid" blast crisis are more likely to reenter a chronic phase after ALL induction therapy. For those whose disease evolves into AML, therapy is largely ineffective in achieving a second chronic phase. Life-threatening infections and bleeding occur frequently in this phase.

Allogeneic stem cell transplantation remains the only curative treatment for CML. However, the efficacy of imatinib in first-line treatment and the treatment-related mortality of stem cell transplant limit the use of transplant to patients with high-risk or relapsed disease or in those patients who are resistant to TKI therapy (Jabbour, 2016). Human leukocyte antigen (HLA)-matched, related donor stem cell transplants result in long-term survival in 45% to 70% of recipients. Patients over 50 years of age have a slightly lower survival rate (30% to 40%) compared with those younger than 30 to 40 years of age (60% to 80%) (O'Brien & Jabbour, 2016).

Nursing Management

The nurse must educate the patient on proper administration of TKI therapy. Some TKIs require timing around meals (nilotinib), and patients may need assistance with optimal scheduling. Antacids, PPIs, and grapefruit juice may interfere with drug absorption, and patients must be counseled to avoid these while on TKI therapy. There are a number of other drug interactions with TKIs, and nurses should collaborate with the pharmacist to review the patient's drug list for potential interactions. Most patients will require lifetime therapy with TKIs. Each TKI has a specific side-effect profile that may interfere with adherence and tolerance. For example, GI side effects and fluid retention are common with some of the TKIs. Patients must be counseled on the individual side-effect profile of the drug and be instructed to notify their health care team promptly with any new symptoms. The nurse's role in side-effect anticipation and management is critical. The nurse also plays an active role in the assessment and promotion of adherence to TKI therapy.

BONE MARROW FAILURE SYNDROMES

Bone marrow failure syndrome is the term for a classification that includes aplastic anemia (AA), paroxysmal nocturnal hemoglobinuria (PNH), and MDS.

APLASTIC ANEMIA (AA)

AA is a rare disease caused by a decrease in or damage to bone marrow stem cells, damage to the microenvironment within the marrow, and replacement of the marrow with fat, resulting in cytopenias (reduction in number of blood cells). Immune effects on marrow function (e.g., viral infection, idiosyncratic drug reactions, direct stem cell toxicity [radiation, chemotherapy]) have been implicated as an underlying etiology (Bagby, 2016). Inherited bone marrow failure has been implicated in 10% to 15% of patients with AA (Bagby, 2016).

Pathophysiology

AA can be congenital or acquired, but most cases are idiopathic (i.e., without apparent cause). Infections and pregnancy can trigger it, or it may be caused by certain medications, chemicals, or radiation damage. Agents that regularly produce marrow aplasia include benzene and benzene derivatives (e.g., airplane glue). Certain toxic materials, such as inorganic arsenic and several pesticides (including dichlorodiphenyltrichloroethane [DDT], which is no longer used or available in the United States), have also been implicated as potential causes. Other possible origins include cytotoxic agents used in cancer chemotherapy: alkylating agents (busulfan, cyclophosphamide) antimetabolites (antifolic compounds), antimitotics (vincristine, vinblastine, colchicine), and some antibiotics (daunorubicin, doxorubicin [Adriamycin]) (Ferri, 2016d). Pregnancy has also been associated with AA, and while the causal relationship is unknown, it may reflect a high level of immunologic activation during pregnancy; the prognosis is poor and associated with bleeding complications (Bagby, 2016).

Clinical Manifestations and Assessment

The manifestations of AA are often insidious. Patients may present with symptoms of anemia or bleeding. Symptoms of anemia, including fatigue, shortness of breath, and decreased activity tolerance, are usually present at the time of diagnosis. Infection at presentation is uncommon even in the setting of severe neutropenia (Ferri, 2016d). CBC may reveal neutropenia, anemia, and/or thrombocytopenia. The MCV is usually elevated. A bone marrow aspirate and biopsy provides the most sensitive evidence for AA. There is an absence of dysplasia, which helps to distinguish between AA and MDS (which is marked by dysplasia) (Bagby, 2016).

Patients with AA should also be tested for PNH because there is an overlap in 40% to 50% of cases. PNH is diagnosed via flow cytometry of the peripheral blood (Bagby, 2016).

Medical Management

Severe AA, defined by the degree of cytopenias, must be treated quickly. Symptomatic anemia and thrombocytopenia can be supported with transfusions of irradiated blood and platelets, respectively. In patients with an absolute neutrophil count (ANC) below 500/μL, prophylactic antibiotics should be considered, and in the presence of fever, empiric antibiotics must be started promptly (Ferri, 2016d).

In patients under 40 years of age who have a matched sibling donor, stem cell transplant is the definitive treatment and is considered curative (Ferri, 2016d). In patients over 40 years of age or those with no matched sibling, immunosuppressive therapy (IST) is the primary treatment. A combination of antithymocyte globulin (ATG) and cyclosporine is employed. ATG, a purified gamma globulin solution, is obtained from horses or rabbits immunized with human T lymphocytes. Infusion reactions are common and may include fever and chills. The sudden onset of a rash or bronchospasm may herald anaphylaxis and requires prompt management (see Chapter 38). Serum sickness, a delayed immune response, evidenced by fever, rash, arthralgias, and pruritus, may develop in some patients; it may take weeks to resolve. Side effects of cyclosporine include hypertension, hirsutism, and gingival hyperplasia. Many patients on cyclosporine require initiation of antihypertensive therapy (Malat & Culkin, 2016). Steroids are used to decrease the risk of serum sickness associated with ATG (Killick et al., 2016). Complete response to IST (development of normal blood counts) can occur, and relapses are uncommon (10% relapse rate), whereas partial responders (blood counts do not normalize, but transfusions are not required) relapse in 40% to 60% of cases within 5 years (Bagby, 2016). If relapse occurs following treatment with IST (i.e., the patient becomes pancytopenic [reduction of RBCs, WBCs, and platelets] again), reinstitution of the same immunologic agents may induce another remission. Corticosteroids are useful as immunosuppressive agents; however, they have significant side effects, including bone complications (i.e., avascular necrosis) and life-threatening infections. For this reason, long-term use of steroids is not recommended.

In patients who do not respond to IST, matched unrelated stem cell transplant should be considered; however, the mortality rate is higher (Ferri, 2016d). Frail elderly patients or those with significant comorbidities may be poor candidates for IST, and alternative therapies, such as androgens or supportive care, should be considered.

Supportive therapy plays a major role in the management of AA. Blood-product support with irradiated products is recommended (Killick et al., 2016). Aspirin is avoided in patients with thrombocytopenia because of its antiplatelet effect, and oral or injectable contraceptives are used to suppress menstruation to prevent menorrhagia (Bagby, 2016). There are no randomized, controlled trials to provide guidance on optimal antimicrobial prophylaxis in patients with AA and no consensus on standards of care (Hochsmann et al., 2013). In patients with a low neutrophil count (below 500) and receiving IST, prolonged neutropenia increases the risk for mold infections; these types of infections are associated with high mortality rates. Therefore, antifungal prophylaxis with agents such as voriconazole or posaconazole is recommended for patients with severe AA and should continue as long as the patient is neutropenic. There remains some controversy related to antibacterial prophylaxis due to concerns for antimicrobial resistance. Patients at highest risk for bacterial sepsis are patients with severe AA, and antibiotic prophylaxis with quinolones can be considered (Hochsmann et al., 2013). Prophylaxis with an antipneumocystis agent (such as aerosolized pentamidine) is essential. Antiviral prophylaxis is routinely recommended for transplant recipients and, in many centers, also considered for those treated with IST (Bagby, 2016).

Death in this population is most commonly caused by hemorrhage or infection.

Nursing Management

Patients with AA are vulnerable to problems related to erythrocyte (RBC), leukocyte (WBC), and platelet deficiencies. They should be assessed carefully for signs of infection and bleeding. Specific nursing interventions are outlined in the sections on neutropenia and thrombocytopenia.

Patients receiving ATG must be educated to promptly report signs and symptoms of hypersensitivity reactions and should be reassured that nurses who administer ATG are properly trained to respond to these reactions. Nurses should educate patients taking cyclosporine regarding the importance of taking the medication as directed and monitoring drug levels and blood pressure as well as reporting signs and symptoms of high blood pressure. The nurse provides anticipatory guidance regarding hirsutism and gingival hyperplasia as these side effects may significantly impact body image and coping.

MYELODYSPLASTIC SYNDROMES (MDSs)

MDS represents a group of heterogeneous diseases with highly variable disease courses, prognosis, treatment strategies, and risk for leukemic transformation. Accurate diagnosis is essential for guiding discussion regarding treatment options and prognosis.

Median age at diagnosis is 71 years; peak incidence is in the seventh and eighth decades of life (Steensma & Stone, 2016). MDS is rare in children, and incidence increases with age. From 2009 through 2013, incidence of MDS was 21,338 with higher incidence in men (U.S. National Cancer Institute's Survey, Epidemiology, and End Results [SEER]).

Pathophysiology

MDS is a group of diseases characterized by ineffective hematopoiesis, dysplasia in at least one cell line (RBC, platelet, or WBC), progressive bone marrow failure, and variable risk for progression to leukemia (Rathore, 2017b).

Clinical Manifestations and Assessment

The majority of symptoms and clinical complications in this population result from cytopenias and the risk for leukemic progression (NCCN, 2016c). Thirty percent of patients with MDS will progress to AML. The risk for leukemia progression varies with the percentage of blasts in the bone marrow, the number and depth of cytopenias, and the presence of high-risk cytogenetic abnormalities and other genetic mutations such as tp53 (Rathore, 2017b; Ousseine et al., 2016). Patients may present with fatigue, dyspnea, activity intolerance, unexplained bruising or bleeding, or recurrent infections. However, many patients are asymptomatic at the time of diagnosis, and in these cases, the diagnosis is suspected based on routine bloodwork alone (Steensma & Stone, 2016).

Diagnosis includes a review of the CBC as well as bone marrow biopsy and aspirate. CBC is evaluated for cytopenias, peripheral blasts, and morphologic abnormalities. The reticulocyte count helps assess the bone marrow response to anemia. Other causes of anemia are ruled out. Serum EPO (erythropoietin) levels are checked to determine the potential role of ESAs in the management of MDS. Aspirate is sent for flow cytometry, cytogenetics, and assessment of genetic mutations. Aspirate is evaluated for evidence of dysplasia, blast count, number of monocytes, ringed sideroblasts, and megakaryocytes, which helps to classify the MDS subtype. The biopsy is evaluated for cellularity and the presence of blasts. Cytogenetics are critical to the prognostic classification of MDS. Favorable cytogenetic abnormalities include deletion of 11q, loss of chromosome Y, or deletion of 5q. Poor cytogenetic abnormalities include a complex karyotype (3 or more cytogenetic abnormalities) (Ridgeway, Fechter, Murray, & Borras, 2012).

Testing for mutations in specific genes has also become important in predicting prognosis in MDS. For example, mutation in TP53 is an independent predictor of poor prognosis in MDS (Rathore, 2017b).

The WHO provides diagnostic categorization of MDS based on morphology and blast percentage. The International Prognostic Scoring System (IPSS) helps to provide prognostic data using number of cytopenias, cytogenetics, and blast percentage, which helped to predict overall survival and risk for transformation to leukemia (Steensma & Stone, 2016). Prognosis can vary greatly; for example, a patient with low-risk MDS has a median overall survival of 5.7 years without therapy compared to a patient with high-risk disease, who has an overall survival of 0.4 months (Ridgeway et al., 2012; NCCN, 2016c).

Medical Management

Treatment strategies depend on the risk category (low risk vs. high risk), performance status, quality of life, and presence of comorbidities (Steensma & Stone, 2016). Strategies for treatment of low-risk MDS focus on minimizing the symptoms associated with cytopenias and minimizing transfusion requirements whereas in high-risk disease, immediate treatment is indicated to improve overall survival since the life expectancy is less than 2 years (Steensma & Stone, 2016). The initial approach to treatment may be to treat symptomatically and monitor the counts over time to assess how quickly the cytopenias progress (NCCN, 2016c).

For symptomatic anemia, transfusions of PRBCs are the mainstay of treatment (Ridgeway et al., 2012; NCCN, 2016c). Long-term transfusion dependence is associated with iron overload so attempts to decrease transfusion requirements with use of other therapies may be considered. Platelet transfusions may be considered in the setting of bleeding (NCCN, 2016c). Granulocyte-colony stimulating factor (GCSF) may be considered in neutropenic patients with recurrent infections. ESAs may be considered in transfusion-dependent patients with a serum EPO less than 500 mU/mL (NCCN, 2016c).

Lenalidomide is also indicated in patients with transfusion-dependent MDS who have low-risk disease and a deletion 5q cytogenetic abnormality with or without other cytogenetic abnormalities. In a phase III study, 57% of patients who took lenalidomide achieved RBC transfusion independence compared to 2% of patients who received a placebo (Giagounidis et al., 2014). Lenalidomide is a pill taken daily; common side effects in MDS include myelosuppression, rash, and diarrhea (Steensma & Stone, 2016). For further discussion of lenalidomide, refer to section on myeloma.

Patients with high-risk disease are at higher risk for transformation to leukemia; decision to treat must consider the patient's performance status and presence of comorbidities in order to predict treatment tolerance. The only cure for MDS is allogeneic stem cell transplant. Many patients may not be eligible due to advanced age, comorbidities, and lack of a suitable donor (Steensma & Stone, 2016).

Azacitidine is a hypomethylating agent approved in the United States for the treatment of MDS with studies demonstrating improved blood counts, prolonged overall survival, prolonged time to progression to AML, and improved quality of life (Steensma & Stone, 2016). Hypomethylating agents are considered low-intensity therapy that are generally well tolerated and can be given in the outpatient setting (NCCN, 2016c).

Response to treatment can take 4 to 6 months of therapy; providing patients anticipatory guidance and setting realistic expectations around this is critical (Kurtin, Demakos, Hayden, & Boglione, 2012; Nazha et al., 2016).

High-intensity therapy includes chemotherapy similar to that used in the treatment of AML, and stem cell transplant. High-intensity therapy is generally reserved for younger patients with no comorbidities. The morbidity and mortality of high-intensity therapies is high with lack of strong supporting evidence; these therapies are recommended in the context of clinical trials (NCCN, 2016c).

Myelosuppression is the most common complication of both MDS and its treatment and cytopenias often get worse with treatment before they improve (Kurtin et al., 2012).

Nursing Management

It is critical that the nurse provides patient education about the disease and management of symptoms, including reportable signs and symptoms of anemia, thrombocytopenia, and infection. The nurse helps the patient to track and trend blood counts and monitor transfusion requirements. The nurse helps the patient understand treatment options and have realistic expectations about timing of response. The majority of care for MDS is provided in the outpatient setting with the patient and family having primary responsibility for care at home. The nurse helps the patient and family with self-care needs and identifies needs for visiting nurse services.

ACUTE LEUKEMIA

Acute leukemia is the result of a series of genetic mutations that occur during hematopoiesis and ultimately reflect the type, quality, and quantity of cells produced (Rose-Inman & Kuehl, 2014). Hematopoiesis is characterized by a rapid, continuous turnover of cells. Normally, production of specific blood cells from their stem cell precursors is regulated carefully according to the body's needs. If the mechanisms that control the production of these cells are disrupted as a result of mutations, the cells proliferate excessively and mature abnormally.

Often hematopoietic malignancies are classified by the cells involved. **Leukemia**, literally "white blood," is a term used to describe neoplastic proliferation of one particular hematopoietic cell type (**granulocyte**s, **monocyte**s, lymphocytes, or, infrequently, erythrocytes or megakaryocytes). The defect originates in the hematopoietic stem cell, in either the myeloid or the **lymphoid** stem cell. Preferential proliferation of leukemia cells leads to decreased production of normal hematopoietic cells (Rose-Inman & Kuehl, 2014).

Thus the common feature of acute leukemias is an unregulated proliferation of leukocytes in the bone marrow and a suppression of other blood cells, including RBCs and platelets. The bone marrow becomes packed with abnormal cells and ultimately begins to release these cells into the circulation prematurely. The increase in the number of leukocytes in the circulation is referred to as *leukocytosis*. Typically, only one specific type of leukocyte is increased, most commonly either the neutrophils (myeloblast) or the lymphocytes (lymphoblast). Extramedullary hematopoiesis is also seen with resultant splenomegaly. With acute leukemias, there can be infiltration of other organs, such as the meninges, lymph nodes, gums, and skin (leukemia cutis).

The cause of leukemia is not fully known, but there is some evidence that genetic influences and viral pathogenesis may be involved. Bone marrow damage from radiation exposure or from chemicals benzene, topoisomerase II inhibitors (such as etoposide) and alkylating agents (e.g., cyclophosphamide [Cytoxan], melphalan [Alkeran]) can cause leukemia.

The leukemias are commonly classified according to the stem cell line involved, either lymphoid (relating to lymphatic tissue) or myeloid (relating to bone marrow myeloid elements). They are also classified as either acute or chronic based on the phase of cell development that is halted, with few leukocytes differentiating beyond that phase.

In acute leukemia, the onset of symptoms is abrupt, often occurring within a few weeks. Leukocyte development is halted at the blast phase so that most leukocytes are undifferentiated, immature cells (blasts). Acute leukemia progresses very rapidly; death can occur within weeks to months without aggressive treatment.

In chronic leukemia, symptoms evolve over a period of months to years. Most of the leukocytes produced are mature and retain some ability to function normally. Chronic leukemia progresses more slowly; the disease trajectory can extend for years.

In 2013, the American Cancer Society estimated close to 6,000 cases of ALL and 14,500 cases of AML (ACS, 2013).

ACUTE MYELOID LEUKEMIA

AML results from a defect in the hematopoietic stem cell that differentiates into all myeloid cells: monocytes, granulocytes (neutrophils, basophils, eosinophils), erythrocytes, and platelets. All age groups are affected; the incidence rises with age, with a peak incidence at age 60 years. Median age of diagnosis is 65 years (Rose-Inman & Kuehl, 2014). AML accounts for 80% of acute leukemias in adults and less than 10% of leukemias in children (Schiffer & Anastasi, 2016).

AML represents a heterogeneous group of clonal myeloid malignancies marked by an excess of myeloid blast cells (greater than 20%). Classification of AML has evolved from a morphologic classification to one based on cytogenetic and molecular abnormalities. The French American British system classifies AML based primarily on morphology and stage of maturation arrest, with eight subtypes. The more recent classification system is that of the WHO, which incorporates cytogenetic and molecular abnormalities, allowing for improved prognostication (Schiffer & Anastasi, 2016). There are cytogenetic abnormalities that may be considered favorable (translocation 15;17, translocation 8;21, and inversion 16), whereas survival is poor in instances of unfavorable cytogenetic abnormalities (deletions of chromosome 5 or 7 and patients with more than three abnormalities [referred to as a complex karyotype]) (Ferri, 2016e). The identification of molecular mutations has further complicated the classification of AML. Mutations in NPM1, FLT3, and CEBPA genes have resulted in the identification of four groups with very different prognoses, with mutations in NPM1 or CEBPA being favorable while mutations in FLT3-ITD are unfavorable (Estey, 2014).

The prognosis of AML is highly variable and related to patient age, performance status, and cytogenetic and molecular characteristics of their disease (Schiffer & Anastasi, 2016). The strongest risk factors for resistant disease, early relapse, and decreased survival include advanced age, poor functional status, and complex cytogenetic abnormalities. Patients over 65 years of age have a poorer response to treatment and a worse prognosis than younger patients. Complete remission rates range from 20% to 90% depending on patient- and disease-specific risk factors (Chen et al., 2015). Those who have leukemia stemming from pre-existing MDS or who previously received alkylating agents or topoisomerase II inhibitors for cancer (secondary AML) have a much worse prognosis; the leukemia tends to be more resistant to treatment, resulting in a much shorter duration of remission. With treatment, patients with secondary AML survive an average of less than 1 year, with death usually a result of infection or hemorrhage. Patients receiving supportive care also usually survive less than 1 year, dying of infection or bleeding.

Clinical Manifestations and Assessment

Most signs and symptoms of AML result from insufficient production of normal blood cells. Fever and infection result from neutropenia, weakness and fatigue from anemia, and bleeding tendencies from thrombocytopenia. The proliferation of leukemic cells within organs leads to a variety of additional symptoms: pain from an enlarged liver or spleen, hyperplasia of the gums, and bone pain from expansion of the bone marrow.

AML develops without warning, with symptoms occurring over a period of weeks to months. The CBC may show a decrease in both erythrocytes and platelets. Although the total leukocyte count can be low, normal, or high, usually the percentage of normal cells is vastly decreased. The differential may reveal the presence of circulating blasts and a decreased neutrophil count.

Diagnosis is established with bone marrow aspirate and biopsy with biopsy revealing more than 20% myeloblasts. Aspirate samples are sent for flow cytometry, analysis of cytogenetic abnormalities, and genetic mutations.

Complications

Complications of AML include bleeding and infection, the major causes of death. The risk of bleeding correlates with the severity of thrombocytopenia. The low platelet count can result in **ecchymoses** (bruises) and **petechiae** (pinpoint red or purple hemorrhagic spots on the skin) (Fig. 20-2). Major spontaneous hemorrhages also may develop when the platelet count drops to less than 10,000/mm^3. The most common sites of bleeding are GI, pulmonary, and intracranial. Fever increases platelet consumption and, therefore, may increase the likelihood of bleeding.

Because of the lack of mature and normal granulocytes, infection is the most common cause of death in patients with acute leukemia. The likelihood of infection increases with the degree and duration of neutropenia; neutrophil counts that persist at less than 100/mm^3 for prolonged periods make the likelihood of systemic infection extremely high. As the

FIGURE 20-2 Petechia and purpura. (From Bickley, L. S. (2013). *Bates' guide to physical examination* (11th ed.). Philadelphia, PA: Lippincott Williams & Wilkins.)

duration of severe neutropenia increases, the patient's risk of developing fungal infection also increases.

Medical Management

When considering approaches to therapy for AML, the first determination is if the patient would be a candidate for allogeneic stem cell transplant. In general, patients who are considered transplant candidates will be treated with an aggressive approach. Patients who are not transplant candidates due to poor performance status, advanced age, or significant comorbidity would be treated with a less aggressive approach focused on optimizing quality of life.

The initial objective of treatment is to achieve complete remission, in which there is no evidence of residual leukemia in the bone marrow. For patients with a good performance status and absence of comorbidities, attempts are made to achieve remission by the aggressive administration of chemotherapy, called *induction therapy*, which usually requires hospitalization for several weeks. Induction therapy typically involves IV administration of cytarabine (Cytosar, Ara-C) and an anthracycline, such as idarubicin (Idamycin) or daunorubicin. The choice of agents is based on the patient's performance status and history of prior antineoplastic treatment. For older patients or patients with poor performance status and comorbidities, less aggressive approaches may be used. Enrollment in clinical trials is always encouraged.

The aim of induction therapy is to eradicate the leukemic cells, but this is often accompanied by the eradication of normal types of myeloid cells. Thus, the patient becomes severely neutropenic (an **absolute neutrophil count** [ANC] of 0 is not uncommon), anemic, and thrombocytopenic (a platelet count of less than 10,000/mm^3 is common). (Refer to Chapter 19 for calculation of the ANC.) During this time, the patient is hospitalized due to high risk for life-threatening complications. Common complications include bacterial, fungal, and, occasionally, viral infections; bleeding; and severe mucositis, which can cause mouth pain and diarrhea as well as a marked decline in the ability to eat and meet nutritional demands.

Supportive care consists of administering blood products (PRBCs and platelets) and promptly treating infections. Prophylactic use of granulocytic growth factors (GCSF or Filgrastim) to minimize the risk of neutropenic fever and infection have not demonstrated the same effects on survival in patients with AML compared to patients with nonhematologic malignancies; therefore, widespread use of GCSF in patients with AML is not recommended (Larson, 2016).

Response to treatment is assessed using bone marrow aspirate and biopsy after induction when blood counts are recovering. The expected result is an absence of leukemic blasts and recovery of normal marrow function. When the patient has recovered from the induction therapy (i.e., the neutrophil and platelet counts have returned to normal and any infection has resolved) and response to induction has been assessed, he or she typically receives *consolidation therapy* (additional postremission chemotherapy) to eliminate any residual leukemia cells that are not clinically detectable and to reduce the chance for recurrence. Multiple treatment cycles of various agents are used, with most regimens using high-dose cytarabine (e.g., Cytosar, Ara-C).

Following consolidation therapy, the next step is determined based on the patient's risk for recurrence. Patients with low- or intermediate-risk leukemia may not require further treatment after they complete consolidation therapy. Patients with high-risk leukemia, or patients who have been treated for a relapse, may be candidates for PBSCT. When a suitable donor is identified (either a sibling or unrelated donor identified in the national registry), the patient embarks on an even more aggressive regimen of chemotherapy (sometimes in combination with total body radiation therapy), with the treatment goal of destroying the hematopoietic function of the patient's bone marrow. The patient is then "rescued" with the infusion of the donor stem cells to reinitiate hematopoiesis. In addition to providing a "rescue" and a healthy source of hematopoiesis, infusion of donor cells also provides protection against disease recurrence. The healthy immune system of the donor kills residual cancer cells and prevents cancer recurrence; this is known as the *graft versus leukemia* effect. Patients who undergo PBSCT have a significant risk for infection, graft-versus-host disease (GVHD, in which the donor's lymphocytes [graft] recognize the patient's body as "foreign" and attack the "foreign" host), and other complications. Refer to Chapter 6 for a detailed discussion of PBSCT.

For patients who are not candidates for transplant, less aggressive approaches to therapy with drugs like hypomethylating agents (decitabine or azacitidine) may be considered (Vasu & Blum, 2013). Both agents have demonstrated response in AML, though further study is required to identify patients most likely to respond. Patients over 65 years of age tend to have poorer prognosis related to treatment-resistant disease (Appelbaum, 2016).

Another important option for the patient to consider is supportive care alone. In fact, supportive care may be the only option if the patient has significant comorbidity, such as extremely poor cardiac, pulmonary, kidney, or liver function; advanced age; or poor performance status. In such cases, aggressive antileukemia therapy is not used; occasionally, hydroxyurea (Hydrea) may be used to control the WBC count and prevent the potential sequelae of leukocytosis. Patients are supported with antimicrobial therapy and transfusions as needed. This treatment approach provides the patient with some additional time at home; however, death frequently occurs within months, typically from infection or bleeding. (Refer to Chapter 3 for a discussion of end-of-life care.)

Treatment of relapsed AML may involve different combinations of chemotherapy if the patient is in good physical condition, or less aggressive therapies or supportive care alone may be used. Clinical trials may also be considered. Relapsed AML is often difficult to treat and overall survival rate is low.

Nursing Management

The priority nursing interventions for the patient with AML include infection prevention, bleeding prevention, promoting comfort, and patient education. Nursing care to prevent infection and bleeding are discussed in detail in Chapters 6 and 19. Patients with a new diagnosis of AML are experiencing a crisis and require an overwhelming amount of education about their disease, self-care, and treatment strategies. The role of the nurse is critical in alleviating anxiety by providing information tailored to the patient's readiness and educational level.

The nurse also assesses for complications of treatment. Massive leukemic cell destruction from chemotherapy results in the release of intracellular electrolytes and fluids into the systemic circulation. Increases in uric acid levels, potassium, and phosphate are seen; this process is referred to as **tumor lysis** syndrome (see Chapter 6). Patients require a high fluid intake and prophylaxis with allopurinol to prevent crystallization of uric acid and subsequent stone formation. Anorexia, nausea, vomiting, diarrhea, and severe mucositis are common.

ACUTE PROMYELOCYTIC LEUKEMIA (APML)

APML is a subtype of AML that is characterized by the cytogenetic abnormality of translocation 15;17, which results in the PML-RARα protein. APML, unlike most other types of AML, is highly curable. APML is often associated with life-threatening DIC, and once the diagnosis is presumed, treatment must start emergently. Diagnosis is established through the detection of the PML-RARα protein, which can be detected in the blood. A bone marrow aspirate and biopsy is also done to establish the diagnosis though detection of PML-RARα protein justifies initiation of treatment. Treatment includes all-trans-retinoic acid (ATRA), an oral agent that stimulates differentiation of the promyelocytes into mature neutrophils. Aggressive supportive care to manage DIC in the initial stages of the disease is critical. Platelets and cryoprecipitate are used to minimize bleeding risk. ATRA has also been shown to decrease the risk of

coagulopathy, which is the leading cause of death in APML (Mantha, Tallman, & Soff, 2016). One fourth of patients treated with ATRA will experience differentiation syndrome in the first 21 days of induction treatment with ATRA. The symptoms include weight gain, shortness of breath, fever, hypotension, effusions, and liver and kidney dysfunction. Risk for differentiation syndrome is increased when the WBC count is over 30. Often steroids are used to prevent and treat this syndrome. Diuretics also may be used to manage volume overload. ATRA may be used in combination with chemotherapy or arsenic trioxide, which is also a differentiating agent (Ferri, 2016f).

Response to treatment is assessed through measurement of PML-RARα protein levels in the blood and bone marrow.

The nursing role in APML is critical; astute assessment skills should be focused on identifying early signs and symptoms of DIC and differentiation syndrome. Daily weights and strict I/Os are important data points in assessing for differentiation syndrome. The nurse also counsels the patient on the importance of adherence to ATRA therapy. For patients on arsenic therapy, monitoring of EKG for prolongation of the QT interval is essential. Other drugs that prolong the QT interval should be minimized (refer to Chapter 17 for drugs associated with prolonged QT).

ACUTE LYMPHOCYTIC LEUKEMIA

Acute lymphocytic leukemia (ALL) results from an uncontrolled proliferation of immature lymphoid cells (lymphoblasts) derived from the lymphoid stem cell. The cell of origin is the precursor to the B lymphocyte in approximately 75% of ALL cases; T-lymphocyte ALL occurs in approximately 25% of ALL cases. The *BCR-ABL* translocation or Philadelphia chromosome (see earlier CML discussion) is found in 20% of ALL blast cells. ALL is most common in young children, with boys affected more often than girls. ALL accounts for 75% of pediatric leukemias and 25% of adult leukemias (NCCN, 2016d). The peak incidence is 4 years of age. After 15 years of age, ALL incidence decreases with a second peak occurring after age 50 (Rose-Inman & Kuehl, 2014). Increasing age appears to be associated with diminished survival; the 5-year event-free survival rate is almost 90% for childhood ALL, but decreases to approximately 60% in adolescents; in young adults (15 to 24 years) survival is nearly 55%, for those 25 years of age to 39, the rate is 42%, 24% for ages 40 to 59 years, and 17.7% for ages 60 to 69 years (Pulte et al., 2014).

Clinical Manifestations and Assessment

Immature lymphocytes proliferate in the marrow and impede the development of normal myeloid cells. As a result, normal hematopoiesis is inhibited, resulting in reduced numbers of leukocytes, erythrocytes, and platelets. Leukocyte counts may be either low or high, but there is always a high proportion of immature cells. Manifestations of leukemic cell infiltration into other organs are more common with ALL than with other forms of leukemia and include pain from an enlarged liver or spleen and bone pain. The testes and central nervous system (CNS) are sanctuary sites where leukemic cells may infiltrate. The patient may exhibit testicular swelling or discomfort, or headache, visual changes, vomiting, and neurologic deficits from CNS invasion. Children are more likely to report musculoskeletal symptoms, including bone and joint pain (Rose-Inman & Kuehl, 2014; NCCN, 2016d).

Diagnosis is established with bone marrow aspirate and biopsy, with bone marrow biopsy demonstrating lymphoblasts at 20% or higher. Aspirate samples are evaluated for flow cytometry as well as cytogenetic and molecular abnormalities. Due to the high incidence of CNS involvement, diagnostic lumbar puncture is also performed. Typically chemotherapy is given into the intrathecal space at the time of initial lumbar puncture to treat or provide prophylaxis for ALL in the CNS (NCCN, 2016d).

Men should have a testicular examination, and abnormalities on examination warrant evaluation with ultrasound as the testes are a sanctuary site for ALL.

Medical and Nursing Management

The expected outcome of treatment is complete remission. Lymphoid blast cells are typically very sensitive to corticosteroids and to vinca alkaloids; therefore, these medications are an integral part of the initial induction therapy. Because ALL frequently invades the CNS, prophylaxis with cranial irradiation or intrathecal (injection of medications into the subarachnoid space [cerebral spinal fluid]) chemotherapy (e.g., methotrexate), or both is also a key part of the treatment plan (Ferri, 2016g).

Treatment protocols for ALL tend to be complex, using a wide variety of chemotherapeutic agents given over a protracted period of time. Treatment includes an induction phase, followed by a consolidation phase, followed by a maintenance phase, when lower doses of medications are given for up to 3 years. Despite the complexity, treatment can often be provided in the outpatient setting.

Imatinib is highly effective in those with Philadelphia chromosome–positive ALL and can be used alone or in combination with chemotherapy, with remission rates exceeding 90%; however, the impact of the addition of imatinib on the duration of remission is not yet known (Appelbaum, 2016). Monoclonal antibodies, in which the antibody specific for the antigens expressed on the ALL blast cell—including CD20, CD22, CD33, and CD52—are a type of targeted therapy used to treat ALL. For example, the CD52 antigen is expressed on approximately 70% of ALL cells; thus, alemtuzumab (Campath), a monoclonal antibody with specific affinity for the CD52 antigen, is effective therapy for this subset of patients.

Infections, especially viral infections, are common. The use of corticosteroids to treat ALL increases the patient's susceptibility to infection. Patients with ALL often require prophylactic antimicrobials to decrease the risk of certain types of infection. Patients with ALL tend to have a better response to treatment than do patients with AML. PBSCT offers a chance for prolonged remission, or even cure, if the illness recurs after therapy.

Nursing Management for Acute Myeloid Leukemia and Acute Lymphocytic Leukemia

Nursing management of the patient with ALL is similar to the care of patients with AML. The nursing priorities include the prevention of infection and bleeding as well as management of symptoms, such as nausea and pain, often resulting from mucositis. As ALL is a disease that most commonly affects children and young adults, fertility preservation should be discussed prior to the initiation of treatment.

Although the clinical picture varies with the type of leukemia as well as the treatment implemented, the health history may reveal a range of subtle symptoms reported by the patient before the problem is detectable on physical examination. Weakness and fatigue are common manifestations, not only of the leukemia but also of the resulting complications of anemia and infection. If the patient is hospitalized, the assessments should be performed daily or more frequently as warranted. Because the physical findings may be subtle initially, a thorough, systematic assessment incorporating all body systems is essential. For example, a dry cough, mild dyspnea, and diminished breath sounds may indicate a pulmonary infection. However, the infection may not be seen initially on the chest x-ray; the absence of neutrophils delays the inflammatory response against the pulmonary infection, and it is the inflammatory response that produces the x-ray changes. The platelet count can become dangerously low, leaving the patient at risk for significant bleeding. The specific body system assessments are delineated in the neutropenic precautions and bleeding precautions found in Chapters 6 and 19, respectively. When serial assessments are performed, current findings are compared with previous findings to evaluate the patient's condition for improvement or worsening.

The nurse also must monitor the results of laboratory studies closely. Flow sheets are particularly useful in tracking the leukocyte count, ANC, hematocrit, platelet, creatinine and electrolyte levels, and liver function tests. During initial treatment for acute leukemia, the ANC often drops below 100/mm^3, placing the patient at very high risk for infection (Andersen et al., 2016; Applebaum, 2016). Empiric antibiotics are used to treat infection preemptively when the patient has a fever of 100.4°F or greater. Culture results need to be reported immediately so that antimicrobial therapy can be modified appropriately based on microbial sensitivity.

LYMPHOMA

The lymphomas are neoplasms (abnormal growth of tissue) of lymphoid tissue, usually derived from B lymphocytes. These tumors usually start in lymph nodes but can involve lymphoid tissue in the spleen, the GI tract (e.g., the wall of the stomach), the liver, or the bone marrow. Often they are classified according to the degree of cell differentiation and the origin of the predominant malignant cell. Lymphomas can be classified into two broad categories: Hodgkin lymphoma and non-Hodgkin lymphoma (NHL). NHLs can be furthered characterized into low grade and high grade.

HODGKIN LYMPHOMA

Hodgkin lymphoma is a relatively rare malignancy that has an impressive cure rate. In 2013, there were 9,290 cases of Hodgkin lymphoma, with more cases in men than women (ACS, 2013).

Pathophysiology

Unlike other lymphomas, Hodgkin lymphoma is unicentric in origin in that it initiates in a single node. The disease spreads by contiguous extension along the lymphatic system. The malignant cell of Hodgkin lymphoma is the Reed–Sternberg cell, a large tumor cell that is morphologically unique and is thought to be of immature lymphoid origin. It is the pathologic hallmark and essential diagnostic criterion for Hodgkin disease. However, the tumor is very heterogeneous and actually may contain few Reed–Sternberg cells. Repeated biopsies may be required to establish the diagnosis.

The cause of Hodgkin lymphoma is unknown, but a viral etiology is suspected. In fact, fragments of the Epstein–Barr virus (EBV) have been found in some Reed–Sternberg cells; however, evidence implicating EBV remains controversial (Ferri, 2016h).

The WHO classifies Hodgkin lymphoma into two groups: classic Hodgkin lymphoma (92% to 97% of cases), which has four main histologic subtypes based on the number of lymphocytes, Reed–Sternberg cells, and the presence of fibrous tissue; and nodular lymphocyte-predominant Hodgkin lymphoma (3% to 8% of cases) (Ferri, 2016h).

Risk Factors

Hodgkin lymphoma is somewhat more common in men than women and has two peaks of incidence: one in the early 20s and the other after 50 years of age. Disease occurrence has a familial pattern: first-degree relatives have a higher-than-normal frequency of disease, but the actual incidence of this pattern is low. Hodgkin lymphoma is seen more commonly in patients receiving chronic IST (e.g., for kidney transplant) and in woodworkers. Also it is seen in veterans of the military who were exposed to the herbicide Agent Orange.

Clinical Manifestations and Assessment

Hodgkin lymphoma usually begins as a painless enlargement of one or more lymph nodes above the diaphragm (most commonly in the cervical or supraclavicular region) (Bartlett & Foyil, 2014). The individual nodes are painless and rubbery or firm but not hard. A mediastinal mass may be seen on chest x-ray; occasionally, the mass is large enough to compress the trachea and cause dyspnea and cough. Pruritus is common; it can be extremely distressing, and the cause is unknown. Rarely patients experience brief but severe pain after drinking alcohol, usually at the site of the tumor (Ferri, 2016h). Again, the cause of this is unknown.

All organs are vulnerable to invasion by Hodgkin lymphoma. The symptoms result from compression of organs by the tumor, such as cough and pulmonary effusion (from pulmonary infiltrates), jaundice (from hepatic involvement or bile duct obstruction), abdominal pain (from splenomegaly or retroperitoneal adenopathy), or bone pain (from skeletal involvement). Herpes zoster infections are common. A cluster of constitutional symptoms has important prognostic implications. Referred to as "B symptoms," they include fever (without chills), drenching sweats (particularly at night), and unintentional weight loss of more than 10%. B symptoms are found in 40% of patients and are more common in advanced disease. An elevated **erythrocyte sedimentation rate** (ESR) represents a poor prognostic indicator (Bartlett & Foyil, 2014).

A mild anemia is the most common hematologic finding. The leukocyte count may be elevated or decreased. The platelet count is typically normal unless the tumor has invaded the bone marrow, suppressing hematopoiesis. Patients with Hodgkin lymphoma have impaired cellular immunity as evidenced by an absent or decreased reaction to skin sensitivity tests (e.g., *Candida*, mumps).

Because many manifestations are similar to those occurring with infection, diagnostic studies are performed to rule out an infectious origin for the disease. The diagnosis is made by means of an excisional lymph node biopsy and the finding of the Reed–Sternberg cell. Once the diagnosis is confirmed and the histologic type is established, it is necessary to assess the extent of the disease, a process referred to as *staging*. See Chapter 6 for discussion of staging.

In addition to a careful physical examination, a chest x-ray; computed tomography (CT) scan of the chest, abdomen, and pelvis; and a positron emission tomography (PET) scan are all obtained to assist with staging. The PET scan may be the most sensitive imaging test in identifying residual disease. Laboratory tests include CBC, platelet count, ESR, lactate dehydrogenase (LDH), and liver and kidney function studies. A bone marrow biopsy is performed if there are signs of marrow involvement, and some physicians routinely perform bilateral biopsies. Bone scans may be performed to identify any involvement in these areas.

Medical Management

The general goal in treatment of Hodgkin lymphoma, regardless of stage, is cure. Data reveal that 90% of patients with early-stage Hodgkin lymphoma and 80% of advanced-stage patients will be cured (Bartlett & Foyil, 2014). Treatment is determined primarily by the stage of the disease, not the histologic type; however, extensive research is ongoing to target treatment regimens to histologic subtypes or prognostic features. Traditionally, early Hodgkin disease was treated by a staging laparotomy followed by radiation therapy. This treatment method has been replaced by a short course (2 to 4 months) of chemotherapy followed by radiation therapy in early-stage disease (I and II). Advanced-stage disease is often treated with chemotherapy alone; the role of radiation in advanced disease remains under investigation (Hutchings, Piris, Baiocchi, & Hertzberg, 2015). When chemotherapy is used alone or with combination radiation therapy for early-stage classical Hodgkin lymphoma, 3- to 5-year progression-free survival rates of 82% to 94.6% have been reported. For advanced-stage classical Hodgkin lymphoma, front-line treatment with combination chemotherapy, such as ABVD [doxorubicin (also known as Adriamycin), bleomycin, vinblastine, and dacarbazine], BEACOPP [bleomycin, etoposide, doxorubicin, cyclophosphamide, vincristine (also known as Oncovin), procarbazine, and prednisone] or the Stanford V regimen (doxorubicin, vinblastine, mechlorethamine, vincristine, bleomycin, etoposide, and prednisone), produces reports of 5-year progression-free survival rates as high as 86.4% (Alinari & Blum, 2016).

Even when Hodgkin lymphoma does recur, the use of high doses of chemotherapeutic agents, followed by autologous PBSCT, can be effective in controlling the disease and extending survival time with progression-free survival rates of up to 60% reported (Alinari & Blum, 2016).

Newer therapies for Hodgkin lymphoma have emerged, including monoclonal antibodies, antibody-drug conjugates (Brentuximab vedotin), and checkpoint inhibitors (nivolumab and pembrolizumab). These new agents offer promising potential alternatives to classical chemotherapy but are currently limited to the relapsed/refractory setting (Rashidi & Bartlett, 2015).

Nursing management is similar to that of NHL and is discussed in that section.

Long-Term Complications of Therapy

Much is now known about the long-term effects of chemotherapy and radiation therapy, primarily from the large numbers of people who were cured of Hodgkin lymphoma by these treatments. Long-term complications include hypothyroidism, immune dysfunction, dental caries, cardiomyopathy, infertility, and secondary malignancies. The incidence of late effects increases over time (NCCN, 2016e). Patients should be followed carefully for late effects, including surveillance for and assessment of risk factors for secondary cancers. Lung cancer and breast cancer are the most common type of secondary malignancy in patients with Hodgkin disease, particularly following combination chemotherapy and radiation (NCCN, 2016e).

Secondary cancers, including lung, breast, lymphoma, and leukemia, as well as cardiovascular disease, including heart failure, valvular disease, coronary artery disease, and MI, are late effects of treatment for Hodgkin lymphoma (van Nimwegen et al., 2015; Hodgson & von Leeuwen, 2015). Secondary cancers are the leading cause of death in survivors of Hodgkin lymphoma. Among female survivors of childhood Hodgkin lymphoma, breast cancer is the most common secondary cancer. There are many contributing risk factors for secondary breast cancer, with age at time of chest radiation being the most important risk factor (Koo, Henderson, Dwyer, & Skandarajah, 2015). For survivors of Hodgkin lymphoma who were treated with radiation to the chest, screening for breast cancer using mammography is recommended beginning 8 years from the time of radiation to the chest or beginning at age 40, whichever comes first (Hodgson & von Leeuwen, 2015). Breast MRI in addition to mammogram is recommended for women treated with radiation to the chest between 10 and 30 years of age (NCCN, 2016e). It is critical that survivors of Hodgkin lymphoma are counseled on their risk for secondary cancers and cardiovascular risk and that the recommended screening tests are adhered to throughout the patient's lifetime (Ferri, 2016h).

Patients should be encouraged to reduce other factors that increase the risk of developing secondary cancers and cardiovascular disease, such as use of tobacco and alcohol and exposure to environmental carcinogens, as well as maintaining an exercise regimen and healthy weight. Revised treatment approaches are under investigation with the goal of minimizing the risk for complications (secondary malignancy and cardiovascular disease) without sacrificing the potential for cure.

NON-HODGKIN LYMPHOMAS

The NHLs are a heterogeneous group of cancers that originate from the neoplastic growth of lymphoid tissue. As in CLL, the neoplastic cells are thought to arise from a single clone of lymphocytes; however, in NHL, the cells may vary morphologically. Most NHLs involve malignant B lymphocytes; only 5% involve T lymphocytes. In contrast to Hodgkin lymphoma, the lymphoid tissues involved in NHL are largely infiltrated with malignant cells. The spread of these malignant lymphoid cells occurs unpredictably, and true localized disease is uncommon. Lymph nodes from multiple sites may be infiltrated as may sites outside the lymphoid system (extranodal tissue).

While the incidence of NHL continues to rise in the United States, it now accounts for approximately 4% of new cancers in the United States and 3% of cancer deaths (Bierman & Armitage, 2016). In 2013, there were 69,740 cases of NHL in the United States with more cases in men (ACS, 2013). The incidence increases with each decade of life, is higher in whites than other ethnic groups, and is diagnosed in patients with an average age of 50 to 60 years. Although no common etiologic factor has been identified, the incidence of NHL has increased in people with immunodeficiencies or autoimmune disorders; treatment with immunosuppressive medications; prior treatment for cancer; prior organ transplant; viral infections (including EBV and HIV); and exposure to pesticides, solvents, dyes, or defoliating agents, including Agent Orange. In addition, some cases may be explained by improved pathology techniques (Bierman & Armitage, 2016). Prognosis varies greatly among the various types of NHL. NHL can be further characterized as low grade or high grade. The most common types of low-grade lymphomas include CLL and follicular lymphoma. High-grade lymphomas include diffuse large B-cell lymphoma, peripheral T-cell lymphomas, and Burkitt lymphoma.

Long-term survival (over 10 years) is commonly achieved in low-grade, localized lymphomas. Even with aggressive disease forms, cure is possible in at least one third of patients who receive aggressive treatment.

Clinical Manifestations and Assessment

Symptoms are highly variable, reflecting the diverse nature of the NHLs. Lymphadenopathy is most common (66%); however, in more indolent (less aggressive) types of lymphomas, the lymphadenopathy can wax and wane. With early-stage disease or with the types that are considered more indolent, there may be no symptoms, and the illness typically is not diagnosed until it progresses to a later stage, when the patient becomes symptomatic. At these stages (III or IV), lymphadenopathy is prominent. One third of patients with NHLs have "B symptoms" (recurrent fever, drenching night sweats, and unintentional weight loss of 10% or more). Lymphomatous masses can compromise organ function. For example, a mass in the mediastinum can cause respiratory distress; abdominal masses can compromise the ureters, leading to kidney dysfunction; and splenomegaly can cause abdominal discomfort, nausea, early satiety, anorexia, and weight loss. Less than 10% of patients will experience CNS involvement at some point in their disease. Certain populations have higher rates of CNS involvement, including patients with HIV or those with testicular, breast, epidural, or sinus involvement.

The actual diagnosis of NHL is categorized into a highly complex classification system based on histopathology, immunophenotyping, and cytogenetic analyses of the malignant cells. The specific histopathologic type of the disease has important prognostic implications. Treatment also varies and is based on these features. Staging, also an important factor, is typically based on data obtained from CT and PET scans, bone marrow biopsy, and, occasionally, cerebrospinal fluid analysis. The stage is based on the site of disease and its spread to other sites. For example, in stage I disease, only one area of involvement is detected; thus, stage I disease is highly localized and may respond well to localized therapy (e.g., radiation therapy). In contrast, in stage IV disease, at least one extranodal site is detected.

Medical Management

Treatment is based on the classification of disease, the stage of disease, prior treatment (if any), and the patient's ability to tolerate therapy. If the disease is not an aggressive form and is truly localized, radiation alone may be the treatment of choice.

Low-grade lymphomas may not require treatment until the disease progresses to a later stage, but historically they have been relatively unresponsive to treatment, and, in most cases, use of therapeutic modalities did not improve overall survival. More aggressive types of NHL (e.g., lymphoblastic lymphoma, Burkitt lymphoma) require prompt initiation of combination chemotherapy; however, these types tend to be more responsive to treatment.

With aggressive types of NHL, aggressive combinations of chemotherapeutic agents are given even in early stages. More intermediate forms are commonly treated with combination chemotherapy and radiation therapy for stage I and II diseases. The advent of the monoclonal antibody, Rituximab, which targets the CD20 antigen on the surface of B cells, has improved survival in patients with NHL significantly. The combination of rituximab with conventional chemotherapy (Cytoxan, doxorubicin, vincristine, and prednisone [CHOP]) is now considered standard treatment for common, aggressive B-cell lymphomas (Bierman & Armitage, 2016). Unfortunately, more than 30% of patients with diffuse large B-cell NHL will experience a relapse. Treatment for relapsed disease includes Rituximab and combination chemotherapy followed by high-dose chemotherapy with stem cell support, which offers the best chance for response. For patients who are not eligible for transplant, chemotherapy may be used alone (Sehn & Gascoyne, 2015). A number of novel therapies are under investigation in an attempt to enhance the efficacy of front-line therapy and improve outcomes in patients with relapsed or refractory disease (Sehn & Gascoyne, 2015). CNS involvement may occur with some aggressive forms of NHL; in this situation, intrathecal chemotherapy is used in addition to systemic chemotherapy. Radiation may be used for palliation of symptoms.

Nursing Management

Lymphoma is a highly complex constellation of diseases. When caring for patients with lymphoma, it is extremely important to know the specific disease type, stage of disease, treatment history, and current treatment plan. Most of the care for patients with Hodgkin lymphoma or NHL takes place in the outpatient setting, unless complications occur (e.g., infection, respiratory compromise due to mediastinal mass). The most commonly used treatment methods are chemotherapy and radiation therapy. Chemotherapy causes systemic side effects (e.g., myelosuppression, nausea, hair loss, risk of infection), whereas radiation therapy causes specific effects that are limited to the area being irradiated. For example, patients receiving abdominal radiation therapy may experience nausea and diarrhea but not hair loss. Regardless of the type of treatment, all patients experience fatigue.

The risk for infection is significant for these patients, not only from treatment-related myelosuppression but also from the defective immune response that results from the disease itself. Patients need to be taught to minimize the risks of infection, to recognize signs of possible infection, and to contact the health care professional should such signs develop (see Chapters 6 and 19). Additional complications depend on the location of the lymphoma. Therefore, it is important for the nurse to know the tumor location so that assessments can be targeted appropriately. For example, patients with lymphomatous masses in the upper chest should be assessed for superior vena cava obstruction or airway obstruction if the mass is near the bronchus or trachea.

Many lymphomas can be cured with current treatments. However, as survival rates increase, the incidence of secondary malignancies, particularly AML or MDS, also increases. Therefore, survivors should be screened regularly for the development of second malignancies.

CHRONIC LYMPHOCYTIC LEUKEMIA (CLL)

CLL is classified as a type of low-grade lymphoma as it is a disease that encompasses both CLL and small lymphocytic lymphoma (SLL). It is the most frequent form of leukemia in Western countries, affecting more than 15,680 people in the Unites States (ACS, 2013). It is a common malignancy of older adults (70% of diagnoses are made in patients over 65 years of age), and the mean age at diagnosis is 65 years (Ferri, 2016i). In general, prognosis is related to the clinical stage (e.g., the average survival in patients with early stage is 10 years, whereas for stage 4 [or Binet stage C] survival is approximately 2½ years). That said, the overall 5-year survival rate has increased to 66% from 60% in the past 10 years largely related to the addition of immunotherapy to combination chemotherapy (Ferri, 2016i).

Pathophysiology

CLL is typically derived from a malignant clone of B lymphocytes (T-lymphocyte CLL is rare). In contrast to the acute forms of leukemia, most of the leukemia cells in CLL are fully mature.

It appears that these cells can escape **apoptosis** (programmed cell death), resulting in an excessive accumulation of the cells in the marrow and circulation. The antigen CD52 is prevalent on the surface of many of these leukemic B cells.

Two classification systems are in regular use to stage CLL; the disease is classified into three (Binet system; stage A, B, C) or five stages (Rai system; stage 0–IV). Both staging systems help to estimate prognosis and assist with treatment stratification (Ferri, 2016i). In the early stage, an elevated lymphocyte count is seen; it can exceed $100,000/mm^3$. Because the lymphocytes are small, they can travel easily through the small capillaries within the circulation, and the pulmonary and cerebral complications of leukocytosis (as seen with myeloid leukemias) typically are not found in CLL.

Lymphadenopathy occurs as the lymphocytes are trapped within the lymph nodes. The nodes can become very large and are sometimes painful. Hepatomegaly and splenomegaly then develop.

In later stages, anemia and thrombocytopenia may develop. Typically treatment is initiated in the later stages; earlier treatment does not appear to increase survival so treatment for limited-stage disease is employed only if the patient is symptomatic (Rai & Stilgenbauer, 2014). Autoimmune complications also can occur at any stage as either AIHA or ITP. ITP is characterized by the destruction of blood platelets due to the presence of antiplatelet autoantibodies, in which antibodies are directed against the patient's own platelets. As the term implies, the platelet level decreases (thrombocytopenia), resulting in visible bruising (purpura) in the skin and mucous membranes. Simply put, in the autoimmune process, the **reticuloendothelial system** (RES) destroys the body's own erythrocytes (hemolytic anemia) or platelets (ITP).

Clinical Manifestations and Assessment

Many patients are asymptomatic and are diagnosed incidentally during routine physical examinations or during treatment for another disease. At the time of diagnosis, lymphadenopathy is seen in 50% to 90% of patients and splenomegaly in 25% to 55% of patients (Rai & Stilgenbauer, 2014). An increased lymphocyte count (lymphocytosis) is always present. The erythrocyte and platelet counts may be normal or, in later stages of the illness, decreased.

Approximately 5% to 10% of patients with CLL present with "B symptoms," a constellation of symptoms including fevers, fatigue, drenching sweats (especially at night), and unintentional weight loss (Rai & Stilgenbauer, 2014). Patients with CLL have defects in their humoral and cell-mediated immune systems; therefore, infections are common. The defect in cellular immunity is evidenced by an absent or decreased reaction to skin sensitivity tests (e.g., *Candida*, mumps), which is known as **anergy**. Life-threatening infections are common. Viral infections, such as herpes zoster, can become widely disseminated.

Medical Management

In early stages, CLL may require no treatment. The decision to treat is triggered by symptom progression, including drenching night sweats, fatigue, weight loss, painful lymphadenopathy or progressive cytopenias, or the development of an associated autoimmune disorder (such as AIHI or ITP) (Wierda, 2015). The period of observation can be as long as several years. Treatment options are selected based on the patient's age, performance status, comorbidities, and risk factors (deletion of chromosome 17 predicts poor response to therapy) (Wierda, 2015; NCCN, 2016f). Five to 10% of patients will experience a transformation from CLL to a more aggressive form of lymphoma. The median survival in this population is 5 months, and often aggressive therapy is employed.

The combination of FCR (fludarabine, cyclophosphamide, and rituxan) remains the standard of care for young patients who have a good performance status (Wierda, 2015; NCCN, 2016f). The major side effect of fludarabine is prolonged bone marrow suppression manifested by prolonged periods of neutropenia, lymphopenia, and thrombocytopenia. Patients are then at risk for infections, such as *Pneumocystis jiroveci*, *Listeria*, mycobacteria, herpes viruses, and cytomegalovirus (CMV). Most patients receive prophylactic antimicrobials to minimize risk for these infections.

For older or more frail patients, newer agents such as the CD20 monoclonal antibodies, obinutuzumab or ofatumumab, or the oral agent, ibrutinib, may be considered (Wierda, 2015; NCCN, 2016f). Ibrutinib targets a tyrosine kinase called Bruton tyrosine kinase, which is responsible for CLL cell growth. It was approved for relapsed or refractory CLL and in patients with CLL who have a deletion of 17p. It has a favorable risk–benefit profile, is taken orally, and shown efficacy even in the refractory setting. Common side effects include diarrhea, fatigue, fever, nausea, and cytopenias (McNally, Long, Brophy, & Badillo, 2015).

Bacterial infections are common in patients with CLL, and treatment with IV immunoglobulin (IVIG) may be given to selected patients with low immunoglobulin levels to decrease the risk for infection.

MULTIPLE MYELOMA (MM)

MM is malignant disease of the plasma cell; it accounts for 10% of all hematologic cancers (Ferri, 2016j). Plasma cells are mature B cells that secrete immunoglobulins, proteins necessary for antibody production (IgG, IgA, IgM, IgD, IgE) to fight infection. Myeloma results in the production of monoclonal antibody proteins (M protein). Incidence in 2013 was 22,350 cases of MM (ACS, 2013). Prevalence is 70,000 in the United States, and the higher prevalence rates are related to more effective therapies, resulting in extended survival (Faiman & Richards, 2014). Median age at diagnosis

is 60 years with the majority of patients over 70 years of age (NCCN, 2016g). The incidence rate is more than twice as high in the black population as compared to white populations. Most patients develop resistance to treatment over time (Faiman & Richards, 2014). The overall survival of MM has improved significantly in the last 15 years from a 2.5-year median survival before 2001 to 4.6 years from 2001 to 2005 and 6.1 years in patients diagnosed between 2006 and 2010 (Rajkumar, 2016). Infection is the leading cause of death.

Pathophysiology

Clonal plasma cells develop as a result of a series of acquired genetic mutations and alterations in the bone marrow microenvironment that create an environment favorable to myeloma cell growth (Falco, Smith, & Sullivan, 2011; Faiman & Richards, 2014). Myeloma cells grow and accumulate in the bone marrow, resulting in bone lesions and bone marrow failure (NCCN, 2016g). In MM, the malignant plasma cells produce an increased amount of a specific immunoglobulin that is nonfunctional. Functional types of immunoglobulin are still produced by nonmalignant plasma cells but in lower-than-normal quantity. The nonfunctional, specific immunoglobulin secreted by the myeloma cells is detectable in the blood and/or urine and is referred to as the *monoclonal protein*, or *M protein*. This protein serves as a useful marker to monitor the extent of disease and the patient's response to therapy. In addition, the presence of light chains (antibodies are made up of light chains and heavy chains) in the urine (sometimes referred to as *Bence–Jones protein*) is considered to be a major criterion in the diagnosis of MM. The monoclonal protein is commonly measured by serum or urine protein electrophoresis. Moreover, the patient's total protein level is typically elevated, again due to the production of M protein.

To establish a diagnosis of myeloma, there must be a measurable M protein in the serum and/or urine; in the absence of measurable M protein, an abnormal serum free light chain ratio may substitute for this criteria. Bone marrow aspirate and biopsy are performed; the presence of more than 10% plasma cells in the bone marrow is another hallmark diagnostic criterion. The diagnosis of myeloma also requires evidence of end-organ damage, including: anemia, hypercalcemia, kidney dysfunction, or bone destruction (Ferri, 2016j). Testing for end-organ damage includes serum creatinine, hemoglobin/hematocrit, calcium, and x-rays of the axial skeleton to detect lytic lesions.

Malignant plasma cells also secrete certain substances to stimulate the creation of new blood vessels to enhance the growth of these clusters of plasma cells; this process is referred to as **angiogenesis**. Occasionally, the plasma cells infiltrate other tissue, in which case they are referred to as *plasmacytomas*. Plasmacytomas can occur in the sinuses, spinal cord, and soft tissues.

Clinical Manifestations and Assessment

As many as 90% of patients with MM develop bone lesions. Although patients can have asymptomatic bone involvement, the most common presenting symptom of MM is bone pain, usually in the back or ribs. Unlike arthritic pain, the bone pain associated with myeloma increases with movement and decreases with rest; patients may report that they have less pain on awakening, but the pain intensity increases during the day. In myeloma, a substance secreted by the plasma cells, osteoclast-activating factor, and other substances (e.g., interleukin-6 [IL-6]) are involved in stimulating osteoclasts. Both mechanisms appear to be involved in the process of bone breakdown. Thus, lytic lesions as well as osteoporosis may be seen on bone x-rays (they are not well visualized on bone scans). The bone destruction can be severe enough to cause vertebral collapse and fractures, including spinal fractures, which can impinge on the spinal cord and result in spinal cord compression. It is this bone destruction that causes significant pain.

If the bone destruction is fairly extensive, excessive ionized calcium is lost from the bone and enters the serum; therefore, hypercalcemia may develop (frequently manifested by excessive thirst, dehydration, constipation, altered mental status, confusion, and, rarely, coma). Kidney failure may also occur; the configuration of the circulating immunoglobulin molecule (particularly the shape of lambda light chains) can damage the renal tubules.

As more and more malignant plasma cells are produced, the marrow has less space for erythrocyte production, and anemia may develop. This anemia is also caused to a great extent by a diminished production of erythropoietin by the kidney. The patient may complain of fatigue and weakness due to the anemia. In the late stage of the disease, a reduced number of leukocytes and platelets may also be seen because the bone marrow is infiltrated by malignant plasma cells.

> **(!) Nursing Alert**
> *Any elderly patient whose chief complaint is back pain and who has an elevated total protein level should be evaluated for possible myeloma. Elderly patients with anemia should also have myeloma on the list of differential diagnoses.*

Medical Management

There is no cure for MM. Even autologous PBSCT is considered to extend remission rather than provide a cure. However, for many patients, it is possible to control the illness and maintain their level of functioning quite well for several years. Initial treatment is dictated by risk level and transplant eligibility. Patients who are transplant eligible are treated with combination therapy, including a proteasome inhibitor (bortezomib in low- and intermediate-risk patients and carfilzomib in high-risk patients), lenalidomide, and dexamethasone for four cycles followed by autologous transplant and maintenance therapy with either lenalidomide (low-risk patients) or a proteasome inhibitor (high-risk patients) (Rajkumar, 2016). Patients who are not eligible for transplant are treated with bortezomib, lenalidomide, and dexamethasone for several cycles followed by maintenance therapy with a proteasome inhibitor for intermediate- and high-risk patients. Frail elderly patients may be treated with lenalidomide and dexamethasone (Rajkumar, 2016).

Recent advances in the understanding of the process of angiogenesis have resulted in new therapeutic options. The sedative thalidomide (Thalomid), initially used as an antiemetic, and the newer agents, Lenalidomide, and Pomalidomide, have significant antimyeloma effects. These agents inhibit the cytokines necessary for new vascular generation, such as vascular endothelial growth factor, and for myeloma cell growth and survival, such as IL-6 and tumor necrosis factor, by boosting the body's immune response against the tumor and by creating favorable conditions for apoptosis (programmed cell death) of the myeloma cells. Thalidomide is effective in refractory myeloma and in "smoldering" disease states and may prevent progression to a more active state. Thalidomide, lenalidomide, and pomalidomide are not typical chemotherapeutic agents and have unique side-effect profiles. Thalidomide commonly causes fatigue, dizziness, constipation, rash, and peripheral neuropathy. Lenalidomide and pomalidomide side-effect profiles are quite different from that of thalidomide: myelosuppression and infections such as pneumonia are more common, whereas sedation, neuropathy, and constipation are not (NCCN, 2016g). Patients who have progressed on thalidomide still can be treated with lenalidomide; lenalidomide is thought to exhibit more antimyeloma activity than thalidomide. Often lenalidomide is used in combination with bortezomib; together, the two drugs are synergistic and may improve outcomes.

Thalidomide, lenalidomide, and pomalidomide are contraindicated in pregnancy because of associated severe birth defects. In addition, due to the risks for birth defects, use of either agent requires registry into a monitoring program that ensures routine pregnancy testing, contraception, and control of drug distribution. Patients must be counseled monthly and agree to use approved methods of birth control prior to taking these drugs.

Newer agents recently approved for the treatment of myeloma include the monoclonal antibodies (MoAb), elotuzumab and daratumumab (Darzalex™). Elotuzumab is a humanized MoAb that targets the CS-1 antigen that is expressed in 97% of cases of myeloma. CS-1 stimulates tumor growth and cell adhesion through interaction with the bone marrow microenvironment; elotuzumab interferes with the activity of CS-1. In the relapsed/refractory setting, elotuzumab, in combination with lenalidomide and dexamethasone, had a response rate of 92% at 18 months (Lonial et al., 2013). Daratumumab is a CD38-targeted MoAb approved in the relapsed/refractory setting in patients treated with at least three prior therapies; overall response rate was 29.2% (Darzalex package insert, 2015).

Radiation therapy is very useful in strengthening the bone at a specific lesion, particularly one at risk for bone fracture or spinal cord compression. It is also useful in relieving bone pain and reducing the size of plasma cell tumors that occur outside the skeletal system. However, because it is a nonsystemic form of treatment, it does not diminish the source of the bone conditions (i.e., the production of malignant plasma cells). Therefore, typically radiation therapy is used in combination with systemic treatment such as chemotherapy.

When lytic lesions result in vertebral compression fractures, vertebroplasty is often performed. This procedure is performed under fluoroscopy. A hollow needle is positioned within the fractured vertebra, and when the precise location is confirmed, an orthopedic cement is injected into the vertebra to stabilize the fracture and strengthen the vertebra. For most patients, relief from pain is almost immediate. This procedure has been enhanced by concomitant kyphoplasty, the use of a special inflatable balloon inserted into the vertebra to increase the height of the vertebra prior to injecting the cement.

All patients with myeloma are at risk for skeletal-related events (SREs), including pathologic fractures and spinal cord compression. Bisphosphonate therapy has been shown to decrease the risk of SREs in patients with and without bone involvement (Munchi & Anderson, 2015). As a result of this data, all patients with symptomatic myeloma should receive bisphosphonate therapy with either pamidronate or zoledronic acid, as an adjunct to their antimyeloma therapy (Terpos, Roodman, Dimopoulos, 2013; NCCN, 2016g). Pamidronate (Aredia) and zoledronic acid (Zometa) have been shown to strengthen bone in MM by diminishing the secretion of osteoclast-activating factor, thus controlling bone pain and potentially preventing bone fracture. These agents are also effective in managing and preventing hypercalcemia. A recent study evaluated survival outcomes and found a survival advantage in patients with myeloma who received bisphosphonate treatment (Morgan et al., 2013). However, a complication associated with IV bisphosphonates is osteonecrosis of the jaw, which can result in intractable pain, swallowing difficulty, sinusitis, soft-tissue abscesses, and extraoral fistulas (a permanent abnormal passageway between the mouth and exterior of the body). Estimates of incidence are from 1% to 12% of patients receiving IV bisphosphonates. Patients should receive a comprehensive dental examination and appropriate dental interventions as needed prior to initiation of bisphosphonate therapy. Throughout the duration of treatment, careful assessment for this complication should be performed.

Hyperviscosity may result from elevations in the M protein levels. When patients have signs and symptoms of hyperviscosity, such as mental status changes or blurred vision, plasmapheresis may be used to lower the immunoglobulin level. Symptoms may be more useful than serum viscosity levels in determining the need for this intervention.

MM increases the risk for the development of VTE. Drugs such as thalidomide, lenalidomide, and pomalidomide are also thrombogenic; the risk for VTE increases when these agents are used in combination with dexamethasone. To minimize the risk for VTE, patients are educated to maintain an active lifestyle including daily exercise. In addition, prophylaxis with aspirin is recommended unless contraindicated.

Nursing Management

Pain management is very important in patients with MM. NSAIDs can be very useful for mild pain or can be administered in combination with opioid analgesics. Because NSAIDs can cause gastritis and kidney dysfunction, kidney function must be monitored carefully. The patient needs to be educated about activity restrictions (e.g., lifting no more than 10 lb, use of proper body mechanics). Braces are needed occasionally to support the spinal column. Patients must understand the importance of reporting any new pain promptly as there is risk for spontaneous pathologic fractures that require prompt intervention to minimize morbidity.

Peripheral neuropathy is a common side effect of the immunomodulatory agents used to treat MM, occurring in as many as 80% of patients. Peripheral neuropathy can significantly impact the patient's quality of life and ability to perform activities of daily living (ADLs). The physical examination should include an assessment of neuropathy using a neurotoxicity assessment tool as well as a subjective assessment of the patient's discomfort. Management of peripheral neuropathy may include decreasing drug doses, holding therapy, treating discomfort with medications such as gabapentin, and involving other disciplines such as occupational and physical therapy to maximize and restore function.

The patient also needs to be instructed about the signs and symptoms of hypercalcemia. Maintaining mobility and hydration is important to minimize risk of exacerbations of this complication; however, the primary cause is the disease itself. Also kidney function should be monitored closely. Kidney failure can become severe, and dialysis may be needed. Maintaining high urine output with aggressive hydration (3 L/day) can be very useful in preventing or limiting this complication.

Because antibody production is impaired, infections, particularly bacterial infections, are common and can be life-threatening. The patient needs to be instructed in appropriate infection-prevention measures, such as hand hygiene and avoiding sick individuals, and should be advised to contact the health care provider immediately if he or she has a fever or other signs and symptoms of infection. The patient should receive vaccines for pneumonia (Pneumovax) and influenza. Sometimes prophylactic antibiotics are used. IVIG can be useful for patients with recurrent infections and low levels of immunoglobulins.

Many patients with MM are treated with high doses of corticosteroids for protracted periods of time. Patients must be monitored for potential short- and long-term effects of steroids, including hyperglycemia and insomnia (short term), and osteopenia, osteoporosis, cataracts, and diabetes (long term).

Gerontologic Considerations

The incidence of MM increases with age; the disease is less common in patients younger than 40 years of age. Due in part to the aging population, incidence is rising. Back pain, which is often a presenting symptom in this disease, should be investigated closely in older patients. In addition, any patient over 40 years of age presenting with anemia should undergo a workup for myeloma, primarily through an evaluation of the serum protein electrophoresis (SPEP). Autologous PBSCT is an option that can prolong remission and potentially cure some patients, but it is unavailable to many older people because of age limitations, poor performance status, and comorbidities.

THERAPIES FOR BLOOD DISORDERS

Splenectomy

Each year 25,000 splenectomies are performed in the United States with the estimated prevalence of asplenic patients reaching 1 million (Rubin & Schaffner, 2014). Removal may be an emergency, in the case of trauma or rupture, or elective in the case of treating selected hematologic disorders. Because the spleen is very vascular, severe hemorrhage can result if the spleen is ruptured. Under such circumstances, splenectomy becomes an emergency procedure.

Splenectomy is also a possible treatment for other hematologic disorders. For example, an enlarged spleen may be the site of excessive destruction of blood cells. If the destruction is life-threatening, surgery may be life-saving. This is the case in AIHA and ITP when these disorders do not respond to more conservative measures, such as corticosteroid therapy. Some patients with grossly enlarged spleens develop severe thrombocytopenia due to the platelets being sequestered in the spleen; splenectomy removes the "trap," and platelet counts may normalize over time.

In general, the mortality rate after splenectomy is low. Laparoscopic splenectomy can be performed in selected patients, with a resultant decrease in postoperative morbidity. The most common complications in patients following splenectomy include infection, thrombosis, bleeding, and wound dehiscence (Matharoo, Afthinos, & Gibbs, 2014; Terreri, 2016). Although young children are at the highest risk after splenectomy, all age groups are vulnerable to overwhelming, lethal infections and should receive recommended vaccinations and be treated promptly for fever or signs of infection (see earlier detailed discussion about splenectomy care in ITP section).

Often, patients with high platelet counts have even higher counts after splenectomy (over 1 million/mm^3), which can predispose them to serious thrombotic or hemorrhagic problems. However, this increase is transient and usually does not warrant additional treatment.

THERAPEUTIC APHERESIS

Apheresis is a Greek word meaning separation. In therapeutic apheresis (or pheresis), blood is taken from the patient and passed through a centrifuge, in which a specific component is separated from the blood and removed. Then the remaining blood is returned to the patient.

The most common apheresis modalities used include therapeutic plasma exchange (e.g., used to treat hyperviscosity in plasma cell disorders), leukocytopheresis (used to treat symptomatic leukocytosis in patients with leukemia), extracorporeal photopheresis (ECP) (used to treat cutaneous T-cell lymphoma, Sezary syndrome, and GVHD), thrombocytopheresis (used to treat symptomatic thrombocytosis with MPNs), and erythrocytapheresis (used in selected cases of PV or ET) (Connelly-Smith & Linenberger, 2015).

The entire system is closed so the risk of bacterial contamination is extremely low. When platelets or leukocytes are removed, the decrease in these cells within the circulation is temporary. However, the temporary decrease provides a window of time until suppressive medications (e.g., chemotherapy) can have therapeutic effects. Sometimes plasma is removed rather than blood cells—typically so that specific, abnormal proteins within the plasma are lowered transiently until a long-term therapy can be initiated.

Also apheresis is used to obtain larger amounts of platelets from a donor than can be provided from a single unit of whole blood. A unit of platelets obtained in this way is equivalent to six to eight units of platelets obtained from six to eight separate donors via standard blood donation methods. Platelet donors can have their platelets apheresed as often as every 14 days.

Leukocytes can be obtained similarly, typically after the donor has received growth factors (G-CSF, GM-CSF) to stimulate the formation of additional leukocytes and thereby increase the leukocyte count. The use of these growth factors also stimulates the release of stem cells within the circulation. Apheresis is used to harvest these stem cells (typically over a period of several days) for use in PBSCT.

THERAPEUTIC PHLEBOTOMY

Therapeutic phlebotomy is the removal of a certain amount of blood under controlled conditions. Usually patients with elevated hematocrits (e.g., those with PV) or excessive iron absorption (e.g., hemochromatosis) can be managed by periodically removing 1 unit (about 500 mL) of whole blood;

however, the elderly, those with small body mass, comorbidities, or women may be able to tolerate only 250 mL (Bacon, 2016; Zubair, 2014). Eventually, this process can produce iron deficiency, leaving the patient unable to produce as many erythrocytes. The actual procedure for therapeutic phlebotomy is similar to that for blood donation (see later discussion).

BLOOD COMPONENT THERAPY

A single unit of whole blood contains 450 mL of blood and 50 mL of an anticoagulant. A unit of whole blood can be processed and dispensed for administration. However, it is more appropriate, economical, and practical to separate that unit of whole blood into its primary components: erythrocytes, platelets, and plasma (leukocytes are rarely used; see later discussion). Because the plasma is removed, a unit of PRBCs is very concentrated (hematocrit approximately 70%). Each component must be processed and stored differently to maximize the longevity of the viable cells and factors within it; each individual blood component has a

different storage life. PRBCs are stored at 4°C. With special preservatives, they can be stored safely for up to 42 days before they must be discarded. In contrast, platelets must be stored at room temperature because they cannot withstand cold temperatures, and they last for only 5 days before they must be discarded. To prevent clumping, platelets are agitated gently while stored. Plasma is frozen immediately to maintain the activity of the clotting factors within; it lasts for 1 year if it remains frozen. Alternatively, plasma can be further pooled and processed into blood derivatives, such as albumin, immune globulin, factor VIII, and factor IX. Table 20-6 describes each blood component and how each is commonly used.

Blood transfusion is discussed in detail on page 617.

Special Preparations

Factor VIII concentrate (antihemophilic factor) is a lyophilized (to dry by freezing in a high vacuum) or freeze-dried concentrate of pooled fractionated human plasma. It is used in treating hemophilia A. Factor IX concentrate (prothrombin complex) is prepared similarly and contains factors II,

TABLE 20-6 Blood and Blood Components Commonly Used in Transfusion Therapy[a]

	Composition	Indications and Considerations
Whole blood	Cells and plasma, hematocrit about 40%	Volume replacement and oxygen-carrying capacity; usually used only in significant bleeding (more than 25% blood volume lost)
Packed red blood cells (PRBCs)	RBCs with little plasma (hematocrit about 70%); some platelets and WBCs remain. Platelets in the unit are not functional; WBCs in the unit may cause reaction and are not functional.	Hemoglobin less than 7–8 g/dL; symptomatic anemia
Platelets—random	Platelets (5.5×10^{10} platelets/unit) Plasma; some RBCs, WBCs survival ↓ in presence of fever, chills, infection Repeated treatment leads to ↓ transfused platelet survival due to alloimmunization	To prevent bleeding in patients with a platelet count below 10,000/mm³ To prevent bleeding in patients with fever or sepsis and platelet count below 20,000/mm³ Prior to major surgery or invasive procedure when platelet count *is less than or equal to 50,000/mm³* Prior to ocular surgery or neurosurgery when platelet count is *less than or equal to 100,000/mm³*
Platelets—single donor	Platelets (3×10^{11} platelets/unit) 1 unit is equivalent to 6–8 units of random platelets	Used to decrease alloimmunization risk by limiting exposure to multiple donors Preferred for patients who will require repeated transfusions over time
Plasma or fresh-frozen plasma (FFP)	Plasma; all coagulation factors Complement	Bleeding in patients with coagulation factor deficiencies To reverse the effects of warfarin in presence of major bleeding
Granulocytes	Neutrophils (greater than 1×10^{10}/unit); lymphocytes; some RBCs and platelets	Severe neutropenia in selected patients; controversial, rarely used
Donor lymphocytes (white blood cells [WBCs])	Lymphocytes (number varies) taken from a donor and infused into a recipient	Stimulate graft-versus-disease effect in a patient who has undergone prior allogeneic stem cell transplant

	Composition	Indications and Considerations
Cryoprecipitate	Fibrinogen 150 or greater mg/bag, Contains high concentrations of factor VIII and fibrinogen; AHF (VIII:C) 80–110 units/bag	von Willebrand disease Hypofibrinogenemia Hemophilia A
Antihemophilic factor (AHF)	Factor VIII	Hemophilia A
Factor IX concentrate	Factor IX	Hemophilia B (Christmas disease)
Factor IX complex	Factors II, VII, IX, X	Hereditary factors VII, IX, X deficiency Hemophilia A with factor VII inhibitors
Albumin	Albumin 5%, 25%	Hypoproteinemia Burns Volume expansion by 5% to ↑ intravascular volume; 25% → ↑ intravascular volume which ↓'s hematocrit due to hemodilution
IV gamma globulin (IVIG)	IgG antibodies	Hypogammaglobulinemia (in CLL, recurrent infections) ITP Primary immunodeficiency states
Antithrombin III concentrate (AT III)	AT III (trace amounts of other plasma proteins)	AT III deficiency with or at risk for thrombosis

AHF, antihemophilic factor; CLL, chronic lymphocytic leukemia; ITP, immune thrombocytopenic purpura.
[a]The composition of each type of blood component is described, as well as the most common indications for using a given blood component. RBCs, platelets, and fresh-frozen plasma are the blood products most commonly used. When transfusing these blood products, it is important to realize that the individual product is always "contaminated" with very small amounts of other blood products (e.g., WBCs mixed in a unit of platelets). This contamination can cause some difficulties, particularly isosensitization, in certain patients.
Shah (2015).

VII, IX, and X. It is used primarily for treatment of factor IX deficiency (hemophilia B). Factor IX concentrate is also useful in treating congenital factor VII and factor X deficiencies. Recombinant forms of factor VIII, such as Humate-P or Alphanate, are also useful. Because they contain vWF, these agents are used in vWD as well as in hemophilia A, particularly when patients develop acquired factor VIII inhibitors (e.g., antibodies).

Plasma albumin is a large protein molecule that usually stays within vessels and is a major contributor to plasma oncotic pressure. This protein is used to expand the blood volume of patients in hypovolemic shock and, rarely, to increase the concentration of circulating albumin in patients with hypoalbuminemia.

Immunoglobulin is a concentrated solution of the antibody IgG; it contains very little IgA or IgM. It is prepared from large pools of plasma. The IV form (IVIG) is used in various clinical situations to replace inadequate amounts of IgG in patients who have experienced recurrent bacterial infection (e.g., those with CLL, BMT or PBSCT recipients) to reduce the risk for future infection. It is also used in certain autoimmune disorders, such as ITP. IVIG, in contrast to all other fractions of human blood, cells, or plasma, can survive being subjected to heating at 60°C (140°F) for 10 hours to free it of the viral contaminants that may be present.

PHARMACOLOGIC ALTERNATIVES TO BLOOD TRANSFUSIONS

Pharmacologic agents that stimulate production of one or more types of blood cells by the marrow are commonly used (Box 20-5).

Researchers continue to seek a blood substitute that is practical and safe (Paul & Nesbitt, 2016). Manufacturing artificial blood is problematic, given the myriad functions of blood components. Research has focused on the role of blood in oxygen transport or its role as an oxygen carrier and the manufacturing of a suitable RBC substitute. The substitutes can be classified as perfluorocarbon emulsions that have a high gas-dissolving capacity for oxygen and hemoglobin-based oxygen carriers (Duke, 2016). Current artificial RBC products have distinct advantages and disadvantages compared with human RBCs. These products can be rendered essentially sterile, resulting in fewer immune-related transfusion problems. They require no refrigeration, have possible unlimited availability, long storage life, and require no cross-matching (Duke, 2016). Potential problems associated with these products include low concentrations of 2,3-DPG, the shifting of the oxyhemoglobin dissociation curve to the left, and a decrease in the off-loading of oxygen at the tissue level. Because the substitutes are also

Pharmacologic Alternatives to Blood Transfusions

Growth Factors

Recombinant technology has provided a means to produce hematopoietic growth factors necessary for the production of blood cells within the bone marrow. By increasing the body's production of blood cells, transfusions and complications resulting from diminished blood cells (e.g., infection from neutropenia or transfusions) may be avoided. However, the successful use of growth factors requires functional bone marrow.

Erythropoietin

Erythropoietin (epoetin alpha/EPO [e.g., Epogen, Procrit]) is an effective alternative treatment for patients with chronic anemia secondary to diminished levels of erythropoietin, as in chronic kidney disease. This medication stimulates erythropoiesis. It also has been used for patients who are anemic from chemotherapy or zidovudine (AZT) therapy and for those who have diseases involving bone marrow suppression, such as myelodysplastic syndrome (MDS). Recent studies have shown that exceeding the recommended Hgb goal of 11 g/dL results in increased risk for cardiovascular events, including stroke and MI. In addition, use of erythropoietin has been associated with decreased survival in certain types of cancer. EPO has been used safely in the preoperative setting to decrease the need for allogeneic blood transfusions. In this setting, erythropoietin also can enable a patient to donate several units of blood for future use (e.g., preoperative autologous donation). The medication can be administered intravenously or subcutaneously, although plasma levels are better sustained with the subcutaneous route. Side effects are rare, but erythropoietin can cause or exacerbate hypertension. If the anemia is corrected too quickly or is overcorrected, the elevated hematocrit can cause headache, hypertension, and, potentially, seizures. These adverse effects are rare except for in patients with kidney failure. Serial CBCs should be performed to evaluate the response to the medication. The dose and frequency of administration are titrated to the hematocrit.

Granulocyte-Colony Stimulating Factor (G-CSF)

G-CSF (filgrastim [Neupogen]) is a cytokine that stimulates the proliferation and differentiation of myeloid stem cells; a rapid increase in neutrophils is seen within the circulation. G-CSF is effective in improving transient but severe neutropenia after chemotherapy or in some MDS subtypes. It is particularly useful in preventing bacterial infections that would be likely to occur with neutropenia. G-CSF is administered subcutaneously on a daily basis. The primary side effect is bone pain; this probably reflects the increase in hematopoiesis within the marrow. Serial CBCs should be performed to evaluate the response to the medication and to ensure that the rise in white blood cells is not excessive. The effect of G-CSF on myelopoiesis is short; the neutrophil count drops once the medication is stopped. There is a long-active formulation, Pegfilgrastim (Neulasta) that is given once per chemotherapy cycle to decrease the risk for infection.

Granulocyte-Macrophage Colony Stimulating Factor (GM-CSF)

GM-CSF (sargramostim [Leukine]) is a cytokine that is naturally produced by a variety of cells, including monocytes and endothelial cells. It works either directly or synergistically with other growth factors to stimulate myelopoiesis. GM-CSF is not as specific to neutrophils as is G-CSF; thus, an increase in erythroid (RBC) and megakaryocytic (platelet) production also may be seen. GM-CSF serves the same purpose as G-CSF. However, it may have a greater effect on macrophage function and, therefore, may be more useful against fungal infections, whereas G-CSF may be better used to fight bacterial infections. GM-CSF is also administered subcutaneously. Side effects include bone pain, fevers, and myalgias.

---

nitric oxide scavengers, vasoconstriction may occur, risking pulmonary hypertension and myocardial ischemia (Duke, 2016). Finally, the solutions may also result in platelet activation (Duke, 2016). Thus, further study is needed to establish safety and efficacy.

PROCURING BLOOD, BLOOD PRODUCTS, AND BLOOD TRANSFUSIONS

Blood Donation

To protect both the donor and the recipients, all prospective donors are examined and interviewed before they are allowed to donate their blood. The intent of the interview is to assess the general health status of the donor and to identify risk factors that might harm a recipient of the donor's blood. Donors should be in good health and meet a number of specific criteria (Box 20-6).

Potential donors should be asked whether they have consumed any aspirin or aspirin-containing medications within the past 3 days. Although aspirin use does not render the donor ineligible, the platelets obtained would be dysfunctional and therefore not useful; aspirin usage within 48 to 72 hours contraindicates platelet donation. Aspirin does not affect the erythrocytes or plasma obtained from the donor.

Directed Donation

At times, friends and family of a patient wish to donate blood specifically for that person. These blood donations are termed *directed donations*. These donations are not any safer than those provided by random donors because directed donors may not be as willing to identify themselves

BOX 20-6
Eligibility Requirements for Blood Donation

All donors are expected to meet the following minimum requirements:

- Be healthy and feeling well
- Be at least 17 years old in most states
- Body weight should exceed 50 kg (110 lb) for a standard 450-mL donation.
- Men must be at least 5'1" tall; women must be at least 5'5"
- No fever or signs/symptoms of infection.
- Blood pressure less than 180/100.
- The hemoglobin level should be at least 12.5 g/dL.

Contraindications to Blood Donation

- A history of viral hepatitis at any time in the past. If the donor lives with or has had sexual contact with a person who has hepatitis, the donor must wait 12 months after the last contact to donate.
- A history of receiving a blood transfusion or an infusion of any blood derivative (other than serum albumin) within 12 months

- A history of untreated malaria because malaria can be transmitted by transfusion even years later
- A history of syphilis or gonorrhea; acceptable if it has been more than 12 months since donor completed treatment for syphilis or gonorrhea
- A history or evidence of IV drug abuse
- A history of possible exposure to HIV
- A recent tattoo within the last 12 months because of the risk of blood-borne infections (e.g., hepatitis, HIV)
- A recent history of asthma, urticaria, or allergy to medications because hypersensitivity can be transferred passively to the recipient
- Recent immunizations (exception: influenza, tetanus, or meningitis, provided that the donor is symptom free and afebrile)
- Pregnancy, because of the nutritional demands of pregnancy on the mother
- A diagnosis of cancer, hemochromatosis, sickle cell disease, or active skin infections at the venipuncture site
- A history of whole blood donation within the past 56 days

For a detailed list of eligibility criteria by topic, visit the American Red Cross website: http://www.redcrossblood.org/donating-blood/eligibility-requirements American Red Cross (2017).

as having a history of any of the risk factors that disqualify a person from donating blood.

Standard Donation

Phlebotomy consists of venipuncture and blood withdrawal. Standard precautions are used. Donors are placed in a semi-recumbent position, and venipuncture with a large bore IV is performed. Withdrawal of 450 mL of blood usually takes less than 15 minutes. After the needle is removed, donors are asked to hold the involved arm straight up, and firm pressure is applied with sterile gauze for 2 to 3 minutes or until bleeding stops. Then a firm bandage is applied. The donor remains recumbent until he or she feels able to sit up, usually within a few minutes.

The donor is instructed to:

- leave the dressing on for a few hours
- avoid heavy lifting or vigorous exercise for the rest of the day
- increase fluid intake by drinking an extra four 8-oz glasses of fluid and avoid alcoholic beverages over the next 24 hours

Specimens from this donated blood are tested to detect infections and to identify the specific blood type (see later discussion).

Autologous Donation

A patient's own blood may be collected for future transfusion; this method is useful for many elective surgeries in which

the potential need for transfusion is high (e.g., orthopedic surgery). Preoperative donations are ideally collected 4 to 6 weeks before surgery. Iron supplements are prescribed during this period to prevent depletion of iron stores. Occasionally, erythropoietin (epoetin-alfa [Epogen, Procrit]) is given to stimulate erythropoiesis, so that the donor's hematocrit remains high enough to be eligible for donation. Typically, one unit of blood is drawn each week; the number of units obtained varies with the type of surgical procedure to be performed (i.e., the amount of blood anticipated to be transfused). Phlebotomies are not performed within 72 hours of surgery.

The primary advantage of autologous transfusions is the prevention of viral infections from another person's blood. It is the policy of the American Red Cross that autologous blood be transfused only to the donor. If the blood is not required, it can be frozen until the donor needs it in the future (for up to 10 years). Wastage rates of autologous transfusions can be up to 40% to 56% (Greenky et al., 2014). The blood is never returned to the general donor supply of blood products to be used by another person.

The disadvantage of autologous donation is that it may be performed even when the likelihood is small that the anticipated procedure will necessitate a transfusion. Needless autologous donation is expensive, takes time, and uses resources inappropriately. Furthermore, although autologous transfusion can eliminate the risk of viral contamination, the risk for bacterial contamination is the same as that in transfusion from random donors.

Contraindications to donation of blood for autologous transfusion are acute infection, severely debilitating chronic disease, hemoglobin level of less than 12.5 g/dL, hematocrit less than 38%, unstable angina, and acute cardiovascular or cerebrovascular disease.

Intraoperative Blood Salvage

This transfusion method provides replacement for patients who cannot donate before surgery and for those undergoing vascular, orthopedic, or thoracic surgery. During a surgical procedure, blood lost into a sterile cavity (e.g., hip joint) is suctioned into a cell-saver machine. The whole blood or PRBCs are washed, often with saline solution, filtered, and then returned to the patient as an IV infusion. The goal of intraoperative salvage is to reduce the need for allogeneic blood transfusions. Studies have demonstrated that intraoperative blood salvage safely and effectively decreases the need for transfusions of donated blood without causing adverse outcomes (Greenky et al., 2014). Devices that collect blood for reinfusion allow for either washing or not washing prior to transfusion. If the blood is washed (with normal saline) to remove lysed RBC debris and contaminants, it can be stored up to 4 hours at room temperature after processing. However, unwashed products must be filtered to remove clots and tissue debris and must be infused within 6 hours from the start of collection due to the risk from other contaminants (Shi, 2013).

Hemodilution

This transfusion method may be initiated before or after induction of anesthesia. About one to two units of blood are removed from the patient through a venous or arterial line and simultaneously replaced with a colloid or crystalloid solution. Then the blood that is obtained is reinfused after surgery. The advantage of this method is that the patient loses fewer erythrocytes during surgery because the added IV solutions dilute the concentration of erythrocytes and lower the hematocrit. However, patients who are at risk of myocardial injury should not be further stressed by hemodilution.

Complications of Blood Donation

The overall incidence of complications secondary to blood donation is very low (2% to 5%) (Greco & Shaz, 2013). The most common complications include bleeding secondary to needle injury (such as hematoma formation) and vasovagal reactions. Excessive bleeding at the donor's venipuncture site is sometimes caused by a bleeding disorder in the donor but more often results from a technique error: laceration of the vein, excessive tourniquet pressure, or failure to apply enough pressure after the needle is withdrawn. A donor who appears pale or complains of faintness should immediately lie down or sit with the head lowered below the knees. He or she should be observed for another 30 minutes.

BLOOD PROCESSING

Samples of the unit of blood are always taken immediately after donation so that the blood can be typed and tested. Each donation is tested for antibodies to HIV 1 and 2, hepatitis B core antibody (anti-HBc), hepatitis C virus (HCV), West Nile virus, and human T-cell lymphotropic virus type I (anti-HTLV-I/II). The blood is also tested for hepatitis B, hepatitis C virus, and Pallidum (Syphilis) (Klineman, 2016). Negative reactions are required for the blood to be used, and each unit of blood is labeled to certify the results. Blood is also screened for Cytomegalovirus (CMV); if it tests positive for CMV, it still can be used except in recipients who are negative for CMV and who are immunocompromised (e.g., BMT or PBSCT recipients).

Equally important to viral testing is accurate determination of the blood type. More than 200 antigens have been identified on the surface of RBC membranes. Of these, the most important for safe transfusion are the ABO and Rh systems. The ABO system identifies which antigens are present on the membrane of a person's erythrocytes: A, B, both A and B, or neither A nor B (type O). Individuals have antibodies in their plasma that are directed against blood group antigens that their RBCs do not express. For example, a person with Type A blood expresses the A antigen on the RBC membrane and has anti-B antibodies. To prevent a significant reaction, the same type of PRBCs should be transfused. In an emergency situation in which the patient's blood type is not known, type O blood may be transfused safely.

The Rh antigen (also called D) is present on the surface of erythrocytes in 85% of the population (Rh-positive). Those who lack the D antigen are called Rh-negative. PRBCs are routinely tested for the D antigen as well as ABO. Patients with Rh positive blood can receive Rh negative blood; however, patients who are Rh negative should only receive Rh negative blood.

The majority of transfusion reactions (other than those due to procedural error) are due to the presence of donor leukocytes within the blood component unit (PRBCs or platelets); the recipient may form antibodies to the antigens present on these leukocytes. PRBC components typically have 1 to 3×10^9 leukocytes remaining in each unit. Leukocytes from the blood product are frequently filtered to diminish the likelihood of developing reactions and refractoriness to transfusions, particularly in patients who have chronic transfusion needs. Filtration can occur at the time the unit is collected from the donor and processed, which achieves better results but is more expensive, or at the time the blood component is transfused by attaching a leukocyte filter to the blood administration tubing. Many centers advocate routinely using leuko-poor filtered blood components for people who have or are likely to develop chronic transfusion requirements.

When a patient is extremely immunocompromised, as in the case of bone marrow or stem cell transplant, any donor lymphocytes must be removed from the blood components. In this situation, the blood component is exposed to low amounts of radiation (25 Gy) that kill any lymphocytes within the blood component. Irradiated blood products are highly effective in preventing transfusion-associated GVHD, which is fatal in most cases. Irradiated blood products have a shorter shelf life.

TRANSFUSION

Administration of blood and blood components requires knowledge of correct administration techniques and possible complications. It is very important to be familiar with the facility's policies and procedures for transfusion therapy.

Setting

Although most blood transfusions are performed in the acute care setting, patients with chronic transfusion requirements often can receive transfusions in other settings, including free-standing infusion centers, ambulatory care clinics, physicians' offices, and, occasionally, even patients' homes. Typically, patients who need chronic transfusions but are otherwise stable physically are appropriate candidates for outpatient therapy. Verification and administration of the blood product are performed as in a hospital setting.

Method

Transfusing blood components are presented in Box 20-7.

Nursing Management

Nursing responsibilities include pretransfusion and posttransfusion assessment.

Pretransfusion Assessment

Patient history is an important component of the pretransfusion assessment to determine the history of previous transfusions as well as previous reactions to transfusion. The history should include the type of reaction, its manifestations, the interventions required, and whether any preventive interventions were used in subsequent transfusions. It is important to assess the number of pregnancies a woman has had because a high number can increase her risk for reaction due to antibodies developed from exposure to fetal circulation. Patients with blood disorders, such as sickle cell anemia or CLL, and patients who have received a stem cell transplant also may be at increased risk for transfusion reactions based on the number of previous transfusions. Other concurrent health problems should be noted, with careful attention to cardiac (particularly congestive heart failure with a decreased left ventricular ejection fraction), pulmonary, and vascular disease.

A systematic physical assessment and measurement of baseline vital signs are important before transfusing any blood product. The respiratory system should be assessed, including careful auscultation of the lungs and the patient's use of accessory muscles. Cardiac system assessment should include careful inspection for any edema as well as other signs of cardiac failure (e.g., jugular venous distention). The skin should be observed for rashes, petechiae, and ecchymoses. The sclera should be examined for icterus. In the event of a transfusion reaction, a comparison of findings can help differentiate between types of reactions.

> **Nursing Alert**
> *To evaluate a patient's response to therapy, the nurse is aware that when administering PRBCs it is expected that one unit of PRBCs will raise the hemoglobin by 1 g and HCT by 3%, if the patient is not bleeding or hemolyzing. If administering platelets (which generally consists of six units of pooled platelets from random donors [random donor platelets or RDP]), the count should increase by approximately 30,000 mm^3 in an adult of average size (Yuan & Goldfinger, 2016).*

Providing Patient Teaching

Reviewing the signs and symptoms of a transfusion reaction is crucial for patients who have not received a transfusion before. Even for patients who have received prior transfusions, a brief review of the signs and symptoms of transfusion reactions is essential. Signs and symptoms of a reaction include fever, chills, itching, hives, respiratory distress, low back pain, nausea, pain at the IV site, or anything "unusual." Although a thorough review is very important, it is also important to reassure the patient that the blood is tested carefully against the patient's own blood (crossmatched) to diminish the likelihood of any adverse reaction. Such assurance can be extremely beneficial in allaying anxiety.

Monitoring and Managing Potential Complications

Any patient who receives a blood transfusion may develop complications from that transfusion. When explaining the reasons for the transfusion, it is important to include the risks and benefits and what to expect during and after the transfusion. Patients must be informed that the supply of blood is not completely risk-free, although it has been tested carefully (Box 20-8). Nursing management is directed toward preventing complications, promptly recognizing complications if they develop, and promptly initiating measures to control complications. The following sections describe the most common or potentially severe transfusion-related complications. Table 20-7 summarizes potential long-term complications.

BOX 20-7 **Transfusion of Packed Red Blood Cells (PRBCs)**

Preprocedure

- Confirm that the transfusion has been prescribed.
- Confirm that a current type and screen of the patient's blood is on file per institution policy.
- Check that patient's blood has been typed and cross-matched.
- Verify that patient has been provided informed consent per institution or agency policy.
- Explain the procedure to the patient. Instruct the patient in signs and symptoms of transfusion reaction (itching, hives, swelling, shortness of breath, fever, chills).
- Take the patient's temperature, pulse, respiration, oxygen saturation, and blood pressure to establish a baseline for comparing vital signs during transfusion.
- Perform hand hygiene and wear gloves in accordance with Standard Precautions.
- Use a 20-gauge or larger needle for insertion in a large vein. Use special tubing that contains a blood filter to screen out fibrin clots and other particulate matter. Do not vent the blood container.

Procedure

- Obtain the PRBCs from the blood bank after the IV line is started and vital signs are assessed. (Institution policy may limit release to only one unit at a time.)
- Double-check the labels with another licensed provider (nurse, advanced practice provider, or physician) to make sure that the ABO group and Rh type agree with the compatibility record. Check to see that the number and type on the donor blood label and on the patient's chart are correct. Check the patient's identification by using two forms of identification (can include the patient's name, date of birth, and medical record number) comparing the blood product label to the patient identification bracelet. Also ask the patient to confirm his or her name and date of birth.
- Check the blood for gas bubbles and any unusual color or cloudiness. (Gas bubbles may indicate bacterial growth. Abnormal color or cloudiness may be a sign of hemolysis.)
- Make sure PRBC transfusion is initiated within 30 minutes after removal of the PRBCs from the blood bank refrigerator.
- For the first 15 minutes, run the transfusion slowly—no faster than 5 mL/min. Observe the patient carefully for adverse effects. If no adverse effects occur during the first 15 minutes, then increase the flow rate unless the patient is at high risk for circulatory overload.
- Monitor the patient closely for 15–30 minutes to detect signs of reaction. Monitor vital signs at regular intervals per institution or agency policy; compare the results with baseline measurements. Increase frequency of measurements based on the patient's condition. Observe the patient frequently throughout the transfusion for any signs of adverse reaction, including restlessness, hives, nausea, vomiting, torso or back pain, shortness of breath, flushing, hematuria, fever, or chills. Should any adverse reaction occur, stop infusion immediately, notify the health care provider, and follow the agency's transfusion reaction policy.
- Note that administration time does not exceed 4 hours because of the increased risk for bacterial growth.
- Be alert for signs of adverse reactions: circulatory overload, sepsis, febrile reaction, allergic reaction, and acute hemolytic reaction.
- Change blood tubing after every 2 units transfused to decrease the chance of bacterial contamination.

Postprocedure

- Obtain vital signs and compare them with baseline measurements.
- Dispose of used materials properly.
- Document the procedure in the patient's medical record, including patient assessment findings and tolerance to procedure.
- Monitor the patient for response to and effectiveness of the procedure.

Note: Never add medications to blood or blood products; if blood is too thick to run freely, normal saline may be added to the unit. If blood must be warmed, use an in-line blood warmer with a temperature monitoring system.

Note: Fresh-frozen platelets (FFP) require ABO but not Rh compatibility. Typically platelets are not cross-matched for ABO compatibility. Never add medications to blood or blood products. Both platelets and FFPs can be infused as rapidly as the patient can tolerate, based on fluid status and cardiac function.

Febrile Nonhemolytic Transfusion Reaction (FNHTR)

A febrile nonhemolytic transfusion reaction is defined by a temperature of 100.4°F or a 1°C (1.8°F) increase in temperature with or without chills during or within 4 hours following completion of a transfusion (Dasararaju & Marques, 2015). An FNHTR is caused by antibodies to donor leukocytes that remain in the unit of blood or blood component; it is the most common type of transfusion reaction, accounting for more than 90% of reactions. It occurs more frequently in patients who have had previous transfusions (exposure to multiple antigens from previous blood products) and in Rh-negative women who have borne Rh-positive children (exposure to an Rh-positive fetus raises antibody levels in the mother). These reactions occur in 1% of PRBC transfusions and 20% of platelet transfusions. Rates have declined since the standardization of leukocyte reduction, which significantly decreases the number of leukocytes in a transfused product, thus decreasing the risk of an antibody-antigen reaction (Silvergleid, 2016a, 2016b). More than 10% of patients with chronic transfusion requirements develop this type of reaction.

The diagnosis of a febrile nonhemolytic reaction is made by excluding other potential causes, such as a hemolytic

BOX 20-8   Diseases Transmitted by Blood Transfusion

Hepatitis (Viral Hepatitis B, C)

- Greater risk from pooled blood products and blood of paid donors than from volunteer donors
- Screening test detects most hepatitis B and C
- Transmittal risk estimated at 1:1 million for hep B and 1: 1.93 million for hep C (Leparc, 2015)

HIV and HTLV

- Donated blood screened for antibodies to HIV
- Transmittal risk estimated at 1:2.135 million (Leparc, 2015)
- People with high-risk behaviors (multiple sex partners, anal sex, IV/injection drug use) and people with signs and symptoms that suggest AIDS should not donate blood

Cytomegalovirus (CMV)

- Transmittal risk greater for premature newborns with CMV antibody-negative mothers and for immunocompromised recipients who are CMV-negative (e.g., those with acute leukemia, organ or tissue transplant recipients)
- Blood products rendered "leukocyte-reduced" help reduce the transmission of virus

Graft-Versus-Host Disease (GVHD)

- Occurs only in severely immunocompromised recipients (e.g., leukemia, bone marrow, and stem cell transplantation)
- Transfused lymphocytes engraft in the recipient and attack host lymphocytes or body tissues; signs and symptoms are fever, diffuse reddened skin rash, nausea, vomiting, diarrhea
- Preventive measures include irradiating blood products to inactivate donor lymphocytes (no known radiation risks to transfusion recipient) and processing donor blood with leukocyte-reduction filters

Creutzfeldt–Jakob Disease (CJD)

- Rare, fatal disease causing irreversible brain damage
- No evidence of transmittal by transfusion, but hemophiliacs and others are concerned that transmittal is possible
- All blood donors must be screened for positive family history of CJD. Those with a blood relative with CJD are not eligible to donate blood.
- Potential donors who spent 6 months or more in the United Kingdom (or Europe) from 1980 to 1996 cannot donate blood; blood products from a donor who develops CJD are recalled.

For more detailed guidelines regarding travel, CJD, and blood donations, please visit the American Red Cross website: http://www.redcrossblood.org/donating-blood/eligibility-requirements

---

reaction, sepsis, or bacterial contamination of the blood product. The signs and symptoms of a febrile nonhemolytic transfusion reaction are chills (minimal to severe) followed by fever. The fever typically begins within 2 hours after the transfusion is begun. Although the reaction is not life-threatening, the fever, and particularly the chills and muscle stiffness, can be frightening to the patient.

This reaction can be diminished, even prevented, by further depleting the blood component of donor leukocyte through filtration. Antipyretics can be given to prevent fever, but routine premedication is not advised because it can mask the beginning of a more serious transfusion reaction. For recurrent FNHTRs despite leukoreduction, washed PRBCs may be indicated (Dasararaju & Marques, 2015).

TABLE **20-7** Common Complications Resulting from Long-Term Packed Red Blood Cell (PRBC) Transfusion Therapy[a]

	Manifestation	Management
Infection	Hepatitis (B, C) Cytomegalovirus (CMV)	May immunize against hepatitis B; give alpha-interferon for hepatitis C; monitor liver function Use WBC filters to protect against CMV
Iron overload	Heart failure Endocrine failure (diabetes, hypothyroidism, hypoparathyroidism, hypogonadism)	Prevent or treat using iron chelation therapy
Transfusion reaction	Sensitization Febrile reactions	Diminish by RBC phenotyping, using WBC-filtered, leukocyte-reduced, or irradiated products

PRBC, packed RBCs; WBC, white blood cell; RBC, red blood cell.
[a]Patients with long-term transfusion therapy requirements are at risk not only for the transfusion reactions discussed in the text but also for the complications noted above. In many cases, the use of WBC-filtered (e.g., leukocyte-poor) blood products is standard for patients who receive long-term PRBC transfusion therapy. Blood product irradiation, which more effectively reduces the leukocytes in the product, is reserved for patients at highest risk for infection, alloimmunization, and GVHD. Iron chelation may be used in select populations to reduce iron burden.

Acute Hemolytic Reaction

The most dangerous, and potentially life-threatening, type of transfusion reaction occurs when the donor blood is incompatible with that of the recipient. Antibodies already present in the recipient's plasma rapidly combine with antigens on donor erythrocytes, and the erythrocytes are hemolyzed (destroyed) in the circulation (intravascular hemolysis). The most rapid hemolysis occurs in ABO incompatibility. This reaction can occur after transfusion of as little as 10 mL of PRBCs. Rh incompatibility often causes a less severe reaction. The most common causes of acute hemolytic reaction are errors in blood component labeling and patient misidentification that result in the administration of an ABO-incompatible transfusion (Dasararaju & Marques, 2015).

Symptoms consist of fever, chills, nausea, vomiting, chest tightness, dyspnea, hypotension, flank pain, hematuria, oliguria, bleeding, and anxiety (Dasararaju & Marques, 2015). As the erythrocytes are destroyed, the hemoglobin is released from the cells and excreted by the kidneys; therefore, hemoglobin appears in the urine (hemoglobinuria). Hypotension, bronchospasm, and vascular collapse may result. Diminished renal perfusion results in acute kidney failure, and DIC also may occur.

The reaction must be recognized promptly and the transfusion discontinued immediately. Blood and urine specimens must be obtained and analyzed for evidence of hemolysis, including DAT testing, haptoglobin, LDH, bilirubin, creatinine, PT/PTT, and fibrinogen. Treatment goals include maintaining blood volume and renal perfusion and preventing and managing DIC if needed. Acute hemolytic transfusion reactions are preventable. Meticulous attention to detail in labeling blood samples and blood components and accurately identifying the recipient cannot be overemphasized.

Delayed Hemolytic Reaction

Delayed hemolytic reactions usually occur within 14 days after transfusion, when the level of antibody has been increased to the extent that a reaction can occur. The hemolysis of the erythrocytes is extravascular via the RES and occurs gradually.

Signs and symptoms of a delayed hemolytic reaction are fever, anemia, increased bilirubin level, decreased or absent haptoglobin, and possibly jaundice. Rarely is there hemoglobinuria. In general, these reactions are not dangerous, but it is useful to recognize them because subsequent transfusions with blood products containing these antibodies may cause a more severe hemolytic reaction. However, recognition is also difficult because the patient may not be in a health care setting to be tested for this reaction, and even if the patient is hospitalized, the reaction may be too mild to be recognized clinically. Because the amount of antibody present can be too low to detect, it is difficult to prevent delayed hemolytic reactions. Fortunately, the reaction is usually mild and requires no intervention.

Allergic Reaction

Allergic reactions occur in 1% to 3% of transfusions. An allergic reaction is marked by the development of urticaria (hives) or generalized itching, rash, or wheezing during a transfusion (Dasararaju & Marques, 2015). The cause of these reactions is thought to be a sensitivity reaction to a plasma protein within the blood component being transfused. The reactions are usually mild and respond to antihistamines. If the symptoms resolve after administration of an antihistamine (e.g., diphenhydramine [Benadryl]), the transfusion may be resumed. Rarely, the allergic reaction is severe, with bronchospasm, laryngeal edema, and shock. These reactions are managed with epinephrine, corticosteroids, and pressor support, if necessary.

Giving the patient antihistamines before the transfusion may prevent future reactions. For severe reactions, future blood components are washed to remove any remaining plasma proteins. Leukocyte filters are not useful to prevent such reactions because the offending plasma proteins can pass through the filter.

Transfusion-Related Acute Lung Injury

Transfusion-related acute lung injury (TRALI) is defined as new-onset lung injury within 6 hours of transfusion with an oxygen saturation of at least 90% on room air and bilateral infiltrates on chest x-ray (Dasararaju & Marques, 2015). TRALI is caused by antibodies to human leukocyte antigens (HLAs) in the transfused blood product. Signs of TRALI include an onset of symptoms within 6 hours of transfusion; symptoms include dyspnea, cyanosis, hypotension, fever, chills, hypoxia, and/or pulmonary artery pressure below 18 mm Hg (and/or no evidence of circulatory overload/left atrial hypertension) (Dasararaju & Marques, 2015). TRALI is often a diagnosis of exclusion because symptoms overlap with other transfusion reaction types (e.g., transfusion-associated circulatory overload [TACO] and FNHTR). Workup should include exclusion of hemolysis, CBC (neutropenia may be seen with TRALI), and chest x-ray, which may reveal bilateral infiltrates. Treatment consists of respiratory support and pressors. Treatment with steroids has not been shown to provide benefits to the patient. Mortality rates are as high as 25%, but with aggressive support, 80% of patients recover within 96 hours (Dasararaju & Marques, 2015).

Transfusion-Associated Circulatory Overload

TACO is the second leading cause of transfusion-related death in the United States (Dasararaju & Marques, 2015). If too much blood is infused too quickly, hypervolemia can occur. Risk factors include older age, the number of units infused, history of CHF, COPD, anemia, or transfusion of plasma products (Dasararaju & Marques, 2015). PRBCs are safer to use than whole blood. If the administration rate is sufficiently slow, circulatory overload may be prevented. Patients receiving fresh-frozen plasma or even platelets may also develop circulatory overload. The infusion rate of these blood components must also be titrated to the patient's tolerance, and concurrent fluid administration should be avoided. Patients at risk must be monitored carefully. For patients who are at risk of, or already in, circulatory overload, diuretics are administered after the transfusion or between units of products (Dasararaju & Marques, 2015).

Nursing Alert
When administering blood products in patients at risk for TACO, the nurse considers all infusing IV solutions and informs the provider so that IV rates can be altered to lower rates while blood is infusing.

Signs of circulatory overload include dyspnea, orthopnea, tachycardia, and sudden anxiety. Jugular vein distention, crackles at the base of the lungs, and an increase in blood pressure can also occur. If the transfusion is continued, pulmonary edema can develop, as manifested by severe dyspnea and coughing up of pink, frothy sputum. These signs and symptoms usually present within 2 hours of initiation of transfusion but may take as long as 6 hours to manifest (Dasararaju & Marques, 2015).

If fluid overload is mild, often the transfusion can be continued after slowing the rate of infusion and administering diuretics. However, if the overload is severe, the patient is placed in an upright position with the feet in a dependent position, the transfusion is discontinued, and the provider is notified. The IV line is kept patent with a very slow infusion of normal saline solution or a saline or heparin lock device to maintain access to the vein in case IV medications are necessary. Oxygen and morphine may be needed to treat severe dyspnea.

Bacterial Contamination

The incidence of bacterial contamination of blood components is very low; however, administration of contaminated products puts the patient at great risk. Gram-negative bacteria, including *Pseudomonas*, *Yersinia*, and *Enterobacter*, are the most common organism found in contaminated RBC products, but *Serratia* can be present also (Spelman & MacLaren, 2016). Contamination can occur at any point during procurement or processing but is usually due to organisms on the donor's skin (Spelman & MacLaren, 2016). Many bacteria cannot survive in the cold temperatures used to store PRBCs, although some organisms can survive cold temperatures. Parasites that infect RBCs, such as *Babesia* or other species of malaria, are more likely to cause infection from RBCs (Dasararaju & Marques, 2015). Platelets are at greater risk of contamination because they are stored at room temperature. Since 2004, blood centers have developed rapid methods of culturing the platelet unit to decrease the risk of using a contaminated platelet unit for transfusion. Despite bacterial

testing, this complication has not been eradicated, thus mandating that nurses remain vigilant for this complication.

Preventive measures include meticulous care in the procurement and processing of blood components. When PRBCs or whole blood is transfused, it should be administered within a 4-hour period because warm room temperatures promote bacterial growth. A contaminated unit of blood product may appear normal, or it may have an abnormal color.

The signs of bacterial contamination are fever, chills, and hypotension, which most commonly occur during the transfusion. Occasionally, the signs of a reaction may occur hours after the transfusion is complete. If the condition is not recognized and treated immediately with fluids and broad-spectrum antibiotics, shock can occur. While these reactions are rare, they can be fatal (Spelman & MacLaren, 2016). The median interval between completion of transfusion and appearance of symptoms is 30 minutes (range 0 to 5 hours) (Spelman & MacLaren, 2016). Patient education must include prompt reporting of any signs of transfusion reaction at home and need for emergent evaluation.

The following steps are taken to determine the type and severity of the reaction:

- Stop the transfusion. Maintain the IV line with normal saline solution through new IV tubing, administered at a slow rate.
- Assess the patient carefully. Compare the vital signs with baseline. Assess the patient's respiratory status carefully. Note the presence of adventitious breath sounds, use of accessory muscles, extent of dyspnea, changes in mental status including anxiety and confusion, and changes in oxygen saturation. Note any chills, diaphoresis, jugular vein distention, and reports of back pain or urticaria.
- Notify the health care provider of the assessment findings, and implement any treatments prescribed. Continue to monitor the patient's vital signs and respiratory, cardiovascular, and renal status.
- Notify the blood bank that a suspected transfusion reaction has occurred.
- Send the blood container and tubing to the blood bank for repeat typing and culture. The identifying tags and numbers are verified.

If a hemolytic transfusion reaction or bacterial infection is suspected, the nurse does the following:

- Obtain appropriate blood specimens from the patient (this usually includes blood cultures, a CBC and a type and screen, LDH, DAT, haptoglobin).
- Collect a urine sample as soon as possible for a hemoglobin determination.
- Document the reaction according to the institution's policy.

CHAPTER REVIEW

Critical Thinking Exercises

1. You are working in a hematology-oncology clinic. The laboratory reports a critical laboratory result for one of your patients with possible acute leukemia: the leukocyte count is 1,200/mm^3 with 10% neutrophils. What other laboratory results would be important to review or consider? The patient is also anemic (hemoglobin 8.2 mg/dL), and platelets are 30,000/mm^3. What observations will you include in your assessment of this patient? Determine the extent to which this patient is neutropenic. What medical treatments would you anticipate? How would you educate the patient about neutropenia and bleeding precautions? What information do you need to obtain about the patient's home setting that will assist you in determining the patient's risk of developing an infection at home?

2. You are caring for a man with a chronic transfusion requirement (typically two to three units of PRBCs each month). He asks you how he should modify his diet so that "I don't need so much blood." How would you respond? What role do iron supplements play in patients with chronic transfusion needs? How would you assess this patient for iron overload?

3. You are caring for a patient who is septic and is now receiving a transfusion of two units of PRBCs. The patient's temperature spikes to 101.3°F (38.5°C) after half of the second unit has been transfused. What are the possible causes of the fever? What are the appropriate nursing interventions?

4. You are caring for a patient with acute leukemia and sepsis who has a declining platelet count of 10,000/mm^3. On assessment, you observe oozing blood from the Hickman catheter site, petechiae to the upper and lower extremities, and epistaxis. What are the potential causes of this patient's bleeding? What other laboratory results would you assess? What further assessments would you perform? What nursing interventions would you implement? What medical interventions would you anticipate?

NCLEX-Style Review Questions

1. A patient's 18-year-old son would like to donate blood. The nurse educates him regarding eligibility requirements for blood donation. Which statement demonstrates that he does not understand the education provided?
   a. "I am so glad that I am old enough to donate."
   b. "Because I just got a tattoo a week ago, I am unable to donate."
   c. "Because I live with a friend with HIV, I cannot donate."
   d. "Because my girlfriend has hepatitis, and we are sexually active, I cannot donate."

2. The nurse is explaining the potential signs and symptoms of a transfusion reaction to a patient who is receiving a first blood transfusion for the first time. How will the nurse ensure safe blood product administration? *Select all that apply.*
   a. Check ABO compatibility by comparing the blood product label to the patient's medical record.
   b. Use two patient identifiers, such as the patient's date of birth and name, to verify the blood product.
   c. Administer the blood product slowly for the first 15 minutes.
   d. Administer acetaminophen and diphenhydramine, which are standard premedications used in all transfused patients.
   e. Obtain baseline vital signs before the transfusion is administered.

3. A patient is being treated for sepsis. On the second day of receiving care, the patient experiences epistaxis and persistent bleeding from a venipuncture site. The nurse suspects DIC. Which laboratory result supports the nurse's suspicion?
   a. Increased fibrinogen, decreased PTT, decreased platelets
   b. Decreased fibrinogen, increased PTT, increased platelets
   c. Decreased fibrinogen, increased PTT, decreased platelets
   d. Increased fibrinogen, increased PTT, increased platelets

4. The nurse provides patient education related to the management of iron deficiency anemia. Which statement made by the patient signifies understanding of the education provided?
   a. "I should take my iron pills with a glass of orange juice."

b. "I should take my iron pills with breakfast to decrease stomach upset."

c. "Iron pills often cause constipation so I should decrease my fluid and fiber intake."

d. "I will need to take these pills for only a few days, and then my problem will be fixed."

5. The nurse is caring for a patient diagnosed with ALL who is receiving initial treatment. The patient has been complaining of a dry cough. The patient also has diminished breath sounds upon auscultation. What should the nurse monitor as priority with regard to potential complications in this patient?

a. Hemoglobin

b. Absolute neutrophil count (ANC)

c. Hematocrit

d. Urine

Try these additional resources, available at **http://thepoint.lww.com/Honan2e**, to enhance your learning and understanding of this chapter:

• NCLEX-Style Student Review Questions
• Journal Articles

REFERENCES AND SELECTED READINGS

References and selected readings associated with this chapter can be found on the website that accompanies the book. Visit **http://thepoint. lww.com/Honan2e** to access the references and other additional resources associated with this chapter.

Problems Related to Digestive, Gastrointestinal, and Metabolic Function

A 55-year-old patient is undergoing bariatric surgery to treat morbid obesity. She is 120 lb over her ideal body weight. The patient also has comorbidities of diabetes and hypertension.

- Discuss patient selection for bariatric surgery.
- What lifestyles changes might the patient expect?
- What complications should the patient be aware of regarding the surgical procedure?

Nursing Assessment: Digestive, Gastrointestinal, and Metabolic Function

Deborah Bains Fahs

Learning Objectives

After reading this chapter, you will be able to:

1. Describe the anatomy and physiology of the gastrointestinal (GI) tract.
2. Identify the metabolic functions of the liver.
3. Discuss important physical assessment findings of the GI tract.
4. Identify the assessment parameters used to determine the status of the upper and lower GI tract.

The gastrointestinal (GI) system performs the functions of ingestion, digestion, and elimination. Its major organs include the esophagus, stomach, small intestines, large intestines, pancreas, gallbladder, spleen, and liver (a most complex organ) (Drake, 2015). An understanding of the structure and function of the biliary tract and pancreas is essential to providing clinical care. Interruption of any of these functions can quickly affect the patient nutritionally and cause myriad fluid, electrolyte, and acid–base imbalances. When performing the GI assessment, the nurse must remember that the majority of people have pre-existing problems and that these problems can be exacerbated or new conditions can develop when illness in other systems occurs.

ANATOMIC AND PHYSIOLOGIC OVERVIEW OF THE DIGESTIVE SYSTEM

Anatomy of the Gastrointestinal Tract

The GI tract is a 23- to 26-foot-long (7 to 7.9 m) pathway that extends from the **mouth** to the esophagus, stomach, small and large intestines, and rectum, to the terminal structure, the **anus** (Fig. 21-1). The **esophagus** is located in the mediastinum, anterior to the spine and posterior to the trachea and heart. This hollow muscular tube, which is approximately 10 in (25 cm) long, passes through the diaphragm at an opening called the *diaphragmatic hiatus* (Reinus & Simon, 2014).

The remaining portion of the GI tract is located within the peritoneal cavity. The **stomach** is situated in the left upper portion of the abdomen under the left lobe of the liver and the diaphragm, overlaying most of the pancreas (see Fig. 21-1). A hollow muscular organ with a capacity of approximately 1,500 mL, the stomach stores food during eating, secretes digestive fluids, and propels the partially digested food into the small intestine. The gastroesophageal junction is the inlet to the stomach. The stomach has four anatomic regions: the cardia (entrance), fundus, body, and pylorus (outlet). Circular smooth muscle in the wall of the pylorus forms the pyloric sphincter and controls the opening between the stomach and the small intestine, allowing for both stomach emptying and prevention of regurgitation of intestinal contents back into the stomach (Porth, 2015).

The **small intestine** is the longest segment of the GI tract, accounting for about two thirds of the total length. It folds back and forth on itself, providing approximately 7,000 cm of surface area for secretion and **absorption,** the process by which nutrients enter the bloodstream through the intestinal walls. It has three sections: the most proximal section is the duodenum, where the common bile duct and pancreatic duct enter at the ampulla of Vater, allowing for the passage of both bile and pancreatic secretions. The middle section of the small intestine is the jejunum, and the distal section is the ileum. They terminate at the ileocecal valve. This valve, or sphincter, controls the flow of digested material from the ileum into the cecal portion of the large intestine, preventing reflux of bacteria into the small intestine. Attached to the cecum is the vermiform appendix, an appendage that has little or no physiologic function.

The **large intestine** consists of an ascending segment on the right side of the abdomen, a transverse segment that extends from right to left in the upper abdomen, and a

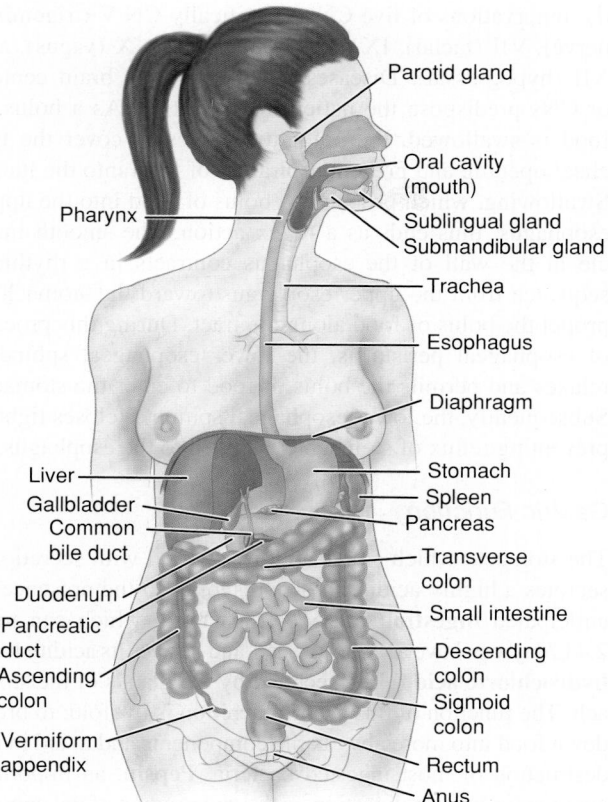

FIGURE 21-1 Organs of the digestive system and associated structures.

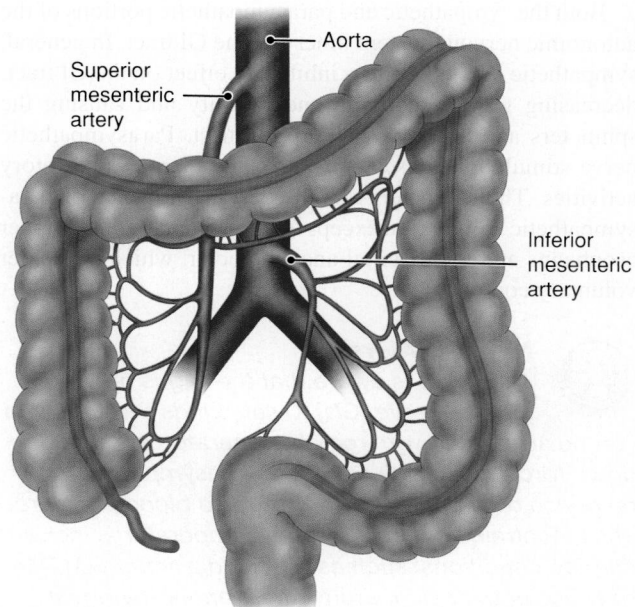

FIGURE 21-2 Anatomy and blood supply of the large intestine.

descending segment on the left side of the abdomen. Completing the terminal portion of the large intestine are the sigmoid colon, the rectum, and the anus. Regulating the anal outlet is a network of striated muscle, which forms both the internal and the external anal sphincters.

Nursing Alert

Since the sigmoid colon lies on the left side of the lower abdomen, the nurse understands that the best position for administration of an enema is left lateral position.

The GI tract receives blood from arteries that originate along the entire length of the thoracic and abdominal aorta and veins that return blood from the digestive organs and the spleen. This portal venous system is composed of five large veins: the superior mesenteric, inferior mesenteric, gastric, splenic, and cystic veins, which eventually form the vena portae that enters the liver. Once in the liver, the blood is distributed throughout and collected into the hepatic veins that then terminate in the inferior vena cava. Of particular importance are the gastric artery and the superior and inferior mesenteric arteries. Oxygen and nutrients are supplied to the stomach by the gastric artery and to the intestine by

the mesenteric arteries (Fig. 21-2). Venous blood is returned from the small intestine, cecum, and the ascending and transverse portions of the colon by the superior mesenteric vein, which corresponds with the distribution of the branches of the superior mesenteric artery. Blood flow to the GI tract is approximately 20% of the total cardiac output and increases significantly after eating.

The internal abdominal cavity is lined with peritoneum, which is the largest serous membrane in the body and which has a surface area similar to that of skin. The peritoneum is a single sheet that has visceral and parietal components. The visceral peritoneum covers the abdominal organs, and the parietal peritoneum lines the walls of the abdominal pelvic cavity. Between these two layers is a potential space containing fluid secreted by the serous membranes (Grossman & Porth, 2014). This space is sometimes accessed for diagnostic procedures, such as peritoneal tap to assess for internal injuries or catheter insertion for peritoneal dialysis. Organs that lie within the peritoneal cavity are called intraperitoneal organs, and include the liver, spleen, and appendix, among others. Structures that lie behind the parietal peritoneum are said to be *retroperitoneal*. A useful mnemonic for retroperitoneal organs is SAD PUCKER which stands for the suprarenal (adrenal) gland, aorta, duodenum, pancreas (except tail), ureters, colon (ascending and descending), kidneys, esophagus, and rectum.

A *mesentery* is a double layer of peritoneum that encircles internal organs such as the intestines and contains blood vessels, nerves, and lymphatic vessels. An *omentum* is a fold of mesentery that passes from the stomach to the organs in the abdominal cavity. It is a sheet that has mobility, cushions the abdominal organs against injury, and provides insulation against loss of body heat.

Both the sympathetic and parasympathetic portions of the autonomic nervous system innervate the GI tract. In general, sympathetic nerves exert an inhibitory effect on the GI tract, decreasing gastric secretion and motility and causing the sphincters and blood vessels to constrict. Parasympathetic nerve stimulation causes peristalsis and increases secretory activities. The sphincters relax under the influence of parasympathetic stimulation except for the sphincter of the upper esophagus and the external anal sphincter, which are under voluntary control.

 Nursing Alert
The nurse is aware that the vagus nerve (cranial nerve [CN] X) surrounds the anus and can be stimulated with rectal temperatures or bearing down forcefully, which causes a parasympathetic response of decreased heart rate and blood pressure. Thus, contraindications to rectal temperatures include cardiac conditions, such as myocardial infarction (MI), because of the risk of bradycardia and arrhythmias. In addition, recent rectal, anal, vaginal, and prostate surgeries would prohibit rectal temperatures because of proximity to the surgical site.

Function of the Digestive System

All cells of the body require nutrients. These nutrients are derived from the diet and need the GI system for digestion, absorption via blood or lymphatic channels, and elimination. Primary functions of the GI tract are the following:

- The breakdown of food particles into the molecular form for **digestion**
- The absorption into the bloodstream of small nutrient molecules produced by digestion
- The **elimination** of undigested unabsorbed foodstuffs and other waste products

After food is ingested, it is propelled through the GI tract, coming into contact with a wide variety of secretions that aid in its digestion, absorption, or elimination.

Chewing and Swallowing

The process of digestion begins with the act of chewing, in which food is broken down into small particles that can be swallowed and mixed with digestive enzymes. Eating—or even the sight, smell, or taste of food—can cause reflex salivation. Approximately 1.5 L of saliva is secreted daily from the parotid, submaxillary, and sublingual glands. Ptyalin, or salivary amylase, is an enzyme that begins the digestion of starches. Water and mucus, also contained in saliva, help lubricate the food as it is chewed, thereby facilitating swallowing.

Swallowing begins as a voluntary act that is regulated by the swallowing center in the medulla oblongata of the central nervous system (CNS). The act of swallowing requires the innervations of five CNs, specifically CN V (trigeminal nerve), VII (facial), IX (glossopharyngeal), X (vagus), and XII (hypoglossal). Diseases that disrupt the brain centers or CNs predispose the patient to aspiration. As a bolus of food is swallowed, the epiglottis moves to cover the tracheal opening and prevent aspiration of food into the lungs. Swallowing, which propels the bolus of food into the upper esophagus, thus ends as a reflex action. The smooth muscle in the wall of the esophagus contracts in a rhythmic sequence from the upper esophagus toward the stomach to propel the bolus of food along the tract. During this process of esophageal peristalsis, the lower esophageal sphincter relaxes and permits the bolus of food to enter the stomach. Subsequently, the lower esophageal sphincter closes tightly, preventing reflux of stomach contents into the esophagus.

Gastric Function

The stomach, which stores and mixes food with secretions, secretes a highly acidic fluid in response to the presence or anticipated **ingestion** of food. This fluid, which can total 2.4 L/day, can have a pH as low as 1 and derives its acidity from **hydrochloric acid** (HCl) secreted by the glands of the stomach. The function of this gastric secretion is twofold: to break down food into more absorbable components and to aid in the destruction of most ingested bacteria. **Pepsin**, an important enzyme for protein digestion, is the end product of the conversion of pepsinogen from the chief cells (Table 21-1). **Intrinsic factor**, also secreted by the gastric mucosa, combines with dietary vitamin B_{12} so that the vitamin can be absorbed in the ileum. In the absence of intrinsic factor, vitamin B_{12} cannot be absorbed and pernicious anemia results.

 Nursing Alert
The nurse is aware that critically ill patients may develop bleeding caused by stress ulceration. Thus it is common prophylactic practice to prescribe medications to suppress acid production of the stomach for patients at risk of stress ulcer bleeding (see Chapter 53 for Curling ulcer).

Peristaltic contractions in the stomach propel the stomach's contents toward the pylorus. Because large food particles cannot pass through the pyloric sphincter, they are churned back into the body of the stomach. In this way, food in the stomach is agitated mechanically and broken down into smaller particles. Food remains in the stomach for a variable length of time, from 30 minutes to several hours, depending on the volume, osmotic pressure, and chemical composition of the gastric contents. Peristalsis in the stomach and contractions of the pyloric sphincter allow the partially digested food to enter the small intestine at a rate that permits efficient absorption of nutrients. This partially digested food mixed with gastric secretions is called **chyme**. Hormones, neuroregulators, and local regulators

TABLE 21-1 The Major Digestive Enzymes and Secretions

Enzyme/Secretion	Enzyme Source	Digestive Action
Action of Enzymes That Digest Carbohydrates		
Ptyalin (salivary amylase)	Salivary glands	Starch → dextrin, maltose, glucose
Amylase	Pancreas and intestinal mucosa	Starch → dextrin, maltose, glucose Dextrin → maltose, glucose
Maltase	Intestinal mucosa	Maltose → glucose
Sucrase	Intestinal mucosa	Sucrose → glucose, fructose
Lactase	Intestinal mucosa	Lactose → glucose, galactose
Action of Enzymes/Secretions That Digest Protein		
Pepsin	Gastric mucosa	Protein → polypeptides
Trypsin	Pancreas	Proteins and polypeptides → polypeptides, dipeptides, amino acids
Aminopeptidase	Intestinal mucosa	Polypeptides → dipeptides, amino acids
Dipeptidase	Intestinal mucosa	Dipeptides → amino acids
Hydrochloric acid	Gastric mucosa	Protein → polypeptides, amino acids
Action of Enzymes Secretions That Digest Fat (Triglyceride)		
Pharyngeal lipase	Pharynx mucosa	Triglycerides → fatty acids, diglycerides, monoglycerides
Steapsin	Gastric mucosa	Triglycerides → fatty acids, diglycerides, monoglycerides
Pancreatic lipase	Pancreas	Triglycerides → fatty acids, diglycerides, monoglycerides
Bile	Liver and gallbladder	Fat emulsification

found in the gastric secretions control the rate of gastric secretions and influence gastric motility (Table 21-2).

Small Intestine Function

The digestive process continues in the duodenum. Duodenal secretions come from the accessory digestive organs—the pancreas, liver, and gallbladder—and the glands in the wall of the intestine itself. These secretions contain digestive enzymes: amylase, lipase, and bile. Pancreatic secretions have an alkaline pH due to their high concentration of bicarbonate. This alkalinity neutralizes the acid entering the duodenum from the stomach. Digestive enzymes secreted by the pancreas include **trypsin**, which aids in digesting protein; **amylase**, which aids in digesting starch; and **lipase**, which aids in digesting fats. These secretions drain into the pancreatic duct, which empties into the duodenum along with the common bile duct at a short dilated tube called the *hepatopancreatic ampulla*, or ampulla of Vater. Bile, secreted by the liver and stored in the gallbladder, aids in emulsifying ingested fats, making them easier to digest and absorb. The sphincter of Oddi (muscle tissue at the confluence of

the common bile duct and the duodenum) controls the flow of bile. When this sphincter is closed, bile will move back into the common bile duct and gallbladder. Hormones, neuroregulators, and local regulators found in these intestinal secretions control the rate of intestinal secretions and also influence GI motility. Intestinal secretions total approximately 1 L/day of pancreatic juice, 0.5 L/day of bile, and 3 L/day of secretions from the glands of the small intestine. Tables 21-1 and 21-2 give further information about the actions of digestive enzymes and GI regulatory substances.

Two types of contractions occur regularly in the small intestine: segmentation contractions and intestinal peristalsis. *Segmentation contractions* produce mixing waves that move the intestinal contents back and forth in a churning motion. *Intestinal peristalsis* propels the contents of the small intestine toward the colon. Both movements are stimulated by the presence of chyme.

Food, initially ingested in the form of fats, proteins, and carbohydrates, is broken down into absorbable particles (constituent nutrients) by the process of digestion. Carbohydrates are broken down into disaccharides (e.g., sucrose, maltose, and galactose) and monosaccharides (e.g., glucose,

TABLE **21-2** The Major Gastrointestinal Regulatory Substances

Substance	Stimulus for Production	Target Tissue	Effect on Secretions	Effect on Motility
Neuroregulators				
Acetylcholine	Sight, smell, chewing food, stomach distention	Gastric glands, other secretory glands, gastric and intestinal muscle	Increased gastric acid	Generally increased; decreased sphincter tone
Norepinephrine	Stress, other various stimuli	Secretory glands, gastric and intestinal muscle	Generally inhibitory	Generally decreased; increased sphincter tone
Hormonal Regulators				
Gastrin	Stomach distention with food	Gastric glands	Increased secretion of gastric juice, which is rich in HCl	Increased motility of stomach, decreased time required for gastric emptying Relaxation of ileocecal sphincter Excitation of colon Constriction of gastroesophageal sphincter
Cholecystokinin	Fat in duodenum	Gallbladder Pancreas Stomach	Release of bile into duodenum Increased production of enzyme-rich pancreatic secretions Inhibits gastric secretion somewhat	Delays gastric emptying
Secretin	pH of chyme in duodenum below 4–5	Stomach Pancreas	Inhibits gastric secretion somewhat Increased production of bicarbonate-rich pancreatic juice	Inhibits stomach contractions
Local Regulator				
Histamine	Unclear; substances in food	Gastric glands	Increased gastric acid production	Increased bowel peristalsis

fructose). Glucose is the major carbohydrate that tissue cells use as fuel. Proteins are a source of energy after they are broken down into amino acids and peptides. Ingested fats become monoglycerides and fatty acid by the process of emulsification, which makes them smaller and, therefore, easier to absorb. Chyme stays in the small intestine for 3 to 6 hours, allowing for continued breakdown and absorption of nutrients.

Small, finger-like projections called villi are present throughout the entire intestine and function to produce digestive enzymes as well as to absorb nutrients. Absorption is the primary function of the small intestine. Vitamins and minerals are not digested but rather absorbed essentially unchanged. The process of absorption begins in the jejunum and is accomplished by both active transport and diffusion across the intestinal wall into circulation. Nutrients are absorbed at specific locations throughout the small intestine and duodenum, whereas fats, proteins, carbohydrates, sodium, and chloride are absorbed in the jejunum. Vitamin B_{12} and bile salts are absorbed in the ileum. Magnesium, phosphate, and potassium are absorbed throughout the small intestine.

Colon Function

Within 4 hours after eating, residual waste material passes into the terminal ileum and slowly into the proximal portion of the right colon through the ileocecal valve. With each peristaltic wave of the small intestine, the valve opens briefly and permits some of the contents to pass into the colon.

It is estimated that there are 300 to 500 different species of intestinal bacteria in the large intestine (Grossman & Porth, 2014), which maintain intestinal homeostasis and are critical to human health (Friedman & Sitaraman, 2012).

Bacteria have many favorable benefits, such as modulating the immune system, producing some vitamins as well as fatty acids (Jensen-Jarolin, 2014). This intestinal flora also provides a critical resistance to potential invading pathogens. The nurse is aware that broad-spectrum antibiotics have the potential to disrupt this normal intestinal flora and place the patient at risk for overgrowth of pathogens, such as *Clostridium difficile*. Probiotics, such as lactobacilli, are live organisms considered healthy for the host organisms and often are administered to restore the microbial balance in the intestines.

Two types of colonic secretions are added to the residual material: an electrolyte solution and mucus. The electrolyte solution is chiefly a bicarbonate solution that acts to neutralize the end products formed by the colonic bacterial action, whereas the mucus protects the colonic mucosa from the interluminal contents.

Slow, weak peristaltic activity moves the colonic contents along the tract. This slow transport allows for efficient reabsorption of water and electrolytes, which is the primary purpose of the colon. The waste materials from a meal eventually reach and distend the rectum, usually in about 12 hours. As much as 25% of the waste materials from a meal may still be in the rectum 3 days after the meal was ingested.

Nursing Alert

Approximately 9 L of fluid are sent through the GI tract daily, and all but 100 mL are reabsorbed; thus the nurse is aware that any process or pathology that increases peristalsis will result in decreased fluid, nutrient, and electrolyte reabsorption, resulting in malnutrition, profound dehydration, and electrolyte depletion.

Waste Products of Digestion

Feces consist of undigested food, inorganic materials, water, and bacteria. Fecal matter is approximately 75% fluid and 25% solid material. The composition is relatively unaffected by alterations in diet because a large portion of the fecal mass is of nondietary origin, derived from the secretions of the GI tract. The brown color of the feces results from the breakdown of bile by the intestinal bacteria. Chemicals formed by intestinal bacteria are responsible in large part for the fecal odor. Gases formed contain methane, hydrogen sulfide, and ammonia, among others. The GI tract normally contains approximately 150 mL of these gases, which are either absorbed into the portal circulation and detoxified by the liver or expelled from the rectum as flatus.

Elimination of stool begins with distention of the rectum, which reflexively initiates contractions of the rectal musculature and relaxes the normally closed internal anal sphincter. The internal sphincter is controlled by the autonomic nervous system; the external sphincter is under the conscious control of the cerebral cortex. During defecation, the external anal sphincter voluntarily relaxes to allow colonic contents to be expelled. Normally, the external anal sphincter is maintained in a state of tonic contraction. Thus, defecation is seen to be a spinal reflex (involving the parasympathetic nerve fibers) that can be inhibited voluntarily by keeping the external anal sphincter closed. Contracting the abdominal muscles (straining) facilitates emptying of the colon. The average frequency of defecation in humans is once daily, but this varies among people.

ACCESSORY DIGESTIVE ORGANS

Liver

The liver, the largest gland of the body, can be considered a chemical factory that manufactures, stores, alters, and excretes a large number of substances involved in metabolism. The location of the liver is essential in this function because it receives nutrient-rich blood directly from the GI tract and then either stores or transforms these nutrients into chemicals that are used elsewhere in the body for metabolic needs. The liver is especially important in the synthesis of glucose, protein, and blood-clotting factors.

An important and unique characteristic of the liver is its ability to regenerate. The normal liver maintains a constant mass regulated by the metabolic needs and size of the person. After removal or injury of liver tissue, hepatocytes proliferate to replace the mass of the liver to its original size (Harvard Stem Cell Institute, 2014). This physiologic feature is important in the event of liver transplant (Cotler, Brown, & Travis, 2015). Thus, the liver displays an extraordinary ability to regenerate cells through matrix remodeling; however, chronic damage results in depletion of this cell pool and subsequent liver failure (Karkampouna, Goumans, Ten Dijke, Dooley, & Kruithof-de Julio, 2014).

The major functions of the liver include glucose metabolism, conversion of ammonia to urea, protein metabolism, fat metabolism, vitamin and iron storage, drug metabolism, bile formation, and bilirubin excretion.

Bile, which is manufactured by the liver and plays a major role in the digestion and absorption of fats in the GI tract, is stored temporarily in the gallbladder until it is needed for digestion, at which time the gallbladder empties and bile enters the intestine (Fig. 21-3). Waste products removed by the liver are secreted into bile. The smallest bile ducts, called *canaliculi*, are located between the lobules of the liver. The canaliculi receive secretions from the hepatocytes and carry them to larger bile ducts, which eventually form the hepatic duct. The hepatic duct from the liver and the cystic duct from the gallbladder join to form the common bile duct, which empties into the small intestine. The sphincter of Oddi, located at the junction where the common bile duct enters the duodenum, controls the flow of bile into the intestine.

The liver is located behind the ribs in the upper right portion of the abdominal cavity and, under normal conditions,

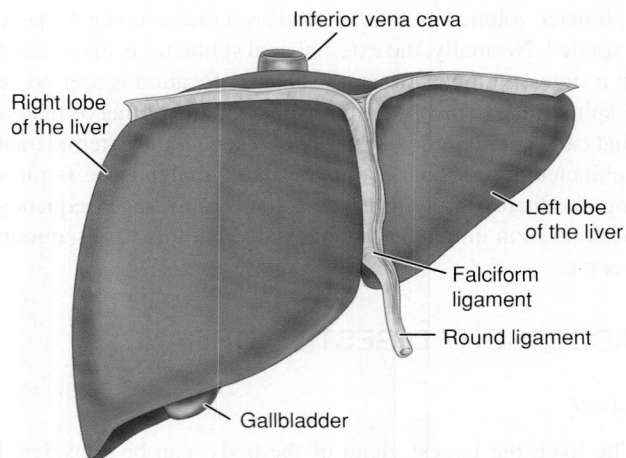

FIGURE 21-3 The liver and biliary system.

FIGURE 21-4 A section of liver lobule showing the location of hepatic veins, hepatic cells, liver sinusoids, and branches of the portal vein and hepatic artery.

cannot be palpated as it lies within the rib cage. It weighs approximately 1,800 g in men and 1,400 g in women and is divided into two large lobes and two smaller lobes. A thin layer of connective tissue surrounds each lobe, extending into the lobe itself and dividing the liver mass into small, functional units called *lobules* (Tortora & Derrickson, 2014).

The circulation of the blood into and out of the liver is of major importance to liver function. The blood that perfuses the liver comes from two sources. Approximately 75% of the blood supply comes from the portal vein, which drains the GI tract and is rich in nutrients. The remainder of the blood supply enters by way of the hepatic artery and is rich in oxygen. Terminal branches of these two blood vessels join to form common capillary beds, which constitute the sinusoids of the liver (Fig. 21-4). Thus, a mixture of venous and arterial blood bathes the liver cells (hepatocytes). The sinusoids empty into venules that occupy the center of each liver lobule and are called the *central veins*. The central veins join to form the hepatic vein, which constitutes the venous drainage from the liver and empties into the inferior vena cava, close to the diaphragm. Thus, there are two sources of blood flowing into the liver and only one exit pathway. Because of the pressure differences between the hepatic and portal veins, the liver normally stores approximately 500 to 1,000 mL of blood (Grossman & Porth, 2014), which can be available in times of hypovolemia. However, in conditions such as right heart failure, in which blood flows back up in the vena cava, additional blood accumulates in the liver.

In addition to hepatocytes, phagocytic cells belonging to the reticuloendothelial system (RES) are present in the liver. Other organs that contain reticuloendothelial cells are the spleen, bone marrow, lymph nodes, and lungs. In the liver, these cells are called *Kupffer cells*. As the most common phagocyte in the human body, their main function is to engulf particulate matter (e.g., bacteria) that enters the liver through the portal blood.

The Gallbladder

The gallbladder, a pear-shaped, hollow, saclike organ, 7.5 to 10 cm (3 to 4 in) long, lies in a shallow depression on the inferior surface of the liver, to which it is attached by loose connective tissue. The capacity of the gallbladder is 30 to 50 mL of bile. Its wall is composed largely of smooth muscle. The gallbladder is connected to the common bile duct by the cystic duct (Fig. 21-5).

The gallbladder functions as a storage area for bile. Between meals, when the sphincter of Oddi is closed, bile

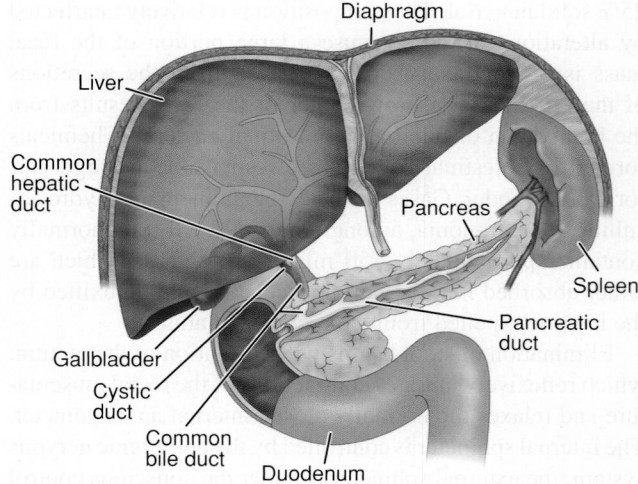

FIGURE 21-5 The liver, biliary system, and pancreas.

produced by the hepatocytes enters the gallbladder. During storage, a large portion of the water in bile is absorbed through the walls of the gallbladder so that gallbladder bile is five to ten times more concentrated than that originally secreted by the liver. When food enters the duodenum, the gallbladder contracts and the sphincter of Oddi relaxes, which allows the bile to enter the intestine. This response is mediated by secretion of the hormone **cholecystokinin-pancreozymin (CCK-PZ)** from the intestinal wall.

Bile is composed of water and electrolytes (sodium, potassium, calcium, chloride, and bicarbonate) along with significant amounts of lecithin, fatty acids, cholesterol, bilirubin, and bile salts. The bile salts, together with cholesterol, assist in emulsification of fats in the distal ileum. Then they are reabsorbed into the portal blood for return to the liver, after which they are excreted into the bile once again. This pathway from hepatocytes to bile to intestine and back to the hepatocytes is called the *enterohepatic circulation*. Because of the enterohepatic circulation, only a small fraction of the bile salts that enters the intestine are excreted in the feces. This decreases the need for active synthesis of bile salts by the liver cells.

Approximately half of the bilirubin, a pigment derived from the breakdown of red blood cells, is converted by the intestinal flora into urobilinogen, a highly soluble substance. Urobilinogen is either excreted in the feces or returned to the portal circulation, where it is re-excreted into the bile.

If the flow of bile is impeded (e.g., by gallstones in the bile ducts), bilirubin does not enter the intestine. As a result, blood levels of bilirubin increase and cause a characteristic yellow hue to the skin, termed *jaundice*, and yellowing of the sclera, termed *icterus*. Increased levels of bilirubin cause increased renal excretion of urobilinogen, resulting in dark-colored urine, which, since bile is a soap, will be frothy when agitated. If the bile is prevented from entering the small intestine, clay-colored stool will be noted. Bile salts are also irritating to the skin, thus the nurse is alert for complaints of itchy skin or pruritus. These changes produce many of the signs and symptoms seen in gallbladder disorders.

The Pancreas

The pancreas, located in the upper abdomen, has **endocrine** as well as **exocrine** functions (see Fig. 21-5). The exocrine functions include secretion of pancreatic enzymes into the GI tract through the pancreatic duct. The endocrine functions include secretion of insulin, glucagon, and somatostatin directly into the bloodstream.

The Exocrine Pancreas

The secretions of the exocrine portion of the pancreas are collected in the pancreatic duct, which joins the common bile duct and enters the duodenum at the ampulla of Vater. Surrounding the ampulla is the sphincter of Oddi, which partially controls the rate at which secretions from the pancreas and the gallbladder enter the duodenum.

The secretions of the exocrine pancreas are digestive enzymes high in protein content and an electrolyte-rich fluid; they include amylase, trypsin, and lipase. The secretions, which are very alkaline because of their high concentration of sodium bicarbonate, are capable of neutralizing the highly acidic gastric juice that enters the duodenum. Hormones originating in the GI tract stimulate the secretion of these exocrine pancreatic juices. The hormone **secretin** is the major stimulus for increased bicarbonate secretion from the pancreas, and the major stimulus for digestive enzyme secretion is the hormone CCK-PZ. The vagus nerve also influences exocrine pancreatic secretion.

The Endocrine Pancreas

The islets of Langerhans, the endocrine part of the pancreas, are collections of cells embedded in the pancreatic tissue. They are composed of alpha, beta, and delta cells. The hormone produced by the beta cells is called *insulin*. The alpha cells secrete glucagon, and the delta cells secrete somatostatin. Refer to Chapter 30 for details on insulin and glucagon secretion.

Somatostatin is a hormone secreted in the pancreas, the stomach, and the small intestine. It decreases GI activity after ingestion of food and also acts in the islets of Langerhans to inhibit the release of insulin and glucagon (Grossman & Porth, 2014). By decreasing the transit time and inhibiting insulin and glucagon, it is proposed that absorption of foodstuffs and nutrients is enhanced.

Spleen

The spleen is a large lymphoid organ located high in the left upper abdominal cavity near ribs 9 and 11 (posterior to the midaxillary line), and rib fractures in this region should alert the nurse to potential splenic laceration. The spleen is highly vascular and is frequently injured in cases of blunt trauma. The spleen filters antigens from the blood, removes old or abnormal RBCs, and is responsible for immune response to infection because it is rich with B- and T-cell lymphocytes. The spleen in a healthy adult is approximately 9 to 13 cm (3.5 to 5.1 in) in length. It cannot be palpated unless significantly enlarged.

Gerontologic Considerations

Although an increased prevalence of several common GI disorders occurs in the elderly population, normal digestion and absorption occurs in the elderly. Thus, aging per se appears to have minimal direct effect on most GI functions, in large part because of the functional reserve of the GI tract (Table 21-3). However, since the rate of cell growth declines and tissues atrophy with aging, there is an increased susceptibility to age-related GI disorders. Common problems in the elderly range from constipation or acid reflux to

TABLE 21-3 GERONTOLOGIC CONSIDERATIONS / Age-Related Changes of the Gastrointestinal System

Component	Structural Changes	Implications
Oral Cavity and Pharynx	• Injury/loss or decay of teeth • Atrophy of taste buds • Decreased saliva production • Reduced ptyalin and amylase in saliva • Atrophy of gingival tissue	Difficulty chewing and swallowing
Esophagus	• Decreased motility and emptying • Weakened gag reflex • Decreased resting pressure of lower esophageal sphincter • Decreased muscle tone and weakness in lower esophageal sphincter	Reflux and heartburn Dysphagia (difficulty swallowing) Dyspepsia (indigestion)
Stomach	• Degeneration and atrophy of gastric mucosal surfaces with decreased production of HCl • Decreased secretion of gastric acids and most digestive enzymes • Decreased motility and emptying	Delayed gastric emptying Food intolerances Malabsorption Decrease in absorption of iron and vitamin B_{12} Anorexia Anemia
Small Intestine	• Atrophy of muscle and mucosal surfaces • Thinning of villi and epithelial cells	Decreased motility and transit time, which lead to complaints of indigestion and constipation
Large Intestine	• Decrease in mucus secretion • Decrease in elasticity of rectal wall • Decreased tone of internal anal sphincter • Slower and duller nerve impulses in rectal area	Decreased absorption of nutrients (dextrose, fats, calcium, and iron), leading to decreased sensation to defecate and increased constipation Fecal incontinence from decrease or loss of sphincter control
Liver	• Decrease in size and weight • Decrease in total hepatic blood flow • Decreased phagocytosis by the Kupffer cells • Decreased drug metabolism	Decreases in size proportional to decreases in body size and weight Increased incidence of hepatitis B Increased incidence of liver abscesses Increased incidence of drug toxicity

life-threatening occurrences of infectious colitis or bowel ischemia. In addition to the increased prevalence of diseases such as diverticulitis and colon cancer in older patients, the role of polypharmacy needs to be considered. The use of non-steroidal anti-inflammatory drugs (NSAIDs), aspirin, or anti-coagulants is a risk factor for ulceration or bleeding. Since symptoms may be subtle, the nurse needs to be alert for a variety of potential GI diseases in the elderly (Hall, 2014).

ASSESSMENT

Health History

A focused GI assessment begins with a complete history. Information about abdominal pain, appetite changes, dyspepsia, gas, nausea and vomiting, diarrhea, constipation, fecal incontinence, and previous GI disease is investigated. Past and current medication use and any previous diagnostic studies, treatments, and surgery are noted.

The initial presentation of a patient with liver disease varies greatly and can range from elevated liver enzymes on routine screening with no clinical signs or symptoms of disease to the patient who presents in liver failure with **jaundice**, **hepatic coma**, or esophageal bleeding. A comprehensive and complete health history is critical to determine exposure to hepatotoxic substances (including alcohol) or infectious agents causing liver dysfunction and to distinguish between acute and chronic liver dysfunction.

Current History

Current nutritional status is ascertained. The nurse and patient discuss changes in appetite or eating patterns and any unexplained weight gain or loss over the past year. A complete metabolic panel, including liver function studies, triglyceride levels, iron studies, and complete blood count (CBC) are obtained.

Questions are raised about the use of tobacco and alcohol and include the need for detailed answers about type, amount, length of use, and the date of discontinuation, if any. It is also important to include questions about psychosocial, spiritual, or cultural factors that may be affecting the patient.

If liver disease is suspected because of clinical manifestations or abnormal liver function tests, the health history focuses on previous exposure of the patient to hepatotoxic substances or infectious agents. Lifestyle behaviors that increase the risk for exposure to infectious agents are identified. The patient's history of alcohol and drug use, including but not limited to the use of IV injection drugs, provides additional information about exposure to toxins and infectious agents. The patient's occupational, recreational, and travel history may assist in identifying exposure to hepatotoxins (e.g., industrial chemicals, other toxins). Travel to endemic areas such as Asia, Africa, the Middle East, and Central America may indicate a risk for hepatitis E (Friedman, Chopra, & Travis, 2015). Sexual practices may be a potential risk factor for liver disease (Grossman & Porth, 2014). The amount and type of alcohol consumption are identified using screening questionnaires that have been developed for this purpose. Men who consume 210 g of alcohol per week and women who consume 140 g per week are estimated to be at high risk for alcoholic cirrhosis; an alcoholic drink generally contains about 14 g of alcohol (Chalasani et al., 2012). The nurse is aware that the impact of alcohol-induced liver injury or disease is increased in the presence of other risk factors, such as hepatitis C (Kasper et al., 2015).

Many medications (including acetaminophen, ketoconazole, and valproic acid) are responsible for liver dysfunction and disease. Acetaminophen overdose can result in **fulminant hepatic failure**, while chronic liver disease is commonly caused by alcohol and viruses, such as hepatitis B or C. A prior history of inflammatory bowel disease or ulcerative colitis may lead to the diagnosis of primary sclerosing cholangitis. Patients with nonalcoholic fatty liver disease (NAFLD) may frequently have a medical history of diabetes, hyperlipidemia, and obesity.

A thorough medication history to assess liver dysfunction should address all current and past prescription medications, over-the-counter medications, herbal remedies, and dietary supplements.

Past History

The history also includes an evaluation of the client's medical history to identify risk factors for liver disease. Current and past medical conditions, including those of a psychological or psychiatric nature, are identified. The family history includes questions about familial liver disorders that may have their origin in alcohol abuse or gallstone disease as well as other familial or genetic diseases, such as hemochromatosis, Wilson disease, or alpha$_1$-antitrypsin disease (Friedman et al., 2014; Kasper et al., 2015). A positive family history of hepatitis B may indicate vertical transmission (infection transmitted from mother to child [embryo, fetus, or baby] during pregnancy or childbirth) (Kubo et al., 2014).

Common Complaints

Pain

Pain can be a major symptom of GI disease. Pain may be described as visceral; that is, nociceptors in the abdominal organs are stimulated and the pain is often described by patients as cramping, aching, squeezing, or colicky and difficult to pinpoint. Parietal pain occurs when the parietal peritoneum is inflamed, as occurs with appendicitis. It is a steady, severe pain that may be localized. Referred pain is pain that travels to a more distant site, where it localizes or presents. The character, duration, pattern, frequency, location, and distribution of referred pain (Fig. 21-6) vary greatly depending on the underlying cause. Other factors such as meals, rest, activity, and defecation patterns may directly affect this pain.

> **! Nursing Alert**
> *The pain of appendicitis initially presents as vague discomfort in the periumbilical area. As the inflammatory process progresses to involve the parietal peritoneum, the pain localizes to the right lower quadrant. The nurse maintains a high degree of suspicion of appendicitis for patients complaining of abdominal pain, nausea, anorexia, and "migratory" pain.*

FIGURE 21-6 Common sites of referred abdominal pain.

Dyspepsia

Dyspepsia, which is upper abdominal discomfort or distress associated with eating (commonly called *indigestion*) is the most common symptom of clients with GI dysfunction. Indigestion is an imprecise term that refers to a host of upper abdominal or epigastric symptoms, such as pain, discomfort, fullness, bloating, early satiety, belching, heartburn, and regurgitation; it occurs in approximately 25% of the adult population. Typically, fatty foods cause the most discomfort because they remain in the stomach for digestion longer than proteins or carbohydrates. Salads and coarse vegetables, as well as highly seasoned foods, may also cause considerable GI distress.

Intestinal Gas

The accumulation of gas in the GI tract may result in belching (expulsion of gas from the stomach through the mouth) or flatulence (expulsion of gas from the rectum). Usually, gases in the small intestine pass into the colon and are released as flatus. Patients often complain of bloating, distention, or feeling "full of gas," with excessive flatulence as a symptom of food intolerance or gallbladder disease.

Nausea and Vomiting

Nausea is a vague, intensely unsettling sensation of sickness or "queasiness" that may or may not be followed by vomiting. It can be triggered by odors, activity, medications, or food intake. The emesis, or vomitus, may vary in color and content and may contain undigested food particles, blood (hematemesis), or bilious material mixed with gastric juices. The causes of nausea and vomiting are many. Nausea and vomiting may result from visceral afferent stimulation (i.e., dysmotility, peritoneal irritation, infections, hepatobiliary or pancreatic disorders, mechanical obstruction); CNS disorders (i.e., vestibular disorders, increased intracranial pressure, infections, psychogenic conditions); and irritation of the chemoreceptor trigger zone from radiation therapy, systemic disorders, and antitumor chemotherapy medications.

Change in Bowel Habits and Stool Characteristics

Changes in bowel habits may signal colonic dysfunction or disease. Diarrhea, an abnormal increase in the frequency of bowel movements and liquidity of the stool or in daily stool weight or volume, commonly occurs when the contents move so rapidly through the intestine and colon that there is inadequate time for the GI secretions and oral contents to be absorbed. Typically this physiologic function is associated with abdominal pain or cramping and nausea or vomiting. Constipation, a decrease in the frequency of bowel movements, or stools that are hard, dry, and of smaller volume than normal, may be associated with anal discomfort and rectal bleeding.

The characteristics of the stool can vary greatly. Stool is normally light to dark brown; however, specific disease processes and ingestion of certain foods and medications

TABLE 21-4 Foods and Medications That Alter Stool Color

Altering Substance	Color
Meat protein	Dark brown
Spinach	Green
Carrots and beets	Red
Cocoa	Dark red or brown
Senna	Yellow
Bismuth, iron, licorice, and charcoal	Black
Barium	Milky white

may change the appearance of stool (Table 21-4). Blood in the stool can present in various ways and must be investigated. If blood is shed in sufficient quantities into the upper GI tract, it produces a tarry-black color (melena), whereas blood entering the lower portion of the GI tract or passing rapidly through will cause the stool to appear bright or dark red. Lower rectal or anal bleeding is suspected if there is streaking of blood on the surface of the stool or if blood is noted on toilet tissue. Other common abnormalities in stool characteristics described by the patient may include:

- Bulky, greasy, foamy stools that are foul in odor and may or may not float
- Light-gray or clay-colored stool, caused by a decrease or absence of conjugated bilirubin
- Stool with mucus threads or pus that may be visible on gross inspection of the stool
- Small, dry, rock-hard masses occasionally streaked with blood
- Loose, watery stool that may or may not be streaked with blood

Nursing Alert

Melena, or black "tarry" stools, occurs in association with upper GI bleeding from the esophagus, stomach, duodenum, or small intestine. Melena can result after blood loss in an amount as small as 60 mL and is caused by stomach acid (hydrochloric acid) or intestinal bacterial conversion of hemoglobin to the black pigment hematin. Pseudomelena, or false melena, is associated with ingestion of iron. The term hematochezia *refers to stools that are maroon or bright red in color, signifying a bleeding below the ligament of Treitz (duodenum level) but may be associated with a rapid upper GI bleed.*

Jaundice

When the bilirubin concentration in the blood is elevated abnormally, all the body tissues, including the sclerae and the skin, become tinged yellow or greenish yellow, a condition called **jaundice**. Jaundice becomes clinically evident when the serum bilirubin level exceeds 2.5 mg/dL (43 μmol/L). The elevated bilirubin stains tissues and fluid, but jaundice is seen most frequently in the sclera (icteris) (Grossman & Porth, 2014). Increased serum bilirubin levels and jaundice may result from impairment of hepatic uptake, conjugation of bilirubin, or excretion of bilirubin into the biliary system. There are several types of jaundice: hemolytic, hepatocellular, and obstructive jaundice, and jaundice due to hereditary hyperbilirubinemia. Hepatocellular and obstructive jaundice are the two types commonly associated with liver disease (refer to Chapter 25).

Pathophysiology Alert

A normal direct bilirubin is 0.0 to 0.3 mg/dL (Hall, 2014). Bilirubin, which gives bile its color, may be reported as direct (conjugated or combined in a molecule similar to glucose) or indirect (termed free or unconjugated). The direct bilirubin reflects bilirubin excreted by the GI tract, whereas indirect bilirubin reflects what normally circulates in the bloodstream (Daniels, 2014). Both are elevated in a variety of disorders since bilirubin is produced in the liver, spleen, and bone marrow.

Ascites

Ascites is an increased accumulation of peritoneal fluid in the abdomen caused by a variety of disorders associated with the liver. One factor associated with development of ascites is portal hypertension and the resulting increase in capillary pressure and obstruction of venous blood flow through the damaged liver. **Portal hypertension** causes an increased pressure gradient (a difference in pressure between the portal vein and the hepatic veins), facilitating fluid accumulation in the peritoneal cavity. Another factor is the decreased synthesis of albumin in liver disease. The hypoalbuminemia results in decreased plasma oncotic pressure, which facilitates fluid accumulation in the abdominal cavity. An obstruction of the normal lymphatic drainage can cause fluid accumulation in the peritoneum, as can cancers or inflammatory processes that stimulate increased production of peritoneal fluid. Ascites also can be associated with nonhepatic etiologies, such as kidney failure and heart failure.

Engorged Veins

Under normal conditions, the veins in the abdominal wall are barely noted unless the skin and subcutaneous fat are thin. When venous pressure increases as a result of obstruction, as in portal hypertension, vessels distal to the inferior vena cava engorge, and distended veins can be seen on the abdomen, chest, and extremities.

Physical Examination

For the purposes of examination and documentation, the abdomen can be divided into either four quadrants or nine regions (Fig. 21-7). The nurse must know the physical proximity of the organs and blood vessels to these quadrants or regions. Choosing one of these mapping methods and using it consistently will ensure a thorough evaluation of the abdomen and appropriate corresponding documentation.

The physical examination includes assessment of the mouth, abdomen, and rectum. Good lighting is necessary, as is full exposure of the abdomen. The patient should be comfortable and relaxed, with an empty bladder. The nurse's hands should be warm and the fingernails short.

The patient lies supine with knees flexed slightly for inspection, auscultation, palpation, and percussion of the abdomen. Arms should not be raised over the head because the abdominal muscles tense in this position. A small pillow may be placed behind the patient's head for comfort. The patient's breasts are covered with a gown, and sheets are rolled down to above the symphysis pubis. Examination of the abdomen is performed with the nurse standing on the patient's right side.

Inspection

The mouth, tongue, buccal mucosa, teeth, and gums are inspected, noting any ulcers, nodules, swelling, discoloration, or inflammation. Dentures should be removed to allow good visualization of the entire oral cavity.

Four quadrants
1 - right upper quadrant (RUQ)
2 - right lower quadrant (RLQ)
3 - left upper quadrant (LUQ)
4 - left lower quadrant (LLQ)

Nine regions
1 - epigastric region
2 - umbilical region
3 - hypogastric or suprapubic region
4 - right hypochondriac region
5 - left hypochondriac region
6 - right lumbar region
7 - left lumbar region
8 - right inguinal region
9 - left inguinal region

FIGURE 21-7 Division of the abdomen into (**A**) four quadrants or (**B**) nine regions.

The nurse inspects the abdominal skin for nodules, lesions, masses, scarring, discolorations, inflammation, bruising, increased vascularity of the abdominal skin, and striae (stretch marks). In the presence of liver disease, the nurse inspects the skin, mucosa, and sclera for jaundice. The extremities are assessed for muscle atrophy, edema, and skin excoriation secondary to scratching. The nurse observes the skin for petechiae or ecchymotic areas (bruises), spider angiomas, and palmar erythema (a diffuse reddening of the palm, particularly near the base of the thumb (thenar eminence) and base of the little finger (hypothenar eminence) that is associated with chronic liver disease. In addition, a male patient is assessed for unilateral or bilateral gynecomastia and testicular atrophy due to hormonal changes associated with liver disease. The patient's cognitive status (recall, memory, abstract thinking) and neurologic status are assessed. The nurse observes for general tremor, asterixis (flapping of the hands when wrists dorsiflexed), weakness, and slurred speech related to elevated ammonia levels secondary to liver failure; the nurse notes the patient's breath for **hepatic fetor,** a sweet, mildly fecal breath odor associated with encephalopathy. The contour and symmetry of the abdomen are noted, and any localized bulging, distention, or peristaltic waves are identified. Under normal circumstances, peristalsis is not noted on the abdominal wall and, if present, usually is associated with early intestinal obstruction. Expected contours of the anterior abdominal wall can be described as flat, rounded, or scaphoid (hollowed or shaped like a boat). The umbilicus is assessed for color, position, and shape. The umbilicus may be everted with increased intra-abdominal pressure. Ecchymoses around the umbilical area is termed *Cullen sign* and is associated with a retroperitoneal bleed due to any cause. Ecchymoses noted on either flank, the groin, or the abdomen, termed *Grey–Turner sign*, is also associated with a retroperitoneal bleed (see Chapter 27, Fig. 27-10). A hernia is a protrusion on the abdominal wall and may be noted anywhere in the abdomen. If ascites is suspected, the nurse notes bulging flanks when the patient is in the supine position as the weight of the fluid flows dependently to the sides.

Nursing Alert

If abdominal distention is noted, the nurse assesses for common causes described as the 6 F's: fetus (pregnancy), feces (constipation), flatulence, fat (obesity), fluid (ascites), and fibroids or full-size tumor.

Auscultation

Auscultation always precedes percussion and palpation since manipulation of the abdomen may alter the frequency and intensity of bowel sounds. The nurse listens to determine the character, location, and frequency of bowel sounds and to identify vascular sounds. Bowel sounds are assessed in all four quadrants using the diaphragm of the stethoscope, which affords greatest auscultation of high-pitched and gurgling sounds. The frequency and character of the sounds are usually heard as clicks and gurgles that occur irregularly and range from 5 to 35 per minute. Frequently the terms *normoactive* (sounds heard about every 2 to 12 seconds), *hypoactive* (fewer than 5 clicks or gurgles per minute), *hyperactive* (more than 35 per minute), or *absent* (no sounds in 3 to 5 minutes) are used in documentation, but these assessments are highly subjective. Hypoactive bowel sounds are associated with decreased bowel function, as occurs in postoperative patients, patients with myxedema, peritonitis, hypokalemia, or mesentery ischemia, and in patients on medications, such as opioid and anticholinergic agents. The nurse must listen for 5 minutes before documenting the absence of bowel sounds, which is suggestive of ileus and can be due to a variety of causes. Hyperactive bowel sounds are associated with diarrhea or gastroenteritis. High-pitched, high-frequency bowel sounds and abdominal cramping are suggestive of a partial intestinal obstruction.

Bruits in the aortic, renal, iliac, and femoral arteries are noted using the bell of the stethoscope. Bruits are associated with turbulent blood flow in an artery. Friction rubs are high-pitched grating sounds heard over the liver or spleen during respiration. These are rare findings but are associated with pathology. Borborygmi, or "stomach growling," is heard as a loud, prolonged gurgle.

Percussion

Percussion is used to assess the size and density of the abdominal organs and to detect the presence of air-filled, fluid-filled, or solid masses. Percussion is used either independently or concurrently with palpation because it can validate palpation findings. All quadrants are percussed for a sense of overall tympany and dullness. Tympany is the predominant sound that results from the presence of air in the stomach and small intestines; dullness is heard over organs and solid masses (Jarvis, 2016).

If ascites is suspected, the nurse can test for shifting dullness, which may help confirm the presence of ascites. This is performed through percussion with the patient in supine position. In this position, the nurse percusses the top of the abdomen and notes tympany, however when the abdomen in percussed laterally, the sound of dullness is noted. The nurse then rolls the patient on their side and will percuss again. Shifting dullness is noted as the fluid flows to the dependent regions when the patient moves to a lateral position (Bickley, 2017).

The nurse estimates the size of the liver by percussing its upper border beginning at lung resonance and changing to liver dullness; then the nurse percusses the lower border by noting the change in sound from abdominal tympany to liver dullness usually at the right costal margin (Jarvis, 2016). The normal liver span is 6 to 12 cm in the midclavicular line

(MCL). A hollow tympanic note over the stomach in the left upper quadrant (LUQ) should be expected. A full bladder elicits dullness above the suprapubic area, whereas abdominal distention increases the area of tympany. If the spleen is enlarged, dullness may be percussed in the LUQ at the area in proximity to the ninth through eleventh ribs (Bickley & Szilagyi, 2013).

Palpation

If a patient complains of abdominal pain, it is important to assess the area of tenderness last. Use of light palpation is appropriate for identifying areas of tenderness or muscular resistance, and deep palpation is used to identify masses. If a mass is noted, the nurse assesses its size, shape, location, consistency, pulsatility, mobility, and tenderness.

A palpable liver has a firm, sharp ridge and a smooth surface (Fig. 21-8). If the liver is palpable, the examiner notes and records its size, its consistency, any tenderness, and whether its outline is regular or irregular. If the liver is enlarged, the degree to which it descends below the right costal margin is recorded to provide some indication of its size. The nurse determines whether the liver's edge is sharp and smooth or blunt and whether the enlarged liver is nodular or smooth. The liver of a patient with cirrhosis is small and hard with a palpable edge, whereas the liver of a patient with acute hepatitis is enlarged and smooth (Jarvis, 2016).

Tenderness of the liver indicates recent acute enlargement with consequent stretching of the liver capsule. The absence of tenderness may imply that the enlargement is of long-standing duration. The liver of a patient with viral hepatitis is tender, whereas that of a patient with alcoholic hepatitis

FIGURE 21-8 Technique for palpating the liver. The examiner places one hand under the right lower rib cage and presses downward with light pressure with the other hand.

is not. Enlargement of the liver is an abnormal finding that requires evaluation (Bickley & Szilagyi, 2013).

The fluid wave test can be conducted if ascites is suspected. A fluid wave can be demonstrated by tapping the patient's flank sharply with one hand while the other hand receives the impulse against the opposite flank. There is a perceptible time lag between the tap and reception of the impulse. Since mesentery fat may produce a similar wave, the patient or an assistant presses the ulnar surface of his or her hand into the midline of the abdomen. A wave passing this hand barrier is usually caused by free fluid. This finding may be negative until ascites is visibly obvious. If both the fluid wave test and the test for shifting dullness are positive and accompanied by peripheral edema, it is three to six times more probable that ascites is present (Bickley, 2017).

Cholecystitis, acute inflammation of the gallbladder, causes pain and tenderness and makes it difficult for the nurse to palpate and percuss the abdomen. The nurse should observe for Murphy sign (the patient's inability to take a deep breath when the examiner's fingers are pressed below the right costal margin).

Testing for rebound tenderness is not performed by many examiners because it can cause severe pain; light percussion is used instead to produce a mild, localized response when peritoneal irritation is present. If testing for rebound tenderness is undertaken, it is done at the end of the examination since the patient's pain will interfere with the remaining examination. Using palpation, the nurse's places his or her hand in the painful quadrant and then releases it quickly. Pain upon releasing is termed *Blumberg sign* and is associated with peritonitis, such as appendicitis.

> ### ⚠ Nursing Alert
> *Guarding, rigidity, and rebound tenderness (Blumberg sign) are reliable indicators of peritonitis, which is inflammation of the peritoneum. Peritonitis can be caused by bacterial invasion (i.e., ruptured appendix, perforated diverticulum), chemical irritation (i.e., perforated ulcer), abdominal trauma, and wounds.*

Rectal Examination

The final part of the physical examination is evaluation of the terminal portions of the GI tract, the rectum, perianal region, and anus. The anal canal is approximately 2.5 to 4 cm in length and opens into the perineum. Concentric rings of muscle, the internal and external sphincters, normally keep the anal canal closed securely. Gloves, water-soluble lubrication, a penlight, and drapes are necessary tools for the evaluation. Although the rectal examination is generally uncomfortable and often embarrassing for the patient, it is a mandatory part of every thorough examination. For women, the rectal examination may be part of the gynecologic examination. Positions for the rectal examination include knee–chest, left lateral with hips and knees flexed, and standing with hips flexed and upper body supported by the examination table. External examination includes inspection for lumps, rashes, inflammation, excoriation, tears, scars, pilonidal dimpling, and tufts of hair at the pilonidal area. The discovery of tenderness, inflammation, or both should alert the examiner to the possibility of a pilonidal cyst, perianal abscess, or anorectal fistula or fissure. The patient's buttocks are carefully spread and visually inspected until the patient has relaxed the external sphincter control. The patient is asked to bear down, thus allowing the ready appearance of fistulas, fissures, rectal prolapse, polyps, and internal hemorrhoids. Internal examination is performed with a lubricated index finger inserted into the anal canal while the patient bears down. The tone of the sphincter is noted, as are any nodules or irregularities of the anal ring. Because this is an uncomfortable part of the examination for most people, the patient is encouraged to focus on deep breathing during the brief examination.

Diagnostic Evaluation

Initial diagnostic tests begin with serum laboratory studies, including but not limited to CBC, a complete metabolic panel, prothrombin time/partial thromboplastin time (PT/PTT), triglycerides, liver function tests, amylase, and lipase, with the possibility of more specific studies, such as carcinoembryonic antigen (CEA), cancer antigen (CA) 19-9, and alpha-fetoprotein, indicating sensitivity and specificity for colorectal and hepatocellular carcinomas, respectively. CEA is a protein that normally is not detected in the blood of a healthy person; therefore, when detected, it indicates that cancer is present but not what type of cancer is present. Practitioners can use CEA results to determine the stage and extent of the disease and the prognosis for patients with cancer, especially colorectal, pancreatic, lung, and stomach cancer (Grossman & Porth, 2014). CA 19-9 is also a protein that exists on the surface of certain cells and is shed by tumor cells, making it useful as a tumor marker to follow the course of the cancer. CA 19-9 levels are elevated in most patients with advanced pancreatic cancer, but it also may be elevated in other conditions, such as colorectal, lung, and gallbladder cancers; gallstones; **pancreatitis**; cystic fibrosis; and liver disease.

Many other modalities are available for diagnostic assessment of the GI tract. Table 21-5 identifies various procedures and their diagnostic uses.

The majority of these tests and procedures are performed on an outpatient basis in special settings designed for this purpose (e.g., endoscopy suite or GI laboratory). In the past, frequently patients who required such tests were elderly; however, within the past 5 years, in part due to heightened media exposure on the subject of early diagnosis of colorectal cancer, the median age of patients evaluated for colorectal

cancer has decreased significantly. Preparation for many of these studies includes clear liquid diets, fasting, ingestion of a liquid bowel preparation, the use of laxatives or enemas, and ingestion or injection of a contrast agent or a radiopaque dye. These measures are poorly tolerated by some patients and are especially problematic in the elderly population or in patients with comorbidities because bowel preparations significantly alter the internal fluid and electrolyte balance. If further assessment or treatment is needed after any outpatient procedure, the patient may be admitted to the hospital. Specific interventions for each diagnostic test are listed in Table 21-6.

General nursing interventions for the patient who is undergoing a GI diagnostic evaluation include:

- Establishing the possible nursing diagnosis
- Providing needed information about the test and the activities required of the patient
- Providing instructions about postprocedure care and activity restrictions
- Providing health information and procedural teaching to patients and significant others
- Helping the patient cope with discomfort and alleviating anxiety
- Informing the physician or nurse practitioner of known medical conditions or abnormal laboratory values that may affect the procedure
- Assessing for adequate hydration before, during, and immediately after the procedure, and providing education about maintenance of hydration

Stool Tests

Basic examination of the stool includes inspecting the specimen for consistency, color, and occult (not visible) blood. Additional studies, including fecal urobilinogen, fecal fat, nitrogen, *Clostridium difficile,* fecal leukocytes, calculation of stool osmolar gap, parasites, pathogens, food residues, and other substances, require laboratory evaluation.

Usually stool samples are collected on a random basis unless a quantitative study (e.g., fecal fat, urobilinogen) is to be performed. Random specimens should be sent promptly to the laboratory for analysis; however, the quantitative 24- to 72-hour collections must be kept refrigerated until transported to the laboratory. Some stool collections require the patient to follow a specific diet or refrain from taking certain medications before the collection. Thorough and accurate patient education regarding a specific stool study prior to collection greatly increases the accuracy of study results.

The stool antigen test is a noninvasive, simple procedure for determining the presence of monoclonal antibodies specific to *Helicobacter pylori*, which places the patient at risk for peptic ulcer disease (Kasper et al., 2015). This test may be performed in the laboratory or, most recently, in the office during a clinic visit (Crowe, Feldman, & Grover, 2015).

Fecal occult blood testing (FOBT) is one of the most commonly performed stool tests. It can be useful in initial

TABLE 21-5 Additional Laboratory Studies for Digestive, Gastrointestinal, and Metabolic Function

Study	Clinical Functions
Abdominal x-ray	To determine gross liver size, assess for intestinal obstruction and/or fecal impaction
Angiography	To visualize liver circulation and detect presence and nature of liver masses
Barium study of esophagus	To identify varices, which indicate increased portal blood pressure
Celiac axis arteriography	To visualize liver and pancreas
Cholecystogram and cholangiogram	To visualize gallbladder and bile duct
Cholesterol levels	Elevated in biliary obstruction; decreased in parenchymal liver disease
Computed tomography (CT) scan	To detect hepatic neoplasms; diagnose cysts, abscesses, and hematomas; and distinguish between obstructive and nonobstructive jaundice. Detects cerebral atrophy in hepatic encephalopathy
Electroencephalogram	To detect abnormalities that occur with hepatic coma
Endoscopic retrograde cholangiopancreatography (ERCP)	To visualize biliary structures and pancreas via endoscopy
Esophagoscopy/endoscopy	To search for esophageal varices and other abnormalities
Gamma-glutamyl transferase (GGT), gamma-glutamyl transpeptidase (GGTP), lactate dehydrogenase (LDH)	Markers for biliary stasis; also elevated in alcohol abuse
Laparoscopy	To directly visualize the anterior surface of liver, gallbladder, and mesentery through a trocar
Liver biopsy (percutaneous or transjugular)	To determine anatomic changes in liver tissue
Liver scan with radio-tagged iodinated rose bengal, gold, technetium, or gallium	To show size and shape of liver; to show replacement of liver tissue with scars, cysts, or tumor
Magnetic resonance imaging (MRI)	To detect hepatic neoplasms; diagnose cysts, abscesses, and hematomas. Detects cerebral atrophy in encephalopathy
Measurement of portal pressure	To detect increased portal pressure, which occurs with cirrhosis of the liver
Serum alkaline phosphatase	In absence of bone disease, to measure biliary tract obstruction
Splenoportogram (splenic portal venography)	To determine adequacy of portal blood flow
Ultrasonography	To show size of abdominal organs and presence of masses

screening for several disorders, although it is used most frequently in early cancer detection programs. FOBT can be performed at the bedside, in the laboratory, or at home. Probably the most widely used in-office or at-home occult blood test is the Hemoccult II. It is inexpensive, noninvasive, and carries minimal risk to the patient.

Breath Tests

H. pylori is a bacteria that can live in the mucosal lining of the stomach, causing peptic ulcer disease (Grossman &

Porth, 2014). The urea breath test is a noninvasive procedure used to detect *H. pylori* based upon the separation of urea by *H. pylori* and creating CO_2 and ammonia. A carbon isotope is administered to the patient by mouth, and the *H. pylori* joins with CO_2 and can be identified via the breath sample (Crowe, Feldman, & Grover, 2015).

Abdominal Ultrasonography

Ultrasonography is a noninvasive diagnostic technique in which high-frequency sound waves are passed into internal

TABLE 21-6 Gastrointestinal Laboratory Tests

Test	Nursing Implications
Abdominal ultrasonography	• The patient is instructed to fast for 8–12 hours before the test to decrease the amount of gas in the bowel. • If gallbladder studies are to be performed, the patient should eat a fat-free meal the evening before the test. • If barium studies are to be performed, they should be scheduled after ultrasonography; otherwise, the barium could interfere with the transmission of the sound waves.
Anoscopy, proctoscopy, and sigmoidoscopy	• Preparation varies according to providers. Patients may receive an enema until the returns are clear. • During the procedure, the nurse monitors vital signs, skin color and temperature, pain tolerance, and vagal response. • After the procedure, the nurse monitors the patient for rectal bleeding and signs of intestinal perforation (i.e., fever, rectal drainage, abdominal distention, and pain). On completion of the examination, the patient can resume regular activities and diet.
Breath tests	• The patient ingests a capsule of carbon-labeled urea, and a breath sample is obtained 10–20 minutes later. Because *Helicobacter pylori* metabolizes urea rapidly, the labeled carbon is absorbed quickly; then it can be measured as carbon dioxide in the expired breath to determine whether *H. pylori* is present. • The patient is instructed to avoid antibiotics and loperamide (Pepto-Bismol) for 1 month before the test; sucralfate (Carafate) and omeprazole (Prilosec) for 1 week before the test; and cimetidine (Tagamet), famotidine (Pepcid), and ranitidine (Zantac) for 24 hours before the test. • *H. pylori* also can be detected by assessing serum antibody levels.
Blood chemistry	• Many electrolytes are altered in GI dysfunction. Calcium is absorbed in the GI tract and may be measured to detect malabsorption. Excessive vomiting or diarrhea causes electrolyte depletion, thus requiring replacement. • Assays of serum enzymes are important in the evaluation of liver damage. AST and ALT are two enzymes found in most patients' livers and other organs. These enzymes are elevated in most liver disorders, but they are highest in conditions that cause necrosis (viral hepatitis). • Conjugated (direct) and unconjugated (indirect) bilirubin are important measurements in the diagnosis of jaundice. • Serum ammonia level is measured to evaluate liver function. • CA 19-9 and CEA are evaluated to diagnose, monitor the success of cancer therapy, and assess for the recurrence of cancer in the GI tract (Daniels, 2014).
Cholecystography	• The patient is asked about allergies to iodine or seafood. If no allergy is identified, the patient receives the oral form of the contrast agent the evening before (10–12 hours) the x-rays are obtained. • After the contrast agent is administered, the patient is permitted nothing by mouth, to prevent contraction and emptying of the gallbladder. • An x-ray of the right upper abdomen is obtained. If the gallbladder is found to fill and empty normally and to contain no stones, gallbladder disease is ruled out. • If gallbladder disease is present, the gallbladder may not be visualized because of obstruction by gallstones. If the gallbladder is not visualized on the first attempt, a repeat of the oral cholecystography with a second dose of the contrast agent may be necessary.
CT	• CT may be performed with or without an oral or IV contrast agent, but the study is far superior with the administration of a contrast agent. • Any allergies to contrast agents, iodine, or shellfish; the patient's current serum creatinine level; and urine levels of human chorionic gonadotropin must be determined before administration of a contrast agent. Patients allergic to the contrast agent may be premedicated with steroids and antihistamines before the scan. • In addition, renal protective measures include the administration of IV sodium bicarbonate 1 hour before and 6 hours after IV contrast and oral acetylcysteine (Mucomyst) before or after the study. Both sodium bicarbonate and Mucomyst are free radical scavengers that sequester the contrast byproducts that are destructive to kidney cells. • The patient is informed that during injection of the contrast medium, a burning sensation may be felt for a few seconds behind the eyes or in the jaw, teeth, tongue, or lips (Daniels, 2014).

Test	Nursing Implications
Endoscopy through ostomy stoma	• Nursing interventions are similar to those for other endoscopic procedures.
ERCP	• Before the procedure, the patient is given an explanation of the procedure and their role in it. • The patient is NPO for several hours before the procedure. • Moderate sedation is used, and the sedated patient must be monitored closely. • It may be necessary to administer medications, such as glucagon or anticholinergics, to make cannulation easier by decreasing duodenal peristalsis. • The nurse observes closely for signs of respiratory and CNS depression, hypotension, oversedation, and vomiting (if glucagon is administered). • During the procedure, the nurse monitors IV fluids, administers medications, and positions the patient. • After the procedure, the nurse monitors the patient's condition, observing vital signs and monitoring for signs of perforation or infection. • The nurse monitors the patient for side effects of any medications received during the procedure and for return of the gag and cough reflexes after the use of local anesthetics.
Fiberoptic colonoscopy	• Adequate colon cleansing provides optimal visualization and decreases the time needed for the procedure. The physician may prescribe a laxative for two nights before the examination and a Fleet's or saline enema until the return is clear the morning of the test. More commonly, polyethylene glycol electrolyte lavage solutions (Go-LYTELY, CoLyte, and Nu-Lytely) are used as intestinal lavages for effective cleansing of the bowel. • The patient maintains a clear liquid diet starting at noon the day before the procedure. Then the patient ingests the lavage solution orally at intervals over 3–4 hours. If necessary, the nurse can give the solution through a feeding tube if the patient cannot swallow. • Patients with a colostomy receive this same bowel preparation. • The use of lavage solutions is contraindicated in patients with intestinal obstruction or inflammatory bowel disease. • Side effects of the electrolyte solutions include nausea, bloating, cramping or abdominal fullness, fluid and electrolyte imbalance, and hypothermia. • The side effects are especially problematic for elderly patients, and sometimes they have difficulty ingesting the required volume of solution. Monitoring elderly patients after a bowel prep is especially important because their physiologic ability to compensate for fluid loss is diminished. • Many elderly people take multiple medications each day; therefore, the nurse's knowledge of their daily medication regimen can prompt assessment for and prevention of potential problems and early detection of physiologic changes.
Gastric analysis, gastric acid stimulation test	• The patient is NPO for 8–12 hours before the procedure. • Any medications that affect gastric secretions are withheld for 24–48 hours before the test. • Smoking is not allowed on the morning of the test because it increases gastric secretions.
Laparoscopy (peritoneoscopy)	• The patient is NPO 12 hours prior to the procedure. An empty stomach lowers the chance of vomiting during or after the procedure. • An enema may be prescribed the day before or several hours prior to the procedure to empty the colon. • The patient should ask the primary care provider if daily medicines should be taken the day of the laparoscopy.
Lower GI series (Barium enema)	• Preparation includes emptying and cleansing the lower bowel. This often necessitates a low-residue diet 1–2 days before the test, a clear liquid diet and a laxative the evening before, NPO after midnight, and cleansing enemas until returns are clear the following morning. • The nurse makes sure that barium enemas are scheduled before any upper GI studies. • If the patient has active inflammatory disease of the colon, enemas are contraindicated. Barium enemas also are contraindicated in patients with signs of perforation or obstruction; instead, a water-soluble contrast study may be performed. • Active GI bleeding may prohibit the use of laxatives and enemas. • Postprocedural patient education includes information about increasing fluid intake, evaluating bowel movements for evacuation of barium, and noting increased number of bowel movements, because barium, due to its high osmolarity, may draw fluid into the bowel, thus increasing the intraluminal contents and resulting in greater output.

(continued on page 644)

TABLE 21-6 **Gastrointestinal Laboratory Tests** (*continued*)

Test	Nursing Implications
MRI	• The patient should be NPO 6–8 hours before the study. • Any ferromagnetic objects (metals that contain iron) can be attracted to the magnet and cause injury. Items that can be problematic or dangerous include jewelry, pacemakers, dental implants, paperclips, pens, keys, IV poles, clips on patient gowns, and oxygen tanks. • The patient and family are informed that the study may take 60–90 minutes; during this time, the technician will instruct the patient to take deep breaths at specific intervals. • The close-fitting scanners used in many MRI facilities may induce feelings of claustrophobia, and the machine will make a knocking sound during the procedure. Patients may choose to wear a headset and listen to music or to wear a blindfold during the procedure. Open MRIs that are less close-fitting eliminate the claustrophobia that many patients experience. • MRI is contraindicated for patients with permanent pacemakers, artificial heart valves and defibrillators, implanted insulin pumps, or implanted transcutaneous electrical nerve stimulation devices because the magnetic field could cause malfunction of the device. • MRI is also contraindicated for patients with internal metal devices (e.g., aneurysm clips) or intraocular metallic fragments. Foil-backed skin patches (e.g., NicoDerm, nitroglycerine [Transderm-Nitro], scopolamine [Transderm-Scop], clonidine [Catapres-TTS]) should be removed before an MRI because of the risk of burns; however, the patient's physician should be consulted before the patch is removed to determine whether an alternate form of the medication should be provided.
PET	• The patient should be NPO for 4 hours on the day of the test. • The patient should refrain from alcohol, caffeine, and tobacco for 24 hours. • Diabetic patients should take their pretest dose of insulin with a meal 3–4 hours before the test. • The patient should be informed that an IV line may be inserted. • After the PET, the patient should change position slowly from lying to standing to avoid postural hypotension. • The patient should be encouraged to drink fluids and urinate frequently to aid in the removal of the radioisotope from the bladder.
pH monitoring	• The patient is NPO for 6 hours before the test. • All medications affecting gastric secretions are withheld for 24–36 hours before the test.
Small-bowel enteroscopy with capsule endoscope (CE)	• The patient must be NPO for 8–10 hours before the test and be NPO for the first 2 hours of the testing. • At the time of the procedure, the patient's abdomen is marked for the location of the sensors, and the 8-lead sensors are applied. The patient wears an abdominal belt that houses a recorder to capture the transmitted images. • After the capsule is taken with a glass of water, the patient may return to normal activity for the remainder of the study. The patient can resume a normal diet 4 hours after the ingestion of the capsule. • During the procedure, the patient may receive a mild sedative and pain medication for comfort. At the end of the procedure, the patient returns to the facility with the receiver for downloading to a central computer. • The procedure lasts approximately 8 hours. • The capsule endoscopy is a single-use device that is propelled through the GI tract by peristalsis and excreted naturally. The patient should be informed that the capsule will be excreted in the stool. • If the patient is concerned about nonevacuation of the capsule, an abdominal x-ray can establish if it has been retained.
Stool tests	• Should not be performed if there is hemorrhoidal bleeding. • Careful assessment of the patient's diet and medication regimen is essential to avoid incorrect interpretation of results. Red meats, fish, turnips, horseradish, and NSAIDs should be avoided for 72 hours prior to the study because they may cause a false-positive result. Ingestion of vitamin C from supplements or foods can cause a false-negative result. • A small amount of the specimen is applied to the guaiac-impregnated paper slide. If the test is performed at home, then the patient mails the slide to the health care provider or laboratory in an envelope provided for that purpose. • Other occult blood tests that may yield more specific and more sensitive readings include Hematest II SENSA and HemoQuant.

Test	Nursing Implications
Ultrasonography	• No fasting is required for ultrasonography of the abdominal aorta, kidney, liver, spleen, or pancreas, but fasting is preferred before ultrasonography of the gallbladder and biliary tree. • During the procedure, the patient is lying down. The patient may be asked to change position so that the health care provider can examine different areas. • The patient also may be asked to hold his or her breath for short periods of time during the examination.
Upper GI fibroscopy/ esophagogastroduodenoscopy	• The patient should be NPO for 8 hours prior to the examination. • A sedative that provides moderate sedation and relieves anxiety during the procedure may be administered at the initiation of the study. • Before the introduction of the endoscope, the patient is given a local anesthetic gargle or spray. • The patient is placed in the left lateral position to facilitate clearance of pulmonary secretions and provide smooth entry of the scope. • After gastroscopy, assessment includes level of consciousness, vital signs, oxygen saturation, pain level, and monitoring for signs of perforation (i.e., pain, bleeding, unusual difficulty swallowing, and rapidly elevated temperature). • After the patient's gag reflex has returned, lozenges, saline gargle, and oral analgesics may be offered to relieve minor throat discomfort. • Patients who were sedated for the procedure must remain in bed until fully alert.
Upper GI series (Barium swallow)	• The patient is instructed to fast after midnight the day before the test. • Smoking, chewing gum, and using mints can stimulate gastric motility; therefore, the nurse advises against these practices. • Typically, oral medications are withheld on the morning of the study and resumed that evening, but each patient's medication regimen should be evaluated on an individual basis. • Follow-up care is provided after the upper GI procedure to ensure that the patient has eliminated most of the ingested barium. Fluids may be increased to facilitate evacuation of stool and barium.
Urine tests	• Amylase can be detected in the urine. There is an increased renal clearance of amylase in patients with acute pancreatitis. Amylase levels in the urine remain high even after serum levels return to normal. • Urine urobilinogen is a form of bilirubin that is converted by the intestinal flora and excreted in the urine. Its measurement is useful in the evaluation of liver and biliary obstruction. The presence of bilirubin in urine often precedes the development of jaundice. For the urine urobilinogen test, some laboratories require keeping the patient NPO after midnight the day of the test, except for water.

ALT, alanine aminotransferase; AST, aspartate aminotransferase; CA 19-9, carbohydrate antigen 19-9; CEA, carcinoembryonic antigen; CT, computed tomography; ERCP, endoscopic retrograde cholangiopancreatography; GI, gastrointestinal tract; IV, intravenous; MRI, magnetic resonance imaging; NSAIDs, nonsteroidal anti-inflammatory drugs; NPO (*nil per os*), nothing by mouth; PET, positron emission tomography.

body structures and the ultrasonic echoes are recorded on an oscilloscope as they strike tissues of different densities. A clear, water-based conducting gel is applied to the skin over the abdomen, which helps with the transmission of the sound waves. Then a handheld probe, called a transducer, is moved over the abdomen. Ultrasonography is particularly useful in the detection of an enlarged gallbladder or pancreas, the presence of gallstones, an enlarged ovary, an ectopic pregnancy, or appendicitis. Most recently this technique has proved useful in diagnosing acute colonic diverticulitis.

Ultrasonography is the diagnostic procedure of choice for gallbladder disease because it is rapid and accurate and can be used in patients with liver dysfunction and jaundice. It does not expose patients to ionizing radiation. The procedure

is most accurate if the patient fasts for 4 to 6 hours prior to the procedure so that the gallbladder is distended (Schiff, Maddrey, & Sorrell, 2012). Ultrasound studies are based on analysis of reflected sound waves. Ultrasound findings include gallbladder sludge, gallbladder wall thickening, and pericholecystic fluid, which are diagnostic for acute cholecystitis. Ultrasonography is diagnostic of calculi in 90% to 95% of cases as it detects thickening of the gallbladder wall, pericholecystic fluid and dilation of the bile duct which are all signs of gallbladder inflammation (Kasper et al., 2015).

Cholescintigraphy (a nuclear medicine test also known as HIDA [hepatobiliary iminodiacetic acid]) or gallbladder scan helps determine if obstruction of the cystic duct is the underlying cause of cholecystitis. The patient is injected with TC-99m HIDA; if the gallbladder is not filled within 60 minutes in response to the injection, it is considered abnormal but not completely diagnostic of acute cholecystitis (Ziessman, O'Malley, & Thrall, 2014). Cholescintigraphy is 90% to 97% sensitive in diagnosing acute cholecystitis but the presence of a stone or tumor-causing cystic duct obstruction without acute cholecystitis may result in a false-positive result (Zakko & Afdhal, 2015).

Endoscopic ultrasonography (EUS) is a specialized enteroscopic procedure that aids in the diagnosis of GI disorders by providing direct imaging of a target area. A small, high-frequency ultrasonic transducer is mounted at the tip of the fiberoptic scope, which displays an image that enables tumor staging and visualization of marginal structures. This procedure delivers results with higher-quality resolution and definition in comparison with regular ultrasonic imaging. EUS may be used for evaluating submucosal lesions, specifically determining their location and depth of penetration. In addition, EUS may aid in the evaluation of Barrett esophagus, portal hypertension, chronic pancreatitis, suspected pancreatic neoplasm, biliary tract disease, and changes in the bowel wall that occur in ulcerative colitis. Intestinal gas, bone, and thick layers of adipose tissue (all of which hamper conventional ultrasonography) are not problematic when EUS is used.

DNA Testing

Researchers have refined methods for genetics risk assessment, preclinical diagnosis, and prenatal diagnosis to identify people who are at risk for certain GI disorders (e.g., gastric cancer, lactose deficiency, inflammatory bowel disease, or colon cancer). In some cases, DNA testing allows providers to prevent (or minimize) disease by intervening before its onset and to improve therapy; however, it is imperative to seek advice from genetics counselors routinely, given the exponential growth of genetics information. People who are identified as at risk of certain GI disorders may choose to undergo genetic counseling to learn about the disease, to understand options for preventing and treating the disease, and to receive support in coping with the situation. Ethical and legal issues are involved in genetic testing, and there are legal protections for clients against discrimination. For instance, false-positive results can create unnecessary worry, alarm, and further testing, typically at the expense of the patient and the family, with potential effects on health-related quality of life (Hidayatallah et al., 2014).

Imaging Studies

Many minimally invasive and noninvasive imaging studies, including x-ray and contrast studies, computed tomography (CT), magnetic resonance imaging (MRI), positron emission tomography (PET), and virtual endoscopy, are available today to aid in the accurate assessment of the many possible causes of GI abnormalities.

Upper Gastrointestinal Tract Study

An upper GI study delineates the entire GI tract after the introduction of a contrast agent. A radiopaque liquid (e.g., barium sulfate) is commonly used; however, thin barium, Hypaque, and, at times, water are used due to their low associated risks. The GI series enables the examiner to detect or exclude anatomic or functional derangement of the upper GI organs or sphincters. It also aids in the diagnosis of ulcers, varices, tumors, regional enteritis, and malabsorption syndromes. The procedure may be extended to examine the duodenum and small bowel (small bowel follow-through). As the barium descends into the stomach, the position, patency, and caliber of the esophagus are visualized, enabling the examiner to detect or exclude any anatomic or functional derangement of that organ. Fluoroscopic examination next extends to the stomach as its lumen fills with barium, allowing observation of stomach motility, thickness of the gastric wall, the mucosal pattern, patency of the pyloric valve, and the anatomy of the duodenum. Multiple x-ray films are obtained during the procedure, and additional images may be taken at intervals for up to 24 hours to evaluate the rate of gastric emptying. Small-bowel x-rays taken while the barium is passing through that area allow for observation of the motility of the small bowel. Obstructions, ileitis, and diverticula can be detected if present.

Variations of the upper GI study include double-contrast studies and enteroclysis (defined below). The double-contrast method of examining the upper GI tract involves administration of a thick barium suspension to outline the stomach and esophageal wall, after which tablets that release carbon dioxide in the presence of water are administered. This technique has the advantage of showing the esophagus and stomach in finer detail, permitting signs of early superficial neoplasms to be noted.

Enteroclysis is a very detailed, double-contrast study of the entire small intestine that involves the continuous infusion, through a duodenal tube, of 500 to 1,000 mL of a thin barium sulfate suspension; after this, methylcellulose is infused through the tube. The barium and methylcellulose fill the intestinal loops and are observed continuously by fluoroscopy and viewed at frequent intervals as they progress through the jejunum and the ileum. This process (even with normal motility) can take up to 6 hours and can be quite uncomfortable for the patient. The procedure aids in the diagnosis of partial small-bowel obstructions or diverticula.

Lower Gastrointestinal Tract Study

Visualization of the lower GI tract is obtained after rectal installation of barium. The barium enema can be used to detect the presence of polyps, tumors, or other lesions of the large intestine and demonstrate any anatomic abnormalities or malfunctioning of the bowel. After proper preparation and evacuation of the entire colon, each portion of the colon may be readily observed. The procedure usually takes about 15 to 30 minutes, during which time x-ray images are obtained.

Other means for visualizing the colon include double-contrast studies and a water-soluble contrast study. A double-contrast, or air-contrast, barium enema involves the instillation of a thicker barium solution, followed by the instillation of air. The patient may feel some cramping or discomfort during this process. This test provides a contrast between the air-filled lumen and the barium-coated mucosa, allowing easier detection of smaller lesions.

If active inflammatory disease, fistulas, or perforation of the colon is suspected, a water-soluble iodinated contrast agent (e.g., Gastrografin) can be used. The procedure is the same as for a barium enema, but the patient must be assessed for allergy to iodine or contrast agent. The contrast agent is eliminated readily after the procedure so there is no need for postprocedure laxatives. Some diarrhea may occur in a few patients until the contrast agent has been totally eliminated.

Computed Tomography

CT provides cross-sectional images of abdominal organs and structures. Multiple x-ray images are taken from numerous angles, digitized in a computer, reconstructed, and then viewed on a computer monitor. The procedure is completely painless, but radiation doses are considerable. New continuous-motion (helical or spiral), three-dimensional CT, which provides very detailed pictures of the GI organs and vasculature, has been developed.

Magnetic Resonance Imaging

MRI is used in gastroenterology to supplement ultrasonography and CT. This noninvasive technique uses magnetic fields and radio waves to produce an image of the area being studied. The use of oral contrast agents to enhance the image has increased the application of this technique for the diagnosis of GI diseases. It is useful in evaluating abdominal soft tissues as well as blood vessels, abscesses, fistulas, neoplasms, and other sources of bleeding.

Positron Emission Tomography

PET produces images of the body by detecting the radiation emitted from radioactive substances. The radioactive substances are injected into the body intravenously and usually are tagged with a radioactive atom, such as carbon-11, fluorine-18, oxygen-15, or nitrogen-13. The atoms decay quickly, do not harm the body, have lower radiation levels than a typical x-ray or CT scan, and are eliminated in the urine or feces. The scanner essentially "captures" where the radioactive substances are in the body, transmits information to a scanner, and produces a scan with "hot spots" for evaluation by the radiologist or oncologist.

Endoscopy Procedures

Endoscopy procedures are performed for a variety of reasons and are associated with a variety of psychological reactions from the patients. Many patients avoid the recommended endoscopies out of fear of the procedure or what the procedure may find. In recent years, propofol has been used increasingly during endoscopy procedures instead of sedation with the combination of an opiate and benzodiazepine. Box 21-1 details nursing responsibilities associated with the use of propofol during a GI endoscopy procedure.

Upper Gastrointestinal Fibroscopy/Esophagogastroduodenoscopy

Fibroscopy of the upper GI tract allows direct visualization of the esophageal, gastric, and duodenal mucosa through

---

| BOX 21-1 | **Sedation and Anesthesia in Gastrointestinal Endoscopy** |

Endoscopy is direct visualization of the GI tract using a flexible fiberoptic endoscope. Visualization of the esophagus, stomach, biliary system, and bowel is possible with an endoscope. Sedation is given to reduce anxiety and diminish the patient's memory of this uncomfortable event. The level of sedation required to perform an endoscopy ranges from minimal sedation to general anesthesia.

In recent years, studies have identified advantages of using propofol during endoscopy procedures over sedation with the combination of an opiate (pethidine and fentanyl are the most popular) and benzodiazepines (midazolam is the benzodiazepine of choice because of its shorter duration of action and better pharmacokinetic profile compared with diazepam). Propofol during GI endoscopy procedures can lead to patient and physician satisfaction, improved patient cooperation, faster recovery, and mild antiemetic properties. Propofol is currently preferred for the endoscopic sedation of patients with advanced liver disease due to its short biologic half-life and lower risk of inducing hepatic encephalopathy. However, there are some disadvantages, including the potential to induce hypotension as it is a cardiovascular depressant and respiratory depression and the fact that there is no pharmacologic antagonist.

The patient should be monitored to detect any changes in pulse, blood pressure, ventilator status (RR, and O_2 saturation), cardiac electrical activity, and neurologic status. An individual with skill sets including certification in basic and advanced cardiac life support should be present to monitor and interpret the patient's status throughout the procedure. The use of an anesthesiologist is recommended in the following situations: endoscopic procedures requiring deep sedation, anticipated intolerance to standard sedatives, multiple comorbidities (obesity; pregnancy; elderly individuals; as well as patients with chronic lung, kidney, or liver disease), and increased risk for airway obstruction because of anatomical variation.

Adapted from American Society for Gastrointestinal Endoscopy, 2008; Triantafillidis et al., 2013.

FIGURE 21-9 Patient undergoing gastroscopy (fibroscopy of the upper GI tract).

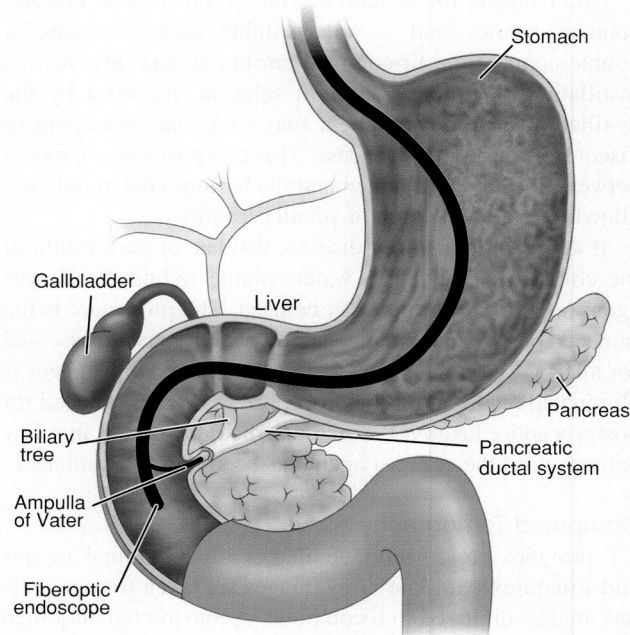

FIGURE 21-10 Endoscopic retrograde cholangiopancreatography (ERCP). A fiberoptic duodenoscope, with side-viewing apparatus, is inserted into the duodenum. The ampulla of Vater is catheterized, and the biliary tree is injected with contrast agent. The pancreatic ductal system is also assessed, if indicated. This procedure is of special value in visualizing neoplasms of the ampulla area and extracting a biopsy specimen.

a lighted endoscope (Fig. 21-9). Esophagogastroduodenoscopy (EGD) is especially valuable when esophageal, gastric, or duodenal abnormalities or inflammatory, neoplastic, or infectious processes are suspected. This procedure also can be used to evaluate esophageal and gastric motility and to collect secretions and tissue specimens for further analysis.

In EGD, the gastroenterologist views the GI tract through a viewing lens and can take still or video photographs through the scope to document findings. Electronic video endoscopes also are available that attach directly to a video processor, converting the electronic signals into pictures on a television screen. This allows larger and continuous viewing capabilities, as well as the simultaneous recording of the procedure.

PillCam ESO2, a pill-sized instrument equipped with two cameras, is available. Each camera takes photographs, and it is used to detect the presence of varices or diseases of the esophageal mucosa. A disadvantage is that it does not allow for obtaining biopsies and cannot be used to perform therapeutic procedures, such as esophageal banding to treat esophageal varices (Cave, Saltzman, & Travis, 2015).

Two additional drawbacks to this method of endoscopy are that it evaluates only the esophagus and that it may become lodged in a previously anastomosed section of bowel and require further endoscopic or surgical intervention for removal.

Side-viewing flexible scopes are used to visualize the common bile duct and the pancreatic and hepatic ducts through the ampulla of Vater in the duodenum. This procedure, called **endoscopic retrograde cholangiopancreatography (ERCP)**, uses the endoscope in combination with x-ray techniques to view the ductal structures of the biliary tract. ERCP is helpful in detecting and treating bile duct stones, bile duct strictures, pancreatic duct disruption, and sphincter of Oddi dysfunction. It should be used carefully in patients diagnosed with acute pancreatitis as it may worsen the severity of the condition (Daniels, 2014). The examination of the hepatobiliary system is carried out via a side-viewing flexible fiberoptic endoscope inserted through the esophagus to the descending duodenum (Fig. 21-10). Multiple position changes are required to pass the endoscope during the procedure, beginning in the left semiprone position. Careful insertion of a catheter through the endoscope into the common bile duct is the most important step in sphincterotomy (division of the muscles of the biliary sphincter) for gallstone extraction via this technique. Although ERCP has been considered the procedure of choice in evaluating biliary disorders, it is now used less frequently as it has been replaced by other imaging methods such as transabdominal and endoscopic ultrasonography, multislice helical CT, and MRI/MRCP (magnetic resonance imaging/cholangiopancreatography) (Hawkey, Bosche, Richter, Garcia-Tsao, & Chan, 2012).

Upper GI fibroscopy also can be a therapeutic procedure when it is combined with other procedures. Therapeutic endoscopy can be used to remove common bile duct stones, dilate strictures, and treat gastric bleeding and esophageal varices. Laser-compatible scopes can be used to provide laser therapy for upper GI neoplasms. Sclerosing solutions can be injected through the scope in an attempt to control upper GI bleeding in cases such as bleeding ulcers and varices.

Colonoscopy   **Sigmoidoscopy**

Ascending colon
Transverse colon
Flexible colonoscope
Descending colon
Presence of polyps
Sigmoid colon
Rectum

FIGURE 21-11 Colonoscopy. The flexible scope is passed through the rectum and sigmoid colon into the descending, transverse, and ascending colon.

Fiberoptic Colonoscopy

Historically, direct visualization of the bowel was the only means to evaluate the colon, but virtual colonoscopy (also known as CT colonography) has brought a more patient-friendly approach to this study. First described by Vining in 1994, virtual colonoscopy provides a computer-simulated endoluminal perspective of the air-filled distended colon using conventional spiral or helical CT scanning (Johnson, 2009). Because it can accurately identify tumor location, nodal, staging, and extent, it may become the diagnostic tool of choice in evaluating colorectal cancers preoperatively (Stagnitti et al., 2015).

Direct visual inspection of the large intestine (anus, rectum, sigmoid, transcending and ascending colon) is possible by means of a flexible fiberoptic colonoscope (Fig. 21-11). These scopes have the same capabilities as those used for EGD but are larger in diameter and longer. Still and video recordings can be used to document the procedure and findings.

This procedure is used commonly as a diagnostic aid and screening device. It is most frequently used for cancer screening (Box 21-2) and for surveillance in patients with previous colon cancer or polyps. In addition, tissue biopsies can be obtained as needed, and polyps can be removed and evaluated. Other uses of colonoscopy include the evaluation of patients with diarrhea of unknown cause, occult bleeding, or anemia; further study of abnormalities detected on barium enema; and diagnosis, clarification, and determination of the extent of inflammatory or other bowel disease.

Therapeutically, the procedure can be used to remove all visible polyps with a special snare and cautery through the colonoscope. Many colon cancers begin with adenomatous

---

BOX 21-2 **Health Promotion**

Guidelines for Colon and Rectal Cancer Screening

- Colorectal screening is currently divided into one of two groups: those tests that primarily detect cancer, including fecal occult blood test (FOBT), fecal immunochemical test (FIT) or stool tests for exfoliated DNA (sDNA), or those that detect cancer and advanced lesions, such as endoscopic and radiologic testing, flexible sigmoidoscopy, colonoscopy, double barium enema, CT colonography, or virtual colonoscopy. Beginning at 50 years of age, both men and women should follow one of these testing schedules:
  - Annual high-sensitivity FOBT
  - sDNA test every 3 years
  - Flexible sigmoidoscopy every 5 years
  - Colonoscopy every 10 years
  - Double-contrast barium enema every 5 years
  - CT colonoscopy every 5 years

  All tests with positive results should be followed up with colonoscopy.

Individuals should talk to their providers about starting colorectal cancer screening earlier and/or undergoing screening more often if they have any of the following risk factors for colorectal cancer:
- A personal history of colorectal cancer or adenomatous polyps
- A strong family history of colorectal cancer or colorectal adenomas found in first-degree relatives (guidelines are based upon relatives' age at diagnosis)
- A personal history of chronic inflammatory bowel disease
- A family history of a hereditary colorectal cancer syndrome (familial adenomatous polyposis or hereditary nonpolyposis colon cancer)
- Patients who have had curative-intent resection of colorectal cancer

Smith et al., 2015.

polyps of the colon; therefore, one goal of colonoscopic polypectomy is early detection and prevention of colorectal cancer. This procedure also can be used to treat areas of bleeding or stricture. Use of bipolar and unipolar coagulators, use of heater probes, and injections of sclerosing agents or vasoconstrictors are all possible during this procedure. Laser-compatible scopes provide laser therapy for bleeding lesions or colonic neoplasms. Bowel decompression (removal of intestinal contents to prevent gas and fluid from distending the coils of the intestine) also can be completed during the procedure.

Colonoscopy is performed while the patient is lying on the left side with the legs drawn up toward the chest. The patient's position may be changed during the test to facilitate advancement of the scope. Biopsy forceps or a cytology brush may be passed through the scope to obtain specimens for histology and cytology examinations. Complications during and after the procedure can include cardiac arrhythmias and respiratory depression resulting from the medications administered, vasovagal reactions, bowel perforation, bleeding from biopsy sites, and circulatory overload or hypotension resulting from overhydration or underhydration during bowel preparation. Therefore, it is important to monitor the patient's cardiac and respiratory function and oxygen saturation continuously, providing supplemental oxygen used as necessary. Typically, the procedure takes about 1 hour, and postprocedure discomfort results from instillation of air to expand the colon and insertion and movement of the scope during the procedure.

Anoscopy, Proctoscopy, and Sigmoidoscopy

Endoscopic examination of the anus, rectum, and sigmoid and descending colon is used to evaluate chronic diarrhea, fecal incontinence, ischemic colitis, and lower GI hemorrhage and to observe for ulceration, fissures, abscesses, tumors, polyps, and other pathologic processes.

Flexible scopes have largely replaced the rigid scopes used in the past for routine examinations. The flexible fiberoptic sigmoidoscope (see Fig. 21-11) permits the colon to be examined up to 40 to 50 cm (16 to 20 in) from the anus, much more than the 25 cm (10 in) that can be visualized with the rigid sigmoidoscope. It has many of the same capabilities as the scopes used for the upper GI study, including the use of still or video images to document findings.

For flexible scope procedures, the patient assumes a comfortable position on the left side with the right leg bent and placed anteriorly. It is important to keep the patient informed throughout the examination and to explain the sensations associated with the examination. Biopsies and polypectomies can be performed during this procedure. Biopsy is performed with small biting forceps introduced through the endoscope; one or more small piece of tissue may be removed. If rectal or sigmoid polyps are present, they may be removed with a wire snare, which is used to grasp the pedicle or stalk. Then an electrocoagulating

current is used to sever the polyp and prevent bleeding. It is extremely important that all excised tissue be placed immediately in moist gauze or in an appropriate receptacle, labeled correctly, and delivered without delay to the pathology laboratory for examination. Monitoring the patient for early signs of cardiac arrhythmias, perforation, and hemorrhage are important considerations.

Endoscopy for Esophageal Varices

Esophageal varices are varicosities that develop from elevated pressure in the veins that drain into the portal system. Varices are associated with cirrhosis of the liver. They are prone to rupture and often are the source of massive hemorrhages from the upper GI tract. Immediate endoscopy is indicated to identify the cause and the site of bleeding; at least 30% of patients with suspected bleeding from esophageal varices are actually bleeding from another source (gastritis, ulcer). Nursing support can be effective in relieving anxiety during this often stressful experience. Careful monitoring can detect early signs of cardiac arrhythmias, perforation, and hemorrhage.

After the examination, fluids are not given until the gag reflex returns. Lozenges and gargles may be used to relieve throat discomfort if the patient's physical condition and mental status permit. If the patient is actively bleeding, oral intake will not be permitted, and the patient will be prepared for further diagnostic and therapeutic procedures.

Laparoscopy (Peritoneoscopy)

With the tremendous advances in minimally invasive surgery, diagnostic laparoscopy is efficient, cost-effective, and useful in the diagnosis of GI disease. After creating a pneumoperitoneum (gas, usually carbon dioxide, is insufflated into the peritoneal cavity to separate the intestines from the pelvic organs, creating a working space for visualization), a small incision is made lateral to the umbilicus, allowing for the insertion of the fiberoptic laparoscope. This allows direct access to the organs and structures within the abdomen, permitting visualization and identification of any growths, anomalies, and inflammatory processes. In addition, biopsy samples can be taken from the structures and organs as necessary. This procedure can be used to evaluate peritoneal disease, chronic abdominal pain, abdominal masses, and gallbladder and liver disease. However, laparoscopy has not become an important diagnostic modality in patients with acute abdominal pain because less invasive tools (i.e., CT and MRI) are readily available. Laparoscopy usually requires general anesthesia and sometimes requires that the stomach and bowel be decompressed. One of the benefits of this procedure is that after visualization of a problem, then excision (e.g., removal of the gallbladder) can be performed at the same time, if appropriate. Patient complaints of shoulder and abdominal pain are associated with residual carbon dioxide effects. Postprocedure standard protocol for postoperative care is followed (see Chapter 5).

Small-Bowel Enteroscopy

Capsule endoscopy is a noninvasive enteroscopy that visualizes the entire small bowel, including the distal ileum. It is used to evaluate the source of GI bleeding. Prior to the development of the capsule endoscopy, visualization of the small intestine was inadequate and physicians relied primarily on barium x-rays for diagnosing disorders of the small intestine. Because the procedure is noninvasive, it has the capability to improve colorectal cancer screening and is useful in those patients where colonoscopy is incomplete (ranges between 10% and 40%) or where colonoscopy is contraindicated (Eliakim & Adler, 2015). The technique consists of the patient swallowing a capsule approximately the size of a vitamin pill that has embedded within it wireless miniature cameras at both ends, a light source, and an image transmission system that takes photographs as it passes through the GI tract (Eliakim & Adler, 2015). The capsule is propelled through the intestines by peristalsis and is excreted naturally in the stool in 1 to 2 days. During the procedure, images are transmitted from the capsule to a data recorder housed in an abdominal belt worn by the patient. In order to achieve accurate results, the bowel-cleansing procedure prior to ingesting the capsule is more rigorous than that of the standard colonoscopy (Sieg, 2011). In addition, the capsule may be retained requiring surgical intervention (Matsui, Matsumoto, Aoyagi, 2014). Colonoscopy remains the preferred method of screening for colorectal cancer as it allows for the removal of polyps and biopsy samples; the nurse must be cognizant that successful screening is dependent upon the quality of the colonoscopy (Sieg, 2011).

Another procedure used to visualize the entire mucosa of the small bowel, as well as to enable diagnostic and therapeutic interventions, is double-balloon enteroscopy (DBE) used with a push and pull method (Matsui et al., 2014). This endoscope has two balloons, one attached to the distal end of the scope and the other attached to the transparent overtube that slides over the endoscope. The endoscope is advanced using a push-and-pull technique that involves inflating and deflating the balloons alternatively. This process causes the telescoping of the small intestine onto the overtube, which enables the endoscope to visualize much more of the small intestine than the length of the scope itself. The procedure takes 1 to 3 hours and requires moderate sedation. DBE is indicated in patients with inflammatory bowel disease, obstruction, neoplastic diseases, hemorrhagic disorders, bile/pancreatic diseases, and for the removal of foreign bodies. It is contraindicated in patients with perforations or severe inflammations (Matsui et al., 2014).

Endoscopy Through Ostomy

Endoscopy using a flexible endoscope through an ostomy stoma is useful for visualizing a segment of the small or large intestine and may be indicated to evaluate the anastomosis for recurrent disease or to visualize and treat bleeding in a segment of the bowel.

Gastric Analysis, Gastric Acid Stimulation Test, and pH Monitoring

Analysis of the gastric juice yields information about the secretory activity of the gastric mucosa and the presence or degree of gastric retention in patients thought to have pyloric or duodenal obstruction. It is also useful for diagnosing **Zollinger-Ellison syndrome**, or atrophic gastritis.

A small nasogastric tube with a catheter tip marked at various points is inserted through the nose. When the tube is at a point slightly less than 50 cm (21 in), it should be within the stomach, lying along the greater curvature. Once in place, the tube is secured to the patient's cheek, and the patient is placed in a semi-reclining position. The entire stomach contents are aspirated by gentle suction into a syringe.

The gastric acid stimulation test usually is performed in conjunction with gastric analysis. Histamine or pentagastrin is administered subcutaneously to stimulate gastric secretions. It is important to inform the patient that this injection may produce a flushed feeling. The nurse monitors the patient's blood pressure and pulse frequently to detect hypotension. Gastric specimens are collected after the injection every 15 minutes for 1 hour and are labeled to indicate the time of specimen collection after histamine injection. The volume and pH of the specimen are measured; in certain instances, cytologic study by the Papanicolaou technique may be used to determine the presence or absence of malignant cells.

Because gastroesophageal reflux with esophageal inflammation may predispose patients to adenocarcinomas of the esophagus, diagnosis of gastroesophageal reflux is important (Fisichella, Allaix, Morino, & Patti, 2014). One method of diagnosing reflux is through ambulatory pH monitoring, considered a valuable method for diagnosing gastroesophageal disease (Fisichella et al., 2014). This may be accomplished by attaching a transmitter sensitive to pH measurement to the esophagus or by inserting a catheter containing a probe through the nose and ending in the distal part of the esophagus to measure pH (Kasper et al., 2015). These measurements are taken while the patient is ambulatory and are measured over 24 to 48 hours (Kasper et al., 2015).

A Bernstein test, developed in the 1950s (Bashashati, Hejazi, Andrews, & Storr, 2014), may be performed to evaluate complaints of acid-related chest or epigastric pain. HCl is instilled through a small feeding tube positioned in the esophagus to try to elicit the reported chest pain. Resultant signs and symptoms are compared with the patient's usual symptoms. To date, the advantage in using this examination to diagnose GERD or functional esophageal disorder is unclear (Bashashati et al., 2014).

Esophageal Manometry

Esophageal manometry is the placement of a catheter via the esophagus that detects pressure and measures esophageal contractility while the patient swallows. It is used to detect motility abnormalities, such as achalasia or esophageal spasms, and to evaluate peristaltic activity of the esophagus prior to surgery (Kasper et al., 2015).

The Bravo pH monitoring system is a newer procedure that offers the advantage of pH monitoring of the esophagus without the transnasal catheter. The Bravo system involves a pH capsule about the size of a gel cap, which is temporarily attached to the wall of the esophagus. The Bravo pH capsule measures pH levels in the esophagus and transmits readings via radio telemetry to the pager-sized receiver worn on the patient's belt or waistband. The patient is instructed to push a button at the onset of symptoms, which then are associated with the presence or absence of acid reflux. If possible, the patient should discontinue using proton pump inhibitors for 5 to 7 days prior to the study. Data are collected for up to 48 hours and then downloaded and analyzed (Bashashati et al., 2014).

Liver Function Tests

Early recognition and assessment of liver dysfunction is critical to provide timely and appropriate care for the patient with acute or chronic liver disease. More than 70% of the parenchyma of the liver may be damaged before liver function test results become abnormal. Function is generally measured in terms of serum enzyme activity (i.e., serum aminotransferases, alkaline phosphatase [ALP], lactic dehydrogenase) and serum concentrations of proteins (albumin and globulins), bilirubin, ammonia, clotting factors, and lipids. Several of these tests may be helpful for assessing patients with liver disease. However, the nature and extent of liver dysfunction cannot be determined by these tests alone because other disorders can affect test results.

Serum aminotransferases (also called transaminases) are enzymes that reflect varying degrees of hepatocellular injury or inflammation of the liver and are useful in detecting acute liver disease, such as hepatitis. Alanine aminotransferase (ALT), aspartate aminotransferase (AST), and gamma-glutamyl transferase (GGT; also called G-glutamyl transpeptidase) are the most frequently used tests for liver damage. ALT levels increase primarily in liver disorders and may be used to monitor the course of hepatitis or cirrhosis or the effects of treatments that may be toxic to the liver. AST is present in tissues that have high metabolic activity; therefore, the level may be increased if there is damage to or death of tissues of organs such as the heart, liver, skeletal muscle, and kidney. Although not specific to liver disease, levels of AST may be increased in cirrhosis, hepatitis, and liver cancer. Abnormal aminotransferases may occur in the absence of any clinical indication of liver disease, and this finding requires further investigation to determine if it is incidental or if hepatic injury is present. The normal ratio of AST to ALT is 0.8. In most cases of hepatocellular damage, the AST is lower than the ALT and the AST/ALT ratio of 2:1 suggests liver injury caused by excessive alcohol ingestion (Friedman et al., 2015).

Increased GGT levels are associated with cholestasis but also can be due to alcoholic liver disease. Although the kidney has the highest level of the enzyme, the liver is considered the source of normal serum activity. Alkaline phosphatase (ALP) elevations may indicate injury to the biliary tree (i.e., biliary obstruction), presence of tumors, primary biliary cirrhosis, and primary sclerosing cholangitis. Elevations of both ALP and GGT indicate disease of the liver or biliary system. Elevation of ALP with normal GGT levels should initiate evaluation for possible bone disease, as this enzyme is also present in bone tissue.

Other important tests to determine the extent of liver dysfunction are serum bilirubin, serum albumin, and prothrombin time as measured by the international normalized ratio (INR). These tests represent the synthetic function of the liver and are used as a prognostic tool to determine the severity of liver disease (Friedman et al., 2015). Common liver function tests are summarized in Table 21-7.

Liver Biopsy

Liver biopsy is considered the gold standard for the diagnosis of liver disease. A small sample of liver tissue is obtained, usually through needle aspiration, for microscopic evaluation of liver cells and architecture. The most common indication is to evaluate diffuse disorders of the parenchyma and to diagnose space-occupying lesions. Liver biopsy is especially useful when clinical findings and laboratory tests are not diagnostic. Bleeding and bile peritonitis after liver biopsy are the major complications; therefore, coagulation studies are obtained, their values are noted, and abnormal results are treated before liver biopsy is performed. Other techniques for liver biopsy are preferred if ascites or coagulation abnormalities exist. A liver biopsy can be performed percutaneously with ultrasound guidance or transvenously through the right internal jugular vein to the right hepatic vein under fluoroscopic control. Liver biopsy also can be performed laparoscopically. Guidelines for assisting with a liver biopsy are found in Box 21-3.

Paracentesis

Paracentesis is the removal of fluid (ascites) from the peritoneal cavity through a puncture or a small surgical incision through the abdominal wall under sterile conditions. Ultrasound guidance may be indicated in some patients who are at high risk for bleeding because of an abnormal coagulation profile and in those who have had previous abdominal surgery and may have adhesions. Also ultrasound guidance is recommended for patients in whom percussion cannot locate the ascites or in whom a first paracentesis attempt does not yield fluid (Garcia-Tsao, 2016). Paracentesis may be used for therapeutic reasons (removal of more than 5 L of fluid) to decrease intra-abdominal pressure resulting in dyspnea, abdominal pain, and abdominal fullness. In addition, paracentesis is appropriate for diagnostic purposes (Runyon, Chopra, & Travis, 2015) in evaluating new-onset ascites, diagnosing spontaneous versus secondary bacterial peritonitis, or detecting the presence of cancer. It is

TABLE **21-7 Common Laboratory Tests to Assess Liver Function**

Test	Normal	Clinical Functions
Pigment Studies		
Serum bilirubin, direct	0–0.3 mg/dL (0–5.1 µmol/L)	These studies measure the ability of the liver to conjugate and excrete bilirubin. Results are abnormal in liver and biliary tract diseases and are associated with jaundice clinically.
Serum bilirubin, total	0–0.9 mg/dL (1.7–20.5 µmol/L)	
Urine bilirubin	0(0)	
Urine urobilinogen	0.05–2.5 mg/24 hr (0.09–4. Ehrlich U/24 hr)	
Fecal urobilinogen (infrequently used)	50–300 mg/24 hr (100–400 Ehrlich U/100 g)	
Protein Studies		
Total serum protein	7.0–7.5 g/dL (70–75 g/L)	Proteins are manufactured by the liver. Their levels may be affected in a variety of liver impairments: albumin is affected in cirrhosis, chronic hepatitis, edema, and ascites; globulins are affected in cirrhosis, liver disease, chronic obstructive jaundice, and viral hepatitis.
Serum albumin	4.0–5.5 g/dL (40–55 g/L)	
Serum globulin	1.7–3.3 g/dL (17–33 g/L)	
Serum protein electrophoresis		
Albumin	4.0–5.5 g/dL (40–55 g/L)	
Alpha$_1$-Globulin	0.15–0.25 g/dL (1.5–2.5 g/L)	
Alpha$_2$-Globulin	0.43–0.75 g/dL (4.3–7.5 g/L)	
Beta-Globulin	0.5–1.0 g/dL (5–10 g/L)	
Gamma-Globulin	0.6–1.3 g/dL (6–13 g/L)	
Albumin/globulin (A/G) ratio	A > G or 1.5:1–2.5:1	A/G ratio is reversed in chronic liver disease (decreased albumin and increased globulin).
Prothrombin Time	100% or 12–16 seconds	Prothrombin time may be prolonged in liver disease. It will not return to normal with vitamin K in severe liver cell damage.
Serum Alkaline Phosphatase	Varies with method: 2–5 Bodansky units 30–50 U/L at 34°C (17–142 U/L at 30°C) (20–90 U/L at 30°C)	Serum alkaline phosphatase is manufactured in bones, liver, kidneys, and intestine and excreted through biliary tract. In the absence of bone disease, it is a sensitive measure of biliary tract obstruction.
Serum Aminotransferase Studies		The studies are based on release of enzymes from damaged liver cells. These enzymes are elevated in liver cell damage.
AST	10–40 units (4.8–19 U/L)	
ALT	5–35 units (2.4–17 U/L)	
GGT, GGTP	10–48 IU/L	Elevated in alcohol abuse. Marker for biliary cholestasis.
LDH	Adults: 140–280 U/L or 2.34–4.68 µkat/L	
Ammonia (plasma)	15–45 µg/dL (11–32 µmol/L)	Liver converts ammonia to urea. Ammonia level rises in liver failure.
Cholesterol		
Ester	60% of total (fraction of total cholesterol: 0.60)	Cholesterol levels are elevated in biliary obstruction and decreased in parenchymal liver disease.
HDL (high-density lipoprotein)	HDL Male: 35–70 mg/dL, Female: 35–85 mg/dL	
LDL (low-density lipoprotein)	LDL <130 µg/dL	

contraindicated in cases of acute abdomen and is generally not used in patients with lower volume ascites (less than 5 L), uncorrected hypovolemia, and those with a platelet count of less than 20,000/uL (Kasper et al., 2015). Paracentesis is used to evaluate patients whose clinical condition has deteriorated or to measure ascitic fluid for cell count, albumin total protein levels, culture, Gram stain, and neutrophilic count (Vincent, Abraham, Moore, Kochanek, & Fink, 2011).

Large-volume (5 to 6 L) paracentesis has been shown to be a safe method for treating patients with severe ascites in those patients with diuretic-resistant ascites or those patients who have been unresponsive to medication or dietary restrictions. This technique may be used in combination with an isotonic albumin solution and sodium (sodium concentrations are dependent upon a hypervolemic or hypovolemic state) (Such, Runyon, Lindor, &

BOX 21-3

GUIDELINES FOR NURSING CARE

Assisting with Percutaneous Liver Biopsy

Equipment

- Liver biopsy tray (contains needles, scalpel, specimen tubes, etc.)
- Sterile gloves
- Antiseptic solution
- Local anesthetic
- Sterile dressing
- Sphygmomanometer to monitor BP

Implementation

NURSING ACTION	RATIONALE
Preprocedure	
1. Ascertain that results of coagulation tests (prothrombin time, partial thromboplastin time, and platelet count) are available and that compatible donor blood is available.	1. Many patients with liver disease have clotting defects and are at risk for bleeding.
2. Check for signed consent; confirm that informed consent has been provided.	2. Ensure that the patient consents to this invasive procedure.
3. Measure and record the patient's pulse, respirations, and blood pressure immediately before biopsy.	3. Prebiopsy values provide a basis on which to compare the patient's vital signs and evaluate status after the procedure.
4. Describe to the patient in advance: steps of the procedure, sensations expected, after-effects anticipated, restrictions of activity, and monitoring procedures to follow.	4. Explanations allay fears and ensure cooperation.
During Procedure	
1. Support the patient during the procedure.	1. Encouragement and support of the nurse enhance comfort and promote a sense of security.
2. Expose the right side of the patient's upper abdomen (right hypochondriac).	2. The skin at the site of penetration will be cleansed and a local anesthetic will be infiltrated.
3. Instruct the patient to inhale and exhale deeply several times, finally to exhale, and to hold breath at the end of expiration. The physician promptly introduces the biopsy needle by way of the transthoracic (intercostal) or transabdominal (subcostal) route, penetrates the liver, aspirates, and withdraws.	3. Holding the breath immobilizes the chest wall and the diaphragm; penetration of the diaphragm thereby is avoided, and the risk of lacerating the liver is minimized.
4. Instruct the patient to resume breathing.	4. The patient often continues holding his or her breath because of anxiety.

Lung · 6th rib · Diaphragm · 7th rib · Liver

NURSING ACTION	RATIONALE
Postprocedure	
1. Immediately after the biopsy, some providers may suggest the patient turn onto the right side with a small pillow under the costal margin (provides extra pressure), and caution the patient to remain in this position, recumbent and immobile, for 2 hours. Instruct the patient to avoid coughing or straining.	1. In this position, the liver capsule at the site of penetration is compressed against the chest wall, and the escape of blood or bile through the perforation is prevented.
2. Measure and record the patient's pulse, respiratory rate, and blood pressure at 10- to 15-minute intervals for the first hour, then every 30 minutes for the next 1–2 hours or until the patient's condition stabilizes.	2. Changes in vital signs may indicate bleeding, severe hemorrhage, or bile peritonitis, rare but serious complications of liver biopsy.
3. If the patient is discharged after the procedure, instruct the patient to avoid heavy lifting and strenuous activity for 1 week.	3. Activity restriction reduces the risk of bleeding at the biopsy puncture site.

BOX 21-4 GUIDELINES FOR NURSING CARE

Assisting with a Paracentesis

Equipment

- Paracentesis tray (contains trocar, syringe, needles, drainage tube)
- Sterile gloves
- Antiseptic solution
- Local anesthetic
- Sterile dressing
- Drainage collection bottles, receptacles
- Sphygmomanometer to monitor BP

Implementation

NURSING ACTION	RATIONALE
Preprocedure	
1. Check for signed consent form.	1. Ensure that patient has agreed to procedure.
2. Prepare the patient by providing the necessary information and instructions and by offering reassurance.	2. Having information increases the patient's understanding of the procedure and the reason for it.
3. Instruct the patient to void.	3. An empty bladder minimizes the risk of inadvertent puncture of the bladder and minimizes discomfort from a full bladder.
4. Gather appropriate sterile equipment and collection receptacles.	4. Sterility of equipment is essential to minimize risk of infection; having equipment available enables the procedure to be performed smoothly.
5. Place the patient in an upright position on the edge of the bed or in a chair with feet supported on a stool. Fowler position should be used by the patient confined to bed.	5. An upright position results in movement of the peritoneal fluid close to the abdominal wall and promotes easier puncture and removal of fluid.
6. Place the sphygmomanometer cuff around the patient's arm.	6. This allows the nurse to monitor the patient's blood pressure during procedure.
During Procedure	
1. The physician, using aseptic technique, inserts the trocar through a puncture below the umbilicus. The trocar, or needle, is connected to a drainage tube, the end of which is inserted into a collecting receptacle. (see the figure next page)	1. Sterile technique minimizes the risk of infection. Bleeding at the puncture site is minimal at this location. The fluid drains by gravity or mild siphon into the container.
2. Help the patient maintain position throughout the procedure.	2. The patient who is fatigued or weak may have difficulty maintaining an optimal position for drainage of fluid.

(continued on page 656)

BOX 21-4

GUIDELINES FOR NURSING CARE (*continued*)

Assisting with a Paracentesis (*continued*)

NURSING ACTION	RATIONALE

Figure on left shows possible sites for insertion of trocar.

3. Measure and record blood pressure at frequent intervals throughout the procedure.

4. Monitor the patient closely for signs of vascular collapse: pallor, increased pulse rate, or decreased blood pressure.

Postprocedure

1. Return the patient to bed or to a comfortable sitting position.
2. Measure, describe, and record the fluid collected.

3. Label samples of fluid and send to laboratory.
4. Monitor vital signs every 15 minutes for 1 hour, every 30 minutes for 2 hours, every hour for 2 hours, and then every 4 hours.
5. Measure the patient's temperature.

6. Assess for hypovolemia, electrolyte shifts, changes in mental status, and encephalopathy.

7. When taking vital signs, check puncture site for leakage or bleeding.

8. Provide patient teaching regarding the need to monitor for bleeding or excessive drainage from the puncture site, the importance of avoiding heavy lifting or straining, the need to change position slowly, and frequency of monitoring for fever.

---

3. Decreased blood pressure may occur with vascular collapse, which can result from removal of the fluid from the peritoneal cavity and fluid shifts.

4. Vascular collapse (hypovolemia) may occur as fluid moves from the vascular system to replace fluid drained from peritoneal cavity.

1. The weak or fatigued patient may have difficulty resuming a comfortable position without assistance.
2. The volume of fluid removed may range from small to very large, and its removal may affect fluid and vascular status; volume should be included in input and output records. The characteristics of the fluid (clear vs. cloudy, red vs. colorless) may be helpful in diagnostic evaluation.
3. Peritoneal fluid is analyzed as part of the diagnostic workup.
4. Vital signs (blood pressure, pulse rate) may change as fluid shifts occur after removal of fluid, especially if a large volume of fluid was removed.
5. An elevated temperature is a sign of infection and should be reported to the patient's provider.
6. Changes in fluid and electrolyte states and mental and cognitive status may occur with removal of fluid and fluid shifts and should be reported.
7. Leakage of fluid may occur because of changes in abdominal pressure and may contribute to further loss of fluid if undetected. Leakage suggests a possible site for infection, and bleeding may occur in patients with altered clotting secondary to liver disease.
8. The patient (or family members) needs to monitor the patient overall and especially the puncture site for bleeding and excessive drainage if the patient is discharged home after the procedure. Heavy lifting or straining is avoided to enable the puncture site to close. Slow changes in position are recommended because of the risk of hypovolemia related to fluid removal. Monitoring for fever is needed to detect infection.

Travis, 2015). Therapeutic paracentesis provides only temporary removal of fluid; ascites rapidly recur, necessitating repeated fluid removal. Guidelines for assisting with paracentesis are found in Box 21-4.

Transjugular Intrahepatic Portosystemic Shunt

Another option to treat patients with ascites who are diuretic resistant or to prevent reoccurrence of hemorrhage is by placement of a transjugular intrahepatic portosystemic shunt (TIPS). This shunt is surgically inserted under radiologic guidance (Kasper et al., 2015), through the internal jugular vein, creating a shunt or opening between the portal and hepatic veins in order to decrease portal pressure (Grossman & Porth, 2014). The nurse should monitor the patient for hepatic encephalopathy, a complication associated with the TIPS. This complication is likely caused by the inability of ammonia and other toxic substances in the gut to pass through the liver (Grossman & Porth, 2014).

Cholecystography

Although cholecystography has been replaced by ultrasonography as the test of choice for gallstones, it is still used if ultrasound equipment is not available or if the ultrasound results are inconclusive. Oral cholecystography may be performed to detect gallstones and to assess the ability of the gallbladder to fill, concentrate its contents, contract, and empty. An iodide-containing contrast agent that is excreted by the liver and concentrated in the gallbladder is administered to the patient. The normal gallbladder fills with this radiopaque substance. If gallstones are present, they appear as shadows on the x-ray film.

The patient is asked about allergies to iodine or seafood. If no allergy is identified, the patient receives the oral form of the contrast agent the evening before the x-rays are obtained. Cholecystography in the obviously jaundiced patient is not useful because the liver cannot excrete the radiopaque dye into the gallbladder in the presence of jaundice.

CHAPTER REVIEW

Critical Thinking Exercises

1. While having blood pressure measurements taken at the adult day care center, one of the patients tells the nurse that this morning after he had a bowel movement, he noticed bright red blood on the toilet tissue. What further data would the nurse need to gather?

2. A 50-year-old female patient is seen in the emergency department complaining of right upper quadrant (RUQ) abdominal pain and cramping for the last 2 days. The symptoms usually began 1 to 2 hours after eating a dinner of fried or spicy foods. As a marketing specialist, she travels extensively and her usual dietary pattern consists of eating at restaurants several times weekly.
   a. For what aspect of the patient's history should the nurse seek additional information or clarification?
   b. What physical assessment findings would the nurse be most likely to find during the abdominal assessment?

NCLEX Style Review Questions

1. Which assessment finding does the nurse expect as a normal consequence of aging?
   a. Increased salivation and drooling
   b. Hyperactive bowel sounds and loose stools
   c. Increased gastric production and heartburn
   d. Decreased sensation to defecate and constipation

2. Which of the following foods could give a false-positive result on the fecal occult blood test (FOBT)? *Select all that apply.*
   a. Red meats
   b. Pasta
   c. Turnips
   d. Fish
   e. Whole-grain bread

3. Which question will best assist the nurse in the assessment of a patient with acute diarrhea?
   a. "Have you had a colonoscopy in the last 3 months?"
   b. "Have you traveled outside the country recently?"
   c. "Do you have any trouble swallowing?"
   d. "Do you have any allergies?"

4. The nurse recognizes that most nutrients and electrolytes are absorbed by which organ?
   a. Esophagus
   b. Stomach
   c. Colon
   d. Small intestine

5. When performing an abdominal assessment on a patient with suspected cholecystitis, how does the nurse palpate the patient's abdomen?
   a. Palpate the right lower quadrant only
   b. Palpate the upper quadrants only
   c. Defer palpation and use percussion only
   d. Palpate the right upper quadrant last

Try these additional resources, available at **http://thepoint.lww.com/Honan2e**, to enhance your learning and understanding of this chapter:

- NCLEX-Style Student Review Questions
- Journal Articles

REFERENCES AND SELECTED READINGS

References and selected readings associated with this chapter can be found on the website that accompanies the book. Visit **http://thepoint. lww.com/Honan2e** to access the references and other additional resources associated with this chapter.

Nursing Management: Patients with Oral and Esophageal Disorders and Patients Receiving Gastrointestinal Intubation, Enteral, and Parenteral Nutrition

Zachary R. Krom

Learning Objectives

After reading this chapter, you will be able to:

1. Describe nursing management of patients with conditions of the oral cavity.
2. Use the nursing process as a framework for care of patients undergoing neck dissection.
3. Describe the various conditions of the esophagus and their clinical manifestations and management.
4. Describe the purposes and types of gastrointestinal intubation.
5. Discuss nursing management of the patient who has a nasogastric or nasoenteric tube.
6. Identify the purposes and uses of parenteral nutrition.

Digestion begins in the mouth; adequate nutrition is closely related to good dental health and the general condition of the mouth. Any discomfort or adverse condition in the oral cavity can affect a person's nutritional status, influencing the type and amount of food ingested as well as the degree to which food particles are exposed to salivary enzymes. Given the close relationship between adequate nutritional intake and the structures of the upper gastrointestinal (GI) tract (lips, mouth, teeth, pharynx, esophagus), nursing assessment and health teaching related to food and fluid intake, general nutritional health, speech, and self-image is warranted. In some patients, certain pathologies impede the function of the GI system, and artificial devices must be placed to support nutritional intake. It is important for the nurse to be familiar with the placement procedures, function, and associated complications when caring for patients receiving supplemental enteral (involving or passing through the intestine, e.g., tube feeding) or parenteral (not involving the GI tract, typically intravenous, e.g., partial parenteral nutrition [PPN]) nutrition.

ORAL DISORDERS

ORAL CARE

The nurse understands that oral health is a very important component of a person's physical and psychological well-being; common oral problems include dental plaque and caries. Healthy teeth must be cleaned conscientiously and effectively on a daily basis. Brushing and flossing are particularly effective in mechanically breaking up the bacterial plaque that collects around teeth. The level of mouth care performed on or by patients is dependent upon patient condition and tolerance of the procedure, with the ideal situation being when patients are able to brush and floss their teeth as they normally would at home. The American Dental Society recommends brushing twice a day and flossing once a day (2014). The primary focus of mouth care is to lessen the amount of bacterial film that accumulates on teeth, around gums, and in saliva (Box 22-1). Normal mastication (chewing) and the normal flow of saliva also aid greatly in

Health Promotion

Preventive Oral Hygiene

Instruct patients to:

- Brush teeth using a soft toothbrush at least twice daily. Hold toothbrush at a 45-degree angle against the gums and teeth. A small brush is better than a large brush. In addition to the teeth, the gums and tongue surface should be brushed.
- Floss at least once daily.
- Use an antiplaque mouth rinse.
- Visit a dentist at least every 6 months or when you have a chipped tooth, a lost filling, an oral sore that persists longer than 2 weeks, or a toothache.
- Avoid alcohol and tobacco products, including smokeless tobacco.
- Maintain adequate nutrition and avoid sweets.
- Replace your toothbrush at the first sign of wear, usually every 2 months.

keeping the teeth clean. Because many ill patients do not eat adequate amounts of food, they produce less saliva, which, in turn, reduces this natural tooth-cleaning process. The nurse may need to assume the responsibility for brushing the patient's teeth. A soft-bristled toothbrush is more effective than a sponge or foam stick. If brushing is not possible, the nurse should wipe the teeth with a gauze pad, and then have the patient swish an antiseptic mouthwash several times before expectorating into an emesis basin. To prevent drying, the nurse can coat the patient's lips with a water-based gel.

Not only is the bacterial film detrimental to the tooth surface and gums, it also can potentially create problems in the respiratory system. This film can translocate to the lungs and cause an infection. A recent systematic review of 35 randomized controlled studies involving medical, surgical, and trauma ICU patients and oral care practices in ventilated patients (Shi et al., 2013) found that the use of chlorhexidine mouthwash or gel had no bearing on morbidity, length of stay, or number of days on a ventilator. Chlorhexidine did decrease the odds of a patient developing ventilator-associated pneumonia (VAP) by 40%. The study also found that toothbrushing in patients who were ventilated had no effect on the reduction of VAP. Despite recent literature that does not directly support the benefit of individual interventions in oral care programs across critical care nursing practice, many hospitals continue to follow the guidelines to prevent VAP as established by the American Association of Critical Care Nurses (2010) (Munroe & Ruggiero, 2014). The guidelines include: oral moisturizing 6 to 12 times a day; brushing teeth, gums, and tongue twice a day; and using oral chlorhexidine gluconate (0.12%) twice a day in patients having cardiac surgery. For more information on VAP, refer to Chapter 10.

TEMPOROMANDIBULAR JOINT DISORDERS

Disorders of the temporomandibular joint (TMJ) can originate within the joint capsule itself or involve the muscle tissue that surrounds and supports the joint. Osteoarthritis, rheumatoid arthritis, and disruption of the joint structures, such as dislocation or disc displacement, occur within the joint.

Clinical Manifestations and Assessment

Pain with mastication and/or pain in the joint itself are the two most common manifestations of a TMJ disorder. Patients have pain ranging from a dull ache to throbbing, debilitating pain that can radiate to the ears, teeth, neck muscles, and facial sinuses. They often have restricted jaw motion and locking of the jaw. There also may be a sudden change in the way the upper and lower teeth fit together. The patient may hear clicking and grating noises, and chewing and swallowing may be difficult (National Institute of Dental and Craniofacial Research, 2014).

Diagnosis is based on the patient's report of pain, limitations in range of motion (ROM), dysphagia, difficulty chewing, difficulty with speech, or hearing difficulties. Magnetic resonance imaging (MRI), x-ray studies, and an arthrogram may be performed.

Medical Management

Conservative and reversible treatment is recommended. If irreversible surgical options are recommended, the patient is encouraged to seek a second opinion.

Nonsurgical Management

Although some practitioners think the role of stress in TMJ disorders is overrated, patient education in stress management may be helpful (to reduce grinding and clenching of teeth). Often occlusal guards are used in conjunction with stress management to prevent further deterioration of the tooth surface and irritation of the joint. Also the patient may benefit from ROM exercises without overextension of the joint. Pain management measures may include nonsteroidal anti-inflammatory drugs (NSAIDs) with the possible addition of opioids, muscle relaxants, or mild antidepressants. Occasionally, intraoral orthotics (a plastic guard worn over the upper and lower teeth) may be worn to reposition the condyle head in the joint space to a more normal position, which, in turn, relieves the stress and pressure of the joint on the tissues. This allows the tissues to heal.

Surgical Management

Correction of mandibular structural abnormalities may require surgery involving repositioning or reconstruction of the jaw. Simple fractures of the mandible without displacement, resulting from a blow on the chin, and planned surgical interventions, as in jaw repositioning (orthognathic) surgical correction to remedy cosmetic and functional jaw problems, may require treatment by these means. Jaw reconstruction may also be necessary in the aftermath of trauma from a severe injury or cancer, both of which can cause tissue and bone loss.

Usually mandibular fractures are closed fractures. Rigid plate fixation (insertion of metal plates and screws into the bone to approximate and stabilize the bone) is the current treatment of choice in many cases of mandibular fracture and in some mandibular reconstructive surgery procedures (Wein, Chandra, Leemans, & Weber, 2014). In some instances, the fracture repair involves wiring the patient's jaw shut for a number of weeks. Bone grafting may be performed to replace structural defects using bones from the patient's own ilium, ribs, or cranial sites. Also rib tissue may be harvested from cadaver donors.

Nursing Management

The patient who has had rigid fixation should be instructed not to chew food in the first 1 to 4 weeks after surgery. A liquid diet is recommended, and dietary counseling should be obtained to ensure optimal caloric and protein intake. To prevent aspiration, these patients should have wire cutters (for rigid fixation) or scissors (for rubber band fixation) at the bedside to release the jaw if the patient begins to vomit. The patient and family members should be instructed before discharge by the surgeon on where and how to cut the wires or rubber bands in an emergency before the patient is discharged. Rigid fixation remains for approximately 6 weeks depending upon the age of the patient, condition of bone, and the extent of the mandible injury.

The patient needs specific guidelines for mouth care and feeding. Any irritated areas in the mouth should be reported to the surgeon. Emphasis is placed on the importance of keeping scheduled appointments to assess the stability of the fixation appliance.

Consultation with a dietitian may be indicated so that the patient and family can learn about foods that are high in essential nutrients and ways in which these foods can be prepared so that they can be consumed through a straw or spoon while remaining palatable. Nutritional supplements may also be recommended.

DISORDERS OF THE SALIVARY GLANDS

About 1,200 mL of saliva is produced daily and swallowed. The three main functions of saliva are lubrication, protection against harmful bacteria, and digestion. The glands that can be affected include the parotids, the submandibulars, and the sublinguals.

Sialadenitis refers to the bacterial or viral infection of the salivary glands. Infection may be caused by dehydration, radiation therapy (RT), stress, malnutrition, salivary gland calculi (stones), or improper oral hygiene. Patients with a

FIGURE 22-1 Parotid gland and duct. (Reprinted from Porth, C. M. (2015). *Essentials of pathophysiology: Concepts of altered states* (4th ed.). Philadelphia, PA: Wolters Kluwer.)

bacterial infection have significant inflammation, pain, swelling, and purulent discharge. Treatment includes antibiotics, massage, hydration, warm compresses, and corticosteroids. Chronic sialadenitis with uncontrolled pain is treated by surgical drainage of the gland or excision of the gland and its ducts.

Parotitis (inflammation of the parotid gland) is the most common inflammatory condition of the salivary glands. The parotids are the largest of the salivary glands. Mumps (epidemic parotitis), a communicable disease caused by viral infection and most commonly affecting children, is an inflammation of a salivary gland, usually the parotid.

People who are elderly, acutely ill, or debilitated with decreased salivary flow from general dehydration or medications are at high risk for parotitis. The infecting organisms travel from the mouth through the salivary duct. The organism is usually *Staphylococcus aureus* (except in mumps). The onset of this complication is sudden, with an exacerbation of both the fever and the symptoms of the primary condition. The gland swells and becomes tense and tender (see Fig. 22-1). The patient feels pain in the ear, and swollen glands interfere with swallowing. The swelling increases rapidly, and the overlying skin soon becomes red and shiny. The patient may have purulent drainage from the site as well.

Medical management includes maintaining adequate nutritional and fluid intake, good oral hygiene, and discontinuing medications (e.g., tranquilizers, diuretics) that can diminish salivation. Antibiotic therapy is necessary, and analgesics may be prescribed to control pain. If antibiotic therapy is not effective, the gland may need to be drained by extraoral pressure applied to the area or by surgical removal of the gland via parotidectomy. Also surgery may be necessary to treat chronic parotitis. The patient is advised to have any necessary dental work performed prior to surgery.

ORAL AND OROPHARYNGEAL CANCER

Cancers of the oral cavity, which can occur in any part of the mouth or throat, are curable if discovered early. Almost 40,000 people were diagnosed with oral cancer in 2015, and close to 20% will die from this disease (American Cancer

Society, 2017). These types of cancers are equally prevalent in blacks and whites, and men have twice the risk of women of being diagnosed (American Cancer Society, 2017).

Pathophysiology

Malignancies of the oral cavity are usually squamous cell cancers. Any area of the oropharynx can be a site of malignant growths, but the lips, the lateral aspects of the tongue, and the floor of the mouth are most commonly affected.

Risk Factors

Oral cancers are often associated with the use of alcohol and all types of tobacco products, which, if used together, have a synergistic carcinogenic effect. Other factors include dietary deficiency, smoked meat ingestion, and prolonged exposure to sun and wind for cancer of the lip.

Cancer of the oral cavity affects men more often than women; however, the incidence of oral cancer in women is increasing, possibly because of increased use of tobacco and alcohol. Cancers of the oral cavity and oropharynx occur more often in African Americans than in Caucasians.

Clinical Manifestations and Assessment

Many oral cancers produce few or no symptoms in the early stages. Later, the most frequent symptom is a painless sore or mass that will not heal. A typical lesion in oral cancer is a painless indurated (hardened) ulcer with raised edges. Tissue from any ulcer of the oral cavity that does not heal in 2 weeks should be examined through biopsy. As the cancer progresses, the patient may complain of tenderness; difficulty in chewing, swallowing, or speaking; coughing of blood-tinged sputum; or enlarged cervical lymph nodes.

Diagnostic evaluation consists of an oral examination as well as an assessment of the cervical lymph nodes to detect possible metastases. Biopsies are performed on suspicious lesions (those that have not healed in 2 weeks). High-risk areas include the buccal mucosa and gingiva in people who use snuff or smoke cigars or pipes. For those who smoke cigarettes and drink alcohol, high-risk areas include the floor of the mouth, the ventrolateral tongue, and the soft palate complex (soft palate, anterior and posterior tonsillar area, uvula, and the area behind the molar and tongue junction).

Medical Management

Management varies with the nature of the lesion, the preference of the physician, and patient choice. Surgical resection, RT, chemotherapy, or a combination of these therapies may be effective.

In cancer of the lip, usually small lesions are excised liberally. RT may be more appropriate for larger lesions involving more than one-third of the lip because of superior cosmetic results. The choice depends on the extent of the lesion and what is necessary to cure the patient while

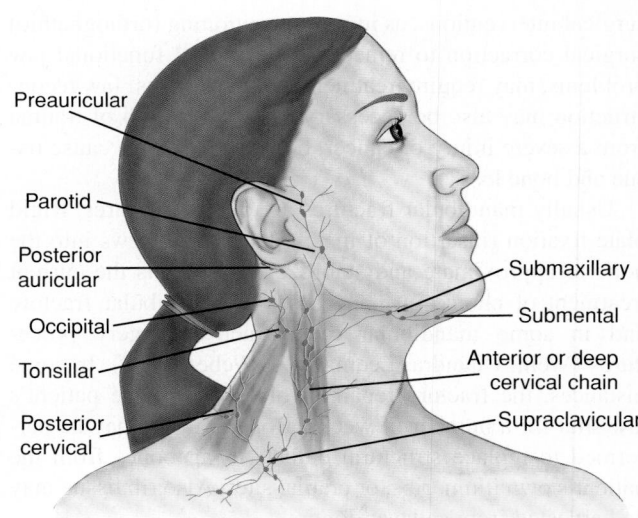

FIGURE 22-2 Lymphatic drainage of the head and neck.

preserving the best appearance. Tumors larger than 4 cm often recur.

In cancer of the tongue, treatment with RT and chemotherapy may preserve organ function and maintain quality of life. A combination of radioactive interstitial implants (surgical implantation of a radioactive source into the tissue adjacent to or at the tumor site) and external beam radiation may be used. Surgical procedures include hemiglossectomy (surgical removal of half of the tongue) and total glossectomy (removal of the tongue).

Neck Dissection

Often cancer of the oral cavity has metastasized through the extensive lymphatic channel in the neck region (Fig. 22-2), requiring a neck dissection and reconstructive surgery of the oral cavity. Surgical treatment often is performed shortly after completion of RT or chemoradiation therapy (CRT). Other malignancies of the head and neck that may metastasize into the lymphatic channel include those of the oropharynx, hypopharynx, nasopharynx, nasal cavity, paranasal sinus, and larynx (Fig. 22-3). There are various types of neck dissection: radical, modified radical, and a selective node dissection (Karakousis, 2015). A radical neck dissection involves removal of all cervical lymph nodes from the mandible to the clavicle and removal of the sternocleidomastoid muscle, internal jugular vein, and spinal accessory muscle on one side of the neck. The associated complications include shoulder drop and poor cosmesis (visible neck depression). Modified radical neck dissection, which preserves one or more of the nonlymphatic structures, is used more often. A selective node dissection (in comparison to a radical dissection) preserves one or more of the lymph node groups, the internal jugular vein, the sternocleidomastoid muscle, and the spinal accessory nerve (Fig. 22-4).

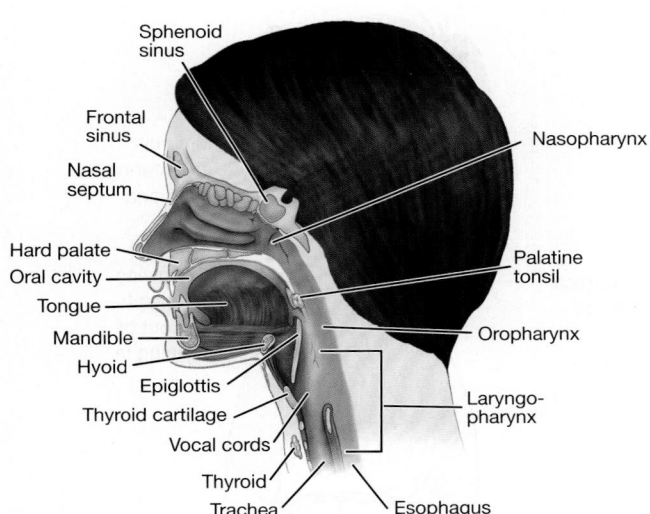

FIGURE 22-3 Anatomy of the head and neck.

> ### Nursing Alert
> *The nurse recognizes that when a laryngectomy (removal of the larynx) is performed, the patient will have a permanent laryngeal stoma (an artificial opening leading to the trachea) (Fig. 22-5). Nursing issues relate to airway management, communication, nutritional and emotional support.*

Reconstructive techniques may be performed with a variety of grafts (Fig. 22-6). A cutaneous flap (skin and subcutaneous tissue), such as the deltopectoral flap, may be used. A myocutaneous flap (subcutaneous tissue, muscle, and skin) is a graft that is used more frequently; the pectoralis major muscle is also used. For large grafts, a microvascular free flap may be used. This involves the transfer of muscle, skin, or bone with an artery and vein to the area of reconstruction, using microinstrumentation. Areas used for a free flap include the scapula, the radial area of the forearm, or the fibula. The fibula, which provides a larger bone area, may be used if mandibular reconstruction is involved. Neck

dissection is discussed in more detail in the nursing process section that follows.

Nursing Management

The nurse assesses the patient's nutritional status preoperatively, and a dietary consultation may be necessary. The patient may require enteral or parenteral feedings before and after surgery to maintain adequate nutrition. If a radial graft is to be performed, an Allen test on the donor arm must be performed to ensure that the ulnar artery is patent. Refer to Chapter 12 for details on the Allen test.

Postoperatively, the nurse monitors the patient's ability to protect the airway by assessing the ability to swallow and manage oral secretions. Suctioning of oral secretions may be necessary, and the patient can be instructed on use of a Yankauer suction device (tonsil tip suction) to remove oral secretions if appropriate. If grafting was part of the surgery, suctioning must be performed with care to prevent damage to the graft. The graft is assessed postoperatively for viability. Although color should be assessed (white may indicate arterial occlusion, and blue mottling may indicate venous congestion), it can be difficult to assess the graft by looking into the mouth. An intermittent Doppler ultrasound device or fiberoptic monitoring device (producing a continuous audible pulse of the graft site), may be used to assess the graft perfusion.

Xerostomia, dryness of the mouth, is a frequent sequela of oral cancer, particularly when the salivary glands have been exposed to radiation or major surgery. Also xerostomia is seen in patients receiving psychopharmacologic agents, patients with HIV infection, patients who cannot close the mouth, patients having endotracheal or tracheostomy tubes, and in patients with poor oral food intake.

The patient's mouth appears red, dry, and tender to palpation. Cracks in the dry oral mucosa may occur in which infection could develop. To minimize this problem, the patient is advised to avoid dry, bulky, and irritating foods and fluids, as well as alcohol and tobacco. Also the patient is encouraged to increase intake of fluids (when not contraindicated) and to use a humidifier during sleep. The use of

FIGURE 22-4 (**A**) A classic radical neck dissection in which the sternocleidomastoid and smaller muscles are removed. All tissue is removed, from the ramus of the jaw to the clavicle. The jugular vein has also been removed. (**B**) The selective neck dissection is similar but preserves the sternocleidomastoid muscle, internal jugular vein, and spinal accessory nerve. The wound is closed (**C**), and portable suction drainage tubes are in place.

A

Intact sternocleidomastoid muscle

B   **C**

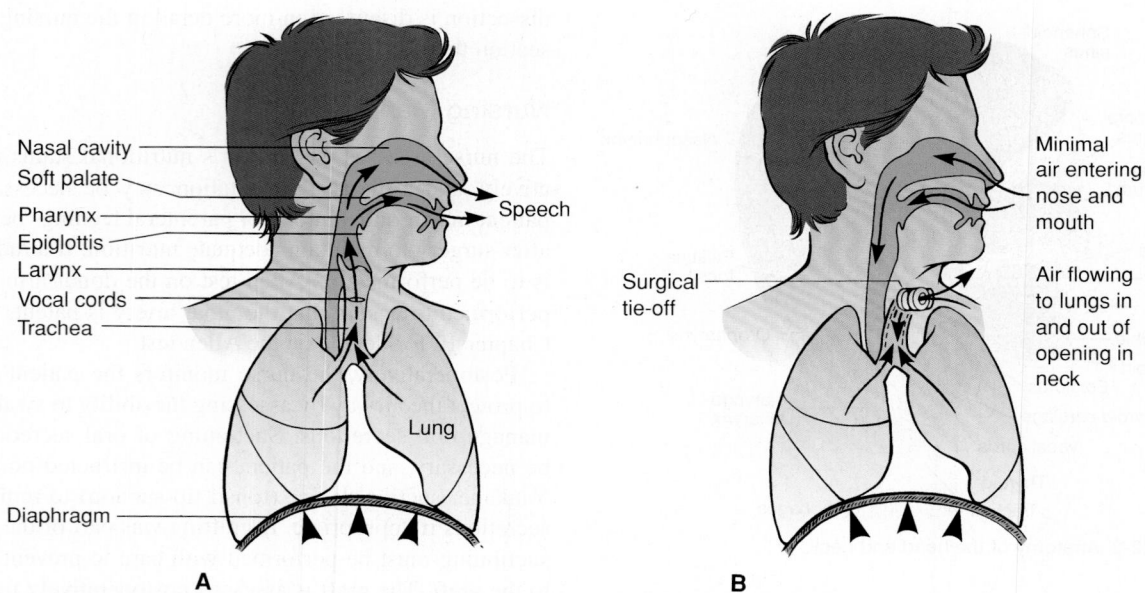

FIGURE 22-5 Airflow after total laryngectomy. After a total laryngectomy the patient breathes through a stoma. **A.** Normal air flow. **B.** Airflow after a total laryngectomy.

FIGURE 22-6 The impact of a radical neck dissection on the appearance of the neck is evident in (**A**) and (**B**). The underlying structures are located immediately deep to the skin and are readily visible. The hollowed appearance of the contour of the neck serves as a constant reminder of the patient's disease. The effect of adjuvant radiation on the soft tissues of the neck serves to produce further fibrosis and contraction, leading to severe scarring and worsening of the contour deformity. The placement of a soft tissue flap deep to the skin helps to ameliorate the usual concave appearance following a radical neck dissection (**C**). The photos that follow demonstrate the technique and the postoperative impact of using a radial forearm free flap with a proximal monitor paddle that is located in a window created in the caudal portion of the neck (**D, E, F**).

E

F

G

FIGURE 22-6 (*Continued*) The intent is to orient the proximal soft tissue flap in the direction of the sterno-cleidomastoid muscle to achieve symmetry with the nonoperated side. The intervening soft tissue helps provide durable improvement in the soft tissue contour, as well as added vascularity to the overlying skin when the procedure is being performed in a patient with prior radiation (**G**). The skin monitor, used to assess the vascularity of the deep portion of the flap, is placed into the lower neck (G, *arrow*). In the latter setting, when removal of the sternocleidomastoid muscle is required, the added soft tissue helps protect the carotid artery and the microvascular pedicle.

synthetic saliva, a moisturizing antibacterial gel such as Oral Balance, or a saliva-production stimulant, such as Salagen, may be helpful.

Stomatitis, or mucositis, which involves inflammation and breakdown of the oral mucosa, is often a side effect of chemotherapy or RT. Mucositis results in decreased oral intake and resultant malnutrition; therefore, the nurse performs routine oral assessments and follows protocols for treatment approaches (see Chapter 6). Prophylactic mouth care is started when the patient begins receiving treatment; however, mucositis may become so severe that a break in treatment is necessary. Often if a patient receiving RT has poor dentition, extraction of the teeth before radiation treatment in the oral cavity is performed to prevent infection. As a result, many RT centers recommend the use of fluoride treatments for patients receiving radiation to the head and neck.

People with cancer of the head and neck frequently have used alcohol or tobacco before surgery; postoperatively, the patient is encouraged to abstain from these substances. Treatment to decrease the likelihood of alcohol and nicotine withdrawal is recommended. Depression and anxiety are also common in this patient population. A recent study found patients undergoing radiotherapy for head and neck cancers returned to their preoperative levels of anxiety 12 months after ending their treatment course and experienced increasing levels of depression posttreatment due to aforementioned symptoms (Neilson et al., 2013).

NURSING PROCESS
The Patient Undergoing a Neck Dissection

ASSESSMENT

Preoperatively, the patient's physical and psychological preparation for major surgery is assessed along with his or her knowledge of the preoperative and postoperative procedures. Postoperatively, the patient is assessed for complications, such as altered respiratory status, wound infection, and hemorrhage. As healing occurs, neck ROM is assessed to determine whether there has been a decrease in ROM due to nerve or muscle damage. A plan of nursing care for a patient who has undergone a neck dissection is available online at http://thepoint.lww.com/Honan2e.

DIAGNOSIS

Nursing diagnoses may include the following:

- Deficient knowledge about preoperative and postoperative procedures
- Ineffective airway clearance related to obstruction by mucus, hemorrhage, or edema
- Acute pain related to surgical incision
- Risk for infection related to surgical intervention secondary to decreased nutritional status, or immunosuppression from chemotherapy or RT

(*continued on page 666*)

- Impaired tissue integrity secondary to surgery and grafting
- Imbalanced nutrition, less than body requirements, related to disease process or treatment
- Situational low self-esteem related to diagnosis or prognosis
- Impaired verbal communication secondary to surgical resection
- Impaired physical mobility secondary to nerve injury
- Anxiety related to cancer diagnosis and surgical dissection

Potential postoperative complications that may develop include the following:

- Hemorrhage
- Chyle fistula
- Nerve injury

PLANNING

The major goals for the patient include participation in the treatment plan, maintenance of respiratory status, attainment of comfort, absence of infection, viability of the graft, maintenance of adequate intake of food and fluids, effective coping strategies, effective communication, maintenance of shoulder and neck motion, and absence of complications.

NURSING INTERVENTIONS

Before surgery, the patient should be informed about the nature and extent of the surgery and what the postoperative period will be like (see Chapter 5 for preoperative education).

For the patient who has had extensive neck surgery, specific postoperative interventions include maintenance of a patent airway and continuous assessment of respiratory status, wound care and oral hygiene, maintenance of adequate nutrition, and observation for hemorrhage or nerve injury.

MAINTAINING THE AIRWAY

After the endotracheal tube or airway has been removed and the effects of the anesthesia have worn off, the patient may be placed in Fowler position to facilitate breathing and promote comfort. This position also increases lymphatic and venous drainage, facilitates swallowing, and decreases venous pressure on the skin flaps.

In the immediate postoperative period, the nurse assesses for stridor (coarse, high-pitched sound on inspiration) by listening frequently over the trachea with a stethoscope. This finding must be reported immediately because it indicates partial obstruction of the airway. Signs of respiratory distress, such as dyspnea, cyanosis, changes in mental status, and changes in vital signs, are assessed because they may suggest edema, hemorrhage, inadequate oxygenation, or inadequate drainage.

Pneumonia may occur in the postoperative phase if pulmonary secretions are not removed. To aid in the removal of secretions, coughing and deep breathing are encouraged. The patient should assume a sitting position, with the nurse supporting the neck so that the patient can bring up excessive secretions. If this is ineffective, the patient's respiratory tract may have to be suctioned. Care is taken to protect the suture lines during suctioning.

If the patient has had a laryngectomy performed, "the laryngeal stoma needs vigilant observation, as the suture material, which secures the trachea, acts as a trap for dried mucus and bronchial secretions and may cause the diameter of the stoma to narrow. A laryngectomy tube is placed in the stoma once the patient is fully recovered from the operative procedure" (Davidson, Lester, & Routt, 2014, p. 69). If a laryngectomy tube is in place, suctioning is performed through the tube. Humidified oxygen or room air decreases the viscosity of secretions and provide moisture to the air (Davidson et al., 2014). Patients and family members are instructed to use a cool mist vaporizer or humidified air compressor to decrease secretion viscosity upon discharge and also should be instructed on care of the stoma and suctioning of the airway. The patient also may be instructed on the use of the Yankauer suction to remove oral secretions. The nurse should not take the patient's temperature orally.

Before a patient takes food or fluid orally, the patient's swallowing function is evaluated to assess for dysphagia; it is important to determine the presence or absence of aspiration, any voice impairment, ease of movement of the larynx, any evidence of gurgling with respiration, pulmonary secretions, lung sounds, and oxygen saturation. Teaching a patient the supraglottic swallowing technique can be effective in reducing the risk of aspiration when surgery impacted the ability of the vocal folds to close (Butler, Pelletier, & Steele, 2013). When the patient is ready to swallow food, the nurse would instruct the patient to inhale deeply, hold their breath, swallow and then finally cough as the swallow was completed. Seeking the guidance of a speech pathologist is recommended when considering aspiration prevention techniques such as this one.

 Nursing Alert
Failure to assess for dysphagia in the patient following postoperative neck dissection may result in severe respiratory compromise, prolonged mechanical ventilation, and aspiration pneumonia.

RELIEVING PAIN

Pain and the patient's fear of pain are assessed and managed. Patients with head and neck cancer often report less pain than do patients with other types of cancer; however, the nurse needs to be aware that each person's pain experience is individual. The nurse administers analgesics as prescribed and assesses their effectiveness.

PROVIDING WOUND CARE

Wound drainage tubes usually are inserted during surgery to prevent the subcutaneous collection of fluid. The drainage tubes are connected to a portable suction device (e.g., Jackson-Pratt) (see Box 33-4), and the container is emptied periodically. Between 80 and 120 mL of serosanguineous secretions may drain over the first 24 hours. Excessive drainage may be indicative of a chyle fistula or hemorrhage (see later discussion). If dressings are present, they may need to be reinforced periodically. Dressings are observed for evidence of hemorrhage and constriction, which impairs respiration and perfusion of the graft. A graft, if present, is assessed for color and temperature and for the presence of a pulse if applicable, to determine viability. The graft should be pale pink and warm to the touch. If lymphatic drainage is obstructed, then edema may develop. The surgical incisions are also assessed for infection, which is reported immediately. Prophylactic antibiotics may be prescribed.

MAINTAINING ADEQUATE NUTRITION

Nutritional status is assessed preoperatively; early intervention to correct nutritional imbalances may decrease the risk of postoperative complications. Frequently, nutrition is less than optimal because of inadequate intake, and the patient often requires enteral or parenteral supplements preoperatively and postoperatively to attain and maintain a positive nitrogen balance.

The patient who can chew may take food by mouth; the level of the patient's chewing ability determines whether some diet modification (e.g., soft, puréed, or liquid foods) is necessary. Also food preferences should be discussed with the patient. Oral care before eating may enhance the patient's appetite, and oral care after eating is important to prevent infection and dental caries.

SUPPORTING COPING MEASURES

Preoperatively, information about the planned surgery is given to the patient and family. Postoperatively, psychological nursing interventions are aimed at supporting the patient who has had a change in body image or who has major concerns regarding the prognosis. The patient may have difficulty communicating and may be concerned about his or her ability to breathe and swallow normally. The nurse supports the patient's family and friends in encouraging and reassuring the patient that adjusting to the results of this surgery will take time.

The person who has had extensive neck surgery often is sensitive about his or her appearance. This can occur when the operative area is covered by bulky dressings, when the incision line is visible, or later after healing has occurred and the appearance of the neck, and possibly the lower face, has been altered significantly. If the nurse accepts the patient's appearance and expresses a positive, optimistic attitude, then the patient is more likely to be encouraged. The patient also needs an opportunity to express concerns regarding the success of the surgery and the prognosis. The American Cancer Society may be a resource to provide a volunteer to meet with the patient either preoperatively or postoperatively.

PROMOTING EFFECTIVE COMMUNICATION

If a laryngectomy was performed, the nurse explores other methods of communicating with the patient and obtains a consultation with a speech/language therapist. Alternatives to verbal communication may include use of a pencil and paper or pointing to needed items on a picture pad. Alternative speech techniques, such as an electrolarynx (a mechanical device held against the neck) or esophageal speech, may be taught by a speech/language therapist.

MAINTAINING PHYSICAL MOBILITY

Excision of muscles and nerves results in weakness at the shoulder that can cause *shoulder drop*, a forward curvature of the shoulder. Many problems can be avoided with a conscientious exercise program. Usually these exercises are begun after the drains have been removed and the neck incision is healed sufficiently. Physical therapists and occupational therapists can assist patients in performing these exercises.

Additionally because lymph node removal can cause nerve damage, and the sternocleidomastoid muscle may have been removed, neck mobility is impaired, thus the neck is supported by the nurse when getting the patient out of bed. Physical therapy can assist with developing a plan for neck and shoulder rehabilitation.

MONITORING AND MANAGING POTENTIAL COMPLICATIONS

Hemorrhage. Hemorrhage may occur from rupture of the carotid artery as a result of necrosis of the graft or damage to the artery itself from tumor or infection. The following measures are indicated:

- Vital signs are assessed. Tachycardia, tachypnea, and hypotension may indicate hemorrhage and impending hypovolemic shock.
- The patient is instructed to avoid the Valsalva maneuver (bearing-down activities such as having a bowel movement) to prevent stress on the graft and carotid artery.
- Signs of impending rupture, such as high epigastric pain or discomfort, are reported.
- Dressings and wound drainage are observed for excessive bleeding.
- If hemorrhage occurs, assistance is summoned immediately.
- Hemorrhage requires the continuous application of pressure to the bleeding site or major associated vessel.
- Close assessment must occur when changing the patient's position to assist in maintaining blood pressure yet minimizing the risk of aspiration and potentially losing airway patency.
- The nurse should maintain a controlled, calm manner to help allay the patient's anxiety.
- The surgeon is notified immediately because a vascular or ligature tear requires surgical intervention.

Chyle Fistula. A chyle fistula (milk-like lymphatic drainage from the thoracic duct into the thoracic cavity) may develop as a result of damage to the lymphatic thoracic duct during surgery. The nurse notes the color of the drainage from the neck drains and notifies the surgeon if milky, odorless discharge is seen since this is suspicious for a chyle leak. The diagnosis is made if there is excess drainage that has a 3% fat content and a specific gravity of 1.012 or greater. Treatment of a small leak (up to 500 mL or less) includes application of a pressure dressing and a diet of medium-chain fatty acids or parenteral nutrition (PN). Surgical intervention to repair the damaged duct is necessary for larger leaks.

(continued on page 668)

Nerve Injury. Nerve injury can occur during a neck dissection procedure due to the location of multiple nerve pathways in and around muscle, lymphatic, and vascular structures. Damage to the accessory nerve can result in shoulder pain and potential dysfunction. The facial nerve can also be damaged which would manifest as poor lower lip function. Tongue movement can be effected with injury to the hypoglossal nerve. If a patient has limited mobility of the arm in the postoperative period a brachial plexus injury is suspected. Damage to the phrenic nerve can affect the respiratory system and the patient's voice can be changed due to injury to the vagus nerve. The nurse assesses the functioning of the anatomic structures mentioned with the knowledge of the corresponding nerve pathways to the appropriate health care provider, such as the surgeon, physical therapist or speech pathologist and recommend interventions.

TEACHING PATIENTS SELF-CARE

The patient and caregiver require instructions about management of the wound, the dressing, and any drains that remain in place. Patients who require oral suctioning or who have a tracheostomy may be very anxious about their care at home; the transition to home can be eased if the caregiver is given several opportunities to demonstrate the ability to meet the patient's needs. Also the patient and caregiver are instructed about possible complications, such as bleeding and respiratory distress, and when to notify the health care provider of signs and symptoms of these complications.

If the patient cannot take food by mouth, detailed instructions and demonstration of enteral or parenteral feedings will be required. Education in techniques of effective oral hygiene is also important.

A referral for home care nursing may be necessary in the early period after discharge. The nurse assesses healing, ensures that feedings are being administered properly, and monitors for any complications. The home care nurse assesses the patient's adjustment to changes in physical appearance and status as well as the patient's ability to communicate and to eat normally. Physical and speech therapy also may be continued at home.

The patient is given information regarding local support groups such as "I Can Cope" or "New Voice Club," if indicated. The local chapter of the American Cancer Society may be contacted for information and equipment needed for the patient.

EVALUATION

Expected patient outcomes may include:
1. Discusses expected course of treatment
2. Demonstrates good respiratory exchange:
   a. Lungs are clear to auscultation
   b. Breathes easily with no shortness of breath
   c. Demonstrates ability to use suction effectively
3. Remains free of infection:
   a. Maintains normal laboratory values
   b. Is afebrile
4. Graft is pink and warm to touch

5. Maintains adequate intake of foods and fluids:
   a. Accepts altered route of feeding
   b. Is well hydrated
   c. Maintains or gains weight
6. Demonstrates ability to cope:
   a. Discusses emotional responses to the diagnosis
   b. Attends support group meetings
7. Verbalizes comfort
8. Attains maximal mobility:
   a. Adheres to physical therapy exercises
   b. Attains maximal ROM
9. Exhibits no complications:
   a. Vital signs stable
   b. No excessive bleeding or discharge
   c. Able to move muscles of lower face

DISORDERS OF THE ESOPHAGUS

The esophagus is a mucus-lined, muscular tube that carries food from the mouth to the stomach. It begins at the base of the pharynx and ends about 4 cm below the diaphragm. Its ability to transport food and fluid is facilitated by two sphincters. The upper esophageal sphincter, also called the *hypopharyngeal sphincter*, is located at the junction of the pharynx and the esophagus. The lower esophageal sphincter, also called the *gastroesophageal sphincter* or *cardiac sphincter*, is located at the junction of the esophagus and the stomach. The lower esophageal sphincter prevents reflux (backward flow) of gastric contents. There is no serosal layer of the esophagus; therefore, if surgery is necessary, it is more difficult to perform suturing or anastomosis.

Disorders of the esophagus include motility disorders achalasia (muscles of the lower part of the esophagus fail to relax), hiatal hernias, diverticula, perforation, esophageal obstruction due to swallowed foreign bodies, chemical burns, gastroesophageal reflux disease, Barrett's esophagus, and carcinoma. **Dysphagia** (difficulty swallowing), the most common symptom of esophageal disease, may vary from an uncomfortable feeling that a bolus of food is caught in the upper esophagus to acute pain on swallowing (**odynophagia**). Obstruction of food (solid and soft) and even liquids may occur anywhere along the esophagus. Often, the patient indicates that the problem is located in the upper, middle, or lower third of the esophagus.

ACHALASIA

Achalasia is absent or ineffective **peristalsis** of the distal esophagus, accompanied by failure of the esophageal sphincter to relax in response to swallowing. Narrowing of the esophagus just above the stomach results in a gradually increasing dilation of the esophagus in the upper chest. Achalasia may progress slowly and occurs most often in people 40 years or older.

FIGURE 22-7 Treatment of achalasia by pneumatic dilation. **A–C.** The dilator is passed, guided by a previously inserted guide wire. **D.** When the balloon is in proper position, it is distended by pressure sufficient to dilate the narrowed area of the esophagus.

Clinical Manifestations and Assessment

The primary symptom is difficulty in swallowing both liquids and solids. The patient has a sensation of food sticking in the lower portion of the esophagus. As the condition progresses, food is regurgitated either spontaneously or intentionally by the patient to relieve the discomfort produced by prolonged distention of the esophagus by food that will not pass into the stomach. The patient may also report chest pain and heartburn (**pyrosis**) that may or may not be associated with eating. Secondary pulmonary complications may result from aspiration of gastric contents.

X-ray studies show esophageal dilation above the narrowing at the gastroesophageal junction. Barium swallow, computed tomography (CT) of the chest, and endoscopy may be used for diagnosis; however, *manometry*, a process in which the esophageal pressure is measured by a radiologist or gastroenterologist, confirms the diagnosis (McQuaid, 2014).

Medical and Nursing Management

The patient is instructed to eat slowly and to drink fluids with meals. As a temporary measure, calcium channel blockers and nitrates have been used to decrease esophageal pressure and improve swallowing. Injection of botulinum toxin (Botox) to quadrants of the esophagus via endoscopy has been helpful because it inhibits the contraction of smooth muscle. Periodic injections are required to maintain remission.

Achalasia may be treated conservatively by pneumatic dilation to stretch the narrowed area of the esophagus (Fig. 22-7). Pneumatic dilation (forcefully dilating the lower esophagus by a balloon) has a high success rate. Although perforation is a potential complication, its incidence is low. The procedure can be painful; therefore, moderate sedation

in the form of an analgesic or tranquilizer, or both, is administered for the treatment. The patient is monitored for perforation. Abdominal tenderness and fever may indicate perforation (see later discussion).

Achalasia may be treated surgically by esophagomyotomy. Usually the procedure is performed laparoscopically, either with a complete lower esophageal sphincter myotomy and an antireflux procedure or without an antireflux procedure. The esophageal muscle fibers are separated to relieve the lower esophageal stricture.

HIATAL HERNIA

In the condition known as hiatus (or hiatal) **hernia**, the opening in the diaphragm through which the esophagus passes becomes enlarged, and part of the upper stomach tends to move up into the lower portion of the thorax. Hiatal hernia occurs more often in women than in men. There are four types of hiatal hernias: sliding, rolling or paraesophageal, a sliding/rolling or mixed, and simultaneous hiatal hernia with another organ (Jobe, Hunter, & Watson, 2014). Sliding, or type I, hiatal hernia occurs when the upper stomach and the gastroesophageal junction are displaced upward and slide in and out of the thorax (Fig. 22-8A). A sliding hernia is the most commonly diagnosed of the four types. A rolling or paraesophageal hernia occurs when all or part of the stomach pushes through the diaphragm beside the esophagus (see Fig. 22-8B). The mixed hernia, or Type III, is characterized by both the cardia and fundus being displaced upward.

Clinical Manifestations and Assessment

The patient with a sliding hernia may have heartburn, regurgitation, and dysphagia, but at least 50% of patients are

FIGURE 22-8 **A.** Sliding esophageal hernia. The upper stomach and gastroesophageal junction have moved upward and slide in and out of the thorax. **B.** Paraesophageal hernia. All or part of the stomach pushes through the diaphragm next to the gastroesophageal junction.

asymptomatic. Often sliding hiatal hernia is implicated in reflux. The patient with a paraesophageal hernia usually feels an uncomfortable sense of fullness after eating or chest pain, or there may be no symptoms. Reflux usually does not occur because the gastroesophageal sphincter is intact. Hemorrhage, obstruction, and strangulation can occur with any type of hernia.

Diagnosis is confirmed by x-ray studies, barium swallow, and fluoroscopy.

Medical and Nursing Management

Management for a sliding hernia includes frequent, small feedings that can pass easily through the esophagus. The patient is advised not to recline for 1 hour after eating, to prevent reflux or movement of the hernia, and to elevate the head of the bed on 4- to 8-in (10- to 20-cm) blocks to prevent the hernia from sliding upward. Surgery is indicated when a patient has significant esophageal injury or when he or she does not respond to medical management. Medical and surgical management of a paraesophageal hernia is similar to that for gastroesophageal reflux; however, people with paraesophageal hernias may require emergency surgery to correct torsion (twisting) of the stomach that can lead to restriction of blood flow to the area.

DIVERTICULUM

A diverticulum is an outpouching of mucosa and submucosa that protrudes through a weak portion of the musculature that can occur at any location in the esophagus.

The most common type of esophageal diverticulum, which is found three times more frequently in men than in women, is *Zenker diverticulum* (also known as pharyngoesophageal pulsion diverticulum or a pharyngeal pouch). It occurs posteriorly through the cricopharyngeal muscle in the midline of the neck. Usually it is seen in people older than 60 years of age. Other types of diverticula include midesophageal (rare), epiphrenic (large), and intramural diverticula (numerous and small; related to stricture).

Clinical Manifestations and Assessment

Symptoms experienced by the patient with a pharyngoesophageal pulsion diverticulum include difficulty swallowing, fullness in the neck, belching, regurgitation of undigested food, and gurgling noises after eating. The diverticulum, or pouch, becomes filled with food or liquid. When the patient assumes a recumbent position, undigested food is regurgitated, and coughing may be caused by irritation of the trachea. Also halitosis and a sour taste in the mouth are common because of the decomposition of food retained in the diverticulum.

Symptoms produced by midesophageal diverticula are less acute. Due to the difficulty these patients have with food passing through their upper GI tract, they often have chest pain and difficulty with swallowing. Some patients experience regurgitation of undigested food, and some do not experience any symptoms at all.

A barium swallow may determine the exact nature and location of a diverticulum. Often pressure studies are performed for patients with epiphrenic diverticula to rule out a motor disorder. Esophagoscopy usually is contraindicated because of the danger of perforation of the diverticulum.

> **Nursing Alert**
> *Blind insertion of NG tubes should be avoided in patients with esophageal diverticulum, esophageal varices, postgastric bypass, and lap banding procedures due to the potential of causing esophageal rupture or surgical site perforation.*

Medical and Nursing Management

Because pharyngoesophageal pulsion diverticulum is progressive, the only means of cure is surgical removal of the diverticulum. During surgery, care is taken to avoid trauma to the common carotid artery and internal jugular veins. The sac is dissected free and amputated flush with the esophageal wall. In addition to a diverticulectomy, often a myotomy of the cricopharyngeal muscle is performed to relieve spasticity of the musculature, which otherwise seems to contribute to a continuation of the previous symptoms. An NG tube may be inserted at the time of surgery. Postoperatively, the surgical incision must be observed for evidence of leakage from the esophagus and a developing fistula. Food and fluids are withheld until radiographic studies indicate that there is no leakage at the surgical site. The diet begins with liquids and is progressively returned to solids as tolerated.

Surgery is indicated for epiphrenic and midesophageal diverticula only if the symptoms are troublesome and becoming worse. Treatment consists of a diverticulectomy and long myotomy. Intramural diverticula usually regress after the esophageal stricture is dilated.

PERFORATION

The esophagus is a common site of injury. Perforation may result from stab or bullet wounds of the neck or chest, trauma from a motor vehicle crash, caustic injury from a chemical burn, inadvertent puncture during a surgical procedure or esophageal dilatation, or from severe retching or vomiting (Boerhaave syndrome).

Clinical Manifestations and Assessment

The patient with a perforated esophagus has persistent pain, followed by dysphagia, fever, leukocytosis (elevated white blood cells), and severe hypotension. In some instances, signs of pneumothorax are observed. X-ray studies and fluoroscopy by either a barium swallow or esophagram are used to identify the site of the injury.

Medical and Nursing Management

Because of the high risk of infection, broad-spectrum antibiotic therapy is initiated. If the perforation is small enough and without symptoms, medical intervention may not be necessary. Nothing is given by mouth; nutritional needs are met by administering nutrition into the intestine, bypassing the stomach, or by the parenteral route. The type of nutritional support depends on the location and the extent of the injury. The enteral or parenteral nutrition lasts for at least 1 month to give the esophagus a chance to heal. A repeat barium swallow study is performed, and the involved area is reevaluated. If there is no evidence of perforation, foods are reintroduced, beginning with liquids and then slowly progressing to solids as tolerated.

Surgery may be necessary to close the wound; in such cases, postoperative nutritional support becomes a primary concern. Depending on the incision site and the nature of surgery, the postoperative nursing management is similar to that for patients who have had thoracic or abdominal surgery.

FOREIGN BODIES

Many swallowed foreign bodies pass through the GI tract without the need for medical intervention. However, some swallowed foreign bodies (e.g., dentures, fish bones, pins, small batteries, items containing mercury or lead) may cause trauma to the esophagus or obstruct its lumen and must be removed. Pain and dysphagia may be present, and dyspnea may occur as a result of pressure on the trachea. The foreign body may be identified by x-ray. Perforation may have occurred (see earlier discussion).

Glucagon, because of its relaxing effect on the esophageal muscle, may be injected intramuscularly. An endoscope (with a covered hood or overtube) may be used to remove the impacted food or object from the esophagus. A mixture consisting of sodium bicarbonate and tartaric acid may be prescribed to increase intraluminal pressure by the formation of a gas, which works to dislodge the foreign body. Caution must be used with this treatment because there is risk of perforation.

CHEMICAL BURNS

The severity of chemical burns to the esophagus is dependent upon the characteristics of the substance: pH, concentration, volume, and duration of contact with mucosa.

Clinical Manifestations and Assessment

Ingestion of the substance can be intentional or unintentional, which is important to consider when assessing the patient or reviewing his or her history. Strongly alkaline substances are more damaging to the esophagus as a result of causing a liquefactive necrosis when they come into contact with the mucosa. Alkalis include lye, chemical strippers, and drain cleaners. In addition, chemical burns of the esophagus also may be caused by undissolved medications in the esophagus. An acute chemical burn of the esophagus may be accompanied by severe burns of the lips, mouth, and pharynx, which can result in airway compromise due to edema or excessive mucus production. Also the patient may experience pain when swallowing.

Medical and Nursing Management

The patient's airway is prioritized, and he or she is treated for pain and possible shock. The patient's injury is evaluated using esophagoscopy. Vomiting and gastric **lavage** are avoided to prevent further exposure of the esophagus to the caustic agent. The patient is given nothing by mouth (NPO status), and IV fluids are administered. An NG tube may be inserted by the medical team. There is no consensus on the use of corticosteroids to reduce inflammation and minimize scarring and stricture formation at this time.

After the acute phase has subsided, the patient may need nutritional support via enteral or parenteral feedings. The patient may require further treatment to prevent or manage strictures of the esophagus. Strictures are repeatedly dilated with progressively larger cylindrical rubber tubes or bougies. For strictures that do not respond to dilation, surgical management is necessary. Reconstruction may be accomplished by esophagectomy and colon interposition to replace the portion of esophagus removed.

GASTROESOPHAGEAL REFLUX DISEASE

Some degree of **gastroesophageal reflux** (back-flow of gastric or duodenal contents into the esophagus) is normal in both adults and children. Excessive reflux may occur because of an incompetent lower esophageal sphincter, pyloric stenosis, or a motility disorder. The incidence of reflux seems to increase with aging.

Clinical Manifestations and Assessment

Symptoms of gastroesophageal reflux disease (GERD) may include pyrosis (burning sensation in the esophagus), dyspepsia (indigestion), regurgitation, dysphagia or odynophagia (pain on swallowing), hypersalivation, and esophagitis. The symptoms may mimic those of acute coronary syndrome. The patient's history aids in obtaining an accurate diagnosis.

Diagnostic testing and evaluation of GERD includes differentiation of other disease processes by proton-pump inhibitor (PPI) treatment and response, ambulatory reflux esophageal monitoring, and endoscopy only with severe symptoms (Katz, Gerson, & Vela, 2013). Barium studies and biopsy are not recommended as diagnostic tools.

Medical and Nursing Management

Management begins with teaching the patient to avoid situations that decrease lower esophageal sphincter pressure or cause esophageal irritation. The patient is instructed to eat a low-fat diet; to avoid caffeine, tobacco, beer, milk, foods containing peppermint or spearmint, and carbonated beverages; to avoid eating or drinking 2 hours before bedtime; to maintain normal body weight; to avoid tight-fitting clothes; to elevate the head of the bed on 6- to 8-in (15- to 20-cm) blocks; and to elevate the upper body on pillows. If reflux persists, the patient may be given antacids or H_2 receptor antagonists, such as famotidine (Pepcid), nizatidine (Axid), or ranitidine (Zantac). PPIs (medications that decrease the release of gastric acid, such as lansoprazole [Prevacid], rabeprazole [AcipHex], esomeprazole [Nexium]) may be used; however, these products may increase intragastric bacterial growth and the risk for infection. In addition, the patient may receive prokinetic agents, which accelerate gastric emptying. These agents include bethanechol (Urecholine), domperidone (Motilium), and metoclopramide (Reglan). Metoclopramide can have extrapyramidal side effects that are increased in certain neuromuscular disorders, such as Parkinson disease. These patients should be monitored carefully.

If medical management is unsuccessful, surgical intervention may be necessary (Katz et al., 2013). Transoral incisionless fundoplication, which involves the reconstruction of the valve at the gastroesophageal junction, is another endoscopic option that was found to have positive results in a recent study of 63 patients (Trad et al., 2015).

BARRETT ESOPHAGUS

Barrett esophagus is a condition in which the lining of the esophageal mucosa is altered. The tissue at the gastroesophageal junction changes from squamous epithelium (flat) to columnar epithelium (elongated). Barrett esophagus is sometimes found in patients being evaluated with a history of chronic regurgitation or heartburn. The disease may lead to esophageal cancer in some patients.

Clinical Manifestations and Assessment

The patient with Barrett esophagus complains of symptoms of GERD, notably frequent heartburn. The patient may also complain of symptoms related to peptic ulcers or esophageal stricture, or both.

An **esophagogastroduodenoscopy (EGD)** is performed. This usually reveals an esophageal lining that is red rather than pink, indicating the cellular change in tissue. With biopsy, cellular changes and goblet cells (mucus producing) are seen.

Medical and Nursing Management

Monitoring for Barrett esophagus varies depending on the extent of cell changes. Some providers recommend a repeat EGD in 6 to 12 months if the cellular changes are minor.

Photodynamic therapy (PDT) may be an alternative for the patient who is considered an operative risk (e.g., at least 70 years of age or older, significant cardiac risk). PDT is a type of laser thermal ablation of the esophageal mucosa that is used to destroy the metaplastic cells once the patient has received a photosensitizing agent, such as sodium porfimer. PDT has been well documented in the literature as a safe and effective treatment.

Ablative techniques including radiofrequency, thermal, and argon plasma coagulation are commonly used with acid suppression treatment. In the past, esophagectomy was the standard of treatment for these patients. Early detection of precancerous changes and the occurrence of high complication rates for surgery have left esophagectomy for treatment of advanced cases.

CANCER OF THE ESOPHAGUS

The American Cancer Society estimates that 16,980 diagnoses of esophageal cancer were made in 2015 as compared with 15,000 estimated diagnoses in 2009 (2015). In the United States, esophageal cancer represents 1% of all cancers diagnosed (American Cancer Society, 2015).

Pathophysiology

Esophageal cancer can be of two cell types: adenocarcinoma and squamous cell carcinoma. The rate of adenocarcinoma is rapidly increasing in the United States as well as in other Western countries. Adenocarcinoma is found in gland cells and is not common to the esophagus except in patients having Barrett esophagus, as described previously. As a result, patients with GERD and Barrett esophagus are at greater risk for developing esophageal cancer.

Tumor cells of adenocarcinoma and of squamous cell carcinoma may spread beneath the esophageal mucosa or directly into, through, and beyond the muscle layers into the lymphatics. In the latter stages, obstruction of the esophagus is noted, with possible perforation into the mediastinum and erosion into the great vessels.

Risk Factors

Esophageal cancer is three to four times more prevalent in men than women (American Cancer Society, 2015).

Chronic irritation is a risk factor for esophageal cancer. In the United States, cancer of the esophagus has been associated with ingestion of alcohol and the use of tobacco. Additional risk factors for squamous cell carcinoma of the esophagus include chronic ingestion of hot liquids or foods, nutritional deficiencies, poor oral hygiene, exposure to nitrosamines in the environment or food, and some esophageal medical conditions, such as caustic injury. Nitrosamines are found in rubber products, cured meats, beer, and pesticides.

Clinical Manifestations and Assessment

Many patients have an advanced ulcerated lesion of the esophagus before symptoms are manifested. Symptoms include dysphagia, initially with solid foods and eventually with liquids; a sensation of a mass in the throat; painful swallowing; substernal pain or fullness; and, later, regurgitation of undigested food with foul breath and hiccups. The patient first becomes aware of intermittent and increasing difficulty in swallowing. As the tumor grows and the obstruction becomes nearly complete, even liquids cannot pass into the stomach. Regurgitation of food and saliva occurs, hemorrhage may take place, and progressive loss of weight and strength occurs from starvation. Later symptoms include substernal pain, persistent hiccup, respiratory difficulty, and foul breath.

The delay between the onset of early symptoms and the time at which the patient seeks medical advice is often 12 to 18 months. Any person having swallowing difficulties should be encouraged to consult a provider immediately.

Currently, diagnosis is confirmed most often by flexible endoscopy with biopsy (Varghese et al., 2013). The biopsy can be used to determine the presence of disease and cell differentiation. At presentation, most patients have moderately differentiated tumors.

Several imaging techniques may provide useful diagnostic information, such as CT, MRI, endoscopic ultrasound, and positron emission tomography (PET). Endoscopic ultrasound is also helpful in determining whether the cancer has spread to the lymph nodes and other mediastinal structures. PET specifically assesses the metabolism of the cells being imaged so that malignant cells can be identified.

Medical Management

If esophageal cancer is detected at an early stage, treatment goals may be directed toward cure; however, it is often detected in late stages, making relief of symptoms the only reasonable goal of therapy. Treatment may include surgery, radiation, chemotherapy, or a combination of these modalities, depending on the type of cell, the extent of the disease, and the patient's condition. A standard treatment plan for a person who is newly diagnosed with esophageal cancer includes the following: preoperative combination chemotherapy/RT for 4 to 6 weeks, followed by a period of no medical intervention for 4 weeks, and, last, surgical resection of the esophagus.

Standard surgical management includes a total resection of the esophagus (esophagectomy) with removal of the tumor plus a wide tumor-free margin of the esophagus and the lymph nodes in the area. The surgical approach may be through the thorax or the abdomen, depending on the location of the tumor. When tumors occur in the cervical or upper thoracic area, esophageal continuity may be maintained by a free jejunal graft transfer, in which the tumor is removed and the area is replaced with a portion of the jejunum (Fig. 22-9). A segment of the colon may be used, or the stomach can be elevated into the chest and the proximal section of the esophagus anastomosed to the stomach.

Tumors of the lower thoracic esophagus are more amenable to surgery than are tumors located higher in the esophagus. GI tract integrity is maintained by anastomosing the lower esophagus to the stomach.

Surgical resection of the esophagus has a relatively high mortality rate because of infection, pulmonary complications, or leakage through the anastomosis. Postoperatively, the patient has an NG tube in place that should not be manipulated. The

FIGURE 22-9 Esophageal reconstruction with free jejunal transfer. A portion of the jejunum is grafted between the esophagus and pharynx to replace the abnormal portion of the esophagus. The vascular structures are also anastomosed. A portion of the graft may be externalized through the neck wound to evaluate graft viability.

patient is given nothing by mouth until x-ray studies confirm that the anastomosis is free from an esophageal leak, there is no obstruction, and there is no evidence of pulmonary aspiration.

Palliative treatment may be necessary to keep the esophagus open, to assist with nutrition, and to control saliva. Palliation may be accomplished with dilation of the esophagus, laser therapy, placement of an endoprosthesis (stent), radiation, or chemotherapy.

Nursing Management

Intervention is directed toward improving the patient's nutritional and physical status in preparation for surgery, RT, or chemotherapy. A program to promote weight gain based on a high-calorie and high-protein diet, in liquid or soft form, is provided if adequate food can be taken by mouth. If this is not possible, parenteral or enteral nutrition is initiated. Nutritional status is monitored throughout treatment. The patient is informed about the nature of the postoperative equipment that will be used, including that required for closed chest drainage, NG suction, parenteral fluid therapy, and gastric intubation.

Immediate postoperative care is similar to that provided for patients undergoing thoracic surgery. It is not uncommon for patients to be placed in an intensive care unit or step-down unit. After recovering from the effects of anesthesia, the patient is placed in a low Fowler position, and later in a Fowler position, to help prevent reflux of gastric secretions. The patient is observed carefully for regurgitation and dyspnea. A common postoperative complication is aspiration pneumonia. Therefore, the patient is placed on a vigorous pulmonary plan of care that includes incentive spirometry (IS), sitting up in a chair, and, if necessary, nebulizer treatments. Chest physiotherapy is avoided due to the risk for aspiration. The patient's temperature is monitored to detect any elevation that may indicate aspiration or seepage of fluid through the operative site into the mediastinum or pleural cavity (depending on the surgeon's approach), which would indicate an esophageal leak. Drainage from the cervical neck wound, usually saliva, is evidence of an early esophageal leak. Typically, no treatment other than NPO and parenteral or enteral support is warranted.

Cardiac complications include atrial fibrillation, which occurs due to irritation of the vagus nerve at the time of surgery. Typical medical management includes digitalization or beta blockade, depending on the patient's response. Cardioversion may be used in rare occasions.

During surgery, an NG tube is inserted and taped or sutured in place. It is connected to low suction.

> **! Nursing Alert**
> *The NG tube is* **not** *manipulated; if displacement occurs, it is not likely to be replaced unless by the surgeon because damage to the anastomosis may occur.*

The NG tube is commonly removed 5 to 7 days after surgery. Then a fiberoptic scope is used, often by a speech pathologist, to evaluate the patient's ability to swallow and to rule out possible aspiration before the patient has a Gastrografin study to assess for an anastomotic leak. If a leak into the mediastinum or pleural cavity is visualized, the study is stopped immediately, the patient returns to being NPO, and the provider is notified.

If the patient completes both procedures successfully, he or she is advanced to a regular diet. Small, frequent feedings (6 to 8 per day) are recommended because large quantities of food overload the stomach and promote gastric reflux. When the patient can increase his or her food and fluid intake to an adequate amount, parenteral fluids are discontinued. After each meal, the patient remains upright for at least 2 hours to allow the food to move through the GI tract. It is a challenge to encourage the patient to eat, because the appetite is usually poor. Family involvement and home-cooked favorite foods may help the patient to eat. Antacids may help patients with gastric distress. Metoclopramide (Reglan) is useful in promoting gastric motility. Daily assessment of weight and nutritional intake is important.

If chemotherapy and radiation are part of the therapy, the patient's appetite will be depressed further, and esophagitis may occur, causing pain when food is eaten. Liquid supplements may be tolerated more easily. However, supplements such as Boost and Ensure should be avoided because they promote *dumping syndrome*, which occurs when large amounts of osmotically active solids and liquids rapidly "dump" into the duodenum. DS involves nausea and diarrhea that can result in symptoms of dehydration effecting the cardiac and respiratory systems. It can occur with each meal or approximately 20 minutes to 2 hours after eating, and although it can be quite disabling, it typically resolves without incident. (Dumping syndrome is discussed in detail later in this chapter.)

When the patient is ready to go home, the family is instructed about how to promote nutrition, what observations to make, what measures to take if complications occur, how to keep the patient comfortable, and how to obtain needed physical and emotional support.

GASTROINTESTINAL INTUBATION

GI intubation involves inserting a tube into the stomach or past the stomach into the duodenum or jejunum. The insertion point can be at the patient's nose, mouth, or the abdominal wall.

Clinical Indications

GI intubation can be done to decompress (remove) stomach fluid or air, lavage the stomach and remove toxins, administer medications and nutrition, treat an obstruction, and to bypass sections of the GI tract to allow them to rest. The size and type of tube used is determined by its purpose.

Tubes

Nasogastric and Orogastric Tubes

Often these types of tubes are used for **decompression** of a stomach that is distended due to air or fluid. These tubes are of large bore and may be single or double lumen. The Levin tube is a single-lumen tube, ranging from 14 to 18 French (Fr) in size and is made of plastic or rubber with multiple distal openings or "eyes" near its tip (1 Fr equals 1/3 of 1 mm, thus an 18 Fr is 6 mm in diameter). Circular markings at specific points on the tube serve as guides for insertion. The Levin tube is connected to low *intermittent* suction (30 to 40 mm Hg) to avoid erosion of gastric mucosa.

Nursing Alert

If a Levine tube is used, it must be on intermittent low wall suction (30 to 40 mm Hg) to prevent gastric erosion or tearing of the stomach lining (which can result after the stomach contents have been drained from suction, and continuous suction causes invagination of the mucosal lining of the stomach into the "eyes" of the tube).

The smaller the French size, the smaller the lumen of the tube. Contraindications to placement of NG tubes include facial and head trauma, severe coagulopathy, deviated septum, esophageal strictures or diverticula, and a history of alkali ingestion (Roberts & Hedges, 2013). Caution is used when inserting NG tubes in patients with esophageal varices

as well as postgastric bypass and lap-banding procedures (Roberts & Hedges, 2013).

A gastric or Salem sump tube (SST) is a double-lumen tube available in 12 to 18 Fr (although typically a 16 to 18 Fr is used for adults); it is marked from the distal end at particular distances indicated by the manufacturer. The larger main lumen tube is intended for suction, and the smaller lumen or *pigtail*, which is typically blue in color, is termed the *venting port*. The venting port ensures that the suction at the distal end of the tube is maintained at a safe level to preserve the mucosa of the stomach by allowing atmospheric air to enter the blue lumen to prevent invagination of stomach into the multiple distal openings. An **antireflux valve** can be placed in the venting port of the tube if gastric fluid leaks through the air vent. The venting tube (blue pigtail) must be higher than the level of the stomach to prevent the siphoning out of gastric contents via this lumen. In the event that leakage has occurred, the larger lumen is irrigated with 30 mL of normal saline, after which air is injected to reestablish a buffer of air between the lumens, and an antireflux valve is applied to the venting lumen. The antireflux valve is a one-way valve that prevents gastric fluid from exiting the SST via the vent lumen (Fig. 22-10). If an SST is used, it must be on continuous low suction.

In the event that gastric decompression is no longer needed, an SST can be used to administer intermittent medications, intermittent liquid feedings, or continuous liquid feedings. However, to do so, the venting tube must be plugged to prevent the instillation fluid from leaking out via

FIGURE 22-10 Gastric sump tube (Salem) equipped with a one-way valve that allows air to enter and can prevent reflux of gastric contents. The antireflux valve is designed with a pressure-activated air buffer (PAAB). The buffer is activated (1) and the valve closes (2) when pressure from gastric contents enters the tubing. (Courtesy of Lippincott's Nursing Procedures and Skills.)

this lumen. Residual volumes of stomach contents in patients receiving continuous tube feedings can be assessed easily with these large-bore tubes (residual volumes are discussed later in the chapter).

Postpyloric Tubes

Tubes that continue past the stomach and enter the duodenum and jejunum are longer, smaller-bore, single-lumen tubes. Duodenal and jejunal tubes are commonly 8 to 10 Fr and 110 to 140 cm long. Most often postpyloric tubes are inserted into the nares and are designed primarily for continuous feeding into the small intestine when gastric feeding is not desired. Examples of contraindications for gastric feedings include patients with a high risk of aspiration and those undergoing gastric surgery. Patients having pancreatitis or pancreatic surgery may have jejunal tubes placed to rest the pancreas by bypassing the hepatopancreatic ampulla, thereby avoiding the release of digestive enzymes into the duodenum.

Postpyloric tubes can be inserted before or during surgery, by interventional radiologists assisted by fluoroscopy, or at the bedside by a trained nurse or health care provider. At the bedside, the tube is advanced past the stomach actively, using a combination of air bolusing and peristalsis-enhancing medications such as metoclopramide, a gastric motility agent. Another method involves electromagnetic tube placement. In addition, self-advancing systems are available, which use a stylet inside the feeding tube that communicates with a receiver on the outside of the patient's body to indicate the position of the tube tip in the patient's GI tract (see Fig. 22-11). A trained nurse or physician is able to determine where the tube terminates in the small intestine. This method of insertion has been found to decrease time between placement and initiation of feedings, decrease the number of x-rays, and decrease instances of misplacement and pneumothorax (Smithard, Barrett, Hargroves, & Elliot, 2015).

Passive advancement involves waiting for the peristaltic movement of the stomach and intestine to facilitate the migration of the tube into the small intestine. Placing the patient on his or her right side may be helpful in advancing the tube because gravity may assist the tube in passing through the pyloric sphincter and into the small intestine.

Nursing Management

Assessing the Patient before Tube Placement

When gastric or enteric/postpyloric intubation is ordered for a patient, it is important for the nurse to review the patient's history to check for contraindications for tube placement. Examples of contraindications include oral or nasal surgery, esophageal varices, esophageal diverticula, and esophageal or gastric surgery, such as a gastric pullup or gastric bypass. Such patients would have a greater risk for perforation, and an altered anatomy would make tube placement difficult if

FIGURE 22-11 All-in-one monitor with integrated visual display terminal, touch screen, and embedded computing system. The tip of the stylet contains an electromagnetic transmitter that generates a real-time signal as the feeding tube is inserted and advanced to the desired placement. The signal from the transmitting stylet is tracked throughout the placement procedure via a lightweight smart receiver unit (SRU) that is placed on the patient's xiphoid process. The real-time tube tip tracking aids confident, safe placement. The all-in-one monitor triangulates the signal from the SRU and displays a real-time representation of the feeding tube tip's passage as it proceeds down the esophagus and into the preferred placement position.

the details of the procedure were not known. It is also important to consider the nutritional status of the patient before a tube is inserted into his or her GI tract; serum prealbumin levels should be assessed. Prealbumin is an excellent marker for malnutrition because it has a shorter half-life (2 days) than does albumin (21 days), and it is not influenced by fluid balance. A normal prealbumin level for people aged 7 years and above is 19 to 38 mg/dL (Fischbach & Dunning, 2014). The likelihood of perforation is higher in patients with severe nutritional deficiencies due to poor tissue integrity.

Passage of an NG tube carries risk for patients with known or suspected cervical injuries and may exacerbate hemorrhage in patients with penetrating neck injuries if coughing and gagging occur during insertion (Roberts & Hedges, 2013). Serious complications include pulmonary misplacement of the NG tube and intracranial placement. Patients with head trauma should be evaluated for basilar skull fracture before an NG tube is placed. The tube could be inserted into the cranial vault inadvertently, if the fracture communicates.

Preparing the Patient

Before the patient is intubated, the nurse explains the purpose of the tube; this information may assist the patient in being cooperative and tolerant of what is often an unpleasant procedure. Then the general activities related to inserting the tube are reviewed, including the fact that the patient may have to breathe through the mouth and that the procedure may cause gagging until the tube has passed the area of the gag reflex.

Inserting the Tube

Before inserting the tube, the nurse determines the length of tubing that will be needed to reach the stomach or the small intestine. A mark is made on the tube to indicate the desired length. This length is determined by measuring the distance from the tip of the **N**ose to the **E**arlobe and from the earlobe to the **X**iphoid process for gastric placement or NEX (Fig. 22-12). A common error in inserting NG tubes is to incorrectly estimate the proper length of the tube that should be inserted, thus NG tubes may be inserted too short (in the lower esophagus) or coiled in the stomach. One additional measurement is noted in the literature: adding 6 in (or 15 cm) to the NEX measurement to prevent high NG tube placement in tall patients (Roberts & Hedges, 2013). The average measurement for adults is 22 to 26 in or 56 to 66 cm (Lippincott Williams & Wilkins, 2013).

Tip of nose to earlobe

Earlobe to xiphoid

Wrap tape around tube here

FIGURE 22-12 Measuring length of nasogastric tube for placement into stomach. To determine how long the NG tube must be to reach the stomach, hold the end of the tube at the tip of the patient's nose. Extend the tube to the patient's earlobe and then down to the xiphoid process (as shown above). (Reprinted with permission from *Nursing Procedures* (4th ed.). Ambler: Lippincott Williams & Wilkins, 2004.)

Insertion of the tube is not a sterile procedure; the nurse and other staff involved should follow Universal Precaution procedures as designated by their facility (gloves, gown, and face mask are recommended). While the tube is being inserted, the patient usually sits upright with a towel or some type of protective barrier spread bib-fashion over the chest. Tissue wipes are made available. Privacy and adequate light are provided. The provider may swab the nostril and spray the oropharynx with tetracaine/benzocaine (Cetacaine) at least 5 minutes before the procedure to numb the nasal passage and suppress the gag reflex. This makes the entire procedure more tolerable. Having the patient gargle with a liquid anesthetic or hold ice chips in the mouth for a few minutes can have a similar effect. Encouraging the patient to breathe through the mouth or to pant often helps, as does swallowing water, if permitted.

A polyurethane tube may need to be warmed to make it more pliable. To make the tube easier to insert, it should be lubricated with a water-soluble lubricant unless it has a dry coating (called *hydromer*), which, when moistened, provides its own lubrication.

The patient is placed in Fowler position, and the nostrils are inspected for any obstruction. The more patent nostril is selected for use. The tip of the patient's nose is tilted, and the tube is aligned to enter the nostril, following the floor of the nose (under the inferior turbinate), not upward toward the nasal bridge. The tube is advanced slowly to avoid pressure on the nasal turbinates until the posterior pharynx is reached. If significant resistance is encountered, the other nostril is tried rather than forcing the tube, which can cause complications of bleeding or dissection into retropharyngeal tissue (Roberts & Hedges, 2013). When the tube reaches the posterior pharynx, the patient is allowed to rest for a few minutes before proceeding. Unless contraindicated, the patient is instructed to flex the neck to facilitate passage into the esophagus and to begin to swallow as the tube is advanced to the predetermined depth. The patient may also sip water through a straw to facilitate advancement of the tube unless drinking is contraindicated. The oropharynx is inspected to ensure that the tube has not coiled in the pharynx or mouth.

Confirming Placement

To ensure patient safety, it is essential to confirm that the tube has been placed correctly: the tube may be inserted in the lungs inadvertently, and this may go undetected in high-risk patients (e.g., those with decreased levels of consciousness, confused mental states, poor or absent cough and gag reflexes, or agitation during insertion). The gold standard for verifying placement of a blindly inserted tube is radiographic or x-ray confirmation (American Association of Critical Care Nurses [AACN, 2016b]). X-ray confirmation is necessary if the patient will be receiving feedings or medications through the tube. When a tube is to be used for removal of air or fluid and not instillation, the nurse can use a combination of visually assessing the aspirate, testing its pH, and using capnographic devices to initially determine placement. Visual assessment of the color of the aspirate may help identify tube placement. The gastric aspirate is most frequently cloudy and green, tan or off-white, or bloody or brown. Intestinal aspirate is primarily clear and yellow to bile-colored. The pleural fluid is usually pale yellow and serous, and tracheobronchial secretions usually consist of mucus that is tan or off-white. The appearance of the aspirate may be helpful in distinguishing between gastric and intestinal placement but is of little value in ruling out respiratory placement.

Determining the pH of the tube aspirate is a more accurate method of confirming tube placement than is maintaining tube length or visually assessing tube aspirate. The pH method also can be used to monitor the advancement of the tube into the small intestine. The pH of gastric aspirate is acidic (1 to 5), typically less than 4. The pH of intestinal aspirate is approximately 6 or higher, and the pH of respiratory aspirate is more alkaline (greater than 6).

Patients who are receiving histamine 2 (H_2)-receptor antagonists or PPIs may demonstrate pH ranges from 0 to 6.0, and pH can be affected by medications or formulas. This alkaline aspirate could falsely confirm a postpyloric tube position (Damm & Gama de Abreu, 2012). Therefore, testing the pH remains an area where further research is warranted. Capnography involves detecting carbon dioxide at the external end of the NG tubes. In a group of 257 patients in medical ICU with NG tube placements, capnography has been found to have 99.4% sensitivity and 91.3% specificity on identifying tubes that did not terminate in the GI tract on first attempt (Smymios et al., 2015).

Placement also must be ensured at regular intervals once the device is placed. These times include when medications or fluids are given and every 4 hours for patients receiving continuous tube feedings. The traditional method has been to inject air through the tube while auscultating the epigastric area with a stethoscope to detect air insufflation. However, studies indicate that this auscultatory method is not particularly accurate in determining whether the tube has been inserted into the stomach, intestines, or respiratory tract (AACN, 2016b). Instead of the auscultation method, a combination of four methods is recommended: assessment of the patient's tolerance to medication and feeding administration, measurement of tube length, visual assessment of aspirate, and assessing the pH measurement of aspirate.

To determine tolerance of the feeding to ascertain placement, the nurse assesses the patient's respiratory status. Coughing, gagging, and decreased pulse oximetry could indicate that the tube has migrated. The nurse also inspects the oral cavity to visualize the tube in the back of the patient's throat. It is possible for a patient to regurgitate the tube into the mouth with frequent gagging and coughing.

After the tube is inserted, the exposed portion of the tube is measured and the length is documented. The nurse measures the exposed tube length every shift and compares it with the original measurement. An increase in the length of exposed tube may indicate dislodgement.

Securing the Tube

After the correct position of the tip of the tube has been confirmed, the NG tube is secured to the nose (Fig. 22-13). A liquid skin barrier can be applied to the skin where the NG tube will be secured. The prepared area is covered with a strip of hypoallergenic tape or Op-Site, and then the tube is placed over the tape and secured with a second piece of tape. Instead of tape, a number of companies have feeding tube device holders that can be placed. A nasal bridle can be used in patients in multiple levels of care who have a history of tube dislodgment due, for example, to impaired mental status related to dementia or traumatic brain injury. Bridling (Fig. 22-14) involves the insertion of a loop of strong but flexible material through the naris, around the nasal septum, and out the other nare as a "bridle" to which the nasoenteric tube is secured. A meta-analysis involving 6 studies and 594 patients found that the use of bridles was significantly effective in reducing dislodgements compared to using tape; however, one drawback was that the incidence of skin breakdown was higher in patients with bridles (Bechtold et al., 2014). In addition, it is wise to secure the NG tube to the patient's gown or pajamas with an elastic band and safety pin or with adhesive tape loops so that a tug on the tube will not pull on the naris. It is crucial that the NG tube is secured without putting undue pressure on the medial or lateral nares in

FIGURE 22-13 Securing nasogastric (NG) tubes. **A.** The NG tube is secured to the nose with tape to prevent injury to the nasopharyngeal passages. **B.** The tubing is secured to the patient's gown with tape attached to a safety pin to prevent tension on the line.

FIGURE 22-14 A bridle nasal tube retaining system. Placement entails: (1) Advance catheter stylet and blue probe in opposite nares until magnets connect. Remove orange stylet from catheter. (2) Slowly remove blue probe, drawing the white catheter around the vomer bone and out the opposite nare. (3) Cut catheter off and discard. (4) Place tube and umbilical tape in clip. (5) Securely close clip 1 cm below nose. Tie two to three knots and cut off excess. (Reprinted with permission from AMT Bridle Nasal Tube Retaining System from Applied Medical Technology, Inc.)

order to prevent tissue necrosis. In addition, the tape securing the tube should be changed daily and the nares inspected for complications such as erosion (Lippincott Williams & Wilkins, 2013). The tube must be looped loosely to prevent tension and dislodgement.

Nursing Alert

If the patient is ambulatory and has an SST, the blue pigtail must be above the level of the stomach to prevent gastric fluid leaking out via this port. The pigtail can be fitted into the larger suction lumen to seal off the NG tube while the patient is ambulating.

Monitoring the Patient and Maintaining Tube Function

It is important to keep an accurate record of all fluid intake, feedings, and irrigation. To maintain patency, the tube is irrigated every 4 to 6 hours with normal saline to avoid electrolyte loss through gastric drainage. Sterile water may be used during medication administration or tube feedings, especially when the access is postpyloric and the acidic environment of the stomach is bypassed (White & Bradnam, 2015). The nurse records the amount, color, and type of all drainage every 8 hours.

When double- or triple-lumen tubes are used, each lumen is labeled according to its intended use: aspiration, feeding, or balloon inflation (refer to Sengstaken-Blakemore tube in Chapter 25).

When feedings or medications are ordered for administration through a GI tube, it is the nurse's responsibility to maintain the patency of the device as well as to assess the patient's tolerance of the feeding or meds. Liquid nutritional solutions are commonly administered at a continuous rate via programmable electronic pump or by syringe in intermittent boluses. With continuous feedings, it is important for the nurse to assess the volume of feed in the bag to ensure it does not run dry.

Administering Medication

When medications are administered through GI tubes, flushing the tube with 30 to 50 mL of (sterile) water may decrease the

risk of tube occlusion (Lippincott Williams & Wilkins, 2013). With NG tubes and small-diameter nasoenteric tubes, thorough crushing of medications in pill form is a necessity. A nurse should collaborate with the medical team and pharmacy to convert medications to liquid forms, if possible. Also the nurse should be aware that administering extended-release tablets that would require crushing through such tubes is prohibited since overdosage can result. However, occasionally, time-released capsules are permitted to be opened (not crushed) and administered, and pharmacy staff should be consulted if any questions or concerns exist related to whether medications can be crushed or opened. The medical team should be notified to have the medications changed to liquid form whenever possible. Table 22-1 discusses administering medications.

TABLE 22-1 Preparing Medication for Delivery by Feeding Tube

Medication Form	Preparation
Liquid	None
Simple compressed tablets	Crush and dissolve in water
Buccal or sublingual tablets	Administer as prescribed
Soft gelatin capsules filled with liquid	Make an opening in the capsule and squeeze the contents out into water to dissolve
Enteric-coated tablets	Do not crush; change in form is required; consult pharmacy department as needed
Timed-release tablets	Do not crush tablets because doing so may release too much drug too quickly (overdose); check with pharmacist for alternative formulation
Timed-release capsules or sustained-release capsules	Some can be opened and contents added to tube-feeding formula; *always* check with pharmacist before doing this

Unclogging Tubes

When a tube becomes clogged with feedings or medications, a number of methods can be used to regain patency of the tube without having to replace it. Smaller-diameter postpyloric tubes can clog if feedings are stopped and the tube is not flushed properly. Warm water can be administered through the tube with caution using varying sizes of syringes; smaller syringes having greater force to dislodge the clog. Cola and cranberry juice have historically been recommended as an effective, noninvasive means of unclogging tubes; however, a more consistently effective method involves instilling a mixture of pancreatic enzymes and sodium bicarbonate into the tube for 20 minutes to digest the clog. The nurse is aware that correct placement of the NG tube must be confirmed before any mixture is injected to unclog the tube.

 Nursing Alert
Currently, a small number of research literature evaluates the nursing considerations and interventions relating to the administration of medications via enteral tubes. The nurse should read current literature and access databases such as the Cochrane library for the most current evidence.

Providing Oral and Nasal Hygiene

Regular and conscientious oral and nasal hygiene is a vital part of patient care because the tube causes discomfort and pressure and may be in place for several days. Moistened cotton-tipped swabs can be used to clean the nose, followed by cleansing with a water-soluble lubricant. Frequent mouth care is comforting for the patient. The nasal tape is changed daily, and the nose is inspected for skin irritation. If the nasal and pharyngeal mucosa is excessively dry, steam or cool vapor inhalations may be beneficial. Throat lozenges, an ice collar, chewing gum, or sucking on hard candies (if permitted) as well as limiting talking also assist in relieving patient discomfort. These activities keep the mucous membranes moist and help prevent inflammation of the parotid glands.

Monitoring and Managing Potential Complications

Patients with NG or nasoenteric intubation are susceptible to a variety of problems, including fluid volume deficit (FVD), pulmonary complications, and tube-related irritations. These potential complications require careful ongoing assessment.

Symptoms of FVD include dry skin and mucous membranes, decreased urinary output, lethargy, orthostatic hypotension, and increased heart rate. Also a nurse can calculate the patient's pulse pressure (systolic blood pressure minus diastolic blood pressure) to predict the patient's volume status. A pulse pressure of less than 30 mm Hg is indicative of FVD. Assessment of FVD involves maintaining an accurate record of intake and output. This includes measuring NG

or nasointestinal (NI) drainage, fluid instilled by irrigation of the NG/NI tube, water taken by mouth, vomitus, water administered with tube feedings, and IV fluids. Laboratory values, particularly blood urea nitrogen and creatinine, are monitored. The nurse assesses 24-hour fluid balance and reports negative fluid balance, increased NG output, interruption of IV therapy, or any other disturbance in fluid intake or output.

Pulmonary complications from NG intubation occur because coughing and clearing of the pharynx are impaired, because gas buildup can irritate the phrenic nerve, and because tubes may become dislodged, retracting the distal end above the esophagogastric sphincter (which places the patient at risk for aspiration, or breathing fluids or foods into the trachea and lungs). Medications such as metoclopramide (Reglan) can be administered to decrease potential problems. Signs and symptoms of complications include coughing during the administration of foods or medications, difficulty clearing the airway, tachypnea, and fever. Assessment includes regular auscultation of lung sounds and routine assessment of vital signs. It is important to encourage the patient to cough and to take deep breaths regularly. The nurse also carefully confirms the proper placement of the tube by assessing tube length before instilling any fluids or medications.

Irritation of the mucous membranes is a common complication of NG/NI intubation. The nostrils, oral mucosa, esophagus, and trachea are susceptible to irritation and necrosis. Visible areas are inspected frequently, and the adequacy of hydration is assessed. When providing oral hygiene, the nurse carefully inspects the mucous membranes for signs of irritation or excessive dryness. The nurse palpates the area around the parotid glands to detect any tenderness or enlarged nodes, indicating parotitis, and observes for any irritation or skin breakdown at the insertion site (e.g., naris) or of the mucous membranes. In order to preserve the skin integrity of the naris, the nurse should rotate the position of the tube on the wall of the naris once every 24 hours. In addition, it is important to assess the patient for esophagitis and tracheitis; symptoms include sore throat and hoarseness.

 Nursing Alert
The nurse alerts the health provider when new frank bleeding is noted in the NG tube drainage or if "coffee-ground material" is noted because it may indicate bleeding. Gastroccult testing is available to assess the presence of blood in gastric drainage. The nurse is aware that hemoccult test for stool cannot be used for evaluation of gastric drainage.

Removing the Tube

Before removing a tube, the nurse may clamp and unclamp it intermittently for a trial period of several hours to ensure that the patient does not experience nausea, vomiting, or distention. Before the tube is removed, it is flushed with 10 mL of water or normal saline to ensure that it is free of debris and away from the gastric lining. Gloves are worn to remove the tube, and a towel or disposable pad is placed on the patient's chest. The tube is withdrawn gently and slowly for 15 to 20 cm (6 to 8 in) until the tip reaches the esophagus; the remainder is withdrawn rapidly from the nostril. If the tube does not come out easily, force should not be used, and the problem should be reported to the provider. As the tube is withdrawn, it is concealed in the disposable pad or towel to prevent secretions from soiling the patient or nurse. After the tube is removed, the nurse provides oral hygiene.

Administering Tube Feedings with Nasogastric and Nasoenteric Devices

Enteral nutrition feedings are given to meet nutritional requirements when oral intake is inadequate or not possible and the GI tract is functioning normally. Tube feedings have several advantages over PN: they are low in cost, safe, well tolerated by the patient, and easy to use both in extended-care facilities and in the patient's home. Other advantages include:

- Preserving GI integrity by delivery of nutrients and medications intraluminally
- Preserving the normal sequence of intestinal and hepatic metabolism
- Maintaining fat metabolism and lipoprotein synthesis
- Maintaining normal insulin/glucagon ratios

Tube feedings are delivered to the stomach (in the case of NG intubation or gastrostomy) or to the distal duodenum or proximal jejunum (in the case of **nasoduodenal** or **nasojejunal tube** feeding). Nasoduodenal or nasojejunal feeding is indicated when the esophagus and stomach need to be bypassed or when the patient is at risk for aspiration. For long-term feedings (longer than 4 weeks), gastrostomy or jejunostomy tubes are preferred for administration of medications or food. The numerous conditions requiring enteral nutrition are summarized in Table 22-2.

Reducing the Risk of Aspiration

To decrease the risk of aspiration, the head of the bed must remain elevated to 30 to 45 degrees at all times if appropriate for the patient's condition (AACN, 2016a). An elevated head of bed may not be appropriate for some patients, such as those with spinal injuries or mobility restrictions due to interventional procedures involving the vasculature of the groin. In these cases, it may be appropriate to adjust the hospital bed to a reverse Trendelenburg position per health care provider's order to decrease aspiration risk. If the patient is on bedrest, the tube feeding must be shut off when bed making, bathing, or anytime the head of the bed must be lowered to below 30 degrees.

TABLE 22-2 Conditions Requiring Enteral Therapy

Condition or Need	Examples
GI problems	Fistula, short-bowel syndrome, mild pancreatitis, Crohn disease, ulcerative colitis, nonspecific maldigestion or malabsorption
Cancer therapy	Radiation, chemotherapy
Convalescent care	Surgery, injury, severe illness
Coma, semi-consciousness[a]	Stroke, head injury, neurologic disorder, neoplasm
Hypermetabolic conditions	Burns, trauma, multiple fractures, sepsis, AIDS, organ transplantation
Chronic illness, psychiatric or neurologic disorder Alcoholism, chronic depression, anorexia nervosa[a]	Alcoholism, chronic depression, anorexia nervosa[a]
Debilitation[a]	Disease or injury
Maxillofacial or cervical surgery	Disease or injury, wired jaw, spinal cord injury
Oropharyngeal or esophageal paralysis[a]	Disease or injury, neoplasm, inflammation, trauma, respiratory failure

[a]Because some of these patients are at risk for regurgitating or vomiting and aspirating administered formula, each condition must be considered individually.

Residual Assessment

Patient tolerance of liquid enteral nutrition is determined by residual measurement, the presence or absence of nausea and vomiting, and increasing abdominal distention. Residual measurement or volume of aspiration is most easily assessed with large-bore GI tubes. Smaller-diameter nasojejunal tubes and duodenal tubes often collapse when suction is applied. The volume of aspirate indicates the rate at which the patient is digesting the feedings and how quickly the chyme is passing into the small intestine. The volume of the stomach is approximately 1 L, with an ability to stretch with increased intake depending on the size of the patient.

To assess gastric residuals, a 60-mL syringe is used to measure volumes from feeding tubes every 4 hours. The nurse slowly applies a steady pressure on the plunger and aspirates the residual volume until no more fluid can be withdrawn into the syringe. Policies vary according to institutions, and the nurse should follow unit guidelines. The American Society of Parenteral and Enteral Nutrition and the Society of Critical Care Medicine recommend that if gastric residual volumes are measured in ICU patients that feedings should be held for volumes over 500 mL, although the societies recognize that evidence to support the practice is poor (McClave et al., 2016). Similar guidelines published in Canada in 2013 support the volume range as well (Dhaliwal, Cahill, Lemieux, & Heyland, 2013). Promotility agents are considered with increasing residual volumes (metoclopramide or erythromycin) (McCarthy & Martindale, 2015). Because individual procedures vary widely, and uncertainty exists regarding the assessment and treatment in high residual volumes, it is important to follow institutional procedures closely and hold feedings as indicated.

Osmosis, Osmolality, and Dumping Syndrome

Osmolality is an important consideration for patients receiving tube feedings through the duodenum or jejunum because feeding formulas with a high osmolality may lead to undesirable effects, such as dumping syndrome.

Fluid balance is maintained by **osmosis**, the process by which water moves through membranes from a dilute solution of lower **osmolality** (ionic concentration) to a more concentrated solution of higher osmolality until both solutions are of nearly equal osmolality. The osmolality of normal body fluids is approximately 300 mOsm/kg. The body attempts to keep the osmolality of the contents of the stomach and intestines at approximately this level.

Highly concentrated solutions and certain foods can upset the normal fluid balance in the body. Individual amino acids and carbohydrates are small particles that have great osmotic effect. Electrolytes, such as sodium and potassium, are comparatively small particles; they have a great effect on osmolality and, consequently, on the patient's ability to tolerate a given solution.

When a concentrated solution of high osmolality is taken in large amounts, water moves to the stomach and intestines from fluid surrounding the organs and the vascular compartment. The patient has a feeling of fullness, nausea, and diarrhea; this causes dehydration, hypotension, and tachycardia, collectively termed **dumping syndrome**. Patients vary in the degree to which they tolerate the effects of high osmolality; usually, debilitated patients are less tolerant. The nurse needs to be knowledgeable about the osmolality of the patient's formula and needs to observe for and take steps to prevent undesired effects. Dumping syndrome can be prevented by the following interventions: using room-temperature feedings (gastric emptying will be faster if temperature of the fluid is too hot or too cold), changing from **bolus** to continuous feedings if appropriate, having the patient remain in a semi-Fowler position for 1 hour after eating to gradually allow the feedings to pass into the intestine, and slowing the rate of feedings to allow more time for digestion.

In the event that a tube feeding uses a high-osmolality formula, the nurse observes the patient's sodium level and expects that free water may be ordered by diluting the tube feeding or by periodic instillation of water by the health care team if rising sodium levels are seen. Response to the free water (either dilution of tube feeding or tap water instilled via the NG/NI tube) is assessed with subsequent electrolyte levels.

Nursing Alert

The nurse understands that administering medication via an enteral tube is not the same as PO (Per Os or by mouth). For example, liquid antibiotics, laxatives, and vitamin and electrolyte solutions far exceed the osmolality of GI secretions (approximately 300 mOsm/kg). The practice of crushing multiple tablets and mixing powders together before administration is an unsafe habit. Mixing drugs together, whether solid or liquid, creates an unknown substance with an unpredictable mechanism of release and bioavailability. Proper flushing of the tube before, between, and after each drug is recommended. Also, enteral feeding needs to be stopped and the feeding tube needs to be flushed before medication is administered. The pharmacist should be consulted regarding medication administration. Refer to the do not crush list at http://www.ismp.org/tools/donotcrush.pdf for specific information.

Tube Feeding Formulas

The choice of formula to be delivered by tube feeding is influenced by the status of the GI tract and the nutritional needs of the patient. Dietitians collaborate with providers and nurses to determine the best formula for the individual patient. The formula characteristics that are considered prior to selection include the chemical composition of the nutrient source (protein, carbohydrates, fat), caloric density, osmolality, residue, bacteriologic safety, vitamins, minerals, and cost.

Various major formula types for tube feedings are available commercially. Commercially prepared polymeric formulas (formulas with high molecular weight) are composed of protein, carbohydrates, and fats in a high–molecular-weight form (e.g., Boost Plus, TwoCal HN, Isosource). Chemically defined formulas (e.g., Peptamen 1.5 or Vivonex) contain predigested and easy-to-absorb nutrients. Modular products contain only one major nutrient, such as protein (Beneprotein). Disease-specific formulas are available for various conditions. For patients with kidney failure, a formula such as Nepro, which is high in calories and low in electrolytes, is ideal because it is formulated to maintain electrolyte and fluid balance. For patients with severe chronic obstructive pulmonary disease, a formula such as Pulmocare may be selected because it is high in fat and low in carbohydrates, has a high density (1.5 calories/mL) that helps maintain fluid restriction, and reduces carbon dioxide production. Excess carbohydrates may increase production of CO_2, and this negatively impacts respiratory status. Fiber is added to some formulas (e.g., Jevity) to decrease the occurrence of diarrhea in some at-risk patients. Blenderized formulas also can be used. They can be made by the patient's family or obtained in a ready-to-use form that is carefully prepared according to directions. Some feedings are given as supplements, and others are designed to meet the patient's total nutritional needs.

Administration Methods and Frequency

The frequency of tube feeding and administration method depends on the location of the tube in the GI tract, patient tolerance, convenience, and cost. Intermittent bolus feedings are administered into the stomach (usually by gastrostomy tube) in large amounts at designated intervals and may be given four to eight times per day. The intermittent gravity drip, another method for administering tube feedings into the stomach, is commonly used when the patient is at home. In this instance, the tube feeding is administered over 30 minutes at designated intervals. Both of these tube feeding methods are practical and inexpensive. However, the feedings delivered at variable rates may be poorly tolerated and time consuming.

Often the continuous infusion method is used when feedings are administered into the small intestine. This method is preferred for patients who are at risk for aspiration or who tolerate tube feedings poorly (Luttikhold et al., 2016; McClave et al., 2016). The feedings are given continuously at a constant rate by means of a pump. This method decreases abdominal distention, gastric residuals, and the risk of aspiration. However, pumps are expensive, and they allow the patient less flexibility than intermittent feedings.

An alternative to the continuous infusion method is **cyclic feeding**. The infusion is administered at a higher hourly volume over the course of 8- to 12-hour intervals with the goal of meeting the prescribed calories and/or macronutrient for a 24-hour period. Feedings may be infused at night to avoid interrupting the patient's lifestyle. Cyclic continuous infusions may be appropriate for patients who are being weaned from tube feedings to an oral diet, as supplements for patients who cannot eat enough, and for patients at home who need day time hours free from the pump. Whichever method is chosen, the head of the bed must be maintained at a minimum of 30 degrees to decrease the risk of aspiration. A wide variety of containers, feeding tubes and catheters, delivery systems, and pumps are available for use with tube feedings.

Complications of Tube Feedings

Diarrhea, the most common complication associated with liquid feedings, is commonly due to the hyperosmolality of the feedings and/or the decreased serum osmolality of the patient's serum. Changing the concentration or type of formula often decreases or stops this complication.

Aspiration pneumonia is an important mechanical complication. Aspiration can occur due to improperly placed tubes or when the patient vomits the formula into the airway. When aspiration occurs or is suspected, it is important for the nurse to stop the feeding, suction the pharynx and trachea, and closely assess the patient's respiratory status while contacting the provider. Aspiration prevention involves keeping the patient's head of bed elevated to at least 30 degrees and verifying the tube placement on insertion, before food or medication administration, and periodically throughout a 24-hour shift.

Patients may have increased blood glucose as a metabolic complication of tube feedings. Carbohydrate content varies between the different types of formula used and should be considered if the patient is hyperglycemic. The nurse should assess the patient's blood sugar frequently especially when initiating a tube feeding. Additional complications of enteral therapy can be found in Table 22-3.

GASTROSTOMY

A **gastrostomy** is a surgical procedure in which an opening is created into the stomach for the purpose of administering foods and fluids via a feeding tube.

Clinical Indications

Gastrostomy is preferred for prolonged enteral nutrition support when the patient's diagnosis makes it difficult to support the nutritional requirements, such as in patients with traumatic brain injury and patients with neurodegenerative diseases (Alzheimer disease). Gastrostomy is also preferred over NG feedings in the patient who is comatose because the gastroesophageal sphincter remains intact. Regurgitation and aspiration are less likely to occur with a gastrostomy than with NG feedings.

Types

Different types of feeding gastrostomies may be used, including the Stamm (temporary and permanent), Janeway (permanent), and **percutaneous endoscopic gastrostomy (PEG)** tube (temporary) systems. The Stamm and Janeway gastrostomies require either an upper abdominal midline incision or a left upper quadrant transverse incision. The Stamm procedure requires the use of concentric pursestring sutures to secure the tube to the anterior gastric wall. To create the gastrostomy, an exit wound is created in the left upper abdomen. The Janeway procedure necessitates the creation of a tunnel (called a *gastric tube*) that is brought out through the abdomen to form a permanent **stoma**.

Insertion of a PEG requires the services of two physicians (or a physician and a nurse with specialty skills). After administering a local anesthetic, one health care provider inserts a cannula into the stomach through an abdominal incision and then threads a nonabsorbable suture through the cannula; the second provider inserts an endoscope via the patient's upper GI tract and uses the endoscopic snare to grasp the end of the suture and guide it up through the patient's mouth. The suture is knotted to the dilator tip at the end of the PEG tube. Then the provider who inserted the endoscope advances the dilator tip through the patient's mouth while the first provider pulls the suture through the cannula site. The attached PEG tube is guided down the

TABLE **22-3** **Complications of Enteral Therapy**

Complications	Causes	Selected Nursing Interventions	
		Treatment	Prevention
Gastrointestinal			
Diarrhea (most common)	Hyperosmolar feedings Rapid infusion/bolus feedings Bacteria-contaminated feedings Lactase deficiency Medications/antibiotic therapy Decreased serum osmolality level Food allergies Cold formula	Assess fluid balance and electrolyte levels; report findings Implement changes in tube feeding formula or rate	Assess rate of infusion and temperature of formula Replace formula every 4 hours; change tube feeding container and tubing daily
Nausea/vomiting	Change in formula or rate Hyperosmolar formula Inadequate gastric emptying	Review medications	Check residuals; if >200 mL consider promotility medications, if >500 mL, check with provider. (Because individual procedures vary widely, it is important to follow institutional procedures closely and to hold feedings as indicated)
Gas/bloating/cramping	Air in tube	Notify provider if persistent	Keep tubing free of air
Dumping syndrome	Bolus feedings/rapid rate Cold formula	Check fiber and water content; report findings Check rate and temperature of formula	Avoid rapid infusion of feeding Administer feeding at or near room temperature
Constipation	High milk (lactose) content Lack of fiber Inadequate fluid intake/dehydration Opioid use	Check fiber and water content; report findings	Administer adequate amount of hydration as flushes
Mechanical			
Aspiration pneumonia	Improper tube placement Vomiting with aspiration of tube feeding Flat in bed Use of large tube	Assess respiratory status and notify provider	Implement reliable method for checking small-bore enteral tube placement (i.e., measuring length of exposed tube) Keep head of bed elevated 30–45 degrees continuously
Tube displacement	Excessive coughing/vomitus Tension on the tube or unsecured tube Tracheal suctioning Airway intubation	Stop feeding and notify provider	Check tube placement before administering feeding
Tube obstruction	Inadequate flushing/formula rate/inadequate medication crushing	Follow policy for declogging feeding tubes	Obtain liquid medications when possible, flush tube and medications adequately
Residue	Inadequate crushing of medications and flushing after administration		Flush tube and crush medications adequately
Nasopharyngeal irritation	Tube position/improper taping Use of large tubes	Assess nasopharyngeal mucous membranes every 4 hours	Tape tube to prevent pressure on nares

		Selected Nursing Interventions	
Complications	Causes	Treatment	Prevention
Metabolic			
Hyperglycemia	Glucose intolerance High carbohydrate content of the feeding	Check blood glucose levels periodically Request dietary consult to reevaluate choice of feeding product	Collaborate with dietician for potential solution changes.
Dehydration and azotemia (excessive urea in the blood)	Hyperosmolar feedings with insufficient fluid intake	Report signs and symptoms of dehydration Implement changes in tube feeding formula, rate, or ratio to water	Provide adequate hydration through flushes or dilution of tube feeding

esophagus, into the stomach, and out through the abdominal incision (Fig. 22-15). The mushroom catheter tip and internal crossbar secure the tube against the stomach wall. An external crossbar or bumper keeps the catheter in place. A tubing adaptor is in place between feedings, and a clamp or plug is used to close or open the tubing.

The initial PEG device can be removed and replaced once the tract is well established (10 to 14 days after insertion). Replacement of the PEG device is indicated to provide long-term nutritional support, to replace a clogged or migrated tube, or to enhance patient comfort. The PEG replacement device should be fitted securely to the stoma to prevent leakage of gastric acid and is maintained in place through traction between the internal and anchoring devices.

An alternative to the PEG device is a **low-profile gastrostomy device (LPGD)** (see Fig. 22-15). The LPGD may be inserted 3 to 6 months after initial gastrostomy tube placement. These devices are inserted flush with the skin; they eliminate the possibility of tube migration and obstruction and have antireflux valves to prevent gastric reflux. Two types of devices may be used—obturated or nonobturated. The obturated devices (G-button) have a dome tip that acts as an internal stabilizer. Only a physician may obturate (insert a tube that is larger than the actual stoma). The nonobturated device (MIC-KEY) has an external skin disk and is inserted into the stoma without force; a balloon is inflated to secure placement. A nurse in the home setting may insert these nonobturated devices. The drawbacks of both types of LPGDs are the inability to assess residual volumes (one-way valve) and the need for a special adaptor to connect the device to the feeding container.

Complications

Reflux from stomach feedings can result in aspiration pneumonia. Therefore, patients at risk for aspiration pneumonia are not ideal candidates for a gastrostomy. A jejunostomy is

FIGURE 22-15 **A.** A detail of the abdomen and the percutaneous endoscopic gastrostomy (PEG) tube, showing catheter fixation. **B.** A detail of the abdomen and the nonobturated low-profile gastrostomy device (LPGD), showing balloon fixation.

preferred, or jejunal feeding through a nasojejunal tube may be recommended.

Other complications of gastrostomy tube placement include premature removal, infection, and leakage around the insertion site. To prevent premature removal, a loosely taped dressing can be placed over the top of the tube flange. A fenestrated drape (split dressing) often used for tracheotomy care works well. In addition, a tube-securing device can be placed on the patient's abdomen or flank to further decrease the tension on the insertion site. These devices use adhesives and Velcro to fix the gastrostomy tube to the patient's skin temporarily. The nurse should educate the patient on how much mobility he or she has with the gastrostomy tube to aid in preventing tension on the device. If the tube is removed inadvertently, the nurse should clean the site, place a dressing, and notify the provider as soon as possible.

Infection is prevented by assessing and cleansing the site daily. Soap and water can be used around the general area. To remove hardened feedings that may accumulate around the insertion site, the nurse can use normal saline. The area should be dried before a dressing is reapplied. Redness, tenderness, and skin breakdown should be documented and the provider notified.

PARENTERAL NUTRITION

Parenteral nutrition (PN) is a method of providing nutrients to the body by a peripheral or central IV route. The solution is composed of a very complex admixture containing proteins, carbohydrates, fats, electrolytes, vitamins, trace minerals, and sterile water in a single container. The goals of PN are to improve nutritional status, establish a positive nitrogen balance (Box 22-2), maintain muscle mass, promote weight maintenance or gain, and support the healing process.

Clinical Indications

In both the home and hospital settings, PN is indicated in the following situations:

- The patient's intake is insufficient to maintain an anabolic state (e.g., severe burns, malnutrition, short bowel syndrome, AIDS, sepsis, cancer).
- The patient's ability to ingest food orally or by tube is impaired (e.g., paralytic ileus, Crohn disease with obstruction, postradiation enteritis, severe hyperemesis gravidarum in pregnancy).
- The patient is unwilling or unable to ingest adequate nutrients (e.g., anorexia nervosa, postoperative elderly patients).
- The underlying medical condition precludes being fed orally or by tube (e.g., acute pancreatitis, high enterocutaneous fistula).
- Preoperative and postoperative nutritional needs are prolonged (e.g., extensive bowel surgery).

BOX 22-2 | **Establishing Positive Nitrogen Balance**

The balance of nitrogen is determined by how much nitrogen is taken into the body versus how much is excreted. Urine contains 90% of the excreted nitrogen while the remaining 10% exits the body through sweat, hair, and stool (Dominiczak & Logue, 2014). When a patient's intake of protein and nutrients is significantly less than that required by the body to meet energy expenditures, a state of negative nitrogen balance results. In response, the body begins to convert the protein found in muscles into carbohydrates to be used to meet energy needs. The result is muscle wasting, weight loss, fatigue, and, if left uncorrected, death.

The suggested daily amount of protein intake for a normal adult is 1.0–1.2 g of protein/kg of body weight (Dominiczak & Logue, 2014). Traditional IV fluids do not provide sufficient calories or nitrogen to meet the body's daily requirements. PN solutions, which supply nutrients such as dextrose, amino acids, electrolytes, vitamins, minerals, and fat emulsions, provide enough calories and nitrogen to meet the patient's daily nutritional needs. In general, PN usually provides 25–35 kcal/kg of ideal body weight and 1.0–1.5 g of protein/kg of ideal body weight.

The patient with fever, trauma, burns, major surgery, or hypermetabolic disease requires additional daily calories. The volume of fluid necessary to provide these calories would surpass fluid tolerance and lead to pulmonary edema or heart failure. To provide the required calories in a small volume, it is necessary to increase the concentration of nutrients and use a route of administration (i.e., a large, high-flow vein, such as the subclavian) that rapidly dilutes incoming nutrients to the proper levels of body tolerance.

When highly concentrated dextrose is administered, caloric requirements are satisfied and the body uses amino acids for protein synthesis rather than for energy. Additional potassium is added to the solution to maintain proper electrolyte balance and to transport glucose and amino acids across cell membranes. To prevent deficiencies and fulfill requirements for tissue synthesis, other elements, such as calcium, phosphorus, magnesium, and sodium chloride, are added.

 Nursing Alert
Cues to malnutrition in patients include a prealbumin level that is less than 16 mg/dL, albumin that is less than 3.5 mg/dL, unintentional weight loss of 10% in 6 months or 5% in 3 months, or a body mass index (BMI) below 18.5. A BMI greater than 19 or less than 22 places a patient at risk for malnutrition (Stewart, 2014).

Preoperatively malnourished patients who are not candidates for enteral feedings should have PN initiated for nutrient resuscitation a week before surgery if possible. PN therapy lasting less than 7 days has been shown to have no effect on nutritional status or was linked to poor outcomes (McClave et al., 2016).

Parenteral Formulas

A total of 2 to 3 L of solution is administered over a 24-hour period using a filter (1.2-micron particulate filter). Before administration, the PN infusion must be inspected for clarity and any precipitate. The label is compared with the provider's order, noting the expiration date. **IV fat emulsions** (IVFEs, Intralipids) may be infused simultaneously with PN through a Y-connector close to the infusion site and *should not* be filtered. Before administration, the IVFE is inspected for frothiness, separation, or oily appearance. If any of these are present, the solution is not used. Usually 500 mL of a 10% emulsion or 250 mL of 20% emulsion is administered over 6 to 12 hours, one to three times a week. IVFEs can provide up to 30% of the total daily calorie intake.

IVFEs can be admixed with other components of PN to create a "three-in-one formulation," commonly called a **total nutrient admixture** (TNA). All the parenteral nutrient components are mixed in one container and administered to the patient over a 24-hour period. A special final filter (1.5-micron filter) is used with this solution. Before administration, the solution is observed for oil droplets that have separated from the solution, forming a noticeable layer ("cracking of lipid emulsion"); such a solution should be discarded.

Initiating Therapy

PN solutions have a higher glucose concentration than do regular IV fluids. As a result, PN is a medium in which bacteria can thrive. It is important for the nurse to use aseptic technique when assessing the catheter port to be used for the PN. The ports should be prepped with an antiseptic wipe. If the PN bag does not come with pre-primed tubing from the pharmacy, the nurse must take great care not to contaminate the bag or tubing. Also the dressing on the catheter should be changed in accordance with the institution's policy to prevent infection at the insertion site. PN solutions are initiated slowly and advanced gradually each day to the desired rate as the patient's fluid and glucose tolerance permits. If the solution is administered too rapidly, the patient could become fluid overloaded. If this occurs, the rate should be decreased, and the patient's respiratory status should be monitored. The patient's laboratory test results and response to PN therapy are monitored on an ongoing basis by the provider and licensed nutrition provider. Standing orders are initiated for weighing the patient; monitoring intake, output, and blood glucose; and baseline and periodic monitoring of complete blood count, platelet count, and chemistry panel, including serum carbon dioxide, magnesium, phosphorus, triglycerides, and prealbumin. A 24-hour urine nitrogen determination may be performed for analysis of nitrogen balance. In most hospitals, the provider prescribes PN solutions on a daily standard PN order form. The formulation of the PN solutions is calculated carefully each day to meet the complete nutritional needs of the individual patient.

Administration Methods

Peripheral Method

A peripheral parenteral nutrition (PPN) formula is prescribed when a patient's oral intake requires supplementation. This type of solution is not as hypertonic as PN or total parenteral nutrition (TPN) so it can be administered peripherally. PPN formulas are not nutritionally complete: there is typically less dextrose content.

Nursing Alert
Any formula with a dextrose concentration of more than 10% should not be administered through peripheral veins because they irritate the intima (innermost walls) of small veins, causing a chemical phlebitis.

Lipids are administered simultaneously to buffer the PPN and to protect the peripheral vein from irritation. For PPN solutions, peripheral access is changed approximately every 3 days to decrease the likelihood of infiltration. These solutions use a *dedicated line*; that is, no other medication or IV solution can be infused other than the PPN solution through this peripheral IV.

Central Method

Because TPN solutions have five or six times the solute concentration of blood (and exert an osmotic pressure of about 2,000 mOsm/L), they are injurious to the intima of peripheral veins. Therefore, to prevent phlebitis and other venous complications, these solutions are administered into the vascular system through a catheter inserted into a high-flow, large blood vessel, such as the subclavian vein. Then concentrated solutions are very rapidly diluted to isotonic levels by the blood in this vessel.

Four types of **central venous access devices (CVADs)** can be used to administer TPN: nontunneled (or percutaneous) central catheters, peripherally inserted central catheters (PICC), tunneled catheters, and implanted ports. Whenever one of these catheters is inserted, catheter tip placement should be confirmed by x-ray studies before PN therapy is initiated. The optimal position is the midproximal third of the superior vena cava at the junction of the right atrium.

Nontunneled Central Catheters
Nontunneled central catheters are used for short-term IV therapy (less than 6 weeks) in acute-care, long-term care, and home-care settings. The provider inserts these catheters. Examples of nontunneled central catheters are Vas-Cath, percutaneous subclavian Arrow, and Hohn catheters. The subclavian vein is the most common vessel used because the subclavian area provides a stable insertion site to which the catheter can be anchored, allows the patient freedom of movement, and provides easy access to the dressing site.

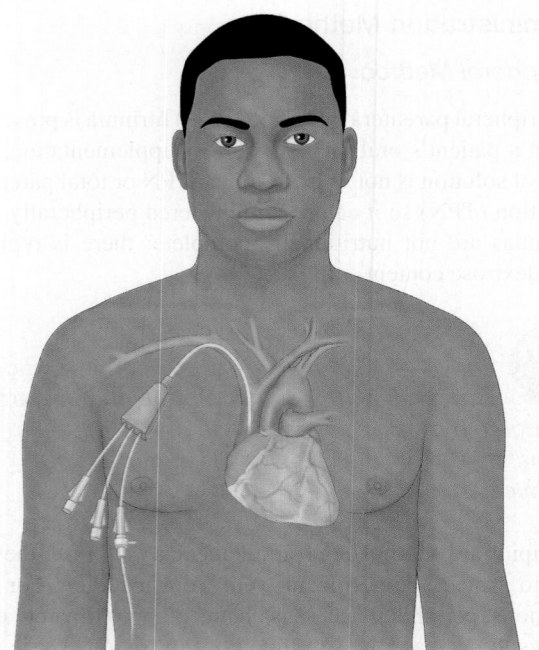

FIGURE 22-16 Subclavian triple-lumen catheter used for parenteral nutrition and other adjunctive therapy. The catheter is threaded through the subclavian vein into the vena cava. Each lumen is an avenue for solution administration. The lumens are secured with threaded needleless adapters or Luer-Lok–type caps when the device is not in use.

The jugular vein should be avoided and only be considered for cannulation if the patient has no other points of access. Jugular access should be used only temporarily for approximately 1 to 2 days.

To ensure accessibility in a patient with limited IV access, a triple-lumen subclavian catheter can be used because it offers three ports for various uses (Fig. 22-16). Blood sampling and administration is commonly done through the distal port. TPN solutions are administered through the medial port. All three ports can be used for medication administration. The nurse may stop an IV solution or medication drip temporarily (if warranted—some solutions cannot be stopped even for brief periods of time, such as a nitroglycerine drip with an acute MI patient) when drawing blood from another lumen on the triple-lumen catheter. Otherwise, these infusions can contaminate the studies ordered and alter the results. The nurse may also waste 5 to 10 cc of blood from the patient before drawing the actual specimen for analysis as an additional method for getting a clean sample.

If a single-lumen central catheter is used for administering TPN, various restrictions apply:

- Blood cannot be drawn from the catheter, and transfusions of blood products cannot be given through the main line because red blood cells may coat the lumen of the catheter, thereby reducing the flow of the nutritional solution.
- Medications cannot be administered through it because the medication may be incompatible with the components

of the nutritional solution (insulin is an exception). If medications must be given, they must be infused through a separate peripheral IV line, not by piggyback into the TPN line.

Once the catheter's position is confirmed, the prescribed TPN solution is started. The initial rate of infusion is usually 50 mL/hr, and the rate is increased gradually to the maintenance rate or predetermined dose (e.g., 100 to 125 mL/hr). An infusion pump is always used for administration of TPN.

Nursing Alert

If, for any reason, there is a delay in the infusion rate, this solution is never increased beyond the hourly ordered rate. There is no "playing catch up" with TPN (Diepenbrock, 2012). If the PN solution is terminated abruptly, a 5% or a 10% dextrose solution is administered for a period of hours to protect against rebound hypoglycemia. Specifically, a 5% solution is administered for PPN, while a 10% solution is administered for TPN at the same rate, owing to the approximate glucose concentration in the two solutions.

An injection site cap is attached to the end of each central catheter lumen, creating a closed system. IV infusion tubing is connected to the insertion site cap of the central catheter with a threaded needleless adapter or Luer-Lok device. Each lumen is labeled by the manufacturer according to location (proximal, middle, and distal). To ensure patency, all lumens are flushed initially, daily when not in use, after each intermittent infusion, after blood drawing, and whenever an infusion is disconnected. A recent systematic review looking at studies comparing the flushing of catheters with saline and heparin found no difference between the two solutions when considering safety and efficacy (Lopez-Briz et al., 2014). Force is never used to flush the catheter. If resistance is met, aspiration may restore lumen patency; if this is not effective, the provider is notified. Low-dose tissue plasminogen activator (alteplase) may be prescribed to dissolve a clot or fibrin sheath. If attempts to clear the lumen are ineffective, the lumen is labeled as "clotted off" and not used again.

Peripherally Inserted Central Catheters

Peripherally inserted central catheters (PICCs) are used for intermediate-term (several days to months) IV therapy in the hospital, long-term care, or home setting. These catheters may be inserted by a specially trained nurse at the bedside or in the outpatient setting. They also can be inserted using fluoroscopy by an interventional radiologist. PICC lines are placed in the arm, specifically the basilic or cephalic vein, via the antecubital space. Then the catheter is threaded to a designated location, depending on the type of solution to be infused (superior vena cava for TPN, which allows dilution of this hypertonic solution). Blood drawing and blood pressure measurement are avoided in the accessed arm.

Tunneled Central Catheters

Tunneled central catheters are for long-term use and may remain in place for many years. These catheters are cuffed and can have single or double lumens; examples are the Hickman, Groshong, and PermCath. These catheters are inserted surgically. They are threaded under the skin (reducing the risk of ascending infection) to the subclavian vein, and the distal end of the catheter is advanced into the superior vena cava.

Implanted Ports

Implanted ports also are used for long-term home IV therapy; examples include the Port-A-Cath, Mediport, Hickman Port, and P.A.S. Port. Instead of exiting from the skin, as do the Hickman and Groshong catheters, the end of the catheter is attached to a small chamber that is placed in a subcutaneous pocket, either on the anterior chest wall or on the forearm. The subcutaneous port requires minimal care and allows the patient complete freedom of activity. Implanted ports are more expensive than the external catheters, and access requires passing a special noncoring needle (Huber-tipped) through the skin into the chamber to initiate IV therapy.

Discontinuing Parenteral Nutrition

The PN solution is discontinued gradually to allow the patient to adjust to decreased levels of glucose. A patient's blood sugar must be followed very closely when weaning a patient off PN, while on a continuous insulin infusion, or when increasing enteral feedings concurrently. Providing oral carbohydrates can shorten the tapering time. Specific symptoms of rebound hypoglycemia include weakness, faintness, diaphoresis, shakiness, feeling cold, confusion, and increased heart rate. Once all IV therapy is completed, the nontunneled central venous catheter or PICC can be removed and an occlusive dressing is applied to the exit site. Once a decision is made to discontinue the line, physicians or nurses who have been deemed competent in the removal procedure and are aware of the potential complications may remove central and PICC lines. Tunneled catheters and implanted ports are removed only by the physician.

CHAPTER REVIEW

Critical Thinking Questions

1. You are the night shift nurse in the intensive care unit and have been assigned a new postoperative patient who has undergone a radical neck dissection. Which form of nutritional support would you most likely see being used, and why? What nursing measures would be used to facilitate breathing and promote comfort? Describe the potential complications of radical neck dissection and the assessment parameters that are used to detect the earliest signs and symptoms of these complications.

2. An elderly woman is brought to the emergency department by paramedics. Her daughter found her on the kitchen floor. A bottle of cleaning fluid with a poison label was open next to the kitchen sink. On admission, the patient was in respiratory distress. Burns were observed around her mouth. What emergency care would be provided for this patient to prevent further trauma to the GI and respiratory tracts? Identify the evidence that supports this care, and evaluate the strength of the evidence.

3. You prepare to administer feedings through a patient's newly placed nasojejunal feeding tube. What methods would you consider to confirm the location of the tube before you initiate feedings? What patients would require postpyloric feedings rather than gastric and why? Before administering medications through the tube, how would you prepare them, and which types of medications would you pay particular attention to?

NCLEX-Style Review Questions

1. A confused patient prematurely removes her NG tube. The nurse knows to observe for which complication?
   a. Constipation
   b. Flatulence
   c. Abdominal distention
   d. Gastric bleeding

2. The nurse is administering liquids to a patient who has recently been changed from NPO to a clear liquid diet. The patient coughs and occasionally gags with sips of water. Which health care team member would the nurse consult?
   a. Physical therapist
   b. Respiratory therapist
   c. Dietician
   d. Speech pathologist

3. A nurse is caring for a patient who is on strict bowel rest and will need IV nutrition. The nurse knows the following devices are appropriate for TPN. Select all that apply.
   a. PICC line
   b. Triple-lumen catheter
   c. Large-bore IV line
   d. Implantable venous assess device (Port-A-Cath)
   e. Arterial line

4. A nurse receives report on a patient experiencing dumping syndrome. The nurse knows that the patient would be displaying which symptom 30 minutes after eating?
   a. Difficulty swallowing
   b. Heartburn
   c. Nausea
   d. Cramping in the abdomen

5. The nurse recognizes which of the following as a cause of xerostomia? Select all that apply.
   a. HIV infection
   b. Oral hypoglycemic medications
   c. Tracheostomy tube
   d. Inability to close the mouth
   e. Kidney failure

Try these additional resources, available at **http://thepoint.lww.com/Honan2e**, to enhance your learning and understanding of this chapter:
- NCLEX-Style Student Review Questions
- Journal Articles

REFERENCES AND SELECTED READINGS

References and selected readings associated with this chapter can be found on the website that accompanies the book. Visit **http://thepoint. lww.com/Honan2e** to access the references and other additional resources associated with this chapter.

Nursing Management: Patients with Gastric and Duodenal Disorders

Jancee Pust-Marcone

Learning Objectives

After reading this chapter, you will be able to:

1. Compare the etiology, clinical manifestations, and management of acute gastritis, chronic gastritis, and peptic ulcer.
2. Describe the management of the patient with gastritis.
3. Describe the dietary, pharmacologic, and surgical treatment of peptic ulcer.
4. Describe the nursing management of patients who undergo surgical procedures to treat obesity.
5. Use the nursing process as a framework for care of patients undergoing gastric surgery.
6. Identify the complications of gastric surgery and their prevention and management.

A person's nutritional status depends not only on the type and amount of intake but also on the functioning of the gastric and intestinal portions of the gastrointestinal (GI) system. This chapter describes disorders of the stomach and duodenum as well as their treatment and related nursing care.

GASTRITIS

Gastritis (inflammation of the **gastric** or stomach mucosa) is a common GI problem. Gastritis may be acute, lasting several hours to a few days, or chronic, resulting from repeated exposure to irritating agents or recurring episodes of acute gastritis.

Acute gastritis is often caused by dietary indiscretion—the person eats food that is irritating, too highly seasoned, or contaminated with disease-causing microorganisms. Other causes of acute gastritis include overuse of aspirin and other nonsteroidal anti-inflammatory drugs (NSAIDs), excessive alcohol intake, bile reflux, and radiation therapy. A more severe form of acute gastritis is caused by the ingestion of strong acid or alkali, which may cause the mucosa to become gangrenous or to perforate. Scarring can occur, resulting in **pyloric stenosis** or obstruction. Acute gastritis also may develop in acute illnesses, especially when the patient has had major traumatic injuries; burns; severe infection; liver,

kidney, or respiratory failure; or major surgery. Gastritis may be the first sign of an acute systemic infection.

Chronic gastritis and prolonged inflammation of the stomach may be caused either by benign or malignant ulcers of the stomach or by the bacteria ***Helicobacter pylori*** (***H. pylori***) (Watari et al., 2014; Yamaoka & Graham, 2014; Venerito, Selgrad, & Malfertheiner, 2013). Also chronic gastritis is sometimes associated with autoimmune diseases, such as pernicious anemia (Varbanova et al., 2014); dietary factors, such as caffeine; the use of medications such as NSAIDs, bisphosphonate (e.g., alendronate [Fosamax], risedronate [Actonel]) or ibandronate (Boniva); alcohol; smoking; or chronic reflux of pancreatic secretions and bile into the stomach.

Pathophysiology

In gastritis, the gastric mucous membrane becomes edematous and hyperemic (congested with fluid and blood) and undergoes superficial erosion (Fig. 23-1). It secretes a scanty amount of gastric juice, containing very little acid but much mucus. Superficial ulceration may occur and can lead to hemorrhage.

Clinical Manifestations and Assessment

The patient with acute gastritis may have a rapid onset of symptoms, such as abdominal discomfort, headache, lassitude,

FIGURE 23-1 Endoscopic view of erosive gastritis (*left*). Damage from irritants (*right*) results in increased intracellular pH, impaired enzyme function, disrupted cellular structures, ischemia, vascular stasis, and tissue death. (Grossman, S., & Porth, C. M. (2014). *Porth's pathophysiology: Concepts of altered health states* (9th ed.). Philadelphia, PA: Wolters Kluwer Health/Lippincott Williams & Wilkins.)

nausea, anorexia, vomiting, and hiccupping, which can last from a few hours to a few days. The patient with chronic gastritis may complain of anorexia, heartburn after eating, belching, a sour taste in the mouth, or nausea and vomiting. Some patients may have only mild epigastric discomfort or report intolerance to spicy or fatty foods or slight pain that is relieved by eating. Patients with chronic gastritis from vitamin deficiency usually have evidence of malabsorption of vitamin B_{12} caused by the production of antibodies that interfere with the binding of vitamin B_{12} to intrinsic factor. However, some patients with chronic gastritis have no symptoms.

Gastritis is sometimes associated with **achlorhydria** or hypochlorhydria (absence or low levels of hydrochloric acid [HCl]) or with hyperchlorhydria (high levels of HCl). Diagnosis can be determined by an upper GI x-ray series or endoscopy and histologic examination of a tissue specimen obtained by biopsy. Diagnostic measures for detecting *H. pylori* infection may be used and are discussed in the section on peptic ulcers.

Medical and Nursing Management

The gastric mucosa is capable of repairing itself after a bout of gastritis. As a rule, the patient recovers in about 1 day, although the appetite may be diminished for an additional 2 or 3 days. Acute gastritis is also managed by instructing the patient to refrain from alcohol and food until symptoms subside. When the patient can take nourishment by mouth, a nonirritating diet is recommended. If the symptoms persist, IV fluids may need to be administered. If bleeding is present,

management is similar to the procedures used to control upper GI tract hemorrhage, discussed later in this chapter.

If gastritis is caused by ingestion of strong acids or alkalis, emergency treatment consists of diluting and neutralizing the offending agent. To neutralize acids, common antacids (e.g., aluminum hydroxide) are used; to neutralize an alkali, diluted lemon juice or diluted vinegar is used. If corrosion is extensive or severe, emetics and lavage are avoided because of the danger of perforation and damage to the esophagus.

Therapy is supportive and may include nasogastric (NG) intubation (see Chapter 22), analgesic agents and sedatives, antacids, and IV fluids. Fiberoptic endoscopy may be necessary. In extreme cases, emergency surgery may be required to remove gangrenous or perforated tissue. A gastric resection or a gastrojejunostomy (anastomosis of jejunum to stomach to detour around the pylorus) may be necessary to treat pyloric obstruction, a narrowing of the pyloric orifice that cannot be relieved by medical management.

Chronic gastritis is managed by modifying the patient's diet, promoting rest, reducing stress, recommending avoidance of alcohol and NSAIDs, and initiating pharmacotherapy. *H. pylori* may be treated with selected drug combinations (Table 23-1).

PEPTIC ULCER DISEASE

A peptic ulcer may be referred to as a gastric, duodenal, or esophageal ulcer, depending on its location. A person who

TABLE 23-1 Pharmacotherapy for Gastritis and Peptic Ulcer Disease

Pharmacologic Agent	Major Action	Nursing Considerations
Antibiotics		
Amoxicillin (Amoxil)	A bactericidal antibiotic that assists with eradicating *H. pylori* bacteria in the gastric mucosa	• May cause diarrhea • Should not be used in patients allergic to penicillin
Clarithromycin (Biaxin)	Exerts bactericidal effects to eradicate *H. pylori* bacteria in the gastric mucosa	• May cause gastrointestinal (GI) upset, headache, altered taste • Many drug–drug interactions (e.g., cisapride, colchicine, lovastatin, warfarin [Coumadin])
Metronidazole (Flagyl)	A synthetic antibacterial and antiprotozoal agent that assists with eradicating *H. pylori* bacteria in the gastric mucosa when administered with other antibiotics and proton pump inhibitors	• Should be administered with meals to decrease GI upset; may cause anorexia and metallic taste • Patient should avoid alcohol; Flagyl increases blood-thinning effects of warfarin (Coumadin)
Tetracycline	Exerts bacteriostatic effects to eradicate *H. pylori* bacteria in the gastric mucosa	• May cause photosensitivity reaction; warn patient to use sunscreen • May cause GI upset • Must be used with caution in patients with kidney or liver impairment • Milk or dairy products may reduce effectiveness
Antidiarrheal		
Bismuth subsalicylate (Pepto-Bismol)	Suppresses *H. pylori* bacteria in the gastric mucosa and assists with healing of mucosal ulcers	• Given concurrently with antibiotics to eradicate *H. pylori* infection • Should be taken on empty stomach
Histamine-2 (H₂) Receptor Antagonists		
Cimetidine (Tagamet)	Decreases amount of HCl produced by stomach by blocking action of histamine on histamine receptors of parietal cells in the stomach	• Least expensive of H_2 receptor antagonists • May cause confusion, agitation, or coma in the elderly or those with kidney or liver insufficiency • Long-term use may cause diarrhea, dizziness, gynecomastia • Many drug–drug interactions (e.g., amiodarone, amitriptyline, benzodiazepines, metoprolol, nifedipine, phenytoin, warfarin [Coumadin])
Famotidine (Pepcid)	Same as for cimetidine	• Best choice for critically ill patients because it is known to have the least risk of drug–drug interactions; does not alter liver metabolism • Prolonged half-life in patients with kidney insufficiency • Short-term relief for GERD
Nizatidine (Axid)	Same as for cimetidine	• Used for treatment of ulcers and GERD • Prolonged half-life in patients with kidney insufficiency • May cause headache, dizziness, diarrhea, nausea/vomiting, GI upset, as well as urticarial
Ranitidine (Zantac)	Same as for cimetidine	• Prolonged half-life in patients with kidney and liver insufficiency • Causes fewer side effects than cimetidine • May cause headache, dizziness, constipation, nausea and vomiting, or abdominal discomfort
Roxatidine (Roxane)	Same as for cimetidine	• Prolonged half-life in patients with kidney and liver insufficiency • Single bedtime dose in combination with PPI to reduce nocturnal acid reflux • May cause headache, dizziness, constipation, nausea and vomiting, or abdominal discomfort

(continued on page 694)

TABLE **23-1** **Pharmacotherapy for Gastritis and Peptic Ulcer Disease** (*continued*)

Pharmacologic Agent	Major Action	Nursing Considerations
Proton Pump Inhibitors of Gastric Acid (PPIs)		
Esomeprazole (Nexium)	Decreases gastric acid secretion by slowing the hydrogen–potassium adenosine triphosphatase (H^+, K^+-ATPase) pump on the surface of the parietal cells of the stomach	• Used mainly for treatment of duodenal ulcer disease and *H. pylori* infection • A delayed-release capsule that is to be swallowed whole and taken before meals—the capsule cannot be crushed or chewed • May increase phenytoin (Dilantin), warfarin (Coumadin) levels. Food decreases absorption by up to 35%. • Most common side effects are headache, diarrhea, nausea, gas, abdominal pain constipation or dry mouth
Lansoprazole (Prevacid)	Decreases gastric acid secretion by slowing the H^+, K^+-ATPase pump on the surface of the parietal cells	• A delayed-release capsule that is to be swallowed whole and taken before meals—the capsule cannot be crushed or chewed • May decrease theophylline levels • Side effects include confusion, dizziness, fast or irregular heart rate, jerky muscle movements, muscle cramps or weakness, bloody diarrhea, cough or seizure
Omeprazole (Prilosec)	Decreases gastric acid secretion by slowing the H^+, K^+-ATPase pump on the surface of the parietal cells	• A delayed-release capsule that is to be swallowed whole and taken before meals • May cause diarrhea, nausea and vomiting, constipation, abdominal pain, headache, or dizziness
Pantoprazole (Protonix)	Decreases gastric acid secretion by slowing the H^+, K^+-ATPase pump on the surface of the parietal cells	• A delayed-release capsule that is to be swallowed whole and taken before meals • May cause diarrhea and hyperglycemia, headache, abdominal pain, and abnormal liver function tests
Rabeprazole (AcipHex)	Decreases gastric acid secretion by slowing the H^+, K^+-ATPase pump on the surface of the parietal cells	• A delayed-release tablet to be swallowed whole • May cause abdominal pain, diarrhea, nausea, and headache • Drug–drug interactions with digoxin, iron, and warfarin (Coumadin)
Prostaglandin E₁ Analog		
Misoprostol (Cytotec)	Synthetic prostaglandin; protects the gastric mucosa from agents that cause ulcers; also increases mucus production and bicarbonate levels	• Used to prevent ulceration in patients using NSAIDs • Administer with food • May cause diarrhea and cramping (including uterine cramping)
Sucralfate (Carafate)	Creates a viscous substance in the presence of gastric acid that forms a protective barrier, binding to the surface of the ulcer, and prevents digestion by pepsin	• Used mainly for the treatment of duodenal ulcers • Should be taken without food but with water • Other medications should be taken 2 hours before or after this medication • May cause constipation or nausea

GERD, gastroesophageal reflux disease; NSAID, nonsteroidal anti-inflammatory drug.

has a peptic ulcer has peptic ulcer disease. A peptic ulcer is an excavation (hollowed-out area) that forms in the mucosal wall of the stomach, in the **pylorus** (the opening between the stomach and duodenum), in the **duodenum** (the first part of small intestine), or in the esophagus. Erosion of a circumscribed area of mucous membrane is the cause (Fig. 23-2). This erosion may extend as deeply as the muscle layers or through the muscle to the **peritoneum**.

Peptic ulcers are more likely to be in the duodenum than in the stomach. As a rule, they occur alone, but they may occur in multiples. Chronic gastric ulcers tend to occur in the lesser curvature of the stomach, near the pylorus. Table 23-2 compares the features of gastric and duodenal ulcers. Esophageal ulcers occur as a result of the backward flow of HCl from the stomach into the esophagus (gastroesophageal reflux disease [GERD]).

Pathophysiology

Peptic ulcers occur mainly in the gastroduodenal mucosa because this tissue cannot withstand the digestive action of gastric acid (HCl) and pepsin. The erosion is caused by

FIGURE 23-2 Deep peptic ulcer. (Strayer, D., & Rubin, E. (2015). *Rubin's pathology: Clinicopathologic foundations of medicine* (7th ed.). Philadelphia, PA: Wolters Kluwer Health.)

the increased concentration or activity of acid–pepsin or by decreased resistance of the mucosa. A damaged mucosa cannot secrete enough mucus to act as a barrier against HCl. The use of NSAIDs inhibits the secretion of mucus that protects the mucosa. Patients with duodenal ulcer disease secrete more acid than normal, whereas patients with gastric ulcer tend to secrete normal or decreased levels of acid. Damage to the gastroduodenal mucosa allows for decreased resistance to bacteria, and, thus, infection from *H. pylori* bacteria may occur.

Zollinger-Ellison syndrome (ZES) is suspected when a patient has several peptic ulcers or an ulcer that is resistant to standard medical therapy (Kim, 2015). ZES is identified by the hypersecretion of gastric juice, duodenal ulcers, and gastrinomas (islet cell tumors) in the pancreas. Ninety percent of tumors are found in the "gastric triangle," which encompasses the cystic and common bile ducts, the second and third portions of the duodenum, and the junction of the head and body of the pancreas. Approximately one third of gastrinomas are malignant. Diarrhea and steatorrhea (unabsorbed fat in the stool) may be evident. The patient may have coexisting parathyroid adenomas (benign tumor of glandular origin) or hyperplasia and, therefore, may exhibit signs of hypercalcemia. The most common symptom is epigastric pain. *H. pylori* is not a risk factor for ZES (Kim, 2015).

Stress-related mucosal disease (SRMD) is a term used to describe the phenomenon of injury to the lining of the stomach and the duodenum during conditions of physiologic stress. Other terms commonly used include *stress erosion, stress ulcer, stress gastritis, erosive gastritis,* and *hemorrhagic gastritis.* These terms also have been given to the acute mucosal ulceration of the duodenal or gastric area that occurs after physiologically stressful events, such as burns, shock, severe sepsis, and multiple organ traumas (Bardou, Quenot, & Barkun, 2015). These ulcers, which are clinically different from peptic ulcers, are most common in ventilator-dependent patients after trauma or surgery. Fiberoptic endoscopy within 24 hours of trauma or surgery reveals shallow erosions of the stomach wall; by 72 hours, multiple gastric erosions are observed. The prevalence of SRMD has been reported to be as high as 74% to 100% in critically ill patients (Bardou, Quenot, & Barkun, 2015). As the stressful condition continues, the ulcers spread. When the patient recovers, the lesions are reversed. This pattern is typical of stress ulceration.

Differences of opinion exist as to the actual cause of mucosal ulceration in stress ulcers, but the etiology is thought to be multifactorial. Usually, the ulceration is preceded by a

TABLE **23-2** Comparison of Duodenal and Gastric Ulcers

Feature	Duodenal Ulcer	Gastric Ulcer
Incidence	30 to 60 years of age Male: female = 2:1 or 3:1 80% of peptic ulcers are duodenal	Usually 50 years of age or older Male: female = 1:1 15% of peptic ulcers are gastric
Symptoms and Clinical Findings	Hypersecretion of stomach acid (HCl) May have weight gain Pain occurs 2 to 3 hours after a meal; often awakened around 1 or 2 AM; ingestion of food relieves pain Vomiting uncommon Hemorrhage less likely than with gastric ulcer, but if present, melena more common than hematemesis More likely to perforate than gastric ulcers	Normal to hyposecretion of stomach acid (HCl) Weight loss may occur Pain occurs ½ to 1 hour after a meal; rarely occurs at night; may be relieved by vomiting; ingestion of food does not help, sometimes increases pain Vomiting common Hemorrhage more likely to occur than with duodenal ulcer; hematemesis more common than melena
Malignancy Possibility	Rare	Occasionally
Risk Factors	*H. pylori*, alcohol, smoking, cirrhosis, stress	*H. pylori*, gastritis, alcohol, smoking, use of nonsteroidal anti-inflammatory drugs (NSAIDs), stress

shock state; often involving hypovolemia and hypoperfusion; leading to decreased gastric mucosal blood flow and gastric ischemia. This hypoperfusion triggers the body's protective mechanisms of activation of the sympathetic nervous system, increased catecholamine release causing further vasoconstriction, and reduced gastric blood flow. Gastric hypoperfusion leads to decreased gastric motility, decreased capacity to neutralize hydrogen ions, and the reflux of duodenal contents into the stomach. In addition, large quantities of pepsin are released. The combination of ischemia, acid, and pepsin creates an ideal climate for ulceration (Kim, 2015).

Stress ulcers should be distinguished from Cushing ulcers and Curling ulcers, two other types of gastric ulcers. Cushing ulcers are common in patients with head injury and brain trauma. They may occur in the esophagus, stomach, or duodenum and usually are deeper and more penetrating than stress ulcers. Curling ulcer is frequently observed about 72 hours after extensive burns and involves the antrum of the stomach or the duodenum.

Risk Factors

Peptic ulcer disease occurs with the greatest frequency in people between 40 and 60 years of age. It is relatively uncommon in women of childbearing age, but it has been observed in children and even in infants. After menopause, the incidence of peptic ulcers in women is almost equal to that in men. Peptic ulcers in the body of the stomach can occur without excessive acid secretion.

In the past, stress and anxiety were thought to be causes of ulcers, but research has documented that peptic ulcers result from infection with the gram-negative bacteria *H. pylori,* which may be acquired through ingestion of food and water. Person-to-person transmission of the bacteria also occurs through close contact and exposure to emesis. Although *H. pylori* infection is common in the United States, most infected people do not develop ulcers. It is not known why *H. pylori* infection does not cause ulcers in all people, but most likely the predisposition to ulcer formation depends on certain factors, such as the type of *H. pylori* and other as yet unknown factors (Kim 2015; Franceschi et al., 2014; Watari et al., 2014).

In addition, excessive secretion of HCl in the stomach may contribute to the formation of peptic ulcers, and stress may be associated with its increased secretion. The ingestion of milk and caffeinated beverages, smoking, and alcohol also may increase HCl secretion. Stress and eating spicy foods may make peptic ulcers worse.

Familial tendency also may be a significant predisposing factor. People with blood type O are more susceptible to peptic ulcers than are those with blood type A, B, or AB; this is another genetic link. There also is an association between peptic ulcers and chronic pulmonary disease or chronic kidney disease. Other predisposing factors associated with peptic ulcer include chronic use of NSAIDs, alcohol ingestion, and excessive smoking.

Peptic ulcers are found in rare cases in patients with tumors that cause secretion of excessive amounts of the hormone gastrin. ZES consists of severe peptic ulcers, extreme gastric hyperacidity, and gastrin-secreting benign or malignant tumors of the pancreas.

Clinical Manifestations and Assessment

Symptoms of an ulcer may last for a few days, weeks, or months and may disappear only to reappear, often without an identifiable cause. Many people with ulcers have no symptoms, and perforation or hemorrhage may occur in 20% to 30% of patients who had no preceding manifestations.

As a rule, the patient with an ulcer complains of dull, gnawing pain or a burning sensation in the midepigastrium or in the back. It is believed that the pain occurs when the increased acid content of the stomach and duodenum erodes the lesion and stimulates the exposed nerve endings. Another theory suggests that contact of the lesion with acid stimulates a local reflex mechanism that initiates contraction of the adjacent smooth muscle. Pain is usually relieved by eating because food neutralizes the acid or by taking alkali; however, once the stomach has emptied or the alkali's effect has decreased, the pain returns. Sharply localized tenderness can be elicited by applying gentle pressure to the epigastrium at or slightly to the right of the midline.

Other symptoms include **pyrosis** (heartburn), vomiting, constipation or diarrhea, and bleeding. Pyrosis is a burning sensation in the esophagus and stomach that moves up to the mouth. Often heartburn is accompanied by sour eructation, or burping, which is common when the patient's stomach is empty.

Although vomiting is rare in uncomplicated duodenal ulcer, it may be a symptom of a complication of an ulcer. It results from obstruction of the pyloric orifice caused by either muscular spasm of the pylorus or mechanical obstruction from scarring or acute swelling of the inflamed mucous membrane adjacent to the ulcer. Vomiting may or may not be preceded by nausea; usually, it follows a bout of severe pain and bloating, which is relieved by vomiting the gastric contents. Emesis often contains undigested food eaten many hours earlier. Constipation or diarrhea may occur, probably as a result of diet and medications.

Fifteen percent of patients with peptic ulcer experience bleeding. The two most relevant risk factors for stress-related GI bleeding include prolonged mechanical ventilation and coagulopathy in the critically ill patient (Bardou et al., 2015). Patients may present with GI bleeding as evidenced by the passage of **melena** (tarry stools). A small portion of patients who bleed from an acute ulcer have only very mild symptoms or none at all (Bardou et al., 2015).

A physical examination may reveal pain, epigastric tenderness, or abdominal distention. A barium study of the upper GI tract may show an ulcer; however, endoscopy is the preferred diagnostic procedure because it allows direct visualization of inflammatory changes, ulcers, and lesions. Through endoscopy, a biopsy of the gastric mucosa and of any suspicious lesions can be obtained. Endoscopy may reveal lesions that, because of their size or location, are not evident on x-ray studies.

Stools may be tested periodically until they are negative for occult blood. Gastric secretory studies are of value in diagnosing achlorhydria and ZES. *H. pylori* infection may be determined by endoscopic and histologic examination of a tissue specimen obtained by biopsy or by a rapid urease test of the biopsy specimen. Other less invasive diagnostic measures for detecting *H. pylori* include serologic testing for antibodies against the *H. pylori* antigen, stool antigen test, and urea breath test (Kim, 2015).

Medical and Nursing Management

Once the diagnosis is established, the patient is informed that the condition can be controlled. Recurrence may develop; however, peptic ulcers treated with antibiotics to eradicate *H. pylori* have a lower recurrence rate than those not treated with antibiotics. The goals are to eradicate *H. pylori* and to manage gastric acidity. Methods used include medications, lifestyle changes, and surgical intervention. The nurse instructs the patient about the factors that will relieve and those that will aggravate the peptic ulcer disease.

Pharmacologic Therapy

Currently, the most commonly used therapy for peptic ulcers is a combination of antibiotics, **proton pump inhibitors** (PPIs), and bismuth salts that suppress or eradicate *H. pylori* (see Table 23-1). Recommended therapy for 10 to 14 days includes triple therapy with two antibiotics (e.g., metronidazole [Flagyl] or amoxicillin [Amoxil] and clarithromycin [Biaxin]) plus a PPI (e.g., lansoprazole [Prevacid], omeprazole [Prilosec], or rabeprazole [Acephex]), or quadruple therapy with two antibiotics (metronidazole [Flagyl] and tetracycline) plus a PPI and bismuth salts (Pepto-Bismol) (den Hollander, 2012). Quadruple therapy is seen more frequently because of increased prevalence of antimicrobial resistance (Kuipers & Blaser, 2016).

Histamine-2 (H₂) receptor antagonists (H₂ blockers) and PPIs are used to treat NSAID-induced ulcers and other ulcers not associated with *H. pylori* infection (Scheiman, 2013; Tuskey & Peura, 2013). Misoprostol (a mucosal protective drug) has similar effects as H₂ blockers in preventing ulcers when given in full doses, but its usefulness is limited due to gastrointestinal side effects. It is not given to pregnant women because it can cause abortion, premature birth, or birth defects. Table 23-3 provides information about the drug regimens used for peptic ulcer disease.

TABLE 23-3 Drug Regimens for Peptic Ulcer Disease

Indications	Drug Regimen	Comments
Ulcer healing	**H₂ receptor antagonists** Ranitidine 150 mg b.i.d. or 300 mg at bedtime Cimetidine 400 mg b.i.d. or 800 mg at bedtime Famotidine 20 mg b.i.d. or 40 mg at bedtime Nizatidine 150 mg b.i.d. or 300 mg at bedtime **Proton pump inhibitors (PPIs)** Omeprazole—20–40 mg daily Lansoprazole—15–30 mg daily Rabeprazole—20 mg daily Pantoprazole—40–80 mg daily Esomeprazole—20–40 mg daily	Should be used for 6 weeks for duodenal ulcer; 8 weeks for gastric ulcer Should be used for 4 weeks for duodenal ulcer and 6 weeks for gastric ulcer Healing occurs in 90% of patients who are compliant with therapy
Initial *Helicobacter pylori* therapy	**First-line therapy, also referred to as "triple therapy"** PPI b.i.d. plus clarithromycin 500 mg b.i.d. plus amoxicillin 1,000 mg b.i.d. *or* metronidazole 500 mg b.i.d. for 10 to 14 days **Second-line therapy, also referred to as "Quadruple therapy"** Bismuth Salt compound 2 tabs q.i.d. plus tetracycline 250 mg q.i.d. plus metronidazole 250 mg q.i.d. PPI b.i.d. daily for 14 days	Efficacy of therapy is approximately 85% QID dosing may decrease compliance
Therapy for retreatment of *H. pylori* therapy failure	Repeat first-line therapy, substitute metronidazole for amoxicillin (or vice versa) for 14 days; may add Bismuth salt compound q.i.d. Add second-line *H. pylori* therapy.	Efficacy of retreatment not known; success of more than two courses of treatment is very low
Prophylactic therapy for NSAID ulcers	Peptic ulcer healing doses of PPIs (above) Misoprostol 200 μg q.i.d.	Prevents recurrent ulceration in approximately 80%–90% of patients

NSAID, nonsteroidal anti-inflammatory drug.
From Kuipers, E. J., & Blaser, M. J. (2016). Acid peptic disease. In L. Goldman & A. I. Schafer (Eds.), *Goldman-Cecil Medicine* (25th ed.). Philadelphia: Elsevier/Saunders; Morgan, D. R., & Crowe, S. E. (2016). Helicobacter pylor infection. In M. Feldman, L. S. Friedman, & L. J. Brandt (Eds.), *Sleisenger & Fordtran's Gastrointestinal and Liver Disease: Pathophysiology, Diagnosis, Management* (10th ed.). Philadelphia: Elsevier/Saunders; den Hollander, W. J., & Kuipers, E. J. (2012). Current pharmacotherapy options for gastritis. *Expert Opinion on Pharmacotherapy, 13*(18), 2625–2636.

Nursing Alert
For patients with peptic ulcer disease who are taking NSAIDs or aspirin, the first step is to ensure the patient understands the need to stop such therapy.

The patient is advised to adhere to and complete the medication regimen to ensure complete healing of the ulcer. Because most patients become symptom-free within a week, it is a nursing responsibility to stress to the patient the importance of following the prescribed regimen so that the healing process can continue uninterrupted and the return of chronic ulcer symptoms can be prevented. Rest, sedatives, and tranquilizers may be added for the patient's comfort and are prescribed as needed. Maintenance dosages of H_2 receptor antagonists are usually recommended for 1 year.

For patients with ZES, hypersecretion of acid may be controlled with high doses of H_2 receptor antagonists. These patients may require twice the normal dose, and dosages usually need to be increased with prolonged use. Octreotide (Sandostatin), a medication that suppresses gastrin levels, also may be prescribed.

Patients at risk for stress ulcers (e.g., patients with head injury or extensive burns) may be treated prophylactically with IV H_2 receptor antagonists and cytoprotective agents (e.g., misoprostol, sucralfate) because of the risk for upper GI tract hemorrhage.

Lifestyle Changes

Lifestyle changes include stress reduction, smoking cessation, and dietary modifications. Reducing environmental stress requires physical and psychological modifications on the patient's part as well as the aid and cooperation of family members and significant others. The nurse assists the patient to identify situations that are stressful or exhausting. A hectic lifestyle and an irregular schedule may aggravate symptoms and interfere with regular meals taken in relaxed settings along with the regular administration of medications. The patient may benefit from regular rest periods during the day, at least during the acute phase of the disease. Biofeedback, hypnosis, behavior modification, massage, or acupuncture may be helpful.

Studies have shown that smoking decreases the secretion of bicarbonate from the pancreas into the duodenum, resulting in increased acidity of the duodenum. Research indicates that continued smoking may significantly inhibit ulcer repair (DiSaverio, 2014). Therefore, the patient is strongly encouraged to stop smoking. Smoking cessation support groups and other smoking cessation approaches should be offered to patients.

The intent of dietary modification for patients with peptic ulcers is to avoid oversecretion of acid and hypermotility in the GI tract. These can be minimized by avoiding extremes of temperature of food and beverage and overstimulation from consumption of meat extracts, alcohol, coffee (including decaffeinated coffee, which also stimulates acid secretion) and other caffeinated beverages, and diets rich in milk and cream (which stimulate acid secretion). In addition, an effort is made to neutralize acid by eating three regular meals a day. Small, frequent feedings are not necessary as long as an antacid or a histamine blocker is taken. Diet compatibility becomes an individual matter: the patient eats foods that are tolerated and avoids those that produce pain.

Surgical Management

The introduction of antibiotics to eradicate *H. pylori* and of H_2 receptor antagonists as treatment for ulcers has greatly reduced the need for surgical intervention. However, surgery usually is recommended for patients with intractable ulcers (those that fail to heal after 12 to 16 weeks of medical treatment), life-threatening hemorrhage, perforation, or obstruction, and for those with ZES not responding to medications (DiSaverio, 2014). Surgical procedures include vagotomy, with or without **pyloroplasty** (transecting nerves that stimulate acid secretion and opening the pylorus) and **antrectomy**, which is removal of the pyloric (antrum) portion of the stomach with anastomosis to either the duodenum (gastroduodenostomy or Billroth I) or jejunum (gastrojejunostomy or Billroth II) procedure (see Table 23-4 and the section on Gastric Surgery, page 699).

Patients who require surgery may have had a long illness. They may be discouraged and have had interruptions in their work role and pressures in their family life that affect their outlook on surgery and resolution of their disease. The nurse provides emotional support regarding the patient and family members altered role and additional responsibilities, and encourages them to express feelings, and ask questions. Referral to support groups or other services may be indicated.

Complications

Several complications may occur for the patient with peptic ulcer disease, including hemorrhage, perforation and penetration, and pyloric obstruction.

Nursing Alert
The nurse reviews with the patient and family the signs and symptoms of complications to be reported. These complications include hemorrhage (cool skin, confusion, increased heart rate, labored breathing, and blood in the stool), penetration and perforation (severe abdominal pain, rigid and tender abdomen, vomiting, elevated temperature, and increased heart rate), and pyloric obstruction (nausea, vomiting, distended abdomen, and abdominal pain).

Hemorrhage

Gastritis and hemorrhage from peptic ulcer are the two most common causes of upper GI tract bleeding (which may also occur with esophageal varices, as discussed in Chapter 22). Hemorrhage, the most common complication, occurs in 28% to 59% of patients with peptic ulcers. Bleeding may be manifested by hematemesis (vomiting blood) or melena (DiSaverio, 2014). The vomited blood can be bright red, or it can have a dark "coffee grounds" appearance from the oxidation of hemoglobin to methemoglobin. When the hemorrhage is large (2,000 to 3,000 mL), most of the blood is vomited.

Because large quantities of blood may be lost quickly, immediate correction of blood loss may be required to prevent hemorrhagic shock. When the hemorrhage is small, much or all of the blood is passed in the stools, which appear tarry black because of the digested hemoglobin. Management depends on the amount of blood lost and the rate of bleeding.

The nurse assesses the patient for faintness or dizziness and nausea, which may precede or accompany bleeding. It

TABLE 23-4 Surgical Procedures for Peptic Ulcer Disease

Operation	Description	Comments
Vagotomy Vagotomy—	Severing of the vagus nerve. Decreases gastric acid by diminishing cholinergic stimulation to the parietal cells, making them less responsive to gastrin. May be performed via open surgical approach, laparoscopy, or thoracoscopy.	May be performed to reduce gastric acid secretion. A drainage type of procedure (see pyloroplasty) is usually performed to assist with gastric emptying (because there is total denervation of the stomach). Some patients experience problems with feeling of fullness, dumping syndrome, diarrhea, and gastritis.
Truncal Vagotomy	Severs the right and left vagus nerves as they enter the stomach at the distal part of the esophagus	This type of vagotomy is most commonly used to decrease acid secretions and reduce gastric and intestinal motility. Recurrence rate of ulcer is 10%–15%.
Selective Vagotomy	Severs vagal innervation to the stomach but maintains innervation to the rest of the abdominal organs	With the availability of excellent acid secretion control with H2-receptor antagonists and proton pump inhibitors, the need for surgical management of PUD has greatly decreased.
Proximal (Parietal Cell) Gastric Vagotomy without Drainage	Denervates acid-secreting parietal cells but preserves vagal innervation to the gastric antrum and pylorus	No dumping syndrome. No need for drainage procedure. Recurrence rate of ulcer is 10%–15%.
Pyloroplasty Pylorus—note longitudinal incision Vertical suture	Longitudinal incision is made into the pylorus and transversely sutured closed to enlarge the outlet and relax the muscle	Usually accompanies truncal and selective vagotomies, which produce delayed gastric emptying due to decreased innervation.

(continued on page 700)

TABLE **23-4** **Surgical Procedures for Peptic Ulcer Disease** (*continued*)

Operation	Description	Comments
Antrectomy		
Billroth I (Gastroduodenostomy) Fundus Body Antrectomy Duodenum Duodenal anastomosis	Removal of the lower portion of the antrum of the stomach (which contains the cells that secrete gastrin) as well as a small portion of the duodenum and pylorus. The remaining segment is anastomosed to the duodenum.	May be performed in conjunction with a truncal vagotomy. The patient may have problems with feeling of fullness, dumping syndrome, and diarrhea. Recurrence rate of ulcer is 1%.
Billroth Ii (Gastrojejunostomy) Fundus Jejunum Body Jejunal anastomosis	Removal of lower portion (antrum) of stomach with anastomosis to jejunum. Dotted lines show portion removed (antrectomy). A duodenal stump remains and is oversewn.	Dumping syndrome, anemia, malabsorption, weight loss. Recurrence rate of ulcer is 10%–15%.

is important to monitor vital signs frequently and to evaluate the patient for tachycardia, hypotension, and tachypnea. Other nursing interventions include monitoring the hemoglobin and hematocrit, testing the stool for gross or occult blood, and recording hourly urinary output to detect anuria or oliguria (absence of or decreased urine production).

Many times, the bleeding from a peptic ulcer stops spontaneously; however, the incidence of recurrent bleeding is high. Because bleeding can be fatal, the cause and severity of the hemorrhage must be identified quickly and the blood loss treated to prevent hemorrhagic shock.

If bleeding cannot be managed by medical therapies (IV infusion of crystalloids and colloids, gastric lavage, and pharmacologic agents), other treatment modalities may be used. Transendoscopic coagulation by laser, heat probe, medication, a sclerosing agent, or a combination of these therapies can halt bleeding and avert surgical intervention. There is debate regarding how soon endoscopy should be performed. Some clinicians believe endoscopy should be performed within the first 24 hours after hemorrhage has been stabilized. Others believe endoscopy may be performed during acute bleeding, as long as the esophageal or gastric area can be visualized (blood may decrease visibility).

For patients who are unable to undergo surgery, selective embolization may be used. This procedure involves forcing emboli of autologous blood clots with or without Gelfoam (absorbable gelatin sponge) through a catheter in the artery to a point above the bleeding lesion. This procedure is performed by an interventional radiologist (DiSaverio, 2014).

Rebleeding may occur and often warrants surgical intervention. The nurse monitors the patient carefully so that bleeding can be detected quickly. Signs of bleeding include tachycardia, tachypnea, hypotension, mental confusion, thirst, and oliguria. If bleeding recurs within 48 hours after medical therapy has been initiated, or more than 6 to 10 units of blood are required within 24 hours to maintain blood volume, the patient may require surgery. Surgery may be recommended if the patient has three or more bleeding episodes. Other indications for surgery are the patient's age (massive hemorrhage is three times more likely to be fatal in people over 60 years of age), a history of chronic duodenal ulcer, and a coincidental gastric ulcer. The area of the ulcer is removed or the bleeding vessels are ligated. Many patients undergo procedures (e.g., vagotomy and pyloroplasty, gastrectomy) aimed at controlling the underlying cause of the ulcers (see Table 23-4).

Perforation and Penetration

Perforation is the erosion of the ulcer through the gastric **serosa** into the peritoneal cavity without warning. It is an abdominal catastrophe and requires immediate surgery. Box 23-1 provides signs and symptoms of perforation. Penetration is erosion of the ulcer through the gastric serosa into adjacent structures such as the pancreas, biliary tract, or gastrohepatic **omentum**. Symptoms of penetration include back and epigastric pain not relieved by medications that had been effective in the past. Like perforation, penetration usually requires surgical intervention.

Because chemical peritonitis develops within a few hours after perforation and is followed by bacterial peritonitis, the perforation must be closed as quickly as possible and the abdominal cavity lavaged of stomach or intestinal contents. In select patients, it may be safe and advisable to perform surgery to treat the ulcer disease in addition to suturing the perforation.

During surgery and postoperatively, the stomach contents are drained by means of an NG tube. The nurse monitors fluid and electrolyte balance and assesses the patient for localized infection or peritonitis (increased temperature, abdominal pain, paralytic ileus, increased or absent bowel sounds, abdominal distention). Antibiotic therapy is administered parenterally as prescribed.

Pyloric Obstruction

Pyloric obstruction, also called **gastric outlet obstruction** (GOO), occurs when the area distal to the pyloric sphincter becomes scarred and stenosed from spasm or edema or from scar tissue that forms when an ulcer alternately heals and breaks down. More than 95% of benign GOO is associated with peptic ulcer disease (duodenal or pyloric) (Ware-McGee & Wheaton, 2013). The patient may have nausea and vomiting, constipation, epigastric fullness, anorexia, and, later, weight loss. On physical examination, abdominal distension may be noted with tympanic left upper quadrant.

In treating the patient with pyloric obstruction, the first consideration is to insert an NG tube to decompress the stomach. Usually, an upper GI study or endoscopy is performed to confirm pyloric obstruction. Decompression of the stomach and management of extracellular fluid volume and electrolyte balances may improve the patient's condition and avert the need for surgical intervention. A balloon dilation of the pylorus via endoscopy may be beneficial. If the obstruction is unrelieved by medical management, surgery (in the form of a vagotomy and **antrectomy** or gastrojejunostomy and vagotomy) may be required. Recently, stent placement has been introduced as an alternative to surgical intervention with initial clinical success but may present problems with recurrent obstruction in patients with malignant gastric outlet obstruction (Goldberg, 2014; Khashab et al., 2013).

MORBID OBESITY

Morbid obesity is a term applied to people who are more than two times their ideal body weight or whose body mass index (BMI) exceeds 30 kg/m^2. Another definition of morbid obesity is body weight that is more than 100 pounds greater than the ideal body weight (Kissler & Setmacher, 2013). In the United States, where morbid obesity is a rapidly growing problem, approximately 65% of the people are overweight (Kissler & Settmacher, 2013), 36.5 percent of adults are obese, and approximately 8 percent are extremely obese (CDC, 2016).

Patients with morbid obesity are at higher risk for health complications, such as diabetes, heart disease, stroke, hypertension, gallbladder disease, osteoarthritis, sleep apnea and other breathing problems, and some forms of cancer (uterine, breast, colorectal, kidney, and gallbladder). They frequently suffer from low self-esteem, impaired body image, and depression. Management for patients with obesity has been outlined in a summary document from the American College of Cardiology and the American Heart Association (2014).

Medical Management

Conservative management of obesity consists of placing the person on a weight loss diet in conjunction with behavioral modification and exercise; however, dietary and behavioral approaches to obesity have had limited success. Depression

---

| BOX 23-1 | **Focused Assessment** |

Perforation

Be alert for the following signs and symptoms:
- Sudden, severe upper abdominal pain (persisting and increasing in intensity); pain may be referred to the shoulders, especially the right shoulder, because of irritation of the phrenic nerve in the diaphragm
- Vomiting
- Collapse (fainting)
- Extremely tender and rigid (boardlike) abdomen
- Hypotension and tachycardia, indicating shock

may be a contributing factor to weight gain, and treatment of the depression with an antidepressant may be helpful (Goritz & Duff, 2014).

Pharmacologic Management

Several medications are approved for treatment of obesity that work as an appetite reduction or inhibition of pancreatic lipase, which results in fat maldigestion. Examples include orlistat (Xenical), Phentermine (Suprenza), and Phentermine and Topiramate extended release (ER) (Qsymia) and Lorcaserin (Belviq). Sibutramine HCL (Meridia) was recently pulled from the European and U.S. markets because of the increased risk of heart attack and stroke associated with this medication. Rimonabant (Acomplia) was pulled from the European markets and has not been approved for use in the U.S. (Hurt, Varayil, & Ebbert, 2014). Orlistat, available by prescription and over the counter as Alli, reduces caloric intake by binding to gastric and pancreatic lipase to prevent digestion of fats. Side effects of orlistat may include increased frequency of bowel movements, increased gas with oily discharge, decreased food absorption, decreased bile flow, and decreased absorption of some vitamins. A multivitamin is usually recommended for patients taking orlistat. These medications are not recommended for pregnant women or those planning to become pregnant as weight loss offers no potential benefit during pregnancy.

Lorcaserin (Belviq) was approved by the FDA in 2012 for weight loss therapy for obesity. Lorcaserin is a selective $5\text{-}HT_{2C}$ agonist with a half-life of about 11 hours. Activation of the serotonin $5\text{-}HT_2$ has been associated with satiety, hypophagia (decreased food intake), and modulations of the side effects of psychostimulant addiction. Previously, the drugs fenfluramine and dexfenfluramine were used because they activated the $5\text{-}HT_{2B}$ receptor, but they were associated with valvular heart disease (Comerma-Steffenson, Grann, Andersen, Rungby, & Simonsen, 2014). In three large phase III studies, there has been no valvular heart disease associated with Lorcaserin (Hurt et al., 2014). Unfortunately, these medications rarely result in loss of more than 10% of total body weight. Furthermore, studies are needed to evaluate their long-term efficacy and risks (Gadde & Yancy, 2015). Studies are currently being undertaken to evaluate additional medication options for the long term treatment of obesity (Aronne, 2014).

Surgical Management

Bariatric surgery, or surgery for morbid obesity, is performed only after other nonsurgical attempts at weight control have failed. The National Institute of Diabetes and Digestive and Kidney Disease reports that the number of bariatric procedures has increased dramatically with 350,000 worldwide procedures done in 2008 (Kissler & Settmacher, 2013). In the United States, 158,000 procedures were performed in 2011 and 196,000 in 2015 (American Society for Metabolic and Bariatric Surgery [ASMBS], 2016). Bariatric surgical procedures work by restricting a patient's ability to eat (restrictive procedure), interfering with ingested nutrient absorption (malabsorptive procedures), or both.

Different bariatric surgical procedures entail different lifestyle modifications, and patients must be well informed about the specific lifestyle changes, eating habits, and bowel habits that may result from a particular procedure. Studies have shown that the average weight loss after bariatric surgery in the majority of patients is approximately 61% of previous body weight; comorbid conditions such as diabetes mellitus, hypertension, and sleep apnea resolve; and dyslipidemia improves (Kissler & Setmacher, 2013). Bariatric surgery has been extended to carefully selected adolescents because of its results in adults (Kissler & Settmacher, 2013).

Patient selection is critical, and the preliminary process may necessitate 6 to 12 months of counseling, education, and evaluation by a multidisciplinary team, including social workers, dietitians, a nurse counselor, and a psychologist or psychiatrist, as well as a surgeon (Table 23-5).

TABLE 23-5 Selection Criteria for Bariatric Surgery

Factor	Criteria
Weight (Adults)	• Body mass index (BMI) of at least 40 kg/m² with no comorbidities • BMI of at least 35 kg/m² with obesity-associated comorbidity (e.g., severe sleep apnea, hypertension, cardiomyopathy related to obesity, severe diabetes mellitus; serious musculoskeletal or neurologic disorders)
Weight loss history	• Failure of previous nonsurgical attempts at weight reduction, including commercial programs (e.g., Weight Watchers, Inc.)
Commitment	• Expectation that patient will adhere to postoperative care • Follow-up visits with provider(s) and team members • Recommended medical management, including the use of dietary supplements • Instructions regarding any recommended procedures or tests
Exclusions	• Reversible endocrine or other disorders that can cause obesity • Current drug or alcohol abuse • Uncontrolled, severe psychiatric illness • Lack of comprehension of risks, benefits, expected outcomes, alternatives, and lifestyle changes required with bariatric surgery

From Mechanick, J, Youdim, A., Jones, D, Timothy Garvey, W., Hurley, D., Molly McMahon, M.,...Brethauer, S. (2013). AACE/TOS/ASMBS: Clinical practice guidelines for the perioperative nutritional, metabolic, and nonsurgical support of the bariatric surgery patient—2013 update. *Surgery for Obesity & Related Diseases, 9*(2), 159–191.

Because bariatric surgery involves such a drastic change in the functioning of the digestive system, body image, and lifestyle adjustments, patients need extensive counseling before and after the surgery (Alegria & Larsen, 2015). Guidelines have been developed to assist physicians and nurses in the care of patients having bariatric surgery (Goritz & Duff, 2014; Kissler & Settmacher, 2013). After bariatric surgery, all patients require lifelong monitoring of weight loss, comorbidities, metabolic and nutritional status, and dietary and activity behaviors because they are at risk for developing malnutrition or weight gain (Goritz & Duff, 2014). Women of childbearing age who have bariatric surgery are advised to use contraceptives for approximately 2 years after surgery to avoid pregnancy until their weight stabilizes.

Procedures

The first surgical procedure used to treat morbid obesity was jejunoileal bypass. This procedure, which resulted in significant complications, has been largely replaced by gastric restriction procedures. Roux-en-Y gastric bypass, gastric banding, vertical banded gastroplasty, laparoscopic sleeve gastrectomy, and biliopancreatic diversion with duodenal switch are the current procedures of choice. These procedures may be performed by laparoscopy or by an open surgical technique. Currently, 90% of all bariatric surgeries are done laparoscopically (Kissler & Settmacher, 2013). Recent studies report long term weight loss success following laparoscopic sleeve gastrectomy at greater than 50% at 5 years or more (Diamantis et al., 2014).

Gastric restrictive procedures, such as adjustable gastric banding (AGB), vertical banded gastroplasty and sleeve gastrectomy (SG), cause early satiety during meals by decreasing the volume of the stomach. Laparoscopic adjustable gastric banding has replaced the vertical gastric banding (VGB) as the favored restrictive procedure. Malabsorptive procedures, such as biliopancreatic diversion with or without duodenal switch (BPD/DS), rely on bypassing various lengths of the small intestine, reducing nutrient absorption. Mixed procedures such as the Roux-en-Y gastric bypass (RYGB) combine gastric restriction with bypass of a short segment of the small intestine.

The Roux-en-Y gastric bypass is recommended for long-term weight loss. It is a combined restrictive and malabsorptive procedure. Biliopancreatic diversion with duodenal switch combines gastric restriction with intestinal malabsorption. See Figure 23-3A–E for additional details about these procedures. After weight loss, the patient may need surgical intervention for body contouring. This may include lipoplasty to remove fat deposits or a panniculectomy to remove excess abdominal skinfolds.

Complications

Bariatric surgical procedures have their own unique complications in addition to those associated with any major abdominal surgery. The most common complications are bleeding, blood clots, bowel obstruction, incisional or ventral hernias, and infection from a leak at the anastomosis. Prevention of complications is critical. Other postoperative problems that may occur include nausea, usually as a result of overfilling the stomach pouch or improper chewing; dumping syndrome associated with the consumption of simple sugars; and changes in bowel function, including diarrhea and constipation. Long-term complications that are related to nutritional deficiency may occur.

Nursing Management

Nursing management focuses on care of the patient after surgery. General postoperative nursing care is similar to that for a patient recovering from a gastric resection but with great attention given to the risks of complications associated with morbid obesity. Complications that may occur in the immediate postoperative period include peritonitis, stomal obstruction, stomal ulcers, atelectasis and pneumonia, thromboembolism, and metabolic imbalances resulting from prolonged vomiting and diarrhea or altered GI function. After bowel sounds have returned and oral intake is resumed, six small feedings consisting of a total of 600 to 800 calories per day are provided, and fluids are encouraged to prevent dehydration.

The patient is usually discharged in 4 days (23 to 72 hours for patients who have had laparoscopic procedures) with detailed dietary instructions (Box 23-2). The nurse instructs the patient to report excessive thirst or concentrated urine, both of which are indications of dehydration. Psychosocial interventions are also essential for these patients. Efforts are directed at helping them modify their eating behaviors and cope with changes in body image. The nurse explains that noncompliance by eating too much or too fast or eating high-calorie liquids and soft foods results in vomiting and painful esophageal distention. The nurse discusses dietary instructions before discharge and emphasizes the importance of routine follow-up outpatient appointments. Long-term side effects may include increased risk of gallstones, nutritional deficiencies (Table 23-6), and potential to regain weight. Factors integral to postsurgical weight loss success include dietary counseling; medication instruction on the importance of taking supplemental vitamin B_{12}, iron, and calcium as well as a standard multivitamin; cognitive-behavioral therapy; and support groups. Obese patients are at risk for vitamin and nutrient deficiencies (Coupaye et al., 2014; Majumder et al., 2013). Nutritional deficits tend to stabilize by 2 years post-procedure (Aquilera, 2014) and do not seem to be affected by type of gastric bypass procedure (Coupaye et al., 2013).

GASTRIC CANCER

The incidence of gastric or stomach cancer continues to decrease in the United States; however, it still accounts for

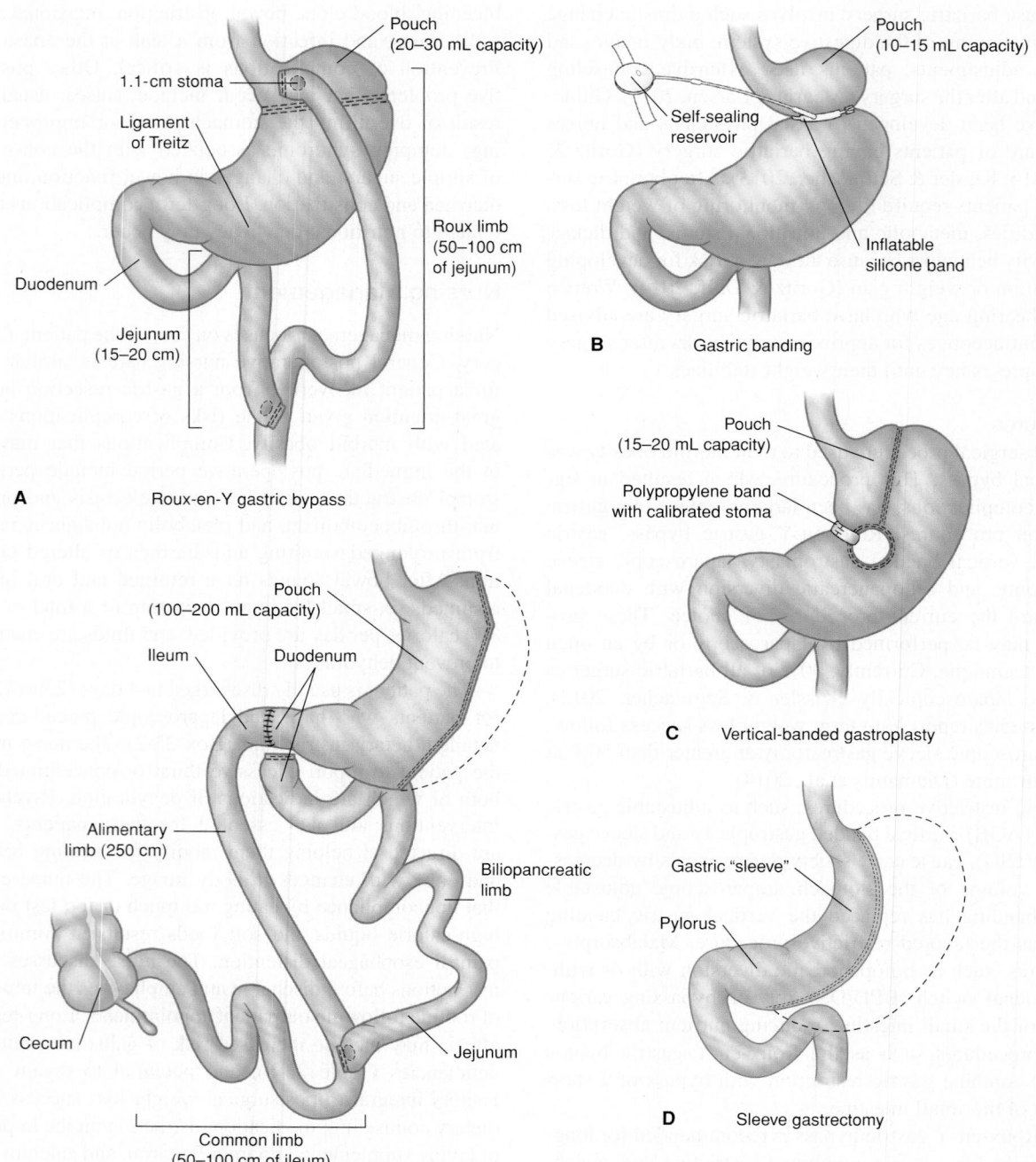

FIGURE 23-3 Surgical procedures for morbid obesity. **A**. Roux-en-Y gastric bypass. A horizontal row of staples across the fundus of the stomach creates a pouch with a capacity of 20 to 30 mL. The jejunum is divided distal to the ligament of Treitz, and the distal end is anastomosed to the new pouch. The proximal segment is anastomosed to the jejunum. **B**. Gastric banding. A prosthetic device is used to restrict oral intake by creating a small pouch of 10 to 15 mL that empties through the narrow outlet into the remainder of the stomach. **C**. Vertical-banded gastroplasty. A vertical row of staples along the lesser curvature of the stomach creates a new, smaller stomach pouch of 10 to 15 mL. **D**. Sleeve gastrectomy. The stomach is incised vertically and up to 85% of the stomach is surgically removed, leaving a "sleeve"-shaped tube that retains intact nervous innervation and does not obstruct or decrease the size of the gastric outlet. The tubular stomach has a limited gastric volume of 60 to 100 mL. **E**. Biliopancreatic diversion with duodenal switch. Half of the stomach is removed, leaving a small area that holds about 60 mL. The entire jejunum is excluded from the rest of the gastrointestinal tract. The duodenum is disconnected and sealed off. The ileum is divided above the ileocecal junction, and the distal end of the jejunum is anastomosed to the first portion of the duodenum. The distal end of the biliopancreatic limb is anastomosed to the ileum. (Reprinted with permission from Hinkle, J. (2013). *Brunner & Suddarth's textbook of medical-surgical nursing* (13th ed.). Philadelphia, PA: Lippincott, Wolters Kluwer Health.)

BOX 23-2
Patient Education

Dietary Guidelines for the Patient Who Has Had Bariatric Surgery

Nutrition:
- Eat six small meals per day (containing protein and fiber), and chew small bites of food thoroughly.
- Consume five daily servings of fresh fruits and vegetables.
- Include two protein snacks per day for a minimum protein intake of 60 g/d.
- Restrict total meal size to less than 1 cup.
- Eat only foods packed with nutrients (e.g., peanut butter, cheese, chicken, fish, beans).
- Do not eat and drink at the same time. Fluids should be consumed slowly.
- Concentrated sweets should be eliminated from the diet to avoid dumping syndrome.

Hydration:
- Fluids should be consumed slowly.
- Drink plenty of water, from 30 minutes after each meal to 15 minutes before the next meal.

- Avoid liquid calories, such as alcoholic beverages, fruit drinks, and regular soda (cola).

Supplements:
- Take 2 chewable multivitamin plus mineral (iron, folic acid, thiamine, copper, zinc) supplements daily.
- Diet/supplements should include 1,200–1,500 mg of elemental calcium.
- Diet/supplements should include:
  - 3,000 IU of vitamin D daily
  - Vitamin B12—1,000 ug/day
- Crushed or liquid rapid-release medications should be used instead of extended-release to maximize absorption.

Exercise:
- Walk for at least 30 minutes per day, minimum of 150 minutes (2½ hours) per week to a goal of 300 minutes (5 hours) per week, supplemented by strength training two to three times per week.

From Bosnic, G. (2014). Nutritional requirements after bariatric surgery. *Critical Care Clinics of North America*, 26(2), 255–262; Mechanick, J., Youdim, A., Jones, D., Timothy Garvey, W., Hurley, D., Molly McMahon, M.,...Brethauer, S. (2013). AACE/TOS/ASMBS: Clinical practice guidelines for the perioperative nutritional, metabolic, and nonsurgical support of the bariatric surgery patient – 2013 update. *Surgery for Obesity & Related Diseases*, 9(2), 159–191.

almost 11,000 deaths annually (American Cancer Society, 2015). The prognosis is generally poor: usually the diagnosis is made late because most patients are asymptomatic during the early stages of the disease. Most cases of gastric cancer are discovered only after local invasion has advanced or metastases are present (Al-Batran & Werner, 2014; Ashraf, Hoffe, & Kim, 2013; Miceli, Tomasello, Bregni, Di Bartolomeo, & Pietrantonio, 2014).

Pathophysiology

Most gastric cancers are adenocarcinomas; they can occur anywhere in the stomach. The tumor infiltrates the surrounding mucosa, penetrating the wall of the stomach and adjacent organs and structures. Often the liver, pancreas, esophagus, and duodenum are affected at the time of diagnosis. Metastasis through lymph to the peritoneal cavity occurs later in the disease.

TABLE **23-6** Nutritional Deficiencies After Bariatric Surgery

Deficiency	Signs and Symptoms
Decreased hemoglobin	Anemia
Decreased ferritin	Anemia
Decreased iron	Fatigue, anemia, lethargy, pallor, and loss of hair
Decreased vitamin B_{12}	Macrocytic anemia, pernicious anemia, leukopenia, thrombocytopenia, paresthesia, neuropathy, muscular pains, weakness, fatigue, dizziness, and brittle nails
Decreased vitamin D_3	Symptoms may include osteopenia, muscle pain, bone fractures
Decreased β-carotene	Reducing the fat-soluble antioxidant capacity, neuropathy
Decreased calcium	Osteopenia, bone fractures
Decreased magnesium	Muscle cramps, muscle pain, constipation, headaches, insomnia, anxiety, hyperactivity
Decreased zinc	Delayed wound healing, altered immune function, mental lethargy, perhaps association with alopecia

From Gletsu-Miller, N., & Wright, B. (2013). Mineral malnutrition following bariatric surgery. *Advances in Nutrition*, 4, 506–517.

Gastrointestinal lymphoma represents a second classification, differing in pathogenesis, treatment and prognosis. Gastric MALT (**m**ucosa-**a**ssociated **l**ymphoid **t**issue) lymphoma is the most common entity with *H. pylori* as the decisive pathogenic factor (Fischbach & Dunning, 2014). MALT is acquired as a secondary process against *H. pylori*. The bacterium is the cause of chronic gastritis and leads to the formation of intramucosal lymph follicles (Fischbach & Dunning, 2014). Eradication of the bacteria results in regression of the lymphoma in 77.5% of Stage I tumors. Chemotherapy or radiation may be required for patients with Stage II disease (Fischbach & Dunning, 2014).

Risk Factors

The typical patient with gastric cancer is between 40 and 70 years of age, but gastric cancer can occur in people younger than 40 years of age. Men have a higher incidence of gastric cancer than do women. Native Americans, Hispanic Americans, and African Americans are twice as likely as Caucasian Americans to develop gastric cancer. The incidence of gastric cancer is much greater in Japan, which has instituted mass screening programs for earlier diagnosis. Diet appears to be a significant factor: a diet high in smoked, salted, or pickled foods and low in fruits and vegetables may increase the risk of gastric cancer. Other factors related to the incidence of gastric cancer include chronic inflammation of the stomach, *H. pylori* infection, pernicious anemia, smoking, achlorhydria, gastric ulcers, previous subtotal gastrectomy (more than 20 years ago), and genetics.

Clinical Manifestations and Assessment

Symptoms of early disease, such as pain relieved by antacids, resemble those of benign ulcers and are seldom definitive because most gastric tumors begin on the lesser curvature of the stomach, where they cause little disturbance of gastric function. Symptoms of progressive disease include dyspepsia (indigestion), early satiety, weight loss, abdominal pain just above the umbilicus, loss or decrease in appetite, bloating after meals, nausea and vomiting, and symptoms similar to those of peptic ulcer disease.

The physical examination is usually not helpful in detecting the cancer because most early gastric tumors are not palpable. Advanced gastric cancer may be palpable as a mass. Ascites, hepatomegaly (enlarged liver), and jaundice may be apparent if the cancer cells have metastasized to the liver. Palpable nodules around the umbilicus, called Sister Mary Joseph's nodules, are a sign of a GI malignancy, usually a gastric cancer. Patients appear cachectic. Esophagogastroduodenoscopy for biopsy and cytologic washings is the diagnostic study of choice, and a barium x-ray examination of the upper GI tract also may be performed. Endoscopic ultrasound is an important tool to assess tumor depth and any lymph node involvement. Computed tomography (CT) completes the diagnostic studies, particularly to assess for surgical resectability of the tumor before surgery is scheduled. CT of the chest, abdomen, and pelvis is valuable in staging gastric cancer.

Medical and Nursing Management

There is no successful treatment for gastric carcinoma except removal of the tumor. If the tumor can be removed while it is still localized to the stomach, the patient may be cured. If the tumor has spread beyond the area that can be excised, cure is less likely. In many patients, effective palliation to prevent discomfort caused by obstruction or dysphagia may be obtained by resection of the tumor (see Gastric Surgery). A diagnostic laparoscopy may be the initial surgical approach to evaluate the gastric tumor, obtain tissue for pathologic diagnosis, and detect metastasis. The patient with a tumor that is deemed resectable undergoes an open surgical procedure to resect the tumor and appropriate lymph nodes. The patient with an unresectable tumor and advanced disease would undergo chemotherapy.

A total gastrectomy may be performed for a resectable cancer in the midportion or body of the stomach. The entire stomach is removed, along with duodenum, the section of esophagus attached to the stomach, supporting mesentery, and lymph nodes. Reconstruction of the GI tract is performed by anastomosing the end of the jejunum to the end of the esophagus, a procedure called an *esophagojejunostomy*.

A radical subtotal gastrectomy is performed for a resectable tumor in the middle and distal portions of the stomach. A Billroth I or Billroth II operation (see Table 23-4) is performed. The Billroth I involves a limited resection and offers a lower cure rate than the Billroth II. The Billroth II procedure is a wider resection that involves removing approximately 75% of the stomach and decreases the possibility of lymph node spread or metastatic recurrence.

A proximal subtotal gastrectomy may be performed for a resectable tumor located in the proximal portion of the stomach or cardia. A total gastrectomy or an esophagogastrectomy is usually performed in place of this procedure to achieve a more extensive resection. A palliative surgical procedure may be required for patients with gastric cancer to achieve a better quality of life (QOL).

Common problems of advanced gastric cancer that often require surgery include pyloric obstruction, bleeding, and severe pain. Gastric perforation is an emergency situation requiring surgical intervention. A gastric resection may be the most effective palliative procedure for advanced gastric cancer. Palliative procedures, such as gastric or esophageal bypass, gastrostomy, or jejunostomy, may alleviate symptoms such as nausea and vomiting temporarily. Palliative rather than radical surgery may be performed if there is metastasis to other vital organs, such as the liver, or to achieve a better QOL. Patients often report a decrease in QOL when the symptom burden of the cancer is prevalent. Symptoms include fatigue, pain, worry, irritability, lack of energy and difficulty sleeping (Deshields, Potter, Olsen, & Liu, 2014; Koornstra, Peters, Donofrio, van den Borne, & de Jong, 2014).

If surgical treatment does not offer cure, treatment with chemotherapy may offer further control of the disease or palliation (Diaz-Neito, Orti-Rodriguez, & Winslet, 2013). A 10 percent increase in cure rate with adjuvant therapies has been reported (Taketa, Sudo, Wadhawa, Blum, & Ajani, 2013). Commonly used chemotherapeutic agents used unaccompanied or in combination include 5-fluorouracil (5-FU), epirubicin (Ellence), cisplatin (Platinol), irinotecan (Camptosar), capecitabine (Xeloda), docetaxel (Taxotere), oxaliplatin (Eloxatin), doxorubicin (Adriamycin), etoposide (Etopophos), and mitomycin-C (Mutamycin). For improved response rates, it is more common to administer combination

therapy, primarily 5-FU–based therapy, with other agents. Studies are being conducted to assess the use of chemotherapy before surgery. Radiation therapy is used mainly for palliation in patients with obstruction, GI bleeding secondary to tumor, and significant pain. Assessment of tumor markers (blood analysis for antigens indicative of cancer), such as carcinoembryonic antigen (CEA), carbohydrate antigen (CA 19–9), and CA 50, may help determine the effectiveness of treatment. If these values were elevated before treatment, they should decrease if the tumor is responding to the treatment (Miceli et al., 2014). Meticulous attention to nutrition (jejunal enteral feedings or total parenteral nutrition [TPN]) is an essential aspect of patient management. Box 23-3 discusses the relationship between the effect of symptoms and QOL for patients with cancer (Deshields et al., 2014).

BOX 23-3 Nursing Research

Bridging the Gap to Evidence-Based Practice

Assessing Symptoms Experienced by Patients with Cancer

McMillan, S., Tofthagen, C., Choe, R., & Rheingans, J. (2015). Assessing symptoms experienced by patients with cancer: Occurrence, intensity, distress, interference, and frequency. *Journal of Hospice & Palliative Nursing, 17*(1), 56–65.

Purpose
Patients with cancer experience multiple symptoms during their disease process. All of these symptoms have the potential to cause significant distress and interfere with the patient's quality of life (QOL). Patients undergoing cancer treatment experience physical, psychosocial, psychological, and economic stressors that may, in turn, affect their QOL. QOL has different meaning for different individuals, reflecting personal values and characteristics. It may be seen as the sum of a whole life or as episodic, a measure of their current state of health and function. Scales to measure QOL reflect this individual diversity, incorporating the physical, psychological, and social dimensions in addition to symptoms of illness and treatment modalities. Many studies have documented the importance of QOL in patients with cancer.

The authors' purpose in conducting this study was to identify the symptom profile of patients being treated for cancer and to validate a new symptom assessment tool for use with persons with cancer, the Cancer Symptom Scale (CSS). In order to manage cancer-related signs and symptoms adequately, nurses caring for patients with cancer need to fully understand each patient's symptom experience. Scales are available for assessing symptoms in patients with cancer, but none of the existing scales include all of the symptoms that patients experience; all four elements that are needed (intensity, distress, interference, and constancy/frequency) can be assessed easily and interpreted on a scale of 0 to 10 using the CSS.

Design
The sample for the study consisted of 234 patients with any cancer diagnosis who were being treated for cancer or

cancer symptoms at one of two facilities in the Southeastern United States: a regional medical center and a National Cancer Institute – designated comprehensive cancer center. Patients had to be adults over 18 years of age and able to read and understand English. Staff nurses referred patients whom they knew to be alert and oriented and able to consent to the study. Patients who were within 3 weeks following surgery were excluded. Consenting patients were accrued during an 18-month period.

Three instruments were used in the study:
1. The CSS was used to assess patient symptoms.
2. The Multidimensional Quality of Life Scale—Cancer (MQOL-C) was used to support the validity of the CSS.
3. Demographic data were also collected.

The CSS assesses the presence, intensity, distress, frequency, and interference of a list of 35 symptoms, each on a scale of 0 to 10 points. The list of symptoms included in the scale was based on the review of literature. Like other scales, the CSS allows the patient to identify whether a symptom has occurred in the past week, and only if the response is "yes" does the patient respond about intensity, distress, frequency, and interference of that symptom. Validity and reliability of this type of scale have been strong. The CSS includes the added assessment of the interference caused by the symptom as well as distress and frequency/constancy. Each dimension is assessed on a scale of 0 to 10 points. Because this is a new study tool, validity and reliability were also studied.

The MQOL-C was used to help assess the construct validity of the new CSS, hypothesizing weak to moderate relationships. QOL is known to be significantly but moderately correlated with symptoms; however, the correlation is not strong because the two instruments are not measuring the same but, rather, related concepts. The MQOL-C has 33 items that measure four dimensions of QOL: physical well-being, psychological well-being, social concerns, and symptoms.

(continued on page 708)

BOX 23-3

Nursing Research (*continued*)

Bridging the Gap to Evidence-Based Practice (*continued*)

Items are scaled from 0 to 10. Validity has been supported by significant correlations with measures of depression as well as social and physical functioning. Cronbach α has been high (0.89–0.91).

Demographic data were collected to describe the sample population, including age, gender, race/ethnicity, and cancer diagnosis. Patients were asked a single item about QOL: "How good has your quality of life been during the past week?" and answered on a scale of 0 (worst) to 10 (best).

Patients were approached in a quiet area within their facilities and asked if they were experiencing any symptoms. If the patient reported any type of symptom, the study was explained, the consent obtained, and questions answered. Consenting patients completed the study questionnaires that were administered to patients by the research assistant who stayed with the patient during the administration. A subset of 15 patients was asked to complete the CSS a second time after a short delay of 1–2 hours. Returning the forms to the research assistant concluded the patient's participation in the study.

Results

The sample consisted of 234 patients with cancer, 55.6% female, 82.9% white, and 63.2% married. The most common type of cancers was leukemia, breast cancer, lymphoma, and colorectal cancer. The mean age of the sample was 60.4 years with a range of 21–90 years of age. The QOL mean score was slightly above the midrange. The symptoms reported most commonly by this group of patients were fatigue/being tired, feeling drowsy, difficulty sleeping, pain, and dry mouth. Patients reported several signs and symptoms to be in the high range of intensity. Highest were feeling irritable, problem with sex, sweats, and diarrhea. All of these had mean scores higher than 6.0. The signs and symptoms causing the most distress were feeling irritable, diarrhea, worrying, and problems with urination; all had mean distress scores higher than 6.0. The signs and symptoms causing the most interference with patients' lives included diarrhea, feeling irritable, fatigue or feeling tired, problems with urination, difficulty sleeping, and shortness of breath. The signs and symptoms reported as occurring most frequently included problems with

urination, problems with sex, difficulty sleeping, rash, poor appetite, numbness and tingling in both the hands and feet, and changes in the skin. All of these had mean scores of 6.4 or higher.

The subscales of the newly developed CSS were correlated with the total scores from the QOL scale and the MQOL-C scale. All correlations were weak to moderate ($r = -0.34–0.56$, $P < 0.001$). Reliability of the CSS was estimated in two ways. First, a small subsample of the patients agreed to complete the CSS twice with a time period between administration of the surveys. Results revealed excellent stability over time in all four of the subscales, with frequency having the highest estimate of reliability. Internal consistency reliability also was estimated using Cronbach α coefficient. All subscale coefficients were greater than 0.70. Reliability of the MQOL-C also was very strong ($\alpha = 0.92$).

Nursing Implications

Cancer outpatients in this study had symptoms of moderate to high intensity that caused distress, caused interference in their lives, and, in some cases, were frequent or long-lasting. Results of this study suggest that nurses need to continue to improve assessment and management of patient symptoms during regular clinic visits. Problems cannot be addressed adequately unless they are thoroughly assessed on an ongoing basis, and this assessment needs to include more than just symptom intensity because distress from symptoms, interference by symptoms, and constancy of symptoms help determine their impact. Patients may not think to tell nurses about all of their symptoms, so nurses must ask. Schools of nursing should emphasize teaching nurses to ask cancer patients about their signs and symptoms at every contact as well as provide teaching on how to manage symptoms. Nurses do assessments for pain frequently, but other symptoms can be neglected. Further research is needed about mechanisms and management of most of the symptoms explored in this study. It should be noted that multisymptom assessment scales, such as the new CSS, allow clinicians to assess symptoms that patients are experiencing simultaneously, with awareness that treating one symptom may lead to the occurrence of others.

GASTRIC SURGERY

Gastric surgery may be performed on patients with peptic ulcers who have life-threatening hemorrhage, obstruction, perforation, or penetration, or whose condition does not respond to medication. It also may be indicated for patients with gastric cancer or trauma. Surgical procedures include a vagotomy and **pyloroplasty** (transecting nerves that stimulate acid secretion and opening the pylorus), a partial gastrectomy, or a total gastrectomy (see Table 23-4).

NURSING PROCESS
The Patient Undergoing Gastric Surgery

ASSESSMENT

Before surgery, the nurse assesses the patient's and family's knowledge of pre- and postoperative surgical routines and the rationale for surgery. The nurse also assesses the patient's nutritional status: Has the patient lost weight? How much? Over how much time? The nurse is aware that a 5% weight loss in 30 days, a 7.5% weight loss in 90 days, or a greater than 10% weight loss in 180 days is associated with significant health risks (Bosnic, 2014). Does the patient have nausea and vomiting? Has the patient had hematemesis? The nurse assesses for the presence of bowel sounds and palpates the abdomen to detect masses or tenderness.

After surgery, the nurse assesses the patient for complications secondary to the surgical intervention, such as hemorrhage, infection, abdominal distention, atelectasis, or impaired nutritional status.

DIAGNOSIS

Nursing diagnoses may include the following:

- Anxiety related to surgical intervention
- Acute pain related to surgical incision
- Deficient knowledge about surgical procedure and postoperative course
- Imbalanced nutrition, less than body requirements, related to poor nutrition before surgery and altered GI system after surgery

PLANNING

The major goals for the patient undergoing gastric surgery may include reduced anxiety, increased knowledge and understanding about the surgical procedure and postoperative course, optimal nutrition and management of the complications that can interfere with nutrition, relief of pain, avoidance of hemorrhage and steatorrhea, and enhanced self-care skills at home.

NURSING INTERVENTIONS

REDUCING ANXIETY

An important part of the preoperative nursing care involves allaying the patient's fears and anxieties about the impending surgery and its implications. The nurse encourages the patient to verbalize fears and concerns and answers the patient's and family's questions. If the patient has an acute obstruction, a perforated bowel, or an active GI hemorrhage, adequate psychological preparation may not be possible. In this event, the nurse caring for the patient after surgery should anticipate the concerns, fears, and questions that are likely to surface and should be available for support and further explanations.

RELIEVING PAIN

After surgery, analgesics may be administered as prescribed to relieve pain and discomfort. It is important to provide adequate pain relief so the patient can perform pulmonary care activities (deep breathing and coughing) and leg exercises, turn from side to side, and ambulate. The nurse assesses the effectiveness of analgesic intervention and consults with other members of the health care team if pain is not controlled adequately. Positioning the patient in the Fowler position promotes comfort and allows emptying of the stomach after gastric surgery.

The nurse maintains functioning of the NG tube to prevent distention and secures the tube to prevent dislocation, which may result in increased pain and tension on the suture line. Normally, the amount of NG drainage after a total gastrectomy is minimal as there is no reservoir where secretions can collect.

PROVIDING TEACHING

The nurse explains routine pre- and postoperative procedures to the patient, which include preoperative medications, NG intubation, IV fluids, abdominal dressings, and the possible need for a feeding tube, pain management, and pulmonary care. These explanations need to be reinforced after surgery, especially if the patient had emergency surgery.

RESUMING ENTERAL INTAKE

The patient's nutritional status is evaluated before surgery. If surgery is performed for gastric cancer, often the patient is malnourished and may require preoperative enteral or, more often, parenteral nutrition. After surgery, parenteral nutrition may be continued to meet caloric needs, to replace fluids lost through drainage and vomiting, and to support the patient metabolically until oral intake is adequate.

After the return of bowel sounds and removal of the NG tube, the nurse may give fluids, followed by food in small portions. Foods are added gradually until the patient is able to eat six small meals a day and drink 120 mL of fluid between meals. The key to increasing the dietary content is to offer food and fluids gradually, as tolerated, and to recognize that each patient's tolerance is different.

RECOGNIZING OBSTACLES TO ADEQUATE NUTRITION

Dysphagia and Gastric Retention. Dysphagia may occur in patients who have had a truncal vagotomy, a surgical procedure that may result in trauma to the lower esophagus. Gastric retention may be evidenced by abdominal distention, nausea, and vomiting. Regurgitation also may occur if the patient has eaten too much or too quickly. It also may indicate that edema along the suture line is preventing fluids and food from moving into the intestinal tract. If gastric retention occurs, it may be necessary to reinstate NPO status and NG suction; pressure must be low in the remaining portion of the stomach to avoid disrupting the sutures.

Bile Reflux. Bile reflux gastritis and esophagitis may occur with the removal of the pylorus, which acts as a barrier to the reflux of duodenal contents. Burning epigastric pain and vomiting of bilious material manifest this condition. Eating or vomiting does not relieve the situation. Agents that bind with bile acid, such as cholestyramine (Questran), may be helpful. Aluminum hydroxide gel (an antacid) and metoclopramide hydrochloride (Reglan) have been used with limited success.

Dumping Syndrome. **Dumping syndrome** is an unpleasant set of vasomotor and GI symptoms that sometimes occur in patients who have had gastric surgery or a form of vagotomy. It is seen

(continued on page 710)

in 10% of all patients having gastric surgery (Ferri, 2016). It may be the mechanical result of surgery in which a small gastric remnant is connected to the jejunum through a large opening. Foods high in carbohydrates and electrolytes must be diluted in the jejunum before absorption can take place, but the passage of food from the stomach remnant into the jejunum is too rapid to allow this to happen. The hypertonic intestinal contents draw extracellular fluid from the circulating blood volume into the jejunum to dilute the high concentration of electrolytes and sugars. The ingestion of fluid at mealtime is another factor that causes the stomach contents to empty rapidly into the jejunum (Bosnic, 2014; Tack & Delosse, 2014).

Early symptoms include a sensation of fullness, weakness, faintness, dizziness, palpitations, diaphoresis, cramping pains, and diarrhea. These symptoms resolve once the intestine has been evacuated. Later, there is a rapid elevation of blood glucose, followed by increased insulin secretion. This results in a reactive hypoglycemia, which also is unpleasant for the patient. Vasomotor symptoms that occur 10 to 90 minutes after eating are pallor, perspiration, palpitations, headache, and feelings of warmth, dizziness, and even drowsiness. These symptoms are thought to be partially due to hypovolemia caused by rapid shifts of fluid from the intravascular space into the lumen of the bowel (Ferri, 2016). Anorexia also may be a result of the dumping syndrome, as the person may be reluctant to eat. There are no symptoms in fasting state.

Steatorrhea (excess fat in feces) also may occur in the patient with gastric surgery. It is partially the result of rapid gastric emptying, which prevents adequate mixing with pancreatic and biliary secretions. In mild cases, reducing the intake of fat and administering an antimotility medication (e.g., loperamide [Imodium]) may control steatorrhea.

Vitamin and Mineral Deficiencies. Other dietary deficiencies that the nurse should be aware of include malabsorption of organic iron, which may require supplementation with oral or parenteral iron, and a low serum level of vitamin B_{12}, which may require supplementation by the intramuscular route. Total gastrectomy results in lack of intrinsic factor, a gastric secretion required for the absorption of vitamin B_{12} from the GI tract. Unless this vitamin is supplied by parenteral injection after gastrectomy, the patient inevitably will suffer vitamin B_{12} deficiency, which eventually leads to a condition identical to pernicious anemia. All manifestations of pernicious anemia, including macrocytic anemia (few, fragile, and larger than normal red blood cells) and combined system disease (neurologic disorders of the central and peripheral nervous systems), may be expected to develop within a period of 5 years or less; they progress in severity thereafter and, in the absence of therapy, are fatal. This complication is avoided by the regular monthly intramuscular injection of vitamin B_{12}. This regimen should be started without delay after gastrectomy. Weight loss is a common long-term problem because the patient experiences early fullness, which suppresses the appetite (Bosnic, 2014; Tack & Delosse, 2014; Majumder, Soriano, Cruz, & Dasanu, 2013).

BOX 23-4 | **Patient Education**

Dietary Management After Gastric Surgery

- To delay stomach emptying and dumping syndrome, assume a low Fowler position (head of bed [HOB] elevated 30 degrees) during mealtime; after the meal, the patient should lie down for 20–30 minutes.
- Take antispasmodics as prescribed to aid in delaying the emptying of the stomach.
- Do not drink fluids with meals; instead, drink fluids up to 1 hour before or 1 hour after mealtime.
- Create meals containing more dry items than liquid items.
- Eat fat as tolerated, but keep carbohydrate intake low and avoid concentrated sources of carbohydrates (sugared soda, pastries).
- Eat smaller but more frequent meals.
- Take dietary supplements of vitamins and medium-chain triglycerides and injections of vitamin B_{12} and iron as prescribed.

TEACHING DIETARY SELF-MANAGEMENT

Because the patient may experience any of the described conditions affecting nutrition, nursing intervention includes proper dietary instruction (Box 23-4). The nurse also gives instructions regarding enteral or parenteral supplementation if it is needed.

MONITORING AND MANAGING POTENTIAL COMPLICATIONS

Occasionally, hemorrhage complicates gastric surgery. The patient has the usual signs of rapid blood loss and shock (see Chapter 54) and may vomit considerable amounts of bright red blood. The nurse assesses NG drainage for type and amount; some bloody drainage for the first 12 hours is expected, but excessive bleeding should be reported. The nurse also assesses the abdominal dressing for bleeding. Because this situation is upsetting to the patient and family, the nurse should remain calm. The nurse performs emergency measures, such as NG lavage and administration of blood and blood products, along with vigilant hemodynamic monitoring.

TEACHING PATIENTS SELF-CARE

Patient teaching is based on the assessment of the patient's physical and psychological readiness to participate in self-care. The nurse provides information about nutrition, enteral or parenteral nutrition if required, nutritional supplements, pain management, and the symptoms of dumping syndrome and measures to prevent or minimize these symptoms.

The patient and caregivers benefit from a team approach to discharge planning. The team members include the patient and caregiver along with the nurse, physician, dietitian, and social worker. Written or video instructions about meals, activities, medications, and follow-up care are helpful. After the patient is discharged from the hospital, the home care nurse helps with the transition to home by supervising the administration of any enteral or parenteral feedings, emphasizing information about detection and prevention of untoward effects or complications related to feedings. Information about community support groups and end-of-life care is provided to the patient, family, or significant other when indicated.

EVALUATION

Expected patient outcomes may include:

1. Reports decreased anxiety; expresses fears and concerns about surgery
2. Demonstrates knowledge regarding postoperative course by discussing the surgical procedure and postoperative course
3. Attains optimal nutrition:
   a. Maintains a reasonable weight
   b. Does not have excessive diarrhea
   c. Tolerates six small meals a day
   d. Does not experience dysphagia, gastric retention, bile reflux, dumping syndrome, or vitamin and mineral deficiencies
4. Attains optimal level of comfort
5. Exhibits no complications

DUODENAL TUMORS

Tumors of the duodenum are uncommon and, when present, usually are benign and asymptomatic. They are most often discovered at autopsy. Malignant tumors are more likely to cause specific signs and symptoms leading to diagnosis. Unfortunately, malignant tumors often are not discovered until they have metastasized to distant sites. Benign tumors may place patients at an increased risk for malignancy. The relative rarity of tumors of the duodenum and the nonspecific nature of their manifestations complicate their diagnosis and treatment.

Clinical Manifestations and Assessment

Duodenal tumors often present insidiously with vague, nonspecific symptoms. Most benign tumors are discovered incidentally on an x-ray study, during surgery, or at autopsy.

When the patient is symptomatic, benign tumors often present with intermittent pain. The next most common presentation is occult bleeding. Malignant tumors often result in symptoms that lead to their diagnosis, although these symptoms may reflect advanced disease. Most patients have sustained weight loss and are malnourished at diagnosis. Bleeding and pain are common. Perforation of the bowel occurs in approximately 10% of patients (di Saverio, 2014).

The traditional approach to diagnosis is an upper GI x-ray series with small bowel follow-through using oral water-insoluble contrast with frequent and detailed x-rays to follow the contrast through the small bowel. A more sensitive examination is an **enteroclysis**, in which an NG tube is advanced into the small bowel to a position above the area in question; then the area is studied by single-contrast and double-contrast techniques. Abdominal CT is used to determine the extent of disease outside the lumen of the duodenum.

Medical and Nursing Management

Benign tumors of the duodenum include adenomas, lipomas, hemangiomas, and hamartomas (a focal malformation that resembles a neoplasm but, unlike a neoplasm, does not result in compression of adjacent tissue). These tumors may be treated endoscopically by excision/resection or electrocautery if the patient is symptomatic. Routine surveillance may be recommended to assess for malignant transformation.

The most common primary malignant tumor of the duodenum is adenocarcinoma; the second and third portions of the duodenum are most often involved. These tumors may present with bleeding or duodenal obstruction (Kordes, Cats, Meijer, & van Laarhoven, 2014). If the tumor is located at the ampulla of Vater, obstructive jaundice is likely. Other rare malignant tumors of the duodenum include carcinoid tumors, lymphoma, and GI stromal tumors. Specialized abdominal surgery may be required to remove these rare tumors. Chemotherapy and radiation therapy may also be part of the treatment regimen.

Nursing care of the patient with a duodenal tumor is similar to that of the patient with gastric cancer. Each patient requires specialized care, astute assessment for complications, prompt interventions, and individualized teaching for self-care.

CHAPTER REVIEW

Critical Thinking Exercises

1. A 45-year-old woman with a history of rheumatoid arthritis and gastritis related to her medication is admitted with abdominal discomfort, headache, lassitude, and nausea and vomiting. What questions should you ask the patient? What signs should be noted during the physical examination? What diagnostic studies should you anticipate for this patient? Describe your nursing interventions, including teaching. How would you modify teaching for this patient if she does not understand English?

2. A 27-year-old woman who is morbidly obese has tried conservative medical management (weight loss diet, behavior modification, exercise, medications for obesity) of her weight condition. She is scheduled for a vertical-banded gastroplasty. Describe the dietary modifications, along with nutritional needs, for this patient during the immediate postoperative period, after discharge from the hospital, and for long-term maintenance. What is the evidence base that supports the use of specific dietary modifications to meet her nutritional needs after surgical procedures to treat obesity? Describe the strength of this evidence and identify the criteria used to evaluate the strength of the evidence that supports the appropriateness of the dietary modifications.

3. A 54-year-old business executive has been admitted with the diagnosis of peptic ulcer disease. As you enter his room, he is vomiting bright red blood. What are the nursing interventions for managing and monitoring this complication? If the bleeding cannot be controlled, what invasive measures may need to be performed? How would you prepare your patient for these? What other complications may occur with a peptic ulcer, and how should they be managed? What teaching interventions are warranted for this patient?

NCLEX-Style Review Questions

1. A 47-year-old man with epigastric pain is being admitted to the hospital. During the admission assessment and interview, what specific information should the nurse obtain from the patient, who is suspected of having peptic ulcer disease?
   a. Any allergies to food or medications
   b. Use of nonsteroidal anti-inflammatory drugs (NSAIDs)
   c. Medical history for two previous generations
   d. History of side effects of all medications

Try these additional resources, available at **http://thepoint.lww.com/Honan2e**, to enhance your learning and understanding of this chapter:
- NCLEX-Style Student Review Questions
- Journal Articles

2. What assessment finding supports a client's diagnosis of gastric ulcer?
   a. Presence of blood in the client's stool for the past month
   b. Complaints of sharp pain in the abdomen after eating a heavy meal
   c. Periods of pain shortly after eating any food.
   d. Complaints of epigastric burning that moves like a wave

3. Which medication should the nurse question before administering it to a patient with peptic ulcer disease?
   a. E-mycin, an antibiotic
   b. Prilosec, a PPI
   c. Flagyl, an antimicrobial agent
   d. Tylenol, a nonnarcotic analgesic

4. The nurse is planning for the discharge of a client with peptic ulcer disease. Which outcome must be included in the plan of care?
   a. The client's pain is controlled with NSAIDs.
   b. The client understands and maintains lifestyle modifications.
   c. The client takes antacids around the clock.
   d. The client has no episodes of GI bleeding.

5. The client with a peptic ulcer is admitted to the hospital's intensive care unit with obvious gastric bleeding. What is the priority intervention for the nurse?
   a. Keep an accurate record of intake and output.
   b. Provide for quiet environment, restrict visitors.
   c. Prepare the client for an endoscopy.
   d. Monitor vital signs and observe for signs of hypovolemia.

REFERENCES AND SELECTED READINGS

References and selected readings associated with this chapter can be found on the website that accompanies the book. Visit **http://thepoint. lww.com/Honan2e** to access the references and other additional resources associated with this chapter.

Nursing Management: Patients with Intestinal and Rectal Disorders

Philip R. Martinez, Jr.

Learning Objectives

After reading this chapter, you will be able to:

1. Describe the health care needs of patients with constipation, diarrhea, or fecal incontinence.
2. Compare the conditions of malabsorption with regard to their pathophysiology, clinical manifestations, and management.
3. Describe diverticular disease and the care of patients with diverticulitis.
4. Compare and contrast regional enteritis and ulcerative colitis regarding their pathophysiology and medical, surgical, and nursing management.
5. Identify the care needs of the patient with inflammatory bowel disease.
6. Describe the responsibilities of the nurse in meeting the needs of the patient with an ileostomy.
7. Describe the various types of intestinal obstructions as well as their medical and nursing management.
8. Describe the pathophysiology, assessment, and management in regard to cancer of the colon or rectum.
9. Describe anorectal conditions including fissures, fistulas, hemorrhoids, and sexually transmitted anorectal diseases.

There are approximately 60 to 70 million people in the United States diagnosed with some type of disease of the gastrointestinal (GI) tract (Peery et al., 2015). These diseases account for more than 104.7 million office visits and approximately 13.5 million hospital admissions annually. A recent study focusing on the economic burden of GI diseases reported more than 15 million emergency room visits in 2007 totaling more than $27 billion in cost (Myer et al., 2013). The types of diseases and disorders that affect the lower GI tract are many and varied.

In all age groups, a fast-paced lifestyle, high levels of stress, irregular eating habits, insufficient intake of fiber and water, and lack of daily exercise contribute to GI disorders. There is a growing understanding of the biopsychosocial implications of GI disease. Nurses can have an impact on these GI disorders by identifying behavior patterns that put patients at risk, by educating the public about prevention and management, and by helping those affected to improve their condition and prevent complications.

DISORDERS RELATED TO FECAL ELIMINATION

Constipation

Constipation is considered an abnormal infrequency or irregularity of defecation, an abnormal hardening of stools that makes their passage difficult and sometimes painful, a decrease in actual stool volume, or retention of stool in the rectum for a prolonged period. Any variation from normal habits may be considered a problem. Symptoms of constipation are extremely common in adults and even more common in people aged 60 years and older (Bharucha, Dorn, Lembo, & Pressman, 2013). The most common complaint is the need to strain in order to pass stool.

Nursing Alert
Hemorrhoids and anal fissures can develop as a result of constipation. Hemorrhoids

713

develop as a result of perianal vascular congestion caused by straining. Anal fissures may result from the passage of the hard stool through the anus, tearing the lining of the anal canal.

Perceived constipation also can be a problem. This subjective problem occurs when a person's bowel elimination pattern is not consistent with what he or she perceives as normal. Chronic laxative use may contribute to this problem and is a major health concern in the United States.

Pathophysiology

The pathophysiology of constipation is poorly understood, but it is thought to include interference with one of three major functions of the colon: mucosal transport (i.e., mucosal secretions facilitate the movement of colon contents), myoelectric activity (i.e., mixing of the rectal mass and propulsive actions), or the processes of defecation.

The urge to defecate is stimulated normally by rectal distention, which initiates a series of four actions: stimulation of the inhibitory rectoanal reflex, relaxation of the internal sphincter muscle, relaxation of the external sphincter muscle and muscles in the pelvic region, and increased intra-abdominal pressure. Interference with any of these processes can lead to constipation.

If all organic causes are eliminated, idiopathic constipation is diagnosed. When the urge to defecate is ignored, the rectal mucous membrane and musculature become insensitive to the presence of fecal masses, and, consequently, a stronger stimulus is required to produce the necessary peristaltic rush for defecation. The initial effect of fecal retention is irritability of the colon, which at this stage frequently goes into spasm, especially after meals, giving rise to colicky midabdominal or low abdominal pains. After several years of this process, the colon loses muscular tone and becomes essentially unresponsive to normal stimuli. **Atony** or decreased muscle tone occurs with aging. This also leads to constipation because the stool is retained for longer periods.

Risk Factors

Constipation can be caused by certain medications (i.e., tranquilizers, anticholinergics, antidepressants, antihypertensives, bile acid sequestrants, opioids, aluminum-based antacids, iron preparations); rectal or anal disorders (e.g., hemorrhoids, fissures); obstruction (e.g., bowel tumors); metabolic, neurologic, and neuromuscular conditions (e.g., Hirschsprung disease, Parkinson disease, multiple sclerosis); endocrine disorders (e.g., diabetes mellitus, hypothyroidism, pheochromocytoma [rare tumor of adrenal medulla]); lead poisoning; and connective tissue disorders (e.g., scleroderma, systemic lupus erythematosus).

Diseases of the colon, such as irritable bowel syndrome (IBS) and diverticular disease, are commonly associated with constipation. Constipation also can occur with any acute disease process in the abdomen (e.g., appendicitis or cholecystitis) or with any abdominal surgery.

Older adults tend to have decreased food intake, reduced mobility, weak abdominal and pelvic muscles, and multiple chronic illnesses requiring medications that can cause constipation. The astute nurse always will check a patient's medication list for those that may exacerbate constipation.

Low-fiber convenience foods are used widely by people who have lost interest in eating. Dentition is important to consider as people with ill-fitting dentures or poor dentition have increased difficulty chewing and frequently will choose softer, processed foods that are lower in fiber. Some older people reduce their fluid intake if they are not eating regular meals. Depression, weakness, or prolonged bed rest also contributes to constipation by decreasing intestinal motility and anal sphincter tone. Nerve impulses are dulled, and there is a decreased urge to defecate. Prolonged bed rest is also a risk factor in constipation; therefore, nursing care for these patients should include ambulation when possible. Many older people overuse laxatives in an attempt to have a daily bowel movement and become dependent on them, which paradoxically can increase the risk of constipation.

Other causes of constipation may include weakness, immobility, debility, fatigue, and an inability to increase intra-abdominal pressure to facilitate the passage of stools, as may occur in patients with emphysema, for instance. Many people develop constipation because they do not take the time to defecate or they ignore the urge to defecate. Additionally, the lack of privacy and interruption of usual bowel regimen are factors associated with constipation in hospitalized patients.

Clinical Manifestations and Assessment

Clinical manifestations of constipation include fewer than three bowel movements per week, abdominal distention, pain and pressure, decreased appetite, headache, fatigue, indigestion, a sensation of incomplete evacuation, straining at stool, and the elimination of small-volume, lumpy, hard, dry stools. Due to the wide range of normal bowel function in people, it is extremely difficult to identify constipation in all patients accurately.

The nurse elicits information about the onset and duration of constipation, current and past elimination patterns, the patient's expectation of normal bowel elimination, and lifestyle information (e.g., exercise and activity level, occupation, food and fluid intake, and stress level) during the health history interview. Medical and surgical history, current medications, and laxative and enema use are important, as is information about the sensation of rectal pressure or fullness, abdominal pain, excessive straining at defecation, and flatulence.

Medical and Nursing Management

Treatment is aimed at the underlying cause of constipation and includes education, bowel habit training, increased fiber and fluid intake, and judicious use of laxatives. Management also may include discontinuing laxative abuse. Routine exercise to strengthen abdominal muscles is encouraged. Inexpensive osmotic agents, such as milk of magnesia or polyethylene glycol, may be prescribed as an early treatment option for patients with chronic constipation prior to the use of stimulant laxatives (Bharucha et al., 2013). Biofeedback has been shown to improve symptoms in many patients with chronic constipation and can be used to help patients learn to relax the sphincter mechanism to expel stool (Woodward, Norton, & Chiarelli, 2014).

Daily dietary intake of 6 to 12 teaspoonfuls of unprocessed bran is recommended, especially for the treatment of the elderly. If laxative use is necessary, one of the following may be prescribed: bulk-forming agents, saline and osmotic agents, lubricants, stimulants, or fecal softeners. The physiologic action and patient education information related to these laxatives are given in Table 24-1. Enemas and rectal suppositories generally are not recommended for treating constipation; they should be reserved for the treatment of impaction. If long-term laxative use is necessary, a bulk-forming agent may be prescribed in combination with an osmotic laxative.

Specific medications may be prescribed to enhance colonic transit by increasing propulsive motor activity. These may include cholinergic agents (e.g., bethanechol [Urecholine]), cholinesterase inhibitors (e.g., neostigmine [Prostigmin]), or prokinetic agents (e.g., metoclopramide [Reglan]).

Patient education and health promotion are important functions of the nurse. Patient education should include establishing a bowel routine, providing dietary information, and reducing patient anxiety. After the health history is

TABLE 24-1 Laxatives: Classification, Agent, Action, and Patient Education

Classification	Sample Agent	Action	Patient Education
Bulk forming	Psyllium hydrophilic mucilloid (Metamucil)	Polysaccharides and cellulose derivatives mix with intestinal fluids, swell, and stimulate peristalsis.	Take with 8-oz water and follow with 8-oz water; do not take dry. Report abdominal distention or unusual amount of flatulence.
Saline agent	Magnesium hydroxide (milk of magnesia)	Nonabsorbable magnesium ions alter stool consistency by drawing water into the intestines by osmosis; peristalsis is stimulated. Action occurs within 2 hours.	The liquid preparation is more effective than the tablet form. Only short-term use is recommended because of toxicity (CNS or neuromuscular depression, electrolyte imbalance). Magnesium laxatives should not be taken by patients with renal insufficiency.
Lubricant	Mineral oil	Nonabsorbable hydrocarbons soften fecal matter by lubricating the intestinal mucosa; the passage of stool is facilitated. Action occurs within 6–8 hours.	Do not take with meals because mineral oils can impair the absorption of fat-soluble vitamins and delay gastric emptying. Swallow carefully, because drops of oil that gain access to the pharynx can produce a lipid pneumonia.
Stimulant	Bisacodyl (Dulcolax)	Irritates the colon epithelium by stimulating sensory nerve endings and increasing mucosal secretions. Action occurs within 6–8 hours.	Catharsis may cause fluid and electrolyte imbalance, especially in the elderly. Tablets should be swallowed, not crushed or chewed. Avoid milk or antacids within 1 hour of taking the medication because the enteric coating may dissolve prematurely.
Fecal softener	Dioctyl sodium sulfosuccinate (Colace)	Hydrates the stool by its surfactant action on the colonic epithelium (increases the wetting efficiency of intestinal water); aqueous and fatty substances are mixed. Does not exert a laxative action.	This can be used safely by patients who should avoid straining (cardiac patients, patients with anorectal disorders).
Osmotic agent	Polyethylene glycol and electrolytes (Colyte)	Cleanses colon rapidly and induces diarrhea	This is a large-volume product. It takes time to consume it safely. It can cause considerable nausea and bloating.

obtained, the nurse sets specific goals for teaching. Goals for the patient include restoring or maintaining a regular pattern of elimination by responding to the urge to defecate, ensuring adequate intake of fluids and high-fiber foods, learning methods to avoid constipation, relieving anxiety about bowel elimination patterns, and avoiding complications.

Complications

Complications of constipation include hypertension, fecal impaction, hemorrhoids (dilated portions of anal veins), fissures (tissue folds), and **megacolon** (abnormal enlargement of the colon). Increased arterial pressure can occur with defecation. Straining at stool, which results in the **Valsalva maneuver** (i.e., forcibly exhaling with the glottis closed), has a striking effect on arterial blood pressure. During active straining, the flow of venous blood in the chest is impeded temporarily because of increased intrathoracic pressure. This pressure tends to collapse the large veins in the chest. The atria and the ventricles receive less blood, and, consequently, less blood is ejected by the left ventricle. Cardiac output is decreased, and there is a transient drop in arterial pressure. Almost immediately after this period of hypotension, an increase in arterial pressure occurs; the pressure is elevated momentarily to a point far exceeding the original level (i.e., *rebound phenomenon*). Thus bowel regimens to prevent constipation frequently are instituted in patients admitted with cardiac and neurologic problems.

> ### Nursing Alert
> *In patients with hypertension, the rebound phenomenon reaction may be exaggerated greatly, and the peak pressure attained may be dangerously high—sufficient to rupture a major artery in the brain or elsewhere.*

Fecal impaction occurs when an accumulated mass of dry feces cannot be expelled. The mass may be palpable on digital examination, may produce pressure on the colonic mucosa that results in ulcer formation, and frequently causes seepage of liquid stools.

Megacolon is caused by a fecal mass that obstructs the passage of colon contents. Symptoms include constipation, liquid fecal incontinence, and abdominal distention. Megacolon can lead to perforation of the bowel.

> ### Nursing Alert
> *Care should be taken when performing digital rectal procedures as vagal nerve stimulation may occur, causing a vasovagal response in the patient. Additionally, straining to stool may also cause a vasovagal response. Signs and symptoms of a vasovagal response include: bradycardia, hypotension, light-headedness, nausea, feelings of hot or cold, confusion, or loss of consciousness.*

Treatment should include reducing the risk of injury during the episode, maneuvers to increase blood flow to the brain (recumbent position with lower extremities elevated), and evaluation of any cardiac and neurologic causes of syncope.

DIARRHEA

Diarrhea is defined as an increased frequency of bowel movements of more than three per day, an increased amount of stool (more than 200 g/day), or abnormally liquid stool. It is usually associated with increased urgency, perianal discomfort, or incontinence. Diarrhea lasting less than 2 weeks is considered acute; conversely, diarrhea lasting more than 4 weeks is considered chronic. Acute diarrhea is associated most often with infection and usually is self-limiting; chronic diarrhea persists for a longer period and may return sporadically. Any condition that causes increased intestinal secretions, decreased mucosal absorption, or altered motility can produce diarrhea. IBS, inflammatory bowel disease (IBD), and lactose intolerance are frequently the underlying disease processes that cause diarrhea.

Pathophysiology

Types of diarrhea include secretory, osmotic, and mixed diarrhea. Secretory diarrhea is usually high-volume diarrhea and is caused by increased production and secretion of water and electrolytes by the intestinal mucosa into the intestinal lumen. Osmotic diarrhea occurs when water is pulled into the intestines by the osmotic pressure of unabsorbed particles, slowing the reabsorption of water. Mixed diarrhea is caused by increased **peristalsis** (usually from IBD) and a combination of increased secretion and decreased absorption in the bowel.

Risk Factors

Diarrhea can be caused by certain medications (e.g., thyroid hormone replacement, stool softeners and laxatives, antibiotics, chemotherapy, magnesium-based antacids), certain tube-feeding formulas, metabolic and endocrine disorders (e.g., diabetes, Addison disease, thyrotoxicosis), and viral or bacterial infectious processes (e.g., dysentery, shigellosis, food poisoning). Other disease processes associated with diarrhea include nutritional and malabsorptive disorders (e.g., celiac disease), anal sphincter defect, Zollinger–Ellison syndrome, paralytic ileus, intestinal obstruction, and AIDS.

Clinical Manifestations and Assessment

In addition to the increased frequency and fluid content of stools, the patient usually has abdominal cramps, distention, intestinal rumbling (**borborygmus**), anorexia, and thirst.

Painful spasmodic contractions of the anus and ineffective straining (**tenesmus**) may occur with defecation. Other symptoms depend on the cause and severity of the diarrhea but are related to dehydration and imbalances of fluid and electrolytes.

Watery stools are characteristic of disorders of the small bowel, whereas loose, semisolid stools are associated more often with disorders of the large bowel. Large, greasy stools suggest intestinal malabsorption, and the presence of mucus and pus in the stools suggests inflammatory enteritis or colitis. Oil droplets on the toilet water are almost always diagnostic of pancreatic insufficiency. Nocturnal diarrhea may be a manifestation of diabetic neuropathy.

Typically, when the source of the diarrhea is not clear, the following diagnostic tests may be performed: complete blood cell count (CBC); serum chemistries; urinalysis; routine stool examination; and stool examinations for infectious or parasitic organisms, bacterial toxins, blood, fat, and electrolytes. Endoscopy or barium enema may assist in identifying the cause.

Nursing Alert

Elderly patients can become dehydrated quickly and develop low potassium levels (i.e., hypokalemia) as a result of diarrhea. The nurse observes for clinical manifestations of muscle weakness, arrhythmias, or decreased peristaltic motility that may lead to paralytic ileus. The older patient taking digitalis (e.g., digoxin [Lanoxin]) must be aware of how quickly dehydration and hypokalemia can occur with diarrhea. The nurse teaches the patient to recognize the symptoms of hypokalemia because low levels of potassium intensify the action of digitalis, leading to digitalis toxicity.

Medical and Nursing Management

Primary management is directed at controlling symptoms, preventing complications, and eliminating or treating the underlying disease. Medications, such as antibiotics (reserved for cases of bacterial overgrowth) and anti-inflammatory agents, may be used to reduce the severity of the diarrhea and treat the underlying disease. The mainstay of treatment in most cases of diarrhea is oral, or, if severe or symptomatic, intravenous rehydration.

The nurse's role includes assessing and monitoring the characteristics and pattern of diarrhea. A health history should address the patient's medication therapy, medical and surgical history, and dietary patterns and intake. Reports of recent exposure to an acute illness or recent travel to another geographic area are important as treatment can change depending on the patient's illness and travel history. Assessment includes abdominal inspection, auscultation (for hyperactive bowel sounds), and palpation for abdominal tenderness. Vital signs are assessed for fever and evidence of fluid volume deficit (weak pulse, hypotension, narrow pulse pressure). Inspection of the mucous membranes and skin is important to determine hydration status. Stool samples are obtained for testing.

During an episode of acute diarrhea, the nurse encourages bedrest and intake of liquids and foods low in bulk until the acute attack subsides. When the patient is able to tolerate food intake, the nurse recommends a bland diet of semisolid and solid foods. The patient should avoid caffeine, carbonated beverages, and very hot and very cold foods due to stimulation of intestinal motility. It may be necessary to restrict milk products, fat, whole-grain products, fresh fruits, and vegetables for several days. Antidiarrheal medications, such as diphenoxylate (Lomotil) or loperamide (Imodium), may be administered as prescribed to reduce the frequency and amount of stools. IV fluid therapy may be necessary for rapid rehydration in some patients, especially in elderly patients and in patients with pre-existing GI conditions, such as IBD. It is important to monitor serum electrolyte levels closely as imbalances such as hypokalemia (K^+ less than 3.5 mEq/L) and acute metabolic acidosis due to a direct loss of bicarbonate (HCO_3^- less than 22 mEq/L) can occur. The nurse immediately reports evidence of arrhythmias, muscular weakness, fatigue or flaccid paralysis, and hyporeflexia (associated with a K^+ less than 2.5 mEq/L).

Nursing Alert

Decreased potassium levels cause cardiac arrhythmias (i.e., atrial and ventricular tachycardia, ventricular fibrillation, premature ventricular contractions) that can lead to death.

The perianal area may become excoriated because diarrheal stool contains digestive enzymes that can irritate the skin. Older individuals have decreased skin turgor and reduced subcutaneous fat layers; therefore, care should be taken to follow a structured perianal skin care routine to reduce irritation and excoriation.

FECAL INCONTINENCE

Fecal incontinence describes the involuntary passage of stool from the rectum. It is estimated that over 40% of residents is extended-care facilities and more than 10% of adults in the community have fecal incontinence. A substantial number of residents in extended-care facilities have what is termed "double incontinence," or difficulties with both urine and stool continence (Shahin & Lohrmann, 2015). Factors that influence fecal continence include the ability of the rectum to sense and accommodate stool, the amount and consistency of stool, the integrity of the anal sphincters and musculature, and rectal motility. It is an embarrassing and socially incapacitating problem that requires a many-tiered approach to treatment and much adaptation on the patient's part.

Nursing Alert
Management of double incontinence should include frequent toileting assistance, identifying patients who may most benefit from targeted toileting programs, and treating underlying fecal disorders including chronic constipation.

Pathophysiology

Continence is maintained by tonic contraction of the muscles around the rectum. During defecation, nerves relax the muscles, causing a straightening of the rectoanal angle. Distension of the rectum causes relaxation of the sphincter. Fecal incontinence is a failure of this process and can occur for a variety of reasons.

Risk Factors

Fecal incontinence can result from trauma (e.g., after surgical procedures involving the rectum), neurologic disorders (e.g., stroke, multiple sclerosis, diabetic neuropathy, dementia), inflammation, infection, chemotherapy, radiation treatment, fecal impaction, pelvic floor relaxation, laxative abuse, medications, or advancing age (i.e., weakness or loss of anal or rectal muscle tone).

Clinical Manifestations and Assessment

Patients may have minor soiling, occasional urgency and loss of control, or complete incontinence. Patients also may experience poor control of flatus, diarrhea, or constipation.

The nurse obtains a thorough health history, including information about previous surgical procedures, chronic illnesses, dietary patterns, bowel habits and problems, and current medication regimen. A visual and digital examination of the rectal area is completed, checking for abnormalities (fecal impaction, hemorrhoids, fissures, and fistulas) that may be contributing to the incontinence.

Diagnostic studies are necessary because the treatment of fecal incontinence depends on the cause. A rectal examination and other endoscopic examinations, such as a flexible sigmoidoscopy, are performed to rule out tumors, inflammation, or fissures. X-ray studies, such as barium enema, computed tomography (CT), anorectal manometry, and transit studies, may be helpful in identifying alterations in intestinal mucosa and muscle tone or in detecting other structural or functional problems.

Medical and Nursing Management

Specific management techniques can help the patient achieve a better quality of life. If fecal incontinence is related to diarrhea, the incontinence may disappear when diarrhea is treated successfully. Frequently fecal incontinence is a symptom of a fecal impaction. After the impaction is removed and the rectum is cleansed, normal functioning of the anorectal area can resume. If the fecal incontinence is related to a more permanent condition, other treatments are initiated. Biofeedback therapy can be of assistance if the problem is decreased sensory awareness or sphincter control. Bowel training programs also can be effective. Surgical procedures include surgical reconstruction, sphincter repair, or fecal diversion.

The nurse initiates a bowel training program that involves setting a schedule to establish bowel regularity. The goal is to help the patient achieve fecal continence. If this is not possible, the goal should be to manage the problem so the person can have predictable, planned elimination. Sometimes, it is necessary to use suppositories to stimulate the anal reflex. After the patient has achieved a regular schedule, the suppository can be discontinued.

Complications

Fecal incontinence may cause problems with perineal skin integrity. Maintaining skin integrity is a priority, especially in the debilitated or elderly patient. Incontinence briefs, although helpful in containing the fecal material, allow for increased skin contact with the feces and may cause excoriation of the skin. The nurse encourages and teaches meticulous skin hygiene, and, in the hospital setting, interventions, such as turning the patient every 2 hours and applying barrier creams or sprays to protect the skin, may be warranted.

Continence sometimes cannot be achieved, and the nurse assists the patient and family to accept and cope with this chronic situation. The patient can use fecal incontinence devices, which include external collection devices and internal drainage systems. External devices are special, drainable pouches. They are attached to a synthetic adhesive skin barrier specially designed to conform to the buttocks. Internal drainage systems can be used to eliminate fecal skin contact and are useful especially when there is extensive excoriation or skin breakdown. A rectal catheter is inserted into the rectum and connected to a drainage system, and stool is collected in order to preserve skin integrity. Rectal catheters are contraindicated in patients who are postoperative from rectal or prostate surgery, recent myocardial infarction, rectal mucosal disease, bleeding dyscrasia, and impaired immune status. It is important to consider that at present, long-term consequences of indwelling fecal collectors have not been studied yet, although some research suggests that some commercially available catheters may be safe for upward of 30 days. A provider's order is required to place these devices.

IRRITABLE BOWEL SYNDROME

IBS is one of the most common GI conditions. Approximately 11% of adults globally report classic symptoms of IBS (Canavan, West, & Card, 2014). Roughly 30% of patients with IBS will consult a health care provider for their symptoms, and patients with IBS have a higher likelihood of other functional GI disorders than those in the general population (Canavan et al., 2014). There is no current evidence that patients with IBS have an increased mortality risk, yet this disorder disrupts daily life for millions of people (Grundmann & Yoon, 2014).

Pathophysiology

IBS results from a functional disorder of intestinal motility. The change in motility may be related to neuroendocrine dysregulation, infection or irritation, or a vascular or metabolic disturbance. The peristaltic waves are affected at specific segments of the intestine and in the intensity with which they propel the fecal matter forward. There is no evidence of inflammation or tissue changes in the intestinal mucosa.

Risk Factors

Although no anatomic or biochemical abnormalities have been found that account for the common symptoms, various factors are associated with the syndrome: heredity, a diet high in fat and stimulating or irritating foods, alcohol consumption, smoking, and psychological stress or conditions such as depression and anxiety. As many as 90% of people diagnosed with IBS present with symptoms of major depression, and it is now suggested that psychotherapy and some antidepressant medications may, in fact, help with symptoms of IBS (Ford et al., 2014).

IBS occurs more commonly in women than in men (Grundmann & Yoon, 2014).

Clinical Manifestations and Assessment

There is a wide variability in symptom presentation. Symptoms range in intensity and duration from mild and infrequent to severe and continuous. The primary symptom is an alteration in bowel patterns—constipation, diarrhea, or a combination of both. Pain and abdominal distention often accompany changes in bowel pattern. Sometimes the abdominal pain is precipitated by eating, and frequently it is relieved by defecation.

A definite diagnosis of IBS requires tests that confirm the absence of structural or other disorders. Stool studies, contrast x-ray studies, and proctoscopy may be performed to rule out other colon diseases. Barium enema and colonoscopy may reveal spasm, distention, or mucus accumulation in the intestine (Fig. 24-1). Manometry and electromyography (EMG) are used to study intraluminal pressure changes generated by spasticity.

Medical and Nursing Management

The goals of treatment are relieving abdominal pain, controlling the diarrhea or constipation, and reducing stress. Restriction and then gradual reintroduction of foods that are possibly irritating may help determine what types of food are acting as irritants (e.g., beans, caffeinated products, fried foods, alcohol, and spicy foods). A high-fiber

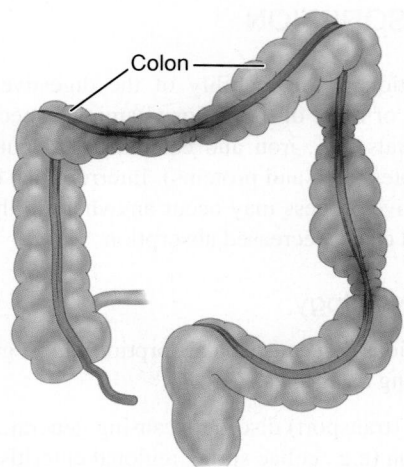

FIGURE 24-1 In irritable bowel syndrome (IBS), the spastic contractions of the bowel can be seen on x-ray contrast studies.

diet is prescribed to help control the diarrhea and constipation. Exercise can assist in reducing anxiety and increasing intestinal motility. Patients often find it helpful to participate in a stress reduction or behavior modification program. Hydrophilic colloids (i.e., bulk) and antidiarrheal agents (e.g., loperamide [Imodium]) may be given to control the diarrhea and fecal urgency. Antidepressants can assist in treating underlying anxiety and depression. Anticholinergics (e.g., propantheline [Pro-Banthine]) may be taken to decrease smooth muscle spasm, thus decreasing cramping and constipation.

Research is ongoing to continue to identify pharmacologic and psychological therapies, including hypnotherapy and cognitive behavioral therapy to lessen the impact of IBS in patients. Current therapies, including antidepressants, hypnotherapy, and various forms of psychotherapy, all are potential effective treatments for IBS (Ford et al., 2014). The role of alternative and complementary therapies for the treatment of IBS is increasing, and research into alternative therapies, such as acupuncture, is ongoing (Halland & Talley, 2013).

The nurse's role is to provide patient and family education. The nurse emphasizes teaching and reinforces good dietary habits. Patients are encouraged to eat at regular times and to chew food slowly and thoroughly. They should understand that although adequate fluid intake is necessary, fluid should not be taken with meals because this results in abdominal distention. Alcohol use and cigarettes should be avoided.

 Nursing Alert
The key to treating IBS in patients is to treat each patient as an individual. Nursing care plans should include interventions that are based on that patient's unique and individual symptoms blending both pharmacologic and psychological-based interventions specific to that particular patient.

MALABSORPTION

Malabsorption is the inability of the digestive system to absorb one or more of the major vitamins (especially A and B_{12}), minerals (i.e., iron and calcium), and nutrients (i.e., carbohydrates, fats, and proteins). Interruptions in the complex digestive process may occur anywhere in the digestive system and cause decreased absorption.

Pathophysiology

The conditions that cause malabsorption can be grouped into the following categories:

- Mucosal (transport) disorders causing generalized malabsorption (e.g., celiac sprue, regional enteritis, radiation enteritis)
- Infectious diseases causing generalized malabsorption (e.g., small bowel bacterial overgrowth, tropical sprue)
- Luminal disorders causing malabsorption (e.g., bile acid deficiency, Zollinger–Ellison syndrome, pancreatic insufficiency)
- Postoperative malabsorption (e.g., after gastric or intestinal resection)
- Disorders that cause malabsorption of specific nutrients (e.g., disaccharidase deficiency leading to lactose intolerance)

Table 24-2 lists the clinical and pathologic aspects of malabsorptive diseases.

Risk Factors

Risk factors predisposing people to malabsorption include any process that interferes with the body's ability to absorb nutrients. These can include pathologic factors, including abdominal diseases or deformities, surgery, radiation therapy, and certain medications that inhibit bacterial growth within the intestine (antibiotics). Bodily fluid losses, from such things as polyuria, emesis, wound drainage, or diarrhea, can decrease absorption. Finally, use of medications, such as mineral oil or laxatives, can decrease absorption by increasing peristalsis.

Clinical Manifestations and Assessment

The hallmarks of malabsorption syndrome are diarrhea or frequent, loose, bulky, foul-smelling stools that have increased fat content and often are grayish in color. Patients often have associated abdominal distention, pain, increased flatus, weakness, weight loss, and a decreased sense of well-being. The chief result of malabsorption is malnutrition, manifested by weight loss and other signs of vitamin and mineral deficiency (e.g., easy bruising [vitamin K deficiency], osteoporosis [calcium deficiency], anemia [iron, vitamin B_{12} deficiency]).

Patients with a malabsorption syndrome, if untreated, become weak and emaciated because of starvation and dehydration. Failure to absorb the fat-soluble vitamins A, D, and K causes a corresponding avitaminosis (chronic or long-term vitamin deficiency).

Several diagnostic tests may be prescribed, including stool studies for quantitative and qualitative fat analysis, lactose tolerance tests, D-xylose absorption tests (absorption of sugar), and Schilling tests (B_{12} deficiency). The hydrogen breath test that is used to evaluate carbohydrate absorption is performed if carbohydrate malabsorption is suspected. This test requires the patient to be fasting before he or she ingests 25 g of carbohydrate dissolved in water. Exhaled breath is assayed for hydrogen content at baseline and at specific intervals for several hours. Since hydrogen is not a normal product of human metabolism, any increase in breath hydrogen concentration suggests bacterial fermentation and indicates that unabsorbed carbohydrate has reached an area with high concentrations of intraluminal bacteria, typically the colon (Schiller & Sellin, 2016).

Endoscopy with biopsy of the mucosa is the best diagnostic tool. Biopsy of the small intestine is performed to assay enzyme activity or to identify infection or destruction of mucosa. Ultrasound studies, CT scans, and x-ray findings can reveal pancreatic or intestinal tumors that may be the cause. A CBC is used to detect anemia. Pancreatic function tests can assist in the diagnosis of specific disorders.

Medical and Nursing Management

Intervention is aimed at avoiding dietary substances that aggravate malabsorption and at supplementing nutrients that have been lost. Common supplements are water-soluble vitamins (e.g., B_{12}, folic acid), fat-soluble vitamins (e.g., A, D, and K), and minerals (e.g., calcium, iron). Primary disease states may be managed surgically or medically. Dietary therapy is aimed at reducing gluten intake in patients with celiac sprue. Folic acid supplements are prescribed for patients with tropical sprue (see Table 24-2). Sometimes antibiotics (e.g., tetracycline [Tetracap, Tetracyn], ampicillin [Polycillin]) are needed in the treatment of tropical sprue and bacterial overgrowth syndromes. Antidiarrheal agents may be used to decrease intestinal spasms. Parenteral fluids may be necessary to treat dehydration.

The nurse provides patient and family education regarding diet and the use of nutritional supplements. It is important to monitor patients with diarrhea for fluid and electrolyte imbalances. The nurse conducts ongoing assessments to determine whether the clinical manifestations related to the nutritional deficits have abated. Patient education includes information about the risk of osteoporosis related to malabsorption of calcium (refer to Chapter 41 for information on osteoporosis).

Pathophysiology Alert
Patients who are severely malnourished are at a higher risk of developing refeeding syndrome if fed too rapidly. Excessively high dextrose administration (e.g., PPN, TPN) stimulates

TABLE **24-2** Characteristics of Diseases of Malabsorption

Diseases/Disorders	Physiologic Pathology	Clinical Features
Gastric resection with gastrojejunostomy	Decreased pancreatic stimulation because of duodenal bypass; poor mixing of food, bile, pancreatic enzymes; decreased intrinsic factor	Weight loss, moderate steatorrhea (presence of fat within the stool), anemia (combination of iron deficiency, vitamin B_{12} malabsorption, folate deficiency)
Pancreatic insufficiency (chronic pancreatitis, pancreatic carcinoma, pancreatic resection, cystic fibrosis)	Reduced intraluminal pancreatic enzyme activity, with maldigestion of lipids and proteins	History of abdominal pain followed by weight loss; marked steatorrhea, azotorrhea (excess of nitrogenous matter in the feces or urine); also frequent glucose intolerance (70% in pancreatic insufficiency)
Ileal dysfunction (resection or disease)	Loss of ileal absorbing surface leads to reduced bile-salt pool size and reduced vitamin B_{12} absorption; bile in colon inhibits fluid absorption	Diarrhea, weight loss with steatorrhea, especially when more than 100 cm resection, decreased vitamin B_{12} absorption
Stasis syndromes (surgical strictures, blind loops, enteric fistulas, multiple jejunal diverticula, scleroderma)	Overgrowth of intraluminal intestinal bacteria, especially anaerobic organisms, to more than 10^6/mL results in deconjugation of bile salts, leading to decreased effective bile-salt pool size, also bacterial utilization of vitamin B_{12}	Weight loss, steatorrhea; low vitamin B_{12} absorption; may have low D-xylose absorption
Zollinger–Ellison syndrome	Hyperacidity in duodenum inactivates pancreatic enzymes	Ulcer; steatorrhea
Lactose intolerance	Deficiency of intestinal lactase results in high concentration of intraluminal lactose with osmotic diarrhea	Varied degrees of diarrhea and cramps after ingestion of lactose-containing foods; positive lactose intolerance test, decreased intestinal lactase
Celiac disease (gluten enteropathy)	Toxic response to a gluten fraction by surface epithelium results in destruction of absorbing surface	Weight loss, diarrhea, bloating, anemia (low iron, folate), osteomalacia, steatorrhea, azotorrhea, low D-xylose absorption; folate and iron malabsorption
Tropical sprue	Unknown toxic factor results in mucosal inflammation, partial villous atrophy	Weight loss, diarrhea, anemia (low folate, vitamin B_{12}); steatorrhea; low D-xylose absorption, low vitamin B_{12} absorption
Whipple disease	Bacterial invasion of intestinal mucosa	Arthritis, hyperpigmentation, lymphadenopathy, serous effusions, fever, weight loss, steatorrhea, azotorrhea
Certain parasitic diseases (giardiasis, strongyloidiasis, coccidiosis, capillariasis)	Damage to or invasion of surface mucosa	Diarrhea, weight loss; steatorrhea; organism may be seen on jejunal biopsy or recovered in stool
Immunoglobulinopathy	Decreased local intestinal defenses, lymphoid hyperplasia, lymphopenia	Frequent association with Giardia: hypogammaglobulinemia or isolated IgA deficiency

insulin release, which rapidly lowers phosphorus, magnesium, and potassium in the blood (due to intracellular shift and use in carbohydrate metabolic pathways). The hyperinsulinemia also tends to cause sodium and fluid retention. Thiamine also is consumed with high carbohydrate loads. The combination of fluid and sodium retention, decrease in blood electrolyte levels (which can cause arrhythmias), and hypermetabolism due to increased calories can result in heart failure. Thus, the complications of refeeding syndrome can include a variety of fluid and electrolyte disturbances, which can include hypoglycemia, cardiac arrhythmias, and death. Risk factors for refeeding syndrome include pre-existing malnutrition, electrolyte depletion, or alcoholism, and after prolonged periods of intravenous hydration therapy (e.g., 5% dextrose) without nutrition support (Chiappetta & Stein, 2016).

TABLE **24-3** Malabsorption of Nutrients, Water, and Electrolytes

Nutrient Malabsorbed	Clinical Manifestation
Protein	Wasting, hypoproteinemic edema
Carbohydrate and fat	Diarrhea, abdominal cramps and bloating, weight loss and growth retardation
Fluid	Kidney stones with volume depletion, weight loss, fluid volume deficit (FVD)
Iron	Anemia
Calcium and vitamin D	Bone pain, fractures, tetany
Magnesium	Paresthesias, tetany
Vitamin B_{12} and folate	Anemia, paresthesias, ataxia (vitamin B_{12} only)
Vitamin E	Paresthesias, ataxia, retinopathy
Vitamin A	Night blindness, diarrhea
Vitamin K	Ecchymoses, bruises easily
Selenium	Cardiomyopathy
Malabsorption of bile salts	Increased colonic fluid secretion and watery diarrhea

Adapted from Semrad, C. (2016). Approach to the patient with diarrhea and malabsorption. In L. Goldman & A. I. Schafer (Eds.), *Goldman-Cecil medicine* (25th ed.). New York: Elsevier/Saunders.

Complications

Complications are related to the underlying disease causing the malabsorption. Depending on the etiology, medical management may include the administration of corticosteroids (for regional enteritis), which may cause a host of adverse effects, such as hypertension, hypokalemia, insomnia, and euphoria. Antibiotics may reduce vitamin K–producing intestinal flora, resulting in a prolonged prothrombin time (PT) and international normalized ratio (INR) if the patient is concurrently taking warfarin (Coumadin). Refer to Table 24-3 for clinical manifestations of malabsorption.

ACUTE INFLAMMATORY CONDITIONS

Appendicitis

The appendix is a small, finger-like appendage about 10 cm (4 in) long that is attached to the cecum just below the ileocecal valve. The appendix fills with food and empties regularly into the cecum. Because it empties inefficiently and its lumen is small, the appendix is prone to obstruction and is particularly vulnerable to infection (i.e., appendicitis).

Appendicitis is the most common reason for emergency abdominal surgery, with an incidence rate in the overall population of 7% to 14% in (Flum, 2015). The disease is most common in patients between 10 and 30 years of age, with a higher incidence in men than women (Flum, 2015).

Pathophysiology

The appendix becomes inflamed and edematous as a result of becoming kinked or occluded by a fecalith (i.e., hardened mass of stool), tumor, or foreign body. The inflammatory process increases intraluminal pressure, initiating a progressively severe, generalized or periumbilical pain that becomes localized to the right lower quadrant of the abdomen within a few hours. Eventually, the inflamed appendix fills with pus.

Risk Factors

Appendicitis is most prevalent in the young, but it can occur at any age. Most cases appear in the winter months although no clear reason as to why has been established. Having a family history of appendicitis may increase a child's risk for the illness, especially in males, and having cystic fibrosis also seems to put a child at higher risk (Lavelle et al., 2015).

Clinical Manifestations and Assessment

Vague epigastric or periumbilical pain progresses to right lower quadrant pain and usually is accompanied by a low-grade fever and nausea and, sometimes, vomiting. Loss of appetite is common. In up to 50% of presenting cases, local tenderness is elicited at McBurney point when pressure is applied (Fig. 24-2). Rebound tenderness (production or intensification of pain when pressure is released) may be present. The extent of tenderness and muscle spasm and the existence of constipation or diarrhea depend not so much on the severity of the appendiceal infection as on the location of the appendix. If the appendix curls around behind the cecum, pain and tenderness may be felt in the lumbar region. If its tip is in the pelvis, these signs may be elicited only on rectal examination. Pain on defecation suggests that the tip of the appendix is resting against the rectum; pain on urination suggests that the tip is near the bladder or impinges on the ureter. Some rigidity of the lower portion of the right rectus muscle may occur. Rovsing sign may be elicited by palpating the left lower quadrant; this paradoxically causes pain to be felt in the right lower quadrant (see Fig. 24-2). If the appendix has ruptured, the pain becomes more diffuse; abdominal distention develops as a result of paralytic ileus, and the patient's condition worsens.

> **Nursing Alert**
> *Constipation also can occur with an acute process, such as appendicitis. Laxatives administered in this instance may result in perforation*

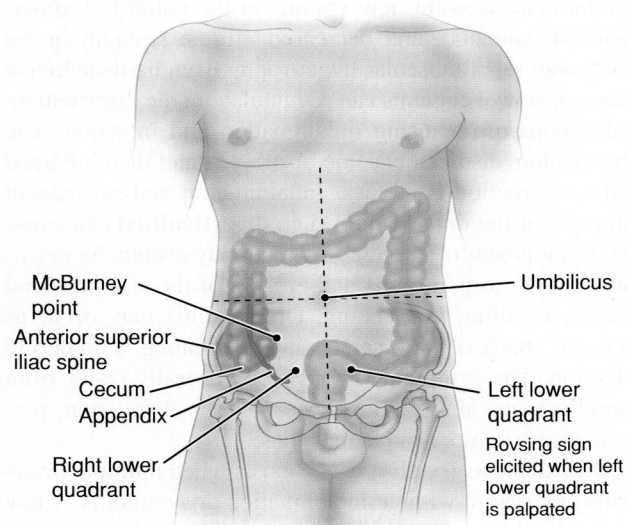

McBurney point

Umbilicus

Anterior superior iliac spine

Cecum

Appendix

Right lower quadrant

Left lower quadrant

Rovsing sign elicited when left lower quadrant is palpated

FIGURE 24-2 When the appendix is inflamed, tenderness can be noted in the right lower quadrant at McBurney point, which is between the umbilicus and the anterior superior iliac spine. Rovsing sign is pain felt in the right lower quadrant after the left lower quadrant has been palpated.

of the inflamed appendix. In general, a laxative or cathartic should never be given when a person has fever, nausea, or pain.

Diagnosis is based on results of a complete physical examination and on laboratory findings and imaging studies. The CBC demonstrates an elevated white blood cell (WBC) count with an elevation of the neutrophils. Abdominal x-ray films, ultrasound studies, and CT scans may reveal a right lower quadrant density or localized distention of the bowel. A diagnostic laparoscopy may be used to rule out acute appendicitis in equivocal cases.

Acute appendicitis is uncommon in the elderly population. When it does occur, classic signs and symptoms are altered and may vary greatly. Pain may be absent or minimal. Symptoms may be vague, suggesting bowel obstruction or another process. Fever and leukocytosis may not be present. As a result, diagnosis and prompt treatment may be delayed, causing complications and mortality. The patient may have no symptoms until the appendix ruptures. The incidence of perforated appendix is higher in the elderly population because many of these patients do not seek health care as quickly as younger patients.

Medical and Nursing Management

Typically, immediate surgery is indicated if appendicitis is diagnosed. To correct or prevent fluid and electrolyte imbalance, dehydration, and sepsis, antibiotics and IV fluids are administered until surgery is performed. Appendectomy (i.e., surgical removal of the appendix) is performed as soon as possible to decrease the risk of perforation. It may

be performed using general or spinal anesthesia with a low abdominal incision (laparotomy) or by laparoscopy. Both laparotomy and laparoscopy are safe and effective in the treatment of appendicitis with perforation. However, generally recovery after laparoscopic surgery is quicker.

When perforation of the appendix occurs, an **abscess** may form. If this occurs, the patient may be treated initially with antibiotics, and the surgeon may place a drain in the abscess during the operative procedure to facilitate drainage. Subsequent surgical procedures may be performed to ensure complete drainage of the abscess. The postoperative care of the patient with a perforated appendix is more complex and complicated due to the risk of developing sepsis and organ damage.

The nurse prepares the patient for surgery, which includes an IV infusion to replace fluid loss and promote adequate kidney function, and antibiotic therapy to prevent infection. If there is evidence or likelihood of paralytic ileus, a nasogastric tube is inserted. An enema is not administered because it can lead to perforation.

After surgery, the nurse places the patient in a high Fowler position. This position reduces the tension on the incision and abdominal organs, helping to reduce pain. An opioid, usually morphine sulfate, is prescribed to relieve pain. When tolerated, oral fluids are administered. Any patient who was dehydrated before surgery receives IV fluids. Food is provided as desired and tolerated on the day of surgery, once normal bowel sounds are present.

The patient may be discharged on the day of surgery if the temperature is within normal limits, there is no undue discomfort in the operative area, and the appendectomy was uncomplicated. Discharge teaching for the patient and family is imperative. The nurse instructs the patient to make an appointment to have the surgeon remove the sutures between the fifth and seventh days after surgery. Incision care and activity guidelines are discussed; usually normal activity can be resumed within 2 to 4 weeks.

If there is a possibility of **peritonitis**, a drain is left in place at the area of the incision. Patients at risk for this complication may be kept in the hospital for several days and are monitored carefully for signs of intestinal obstruction or secondary hemorrhage. Secondary abscesses may form in the pelvis, under the diaphragm, or in the liver, causing elevation of the temperature, pulse rate, and WBC count.

When the patient is ready for discharge, the nurse teaches the patient and family to care for the incision and perform dressing changes and irrigations as prescribed. A home care nurse may be needed to assist with this care and to monitor the patient for complications and wound healing.

Complications

The major complication of appendicitis is perforation of the appendix, which can lead to peritonitis, abscess formation (collection of purulent material), or portal pylephlebitis, which is septic thrombosis of the portal vein caused by

TABLE **24-4** Potential Complications and Nursing Interventions After Appendectomy

Complication	Nursing Interventions
Peritonitis	Observe for abdominal tenderness, fever, vomiting, abdominal rigidity, and tachycardia. Employ nasogastric suction. Correct dehydration as prescribed. Administer antibiotic agents as prescribed.
Pelvic abscess	Evaluate for anorexia, chills, fever, and diaphoresis. Observe for diarrhea, which may indicate pelvic abscess. Prepare patient for rectal examination. Prepare patient for surgical drainage procedure.
Subphrenic abscess (abscess under the diaphragm)	Assess patient for chills, fever, and diaphoresis. Observe for Hiccups because of diaphragmatic irritation. Prepare for x-ray examination. Prepare for surgical drainage of abscess.
Ileus (paralytic and mechanical)	Assess for bowel sounds. Employ nasogastric intubation and suction. Replace fluids and electrolytes by intravenous route as prescribed. Prepare for surgery if diagnosis of mechanical ileus is established.

vegetative emboli that arise from septic intestines. Perforation generally occurs 24 hours after the onset of pain if no intervention has occurred. Symptoms include a fever of 37.7°C (100°F) or greater, a toxic appearance, and continued abdominal pain or tenderness. Other complications of appendectomy are listed in Table 24-4.

DIVERTICULAR DISEASE

A diverticulum is a sac-like herniation of the lining of the bowel that extends through a defect in the muscle layer. Diverticula may occur anywhere in the small intestine or colon but occur most commonly in the distal sigmoid colon. The incidence of diverticular disease of the colon is 35% to 50%, and increases with age. For example, the incidence is less than 10% under age 40, but rises to 80% when over 85 (Ferri, 2017). The health care cost of diverticular disease is estimated at more than $2 billion (Perry et al., 2012).

Pathophysiology

Diverticula form when the mucosa and submucosal layers of the colon herniate through the muscular wall because of high intraluminal pressure, low volume in the colon (i.e., fiber-deficient contents), and decreased muscle strength in the colon wall (e.g., muscular hypertrophy from hardened fecal masses). Bowel contents can accumulate in the diverticulum and decompose, causing inflammation and infection. The diverticulum also can become obstructed and then inflamed if the obstruction continues. Inflammation and subsequent infection of the diverticulum (i.e., **diverticulitis**) can cause the development of abscesses, which may eventually perforate, leading to peritonitis and erosion of the arterial blood vessels, resulting in bleeding. Diverticulitis may occur as an acute attack or may persist as a continuing, smoldering infection. The symptoms manifested generally result from complications: abscess, fistula formation, obstruction, perforation, peritonitis, and hemorrhage.

Diverticulosis (see Fig. 24-3) exists when multiple diverticula are present without inflammation or symptoms. A low intake of dietary fiber is considered a predisposing factor, but the exact cause has not been identified. Most patients with diverticular disease are asymptomatic, so its exact prevalence is unknown.

Risk Factors

It is estimated that 10% to 25% of people with diverticulosis have diverticulitis at some point in their lives (Shahedi et al., 2013). A congenital predisposition is suspected when the disorder occurs in those younger than 40 years of age.

Clinical Manifestations and Assessment

Chronic constipation often precedes the development of diverticulosis, sometimes by many years. Frequently, no problematic symptoms occur with diverticulosis. Signs and symptoms of diverticulosis are relatively mild and include bowel irregularity with intervals of diarrhea, nausea, anorexia, and abdominal distention. Abdominal pain may radiate to the back, flank,

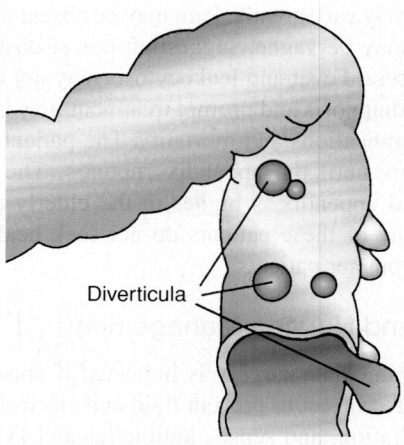

FIGURE 24-3 (Top) Location of diverticula in the sigmoid colon; (Bottom left) Diverticulosis; (Bottom right) Diverticulitis. (Reprinted with permission from Diepenbrock, N. (2011). *Quick reference to critical care* (4th ed.). Philadelphia, PA: Wolters Kluwer.)

or suprapubic region. With repeated local inflammation of the diverticula, the large bowel may narrow with fibrotic strictures, leading to cramps, narrow stools, and increased constipation or, at times, intestinal obstruction. Weakness, fatigue, and anorexia are common symptoms. With diverticulitis, the patient reports an acute onset of mild to severe pain in the lower left quadrant, accompanied by nausea, vomiting, fever, chills, and leukocytosis (elevated WBC). Rebound tenderness is suggestive of perforation. The condition, if untreated, can lead to septicemia (see Chapter 54).

Typically diverticulosis is diagnosed by colonoscopy, which permits visualization of the extent of diverticular disease and allows the clinician to biopsy tissue to rule out other diseases as needed. Until recently, barium enema had been the preferred diagnostic test, but now it is used less frequently than colonoscopy. However, if acute diverticulosis is suspected or there are symptoms of peritoneal irritation, a colonoscopy or barium enema is contraindicated because of potential for perforation. CT scan is the diagnostic test of choice if the suspected diagnosis is diverticulitis; it also can reveal one or more abscesses. Abdominal x-rays may demonstrate free air under the diaphragm if a perforation has occurred from the diverticulitis, which causes peritonitis. Laboratory tests that assist in diagnosis include a CBC, revealing an elevated WBC count, and elevated erythrocyte sedimentation rate (ESR).

Gerontologic Considerations

The incidence of diverticular disease increases with age because of degeneration and structural changes in the circular muscle layers of the colon and because of cellular hypertrophy. The symptoms are less pronounced in the elderly than in other adults. The elderly may not have abdominal pain until infection occurs. They may delay reporting symptoms because they fear surgery or are afraid that they may have cancer. Frequently blood in the stool is overlooked, especially in the elderly because of a failure to examine the stool or the inability to see changes if vision is impaired.

Medical and Nursing Management

Usually diverticulitis can be treated on an outpatient basis with diet and medication. When symptoms occur, rest, analgesics, and antispasmodics are recommended. Initially, the diet is clear liquid until the inflammation subsides; then a high-fiber, low-fat diet is recommended. This type of diet helps increase stool volume, decrease colonic transit time, and reduce intraluminal pressure. Antibiotics are prescribed for 7 to 10 days. A bulk-forming laxative also is prescribed.

> **Nursing Alert**
> *High-fiber foods include items such as potatoes, rice, artichoke, and split peas. In addition, patient teaching can include adding foods*

such as raspberries and pears as snacks to help increase fiber intake. In the past, it was recommended that people with diverticular disease (diverticulosis or diverticulitis) avoid nuts, corn, popcorn, and seeds for fear that these foods would become lodged in the diverticula and lead to inflammation. However, there is no convincing evidence to support any particular foods that should be favored or avoided (Wilkins, Embry, & George, 2013).

In acute cases of diverticulitis hospitalization may be required for patients who cannot tolerate PO fluids and food. Measures taken to rest the bowel include withholding oral intake, administering IV fluids and antibiotics, and instituting nasogastric suctioning if vomiting or abdominal distention are present. An opioid is prescribed for pain relief. Historically, morphine was considered to be contraindicated because of a claim that it could increase intraluminal pressure in the colon, thus exacerbating symptoms; however, no research evidence is available to support this claim. Uncomplicated acute diverticulitis can be managed with oral antibiotics for 7 to 10 days in the outpatient setting. Nonsteroidal anti-inflammatory drugs (NSAIDs) are associated with increased risk of perforation and should be avoided.

More often than not, acute diverticulitis will subside with medical management. Immediate surgical intervention is necessary if complications (e.g., perforation, peritonitis, hemorrhage, obstruction) occur. In cases of abscess formation without peritonitis, hemorrhage, or obstruction, CT-guided percutaneous drainage may be performed to drain the abscess, and IV antibiotics are administered. Stabilization of the patient by drainage of the abscess and resolution of the inflammation is complete after approximately 6 weeks; surgery may be recommended to prevent repeated episodes. Typically two types of surgery are considered either to treat acute complications or to prevent further episodes of inflammation:

- One-stage resection, in which the inflamed area is removed and a primary end-to-end anastomosis is completed
- Multiple-stage procedures for complications such as obstruction or perforation (Fig. 24-4)

The type of surgery performed depends on the extent of complications found during surgery. When possible, the area of diverticulitis is taken out and the remaining bowel is joined end-to-end (i.e., primary resection and end-to-end anastomosis). This is performed through traditional surgical or laparoscopically assisted colectomy. A two-stage resection may be performed in which the diseased colon is removed (as in a one-stage procedure) but no anastomosis is performed; both ends of the bowel are brought out onto the abdomen as stomas. Then this "double-barrel" temporary colostomy is reanastomosed in a later procedure. Fecal diversion procedures are discussed later in this chapter.

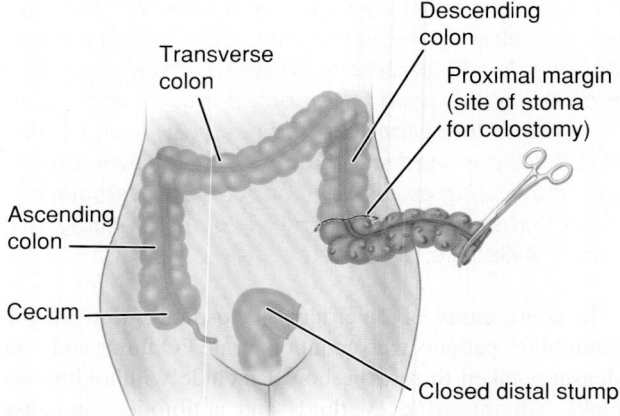

FIGURE 24-4 The Hartmann procedure for diverticulitis: primary resection for diverticulitis of the colon. The affected segment (*clamp attached*) has been divided at its distal end. In a primary anastomosis, the proximal margin (*dotted line*) is transected and the bowel attached end-to-end. In a two-stage procedure, a colostomy is constructed at the proximal margin with the distal stump oversewn (Hartmann procedure, as shown) or brought to the outer surface as a mucous fistula. The second stage consists of colostomy takedown and anastomosis.

Complications

Complications of diverticulitis include peritonitis (see below), abscess formation, and bleeding. If an abscess develops, the associated findings are tenderness, a palpable mass, fever, and leukocytosis. An inflamed diverticulum that perforates results in abdominal pain localized over the involved segment, usually the sigmoid; local abscess or peritonitis follows. Abdominal pain, a rigid board-like abdomen, loss of bowel sounds, and signs and symptoms of shock occur with peritonitis. Noninflamed or slightly inflamed diverticula may erode areas adjacent to arterial branches, causing massive rectal bleeding.

PERITONITIS

Peritonitis is inflammation of the peritoneum, the serous membrane lining the abdominal cavity and covering the viscera. Peritonitis is typically a life-threatening emergency that requires prompt surgical intervention and typically involves postoperative critical care monitoring due to the risk of sepsis, organ failure, and subsequent infections.

> ### Nursing Alert
> The development of peritonitis can include a variety of signs and symptoms in patients, including a firm and distended abdomen, rebound tenderness, and guarding by the patient of the abdomen during the examination. These signs and symptoms should cue nurses into suspecting peritonitis in their patients.

Pathophysiology

Peritonitis is caused by leakage of contents from abdominal organs into the abdominal cavity, usually as a result of inflammation, infection, ischemia, trauma, or tumor perforation. Bacterial proliferation occurs. Edema of the tissues ensues, and exudation of fluid develops in a short time. Fluid in the peritoneal cavity becomes turbid with increasing amounts of protein, WBCs, cellular debris, and blood. The immediate response of the intestinal tract is hypermotility, soon followed by paralytic ileus with an accumulation of air and fluid in the bowel.

Risk Factors

Usually, peritonitis is a result of bacterial infection; the organisms come from diseases of the GI tract or, in women, from the internal reproductive organs. Peritonitis also can result from external sources, such as injury or trauma (e.g., gunshot wound, stab wound) or an inflammation that extends from an organ outside the peritoneal area, such as the kidney. The most common bacteria implicated are gram-negative organisms (*Escherichia coli*, *Klebsiella*, *Proteus*), gram-positive bacteria (enterococci, streptococci, staphylococci), anaerobic bacteria (*Bacteroides*, *Clostridium*), and fungi (Ferri, 2016). Inflammation and paralytic ileus are the direct effects of the infection. Other common causes of peritonitis are appendicitis, perforated ulcer, diverticulitis, and bowel perforation (Fig. 24-5). Peritonitis also may be associated with abdominal surgical procedures and peritoneal dialysis.

Clinical Manifestations and Assessment

Symptoms depend on the location and extent of the inflammation. The early clinical manifestations of peritonitis

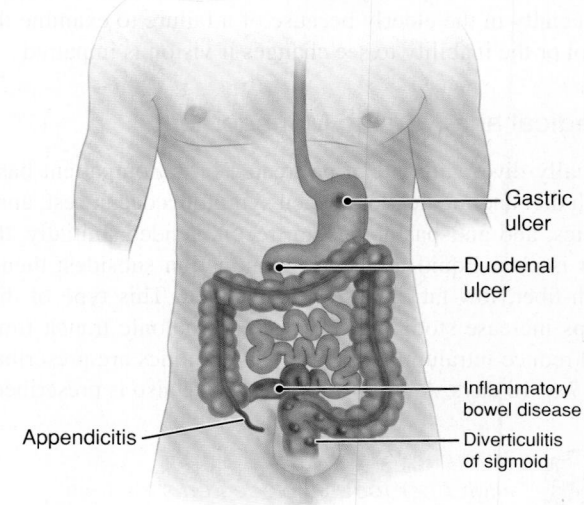

FIGURE 24-5 Common gastrointestinal causes of peritonitis.

frequently are the symptoms of the disorder causing the condition, aptly nicknamed an "acute abdomen." At first, a diffuse type of pain is felt. The pain tends to become constant, localized, and more intense near the site of the inflammation. Movement usually aggravates it. The affected area of the abdomen becomes extremely tender and distended, and the muscles become rigid. Rebound tenderness and paralytic ileus may be present. Diminished perception of pain in peritonitis can occur in people receiving corticosteroids or analgesics. Patients with diabetes who have symptoms of advanced neuropathy and patients with cirrhosis who have signs of ascites may not experience pain during an acute bacterial episode. Usually, nausea and vomiting occur, and peristalsis is diminished (decreased bowel sounds). A temperature of 100° to 101°F (37.8° to 38.3°C) can be expected, along with an increased pulse rate, tachypnea, dyspnea, and hypotension.

The WBC count is almost always elevated. The hemoglobin and hematocrit levels may be low if blood loss has occurred. Serum electrolyte studies may reveal altered levels of potassium, sodium, and chloride.

An abdominal x-ray study may show air and fluid levels as well as distended bowel loops. A CT scan of the abdomen may show abscess formation, acute inflammation or infection of one of the major abdominal organs, or a perforation of the small or large bowel. Peritoneal aspiration and culture and sensitivity studies of the aspirated fluid may reveal infection and identify the causative organisms.

Medical and Nursing Management

Fluid, colloid, and electrolyte replacement is the major focus of medical management. The administration of several liters of an isotonic solution is emergently prescribed. Hypovolemia occurs because massive amounts of fluid and electrolytes move from the intestinal lumen into the peritoneal cavity and deplete the fluid in the vascular space.

Analgesics are prescribed for pain. Antiemetics are administered as prescribed for nausea and vomiting. Placement of a nasogastric tube is warranted, and suction is maintained to assist in relieving abdominal distention. Fluid in the abdominal cavity can cause pressure that restricts expansion of the lungs and causes respiratory distress. Oxygen therapy by nasal cannula or mask generally promotes adequate oxygenation, but airway intubation and ventilatory assistance occasionally are required due to the patient's inability to compensate for the metabolic acidosis that typically occurs with peritonitis.

Antibiotic therapy is initiated early in the treatment of peritonitis. Large doses of a broad-spectrum antibiotic and antifungicide are administered IV until the specific organism causing the infection is identified and appropriate antibiotic therapy can be initiated.

Surgical objectives include removing the infected material and correcting the cause. Surgical treatment is directed toward excision (i.e., appendix), resection with or without anastomosis (i.e., intestine), repair (i.e., perforation), and/or drainage (i.e., abscess). With sepsis accompanying the peritonitis, a fecal diversion may need to be created.

The two most common postoperative complications are wound evisceration and abscess formation. Any suggestion from the patient that an area of the abdomen is tender or painful or "feels as if something just gave way" must be reported. The sudden occurrence of serosanguineous wound drainage strongly suggests wound dehiscence and is a surgical emergency that must be reported promptly to the on-call provider.

Often intensive care is needed. The blood pressure is monitored by arterial line if shock is present. Accurate recording of all intake and output and central venous pressures and/or pulmonary artery pressures assists in calculating fluid replacement. The nurse administers and closely monitors IV fluids response.

In addition, ongoing assessment of pain, GI function, and fluid and electrolyte balance is important. Bladder pressure also is measured routinely to identify abdominal compartment syndrome (refer to Chapter 53, Fig. 53-4). The nurse reports the nature of the pain, its location in the abdomen, and any changes in location. Administering analgesic medication and positioning the patient for comfort are helpful in decreasing pain. The patient is placed on the side with knees flexed; this position decreases tension on the abdominal organs.

Signs that indicate that peritonitis is subsiding include a decrease in temperature and pulse rate, softening of the abdomen, return of peristaltic sounds, and passing of flatus and bowel movements. The nurse increases fluid and food intake gradually and reduces parenteral fluids as prescribed. A worsening clinical condition may indicate a complication, and the nurse must prepare the patient for emergency surgery.

Frequently drains are inserted during the surgical procedure, and the nurse must observe and record the character of the drainage postoperatively. Care must be taken when moving and turning the patient to prevent the drains from being dislodged. It is prudent to safety-pin the drains to the patient's gown to limit the chance of accidental dislodgement. Also it is important for the nurse to prepare the patient and family for discharge by teaching the patient to care for the incision and drains if the patient will be sent home with the drains still in place. Referral for home care or rehabilitation may be indicated for further monitoring and patient and family teaching.

Complications

Frequently, the inflammation is not localized, and the entire abdominal cavity shows evidence of widespread infection. Sepsis is the major cause of death from peritonitis. Shock may result from septicemia or hypovolemia. The inflammatory process may cause intestinal obstruction, primarily from the development of bowel adhesions, and care must be made to monitor the patient's nasogastric tube drainage and input and output closely. The patient is also at high risk of developing pulmonary emboli, and compression stockings, sequential-compression boots, and subcutaneous anticoagulation may be prescribed.

INFLAMMATORY BOWEL DISEASE

IBD refers to two chronic inflammatory GI disorders: regional enteritis (i.e., Crohn disease) and ulcerative colitis (UC). Both disorders have striking similarities but also several differences (Table 24-5); medical and nursing management for both types is similar and discussed jointly.

The incidence of IBD in the United States has increased to well over 1 million cases (Kaplan, 2015). Typically IBD presents during childhood or later in life and is attributed to a high morbidity and a decreased quality of life (Kaplan & Jess, 2016). Women and men tend to be affected equally, and family history appears to predispose people to develop IBD, particularly if a first-degree relative has the disease.

Despite extensive research, the cause of IBD is still unknown. Researchers theorize that it is triggered by environmental agents, such as pesticides, food additives, tobacco, and radiation (Kaplan & Jess, 2016). NSAIDs have been found to exacerbate IBD. Allergies and immune disorders also have been suggested as causes. Abnormal response to dietary or bacterial antigens has been studied extensively, and genetic factors also are being examined.

REGIONAL ENTERITIS (CROHN DISEASE)

Usually regional enteritis (Crohn disease) is diagnosed first in adolescents or young adults but can appear at any time in a person's life. The incidence of regional enteritis has risen both nationally and internationally, suggesting that Crohn disease is emerging as a disease of global

TABLE 24-5 Comparison of Regional Enteritis and Ulcerative Colitis

Factor	Regional Enteritis	Ulcerative Colitis
Course	Prolonged, variable	Exacerbations, remissions
Pathology		
Early	Transmural thickening	Mucosal ulceration
Late	Deep, penetrating granulomas	Minute, mucosal ulcerations
Clinical Manifestations		
Location	Ileum, ascending colon (usually)	Rectum, descending colon
Bleeding	Usually not, but if it occurs, it tends to be mild	Common—severe
Perianal involvement	Common (seen in 30–45% of patients)	Rare—mild
Fistulas	Common	Rare
Rectal involvement	About 20%	Almost 100%
Diarrhea	Less severe	Severe
Diagnostic Study Findings		
Barium series	Regional, discontinuous lesions Narrowing of colon Thickening of bowel wall Mucosal edema Stenosis, fistulas, fissures "String sign" of the terminal ileum, indicating the constriction of a segment of intestine. Ulcerations (the cobblestone appearance)	Diffuse involvement No narrowing of colon No mucosal edema Rare occurrence of stenosis Shortening of colon
Sigmoidoscopy	May be unremarkable unless accompanied by perianal fistulas	Abnormal inflamed mucosa
Colonoscopy	Distinct ulcerations separated by relatively normal mucosa in ascending colon	Friable mucosa with pseudopolyps or ulcers in descending colon

Factor	Regional Enteritis	Ulcerative Colitis
CT scan*	May show bowel-wall thickening and fistula formation in regional enteritis (Crohn disease)	Depicts bowel-wall thickening, abscesses, fistulas, and obstructions
Therapeutic Management	Corticosteroids, sulfonamides (sulfasalazine [Azulfidine]) Antibiotics Parenteral nutrition Partial or complete colectomy with ileostomy or anastomosis Rectum can be preserved in some patients Recurrence common	Corticosteroids, sulfonamides; sulfasalazine useful in preventing recurrence Bulk hydrophilic agents Antibiotics Proctocolectomy, with ileostomy Rectum can be preserved in only a few patients "cured" by colectomy
Systemic Complications	Small bowel obstruction Right-sided hydronephrosis Nephrolithiasis Cholelithiasis Arthritis Retinitis, iritis Erythema nodosum	Toxic megacolon Perforation Hemorrhage Malignant neoplasms Pyelonephritis Nephrolithiasis Cholangiocarcinoma Arthritis Retinitis, iritis Erythema nodosum

*can reveal acute inflammation or infection of one of the major abdominal organs or a perforation of the small or large bowel.

significance (Conley & Redeker, 2016). The most popular theory is that the body's immune system reacts abnormally in people with Crohn disease, mistaking bacteria, foods, and other substances for dangerous foreign substances (National Institutes of Health [NIH], U.S. Department of Health and Human Services, 2009; Targownik, Coneys, & Dhillon, 2016). Recent research also has suggested that lower levels of vitamin D may play a role in the increasing incidence of regional enteritis and warrants further study (Holmes, Xiang, & Lucas, 2015).

Pathophysiology

Regional enteritis is a subacute and chronic inflammation of the GI tract wall that extends through all layers (i.e., transmural lesion). Although it can occur anywhere in the GI tract, it most commonly occurs in the distal ileum but can be seen in the ascending colon. It is characterized by periods of remission and exacerbation. The disease process begins with edema and thickening of the mucosa. Ulcers begin to appear on the inflamed mucosa. The ulcerations in regional enteritis differ from UC in that they are not continuous or in contact with each other and are separated by normal tissue. Hence, these clusters of ulcers tend to take on a classic "cobblestone" appearance on colonoscopy. Fistulas, fissures, and abscesses form as the inflammation extends down into the peritoneum. **Granulomas** (localized nodular inflammation) occur in 50% of patients. As the disease advances, the bowel wall thickens and becomes fibrotic, and the intestinal lumen narrows. Diseased bowel loops sometimes stick to other loops surrounding those developing adhesions.

Clinical Manifestations and Assessment

Usually the onset of symptoms is insidious in regional enteritis, with prominent lower right quadrant abdominal pain unrelieved by defecation, fatigue, diarrhea, and weight loss. Scar tissue and the formation of granulomas interfere with the ability of the intestine to transport products of the upper intestinal digestion through the constricted lumen, resulting in crampy abdominal pains. There is abdominal tenderness and spasm. Because eating stimulates intestinal peristalsis, the crampy pain typically occurs after meals. The patient will tend to limit food intake in order to reduce the crampy pain and, in fact, can reduce the amount and type of food to such a degree that normal nutritional requirements often are not met. As a result, weight loss, malnutrition, and secondary anemia occur.

Ulcers in the membranous lining of the intestine and other inflammatory changes result in a weeping, edematous intestine that continually empties a colonic- and skin-irritating discharge. Disrupted absorption causes chronic diarrhea and associated fluid and electrolyte imbalances (hypokalemia, hypomagnesemia, hypocalcemia, and low albumin) as well as nutritional deficits. In some patients, the inflamed intestine may perforate, leading to intra-abdominal and anal abscesses. Fever and leukocytosis may occur. Chronic symptoms of regional enteritis may **include steatorrhea** (i.e., excessive fat in the feces).

Abscesses, fistulas, and fissures are common. Manifestations may extend beyond the GI tract and commonly include joint disorders (e.g., arthritis), skin lesions (e.g., erythema nodosum), ocular disorders (e.g., conjunctivitis), and oral ulcers. The clinical course and symptoms can vary; in some patients, periods of remission and exacerbation occur, but in others, the disease follows a fulminating course.

Usually a proctosigmoidoscopy is performed initially to determine whether the rectosigmoid area is inflamed. A stool examination also is performed; the result may be positive for occult blood and steatorrhea. Endoscopy, colonoscopy, and intestinal biopsies may be used to confirm the diagnosis. A CT scan may show bowel-wall thickening and fistula formation.

A CBC is performed to assess hematocrit and hemoglobin levels (usually decreased) as well as the WBC count (may be elevated). Usually the ESR is elevated in relation to the inflammation. Albumin (the long-term marker of nutrition) and protein levels may be decreased, indicating malnutrition.

Complications

Complications of regional enteritis include intestinal obstruction or stricture formation, perianal disease, fluid and electrolyte imbalances, malnutrition from malabsorption, and formation of fistulas and abscesses. The most common type of small bowel fistula caused by regional enteritis is the enterocutaneous fistula (i.e., an abnormal opening between the small bowel and the skin). Abscesses can be the result of an internal fistula that results in fluid accumulation and infection. Patients with regional enteritis are also at increased risk of colon cancer.

ULCERATIVE COLITIS

UC is a recurrent ulcerative and inflammatory disease of the mucosal and submucosal layers of the colon and rectum. The prevalence of UC is highest in Caucasians and people of Jewish heritage (Centers for Disease Control [CDC], 2016). It affects men and women equally. It is a serious disease, accompanied by systemic complications and a high mortality rate. Approximately 3% of patients with UC develop colon cancer (Desai et al., 2015; NIH, U.S. Department of Health and Human Services, 2009). Worldwide incidence of UC is more common than incidence of Crohn disease (Ferri, 2016).

Pathophysiology

UC affects the superficial mucosa of the colon and is characterized by multiple ulcerations, diffuse inflammations, and desquamation or shedding of the colonic epithelium. Bleeding occurs as a result of the ulcerations. The mucosa becomes edematous and inflamed. The lesions are contiguous, occurring one after the other. Abscesses form, and infiltrate is seen in the mucosa and submucosa, with clumps of neutrophils found in the lumens of the crypts (i.e., crypt abscesses) that line the intestinal mucosa (Porth, 2015). The disease process usually begins in the rectum and spreads proximally to involve the entire colon. Eventually, the bowel narrows, shortens, and thickens because of muscular hypertrophy and fat deposits.

Clinical Manifestations and Assessment

The clinical course is usually one of intermittent exacerbations and remissions. The predominant symptoms of UC include bloody diarrhea, passage of mucus, urgency, lower left quadrant abdominal pain, intermittent tenesmus, and fever. Symptoms will differ according to the extent of disease. The bleeding may be mild or severe, and pallor, anemia, and fatigue are the result. The patient may have anorexia, weight loss, vomiting, and dehydration, as well as cramping, the feeling of an urgent need to defecate, and the passage of 10 to 20 liquid stools each day. The disease is classified as mild, severe, or fulminant, depending on the severity of the symptoms. Hypocalcemia and anemia frequently develop. Rebound tenderness may occur in the right lower quadrant. Extraintestinal manifestations include skin lesions (e.g., erythema nodosum), eye lesions (e.g., uveitis), joint abnormalities (e.g., arthritis), and liver disease.

The patient should be assessed for tachycardia, hypotension, tachypnea, fever, and pallor (hypovolemic shock) from rectal bleeding. UC bleeding is painless and stops spontaneously in approximately 60% of patients (Ferri, 2016). Treatment is aimed at blood replacement and correction of volume and any clotting abnormalities. Other assessments address level of hydration and nutritional status. The abdomen is examined for bowel sounds, distention, and tenderness. Peripheral edema can occur secondary to hypoalbuminemia. These findings assist in determining the severity of the disease.

The stool can be positive for blood, and laboratory test results reveal low hematocrit and hemoglobin levels in addition to an elevated WBC count, low albumin levels, and an electrolyte imbalance. Iron-deficiency anemia may be present because of chronic blood loss. Hypokalemia, metabolic alkalosis, and elevated serum levels of blood urea nitrogen and creatinine may be present in severe flares of UC, reflecting volume depletion (Osterman & Lichtenstein, 2016). Abdominal x-ray studies are useful for determining the cause of symptoms. Free air in the peritoneum and bowel dilation or obstruction should be excluded as a source of the presenting symptoms, as peritonitis also can occur.

Colonoscopy should be avoided during acute diverticulitis due to the risk of perforation. In general, it can be performed after 6 weeks to rule out the presence of cancer and IBD (Ferri, 2016). Colonoscopy may reveal friable, inflamed mucosa with exudate and ulcerations. This procedure assists in defining the extent and severity of the disease. With the advent of endoscopy, barium studies have been used less often but remain important for certain specific scenarios, such as evaluation of colonic strictures;

LOCAL COMPLICATIONS

Inflammatory polyps (pseudopolyps) Colonic carcinoma

Toxic megacolon Perforation Hemorrhage

FIGURE 24-6 Ulcerative colitis. A schematic representation of the major features of ulcerative colitis in the colon. (Reprinted with permission from Strayer, D. S., & Rubin, E. (2014). *Rubin's pathology* (7th ed.). Philadelphia, PA: Wolters Kluwer.)

barium enema provides information on their location, length, and diameter and allows visualization of the entire colon when the presence of strictures precludes advancement of the colonoscope (Osterman & Lichtenstein, 2016). CT scanning can identify acute diverticulitis and diverticulosis, abscesses, and perirectal involvement. Arteriography may be performed with significant rectal bleeding, in which case vasopressin may be infused directly into the arteries supplying the bleeding, as well as selective arterial embolization (Ferri, 2016).

Careful examination of the patient's stool for parasites and other microbes is performed to rule out dysentery caused by common intestinal organisms, especially *Entamoeba histolytica* and *Clostridium difficile*.

Complications

Complications of UC include toxic megacolon, perforation and bleeding as a result of ulceration, vascular engorgement, and highly vascular granulation tissue (Fig. 24-6). In toxic megacolon, the inflammatory process extends into the muscularis, inhibiting its ability to contract and resulting in colonic distention. Symptoms include fever, abdominal pain and distention, vomiting, and fatigue. If the patient with toxic megacolon does not respond within 24 to 72 hours to medical management with nasogastric suction, IV fluids with electrolytes, corticosteroids, and antibiotics, then surgery is required. Then total colectomy is indicated. For many patients, surgery becomes necessary to relieve the effects of the disease and to treat these serious complications; an ileostomy usually is performed. The surgical procedures involved and the care of patients with this type of fecal diversion are discussed later in this chapter. In addition, hypercoagulability is a well-recognized complication of UC, resulting in deep vein thrombosis and pulmonary emboli. The mechanism of increased thrombotic risk is unclear. Standard anticoagulants would be administered. Episcleritis (painless hyperemia of the sclera and conjunctiva without loss of vision) and uveitis (acute or subacute pain in the eye with visual blurring often accompanied by photophobia and headache) occurs in 5% to 8% of patients with UC. Episcleritis parallels the level of bowel disease and generally responds to anti-inflammatory therapy. In contrast, the occurrence of uveitis increases with the dose and duration of glucocorticoid use. Patients

with uveitis should receive prompt ophthalmologic examination and treatment with glucocorticoid ocular drops to prevent progression to blindness. Steroid therapy also can lead to cataracts. Thus, patients receiving glucocorticoid therapy should undergo annual ophthalmologic examination (Osterman & Lichtenstein, 2016).

Patients with IBD also have a significantly increased risk of osteoporotic fractures due to decreased bone mineral density. Corticosteroid therapy also may contribute to the diminished bone density.

MEDICAL AND NURSING MANAGEMENT OF INFLAMMATORY BOWEL DISEASE

Medical treatment for regional enteritis and UC is aimed at reducing inflammation, suppressing inappropriate immune responses, providing rest for a diseased bowel so that healing may take place, improving quality of life (Box 24-1), and preventing or minimizing complications. Most patients have long periods of well-being interspersed with short intervals of illness, and management depends on the disease location, severity, and complications.

Oral fluids and a diet that is low residue, high protein, and high calorie with supplemental vitamin therapy and iron replacement are prescribed to meet nutritional needs, reduce inflammation, and control pain and diarrhea. Fluid and electrolyte imbalances from dehydration caused by diarrhea are corrected by IV therapy as necessary if the patient is hospitalized or by oral fluids if the patient is managed at home. Any foods that exacerbate diarrhea are avoided. Milk may contribute to diarrhea in those with lactose intolerance. Smoking is avoided because of increased intestinal motility. Consultation with a dietitian is highly recommended regarding oral diet or enteral feeding; parenteral nutrition has not yielded clinical benefit in this patient population (see Chapter 22).

Aminosalicylate formulations, such as sulfasalazine (Azulfidine), often are effective for mild or moderate inflammation and are used to prevent or reduce recurrences in long-term maintenance regimens. Sulfa-free aminosalicylates (e.g., mesalamine [Asacol, Pentasa]) are effective in preventing and treating recurrence of inflammation. Antibiotics (e.g., metronidazole [Flagyl]) are used for secondary infections, particularly for purulent complications, such as abscesses, perforation, and peritonitis.

BOX 24-1 Nursing Research

Bridging the Gap to Evidence-Based Practice

The Effect of Abdominal Massage on Constipation and Quality of Life

Does Abdominal Massage have an effect on GI function, quality of life (QOL), and the use of laxatives in patients who have not had a bowel movement in the first 3 days after surgery?

Turan, N., & Atabek Asti, T. (2016). The effect of abdominal massage on constipation and quality of life. *Gastroenterology Nursing*, *39*(1), 48–59.

Purpose

Constipation is a common problem that has a profound effect on people's health and well-being. There are few existing studies related to nursing interventions regarding abdominal massage. Therefore, the purpose of this study was to identify the effects of abdominal massage in patients with constipation related to their GI function, QOL, and the use of laxatives.

Design

A randomized controlled study was conducted. Sample criteria included patients 18 years of age or older, who had surgery and were hospitalized for treatment, and who had not had a bowel movement for the first 3 days after surgery. A total of 60 patients (30 in the control group and 30 in the experimental group) fit criteria and agreed to be in the study. Abdominal massage was defined for this study as applied daily for 15 minutes in a clockwise fashion using four basic strokes: stroking, effleurage, kneading, and vibration.

Several data collection instruments were used to measure gastrointestinal symptom ratings, constipation severity scores, and the general health of the patient. Analysis of the data showed that patients who had abdominal massage completed defecation more often, had decreased symptoms of constipation, and stated there was improvement in their QOL. The study also showed that abdominal massage decreased the symptoms of constipation more than the use of laxatives, suppositories, or enemas.

Nursing Implications

This study has shown that abdominal massage is an effective tool in decreasing the symptoms of constipation and increasing the QOL for patients who are constipated. The nurse plays an important role in the treatment of constipation in postoperative patients. Implementing abdominal massage, in conjunction with dietary changes and increasing exercise, provide nonpharmacologic treatments for patients that can be implemented by the nurse in the early postoperative period. Future studies should analyze other patient groups to determine the ability of abdominal massage to treat patients with constipation in other clinical settings.

Corticosteroids are used to treat severe and fulminant disease and can be administered orally (e.g., prednisone [Deltasone]) in outpatient treatment or parenterally (e.g., hydrocortisone [Solu-Cortef]) in hospitalized patients. Topical (i.e., rectal administration) corticosteroids (e.g., hydrocortisone enema, budesonide [Entocort]) also are used widely in the treatment of distal colon disease. When the dosage of corticosteroids is reduced or stopped, the symptoms of disease may return. If corticosteroids are continued, adverse sequelae, such as hypertension, fluid retention, cataracts, hirsutism (i.e., abnormal hair growth), adrenal suppression, steroid-induced diabetes mellitus (secondary to the hyperglycemia associated with glucocorticoid therapy), poor wound healing, and loss of bone density, may occur.

Immunomodulators (e.g., azathioprine [AZA], 6-mercaptopurine [6-MP], methotrexate, and cyclosporine) and antitumor necrosis factor agents have been used to alter the immune response. The exact mechanism of action of these medications in treating IBD is unknown. These medications are useful in maintenance regimens to prevent relapses. Biologic therapies using monoclonal antibodies, such as natalizumab (Tysabri), continue to be used to treat Crohn disease (Scott & Osterman, 2015) and infliximab (Remicade) for treating UC (Bressler et al., 2015). Initial reports from clinical trials appear promising for both these medications (Arias et al., 2015; Scott & Osterman, 2015), although the use of natalizumab is limited currently to patients who have not tolerated or failed treatment with other biologic agents (Scott & Osterman, 2015).

When nonsurgical measures fail to relieve the severe symptoms of IBD, surgery may be necessary. Approximately 75% of all patients with regional enteritis who have had the disease for 20 years required some type of surgery. Fortunately, this number has been decreasing steadily with the increased use of infliximab therapy (Bressler et al., 2015). The most common indications for surgery are medically intractable disease, poor quality of life, or complications from the disease or its treatment. Recurrence of inflammation and disease after surgery in regional enteritis is inevitable.

A common procedure performed for strictures of the small intestines is laparoscope-guided strictureplasty, in which the blocked or narrowed sections of the intestines are widened, leaving the intestines intact. In some cases, a small bowel resection is performed: diseased segments of the small intestines are resected, and the remaining portions of the intestines are anastomosed. Surgical removal of up to 50% of the small bowel usually can be tolerated. In cases of severe regional enteritis of the colon, a total colectomy and ileostomy may be the procedure of choice.

A newer surgical procedure developed for patients with severe regional enteritis is intestinal transplant. Now this technique is available to children and to young and middle-aged adults who have lost intestinal function from disease. Although this procedure is not a cure, eventually it may provide improvement in quality of life for some patients. The associated technical and immunologic problems remain formidable, and the costs and mortality rates remain high.

Long-term colectomy rates for patients with UC for 3 years ranges from 50% to 62% (Seah & De Cruz, 2016). When the colon is surgically removed, the patient is considered "cured" in that extraintestinal manifestations subside and the disease process is otherwise limited to the colon. Indications for surgery include lack of improvement and continued deterioration, profuse bleeding, perforation, continued stricture formation, and cancer. Surgical excision usually improves quality of life. Proctocolectomy with ileostomy (i.e., complete excision of colon, rectum, and anus) is recommended when the rectum is severely diseased. If the rectum can be preserved, the procedure of choice is restorative proctocolectomy with ileal pouch anal anastomosis (IPAA).

ILEOSTOMY

Procedures

An **ileostomy**, the surgical creation of an opening into the ileum or small intestine (usually by means of an ileal stoma on the abdominal wall), is commonly performed after a total colectomy (i.e., excision of the entire colon). It allows for drainage of fecal matter (i.e., effluent) from the ileum to the outside of the body. The drainage is typically loose to semiformed and may occur at frequent intervals.

Another procedure involves the creation of a continent ileal reservoir (i.e., **Kock pouch**) by diverting a portion of the distal ileum to the abdominal wall and creating a stoma (Fig. 24-7). This procedure eliminates the need for an external fecal collection bag. Approximately 30 cm of the distal ileum is reconstructed to form a reservoir with a nipple valve that is created by pulling a portion of the terminal ileal loop back into the ileum. GI effluent can accumulate in the pouch for several hours and then be removed by means of a catheter inserted through the nipple valve. In many patients, a total colectomy also is performed with the Kock pouch. Possible indications for a total colectomy with Kock pouch placement (rather than a restorative proctocolectomy with IPAA) include a badly diseased rectum, lack of rectal sphincter tone, or inability to achieve fecal continence post-IPAA.

The major problem with the Kock pouch is malfunction of the nipple valve. The ileocecal nipple valve is used commonly to create a continent, catheterizable channel. Another surgical option is the appendicovesicostomy, which repurposes the appendix to create a tunneled channel (Levy & Elliott, 2016).

A restorative proctocolectomy with IPAA is the surgical procedure of choice in cases in which the rectum can be preserved in that it eliminates the need for a permanent ileostomy. It establishes an ileal reservoir, and anal sphincter control of elimination is retained. The procedure involves connecting a portion of the ileum to the anus (i.e., ileoanal anastomosis) in conjunction with removal of the colon

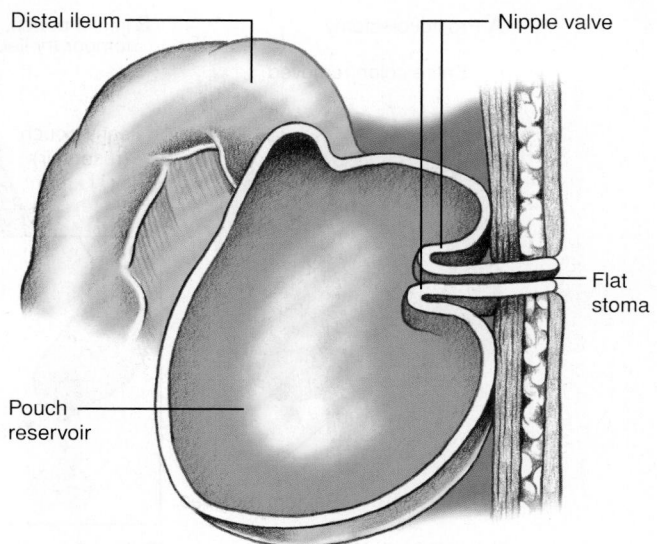

FIGURE 24-7 Anatomy of a Kock pouch. A Kock pouch is formed by surgically looping part of the distal ileum, stapling the loops together, and opening the inner canals to form a reservoir for the soft, watery stool to be held until catheterized for removal. The nipple valve is formed as shown, by pulling part of the pouch tissue back over the terminal end of the ileum and stapling it closed to reduce the size of the opening and form a canal for the catheter. The length and smaller diameter of the nipple valve prevents waste products from escaping, although some mucus drainage may be expected. (Reprinted with permission from *Lippincott's Nursing Advisor.* (2009), Wolters Kluwer.)

and the rectal mucosa (i.e., total abdominal colectomy and mucosal proctectomy) (Fig. 24-8). A temporary diverting loop ileostomy is constructed at the time of surgery and closed about 3 months later.

With ileoanal anastomosis, the diseased colon and rectum are removed, voluntary defecation is maintained, and anal continence is preserved. The ileal reservoir decreases the number of bowel movements by 50%, from approximately 14 to 20 per day to seven to 10 per day. Nighttime elimination is reduced gradually to one bowel movement. Complications of ileoanal anastomosis include irritation of the perianal skin from leakage of fecal contents, stricture formation at the anastomosis site, and small bowel obstruction.

Nursing management of patients with IBD may be medical, surgical, or both. Patients in the community setting or those recently diagnosed may require education about diet and medications as well as referral to support groups. Hospitalized patients with longstanding or severe disease also require careful monitoring, parenteral nutrition, fluid replacement, and possibly emergent surgery. The surgical procedures may involve a fecal diversion with attendant needs for physical care, emotional support, and extensive teaching about management of the ostomy.

Nursing Management for Ileostomy

Some patients with IBD eventually require a permanent fecal diversion with creation of an ileostomy to manage symptoms

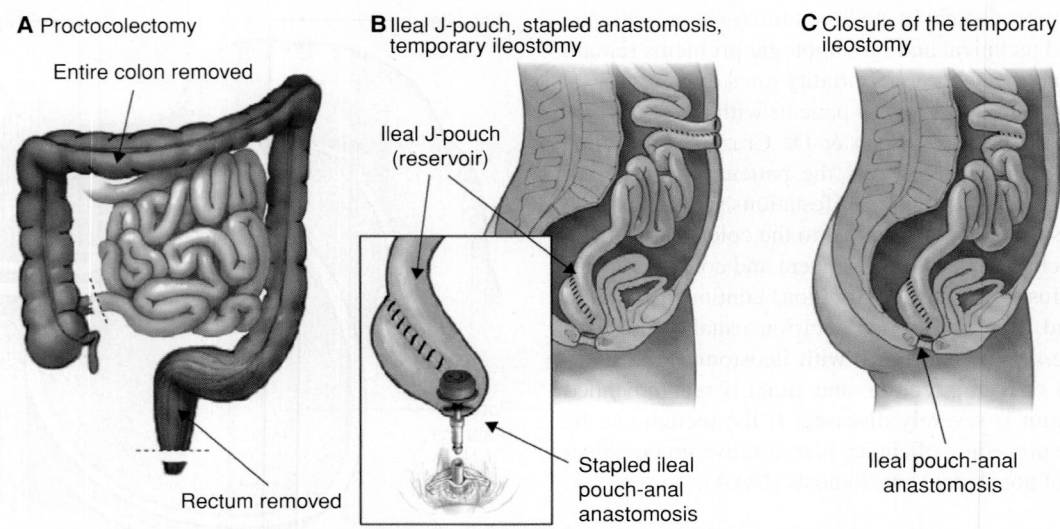

A Proctocolectomy

Entire colon removed

Rectum removed

B Ileal J-pouch, stapled anastomosis, temporary ileostomy

Ileal J-pouch (reservoir)

Stapled ileal pouch-anal anastomosis

C Closure of the temporary ileostomy

Ileal pouch-anal anastomosis

FIGURE 24-8 **(A)** Proctocolectomy. **(B)** Ileal J-pouch, stapled anastomosis, and temporary ileostomy. **(C)** Closure of the temporary ileostomy. The entire surgical procedure is based on four steps: removal of the colon; pelvic dissection and rectum removal sparing the pelvic nerves and the anal sphincter; construction of the ileal pouch, usually with the last 30 to 40 cm of the terminal ileum; and anastomosis of the pouch to the canal anal. (Reprinted with permission from Holzman, R. S., Mancuso, T. J., & Polaner, D. M. (2015). *A practical approach to pediatric anesthesia* (2nd ed.). Philadelphia, PA: Wolters Kluwer.)

and to treat or prevent complications. Ileostomy education can be started while the patient is still in the hospital, and with a small amount of planning and care, the patient lives a very normal life. A plan of nursing care for a patient undergoing ostomy surgery is available online at http://thepoint. lww.com/Honan2e.

Providing Preoperative Care

A period of preparation with intensive replacement of fluid, blood, and protein is necessary before surgery is performed. Antibiotics may be prescribed. If the patient has been taking corticosteroids, they will be continued during the surgical phase to prevent steroid-induced adrenal insufficiency. Usually, the patient is provided with frequent, small feedings. All other preoperative measures are similar to those for general abdominal surgery. The abdomen is marked for the proper placement of the stoma by the surgeon or the enterostomal therapist. Care is taken to ensure that the stoma is placed in a convenient location—usually in the right lower quadrant about 2 in below the waist, in an area away from previous scars, bony prominences, skin folds, or fistulas.

The patient must have a thorough understanding of the surgery to be performed and what to expect after surgery. Information about an ileostomy is presented to the patient by means of written materials, models, and discussion. Preoperative teaching includes management of drainage from the stoma, the nature of drainage, and the need for nasogastric intubation, parenteral fluids, and, possibly, perineal packing.

Providing Postoperative Care

Nursing Alert

A healthy stoma appears pink or red and moist; the nurse alerts the surgeon if the stoma is dusky, white, or dark since circulation may be compromised.

General abdominal surgery wound care is required. The nurse observes the stoma for color and size. It should be pink to bright red and shiny. Typically, a temporary plastic bag with an adhesive facing is placed over the ileostomy in the operating room and firmly pressed onto the surrounding skin. The nurse monitors the ileostomy for fecal drainage, which should begin about 72 hours after surgery. The drainage is a continuous liquid from the small intestine because the stoma does not have a controlling sphincter. The contents drain into the plastic bag and thus are kept from coming into contact with the skin. They are collected and measured when the bag becomes full. If a continent ileal reservoir was created, as described for the Kock pouch, continuous drainage is provided by an indwelling reservoir catheter for 2 to 3 weeks after surgery. This allows the suture lines to heal.

As with other patients undergoing abdominal surgery, the nurse encourages those with an ileostomy to engage in early ambulation. It is important to administer prescribed pain medications as required.

Because these patients lose much fluid in the early postoperative period, an accurate record of fluid intake, urinary output, and fecal discharge is necessary to help gauge the fluid needs of the patient. There may be up to 1 L of fluid lost each day, in addition to expected fluid loss through urine, perspiration, respiration, and other sources. With this loss, sodium and potassium are depleted. The nurse monitors laboratory values and administers electrolyte replacements as prescribed. Fluids are administered IV for 4 to 5 days to replace lost fluids.

Nasogastric suction is also a part of immediate postoperative care, with the tube requiring frequent irrigation as prescribed. The purpose of nasogastric suction is to prevent a buildup of gastric contents. After the tube is removed, the nurse offers sips of clear liquids and gradually progresses the diet. It is important to report nausea and abdominal distention immediately because they may indicate intestinal obstruction.

By the end of the first week, rectal packing is removed. Because this procedure may be uncomfortable, the nurse may administer an analgesic an hour before its removal. After the packing is removed, the perineum is irrigated two or three times daily until full healing takes place.

The patient with a traditional ileostomy cannot establish regular bowel habits because the contents of the ileum are fluid and are discharged continuously. The patient must wear a pouch at all times. Stomal size and pouch size vary initially; the stoma should be rechecked 3 weeks after surgery, when the edema has subsided. The final size and type of appliance is selected in 3 months, after the patient's weight has stabilized and the stoma shrinks to a stable shape.

The location and length of the stoma are significant in the management of the ileostomy by the patient. The surgeon positions the stoma as close to the midline as possible and at a location where even an obese patient with a protruding abdomen can care for it easily. Usually, the ileostomy stoma is about 2.5 cm (1 in) long, which makes it convenient for the attachment of an appliance.

Skin excoriation around the stoma can be a persistent problem. Peristomal skin integrity may be compromised by several factors, such as an allergic reaction to the ostomy appliance, skin barrier, or paste; chemical irritation from the effluent; mechanical injury from the removal of the appliance; and infection. If irritation and yeast growth occur, nystatin powder (Mycostatin) is dusted lightly on the peristomal skin.

Changing an Appliance

A regular schedule for changing the pouch before leakage occurs must be established for those with a traditional ileostomy. The amount of time a person can keep the appliance sealed to the body surface depends on the location of the stoma and on body structure. The usual wearing time is 5 to 7 days. The appliance is emptied every 4 to 6 hours or at the same time the patient empties the bladder. An emptying spout at the bottom of the appliance is closed with a special clip made for this purpose.

Most pouches are disposable and odor-proof. Foods such as spinach and parsley act as deodorizers in the intestinal tract; foods that cause odors include cabbage, onions, and fish. Bismuth subcarbonate tablets, which may be prescribed

and taken orally three or four times each day, are effective in reducing odor. Oral diphenoxylate (Lomotil) also can be prescribed to diminish intestinal motility, thereby thickening the stool and assisting in odor control.

Changing an ileostomy appliance also allows for examination of the skin around the stoma, and assists in controlling odor if this becomes a problem. The appliance should be changed at any time that the patient complains of burning or itching under the disk or pain in the area of the stoma; routine changes should be performed early in the morning before breakfast or 2 to 4 hours after a meal, when the bowel is least active. See Box 24-2 for guidelines on changing an ostomy appliance.

Managing Dietary and Fluid Needs

A low-residue diet is followed for the first 6 to 8 weeks. Strained fruits and vegetables are given. These foods are important sources of vitamins A and C. Foods are reintroduced one at a time. The nurse assesses the patient's tolerance for these foods and reminds him or her to chew food thoroughly.

Fluids may be a problem during the summer when fluid lost through perspiration adds to the fluid loss through the ileostomy. Fluids such as Gatorade are helpful in maintaining electrolyte balance.

Preventing Complications

Monitoring for complications is an ongoing activity for the patient with an ileostomy. Peristomal skin irritation, which results from leakage of effluent, is the most common complication of an ileostomy. A drainable pouching system that does not fit well is often the cause. Components of the drainable pouching system include the pouch, a solid skin barrier, and adhesive. The enterostomal therapist typically recommends the appropriate drainable pouching system. The solid skin barrier is the component of this system that is most important in ensuring healthy peristomal skin. Solid skin barriers typically are shaped as rectangular or elliptical wafers and are composed of polymers and hydrocolloids. They protect the skin around the stoma from effluent from the stoma and provide a stable interface between the stoma and the pouch.

Other common complications include fluid volume deficit, stomal stenosis, urinary calculi, and cholelithiasis. Even in the presence of a properly fitted drainable pouching system, loose watery effluent can be problematic, often filling the pouch (every hour or sooner), which can quickly lead to dehydration and electrolyte losses. Supplemental water, sodium, and potassium are administered to prevent hypovolemia and hypokalemia. Antidiarrheal agents or bile salt sequestrants may be administered to decrease the watery effluent.

Stenosis is caused by circular scar tissue that forms at the stoma site. The scar tissue must be released surgically. Urinary calculi may occur in patients with ileostomies and are attributed, at least partly, to dehydration from decreased fluid intake. Intense lower abdominal pain that radiates to the legs,

BOX 24-2 GUIDELINES FOR NURSING CARE

Changing an Ileostomy Appliance

Equipment Needed

- Mild soap
- Clean cloths or towels
- Skin barrier (stoma adhesive, Convatec)
- Cutting guide
- Appliance pouch

Optional Equipment

- Barrier powder
- Antifungal spray or powder
- Barrier washer

Implementation

NURSING ACTION	RATIONALE

1. Promote patient comfort and involvement in the procedure.
   a. Have the patient assume a relaxed position.
   b. Provide privacy.
   c. Explain details of the procedure.
   d. Expose the ileostomy area; remove the ileostomy belt (if worn).
	1. Providing a relaxed atmosphere and adequate explanations help the patient to become an active participant in the procedure.

2. Remove the appliance.
   a. Have the patient sit on the toilet or on a chair facing the toilet. A patient who prefers to stand should face the toilet.
   b. The appliance (pouch) can be removed by gently pushing the skin away from the adhesive.
	2. These positions facilitate disposal or drainage.

3. Cleanse the skin:
   a. Wash the skin gently with a soft cloth moistened with tepid water and mild soap; the patient may prefer to bathe before putting on a clean appliance.
   b. Rinse the soap and dry the skin thoroughly after cleansing.
	3. The patient may shower with or without the pouch.
	   a. Micropore or waterproof tape applied to the sides of the faceplate keeps it secure during bathing.
	   b. Moisture or soap residue interferes with appliance adhesion.

Pouching options

One-piece systems

Skin barrier
Starter opening
Cut-to-fit skin barrier
Tape collar
Comfort panel
Tail

In a one-piece system, the pouch and skin barrier are a single unit.

Tail clip

Two-piece systems

Tape collar
Flange
Skin barrier
Starter opening
Flange
Comfort panel
Tail

In a two-piece system, the pouch attaches to a skin barrier with flange.

Tail clip

NURSING ACTION	RATIONALE

4. Apply appliance:
When there is *no* skin irritation:
  a. An appropriate skin barrier is applied to the peristomal skin before the appliance is applied.
  b. Remove cover from adherent surface of disk of disposable plastic appliance and apply directly to the skin.
  c. Press firmly in place for 30 seconds to ensure adherence.
When there is skin irritation:
  a. Cleanse the skin thoroughly but gently; pat dry. Apply barrier powder.
  b. If more irritation developed, apply Kenalog spray; blot excess moisture with a cotton pledget, and dust lightly with nystatin (Mycostatin) powder.
    OR
    Place the sizing guide directly on the skin around the stoma, leaving as little skin as possible around the stoma uncovered. Then, using the guide, cut the appropriate hole in the disk. At times, the stoma site is irregular; if this is the case, the hole should be cut approximating the stoma site as closely as possible.
    Apply as an alternative a wafer or barrier (Stomahesive, ConvaTec), which is commercially available. The stomal opening should be the same size as the stoma; use a cutting guide (supplied with appliance as indicated). The wafer is applied directly to the skin. Barrier powder can be used to dry irritated skin before barrier application.
  c. Another alternative is to apply a special barrier washer (e.g., Eakin's Seal). The special barrier adheres well to irritated skin.
  d. Then the pouch is applied to the treated skin.
5. Check the pouch bottom for closure; use clamp, Velcro closure, or clip provided.
	4. Many appliances have a built-in skin barrier. The skin should be dried thoroughly before applying the appliance.
	  a. Cleansing removes debris and protects irritated skin under the wafer.
	  b. The corticosteroid preparation (Kenalog) helps decrease inflammation. The antifungal agent (nystatin) treats those types of infections that are common around stomas. A prescription is required for either medication. A skin barrier is a substance that facilitates healing of excoriated skin. It adheres well even to moist, irritated skin.
	  c. A special barrier protects skin from effluent, promotes healing, and helps with adherence.
	  d. This allows skin to heal while the appliance is in place.
	
	5. Proper closure controls leakage.

hematuria, and signs of dehydration indicate that the urine should be strained. Fluid intake is encouraged. Sometimes, small stones are passed during urination; otherwise, treatment is necessary to crush or remove the calculi (see Chapter 28).

Cholelithiasis (i.e., gallstones) occurs more commonly in patients with an ileostomy than in the general population because of changes in the absorption of bile acids that occur postoperatively. Spasm of the gallbladder causes severe upper right abdominal pain that can radiate to the back and right shoulder (see Chapter 25).

MASSES IN THE COLON AND RECTUM

A *polyp* is a mass of tissue that protrudes into the lumen of the bowel. Polyps can occur anywhere in the intestinal tract and rectum. They can be classified as neoplastic (i.e., adenomas and carcinomas) or nonneoplastic (i.e., mucosal and hyperplastic).

NONNEOPLASTIC POLYPS

Although most polyps do not develop into invasive neoplasms, they must be identified and followed closely.

Risk Factors

Nonneoplastic polyps, which are benign epithelial growths, are common in the Western world. They occur more commonly in the large intestine than in the small intestine. Adenomatous (benign) polyps are more common in men. The proportion of these polyps arising in the proximal part of the colon increases with age (after 50 years of age). Prevalence rates vary from 25% to 60%, depending on age. Nonneoplastic polyps occur in 80% of the population, and their frequency increases with age.

Clinical Manifestations and Assessment

Clinical manifestations depend on the size of the polyp and the amount of pressure it exerts on intestinal tissue. The most common symptom is rectal bleeding. Lower abdominal pain also may occur. If the polyp is large enough, symptoms of obstruction occur. The diagnosis is based on history and digital rectal examination, barium enema studies, sigmoidoscopy, or colonoscopy.

Medical and Nursing Management

After a polyp is identified, it should be removed. There are several methods: colonoscopy with the use of special equipment (i.e., biopsy forceps and snares), laparoscopy, or colonoscopic excision with laparoscopic visualization. The latter technique enables immediate detection of potential problems and allows laparoscopic resection and repair of the major complications of perforation and bleeding that may occur with polypectomy. Microscopic examination of the polyp then identifies the type of polyp and indicates what further surgery is required, if any.

COLORECTAL CANCER

Tumors of the colon and rectum are relatively common; the colorectal area (the colon and rectum combined) is now the third most common site of new cancer cases and deaths in the United States. Colorectal cancer is the second most common cause of cancer death among men who are 40 to 79 years of age (Siegel, Miller, & Jemal, 2016). Improved screening strategies have helped reduce the number of deaths from colon cancer in recent years. Of the approximately 150,000 people diagnosed each year, fewer than half that number dies annually (American Cancer Society [ACS], 2015).

Early diagnosis and prompt treatment could save almost three of every four people. If the disease is detected and treated at an early stage, the 5-year survival rate is 90%; however, in the more distal stages of disease, the 5-year survival rate is only approximately 13% (ACS, 2015). Most people are asymptomatic for long periods and seek health care only when they notice a change in bowel habits or rectal bleeding. Prevention and early screening are the keys to detection and reduction of mortality rates.

Pathophysiology

Cancer of the colon and rectum is predominantly (95%) adenocarcinoma (i.e., arising from the epithelial lining of the intestine) (ACS, 2015). It may start as a benign polyp but may become malignant, invade and destroy normal tissues, and extend into surrounding structures. Cancer cells may migrate away from the primary tumor and spread to other parts of the body (most often to the liver).

Risk Factors

Colorectal cancer is a disease of Western cultures. The incidence increases with age (the incidence is highest in people over 85 years of age) and is higher in people with a family history of colon cancer and those with IBD or polyps. In men, only the incidence of prostate cancer and lung cancer exceeds that of colorectal cancer. In women, only the incidence of breast and lung cancer exceeds that of colorectal cancer.

Colon cancer in the elderly has been closely associated with dietary carcinogens. High-fiber intake, particularly from fruits and cereals, reduces the risk of colorectal cancer (Kunzmann et al., 2015). Excess dietary fat, high alcohol consumption, and smoking all increase the incidence of colorectal tumors. Physical activity and dietary folate have protective effects (Siegel et al., 2016).

Clinical Manifestations and Assessment

Symptoms are often insidious. Patients with colorectal cancer usually report fatigue, which is caused primarily by iron-deficiency anemia. In early stages, minor changes in bowel patterns and occasional bleeding may occur. The later symptoms reported most commonly by the elderly are abdominal pain, obstruction, tenesmus, and rectal bleeding.

The symptoms are greatly determined by the location of the cancer, the stage of the disease, and the function of the intestinal segment in which it is located. The most common presenting symptom is a change in bowel habits. The passage of blood in the stools is the second most common symptom. Symptoms also may include unexplained anemia, anorexia, weight loss, and fatigue.

The symptoms most commonly associated with right-sided lesions are dull abdominal pain and melena (black, tarry stools). The symptoms most commonly associated with left-sided lesions are those associated with obstruction (abdominal pain and cramping, narrowing stools, constipation, distention), as well as bright red blood in the stool. Symptoms associated with rectal lesions are tenesmus (ineffective, painful straining at stool), rectal pain, the feeling of incomplete evacuation after a bowel movement, alternating constipation and diarrhea, and bloody stool.

Along with an abdominal and rectal examination, the most important diagnostic procedures for cancer of the colon are fecal occult blood testing, barium enema, proctosigmoidoscopy, and colonoscopy (see Chapter 21). The majority of colorectal cancer cases can be identified by colonoscopy with biopsy or cytology smears.

Carcinoembryonic antigen (CEA) studies also may be performed. Although CEA may not be a highly reliable indicator in diagnosing colon cancer because not all lesions secrete CEA, studies show that CEA levels are reliable prognostic predictors. With complete excision of the tumor, the elevated levels of CEA should return to normal within 48 hours. Elevations of CEA at a later date suggest recurrence.

Medical and Nursing Management

The patient with symptoms of intestinal obstruction is treated with IV fluids and nasogastric suction. If there has been significant bleeding, blood component therapy may be required.

Treatment for colorectal cancer depends on the stage of the disease and consists of surgery to remove the tumor, supportive therapy, and adjuvant therapy. Patients who receive some form of adjuvant therapy, which may include chemotherapy, radiation therapy, immunotherapy, or multimodality therapy, typically demonstrate delays in tumor recurrence and increases in survival time.

Radiation therapy is used before, during, and after surgery to shrink the tumor, to achieve better results from surgery, and to reduce the risk of recurrence. For inoperative or unresectable tumors, radiation is used to provide significant relief from symptoms. Intracavitary and implantable devices are used to deliver radiation to the site. The response to adjuvant therapy varies.

Surgery is the primary treatment for most colon and rectal cancers. It may be curative or palliative. Advances in surgical techniques can enable the patient with cancer to have sphincter-saving devices that restore continuity of the GI tract. The type of surgery recommended depends on the location and size of the tumor. Cancers limited to one site can be removed through the colonoscope. Laparoscopic colotomy with polypectomy minimizes the extent of surgery needed in some cases. A laparoscope is used as a guide in making an incision into the colon; then the tumor mass is excised. Use of the neodymium/yttrium-aluminum-garnet (Nd:YAG) laser has proved effective with some lesions as well.

Surgical procedures include the following:

- Segmental resection with anastomosis (i.e., removal of the tumor and portions of the bowel on either side of the growth, as well as the blood vessels and lymphatic nodes) (Fig. 24-9)
- Abdominoperineal resection with permanent sigmoid colostomy (i.e., removal of the tumor and a portion of the sigmoid and all of the rectum and anal sphincter) (Fig. 24-10)
- Temporary colostomy followed by segmental resection and anastomosis and subsequent reanastomosis of the colostomy, allowing initial bowel decompression and bowel preparation before resection
- Permanent colostomy or ileostomy for palliation of unresectable obstructing lesions
- Construction of a coloanal reservoir called a *colonic J pouch*, which is performed in two steps. A temporary loop ileostomy is constructed to divert intestinal flow, and the newly constructed J pouch (made from 6 to 10 cm of colon) is reattached to the anal stump. About 3 months after the initial stage, the ileostomy is reversed and intestinal continuity is restored. The anal sphincter and, therefore, continence are preserved.

A colostomy is the surgical creation of an opening (i.e., stoma) into the colon. It can be created as a temporary or permanent fecal diversion. It allows the drainage or evacuation of colon contents to the outside of the body. The consistency

Cecum and lower ascending colon

Descending colon and upper sigmoid

Low sigmoid and upper rectum

Rectal sigmoid resection

FIGURE 24-9 Examples of areas where cancer can occur, the area that is removed, and how the anastomosis is performed (*small diagrams*).

of the drainage is related to the placement of the colostomy, which is dictated by the location of the tumor and the extent of invasion into surrounding tissues (Fig. 24-11). With improved surgical techniques, colostomies are performed in less than one third of patients with colorectal cancer.

Complications

Tumor growth may cause partial or complete bowel obstruction. Extension of the tumor and ulceration into the surrounding blood vessels result in hemorrhage. Perforation, abscess formation, peritonitis, sepsis, and shock may occur.

The elderly are at increased risk of complications after surgery and may have difficulty managing colostomy care. Some elderly patients may have decreased vision, impaired hearing, and difficulty with fine motor coordination. It may be helpful for patients to handle ostomy equipment and simulate cleaning the peristomal skin and irrigating the stoma

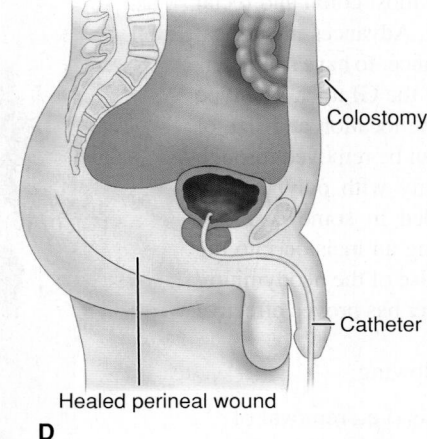

FIGURE 24-10 Abdominoperineal resection for carcinoma of the rectum. **A.** Prior to surgery. Note tumor in rectum. **B.** During surgery, the sigmoid is removed and the colostomy is established. The distal bowel is dissected free to a point below the pelvic peritoneum, which is sutured over the closed end of the distal sigmoid and rectum. **C.** Perineal resection includes removal of the rectum and free portion of the sigmoid from below. A perineal drain is inserted. **D.** The final result after healing. Note the healed perineal wound and the permanent colostomy.

before surgery. Skin care is a major concern in older patients with a colostomy because of the skin changes that occur with aging—the epithelial and subcutaneous fatty layers become thin, and the skin is irritated easily. To prevent skin breakdown, special attention is paid to skin cleansing and the proper fit of an appliance. Arteriosclerosis causes decreased blood flow to the wound and stoma site. As a result, transport of nutrients is delayed, and healing time may be prolonged. Some patients have delayed elimination after irrigation because of decreased peristalsis and mucus production. Most patients require 6 months before they feel comfortable with their ostomy care.

INTESTINAL OBSTRUCTION

Intestinal obstruction exists when blockage prevents the normal flow of intestinal contents through the intestinal tract. In mechanical obstruction, intraluminal or mural obstructions secondary to pressure on the intestinal wall occur. Examples are intussusception (telescoping of a portion of the intestine within another immediately adjacent portion of intestine),

polypoid tumors and neoplasms, stenosis, strictures, adhesions, hernias, and abscesses. Figure 24-12 depicts additional causes of obstruction. In functional obstruction, intestinal musculature cannot propel the contents along the bowel thereby causing a blockage within the intestine. Examples are amyloidosis, muscular dystrophy, endocrine disorders such as diabetes mellitus, or neurologic disorders such as Parkinson disease. The blockage also can be temporary and the result of the manipulation of the bowel during surgery.

The obstruction can be partial or complete. Its severity depends on the region of bowel affected, the degree to which the lumen is occluded, and especially the degree to which the vascular supply to the bowel wall is disturbed.

Most bowel obstructions occur in the small intestine. Adhesions are the most common cause of small bowel obstruction, followed by hernias and neoplasms. Other causes include intussusception, **volvulus** (i.e., twisting of the bowel), and paralytic ileus. Most obstructions in the large bowel occur in the sigmoid colon. The most common causes are carcinoma, diverticulitis, inflammatory bowel disorders, and benign tumors. Table 24-6 and Figure 24-12 list mechanical causes of obstruction and describe how they occur.

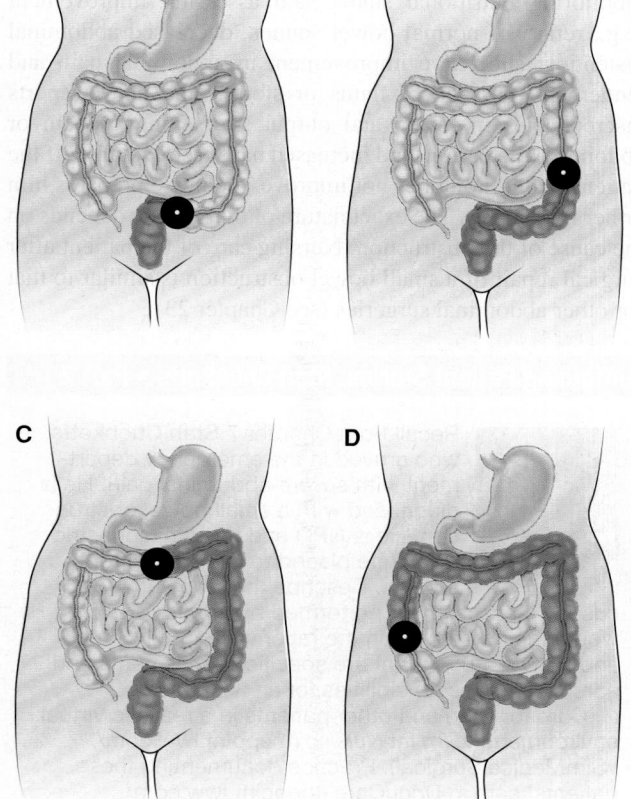

FIGURE 24-11 Placement of permanent colostomies. The nature of the discharge varies with the site. Shaded areas show sections of bowel removed. With a sigmoid colostomy (**A**), the feces are solid. With a descending colostomy (**B**), the feces are semiformed. With a transverse colostomy (**C**), the feces are unformed. With an ascending colostomy (**D**), the feces are fluid.

Small intestine
Hernial sac
Peritoneum
Testicle

FIGURE 24-12 Three causes of intestinal obstruction. **A.** Intussusception invagination or shortening of the colon caused by the movement of one segment of bowel into another. **B.** Volvulus of the sigmoid colon; the twist is counterclockwise in most cases. Note the edematous bowel. **C.** Hernia (inguinal). The sac of the hernia is a continuation of the peritoneum of the abdomen. The hernial contents are intestine, omentum, or other abdominal contents that pass through the hernial opening into the hernial sac.

SMALL BOWEL OBSTRUCTION

Pathophysiology

Intestinal contents, fluid, and gas accumulate above the intestinal obstruction. The abdominal distention and retention of fluid reduce the absorption of fluids and stimulate more gastric secretion. Increases in intestinal lumen pressure

TABLE 24-6 Mechanical Causes of Intestinal Obstruction

Cause	Course of Events	Result
Adhesions	Loops of intestine become adherent to areas that heal slowly or scar after abdominal surgery.	After surgery, adhesions produce a kinking of an intestinal loop.
Intussusception	One part of the intestine slips into another part located below it (like a telescope shortening).	The intestinal lumen becomes narrowed.
Volvulus	Bowel twists and turns on itself.	Intestinal lumen becomes obstructed. Gas and fluid accumulate in the trapped bowel.
Hernia	Protrusion of intestine through a weakened area in the abdominal muscle or wall.	Intestinal flow may be obstructed completely. Blood flow to the area may be obstructed as well.
Tumor	A tumor that exists within the wall of the intestine extends into the intestinal lumen, or a tumor outside the intestine causes pressure on the wall of the intestine.	Intestinal lumen becomes partially obstructed; if the tumor is not removed, complete obstruction results.

causes occlusion of capillary blood flow and compromise of venous return and arterial flow. This causes edema, congestion, necrosis, and eventual rupture or perforation of the intestinal wall, with resultant peritonitis.

Reflux vomiting may be caused by abdominal distention. Vomiting results in loss of hydrochloric acid (HCl) and potassium from the stomach, leading to reduction of chlorides and potassium in the blood and to metabolic alkalosis. Dehydration develops from loss of water and sodium. With acute fluid losses, hypovolemic shock may occur.

Clinical Manifestations and Assessment

The initial symptom is usually crampy pain that is wavelike and colicky. The patient may pass blood and mucus but no fecal matter and no flatus. Vomiting occurs. If the obstruction is complete, the peristaltic waves initially become extremely vigorous and eventually assume a reverse direction, with the intestinal contents propelled toward the mouth instead of toward the rectum. If the obstruction is in the ileum, fecal vomiting takes place. First, the patient vomits the stomach contents, then the bile-stained contents of the duodenum and the jejunum, and finally, with each paroxysm of pain, the darker, fecal-like contents of the ileum. The signs of dehydration become evident: intense thirst, drowsiness, generalized malaise, aching, and a parched tongue and mucous membranes. The abdomen becomes distended. The lower the obstruction is in the GI tract, the more marked the abdominal distention. If the obstruction continues uncorrected, hypovolemic shock occurs from dehydration and loss of plasma volume.

Diagnosis is based on the symptoms described previously and on imaging studies. Abdominal x-ray and CT findings include abnormal quantities of gas, fluid, or both in the intestines. Laboratory studies (i.e., electrolyte studies and a CBC) reveal a picture of dehydration, loss of plasma volume, and possible infection.

Medical and Nursing Management

Decompression of the bowel through a nasogastric tube (see Chapter 22) is successful in most cases. When the bowel is obstructed completely, the possibility of strangulation warrants surgical intervention. Before surgery, IV therapy is necessary to replace the depleted water, sodium, chloride, and potassium.

The surgical treatment of intestinal obstruction depends largely on the cause of the obstruction. In the most common causes of obstruction, such as hernia and adhesions, the surgical procedure involves repairing the hernia or dividing the adhesion to which the intestine is attached. In some instances, the portion of affected bowel may be removed and an anastomosis performed. The complexity of the surgical procedure for intestinal obstruction depends on the duration of the obstruction and the condition of the intestine.

Nursing management of the nonsurgical patient with a small bowel obstruction includes maintaining the function of the nasogastric tube, assessing and measuring the nasogastric output, assessing for fluid and electrolyte imbalance, monitoring nutritional status, and assessing improvement (e.g., return of normal bowel sounds, decreased abdominal distention, subjective improvement in abdominal pain and tenderness, passage of flatus or stool). The nurse reports discrepancies in intake and output, worsening of pain or abdominal distention, and increased nasogastric output. If the patient's condition does not improve, the nurse prepares him or her for surgery. The exact nature of the surgery depends on the cause of the obstruction. Nursing care of the patient after surgical repair of a small bowel obstruction is similar to that for other abdominal surgeries (see Chapter 23).

Unfolding Patient Stories: Stan Checketts • Part 2

Recall from Chapter 7 Stan Checketts, who arrived in the emergency department with severe abdominal pain. He is diagnosed with a small bowel obstruction. He is NPO and has a nasogastric (NG) tube placed to low intermittent suction. Describe the steps of a focused GI assessment performed by the nurse. How would the nurse explain the rationale for an NG tube and NPO status? What are specific assessments and nursing care responsibilities for an NG tube?

Care for Stan and other patients in a realistic virtual environment: *vSim for Nursing* (thepoint.lww.com/vSimMedicalSurgical). Practice documenting these patients' care in DocuCare (thepoint.lww.com/DocuCareEHR).

LARGE BOWEL OBSTRUCTION

Pathophysiology

As in small bowel obstruction, large bowel obstruction results in an accumulation of intestinal contents, fluid, and gas proximal to the obstruction. Obstruction in the large bowel can lead to severe distention and perforation unless some gas and fluid can flow back through the ileal valve. Large bowel obstruction, even if complete, may be without catastrophic issue if the blood supply to the colon is not disturbed. However, if the blood supply is cut off, intestinal strangulation and necrosis (i.e., tissue death) occur; this condition is life threatening. In the large intestine, dehydration occurs more slowly than in the small intestine because the colon can absorb its fluid contents and can distend to a size considerably beyond its normal full capacity.

Adenocarcinoid tumors account for the majority of large bowel obstructions. Most tumors occur beyond the splenic flexure, making them accessible with a flexible sigmoidoscope.

Clinical Manifestations and Assessment

Large bowel obstruction differs clinically from small bowel obstruction in that the symptoms develop and progress relatively slowly. In patients with obstruction in the sigmoid colon or the rectum, constipation may be the only symptom for months. The shape of the stool is altered as it passes the obstruction that is gradually increasing in size. Blood in the stool may result in iron-deficiency anemia. The patient may experience weakness, weight loss, and anorexia. Eventually, the abdomen becomes markedly distended, loops of large bowel become visibly outlined through the abdominal wall, and the patient has crampy lower abdominal pain. Finally, fecal vomiting develops. Symptoms of shock may occur.

Diagnosis is based on symptoms and on imaging studies. Abdominal x-ray and abdominal CT or MRI findings reveal a distended colon and pinpoint the site of the obstruction. Barium studies are contraindicated because of risk of perforation.

Medical and Nursing Management

Restoration of intravascular volume, correction of electrolyte abnormalities, and nasogastric aspiration and decompression are instituted immediately. A colonoscopy may be performed to untwist and decompress the bowel. A cecostomy, in which a surgical opening is made into the cecum, may be performed in patients who are poor surgical risks and urgently need relief from the obstruction. The procedure provides an outlet for releasing gas and a small amount of drainage. A rectal tube may be used to decompress an area that is lower in the bowel. However, the usual treatment is surgical resection to remove the obstructing lesion. A temporary or permanent colostomy may be necessary. An ileoanal anastomosis may be performed if it is necessary to remove the entire large bowel.

The nurse's role is to monitor the patient for symptoms that indicate that the intestinal obstruction is worsening and to provide emotional support and comfort. The nurse administers IV fluids and electrolytes as prescribed. If the patient's condition does not respond to nonsurgical treatment, the nurse prepares the patient for surgery. This preparation includes preoperative teaching as the patient's condition indicates. After surgery, general abdominal wound care and routine postoperative nursing care are provided.

DISEASES OF THE ANORECTUM

Diseases of the anorectum include anal fistulas and fissures, hemorrhoids, sexually transmitted anorectal diseases, and pilonidal cysts. Nursing management of these conditions is discussed in Box 24-3.

ANAL FISTULA

An anal fistula is a tiny, tubular, fibrous tract that extends into the anal canal from an opening located beside the anus (Fig. 24-13A). Fistulas usually result from an infection. They also may develop from trauma, fissures, or regional enteritis. Pus or stool may leak constantly from the cutaneous opening. Other symptoms may be the passage of flatus or feces from the vagina or bladder, depending on the fistula tract. Untreated fistulas may cause systemic infection with related symptoms.

Surgery is always recommended because few fistulas heal spontaneously. A fistulectomy (i.e., excision of the fistulous tract) is the recommended surgical procedure. The lower bowel is evacuated thoroughly with several prescribed enemas. The fistula is dissected out or laid open by an incision from its rectal opening to its outlet. The wound is packed with gauze.

ANAL FISSURE

An anal fissure is a longitudinal tear or ulceration in the lining of the anal canal (see Fig. 24-13B). Usually fissures

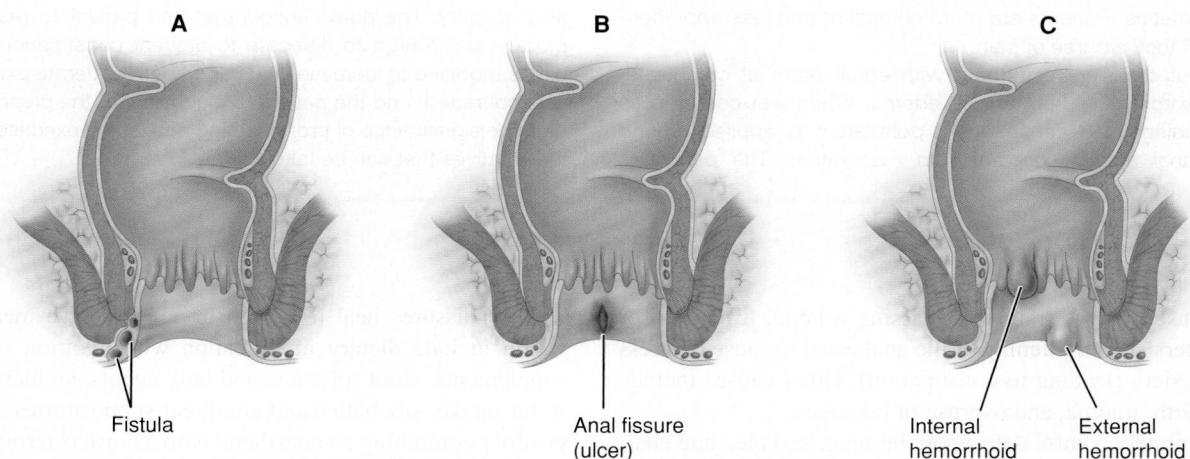

A   **B**   **C**

Fistula   Anal fissure (ulcer)   Internal hemorrhoid   External hemorrhoid

FIGURE 24-13 Various types of anal lesions. **A.** Fistula. **B.** Fissure. **C.** External and internal hemorrhoids.

BOX 24-3 **Nursing Management of Anorectal Disorders**

Relieving Constipation

The nurse encourages intake of at least 2 L of water daily to provide adequate hydration; in addition, the nurse recommends high-fiber foods to promote bulk in the stool and to make it easier to pass fecal matter through the rectum. In patients with pre-existing cardiopulmonary or kidney disease, consultation with the patient's provider regarding fluid intake should occur. Bulk laxatives such as psyllium (Metamucil) and stool softeners (e.g., docusate [Colace]) are administered as prescribed. The patient is advised to set aside a time for bowel movements and to heed the urge to defecate as promptly as possible. It may be helpful to have the patient perform relaxation exercises before defecating to relax the abdominal and perineal muscles, which may be constricted or in spasm. Administering an analgesic before a bowel movement is beneficial.

Reducing Anxiety

Patients facing rectal surgery may be upset and irritable because of discomfort, pain, and embarrassment. The nurse identifies specific psychosocial needs and individualizes the plan of care. The nurse maintains the patient's privacy while providing care and limits visitors, if the patient desires. Soiled dressings are removed from the room promptly to prevent unpleasant odors; room deodorizers may be needed if dressings are foul smelling.

Relieving Pain

During the first 24 hours after rectal surgery, painful spasms of the sphincter and perineal muscles may occur. Control of pain is a prime consideration. The patient is encouraged to assume a comfortable position. Flotation pads under the buttocks when sitting help decrease the pain, as may ice and analgesic ointments. Warm compresses may promote circulation and soothe irritated tissues. Sitz baths taken three or four times each day can relieve soreness and pain by relaxing sphincter spasm. Twenty-four hours after surgery, topical anesthetic agents may be beneficial in relieving local irritation and soreness. Medications may include topical anesthetics (i.e., suppositories), astringents, antiseptics, tranquilizers, and antiemetics. Patients are more compliant and less apprehensive if they are free of pain.

Wet dressings saturated with equal parts of cold water and witch hazel help relieve edema. When wet compresses are being used continuously, petrolatum is applied around the anal area to prevent skin maceration. The patient is instructed to assume a prone position at intervals because this position reduces edema of the tissue.

Promoting Urinary Elimination

Voiding may be a problem after surgery because of a reflex spasm of the sphincter at the outlet of the bladder and a certain amount of muscle guarding from apprehension and pain. The nurse tries all methods to encourage voluntary voiding (i.e., increasing fluid intake, listening to running water, and pouring warm water over the urinary meatus) before resorting to catheterization. After rectal surgery, urinary output is monitored closely.

Monitoring and Managing Complications

The operative site is examined frequently for rectal bleeding. The nurse assesses the patient for systemic indicators of excessive bleeding (i.e., tachycardia, hypotension, restlessness, and thirst). After hemorrhoidectomy, hemorrhage may occur from the veins that were cut. If a tube has been inserted through the sphincter after surgery, blood may be visible on the dressings. If bleeding is obvious, direct pressure is applied to the area, and the surgeon is notified. It is important to avoid using moist heat because it encourages vessel dilation and bleeding.

Promoting Home and Community-Based Care

Teaching Patients Self-Care

Most patients with anorectal conditions are not hospitalized. Those who undergo surgical procedures to correct the condition often are discharged directly from the outpatient surgical center. If they are hospitalized, it is for a short time, usually only 24 hours.

The nurse instructs the patient to keep the perianal area as clean as possible by gently cleansing with warm water and then drying with absorbent cotton wipes. The patient should avoid rubbing the area with toilet tissue. Instructions are provided about how to take a sitz bath and how to test the temperature of the water.

Continuing Care

Sitz baths should follow each bowel movement for 1–2 weeks after surgery. The nurse encourages the patient to respond quickly to the urge to defecate to prevent constipation. The diet is modified to increase fluids and fiber. Moderate exercise is encouraged, and the patient is taught about the prescribed diet, the significance of proper eating habits and exercise, and the laxatives that can be taken safely.

---

are caused by the trauma of passing a large, firm stool or from persistent tightening of the anal canal because of stress and anxiety (leading to constipation). Other causes include childbirth, trauma, and overuse of laxatives.

Extremely painful defecation, burning, and bleeding characterize fissures. Bright red blood may be seen on the toilet tissue after a bowel movement.

Most fissures heal if treated by conservative measures, which include dietary modification with addition of fiber supplements, stool softeners and bulk agents, an increase in water intake, sitz baths, and emollient suppositories. A suppository combining an anesthetic with a corticosteroid helps relieve the discomfort. Anal dilation under anesthesia may be required.

If fissures do not respond to conservative treatment, surgery is indicated. Most surgeons consider the procedure of choice to be the lateral internal sphincterotomy with excision of the fissure.

HEMORRHOIDS

Hemorrhoids are dilated portions of veins in the anal canal. They are very common: by 50 years of age, about 50% of people have hemorrhoids, although the prevalence is hard to estimate as many people do not report having hemorrhoids and rely on over-the-counter treatments (Ganz, 2013; NIH, U.S. Department of Health and Human Services, 2009). Shearing of the mucosa during defecation results in the sliding of the structures in the wall of the anal canal, including the hemorrhoidal and vascular tissues. Increased pressure in the hemorrhoidal tissue due to pregnancy may initiate hemorrhoids or aggravate existing ones. Hemorrhoids are classified as one of two types: those above the internal sphincter are called *internal hemorrhoids*, and those appearing outside the external sphincter are called *external hemorrhoids* (see Fig. 24-13C).

Hemorrhoids cause itching and pain and are the most common cause of bright red bleeding with defecation. External hemorrhoids are associated with severe pain from the inflammation and edema caused by thrombosis (i.e., clotting of blood within the hemorrhoid). This may lead to ischemia of the area and eventual necrosis. Internal hemorrhoids usually are not painful until they bleed or prolapse when they become enlarged.

Hemorrhoid symptoms and discomfort can be relieved by good personal hygiene and by avoiding excessive straining during defecation. A high-residue diet that contains fruit and bran along with an increased fluid intake may be all the treatment necessary to promote the passage of soft, bulky stools to prevent straining. If this treatment is not successful, the addition of hydrophilic bulk-forming agents such as psyllium (Metamucil) may help. Warm compresses, sitz baths, analgesic ointments and suppositories, astringents (e.g., witch hazel), and bed rest allow the engorgement to subside.

> ⓘ **Nursing Alert**
> *In addition to increasing fiber and good personal hygiene, light exercise should be included in patient teaching in order to help improve peristalsis and improve defecation.*

There are several types of nonsurgical treatments for hemorrhoids. Infrared photocoagulation, bipolar diathermy, and laser therapy are used to affix the mucosa to the underlying muscle. Injection of sclerosing agents is also effective for small, bleeding hemorrhoids. These procedures help prevent prolapse.

A conservative surgical treatment of internal hemorrhoids is the rubber-band ligation procedure. The hemorrhoid is visualized through the anoscope, and its proximal portion above the mucocutaneous lines is grasped with an instrument. Then a small rubber band is slipped over the hemorrhoid. Tissue distal to the rubber band becomes necrotic after several days and sloughs off. Fibrosis occurs; the result is that the lower anal mucosa is drawn up and adheres to the underlying muscle. Although this treatment has been satisfactory for some patients, it has proven painful for others and may cause secondary hemorrhage. It also has been known to cause perianal infection.

Cryosurgical hemorrhoidectomy, another method for removing hemorrhoids, involves freezing the hemorrhoid for a sufficient time to cause necrosis. Although it is relatively painless, this procedure is not used widely because the discharge is very foul smelling and wound healing is prolonged. The Nd:YAG laser is useful in excising hemorrhoids, particularly external hemorrhoidal tags. The treatment is quick and relatively painless. Hemorrhage and abscess are rare postoperative complications.

The previously described methods of treating hemorrhoids are not effective for advanced thrombosed veins, which must be treated by more extensive surgery. Hemorrhoidectomy, or surgical excision, can be performed to remove all the redundant tissue involved in the process. During surgery, usually the rectal sphincter is dilated digitally and the hemorrhoids are removed with a clamp and cautery or are ligated and then excised. After the surgical procedures are completed, a small tube may be inserted through the sphincter to permit the escape of flatus and blood; pieces of Gelfoam or Oxycel gauze may be placed over the anal wounds.

SEXUALLY TRANSMITTED ANORECTAL DISEASES

Three infectious syndromes that are related to sexually transmitted infections (STIs) have been identified: proctitis, proctocolitis, and enteritis. Proctitis involves the rectum. It is commonly associated with recent anal-receptive intercourse with an infected partner. Symptoms include a mucopurulent discharge or bleeding, pain in the area, and diarrhea. The pathogens most frequently involved are *Neisseria gonorrhoeae*, *Chlamydia*, herpes simplex virus, and *Treponema pallidum*. Proctocolitis involves the rectum and lowest portion of the descending colon. The most common pathogens causing proctocolitis are *Campylobacter*, *Shigella*, *Entamoeba histolytica*, and *Chlamydia trachomatis*. Symptoms are similar to proctitis but also may include watery or bloody diarrhea, cramps, and abdominal tenderness. Enteritis involves more of the descending colon, and symptoms include watery, bloody diarrhea; abdominal pain; and weight loss. The most common pathogens causing enteritis are *E. histolytica*, *Giardia lamblia*, *Shigella*, and *Campylobacter*.

Sigmoidoscopy is performed to identify portions of the anorectum involved. Samples are taken with rectal swabs, and cultures are obtained to identify the pathogens involved. Antibiotics (i.e., cefixime [Suprax], doxycycline [Vibramycin], and penicillin G) are the treatment of choice for bacterial infections. Acyclovir [Zovirax] is given to patients with viral infections. Antiamebic therapy (i.e., metronidazole [Flagyl]) is appropriate for infections with *E. histolytica* and *G. lamblia*. Ciprofloxacin (Cipro) is effective for *Shigella*. The antibiotics erythromycin (E-Mycin) and ciprofloxacin are the treatment of choice for *Campylobacter* infection.

PILONIDAL SINUS OR CYST

A pilonidal sinus or cyst is found in the intergluteal cleft on the posterior surface of the lower sacrum (Fig. 24-14). Current theories suggest that it results from local trauma, causing the penetration of hairs into the epithelium and subcutaneous tissue. It also may be formed congenitally by an infolding of epithelial tissue beneath the skin, which may communicate with the skin surface through one or several small sinus openings. Hair frequently is seen protruding from these openings, and this gives the cyst its name, *pilonidal* (i.e., a nest of hair). The cysts rarely cause symptoms until adolescence or early adult life, when infection produces an irritating drainage or an abscess. Perspiration and friction easily irritate this area.

FIGURE 24-14 **A.** Pilonidal sinus on lower sacrum about 5 cm (2 in) above the anus in the intergluteal cleft. **B.** Hair particles emerge from the sinus tract, and localized indentations (pits) can appear on the skin near the sinus openings.

In the early stages of the inflammation, the infection may be controlled by antibiotic therapy, but after an abscess has formed, surgery is indicated. The abscess is incised and drained under local anesthesia. After the acute process resolves, further surgery is performed to excise the cyst and the secondary sinus tracts. The wound is allowed to heal by granulation. Gauze dressings are placed in the wound to keep its edges separated while healing occurs.

CHAPTER REVIEW

Critical Thinking Exercises

1. Discuss the antibiotic choices for spontaneous bacterial peritonitis using the current evidence-based practice.

2. Compare and contrast the pathophysiologic differences between Crohn disease and ulcerative colitis in their presentation, course of disease, and treatment regimens.

NCLEX-Style Review Questions

1. A patient returns to his room following a diagnostic colonoscopy after radiologic evidence of diverticulosis. He reports an increase in abdominal pain, fever, and chills. Which clinical condition is most concerning to the nurse?
   a. Colon cancer
   b. Hemorrhoids
   c. Bowel perforation
   d. Anal fissure

2. A patient is complaining of right lower quadrant pain, fever, and decreased appetite. What does the nurse suspect is the most likely cause?
   a. Diverticulitis
   b. Appendicitis
   c. Small bowel obstruction
   d. Sigmoid colon cancer

3. A patient complains of abdominal pain unrelieved by defecation, that typically occurs after meals along with diarrhea. What does the nurse recognize as the most likely diagnosis?
   a. Ulcerative colitis
   b. Regional enteritis
   c. Cholecystitis
   d. Diverticulosis

4. A patient complains of abdominal pain and distention, fever, tachycardia, and diaphoresis. An abdominal x-ray shows free air under the diaphragm. The emergency department nurse should suspect which condition?
   a. Intestinal obstruction
   b. Malabsorption
   c. Intestinal perforation
   d. Acute cholelithiasis

5. A patient has a bowel perforation from a recent surgery and now has been diagnosed with peritonitis. The patient has hypoactive bowel sounds, a temperature of 100.5°F, and an elevated WBC count. What is the most serious potential complication of peritonitis for which the nurse should monitor?
   a. Nausea
   b. Diarrhea
   c. Sepsis
   d. Abdominal tenderness

Try these additional resources, available at **http://thepoint.lww.com/Honan2e**, to enhance your learning and understanding of this chapter:
- NCLEX-Style Student Review Questions
- Journal Articles

REFERENCES AND SELECTED READINGS

References and selected readings associated with this chapter can be found on the website that accompanies the book. Visit **http://thepoint. lww.com/Honan2e** to access the references and other additional resources associated with this chapter.

Nursing Management: Patients with Hepatic and Biliary Disorders

Honore Kotler

Learning Objectives

After reading this chapter, you will be able to:

1. Relate jaundice, portal hypertension, ascites, varices, nutritional deficiencies, and hepatic coma to pathophysiologic alterations of the liver.
2. Describe the medical, surgical, and nursing management of patients with esophageal varices.
3. Compare the various types of hepatitis and their causes, prevention, clinical manifestations, management, prognosis, and home health care needs.
4. Discuss medical and nursing management of patients with cancer of the liver.
5. Describe the postoperative nursing care of the patient undergoing liver transplantation.
6. Discuss management of cholelithiasis.
7. Differentiate between acute and chronic pancreatitis.
8. Discuss nursing management of patients with acute pancreatitis.

Liver function is complex, and liver dysfunction affects all body systems. Liver disorders are common and may result from a virus, exposure to toxic substances such as alcohol, or tumors. Disorders of the biliary tract and pancreas also are common and include gallbladder stones and pancreatic dysfunction. An understanding of how biliary tract disorders are closely linked with liver disease is necessary to adequately care for patients.

HEPATIC DISORDERS

Understanding and managing liver disorders requires expert clinical assessment and management skills. Box 25-1 highlights important considerations for hepatic assessment.

MANIFESTATIONS OF HEPATIC DYSFUNCTION

JAUNDICE

Yellowing of the skin and sclerae of the eyes are caused by impairment of the liver's ability to metabolize and secrete bilirubin. Jaundice is apparent when the serum bilirubin level exceeds 3 mg/dL. Elevations of serum bilirubin levels can result from either acute or chronic liver injury. The differential diagnosis of jaundice can result from the following causes:

- Hepatocellular jaundice caused by viral hepatitis, hepatotoxins (including drugs, alcohol), metabolic disorders, ischemia, autoimmune hepatitis, or pregnancy
- Obstructive jaundice caused by obstruction of the bile ducts; gallstones; inflammation of bile ducts caused by primary sclerosing cholangitis, biliary strictures, malignancies of the biliary system, pancreatic cancer, liver cancer, or pancreatitis
- Hemolytic jaundice caused by increased production of bilirubin due to hemolysis, hematologic disorders, resorption of a hematoma, or multiple transfusions
- Hereditary hyperbilirubinemia caused by the inherited disorders of bilirubin metabolism, including various syndromes, some of which may require transplantation

PORTAL HYPERTENSION

Portal hypertension is caused by increased resistance to blood flow through the liver and increased blood flow due to vasodilatation in the splanchnic circulation (see Fig. 25-1). The two major complications of portal hypertension are **ascites** and gastroesophageal varices (discussed below) (Garcia-Tso, 2016).

BOX 25-1
Review of Hepatic Assessment

The initial presentation of a patient with liver disease varies greatly and can range from elevated liver enzymes on routine screening with no clinical signs or symptoms of disease to the patient who presents in liver failure with jaundice, hepatic coma, or esophageal bleeding. A comprehensive and complete health history is critical to determine exposure to hepatoxic substances (including alcohol) or infectious agents causing liver dysfunction and to distinguish between acute and chronic hepatic dysfunction.

Health History Findings
Common Symptoms
- General: Lethargy, weakness, fatigue, fever, jaundice, pruritus (itching)
- Neurologic: Changes in mental acuity, personality changes, sleep disturbances, confusion, and outright coma in advanced chronic liver disease or acute failure
- Cardiopulmonary: Dyspnea resulting from increased fluid retention
- GI: Abdominal pain, increasing abdominal girth, anorexia, nausea, vomiting, hematemesis (vomiting blood), melena (black, tarry stool), hematochezia (stool that contains blood)
- Hematologic/Circulatory: Increased bruising, spontaneous bleeding, dependent and or/pedal edema
- Endocrine: Decreased libido in both men and women

Past Medical History
A prior history of inflammatory bowel disease or ulcerative colitis may lead to the diagnosis of primary sclerosing cholangitis (inflammation of the bile ducts). Chronic liver disease is commonly caused by alcohol and viruses, such as hepatitis B or C. Frequently patients with nonalcoholic fatty liver disease (NAFLD) may have prior medical history of diabetes, hyperlipidemia, and obesity.

Family History
Wilson disease, hemochromatosis, and autoimmune liver disease are genetically based. A positive family history of hepatitis B may indicate vertical transmission (Greenberger, 2012).

Social History
- Lifestyle: Current and prior drug use (i.e., IV drug abuse, inhalation of drugs), sexual practices, tattoos, piercings, blood transfusions, needlestick injury, shared razors, toothbrushes
- Occupational: Exposure to toxins in workplaces; health care worker exposure to patients in trauma areas, operating rooms, Hemodialysis unit or Center

- Travel history: Recent travel to endemic areas such as Mexico, Africa, India, or Latin America with ingestion of contaminated food or water, and raw shellfish
- Alcohol use: Information regarding current and prior alcohol use should be obtained from both patient and family (i.e., amount of alcohol ingested daily). Intake of 60 g/day for men and 30 g/day for women (10 g of alcohol is equivalent to 1-oz bourbon, or 12-oz beer, or 4-oz red wine) is sufficient to cause liver injury. The impact of alcohol-induced liver injury or disease is increased in the presence of other risk factors, such as hepatitis C (Greenberger, 2012).
- Medications: Review all prescription medications, over-the-counter, herbal supplements or home remedies, and intake of vitamins (especially vitamin A). Medications are frequent culprits in acute hepatic dysfunction and may lead to fulminant hepatic failure (e.g., acetaminophen overdose).

Physical Examination Findings
- Integumentary and oral: Jaundice, ecchymosis, spider angiomas and palmar erythema, scleral icterus or yellowing of the sclerae, leukonychia of the nails (white spots on nails), and clubbing of the fingers
- Oral: Hepatic fetor, a sweet, mildly fecal breath odor associated with encephalopathy
- Neurologic: Impairment of the patient's neurologic or cognitive status (slurred speech, confusion, poor recall, or slowed responses)
- Musculoskeletal: Muscle wasting; tremors or asterixis (flapping of the hands when wrists dorsiflexed) with altered mental status indicate hepatic encephalopathy.
- Abdominal: Signs of abdominal distention indicating ascites, or prominent dilated veins visible through the skin. Umbilical hernia or ventral hernias also may be observed. The patient with liver disease may also show striae, excoriations, or petechiae of the abdominal skin. Palpation of the liver is important to determine its size, shape, and consistency, and percussion is necessary to assess for ascites. The normal liver has a sharp, smooth edge and is firm, but not hard, with a nonpalpable left lobe. Presence of an enlarged liver indicates liver disease (Greenberger, 2012).
- Other: Pitting edema of the lower extremities; males may demonstrate gynecomastia and testicular atrophy (Greenberger, 2012).

Diagnostic Evaluation
Diagnostic evaluation includes liver biopsy, liver function tests, and ultrasound (see Chapter 21).

ASCITES

In ascites, fluid accumulates in the peritoneal cavity. Increased blood flow in the veins draining the portal system results in dilation and the development of varicose veins.

Pathophysiology

The mechanisms responsible for the development of ascites are not completely understood. Portal hypertension and the resulting increase in capillary pressure and obstruction of

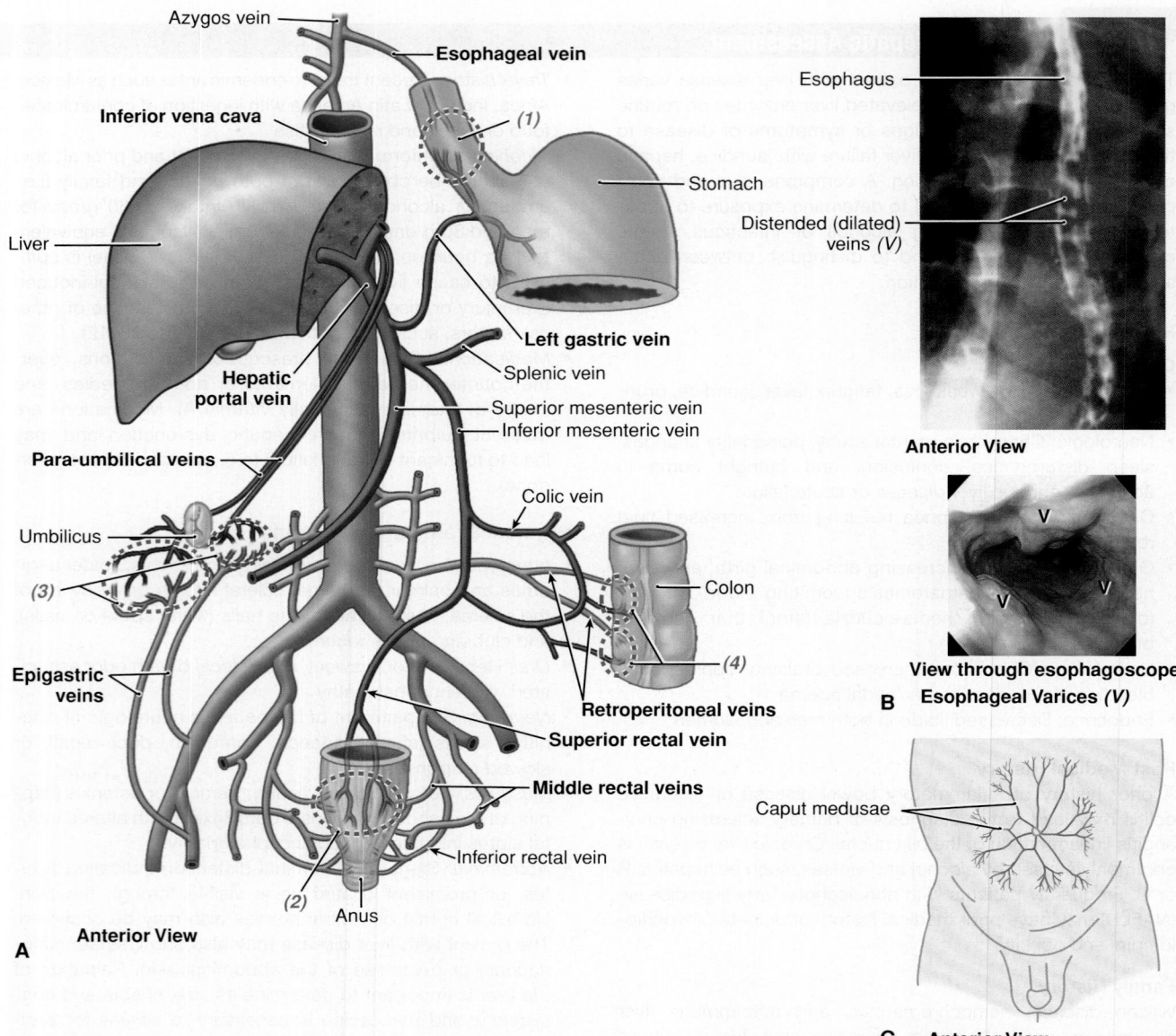

FIGURE 25-1 **A.** Portacaval system. In this diagram, portal tributaries (*dark blue*) and systemic tributaries and communicating veins (*light blue*). In portal hypertension (as in hepatic cirrhosis), the portal
blood cannot pass freely through the liver, and the portacaval anastomoses become engorged,
dilated, or even varicose; as a consequence, these veins may rupture. The sites of the portocaval
anastomosis shown are between (1) esophageal veins draining into the azygos vein (systemic) and
left gastric vein (portal), which when dilated are esophageal varices; (2) the inferior and middle rectal
veins, draining into the inferior vena cava (systemic), and the superior rectal vein continuing as the
inferior mesenteric vein (portal) (hemorrhoids result if the vessels are dilated); (3) paraumbilical veins
(portal) and small epigastric veins of the anterior abdominal wall (systemic), which when varicose
form "caput medusae" (so named because of the resemblance of the radiating veins to the serpents
on the head of Medusa, a character in Greek mythology); and (4) twigs of colic veins (portal) anastomosing with systemic retroperitoneal veins. **B.** Esophageal varices. **C.** Caput medusae. (Grant's Atlas
of Anatomy, Anne M. R. Agur; Arthur F Dalley.)

venous blood flow through the damaged liver are contributing factors. The vasodilation that occurs in the splanchnic
circulation is also a suspected causative factor. The failure
of the liver to metabolize aldosterone increases sodium and
water retention by the kidney. Sodium and water retention,
increased intravascular fluid volume, increased lymphatic

flow, and decreased synthesis of albumin by the damaged
liver all contribute to the movement of fluid from the vascular system into the peritoneal space. The process becomes
self-perpetuating as loss of fluid into the peritoneal space
causes further sodium and water retention by the kidney in
an effort to maintain the vascular fluid volume. As a result

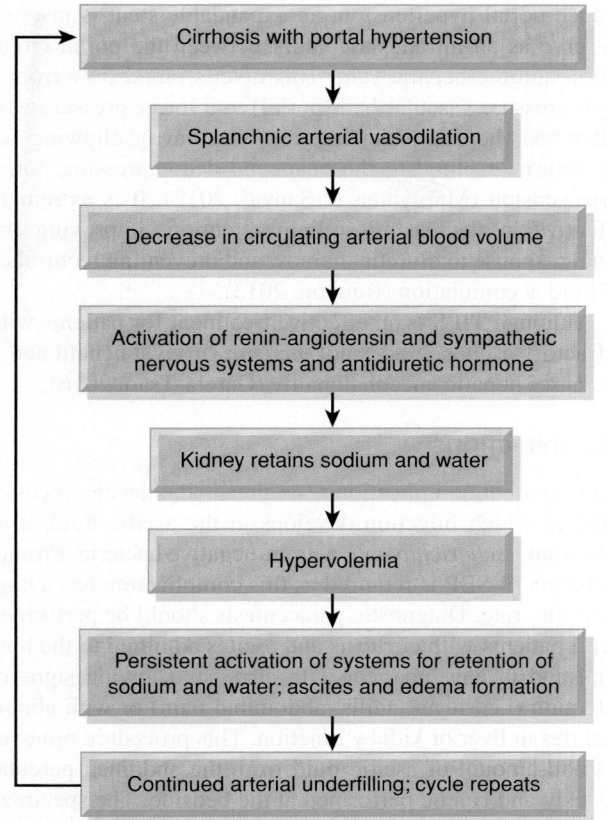

FIGURE 25-2 Pathogenesis of ascites (arterial vasodilation theory).

of liver damage, large amounts of albumin-rich fluid, 15 L or more, may accumulate in the peritoneal cavity as ascites (Runyon, 2013). Figure 25-2 illustrates the pathogenesis of ascites.

Clinical Manifestations and Assessment

Common symptoms of the patient presenting with ascites include increased abdominal girth, weight gain, and swelling of the lower extremities (pedal edema). Dyspnea may be present as the result of abdominal distention or pleural effusions. Abdominal hernias due to increased intra-abdominal pressure may be visible as well as visible collateral veins and striae (stretch marks). The patient also may experience early satiety, anorexia, and general weakness (Runyon, 2013).

The detection of ascites by physical examination can be assessed by percussion for shifting dullness. With the patient supine, the free fluid in the abdomen will accumulate in the flanks; percussion of the abdomen will reveal tympany over the anterior abdomen and dullness over the flanks. Turning the patient to one side with repeat percussion will reveal shifting dullness (the uppermost area will sound tympanic while the lower area will sound dull to percussion). Assessing for abdominal fluid wave also detects ascites (Fig. 25-3). Bulging flanks also may reveal the presence of ascites. Accurate physical assessment of ascites through examination may

be decreased if ascitic fluid is less than 1,500 mL or if the patient is obese (Runyon, 2013).

Ultrasonography of the liver and abdomen will definitively confirm the presence of ascites (Runyon, 2013). Diagnostic paracentesis (discussed in Chapter 21) is performed routinely on patients presenting with ascites upon hospital admission to detect the presence of spontaneous bacterial peritonitis (SBP). This complication of cirrhosis has a high mortality rate and will be discussed later in the chapter (Runyon, 2013).

Medical and Nursing Management

Dietary Modification

Dietary restriction of salt intake is the mainstay of treatment of ascites to achieve a negative sodium balance to reduce fluid retention. The recommended daily sodium intake of patients with ascites should be 2,000 mg or less (Runyon, 2013). Patients on sodium-restricted diets should receive nutritional education and guidance on foods that contain high sodium content (i.e., all processed foods, frozen and canned foods not indicated as low sodium) and avoid the use of added salt in meals and food preparation. Ongoing patient education and referral to a licensed nutritionist will facilitate dietary adherence.

Diuretics

The addition of diuretics with sodium restriction will result in decreased ascites in approximately 90% of patients.

FIGURE 25-3 Assessing for abdominal fluid wave. The examiner places the hands along the sides of the patient's flanks and then strikes one flank sharply, detecting any fluid wave with the other hand. An assistant's hand is placed (ulnar side down) along the patient's midline to prevent the fluid wave from being transmitted through the tissues of the abdominal wall.

Combination drug therapy using spironolactone (Aldactone), an aldosterone-blocking agent, and furosemide (Lasix), a loop diuretic agent, is the most effective regimen to control ascites and pedal edema. Patients should be monitored for daily weight changes (not to exceed 0.5 kg/day (1.1 lb) gain or loss in patients without peripheral edema, whereas in patients with peripheral edema, there may be no limit on daily weigh loss (Runyon, 2013). Frequently failure to achieve weight reduction and decrease in ascites with the use of therapeutic doses of diuretics is due to insufficient salt restriction (Runyon, 2013).

Possible complications of diuretic therapy are dehydration, volume depletion, and electrolyte abnormalities, such as hypokalemia or hyperkalemia, hyponatremia, kidney impairment, and hepatic encephalopathy. Gynecomastia is a common side effect caused by Spironolactone. If patients with ascites develop dilutional hyponatremia (serum sodium below 134 mmol/L), then diuretics should be discontinued and fluid restriction initiated. Dietary salt restriction to less than 2,000 mg daily should be reinforced (Runyon, 2013).

Paracentesis

Paracentesis is the removal of fluid (ascites) from the peritoneal cavity through a puncture or a small surgical incision through the abdominal wall under sterile conditions. Therapeutic paracentesis provides only temporary removal of fluid; ascites rapidly recurs, necessitating repeated fluid removal. See Chapter 21 for detailed discussion of paracentesis.

Transjugular Intrahepatic Portosystemic Shunt

Transjugular intrahepatic portosystemic shunt (TIPS) is a method of treating ascites in which a cannula is threaded into the portal vein by the transjugular route (Fig. 25-4). To reduce portal hypertension, an expandable stent is inserted to serve as an intrahepatic shunt between the portal circulation and the hepatic vein. This diverts blood flow from a high-pressure vascular bed (portal) to a lower-pressure vascular bed (hepatic veins/inferior vena cava), allowing for the return of blood to the heart and decompressing portal hypertension (Maruyama & Sanyal, 2012). It is extremely effective in decreasing sodium retention, improving the renal response to diuretic therapy, and preventing recurrence of fluid accumulation (Runyon, 2013).

Although TIPS is an effective treatment for patients with refractory ascites, it does not increase survival benefit and it increases hepatic encephalopathy (Garcia-Tsao, 2016).

Complications

An important complication of ascites is the development of SBP, in which infection develops in the ascitic fluid, usually from *Escherichia coli*, a gram-negative bacteria. Prompt detection of SBP is required as this complication has a high mortality rate. Diagnostic paracentesis should be performed in all patients with cirrhosis and ascites admitted to the hospital and in any inpatient with cirrhosis showing signs of infection (i.e., fever, chills, abdominal pain) or with abnormalities in liver or kidney function. This procedure removes a small amount of ascitic fluid from the abdomen percutaneously and can be performed at the bedside. The specimen is analyzed for cell count and differential, albumin, total protein, and susceptible organisms (Runyon, 2013). The treatment of SBP includes the use of IV antibiotics or oral treatment if tolerated. Long-term prophylaxis with oral antibiotic therapy is recommended to prevent future infection in patients who have had a diagnosis of SBP (Garcia-Tsao, 2016; Runyon, 2013).

ESOPHAGEAL VARICES

Gastroesophageal varices are present in 50% of patients with cirrhosis and are the most life-threatening complication in patients with chronic liver disease. Bleeding or hemorrhage from esophageal varices is associated with significantly decreased overall lifespan with a mortality rate as high as 20% within the first 6 weeks of initial bleeding episode (Garcia-Tsao, 2016).

Pathophysiology

Esophageal varices are dilated, tortuous veins that usually are found in the submucosa of the lower esophagus but may develop higher in the esophagus or extend into the stomach. Portal hypertension is the primary mechanism by which collateral circulation develops.

Because of increased obstruction of the portal vein, venous blood from the intestinal tract and spleen seeks an outlet through collateral circulation (new pathways for return of blood to the right atrium). The effect is increased

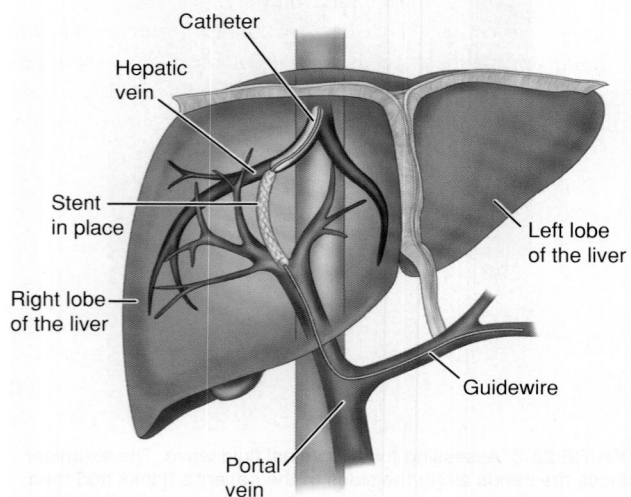

FIGURE 25-4 Transjugular intrahepatic portosystemic shunt (TIPS). A stent is inserted via catheter to the portal vein to divert blood flow and reduce portal hypertension.

Catheter

Hepatic vein

Stent in place

Right lobe of the liver

Left lobe of the liver

Guidewire

Portal vein

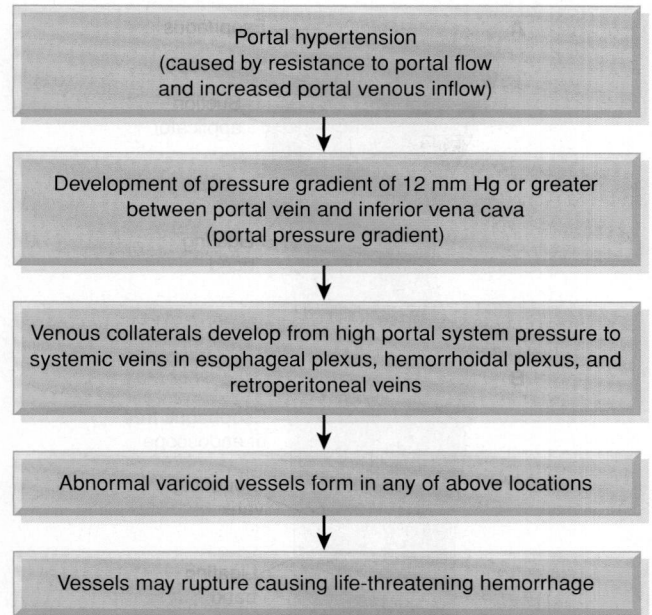

FIGURE 25-5 Pathogenesis of bleeding esophageal varices.

pressure, particularly in the vessels in the submucosal layer of the lower esophagus and upper part of the stomach. These collateral vessels are not very elastic; rather, they are tortuous and fragile, and they bleed easily (Maruyama & Sanyal, 2012). Gastroesophageal bleeding (Fig. 25-5) is due to high portal pressure and increased collateral blood flow, causing dilation and thinning of varices. Any additional increase in pressure or defect in the varices will cause rupture and hemorrhage. Factors that may precipitate hemorrhage are alcohol intake, physical exercise, and any activity that would increase intra-abdominal pressure (e.g., lifting, straining to pass stool, vomiting, coughing) (Maruyama & Sanyal, 2012).

Bleeding esophageal varices are life-threatening and can result in hemorrhagic shock that produces decreased cerebral, hepatic, and renal perfusion. In turn, there is an increased nitrogen load from bleeding into the GI tract and an increased serum ammonia level, increasing the risk for encephalopathy.

Clinical Manifestations and Assessment

The patient with bleeding esophageal varices may present with hematemesis, melena, or general deterioration in mental or physical status and often has a history of alcohol abuse. Signs and symptoms of shock (cool clammy skin, hypotension, tachycardia) may be present. Endoscopic evaluation (or esophagogastroduodenoscopy [EGD]) is used in the diagnosis and treatment of varices, in both the acute and outpatient settings. Assessment of variceal size, location, and features are used to predict the risk of bleeding. Variceal size is an important factor that determines both pharmacologic and endoscopic therapies to prevent and manage risk of bleeding. In the acute setting, endoscopy should take place within 12 hours after stabilization of the patient (Garcia-Tsao, 2016).

Medical Management

Acute bleeding from esophageal varices is an emergency that can quickly lead to hemorrhagic shock. The patient is critically ill, requiring aggressive medical care and expert nursing care, and he or she should be transferred to the intensive care unit (ICU) for close monitoring and management. Assessment and protection of the patient's airway and peripheral venous access is required. Endotracheal intubation may be necessary to prevent aspiration of blood (Garcia-Tsao, 2016).

The extent of bleeding is evaluated, and vital signs are monitored continuously if hematemesis and melena are present. Signs of potential hypovolemia are noted, such as cold clammy skin, tachycardia, a drop in blood pressure, decreased urine output, restlessness, and weak peripheral pulses. The volume of circulating blood is estimated and monitored with a central venous catheter or pulmonary artery catheter. Blood pressure is monitored noninvasively or via an arterial catheter. Oxygen is administered to prevent hypoxia and to maintain adequate blood oxygenation, which is evaluated via pulse oximetry or arterial blood gases (ABGs).

Because patients with bleeding esophageal varices have intravascular volume depletion and are subject to electrolyte imbalance, IV fluids with electrolytes and volume expanders are provided to restore fluid volume and replace electrolytes. Transfusion of blood components also may be required to maintain hemodynamic stability and correct coagulopathy. Caution must be taken with volume resuscitation so that overhydration does not occur because this would raise portal pressure and increase bleeding (Maruyama & Sanyal, 2012; Garcia-Tsao, 2016). Usually an indwelling urinary catheter is inserted to permit frequent monitoring of urine output.

Although a variety of pharmacologic, endoscopic, and surgical approaches are used to treat bleeding esophageal varices, none is ideal, and most are associated with considerable risk to the patient. Nonsurgical treatment of bleeding esophageal varices still is preferable because of the high mortality rate of emergency surgery to control bleeding esophageal varices and because of the poor physical condition that is typical of the patient with severe liver dysfunction.

Pharmacologic Therapy

The medical management of the patient with acute variceal hemorrhage includes the use of antibiotic therapy (IV ciprofloxacin, or ceftriaxone in patients with advanced cirrhosis) to prevent infection and improve survival. The most effective specific therapy for the control of active variceal hemorrhage is the combination of a vasoconstrictor with endoscopic therapy. Vasoconstrictors include somatostatin or octreotide because they decrease the splanchnic arterial blood and decrease portal pressure with fewer side effects and equal efficacy compared with vasopressin (discussed below). Octreotide has a longer half-life than somatostatin (100 minutes vs. 2 to 3 minutes) and, as a result, has become the agent of choice in managing acute variceal hemorrhage (Rigberg & Gelabert, 2013). Octreotide is maintained for 2 to 5 days in conjunction with endoscopic therapy (discussed below). Nonselective beta blockers are used for the prevention of variceal bleeding in patients with cirrhosis and also to reduce episodes of rebleeding after an initial episode (Garcia-Tsao, 2016).

In a patient who is actively bleeding, medications are administered initially because other therapies take longer to take effect. Although vasopressin (pitressin) is no longer considered first-line therapy in the management of active bleeding varices, it may be used to slow variceal hemorrhage because it produces constriction of the splanchnic arterial bed and decreases portal pressure (Rigberg & Gelabert, 2013). It may be administered by IV infusion. Stable vital signs and the decreasing presence or absence of blood in the gastric aspirate indicate the effectiveness of vasopressin. Monitoring of fluid intake and output and electrolyte levels is necessary because hyponatremia may develop, and vasopressin may have an antidiuretic effect.

The use of vasopressin may be used in conjunction with nitroglycerin or isoproterenol to prevent the side effects of vasoconstriction, including cardiac ischemia, arrhythmias, and hypertension (Maruyama & Sanyal, 2012; Rigberg & Gelabert, 2013).

Nursing Alert
If vasopressin is administered in acute esophageal bleed (because of its vasoconstrictive properties in the splanchnic, portal, and intrahepatic vessels), the nurse understands that this medication also causes coronary artery constriction that may dispose patients with coronary artery disease to cardiac ischemia. Thus the nurse observes the patient for evidence of chest pain, electrocardiogram (ECG) changes, and vital sign changes. A high degree of suspicion is maintained as many patients may have silent ischemia. Nitroglycerine may be administered concurrently with vasopressin.

Endoscopic Therapies

Esophageal Banding Therapy (Variceal Band Ligation)
In **variceal banding** (Fig. 25-6), an esophagogastroduodenoscopy is performed using a modified endoscope loaded with an elastic rubber band that is passed through an overtube directly onto the varix (or varices) to be banded. After the bleeding varix is suctioned into the tip of the endoscope, the rubber band is slipped over the tissue, causing necrosis, ulceration, and eventual sloughing of the varix. Complications include superficial ulceration and dysphagia (difficulty

FIGURE 25-6 Esophageal banding. **A.** A rubber band–like ligature is slipped over an esophageal varix via an endoscope. **B.** Necrosis results, and the varix eventually sloughs off.

swallowing), transient chest discomfort, and, rarely, esophageal strictures (Maruyama & Sanyal, 2012).

Esophageal banding is the most effective therapy to treat acute hemorrhage. After an acute episode of bleeding, the combination of beta-blocker therapy and routine esophageal banding is the treatment of choice and has been shown to effectively prevent rebleeding and improve survival (Garcia-Tsao, 2016).

Endoscopic Injection Sclerotherapy
In endoscopic injection **sclerotherapy** (EIS), a sclerosing agent is injected through a fiberoptic endoscope into the bleeding esophageal varices to promote thrombosis and eventual sclerosis (Fig. 25-7). This therapy is used only to treat an acute variceal bleed if esophageal banding is not feasible. Because of unproven efficacy and a high incidence

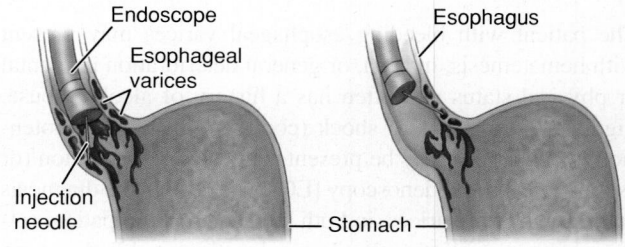
FIGURE 25-7 Endoscopic injection sclerotherapy. Injection of sclerosing agent into esophageal varices through an endoscope promotes thrombosis and eventual sclerosis, thereby obliterating the varices.

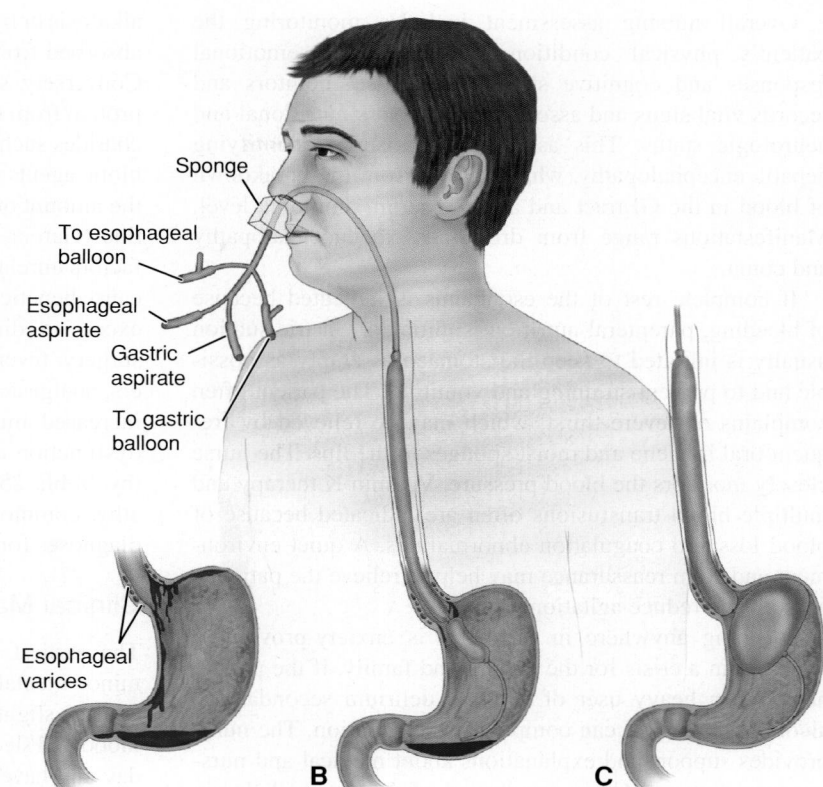

FIGURE 25-8 Balloon tamponade to treat esophageal varices. **A.** Dilated, bleeding esophageal veins (varices) of the lower esophagus. **B.** A four-lumen esophageal tamponade tube with balloons (uninflated) in place. **C.** Compression of bleeding esophageal varices by inflated esophageal and gastric balloons. The gastric and esophageal outlets permit the nurse to aspirate secretions.

of complications, endoscopic variceal sclerotherapy use is limited (Maruyama & Sanyal, 2012).

Balloon Tamponade

Balloon tamponade may be used as a temporary measure to control bleeding in an active hemorrhage. In this procedure, pressure is exerted on the cardia (upper orifice of the stomach) and against the bleeding varices by a double-balloon tamponade (Sengstaken-Blakemore tube) (Fig. 25-8). The tube has four openings, each with a specific purpose: gastric aspiration, esophageal aspiration, gastric balloon inflation, and esophageal balloon inflation. This method is effective in controlling bleeding in 80% of patients; however, it is associated with lethal complications, including esophageal rupture, aspiration, and rebleeding, and it carries a high risk of mortality. Its use is restricted to patients with uncontrolled bleeding and as a temporary bridge to other treatments, such as TIPS or endoscopy (Maruyama & Sanyal, 2012).

> **⚠ Nursing Alert**
> *The patient being treated with balloon tamponade must remain under close observation in the ICU because of the risk for serious complications. The patient must be monitored closely and continuously. Precautions must be taken to ensure that the patient does not pull on or inadvertently displace the tube.*

Transjugular Intrahepatic Portosystemic Shunting

A TIPS procedure is indicated for the treatment of an acute episode of variceal bleeding refractory to pharmacologic or endoscopic therapy. In 10% to 20% of patients for whom urgent band ligation and medications are not successful in eradicating bleeding, a TIPS procedure can control acute variceal hemorrhage effectively by rapidly lowering portal pressure. TIPS is also indicated for those patients who rebleed after pharmacologic or endoscopic prophylaxis has failed. This technique also is used as a bridge to liver transplantation. Potential complications include bleeding, sepsis, increased hepatic encephalopathy, heart failure, organ perforation, shunt thrombosis, and progressive liver failure (Maruyama & Sanyal, 2012).

Nursing Management

After treatment for acute hemorrhage, the patient must be observed for bleeding, perforation of the esophagus, aspiration pneumonia, and esophageal stricture. Antacids, histamine-2 antagonists such as cimetidine (Tagamet), or proton pump inhibitors such as pantoprazole (Protonix) may be administered after the procedure.

After the examination, fluids are not given until the gag reflex returns. Lozenges and gargles may be used to relieve throat discomfort if the patient's physical condition and mental status permit. If the patient is actively bleeding, oral intake will not be permitted, and the patient will be prepared for further diagnostic and therapeutic procedures.

Overall nursing assessment includes monitoring the patient's physical condition and evaluating emotional responses and cognitive status. The nurse monitors and records vital signs and assesses the patient's nutritional and neurologic status. This assessment assists in identifying hepatic encephalopathy, which results from the breakdown of blood in the GI tract and a rising serum ammonia level. Manifestations range from drowsiness to encephalopathy and coma.

If complete rest of the esophagus is indicated because of bleeding, parenteral nutrition is initiated. Gastric suction usually is initiated to keep the stomach as empty as possible and to prevent straining and vomiting. The patient often complains of severe thirst, which may be relieved by frequent oral hygiene and moist sponges to the lips. The nurse closely monitors the blood pressure. Vitamin K therapy and multiple blood transfusions often are indicated because of blood loss and coagulation abnormalities. A quiet environment and calm reassurance may help to relieve the patient's anxiety and reduce agitation.

Bleeding anywhere in the body is anxiety-provoking, resulting in a crisis for the patient and family. If the patient has been a heavy user of alcohol, delirium secondary to alcohol withdrawal can complicate the situation. The nurse provides support and explanations about medical and nursing interventions. Close monitoring of the patient helps in detecting and managing complications. Management modalities and nursing care of the patient with bleeding esophageal varices are summarized in Table 25-1.

Hepatic Encephalopathy and Coma

Hepatic encephalopathy, a life-threatening complication of liver disease, occurs with profound liver failure and may result from the accumulation of ammonia and other toxic metabolites in the blood. Hepatic coma represents the most advanced stage of hepatic encephalopathy.

Pathophysiology

Ammonia is produced in the liver as a by-product of protein and amino acid breakdown. The colon and small intestine are also sites of ammonia production resulting from bacterial action. The liver converts ammonia into urea, which is excreted into the urine. In normal liver function, this process prevents the toxic buildup of ammonia in the blood (Porth, 2015). Damaged liver cells fail to detoxify and convert the ammonia to urea, and the elevated quantity of ammonia enters the bloodstream.

Circumstances that increase serum ammonia levels tend to aggravate or precipitate hepatic encephalopathy. The largest source of ammonia is the enzymatic and bacterial digestion of dietary and blood proteins in the GI tract. Ammonia from these sources increases as a result of GI bleeding (i.e., bleeding esophageal varices, chronic GI bleeding), a high-protein diet, bacterial infection, or uremia. In the presence of alkalosis or hypokalemia, increased amounts of ammonia are absorbed from the GI tract and from the renal tubular fluid. Conversely, serum ammonia is decreased by elimination of protein from the diet, administration of nonabsorbable disaccharides such as lactulose, and by the administration of antibiotic agents such as rifaximin or neomycin sulfate, reducing the amount of ammonia produced and absorbed in the intestine (Garcia-Tsao, 2016; Prakash & Mullen, 2012). Other factors unrelated to increased serum ammonia levels that can cause hepatic encephalopathy in susceptible patients include excessive diuresis, dehydration, infections, constipation, surgery, fever, and some medications (sedatives, tranquilizers, analgesics, and diuretics that cause potassium loss). The increased ammonia concentration in the blood causes brain dysfunction and damage, resulting in hepatic encephalopathy. Table 25-2 presents the stages of hepatic encephalopathy, common signs and symptoms, and potential nursing diagnoses for each stage (Garcia-Tsao, 2016).

Clinical Manifestations and Assessment

The earliest symptoms of hepatic encephalopathy include minor mental changes and motor disturbances. The patient appears slightly confused and unkempt and has alterations in mood and sleep patterns. The patient tends to sleep during the day and have restlessness and insomnia at night. As hepatic encephalopathy progresses, the patient may become difficult to awaken, eventually resulting in coma (Garcia-Tsao, 2016).

Asterixis (flapping tremor of the hands) may occur (Fig. 25-9). Simple tasks, such as handwriting, become difficult. A handwriting or drawing sample (e.g., star figure), taken daily, may provide graphic evidence of progression or reversal of hepatic encephalopathy; *constructional apraxia* is the inability to reproduce a simple figure (Fig. 25-10). In the early stages of hepatic encephalopathy, the deep tendon reflexes are hyperactive; with worsening of the encephalopathy, these reflexes disappear and the extremities may become flaccid (Vilstrup et al., 2014).

The electroencephalogram (EEG) shows generalized slowing, an increase in the amplitude of brain waves, and characteristic triphasic waves (Garcia-Tsao, 2016). Occasionally, **fetor hepaticus**, a sweet, slightly fecal odor to the breath that is presumed to be of intestinal origin, may be noticed (Greenberger, 2012). The odor also has been described as similar to that of freshly mowed grass, acetone, or old wine. Fetor hepaticus is prevalent with extensive collateral portal circulation in chronic liver disease. In a more advanced stage, there are gross disturbances of consciousness and the patient is completely disoriented with respect to time and place (Vilstrup et al., 2014).

Medical Management

Medical management of hepatic encephalopathy focuses on identifying and correcting the precipitating cause if possible. Lactulose (Cephulac) is administered to reduce serum

TABLE **25-1** Management Modalities and Nursing Care for the Patient with Bleeding Esophageal Varices

Treatment Modality[a]	Action	Nursing Priorities
Nonsurgical Modalities		
Pharmacologic Agents		
Propranolol (Inderal)/nadolol (Corgard)	Reduces portal pressure by beta-adrenergic blocking action	*Propranolol* and *nadolol*—decreased pulse pressure, impaired cardiovascular response to hemorrhage.
Somatostatin/octreotide (Sandostatin)	Reduces portal pressure by selective vasodilation of portal system	Support patient during treatment.
Vasopressin (Pitressin)	Reduces portal pressure by constricting splanchnic arteries	Observe response to therapy. Monitor for side effects: *vasopressin*—angina; nitroglycerin may be prescribed to prevent or treat angina.
Balloon tamponade	Exerts pressure directly to bleeding sites in esophagus and stomach	Explain procedure to patient briefly to obtain cooperation with insertion and maintenance of esophageal/gastric tamponade tube and reduce patient's fear of the procedure. Monitor closely to prevent inadvertent removal or displacement of tube, subsequent airway obstruction, and aspiration. Provide frequent oral hygiene.
Room-temperature saline lavage	Clears blood and secretions before endoscopy and other procedures	Ensure patency of the nasogastric tube to prevent aspiration. Observe gastric aspirate for blood and cessation of bleeding.
Injection sclerotherapy	Promotes thrombosis and sclerosing of bleeding sites by injection of sclerosing agent into the esophageal varices	Observe for aspiration, perforation of the esophagus, and recurrence of bleeding after treatment.
Variceal banding	Provides thrombosis and mucosal necrosis of bleeding sites by band ligation	Observe for recurrence of bleeding, esophageal perforation.
Surgical Modalities		
Transjugular intrahepatic portosystemic shunt (TIPS)	Reduces portal pressure by creating a shunt within the liver between the portal and systemic venous systems	Observe for rebleeding and signs of infection. Observe for development of portal-systemic encephalopathy (altered mental status, neurologic dysfunction), liver failure, hypertension due to increased volume after surgery, and coagulopathy. Requires intensive, expert nursing care for prolonged period. Follow-up may include ultrasound with Doppler to evaluate for shunt patency.
Surgical ligation of varices	Ties off blood vessels at the site of bleeding	Observe for rebleeding.
Esophageal transection and devascularization	Separates bleeding site from portal system	Observe for rebleeding.

[a]Several modalities may be used concurrently or in sequence.

TABLE **25-2** Stages of Hepatic Encephalopathy and Possible Nursing Diagnoses[a]

Stage	Clinical Symptoms	Clinical Signs	Electroencephalogram (EEG) Changes	Selected Potential Nursing Diagnoses
1	Normal level of consciousness with periods of lethargy and euphoria; reversal of day–night sleep patterns	Asterixis; impaired writing and ability to draw line figures	Normal EEG	Activity intolerance Self-care deficit Disturbed sleep pattern
2	Increased drowsiness; disorientation; inappropriate behavior; mood swings; agitation	Asterixis; fetor hepaticus	Abnormal EEG with generalized slowing	Impaired social interaction Ineffective role performance Risk for injury
3	Stuporous; difficult to rouse; sleeps most of time; marked confusion; incoherent speech	Asterixis; increased deep tendon reflexes; rigidity of extremities	EEG markedly abnormal	Imbalanced nutrition Impaired mobility Impaired verbal communication
4	Comatose; may not respond to painful stimuli	Absence of asterixis; absence of deep tendon reflexes; flaccidity of extremities	EEG markedly abnormal	Risk for aspiration Impaired gas exchange Impaired tissue integrity Disturbed sensory perception

[a]Nursing diagnoses are likely to progress so that most nursing diagnoses present at earlier stages will continue during later stages as well.

ammonia levels. It acts by several mechanisms that promote the excretion of ammonia in the stool:

- Ammonia is kept in the ionized state, resulting in a decrease in colon pH, reversing the normal passage of ammonia from the colon to the blood.
- Evacuation of the bowel takes place, which decreases the ammonia absorbed from the colon.
- Fecal flora are changed to organisms that do not produce ammonia from urea.

Two or three soft stools per day are desirable; this indicates that lactulose is performing as intended.

Possible side effects include intestinal bloating and cramps, which usually disappear within a week. To mask the sweet taste, which some patients dislike, lactulose can be diluted with fruit juice. The patient is monitored closely for hypokalemia (due to GI loss of potassium) and dehydration. Other laxatives are not prescribed during lactulose administration because their effects disturb dosage regulation.

FIGURE 25-9 Asterixis or "liver flap" may occur in hepatic encephalopathy. The patient is asked to hold the arm out with the hand held upward (dorsiflexed). Within a few seconds, the hand falls forward involuntarily and then quickly returns to the dorsiflexed position.

FIGURE 25-10 Effects of constructional apraxia. Deterioration of handwriting and inability to draw a simple star figure occurs with progressive hepatic encephalopathy. (With permission from Sherlock, S., & Dooley, J. (2002). *Diseases of the liver and biliary system* (11th ed.). Oxford, UK: Blackwell Scientific Ltd.)

Lactulose may be administered by nasogastric (NG) tube or enema for patients who are comatose or for those in whom oral administration is contraindicated or impossible (Vilstrup et al., 2014).

Nursing Alert
The patient receiving lactulose is monitored closely for the development of watery diarrheal stools because they indicate a medication overdose.

The addition of antibiotic therapy to alter the intestinal flora and reduce nitrogenous waste from the gut can be used as adjunct therapy to lactulose. Agents such as neomycin and rifaximin have been used; only short-term use (less than 2 weeks) of neomycin is recommend due to possible auditory loss and nephrotoxicity (Vilstrup et al., 2014).

Other aspects of management include IV administration of glucose to minimize protein breakdown, administration of vitamins to correct deficiencies, and correction of electrolyte imbalances (especially potassium). Additional principles of management of hepatic encephalopathy include the following (Garcia-Tsao, 2016; Prakash & Mullen, 2012; Vilstrup et al., 2014):

- Therapy is directed toward treating or removing the cause.
- Neurologic status is assessed frequently.
- Mental status is monitored by keeping a daily record of handwriting and arithmetic performance.
- Fluid intake and output and body weight are recorded each day.
- Vital signs are measured and recorded every 4 hours.
- Potential sites of infection (peritoneum, lungs) are assessed frequently, and abnormal findings are reported promptly.
- Serum ammonia level is monitored.
- Protein intake is moderately restricted in patients who are comatose or who have encephalopathy that is refractory to lactulose and antibiotic therapy (Box 25-2).
- Reduction in the absorption of ammonia from the GI tract is accomplished by the use of gastric suction, enemas, or oral antibiotics.
- Electrolyte status is monitored and corrected if abnormal.
- Sedatives, tranquilizers, and analgesic medications are discontinued.
- Benzodiazepine antagonists, such as flumazenil (Romazicon), may be administered to improve encephalopathy, whether or not the patient has taken benzodiazepines previously.

Nursing Management

The nurse is responsible for maintaining a safe environment to prevent injury, bleeding, and infection. The nurse administers the prescribed treatments and monitors the patient for

---

BOX 25-2   **Nutrition Alert**

Management of Hepatic Encephalopathy

- Prevent the formation and absorption of toxins, principally ammonia, from the intestine.
- Keep daily protein intake between 1.0 and 1.5 g/kg, depending on the degree of decompensation.
- Avoid protein restriction if possible, even in those with encephalopathy. If necessary, implement temporary restriction of 0.5–0.8 g/kg.
- For patients who are truly protein-intolerant, provide additional nitrogen in the form of an amino acid supplement. Use of branched-chain amino acids is still controversial.
- Provide small, frequent meals and an evening snack of complex carbohydrates to avoid protein loading.
- Substitute vegetable protein for animal protein in as high a percentage as possible.

---

the numerous potential complications. The nurse also communicates with the patient's family, to inform them about the patient's status, and supports them by explaining the procedures and treatments that are part of the patient's care. If the patient recovers from hepatic encephalopathy and coma, rehabilitation is likely to be prolonged. Therefore, the patient and family will require assistance to understand the causes of this severe complication and to recognize that it may recur.

Vitamin Deficiency

Decreased production of several clotting factors may be due in part to deficient absorption of vitamin K from the GI tract. This probably is caused by the inability of liver cells to use vitamin K to make prothrombin. Absorption of the other fat-soluble vitamins (vitamins A, D, and E) as well as dietary fats also may be impaired because of decreased secretion of bile salts into the intestine.

Another group of problems common to patients with severe chronic liver dysfunction results from inadequate intake of sufficient vitamins. These include the following:

- Vitamin A deficiency, resulting in night blindness and eye and skin changes
- Thiamine deficiency, leading to beriberi, polyneuritis, and Wernicke–Korsakoff psychosis
- Riboflavin deficiency, resulting in characteristic lesions of the skin and mucous membrane
- Vitamin B_6 deficiency, resulting in lesions of the skin and mucous membrane and neurologic changes
- Vitamin C deficiency, resulting in the hemorrhagic lesions of scurvy
- Vitamin K deficiency, resulting in hypoprothrombinemia, characterized by spontaneous bleeding and ecchymosis
- Folic acid deficiency, resulting in macrocytic anemia

Because of these avitaminoses (vitamin deficiencies), the diet of patients with chronic liver disease (especially if alcohol-related) is supplemented with vitamins.

 Nursing Alert
Patients with liver disease frequently have abnormal bleeding times. If the prolonged prothrombin time (PT) is due to a vitamin K deficiency, generally the PT will normalize within 24 to 48 hours after parenteral repletion. However, if the etiology of the prolonged PT is due to decreased synthesis of clotting factors (which is reflective of hepatocyte dysfunction), there may be little or no response to vitamin K (Berk & Korenblat, 2016).

Other Manifestations

The patient with advanced chronic liver disease and cirrhosis frequently will develop other systemic complications, such as altered respiratory or cardiac function, resulting from hepatopulmonary syndrome (HPS) and renal function hepatorenal syndrome (HRS). HPS symptoms include exertional dyspnea, clubbing, and cyanosis; in addition, vascular spiders may be observed on physical examination. HPS is related to pulmonary capillary dilatation. Normally one red blood cell fits through the pulmonary capillary, facilitating oxygenation; with pulmonary dilation, many RBCs are passing through the capillary, resulting in a large number of red cells that are not oxygenated. This is equivalent of a right-to-left shunt (see Chapter 10). HRS is a type of prerenal kidney injury that occurs in patients with cirrhosis and ascites. It is the result of maximal peripheral vasodilation and maximal activation of hormones that cause the retention of sodium and water and intense vasoconstriction of the renal arteries (Garcia-Tsao, 2016, p. 1026).

Hematologic abnormalities in patients with cirrhosis are common due to a decrease in clotting factors, resulting from vitamin K deficiency, decreased platelets (thrombocytopenia), anemia, and decreased white cells (neutropenia). The patient with cirrhosis will demonstrate easy bruising and bleeding as well as increased susceptibility to infection (Garcia-Tsao, 2016; Martin, 2016). Endocrine dysfunction in the regulation of glucose control and altered synthesis of sex hormones by the liver result in gynecomastia, testicular atrophy, and decreased libido and impotence in men. Women may have irregular or absent menstrual cycles and decreased sexual function as well.

VIRAL HEPATITIS

Viral hepatitis is a systemic, viral infection in which necrosis and inflammation of liver cells produce a characteristic cluster of clinical, biochemical, and cellular changes. To date, several types of viral hepatitis have been identified: hepatitis A, B, C, D, and E (Pawlotsky, 2016a) (Table 25-3). These viruses infect the liver and can result in either acute or chronic liver dysfunction and disease. Initial presentation of viral hepatitis may be asymptomatic or result in fulminant liver failure or chronic liver disease. Patients may have nonspecific symptoms of malaise, GI distress, or present with frank jaundice and elevations of aminotransferases (Pawlotsky, 2016a). Terms associated with viral hepatitis are listed in Box 25-3.

Hepatitis A Virus

Pathophysiology

The mode of transmission of hepatitis A virus (HAV) occurs through the fecal–oral route, primarily through person-to-person contact and/or ingestion of fecally contaminated food or water. Uncooked food or poor food-handling practices are common methods of transmission of HAV.

HAV replicates in the liver, is excreted in bile, and is shed in the stool. The incubation period is 2 to 4 weeks, with signs and symptoms typically lasting less than 2 months (although in some patients, these can extend up to 6 months). The peak period for transmission of HAV from one person to another occurs in the 2-week period prior to development of jaundice or symptoms, when the concentration of virus in the stool is highest (Watson & Sjogren, 2012). Typically, persons infected with HAV spontaneously recover; however, adults over 50 years of age or those with chronic liver disease may progress to fulminant liver failure (Pawlotsky, 2016a).

Clinical Manifestations and Assessment

Infection by HAV can present either asymptomatically or with acute symptoms such as fever, malaise, anorexia, nausea, diarrhea, vomiting, abdominal pain, and jaundice. Jaundice presents in over 70% of patients, primarily in adults. Serologic testing is required for accurate diagnosis of hepatitis A infection. A positive anti-HAV (IgM) signifies serum IgM antibodies that are reactive to the HAV and confirms an acute infection.

Anti-HAV (IgG) becomes positive shortly after the onset of infection, will remain positive throughout the person's life, and confers immunity. Total positive anti-HAV and negative anti-HAV (IgM) indicate exposure or vaccination (Pawlotsky, 2016a).

Prevention

Current recommendations to prevent the transmission of HAV are to vaccinate all children routinely, to identify and vaccinate persons at high risk for contracting HAV, and to vaccinate any person who wishes to prevent HAV (Pawlotsky, 2016a).

TABLE **25-3** Comparison of Major Forms of Viral Hepatitis

	Hepatitis A	Hepatitis B	Hepatitis C	Hepatitis D	Hepatitis E
Previous names	Infectious hepatitis	Serum hepatitis	Non-A, non-B hepatitis		
Epidemiology					
Cause	Hepatitis A virus (HAV)	Hepatitis B virus (HBV)	Hepatitis C virus (HCV)	Hepatitis D virus (HDV)	Hepatitis E virus (HEV)
Mode of transmission	Fecal–oral route; poor sanitation. Person-to-person contact Waterborne; foodborne Transmission possible with oral–anal contact during sex	Parenterally; by intimate contact with carriers or those with acute disease; sexual and oral–oral contact Perinatal transmission from mothers to infants An important occupational hazard for health care personnel	Transfusion of blood and blood products; exposure to contaminated blood through equipment or drug paraphernalia Transmission possible with sex with infected partner; risk increased with STD	Same as HBV HBV surface antigen necessary for replication; pattern similar to that of hepatitis B	Fecal–oral route; person-to-person contact may be possible, although risk appears low
Incubation (days)	14–35 days	60–150 days	14–160 days	21–140 days	14–65 days
Immunity	Average: 30 days Homologous	Average: 70–80 days Homologous	Average: 50 days Second attack may indicate weak immunity or infection with another agent.	Average: 35 days Homologous	Average: 42 days Unknown
Nature of Illness					
Signs and symptoms	May occur with or without symptoms; flulike illness *Preicteric phase:* Headache, malaise, fatigue, anorexia, fever *Icteric phase:* Dark urine, jaundice of sclera and skin, tender liver	May occur without symptoms May develop arthralgias, rash	Similar to HBV; less severe and anicteric	Similar to HBV	Similar to HAV; very severe in pregnant women
Outcome	Usually mild with recovery. Fatality rate: less than 1% No carrier state or increased risk of chronic hepatitis, cirrhosis, or hepatic cancer	May be severe. Fatality rate: 1–10%. Carrier state possible Increased risk of chronic hepatitis, cirrhosis, and hepatic cancer	Frequent occurrence of chronic carrier state and chronic liver disease Increased risk of hepatic cancer	Similar to HBV but greater likelihood of carrier state, chronic active hepatitis, and cirrhosis	Similar to HAV except very severe in pregnant women

---

BOX 25-3 **Hepatitis Terms and Abbreviations**

Hepatitis A

HAV	Hepatitis A virus; etiologic agent of hepatitis A (formerly infectious hepatitis)
IgG anti-HAV	Antibody to hepatitis A virus; appears in serum soon after onset of symptoms; persists indefinitely, indicates life-
IgM anti-HAV	long immunity: IgM antibody to HAV; indicates recent infection with HAV; positive up to 6 months after infection

Hepatitis B

HBV	Hepatitis B virus; etiologic agent of hepatitis B (formerly serum hepatitis)
HBsAG	Hepatitis B surface antigen (Australian antigen); indicates acute or chronic hepatitis B or carrier state; indicates infectious state
Anti-HBs	Antibody to hepatitis B surface antigen; indicates prior exposure and immunity to hepatitis; may indicate passive antibody from HBIG or immune response from hepatitis B vaccine
HBeAg	Hepatitis B e-antigen; present in serum early in course; indicates highly infectious stage of hepatitis B; persistence in serum indicates progression to chronic hepatitis
Anti-HBe	Antibody to hepatitis B e-antigen; suggests low titer of HBV
HBcAg	Hepatitis B core antigen; found in liver cells; not easily detected in serum
Anti-HBc	Antibody to hepatitis B core antigen; most sensitive indicator of hepatitis B; appears late in the acute phase of the disease; indicates infection of HBV at some time in the past
IgM anti-HBc	IgM antibody to HBcAg; present for up to 6 months after HBV infection

Hepatitis C

HCV	Hepatitis C virus (formerly non-A, non-B virus); may be more than one virus

Hepatitis D

HDV	Hepatitis D virus (delta agent); etiologic agent to hepatitis D; HBV required for replication
HDAg	Hepatitis delta antigen; detectable in early acute HDV infection
Anti-HDV	Antibody to HDV; indicates past or present infection with HDV

Hepatitis E

HEV	Hepatitis E virus; etiologic agent of hepatitis E

At-risk persons who should be vaccinated include:

- Travelers or visitors to countries with increased incidence of HAV (Mexico, Latin America, Africa, Middle East, Asia, India)
- Men having sex with men
- Illicit drug users
- Persons with occupational risk (e.g., research with primates or HAV in laboratory settings)
- Persons with clotting factor disorders
- Persons with chronic liver disease

Active immunization for HAV is through vaccination with hepatitis A antigen in two dose schedules and is administered intramuscularly in the deltoid muscle. Passive immunization is achieved through administration of immune globulin–containing hepatitis A antibodies to persons for prophylaxis after exposure to the virus. Its use is indicated for patients with no evidence of immunity (Robinson & Advisory Committee on Immunization Practices [ACIP], 2016).

Box 25-4 discusses community prevention of hepatitis A.

Medical Management

Acute HAV infection in most patients is managed with supportive care. The patient may experience decreased appetite due to alterations in GI function. Dehydration should be prevented; if necessary, IV fluids may be administered. Patients can participate in physical activity as tolerated. Signs and symptoms indicating possible fulminant liver failure, such as altered mental status or severe vomiting, should be identified promptly with referral to a liver transplant center (Watson & Sjogren, 2012).

BOX 25-4 **Community Prevention of Hepatitis A**

- Proper community and home sanitation
- Conscientious individual hygiene
- Safe practices for preparing and dispensing food
- Effective health supervision of schools, dormitories, extended-care facilities, barracks, and camps
- Community health education programs
- Mandatory reporting of viral hepatitis to local health departments
- Vaccination for travelers to developing countries, illegal drug users (injection and noninjection drug users), men who have sex with men, and persons with chronic liver disease
- Vaccination to interrupt community-wide outbreaks

Nursing Management

Management usually occurs in the home unless symptoms are severe. Therefore, the nurse assists the patient and family in coping with the temporary disability and fatigue that are common in hepatitis and instructs them to seek additional health care if the symptoms persist or worsen. The patient and family also need specific guidelines about diet, rest, follow-up blood work, and the importance of avoiding alcohol, as well as sanitation and hygiene measures (particularly hand washing after bowel movements and before eating) to prevent spread of the disease to other family members, environmental sanitation (safe food and water supply, effective sewage disposal), proper food storage, and thorough cooking of foods to recommended temperatures.

HEPATITIS B VIRUS

Hepatitis B virus (HBV) infection is an important public health problem with as many as 350 million people worldwide diagnosed with chronic infection (Pawlotsky, 2016a). HBV is highly prevalent in Asia, Africa, Middle East, parts of Europe, the Caribbean, and Central and South America (Lok & Negro, 2012).

Pathophysiology

HBV is transmitted primarily through blood (percutaneous and mucosal routes). HBV can be found in blood, saliva, and semen and can be transmitted through mucous membranes and breaks in the skin. HBV is also transferred from carrier mothers to their babies, especially in areas with a high incidence (Pawlotsky, 2016a). HBV is primarily transmitted by perinatal, percutaneous, sexual exposure, and close person-to-person contact via contact with open cuts or sores or by use of shared razors or toothbrushes. HBV-contaminated surfaces also are possible sources of infection as the virus can survive outside of the body for extended periods (Pawlotsky, 2016a).

HBV has a long incubation period. It replicates in the liver and remains in the serum for relatively long periods, allowing transmission of the virus. Most people (more than 95%) who contract HBV infection develop antibodies and recover spontaneously (Pawlotsky, 2016a). The risk of developing chronic HBV infection is significantly higher in persons from endemic countries and when infected from birth (e.g., chronicity rate higher than 95% among patients infected at birth) (Pawlotsky, 2016a). Acute HBV infection can result in fulminant liver failure or progress to chronic infection. Patients with chronic HBV infection eventually may develop cirrhosis, end-stage liver disease, and cancer of the liver (Lok & Negro, 2012; Pawlotsky, 2016a).

Risk Factors

Those at risk for development of hepatitis B include individuals born in areas with high rates of HBV infection.

BOX 25-5 Risk Factors for Hepatitis B

- Frequent exposure to blood, blood products, or other body fluids
- Being a health care worker: hemodialysis staff, oncology and chemotherapy nurses, personnel at risk for needlesticks, operating room staff, respiratory therapists, surgeons, dentists
- Hemodialysis
- Male homosexual and bisexual activity
- IV/injection drug use
- Close contact with carrier of HBV
- Travel to or residence in area with uncertain sanitary conditions
- Multiple sexual partners
- Recent history of sexually transmitted disease
- Receipt of blood or blood products (e.g., clotting factor concentrate)

Risk factors for HBV infection are summarized in Box 25-5 (Pawlotsky, 2016a).

Clinical Manifestations and Assessment

Signs and symptoms of acute hepatitis B may be insidious and variable. The patient may have anorexia, sleep disturbances, fevers, dyspepsia, pain in the upper right quadrant, generalized aching, malaise, and weakness. Jaundice may or may not be evident. Skin rashes and arthralgias (pain in the joints) may occur (Ferri, 2016a). Chronic hepatitis B may remain largely asymptomatic until the development of cirrhosis and signs of hepatic decompensation (Pawlotsky, 2016a).

The evaluation of a patient with HBV infection includes a complete history and physical examination, a family history of liver disease, and potential risk factors for disease transmission.

Laboratory testing should include complete blood counts (CBC with platelets), hepatic function panel, and prothrombin time and international normalized ratio (INR). Laboratory tests to detect hepatitis B replication and other viral coinfections (HAV, HCV, HIV) should be included in the assessment (Terrault et al., 2015).

Prevention

The goals of prevention are to interrupt the chain of transmission, to protect people who are at high risk by active immunization through the use of hepatitis B vaccine, and to use passive immunization for unprotected people exposed to HBV.

Preventing Transmission

Recommendations to prevent transmission of hepatitis B include vaccination of sexual contacts of individuals with chronic hepatitis B, use of barrier protection during sexual intercourse, avoidance of sharing toothbrushes and razors with others, and covering of open sores or skin lesions. Blood spills should be cleaned with bleach diluted to a 10:1 concentration. Persons with HBV infection should be advised to avoid donation of blood, organs, or sperm.

Active Immunization: Hepatitis B Vaccine

The most effective strategy to prevent hepatitis B infection is through vaccination. Current prevention recommendations include:

- Universal vaccination of infants at birth
- Screening of pregnant women for hepatitis B surface antigen (HBsAg)
- Prophylaxis of infants with HBsAg-positive mothers or those with unknown HBsAg status
- Vaccination of unvaccinated children and adolescents
- Vaccination of unvaccinated adults at risk for HBV infection (i.e., health care workers, sexual or household contacts of HBV carriers) (Pawlotsky, 2016a)

The hepatitis B vaccine series is administered in three doses intramuscularly: the initial injection, then 1-month, and 6-month intervals for adults (Robinson & ACIP, 2016).

Nursing Alert

The U.S. Food and Drug Administration (FDA) has approved a combined vaccine for both hepatitis A and B (Twinrix) for vaccination of people 18 years of age and older with indications for both hepatitis A and B vaccination. Vaccination consists of three doses on the same schedule as that used for single-antigen hepatitis B vaccine (Robinson & ACIP, 2016).

Passive Immunity: Hepatitis B Hyperimmune Globulin

Hepatitis B hyperimmune globulin (HBIG) provides passive immunity to hepatitis B and is indicated for people exposed to HBV who have never had hepatitis B, who have had sexual exposure (within 14 days), infants who have had exposure at birth, and those who have never received hepatitis B vaccine. A second dose of HBIG is given in 28 days for those refusing vaccine or vaccine nonresponders (Ferri, 2016a). It has demonstrated efficacy in the prevention of HBV infection in high-risk persons (exposure to blood-containing HBV, sexual partners of patients with hepatitis B, and newborn infants of HBsAg-positive mothers) (Gold Standard, 2015).

Medical Management

The goals of treatment for hepatitis B are to prevent replication of active HBV (viral suppression) and reduce the effects of chronic liver inflammation. The ultimate goal of medical management of hepatitis B is to prevent cirrhosis, liver failure, and hepatocellular carcinoma (HCC) (Pawlotsky,

2016a). Multiple antiviral therapies are available to treat hepatitis B; of these, pegylated interferon alfa, adefovir, entecavir, telbivudine, lamivudine, and tenofovir are the preferred medications, either as single agents or in combination. Patients with HBV infection should have periodic laboratory testing to assess elevations in liver function and replication of HBV DNA. Patients at high risk for HCC (discussed later in this chapter), including patients with cirrhosis, should receive ultrasound screening every 6 months (Terrault et al., 2015).

Nursing Management

In patients with acute hepatitis B, management of the symptoms of malaise, anorexia, nausea, vomiting, and fever primarily is supportive to maintain nutrition, fluid intake, and adequate rest during recovery. The nurse must be vigilant for signs of progression to fulminant liver failure (discussed later in the chapter); however, alterations in mental status, severe vomiting, and increasing jaundice should initiate referral to a tertiary care center or liver transplant center. In patients with chronic hepatitis B, the nursing role is geared to patient education in the prevention of transmission and avoidance of lifestyle factors that may exacerbate existing liver disease.

HEPATITIS C VIRUS

Hepatitis C virus (HCV) infection is the leading cause of liver disease and is the primary indication for liver transplantation.

Pathophysiology

HCV is a blood-borne RNA virus and is avidly replicated in the liver. Transmission of hepatitis C occurs primarily through injection of drugs and through transfusion of blood products prior to 1992. Its route is through parenteral contact with blood. Sexual transmission also may occur, with high risk associated with multiple sex partners. Other less common modes of transmission include via hemodialysis, health care worker exposure to needlestick injury or contaminated blood, and tattooing (AASLD/IDSA HCV Guidance Panel, 2015; Pawlotsky, 2016a). Box 25-6 summarizes risk factors for hepatitis C.

Patients infected with this virus spontaneously clear the acute infection in 20% to 50% of cases; the majority of individuals will develop chronic infection, with evidence of hepatitis C RNA viremia (Pawlotsky, 2016b). Unlike other hepatitis viruses, the acute stage of hepatitis C often is asymptomatic for decades. Hepatitis C infection with progression to cirrhosis occurs in up to 20% of patients over a period of 20 years or longer if untreated. Factors contributing to the severity of liver disease include increased alcohol use, male gender, older age at infection, HIV or HBV coinfection, and obesity (AASLD/IDSA HCV Guidance Panel, 2015; Pawlotsky, 2016b). Individuals with HCV cirrhosis are at higher risk of developing hepatic decompensation and

Risk Factors for Hepatitis C

- Receiving blood products or organ transplant before 1992 or clotting factor concentrates before 1987
- Being a health care or public safety worker (needlestick injuries or mucosal exposure to blood)
- Being a child born to a woman infected with hepatitis C virus
- Past/current illicit IV/injection drug use
- Past treatment with chronic hemodialysis
- Multiple sex partners, history of sexually transmitted disease, unprotected sex

HCC, and in industrialized countries, hepatitis C remains the most common cause of HCC (Pawlotsky, 2016b).

Clinical Manifestations and Assessment

Most patients with acute or chronic hepatitis C are asymptomatic. Some patients will develop jaundice, nausea, vomiting, and malaise during the acute stage (Pawlotsky, 2016a) (Box 25-7). Patients with chronic hepatitis C frequently will be diagnosed incidentally during routine laboratory testing or not until cirrhosis develops. Extrahepatic signs of hepatitis C are common, such as skin rashes, joint aches, and purpura (small blood vessels leaking under the skin and causing purple bruising) (Pawlotsky, 2016a).

The diagnosis of HCV infection is confirmed by serology with anti-HCV antibodies present and measurement

of viremia through HCV RNA. Genotype testing and liver biopsy will provide information to assist in the management and treatment of hepatitis C as well as to stage the severity of disease. Other tests to assess the extent of liver disease include laboratory tests (i.e., bilirubin, albumin, aminotransferases, prothrombin time, and INR). Ultrasound or other imaging may be used to assess for cirrhosis or the presence of lesions (AASLD/IDSA HCV Guidance Panel, 2015).

Medical and Nursing Management

Treatment of hepatitis C aims to reduce mortality by preventing the progression of fibrosis and evolution to cirrhosis by reducing HCV RNA levels to nondetectable levels. A nondetectable viral load or HCV RNA 12 weeks after completion of therapy is considered curative. This is called a *sustained viral response (SVR)*. New antiviral therapies with direct acting agents (DAA), called protease inhibitors, have revolutionized treatment of hepatitis C. Use of these drugs and drug combinations is evolving rapidly, resulting in SVR in genotypes or comorbidities that previously had been difficult to treat. Clinical trial evidence has demonstrated protease inhibitor therapy is well tolerated with less to no symptomatic complaints from patients during treatment course unlike its predecessor, pegylated interferon, given weekly by injection and associated with many side effects (AASLD/IDSA HCV Guidance Panel, 2015). The specific protease inhibitor or drug combination, dosage, and length of therapy are determined by HCV genotype, history or prior HCV treatment, and presence of cirrhosis and level

Nursing Research

Bridging the Gap to Evidence-Based Practice

Incidence of Preventable Postoperative Readmissions Following Pancreaticoduodenectomy: Implications for Patient Education. Hari, M., & Rosenzweig, M. (2012). *Oncology Nursing Forum, 39*(4), 408–412.

Purpose
The purpose of this article is to determine readmission rates post-pancreaticoduodenectomy (PD), readmission reasons following PD, and patients' postoperative education prior to discharge.

Design
A retrospective, descriptive study was conducted using established medical records of patients who had undergone PD from 2006 to 2008. Records were reviewed from the PD cohort within a pancreatic cancer program where there were 62 patients aged 18 years or older diagnosed with pancreatic cancer who had PD. Data were abstracted from inpatient and outpatient electronic records per study protocol and entered into an Excel® spreadsheet for analysis. Incidences of and reasons for readmissions post the PD procedure were reviewed. Discharge education given to patients prior to discharge was reviewed.

Findings
Patients were discharged at mean postoperative day 11.3. Readmission rate was 28%. Reasons for readmission were dehydration or malnutrition (n = 10, 16%) and surgical site infection (n = 7, 11%); 10% of patients (n = 6) had documented difficulties with dehydration, malnutrition, and failure to thrive noted at follow-up. PD discharge teaching was documented in a mandatory discharge form. No standard curriculum was used. Conclusions: Patients undergoing PD experienced an increase in self-care demand postdischarge. Poor discharge education can lead to high rates of readmission, specifically for dehydration and malnutrition, mandating an assessment of patient education prior to discharge.

Nursing Implications
Close attention must be given to the needs of patients with pancreatic cancer postdischarge. Trying to identify the areas of educational deficit at patient readmission could help nurses identify what they can do to minimize preventable complications. Educational focus for patients undergoing PD should be on prevention of dehydration, malnutrition, and surgical site infections.

of decompensation. Patients who previously failed therapy with interferon and/or other types of protease inhibitors and patients with recurrent HCV after liver transplant are eligible to receive alternative regimens in hopes of achieving SVR as well. Patients are monitored with serum laboratory testing, including CBC, metabolic panel, hepatic function panel, and HCV viral load testing at prescribed intervals in conjunction with telephone and monitoring visits to evaluate adherence, tolerance, and compliance (AASLD/IDSA HCV Guidance Panel, 2015).

HEPATITIS D VIRUS

Hepatitis D virus (delta agent) (HDV) infection occurs in some cases of hepatitis B. Because the virus requires hepatitis B surface antigen for its replication, only individuals with hepatitis B are at risk for hepatitis D. Anti-HDV antibodies (IGg) in patients with chronic hepatitis B confirms the diagnosis (Pawlotsky, 2016b; Lok & Negro, 2012).

The symptoms of hepatitis D are similar to those of hepatitis B, except that patients are more likely to develop fulminant hepatitis and to progress to chronic active hepatitis and cirrhosis. Current treatment for hepatitis D is the use of interferon or pegylated interferon alfa for 12 months (Pawlotsky, 2016b).

HEPATITIS E VIRUS

It is believed that hepatitis E virus (HEV) is transmitted by the fecal–oral route, principally through contaminated water in endemic areas with poor sanitation. This form of hepatitis usually is self-limiting, with acute onset and subsequent recovery with no chronicity. HEV is responsible for most cases of fulminant hepatitis in India. Pregnant women infected with hepatitis E infection have a high mortality rate (between 15% and 25%); this is increased during the last trimester (Watson & Sjogren, 2012). Currently, there is no vaccine or specific treatment for HEV; however, research in vaccine development may be promising in the near future.

Prevention of transmission is focused on improvement of sanitation, development of clean water supplies in endemic countries, and safe food-handling practices (Pawlotsky, 2016a).

NONVIRAL HEPATITIS

Liver inflammation and disease can be caused by nonviral etiologies, such as toxins, infections, alcoholic overuse, and autoimmune disorders.

ALCOHOLIC LIVER DISEASE (ALCOHOLIC HEPATITIS)

Excessive ingestion or abuse of alcohol is a common cause of acute hepatitis, and chronic use results in cirrhosis.

Alcoholic liver disease (ALD) is a major public health problem and accounts for approximately 40% of deaths related to cirrhosis of the liver. It is estimated that fatty liver results from alcohol in 80% to 90% of heavy drinkers, while 30% to 40% of that population progress toward more problematic forms of liver disease, such as fibrosis, cirrhosis, and HCC (Chalasani, 2016; Dasarathy & McCullough, 2012; Orman, Odena, & Batallar, 2013).

The impact of alcohol ingestion upon the liver is dose-dependent; women will develop advanced liver disease at lower amounts of alcohol than will men. Other cofactors contributing to the development of cirrhosis in ALD is hepatitis C infection, smoking, and obesity. The amount of alcohol consumed to result in significant liver disease is more than 20 g of alcohol daily over a 10-year period in females and 60 to 80 g of alcohol daily in men (Dasarathy & McCullough, 2012; Singal et al., 2014).

Pathophysiology

Ethanol (alcohol) is metabolized by the liver by alcohol dehydrogenases, cytochrome P450, and catalase. The resultant product, acetaldehyde, is toxic to the liver, resulting in impairment of liver function and cells. Other factors contributing to the pathogenesis of ALD are oxidative stress, hypoxia or oxygen depletion of cells, and mitochondrial injury. Fatty infiltration of liver cells (hepatic steatosis) is a common finding in liver biopsies of patients with ALD (Chalasani, 2016; Dasarathy & McCullough, 2012).

Clinical Manifestations and Assessment

Patients presenting with alcoholic hepatitis are universally jaundiced. The patient may have symptoms of anorexia, nausea, vomiting, and abdominal pain. Fever, muscle wasting, and *stigmata*—such as spider angiomas (Fig. 25-11) or palmar erythema (redness of the palm)—are common findings. The liver may be enlarged, or hard and small. The spleen

FIGURE 25-11 Spider angioma. This vascular (arterial) spider appears on the skin. Beneath the elevated center and radiating branches, the blood vessels are looped and tortuous.

will be enlarged, and late signs of hepatic decompensation may be evident, such as ascites, pedal edema, and hepatic encephalopathy (Chalasani, 2016).

There is no specific evaluation or test for the diagnosis of ALD; the clinical history and physical presence of liver disease correlated with information regarding alcohol overuse is diagnostic. An AST/ALT ratio of greater than two indicates ALD in over 70% of cases (Chalasani, 2016).

A complete history and physical examination is important in the assessment of patients with ALD. Patients should be screened for frequency, amount of alcohol use, type of alcohol, and patterns of alcohol use. Several evidence-based screening instruments for assessment of alcohol dependence exist, such as the CAGE and AUDIT tools to assist clinicians with detection and diagnosis (Dasarathy & McCullough, 2012). Additional information regarding the negative impact of alcohol abuse upon employment, health (i.e., falls, fractures), or driving status provides more data to assess the extent of alcohol use (Dasarathy & McCullough, 2012).

Nursing Alert

CAGE (Cut down, Annoyed, Guilty, and Eye-opener)

Ask your patients these four questions and use the scoring method described below to determine if substance abuse exists and needs to be addressed.

CAGE Questions

1. *Have you ever felt you should cut down on your drinking?*
2. *Have people annoyed you by criticizing your drinking?*
3. *Have you ever felt bad or guilty about your drinking?*
4. *Have you ever had a drink first thing in the morning to steady your nerves or to get rid of a hangover (eye-opener)?*

Scoring: Item responses on the CAGE questions are scored 0 for "no" and 1 for "yes" answers, with a higher score being an indication of alcohol problems. A total score of two or greater is considered clinically significant.

Medical Management

The mainstay of treatment for ALD is abstinence and either oral or enteral nutritional therapy. Patients with ALD frequently are malnourished, with depleted protein stores and vitamin deficiencies; the complex nutritional management of these patients is best suited to clinical nutritionists with expertise in this area. In patients with severe alcoholic hepatitis, prednisolone may be used. Clinical trials have demonstrated improved survival of patients treated for severe alcoholic hepatitis with corticosteroids; however, this remains controversial and is contraindicated in the presence of infection, bleeding, or renal impairment (Orman et al., 2013; Dasarathy & McCullough, 2012). Box 25-8 reviews dietary management appropriate for patients with hepatitis.

> **BOX 25-8** **Nutrition Alert**
>
> **Dietary Management of Viral or Drug-Related Hepatitis**
>
> - Recommend small, frequent meals.
> - Provide intake of 2,000–3,000 kcal/day during acute illness.
> - Although early studies indicate that a high-protein, high-calorie diet may be beneficial, advise patient not to force food and to restrict fat intake.
> - Carefully monitor fluid balance.
> - If anorexia and nausea and vomiting persist, enteral feedings may be necessary.
> - Instruct patient to abstain from alcohol during acute illness and for at least 6 months after recovery.
> - Advise patient to avoid substances (medications, herbs, illicit drugs, and toxins) that may affect liver function.

General management includes supportive care with adequate rest, correction of bleeding abnormalities, treatment of infection, and management of fluid overload. Providers trained in alcohol addiction should be employed once the patient is able to engage in therapy to maintain abstinence.

DRUG-INDUCED LIVER DISEASE (DRUG-RELATED HEPATITIS)

Drug-induced hepatotoxicity is very common and can range from mild elevations in aminotransferases to fulminant liver failure due to ingestion or exposure to medications, toxins, or herbal remedies alone or in combination (Larson, 2012). It is the most common cause of acute liver failure, accounting for more than 50% of all cases in the United States and the United Kingdom (Lee, 2016).

Pathophysiology

Although any medication can affect liver function, use of acetaminophen (found in many over-the-counter medications used to treat fever and pain) has been identified as a leading cause of acute liver failure (Everson, 2016). Other medications commonly associated with liver injury include antibiotics, anticonvulsants, NSAIDs, and antituberculosis agents (Lee, 2016).

Clinical Manifestations and Assessment

Manifestations of sensitivity to a medication may occur on the first day of its use or not until several months later, depending on the medication. Usually the onset is abrupt, with chills, fever, rash, pruritus, arthralgia, anorexia, and nausea. Later, there may be jaundice, dark urine, and an enlarged and tender liver. After the offending medication is withdrawn, symptoms may subside gradually. However, reactions can be severe, or even fatal, even if the medication is stopped. If fever, rash, or pruritus occurs from any medication, its use should be stopped immediately. A thorough history of all medications, over-the-counter medications, and supplements should be obtained from all patients presenting with signs or symptoms of acute or chronic liver disease.

Medical and Nursing Management

The management of drug-induced liver injury includes discontinuation of the suspected medication or medications; evaluation of liver damage, including hospitalization if jaundice or impaired hepatic function is present; and, in cases of fulminant or acute liver failure, referral to a liver transplant center. Antidotes should be delivered if available. N-acetylcysteine (Mucomyst) is administered routinely in the setting of overdose of acetaminophen by restoring hepatic concentration of glutathione (Lee, 2016).

Although its efficacy is uncertain, a short course of high-dose corticosteroids may be used in patients with severe hypersensitivity (Chitturi & Farrell, 2012).

 Nursing Alert
The liver metabolizes many medications, such as barbiturates, opioids, sedative agents, anesthetics, and amphetamines. Metabolism generally results in inactivation of the medication, although in some cases activation of the medication may occur. One of the important pathways for medication metabolism involves conjugation (binding) of the medication with a variety of compounds to form more soluble substances that may be excreted in the feces or urine, similar to bilirubin excretion. Bioavailability is the fraction of the administered medication that actually reaches the systemic circulation. The bioavailability of an oral medication (absorbed from the GI tract) can be decreased if the medication is metabolized to a great extent by the liver before it reaches the systemic circulation; this is known as first-pass effect. *Some medications have such a large first-pass effect that their use is limited essentially to the parenteral route, or oral doses must be substantially larger than parenteral doses to achieve the same effect. If medications are administered that have a high hepatic metabolism, bioavailability increases and hepatic clearance decreases in liver disease. It is important for the nurse to understand the clearance of medications and to observe patients for signs of further deterioration.*

FULMINANT HEPATIC FAILURE

Fulminant hepatic failure is the clinical syndrome of sudden and severely impaired liver function in a previously healthy person.

Pathophysiology

Fulminant liver failure is caused by many different etiologies. Viral hepatitis caused by A, B, and E is a common culprit worldwide. Acetaminophen overdose, drug-induced liver injury, autoimmune hepatitis, metabolic disorders such as Wilson disease, poisonous mushroom ingestion, and obstruction to hepatic blood flow (**Budd–Chiari syndrome**) are the most common causes of acute liver failure in the United States (Everson, 2016).

Clinical Manifestations and Assessment

The clinical manifestations of fulminant liver failure are **hepatic encephalopathy**, jaundice, nausea, anorexia, vomiting, and coagulopathy in a patient with no history of prior liver disease (Larson, 2012). The onset is abrupt, and the patient or family may or may not be able to identify the precipitating event.

Medical and Nursing Management

The clinical decision whether a patient will recover from acute liver injury with intense medical management or require liver transplantation typically is made on a case-by-case basis after careful evaluation of the patient. Multiple selection criteria have been developed to determine survival outcome (i.e., risk of death with or without transplant) and assist in the selection of patients appropriate for liver transplant, including time from jaundice to encephalopathy, prothrombin time, and levels of bilirubin, arterial pH, and creatinine (Everson, 2016).

Currently, in the United States, the United Network for Organ Sharing (UNOS) has defined criteria to determine which patients qualify for urgent transplant listing for fulminant liver failure:

- Onset of hepatic encephalopathy within 8 weeks of first symptoms of liver disease
- Absence of pre-existing liver disease
- Transaminases ALT/AST of greater than 3,000
- INR greater than 2.0

Patients may require one of the following interventions:

- Ventilator dependence
- Dialysis or continuous veno-venous hemofiltration (CVVH) or continuous veno-venous hemofiltration with dialysis (CVVD) (refer to Chapter 27)
- Care within an ICU

Patients with fulminant liver failure must have a life expectancy of less than 7 days without liver transplant to qualify for the highest active status for liver allocation, status 1A (United Network of Organ Sharing [UNOS], 2016).

The key to optimized treatment is rapid recognition of acute liver failure and intensive intervention. Supporting the patient in the ICU and assessing the indications for and feasibility of liver transplantation are hallmarks of management in this population. Often fulminant hepatic failure is accompanied by coagulation defects, kidney failure and electrolyte disturbances, cardiovascular abnormalities, infection, hypoglycemia, encephalopathy, and cerebral edema. The use of antidotes for certain conditions may be indicated, such as *N*-acetylcysteine for acetaminophen toxicity.

In patients who have fulminant liver failure with stage three (somnolent but can be aroused) or four (coma) encephalopathy, or elevated serum ammonia, there is a high risk for cerebral edema, a life-threatening complication. These patients may require intracranial pressure monitoring, although its use remains controversial. Measures to promote adequate cerebral perfusion include careful fluid balance and hemodynamic assessments, a quiet environment, and diuresis with mannitol, an osmotic diuretic. Use of barbiturate anesthesia or pharmacologic paralysis and sedation is indicated to prevent surges in intracranial pressure related to agitation. Other support measures include monitoring for and treating hypoglycemia, coagulopathy, kidney impairment, and infection. Despite these treatment modalities, the mortality rate remains high. Consequently, liver transplantation (discussed later) has become the treatment of choice for fulminant hepatic failure (Everson, 2016).

CIRRHOSIS

The most common causes of chronic liver disease are viral hepatitis B and C, ALD, nonalcoholic fatty liver disease (NAFLD), primary biliary cirrhosis, and autoimmune disorders of the liver. Acute forms of liver dysfunction and failure can occur from viral agents, drug hepatotoxicity, toxins, parasites, or metabolic disorders, such as Wilson disease (Garcia-Tsao, 2016). The development of cirrhosis is the final stage of all chronic liver disease and is one of the leading causes of death in the United States (Runyon, 2013).

Pathophysiology

Cirrhosis of the liver occurs when the normal liver tissue is replaced by fibrotic tissue in response to damage to liver cells, resulting in accumulation of extracellular matrix or "scar." The progression from fibrosis to cirrhosis results in the loss of normal structure and function in the liver (Schiff et al., 2012). The progression and severity of chronic liver disease can be classified as either compensated or decompensated cirrhosis.

Clinical Manifestations and Assessment

Typically compensated cirrhosis is asymptomatic. The transition from compensated cirrhosis to decompensated cirrhosis results in the development of jaundice, ascites, GI bleeding from esophageal varices, and hepatic encephalopathy. Box 25-9 provides guidelines for assessing cirrhosis. The development of any of these complications of hepatic dysfunction

---

BOX 25-9

Focused Assessment

Cirrhosis

Be alert for the following signs and symptoms:

Compensated Cirrhosis

- Intermittent mild fever
- Vascular spiders
- Palmar erythema (reddened palms)
- Unexplained epistaxis
- Ankle edema
- Vague morning indigestion
- Flatulent dyspepsia
- Abdominal pain
- Firm, enlarged liver
- Splenomegaly

Decompensated Cirrhosis

- Ascites
- Jaundice
- Weakness
- Muscle wasting
- Weight loss
- Continuous mild fever
- Clubbing of fingers
- Purpura (due to decreased platelet count)
- Spontaneous bruising
- Epistaxis
- Hypotension
- Sparse body hair
- White nails
- Gonadal atrophy

---

signals that the patient has progressed to decompensated cirrhosis. The hallmarks of decompensated cirrhosis are the development of jaundice, ascites (fluid collection in the peritoneum), pedal edema, gastroesophageal varices, and hepatic encephalopathy. Other complications, such as spontaneous bacterial peritonitis, hepatorenal syndrome (kidney dysfunction), and hepatopulmonary syndrome (causes symptoms such as shortness of breath and hypoxemia) may occur as well (Garcia-Tsao, 2016; Runyon, 2013).

Medical Management

NURSING PROCESS
The Patient with Cirrhosis

ASSESSMENT

Nursing assessment focuses on the onset of symptoms and the history of precipitating factors, particularly long-term alcohol abuse, as well as dietary intake and changes in the patient's

(*continued on page 770*)

physical and mental status. The patient's past and current patterns of alcohol use (duration and amount) are assessed and documented. It is also important to document any exposure to toxic agents encountered in the workplace or during recreational activities. The nurse documents and reports exposure to potentially hepatotoxic substances, including medications, illicit IV/injection drugs, inhalants, and general anesthetic agents.

The nurse assesses the patient's mental status during the interview and other interactions with the patient; orientation to person, place, and time is noted. The patient's ability to carry out a job or household activities provides some information about physical and mental status. The patient's relationships with family, friends, and coworkers may give some indication about incapacitation secondary to alcohol abuse and cirrhosis. Abdominal distention, GI bleeding, bruising, and weight changes are noted.

The nurse assesses nutritional status, which is of major importance in cirrhosis, by obtaining daily weights and monitoring plasma proteins, transferrin, and creatinine levels. A plan of nursing care for a patient with impaired liver function is available online at http://thepoint.lww.com/Honan2e.

DIAGNOSIS

Nursing diagnoses may include the following:
- Activity intolerance related to fatigue, general debility, muscle wasting, and discomfort
- Imbalanced nutrition, less than body requirements, related to chronic gastritis, decreased GI motility, and anorexia
- Impaired skin integrity related to compromised immunologic status, edema, and poor nutrition
- Risk for injury and bleeding related to altered clotting mechanisms

Potential complications may include the following:
- Bleeding and hemorrhage
- Hepatic encephalopathy
- Fluid volume excess

PLANNING

The goals for the patient may include increased participation in activities, improvement of nutritional status, improvement of skin integrity, decreased potential for injury, improvement of mental status, and absence of complications.

NURSING INTERVENTIONS

PROMOTING REST

The patient with active liver disease requires rest and other supportive measures to permit the liver to reestablish its functional ability. If the patient is hospitalized, weight and fluid intake and output are measured and recorded daily. The nurse adjusts the patient's position in bed for maximal respiratory efficiency, which is especially important if ascites is marked because it interferes with adequate thoracic excursion. Oxygen therapy may be required in liver failure.

Rest reduces the demands on the liver and increases the liver's blood supply. Because the patient is susceptible to the hazards of immobility, efforts to prevent respiratory, circulatory, and vascular disturbances are initiated, such as range-of-motion exercises, turning every 2 hours, and the use of an incentive spirometer (IS) every hour while awake. These measures may help prevent such problems as pneumonia, thrombophlebitis, and pressure ulcers. After nutritional status improves and strength increases, the nurse encourages the patient to increase activity gradually. Activity and mild exercise, as well as rest, are planned.

IMPROVING NUTRITIONAL STATUS

The patient with cirrhosis who has no ascites or edema and exhibits no signs of impending hepatic coma should receive a nutritious, high-protein diet, if tolerated, supplemented by vitamins of the B complex and others as indicated (including vitamins A, C, K, and folic acid). Because proper nutrition is so important, the nurse makes every effort to encourage the patient to eat. Proper nutrition is as important as any medication. Often, small, frequent meals are better tolerated than three large meals because of the abdominal pressure exerted by ascites. Protein supplements also may be indicated.

Patient preferences are considered. Patients with prolonged or severe anorexia and those who are vomiting or eating poorly for any reason may receive nutrients by the enteral or parenteral route.

Patients with fatty stools (**steatorrhea**) should receive water-soluble forms of fat-soluble vitamins—A, D, and E (Aquasol A, D, and E). Folic acid and iron are prescribed to prevent anemia. If the patient shows signs of impending or advancing coma, the amount of protein in the diet is decreased temporarily. In the absence of hepatic encephalopathy, a moderate-protein, high-calorie intake is provided, with protein foods of high biologic value. A diet containing 1 to 1.5 g of protein per kilogram of body weight per day is required unless the patient is malnourished. Protein is restricted if encephalopathy develops. Incorporating vegetable protein to meet protein needs may decrease the risk for encephalopathy. Also sodium restriction is indicated to prevent ascites.

PROVIDING SKIN CARE

Providing careful skin care is important because of subcutaneous edema, the patient's immobility, jaundice, and increased susceptibility to skin breakdown and infection. Frequent changes in position are necessary to prevent pressure ulcers. To prevent trauma to the skin, it is important to avoid irritating soaps and the use of adhesive tape. Lotion may be soothing to irritated skin; the nurse takes measures to minimize scratching by the patient.

REDUCING RISK OF INJURY

The nurse protects the patient with cirrhosis from falls and other injuries. The side rails should be in place and padded with blankets or other materials in case the patient becomes agitated or restless. To minimize agitation, the nurse orients the patient to time and place and explains all procedures. The nurse instructs the patient to ask for assistance to get out of bed. The nurse carefully evaluates any injury because of the possibility of internal bleeding.

> ⚠ **Nursing Alert**
> *Because of the risk for bleeding from abnormal clotting, the patient should use an electric razor rather than a safety razor. A soft-bristled toothbrush helps minimize bleeding gums, and pressure applied to all venipuncture sites helps minimize bleeding.*

MONITORING AND MANAGING POTENTIAL COMPLICATIONS

Bleeding and Hemorrhage. The patient is at increased risk for bleeding and hemorrhage because of decreased production of prothrombin and decreased ability of the diseased liver to synthesize the necessary substances for blood coagulation. Precautionary measures include protecting the patient with padded side rails, applying pressure to injection sites, and avoiding injury from sharp objects. The nurse observes for melena and assesses stools for blood (signs of possible internal bleeding). Vital signs are monitored regularly. Precautions are taken to minimize rupture of esophageal varices by avoiding further increases in portal pressure (see earlier discussion). Dietary modification and appropriate use of stool softeners may help prevent straining during defecation. The nurse closely monitors the patient for GI bleeding and keeps readily available equipment (e.g., balloon tamponade tube), IV fluids, and medications needed to treat hemorrhage from esophageal and gastric varices.

If hemorrhage occurs, the nurse helps the provider initiate measures to halt the bleeding and administers fluid and blood component therapy and medications. The patient with massive hemorrhage from bleeding esophageal or gastric varices is transferred to the ICU and requires emergency surgery or other treatment modalities. The patient and family require explanations about the event and the necessary treatment.

HEPATIC ENCEPHALOPATHY

Hepatic encephalopathy and coma, possible complications of cirrhosis, may manifest as deteriorating mental status and dementia or as physical signs, such as abnormal voluntary and involuntary movements. Hepatic encephalopathy is caused mainly by the accumulation of ammonia in the blood and its effect on cerebral metabolism. Many factors predispose the patient with cirrhosis to hepatic encephalopathy. Therefore, the patient may require extensive diagnostic testing to identify hidden sources of bleeding and increased ammonia production.

Treatment may include the use of lactulose and nonabsorbable intestinal tract antibiotics to decrease ammonia levels, modification of medications to eliminate those that may precipitate or worsen hepatic encephalopathy, and bed rest to minimize energy expenditure.

Monitoring is an essential nursing function to identify early deterioration in mental status. The nurse monitors the patient's mental status closely and reports changes, so that treatment of encephalopathy can be initiated promptly. Because electrolyte disturbances can contribute to encephalopathy, serum electrolyte levels are carefully monitored and corrected if abnormal. Oxygen is administered if oxygen desaturation occurs. The nurse monitors for fever or abdominal pain, which may signal the onset of bacterial peritonitis or other infection (see earlier discussion of hepatic encephalopathy).

> ⚠ **Nursing Alert**
> *Signs and symptoms of bacterial peritonitis include fever with abdominal pain, nausea, vomiting, and diarrhea; however, in patients with cirrhosis, a low-grade temperature with or without abdominal pain may be noted (Ferri, 2016b).*

Fluid Volume Excess. Patients with advanced chronic liver disease develop cardiovascular abnormalities. These occur due to an increased cardiac output and decreased peripheral vascular resistance, possibly resulting from the release of vasodilators. A hyperdynamic circulatory state develops in patients with cirrhosis, and plasma volume increases. The greater the degree of hepatic decompensation, the more severe the hyperdynamic state. Close assessment of cardiovascular and respiratory status is of key importance for the care of patients with this disorder. Pulmonary compromise, which is always a potential complication of ESLD because of plasma volume excess, makes prevention of pulmonary complications an important role for the nurse. Administering diuretics, implementing fluid restrictions, and enhancing patient positioning can optimize pulmonary function. Fluid retention may be noted in the development of ascites, lower extremity swelling, and dyspnea. Monitoring of intake and output, daily weight changes, changes in abdominal girth, and edema formation is part of nursing assessment in the hospital or in the home setting. Patients also are monitored for any changes in kidney function.

PROMOTING HOME AND COMMUNITY-BASED CARE

During the hospital stay, the nurse and other health care providers prepare the patient with cirrhosis for discharge, focusing on dietary instruction. Of greatest importance is the exclusion of alcohol from the diet. The patient may need referral to Alcoholics Anonymous, psychiatric care, or counseling or may benefit from support from a spiritual advisor. Also the patient should avoid the consumption of raw meats and shellfish due to the increased risk of foodborne illness in immunosuppressed patients.

Sodium restriction will continue for a considerable time, if not permanently. The patient will require written instructions, teaching, reinforcement, and support from the staff as well as family members.

Successful treatment depends on convincing the patient of the need to adhere completely to the therapeutic plan. The nurse also instructs the patient and family about symptoms of impending encephalopathy, possible bleeding tendencies, and susceptibility to infection.

(continued on page 772)

Recovery is neither rapid nor easy; there are frequent setbacks and apparent lack of improvement. Many patients find it difficult to refrain from using alcohol for comfort or escape. The nurse plays a significant role in offering support and encouragement to the patient.

EVALUATION

Expected patient outcomes may include the following:
1. Participates in activities:
   a. Plans activities and exercises to allow alternating periods of rest and activity
   b. Reports increased strength and well-being
   c. Participates in hygiene care
2. Increases nutritional intake:
   a. Demonstrates intake of appropriate nutrients and avoidance of alcohol as reflected by diet log
   b. Gains weight without increased edema and ascites formation
   c. Reports decrease in GI disturbances and anorexia
   d. Identifies foods and fluids that are nutritious and allowed on or restricted from the diet
   e. Adheres to vitamin therapy regimen
   f. Describes the rationale for small, frequent meals
3. Exhibits improved skin integrity:
   a. Has intact skin without evidence of breakdown, infection, or trauma
   b. Demonstrates normal turgor of skin of the extremities and trunk, and decreased edema
   c. Changes position frequently and inspects bony prominences daily
   d. Uses lotions to decrease pruritus
4. Avoids injury:
   a. Is free of ecchymotic areas or hematoma formation
   b. States rationale for side rails and asks for assistance to get out of bed
   c. Uses measures to prevent trauma (e.g., uses electric razor and soft toothbrush, blows nose gently, arranges furniture to prevent bumps and falls, avoids straining during defecation)
5. Is free of complications:
   a. Reports absence of frank bleeding from the GI tract (i.e., absence of melena and hematemesis)
   b. Is oriented to time, place, and person and demonstrates normal attention span
   c. Has a serum ammonia level within normal limits
   d. Identifies early, reportable signs of impaired thought processes

HEPATOCELLULAR CARCINOMA

HCC is the most common hepatic malignancy. It is the third leading cause of cancer death worldwide and the ninth leading cause of cancer death in the United States (Crissien & Frenette, 2014).

Risk Factors

HCC is strongly linked to cirrhosis and chronic hepatitis B and C infections. ALD, nonalcoholic steatohepatitis (inflammation and fat accumulation of the liver), primary biliary cirrhosis, and hemochromatosis (excessive retained iron in the body) also are thought to increase risk for HCC. Persons over 50 years of age and male gender also increase the likelihood of HCC developing in patients with cirrhosis (Forner, Ayuso, & Bruix, 2012). HCC may arise in patients without cirrhosis; typically these are individuals with chronic hepatitis B infection.

Clinical Manifestations and Assessment

Usually the clinical manifestations of HCC are found in the context of the patient with known cirrhosis: jaundice, ascites, varices, and the stigmata of chronic liver disease are common features. Unintentional weight loss, anorexia, and right upper quadrant pain may be additional presenting signs. In late cases, the patient may present with intra-abdominal bleeding from tumor rupture. In patients deemed high risk, routine screening with abdominal ultrasound and measurement of alpha fetoprotein levels has improved the detection of liver cancer (Bruix & Sherman, 2011; Crissien & Frenette, 2014).

The diagnosis of liver cancer is based on clinical signs and symptoms, the history and physical examination, and the results of laboratory and imaging studies. Increased serum levels of bilirubin, alkaline phosphatase, GGT, and alpha fetoprotein may occur. Anemia is a common finding, and leukocytosis (increased white blood cells [WBCs]), hypercalcemia, hypoglycemia, and hypocholesterolemia also may be seen on laboratory assessment.

Confirmation of the diagnosis of HCC is made radiologically with use of computed tomography (CT) scan imaging or magnetic resonance imaging (MRI) to determine the number, size, and location of tumors and if vascular invasion has occurred. In equivocal cases, liver biopsy may be used to obtain tissue samples of the lesion to determine malignancy (Crissien & Frenette, 2014).

Medical and Nursing Management

Currently there are multiple treatment options for the patient with HCC. Surgical resection is the preferred treatment for patients without cirrhosis and with adequate hepatic reserve; average 5-year survival outcomes after resection now exceed 50%; however, recurrence rates are as high as 70% at 5 years (Crissien & Frenette, 2014). In patients with HCC and cirrhosis, liver transplantation (discussed in detail below) is the treatment of choice. Liver transplantation is curative for patients with both HCC and ESLD; however, careful patient selection is critical to achieve good outcomes (Crissien & Frenette, 2014; Bruix & Sherman, 2011).

Other treatments for HCC are percutaneous ethanol injection (PEI) and radiofrequency (RFA) or microwave ablation (MWA), which directly induce tumor necrosis. Transarterial chemoembolization (TACE) is used to block the hepatic blood flow feeding the tumor and is used in combination with chemotherapeutic agents (Crissien & Frenette, 2014; Bruix & Sherman, 2011). Systemic chemotherapy includes sorafenib and other agents; currently multiple clinical trials are underway to study the effectiveness of chemotherapeutic agents to treat HCC (Crissien & Frenette, 2014).

LIVER TRANSPLANTATION

With recent advances in surgical techniques, immunosuppressant medications, and increased knowledge of immunology, liver transplantation has become the treatment of choice for patients with ESLD and acute liver failure. Because liver transplantation now is recognized as an established therapeutic modality, rather than an experimental procedure to treat these disorders, the number of liver transplantation centers is increasing. Often patients requiring transplantation are referred from distant hospitals to these sites. To prepare the patient and family for liver transplantation, nurses in all settings must understand the processes and procedures of liver transplantation.

The transplantation procedure involves total surgical removal of the diseased liver and replacement with a healthy donor organ in the same anatomic location (**orthotopic liver transplantation** [OLT]). The efficacy of this therapeutic modality is demonstrated by survival outcomes of 70.5% at 5 years (Kim et al., 2014). The important benefit of this option for patients with ESLD or fulminant liver failure is limited by the shortage of cadaveric donor organs. As of 2016, 14,000 patients were on the national UNOS transplant list awaiting liver transplant (HRSA/OPTN, 2016).

Indications and Contraindications

Indications for liver transplantation include:

- Advanced chronic liver disease
- Fulminant hepatic failure
- Metabolic liver diseases
- HCC
- Hepatocellular liver diseases (e.g., viral hepatitis, drug- or alcohol-induced liver disease, Wilson disease)
- Cholestatic diseases (interruption in bile flow seen in primary biliary cirrhosis, sclerosing cholangitis, and biliary atresia)

Other less common diseases requiring liver transplantation are polycystic liver disease, vascular disease (Budd–Chiari), and rare metabolic disorders (Everson, 2016).

Medical contraindications for liver transplant include uncontrolled infection, extrahepatic malignancy or advanced hepatobiliary metastatic disease, irreversible brain damage, anatomic difficulties, and multiorgan failure. Psychosocial

contraindications include active substance use, medical nonadherence, and severe psychiatric instability (Everson, 2016; Martin et al., 2014). Other factors that may present obstacles to successful transplant are comorbidities, such as advanced cardiac or pulmonary disease, and poor psychosocial support.

Selection and Evaluation for Liver Transplant

The selection and evaluation of a patient for liver transplantation is a multidisciplinary process that requires a complete assessment of the patient, including etiology and stage of liver disease, and evaluation of comorbidities and/or contraindications, psychosocial status, and any medical or surgical issues. The patient being considered for liver transplantation frequently has many systemic problems that influence preoperative and postoperative care. The medical condition of the patient must be optimized as well as possible to prevent complications and to ensure good outcomes. Patients must undergo complete medical, surgical, and psychosocial testing to determine if liver transplant is feasible, and for organ matching.

Once the patient is evaluated and deemed appropriate for liver transplant by the transplant center, he or she is placed on the national transplant wait-list administered by the UNOS. The priority for obtaining a cadaveric liver organ is determined by the Model of End Stage Liver Disease (MELD) score, which stratifies the level of illness of those awaiting a liver transplant. The MELD score is derived from a complex formula incorporating sodium levels, bilirubin levels, prothrombin time (reported as INR), and creatinine levels. The MELD score is an indicator of short-term mortality for those with ESLD. Additional priority beyond the patient's physiologic MELD score may be provided for selected diseases that increase the patient's mortality risk, such as HCC, HPS, and metabolic diseases of the liver. The highest priority on the transplant wait-list is provided to patients with acute or fulminant liver failure (HRSA/OPTN, 2016).

Surgical Procedure

The transplant operation involves total removal of the diseased liver, or hepatectomy, replacement with the donor organ, vascular anastomoses of the donor liver to the recipient, and biliary reconstruction. This complex surgical procedure is divided in three stages or phases: hepatectomy, anhepatic (no liver) phase, and reperfusion phase.

The first stage involves the total removal of the diseased liver. Vascular clamps are placed on the portal vein and the inferior vena cava above and below the liver, and the native liver is dissected from the recipient. Hemostasis is maintained using sutures and cauterization of bleeding vessels. After preparation of the donor liver, anastomoses of the suprahepatic inferior vena cava, infrahepatic inferior vena cava, and portal vein surgically connect the donor liver to the recipient. Reperfusion of the new donor liver is achieved by removal of vascular clamps and perfusion of portal venous blood. Then hepatic artery anastomosis is performed and, last, biliary reconstruction.

Multiple surgical innovations have been developed to prevent complications, such as bleeding, bile leaks, and reperfusion injury of the new graft, to improve outcomes (Eghtesad & Fung, 2012).

Liver transplantation is a long surgical procedure, partly because the patient with liver failure often has portal hypertension that requires the ligation of many venous collateral vessels. Blood loss during the surgical procedure may be extensive. If the patient has adhesions from previous abdominal surgery, lysis of adhesions is often necessary. If a shunt procedure was performed previously, it must be surgically reversed to permit adequate portal venous blood supply to the new liver. During the lengthy surgery, it is helpful to provide regular updates to the family about the progress of the operation and the patient's status.

Complications

Immediate postoperative complications may include bleeding, infection, rejection, and delayed graft function. Other complications include biliary leaks and obstruction, hepatic artery thrombosis, and portal vein thrombosis (Everson, 2016).

Primary Graft Nonfunction

Primary graft nonfunction is the most severe complication of liver transplant and occurs in up to 8.5% of cases. Ongoing encephalopathy, coagulopathy, jaundice, metabolic acidosis, and hemodynamic instability are clinical indications of primary graft nonfunction (Everson, 2016). Transplant recipients with primary graft nonfunction require immediate retransplantation and receive priority on the transplant waitlist (HRSA/OPTN, 2016).

Bleeding

Bleeding is common in the postoperative period and may result from coagulopathy, portal hypertension, and fibrinolysis (breakdown of fibrin clots) caused by ischemic injury to the donor liver. Hypotension may occur in this phase, secondary to blood loss. Administration of platelets, fresh-frozen plasma, or other blood products may be necessary. Hypertension is more common, although its cause is uncertain. Blood pressure elevation that is significant or sustained is treated.

Infection

Infection is a life-threatening complication after liver transplantation. Pulmonary and fungal infections are common; susceptibility to infection is increased by the immunosuppressive therapy that is needed to prevent rejection (Everson, 2016). Therefore, precautions must be taken to prevent health care–associated infections. The nurse uses strict asepsis

when manipulating central venous catheters, arterial lines, and drainage systems for urine, bile, and any body fluids; when obtaining specimens; and when changing dressings. Meticulous hand hygiene and contact precautions are crucial to prevent infection in the recipient of a liver transplant.

Rejection

Rejection is a primary concern. A transplanted liver is perceived by the immune system as a foreign antigen. This triggers an immune response, leading to the activation of T lymphocytes that attack and destroy the transplanted liver. Immunosuppressive agents are used as long-term therapy to prevent this response and rejection of the transplanted liver. These agents inhibit the activation of immunocompetent T lymphocytes to prevent the production of effector T cells. Most transplant centers use two or three immunosuppressants in combination to prevent rejection (Lucey et al., 2013; Wiesner, 2012). The recipient of the liver transplant requires intensive education in dosing, side effects, and the drug interactions of these medications and will require lifelong immunosuppression.

Although the 1- and 5-year survival rates have increased dramatically with the use of new immunosuppressive therapies, these therapies are not without side effects. Both cyclosporine and tacrolimus have important side effects, such as kidney dysfunction, hypertension, hyperlipidemia, and hyperkalemia. Neurotoxicity may occur with use of tacrolimus, and patients may experience tremors to more severe complications, such as psychosis or seizures. Optimal dosing of immunosuppression must be monitored carefully to prevent rejection and to reduce side effects (Lucey et al., 2013).

Despite the success of immunosuppression in reducing the incidence of rejection of transplanted organs, liver transplantation is not routine and may be accompanied by complications related to the lengthy surgical procedure, immunosuppressive therapy, infection, and the technical difficulties encountered in reconstructing the blood vessels and biliary tract.

Nursing Management

The patient considering transplantation, together with the family, must make difficult choices about treatment, use of financial resources, and relocation to another area to be closer to the medical center. They also must cope with the patient's longstanding health problems and any social and family problems associated with behaviors that may have caused the patient's liver failure. As a result, considerable emotional stress occurs while the patient and family consider liver transplantation and wait for an available liver. The nurse must be aware of these issues and attuned to the emotional and psychological status of the patient and family. Referral to a psychiatric liaison nurse, psychologist, psychiatrist, or spiritual advisor may help them cope with the stressors associated with ESLD and liver transplantation.

Preoperative Nursing Interventions

The nurse, surgeon, hepatologist, and other members of the health care team provide the patient and family with full explanations about the procedure, the chances of success, and the risks, including the side effects of long-term immunosuppression. The need for close follow-up and lifelong compliance with the therapeutic regimen, including immunosuppression, is explained to the patient and family.

The nurse coordinator is an integral member of the transplant team and plays an important role in preparing the patient for liver transplantation. The nurse serves as advocate for the patient and family and assumes the important role of liaison between the patient and the other members of the transplant team. The nurse also serves as a resource to other nurses and members of the health care team involved in evaluating and caring for the patient.

Postoperative Nursing Interventions

The patient is maintained in an environment as free from bacteria, viruses, and fungi as possible because immunosuppressive medications reduce the body's natural defenses. In the immediate postoperative period, cardiovascular, pulmonary, renal, neurologic, and metabolic functions are monitored continuously. Mean arterial pressures and pulmonary artery pressures (PAPs) also are monitored. Ventilator support and airway management are priorities. Cardiac output (CO), central venous pressure (CVP), PAPs, pulmonary capillary wedge pressure (PCWP), arterial and mixed venous blood gases, oxygen saturation, oxygen demand and delivery, urine output, heart rate, and blood pressure are used to evaluate the patient's hemodynamic status and intravascular fluid volume. Liver function tests, electrolyte levels, the coagulation profile, chest x-ray, electrocardiogram, and fluid output (including urine, bile from the T tube, and output from NG and drainage tubes) are monitored closely. Because the liver is responsible for the storage of glycogen and the synthesis of protein and clotting factors, these substances need to be monitored and replaced in the immediate postoperative period. The nurse monitors for signs of excess bleeding in the immediate postoperative period and notifies the provider immediately if bleeding is suspected (hypotension, tachycardia, tachypnea, decreasing CO, melena, increasing abdominal girth, bloody NG drainage, etc.).

There is a high risk for atelectasis and an altered ventilation–perfusion ratio, caused by insult to the diaphragm during the surgical procedure, prolonged anesthesia, immobility, and postoperative pain. Because of this risk, the patient will have an endotracheal tube in place and will require mechanical ventilation during the initial postoperative period. Suctioning is performed as required, and sterile humidification is provided.

As the vital signs and condition stabilize, efforts are made to assist the patient to recover from the trauma of this complex surgery. After removal of the endotracheal tube, the nurse encourages the patient to use an IS to decrease the risk for atelectasis. Once the arterial lines and the urinary catheter are removed, the patient is assisted to get out of bed, to ambulate as tolerated, and to participate in self-care to prevent the complications associated with immobility. Close monitoring for signs and symptoms of liver dysfunction and rejection continue throughout the hospital stay. Plans are made for close follow-up after discharge as well. Teaching is initiated during the preoperative period and continues after surgery.

Promoting Home and Community-Based Care

Teaching the patient and family about long-term measures to promote health is crucial for the success of transplantation and represents an important role of the nurse. The patient and family must understand why they need to adhere continuously to the therapeutic regimen, with special emphasis on the methods of administration, rationale, and side effects of the prescribed immunosuppressive agents. The nurse provides written as well as verbal instructions about how and when to take the medications. To avoid running out of medication or skipping a dose, the patient must make sure that an adequate supply of medication is available. Also instructions are provided about the signs and symptoms that indicate problems necessitating consultation with the transplant team.

The nurse emphasizes the importance of follow-up blood tests and appointments with the transplant team. Trough blood levels (the lowest concentration reached by a medication before the next dose is administered) of immunosuppressive agents are obtained along with other blood tests that assess the function of the liver and kidneys. During the first months, the patient is likely to require blood tests two or three times a week. As the patient's condition stabilizes, blood studies and visits to the transplant team are less frequent. The importance of routine ophthalmologic examinations is emphasized because of the increased incidence of cataracts and glaucoma associated with the long-term corticosteroid therapy used with transplantation. Regular oral hygiene and follow-up dental care, with administration of prophylactic antibiotics before dental examinations and treatments, are recommended because of the immunosuppression.

The nurse reminds the patient that preventing rejection and infection leads to a successful transplantation and increases the chances for survival and living a more normal life than before transplantation. Many patients have lived successful and productive lives after receiving a liver transplant.

DISORDERS OF THE GALLBLADDER

Several disorders affect the biliary system and interfere with normal drainage of bile into the duodenum. These disorders include inflammation of the biliary system and carcinoma that obstructs the biliary tree. Gallbladder disease with gall-stones is the most common disorder of the biliary system. Although not all occurrences of gallbladder inflammation (**cholecystitis**) are related to gallstones (**cholelithiasis**), more than 90% of patients with acute cholecystitis have gallstones. However, most of the 20 million Americans with gallstones have no pain and are unaware of the presence of stones.

CHOLELITHIASIS

Calculi, or gallstones, usually form in the gallbladder from the solid constituents of bile; they vary greatly in size, shape, and composition (Fig. 25-12).

Pathophysiology

There are two major types of gallstones: those composed predominantly of pigment and those composed primarily of cholesterol. Pigment stones form when unconjugated pigments in the bile precipitate to form stones. The risk of developing such stones is increased in patients with cirrhosis, hemolysis, and infections of the biliary tract. Pigment stones cannot be dissolved and must be removed surgically.

Cholesterol stones account for over 70% to 80% of gall-bladder disease in the United States. Cholesterol, a normal constituent of bile, is insoluble in water. Its solubility depends on bile acids and lecithin (phospholipids) in bile.

In patients who are gallstone prone, there is decreased bile acid synthesis and increased cholesterol synthesis in the liver, resulting in bile supersaturated with cholesterol, which precipitates out of the bile to form stones. The cholesterol-saturated bile predisposes to the formation of gallstones and acts as an irritant that produces inflammatory changes in the gallbladder (Fogel & Sherman, 2016).

Risk Factors

Gallstones are uncommon in children and young adults but become increasingly prevalent after 40 years of age, especially in women (Box 25-10).

Clinical Manifestations and Assessment

Gallstones may be silent, producing no pain and only mild GI symptoms. Such stones may be detected incidentally during surgery or evaluation for unrelated problems.

The patient with gallbladder disease resulting from gall-stones may develop two types of symptoms: those due to disease of the gallbladder itself, and those due to obstruction of the bile passages by a gallstone. The symptoms may be acute or chronic. Epigastric distress, such as fullness, abdominal distention, and vague pain in the right upper quadrant of the abdomen, may occur. This distress may follow a meal rich in fried or fatty foods. Clinical manifestations of gallstones are largely asymptomatic; however, 15% to 20% of patients with gallstones will develop pain and biliary colic with repeated

FIGURE 25-12 Examples of cholesterol gallstones (*left*) made up of a coalescence of multiple small stones and pigment gallstones (*right*) composed of calcium bilirubinate. (From Rubin, R., & Strayer, D. S. (2008). *Rubin's Pathology* (5th ed). Philadelphia, PA: Lippincott Williams & Wilkins.)

Risk Factors for Cholelithiasis

- Obesity
- Female gender, especially women who have had multiple pregnancies or who are of Native American or U.S. Southwestern Hispanic ethnicity
- Frequent changes in weight
- Rapid weight loss (leads to rapid development of gallstones and high risk of symptomatic disease)
- Treatment with high-dose estrogen (e.g., in prostate cancer)
- Low-dose estrogen therapy; a small increase in the risk of gallstones
- Ileal resection or disease
- Gastric bypass
- Total parental nutrition
- Cystic fibrosis
- Diabetes mellitus
- Family history

episodes of obstruction. Increased frequency of biliary colic typically will result in cholecystitis. If the gallstone is dislodged and no longer obstructs the cystic duct, the gallbladder drains and the inflammatory process subsides after a relatively short time. If the gallstone continues to obstruct the duct, abscess, necrosis, and perforation with generalized peritonitis may result.

Nursing Alert
The nurse is alert to the signs and symptoms of peritonitis, including abdominal pain that initially may be vague and generalized but becomes increasingly severe and constant; abdominal distention and tenderness with rebound tenderness; anxiety, paleness, and diaphoresis; anorexia; nausea; vomiting; inability to pass feces and flatus; rigidity of the abdomen; an absence of bowel sounds; cautious movement; and knee–chest position for comfort.

If a gallstone obstructs the cystic duct, the gallbladder becomes distended, inflamed, and, eventually, infected (acute cholecystitis). The patient develops a fever and may have a palpable abdominal mass. The patient may have biliary colic with excruciating upper right abdominal pain that radiates to the back or right shoulder. Usually biliary colic is associated with nausea and vomiting, and it is noticeable several hours after a heavy meal. The patient moves about restlessly, unable to find a comfortable position. The pain will fluctuate, lasting from 30 minutes to up to 6 hours. The patient may experience other symptoms, including nausea, chills, and gastric distress, including belching and bloating.

Such a bout of biliary colic is caused by contraction of the gallbladder, which cannot release bile because of obstruction by the stone. This produces marked tenderness in the

right upper quadrant on deep inspiration and prevents full inspiratory excursion when the examiner's fingers are under the liver border, known as *Murphy sign* (Fogel & Sherman, 2016). See management under cholecystitis.

CHOLECYSTITIS

Cholecystitis is acute inflammation of the gallbladder. An empyema of the gallbladder develops if the gallbladder becomes filled with purulent fluid (pus). Repeated episodes of obstruction of the cystic duct by gallstones will cause cholecystitis.

Pathophysiology

Calculous cholecystitis is the cause of more than 90% to 95% of cases of acute cholecystitis (Fogel & Sherman, 2016). In calculous cholecystitis, a gallbladder stone obstructs bile outflow. Bile remaining in the gallbladder initiates a chemical reaction; autolysis and edema occur. The gallbladder becomes inflamed and distended due to increased pressure and vascular compromise, resulting in ischemia and necrosis. The release of inflammatory agents additionally plays a role in the pathophysiology of acute cholecystitis. Secondary infection with bacteria complicates the course of this disorder in up to 50% of patients (Fogel & Sherman, 2016).

Acalculous cholecystitis describes acute gallbladder inflammation in the absence of obstruction by gallstones. It occurs after major surgical procedures, severe trauma, or burns. Other factors associated with this type of cholecystitis include congestive heart failure, diabetes mellitus, cystic artery embolism, immunosuppression, abdominal vasculitis, multiorgan failure, and acute renal failure. It is speculated that acalculous cholecystitis is caused by further progression of multiple systemic failures, resulting in gallbladder stasis, increased bacterial colonization, and ischemia. Bile stasis (lack of gallbladder contraction) and increased viscosity of the bile are also thought to play a role (Fogel & Sherman, 2016; Treinen et al., 2015).

Clinical Manifestations and Assessment

Cholecystitis causes pain, tenderness, and rigidity of the upper right abdomen; usually the pain radiates to the back or right shoulder or scapula. Nausea and vomiting are common. The patient will have leukocytosis (elevated WBCs), and physical examination may reveal a positive Murphy sign (right subcostal tenderness) (Fogel & Sherman, 2016).

Medical Management

The major objectives of medical therapy are to reduce the incidence of acute episodes of gallbladder pain and cholecystitis by supportive and dietary management and, if possible, to remove the cause of cholecystitis by pharmacologic therapy, endoscopic procedures, or surgical intervention. Asymptomatic cholelithiasis can be treated with prophylactic cholecystectomy, especially with findings of large gallstones (greater than 3 cm) due to their malignant potential. Initial management of cholecystitis involves bowel rest (i.e., nothing by mouth [NPO]), management of fluids and electrolyte balance, pain management, and antibiotic coverage (Fogel & Sherman, 2016).

Pharmacologic Therapy

Ursodeoxycholic acid (UDCA) and chenodeoxycholic acid (chenodiol or CDCA) have been used to dissolve small, radiolucent gallstones composed primarily of cholesterol in patients with symptomatic cholecystitis. Because of the high long-term risk of recurrence, laparoscopic cholecystectomy (50% within 5 years), and widespread availability of laparoscopic cholecystectomy, rarely is this method of treatment used today. However, it may be beneficial in prevention of gallstone disease during periods of rapid weight loss (EASL, 2016; Fogel & Sherman, 2016).

Surgical Management

Laparoscopic or open cholecystectomy is more appropriate for symptomatic patients with acceptable operative risk. Removal of the gallbladder (**cholecystectomy**) through

traditional surgical approaches was considered the standard treatment for more than 100 years. There is now widespread use of **laparoscopic cholecystectomy** (removal of the gallbladder through a small incision through the umbilicus). As a result, surgical risks have decreased, along with the length of hospital stay and the long recovery period required after standard surgical cholecystectomy (Fogel & Sherman, 2016).

Laparoscopic Cholecystectomy

Laparoscopic cholecystectomy (Fig. 25-13) has dramatically changed the approach to the management of cholecystitis. It has become the new standard for therapy of symptomatic gallstones. Approximately 750,000 patients in the United States require surgery each year for removal of the gallbladder, and greater than 90% of them are candidates for laparoscopic cholecystectomy (Fogel & Sherman, 2016).

Before the procedure, the patient is informed that an open abdominal procedure may be necessary, and general anesthesia is administered. Laparoscopic cholecystectomy is performed through a small incision or puncture made through the abdominal wall at the umbilicus. The abdominal cavity is insufflated with carbon dioxide (pneumoperitoneum) to assist in inserting the laparoscope and to aid in visualizing the abdominal structures. The fiberoptic scope is inserted through the small umbilical incision. Several additional punctures or

A

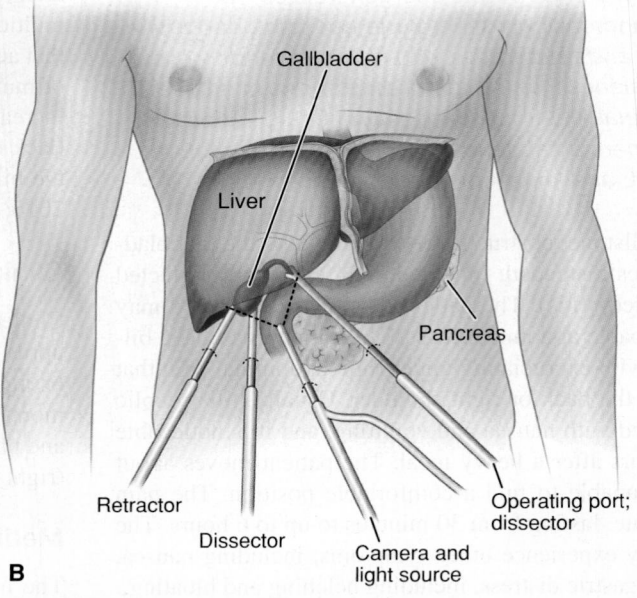

B

FIGURE 25-13 In laparoscopic cholecystectomy (**A**), the surgeon makes four small incisions (less than 12 in each) in the abdomen (**B**) and inserts a laparoscope with a miniature camera through the umbilical incision. The camera apparatus displays the gallbladder and adjacent tissues on a screen, allowing the surgeon to visualize the sections of the organ for removal.

small incisions are made in the abdominal wall to introduce other surgical instruments into the operative field. The surgeon visualizes the biliary system through the laparoscope; a camera attached to the scope permits a view of the intra-abdominal field to be transmitted to a television monitor. After the cystic duct is dissected, the common bile duct can be visualized by ultrasound or cholangiography (imaging of the bile ducts with contrast medium) to evaluate the anatomy and identify stones. The cystic artery is dissected free and clipped. The gallbladder is separated from the hepatic bed and dissected. Then the gallbladder is removed from the abdominal cavity after bile and small stones are aspirated. Stone forceps also can be used to remove or crush larger stones.

Advantages of the laparoscopic procedure are that the patient does not experience the paralytic ileus that occurs with open abdominal surgery and has less postoperative abdominal pain. Early laparoscopic cholecystectomy (within 24 of symptoms) is the preferred intervention for treatment of acute cholecystitis and results in reduced length of stay, fewer surgical complications, and faster recovery for the patient (Fogel & Sherman, 2016; Gurusamy et al., 2013).

Conversion to a traditional abdominal surgical procedure may be necessary if problems are encountered during the laparoscopic procedure; this occurs in 3% of reported surgical cases (Fogel & Sherman, 2016). Careful screening of patients and identification of those at low risk for complications limit the frequency of conversion to an open abdominal procedure. However, with increasing use of laparoscopic procedures, the number of such conversions may increase. The most serious complication after laparoscopic cholecystectomy is a bile duct injury, which may be identified and corrected at the time of the procedure. A bile leak that develops from an unrecognized injury may result in fluid collections that usually can be managed by endoscopic stent placement. Bile peritonitis, a more serious but rare complication, may result in critical illness or death.

Because of the short hospital stay with uncomplicated laparoscopic cholecystectomies, it is important to provide written and verbal instructions about managing postoperative pain and reporting signs and symptoms of intra-abdominal complications, including loss of appetite, vomiting, pain, distention of the abdomen, and temperature elevation. Although recovery from laparoscopic cholecystectomy is rapid, patients are drowsy afterward. The patient must have assistance at home during the first 24 to 48 hours. Box 25-11 details patient self-care after a laparoscopic cholecystectomy.

Cholecystectomy

In cholecystectomy, the gallbladder is removed through an abdominal incision (usually right subcostal) after the cystic duct and artery are ligated. The procedure is performed for acute and chronic cholecystitis. In some patients, a drain is placed close to the gallbladder bed and brought out through a puncture wound if there is a bile leak. A small leak should

BOX 25-11 | **Patient Education**

Managing Self-Care After Laparoscopic Cholecystectomy

Resuming Activity
- Begin light exercise (walking) immediately.
- Take a shower or bath after 1 or 2 days.
- Wait to drive a car for 3 or 4 days.
- Avoid lifting objects exceeding 5 lb after surgery, usually for 1 week.
- Resume sexual activity when cleared by surgical team.

Caring for the Wound
- Check puncture site daily for signs of infection.
- Wash puncture site with mild soap and water.
- Allow special adhesive strips on the puncture site to fall off. Do not pull them off.

Resuming Eating
- Resume your normal diet.
- If you had fat intolerance before surgery, gradually add fat back into your diet in small increments.

Managing Pain
- You may experience pain or discomfort in your right shoulder from the gas used to inflate your abdominal area during surgery. Sitting upright in bed or a chair, walking, or use of a heating pad may ease the discomfort.
- Take analgesics as needed and as prescribed. Report to surgeon if pain is unrelieved even with analgesic use.

Managing Follow-Up Care
- Make an appointment with your surgeon for 7–10 days after discharge.
- Call your surgeon if you experience any signs or symptoms of infection at or around the puncture site: redness, tenderness, swelling, heat, or drainage.
- Call your surgeon if you experience a fever of 37.7°C (100°F) or more for 2 consecutive days.
- Call your surgeon if you develop nausea, vomiting, or abdominal pain.

close spontaneously in a few days, with the drain preventing accumulation of bile. Usually, only a small amount of serosanguineous fluid drains in the initial 24 hours after surgery; afterward, the drain is removed. Typically the drain is maintained if there is excess oozing or bile leakage. Bile duct injury is a rare but serious complication of cholecystectomy, but it occurs less frequently than with the laparoscopic approach. Patients with multiple comorbidities or with high surgical risk may be treated with the open cholecystectomy (Fogel & Sherman, 2016).

DISORDERS OF THE PANCREAS

Pancreatitis

Pancreatitis (inflammation of the pancreas) is a serious disorder. The most basic classification system used to describe or categorize the various stages and forms of pancreatitis divides the disorder into acute and chronic forms. Acute pancreatitis can be a medical emergency associated with a high risk for life-threatening complications and mortality, whereas chronic pancreatitis may not be detected until significant **exocrine** and endocrine tissue is destroyed. Approximately 10% of patients with acute pancreatitis will develop chronic pancreatitis, which can be characterized by acute episodes or may be subclinical (Forsmark, 2016). Frequently common causes for pancreatitis are due to alcohol abuse or gallstones; however, drugs, trauma, infection, autoimmune disease, or infection also may result in pancreatitis (Forsmark, 2016; Ito et al., 2015).

Although the mechanisms causing pancreatic inflammation are unknown, pancreatitis is commonly described as autodigestion of the pancreas. It is believed that the pancreatic duct becomes temporarily obstructed, accompanied by hypersecretion of the exocrine enzymes of the pancreas. These enzymes enter the bile duct, where they are activated and, together with bile, back up (reflux) into the pancreatic duct, causing pancreatitis.

ACUTE PANCREATITIS

Acute pancreatitis ranges from a mild, self-limited disorder to a severe, rapidly fatal disease that does not respond to any treatment. Mild acute pancreatitis is characterized by edema and inflammation confined to the pancreas. Minimal organ dysfunction is present, and return to normal function usually occurs within 6 months. Although this is considered the milder form of pancreatitis, the patient is acutely ill and at risk for hypovolemic shock, fluid and electrolyte disturbances, and sepsis. A more widespread and complete enzymatic digestion of the gland characterizes severe acute pancreatitis. Enzymes damage the local blood vessels, and bleeding and thrombosis can occur. The tissue may become necrotic, with damage extending into the retroperitoneal tissues. Local complications consist of pancreatic cysts or abscesses and acute fluid collections in or near the pancreas. Patients who develop systemic complications with organ failure, such as pulmonary insufficiency with hypoxia, shock, kidney failure, and GI bleeding, also are characterized as having severe acute pancreatitis (Forsmark, 2016). The severity of acute pancreatitis and its outcomes can be predicted based on clinical and laboratory data (Box 25-12).

Pathophysiology

Self-digestion of the pancreas by its own proteolytic enzymes, principally **trypsin** in a critical initial step, causes acute pancreatitis. Activation of the enzymes can lead to, inflammation, necrosis, erosion, and hemorrhage. This cascade of events also may result in multiorgan failure (Forsmark, 2016).

Long-term use of alcohol is commonly associated with acute episodes of pancreatitis, but the patient usually has had

---

BOX 25-12 **Criteria for Predicting Severity of Pancreatitis**[a]

Criteria on Admission to Hospital
- Age over 55 years
- WBC more than 16,000 mm^3
- Serum glucose greater than 200 mg/dL (greater than 11.1 mmol/L)
- Serum LDH greater than 350 IU/L (greater than 350 U/L)
- AST greater than 250 U/mL (120 U/L)

Criteria within 48 Hours of Hospital Admission
- Fall in hematocrit greater than 10% (greater than 0.10)
- Blood urea nitrogen (BUN) increase greater than 5 mg/dL (greater than 1.7 mmol/L)
- Serum calcium less than 8 mg/dL (less than 2.0 mmol/L)
- Base deficit greater than 4 mEq/L (greater than 4 mmol/L)
- Fluid retention or sequestration greater than 6 L
- PO$_2$ less than 60 mm Hg
- Two or fewer signs, 1% mortality; three or four signs, 15% mortality; five or six signs, 40% mortality; more than six signs, 100% mortality

[a]The more risk factors a patient has, "the greater the severity and likelihood of complications or death".

undiagnosed chronic pancreatitis before the first episode of acute pancreatitis occurs.

Other, less common causes of pancreatitis include bacterial or viral infection, with pancreatitis occasionally developing as a complication of a virus, such as cytomegalovirus (CMV) and mumps (Forsmark, 2016). Blunt abdominal trauma, peptic ulcer disease, ischemic vascular disease, hyperlipidemia, hypercalcemia, and the use of corticosteroids, thiazide diuretics, oral contraceptives, and other medications also have been associated with an increased incidence of pancreatitis. Acute pancreatitis may develop after surgery on or near the pancreas or after instrumentation of the pancreatic duct. Acute idiopathic pancreatitis accounts for up to 10% of the cases of acute pancreatitis. In addition, there is a small incidence of hereditary pancreatitis (Forsmark, 2016).

Clinical Manifestations and Assessment

Severe abdominal pain is the major symptom of pancreatitis that causes the patient to seek medical care. Typically, the pain occurs in the midepigastrium. Frequently pain is acute in onset, occurring 24 to 48 hours after a very heavy meal or alcohol ingestion, and it may be diffuse and difficult to localize. In general, it is more severe after meals and is unrelieved by antacids. Pain may be accompanied by abdominal distention; a poorly defined, palpable abdominal mass; and decreased peristalsis. Pain caused by pancreatitis is accompanied frequently by vomiting that fails to relieve the pain or nausea.

The patient appears acutely ill. Abdominal guarding is present. A rigid or board-like abdomen may develop and is generally an ominous sign; the abdomen may remain soft in the absence of peritonitis. Ecchymosis (bruising) in the flank (Grey–Turner sign) or around the umbilicus (Cullen sign) may indicate severe pancreatitis with retroperitoneal hemorrhage (see Chapter 27, Fig. 27-10). Nausea and vomiting are common in acute pancreatitis. The emesis is usually gastric in origin but also may be bile-stained. Fever, jaundice, mental confusion, and agitation also may occur.

Hypotension is typical and reflects hypovolemia and shock caused by the loss of large amounts of protein-rich fluid into the tissues and peritoneal cavity. In addition to hypotension, the patient may develop tachycardia, cyanosis, and cold, clammy skin. Respiratory distress and peritonitis also are associated with acute pancreatitis (Forsmark, 2016). In addition, the patient may develop a pleural effusion which would present as dullness to percussion on the affected lung.

The diagnosis of acute pancreatitis is based on a history of abdominal pain, the presence of known risk factors, and findings from the physical examination and diagnostics. Serum **amylase** and **lipase** levels are used in making the diagnosis of acute pancreatitis. Serum amylase and lipase levels will be elevated three times the upper limit of normal in most cases. The lipase remains elevated longer than amylase. A history of gallstones, alcohol use, and viral infection is used to diagnose acute pancreatitis. Usually the WBC count is elevated; hypocalcemia is present in many patients and correlates well with the severity of pancreatitis. Transient hyperglycemia and glucosuria and elevated serum bilirubin levels occur in some patients with acute pancreatitis. Plasma lipids and calcium are additional laboratory tests used to diagnose acute pancreatitis.

Ultrasound and contrast-enhanced CT or MRI scans are used to identify an increase in the diameter of the pancreas and to detect pancreatic cysts, abscesses, or pseudocysts. CT or MRI imaging is the modality of choice for the assessment of both acute and chronic pancreatitis (Forsmark, 2016).

Medical Management

The overall mortality rate of patients with severe acute pancreatitis is high because of shock, anoxia, hypotension, or fluid and electrolyte imbalances. Attacks of acute pancreatitis may result in complete recovery, may recur without permanent damage, or may progress to chronic pancreatitis. The patient who is admitted to the hospital with a diagnosis of pancreatitis is acutely ill and needs expert nursing and medical care (Forsmark, 2016).

Management of acute pancreatitis is directed toward relieving symptoms and preventing or treating complications. All oral intake is withheld to inhibit stimulation of the pancreas and its secretion of enzymes. The current recommendation is that, whenever possible, the enteral route should be used to meet nutritional needs in patients with pancreatitis. This strategy also has been found to prevent infectious complications and is safe and cost effective in doing so.

The mainstay of therapy for acute pancreatitis is analgesic management of pain, IV fluids to maintain intravascular volume, and elimination of oral intake. Aggressive IV therapy will be needed in patients with severe pancreatitis; however, it is important to prevent fluid overload because of the potential development of abdominal compartment syndrome (refer to Chapter 53). In cases of severe or necrotizing acute pancreatitis, the use of antibiotics is recommended (Forsmark, 2016; Gurusamy et al., 2013).

Although surgery is often risky because the acutely ill patient is a poor surgical risk, it may be performed to assist in the diagnosis of pancreatitis (diagnostic laparotomy), to establish pancreatic drainage, or to resect or débride a necrotic pancreas (Forsmark, 2016; Gurusamy et al., 2013).

Nursing Management

A plan of nursing care for a patient with acute pancreatitis is available online at http://thepoint.lww.com/Honan2e.

Relieving Pain and Discomfort

Because the pathologic process responsible for pain is auto-digestion of the pancreas, the objectives of therapy are to relieve pain and decrease secretion of pancreatic enzymes. The pain of acute pancreatitis is often very severe, necessitating the liberal use of analgesics. The current recommendation for pain management in this population is parenteral narcotics, such as hydromorphone (Forsmark, 2016). Oral feedings are withheld to decrease the formation and secretion of **secretin**. The patient is maintained on parenteral fluids and electrolytes to restore and maintain fluid balance. NG suction may be used to relieve nausea and vomiting or to treat abdominal distention and paralytic ileus (refer to Chapter 22 for care of NG tube). The nurse provides frequent oral hygiene and care to decrease discomfort from the NG tube and relieve dryness of the mouth.

The acutely ill patient is maintained on bed rest to decrease the metabolic rate and reduce the secretion of pancreatic and gastric enzymes. If the patient experiences increasing severity of pain, the nurse reports this to the provider because the patient may be experiencing hemorrhage of the pancreas or the dose of analgesic may be inadequate.

The patient with acute pancreatitis often has a clouded sensorium because of severe pain, fluid and electrolyte disturbances, and hypoxia. Therefore, the nurse provides frequent and repeated but simple explanations about the need for withholding fluids, maintenance of gastric suction, and bed rest.

Improving Breathing Pattern

The nurse maintains the patient in a semi-Fowler position to decrease pressure on the diaphragm by a distended abdomen and to increase respiratory expansion. Frequent changes of position are necessary to prevent atelectasis and pooling of respiratory secretions. Pulmonary assessment and monitoring of pulse oximetry or ABGs are essential to detect changes in respiratory status so that early treatment can be initiated. The nurse instructs the patient in techniques of deep breathing and in the use of an IS to improve respiratory function, and the nurse encourages and assists the patient to perform these activities every hour. Intubation may be necessary to support ventilation.

Improving Nutritional Status

In general, the patient with acute pancreatitis has not been permitted food or oral fluid intake. However, recent studies suggest that maintaining NPO but use of enteral feedings with nasojejunum tubes, thereby preventing pancreatic enzyme release maintains gut integrity, enhances immune system functioning, and demonstrates lower complication rates when compared to parenteral feedings (Wu & Banks, 2013). It is important to assess the patient's nutritional status and to note factors that alter the patient's nutritional requirements (e.g., temperature elevation, surgery, drainage). Laboratory test results and daily weights are useful to monitor the nutritional status.

In addition to administering enteral or parenteral nutrition, the nurse monitors serum glucose levels every 4 to 6 hours. As the acute symptoms subside, the nurse gradually reintroduces oral feedings. Between acute attacks, the patient receives a diet that is high in carbohydrates and low in fats and proteins. The patient should avoid heavy meals and alcoholic beverages.

Improving Skin Integrity

The patient is at risk for skin breakdown because of poor nutritional status, enforced bed rest, and restlessness, which may result in pressure ulcers and breaks in tissue integrity. In addition, the patient who has undergone surgery may have multiple drains or an open surgical incision and is at risk for skin breakdown and infection. The nurse carefully assesses the wound, drainage sites, and skin for signs of infection, inflammation, and breakdown. The nurse carries out wound care as prescribed and takes precautions to protect intact skin from contact with drainage. It is important to turn the patient every 2 hours; use of specialty beds may be indicated to prevent skin breakdown. Often consultation with an **enterostomal therapist** (also referred to as a wound care specialist or wound-ostomy-continence nurse) is helpful in identifying appropriate skin care devices and protocols.

Monitoring and Managing Potential Complications

Fluid and electrolyte disturbances are common complications because of nausea, vomiting, movement of fluid from the vascular compartment to the peritoneal cavity, diaphoresis, fever, and the use of gastric suction. The nurse assesses the patient's fluid and electrolyte status by noting skin turgor and moistness of mucous membranes. The nurse weighs the patient daily and carefully measures fluid intake and output, including urine output, NG secretions, and diarrhea. In addition, it is important to assess for other factors that may affect fluid and electrolyte status, including increased body temperature and wound drainage. Inflammation can lead to significant fluid depletion as well as extravasation of fluid into the retroperitoneal space and abdominal cavity.

The nurse assesses the patient for ascites and measures abdominal girth daily if ascites is suspected.

Fluids are administered intravenously and may be accompanied by infusion of blood or blood products to maintain the blood volume and to prevent or treat hypovolemic shock. It is important to keep emergency medications readily available because of the risk for circulatory collapse and shock. The nurse promptly reports decreased blood pressure and reduced urine output because these signs may indicate hypovolemia and shock or kidney failure. Low serum calcium and magnesium levels may occur and require prompt treatment.

Pancreatic necrosis is a major cause of morbidity and mortality in patients with acute pancreatitis. The patient who develops necrosis is at risk for hemorrhage, septic shock, and multiple organ failure. The patient may undergo diagnostic procedures to confirm pancreatic necrosis; surgical débridement or insertion of multiple drains may be performed. The patient with pancreatic necrosis is usually critically ill and requires expert medical and nursing management, including hemodynamic monitoring in the ICU.

In addition to carefully monitoring vital signs and other signs and symptoms, the nurse is responsible for administering prescribed fluids, medications, and blood products; assisting with supportive management, such as use of a ventilator; preventing additional complications; and attending to the patient's physical and psychological care.

Shock and multiple organ failure may occur with acute pancreatitis. Hypovolemic shock may occur as a result of hypovolemia and sequestering of fluid in the peritoneal cavity. Hemorrhagic shock may occur with hemorrhagic pancreatitis. Septic shock may occur with bacterial infection of the pancreas. Cardiac dysfunction may occur as a result of fluid and electrolyte disturbances, acid–base imbalances, and release of toxic substances into the circulation.

The nurse closely monitors the patient for early signs of neurologic, cardiovascular, renal, and respiratory dysfunction. The nurse must be prepared to respond quickly to rapid changes in the patient's status, treatments, and therapies. In addition, it is important to inform the family about the status and progress of the patient and to allow them to spend time with the patient.

Promoting Home and Community-Based Care

The patient who has survived an episode of acute pancreatitis has been acutely ill. A prolonged period is needed to regain strength and return to the previous level of activity. Often the patient is still weak and debilitated for weeks or months after an acute episode of pancreatitis. Because of the severity of the acute illness, the patient may not recall many of the explanations and instructions given during the acute phase. Teaching often needs to be repeated and reinforced. The nurse instructs the patient about the factors implicated in the onset of acute pancreatitis and about the need to avoid high-fat foods, heavy meals, and alcohol. It is important to give the patient and family verbal and written instructions about signs and symptoms of acute pancreatitis and possible complications that should be reported promptly to the provider.

If acute pancreatitis is a result of biliary tract disease, such as gallstones and gallbladder disease, additional explanations are needed about required dietary modifications. If the pancreatitis is a result of alcohol abuse, the nurse reminds the patient of the importance of eliminating all alcohol.

Often a referral for home care is indicated. This enables the nurse to assess the patient's physical and psychological status and adherence to the therapeutic regimen. The nurse also assesses the home situation and reinforces instructions about fluid and nutrition intake and avoidance of alcohol. The nurse provides specific information about resources and support groups that may be of assistance in avoiding alcohol in the future. Referral to Alcoholics Anonymous or other appropriate support groups is essential.

CHRONIC PANCREATITIS

Chronic pancreatitis is an inflammatory disorder that is characterized by progressive anatomic and functional destruction of the pancreas.

Pathophysiology

As cells are replaced by fibrous tissue with repeated attacks of pancreatitis, pressure within the pancreas increases. The end result is mechanical obstruction of the pancreatic and common bile ducts and the duodenum. In addition, there is atrophy of the epithelium of the ducts, inflammation, and destruction of the secreting cells of the pancreas.

Alcohol consumption in Western societies and malnutrition worldwide, frequently associated with cigarette smoking, are the major causes of chronic pancreatitis. Excessive and prolonged consumption of alcohol accounts for 40% of cases of chronic pancreatitis in the United States, although 25% of cases may be attributed to smoking alone (Forsmark, 2016). Long-term alcohol consumption causes hypersecretion of protein in pancreatic secretions, resulting in protein plugs and calculi within the pancreatic ducts. Alcohol also has a direct toxic effect on the cells of the pancreas. Some

research suggests that hypertriglyceridemia, dyslipidemia, and diet also may contribute to the development of chronic pancreatitis. Less common causes of chronic pancreatitis are due to genetic mutations, autoimmune pancreatitis, duct obstruction, and idiopathic pancreatitis. Patients with chronic pancreatitis are at increased risk for the development of pancreatic cancer (Forsmark, 2016).

Clinical Manifestations and Assessment

Chronic pancreatitis is characterized by recurring attacks of severe upper abdominal and back pain, accompanied by vomiting. Often attacks are so painful that opioids, even in large doses, do not provide relief. As the disease progresses, recurring attacks of pain are more severe, more frequent, and of longer duration. Some patients experience continuous severe pain, others have a dull, nagging constant pain, and a small percentage of other patients does not have pain and instead presents with exocrine (steatorrhea, weight loss) or endocrine (diabetes) pancreatic insufficiency (Forsmark, 2016, p. 964). The risk of opioid dependence is increased in pancreatitis because of the chronic nature and severity of the pain.

Weight loss is a major problem in chronic pancreatitis: more than 75% of patients experience significant weight loss, usually caused by decreased dietary intake secondary to anorexia or fear that eating will precipitate another attack. Malabsorption occurs late in the disease due to decreases in lipase production. As a result, digestion, especially of proteins and fats, is impaired. The stools become frequent, frothy, and foul-smelling because of impaired fat digestion, which results in stools with a high fat content (referred to as **steatorrhea**). As the disease progresses, calcification of the gland may occur, and calcium stones may form within the ducts. Diabetes mellitus occurs due to loss of pancreatic beta cells.

Various imaging procedures, including MRI, CT scans, and ultrasound, have been useful in the diagnostic evaluation of patients with suspected pancreatic disorders. A CT scan or ultrasound study also is helpful to detect pancreatic cysts. Steatorrhea can be confirmed by laboratory analysis of fecal fat content and determination of exocrine pancreatic insufficiency via the secretin-cholecystokinin test. In most cases, the diagnosis of chronic pancreatitis is based upon clinical findings, history, and imaging modalities such as ERCP, CT, and MRI to detect abnormalities of the pancreas (Forsmark, 2016).

Nursing Alert
Endoscopic retrograde cholangiopancreatography (ERCP) provides detail about the anatomy of the pancreas and the pancreatic and biliary ducts, and it is helpful in obtaining tissue for analysis and differentiating pancreatitis from other conditions, such as carcinoma. However, because of its risk, ERCP should be undertaken only when therapy involving the pancreatic duct is appropriate.

Medical Management

Nonsurgical Management

Nonsurgical approaches are focused primarily on complete abstinence of alcohol and tobacco, pain management, nutritional management, and treatment of diabetes mellitus. Pain management is achieved through use of analgesics as first-line therapy and for refractory pain. Pancreatic enzyme replacement is indicated for the patient with malabsorption and steatorrhea. A proton pump inhibitor (omeprazole [Prilosec], lansoprazole [Prevacid]) is administered with enzyme therapy to reduce gastric acid inactivation of enzymes. Also supplementation of fat-soluble vitamins is indicated. Improved nutrition and resolution of steatorrhea usually are indicators of clinical improvement in the patient with chronic pancreatitis.

Diabetes mellitus resulting from dysfunction of the pancreatic islet cells is treated with diet, insulin, or oral antidiabetic agents. Use of insulin is the preferred therapy; however, administration should be adjusted carefully to avoid hypoglycemic events (Forsmark, 2016).

Surgical Management

Surgery or interventional therapies are used primarily to address complications of pancreatitis and to relieve abdominal pain and discomfort, restore drainage of pancreatic secretions, and reduce the frequency of acute attacks of pancreatitis. The type of surgery that is performed depends on the anatomic and functional abnormalities of the pancreas, including the location of disease within the pancreas, the presence of diabetes, exocrine insufficiency, biliary stenosis, and pseudocysts of the pancreas.

Pancreaticojejunostomy (also referred to as Roux-en-Y), with a side-to-side anastomosis or joining of the pancreatic duct to the jejunum, allows drainage of the pancreatic secretions into the jejunum. Other surgical procedures may be performed for different degrees and types of underlying disorders. These procedures include revision of the sphincter of the ampulla of Vater, internal drainage of a pancreatic cyst into the stomach, insertion of a stent, and wide resection or removal of the pancreas. A Whipple resection (pancreaticoduodenectomy) can be carried out to relieve the pain of chronic pancreatitis. Endoscopic therapy is used for pancreatic duct stones and strictures. The use of surgical and endoscopic treatment is based upon patient presentation, complications, and the availability of surgical expertise (Forsmark, 2016).

PANCREATIC CANCER

Pancreatic cancer is the fourth leading cause of cancer death in the United States. Cancer may develop in the head, body, or tail of the pancreas; most pancreatic cancers originate in the head of the pancreas. Patients usually do not seek medical attention until late in the disease; most patients have an advanced, unresectable tumor when first detected. In fact, pancreatic carcinoma has a survival rate of only 6% at 5 years regardless of the stage of disease at diagnosis or treatment, the lowest among all cancers (Muniraj, Jamidar, & Aslanian, 2013).

Risk Factors

The average patient age at diagnosis of most pancreatic cancers is 71 years old, with higher prevalence in men and African Americans. Use of tobacco, obesity, and nonhereditary chronic pancreatitis are risk factors for pancreatic cancer. Diabetes mellitus is also associated with pancreatic cancer; however, whether it is a cause or a result of pancreatic cancer is unclear. Genetic predisposition also may play a role; up to 10% of patients with this cancer have a first-degree relative diagnosed with pancreatic cancer (Muniraj et al., 2013).

Clinical Manifestations and Assessment

The majority of patients present with pain and/or jaundice, which, along with weight loss, are considered classic signs of pancreatic carcinoma. However, they often do not appear until the disease is far advanced. Other signs include rapid, profound, and progressive weight loss as well as vague upper or midabdominal pain or discomfort that is unrelated to any GI function and is often difficult to describe. Such discomfort radiates as a boring pain in the midback and is unrelated to posture or activity. Often it is progressive and severe, requiring the use of opioids. The formation of ascites is common. An important sign, if it is present, is the onset of symptoms of insulin deficiency: glucosuria, hyperglycemia, and abnormal glucose tolerance. Therefore, diabetes may be an early sign of carcinoma of the pancreas. Meals often aggravate epigastric pain, which usually occurs before the appearance of jaundice and pruritus. Diarrhea and steatorrhea also commonly are present in pancreatic cancer (Muniraj et al., 2013).

CT and MRI imaging are currently the most useful preoperative imaging technique. CT or MRI can accurately image pancreatic masses, show dilatation of pancreatic duct, and indicate if metastases are present in the liver or peritoneum. Endoscopic retrograde pancreatography (ERCP), endoscopic ultrasound (EUS), and magnetic resonance cholangiopancreatography (MRCP) also are used to diagnose pancreatic cancer. Cells obtained during ERCP/EUS are sent to the laboratory for histologic analysis. Although cancer-associated antigen (CA 19-9) serum levels may be elevated, this tumor marker is used primarily to monitor disease progression and treatment efficacy (Muniraj et al., 2013).

Medical Management

Only 10% to 20% of patients with pancreatic cancer benefit from surgical resection; the majority of patients present

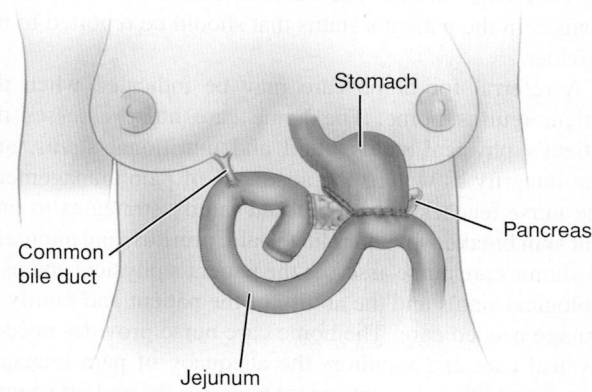

FIGURE 25-14 Pancreatoduodenectomy (Whipple procedure or resection). End result of resection of carcinoma of the head of the pancreas or the ampulla of Vater. The common duct is sutured to the end of the jejunum, and the remaining portion of the pancreas and the end of the stomach are sutured to the side of the jejunum.

at a late stage, frequently with metastatic spread to other organs or vascular invasion. In patients with early-stage disease, the Whipple procedure (pancreaticoduodenectomy) is used to remove the pancreatic head, duodenum, part of the jejunum, common bile duct, and gallbladder (Fig. 25-14). Use of adjuvant therapy (i.e., chemotherapy) continues to be controversial and nonstandard in this small group of surgical patients, with ongoing clinical trials to evaluate potential benefits of treatment. The chemotherapy agent gemcitabine alone or in combination with other chemotherapeutic agents remains the treatment of choice for most patients with pancreatic cancer. Overall, patients with pancreatic cancer have a high mortality rate and poor survival outcomes even with chemotherapy or surgical treatment. Palliative measures to address symptoms of pancreatic cancer include nutritional support and pain management (Muniraj et al., 2013).

Nursing Management

Pain management and attention to nutritional requirements are important nursing measures that improve the level of patient comfort. Refer to Chapter 7 for treatment of cancer pain. Skin care and nursing measures are directed toward relief of pain and discomfort associated with jaundice, anorexia, and profound weight loss. Specialty mattresses are beneficial and protect bony prominences from pressure. Pain associated with pancreatic cancer may be severe and may require liberal use of opioids; patient-controlled analgesia should be considered for the patient with severe, escalating pain.

Because of the poor prognosis and likelihood of short survival, end-of-life preferences are discussed and honored. If appropriate, the nurse refers the patient to hospice care (see Chapter 3 for further discussion).

The postoperative management of patients who have undergone a pancreaticoduodenectomy is similar to the management of patients after extensive GI or biliary surgery. The patient's physical status is often suboptimal, increasing the risk for postoperative complications. Hemorrhage, vascular collapse, and hepatorenal failure remain the major complications of these extensive surgical procedures. The mortality rate associated with these procedures has improved because of advances in nutritional support and improved surgical techniques. An NG tube with suction, NPO status, and nutrition that allows the GI tract to rest while promoting adequate nutrition is anticipated (Fig. 25-15).

Preoperatively and postoperatively, nursing care is directed toward promoting patient comfort, preventing complications, and assisting the patient to return to and maintain as normal and comfortable a life as possible. The nurse closely monitors the patient in the ICU after surgery; in the immediate postoperative period, multiple IV and arterial

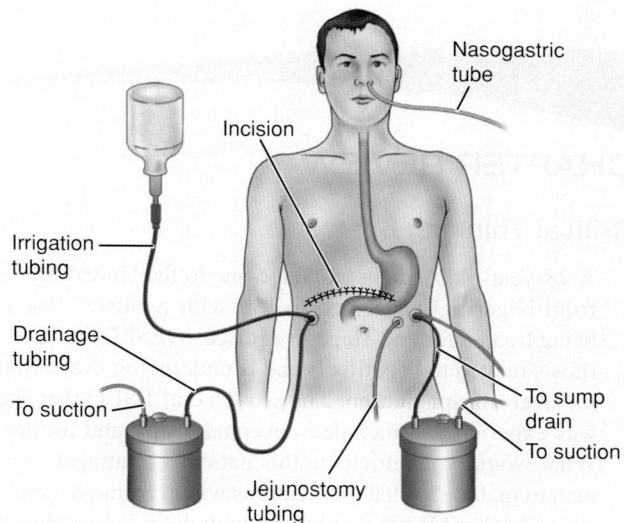

FIGURE 25-15 Multiple sump tubes are used after pancreatic surgery. Triple-lumen tubes consist of ports that provide tubing for irrigation, air venting, and drainage.

lines are used for fluid and blood replacement and hemodynamic monitoring, and a mechanical ventilator is used. It is important to note and report changes in vital signs, ABGs and pressures, pulse oximetry, laboratory values, and urine output. The nurse also must consider the patient's compromised nutritional status and risk for bleeding. Depending on the type of surgical procedure performed, malabsorption syndrome and diabetes mellitus are likely; the nurse must address these issues during acute and long-term patient care.

Although the patient's physiologic status is the focus of the health care team in the immediate postoperative period, the patient's psychological and emotional state must be considered, along with that of the family. The patient has undergone a major high-risk surgery and is critically ill; anxiety and depression may affect recovery. The immediate and long-term outcomes of this extensive surgical resection are uncertain, and the patient and family require emotional support and understanding in the critical and stressful preoperative and postoperative periods.

Promoting Home and Community-Based Care

The specific teaching for the patient and family varies with the stage of disease and the treatment choices made by the patient. The patient who has undergone this extensive surgery requires careful and thorough preparation for self-care at home. The nurse instructs the patient and family about the need for modifications in the diet because of malabsorption and hyperglycemia resulting from the surgery. It is important to instruct the patient and family about the continuing need for pancreatic enzyme replacement, a low-fat diet, and vitamin supplementation.

The nurse teaches the patient and family strategies to relieve pain and discomfort, along with strategies to manage drains, if present, and to care for the surgical incision. The patient and family members may require instruction about use of patient-controlled analgesia, enteral/parenteral nutrition, wound care, skin care, and management of drainage. It is important to describe, verbally and in writing, the signs and symptoms of complications and to teach the patient and family about indicators of complications that should be reported promptly.

Discharge of the patient to a long-term care or rehabilitation facility may be warranted after surgery as extensive as a pancreaticoduodenectomy, particularly if the patient's preoperative status was not optimal. Information about the teaching that has been provided is shared with the long-term care staff so that instructions can be clarified and reinforced.

If the patient elects to receive chemotherapy, the nurse focuses teaching on prevention of side effects and complications of the agents used. If surgery is performed to relieve obstruction and establish biliary drainage, teaching addresses management of the drainage system and monitoring for complications. The nurse instructs the family about changes in the patient's status that should be reported to the provider.

A referral for home care may be indicated when the patient returns home. The home care nurse assesses the patient's physical status, fluid and nutritional status, and skin integrity as well as the adequacy of pain management. The nurse teaches the patient and family strategies to prevent skin breakdown and relieve pain, pruritus, and anorexia. The home care nurse assesses the patient's physical and psychological status and the ability of the patient and family to manage needed care. The home care nurse provides needed physical care and monitors the adequacy of pain management. In addition, it is important to assess the patient's nutritional status and monitor the use of parenteral nutrition. The nurse discusses the use of hospice services with the patient and family and makes a referral if indicated.

CHAPTER REVIEW

Critical Thinking Exercises

1. A 28-year-old African woman came to the United States from Nigeria 3 years ago to live with relatives. She is being treated for end-stage liver disease (ESLD) with cirrhosis related to hepatitis B and is undergoing evaluation for liver transplantation. The sequelae of ESLD that she was experiencing included encephalopathy and ascites. What would you anticipate this patient's treatment regimen to include? What medications would be most appropriate for her? What would you include in your cultural assessment when you develop a preoperative teaching plan for this patient? What alternative therapies might be employed preoperatively? Once the patient receives a liver transplant, what medications would you expect to be prescribed for her in addition to an immunosuppressant regimen?

2. A 64-year-old man is admitted to the hospital with end-stage liver disease (ESLD), ascites, and impending hepatic encephalopathy. Dietary modifications and lactulose (Cephulac) are prescribed to minimize hepatic encephalopathy. What is the evidence base for use of dietary measures and lactulose in reducing or reversing hepatic encephalopathy? What is the strength of that

evidence? What are the nursing implications associated with prescribed dietary modifications, lactulose, and other measures to reduce the severity and progression of hepatic encephalopathy?

3. A 34-year-old woman is scheduled for a cholecystectomy. Since undergoing bariatric surgery a year ago, she has lost 150 lb. What postoperative care is indicated for this patient? What impact, if any, does her previous surgical procedure have on her postoperative recovery?

4. A 56-year-old man with a history of alcoholism and cirrhosis is admitted to your unit with a diagnosis of pancreatitis. He is complaining of severe epigastric pain, vomiting, and diarrhea. What medications and laboratory tests would you expect to see prescribed for this patient? What physical assessment findings will you see? Describe nursing care for this patient, and compare and contrast care with and without the diagnosis of cirrhosis. What issues would be of high priority in caring for this patient during his hospital stay? What issues would be of high priority in preparing him for hospital discharge?

NCLEX-Style Review Questions

1. The nurse is caring for a patient diagnosed with ascites. What would the nurse expect to be restricted from the patient's diet?
   a. Potassium
   b. Calcium
   c. Sodium
   d. Magnesium

2. A patient diagnosed with hepatic encephalopathy is receiving lactulose. When preparing to administer this medication, the nurse understands that it is used to decrease which serum level?
   a. Calcium
   b. Ammonia
   c. Potassium
   d. Sodium

3. Patients with severe chronic liver dysfunction often have problems related to inadequate intake of sufficient vitamins. What vitamin deficiency would result in hemorrhagic lesions of scurvy?
   a. Riboflavin
   b. Vitamin C
   c. Vitamin A
   d. Vitamin K

4. A patient with hepatitis A is admitted to a general medical-surgical floor. The nurse knows that this type of hepatitis is spread through which mode of transmission?
   a. Injection of drugs
   b. Blood
   c. Semen
   d. Fecal–oral

5. A patient is being seen in the clinic to rule out pancreatitis. The nurse expects which diagnostic test will be performed to diagnose this disease process? *Select all that apply.*
   a. MR/CT
   b. Abdominal ultrasound
   c. Lumbar puncture
   d. Endoscopy
   e. Amylase and lipase

Try these additional resources, available at **http://thepoint.lww.com/Honan2e**, to enhance your learning and understanding of this chapter:
- NCLEX-Style Student Review Questions
- Journal Articles

REFERENCES AND SELECTED READINGS

References and selected readings associated with this chapter can be found on the website that accompanies the book. Visit **http://thepoint. lww.com/Honan2e** to access the references and other additional resources associated with this chapter.

Problems Related to Urinary Tract Function

A nurse is caring for a patient diagnosed with kidney failure. He is currently receiving hemodialysis three times a week. He is very anxious about the lifestyle change that is occurring due to his health problems.

- What areas of teaching would be important for the nurse to emphasize for this patient?
- Explain the various treatment modalities available for this patient population.
- Discuss areas of nursing management that would apply to this patient.

Nursing Assessment: Renal and Urinary Tract Function

Deborah Bain Fahs

Learning Objectives

After reading this chapter, you will be able to:

1. Describe the anatomy and physiology of the renal and urinary systems.
2. Discuss the role of the kidney in regulating fluid and electrolyte balance, acid–base balance, and blood pressure.
3. Identify the assessment parameters used for determining the status of upper and lower urinary tract function.
4. Describe the diagnostic studies used to determine upper and lower urinary tract function.

Proper function of the renal and urinary systems is essential to life. Dysfunction of the kidneys and lower urinary tract is common and may occur at any age and with varying degrees of severity. Assessment of upper and lower urinary tract function is part of every health examination and necessitates an understanding of the anatomy and physiology of the urinary system as well as of the effects of changes in the system on other physiologic functions.

ANATOMIC AND PHYSIOLOGIC OVERVIEW

The primary function of the renal and urinary systems is to maintain the body's state of homeostasis by carefully regulating fluid and electrolytes, removing wastes, and providing hormones that are involved in red blood cell (RBC) production, bone metabolism, and blood pressure. A thorough understanding of the renal and urinary systems is necessary for assessing people with acute or chronic dysfunction and implementing appropriate nursing care.

Anatomy of the Renal and Urinary Systems

The renal and urinary systems include the kidneys, ureters, bladder, and urethra. Urine is formed by the kidney and flows through the other structures to be eliminated from the body.

Kidneys

The kidneys are a pair of bean-shaped, brownish-red structures located retroperitoneally (behind and outside the peritoneal cavity) on the posterior wall of the abdomen—from the

12th thoracic vertebra to the 3rd lumbar vertebra in the adult (Fig. 26-1A). The average adult kidney weighs approximately 113 to 170 g (about 4.5 oz) and is 10 to 12 cm long, 6 cm wide, and 2.5 cm thick (Tortora & Derrickson, 2014). The right kidney is slightly lower than the left due to the location of the liver.

The kidneys are well protected by the ribs and by the muscles of the abdomen and back. Internally, fat deposits surround each kidney, providing protection against jarring. The kidneys and surrounding fat are suspended from the abdominal wall by renal fascia made of connective tissue. The fibrous connective tissue, blood vessels, and lymphatics surrounding each kidney are known as the *renal capsule* (Grossman & Porth, 2014) (Fig. 26-1B).

An adrenal gland lies on top of each kidney. Each organ is independent in terms of its function, blood supply, and innervation.

The renal parenchyma (organ tissue) is divided into two parts: the cortex and the medulla. The medulla is the inner portion of the kidney. It contains the loops of Henle, the vasa recta, and the collecting ducts of the juxtamedullary nephrons. The collecting ducts from both the juxtamedullary and the cortical nephrons connect to the renal pyramids, which are triangular and are situated with the base facing the concave surface of the kidney and the point (papilla) facing the hilum, or pelvis. Each kidney contains approximately 8 to 18 pyramids. The pyramids drain into 4 to 13 minor calices, which drain into 2 to 3 major calices that open directly into the renal pelvis. The renal pelvis is the beginning of the collecting system and is composed of structures that are designed to collect and transport urine. Once the urine leaves the renal pelvis, the composition or amount of urine does not change.

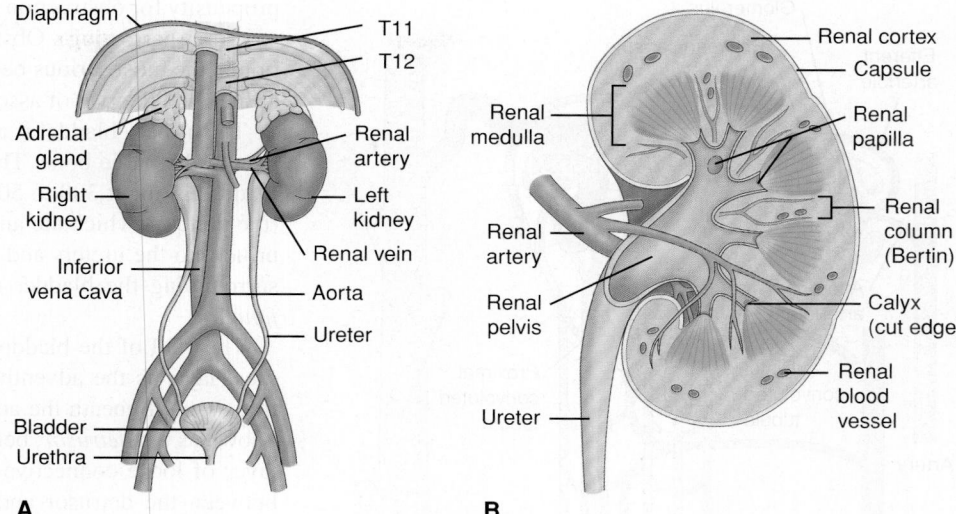

FIGURE 26-1 **A.** Kidneys, ureters, and bladder. (The right kidney is usually lower than the left.) **B.** Internal structure of the kidney. (Grossman, S., & Porth. C. M. (2014). *Porth's pathophysiology concepts of altered health states* (9th ed.). Philadelphia, PA: Wolters Kluwer/Lippincott Williams & Wilkins.)

The cortex, which is approximately 1 cm wide, is located farthest from the center of the kidney and around the outermost edges. It contains the **nephrons** (the functional units of the kidney), which are discussed below.

Blood Supply to the Kidneys

The hilum, or pelvis, is the concave portion of the kidney through which the renal artery enters and the ureters and renal vein exit. The kidneys receive 20% to 25% of the total cardiac output; all of the body's blood circulates through the kidneys approximately 12 times per hour. The renal artery arises from the abdominal aorta and divides into smaller and smaller vessels, eventually forming the afferent arterioles. Each afferent arteriole branches to form a **glomerulus**, which is the capillary bed responsible for glomerular filtration. Blood leaves the glomerulus through the efferent arteriole and flows back to the inferior vena cava through a network of capillaries and veins.

Nursing Alert

The nurse auscultates for renal artery bruits, which indicate turbulent blood flow and are associated with a narrowing of the blood vessel or increased flow. Any patient with hypertension should be evaluated for bruits. Typically they are noted with renal artery stenosis just above (2 cm) and to the right or left of the umbilicus. A whooshing sound is indicative of a bruit.

Nephrons

Each kidney has 1 million nephrons, which usually allow for adequate kidney function even if the opposite kidney is damaged or becomes nonfunctional. The nephrons are the structures located within the renal parenchyma that are responsible for the initial formation of urine. If the total number of functioning nephrons is less than 20% of normal, renal replacement therapy needs to be considered.

There are two kinds of nephrons. The cortical nephrons, making up 80% to 85% of the total number, are located in the outermost part of the cortex. The juxtamedullary nephrons, distinguished by long loops of Henle, make up the remaining 15% to 20%, are located deeper in the cortex, and are surrounded by long capillary loops called *vasa recta* that dip into the medulla of the kidney. The length of the tubular component of the nephron is related directly to its ability to concentrate urine.

Nephrons are made up of two basic components: a filtering element composed of an enclosed capillary network (the glomerulus) and the attached tubule (Fig. 26-2). The glomerulus is a unique network of capillaries suspended between the afferent and efferent blood vessels, which are enclosed in an epithelial structure called *Bowman capsule*. The glomerular membrane is composed of three filtering layers: the capillary endothelium, the basement membrane, and the epithelium. This membrane normally allows filtration of fluid and small molecules yet limits passage of larger molecules, such as blood cells and albumin. Pressure changes and the permeability of the glomerular membrane of Bowman capsule facilitate the passage of fluids and various substances from the blood vessels, filling the space within Bowman capsule with this filtered solution.

The tubular component of the nephron begins in the Bowman capsule. The filtrate created in the Bowman capsule travels first into the proximal tubule, then the loop of Henle, the distal tubule, and either the cortical or medullary collecting ducts. Changes are made continually as the filtrate travels through the tubules until it enters the collecting system and is expelled as urine from the body (see Fig. 26-2).

The structural arrangement of the tubule allows the distal tubule to lie in close proximity to where the afferent and efferent arteriole, respectively, enter and leave the glomerulus.

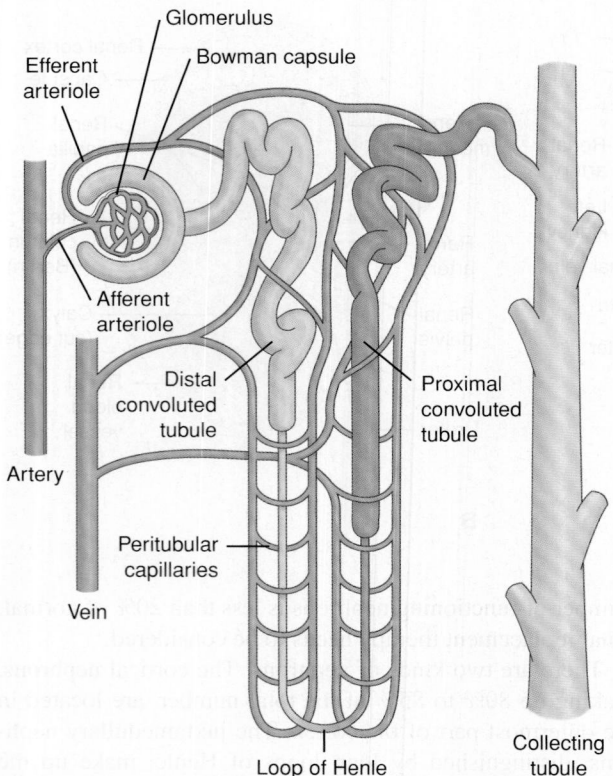

FIGURE 26-2 Representation of a nephron. Each kidney has about 1 million nephrons, which take two forms: cortical and juxtamedullary. Cortical nephrons are located in the cortex of the kidney; juxtamedullary nephrons are adjacent to the medulla.

The distal tubular cells located in this area, known as the *macula densa*, function with the adjacent afferent arteriole and create what is known as the *juxtaglomerular apparatus*. This is the site of renin production. Renin is a hormone involved directly in the control of arterial blood pressure; it is essential for proper functioning of the glomerulus (see later discussion).

Ureters, Bladder, and Urethra

The urine formed in the nephrons flows into the renal pelvis and then into the ureters, which are long fibromuscular tubes that connect each kidney to the bladder. Each is 24 to 30 cm long, originates at the lower portion of the renal pelvis, and terminates in the trigone of the bladder wall.

The lining of the ureters is made up of transitional cell epithelium called *urothelium*. The urothelium maintains bladder and blood impermeability as well as monitors for the presence of foreign substances or bacteria (Lu & Chai, 2014). The movement of urine from each renal pelvis through the ureter into the bladder is facilitated by peristaltic contraction of the smooth muscles in the ureter wall. There are three narrowed areas of each ureter: the ureteropelvic junction, the ureteral segment near the sacroiliac junction, and the ureterovesical junction. These three areas of the ureters have a propensity for obstruction by renal calculi (kidney stones) or stricture (narrowing). Obstruction of the ureteropelvic junction is the most serious because of its close proximity to the kidney and the risk of associated kidney dysfunction.

The urinary bladder is a muscular, hollow sac located just behind the pubic bone. The functional capacity of the adult bladder is about 300 to 500 mL. The bladder has two inlets (the ureters), which are angled to prevent retrograde flow of urine into the ureters and one outlet (the urethra). The area surrounding the bladder neck is called the *urethrovesical junction*.

The wall of the bladder contains four layers. The outermost layer is the adventitia, which is made up of connective tissue. Beneath the adventitia is a smooth muscle layer known as the *detrusor*; beneath the detrusor is a submucosal layer of loose connective tissue that serves as an interface between the detrusor and the innermost layer, a mucosal lining. This inner layer contains specialized transitional cell epithelium, a membrane that is impermeable to water and prevents reabsorption of urine stored in the bladder.

When the detrusor muscle contracts, urine is released from the bladder; thus, the detrusor is responsible for **micturition** (voiding). This muscle is continuous with the bladder neck, which forms a portion of the urethral sphincter often referred to as the *internal urethral sphincter*. When the bladder is relaxed, the muscle fibers are closed and functions as a sphincter (Grossman & Porth, 2014). The sphincteric mechanism helps maintain continence. Another muscle involved in continence is the external urinary sphincter at the anterior urethra, the segment most distal from the bladder (Grossman & Porth, 2014). During micturition, increased intravesical pressure keeps the ureterovesical junction closed and keeps urine within the ureters. As soon as micturition is completed, intravesical pressure returns to its normal low baseline value, allowing efflux of urine to resume. The only time that the bladder is completely empty is in the last seconds of micturition, before efflux of urine resumes.

The urethra arises from the base of the bladder: In the male, it passes through the penis; in the female, it opens just anterior to the vagina. In the male, the prostate gland, which lies just below the bladder neck, surrounds the urethra posteriorly and laterally.

Functions of the Upper and Lower Urinary Tracts

Urine Formation

The healthy human body is composed of approximately 60% water. Water balance is regulated by the kidneys and results in the formation of urine. Urine is formed in the nephrons through a complex three-step process: glomerular filtration, **tubular reabsorption**, and **tubular secretion** (Fig. 26-3). The various substances normally filtered by the glomerulus, reabsorbed by the tubules, and excreted in the urine include sodium, chloride, bicarbonate, potassium, glucose, urea,

FIGURE 26-3 Urine is formed in the nephrons in a three-step process: filtration, reabsorption, and excretion. Water, electrolytes, and other substances, such as glucose and creatinine, are filtered by the glomerulus; varying amounts of these substances are reabsorbed in the renal tubule or excreted in the urine. Approximate normal volumes of these substances during the steps of urine formation are shown at the top. Wide variations may occur in these values depending on diet.

creatinine, and uric acid. Within the tubule, some of these substances are reabsorbed selectively into the blood to maintain electrolyte and acid–base balance. Others are secreted from the blood into the filtrate as it travels down the tubule.

Usually amino acids and glucose are filtered at the level of the glomerulus and reabsorbed so that neither is excreted in the urine. Normally, glucose does not appear in the urine. However, glycosuria occurs if the amount of glucose in the blood and glomerular filtrate exceeds the amount that the tubules are able to reabsorb. **Renal glycosuria** occurs in cases of diabetes and is the most common clinical expression of a blood glucose level exceeding the kidneys' reabsorption capacity. In general, the serum glucose level is greater than 180 to 200 mg/dL when glycosuria is seen.

Protein molecules also are not usually found in the urine; however, low–molecular-weight proteins (globulins and albumin) may be excreted periodically in small amounts. Recall that the glomerulus filters the blood, similar to a strainer. Therefore, when significant **proteinuria** is found, glomerular disease is suspected. Levels of greater than 3.5 g/day are indicative of severe proteinuria and are associated with nephrotic syndrome as well as a variety of glomerular disorders (see Chapter 27).

Glomerular Filtration

The normal blood flow through the kidneys is about 1,200 mL/min. As blood flows into the glomerulus from an afferent arteriole, filtration occurs. The filtered fluid enters the renal tubules. Under normal conditions, about 20% of the blood passing through the glomeruli is filtered into the nephron, amounting to about 180 L/day of filtrate. The filtrate normally consists of water, electrolytes, and other small molecules, whereas larger molecules stay in the bloodstream. Efficient filtration depends on adequate blood flow that maintains a consistent pressure through the glomerulus. Many factors can alter this blood flow and pressure, including hypotension, decreased oncotic pressure in the blood, and increased pressure in the renal tubules from an obstruction.

Tubular Reabsorption and Tubular Secretion

The second and third steps of urine formation occur in the renal tubules. In tubular reabsorption, a substance moves from the filtrate back into the peritubular capillaries or vasa recta. In tubular secretion, a substance moves from the peritubular capillaries or vasa recta into tubular filtrate. Of the 180 L (45 gallons) of filtrate that the kidneys produce each day, 99% is reabsorbed into the bloodstream, resulting in the formation of 1,000 to 1,500 mL of urine each day. Although most reabsorption occurs in the proximal tubule, reabsorption does occur along the entire tubule. Reabsorption and secretion in the tubule frequently involve passive and active transport. Filtrate becomes concentrated in the distal tubule and collecting ducts under hormonal influence and becomes urine, which then enters the renal pelvis.

Osmolarity and Osmolality

Osmolarity and osmolality refer to the ratio of solute (e.g., sodium, chloride, potassium, urea, and glucose) to water in blood or urine. While osmolarity refers to measuring the ratio of the amount of solutes (milliosmoles) to water using liters (expressed as mOsm/L), osmolality calculates the ratio of the amount of solutes (milliosmoles) to water using weight or kilograms (expressed as mOsm/kg). The terms are confusing and often misused; what is important to remember is that clinicians are attempting to determine the concentration of blood or urine. Because 1 L is roughly equivalent to 1 kg, generally they are similar. The regulation of salt and water is paramount for control of the extracellular volume and both serum and urine osmolarity. Controlling either the amount of water or the amount of solute can change the concentration of blood and urine. Osmolarity and ionic composition are maintained by the body within very narrow limits. Sodium levels elevated 2 mEq/L above normal cause a change in the serum osmolarity (increased number of solute atoms or molecules), causing a conscious desire to drink and conservation of water by the kidneys (Hall, 2016). It is important for nurses to recognize that cognitive impairments can interfere with recognition of cues of thirst and predispose a patient to dehydration.

> **! Nursing Alert**
> *The terms* isotonic, hypotonic, *and* hypertonic *refer to the osmolarity of body fluids (measure of the number of dissolved particles).*

A serum osmolality test measures the amount of chemicals dissolved in the fluid portion of blood (serum). It could be imagined visually as the total number of molecules floating in the fluid. Normal serum osmolality equals 280 to 303 mOsm/kg of body weight (Fischbach & Dunning, 2014). When a hypotonic solution is administered intravenously (IV), the RBCs will swell; conversely, a hypertonic solution will cause the cells to shrink (Reddi, 2014). An isotonic solution will not cause a change in the size of the RBCs. Sodium chloride 0.9% (AKA normal saline) is an example of an IV isotonic solution, sodium chloride 0.45% (AKA half saline) is an example of a hypotonic solution, and sodium chloride 3% is an example of a hypertonic solution.

Nursing Alert
Nurses need to have some understanding of the concentration of an intravenous (IV) solution's osmolarity and its relationship to clinical practice. Isotonic solutions are equal to normal osmolarity (approximately 300 mOsm/L; e.g., lactated Ringer's [275 mOsm/L] and normal saline [308 mOsm/L]); hypotonic solutions have fewer molecules and more water in the solution (less than 275 mOsm/L; e.g., half-normal saline [154 mOsm/L]); and hypertonic solutions have a higher number of molecules and are more concentrated solutions (over 300 mOsm/L; e.g., dextrose 5% in half-normal saline [405 mOsm/L]). Any fluid or medication with an osmolarity greater than 600 mOsm/L should not be infused through a peripheral catheter; instead a peripherally inserted central catheter (PICC) is recommended by the Infusion Nurses Society (Wojnar & Beaman, 2013).

Regulation of Water Excretion

Regulation of the amount of water excreted is an important function of the kidney. **Antidiuretic hormone (ADH)**, also known as *vasopressin*, plays a key role in the regulation of extracellular fluid by excreting or retaining water. ADH is secreted by the posterior portion of the pituitary gland and acts on the kidney in response to changes in osmolality of the blood; that is, ADH is secreted or suppressed depending on blood concentration or dilution, respectively. An increase in blood osmolality is seen with decreased water intake or increased water loss, stimulating ADH release. Consequently, a small volume of concentrated urine is excreted. ADH increases reabsorption of water and returns the osmolality of the blood to normal. With excess water intake or increased retention of water, as occurs in many disease states such as kidney failure, the blood becomes dilute, resulting in suppression of ADH secretion, causing less water to be

TABLE **26-1** 24-hour Balance of Intake and Output for Adults

Water Input	Input Volume (mL)	Output	Output Volume (mL)
Liquid	800–1,500	Urine	800–1,500
Solid	500–700	Lung/Skin	600–700
Oxidative metabolism	150–250	Sweat Stool	0–100 100–200
Total ~1,500–2,500 mL per day		**Total ~ 1,500–2,500 mL**	

reabsorbed by the kidney tubule. Assuming maintenance of kidney function, this would result in increased urine volume (diuresis).

In general, individuals require about 100 mL of water per 100 calories metabolized in order to rid the body of metabolic waste products. In other words, if a person uses 1,800 calories for energy, he/she will require 1,800 mL of water to metabolize them (Grossman & Porth, 2014). Fevers increase the metabolic and respiratory rate; therefore, the patient will lose additional water via the lungs and perspiration (Grossman & Porth, 2014). The greatest source of body water is through liquid (1,000 mL) and solid (700 mL) oral intake with an additional 200 mL gained through oxidation. Of the fluid ingested, the main source of loss is through the urine (1,500 mL); approximately 800 mL is lost through the skin and lungs (called *insensible loss*), and 200 mL through feces (Grossman & Porth, 2014). Normal urine output is approximately 1.5 L in 24 hours (Grossman & Porth, 2014) and intake is roughly equivalent to output in a healthy person (see Table 26-1). It is important to consider all fluid gained and lost when evaluating total fluid status. Daily weight measurements are a reliable means of determining overall fluid status. One pound equals approximately 500 mL so a weight change of as little as 1 lb could suggest an overall fluid gain or loss of 500 mL. The nurse is aware that edema is not present until 2.5 to 3 L of interstitial fluid has been retained (Sterns, 2015).

Nursing Alert
It is important to maintain consistency when assessing daily weight: the nurse uses the same scale, with the patient wearing the same clothes at the same time daily.

Regulation of Electrolyte Excretion

When the kidneys are functioning normally, the volume of electrolytes excreted per day is equal to the amount ingested. For example, the average American daily diet contains 6 to 8 g of sodium chloride (salt) and approximately the same amount is excreted in the urine.

Sodium

Normal serum sodium levels are between 135 and 145 mmol/L, making sodium the most plentiful extracellular ion (see Chapter 4). Sodium plays an important role in controlling the fluid and electrolyte balance: where sodium goes, water follows. Sodium is linked inseparably to both blood volume and blood pressure. The kidneys are responsible for regulating electrolyte loss, and approximately 65% to 80% of sodium is reabsorbed by the proximal tubule and 20% to 25% in the loop of Henle (Grossman & Porth, 2014).

As water from the filtrate follows the reabsorbed sodium, the body's osmotic balance is maintained. If more sodium is excreted than ingested, fluid deficit results; if less sodium is excreted than ingested, fluid retention results. Under normal circumstances, the kidneys are quite efficient at preserving or excreting sodium depending on its loss via the gastrointestinal (GI) tract or skin as well as its gain via diet, medications, or IV therapy.

The regulation of sodium volume excreted depends on **aldosterone**, a hormone synthesized and released from the adrenal cortex. With increased aldosterone in the blood, less sodium is excreted in the urine, as aldosterone causes renal reabsorption of sodium. The release of aldosterone from the adrenal cortex is largely under the control of angiotensin II, the most effective physiologic vasoconstrictor known. Angiotensin II levels are controlled by renin, a proteolytic enzyme released from specialized juxtaglomerular cells in the renal afferent arteriole (see Fig. 26-4). Renin secretion is controlled by three distinct but overlapping regulatory systems: (1) renal afferent arteriolar pressure (if it

decreases renin secretion increases); (2) cardiopulmonary baroreceptors that are capable of modulating sympathetic nervous system outflow (a fall in blood pressure increases renin secretion by increasing sympathetic tone); and (3) the delivery of NaCl to the macula densa, a group of modified distal tubular cells (a decrease in NaCl delivery to these cells increases renin secretion while an increase in NaCl delivery has the opposite effect). Activation of this system (by dehydration, e.g., shock or hypotension) will increase NaCl reclamation and, pari passu, water retention culminating in an expansion of the intravascular fluid volume. The net result is the maintenance of pressure within the glomerulus to ensure adequate glomerular filtration pressure and renal function.

 Nursing Alert
The nurse recognizes that a mean arterial pressure (MAP) should be at least 65 mm Hg or higher in order to maintain renal perfusion.

Potassium

Potassium is the most abundant intracellular ion; about 98% of the total body potassium is located intracellularly. To maintain a normal serum potassium balance (see Chapter 4), the kidneys are responsible for excreting more than 90% of the total daily potassium intake. Aldosterone causes the kidneys to excrete potassium, in contrast to its effects on sodium. The acid–base balance, the amount of dietary potassium intake, and the flow rate of the filtrate in the distal tubule also influence the amount of potassium secreted into the urine. Retention of potassium is the most life-threatening effect of kidney failure.

 Nursing Alert
When the level of potassium is above 6.5 mEq/L, it represents a medical emergency, primarily due to its effect on the heart. Renal perfusion is essential for excretion of potassium; when the MAP decreases to less than 70 mm Hg, urine volumes begin to decrease, resulting in impaired potassium excretion. Therefore, the nurse is alert to minimal urinary output hourly (0.5 to 1.0 mL/kg/hr) and its effect on K^+. The nurse is aware that EKG changes include a progression from peaked T waves to a prolonged PR interval, and then to a widened QRS and heart block; a K^+ level above 7 mEq/L is associated with serious arrhythmias.

Regulation of Acid–Base Balance

The normal serum pH is about 7.35 to 7.45 and must be maintained within this narrow range for optimal physiologic function. The kidney reabsorbs and returns bicarbonate from the urinary filtrate to the body's circulation. It also excretes acid in the urine. Because bicarbonate is a small ion, it is

FIGURE 26-4 The renin–angiotensin system. ADH, antidiuretic hormone; GFR, glomerular filtration rate.

filtered freely at the glomerulus and reabsorbed in the urinary filtrate. To replace any lost bicarbonate, new bicarbonate is generated by the renal tubular cells and then reabsorbed by the tubules and returned to the body.

The body's acid production is the result of the breakdown of proteins, which produces acid compounds. The normal daily diet also includes a certain amount of acid materials. Unlike carbon dioxide (CO_2), the phosphoric and sulfuric acids produced are nonvolatile (solid) and cannot be eliminated by the lungs. If these acids were not excreted in the urine, accumulation of these acids in the blood would lower its pH and inhibit cell function. A person with normal kidney function excretes about 70 mEq of acid each day. The kidney is able to excrete some of this acid directly into the urine until the urine pH reaches 4.5, which is 1,000 times more acidic than blood.

More acid may need to be eliminated from the body than can be secreted directly as free acid in the urine. These excess acids are bound to chemical buffers so that they can be excreted in the urine. Two important chemical buffers are phosphate ions and ammonia (NH_3). Through the buffering process, the kidney is able to excrete large quantities of acid in a bound form, without further lowering the pH of the urine.

Autoregulation of Blood Pressure

Regulation of blood pressure is also a function of the kidney. Specialized vessels of the kidney, called the *vasa recta*, constantly monitor blood pressure as blood begins its passage into the kidney. When the vasa recta detect a decrease in blood pressure, specialized juxtaglomerular cells near the afferent arteriole, distal tubule, and efferent arteriole secrete the hormone renin. Renin does not affect blood pressure directly. It converts a circulating plasma protein named angiotensinogen to angiotensin I, which is converted to angiotensin II and causes the blood pressure to increase by its vasoconstrictor properties and secretion of aldosterone (Grossman & Porth, 2014). Aldosterone causes renal reabsorption of sodium and water by the distal tubules and collecting ducts, thus volume is returned to systemic circulation. Any etiology that results in poor perfusion or increasing serum osmolality, such as hemorrhage or diarrhea, will cause activation of renin, which leads to activation of angiotensin II and aldosterone secretion. The result is an increase in blood pressure. When the vasa recta recognize the increase in blood pressure, renin secretion stops. Failure of this feedback mechanism is one of the primary causes of hypertension.

Renal Clearance

Renal clearance refers to the ability of the kidneys to clear solutes from the plasma. A 24-hour collection of urine is the primary test of renal clearance. Renal clearance depends on several factors: how quickly the substance is filtered across the glomerulus, how much of the substance is reabsorbed along the tubules, and how much of the substance is secreted into the tubules. It is possible to measure the renal clearance of any substance, but the one measure that is particularly useful is the creatinine clearance: as renal function declines, creatinine clearance decreases; that is, the patient's serum creatinine rises.

Creatinine is an endogenous waste product of skeletal muscle that is filtered at the glomerulus, passed through the tubules with minimal change, and excreted in the urine, making creatinine clearance a good measure of the **glomerular filtration rate (GFR)**. To calculate creatinine clearance, a 24-hour urine specimen is collected. Midway through the collection, the serum creatinine level is measured.

The GFR in a young, healthy individual is 120 to 130 mL/min/1.73 m^2 (Grossman & Porth, 2014).

Regulation of Red Blood Cell Production

When the kidneys sense a decrease in the oxygen tension in renal blood flow, they release erythropoietin. Erythropoietin stimulates the bone marrow to produce RBCs, thereby increasing the number of circulating RBCs, raising the O_2 carrying capacity of the blood. Some conditions, such as chronic kidney disease, require that patients receive exogenous erythropoietin in order to maintain RBC production.

Vitamin D Synthesis

The kidneys also are responsible for the final conversion of inactive vitamin D to its active form, 1,25-dihydroxycholecalciferol. Vitamin D is necessary for maintaining normal calcium balance in the body.

Secretion of Prostaglandins

The kidneys also produce prostaglandin E and prostacyclin, which have a vasodilatory effect and are important in maintaining renal blood flow.

Excretion of Waste Products

The kidney functions as the body's main excretory organ, eliminating the body's metabolic waste products. The major waste product of protein metabolism is urea, of which about 25 to 30 g are produced and excreted daily. All of this urea must be excreted in the urine; otherwise it accumulates in body tissues. Other waste products of metabolism that must be excreted are creatinine, phosphates, and sulfates. Uric acid, formed as a waste product of purine metabolism, also is eliminated in the urine. The kidneys serve as the primary mechanism for excreting drug metabolites.

Nursing Alert

The kidneys are responsible for excretion of waste products that account for a daily solute load of approximately 600 mOsm. It is approximated that 500 cc of urine is required daily to excrete that solute load. Without that excretion of 500 cc, toxins and waste products will rise in the serum or blood value. The term azotemia *refers to the buildup of excessive nitrogenous wastes in the blood (refer to Chapter 27 for additional detail).*

Urine Storage

The bladder is a hollow, distensible, muscular organ whose size, shape, and position vary in relation to the amount of urine it contains. Both filling and emptying of the bladder are mediated by coordinated sympathetic and parasympathetic nervous system control mechanisms involving the detrusor muscle and the bladder sphincters. Conscious awareness of bladder filling occurs as a result of sympathetic neuronal pathways that travel via the spinal cord to the level of T10 through T12, where peripheral, hypogastric nerve innervation allows for continued bladder filling. As bladder filling continues, stretch receptors in the bladder wall are activated, coupled with the desire to void. This information from the detrusor muscle is relayed back to the cerebral cortex via the parasympathetic pelvic nerves at the level of S1 through S4. Overall bladder pressure remains low due to the bladder's compliance (ability to expand or collapse) as urine volume changes.

Bladder compliance is due to the smooth muscle lining of the bladder and collagen deposits within the wall of the bladder, as well as to neuronal mechanisms that inhibit the detrusor muscle from contracting (specifically, adrenergic receptors that mediate relaxation). To maintain adequate kidney filtration rates, bladder pressure during filling must remain lower than 40 cm H_2O. This low pressure allows the urine to leave the renal pelvis and enter the ureters freely. The bladder is capable of holding 1,500 to 2,000 mL of urine. This is referred to as the *anatomic capacity* of the bladder. The sensation of bladder fullness is transmitted to the central nervous system when the bladder has reached about 150 to 250 mL in adults, and an initial desire to void occurs (Grossman & Porth, 2014). A marked sense of fullness and discomfort with a strong desire to void usually occurs when the bladder contains 350 mL or more of urine, referred to as the *functional capacity*. Neurologic changes to the bladder at the level of the supraspinal nerves, the spinal nerves, or the bladder wall itself can cause abnormally high volumes of urine to be stored due to a decreased or absent urge to void.

The bladder should be able to store urine for periods of 2 to 4 hours at a time during the day. At night, the release of vasopressin in response to decreased fluid intake causes a decrease in the production of urine and makes it more concentrated. It allows the bladder to continue filling for periods of 6 to 8 hours in adolescents and adults, making them able to sleep for longer periods before needing to void. This process, which is less pronounced in the elderly, coupled with decreasing bladder compliance and decreased vasopressin (ADH) levels, often causes **nocturia**.

Bladder Emptying

Micturition normally occurs approximately eight times in a 24-hour period. It is activated via the micturition reflex arc within the sympathetic and parasympathetic nervous system, which causes a coordinated sequence of events. Initiation of voiding occurs when the efferent pelvic nerve, which originates at S1 to S4, stimulates the bladder to contract, resulting in complete relaxation of the striated urethral sphincter. This is followed by a decrease in urethral pressure, contraction of the detrusor muscle, opening of the vesicle neck and proximal urethra, and flow of urine. This coordinated effort by the parasympathetic system is mediated by muscarinic and, to a lesser extent, cholinergic receptors within the detrusor muscle. The pressure generated in the bladder during micturition is about 20 to 40 cm H_2O in females. It is somewhat higher and more variable in males 45 years of age and older due to the normal hyperplasia of the lobes of the prostate gland, which surround the proximal urethra. Any obstruction of the bladder outlet, such as in advanced benign prostatic hyperplasia (BPH), results in a high voiding pressure. High voiding pressures make it more difficult to start urine flow and maintain it.

If the spinal pathways from the brain to the urinary system are destroyed (e.g., after a spinal cord injury), reflex contraction of the bladder is maintained, but voluntary control over the process is lost. In both situations, the detrusor muscle can contract and expel urine, but generally the contractions are insufficient to empty the bladder completely so residual urine (urine left in the bladder after voiding) remains. Normally, residual urine amounts to no more than 50 mL in the middle-aged adult and less than 50 to 100 mL in the older adult.

> ### Nursing Alert
> *Any anatomical or functional disorder causing urinary obstruction or stasis places the individual at risk for urinary tract infections (UTIs) (Kasper et al., 2015). A post-void residual (PVR) of less than 50 cc is considered normal bladder emptying, whereas a PVR of over 200 cc is a risk factor for a UTI (Grossman & Porth, 2014).*

Gerontologic Considerations

Upper and lower urinary tract function changes with age (Table 26-2). The GFR decreases, starting between 35 and 40 years of age, and a yearly decline of about 1 mL/min continues thereafter (Kasper et al., 2015). In patients 80 years of age and over, system function is about one half to two thirds less efficient than in young adults (Griebling, 2014). The elderly are more susceptible to acute and chronic kidney failure due to the structural and functional changes in the kidney. As one ages, there is a decline in organ functioning but, in particular, in those organs that are paired, such as the lungs and the kidneys (Griebling, 2014). Examples include

TABLE 26-2 GERONTOLOGIC CONSIDERATIONS / Age-Related Changes in the Renal System

Component	Structural and Functional Changes	History and Physical Findings
Kidney	Kidney weight and volume (primarily of the cortex) declines after age 40	Progressive decline of kidney reserve (the ability to respond to changes in water or electrolyte imbalances)
Renal blood flow	Blood flow decreases approximately 10% per decade Renal arteries thicken (similar to other vascular changes) Sclerosis of the glomerulus results in atrophy of the afferent and efferent arteriole	Increased risk for kidney failure due to polypharmacy, comorbidities, and decreased kidney function
Nephron	The number of nephrons declines after the age of 40 and is associated with decline in GFR The glomerular basement membrane thickens	Yearly decline in GFR of 1 mL per minute (after age 40) The elderly are at risk for altered drug excretion and drug–drug interaction
Tubule system	Degeneration of the tubule system, replaced with connective tissue Decrease in the length of the proximal tubule	Ability to conserve sodium or excrete hydrogen is decreased, predisposing the elderly to fluid and electrolyte and acid–base disturbances. Decline in maximal concentrating capacity, with increased difficulty in excreting a salt load or conserving water in the face of dehydration
Bladder	Reduced bladder tone Residual bladder urine volume increases Decreased bladder capacity In women, decreased estrogen causes changes to the urethral sphincter	Increased sense of urgency In women, increased risk of urinary incontinence Incomplete emptying of bladder, leading to urinary tract infection Increased irritability of bladder with advancing age and may generate less power, which is a problem especially in men with prostatic hypertrophy
Prostate	Enlargement of the prostate	Obstruction to urine flow, leading to frequency, oliguria, anuria
General	Decrease in muscle mass results in decreased production of creatinine Decreased vitamin D synthesis Vaginal and urethral atrophy	Serum creatinine levels remain constant; creatinine clearance is a better indicator of kidney function Osteomalacia Predisposition of women to urinary tract infections

Adapted from Criddle, L. (2009). Caring for the critically ill elderly patient. In K. Carlson (Ed.). *Advanced critical care nursing, American Association of Critical-Care Nursing.* St. Louis, MO: Saunders, Elsevier; Grossman, S., & Porth. C. M. (2014). *Porth's pathophysiology concepts of altered health states* (9th ed.). Philadelphia, PA: Wolters Kluwer/ Lippincott Williams & Wilkins; and Walston, J. (2015). Common clinical sequelae of aging. In *Cecil textbook of medicine* (25th ed.). Philadelphia, PA: Saunders.

sclerosis of the glomerulus and renal vasculature, decreased blood flow, decreased GFR, altered tubular function, and acid–base imbalance. In addition, nephrons lose their ability to compensate as one becomes older (Greibling, 2014). Although kidney function usually remains adequate despite these changes, renal reserve is decreased and may reduce the kidneys' ability to respond effectively to drastic or sudden physiologic changes. This steady decrease in glomerular filtration, combined with the use of multiple medications in which metabolites are cleared by the kidneys, puts the older person at higher risk for adverse drug effects and drug–drug interactions (Greibling, 2014).

The elderly are more prone to develop hypernatremia and fluid volume deficit because increasing age also is associated with diminished osmotic stimulation of thirst (Greibling, 2014). Thirst is a subjective sensory symptom that is defined as an awareness of the desire to drink. The elderly, because of both decreased thirst and/or diminished access to fluids and/or impaired urinary concentrating ability, are at the highest risk of developing hypernatremia (an increase in the plasma Na⁺ concentration to at least 145 mEq/L).

Likewise, many older adults may be placed on diuretics, such as furosemide, to control congestive heart failure (CHF) meaning excess sodium may be lost in the urine. This sodium loss results in hyponatremia and a decrease in both central venous pressure (CVP) and arterial blood pressure, causing prerenal failure (Greibling, 2014). In addition, hypervolemic hyponatremia commonly occurs when patients have excess free water relative to serum sodium levels (e.g., kidney failure, cardiac failure, liver failure). Therefore the nurse is alert to sodium levels (hypernatremia or hyponatremia) and is aware of common causes and clinical presentation in order to alert practitioners to reverse this potentially life-threatening condition.

Structural or functional abnormalities that occur with aging also may prevent complete emptying of the bladder. This may be due to decreased bladder wall contractility, secondary to myogenic or neurogenic factors, or it may be related to bladder outlet obstruction, such as in BPH (Grossman & Porth, 2014). Vaginal and urethral tissues atrophy (become thinner) in aging women due to decreased estrogen levels, resulting in decreased blood supply to the urogenital tissues, with subsequent urethral and vaginal irritation and possible urinary incontinence.

UTIs are common in individuals aged 65 years and over. Risk factors include patients residing in convalescent facilities as well as patients with chronic catheterizations and increasing antibiotic resistance. Symptoms present differently and more subtly than in younger adults and may include increasing confusion, falls, and a loss of appetite. In addition, older adults with impaired cognitive functioning may have difficulty communicating symptoms (Griebling, 2014).

Also nocturia is common in older adults, resulting in disturbed sleep that impacts daytime fatigue. Because the individual must awaken at night to void, the risk of falls increases and may results in fractures. Other urologic disorders affected by aging are prostate and bladder cancers, BPH, and urinary incontinence, which is the most prevalent urologic disorder in the older adult (Griebling, 2014).

As individuals age, the density of smooth muscle to connective tissue in the bladder decreases, increasing the likelihood of detrusor fibrosis. Because bladder capacity is reduced, patients may experience a decrease in the force of urinary stream, increased hesitancy, inability to empty the bladder fully, and urinary dribbling; although it may be unclear which symptoms are caused by comorbidities or are a result of aging (Griebling, 2014).

Hypertension increases in the geriatric population, contributing to kidney disease and erectile dysfunction. Polypharmacy is another factor impacting urologic health, resulting in drug-induced urgency, frequency, retention, and urinary incontinence (Griebling, 2014). Urinary incontinence is common in the older adult, particularly in females, negatively impacting quality of life; frailty is a major risk factor. About half of all American females experience incontinence at some point in their lives. The nurse should teach bladder-training exercises, such as Kegel maneuvers (refer to Chapter 33, Box 33-9). Incontinence caused by urinary or vaginal prolapse should be referred to a specialist. UTIs always should be considered as a cause of incontinence along with the use of medications, such as diuretics, antidepressant medications, sedative hypnotics, adrenergic agonists, anticholinergics, and calcium channel blockers. Whether estrogen replacement improves incontinence remains controversial. The nurse must become familiar with resources addressing the medical, social, and functional needs of the older adult, such as rehabilitative services, Medicare/Medicaid reimbursement in both in- and outpatient settings, home care services, assisted care facilities, day programs, and long-term care facilities. Also it is necessary to address other lifestyle changes:

- proper exercise (at least 150 minutes of brisk walking or other moderate forms of exercise per week),
- proper nutrition (increased consumption of fruits and vegetables),
- adequate fluid intake of at least 1,000 mL/day,
- consumption of fat-free and low-fat dairy products,
- decreased intake of sugar and sodium,
- moderate alcohol intake (1 drink per day), and
- increased dietary fiber (Kasper et al., 2015).

Treatment modalities for urinary incontinence are described in further detail in Chapter 28.

ASSESSMENT

Obtaining a comprehensive health history is the first step in assessing a patient with upper or lower urinary tract dysfunction.

Health History

Obtaining a urologic health history requires excellent communication skills because many patients are embarrassed or uncomfortable discussing genitourinary function or symptoms. It is important to use language the patient can understand and to avoid medical jargon while reviewing risk factors, particularly for those patients who are at high risk.

When obtaining the health history specific to the renal and urinary systems, the nurse should inquire about the following:

- The patient's chief concern or reason for seeking health care, the onset of the problem, and its effect on the patient's quality of life
- The location, character, and duration of pain, if present, and its relationship to voiding; factors that precipitate pain and those that relieve it
- History of UTIs, including past treatment or hospitalization for UTI

- Presence of fever or chills
- Previous renal or urinary diagnostic tests
- Use of indwelling urinary catheters, suprapubic tubes, condom catheters, or intermittent catheterization
- Dysuria or painful urination which may occur at initiation or termination of voiding
- Hesitancy, straining, or pain during or after urination
- Urinary incontinence (stress incontinence, urge incontinence, overflow incontinence, or functional incontinence)
- Hematuria (blood in urine) or change in color or volume of urine
- The presence of nocturia and number of episodes nightly
- Renal calculi (kidney stones), passage of stones or gravel in urine
- Female patients: Number and type (vaginal or cesarean) of deliveries; use of forceps; vaginal infection, discharge, or irritation; contraceptive practices
- History of anuria (less than 50 cc of urine a day) (Liangos & Jaber, 2015) or other renal problem
- Presence or history of genital lesions or sexually transmitted diseases
- Use of tobacco, alcohol, or recreational drugs
- Any prescription and over-the-counter medications (including those prescribed for renal or urinary problems)

Common Complaints

Fatigue, pain, changes in voiding, and GI symptoms are particularly suggestive of urinary tract disease. Dysfunction

of the kidney can produce a complex array of symptoms throughout the body.

Fatigue

Gradual kidney dysfunction can be insidious in its presentation, although fatigue is a common symptom. Fatigue, shortness of breath, and exercise intolerance all result from the condition known as *anemia of chronic disease.* Although historically hematocrit has been the blood test of choice when assessing a patient for anemia, currently the use of the hemoglobin level rather than hematocrit is recommended because that measurement is a better assessment of the oxygen transport ability of the blood.

Pain

Usually genitourinary pain is caused by distention of some portion of the urinary tract as a result of obstructed urine flow or inflammation and swelling of tissues. Severity of pain is related to the sudden onset rather than the extent of distention.

Table 26-3 lists the various types of genitourinary pain, characteristics of the pain, associated signs and symptoms, and possible causes. Initially a gradual decline in kidney functioning may be asymptomatic and only noted when the patient presents for routine examination; an elevation in serum creatinine or abnormal urinalysis may be the first clue to kidney disease. However, some patients present with flank pain or extrarenal symptoms, such as edema, hypertension, hematuria, and signs of uremia (Rosenberg, 2015), leading the nurse to further explore kidney function.

TABLE **26-3** Identifying Characteristics of Genitourinary Pain

Type	Location	Character	Associated Signs and Symptoms	Possible Etiology
Kidney	Costovertebral angle, may extend to umbilicus	Dull constant ache; if sudden distention of capsule, pain is severe, sharp, stabbing, and colicky in nature	Nausea and vomiting, diaphoresis, pallor, signs of shock	Acute obstruction, kidney stone, blood clot, acute pyelonephritis, trauma
Bladder	Suprapubic area	Dull, continuous pain, may be intense with voiding, may be severe if bladder full	Urgency, pain at end of voiding, painful straining	Overdistended bladder, infection, interstitial cystitis; tumor
Ureteral	Costovertebral angle, flank, lower abdominal area, testis, or labium	Severe, sharp, stabbing pain, colicky in nature	Nausea and vomiting, paralytic ileus	Ureteral stone, edema or stricture, blood clot
Prostatic	Perineum and rectum	Vague discomfort, feeling of fullness in perineum, vague back pain	Suprapubic tenderness, obstruction to urine flow; frequency, urgency, dysuria, nocturia	Prostatic cancer, acute or chronic prostatitis
Urethral	Male: along penis to meatus; female: urethra to meatus	Pain variable, most severe during and immediately after voiding	Frequency, urgency, dysuria, nocturia, urethral discharge	Irritation of bladder neck, infection of urethra, trauma, foreign body in lower urinary tract

Changes in Voiding

Micturition is normally a painless function that occurs approximately eight times in a 24-hour period. The average person voids approximately 1,500 mL of urine in 24 hours, although this amount varies depending on fluid intake, sweating, environmental temperature, vomiting, or diarrhea. Common problems associated with voiding include **frequency**, urgency, dysuria, hesitancy, incontinence, enuresis (bed wetting), **polyuria** (more than 3 L/day of urine), **oliguria** (less than 400 mL/day), and hematuria (two to five RBCs per high-powered field or a positive dipstick) (Kasper et al., 2015) (Table 26-4). Pain that may be associated with an overdistended bladder, difficulty starting the stream of urine or decrease in amount of urine, or straining to void all may be symptoms of urinary retention (Bickley, 2013) and should be evaluated.

Gastrointestinal Symptoms

GI symptoms may occur with urologic conditions because of shared autonomic and sensory innervation and renointestinal reflexes (Tortora & Derrickson, 2014). For example, afferent stimulation from the renal pelvis may cause spasms of the pylorus of the stomach; thus the patient may experience symptoms similar to peptic ulcer disease (Tanagho & McAninch, 2012). The most common signs and symptoms are nausea, vomiting, diarrhea, abdominal discomfort, and abdominal distention.

Risk Factors

Various diseases or clinical situations can increase a patient's risk for renal and urinary tract dysfunction. Data collection about previous health problems or diseases provides the health care team with useful information for evaluating the patient's

TABLE 26-4 Problems Associated with Changes in Voiding

Problem	Definition	Possible Etiology
Frequency	Frequent voiding; more than every 3 hours	Infection, obstruction of lower urinary tract leading to residual urine and overflow, anxiety, diuretics, benign prostatic hyperplasia, urethral stricture, diabetic neuropathy, interstitial cystitis (IC), neurologic conditions
Urgency	Strong desire to void	Infection, chronic prostatitis, urethritis, obstruction of lower urinary tract leading to residual urine and overflow, anxiety, diuretics, benign prostatic hyperplasia, urethral stricture, diabetic neuropathy, IC, neurologic conditions
Dysuria	Painful or difficult voiding	Lower urinary tract infection, inflammation of bladder or urethra, acute prostatitis, stones, foreign bodies, tumors in bladder, IC
Hesitancy	Delay, difficulty in initiating voiding	Benign prostatic hyperplasia, compression of urethra, outlet obstruction, neurogenic bladder, DSD (detrusor sphincter dyssynergia: the sphincter and bladder do not coordinate)
Nocturia	Wakening from sleep to void more than twice a night	Decreased renal concentrating ability, heart failure, diabetes mellitus, incomplete bladder emptying, excessive fluid intake at bedtime, nephrotic syndrome, cirrhosis with ascites
Incontinence	Involuntary loss of urine	External urinary sphincter injury, obstetric injury, lesions of bladder neck, detrusor dysfunction, infection, neurogenic bladder, medications, neurologic abnormalities
Enuresis	Involuntary voiding during sleep	Delay in functional maturation of central nervous system (bladder control usually achieved by 5 years of age), obstructive disease of lower urinary tract, genetic factors, failure to concentrate urine, urinary tract infection, psychological stress, neurologic conditions
Polyuria	Increased volume of urine voided (generally over 3 L/day)	Diabetes mellitus, diabetes insipidus, use of diuretics, excess fluid intake, lithium toxicity, some forms of kidney disease (hypercalcemic and hypokalemic nephropathy)
Oliguria	Urine output less than 400 mL/day	Acute or chronic kidney failure (see Chapter 27), inadequate fluid intake
Anuria	Urine output less than 50 mL/day	Acute or chronic kidney failure (see Chapter 27), complete obstruction
Hematuria	Red blood cells in the urine	Cancer of genitourinary tract, acute glomerulonephritis, kidney stones, renal tuberculosis, blood dyscrasia, trauma, extreme exercise, rheumatic fever, hemophilia, leukemia, sickle cell trait or disease
Proteinuria	Abnormal amounts of protein in the urine	Acute and chronic kidney disease, nephrotic syndrome, vigorous exercise, heat stroke, severe heart failure, diabetic nephropathy, multiple myeloma

current urinary status. For example, the nurse needs to be aware that multiparous women delivering their children vaginally have a high risk for stress **urinary incontinence**. Elderly women and people with neurologic disorders, such as diabetic neuropathy, multiple sclerosis (MS), or Parkinson disease, often have incomplete emptying of the bladder and urinary stasis, which may result in UTI or increasing bladder pressure, leading to overflow incontinence, hydronephrosis, pyelonephritis, or renal insufficiency. People with diabetes who have consistent hypertension and those with primary hypertension are at risk for renal dysfunction as are those who suffer from autoimmune diseases, such as systemic lupus erythematosus (SLE). Older men are at risk for prostatic enlargement, which causes urethral obstruction and can result in UTIs and renal failure.

Risk factors for specific disorders and kidney and lower urinary tract dysfunction are summarized in Table 26-5 and discussed in Chapters 27 and 28.

Family History

People with a family history of urinary tract problems are at increased risk for renal disorders, such as autosomal dominant polycystic kidney disease (which occurs in 1 of 400 to 1,000 people) (Torres & Bennett, 2015), heredity nephritis, or urolithiasis (Scheinman, 2015).

Social History

It is especially important to obtain a thorough medication history when assessing elderly patients, for whom the increased occurrence of chronic illness often leads to polypharmacy (concurrent use of multiple medications). Aging affects the way the body absorbs, metabolizes, and excretes drugs, placing the elderly patient at risk for adverse reactions. Aging also affects the genitourinary system, leading to compromise and dysfunction in the renal and urinary systems.

Other key information to obtain includes an assessment of the patient's psychosocial status, level of anxiety, perceived threats to body image, available support systems, and sociocultural patterns. Obtaining this information during the initial and subsequent nursing assessments enables the nurse to uncover special needs, misunderstandings, lack of knowledge, and need for patient teaching.

TABLE 26-5 Risk Factors for Selected Renal or Urologic Disorders

Risk Factor	Possible Renal or Urologic Disorder
Childhood diseases: "strep throat" impetigo, nephrotic syndrome	Chronic kidney failure
Advanced age	Incomplete emptying of bladder, leading to urinary tract infection
Instrumentation of urinary tract, cystoscopy, catheterization	Urinary tract infection, incontinence
Immobilization	Kidney stone formation
Occupational, recreational, or environmental exposure to chemicals (plastics, pitch, tar, rubber)	Acute kidney failure
Diabetes mellitus	Chronic kidney failure, neurogenic bladder
Hypertension	Renal insufficiency, chronic kidney failure
Multiple sclerosis	Incontinence, neurogenic bladder
Parkinson disease	Incontinence, neurogenic bladder
Systemic lupus erythematosus	Nephritis, chronic kidney failure
Gout, hyperparathyroidism, Crohn disease, ileostomy	Kidney stone formation
Sickle cell anemia, multiple myeloma	Chronic kidney failure
Benign prostatic hyperplasia	Obstruction to urine flow, leading to frequency, oliguria, anuria
Radiation therapy to pelvis	Cystitis, fibrosis of ureter, or fistula in urinary tract, frequency, hematuria
Recent pelvic surgery	Inadvertent trauma to ureters or bladder
Pregnancy	Proteinuria, frequent voiding
Obstetric injury, tumors	Incontinence, fistulas
Spinal cord injury	Neurogenic bladder, urinary tract infection, incontinence

FIGURE 26-5 Technique for palpating the right kidney (*top*). Place one hand under the patient's back with the fingers under the lower rib. Place the palm of the other hand anterior to the kidney with fingers above the umbilicus. Push the hand on top forward as the patient inhales deeply. The left kidney (*bottom*) is palpated similarly by reaching over to the patient's left side and placing the right hand beneath the patient's lower left rib. (From Weber, J. W., & Kelley, J. (2013). *Health assessment in nursing* (4th ed.). Philadelphia, PA: Lippincott Williams & Wilkins.)

Physical Examination

Several body systems can affect upper and lower urinary tract dysfunction, and that dysfunction can affect several end organs; therefore, a head-to-toe assessment is indicated. Areas of emphasis include the abdomen, suprapubic region, genitalia, lower back, and lower extremities.

Palpation of the Kidneys

A normal right kidney may be palpable especially in very thin patients with relaxed abdominal muscles; however, a left kidney is not usually palpated. Palpation of the kidneys may detect an enlargement that could prove to be very important (Bickley, 2013). The correct technique for palpation is illustrated in Figure 26-5. Renal dysfunction may produce tenderness over the costovertebral angle, which is the angle formed by the lower border of the 12th rib and the spine (Fig. 26-6).

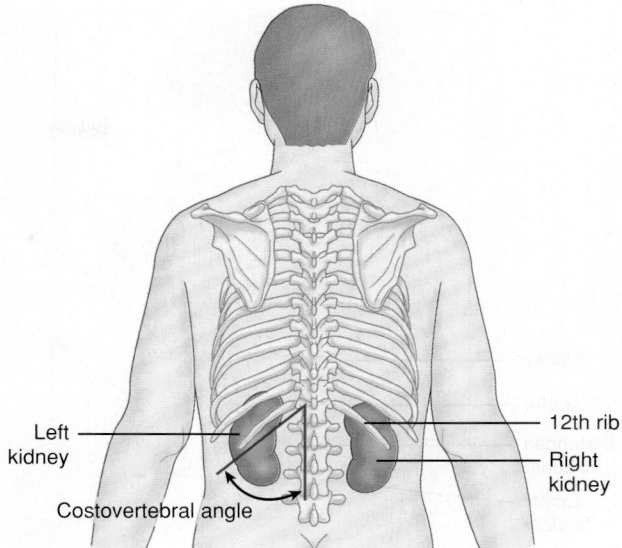

FIGURE 26-6 Location of the costovertebral angle.

Inspection, Palpation, Percussion, and Auscultation of the Abdomen

The abdomen (just slightly to the right and left of midline in both upper quadrants) is auscultated to assess for bruits (low-pitched murmurs that indicate renal artery stenosis or an aortic aneurysm) (Fig. 26-7). The abdomen also is assessed for the presence of ascites (accumulation of fluid in the peritoneal cavity), which may occur with dysfunction of the kidney as well as the liver. On inspection, with the patient lying down, a distended abdomen is noted with bulging flanks (sides) due to the weight of fluid accumulation pressing against the flanks. On percussion, dullness is noted on the flank area (where the water is), whereas tympanic sounds are heard on the upper abdomen as the gas-filled intestines rise above the ascites fluid (refer to Chapter 21 for further details and techniques).

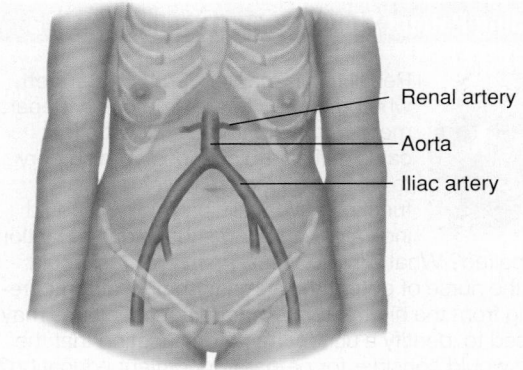

FIGURE 26-7 Arterial bruits with both systolic and diastolic components suggest partial occlusion of the aorta or large arteries. Partial occlusion of a renal artery may cause and explain hypertension. (From Bickley, L. S., & Szilagyi, P. (2003). *Bates' guide to physical examination and history taking* (8th ed.). Philadelphia, PA: Lippincott Williams & Wilkins.)

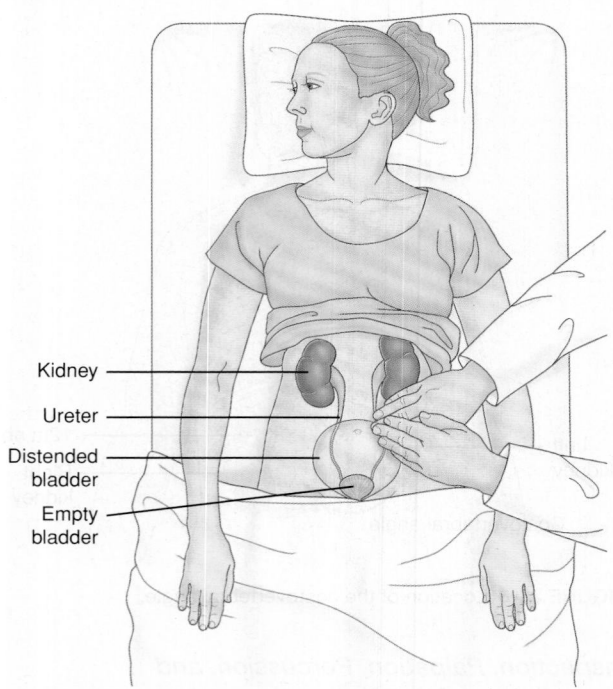

FIGURE 26-8 Palpation of the bladder.

Percussion of the Bladder

To check for residual urine, the bladder may be percussed after the patient voids. Percussion of the bladder begins at the midline just above the umbilicus and proceeds downward. The sound changes from tympanic to dull when percussing over the bladder. If dullness is noted, the bladder volume is typically 400 to 500 mL (Bickley, 2013). The bladder, which can be palpated only if it is moderately distended, feels like a smooth, firm, round mass rising out of the abdomen, usually at midline (Fig. 26-8). Dullness to percussion of the bladder after voiding indicates incomplete bladder emptying. A bladder scan can be performed to assess volume of urine retained after voiding.

Unfolding Patient Stories: Lloyd Bennett • Part 2

Recall from Chapter 19 **Lloyd Bennett,** who presented to the emergency department with a hip fracture. What effect can significant blood loss from surgery to repair the fracture have on renal function? What clinical findings would indicate to the nurse that kidney function is impaired? What clinical assessment findings would alert the nurse of potential trauma to the urinary tract resulting from the hip fracture? What diagnostic tests may be used to identify a urinary tract complication that the nurse would consider for preparatory patient education?

Care for Lloyd and other patients in a realistic virtual environment: *v****Sim*** *for Nursing* (thepoint.lww.com/vSimMedicalSurgical). Practice documenting these patients' care in DocuCare (thepoint.lww.com/DocuCareEHR).

Palpation of the Prostate and Inguinal Area

In older men, BPH or prostatitis can cause difficulty with urination. The prostate gland is palpated by digital rectal examination (DRE) as part of the yearly physical examination in men 50 years of age and older (see Chapters 32 and 34). A blood specimen to test the prostate-specific antigen (PSA) level is recommended for younger men (40 to 45 years of age) if they are at high risk for prostate cancer; namely, African American men and men who have a first-degree relative (father, brother, or son) diagnosed with prostate cancer at an early age (under 65 years of age) (American Cancer Society, 2015); then the results of the DRE and PSA are correlated. If a PSA is to be drawn, the sample should be obtained before the DRE because manipulation of the prostate can cause the PSA level to increase temporarily. Refer to Chapter 34 for further details on prostate cancer. The inguinal area is examined for enlarged nodes or an inguinal or femoral hernia.

Inspection and Palpation of the Female Genitalia

In women, the vulva, urethral meatus, and vagina are examined; refer to Chapter 33 for additional details regarding the vaginal examination. The urethra is palpated for diverticula, and the vagina is assessed for adequate estrogen effect and any evidence of herniation. A *urethrocele* is the bulging of the anterior vaginal wall into the urethra. When the pelvic floor muscles, fascia, or supporting ligaments fail, pelvic organs may fall through the vagina. A *cystocele* is the herniation of the bladder wall into the anterior vaginal vault. Urinary stasis with a cystocele is a risk factor for the development of UTIs. A *rectocele* is herniation of the terminal rectum into the posterior vagina (LeBlond, Brown, Suneja, & Szot, 2015).

Assessment for Edema and Body Weight

The patient is assessed for edema and changes in body weight. Edema may be observed, particularly in the face and dependent parts of the body, such as the ankles and sacral areas, and suggests fluid retention. An increase in body weight commonly accompanies edema. A weight gain of 1 kg equals approximately 1,000 mL of fluid (1 lb ≈ 500 mL).

Assessment of Lower Extremities

The deep tendon reflexes of the knee are assessed for quality and symmetry. This is an important part of testing for neurologic causes of bladder dysfunction because the sacral area, which innervates the lower extremities, is the same peripheral nerve area responsible for urinary continence. The gait pattern of the person with bladder dysfunction is also noted, as well as the patient's ability to walk heel to toe. These tests evaluate possible supraspinal causes for urinary incontinence.

Diagnostic Evaluation

A comprehensive health history and physical examination are used to determine the appropriate laboratory and diagnostic tests. Most patients undergoing urologic testing or imaging studies are apprehensive, even those who have had these tests in the past. Patients frequently feel discomfort and embarrassment about such a private and personal function as voiding. Voiding in the presence of others frequently can cause guarding, a natural reflex that inhibits voiding due to situational anxiety. Because the outcomes of these studies determine the plan of care, the nurse must help the patient relax by providing as much privacy and explanation about the procedure as possible. The following sections review some of the tests that might be used.

Urinalysis and Urine Culture

The urinalysis provides important clinical information about kidney function and helps diagnose other diseases, such as diabetes. The urine culture determines whether bacteria are present in the urine, as well as their strains and concentration. Urine culture and sensitivity (C&S) also identify the antimicrobial therapy that is best suited for the particular strains identified, taking into consideration the antibiotics that have the best rate of resolution in that particular geographic region. Appropriate evaluation of any abnormality can assist in detecting serious underlying diseases. Refer to Table 26-6 for the details regarding urinalysis components and potential significance.

Renal Function Tests

Renal function tests are used to evaluate the severity of kidney disease and to assess the status of the patient's kidney function. These tests also provide information about the effectiveness of the kidney in carrying out its excretory function. Renal function test results may be within normal limits

TABLE 26-6 Select Urinalysis Components

Component	Discussion
Color	Colorless to pale yellow (possible causes: Dilute urine due to diuretics, alcohol consumption, diabetes insipidus, glycosuria, excess fluid intake, renal disease) Yellow to milky white (possible causes: Pyuria, infection, vaginal cream) Bright yellow (possible causes: Multiple vitamin preparations) Pink to red (possible causes: Hemoglobin breakdown, red blood cells, gross blood, menses, bladder or prostate surgery, beets, blackberries, medications [phenytoin, rifampin, phenothiazine, cascara, senna products]) Blue, blue green (possible causes: Dyes, methylene blue, *Pseudomonas* species organisms, medications [amitriptyline, triamterene, phenyl salicylate]) Orange to amber (possible causes: Concentrated urine due to dehydration, fever, bile, excess bilirubin or carotene, medications [phenazopyridium HCl, nitrofurantoin, sulfasalazine, docusate calcium, thiamine]) Brown to black (possible causes: Old red blood cells, urobilinogen, bilirubin, melanin, porphyrin, extremely concentrated urine due to dehydration, medications [cascara, metronidazole, iron preparations, quinine, senna products, methyldopa, nitrofurantoin]; myoglobinuria)
Specific gravity	Evaluates ability of kidneys to concentrate solutes in urine and is altered by the presence of blood, protein, and casts in the urine. Disorders or conditions that cause *decreased* urine-specific gravity (i.e., dilute urine) include diabetes insipidus, glomerulonephritis, and severe kidney damage, which may cause a fixed specific gravity of 1.010. Glucose, protein, or dyes excreted in the urine *increase* the specific gravity (concentrated urine); therefore, etiologies include diabetes mellitus, patients who recently received high-density radiopaque dyes, and fluid deficit.
Osmolality	Concentrating ability is lost early in kidney disease; these test findings may disclose early defects in kidney function.
Red blood cells (hematuria)	Can develop from an abnormality anywhere along the genitourinary tract and is more common in women than in men. Common causes include acute infection (cystitis, urethritis, or prostatitis), renal calculi, and neoplasm. Other causes include systemic disorders, such as bleeding disorders; malignant lesions; and medications, such as warfarin and heparin.
White blood cells	Should be very few; increased numbers indicate infection or inflammation.
Protein	Occasional loss of up to 150 mg/day of protein in the urine primarily is considered normal and usually does not require further evaluation. Urine concentration, pH, hematuria, and radiocontrast materials all affect the results. Microalbuminuria (excretion of 20–200 mg/dL of protein in the urine) is an early sign of diabetic nephropathy. Common benign causes of transient proteinuria are fever, strenuous exercise, and prolonged standing. Causes of persistent proteinuria include glomerular diseases, malignancies, collagen diseases, diabetes mellitus, pre-eclampsia, UTI, hyperthyroidism, hypertension, heart failure, and use of a wide variety of medications (Fischbach & Dunning, 2014).
Glucose	Should be absent; its presence is suspicious for diabetes.

TABLE 26-7 Additional Tests of Renal Function

Test	Description	Normal Range
Creatinine clearance	Detects and evaluates progression of kidney disease. Test measures volume of blood cleared of endogenous creatinine in 1 minute, which provides an approximation of the glomerular filtration rate. Sensitive indicator of kidney disease used to follow progression of disease.	Measured in mL/min/1.73 m² Age — Male — Female Under 30 years — 88–146 — 81–134 30–40 years — 82–140 — 75–128 40–50 years — 75–133 — 69–122 50–60 years — 68–126 — 64–116 60–70 years — 61–120 — 58–110 70–80 years — 55–113 — 52–105
Creatinine level	Measures effectiveness of kidney function. In normal function, the level of creatinine remains fairly constant in the body.	0.6–1.2 mg/dL (50–110 mmol/L)
Urea nitrogen (blood urea nitrogen [BUN])	Serves as index of kidney function. Urea is a nitrogenous end product of protein metabolism. Test values are affected by protein intake, tissue breakdown, and fluid volume changes.	7–18 mg/dL Patients over 60 years: 8–20 mg/dL
BUN to creatinine ratio	Evaluates hydration status. An elevated ratio is seen in hypovolemia (may rise to 20:1); a normal ratio with an elevated BUN and an elevated creatinine is seen with intrinsic kidney disease.	About 10:1

until the GFR is reduced to less than 50% of normal. Renal function can be assessed most accurately if several tests are performed and their results are analyzed together. Common tests of renal function include renal concentration tests, creatinine clearance, and serum creatinine and **blood urea nitrogen** (BUN) levels. Table 26-7 describes the purpose and gives the normal range for each test. Other tests for evaluating kidney function that may be helpful include serum electrolyte levels (see Chapter 4). A plan of nursing care for a patient undergoing diagnostic testing of the renal/urologic system is available online at http://thepoint.lww.com/Honan2e.

Nursing Alert

The nurse understands that a normal BUN/ creatinine (Cr) ratio is approximately 10:1. As kidney function declines, both the BUN and the Cr rise, thus although elevated the ratio remains within normal limits. If a BUN is elevated but the creatinine is normal (BUN/Cr greater than 20:1), the nurse must assess for causes excluding renal dysfunction. Reasons may include GI bleeding such as gastric ulcers, duodenal ulcers, and gastric cancer (digestion of RBCs elevates the protein level which is transported to the liver and metabolized to BUN), or dehydration (less water available in the intravascular space) where the BUN may increase in a higher proportion than the creatinine, thus indicators of intravascular depletion include an elevated hematocrit value, and a BUN/Cr ratio of greater than 20:1. In situations where the BUN/Cr ratio is less than 10:1, the nurse considers conditions where there is decreased urea

synthesis such as severe liver disease or starvation, syndrome of inappropriate ADH (increased water in the intravascular space), and pregnancy (since the GFR increases 50% in pregnancy, there is a resultant decrease in serum creatinine).

Imaging Modalities

Several imaging modalities play a vital role in the evaluation of renal and urologic disease.

X-Ray: Kidneys, Ureters, Bladder (KUB)

This x-ray delineates the size, shape, and position of the kidneys and reveals abnormalities, such as calculi in the kidneys or urinary tract, hydronephrosis, cysts, tumors, or kidney displacement by abnormalities in surrounding tissues.

Computed Tomography and Magnetic Resonance Imaging

Computed tomography (CT) scans and magnetic resonance imaging (MRI) are noninvasive techniques that provide excellent cross-sectional views of the kidney and urinary tract. They are used to evaluate genitourinary masses, nephrolithiasis, chronic kidney infections, renal or urinary tract trauma, metastatic disease, and soft tissue abnormalities. Occasionally, an oral or IV radiopaque contrast agent is used in CT scanning to enhance visualization, although the use of a CT scan should take into account the patient's previous exposures to radiation via imaging studies. In addition, the risks associated with contrast agents should be considered. Contrast-induced nephropathy is associated with a pre-existing renal insufficiency, history of diabetes, and reduced intravascular volume (Reekers, 2015). Preprocedure hydration, along with recognition of the lowest dose of contrast as possible for the study, is recommended.

Intravenous Urography

This test shows the kidneys, ureters, and bladder via x-ray imaging as a radiopaque contrast agent that is administered intravenously moves through the upper and then the lower urinary system. It may be used as the initial assessment of many suspected urologic problems, especially lesions in the kidneys and ureters and provides an approximate estimate of kidney function.

Retrograde Pyelography

If an IV urography provides inadequate visualization of the collecting systems, a retrograde pyelography may be performed. It involves advancing catheters through the ureters into the renal pelvis by means of cystoscopy, followed by injection of a contrast agent.

Cystography

In cystography, a catheter is inserted into the bladder, and a contrast agent is instilled to outline the bladder wall. This study aids in evaluating vesicoureteral reflux (backflow of urine from the bladder into one or both ureters) and in assessing for bladder injury.

Voiding Cystourethrography

In a voiding cystourethrography, a urethral catheter is inserted, and a contrast agent is instilled into the bladder. When the bladder is full and the patient feels the urge to void, the catheter is removed, and the patient voids. This study uses fluoroscopy to visualize the lower urinary tract and assess urine storage in the bladder. It is used as a diagnostic tool to identify vesicoureteral reflux. Retrograde urethrography, in which a contrast agent is injected retrograde into the urethra, is always performed before urethral catheterization if urethral trauma is suspected.

> ### ! Nursing Alert
> *The presence of urethral injury should be ruled out prior to Foley catheter placement in patients with blood at the urethra and suspicion of injury to the lower urinary tract. Catheter placement may potentially convert a partial urethral tear to a complete urethral disruption (Tibbles, 2015, p. 232).*

Nuclear Scans

A nuclear scan requires injection of a radioisotope into the circulatory system; then the isotope is monitored as it moves through the blood vessels of the kidneys. The test provides information about kidney perfusion and function. It is used to evaluate acute and chronic kidney failure, renal masses, and blood flow before and after kidney transplantation.

Renal Angiography

In renal angiography, a catheter is threaded up through the femoral and iliac arteries into the aorta or renal artery. A contrast agent is injected to opacify the renal arterial supply. Angiography is used to evaluate renal blood flow, to differentiate renal cysts from tumors, to evaluate hypertension, and preoperatively, for renal transplantation.

Bladder Ultrasonography

Ultrasonography is a noninvasive procedure that uses sound waves passed into the body through a transducer to detect abnormalities of internal tissues and organs. A bladder ultrasonography is a noninvasive method of measuring urine volume in the bladder; it automatically calculates and displays urine volume. The test requires a full bladder; therefore, fluid intake should be encouraged before the procedure. This test also can be used to determine if a patient is emptying the bladder after urination.

Urologic Endoscopic Procedures

Endourology, or urologic endoscopic procedures, can be performed in one of two ways: using a cystoscope (Fig. 26-9) inserted into the urethra, or percutaneously, through a small incision (Table 26-8).

Bladder Scan

A portable ultrasound device provides a 3D image of the bladder and measures bladder volume noninvasively, providing immediate details on the volume of urine retained within the bladder.

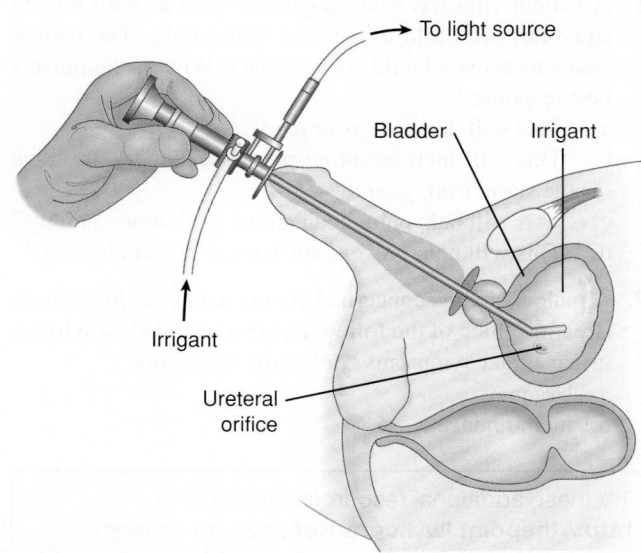

FIGURE 26-9 Cystoscopic examination. A rigid or semirigid cystoscope is introduced into the bladder. The upper cord is an electric line for the light at the distal end of the cystoscope. The lower tubing leads from a reservoir of sterile irrigant that is used to inflate the bladder.

TABLE **26-8** **Common Urologic Procedures**

Procedure	Description	Purpose
Cystoscopy	Cystoscope is inserted through the urethra into the bladder.	Used to visualize the urethra and bladder directly, as well as the urethral orifices and prostatic urethra. Calculi may be removed from the urethra, bladder, and ureter.
Renal and ureteral brush biopsy	Ureteral catheter is introduced via cystoscope, followed by a biopsy brush that is passed through the catheter.	Suspected lesion is brushed back and forth to obtain cells and surface tissue fragments for histologic analysis.
Kidney biopsy	Small section of renal cortex is obtained either percutaneously (needle biopsy) or by open biopsy through small flank incision.	Helps diagnose and evaluate the extent of kidney disease. Indications for biopsy include unexplained acute kidney failure, persistent proteinuria/hematuria, transplant rejection, glomerulopathies.

CHAPTER REVIEW

Critical Thinking Exercises

1. Discuss the changes to kidney function in an otherwise healthy 28-year-old female patient who becomes dehydrated during a marathon.

2. Discuss some of the changes that are likely to be seen when examining the urine of a diabetic patient with poor control of his or her blood sugar. How do you explain each finding?

NCLEX-Style Review Questions

1. A patient who has been diagnosed with a small kidney stone has been told to increase fluid intake. The patient wants to know why this is necessary. What is the nurse's best response?
   a. "This will decrease your pain."
   b. "This will increase urine production and help move the stone from your system."
   c. "This will help pain medications work more quickly."
   d. "This will help prevent any nausea you are having."

2. A male patient is concerned about changes to his urinary stream. Which of the following are associated with lower urinary tract symptoms? *Select all that apply.*
   a. Urgency
   b. Incontinence

   c. Frequency
   d. Dribbling
   e. Costovertebral angle (CVA) tenderness

3. The nurse recognized that a patient with chronic kidney disease will need which hormone replaced?
   a. Anterior pituitary
   b. Parathyroid
   c. Erythropoietin
   d. Corticotropin-releasing

4. The nurse knows that a frequent cause of white blood cells (WBCs) in the patient's urine is which condition?
   a. Prostate enlargement
   b. Hypertension
   c. Bladder cancer
   d. Genitourinary infection

5. A 42-year-old male patient complains of nausea, vomiting, and right flank pain. What is the most likely cause of these symptoms?
   a. Interstitial cystitis
   b. Renal colic
   c. Ureterocele
   d. Nephritic syndrome

Try these additional resources, available at **http://thepoint.lww.com/Honan2e**, to enhance your learning and understanding of this chapter:
• NCLEX-Style Student Review Questions
• Journal Articles

REFERENCES AND SELECTED READINGS

References and selected readings associated with this chapter can be found on the website that accompanies the book. Visit **http://thepoint. lww.com/Honan2e** to access the references and other additional resources associated with this chapter.

Nursing Management: Patients with Renal Disorders

Andrea Rothman Mann

Learning Objectives

After reading this chapter, you will be able to:

1. Compare and contrast the pathophysiology, assessment, nursing management, and medical management of the glomerular diseases.
2. Identify the causes of acute and chronic renal failure.
3. Summarize the nursing management of the patient with renal failure.
4. Describe renal replacement therapies.
5. Provide patient education for the patient undergoing kidney transplantation.
6. Describe care for the patient sustaining renal trauma.
7. Evaluate outcomes of care for the patient with renal disorders.

The renal system is an important regulator of the body's internal environment and is essential for the maintenance of life. The kidneys regulate fluid volume and electrolyte balance; they also play a role in acid–base balance, excrete waste products, regulate blood pressure (BP) and blood osmolarity, and contribute to red blood cell (RBC) production and vitamin D metabolism. Kidney dysfunction may be acute or chronic and can affect all body systems. Renal disease is often asymptomatic or presents with nonspecific complaints. Its presence is frequently first noted on abnormal routine laboratory data (Godara, Hirbe, Nassif, Otepka, & Rosenstock, 2014). Various factors contribute to kidney dysfunction; Box 27-1 addresses gerontologic considerations. This chapter addresses glomerular dysfunction, acute kidney injury (AKI), chronic kidney failure, and treatment options, as well as kidney trauma and transplant.

GLOMERULAR DISEASES

Acute Glomerulonephritis

Glomerulonephritis is an inflammation of the glomerular capillaries. Acute glomerulonephritis is more common in children older than 2 years of age, but it can occur at any age.

Pathophysiology

Acute glomerulonephritis (GN) comprises a specific set of renal diseases in which an immunologic mechanism triggers inflammation and proliferation of glomerular tissue that can result in damage to the basement membrane, mesangium (thin membrane supporting the capillary loops in renal glomeruli), or capillary endothelium. Acute poststreptococcal glomerulonephritis (PSGN) is the archetype of acute GN (Parmar & Batuman, 2015; Ballestas & Caico, 2014). Examples of primary diseases are postinfectious glomerulonephritis, rapidly progressive glomerulonephritis, membrane proliferative glomerulonephritis, and membranous glomerulonephritis. HIV-associated nephropathy also may occur (Godara et al., 2014). Acute nephritic syndrome is the clinical manifestation of glomerular inflammation. In acute glomerulonephritis, the kidneys become large, edematous, and congested. All renal tissues, including the glomeruli, tubules, and blood vessels, are affected to varying degrees. Box 27-2 depicts the pathophysiology of glomerulonephritis.

Acute GN may occur after infections of the pharynx or skin (i.e., impetigo) caused by certain strains of group A beta-hemolytic streptococcal infections; this is referred to as PSGN. Systemic lupus erythematosus (SLE), vascular injury, disseminated intravascular coagulation (DIC), or diabetes may be additional causes (Ballestas & Caico, 2014). An immune-mediated antigen–antibody reaction and inflammation causes insoluble immune complexes to become trapped in the glomeruli, causing protein and RBCs to enter the urine (Ballestas & Caico, 2014). Sudden onset of hematuria, proteinuria, and RBC casts in the urine define the disease and cause the smoky or coffee-colored urine typically seen in acute GN. Often this clinical picture is accompanied by hypertension, edema, azotemia (i.e., decreased glomerular filtration rate [GFR], rising blood urea nitrogen [BUN], and creatinine), and retention of renal salt and water.

Treatment of PSGN is mainly supportive. The inflammation typically lasts about 2 weeks, with individuals rarely developing chronic disease (Ballestas & Caico, 2014). When acute GN is associated with chronic infections, the underlying infections must be treated (Parmar & Batuman, 2015). Hyalinization (deterioration of normal tissue) or sclerosis indicates irreversible injury.

Risk Factors

Risk factors include a family history of glomerulonephritis; a pre-existing history of known diseases, such as a streptococcal infection (27.9%) of the upper respiratory tract; other infections with organisms (Parmar & Batuman, 2015) and viral infectious diseases, such as hepatitis, mumps, and varicella zoster. Additionally, other diseases, such as Goodpasture syndrome, Wegener granulomatosis, SLE, subacute bacterial endocarditis, and sepsis, have been implicated as risk factors.

PSGN usually develops 1 to 3 weeks after acute infection with group A beta-hemolytic streptococcus. The incidence of GN is approximately 5% to 10% in persons with pharyngitis and 25% in those with skin infections. GN comprises 25% to 30% of all cases of end-stage kidney failure. About one fourth of patients present with acute nephritic syndrome. Most cases that progress do so relatively quickly, and kidney failure may occur within weeks or months of the onset of acute nephritic syndrome. Asymptomatic episodes of PSGN exceed symptomatic episodes by a ratio of 3–4:1 (Parmar & Batuman, 2015).

Clinical Manifestations and Assessment

The primary presenting features of acute glomerulonephritis are hematuria, edema, **azotemia** (excessive nitrogenous wastes in the blood), and proteinuria (over 3 to 5 g/day). The hematuria may be microscopic or macroscopic (visible to the eye). The urine with myoglobin (myoglobinuria) is dark and may be described as brown in color. Cola-colored or coffee colored urine develops when the released myoglobin from skeletal muscle is quickly cleared from the serum into the urine. RBC and cellular debris called casts, indicate microscopic amount of bleeding from the kidney and may be associated with glomerular injury. Glomerulonephritis may be mild, and the hematuria may be discovered incidentally through a routine microscopic urinalysis, or the disease may be severe, with AKI, oliguria (less than 400 mL), and shortness of breath. Additional assessments to detect underlying cause include assessing for pharyngitis, impetigo, or a heart murmur (endocarditis) (Parmar & Batuman, 2015).

Some degree of edema and hypertension is present in most patients. Marked proteinuria due to the increased permeability of the glomerular membrane also may occur, with associated pitting edema, and hypoalbuminemia. BUN and serum creatinine levels may increase as urine output decreases. In addition, anemia may be present.

In the more severe form of the disease, patients also complain of headache, malaise, and flank pain (pain on sides below ribs and above the pelvis). Elderly patients may experience circulatory overload with dyspnea, engorged neck veins, cardiomegaly, and pulmonary edema. Atypical symptoms include confusion, somnolence, and seizures, which often are confused with the symptoms of a primary neurologic disorder.

Cultures of throat and skin lesions to rule out Streptococcus species may be obtained. Diagnostic tests include assessing for increasing antistreptolysin O (ASO) titer, which confirms recent infection. This is elevated in 60% to 80% of patients. Titers begin to increase in 1 to 3 weeks, peak in 3 to 5 weeks, and then return to normal in 6 months. ASO titer is unrelated to severity, duration, or prognosis of disease. In patients with skin infection, anti-DNAase B (ADB) titers are more sensitive than ASO titers for infection with *Streptococcus*. The antinuclear antibody test is useful for patients with acute GN and symptoms of underlying systemic illness, such as SLE and polyarteritis nodosa. Blood culture is indicated in patients with fever, immunosuppression, history of intravenous (IV) drug use, indwelling shunts, or catheters. Other laboratory testing may reveal elevations in complement C3 and C4, hypertriglyceridemia, decreased GFR, or anemia (Parmar & Batuman, 2015).

BOX 27-2

Focus on Pathophysiology

Acute Glomerulonephritis

Acute glomerulonephritis is an inflammatory disease of the glomeruli associated with an antigen–antibody response to infection. One postinfectious cause is group A beta-hemolytic streptococcal infection of the throat that precedes the onset of glomerulonephritis by 2 to 3 weeks. It may also follow impetigo (infection of the skin), visceral abscesses, and acute viral infections (upper respiratory tract infections, mumps, varicella zoster virus, Epstein–Barr virus, hepatitis, and HIV infection). In some patients, antigens outside the body (e.g., medications, foreign serum) initiate the process, resulting in antigen–antibody complexes being deposited in the glomeruli. In other patients, the kidney tissue itself serves as the inciting antigen.

From the antigen, the below sequence occurs and results in decreased glomerular filtration rate (GFR).

Antigen (group A beta-hemolytic streptococcus)

↓

Antigen–antibody product

↓

Deposition of antigen–antibody complex in glomerulus

↓

Increased production of epithelial cells lining the glomerulus

↓

Leukocyte infiltration of the glomerulus

↓

Thickening of the glomerular filtration membrane

↓

Scarring and loss of glomerular filtration membrane

↓

Decreased glomerular filtration rate (GFR)

Renal biopsy may be performed in patients with an individual or family history of kidney disease and patients with an atypical presentation, including massive proteinuria, nephrotic syndrome (discussed later in this chapter), or a rapid rise in creatinine level without resolution (Parmar & Batuman, 2015).

If the patient improves, the amount of urine increases and the urinary protein and sediment diminish. The percentage of adults who recover is not well known. Some patients develop severe **uremia** within weeks and require dialysis for survival. Others, after a period of apparent recovery, insidiously develop chronic glomerulonephritis.

Medical and Nursing Management

Management consists primarily of treating symptoms, attempting to preserve kidney function, and treating compli-cations promptly. When there is no evidence of malnutrition, dietary protein is restricted when renal insufficiency and nitrogen retention (elevated BUN) develop. Carbohydrates are given liberally to provide energy and reduce the catabolism of protein. Sodium is restricted when the patient has hypertension, edema, or heart failure (Parmar & Batuman, 2015). Diuretic and antihypertensive medications may be prescribed to control hypertension. Glomerular disease presenting with proteinuria should rely on treatment with ACE inhibitors or ARBs (Godara et al., 2014). Additionally, vasodilator drugs (e.g., nitroprusside, nifedipine, hydralazine, diazoxide) may be used in the presence of severe hypertension or encephalopathy. Early plasmapheresis may be used to remove antibodies and mediators of inflammation when antiglomerular basement antibodies are present (Swiatecka-Urban et al., 2014).

The nurse teaches the patient about fluid restriction for treatment of signs and symptoms of fluid retention (e.g., edema, pulmonary edema). Bed rest is recommended until signs of glomerular inflammation and circulatory congestion subside.

Pharmacologic therapy is focused on the cause of acute glomerulonephritis. If residual streptococcal infection is suspected, penicillin or erythromycin is used but does not appear to prevent the development of GN, unless given within the first 36 hours (Parmar & Batuman, 2015). Other antibiotic agents may be prescribed. Corticosteroids and immunosuppressant medications may be prescribed for patients with acute glomerulonephritis that is rapidly progressive.

Intake and output (I&O) are measured and recorded carefully. Fluids are given according to the patient's fluid losses and daily body weight. Insensible fluid loss of approximately 1 L (lungs and skin) is considered when estimating fluid loss. Diuresis usually begins about 1 week after the onset of symptoms, with a decrease in edema and BP. Proteinuria and microscopic hematuria may persist for many months. Recovery from acute glomerulonephritis occurs as inflammation abates, which takes about 2 weeks. Some patients may develop chronic glomerulonephritis characterized by oliguria, shortness of breath, weakness, and periorbital and generalized edema (anasarca). The patient should be instructed to report these symptoms to the health care provider immediately.

Nursing Alert
The most accurate indicator of fluid loss or gain in an acutely ill patient is weight, as accurate I&O and assessment of insensible losses may be difficult. A weight gain of 1 kg is equal to 1,000 mL of retained fluid (Grossman & Porth, 2014).

Nursing interventions focus on patient education about the disease process, explanations of laboratory and other diagnostic tests, and preparation for safe and effective self-care at home. Patient education is directed toward symptom management and monitoring for complications. The nurse emphasizes fluid and diet restrictions to avoid worsening of edema and hypertension. The patient is instructed to notify the primary care provider (PCP) if symptoms of kidney failure occur, including fatigue, nausea, vomiting, diminishing urine output, or at the first sign of any infection. Information for patient education should be given verbally and in writing.

The nurse educates the patient on the importance of follow-up evaluations of BP, urinalysis for protein, and serum BUN and serum creatinine levels to evaluate for disease progression in the patient. A referral for home care may be indicated, giving the nurse an opportunity for assessment and detection of early signs and symptoms of renal insufficiency. If corticosteroids, immunosuppressant agents, or antibiotic medications are prescribed, the nurse uses the opportunity to review the dosage, desired actions, and adverse effects of medications and the precautions to be taken.

Complications

Complications of acute glomerulonephritis include hypertensive encephalopathy, heart failure, and pulmonary edema. Hypertensive encephalopathy is a medical emergency, and therapy is directed toward reducing the BP without impairing kidney function. Rapidly progressive glomerulonephritis is characterized by a rapid decline in kidney function. Without treatment, kidney failure develops in a matter of weeks or months. Signs and symptoms are similar to those of acute glomerulonephritis (hematuria and proteinuria), but the course of the disease is more severe and rapid. Crescent-shaped cells accumulate in Bowman space (the filter within the glomerulus), disrupting the filtering process. Plasma exchange (plasmapheresis) and treatment with high-dose corticosteroids and cytotoxic agents have been used to reduce the inflammatory response. Dialysis is initiated in acute glomerulonephritis if signs and symptoms of uremia are severe. The prognosis for patients with acute glomerulonephritis is favorable, with most patients recovering; however, 20% may have proteinuria for up to 1 year (Grossman & Porth, 2014).

Nursing Alert
Azotemia refers to the accumulation of nitrogen-combining compounds (BUN, creatinine) in the blood. It usually occurs before symptoms are noted. Uremia describes the clinical manifestations of kidney failure (altered fluid, electrolyte, acid–base balance; impaired body function [hypertension, anemia, pruritus, osteodystrophy, etc.]).

CHRONIC GLOMERULONEPHRITIS

Pathophysiology

Chronic glomerulonephritis is characterized by proteinuria, usually caused by repeated episodes of glomerular injury that results in renal destruction. The kidneys are reduced to as little as one fifth their normal size, consisting largely of fibrous tissue. The glomeruli and their tubules become scarred, and the branches of the renal artery are thickened. The result is severe glomerular damage that can progress to kidney failure.

Risk Factors

Risk factors include acute glomerulonephritis, diabetes, hypertensive **nephrosclerosis** (sclerosis [hardening] of the small blood vessels in the kidneys), hyperlipidemia, chronic tubulointerstitial injury, or hemodynamically mediated glomerular sclerosis. Secondary glomerular diseases that can have systemic effects include SLE and Goodpasture syndrome (autoimmune diseases), diabetic glomerulosclerosis, and amyloidosis (a rare disease characterized by the buildup of the protein amyloid in tissues and organs).

Clinical Manifestations and Assessment

The symptoms of chronic glomerulonephritis vary. Some patients with severe disease are asymptomatic for many years. Their condition may be discovered when hypertension is found, elevated BUN and serum creatinine levels are detected, or during a routine eye examination when vascular changes or retinal hemorrhages are discovered. The first indication of disease may be a sudden, severe nosebleed, a stroke, or a seizure. Many patients report that their feet are slightly swollen (edematous) at night. Most patients also have general symptoms, such as loss of weight and strength, increasing irritability, and an increased need to urinate at night (nocturia). Headaches, dizziness, and digestive disturbances are common.

As chronic glomerulonephritis progresses, signs and symptoms of chronic kidney failure may develop. The patient appears poorly nourished, with a yellow-gray pigmentation of the skin due to uremia. Periorbital and peripheral (dependent) edema with a normal or severely elevated BP may be noted. Mucous membranes are pale due to anemia. Cardiomegaly, a gallop rhythm, distended neck veins, and other signs and symptoms of heart failure may be present. Crackles can be heard in the lungs.

Peripheral neuropathy with diminished deep tendon reflexes and neurosensory changes occur late in the disease. The patient becomes confused and demonstrates a limited attention span. An additional late finding includes evidence of pericarditis with or without a pericardial friction rub (see Chapter 16).

A number of laboratory abnormalities occur. Urinalysis reveals a fixed specific gravity of about 1.010, variable proteinuria, and **urinary casts**, which are proteins secreted by damaged kidney tubules. As kidney failure progresses and the GFR falls, the following changes occur:

- Hyperkalemia due to decreased potassium excretion, acidosis, catabolism, and excessive potassium intake from food and medications
- Metabolic acidosis from decreased acid secretion by the kidney and inability to regenerate and reabsorb bicarbonate
- Anemia secondary to decreased erythropoiesis (production of RBCs)
- Hypoalbuminemia with edema secondary to protein loss through the damaged glomerular membrane
- Increased serum phosphorus level due to its decreased renal excretion
- Decreased serum calcium level (calcium and phosphorus exist in an inverse ratio in the body) and decreased vitamin D activation
- Mental status changes due to buildup of nitrogenous wastes
- Impaired nerve conduction due to electrolyte abnormalities and uremia

Nursing Alert
Microalbuminuria refers to urinary albumin excretion greater than the normal rate of 30 mg/24 hours and may precede the development of nephropathy by 5 to 7 years. A 24-hour urine check for protein is performed; dipsticks are not accurate until more than 300 to 500 mg/day protein are excreted.

The signs and symptoms of common fluid and electrolyte disturbances that can occur in patients with renal disorders and their general management strategies are listed in Table 27-1.

Chest x-rays may show cardiac enlargement and pulmonary edema. The electrocardiogram (ECG) may be normal or may indicate left ventricular hypertrophy (LVH) associated with hypertension. Signs of electrolyte disturbances, such as tall, tented T waves associated with hyperkalemia or dysrhythmia may appear. Computed tomography (CT) and magnetic resonance imaging (MRI) scans reveal a decrease in the size of the renal cortex.

Medical and Nursing Management

Treatment is directed toward reversing the renal impairment and eliminating the underlying cause, if possible. Changes in fluid and electrolyte status and in cardiac and neurologic status are reported promptly to the PCP. Often anxiety levels are extremely high for both the patient and family. Throughout the course of the disease and treatment, the nurse gives emotional support by providing opportunities for the patient and family to verbalize their concerns, have their questions answered, and explore their options for treatment if the kidneys fail.

Instructions to the patient include explanations and scheduling for follow-up evaluations of BP, urinalysis for protein and casts, serum BUN and creatinine levels. If long-term dialysis is needed, the patient and family are taught about the procedure, how to care for the access site, dietary restrictions, and other necessary lifestyle modifications. These topics are discussed later in this chapter.

The nurse in the hospital and community setting educates the patient and reinforces the importance of notifying the health care provider for worsening signs and symptoms of kidney failure, including nausea, vomiting, and diminished urine output. Specific teaching includes explanations about recommended diet and fluid modifications and medications (purpose, desired effects, adverse effects, dosage, and administration schedule). The patient is instructed to inform all health care providers about the diagnosis of glomerulonephritis so that all medical management, including pharmacologic therapy, is based on altered kidney function.

Complications

The major complication of chronic glomerulonephritis is chronic kidney failure. Glomerulonephritis is the third most common disease causing kidney failure (National Kidney Foundation, 2017).

TABLE **27-1** Common Fluid and Electrolyte Disturbances in Renal Disorders

Disturbance	Manifestations	General Management Strategies
Fluid volume excess	Acute weight gain of at least 5%, edema, crackles, shortness of breath, decreased BUN, decreased hematocrit, distended neck veins	Fluid and sodium restriction, diuretics, dialysis
Sodium deficit (often dilutional)	Nausea, malaise, lethargy, headache, abdominal cramps, apprehension, seizures	Low-sodium diet, fluid restriction, normal saline or hypertonic saline solutions during dialysis
Sodium excess	Dry, sticky mucous membranes; thirst; rough dry tongue; fever; restlessness; weakness; disorientation	Fluids, diuretics, dietary restriction
Potassium excess	Diarrhea, colic, nausea, irritability, muscle weakness, electrocardiogram (ECG) changes (tall tented T waves is usually the earliest sign on the ECG)	Dietary restriction, diuretics, IV glucose and insulin and sodium bicarbonate, cation exchange resin, calcium gluconate, dialysis
Calcium deficit	Abdominal and muscle cramps, stridor, hyperactive reflexes, tetany, positive Chvostek or Trousseau sign, tingling of fingers and around mouth, ECG changes	Diet, phosphate binders, oral or parenteral calcium salt replacement
Bicarbonate deficit	Headache, confusion, drowsiness, increased respiratory rate and depth, nausea and vomiting, warm flushed skin	Citric acid–sodium citrate, bicarbonate replacement (rare), dialysis
Protein deficit	Chronic weight loss, emotional depression, pallor, fatigue, soft flabby muscles	Diet, dietary supplements, total parenteral nutrition, albumin
Magnesium excess	Facial flushing, nausea and vomiting, sensation of warmth, drowsiness, depressed deep tendon reflexes, muscle weakness, respiratory depression, cardiac arrest	Calcium gluconate, mechanical ventilation, dialysis
Phosphorus excess	Tetany, tingling of fingers and around mouth, muscle spasms, soft tissue calcification	Diet restriction, phosphate binders

NEPHROTIC SYNDROME

Nephrotic syndrome is a cluster of clinical findings reflecting underlying damage to the glomerular capillary membrane. Nephrotic syndrome can occur with diseases or medications that affect the kidney. Although generally considered a disorder of childhood, nephrotic syndrome does occur in adults, including the elderly (Ballestas & Caico, 2014).

Pathophysiology

Nephrotic syndrome results from damage to the glomerular capillary membrane, increasing capillary permeability, which allows protein to leak out into the urine (proteinuria). The patient may lose as much as 40 g of urinary protein per day, of which 80% is albumin. Hypoalbuminemia, hyperlipidemia, and edema are typical findings. The patient becomes vulnerable to infection and may develop thrombolytic complication related to decreased albumin and loss of antithrombin (Ballestas & Caico, 2014). Figure 27-1 depicts the pathophysiology of nephrotic syndrome.

FIGURE 27-1 Sequence of events in nephrotic syndrome.

Pathophysiology Alert
The classic symptoms of nephrotic syndrome are proteinuria, edema, and hyperlipidemia. Proteinuria results primarily from damage to the glomerular capillary membrane.

The edema of nephrotic syndrome results from the loss of plasma proteins, primarily in the form of albumin into the urine, resulting in serum hypoalbuminemia. This loss of protein causes a decrease in serum colloid osmotic pressure (COP); since there is "less particles to pull fluid into the intravascular space," the fluid stays in the tissue (edema). Additionally, renal disease itself may cause sodium retention due to enhanced sodium reabsorption by the collecting duct. The hyperlipidemia results from an increase in hepatic synthesis of lipoproteins and decreased catabolism of circulating lipoproteins (Rennke & Denker, 2013).

Risk Factors

Diabetic nephropathy is the most common cause of nephrotic syndrome; however, other glomerular diseases may be implicated. Such causes include SLE, infections/chronic glomerulonephritis, cancers, preeclampsia, drug addiction, and nephrotoxic drugs (Ballestas & Caico, 2014). Occasionally, amyloidosis of the kidney, multiple myeloma, and renal vein thrombosis may be seen.

Clinical Manifestations and Assessment

Proteinuria, predominately in the form of albuminuria, where albumin excretion exceeds 3.5 g/day, is the hallmark of nephrotic syndrome. Hypoalbuminuria is the result, leading to edema, periorbital edema, scrotal swelling, abdominal distention, weight gain, or anasarca. Fatigue and anorexia may be reported, as well as shortness of breath, pulmonary edema, or hypertension (Ballestas & Caico, 2014). The urine may contain increased white blood cells (WBCs) as well as granular and epithelial casts. The presence of hypoimmunoglobulinemia places the patient at risk for infections. Hyperlipidemia with increased high-density lipoproteins (HDL) occurs and places the patient at risk for cardiovascular disease. Hypertension, irritability, headache, and malaise occur.

The nurse can expect a variety of diagnostic tests will be performed, including urinalysis, blood chemistries including albumin and lipid levels, complete blood count (CBC), coagulation studies, renal function tests, blood glucose to exclude a diagnosis of diabetes, or renal ultrasound to evaluation for structural abnormalities (Ballestas & Caico, 2014).

Drug Alert!
Decreased serum albumin level presents decreased protein-binding sites for medications. Patients with hypoalbuminemia must be observed closely for signs of drug toxicity as the amount of free or unbound drug is increased (Grossman & Porth, 2014).

A needle biopsy of the kidney may be performed for histologic examination of renal tissue to confirm the diagnosis.

Medical and Nursing Management

Patients with nephrotic syndrome need instruction about the importance of following medication and dietary regimens so that their condition can remain stable for as long as possible. The patient who does not have hyperkalemia may be placed on a low-sodium diet containing liberal amounts of potassium. This type of diet enhances the sodium–potassium pump mechanism and assists in elimination of sodium to reduce edema. Reduction in dietary cholesterol and saturated fats helps with lipidemia. Protein intake should be moderate, sufficient to meet protein needs while avoiding excessive intake, which may accelerate renal deterioration and increase urinary protein losses. An intake of 0.7 to 0.8 g/kg/day is suggested with at least half of the protein from high biologic value (HBV) sources, such as meat, fish, poultry, milk, eggs, and soy (Dudek, 2014).

The patient is taught to report any signs of acute infection promptly (recall they have decreased immunoglobulin), such as a respiratory tract infection, to prevent further glomerular damage. For example, an untreated streptococcal infection may be a risk factor for acute poststreptococcal glomerulonephritis; pathogens in the bloodstream may lead to sepsis with resulting decreased renal perfusion. Diuretics may be prescribed for the patient with severe edema; however, caution must be used because of the risk of reducing the plasma volume to the point of impaired circulation with subsequent prerenal AKI (discussed later in the chapter). The use of angiotensin-converting enzyme (ACE) inhibitors or angiotensin receptor blocking agents, in combination with diuretics, often reduces the degree of proteinuria (Ballestas & Caico, 2014). Statin medications have been shown to improve endothelial function and decrease proteinuria (Ballestas & Caico, 2014).

Other medications used to treat nephrotic syndrome include corticosteroids, antineoplastic agents (cyclophosphamide [Cytoxan]) or immunosuppressant medications (azathioprine [Imuran], chlorambucil [Leukeran], or cyclosporine [Neoral]). It may be necessary to repeat treatment with corticosteroids if relapse occurs. Patients should be taught to protect themselves from infection and to report any infections promptly due to immunosuppression.

Complications

Complications of nephrotic syndrome include infection secondary to loss of immunoglobulins, accelerated atherosclerosis secondary to hyperlipidemia, and a hypercoagulable state that may result in thromboembolism (Ballestas & Caico, 2014). Body image may be altered due to anasarca and edema, causing a change in appearance.

KIDNEY FAILURE

Kidney failure results when the kidneys cannot remove the body's metabolic wastes or perform their regulatory functions. This process may be acute, developing over hours to days, or chronic, developing over months to years. Kidney failure results in azotemia, metabolic derangements, acid–base disturbances, and electrolyte imbalances. Kidney failure is a systemic disease and is a final common pathway of many different kidney and urinary tract diseases. Each year, the number of deaths from irreversible renal failure increased until 2009, at which point it began to decline somewhat (National Institute of Diabetes and Digestive and Kidney Diseases [NIDDK], 2016a).

ACUTE KIDNEY INJURY (FORMERLY KNOWN AS ACUTE RENAL FAILURE)

AKI is a clinical syndrome that is typically reversible; it is marked by an abrupt loss of kidney function and GFR over a period of hours to days. AKI occurs in 5% to 7% of patients who are hospitalized and up to 20% of patients who are critically ill. The mortality rate of 40% in patients who are critically ill has not appreciably changed over the last several decades due to an aging population, development of multisystem failure, and associated increased comorbidities (Dirkes, 2015).

In recent years, AKI has gained increasing recognition as a major risk factor for the development of chronic kidney disease (CKD). The clearest example of this relationship comes in cases of severe dialysis-requiring AKI where patients fail to recover kidney function. **Acute tubular necrosis (ATN)** without recovery is the primary diagnosis for 2% to 3% of cases of kidney failure annually (USRDS, 2014). AKI is frequently superimposed on CKD and, therefore, plays a key role in progression of CKD (discussed shortly).

Manifestations of AKI include oliguria or anuria with resulting azotemia (increased serum creatinine, BUN, and other nitrogenous waste products). Acidemia, fluid volume excess, alterations in calcium and phosphorus balance and BP alterations develop rapidly. Erythropoiesis fails with resulting anemia.

Pathophysiology

Although the exact pathogenesis of AKI is not always known, this condition may be reversible if identified and treated before kidney function is impaired permanently. AKI is classified by its etiology, which helps to focus the treatment.

Classification of Acute Kidney Injury

The major classifications of AKI are prerenal azotemia caused by hypoperfusion of the kidney; intrarenal or intrinsic causes, in which the renal parenchyma or nephron is damaged; and postrenal causes, in which outflow of urine is obstructed. Common causes of each type of AKI are summarized in Box 27-3.

BOX 27-3 **Causes of Acute Kidney Injury**

Prerenal Failure

- Volume depletion resulting from:
  - Hemorrhage
  - Renal losses (diuretics, osmotic diuresis)
  - GI losses (vomiting, diarrhea, nasogastric suction)
- Impaired cardiac efficiency resulting from:
  - Myocardial infarction
  - Heart failure
  - Dysrhythmias
  - Cardiogenic shock
- Vasodilation resulting from:
  - Sepsis
  - Anaphylaxis
  - Antihypertensive medications or other medications that cause vasodilation

Intrarenal Failure

- Prolonged renal ischemia resulting from:
  - Pigment nephropathy (associated with the breakdown of blood cells containing pigments that occlude kidney structures)
  - Myoglobinuria (trauma, crush injuries, burns)

- Hemoglobinuria (transfusion reaction, hemolytic anemia)
- Rhabdomyolysis
- Nephrotoxic agents such as:
  - Aminoglycoside antibiotics (gentamicin, tobramycin)
  - Antirejection medications (cyclosporine, tacrolimus)
  - Radiopaque contrast agents
  - Heavy metals (lead, mercury)
  - Solvents and chemicals (ethylene glycol, carbon tetrachloride, arsenic)
  - NSAIDs
  - ACE inhibitors
- Infectious processes such as:
  - Acute pyelonephritis
  - Acute glomerulonephritis

Postrenal Failure

- Urinary tract obstruction, including:
  - Calculi (stones)
  - Tumors
  - Benign prostatic hyperplasia (BPH)
  - Strictures
  - Blood clots

Prerenal AKI, which occurs in 60% of cases, is caused by reduced blood flow to the kidney with resulting decrease in the GFR and urine output (Dirkes, 2015). Common clinical situations are volume-depletion states, which include dehydration; hemorrhage or gastrointestinal (GI) losses; decreased cardiac output such as occurs with myocardial infarction, heart failure, or cardiogenic shock; and vasodilated states, such as sepsis or anaphylaxis. To maintain adequate renal perfusion the mean arterial pressure (MAP) must be 65 mm Hg (Dirkes, 2015). For patients with a history of hypertension and/or renal vascular diseases, higher pressures may be required to maintain renal perfusion.

Intrarenal or intrinsic AKI is the result of actual parenchymal damage to the glomeruli or kidney tubules. ATN is the most common cause of intrarenal AKI in the patient who is hospitalized. Ischemia due to decreased renal perfusion and MAP below 65 mm Hg (Dirkes, 2015), accounts for more than 50% of cases of ATN. In the early period of renal ischemia, kidney function can be restored completely by improving renal blood flow, typically with IV fluids. If left untreated or when fluid resuscitation is inadequate, ATN will ensue (Wolfson, 2014, p. 1298). Additionally, nephrotoxic agents, such as aminoglycosides and radiocontrast agents, may cause ATN through direct damage to the nephron. Conditions such as burns, crush injuries, infections, and severe blood transfusion reactions can lead to rhabdomyolysis with **myoglobinuria**. With burns and crush injuries, myoglobin (a protein released from muscle when injury occurs) and hemoglobin are liberated, causing obstruction of renal tubules, renal toxicity, and ischemia. The term **rhabdomyolysis**, in which breakdown of skeletal muscle is seen, may be used to describe this event. Severe transfusion reactions may also cause intrarenal failure; hemoglobin released through hemolysis filters through the glomeruli and becomes concentrated in the kidney tubules to such a degree that precipitation of hemoglobin occurs. Additionally, hyperglycemic hyperosmolar nonketotic coma (see Chapter 30), in which as much as 25% of total body water can be lost, is associated with ATN as well as conditions where there is third spacing of fluids (fluid sequestered in a nonfunctional area) such as in pancreatitis and peritonitis (Wolfson, 2014). Certain medications, especially nonsteroidal anti-inflammatory drugs (NSAIDs) and ACE inhibitors or ARBs, also may predispose a patient to intrarenal damage. These medications interfere with the normal autoregulatory mechanisms of the kidney and may cause hypoperfusion and eventual ischemia.

Postrenal AKI is the result of a mechanical obstruction that develops anywhere in the renal system. This may result from ureteral blockage, such as from bilateral renal calculi, benign prostatic hyperplasia (BPH), strictures, tumors, or congenital defects (Dirkes, 2015). Pressure rises in the kidney tubules and hydronephrosis occurs, compressing normal renal tissue and resulting in a decrease in the GFR. Any sudden or complete cessation of urine output with an indwelling catheter should alert the nurse to possible obstruction. The catheter should be inspected and kinks removed or the catheter irrigated or changed to reestablish urine flow.

Phases of AKI

There are four clinical phases of AKI: initiation or onset, oliguric, diuretic, and recovery. The onset phase begins with the triggering event and ends when cellular injury and oliguria develop. Common events include significant fluid or blood loss, burns, or diabetes insipidus (Dirkes, 2015). A small number of patients develop nonoliguric renal failure, usually associated with nephrotoxic agents; it may also occur with burns, traumatic injury, and the use of halogenated anesthetic agents.

The oliguric period is accompanied by fluid overload and an increase in the serum concentration of wastes, such as urea, creatinine, organic acids, and the electrolytes potassium, phosphorous, and magnesium. The average time period for oliguria is 8 to 14 days, but it may last longer (Dirkes, 2015). Because the minimum amount of urine needed to rid the body of fluid and metabolic waste products is 500 mL in 24 hours (Hall, 2016), renal replacement therapy (RRT), such as dialysis, may be needed until kidney function returns.

The diuretic phase occurs when the cause of acute renal failure (ARF) is corrected. This phase is marked by a gradual increase in urine output, which signals that glomerular filtration has started to recover. Urine output may be normal, or the patient may excrete large amounts of dilute urine along with electrolytes. The patient should be observed closely for dehydration, which may damage the kidney further, as well as for hypokalemia (Dirkes, 2015). Abnormal laboratory values plateau and begin to decline.

The recovery period is signaled by the improvement of kidney function and energy level and may take 6 to 12 months (Grossman & Porth, 2014). If residual damage to the glomerular basement membrane occurs, residual renal impairment may result.

Clinical Manifestations and Assessment

Almost every system of the body is affected when there is failure of the renal regulatory mechanisms. The patient may appear critically ill and lethargic. Table 27-2 summarizes common clinical findings in all three categories of AKI.

Assessment of the patient with AKI includes evaluation for changes in the urine output, diagnostic tests that evaluate the kidney contour and function, and a variety of laboratory values. See Chapter 26 for information about the normal characteristics of urine, diagnostic findings, and laboratory values in the renal system.

TABLE **27-2** Comparing Clinical Findings Among Categories of Acute Kidney Injury

Characteristics	Categories		
	Prerenal	Intrarenal	Postrenal
Etiology	Hypoperfusion	Parenchymal damage	Obstruction
Blood urea nitrogen value	Increased proportion (greater than 20:1) blood urea nitrogen (BUN) to creatinine	Increased	Increased
Creatinine	Normal or slightly increased	Increased	Increased
Urine output	Decreased	Varies, often decreased	Varies, may be decreased, or sudden anuria
Urine sodium	Typically decreased	Typically increased	Varies
Urinary sediment	Normal, few hyaline casts	Abnormal casts and debris	Usually normal
Urine osmolality	Increased to 500 mOsm	Approximately 350 mOsm, similar to serum	Varies, increased or equal to serum
Urine-specific gravity	Increased	Low normal	Varies

In AKI, oliguria (less than 400 mL a day) is typically present. Hematuria may be present, and the urine has a low specific gravity due to the kidney's inability to concentrate the urine (Grossman & Porth, 2014). Patients with AKI have decreased urine sodium levels and urinary casts, and other cellular debris may be present.

The BUN level increases steadily at a rate dependent on the degree of protein catabolism, renal perfusion, and fluid or protein intake. Nausea, vomiting, lethargy, headache, muscle twitching, and seizures may occur. Serum creatinine, a more sensitive indicator of kidney function than BUN, increases with glomerular damage and is used to monitor kidney function and disease progression.

Patients with oliguria and **anuria** (less than 50 mL/day) are at high risk for hyperkalemia, a potassium level of more than 5.1 mEq/L (5.1 mmol/L). Hyperkalemia develops as the damaged kidney cannot excrete potassium; protein catabolism and acidosis result in the release of intracellular potassium into the serum, worsening hyperkalemia. The ECG may reveal changes, including tall, tented, or peaked T waves, absent P wave, widened QRS, or bradydysrhythmia. Additional symptoms of hyperkalemia may include weakness, diarrhea, dysrhythmias, and cardiac arrest. The nurse should be aware of exogenous sources of potassium, such as IV infusions, or medications, such as potassium penicillin, as well as dietary sources (avocado, brussels sprouts, okra, spinach (green leafy vegetables), potatoes, pumpkin, spinach, sweet potatoes, tomatoes, yams, apricots, bananas, nectarines, orange juice, prune juice) (Dudek, 2014).

As metabolic acidosis develops, normal renal buffering mechanisms fail, resulting in hyperventilation. The patient may breathe more rapidly and deeply to "blow off" CO_2 in an attempt to restore normal serum pH. Hyperventilation as compensation for acidosis may lead to respiratory fatigue or failure, requiring mechanical ventilation.

Serum phosphate levels increase. Calcium levels may decrease in response to decreased absorption of calcium from the intestine as well as a compensatory mechanism for the elevated blood phosphate levels. Anemia is another common laboratory finding in AKI, as a result of reduced erythropoietin production, uremic GI lesions, reduced RBC lifespan, and blood loss, usually from the GI tract.

 Nursing Alert
Monitor urine output hourly; output should measure at least 0. 5 mL/kg/hr. Urine output directly reflects GFR in the kidney and, therefore, is a sensitive and early biomarker of AKI (Dirkes, 2015).

Prevention

Prevention of AKI is essential as AKI mortality rates as high as 60% or more, especially in patients where multisystem failure is observed (Box 27-4).

The nurse assesses for use of potentially nephrotoxic agents and exposure to environmental toxins. Patients taking nephrotoxic medications, such as aminoglycosides (gentamicin, tobramycin, neomycin), amphotericin B, vancomycin, cyclosporine, certain antineoplastics (Adams & Urban, 2016) or anesthetics, heavy metals such as cisplatin or bismuth, or radiologic contrast agents, should be monitored closely for changes in kidney function. BUN and serum creatinine levels should be obtained at baseline, during treatment, and after therapy is complete, if indicated.

Chronic use of analgesics, particularly NSAIDs, may cause **interstitial nephritis** (inflammation within the renal

Health Promotion

Preventing Acute Kidney Injury

- Provide adequate hydration to patients at risk of dehydration:
  - Perioperative patients
  - Patients on fluid restriction
  - Patients undergoing diagnostic studies with or requiring contrast agents (e.g., barium enema, intravenous pyelograms, angiography), especially elderly patients who may have marginal renal reserve
  - Patients with neoplastic disorders and those receiving chemotherapy
  - Patients with metabolic disorders, such as gout, glycosuria
- Prevent and treat hypotension or shock promptly with blood and fluid replacement
- Monitor hourly urine output of patients who are critically ill to detect the onset of kidney failure as early as possible. When available, monitor central venous and arterial pressures
- Continually assess renal laboratory values
- Properly identify patients to prevent transfusion reactions, which can precipitate myoglobinuria
- Prevent and treat infections promptly. Infections can lead to sepsis and renal damage
- Intervene promptly with wounds, burns, and other precursors of sepsis
- To prevent infections from ascending in the urinary tract, give meticulous care to patients with indwelling catheters. Remove catheters as soon as possible
- To prevent toxic drug effects, closely monitor dosage, duration of use, and blood levels of all medications metabolized or excreted by the kidneys

tissue) and papillary necrosis. Patients with heart failure or cirrhosis with ascites are at particular risk for NSAID-induced kidney failure. Increased age, pre-existing kidney disease, and the coadministration of nephrotoxic agents increase the risk for kidney damage.

Radiocontrast-induced nephropathy is a major cause of hospital-acquired AKI (Adams & Urban, 2016); therefore, those at risk should be identified prior to procedures where contrast media is used (BUN and serum creatinine should be assessed before contrast dye is administered). Patients with creatinine levels greater than 2 mg/dL should receive pre-procedure hydration and receive as low a dose of contrast as possible for the study. *N*-acetylcysteine given before and after contrast administration appears to decrease the incidence of contrast nephropathy (Wolfson, 2014, p. 1300). The nurse should withhold Metformin prior to procedures requiring IV contrast. While metformin is not nephrotoxic, if AKI occurs after a procedure, the acidosis associated with kidney failure may worsen in the presence of this medication.

Promising diagnostic biomarkers allow early detection of AKI. The level of urine or serum neutrophil gelatinase-

associated lipocalin (NGAL) increases after an episode of poor kidney perfusion. NGAL levels increase 24 to 48 hours before serum creatinine rises, indicating renal dysfunction before kidney failure. Cystatin C level, assessed in urine and serum, is considered an early predictor of AKI as well as of increased mortality. Tissue inhibitor metalloproteinase-2 (TIMP-2) appears in urine within 12 hours of an injury due to ischemia or sepsis, indicating a seven-fold risk of AKI (Dirkes, 2015). Currently, studies are underway to determine the application of these biomarkers.

Medical and Nursing Management

The kidneys have a remarkable ability to recover from insult. Management includes maintaining fluid and electrolyte balance, avoiding fluid excesses, and supporting the patient until repair of renal tissue and restoration of function occur. Dialysis may be used on a temporary basis to restore homeostasis.

The underlying cause is identified, treated, and eliminated when possible. If the cause of AKI is related to prerenal factors, then treatment consists of optimizing renal perfusion by repletion of intravascular volume with fluids or treating decreased cardiac output (keeping the MAP above 65 mm Hg). Adequate blood flow to the kidneys in patients with prerenal causes of AKI may be restored by IV fluids or transfusions of blood products. If AKI is caused by hypovolemia secondary to hypoproteinemia, an infusion of albumin may be prescribed. Treatment of postrenal failure is aimed at restoring normal outflow of urine by relieving the obstruction. Surgery, such as prostatectomy, percutaneous nephrostomy tubes, stents or indwelling catheters, may be used. Intrarenal azotemia is treated with supportive therapy, removal of causative agents, and aggressive fluid resuscitation in cases of shock, infection, and rhabdomyolysis. Early dialysis may be required to control rapidly developing complications, such as fluid volume excess (hypertension, CHF, pericarditis, and pulmonary edema), metabolic acidosis, or hyperkalemia. While this is expected to be a temporary intervention, a small portion of patients do not recover kidney function and may develop chronic kidney failure.

The nurse observes for fluid excess manifested by dyspnea, crackles, tachycardia, hypertension, and distended neck veins, as well as generalized edema in the presacral and pretibial areas and any dependent region of the body. The central venous pressure (CVP), where measured, will be elevated. Fluid and sodium should be restricted in patients with FVE and oliguria or anuria to prevent fluid overload and pulmonary edema. The nurse observes for signs and symptoms of pericarditis (chest pain that increases when lying down or fever and pericardial friction rub) or pericardial effusion (feeling of pressure in the chest, engorged neck veins, distant [muffled] heart sounds, equalizing pressure in heart chambers, pulsus paradoxus), which generally is associated with the need to initiate dialysis. Emergency pericardiocentesis may be required (refer to Chapter 15). Diuretics, such as furosemide (Lasix), may be prescribed to initiate diuresis and maintain renal perfusion when intravascular volume deficits have been corrected. Careful attention to intake and output is required as well as cautious estimates of insensible loss (refer to Chapter 4).

Pharmacologic Therapy

Hyperkalemia may be reduced by administering polystyrene sulfonate (Kayexalate) orally, via NG tube, or by retention enema (Adams & Urban, 2016). Kayexalate, a cation-exchange resin which works by exchanging sodium ions for potassium ions in the intestinal tract. Typically Sorbitol is combined with Kayexalate to draw water into the bowel, inducing diarrhea and excretion of potassium. The patient should retain the Kayexalate enema for 30 to 45 minutes. For symptomatic hyperkalemia, IV insulin, given with glucose to prevent hypoglycemia, may be administered to temporarily shift potassium back into the cells. Calcium may be administered to treat the cardiotoxicity that has developed secondary to hyperkalemia since it directly antagonizes the membrane effects of hyperkalemia. Albuterol sulfate (Ventolin HFA) by nebulizer can lower plasma potassium concentration by 0.5 to 1.5 mEq/L. It is important to understand that hyperkalemia is the most common metabolic cause of death in patients with AKI (Wolfson, 2014).

High anion-gap acidosis may require sodium bicarbonate therapy—if the serum bicarbonate concentration is below 15 mmol/L or arterial pH is less than 7.2 (Longo et al., 2015)—or dialysis. Phosphate-binding agents, such as calcium acetate (PhosLo) or aluminum hydroxide gel (short term only), are given to decrease the absorption of phosphate from the intestinal tract.

Because kidney failure alters the metabolism and action of many drugs, often in ways that are not predictable, medications that are excreted via the kidney require dosage adjustment to prevent toxicity. Commonly used agents requiring adjustment are antibiotics, especially aminoglycosides, digoxin, ACE inhibitors, and magnesium-containing agents.

Nutritional Therapy

AKI causes impaired glucose use and protein synthesis and increased tissue catabolism. Azotemia may cause nausea and vomiting. Weight loss may result from negative nitrogen balance. Dietary proteins are restricted (Dudek, 2015), and caloric requirements are met with high-carbohydrate meals due to their protein-sparing effect. Dietary restrictions include foods and fluids containing potassium, such as bananas, citrus, tomatoes, or melons. Foods containing phosphorus, including dairy products, beans, nuts, legumes, and carbonated beverages, are restricted as well. Caffeine also is restricted. The patient may require enteral or parenteral nutrition.

Suspect fluid retention if the patient develops hypertension, crackles, edema, or weight gain. Administering fluids (PO or IV) may require replacing both sensible and insensible loss. Insensible loss is estimated at 1 L. Fluid replacement in kidney disease may be based on urine output, any GI losses (gastric drainage or diarrhea), plus insensible losses, thus meticulous attention is paid to accurate intake and output. Metabolism and the oxidation process produce about 200 to 500 mL of fluid per day, which may decrease the fluid requirements, whereas fever may increase the fluid requirement (Dudek, 2015). As AKI resolves, results of blood chemistry tests are used to determine the amounts of sodium, potassium, and water needed for replacement. Following the diuretic phase, the patient is placed on a high-carbohydrate diet with sufficient protein to promote nitrogen balance. The patient is encouraged to resume activities gradually.

> **Nursing Alert**
> If the caloric intake is insufficient to prevent the breakdown of body protein, accumulation of additional nitrogenous waste develops, which may increase uremic symptoms.

The nurse monitors for complications, participates in emergency treatment of imbalances of fluids and electrolytes, assesses the patient's progress and response to treatment, and provides physical and emotional support. Additionally, the nurse keeps family members informed about the patient's condition, helps them understand the treatments, and provides psychological support. AKI is a serious problem, and the nurse must continue to provide interventions for the underlying disorder (e.g., burns, shock, trauma, obstruction of the urinary tract, etc.).

Reducing Metabolic Rate

Bed rest may be indicated to reduce exertion and the metabolic rate during the most acute stage of the disorder. Fever and infection, both of which increase the metabolic rate and catabolism, are prevented or treated promptly.

> **Nursing Alert**
> Fever increases the insensible water loss by increasing water vapor in the lungs and allowing more water to be lost from the respiratory mucosa (Grossman & Porth, 2014).

Promoting Pulmonary Function

Attention is given to pulmonary function, and the patient is assisted to turn, cough, and deep breathe frequently to prevent atelectasis and respiratory tract infection. Drowsiness and lethargy may prevent the patient from moving and turning without encouragement and assistance. Maintaining a patent airway through oral or endotracheal suction may be necessary.

Preventing Infection

Asepsis is essential with invasive lines and catheters to minimize the risk of infection and subsequent increased metabolism. Uremia impairs host defenses, particularly leukocyte function, and infection is a significant cause of morbidity and mortality in patients with AKI (Wolfson, 2014, p. 1301). Any fever warrants an assessment and notification of the provider. Sepsis disrupts blood flow, causing cell ischemia and death (Dirkes, 2015). An indwelling urinary catheter is avoided whenever possible because of the high risk of urinary tract infection (UTI) associated with its use.

Providing Skin Care

The skin may be dry or susceptible to breakdown as a result of edema; therefore, meticulous skin care is important. Additionally, excoriation and itching of the skin may result from the deposit of uremic toxins in the patient's tissues. Turning the patient frequently, bathing the patient with cool water, and keeping the patient's skin clean and well moisturized and the fingernails trimmed to avoid excoriation are comforting and prevent skin breakdown.

Nursing Alert

The nurse recognizes that edematous tissue is fragile and must assess any edematous area for evidence of erythema to prevent skin breakdown.

Providing Support

While AKI is considered potentially reversible, there is variability in the length of time that the patient is ill and the duration of treatment. The patient and family need assistance, explanation, and support during this period. The nurse provides frequent explanations of the purpose and rationale of the treatments, as rising BUN leads to confusion and lethargy. Both the patient and family are included in teaching to allay anxiety and fear. Consistent with the goal of Healthy People 2020, which is to increase the number of patients hospitalized with AKI who receive a renal evaluation within 6 months of discharge, the nurse explains the importance of follow-up with a nephrologist (Healthy People 2020, 2017).

Gerontologic Considerations

The prevalence of renal dysfunction in Americans older than 70 years of age is 15% (Dirkes, 2015). The incidence and mortality of AKI is increased in older patients who are hospitalized due to a decrease in the number of functional nephrons and renal blood flow as well as to atherosclerosis of the renal arteries. This is especially so in those with comorbidities, such as diabetes, hypertension, and heart disease (Dirkes, 2015). The older individual is particularly susceptible to AKI due to limited renal reserve to counteract insults to their kidney function, such as sepsis and hydration.

Diuretics and NSAIDs increase the risk of AKI threefold, as do ACE inhibitors (Lewis, 2013). It is estimated that 50% of hospitalizations are avoidable; hospitalization is associated with increased mortality (Lewis, 2013). The older patient with systemic infection accompanied by vomiting or diarrhea should be kept hydrated, and NSAIDs, diuretics, ACE inhibitors or ARBs should be withheld (Lewis, 2013).

Nurses need to be aware of the risk of AKI in elderly patients, especially those undergoing diagnostic testing or procedures that can result in dehydration. Suppression of thirst, decreased mobility with lack of access to drinking water, and confusion contribute to the older patient's failure to consume adequate fluids, which may lead to dehydration and further compromise of kidney function.

Nursing Alert

Muscle mass and GFR can decrease with age; therefore, even small elevations in creatinine may indicate significant renal impairment in the elderly and should be investigated.

CHRONIC KIDNEY DISEASE AND END-STAGE KIDNEY DISEASE

Kidney failure is a progressive and irreversible deterioration in renal function taking place over months to years. Kidney failure results in the body's inability to maintain metabolic and fluid and electrolyte balance, resulting in azotemia and subsequent uremia. CKD is the term used with kidney damage or decreased renal function for 3 months or more with evidence of irreversible nephron loss and scarring. More than 10% of adults in the United States—over 20 million people—may have CKD, of varying levels of progression which may lead to ESKD (CDC, 2015). When end-stage kidney failure is reached, RRT with dialysis or kidney transplant is needed to sustain life. Chronic renal insufficiency (CRI) occurs when the GFR has been reduced moderately but not to a degree sufficient to cause clear-cut clinical symptoms (Wolfson, 2014).

There were 114,813 new cases of kidney failure reported in 2012, representing a decrease of 3.7% from the previous year. Despite this decrease, at the end of 2012, there were 636,905 dialysis and transplant patients receiving treatment; 449,342 individuals are receiving hemodialysis or peritoneal dialysis (PD) and 186,303 have functioning renal transplants (USRDS, 2014). Healthy People 2020 has set goals related to kidney failure, including:

- Decreasing the percentage of the US population with CKD,
- Increasing awareness of kidney disease among people with reduced kidney function,
- Decreasing the number of new individuals requiring dialysis, and
- Decreasing morbidity and mortality related to CKD (Healthy People 2020.gov).

Stages of Chronic Kidney Disease

Stages are based on the GFR. The normal GFR is 120–130 mL/min corrected for body size (per 1.73 m²).
Stage 1: GFR ≥90 mL/min; hematuria, proteinuria, or abnormal renal anatomy
Stage 2 (Mild CKD): GFR = 60–89 mL/min; hematuria, proteinuria or abnormal renal anatomy; nephrons highly susceptible to failure
Stage 3a (Moderate CKD): 45–59 mL
Stage 3b (Moderate CKD): GFR = 30–44 mL/min;
Stage 4 (Severe CKD): GFR = 15–29 mL/min;
Stage 5 (End Stage CKD): GFR <15 mL/min/1.73 m² or dialysis dependent

Adapted from Lewis, R. (2013). An overview of chronic kidney disease in older people. *Nursing Older People, 25*(10), 31–38.

The incidence of CKD is increasing most rapidly in people who are 65 years of age and above, more than doubling between 2000 and 2008, while the incidence of recognized CKD among those who are 20 to 64 years of age is less than 0.5%. CKD in African Americans is three times higher than in Caucasians; incidence rates for Native Americans have started to decline (NIDDK, 2016b).

Pathophysiology

As renal function declines, the end products of protein metabolism, normally excreted in urine, accumulate in the blood. Uremia develops and adversely affects every system in the body. The greater the buildup of waste products, the more severe the symptoms. Box 27-5 outlines stages of CKD. The disease tends to progress in patients who excrete significant amounts of protein or those who have elevated BP more rapidly than in those without these conditions.

Risk Factors

While the number of new patients with end-stage kidney failure appears to be stabilizing in the United States, the need to reduce both the incidence and prevalence of this devastating complication of kidney disease even further cannot be overemphasized. Undoubtedly the key to success is prevention of both CKD and AKI (USRDS, 2014). Healthy People 2020 identifies five risk factors for kidney failure:

1. Diabetes
2. Hypertension
3. Proteinuria
4. Family history
5. Increasing age

It also identifies diabetes (36%) and hypertension (24%) as the two major causes. Other causes include chronic glomerulonephritis, **pyelonephritis**, obstruction of the urinary tract, hereditary lesions such as in polycystic kidney disease, vascular and autoimmune disorders (such as SLE), infections, medications, or toxic agents. Men are 50% more likely to develop CKD than are women (CDC, 2014). Comorbid conditions that develop during CKD contribute to the high morbidity and mortality among patients with kidney failure (CDC, 2014). Environmental and occupational agents that have been implicated in kidney failure include lead, cadmium, mercury, and chromium.

When targeting health education for prevention of CKD, the nurse includes evidence that early detection and treatment of kidney disease may prevent—or at least delay—the progression of chronic kidney failure to end-stage kidney failure. ACE inhibitors or angiotensin receptor blockers (ARBs) are used to slow the progression of kidney failure. Strict control of blood glucose delays and possibly even prevents the progression of diabetic nephropathy (Lewis, 2013).

Clinical Manifestations and Assessment

Patients with significant kidney damage may be asymptomatic until the GFR reaches 20% to 50% (Adams & Urban, 2016; Grossman & Porth, 2014). Virtually every body system is affected by CKD. Severity of signs and symptoms depends on the degree of renal impairment, other underlying conditions, and the patient's age. Clinical manifestations of uremia do not generally appear until the GFR is reduced to approximately 15% to 20% of normal (Wolfson, 2014). Uremia has particular effects on a variety of organ systems that are detailed below. Some can be managed with dialysis while others cannot.

Systemic Manifestations

- *Neurologic manifestations:* Neurologic changes include lethargy, altered level of consciousness, inability to concentrate, muscle twitching, agitation, confusion, and seizures. Peripheral neuropathy and cramps are present in some patients. Restless leg syndrome and painful or "burning" feet can occur in the early stage of uremic peripheral neuropathy.
- *Cardiovascular manifestations:* Hypertension results from retention of sodium and water due to activation of the renin–angiotensin–aldosterone system; fluid volume excess causes heart failure and pulmonary edema. Pericarditis (with or without pericardial fluid accumulation) is caused by irritation of the pericardium by uremic toxins and may require dialysis. Cardiovascular disease is the predominant cause of death in patients with kidney failure (Wolfson, 2014). In patients receiving chronic hemodialysis, approximately 45% of overall mortality is attributable to cardiac disease, and about 20% of these cardiac deaths are due to acute myocardial infarction (Choi, Park, & Ha, 2014).

![Nursing Alert icon] **Nursing Alert**
Abrupt weight gain or a body weight considerably over "dry weight" (typically more than 5 lb) is the most reliable clue of fluid volume excess (Wolfson, 2014).

- *GI manifestations:* GI signs and symptoms are common and include anorexia, nausea, vomiting, and hiccups. The patient's breath may have the odor of ammonia or urine (uremic fetor), or the patient may complain of a metallic taste in the mouth.
- *Immunologic manifestations:* Defective granulocytes, B- and T-cell function, and impaired phagocytosis can lead to impaired immune and inflammatory response.
- *Hematology manifestations:* Anemia, secondary to decreased erythropoietin (hormone that stimulates RBC production by the bone marrow) production. Increased bleeding risk because of defective platelet adhesiveness. In general, a normal amount of

platelets are seen; however, bleeding time is prolonged.
- *Genitourinary manifestations:* Erectile dysfunction, decreased libido, pain during intercourse (women), and amenorrhea may result.
- *Dermatologic manifestations:* Pruritus is common. Uremic frost, the deposit of urea crystals on the skin, is uncommon today because of early and aggressive treatment of kidney failure with dialysis. The skin may be bronze or waxy yellow or gray, particularly in dark-skinned individuals. The precise mechanisms have not been identified for many of these diverse signs and symptoms.

Musculoskeletal manifestations: Bone and joint problems are associated with disturbances of calcium and phosphate metabolism, resulting in renal osteodystrophy, a clinical entity encompassing several overlapping varieties of bone disease that can cause bone pain or frank fractures (Wolfson, 2014). Box 27-6 summarizes the signs and symptoms seen in kidney failure.

BOX 27-6 **Focused Assessment**

Chronic Kidney Failure

Be alert for the following signs and symptoms:

Neurologic
- Weakness and fatigue
- Confusion or behavior changes
- Inability to concentrate
- Disorientation
- Tremors
- Seizures
- Asterixis
- Restless leg syndrome
- Burning of soles of feet

Integumentary
- Gray-bronze skin color
- Dry, flaky skin
- Pruritus
- Ecchymosis or purpura
- Thin, brittle nails
- Coarse, thinning hair

Cardiovascular
- Hypertension
- Pitting edema (feet, hands, sacrum)
- Periorbital edema
- Engorged neck veins
- Pericarditis/pericardial friction rub
- Pericardial effusion or tamponade
- Hyperkalemia
- Hyperlipidemia

Pulmonary
- Crackles
- Thick, tenacious sputum

- Depressed cough reflex
- Pleuritic pain
- Shortness of breath
- Tachypnea
- Kussmaul-type respirations
- Uremic pneumonitis

Gastrointestinal
- Ammonia odor to breath ("uremic fetor")
- Metallic taste
- Mouth ulcerations and bleeding
- Anorexia, nausea, and vomiting
- Hiccups
- Constipation or diarrhea
- Bleeding from GI tract

Hematologic
- Anemia
- Thrombocytopenia

Reproductive
- Erectile dysfunction
- Amenorrhea
- Testicular atrophy
- Infertility
- Decreased libido

Musculoskeletal
- Muscle cramps
- Loss of muscle strength
- Renal osteodystrophy
- Bone pain
- Bone fractures
- Foot drop

Glomerular Filtration Rate

As glomerular filtration decreases, the serum creatinine and BUN levels increase; the creatinine clearance decreases. Serum creatinine is the more sensitive indicator of kidney function because of its constant production in the body. The BUN is affected not only by kidney disease but also by protein intake in the diet, tissue catabolism, fluid intake, parenteral nutrition, and medications such as corticosteroids. Calculation of GFR is discussed in Chapter 26, and the stages of CKD based on GFR can be found in Box 27-5.

Sodium and Water Retention

Some patients retain sodium and water, thus increasing the risk for edema, heart failure, and hypertension. Dilutional hyponatremia typically occurs. Hypertension also may result from activation of the renin–angiotensin–aldosterone system and the concomitant increased secretion of aldosterone. Episodes of vomiting and diarrhea may cause sodium and water depletion, which worsens the uremic state.

Acidosis

In advanced kidney disease, metabolic acidosis occurs because the kidneys are unable to excrete hydrogen ions (H^+). Decreased acid secretion results from the inability of the kidney tubules to excrete ammonia (NH_3^-) and to reabsorb bicarbonate (HCO_3^-). There is also decreased excretion of phosphates and other organic acids.

Anemia

Anemia is caused by inadequate production of erythropoietin by the damaged kidney. Erythropoietin, normally produced by the kidneys, stimulates bone marrow to produce RBCs. Anemia is exacerbated further by the shortened lifespan of RBCs due to uremia, nutritional deficiencies, and the patient's tendency to bleed, particularly from the GI tract. The nurse should assess for fatigue, shortness of breath, and chest pain.

Calcium and Phosphorus Imbalance

Hyperphosphatemia with resulting hypocalcemia develops in kidney failure. The decreased serum calcium level causes increased secretion of parathormone from the parathyroid glands, causing calcium to leave the bone. Bone weakness and fractures may result. The active metabolite of vitamin D (1,25-dihydroxycholecalciferol), normally manufactured by the kidney, decreases as kidney failure progresses, impairing calcium absorption. Uremic bone disease or renal osteodystrophy develops from the complex changes in the balance of calcium, phosphate, and parathormone.

Medical Management

The goal of management is to maintain kidney function and homeostasis for as long as possible while continuing to treat the underlying disorder(s). Avoidance of risk factors, dietary modification, BP control, adequate treatment of the associated conditions, and where needed, preparation for RRT, are utilized (Godara et al., 2014). **Renal replacement therapy** is planned for as kidney disease progresses and is discussed in detail later in the chapter.

Pharmacologic Therapy

Complications can be prevented or delayed by administering prescribed phosphate-binding agents, calcium supplements, antihypertensive and cardiac medications, anticonvulsants, and erythropoietin (Epogen/Procrit).

Calcium and Phosphorus Binders
Hyperphosphatemia and hypocalcemia are treated with medications that bind dietary phosphorus in the GI tract. Binders, such as calcium carbonate (Os-Cal) or calcium acetate (PhosLo), are prescribed. If the calcium–phosphorus product exceeds 55 mg/dL, a polymeric phosphate binder, such as sevelamer hydrochloride (Renagel) or sevelamer carbonate (Renvela), may be used. The calcium-phosphorus product is calculated by multiplying the serum calcium (corrected for albumin—see Nursing Alert below) by the phosphate level. The nurse plans to administer phosphate binders with food for them to be effective. Parathyroid agents, such as cinacalcet (Sensipar), which mimics calcium, may be given for secondary hyperparathyroidism of kidney failure. The medication "tricks" the parathyroid glands into sensing high calcium levels, causing reduced production of parathyroid hormone (PTH). When PTH decreases, bone resorption diminishes (Adams & Urban, 2016).

> **Nursing Alert**
> Calcium exists as either bound to albumin or in its free form, which is termed ionized. Ionized calcium is physiologically active whereas calcium bound to albumin is inactive. Standard laboratory tests measure the total calcium (ionized and bound). If serum albumin is low, as it is in patients with nephrotic syndrome and other processes such as starvation or renal cachexia, a lower total calcium is seen on laboratory results. An ionized calcium level may be ordered or a correction for this perceived calcium deficit may be used.
>
> To correct the calcium level, the nurse adds 0.8 g/dL to the total calcium value for every gram of albumin below 4.0 g/dL, using this formula:
>
> Corrected calcium = serum total calcium (mg/dL) + 0.8 × (4 − serum albumin [g/dL])
>
> Note: a normal serum calcium level is 8 to 10 mg/dL, which may vary slightly by laboratory; a normal serum albumin is 3.5 to 5.2 g/dL.
>
> Example: Patient has albumin of 2 g/dL (20 g/L), and total serum calcium concentration of 8 mg/dL.

Formula: 8 mg/dL + 0.8 (4 – 2 g/dL)

> *8 + 0.8(2)*
> *8 + 1.6*
> *9.6 mg/dL = corrected calcium level*

Pathophysiology Alert

The parathyroid glands regulate blood calcium. Secondary hyperparathyroidism may develop in patients with kidney failure. The parathyroid glands respond to hypocalcemia by increasing the secretion of PTH. PTH attempts to elevate the blood calcium by stimulating the release of calcium from the bones. Thus, the nurse should observe for bone pain, osteoporosis, and pathologic bone fractures.

Pathophysiology Alert

Under normal circumstances, hypocalcemia results in enhanced calcium uptake by renal collecting tubules. However in kidney failure, the collecting tubes are unable to reabsorb calcium, and activation of vitamin D also is impaired. With decreased renal synthesis of 1,25-dihydroxyvitamin D (also known as calcitriol, the active form of vitamin D), the intestinal absorption of calcium is decreased. Thus kidney diseases place patients at risk for hypocalcemia, secondary hyperparathyroidism, and hyperphosphatemia.

Antihypertensive and Cardiovascular Agents

Hypertension is managed by restriction of sodium and fluids as well as antihypertensive agents. Diuretics (in patients with some residual kidney function) and inotropics, such as digoxin (Lanoxin) or dobutamine (Dobutrex), may be used. Care must be taken to prevent digoxin toxicity in patients with renal impairment.

Nursing Alert

A therapeutic serum level of digoxin is 0.8 to 2 ng/mL (1.0 to 2.6 nmol/L) for patients with congestive heart failure (CHF) and 1.5 to 2.5 ng/mL (2.0 to 3.2 nmol/L) for patients with arrhythmias. The nurse is aware that signs and symptoms of digoxin toxicity may include nausea, vomiting, anorexia, green/yellow visual distortion (a commonly reported symptoms in hospitalized patients) (Fischbach & Dunning, 2014).

Anticonvulsants Agents

IV diazepam (Valium), lorazepam (Ativan), or phenytoin (Dilantin) usually is administered to control seizures, which may develop as azotemia worsens. The side rails of the bed should be raised and bed in low position to protect the patient. If a seizure occurs, the nurse protects the patient's head, loosens constrictive clothing, and removes patient's eyeglasses. The nursing management of the patient with seizures is discussed in Chapter 46.

Erythropoietin

Anemia associated with CKD is treated with recombinant human erythropoietin (e-poietin, Epogen/Procrit) or darbepoetin alfa (Aranesp). Therapy is initiated to achieve a hematocrit of 33% to 38% and a target hemoglobin of >11 g/dL, to alleviate the symptoms of anemia (Adams & Urban, 2016). Hemoglobin values above 12 g increase the risk of death and serious thromboembolic and cardiovascular events. E-poietin is administered intravenously at the end of dialysis or subcutaneously. Blood transfusions are indicated for patients with chest pain or extreme dyspnea. Adverse effects seen with erythropoietin therapy include headache, arthralgia, nausea, hypertension, increased clotting, seizures, and depletion of body iron stores (Adams & Urban, 2016). The expected outcome for patients receiving e-poietin is decreased fatigue, higher-energy levels, increased feeling of well-being, better tolerance of dialysis, and improved tolerance of exercise.

Nursing Alert

The use of erythropoietin (Epogen/Procrit) has been shown to have a significant effect on hematocrit levels. Patients with CKD whose anemia is untreated typically have hemoglobin concentrations in the range of 6 to 8 g/dL, and erythropoietin administration has demonstrated success in correcting the anemia. However, a black-box warning about erythropoietin-stimulating agents (ESAs) suggests that clinicians and patients with CKD "weigh the benefits of ESAs to decrease the need for transfusions against the increased risks for serious, adverse cardiovascular events" associated with ESAs (FDA, 2017; Berns, 2016). The lowest dose of ESA sufficient to reduce the need for transfusion is recommended. Although a target Hgb range is not provided, it is suggested that for dialysis patients receiving ESA treatment should be initiated when the Hgb level is below 10 g/dL and dose interrupted or reduced for Hb >11 gm (or >10 gm in non dialysis patients) (fda.gov, 2017). Hgb levels >11 g/dL are associated with adverse cardiovascular events which include hypertension, increased risk for stroke, and vascular thrombosis (FDA, 2017).

Iron, in the form of iron sucrose (Venofer) and ferric gluconate (Ferrlecit), may be prescribed to promote an adequate response to erythropoietin. Hypertension that cannot be controlled is a contraindication to recombinant erythropoietin therapy.

Nutritional Therapy

The diet for patients with kidney disorders includes limiting protein as well as restrictions on fluids, sodium, potassium, and phosphorus. Protein restriction to 0.8 g/kg/day of ideal body weight can slow the progression of renal disease and improve the symptoms of uremia, including nausea and vomiting. At least 50% of the allowed protein must be of high biologic value (HBV), including eggs, meats, and plant-based proteins. There is controversy over the degree of protein restriction: too little protein and malnutrition can cause loss of strength, muscle mass, and weight (Grossman & Porth, 2014). Protein restriction is difficult for most patients; the nurse should give positive feedback and express confidence in the patient's ability to adhere to the eating plan. Dietary protein is increased slightly during dialysis to compensate for loss of protein and amino acids in the dialysate. At the same time, adequate caloric intake and vitamin supplementation must be ensured because a protein-restricted diet does not provide the necessary complement of vitamins, and dialysis results in loss of water-soluble vitamins. Calories are supplied by carbohydrates and fat to prevent wasting.

The patient must adhere to a daily fluid allowance of approximately 500 to 800 mL plus the previous day's 24-hour urine output (recall insensible loss is 1 L per day). WE CAN GO WITH TYPICAL FLUID ALLOWANCE OF 1000 ML/DAY (COULD VARY). OK TO LEAVE OFF PREVIOUS DAY'S OUTPUT. The nurse teaches the patient different strategies to control intake and thirst, such as sucking on hard candies or mints, chewing gum, rinsing the mouth with refrigerated water, sucking on a lemon wedge, using small glasses instead of large ones, and moisturizing the lips.

Potassium restriction involves limiting citrus, tomatoes, melons, green leafy vegetables, and potatoes. Also phosphorus is restricted; this is contained in dairy, peas, beans, nuts (including peanut butter), and cola products. Sodium is contained in many canned and processed foods and in smoked foods lunchmeats, as well as in MSG.

Nursing Alert
Patients with kidney disease must be aware that some salt substitutes contain potassium chloride and should be avoided.

Dialysis

The patient with increasing symptoms of kidney failure is referred to a dialysis or transplantation center early in the course of progressive disease. Dialysis is initiated when the patient cannot maintain homeostasis with conservative treatment; dialysis is discussed in detail later in the chapter.

Nursing Management

The patient with CKD requires astute nursing care to avoid the complications of reduced kidney function and the stresses and anxieties of dealing with a life-threatening illness.

Nursing care and education are directed toward fluid and electrolyte imbalance, dietary management, and promoting positive feelings by encouraging increased self-care and greater independence. It is extremely important to provide frequent, clear explanations and information to the patient and family concerning kidney failure, treatment options, and potential complications. A plan of nursing care for a patient with kidney failure is available online at http://thepoint.lww.com/Honan2e.

Teaching Patients Self-Care

Encouraging self-management is an essential role of the nurse when caring for patients with kidney failure. Nurses in home care, dialysis centers, hospitals, and outpatient settings all provide ongoing education and reinforcement while monitoring the patient's progress and adherence to the treatment regimen. The nurse includes the patient's beliefs, values, and concerns in the treatment regimen to improve patient outcomes.

The nurse and dietician reinforce the diet parameters for patients with renal disorders as well as fluid restrictions, explaining the correlation between symptoms and nonadherence. The patient can be encouraged to take BP measurements and daily weights at home to illustrate the effect of prescribed antihypertensives and fluid restriction with BP elevations or SOB.

The patient and family should report the following symptoms of worsening kidney function to the health care provider:

- Signs and symptoms of worsening kidney failure, including nausea, vomiting, change in usual urine output, or ammonia/urine odor to the breath
- Signs and symptoms of hyperkalemia, including muscle weakness, diarrhea, abdominal cramps
- If receiving dialysis, signs and symptoms of access problems, such as clotted fistula or graft or signs of infection at the site

Continuing Care

The nurse teaches the patient to follow-up with examinations and treatments to prevent and detect progression of renal disease as well as reinforce care for the primary disorder. The patient and family should be alerted to symptoms of worsening condition, have treatment options explained, and be offered psychoemotional support. The home care nurse has the opportunity to assess the patient's environment, emotional status, and the coping strategies used by the patient and family to deal with the changes in family roles often associated with chronic illness. Assessment, ongoing education, and reinforcement of the diet for patients with renal disorders are performed. Reminders about the need for health-promoting activities and health screening, particularly cardiovascular health, are important when caring for the patient with kidney failure.

Gerontologic Considerations

The age and number of patients with CKD over 60 years of age have increased steadily each year, while the incidence of those under 40 years of age remains at 0.5% (USRDS, 2014). The number of patients aged 75 years and older being treated for end-stage kidney failure has doubled. The increased incidence of diabetes and hypertension is one cause of this increase. Other common causes of kidney failure in the elderly population include renovascular disease (27%) and urinary tract obstruction by the prostate (22%) (Lewis, 2013). The signs and symptoms of renal disease in the elderly may be nonspecific. Comorbid disorders, such as heart failure or dementia, can delay diagnosis and complicate treatment. Hemodialysis and PD have been used effectively in treating elderly patients. Although there is no specific age limitation for renal transplantation, concomitant disorders, such as coronary artery disease or peripheral vascular disease, have made that treatment less common for the elderly. Treatment for those with CKD should be adapted to suit the patient's comorbidities and life expectancy (Lewis, 2013). Older persons are more prone to "white coat hypertension" (refer to Chapter 13); therefore 24-hour monitors should be used to validate a diagnosis of hypertension. Systolic hypertension also is common in the elderly; overtreatment can result in diastolic hypotension or orthostatic hypotension, which may lead to dizziness, falls, and risk for fracture (Lewis, 2013).

ACE inhibitors and ARBs have renal protective effects, yet the use of these medications in the elderly should be undertaken with caution. If the patient's serum creatinine increases by 25% or more with the use of these agents, then the medication should be discontinued (Lewis, 2013).

Knowing that CKD is a risk factor for cardiovascular disease, the elderly should receive advice on lifestyle modification and medications, such as antiplatelet and lipid-lowering medications.

Only 1% of older individuals with stage 3 kidney disease progress to kidney failure (Lewis, 2013); rather, they die from other causes. Of those over 75 years of age who choose RRT, 50% die within a year of starting treatments. The patient and family must be aware that RRT cannot restore health (Lewis, 2013).

Available diagnostic criteria and treatment guidelines are not tailored specifically to the older adult. Tight control of BP and polypharmacy may place the elderly and infirm at risk for complications. Individuals over 75 years of age without proteinuria and stable estimated glomerular filtration rates (eGFR) of 45 to 60 mL/min should be managed as are those without CKD (Lewis, 2013).

> **Nursing Alert**
> The eGFR is a calculation based on blood creatinine level and other variables such as age, sex, and race (e.g., African American vs. non–African American), whereas the GFR requires a creatinine clearance test (timed urine collection of 24 hours) and the serum creatinine in order to compare blood and urine creatinine concentrations.

When an elderly patient refuses dialysis or transplantation, conservative management with nutritional therapy, fluid control, and medications may be used. Advanced directives and end-of-life care based on quality of life should be explored. This end-of-life care may be in order for those for whom conservative management is no longer effective or those who choose to withdraw from RRT (Lewis, 2013).

Complications

Complications of chronic kidney failure necessitate a collaborative approach to care and include the following:

- Hyperkalemia due to decreased excretion, metabolic acidosis, catabolism, and excessive intake (diet, medications, fluids)
- Pericarditis, pericardial effusion, and pericardial tamponade due to retention of uremic waste products and inadequate dialysis
- Hypertension due to retention of sodium and water and malfunction of the renin–angiotensin–aldosterone system
- Anemia due to decreased production of erythropoietin, decreased RBC lifespan, bleeding in the GI tract from irritating toxins and ulcer formation, and blood loss during hemodialysis
- Bone disease and metastatic and vascular calcifications due to retention of phosphorus, low levels of serum calcium, abnormal metabolism of vitamin D, and elevated levels of aluminum

RENAL REPLACEMENT THERAPIES

Renal replacement therapy is a term used to encompass life-supporting treatments for kidney failure, including hemodialysis, PD, hemofiltration, and renal transplantation. While these treatment modalities are discussed within the context of kidney failure, hemodialysis and PD may be employed to restore homeostasis in patients with AKI as well.

As end-stage kidney disease (ESKD) approaches, the patient's very survival is threatened. Choosing a treatment option for kidney failure can be overwhelming. Applying best practices and health care navigation for patient with end-stage renal disease may improve their ability to make informed decisions and increase the numbers of those pursuing transplant (Skelton, Waterman, Davis, Peipert, & Fish, 2015). The *My Life, My Dialysis Choice Decision Aid* from the nonprofit Medical Education Institute, Inc. shifts the discussion from *how* to do dialysis to *why* a particular RRT option may be a better fit for the patient's lifestyle (Schatell, 2015). Additionally, there is a need to normalize discussions about concerns, fears, preferences, priorities, and future care for those with kidney failure throughout the disease process. For individuals struggling to maintain career and family life and roles while undergoing hemodialysis, there is a need for advanced care planning early in the trajectory of the disease to facilitate development of realistic goals. For those over 65 years of age receiving hemodialysis, recognizing that 25% will die within the year means preferences and priorities for future care should be elicited (Bristowe et al., 2015).

DIALYSIS

Dialysis is used to remove fluid and uremic waste products from the body when the kidneys are unable to do so. Methods of therapy include hemodialysis, PD, and continuous renal replacement therapy (CRRT).

Whether kidney disease is acute or chronic, dialysis becomes necessary in uremia upon the development of hyperkalemia, fluid overload, or impending pulmonary edema, acidosis, pericarditis, or severe confusion/encephalopathy. It also may be used to remove certain medications or other toxins due to poisoning or medication overdose.

The decision to initiate dialysis is reached after thoughtful discussion with the patient, family, providers, and others (social work, spiritual adviser, etc.), as appropriate. Many potentially life-threatening issues are associated with the need for dialysis. The nurse can assist the patient and family by answering their questions, clarifying the information provided, and supporting their decision. Often the lifestyle changes that patients requiring long-term hemodialysis need to make are overwhelming.

Although the costs of dialysis usually are reimbursable, limitations on the patient's ability to work, resulting from illness and dialysis, usually impose a great financial burden on the patient and family.

HEMODIALYSIS

Hemodialysis is the most common method of dialysis. Treatments usually occur three times a week and take about 3 to 5 hours per treatment. The trend in managing CKD is to initiate treatment before the signs and symptoms associated with uremia become severe.

Description

Hemodialysis functions as an artificial kidney, removing toxic nitrogenous substances and excess water from the blood. The patient's blood is diverted to a machine, where toxins are removed, and then the blood is returned to the patient's body. Hemodialysis requires a semipermeable membrane found in the hollow fiber **dialyzer**, or artificial kidney, to replace the function of the impaired kidneys. The dialyzer contains thousands of tiny cellophane tubules through which the blood flows; a **dialysate** solution circulates around the tubules. The exchange of wastes from the blood to the dialysate occurs through the semipermeable membrane by way of **osmosis**, **diffusion**, and **ultrafiltration** (Fig. 27-2). The toxins and wastes in the blood are removed by diffusion, in which particles move from an area of higher concentration in the blood to an area of lower concentration in the dialysate. The dialysate is a solution made up of electrolytes in their ideal extracellular concentrations. The electrolyte level in the patient's blood can be brought under control by adjusting the dialysate. The semipermeable membrane impedes the diffusion of large molecules, such as RBCs and proteins, keeping them in the bloodstream.

Excess water is removed from the blood by osmosis, in which water moves from an area of lower concentration of particulates in the blood (dilute) toward an area of higher concentration of particulates in the dialysate. In ultrafiltration, water moves under high pressure to an area of lower pressure to facilitate water removal. This process is accomplished by applying negative pressure or a suctioning force to the dialysis membrane.

The anticoagulant heparin is administered to keep blood from clotting in the dialysis circuit. When this is dangerous to the patient, such as in patients with thrombocytopenia, saline flushes may be used. At the end of the treatment, the dialysate, excess fluid, and waste products are discarded.

Vascular Access

Access to the patient's vascular system must be established to allow blood to be removed, cleansed, and returned to the patient's vascular system at rates between 300 and 550 mL/min. Several types of access are available.

Temporary Vascular Access Devices

Immediate access to the patient's circulation for emergency hemodialysis is achieved by inserting a double-lumen large-bore catheter into the subclavian, internal jugular, or femoral vein (Fig. 27-3). This method of vascular access involves some risk, such as hematoma, pneumothorax, infection, thrombosis of the subclavian vein, or inadequate flow. For the patient with end-stage kidney failure, the nurse should emphasize that these are "bridge" catheters and not permanent access; they are used while a method for permanent vascular access is created and heals.

> **(!) Nursing Alert**
> *Temporary vascular access devices for dialysis (e.g., Quinton catheter or permacath) typically are flushed with heparin by the dialysis nurse at the end of the treatment to maintain device patency. Typically the nurse should not use these devices for routine access. If, however, a life-threatening emergency occurs and no other access is available, the nurse MUST know that the catheter is NEVER flushed before ASPIRATING THE CATHETER PORTS to prevent systemic anticoagulation.*

The Fistula First Project (National Vascular Access Improvement Initiative) was designed to increase permanent

FIGURE 27-2 Hemodialysis system. **A.** Blood from an artery is pumped into (**B**) a dialyzer where it flows through the cellophane tubes, which act as the semipermeable membrane (*inset*). The dialysate, which has the same chemical composition as the blood except for urea and waste products, flows in around the tubules. The waste products in the blood diffuse through the semipermeable membrane into the dialysate.

access with AV fistula placement in 66% of long-term dialysis patients by 2009. The AVF First Breakthrough Initiative (FFBI) has made dramatic progress, increasing permanent access to nearly 60% by 2011 (Vassalotti et al., 2012).

Arteriovenous Fistula

The gold standard for permanent access is a surgically created **arteriovenous fistula**, usually placed in the forearm. The fistula is created by joining (anastomosing) an artery to a vein (Fig. 27-4). The venous segment of the fistula will dilate in response to increased arterial pressure to provide for rapid removal and return of blood. When performing dialysis, two large-bore (14- to 16-gauge) needles are inserted into the fistula; the arterial segment of the fistula is used for flow to the dialyzer and the venous segment for reinfusion of the dialyzed blood. The fistula should be given heal and mature (4 to 6 weeks is preferable). The patient is encouraged to perform exercises, such as squeezing a rubber ball, to help the access mature and to increase the size of these vessels.

Arteriovenous Graft

An **arteriovenous graft** can be created by subcutaneously inserting synthetic graft material between an artery and vein (see Fig. 27-4). The synthetic graft material that is used most commonly is expanded polytetrafluoroethylene (Gortex). Usually, a graft is created when the patient's vessels are not suitable for creation of a fistula, such as in the patient with diabetes. Infection and thrombosis are the most common complications of arteriovenous grafts.

Ideally, the surgical access is created 2 to 3 months before the need for RRT so the access can mature (niddk.nih.gov, 2014). Patients should be given information about the access and about potential changes in body image, which can trigger noncompliance or depression.

Nursing Alert

Failure of the permanent dialysis access (fistula or graft) accounts for most hospital admissions of patients undergoing chronic hemodialysis. Thus, protection of the dialysis access is of high priority.

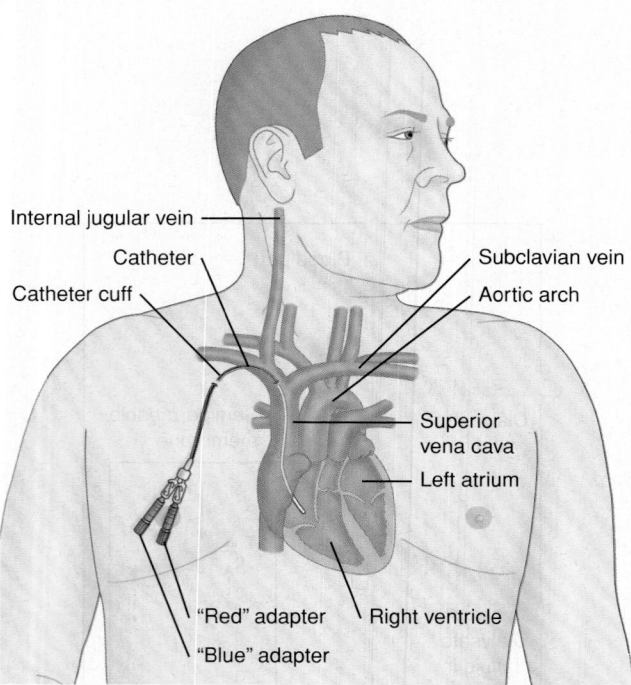

FIGURE 27-3 Double-lumen, cuffed hemodialysis catheter used in acute hemodialysis. The red adapter is attached to a blood line through which blood is pumped from the patient's body to the dialyzer. After the blood passes through the dialyzer (artificial kidney), it returns to the patient's body through the blue adapter.

Patient Education

The nurse teaches the patient with a fistula or graft to check daily for a thrill, a vibrating or buzzing sensation, over the graft and to notify the health care provider or dialysis center if this is absent. The nurse assesses for a thrill and a bruit, a

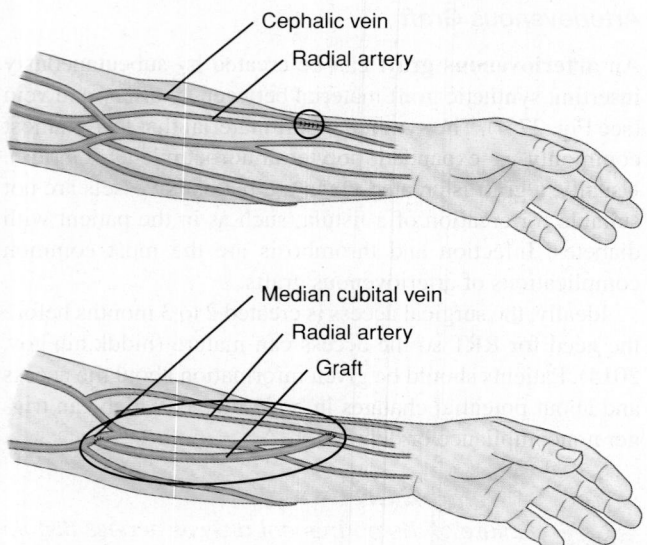

FIGURE 27-4 An internal arteriovenous fistula (**top**) is created by a side-to-side anastomosis of the artery and vein. A graft (**bottom**) can also be established between the artery and vein.

swishing sound heard with the stethoscope. Further teaching includes avoiding compression of the site; not permitting blood to be drawn, an IV to be inserted, or BP to be taken on the extremity with the dialysis access; not to wear tight clothing or carry bags or pocketbooks on that side; and not to lie on or sleep on the area. The patient is taught to observe the site daily for redness, swelling, bleeding, drainage, heat, or pain and to report these promptly to the health care provider.

Clotting of the dialysis access increases the risk of life-threatening imbalance of fluids and electrolytes as lack of patency means dialysis cannot be performed. If this occurs, fibrinolysis, surgical thrombectomy, or revision is indicated.

Medical and Nursing Management

During dialysis, the patient, the dialyzer, and the dialysate bath require constant monitoring for complications. The dialysis nurse uses this time for assessing, monitoring, supporting, and educating the patient. The nurse may use this time to discuss the diet for patients with renal disorders or to reinforce fluid restriction, which may cause interdialytic weight gain (Box 27-7). The nurse palpates the fistula or graft for a thrill and auscultates for a bruit or swishing sound, indicating patency of the access.

Pharmacologic Therapy

Just as many medications are excreted wholly or in part by the kidneys, many medications are removed from the blood during hemodialysis; therefore, dosage adjustments may be needed. Metabolites of drugs that are bound to protein are not removed during dialysis. Removal of other drug metabolites depends on the weight and size of the molecule.

Patients undergoing hemodialysis who require medications, for example, cardiac glycosides, antibiotic agents, antiarrhythmic medications, or antihypertensive agents, are monitored closely to ensure that the blood and tissue levels of these medications are maintained without toxic accumulation. The nurse plans to administer these medications after dialysis to avoid their removal.

Evaluating for medications that may promote complications during dialysis is part of nursing care. For example, if an antihypertensive agent is taken prior to dialysis, dangerous hypotension may occur during dialysis. Administration of many medications that are taken once daily can be delayed until after the dialysis treatment. Collaboration with the hospital pharmacist is important.

Nutritional and Fluid Therapy

Diet is an important factor for patients on hemodialysis because of the effects of uremia. With the initiation of hemodialysis, the patient usually requires restriction of dietary protein, sodium, potassium, phosphorous, and fluid. Protein intake is more liberal during hemodialysis but still restricted to about 1.2 to 1.3 g/kg/day of ideal body weight; therefore,

BOX 27-7

Nursing Research

Bridging the Gap to Evidence-Based Practice

Interdialytic Laughter Yoga Therapy for haemodialysis patients: a pre-post intervention feasibility study

Bennet, P., Parsons, T., Ben-Moshe, R., Neal, M., Weinberg, M., Gilbert, K., ... Hutchinson, M. (2015). Interdialytic laughter yoga therapy for haemodialysis patients: A pre-post intervention feasibility study. *BMC Complementary and Alternative Medicine, 15*, 176.

Purpose
Laughter can provide a positive respite from negative emotional effects associated with illness by improving mood and quality of life and reducing depression. The effects of laughter have been manifested as the same outcome whether the laughter is spontaneous or simulated. The authors undertook a feasibility study to determine if laughter yoga, which incorporates clapping, movement of the extremities, deep breathing, neck and shoulder stretches, smiling, and laughter as well as meditation-relaxation, can improve life satisfaction and reduce stress and anxiety in healthy participants receiving hemodialysis.

Design
A 4-week feasibility study was developed with 18 participants with end-stage kidney disease who had been receiving hemodialysis for at least 3 months. Of individuals who completed the study, there were 10 men and seven women, 20 to 89 years of age. The interdialytic intervention was offered by yoga therapists for 30 minutes, three times weekly. Primary outcomes measured at the first and last Laughter Yoga sessions included quality of life, subjective mood, depression, anxiety, and stress. Secondary outcomes were blood pressure, intradialytic hypotensive episodes, and lung function in the form of forced expiratory volume (FEV). Dialysis nurses exposed to

the intervention also rated the outcomes using a survey of attitudes and perceptions.

Findings
The authors found nonsignificant increases in happiness, mood, and optimism with a decrease in stress. Of note is that only 13 of 17 individuals completed the first questionnaire, while nine individuals completed the second questionnaire; the researchers' decision was to not pursue the data further and burden those with chronic illness more. Additional findings revealed episodes of intradialytic hypotension decreased by 80%. There were no changes in lung function; however, there was no pulmonary compromise, which is common in those receiving dialysis. The nurses' feedback revealed Laughter Yoga had a positive impact on patients' mood, and they would recommend this to their patients. The authors determined a minimum of 207 participants would be required to detect key changes in the psychological variables measured.

Nursing Implications
Laughter Yoga is a safe, low-intensity and inexpensive form of intradialytic physical activity that has the potential to improve mood and decrease anxiety in hemodialysis settings. Nurses spontaneously participated in the Laughter Yoga sessions as well; engagement of nurses is important in connection with long-term use of this intervention. A strong sense of humor has been shown to assist patients with coping with stressful life events and increasing the likelihood of survival into old age. While the sample size was small, further studies with larger groups may be of benefit as sustained intradialytic physical activity has been rarely successful in groups with end-stage kidney disease.

---

protein must be of high biologic quality and consist of the essential amino acids to prevent poor protein use and to maintain a positive nitrogen balance (Dudek, 2014). Examples of foods high in biologic protein content are typically from animal sources and include eggs, meat, milk, cheese, poultry, and fish. Usually sodium is restricted to 1 to 3 g/day; fluids are restricted to replace insensible losses (Grossman & Porth, 2014). The goal for patients on hemodialysis is to keep their interdialytic weight gain under 1.5 kg (recall dialysis is typically every 2 to 3 days). Water-soluble vitamins may need to be replaced as they are dialyzed out; these are available in a single gelcap containing vitamins B, C, pyridoxine, folate, riboflavin, biotin, and other supplements (Nephrocaps) (USNLM, n.d.).

Dietary restriction is a difficult lifestyle change for many patients with kidney failure. Patients often feel stigmatized in social situations because they may feel there are few food choices available for their diet. If the restrictions are ignored, life-threatening complications, such as hyperkalemia, hypertension, and pulmonary edema, may result. The nurse who cares for a patient with symptoms or

complications resulting from dietary indiscretion should avoid harsh, judgmental, or punitive tones when communicating with the patient. Rather, the nurse emphasizes the correlation between dietary indiscretion and the outcome, such as hypertension or dyspnea, and promotes self-management of the disease.

Providing Psychosocial Care

Often patients requiring long-term hemodialysis are concerned about the unpredictability of the illness and the disruption to their lives. Financial problems, difficulty working, waning sexual desire and impotence, poor-quality sleep, depression from chronic illness, and fear of dying may occur. Younger patients have concerns about marriage, having children, and the burden on their families. Dialysis treatments and restrictions in food and fluid intake often impose challenges to the patient and family. The time required for dialysis and physician visits as well as fatigue and chronic illness can create conflict, frustration, guilt, and depression. The nurse can encourage caregivers and patients to express concerns, anger, or negative feelings; if not expressed, anger may be directed inward and lead to depression, despair, or suicide. If anger is projected outward to other people, it may destroy already-threatened family relationships.

Depression is a common comorbidity in patients receiving dialysis. Inflammation, uremic toxins, sleep disturbances, pain, fatigue, anorexia, adverse medication effects, dietary constraints, changes in sexual function, role strain, and fear of death may contribute to the development of depression. Depression has been linked to nonadherence to dialysis treatment. Counseling, therapy, and pharmacologic treatment as well as deep slow breathing as a relaxation technique may relieve depression (Tsai et al., 2015). Also a mental health provider with expertise in the care of patients receiving dialysis may be helpful. The sense of loss that the patient experiences cannot be underestimated because every aspect of a "normal life" is disrupted.

Some patients use denial to deal with the overwhelming array of medical issues. Labeling a patient "noncompliant" does not demonstrate respect for the impact of kidney failure and its treatment on the patient and family, nor does it encourage positive coping strategies. The idea of "perfect compliance" should be replaced with the term *adherence*, which is more neutral and encourages the patient to share difficulties, such as indiscretion in fluid intake, so it can be dealt with during dialysis.

Patients and their families should be encouraged to discuss end-of-life options. Only between 21% and 25% of patients on hemodialysis have an advanced directive or living will. The ANNA Ethics Committee has developed an end-of-life module to foster the nurse's role in these discussions (ANNA, 2017).

Teaching Self-Care

The diagnosis of CKD and the need for dialysis may be overwhelming. Many patients with kidney failure have depressed mentation, a shortened attention span, a decreased level of concentration, and altered perception. Therefore, teaching should occur in brief, 10- to 15-minute sessions, with time added for clarification, repetition, reinforcement, and questions from the patient and family. The nurse needs to convey a nonjudgmental attitude to enable the patient and family to discuss feelings about those treatment options and the material taught.

One study indicated that higher levels of knowledge and greater degree of self-management were associated with significant improvement of function and well-being. Teaching materials at all reading levels are available on the National Kidney Foundation and National Institute of Health web sites (www.kidney.org, 2015).

Home Hemodialysis

Although most patients who require hemodialysis undergo the procedure in an outpatient setting, home hemodialysis is an option for some. Patients delivering their own hemodialysis have been shown to increase emotional wellness, energy level, and social functioning. Home hemodialysis allows the patient set the schedule, decreases travel and wait times at the dialysis center, and, if done slowly through the night, increases removal of more phosphorus and wastes. Thus, the patient may not require as much dietary restriction or antihypertensive therapy (NIDDK, nd).

According to the NIDDK, a patient learns to perform treatments at the dialysis center, working with a dialysis nurse. Most people who do home hemodialysis have a family member, neighbor, or close friend who trains with them at the clinic. The dialysis center supplies the machine and equipment, such as dialysis solution, that will be delivered to the home once or twice a month. The training staff makes sure the patient is confident about performing each task before doing home hemodialysis. Someone from the clinic will be available to answer phone calls 24 hours a day. The health care team never forces a patient to use home hemodialysis because this treatment requires significant changes in the home and family. Home hemodialysis must be the patient's and family's decision. During training, the patient and caregiver learn to:

- Prepare equipment and supplies
- Place the needle in the vascular access
- Monitor the machine
- Check BP and pulse
- Keep records of the treatments
- Clean the equipment and the room where dialysis is done
- Order supplies

In addition, training includes how to prepare, operate, and disassemble the dialysis machine; maintain and clean the equipment; administer medications (e.g., heparin) into the machine lines; and handle emergency problems, such as hemodialysis dialyzer rupture, electrical or mechanical problems, hypotension, shock, and seizures.

Before home hemodialysis is initiated, resources are assessed in the home environment, household, and community. The home is surveyed to see if electrical outlets, plumbing facilities, and storage space are adequate. The home must have room for the HD machine, supplies, and, in some cases, a water purification machine. Modifications may be needed to enable the patient and caregiver to perform dialysis safely and to deal with emergencies.

Once home dialysis is initiated, the home care nurse visits periodically to evaluate adherence with the recommended techniques, to assess the patient for complications, to reinforce previous teaching, and to provide reassurance. The patient may report to the dialysis center monthly to see the nephrologist, dialysis nurse, and dietitian. Blood tests will be done to evaluate and adjust hemodialysis treatments.

Continuing Care

The health care team's goal in treating patients undergoing hemodialysis is to maximize the patients' vocational potential, functional status, and quality of life. Many patients can resume relatively normal lives, doing the things that are important to them: traveling, exercising, working, or actively participating in family activities. Outcome goals for renal rehabilitation include employment for those able to work, improved physical functioning of all patients, improved understanding about adaptation and options for living well, increased control over the effects of kidney disease and dialysis, and resumption of activities enjoyed before dialysis. Nurses must shift patient care away from the traditional paradigm of management by the health care team to one of self-management.

Complications

Although hemodialysis can prolong life, it does not alter the natural course of the underlying kidney disease, nor does it completely replace kidney function. The patient is subject to a number of problems and complications. A leading cause of death among patients undergoing maintenance hemodialysis is atherosclerotic cardiovascular disease (USRDS, 2014). Disturbances of lipid metabolism (hypertriglyceridemia) appear to be accentuated by hemodialysis. Anemia and fatigue contribute to diminished physical and emotional well-being, lack of energy and drive, and apathy. Gastric ulcers and other GI problems result from the physiologic stress of chronic illness, medication, and related problems. Disturbed calcium metabolism leads to renal osteodystrophy that produces bone pain and fractures. Other problems include fluid overload associated with heart failure, malnutrition, infection, neuropathy, and pruritus.

Up to 85% of people undergoing hemodialysis experience major sleep problems that further complicate their overall health status. Early-morning or late-afternoon dialysis may be a risk factor for developing sleep disturbances. Interventions, such as changing the temperature of the dialysate bath, may prevent temperature elevation, and limiting napping during dialysis may reduce sleep problems in people receiving hemodialysis. Some centers are offering nocturnal dialysis for 6 to 8 hours nightly.

Other complications during dialysis may include:

- Hypotension associated with nausea and vomiting, diaphoresis, tachycardia, and dizziness due to acute reduction in circulating intravascular volume and the failure of the patient's homeostatic mechanisms to compensate for it
- Painful muscle cramping, usually late in dialysis, as fluid and electrolytes rapidly leave the extracellular space
- Exsanguination if blood lines separate or dialysis needles become dislodged
- Dysrhythmias resulting from changes in electrolytes and pH or from removal of dysrhythmia medications during dialysis
- Air embolism, a rare circumstance, but can occur if air enters the vascular system

- Chest pain, particularly in patients with anemia or arteriosclerotic heart disease
- Dialysis disequilibrium resulting from shifts of cerebral fluid, resulting in headache, nausea and vomiting, restlessness, decreased level of consciousness, and seizures. This is more likely to occur in patients with AKI or when BUN levels are very high.
- Dialyzer clotting, which can be prevented by adjusting heparin doses

ADDITIONAL RENAL REPLACEMENT THERAPIES

Continuous RRT (Joannidis & Forni, 2015) is used with patients demonstrating hemodynamic instability such as hypotension, or in those who cannot tolerate the rapid fluid shifts that may occur with hemodialysis. CRRT (Fig. 27-5) circulates the blood outside the body through a filter similar to the hemodialysis filter. A pump is used to assist blood flow. The types of CRRT include continuous venovenous hemofiltration (CVVH), continuous venovenous hemofiltration with dialysis (CVVHD), and continuous venovenous hemodiafiltration (CVVHDF). Slow, continuous ultrafiltration (SCUF) is performed primarily to remove fluid (Richardson & Whatmore, 2014).

Continuous Venovenous Hemofiltration

CVVH is used to manage AKI. Blood from a double-lumen venous catheter is pumped through a hemofilter and then returned to the patient's body through the same catheter. CVVH provides continuous, slow fluid removal (ultrafiltration); therefore, hemodynamic effects are mild and better

FIGURE 27-5 Diapact® CRRT System.

tolerated by patients with unstable conditions. CVVH does not require arterial access, and critical care nurses can set up, initiate, maintain, and terminate the system.

Continuous Venovenous Hemofiltration with Dialysis

CVVHD is similar to CVVH. Blood is pumped from a double-lumen venous catheter through a hemofilter and then returned to the patient's body through the same catheter. In addition to the benefits of ultrafiltration, CVVHD uses a dialysate to create a concentration gradient, thus facilitating the removal of uremic toxins and fluid. The access required is the same as for emergency hemodialysis (Richardson & Whatmore, 2014). Critical care nurses perform this procedure after competency has been validated.

Continuous Venovenous Hemodiafiltration

An additional modification of the techniques described previously is called CVVHDF. In this technique patients are connected to the CRRT machine, and their blood is pumped through the filter with dialysate running in a counter current flow outside of the hemofilter. Replacement fluid is pumped in after the filter. Using this technique, the end products of nitrogen metabolism (urea, creatinine, uric acid) are removed as well as the ultrafiltrate, which refers to the fluid removed through a semipermeable membrane.

RRT may be intermittent or continuous and described as IRRT or CRRT, respectively. There is some evidence suggesting a worse renal outcome when intermittent therapies are used (Joannidis & Forni, 2015).

Continuous Ultrafiltration

During SCUF, the patient is connected to a machine with a highly permeable filter that primarily removes water (ultrafiltration). This treatment is indicated when the patient has significant fluid overload (Richardson & Whatmore, 2014), such as a patient with heart failure (HF) refractory to diuretics. Since the ultrafiltrate is not replaced it corresponds to fluid loss in the patient.

 Nursing Alert
It is important to secure the central venous catheter used for CRRT to prevent dislodgement. The catheter may be sutured and covered with secure dressing (Richardson & Whatmore, 2014).

PERITONEAL DIALYSIS

The goals of PD are to remove toxic substances and metabolic wastes and to reestablish normal balance of fluids and electrolytes. PD may be performed chronically on an outpatient basis or for patients who are acutely ill, although the latter is falling out of favor. Patients who are unable or unwilling to undergo hemodialysis or renal transplantation, or who do not have access to the bloodstream, can benefit from PD. In addition, patients who do not tolerate the rapid changes in fluids, electrolytes, and metabolism that occur during hemodialysis experience fewer of these problems with the slower rate of PD. Therefore, patients with diabetes or cardiovascular disease, many older patients (Lewis, 2013), and those who may be at risk for adverse effects of systemic heparin are likely candidates for PD. Additionally, severe hypertension, heart failure, and pulmonary edema not responsive to usual treatment regimens have been treated successfully with PD.

During PD, the thin, serous peritoneal membrane that covers the abdominal organs and lines the abdominal wall serves as the semipermeable or dialyzing membrane (Porth, 2015). Sterile dialysate fluid is introduced into the peritoneal cavity through a peritoneal or Tenckhoff catheter (Fig. 27-6). Diffusion across the semipermeable membrane removes urea creatinine and metabolic end products normally excreted by the kidneys. Excess fluid is removed through osmosis as water moves from an area of lower particle concentration in the patient's blood to an area of higher concentration across a semipermeable membrane into the dialysate. Dialysis solutions are available in concentrations of 1.5%, 2.5%, and 4.25% dextrose. This concentration gradient for fluid removal is created by varying concentrations of glucose; the higher the dextrose concentration, the greater the osmotic gradient and the more water will be removed. PD is a slower process than hemodialysis; therefore, it takes longer to reach equilibrium.

FIGURE 27-6 In peritoneal dialysis (PD) and in acute intermittent PD, dialysate is infused into the peritoneal cavity by gravity, after which the clamp on the infusion line is closed. After a dwell time (when the dialysate is in the peritoneal cavity), the drainage tube is unclamped and the fluid drains from the peritoneal cavity, again by gravity. A new container of dialysate is infused as soon as drainage is complete. The duration of the dwell time depends on the type of PD.

When assessing a patient for suitability for PD, the nurse must evaluate whether the patient's home is clean and has space for storage of equipment. Patients or caregivers must be able to lift dialysate bags, have appropriate cognitive function and dexterity to work the machine, and maintain asepsis (Lewis, 2013). Therefore, PD, while gentler on the cardiovascular system, is offered less often to the elderly than hemodialysis.

Procedure

Preparing the Patient

Insertion of the peritoneal catheter may be performed at the bedside or in the operating room, depending on acuity of the patient. A broad-spectrum antibiotic may be administered prior to the procedure to prevent postoperative infection. The patient is encouraged to empty the bladder and bowel prior to catheter insertion to reduce the risk of puncturing internal organs. Baseline vital signs, weight, and serum electrolyte levels are recorded. The nurse also assesses the patient's anxiety about the procedure and provides support and instruction.

Preparing the Equipment

Aseptic technique is imperative during PD. The nurse assembles the equipment, including the dialysate and any medications to be added. Heparin may be added to prevent occlusion of the peritoneal catheter, potassium chloride to prevent hypokalemia, and antibiotics to prevent or treat **peritonitis**. The osmotic agent in the dialysate is glucose, which may be absorbed; therefore, regular insulin may be added.

> **Nursing Alert**
> *It is important to remember that peritoneal solutions contain varying concentrations of glucose. Because 30% to 40% of patients receiving PD are diabetic, glycemic monitoring is critical.*

Before medications are added, the dialysate is warmed to the temperature dictated by hospital policy to prevent abdominal discomfort and to dilate the vessels of the peritoneum to increase urea clearance. Dry heating with a heating cabinet or incubator is recommended. Microwave heating of the fluid is *not* recommended because of the danger of burning the peritoneum. The nurse primes the PD tubing with the dialysate to prevent air from entering the peritoneal cavity.

Catheters used for long-term PD (i.e., Tenckhoff) usually are made of silicone and are radiopaque to permit visualization on x-ray. The catheter has two cuffs, which stabilize the catheter, limit movement, prevent leaks, and provide a barrier against microorganisms. One cuff is placed just distal to the peritoneum, and the other cuff is placed subcutaneously. The subcutaneous tunnel (5 to 10 cm long) further protects against bacterial infection (Fig. 27-7).

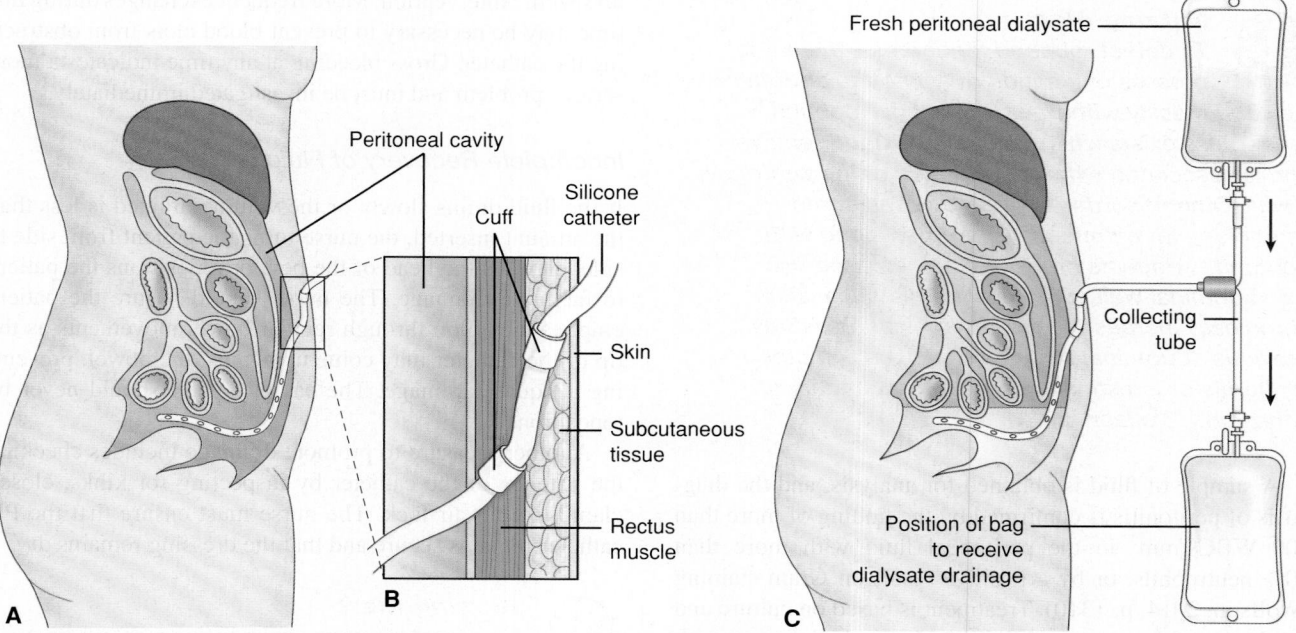

FIGURE 27-7 Continuous ambulatory peritoneal dialysis. **A.** The peritoneal catheter is implanted through the abdominal wall. **B.** Dacron cuffs and a subcutaneous tunnel provide protection against bacterial infection. **C.** Dialysate flows by gravity through the peritoneal catheter into the peritoneal cavity. After a prescribed period of time, the fluid is drained by gravity and discarded. Then new solution is infused into the peritoneal cavity until the next drainage period. Dialysis thus continues on a 24-hour-a-day basis during which the patient is free to move around and engage in his or her usual activities.

Performing the Exchange

PD involves a series of exchanges or cycles. An exchange is defined as the infusion, dwell, and drainage of the dialysate. This cycle is repeated throughout the course of the dialysis. The dialysate is infused by gravity into the peritoneal cavity. Usually a period of about 5 to 10 minutes is required to infuse 2 L of fluid. The prescribed dwell, or equilibration time, allows both diffusion and osmosis to occur. At the end of the dwell time, the drainage portion of the exchange begins. The solution drains from the peritoneal cavity by gravity through a closed, sterile system. Usually drainage is completed in 10 to 30 minutes. The effluent or drainage fluid is normally clear, colorless, or straw-colored. Bloody drainage may be seen in the first few exchanges after insertion of a new catheter but should not occur after that time. Cloudy drainage may indicate infection.

The number of cycles or exchanges, their frequency, and concentration of dialysate solution are prescribed based on the patient's physical status, fluid balance, and acuity of illness.

Complications

Peritonitis

Peritonitis is the most serious complication of PD. The nurse assesses for cloudy drainage or effluent, low-grade fever, abdominal pain, malaise (Wolfson, 2014), and rebound tenderness.

 Nursing Alert
To detect rebound tenderness, the nurse presses one hand firmly into the abdominal wall and quickly withdraws the hand. Rebound tenderness exists when pain occurs upon removal and is associated with inflammation of the peritoneal cavity. Other disorders should be considered as etiology for a patient's symptoms along with peritonitis. Patients on PD are at increased risk for abdominal wall or inguinal hernia because of chronically increased intra-abdominal pressures; previous abdominal surgery is also a risk factor for hernia or intestinal obstruction secondary to adhesions (Wolfson, 2014).

A sample of fluid is obtained for analysis, and the diagnosis of peritonitis is confirmed by the finding of more than 100 WBCs/mm^3 in the peritoneal fluid with more than 50% neutrophils, or by a positive result on Gram staining (Wolfson, 2014, p. 1310). Treatment is based on culture and sensitivity of the peritoneal fluid. Antimicrobial therapy with a cephalosporin or aminoglycoside may be administered intravenously and/or added to the dialysate. Hypotension and other signs of shock may occur. Regardless of which organism causes peritonitis, the patient with peritonitis loses large amounts of protein through the peritoneum. Acute malnutrition

and delayed healing may result. Therefore, attention must be given to detecting and treating peritonitis promptly.

Leakage

Leakage of dialysate around the catheter site must be corrected because the area acts as a pathway for bacteria to enter the peritoneal cavity. Usually, the leak stops spontaneously if dialysis is withheld for several days to give the incision and exit site time to heal. If necessary, leakage of dialysate around the catheter site may be managed with extra sutures and a decrease in the amount of dialysate used. Increases in intra-abdominal pressure, such as vomiting, coughing, and straining during bowel movements, should be avoided as these may delay healing. Leakage through the exit site or into the abdominal wall can occur for months or years after catheter placement.

Bleeding

A bloody effluent (drainage) may be expected in the initial outflow or observed occasionally in young, menstruating women (retrograde menstruation, or endometriosis). Bleeding is common during the first few exchanges after a new catheter insertion because some blood enters the abdominal cavity following insertion. During menstruation, the hypertonic fluid pulls blood from the uterus, through the opening in the fallopian tubes, into the peritoneal cavity. Some patients have had bloody effluent after an enema or from minor trauma. Invariably, bleeding stops in 1 to 2 days and requires no specific intervention. More frequent exchanges during this time may be necessary to prevent blood clots from obstructing the catheter. Gross bleeding at any time indicates a more serious problem and must be investigated immediately.

Incomplete Recovery of Fluid

If the fluid drains slowly or the volume drained is less than the amount inserted, the nurse turns the patient from side to side, elevates the head of the bed, or repositions the patient to facilitate drainage. The nurse should ensure the patient empties the colon through regular bowel movements as the tip of the catheter may come up against the bowel, preventing adequate drainage. The catheter itself should never be repositioned.

Another measure to promote drainage includes checking the patency of the catheter by inspecting for kinks, closed clamps, or an air lock. The nurse must ensure that the PD catheter remains secure and that the dressing remains dry.

 Nursing Alert
The most common reason for outflow delay or failure to drain dialysate is constipation, which typically is treated with oral laxatives or an enema. There is an increased risk of constipation for patients on PD because of restrictions on fluid or diet as well as the administration of medications,

BOX 27-8

Assessing Suitability for Continuous Ambulatory Peritoneal Dialysis (CAPD)

Although CAPD is not suitable for all patients with kidney failure, it is a viable therapy for those who can perform self-care and exchanges and who can fit therapy into their own routines. Often, patients report having more energy and feeling healthier once they begin CAPD. Nurses can be instrumental in helping patients with kidney failure find the dialysis therapy that best suits their lifestyle. Those considering CAPD need to investigate the advantages and disadvantages along with the indications and contraindications for this form of therapy.

Advantages

- Freedom from a dialysis machine
- Control over daily activities
- Opportunities to avoid dietary restrictions, increase fluid intake, raise serum hematocrit values, improve BP control, avoid venipuncture, and gain a sense of well-being

Disadvantages

- Continuous dialysis 24 hours a day, 7 days a week

Indications

- Patient's willingness, motivation, and ability to perform dialysis at home
- Strong family or community support system (essential for success), particularly if the patient is an older adult

- Special problems with long-term hemodialysis, such as dysfunctional or failing vascular access devices, excessive thirst, severe hypertension, postdialysis headaches, and severe anemia requiring frequent transfusion
- Interim therapy while awaiting kidney transplantation
- Kidney failure secondary to diabetes because hypertension, uremia, and hyperglycemia are easier to manage with CAPD than with hemodialysis

Contraindications

- Adhesions from previous surgery (adhesions reduce clearance of solutes) or systemic inflammatory disease
- Chronic backache and pre-existing disc disease, which could be aggravated by the pressure of dialysis fluid in the abdomen
- Risk of complications, for example, in patients receiving immunosuppressive medications, which impede healing of the catheter site, and in patients with a colostomy, ileostomy, nephrostomy, or ileal conduit because of the risk of peritonitis. The risk for complications is not an absolute contraindication for CAPD therapy but must be taken into consideration.
- Diverticulitis, because CAPD has been associated with rupture of the diverticulum
- Severe arthritis or poor hand strength, necessitating assistance in performing the exchange; however, patients who are blind or partially blind and those with other physical limitations can learn to perform CAPD.

such as phosphate binders. After resolution of the constipation, the nurse should educate the patient about monitoring his or her bowel pattern and having an established bowel regimen. Current studies on constipation in PD patients are limited; best practice has yet to be established.

Other Complications

Hypertriglyceridemia is common in patients undergoing long-term PD as well as in long-term hemodialysis. Cardiovascular disease is a major cause of morbidity and mortality and is managed with beta blockers, ACE inhibitors, aspirin, and statins.

Other complications that may occur with long-term PD include abdominal hernias (incisional, inguinal, diaphragmatic, and umbilical). The persistently elevated intra-abdominal pressure also aggravates symptoms of hiatal hernia and hemorrhoids. Low back pain and anorexia from fluid in the abdomen and a constant sweet taste related to glucose absorption also may occur.

Approaches to Peritoneal Dialysis

PD can be performed using several different approaches: acute continuous or intermittent PD, continuous ambulatory PD (CAPD), and continuous cyclic PD (CCPD).

Continuous Ambulatory Peritoneal Dialysis

CAPD works on the same principles as other forms of PD; however, there are less extreme fluctuations in the patient's laboratory values with CAPD than with intermittent PD or hemodialysis because the dialysis is constantly in progress. CAPD is performed at home by the patient or a trained caregiver; the procedure allows the patient reasonable freedom and control of daily activities (Box 27-8).

The patient performs exchanges four or five times a day, 24 hours a day, 7 days a week, at intervals scheduled throughout the day. The dialysate dwells for the prescribed period of time; 4 to 6 hours is common. The patient is free to ambulate and participate in activities of daily living. At the end of the dwell time, the dialysate is drained from the peritoneal cavity into the empty sterile bag. Box 27-9 provides nursing management for CAPD.

Continuous Cyclic Peritoneal Dialysis

CCPD combines overnight intermittent PD with a prolonged dwell time during the day. The peritoneal catheter is connected to a cycler machine every evening, and the patient receives three to five exchanges during the night. In the morning, the patient caps off the catheter after infusing 1.5 to 2.5 L of fresh dialysate. This dialysate remains in the

BOX 27-9 **Nursing Management for Peritoneal Dialysis**

Caring for the Catheter Site

To reduce the risk of peritonitis in the patient using peritoneal dialysis (PD), the patient must use meticulous care to avoid contaminating the catheter, fluid, or tubing and to avoid accidentally disconnecting the catheter from the tubing. Excess manipulation is avoided, and meticulous care of the catheter entry site is provided using a standardized protocol. The patient and other caregivers who are present wear a mask and use strict aseptic technique for preparation of the dialysate and dressing changes.

The nurse uses every opportunity to assess technique of catheter care and correct the patient's technique. Routine catheter site care, recommended daily or three or four times weekly, typically is performed during showering or bathing. The exit site should not be submerged in bath water. The most common cleaning method is soap and water; liquid soap is recommended. During care, the nurse and patient need to make sure that the catheter remains secure to avoid tension and trauma. The patient may wear a gauze or semitransparent dressing over the exit site.

Meeting Psychosocial Needs

In addition to the complications of PD previously described, patients who elect to use continuous ambulatory peritoneal dialysis (CAPD) may experience altered body image because of the abdominal catheter and the bag and tubing. Waist size increases from 1 to 2 in (or more) with fluid in the abdomen. This affects clothing selection and may make the patient feel "fat." Body image may be so altered that patients do not want to look at or care for the catheter for days or weeks. The nurse may arrange for the patient to talk with other patients who have adapted well to CAPD. Although some patients have no psychological problems with the catheter—they think of it as their lifeline and as a life-sustaining device—other patients feel they are doing exchanges all day long and have no free time, particularly in the beginning. They may experience depression because they feel overwhelmed with the responsibility of self-care.

Patients undergoing CAPD also may experience altered sexuality patterns and sexual dysfunction. The patient and partner may be reluctant to engage in sexual activities, partly because of the catheter being psychologically "in the way" of sexual performance. The peritoneal catheter, drainage bag, and about 2 L of dialysate may interfere with the patient's sexual function and body image as well. Although these problems may resolve with time, some problems may warrant special counseling. Questions by the nurse about concerns related to sexuality and sexual function often provide the patient with a welcome opportunity to discuss these issues and provide a first step toward their resolution.

Teaching Patients Self-Care

Patients are taught to perform PD according to their own learning ability and knowledge level and are given only as much information at one time as they can handle without feeling uncomfortable or becoming overwhelmed.

Because protein loss is higher with PD than with hemodialysis, the patient is instructed to eat a well-balanced diet that is high in protein. Also the patient is encouraged to increase his or her daily fiber intake to help prevent constipation, which can impede the flow of dialysate into or out of the peritoneal cavity. Many patients gain 3 to 5 lb within a month of initiating CAPD so they may be asked to limit their carbohydrate intake to avoid excessive weight gain. Usually restrictions on potassium, sodium, and fluids are not needed. Patients commonly lose about 2 to 3 L of fluid over and above the volume of dialysate infused into the abdomen during a 24-hour period, permitting a more normal fluid intake.

Continuing Care

The nurse assesses that strict aseptic technique is being followed. Blood chemistry values are followed closely to make certain the therapy is adequate for the patient. The home care nurse assesses the home environment and suggests modifications to accommodate the equipment and facilities needed to carry out CAPD. Additional assessments include checking for changes related to kidney disease, complications such as peritonitis, and treatment-related problems such as heart failure, inadequate drainage, and weight gain or loss. The nurse continues to reinforce and clarify teaching about kidney failure and kidney disease while assessing the patient's and family's progress in coping with the procedure.

---

abdominal cavity until the tubing is reattached to the cycler machine at bedtime.

CCPD has a lower rate of infection than other forms of PD because there are fewer opportunities for contamination with bag changes and tubing disconnections. It also allows the patient to be free from exchanges throughout the day, making it possible to engage more freely in work and activities of daily living.

KIDNEY TRANSPLANTATION

Kidney transplantation has become the treatment of choice for most patients with end-stage kidney failure. Each year, between 17,000 and 18,000 total renal transplants, including combined kidney–pancreas, kidney–liver, and kidney–heart, are performed in the United States (Cohen & Valeri, 2016). Waiting times for transplantation across the country continue to increase; the active waiting list is three times longer than the supply of donor kidneys (USRDS, 2014). The median waiting time for a patient awaiting kidney transplantation is currently 4.3 years (Cohen & Valeri, 2016). Healthy People 2020 calls to increase the proportion of patients with kidney failure who receive a transplant within 3 years. A second goal is to increase the proportion of patients who receive a preemptive transplant at the start of kidney failure. Unfortunately, approximately 10% of newly listed candidates for kidney transplants will die within three years waiting for the organ (Cohen & Valeri, 2016). See Box 27-10 regarding kidney donation.

Kidney Donation

An inadequate number of available kidneys remain the greatest limitation to treating patients with end-stage kidney disease successfully. For those interested in donating a kidney, the National Kidney Foundation provides written information describing the organ donation program and a card specifying the organs to be donated in the event of death.

The organ donation card is signed by the donor and two witnesses and should be carried by the donor at all times. Procurement of an adequate number of kidneys for potential recipients is still a major problem despite national legislation that requires relatives of deceased patients or patients declared brain-dead to be asked if they would consider organ donation.

In some states in the United States, drivers can indicate their desire to be organ donors on their driver's license application or renewal.

https://www.google.com/search?q=sample+organ+donation+drivers+license

Patients choose kidney transplantation for various reasons, such as the desire to avoid dialysis or to improve their sense of well-being and the wish to lead a more normal life. Additionally, the cost of maintaining a successful transplantation is one third the cost of dialysis treatment. Patients on dialysis have an adjusted all-cause mortality rate that is 6.5 to 7.4 times higher than that of the general population; the rate is 1.1 to 1.6 times higher for transplant patients (www.kidneyfund.org.).

Kidney transplantation involves transplanting a kidney from a living donor or heartbeat-only donor (one who has been pronounced brain dead but whose cardiopulmonary system is maintained artificially) to a recipient who has end-stage kidney failure (Box 27-10). Kidney transplant donors had traditionally been blood relatives; however, living donor kidney transplant (LDKT) between spouses, friends, and those on organ registries may be performed. The LDKT provides a better quality kidney more quickly than from a heart beat only donor (Skelton et al., 2015). The success rate increases if kidney transplantation from a living donor is performed before dialysis is initiated; this is referred to as *preemptive transplant*.

Depending on the cause and symptoms of kidney failure, occasionally a nephrectomy of the patient's own native kidneys may be performed before transplantation. The transplanted kidney is placed in the patient's iliac fossa anterior to the iliac crest. The renal artery of the donor is anastomosed to the hypogastric, renal, or iliac artery of the recipient. The ureter of the newly transplanted kidney is anastomosed to the ureter of the recipient, and the renal vein is anastomosed to the renal vein of the recipient (Fig. 27-8). The left donor kidney is preferred because the left renal vein is longer than the right (6 to 7 cm vs. 2 to 4 cm).

Medical and Nursing Management

Preoperative Management

Preoperative management goals include bringing the patient's metabolic state to a level as close to normal as possible, making sure that the patient is free of infection, and preparing the patient for surgery and the postoperative course. Preoperatively,

FIGURE 27-8 Kidney transplantation: (*1*) The diseased kidney may be removed and the renal artery and vein tied off. (*2*) The transplanted kidney is placed in the iliac fossa. (*3*) The renal artery of the donated kidney is sutured to the iliac artery, and the renal vein is sutured to the iliac vein. (*4*) The ureter of the donated kidney is sutured to the bladder or to the patient's ureter.

immunosuppressant medication is initiated prior to the transplant to prevent rejection of the new kidney.

A complete physical examination is performed to detect and treat any conditions that could cause complications after transplantation. Tissue typing, blood typing, and antibody screening are performed to determine compatibility of the tissues and cells of the donor and recipient. Other diagnostic tests must be completed to identify conditions requiring treatment before transplantation. The lower urinary tract is studied to assess bladder neck function and to detect urethral reflux.

The patient must be free of infection and cancers at the time of renal transplantation because medications to prevent transplant rejection suppress the immune response, leaving the patient at risk for infection. Therefore, the patient is evaluated and treated for any infections, including gingival (gum) disease and dental caries.

A psychosocial evaluation is conducted to assess the patient's ability to adjust to the transplant, coping styles, social history, social support available, and financial resources. A history of psychiatric illness is important to obtain because often psychiatric conditions are aggravated by the corticosteroids needed for immunosuppression after transplantation. If a dialysis routine has been established, hemodialysis is performed the day before the scheduled transplantation procedure to optimize the patient's physical status.

The nursing aspects of preoperative care for the patient undergoing renal transplant are similar to those for patients undergoing other types of elective abdominal surgery. Preoperative teaching addresses postoperative pulmonary hygiene, pain management options, dietary restrictions, IV and arterial lines, tubes such as an indwelling catheter and possibly a nasogastric tube, and early ambulation. The patient who receives a kidney from a living-related donor often expresses concern about the donor and how the donor will handle the procedure as well as long-term consequences of donation (Sierverdes et al., 2014).

Most patients have been on dialysis for months or years before transplantation. Many have waited months to years for a kidney transplant and are anxious about the surgery, possible rejection, and the need to return to dialysis. Helping the patient to deal with these concerns is part of the nurse's role in preoperative management as is teaching the patient about what to expect after surgery. A plan of nursing care for a patient undergoing kidney surgery is available online at http://thepoint.lww.com/Honan2e.

Postoperative Management

The goal of care is to maintain homeostasis until the transplanted kidney is functioning well. The patient whose transplanted kidney functions immediately has a more favorable prognosis than does the patient whose transplanted kidney does not.

Antirejection Medication

The survival of a transplanted kidney depends on the ability to prevent the body's immune response to the transplanted kidney. To overcome or minimize the body's defense mechanism, immunosuppressive agents are administered. Corticosteroids are initially part of the immunosuppression regimen but are frequently tapered due to long-term side effects (Wright, 2014). Cyclosporine is available in a microemulsion form (Neoral) that delivers the medication reliably, thus producing a steady-state serum concentration. Tacrolimus (Prograf) is similar to cyclosporine, is about 100 times more potent, and may be more effective in some patients at preventing transplant rejection. Tacrolimus and cyclosporine have received a pregnancy category C designation. This designation means that animal studies have shown an adverse effect and there are no adequate well-controlled studies in pregnant women or no studies have been conducted on animals or humans. Mycophenolate mofetil (CellCept), sirolimus (Rapamune), and antithymocyte globulin (Thymoglobulin), as well as tacrolimus, are used in various combinations to prevent transplant rejection. Treatment with combinations of these new agents has improved survival rates dramatically (Adams & Urban, 2016).

Doses of corticosteroid agents are tapered gradually over a period of several weeks, depending on the patient's immunologic response to the transplant. Corticosteroids may be discontinued, but the nurse reinforces that the patient must take some form of immunosuppressive therapy for the life of the transplanted kidney (Wright, 2014).

The side effects and risks associated with these medications include nephrotoxicity, hypertension, hyperlipidemia, hirsutism, headache, tremor, and several types of cancers (Adams & Urban, 2016).

> ### Drug Alert!
> Long-term use of corticosteroids is associated with hypertension, hyperlipidemia, diabetes, infection, osteoporosis, avascular necrosis, weight gain, cataracts, and mood changes and may contribute to development or worsening of cardiovascular disease (Wright, 2014).

> ### Drug Alert!
> Echinacea, often used to treat the common cold and influenza, may interfere with the action of immunosuppressant medications, resulting in subtherapeutic levels (Adams & Urban, 2016).

Assessing the Patient for Transplant Rejection

After kidney transplantation, the nurse assesses the patient for signs and symptoms of transplant rejection: oliguria, edema, fever, increasing BP, weight gain, and swelling or tenderness over the transplanted kidney or graft. Leukocytosis and increasing BUN and creatinine levels should be evaluated. Patients receiving cyclosporine may not exhibit the usual signs and symptoms of acute rejection. In these patients, the only sign may be an asymptomatic rise in the serum creatinine level (a rise of more than 20% is considered

Renal Transplant Rejection and Infection

Renal graft rejection and failure may occur immediately (hyperacute), within the first 2 weeks, or later. Failure is potentially reversible (acute), or the transplanted kidney may steadily lose function after many years (chronic). It is not uncommon for rejection to occur during the first year after transplantation.

Detecting Rejection

Ultrasonography may be used to detect enlargement of the kidney; percutaneous renal biopsy (most reliable) and x-ray techniques are used to evaluate transplant rejection. If the body rejects the transplanted kidney, the patient needs to return to dialysis. The rejected kidney might not be removed, depending on the risk for infection if the kidney is left in place.

Risk for Infection

About 75% of recipients of kidney transplant have at least one episode of infection in the first year after transplantation because of immunosuppressant therapy. Immunosuppressants of the past made the transplant recipient more vulnerable to opportunistic infections (candidiasis, cytomegalovirus, *Pneumocystis* pneumonia) and infection with other relatively nonpathogenic viruses, fungi, and protozoa, which can be a major hazard. Cyclosporine therapy has reduced the incidence of opportunistic infections because it selectively exerts its effect, sparing T cells that protect the patient from life-threatening infections. In addition, combination immunosuppressant therapy and improved clinical care have produced 1-year patient survival rates approaching 100% and graft survival exceeding 90%. Infections, however, remain a major cause of death at all points in time for recipients of kidney transplant.

acute rejection). Box 27-11 discusses renal transplant rejection and infection.

Preventing Infection

The patient is monitored closely for infection because of susceptibility to impaired healing and infection related to immunosuppressive therapy and complications of kidney failure. Clinical manifestations of infection include shaking, chills, fever, tachycardia, and tachypnea as well as either an increase or a decrease in WBCs (leukocytosis or leukopenia).

Infection may be introduced through the urinary tract, the respiratory tract, the surgical site, or other sources. Urine cultures are performed frequently because of the high incidence of bacteriuria during early and late stages of transplantation. Any type of wound drainage should be viewed as a potential source of infection because drainage is an excellent culture medium for bacteria. Catheter and drain tips should be cut with sterile scissors, placed in a sterile container, and sent to the laboratory for culture.

The nurse ensures that the patient is protected from exposure to infection by hospital staff, visitors, and other patients with active infections. Careful hand hygiene is imperative for all who come in contact with the patient.

Monitoring Urinary Function

A kidney from a living donor related to the patient usually begins to function immediately after surgery and may produce large quantities of dilute urine. A kidney from a nonliving donor may undergo ATN and, therefore, may not function for 2 or 3 weeks, during which time anuria, oliguria, or polyuria may be present. During this stage, the patient may experience significant changes in fluid and electrolyte status. Therefore, careful monitoring of hourly urine output should be performed. IV fluids are administered on the basis of urine volume and serum electrolyte levels and as prescribed by the provider. Hemodialysis may be necessary postoperatively to maintain homeostasis until the transplanted kidney is functioning well.

Addressing Psychological Concerns

The rejection of a transplanted kidney remains a matter of great concern to the patient, the family, and the health care team. The fears of kidney rejection and the complications of immunosuppressive therapy, which include Cushing syndrome, diabetes, capillary fragility, osteoporosis, glaucoma, cataracts, acne, and nephrotoxicity, place tremendous psychological stresses on the patient. Often anxiety and uncertainty about the future and difficult posttransplantation adjustment are sources of stress for the patient and family.

An important nursing function is the assessment of the patient's stress and coping. The nurse uses each visit with the patient to determine if the patient and family are coping effectively and if the patient is adhering to the prescribed medication regimen. If indicated or requested, the nurse refers the patient for counseling.

Monitoring and Managing Potential Complications

The patient undergoing kidney transplantation is at risk for the postoperative complications that are associated with any surgical procedure. In addition, the patient's physical condition may be compromised because of the complications associated with longstanding kidney failure and its treatment. Therefore, careful assessment for the complications related to kidney failure and corticosteroid use, such as poor wound healing, is an important aspect of nursing care.

GI ulceration and corticosteroid-induced bleeding may occur. Fungal colonization of the GI tract, especially the mouth and urinary bladder, may occur secondary to corticosteroid and antibiotic therapy. Closely monitoring the patient and notifying the provider about the occurrence of these complications are important nursing interventions. In addition, the patient is monitored closely for adverse effects of corticosteroids or signs of adrenal insufficiency when these medications are discontinued.

Teaching Patients Self-Care

The nurse works closely with the patient and family to be sure that they understand the need for continuing immunosuppressive therapy as prescribed. Additionally, the patient and family are instructed to assess for and report signs and symptoms of transplant rejection, infection, or significant adverse effects of the immunosuppressive regimen. These include decreased urine output; weight gain; malaise; fever; respiratory distress; tenderness over the transplanted kidney; anxiety; depression; changes in eating, drinking, or other habits; and changes in BP. The patient is instructed to inform other health care providers (e.g., dentist) about the kidney transplant and the use of immunosuppressive agents.

Continuing Care

Follow-up care with the transplant team is a lifelong necessity. Individual verbal and written instructions are provided concerning diet, medication, fluids, daily weight, daily measurement of urine, management of intake and output, prevention of infection, resumption of activity, and avoidance of contact sports in which the transplanted kidney may be injured. Cardiovascular disease is the major cause of morbidity and mortality after transplantation, due in part to the increasing age of patients with transplants.

Malignancy develops more frequently in patients receiving long-term immunosuppressive therapy. Posttransplant, patients are at increased risk for various conditions: a "20-fold increase for non-Hodgkin lymphomas, nonmelanoma skin cancers, and Kaposi sarcoma; a 15-fold increase for kidney cancers; a 5-fold increase for melanoma, leukemia, hepatobiliary tumors, cervical tumors, and vulvovaginal tumors; a 3-fold increase for testicular and bladder cancers; and a 2-fold increase for most common tumors (e.g., colon, lung, prostate, stomach, esophagus, pancreas, ovary, and breast)" (Flechner, 2013). The patient is reminded of the importance of health-promotion activities, such as using sunscreen and health screenings, including regular PAP smears, mammogram, colonoscopy, and breast or testicular self-examination as appropriate.

The American Association of Kidney Patients (see Resources) is a nonprofit organization that serves the needs of those with kidney disease. It can provide many helpful suggestions for patients and family members learning to cope with dialysis and transplantation.

RENAL TRAUMA

The kidneys are protected by the rib cage and musculature of the back posteriorly and by a cushion of abdominal wall and viscera anteriorly. They are highly mobile and are fixed only at the renal pedicle (stem of renal blood vessels and the ureter). With traumatic injury, the kidneys can be thrust against the lower ribs, resulting in contusion and rupture. Renal trauma occurs in approximately 10% of abdominal injuries,

and 90% of renal trauma is due to blunt injury (automobile and motorcycle collisions, falls, athletic injuries, assaults) (Coburn, 2013). The nurse should suspect renal injury when the patient presents with blunt abdominal or penetrating flank and back wounds (gunshot wounds, stabbings); nearly all patients with renal gunshot wounds have associated injuries of other internal organs. For renal stab wounds, approximately 60% of have additional intra-abdominal injuries (Coburn, 2013).

Blunt renal trauma is classified into one of four groups, as follows:

- *Contusion:* Bruises or hemorrhages under the renal capsule; capsule and collecting system intact
- *Minor laceration:* Superficial disruption of the cortex; renal medulla and collecting system are not involved
- *Major laceration:* Parenchymal disruption extending into cortex and medulla, possibly involving the collecting system
- *Vascular injury:* Tears of renal artery or vein

The most common renal injuries are contusions, lacerations, ruptures, and renal pedicle injuries or small internal lacerations of the kidney (Fig. 27-9). The kidneys receive half of the blood flow from the abdominal aorta; therefore, even a fairly small renal laceration can produce massive bleeding. The nurse should consider hemorrhage is likely present when gross hematuria or microscopic hematuria occurs. Additional signs of hemorrhage include a decreasing BP, MAP below 65 mm Hg, or tachycardia without a discernible cause, such as pain.

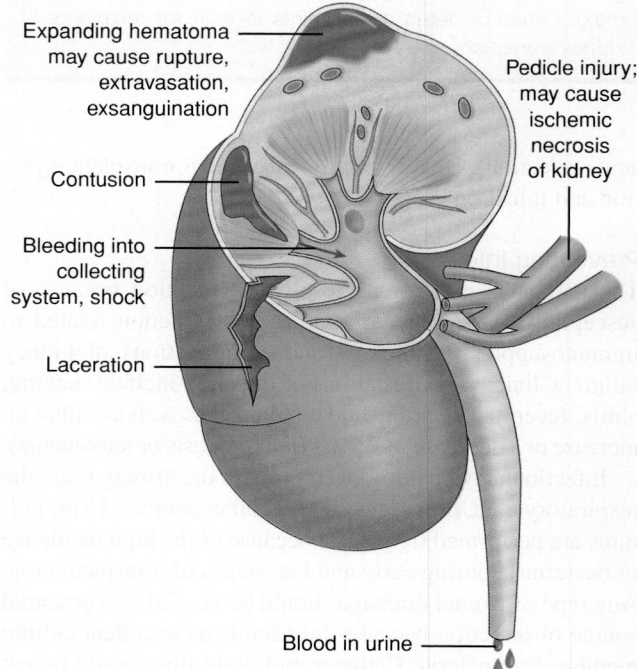

FIGURE 27-9 Types and pathophysiologic effects of renal injuries: contusions, lacerations, rupture, and pedicle injury.

FIGURE 27-10 Ecchymosis with renal trauma. **A.** Grey–Turner sign. **B.** Cullen sign. (A from D. Berg, & K. Worzala. (2006). *Atlas of adult physical diagnosis*. Philadelphia, PA: Lippincott Williams & Wilkins.)

Clinical Manifestations and Assessment

Clinical manifestations of renal injury include pain, renal colic (due to blood clots or fragments obstructing the collecting system), hematuria, mass or swelling in the flank, ecchymosis, and lacerations or wounds of the lateral abdomen and flank. While hematuria is the most common manifestation of renal trauma, there is no relationship between the degree of hematuria and the degree of injury.

The nurse assesses for ecchymosis over the flank (Grey–Turner sign) and periumbilical area (Cullen sign) as well as flank tenderness with palpation and gross hematuria (Fig. 27-10).

> ### Nursing Alert
> *Grey–Turner sign and Cullen sign are associated with retroperitoneal bleeds.*

Microscopic hematuria may be present; therefore, evaluation of hemoglobin and hematocrit is critical. A CT scan of the abdomen may be done to assess penetrating trauma. Free air, injury to the kidney, or a penetrating object is assessed. Any patient with gross hematuria will need to be evaluated, although the nurse should recognize that the amount of hematuria correlates poorly with the magnitude of injury (Coburn, 2013).

Medical and Nursing Management

The goals of management in patients with renal trauma are to control hemorrhage and pain, to prevent infection, and to preserve and restore kidney function. The patient is monitored for oliguria and signs of hemorrhagic shock because a pedicle injury or shattered kidney can lead to rapid exsanguination and death. An expanding hematoma may cause rupture of the kidney capsule. A palpable flank or abdominal mass with local tenderness, swelling, and ecchymosis suggests renal hemorrhage. The area of the original mass can be outlined with a marking pen so that the examiner can evaluate the area for change.

Often renal trauma is associated with other injuries to nearby organs; therefore, the patient is assessed for skin abrasions, lacerations, and entry and exit wounds of the upper abdomen and lower thorax because these may be associated with renal injury. Trauma to the right kidney may be associated with liver injury while trauma to the left kidney may involve injury to the spleen. In rare cases, damage to the adrenal gland may result in adrenal insufficiency and death.

With a contusion of the kidney, healing may take place with conservative measures. If the patient has microscopic hematuria and a normal IV urogram, bed rest will allow the contusion to resolve with time (Coburn, 2013), and outpatient management is possible. If gross hematuria or a minor laceration is present, the patient is hospitalized and kept on bed rest until the hematuria clears. Antimicrobial medications may be prescribed to prevent infection from perirenal hematoma or urinoma (a cyst containing urine). Patients with retroperitoneal hematomas may develop low-grade fever as absorption of the clot takes place.

> ### Nursing Alert
> *When caring for a trauma patient, if the patient presents with blood at the urethral meatus, an inability to void, and a perineal hematoma, a urethral injury should be suspected. Insertion of a urinary catheter should NOT be undertaken until the patient is evaluated by the provider.*

Surgical Management

In renal trauma, any sudden change in the patient's condition suggests hemorrhage and requires rapid surgical intervention within 12 hours to reestablish blood flow to the ischemic kidney (Eswara, 2015). The patient is often in shock and requires aggressive fluid resuscitation. The damaged kidney may have to be removed (nephrectomy).

Early postoperative complications (within 6 months) include rebleeding, formation of a perinephritic abscess, sepsis, urine extravasation, and formation of a fistula. Other complications include formation of stones, infection or abscess, cysts, chronic pyelonephrosis, vascular aneurysms, and loss of kidney function. Hypertension can be a complication of any renal surgery but usually is a late complication of renal injury.

The patient who has undergone surgery is instructed about care of the incision and the importance of an adequate fluid intake. In addition, instructions about changes that should be reported to the provider, such as fever, hematuria, flank pain, or any signs and symptoms of decreasing kidney function, are provided. Also guidelines for gradually increasing activity, lifting, and driving are provided in accordance with the provider's prescription.

Follow-up nursing care includes monitoring the BP to detect hypertension and advising the patient to restrict activities for about 1 month after trauma to minimize the incidence of delayed or secondary bleeding. The patient should be advised to schedule periodic follow-up assessments of renal function (creatinine clearance, BUN, and serum creatinine analyses). If a nephrectomy was necessary, the patient is advised to wear medical identification.

Gerontologic Considerations

Care for this population is essentially the same; however, the elderly may have chronic disease processes that must be considered. Older adults often have higher mortality following traumatic injury than do younger adults, including alterations in the cardiac and respiratory systems that reduce physiologic reserve needed to respond to shock and hypoxia.

CHAPTER REVIEW

Critical Thinking Exercises

1. As the primary nurse for a 50-year-old man with kidney failure secondary to poorly controlled diabetes, develop a teaching plan to explain the different types of renal replacement therapies. Include the level of involvement on the part of the patient and family for self-management required for each. How would you modify the approach if the patient is distraught and does not seem to hear what you are saying?

2. A 45-year-old married woman with three teenage children visits the nephrology department to discuss options for dealing with her kidney failure. Her healthy twin sister wants to donate her kidney, and the preliminary reports show that a match is possible. The patient states that she does not want her sister to go through the process of kidney donation if dialysis is possible. Identify the pros and cons of her wishes based on current evidence regarding outcomes of dialysis compared to kidney transplantation.

3. You are treating a 35-year-old woman who is in the emergency department following a motor vehicle crash; she is complaining of severe left-sided flank pain. Identify possible causes of her pain and laboratory tests that would be indicated. What nursing assessment and interventions should you make at this time? What explanations would you give the patient while awaiting the results of laboratory tests?

NCLEX-Style Review Questions

1. The nurse is receiving report on a client with AKI. What should the nurse follow up on first?
   a. Potassium value of 5.0 mEq/L
   b. Patient refused fingerstick blood glucose
   c. Crackles throughout lung fields
   d. Patient reports itching skin

2. When caring for the patient with kidney failure, the nurse teaches the patient to manage his diet by avoiding which foods?
   a. Green leafy vegetables and citrus
   b. Apples and pears
   c. Proteins of high biologic value
   d. Oat, wheat, and rye-containing products

3. The nurse recognizes the patient comprehends the signs and symptoms of renal transplant rejection when the patient states he will monitor for which of these signs and symptoms? Select all that apply.
   a. Thrill and bruit over the fistula
   b. Weight gain and fever
   c. Palpitations and thirst
   d. Flank pain and pyuria
   e. Swelling of the ankles and around the eyes

4. When planning care for the patient with kidney trauma, the nurse notifies the physician immediately for which of these findings?
   a. Laboratory reports microscopic hematuria
   b. Tachycardia and hypotension
   c. Patient is upset and crying
   d. Scar noted on patient's left flank

5. When caring for the patient with nephrotic syndrome, what is appropriate to include in the patient teaching plan to prevent long-term?
   a. Observe for dark urine and clay-colored stool.
   b. Void every 2 hours on schedule.
   c. Avoid driving at night.
   d. Minimize the intake of saturated fat.

Try these additional resources, available at **http://thepoint.lww.com/Honan2e**, to enhance your learning and understanding of this chapter:
- NCLEX-Style Student Review Questions
- Journal Articles

REFERENCES AND SELECTED READINGS

References and selected readings associated with this chapter can be found on the website that accompanies the book. Visit **http://thepoint. lww.com/Honan2e** to access the references and other additional resources associated with this chapter.

Nursing Management: Patients with Urinary Disorders

Susanne A. Quallich • Michelle J. Lajiness

Learning Objectives

After reading this chapter, you will be able to:

1. Identify factors contributing to upper and lower urinary tract infections (UTIs).
2. Describe nursing care of the patient with a UTI.
3. Differentiate between the various adult dysfunctional voiding patterns.
4. Develop a patient education plan for a patient who has mixed (stress and urge) urinary incontinence.
5. Identify potential causes of an obstruction of the urinary tract, and management of the patient with this condition.
6. Develop a teaching plan for the patient undergoing treatment for renal calculi (kidney stones).
7. Discuss the available options for management of urinary cancers.
8. Identify issues relevant to the initial management of trauma to the urinary tract.
9. Identify issues important to patient self-care of urinary diversions.

The urinary system is responsible for providing the route for drainage of urine formed by the kidneys. Nursing requires an understanding of the anatomy, physiology, diagnostic testing, nursing care, and rehabilitation of patients with the multiple processes that interfere with the urinary system. This chapter focuses on the nursing management of patients with common urinary conditions.

INFECTIONS OF THE URINARY TRACT

Urinary tract infections (UTIs) are caused by pathogenic microorganisms in the urinary tract (the normal urinary tract is sterile above the urethra). Lower UTIs include bacterial **cystitis** (inflammation of the bladder), bacterial **prostatitis** (inflammation of the prostate), and bacterial **urethritis** (inflammation of the urethra). Acute or chronic nonbacterial causes of inflammation in any of these areas can be misdiagnosed as bacterial infections. Upper UTIs are much less common and include acute or chronic **pyelonephritis** (inflammation of the kidney and renal pelvis), interstitial nephritis (inflammation of the spaces between the kidney tubules), and renal abscesses (pus-filled cavity of the kidney) (Fig. 28-1). Upper and lower UTIs are further classified as uncomplicated or complicated, depending on other patient-related conditions (Box 28-1) (e.g., whether the UTI is recurrent and the duration of the infection). Most uncomplicated UTIs are community-acquired, while complicated UTIs usually occur in people with urologic abnormalities, comorbidities such as diabetes, or recent catheterization.

A UTI is the most common bacterial infection encountered in the ambulatory care setting in the United States (Ferri, 2016), and the second most common reason patients seek health care (Grossman & Porth, 2014). Most cases occur in women; one out of every five women in the United States will develop a UTI sometime during her lifetime, and by the age of 32 years half of all women report having had at least one UTI (Ferri, 2016). The urinary tract is the most common site of nosocomial infection, accounting for greater than 3% of the total number reported by hospitals each year (Centers for Disease Control and Prevention [CDC], 2015). In most of these hospital-acquired UTIs, instrumentation of the urinary tract or catheterization is the precipitating cause.

LOWER URINARY TRACT INFECTIONS

Pathophysiology

For infection to occur, bacteria must gain access to the bladder, attach to and colonize the epithelium of the urinary tract,

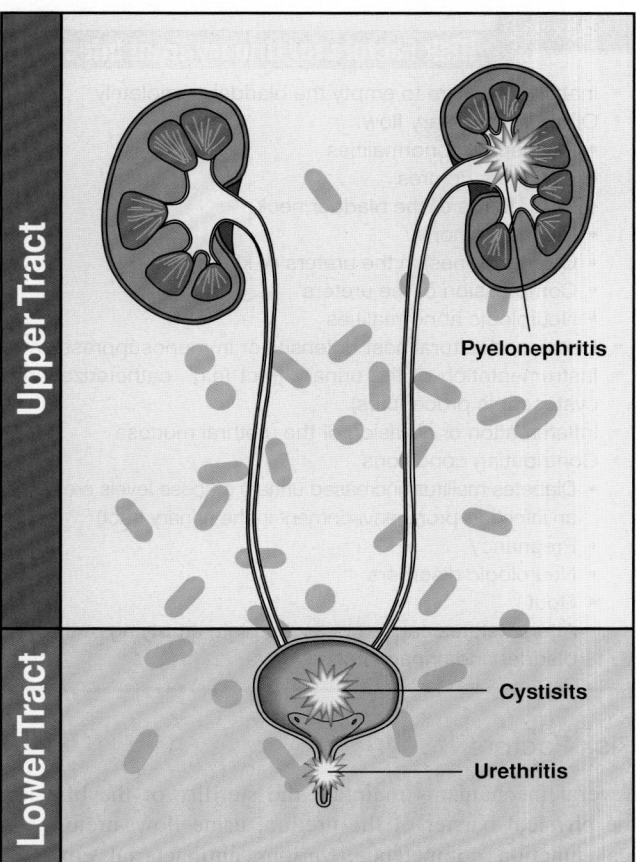

FIGURE 28-1 Urinary Tract Infection. (Courtesy of LifeArt, Lippincott, Wolters Kluwer.)

BOX 28-1

Classifying Urinary Tract Infections

Urinary tract infections (UTIs) are classified by location: the lower urinary tract (which includes the bladder and structures below the bladder) or the upper urinary tract (which includes the kidneys and ureters). They can also be classified as uncomplicated or complicated UTIs.

Lower UTIs

Cystitis, prostatitis, urethritis

Upper UTIs

Acute pyelonephritis, chronic pyelonephritis, renal abscess, interstitial nephritis, perirenal abscess

Uncomplicated Lower or Upper UTIs

Community-acquired infection; common in young women and not usually recurrent

Complicated Lower or Upper UTIs

Often nosocomial (acquired in the hospital) and related to catheterization; occur in patients with urologic abnormalities, pregnancy, immunosuppression, diabetes mellitus, and obstructions and are often recurrent

---

evade host defense mechanisms, and initiate inflammation. Many UTIs result from fecal organisms that ascend from the perineum to the urethra and the bladder and then adhere to the mucosal surfaces.

Bacterial Invasion of the Urinary Tract

By increasing the normal slow shedding of bladder epithelial cells (resulting in bacteria removal), the bladder can clear even large numbers of bacteria. Glycosaminoglycan (GAG), a hydrophilic protein, normally exerts a nonadherent protective effect against various bacteria by attracting water molecules and forming a water barrier that serves as a defensive layer between the bladder and the urine. GAG may be impaired by certain agents (cyclamate, saccharin, aspartame, and tryptophan metabolites). The normal bacterial flora of the vagina and urethral area also interfere with adherence of *Escherichia coli*.

Reflux

An obstruction to free-flowing urine is a problem known as **urethrovesical reflux**, which is the reflux of urine from the urethra into the bladder (Fig. 28-2). With coughing, sneezing, or straining, the bladder pressure increases, which may

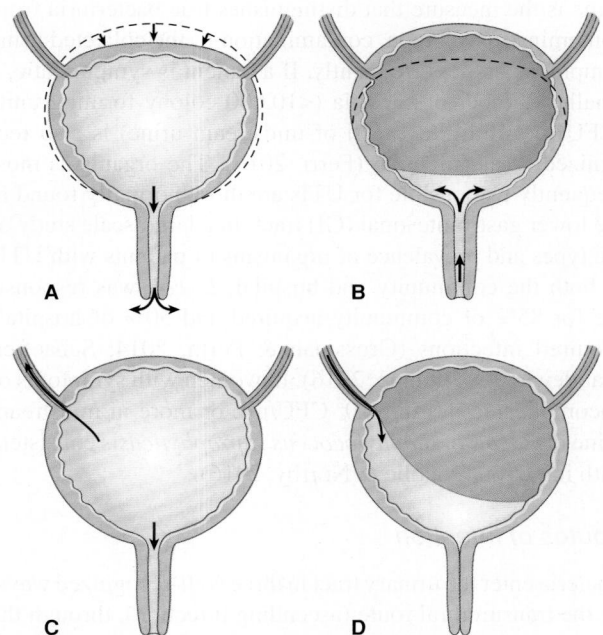

FIGURE 28-2 Mechanisms of urethrovesical and ureterovesical reflux may cause urinary tract infection. Urethrovesical reflux: With coughing and straining, bladder pressure rises, which may force urine from the bladder into the urethra. (**A**) When bladder pressure returns to normal, the urine flows back to the bladder (**B**), which introduces bacteria from the urethra to the bladder. Ureterovesical reflux: With failure of the ureterovesical valve, urine moves up the ureters during voiding (**C**) and flows into the bladder when voiding stops (**D**). This prevents complete emptying of the bladder. It also leads to urinary stasis and contamination of the ureters with bacteria-laden urine.

force urine from the bladder into the urethra. When the pressure returns to normal, the urine flows back into the bladder, bringing into the bladder bacteria from the anterior portions of the urethra. Urethrovesical reflux is also caused by dysfunction of the bladder neck or urethra. The urethrovesical angle and urethral closure pressure may be altered with menopause, increasing the incidence of infection in postmenopausal women.

Ureterovesical or **vesicoureteral reflux** refers to the backward flow of urine from the bladder into one or both ureters (see Fig. 28-2). The ureters tunnel into the bladder wall, so that the bladder musculature compresses a small portion of the ureter during normal voiding. When the ureterovesical valve is impaired by congenital causes or ureteral abnormalities, the bacteria may reach the kidneys (Grossman & Porth, 2014).

Uropathogenic Bacteria

Bacteriuria is generally defined as more than 10^5 colonies of bacteria per milliliter of urine, which distinguishes true bacteriuria from contamination, and is a major criterion for infection (Grossman & Porth, 2014). Because urine samples (especially in women) are commonly contaminated by the bacteria normally present in the urethral area, a bacterial count exceeding 10^5 colonies/mL of clean-catch midstream urine is the measure that distinguishes true bacteriuria from contamination. In men, contamination of the collected urine sample occurs less frequently. If a patient is symptomatic, a smaller number of bacteria (<10,000 colony-forming units [CFU] per milliliter [mL] of midstream urine) is also recognized as an infection (Ferri, 2016). The organisms most frequently responsible for UTIs are those normally found in the lower gastrointestinal (GI) tract. In a large-scale study of the types and prevalence of organisms of patients with UTIs in both the community and hospital, *E. coli* was responsible for 85% of community-acquired and 50% of hospital-acquired infections (Grossman & Porth, 2014; Schaeffer, Matulewicz, & Klumpp, 2016). In women with symptoms of uncomplicated cystitis, 10^2 CFU/mL or more in midstream urine of *E. coli* or *Staphylococcus saprophyticus* is consistent with infection (Nicolle & Norrby, 2016).

Routes of Infection

Bacteria enter the urinary tract in three well-recognized ways: by the transurethral route (ascending infection), through the bloodstream (hematogenous spread), or by means of a fistula (direct extension). The most common route of infection is transurethral, in which bacteria (often from fecal contamination) colonize the periurethral area and subsequently enter the bladder by means of the urethra. In women, the short urethra offers little resistance (Grossman & Porth, 2014). Sexual intercourse or massage of the urethra forces the bacteria up into the bladder, accounting for the increased incidence of UTIs in sexually active women.

BOX 28-2 | **Risk Factors for Urinary Tract Infection**

- Inability or failure to empty the bladder completely
- Obstructed urinary flow:
  - Congenital abnormalities
  - Urethral strictures
  - Contracture of the bladder neck
  - Bladder tumors
  - Calculi (stones) in the ureters or kidneys
  - Compression of the ureters
  - Neurologic abnormalities
- Decreased natural host defenses or immunosuppression
- Instrumentation of the urinary tract (e.g., catheterization, cystoscopic procedures)
- Inflammation or abrasion of the urethral mucosa
- Contributing conditions:
  - Diabetes mellitus (increased urinary glucose levels create an infection-prone environment in the urinary tract)
  - Pregnancy
  - Neurologic disorders
  - Gout
  - Altered states caused by incomplete emptying of the bladder and urinary stasis

---

Risk Factors

Several mechanisms maintain the sterility of the bladder: the physical barrier of the urethra, urine flow, ureterovesical junction competence, various antibacterial enzymes and antibodies, and antiadherent effects mediated by the mucosal cells of the bladder. Abnormalities or dysfunctions of these mechanisms are contributing risk factors for lower UTIs (Box 28-2).

The American College of Obstetricians and Gynecologists (ACOG) recommends that all pregnant women be screened for asymptomatic bacteriuria, because pregnancy itself is a risk factor for UTIs; the bladder does not empty as well as it normally does.

Clinical Manifestations and Assessment

Signs and Symptoms

A variety of signs and symptoms are associated with UTI but about half of all patients with bacteriuria have no symptoms, and may not need treatment. Signs and symptoms of an uncomplicated lower UTI include **dysuria** (painful or difficult urination), burning on urination, **frequency**, urgency, **nocturia** (excessive urination at night), and incontinence. Suprapubic or pelvic pain, hematuria (bloody urine) and back pain are less common symptoms (Bickley, 2013; Schaeffer et al., 2016). In older people, these symptoms are less common.

(!) Nursing Alert
Elderly patients often lack the typical symptoms of UTI and sepsis. Although frequency, urgency, and dysuria may occur,

nonspecific symptoms, such as altered sensorium, lethargy, anorexia, new incontinence, hyperventilation, and low-grade fever, may be the only clues.

> **Nursing Alert**
> *Often clinicians confuse asymptomatic bacteriuria (ASB, which is bacteria in the urine without any symptoms), with a UTI, resulting in unnecessary antibiotic treatment (Cortes-Penfield, Trautner, & Jump, 2017). The Infectious Diseases Society of America Guidelines for the Diagnosis and Treatment of Asymptomatic Bacteriuria (ASB) in Adults (2016) do not recommend treatment of asymptomatic elderly patients with bacteriuria if the patient is asymptomatic the nurse consider the method of urine collection. For example, a "clean-catch" or mid-stream urine collection in an asymptomatic female should necessitate a repeat sampling to confirm a UTI.*

In patients with complicated UTIs, such as those with indwelling catheters, manifestations can range from asymptomatic bacteriuria to gram-negative sepsis with shock. Complicated UTIs often are due to a broader spectrum of organisms, have a lower response rate to treatment, and tend to recur. Many patients with catheter-associated UTIs are asymptomatic and do not need to be treated because administration of antimicrobials to catheterized patients with asymptomatic bacteriuria inevitably results in reinfection with more resistant organisms (Nicolle & Norrby, 2016). However, any patient with a catheter who suddenly develops signs and symptoms of septic shock should be evaluated for **bacteremia** (the presence of bacteria in blood) **from a UTI**. The kidneys receive approximately 25% of the cardiac output every minute. When a patient has pyelonephritis, the infection is in the kidney parenchyma and can travel from the kidney into the bloodstream, which is termed *bacteremia*. *Septicemia* is the clinical syndrome associated with the bacteremia that results in vasodilatation, microvascular permeability, and massive inflammatory response. Nurses should be alert for signs and symptoms of bacteremia from UTI, including hypothermia or hyperthermia, tachycardia, tachypnea, leukocytosis or leukopenia, and greater than 10% immature (band) forms (bands are immature neutrophils that contain a nucleus, indicating infection). Under normal circumstances only 1% to 3% of neutrophils are band forms. Refer to Chapter 54 for further discussion of sepsis and septic shock.

Diagnostic Tests

Results of various tests such as urine cultures and sensitivities help confirm the diagnosis of UTI. In an uncomplicated UTI, the strain of bacteria determines the antibiotic of choice. Urine cultures are useful for documenting a UTI and can identify the specific organism present. UTI and subsequent sepsis can occur with lower bacterial colony counts. About one third of women with symptoms of acute infections have negative midstream urine culture results and may go untreated if 10^5 CFU/mL is used as the only criterion for infection. The presence of any bacteria in specimens obtained by catheterization (insertion of a tube into the urinary bladder) is considered indicative of infection. If a urine dipstick is used, a positive nitrite and positive leukocyte esterase usually is indicative of UTI in a symptomatic patient (if urine collection was from clean catch or midstream collection or urinary catheterization) (Ferri, 2016).

The following groups of patients may need urine cultures when bacteriuria and symptoms are present:

- All men (because of the likelihood of structural or functional abnormalities)
- Women with a history of compromised immune function or renal problems
- Patients with diabetes mellitus
- Patients who have undergone recent instrumentation (including catheterization) of the urinary tract
- Patients who have been recently hospitalized or who live in long-term care facilities
- Patients with prolonged or persistent symptoms
- Patients with three or more UTIs in the past year
- Pregnant women
- Postmenopausal women
- Sexually active women that use a spermicide for birth control

A multiple-test dipstick often includes testing for white blood cells (WBCs), known as the *leukocyte esterase test*, and nitrite testing (Griess nitrate reduction test). If the leukocyte esterase test is positive, it is assumed that the patient has pyuria (pus in the urine), since esterase is an enzyme released from WBCs; a UTI is suspected and should be treated. The Griess nitrate reduction test is considered positive if bacteria that reduce normal urinary nitrates to nitrites are present. Most Gram-negative bacteria metabolize nitrate to nitrite, however Gram-positive bacteria and fungi do not metabolize nitrate. This rapid (<1 minute) and inexpensive test has a high degree of specificity but is insensitive because it does not detect infections caused by gram-positive organisms (Nicolle & Norby, 2016, page 1874).

> **Nursing Alert**
> *The nurse is aware that false-positive leukocyte esterase tests can occur if the clean-catch midstream urine collection was not performed correctly or there was contamination from the vagina in the specimen.*

Tests for sexually transmitted infections (STIs) may be performed (see Chapter 35) because acute urethritis caused by sexually transmitted organisms or acute vaginitis infections may be responsible for symptoms similar to those of UTIs.

BOX 28-3

Patient Education

Preventing Recurrent Urinary Tract Infections

Hygiene
- Shower rather than bathe in tub because bacteria in the bath water may enter the urethra.
- After each bowel movement, clean the perineum and urethral meatus from front to back. This will help reduce concentrations of pathogens at the urethral opening and, in women, the vaginal opening.

Fluid Intake
- Drink liberal amounts of fluids daily to flush out bacteria.
- Avoid coffee, tea, colas, alcohol, and other fluids that are urinary tract irritants.

Voiding Habits
- Void every 2–3 hours during the day and completely empty the bladder. This prevents overdistention of the bladder and compromised blood supply to the bladder wall. Both predispose the patient to UTI. Precautions expressly for women include voiding immediately after sexual intercourse.

Therapy
- Take medication *exactly* as prescribed.
- If bacteria continue to appear in the urine, long-term antimicrobial therapy may be required to prevent colonization of the periurethral area and recurrence of infection.
- Special timing of administration may be required.
- If prescribed, test urine for presence of bacteria following manufacturer's and health care provider's instructions.
- Notify the primary health care provider if fever occurs or if signs and symptoms persist.
- Consult the primary health care provider regularly for follow-up.

Imaging studies are rarely indicated for the evaluation of UTIs, except with suspected anatomic issues or if additional pathology, such as renal lithiasis (stone formation or calculi) or fistula (a false track or abnormal passageway), is suspected.

Medical and Nursing Management

Management of UTIs typically involves pharmacologic therapy and patient education. The nurse teaches the patient about medication regimens and infection prevention measures (Box 28-3).

Nursing Alert
Patients who are asymptomatic do not require screening for bacteriuria. It is important to consider that treatment of asymptomatic bacteriuria has not been associated with improved outcomes but is uniformly followed by reinfection with organisms of increasing antimicrobial resistance. There are two exceptions to treatment of asymptomatic bacteriuria: pregnant women or when antimicrobials are given as perioperative prophylaxis before a urologic procedure where trauma to the genitourinary mucosa is anticipated (Nicolle & Norrby, 2016).

Initial Pharmacologic Therapy

The ideal medication for treatment of UTI is an antibacterial agent that eradicates bacteria from the urinary tract with minimal effects on GI and vaginal flora, minimizing the incidence of vaginal yeast infections. (Yeast vaginitis occurs in as many as 25% of patients treated with antimicrobial agents that affect vaginal flora, causes more symptoms, and is more difficult and, thus, more costly to treat than the UTI.) The antibacterial agent should be affordable, have few adverse effects, and produce low resistance in the targeted organisms.

Because the organism in initial, uncomplicated UTIs is most likely *E. coli* or other fecal flora, the agent should be effective against these organisms.

Various treatment regimens have been successful in treating uncomplicated lower UTIs in women: single-dose administration, short-course (3 to 4 days) regimens, or 7- to 10-day regimens. The trend is toward a shortened course of antibiotic therapy for uncomplicated UTIs, because most cases are cured after 3 days of treatment (Nicolle & Norrby, 2016). Phenazopyridine, a urinary analgesic, may be prescribed to relieve the discomfort associated with the infection (Karch, 2015). Patients should be informed that their urine will turn dark orange with this medication. Regardless of the regimen prescribed, the patient is instructed to take all the doses prescribed, even if relief of symptoms occurs promptly.

A fluoroquinolone is a routine choice for short-course therapy of uncomplicated, mild to moderate UTIs. There is high patient adherence (95.6%) to the 3-day regimen and a high eradication rate (96.4%) for all pathogens. Before using a fluoroquinolone in patients with complicated UTIs, the causative pathogen should be identified; fluoroquinolone is used only when generic and less costly antibiotics are likely to be ineffective (Vallerand & Sanoski, 2015).

Drug Alert!
Fluoroquinolones are associated with an increased risk of tendinitis and tendon rupture. This risk is further increased in those over age 60, in kidney, heart, and lung transplant recipients, and with use of concomitant steroid therapy. Providers should advise patients, at the first sign of tendon pain, swelling, or inflammation, to stop taking the fluoroquinolone, to avoid exercise and use of the affected area, and to promptly contact their provider about changing to a nonfluoroquinolone antimicrobial drug (U.S. Food and Drug Administration, 2017).

Nitrofurantoin should not be used in patients with renal insufficiency because it is ineffective at glomerular filtration rates of less than 50 mL/min, and may cause peripheral neuropathy.

In a complicated UTI (i.e., pyelonephritis), the general treatment of choice is usually a cephalosporin or an ampicillin/aminoglycoside combination; ideally, the choice is based on culture results. Patients in institutional settings may require 7 to 10 days of medication for the treatment to be effective. Medications such as ampicillin or amoxicillin can be used, but *E. coli* has developed resistance. Because of this problem of resistance, the fluoroquinolone ciprofloxacin is often used as a first-line agent (Heinz, 2016). Longer medication courses are indicated for men, pregnant women, and women with pyelonephritis and other types of complicated UTIs. Hospitalization and IV antibiotics are occasionally needed.

Long-Term Pharmacologic Therapy

Although brief pharmacologic treatment of UTIs for 3 days is usually adequate in women, infection recurs in about 20% of women treated for uncomplicated UTIs. Infections that recur within 2 weeks of therapy do so because organisms of the original offending strain remain in the vagina. Relapses suggest that the source of bacteriuria may be the upper urinary tract or that initial treatment was inadequate or administered for too short a time. Recurrent infections in men are usually due to persistence of the same organism; further evaluation and treatment are indicated.

If infection recurs after completing antimicrobial therapy, another short course (3 to 4 days) of full-dose antimicrobial therapy, followed by a regular bedtime dose of an antimicrobial agent may be prescribed. In addition, continuous prophylaxis via a 4- to 12-month course of antibiotics may be considered, either nightly or every other night (Heinz, 2016). Long-term use of antimicrobial agents decreases the risk of reinfection and may be indicated in patients with recurrent infections. Choice of antibiotic will be based upon the organism involved, previous UTI strains, and allergic drug history of the patient. Development of microbial resistance to prolonged antibiotic administration is always a concern, therefore the nurse is alert for signs and symptoms of a UTI despite antibiotic therapy.

Reinfection with new bacteria is the reason for more than 90% of recurrent UTIs in women. If the diagnostic evaluation reveals no structural abnormalities in the urinary tract, the woman with recurrent UTIs may be instructed to begin self-treatment when symptoms occur and to contact her health care provider only when symptoms persist, fever occurs, or the number of treatment episodes exceeds three of more episodes in a 6-month period (Ferri, 2016).

If recurrence is caused by persistent bacteria from preceding infections, the cause (i.e., kidney stone, abscess) must be treated. After treatment and sterilization of the urine, low-dose preventive therapy (trimethoprim with or without sulfamethoxazole) each night at bedtime may be prescribed. Finally, for those women who develop UTI after sexual intercourse, postcoital prophylaxis with low-dose antimicrobials may be prescribed.

The patient is encouraged to drink liberal amounts of fluids (water is the best choice) to promote renal blood flow and to flush the bacteria from the urinary tract. Current evidence about the effectiveness of daily intake of cranberry juice to prevent UTIs has shown that it is no better than placebo for preventing UTIs (Ferri, 2016). However, patients who like cranberry juice can be encouraged to include it in their increased fluid intake that will assist to flush bacteria. Cranberry pill supplement may be recommended, although current evidence is inconclusive regarding its efficacy. It should not be administered to patients on anticoagulants or antiplatelet drugs because of potential to affect coagulation or platelet aggregation. Urinary tract irritants (e.g., coffee, tea, citrus, spices, colas, alcohol) are avoided.

The pain associated with UTI is quickly relieved once effective antimicrobial therapy is initiated. Analgesic agents and the application of heat to the perineum help relieve pain and spasm.

Frequent voiding (every 2 to 3 hours) is encouraged to empty the bladder completely because this can significantly lower urine bacterial counts, reduce urinary stasis, and prevent reinfection.

Gerontologic Considerations

The incidence of bacteriuria in the elderly differs from that in younger adults. Bacteriuria increases with age and disability, and women are affected more frequently than men. UTI is the most common cause of acute bacterial sepsis in patients older than 65 years, in whom gram-negative sepsis carries a mortality rate exceeding 50%. Urologists see many asymptomatic older patients with bacteriuria, and 20% are women older than 65 years. In long-term care facilities, up to 50% of females have asymptomatic bacteriuria (Nicolle & Norrby, 2016). When indwelling catheters are used, the risk for UTI increases dramatically.

In the elderly population at large, structural abnormalities secondary to decreased bladder tone and neurogenic bladder secondary to stroke or autonomic neuropathy of diabetes may prevent complete emptying of the bladder and increase the risk for UTI (Nicolle & Norby, 2016). Elderly women often have incomplete emptying of the bladder and urinary stasis. In the absence of estrogen, postmenopausal women are susceptible to colonization and increased adherence of bacteria to the vagina and urethra. Oral or topical estrogen has been used to restore the glycogen content of vaginal epithelial cells and an acidic pH for some postmenopausal women with recurrent cystitis.

The antibacterial activity of prostatic secretions that protect men from bacterial colonization of the urethra and bladder decreases with aging. Although UTIs are rare in men, the prevalence of infection in men older than 50 years approaches that of women in the same age group. The increase of UTIs in men as they age is due largely to prostatic hyperplasia, strictures of the urethra, and neuropathic bladder. Catheterization may also contribute to the higher incidence of UTI in this group. The incidence of bacteriuria increases in men with confusion, dementia, or bowel or bladder incontinence. The most common cause of recurrent UTIs in elderly males is chronic bacterial prostatitis. In institutionalized elderly patients, such as those in long-term care facilities, infecting pathogens are often resistant to many antibiotics.

Diligent hand hygiene, careful perineal care, and frequent toileting may decrease the incidence of UTIs seen in patients in long-term care facilities. The organisms responsible for UTIs in the institutionalized elderly may differ from those found in patients residing in the community; this may be due to the frequent use of antibiotic agents by patients in long-term care facilities. *E. coli* is the most common organism seen in elderly patients in the community or hospital. However, patients with indwelling catheters are more likely to be infected with *Proteus, Klebsiella, Pseudomonas*, or *Staphylococcus* species. Patients who have been previously treated with antibiotics may be infected with *Enterococcus* species. Controversy continues about the need for treatment of asymptomatic bacteriuria in institutionalized elderly patients, because resulting antibiotic-resistant organisms and sepsis may be greater threats to patients. Treatment regimens are generally the same as those for younger adults, although age-related changes in the intestinal absorption of medications and decreased renal function and hepatic flow may necessitate alterations in dose.

UPPER URINARY TRACT INFECTIONS

Pyelonephritis is a bacterial infection of the renal pelvis, tubules, and interstitial tissue of one or both kidneys. Causes involve either the ascending spread of bacteria from the bladder or proliferation of bacteria from systemic sources reaching the kidney via the bloodstream. It is not uncommon for bacteria that are causing a bladder infection to ascend into the kidney, causing pyelonephritis. An incompetent ureterovesical valve or obstruction occurring in the urinary tract increases the susceptibility of the kidneys to infection (see Fig. 28-1) because static urine provides a good medium for bacterial growth. Bladder tumors, strictures, benign prostatic hyperplasia (BPH), and urinary stones are some potential causes of obstruction that can lead to infections.

Pyelonephritis may be acute or chronic. Acute pyelonephritis is usually manifested by enlarged kidneys with interstitial infiltrations of inflammatory cells. Abscesses may be noted on the renal capsule and at the corticomedullary junction. Atrophy and destruction of tubules and the glomeruli may result.

When pyelonephritis becomes chronic, the kidneys become scarred, contracted, nonfunctional, and cause chronic kidney disease that can result in the need for therapies such as transplantation or dialysis.

ACUTE PYELONEPHRITIS

More than 250,000 cases of acute pyelonephritis occur in the United States each year, with 100,000 patients requiring hospitalization.

Clinical Manifestations and Assessment

The patient with acute pyelonephritis is acutely ill with chills, fever, leukocytosis (elevated WBCs), bacteriuria, and pyuria. Low back pain, flank pain (resulting from inflammation and edema of the renal parenchyma), nausea and vomiting, headache, malaise, and painful urination are common findings. Physical examination reveals pain and tenderness in the area of the costovertebral angle (see Chapter 26, Fig. 26-6). In addition, symptoms of lower urinary tract involvement, such as dysuria and frequency, are common. An ultrasound study or a computed tomography (CT) scan may be performed to locate any obstruction in the urinary tract. Relief of obstruction is essential to prevent the complications and eventual kidney damage. Urine culture and sensitivity tests are performed to determine the causative organism so that appropriate antimicrobial agents can be prescribed.

Medical and Nursing Management

Patients with acute uncomplicated pyelonephritis are treated on an outpatient basis if they are not exhibiting dehydration, nausea or vomiting, or symptoms of sepsis. A 2-week course of antibiotics is recommended because renal parenchymal disease is more difficult to eradicate than mucosal bladder infections. Commonly prescribed agents for stable patients who can tolerate oral medications with sensitive pathogens include ciprofloxacin or Levaquin for 10 to 14 days, however recent trials reveal a 7-day course is not inferior to a 14-day course of treatment in women with uncomplicated pyelonephritis (Ferri, 2016). Whereas intravenous (IV) medications are indicated for symptomatic complicated patients, and treatment includes IV Cipro, or Levaquin; piperacillin/tazobactam, carbapenems; aminoglycosides such as gentamicin with or without ampicillin, or a third-generation cephalosporin (Ferri, 2016). Treatment will be based upon urine culture and sensitivity results. These medications must be used with great caution if the patient has renal or liver dysfunction. Pregnant women may be hospitalized for 2 or 3 days of parenteral antibiotic therapy. Oral antibiotic agents may be prescribed once the patient is afebrile and showing clinical improvement. Hydration is essential in all patients with UTIs when there is adequate kidney function; this helps facilitate "flushing" of the urinary tract and reduces pain and discomfort.

A possible issue in acute pyelonephritis treatment is a chronic or recurring symptomless infection persisting for months or years. After the initial antibiotic regimen, the patient may need antibiotic therapy for up to 6 weeks if evidence of a relapse is seen. A follow-up urine culture is obtained 2 weeks after completion of antibiotic therapy to document clearing of the infection.

CHRONIC PYELONEPHRITIS

Repeated bouts of acute pyelonephritis may lead to chronic pyelonephritis.

Clinical Manifestations and Assessment

The patient with chronic pyelonephritis usually has no symptoms of infection unless an acute exacerbation occurs. Noticeable signs and symptoms may include fatigue, headache, poor appetite, polyuria, excessive thirst, and weight loss. Persistent and recurring infection may produce progressive scarring of the kidney resulting in kidney failure (see Chapter 27).

The extent of the disease is assessed by an IV urogram and degree of renal dysfunction via measurements of creatinine clearance, blood urea nitrogen, and creatinine levels. Bacteria, if detected in the urine, are eradicated if possible.

Medical and Nursing Management

Long-term use of prophylactic antimicrobial therapy may help limit recurrence of infections and renal scarring (Kumar, 2015). Impaired renal function alters the excretion of antimicrobial agents and necessitates careful monitoring of renal function, especially if the medications are potentially toxic to the kidneys.

The patient may require hospitalization or may be treated as an outpatient. When the patient requires hospitalization, fluid intake and output are carefully measured and recorded. Unless contraindicated, 3 to 4 L of fluids per day is encouraged to dilute the urine, decrease burning on urination, and prevent dehydration. The nurse assesses the patient's temperature every 4 hours and administers antipyretic and antibiotic agents as prescribed. Symptomatic patients are often more comfortable on bedrest. Patient teaching focuses on prevention of further infection by consuming adequate fluids, emptying the bladder regularly, and performing recommended perineal hygiene. The importance of taking antimicrobial medications exactly as prescribed is stressed, as is the need for keeping follow-up appointments.

Complications

Complications of chronic pyelonephritis include end-stage kidney disease (ESKD) from progressive loss of nephrons secondary to chronic inflammation and scarring.

ADULT VOIDING DYSFUNCTION

Both neurogenic and nonneurogenic disorders can cause adult voiding dysfunction (Table 28-1). The **micturition** process involves several highly coordinated neurologic responses that mediate bladder function. A functional urinary system allows for appropriate bladder filling and complete bladder emptying (see Chapter 26). If voiding dysfunction goes undetected and untreated, the upper urinary system may be compromised. Chronic incomplete bladder emptying from poor detrusor pressure results in recurrent bladder infection. Incomplete bladder emptying due to bladder outlet obstruction (such as BPH), causing high-pressure detrusor contractions, can result in hydronephrosis from the high detrusor pressure that radiates up the ureters to the renal pelvis.

OVERACTIVE BLADDER

It is estimated that over 33 million Americans have overactive bladder (OAB). OAB is a condition in which a person has urgency, frequency, and nocturia that may or may not be associated with urinary incontinence (Drake, 2016). Normal frequency is seven voids per day and once at night up until the age of 70 years. OAB can have a significant impact on quality-of-life indicators. Treatment for OAB is similar to urge incontinence, discussed later in the chapter.

URINARY INCONTINENCE

More than 17 million adults in the United States are estimated to have **urinary incontinence**, with most of them experiencing OAB syndrome, making this disorder more prevalent than diabetes or ulcer disease. Despite widespread media coverage, urinary incontinence remains underdiagnosed and underreported. Patients may be too embarrassed to seek help, causing them to ignore or conceal symptoms. Many patients resort to using absorbent pads or other devices without having their condition properly diagnosed and treated. Health care providers must be alert to subtle cues of urinary incontinence and stay informed about current management strategies. Subtle cues include avoidance of social situations, perineal dermatitis, and depression. The costs of care for patients with urinary incontinence include cost of absorbent products, medications, and surgical or nonsurgical treatment modalities, as well as the psychosocial costs of urinary incontinence, including embarrassment, loss of self-esteem, and social isolation.

Risk Factors

Urinary incontinence affects people of all ages but is particularly common among the elderly and can decrease an elderly person's ability to maintain an independent lifestyle. This

TABLE **28-1** **Conditions Causing Adult Voiding Dysfunction**

Condition	Voiding Dysfunction	Treatment
Neurogenic Disorders		
Cerebellar ataxia	Incontinence or dyssynergia	Timed voiding; anticholinergics
Cerebrovascular accident	Retention or incontinence	Anticholinergics; bladder retraining
Dementia	Incontinence	Prompted voiding
Diabetes mellitus	Incontinence and/or incomplete bladder emptying	Timed voiding; electromyelogram (EMG)/biofeedback; pelvic floor nerve stimulation; anticholinergics/antispasmodics; well-controlled blood glucose levels
Multiple sclerosis	Incontinence or incomplete bladder emptying	Timed voiding; EMG/biofeedback to learn pelvic muscle exercises and urge inhibition; pelvic floor nerve stimulation; antispasmodics
Parkinson disease	Incontinence	Anticholinergics/antispasmodics
Spinal Cord Dysfunction		
Acute injury	Urinary retention	Indwelling catheter
Degenerative disease	Incontinence and/or incomplete bladder emptying	EMG/biofeedback; pelvic floor nerve stimulation; anticholinergics
Nonneurogenic Disorders		
"Bashful bladder"	Inability to initiate voiding in public bathrooms	Relaxation therapy; EMG/biofeedback
Overactive bladder	Urgency, frequency, and/or urge incontinence	EMG/biofeedback; pelvic floor nerve stimulation; anticholinergics
Post general surgery	Acute urine retention	Catheterization
Post-prostatectomy	Incontinence	*Mild:* biofeedback; pelvic floor nerve stimulation *Moderate/severe:* surgery—artificial sphincter
Stress incontinence	Incontinence with cough, laugh, sneeze, position change	*Mild:* biofeedback: periurethral bulking with collagen *Moderate/severe:* surgery

increases dependence on caregivers and may lead to institutionalization. More than half of all nursing home residents have urinary incontinence. Although urinary incontinence is not a normal consequence of aging, age-related changes in the urinary tract predispose the older person to incontinence.

Although it is commonly regarded as a condition that occurs in older multiparous women, it is also seen in young nulliparous women, especially during vigorous high-impact activity. Age, gender, and number of vaginal deliveries are established risk factors (Box 28-4) that explain, in part, the increased incidence in women.

Types of Incontinence

Only with appropriate recognition of the problem, assessment, and referral for diagnostic evaluation and treatment can the outcome of incontinence be determined. All patients with incontinence should be considered for evaluation and treatment. Urinary incontinence may be transient or

---

BOX 28-4 **Risk Factors for Urinary Incontinence**

- Pregnancy: vaginal delivery, episiotomy
- Menopause
- Genitourinary surgery
- Pelvic muscle weakness
- Incompetent urethra due to trauma or sphincter relaxation
- Immobility
- High-impact exercise
- Diabetes mellitus
- Stroke
- Age-related changes in the urinary tract
- Morbid obesity
- Cognitive disturbances: dementia, Parkinson disease
- Medications: diuretics, sedatives, hypnotics, opioids
- Caregiver or toilet unavailable

Causes of Transient Incontinence: DIAPPERS

Delirium
Infection of urinary tract
Atrophic vaginitis, urethritis
Pharmacologic agents (anticholinergics, sedatives, alcohol, analgesics, diuretics, muscle relaxants, adrenergic agents)
Psychological factors (depression, regression)
Excessive urine production (increased intake, diabetes insipidus, diabetic ketoacidosis)
Restricted activity
Stool impaction

reversible if the underlying cause is successfully treated and the voiding pattern reverts to normal (Box 28-5).

Stress incontinence is the involuntary loss of urine through an intact urethra as a result of sneezing, coughing, or changing position. It predominantly affects women who have had vaginal deliveries and is thought to be the result of decreasing ligament and pelvic floor support (pelvic floor dysfunction) of the urethra and decreasing or absent estrogen levels within the urethral walls and bladder base. In men, stress incontinence is often experienced after a radical prostatectomy for prostate cancer because of the loss of urethral compression that the prostate had supplied before the surgery.

Urge incontinence is the involuntary loss of urine associated with a strong urge to void that cannot be suppressed. The patient is aware of the need to void but is unable to reach a toilet in time. An uninhibited detrusor contraction is the precipitating factor. This can occur in a patient with neurologic dysfunction that impairs inhibition of bladder contraction or in a patient without overt neurologic dysfunction.

Reflex incontinence is the involuntary loss of urine due to hyperreflexia in the absence of normal sensations usually associated with voiding. This commonly occurs in patients with spinal cord injury because they have neither neurologically mediated motor control of the detrusor nor sensory awareness of the need to void (see Chapter 45).

Overflow incontinence is the involuntary loss of urine associated with overdistention of the bladder. Such overdistention results from the bladder's inability to empty normally, despite frequent urine loss. Neurologic abnormalities (e.g., spinal cord lesions), factors that obstruct the outflow of urine (e.g., tumors, strictures, and prostatic hyperplasia), and myogenic abnormalities (problems with bladder contractions) can cause overflow incontinence.

Functional incontinence refers to those instances in which lower urinary tract function is intact but other factors, such as severe cognitive impairment (e.g., Alzheimer dementia), make it difficult for the patient to identify the need to void or physical impairments make it difficult or impossible for the patient to reach the toilet in time for voiding.

Iatrogenic incontinence refers to the involuntary loss of urine due to extrinsic medical factors, predominantly medications. One such example is the use of alpha-adrenergic agents to decrease blood pressure. In some people with an intact urinary system, these agents adversely affect the alpha receptors responsible for bladder neck closing pressure; the bladder neck relaxes to the point of incontinence with a minimal increase in intra-abdominal pressure, thus mimicking stress incontinence. As soon as the medication is discontinued, the apparent incontinence resolves.

Some patients have several types of urinary incontinence. This mixed incontinence is usually a combination of stress and urge incontinence (Drake, 2016).

Clinical Manifestations and Assessment

Once incontinence is recognized, a thorough history is necessary. This includes a detailed description of the problem and a history of medication use, noting those associated with urinary incontinence such as loop diuretics, ACE inhibitors, calcium channel blockers, narcotics, sedatives–hypnotics (including alcohol), anticholinergics, and NSAIDs (Resnick, 2016). The patient's voiding history, a diary of fluid intake and output, and bedside tests (e.g., residual urine, stress maneuvers) may be used to help determine the type of urinary incontinence involved. Extensive urodynamic tests may be performed. In addition, urinalysis and urine culture are performed to identify infection.

Medical Management

Management depends on the type of urinary incontinence and its causes. Strategies for promoting urinary continence can be found in Box 28-6. Management of urinary

Patient Education

Strategies for Promoting Urinary Continence

- Increase your awareness of the amount and timing of all fluid intake.
- Avoid taking diuretics after 4 PM.
- Avoid bladder irritants, such as caffeine, alcohol, and aspartame (NutraSweet).
- Take steps to avoid constipation: Drink adequate fluids, eat a well-balanced diet high in fiber, exercise regularly, and take stool softeners if recommended.
- Void regularly, 5–8 times a day (about every 2–3 hours at first, and increasing duration between voids):
  - First thing in the morning
  - Before each meal
  - Before retiring to bed
  - Once during night if necessary
- Perform all pelvic floor muscle exercises as prescribed, every day.
- Stop smoking (smokers usually cough frequently, which increases incontinence).

incontinence may be behavioral, pharmacologic, or surgical in nature.

Behavioral Therapy

Behavioral therapies are the first choice to decrease or eliminate urinary incontinence and or symptoms of OAB (Box 28-7). In using these techniques, health care professionals help patients avoid potential adverse effects of pharmacologic or surgical interventions.

Pharmacologic Therapy

Pharmacologic therapy works best when used as an adjunct to behavioral interventions. Anticholinergic agents inhibit bladder contraction and are considered first-line medications for urge incontinence. Oxybutynin (Ditropan) is frequently prescribed and has dual actions of relaxing the detrusor muscle and inhibiting bladder contraction. Hormone therapy (e.g., estrogen) taken orally, transdermally, or topically was once the treatment of choice for urinary incontinence in

---

BOX 28-7 | **Behavioral Interventions for Urinary Incontinence**

Behavioral strategies are largely carried out, coordinated, and monitored by the nurse. These interventions may or may not be augmented by the use of medications.

Fluid Management

One of the most common approaches is fluid management because adequate daily fluid intake of approximately 50–60 oz (1,500–1,800 mL), taken as small increments between breakfast and the evening meal, helps to reduce urinary urgency related to concentrated urine production, decreases the risk of urinary tract infection, and maintains bowel functioning. (Constipation, resulting from inadequate daily fluid intake, can increase urinary urgency and/or urine retention.) The best fluid is water. Fluids containing caffeine, carbonation, alcohol, or artificial sweetener should be avoided because they irritate the bladder wall, thus resulting in urinary urgency. Some patients who have coexisting medical diagnoses, such as heart failure or end-stage kidney disease, need to discuss their daily fluid limit with their primary health care provider.

Weight Management

Obesity is associated with OAB and urinary incontinence, thus weight control should be considered as a first-line intervention, particularly when the body mass index (BMI) is greater than 27. Studies reveal that weight loss leads to a significant reduction of the frequency and severity of urge incontinence episodes (Krhut et al., 2016).

Standardized Voiding Frequency

After establishing a patient's natural voiding and urinary incontinence tendencies, voiding on a schedule can be very effective in those with and without cognitive impairment, although patients with cognitive impairment may require assistance with this technique from nursing personnel or family members. The object is to purposely empty the bladder before the bladder reaches the critical volume that would cause an urge or stress incontinence episode. This approach involves the following:

- **Timed voiding** involves establishing a set voiding frequency (such as every 2 hours if incontinent episodes tend to occur 2 or more hours after voiding). The individual chooses to "void by the clock" at the given interval while awake, rather than wait until a voiding urge occurs.
- **Prompted voiding** is timed voiding that is carried out by staff or family members when the individual has cognitive

difficulties that make it difficult to remember to void at set intervals. The caregiver checks the patient to assess if he or she has remained dry and, if so, assists the patient to use the bathroom while providing positive reinforcement for remaining dry.

- **Habit retraining** is timed voiding at an interval that is more frequent than the individual would usually choose. This technique helps to restore the sensation of the need to void in individuals who are experiencing diminished sensation of bladder filling due to various medical conditions such as a mild cerebrovascular accident (CVA).
- **Bladder retraining** incorporates a timed voiding schedule and urinary urge inhibition exercises to inhibit voiding, or leaking urine, in an attempt to remain dry for a set time. When the first timing interval is easily reached on a consistent basis without urinary urgency or incontinence, a new voiding interval, usually 10–15 minutes beyond the last, is established. Again, the individual practices urge inhibition exercises to delay voiding or avoid incontinence until the next preset interval arrives. When an acceptable voiding interval is reached, the patient continues that timed voiding sequence throughout the day.

Pelvic Muscle Exercise

Pelvic muscle exercise (PME) aims to strengthen the voluntary muscles that assist in bladder and bowel continence in both men and women. Research shows that written and/or verbal instruction alone is usually inadequate to teach an individual how to identify and strengthen the pelvic floor for sufficient bladder and bowel control. Biofeedback-assisted PME uses either electromyography or manometry to help the individual identify the pelvic muscles as he or she attempts to learn which muscle group is involved when performing PME. The biofeedback method also allows assessment of the strength of this muscle area.

PME involves gently tightening the same muscles used to stop flatus or the stream of urine for 5- to 10-second increments, followed by 10-second resting phases. To be effective, these exercises need to be performed 2 or 3 times a day for at least 6 weeks. Depending on the strength of the pelvic musculature when initially evaluated, anywhere from 10 to 30 repetitions of PME are prescribed at each session. Elderly patients may need to exercise for an even longer time to strengthen the pelvic floor muscles. Pelvic muscle exercises are helpful for women with stress, urge, or mixed incontinence and for men who have undergone prostate surgery.

Vaginal Cone Retention Exercises

Vaginal cone retention exercises are an adjunct to the pelvic muscle (Kegel) exercises. Vaginal cones of varying weight are inserted intravaginally twice a day. The patient tries to retain the cone for 15 minutes by contracting the pelvic muscles.

Transvaginal or Transrectal Electrical Stimulation

Commonly used to treat urinary incontinence, electrical stimulation is known to elicit a passive contraction of the pelvic floor musculature, thus re-educating these muscles to provide enhanced levels of continence. This modality is often used with biofeedback-assisted pelvic muscle exercise training and voiding schedules. At high frequencies, it is effective for stress incontinence. At low frequencies, electrical stimulation can also relieve symptoms of urinary urgency, frequency, and urge incontinence. Intermediate ranges are used for mixed incontinence.

Neuromodulation

Neuromodulation via transvaginal or transrectal nerve stimulation of the pelvic floor inhibits detrusor overactivity and hypersensory bladder signals and strengthens weak sphincter muscles.

postmenopausal women, however evidence now exists that oral estrogen may worsen incontinence (Resnick, 2016) and is not recommended (Lukacz, 2016). Topical estrogen can be useful for peri- or postmenopausal women with either stress or urgency incontinence and vaginal atrophy which can contribute to incontinence (Lukacz, 2016).

Surgical Management

Surgical correction may be indicated in patients who have not achieved continence using behavioral and pharmacologic therapy. Surgical options vary according to the underlying anatomy and the physiologic problem. Most procedures involve lifting and stabilizing the bladder or urethra to restore the normal urethrovesical angle or to lengthen the urethra (Dmochowski, Osborn, & Reynolds, 2016). Urethral slings are currently the procedure of choice for the surgical correction of female stress urinary incontinence. Women with stress incontinence may undergo an anterior vaginal repair, retropubic suspension, or needle suspension to reposition the urethra. Procedures to compress the urethra and increase resistance to urine flow include sling procedures and placement of periurethral bulking agents such as artificial collagen.

Periurethral bulking is a semipermanent procedure in which small amounts of artificial collagen (or other substances) are placed within the walls of the urethra to enhance the closing pressure of the urethra. This procedure takes only 10 to 20 minutes and may be performed under local anesthesia or moderate sedation. A cystoscope is inserted into the urethra, and a small amount of collagen is injected into the urethral wall. The patient is usually discharged home after voiding. More than one collagen bulking session may be necessary if the initial procedure did not halt the stress urinary incontinence. Periurethral bulking with collagen offers an alternative to surgery, as in a frail, elderly person. It is also an option for people who are seeking help with stress urinary incontinence who prefer to avoid surgery and who do not have access to behavioral therapies. Although limited evidence exists to date for the benefit of these agents, because of the low risk of side effects associated with periurethral bulking agents, it is considered an option for those not ready to undergo a more invasive surgical procedure (Dmochowski et al., 2016).

An artificial urinary sphincter can be used to close the urethra and promote continence. Two types of artificial sphincters are a periurethral cuff and a cuff inflation pump. This therapy is approved for men only and is often used after treatment for prostate cancer (Fig. 28-3).

Men with overflow and urge incontinence may undergo a transurethral resection to relieve symptoms of prostatic enlargement.

Nursing Management

Nursing management is based on the premise that incontinence is not inevitable with illness or aging and that it is often reversible and treatable. The nursing interventions are

FIGURE 28-3 Male artificial urinary sphincter. An inflatable cuff is inserted surgically around the urethra or neck of the bladder. To empty the bladder, the cuff is deflated by squeezing the control pump located in the scrotum.

determined by the type of treatment that is undertaken. For behavioral therapy to be effective, the nurse must provide support and encouragement because it is easy for the patient to become discouraged if therapy does not quickly improve the level of continence. Patient teaching is important and should be provided verbally and in writing (see Box 28-6). The patient should be taught to develop and use a log or diary to record timing of pelvic floor muscle exercises, frequency of voiding, any changes in bladder function, and any episodes of incontinence (Drake, 2016; Resnick, 2016).

If pharmacologic treatment is used, it is important to educate patients who have mixed incontinence (both stress and urge incontinence) that anticholinergic and antispasmodic agents can help decrease urinary urgency and frequency and urge incontinence, but they do not decrease the urinary incontinence related to stress incontinence. If surgical correction is undertaken, the procedure and its desired outcomes are described to the patient and family. Follow-up contact with the patient enables the nurse to answer the patient's questions and to provide reinforcement and encouragement.

Gerontologic Considerations

Many older people experience transient episodes of incontinence that tend to be abrupt in onset. When this occurs, the nurse should question the patient, as well as the family if possible, about the onset of symptoms and any signs or symptoms of a change in other organ systems. Acute UTI, infection elsewhere in the body, constipation, stool impaction, a change in a chronic disease pattern, such as elevated blood glucose levels in patients with diabetes or decreased estrogen levels in menopausal women, can provoke the onset of urinary incontinence. If the cause is identified and modified or eliminated early at the onset of incontinence, the incontinence itself may be eliminated. Although the bladder of the older person is more vulnerable to altered detrusor activity (bladder capacity does not change, but sensation and contractility decrease), age alone is not a risk factor for urinary incontinence (Resnick, 2016). Decreased bladder muscle tone is a normal age-related change found in the elderly, which can lead to, increased residual urine, and an increase in urgency (Resnick, 2016).

URINARY RETENTION

Urinary retention is the inability to empty the bladder completely during attempts to void. Acute urinary retention in men is frequently associated with obstruction such as BPH or acute prostatitis. Acute retention occurs infrequently in women, with the exception of postoperatively due to anesthesia effects; it can also occur due to organ prolapse. Chronic urine retention often leads to overflow incontinence (from the pressure of the retained urine in the bladder). **Residual urine** is urine that remains in the bladder after voiding. In a healthy adult younger than 60 years, complete bladder emptying should occur with each voiding. In adults older than 60 years, 50 to 100 mL of residual urine may remain after each voiding because of the decreased contractility of the detrusor muscle.

Urinary retention can occur postoperatively in any patient who received spinal or general anesthesia. General anesthesia reduces bladder muscle innervation and suppresses the urge to void, impeding bladder emptying. A number of medications have been implicated in the development of urinary retention and are briefly discussed below. Other etiologies that should be considered in acute urinary retention are trauma, infection (prostatitis, cystitis), and neurologic and psychiatric disorders.

Pathophysiology

Urinary retention may result from diabetes, prostatic enlargement, urethral pathology (infection, urethral strictures, tumor, calculus), trauma (pelvic injuries), pregnancy, or neurologic or myogenic disorders such as stroke, spinal cord injury, multiple sclerosis (MS), Guillain–Barré syndrome, or Parkinson disease.

Some medications cause urinary retention, either by inhibiting bladder contractility or by increasing bladder outlet resistance, namely anticholinergics and sympathomimetic agents. Medications that cause retention by inhibiting bladder contractility include antispasmodic agents (oxybutynin chloride, belladonna, and opioid suppositories) and tricyclic antidepressant medications (imipramine, doxepin). Medications that cause urine retention by increasing bladder outlet resistance include alpha-adrenergic agents (ephedrine sulfate, pseudoephedrine), beta-adrenergic blockers (propranolol), and estrogens.

Sympathomimetics "mimic" the sympathetic nervous system and therefore have the anticipated result of increasing heart rate and contractility, dilating bronchioles and pupils, and—pertinent to this chapter—relaxing the bladder wall and thus closing the sphincter, affecting urinary retention. Anticholinergics work by blocking the parasympathetic nervous system response, which causes contraction of the bladder and relaxation of the sphincter. Thus since this response is blocked, clinically the effects are similar to the sympathomimetics; hence, both drugs are implicated in urinary retention.

Clinical Manifestations and Assessment

The assessment of a patient for urinary retention is multifaceted because the signs and symptoms may be easily overlooked. The following questions serve as a guide in assessment:

- What was the time of the last voiding, and how much urine was voided?
- Is the patient voiding small amounts of urine frequently?
- Is the patient dribbling urine?

- Does the patient complain of pain or discomfort in the lower abdomen? (Discomfort may be relatively mild if the bladder distends slowly.)
- Is the pelvic area rounded and swollen, indicating urine retention and a distended bladder?
- Does percussion of the suprapubic region elicit dullness, possibly indicating urine retention and a distended bladder?
- Are other indicators of urinary retention present, such as restlessness and agitation?
- Does a postvoid bladder ultrasound test reveal residual urine?

The patient may verbalize an awareness of bladder fullness and a sensation of incomplete bladder emptying. Signs and symptoms of UTI (hematuria, urgency, frequency, nocturia, and dysuria) may be present. A series of urodynamic studies, described in Chapter 26, may be performed to identify the type of bladder dysfunction and to aid in determining appropriate treatment. The patient may complete a voiding diary to provide a written record of the amount of urine voided and the frequency of voiding. Postvoid residual urine may be assessed either using straight catheterization or an ultrasound bladder scanner and is considered diagnostic of urinary retention if there is more than 100 mL of residual urine.

Medical Management

Management strategies are instituted to prevent overdistention of the bladder and to treat infection or correct underlying etiology for the retention. Immediate management involves decompression of the bladder via catheterization, which is discussed later in this chapter.

Nursing Management

Many problems can be prevented with careful assessment and appropriate nursing interventions. The nurse explains why normal voiding is not occurring and monitors urine output closely. The nurse also provides reassurance about the temporary nature of retention and successful management strategies.

In the case of acute urinary retention, decompression with a urethral catheter is commonly required. Nurses need to assess, however, if the patient recently underwent surgery, such as a radical prostatectomy or urethral reconstruction, since catheterization via urethra would be contraindicated. Barring no contraindications to urinary catheterization, the nurse chooses a 14- to 18-French Foley catheter, and if the patient has a past history of prostatic disease a *coude* catheter is recommended to facilitate passage through the posterior urethra. A complication associated with emergent catheterization for urinary retention is hypotension and hematuria.

Promoting Urinary Elimination

Nursing measures to encourage normal voiding patterns include providing privacy, ensuring an environment and a position conducive to voiding, and assisting the patient with the use of the bathroom or bedside commode, rather than a bedpan, to provide a more natural setting for voiding. The male patient may stand beside the bed while using the urinal; most men find this position more comfortable and natural.

Additional measures include applying warmth to relax the sphincters (i.e., sitz baths, warm compresses to the perineum, showers), giving the patient hot tea, and offering encouragement and reassurance. Simple trigger techniques, such as turning on the water faucet while the patient is trying to void, may also be used. After surgery or childbirth, prescribed analgesics should be administered because pain in the perineal area can make voiding difficult.

When the patient cannot void, catheterization is used to prevent overdistention of the bladder (see later discussion of neurogenic bladder and catheterization). Rarely is a suprapubic tube used for BPH. After urinary drainage is restored, bladder retraining is initiated for the patient who cannot void spontaneously.

Promoting Home Care

Modifications to the home environment can provide simple and effective ways to assist in treating urinary incontinence and retention. For example, the patient may need to remove obstacles, such as throw rugs or other objects, to provide easy, safe access to the bathroom. Other modifications that the nurse may recommend include installing support bars in the bathroom; placing a bedside commode, bedpan, or urinal within easy reach; leaving lights on in the bedroom and bathroom; and wearing clothing that is easy to remove quickly.

Complications

Urine retention can lead to chronic infection and, if left unresolved, predispose the patient to renal calculi (urolithiasis or nephrolithiasis), pyelonephritis, and sepsis. Acute or chronic kidney failure may develop secondary to renal obstruction (refer to Chapter 27). If hydronephrosis has occurred due to large volumes of retained urine, renal insufficiency may develop and progress to kidney failure.

NEUROGENIC BLADDER

Neurogenic bladder is a dysfunction that results from a lesion of the nervous system and leads to urinary incontinence. It may be caused by spinal cord injury, spinal tumor, herniated vertebral disk, MS, congenital disorders (spina bifida or myelomeningocele), myogenic disorders, infection, or diabetes mellitus.

Pathophysiology

The two types of neurogenic bladder are spastic (or reflex) bladder and flaccid bladder. Spastic bladder is more common and is caused by any spinal cord lesion above the voiding reflex arc (upper motor neuron lesion). The result is a loss of conscious sensation and cerebral motor control. A spastic bladder empties on reflex, with minimal or no controlling influence to regulate its activity.

Flaccid bladder is caused by a lower motor neuron lesion, commonly resulting from trauma, but increasingly recognized in patients with diabetes mellitus. The bladder continues to fill and becomes greatly distended, and overflow incontinence occurs. The bladder muscle does not contract forcefully at any time. Because sensory loss may accompany a flaccid bladder, the patient feels no discomfort. This can also occur in men with BPH with obstructive component.

Clinical Manifestations and Assessment

Evaluation for neurogenic bladder involves measurement of fluid intake, urine output, and residual urine volume, urinalysis, and assessment of sensory awareness of bladder fullness and degree of motor control. Comprehensive urodynamic studies are also performed.

Medical Management

The problems resulting from neurogenic bladder disorders vary considerably from patient to patient. Several long-term objectives are appropriate for all types of neurogenic bladders:

- Preventing overdistention of the bladder
- Emptying the bladder regularly and completely
- Maintaining urine sterility with no stone formation
- Maintaining adequate bladder capacity with no reflux

Specific interventions include continuous or intermittent self-catheterization (ISC), use of an external condom-type catheter, and encouragement of mobility and ambulation. A liberal fluid intake is encouraged to reduce the urinary bacterial count, reduce stasis, decrease the concentration of calcium in the urine, and minimize the precipitation of urinary crystals and subsequent stone formation.

A bladder retraining program may be effective in treating a spastic bladder or urine retention. Use of a timed voiding schedule may be established. The patient may be taught to "double void": after each voiding, the patient is instructed to remain on the toilet, relax for 1 to 2 minutes, and then attempt to void again in an effort to further empty the bladder.

Pharmacologic Therapy

Alpha blockers were originally developed for hypertension; these drugs block the adrenergic system and help patients with BPH by relaxing smooth muscle tissue found in the prostate and the bladder neck, thereby facilitating urine outflow. The four alpha medications approved by the U.S. Food and Drug Administration (FDA) are: terazosin (Hytrin), doxazosin (Cardura), tamsulosin (Flomax), and alfuzosin (Uroxatral).

Surgical Management

In some cases, surgery may be carried out to correct bladder neck contractures, prostatic obstruction, vesicoureteral reflux, or to perform some type of urinary diversion procedure.

Catheterization

In patients with a urologic disorder or with marginal kidney function, care must be taken to ensure that urinary drainage is adequate and that kidney function is preserved. When urine cannot be eliminated naturally and must be drained artificially, catheters may be inserted directly into the bladder, the ureter, or the renal pelvis. Catheters vary in size, shape, length, material, and configuration. The type of catheter used depends on its purpose, and catheterization is performed to achieve the following:

- Relieve urinary tract obstruction
- Assist with postoperative drainage in urologic and other surgeries
- Provide a means to monitor accurate urine output in critically ill patients
- Promote urinary drainage in patients with neurogenic bladder dysfunction or urine retention
- Prevent urinary leakage in patients with stage III to IV pressure ulcers (see Chapter 52)

A patient should be catheterized only if necessary, because instrumentation can lead to UTI. Catheters impede most of the natural defenses of the lower urinary tract by obstructing the periurethral ducts, irritating the bladder mucosa, and providing an artificial route for organisms to enter the bladder. Organisms may be introduced from the urethra into the bladder during catheterization, or they may migrate along the epithelial surface of the urethra or external surface of the catheter.

Indwelling Catheters

Approximately 50,000 long-term care patients each year have an indwelling catheter (CDC, 2015). When an indwelling catheter cannot be avoided, a closed drainage system is essential. This drainage system is designed to prevent any disconnections, thereby reducing the risk of contamination. The spout (or drainage port) of any urinary drainage bag can become contaminated when opened to drain the bag. Bacteria enter the urinary drainage bag, multiply rapidly, and then migrate to the drainage tubing, catheter, and bladder. By keeping the drainage bag lower than the patient's bladder and not allowing urine to flow back into the bladder, this risk is minimized.

Triple-lumen catheters are commonly used after transurethral prostate surgery (TURP) (see Chapter 34). This system has a triple-lumen indwelling urethral catheter attached to a closed sterile drainage system. With the triple-lumen catheter, urinary drainage occurs through one channel. The retention balloon of the catheter is inflated with water or air through the second channel, and the bladder is continuously irrigated with sterile irrigating solution through the third channel.

> ### Nursing Alert
> *After a patient undergoes a TURP, he will have a three-way catheter system in place that fulfills several roles: irrigation, tamponade, drainage, and traction. Precise intake and output records must be maintained, especially if total resection time was greater than 90 minutes. These men are at risk for TUR syndrome, a result of the absorption of irrigation fluid intraoperatively, which can lead to hyponatremia, bradycardia, and confusion.*

Accurate intake and output and patient assessment are essential to avoid the complication of hyponatremia and volume overload associated with instillation of large volumes of irrigating solution. Solutions used for urinary irrigation are electrolyte-free, thus hypo-osmotic and in general are glycine, sorbitol, and mannitol. During a TURP, the hypotonic solution can be absorbed into the prostatic veins with resultant volume overload and dilutional hyponatremia. The nurse is alert for signs of fluid overload such as dyspnea, decreasing O_2 saturation, jugular vein distention, development of S_3 gallop, hypertension or hypotension (with the development of congestive heart failure [CHF]), and arrhythmias. Early signs of dilutional hyponatremia are mental status changes, headache, nausea and vomiting, muscle twitching, and respiratory distress. The provider is notified of any change in patient condition. The rate of irrigant infusion is aimed at maintaining clear to pink-colored urine. When clots are present, the rate of infusion is increased to prevent clot retention. Since the draining irrigant and urine are both returning to the urinary drainage bag, the nurse must keep an accurate record of amount of irrigant solution instilled and subtract the volume of the irrigant from the total drainage amount in the urinary drainage bag, which is recorded as urine. Thus, if 2 L were instilled over the past 4 hours and the urinary drainage bag contained 2,150 mL, the urine output for the past 4 hours is recorded as 150 mL.

Suprapubic Catheters
Suprapubic catheterization allows bladder drainage by inserting a catheter or tube into the bladder through a suprapubic (above the pubis) incision or puncture (Fig. 28-4). The catheter or suprapubic drainage tube is then threaded into the bladder and secured with sutures or tape, and the area around the catheter is covered with a sterile dressing. The catheter is connected to a sterile closed drainage system, and the tubing is secured to prevent tension on the catheter. This may be a temporary or permanent measure to divert the flow of urine from the urethra when the urethral route is impassable (because of injuries, strictures, prostatic obstruction),

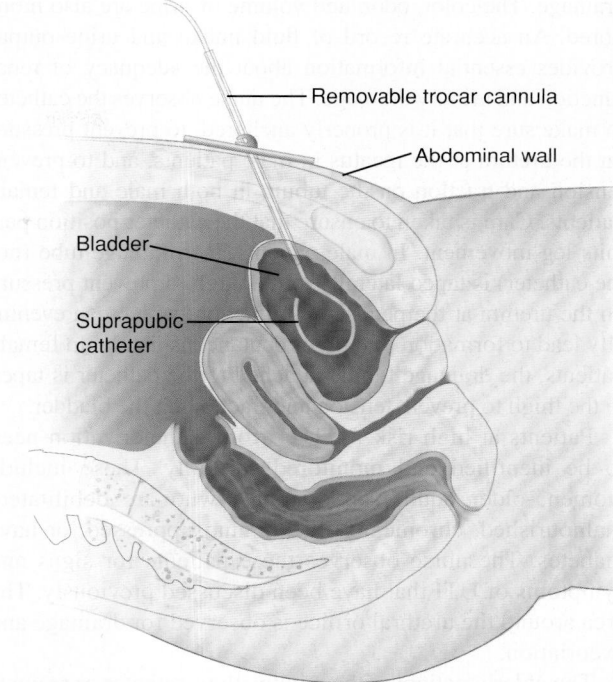

FIGURE 28-4 Suprapubic bladder drainage. A trocar cannula is used to puncture the abdominal and bladder walls. The catheter is threaded through the trocar cannula, which is then removed, leaving the catheter in place. The catheter is secured by tape or sutures to prevent unintentional removal.

after gynecologic or other abdominal surgery when bladder dysfunction is likely to occur, and occasionally after pelvic fractures. Suprapubic bladder drainage may be maintained continuously for several weeks.

Suprapubic drainage offers certain advantages. Patients can usually void sooner after surgery than can those with urethral catheters, and they may be more comfortable. The catheter allows greater mobility, permits measurement of residual urine without urethral instrumentation, and presents less risk of bladder infection. The suprapubic catheter is removed when it is no longer required, and a sterile dressing is placed over the site.

The patient requires liberal amounts of fluid to prevent encrustation around the catheter. Other potential problems include the formation of bladder stones, acute and chronic infections, and problems collecting urine. A **wound care specialist**/enterostomal therapist, also referred to as a wound-ostomy-continence nurse, may be consulted to assist the patient and family in selecting the most suitable urine collection system and to teach them about its use and care.

Nursing Management During Catheterization

Assessing the Patient and the System

For patients with indwelling catheters, the nurse assesses the drainage system to ensure that it provides adequate urinary drainage. The color, odor, and volume of urine are also monitored. An accurate record of fluid intake and urine output provides essential information about the adequacy of renal function and urinary drainage. The nurse observes the catheter to make sure that it is properly anchored, to prevent pressure on the urethra at the meatus in male patients, and to prevent tension and traction on the tubing in both male and female patients. Care is taken to ensure that the catheter position permits leg movement. In male patients, the drainage tube (not the catheter) is taped laterally to the thigh to prevent pressure on the urethra at the penoscrotal junction, which can eventually lead to formation of a urethrocutaneous fistula. In female patients, the drainage tubing attached to the catheter is taped to the thigh to prevent tension and traction on the bladder.

Patients at high risk for UTI from catheterization need to be identified and monitored carefully. These include women, older adults, and patients who are debilitated, malnourished, chronically ill, immunosuppressed, or have diabetes. The nurse observes these patients for signs and symptoms of UTI that have been discussed previously. The area around the urethral orifice is observed for drainage and excoriation.

The elderly patient with an indwelling catheter or patients with neurologic conditions (MS, stroke, spinal cord injury) may not exhibit the typical signs and symptoms of infection. Any subtle change in physical condition or mental status must be considered a possible indication of infection and promptly investigated because sepsis may occur before the infection is diagnosed. Figure 28-5 summarizes the sequence of events leading to infection and leakage of urine that often follow long-term use of an indwelling catheter in an elderly patient.

Preventing Infection

Certain principles of care are essential to prevent infection in patients with a closed urinary drainage system (Box 28-8). The catheter is a foreign body in the urethra and produces a reaction in the urethral mucosa with some urethral discharge.

Bacteriuria is considered inevitable in patients with indwelling catheters. Continual observation for fever, chills, and other signs and symptoms of systemic infection is necessary; these symptoms are generally treated aggressively.

Minimizing Trauma

Trauma to the urethra during catheterization can be minimized by:

- Using an appropriate-sized catheter
- Lubricating the catheter adequately with a water-soluble lubricant during insertion
- Inserting the catheter far enough into the bladder to prevent trauma to the urethral tissues when the retention balloon of the catheter is inflated

Manipulation of the catheter is the most common cause of trauma to the bladder mucosa in the catheterized patient.

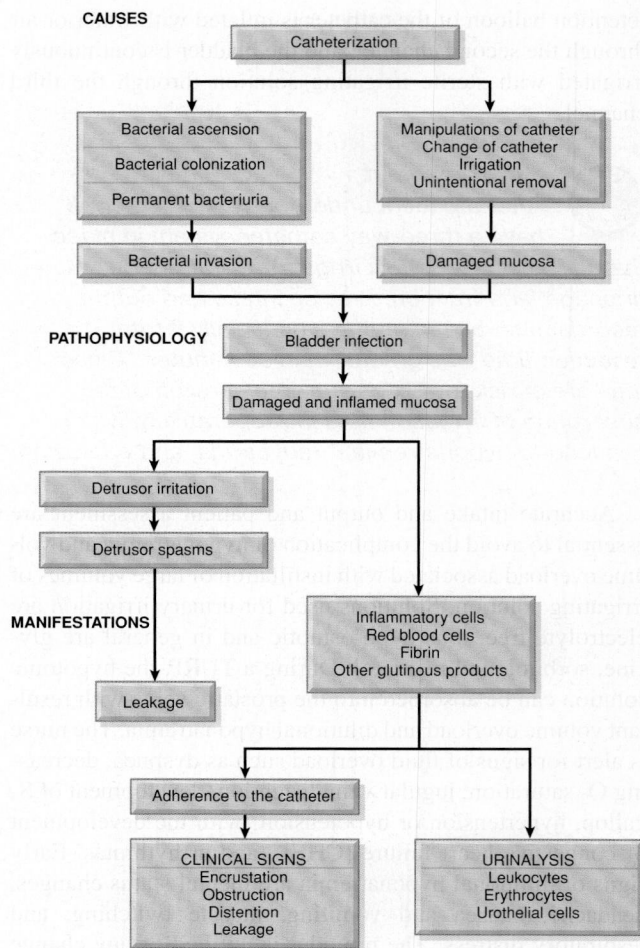

FIGURE 28-5 Pathophysiology and manifestations of bladder infection in long-term catheterized patients.

Infection can occur when urine invades the damaged mucosa. Special care should be taken to ensure that any patient who is confused does not remove the catheter with the retention balloon still inflated, because this could cause bleeding and considerable injury to the urethra.

Retraining the Bladder

When an indwelling urinary catheter is in place, the detrusor muscle does not actively contract the bladder wall to stimulate emptying because urine is continuously draining from the bladder. The detrusor may not immediately respond to bladder filling when the catheter is removed, resulting in either urine retention or urinary incontinence. This condition, known as *postcatheterization detrusor instability*, can be managed with bladder retraining (Box 28-9).

Immediately after the indwelling catheter is removed, the patient is placed on a timed voiding schedule, usually every 2 to 3 hours. After voiding, the bladder is scanned using a portable ultrasonic bladder scanner. If 100 mL or more of urine remains in the bladder, straight catheterization may

BOX 28-8

Preventing Infection in the Catheterized Patient

- Use scrupulous aseptic technique during insertion of the catheter. Use a preassembled, sterile, closed urinary drainage system.
- To prevent contamination of the closed system, *never* disconnect the tubing. The drainage bag must *never* touch the floor. The bag and collecting tubing are changed if contamination occurs, if urine flow becomes obstructed, or if tubing junctions start to leak at the connections.
- If the collection bag *must* be raised above the level of the patient's bladder, clamp the drainage tube. This prevents backflow of contaminated urine into the patient's bladder from the bag.
- Ensure a free flow of urine to prevent infection. Improper drainage occurs when the tubing is kinked or twisted, allowing pools of urine to collect in the tubing loops.
- To reduce the risk of bacterial proliferation, empty the collection bag at least every 8 hours through the drainage spout—more frequently if there is a large volume of urine.
- Avoid contamination of the drainage spout. A receptacle in which to empty the bag is provided for each patient.
- Never irrigate the catheter routinely. If the patient is prone to obstruction from clots or large amounts of sediment, use a three-way system with continuous irrigation.
- Never disconnect the tubing to obtain urine samples, to irrigate the catheter, or to ambulate or transport the patient.
- Never leave the catheter in place longer than is necessary.
- Avoid routine catheter changes. The catheter is changed only to correct problems such as leakage, blockage, or encrustations.

- To remove obvious encrustations from the external catheter surface, the area can be washed gently with soap during the daily bath. Using silicone catheters results in significantly less crust formation. A liberal fluid intake, within the limits of the patient's cardiac and renal reserve, and an increased urine output must be ensured to flush the catheter and to dilute urinary substances that might form encrustations.
- Avoid unnecessary handling or manipulation of the catheter by the patient or staff.
- Carry out hand hygiene before and after handling the catheter, tubing, or drainage bag.
- Wash the perineal area with soap and water at least twice a day; avoid a to-and-fro motion of the catheter. Vigorous cleansing of the meatus while the catheter is in place is discouraged because the cleansing action can move the catheter back and forth, increasing the risk of infection. Dry the area well, but avoid applying powder because it may irritate the perineum.
- Monitor the patient's voiding when the catheter is removed. The patient must void within 8 hours; if unable to void, the patient may require catheterization with a straight catheter.
- Urine cultures are obtained as prescribed or indicated when monitoring the patient for infection; many catheters have an aspiration (puncture) port from which a specimen can be obtained.

BOX 28-9

Bladder Retraining After Indwelling Catheterization

- Instruct the patient to drink a measured amount of fluid from 8 AM to 10 PM to avoid bladder overdistention. Offer no fluids (except sips) after 10 PM.
- At specific times, ask the patient to void by applying pressure over the bladder, tapping the abdomen, or stretching the anal sphincter with a finger to trigger the bladder.
- Immediately after the voiding attempt, assess the postvoid residual (PVR) urine either using straight catheterization or an ultrasound bladder scanner. Residual urine of more than 100 mL is considered diagnostic of urinary retention.
- Measure the volumes of urine voided and obtained by catheterization if indicated.
- Palpate the bladder at repeated intervals to assess for distention. If there is suspicion of urinary retention, percuss the bladder (refer to Chapter 26).
- Instruct the patient who has no voiding sensation to be alert for any signs that indicate a full bladder, such as perspiration, cold hands or feet, or feelings of anxiety.
- Lengthen the intervals between catheterizations as the volume of residual urine decreases. Catheterization is usually discontinued when the volume of residual urine is less than 100 mL.

be performed for complete bladder emptying. After a few days, as the nerve endings in the bladder wall become aware of bladder filling and emptying, bladder function usually returns to normal. If the person has had an indwelling catheter in place for an extended period, bladder retraining will take longer.

Assisting with Intermittent Self-Catheterization (ISC)

ISC provides periodic drainage of urine from the bladder. By promoting drainage and eliminating excessive residual urine, intermittent catheterization protects the kidneys, reduces the incidence of UTIs, and improves continence. It is the treatment of choice in patients with spinal cord injury and other neurologic disorders, such as MS, when the ability to empty the bladder is impaired. Self-catheterization promotes independence, results in few complications, and enhances self-esteem and quality of life.

When teaching the patient how to perform self-catheterization, the nurse must use aseptic technique to minimize the risk of cross-contamination. However, the patient may use a "clean" (nonsterile) technique at home, where the risk of cross-contamination is reduced. In teaching the patient, the nurse emphasizes the importance of frequent catheterization

Patient Education

Intermittent Self-Catheterization[a]

Females:
- Assume a sitting position.
- Use a mirror to help locate the urinary meatus once, and then after that feel for the appropriate location.
- Insert the lubricated catheter 7.5 cm (3 in) into the urethra, in a downward and backward direction until urine begins to flow.
- After removal, discard the catheter.
- Consult a primary health care provider at regular intervals to assess urinary function and to detect complications.

Males:
- Assume a Fowler's or sitting position.
- Lubricate the catheter.
- Retract the foreskin of the penis (if necessary) with one hand.
- Grasp the penis and hold it at a right angle to the body. (This maneuver straightens the urethra and makes it easier to insert the catheter.)
- Insert the catheter 15–25 cm (6–10 in) until urine begins to flow.
- After removal, discard the catheter.
- Consult a primary health care provider at regular intervals to assess urinary function and to detect complications.

[a]If the patient cannot perform intermittent self-catheterization, a family member may be taught to carry out the procedure at regular intervals during the day.

and emptying the bladder at the prescribed time. The average daytime clean intermittent catheterization schedule is every 4 to 6 hours and just before bedtime. If the patient is awakened at night with an urge to void, catheterization may be performed after an attempt is made to void normally. Refer to Box 28-10 for details regarding ISC teaching.

Complications

The most common complication of neurogenic bladder is infection resulting from urinary stasis and catheterization. Long-term complications include urolithiasis (stones in the urinary tract), vesicoureteral reflux, and hydronephrosis, all of which can lead to destruction of the kidney.

UROLITHIASIS AND NEPHROLITHIASIS

Urolithiasis and nephrolithiasis refer to stones (calculi) in the urinary tract and kidney, respectively. Urinary stones are a common condition with almost 2 million outpatient visits for a primary diagnosis of urolithiasis recorded in 2000, and over 80% of these stones will contain calcium, usually as calcium oxalate (Preminger & Curhan, 2016). Additionally, the

incidence of asymptomatic renal stones has been reported in approximately 10% of screened populations (Leavitt, de la Rosette, & Hoenig, 2016).

Pathophysiology

Stones are formed in the urinary tract when urinary concentrations of substances such as calcium oxalate, calcium phosphate, and uric acid increase. Referred to as *supersaturation*, this is dependent on the amount of the substance, ionic strength, and pH of the urine (an acid environment promotes calcium excretion). Stones may be found anywhere from the kidney to the bladder (Fig. 28-6) and may vary in size from minute granular deposits, called sand or gravel, to bladder stones as large as an orange.

Stone formation is not clearly understood, and there are a number of theories about their causes and links to systemic conditions such as obesity, hypertension and diabetes. Although it is not clear if stone disease is a direct cause of these disorders or if it is a consequence of the same conditions that lead to these disorders (Pearle et al., 2014, p. 316). Another theory relates to fluid volume status of the patient (stones tend to occur more often in dehydrated patients). Certain factors favor the formation of stones; however, in many patients, no cause may be found.

Risk Factors

Urinary stones occur predominantly in the third to fifth decades of life and affect men more than women (13% in men and 7% in women, annually), although an increased prevalence is observed across all age groups and in both sexes (Ferri, 2016). About half of patients with a single renal stone have another episode within 5 years. Anatomical

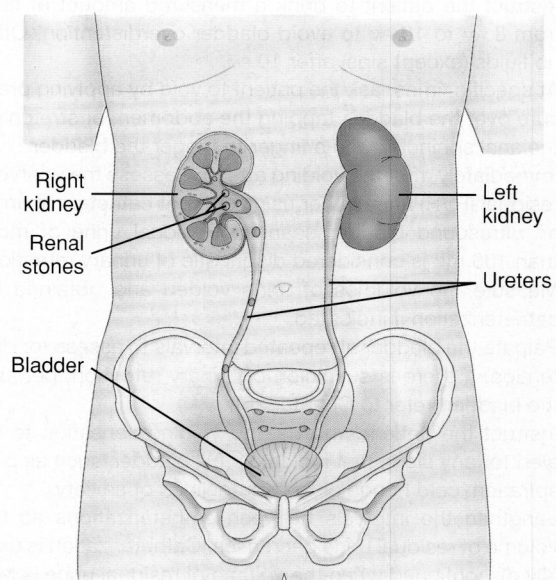

FIGURE 28-6 Examples of potential sites of calculi formation (urolithiasis) in the urinary tract.

structure of the upper and lower urinary tract may pose a risk as UTIs (struvite calculi) or stasis is associated with stone formation. Metabolic defects such as hyperparathyroidism and hyperuricemia (gout) are also associated with stone formation. Genetic predisposition, such as familial renal tubule acidosis, is strongly associated with nephrolithiasis. Spring and summer season are associated with a higher incidence of stone formation, most likely due to dehydration.

Clinical Manifestations and Assessment

Signs and symptoms of stones in the urinary system depend on the presence of obstruction, infection, and edema. When stones block the flow of urine, obstruction develops, producing an increase in hydrostatic pressure and distending the renal pelvis and proximal ureter. Infection (pyelonephritis and UTI with chills, fever, and dysuria) can be a contributing factor with struvite stones (Pearle et al., 2014). Some stones cause few symptoms while slowly destroying the nephrons of the kidney; others cause excruciating pain and discomfort.

Stones in the renal pelvis may be associated with an intense, deep ache in the costovertebral region (see Fig. 26-7). Hematuria is often present; pyuria may also be noted. Pain originating in the renal area radiates anteriorly and downward toward the bladder in the female and toward the testis in the male. If the pain suddenly becomes acute, with tenderness over the costovertebral area, and nausea and vomiting appear, the patient is having an episode of renal colic. Diarrhea and abdominal discomfort may occur. Stones lodged in the ureter (ureteral obstruction) cause ureteral colic: acute, excruciating, colicky, wavelike pain, radiating down the thigh and to the genitalia. Often, the patient has a desire to void, but little urine is passed, and it usually contains blood because of the abrasive action of the stone. In general, the patient spontaneously passes stones 0.5 to 1 cm in diameter. Stones larger than 1 cm in diameter usually must be removed or fragmented so that they can be removed or passed spontaneously. Stones lodged in the bladder usually produce symptoms of irritation and may be associated with UTI and hematuria. If the stone obstructs the bladder neck, urinary retention occurs.

The diagnosis is confirmed by x-rays of the kidneys, ureters, and bladder (KUB) or by ultrasonography, IV urography, or retrograde pyelography. Blood chemistries and a 24-hour urine test for measurement of calcium, uric acid, creatinine, sodium, pH, and total volume are part of the diagnostic workup. Dietary and medication histories and family history of renal stones are obtained to identify factors predisposing the patient to the formation of stones.

When stones are recovered (stones may be freely passed by the patient or removed through special procedures), chemical analysis is carried out to determine their composition.

Stone analysis can provide a clear indication of the underlying disorder (Table 28-2, p. 866).

Medical Management

The goals of management are to eradicate the stone, determine the stone type, prevent nephron destruction, control infection, and relieve any obstruction that may be present. The immediate objective of treatment of renal or ureteral colic is to relieve the pain until its cause can be eliminated. Opioid analgesics are administered; nonsteroidal anti-inflammatory drugs (NSAIDs) also have demonstrated efficacy in treating renal stone pain. In addition, NSAIDs also inhibit the synthesis of prostaglandin E, reducing swelling and facilitating passage of the stone. Hot baths or moist heat to the flank areas may also be useful. Fluids are encouraged to increase the hydrostatic pressure behind the stone, assisting it in its downward passage.

Nutritional Therapy

Nutritional therapy plays an important role in preventing renal stones (Pearle et al., 2014). Fluid intake is the mainstay of most medical therapy for renal stones. Unless fluids are contraindicated, patients with renal stones should drink eight to ten 8-oz glasses of water daily or have IV fluids prescribed to keep the urine dilute. A urine output exceeding 2 L a day is advisable.

Procedures for Treatment of Stone Disease

If the stone does not pass spontaneously or if complications occur, common interventions include endoscopic or other procedures—for example, ureteroscopy, extracorporeal shock wave lithotripsy (ESWL), or endourologic (percutaneous) stone removal (Fig. 28-7). Refer to discussion of surgical treatment in Table 28-3 on page 868.

Open surgical removal was the major mode of therapy before the advent of lithotripsy and improved endoscopic techniques. Today, open procedures are performed in only 1% to 2% of patients. Surgical intervention is indicated if the stone does not respond to other forms of treatment, and to correct anatomic abnormalities within the kidney to improve urinary drainage. If the stone is in the kidney, the surgery performed may be a nephrolithotomy (incision into the kidney with removal of the stone) or a nephrectomy, if the kidney is nonfunctional secondary to infection or hydronephrosis. Stones in the kidney pelvis are removed by a pyelolithotomy, those in the ureter by ureterolithotomy, and those in the bladder by cystotomy. If the stone is in the bladder, an instrument may be inserted through the urethra into the bladder, and the stone is crushed in the jaws of this instrument. Such a procedure is called a cystolitholapaxy. Nursing management following kidney surgery is discussed in Chapter 27.

TABLE **28-2** Comparison of Renal Stones

Stone Type	Causes	Treatment
Calcium (~75% of renal stones)	• Hypercalcemia (high serum calcium) and hypercalciuria (high urine calcium) • Hyperparathyroidism • Renal tubular acidosis • Cancers • Granulomatous diseases (e.g., sarcoidosis, tuberculosis), which may cause increased vitamin D production by the granulomatous tissue • Excessive intake of vitamin D • Excessive intake of milk and alkali • Myeloproliferative diseases (leukemia, polycythemia vera, multiple myeloma), which produce an unusual proliferation of blood cells from the bone marrow • Insufficient fluid intake	• If type II absorptive hypercalciuria (half of all patients with calcium stones), restricted calcium intake. • Liberal fluid intake encouraged. • Dietary restriction of protein and sodium. • Medications, such as ammonium chloride, may be used. • Thiazide diuretics may be beneficial in reducing calcium loss in the urine and lowering elevated parathormone levels.
Uric acid (~5–10% of stones) • Gout • Myeloproliferative disorders	• Low-purine diet • Foods high in purine (shellfish, anchovies, asparagus, mushrooms, and organ meats) are avoided. • Allopurinol may be prescribed to reduce serum uric acid levels and urinary uric acid excretion.	• Dietary management is key. • Sustained alkalization of urine with potassium citrate or sodium bicarbonate results in dissolution of existing stones. • Recommended urine output 30 mL/kg/24 hr.
Struvite (~15% of stones)	• Form in persistently alkaline, ammonia-rich urine caused by the presence of urease-splitting bacteria such as *Proteus, Pseudomonas, Klebsiella, Staphylococcus,* or *Mycoplasma* species • Predisposing factors for struvite stones include neurogenic bladder, foreign bodies, and recurrent urinary tract infections (UTIs).	• Fluid intake is increased.
Cystine (1–2% of all stones)	• Occur exclusively in patients with a rare inherited defect in renal absorption of cystine (an amino acid)	• Low-protein diet. • Urine is alkalinized. • Fluid intake is increased.
All stone types	• Infection, urinary stasis, and periods of immobility, all of which slow renal drainage and alter calcium metabolism • Anatomic derangements such as polycystic kidney disease, horseshoe kidneys, chronic strictures, and medullary sponge disease; also inflammatory bowel disease and in ileostomy or bowel resection (patients absorb more oxalate).	• Cessation of medications that cause stones including antacids, acetazolamide, Amphotericin B, vitamin D, loop diuretics, theophylline and high doses of aspirin (Bose, Monk, & Bushinsky, 2016). • A sodium intake of 3–4 g/day is recommended. Table salt and high-sodium foods should be reduced, because sodium competes with calcium for reabsorption in the kidneys. • Avoid intake of oxalate-containing foods (e.g., spinach, strawberries, rhubarb, tea, peanuts, wheat bran). • Drink two glasses of water at bedtime and an additional glass at each nighttime awakening to prevent urine from becoming too concentrated during the night. • Avoid activities leading to sudden increases in environmental temperatures that may cause excessive sweating and dehydration. • Contact your primary health care provider at the first sign of a UTI.

FIGURE 28-7 Methods of treating renal stones. **A.** During a cystoscopy, which is used for removing small stones located in the ureter close to the bladder, a ureteroscope is inserted into the ureter to visualize the stone. The stone is then fragmented or captured and removed. **B.** Extracorporeal shock wave lithotripsy (ESWL) may be used for symptomatic, nonpassable upper urinary tract stones. Electromagnetically generated shock waves are focused over the area of the renal stone. The high-energy dry shock waves pass through the skin and fragment the stone. **C.** Percutaneous nephrolithotomy is used to treat larger stones. A percutaneous tract is formed and a nephroscope is inserted through it. Then the stone is extracted or pulverized.

TABLE 28-3 Surgical Treatment of Renal Stones

Procedure	Description	Postprocedure Care
Ureteroscopy (see Fig. 28-7A)	Access to the stone is accomplished by inserting a ureteroscope into the ureter and then, depending on the size of the stone, either basketing or inserting a laser, electrohydraulic lithotripter, or ultrasound device through the ureteroscope to fragment and remove the stones. A stent may be inserted and left in place for 48 hours or more after the procedure to keep the ureter patent.	*For all procedures:* • Increase fluid intake to assist in the passage of stone fragments. • Monitor for signs and symptoms that indicate complications, such as fever, decreasing urine output, and pain. *For all procedures except electrohydraulic lithotripsy:* • Expect hematuria (it is anticipated in all patients), but it should disappear within 4–5 days.
Extracorporeal shock wave lithotripsy (ESWL) (see Fig. 28-7B)	A high-energy amplitude of pressure, or shock wave, is generated by the abrupt release of energy and transmitted through water and soft tissues; noninvasive procedure used to break up stones in the calyx of the kidney. After the stones are fragmented to the size of grains of sand, the remnants of the stones are spontaneously voided. The patient is observed for obstruction and infection resulting from blockage of the urinary tract by stone fragments.	
Endourologic methods (see Fig. 28-7C) percutaneous nephrostomy; percutaneous nephrolithotomy	A nephroscope is introduced through a percutaneous route into the renal parenchyma. Depending on its size, the stone may be extracted with forceps or by a stone retrieval basket.	
Electrohydraulic lithotripsy	An electrical discharge is used to create a hydraulic shock wave to break up the stone. A probe is passed through the cystoscope, and the tip of the lithotripter is placed near the stone. After the stone is extracted, the percutaneous nephrostomy tube is left in place for a time to ensure that the ureter is not obstructed by edema or blood clots.	

NURSING PROCESS
The Patient with Kidney Stones

ASSESSMENT

The patient with suspected renal stones is assessed for pain and discomfort as well as associated symptoms, such as nausea, vomiting, diarrhea, and abdominal distention. The severity and location of pain are determined, along with any radiation of the pain. Nursing assessment also includes observing for signs and symptoms of UTI and obstruction. The urine is inspected for blood and is strained for stones or gravel. The history focuses on factors that predispose the patient to urinary tract stones or that may have precipitated the current episode of renal or ureteral colic. The patient's knowledge about renal stones and measures to prevent their occurrence or recurrence is also assessed.

DIAGNOSIS

Appropriate nursing diagnoses of the patient with kidney stones may include:

• Acute pain related to inflammation, obstruction, and abrasion of the urinary tract
• Deficient knowledge regarding prevention of recurrence of renal stones
• Deficient knowledge regarding the role of diet in the treatment of renal stones
• Impaired urinary elimination due to presence of renal stones

Potential complications may include the following:

• Infection and urosepsis (from UTI and pyelonephritis)
• Obstruction of the urinary tract by a stone or edema with subsequent acute kidney failure

PLANNING

The major goals for the patient may include relief of pain and discomfort, prevention of recurrence of renal stones, and absence of complications.

NURSING INTERVENTIONS

RELIEVING PAIN

Severe and acute pain is often the presenting symptom of a patient with renal and urinary calculi and requires immediate attention. Opioid analgesic agents (IV or intramuscular) may be prescribed and administered to provide rapid relief along with an IV NSAID. The patient is encouraged and assisted to assume a position of comfort. If activity brings pain relief, the patient is assisted to ambulate. The pain level is monitored closely, and an increase in severity is reported promptly so that relief can be provided and additional treatment initiated.

MONITORING AND MANAGING POTENTIAL COMPLICATIONS

Increased fluid intake is encouraged to prevent dehydration and increase hydrostatic pressure within the urinary tract to promote passage of the stone. If the patient cannot take adequate fluids orally, IV fluids are prescribed. The total urine output and patterns of voiding are monitored. Ambulation is encouraged as a means of moving the stone through the urinary tract.

All urine is strained because uric acid stones may crumble. Any blood clots passed in the urine should be crushed and the sides of the urinal and bedpan inspected for clinging stones. Because renal stones increase the risk of infection, sepsis, and obstruction of the urinary tract, the patient is instructed to report decreased urine volume and bloody or cloudy urine.

Patients with calculi require frequent nursing observation to detect the spontaneous passage of a stone. The patient is instructed to immediately report any sudden increases in pain intensity because of the possibility of a stone fragment obstructing a ureter. Vital signs, including temperature, are monitored closely to detect early signs of infection. UTIs may be associated with renal stones due to an obstruction from the stone or from the stone itself. All infections should be treated with the appropriate antibiotic agent before efforts are made to dissolve the stone.

Because the risk of recurring renal stones is high, the nurse provides education about the causes of kidney stones and recommendations to prevent their recurrence (see Table 28-2). The patient is encouraged to follow a regimen to avoid further stone formation, including maintaining a high fluid intake because stones form more readily in concentrated urine. A patient who has shown a tendency to form stones should drink enough fluid to excrete greater than 2,000 mL for the rest of his or her life.

CONTINUING CARE

The patient is monitored closely in follow-up care to ensure that treatment has been effective and that no complications, such as obstruction, infection, renal hematoma, or hypertension, have developed.

The patient's ability to monitor urinary pH and interpret the results is assessed during follow-up visits to the clinic or health care provider's office. Because of the high risk of recurrence, the patient with renal stones needs to understand the signs and symptoms of stone formation, obstruction, and infection, and the importance of reporting these signs promptly. If medications are prescribed for the prevention of stone formation, the actions and importance of the medications are explained to the patient.

EVALUATION

Expected patient outcomes may include:
1. Reports relief of pain
2. States increased knowledge of health-seeking behaviors to prevent recurrence:
   a. Consumes increased fluid intake (at least eight 8-oz glasses of fluid per day)
   b. Participates in appropriate activity
   c. Consumes diet prescribed to reduce dietary factors predisposing to stone formation
   d. Recognizes symptoms (fever, chills, flank pain, hematuria) to be reported to health care provider
   e. Monitors urinary pH as directed
   f. Takes prescribed medication as directed to reduce stone formation
3. Experiences no complications:
   a. Reports no signs or symptoms of infection or urosepsis
   b. Voids 200 to 400 mL per voiding of clear urine without evidence of bleeding
   c. Experiences absence of dysuria, frequency, and hesitancy
   d. Maintains normal body temperature

GENITOURINARY TRAUMA

Various types of injuries of the flank, back, or upper abdomen may result in trauma to the ureters, bladder, or urethra. Renal injury occurs in 8% to 10% of cases of blunt and penetrating trauma, of which approximately 90% result from blunt force and 10% from penetrating injuries (gunshot or stabbing) (Miller & Mirvis, 2015). Approximately 10% of all injuries seen in the emergency department involve the genitourinary system (Runyon, 2014).

 Nursing Alert

If a patient is admitted with pelvic fractures, blunt trauma, with trauma related to motor vehicle accidents (MVAs), or with penetrating injuries, or has recently had urethral or bladder neck surgery, do not perform a urinary catheterization unless the provider has evaluated the patient for urethral tear.

Specific Injuries and Clinical Manifestations

Urethral Trauma

Urethral injuries usually occur with blunt trauma to the lower abdomen or pelvic region. Many patients also have associated pelvic fractures. Classic symptoms include blood at the urinary meatus (present in 80% to 90% of patients with urethral injury), penile, scrotal, or perineal, an inability to void, and a distended bladder. The nurse is aware that urinary catheterization is contraindicated if blood is noted at the urinary meatus, until urethral tear has been ruled out.

Ureteral Trauma

Penetrating trauma and unintentional injury during surgery are the major causes of trauma to the ureters. Gunshot wounds account for 95% of ureteral injuries, which may range from contusions to complete transection. Unintentional injury to the ureter may occur during gynecologic or urologic surgery. There are no specific signs or symptoms of ureteral injury; many traumatic injuries are discovered during exploratory surgery. If the ureteral trauma is not detected and urine leakage continues, fistulas can develop. IV urography detects 90% of ureteral injuries and can be performed on the operating table in patients undergoing emergent surgery. Surgical repair with placement of stents (to divert urine away from an anastomosis) is usually necessary.

Bladder Trauma

Injury to the bladder may occur with pelvic fractures and multiple traumas or from a blow to the lower abdomen when the bladder is full (lap belt or steering wheel injuries). Gross hematuria is present in more than 95% of patients with bladder rupture (Biffl, 2015). Blunt trauma may result in contusion, evident as an ecchymosis—a large, discolored bruise resulting from escape of blood into the tissues and involving a segment of the bladder wall—or in rupture of the bladder extraperitoneally, intraperitoneally, or both. Complications from these injuries include hemorrhage, shock, sepsis, and extravasation of blood into the tissues.

Medical Management

The goals of management in patients with genitourinary trauma are to control hemorrhage, pain, and infection and to maintain urinary drainage. Genitourinary trauma is frequently associated with renal trauma. Hematocrit and hemoglobin levels are monitored closely; decreasing values may indicate hemorrhage within the genitourinary system. The patient is also monitored for oliguria, signs of hemorrhagic shock, and signs and symptoms of acute peritonitis.

Surgical Management

Surgery is indicated for hemodynamic instability, ongoing bleeding, or urinary extravasation. However, minimally invasive techniques, such as angiographic embolization for hemorrhage and stenting for urinary extravasation, may allow renal salvage (Biffl, 2015, p. 589). In the case of urethral trauma, unstable patients who need monitoring of urine output may need a suprapubic catheter inserted. The patient is catheterized after urethrography is performed to minimize the risk of urethral disruption and extensive, long-term complications, such as stricture, incontinence, and impotence. Surgical repair may be performed immediately; delayed surgical repair tends to be the favored procedure because it is associated with fewer long-term complications. After surgery, an indwelling urinary catheter may remain in place for up to 1 month.

Nursing Management

The patient with genitourinary trauma should be assessed frequently during the first few days after injury to detect flank and abdominal pain, muscle spasm, and swelling over the flank.

During this time, patients can be instructed about care of the incision and the importance of an adequate fluid intake. In addition, instructions about changes that should be reported to the physician, such as fever, hematuria, flank pain, or any signs and symptoms of decreasing kidney function, are provided. The patient with a ruptured bladder may have gross bleeding for several days after repair. Guidelines for increasing activity gradually, lifting, and driving are also provided in accordance with the physician's prescription.

Follow-up nursing care includes monitoring the blood pressure to detect hypotension and advising the patient to restrict activities for about 1 month after trauma to minimize the incidence of delayed or secondary bleeding.

CANCER OF THE BLADDER

Urinary tract cancers include those of the urinary bladder, kidney and renal pelvis, ureters, and other urinary structures, such as the prostate. Approximately 380,300 cases of bladder cancer are diagnosed annually worldwide; in the United States it is the sixth most common cancer with an estimated 73,510 diagnoses and 13,750 deaths in 2012 (Smith, Balar, Milowsky, & Chen, 2013). Bladder cancer can span the spectrum from non–life-threatening, to invasive tumors that have metastasized at the time of diagnosis. The three types of bladder cancer are transitional cell carcinoma (TCCa) (93%), squamous cell carcinoma (6%), and adenocarcinoma (1%) (Ferri, 2016).

Risk Factors

Bladder cancer has a high worldwide incidence, and when combined with prostatic cancer, is the most common urologic malignancy, accounting for 90% of all tumors seen. Cancers arising from the prostate, colon, and rectum in males

Risk Factors for Bladder Cancer

- Cigarette smoking: risk proportional to number of packs smoked daily and number of years of smoking (associated with 50% of bladder cancers in the United States)
- Exposure to environmental carcinogens: Dyes, rubber, leather, ink, paint, metals, and petroleum
- Recurrent or chronic bacterial infection of the urinary tract
- Bladder stones
- High urinary pH
- High cholesterol intake
- Pelvic radiation therapy
- Cancers arising from the prostate, colon, and rectum in males
- Diets rich in beef, pork, and animal fat increase risk of bladder cancer (Ferri, 2016)
- Age, incidence increases with age: higher after the age 60 years, uncommon younger than 40 years median age at diagnosis is 73–74 years (Ferri, 2016)

and from the lower gynecologic tract in females may metastasize to the bladder. Box 28-11 summarizes risk factors.

Clinical Manifestations and Assessment

Bladder tumors usually arise at the base of the bladder and involve the ureteral orifices and bladder neck. Painless gross hematuria is the most common symptom of bladder cancer. Infection of the urinary tract is a common complication, producing frequency, urgency, and dysuria. Any alteration in voiding or change in the urine may indicate cancer of the bladder. Pelvic or back pain may occur with metastasis.

The diagnostic evaluation includes cystoscopy (the mainstay of diagnosis), excretory urography, CT, ultrasonography, and bimanual examination with the patient anesthetized. Biopsies of the tumor and adjacent mucosa are the definitive diagnostic procedures. TCCAs and carcinomas in situ shed recognizable cancer cells. Cytologic examination of fresh urine and saline bladder washings provide information about the prognosis and staging, especially for patients at high risk for recurrence of primary bladder tumors (Ferri, 2016).

Although the current diagnostic tools such as cytology and CT have a high detection rate, they are costly. Newer diagnostic tools such as bladder tumor antigens, nuclear matrix proteins, adhesion molecules, cytoskeletal proteins, and growth factors are being studied to support the early detection and diagnosis of bladder cancer. For example, urine telomerase in voided urine or bladder washings determined by the telomeric repeat amplification protocol (TRAP) assay has been reported to accurately detect the presence of bladder tumors in men (Ferri, 2016). It may represent a useful noninvasive diagnostic innovation for bladder cancer detection in high-risk groups such as habitual smokers or

in symptomatic patients (Ferri, 2016). To date, no universal screening test has been promoted.

Medical and Nursing Management

Treatment of bladder cancer depends on the grade of the tumor (the degree of cellular differentiation), the stage of tumor growth (the degree of local invasion and the presence or absence of metastasis), and the multicentricity (having many centers) of the tumor. Refer to Chapter 6 for further details on cancer. The patient's age and physical, mental, and emotional status are considered when discussing treatment modalities. Specific nursing care will be dictated by the treatment plan (e.g., relaying instructions with intravesical treatments).

Surgical Management

Transurethral resection or fulguration (cauterization) may be performed for simple papillomas (benign epithelial tumors). These procedures eradicate the tumors through surgical incision or electrical current with the use of instruments inserted through the urethra. After this surgery, intravesical administration of bacille Calmette-Guérin (BCG) may be appropriate. BCG is an attenuated live strain of *Mycobacterium bovis*, the causative agent for tuberculosis. The exact action of BCG is unknown, but it is has shown antitumor activity in multiple cancers, including urothelial carcinoma (Smith et al., 2013).

Management of superficial bladder cancers presents a challenge because there are usually widespread abnormalities in the bladder mucosa. The entire lining of the urinary tract, or urothelium, is at risk because carcinomatous changes can occur in the mucosa of the bladder, renal pelvis, ureter, and urethra. About 25% to 40% of superficial tumors recur after transurethral resection or fulguration. Patients with benign papillomas should undergo cytology and cystoscopy periodically for the rest of their lives.

A simple **cystectomy** or a radical cystectomy is performed for invasive or multifocal bladder cancer. Radical cystectomy in men involves removal of the bladder, prostate, and seminal vesicles and immediate adjacent perivesical tissues. In women, radical cystectomy involves removal of the bladder, lower ureter, uterus, fallopian tubes, ovaries, anterior vagina, and urethra. Removal of the bladder requires a urinary diversion procedure. Radical cystectomy remains the standard of care for invasive bladder cancer in the United States.

Pharmacologic Therapy

Chemotherapy with a combination of methotrexate, 5-fluorouracil, vinblastine, doxorubicin (Adriamycin), and cisplatin has been effective in producing partial remission of TCCa of the bladder in some patients. Topical chemotherapy (intravesical chemotherapy or instillation of antineoplastic agents into the bladder, resulting in contact of the agent with the bladder wall) is considered when there is a high risk of recurrence, when cancer in situ is present, or when tumor resection has been incomplete, and it delivers a high concentration of medication to the tumor to promote tumor destruction.

BCG is now considered the most effective intravesical agent for recurrent bladder cancer, especially superficial TCCa, because it is an immunotherapeutic agent that enhances the body's immune response to cancer. BCG is particularly effective in the treatment of carcinoma in situ, eradicating it in more than 80% of cases. Once the bladder is full, the patient must retain the intravesical solution for 2 hours before voiding. At the end of the procedure, the patient is encouraged to void and to drink liberal amounts of fluid to flush the medication from the bladder.

Radiation Therapy

Radiation of the tumor may be performed preoperatively to reduce microextension of the neoplasm and viability of tumor cells, thus reducing the chances that the cancer may recur in the immediate area or spread through the circulatory or lymphatic systems. Radiation therapy is also used in combination with surgery or to control the disease in patients with inoperable tumors.

URINARY DIVERSIONS

Urinary diversion procedures are performed to divert urine from the bladder to a new exit site, usually through a surgically created opening (stoma) in the skin. These procedures are primarily performed when a bladder tumor necessitates cystectomy. Urinary diversion has also been used in managing pelvic malignancy, birth defects, strictures, trauma to the ureters and urethra, neurogenic bladder, chronic infection causing severe ureteral and renal damage, and intractable **interstitial cystitis**.

Controversy exists about the best method of establishing permanent diversion of the urinary tract. New techniques are frequently introduced in an effort to improve patient outcomes and quality of life. The age of the patient, condition of the bladder, body build, degree of obesity, degree of ureteral dilation, status of renal function, and the patient's learning ability and willingness to participate in postoperative care are all taken into consideration when determining the appropriate surgical procedure. Acceptance of a urinary diversion depends to a large degree on the location or position of the stoma, whether the drainage device (pouch or bag) establishes a watertight seal to the skin, and the patient's ability to manage the pouch and drainage apparatus.

There are two types of urinary diversion. In a cutaneous urinary diversion, urine drains through an opening created in the abdominal wall and skin (Fig. 28-8, p. 873). In a **continent urinary diversion**, a portion of the intestine is used to create a new reservoir for urine (Fig. 28-9, p. 874).

CUTANEOUS URINARY DIVERSIONS

ILEAL CONDUIT

The **ileal conduit**, or ileal loop, is the oldest and most common of the urinary diversion procedures in use, because of the low number of complications and surgeons' familiarity with the procedure. The urine is diverted by implanting the ureters into a 12-cm loop of ileum that is led out through the abdominal wall. This loop of ileum is a simple conduit (passageway) for urine from the ureters to the surface. The resected (cut) ends of the remaining intestine are anastomosed (connected) to provide an intact bowel. A loop of the sigmoid colon may also be used. An ileostomy bag is used to collect the urine.

Stents are placed in the ureters to prevent occlusion secondary to postsurgical edema. Bilateral ureteral stents allow urine to drain from the kidney to the stoma and provide a method for accurate measurement of urine output. They may be left in place 10 to 21 days postoperatively. Jackson–Pratt tubes or other types of drains are inserted to prevent the accumulation of fluid in the space created by removal of the bladder.

After surgery, a skin barrier and a transparent, disposable urinary drainage bag are applied around the conduit and connected to drainage. A custom-cut appliance is used until the edema subsides and the stoma shrinks to its final size. The clear bag allows the stoma to be inspected and the patency of the stent and the urine output to be monitored. The ileal bag drains urine (not feces) continuously. The appliance usually remains in place as long as it is watertight; it is changed when necessary to prevent leakage of urine.

 Nursing Alert
The stoma should be pink or red in color. If it appears dusky, the nurse suspects impaired perfusion and alert the surgeon.

Complications

Complications that may follow placement of an ileal conduit include wound infection or wound dehiscence, urinary leakage, ureteral obstruction, hyperchloremic acidosis, small-bowel obstruction, ileus, and gangrene of the stoma. Delayed complications include ureteral obstruction, contraction or narrowing of the stoma (stenosis), renal deterioration due to chronic reflux, pyelonephritis, and renal calculi. Approximately 10% of patients with ileal conduits will demonstrate hyperchloremic acidosis; it can occur both shortly after the procedure or as a longer-term consequence due to retention of urinary ammonium from the mucosa of the colon and loss of bicarbonate.

Stoma Ischemia and Necrosis

The stoma is monitored because ischemia and necrosis of the stoma can result from tension on the mesentery blood vessels,

A Conventional ileal conduit.
The surgeon transplants the ureters to an isolated section of the terminal ileum (ileal conduit), bringing one end to the abdominal wall. The ureter may also be transplanted into the transverse sigmoid colon (colon conduit) or proximal jejunum (jejunal conduit).

B Cutaneous ureterostomy.
The surgeon brings the detached ureter through the abdominal wall and attaches it to an opening in the skin.

C Vesicostomy.
The surgeon sutures the bladder to the abdominal wall and creates an opening (stoma) through the abdominal and bladder walls for urinary drainage.

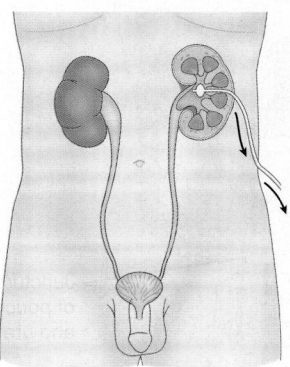

D Nephrostomy.
The surgeon inserts a catheter into the renal pelvis via an incision in the flank or by percutaneous catheter placement into the kidney.

FIGURE 28-8 Types of cutaneous diversions include (**A**) the conventional ileal conduit, (**B**) cutaneous ureterostomy, (**C**) vesicostomy, and (**D**) nephrostomy.

twisting of the bowel segment (conduit) during surgery, or arterial insufficiency. The new stoma must be inspected at least every 4 hours to assess the adequacy of its blood supply. The stoma should be red or pink. If the blood supply to the stoma is compromised, the color changes to purple, brown, or black. These changes are reported immediately to the surgeon. The surgeon or wound care specialist/enterostomal therapist may insert a small, lubricated tube into the stoma and shine a flashlight into the lumen of the tube to assess for superficial ischemia or necrosis. A necrotic stoma requires surgical intervention, but if the ischemia is superficial, the dusky stoma is observed and may slough its outer layer in several days.

Stoma Retraction and Separation

Stoma retraction and separation of the mucocutaneous border can occur as a result of trauma or tension on the internal bowel segment used for creation of the stoma. Mucocutaneous

separation can occur if the stoma does not heal as a result of accumulation of urine on the stoma and mucocutaneous border. Using a collection drainage pouch with an antireflux valve is helpful because the valve prevents urine from pooling on the stoma and mucocutaneous border. Meticulous skin care to keep the area around the stoma clean and dry promotes healing. If a separation of the mucocutaneous border occurs, surgery is not usually needed. The separated area is protected by applying karaya powder, stoma adhesive paste, and a properly fitted skin barrier and pouch. By protecting the separation, healing is promoted. If the stoma retracts into the peritoneum, surgical intervention is mandatory.

If surgery is needed to manage these complications, the nurse provides explanations to the patient and family. The need for additional surgery is usually perceived as a setback by the patient and family. Emotional support of the patient and family is provided along with physical preparation of the patient for surgery.

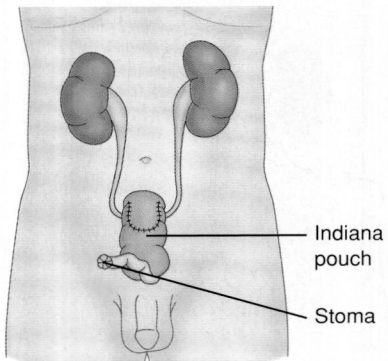

A Indiana pouch.
The surgeon introduces the ureters into a segment of ileum and cecum. Urine is drained periodically by inserting a catheter into the stoma.

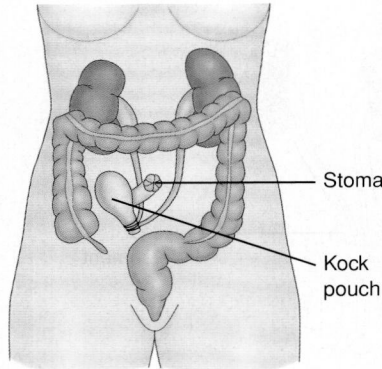

B Continent ileal urinary diversions (Kock pouch).
The surgeon transplants the ureters to an isolated segment of small bowel, ascending colon, or ileocolonic segment and develops an effective continence mechanism or valve. Urine is drained by inserting a catheter into the stoma.

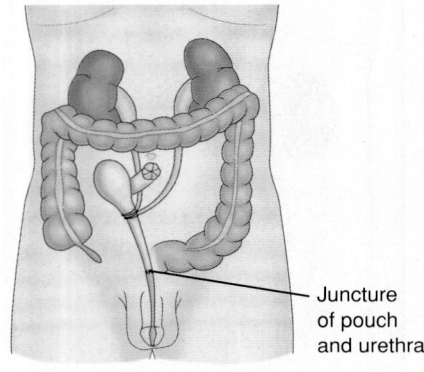

C
In male patients, the Kock pouch can be modified by attaching one end of the pouch to the urethra, allowing more normal voiding. The female urethra is too short for this modification.

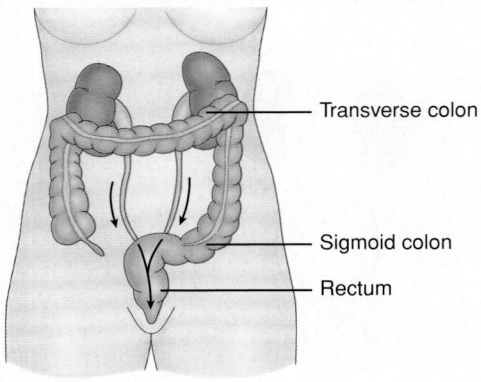

D Ureterosigmoidostomy.
The surgeon introduces the ureters into the sigmoid colon, thereby allowing urine to flow through the colon and out of the rectum.

FIGURE 28-9 Types of continent urinary diversions include (**A**) the Indiana pouch, (**B**) and (**C**) the Kock pouch, also called a continent ileal diversion, and (**D**) a ureterosigmoidostomy.

Nursing Management

Teaching Patients Self-Care

A major postoperative objective is to assist the patient to achieve the highest level of independence and self-care possible. The nurse and wound care specialist/enterostomal therapist work closely with the patient and family to instruct and assist them in all phases of managing the ostomy. Adequate supplies and complete instruction are necessary to enable the patient and a family member to develop competence and confidence in their skills. Written and verbal instructions are provided, and the patient is encouraged to contact their provider with follow-up questions. Follow-up telephone calls from the nurse to the patient and family after discharge may provide added support and provide another opportunity to answer their questions. Follow-up visits and reinforcement of correct skin care and appliance management techniques also promote skin integrity. Specific techniques for managing the appliance are described in Box 28-12.

The patient is encouraged to participate in decisions regarding the type of collecting appliance and the time of day to change the appliance. The patient is assisted and encouraged to look at and touch the stoma early to overcome any fears. The patient and family need to know the characteristics of a normal stoma:

- Pink and moist, like the inside of the mouth
- Insensitive to pain because it has no nerve endings
- Vascular and may bleed when cleaned

Additionally, if a segment of the GI tract was used to create the urinary diversion, mucus may be visible in the urine. By learning what is normal, the patient and family become familiar with what signs and symptoms they should report to the health care provider or nurse and what problems they can handle themselves.

BOX 28-12
Patient Education

Using Urinary Diversion Collection Appliances

Applying a Reusable Pouch System

1. Gather all necessary supplies.
2. Prepare new appliance according to the manufacturer's directions: Apply double-faced adhesive disk that has been properly sized to fit the reusable pouch faceplate. Remove paper backing and set pouch aside, or apply thin layer of contact cement to one side of the reusable pouch faceplate. Set pouch aside.
3. Remove soiled pouch gently. Lay aside to clean later.
4. Clean peristomal skin (skin around stoma) with small amount of soap and water. Rinse thoroughly and dry. If a film of soap remains on the skin and the site does not dry, the appliance will not adhere adequately.
5. Inspect peristomal skin for irritation.
6. Use a wick (rolled gauze pad or tampon) over the stoma to absorb urine and keep the skin dry throughout the appliance change.
7. A skin protector wipe or barrier ring may be applied before centering the faceplate opening directly over the stoma.
8. Position appliance over stoma and press gently into place.
9. If desired, use a pouch cover or apply cornstarch under the pouch to prevent perspiration and skin irritation.
10. Clean soiled pouch and prepare for reuse.

Applying a Disposable Pouch System

1. Gather all necessary supplies.
2. Measure stoma and prepare an opening in the skin barrier about 1/8-in larger than the stoma and the same shape as the stoma.
3. Remove paper backing from skin barrier and set aside.
4. Gently remove old appliance and set aside.
5. Clean peristomal skin with warm water and dry thoroughly.
6. Inspect peristomal skin (skin around stoma) for irritation.
7. Use a wick (rolled gauze pad or tampon) over the stoma to absorb urine and keep the skin dry during the appliance change.
8. Center opening of skin barrier over stoma and apply with firm, gentle pressure to attain a watertight seal.
9. If using a two-piece system, snap pouch onto the flanged wafer that adheres to skin.
10. Close drainage tap or spout at bottom of pouch.
11. A pouch cover can be used or cornstarch applied under pouch to prevent perspiration and skin irritation.
12. Apply hypoallergenic tape around the skin barrier in a picture-frame manner.
13. Dispose of soiled appliance.

Information provided to the patient and the extent of involvement in self-care are determined by the patient's physical recovery and ability to accept and acquire the knowledge and skill needed for independence. The patient is given the opportunity to practice and demonstrate the knowledge and skills needed to manage urinary drainage.

Continuing Care

Follow-up care is essential to determine how the patient has adapted to the body image changes and lifestyle adjustments. Visits from a home care nurse are important to assess the patient's adaptation to the home setting and management of the ostomy. Teaching and reinforcement may assist the patient and family to cope with altered urinary function. It is also necessary to assess for long-term complications that may occur, such as pouch leakage or rupture, stone formation, stenosis of the stoma, deterioration in renal function, or incontinence.

Long-term monitoring for anemia is performed to identify vitamin B deficiency, which may occur when a significant portion of the terminal ileum is removed. This may take several years to develop and can be treated with vitamin B injections. The patient and family are informed of the United Ostomy Association and any local ostomy support groups to provide ongoing support, assistance, and education.

CUTANEOUS URETEROSTOMY

A cutaneous ureterostomy (see Fig. 28-8, p. 873), in which the ureters are directed through the abdominal wall and attached to an opening in the skin, is used for selected patients with ureteral obstruction (i.e., advanced pelvic cancer) because it requires less extensive surgery than other urinary diversion procedures. It is also an appropriate procedure for patients who have had previous abdominal irradiation.

A urinary appliance is fitted immediately after surgery. The management of the patient with a cutaneous ureterostomy is similar to the care of the patient with an ileal conduit, although the stomas are usually flush with the skin or retracted.

CONTINENT URINARY DIVERSIONS

CONTINENT ILEAL URINARY RESERVOIR (INDIANA POUCH)

The most common continent urinary diversion is the Indiana pouch, created for the patient whose bladder is removed or no longer functions. The Indiana pouch uses a segment of the ileum and cecum to form the reservoir for urine (see Fig. 28-9A, p. 874). The ureters are tunneled through the muscular bands of the intestinal pouch and anastomosed. The reservoir is made continent by narrowing the efferent portion of the ileum and sewing the terminal ileum to the subcutaneous tissue, forming a continent stoma flush with the skin. The pouch is sewn to the anterior abdominal wall around a cecostomy tube. Urine collects in the pouch until a catheter is inserted and the urine is drained (Skinner & Daneshmand, 2016).

The pouch must be drained at regular intervals by a catheter to prevent absorption of metabolic waste products from the urine, reflux of urine to the ureters, and UTI. Postoperative nursing care of the patient with a continent ileal urinary pouch is similar to nursing care of the patient with an ileal conduit. These patients usually have additional drainage tubes (cecostomy catheter from the pouch, stoma catheter exiting from the stoma, ureteral stents, Penrose drain, as well as a urethral catheter). All drainage tubes must be carefully monitored for patency and amount and type of drainage. In the immediate postoperative period, the cecostomy tube is irrigated two or three times daily to remove mucus and prevent blockage.

Other variations of continent urinary reservoirs include the Kock pouch (U-shaped pouch constructed of ileum,

with a nipple-like one-way valve; see Fig. 28-9B,C) and the Charleston pouch (uses the ileum and ascending colon as the pouch, with the appendix and colon junction serving as the one-way valve mechanism).

URETEROSIGMOIDOSTOMY

Ureterosigmoidostomy, another form of continent urinary diversion, is an implantation of the ureters into the sigmoid colon (see Fig. 28-8D). It is usually performed in patients who have had extensive pelvic irradiation, previous small bowel resection, or coexisting small bowel disease.

After surgery, voiding occurs from the rectum (for life), and an adjustment in lifestyle will be necessary because of urinary frequency. Drainage has a consistency equivalent to watery diarrhea, and the patient has some degree of nocturia. Patients usually need to plan activities around the frequent need to urinate, which in turn may affect the patient's social life. However, this provides the advantage of urinary control without having to wear an external appliance.

CHAPTER REVIEW

Critical Thinking Exercises

1. As the head nurse in a long-term care facility, you are approached by the daughter of one of the residents. She requests that her mother, who can ambulate with assistance, undergo bladder retraining in order to increase her level of independence. What should your response be to this request? What is the evidence base that supports your response? Identify the criteria used to evaluate the strength of the evidence.

2. As one of the nurses in a busy urology practice, you are performing telephone triage. A 62-year-old man who underwent a ureteroscopy for stone disease 2 days ago complains of increasing urinary frequency, dysuria, and increasing abdominal pain. Explain the instructions you would provide. What medical and nursing interventions would you anticipate?

NCLEX-Style Review Questions

1. A sexually active, 23-year-old woman presents with a history of three UTIs in the past 12 months. What is the first step in her evaluation?
   a. A urine culture
   b. An intravenous pyelogram to look for an anatomic abnormality

   c. A history and physical examination
   d. A 3-day course of antibiotics
   e. A pregnancy test

2. A 55-year-old woman reports stress incontinence when sneezing and playing tennis. She asks what she can do to prevent this from happening. Which of the following is the nurse's best response?
   a. Start an anticholinergic medication.
   b. Void immediately prior to playing tennis to try and decrease urine loss while playing.
   c. Decrease overall fluid intake so this is unlikely to happen at any time.
   d. Restrict intake of calcium-containing foods.
   e. Choose more supportive undergarments.

3. Mrs. Andersen has an indwelling catheter after an open cholecystectomy. She develops cramping in the suprapubic area and urinary leakage. What is the nurse's first intervention?
   a. Make certain the catheter is not kinked
   b. Evaluate for incisional pain
   c. Explain that her symptoms are due to peristalsis
   d. Irrigate the urinary catheter to assess for blockage of flow
   e. Provide an antispasmodic medication

4. Traci, a 29-year-old married woman, frequently experiences a UTI after sexual intercourse. In addition to instruction regarding voiding after intercourse, her initial management may include which of the following?
   a. A recommendation for abstinence
   b. Testing for anatomic abnormalities
   c. A prescription for antibiotics to be used post-coitus
   d. Boric acid suppositories
   e. Wipe the vagina from back to front after voiding

5. When being instructed on methods for managing the mucus in their urinary diversion, patients should be reminded to do which of the following?
   a. Increase fiber intake
   b. Consume high levels of citrus fruits and juices
   c. Increase consumption of cranberry juice
   d. Avoid caffeine consumption
   e. Increase intake of dairy products

Try these additional resources, available at **http://thepoint.lww.com/Honan2e**, to enhance your learning and understanding of this chapter:
• NCLEX-Style Student Review Questions
• Journal Articles

REFERENCES AND SELECTED READINGS

References and selected readings associated with this chapter can be found on the website that accompanies the book. Visit **http://thepoint. lww.com/Honan2e** to access the references and other additional resources associated with this chapter.

Problems Related to Endocrine Function

A 70-year-old patient with type 1 diabetes is being seen in the endocrinology clinic because of a foot wound that will not heal. The patient states that his blood sugar levels have been ranging from 78 to 350 mg/dL and that he eats "sweets" at every meal. A culture of the wound was sent to the laboratory.

- What questions are pertinent to ask the patient regarding his fluctuating blood sugar levels?
- What teaching areas would you reinforce regarding wound healing in this patient?
- What would help the patient keep an accurate record of his blood sugar times and levels?

Nursing Assessment: Endocrine Function

Gayge J. Maggio

Understanding the function of the endocrine glands and the consequences of dysfunction enables the health care professional to anticipate physiologic changes. Symptoms of endocrine disorders usually manifest according to hormone over- or under-secretion. The assessment of the endocrine system is not as straightforward as the other systems because it is difficult to inspect and palpate these glands due to their anatomic location, and patients present with a wide variety of symptoms. The health care professional must understand the function of endocrine hormones and attentively assess a patient's symptoms and diagnostic findings to detect an endocrine disorder.

ANATOMIC AND PHYSIOLOGIC OVERVIEW

Function and Regulation of Hormones

The **endocrine** system consists of groups of organs involved in regulating metabolism, tissue function, reproduction, growth, and development by synthesizing and releasing specific hormones. The **hormones** are chemical messengers that, when released, have specific "target" tissue, where the hormone binds and impacts the cells' functions and reactions (Fig. 29-1). The endocrine system maintains optimal internal functional cell integrity, thus its influence impacts almost every cell, organ, and function of the body. The endocrine glands include the pituitary, thyroid, parathyroids, adrenals, pancreatic islets, ovaries, and testes (Fig. 29-2). Endocrine glands secrete their hormones directly into the bloodstream, which differentiates them from **exocrine** glands, such as sweat glands, which secrete their products through ducts onto epithelial surfaces of the skin, or the salivary glands, which secrete directly into the digestive tract. The endocrine glands are composed of secretory cells arranged in minute clusters known as *acini*. No ducts are present, but the glands have a rich blood supply so the hormones they produce enter the bloodstream rapidly.

The hypothalamus is the link between the nervous system and the endocrine system. The hypothalamus controls the pituitary, which secretes hormones to influence the target glands through the action of the secreting hormones. Table 29-1 lists the major hormones, their target tissue, and some of their properties.

In the healthy physiologic state, hormone concentration in the bloodstream is maintained at a relatively constant level

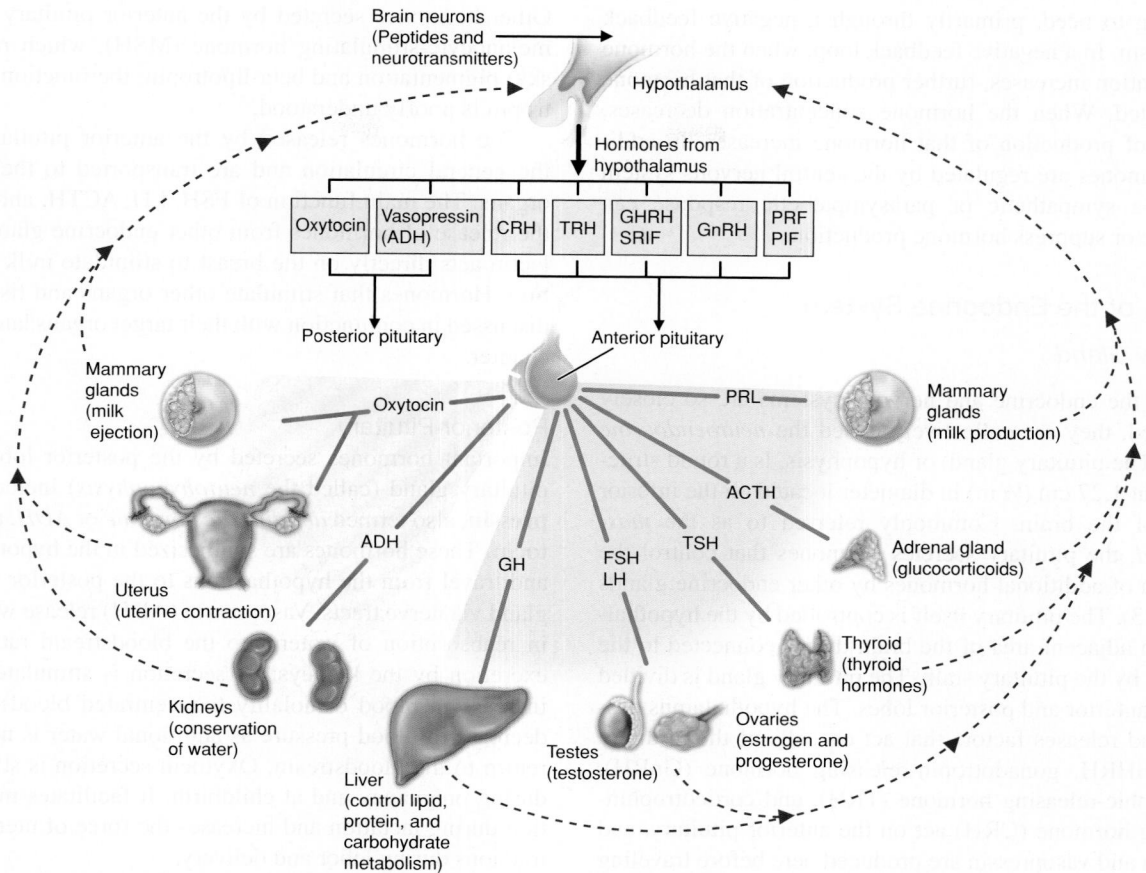

FIGURE 29-1 Hypothalamic and pituitary hormones and their target organs. The hypothalamus produces hormones that act on the anterior pituitary or are stored in the posterior pituitary. The anterior pituitary produces hormones that act on various body tissues and stimulate production of other hormones. T3, triiodothyronine; T4, thyroxine; TRH, thyrotropin-releasing hormone; TSH, thyroid-stimulating hormone.

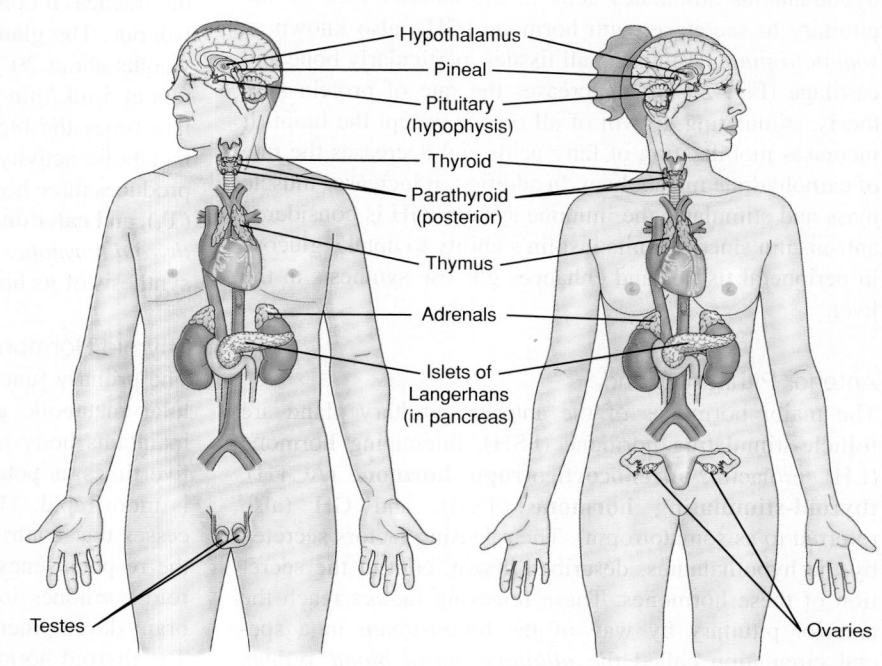

FIGURE 29-2 Major hormone-secreting glands of the endocrine system.

according to need, primarily through a negative feedback mechanism. In a negative feedback loop, when the hormone concentration increases, further production of that hormone is inhibited. When the hormone concentration decreases, the rate of production of that hormone increases. In addition, hormones are regulated by the central nervous system (CNS)—a sympathetic or parasympathetic response can stimulate or suppress hormone production.

Glands of the Endocrine System

Pituitary Gland

Because the endocrine and nervous systems are so closely associated, they are collectively called the *neuroendocrine system*. The pituitary gland, or hypophysis, is a round structure about 1.27 cm (½ in) in diameter located on the inferior aspect of the brain. Commonly referred to as the *master gland*, the pituitary secretes hormones that control the secretion of additional hormones by other endocrine glands (Fig. 29-3). The pituitary itself is controlled by the hypothalamus, an adjacent area of the brain that is connected to the pituitary by the pituitary stalk. The pituitary gland is divided into the anterior and posterior lobes. The hypothalamus produces and releases factors that act on cells of the pituitary gland: GHRH, gonadotropin-releasing hormone (GnRH), thyrotrophic-releasing hormone (TRH), and corticotrophin-releasing hormone (CRH) act on the anterior pituitary, and oxytocin and vasopressin are produced here before traveling to the posterior pituitary.

Growth Hormone

Growth hormone–releasing hormone (GHRH) from the hypothalamus stimulates cells in the anterior lobe of the pituitary to secrete growth hormone (GH), also known as *somatotropin*. GH impacts all tissues, particularly bone and cartilage (Fig. 29-4). It increases the rate of protein synthesis, stimulating growth of all organs except the brain. It increases mobilization of fatty acids and decreases the rate of carbohydrate metabolism. In addition, it increases muscle mass and stimulates the immune system. GH is considered anti-insulin since it limits insulin's ability to uptake glucose in peripheral tissues and enhances glucose synthesis in the liver.

Anterior Pituitary Gland

The major hormones of the anterior pituitary gland are follicle-stimulating hormone (FSH), luteinizing hormone (LH), prolactin, **adrenocorticotropic hormone** (ACTH), **thyroid-stimulating hormone** (TSH), and GH (also referred to as somatotropin). The releasing factors secreted by the hypothalamus, described above, control the secretion of these hormones. These releasing factors reach the anterior pituitary by way of the bloodstream in a special circulation called the *pituitary portal blood system*.

Other hormones secreted by the anterior pituitary include melanocyte-stimulating hormone (MSH), which regulates skin pigmentation and beta-lipotropin; the function of lipotropin is poorly understood.

The hormones released by the anterior pituitary enter the general circulation and are transported to their target organs. The main function of FSH, LH, ACTH, and TSH is the release of hormones from other endocrine glands. Prolactin acts directly on the breast to stimulate milk production. Hormones that stimulate other organs and tissues are discussed in conjunction with their target organs later in this chapter.

Posterior Pituitary

Important hormones secreted by the posterior lobe of the pituitary gland (called the *neurohypophysis*) include **vasopressin**, also termed *antidiuretic hormone* or *ADH*, and **oxytocin**. These hormones are synthesized in the hypothalamus and travel from the hypothalamus to the posterior pituitary gland via nerve tracts. Vasopressin (ADH) release will result in reabsorption of water into the bloodstream rather than excretion by the kidneys; its secretion is stimulated by an increase in blood osmolality (concentrated blood) or by a decrease in blood pressure as additional water is needed to return to the bloodstream. Oxytocin secretion is stimulated during pregnancy and at childbirth. It facilitates milk ejection during lactation and increases the force of uterine contractions during labor and delivery.

Thyroid Gland

TSH (also called *thyrotropin*) acts on the thyroid gland, a butterfly-shaped organ located in the lower neck, anterior to the trachea. It consists of two lateral lobes connected by an isthmus. The gland is about 5 cm long and 3 cm wide and weighs about 30 g. Blood flow to the thyroid is very high (about 5 mL/min per gram of thyroid tissue, approximately five times the blood flow to the liver), reflecting the high metabolic activity of the thyroid gland. The thyroid gland produces three hormones: **thyroxine (T_4), triiodothyronine (T_3),** and **calcitonin**. T_4 and T_3 are referred to collectively as *thyroid hormone*. Iodine is essential to the thyroid gland for synthesis of its hormones.

Thyroid Hormone

The primary function of thyroid hormone is to control cellular metabolic activity. T_4, a relatively weak hormone, maintains body metabolism in a steady state. T_3 is about five times as potent as T_4 and has a metabolic action that is more rapid. These hormones accelerate all bodily processes that contribute to oxygen consumption and altering the responsiveness of tissues to other hormones. The thyroid hormones influence cell replication, are important in brain development, and are necessary for normal growth. The thyroid hormones influence every major organ system

TABLE **29-1** Major Action and Source of Selected Hormones

Source	Hormone	Major Action
Hypothalamus	Releasing and inhibiting hormones	Controls the release of pituitary hormones
	Corticotrophin-releasing hormone (CRH)	ACTH secretion stimulated by CRH
	Thyrotropin-releasing hormone (TRH)	Stimulates the release of TSH
	Growth hormone–releasing hormone (GHRH)	GH secretion stimulated by GHRH
	Gonadotropin-releasing hormone (GnRH)	Stimulates secretion of LH and FSH
	Somatostatin	Inhibits GH and TSH
	Dopamine	Inhibits secretion of prolactin
Anterior pituitary	Growth hormone (GH)	Stimulates growth of bone and muscle, promotes protein synthesis and fat metabolism, decreases carbohydrate metabolism
	Adrenocorticotropic hormone (ACTH)	Stimulates synthesis and secretion of adrenal cortical hormones
	Thyroid-stimulating hormone (TSH)	Stimulates synthesis and secretion of adrenal cortical hormones
	Follicle-stimulating hormone (FSH)	Stimulates synthesis and secretion of thyroid hormone Female: stimulates growth of ovarian follicle, ovulation Male: stimulates sperm production
	Luteinizing hormone (LH)	Female: stimulates development of corpus luteum, release of oocyte, production of estrogen and progesterone Male: stimulates secretion of testosterone, development of interstitial tissue of testes
	Prolactin	Prepares female breast for breast-feeding
Posterior pituitary	Antidiuretic hormone (ADH)	Increases water reabsorption by kidney
	Oxytocin	Stimulates contraction of pregnant uterus, milk ejection from breasts after childbirth
Adrenal cortex	Mineralocorticosteroids, mainly aldosterone	Increases sodium absorption, potassium loss by kidney
	Glucocorticoids, mainly cortisol	Affects metabolism of all nutrients; regulates blood glucose levels, affects growth, has anti-inflammatory action, and decreases effects of stress
	Adrenal androgens, mainly dehydroepiandrosterone (DHEA) and androstenedione	Have minimal intrinsic androgenic activity; they are converted to testosterone and dihydrotestosterone in the periphery
Adrenal medulla	Epinephrine Norepinephrine	Serve as neurotransmitters for the sympathetic nervous system; the flight or fight response specifically increases heart rate, blood flow to skeletal muscle and production of glucose
Thyroid (follicular cells)	Thyroid hormones: triiodothyronine (T_3), thyroxine (T_4)	Increase the metabolic rate; increase protein and bone turnover; increase responsiveness to catecholamines; necessary for fetal and infant growth and development
Thyroid C cells	Calcitonin	Lowers blood calcium and phosphate levels
Parathyroid glands	Parathormone (PTH, parathyroid hormone)	Regulates serum calcium
Pancreatic islet cells	Insulin	Lowers blood glucose by facilitating glucose transport across cell membranes of muscle, liver, and adipose tissue
	Glucagon	Increases blood glucose concentration by stimulation of glycogenolysis and glyconeogenesis
	Somatostatin	Delays intestinal absorption of glucose
Kidney	1,25-Dihydroxyvitamin D	Stimulates calcium absorption from the intestine
	Renin	Activates renin–angiotensin–aldosterone system
	Erythropoietin	Increases red blood cell production

(continued on page 884)

TABLE **29-1** Major Action and Source of Selected Hormones (*continued*)

Source	Hormone	Major Action
Ovaries	Estrogen	Affects development of female sex organs and secondary sex characteristics
	Progesterone	Influences menstrual cycle; stimulates growth of uterine wall; maintains pregnancy
Testes	Androgens, mainly testosterone	Affect development of male sex organs and secondary sex characteristics; aid in sperm production

Grossman, S., & Porth, C. M. (2014). *Pathophysiology: Concepts of altered health states* (9th ed.). Philadelphia, PA: Lippincott Williams & Wilkins.

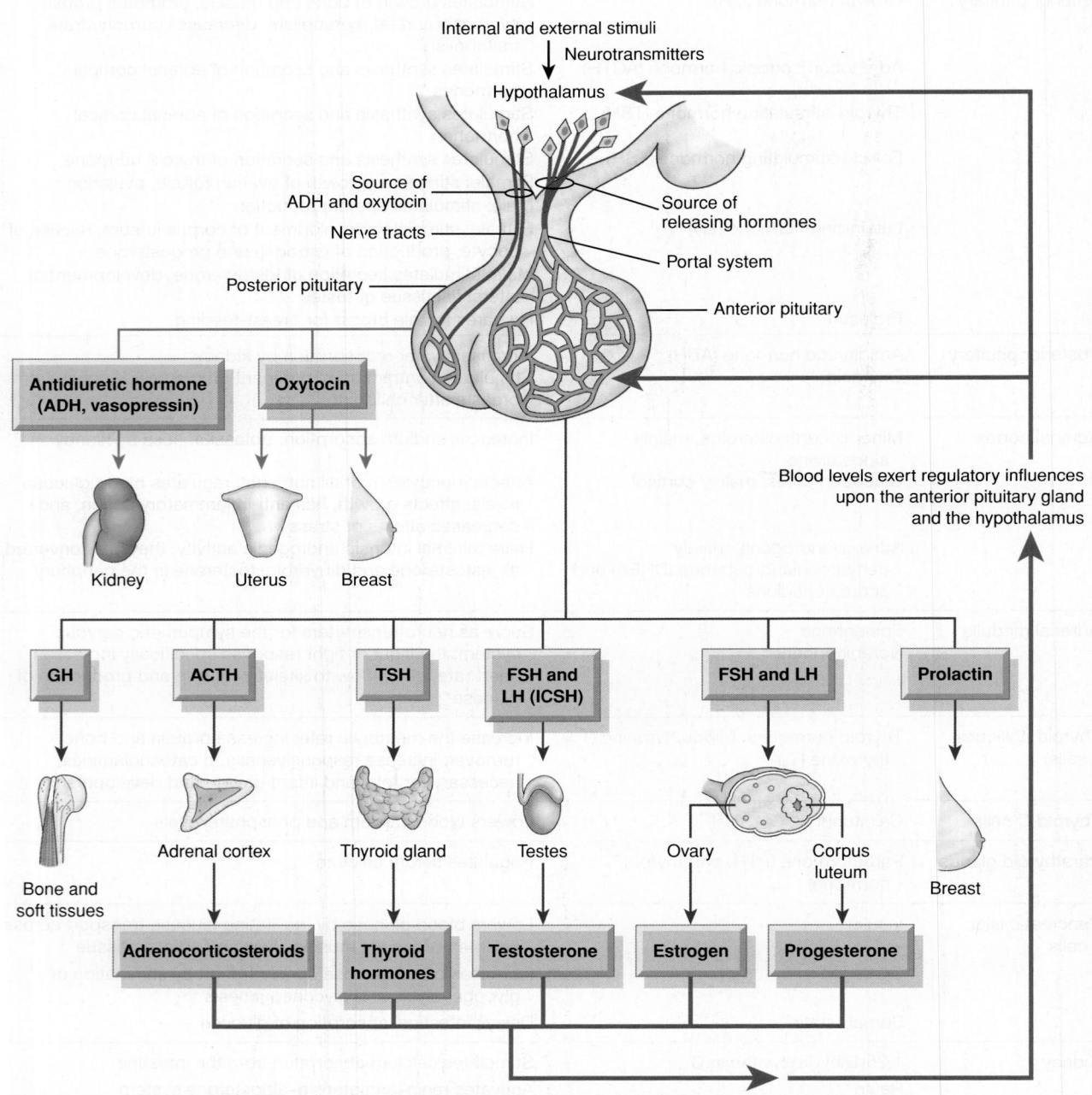

FIGURE **29-3** The pituitary gland, the relationship of the brain to pituitary action, and the hormones secreted by the anterior and posterior pituitary lobes.

FIGURE 29-4 Feedback mechanism for growth stimulation. Regulation of growth hormone by growth hormone–releasing hormone (GHRH) promotes growth through the action of insulin-like growth factor 1 (IGF-1). Increases in IGF-1 trigger an increase in somatostatin to inhibit growth. Dysregulation can result in gigantism or acromegaly. (Reprinted with permission from Felner, E. I., & Umpierrez, G. E. (2014). *Endocrine pathophysiology.* Philadelphia, PA: Lippincott Williams & Wilkins.)

through their widespread effects on cellular metabolism. The secretion of T_3 and T_4 by the thyroid gland is controlled by TSH from the anterior pituitary gland. TSH controls the rate of release of thyroid hormone. In turn, the level of thyroid hormone in the blood determines the release of TSH. If the concentration of thyroid hormone in the blood decreases, the release of TSH increases, which causes increased output of T_3 and T_4 (this is an example of negative feedback). The term **euthyroid** refers to thyroid hormone production that is within normal limits. Thyrotropin-releasing hormone (TRH) exerts a modulating influence on the release of TSH from the pituitary. Environmental factors, such as a decrease in temperature, may lead to increased secretion of TRH, resulting in elevated secretion of thyroid hormones. Figure 29-5 shows the hypothalamic–pituitary–thyroid axis, which regulates production of thyroid hormone.

Parathyroid Glands

The parathyroid glands (normally four in number) are situated in the neck and embedded in the posterior aspect of the thyroid gland (Fig. 29-6). Parathormone (parathyroid hormone), the protein hormone produced by the parathyroid glands, regulates metabolism of calcium and phosphorus. Increased secretion of parathormone results in osteoclast growth and bone resorption. When bone resorption is increased, calcium

is released from the bone into the blood, thereby increasing the serum or blood calcium level. Some actions of this hormone are increased by the presence of vitamin D. Parathormone also tends to lower the level of phosphorus in the blood. The serum level of ionized calcium regulates the output of parathormone. Increased serum calcium results in decreased parathormone secretion, another example of a negative feedback system (Fig. 29-7).

Calcitonin

Calcitonin is secreted in response to high plasma levels of calcium, and it reduces the plasma level of calcium by increasing its deposition in bone.

Adrenal Glands

There are two adrenal glands, one attached to the upper portion of each kidney. CRH from the hypothalamus stimulates the pituitary gland to secrete ACTH, which, in turn, stimulates the adrenal cortex to secrete the adrenal hormones (glucocorticoids, mineralocorticoids, and androgens). Increased levels of the adrenal hormones then inhibit the production or secretion of CRH and ACTH. Each adrenal gland is, in reality, two endocrine glands with independent functions. The adrenal medulla at the center of the gland secretes catecholamines, and the outer portion

FIGURE 29-5 Thyroid hormone regulation. (1). TRH is secreted by the hypothalamus when thyroid hormone levels in the blood decline. (2). TSH is released by the anterior lobe of the pituitary gland. (3). In response to TSH, the thyroid gland releases thyroid hormones into the bloodstream. Elevated thyroid hormone levels provide the negative feedback signal to the hypothalamus, causing TRH to be reduced. (Reprinted with permission from Wingerd, B. (2014). *The human body*. Philadelphia, PA: Lippincott Williams & Wilkins.)

of the gland, the adrenal cortex, secretes glucocorticoids, mineralocorticoids, and sex hormones (Fig. 29-8). The hypothalamic–pituitary–adrenal axis regulates secretion of hormones from the adrenal glands.

Adrenal Medulla

The adrenal medulla functions as part of the autonomic nervous system. Stimulation of preganglionic sympathetic nerve fibers, which travel directly to the cells of the adrenal medulla, causes release of the catecholamine hormones epinephrine and norepinephrine. About 90% of the secretion of the human adrenal medulla is epinephrine (also called

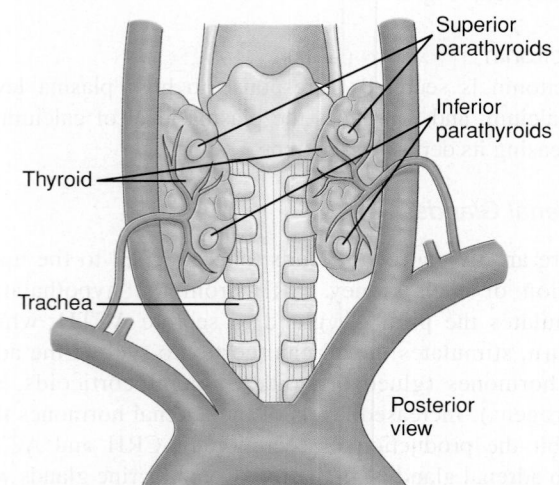

FIGURE 29-6 The parathyroid glands are located behind the thyroid gland. The parathyroids may be embedded in the thyroid tissue.

adrenaline). The major effect of epinephrine release is to prepare to meet a challenge (fight-or-flight response). This causes decreased blood flow to tissues that are not needed in emergency situations, such as the gastrointestinal (GI) tract, and increased blood flow to tissues that are important for effective fight or flight, such as cardiac and skeletal muscle. Catecholamines regulate metabolic pathways to promote catabolism of stored fuels to meet caloric needs from endogenous sources, induce the release of free fatty acids, increase the basal metabolic rate, and elevate the level of blood glucose.

Adrenal Cortex

A functioning adrenal cortex is necessary for life; adrenocortical secretions make it possible for the body to adapt to stress of all kinds. The adrenal cortex secretes three types of steroid hormones produced by the adrenal cortex: **glucocorticoids**, the prototype of which is hydrocortisone; **mineralocorticoids**, mainly aldosterone (important in NA^+/K^+ regulation); and sex hormones, mainly **androgens** (male sex hormones).

Glucocorticoids. The adrenal cortex secretes glucocorticoids in response to the release of ACTH from the anterior lobe of the pituitary gland. Glucocorticoids have major effects on the metabolism of almost all organs because of their influence on glucose metabolism (elevation of blood glucose levels) as well as their ability to inhibit the inflammatory response to tissue injury and suppress allergic manifestations. Without the adrenal cortex, severe stress would cause peripheral circulatory failure, circulatory shock, and prostration.

FIGURE 29-7 As extracellular calcium decreases, the parathyroid gland increases secretion of its hormone, P.T.H., which acts on bone tissue to release calcium into the blood. It also acts on the kidneys and intestines to increase the reabsorption of calcium. Calcitonin, which is produced and secreted by the thyroid gland, decreases serum calcium levels by opposing bone resorption. A low calcium level is called hypocalcemia. A high calcium level is called hypercalcemia.

Survival in the absence of a functioning adrenal cortex is possible only with replacement of nutritional components, electrolytes, fluids, and appropriate exogenous adrenocortical hormone.

Mineralocorticoids. **Mineralocorticoids** exert their major effects on electrolyte metabolism. Aldosterone is the primary mineralocorticoid and is the primary hormone for the long-term regulation of sodium balance. It influences fluid balance through the renin–angiotensin–aldosterone system. When sensing decreased perfusion pressure in the body, renin is released from the kidney into the bloodstream. The renin cascade results in an increase in angiotensin II, which stimulates the release of aldosterone and elevates the blood pressure by constricting arterioles. Increased aldosterone levels act principally on the renal tubule to cause increased absorption of sodium ions in exchange for excretion of potassium or hydrogen ions. This tends to restore blood pressure to normal and increases renal excretion of potassium. Therefore, the release of aldosterone also can be increased in the presence of hyperkalemia.

Sex Hormones. ACTH controls the secretion of adrenal androgens which exert effects similar to those of male sex hormones. The adrenal cortex also may secrete small amounts of some estrogens, or female sex hormones. When secreted in normal amounts, the adrenal androgens appear to have little effect, but when secreted in excess, as in certain inborn enzyme deficiencies, masculinization may result. This is termed the **adrenogenital syndrome**.

Pancreatic Islets

The pancreas lies transversely in the upper abdomen, with the head of the pancreas resting at the curve of the duodenum and the body beneath the stomach. The beta cells of the pancreas secrete insulin, which facilitates glucose transport into body cells, thus lowering the blood glucose levels when they are above normal. When blood glucose levels are low, alpha cells of the pancreas secrete the hormone glucagon. It promotes gluconeogenesis to raise the blood glucose level. Because its action is opposite to insulin, it may be termed a *counter-regulatory hormone*. The delta cells of the pancreas secrete somatostatin, which reduces the rate at which food is absorbed from the GI tract. See Chapter 30 for more detailed discussion of insulin.

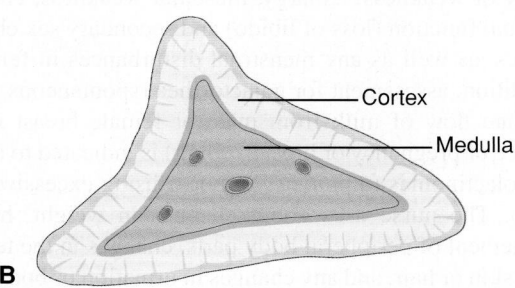

FIGURE 29-8 **A.** The adrenal glands sit on top of the kidneys. **B.** Each gland is composed of an outer cortex and an inner medulla. Each area secretes specific hormones. The adrenal medulla secretes catecholamines—epinephrine and norepinephrine; the adrenal cortex secretes glucocorticoids, mineralocorticoids, and sex hormones.

TABLE 29-2 GERONTOLOGIC CONSIDERATIONS / Age-Related Changes to the Endocrine System

Endocrine Gland	Age-Related Changes	History and Physical Findings
Thyroid	Atrophy and fibrosis of the thyroid gland with decreased activity of the thyroid gland, resulting in decreased basal metabolic rate Reduced uptake of radioactive iodine and decreased secretion and release of thyrotropin Increased nodularity of the thyroid	Cold intolerance Decreased appetite Decreased vital signs
Parathyroid gland	Decreased absorption and activation of vitamin D, which can lead to increased loss of bone minerals and decreased bone mass	Increased risk for fractures
Adrenal gland	Decreased adrenal function; adrenocorticotropic hormone (ACTH) secretion decreases with age with resultant decreased estrogen, progesterone, androgen, and glucocorticoids	Increased incidence of osteoporosis Perineal and vaginal dryness Fragile skin tissue
Pituitary gland	The volume of the pituitary decreases Decreased ACTH, thyroid-stimulating hormone (TSH), follicle-stimulating hormone (FSH), luteinizing hormone (LH)	Decreased muscle mass Decreased strength and energy tolerance Thin and dry skin
Pancreas	Decreased secretion of insulin and decreased sensitivity to circulating insulin, resulting in reduced ability to metabolize glucose	

Adapted from Elipoulos, C. (2013). *Gerontological nursing* (8th ed.). Philadelphia, PA: Lippincott Williams & Wilkins.

Gerontologic Considerations

As a result of aging, the endocrine glands have decreased ability to secrete hormones, or the target organs lose their ability to respond to the hormones produced by the different glands.

These gerontologic changes are summarized in Table 29-2.

ASSESSMENT OF THE ENDOCRINE SYSTEM

Health History

The nurse assesses the patient's history for the presence of pre-existing endocrine disorders, compliance with medications, and the presence of coexisting medical problems.

Endocrine disorders often manifest with nonspecific, atypical symptoms or common complaints that can be attributed to a variety of disorders. Symptoms include weight gain or loss, constipation or diarrhea, tachycardia or bradycardia, hypotension or hypertension, depression or anxiety, heat or cold intolerance, etc. Additionally, endocrine disease may be masked or associated with other comorbidities. For example, the symptoms of an elderly patient admitted with congestive heart failure (CHF) may be attributed to pre-existing cardiac disease without considering thyroid disease. Because the endocrine system impacts nearly all cells and organs, the nurse must have a suspicion of potential endocrine disorders

in all hospitalized patients. Additionally, it is the clustering of signs and symptoms, correlated with the nurse's knowledge of normal physiologic endocrine function, that will alert the nurse to an underlying endocrine disorder. Clinical presentations of endocrine disorders are discussed below according to specific endocrine glands.

Pituitary Dysfunction

Hormonal imbalances of the pituitary involve FSH, LH, ACTH, GH (somatotropin), TSH, MSH, and prolactin from the anterior pituitary as well as ADH and oxytocin from the posterior pituitary.

During the health history, the nurse asks the patient about history of weakness, lethargy, muscular weakness, changes in sexual function (loss of libido) and secondary sex characteristics, as well as any menstrual disturbances in females. In addition, assessment for galactorrhea (spontaneous, inappropriate flow of milk from male or female breast in the absence of pregnancy or breastfeeding) is indicated to assess for prolactinomas (a pituitary tumor causing excessive prolactin). The nurse asks about changes in weight, height, enlargement of peripheral body parts, changes in the texture of the skin or hair, and any changes in urination or body temperature. Owing to the proximity of the pituitary to the optic chiasm, complaints of headaches and visual disturbances are not uncommon and should be evaluated. Neurologic assessment data should consider the patient's level of consciousness, orientation, ability to obey commands, and appropriate response to stimuli. The nurse also inquires about symptoms of hyper/hypotension, heat or cold intolerance, palpitations, tremors, and mood changes.

Growth Hormone Dysfunction

Males and females are affected equally. In adults, assess for bony changes, such as increase in the width and thickness of bones—enlarged hands, feet, sinuses, spine, and mandible (protruding jaw), increase in the size of nose. If there is pressure on the optic nerve, changes in vision and headaches may occur. As GH can cause complications with insulin secretion, including glucose intolerance, leading to diabetes, the blood sugar should be assessed.

Thyroid Gland Dysfunction

During the health history, the nurse asks the patient about changes in weight and appetite, bowel movements, heart rate and respiration, any marked tremors, nervousness, excitability, apprehension or impaired memory, decreased initiative, and slow thought processes. The nurse also asks about changes in the patient's tolerance to heat and cold as well as excessive sweating or feeling very cold, lethargy or apathy, and changes in hair and skin. The presence of exophthalmos, which is an abnormal protrusion of one or both eyeballs that produces a startled expression, also should be assessed (Freedman, 2015).

Parathyroid Dysfunction

During the health history, the nurse considers that hypofunction of the parathyroids is associated with hypocalcemia. Calcium and phosphorus have an inverse relationship, thus when serum calcium levels are low (as a result of parathyroid hyposecretion), phosphate levels rise. If hypofunction is suspected, the nurse assesses for neuromuscular irritability since nerve cells become excited and overstimulate muscle cells in the presence of hypocalcemia. Clinical manifestations include complaints of paresthesias (perioral, extremities) and fasciculations (muscle twitching); therefore, the nurse asks the patient about neuromuscular manifestations. In addition, hypocalcemia has an impact on cardiac function and can prolong the QT interval, causing cardiac arrhythmias, hypotension, and potential cardiac failure. The nurse inquires about complaints of palpitations, shortness of breath, dizziness, and presence of peripheral edema. In addition, since chronic hypocalcemia is associated with cataract formation, the nurse asks about visual changes. The mechanism for the development of cataract may be related to changes in the surface tension of the lens and instability of aqueous humor leading to the development of cataracts in the presence of low calcium.

Hyperfunction of the parathyroids may result in hypercalcemia, as excessive parathyroid hormone causes the release of calcium from bones (Porth, 2015). If hyperfunction of the parathyroid is suspected, the nurse understands that symptoms of hypercalcemia may be vague and include complaints in the following systems: GI (anorexia, nausea, vomiting, bowel hypomotility, and constipation), musculoskeletal (muscle weakness, bone pain), neurologic (fatigue, decreased concentration), or renal (polyuria as hypercalcemia decreases the concentrating ability in the distal tubule). Also the patient may make complaints that are more severe. For example, hyperparathyroidism is associated with an increased incidence of peptic ulcer disease; therefore, the nurse should ask about the presence of melena (dark tarry stools containing decomposing blood). Additionally, the patient is asked about cardiac complaints since hypercalcemia is associated with shortened QT interval, bradycardia, and hypertension. Finally, the formation of stones in one or both kidneys may cause symptoms due to renal calculi, such as back or flank pain, nausea, vomiting, and dysuria.

Adrenal Dysfunction

The nurse asks the patient about symptoms of fluid imbalance (related to aldosterone), symptoms of hyper/hypoglycemia (related to cortisol), and changes in voice, hair, and sexual drive (related to androgens).

To address hypersecretion of the adrenal cortex (known as Cushing disease, covered in Chapter 32), the nurse should inquire about problems with acne or hirsutism (related to hypersecretion of androgens), muscle weakness and paresthesia (hypersecretion of aldosterone), or history of fractures (hypersecretion of cortisol). When considering failure of the adrenal cortex (known as Addison disease, covered in Chapter 32), the nurse asks about symptoms of weakness, fatigue, poor appetite, and weight loss. If a problem with the adrenal medulla is suspected, the nurse assesses the patient's level of stress (related to catecholamines), such as headache, anxiety, nervousness, complaints of a racing heart, and sweating.

Physical Examination

General Appearance

To assess for endocrine dysfunctions, the nurse notes the appearance of facial features, presence of hair, skin condition, and overall proportion. Excessive adrenocortical hormones may cause facial hair in women, "moon face" (swollen and round face), "buffalo hump" (accumulation of fatty deposits at the base of the neck), thinning of the skin, obesity of the trunk and thinness of the extremities, purple striae (stretch marks), and slow healing of minor cuts and bruises. Masculinization in females and truncal obesity may be seen with adrenal hypersecretion as well as a bronze skin color in the creases of the hands or over the metacarpophalangeal (finger) joints, elbows, and knees. This increased pigmentation is associated with excessive MSH.

FIGURE 29-9 Palpating the thyroid. **A.** Posterior approach. **B.** Anterior approach. (From Rhoads, J. (2006). *Advanced health assessment and diagnostic reasoning*. Philadelphia, PA: Lippincott Williams & Wilkins.)

Vital Signs

The nurse performs a thorough cardiac assessment, including vital signs, noting rate and rhythm of the heart and auscultation of heart sounds. Bradycardia is associated with hypothyroidism; tachycardia is associated with hyperthyroidism. Diabetes insipidus, which causes profound polyuria, may cause clinical signs of volume depletion, such as tachycardia and hypotension.

Parathyroid problems may cause calcium derangements, which profoundly impact the cardiac system. Hypocalcemia decreases myocardial contractility, prolongs the QT interval (predisposing patients to ventricular arrhythmias), and is associated with hypotension secondary to reduced cardiac output. Hypercalcemia alters myocardial function; causes rhythm disturbances, such as bradycardia, first-, second-, and third-degree heart blocks, and a shortened QT interval; and is associated with hypertension. When a parathyroid problem is suspected, the nurse should assess for pathologic fractures or symptoms due to renal calculi. Assess for neuromuscular irritability (tetany) related to hypocalcemia (refer to Chapter 32 for assessment cues). Pheochromocytoma, a tumor of the adrenal medulla that causes excess secretion of catecholamines, results in episodic severe hypertension and tachycardia.

Thyroid

The nurse inspects and palpates the thyroid gland routinely in all patients. Inspection begins with identification of landmarks. The nurse inspects the lower neck region between the sternocleidomastoid muscles for swelling or asymmetry. The nurse instructs the patient to extend the neck slightly and swallow. Thyroid tissue rises normally with swallowing. The thyroid is palpated for size, shape, consistency, symmetry, and the presence of tenderness. Each of the lobes is palpated in detail. The nurse may examine the thyroid from an anterior or a posterior position (Fig. 29-9). If palpation discloses an enlarged thyroid gland, check for thrills and auscultate both lobes using the bell of the stethoscope to identify any bruits (Box 29-1).

Eyes and Vision

Assess central vision and visual fields. Loss of color discrimination, diplopia (double vision), or blindness in a portion of a field of vision may be related to pressure of a pituitary tumor on the optic chiasm (located anterior to the pituitary stalk). See Chapter 49 for information on assessing vision and extraocular movements (EOM). Exophthalmos or *proptosis* is an anterior bulging of the eyeballs associated with hyperthyroidism.

Diagnostic Evaluation

Diagnostic evaluation is described related to the glands.

Anterior Pituitary Gland Tests

Computed tomography (CT) scan and magnetic resonance imaging (MRI) can be done to identify the presence or extent

---

BOX 29-1

Physical Assessment of an Enlarged Thyroid

In Graves disease, hypertrophy (enlarged cells) and hyperplasia (increased number of cells) of the thyroid may cause the gland to grow to two to three times its normal size. If the thyroid is retrosternal, goiters may not be visual so it is important to assess for difficulty in swallowing. When the nurse places the hands on the thyroid, he or she feels increased blood flow to the thyroid (thrills). Often thrills are described as sensation of a purring cat. Auscultation using a stethoscope assesses for a bruit (blowing or whooshing sound), which signifies turbulent blood flow and may be found on one side or on the entire gland.

of tumors. Serum levels of pituitary hormones, along with hormones of target glands, may be indicated to evaluate for increased or decreased activity of each gland. For example, an increased thyrotrophic hormone–releasing factor (TRF), which targets the thyroid, is associated with hyperthyroidism. An increase in ACTH, which targets the adrenal cortex, is found in Cushing disease, whereas a decrease in ACTH will be seen in adrenal insufficiency or Addison disease.

Posterior Pituitary Gland Tests

Plasma levels of ADH can indicate increased or decreased levels. A fluid deprivation test may be indicated for diabetes insipidus. In this test, plasma and urine osmolality are measured, and these levels may be altered in disease. Refer to Chapter 31 for more details on this test.

Urine osmolality is assessed for syndrome of inappropriate secretion of antidiuretic hormone (SIADH). Because patients with SIADH do not excrete dilute urine, the urine osmolality will be increased. Also serum sodium levels will be recorded as low because of the retention of water. SIADH will be covered in Chapter 32.

Thyroid Gland Tests

Several tests can be performed to test the functioning of the thyroid gland. Serum TSH is the best screening test for thyroid disorders and helps differentiate between disorders of the thyroid gland itself and disorders of the pituitary and hypothalamus. High levels of serum TSH will indicate normal function or hypothyroidism, whereas low values indicate hyperthyroidism. This is an example of the negative feedback system. If the thyroid hormones (T_3 and T_4) are not secreted by the thyroid, TSH is increased to help stimulate the thyroid to produce these hormones. If T_3 and T_4 are excreted in large amounts, as occurs in hyperthyroidism, TSH is decreased. Also TSH is used to monitor thyroid replacement regimen.

Free T_4 levels measure the unbound thyroxine levels in the blood that is free to enter cells and produce its effects (Porth, 2015). More than 99% of T_3 and T_4 are bound to proteins. Thus, levels of serum-free T_4 will be increased in hyperthyroidism. T_4 decreases in hypothyroidism. Total levels of T_3 or T_4–T_3 increase in hyperthyroidism.

Antithyroid antibodies will be seen in autoimmune thyroid disease, like Hashimoto thyroiditis and Graves disease. A radioactive iodine uptake test also can be done. This indicates the rate of iodine uptake by thyroid gland. It increases in hyperthyroidism and decreases in hypothyroidism. Needle aspiration biopsy can be done to evaluate thyroid cell structure.

Thyroid imaging can be used in the differential diagnosis of masses. Often increased functioning of nodules or "hot" nodules is associated with benign adenomas, whereas "cold" areas refer to decreased functioning. Cancer of the thyroid often manifests as a "cold" area.

Parathyroid Tests

Serum calcium and PTH levels, as well as bone density tests, may be ordered.

In hyperparathyroidism, the serum PTH and calcium will increase, whereas the serum PTH will decrease with hypercalcemia that is related to an etiology other than the parathyroid hypersecretion. Phosphate levels may be decreased but, in general, are in the lower range of normal. Bone density tests may reveal decreased density owing to the increased osteoclast activity.

In hypoparathyroidism, the levels of serum calcium will be lower and phosphate levels elevated.

Adrenal Medulla Tests

With pheochromocytoma, a rare tumor of the adrenal medulla, there will be increased levels of catecholamine and metanephrine in urine and plasma and elevated serum levels of epinephrine and norepinephrine.

A urine vanillylmandelic acid (VMA) level test is performed when pheochromocytoma is suspected. A 24-hour urine specimen will show the level of urine VMA as high as two times the normal level.

Clonidine suppression test, CT, MRI, ultrasound, and scintigraphy are other tests that can be ordered.

Adrenal Cortex Tests

In adrenal insufficiency (Addison disease), the adrenal glands produce too little cortisol, reducing serum cortisol and blood glucose. Reduced levels of aldosterone cause decreased serum sodium and increased potassium levels. A patient with primary adrenal insufficiency will present with a low serum cortisol level and a simultaneously high serum ACTH level. A patient with secondary adrenal insufficiency (pituitary disease) will reveal low serum cortisol and ACTH levels. Refer to Chapter 32 for more details of primary versus secondary adrenal insufficiency.

To assess for adrenal hypersecretion (Cushing syndrome), a variety of test can evaluate the functioning of the adrenal cortex such as: an overnight dexamethasone suppression test, plasma ACTH, plasma and urinary cortisol, and 24-hour urinary free cortisol level.

CHAPTER REVIEW

Critical Thinking Exercises

1. Explain the mechanism by which the hypothalamic–pituitary–thyroid axis regulates thyroid hormone production.

2. Summarize the functions of the three major types of hormones secreted by the adrenal cortex.

NCLEX-Style Review Questions

1. A client complains of nervousness and palpitations. Upon assessing the patient's heart rate, the nurse notes a heart rate of 120 bpm. Which of the following endocrine disorders is associated with palpitations and increased heart rate?
   a. Hypothyroidism
   b. Hyperthyroidism
   c. SIADH
   d. Hypoparathyroidism

2. While assessing a client with Cushing syndrome, the nurse should expect high blood glucose reading due to increased secretion of which of the following?
   a. The thyroid gland
   b. The parathyroid glands
   c. The adrenal glands
   d. The pituitary gland

3. An elderly woman complaining of weight gain, depression, and lethargy is diagnosed with hypothyroidism, and thyroid replacement is prescribed. During initiation of thyroid replacement therapy for the patient, the priority assessment for the nurse is to evaluate which of the following?
   a. Mental status
   b. Nutritional status
   c. Cardiovascular function
   d. Bowel function

4. A 47-year-old woman presents to her primary care provider complaining of bone pain. Routine laboratory studies reveal a high serum calcium of 12.0 mg/dL and increased PTH levels. Which of the following is the most likely diagnosis?
   a. Graves disease
   b. Cushing disease
   c. Addison disease
   d. Hyperparathyroidism

5. The nurse is assessing a client for acromegaly at the clinic. Besides asking about changes in shoe size and facial features, the nurse should also inquire about changes in which of the following?
   a. Hearing
   b. Bowel habits
   c. Vision
   d. Taste of foods

Try these additional resources, available at **http://thepoint.lww.com/Honan2e**, to enhance your learning and understanding of this chapter:
• NCLEX-Style Student Review Questions
• Journal Articles

REFERENCES AND SELECTED READINGS

References and selected readings associated with this chapter can be found on the website that accompanies the book. Visit **http://thepoint.lww.com/Honan2e** to access the references and other additional resources associated with this chapter.

Nursing Management: Diabetes Mellitus

Kathryn W. Tierney

Learning Objectives

After reading this chapter, you will be able to:

1. Differentiate between type 1 and type 2 diabetes.
2. Describe etiologic factors associated with diabetes.
3. Relate the clinical manifestations of diabetes to the associated pathophysiologic alterations.
4. Identify the diagnostic and clinical significance of blood glucose test results.
5. Explain the dietary modifications used for management of people with diabetes.
6. Describe the relationships among diet, exercise, and medication for people with diabetes.
7. Develop a plan for teaching insulin self-management.
8. Identify the role of non-insulin antidiabetic agents in diabetic therapy.
9. Differentiate between hyperglycemia with diabetic ketoacidosis and hyperosmolar nonketotic syndrome.
10. Describe management strategies for a person with diabetes to use during "sick days."
11. Describe the major macrovascular, microvascular, and neuropathic complications of diabetes.
12. Use the nursing process as a framework for care of hospitalized patients with diabetes.

Diabetes mellitus is a group of metabolic diseases characterized by elevated levels of glucose in the blood (**hyperglycemia**). Diabetes is a chronic illness that requires medical care and patient self-management to prevent or decrease the risk of complications (American Diabetes Association [ADA], 2017a). It affects many body systems and has potentially far-reaching and devastating physical, social, and economic consequences. It is a significant risk factor in the development of heart disease and stroke, and it is the leading cause of nontraumatic amputations, blindness in working-age adults, and end-stage kidney disease (ESKD) (Centers for Disease Control and Prevention [CDC], 2014).

The economic cost of diabetes continues to rise because of increasing health care costs and an aging population. Costs related to diabetes are estimated to be $245 billion annually, including direct medical care expenses and indirect costs attributable to disability and premature death (CDC, 2014).

Nursing management of patients with diabetes can involve treatment of a wide variety of physiologic disorders, depending on the patient's health status and whether the patient is newly diagnosed or seeking care for an unrelated health problem. Because all patients with diabetes must master the concepts and skills necessary for long-term management and avoidance of potential complications of diabetes, patient education is necessary for competent self-care and is an ongoing focus of nursing care.

DIABETES MELLITUS

Diabetes affects more than 29 million people in the United States, or approximately 9.3% of the population (CDC, 2014). Of this number, 21 million are diagnosed with diabetes, and an estimated 8.1 million are undiagnosed. As many as 86 million people are thought to have **prediabetes**, a condition that puts people at increased risk for the development of diabetes (CDC, 2014). The occurrence of diabetes, especially type 2 diabetes, is increasing in all age groups. Diabetes is especially prevalent in persons over 60 years of age (CDC, 2014).

Classification

The major classifications of diabetes are type 1 diabetes, type 2 diabetes, and gestational diabetes. Other types of diabetes, comprising 1% to 5% of all diagnosed cases, are caused by genetic conditions, surgery, medications, pancreatic disease, and other illnesses (ADA, 2017b).

Table 30-1 summarizes the major classifications of diabetes, current terminology, and major clinical characteristics. This classification system is dynamic in two ways. First, there can be many differences among individuals within each category. Second, except for people with type 1 diabetes, patients may move from one category to another. For example, a woman with gestational diabetes may, after delivery, move into the type 2 category. Also, metabolic processes typically associated with one diagnosis, such as insulin resistance in type 2 diabetes, may be present in other settings, such as type 1 diabetes. Older terms, such as "insulin-dependent diabetes," "non–insulin-dependent diabetes," "juvenile diabetes," "adult-onset diabetes," and others have been eliminated to reduce confusion.

TABLE **30-1** Classification of Diabetes Mellitus and Related Glucose Intolerances

Current Classification	Previous Classifications	Clinical Characteristics and Clinical Implications
Type 1 (5–10% of all diabetes)	Juvenile diabetes Juvenile-onset diabetes Ketosis-prone diabetes Brittle diabetes Insulin-dependent diabetes mellitus (IDDM)	Onset any age, but usually young (under 30 years of age) Usually thin at diagnosis; recent weight loss Etiology includes genetic, immunologic, and environmental factors (e.g., virus) Often have positive islet cell or GAD (glutamic acid decarboxylase) antibodies Little or no endogenous insulin Need insulin to preserve life Ketosis-prone when insulin absent Acute complication of hyperglycemia: diabetic ketoacidosis
Type 2 (90–95% of all diabetes: obese— 80% of type 2; nonobese—20% of type 2)	Adult-onset diabetes Maturity-onset diabetes Ketosis-resistant diabetes Stable diabetes Non–insulin-dependent diabetes (NIDDM)	Onset any age, usually over 30 years of age Usually obese at diagnosis Causes include obesity, heredity, and environmental factors No islet cell antibodies Decrease in endogenous insulin, or increased with insulin resistance Most patients can improve blood glucose through weight loss if obese Oral antidiabetic agents may improve blood glucose levels if dietary modification and exercise are unsuccessful May need insulin on a short- or long-term basis to prevent hyperglycemia Ketosis uncommon, except in stress or infection Acute complication: hyperglycemic hyperosmolar nonketotic syndrome
Diabetes mellitus associated with other conditions or syndromes	Secondary diabetes	Accompanied by conditions known or suspected to cause the disease: pancreatic diseases, hormonal abnormalities, medications such as corticosteroids and estrogen-containing preparations Depending on the ability of the pancreas to produce insulin, the patient may require treatment with insulin
Gestational diabetes	Gestational diabetes	Onset during pregnancy, usually in the second or third trimester Due to hormones secreted by the placenta, which inhibit the action of insulin Above-normal risk for perinatal complications, especially macrosomia (abnormally large babies) Treated with diet and, if needed, insulin to strictly maintain normal blood glucose levels Occurs in about 2–5% of all pregnancies Glucose intolerance transitory but may recur: • In subsequent pregnancies • 30–40% will develop overt diabetes (usually type 2) within 10 years (especially if obese) • Risk factors include obesity, over 30 years of age, family history of diabetes, previous macrosomia (over 9 lb) All pregnant women between 24 and 28 weeks of gestation should be screened with oral glucose tolerance test

Current Classification	Previous Classifications	Clinical Characteristics and Clinical Implications
Impaired glucose tolerance	Borderline diabetes Latent diabetes Chemical diabetes Subclinical diabetes Asymptomatic diabetes	Oral glucose tolerance test value between 140 mg/dL (7.7 mmol/L) and 200 mg/dL (11 mmol/L) Impaired fasting glucose is defined as a fasting plasma glucose between 110 mg/dL (6 mmol/L) and 126 mg/dL (7 mmol/L) 29% eventually develop diabetes Above-normal susceptibility to atherosclerotic disease Renal and retinal complications usually not significant May be obese or nonobese Should be screened for diabetes periodically
Prediabetes	Previous abnormality of glucose tolerance (PrevAGT)	Current normal glucose metabolism Previous history of hyperglycemia (e.g., during pregnancy or illness) Periodic blood glucose screening after age 40 if there is a family history of diabetes or if symptomatic Encourage ideal body weight, because loss of 10–15 lb may improve glycemic control
Prediabetes	Potential abnormality of glucose tolerance (PotAGT)	No history of glucose intolerance Increased risk of diabetes if: • Positive family history • Obesity • Mother of babies over 9 lb at birth • Member of certain Native American tribes (e.g., Pima) with high prevalence of diabetes Screening and weight advice as in PrevAGT

Pathophysiology

Insulin is a hormone produced by the pancreas that controls blood glucose levels by regulating the production, use, and storage of glucose. It is secreted by beta cells, in the islets of Langerhans of the pancreas. In patients with diabetes, cells may respond inadequately to insulin or the pancreas may decrease insulin secretion or stop insulin production completely. Insulin is an anabolic, or storage hormone. When a person eats a meal, insulin secretion increases and moves glucose from the blood into muscle, liver, and fat cells. Once inside the cells, insulin functions in the following ways:

• Transports and metabolizes glucose for energy
• Stimulates storage of glucose as glycogen in the liver and muscle cells
• Signals liver cells to stop the release of glucose
• Enhances storage of dietary fat in adipose tissue
• Accelerates transport of amino acids into cells
• Facilitates the transport of potassium into the cells
• Inhibits the breakdown of stored glucose, protein, and fat (Porth, 2015)

During fasting periods, for example, between meals and overnight, the pancreas continuously releases a small amount of "basal" insulin. If the blood sugar becomes too low, another pancreatic hormone, *glucagon*, is secreted by the alpha cells of the islets of Langerhans. Glucagon stimulates the liver to release stored glucose, thereby increasing the blood sugar. In short, insulin promotes hypoglycemia; glucagon promotes hyperglycemia. They work in tandem to maintain a constant level of glucose in the blood.

 Nursing Alert
Approximately 50% of the total insulin secreted daily by the pancreas is secreted under basal conditions, and the remainder is in response to meals. The estimated secretion rate of basal insulin in the average adult (assume a weight of 70 kg) ranges from 18 to 32 units/24 hours (0.7 to 1.3 mg) (Kahn et al., 2005). Minutes after eating, the serum insulin level rises, peaking in 3 to 5 minutes and returning to baseline within 2 to 3 hours (Porth, 2015). To attain glycemic control, nurses may be required to manage insulin drips based upon the secretion rate of basal insulin.

The liver assists with glucose control by storing glucose in the form of glycogen. As the level of glucose in the blood begins to drop, the liver produces glucose through the breakdown of glycogen (glycogenolysis). After 8 to 12 hours without food, the liver forms glucose from the breakdown of noncarbohydrate substances, including amino acids (gluconeogenesis).

Type 1 Diabetes

Type 1 diabetes affects approximately 5% to 10% of people with the disease. It is often characterized by an acute onset and most commonly affects children and young adults, although it can occur at any age (ADA, 2017b). Type 1 diabetes is characterized by destruction of the pancreatic beta cells. The diagnosis is further defined as type 1a, or immune-mediated diabetes, and type 1b, or idiopathic (Porth, 2015). The etiology of type 1a diabetes is primarily autoimmune. Autoimmune diseases are caused by abnormal immune responses in which antibodies are directed against normal tissues of the body, responding to those tissues as if they were foreign. Immune destruction of the beta cells, caused by autoantibodies against islet cells and insulin, is associated with certain types of human leukocyte antigen (HLA). It is believed that destruction by the immune system of the beta cells is initiated by a combination of genetic, immunologic, and environmental factors, such as viruses or toxins. The risk of developing type 1 diabetes is three to five times higher in people with certain types of HLA. People do not inherit type 1 diabetes itself, but rather they may have a genetic predisposition, or tendency, toward development of the disease.

Type 1b diabetes represents beta cell failure without an immune-mediated etiology. Whereas there is genetic susceptibility in type 1a diabetes, those with type 1b diabetes have a very strong hereditary component (Porth, 2015).

Regardless of the specific cause, beta cell destruction results in decreased insulin production, unchecked glucose production by the liver, and hyperglycemia. In addition, glucose derived from food cannot be stored in the liver but instead remains in the blood and contributes to postprandial (after meals) hyperglycemia. If the concentration of glucose in the blood exceeds the renal threshold for glucose, usually 180 to 200 mg/dL, the kidneys cannot reabsorb all of the filtered glucose; glucose then appears in the urine (glycosuria). Glucose is an osmotic agent; water follows it. As the glucose is excreted in the urine, it is accompanied by excessive loss of fluids and electrolytes. This is termed *osmotic diuresis*.

Because insulin normally inhibits glycogenolysis (breakdown of stored glucose) and gluconeogenesis (production of new glucose from amino acids and other substrates), these processes occur unrestrained in people with insulin deficiency and contribute further to hyperglycemia. In addition, fat breakdown occurs, resulting in an increased production of **ketones**, which are organic acids. If excessive amounts of ketones are present in the blood, ketoacidosis develops.

Glucose levels can be measured in several ways, including serum levels, capillary glucose, glycated hemoglobin (A1c), and continuous glucose sensing. Serum levels are measured by laboratory testing after a venous blood draw. Capillary glucose is measured using blood from a fingerstick that is placed on a glucose test strip. This type of testing is available to patients at home and is used most frequently to determine glucose levels day to day. The hemoglobin A1c is a measure of average glucose levels over a period of 2 to 3 months. Because it is an average, it does not give any information regarding patterns of blood sugar or periods of hyper

or hypoglycemia, but it is useful to track overall control over time. Continuous glucose monitors (CGM) measure subcutaneous glucose levels and provide real-time data on glucose levels and direction and rate of change. Each of these methods of measuring glucose control has pros and cons as well as situations in which they are not as accurate.

Type 2 Diabetes

Type 2 diabetes affects approximately 90% to 95% of people with the disease. Although type 2 diabetes is commonly associated with older age and obesity, its incidence is increasing in younger people because of the growing epidemic of obesity in children, adolescents, and young adults (CDC, 2014). The two main problems related to insulin in type 2 diabetes are insulin resistance and impaired insulin secretion. *Insulin resistance* refers to decreased tissue sensitivity to insulin. Normally, insulin binds to special receptors on cell surfaces and initiates a series of reactions involved in glucose metabolism. In type 2 diabetes, these intracellular reactions are diminished, making insulin less effective in stimulating glucose uptake by the cells and at regulating glucose release by the liver (Fig. 30-1). The exact mechanisms that lead to insulin resistance and impaired insulin secretion in type 2 diabetes are unknown, although increasing age, obesity, and lack of physical exercise as well as genetic factors are thought to play a role (ADA, 2017b).

To overcome insulin resistance and prevent the buildup of glucose in the blood, increased amounts of insulin must be secreted to maintain the glucose level. However, if the beta cells cannot keep up with the increased demand for insulin, the glucose level rises, and type 2 diabetes develops.

Despite the impaired insulin secretion that is characteristic of type 2 diabetes, there is enough insulin present to prevent the breakdown of fat and the accompanying production of ketone acids. Therefore, diabetic ketoacidosis (DKA) does not typically occur in type 2 diabetes. However,

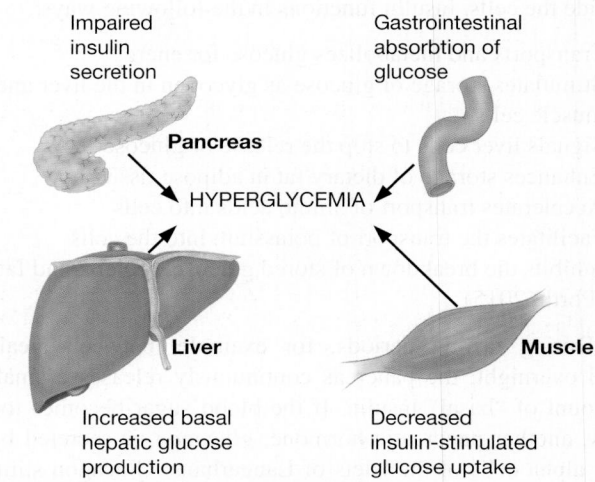

FIGURE 30-1 Pathogenesis of type 2 diabetes.

uncontrolled type 2 diabetes may lead to *hyperglycemic hyperosmolar nonketotic syndrome* (HHNS), another acute complication of diabetes discussed later in this chapter.

Because type 2 diabetes is usually associated with slow, progressive glucose intolerance, its onset may go undetected for many years. If the patient experiences symptoms, they are frequently mild and may include fatigue, irritability, increased urination, increased thirst, poor wound healing, frequent infections, or changes in vision.

Many patients with type 2 diabetes are diagnosed as a result of routine laboratory tests or during ophthalmoscopic examinations. One consequence of undetected diabetes is that long-term microvascular (diabetic retinopathy, neuropathy, and nephropathy) and macrovascular complications (peripheral vascular, coronary disease, and stroke) may have developed before the actual diagnosis of diabetes is made (ADA, 2017b).

Gestational Diabetes

Gestational diabetes mellitus (GDM) is any degree of glucose intolerance with onset occurring during pregnancy. Hyperglycemia can develop during pregnancy because of the secretion of placental hormones, which causes insulin resistance. It also can develop when the physiologic stress of pregnancy reveals glucose tolerance abnormalities that were not apparent prior to pregnancy. Gestational diabetes occurs in around 9% of pregnant women (DeSisto, 2014). Having hyperglycemia increases the risk for congenital anomalies and other complications during pregnancy (ADA, 2017h).

Risk assessment for gestational diabetes should be completed during the first prenatal visit. Women at high risk for GDM include those with marked obesity, personal history of GDM, glycosuria, or a strong family history of diabetes. Those at high risk should have their blood glucose tested as soon as possible in the first trimester and retested between 24 and 28 weeks of gestation, if initial glucose was normal. Women at low to moderate risk for gestational diabetes should be tested between 24 and 28 weeks of pregnancy (ADA, 2017b).

Initial management of gestational diabetes includes diet and exercise changes as well as blood glucose monitoring. If hyperglycemia persists despite lifestyle changes, then medication is prescribed. Goals for blood glucose levels during pregnancy are 95 mg/dL or less before meals, less than or equal to 140 mg/dL 1 hour after meals, and less than or equal to 120 mg/dL 2 hours after meals (ADA, 2017h).

After delivery, blood glucose levels in women with GDM usually return to normal. However, women who have had GDM are at risk for developing type 2 diabetes later in life and should be screened at least every 3 years. A woman who has had GDM should be counseled to maintain her ideal body weight and to exercise regularly to reduce her risk for type 2 diabetes.

BOX 30-1 | **Risk Factors for Diabetes Mellitus**

- Family history of diabetes (i.e., parents or siblings with diabetes)
- Obesity (i.e., BMI at least 25 kg/m^2)
- Ethnicity (e.g., African American, Latino, Native American, Asian American, Pacific Islanders)
- Age 45 years of age or older
- Previously identified impaired glucose tolerance or impaired fasting glucose
- Hypertension (at least 140/90 mm Hg)
- HDL cholesterol level at least 35 mg/dL (0.90 mmol/L) and/or triglyceride level at least 250 mg/dL (2.82 mmol/L)
- History of gestational diabetes or delivery of babies over 9 lb

Adapted from American Diabetes Association. (2015). Standards of medical care in diabetes. *Diabetes Care, 30*(S1), S6.

Risk Factors

Because diabetes is sometimes not diagnosed until complications are present, screening is recommended for overweight adults and children with risk factors for type 2 diabetes. Box 30-1 summarizes risk factors for diabetes mellitus.

Because of the increased incidence of type 2 diabetes in children, screening is recommended for at-risk children beginning at 10 years of age (ADA, 2017b).

Ethnic groups and minority populations are disproportionately affected by diabetes. Age-adjusted population differences demonstrate the highest incidence among Native Americans and Alaska Natives (15.9%), followed by blacks (13.2%) and Hispanics (12.8%), compared with 9% for Asian Americans and 7.6% for whites (CDC, 2014). By 2050, nearly half of the population in the United States will be of an ethnicity other than white. Because the racial and ethnic groups noted above are at greater risk for diabetes and because of increasing obesity and inactivity in the general population, the incidence of diabetes is expected to continue to rise well into the 21st century.

Clinical Manifestations and Assessment

Clinical manifestations depend on the patient's level of hyperglycemia. Classic clinical manifestations of all types of diabetes include the "three Ps": polyuria, polydipsia, and polyphagia. Polyuria (increased urination) and polydipsia (increased thirst) occur as a result of the excess loss of fluid associated with osmotic diuresis. Patients may experience polyphagia (increased appetite) resulting from the catabolic state induced by insulin deficiency and the breakdown of proteins and fats. Other symptoms include dehydration, weight loss, fatigue and weakness, vision changes (the accumulation of glucose on the lens causes refractive error but resolves with glucose control, [Crandall & Shamoon, 2016]), tingling or numbness in the hands or feet, dry skin, skin lesions or wounds that are slow to heal, and recurrent infections.

Nursing Alert

Hyperglycemia impairs immune function (decreases white blood cell function), promotes inflammation, increases blood viscosity, favors the growth of yeast organisms, and is associated with changes in the blood vessel walls, resulting in increased risk for infection, microvascular and macrovascular complications, and foot ulcers.

A blood glucose level that is abnormally high is the basic criterion for the diagnosis of diabetes. There are three ways to diagnose diabetes: fasting plasma glucose (FPG) levels of 126 mg/dL or higher, a random plasma glucose level exceeding 200 mg/dL in a patient with classic symptoms of hyperglycemia, or an A1c level of 6.5% or higher (ADA, 2017b). It is recommended that in the absence of overt symptoms of hyperglycemia, the tests should be repeated or two of the three tests should be used simultaneously to confirm the diagnosis (ADA, 2017b). Normal fasting glucose for a nondiabetic is 80 to 90 mg/dL with a range of 70 to 120 mg/dL. Prediabetes is diagnosed when the FPG is 100 to 125 mg/dL. The oral glucose tolerance test (OGTT) is no longer recommended for routine clinical use in nonpregnant adults. See Box 30-2 for ADA diagnostic criteria for diabetes mellitus.

In addition to assessment and diagnostic evaluation to diagnose diabetes, other important components of care include ongoing specialized assessment of patients with known

---

BOX 30-2

Criteria for the Diagnosis of Diabetes Mellitus

1. A1c of 6.5% or greater
   or
2. Symptoms of diabetes plus casual plasma glucose concentration equal to or greater than 200 mg/dL (11.1 mmol/L). "Casual" is defined as any time of day without regard to time since last meal. The classic symptoms of diabetes include polyuria, polydipsia, and unexplained weight loss.
   or
3. Fasting plasma glucose greater than or equal to 126 mg/dL (7.0 mmol/L). Fasting is defined as no caloric intake for at least 8 hours.
   or
4. Two-hour postload glucose equal to or greater than 200 mg/dL (11.1 mmol/L) during an oral glucose tolerance test. The test should be performed as described by the World Health Organization, using a glucose load containing the equivalent of 75 g anhydrous glucose dissolved in water.

In the absence of unequivocal hyperglycemia with acute metabolic decompensation, these criteria should be confirmed by repeat testing on a different day. The fourth measure is not recommended for routine clinical use.

Used with permission of American Diabetes Association. (2016). Report of the expert committee on the diagnosis and classification of diabetes mellitus. *Diabetes Care, 30*(1), S46.

---

diabetes and evaluation for complications in patients with newly diagnosed diabetes. Parameters that should be assessed regularly are shown in Box 30-3.

Gerontologic Considerations

The overall incidence of diabetes is increasing, with the greatest increase occurring in the aging population (CDC, 2014), necessitating assessment in the elderly. The cause of age-related changes in carbohydrate metabolism is not clear. Possibilities include poor diet, physical inactivity, altered insulin secretion, and insulin resistance.

Elevated levels of blood glucose commonly appear in the fifth decade of life and increase in frequency with advancing age. Almost 27% of people over 65 years of age have diabetes (CDC, 2014). This number is expected to grow (ADA, 2017g). Because people with diabetes are living longer, both type 1 and type 2 diabetes are seen more frequently in the elderly population.

Older patients with diabetes are likely to have coexisting illnesses, such as hypertension, heart disease, stroke, and other health care problems that complicate diabetes management. Normal physiologic changes of aging may mask the symptoms of diabetes, making diagnosis more difficult. Finally, age-related health problems, such as polypharmacy, depression, cognitive impairment, urinary incontinence, falls, and chronic pain increase the risk for complications of diabetes (ADA, 2017f).

Regardless of the type or duration of diabetes, the goals of diabetes treatment may need to be altered when caring for elderly patients. The focus is on quality-of-life issues, such as maintaining independent functioning and promoting general well-being. Although striving for strict control of blood glucose levels may not be safe or appropriate, prolonged hyperglycemia should be avoided. Box 30-4 presents age-related changes that may affect diabetes and its management.

Medical Management

The therapeutic goal for diabetes management is to achieve normal levels of blood glucose (euglycemia) without hypoglycemia while maintaining a high quality of life. Diabetes management has five components:

- Nutrition
- Exercise
- Monitoring
- Medication
- Education

Patients with type 1 diabetes produce little or no insulin and require daily insulin injections to control levels of blood glucose. The primary treatment of type 2 diabetes is decreasing insulin resistance, most commonly with weight loss. Exercise is also important in enhancing the effectiveness of insulin for all patients with diabetes. In patients with type 2 diabetes, non-insulin antidiabetic agents may be added if

BOX 30-3

Assessing the Patient with Diabetes

History

- Symptoms related to the diagnosis of diabetes:
  Symptoms of hyperglycemia
  Symptoms of hypoglycemia
  Frequency, timing, severity, and resolution
- Results of monitoring of blood glucose
- Status, symptoms, and management of chronic complications of diabetes:
  Eye, kidney, nerve, genitourinary and sexual, bladder, and gastrointestinal
- Cardiac, peripheral vascular, foot complications associated with diabetes:
- Adherence to/ability to follow prescribed dietary management plan
- Adherence to prescribed exercise regimen
- Adherence to/ability to follow prescribed pharmacologic treatment (insulin or oral antidiabetic agents)
- Use of tobacco, alcohol, and prescribed and over-the-counter medications/drugs
- Lifestyle, cultural, psychosocial, and economic factors that may affect diabetes treatment
- Effects of diabetes or its complications on functional status (e.g., mobility, vision)

Physical Examination

- Blood pressure (sitting and standing to detect orthostatic changes)

- Body mass index (height and weight)
- Fundoscopic examination and visual acuity
- Foot examination (lesions, signs of infection, pulses)
- Skin examination (lesions and insulin-injection sites)
- Neurologic examination:
  Vibratory and sensory examination using monofilament
  Deep tendon reflexes
- Oral examination

Laboratory Examination

- A1c (glycated hemoglobin)
- Fasting lipid profile
- Test for microalbuminuria
- Serum creatinine level
- Urinalysis
- Electrocardiogram

Need for Referrals

- Ophthalmology
- Podiatry
- Dietitian
- Diabetes educator
- Others if indicated

BOX 30-4

Gerontologic Considerations

Age-Related Changes that May Affect Diabetes and Its Management

Sensory Changes
- Decreased vision
- Decreased smell
- Taste changes
- Decreased proprioception
- Diminished thirst

Gastrointestinal Changes
- Dental problems
- Appetite changes
- Delayed gastric emptying
- Decreased bowel motility

Activity/Exercise Pattern Changes
- More sedentary

Kidney Function Changes
- Decreased function
- Decreased drug clearance

Affective/Cognitive Changes
- Medications/meals omitted or taken erratically

Socioeconomic Factors
- Fad diets
- Loneliness/living alone
- Lack of money/lack of support system

Chronic Diseases
- Hypertension
- Arthritis
- Neoplasms
- Acute/chronic infections

Potential Drug Interactions
- Use of another person's medications
- Consulting multiple health providers for different illnesses
- Alcohol use/abuse

meal planning, diet therapy, and exercise are not successful in controlling blood glucose levels. If maximum doses of a single category of non-insulin agents fail to reduce glucose to satisfactory levels, additional agents may be used. Insulin may be added to other therapies, or the patient may be changed to insulin therapy entirely. Some patients require insulin on an ongoing basis; others require insulin on a temporary basis during periods of acute physiologic stress, such as illness or surgery. The types and number of agents used initially depend on the severity of the hyperglycemia at the time of diagnosis.

Nursing Alert

The stress response results in hyperglycemia because it activates the sympathetic nervous system. The ensuing increase in catecholamines, systemically derived from the adrenal gland or released locally at the level of the liver, increases hepatic glycogenolysis and the release of large quantities of glucose into the bloodstream while inhibiting the release of insulin. Thus, all patients who are stressed are at risk for hyperglycemia.

Treatment varies because of changes in lifestyle and physical and emotional status as well as because of advances in treatment methods. Therefore, diabetes management involves ongoing assessment and modification of the treatment plan as needed. Although the health care team directs treatment, it is the individual patient who must manage the complex therapeutic regimen. For this reason, education of the patient and family is an essential component of diabetes treatment.

Nutrition

Nutrition is the foundation of diabetes management. Nutrition management alone can be associated with reversal or significant improvement of hyperglycemia in type 2 diabetes. The most important objectives in the dietary management of diabetes are control of total caloric intake to attain or maintain a reasonable body weight, control of blood glucose levels, and normalization of lipids and blood pressure to prevent heart disease. However, achieving these goals is not always easy. Because medical nutrition therapy (nutritional therapy) for diabetes is complex, a registered dietitian who understands diabetes management has the primary responsibility for designing and teaching this aspect of the therapeutic plan. Nurses and other members of the health care team must be knowledgeable about nutrition therapy and supportive of patients who need to implement diet and lifestyle changes. Nutrition management of diabetes includes the following guidelines (ADA, 2017c):

- Promote eating patterns that help improve glucose, blood pressure, and lipid control.
- Tailor therapy to each person's individual cultural and behavioral needs.

- Emphasize the pleasure of eating while changing eating habits.
- Provide practical tools for healthy eating.

For patients who require insulin to help control blood glucose levels, maintaining as much consistency as possible in the amounts of calories and carbohydrates ingested at each meal is essential. In addition, consistency in the approximate time intervals between meals, with the addition of snacks if necessary, helps prevent hypoglycemic reactions and maintain overall control of blood glucose.

For patients who are overweight and obese and have type 2 diabetes, weight loss is an important part of treatment. Weight loss of more than 5% of total weight may improve blood glucose levels (Franz, 2015). Some patients with type 2 diabetes who require insulin or other agents to control blood glucose levels may be able to reduce or eliminate the need for medication through weight loss.

Consistently following a meal plan is one of the most challenging aspects of diabetes management. However, pacing food intake throughout the day and decreasing overall caloric intake places more manageable demands on the pancreas and can lead to weight loss. For obese patients with diabetes who do not take insulin or other agents, consistent meal content or timing is important but not as critical.

Nursing Alert

It is important to assess the patient's blood sugar BEFORE meals when insulin coverage is ordered since the patient's blood sugars will rise after ingesting food.

Meal Planning

For all patients with diabetes, the meal plan must consider the patient's food preferences, lifestyle, usual eating times, and ethnic and cultural background. Advances in diabetes management and insulin therapy allow greater flexibility in the timing and content of meals. This contrasts with the older concept of maintaining a constant dose of insulin, which required patients to adjust their schedule to the actions and duration of the insulin.

When teaching about meal planning, clinical dietitians use various educational tools, materials, and approaches. Initial education addresses the importance of consistent eating habits, the relationship of food and insulin, and the provision of an individualized meal plan. In-depth follow-up education then focuses on management skills, such as eating at restaurants, reading food labels, and adjusting the meal plan for exercise, illness, and special occasions. The nurse plays an important role in communicating pertinent information to the dietitian and reinforcing the patient's understanding.

For some patients, certain aspects of meal planning may be difficult to learn. This may be related to limitations in the patient's intellectual level or to emotional issues, such as difficulty accepting the diagnosis of diabetes or feelings of deprivation. In any case, it helps to emphasize that nutritional management of diabetes provides a new way of thinking about food, rather than a new way of eating. It is also important to simplify information as much as possible and to provide opportunities for the patient to practice and repeat activities and information.

Caloric Requirements and Distribution. Calorie-controlled diets are planned by first calculating a person's energy needs and caloric requirements based on age, gender, height, and weight. Then an activity element is factored in to provide the actual number of calories required for weight maintenance. To promote a 1- to 2-lb weight loss per week, 500 to 1,000 calories are subtracted from the daily total. The calories are distributed into carbohydrates, proteins, and fats, and a meal plan is developed with consideration of the patient's lifestyle and food preferences. Currently, the ADA and the American Dietetic Association recommend that the percentages of carbohydrate, protein, and fat of any diet be tailored specifically to each individual (ADA, 2017c).

Carbohydrates. Carbohydrates are an important source of energy. In general, carbohydrates have the greatest effect on blood glucose levels because they are more quickly digested than other foods and are converted into glucose rapidly.

Sources of carbohydrates include grains, fruits, vegetables, legumes, and milk. The majority of carbohydrate selections in the diabetic diet should come from these sources. Foods containing sucrose (sugar) may be included in the diabetic diet. However, because they are typically high in fat and lack vitamins, minerals, and fiber, sucrose-containing foods and beverages should be limited. All carbohydrates should be eaten in moderation to avoid high postprandial (after meal) levels of blood glucose (ADA, 2017c).

Fats. The current recommendations regarding fat content of the diabetic diet is the same as that for the general population. Increased intake of foods, such as fish, containing long-chain omega-3 fatty acids is recommended (ADA, 2017c).

Protein. The amount of protein intake in people with diabetes should be tailored to their specific needs. Because protein appears to have minimal effect on glucose level, foods with significant protein content should be avoided for treatment of hypoglycemia (ADA, 2017c).

Food Classification Systems. To teach diet principles and to help patients with meal planning, several systems have been developed in which foods are organized into groups with common characteristics, such as number of calories, composition of foods, or effect on blood glucose levels. Food intake can be managed several ways, including carbohydrate counting, exchange lists, food lists, and calorie counting.

Carbohydrate Intake. Because carbohydrates are the main nutrients in food that influence blood glucose, monitoring carbohydrate intake by carbohydrate counting, exchange lists, or experienced-based estimation can be effective ways to achieve control of blood glucose (ADA, 2017c).

Carbohydrate counting provides flexibility in food choices and can be less complicated to understand than other systems. It also allows for more accurate management with medication and exercise, particularly with insulin. Insulin-to-carbohydrate (I:C) ratios are patient specific and can change over time with changes in weight and other health issues. For example, a patient with an I:C ratio of 1:15 would take 1 unit of insulin for every 15 g of carbohydrate consumed. All food sources of carbohydrates should be considered when developing a diabetic meal plan using carbohydrate counting. Patients who can manage insulin-to-carbohydrate calculations have the potential to enjoy a more flexible lifestyle and more predictable diabetes control.

Exchange lists also are used for the nutritional management of diabetes but have largely been replaced by carbohydrate counting. The Exchange Lists for Meal Planning (ADA, 1995; Oh, Rastogi Kalyani, & Dobs, 2014) consist of six main exchange lists: (1) starch, (2) fruit, (3) milk (4) vegetable, (5) meat, and (6) fat. Foods included on each list, in the amounts specified, contain equal numbers of calories and are approximately equal in grams of protein, fat, and carbohydrate. Meal plans are based on a recommended number of choices from each exchange list. Foods on one list may be interchanged with one another, allowing the patient to choose a variety while maintaining as much consistency as possible in the nutrient content of foods eaten. Table 30-2 presents three sample lunch menus that are interchangeable in terms of carbohydrate, protein, and fat content.

Other Dietary Concerns

Alcohol. Patients with diabetes do not need to give up alcoholic beverages entirely, but they must be aware of the potential adverse effects of alcohol specific to diabetes. Alcohol is absorbed before other nutrients and does not require insulin for absorption. Large amounts can be converted to fats, increasing the risk for DKA. In general, the same precautions regarding the use of alcohol by people without diabetes should be applied to patients with diabetes. Patient teaching about alcohol intake must emphasize moderation in the amount of alcohol consumed. Moderate intake is considered to be one alcoholic beverage per day for women and two per day for men (ADA, 2017c).

A major danger of alcohol consumption by the patient with diabetes is hypoglycemia, especially for patients who take insulin or secretagogues (an agent that stimulates secretion of another substance; in relation to diabetes, secretagogues stimulate insulin secretion). Alcohol may decrease the normal physiologic reactions in the body that produce glucose (gluconeogenesis). Therefore, if a patient with diabetes consumes alcohol on an empty stomach, there is an increased likelihood of hypoglycemia. In addition, excessive alcohol intake may impair the patient's ability to recognize and treat hypoglycemia or to follow a prescribed meal plan

TABLE **30-2** Selected Sample Lunch Menus from Exchange Lists

Exchanges	Sample Lunch #1	Sample Lunch #2	Sample Lunch #3
2 starch	2 slices bread	Hamburger bun	1 cup cooked pasta
3 meat	2-oz sliced turkey and 1-oz low-fat cheese	3-oz lean beef patty	3-oz boiled shrimp
1 vegetable	Lettuce, tomato, onion	Green salad	½ cup plum tomatoes
1 fat	1-tsp mayonnaise	1-tbsp salad dressing	1-tsp olive oil
1 fruit	1 medium apple	1¼ cup watermelon	1¼ cup fresh strawberries
"Free" items (optional)	Unsweetened iced tea Mustard, pickle, hot pepper	Diet soda 1-tbsp catsup, pickle, onions	Ice water with lemon Garlic, basil

to prevent hypoglycemia. To reduce the risk of hypoglycemia, the patient should be cautioned to consume food with alcohol.

Sweeteners. There are two main types of sweeteners: nutritive and non-nutritive. Nutritive sweeteners contain calories; non-nutritive sweeteners have few or no calories in the amounts normally used. It is unclear whether the use of non-nutritive sweeteners is acceptable for patients with diabetes. While non-nutritive sweeteners lack calories, which would potentially aid in weight loss and glucose control, recent studies suggest that non-nutritive sweeteners have similar metabolic effects as sugar (Pepino, 2015). Moderation in the amount of any type of sweetener that is used is encouraged to avoid potential adverse effects (Shankar, Ahuja, & Sriram, 2013).

Misleading Food Labels. Food manufacturers are required to include the nutrition content of foods on package labels. Reading food labels is an important skill for patients to learn and use when food shopping.

Foods labeled "sugarless" or "sugar-free" may still provide calories equal to those of the equivalent sugar-containing products if they are made with nutritive sweeteners. Therefore, for weight loss, these products may not always be useful. In addition, patients must not consider them "free" foods to be eaten in unlimited quantity because they can elevate blood glucose levels.

Foods labeled "dietetic" are not necessarily reduced-calorie foods. They may be lower in sodium or have other special dietary uses. Patients are advised that foods labeled "dietetic" still may contain significant amounts of sugar or fat.

Patients also must be taught to read the labels of "health foods"—especially snacks—because they often contain carbohydrates, such as honey, brown sugar, and corn syrup. In addition, these supposedly healthy snacks frequently contain saturated vegetable fats (e.g., coconut or palm oil), hydrogenated vegetable fats, or animal fats, which may be contraindicated in people with elevated blood lipid levels.

Exercise

Benefits
Exercise is extremely important in diabetes management because of its effects on lowering blood glucose, aiding in weight loss, and reducing cardiovascular risk factors. Exercise lowers blood glucose levels by increasing the uptake of glucose by body muscles and by improving insulin utilization. These effects are useful in patients with diabetes in relation to losing weight, easing stress, and maintaining a feeling of well-being. Exercise also alters blood lipid concentrations, increasing levels of high-density lipoproteins (HDLs) and decreasing levels of total cholesterol and triglycerides. This is especially important for people with diabetes because of their increased risk of cardiovascular disease.

Exercise Precautions
Exercise in the setting of insulin deprivation and acute ketosis can lead to worsening hyperglycemia and ketosis. Patients should monitor urine ketones prior to exercise and should not begin exercising until urine test results are negative for ketones. Hyperglycemia in the absence of ketonuria is not a contraindication for exercise.

Exercising facilitates glucose uptake via intracellular means; therefore, patients also should be instructed to avoid unexpected hypoglycemia. Patients who require insulin or insulin secretagogues should be taught to check a blood glucose level prior to exercising. If the blood glucose is less than 100 mg/dL (5.6 mmol/L), carbohydrate should be consumed prior to starting the exercise (ADA, 2017c). Insulin doses also may need to be altered around the time of exercise to avoid hypoglycemia. The exact change in insulin dose and amount of food needed varies from person to person and should be determined by monitoring blood glucose. Another potential problem for patients who take insulin is hypoglycemia that occurs many hours after exercise. To avoid postexercise hypoglycemia, especially after strenuous or prolonged exercise, the patient may need to eat a snack at the end of the exercise session and at bedtime as well as monitor the blood glucose level more frequently. Other participants or observers should be aware that the person exercising has diabetes, and they should know how to assist if hypoglycemia occurs.

Regular daily exercise, rather than sporadic exercise, should be encouraged. Exercise recommendations must be altered as necessary for patients with diabetic complications, such as retinopathy, autonomic neuropathy, sensorimotor neuropathy, and cardiovascular disease (ADA, 2017c). Increased blood pressure associated with exercise may aggravate diabetic retinopathy and increase the risk of a hemorrhage into the vitreous or retina. Patients with ischemic heart disease risk triggering angina or a myocardial infarction. Avoiding trauma to the lower extremities is especially important in patients with numbness related to neuropathy.

In general, a slow, gradual increase in the exercise period is encouraged. For many patients, walking is a safe and beneficial form of exercise that, other than proper shoes, requires no special equipment and can be performed anywhere. People with diabetes should discuss exercise with their health care providers and undergo medical evaluation before starting an exercise program (ADA, 2017c).

Monitoring Glucose Levels and Ketones

Self-Monitoring of Blood Glucose

Blood glucose monitoring is a cornerstone of diabetes management. **Self-monitoring of blood glucose (SMBG)** levels by patients has altered diabetes care dramatically. Using frequent SMBG and learning how to respond to the results enable people with diabetes to adjust their treatment regimen to obtain optimal control of blood glucose. This allows for detection and prevention of hypoglycemia and hyperglycemia and plays a crucial role in normalizing blood glucose levels, which, in turn, may reduce the risk of long-term diabetic complications.

SMBG is a key component of treatment for any intensive regimen of insulin therapy and for diabetes management during pregnancy. It is also recommended for patients with unstable diabetes, those with a tendency to develop severe ketosis or hypoglycemia, and for patients who experience hypoglycemia without warning symptoms.

Various methods for SMBG are available. Most involve applying a drop of blood to a special reagent strip and allowing the blood to stay on the strip for the amount of time specified by the manufacturer. Blood glucose meters give a digital readout of the blood glucose value.

Advantages and Disadvantages of SMBG Systems. Methods for SMBG must match the skill level of patients. Factors affecting SMBG performance include visual acuity, fine motor coordination, cognitive ability, comfort with technology and willingness to use it, and cost.

The use of meters to monitor blood glucose is recommended because meters have become much less expensive and less dependent on technique, making the results more accurate. Most insurance companies cover some or all of the costs of meters and strips.

Nurses play an important role in providing initial teaching about techniques for SMBG. Equally important is evaluating the techniques of patients who are experienced in self-monitoring. Patients should be discouraged from purchasing SMBG products from stores or catalogs that do not provide direct education. The accuracy of the meter and strips also should be assessed with control solutions specific to that meter whenever a new vial of strips is used and whenever the validity of the reading is in doubt.

Frequency. For most patients who require insulin, SMBG is recommended two to four times daily, usually before meals and at bedtime. For patients on intensive insulin regimens, such as those on pump therapy or basal-bolus insulin regimens, SMBG is recommended up to 6 to 10 times per day (ADA, 2017d). Patients not receiving insulin may be instructed to assess their blood glucose levels at least two or three times a week, including a 2-hour postprandial test. For all patients, testing is recommended whenever hypoglycemia or hyperglycemia is suspected. Patients should increase the frequency of SMBG with changes in medications, activity, or diet and with stress or illness. Patients are asked to keep a record or logbook of blood glucose levels so that patterns can be detected. SMBG instruction should include parameters for contacting the primary care or endocrine provider.

Continuous Glucose Monitoring System

A **continuous glucose monitoring system (CGMS)** uses technology capable of monitoring blood glucose continuously. A sensor capable of measuring glucose in the interstitial fluid is inserted subcutaneously, and the information is transmitted to a receiver or blue-tooth enabled device. The glucose is measured approximately every 3 to 5 minutes, providing real-time information regarding glucose level and rate of change in either direction. Information from the CGMS is especially useful for patients using insulin pumps and intensive insulin regimens in that it can warn the patient of hypoglycemia and hyperglycemia, as well as provide information regarding patterns of diabetes control over specific periods of time. Figure 30-2 shows a CGMS.

Measuring Glycated Hemoglobin

A1c is a blood test that reflects average blood glucose levels over a period of several months (ADA, 2017d). When blood glucose levels are elevated, glucose molecules attach to hemoglobin in red blood cells. The longer the amount of glucose in the blood remains above normal, the more glucose binds to hemoglobin and the higher the glycated hemoglobin level becomes. The glucose remains attached to the hemoglobin for the life of the individual red blood cell, approximately 90 to 120 days. If near-normal blood glucose levels are maintained, with only occasional increases, the overall value will not be elevated greatly. However, if

FIGURE 30-2 MiniMed CGMS System Gold Continuous Glucose Monitoring System (Medtronic, Northridge, CA).

the blood glucose values are consistently high, then the test result also is elevated. If the patient reports mostly normal results of SMBG but the glycated hemoglobin is high, there may be errors in the methods used for glucose monitoring, errors in recording results, or frequent elevations in glucose levels at times during the day when the patient is not usually monitoring blood sugar levels. Normal values differ slightly from test to test and from laboratory to laboratory but typically range from 4% to 6%. Values within the normal range indicate consistently near-normal concentrations of blood glucose, a goal made easier by SMBG.

It should be noted that the A1c can be affected by changes in red blood cell turnover and that A1c levels do not correlate with SMBG in some patients. Also, because the A1c represents average glucose levels, it does not provide any information regarding the variability in a particular patient's blood glucose (ADA, 2017d).

Urine Glucose Testing

Before SMBG was available, urine glucose testing was the only way to monitor diabetes on a daily basis. Its advantages are that it is less expensive than SMBG, noninvasive, and painless. However, urine glucose testing is not recommended because the results do not accurately reflect blood glucose level at the time of the test and because the renal threshold for glucose, 180 to 200 mg/dL, is far above target blood glucose levels.

Furthermore, because age and kidney function can affect the renal threshold, it is not an accurate measure of blood glucose control. Finally, urine testing for glucose cannot detect or measure hypoglycemia.

Testing for Ketones

Ketones (or ketone bodies) are by-products of fat breakdown that accumulate in the blood and urine. Ketones in the urine signal that control of type 1 diabetes is deteriorating and that the risk of DKA is high. When there is little or no effective insulin available, the body starts to break down stored fat for energy. Urine testing is the most common method used for self-testing of ketone bodies by patients. A urine dipstick (Ketostix or Chemstrip uK) is used to detect ketonuria. Other strips are available for measuring both urine glucose and ketones (Keto-Diastix or Chemstrip uGK).

Urine ketone testing should be performed whenever patients with type 1 diabetes have glycosuria, persistently elevated blood glucose levels, or are symptomatic for DKA, as well as during illness and pregnancy.

Pharmacologic Therapy

As previously stated, insulin is secreted by the beta cells of the islets of Langerhans and works to lower the blood glucose level after meals by facilitating the uptake and utilization of glucose by muscle, fat, and liver cells. In the absence of adequate insulin levels or utilization, pharmacologic therapy is essential.

Insulin Therapy

In type 1 diabetes, exogenous insulin must be administered daily for life because the body no longer produces adequate insulin. In type 2 diabetes, insulin may be necessary on a long-term basis to control glucose levels if meal planning and other agents are ineffective. In addition, some patients with type 2 diabetes who usually are controlled by meal planning alone, or by meal planning and an antidiabetic agent, may require insulin temporarily during illness, infection, pregnancy, surgery, or other stressful events.

Sources of Insulin. In the past, all insulins were obtained from pork and beef pancreas. Currently, recombinant DNA technology or genetic engineering is used to create "human" insulin. Human source insulin, which is designed to act more like insulin from the human pancreas, is now standard therapy.

Insulin Preparations. Insulin is available in the following preparations: rapid-acting, short-acting, intermediate-acting, and long-acting. In general, the rapid- and short-acting insulins are expected to cover the increase in glucose levels after meals soon after injection; the intermediate-acting insulins are expected to cover subsequent meals; and the long-acting insulins provide a relatively constant (or basal) level of insulin. Table 30-3 summarizes categories of insulin.

Rapid-acting or "bolus" insulins, such as insulin lispro (Humalog), insulin aspart (NovoLog), and insulin glulisine

TABLE **30-3** Categories of Subcutaneous Insulin

Time Course	Agent	Onset	Peak	Duration	Indications
Rapid-acting	Lispro (Humalog) Aspart (Novolog) Glulisine (Apidra)	15 minutes 15 minutes 15 minutes	1 h 40–50 minutes 1 hour	3–5 hours 3–5 hours	Used for rapid reduction of glucose level, to treat postprandial hyperglycemia, and/or to prevent nocturnal hypoglycemia "Meal-time insulin"
Short-acting	Regular (Humulin-R, Novolin-R)	½–1 hour	2–3 hours	4–6 hours	Usually administered 20–30 minutes before a meal; may be taken alone or in combination with longer-acting insulin
Intermediate-acting	NPH (Humulin N, Novolin N)	2–4 hours	6–8 hours	12–16 hours	Usually taken after food
Long-acting	Glargine (Lantus, Basaglar) Glargine U-300 (Toujeo) Detemir (Levemir) Degludec (Tresiba)	2 hours	Continuous (no defined onset or peak)	24 hours 42 hours	Used for basal dose

(Apidra), produce a rapid effect that attempts to mimic the normal physiologic response of the pancreas to food intake. These insulins must be timed to the meal because of their rapid onset. The patient should be instructed to eat within 15 minutes of taking the insulin. The short duration of action of these insulins usually requires that patients with type 1 diabetes and some patients with type 2 or gestational diabetes receive additional longer-acting insulin to maintain glucose control.

Short-acting insulin, called regular insulin and marked "R" on the vial, is an unmodified clear solution that usually is administered 20 to 30 minutes before a meal. **Regular insulin is the only insulin that can be given intravenously** and is used to treat DKA. It can be given either alone or in combination with modified longer-acting insulins. Humulin R and Novolin R are examples of regular insulin.

Intermediate-acting insulin is NPH insulin, marked "N" on the vial. Intermediate-acting insulin is cloudy and white in appearance and frequently is used in combination with rapid-acting insulin. To avoid hypoglycemia, it is important that patients eat around the time of the onset and peak of intermediate-acting insulin. Humulin N and Novolin N are examples of NPH insulins.

Basal insulins are long-acting insulins that act consistently over 24 hours. They are given subcutaneously, once a day, and do not have a peak time of effect. Examples of basal insulins are insulin glargine (Lantus), insulin detemir (Levemir), and insulin degludec (Tresiba). Although these insulins are clear and colorless, mixing them with other insulins may cause a dangerous precipitation or diminish the effect of the insulin. Basal insulins can be given once a day and should be given at approximately the same time each day.

Most insulins are considered U-100 insulin, which refers to the concentration of the insulin per volume. In other words,

every 1 mL of insulin contains 100 units. This allows for standardization and accuracy in dosing. There are, however, other insulins that are more concentrated for those patients with significant insulin resistance who require larger volumes of insulin each day. Toujeo is insulin glargine U-300. That is, it is modified to be three times more concentrated than U-100 Lantus. Tresiba is available as both U-100 and U-200 concentrations. Humulin R U-500 is five times more concentrated than conventional insulins. A 10-unit dose change in Humulin R U-500 is equivalent to a 50-unit dose change in conventional U-100 insulin. Humalog is also available as U-200 insulin.

Afrezza is the only inhaled insulin approved for use in the United States. This insulin is used as a pre-meal dose and is delivered through an inhaler device. Afrezza is a rapid-acting or bolus insulin and is available in 4- and 8-unit cartridges. Multiple cartridges can be used consecutively for higher insulin requirements. Patients must undergo spirometry testing prior to using inhaled insulin. Afrezza is contraindicated in patients with chronic lung disease, and only patients who do not smoke or who have not smoked for at least 6 months can use the medication.

Insulin Regimens. Insulin regimens vary from one to four or more injections a day. Usually there is a combination of short-acting insulin and longer-acting insulin in order to more closely approximate insulin secretion in a system without diabetes. The normally functioning pancreas continuously secretes small amounts of insulin during the day and night. In addition, whenever blood glucose increases after ingestion of food, there is a rapid burst of insulin secretion in proportion to the glucose-raising effect of the food. The goal of all but the simplest, one-injection insulin regimens is to mimic this normal pattern of insulin secretion in response to food intake

TABLE 30-4 Insulin Regimens

Schematic Representation	Description	Advantages	Disadvantages
Normal pancreas 100 µU/mL — 0 BR LU DI SN BR	Release of insulin increases when levels of blood glucose rise and continues at a low, steady rate between meals.		
One injection per day Insulin effect Rapid-acting insulin / NPH BR LU DI SN BR	Morning or night • Long-acting (basal) insulin	Simple regimen	Afternoon hypoglycemia may result from attempts to control the level of fasting glucose by increasing NPH dose
Two injections per day-mixed Insulin effect Rapid-acting insulin / NPH Rapid-acting insulin / NPH BR LU DI SN BR	Before breakfast and dinner: • NPH or • NPH with rapid-acting insulin or • Premixed (rapid-acting insulin) insulin	Simplest regimen that attempts to mimic normal pancreas	Need relatively fixed schedule of meals and exercise Cannot independently adjust NPH or regular insulin if premixed insulin is used
Three or four injections per day Insulin effect Rapid-acting insulin Rapid-acting insulin Rapid-acting insulin / NPH BR LU DI SN BR Insulin effect Rapid-acting insulin Rapid-acting insulin Rapid-acting insulin / Glargine BR LU DI SN BR	Rapid-acting insulin before each meal with: • Glargine one or two times per day	More closely mimics normal pancreas than two-injection regimen Each premeal dose of bolus insulin is determined independently More flexibility with meals and exercise	Requires more injections than other regimens Requires multiple blood glucose tests on a daily basis Requires intensive education and follow-up
Insulin pump BOLUS Insulin effect Rapid-acting insulin Rapid-acting insulin Rapid-acting insulin BASAL RATE Rapid-acting insulin BR LU DI SN BR	Uses ONLY rapid-acting insulin (lispro, aspart, glulisine) infused at continuous, low rate called *basal rate* (commonly 0.5–1.5 units/hr) and premeal *bolus doses* activated by pump wearer	Most closely mimics normal pancreas Decreases unpredictable peaks of intermediate-acting and long-acting insulins Increases flexibility around meals and exercise	Requires intensive training and frequent follow-up Potential for mechanical problems Requires multiple blood glucose tests on a daily basis Potential increase in expenses (depending on insurance coverage)

BR, breakfast; LU, lunch; DI, dinner; SN, snack. Rapid-acting insulin; lispro, aspart, or glulisine.

and activity patterns. Table 30-4 illustrates several insulin regimens, including the advantages and disadvantages of each.

The more intensive regimens require significant education and close follow-up by the health care team. There is a greater risk of hypoglycemia with the intensive regimens, but often they are more effective at controlling glucose more closely.

Conventional Insulin Therapy. One approach to insulin use is to simplify the regimen as much as possible, with the goal of avoiding acute complications of diabetes (hypoglycemia and symptomatic hyperglycemia). Conventional insulin therapy typically involves one injection per day of long-acting insulin, but other insulins, such as short-acting or mixed insulins, can be used depending on the patient's blood glucose pattern.

Intensive Insulin Therapy. A second approach is to use a more complex insulin regimen to achieve levels of blood glucose that are as close to normal as is safe and practical. An intensive insulin therapy regimen involves three to four injections of insulin a day using both long-acting and short-acting insulin or using insulin pump therapy. Although intensive treatment is beneficial in reducing the risk of complications, not all people with diabetes are candidates for this approach to diabetes management.

> ### Nursing Alert
> *When administering insulin, it is very important to read the label carefully and to be sure that the correct type of insulin is administered. Take care to avoid mistaking Lantus insulin for Lispro insulin (because both begin with "L") or Lantus for regular insulin because both are clear.*

Teaching Patients to Self-Administer Insulin. Insulin injections are self-administered into the subcutaneous tissue with the use of insulin-specific syringes. A variety of syringes, insulin pens, and injection-aid devices is available.

Storing Insulin. All insulin, including spare pens and vials not in use, should be refrigerated. Extremes of temperature should be avoided; insulin should not be allowed to freeze and should not be kept in direct sunlight or in high temperatures. The insulin pen or vial in use should be kept at room temperature to reduce local irritation at the injection site, which may occur if cold insulin is injected. Typically, insulin can be kept at room temperature for 1 month, but the patient should consult the package insert for individual instructions for each type of insulin.

Vials of intermediate-acting insulin also should be inspected for flocculation, which is a frosted, whitish coating inside the bottle. If a frosted, adherent coating is present, some of the insulin is bound and should not be used. Pens or vials of insulin that have been open for more than 1 month or those that have passed the expiration date also should be discarded.

Selecting Syringes. Syringes must be matched with the insulin concentration (e.g., U-100). Currently, three sizes of U-100 insulin syringes are available:

- 1-mL syringes that hold 100 units
- 0.5-mL syringes that hold 50 units
- 0.3-mL syringes that hold 30 units

Insulin syringes are disposable and have a 31-gauge needle that is 6 mm, 8 mm, or 12.7 mm long. The smaller syringes are marked in 1-unit increments and may make it easier for patients with visual deficits and those taking very small doses of insulin to get a dose that is more accurate. The 1-mL syringes are marked in 1- and 2-unit increments.

Preparing the Injection: Mixing Insulins. Regular and NPH insulins can be mixed together in the same syringe. Regular insulin must be inspected for clarity and not used unless it is crystal clear. NPH will be cloudy and should be mixed carefully by rolling the vial gently. The regular insulin is drawn into the syringe first, followed by the NPH. Injecting cloudy insulin into a vial of clear insulin contaminates the entire vial of clear insulin and alters its action.

Patients who have difficulty mixing insulins have two options. They may use premixed insulin in a vial or in a prefilled syringe. A prefilled syringe is shown in Figure 30-3; it is also discussed in detail below. Premixed insulins are

FIGURE 30-3 Prefilled insulin syringe.

FIGURE 30-4 Suggested areas for insulin injection.

available in different ratios of NPH insulin to regular insulin. The ratio of 70/30 (70% NPH and 30% regular insulin in one vial) is most common; this combination is available as Novolin 70/30 (Novo-Nordisk) and Humulin 70/30 (Lilly). Humulin is also available in a 50/50 ratio (Humulin 50/50).

For patients who can inject insulin but who have difficulty drawing up a single or mixed dose, syringes may be prefilled with the help of home care nurses or family and friends. A 3-week supply of insulin syringes may be prepared and kept in the refrigerator. Prefilled syringes should be stored with the needle in an upright position to avoid clogging of the needle. Like insulin in vials, prefilled syringes should be rotated gently between the hands to mix and warm the insulin before injection.

Selecting and Rotating the Injection Site. As shown in Figure 30-4, the four main areas for injection are the abdomen, the posterior surface of the upper arms, the anterior surface of the thighs, and the flank area. Insulin is absorbed faster in some areas of the body than in others. The rate of absorption is greatest in the abdomen and decreases progressively in the arm, thigh, and hip, respectively.

Systematic rotation of injection sites within an anatomic area is recommended to prevent localized changes in fatty tissue (lipodystrophy). To promote consistency in insulin absorption, the patient should be encouraged to use all available injection sites within one area rather than randomly rotating sites from area to area (ADA, 2004d). Another approach to site rotation is always to use the same area at the same time of day. For example, patients may inject morning doses into the abdomen and evening doses into the arms or legs.

> ### Nursing Alert
> *If the patient plans to exercise, insulin should not be injected into the limb that will be exercised because this can cause faster absorption and may result in hypoglycemia.*

Insulin Injection. The injection site is cleansed prior to insertion of the needle. To inject insulin, the skin is gently pinched and the needle inserted at a 90-degree angle. For patients with a lower BMI, a 45-degree angle can be used to avoid inadvertently injecting into muscle. Injection sites should be at least 1 inch apart. An injection that is too deep or too shallow may affect the rate of absorption. Because insulin is injected into subcutaneous tissue, routine aspiration to assess for blood being drawn into the syringe is not necessary. Box 30-5 illustrates patient education for insulin injection. Box 30-6 details how to evaluate the effectiveness of self-injection of insulin education.

> ### Nursing Alert
> *When administering insulin subcutaneously, the injection site should **not** be massaged because massaging can interfere with insulin absorption.*

Insulin Pens. Insulin pens are prefilled devices for insulin delivery that provide more accurate insulin delivery. Each pen typically holds 300 units of insulin. Rather than having to measure the insulin in a syringe, the pen device allows the patient to select the correct number of units by turning a knob on the end of the pen. A one-time-use pen needle is attached to the pen prior to using and can be discarded the same way as insulin syringes. Insulin pens are generally more convenient than insulin syringes, particularly during travel or eating out. They also are useful for patients with impaired manual dexterity, vision, or cognitive function that makes the use of traditional syringes difficult. Insulin injection technique is the same with the insulin pen as it is for insulin syringe. Insulin pens should not be used for more than one person as blood and other biologic material may transfer into the insulin and cause transmission of blood-borne pathogens between patients.

Selecting Insulin Pen Needles. There are a variety of sizes of pen needles available. In general, all brands are interchangeable and can be used on all insulin pens. Sizes range from 4 mm/32-gauge to 12.7 mm/29-gauge. For most patients, the smaller needles will allow for equivalent glucose control but less pain on injection compared to the larger needles (Bergenstal et al., 2015).

Alternative Methods of Insulin Delivery. Alternative methods of insulin delivery include the use of insulin pumps and jet injectors.

Continuous Subcutaneous Insulin Infusion (CSII): Insulin Pumps. Continuous subcutaneous insulin infusion (CSII), or insulin pump therapy, involves the use of small devices worn externally that more closely mimic the functioning of the normal pancreas. Insulin pumps contain a special syringe, called a reservoir, and are connected to a subcutaneous needle by a thin, narrow-lumen tube with a needle or Teflon catheter attached to the end. The patient inserts the needle or

BOX 30-5 Patient Education

Self-Injection of Insulin

1. With one hand, stabilize the skin by spreading it or pinching up a large area.

Pinching the skin

2. Pick up the syringe with the other hand and hold it as you would a pencil. Insert the needle straight into the skin.[a]

Inserting the needle into the skin

3. To inject the insulin, push in the plunger all the way.

Injecting the insulin

4. Pull the needle straight out of the skin. Press a cotton ball over the injection site for several seconds.

Removing the needle and holding cotton ball over site

5. Use a disposable syringe *only once* and discard it into a hard plastic container (with a tight-fitting top), such as an empty bleach or detergent container. Follow state regulations for disposal of syringes and needles.

Disposing of syringe

[a]Some patients may be taught to insert the needle at a 45-degree angle.

---

catheter into subcutaneous tissue, usually on the abdomen, and secures it with tape or a transparent dressing. The needle or catheter is changed and the reservoir is refilled at least every 2 to 3 days. Figure 30-5 illustrates CSII equipment.

In order to more closely approximate the action of a pancreas that is functioning normally, the insulin pump is programmed to deliver rapid-acting insulin in both a basal and bolus manner. The basal rate is infused continuously over 24 hours, though the rate itself can be tailored to the patient's specific needs at specific times of day. For instance, the basal rate is set at a higher rate overnight if the patient has a history of dawn phenomenon (abnormal early-morning increase in blood sugar—usually between 3 and 8 AM) or abnormal nocturnal rise in blood glucose due to release of hormones. Boluses at meals can be calculated by the pump after the patient inputs the blood glucose at the time of the bolus and the amount of carbohydrate that he or she intends to consume. Because the pump is infusing rapid-acting insulin, the patient

has increased control over delivery of the insulin and, therefore, has more flexibility regarding meal times, food choices, and exercise timing. The pump can easily be disconnected for limited periods for showering, exercise, or sexual activity.

In general, only rapid-acting insulins, such as lispro, aspart, and glulisine, are used in the insulin pump. In rare cases, Humulin R U-500 insulin may be used for patients who have extreme insulin resistance.

One disadvantage of insulin pumps is that unexpected disruptions in the flow of insulin from the pump may happen if the tubing or needle becomes occluded, if the supply of insulin runs out, or if the battery is depleted. These occurrences increase the risk of DKA. Another disadvantage is the potential for infection at the sites of needle insertion. Effective patient teaching minimizes these risks. Hypoglycemia also may occur with insulin pump therapy; however, this usually is related to the lowered level of blood glucose achieved by many patients rather than to a specific problem with the pump itself.

| BOX 30-6 | **Outcome Criteria for Determining Effectiveness of Self-Injection of Insulin Education** |

Equipment

Insulin

1. Identifies information on label of insulin vial or pen:
   - Type (e.g., NPH, regular, 70/30)
   - Species (human, biosynthetic, pork)
   - Manufacturer (Lilly, Novo Nordisk)
   - Concentration (e.g., U-100)
   - Expiration date
2. Checks appearance of insulin:
   - Clear or milky white
   - Checks for flocculation (clumping, frosted appearance)
3. Identifies where to purchase and store insulin:
   - Indicates approximately how long vial or pen will last (1,000 units per bottle U-100 insulin)
   - Indicates how long opened vials or pens can be used

Syringes

1. Identifies concentration (U-100) marking on syringe; U-100 = 100 units per 1 mL.
2. Identifies size of syringe (e.g., 500-unit 100-unit, 50-unit, 30-unit). The most common syringe used for insulin administration is a U-100. However, in the event that very small or large doses of insulin are required, syringe size may be varied. For example, a U-30 syringe = 30 units per mL, allowing for accurate withdrawal of small dosages; however, a U-500 syringe = 500 units per 1 mL, which may be required in patients with insulin resistance.
3. Describes appropriate disposal of used syringe.

Preparation and Administration of Insulin Injection

1. Draws up correct amount and type of insulin
2. Properly mixes two insulins if necessary
3. Inserts needle and injects insulin
4. Describes site rotation:
   - Demonstrates injection with all anatomic areas to be used
   - Describes pattern for rotation, such as using abdomen only or using certain areas at the same time of day
   - Describes system for remembering site locations, such as horizontal pattern across the abdomen as if drawing a dotted line

Knowledge of Insulin Action

1. Lists prescription:
   - Type and dosage of insulin
   - Timing of insulin injections
2. Describes approximate time course of insulin action:
   - Identifies long- and short-acting insulins by name
   - States approximate time delay until onset of insulin action
   - Identifies need to delay food consumption until 5–15 minutes after injection of rapid-acting insulin (lispro, aspart, glulisine)

Incorporation of Insulin Injections into Daily Schedule

1. States proper order of premeal diabetes activities:
   - May use mnemonic device such as the word "tie," which helps the patient remember the order of activities ("t" = test [blood glucose], "i" = insulin injection, "e" = eat).
   - Describes daily schedule, such as test, insulin, eat before breakfast and dinner; test and eat before lunch and bedtime.
2. Describes information regarding hypoglycemia:
   - Symptoms: shakiness, sweating, nervousness, hunger, weakness
   - Causes: too much insulin, too much exercise, not enough food
   - Treatment: 15-g concentrated carbohydrate, such as two or three glucose tablets, 1 tube glucose gel, or ½ cup of juice
   - After initial treatment, follow with snack that includes starch and protein, such as cheese and crackers, milk and crackers, half sandwich
3. Describes information regarding prevention of hypoglycemia:
   - Avoids delays in meal timing
   - Eats a meal or snack approximately every 4–5 hours (while awake)
   - Does not skip meals
   - Increases food intake before exercise if blood glucose level is less than 100 mg/dL
   - Checks blood glucose regularly
   - Identifies safe modification of insulin doses consistent with management plan
   - Carries a form of fast-acting sugar at all times
   - Wears a medical identification bracelet
   - Teaches family, friends, coworkers about signs and treatment of hypoglycemia
   - Has family, roommates, traveling companions who learn to use injectable glucagon for severe hypoglycemic reactions
4. Maintains regular follow-up for evaluation of diabetes control:
   - Keeps written record of blood glucose, insulin doses, hypoglycemic reactions, variations in diet
   - Keeps all appointments with health professionals
   - Sees health care provider regularly (usually two to four times per year)
   - States how to contact health care provider in case of emergency
   - States when to call health care provider to report variations in blood glucose levels

FIGURE 30-5 Medtronic (Northridge, CA) insulin pump system.

Candidates for the insulin pump must be willing to assess their blood glucose level several times daily. In addition, they must be psychologically stable and open about having diabetes because the insulin pump is a visible sign to others and a constant reminder to patients that they have diabetes. Most important, patients using insulin pumps must have extensive education in the use of the pump and in self-management of blood glucose and insulin doses.

The newest insulin pumps have increased decision-making capability. They combine continuous glucose sensing with insulin infusions and are able to stop the insulin infusion in the setting of unchecked hypoglycemia. Current research is focused on closed-loop systems that include dual hormone infusions with both insulin and glucagon that have the potential to be able to control blood glucose levels with limited input from the patient.

Jet Injectors. Jet injection devices deliver insulin through the skin under pressure in an extremely fine stream. These devices are more expensive than other methods of insulin administration and require thorough training and supervision when first used. In addition, patients should be cautioned that absorption rates, peak insulin activity, and insulin levels may be different when using a jet injector.

Disposing of Syringes and Needles. Insulin syringes and pens, needles, and lancets should be disposed of according to local regulations. Some areas have special programs for needle disposal to prevent sharps from being discarded in the main waste disposal system. If community disposal programs are unavailable, used sharps should be placed in a puncture-resistant container. The patient should contact local authorities for instructions about proper disposal of filled containers; containers of sharps should never be mixed with containers to be recycled.

Complications of Insulin Therapy. Reactions to insulin therapy and other complications may occur.

Local Allergic Reactions. A local allergic reaction (redness, swelling, tenderness, and induration) may appear at an injection site 1 to 2 hours after insulin administration. These reactions are becoming rare because of the increased use of human insulins.

Systemic Allergic Reactions. Systemic allergic reactions to insulin also are rare. When they do occur, there is an immediate local skin reaction that gradually spreads into generalized urticaria (hives). Treatment is desensitization with the administration of small doses of purified pork or human insulin in gradually increasing amounts. Occasionally, these rare reactions are associated with generalized edema or anaphylaxis.

Insulin Lipodystrophy. Lipodystrophy refers to a localized reaction at the insulin injection site, in the form of either lipoatrophy or lipohypertrophy. Lipoatrophy is loss of subcutaneous fat; it appears as slight dimpling or pitting of subcutaneous fat. Lipohypertrophy is the development of a fibrofatty mass; it appears as raised, hardened tissue. Because injection into a damaged site may delay absorption of insulin, use of these areas should be delayed until the lipodystrophy is resolved. The use of human insulin, site rotation, and administration of insulin at room temperature decreases the risk of lipodystrophy.

Resistance to Injected Insulin. Many patients have some degree of insulin resistance at one time or another for various reasons, the most common being obesity, which can be moderated by weight loss. Clinical insulin resistance has been defined as a daily insulin requirement of 200 units or more. Approaches to increased insulin requirements include using insulin sensitizers or using a more concentrated insulin preparation, such as U-500.

Fasting Hyperglycemia. An elevated level of blood glucose upon arising in the morning or after a period of fasting is caused by an insufficient level of insulin or lack of suppression of glucagon. Particular processes, including dawn phenomenon, the Somogyi effect, or insulin waning, also may be present. The *dawn phenomenon* is characterized by a blood glucose level that is relatively normal until approximately 3 AM, when blood glucose levels begin to rise. This phenomenon is thought to result from nocturnal surges in growth hormone secretions, which create a greater need for insulin in the early morning hours in patients with type 1 diabetes. The dawn phenomenon must be distinguished from *insulin waning* (the progressive increase in blood glucose from bedtime to morning) and from the *Somogyi effect* (nocturnal hypoglycemia followed by rebound hyperglycemia).

It may be difficult to tell from a patient's history which of the above causes is responsible for morning hyperglycemia. To determine the cause, the patient must be awakened once or twice during the night to test blood glucose levels, or a continuous glucose sensor may be used. Testing at bedtime, at 3 AM, and on awakening or reviewing glucose patterns provided by a glucose sensor provides information that can be

TABLE **30-5** Causes of Morning Hyperglycemia

Characteristic	Treatment
Insulin Waning	
Progressive rise in blood glucose from bedtime to morning	Increase evening (predinner or bedtime) dose of intermediate- or long-acting insulin, or institute a dose of insulin before the evening meal if one is not already part of the treatment regimen.
Dawn Phenomenon	
Relatively normal blood glucose until about 3 AM, when the level begins to rise	Change time of injection of evening intermediate-acting insulin from dinnertime to bedtime.
Somogyi Effect	
Normal or elevated blood glucose at bedtime, a decrease at 2–3 AM to hypoglycemic levels, and a subsequent increase caused by the production of counterregulatory hormones	Decrease evening (predinner or bedtime) dose of intermediate-acting insulin, or increase bedtime snack.

used to make adjustments in insulin to avoid morning hyperglycemia. Table 30-5 summarizes the differences among insulin waning, the dawn phenomenon, and the Somogyi effect.

Non-insulin Antidiabetic Agents

Non-insulin antidiabetic agents may be effective for patients with type 2 diabetes who cannot be treated effectively with diet and exercise alone. These agents include biguanides, dipeptidyl peptidase 4 (DPP-4) inhibitors, glucagon-like peptide 1 (GLP-1) analogs, sodium-glucose transporter 2 (SGLT-2) inhibitors, sulfonylureas, alpha-glucosidase inhibitors, nonsulfonylurea insulin secretagogues (meglitinides and phenylalanine derivatives), and thiazolidinediones (glitazones). Sulfonylureas and meglitinides are known as *insulin secretagogues* because their action increases the secretion of insulin by the pancreatic beta cells. Table 30-6 provides a summary of antidiabetic agents with nursing implications.

Patients must understand that antidiabetic agents are prescribed as an addition to, not as a substitute for, diet and exercise. Use of antidiabetic medications may need to be stopped temporarily and insulin prescribed during illness, pregnancy, or hospitalization.

In time, as beta cells continue to decline, non-insulin antidiabetic agents may no longer be adequate in controlling type 2 diabetes. In such cases, the patient is treated with insulin. Approximately half of all patients who initially use non-insulin antidiabetic agents eventually require insulin. Because mechanisms of action vary, use of multiple medications with different actions is common. For some patients with type 2 diabetes, the use of non-insulin agents in combination with insulin is indicated. Mechanisms of action for non-insulin antidiabetic agents are shown in Figure 30-6.

Biguanides. Metformin, the most commonly used biguanide, produces its antidiabetic effects by decreasing hepatic production of glucose and facilitating the action of insulin on peripheral receptor sites. Biguanides have no effect on pancreatic beta cells. Metformin is contraindicated in patients with kidney impairment and in those at risk for acute kidney dysfunction. Metformin-induced lactic acidosis is a serious complication of biguanide therapy in patients with kidney failure. Metformin should not be administered for 2 days before any diagnostic testing that may require use of a contrast agent, and normal kidney function should be confirmed before the medication is restarted after the procedure.

DPP-4 Inhibitors. The DPP-4 inhibitors act by reducing the activity of the DPP-4 enzyme, whose primary action is to degrade glucagon-like peptide 1 (GLP-1). This prolongs the availability of GLP-1, whose actions are to stimulate insulin production, slow gastric emptying, and suppress glucagon secretion.

GLP-1 Agonists. GLP-1 agonists are a class of medications that work to increase insulin secretion, delay gastric emptying, promote satiety, and suppress glucagon secretion. All GLP-1 medications are injected once daily or once weekly depending on the preparation. Whereas most other non-insulin antidiabetic agents are weight neutral or cause weight gain, GLP-1 agonists promote weight loss. They also are glucose dependent and generally do not cause hypoglycemia unless combined with other medications or insulin. Usually side effects are mild but can include nausea.

SGLT-2 Inhibitors. Sodium glucose co-transporter-2 (SGLT-2) inhibitors are oral medications that work primarily by inhibiting reabsorption of glucose in the proximal renal tubules, which promotes loss of glucose through the urine, thereby reducing blood glucose levels. Weight loss and improved blood pressure also are seen with these medications. Common side effects include increased urinary frequency and genital mycotic infections, and some patients have developed DKA while taking the medication.

TABLE **30-6** Antidiabetic Agents

Generic (Trade) Name	Action/Indications	Side Effects	Implications
Sulfonylureas			
First- and Second-Generation Sulfonylureas	Used in type 2 diabetes to control blood glucose levels Stimulate beta cells of the pancreas to secrete insulin; may improve binding between insulin and insulin receptors or increase the number of insulin receptors	Hypoglycemia Mild GI symptoms Weight gain Drug–drug interactions (nonsteroidal anti-inflammatory drugs, warfarin, sulfonamides) Sulfa allergy	Monitor patient for hypoglycemia Monitor blood glucose and urine ketone levels to assess effectiveness of therapy Patients at high risk for hypoglycemia: advanced age, renal insufficiency When taken with beta-adrenergic blocking agents, may mask usual warning signs and symptoms of hypoglycemia Instruct patients to avoid use of alcohol
Second-Generation Sulfonylureas Glipizide (Glucotrol, Glucatrol XL) Glyburide (Micronase, Glynase, Dia-Beta) Glimepiride (Amaryl)	Have more potent effects than first-generation sulfonylureas May be used in combination with metformin or insulin to improve glucose control	Same as above	Same as above
First-Generation Sulfonylureas Chlorpropamide (Diabinese) Tolazamide (Tolinase) Tolbutamide (Orinase)	Used infrequently in the United States today		
Biguanides			
Metformin (Glucophase, Glucophage XL, Fortamet)	Inhibit production of glucose by the liver Increase body tissues' sensitivity to insulin Decrease hepatic synthesis of cholesterol Used in type 2 diabetes to control blood glucose levels Metformin has been effective in preventing type 2 diabetes related to obesity in young adults	Lactic acidosis Hypoglycemia if metformin is used in combination with insulin or other antidiabetic agents Drug–drug interactions GI disturbances Contraindicated in patients with impaired kidney or liver function, respiratory insufficiency, severe infection, or alcohol abuse	Monitor for lactic acidosis and hypoglycemia Patients taking metformin are at increased risk of acute kidney failure and lactic acidosis with use of iodinated contrast material for diagnostic studies; metformin should be stopped 48 hours prior to and for 48 hours after use of contrast agent or until kidney function is evaluated and normal.
Alpha-Glucosidase Inhibitors			
Acarbose (Precose) Miglitol (Glyset)	Delay absorption of complex carbohydrates in the intestine and slow entry of glucose into systemic circulation Do not increase insulin secretion Used in type 2 diabetes to control blood glucose levels Can be used alone or in combination with sulfonylureas, metformin, or insulin to improve glucose control	Hypoglycemia (risk increased if used with insulin or other antidiabetic agents) GI side effects (abdominal discomfort or distention, diarrhea, flatulence) Drug–drug interactions	Must be taken with first bite of food to be effective Monitor for GI side effects (diarrhea, abdominal distention) Monitor for blood glucose levels to assess effectiveness of therapy Monitor liver function studies every 3 months for 1 year, then periodically afterward Contraindicated in patients with GI or renal dysfunction or cirrhosis

(continued on page 914)

TABLE **30-6** Antidiabetic Agents (*continued*)

Generic (Trade) Name	Action/Indications	Side Effects	Implications
Nonsulfonylurea Insulin Secretagogues			
Repaglinide (Prandin) categorized as a meglitinide Neteglide (Starlix) categorized as a D-phenylalanine derivative	Stimulate rapid and short insulin secretion from the pancreas Used in type 2 diabetes to control blood glucose levels by decreasing postprandial increases in blood glucose Can be used alone or in combination with metformin or thiazolidinediones to improve glucose control	Hypoglycemia/weight gain less likely than with sulfonylureas Drug–drug interactions (with ketoconazole, fluconazole, erythromycin, rifampin, isoniazid)	Monitor blood glucose levels to assess effectiveness of therapy Has rapid action and short half-life Monitor patients with impaired liver function and renal impairment Has no effect on plasma lipids Is taken before each meal
Thiazolidinediones (or Glitazones)			
Pioglitazone (Actos)	Sensitize body tissue to insulin; stimulate insulin receptor sites to lower blood glucose and improve action of insulin May be used alone or in combination with sulfonylurea, metformin, or insulin	Hypoglycemia (risk increased with use of insulin or other antidiabetic agents) Anemia Weight gain, edema Decrease effectiveness of oral contraceptives Possible liver dysfunction Drug–drug interactions Hyperlipidemia (has variable effect on lipids; pioglitazone may be preferred choice in patients with lipid abnormalities) Impaired platelet function	Monitor blood glucose levels to assess effectiveness of therapy Monitor for signs of fluid overload Monitor liver function Arrange dietary teaching to establish weight control program
DPP-4 Inhibitors			
Sitagliptin (Januvia) Saxagliptin (Onglyza) Linagliptin (Tradjenta)	Used in type 2 diabetes to control blood glucose levels Indirectly stimulates release of insulin; prevents secretion of glucagon	Nasopharyngitis Possible acute pancreatitis	Can be used with metformin or sulfonylureas to achieve improved blood glucose control
GLP-1 Agonists			
Exenatide and exenatide extended release (Byetta, Bydureon) Liraglutide (Victoza) Albiglutide (Tanzeum) Dulaglutide (Trulicity)	Simulates release of insulin; prevents secretion of glucagon; slow gastric emptying; promotes weight loss	GI side effects, including nausea and diarrhea Possible acute pancreatitis	Use with caution in patients with gastroparesis
SGLT-2 Inhibitors			
Canagliflozin (Invokana) Dapagliflozin (Farxiga) Empagliflozin (Jardiance)	Promotes insulin-independent renal excretion of glucose	Polyuria; mycotic infection; possible DKA	Helpful in controlling blood pressure and improving weight loss; avoid use in renal insufficiency

Sulfonylureas. The sulfonylureas exert their primary action by stimulating the pancreas directly to secrete insulin. Therefore, a functioning pancreas is necessary for these agents to be effective, and they are not indicated in patients with type 1 diabetes.

Sulfonylureas improve insulin action at the cellular level and also may directly decrease glucose production by the liver.

The most common side effect of sulfonylureas is hypoglycemia. Second-generation sulfonylureas (glipizide,

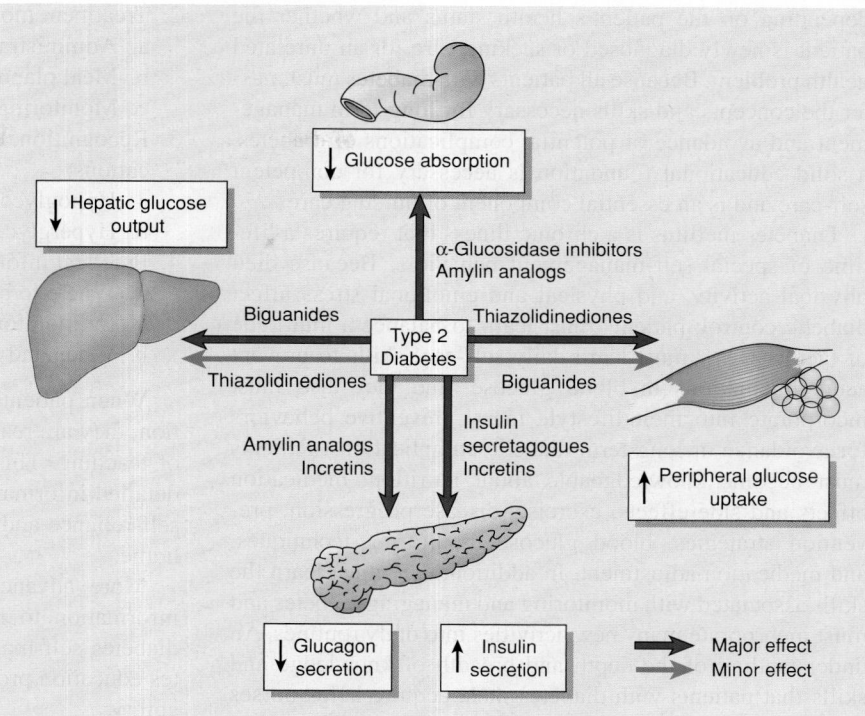

FIGURE 30-6 Sites of action of oral antidiabetic agents.

glyburide, glimepiride) have fewer side effects and drug interactions than do first-generation sulfonylureas since they are excreted by both the liver and the kidneys, thus making them safer to use in the elderly. However, if renal or hepatic insufficiency is suspected, patients must be monitored for hypoglycemia. Because the second-generation drugs are a safer option, first-generation sulfonylureas are seldom used today.

Nonsulfonylurea Insulin Secretagogues. Repaglinide (Prandin) and naglitinide (Starlix) act similarly to sulfonylureas but have a different chemical structure. Both lower the blood glucose level by stimulating insulin release from the pancreatic beta cells. These drugs have a very rapid onset and a short duration and *must be taken with meals*; they should not be taken if a meal is skipped.

Alpha-Glucosidase Inhibitors. Acarbose (Precose) and miglitol (Glyset) are alpha-glucosidase inhibitors. They work by delaying the absorption of glucose in the intestines, which results in a lower level of postprandial blood glucose. Reduction in plasma glucose results in improved diabetes control and lower A1c levels.

The advantage of alpha-glucosidase inhibitors is that they are not systemically absorbed, making them safer to use. Side effects include diarrhea and flatulence. These effects may be minimized by starting at a very low dose and increasing the dose gradually. Because acarbose and miglitol affect food absorption, they must be taken immediately before a meal, making therapeutic adherence a potential problem.

Thiazolidinediones (TZDs). Pioglitazone (Actos) is an oral antidiabetic medication categorized as a thiazolidinedione (TZD). This class of medication enhances insulin action at receptor sites without increasing insulin secretion from the beta cells of the pancreas. These medications can be used alone or in combination with other antidiabetic agents. These medications may impair liver function and also may increase the risk of myocardial infarction and congestive heart failure. Liver function studies must be performed at baseline and at frequent intervals throughout treatment.

Other Pharmacologic Therapy

Pramlintide (Symlin) is a synthetic analog of human amylin, a hormone that is secreted by the beta cells of the pancreas. It is used as an adjunct in the treatment of type 1 and type 2 diabetes when insulin alone cannot control blood glucose levels. Pramlintide is used with insulin, not in place of insulin.

Transplantation of Pancreatic Cells

Transplantation of the whole pancreas or a segment of the pancreas is being performed on a limited population, mostly in patients with diabetes who are receiving kidney transplantation simultaneously. The main issue involves weighing the risks of antirejection medications against the advantages of pancreas transplantation.

Nursing Management

Nursing management of patients with diabetes can involve treatment of a wide variety of physiologic disorders, depending on the patient's health status and whether the patient is newly diagnosed or seeking care for an unrelated health problem. Because all patients with diabetes must master the concepts and skills necessary for long-term management and avoidance of potential complications of diabetes, a solid educational foundation is necessary for competent self-care and is an essential component of nursing care.

Diabetes mellitus is a chronic illness that requires a lifetime of special self-management behaviors. Because diet, physical activity, and physical and emotional stress affect diabetic control, patients must learn to balance a multitude of factors. They must learn daily self-care skills to prevent acute fluctuations in blood glucose, and they also must incorporate into their lifestyle many preventive behaviors for avoidance of long-term diabetic complications. Patients must become knowledgeable about nutrition, medication effects and side effects, exercise, disease progression, prevention strategies, blood glucose monitoring techniques, and medication adjustment. In addition, they must learn the skills associated with monitoring and managing diabetes and must incorporate many new activities into daily routines. An understanding of the depth and breadth of knowledge and skills that patients with diabetes must acquire helps nurses provide effective patient education and counseling.

Developing a Diabetic Teaching Plan

Changes in the health care system as a whole have had a major impact on education and training for patients with diabetes. Patients with new-onset type 1 diabetes are hospitalized for much shorter periods or may be managed completely on an outpatient basis. Patients with new-onset type 2 diabetes are rarely hospitalized for initial care. Because many patients with diabetes are admitted to the hospital for reasons other than diabetes or its complications, all nurses play a vital role in identifying patients with diabetes, assessing self-care skills, providing basic education, reinforcing teaching, and referring patients for follow-up care after discharge. Regardless of the setting, all encounters with patients with diabetes are opportunities for reinforcement of self-management skills.

Patients with newly diagnosed diabetes and those who have had diabetes for several years should be assessed for self-care needs. The ADA recommends that teaching include three levels of care. The first, survival skills, provides the patient with basic knowledge and skills for diabetes management. An outline of survival information includes the following:

1. Simple pathophysiology:
   a. Basic definition of diabetes
   b. Normal blood glucose ranges and target blood glucose levels
   c. Effect of insulin and exercise
   d. Effect of food and stress, including illness and infections
   e. Basic treatment approaches

2. Treatment modalities:
   a. Administration of insulin and oral medications
   b. Meal planning
   c. Monitoring of blood glucose and urine ketones
3. Recognition, treatment, and prevention of acute complications:
   a. Hypoglycemia
   b. Hyperglycemia
4. Practical information:
   a. Where to buy and store insulin, syringes, and supplies for monitoring glucose
   b. When and how to contact the primary care provider

When patients have mastered basic skills and information, they are ready for home management, the second level of teaching. This level involves providing the patient with detailed information, beyond basic survival skills, to foster self-reliance and independence for diabetes management at home.

More advanced patient education includes skills and information to improve lifestyle and individualization of diabetes self-management. The degree of advanced diabetes education provided depends on the patient's interest and ability.

Unfolding Patient Stories: Skyler Hansen • Part 2

Recall from Chapter 3 **Skyler Hansen**, a high school student recently diagnosed with type 1 diabetes. Outline a diabetes education plan for Skyler and his parents. What are important patient education topics, resources, and methods for the nurse to consider? How would the nurse evaluate whether the patient and his family understand the education provided?

Care for Skyler and other patients in a realistic virtual environment: *vSim for Nursing* (thepoint.lww.com/vSimMedicalSurgical). Practice documenting these patients' care in (thepoint.lww.com/DocuCareEHR).

Assessing Readiness to Learn

The nurse must assess the patient's readiness to learn before initiating diabetes education. When patients are first diagnosed with diabetes, or first told of the need for insulin, they often go through various stages of the grieving process. The amount of time it takes for the patient and family members to accept the realities of living with diabetes varies.

Once the patient's questions have been answered and possible misconceptions are corrected, the nurse focuses attention on concrete survival skills. Because of the immediate need for multiple new skills, teaching is initiated as soon as possible after diagnosis. Nurses whose patients are in the hospital rarely have the luxury of waiting until the patient feels ready to learn; short hospital stays necessitate initiation of survival skill education as early as possible. This gives the patient the opportunity to practice skills with supervision by the nurse before discharge. Follow-up by home health nurses often is necessary for reinforcement of survival skills.

Determining Teaching Methods

Patient teaching must be flexible and planned to meet the needs of the individual patient. Teaching skills and providing information in a logical sequence is not always the most helpful approach for patients. For example, many patients fear self-injection. Before they learn how to prepare insulin, patients should be taught to insert the needle and inject insulin. Once they have actually performed injections, most patients are better prepared to hear and to comprehend other information necessary for insulin administration. Ample opportunity should be provided for patients and families to practice skills under supervision. Refer to Chapter 2 for details on Teaching Techniques and Learning Readiness.

Implementing the Plan

Teaching Experienced Patients

Nurses should continue to assess the skills and self-care behaviors of patients who have had diabetes for many years. Assessment of experienced patients must include direct observation of skills, not just the patient's self-report of self-care behaviors. In addition, these patients must be fully aware of preventive measures related to foot care and eye care as well as management of risk factors.

Teaching Patients Self-Care

Patient teaching and support for diabetes self-management is an important nursing responsibility. Patients who are having difficulty following the diabetes treatment plan must be approached with care and understanding. If problems with glucose control or with the development of preventable complications exist, the nurse should assess the patient to determine possible reasons. Often problems can be corrected simply by providing complete information and ensuring that the patient understands the information. The focus of diabetes education is on patient empowerment, highlighting the knowledge, skills, and attitudes needed to maintain and improve one's health.

If knowledge deficit is not the problem, certain physical or emotional factors may be impairing the patient's ability to perform self-care skills. For example, decreased visual acuity may interfere with the patient's ability to administer insulin accurately, measure the blood glucose level, or inspect the skin and feet. Decreased joint mobility or other disability also may impair a patient's ability to inspect the bottom of the feet. Emotional factors, such as depression or denial of the diagnosis, may impair the patient's ability to carry out multiple daily self-care measures. Sometimes family, personal, or work problems are given priority over diabetes management. It is also important to assess the patient for infection or emotional stress, which can lead to elevated blood glucose levels despite adherence to the treatment regimen.

Providing Continuing Care

Continuing care of patients with diabetes is critical in managing and preventing complications. The degree to which patients interact with health care providers to obtain ongoing care depends on many factors. Age, socioeconomic level, existing complications, type of diabetes, and other health problems all may influence the frequency of follow-up visits. Home health nurses are an excellent resource for ongoing diabetes education, wound care, insulin preparation, or assistance with glucose monitoring. Even patients who achieve excellent glucose control and have no complications should see their primary health care provider at least twice a year for ongoing evaluation. In addition, the nurse should remind the patient about the importance of participating in other health promotion activities, such as immunizations and recommended age-appropriate health screenings. Participation in support groups is encouraged for patients who have had diabetes for many years as well as for those who are newly diagnosed. Those who participate in support groups often have an opportunity to share valuable information and experiences and to learn from others.

ACUTE COMPLICATIONS OF DIABETES

The three major acute complications of diabetes are caused by short-term imbalances in blood glucose levels. They are hypoglycemia, DKA, and HHNS, also called hyperglycemic hyperosmolar syndrome (HHS).

HYPOGLYCEMIA (INSULIN REACTION)

Hypoglycemia (low blood glucose) occurs when the blood glucose falls below the range of 50 to 60 mg/dL.

Pathophysiology

Hypoglycemia is caused primarily by medication, such as insulin or oral hypoglycemic agents. Common factors that affect the action of those medications include inadequate food intake or increased physical activity. Hypoglycemia may occur at any time of the day or night. It often occurs before meals, especially if meals are delayed or snacks are omitted. For example, midmorning hypoglycemia may occur when the morning regular insulin is peaking, while hypoglycemia that occurs in the late afternoon often coincides with the peak of the morning NPH insulin. Nocturnal hypoglycemia may occur because of peaking late afternoon NPH insulin, especially in patients who have not eaten a bedtime snack.

Clinical Manifestations and Assessment

The clinical manifestations of hypoglycemia are grouped into two categories, based on where they are apparent; they are symptoms of the autonomic nervous system (ANS) and of the central nervous system (CNS).

At the onset of hypoglycemia, the parasympathetic system is activated, causing hunger (Porth, 2015). This is followed by activation of the sympathetic nervous system, resulting in a surge of epinephrine and norepinephrine. This causes symptoms, such as diaphoresis, tremor, tachycardia, palpitation, anxiety, and hunger.

In moderate hypoglycemia, the fall in blood glucose level deprives the brain cells of needed fuel for functioning. Signs of impaired function of the CNS may include inability to concentrate, headache, lightheadedness, confusion, memory lapses, numbness of the lips and tongue, slurred speech, impaired coordination, emotional changes, irrational or combative behavior, diplopia (double vision), and drowsiness. Any combination of these symptoms may occur.

In patients with severe cases of hypoglycemia, CNS function is so impaired that the patient needs the assistance of another person for treatment of hypoglycemia. Symptoms may include disoriented behavior, seizures, difficulty arousing from sleep, or loss of consciousness.

> **Nursing Alert**
> The brain relies almost entirely on glucose for energy. Since, the brain cannot synthesize or store more than a few minutes' supply of glucose, symptoms of cerebral function deterioration are noted with hypoglycemia (Porth, 2015).

Symptoms of hypoglycemia may occur suddenly and unexpectedly and vary considerably from person to person. To some degree, this may be related to the actual level to which the blood glucose falls or to the rate at which it falls. For example, patients who usually have a blood glucose level in the hyperglycemic range (e.g., 200 mg/dL or greater) may feel hypoglycemic symptoms when the blood glucose falls rapidly to 120 mg/dL or less. This is commonly referred to as *relative hypoglycemia*. Conversely, patients who frequently have a glucose level in the low range of normal (e.g., 80 to 100 mg/dL) may be asymptomatic until the blood glucose falls to less than 50 mg/dL. Some patients who have had diabetes for many years experience hypoglycemic unawareness. This condition occurs when the normal compensatory response to low blood sugar fails to cause symptoms, thus the patient is unaware of the problem and may experience profound hypoglycemia without any warning.

Medical and Nursing Management

Giving Carbohydrates

Immediate treatment must be given when hypoglycemia occurs. The usual recommendation is that 15 to 20 g of a fast-acting concentrated source of glucose be taken orally. Sources of glucose for the treatment of hypoglycemia include:

- Three or four commercially prepared glucose tablets
- 4 to 6 oz of fruit juice or regular soda
- 6 to 10 hard candies
- 2 to 3 teaspoons of sugar or honey

Sugar should *not* be added to juice, even if it is labeled as unsweetened juice. Adding table sugar to fruit juice may cause a sharp increase in the blood glucose level, causing prolonged hyperglycemia.

The blood glucose level should be retested in 15 minutes and retreated with another 15 g of carbohydrate if the patient is still hypoglycemic. If the symptoms persist for longer than 15 minutes after initial treatment, the treatment is repeated even if blood glucose testing is not possible. Once the blood glucose has returned to normal, a snack or meal containing protein and starch (e.g., milk or cheese and crackers) is recommended to prevent recurrent hypoglycemia (ADA, 2017d). It is important that people with diabetes, especially those receiving insulin or oral hypoglycemic agents, have a source of carbohydrate readily available at all times.

> **Nursing Alert**
> If a patient with hypoglycemia is unresponsive, a glucagon injection or bolus of IV dextrose according to hospital protocol is administered rather than risking aspiration with carbohydrates by mouth.

Initiating Emergency Measures

For adult patients experiencing hypoglycemia who are unconscious or unable to swallow safely, an injection of glucagon 1 mg can be administered either subcutaneously or intramuscularly. **Glucagon** is a hormone produced by the alpha cells of the pancreas that stimulates the liver to convert glycogen to glucose. Because of glycogen's short duration of action, the patient should be given both a concentrated source of carbohydrate followed by a snack once he or she regains consciousness. This will prevent recurrence of hypoglycemia and help replenish the glucose stored in the liver.

Glucagon is sold by prescription only and should be part of the emergency supplies available to patients with diabetes who require insulin. Family members, friends, and coworkers should be instructed in the use of glucagon, especially for patients who have little or no warning of hypoglycemic episodes.

Patients who are hospitalized and experience severe hypoglycemia are generally given 25 to 50 mL of 50% dextrose in water ($D_{50}W$) via IV push at a rate of 10 mL/min, but actual amounts are dictated by hospital protocol. This intervention is effective in achieving an increase in the blood glucose within minutes.

DIABETIC KETOACIDOSIS

DKA is caused by an absence or markedly inadequate amount of insulin. This deficit of insulin results in disorders in the metabolism of carbohydrates, proteins, and fats. The primary clinical features of DKA are hyperglycemia, ketosis, dehydration, electrolyte loss, and metabolic acidosis.

Pathophysiology

Without insulin, the amount of glucose entering the cells is reduced, and production and release of glucose by the liver is increased. Both factors lead to hyperglycemia. In an attempt to rid the body of the excess glucose, the kidneys excrete excess glucose, causing an osmotic diuresis, leading to dehydration and marked loss of electrolytes. The hyperosmolality of the extracellular fluid leads to the stimulation of thirst, resulting in polydipsia and fluid shifting from intracellular to extracellular space. This fluid shifting causes low or normal levels of serum sodium despite water losses with polyuria. This low serum sodium level is referred to as *pseudohyponatremia*.

Another effect of insulin deficiency is the breakdown of fat (lipolysis) into free fatty acids and glycerol. The free fatty acids are converted into ketone bodies by the liver. In DKA, the excessive production of ketone bodies leads to the development of metabolic acidosis. A characteristic response to this acidemia is for the respiratory center to blow off its respiratory acid, leading to rapid deep respirations known as **Kussmaul respirations**.

> **Nursing Alert**
> *Since ketones are a volatile acid, as they are exhaled, they may manifest as acetone breath that has a fruity odor similar to overripe apples.*

Causes of DKA include insufficient or missed doses of insulin, physical or emotional stress, and illness or infection. An insulin deficit may result from an insufficient dosage of insulin prescribed or from insufficient insulin being administered by the patient. Physical and emotional stress increases the level of the counter regulatory ("stress") hormones—glucagon, epinephrine, norepinephrine, and cortisol—all of which cause an increase in blood glucose. Finally, illness and infection are associated with insulin resistance, which puts the patient at risk for hyperglycemia. If insulin is not increased during times of stress, illness, and infection, hyperglycemia may progress to DKA. For some patients with undiagnosed or untreated type 1 diabetes, DKA is the initial manifestation of diabetes.

Clinical Manifestations and Assessment

Hyperglycemia leads to polyuria, polydipsia, weakness, and malaise. In addition, the patient may experience blurred vision due to osmotic changes on the lens related to hyperglycemia. Clinical manifestations of DKA are depicted in Figure 30-7. Patients with marked intravascular volume depletion may present with orthostatic hypotension; warm, dry skin; decreased skin turgor; flat neck veins; and dry mucous membranes. Volume depletion also may lead to frank hypotension and a weak, rapid pulse.

The ketosis and acidosis of DKA lead to gastrointestinal (GI) symptoms, such as anorexia, nausea, vomiting, and abdominal pain. The patient may have acetone breath (a fruity odor) as well as Kussmaul respirations representing the body's attempt to decrease the acidosis, counteracting the effect of ketone accumulation. Mental status changes in DKA vary widely; the patient may be alert, lethargic, or comatose, usually depending on the severity of the abnormality of plasma osmolality.

> **Nursing Alert**
> *Ketone bodies are acids that disturb the acid–base balance of the body when they accumulate in excessive amounts. The resulting DKA may cause signs and symptoms, such as abdominal pain, nausea, vomiting, hyperventilation, a fruity breath odor, and, if left untreated, altered level of consciousness, coma, and death. Initiation of insulin treatment, along with fluid and electrolytes as needed, is essential to treat hyperglycemia and DKA and rapidly improves the metabolic abnormalities.*

Diagnostic findings include:

- Blood glucose levels greater than 250 mg/dL
- Low serum pH (6.8 to 7.3)
- Low serum bicarbonate (0 to 15 mEq/L)
- Accumulation of serum and urine ketones
- Presence of glucose in the urine
- Abnormal levels of serum electrolytes (sodium, potassium, and chloride)

> **Pathophysiology Alert**
> *Plasma ketones are used by the body as an energy source when glucose is low or unavailable for cellular metabolism. With the breakdown of stored fat (lipolysis), liberated fatty acids are oxidized to ketone bodies, such as acetone (least abundant of all serum ketones), acetoacetate (a ketoacid), and beta-3-hydroxybutyrate (hydroxy acid). Testing urine for ketones evaluates only acetoacetate and acetone but NOT hydroxybutyrate. Elevated plasma beta-3-hydroxybutyrate is associated with high anion gap metabolic acidosis. Bedside testing or point of care testing (such as glucose finger sticks) for plasma beta-3-hydroxybutyrate is recommended rather than a urine dip test for ketones as a screening for DKA. The technology to do capillary blood testing for beta-3-hydroxybutyrate is currently in development and testing, and nurses can expect this to be available in the future.*

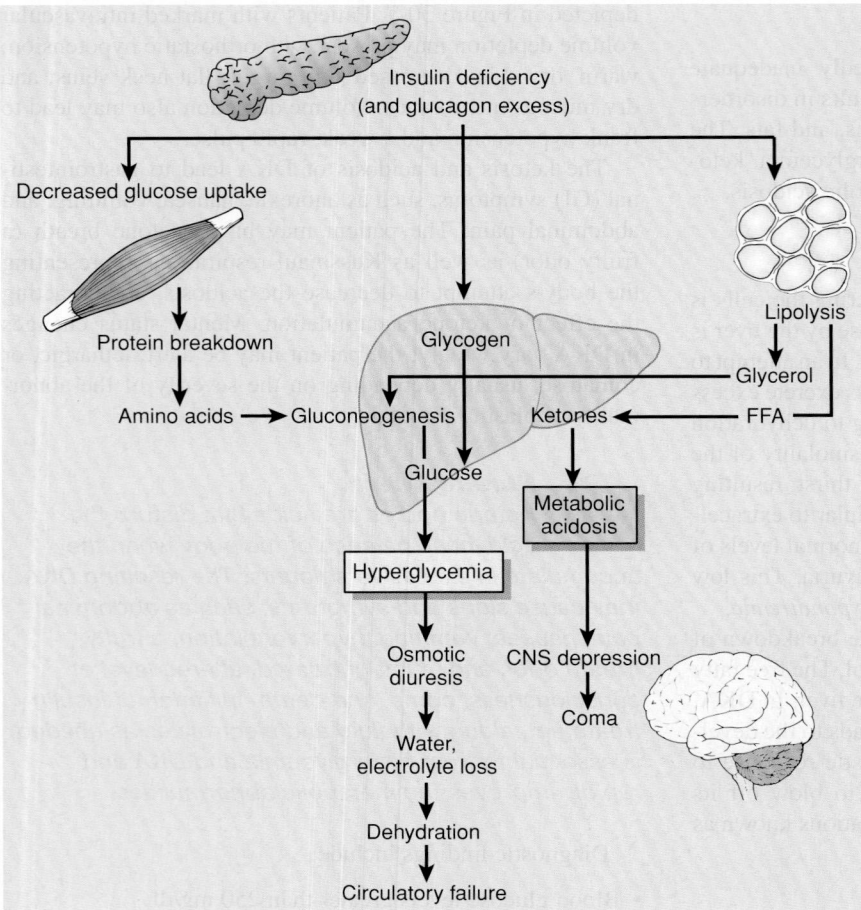

FIGURE 30-7 Mechanisms of diabetic keto-acidosis (DKA). DKA is associated with very low levels of insulin and extremely high levels of glucagon, catecholamines, and other counterregulatory hormones. Increased levels of glucagon and the catecholamines lead to mobilization of substrates for gluconeogenesis and ketogenesis by the liver. Gluconeogenesis in excess of that needed to supply glucose for the brain and other glucose-dependent tissues produces a rise in blood glucose levels. Mobilization of free fatty acids from triglyceride stores in adipose tissue leads to accelerated production of ketones and ketosis. FFA, free fatty acids; CNS, central nervous system. (From Porth, C. M. (2015). *Essentials of pathophysiology* (4th ed.). Philadelphia, PA: Lippincott Williams & Wilkins.)

Prevention

For prevention of DKA related to illness, patients must be taught "sick day" rules for managing their diabetes when ill. Box 30-7 lists sick day rules. The most important concept to teach patients is not to eliminate insulin doses when nausea and vomiting occur. Instead, the patient should take the usual insulin dose, or previously prescribed "sick day" doses, and then attempt to consume frequent small portions of carbohydrates. Drinking fluids every hour is important to prevent dehydration. Blood glucose and urine ketones must be assessed every 3 to 4 hours.

If the patient cannot take fluids without vomiting, or if elevated glucose or ketone levels persist, the patient must contact his or her health care provider. After the acute phase of DKA has been resolved, the patient should be assessed for the underlying cause.

Medical and Nursing Management

In addition to treating hyperglycemia, management of DKA is directed toward correcting dehydration, electrolyte loss, and acidosis.

BOX 30-7 · Patient Education

Guidelines to Follow During Periods of Illness ("Sick Day Rules")

- Take insulin or oral antidiabetic agents as usual.
- Test blood glucose and test urine ketones every 3–4 hours.
- Report elevated glucose levels (over 300 mg/dL [16.6 mmol/L] or as otherwise specified) or urine ketones to your health care provider.
- If you take insulin, you may need supplemental doses of regular insulin every 3–4 hours.
- If you cannot follow your usual meal plan, substitute soft foods (e.g., 3 cup regular gelatin, 1 cup cream soup, 2 cup custard, 3 squares graham crackers) six to eight times per day.
- If vomiting, diarrhea, or fever persists, take liquids (e.g., 2 cup regular cola or orange juice, 2 cup broth, 1 cup Gatorade) every 1–2 hours to prevent dehydration and to provide calories.
- Report nausea, vomiting, and diarrhea to your health care provider because extreme fluid loss may be dangerous.
- If you are unable to retain oral fluids, you may require hospitalization to avoid diabetic ketoacidosis and, possibly, coma.

Rehydration

In patients who are dehydrated, rehydration is important for maintaining tissue perfusion. In addition, fluid replacement enhances the excretion of excessive glucose by the kidneys. The patient may need as much as 6 to 9 L of IV fluid to replace fluid losses caused by polyuria, hyperventilation, diarrhea, and vomiting.

Initially, 0.9% sodium chloride (normal saline) is the IV solution selected for patients admitted with DKA. Many protocols call for administration of 1 to 2 L in the first 1 to 2 hours and then 1 L/hour for 3 to 4 hours, depending on the patient's response. The rate of administration varies; however, the ADA suggests a rate of 15 to 20 mL/kg/hr or 1 to 1.5 L during the first hour. Another calculation recommended by Maletkovic and Drexler (2013) is 10 to 15 mL/kg/hr, reducing to a rate of 4 to 14 mL/kg and changing the solution to 0.45% sodium chloride (½ NS) once the patient is euvolemic (has appropriate water balance). The subsequent IV fluid replacement will depend on the sodium level and level of dehydration; typically it will be either normal saline or half-strength normal saline solution. Moderate to high rates of infusion (200 to 500 mL/hr) may continue for several more hours, depending on the patient's vital signs, physical assessment findings, and urinary output. The nurse follows the institutions protocol regarding IV rate of administration. Administration of IV fluid that is too rapid increases the risk of cerebral edema, and while the patient clinically may present with hypovolemic shock, it is essential to monitor the patient closely to avoid cerebral edema while correcting the fluid volume deficit. When the blood glucose level reaches 250 mg/dL or less, change to IV solutions containing glucose (D_5NS, $D_5$1/2NS) to prevent a precipitous decline in the blood glucose level with insulin administration (Gosmanov et al., 2014).

> **Nursing Alert**
> *The intravenous administration of regular insulin is faster than subcutaneous administration. In general, when regular insulin is administered IV, its half-life is about 9 minutes, and steady state is reached in approximately 45 minutes. Therefore, when monitoring blood glucose levels, the nurse is aware that the IV regular insulin is continuing to exert its action. Once the blood glucose level reaches 250 mg/dL or less, prevention of hypoglycemia necessitates changing the IV solution to one containing glucose. Typically, the initial insulin infusion rate is 0.1 U/kg/hr (Gosmanov et al., 2014).*

Monitoring of fluid volume status involves frequent measurements of vital signs; respiratory, cardiac, and neurologic assessment; and evaluation of intake and output. Monitoring for signs of fluid overload is especially important for patients who are older, have renal impairment, or who are at risk for heart failure. Signs include crackles, distended neck veins, edema, weight gain, shortness of breath, orthopnea, paroxysmal nocturnal dyspnea, hypertension, moist mucous membranes, and a full and bounding pulse.

Restoring Electrolytes

Potassium is the major electrolyte of concern during treatment of DKA. The initial plasma concentration of potassium may be low because of renal loss due to osmotic diuresis. Conversely, it may be normal or high because of the shifting of potassium out of the cell to accompany the movement of hydrogen into the cells because of acidemia. If the potassium level is elevated, potassium replacement is withheld until serum levels fall to normal; this prevents the possibility of cardiac arrest from hyperkalemia. The serum level of potassium will decrease with insulin administration as insulin facilitates the movement of potassium intracellularly. Additionally, rehydration leads to increased plasma volume and subsequent decreases in the concentration of serum potassium as well as increased urinary excretion of potassium. It is critical that serum potassium levels be monitored carefully during treatment for DKA.

> **Nursing Alert**
> *Potassium levels must be assessed prior to starting insulin therapy in the acute care setting. Insulin facilitates movement of potassium into the cell and, therefore, can exacerbate hypokalemia. Potassium must be replaced prior to starting insulin. Every 10 mEq of parenteral potassium should increase the serum level by approximately 0.1 mEq/L. Most protocols require the serum potassium level be greater than 3.3 mEq/L prior to starting insulin. Cautious but timely potassium replacement is vital to avoid arrhythmias that may occur with hypokalemia. An ECG should be done on admission, and continuous cardiac monitoring is anticipated until the crisis is resolved. To prevent hyperkalemia, urine output is monitored to ensure adequate kidney function before potassium is administered. If the K^+ is higher than 5.3 or the patient is anuric, potassium replacement is withheld. Frequent laboratory measurements of potassium levels are expected.*

> **Nursing Alert**
> *Signs and symptoms of hypokalemia generally are not seen until the serum level is less than 3.0 mEq/L. The most profound effects are on cardiac function and may lead to cardiac arrhythmias, predisposition to digitalis toxicity, and electrocardiographic (ECG) changes, such as prolonged PR interval and the development of a U wave. In addition, patients complain of muscle weakness and fatigue. If the potassium is less than 2.5 mEq/L, muscle weakness and paralysis of the respiratory muscles can occur (Porth, 2015).*

Reversing Acidosis

Accumulation of ketone (acetone) bodies occurs as a result of fat breakdown. The acidosis that occurs in DKA is reversed with insulin, which inhibits fat breakdown. Regular insulin is added to a saline solution and infused intravenously at a slow, continuous rate (e.g., 0.1 U/kg/hr) (Gosmanov et al., 2014). Hourly blood glucose values must be measured to avoid precipitous drops in glucose or an inadequate decline. The goal is to decrease the serum glucose level by 50 to 100 mg/dL/hr to prevent complications, such as cerebral edema. When the serum osmolality is decreased too rapidly, fluid shifts into the CNS, causing cerebral edema. Patients may complain of headache and exhibit changes in level of consciousness and cranial nerve function.

To avoid a rapid drop in the level of blood glucose during treatment, normal saline (NS) solutions with higher concentrations of glucose (e.g., D5NS, D5.45NS) are administered when blood glucose levels reach 250 mg/dL.

Intravenous regular insulin is the insulin used most commonly to treat DKA (Gosmanov et al., 2014). The nurse must convert hourly rates of insulin infusion (frequently prescribed as "units per hour") to IV drip rates. For example, if 100 units of regular insulin are mixed in 500 mL of 0.9% NS, then 1 unit of insulin equals 5 mL; therefore, an initial insulin infusion rate of 5 units/hr would equal 25 mL/hr. The insulin solution is infused separately from rehydration solutions to allow for the frequent changes in the rate and concentration of the latter.

Insulin is infused continuously until subcutaneous administration of insulin can be resumed. Even if blood glucose levels are decreasing and returning to normal, the insulin drip must not be stopped until subcutaneous insulin therapy has been started. Instead, the rate or concentration of the dextrose infusion can be increased. Usually blood glucose levels are corrected before acidosis is corrected. Therefore, IV insulin must be continued until the serum bicarbonate level improves to at least 15 mEq/L and the anion gap is 12 or less (Gosmanov et al., 2014).

Nursing Alert
To minimize the effect of adsorption of insulin to the IV container or tubing, it is recommended that the nurse "coat the IV line" by flushing the tubing with the insulin solution. When using a standard IV insulin infusion of 100 U of regular human insulin in 100 mL of normal saline, a priming volume of 20 mL is sufficient to saturate the binding sites before connecting it to the patient (Thompson, Vital-Carona, & Faustino, 2012).

HYPERGLYCEMIC HYPEROSMOLAR NONKETOTIC SYNDROME

HHNS is a serious life-threatening condition characterized by hyperosmolality (at least 340 mOsm/L) and hyperglycemia (at least 600 mg/dL) with alterations in level of consciousness. Ketosis is minimal or absent. Persistent hyperglycemia causes osmotic diuresis, which results in losses of water and electrolytes. The higher the serum glucose, the more profound the dehydration, and the greater the risk for renal impairment and mental status changes. Table 30-7 compares DKA and HHNS.

TABLE 30-7 Comparison of Diabetic Ketoacidosis (DKA) and Hyperglycemic Hyperosmolar Nonketotic Syndrome (HHNS)

Characteristics	DKA	HHNS
Patients most commonly affected	Can occur in type 1 or type 2 diabetes; more common in type 1 diabetes	Can occur in type 1 or type 2 diabetes; more common in type 2 diabetes, especially elderly patients with type 2 diabetes
Precipitating event	Omission of insulin; physiologic stress (infection, surgery, stroke, MI)	Physiologic stress (infection, surgery, stroke, MI)
Onset	Rapid (less than 24 hours)	Slower (over several days)
Blood glucose levels	Usually over 250 mg/dL (over 13.9 mmol/L)	Usually over 600 mg/dL (over 33.3 mmol/L)
Arterial pH level	Below 7.3	Normal
Serum and urine ketones	Present	Absent
Serum osmolality	300–350 mOsm/L	Greater than 350 mOsm/L
Plasma bicarbonate level	Less than 15 mEq/L	Normal
BUN and creatinine levels	Elevated	Elevated
Mortality rate	Less than 5%	10–40%

MI, myocardial infarction.

Pathophysiology

HHNS occurs most often in older people between 50 and 70 years of age who have no known history of diabetes or who have type 2 diabetes. HHNS often can be traced to a precipitating event, such as infection, acute or chronic illness (e.g., pneumonia, stroke), medications that exacerbate hyperglycemia, or therapeutic procedures, such as surgery or dialysis. The history may include days to weeks of polyuria and polydipsia. What distinguishes HHNS from DKA is that ketosis and acidosis generally do not occur in HHNS, partly because of differences in insulin levels. In DKA, no insulin is present, and this promotes the breakdown of stored glucose, protein, and fat, which leads to the production of ketone bodies and ketoacidosis. In HHNS, the insulin level is too low to prevent hyperglycemia and subsequent osmotic diuresis, but it is high enough to prevent fat breakdown.

Clinical Manifestations and Assessment

The clinical picture of HHNS is one of hypotension, profound dehydration (dry mucous membranes, poor skin turgor), tachycardia, and variable neurologic signs (e.g., alteration of sensorium, seizures, hemiparesis). As HHNS tends to occur in the elderly, many of whom have coexisting cardiac and renal disease, the mortality rate ranges from 10% to 40%, usually related to an underlying illness, the vulnerability of the elderly patient, and the severity of HHNS.

Diagnostic assessment reveals very high blood glucose, usually 600 to 1,200 mg/dL, and high serum osmolality, often exceeding 350 mOsm/kg. Levels of electrolytes and blood urea nitrogen (BUN) are consistent with the clinical picture of profound dehydration. Mental status changes and neurologic deficits are common secondary to cerebral dehydration that results from extreme hyperosmolality. Postural hypotension results from the dehydration.

Medical Management

The overall approach to the treatment of HHNS is similar to that of DKA: replacement of fluids, correction of electrolyte imbalances, and administration of insulin. Because patients with HHNS are typically older, close monitoring of volume and electrolyte status is important for prevention of fluid overload, heart failure, and cardiac dysrhythmias. Fluid treatment is started with 0.9% or 0.45% NS, depending on the patient's sodium level and the severity of volume depletion. Fluid replacement is guided by central venous or hemodynamic pressure monitoring. Potassium is added to IV fluids when urinary output is adequate and is guided by continuous ECG monitoring and frequent laboratory determinations of potassium.

Extremely elevated concentrations of blood glucose decrease as the patient is rehydrated. Insulin plays a less important role in the treatment of HHNS as opposed to DKA because it is not needed for reversal of acidosis, and,

therefore, the patient may have lower insulin requirements. Insulin is administered at a continuous low rate to treat hyperglycemia.

As in DKA, replacement IV fluids with dextrose are administered after the glucose level has decreased to the range of 250 to 300 mg/dL (Maletkovic & Drexler, 2013).

Other therapeutic modalities are determined by the underlying illness and the results of continuing clinical and laboratory evaluation. It may take 3 to 5 days for neurologic symptoms to resolve; treatment of HHNS usually continues well after metabolic abnormalities are resolved. After recovery from HHNS, many patients can control their diabetes with diet alone or with diet and oral antidiabetic medications. Insulin may not be needed once the patient has recovered from the acute hyperglycemic episode. Frequent self-blood glucose monitoring (SBGM) is important in preventing recurrence of HHNS.

Nursing Management

Nursing care of patients with HHNS includes close monitoring of vital signs, fluid status, and laboratory values. In addition, strategies are implemented to maintain safety and prevent injury related to changes in the sensorium secondary to HHNS. Fluid status and urine output are monitored closely because of the high risk of kidney failure secondary to severe dehydration. In addition, the nurse must direct care to the condition that may have precipitated the onset of HHNS, such as MI, infection, illness, or extreme stress (burns, trauma, etc.), or consider iatrogenic treatments, such as TPN/PPN, enteral feedings, or sympathomimetics. Because HHNS tends to occur in older patients, the physiologic changes that occur with aging should be noted. Careful assessment of cardiovascular, pulmonary, and renal function throughout the acute and recovery phases of HHNS is important.

LONG-TERM COMPLICATIONS OF DIABETES

Long-term complications, which are becoming more common as people live longer with diabetes, can affect almost every organ system of the body and are a major cause of death and disability. The general categories of long-term diabetic complications are macrovascular disease, microvascular disease, and neuropathy.

The specific causes and pathogenesis of each type of complication are not thoroughly understood. However, it appears that increased levels of blood glucose predispose patients with diabetes to microvascular complications and risk factors contributing to macrovascular complications. Hypertension is most likely another contributing factor, especially in both macrovascular and microvascular diseases.

Long-term complications are seen in both patients with type 1 and type 2 diabetes. Because patients with type 2 diabetes can go undiagnosed for many years, evidence of complications may be present at the time of diagnosis.

MACROVASCULAR COMPLICATIONS

Diabetic macrovascular (macroangiopathy) complications result from changes in medium to large blood vessels. Blood vessel walls thicken, sclerose, and become occluded by plaque that adheres to the vessel walls. Eventually, blood flow is blocked. These atherosclerotic changes tend to occur more often and at an earlier age in patients whose diabetes is poorly controlled. Coronary artery disease, cerebrovascular disease, and peripheral vascular disease are the three main types of macrovascular complications that occur frequently in the diabetic population.

Cardiovascular disease is the major cause of illness and death for people with diabetes (ADA, 2017e). One unique feature of coronary artery disease in patients with diabetes is that typical ischemic symptoms may be absent. Therefore, the patient may not experience the early warning signs of decreased coronary blood flow and may have a "silent" myocardial infarction. This lack of ischemic symptoms may be secondary to autonomic neuropathy. Cardiac disease is discussed in detail in Chapter 14.

Cerebral blood vessels are affected similarly by accelerated atherosclerosis. Occlusive changes or an embolus elsewhere in the vasculature that lodges in a cerebral blood vessel can lead to transient ischemic attacks and strokes. People with diabetes have three times the risk of developing cerebrovascular disease and a greater likelihood of death (Powers, 2016). Recovery from a stroke is likely to be more difficult for patients with elevated blood glucose levels at the time of, and immediately after, a stroke. Because symptoms of cerebrovascular disease may be similar to symptoms of acute diabetic complications (HHNS or hypoglycemia), it is very important to assess the blood glucose level and treat abnormal levels rapidly so that testing and treatment of cerebrovascular disease can be initiated promptly, if indicated.

Atherosclerotic changes in the large blood vessels of the lower extremities are responsible for a two to three times higher incidence of occlusive peripheral arterial disease in people with diabetes. Signs and symptoms of peripheral vascular disease include diminished peripheral pulses and intermittent claudication (pain in the buttock, thigh, or calf during walking). Severe arterial occlusive disease in the lower extremities is largely responsible for the increased incidence of gangrene and subsequent amputation in patients with diabetes. Refer to Chapter 12 for assessment of ankle-brachial index (ABI).

Medical and Nursing Management

The focus of management is aggressive modification and reduction of risk factors. Diet and exercise are important in managing diabetes, obesity, hypertension, and hyperlipidemia. Smoking cessation is essential. If blood pressure goals are not met within 3 months of lifestyle changes, angiotensin-converting enzyme (ACE) inhibitors or angiotensin receptor blockers (ARBs) are recommended for blood pressure control. Antilipidemic medications (e.g., statins) may be added. Aspirin therapy is recommended as a primary prevention strategy in those patients who have a 10-year risk for cardiovascular disease of at least 10%. Aspirin is not recommended routinely for all patients (ADA, 2017e).

When macrovascular complications do occur, patients may require medication changes or intensification of their regimen to get glucose levels to goal. Target A1c and blood glucose goals are patient-dependent and should be modified to avoid hypoglycemia, with higher A1c targets particularly in those patients who are elderly or have known coronary artery disease.

MICROVASCULAR COMPLICATIONS

Diabetic microvascular disease (microangiopathy) is characterized by thickening of the membrane of the capillary basement. The basement membrane surrounds the endothelial cells of the capillary. Increased blood glucose levels react through a series of biochemical responses to thicken the basement membrane to several times its normal thickness. Two areas affected by these changes are the retina and the kidneys.

Diabetic Retinopathy

Diabetic retinopathy is the leading cause of blindness in the United States among people between 20 and 74 years of age; it occurs in patients with both type 1 and type 2 diabetes. Glaucoma, cataracts, and other disorders of the eye occur earlier and more frequently in people with diabetes (ADA, 2017f). Table 30-8 summarizes the complications of diabetes that affect vision.

Diabetic retinopathy is caused by changes in the small blood vessels in the retina, the area of the eye that receives images and sends information about the images to the brain. The retina is richly supplied with blood vessels of all kinds: small arteries and veins, arterioles, venules, and capillaries. Figure 30-8 shows the difference between a healthy retina and a retina affected by diabetes.

The risk for retinopathy increases with the length of time a person has had diabetes. Chronic hyperglycemia and hypertension also increase the risk for retinopathy (ADA, 2017f). Changes in the microvasculature include microaneurysms, intraretinal hemorrhage, hard exudates, and focal capillary closure.

Retinopathy has three stages: nonproliferative, preproliferative, and proliferative.

- *Stage I:* Nonproliferative retinopathy is characterized by macular edema and occurs in approximately 10% of people with type 1 or type 2 diabetes. It may lead to visual distortion and loss of central vision.

TABLE 30-8 Ocular Complications of Diabetes

Eye Disorder	Characteristics
Retinopathy	Deterioration of the small blood vessels that nourish the retina
Nonproliferative (Background)	Early-stage, asymptomatic retinopathy. Blood vessels within the retina develop microaneurysms that leak fluid, causing swelling and forming deposits (exudates). In some cases, macular edema causes distorted vision.
Preproliferative	Represents increased destruction of retinal blood vessels
Proliferative	Abnormal growth of new blood vessels on the retina. New vessels rupture, bleeding into the vitreous and blocking light. Ruptured blood vessels in the vitreous form scar tissue, which can pull on and detach the retina.
Cataracts	Opacity of the lens of the eye; cataracts occur at an earlier age in patients with diabetes.
Lens changes	The lens of the eye can swell when blood glucose levels are elevated. For some patients, visual changes related to lens swelling may be the first symptoms of diabetes. It may take up to 2 months of improved blood glucose control before hyperglycemic swelling subsides and vision stabilizes. Therefore, patients are advised not to change eyeglass prescriptions during the 2 months after discovery of hyperglycemia.
Glaucoma	Results from occlusion of the outflow channels by new blood vessels. Glaucoma may occur with slightly higher frequency in the diabetic population.

- *Stage II:* Preproliferative retinopathy involves more widespread vascular changes and loss of nerve fibers. Approximately 10% to 50% of patients with preproliferative retinopathy develop proliferative retinopathy in a short time, some within a year.
- *Stage III:* Proliferative retinopathy is characterized by production of new blood vessels and formation of scar tissue. The new vessels are prone to bleeding. Fibrous scar tissue places traction on the retina that may cause hemorrhage or retinal detachment, with subsequent loss of vision.

Clinical Manifestations and Assessment

Retinopathy is a painless process. In nonproliferative and preproliferative retinopathy, blurry vision secondary to macular edema occurs in some patients, although many patients are asymptomatic. Even patients with a significant degree of proliferative retinopathy and some hemorrhaging may not experience major visual changes. Symptoms indicative of hemorrhaging include floaters or cobwebs in the visual field,

sudden visual changes including spotty or hazy vision, or complete loss of vision.

Diagnosis of retinopathy is made by direct visualization of the retina through dilated pupils with an ophthalmoscope by an ophthalmologist or optometrist.

Medical Management

The primary focus of the management of retinopathy is prevention through blood glucose control. Other strategies that may slow the progression of diabetic retinopathy include control of hypertension and smoking cessation. Laser photocoagulation in patients with retinopathy is effective at preventing vision loss. Routine screening for diabetic retinopathy allows for earlier access to this important procedure (ADA, 2017f).

Nursing Management

Nursing management of patients with diabetic retinopathy or other eye disorders focuses on patient education about the

FIGURE 30-8 Diabetic retinopathy. (**A**) In the fundus photograph of a normal eye, the light circular area over which a number of blood vessels converge is the optic disc, where the optic nerve meets the back of the eye. (**B**) The fundus photograph of a patient with diabetic retinopathy shows characteristic waxy-looking retinal lesions, microaneurysms of the vessels, and hemorrhages. (Courtesy of American Optometric Association.)

importance of prevention through regular ophthalmologic examinations and control of blood glucose. The effectiveness of early diagnosis and prompt treatment is emphasized. If vision loss occurs, nursing care also must address the patient's adjustment to impaired vision and use of adaptive devices for diabetes self-care as well as activities of daily living. Nursing care for patients with low vision or loss of vision is discussed in detail in Chapter 49.

Diabetic Nephropathy

Diabetic nephropathy, or renal disease secondary to microvascular changes in the kidney occurs in 20% to 40% of patients with diabetes and is the single leading cause of End Stage Kidney Disease (ESKD) (ADA 2017f). It is characterized by albuminuria (albumin in the urine), hypertension, and progressive renal insufficiency. Some patients eventually require dialysis or kidney transplantation.

Patients with type 1 diabetes frequently show initial signs of renal disease after 10 to 15 years, while patients with type 2 diabetes may develop renal disease within 10 years after diagnosis. However, because many patients with type 2 diabetes have had diabetes for many years before diagnosis, there can be evidence of nephropathy at the time of diagnosis.

Pathophysiology

If blood glucose levels are elevated consistently for a significant period of time, the kidney's filtration mechanism is stressed, allowing blood proteins to leak into the urine. As a result, the pressure in the blood vessels of the kidney increases. It is thought that this elevated pressure serves as the stimulus for the development of nephropathy.

Clinical Manifestations and Assessment

Most of the signs and symptoms of renal dysfunction in patients with diabetes are similar to those seen in patients without diabetes. For patients with diabetes, as kidney failure progresses, the catabolism (breakdown) of both exogenous and endogenous insulin decreases, causing increased risk for hypoglycemic episodes. Insulin needs change as a result of changes in the catabolism of insulin, changes in diet related to the treatment of nephropathy, and changes in insulin clearance that occur with decreased kidney function. Other medications excreted through the kidney, such as sulfonylureas, may also need to be adjusted to avoid hypoglycemia.

Nephropathy is characterized by the presence of albumin in the urine. Routine urine screening can detect even slight elevations in albumin levels. Albuminuria of ≥30 mg/g is abnormal and signals early nephropathy. People with diabetes should have their urine checked at least annually for the presence of albumin (ADA, 2017f).

Hypertension, whether it is a downstream effect of diabetic nephropathy or a comorbid condition, should be managed aggressively.

Medical Management

In addition to achieving and maintaining near-normal blood glucose levels, management for all patients with diabetes should include careful attention to control of hypertension and promoting smoking cessation to decrease or delay the onset of early albuminuria. Other concerns include prevention or vigorous treatment of urinary tract infections and avoidance of nephrotoxic medications. As kidney function changes, adjustment of medications may be necessary.

For patients who have developed albuminuria, an ACE inhibitor or angiotensin receptor blocker (ARB) should be prescribed. These medications lower blood pressure and reduce albuminuria, thereby protecting the kidney. This preventive strategy should be part of the standard of care for all people with diabetes. In chronic or end-stage kidney failure, two types of treatment are available: dialysis (hemodialysis or peritoneal dialysis) and kidney transplantation.

Diabetic Neuropathy

Diabetic neuropathy refers to a group of diseases that affect all types of nerves, including peripheral (sensorimotor) and autonomic nerves. The disorders are clinically diverse and depend on the location of the affected nerve cells. They may be focal or diffuse (ADA, 2017f).

The etiology of neuropathy appears to be related to elevated levels of blood glucose over a period of years. The pathogenesis of neuropathy may be attributed to either vascular or metabolic mechanisms, or both. Thickening of the membrane of the capillary basement and closure of capillaries disrupt blood supply to nerves. Also, demyelinization of nerves, which is thought to be related to hyperglycemia, and accumulation of sorbitol in nerve cells slow nerve conduction.

The two most common types of diabetic neuropathy are sensorimotor polyneuropathy and autonomic neuropathy. Sensorimotor polyneuropathy, also called *peripheral neuropathy*, most commonly affects the distal portions of the nerves, especially the nerves of the lower extremities. Mononeuropathies (e.g., cranial neuropathies affecting the oculomotor nerve) affect a single nerve. Autonomic neuropathies cause a variety of clinical manifestations, depending on the area involved.

Peripheral Neuropathy

Clinical Manifestations and Assessment

Initial symptoms of neuropathy may include paresthesias (numbness or tingling) and aching or burning sensations, especially at night. A decrease in proprioception (awareness of posture and movement of the body and of position and weight of objects in relation to the body) and a decreased sensation of light touch may lead to an unsteady gait. Decreased sensations of pain and temperature place patients with neuropathy at increased risk for injury and undetected

FIGURE 30-9 Use of a monofilament in testing for impaired sensation in the foot of a person with diabetes. (From Porth, C. M. (2015). *Pathophysiology* (4th ed.). Philadelphia, PA: Lippincott Williams & Wilkins.)

foot infections. Joint deformities may result from abnormal weight distribution on joints, resulting from lack of proprioception. Sensation can be assessed using a monofilament device (see Fig. 30-9).

On physical examination, there may be a decrease in deep tendon reflexes and vibratory sensation. For patients who have few or no symptoms of neuropathy, these physical findings may be the only indication of neuropathic changes.

Medical and Nursing Management

Pain, particularly of the lower extremities, is a disturbing symptom for many people with neuropathy due to diabetes. The first step in pain management is to achieve optimal control of blood glucose. Pharmacologic treatment of pain may include nonopioid analgesics, opioid analgesics, antidepressants, and antiseizure medications, as well as use of transcutaneous electrical nerve stimulation (TENS).

Autonomic Neuropathies

Neuropathy of the ANS can result in a broad range of dysfunctions affecting many organ systems. Three manifestations of autonomic neuropathy are related to the cardiac, GI, and urogenital systems. Cardiovascular symptoms may range from resting tachycardia, exercise intolerance, and orthostatic hypotension to silent, or painless, myocardial ischemia and infarction.

GI symptoms of early satiety, bloating, nausea, vomiting, and constipation or diarrhea may occur as a result of delayed gastric emptying. Decreased gastric motility may result in poor control of blood glucose caused by delayed absorption of glucose from ingested foods, which leads to increased variability in blood glucose levels and increased risk of hypoglycemia.

Urinary retention, a decreased sensation of bladder fullness, and other urinary symptoms of neurogenic bladder may result from autonomic neuropathy. The patient with a neurogenic bladder is predisposed to development of urinary tract infections because of the inability to empty the bladder completely. This is especially true of patients with poorly controlled diabetes because hyperglycemia impairs resistance to infection.

Sexual dysfunction, especially erectile dysfunction and ejaculatory changes in men, is a complication of diabetes. Impotence occurs with greater frequency in men with diabetes. Some men with autonomic neuropathy have normal erectile function and can experience orgasm but do not ejaculate normally. The effects of autonomic neuropathy on female sexual functioning include reduced vaginal lubrication, decreased libido, and lack of orgasm. Vaginal infection, which is more common in women with diabetes, may be associated with decreased lubrication, itching, and tenderness.

Medical and Nursing Management

Management strategies depend on symptoms and focus on modification and management of risk factors. Early recognition and appropriate management of neuropathy is important. Effective treatment options for symptomatic diabetic neuropathy are available and may relieve symptoms.

For example, treatment of delayed gastric emptying includes a low-fat diet, frequent small meals, and close monitoring of blood glucose. Metoclopramide is now reserved for the most severe cases of gastroparesis, and treatment duration should be limited (ADA, 2017f). Treatment of diabetic diarrhea may include bulk-forming laxatives or antidiarrheal agents. Constipation is treated with a high-fiber diet and adequate hydration; medications, laxatives, and enemas may be necessary if constipation is severe. Treatment of erectile dysfunction may include medication (e.g., phosphodiesterase type 5 inhibitors) and mechanical devices (ADA, 2017f).

COMPLICATIONS OF THE FEET AND LEGS

Amputation and foot ulcers, consequences of diabetic neuropathy and/or peripheral artery disease, are common and major causes of death and disability in people with diabetes. Early recognition and management of risk factors can prevent or delay these complications of diabetes (ADA, 2017f).

As shown in Figure 30-10, the typical sequence of events in the development of a diabetic foot ulcer begins with a soft tissue injury of the foot, formation of a fissure between the toes or in an area of dry skin, or formation of a callus. Patients with an insensitive foot do not feel injuries, which may be thermal (e.g., from using heating pads, walking barefoot on hot concrete, testing bath water with the foot), chemical (e.g., burning the foot while using caustic agents on calluses, corns, or bunions), or traumatic (e.g., injuring skin while cutting nails, walking with an undetected foreign object in the shoe, or wearing ill-fitting shoes and socks).

FIGURE 30-10 Neuropathic ulcers occur on pressure points in areas with diminished sensation in diabetic polyneuropathy. The ulcer may go unnoticed if pain is absent.

If the patient is not in the habit of thoroughly inspecting both feet on a daily basis, the injury or fissure may go unnoticed until a serious infection has developed. Drainage, swelling, redness of the leg, or gangrene may be the first sign of foot problems that the patient notices. Treatment of

foot ulcers typically involves antibiotics and debridement. Controlling glucose levels, which tend to increase when infections occur, is important for promoting wound healing. In addition, smoking cessation should be promoted aggressively. In patients with peripheral vascular disease, foot ulcers may not heal because of the decreased ability of oxygen, nutrients, and antibiotics to reach the injured tissue due to decreased circulation. Amputation may be necessary to prevent the spread of infection.

The risk of amputation and other problems involving the lower extremities is especially high for patients who have had diabetes for more than 10 years, those with poor blood glucose control, and those with peripheral vascular disease and peripheral neuropathy. Foot assessment and foot care instructions are vitally important for patients who are at high risk for foot infections.

Medical and Nursing Management

Teaching patients proper foot care is a nursing intervention that can prevent costly and painful complications that result in disability. Box 30-8 provides foot care tips for patient education. Preventive foot care begins with careful daily assessment of the feet. The feet must be inspected for redness, blisters, fissures, calluses, ulcerations, changes in

---

BOX 30-8 **Patient Education**

Foot Care Tips

- Take care of your diabetes:
  - Work with your health care team to keep your blood glucose level within a normal range.
- Inspect your feet every day:
  - Look at your bare feet every day for cuts, blisters, red spots, and swelling.
  - Use a mirror to check the bottoms of your feet, or ask a family member for help if you have trouble seeing.
  - Check for changes in temperature.
- Wash your feet every day:
  - Wash your feet in warm, not hot, water.
  - Dry your feet well. Be sure to dry between the toes.
  - Do not soak your feet.
  - Do not check water temperature with your feet; use a thermometer or your elbow.
- Keep the skin soft and smooth:
  - Rub a thin coat of skin lotion over the tops and bottoms of your feet but not between your toes.
  - Have corns and calluses trimmed by a podiatrist.
- Inspect toenails. All diabetic individuals should seek a qualified podiatrist for maintenance of feet and nails.
- Wear shoes and socks at all times:
  - Never walk barefoot.
  - Wear comfortable closed-toe shoes that fit well and protect your feet.
  - Stockings should fit well (without folds, wrinkles, or seams), be comfortable, and be changed daily.

- Feel inside your shoes before putting them on each time to make sure the lining is smooth and there are no objects inside.
  - Wear sandals in public showers.
- Protect your feet from hot and cold:
  - Wear shoes at the beach or on hot pavement.
  - Wear socks at night if your feet get cold.
- Keep the blood flowing to your feet:
  - Put your feet up when sitting.
  - Wiggle your toes and move your ankles up and down for 5 minutes, two or three times a day.
  - Do not cross your legs for long periods of time.
  - Do not smoke.
- Check with your health care provider:
  - Have your health care provider check your bare feet and find out whether you are likely to have serious foot problems. Remember that you may not feel the pain of an injury.
  - Call your health care provider right away if there is a cut, sore, blister, or bruise on your foot that does not begin to heal after 1 day.
  - Follow your health care provider's advice about foot care.
  - Do not self-medicate or use home remedies or over-the-counter agents to treat foot problems.

FIGURE 30-11 The monofilament test is used to assess the sensory threshold in patients with diabetes. The test instrument—a monofilament (A, B, and C are examples of monofilaments)—is gently applied to about five pressure points on the foot (as shown in image on left). The examiner applies the monofilament to the test area to determine whether the patient feels the device. (Adapted with permission from Cameron, B. L. (2002). Making diabetes management routine. *American Journal of Nursing, 102*(2), 26–32.)

skin temperature, or development of foot deformities. For patients with visual impairment or decreased joint mobility, use of a mirror or the help of a family member to inspect the bottoms of both feet may be necessary. The interior surfaces of shoes also should be inspected for any rough spots or foreign objects. In addition to daily visual and manual inspection of the feet, the feet should be examined during every health care visit or at least once a year by a health care provider. Patients with diabetes also should undergo neurologic and circulatory evaluation by an experienced examiner. Neurologic examination can be done using a monofilament device, shown in Figure 30-11. Circulation can be assessed by palpating for pulses in the lower extremities or by Doppler ultrasound. Patients with pressure areas, such as calluses, or thick toenails should be treated by a podiatrist.

Blood glucose control is important for preventing infection and diabetic neuropathy. The patient may be referred by the health provider to a wound care center for management of persistent wounds of the feet or legs.

SPECIAL ISSUES IN DIABETES CARE

Patients with Diabetes Who Are Undergoing Surgery

During periods of physiologic stress, such as surgery, blood glucose levels tend to increase because of changes in stress hormones. If hyperglycemia is not controlled during surgery, the resulting osmotic diuresis may lead to excessive loss of fluids and electrolytes. Patients with type 1 diabetes also are at risk of developing ketoacidosis during periods of stress.

Hypoglycemia is a concern in patients with diabetes who are undergoing surgery. This is a concern especially during the preoperative period if surgery is delayed beyond the morning when the patient received a morning injection of long-acting insulin.

There are various approaches to managing glucose levels during the perioperative period. Frequent monitoring of blood glucose is essential throughout the preoperative and postoperative periods, regardless of the method used for glucose control.

During the postoperative period, patients with diabetes also must be monitored closely for cardiovascular complications because of the increased prevalence of atherosclerosis, wound infection, and skin breakdown.

Patients with Diabetes Who Are Hospitalized

At any one time, 10% to 20% of hospitalized general medical-surgical patients have diabetes. This number may increase as elderly patients make up an increasing proportion of the hospitalized population.

Often, diabetes is not the primary medical diagnosis, yet problems with control of diabetes frequently result from changes in the patient's normal routine or from surgery or illness. Some of the main issues pertinent to nursing care of patients with diabetes who are hospitalized are presented below.

Self-Care Issues

All patients admitted to the hospital must relinquish control of some aspects of their daily care to the hospital staff. For patients with diabetes who are actively involved in diabetes self-management, relinquishing control over meal timing, insulin timing, and insulin dosage can be particularly difficult.

It is important for the nurse to acknowledge the patient's concerns and involve the patient in the plan of care as much as possible. If the patient disagrees with certain aspects of nursing or medical care related to diabetes, the nurse must communicate this to other members of the health care team and, where appropriate, make changes in the plan to meet the patient's needs.

Hyperglycemia During Hospitalization

Hyperglycemia may occur in patients who are hospitalized as a result of the illness that precipitated the hospitalization. Other factors that may contribute to hyperglycemia during hospitalization include:

- Changes in usual treatment regimen
- Use of medications and IV fluids, such as partial parenteral nutrition (PPN) and total parenteral nutrition (TPN), that increase blood sugar
- Inappropriate withholding of insulin or inappropriate use of "sliding scales," or the progressive increase in **insulin** doses based on predefined blood glucose ranges
- Mismatched timing of meals and insulin

Nursing actions to correct or manage these factors are important for avoiding hyperglycemia.

Hypoglycemia During Hospitalization

Hypoglycemia in hospitalized patients is often the result of too much insulin or delays in eating. Causes of hypoglycemia in hospitalized patients include:

- Overuse of "sliding scale" insulin
- Lack of change in insulin dosage when dietary intake is changed
- Overly vigorous treatment of hyperglycemia
- Delayed meal after insulin administration
- Heart failure or kidney or liver disease

The nurse must assess the pattern of glucose values and avoid giving doses of insulin that repeatedly lead to hypoglycemia. Successive doses of subcutaneous rapid-acting insulin should be administered no more frequently than every 3 to 4 hours. To avoid hypoglycemic reactions caused by delayed food intake, the nurse should arrange for snacks to be given to the patient if meals are postponed because of procedures, physical therapy, or other activities.

Assisting with Hygiene

Nurses caring for patients with diabetes who are hospitalized must focus attention on oral hygiene and skin care. Because these patients are at increased risk for periodontal disease, it is important for the nurse to assist the patient with daily dental care. The patient also may require assistance in keeping the skin clean and dry, especially in the groin and axillary areas and under the breasts, where chafing and fungal infections tend to occur.

For patients who are confined to bed, nursing care must emphasize the prevention of skin breakdown at pressure points. The heels are particularly susceptible to breakdown because of loss of sensation of pain and pressure associated with sensory neuropathy.

Feet should be cleaned, dried, lubricated with lotion, and inspected frequently. If the patient is in the supine position, pressure on the heels can be alleviated by elevating the lower legs on a pillow, with the heels positioned over the edge of the pillow. When the patient is seated in a chair, the feet should be positioned so that pressure is not placed on the heels. If the patient has an ulcer on one foot, it is important to provide preventive care to the unaffected foot as well as to give special care to the affected foot. As always, every opportunity should be taken to teach the patient about diabetes self-management, including daily oral, skin, and foot care.

Managing Stress

Physiologic stress, such as infections and surgery, contributes to hyperglycemia and may precipitate DKA or HHNS. Emotional stress can have a negative impact on diabetes control as well. An increase in stress hormones leads to an increase in glucose levels, especially if intake of food and insulin remains unchanged. In addition, during periods of emotional stress, people with diabetes may alter their usual pattern of meals, exercise, and medication. This can contribute to hyperglycemia or hypoglycemia.

People with diabetes must be made aware of the potential deterioration in diabetic control that can accompany emotional stress. Nursing care must include encouraging the patient to follow the diabetes treatment plan as much as possible during times of stress. In addition, learning strategies for minimizing stress and coping with stress are important aspects of diabetes education.

NURSING PROCESS
The Patient with Diabetes as a Secondary Diagnosis

Patients with diabetes frequently seek medical attention for problems not directly related to control of blood glucose. However, during the course of treatment for the primary medical diagnosis, blood glucose control may worsen. Therefore, it is important for nurses caring for patients with diabetes to focus attention on the diabetes as well as on the primary health issue.

NURSING ASSESSMENT

In addition to nursing assessment for the primary problem, assessment of the patient with diabetes also must focus on hypoglycemia and hyperglycemia, skin assessment, and diabetes self-care skills, including survival skills and measures for prevention of long-term complications. In addition, the nurse should ask about the use of alternative and complementary therapies.

Assessment for hypoglycemia and hyperglycemia involves frequent monitoring of blood glucose, usually before meals and at bedtime, and monitoring for signs and symptoms of hypoglycemia or prolonged hyperglycemia, including DKA or HHNS.

Careful assessment of the skin, especially at pressure points and on the lower extremities, is important. The skin is assessed for dryness, cracks, skin breakdown, and redness. The patient is asked about symptoms of neuropathy, such as tingling and pain or numbness of the feet. Deep tendon reflexes are assessed.

The nurse should assess the patient's diabetes self-care skills as soon as possible to determine whether further diabetes teaching is required. The nurse observes the patient preparing and injecting the insulin, monitoring blood glucose, and performing foot care. The patient's knowledge about diet can be assessed with the help of a dietitian through direct questioning and review of the patient's menu choices. The patient is asked about signs and symptoms, treatment, and prevention of hypoglycemia and hyperglycemia. The patient's knowledge of risk factors for microvascular and macrovascular disease, including hypertension, increased lipids, and smoking, is assessed. In addition, the patient is asked the date of the last eye examination, which included dilation of the pupils. Also it is important to assess the patient's use of preventive health measures, such as an annual influenza vaccination, date of the most recent pneumonia vaccination, as well as current medication regimen.

NURSING DIAGNOSIS

Appropriate nursing diagnoses may include:

- Imbalanced nutrition related to increase in stress hormones secondary to the primary medical problem and imbalances in insulin, food, and physical activity
- Risk for impaired skin integrity related to immobility and decreased sensation
- Deficient knowledge about diabetes self-care skills related to new diagnosis, lack of basic diabetes education, or lack of continuing in-depth diabetes education

Potential complications from inadequate control of blood glucose may include:

- Hyperglycemia, hypoglycemia
- DKA or HHNS

PLANNING AND GOALS

The major goals for the patient may include improved nutritional status, maintenance of skin integrity, and ability to perform basic diabetes self-care skills as well as preventive care for the avoidance of chronic complications of diabetes and absence of complications.

NURSING INTERVENTIONS

IMPROVING NUTRITIONAL STATUS

The patient's food intake is planned with the primary goal of glucose control. The dietary prescription also must consider the primary health problem in addition to lifestyle, cultural background, activity level, and food preferences. Alterations may be required because of the patient's primary health problem. The patient may be NPO in preparation for diagnostic or surgical procedures. Other common alterations for the patient who is hospitalized include special diets, tube feedings, and parenteral fluids. All of these treatments require special consideration for the patient with diabetes. The patient's nutritional intake is monitored carefully along with blood glucose and daily weight.

MAINTAINING SKIN CARE

The skin is assessed daily for dryness or breaks. The feet are cleaned with warm water and soap. Excessive soaking of the feet is avoided. The feet are dried thoroughly, especially between the toes, and lotion is applied to the entire foot, except between the toes. For patients who are confined to bed, the heels are elevated off the bed with a pillow placed under the lower legs and the heels resting over the edge of the pillow. Dermal ulcers are treated as indicated and prescribed. The nurse promotes optimal control of blood glucose in the patient with skin breakdown.

ADDRESSING KNOWLEDGE DEFICITS

Hospital admission of the patient with diabetes provides an ideal opportunity for the nurse to assess the patient's level of knowledge about diabetes and its management. The nurse uses this opportunity to assess the patient's understanding of diabetes management, including blood glucose monitoring, administration of medications, meal planning, exercise, and strategies to prevent long- and short-term complications of diabetes. The nurse also assesses the adjustment of the patient and family to diabetes and its management and identifies any misconceptions they may have.

MONITORING AND MANAGING POTENTIAL COMPLICATIONS

Inadequate control of blood glucose levels may hinder recovery from the primary health problem. Blood glucose levels are monitored, and insulin is administered as prescribed. It is important for the nurse to ensure that the prescribed insulin dosage is modified as needed to compensate for changes in the patient's schedule or eating pattern. Treatment is given for hypoglycemia or hyperglycemia. Blood glucose records are assessed for patterns of hypoglycemia and hyperglycemia at the same time of day, and findings are reported to the primary care provider. In the patient with prolonged elevations in blood glucose, laboratory values, and the patient's physical condition are monitored for signs and symptoms of DKA or HHNS.

Development of acute complications of diabetes secondary to inadequate control of blood glucose levels may be associated with other health care problems because of changes in activity level and diet, and physiologic alterations related to the primary health problem itself. Therefore, the patient must be monitored for hyperglycemia and hypoglycemia, and measures must be implemented for their prevention and early treatment.

PROVIDING CONTINUING CARE

A patient who is hospitalized for another health problem may require referral for home care for that problem or if gaps in knowledge about self-care are found. The home care nurse reinforces the teaching provided during hospitalization and assesses the home care environment to determine its adequacy for self-care and safety.

EVALUATION

Expected patient outcomes may include the following:
1. Achieves optimal control of blood glucose:
   a. Avoids extremes of hypoglycemia and hyperglycemia
   b. Takes steps to resolve rapidly any hypoglycemic episodes
2. Maintains skin integrity:
   a. Maintains intact skin without dryness and cracking
   b. Avoids ulcers caused by pressure and neuropathy

(continued on page 932)

3. Demonstrates/verbalizes diabetes survival skills and preventive care
4. Exhibits understanding of treatment modalities:
   a. Demonstrates correct technique for administering insulin or other antidiabetic medications and assessing blood glucose
   b. Demonstrates appropriate knowledge of diet through proper menu selections and identification of pattern used for selecting foods at home
   c. Verbalizes signs and symptoms, appropriate treatment, and prevention of hypoglycemia and hyperglycemia
5. Demonstrates proper foot care:
   a. Inspects feet, including inspection for cracks or infections between toes
   b. Washes feet with warm water and soap; dries feet thoroughly
   c. Applies lotion to entire foot, except between toes
   d. Identifies strategies that decrease the risk of foot ulcers, including wearing shoes at all times; using hand or elbow, not foot, to test temperature of bath water; avoiding use of heating pad on feet; avoiding constrictive shoes; wearing new shoes for brief periods only; avoiding home remedies for treatment of corns and calluses; having feet examined at every appointment with the health care provider; and consulting a podiatrist for regular nail care if necessary

6. Takes steps to prevent eye disease:
   a. Verbalizes need for yearly or more frequent thorough eye examinations with pupil dilation by an ophthalmologist
   b. Verbalizes that retinopathy usually does not cause change in vision until serious damage to the retina has occurred
   c. States that early laser treatment along with good control of blood glucose and blood pressure may prevent visual loss from retinopathy
   d. Identifies hypoglycemia and hyperglycemia as two causes of temporary blurred vision
7. States measures to control risk factors:
   a. Smoking cessation
   b. Limitation of fats and cholesterol
   c. Control of hypertension
   d. Exercise
   e. Regular monitoring of kidney function
8. Reports absence of acute complications:
   a. Maintains blood glucose and urine ketones within normal limits
   b. Experiences no signs or symptoms of hypoglycemia or hyperglycemia
   c. Identifies signs and symptoms of hypoglycemia or hyperglycemia
   d. Reports appearance of symptoms so that treatment can be initiated

CHAPTER REVIEW

Critical Thinking Exercises

1. A 65-year-old man with type 2 diabetes is scheduled for surgical repair of an abdominal aortic aneurysm. What modifications in nursing assessment and care before, during, and after surgery are indicated because of the diagnosis of type 2 diabetes? How would these differ if the patient had type 1 diabetes?

2. You are providing discharge instructions for a patient being discharged from the hospital after coronary artery bypass surgery. The 52-year-old man was overweight before surgery and smoked two packs of cigarettes daily for 20 years. He states that he neglected his health and his type 2 diabetes for two reasons: (1) the stress of his work, and (2) his belief that his diabetes was not serious because he never required insulin. Identify the areas of patient teaching you would provide for this patient and the rationale for each topic as it relates to the complications of diabetes.

3. A 28-year-old patient is newly diagnosed with type 1 diabetes. Identify the major nursing assessment issues and

nursing interventions in each of the following situations: (1) the patient is in the first trimester of pregnancy; (2) the patient has a phobia about use of needles; (3) the patient has been blind from birth; and (4) the patient speaks very little English.

4. A 48-year-old woman is brought to the emergency department by her coworkers because she has become drowsy and has had slurred speech for the past hour. Her coworkers report that she lives alone and has no family nearby. They state that they think she has diabetes but can provide no additional information, including the type of diabetes or the name of her health care provider. What would be your initial actions? What assessment data would you obtain initially? What diagnostic tests and treatments would you anticipate? Provide the rationale for those tests and treatments.

5. A 45-year-old man who has three children has had diabetes for 5 years and has not followed the prescribed treatment regimen. He says, "My father and grandfather both died from diabetes. I don't see any point in modifying

my life if I'm going to die from diabetes anyway." How would you approach this patient? What resources would you use? How would you alter your approach if your first efforts to convince him of the benefits of treatment were unsuccessful? How would you modify your teaching plan if the patient understands little English?

6. You are caring for a patient with diabetes, for whom self-blood glucose monitoring is recommended. Identify teaching approaches to instruct the patient about blood glucose monitoring. What is the evidence base for the teaching approach or strategy that you selected? What is the strength of the evidence, and what criteria do you use to select the approach? How would you evaluate the effectiveness of your teaching to this patient? Explain how the results of monitoring are used in the management of type 1 and type 2 diabetes.

NCLEX-Style Review Questions

1. Which should be included when teaching a newly diagnosed patient about the dietary management of diabetes?
   a. Food intake should be decreased before exercise.
   b. Consistency between food intake and activity is important.
   c. Carbohydrates are strictly limited.
   d. Insulin and other antidiabetic agents decrease the need for dietary management.

2. A morning dose of NPH insulin is given at 7:30 AM. What is the timeframe in which the nurse can expect it to peak?
   a. 11:30 AM and 1:30 PM
   b. 1:30 PM and 3:30 PM
   c. 3:30 PM and 9:30 PM
   d. 5:30 PM and 11:30 PM

3. The nurse would expect that insulin may be substituted for other antidiabetic agents in which of the following patients?
   a. In a patient with a history of DM hospitalized for an acute infection
   b. In a patient having difficulty with weight management
   c. In a patient experiencing hypoglycemia
   d. In a patient who is newly diagnosed with borderline hyperglycemia

4. The nurse anticipates that during the initial treatment of diabetic ketoacidosis, the provider will order which solution?
   a. D_5W
   b. $D_5.45\%$ saline
   c. Lactated Ringer solution
   d. 0.9% saline

5. Which does the nurse recognize as an early indicator of nephropathy?
   a. Hematuria
   b. Glycosuria
   c. Albuminuria
   d. Polyuria

Try these additional resources, available at **http://thepoint.lww.com/Honan2e**, to enhance your learning and understanding of this chapter:
- NCLEX-Style Student Review Questions
- Journal Articles

REFERENCES AND SELECTED READINGS

References and selected readings associated with this chapter can be found on the website that accompanies the book. Visit **http://thepoint. lww.com/Honan2e** to access the references and other additional resources associated with this chapter.

Nursing Management: Patients with Endocrine Disorders

Elaine Siow

Learning Objectives

After reading this chapter, you will be able to:

1. Identify the disorders associated with each of the endocrine glands.
2. Describe the underlying pathophysiology of each of the endocrine disorders.
3. Identify the risk factors associated with each of the endocrine disorders.
4. Describe the clinical manifestations and assessment of each of the endocrine disorders.
5. Summarize the medical and nursing management of each of the endocrine disorders.

Disorders of the endocrine system are common and have the potential to affect the function of every organ system in the body, such as growth, development, metabolism, and fluid and electrolyte balances. When considering pathology of the endocrine system, it is helpful to consider that disorders commonly reflect either too little hormone (undersecretion), too much hormone (oversecretion), or tumors. Refer to Table 31-1 for a list of disorders associated with hormone oversecretion and undersecretion (each will be presented in this chapter). Endocrine disorders can occur from a primary condition or from a secondary disorder that resulted in altered endocrine function.

PITUITARY DISORDERS

Oversecretion (hypersecretion) is the most common cause of pituitary disorders. It usually involves hypersecretion of adrenocorticotropic hormone (ACTH) that leads to Cushing syndrome or hypersecretion of growth hormone leading to **acromegaly** or **gigantism**. While oversecretion of the pituitary may affect a singular hormone, such as growth hormone, undersecretion (hyposecretion) usually involves all of the **anterior pituitary hormones** and is termed *panhypopituitarism*. In this condition, the thyroid gland, the adrenal cortex, and the gonads atrophy because of loss of the trophic-stimulating hormones (influencing the activity of a gland). Hypopituitarism can result from destruction of the anterior lobe of the pituitary gland.

Recall that the **posterior lobe of the pituitary gland** secretes antidiuretic hormone (ADH), also known as *vasopressin*;

too little ADH results in diabetes insipidus (DI), while too much ADH leads to **syndrome of inappropriate ADH (SIADH)**.

PITUITARY TUMORS

Pathophysiology

Pituitary tumors are usually benign, although their location and effects on hormone production by target organs can cause life-threatening effects. Although local symptoms, such as headache and visual changes, may be seen as the tumor causes pressure within the brain, systemic effects are varied depending on the over/undersecretion of particular hormones. Prolactinomas are the most common form of pituitary tumor, causing a hypersecretion of prolactin that may lead to amenorrhea (loss of menstruation), galactorrhea (spontaneous, inappropriate flow of milk from male or female breasts in the absence of pregnancy/breastfeeding), and infertility in females. In males, these tumors can cause hypogonadism, decreased libido, and impotence. Because the disorder is not diagnosed early, generally the tumor is large; therefore, visual complaints from pressure on the optic chiasm (Fig. 31-1) and headaches are common findings.

Risk Factors

Multiple endocrine neoplasia, type 1 (MEN1), also known as *Wermer syndrome*, is an autosomal dominant hereditary condition that is strongly associated with developing pituitary tumors (National Cancer Institute, 2015).

TABLE **31-1** Disorders Associated with Hormone Oversecretion and Undersecretion

Hormone	Disorders Caused by Oversecretion	Disorders Caused by Undersecretion
Adrenocorticotropic hormone (ACTH)	Cushing syndrome	Addison disease
Thyroid-stimulating hormone (TSH)	Hyperthyroidism	Hypothyroidism
Growth hormone	In adults: acromegaly In children: gigantism	In children: dwarfism
Antidiuretic hormone (ADH; vasopressin)	Syndrome of inappropriate antidiuretic hormone (SIADH) secretion	Diabetes insipidus
Thyroid hormone	Hyperthyroidism	In children and adults: hypothyroidism or myxedema During fetal and neonatal development: cretinism (stunted body growth and mental development)
Parathormone	Hyperparathyroidism	Hypoparathyroidism
Insulin	Hypoglycemia	Diabetes mellitus

Clinical Manifestations and Assessment

A normal anterior pituitary gland is formed by multiple cell types, including eosinophilic, basophilic, and chromophobic cells. Eosinophilic tumors that develop early in life can result in gigantism, as the epiphyseal plates have not yet fused. The affected person may be more than 7 ft tall and large in all proportions, but the person may be so weak and lethargic that he or she can hardly stand. If the disorder begins during adult life, the excessive skeletal growth occurs only in the feet, the hands, and the superciliary ridge (bony ridge located above the eye sockets); facial features (nose, lips, ears, and forehead) become broader and larger, the tongue enlarges, the space between the teeth increases, and the lower jaw grows, resulting in an underbite and extended lower jaw (Melmed & Synder, 2016), which is called *acromegaly.* Enlargement also can involve all tissues and organs of the body. As an example, because of soft tissue enlargement, carpal tunnel syndrome

is noted frequently in patients with acromegaly when carpal tunnel growth compresses on the median nerve. Patients typically suffer from severe headaches and visual disturbances because the growth of tumors exerts pressure on the optic nerves (Porth, 2015). Assessment of central vision and visual fields may indicate loss of color discrimination, diplopia (double vision), or temporal hemianopia (loss of vision of one half of the visual field). These tumors promote protein synthesis, which stimulates the growth of all organs; liver gluconeogenesis, causing hyperglycemia; decalcification of the skeleton; muscular weakness; and endocrine disturbances. Skeletal changes that occur with acromegaly are not reversible, whereas soft tissue changes may be.

Basophilic tumors that give rise to Cushing disease have manifestations that are associated with excessive secretion of ACTH in the pituitary gland. This can lead to masculinization and amenorrhea in females, truncal obesity, hypertension, thin skin, moon face, purple skin striae, and osteoporosis.

Chromophobic tumors represent 90% of pituitary tumors. These tumors usually produce no hormones but destroy the rest of the pituitary gland, causing hypopituitarism. Because the pituitary gland releases growth hormone, thyroid-releasing hormone (TRH), ACTH, luteinizing hormone, follicle-stimulating hormone, and prolactin, signs and symptoms vary depending on the specific hormones that are deficient but may include weight loss; somnolence; fine, scant hair; dry, soft skin; a pasty complexion; short stature; and small bones. Patients also experience headaches, loss of libido, and visual defects progressing to blindness. Other signs and symptoms include polyuria, polyphagia, a lowering of the **basal metabolic rate**, and a subnormal body temperature.

Diagnosis requires a careful history and physical examination, including assessment of visual acuity and visual fields. Computed tomography (CT) and magnetic resonance imaging (MRI) reveal the presence and extent of pituitary tumors. If other information is inconclusive, serum levels of

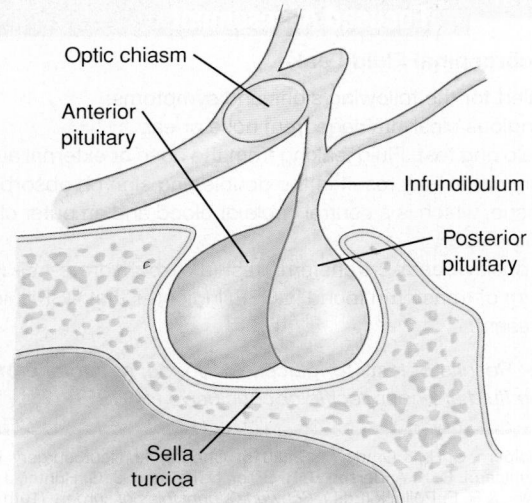

Optic chiasm

Anterior pituitary

Infundibulum

Posterior pituitary

Sella turcica

FIGURE 31-1 Relationship of the pituitary gland to the optic chiasm.

pituitary hormones may be obtained, along with measurements of hormones of target organs (e.g., thyroid and adrenal) to assist in diagnosis.

Medical Management

Hypophysectomy using a transsphenoidal approach is the treatment of choice for patients with a pituitary tumor, as the approach offers direct access to the sella turcica with minimal risk of trauma and hemorrhage. Tumors within the sella turcica and small adenomas of the pituitary can be removed through a transsphenoidal approach: an incision is made beneath the upper lip (sublabial) or via an endonasal approach, in which entry is gained successively into the nasal cavity, sphenoidal sinus, and sella turcica with minimal risk of trauma and hemorrhage. Microsurgical techniques used in the transsphenoidal approach provide improved illumination, magnification, and visualization so that nearby vital structures can be avoided. The transsphenoidal approach also avoids the risks of craniotomy, and the postoperative discomfort is similar to that of other transnasal surgical procedures.

Preoperatively, the patient undergoes a series of typical baseline endocrine tests, such as measurement of serum prolactin, assessment of hypercortisolism (excessive corticosteroids) for Cushing syndrome, and assessment of hypersecretion of insulin-like growth factor for acromegaly (Woodmansee, Carmichael, Kelly, & Katznelson, 2015). Funduscopic and visual field examination are performed because sometimes the pituitary tumor may create localized pressure on the optic nerve or chiasm. In addition, the nasopharyngeal secretions are cultured to detect a sinus infection, which is a contraindication to using the transsphenoidal approach.

Corticosteroids may be administered before and after surgery because the pituitary is the source of ACTH. In addition, the absence of the pituitary gland can alter the function of many body systems. For instance, cessation of menstruation and infertility can occur after total or near-total ablation of the pituitary gland. Corticosteroid replacement therapy and thyroid hormone replacement is necessary. In addition, prior to surgery, octreotide may be used to shrink the pituitary tumor and inhibit the production or release of growth hormone, improving the patient's clinical condition.

The initial postoperative management focuses on preventing infection and promoting healing because the procedure disrupts the oral and nasal mucous membranes. Antimicrobial agents are continued until removal of the nasal packing. Other medications include corticosteroids, analgesic agents for discomfort, and agents for the control of diabetes insipidus (insufficiency of ADH leading to diabetes insipidus) (Woodmansee et al., 2015).

Nursing Management

Preoperative nursing care of patients undergoing transsphenoidal removal of the pituitary tumor includes teaching deep-breathing exercises before surgery and instructing the patient to avoid vigorous coughing, blowing the nose, sucking through a straw, or sneezing because these actions may place increased pressure at the surgical site and cause a leak of cerebrospinal fluid (CSF). A leak represents a tear in the tough outermost meningeal dura, the membrane that surrounds the brain and spinal cord that contains CSF. If CSF can descend and escape via the nares, so too can bacteria ascend into the meninges. Therefore, the nurse assesses for signs of meningeal irritation, such as nuchal rigidity, temperature elevation, and changes in mental status (see Chapter 46). The nurse teaches patients to avoid activities, such as bending over or straining during urination or defecation, because they can raise intracranial pressure (ICP).

Postoperative nursing care includes monitoring vital signs, such as hemodynamic, cardiac, and respiratory status. The nurse assesses visual acuity and visual fields at regular intervals because of the close anatomic proximity of the pituitary gland to the optic chiasm. One method is to ask the patient to count the number of fingers held up by the nurse. Evidence of decreasing visual acuity may suggest an expanding hematoma. In addition, the nurse raises the head of the bed to 15 to 30 degrees with the patient's head in the midline position to limit neck vein compression, decrease pressure on the sella turcica, and promote cerebral venous drainage (reducing potential for elevated ICP). Measurement of the patient's serum electrolytes and intake and output guide replacement of fluid and electrolytes and assess for diabetes insipidus. The urine-specific gravity is measured after each voiding. The patient's daily weight is monitored to determine fluid status. Usually fluids are given after nausea ceases, after which the patient may be able to progress to a regular diet.

The nurse should check the nasal packing inserted during surgery frequently for blood or CSF drainage (Box 31-1). Often patients are instructed to breathe through their mouth instead of the nose, and oral care should be offered every 4 hours or more frequently as the patient can experience

---

BOX 31-1 | **Focused Assessment**

Cerebrospinal Fluid Leak

Be alert for the following signs and symptoms:

- Copious clear drainage from nose or ear.
- Halo ring test: Fluid leaking from the nose or external auditory canal may result in the double ring sign on absorbent tissue, which is a central circle of blood and an outer clear ring of CSF.
- A positive beta-2-transferrin test (a carbohydrate-free isoform of transferrin found in CSF) indicates that CSF fluid is present.

Note: Results of tests for glucose, chloride, and total protein of the fluid are not specific or conclusive for CSF.

From Halpern, C. H., & Grady, M. S. (2015). Chapter 42: Neurosurgery. In F. C. Brunicardi, D. K. Andersen, T. R. Billiar, D. L. Dunn, J. G. Hunter, J. B. Matthews, & R. E. Pollock (Eds.), *Schwartz's principles of surgery* (10th ed.). New York: McGraw Hill Professional.

excessive mouth dryness. If a sublabial approach is used, the patient is advised not to brush his or her teeth until the incision above the teeth has been healed. Measures to help patient maintain oral care and moist mucous membranes include offering warm saline mouth rinses, using a mist vaporizer, applying lip balm, and using a room humidifier. Often nasal packing is removed 3 to 4 days postoperatively, and only then can the area around the nares be cleaned with the prescribed solution to remove crusted blood and moisten the mucous membranes (Hickey, 2014). In addition, IV antibiotics are administered as ordered to protect the patient from infection.

DIABETES INSIPIDUS

Diabetes insipidus is a disorder of the posterior lobe of the pituitary gland that is characterized by a deficiency of ADH, also known as *vasopressin*. In general, this disorder is characterized by excessive thirst (polydipsia) and large volumes of dilute urine. It is helpful to remember the three D's: **D**iabetes insipidus, **D**ecreased ADH, and **D**iuresis. There are three types of diabetes insipidus: neurogenic, nephrogenic, and psychogenic polydipsia.

Pathophysiology

Neurogenic diabetes insipidus is characterized by an acute onset resulting from the destruction of the posterior pituitary gland, resulting in a lack of vasopressin. Nephrogenic diabetes insipidus generally results from drug-related damage to the renal tubules, resulting in the inability to conserve water. Psychogenic diabetes insipidus is caused by excessive water intake.

Risk Factors

Diabetes insipidus may develop as a result of head trauma, brain tumor, surgical ablation, or irradiation of the pituitary. It also may occur with infections of the central nervous system (CNS) (e.g., meningitis, encephalitis, or tuberculosis) or with tumors (e.g., metastatic disease and lymphoma of the breast or lung). Another cause of diabetes insipidus is failure of the renal tubules to respond to ADH. This nephrogenic form of diabetes insipidus may be related to hypokalemia, hypercalcemia, or medications that impair the kidneys' ability to reabsorb water. The incidence of acute diabetes insipidus in patients with a severe head injury is high, especially in penetrating injuries. Independent risk factors for diabetes insipidus include a Glasgow Coma Scale (GCS) of 8 or less, and cerebral edema. See Chapter 45 for details on GSC (Table 45-6). Often acute diabetes insipidus after traumatic brain injury is associated with significantly increased mortality (Hannon et al., 2013).

Clinical Manifestations and Assessment

Without the action of ADH on the distal nephron of the kidney, a patient with ADH likely will have an enormous daily output of very dilute urine (3 to 20 L) with nocturia, frequency, and a specific gravity of 1.001 to 1.005 occurs. Signs and symptoms of fluid volume deficit that occur as patients are unable to compensate for the massive urinary loss include:

- Weight loss
- Poor skin turgor
- Dry mucous membranes
- Increased heart rate
- Hypotension

Due to intense thirst, the patient tends to drink 2 to 20 L of fluid daily and often prefers cold water. The onset of diabetes insipidus may be abrupt or insidious. The disease cannot be controlled by limiting fluid intake because the high-volume loss of urine continues even without fluid replacement. Fluid restriction can cause the patient to experience an insatiable craving for fluid and to develop hypernatremia and severe dehydration.

To diagnose diabetes insipidus, an accurate 24-hour urine collection is obtained to measure for volume and creatinine. A urine volume of less than 2 L/24 hours (without hypernatremia) rules out diabetes insipidus.

If central diabetes insipidus is suspected, a *vasopressin challenge test* may be used (Box 31-2). Desmopressin (DDAVP; desamino-arginine vasopressin) is administered intranasally, subcutaneously, or intravenously (IV) with subsequent measurement of urine volumes, specific gravity, and/or urine osmolality. If diabetes insipidus is secondary to central or neurogenic diabetes insipidus, administration of ADH results in an elevation of urine osmolality by more than 50%. However, if the etiology is nephrogenic, there is a small or no increase in urine osmolality as the kidneys are not responsive to ADH. In addition, levels of serum plasma are obtained to screen for diabetes mellitus (DM) (glucose),

---

BOX 31-2 Vasopressin Challenge Test

1. Typically vasopressin test is performed in the morning with the patient having fasted.
2. An IV line has to be inserted to facilitate delivery of medications.
3. Blood samples were obtained to measure serum corticotropin (ACTH) and serum cortisol.
4. The vasopressin test involves administration of intramuscular arginine-vasopressin (AVP; 10 pressor units) or intravenous desmopressin (10 mcg).
5. Before administration of vasopressin, blood samples were obtained 15 minutes before, immediately before, and then afterward at the following intervals: 15, 30, 45, 60, 90, and 120 minutes.

From Lacroix, A., Nieman, L. K., & Martin, K. A. (2013). Vasopressin and desmopressin simulation test. *UpToDate*. Retrieved from http://www.uptodate.com/contents/vasopressin-and-desmopressin-stimulation-test.

TABLE **31-2** Laboratory Tests for Diabetes Insipidus

Test	Normal Values	Critical Values	Nursing Implications
Serum osmolality Urine osmolality Urine-specific gravity	288–291 mOsm/Kg 700–1,400 mOsm/Kg At least 1.015	Over 295 mOsm/kg Under 200 mOsm/kg 1.001–1.005	Patients will not be given fluid intake for 4–18 hours. The nurse will measure hourly urine osmolality, urine-specific gravity, and weigh patient. If patient loses at least 3% of body weight, the nurse will measure serum osmolality.
Plasma sodium	135–145 mEq/L	Over 145 mEq/L	Patient will be monitored for hypernatremia due to hypothalamic lesions, which cause impaired osmotic regulation but intact volume regulation of ADH secretion.
Serum ADH levels	1.3–4.1 pg/mL (values may vary slightly among different laboratories)	Look for low serum ADH levels in diabetes insipidus; e.g., in central diabetes insipidus, look for values below 1.1 pg/mL. High serum ADH levels are seen in nephrogenic diabetes insipidus.	If three successive hourly tests of urine osmolality indicate no change, administer 5 units of vasopressin and measure urine osmolality 1 hour later. Serum ADH is used to determine type of diabetes insipidus; e.g., primary diabetes insipidus ranges from 3 to 7.5 pg/mL, and nephrogenic diabetes insipidus ranges from 12 to 13 pg/mL. The nurse should be aware that serum ADH levels are always interpreted relative to serum osmolality.

Adapted from Williamson, M. A., & Snyder, L. M. (2015). *Wallach's interpretation of diagnostic tests*. Philadelphia, PA: Lippincott Williams & Wilkins.

dehydration and azotemia (urea nitrogen), hypercalcemia (calcium), hypokalemia (potassium), and hyperuricemia (uric acid).

Other diagnostic procedures include concurrent measurements of plasma levels of ADH and plasma and urine osmolality. Table 31-2 summarizes laboratory findings. A fluid deprivation test may be considered, but it is contraindicated if the patient's serum sodium is elevated. This test involves withholding fluids for 8 to 12 hours or until 3% to 5% of the body weight is lost, and plasma and urine osmolality studies are performed at the beginning and end of the test. Diabetes insipidus is likely if the patient continues to excrete large volumes of urine with low specific gravity and osmolality or experiences weight loss, increasing serum osmolality, and elevated levels of serum sodium. During the deprivation test, ADH or vasopressin can be given subcutaneously as described previously. However, the patient's condition needs to be monitored frequently due to the risk of severe dehydration. The test will be terminated if the patient develops tachycardia, excessive weight loss, or hypotension.

Once the diagnosis is confirmed but the cause (e.g., head injury) is unclear, the patient will be assessed further for presence of tumors that may be causing the disorder.

Pathophysiology Alert

ADH is also known as vasopressin or by its chemical name, arginine vasopressin or AVP. When ADH activity is present, small volumes of concentrated urine are excreted; whereas if ADH is absent, large amounts of diluted urine are excreted. Increased ADH is associated with SIADH while decreased levels are associated with DI (central). Normal levels are below 2.5 pg/mL or below 2.3 pmol/L (Fischbach & Dunning, 2014).

Medical Management

The objectives of medical therapy are to replace ADH (which is usually a long-term therapeutic program), to ensure adequate fluid replacement, and to identify and correct the underlying intracranial pathology.

Desmopressin/DDAVP, a synthetic vasopressin, is used to control fluid balance and prevent dehydration. Desmopressin does not have the vascular effects of natural ADH. Thus, it is particularly valuable due to its longer duration of action and fewer adverse effects compared to other preparations previously used to treat the disease. Desmopressin can be administered orally as tablets or intranasally using a spray or a flexible calibrated plastic tube. Usually one or two administrations daily (every 12 to 24 hours) are needed to control the symptoms. However, sometimes nasal decompression can cause rhinitis or conjunctivitis (Fitzgerald, 2015).

Other medications used to treat patients with diabetes insipidus include intramuscular administration of vasopressin, chlorpropamide (Diabinese), thiazide diuretics (potentiate the action of vasopressin), and/or prostaglandin inhibitors (e.g., ibuprofen, indomethacin, and aspirin). Intramuscular administration of ADH, vasopressin tannate in oil, is used if the intranasal route is not possible. The medication is administered every 24 to 96 hours. The vial of medication should be warmed or shaken vigorously before administration. The injection is administered in the evening so that maximum results are obtained during sleep. Abdominal cramps are a side effect of this medication. Rotation of injection sites is necessary to prevent lipodystrophy. The patient receiving chlorpropamide should be warned of the possibility of hypoglycemic reactions. If the diabetes insipidus is renal in origin, the previously described treatments are ineffective. Thiazide diuretics, mild salt depletion, and prostaglandin inhibitors (ibuprofen, indomethacin, and aspirin) are used to treat the nephrogenic form of diabetes insipidus. There is no effective treatment for psychogenic diabetes insipidus, and sometimes the only help for these patients is to prevent water intoxication by limiting use of drugs that impair free water excretion, such as thiazide diuretics and carbamazepine (Tegretol) (Robertson, 2015).

Nursing Management

The nursing management of the patient with diabetes insipidus includes maintaining adequate fluid volume, monitoring patient's weight, administering vasopressin, monitoring vital signs, and monitoring patient's intake and output. Due to vasoconstrictive properties, vasopressin should be avoided in patients with pre-existing coronary artery disease (CAD) or vascular disease. The patient with possible diabetes insipidus needs support while undergoing studies for a possible cranial lesion. Prior to discharge, the nurse informs the patient and family about follow-up care and emergency measures, provides specific verbal and written instructions, demonstrates how to administer the medications, and observes return demonstrations as appropriate. The nurse should provide instructions on measuring daily weights to determine how much body fluid has been gained or lost. This information will allow the provider to titrate the dosage of vasopressin accordingly to avoid doses that are too high or too low. For instance, high dose of vasopressin will lead to fluid retention and weight gain. On the other hand, insufficient or low dose of vasopressin will lead to excess urine production (polyuria) and weight loss. In addition, the nurse should advise the patient to wear a medical identification bracelet and to carry medication and information about this disorder at all times.

SYNDROME OF INAPPROPRIATE ANTIDIURETIC HORMONE

SIADH is a syndrome characterized by excessive secretion of ADH, causing significant retention of water. As a result, the sodium level becomes dilute, and hyponatremia ensues. It is the most frequently cited cause of euvolemic hyponatremia. In patients hospitalized with hyponatremia, over 50% of cases can be attributed to SIADH (Ferri, 2016a). Table 31-3 details the characteristics of DI versus SIADH.

TABLE 31-3 Differentiating Features of DI versus SIADH

Value	Diabetes Insipidus	SIADH
ADH	⇓	⇑
Serum sodium (Na)	⇑	⇓
Urine output	⇑ urine output	⇓ urine output
Urine osmolality	⇓ (for what would be expected)	⇑ (for what would be expected)
Specific gravity	⇓ <1.005	⇑ >1.030

Pathophysiology

SIADH is a disorder of impaired water excretion caused by the inability to stop the secretion of ADH. As a result, excessive ADH can be secreted from the pituitary gland directly into the bloodstream, or by abnormal synthesis and secretion of vasopressin by tumors. Patients with this disorder cannot excrete diluted urine. They retain water and develop a subsequent sodium deficiency known as **dilutional hyponatremia**. With too much H_2O in the bloodstream, the kidneys cannot excrete dilute urine, and the water moves from the extracellular compartment to the intracellular region, causing brain cells to swell. This has a significant impact on the CNS (brain and spinal cord) because of brain edema and increased ICP. If the sodium level becomes low enough (approximately 115 mEq/L), seizures may occur.

Risk Factors

SIADH is often of nonendocrine origin. For instance, the syndrome may occur in patients with malignancies, pulmonary disorders, disorders of the nervous system, and medication use. Carcinomas (lung, GI tract [stomach, duodenum, pancreas], GU tract [ureter, bladder, prostate, endometrium], and lymphoma) that synthesize and release ADH can lead to SIADH. SIADH has occurred in patients with pulmonary disease, such as advanced tuberculosis, severe pneumonia, positive-pressure ventilation, and other disorders of the lungs (Porth, 2015). Disorders of the CNS, such as head injury, brain surgery or tumor, vascular (stroke, subdural hematoma, subarachnoid hemorrhage), and infection (brain abscess, meningitis, encephalitis), can produce SIADH by direct stimulation of the pituitary gland. HIV infection is also associated with the development of SIADH and may be related to an underlying infection of the pulmonary (pneumocystic pneumonia) or CNS or malignancy (Porth, 2015). Medications, such as vincristine, phenothiazines, tricyclic antidepressants (SSRIs, tricyclic, MAOI), thiazide diuretics, anticonvulsants, antidiabetic drugs, and nicotine, can cause SIADH, either by directly stimulating the pituitary gland or by increasing the sensitivity of renal tubules to circulating ADH.

Clinical Manifestations and Assessment

The clinical manifestations of SIADH include the following:

- Hyponatremia (sodium below 134 mEq/L),
- Decreased serum osmolality (less than 280 mOsm/kg) with inappropriately increased urine osmolality (greater than 100 mOsm/kg—reveals impaired ability of the kidneys to dilute the urine),
- Urine sodium over 20 mEq/L,
- Low blood urea nitrogen (BUN) (below 10 mg/dL), and
- Hypouricemia (uric acid below 4 mg/dL) (Cho, 2015).

Obtain a detailed history to rule out other causes of hyponatremia, such as heart failure, adrenal insufficiency, and kidney failure. On assessment, patients usually present with normal vital signs, moist mucous membranes, normal skin turgor, and no edema. The reabsorbed water tends to be intracellular rather than interstitial, and, therefore, patients appear euvolemic (normal volume). Patients with SIADH resulting in severe hyponatremia often exhibit more acute symptoms, such as confusion, lethargy, weakness, myoclonus, asterixis, depressed reflexes, generalized seizures, and coma related to ensuing cerebral edema.

Medical Management

Medical management includes identifying and eliminating the underlying cause. Brain and chest imaging may be obtained to identify a potential etiology, such as CNS or lung pathology. Laboratory testing is performed to rule out other cause of hyponatremia, such as infection (white blood cell [WBC] count) or dysfunction of a number of systems: thyroid (thyroid-stimulating hormone [TSH] level), adrenal (cortisol), cardiac (EKG, echocardiogram, brain natriuretic peptide [BNP]), liver (liver function tests), and kidney (BUN and serum creatinine). Elevated plasma arginine vasopressin (AVP) level is expected. Treatment will depend on the speed of onset of the hyponatremia and the clinical presentation. In asymptomatic patients, fluid restriction is the treatment of choice (less than 1 L water per day), whereas in acutely symptomatic patients (profound hyponatremia is present with Na below 120 mEq/L), an IV of 3% sodium chloride (hypertonic saline) will be infused slowly via a central line and IV pump. Diuretics, such as furosemide (Lasix) IV, will prevent extracellular fluid volume expansion by causing diuresis. Because retained water is excreted slowly through the kidneys, the extracellular fluid volume contracts and the serum sodium concentration gradually increases toward normal. It is important not to correct the sodium level too rapidly; the rate of correction aims to increase the serum sodium 8 to 10 mEq/L during the first 24 hours (Ferri, 2016a; Spasovski et al., 2014) since rapid correction can cause demyelination and permanent damage to the CNS.

Nursing Management

Nursing management includes close monitoring of fluid intake and output (fluid restriction is a mainstay of therapy

---

BOX 31-3

Focus on Pathophysiology

Central Pontine Myelinolysis

Central pontine myelinolysis (CMP) is a serious complication that develops after aggressive treatment of hyponatremia. The rapid rise in serum sodium with resultant change in serum osmolality causes water to be pulled from the brain cells. The changes in the brain cell volume (shift in water out of brain cells) causes injury to the myelin sheath (myelin sheath protects the nerves). These changes can result in significant neurologic morbidity and mortality. The most common presentation of CMP is a decreased level of consciousness.

---

in most patients with SIADH, with a suggested goal intake of less than 800 mL/day), daily weight, urine and blood chemistries, and neurologic status. The sodium level will be evaluated at regular intervals—typically every 4 to 6 hours with any active treatment—until the sodium level stabilizes. The nurse assesses for neurologic signs caused by hyponatremia, such as confusion, seizures, and delirium as well as cardiopulmonary status (hypervolemia, including hypertension, pulmonary crackles, pleural effusions, tachypnea, decreased O_2 saturation, ascites, JVD, and peripheral edema). If ordered, the nurse carefully monitors hypertonic saline administration because a complication of overaggressive treatment with 3% saline is central pontine myelinolysis (CMP) (Box 31-3). Providing supportive measures and explanations of procedures helps the patient with this disorder.

> **Nursing Alert**
> As appropriate, use seizure precautions to protect the patient from injury and prevent aspiration. Keep oxygen and suctioning equipment at the bedside. See Box 46-2 on page 1319 for details on seizure precautions. In the event of a seizure, lower the head of the bed and place the patient on his or her side to prevent aspiration and protect the airway.

DISORDERS OF THE THYROID GLAND

The thyroid gland controls cellular metabolic activity, refer to Box 31-4 for symptoms of undersecretion (hypothyroidism) and oversecretion (hyperthyroidism).

HYPOTHYROIDISM

Hypothyroidism results from insufficient levels of thyroid hormone. Thyroid deficiency can affect all body functions, and symptoms range from mild, subclinical forms to myxedema coma, a life-threatening hypothyroidism.

Often patients with hypothyroidism may have *primary* or *thyroidal hypothyroidism*, which refers to dysfunction of

Focused Assessment

Hyperthyroidism versus Hypothyroidism

Be alert for the following signs and symptoms of hyperthyroidism:

- Weight loss
- Warm, moist, flushed skin
- Tremors, emotionally hyperexcitable
- Tachycardia, irregular pulse
- Heat intolerance, hyperthermia
- Increased GI function
- Thinning of hair
- Exophthalmos (visual protrusion of the eye), corneal ulcerations
- Patients may have a staring gaze, a rim of sclera visible between the upper eyelid and the superior margin of the iris during downward gaze (lid lag)
- Systolic murmur, thrill, bruit

Be alert for the following signs and symptoms of hypothyroidism:

- Weight gain
- Dry skin, nonpitting edema
- Fatigue, mental and physical sluggishness
- Bradycardia
- Cold intolerance
- Constipation
- Coarse hair, loss of eyebrows
- Carpal tunnel syndrome
- Pleural and pericardial effusions

the thyroid gland itself. If the cause of the thyroid dysfunction is failure of the pituitary gland, the hypothalamus, or both, then the hypothyroidism is known as *central hypothyroidism*. If the cause is entirely a pituitary disorder, then it may be referred to as *pituitary* or *secondary hypothyroidism*. If the cause is a disorder of the hypothalamus resulting in inadequate secretion of TSH due to decreased stimulation by TRH, then it is referred to as *hypothalamic* or *tertiary*

hypothyroidism. If thyroid deficiency is present at birth, then the hypothyroidism is known as *cretinism*. In such instances, the mother also may have thyroid deficiency. See Figure 31-2 and Table 31-4.

Pathophysiology

In hypothyroidism, the decreased production of thyroxine (T_4) leads to the stimulation of TSH in the pituitary gland. Subsequently, TSH stimulates the secretion of triiodothyronine (T_3) to increase production of T_4, leading to hypertrophy of the thyroid gland. Laboratory findings include decreased T_3 and T_4 and an increased TSH.

Risk Factors

The most common cause of hypothyroidism in adults is autoimmune thyroiditis (**Hashimoto disease**), in which the immune system attacks the thyroid gland. Hypothyroidism can occur in patients with previous hyperthyroidism treated with radioiodine or antithyroid medications or **thyroidectomy**. There is an increased incidence of hypothyroidism in patients who have undergone radiation therapy for head and neck cancer. Therefore, thyroid function tests are recommended for all patients who receive such treatment.

Hypothyroidism has been shown to affect women five times more frequently than men and occurs most often in people between 30 and 60 years of age. Additionally, long-standing mild to moderate hypothyroidism often is seen in the elderly. The explanation for the higher prevalence of hypothyroidism among elderly people may be related to alterations in immune function with age. Subclinical disease is common among older women and can be asymptomatic or mistaken for other medical conditions. For instance, subtle symptoms of hypothyroidism, such as fatigue, muscle aches, and mental confusion, may be attributed to the normal aging process by the patient, family, and health care provider. Hence, screening of TSH levels over a 3- to 6-month interval

FIGURE 31-2 Algorithm for diagnosis of hypothyroidism. The sensitive thyroid-stimulating hormone (TSH) test is the preferred primary screening test for thyroid disease. Low TSH obviates the need for the thyroid-releasing hormone (TRH) test in most patients. T4, thyroxine; T3, triiodothyronine; FTI, free thyroxine index. (From, Talreia, D. T., Talreia, R. R., & Talreia, R. S. (2005). *Internal medicine peripheral brain*. Philadelphia, PA: Lippincott Williams & Wilkins.)

TABLE **31-4** Varieties of Hypothyroidism and their Causes

Name	Cause
Primary or *thyroidal* hypothyroidism	Dysfunction of the thyroid gland itself
Central hypothyroidism	Failure of the pituitary gland, the hypothalamus, or both
Pituitary or *secondary* hypothyroidism	A pituitary disorder
Hypothalamic or *tertiary* hypothyroidism	Disorder of the hypothalamus resulting in inadequate secretion of TSH due to decreased stimulation by TRH
Cretinism	Thyroid deficiency present at birth, the mother also may have thyroid deficiency

is recommended for nonpregnant adults to confirm or rule out abnormal findings before making a diagnosis or considering any treatment strategies (LeFevre, 2015). Gerontologic considerations are discussed in Box 31-5.

Clinical Manifestations and Assessment

Clinical manifestations of hypothyroidism are divided into early and late symptoms and represent slowing of the metabolic process. The early symptoms of hypothyroidism are nonspecific and can range from fatigue to somnolence, loss of libido to amenorrhea, apathy to mental and physical sluggishness, nonpitting edema to pleural and pericardial effusions. Reports of hair loss, brittle nails, and dry skin are common. The patient frequently complains of constipation. Paresthesia (numbness and tingling of the fingers) and nerve entrapment syndrome have been linked with endocrine disorders, such as hypothyroidism, but the etiology is poorly understood. Also hearing loss may occur.

Late symptoms include slow speech, subdued emotional responses, apathy, absence of sweating, cold intolerance, constipation, thickening of skin (due to accumulation of mucopolysaccharides in subcutaneous tissues), dyspnea, weight gain, thinning of hair, alopecia, and deafness. On assessment, patients usually present with swelling of eyelids, pitting edema, bradycardia, hypotension, and hypothermia. Figure 31-3 illustrates clinical manifestations of hypothyroidism.

Advanced hypothyroidism may produce personality and cognitive changes that are characteristic of dementia. Respiratory manifestations include pleural effusion, respiratory muscle weakness, inadequate ventilation, and sleep apnea.

Severe hypothyroidism is associated with an elevated level of serum cholesterol, atherosclerosis, CAD, poor left ventricular function, and pericardial effusion. In addition, the patient with severe hypothyroidism often presents with subnormal temperature and pulse rate. The patient usually begins to gain

BOX 31-5 **Gerontologic Considerations**

Hypothyroidism

The elderly often present with atypical signs and symptoms of hypothyroidism. For instance, the elderly patient may have few or no symptoms until the dysfunction is severe. Depression, apathy, and decreased mobility are major initial symptoms that may be accompanied by significant weight gain despite a poor appetite. In addition, constipation is common and affects one fourth of elderly patients with hypothyroidism. In the elderly patient with mild to moderate hypothyroidism, thyroid hormone replacement must be started with low dosages and increased gradually to prevent serious cardiovascular and neurologic side effects. (Remember "start low and go slow.") In general, thyroid replacement begins at one fourth to one half the expected dose and is increased in small increments no sooner than 4 to 6 weeks apart. Angina may occur with rapid thyroid replacement in the presence of coronary artery disease secondary to the hypothyroid state or pre-existing atherosclerosis. Heart failure and tachyarrhythmias may worsen during the transition from the hypothyroid state to the normal metabolic state. Dementia may become more apparent during early replacement of thyroid hormone in the elderly patient.

Elderly patients with severe hypothyroidism and atherosclerosis may become confused and agitated if their metabolic rate is increased too quickly. Marked clinical improvement follows the administration of hormone replacement; such medication must be continued for life. The elderly patient requires periodic follow-up monitoring of levels of serum TSH. In addition, the elderly should be reminded that failure to comply with current therapy may lead to complications. A careful history can identify the need for further teaching about the importance of safe medication administration.

Complications, such as myxedema and myxedema coma, usually occur exclusively in patients older than 50 years of age. The high mortality rate of myxedema coma mandates immediate IV administration of thyroid hormone as well as supportive care and monitoring for cardiac complications, particularly in patients with ischemic heart disease.

weight even without an increase in food intake, although he or she may be cachectic. The hair thins and falls out, and the face becomes expressionless and masklike. The patient often complains of being cold, even in a warm environment.

 Nursing Alert
The patient with advanced hypothyroidism is profoundly hypothermic (91°F to 95°F) and abnormally sensitive to sedatives, opioids, and anesthetic agents. Therefore, these medications are administered with extreme caution. If these medications are used, closely monitor the patient's vital signs (heart rate, blood pressure, body temperature, and respiration rate).

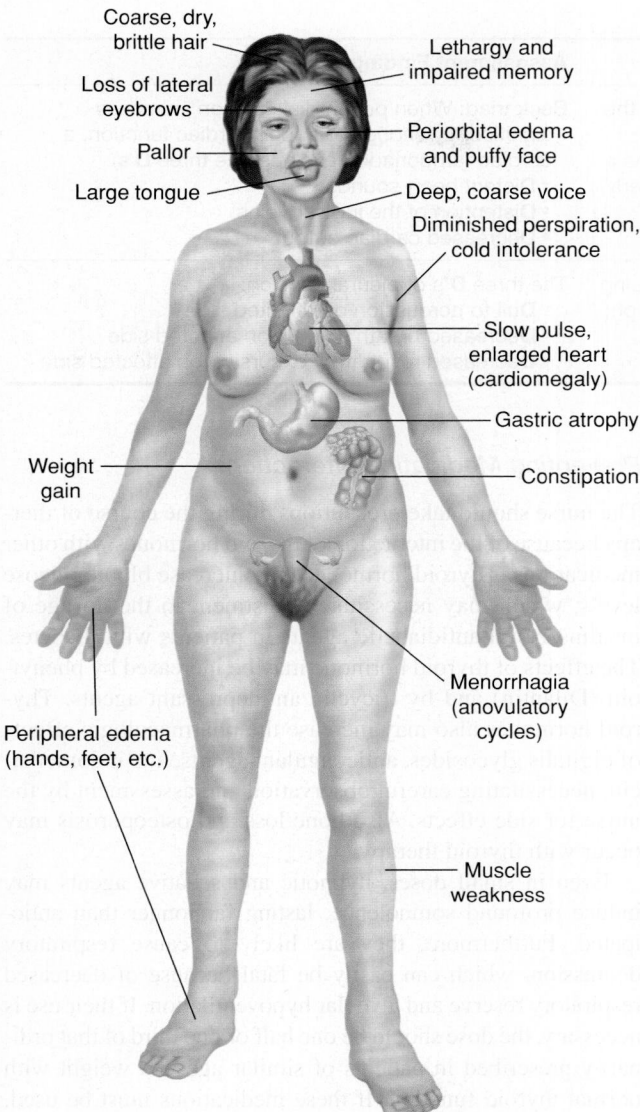

Coarse, dry, brittle hair

Loss of lateral eyebrows

Pallor

Large tongue

Weight gain

Peripheral edema (hands, feet, etc.)

Lethargy and impaired memory

Periorbital edema and puffy face

Deep, coarse voice

Diminished perspiration, cold intolerance

Slow pulse, enlarged heart (cardiomegaly)

Gastric atrophy

Constipation

Menorrhagia (anovulatory cycles)

Muscle weakness

FIGURE 31-3 Dominant clinical features of hypothyroidism. (From Porth, C. M. (2015). *Essentials of pathophysiology: Concepts of altered health states* (4th ed.). Philadelphia, PA: Lippincott Williams & Wilkins.)

Myxedema coma describes the most extreme, severe stage of hypothyroidism, in which the patient is hypothermic and unconscious. Increasing lethargy may progress to stupor and then to coma. Myxedema leads to the accumulation of mucopolysaccharides in subcutaneous and other interstitial tissues; this causes nonpitting edema and doughy skin. The fluid accumulation causes a characteristic puffy appearance to the face and eyes (periorbital edema). The patient's tongue can be enlarged, and his or her voice becomes hoarse and husky. Sometimes myxedematous fluid can cause pericardial and pleural effusions (Porth, 2015). Myxedema coma may also develop with undiagnosed hypothyroidism and may be precipitated by infection, systemic disease, or the use of sedatives or opioid analgesic agents. The patient's respiratory drive is depressed, resulting in alveolar hypoventilation, progressive carbon dioxide retention, narcosis, and coma. These symptoms, along with cardiovascular collapse and shock, require aggressive and intensive therapy if the patient is to survive. Myxedema coma is a medical emergency; even with early vigorous therapy, mortality rate is high.

Medical Management

Hormone Replacement

The primary objective in the medical management of hypothyroidism is to restore a normal metabolic state by replacing the missing hormone, levothyroxine (thyroxine; T_4). Synthetic levothyroxine (Synthroid or Levothroid) is the preferred preparation for treating hypothyroidism and suppressing nontoxic **goiters** (enlargements of the thyroid gland). The dosage for hormone replacement is based on the concentration of the patient's serum TSH. If replacement therapy is adequate, the symptoms of myxedema disappear and normal metabolic activity is resumed.

Cardiac Management

The patient who has lived with hypothyroidism for a long period of time is likely to have coronary-related diseases, such as atherosclerosis and CAD. Recall that there is elevated serum cholesterol in hypothyroidism, which is largely accounted for by an increase of LDL-cholesterol, which is a risk factor for coronary heart disease. As long as metabolism is subnormal and the tissues, including the myocardium, require relatively little oxygen, a reduction in blood supply is tolerated without overt symptoms of CAD. When thyroid hormone is administered, the myocardial oxygen demand increases without increasing the myocardial oxygen supply; therefore, patients should be monitored for cardiac complications, such as chest pain and congestive heart failure. Patients also may be treated for angina or arrhythmias due to the release of catecholamines that may be activated during thyroid replacement therapy. In the event of angina or arrhythmias, the nurse should notify the primary care provider immediately and discontinue administration of the thyroid hormone. The thyroid hormone replacement can be resumed at a later time at a lower prescribed starting dosage under the close observation of the prescribing provider and the nurse.

Nursing Management

A plan of nursing care for a patient with hypothyroidism is available online at http://thepoint.lww.com/Honan2e.

Monitoring Physical Status

The nurse closely monitors the patient's vital signs and cognitive level to detect any deterioration of physical and mental status, signs and symptoms indicating that treatment

TABLE **31-5** Pericardial and Pleural Effusion

Effusion	Description	Assessment Findings
Pericardial effusion	When fluid accumulates in the pericardium, the intrapericardial pressure increases around the heart, causing a cardiac tamponade. As a result, the ventricles are unable to fill properly, leading to a low stroke volume.	Beck triad: When pericardial effusion increases significantly enough to impair cardiac function, a cardiac tamponade develops (the three **D**'s): • **D**istant heart sounds • **D**istention of the jugular veins • **D**ecreased cardiac output
Pleural effusion	Fluid accumulates in the pleural space, causing symptoms of dyspnea, nonproductive cough, and pleuritic chest pain.	The three **D**'s of pleural effusion: • **D**ull to percussion on affected side • **D**ecreased breath sounds on affected side • **D**ecreased respiratory excursion on affected side

has resulted in a metabolic rate exceeding the ability of the cardiovascular and pulmonary systems to respond, and continued limitations or pleural and pericardial effusions (complications of myxedema). The normal levels of pericardial fluid are from 15 to 50 mL and pleural fluid of less than 10 to 20 mL (Porth, 2015). Table 31-5 discusses pleural and pericardial effusions.

Providing Supportive Management

In severe hypothyroidism and myxedema coma, nursing care includes maintaining vital functions, such as managing cardiopulmonary status, hyponatremia, and hypoglycemia (Porth, 2015). Arterial blood gases (ABGs) may be measured to determine retention of carbon dioxide and to guide the use of assisted ventilation to combat hypoventilation. Pulse oximetry also may be helpful in monitoring oxygen saturation levels. The nurse should administer fluids cautiously because of the danger of water intoxication. The patient's blood glucose levels will be monitored closely, especially when on thyroid replacement therapy.

Nursing Alert
Hypoglycemia may be seen with hypothyroidism. The etiology of this finding is associated with a sluggish liver, increasing the patient's susceptibility to low blood sugar. Hyponatremia is associated with approximately 50% of patients with myxedema coma and is thought to be associated with impairment of free water excretion by the kidneys, excess ADH release, or renal impairment (Ross, 2015).

Nursing Alert
If hypoglycemia is evident, concentrated glucose may be prescribed to provide glucose without precipitating fluid overload. Oral antidiabetic agents or insulin may be administered to reduce the effect of hyperglycemia that results from thyroid replacement therapy.

Preventing Medication Interactions

The nurse should take precautions during the course of therapy because of the interaction of thyroid hormones with other medications. Thyroid hormones may increase blood glucose levels, which may necessitate adjustment in the dosage of insulin or oral antidiabetic agents in patients with diabetes. The effects of thyroid hormone may be increased by phenytoin (Dilantin) and by tricyclic antidepressant agents. Thyroid hormones also may increase the pharmacologic effects of digitalis glycosides, anticoagulant agents, and indomethacin, necessitating careful observation and assessment by the nurse for side effects. Also bone loss and osteoporosis may occur with thyroid therapy.

Even in small doses, hypnotic and sedative agents may induce profound somnolence, lasting far longer than anticipated. Furthermore, they are likely to cause respiratory depression, which can easily be fatal because of decreased respiratory reserve and alveolar hypoventilation. If their use is necessary, the dose should be one half or one third of that ordinarily prescribed in patients of similar age and weight with normal thyroid function. If these medications must be used, the patient must be monitored closely for signs of impending narcosis (stupor-like condition) or respiratory failure.

Encouraging Mobility

Encouraging participation in activities within established tolerance can help prevent complications of immobility. The patient with hypothyroidism experiences decreased energy and moderate to severe lethargy. As a result, the risk of complications from immobility increases. The patient's ability to exercise and to participate in activities is further limited by the changes in cardiovascular and pulmonary status that occur secondary to hypothyroidism. The nurse assists the patient with care and hygiene while encouraging the patient to participate within his or her ability.

Promoting Comfort and Safety

The patient often experiences chilling and extreme intolerance to cold, even if the room feels comfortable or hot to others. The nurse provides extra clothing and blankets and protects the patient from drafts. Heating pads and electric blankets should be avoided because of the risk for peripheral vasodilatation, further loss of body heat, and vascular collapse. In addition, the patient is at risk of experiencing burns from these items without being aware of it because of his or her delayed responses and decreased mental status associated with hypothyroidism.

Enhancing Coping Mechanisms

The patient with moderate to severe hypothyroidism may experience severe emotional reactions to changes in appearance and body image and the frequent delay in diagnosis. The nonspecific, early symptoms may have produced negative reactions by family members and friends, who may have labeled the patient mentally unstable, uncooperative, or unwilling to participate in self-care activities. As hypothyroidism is treated successfully and symptoms subside, the patient may experience depression and guilt as a result of the progression and severity of symptoms that occurred. The nurse informs the patient and family that the symptoms and inability to recognize them are common and are part of the disorder itself. The patient and family may require assistance and counseling to deal with the emotional concerns and reactions that result.

HYPERTHYROIDISM

Hyperthyroidism is the second most prevalent endocrine disorder, after DM.

Pathophysiology

Hyperthyroidism occurs as a result of the overproduction of T_3, T_4, or both from the thyroid gland. Oversecretion of thyroid hormones (hyperthyroidism) is manifested by a greatly increased metabolic rate. Other characteristics of hyperthyroidism result from the increased response to circulating catecholamines (epinephrine and norepinephrine). Refer to Box 31-4. Usually oversecretion of thyroid hormones is associated with an enlarged thyroid gland (goiter).

Graves disease is a common cause of hyperthyroidism. It is an autoimmune disease of the thyroid gland that results in the binding of antibodies to TSH, which causes the overproduction of thyroid hormones T_3 and T_4. Women are eight times more likely to be affected with this disease than men, with an onset usually between 20 and 40 years of age (Fitzgerald, 2015). Symptoms may appear after an emotional shock, stress, or an infection, but the exact significance of these relationships is not understood. Other less common causes of hyperthyroidism include thyroiditis (inflammation of the thyroid), overmedication with synthetic thyroid hormone, and thyroid nodules. Symptoms of hyperthyroidism also may occur with the release of excessive amounts of thyroid hormone as a result of inflammation after irradiation of the thyroid or destruction of thyroid tissue by tumor.

Patients with well-developed hyperthyroidism exhibit a typical group of signs and symptoms associated with hypermetabolism (the basal metabolic rate can increase 60% to 100% above normal when in hyperthyroid state where large amounts of T_4 are present [Porth, 2015]). The course of the disease may be mild, characterized by remissions and exacerbations and terminating with spontaneous recovery in a few months or years. When untreated, the disease may progress relentlessly, leading to emaciation, nervousness, delirium, disorientation, and heart failure. The term **thyrotoxicosis** refers to *symptomatic* hyperthyroxinemia. While hyperthyroidism is a type of thyrotoxicosis, they are not the same. Although thyrotoxicosis can be caused by hyperthyroidism, other examples of thyrotoxicosis are associated with inflammation of the thyroid gland or ingestion of thyroid hormone. In these circumstances, there is an increased in either release of stored thyroid hormone or ingestion of exogenous hormone but not accelerated synthesis. Finally, a life-threatening complication of hyperthyroidism, in which profound hypermetabolism involves multiple systems, is called *thyrotoxic crisis* or *thyroid storm*.

Clinical Manifestations and Assessment

Patients with hyperthyroidism often present with symptoms of nervousness. Often these patients are emotionally hyperexcitable, irritable, and apprehensive. They cannot sit quietly. Cardiac complaints may include palpitations. Rapid resting pulse rates typically range between 90 and 160 beats per minute. The systolic blood pressure is elevated; and electrocardiogram (ECG) findings may reveal sinus tachycardia or atrial fibrillation. Patients tolerate heat poorly and perspire unusually freely (hyperhydrosis–excessive sweating). The skin appears flushed and feels warm, soft, and moist. The elderly may report dry skin and diffuse pruritus. A fine tremor of the hands and tongue may be observed. Patients typically exhibit **exophthalmos** (bulging eyes associated with abnormal fluid accumulation behind the eyes), which produces a startled facial expression. Other manifestations include increased dietary intake, progressive weight loss, abnormal muscular fatigability, weakness (e.g., difficulty climbing stairs and rising from a chair), amenorrhea, decreased fertility, and changes in bowel patterns (increased peristalsis). Also osteoporosis and fracture are associated with hyperthyroidism because of increased loss of bone minerals.

On physical assessment, the thyroid gland is enlarged, feels soft, and may pulsate; often a thrill can be palpated, and a bruit is heard over the thyroid arteries. These are signs of increased blood flow through the thyroid gland. If the thyroid becomes hypertrophied, compression may be noted on the trachea or esophagus. Assess for respiratory distress, stridor, or dysphagia. Cardiac effects on the ECG may include sinus tachycardia or arrhythmias. In addition, the physical examination may reveal increased pulse pressure and palpitations. These changes may occur due to the increased sensitivity to

BOX 31-6

Gerontologic Considerations

Hyperthyroidism

Hyperthyroidism is less common in the elderly than hypothyroidism. Patients older than 60 years of age account for 10% to 15% of the cases of hyperthyroidism. Clinical manifestations may be as vague as anorexia and weight loss or isolated atrial fibrillation with an absence of ocular signs, making disorders difficult to detect. New or worsening heart failure or angina is more likely to occur in elderly than in younger patients. Patients also may report other cardiovascular symptoms and difficulty climbing stairs or rising from a chair due to muscle weakness.

Spontaneous remission of hyperthyroidism is rare in the elderly. Assessment of TSH levels are indicated in the elderly who have unexplained physical or mental deterioration. In general, the use of radioactive iodine is recommended for treatment of thyrotoxicosis in the elderly unless an enlarged thyroid gland is pressing on the airway. The hypermetabolic state of thyrotoxicosis must be controlled by antithyroid medications before radioactive iodine is administered because radiation therapy may precipitate thyroid storm by increasing the release of thyroid hormones.

In general, antithyroid medications are not recommended for elderly patients because of the increased incidence of side effects, such as granulocytopenia, and the need for frequent monitoring. The dosage of other medications used to treat other chronic illnesses in elderly patients may need to be modified because of the altered rate of metabolism in hyperthyroidism. In addition, antithyroid medications are considered to be less effective in the treatment of toxic nodular goiter, the most common cause of thyrotoxicosis in the elderly.

Use of beta-adrenergic blocking agents (e.g., propranolol) may be indicated to decrease the cardiovascular and neurologic signs and symptoms of thyrotoxicosis. These agents must be used cautiously in the elderly to minimize adverse effects on cardiac function, such as heart failure.

catecholamines or to changes in neurotransmitter turnover. Myocardial hypertrophy and heart failure may occur if the hyperthyroidism is severe and untreated. Systolic murmurs may be noted. Cardiac decompensation in the form of heart failure is common, especially in the elderly; note the presence of dyspnea, crackles, peripheral edema, jugular vein distention, and the S_3 heart sound. See Box 31-6 for additional gerontologic considerations. Laboratory findings include a decrease in serum TSH (with primary disease), increased T_3 and T_4, and an increase in radioactive iodine uptake.

Medical Management

Appropriate treatment of hyperthyroidism depends on the underlying cause and often consists of a combination of therapies, including radioactive iodine, antithyroid agents, and surgery. Treatment of hyperthyroidism aims to reduce thyroid

hyperactivity, relieve symptoms, and prevent complications. The use of radioactive iodine (^{131}I) is the most common form of treatment for Graves disease due to the small risk of developing thyrotoxic crisis (thyroid storm) that can be minimized with 1 month's dosing of antithyroid drugs before radioiodine treatment (Jameson & Weetman, 2015).

Radioisotope Iodine 131 (^{131}I) Therapy

The goal of radioactive iodine therapy (^{131}I) is to destroy the overactive thyroid cells. Almost all the iodine that enters and is retained in the body becomes concentrated in the thyroid gland. Therefore, the radioactive isotope of iodine becomes concentrated in the thyroid gland, where it destroys thyroid cells without jeopardizing other radiosensitive tissues. Over a period of several weeks, thyroid cells exposed to the radioactive iodine are destroyed, resulting in reduction of the hyperthyroid state and, inevitably, hypothyroidism.

The patient is instructed about what to expect with this tasteless, colorless radioiodine, which may be administered by the radiologist. About 95% of patients are cured by one dose of radioactive iodine. The additional 5% of patients require two doses; rarely is a third dose necessary. Radioactive iodine ablation initially causes an acute release of thyroid hormone from the thyroid gland and may cause an increase of symptoms. The patient is observed for signs of **thyroid storm** (Box 31-7). The use of beta-adrenergic blocking agents, such as propranolol (Inderal), is helpful in controlling these symptoms. Because a higher rate of treatment failure was reported among patients taking Methimazole, it is sometimes discontinued at least 4 days before radioisotope therapy (Fitzgerald, 2015).

After treatment with radioactive iodine, the patient is monitored closely until a **euthyroid** state is reached. Sometimes the symptoms of hyperthyroidism can persist for 2 to 3 months before radioactive iodine takes effect. Close follow-up is required to evaluate thyroid function because the incidence of hypothyroidism after this form of treatment is very high. Approximately 10% to 20% of patients become hypothyroid within the first year of treatment and another 5% of patients each year thereafter (Jameson & Weetman, 2015). Thus, patients are informed of this possibility before treatment and require close follow-up during the first year and annually for thyroid function tests. When necessary, small doses of thyroid hormone replacement are prescribed with gradual increasing doses over a period of months (up to about 1 year) until the free T_4 and TSH levels stabilize within normal ranges.

Radioactive iodine has been used to treat toxic adenomas, multinodular goiter, and most varieties of thyrotoxicosis (rarely with permanent success); it is preferred for treating patients beyond the childbearing years who have diffuse toxic goiter. Radioiodine treatment is contraindicated during pregnancy for fear of fetal irradiation and risk of fetal/neonatal hyperthyroidism from the mother's TSH-receptor

BOX 31-7

Thyroid Storm (Thyrotoxic Crisis, Thyrotoxicosis)

Thyroid storm (thyrotoxic crisis) is a form of severe hyperthyroidism, usually of abrupt onset. It is fatal if left untreated, but with proper treatment, the mortality rate is reduced substantially. The patient with thyroid storm or crisis is critically ill and requires astute observation and aggressive and supportive nursing care during and after the acute stage of illness.

Clinical Manifestations

Thyroid storm is characterized by:
- High fever (hyperpyrexia) above 38.5°C (101.3°F)
- Extreme tachycardia (more than 130 bpm)
- Exaggerated symptoms of hyperthyroidism with disturbances of a major system—e.g., GI (weight loss, diarrhea, abdominal pain) or cardiovascular (edema, chest pain, dyspnea, palpitations)
- Altered neurologic or mental state, which frequently appears as delirium, psychosis, somnolence, or coma

Usually life-threatening thyroid storm is precipitated by stress, such as injury, infection, thyroid and nonthyroidal surgery, tooth extraction, insulin reaction, diabetic ketoacidosis, pregnancy, digitalis intoxication, abrupt withdrawal of antithyroid medications, extreme emotional stress, or vigorous palpation of the thyroid. These factors can precipitate thyroid storm in a patient whose hyperthyroidism is partially controlled or completely untreated. Current methods of diagnosis and treatment for hyperthyroidism have greatly decreased the incidence of thyroid storm, making it uncommon today.

Management

Immediate objectives are reduction of body temperature and heart rate and prevention of vascular collapse. Measures to accomplish these objectives include:
- A hypothermia mattress or blanket, ice packs, a cool environment, hydrocortisone, and acetaminophen (Tylenol). Salicylates (e.g., aspirin) are not used because they displace thyroid hormone from binding proteins and worsen the hypermetabolism.
- Humidified oxygen is administered to improve tissue oxygenation and meet the high metabolic demands. ABG levels or pulse oximetry may be used to monitor respiratory status.
- IV fluids containing dextrose are administered to replace liver glycogen stores that have been decreased in the hyperthyroid patient.
- PTU or methimazole is administered to impede formation of thyroid hormone and block conversion of T_4 to T_3, the more active form of thyroid hormone.
- Hydrocortisone is prescribed to treat shock or adrenal insufficiency.
- Iodine is administered to decrease output of T_4 from the thyroid gland. For cardiac problems, such as atrial fibrillation, arrhythmias, and heart failure, sympatholytic agents may be administered. Propranolol, combined with digitalis, has been effective in reducing severe cardiac symptoms.

---

stimulating antibodies, which increases during radioiodine therapy (Ferri, 2016b). Pregnancy should be postponed for at least 6 months after treatment.

A major advantage of treatment with radioactive iodine is that it avoids many of the side effects associated with antithyroid medications. However, some patients and their families fear medications that are radioactive. For this reason, patients may elect to take antithyroid medications rather than radioactive iodine.

Antithyroid Drug Therapy

Antithyroid medications are summarized in Table 31-6. The objective of pharmacotherapy is to inhibit one or more stages in thyroid hormone synthesis or hormone release. Antithyroid agents block the utilization of iodine by interfering with the iodination of tyrosine and the coupling of iodotyrosines in the synthesis of thyroid hormones. This prevents the synthesis of thyroid hormone. Most commonly, propylthiouracil (PTU) or methimazole (Tapazole) is used until the patient is euthyroid. These medications block the conversion of T_4 to T_3. T_3 is about four times more potent than T_4.

The therapeutic dose is determined on the basis of clinical criteria, including changes in pulse rate, pulse pressure, body weight, size of the goiter, and results of laboratory studies

of thyroid function. Antithyroid medications do not interfere with release or activity of thyroid hormones that were formed previously. As a result, it may take several weeks until relief of symptoms occurs. At that time, the maintenance dose is established, and a gradual withdrawal of the medication over the next several months follows.

Toxic complications of antithyroid medications are relatively uncommon. Nevertheless, the importance of periodic follow-up is emphasized because of medication sensitization, such as fever, rash, urticaria, or even agranulocytosis (a marked decrease in the number of granulocytes) and thrombocytopenia (decreased platelets) may develop. With any sign of infection, especially pharyngitis and fever or the occurrence of mouth ulcers, the patient is advised to notify the provider immediately and undergo hematologic studies. Agranulocytosis, the most serious toxic side effect, occurs in approximately 0.5% of patients. Its incidence is higher in patients older than 40 years of age. It usually occurs within the first 3 months but may occur up to 1 year after therapy is started.

Patients taking antithyroid medications are instructed not to use decongestants for nasal stuffiness because these agents are poorly tolerated. PTU is the treatment of choice during the first trimester of pregnancy, and then Methimazole is administered in the second trimester of pregnancy

TABLE **31-6** Pharmacologic Agents Used to Treat Hyperthyroidism

Agent	Action	Nursing Considerations
Propylthiouracil (PTU)	Blocks synthesis of hormones (conversion of T_4 to T_3)	Monitor cardiac parameters. Observe for conversion to hypothyroidism. Must be given by mouth. Watch for rash, nausea, vomiting, agranulocytosis, lupus syndrome.
Methimazole	Blocks synthesis of thyroid hormone	More toxic than PTU Watch for rash and other symptoms as for PTU.
Sodium iodide	Suppresses release of thyroid hormone	Given 1 hour after PTU or methimazole. Watch for edema, hemorrhage, GI upset.
Potassium iodide	Suppresses release of thyroid hormone	Discontinue for rash. Watch for signs of toxic iodine levels.
Saturated solution of potassium iodide (SSKI)	Suppresses release of thyroid hormone	Mix with juice or milk. Give by straw to prevent staining of teeth.
Dexamethasone	Suppresses release of thyroid hormone	Monitor input and output. Monitor glucose. May cause hypertension, nausea, vomiting, anorexia, infection.
Beta-blocker (e.g., propranolol)	Beta-adrenergic blocking agent	Monitor cardiac status. Hold for patients with bradycardia or decreased cardiac output. Use with caution in patients with heart failure.

Adapted from Morton, P. G., & Fontaine, D. K. (2013). *Essentials of critical care nursing: A holistic approach.* Philadelphia, PA: Wolters Kluwer Health/Lippincott Williams & Wilkins.

(Stagnaro-Green, 2015). As thyroid function improves, the dose is tapered as antithyroid medications in late pregnancy can cause fetal hypothyroidism, fetal bradycardia, goiter, and cretinism as well as maternal side effects, such as rash (5%), purities, hepatitis, lupus-like syndrome, drug fever, and bronchospasm (Mandel & Cooper, 2013).

Another goal of therapy is to reduce the amount of thyroid tissue, with resulting decreased production of thyroid hormone. Occasionally thyroid hormone is administered with antithyroid medications to put the thyroid gland at rest. In this approach, hypothyroidism from excess antithyroid medication is avoided, as is stimulation of the thyroid gland by TSH. Levothyroxine sodium (Synthroid) is the most common thyroid hormone preparation used. It takes approximately 10 days of its administration to achieve full effect. Liothyronine sodium (Cytomel) has a more rapid onset, and its action is of short duration.

Adjunctive Therapy

Iodine or iodide compounds, once the only therapy available for patients with hyperthyroidism, are no longer used as the sole method of treatment. Such compounds decrease the release of thyroid hormones from the thyroid gland and reduce the vascularity and size of the thyroid. Compounds, such as potassium iodide (KI), Lugol's solution, and saturated solution of potassium iodide (SSKI), may be used in combination with antithyroid agents or beta-adrenergic blockers to prepare the patient with hyperthyroidism for surgery. These agents reduce the activity of the thyroid hormone and the vascularity of the thyroid gland, making the surgical procedure safer. Solutions of iodine and iodide compounds are more palatable in milk or fruit juice and are administered through a straw to prevent staining of the teeth. These compounds reduce the metabolic rate more rapidly than antithyroid medications, but their action does not last as long. Beta-adrenergic blocking agents are important in controlling the effects of hyperthyroidism on the sympathetic nervous system. For example, propranolol generally is used to control nervousness, tachycardia, tremor, anxiety, and heat intolerance. The patient continues taking propranolol until the free T_4 is within the normal range and the TSH level approaches normal.

Thyroidectomy

Thyroidectomy, the surgical removal of most of the thyroid gland, was once the primary method of controlling hyperthyroidism (Fig. 31-4). The surgical removal of about five sixths of the thyroid tissue (subtotal thyroidectomy) reliably results in a prolonged remission in most patients with exophthalmic goiter. Presently, the surgical option is reserved only

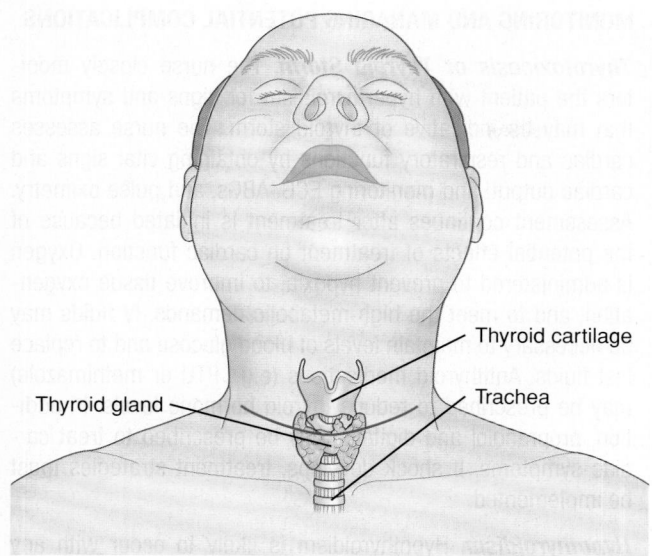

FIGURE 31-4 Thyroidectomy incision.

for special circumstances, such as for patients with nodular goiters with suspicion of malignancy, pregnant women with thyrotoxicosis not controlled with low doses of thioureas, women who desire to become pregnant in the future (Fitzgerald, 2015), and patients who are allergic to or unable to take antithyroid medications. Surgery for the treatment of hyperthyroidism is performed soon after the thyroid function has returned to normal (4 to 6 weeks).

Preoperatively, PTU is administered until signs of hyperthyroidism have disappeared. A beta-adrenergic blocking agent (propranolol) may be used to reduce the heart rate and other signs and symptoms of hyperthyroidism; however, this does not create a euthyroid state. Iodine (Lugol's solution or KI) may be prescribed in an effort to reduce blood loss; however, the effectiveness of this treatment is unknown.

NURSING PROCESS
The Patient with Hyperthyroidism

ASSESSMENT

The patient history assessment focuses on symptoms related to accelerated or exaggerated metabolism. These include reports of irritability, increased emotional reaction, and changes in the patient's interactions with family, friends, and co-workers. Additional symptoms include anxiety, sleep disturbances, apathy, and lethargy. The family can provide useful information about the recent changes in the patient's emotional status.

The history-taking also includes probing for other stressors and the patient's ability to cope with stress. The nurse assesses the nutritional status of the patient by obtaining the typical dietary habits of patient and recording the height and weight of the patient. In addition, the nurse assesses for symptoms related to excessive nervous system output and changes in vision and appearance of the eyes. Periodically, the nurse should assess and monitor the patient's cardiac status, including heart rate, heart sounds, blood pressure, and peripheral pulses.

DIAGNOSIS

Appropriate nursing diagnoses may include:

- Altered nutrition, less than body requirements, related to exaggerated metabolic rate, excessive appetite, and increased gastrointestinal (GI) activity
- Ineffective coping related to irritability, hyperexcitability, apprehension, and emotional instability
- Low self-esteem related to changes in appearance, excessive appetite, and weight loss
- Altered body temperature related to hypermetabolic status
- Discomfort related to eye changes secondary to hyperthyroidism

Potential complications may include the following:

- Thyrotoxicosis or thyroid storm
- Hypothyroidism

PLANNING

The goals for the patient may be improved nutritional status, improved coping ability, improved self-esteem, maintenance of normal body temperature, and absence of complications.

NURSING INTERVENTIONS

IMPROVING NUTRITIONAL STATUS

Hyperthyroidism affects all body systems, including the GI system. The appetite is increased but may be satisfied by several well-balanced meals of small size, up to six meals a day. Foods and fluids are selected to replace fluid lost through diarrhea and diaphoresis and to control the diarrhea that results from increased peristalsis. Rapid movement of food through the GI tract may result in nutritional imbalance and further weight loss. The nurse should monitor fluid and electrolytes to assess for unusual loss due to increased GI motility. To reduce diarrhea, highly seasoned foods and stimulants such as coffee, tea, cola, and alcohol are discouraged. The nurse encourages high-calorie, high-protein foods. A quiet atmosphere during mealtime may aid digestion. The nurse records weight (500 mL = 1 lb), dietary intake, and input/output (I&O) to monitor nutritional status.

ENHANCING COPING MEASURES

The patient with hyperthyroidism needs reassurance that the emotional reactions being experienced are a result of the disorder and that, with effective treatment, those symptoms will be controlled. Because of the negative effect these symptoms have on family and friends, they too need reassurance that the symptoms are expected to disappear with treatment. It is

(continued on page 950)

important to use a calm, unhurried approach with the patient and to minimize stressful experiences. For instance, the patient should not be placed in a room with other patients who are very ill or talkative. The nurse introduces relaxing activities, such as listening to soft music, or keeps the room quiet. The nurse minimizes noises, such as loud music, conversation, and equipment alarms, as much as possible. If thyroidectomy is planned, the patient needs to know that pharmacologic therapy is necessary to prepare the thyroid gland for surgical treatment. The nurse reminds the patient to take the medications as prescribed. Because of hyperexcitability and shortened attention span, the patient may require repetition of this information and written instructions.

IMPROVING SELF-ESTEEM

The patient with hyperthyroidism is likely to experience changes in appearance, appetite, and weight. These factors, along with the patient's inability to cope well with family and the illness, may result in loss of self-esteem. The nurse must convey an understanding of the patient's concern about these problems and assist the patient in developing effective coping strategies. The patient and family need to know that these changes are a result of the thyroid dysfunction and are, in fact, out of the patient's control.

If changes in appearance are very disturbing to the patient, mirrors may be covered or removed. In addition, the nurse reminds family members and personnel to avoid bringing these changes to the patient's attention. The nurse explains to the patient and family that these physical changes are expected to disappear with effective treatment.

MAINTAINING NORMAL BODY TEMPERATURE

It is important for the patient to maintain a normal body temperature. The patient with hyperthyroidism frequently finds a normal room temperature too warm because of an exaggerated metabolic rate and increased heat production. To ensure a normal body temperature, the nurse maintains the environment at a cool, comfortable temperature and changes bedding and clothing as needed. Instructions to the patient and family emphasize that cool baths and cool or cold fluids may provide relief. However, shivering is to be avoided as it increases metabolic energy expenditure. The nurse explains the reason for the patient's discomfort and the importance of providing a cool environment to the family and staff.

PROVIDING EYE CARE

Relief of symptoms related to excessive output by the nervous system and changes in vision and appearance of the eyes is indicated when necessary. For instance, if the patient experiences eye changes secondary to hyperthyroidism, eye care and protection may be necessary. The patient may need instructions about instillation of eye drops or ointment prescribed to soothe the eyes and protect the exposed cornea.

MONITORING AND MANAGING POTENTIAL COMPLICATIONS

Thyrotoxicosis or Thyroid Storm. The nurse closely monitors the patient with hyperthyroidism for signs and symptoms that may be indicative of thyroid storm. The nurse assesses cardiac and respiratory functions by obtaining vital signs and cardiac output, and monitoring ECG, ABGs, and pulse oximetry. Assessment continues after treatment is initiated because of the potential effects of treatment on cardiac function. Oxygen is administered to prevent hypoxia, to improve tissue oxygenation, and to meet the high metabolic demands. IV fluids may be necessary to maintain levels of blood glucose and to replace lost fluids. Antithyroid medications (e.g., PTU or methimazole) may be prescribed to reduce thyroid hormone levels. In addition, propranolol and digitalis may be prescribed to treat cardiac symptoms. If shock develops, treatment strategies must be implemented.

Hypothyroidism. Hypothyroidism is likely to occur with any of the treatments used for hyperthyroidism; periodically monitor the patient for signs and symptoms of hypothyroidism. In addition, as part of the teaching for the patient and family, include instructions on the importance of continuing therapy indefinitely after discharge and a discussion of the consequences of failing to take medication.

EVALUATION

Expected patient outcomes may include the following:
1. Demonstrates improvement in nutritional status:
   a. Reports adequate dietary intake and decreased hunger
   b. Identifies high-calorie, high-protein foods; identifies foods to be avoided
   c. Avoids use of alcohol and other stimulants
   d. Reports decreased episodes of diarrhea
2. Demonstrates effective coping methods in dealing with family, friends, and coworkers:
   a. Explains reasons for irritability and emotional instability
   b. Avoids stressful situations, events, and people
   c. Participates in relaxing, nonstressful activities
3. Achieves increased self-esteem:
   a. Verbalizes feelings about self and illness
   b. Describes feelings of frustration and loss of control
   c. Describes reasons for increased appetite
4. Maintains normal body temperature
5. Experiences relief of symptoms
6. Absence of complications:
   a. Has levels of serum thyroid hormone and TSH within normal limits
   b. Identifies signs and symptoms of thyroid storm and hypothyroidism
   c. Vital signs, ECG, ABGs, and pulse oximetry are within normal limits
   d. States importance of regular follow-up and lifelong maintenance of prescribed therapy

THYROIDITIS

Thyroiditis refers to the inflammation of the thyroid gland that may result in abnormalities in its functioning. The clinical classification of thyroiditis is based on the onset and duration of the disease, resulting from causes that are acute, subacute, or chronic. Thyroiditis can result in the swelling of the thyroid gland, manifesting symptoms in the form of acute and subacute thyroiditis. The chronic form of thyroiditis often presents with painless enlargement of the thyroid gland.

Pathophysiology

Acute thyroiditis is a rare disorder caused by infection of the thyroid gland by bacteria, fungi, mycobacteria, or parasites. The most common cause of acute thyroiditis is *Staphylococcus aureus* and other staphylococci. Chronic thyroiditis occurs frequently in women between 30 and 50 years of age. It has been termed as *Hashimoto disease* or *chronic lymphocytic thyroiditis*. The diagnosis is based on the histologic appearance of the inflamed gland. Cell-mediated immunity may play a significant role in the pathogenesis of chronic thyroiditis, and there may be a genetic predisposition to it. If left untreated, the disease runs a slow, progressive course, eventually leading to hypothyroidism.

Clinical Manifestations and Assessment

In acute thyroiditis, often pharyngitis or pharyngeal pain is present. Physical examination may reveal warmth, erythema (redness), and tenderness over the thyroid gland. The condition manifests as a painful swelling in the anterior neck that lasts between 1 and 2 months and then disappears spontaneously without residual effect. It often follows a respiratory infection. The thyroid enlarges symmetrically and may be painful. The overlying skin is often red and warm. Swallowing may be difficult and uncomfortable. Irritability, nervousness, insomnia, weight loss, chills, fever, and manifestations of hyperthyroidism are common. In contrast to acute thyroiditis, the chronic forms are not accompanied by pain, pressure symptoms, or fever, and thyroid activity is normal or low rather than increased. The most common presentation in a patient suspected to have chronic thyroiditis is a palpable, enlarged, and painless firm mass over the thyroid gland. In addition, patients are likely to present with symptoms of hypothyroidism (Fitzgerald, 2015).

Medical Management

The medical management of acute thyroiditis includes antimicrobial agents and fluid replacement. Surgical incision and drainage may be needed if an abscess is present. In subacute thyroiditis, the treatment aims to control the inflammation. Nonsteroidal anti-inflammatory drugs are commonly used to relieve neck pain. Acetylsalicylic acid (aspirin) is avoided if symptoms of hyperthyroidism occur because aspirin displaces thyroid hormone from its binding sites and increases the amount of circulating hormone. Beta-adrenergic blocking agents (e.g., propranolol) may be used to control symptoms of hyperthyroidism. Antithyroid agents that block the synthesis of T_3 and T_4 are not effective in thyroiditis because the associated thyrotoxicosis results from the release of stored thyroid hormones rather than from their increased synthesis. In more severe cases, oral corticosteroids may be prescribed to reduce swelling and relieve pain. In some cases, temporary hypothyroidism may develop and may necessitate thyroid hormone therapy.

In chronic thyroiditis, the objective of the treatment is to reduce the size of the thyroid gland and prevent hypothyroidism. Thyroid hormone therapy is prescribed to reduce thyroid activity and the production of thyroglobulin. If hypothyroid symptoms are present, thyroid hormone therapy is prescribed. Surgery may be required if pressure symptoms persist.

Nursing Management

The nursing management of patients with thyroiditis includes educating patients about their condition, specifically on pain management and the use of medications. Most patients who present with thyroiditis are given patient education on how to manage the symptoms of the disease and usually do not require in-patient admission.

THYROID TUMOR AND CANCER

Classification of tumors of the thyroid gland includes benign or malignant, presence or absence of associated thyrotoxicosis, and diffuse or irregular quality of the glandular enlargement. A goiter is present if the enlargement is sufficient to cause a visible swelling in the neck. All grades of goiter may occur, from barely visible to those producing disfigurement. The histopathology differs depending on the etiology of goiter. For instance, some are symmetric and diffuse; others are nodular. Often toxic goiters are accompanied by hyperthyroidism. Nontoxic goiters, on the other hand, are associated with a euthyroid (normal) state that does not result from an inflammatory or neoplastic cause.

Thyroid cancer is less prevalent than other forms of cancer; only about 1 in 20 thyroid nodules is cancerous. According to the American Cancer Society, an estimated 62,450 new cases of thyroid cancer are diagnosed each year, 47,230 in women and 15,220 in men. About 1,080 women and 870 men die annually from this malignancy (American Cancer Society, 2015a). Exposure to radiation of the head, neck, or chest in childhood increases the risk for thyroid carcinoma (American Cancer Society, 2015b).

Pathophysiology

The most common type of goiter, a simple or colloid goiter, often is encountered in geographic regions where there is lack of iodine (e.g., the Great Lakes areas of the United States). If too little iodine exists, the level of T_4 will decrease, causing the stimulation of TSH from the anterior pituitary. This stimulation causes the enlargement of the thyroid. Simple goiter also may be caused by an intake of large quantities of goitrogenic substances in patients with unusually susceptible glands. These substances include excessive amounts of iodine or lithium, often used in the treatment of bipolar disorders. Too much iodine can cause enlargement of the thyroid, resulting in the development of excess secretion of thyroid hormone. Keep in mind that many patients receive IV iodine in the hospital as a result of diagnostic studies that require contrast, such as cardiac catheterization and CT scans.

Simple goiter represents a compensatory hypertrophy of the thyroid gland, caused by stimulation by the pituitary gland. Such goiters usually cause no symptoms, except for the swelling in the neck, which may result in tracheal compression when excessive. Many goiters of this type recede after the iodine imbalance is corrected. Supplementary iodine, such as SSKI, is prescribed to suppress the pituitary's thyroid-stimulating activity.

Some thyroid glands are nodular because of areas of hyperplasia (overgrowth). No symptoms may arise unless these nodules increase in size and descend into the thorax, where symptoms of local pressure may manifest. Some nodules become malignant, and some are associated with a hyperthyroid state. The patient with many thyroid nodules eventually may require surgery.

Clinical Manifestations and Assessment

Most patients with simple goiters are asymptomatic and may complain of pressure in the neck. On assessment, the patient may present with a soft, diffusely enlarged nodule over the neck. As the goiter progresses, the patient may experience symptoms, such as difficulty breathing and swallowing. Patients usually present in euthyroid state with normal levels of TSH and T_4.

On the other hand, lesions that are single, hard, and fixed on palpation or associated with cervical lymphadenopathy suggest malignancy. Although thyroid function tests may be helpful in evaluating thyroid nodules and masses, the results are rarely conclusive. Fine-needle biopsy (FNB) of the thyroid gland often is used to establish the diagnosis of thyroid cancer. The purpose of the biopsy is to differentiate cancerous thyroid nodules from noncancerous nodules and to stage the cancer if detected. The procedure is safe and usually requires only a local anesthetic. Another type of aspiration or biopsy uses a large-bore needle rather than the fine needle. This method often is used to detect rapid-growing tumors or when the results of the FNB are inconclusive. Other diagnostic studies include ultrasound, MRI, CT, thyroid scans, radioactive iodine uptake studies, and thyroid suppression tests.

Medical Management

Most patients with small, simple goiters and euthyroid states do not require treatment. Patients with large goiters generally receive exogenous thyroid hormones and iodine to reduce thyroid growth. Surgery is not required unless the goiter continues to grow (1) despite pharmacologic treatment, (2) causing airway difficulties, and (3) leading to suspected malignancy.

Surgical removal, however, is the treatment of choice for thyroid cancers. Total or near-total thyroidectomy is performed if possible. Patients whose thyroid cancer is detected early and who are appropriately treated usually do very well. Patients who have had papillary cancer, the most common and least aggressive tumor, have a 10-year survival rate of 97% (Fitzgerald, 2015). Mortality rates associated with follicular thyroid cancer are less favorable due to more patients presenting with later stages of the disease (Jameson & Weetman, 2015). Hence, continuing thyroid hormone therapy and periodic follow-up with diagnostic testing are important to ensure the patient's well-being.

A modified neck dissection or more extensive radical neck dissection is performed if there is lymph node involvement. Efforts are made to spare parathyroid tissue to reduce the risk of postoperative hypocalcemia with resultant tetany. Ablation procedures are carried out with radioactive iodine to eradicate residual thyroid tissue if the tumor is radiosensitive.

Postoperatively, the patient is instructed to take exogenous thyroid hormone to prevent hypothyroidism. If the remaining thyroid tissue is inadequate to produce sufficient thyroid hormone, thyroxine is required permanently. Free T_4, TSH, and levels of serum calcium and phosphorus are monitored to determine whether the thyroid hormone supplementation is adequate and to note whether calcium balance is maintained. Although local and systemic reactions to radiation may occur and may include neutropenia or thrombocytopenia, these complications are rare when radioactive iodine is used. Patients who undergo surgery that is combined with radioactive iodine have a higher survival rate than do those who undergo surgery alone (Jameson & Weetman, 2015).

Posthospitalization follow-up includes clinical assessment for recurrence of nodules or masses in the neck and signs of hoarseness, dysphagia, or dyspnea. Total-body scans are performed 2 to 4 months after surgery to detect residual thyroid tissue or metastatic disease. Thyroid hormones are stopped for about 6 weeks before the tests. Care must be taken to avoid iodine-containing foods and contrast agents. A repeat scan is performed 1 year after the initial surgery. If measurements are stable, a final scan is obtained in 3 to 5 years.

Nursing Management

Providing Preoperative Teaching

Preoperative patient education is important to gain the patient's confidence and reduce anxiety. The nurse instructs the patient about the importance of eating a diet high in carbohydrates and proteins. A high daily caloric intake is necessary because of the increased metabolic activity and rapid depletion of glycogen reserves. Supplementary vitamins, particularly thiamine and ascorbic acid, may be prescribed. The nurse advises the patient to avoid tea, coffee, cola, and other stimulants. The nurse explains the purpose of preoperative tests and what preoperative preparations to expect. In addition, special efforts are made to ensure a good night's rest before surgery, although many patients are admitted to the hospital on the day of surgery. Preoperative teaching includes demonstrating to the patient how to support the neck with the hands after surgery to prevent stress on the incision. This involves raising the elbows and placing the hands behind the neck to provide support and reduce strain and tension on the neck muscles and the surgical incision.

Assessing the Postoperative Patient

Postoperatively, the nurse periodically assesses the surgical dressings and reinforces them if necessary. The nurse observes the sides and the back of the neck as well as the anterior dressing for bleeding. In addition to monitoring the pulse and blood pressure for any indication of internal bleeding, it is important to be alert for complaints of a sensation of pressure or fullness at the incision site, frequent swallowing, or choking. Such symptoms may indicate subcutaneous hemorrhage and hematoma formation. In addition, the nurse notes vocal changes or hoarseness, as this may indicate injury to the laryngeal nerve or laryngeal edema, which may develop postoperatively. If drains are inserted intraoperatively, the nurse records the color, amount, and consistency of the drainage and maintains function of the device.

Maintaining the Airway

Respiratory difficulties can occur as a result of edema of the glottis, hematoma formation, or injury to the recurrent laryngeal nerve. This complication requires insertion of an airway. It is vital to have a tracheostomy set by the bedside at all times because, in the event of significant edema, placement of an endotracheal tube is unlikely because of narrowing of the airway. If the respiratory distress is caused by hematoma, a surgical evacuation is required.

Managing Pain

The nurse assesses the intensity of pain and administers analgesic agents as prescribed. The nurse should anticipate apprehension in the patient and inform the patient that oxygen will assist breathing. When moving and turning the patient, the nurse must carefully support the patient's head and avoid tension on the sutures. The most comfortable patient position is the semi-Fowler position, with the head elevated and supported by pillows.

Administering Hydration Therapy

IV fluids are administered during the immediate postoperative period. Nurses can anticipate that when PO fluids are allowed, patients report little difficulty in swallowing. Serving small amounts of cold fluids and ice is recommended.

Managing Safety

The nurse advises the patient to talk as little as possible to reduce edema to the vocal cords. Items that are needed frequently are kept within easy reach so the patient does not need to turn the head to reach for them. An overbed table provides easy access to items, such as tissues, a water pitcher and glass, and a small emesis basin. It is also convenient to use this table when vapor-mist inhalations are prescribed for the relief of excessive mucus accumulation.

Encouraging Nutrition and Physical Activity

The patient is permitted to get out of bed as soon as possible but must support his or her neck to reduce strain on the neck muscles. The nurse encourages the patient to eat soft foods. A well-balanced diet high in calories and protein may be prescribed to promote weight gain.

Providing Postoperative Patient Education

Patient teaching emphasizes the importance of taking prescribed medications, discusses postoperative appointment(s), describes suture removal, and provides postoperative recommendations for follow-up. Usually the patient is discharged from the hospital on the day of surgery or soon afterward if the postoperative course is uncomplicated. Also the patient who is undergoing radiation therapy is instructed in how to assess and manage side effects of treatment.

Managing Post-Thyroidectomy Complications

Hemorrhage, hematoma formation, edema of the glottis, and injury to the recurrent laryngeal nerve are complications discussed above. Recall that parathyroid hormone regulates the level of calcium within the blood. Sometimes the parathyroid glands are removed during thyroid surgery, resulting in altered calcium metabolism. As the blood calcium level falls (hypocalcemia), hyperirritability of the nerves occurs, with spasms of the hands and feet and muscle twitching. This group of symptoms is termed *tetany*. Ensure adequate opening of the airway because laryngospasm, although rare, may occur and obstruct the airway. *Usually* tetany is treated with IV calcium gluconate. Hypocalcemia is temporary after thyroidectomy unless all parathyroid tissue was removed.

DISORDERS OF THE PARATHYROID GLANDS

HYPERPARATHYROIDISM

Pathophysiology

Hyperparathyroidism is characterized by having excess parathormone (PTH), leading to a markedly increased level of serum calcium that can present as a potentially life-threatening situation.

Nursing Alert
Hypercalcemia is a total calcium concentration greater than 10.5 mg/dL; hypocalcemia is a total calcium concentration of less than 8.5 mg/dL.

The actions of PTH are increased by the presence of vitamin D. The serum level of ionized calcium regulates the output of parathormone (Fig. 31-5). Increased serum calcium leads to a decreased secretion of parathormone, thus creating a negative feedback system. When the product of serum calcium and serum phosphorus rises, calcium phosphate may precipitate and calcify in various organs of the body, such as the kidneys.

Risk Factors

About 100,000 new cases of hyperparathyroidism are detected each year in the United States. The incidence of this

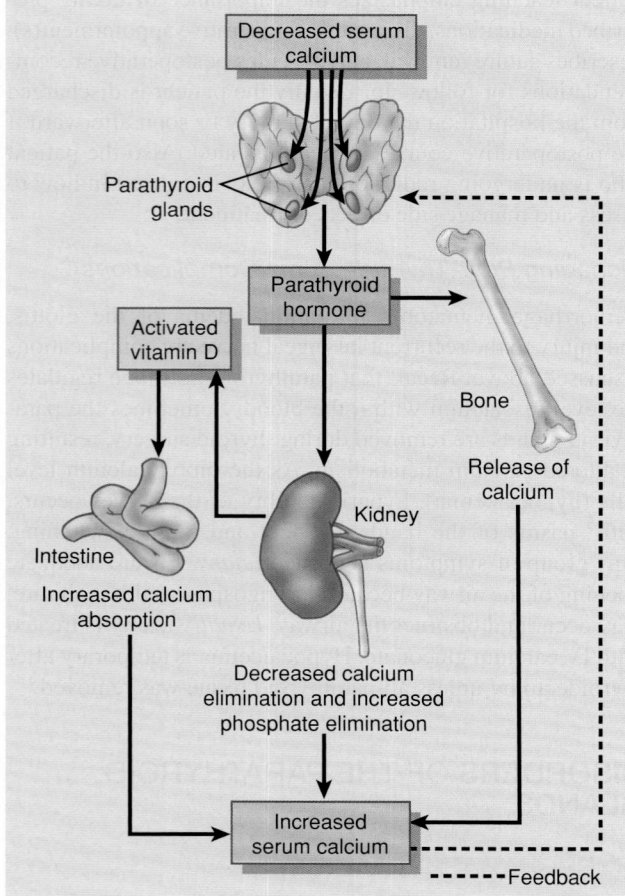

FIGURE 31-5 Regulation of serum calcium concentration by parathyroid hormone. (From Porth, C. M. (2015). *Essentials of pathophysiology: Concepts of altered health states* (4th ed.). Philadelphia, PA: Lippincott Williams & Wilkins.)

Kidney Failure and Secondary Hyperparathyroidism

Phosphate excretion becomes impaired when kidney function deteriorates, resulting in an elevated level of serum phosphate. There is an inverse relationship between calcium and phosphorus: as the level of serum phosphate rises, the level of serum calcium falls.

This hypocalcemia stimulates PTH release with resultant increase in calcium release from the bone. In kidney failure, the kidneys' ability to synthesize vitamin D becomes impaired, which leads to decreased intestinal absorption of calcium. Hypocalcemia in this situation will stimulate the release of PTH, leading to hyperparathyroidism.

---

disorder increases 10-fold between 15 and 65 years of age. Primary hyperparathyroidism (tumor or hyperplasia of the parathyroids) occurs two to four times more often in women than in men and is most common in people between 60 and 70 years of age. Secondary hyperparathyroidism is seen most often in patients with chronic kidney failure (Box 31-8).

Clinical Manifestations and Assessment

Half of the people diagnosed with hyperparathyroidism are asymptomatic. Most cases were detected by high levels of serum calcium during routine blood tests. Secondary hyperparathyroidism manifests signs and symptoms similar to those of primary hyperparathyroidism.

The patient may experience signs and symptoms resulting from involvement of several body systems; Box 31-9 summarizes symptoms of hypercalcemia. Apathy, fatigue, muscle weakness, nausea, vomiting, and constipation may occur due to the increased concentration of calcium in the blood. The direct effect of calcium on the brain and nervous system can cause psychological manifestations, such as irritability, neurosis, or psychoses. Cardiac responses to elevated serum calcium levels include increased cardiac contractility and the development of ventricular arrhythmias. It is important for the nurse to assess patients on digitalis as this drug accentuates the cardiac response of hypercalcemia.

The formation of stones in one or both kidneys, related to the increased urinary excretion of calcium and phosphorus,

---

BOX 31-9 **Focused Assessment**

Hypercalcemia

Be alert for the following signs and symptoms:
- **Stones:** Kidney
- **Bones:** Bone pain, osteoporosis, pathologic fractures
- Abdominal **Moans:** Nausea, vomiting, and abdominal pains (hypercalcemia can lead to development of peptic ulcer and acute pancreatitis)
- Psychic **Groans:** Mental irritability, neurosis, confusion

occurs in 55% of patients with primary hyperparathyroidism. Renal damage results from the precipitation of calcium phosphate in the renal pelvis and parenchyma, which causes renal calculi (kidney stones), obstruction, pyelonephritis, and kidney failure.

Musculoskeletal symptoms accompanying hyperparathyroidism—such as skeleton pain and tenderness, especially of the back and joints, pain on weight bearing, pathologic fractures, deformities, and shortening of body stature—may be caused by demineralization of the bones or by bone tumors composed of benign giant cells, resulting from overgrowth of osteoclasts. Oversecretion of PTH causes excessive osteoclast growth, which, in turn, promotes bone resorption. The resultant loss of calcium from the bone or demineralization causes kyphosis, compression fractures, and bony cysts that produce fragile bones, increasing the risk for fracture. Hypercalcemia may stimulate gastric secretions, causing an increased incidence of peptic ulcer and abdominal pain. Pancreatitis may develop as a result of stones in the pancreatic ducts.

Primary hyperparathyroidism is diagnosed by persistent elevation of serum calcium levels and an elevated concentration of PTH. **Radioimmunoassay** for PTH is sensitive and differentiates primary hyperparathyroidism from other causes of hypercalcemia in more than 90% of patients with elevated serum calcium levels. An elevated serum calcium level alone is a nonspecific finding because serum levels may be altered by diet, medications, and kidney disease and bone changes. Bone changes on x-ray or bone scans indicates advanced disease. The double-antibody parathyroid hormone test distinguishes between primary hyperparathyroidism and malignancy as a cause of hypercalcemia. Ultrasound, MRI, thallium scan, and FNB evaluate the parathyroid functions and localize parathyroid cysts, adenomas, or hyperplasia.

Medical and Nursing Management

The recommended treatment of primary hyperparathyroidism is the surgical removal of abnormal parathyroid tissue (parathyroidectomy). In some patients who are without symptoms and have serum calcium concentrations that are only mildly elevated and normal kidney function, surgery may be delayed, and the patient is monitored closely for worsening of hypercalcemia, bone deterioration, renal impairment, or the development of kidney stones. Nursing management involves providing hydration, encouraging mobility, administering nutrition and medications, providing emotional support, and observing for and managing hypercalcemic crisis.

Providing Hydration Therapy

Patients with hyperparathyroidism are at risk for renal calculi because kidney involvement is possible. Strict intake and output measurements are monitored in hospitalized patients. The nurse encourages a daily fluid intake of 2,000 mL

or more (unless contraindicated) to help prevent calculus formation. Cranberry juice or cranberry extract tablets are suggested as alternatives because it may lower the urinary pH. The nurse instructs the patient to report symptoms of renal calculi, such as abdominal pain and hematuria. Thiazide diuretics are avoided because they decrease the renal excretion of calcium and further elevate levels of serum calcium. Because of the risk for hypercalcemic crisis, the nurse should instruct the patient to avoid dehydration and to seek immediate attention if conditions that commonly produce dehydration (e.g., vomiting and diarrhea) occur.

Encouraging Mobility

The nurse encourages the patient to ambulate using a walker. For those with limited mobility, use a rocking chair because bones that are subjected to normal stress give up less calcium. Bedrest increases calcium excretion and the risk for renal calculi. Oral phosphates lower the serum calcium level in some patients; however, long-term use is not recommended due to the risk of ectopic calcium phosphate deposition into the soft tissues.

Administering Nutrition and Medication

Dietary calcium will be restricted or increased depending on the patient's serum calcium level. If the patient has a coexisting peptic ulcer, prescribed antacids and protein feedings are necessary. Measures to prevent constipation (a common occurrence postoperatively) include offering prune juice or stool softeners (e.g., Colace or Senna) and increasing physical activity and fluid intake.

Providing Emotional Support

The insidious and chronic onset of hyperparathyroidism together with diverse and vague symptoms may lead to depression and frustration. The family may have considered the patient's illness to be psychosomatic. Increasing awareness of the course of the disorder with patient education may help the patient and family deal with their reactions and feelings.

Managing Hypercalcemic Crisis

Acute hypercalcemic crisis can occur with extreme elevation of serum calcium levels. Serum calcium levels of greater than 15 mg/dL (3.7 mmol/L) result in neurologic, cardiovascular, and renal symptoms that can be life-threatening. Treatment involves rehydration with large volumes of IV fluids to keep urine output above 100 mL/hr (normal saline expands volume and inhibits calcium resorption), diuretic agents (to promote renal excretion of excess calcium), and phosphate therapy (to correct hypophosphatemia and decrease serum calcium levels by promoting calcium deposition in bone and reducing the GI absorption of calcium). Cytotoxic agents (e.g., mithramycin), calcitonin, and dialysis may be used in emergency situations to decrease serum calcium levels quickly. Effective results occur within 24 hours but last only about 1 to 2 weeks. A combination of calcitonin and corticosteroids has been administered in emergencies to reduce the serum calcium level by increasing calcium deposition in bone. Other agents that may be administered to decrease serum calcium levels include bisphosphonates (e.g., etidronate [Didronel], pamidronate [Aredia]). Refer to Chapter 6 for more details on hypercalcemia.

Careful assessment and care are required to minimize complications and reverse the life-threatening hypercalcemia. Particular attention to cardiac function is advised since often death from hypercalcemic crisis is caused by cardiac arrest (Porth, 2015). Medications are administered with care, and attention is given to fluid and electrolyte balance. Supportive measures are necessary for the patient and family.

HYPOPARATHYROIDISM

Pathophysiology

Hypoparathyroidism results from hyposecretion of the parathyroid glands, leading to low levels of PTH that eventually results in hypocalcemia and hyperphosphatemia. In the absence of PTH, there is increased blood phosphate (hyperphosphatemia) and a resultant decreased level of blood calcium (hypocalcemia) due to the inverse relationship between serum phosphorus and calcium described in Box 31-8. Without PTH, there is also decreased intestinal absorption of dietary calcium as well as decreased resorption of calcium from bone and through the renal tubules, causing hypocalcemia.

The most common cause of hypoparathyroidism is from surgical removal of parathyroid gland tissue during thyroidectomy, parathyroidectomy, or radical neck dissection. These small glands are easily overlooked and can be removed inadvertently during thyroid surgery.

Hypoparathyroidism also may occur in patients who have undergone a subtotal resection or total parathyroidectomy with parathyroid autotransplantation. Other risk factors include genetic predisposition, exposure to radiation, and magnesium depletion (hypomagnesemia: less than 0.4 mmol/L; less than 0.8 mEq/L) (Jameson & Weetman, 2015).

Clinical Manifestations and Assessment

Hypocalcemia causes irritability of the neuromuscular system and contributes to the chief symptom of hypoparathyroidism, tetany. Tetany is a general muscle hypertonia, with tremor and spasmodic or uncoordinated contractions occurring with or without efforts to make voluntary movements. Symptoms of latent tetany are numbness, tingling, and cramps in the extremities, and the patient complains of stiffness in the hands and feet. In overt tetany, the signs include

FIGURE 31-6 Tetany is caused by tonic spasm of the intrinsic hand muscles. Evaluate the patient for Trousseau sign (**A**) or Chvostek sign (**B**).

bronchospasm, laryngeal spasm, carpopedal spasm (flexion of the elbows and wrists and extension of the carpophalangeal joints and dorsiflexion of the feet), dysphagia, photophobia, cardiac arrhythmias, and seizures. Other symptoms include anxiety, irritability, depression, and even delirium. ECG changes, such as prolonged QT intervals, and hypotension also may occur.

A positive **Trousseau sign** or a positive **Chvostek sign** on physical assessment suggests latent tetany (Fig. 31-6). Trousseau sign is positive when carpopedal spasm is induced by occluding the blood flow to the arm for 3 minutes with a blood pressure cuff. Chvostek sign is positive when a sharp tapping over the facial nerve just in front of the parotid gland and anterior to the ear causes spasm or twitching of the mouth, nose, and eye.

The diagnosis of hypoparathyroidism often is difficult because of the vague symptoms, such as aches and pains. Therefore, laboratory studies are especially helpful. Tetany develops at serum calcium levels of 5 to 6 mg/dL (1.2 to 1.5 mmol/L) or lower. Serum phosphate levels are increased, and x-rays of bone show increased density. Calcification is detected on x-rays of the subcutaneous or paraspinal basal ganglia of the brain.

Medical Management

The goal is to increase the serum calcium level to 8 to 9 mg/dL (2.0 to 2.25 mmol/L) and to eliminate the symptoms of hypoparathyroidism and hypocalcemia. When hypocalcemia and tetany occur after a thyroidectomy, the immediate treatment is administration of IV 10% calcium gluconate. If this does not decrease neuromuscular irritability and seizure activity immediately, sedative agents, such as pentobarbital, may be administered. Parenteral PTH can be administered to treat acute hypoparathyroidism with tetany. The patient receiving PTH is monitored closely for allergic reactions and changes in serum calcium levels.

Treatment for chronic hypoparathyroidism is determined after serum calcium levels are obtained. A diet high in calcium and low in phosphorus is prescribed (Box 31-10). Oral calcium salts, such as calcium gluconate, may be used

BOX 31-10 Nutrition Alert

Hypoparathyroidism

Patients with hypoparathyroidism are prescribed a diet high in calcium and low in phosphorus. The following foods are recommended:

- Rice milk or nondairy creamer
- Refined white bread
- Green beans, broccoli, cucumbers
- Fish

The following foods are restricted:

- Egg yolks
- Milk and milk products (although high in calcium, these are restricted because they also contain high levels of phosphorus)
- Spinach (contains oxalate that forms insoluble calcium substances)

to supplement the diet. Aluminum hydroxide gel or aluminum carbonate (Gelusil, Amphojel) may be used after meals to bind phosphate and promote its excretion through the GI tract. Other variable dosages of a vitamin D preparation—dihydrotachysterol (AT 10 or Hytakerol), ergocalciferol (vitamin D), or cholecalciferol (vitamin D)—are usually required and enhance calcium absorption from the GI tract.

If the patient develops respiratory distress resulting from neuromuscular irritability, the patient may require tracheostomy or mechanical ventilation along with bronchodilating medications.

Nursing Management

Nursing management of the patient with acute hypoparathyroidism includes the care of patients who have undergone thyroidectomy, parathyroidectomy, or radical neck dissection. Care is directed toward detecting early signs of hypocalcemia and anticipating signs of tetany, seizures, and respiratory difficulties. To anticipate emergencies, calcium gluconate should be kept at the bedside in a locked container or in a place where it is readily available along with equipment necessary for IV administration. Calcium gluconate is administered slowly in patients who have a current cardiac disorder, such as arrhythmias, and in patients who are currently receiving digitalis.

The patient requires continuous cardiac monitoring and careful assessment because calcium and digitalis increase systolic contraction and also potentiate each other, which can produce potentially fatal arrhythmias.

Patient education about medications and diet therapy is essential. The patient needs to know the reason for high calcium and low phosphate intake and the symptoms of hypocalcemia and hypercalcemia. In addition, the nurse teaches the patient to contact the primary care provider if these symptoms occur.

DISORDERS OF THE ADRENAL GLANDS

PHEOCHROMOCYTOMA

Pheochromocytoma is a rare disease, found in two to four new cases per million annually (Fitzgerald, 2015). Although around 0.1% of patients with high blood pressure have this tumor, it can cause severe hypertensive crisis (Neumann, 2015).

Pathophysiology

Pheochromocytoma begins with benign growth of a tumor inside the adrenal medulla and usually secretes epinephrine and norepinephrine (Fitzgerald, 2015). In 90% of patients, the tumor arises in the medulla but can arise in other extra-adrenal chromaffin tissue located in or near the aorta, ovaries, spleen, or other organs. This clinical syndrome is characterized by a massive release of catecholamines that causes severe hypertension. The release may be paroxysmal rather than continuous, causing intermittent episodes of headaches, tremor, nervousness, and marked variability in blood pressure (Porth, 2015).

Risk Factors

Around 30% of patients with pheochromocytoma have a positive family history that makes them prone to developing the tumor (Fitzgerald, 2015). In most cases, 10% of the tumors are bilateral, and 10% are malignant. Although rare, there has been evidence that multiple endocrine neoplasia type 2 (MEN-2) may predispose one to having pheochromocytoma (Neumann, 2015). MEN type 2 is a rare inherited disease that leads to overactivity and enlargement of the endocrine glands (e.g., overproduction of adrenaline in the adrenal glands). Because of the risk of pheochromocytoma in family members of affected people, the patient's family members should be alerted and examined for pheochromocytoma.

Clinical Manifestations and Assessment

The nature and severity of symptoms of functioning tumors of the adrenal medulla depend on the relative proportions of epinephrine and norepinephrine secretion (Table 31-7). Typical presentation of a patient with pheochromocytoma includes the five **H**'s:

- **H**ypertension (severe),
- **H**eadache,
- **H**yperhydrosis (excessive sweating),
- **H**ypermetabolism, and
- **H**yperglycemia (conversion of liver and muscle glycogen to glucose due to epinephrine secretion).

Other symptoms may include tremor, flushing, and anxiety. Approximately 8% of patients are completely asymptomatic.

TABLE **31-7** Laboratory Tests for Epinephrine and Norepinephrine

Test	Normal Values	Critical Values	Nursing Implications
Plasma level of epinephrine Plasma level of norepinephrine	100 pg/mL (590 pmol/L) Less than 100–550 pg/mL (590–3,240 pmol/L)	Greater than 400 pg/mL (2,180 pmol/L) diagnostic of pheochromocytoma Greater than 2,000 pg/mL (11,800 pmol/L) diagnostic of pheochromocytoma	The nurse should ensure that patients should not be on epinephrine drugs, such as nose drops and cough mixtures, and norepinephrine drugs, such as Levophed, because these drugs may lead to false increases in levels of plasma epinephrine and norepinephrine. In addition, the patient's blood should be drawn in a nonstressful environment.

Paroxysmal symptoms of pheochromocytoma usually develop in the fifth decade of life.

Typically, pheochromocytoma is characterized by acute, unpredictable attacks lasting seconds or several hours. The attacks can be triggered by events, such as use of intravenous contrast dyes or glucagon injection, needle biopsy of the mass, anesthesia, or surgical procedures, exercise, bending, lifting, emotional stress, and drugs (e.g., MAO inhibitors, caffeine, nicotine, decongestions, and amphetamines) (Fitzgerald, 2015). Symptoms usually begin abruptly and subside slowly. During these attacks, the patient is extremely anxious, tremulous, and weak. The patient may experience headache, vertigo, blurring of vision, tinnitus, air hunger, and dyspnea. Other symptoms include polyuria, nausea, vomiting, diarrhea, abdominal pain, and a feeling of impending doom. Headache is the most common symptom and can be quite severe (Porth, 2015). Blood pressures exceeding 250/150 mm Hg have been recorded. Such elevations in blood pressure are life-threatening and can cause severe complications, such as cardiac arrhythmias, dissecting aneurysm, stroke, and acute kidney failure. Postural hypotension (decrease in systolic blood pressure, lightheadedness, dizziness on standing) occurs in 70% of patients with untreated pheochromocytoma.

Diagnostic measurements of urine and plasma levels of catecholamine and their metabolites (metanephrine [MN], vanillylmandelic acid [VMA]) are the most direct and conclusive tests for overactivity of the adrenal medulla. CT and MRI studies detect tumors and possible metastases. A negative test result for catecholamines virtually excludes pheochromocytoma; however, increased levels of at least one catecholamine or MN can occur in 10% of patients with essential hypertension. In most cases, pheochromocytoma can be diagnosed or confirmed based on a properly collected 24-hour urine sample of free catecholamine, MN, and VMA; levels as high as twice the normal level may be found. The use of combined serum and urine tests increases the diagnostic accuracy of testing. A number of medications and foods, such as coffee and tea (including decaffeinated varieties), bananas, chocolate, vanilla, and aspirin, may alter the results of these tests. Therefore, the patient must be given instructions to avoid such items.

The total concentration of plasma catecholamine (epinephrine and norepinephrine) is measured with the patient supine and at rest for 30 minutes. To prevent elevation of catecholamine levels resulting from the stress of venipuncture, a butterfly needle, scalp vein needle, or venous catheter may be inserted 30 minutes before the blood specimen is obtained. Factors that may elevate catecholamine concentrations must be controlled to obtain valid results; these factors include the dietary items noted earlier, use of tobacco, emotional and physical stress, and use of many prescription and over-the-counter medications (e.g., amphetamines, nose drops or sprays, decongestant agents, bronchodilators).

Medical Management

Although uncommon, other conditions may be associated with this tumor, including cardiac complications, hypotension, shock, and sudden death. Once pheochromocytoma is diagnosed, the main goal of surgical treatment is the removal of primary tumors and, if possible, the resection of local and distant metastases (Parenti et al., 2012). A laparoscopic removal of the tumor is often the treatment of choice, but open laparotomy is required if tumors are large and invasive in nature (Fitzgerald, 2015).

The patient will be admitted to the intensive care unit for close monitoring (especially ECG) and careful administration of alpha-adrenergic blocking agents (e.g., phentolamine [Regitine]) or smooth muscle relaxants (e.g., sodium nitroprusside [Nipride]) to lower the blood pressure quickly. Phenoxybenzamine (Dibenzyline), a long-acting alpha blocker, may be used after the blood pressure is stable to prepare the patient for surgery. Calcium-channel blockers, such as nifedipine (Procardia) usually are well tolerated by patients and have reduced requirements for perioperative fluids. Although the use of calcium-channel blockers in the management of patients with catecholamine-secreting tumors does not prevent hemodynamic changes, their use was found to be associated with low morbidity and mortality (Lebuffe et al., 2005). However, using calcium-channel blockers alone is not recommended unless patients have very mild preoperative hypertension or have severe orthostatic hypotension (Lenders et al., 2014). Usually calcium-channel blockers are co-administered with alpha-adrenergic blocking agents. Beta-adrenergic blocking agents, such as propranolol (Inderal), may be used in patients with cardiac arrhythmias and in those not responsive to alpha blockers. Alpha-adrenergic and beta-adrenergic blocking agents must be used with caution because patients with pheochromocytoma may have increased sensitivity to them. Catecholamine synthesis inhibitors, such as alpha-methyl-*p*-tyrosine (metyrosine), also may be used preoperatively if adrenergic blocking agents do not reduce the effects of catecholamines. Insulin may be required to maintain normal serum glucose levels.

Nursing Management

The nursing management of the patient includes close monitoring of the patient's vital signs (especially heart rate and blood pressure) for several days in the intensive care unit. Most importantly, the nurse monitors the patient closely for excessive rapid decrease in blood pressure that may cause underperfusion to the vital organs (e.g., brain and kidneys). Other management includes monitoring of patient's mental status, acute ECG changes, arterial pressures, fluid and electrolyte balance, and blood glucose levels. Several IV lines are inserted for administration of fluids and medications. Despite large doses of medications used to lower the blood pressure, some patients may continue to be hypertensive. This is due to the effect of poor elasticity of the damaged blood vessels from chronic hypertension.

During the phases of care, the nurse informs the patient about the importance of follow-up monitoring to ensure that pheochromocytoma does not recur undetected. For instance, due to the risk for recurrence of hypertension, periodic checkups are required, especially in young patients and in those whose families have a history of pheochromocytoma. The patient is scheduled for periodic follow-up appointments to observe for return of normal blood pressure and plasma and urine levels of catecholamines.

ADDISON DISEASE

Addison disease, or primary adrenocortical insufficiency, occurs when adrenal cortex function is inadequate to meet the patient's need for cortical hormones. The three adrenal corticosteroids are glucocorticoids (primarily cortisol, which decreases inflammatory reaction, decreases WBC migration to inflamed area, increases fat metabolism, and raises serum glucose), mineralocorticoids (primarily aldosterone, which causes sodium reabsorption and, with it, water, along with renal excretion of potassium), and androgens (sex hormones).

Pathophysiology

A primary adrenal insufficiency originates in the adrenal glands themselves and is likely associated with autoimmune or idiopathic atrophy of the adrenal cortex when cell-mediated immune mechanisms result in decreased production of adrenocortical hormones (e.g. cortisol and aldosterone). While primary adrenal insufficiency is an uncommon disorder, autoimmunity is responsible for about 80% of spontaneous cases

in the United States (Fitzgerald, 2015). In contrast, secondary adrenal insufficiency can be due to either a lack of pituitary ACTH secretion, or Hypothalamic corticotropin-releasing hormone (CRH) dysfunction. This causes a resultant decrease production of cortisol but not aldosterone. ACTH only minimally influences aldosterone secretion, as it is secreted primarily in response to the presence of angiotensin II in the bloodstream.

Risk Factors

The risk factors for Addison disease include surgical removal of both adrenal glands and infection of the adrenal glands. Tuberculosis, cytomegalovirus, and bacterial infections (such as Neisseria meningitidis) are common infections that destroy adrenal gland tissue (National Institute of Diabetes and Digestive and Kidney Disease [NIDDK], 2014). Although autoimmune destruction has replaced tuberculosis as the principal cause of Addison disease, tuberculosis should be considered in the diagnostic workup because of its increasing incidence. Inadequate secretion of ACTH from the pituitary gland results in secondary adrenal insufficiency because of decreased stimulation of the adrenal cortex. Symptoms of adrenocortical insufficiency also may result from the sudden cessation of exogenous adrenocortical hormonal therapy, which suppresses the body's normal response to stress and interferes with normal feedback mechanisms. Hence, corticosteroids should never be stopped abruptly. Daily administration of corticosteroids has the potential to suppress function of the adrenal cortex. It has been shown that a patient who is acutely ill receiving more than 30 mg/day of hydrocortisone, 7.5 mg/day of prednisolone, or 0.75 mg/day of dexamethasone for more than 3 weeks can experience suppression of adrenal cortex function (Cooper & Stewart, 2003).

Clinical Manifestations and Assessment

Addison disease is characterized by muscle weakness, anorexia, GI symptoms, fatigue, emaciation, skin pigmentation changes (Box 31-11), and hypotension as well as low blood glucose, low serum sodium, and high serum potassium levels. Depression, emotional lability, apathy, and confusion are present in 60% to 80% of patients. With decreased glucocorticoids, mineralocorticoids, and androgens, there is a stimulation of the anterior pituitary to increase ACTH. This releases the melanocyte hormone, which results in a bronze-pigmented rash (Fig. 31-7). Figure 31-7 details the clinical manifestations of Addison disease and diagram specifies the relationship of signs and symptoms to specific hormone deficiency.

In severe cases, the disturbance of the metabolism of sodium and potassium may be marked by depletion of sodium and water and severe chronic dehydration. **Addisonian crisis** is an acute life-threatening event that develops with disease progression. Acute hypotension is characterized

Focused Assessment

Skin Changes in Addison Disease

Be alert for the following signs and symptoms:

- Skin pigmentation changes of bronzed or suntanned appearance (seen in primary Addison disease because the persistently low levels of cortisol cause hypersecretion of ACTH from the pituitary gland; increased melanin synthesis is associated with an increase in ACTH, thus hyperpigmentation occurs)
- Increased pigmentation at skin creases, pressure points (knuckles, elbows, knees) and buccal mucosa

by cyanosis and the classic signs of circulatory shock: pallor, apprehension, rapid and weak pulse, rapid respirations, and low blood pressure. In addition, the patient may complain of headache, nausea, abdominal pain, and diarrhea and may show signs of confusion and restlessness. Even slight overexertion, exposure to cold, acute infection, or a decrease in salt intake may lead to circulatory collapse, shock, and death if untreated. The stress of surgery or dehydration resulting from preparation for diagnostic tests may precipitate an addisonian or hypotensive crisis.

Symptoms of secondary adrenal insufficiency are the same as those for primary adrenal insufficiency with a few exceptions, most notably the lack of hyperpigmentation, as

FIGURE 31-7 (**A**) Clinical manifestations of Addison disease. (From Porth, C. M. (2015). *Essentials of pathophysiology: Concepts of altered health states* (4th ed.). Philadelphia, PA: Lippincott Williams & Wilkins.) (**B**) Chart detailing the signs and symptoms of Addison disease and relationship to specific hormone deficiencies. (Reprinted with permission from Diepenbrock, N. H. (2015). *Quick reference to critical care* (5th ed.). Philadelphia, PA: Lippincott Williams & Wilkins.)

ACTH secretion is not increased. In addition, symptoms are due to glucocorticoid rather than mineralocorticoid deficiency. Therefore, signs of hypoglycemia are present, while signs of hyperkalemia are not because of the continued presence of aldosterone.

The diagnosis is confirmed by laboratory test results. Combined measurements of early-morning serum cortisol and plasma ACTH are performed to differentiate patients with primary adrenal insufficiency from those with secondary adrenal insufficiency.

Patients with primary insufficiency have a plasma ACTH level that is greatly increased (over 22.0 pmol/L) and a serum cortisol concentration lower than the normal range (less than 165 nmol/L) or in the low-normal range. Other laboratory findings include decreased levels of blood glucose (hypoglycemia) and sodium (hyponatremia), an increased concentration of serum potassium (hyperkalemia), and an increased WBC count (leukocytosis). If the adrenal cortex is destroyed, baseline cortisol values become low, and ACTH administration fails to cause the normal increase in plasma cortisol and urinary 17-hydroxycorticosteroids. Secondary adrenal insufficiency is characterized by low pituitary dysfunction. The adrenal gland is a healthy, but it is not being stimulated properly by the pituitary. In this situation, low levels of adrenocortical hormones in the blood or urine and decreased serum cortisol levels are seen. A normal response to repeated doses of exogenous ACTH is seen (adrenal gland is normal), but no response occurs after the administration of metyrapone, which stimulates endogenous ACTH.

Medical Management

Immediate treatment is directed toward combating circulatory shock: restoring blood circulation, administering fluids and corticosteroids, monitoring vital signs, and placing the patient in a recumbent position with the legs elevated. Corticosteroid use is discussed in Box 31-12 and Table 31-8. Hydrocortisone (Solu-Cortef) is administered intravenously, followed by 5% dextrose in normal saline. Oral hydrocortisone replacement is resumed once intravenous infusion is discontinued. Vasopressor amines may be required if hypotension persists. Broad-spectrum antibiotics may be administered if infection has precipitated adrenal crisis in a patient with chronic adrenal insufficiency. In addition, the patient is assessed closely to identify other factors, stressors, or illnesses that led to the acute episode.

Nursing Management

Restoring Fluid Status

Along with dietitian referral, the nurse encourages the patient to consume foods and fluids that assist in restoring and maintaining fluid and electrolyte balance and teaches the patient to select foods that are high in sodium during GI disturbances and in very hot weather. The nurse instructs the patient and family to administer hormone replacement as prescribed and to modify the dosage during illness and other stressful situations. Written and verbal instructions are provided about the administration of mineralocorticoid (Florinef) or corticosteroid (prednisone).

Prior to fluid replacement therapy, the nurse monitors the patient for any signs and symptoms of fluid imbalances by monitoring the blood pressure and pulse rate as the patient moves from a lying to a standing position. A decrease in systolic pressure (20 mm Hg or more) indicates fluid volume deficit, as evidenced by the patient's narrowed pulse pressure, delayed capillary filling, and flat neck veins. The nurse monitors the patient for manifestations of hypovolemic shock: hypotension, rapid weak pulse, rapid respiratory rate, pallor, and extreme weakness. Other key considerations include checking for weight loss, measuring intake and output, assessing for muscle weakness and fatigue, and investigating any illness or stress that may have precipitated the acute crisis.

Reducing Stress

Until the patient's condition is stabilized, unnecessary activity and stress that could precipitate another hypotensive episode are avoided. The nurse assesses for signs of infection or the presence of other stressors. Even minor events or stressors may be excessive in patients with adrenal insufficiency. During the acute crisis, the nurse maintains a quiet, nonstressful environment and performs all activities (e.g., bathing, turning) for the patient. Maintaining communication and explaining all procedures to the patient and family can help reduce their anxiety. During stressful procedures or significant illnesses, additional supplementary therapy or higher doses of glucocorticoids are required to prevent an addisonian crisis.

Maintaining Self-Care

Because of the need for lifelong replacement of adrenal cortex hormones to prevent addisonian crises, the patient and family members receive explicit verbal and written instructions about the rationale for replacement therapy and proper dosage. In addition, they learn about how to modify the medication dosage and increase salt intake in times of illness, very hot weather, and other stressful situations. The patient also learns how to modify diet and fluid intake to help maintain fluid and electrolyte balance.

The patient and family are prescribed preloaded, single-injection syringes of corticosteroid for use in emergencies. Specific instructions on how and when to use the injection also are provided. It is important to instruct the patient to inform other health care providers, such as dentists, about the use of corticosteroids, to wear a medical alert bracelet, and to carry information at all times about the need for corticosteroids. The patient and family need to know the

BOX 31-12 **Using Corticosteroids in the Treatment of Adrenal Disease**

Synthetic corticosteroids are administered for a variety of clinical conditions, including adrenal insufficiency, suppressing inflammation and autoimmune reactions, controlling allergic reactions, and reducing the rejection process in transplantation. Choices for corticosteroids include: prednisone, methylprednisolone, and dexamethasone which are all synthetic compositions of cortisol (hydrocortisone). The dosage of corticosteroids is determined by the nature and chronicity of the illness as well as the patient's other medical conditions. Side effects include the development of diabetes mellitus, osteoporosis, peptic ulcer, increased protein breakdown resulting in muscle wasting and poor wound healing, and redistribution of body fat. Therefore, the adverse effects of corticosteroids must be weighed against the benefits to the patient's current condition.

Depending on the severity of disease, corticosteroids may be used for a period of time and gradually reduced or tapered as the symptoms subside so as to avoid undesirable effects, such as adrenal suppression. Traditionally, adrenal suppression was anticipated in individuals who received more than 30 mg of hydrocortisone or its equipotent dosage of 7.5 mg of prednisolone per day (the average daily equivalent output of the adrenal glands) for more than 3 weeks. However, this practice has been questioned since doses of exogenous glucocorticoids do not correlate directly with endogenous production.

Once the primary disorder is resolved, corticosteroid dosages are tapered to allow the return of normal adrenal function and to prevent steroid-induced adrenal insufficiency. However, up to 1 year or longer after use of corticosteroids, the patient still may be at risk for adrenal insufficiency in times of stress. If surgery is necessary, the patient is likely to require IV corticosteroids during and after surgery to reduce the risk for acute adrenal crisis. The nurse plays an important role in providing education about the dosage, taper schedule, and side effects of corticosteroids. Table 31-7 provides an overview of the effects of corticosteroid therapy and their nursing implications.

In keeping with the natural secretion of cortisol, the best time of day for the total corticosteroid dose is in the early morning, between 7 and 8 AM. The half-life of synthetic steroids is approximately 8 hours. Therefore, if a large-dose therapy is administered at 8 AM (when the adrenal gland is most active), maximal suppression of the adrenal gland occurs. The adrenal suppressive effect can last for 12 to 24 hours. If symptoms of the disorder being treated are suppressed, alternate-day therapy may be helpful in reducing pituitary–adrenal suppression in patients requiring prolonged therapy. Since large amounts of glucocorticoids administered exogenously in the blood inhibit the release of ACTH and endogenous glucocorticoids, atrophy of the adrenal cortex can develop with long-term use. If exogenous glucocorticoid administration is discontinued suddenly, adrenal insufficiency can occur due to the inability of the atrophied cortex to respond adequately.

Although the synthetic corticosteroids are safe for some patients because of relative freedom from mineralocorticoid activity, most natural and synthetic corticosteroids produce similar kinds of side effects. Mineralocorticoids have major effects on electrolyte metabolism, acting principally on the renal tubular and GI epithelium to cause increased absorption of sodium ions in exchange for excretion of potassium or hydrogen ions. ACTH only minimally influences aldosterone secretion. It is primarily secreted in response to the presence of angiotensin II in the bloodstream. Angiotensin II is a substance that elevates the blood pressure by constricting arterioles. Its concentration is increased when renin is released from the kidney in response to decreased perfusion pressure. The resultant increased levels of aldosterone promote sodium reabsorption by the kidney and the GI tract, which tends to restore blood pressure to normal. The release of aldosterone also is increased by hyperkalemia.

---

signs of excessive or insufficient hormone replacement. The development of edema or weight gain may signify the dose is too high; postural hypotension and weight loss frequently signify the dose is too low.

Monitoring and Managing Addisonian Crisis

Physical and psychological stressors must be avoided since the patient with Addison disease is at risk for an addisonian crisis, which presents as complete circulatory collapse and shock. Triggers include exposure to cold, overexertion, infection, and emotional distress. The patient with an addisonian crisis requires immediate treatment with IV administration of fluid, glucose, and electrolytes, especially sodium; replacement of missing steroid hormones; and vasopressors. Additionally, the patient must avoid exertion; therefore, the nurse must anticipate the patient's needs and take measures to meet them. Careful monitoring of symptoms, vital signs, weight, and status of fluids and electrolytes is essential to assess the patient's progress and return to a precrisis state. To reduce the risk of future episodes of an addisonian crisis, efforts are made to identify and reduce the factors that may have led to the crisis.

CUSHING SYNDROME/DISEASE

Pathophysiology

Cushing syndrome, or hypercortisolism, is a disorder characterized by high levels of serum cortisol—too much ACTH is at work in the body. Three important causes of Cushing syndrome are:

- A pituitary tumor that overproduces ACTH, termed Cushing disease
- An adrenal tumor that overproduces ACTH, termed Cushing syndrome
- Long-term glucocorticoid pharmacologic therapy, termed iatrogenic

TABLE **31-8** Side Effects of Corticosteroid Therapy and Implications for Nursing Practice

Side Effects	Collaborative Interventions
Cardiovascular Effects	
Hypertension	Monitor for elevated blood pressure.
Thrombophlebitis	Assess for signs and symptoms of deep venous thrombosis (DVT): redness, warmth,
Thromboembolism	tenderness, and unilateral edema of an extremity.
Accelerated atherosclerosis	Remind the patient to avoid positions and situations that restrict blood flow (e.g., crossing
	legs, prolonged sitting in same position, use of knee highs or girdles).
	Encourage foot and leg exercises when recumbent.
	Encourage low sodium intake.
	Encourage limited intake of fat.
Immunologic Effects	
Increased risk of infection and	Assess for subtle signs of infection and inflammation.
masking of signs of infection	Encourage the patient to avoid exposure to others with upper respiratory infection.
	Monitor the patient for fungal infections.
	Encourage handwashing.
Ophthalmologic Changes	
Glaucoma	Encourage frequent eye examinations.
Corneal lesions	Refer the patient to an ophthalmologist if changes are detected in visual acuity.
Musculoskeletal Effects	
Muscle wasting	Encourage high intake of protein and vitamin C or supplementation of protein and vitamin C,
Poor wound healing	if indicated.
Osteoporosis with vertebral	Encourage a diet high in calcium and vitamin D or supplementation of calcium and vitamin D,
compression fractures,	if indicated.
pathologic fractures of long	Take measures to avoid falls and other trauma.
bones, aseptic necrosis of	Use caution in moving and turning patient.
head of the femur	Encourage postmenopausal women on corticosteroids to consider bone mineral density
	testing and treatment, if indicated.
	Instruct the patient to rise slowly from the bed or chair to avoid falling.
Metabolic Effects	
Alterations in glucose	Monitor blood glucose levels at periodic intervals.
metabolism	Instruct the patient about medications, diet, and exercise prescribed to control blood
Steroid withdrawal syndrome	glucose level.
	Report signs of adrenal insufficiency.
	Administer corticosteroids and mineralocorticoids as prescribed.
	Monitor fluid and electrolyte balance.
	Administer fluids and electrolytes as prescribed.
	Instruct the patient about the importance of taking corticosteroids as prescribed without
	stopping therapy abruptly.
	Encourage the patient to obtain and wear a medical identification bracelet.
	Advise the patient to notify all health care providers (e.g., dentist) about the need for
	corticosteroid therapy.
Changes in Appearance	
Moon face	Encourage a low-calorie, low-sodium diet.
Weight gain	Assure the patient that most changes in appearance are temporary and will disappear if and
Acne	when corticosteroid therapy is no longer necessary.

Pathophysiology

Cushing syndrome is commonly caused by chronic use of synthetic corticosteroid medications and infrequently is due to excessive production of corticosteroid secondary to hyperplasia or tumor of the adrenal cortex. Overproduction of endogenous corticosteroids may be caused by several mechanisms, including a tumor of the pituitary gland that produces ACTH and stimulates the adrenal cortex to increase its hormone secretion despite production of adequate amounts (as noted earlier, technically termed *Cushing disease*). Primary hyperplasia of the adrenal glands in the absence of a pituitary tumor is less common. Another less common cause of Cushing syndrome is the ectopic production of ACTH by malignancies; bronchogenic carcinoma is the most common type of these malignancies. Regardless of the cause, the normal feedback mechanisms that control the function of the adrenal cortex become ineffective, and the usual diurnal pattern of cortisol is lost.

Risk Factors

The chronic use of corticosteroids is a common risk factor of developing Cushing syndrome. Females are three times more likely than males to develop Cushing syndrome, and the median age of onset or diagnosis was 41.4 years of age (Lacroix, Feelders, Stratakis, & Nieman, 2015). Other less common risk factors that may result in Cushing syndrome include primary hyperplasia of the adrenal glands in the absence of a pituitary tumor and ectopic production of ACTH by malignancies.

Clinical Manifestations and Assessment

The signs and symptoms of Cushing syndrome are primarily due to oversecretion of glucocorticoids and androgens (sex hormones), although mineralocorticoid secretion also may play a role. Overproduction of the adrenal cortical hormone leads to an arrest of height, obesity, musculoskeletal changes, and glucose intolerance. Altered fat metabolism results in a classic picture of Cushing syndrome in the adult: central-type obesity, a protruding abdomen, a fatty "buffalo hump" in the neck and supraclavicular areas, and a round "moon-faced" appearance (Fig. 31-8). The skin is thin, fragile, and easily traumatized; ecchymoses (bruises) and purple striae develop (secondary to stretching of the weakened skin). The patient complains of weakness and lassitude. Sleep is disturbed due to altered diurnal secretion of cortisol.

Muscle weakness, wasting, and thin extremities are caused by protein wasting. Excessive catabolism of bone protein can result in osteoporosis. Kyphosis, backache, and compression fractures of the vertebrae may result.

Retention of sodium and water occurs as a result of increased mineralocorticoid activity, producing hypertension, hypokalemia, and heart failure. Hyperglycemia or overt diabetes may develop. The patient may report weight gain, increased susceptibility to infection, and slow healing of minor cuts.

In females of all ages, virilization may occur as a result of excess androgens. Virilization is characterized by the appearance of masculine traits and the recession of feminine traits. There is an excessive growth of hair on the face (hirsutism), the breasts atrophy, menses cease, the clitoris enlarges, and the voice deepens. Libido is lost in men and women.

Changes occur in mood and mental activity, and psychosis may develop. Distress and depression are common and are

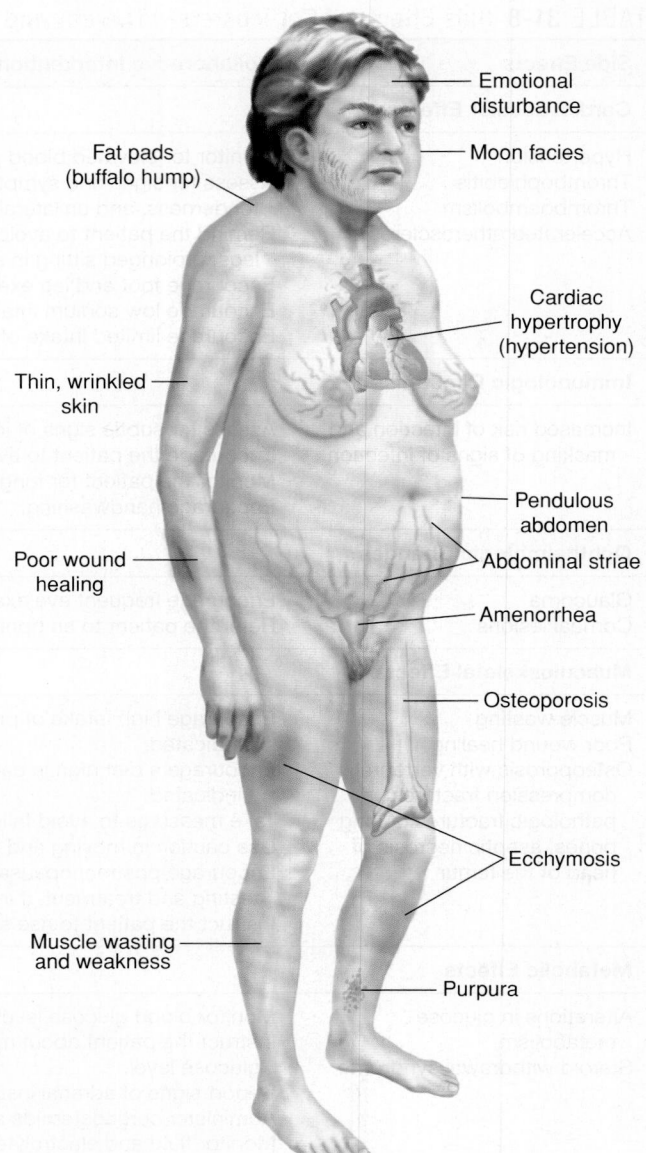

FIGURE 31-8 Major clinical manifestations of Cushing syndrome. (From Porth, C. M. (2015). *Essentials of pathophysiology: Concepts of altered health states* (4th ed.). Philadelphia, PA: Lippincott Williams & Wilkins.)

increased by the severity of the physical changes that occur with this syndrome. If Cushing disease is a consequence of a pituitary tumor, visual disturbances may occur because of pressure of the growing tumor on the optic chiasm.

The initial diagnostic assessment involves:

  i. urine free cortisol (2 measurements),
 ii. late night salivary cortisol (2 measurements), and
iii. dexamethasone suppression test: 1 mg overnight or 2 mg over 2 days (Nieman et al., 2008).

The 1 mg overnight dexamethasone suppression test is widely used and the most sensitive screening for the diagnosis of pituitary and adrenal causes of Cushing disease (Porth, 2015). In general, 1 mg of dexamethasone is administered orally at 11:00 PM, and a plasma cortisol level is obtained at 8:00 AM the next morning. Suppression of cortisol to less than 5 mg/dL indicates that the hypothalamic–pituitary–adrenal axis is functioning properly. Stress, obesity, depression, and medications, such as antiseizure agents, estrogen (during pregnancy or as oral medications), and rifampin, can falsely elevate cortisol levels. Studies have shown that nighttime salivary cortisol levels show promise in screening effectively for Cushing syndrome. Although not a routine diagnostic test in the United States, salivary cortisol concentrations are shown to be reflective of active free cortisol in plasma. Usually a saliva sample is collected on two separate evenings either by passive drooling into a plastic tube or by chewing a piece of cotton salivette for 1 to 2 minutes (Nieman et al., 2008). Saliva samples can be obtained easily in a nonstressful environment (e.g., at home); the test is relatively safe and easy to administer, with a sensitivity of 92% to 100% and a specificity of 93% to 100% (Carroll, Raff, & Findling, 2008).

Indicators of Cushing syndrome include an increase in levels of serum sodium (hypernatremia) and blood glucose (hyperglycemia), a decrease in serum potassium (hypokalemia), a reduction in the number of blood eosinophils, and disappearance of lymphoid tissue. Measurements are obtained of plasma and urinary cortisol levels. Several blood samples may be collected to determine whether the normal diurnal variation in plasma levels is present; frequently this variation is absent in adrenal dysfunction. If several blood samples are required, they must be collected at the times specified, and the time of collection must be noted on the requisition slip.

Radioimmunoassay measurement of plasma ACTH is used together with the high-dose suppression test to distinguish pituitary tumors from ectopic sites of ACTH production. Elevation of ACTH and cortisol indicates pituitary or hypothalamic disease. Low ACTH with high cortisol level indicates adrenal disease. CT, ultrasound, or MRI is performed to localize adrenal tissue and detect tumors of adrenal gland.

Medical Management

Treatment is directed at the pituitary gland if Cushing's is caused by pituitary tumors rather than tumors of the adrenal cortex. Successful surgical removal of the tumor by transsphenoidal hypophysectomy is the treatment of choice, and it has early postoperative remission rates between 67% and 95% (Pendharkar, Sussman, Ho, Hayden Gephart, & Katznelson, 2015). In addition, radiation of the pituitary gland has been successful, but it may take several months for control of the symptoms. **Adrenalectomy** is the treatment of choice in patients with primary adrenal hypertrophy or when other therapies have failed.

Postoperatively, symptoms of adrenal insufficiency may begin to appear 12 to 48 hours after surgery because of the reduction of high levels of circulating adrenal hormones. Temporary replacement therapy with hydrocortisone may be necessary for several months, until the adrenal glands begin to respond normally to the body's needs. If both adrenal glands have been removed (bilateral adrenalectomy), patients should be educated that a lifetime replacement of adrenal cortex hormones is necessary, and they should be taught how to identify signs of acute addisonian crisis.

Adrenal enzyme inhibitors, such as metyrapone, aminoglutethimide, mitotane, and ketoconazole, are used to reduce hyperadrenalism if the syndrome is caused by ectopic ACTH secretion by a tumor that cannot be eradicated. Close monitoring is necessary because symptoms of inadequate adrenal function may result due to possible side effects of these medications.

If Cushing syndrome is a result of the administration of corticosteroids, an attempt is made to reduce or taper the medication to the minimum dosage needed to treat the underlying disease process (e.g., autoimmune, allergic disease, or rejection of transplanted organ). Frequently, alternate-day therapy decreases the symptoms of Cushing syndrome and allows recovery of the adrenal glands' responsiveness to ACTH.

Nursing Management

Decreasing Risk of Injury

Establishing a protective environment helps prevent falls, fractures, and other injuries to bones and soft tissues. The patient who is very weak may require assistance in ambulating to avoid falling or bumping into sharp corners of furniture. Foods high in protein, calcium, and vitamin D are recommended to minimize muscle wasting and osteoporosis. Referral to a dietitian may assist the patient in selecting appropriate foods that are also low in sodium and calories.

Decreasing Risk of Infection

The patient should avoid unnecessary exposure to others with infections. The nurse frequently assesses the patient for subtle signs of infection because the anti-inflammatory effects of corticosteroids may mask the common signs of inflammation and infection.

Encouraging Rest and Activity

Weakness, fatigue, and muscle wasting make it difficult for the patient with Cushing syndrome to carry out normal activities; however, the nurse encourages moderate activity to prevent complications of immobility and promote increased self-esteem. Insomnia often contributes to the patient's fatigue. It is important to help the patient plan and space rest periods throughout the day. Efforts are made to promote a relaxing, quiet environment for rest and sleep.

Promoting Skin Integrity

Proper skin care is necessary to avoid traumatizing the patient's fragile skin. The nurse avoids use of adhesive tape because it can irritate and tear the fragile skin when the tape is removed. The nurse frequently assesses the skin and bony prominences and encourages and assists the patient to change positions frequently to prevent skin breakdown.

Improving Body Image

If the cause of Cushing syndrome can be treated successfully, the major physical changes disappear in time. The patient may benefit from discussion of the effect the changes have had on his or her self-concept and relationships with others. Weight gain and edema may be modified by recommending a low-carbohydrate, low-sodium, and high-protein diet.

Improving Thought Processes

Explanations to the patient and family members about the cause of emotional instability are important in helping them cope with the mood swings, irritability, and depression that may occur. Psychotic behavior may occur in a few patients and should be reported. The nurse encourages the patient and family members to verbalize their feelings and concerns.

Monitoring and Managing Addisonian Crisis

The patient with Cushing syndrome whose symptoms are treated by the withdrawal of corticosteroids, by adrenalectomy, or by removal of a pituitary tumor is at risk for adrenal hypofunction and addisonian crisis. If high levels of circulating adrenal hormones have suppressed the function of the adrenal cortex, atrophy of the adrenal cortex is likely. If the level of circulating hormones is decreased rapidly because of surgery or abrupt cessation of corticosteroid agents, manifestations of adrenal hypofunction and addisonian crisis may develop. The nurse monitors the patient closely for hypotension, rapid weak pulse, rapid respiratory rate, pallor, and extreme weakness. Efforts are made to identify factors that may have led to the crisis. The patient may require IV administration of fluid, electrolytes, and corticosteroids before, during, and after treatment or surgery. The nurse assesses the status of fluid and electrolytes by monitoring laboratory values and daily weights. Retention of sodium and water may result in the development of edema and hypertension; therefore, assessment of vital signs and fluid volume excess is warranted. In addition, observe for signs and symptoms of hypokalemia (K$^+$ below 3.5 mEq/L), which can have a profound impact on cardiac and neurologic function. Blood glucose monitoring should be followed closely because of the increased risk for glucose intolerance and hyperglycemia with Cushing syndrome and hypoglycemia if the patient is now at risk for adrenal hypofunction due to interventions to treat Cushing syndrome. If addisonian crisis occurs, the patient is treated for circulatory collapse and shock.

Teaching Self-Care Measures

Upon discharge, the patient and family should understand that stopping the use of the corticosteroid abruptly and without medical supervision is likely to result in acute adrenal insufficiency as well as reappearance of the underlying symptoms of the chronic disease. The nurse emphasizes the need to ensure an adequate supply of the corticosteroid because running out of the medication or skipping doses can precipitate adrenal insufficiency and addisonian crisis. The need for dietary modifications is stressed; the nurse reminds the patient and family that it is important to ensure adequate calcium intake without increasing the risks for hypertension, hyperglycemia, and weight gain. The patient and family may be taught to monitor blood pressure, blood glucose levels, and weight. Wearing a medical alert bracelet and notifying health care providers (e.g., dentist) of the patient's condition are important.

PRIMARY ALDOSTERONISM

Pathophysiology

Primary aldosteronism, also known as *Conn syndrome*, is a condition in which the adrenal cortex produces too much aldosterone because of hyperplasia or tumor. The principal action of aldosterone is to conserve body sodium, thus excessive aldosterone will result in increased renal reabsorption of sodium and an increase in extracellular fluids and blood pressure.

Secondary hyperaldosteronism also can occur from a nonadrenal cause of elevated aldosterone and/or nonsuppressed plasma renin activity, such as renal artery stenosis, renin-secreting tumors, kidney disease, and malignant hypertension.

Risk Factors

Excessive production of aldosterone occurs in some patients with functioning tumors of the adrenal gland. The peak incidence is between 30 and 60 years of age (Fitzgerald, 2015). Other risk factors for primary aldosteronism include unilateral or bilateral adrenal hyperplasia (caused by overactivity of one or both adrenal glands), familial hyperaldosteronism, and aldosterone-producing adrenal adenoma (Fitzgerald, 2015).

Clinical Manifestations and Assessment

Patients with hyperaldosteronism exhibit a profound decline in the serum levels of potassium (hypokalemia) and hydrogen ions (alkalosis, leading to tetany) as demonstrated by an increase in pH and serum bicarbonate concentration. The serum sodium level is normal or typically elevated depending on the amount of water reabsorbed with the sodium or water loss in the urine. Hypertension is the most prominent and almost universal sign of aldosteronism and accounts for 10% of cases of hypertension (Piaditis, Markou, Papanastasiou, Androulakis, & Kaltsas, 2015).

Hypokalemia leads to muscle weakness, cramping, and fatigue as well as an inability on the part of the kidneys to acidify or concentrate the urine, leading to polyuria. Serum sodium becomes abnormally concentrated, contributing to excessive thirst (polydipsia) and arterial hypertension. A secondary increase in blood volume and possible direct effects of aldosterone on nerve receptors, such as the carotid sinus, result in hypertension.

Hypokalemic alkalosis may decrease the level of ionized serum calcium and predispose the patient to tetany and paresthesia. Glucose intolerance may occur because hypokalemia interferes with insulin secretion from the pancreas.

In addition to a high or normal serum sodium level and a low serum potassium level, diagnostic studies indicate high serum aldosterone and low serum renin levels. The measurement of the aldosterone excretion rate after salt loading is a useful diagnostic test for hyperaldosteronism. The renin–aldosterone stimulation test and bilateral adrenal venous sampling are useful in differentiating the cause of primary aldosteronism. Antihypertensive medication may be discontinued up to 2 weeks before testing.

Medical Management

Treatment of primary aldosteronism usually involves surgical removal of the adrenal tumor through adrenalectomy.

Adrenalectomy is performed through an incision in the flank or the abdomen using laparoscopic techniques. In general, postoperative care resembles that for other abdominal surgeries. The patient is susceptible to fluctuations in adrenocortical hormones and requires administration of corticosteroids, fluids, and other agents to maintain blood pressure and prevent acute complications. If the adrenalectomy is bilateral, lifetime replacement of corticosteroids will be necessary. If one adrenal gland is removed, the replacement therapy may be only temporary because of the suppression of the remaining adrenal gland by high levels of adrenal hormones. A normal level of serum glucose is maintained with insulin, IV fluids, and dietary modifications. Hypokalemia resolves for all patients after surgery, but hypertension may persist. Spironolactone (potassium-sparing diuretic) and Eplerenone may be prescribed to control hypertension and minimize hypokalemia.

Nursing Management

The nursing management during the postoperative period includes frequent assessment of vital signs to detect early signs and symptoms of adrenal insufficiency and crisis or hemorrhage. Explaining all treatments and procedures, providing comfort measures, and providing rest periods can reduce the patient's stress and anxiety level.

CHAPTER REVIEW

Critical Thinking Exercises

1. A 65-year-old woman has just been diagnosed with thyroid cancer. She is scheduled for a total thyroidectomy in 1 week. What preoperative and postoperative nursing care is necessary for her recovery? What long-term follow-up would you anticipate, and what issues should you discuss with the patient and her family?

2. A 70-year-old man has a diagnosis of bronchogenic carcinoma. He is being evaluated for possible SIADH. The patient and his family are asking for explanations about the syndrome and about methods of managing it. What nursing interventions and patient and family teaching are warranted when caring for this patient? Compare and contrast the clinical picture and symptoms of SIADH with those of diabetes insipidus.

3. A 14-year-old girl was diagnosed recently with Addison disease. The patient is overly concerned that she will not be able to lead a normal life as a result of this disease. What advice/patient education should the nurse give to the patient? Describe and provide rationale on how each piece of advice will benefit the patient.

NCLEX-Style Review Questions

1. Upon evaluation of the patient's laboratory data and clinical signs and symptoms, the nurse suspects that the patient may have pheochromocytoma. Which of the following is directly related with pheochromocytoma? Select all that apply.
   a. Severe headache; pain score of 9 out of 10
   b. Perspiration
   c. Blood pressure 80/90 mm Hg
   d. Pallor
   e. Lethargy

2. A 70-year-old female patient is admitted to the unit with enlargement of thyroid gland, hypertension, high TSH levels, and bulging eyes. What nursing intervention is most appropriate for this patient?
   a. Providing a blanket
   b. Instilling eye ointment
   c. Providing a warm bath
   d. Keep room temperature comfortable at 85°F

3. A patient presented to the unit with an ADH-secreting tumor. Upon diagnostic and physical evaluation, the

nurse suspects the patient is experiencing SIADH. Which of the following is a clinical manifestation of SIADH? Select all that apply.

a. Hyponatremia
b. Hypernatremia
c. Increased serum osmolality
d. Reduced serum osmolality
e. Dry mucous membranes
f. Low urine output

4. The nursing management of a patient who underwent transsphenoidal removal of a pituitary tumor yesterday includes which of the following actions? Select all that apply.

a. Maintaining oral care
b. Removing nasal pack to check for bleeding and CSF leak
c. Giving fluid after nausea, and then slowly progressing to normal diet
d. Raising the head of the bed to promote drainage
e. Brush teeth to prevent bacterial overgrowth with hard toothbrush

5. A 55-year-old female presents to the clinic with complaints of fatigue and tiredness. The nurse notices that the patient's skin is thin, fragile, and easily traumatized. Ecchymosis and purple striae are noted over the thighs and abdomen. She presents with a slight kyphosis and a protruding abdomen. Which of the following methods of management might be appropriate for her?

a. Increase dose of corticosteroids
b. Unilateral or bilateral adrenalectomy
c. Increase dose of Spironolactone
d. Diet that is high in carbohydrates and low in protein

Try these additional resources, available at **http://thepoint.lww.com/Honan2e**, to enhance your learning and understanding of this chapter:
- NCLEX-Style Student Review Questions
- Journal Articles

REFERENCES AND SELECTED READINGS

References and selected readings associated with this chapter can be found on the website that accompanies the book. Visit **http://thepoint. lww.com/Honan2e** to access the references and other additional resources associated with this chapter.

Problems Related to Reproductive Function

A 40-year-old mother of three children has been diagnosed with squamous cell carcinoma of the cervix following an abnormal Pap smear and colposcopy. She is being seen in the gynecologist office for follow-up treatment. She is very worried about her prognosis.

- Discuss risk factors associated with this type of cancer.
- What clinical manifestations may this patient have had prior to this diagnosis?
- What is the purpose of a colposcopy?
- Discuss medical management of cervical cancer.

Nursing Assessment: Female and Male Reproductive Function

Jennifer L. Mosher • Susanne A. Quallich

Learning Objectives

After reading this chapter, you will be able to:

1. Describe female reproductive function.
2. Discuss components of female reproductive assessment.
3. Identify the diagnostic examinations and tests used to determine alteration in female reproductive function and breast disorders.
4. Describe structures and function of the male reproductive system.
5. Discuss nursing assessment of the male reproductive system and identify diagnostic tests that complement assessment.

FEMALE REPRODUCTIVE SYSTEM

Statistically women utilize the health care system more often than do men (Blackwell, Lucas, & Clarke, 2014), often seeking health care during the changes involving the reproductive system from the onset of menarche to menopause. An understanding of the normal anatomy and physiology of the female reproductive system is a necessary and important function of the nurse. It is integral to recognizing the complex issues that can occur within the female reproductive system.

ANATOMIC AND PHYSIOLOGIC OVERVIEW

Anatomy of the Female Reproductive System

The female reproductive system consists of the external and internal genital structures as well as the mammary glands located in the female breast. Hormonal influences on the female reproductive system are driven by the hypothalamus and pituitary gland. These influences cause the cyclical changes throughout the reproductive life of women, and the cessation of the changes results in menopause.

External Genitalia

The external genital structures, referred to as the vulva, consist of the mons pubis; labia majora; labia minora; clitoris;

and the vestibule of the vagina, which contains the hymen, the urethral and vaginal orifice, and the paraurethral (Skene) and Bartholin glands (Fig. 32-1). The mons pubis is the fatty tissue at the junction of the thighs and torso, while the labia majora are two thick folds of tissue that form the outer border of the vulva. Both are covered by pubic hair after puberty. The upper portions of the labia minora unite anteriorly to form a partial covering for the clitoris, a highly sensitive organ composed of erectile tissue. The labia minora are thinner folds of tissue internal to the majora that cover the urethral meatus and vaginal **introitus**. The urethral meatus lies below and posterior to the clitoris, and the vaginal introitus lies just posterior to the urethral meatus. The mucus-secreting structures that are set in the wall of the urethra are termed *Skene glands*. The Bartholin glands, bean-sized structures that also secrete mucus, lie on each side of the vaginal orifice. The area between the vagina and rectum is called the perineum.

Internal Reproductive Structures

The internal structures of the female reproductive system are the vagina, uterus, ovaries, and fallopian tubes (Fig. 32-2).

The vagina is a canal that is lined with a mucous membrane and that extends from the vulva to the cervix. The upper part of the vagina, the **fornix**, surrounds the **cervix** (the inferior part of the uterus).

The uterus is a pear-shaped, muscular organ, which can vary in size depending on parity (number of viable births) and uterine abnormalities (e.g., fibroids). The uterus lies posterior to the bladder and is held in position by several

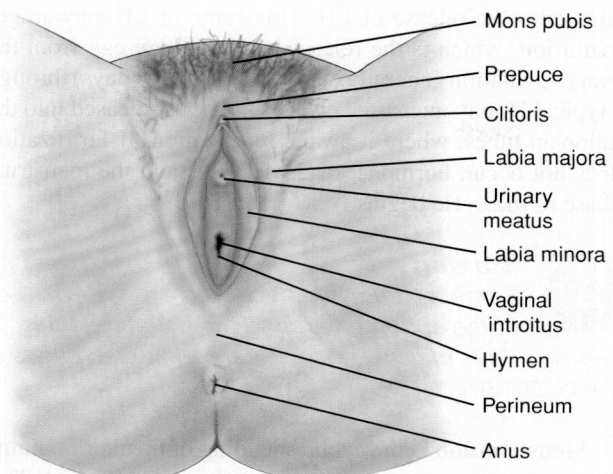

FIGURE 32-1 External female genitalia.

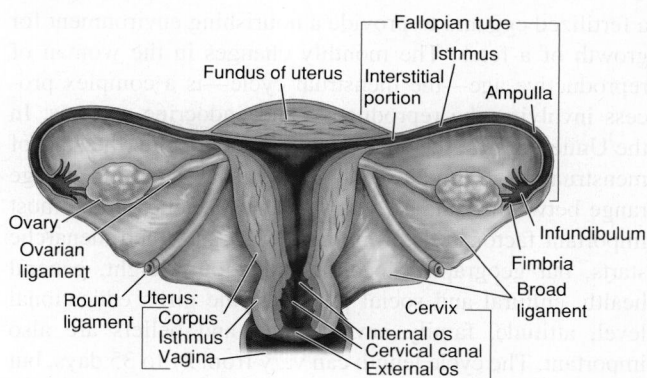

FIGURE 32-2 Internal female reproductive structures.

ligaments. The uterus consists of the cervix, which projects into the vagina, and the **fundus** or body. The triangular inner portion of the fundus narrows to a small canal in the cervix that has constrictions at each end, referred to as the *external os* and *internal os*. The upper lateral parts of the uterus are called the *cornua*. From here, the oviducts, or fallopian tubes, extend outward to meet the ovaries.

The **ovaries** lie behind and below the fallopian tubes. They are oval bodies about 3 cm long. When a girl is born, her ovaries contain thousands of tiny egg cells or *ova*. The ovaries and the fallopian tubes together are referred to as the **adnexa**.

Breasts

The breasts lie over the pectoralis muscle from the sternum to the midaxillary line. An area of breast tissue, called the

tail of Spence, extends into the axilla. Cooper's ligaments support the breast on the chest wall. During puberty, estrogen and other hormones in the female body stimulate breast development. This development usually occurs from 10 to 16 years of age, although the range can vary from 9 to 18 years of age.

Each fully developed breast (Fig. 32-3) is made up of glandular lobules and ducts bound and separated by fibrous tissue and fat. Approximately 15 to 20 lobules are grouped together to form cone-shaped lobes. Fibrous tissue surrounds the lobes and ducts. Fatty tissue fills the spaces between lobes and ducts and gives the breast a soft texture. During lactation, milk is produced in the lobules and is carried through the ducts to the nipple.

Function of the Female Reproductive System

The main function of the female reproductive system is to prepare the woman's body each month to be ready to accept

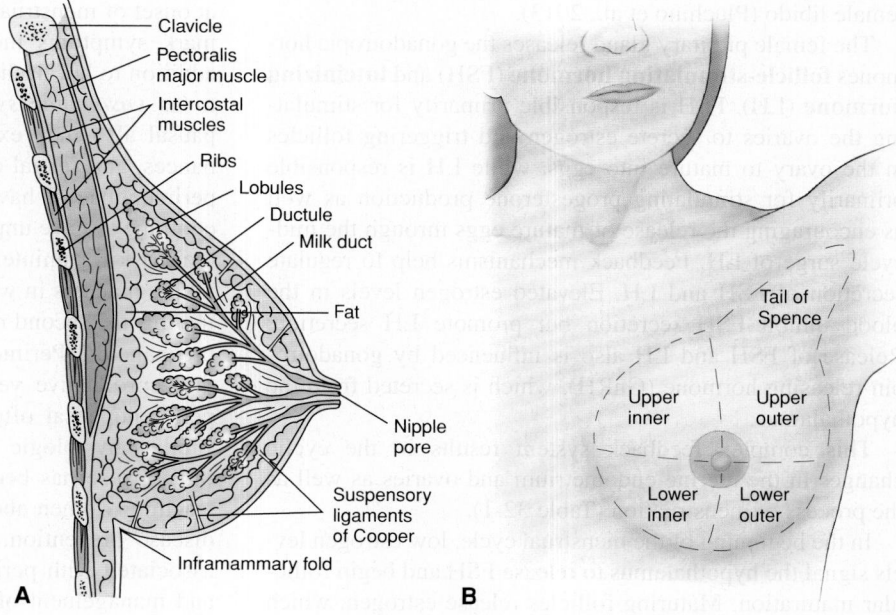

FIGURE 32-3 **A.** Anatomy of the breast. **B.** Areas of breast, including the tail of Spence.

a fertilized egg and to provide a nourishing environment for growth of a fetus. The monthly changes in the woman of reproductive age—the menstrual cycle—is a complex process involving the reproductive and endocrine systems. In the United States, the average age at **menarche** (the start of menstruation in females) is 12.8 years of age, with an age range between 8 and 18 years of age. Genetics is the most important factor in determining the age at which menarche starts, but geographic location, nutrition, weight, general health, cultural and social practices, the girl's educational level, attitude, family environment, and beliefs are also important. The cycle length can vary from 21 to 35 days, but the average length is 28 days (Ricci, 2013).

The woman's reproductive cycle consists of a complex series of interactions among the hypothalamic–pituitary system, the ovarian system, the endometrial system, and the various hormones secreted by each of those systems.

The Menstrual Cycle

Estrogen and progesterone are two hormones integral to proper functioning of the female reproductive system. The ovaries produce several types of **estrogen** as well as progesterone. Estrogen is responsible for development and maintenance of the female reproductive organs, secondary sex characteristics of the adult female, breast development, and the monthly uterine changes associated with menstruation. **Progesterone** plays a role in regulating uterine changes during the menstrual cycle, preparing the **endometrium** (via the **corpus luteum**) for implantation of a fertilized ovum, and maintaining (via the placenta) a normal pregnancy. Together, progesterone and estrogen help prepare the breasts for lactation. **Androgens** are hormones that are produced by the ovaries and the adrenals in small amounts; they influence early follicular development (Nathan, 2013) as well as the female libido (Pluchino et al., 2013).

The female pituitary gland releases the gonadotropic hormones **follicle-stimulating hormone** (FSH) and **luteinizing hormone** (LH). FSH is responsible primarily for stimulating the ovaries to secrete estrogen and triggering follicles in the ovary to mature into eggs, while LH is responsible primarily for stimulating progesterone production as well as encouraging the release of mature eggs through the midcycle surge of LH. Feedback mechanisms help to regulate secretion of FSH and LH. Elevated estrogen levels in the blood inhibit FSH secretion but promote LH secretion. Release of FSH and LH also is influenced by gonadotropin-releasing hormone (GnRH), which is secreted from the hypothalamus.

This complex feedback system results in the cyclic changes in the uterine endometrium and ovaries as well as the process of menstruation (Table 32-1).

In the beginning of the menstrual cycle, low estrogen levels signal the hypothalamus to release FSH and begin follicular maturation. Maturing follicles release estrogen, which

stimulates the release of LH. This surge of LH encourages **ovulation**, which is the release of the mature egg from the ovary. Ovulation generally occurs mid-way (14 days) through a typical 28-day menstrual cycle. The egg is released into the fallopian tubes, where it awaits fertilization. If fertilization does not occur, hormone levels decrease and the menstrual phase of the cycle begins.

 Nursing Alert
Some women can feel a pain on one side of the abdomen around the time the egg is released. This midcycle pain is called mittelschmerz (Ricci, 2013).

Menstruation is the cyclic shedding of the uterine lining that occurs when pregnancy has not been established. This menstrual flow is discharged through the cervix and into the vagina, and it usually lasts an average of 3 to 7 days. The amount of menstrual flow varies but averages 1 oz or a range of approximately 2/3 to 2-2/3 oz in volume per cycle. The beginning of the menstrual flow marks the end of one menstrual cycle and the start of a new one (Ricci, 2013).

 Nursing Alert
Regardless of cycle length, ovulation typically occurs 14 days prior to menses (Costanzo, 2014).

Perimenopause

Perimenopause is a transitional time late in a woman's reproductive life before the final menstrual period. Menopause is defined retrospectively by 12 months of amenorrhea and loss of ovarian follicular activity. The mean duration of perimenopause is 5 years, but symptoms may begin 8 years or more before the final menstrual period. The average age at onset of menstrual irregularity is 47.5 years of age. Hallmark symptoms include irregular menstrual bleeding in addition to hot flashes and night sweats, which are referred to as *vasomotor symptoms*. Women who are perimenopausal also may experience mood changes, sleep disturbances, and sexual dysfunction. Although women who are perimenopausal have declining estrogen levels, they may continue to have unpredictable ovulatory cycles, increasing their risk for unintended pregnancy. Forty-eight percent of all pregnancies in women in their 40s are unplanned, making this the second most common age cohort for unplanned pregnancies. Perimenopause marks a transition between the reproductive years and menopause. Women who are perimenopausal often benefit from information about the subtle physiologic changes they are experiencing. Perimenopause has been described as an opportune time for teaching women about strategies for health promotion and disease prevention. Awareness of the hormonal changes associated with perimenopause helps with the recognition and management of symptoms, including menstrual cycle

TABLE **32-1** Hormonal Influences and Menstrual Cycle

(Times approximate) Phase	Menstrual	Follicular	Ovulation	Luteal	Premenstrual
Days	1 2 3 4 5 6 7 8 9 10	11 12 13 14 15 16	17 18 19 20	21 22 23 24 25	26 27 28 1 2
Ovary					
	Degenerating corpus luteum; beginning follicular development	Growth and maturation of follicle	Ovulation	Active corpus luteum	Degenerating corpus luteum
Estrogen Production					
	Low	Increasing	High	Decreasing, then a secondary rise	Decreasing
Progesterone Production					
	None	Low	Low	Increasing	Decreasing
FSH Production					
	Increasing	High, then decreasing	Low	Low	Increasing
LH Production					
	Low	Low, then increasing	High	High	Decreasing
Endometrium					
	Degeneration and shedding of superficial layer. Coiled arteries dilate and then constrict again.	Reorganization and proliferation of superficial layer	Continued growth	Active secretion and glandular dilation; highly vascular; edematous	Vasoconstriction of coiled arteries; beginning degeneration

irregularity, VMS, mood and sleep disorders, and sexual dysfunction. For many patients, hormonal contraception (with appropriate counseling) treats these symptoms and prevents the real risk for pregnancy (McNamara, Batur, & DeSapri, 2015).

Menopause

Menopause marks the end of a woman's reproductive capacity and generally occurs between 45 and 52 years of age. With menopause, the ovaries are no longer active and the reproductive organs become smaller. Menopause is not a pathologic phenomenon but a normal part of aging and maturation. In addition to the effects of reduced estrogen on the reproductive system, neuroendocrinologic, biochemical, and metabolic changes related to aging occur throughout the woman's body (Table 32-2). Early menopause may occur if the ovaries are surgically removed, are destroyed by radiation or chemotherapy, or because of an unknown etiology. Menopause offers a unique opportunity for dialogue between women and their health care providers to evaluate and improve health-related practices. By considering a woman's concerns, values, and preferences, nurses have the potential to enhance a woman's sense of well-being, not only at menopause but for the rest of their lives (Shifren & Gass, 2014). Box 32-1 discusses nursing care of patients experiencing menopause.

ASSESSMENT

Nurses obtaining health history information and performing physical assessments are in ideal positions to discuss women's general health issues, health promotion, and health-related concerns. Relevant topics include fitness, nutrition, cardiovascular risks, health screening, sexuality, menopause, abuse, health risk behaviors, and immunizations. Recommendations for health screening are summarized in Table 32-3. Many problems can be corrected if treated early, while allowing them to go untreated may result in serious health problems.

Although sexuality and sexual function are discussed more often with gynecologic or women's health care providers, any nurse caring for women should consider these issues part of a routine health assessment.

Health History

In addition to obtaining a general health history, information related to past illnesses and experiences specific to women's

TABLE 32-2 GERONTOLOGIC CONSIDERATIONS / Age-Related Changes in the Female Reproductive System

Structural Change	Functional Change	History and Physical Findings
Cessation of ovarian function and decreased estrogen production; thinning of urinary and genital tracts; thinning of pubic hair and shrinking of labia	Decreased ovulation Onset of menopause Vasomotor instability and hormonal fluctuations Decreased bone formation Decreased vaginal lubrication Increased vaginal pH	Decreased/loss of ability to conceive; increased infertility Irregular menses with eventual cessation of menses Hot flashes or flushing; night sweats, sleep disturbances; mood swings; fatigue Bone loss and increased risk for osteoporosis and osteoporotic fractures; loss of height Dyspareunia, resulting in lack of interest in sex Increased risk for urinary tract infection Increased incidence of inflammation (atrophic vaginitis) with discharge, itching, and vulvar burning
Relaxation of pelvic musculature	Prolapse of uterus, cystocele, rectocele	Dyspareunia, incontinence, feelings of perineal pressure

---

BOX 32-1 Management During Menopause

Clinical Manifestations and Assessment

Long before menopause occurs, hormonal changes contribute to common symptoms of menopause, including irregular menses, breast tenderness, mood changes, hot flashes, and night sweats. Thought to be due to hormonal changes, hot flashes denote vasomotor instability and vary in intensity from a barely perceptible warm feeling to a sensation of extreme warmth accompanied by profuse sweating, causing discomfort, sleep disturbances, and subsequent fatigue. Also osteoporosis can be a manifestation of menopause.

Reduced estrogen levels affect the entire genitourinary system. Changes in the vulvovaginal area include gradual thinning of pubic hair and a shrinking of the labia. Vaginal secretions decrease, and women may report dyspareunia (discomfort during intercourse). The vaginal pH increases during menopause, predisposing women to bacterial infections and atrophic vaginitis. Some women report fatigue, forgetfulness, weight gain, irritability, feeling "blue," and feelings of panic. Menopausal complaints need to be evaluated carefully because they also may indicate other disorders.

Women's reactions and feelings related to loss of reproductive capacity may vary. Some women may experience role confusion, whereas others experience a sense of sexual and personal freedom. Each woman's experience must be considered on an individual basis, and nurses need to be sensitive to all possibilities.

Medical Management

Women approaching menopause often have many concerns about their health. Some have concerns based on a family history of heart disease, osteoporosis, or cancer. Each woman needs to be as knowledgeable as possible about her options and should be encouraged to discuss her concerns with her primary health care provider in order to make an informed decision about managing menopausal symptoms and maintaining her health. Postmenopausal bleeding, or bleeding 1 year after menses cease at menopause, must be investigated as a malignant condition must be considered until proved otherwise.

Seventy-five percent of women who are menopausal experience vasomotor symptoms, such as hot flashes and night sweats. Eighty percent of these women will endure these symptoms for longer than 1 year and 50% for longer than 5 years. Hormone therapy (HT) is first-line treatment. Current recommendations are that HT use should be limited to the lowest effective dose for the shortest treatment duration and that ongoing use should be re-evaluated periodically (Washington & Zacur, 2015).

HT has risks as well as benefits. Extended follow-up data from the Women's Health Initiative (WHI) trials do not support the use of HT for chronic disease prevention (Boardman, 2014). The U.S. Preventive Services Task Force (USPSTF) has found convincing evidence to support combined estrogen/progestin therapy in the reduction of risk for fractures in women who are postmenopausal. However, evidence also indicates an association with moderate harms, including an increase in instances of stroke, dementia, gallbladder disease, deep venous thrombosis (DVT), pulmonary embolism, and a small increase in breast cancer deaths. Combined therapy does not have a beneficial effect on coronary heart disease (CHD) and probably increases the risk of its occurrence. The USPSTF has concluded with high certainty that the chronic disease prevention benefits of combined estrogen and progestin do not outweigh the harms in most women who are postmenopausal (Moyer, 2013).

There are several different treatment methods for those women who do elect to take HT. Both estrogen and progestin pills are prescribed for women who still have a uterus.

Progestin prevents proliferation of the uterine lining and hyperplasia, which are factors that increase the risk for uterine cancer. Women without a uterus can take estrogen without progestin (unopposed estrogen).

Patches are another option. Estrogen patches are replaced once or twice weekly but will require a progestin pill along with them if the woman still has a uterus. Another type of patch provides both estrogen and progestin treatment. Vaginal symptoms can be treated with an estrogen cream or suppository, or an estradiol vaginal ring may be used for vaginal dryness or atrophic vaginitis. The selective estrogen receptor modulator, ospemifene, is another option for women with moderate to severe dyspareunia (painful intercourse).

HT is contraindicated in women with a history of breast cancer, vascular thrombosis, impaired liver function, some cases of uterine cancer, and undiagnosed abnormal vaginal bleeding. Because HT increases the risk for thromboembolic phenomena, women who elect to take HT must be taught the signs and symptoms of DVT and pulmonary embolism (i.e., unilateral leg redness, tenderness, and edema; chest pain, and sudden onset shortness of breath) and told to report these signs and symptoms immediately.

Alternatives to HT for vasomotor symptoms are for women who cannot tolerate or who have contraindications to estrogen use. Selective serotonin and norepinephrine reuptake inhibitors (SSRIs, SNRIs) may reduce hot flashes by up to 61%. Behavioral modifications also have been recommended in the reduction of hot flashes. These include the use of a fan or drinking cool beverages; relaxation techniques, such as slow breathing and yoga; and exercise. Alternate treatment options for vaginal symptoms include moisturizers and lubricants to relieve symptoms of vaginal dryness and dyspareunia (Washington & Zacur, 2015).

Although the results of the WHI study may make the decision about use of HT easy for some women, it remains a difficult decision for those who could benefit from it because of the disruptive symptoms of menopause and evidence of bone loss. HT may be useful for women for short periods of time when no other therapy has been able to reduce their vasomotor symptoms. Women often seek information about alternative therapies to the use of HT, but often these therapies are not regulated or research-proven methods and must be used with caution. Assessment of patients who are menopausal should address their use of complementary and alternative therapies and supplements.

The decisions women make related to the use of HT must be individualized and based on each woman's current health, risk factors, family history, and severity of symptoms.

Nursing Management

Nurses can encourage women to view menopause as a natural change resulting in freedom from symptoms related to menses and pregnancy. Measures should be taken to promote general health. The nurse can explain to the patient that cessation of menses is normal and rarely is accompanied by illness. Many symptoms can even be controlled with lifestyle factors. The current expected lifespan after menopause for the average woman is 30 to 35 years, and women retain their usual response to sex long after menopause. The individual woman's evaluation of herself and her worth, now and in the future, is likely to affect her emotional reaction to menopause. Patient teaching and counseling regarding healthy lifestyles, health promotion, and health screening are of paramount importance.

---

health are necessary. In addition to basic information related to medical and surgical history, data should be collected about the following:

- Menstrual history (including menarche, length of cycles, length and amount of flow, presence of cramps or pain, bleeding between periods or after intercourse, bleeding after menopause), pain with menses, pain with intercourse, pelvic pain
- Sexual history, including past and present contraceptive use
- Pregnancy history (number of pregnancies, outcomes of pregnancies)
- Exposure to medications (diethylstilbestrol [DES], immunosuppressive agents, others) and present medication use (vitamins, prescriptions, herbs)
- History of vaginal discharge and odor or itching
- History of problems with urinary function, including frequency, urgency, and incontinence
- History of bowel problems
- History of sexually transmitted diseases (STDs) and methods of treatment
- History of fertility treatments or hormone therapy
- History of breast health, including family history of breast disease

- History of sexual or physical abuse
- History of surgery or other procedures on structures within the reproductive tract (including female genital mutilation [FGM] or female circumcision)
- History of chronic illness or disability that may affect health status, reproductive health, need for health screening, or access to health care
- Psychosocial information (availability of resources and support)

Sexual History

Incorporation of the sexual history into the general health history can provide the opportunity to clarify myths and explore areas of concern that the patient may not have felt comfortable discussing in the past. The nurse can begin by explaining the purpose of obtaining a sexual history. History-taking includes gathering data about present and past sexual activity, sexual orientation, and possible sexual dysfunction. Sexual problems may be related to medication, life changes, disability, or the onset of physical or emotional illness. By initiating an assessment about sexual concerns, the nurse can provide a safe environment for discussing sensitive topics

TABLE **32-3** Summary of Health Screening and Counseling Issues for Women[a]

Component	Screening and Counseling		
	Ages 19–39	Ages 40–64	Ages 65+
Sexuality and reproductive issues	Annual pelvic examination Annual clinical breast examination Contraceptive options High-risk sexual behaviors	Annual pelvic examination Annual clinical breast examination Contraceptive options High-risk sexual behaviors Menopausal concerns	Annual pelvic examination Annual clinical breast examination High-risk sexual behaviors
Health and risk behaviors	Hygiene Injury prevention Nutrition Exercise patterns Risk for domestic abuse Use of tobacco, drugs, and alcohol Life stresses Immunizations	Hygiene Bone loss and injury prevention Nutrition Exercise patterns Risk for domestic abuse Use of tobacco, drugs, and alcohol Life stresses Immunizations	Hygiene Injury prevention Nutrition Exercise patterns Risk for domestic abuse Use of tobacco, drugs, and alcohol Life stresses Immunizations
Diagnostic testing	Pap smear[b] Screening for sexually transmitted diseases (STD) as indicated	Pap smear Mammography[c] Cholesterol and lipid profile Colorectal cancer screening Bone mineral density testing Thyroid-stimulating hormone testing Hearing and eye examinations	Pap smear Mammography Cholesterol and lipid profile Colorectal cancer screening Bone mineral density testing Thyroid-stimulating hormone testing Hearing and eye examinations

[a]Each individual's risks (family history, personal history) influence the need for specific assessments and their frequency.
[b]Recommendations state that cytology screening (Pap smear) should not start before 21 years of age and should be done every 3 years until 30 years of age, when they can continue with cytology only every 3 years or cytology with HPV testing every 5 years.
[c]Recent recommendations include regular screening with mammography at age 50 and then every 2 years through 74 years of age.
http://www.ahrq.gov/professionals/clinicians-providers/guidelines-recommendations/guide/cpsguide.pdf

as well as validation that these topics are appropriate for discussion.

Sexually Transmitted Infections

Individual risk for sexually transmitted infections (STIs) can be assessed by determining the number of partners a patient has had in the past year or in her lifetime as well as whether or not she is taking proper protective precautions with her partner(s). Women must understand that certain STIs (e.g., chlamydia and gonorrhea), especially if left untreated, can result in pelvic inflammatory disease, ectopic pregnancy, and infertility (Workowski & Bolan, 2015). (For further details, refer to Chapter 35.)

Female Genital Mutilation

Female genital mutilation (FGM) includes procedures that intentionally alter or cause injury to the female genital organs for nonmedical reasons, including partial or total removal of the external female genitalia. FGM is carried out mostly on young girls sometime between infancy and age 15. There are more than 125 million girls and women alive today who have experienced FGM in the 29 countries in Africa and the Middle East where FGM is concentrated. FGM is carried out mostly by traditional circumcisers, who often play other central roles in communities, such as attending childbirths; however, more than 18% of all FGM is performed by health care providers, and the trend toward medicalization is increasing. The causes of FGM include a mix of cultural, religious, and social factors within families and communities. FGM is a rite of passage to womanhood and is a culturally acceptable practice as it is believed to promote hygiene, protect virginity and family honor, prevent promiscuity, improve female attractiveness and male sexual pleasure, and enhance fertility (World Health Organization [WHO], 2014). There are four types of FGM (Table 32-4).

From a medical perspective, FGM has no health benefits, and it harms girls and women in many ways. Immediate complications can include severe pain, shock, hemorrhage, tetanus or sepsis, urinary retention, open sores in the genital region, and injury to nearby genital tissue. Long-term consequences

TABLE 32-4 Types of Female Genital Mutilation (FGM)

Type	Description
Type 1 FGM (Clitoridectomy)	Partial or total removal of the clitoris (a small, sensitive, and erectile part of the female genitals) and, rarely, the prepuce (the fold of skin surrounding the clitoris) as well
Type II FGM (Excision)	Clitoridectomy with partial or total excision of the labia minora, with or without excision of the labia majora
Type III FGM (Infibulation)	Narrowing of the vaginal opening through the creation of a covering seal, formed by cutting and repositioning the inner or outer labia, with or without the removal of the clitoris. Type III is more likely than other types of FGM to result in infertility.
Type IV FGM (Other)	All other harmful procedures to the female genitalia for nonmedical purposes, e.g., pricking, piercing, incising, scraping, and cauterizing the genital area.

From World Health Organization. (2014). *Female genital mutilation*. Retrieved from http://www.who.int/mediacentre/factsheets/fs241/en/#

can include recurrent infections in the bladder and urinary tract, cysts, infertility, an increased risk of childbirth complications and newborn deaths as well as the need for later surgeries. Women who have undergone FGM may not think of themselves as mutilated. Nurses who care for these women must be sensitive, knowledgeable, culturally competent, and nonjudgmental. Respect for others' health beliefs, practices, and behaviors as well as recognition of the complexity of issues involved is crucial (WHO, 2014).

Domestic Violence

Domestic violence is a broad term that includes child abuse, elder abuse, and abuse of women and men. Abuse can be emotional, physical, sexual, or economic, and it involves fear of one partner by another and control by threats, intimidation, and physical abuse. Nearly 31% of women report having been the victim of some form of violence from an intimate partner in their lifetime. This estimate is likely underrepresentative of actual rates due to underreporting. Although all women are at potential risk for abuse, factors that elevate risk include young age, substance abuse, marital difficulties, and economic hardships (Moyer, 2013). Violence is rarely a one-time occurrence in a relationship; it usually continues and escalates in severity.

All women should be screened for domestic violence. For women who are not pregnant, screening should occur at routine visits. For women who are pregnant, screening should occur over the course of the pregnancy, including at the first prenatal visit, at least once per trimester, and at the

postpartum checkup. Abuse should be considered a factor in the presentation of medical complaints because experiences with abuse may adversely affect health status or the ability to comply with medical recommendations (Moyer, 2013). See Box 32-2.

Incest and Childhood Sexual Abuse

Sexual assault is one of the most underreported crimes (Rape, Abuse, & Incest National Network [RAINN], 2015). Strangers do molest children. But in at least 80% of cases, the perpetrators of sexual abuse are known to the child and often are authority figures that the child trusts (American Academy of Pediatrics, 2015). Victims of sexual assault are more likely to suffer from depression or posttraumatic stress disorder, abuse alcohol or drugs, and contemplate suicide (RAINN, 2015). The nurse should plan to offer support and appropriate referrals to psychologists, community resources, and self-help groups.

Rape and Sexual Assault

In 2013, there were an average of 293,066 victims of rape and sexual assault. That means every 107 seconds, another American was sexually assaulted (RAINN, 2015a,b). Screening for abuse, rape, and violence should be part of routine assessment because women often do not report or seek treatment for assault. Often, the assailant is a partner, husband, or date. Nurses may encounter women with infections or pregnancies related to sexual assault who require support, understanding, and comprehensive care. Women who have experienced rape or sexual abuse may be very anxious about pelvic examinations, labor, pelvic or breast irradiation, or any treatment or examination that involves hands-on treatment or requires removal of clothing.

Physical Assessment

The nurse can use the physical assessment time to educate patients on their reproductive health, including normal physiologic processes, like menstruation and menopause, and to assess possible abnormalities. This section focuses on physical assessment, including gynecologic and breast examinations. Annual breast and pelvic examinations are important for all women 18 years of age or older and for those who are sexually active, regardless of age. Most women have a gynecologic examination as part of their annual physical. The gynecologic portion is often the last portion of the physical examination as care providers tend to move from less sensitive areas to more sensitive ones. This also gives the patient a chance to become comfortable with the examination and her provider.

Pelvic Examination

The pelvic portion of the assessment consists of external and internal inspection and palpation or structures and

BOX 32-2

GUIDELINES FOR NURSING CARE

Managing Domestic Violence

Equipment

- Appropriate documentation forms
- Camera
- Appropriate patient teaching materials

Procedure

ACTIONS	RATIONALE
1. Reassure the woman that she is not alone.	1. Women often believe that they are alone in experiencing abuse at the hands of their partners.
2. Express your belief that no one should be hurt, that abuse is the fault of the abuser, and that it is against the law.	2. Sharing these beliefs lets the woman know that no one deserves to be abused and that she has not caused the abuse.
3. Assure the woman that her information is confidential, although it does become part of her medical record. *If children are suspected of being abused or are being abused, the law requires that this be reported to the authorities.* Some states require reporting of spousal or partner abuse. Domestic violence agencies and medical and nursing groups disagree with this policy and are trying to have it changed. Serious opposition is based on the fact that reporting does not and cannot currently guarantee a woman's safety and may place her in more danger. It also may interfere with a patient's willingness to discuss her personal life and concerns with care providers. This places a serious barrier in the way of comprehensive nursing care. If nurses are in doubt about laws on reporting abuse, they need to check with their local or state domestic violence agency.	3. Often women are afraid that their information will be reported to the police or protective services and their children may be taken away.
4. Document the woman's statement of abuse, and take photographs of any visible injuries if written formal consent has been obtained. (Emergency departments usually have a camera available if one is not on the nursing unit.)	4. The written statement and photographic proof provide documentation of injuries that may be needed for later legal or criminal proceedings.
5. Provide teaching: • Inform the woman that shelters are available to ensure safety for her and her children. (Lengths of stay in shelters vary by state but often are up to 2 months. Staff often assist with housing, jobs, and the emotional distress that accompanies the break-up of the family.) Provide a list of shelters. • Inform the woman that violence gets worse, not better. • If the woman chooses to go to a shelter, let her make the call. • If the woman chooses to return to the abuser, remain nonjudgmental and provide information that will make her safer than she was before disclosing her situation. • Make sure that the woman has a 24-hour hotline telephone number that provides information and support (Spanish translation and a device for the deaf are also available) as well as contact information for her local police (and a reminder about the availability of 911 service). • Assist her to set up a safety plan in case she decides to return home. (A safety plan is an organized plan for departure with packed bags and important papers hidden in a safe spot.)	5. These options may be life-saving for the woman and her children.

Patient Education

Pelvic Examination

A pelvic examination includes assessment of the appearance of the vulva, vagina, and cervix and the size and shape of the uterus and ovaries to ensure reproductive health and absence of illness. The nurse should share the following information with the patient in order to help make the examination proceed more smoothly:

- You may have a feeling of fullness or pressure during the examination, but you should not feel pain. It is important to relax because if you are very tense, you may feel discomfort.
- It is normal to feel uncomfortable and apprehensive.
- A narrow, warmed speculum will be inserted to visualize the cervix.
- A Papanicolaou (Pap) smear will be obtained and should not be uncomfortable.
- You may watch the examination with a mirror if you choose.
- The examination usually takes no longer than 5 minutes.
- Draping will be used to minimize exposure and reduce embarrassment.

organs. Gynecologic examinations may be uncomfortable or even distressing for some women. It is important, then, that the nurse employs assessment techniques that help patients feel more comfortable and less vulnerable. Patient education is essential as appropriate and accurate information can help to minimize the fear and negative feelings that some women associate with gynecologic examinations (Box 32-3).

Before the examination begins, the patient should be asked to empty her bladder. This can aid the examination as a full bladder can make palpation of pelvic organs difficult for the examiner, which may increase discomfort to the patient.

Positioning

Although several positions may be used for the pelvic examination, the supine lithotomy position is used most commonly. In this position, the patient lies on the table with her feet in stirrups, buttocks at the edge of the table, and thighs spread as widely apart as possible. Supine lithotomy offers several advantages as it is more comfortable for most women and allows better eye contact between patient and examiner. It may also facilitate the bimanual examination as well. However, it may be uncomfortable for some women, and some patients may need to be reminded to keep their legs in the proper position. Sims' position (patient on left side with her right leg bent at a 90-degree angle) may be used with a patient who is unable to maintain the supine lithotomy position due to acute illness or disability. The presence of a disability does not justify skipping any parts of the physical assessment, including the pelvic examination.

Inspection

After the patient is positioned, the examiner inspects the external genitalia. Lesions of any type are evaluated. In the nulliparous woman, the labia minora come together at the opening of the vagina. In a woman who has delivered children vaginally, the labia minora may gape and vaginal tissue may protrude. Structural changes from childbirth include **cystocele** (bulging of bladder into the vagina), **rectocele** (bulging of rectum into the vagina), or **uterine prolapse** (uterus falling out of normal position). The examiner may ask the patient to bear down in order to visualize these changes.

Palpation

Using the fingers of a gloved hand, the examiner gently separates the labia and palpates the lower part of the vagina. In many women who have not had vaginal intercourse, the **hymen** can be palpated within the vaginal opening. In the sexually active woman, remnants of the hymen may be palpated as a rim of scar tissue. The greater vestibular glands (Bartholin glands) lie between the labia minora and the hymenal ring and should be free of abscess and drainage.

Speculum Examination

The speculum is an instrument used to open the vaginal walls for internal inspection of the vagina and cervix as well as for performance of the Papanicolaou (Pap) smear. Warming the speculum prior to insertion can be more comfortable for the patient. Lubrication of the outer superior and inferior blade of the plastic vaginal speculum with a small amount of a water-soluble lubricant gel decreases the pain associated with insertion and opening of the vaginal speculum in both premenopausal and postmenopausal women without affecting the quality of the cytology results during the collection of Pap test specimens (Simavli, Kaygusuz, Kinay, & Cukur, 2014). When the speculum is positioned properly, it is opened slowly to visualize the cervix and then tightened to hold it in place for inspection of the cervix (Fig. 32-4). The examiner inspects the cervical surface for any lesions or anomalies. The cervix typically is 2 to 3 cm wide and pink in color with a smooth appearance. Discharge from the cervical os may be cultured to rule out infection or disease.

While withdrawing the speculum, the practitioner inspects the vagina. Vaginal discharge, which may be normal or may result from vaginitis, may be present (Table 32-5). Purulent material appearing at the cervical os is obtained for culture with a sterile applicator. In patients at high risk for infection, routine cultures for gonococcal and chlamydial organisms are recommended.

While the speculum is in place, a **Papanicolaou** (Pap) smear is obtained (this test is discussed in detail under diagnostic evaluation).

Bimanual Palpation

After the internal inspection, a bimanual examination of the pelvic organs may be conducted. The practitioner inserts two

FIGURE 32-4 Technique for speculum examination of the vagina and cervix. (**A**) The labia are spread apart with a gloved left hand while the speculum is grasped in the right hand and turned counterclockwise before being inserted into the vagina. Once the speculum is inserted, the blades are spread apart (**B**) to reveal the cervical os (**C**).

lubricated fingers from one hand into the vagina of the patient while the other hand compresses from the outside to assess the reproductive organs. The practitioner assesses size and position of the uterus and ovarian structures while looking for any tenderness upon movement of the organs. Some mild discomfort is not unusual when palpating the ovaries. Many practitioners also perform a rectal examination at this time.

Breast Examination

The American Cancer Society (ACS) recommends that women at average risk for breast cancer undergo a clinical breast examination at least every 3 years while in their 20s and 30s and then annually thereafter (see Chapter 33). In the normal progression of a general physical examination, the

TABLE 32-5 Vaginal Discharge Characteristics

Cause of Discharge	Symptoms	Odor	Consistency/Color
Physiologic	None	None	Mucus/white
Candida infection	Itching, irritation	Yeast odor or none	Thin to thick, curd-like/white
Bacterial vaginosis	Odor	Fishy, often noticed after intercourse	Thin/grayish or yellow
Trichomonas infection	Irritation, odor	Malodorous	Copious, often frothy/yellow-green
Atrophic	Vulvar or vaginal dryness	Occasional mild malodor	Usually scant and mucoid/may be blood-tinged

breasts would be examined before the genitals as the provider moves from "head to toe." Before the examination, the patient should be asked if she has any known, palpable masses and if there is any associated pain, swelling, redness, nipple discharge, or skin changes.

Research has not shown a clear benefit of regular physical breast exams done by either a health professional (clinical breast exams) or by the woman herself (breast self-exams). There is very little evidence that these tests help find breast cancer early when women also get screening mammograms. Most often when breast cancer is detected because of symptoms (such as a lump), a woman discovers the symptom during usual activities such as bathing or dressing. Women should be familiar with how their breasts normally look and feel and report any changes to a health care provider right away (ACS, 2017). Breast cancers that are found because they are causing symptoms tend to be larger and more likely to have already spread beyond the breast. In contrast, breast cancers found during screening examinations are more likely to be smaller and still confined to the breast (ACS, 2015).

Inspection

Examination begins with inspection. The patient disrobes to the waist and sits in a comfortable position facing the examiner. The breasts are inspected for size and symmetry. A slight variation in size between the breasts is common and generally normal. Inspect the skin for color, venous pattern, thickening, or edema. Nipple inversion of one or both breasts is not uncommon and is significant only when of recent origin. Ulceration or rashes require evaluation. Then the breasts are inspected while the patient raises both arms overhead and again while she places her hands on her waist, pushing her shoulders in. These movements cause contraction of the pectoral muscles and should not alter the breast contour or nipple direction. Dimpling or retraction observed during these position changes suggests an underlying mass. The nurse observes for deep pin-point dimpling of the skin similar to an orange's skin (termed *peau d'orange*), which is associated with carcinoma. The clavicular and axillary regions are visually inspected before palpation.

Two of the more common issues providers may find affecting the nipple are nipple discharge and fissures.

Nipple Discharge. Nipple discharge in a woman who is not lactating may be related to many causes (Table 32-6), although any discharge that is spontaneous, persistent, or unilateral is of concern. Clear discharge on expression is usually normal, while green discharge could indicate an infection. Bloody discharge does not always indicate malignancy. Tumors of the pituitary or thyroid gland or brain, encephalitis (a brain infection), and head injuries also can cause a nipple discharge. Oral contraceptives, pregnancy,

TABLE 32-6 Nipple Discharge and Associated Causes

Description of Discharge	Associated Conditions
Clear discharge	Galactorrhea, blunt injury, fibrocystic changes
Bloody discharge	Noncancerous breast tumor (intraductal papilloma), breast cancer (less common), blunt injury, a blocked duct (mammary duct ectasia)
Greenish discharge	Fibroadenoma (a noncancerous solid lump), galactorrhea, a blocked duct (mammary duct ectasia)
Pus discharge	Breast infection, abscess
Milky discharge	Galactorrhea (in women who are not breastfeeding)

hypertension, chlorpromazine-type medications, and frequent breast stimulation may be contributing factors. Among women who have an abnormal discharge, benign conditions are much more common than breast cancer; in fact, breast cancer is the cause in fewer than 12% of cases (Patel, Falcon, & Drukteinis, 2014).

A discharge from one breast is likely to be caused by a problem with that breast, such as a noncancerous or cancerous breast tumor. A discharge from both breasts is more likely to be caused by a problem outside the breast, such as an imbalance of hormones made by the pituitary or thyroid gland, or by drugs. If a nipple discharge persists for more than one menstrual cycle or seems unusual to the woman, she should seek evaluation. Postmenopausal women who have a nipple discharge should seek evaluation promptly.

Fissure. A fissure is a longitudinal ulcer that may develop in breastfeeding women. Improper infant positioning may irritate the nipple and may form a painful, raw area, which can be a site of infection. Comfort care measures include daily washing with water, massage with breast milk or lanolin, and exposure to air.

 Nursing Alert

Very small erosions (1 to 2 mm) of the nipple epithelium may be the only manifestation of Paget carcinoma (a rare type of breast cancer that occurs in the ducts adjacent to the nipple and areola and spreads to the skin of the nipple and the areola) (Karam, 2013). It accounts for only 1% of breast cancers and may be associated with ductal carcinoma in situ (DCIS) (Karam, 2013). See Chapter 33 for more information.

FIGURE 32-5 Breast examination with the woman in a supine position. The entire surface of the breast is palpated from the outer edge of the breast to the nipple; palpation patterns are circular or clockwise, wedge, and vertical strip.

Palpation

Both breasts are palpated with the patient sitting up (upright) and lying down (supine). The entire surface of the breasts and axillary tails are palpated systematically in dime-sized circles, from the outer limits of the breast toward the nipple in a clockwise direction (Fig. 32-5). If a mass is detected, it is described by its location (e.g., left breast, 2 cm from the nipple at 2 o'clock position). Size, shape, consistency, border delineation, and mobility are included in the description. Different phases of the menstrual cycle cause changes in the breast tissue.

Special Considerations in Health Assessment

Cultural Considerations

The health care system is an area in which cultural divisions are notable. Cultural views and beliefs differ, and traditional cultural beliefs can affect women's health care encounters. A nurse who is culturally competent is able to deliver services that are respectful of and responsive to the health beliefs, practices, and cultural and linguistic needs of diverse patients. Cultural competency is critical to reducing health disparities and improving access to high-quality health care, health care that is respectful of and responsive to the needs of diverse patients (National Institutes of Health [NIH], 2015). Refer to Chapter 2 for further details on cultural competency. The nurse should refrain from making assumptions about patients from any ethnic group. Instead, the nurse should feel comfortable asking the patient questions about how she perceives her health care and what she needs in order to make her feel comfortable and confident in the health care setting. A number of social, cultural, and gender-related obstacles can prevent a woman from realizing her preferences (Lewis, Doshi, de Leon, & Refaat, 2014). Knowledge of various cultures can help nurses adapt to the multiple personal preferences and cultural perspectives of patients whose ethnicity, race, age, sex, sexual orientation, religion, language, and/or socioeconomic status differ from their own. Effective communication and positive relationships are essential to developing collaborative culturally competent care and shared decision-making that result in women's greater understanding of their health care plans, satisfaction, and improved health outcomes (Jesse & Kirkpatrick, 2013).

Women with Disabilities

About 27 million women in the United States have disabilities—and the number is growing. More than 50% of women older than 65 years of age are living with a disability. Women with disabilities may need special care to address their individual needs. In addition, they need the same general health care as women without disabilities, and they also may need additional care to address their specific needs. However, research has shown that many women with disabilities may not receive regular health screenings within recommended guidelines (Centers for Disease Control and Prevention [CDC], 2014a). Nurses

Assessment of Women with Disabilities

Health History

Address questions directly to the woman herself rather than to people accompanying her. Ask about:

- Self-care limitations resulting from her disability (ability to feed and dress herself, use of assistive devices, transportation requirements, other assistance needed)
- Sensory limitations (lack of sensation, low vision, deaf or hard of hearing)
- Accessibility issues (ability to get to health care provider, transfer to examination table, accessibility of office/clinic of health care provider, previous experiences with health care providers, health screening practices, her understanding of physical examination)
- Cognitive or developmental changes that affect understanding
- Limitations secondary to disability that affect general health issues and reproductive health and health care
- Sexual function and concerns (those of all women and those who may be affected by the presence of a disabling condition)
- Menstrual history and menstrual hygiene practices
- Physical, sexual, or psychological abuse (including abuse by care providers; abuse by neglect or withholding or withdrawing assistive devices or personal health care)
- Presence of secondary disabilities (i.e., those resulting from the patient's primary disability: pressure ulcers, spasticity, osteoporosis, etc.)
- Health concerns related to aging with a disability

Physical Assessment

Provide instructions directly to the woman herself rather than to people accompanying her; provide written or audiotaped instructions.

Ask the woman what assistance she needs for the physical examination, and provide assistance if needed:

- Undressing and dressing
- Providing a urine specimen
- Standing on scale to be weighed (provide alternative means of obtaining weight if she is unable to stand on scale)
- Moving on and off the examination table
- Assuming, changing, and maintaining positions

Consider the fatigue experienced by the woman during a lengthy examination and allow her time to rest.

Provide assistive devices and other aids/methods needed to allow adequate communication with the patient (interpreters, signers, large-print written materials).

Complete the examination as it would be indicated for any other woman; having a disability is never justification for omitting parts of the physical examination, including the pelvic examination.

---

assessing women with disabilities may require additional time to complete an assessment (Box 32-4) in a sensitive and unhurried manner.

Breast cancer is a major public health concern for all women, including women with disabilities. Women who have disabilities less likely to have had a mammogram compared to able-bodied women and are significantly less likely to have been screened within the recommended guidelines women (CDC, 2014b). Studies also show higher rates of death related to breast cancer among women with a disability, even when diagnosed at the same stage as women without a disability. Having regular mammograms can lower the risk of dying from breast cancer (CDC, 2014a). Reminding women of the need for recommended and regular checkups, clinical breast examinations, and mammograms is an important part of nursing care.

Gerontologic Considerations

Women represent the majority of the population 65 years of age and over. On average, women live 6 to 8 years longer than men and, therefore, encounter and live with more physical and medical limitations with aging (Lewis et al., 2014). Elderly women are more likely to place value on screening services, such as mammography, instead of preventative health care counseling regarding things like the effects of diet and exercise on longevity. While diagnostic screening measures are appropriate, preventative health issues may be more likely to positively impact quality and longevity of life in the elderly woman and, therefore, may be appropriate for the practitioner to discuss with elderly patient (McNamara & Walsh, 2015). However, nurses should encourage all aging women to undergo an annual gynecologic examination, and they should use this time to educate and reassure their aging patients.

Caring for older women with gynecologic concerns requires the nurse to be prepared for a wide spectrum of issues. A clinical approach to older women goes beyond a traditional history and physical examination; nurses need to include functional, social, and psychosocial elements that affect the older woman's well-being and quality of life (Johnson & Reuben, 2014). The optimal treatment modality for the elderly patient should not be based on age alone. Many older women, regardless of advancing chronologic age, remain in excellent health. Therefore, the woman's treatment preferences must play a role in the decision-making process, and this should include making her aware of preventative health activities that may be just as important to her continued health as diagnostic procedures (Chang & Williams, 2014).

Abnormal gynecologic findings in the elderly woman include perineal pruritus, which may indicate a disease process, and vulvar dystrophy, characterized by thickened or whitish discoloration of tissue. With relaxing pelvic musculature, uterine prolapse and relaxation of the vaginal walls can occur. Performance of Kegel exercises to strengthen the pelvic floor is frequently recommended. Refer to Chapter 33, Box 33-9 for details regarding Kegel exercises.

Diagnostic Evaluation

Papanicolaou (Pap) Cytologic Test for Cervical Cancer

Often cervical cancer can be found early, and sometimes even prevented entirely, by having regular Pap tests. If detected early, cervical cancer is one of the most successfully treatable cancers. Deaths from cervical cancer are higher in populations around the world where women do not have routine screening for cervical cancer. In fact, cervical cancer is the major cause of cancer deaths in many women in developing countries. Usually these women are diagnosed with late-stage cancers rather than precancers or early cancers. In the United States, however, the death rate from cervical cancer has declined by more than 50% over the last 30 years. This is thought to be mainly related to the effectiveness of Pap test screening (ACS, 2014). Incorporation of the Pap test into routine well-woman care has decreased the incidence of cervical cancer to levels lower than that of breast or ovarian cancer.

During the Pap test, a sample of cells and mucus is lightly scraped or brushed from the cervix. If the cervix has been removed, the cells will be sampled from the upper part of the vagina, known as the vaginal cuff. This test should not be performed when a patient is menstruating as blood can interfere with interpretation. Although the Pap test is an excellent screening system, it is not a diagnostic test; both false-positive and false-negative results may occur. The Bethesda Classification system has been developed to promote consistency in reporting Pap results.

Nursing Alert
To make a Pap test as accurate as possible, patients are informed to:

- *Try not to schedule an appointment for a time during your menstrual period. The best time is at least 5 days after your menstrual period stops.*
- *Don't use tampons; birth-control foams or jellies; other vaginal creams, moisturizers, or lubricants; or vaginal medicines for 2 to 3 days before the test.*
- *Don't douche for 2 to 3 days before the test.*
- *Don't have sexual intercourse for 2 days before the test (ACS, 2014).*

Although patients may assume (incorrectly) that an abnormal Pap smear signifies cancer, this is not generally the case. It simply means just that, it is abnormal: Under the microscope, the appearance of a few cells differs in some way from the classic appearance of healthy, intact cervical cells. The difference could be due to local irritation, a non-HPV

BOX 32-5 | **Follow-up According to Pap Test Results**

- 21–29 years of age:
  - HPV testing should not be used for screening in this age group. It is done as secondary testing for management decisions.
  - HPV-positive ASC-US: Repeat cytology in 12 months.
  - Cytology of LSIL: Repeat cytology in 12 months.
  - Cytology more severe than LSIL: Colposcopy is recommended.
  - Cytology negative or HPV-Negative ASC-US: Rescreen with cytology in 3 years.
- 30–65 years of age:
  - HPV and cytology "co-testing" every 5 years (preferred screening) results
    - HPV-positive ASC-US or cytology of LSIL or more severe: Colposcopy is recommended.
    - HPV-positive, cytology negative:
      - Option 1: 12-month follow-up with co-testing.
      - Option 2: Test for HPV16 or HPV16/18 genotypes.
        - If HPV16 or HPV16/18 positive: Refer for colposcopy.
        - If HPV16 or HPV16/18 negative: 12-month follow-up with co-testing.
    - Co-test negative or HPV-negative ASC-US: Rescreen with co-testing in 5 years.
  - Cytology alone every 3 years (acceptable screening) results
    - HPV-positive ASC-US or cytology of LSIL or more severe: Colposcopy is recommended.
    - Cytology negative or HPV-negative ASC-US: Rescreen with cytology in 3 years
- Over 65 years of age:
  - No screening following adequate negative prior screening.
  - Women with a history of CIN2 or more severe diagnosis should continue routine screening for at least 20 years.
- After hysterectomy:
  - No screening. This applies to women without a cervix and without history of CIN2 or a more severe diagnosis in the past 20 years or cervical cancer ever.

CIN, cervical intraepithelial neoplasia; LSIL, low-grade squamous intraepithelial lesions; ASC-US, atypical squamous cells of undetermined significance; HPV, human papillomavirus. Adapted from American Society for Colposcopy and Cervical Pathology. (2013). Algorithms: Updated consensus guidelines for managing abnormal cervical cancer screening tests and cancer precursors http://www.asccp.org/Portals/9/docs/ASCCP%20 Management%20Guidelines_August%202014.pdf infection, a low-risk or high-risk HPV type, or even a mistake in the preparation of the cell sample (National Cervical Cancer Coalition, 2015). Abnormal Pap results require prompt notification and follow-up as abnormalities detected in a Pap test may signify cellular changes that may lead to cancer if left untreated (Box 32-5). Factors associated with poor adherence to recommendations or lack of follow-up include young age, nonwhite race/ethnicity, less than high school education, lack of health insurance, less knowledge about HPV, and physiologic distress (Fish et al., 2013). The nurse should provide simple and clear explanations as well as emotional support designed to meet the needs of the specific patients that may encourage appropriate and timely follow-up. The message should be persuasive enough to convince women of the importance of follow-up while at the same time minimizing anxiety and distress (Box 32-6).

Uterine Diagnostics

Certain uterine conditions, such as dysfunctional uterine bleeding, may require diagnostic testing as well. Diagnostic tests performed on uterine and peritoneal tissues include endometrial (aspiration) biopsy, dilation and curettage (D&C), laparoscopy, hysteroscopy, and **endometrial ablation**. For information on these procedures, refer to Table 32-7.

Mammography

Mammography is a breast-imaging technique that takes about 20 minutes and is performed in a hospital radiology department or independent imaging center that can detect nonpalpable lesions and assist in diagnosing palpable masses. The breast is mechanically compressed from top to bottom (craniocaudal view) and side to side (mediolateral oblique view) (Fig. 32-6). Although usually two views of each breast are taken for a screening mammogram, for some women, such as those with breast implants or large breasts, additional pictures may be needed. Experiences of slight discomfort are due to the maximum compression necessary for proper visualization. Although mammography may detect a breast tumor before it is clinically palpable (i.e., smaller than 1 cm), mammography has limitations. Overall, screening mammograms do not find about one in five instances of breast cancer. They do not work as well in women with

---

BOX 32-6

Diagnostic Testing Indicated by Abnormal Pap Test Results

Colposcopy

All suspicious Pap smears should be evaluated by colposcopy. Nurse practitioners and gynecologists require special training in this diagnostic technique.

The colposcope is a portable microscope used to visualize the cervix and obtain samples of abnormal tissue for analysis. The examiner applies acetic acid (similar to vinegar) to the cervix to outline suspect areas.

A cervical biopsy or endocervical curettage may be performed during colposcopy. Tissue analysis is used to determine whether abnormal changes have occurred. If these biopsy specimens show premalignant cells, cervical dysplasia, or cervical intraepithelial neoplasia (CIN), the patient usually requires further intervention (cryotherapy, laser therapy, or a cone biopsy).

Cervical Biopsy

Abnormal colposcopy findings indicating the need for biopsy include leukoplakia (white plaque visible before applying acetic acid), acetowhite tissue (white epithelium after applying acetic acid), punctation (dilated capillaries occurring in a dotted or stippled pattern), mosaicism (a tile-like pattern), and atypical vascular patterns.

Biopsy involves taking a sample of tissue from the cervix for further analysis.

Cryotherapy and Laser Therapy

Both are outpatient procedures. Cryotherapy is the freezing of suspect cervical tissue with nitrous oxide. It is good for small areas of mild to moderate dysplasia. It can be used to treat carcinoma in situ of the cervix (stage 0) but not invasive cancer.

Cryotherapy may result in cramping and occasional feelings of faintness (vasovagal response). A watery discharge is normal for a few weeks after the procedure as the cervix heals. It is not precisely controlled so abnormal cells may be left behind.

Laser treatment uses a tiny beam of light to vaporize abnormal cervical cells. The laser beam is directed through a colposcope, is more precise than cryosurgery, and has the benefit of targeting only the diseased cervical tissues. Healing is much faster than with freezing. Not all offices have lasers, thus increasing costs to patient if treatment is carried out in the hospital. This, too, can be used to treat carcinoma in situ of the cervix (stage 0) but not invasive cancer.

Cone Biopsy and Loop Electrosurgical Excision Procedure

If endocervical curettage findings indicate abnormal changes or if the lesion extends into the canal, the patient may undergo a cone biopsy. The cone biopsy can be performed surgically or with a procedure called loop electrosurgical excision procedure (LEEP).

LEEP can be performed in the outpatient setting and has a high success rate in removal of abnormal cervical tissue. The provider uses a fine wire loop with electrical energy flowing through it to remove abnormal cervical tissue. Samples are sent to pathology.

Usually cone biopsy is done in an operating room with a laser or conventional surgical instruments (cold-cone). A cone- or cylinder-shaped piece of the cervix is removed. Also a diagnostic cone may treat the problem.

TABLE **32-7** Uterine Diagnostic Tests

Test	Description
Endometrial (aspiration) biopsy	Method of obtaining endometrial tissue by placing a flexible suction tube through the cervix into the uterus. This tissue sample permits diagnosis of cellular changes in the endometrium. Indicated in cases of midlife irregular bleeding, postmenopausal bleeding, and irregular bleeding while taking hormone therapy or tamoxifen.
Dilation and curettage (D&C)	Can be used as a diagnostic or therapeutic tool. Cervical canal is dilated and the endometrium is scraped. Can be used to gather endometrial tissue for cytologic examination, control abnormal uterine bleeding, and as a therapeutic measure for incomplete miscarriage.
Laparoscopy (pelvic peritoneoscopy)	Involves inserting laparoscope into peritoneal cavity through small incision below the umbilicus to allow visualization of the pelvic structures. Used for diagnostic purposes (e.g., in cases of pelvic pain when no cause can be found) as well as for surgical procedures, including tubal ligation, ovarian biopsy, hysterectomy, and adhesion lysis.
Hysteroscopy (transcervical intrauterine endoscopy)	Allows direct visualization of all parts of the uterine cavity by means of a lighted optical instrument. Under a local anesthetic, the hysteroscope is passed into the cervical canal and advanced 1 or 2 cm under direct vision. Uterine-distending fluid is infused through the instrument to dilate the uterine cavity and enhance visibility.
Endometrial ablation (destruction of the uterine lining)	Performed in cases of severe bleeding not responsive to other therapies. Performed in an outpatient setting under general, regional, or local anesthesia, the uterus is distended with a fluid infusion. Providers use a hysteroscope and resector (cutting loop), roller ball (a barrel-shaped electrode), or laser beam to destroy the lining of the uterus. Hemorrhage, perforation, and burns can occur. This rapid procedure is an alternative to hysterectomy for some patients.
Hysterosalpingography (HSG)	Radiographic study of the uterus and fallopian tubes performed to evaluate infertility or tubal patency and to detect abnormal conditions in the uterine cavity. With the patient in lithotomy position, the cervix is exposed with a speculum. A cannula is inserted into the cervix, and a contrast agent is injected into the uterine cavity and the fallopian tubes. Then x-rays are taken to show the path and the distribution of the contrast agent.
Ultrasonography (ultrasound [US])	Useful adjunct to the physical examination for patients with abnormal pelvic findings. Based on transmission of pulsed ultrasonic sound waves via a transducer that is either placed on the abdomen (abdominal scan) or through a vaginal probe (vaginal US). The entire procedure takes usually less than 10 minutes and involves no ionizing radiation.
Computed tomography (CT)	More effective than US for obese patients or for those with a distended bowel; demonstrates tumor and any extension into the retroperitoneal lymph nodes and skeletal tissue. Does expose the patient to radiation. More costly than US procedures.
Magnetic resonance imaging (MRI)	Produces patterns that are finer and more definitive than other imaging procedures; does not expose patients to radiation. High cost is the major drawback.

dense breasts since dense breasts can hide a tumor. Dense breasts are more common in younger women, pregnant women, and women who are breastfeeding, but any woman can have dense breasts.

Current screening guidelines of the ACS recommend a mammogram every year beginning at 40 years of age. The ACS also has guidelines for older women and women at increased risk of breast cancer. Three other diagnostic tests to detect/view breast masses are ductogram (galactogram), ultrasound (US), and magnetic resonance imaging (MRI) (Table 32-8).

Other Radiologic Tests for Breasts Masses

Ductogram, also called a galactogram, is used sometimes to help find the cause of any worrisome nipple discharge. In this test, a very thin tube is inserted into the opening of a duct in the nipple where the discharge is coming from and a small amount of contrast material is injected. The contrast material outlines the shape of the duct on x-ray and can show whether there is a mass inside the duct.

Ultrasound (US), also known as sonography, uses sound waves to look inside a part of the body. This test is painless and has no radiation exposure. Breast US is used most often to evaluate breast problems that are found during a mammogram or physical examination and to guide a needle biopsy of a suspicious mass. In someone with a breast tumor, US also may be used to assess lymph nodes under the arm. Breast US may be helpful to use along with a mammogram when screening a woman with dense breast tissue.

Magnetic resonance imaging (MRI) of the breast is a highly sensitive technology that uses magnets and radio waves instead of x-rays to produce very detailed, cross-sectional

X-ray tube

X-ray

Compression paddle

X-ray film cassette

A **B**

FIGURE 32-6 The mammography procedure (**A**) relies on x-ray imaging to produce the mammogram (**B**), which, in this case, reveals a breast lump.

pictures. It is a useful diagnostic adjunct to mammography without exposure to radiation. The procedure cannot always distinguish accurately between malignant and benign breast conditions. This is why MRI is not recommended as a screening test for women at average risk of breast cancer as it would result in unneeded biopsies and other tests in many of these women.

MRI is most useful when assessing for disease that is either multifocal (more than one tumor in the same quadrant of the breast) or multicentric (more than one tumor in different quadrants of the breast), chest wall involvement, tumor recurrence, or response to chemotherapy.

MRI also can identify occult (undetectable) breast cancer and determine the integrity of saline or silicone breast implants.

Disadvantages of MRI include high cost, variations in technique and interpretation, and the potential for patient claustrophobia.

Breast Tissue Analysis

Diagnostic tests performed on breast tissue are described in Table 32-8.

MALE REPRODUCTIVE SYSTEM

In the male, several organs serve as parts of both the urinary tract and the reproductive system. Disorders in the male reproductive organs may interfere with the functions of one or both of these systems. As a result, diseases of the male reproductive system are commonly treated by a urologist.

TABLE **32-8 Procedures for Breast Tissue Analysis**

Procedure	Description
Percutaneous biopsy	Samples palpable and nonpalpable lesions via needle or core biopsy that obtains tissue by making a small puncture in the skin. It is less invasive than a surgical biopsy.
Fine-needle aspiration (FNA)	Small-gauge needle with a syringe is inserted into the mass or area of nodularity. Cellular material obtained during the procedure is spread on a glass slide or placed in a preservative and sent for analysis.
Core needle biopsy	Similar to FNA except that a needle with a larger gauge is used (usually 14 gauge). It allows for a more definitive diagnosis than FNA because actual tissue, not just cells, is removed. Often performed for relatively large tumors that are close to the skin surface.
Stereotactic core biopsy	Performed on nonpalpable lesions detected by mammography. After using digital mammography to determine the exact coordinates of the lesion, a core needle is inserted to retrieve samples of the tissue for pathologic examination. Stereotactic biopsy often allows the patient to avoid a surgical biopsy.
Ultrasound-guided core biopsy	Performed on nonpalpable lesions found by ultrasound; does not use radiation and is faster and less expensive than stereotactic core biopsy.
Excisional biopsy (lumpectomy)	Standard procedure for complete pathologic assessment of a palpable breast mass. The entire mass, plus a margin of surrounding tissue, is removed.
Incisional biopsy	Surgical removal of a portion of a mass when complete excision of the area may not be possible or immediately beneficial to the patient. Incisional biopsy is becoming less common as pathologic information can be obtained from core needle biopsy.
Wire needle localization	Technique used to precisely locate nonpalpable masses detected on a mammogram, ultrasound, or MRI that require an excisional biopsy. A long, thin wire is inserted through a needle and guided into the area of abnormality using x-ray or ultrasound. The needle is withdrawn, and the wire is left in place to ensure the precise location.

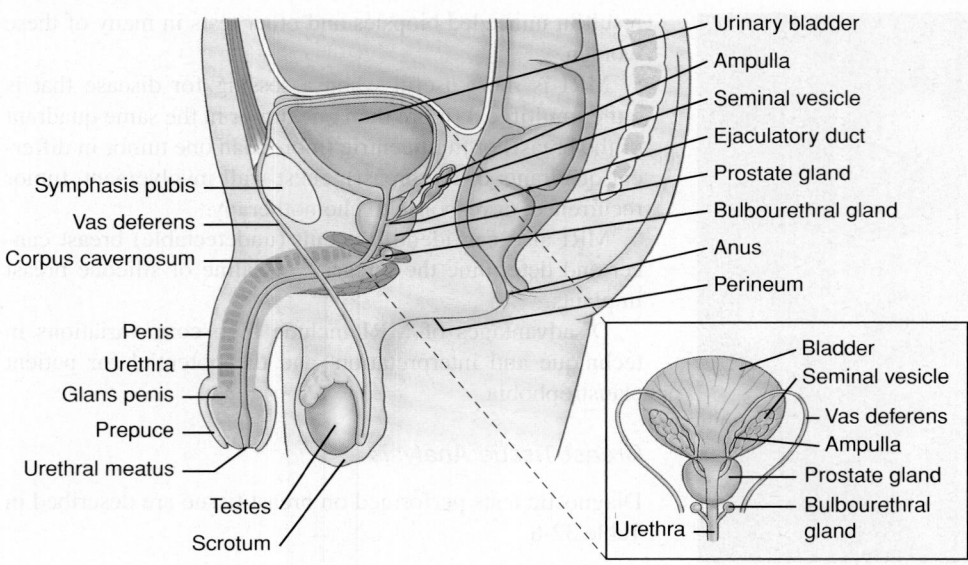

FIGURE 32-7 Structures of the male reproductive system.

ANATOMIC AND PHYSIOLOGIC OVERVIEW

The structures in the male reproductive system include the testes, the vas deferens (ductus deferens) and seminal vesicles, the penis, and certain accessory glands, such as the prostate gland and Cowper gland (bulbourethral gland) (Fig. 32-7).

The testes are formed in the embryo, within the abdominal cavity, near the kidney. During the last month of fetal life, the testes descend posterior to the peritoneum, pierce the abdominal wall in the groin, and progress along the inguinal canal into the scrotum. In this descent, they are accompanied by blood vessels, lymphatics, nerves, and ducts, all of which support the tissue and make up the spermatic cord. This cord extends from the internal inguinal ring through the abdominal wall and the inguinal canal to the scrotum. As the testes descend into the scrotum, a tubular extension of peritoneum accompanies them. This tissue is obliterated during fetal development; the only remaining portion is that which covers the testes, the tunica vaginalis.

The testes are encased in the scrotum, which keeps them at a slightly lower temperature than the rest of the body to facilitate spermatogenesis. The **testes** have a dual function: **spermatogenesis** (production of sperm) and secretion of the male sex hormone **testosterone**, which induces and preserves the male sex characteristics. The testes consist of numerous seminiferous tubules in which the spermatozoa form. Collecting tubules transmit the spermatozoa into the epididymis, a hood-like structure lying on the testes and containing winding ducts that lead into the vas deferens. This firm, tubular structure passes upward through the inguinal canal as part of the spermatic cord to enter the abdominal cavity behind the peritoneum. It then extends downward toward the base of the bladder. An outpouching from this

structure is the seminal vesicle. The tract is continued as the ejaculatory duct, which passes through the prostate gland to enter the urethra. Secretions from the seminal vesicles join secretions from the prostate and exit the penis during ejaculation.

The **penis** has a dual function: it is the organ for copulation and for urination. Anatomically, it consists of the glans penis, the body, and the root. The glans penis is the soft, rounded portion at the distal end of the penis. The urethra opens at the tip of the glans. The glans is naturally covered or protected by elongated penile skin—the foreskin—which may be retracted to expose the glans. However, many men have had the foreskin removed (circumcision) as newborns. The body of the penis is composed of erectile tissues containing numerous blood vessels that become distended, leading to an erection during sexual excitement. The urethra, which passes through the penis, extends from the bladder through the prostate to the distal end of the penis, ending at the meatal opening.

The **prostate gland** lies just below the neck of the bladder. It surrounds the urethra and is traversed by the ejaculatory duct, a continuation of the vas deferens. This gland produces a secretion that is suitable both chemically and physiologically to the needs of the spermatozoa in their passage from the testes. The Cowper gland lies below the prostate, within the posterior aspect of the urethra. This gland empties its secretions into the urethra during ejaculation, providing lubrication.

Gerontologic Considerations

As men age, the prostate gland enlarges, prostate secretion decreases, the scrotum hangs lower, the testes become smaller and less firm, and pubic hair becomes sparser. Changes in gonadal function include a decline in plasma testosterone

TABLE 32-9 GERONTOLOGIC CONSIDERATIONS / Age-Related Changes in the Male Reproductive System

Structural Change	Functional Change	History and Physical Findings
Decrease in secretion of sex hormones, especially testosterone Decreased muscle strength and sexual energy Shrinkage and loss of firmness of testes; thickening of seminiferous tubules Enlargement of prostate gland	Changes in sexual response: prolonged time to reach full erection, rapid penile detumescence (decreased rigidity) and prolonged refractory period Possible decline in libido Decrease in number of viable sperm	Smaller testes Erectile dysfunction Weakening of prostatic contractions Hyperplasia of prostate gland Signs and symptoms of obstruction of lower urinary tract (urgency, frequency, nocturia)

levels and reduced production of progesterone (Table 32-9). Other potential changes include decreased sexual function, slowed sexual responses, an increased incidence of cancer of the genitourinary tract, and possible urinary incontinence or retention.

Male reproductive capability is maintained with advancing age. Although degenerative changes occur in the seminiferous tubules, spermatogenesis continues. However, libido (sexual desire) and potency decrease (Moskovic, Araujo, Lipshultz, & Khera, 2013).

> **Nursing Alert**
> *If the patient is concerned about impotence, the nurse can ask about whether the patient on waking has an early morning erection. If he does, this argues against an organic cause (neurologic, vascular, or endocrinologic) and suggests a functional problem. A thorough history focusing on the onset and progression of symptoms, libido, medications, surgery, and psychosocial issues is important in the evaluation. Screening for depression, hypothyroidism, hypogonadism, and diabetes can be considered (LeBlond, Brown, & DeGowin, 2015).*

Hypogonadism occurs in up to one fourth of older men. This decline is more evident in men older than 60 years of age (Moskovic et al., 2013). In older men, the sexual response slows, attaining an erection takes longer, and full erections may not be attained until climax. Sexual function can be affected by several factors, such as:

- Psychological problems,
- Comorbidities (vasculogenic [atherosclerotic disease, occlusions to vasculature after pelvic trauma, liver failure]),
- Neurogenic (spinal cord injury, Parkinson disease, stroke, tumors, trauma),
- Endocrine (hypogonadism, hyper- and hypothyroidism),
- Mixed causation (diabetes, uremia), and
- Medication related (opioids, alcohol, antihypertensive, antidepressants among others) (Mullins, 2013).

Cancers of the kidney, bladder, prostate, and penis all have increased incidence in men older than 50 years of age. Digital rectal examination (DRE) and screening tests for hematuria may uncover a higher percentage of malignancies at earlier stages and lead to lower morbidity associated with treatment as well as a lower mortality rate.

Urinary incontinence or retention in the elderly man may have many causes, including medications and age-related conditions, such as neurologic disease or benign prostatic hyperplasia (BPH). Diagnostic tests are performed to exclude reversible causes of urinary incontinence.

ASSESSMENT

Health History

Male sexuality is a complex phenomenon that is strongly influenced by personal, cultural, and social factors. Sexuality and male reproductive function become concerns in the presence of illness (Davis, Binik, Amsel, & Carrier, 2013). Assessment of male reproductive function begins with an evaluation of urinary function and symptoms. This assessment also includes a focus on sexual function as well as on manifestations of sexual dysfunction.

The patient is asked about his usual state of health and any recent change in general physical and sexual activity. Any symptoms or changes in function are explored fully and described in detail. These symptoms may include those associated with an obstruction caused by an enlarged prostate gland: increased urinary frequency, decreased force of urine stream, or "double" voiding (the patient needs to urinate two or three times over a period of several minutes to completely empty his bladder). The patient also is assessed for dysuria (painful urination) and hematuria (blood in the urine).

Assessment of sexual function is an essential part of every health history. The extent of the history depends on the patient's presenting symptoms and the presence of factors that may affect sexual function: chronic illnesses (e.g., diabetes, multiple sclerosis, stroke, cardiac disease), use of medications that affect sexual function (e.g., many antihypertensive and anticholesterolemic medications, psychotropic agents), stress, and alcohol use.

Often patients are hesitant to initiate a discussion about sexual issues with their health care providers. By initiating an assessment about sexual concerns, the nurse demonstrates that changes in sexual functioning are valid topics for discussion and provides a safe environment for discussing these sensitive topics.

Physical Assessment

Physical assessment includes examination of the penis and scrotum, the DRE, and assessment of the male breasts.

Penis and Scrotal Examination

The male genitalia are inspected for abnormalities and palpated for masses. The scrotum is palpated carefully for nodules, masses, or inflammation. Examination of the scrotum can reveal such disorders as hydrocele (accumulation of serous fluid in the scrotal sac), varicocele (enlargement of the veins of the spermatic cord), or tumor of the testis. The penis is inspected and palpated for ulcerations, plaques, inflammation, and discharge. The testicular examination provides an excellent opportunity to instruct the patient about techniques for testicular self-examination (TSE) and its importance in early detection of testicular cancer (see Chapter 34). TSE could begin during adolescence, although recently this practice has been called into question with recommendations that TSE not be emphasized due to the low incidence of testicular cancer and the high rate of anxiety associated with self-examination (O'Reilly, Le, Sinyavskaya, & Mandel, 2016).

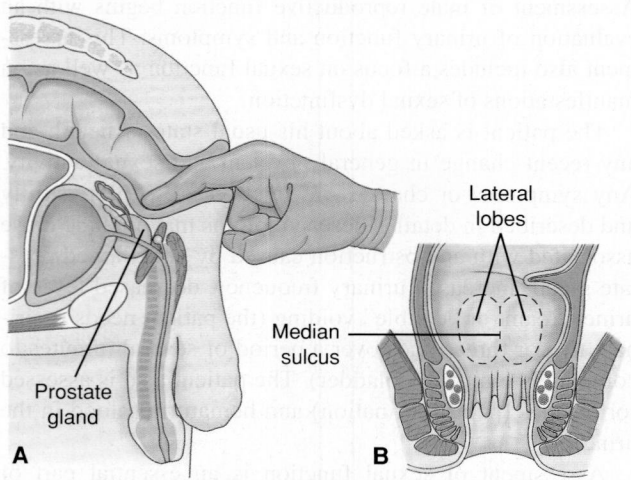

FIGURE 32-8 **A.** Palpation of the prostate gland during digital rectal examination (DRE) enables the examiner to assess the size, shape, and texture of the gland. **B.** The prostate is round, with a palpable median sulcus or groove separating the lateral lobes. It should feel rubbery and free of nodules and masses.

Digital Rectal Examination

The DRE is recommended as part of the regular health checkup for every man older than 50 years of age; it is invaluable in screening for cancer of the prostate gland. The DRE enables the examiner to estimate the size, shape, and consistency of the prostate gland (Fig. 32-8). Tenderness of the prostate gland on palpation and the presence and consistency of any nodules are noted. Although this examination may be embarrassing for the patient, it is an important screening tool.

Assessment of the Male Breasts

Breast cancer can occur in men. Examination of the male breasts and axillae should be included in a physical examination. The nipple and areola are inspected for masses and nipple discharge.

Gynecomastia is the firm enlargement of glandular tissue beneath and immediately surrounding the areola of the male. This is different from the enlargement of soft, fatty tissue, which is caused by obesity.

Diagnostic Evaluation

Prostate-Specific Antigen Test

The prostate gland produces a substance known as prostate-specific antigen (PSA). It can be measured in a blood specimen, and levels increase with certain pathologies: prostate cancer, BPH, acute urinary retention, and acute prostatitis are the most common examples. In most laboratories, the range of values generally considered normal is 0.2 to 4.0 ng/mL, with levels greater than 4.0 considered elevated. The use of age-specific reference ranges for populations helps minimize unnecessary biopsies (American Urological Association [AUA], 2013a, 2013b).

Prostate cancer screening with serum PSA testing has become common practice although its overall utility has recently come into question (AUA, 2013a). The AUA recommends a PSA test beginning at 55 years of age, along with DRE, and then screening at 2- to 4-year intervals, although screening needs to be discussed with each man individually, based on his history and risk. Screening should begin at 40 years of age for men at high risk, including those with a family history of prostate cancer (first-degree relative [father, brother, or son] diagnosed with prostate cancer at an early age [under 65 years of age]) and African-American men (AUA, 2013a). Also PSA is useful to monitor patients for recurrence after treatment for cancer of the prostate.

Ultrasonography

Transrectal ultrasound (TRUS) may be offered to patients with abnormalities detected by DRE and in those with elevated PSA levels; a lubricated, condom-covered rectal probe transducer is inserted into the rectum, along the anterior wall. Needle biopsies of the prostate are commonly guided by TRUS.

Prostate Fluid or Tissue Analysis

Specimens of prostate fluid or tissue may be obtained for culture if disease or inflammation of the prostate gland is suspected, but this is uncommonly performed.

Tests of Male Sexual Function

If the patient cannot engage in sexual intercourse to his satisfaction, a detailed history is obtained. A Rigiscan® test may be ordered, or nocturnal penile tumescence tests may be conducted in a sleep laboratory to monitor changes in penile circumference during sleep. The results help identify the cause of erectile dysfunction. Additional tests, including penile Doppler studies or psychological evaluations, also can be part of the diagnostic workup and usually are conducted by a specialized team of health care providers.

CHAPTER REVIEW

Critical Thinking Exercises

1. While you are preparing a male patient to be evaluated by his provider, he confides that his interest in sexual activity and overall energy level have lessened. Explain the information you would provide. What medical and nursing interventions would you anticipate?

2. A 55-year-old woman who is postmenopausal comes to you with concerns regarding vaginal bleeding. She has not had a period in 3 years and is not currently on HR therapy. Vaginal bleeding is noted most significantly after intercourse. What lifestyle questions would you ask this patient? How would you prioritize her plan of care? What types of tests might you order to rule out disease processes?

NCLEX-Style Review Questions

1. A 61-year-old male patient who has been given written information asks why it has been recommended he have a PSA test. What is the nurse's best response?
   a. It will measure his sperm count.
   b. It will measure his response to testosterone replacement.
   c. It is a useful test to screen for cancer of the prostate.
   d. It is a useful test to screen for sexual function.

2. A 21-year-old man asks how long he will continue to produce sperm since he "knows that women can't have babies after they're 43." What is the nurse's best response?
   a. "That is correct; men and women lose their reproductive capacity at roughly the same time."
   b. "Men continue to produce sperm despite advanced age."
   c. "Current literature does not provide this information for men."
   d. "Men stop sperm production at 60 years of age."

3. A 19-year-old girl complains of vaginal irritation. She says she was out for an evening a week ago at a club with friends but doesn't remember leaving the club. She states that she has never been sexually active but is afraid she may have been assaulted. What are the appropriate steps for the nurse to take?
   a. Tell her you are sure nothing bad happened to her if she left willingly with a man. If he was a bad guy, her friends would not have let her leave with him.
   b. Tell her you believe her, this is not her fault, and you want to help her.
   c. Tell her she probably decided to have sex with a man, now she has an STD, and she needs to accept the responsibility for her own actions.
   d. Offer emotional support and referral for counseling, but medical treatment at this time is not necessary as it has been too long since the incident.

4. A 61-year-old male is complaining of erectile dysfunction. The nurse reviews the patient's medical/surgical history. What data in the patient's chart are associated with erectile dysfunction? Select all that apply.
   a. Hypertension
   b. Hyperlipidemia
   c. GERD
   d. Asthma
   e. Pelvic fracture 15 years ago
   f. Appendectomy
   g. ORIF of the left arm

5. A 35-year-old woman has an abnormal Pap test. She will undergo cryotherapy for treatment of moderate dysplasia. What should be included in the teaching plan for this patient?
   a. All abnormal cells will be removed.
   b. The procedure involves freezing of cervical tissue.
   c. Discharge following the procedure is considered abnormal.
   d. A tiny beam of light is used to vaporize abnormal cervical cells.

Try these additional resources, available at **http://thepoint.lww.com/Honan2e**, to enhance your learning and understanding of this chapter:

- NCLEX-Style Student Review Questions
- Journal Articles

REFERENCES AND SELECTED READINGS

References and selected readings associated with this chapter can be found on the website that accompanies the book. Visit **http://thepoint. lww.com/Honan2e** to access the references and other additional resources associated with this chapter.

Nursing Management: Patients with Breast and Female Reproductive Disorders

Edith Caroline Smith • Vanessa Pomarico-Denino

Learning Objectives

After reading this chapter, you will be able to:

1. Describe common benign breast problems.
2. Identify risk factors for breast cancer.
3. Identify screening and diagnostic tests used to detect breast disorders.
4. Describe different treatment modalities for breast cancer.
5. Use the nursing process as a framework for care of the patient undergoing breast cancer treatment.
6. Describe the various types of menstrual disorders and their management.
7. Differentiate between bacterial vaginosis and candidiasis.
8. Identify factors associated with pelvic organ prolapse.
9. Understand risk factors for gynecologic cancers.
10. Describe differences between the types of hysterectomies.
11. Identify appropriate care for the transgendered client.

The breast and female reproductive organs play a significant role in normal and abnormal physiology as well as in a woman's sexuality and body image. Disorders of the breast or reproductive system, whether minor or serious, can cause great anxiety. Some disorders require only modest management, while others require significant intervention and may even be life-threatening. All disorders necessitate nurses to have knowledge, understanding, and skill in patient teaching involving all aspects of care, including prevention, etiology, and treatment.

BREAST DISORDERS

Benign Conditions of the Breast

Most benign breast disorders result from normal physiologic processes. They represent a spectrum of conditions that receive clinical attention and may present as imaging abnormalities, palpable lesions, irregularities found on physical examination, or pain. Once a benign diagnosis has been confirmed, treatment typically focuses on symptom management and patient education. Benign epithelial breast lesions are classified in three categories: nonproliferative, proliferative without atypia, and **atypical hyperplasia**. The latter confers a mild to moderate increase in a patient's risk for developing breast cancer and indicates the need for further evaluation, increased screening recommendations, and a discussion of risk-reduction strategies (Sabel, 2015). The nurse should work as an integral member of the interdisciplinary team to ensure a thorough history and physical examination are completed and that all diagnostic and treatment options are made available to the patient. In addition, the nurse is an invaluable resource and provider of patient education. Table 33-1 compares various types of benign and malignant breast masses.

BREAST PAIN

Mastalgia, or breast pain, is one of the most common breast complaints. Cyclical breast pain, the most common type of breast pain, accounts for nearly 75% of all complaints. It is usually related to hormonal fluctuations during the **luteal phase** of the menstrual cycle that stimulate the proliferation of normal glandular tissue and subsequently cause pain. Noncyclical pain is far less common, can be constant or intermittent, and does not vary with the menstrual cycle.

993

TABLE 33-1 Comparison of Various Breast Masses

The most common breast masses are due to cysts, fibroadenomas, or malignancy. Biopsy is usually needed for confirmation, but the following characteristics are diagnostic clues:

Characteristics	Cysts	Fibroadenomas	Malignancy
Age	30–55 years of age, regress after menopause except with use of estrogen therapy	Puberty to menopause	At least 30–90+ years of age, most common in postmenopausal years
Number	Single or multiple	Usually single, may be multiple	Usually single
Shape	Round	Round, disk, or lobular	Irregular or stellate
Consistency	Soft to firm, usually elastic	Usually firm	Firm or hard
Mobility	Mobile	Mobile	May be fixed to skin or underlying tissues
Tenderness	Usually tender	Usually nontender	Usually nontender
Retraction signs	Absent	Absent	May be present

Women who experience muscle strain or trauma to the breast may experience noncyclical pain. Patients should be reassured that breast pain is rarely indicative of cancer. A patient should seek attention from her health care provider for persistent pain. Elimination of methylxanthines, including caffeine, theophylline, and theobromine may alleviate breast pain. These substances are found in coffee, tea, chocolate, and cola beverages. Lowering dietary fat also may improve cyclic pain, and nonsteroidal anti-inflammatory drugs (NSAIDs) often are initiated. There is some evidence that evening primrose oil, vitamin E, and flaxseed may provide some relief for patients who prefer remedies that are more natural. The attenuated androgen, danazol, may be implemented for severe, persistent pain and is effective due to its ability to suppress pituitary gonadotropins. However, there are significant side effects to this treatment option, and it is not easily tolerated. Because of this, it is rarely used. Similarly, Tamoxifen (a selective estrogen receptor modulator) is an option to treat severe symptoms, but it also carries with it a host of often intolerable side effects, thus it too is not prescribed often. The nurse may recommend that the patient wear a supportive bra both day and night, decrease caffeine intake, and take NSAIDs as needed for breast pain. Oftentimes, this combination of therapies alleviates symptoms significantly (Giuliano & Hurvitz, 2014; Sabel, 2015).

BREAST CYSTS

Cysts are the most common nonproliferative breast lesions. They do not increase a woman's risk for developing breast cancer. They are fluid-filled, round or ovoid masses, derived from the terminal duct lobular unit, that develop due to cystic lobular involution (regression of breast lobules). Cysts occur most commonly in women of childbearing age and may be exacerbated during perimenopause when hormonal fluctuations increase. Acute enlargement of cysts, which may occur immediately prior to menses, may cause sudden-onset severe, localized pain.

Simple Cysts

Simple cysts are benign by definition and do not require intervention. On ultrasound, they are well circumscribed, anechoic (low degree of sound reverberation), and have posterior acoustic enhancement and an absence of solid components. Often aspiration is performed to relieve discomfort, but simple, nonpainful cysts identified incidentally on ultrasound do not require intervention.

Complicated Cysts

Complicated cysts meet most, but not all, criteria for simple cysts on ultrasound examination. They may have internal echoes, fluid or debris components, and an imperceptible wall and may lack posterior acoustic enhancement. They are very rarely malignant but should be aspirated to confirm diagnosis or are followed with repeat imaging.

Complex Cysts

Complex cysts have mixed components that are both cystic and solid in nature with a thick wall and/or internal septa (thin wall or partition) and do require core biopsy to rule out malignancy. These lesions are more likely than simple or complicated cysts to be cancerous. The nurse should educate the patient as to the diagnostic workup process and provide support to alleviate anxiety (Athanasiou et al., 2014).

FIBROCYSTIC BREAST CONDITIONS

Often breast pain is attributed to **fibrocystic breast changes** and may be the patient's presenting complaint. Fibrocystic breast condition also can produce a transient breast mass. Both breast discomfort and breast nodularity are very common and are often a normal response to hormonal changes during the menstrual cycle, with estrogen primarily being the underlying causative factor. Pathologists also may use the term "fibrocystic" in reference to microscopic findings, such as fibrosis, adenosis, papillomatosis, ductal epithelial hyperplasia, and cysts (Giuliano & Hurvitz, 2014).

FIBROADENOMAS

Fibroadenomas are proliferative lesions without atypia (cell abnormalities) in which the underlying etiology is the estrogenic effects on breast tissue. They usually present as firm, round, movable, benign tumors that contain glandular and stromal tissue (connective tissue cells). In many cases, multiple fibroadenomas will occur in the same breast or bilaterally. They can occur from puberty to menopause and are most common from the late teens through the early 30s. Fibroadenomas usually do not require treatment. Diagnosis is best confirmed through a "triple test": clinical examination, imaging, and tissue biopsy. Fibroadenomas larger than 2 cm are more likely to persist and commonly are excised. Fibroadenomas also are sometimes excised when they are painful or when the presence of a palpable mass is too anxiety-provoking for the patient to tolerate. Patients with a negative "triple test" (nonsuspicious clinical examination, benign appearance on imaging, and benign pathology results)

do not require treatment but should have short-term interval follow-up with clinical examination and age-appropriate imaging (Giuliano & Hurvitz, 2014; American Cancer Society [ACS], 2015).

ATYPICAL DUCTAL HYPERPLASIA

Atypical ductal hyperplasia (ADH) is usually an incidental finding from biopsy of a radiographic abnormality or palpable mass. It is characterized by an abnormal growth of ductal cells in the breast and the presence of atypia (structural abnormality in a cell) without either the cytologic or architectural criteria necessary for a diagnosis of ductal carcinoma in situ (DCIS). The presence of ADH increases a woman's risk for breast cancer to four to five times that of the general population. Multifocal ADH lesions can present an even higher risk for developing breast cancer (ACS, 2015; Hartmann et al., 2015).

LOBULAR CARCINOMA IN SITU

Lobular carcinoma in situ (LCIS) is characterized by an abnormal proliferation of cells within the breast lobules. LCIS is usually found incidentally from a breast biopsy as it cannot be seen mammographically and may not form a palpable mass. Actually the term is a bit misleading because this condition is not "carcinoma," or cancer. Historically, LCIS was considered a premalignant condition but is now considered more of a marker of increased risk for invasive breast cancer. The subsequent invasive carcinoma can be either ductal or lobular in origin and can develop in either breast. LCIS increases a woman's risk of breast cancer about 7 to 11 times when compared with that of the general population (ACS, 2016). Patients with LCIS should be referred to a breast cancer specialist for full discussion of treatment options due to the significantly higher risk for developing breast cancer. These options include increased surveillance, chemoprevention to reduce the risk of developing breast cancer, and consideration for enrollment in breast cancer prevention trials. Patients also may consider bilateral **prophylactic mastectomy** dependent upon the level of risk, family history, and other factors (Sabel, 2014; National Comprehensive Cancer Network [NCCN], 2015).

MALIGNANT CONDITIONS OF THE BREAST

Breast cancer occurs when cells in the breast change and grow out of control. Some breast cancers are in situ, meaning confined within the walls of the ducts of the breast, but the majority are invasive or infiltrating. Invasive cancers have extended through the ducts or glandular walls and invaded the surrounding breast tissue. The expected prognosis for invasive breast cancer depends largely on the extent to which it has spread when it is first diagnosed. Breast cancer is the most commonly diagnosed malignancy in women, except for nonmelanoma skin cancer. The ACS estimates that 231,840 new cases of invasive breast cancer were diagnosed in the United States in 2015 as well as an additional estimated 60,290 cases of in situ breast cancer; 39,620 women were expected to die from breast cancer in the United States in 2013. Lung cancer is the only cancer that causes more deaths in women. Although much more rare, males can develop breast cancer. In 2015, it was estimated that 2,350 men were diagnosed with breast cancer, accounting for about 1% of all breast cancer diagnoses. In 2015, there were approximately 2.8 million women living with a history of breast cancer or currently undergoing treatment for the disease (ACS, 2015; Breastcancer.org, 2015).

Risk Factors

The two most significant risk factors for developing breast cancer are being female and growing older. Eighty-five percent of women who develop breast cancer have no risk factors other than age and gender. Whereas most breast cancers are "sporadic," a small percentage (5% to 10%) are due to having an inherited genetic mutation, such as in the ***BRCA1*** or ***BRCA2*** genes. Women who carry these mutations have a lifetime risk of 41% to 90% of developing breast cancer (NCCN, 2015). Box 33-1 lists other risk factors for developing breast cancer.

Screening and Prevention

Breast cancer is primarily a disease of early detection, but it also can be one of prevention, especially in high-risk women. Though some risk factors for breast cancer are modifiable, the two greatest risk factors, being female and growing older, are not modifiable. This is why screening mammograms and prompt attention for any breast abnormality are extremely important.

Men can experience breast cancer, as well, with the risk being 1 in 1,000 males, The disease is 100 times more likely to occur in women than in men. Since it is so rare in men, they are not offered routine screening, and male breast cancer is not addressed in detail in this chapter. Any breast mass or abnormality should be evaluated in men, and male BRCA mutation carriers, due to their increased risk of developing breast cancer, are followed with increased breast cancer surveillance. Upon diagnosis, male breast cancer is treated similarly to breast cancer in females (ACS, 2015; NCCN, 2015).

Protective Factors

Women can choose to maximize their overall health by maintaining a normal weight, particularly after menopause, engaging in regular physical activity, and avoiding or limiting alcohol consumption. Women who breastfeed for an extended period of time (for a year or longer) may have

---

BOX 33-1 Risk Factors for Breast Cancer

- Being a woman
- Increasing age
- Inherited genetic mutation for breast cancer, such as BRCA1 and/or BRCA2 or other cancer susceptibility genes
- Family history of breast cancer, particularly with a first-degree relative diagnosed with breast cancer at an early age (under 50 years of age)
- Personal history of breast cancer
- History of benign proliferative breast disease, especially those with atypia
- History of high-dose radiation therapy to the chest, such as patients who have undergone treatment for Hodgkin's disease or non-Hodgkin lymphoma
- Hormonal factors:
  - Early menarche (before 12 years of age)
  - Late menopause (after 55 years of age)
  - Nulliparity or no full-term pregnancies
  - Late age at first full-term pregnancy (after 30 years of age)
  - Recent contraceptive use
  - Long-term use of estrogen and progestin (hormone replacement therapy)
- History of ovarian cancer or endometrial cancer
- Obesity, particularly postmenopausal
- Alcohol consumption
- Ashkenazi Jewish ethnicity related to BRCA1/2 mutation carrier risk

---

some added protection. Women at high risk for breast cancer may be candidates for chemoprevention and opt to take medications such as tamoxifen, raloxifene, or exemestane to reduce their risk (ACS, 2013; NCCN, 2015).

Screening Recommendations

The ACS recommends that women at population risk for breast cancer begin annual screening mammography at age 40. Women also should have a clinical breast examination every 1 to 3 years beginning in their 20s and then annually beginning at 40 years of age, and they should practice breast self-awareness. Women who are at increased risk for breast cancer should talk with their health care provider to establish the optimal age to begin screening as women at high risk often begin clinical breast examinations and breast imaging at younger ages (ACS, 2013; NCCN, 2015).

Prevention Strategies in the High-Risk Patient

By identifying the population of women who are at highest risk for breast cancer, prevention and earlier detection are possible. Women who have risk factors should talk with their health care provider to assess their risk and implement an individualized plan for surveillance and risk reduction. The decision whether or not to undergo genetic testing and the risks and benefits of prevention strategies should be discussed in detail, weighing the potential benefits with the risks of the interventions.

Long-Term Surveillance

Some women at high risk choose a conservative approach, with more frequent or earlier screening and additional imaging modalities, such as magnetic resonance imaging (MRI). More frequent clinical breast examinations and breast self-awareness are emphasized. The NCCN Clinical Practice Guidelines in Oncology offer patient-specific recommendations for screening in this population (2015).

Chemoprevention

Chemoprevention with a variety of medications has demonstrated significant reduction in breast cancer in women at high risk. The National Surgical Adjuvant Breast and Bowel Project (NSABP) Breast Cancer Prevention Trial showed that treatment with tamoxifen resulted in a 49% decrease in short-term risk for breast cancer in healthy women at increased risk. Raloxifene has also demonstrated effectiveness in risk reduction and has a lower side-effect profile than tamoxifen. Both tamoxifen and raloxifene, which are categorized as selective estrogen receptor modulators (SERMs), are FDA approved for chemoprevention. Another medication, Exemestane, an aromatase inhibitor, also has demonstrated effectiveness in reducing the risk for breast cancer in healthy women who are high risk. Though its use is recognized by the NCCN and the American Society of Clinical Oncology (ASCO), exemestane is not FDA approved for that use (Visvanathan et al., 2013; Giuliano & Hurvitz, 2014; NCCN, 2015). When considering chemoprevention, the risks and benefits should be weighed carefully by the patient and her health care provider.

Prophylactic Mastectomy

Prophylactic bilateral **total mastectomy** is an option for carefully selected women with significant breast cancer risk and/or extreme anxiety associated with potential diagnosis. This surgery as a method of breast cancer prevention has demonstrated a significant risk reduction in women who are known to have *BRCA1* or *BRCA2* mutations. The decision to undergo prophylactic mastectomy should be made carefully and with the input of the multidisciplinary team. All breast tissue should be removed, but lymph node dissection is not necessary unless breast cancer is detected upon pathologic examination of the tissue (NCCN, 2015).

Clinical Manifestations

Breast cancers can occur anywhere in the breast but usually are found in the upper outer quadrant, where the most breast tissue is located. In general, the lesions are nontender, tend to be fixed rather than mobile, and may be harder with irregular borders.

With the increased use of screening mammography, more women are being diagnosed early and are seeking treatment for earlier-stage disease. These women often present with no signs or symptoms other than having a mammographic abnormality. Unfortunately, some women seek initial treatment after ignoring symptoms. Oftentimes, those women present with advanced stage disease. Advanced signs may include skin dimpling, nipple retraction, or skin ulceration.

Breast Imaging

Breast imaging includes all of the radiographic imaging modalities used to detect and diagnose breast abnormalities and diseases. Mammography is the most common imaging modality and has improved dramatically over the past several decades. Other common imaging modalities include ultrasound and MRI.

Mammography

Mammography is a specific type of radiographic imaging that utilizes low-dose x-ray for examination of the breasts. Mammography is the best and most universally accepted screening tool available to detect breast cancer at its earliest and most treatable stages, and it is currently the only imaging modality recommended for routine breast cancer screening in the general population.

There are two types of mammograms: screening and diagnostic. Screening mammograms are for routine use at recommended intervals to detect unanticipated breast cancer in asymptomatic women. Screening mammography must be performed on a regular basis in order to reduce breast cancer mortality. Diagnostic mammograms are performed either when a radiographic abnormality is detected on a screening mammogram or when the patient or her caregiver notices a change or a problem in her breast. Also mammography is used to assist in interventional breast procedures, such as stereotactic breast biopsy and needle localization.

Newer, digital mammography techniques provide dramatic improvements in the visualization of lesions for interpreting physicians and greater ease of examination for the patient.

The mammography examination takes only a few minutes and has minimal radiation exposure. During a mammogram, the breast is manually compressed in the mammography unit by a registered mammography technologist in two different views: the craniocaudal view (compression from top to bottom) and the mediolateral oblique view (from side to side). Other views may be obtained when a patient has a palpable or image-detected abnormality requiring more focused or directed examination. The nurse should educate the patient on the importance of regular screening mammography, immediate pursuit of attention upon discovery of any palpable abnormality, and the availability of comfort options, such as disposable foam pads to ease discomfort during compression.

Ultrasound

Ultrasonography (ultrasound) is used as a screening or diagnostic adjunct to mammography. The procedure consists of a thin coating of lubricating jelly spread over the area to be imaged. Then a transducer is placed on the breast. The transducer transmits high-frequency sound waves through the skin toward the area of concern. The sound waves that are reflected back form a two-dimensional image, which is then displayed on a computer screen. No radiation is emitted during the procedure. The technique is used often to determine if a mass is cystic versus solid but cannot rule out malignant lesions definitively. Due to its limited specificity, ultrasound should not be used for routine screening but has recently been advocated as a valuable screening tool in women who have mammographically dense breasts (ACS, 2015).

Magnetic Resonance Imaging

MRI of the breast produces very detailed cross-sectional images using magnetic fields rather than x-rays. An IV injection of gadolinium, a contrast dye, is given to improve visibility. The patient lies face down and the breast is placed through a depression in the table. A coil is placed around the breast, and the patient is placed inside the MRI machine. The entire procedure takes about 30 to 40 minutes.

MRI is most useful in patients with proven breast cancer, when assessing for multifocal (more than one tumor in the same quadrant of the breast) or multicentric (more than one tumor in different quadrants of the breast), or bilateral disease, chest wall involvement, tumor recurrence, or response to chemotherapy. The procedure also can identify occult (undetectable) breast cancer and determine the integrity of saline or silicone breast implants. It is not recommended for routine screening in the general population, but it is recommended for individuals who have a lifetime risk of greater than 20% to 25% based on predictive models, who have a known or suspected genetic predisposition to breast cancer, or those with other elevating risk factors, such as prior radiation exposure. The risks of false-positive and false-negative examination results should be addressed, and MRI screening should be performed after a detailed discussion with the patient (Giuliano & Hurvitz, 2014).

Some disadvantages of MRI include high cost, variations in technique and interpretation, and the potential for patient claustrophobia. Breast MRI is highly sensitive but has low specificity so the procedure cannot always distinguish between malignant and benign breast conditions accurately. MRI is contraindicated in patients with implantable metal devices, such as aneurysm clips, pacemakers, and ports of tissue expanders, because of the magnetic force acting on metallic objects. Foil-backed medication patches should be removed prior to MRI to avoid burns to the skin (Giuliano & Hurvitz, 2014).

Breast Biopsy

Percutaneous needle biopsy, either by fine-needle aspiration (FNA) or by tissue core biopsy, is the simplest biopsy technique and should always be the first modality considered for breast tissue sampling. This type of biopsy allows for definitive diagnosis with lower morbidity than open surgical biopsy and a lower cost for the procedure. The nurse educates the patient prior to the procedure, answers questions, and offers emotional support.

Fine-Needle Aspiration

Fine-needle aspiration (FNA) is a noninvasive biopsy technique that is generally well tolerated by most women. A local anesthetic may or may not be used. For palpable masses, a surgeon performs the procedure. A small-gauge needle (25- or 22-gauge) attached to a syringe is inserted into the mass or area of nodularity. Suction is applied to the syringe, and multiple passes are made through the mass. A simple cyst often disappears on aspiration, and the fluid is usually discarded, though it may be sent for pathologic examination. If no fluid is obtained on aspiration, then any cellular material obtained in the hub of the needle is spread on a glass slide or placed in a preservative and sent to the laboratory for analysis. For nonpalpable masses, the same procedure can be performed by a radiologist or surgeon using ultrasound guidance.

FNA is less expensive than other diagnostic methods, and usually results are available quickly; however, due to risk of a false-negative result, close clinical correlation is necessary (Giuliano & Hurvitz, 2014).

Ultrasound-Guided Breast Biopsy

Ultrasound-guided breast biopsy is a minimally invasive procedure wherein the physician uses the ultrasound to visualize the lesions and guide the needle for sampling (Fig. 33-1). It is the preferred biopsy modality for all lesions visible by ultrasound. For the procedure, the patient lies supine on a table and the physician inserts a needle to obtain specimens after

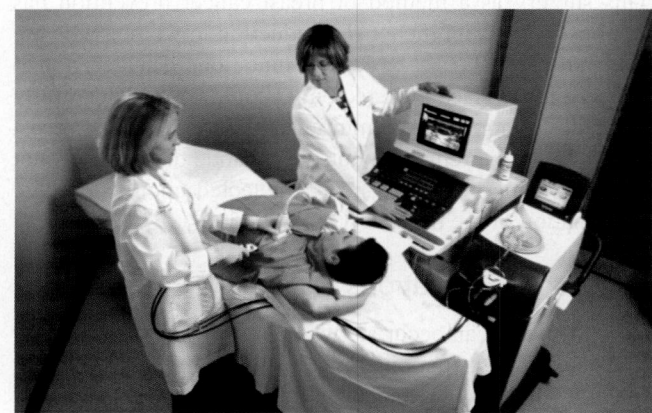

FIGURE 33-1 Ultrasound-guided breast biopsy. (Courtesy of Mammotome.)

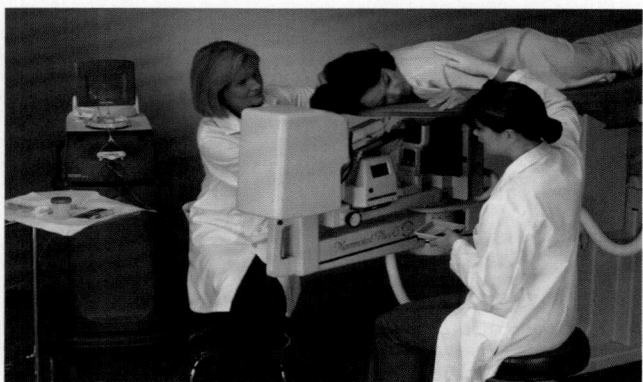

FIGURE 33-2 Stereotactic breast biopsy. (Courtesy of Mammotome.)

thoroughly cleaning the skin, injecting subcutaneous analgesia such as lidocaine, and making a small nick in the skin. The needle may or may not have vacuum assistance to help obtain adequate specimens. The biopsy needle is typically 12- to 18-gauge without vacuum assistance and 7- to 12-gauge with vacuum assistance. Several tissue samples are obtained and sent to the laboratory for analysis. A small titanium clip should be placed in the biopsy cavity for documentation of correct sampling site, for future mammogram evaluation, and for locating the site should further treatment be warranted.

Stereotactic Breast Biopsy

Stereotactic core biopsy is another minimally invasive procedure that uses x-ray guidance to obtain breast tissue samples (Fig. 33-2). It is the preferred biopsy modality for microcalcifications and lesions not visible by ultrasound. The patient lies prone on the stereotactic table, and the breast is suspended through an opening and compressed between two x-ray plates. Digital mammography images are obtained, and the exact coordinates of the lesion to be sampled are located with the aid of a computer. After sterilizing the skin, a local anesthetic is injected into the entry site on the breast. A small nick is made in the skin, a core needle is inserted, and samples of the tissue are taken for pathologic examination. Often, several passes are taken to ensure adequate tissue sampling. Clip placement is necessary for this type of biopsy as well.

Magnetic Resonance Imaging–Guided Breast Biopsy

MRI-guided breast biopsy is logistically similar to **stereotactic biopsy** and is used increasingly for lesions that cannot be visualized under mammography or ultrasound. Special concern is necessary for equipment safety in the magnetic field, and MRI-specific biopsy equipment is used.

Surgical Biopsy

When minimally invasive breast biopsy is not feasible, an excisional or surgical biopsy may be used to remove an entire lesion and a surrounding margin of breast tissue that appears normal. This type of biopsy also may be referred to as a *lumpectomy*. Depending on the clinical situation, a frozen-section analysis of the specimen may be performed at the time of the biopsy by the pathologist, who does an immediate intraoperative reading and provides a provisional diagnosis. Surgical biopsy is usually performed using local anesthesia and IV sedation and often follows *wire needle localization*, wherein mammography or ultrasonography are used to locate the lesion and place a guidewire through the skin and into the area of suspicion. Then the surgeon may follow the guidewire down to the lesion for precise removal and minimal tissue loss.

The nurse plays an important role in surgical breast biopsy. During the preoperative visit, the nurse assesses the patient for specific educational, physical, or psychosocial needs. The nurse should review medical and psychosocial history and facilitate conversation regarding fears, concerns, and questions. Often patients are worried not only about the procedure but also about the potential implications of the pathology results. The nurse should provide a thorough explanation and written materials to reinforce education.

The patient should discontinue any anticoagulant therapy prior to the procedure. The patient may be instructed not to eat or drink for several hours or after midnight the night before the procedure, depending on the type of biopsy planned. Most breast biopsy procedures today are performed with the use of moderate sedation and local anesthesia.

Immediate postoperative assessment includes monitoring the effects of the anesthesia and inspecting the surgical dressing for any signs of bleeding. Once the sedation has worn off, the nurse reviews the care of the biopsy site, pain management, and activity restrictions with the patient. Prior to discharge from the ambulatory surgical center or the office, the patient must be able to tolerate fluids, ambulate, and void. The patient must have someone to drive her home. Usually the dressing covering the incision is removed after 48 hours, but the Steri-Strips, which are applied directly over the incision, should remain in place for approximately 7 to 10 days. The use of a supportive bra following surgery is encouraged to limit movement of the breast and to reduce discomfort. A follow-up telephone call from the nurse 24 to 48 hours after the procedure can provide the patient with the opportunity to ask any questions and can be a source of great comfort and reassurance.

Most women return to their usual activities the day after the procedure but are encouraged to avoid jarring or high-impact activities for 1 week to promote healing of the biopsy site. Usually discomfort is minimal, and most women find acetaminophen sufficient for pain relief, although a mild opioid may be prescribed if needed. Follow-up after the biopsy includes a return visit to the surgeon for discussion of the final pathology report and assessment of the healing of the biopsy site.

Staging

There are three primary staging systems for cancer. The most clinically relevant, the American Joint Committee on Cancer (AJCC)'s TNM system classifies tumors using information on the size of the tumor and the extent of spread within the breast (T), involvement in lymph nodes (N), and spread to distant organs (M). Refer to Chapter 6 for more information on staging of cancer. This staging system is used very commonly in clinical settings and assigns a stage of I, II, III, or IV according to the determined T, N, and M classification. Stage I indicates an early-stage breast cancer, and IV indicates the most advanced. The Extent of Disease system used by the National Cancer Institute's Surveillance, Epidemiology, and End Results (SEER) program and the Summary Stage system are other classification systems that are used most often in data reporting and state tumor registries (Le-Petross & Caudle, 2015).

Prognosis

The two most important prognostic factors associated with breast cancer are tumor size and axillary lymph node involvement.

In general, a smaller tumor is associated with a better prognosis. Prognosis also depends on the extent that the breast cancer has spread. Women who are diagnosed at a more advanced stage have a lower 5-year relative survival rate, as do women with larger tumor size at diagnosis. The 5-year relative survival rate for localized disease (stages 0–I) is near or equal to 100%, for regional disease (stages II–III) it is 72% to 93%, and for distant-stage disease (stage IV) it is 22% (ACS, 2015). The most common route of regional spread is to the axillary lymph nodes (Fig. 33-3). Other sites of lymphatic spread include the internal mammary and supraclavicular nodes. Distant metastasis can affect any organ, but the most common sites are bone, lung, liver, pleura, adrenals, skin, and brain. Amplification of certain genes, such as *HER2/neu* (discussed later in this chapter), or excessive amounts of their protein product may represent a poorer prognosis. Box 33-2 lists other prognostic factors.

Types

Ductal Carcinoma in Situ

Ductal carcinoma in situ (DCIS) is characterized by the proliferation of malignant cells inside the milk ducts without invasion into the surrounding tissue. Frequently DCIS is manifested on a mammogram with the appearance of calcifications, and it is considered stage 0 breast cancer. Treatment options include breast-conserving surgery and radiation therapy with or without tamoxifen, total mastectomy with or without tamoxifen, and breast-conserving surgery without radiation therapy (NCI, 2015).

Infiltrating Ductal Carcinoma

Infiltrating ductal carcinoma (IDC), the most common histologic type of breast cancer, accounts for 80% of all cases. The tumors arise from the duct system and invade the surrounding tissues. They often present as a solid mass in the breast.

Infiltrating Lobular Carcinoma

Infiltrating lobular carcinoma (ILC) accounts for approximately 10% of breast cancers and is the second most common type of breast cancer after IDC. These tumors arise from the lobular epithelium and typically occur as an area of ill-defined thickening in the breast. They are often multicentric and can be bilateral.

Medullary Carcinoma of the Breast

Medullary carcinoma is a rare subtype of IDC and accounts for about 5% of breast cancers. It tends to be diagnosed more often in women in their 40s to early 50s. The tumor is usually a soft, fleshy mass that tends to be low grade, and it is not likely to spread outside of the breast tissue. Because of this, the prognosis is often favorable.

Medical and Nursing Management

A multidisciplinary team approach to treatment for breast cancer allows for an individualized plan of care based upon careful consideration of the optimal treatment for the stage and biologic characteristics of the tumor; the patient's personal preference, performance status, and age; and the potential risks and benefits of all treatment options. Treatment decisions should be made by the patient and her physician. Most women who are diagnosed with breast cancer will undergo some type of surgery, and many also will have radiation therapy, chemotherapy, hormone therapy, and/or biologic therapy. The treatment guidelines for breast cancer are available via free registration from the NCCN at nccn.org/professionals/physician_gls/PDF/breast.pdf (NCCN, 2017).

Surgical Management

The primary goal of surgery is to obtain local control of the disease by removing the cancer from the breast and to determine the stage and extent of disease. Because breast cancer is now diagnosable at earlier stages, options for less invasive surgical procedures are available.

Procedures

Lumpectomy. In a lumpectomy, the surgeon removes the cancerous tissue and a border of normal tissue. This usually follows a wire needle localization procedure to mark the tumor or the metallic clip left from the biopsy. Patients who undergo lumpectomy almost always undergo 5 to 7 weeks of radiation therapy afterward. Patients who have a lumpectomy

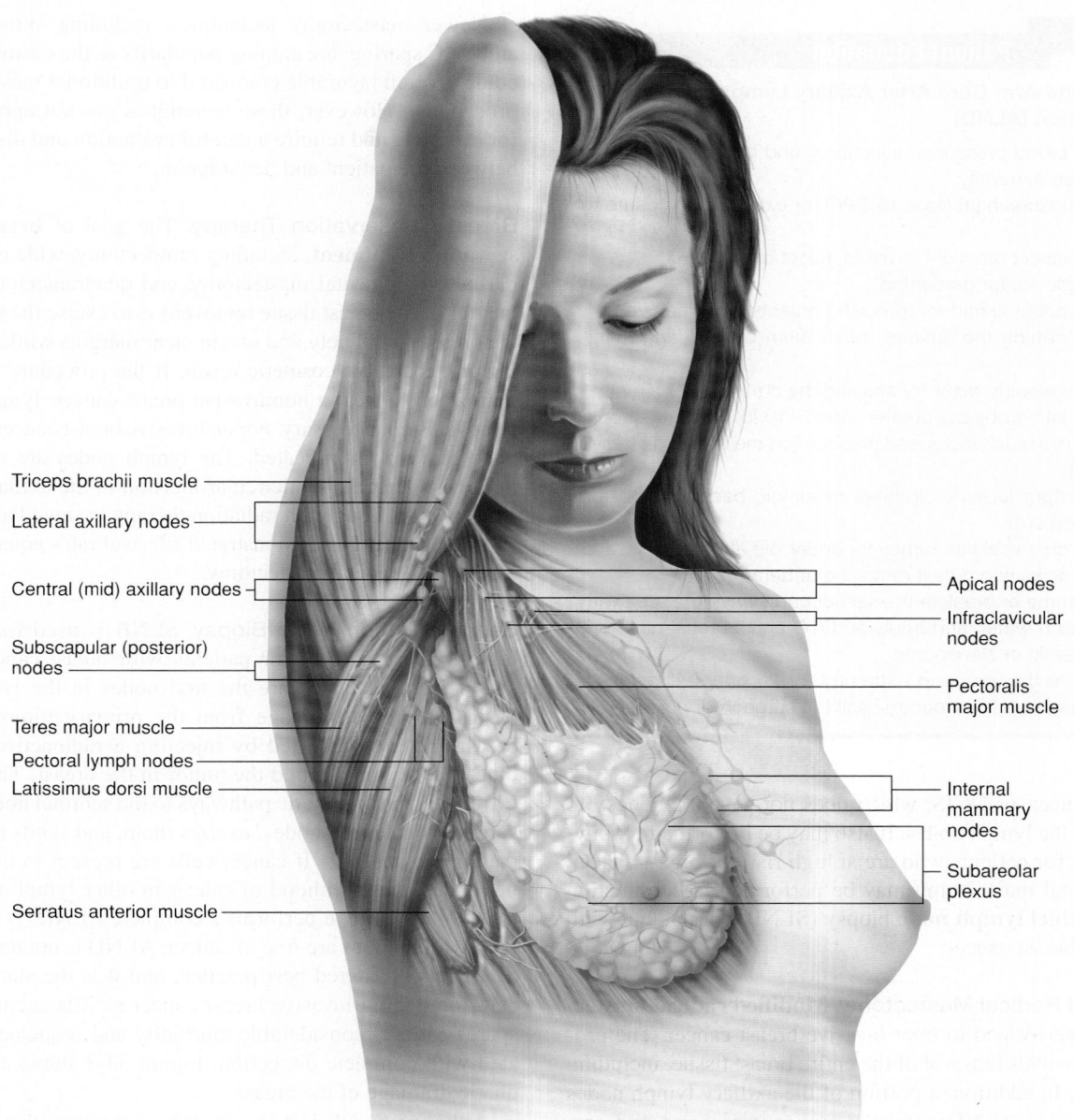

Triceps brachii muscle

Lateral axillary nodes

Central (mid) axillary nodes

Subscapular (posterior) nodes

Teres major muscle

Pectoral lymph nodes

Latissimus dorsi muscle

Serratus anterior muscle

Apical nodes

Infraclavicular nodes

Pectoralis major muscle

Internal mammary nodes

Subareolar plexus

FIGURE 33-3 Lymphatic drainage of the breast. (Reprinted from Health assessment made incredible visual, Lippincott, Wolters, Kluwer.)

BOX 33-2

Factors Affecting Prognosis for Breast Cancer

- Age and menopausal status of the patient
- Stage of disease
- Histologic and nuclear grade of the primary tumor
- Estrogen and progesterone receptor status of the primary tumor
- Proliferative capacity of the tumor
- *HER2/neu* gene amplification

From *Breast Cancer Treatment*, NCI. https://www.cancer.gov/types/breast/patient/breast-treatment-pdq

or breast conservation surgery followed by radiation therapy have the same predicted long-term survival as patients who choose to undergo mastectomy (Giuliano & Hurvitz, 2014). Appropriate patient selection is critical when planning surgical intervention. A woman who undergoes lumpectomy also may have regional lymph nodes removed to determine if the cancer has spread beyond the breast.

Simple Mastectomy. In a simple or total mastectomy, the entire breast and nipple–areola complex (NAC) are removed, without axillary lymph node dissection (ALND). Total mastectomy may be performed for patients with noninvasive

---

BOX 33-3   Patient Education

Hand and Arm Care After Axillary Lymph Node Dissection (ALND)

- Avoid blood pressures, injections, and blood draws in the affected extremity.
- Use sunscreen (at least 15 SPF) for extended exposure to sun.
- Apply insect repellent to avoid insect bites.
- Wear gloves for gardening.
- Use a cooking mitt for removing objects from the oven.
- Avoid cutting the cuticles; push them back during manicures.
- Use an electric razor for shaving the armpit.
- Avoid lifting objects greater than 5–10 lb. Patients should avoid too much increased pressure on the arm (e.g., heavy purse).
- Avoid tight jewelry, clothing, or elastic bandages on the affected arm.
- Avoid chemical hair removers under the affected arm, and avoid nicks and cuts if removing underarm hair.
- If a trauma or break in the skin occurs, wash the area with soap and water, and apply an OTC antibacterial ointment (Bacitracin or Neosporin).
- Observe the area and extremity for 24 hours; if redness, swelling, or a fever occurs, call the surgeon or nurse.

---

breast cancer, or DCIS, which does not have a tendency to spread to the lymph nodes. It also may be performed prophylactically for patients who are at high risk for breast cancer. Also a total mastectomy may be performed in conjunction with **sentinel lymph node** biopsy (SLNB) for patients with invasive breast cancer.

Modified Radical Mastectomy. Modified radical mastectomy is performed to treat invasive breast cancer. The procedure involves removal of the entire breast tissue, including the NAC. In addition, a portion of the axillary lymph nodes are removed (ALND). Box 33-3 discusses hand and arm care after ALND.

If immediate breast reconstruction is desired, the patient is referred to a plastic surgeon prior to the mastectomy so that she has the opportunity to explore all available options. In modified radical mastectomy, the pectoralis major and pectoralis minor muscles are left intact, unlike in radical mastectomy, in which the muscles are removed.

Radical Mastectomy. Radical mastectomy includes removal of the entire breast and lymph nodes under the arm as well as removal of the underlying pectoralis major and minor muscles. This technique is currently used very rarely due to the proven effectiveness and significantly decreased morbidity associated with less aggressive procedures, such as modified radical mastectomy, total mastectomy, and lumpectomy.

Newer mastectomy techniques, including skin-sparing and NAC sparing, are gaining popularity as the cosmetic outcome is often favorable compared to traditional mastectomy procedures. However, these techniques are not appropriate for everyone and require a careful evaluation and discussion between the patient and her surgeon.

Breast Conservation Therapy. The goal of **breast conservation treatment**, including lumpectomy, wide excision, partial or segmental mastectomy, and quadrantectomy (one quarter of the breast tissue removed) is to excise the tumor in the breast completely and obtain clear margins while achieving an acceptable cosmetic result. If the procedure is being performed to treat a noninvasive breast cancer, lymph node removal is not necessary. For an invasive breast cancer, lymph node removal is indicated. The lymph nodes are removed through a separate semicircular incision in the axilla. Breast conservation along with radiation therapy in stage I and stage II breast cancer has demonstrated survival rates equal to that of modified radical mastectomy.

Sentinel Lymph Node Biopsy. SLNB is used for pathologic axillary staging for patients with breast cancer. The sentinel lymph nodes are the first nodes in the lymphatic basin to receive drainage from the primary tumor in the breast and are identified by injecting a radioactive tracer, blue dye, or both around the tumor in the breast. The tracer travels via the lymphatic pathways to the sentinel nodes. The surgeon locates the nodes, excises them, and sends them for pathologic analysis. If cancer cells are present in the sentinel nodes, the likelihood of cancer in other lymph nodes is high so the surgeon performs a complete ALND. If the sentinel lymph nodes are free of cancer, ALND is not necessary. SLNB is considered best practice, and it is the standard of care for staging invasive breast cancer as it is accurate and spares patients considerable morbidity and sequelae associated with complete dissection. Figure 33-3 shows the lymphatic drainage of the breast.

Although SLNB is a less invasive procedure than ALND and results in a shorter recovery period, a patient who has undergone SLNB still may experience complications, such as lymphedema, related to the procedure. The nurse's role is to listen to the patient's concerns, provide emotional support, and refer the patient to appropriate specialists when indicated.

Complications for the Surgical Patient

Lymphedema. Lymphedema results from impaired flow of lymph fluid through the draining lymphatic vessels after lymph node dissection. An accumulation of lymph fluid develops in the surrounding and dependent tissues, leading to swelling, fibrosis of the soft tissues, neurologic complications such as pain and paresthesias, and infection. Continuous assessment and early identification of signs and symptoms of lymphedema should be integral in the care of patients undergoing therapy for breast cancer. Risk for lymphedema depends on the type of therapy received and is more common in patients who undergo ALND. Referral to a lymphedema specialist is key to management of this complication (ACS, 2013).

> **Nursing Alert**
> *To prevent lymphedema or lymphangitis (infection of the lymph vessels), nurses should place a sign above the bed of a patient following mastectomy or node dissection not to perform blood pressures, blood draws, injections, or IV insertions on the side where the operation was performed. Lymphatic drainage is altered due to node dissection, causing the potential for fluid to accumulate in the affected extremity. Complications of infiltration, phlebitis, or trauma can result if the affected extremity is used. Some patients will obtain a medical alert bracelet with this warning.*

Hematoma and Seroma Formation. Hematoma, a collection of blood inside the surgical cavity, may occur after either mastectomy or breast conservation and usually develops within the first 12 hours after surgery. The nurse assesses for signs and symptoms of hematoma at the surgical site, which may include swelling, tightness, pain, and bruising of the skin. The surgeon should be notified immediately for gross swelling or increased bloody output from the drain, typically a Jackson Pratt. While most hematomas are small and resolve without intervention, some must be evacuated surgically. Refer to Box 33-4 for drain care.

A seroma, a collection of serous fluid, may accumulate under the breast incision after mastectomy or breast conservation or in the axilla. Signs and symptoms include swelling, heaviness, discomfort, and a sloshing of fluid. Seromas may develop temporarily after the drain is removed or if the drain is in place and becomes obstructed. Seromas rarely pose a threat and the surgeon or health care provider may unclog the drain or manually aspirate the fluid with a needle and syringe.

Infection. Infection is a risk after any surgical procedure. This risk may be higher in patients with accompanying conditions, such as diabetes, immune disorders, and advanced age, as well as in those with poor hygiene. Patients are taught to monitor for signs and symptoms of infection, such as redness, warmth around the incision, tenderness, foul-smelling drainage, temperature greater than 100.4°F, and chills and to contact the surgeon or nurse for evaluation should they notice any of these. For more severe infections, treatment consists of oral or IV antibiotics for 1 or 2 weeks.

Nursing management for patients undergoing surgery is discussed in the nursing process section later in this chapter.

Reconstructive Surgery

A variety of reconstructive options is available today for women who desire a correction in the size or the shape of the breast, including reduction **mammoplasty**, augmentation mammoplasty, and mastopexy (discussed shortly). Several options are also available to reconstruct the breast after a mastectomy.

Reconstructive Surgeries for Lumpectomy. Reconstructive surgeries include reduction mammoplasty, augmentation mammoplasty, and mastopexy.

Usually reduction mammoplasty is performed on women who have large breasts. It is an outpatient procedure that is performed under general anesthesia. Most commonly, an anchor-shaped incision that circles the areola is made, extending downward and following the natural curve of the inframammary fold. Depending on the size of the breast, the nipple may be moved up to a higher position while still attached to the breast tissue, or it may be separated and transplanted to a new location. Drains are placed in the incision and remain for 2 to 5 days.

Augmentation mammoplasty is performed on women who desire larger or fuller breasts. Usually this procedure is performed by placing a silicone or saline breast implant under the pectoralis muscle. The incision line can be placed in the inframammary fold, in the axilla, or around the areola. The procedure is performed as an outpatient procedure under general anesthesia. A drain is not necessary.

Mastopexy is performed when the patient is content with the size of her breasts but wishes to have the shape improved and a lift performed. The procedure is also an outpatient surgery.

Reconstructive Procedures After Mastectomy. Breast reconstruction can provide a significant psychological benefit for women who are already struggling with the emotional distress of losing a breast. A consultation with a plastic surgeon can help the patient understand procedures for which she is a candidate and the pros and cons of each option. Factors to consider include body size and shape; comorbidities, such as hypertension, diabetes mellitus, or obesity; personal habits, such as smoking; and patient preference. The patient must be informed that although breast reconstruction can provide a good cosmetic result, it will never precisely duplicate the natural breast. Realistic preparation can help the patient avoid unrealistic expectations. Reconstruction is considered an integral component in the surgical treatment of breast cancer and is usually covered by insurance companies.

Many women elect immediate reconstruction at the time of the mastectomy operation. Delayed reconstruction may be preferable to women who are having a difficult time deciding on whether reconstruction is desired at all or if they are unsure as to the type of reconstruction they prefer. In patients with advanced disease, such as in inflammatory breast cancer, treatments should be given without delay so immediate reconstruction is not recommended. Delays in healing after immediate reconstruction may interfere with the initiation of treatment, particularly radiation therapy.

BOX 33-4   Surgical Breast Cancer Patient with a Drainage Device

A drain is placed in the surgical wound at the time of surgery to evacuate drainage from the surgical site. The tubing has multiple perforations on the distal end (in the wound site), and the tubing is attached to a device externally that collects the drainage. Suction is maintained by compression of the device. Usually the drain is sutured to the skin. The typical device used for breast surgery is called a *Jackson Pratt* (JP), a bulb-like device (see the figure below).

The nurse and patient or caregiver are aware that the device must be compressed to maintain suction at the wound bed. If the device is inflated fully, it must be emptied to maintain the vacuum necessary to facilitate drainage away from the wound bed.

The nurse explains the procedure to the patient and/or caregiver, brings a measuring device such as an ounce medicine cup (if limited drainage is expected) or a graduated cylinder, and explains the importance of hand washing before the procedure (maximum capacity of the JP is approximately 100 mL). Nonsterile gloves are donned.

The JP drainage device is unclipped from the patient's gown, and, using sterile technique, the spout plug is opened on the JP bulb. The device will expand fully since the suction has been released (image above reveals fully expanded JP; no vacuum exists). The nurse is careful not to touch the inside of the spout or plug and teaches this to the patient and/or caregiver. The device is emptied by turning the bulb over and squeezing the bulb so that the contents can escape from the device. The amount and appearance of the drainage is recorded. The JP bulb is NEVER squeezed unless the spout plug is released.

An alcohol wipe can be used to clean the spout and plug. Maintaining sterile technique, the JP is compressed completely flat with one hand, and, while compression is maintained, the plug is reattached with the other hand.

The nurse is aware that the system must be airtight to function. If rapid reinflation is noted after plugging the spout, an air leak should be suspected; the nurse attempts to compress and plug the device again and if the device remains inflated, the provider should be notified. The nurse secures the device to the patient's gown, below the wound (to facilitate drainage) to prevent pulling on the wound site and/or potential dislodgment. The nurse removes and discards gloves and washes hands thoroughly.

If multiple drains are used, they are labeled numerically (1, 2) or alphabetically (a, b), and drainage per drain is recorded as deemed by institutional policy or surgeon protocol.

Depending on surgeon preference and quality of the drainage, the patient may be instructed on how to "milk clots" through the tubing of the drainage device, which requires gentle compression of the tubing between the thumb and index finger while stabilizing the exit site to prevent dislodgment of the tubing with the nondominant hand. Holding the tube securely above the obstruction is necessary to avoid pulling the tube out of the incision. *Note: This is only done depending on surgeon preference.*

The nurse teaches the patient and/or caregiver which observations of the drain site require contacting the physician or nurse (e.g., sudden change in color of drainage, sudden cessation of drainage, signs or symptoms of an infection) as per the surgeon's recommendation.

The nurse reinforces that the drain is typically ready for removal by the surgeon when draining is less than 30 mL for a 24-hour period.

Tissue Expander Followed by Permanent Implant. Breast reconstruction using a tissue expander followed by a permanent implant is commonly used. To accommodate an implant, the skin remaining after a mastectomy and the underlying muscle must be stretched gradually by a process called *tissue expansion.* The surgeon places a balloon-like device through the mastectomy incision underneath the pectoralis muscle. A small amount of saline is injected through a metal port intraoperatively to partially inflate the expander, followed by additional saline injections through the port at weekly intervals until the expander is fully inflated. It remains fully expanded for about 6 weeks to allow the skin to loosen. Then the expander is exchanged for a permanent implant.

Advantages are a shorter operating time and a shorter recuperation period than for autologous (using the patient's own tissue) reconstruction. A disadvantage is a tendency for the implant to feel firm and round, with little natural ptosis, or sag. Women with a small to medium contralateral breast with little ptosis are good candidates for this procedure. Women who have had prior radiation or who have connective tissue disease are not good candidates because of the decreased elasticity of the skin.

The patient may be instructed not to have an MRI while the tissue expander is in place as often the port contains metal. This is not an issue once the permanent implant is in place. Figure 33-4 shows breast reconstruction with a tissue expander.

FIGURE 33-4 Breast reconstruction with tissue expander. **A.** Mastectomy incision line prior to tissue expansion. **B.** The expander is placed under the pectoralis muscle and is filled gradually with saline solution through a port to stretch the skin enough to accept a permanent implant. **C.** The breast mound is restored. Although permanent, scars will fade with time. The nipple and areola are reconstructed later. (Adapted from American Society of Plastic and Reconstructive Surgeons. *Breast reconstruction*. Arlington Heights, IL: Author.)

Tissue Transfer Procedures. Autologous reconstruction is the use of the patient's own tissue to create a breast mound. A flap of skin, fat, and muscle with its attached blood supply is rotated to the mastectomy site to create a mound that simulates the breast. Donor sites may include the **transverse rectus abdominis myocutaneous (TRAM) flap** (Fig. 33-5), gluteal flap, or the latissimus dorsi flap (Fig. 33-6). The results more closely resemble a real breast because the skin and fat from the donor sites are similar in consistency to a natural breast. These procedures are far more complex and involve longer recuperation than a procedure with a tissue expander. The risk for potential complications, such as infection, bleeding, and flap necrosis, is also greater.

The TRAM flap is the tissue transfer procedure that is performed most commonly. This involves completely detaching the skin, fat, muscle, and blood supply from the body and then transplanting them to the mastectomy site using microvascular surgery. Postoperatively, patients who have undergone TRAM procedures often face a lengthy recovery of 8 to 10 weeks and have incisions both at the mastectomy site and at the donor site in the abdomen. The nurse must assess the newly constructed breast site for changes in color, circulation, and temperature because flap loss is a potential complication. Mottling or an obvious decrease in skin temperature is reported to the surgeon immediately. Breathing and leg exercises are essential because the patient is more limited

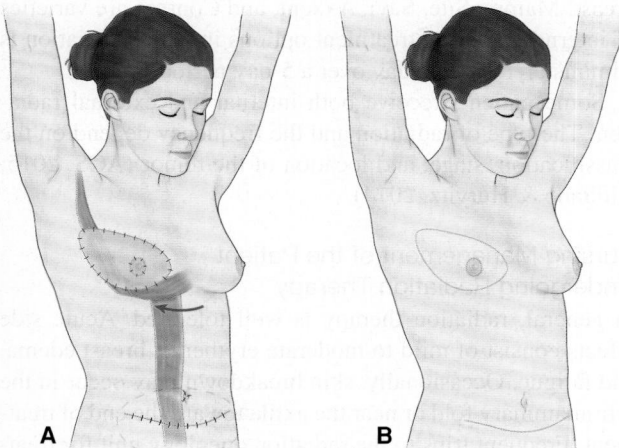

FIGURE 33-5 Breast reconstruction: transverse rectus abdominis myocutaneous (TRAM) flap. **A.** A breast mound is created by tunneling abdominal skin, fat, and muscle to the mastectomy site. **B.** Final location of scars. (Adapted from American Society of Plastic and Reconstructive Surgeons. *Breast reconstruction.* Arlington Heights, IL: Author.)

FIGURE 33-6 Breast reconstruction: latissimus dorsi flap. **A.** The latissimus muscle with an ellipse of skin is rotated from the back to the mastectomy site. **B.** Because the flap usually is not bulky enough to provide an adequate breast mound, often an implant is also required. (Adapted from American Society of Plastic and Reconstructive Surgeons. *Breast reconstruction.* Arlington Heights, IL: Author.)

in her activity and is at greater risk for respiratory complications and deep vein thrombosis (DVT). Measures to help the patient reduce tension on the abdominal incision during the first postoperative week include elevating the head of the bed 45 degrees. Once the patient is able to ambulate, she can protect the surgical incision by splinting it and gradually will achieve a more upright position. The patient is instructed to avoid high-impact activities and lifting to prevent stress on the incision.

Nipple–Areolar Reconstruction. After the breast mound has been created and the site has healed, some women choose to have nipple–areolar reconstruction. This is a minor surgical procedure carried out either in the physician's office or at an outpatient surgical facility. The most common method of creating a nipple is with the use of local flaps of skin and fat from the center of the new breast mound, which are wrapped around each other to create a projecting nipple. The areola is created using a skin graft. The most common donor site is the upper inner thigh, because this skin has darker pigmentation than the skin on the reconstructed breast. After the nipple graft has healed, micropigmentation or tattooing can be performed to achieve a more natural color. Usually the surgeon can match the reconstructed nipple–areola complex with that of the contralateral breast for an acceptable cosmetic result.

Prosthetics. A breast prosthesis, an external form that simulates the breast, is an option for women who are not candidates for or do not desire breast reconstruction. Prosthetics are available in different shapes, sizes, colors, and materials and can be placed inside a bra.

Prior to discharge from the hospital, the nurse usually provides the patient with a temporary, lightweight, cotton-filled form that can be worn until the surgical incision is well healed. Then the patient can be fitted for a prosthesis. Insurance companies generally cover the cost of the prosthesis and the special bras that hold it in place. A breast prosthesis can provide a psychological benefit and assist the woman in resuming proper posture by balancing the weight of the remaining breast.

Radiation

Patients may undergo radiation therapy to destroy any residual microscopic cancer cells in the breast, the chest wall, axilla, internal mammary, or supraclavicular nodes following surgery.

Breast conservation treatment followed by radiation therapy for stage I and II breast cancer results in a survival rate equal to that of a modified radical mastectomy. If radiation therapy, a component of breast conservation treatment, were contraindicated, then a mastectomy would be indicated. Also radiation treatment is recommended after mastectomy in women whose breast cancer tumors were large (greater than 5 cm) or when the lymph nodes were involved.

Types

Patients may undergo external beam radiation (EBR) therapy or internal radiation, also known as **brachytherapy**.

External Beam Radiation. EBR typically begins about 6 weeks after breast conservation surgery to allow the surgical site to heal. If systemic chemotherapy is indicated, radiation therapy usually begins after its completion. Before radiation begins, the patient undergoes a planning session called a *simulation*, in which the anatomic areas to be treated are mapped out and then identified with small permanent ink markings. EBR delivers high-energy photons from a linear accelerator and usually is administered to the entire breast region. Each treatment lasts only a few minutes and generally is given 5 days a week for 5 to 7 weeks. In women whose surgery consisted of breast conservation, after completion of radiation to the entire breast, many patients receive a "boost," a dose of radiation to the lumpectomy site where the cancer was removed. If a mastectomy was performed, radiation treatments are targeted at the chest wall. The treatments are not painful.

Accelerated breast irradiation is a newer technique that is gaining favor. It is similar to standard EBR, but it is given at a slightly higher dose over a 3-week period as opposed to 5 to 6 weeks. Breast cancer recurrence rates at 10 years are equal in both groups. Even more accelerated approaches in radiation treatment are being implemented in some settings. These include even larger doses of radiation over a 5-day period as well as intraoperative radiation therapy (IORT), which is single-dose treatment given in the operating room after lumpectomy is performed.

Internal Radiation Therapy. Internal radiation therapy, or brachytherapy, involves inserting a radioactive substance sealed in needles, seeds, catheters, or wires directly into the breast. MammoSite, Savi, Axxent, and Contura are varieties of internal radiation treatment options in which radiation is administered twice a day over a 5-day period.

Some patients receive both internal and external radiation. The type of radiation and the frequency depend on the classification, stage, and location of the tumor (ACS, 2015; Giuliano & Hurvitz, 2014).

Nursing Management of the Patient Undergoing Radiation Therapy

In general, radiation therapy is well tolerated. Acute side effects consist of mild to moderate erythema, breast edema, and fatigue. Occasionally, skin breakdown may occur in the inframammary fold or near the axilla toward the end of treatment. Frequent trips to the radiation oncology unit for treatment can exacerbate fatigue and may be accompanied by depression. The patient needs to be reassured that the fatigue is normal and not a sign of recurrence. Side effects usually resolve within a few weeks to a few months after treatment is completed. Rare long-term effects of radiation therapy include pneumonitis, rib fracture, breast fibrosis, and lymphedema (if radiation treatment also included the axilla).

Self-care instructions for patients receiving radiation are provided to assist in the maintenance of skin integrity during the treatments and for several weeks after completion. They pertain only to the area being treated and not to the rest of the body.

- Use mild soap with minimal rubbing.
- Avoid perfumed soaps or deodorants.
- Use hydrophilic lotions (Lubriderm, Eucerin, Aquaphor) for dryness.
- Use a nondrying, antipruritic soap (Aveeno) if pruritus occurs.
- Avoid tight clothes, underwire bras, excessive temperatures, and ultraviolet light.

Follow-up care includes teaching the patient to minimize sun exposure to the treated area, such as using sunblock with an SPF of 15 or above, and reassuring the patient that minor twinges and shooting pain in the breast are normal after radiation treatment.

Systemic Therapy

Systemic treatment uses anticancer, or antineoplastic, drugs that are given intravenously or orally and travel throughout the body in the bloodstream with the goal of destroying cancer cells that have escaped the breast and axillary lymph nodes before they metastasize. Chemotherapy and targeted therapy are two types of systemic treatment. **Neoadjuvant therapy** (drug treatment given prior to surgery) allows for assessment of the tumor's response to the chemical agent and is used to shrink a tumor before surgery. When successful tumor shrinkage occurs, breast conservation surgery without the need for mastectomy can be performed. **Adjuvant therapy** is administered after surgery and is used to eradicate any residual cancer cells in the body. The type of systemic therapy used depends on the tumor type/grade, size, lymph node status, and angiolymphatic invasion (cancer cells seen in small blood or lymph vessels), as well as the age and performance status of the patient.

For some patients who have metastatic disease, or breast cancer that has traveled beyond the breast and into other organs or parts of the body, surgery may no longer be advisable, and systemic therapy is the primary treatment of choice.

Targeted therapy includes both biologic therapy and endocrine (hormone) therapy.

Biologic Therapy

HER2/neu is a growth-promoting protein that is present in about 15% to 30% of breast cancers and results in faster growth and a higher recurrence rate than in tumors that do not overproduce it. Trastuzumab is a monoclonal antibody that targets this protein and reduces the recurrence rate and mortality in women with both metastatic and early-stage breast cancer. Lapatinib, bevacizumab, and pertuzumab are other biologic therapies that are used to treat advanced breast cancer in appropriate patients.

Endocrine (Hormone) Therapy

Estrogen is a hormone produced in the ovaries that can promote breast cancer growth. Women whose breast cancers have positive hormone receptors may take hormone therapy to block the effects of estrogen on tumor growth. Both premenopausal and postmenopausal women may take tamoxifen if their tumors test positive for hormone receptors. Tamoxifen works by blocking the effects of estrogen on breast tissue. Tamoxifen is recommended for a 5- to 10-year course of therapy after surgery and has demonstrated significant reduction in the recurrence rate and improved survival. Sequelae of tamoxifen include menopausal symptoms, fatigue, mood swings, and an increased risk of endometrial cancer and blood clots.

Aromatase inhibitors, such as letrozole, anastrozole, and exemestane, are another hormone therapy option for postmenopausal women. These drugs work by blocking aromatase, an enzyme whose role is to convert the hormone androstenedione to estrogen in the body after menopause, thus decreasing levels of circulating estrogen. Aromatase inhibitors cannot stop the ovaries from making estrogen so they are not effective in premenopausal women. They are prescribed for a 5-year course of therapy and may be given alone or following a course of tamoxifen. Aromatase inhibitors have a lower side-effect profile than tamoxifen but can cause osteoporosis, bone fractures, and musculoskeletal problems (ACS, 2015). Table 33-2 lists potential adverse effects of different hormonal therapies for breast cancer. Box 33-5 addresses side-effect management of hormonal agents.

Chemotherapy

The indication for chemotherapy depends on the size of the tumor, lymph node involvement, the presence or absence of hormone receptors in the tumor, and the amount of HER2/neu present in the breast cancer cells. Combination chemotherapy, or the use of more than one drug, has proven to be more effective than single-drug regimens. The most common drugs recommended for use in breast cancer are cyclophosphamide, docetaxel, doxorubicin, epirubicin, fluorouracil, and paclitaxel. Most chemotherapy regimens are given in 2- to 3-week cycles for a total of 3 to 6 months of therapy (ACS, 2015).

Nursing Management of the Patient Undergoing Chemotherapy

Common physical side effects of chemotherapy for breast cancer vary with the type of treatment given and may include nausea, vomiting, bone marrow suppression, taste changes, alopecia (hair loss), mucositis (painful inflammation and ulcerations of the mucous membranes in the digestive tract),

TABLE **33-2** Adverse Reactions Associated with Adjuvant Hormonal Therapy Used to Treat Breast Cancer

Therapeutic Agent	Adverse Reactions/Side Effects
Selective Estrogen Receptor Modulator	
Tamoxifen	Hot flashes, vaginal dryness/discharge/bleeding, irregular menses, nausea, mood disturbances; increased risk for endometrial cancer; increased risk for thromboembolic events (deep vein thrombosis, pulmonary embolism, superficial phlebitis)
Aromatase Inhibitors	
Anastrozole Letrozole Exemestane	Musculoskeletal symptoms (arthritis, arthralgia [joint pain], myalgia [muscle pain]), increased risk of osteoporosis/fractures, nausea/vomiting, hot flashes, fatigue, mood disturbances

skin changes, and fatigue. A weight gain of more than 10 lb occurs in about half of all patients; the cause is unknown. Premenopausal women also may experience temporary or permanent **amenorrhea** (absence of menstrual period) leading to sterility. Nurses play an important role in helping patients manage the physical and psychosocial sequelae of chemotherapy. Instructing the patient about the use of antiemetics and reviewing the optimal dosage schedule can help minimize nausea and vomiting. Measures to ease the symptoms of mucositis may include rinsing with normal saline solution, avoiding hot and spicy foods, and using a soft toothbrush. Some patients may require hematopoietic growth factors to minimize the effects of chemotherapy-induced neutropenia and anemia. Granulocyte colony–stimulating factors (G-CSFs) boost the white blood cell count, helping reduce the incidence of neutropenic fever and infection. Erythropoietin growth factor increases the production of red blood cells, thus decreasing the symptoms of anemia. The nurse instructs the patient and family on proper injection technique of hematopoietic growth factors and about symptoms that require follow-up with their provider.

The nurse may assist the patient in finding a wig prior to hair loss to alleviate the stress associated with alopecia. The nurse may provide a list of wig suppliers in the patient's geographic region. Also familiarity with creative ways to use scarves and turbans may help minimize the patient's distress. The patient needs reassurance that new hair will grow back when treatment is completed, although the color and texture may be different. The ACS offers a program called "Look Good, Feel Better" that provides useful tips for applying cosmetics during chemotherapy.

BOX 33-5 **Patient Education**

Managing Side Effects of Adjuvant Hormonal Therapy in Breast Cancer

Hot Flashes
- Wear breathable, layered clothing.
- Avoid caffeine and spicy foods.
- Perform breathing exercises (paced respirations).
- Consider medications (vitamin E, antidepressants) or acupuncture.

Vaginal Dryness
- Use vaginal moisturizers for everyday dryness (e.g., Replens, vitamin E suppository).
- Apply vaginal lubrication during intercourse (e.g., Astroglide, K-Y jelly).

Nausea and Vomiting
- Consume a bland diet.
- Try to take medication in the evening.

Musculoskeletal Symptoms
- Take nonsteroidal analgesics as recommended.
- Take warm baths.

Risk of Endometrial Cancer
- Report any irregular bleeding to a gynecologist for evaluation.

Risk for Thromboembolic Events
- Report any redness, swelling, or tenderness in the lower extremities or any unexplained shortness of breath.

Risk for Osteoporosis or Fractures
- Undergo a baseline bone density scan.
- Perform regular weight-bearing exercises.
- Take calcium supplements with vitamin D.
- Take bisphosphonates (e.g., alendronate) or calcitonin as prescribed.

Chemotherapy may negatively affect the patient's self-esteem, sexuality, and sense of well-being. This, combined with the stress of a potentially life-threatening disease, can be overwhelming. Providing support and promoting open communication are important aspects of nursing care. Referring the patient to the dietitian, social worker, psychiatrist, or spiritual advisor can provide additional support. Numerous community support and advocacy groups are available for patients and their families. Complementary therapies, such as guided imagery, meditation, and relaxation exercises, also can be used in conjunction with conventional treatments. Refer to Chapter 6 for details on cancer care.

Nursing Alert

The nurse recognizes that many patients will experience chemotherapy-induced nausea and vomiting (CINV) which may persist for several days after chemotherapy. For patients at high risk for CINV, antiemetics are given prior to initiation of treatment, and the nurse reviews the discharge medication plan for breakthrough nausea and vomiting. Refer to Chapter 6 for details on CINV.

Treatment for Recurrent or Metastatic Breast Cancer

Breast cancer may recur locally (on the chest wall or in the conserved breast), regionally (in the remaining lymph nodes), or systemically (in distant organs). In metastatic disease, the bone, usually the hips, spine, ribs, or pelvis, is the most common site of spread. Other sites of metastasis include the lungs, liver, pleura, and brain.

The overall prognosis and optimal treatment are determined by a variety of factors, such as the site and extent of recurrence, the time to recurrence from the original diagnosis, history of prior treatments, the patient's performance status, and any existing comorbid conditions. Patients with bone metastases generally have a longer overall survival compared with metastases in visceral organs.

Local recurrence in the absence of systemic disease is treated aggressively with surgery, radiation, and hormonal therapy. Chemotherapy also may be used for tumors that are not hormonally sensitive. Local recurrence may be an indicator that systemic disease will develop in the future, particularly if it occurs within 2 years of the original diagnosis.

Metastatic breast cancer involves control of the disease rather than cure. Treatment includes hormonal therapy, chemotherapy, and targeted therapy. Surgery or radiation may be indicated in select situations. Premenopausal women who have hormonally dependent tumors may eliminate the production of estrogen by the ovaries through **oophorectomy** or suppression of estrogen synthesis by luteinizing hormone–releasing hormone (LHRH) agonists, such as leuprolide or goserelin.

Patients with advanced breast cancer are monitored closely for signs of disease progression. Baseline studies are obtained at the time of recurrence. These may include complete blood count; comprehensive metabolic panel; tumor markers; bone scan; CT of the chest, abdomen, and pelvis; and MRI of symptomatic areas. Additional x-rays may be performed to evaluate areas of pain or abnormal areas seen on bone scan. These studies are repeated at regular intervals to assess for effectiveness of treatment and to monitor progression of disease.

Nursing Management of the Patient with Recurrent or Metastatic Breast Cancer

Nurses play an important role in not only educating patients and managing their symptoms but also in providing emotional support. Many patients find that recurrence of the disease is more distressing than the initial cancer diagnosis. In addition to coping with further treatments, they are faced with a greater uncertainty about their future and long-term survival. The nurse can help the patient identify coping strategies and set priorities to optimize quality of life (QOL). Family members and significant others should be included in the treatment plan and follow-up care. Referrals to support groups, psychiatry, social work, and complementary medicine programs, such as guided imagery, meditation, and yoga, should be made as indicated.

Nurses are also key members of the interdisciplinary team providing palliative care. The highest priorities should include alleviating pain and providing comfort measures. A frank discussion with the patient and family regarding their preferences for end-of-life care should occur before the need arises, to ensure a smooth transition without disruption of care. Referrals to hospice and home health care should be initiated as necessary.

Survivorship and Quality of Life

With increased early detection and improved treatment modalities, women with breast cancer have become the largest group of cancer survivors. Sequelae of diagnosis and treatment may affect the patient and her family for an extended period of time. It is important that nurses learn about these long-term effects and intervene appropriately to optimize QOL. The nurse can be pivotal in providing education and support to the patient as she makes very difficult and emotional decisions. The patient should be prepared early for the potential long-term complications of the disease and its treatments so that she can make informed decisions, has realistic expectations, and can be proactive in obtaining the support she needs.

Many breast cancer survivors have difficulty with issues pertaining to sexuality and menopausal symptoms. Estrogen withdrawal due to chemotherapy-induced menopause and hormone therapy can cause a variety of symptoms, including hot flashes, vaginal dryness, urinary tract infections (UTIs), weight gain, decreased sex drive, and increased risk for osteoporosis. Some of these symptoms also can lead to fatigue and sleep disturbances. Hormone replacement therapy (HRT) to alleviate menopausal symptoms is contraindicated in women with breast cancer so women need to rely on alternative remedies. Certain chemotherapeutic agents can cause long-term cardiac effects and impaired cognitive functioning, such as difficulty concentrating. Rare long-term effects of radiation can include pneumonitis and rib fractures. Long-term sequelae after breast surgery may include lymphedema (mainly after ALND), pain, and sensory disturbances.

Nursing Alert
Cardiac function must be assessed in patients undergoing chemotherapy and/or radiation since impaired aortic elasticity and stiffness have been noted in patients with breast cancer undergoing radiation (Kilicaslan et al., 2013), and cardiotoxicity is associated with some chemotherapy agents (Vasiliadis, Kolovou, & Mikhailidis, 2013). The nurse is aware that echocardiography, holter monitoring, cardiac and pulmonary assessments, and laboratory work, such as brain natriuretic peptide (BNP) and troponin levels, may be monitored.

Long-term psychosocial ramifications may include anxiety, depression, uncertainty about the future, and fear of recurrence. Many of these sequelae can affect the patient's partner and children. In the workplace, the patient may suffer from fear of discrimination, concern over coworkers' reactions, fear of losing benefits, and lack of physical stamina. The nurse should facilitate open conversation with the patient about her fears and concerns and provide referrals to support groups and counseling as needed.

NURSING PROCESS
The Patient Undergoing Surgery for Breast Cancer

ASSESSMENT

The health history is a valuable tool to assess the patient's reaction to the diagnosis and her ability to cope with it. Pertinent questions include the following:

- How is the patient responding to the diagnosis?
- What coping mechanisms does she find most helpful?
- What psychological or emotional supports does she have and use?
- Is there a partner, family member, or friend available to assist her in making treatment choices?
- What are her educational needs?
- Is she experiencing any pain or discomfort?

DIAGNOSIS

Major preoperative nursing diagnoses may include the following:

- Deficient knowledge about the planned surgical treatments
- Anxiety related to the diagnosis of cancer
- Fear related to specific treatments and body image changes
- Risk for ineffective coping (individual or family) related to the diagnosis of breast cancer and related treatment options
- Decisional conflict related to treatment options

Major postoperative nursing diagnoses may include the following:

- Pain and discomfort related to surgical procedure
- Disturbed sensory perception related to nerve irritation in affected arm, breast, or chest wall
- Disturbed body image related to loss or alteration of the breast
- Risk for impaired adjustment related to the diagnosis of cancer and surgical treatment
- Self-care deficit related to partial immobility of upper extremity on operative side
- Risk for sexual dysfunction related to loss of body part, change in self-image, and fear of partner's responses
- Deficient knowledge:
  - Drain management after breast surgery
  - Arm exercises to regain mobility of affected extremity
  - Hand and arm care after an ALND

Potential complications may include the following:

- Lymphedema
- Hematoma/seroma formation
- Infection

PLANNING

The major goals may include increased knowledge about the disease and its treatment; reduction of preoperative and postoperative fear, anxiety, and emotional stress; improvement of decision-making ability; pain management; improvement in coping abilities; improvement in sexual function; and the absence of complications.

INTERVENTIONS

Both pre- and postoperative nursing care greatly impact the patient's surgical experience.

PREOPERATIVE NURSING INTERVENTIONS

Providing Education and Preparation About Surgical Treatments. Patients with newly diagnosed breast cancer are expected to absorb an abundance of new information during a very emotionally difficult time. The nurse plays a key role in reviewing treatment options by reinforcing information provided to the patient and answering any questions. The nurse fully prepares the patient for what to expect before, during, and after surgery. Patients undergoing breast conservation with ALND, or a total or modified radical mastectomy, generally remain in the

BOX 33-6

Patient Education

Exercise After Breast Surgery

1. *Wall handclimbing.* Stand facing the wall with feet apart and toes as close to the wall as possible. With elbows slightly bent, place the palms of the hand on the wall at shoulder level. By flexing the fingers, work the hands up the wall until arms are fully extended. Then reverse the process, working the hands down to the starting point.

2. *Rope turning.* Tie a light rope to a doorknob. Stand facing the door. Take the free end of the rope in the hand on the side of surgery. Place the other hand on the hip. With the rope-holding arm extended and held away from the body (nearly parallel with the floor), turn the rope, making as wide swings as possible. Begin slowly at first; speed up later.

3. *Rod or broomstick lifting.* Grasp a rod with both hands, held about 2 ft apart. Keeping the arms straight, raise the rod over the head. Bend elbows to lower the rod behind the head. Reverse the maneuver, raising the rod above the head, and then return to the starting position.

4. *Pulley tugging.* Toss a light rope over a shower curtain rod or doorway curtain rod. Stand as nearly under the rope as possible. Grasp an end in each hand. Extend the arms straight and away from the body. Pull the left arm up by tugging down with the right arm, then the right arm up and the left down in a see-sawing motion.

hospital overnight (or longer if they have immediate reconstruction). Surgical drains will be inserted in the mastectomy incision and in the axilla if the patient undergoes an ALND. The patient should be informed that she will go home with the drain(s) and that complete instructions about drain care will be provided prior

to discharge. In addition, the patient should be informed that often she will have decreased arm and shoulder mobility after an ALND and that she will be shown range-of-motion exercises prior to discharge. Refer to Box 33-6 for exercises after breast surgery. The patient also should be reassured that appropriate

(continued on page 1012)

analgesia and comfort measures will be provided to alleviate any postoperative discomfort.

Reducing Fear and Anxiety and Improving Coping Ability. The nurse must help the patient cope with the physical as well as the emotional effects of surgery. Many fears may emerge during the preoperative phase. These can include fear of pain, mutilation (after mastectomy), and loss of sexual attractiveness; concern about inability to care for oneself and one's family; concern about taking time off from work; and coping with an uncertain future. Providing the patient with realistic expectations about the healing process and expected recovery can help alleviate fears. Maintaining open communication and assuring the patient that she can contact the nurse at any time with questions or concerns can be a source of comfort. The patient also should be made aware of available resources at the treatment facility as well as in the breast cancer community, such as social workers, psychiatrists, and support groups. Some women find it helpful and reassuring to talk to a breast cancer survivor who has undergone similar treatments.

Promoting Decision-Making Ability. Choosing the optimal treatment can be very overwhelming for patients. The nurse can be instrumental in ensuring that the patient and family members truly understand their options and can weigh the risks and benefits of each option. The patient may be presented with the option of having breast conservation treatment followed by radiation or a mastectomy. The nurse can explore the issues with the individual patient by asking questions such as the following:

- How would you feel about losing your breast?
- Are you considering breast reconstruction?
- If you choose to retain your breast, would you consider undergoing radiation treatments 5 days a week for 5 to 6 weeks?

Questions such as these can help the patient focus. Once the patient's decision is made, it is very important to support it.

POSTOPERATIVE NURSING INTERVENTIONS

Relieving Pain and Discomfort. Many patients tolerate the breast surgery quite well and have minimal pain during the postoperative period. Patients who have had more invasive procedures, such as a modified radical mastectomy with immediate reconstruction, may have considerably more pain. All patients are discharged home with analgesic and are encouraged to take it if needed. Sometimes patients complain of a slight increase in pain after the first few days of surgery as they regain sensation around the surgical site and become more active. Patients who report severe pain must be evaluated to rule out any potential complications. Alternative methods of pain management, such as taking warm showers and using distraction methods such as guided imagery, also may be helpful.

Managing Postoperative Sensations. Because nerves in the skin and axilla often are cut or injured during breast surgery, patients experience a variety of sensations, such as tenderness, soreness, numbness, tightness, pulling, and twinges along the chest wall, in the axilla, and along the inside aspect of the upper arm. After mastectomy, some patients experience phantom sensations and report a feeling that the breast and/or nipple are still present. Sensations usually persist for several months and then begin to diminish. Patients should be reassured that this is a normal part of healing and that these sensations are not indicative of a problem.

Promoting Positive Body Image. Patients who have undergone mastectomy often find it very difficult to view the surgical site for the first time. No matter how prepared the patient may think she is, the appearance of an absent breast can be very emotionally distressing. Some patients who have undergone breast conservation treatment may find it difficult to view their surgical incisions, although this is rare. Ideally, the patient sees the incision for the first time when she is with the nurse or another health care provider who is available for support. The nurse first assesses the patient's readiness and provides gentle encouragement and a private setting.

Promoting Positive Adjustment and Coping. Providing ongoing assessment of how the patient is coping with her diagnosis of breast cancer and her surgical treatment is important in determining her overall adjustment. Assisting the patient in identifying and mobilizing her support systems can be beneficial to her well-being. The patient's spouse or partner may need guidance, support, and education as well. The patient and partner may benefit from a wide network of available community resources, including the Reach to Recovery program of the ACS, advocacy groups, or a spiritual advisor. Encouraging the patient to discuss issues and concerns with other patients who have had breast cancer may help her to understand that her feelings are normal and that other women who have had breast cancer can provide invaluable support and understanding.

The patient also may have considerable anxiety about the treatments that will follow surgery and their implications. Providing her with information about the plan of care and referring her to the appropriate members of the health care team also promote coping during recovery. Some women require additional support to adjust to their diagnosis and the changes that it brings. Box 33-7 lists talking points for patients and partners.

Improving Sexual Function. Once discharged from the hospital, most patients are physically allowed to engage in sexual activity. However, any change in the patient's body image, self-esteem, or the response of her partner may increase her anxiety level and affect sexual function. Some partners may have difficulty looking at the incision, whereas others may be completely unaffected. Encouraging the patient to openly discuss how she feels about herself and about possible reasons for a decrease in libido, such as fatigue, anxiety, and self-consciousness, may help clarify issues for her. Helpful suggestions for the patient may include varying the time of day for sexual activity, such as when the patient is less tired, assuming positions that are more comfortable, and expressing affection using alternative measures such as hugging, kissing, and manual stimulation.

BOX 33-7
Talking with Patients and Partners

For patients in the diagnostic phase: We've talked about your recent breast cancer diagnosis. It's natural for you to be full of feelings, concerns, and fears for yourself and your family. Sometimes it's hard to find someone to speak freely with. Would you like to share what you've been thinking about, feeling, and worrying about recently?

For partners in the diagnostic phase: We've talked about your partner's recent breast cancer diagnosis. It's natural for you to have a lot of feelings, concerns, and fears for your partner, yourself, and your family. Partners often feel that they have to be strong for the patient or for others and that they aren't entitled to express their own concerns. Would you like to share what you've been thinking about, feeling, or worrying about recently?

For patients in the postsurgical phase: Many women who have had breast surgery, especially mastectomy or extensive lumpectomy, are concerned not only with their own loss but also with how their partner will accept it. How have you felt about losing [part of] your breast? How has it changed your body image? Your sense of your sexuality? Your desire for intimacy?

For partners in the postsurgical phase: Many partners of women who have had breast surgery are concerned, as are the women themselves, about how they'll respond to the loss. How have you felt about your partner's losing [part of] her breast? How has it changed her attractiveness for you? Your sexual feelings toward her? Your desire for intimacy?

For patients in the adjuvant therapy phase: Given the type of therapy (radiation, chemotherapy, hormone therapy) you're going to have, what side effects do you anticipate? What do you know about them? Let's talk about ways to reduce and handle potential side effects.

For partners in the adjuvant therapy phase: Given the type of therapy (radiation, chemotherapy, hormone therapy) your partner is going to have, what side effects do you anticipate? What do you know about them? Let's talk about ways to reduce and handle potential side effects and how it might help you to be familiar with them.

For patients in the ongoing recovery phase: As you plan your return to a full work schedule, what measures—setting priorities, delegating responsibility, managing stress—might help you make the necessary physical and emotional adjustments? What have you learned about balancing work, family, and play in your life?

For partners in the ongoing recovery phase: As your partner plans her return to a full work schedule, what strategies have you thought about using to make your own physical and emotional adjustments so that you don't continue to be overburdened at work and at home?

From Hoskins, C. N., & Haber, J. (2000). Adjusting to breast cancer. *American Journal of Nursing*, 100(4), 26–32.

Most patients and their partners adjust with minimal difficulty if they openly discuss their concerns. However, if issues cannot be resolved, a referral may be helpful. The ambulatory care nurse in the outpatient clinic or hospital should inquire whether the patient is having difficulty with sexuality issues because many patients are reluctant or embarrassed to bring it up themselves.

EVALUATION

Expected preoperative patient outcomes may include:
1. Exhibits knowledge about diagnosis and surgical treatment options:
   a. Asks relevant questions about diagnosis and available surgical treatments
   b. States rationale for surgery
   c. Describes advantages and disadvantages of treatment options
2. Verbalizes willingness to deal with anxiety and fears related to the diagnosis and the effects of surgery on self-image and sexual functioning
3. Demonstrates ability to cope with diagnosis and treatment:
   a. Verbalizes feelings appropriately and recognizes normalcy of mood lability
   b. Proceeds with treatment in timely fashion
   c. Discusses impact of diagnosis and treatment on family and work

4. Demonstrates ability to make decisions regarding treatment options in timely fashion

Expected postoperative patient outcomes may include:
1. Reports that pain has decreased and states that pain and discomfort management strategies are effective
2. Identifies postoperative sensations and recognizes that they are a normal part of healing
3. Exhibits clean, dry, and intact surgical incisions without signs of inflammation or infection
4. Lists the signs and symptoms of infection to be reported to the nurse or surgeon
5. Verbalizes feelings regarding change in body image
6. Discusses meaning of the diagnosis, surgical treatment, and fears appropriately
7. Participates actively in self-care activities:
   a. Performs exercises as prescribed
   b. Participates in self-care activities as prescribed
8. Discusses issues of sexuality and resumption of sexual relations
9. Demonstrates knowledge of postdischarge recommendations and restrictions:
   a. Describes follow-up care and activities
   b. Demonstrates appropriate care of incisions and drainage system
   c. Demonstrates arm exercises and describes exercise regimen and activity limitations during postoperative period

(continued on page 1014)

d. Describes care of affected arm and hand and lists indications to contact the surgeon or nurse
10. Experiences no complications:
    a. Identifies signs and symptoms of reportable complications (e.g., redness, heat, pain, edema)
    b. Explains how to contact appropriate health care providers in case of complications

REPRODUCTIVE DISORDERS

Menstrual Disorders

Menstrual disorders consist of any irregularity within the menstrual cycle. Previous terminology used to describe deviations in uterine bleeding has included: **amenorrhea** (absence of menses), **dysmenorrhea** (painful menses), **menorrhagia** (excessive menstrual bleeding), **metrorrhagia** (excessive and prolonged menstrual bleeding), irregular bleeding patterns, **premenstrual syndrome** (PMS), and **premenstrual dysphoric disorder** (PMDD). Normal menstrual cycles typically occur every 21 to 35 days (Klein & Poth, 2013).

Any menstrual cycle changes should be discussed with the patient's health care provider, so that appropriate diagnosis, management, and treatment can occur.

AMENORRHEA

Amenorrhea is divided into two types: primary, which is the absence of menses until age 16 or absence of secondary sex characteristics and menarche by age 14; and secondary, which is more common and occurs after a regular pattern of menstrual cycles has been established already (Papadakis & McPhee, 2014).

Pathophysiology

Primary amenorrhea is caused by hypothyroidism, **Turner syndrome**, pituitary disorders, hyperandrogenism, disorders of sexual development, pregnancy, anatomic abnormalities or in utero exposure to DES (diethylstilbestrol) (Klein & Poth, 2013; Papadakis & McPhee, 2014). Those with Turner syndrome have only one normal "X" chromosome and have absence of breast or pubic hair development. DES was a drug given to pregnant women between 1938 and 1970 to help prevent miscarriages. It was discovered later that the drug affected the reproductive organs of the female offspring, causing infertility. These patients will have secondary sex characteristics but incomplete development of reproductive organs (Centers for Disease Control and Prevention [CDC], 2012a).

When menses do not occur for 6 months or more after a regular pattern of cycles has been established, it is considered **secondary amenorrhea**. Pathologic causes of secondary amenorrhea include eating disorders, pregnancy, excessive weight loss, low body mass index (BMI) of less than 22% of average, excessive exercise, endocrine dysfunction such as polycystic ovarian syndrome (PCOS), hypothalamic or pituitary dysfunction, medications, or anatomical deviations such as **cervical stenosis** or **imperforate hymen** (Klein & Poth, 2013; Papadakis & McPhee, 2014).

This type of amenorrhea is common among athletes and those with rapid weight loss due to bariatric surgery or starvation dieting. Amenorrhea also may be caused by hormonal contraceptives, such as oral contraception, Depo-Provera, implanted long-term progesterone contraception, or the presence of a progesterone-only intrauterine device (IUD). Patients with eating disorders are at risk for developing menstrual irregularities due to suppression in the hypothalamic–pituitary–ovarian axis (Snyder, 2014).

❤ *Pathophysiology Alert*
The female athlete triad is an association between low-energy availability (with or without eating disorders), amenorrhea, and osteoporosis. It is a state of insufficient caloric intake (excessive exercise or reduced energy intake), low estrogen, and elevated cortisol. The elevated cortisol inhibits the release of gonadotropins which results in suppression of ovulation and decreased estrogen production. The negative impact on bone density occurs because of the decreased estrogen availability and suppression of hormones that stimulate bone growth. As a result, amenorrhea, and decreased bone mineral density is seen (Casey & Chen, 2017; Griffin, 2015).

Clinical Manifestations and Assessment

Patients who have an established menstrual cycle pattern will report a history of the absence of menstruation or other symptoms that are associated with the underlying cause of amenorrhea. Those patients 16 years of age who have developed secondary sex characteristics generally will seek medical evaluation if they have not experienced any menstruation as will 14-year-olds who have not developed any secondary sex characteristics. A detailed menstrual history is critical in determining abnormality in menstrual patterns and should be accompanied by pregnancy and sexual histories, contraception use, medications, exercise patterns, and detailed history on any intentional or unintentional changes in weight.

Once pregnancy has been excluded, appropriate labs should include thyroid-stimulating hormone (TSH) and prolactin levels, follicle-stimulating hormone (FSH), luteinizing hormone (LH, also known as lutropin), dehydroepiandrosterone sulfate (DHEAS), and serum testosterone. If the patient is short in stature, genetic testing for Turner syndrome should be considered (Klein & Poth, 2013; Papadakis & McPhee, 2014). Physical examination of the external and internal genitalia by a health care provider will determine any anatomical deviations that may cause obstruction of the vaginal outlet.

Medical and Nursing Management

A withdrawal bleed occurs with the administration of medroxyprogesterone acetate (MPA) (Provera) 10 mg for 7 to 10 days. Depending upon risk factors, an oral contraceptive pill (OCP) then can be initiated to assist with regulation of the menstrual cycle. Alternatively, the patient can be prescribed progesterone the first week of each month or every 3 months for a withdrawal bleed. It is important to instruct the patient that if she has not had a menstrual period for several months, she can expect a heavy flow after taking MPA and may experience severe cramping as a result. Therapies for painful menstruation are listed below.

Also a pelvic ultrasound may be ordered to confirm the absence or presence of a uterus or any other structural abnormalities that may be a contributing factor in amenorrhea (Klein & Poth, 2013).

DYSMENORRHEA

Painful menstruation, or dysmenorrhea, has two classifications: primary and secondary. Primary dysmenorrhea occurs at the onset of menarche and the early following years after establishing a cycle and may become more severe over time (Papadakis & McPhee, 2014). It is considered one of the most common causes of pelvic pain with rates as high as 90% (Osayande & Mehulic, 2014). Approximately 10% to 15% of adolescent females report severe pain from their menstrual cycles, resulting in lost time from work or school (Yu, 2014). Secondary dysmenorrhea begins well after the menstrual cycle has been established and is typically caused by some organic or structural causes (Papadakis & McPhee, 2014).

Pathophysiology

The classic characterization of primary dysmenorrhea is crampy pain in the abdomen and/or lower back just before the onset of bleeding and persisting for the first few days into the menstrual flow. It is due to an excessive production of **prostaglandins** in the lining of the uterus, which causes contractions of the smooth muscle (Yu, 2014). The onset of primary dysmenorrhea typically occurs 6 to 12 months after the menstrual cycle has been established (Osayande & Mehulic, 2014).

Secondary dysmenorrhea begins well after the onset of menarche, usually after age 20, but can occur as late as the third or fourth decade of life and is suggestive of an underlying pathology, such as **endometriosis** (most common cause), fibroids (discussed later in this chapter), or a pelvic infection. It may be related to IUDs, congenital anomalies, ovarian cysts, or benign or malignant tumors (Papadakis & McPhee, 2014).

Clinical Manifestations and Assessment

Often primary dysmenorrhea is characterized by sharp, intermittent abdominal pain that is accompanied by headache, fatigue, backache, nausea, diarrhea, or constipation. The gastrointestinal (GI) symptoms are caused by prostaglandins triggering uterine vasoconstriction and prolonged contractions or cramping (Papadakis & McPhee, 2014). Symptoms for secondary dysmenorrhea begin earlier in the cycle and last longer. There is also a change in bowel habits, rectal pressure, and painful defecation due to the influence production of prostaglandins. Table 33-3 compares primary and secondary dysmenorrhea.

Medical Management

Nonsteroidal anti-inflammatories (NSAIDs) and hormonal contraceptives are the mainstay and first-line therapy for treating primary dysmenorrhea due to their antiprostaglandin effect (Osayande & Mehulic, 2014; Papadakis & McPhee, 2014).

Ibuprofen and naproxen are available over the counter (OTC). Other NSAIDs available by prescription include mefenamic acid (Ponstel), prescription-strength ibuprofen and naproxen, and cyclooxygenase (COX)-2 inhibitors (Celebrex). By blocking the production of prostaglandin, pain usually will not occur or will be mild in comparison.

While effective, NSAIDs can have a negative impact on the GI system; therefore, care must be taken to avoid long-term use of these medications. Combined oral contraceptives (COCs) are very beneficial in treatment for this condition as the combined hormones inhibit ovulation as well as decrease uterine flow and thereby decrease uterine contractility (Osayande & Mehulic, 2014). COCs are a good choice for sexually active women who desire birth control as well as relief from dysmenorrhea.

TABLE 33-3 Comparing Primary and Secondary Dysmenorrhea

Aspect	Primary Dysmenorrhea	Secondary Dysmenorrhea
Quality of pain	Sharp, intermittent pain	Recurrent, crampy, suprapubic pain
Timing	Begins with onset of menarche	Symptoms begin earlier in cycle and last longer
Age of onset	Occurs with menarche	Occurs between 30 and 40 years of age
Additional symptoms	Headache, fatigue, backache, dizziness, nausea, diarrhea, and constipation	Change in bowel habits, rectal pressure, painful defecation, dyspareunia

Management of secondary dysmenorrhea is aimed at identification of the causative factor through the use of the appropriate diagnostic tests. The same medications listed above also may be used to alleviate pain.

Nursing Management

Nurses can teach patients how to accurately keep a menstrual diary that will assist in tracking patterns of menstrual discomfort and pain (Fig. 33-7). Advising the patient to take an OTC NSAID 1 to 2 days prior to the onset of menses will help to inhibit prostaglandin production and help to decrease the amount of abdominal pain and cramping. Patients who

take proton pump inhibitors (PPIs), which are available OTC or by prescription, need to be instructed on the proper administration of these drugs, which will help to protect the lining of the stomach from the effects of the NSAIDs. It is recommended that PPIs be taken on an empty stomach. The patient should eat something 30 to 60 minutes after taking the PPI to allow the medication to start working. Also, taking the NSAID with food will help to minimize stomach upset.

Nonpharmacologic therapy includes supplementation with magnesium, calcium, and vitamins B and E, but further studies are needed to accurately define appropriate dosages and outcomes (Yu, 2014). Low-level localized heat, such as a heating pad or wrap, for 15 to 20 minutes intermittently

Menstrual Cycle Log

Month and Date	Bleeding Y/N	Symptoms	Length of Time	Intensity	Treatment	Impact
1						
2						
3						
4						
5						
6						
7						
8						
9						
10						
11						
12						
13						
14						
15						
16						
17						
18						
19						
20						
21						
22						
23						
24						
25						
26						
27						
28						
29						
30						
31						

KEY:
Symptoms:
NS, no symptoms
N/V, nausea/vomiting
TS, trouble sleeping
S, sensitive to light, sight, or sound
D, disturbances in sight/vision
B, bleeding: heavy, moderate, light
GI, diarrhea or constipation
BE, binge eating
FC, food cravings

I-irritable
FN-feeling nervous
T-tired
C-abdominal cramping or pain
H-headache
M-mood: depressed, anxious

Intensity:
Mild
Moderate
Severe

Treatment:
M-medicine
BR-bed rest
HCP-contacted health care professional

FIGURE 33-7 Menstrual log.

can be beneficial in easing uterine contractility. It is important to instruct the patient not to use heat that is too high or for prolonged periods of time due to the risk of burns.

ABNORMAL UTERINE BLEEDING

Any uterine bleeding that deviates from a patient's usual pattern is considered abnormal uterine bleeding (AUB). This includes bleeding between periods, postmenopausal bleeding, postcoital bleeding, bleeding heavier than usual or for greater length of time, or bleeding between menstrual cycles (American College of Obstetricians and Gynecologists [ACOG], 2013). Approximately 1.4 million women report AUB annually (Carcio & Secor, 2015). The ACOG introduced new terminology recommendations for a universal classification system describing deviations in menstrual bleeding that will lend itself to easier classification. The new classification system is called PALM-COEIN, which is an acronym that refers to polyps, adenomyosis, leiomyoma, malignancies, coagulopathies, ovulatory dysfunction, iatrogenic, not yet classified (ACOG, 2013; Twiss, 2013). This classification system refers to the identification of structural or nonstructural etiologies that contribute to the development of AUB. Despite the new classification recommendations, much of the literature still uses the following terms to describe and categorize abnormal bleeding patterns:

- Any change in a normal menstrual cycle is referred to as *abnormal uterine bleeding* (AUB) (Twiss, 2013).
- Bleeding that occurs at regular intervals but is in excessive amounts and/or duration is known as *menorrhagia* or *heavy menstrual bleeding (HB)*.
- "*Excessive menstrual blood loss* is that which interferes with the woman's physical, emotional, social, and material QOL and can occur alone or in combination with other symptoms" (ACOG, 2013).
- Unpredictable bleeding patterns are considered to be *anovulatory bleeding* (Twiss, 2013).

Bleeding that occurs frequently but irregularly is known as *metrorrhagia. Menometrorrhagia* is now the term used to refer to heavy and prolonged menstrual bleeding (HPMB) and is heavy bleeding of prolonged duration occurring at irregular intervals. Any persistent AUB can lead to iron-deficiency anemia if left undiagnosed and untreated. Cycles greater than 35 days are known as **oligomenorrhea**, and cycles occurring in less than 21 days are known as **polymenorrhea**.

Causes

Coagulation disorders, such as thrombocytopenia (low platelet count) or Von Willebrand disease (most common inherited bleeding disorder in humans, refer to Chapter 20), are causes of AUB and should be ruled out as an underlying factor. Women who take unopposed estrogen are likely to develop AUB, as well as those with liver diseases that impair fibrinogen synthesis. Certain endocrine disorders, including Cushing syndrome, Addison disease, thyroid disorders, and PCOS; extreme fluctuations in weight; or excessive exercise can cause irregular uterine bleeding. Pregnancy should always be excluded when AUB is present (Papadakis & McPhee, 2014).

Other causes include pelvic infections caused by sexually transmitted infections (STIs; gonorrhea, *Chlamydia*, trichomonas), weight loss or weight gain, recent systemic infections, endometriosis, trauma, benign tumors, or lesions (Papadakis & McPhee, 2014). Refer to Chapter 35 for details on STIs.

Medical and Nursing Management

Nursing care must include vital signs, including orthostatic blood pressures, pulse rate to evaluate for tachycardia or arrhythmias, and a BMI (Carcio & Secor, 2015). Menstrual pad counts assist the health care provider in determining the approximate amount of blood loss through the description of the saturation of sanitary pads or tampons on an hourly basis. Characteristics of the flow, such as the color of blood and presence of clots, are to be noted as well. Physical examination of the genitalia and a Pap smear are performed. It is important that the patient undergo appropriate diagnostic testing to determine underlying pathology of AUB prior to treatment. This may include a pelvic ultrasound and endocrine tests, as described earlier. A CBC with differential, TSH, prothrombin time (PT), and partial prothrombin time (PTT) are indicated in the workup for AUB. Also an iron panel should be included to determine the presence of iron-deficiency anemia (Papadakis & McPhee, 2014). An endometrial biopsy is considered the first-line diagnostic test to rule out endometrial hyperplasia or malignancy in women over 35 years of age or in those under 35 years of age who are morbidly obese or who have chronic anovulation or PCOS (Twiss, 2013).

Once any pathology has been ruled out, it is appropriate for the patient to be treated with hormonal contraception that will regulate the menstrual cycle, decrease bleeding and cramping associated with heavy bleeding, and decrease any incidence of anemia associated with excessive blood loss. Progestin-releasing IUDs reduce blood flow, as does implanted progesterone (Papadakis & McPhee, 2014; Twiss, 2013).

PREMENSTRUAL SYNDROME AND PREMENSTRUAL DYSPHORIC DISORDER

PMS is the name given to a cluster of behavioral, emotional, and physical symptoms that typically occur the week prior to menstruation and may continue into the first week of the menstrual cycle (Papadakis & McPhee, 2014). Symptoms usually resolve with the onset of menstrual flow but can persist for the first few days of bleeding. PMDD is a more severe form of PMS and is recognized by diagnostic criteria developed by the American Psychiatric Association (APA), ACOG, and the World Health Organization (WHO). Symptoms must be present consistently during the luteal phase (second half of the menstrual cycle) and have a negative impact to some degree on the woman's life. The severity of the symptoms experienced by the patient and the impact on daily functioning are what delineates PMDD from PMS (Kelderhouse & Taylor, 2013).

It is estimated that approximately 40% of women of reproductive age are affected by symptoms related to menstrual cycle changes that interfere with daily lifestyle and relationships (Papadakis & McPhee, 2014). There is no known cause of PMS/PMDD, although research indicates these symptoms are most likely due to fluctuating levels of estrogen, progesterone, and serotonin.

Clinical Manifestations and Assessment

More than 100 physical and behavioral symptoms are associated with PMS/PMDD and range from mild to severely disabling (Box 33-8).

Symptoms may be misdiagnosed as menopause, anxiety, bipolar disorder, metabolic disorders (such as diabetes), chronic fatigue syndrome, or rheumatologic diseases. It is important that health care providers take a comprehensive, systematic approach to properly diagnosing patients with PMS/PMDD so that appropriate therapy may be initiated.

BOX 33-8 **Focused Assessment**

Premenstrual Syndrome

Be alert for the following signs and symptoms:
Physical:
- Weight gain
- Abdominal bloating
- Constipation or diarrhea
- Breast tenderness
- Acne
- Headache
- Heart palpitations

Behavioral:
- Irritability
- Depression
- Mood swings
- Increased appetite
- Overwhelming fatigue
- Insomnia
- Crying spells

Cognitive:
- Decreased concentration
- Paranoia
- Indecision
- Sensitivity to rejection
- Suicidal ideation

Women may experience some of the symptoms or a constellation of symptoms at any one time during the luteal phase, including breast pain, bloating, ankle swelling, perceived weight gain, food cravings, and functional and cognitive impairments (Papadakis & McPhee, 2014).

Medical Management

Menstrual cycle diaries (see Fig. 33-7) are kept for two to three menstrual cycles (Kelderhouse & Taylor, 2013). The presence or absence of symptoms is to be noted daily, along with the impact of symptoms on daily activities. Providers are able to view trends of symptoms based on these logs that correlate with the menstrual cycle. Nurses can encourage lifestyle changes that will impact the severity of symptoms. These lifestyle changes include regular exercise, which promotes increased circulation of endorphins released from exercise; avoidance of excessive caffeine (coffee, soda, tea, energy drinks, and chocolate) and sodium-rich foods; decreased alcohol intake; and smoking cessation. Randomized trials of patients taking increased complex carbohydrates during the luteal phase have revealed a decrease in the severity of PMS symptoms (Kelderhouse & Taylor, 2013). Low serum calcium can cause muscle irritability; therefore, it is recommended that the patient ensure a daily intake of 1,200 to 1,600 mg of calcium daily.

Use of vitamin B_6 from 50 to 500 mg/day has been met with mixed success. Other nonpharmacologic therapies include oral magnesium, vitamin E supplements, and evening primrose oil. Due to flaws in recent studies of evening primrose oil, results of previous randomized control trials have demonstrated that it does not appear to provide any significant improvement of symptoms (Nevatte et al., 2013).

There are some results on the use of chasteberry for its dopaminergic effects on the emotional and physical symptoms of PMS and PMDD, but the exact mechanism is unknown (Nevatte et al., 2013). For women who do not respond to nonpharmacologic therapy, pharmacologic management is considered. The use of oral contraceptives has proven to be of great benefit for those with physical and emotional symptoms of PMS. Continuous contraception for 3 months' duration or longer often alleviates PMS symptoms (Nevatte et al., 2013; Papadakis & McPhee, 2014).

Selective serotonin reuptake inhibitors (SSRIs) and serotonin-norepinephrine reuptake inhibitors (SNRIs) have shown efficacy in mood stabilization. Pulsed or cyclical dosing of SSRIs also can be used during the 2 weeks prior to and including the week of menstrual flow (Papadakis & McPhee, 2014).

Gonadotropin-releasing hormone (GnRH) agonists (Lupron or Depo-Provera) suppress the menstrual cycle, but long-term use can produce consequences of menopause due to the lack of estrogen, which may lead to irreversible osteoporosis. NSAIDs are beneficial for physical symptoms, including headache and dysmenorrhea.

Nursing Management

Nurses must take accurate and detailed health and nutritional histories and screen for symptoms of anxiety and/or depression as well as assess for current or past suicidal and homicidal ideation.

If the nurse recognizes any signs of an inability to manage anger, suicide/homicide ideation, depression, or anxiety, he or she should encourage the patient to seek evaluation by an appropriate health care provider. Nurses also may help patients with stress reduction and management techniques, compliance with medication, and therapeutic lifestyle changes (such as smoking cessation, regular exercise, and eating a low-fat, low-cholesterol, low-sodium diet). Pain management is similar to that discussed under dysmenorrhea (NSAIDs, PPIs, and heat pad use).

VULVOVAGINAL INFECTIONS

Fungal and bacterial infections in the vagina are common, self-limited gynecologic conditions that occur in women of all ages due to a disruption in the normal pH of the vagina (CDC, 2014a). The pH of the vagina is 3.5 to 4.5 and provides the normal environment for *Lactobacillus acidophilus* to exist. This is a healthy bacterium that thrives in the vaginal ecosystem and provides protection against infections by inhibiting growth of anaerobes (Cibulka & Barron, 2013).

Lactobacillus metabolizes glycogen to lactic acid in the vagina and maintains normal vaginal pH. Antibiotics, menopause (or estrogen deficiency), oral contraceptives, spermicides, diabetes, douching, frequent intercourse, and smoking are known to decrease the number of healthy lactobacilli (Miller, 2014).

Without the lactobacillus, there is a proliferation of anaerobic activity, the pH of the vagina is altered, and an overgrowth of bacteria is produced. Table 33-4 summarizes types of vaginal infections and vaginitis. **Bacterial vaginosis** (BV) and **vulvovaginal candidiasis** (VVC) are discussed in detail below.

Nurses play a vital role in helping patients to understand the mode of infection, treatment, and self-care modalities. Although not considered STIs, BV and VVC can coexist with STIs; therefore, appropriate screening for these infections is important (Carcio & Secor, 2015). Also it is important to note that the creams and suppositories used in the treatment of VVC and BV have been known to weaken latex condoms, diaphragms, and cervical caps; therefore, caution should be taken to avoid sexual intercourse during treatment.

BACTERIAL VAGINOSIS

The most common vaginal infection is BV or Gardnerella, occurring in approximately 40% to 50% of all cases of vaginitis when there is a decrease in lactobacilli (Cibulka & Barron, 2013; CDC, 2014b, 2015a).

Risk Factors

Risk factors for developing BV include new or multiple sexual partners, douching, an increase in sexual activity, retained foreign body in the vagina (such as a tampon, broken condom, or sex toy) and coexisting STIs (Raphaelidis, 2015). BV also may be present after a menstrual cycle due to the increase in the vaginal pH. If left untreated in patients who are pregnant, BV is a risk factor for premature labor as well as post-abortion endometritis and cuff cellulitis (infection) after hysterectomy.

Clinical Manifestations and Assessment

Approximately 50% of women who have BV are asymptomatic (Carcio & Secor, 2015). Patients with symptomatic BV will report an increased malodorous, vaginal discharge, or leukorrhea that is grayish white in color. Amines commonly found in the vagina become unstable when the pH is altered and release the characteristic "fishy" odor. The odor is generally more noticeable after sexual intercourse, sexual activity, or menses. Unprotected intercourse will produce the malodorous discharge due to the interaction of semen and normal vaginal amines. Sometimes women will report vaginal itching, dysuria, or pelvic pressure similar to that of a UTI due to the localized irritation of the urinary meatus from the discharge (Cibulka & Barron, 2013).

A swab of vaginal discharge taken from the vaginal walls and applied to two glass slides is known as a *wet mount*. One slide has saline added; the other slide has potassium hydroxide (KOH) added and then is viewed under a microscope. The presence of *clue cells* (vaginal epithelial cells that are coated with bacteria) on the saline slide is a hallmark for diagnosing BV. The KOH-prepared slide will release amines and is known as a "whiff test." The presence of a fishy odor on the whiff test suggests BV. Nitrazine paper determines the pH, which will be greater than 4.5 for BV (Carcio & Secor, 2015).

Medical and Nursing Management

The preferred medication for treatment of BV is metronidazole 500 mg twice daily for 7 days. If the patient is noncompliant, a single 2-g dose may be administered, although higher cure rates occur with the 7-day dose (Papadakis & McPhee, 2014). The CDC no longer recommends the single-dose therapy due to its low efficacy (CDC, 2015a). Metronidazole gel 0.75% administered in one 5-g applicator vaginally at bedtime for 7 nights is an alternative and is preferred to avoid any GI upset caused by oral medications. If an allergy to metronidazole exists, alternative therapies are oral clindamycin 300 mg twice daily for 7 days; clindamycin 2% cream, one 5-g application vaginally at bedtime for 7 days; or clindamycin ovules 100 mg intravaginally

TABLE **33-4** Vaginal Infections and Vaginitis

Infection	Cause	Clinical Manifestations	Management Strategies
Candidiasis	*Candida albicans, glabrata,* or *tropicalis*	Inflammation of vaginal epithelium, producing itching, reddish irritation White, cheese-like discharge clinging to epithelium	Eradicate the fungus by administering an antifungal agent. Frequently used brand names of vaginal creams and suppositories are Monistat, Femstat, Terazol, and Gyne-Lotrimin. Review other causative factors (e.g., antibiotic therapy, nylon underwear, tight clothing, pregnancy, oral contraceptives). Assess for diabetes and HIV infection in patients with recurrent infections
Gardnerella-associated bacterial vaginosis	*Gardnerella vaginalis* and vaginal anaerobes	Usually no edema or erythema of vulva or vagina Gray-white to yellow-white discharge clinging to external vulva and vaginal walls	Administer metronidazole (Flagyl) with instructions about avoiding alcohol while taking this medication. If infection is recurrent, may treat partner.
Trichomonas vaginalis vaginitis (STD)	*Trichomonas vaginalis*	Inflammation of vaginal epithelium, producing burning and itching Frothy yellow-white or yellow-green vaginal discharge	Relieve inflammation, restore acidity, and reestablish normal bacterial flora; provide oral metronidazole for patient and partner.
Bartholinitis (infection of greater vestibular gland)	*Escherichia coli* *Trichomonas vaginalis* *Staphylococcus* *Streptococcus* *Gonococcus*	Erythema around vestibular gland Swelling and edema Abscessed vestibular gland	Drain the abscess; provide antibiotic therapy; excise gland of patients with chronic bartholinitis.
Cervicitis: acute and chronic	*Chlamydia* *Gonococcus* *Streptococcus* Many pathogenic bacteria	Profuse purulent discharge Backache Urinary frequency and urgency	Determine the cause: perform cytologic examination of cervical smear and appropriate cultures. Eradicate the gonococcal organism, if present: penicillin (as directed), or spectinomycin or tetracycline if patient is allergic to penicillin. Tetracycline or doxycycline (Vibramycin) to eradicate chlamydia. Eradicate other causes.
Atrophic vaginitis	Lack of estrogen; glycogen deficiency	Discharge and irritation from alkaline pH of vaginal secretions	Provide topical vaginal estrogen therapy; improve nutrition if necessary; relieve dryness through use of moisturizing medications.

once at bedtime for 3 days. Tinidazole, a newer-generation medication that is chemically related to metronidazole, was approved in 2007 by the U.S. Food and Drug Administration (FDA) for treatment of BV. Improved patient adherence due to once-a-day dosing and shorter duration of therapy is observed (CDC, 2015a).

It is extremely important that the nurse educate the patient on avoidance of all alcoholic use while taking metronidazole and for 3 days after the last dose due to the disulfiram (Antabuse)-type reaction that is induced; this causes nausea, vomiting, flushing of the skin, chest pain, blurred vision, mental confusion, sweating, breathing difficulty, and anxiety.

VULVOVAGINAL CANDIDIASIS

VVC is caused predominantly by *Candida albicans*. Other nonalbicans species that cause VVC include *C. tropicalis* and *C. glabrata* (Miller, 2014). It is estimated that approximately 25% of all vaginal infections are VVC, but that number is difficult to determine because it is not a reportable condition and because the availability of OTC treatments makes it hard to determine how many women are affected.

Risk Factors

Risk factors include use of broad-spectrum antibiotics (such as penicillins, cephalosporins, and tetracyclines), exogenous hormones, or corticosteroids as well as pregnancy (Papadakis & McPhee, 2014). Other risk factors for VVC include uncontrolled diabetes, obesity, and diets high in sugars or artificial sweeteners (Carcio & Secor, 2015). New sexual partners, contaminated sex toys, or an increase in sexual activity also may change the pH of the vagina, making it more susceptible to infection. Males who are uncircumcised and do not practice good hygiene may harbor yeast and pass on the infection to their partners.

Clinical Manifestations and Assessment

The most common complaint is vulvar pruritus (Miller, 2014). Patients also complain of dysuria related to inflammation of the urinary meatus by means of the vaginal discharge. A urine specimen should be obtained to rule out any other source of infection. **Dyspareunia**, or pain with intercourse, may also be reported.

VVC differs from BV in that the discharge is generally thick; white; and curd-like, much like the appearance of cottage cheese; and is odorless. It is adherent to the vaginal walls on speculum examination. On physical examination, the external genitalia are erythematous, and adherent white discharge may be noted on the vaginal walls and labia. Diagnosis is established based on a wet mount (a swab of the vaginal discharge on a glass slide that has been mixed with KOH). Under microscopic examination, the presence of hyphae is visible, and Nitrazine will reveal a normal pH of 4.0 to 4.5. If there are clue cells or trichomonads present, it is indicative of a coexisting BV or trichomonas infection (Cibulka & Barron, 2013). A 48-hour culture will diagnose the predominant causative factor definitively.

Medical Management

Many women will self-diagnose and treat based on symptoms with OTC topical preparations containing azole (Monistat or Gyne-Lotrimin). This practice is not encouraged as patients may be self-treating for an infection that may not be VVC or that the yeast will become resistant to the OTC treatment (CDC, 2015). It is important to educate patients to seek evaluation by a health care professional who can diagnose and treat any vaginal infection appropriately.

Topical antifungal agents that are used vaginally offer the most rapid relief. Terconazole (Terazol) cream is available in both 3- and 7-day preparations. This medication covers all three species of yeast, whereas the OTC preparations cover only *C. albicans*. Fluconazole (Diflucan) is a single-dose oral medication that is effective against *Candida*, but there is a delay in symptom relief of up to 3 days. It is, however, an effective treatment, particularly when treating a patient with coexisting BV who is using a vaginal preparation of metronidazole. Oral fluconazole (Diflucan) is a category C drug and should be used with caution during the first trimester of pregnancy. There have

been some reports of formation of congenital defects when oral fluconazole is used repeatedly during the first trimester (Cibulka & Barron, 2013).

Nursing Management

The nurse's role in educating a patient with BV or VVC includes assessing for high-risk behaviors, such as multiple sexual partners and unprotected sexual intercourse. If a patient is having recurrent vaginal infections, it is important for the patient to be evaluated by a health care professional to determine the cause.

Recurrent infections can be caused by nonadherence with medication therapy and poor hygiene (Miller, 2014). Also it is important to assess any cross-contamination with sexual toys. Teaching patients and their partners about proper hygiene in addition to sterilization of sex toys can decrease recurrent infections.

If the cause is determined to be from diabetes, the nurse can assist the patient with compliance with dietary guidelines, proper management of blood glucose, and hygienic practices as well as referral to appropriate health care providers for further management.

STRUCTURAL DISORDERS

Physical strain and hormone deficiencies compromise the ability of the pelvic musculature to support pelvic organs. Weakening of this musculature causes pelvic organs to displace downward into the pelvic cavity to varying degrees (Figure 33-8).

PROLAPSE

The pelvic organs are supported by a complex system of ligaments and muscles that are protected by the bony pelvis. The bony pelvis serves as an attachment site for these ligaments and muscles. The uterus is located deep within the bony pelvis but is freely movable during physical examination. A series of muscles known as the pubococcygeal muscles extend from the pubic bone to the coccyx, encompassing the urethra, vagina, anus, and rectum (Carcio & Secor, 2015).

If the muscles and ligaments are weakened, the uterus and bladder prolapse or herniate into the vaginal canal. Patients may or may not be aware of these structural defects until they become symptomatic or are discovered on physical examination. Types of prolapse include:

- *Cystocele:* The herniation of the bladder into the anterior vagina (Fig. 33-8A)
- *Rectocele:* The extrusion of the rectum into the posterior vagina (Fig. 33-8B)
- *Enterocele:* The descent of the small intestine into the vaginal vault (Fig. 33-8C)

FIGURE 33-8 Diagrammatic representation of the three most common types of pelvic floor relaxation: **(A)** cystocele, **(B)** rectocele, and **(C)** enterocele. *Arrows* depict sites of maximum protrusion.

- *Uterine prolapse:* Downward descent of the uterus into the vagina (Fig. 33-9)
- *Vault prolapse:* Top of the vagina prolapses after a hysterectomy

Pelvic organ prolapse increases with age. More than 225,000 surgical procedures are performed annually to correct these defects (Nygaard et al., 2013). Patients are more likely to develop prolapse once the muscles and ligaments begin to loosen or relax.

Risk Factors

Increased pressure on the abdomen and pelvic floor from pregnancy or obesity causes the ligaments of the pelvic floor to weaken. Direct injury to the levator ani or the stretching of the pudendal nerves during childbirth impairs the elasticity of the pelvic floor muscles (Carcio & Secor, 2015). Women who have more than one vaginal birth are at higher risk for developing prolapse, with risk increasing with each subsequent vaginal delivery (Karatayli et al., 2013). Estrogen helps with maintaining pelvic structure; therefore, patients who are menopausal are more likely to develop a prolapse due to lack of estrogen. Other predisposing factors for developing pelvic organ prolapse include connective tissue disease and neurologic disorders. Increasing strength of the pelvic floor can be correlated to the strengthening effect of exercising the core and abdominal muscles; this can prevent pelvic organs from displacement (Overby, Persons, Carrillo, & Martin, 2014).

Regardless of age, straining from constipation and increased intra-abdominal pressure from coughing are other risk factors for prolapse.

Clinical Manifestations and Assessment

Many patients who have a uterine or bladder prolapse will be asymptomatic, while others may seek evaluation by a health care provider because of a noticeable "bulge" in the vaginal area. Back pain in the absence of trauma may be present. Urinary incontinence is a common complaint with a bladder prolapse accompanied by pelvic pressure. Frequently women will complain of a UTI when, in fact, it is the prolapse that is producing the symptoms. Patients also may report difficulty having a bowel movement and often will need to place pressure on their perineal or vaginal areas in order to facilitate a bowel movement. Incomplete rectal evacuation or fecal incontinence may occur as a result of prolapse (Papadakis & McPhee, 2014).

Medical and Nursing Management

Treatment depends upon the severity of the symptoms and degree of prolapse involved. Patients' general state of health and activity is also of concern if considering surgical intervention. Urodynamic testing evaluates bladder function. For mild uterine prolapse, a **pessary** is the first line of treatment. Pessaries are removable devices made of silicone, latex, plastic, or rubber that are inserted into the vagina to provide support. A variety of styles is available, and they are cost-effective while providing immediate relief of symptoms (Lewthwaite, Staley, Girouard, & Maslow, 2013) (Fig. 33-10).

FIGURE 33-9 Complete prolapse of the uterus through the introitus.

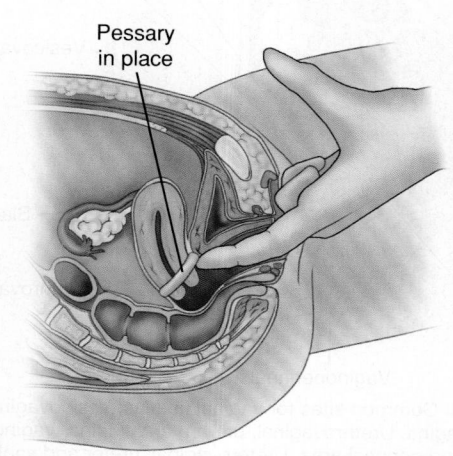

Pessary in place

FIGURE 33-10 Examples of pessaries. **A.** Various shapes and sizes of pessaries available. **B.** Insertion of one type of pessary.

Pelvic floor rehabilitation or pelvic floor muscle training (PFMT) offers a nonsurgical approach to patients who are motivated to adhere to the exercise schedule (Overby et al., 2014). **Kegel exercises** are a form of PFMT (Box 33-9). Physical therapists or urogynecologists who are specifically trained in PFMT teach the patient exercises that increase the strength of the pelvic floor muscle. Biofeedback programs feature assisted pelvic floor exercises utilizing a functional electrical stimulator (FES) and are used to help patients contract the appropriate pelvic muscles. Nurses can become trained in PFMT and are able to effectively teach patients about proper use of FES equipment.

Reconstructive pelvic surgery depends upon the impact of the severity of symptoms on the patients' daily living. Sacrospinous fixation, also referred to as an *anterior-posterior repair*, utilizes the surrounding ligaments to tighten and attach lax musculature onto the bony pelvis (van der Ploeg, van der Steen, Rengerink, van der Vaart, & Roovers, 2014). Vaginal hysterectomy is the most common surgical treatment for women beyond childbearing age who have a uterovaginal prolapse (Karatayli et al., 2013). There are some studies that suggest a failure rate 2 to 5 years after surgery for pelvic organ prolapse due to cystocele or rectocele formation (Nygaard et al., 2013).

Nurses provide important patient teaching. Educating the patient on weight loss, smoking cessation, and avoiding heavy lifting enables the patient to care for herself. Proper insertion, removal, and cleaning of pessary devices will help the patient to avoid vaginal infections. Nurses can discuss appropriate ways to avoid unnecessary straining and constipation. Anticipatory guidance regarding procedures or surgery will help to alleviate any patient anxiety about the surgical process.

FISTULAS

A fistula is an abnormal, tortuous opening between two internal organs or between an internal hollow organ and the exterior of the body. Fistulas may be simple or complex. Figure 33-11 depicts vaginal fistulas. Rectovaginal fistulas (RVFs) are abnormal openings that occur between the vagina and the rectum, allowing fecal material and flatulence to leak into the vagina, causing fecal incontinence. Anal fistulas generally develop as a result of an anal abscess and may be an indication of some other disorder, such as lymphogranuloma venereum (a sexually transmitted systemic disease that affects the lymph nodes and rectal area, as well as the genitals), rectal tuberculosis, or neoplasm (Papadakis & McPhee, 2014; Nasser, Mendes, Zein, Tanios, & Berjaoui, 2014). Vesicovaginal fistulas occur between the bladder and

---

BOX 33-9   **Patient Education**

Performing Kegel (Pelvic Muscle) Exercises

Purposes: To strengthen and maintain the tone of the pubococcygeal muscle, which supports the pelvic organs; to reduce or prevent stress incontinence and uterine prolapse; to enhance sensation during sexual intercourse; and to hasten postpartum healing:

1. Become aware of pelvic muscle function by "drawing in" the perivaginal muscles and anal sphincter as if to control urine or defecation, but not contracting the abdominal, buttock, or inner thigh muscles.
2. Sustain contraction of the muscles for up to 10 seconds, followed by at least 10 seconds of relaxation.
3. Perform these exercises 30–80 times a day.

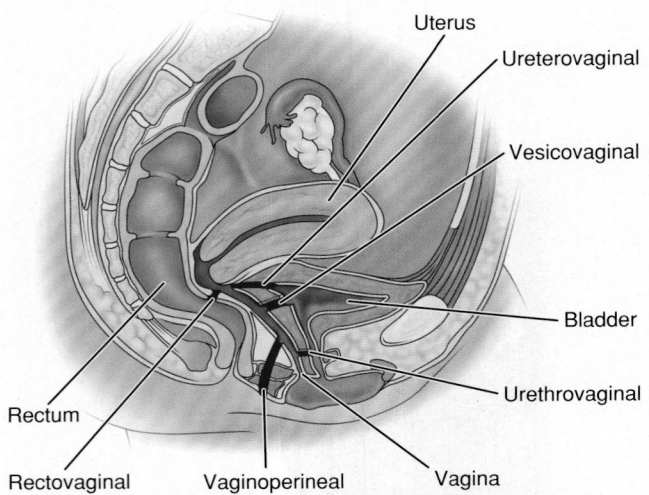

FIGURE 33-11 Common sites for vaginal fistulas: Vesicovaginal, bladder and vagina. Urethrovaginal, urethra and vagina. Vaginoperineal, vagina and perineal area. Ureterovaginal, ureter and vagina. Rectovaginal, rectum and vagina.

the vagina and cause urinary incontinence. These conditions occur as a result of congenital anomalies, trauma due to childbirth or surgery, radiation therapy, Crohn disease, diverticular diseases, or neoplasm of the rectum or vagina. Postpartum infections also may result in fistula formation due to third- and fourth-degree perineal tears or tissue breakdown (Brincat, Crosby, McLeod, & Fenner, 2014). This condition causes severe pain and risk for urosepsis due to recurrent UTIs and has social ramifications related to urinary and fecal incontinence (Ma et al., 2015).

Clinical Manifestations and Assessment

Depending upon the type of fistula, symptoms will vary. If caused by an obstetric or surgical complication, fistulas may not be apparent for up to 30 days after the initial injury or may be discovered incidentally during the 6-week postpartum follow-up visit (Ma et al., 2015). Urinary or fecal incontinence are the main reasons why women will seek evaluation by a health care provider. Fecal discharge through the vagina produces a malodorous discharge and may be mistaken for a vaginal infection. An accurate history of onset, timing, and location, along with symptoms the patient is experiencing, is important to help locate the structural abnormality. Physical assessment of the genital area will help to identify the affected area. The fistula may be palpable on digital rectal examination or vaginal examination. A sigmoidoscopy, colonoscopy, small bowel imaging, cystoscopy, or intravenous pyelography will aid in definitive diagnosis.

Medical and Nursing Management

If the fistula is due to Crohn disease or diverticular disease, treatment is aimed at the causative disease and should be followed by a gastroenterologist.

Surgical repair is the only option if the fistula does not heal spontaneously. There is a high rate of recurrence of fistulas in spite of surgical repair. Nurses play an important role in helping the patient to understand the importance of cleanliness and hygiene and to understand the signs and symptoms of recurrent infection or surgical failure to repair the fistula. Regular sitz baths and changing of perineal pads help prevent infection. It is important for the nurse to inspect the patient's skin for any signs of erythema or breakdown.

It is also imperative that nurses assess the impact fistulas play on the patient's psychological state. Many patients suffer from physical and social distress as well as sexual dysfunction as a result of urinary and fecal incontinence due to fistulas (Ma et al., 2015). Assessing the patient's support system as well as appropriate referrals to pain management and surgeons familiar with this type of surgery is imperative.

BENIGN DISORDERS

OVARIAN CYSTS

Ovaries produce estrogen, progesterone, and a small amount of testosterone necessary for female reproductive function as well as formation of oocytes or eggs. Follicles are structures within the ovary containing a single ovum or egg. Follicular growth is stimulated by FSH once a month. After ovulation occurs (release of the egg), the graafian follicle that houses the ovum becomes the corpus luteum. This structure undergoes transformation and regresses with the onset of menses. Ovaries are a common site for cysts to form as a result of hormonal influence on the formation of the **graafian follicle** and subsequent corpus luteum. When this series of hormonal transitions does not occur, a cyst may develop (Carcio & Secor, 2015). Any graafian follicle that is over 2 cm is considered a cyst. Ovarian cysts are classified as functional or nonfunctional. Statistically, women under age 50 are more likely to have a benign cyst, whereas women over age 50 are more likely to have a cyst that is malignant (McGahan, Corwin, & Gerscovich, 2014).

Types

Functional cysts are also known as *simple cysts* due to their appearance on ultrasound.

These types of cysts rupture and hemorrhage and occasionally cause pain. The condition is self-limiting. Pain that occurs during ovulation, known as **mittelschmerz**, also produces unilateral ovarian pain and generally is relieved with symptomatic treatment, such as OTC NSAIDs. Ovarian follicles that rupture during ovulation release fluid, cause pain, and may be noted on ultrasound (McGahan et al., 2014).

Nonfunctional cysts, or endometriomas, are also known as "chocolate cysts" due to their characteristic appearance on ultrasound. The cysts develop as a result of sloughed off endometrial tissue that has formed a cystic mass on the ovary; they are brown in appearance. Dermoid cysts are non-functional and are comprised of embryonic cells containing hair, teeth, bone, and nails. Since the histologic features and clinical behaviors of dermoid cysts or germ-cell tumors have been well established, there has been little new research performed in this area for the past two decades (Nogales, Dulcey, & Preda, 2014).

Patients with nonfunctional dermoid cysts are diagnosed by pelvic ultrasound after they have had a missed menstrual cycle and have a false-positive pregnancy test. These cysts have characteristic microscopic fat detected within the mass on MRI (McGahan et al., 2014).

Ovaries with multiple cysts due to chronic anovulatory cycles and hyperandrogenism are known as *polycystic ovarian syndrome* (PCOS). PCOS is the most common endocrine disorder that affects approximately 5% to 10% of women of reproductive age (Papadakis & McPhee, 2014). It is a complex disorder of androgen excess, insulin resistance, and an imbalance in the ratios of luteinizing hormone and FSH, causing **anovulation** (lack of ovulation). Androgen excess coupled with disproportionate amounts of LH and FSH, and decreased sex hormone–binding globulins (SHBG), causes the occurrence of anovulatory cycles. This fluctuation in the normal levels of hormones results in insulin resistance due to the influence of hormone production from the pituitary. Women affected by PCOS are at risk for developing type 2 diabetes, acne, endometrial cancer, hyperlipidemia, obesity, hirsutism, and infertility (Carcio & Secor, 2015; Mahoney, 2014).

Clinical Manifestations and Assessment

Patients experiencing rupture of functional cysts present with a sudden onset of unilateral lower abdominal pain. Nausea and vomiting may be present. Pain typically increases with movement. A typical presentation of PCOS will include a history of irregular menstrual cycles (can be over 35 days per cycle or fewer than eight menses annually). Characteristics of bleeding include heavy flow with increased abdominal cramping and also may include large clots. The patient may be hirsute on the face and chest or between the breasts and demonstrate mild to severe acne. Male pattern baldness or alopecia may be present. Forty to 60% of women with PCOS have central obesity (Mahoney, 2014). **Acanthosis nigricans** is a hyperpigmentation of the skin around the neck (see Figure 33-12) but also may be noted in the axilla, groin, or the dorsal aspect of hands, and the patient also may have an excessive number of skin tags around the neck, under the arms and breasts, or in the groin (Buttaro et al., 2013). It is commonly associated with insulin resistance. See Figure 33-12. Pelvic ultrasound utilizing color Doppler will reveal follicles varying in size from 2 to 9 mm or will show an increase in ovarian volume unilaterally (Carcio & Secor, 2015). Patients with unilateral right lower quadrant pain must be evaluated for the potential of appendicitis.

FIGURE 33-12 Acanthosis nigricans. Hyperpigmentation of skin folds, velvety in appearance commonly seen in axilla, groin, and neck. (From *Danforth obstetrics and gynecology*. Philadelphia, PA: Lippincott Williams & Wilkins.)

Medical and Nursing Management

Functional cysts are self-limiting and generally respond to the use of OTC NSAIDs, such as ibuprofen or naproxen. Once a diagnosis of ovarian cysts is made, and depending upon the size of the cyst, hormonal contraception is recommended to induce suppression of FSH. This decreases the incidence of formation of ovarian follicles, limits or halts an increase in the size of any established cysts, and halts the future formation of cysts. If pain persists longer than 48 hours, an exploratory laparoscopy may be performed to rule out the presence of ovarian torsion (twisting of the ovary, primarily affecting the right ovary).

Patients with PCOS require extensive blood work and a transvaginal ultrasound to rule out any other causative factors. Labs include FSH, LH, beta human chorionic gonadotropin (β-hCG), SHBG, free testosterone, prolactin, lipid panel, thyroid studies, and a fasting glucose. A 2-hour glucose tolerance test is useful in determining glucose intolerance. The LH-to-FSH ratio in patients with PCOS is usually greater than 2:1 or 3:1, but a normal ratio is not a diagnosis of exclusion (Buttaro et al., 2013).

It is important that blood work not be performed while the patient is currently taking oral contraceptives as this will alter the accuracy of results and delay diagnosis.

Treatment of PCOS is aimed at the primary concerns (acne, infertility, obesity). Due to the incidence of insulin resistance with PCOS, patients should follow a regular program of exercise and eat a low-fat diet. If, in spite of therapeutic lifestyle changes, the patient is unable to lose weight or ovulate, metformin or Glucophage is initiated to assist with decreasing insulin resistance and allow for spontaneous ovulation. Metformin is an insulin-sensitizing agent that lowers testosterone levels and induces ovulation once hormone levels are balanced. The most common side effect of this medication is transient nausea and diarrhea. Slowly increasing the dosage of metformin and dosing at mealtime will help alleviate these side effects and increase patient compliance. It is estimated that a 1% reduction in BMI has shown a reduction in insulin resistance (Mahoney, 2014). The method of birth control used while on metformin should be discussed with the patient because treatment can restore fertility. Patients with PCOS should be evaluated by a reproductive endocrinologist.

COCs help patients with PCOS regulate menstrual cycles and decrease blood flow with menses and the cramping associated with heavy menses. Additionally, COCs improve SHBG production, which helps bind-free testosterone. This improves acne, hirsutism, and alopecia. Women who do not have regular menstrual cycles are at risk for endometrial cancer due to the prolonged exposure of estrogen and overgrowth of the endometrial lining and, therefore, may need to have an endometrial biopsy if there has not been a menses in 1 year (Valentin, 2014).

Spironolactone is a blood pressure medication that has antiandrogenic effects that is beneficial to those who experience hirsutism (Carcio & Secor, 2015). Because this is a potassium-sparing diuretic, patients with PCOS should have their electrolytes monitored periodically, particularly the potassium level. Two COCs, Yaz and Yasmin, are available that contain *drospirenone*, a newer-generation progesterone that has the same antiandrogenic effects as spironolactone.

Nurses can assist patients with weight loss and exercise guidelines as well as with adherence with medications. It is important to help patients understand the implications of this disease on QOL and infertility. Nurses play an important role in supporting patients with this disease and recognizing if patients need referral to a dietician or for psychological support.

UTERINE FIBROIDS

Leiomyomas or myomas are common, benign growths of the uterus (Fig. 33-13). Approximately 25% of women over 35 years of have a uterine leiomyomata (Tulandi & As-Asmari, 2015). Risk factors include being African American or being overweight (CDC, 2014d). The high prevalence of uterine fibroids is the cause of high disease burden at the cost of approximately $5.9 to $34.4 billion in the United States annually (Falcone & Parker, 2013; Xuping et al., 2014). Approximately 50% of cases will require surgical intervention. Symptoms largely depend on the size and number of fibroids. The incidence of fibroids increases with age. Box 33-10 describes the types of uterine fibroids.

Clinical Manifestations and Assessment

The majority of women with fibroids are asymptomatic until the fibroid has enlarged and is impeding on other organs. Fibroids cause significant symptoms, including heavy menstrual bleeding, dyspareunia, disabling pelvic pain, rectal pressure, and infertility (Xuping et al., 2014). Diagnosis is made with pelvic ultrasound, which confirms the presence,

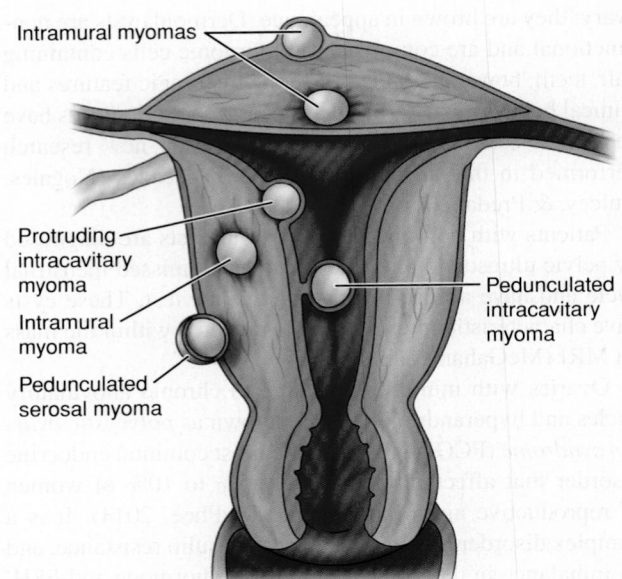

FIGURE 33-13 Myomas (fibroids). Those that impinge on the uterine cavity are called intracavitary myomas.

size, and location of fibroids (Papadakis & McPhee, 2014). Fibroids may be palpated initially on bimanual pelvic examination. Often the uterus is enlarged as a result of the growth.

It is important to rule out pregnancy with a woman who is experiencing these signs and symptoms. There is a risk for miscarriage as the fibroid distorts the uterus impacting on fetal growth. It is estimated that approximately one third of fibroids grow during pregnancy (Lee, Norwitz, & Shaw, 2010).

Medical Management

There are several treatments for fibroids. Medical management is indicated for those women who are considered surgical risks or who decline surgical intervention (Tulandi & Al-Asmari, 2015). GnRH agonists, such as Lupron, are used to decrease the size of the fibroid by effectively suppressing the hormonal production that feeds the fibroid. Hysterectomy is another treatment (see discussion later in the chapter). For patients who have fibroids and want to preserve their fertility, a **myomectomy** is performed. This is a

BOX 33-10 | **Types of Uterine Fibroids**

- *Subserosal fibroids* lie underneath the outermost layer of the uterus and grow toward the pelvic cavity.
- *Intramural fibroids* grow within the wall of the uterine muscle and are the most common type.
- *Submucosal fibroids* grow immediately below the inner uterine surface and into the uterine cavity.
- *Pedunculated fibroids* arise from inside or outside the surface of the uterine muscle and project outward.

surgical procedure that removes the fibroid but leaves the uterus intact. Myomectomies can be performed laparoscopically, hysteroscopically (inspection of the uterine cavity by laparoscopy), or via robotic-assisted laparoscopy (Falcone & Parker, 2013).

Uterine artery embolization (UAE) uses minimally invasive plastic or gelatin particles that are injected into the uterine arteries to occlude blood flow to the fibroid (Ananthakrishnan et al., 2013). The fibroid then shrinks over time. This type of procedure is used only on women who have completed childbearing. Magnetic resonance–guided high-frequency focused ultrasound energy (MRgFUS) uses high-intensity ultrasound with increased temperature to destroy fibroid cells without damaging collateral tissue (Hesley, Gorny, & Woodrum, 2013). In general, this type of procedure is confined to only premenopausal women with symptomatic fibroids. The advantage to this procedure is that patients generally can return to normal activities the day after treatment. Cryoablation, or radiofrequency of individual fibroids, is now FDA approved and is proven safe and effective in reducing the size of fibroids. Cryoablation also has been found to provide a reduction in severity of symptoms 12 months after the procedure without concerns of postembolization syndrome commonly found with patients who have undergone UAE (Chudnoff et al., 2013). Patients typically return to normal activities approximately 5 days postprocedure. Some women undergoing UAE may develop postembolization syndrome: fever, pain, and leukocytosis due to the degenerating fibroid. This is a normal response to treatment, but patients must be monitored for worsening symptoms (Chudnoff et al., 2013).

Nursing Management

Patients experience heightened anxiety when diagnosed with a fibroid. Nurses can reassure patients of the benign nature of fibroids and the potential side effects of medications and surgical procedures. The use of GnRH agonists induces temporary menopause and vasomotor symptoms associated with menopause. The patient may experience hot flashes, sleep disruption, and vaginal dryness as a result of loss of estrogen. These symptoms are reversible once the medication has been discontinued. Due to the high level of bleeding associated with any myomectomy or surgical procedure, all aspirin and aspirin-containing products should be discontinued 3 to 4 weeks before the procedure is performed. Aggressive pain management is advised due to the increased amount of cramping from the infarction of the fibroid. Instructing patients on the patient-controlled analgesia (PCA) pumps and regular administration of NSAIDs and antiemetics will ensure adequate pain control. Patients are coping not only with the physical loss but also the psychological loss of fertility if the patient is not undergoing fertility-sparing surgery so nurses need to address those concerns and offer referrals to therapists if needed.

ENDOMETRIOSIS

Endometriosis is a progressive, benign gynecologic disorder affecting women in their childbearing years and causing chronic inflammation and formation of adhesions. It does not continue after menopause. Approximately 6% to 10% of women suffer from endometriosis, with as high as 80% of these women reporting chronic pelvic pain (Papadakis & McPhee, 2014). This disease may be disabling and chronic. It impacts the woman's sexual relations as well as her physical, social, and psychological well-being.

Pathophysiology

Endometriosis is the presence of endometrial-like tissue that proliferates outside of the uterine cavity, causing persistent pelvic pain and scarring that leads to infertility. The pathophysiology of this disease is largely unknown, but many theories exist (ACOG, 2014). It is thought to be caused by the retrograde flow during menses of endometrial tissue through the fallopian tubes and into the peritoneal cavity, where this tissue seeds, forming adhesions in the pelvic, bladder, and bowel areas. The peritoneal endometrial tissues are influenced by the hormonal changes of the menstrual cycle and, therefore, swell, break down, and bleed; typically, the patient's symptoms worsen during the premenstrual phase. A significant number of women are asymptomatic and may have a normal pelvic examination (Papadakis & McPhee, 2014).

Clinical Manifestations and Assessment

Chronic pelvic pain is the most frequent presentation of endometriosis, but clinical manifestations of the disease are variable in presentation and course of progression (Papadakis & McPhee, 2014). Low back pain, dyspareunia, dysuria, **dyschezia** (pain with defecation), dysmenorrhea, and menorrhagia are among the common complaints. The level of pain associated with endometriosis is not necessarily correlated with the stage of endometriosis. The cyclical bowel and bladder symptoms of endometriosis are similar to those found in irritable bowel syndrome (IBS) or interstitial cystitis (IC), making it difficult to differentiate among the disorders.

A detailed health history regarding the patient's symptoms in relation to her menstrual cycle will help the health care provider establish a pattern. Any tenderness of the fallopian tubes, ovaries, or uterus on bimanual examination is an indication for further evaluation. The most common finding is tenderness with palpation of the posterior vaginal fornix, but a definitive diagnosis cannot be established without further diagnostic testing. Transvaginal ultrasound visualizes the uterine cavity and endometrium for any adhesions. This examination is unable to visualize smaller lesions; therefore, misdiagnosis may be made. Currently, direct visualization of the adhesions through surgical intervention remains the preferred method for definitive diagnosis (ACOG, 2014).

Medical and Nursing Management

The first line of treatment for endometriosis consists of the use of NSAIDs for pain and COCs to treat the condition. The combined hormones in COCs suppress ovulation and growth of endometrial implants, thereby decreasing inflammation and pain. GnRH agonists (such as Lupron), androgenic agents (Danazol), depot MPA, and levonorgestrel IUD are considered second-line therapy for 3 months (ACOG, 2014). Any of these medications suppresses ovulation and endometrial growth and reduces or eliminates menses, thus alleviating the chance of retrograde flow into the pelvic cavity. Use of continuous contraception provides prolonged suppression of ovulation, inhibiting growth of endometrial tissue. There are no differences in the outcomes of the use of COCs over GnRH, although patients given GnRH agonists have higher incidence of complaints of hot flashes, vaginal dryness, and other vasomotor symptoms associated with menopause. These symptoms are reversible once GnRH therapy has been discontinued.

Surgical intervention is considered the last line of therapy especially if it follows a 24-month use of OCPs (ACOG, 2014). Exploratory laparoscopy with lysis of adhesions is considered the gold standard and temporarily decreases the pain and bleeding associated with endometriosis, although approximately 44% of women will have a recurrence 1 year after surgery (ACOG, 2014). Total abdominal hysterectomy (TAH) remains the definitive therapy for those women who have completed their childbearing and is effective for those women who suffer from debilitating pain (Papadakis & McPhee, 2014).

Complementary and alternative therapies are useful in women who suffer from endometriosis and should be a part of the plan of care for these women. Due to the issues surrounding loss of fertility with this disease, stress management should be included. Yoga may help with stress reduction and also increases core and abdominal strength, which will help patients who undergo surgical intervention to have an easier recovery. Specifically trained physical therapists can help alleviate and manage the symptoms associated with chronic pelvic pain.

Educating the woman affected by endometriosis and her family and support network will help them to understand the significant impact of this disease on the woman and her physical and psychological health. Many women have sought the opinions of multiple medical providers regarding the treatment of endometriosis, and many have had a negative experience or may be in denial of the ramifications of the disease; therefore, establishing trust between the patient and the health care provider is crucial. A collaborative effort among all members of the health care team, including the nurse, health care provider, pharmacist, pain management specialist, and social worker, must exist to help improve the patient's outcome.

MALIGNANT CONDITIONS

CANCER OF THE CERVIX

The most common reproductive cancer among women is cervical cancer; it is the second most common cancer among women. Over 12,000 new cases of cervical cancer were diagnosed in 2011 (the most recent information available), and approximately 4,000 women died of cervical cancer that year (CDC, 2014b). The incidence and mortality of cervical cancer has decreased dramatically over the past 50 years due to the development and subsequent acceptance and use of the Pap smear (Waterman & Voss, 2015).

The most common type of cervical cancer is squamous cell carcinoma (SCC), accounting for approximately 85% of all cervical cancer cases, but the incidence of SCC is decreasing while the incidence of cervical adenocarcinoma is on the rise (Papadakis & McPhee, 2014). Scientists researching triggers to changes in the cervical tissue that lead to cancer have implicated human papilloma virus (HPV) as the most common causative factor in development of cervical cancer (CDC, 2014b). Cervical cancer has a slow progression from certain strains of oncogenic HPV to invasive cervical cancer and may take years to progress. HPV comprises over 100 strains, some of which have oncogenic potential and are known to cause cervical abnormalities. Women are asymptomatic unless they have external genital warts, or **condyloma**. In general, infection with HPV during a woman's younger years is cleared spontaneously or is suppressed to undetectable levels. The HPV vaccine was developed in 2006, and the quadrivalent vaccine covers four of the oncogenic strains (6, 11, 16, 18) while the bivalent vaccine covers two of the oncogenic strains. This is a primary prevention measure to reduce cervical cancer cases and deaths, but the literature shows that the vaccine continues to be underused (CDC, 2014c).

Screening and Prevention

The Pap smear is a screening tool used to detect any abnormalities of the cervix (Table 33-5). In recent years, liquid-based cytology has been developed to improve specimen adequacy, making it superior to traditional glass slide specimens.

Cytologic screening tests are the most effective preventative measure for screening and diagnosing invasive cervical cancer.

Risk Factors

Lesbian women are at higher risk for HPV and cervical cancer due to misinformation as well as insufficient knowledge and screening. Lesbians are underrepresented in current

TABLE **33-5** American Congress of Obstetricians and Gynecologists (ACOG) Cervical Cytology Screening Guidelines

Patient Population	Frequency
21–29 years of age	Every 3 years
30–65 years of age	Every 3 years with HPV cotesting every 5 years
65 years of age and older	Discontinue if no abnormal Pap tests for 10 years and no previous history of moderate–severe dysplasia or cancer
Patients having had a hysterectomy for noncancerous reasons	Discontinue after hysterectomy *unless* patient has had a supracervical hysterectomy, then above guidelines would apply
Patients with high-risk factors: HIV, diethylstilbestrol (DES) exposure, or cervical intraepithelial neoplasm (CIN) 2 or 3	Every 6 months or as directed by health care provider

ACOG. (2013). *Cervical cancer screening*; AP085, January 2013.

research due to privacy concerns, lack of inquiries of the part of the health care provider regarding sexual orientation, or fear of repercussions (Waterman & Voss, 2015). Box 33-11 lists other risk factors for cervical cancer.

Clinical Manifestations and Assessment

Routine screening for cervical cancer increases a woman's chances of being diagnosed at an earlier stage. Advanced disease will manifest itself with irregular vaginal bleeding as well as pelvic pain and pressure. Malodorous vaginal discharge occurs as a result of tumor necrosis. Dyspareunia and rectal pressure also are common as the tumor increases in size and extent, invading surrounding tissue and causing other symptoms to develop. The standard of care for an abnormal Pap test is to follow-up with a **colposcopy** and directed biopsy. Colposcopy is a high-powered magnification of the

BOX 33-11
Risk Factors for Cervical Cancer

- Intercourse with an uncircumcised male
- Early age of first coitus
- Multiple sexual partners
- High parity
- STIs
- Cigarette smoking
- Exposure to human papillomavirus (HPV)

cervix, which has had an acetic acid solution applied to it to help differentiate the cervical cells. Biopsies are taken in areas of visible abnormal vascular patterns.

The squamocolumnar junction of the cervix is rich with squamous cells; this is known as the transformational zone. Cellular abnormalities develop over time, leading to the development of squamous cell dysplasia or cervical intraepithelial neoplasia (CIN) (Papadakis & McPhee, 2014). There are no overt signs or symptoms of CIN, and it is strictly diagnosed via liquid cytology, which provides superior sensitivity to detection of cancer cells. Low-grade lesions correlate with CIN 1, which is mild dysplasia that generally resolves spontaneously without treatment and is monitored through serial cytology to determine any progression to a higher-grade lesion. High-grade lesions are consistent with CIN 2 and CIN 3 and are considered precancerous lesions (Massad et al., 2013). High-grade lesions (severe dysplasia) are more likely to progress to cervical cancer if not treated. Biopsy confirms whether or not the lesion is SCC or adenocarcinoma. Cervical cancer screening should begin at 21 years of age, regardless of sexual debut (ACOG, 2014). Between 21 and 29 years of age, women should have cervical cytology screening without HPV testing every 3 years. All women over 30 years of age should have cervical cytology screening and cotesting for HPV every 3 to 5 years, unless an abnormality is detected. If an abnormal cytology is detected, then appropriate follow-up should occur based on current algorithm guidelines for abnormal cytology. All women 65 years of age and older who have had normal cervical cytology without prior history of CIN should no longer undergo cervical cytology due to the low incidence of disease in this age group (American Society for Colposcopy and Cervical Pathology [ASCCP], 2014).

Delayed diagnosis of cervical cancer will result in a more advanced disease state.

Staging is the next step, once the diagnosis for invasive cervical cancer has been made. Staging is performed on a scale of 0 to IVB. Stage 0 is known as carcinoma in situ (CIS). Stage IVB is consistent with distant metastasis when the disease has spread to the remainder of the reproductive organs, bladder, rectum, liver, and/or lungs. Treatment is dependent upon type of carcinoma and extent of disease. As the tumor size increases, so does the risk of treatment failure. Pelvic ultrasound is an easy and noninvasive way to evaluate any cervical pathology due to its ability to visualize the size and location of a cervical mass. A chest x-ray and abdominal/pelvic imaging, such as CT scan or MRI, are performed to rule out metastasis to other areas of the body.

Medical Management

Abnormal Pap smears that reveal high- or low-grade squamous intraepithelial lesions (HGSIL or LGSIL) are followed up with a colposcopy and cervical biopsy. Once diagnosis has been established, a cervical *conization* or cone biopsy is performed. Cold knife conization and loop electrosurgical excision procedure (LEEP) are other procedures that may be performed to treat HGSIL or LGSIL, which are precursors to cervical cancer. These types of procedures remove cone-shaped wedges high in the cervical canal with enough surrounding tissue to ensure clear margins. This is accomplished using a surgical scalpel, laser, or electrocautery. Prognosis is excellent for patients treated with these types of procedures. Cervical conization alone is adequate for those women who want to preserve childbearing ability (Massad et al., 2013). Invasive cervical cancer is rare under the age of 20, but there has been a documented increased risk for premature births among women who have had excisional cervical procedures for dysplasia prior to conception.

Patients diagnosed with a stage of IB or IIA undergo a radical hysterectomy: removal of the uterus and upper one third of the vagina, including the cervix, but sparing the ovaries. Bilateral pelvic lymph node sampling is also done. Pelvic radiation and chemotherapy may follow depending upon the size and extent of the tumor. Stage IB carries an increased risk of recurrence. Neoadjuvant chemotherapy has demonstrated success in decreasing tumor size and increasing survival when used prior to a radical hysterectomy. Survival rates for patients diagnosed with locally advanced cervical cancer have a higher rate of recurrence than those patients diagnosed with early-stage disease. The survival rate for a patient diagnosed with stage IB is approximately 80% (Straughn & Yashar, 2016).

The HPV vaccine could prevent 95% to 100% of CIN and adenocarcinoma in situ, 99% of genital warts, and 70% of cervical cancer cases worldwide (Papadakis & McPhee, 2014). There are currently two HPV vaccines available: bivalent, which prevents types 16 and 18, and quadrivalent, which prevents types 6, 11, 16, and 18. Routine vaccination should be administered as follows:

- For both males and females at 11 or 12 years of age, and
- For females through 26 years of age and males through 21 years of age who have not been vaccinated previously or who have not completed the 3-dose series (CDC, 2012b).

The HPV vaccines are a series of three vaccines administered at 2 and 6 months after the initial injection. It is important to receive the entire series of three vaccinations. It is recommended that patients remain in the office for at least 15 minutes after administration of the vaccine to ensure there is no reaction.

For women over age 26 years, the best way to prevent cervical cancer is to get routine cervical cancer screening, as recommended.

Nursing Management

Nurses working in a variety of settings have the opportunity to educate women on cervical cancer screenings. Availability of access to care is prevalent with federally funded cervical cancer screening programs through public health departments, hospital-based primary care centers, and community health care clinics. Educating parents and young women about HPV vaccination is important when considering that vaccination is so efficacious. Clinical trials of the vaccine demonstrated a 93% efficacy in prevention of cervical precancers of types 16 and 18 in women who were exposed to HPV. There is a reported 99% antibody response in all studies of the bivalent vaccine 1 month after completion of the series (CDC, 2015b).

If a woman has undergone any cervical biopsy procedures, it is important to instruct her on the importance of pelvic rest (such as abstinence and no vaginal penetration) as well as observing and reporting to her provider if fever, increased bleeding, pelvic pain, or malodorous vaginal discharge is noted. Ensure that the patient has the phone number of her health care provider or local hospital in the event that any of these symptoms occur after her procedure.

CANCER OF THE UTERUS

Cancer of the endometrium or uterus is the most commonly reported female reproductive cancer and comprises approximately 6% of all reproductive cancers in the United States (Park & Nam, 2015). The 5-year survival rate is 67% with localized disease. Usually it is diagnosed early, and better outcomes are reported with surgical intervention. It is rarely diagnosed in women under 40 years of age (CDC, 2014d). Cervical cytology may show atypical endometrial cells but are considered poor predictors of pathology. Endocervical and endometrial sampling is considered the gold standard for diagnosis of this type of cancer (Papadakis & McPhee, 2014).

Most endometrial cancers are considered endometrioid. Less common are the nonendometrioid lesions, including serous, clear cell, and carcinosarcomas. Nonendometrioid cancers are more aggressive, with an increased mortality rate.

Unopposed estrogen causes endometrial hyperplasia, or an overgrowth of the uterine lining. Simple hyperplasia often spontaneously regresses, but complex hyperplasia and atypical hyperplasia are more likely to progress to cancer (ACOG, 2014). The prognosis for type 1 endometrial cancer is good as opposed to type 2, which carries a higher mortality rate. Fertility-sparing progestin therapy is recommended for those who wish to preserve fertility and presumably have type 1 endometrial adenocarcinoma (Park & Nam, 2015). Oral MPA is the most commonly used progestin in this population and should be used for 12 weeks prior to evaluating response to treatment.

Risk Factors

Risk factors are discussed in Box 33-12. Nurses should encourage those with hereditary nonpolyposis colorectal cancer (HNPCC) (Box 33-13) or who are high risk for it

BOX 33-12
Risk Factors for Endometrial Cancer

- Unopposed estrogen use
- Early onset of menarche (under 12 years of age) or late menopause (over 50 years of age)
- Nulliparous
- Polycystic ovarian syndrome (PCOS)
- Use of tamoxifen
- Obesity
- Diabetes
- Prior pelvic radiation
- Personal or family history of breast, uterine, ovarian, or colon cancer
- Previous history of atypical hyperplasia

to begin annual screening with endometrial biopsies and transvaginal ultrasound beginning at 25 years of age. Some women may reduce their risk of endometrial cancer through the use of OCPs or cyclic progestin therapy (Papadakis & McPhee, 2014).

Clinical Manifestations and Assessment

Abnormal vaginal bleeding is the most common early symptom of endometrial cancer; 80% of women will present with abnormal vaginal bleeding as their chief complaint (Papadakis & McPhee, 2014). Postmenopausal women also may present with complaints of vaginal bleeding well after menses has ceased. Any unexplained vaginal bleeding or an irregularity in menstrual cycle should be evaluated by a health care professional.

Traditionally diagnosis has been made based on the tissue pathology from a dilation and curettage (D&C); however, endometrial biopsy is the preferred method since it is a simple procedure performed in the health care provider's office and does not involve anesthesia. If the biopsy is inconclusive or suggests endometrial cancer, a D&C is the gold standard. Hysteroscopic-directed biopsy is another alternative that is performed with the insertion of a scope through the cervix and directly into the uterus, allowing for complete

BOX 33-13
Hereditary Nonpolyposis Colorectal Cancer (HNPCC) Syndrome

Hereditary nonpolyposis colorectal cancer (HNPCC) syndrome increases women's risk of developing ovarian, colon, endometrial, renal, bladder, brain, and stomach cancer.

It is an inherited cancer susceptibility syndrome occurring in approximately 5% of all cancers.

A woman is at higher risk for HNPCC if she has three or more first-degree relatives with colon or endometrial cancer, with at least two of them having been diagnosed with colon cancer at age 50 or younger.

Genetic testing for HNPCC is available and recommended to those at risk.

visualization of the endometrium. A transvaginal ultrasound may be performed as well as measurements taken of the endometrial thickness. Greater than 16 mm is a predictor of abnormal pathology; in postmenopausal women, greater than 5 mm is considered pathologic (Valentin, 2014).

Nursing Alert
A D&C is brief surgical procedure that can be performed in a medical office or outpatient surgical center in which the cervix is dilated and a special instrument called a curette, or by a suction curettage (also called vacuum aspiration for evacuations for terminations or abortions), is used to scrape the uterine lining. An anesthetic is administered (spinal, general, or local anesthetizing of the cervix) and a sample of the uterine contents may be sent for analysis.

Medical Management

Once the diagnosis has been established, the standard treatment is a TAH with bilateral salpingo-oophorectomy (BSO) (removal of fallopian tubes and ovaries). There is questionable value in pelvic lymph node removal; it is a current source of debate (Valentin, 2014). Type of hysterectomy has little bearing on outcome, although some believe that an open hysterectomy is optimal in visualizing the peritoneum over a laparoscopic-assisted vaginal hysterectomy, in which the peritoneum is not as well visualized; however, this has not been proven in the literature. Laparoscopic vaginal hysterectomy decreases morbidity in women who are morbidly obese or those with high rates of comorbid conditions (ACOG Committee Opinion, 2015). Surgical staging is the most precise method to determine metastasis to surrounding tissues and organs; it involves abdominal and pelvic washings and periaortic lymph node evaluation.

Stage I is curable by surgery alone as it is considered low risk and the disease is confined to the uterus. High-risk stage I and some stage II cancers will require postoperative adjuvant radiation therapy or vaginal brachytherapy as the disease has lymph node involvement, is outside of the uterus, or contains high-risk cell types (papillary or clear cell). Radiation affects the ability of cells to proliferate and decreases growth of cancer cells (ACOG, 2015a). Vaginal brachytherapy consists of the placement of a device containing sealed radioactive material into the vagina postoperatively for 3 to 4 days and then removed. This method is preferred over EBR due to its lessened side effects. It delivers low- or high-dose radiation directly into the tumor. Brachytherapy decreases the incidence of regional recurrence and offers less toxicity than EBR (Klopp et al., 2014). During this time, the patient is on strict bed rest for the entire duration of therapy. Patients are isolated from other patients, and a camera mounted on the wall of the room allows monitoring of the patient while minimizing caregivers' exposure to radiation. Lead absorbs more radiation than any other material; therefore, a portable lead shield is placed at the bedside behind which all caregivers stand to administer medications, change IV bags, or deliver food trays. Nurses wear film badges or dosimeters to measure the amount of radiation exposure.

Patients are kept on a diet of clear liquid or low-residue foods to avoid stool formation. Stool softeners and medications to decrease peristalsis are administered.

Patients with diseases in high-risk stages II and III will receive both radiation and chemotherapy. The role of adjuvant chemotherapy alone or with concurrent radiation is currently under investigation (Papadakis & McPhee, 2014). High-risk features stage IC or poorly differentiated adenocarcinoma, clear cell carcinoma, and papillary serous carcinoma.

Nursing Management

Educating women who have high-risk factors and discussing strategies to reduce risk factors is considered primary prevention. Decreasing obesity and controlling diabetes are two ways to decrease the risk of the development of endometrial cancer.

Nurses can stress the importance of evaluation for any abnormal vaginal bleeding. Use of oral contraceptives as a younger adult also provides some protection against developing endometrial cancer.

Nurses caring for patients receiving brachytherapy must take precautions against occupational exposure to radioactive material. **Time**, **distance**, and **shielding** make up the rules for protecting against unnecessary exposure. A long-handled forceps and lead container are kept in the patient's room after the radioactive material has been placed into the patient. It is imperative that staff never pick up the radioactive source with their bare hands if it becomes displaced from the patient's vagina. The institution's radiation safety team should be notified in the event this occurs. Also patients should be made aware of the side effects of radiation therapy, including radiation enteritis, nausea, loss of appetite, bladder irritation, early menopause, vaginal dryness, and loss of interest in sexual intercourse (Gray & Koh, 2014). Refer to Chapter 6 for more details on radiation therapy.

CANCER OF THE OVARY

Ovarian cancer is referred to as a cancer that "whispers" because its clinical manifestations are not apparent until the tumor has invaded surrounding structures and is causing symptoms. It is the leading cause of death from cancers of the reproductive tract. Approximately 75% of women with ovarian cancer are diagnosed with advanced disease (Papadakis & McPhee, 2014). It carries a high fatality rate due to the aggressiveness of the malignancy. Five-year survivorship rate is not unforeseeable if the cancer is diagnosed at an early stage, but only 20% of women with ovarian cancer are diagnosed at that stage (ACS, 2015). Eighty-five percent of

---

BOX 33-14 | **Risk Factors for Cancer of the Ovary**

- Age over 40 or postmenopausal
- Nulliparous
- Northern American or Northern European descent
- Personal history of breast, colon, or endometrial cancer
- Obesity (BMI over 30)
- Use of fertility drugs
- Long-term use of hormone replacement therapy (HRT)
- Genetic predisposition; positive family history of ovarian cancer

---

women diagnosed are over 50 years of age; 15% have genetic links, 10% have *BRCA1* and *BRCA2* mutations, and 5% have HNPCC risk factors. See Box 33-14 for additional risk factors. Use of oral contraceptives has been proven to decrease risk of developing ovarian cancer by 50% with long-term protection benefits. Hormonal contraception causes reversible anovulation, thus decreasing the cumulative cycles of the ovary over a woman's lifetime. The longer the duration of use of OCPs means a decrease to the risk of ovarian cancer; every 5 years of use of oral contraceptives equates to a risk reduction of approximately 20% (ACS, 2015).

Cancers of the ovary occur in the epithelial cells lining the ovary. There are several different types of ovarian tumors: those that are germ cell tumors, originating from cells that produce eggs from the ovary; surface cell tumors; and sex cord stromal tumors. Malignant ovarian cells shed from the ovary implant onto the surfaces of the peritoneal cavity. Then these cancerous cells undergo transformation into ovarian surface epithelium (Rooth, 2013). Newer theories point to endometriosis as the predisposing factor for development of ovarian cancer due to damage from inclusion cysts on the ovary or exposure to mullerian factors (specific sensitive tumor marker for ovaries) during menstruation (Tellawi & Morozov, 2014).

Clinical Manifestations and Assessment

Symptoms of ovarian cancer are subtle and start with persistent bloating, early satiety, or a change in bowel or bladder habits. Typically women will complain of weight gain confined to their abdominal area. Due to the close proximity of the ovaries to the intestines, patients will complain of GI symptoms, and, as a result, this cancer carries a high rate of misdiagnosis, with patients commonly receiving treatment for a variety of disorders, including IBS, gastroesophageal reflux (GERD), menopause, or UTIs. Ascites (fluid accumulation in the peritoneal cavity) is considered a late-stage symptom, and prognosis is poor (Rooth, 2013).

No reliable screening tools are available for this disease. Treatment is hindered by late diagnosis, when the disease has already invaded peritoneal tissues and surrounding structures.

Bimanual examinations diagnose approximately one third of ovarian masses. Pelvic ultrasounds and blood tests for CA 125, a tumor marker, are the first diagnostics performed when ruling out an ovarian mass. If either of these tests is suggestive of a tumor, an abdominal and pelvic CT scan is performed. Patients are always referred to an oncologic gynecologist for management of this disease.

Medical Management

Surgical staging identifies tumor histologic grade and volume, which allows for the identification of treatment options and determines the prognosis based on tumor type (Table 33-6). During surgery, the suspicious tissue that is removed and sent to the laboratory for immediate analysis is known as a *frozen section*. If positive, the surgeon then performs extensive cytoreduction surgery or **debulking** to obtain clean tissue margins. This includes a TAH with BSO, removal of the omentum, peritoneal washings, and partial colectomy if there is any colon involvement (Rooth, 2013).

Stage IA or IB tumors are considered low risk and favorable to treatment, if well- or moderately well-differentiated tumors are confined to the ovary. Absence of tumor on the external surfaces, absence of ascites, and negative peritoneal washings are also favorable signs. Stage IA or IB with poorly differentiated tumors, tumors notable on the external surface of the ovary, ruptured tumor capsule, and positive peritoneal washings all are considered high risk and unfavorable. Advanced stages III and IV require combination chemotherapy after surgical staging has been performed to determine tumor sensitivity to a particular chemotherapeutic agent.

Chemotherapy treats residual tumor and helps to control any metastatic disease. Advance tumors receive chemotherapy first to decrease the size of the tumor; then the patient undergoes surgical debulking to remove as much tumor as possible. First-line chemotherapy consists of platinum and paclitaxel. Seventy-five percent of women respond to initial treatment, but there is an 85% relapse rate with a median survival of 3 years after platinum therapy. Carboplatin and paclitaxel are considered the gold standard for treatment of ovarian cancer. Carboplatin has recently replaced cisplatin due to its ability to be administered on an outpatient basis and its lesser toxicity. Patients undergo two or three cycles to evaluate their response and toxicity before proceeding with

TABLE 33-6 Stages of Ovarian Cancer

Stage	Description
Stage I	Tumor confined to ovary
Stage II	Involves one or both ovaries and extends into pelvis
Stage III	Involves one or both ovaries, as well as peritoneal metastasis and/or lymph node involvement
Stage IV	Distant metastasis beyond peritoneal cavity, including the liver

further treatment. Carboplatin combined with gemcitabine yields a higher response rate that has a longer median progression-free survival (ACS, 2015). Patients whose tumors are resistant to platinum receive single-agent therapy. A blood test for CA 125 is a sensitive indicator of disease relapse.

Nursing Management

Education and support begin preoperatively and continue through discharge (Rooth, 2013). Care must be individualized based on the patient's psychological and physical status, stage of illness, and treatment plan. Patients will need anticipatory guidance regarding postoperative infections, pain management, and potential side effects from chemotherapeutic agents. Postoperatively, patients will need to be monitored for signs and symptoms of infection, ileus, DVT, pulmonary embolus (PE), and bleeding. Encouraging the patient in the regular use of incentive spirometry, as well as regular ambulation, will help to decrease the development of DVT and atelectasis.

Emotional support is extremely important as the patient recovers from surgery and has to cope with a diagnosis of cancer. Side effects from chemotherapy should be discussed with the patient and her support system. Hair loss, nutrition, neuropathies, and nausea and vomiting as well as self-image alterations should be addressed regularly with the patient during her preoperative assessment and should be ongoing during her treatment. Refer to Chapter 6 for details on cancer care.

CANCER OF THE VULVA

Vulvar cancer is rare and represents just 5% of all cancers of the female reproductive tract (Rauh-Hain et al., 2014). Its incidence has been increasing slowly since 1973, however, and this is thought to be due to its link with HPV. There is increased evidence of young women with HPV being diagnosed with vulvar intraepithelial neoplasia (VIN), but the disease has a high cure rate after surgical resection and radiotherapy. Women diagnosed with vulvar cancer are usually between 65 and 70 years of age; however, studies now show that age is decreasing to 55 to 60 years of age at diagnosis (Rauh-Hain et al., 2014). Approximately 60% of women will be diagnosed with localized disease (Carcio & Secor, 2015).

The majority (90%) of cases of vulvar cancer is SCC, and approximately 40% to 60% of subtypes are largely due to high-risk strains of HPV (Papadakis & McPhee, 2014). VIN is more complex, deeply invasive, and is considered the precancerous condition of HPV types 16, 18, 31, and 33. Women who have been treated for condyloma, HPV, or abnormal cervical cytology, and those who smoke cigarettes or have an increased number of sexual partners have increased risk of developing cancer of the vulva.

Clinical Manifestations and Assessment

Longstanding external labial itching or burning of the external genitalia are early signs often self-treated by patients with OTC cortisone or anti-itch creams. Only about half of women will present with dyspareunia, vulvar edema, or pain. Later-stage manifestations include ulcerated lesions that are indicative of cancer. Older women are more likely to have advanced disease at the time of diagnosis (Rauh-Hain et al., 2014). Lesions occur in the vulvar area but may extend into the perianal and rectal areas, and lesions occur most commonly in areas that do not have hair. A Keyes punch biopsy or tissue biopsy is the gold standard for diagnosing vulvar cancer.

Medical Management

As with all cancerous lesions, early diagnosis of vulvar cancer is paramount. Vulvar biopsy can be performed in the office if short-term medical therapies have been proven unsuccessful or if there is a high index of suspicion for cancer. Vulvar colposcopy may be performed, but laser ablation or a wide excision of the affected area or a vulvectomy (removal of the vulva) with lymph node sampling for clear margins is dependent upon the size, depth, and focality of lesions. As a result, preservation of the clitoral area may or may not occur (Papadakis & McPhee, 2014). An alternative to surgery for early-stage lesions is the use of imiquimod (Aldara), which is a topical immune-response modifier with antiviral and antitumor properties typically used for the treatment of external genital warts. Depending upon the extent of the vulvectomy, use of chemotherapy, biologics, and radiation treatments also may be indicated. If there is evidence of disease spread to adjacent organs or regional lymph nodes, lymphadenectomy will be performed. There is a statistically significant correlation between extent of reconstructive surgery and disease outcomes, with local reconstructive surgery demonstrating a better prognosis with significant reduction in relapse rate.

Nursing Management

Patients are at higher risk for infection depending upon the size and extent of the surgical site. Monitoring patients postoperatively for wound infections, fever, discharge, and pain is a priority. Avoidance of cross-contamination of body fluids (such as urine or feces) will help to decrease infection. Foley care and assessment of skin are important in identifying any potential site of entry for infection.

Nursing Alert

Catheter-associated urinary tract infection (CAUTI) is one of the most common causes of hospital-acquired infection (HAI); therefore, the nurse plays a key role in detection and prevention of UTIs. The following interventions are recommended:

- *Insert catheters only for appropriate indications, and remove them as soon as possible.*
- *Ensure that only properly trained persons insert and maintain catheters; insert catheters using sterile technique and sterile equipment. Use as small a catheter as possible to minimize urethral trauma.*
- *Maintain a closed drainage system. Empty the collecting bag regularly using a separate collecting container for each patient. Avoid touching the draining spigot to the collecting container.*
- *Maintain unobstructed urine flow (keep the collecting bag below the level of the bladder at all times; do not place the bag on the floor; keep the catheter and collecting tube free from kinking).*
- *Maintain hand hygiene and follow standard (or appropriate isolation) precautions.*
- *If a urine specimen is needed, collect a small sample by aspirating urine from the needleless sampling port with a sterile syringe/cannula adaptor after cleansing the port (Lo et al., 2014; CDC, 2015d).*

Postoperative requirements for prolonged bed rest underscore the importance of assessing the patient for the development of DVT and PE to avoid tension on the surgical site and promote healing. Frequent position changes, and the use of compression stockings and intermittent pneumatic compression boots, along with regular use of incentive spirometry, will aid in avoiding the formation of DVTs and PEs.

Patients who have undergone a vulvectomy may suffer from distorted body images as a result of surgical resection; however, there are gaps in the literature that supports this theory (McCallum et al., 2014). Decreased sensation, vaginal dryness, and dyspareunia all affect a woman's ability to enjoy sexual relations. There is also a risk of pelvic floor dysfunction due to the severing of the delicate nerve supply in the vulvar area. Discussion with the surgeon regarding the extent of surgery will help the nurse to answer any questions the patient may have postoperatively. One of the most frequently reported concerns of patients with gynecologic cancer is the fear of recurrence and difficulty with changes in their sexual health (McCallum et al., 2014). Partner involvement and a social work or mental health referral are beneficial to help patients and their partners understand what to expect after discharge from the hospital.

HYSTERECTOMY

Surgical removal of the female reproductive organs is performed for a variety of reasons: dysfunctional uterine bleeding, benign or malignant masses, pelvic organ prolapse, pelvic pain, endometriosis, or trauma. Hysterectomies are the most common nonobstetric major surgery performed in the United States. Over 600,000 hysterectomies are performed annually (CDC, 2015e). The majority of hysterectomies are performed for benign uterine disorders that impact the QOL for women suffering from uterine disease or menstrual disorder.

Minimally invasive surgical techniques are now preferred due to reduced blood loss, decreased postoperative complications, and quicker recovery time (Mikhail et al., 2015). Hysterectomies consist of surgical removal of the uterus and fallopian tubes; however, conservation of the ovaries and cervix may be considered depending upon the patient's age and reason for surgery. Bilateral oophorectomy is associated with a decreased risk of breast and ovarian cancer. Fifty percent of women who undergo hysterectomy between 40 and 44 years of age will have both ovaries removed at the time of surgery. That percentage increases to 78% for women between 45 and 64 years of age. Surgical removal of the ovaries results in immediate cessation of production of both estrogen and androgen, causing surgical menopause. Subtotal hysterectomy or sparing of the cervix has no proven benefits (Saccardi et al., 2015). It is important for women to know if they have not had their cervix removed; women with an intact cervix will need to continue to undergo annual Pap smear screening for cervical cancer.

Types

Deciding on whether a TAH versus a total vaginal hysterectomy (TVH) should be performed is largely dependent upon a patient's BMI and other comorbid conditions. TVH allows for less blood loss, quicker recovery, shorter hospital stays, fewer infections, and less pain than the abdominal approach, which requires incisions through the abdominal musculature. TVH and laparoscopic-assisted vaginal hysterectomy (LAVH) can be done in a 1-day surgery center, whereas TAH and radical hysterectomies require a longer hospital stay. The use of laparoscopic and hysteroscopic (inspection of the uterine cavity by endoscopy) approaches are other alternatives to be considered and are dependent upon the surgeons' skill and experience with the equipment, as is robotic-assisted surgery. LAVH seems to be a safe alternative to TAH for patients who are obese (Mikhail et al., 2015). Radical hysterectomies, performed for malignant conditions, consist of the complete removal of all the reproductive organs, including the surrounding tissue margins, the upper one third of the vagina, and pelvic lymph node sampling. The number of hysterectomies performed overall is less now due to the development and use of endometrial ablation, progestin IUDs, and UAE.

Nursing Management

All patients with hysterectomies are surgical patients and, therefore, must be cared for like any other surgical patient. Attention to pain management; postoperative complications, such as DVT, PE, wound infections, and UTIs; and return of bowel function are the primary concerns for nurses. The nurse assesses the patient's lung sounds and encourages regular use of incentive spirometry. The nurse also monitors for return of bowel functions, as an ileus may occur due to manipulation of the bowel during surgery and the effects of anesthesia and analgesia on peristalsis.

Encouraging patients to walk with assistance as soon as the effects from general anesthesia have resolved helps with circulation and prevents formation of blood clots. Many patients undergoing hysterectomy also are dealing with the loss of fertility and, possibly, a cancer diagnosis. The nurse allows patients to verbalize their concerns and feelings and makes referrals to mental health providers if needed.

Discharge planning should include pelvic rest for 4 to 6 weeks and teaching the patient wound care and signs and symptoms of infection. Patients are allowed to shower and should be encouraged to resume regular activity gradually as per the surgeon's recommendation. Patients who have had a TAH generally are not permitted to drive for 4 to 6 weeks. They should avoid any heavy lifting, pushing, or pulling (such as vacuum cleaning) until their surgeon clears them to resume those activities. It is normal for women who have had hysterectomies to have some vaginal discharge. Patients who have undergone TAH normally will have some vaginal bleeding for up to 1 week postoperatively; patients who have undergone TVH and LAVH may have some vaginal discharge consisting of blood and mucus for several weeks postoperatively. Any foul-smelling vaginal discharge, unusual pain, or fever should be reported to the surgeon immediately. If there is evidence of unilateral swelling of the lower extremities, shortness of breath, or any discharge or redness around their incision sites, patients should contact their health care provider.

Unfolding Patient Stories: Doris Bowman • Part 2

Recall from Chapter 6 **Doris Bowman**, who is undergoing a TAH with BSO. What are potential postoperative complications that the nurse should consider? What assessments and interventions are done by the nurse to monitor for early detection or to prevent these complications? Describe the discharge education provided by the nurse on self-care monitoring required of the patient at home and what should be reported to the health care provider.

Care for Doris and other patients in a realistic virtual environment: *vSim for Nursing* (thepoint.lww.com/vSimMedicalSurgical). Practice documenting these patients' care in DocuCare (thepoint.lww.com/DocuCareEHR).

TRANSGENDER HEALTH CARE

Health Care Disparities

There is an increasing awareness of **transgender** patients and their lack of access to health care. As more people identify as transgender, it is paramount that nurses and health care providers educate themselves in the care of this underserved and sexually marginalized population (Zuzelo, 2014). This patient population is largely uninsured, experiences social stigmatization, and is at higher risk for PCOS, HIV exposure, interpersonal violence, and suicide. Transgender individuals are persons whose gender identity differs from their birth sex or their gender expression is different from what is typically considered to be societal norms. *Gender dysphoria* is a term used to describe the physical and emotional discomfort in one's assigned birth sex (IOM, 2011). If left untreated or if a person was unable to express or live as the gender one identifies with, that could lead to increased depression and, often, suicide. There are a disproportionate number of transgender individuals, especially teens and young adults, who become homeless due to familial isolation, loss of income, and inability to secure employment or housing. They may be placed inappropriately in emergency shelters and become victims of violence.

In 2010, the National Center for Transgender Equality and the National Gay and Lesbian Task Force performed a survey, "National Transgender Discrimination Survey Report on health and health care" (National Center for Transgender Equality, 2010). The results of this survey revealed that 50% of the respondents reported having to teach their health care provider about transgender care. Forty-one percent of transgender individuals reported suicide attempts versus the national average of 1.6%; this population also reported HIV rates that are four times that of the national average. The results also include that a staggering 24% have been discriminated against by a health care provider, and 19% were denied care from a health care provider completely. All patients deserve the same respect regardless of gender identity, preference, or expression.

When an individual identifies as transgender, he or she begins to live socially as a member of the sex identified with, through clothing and perhaps a name change. This is known as "transition." Some will choose to take hormones, such as testosterone or estrogen, for the desired physical effects of the gender they identify with. Many insurance companies deny coverage of hormone therapy for these patients. Others may have gender-affirming surgery, such as chest reconstruction (i.e., bilateral mastectomy), breast implants, orchiectomy, vaginoplasty, or phalloplasty while others may never have surgery at all. Some transgender persons may or may not choose to take hormones. Many patients who are in transition do not qualify for health care insurance, nor will current insurance pay for any procedures related to patients' transitions, mental health therapy, facial-feminization, or gender-affirming surgery. As a result, many patients will purchase hormones via the Internet or from unreliable sources. If patients become hospitalized, they may be anxious that they will not receive their hormones. Frequently they are discriminated against by those in the health care profession due to lack of knowledge, training, or personal bias on the part of the provider. The patient's level of anxiety may be escalated, and he or she may be perceived as a "difficult" patient. A person who has had to turn to prostitution to survive or who has been discriminated against repeatedly throughout life may turn to negative behaviors in times of crisis. Elder transgender persons are increasingly at risk for death from treatable chronic diseases or cancer due to their fear of stigmatization and previous discrimination or lack of health insurance. End-of-life issues and health care directives become a worrisome issue for elder transgender persons due to the absence of a legal marriage and subsequent legal inability to allow partners to make health care decisions (Kimmel, 2014). Many states that do not recognize same-sex marriage also do not allow partners to make health care decisions so it falls onto the next of kin. This becomes a legal debate especially in the context of end-of-life care especially if the patient does not have a living will or if the patient lives in a state that does not recognize domestic partnerships or same-sex marriages.

These behaviors will dissipate once a relationship of trust with care providers has been formed. It is difficult to find culturally competent and compassionate providers who have experience with transgender clients. The nurse is reminded that Healthy People 2020 states "access to quality health care and related services is important in order to eliminate health disparities and increase the quality and years of healthy life for all persons in the United States" (Healthy People 2020).

Nursing Management

It is important for nurses to be culturally diverse at all levels of practice. Nurses need to understand the specific needs of transgender patients and demonstrate acceptance with increased sensitivity and remain nonjudgmental while delivering care. It is equally as important for nurses to educate other members of the health care team who may not have experience with this population to avoid any compromise in patient care due to bias or ignorance. Any bias or ignorance should not be tolerated by any member of the health care team.

Due to the historically poor treatment of the transgender population by the health care profession, many will seek care only in an emergency and when routine health conditions have exacerbated into a serious condition. It is vital that nurses treat the patient, not the gender, and accept and encourage involvement of the client's domestic partner, significant other, and any other person who is considered family by that patient. Nurses also must be familiar with individual institution policies regarding nonblood relatives as next-of-kin for patients.

Nurses are in a unique position to establish a trusting relationship with patients. It is important to use gender-neutral terms and to ask the patient for the preferred name and pronoun. Other important interventions for this patient population include:

- Assessing the patient for high-risk behaviors, including IV drug abuse, prostitution, or use of hormones obtained via the Internet, on the street, or from the patient's friends.
- Offering to help **female-to-male** (FTM or transman) patients with their breast binder (if they wear one) after a

shower, or assisting with padded bras and undergarments for **male-to-female** (MTF or transwoman) patients.
- Offering support and reassurance for those undergoing invasive examinations, such as a breast or pelvic examination, as transgender clients have a lot of emotional conflict between their actual body and what they perceive their body to be.

Hysterectomies are routine gynecologic procedures performed for specific medical and surgical needs, as previously discussed in this chapter. In order to be considered a surgical candidate for a hysterectomy, the client will need to undergo a gynecologic examination. It is important to note that almost all transgender patients undergoing this surgery are either nulliparous or have never had vaginal penetration. If the client has been using testosterone, a significant amount

of vaginal atrophy will occur. If a client is taking estrogen therapy, penile and scrotal atrophy will be present. A digital rectal examination is still mandatory on any MTF (transwoman) patients over 50 years of age due to the presence of the prostate gland. Any FTM (transman) patient who has not had a hysterectomy or has had a supracervical hysterectomy will need to continue with routine cervical screening. ACOG (2011) recommends routine age-appropriate preventative screenings, including prostate and breast examinations, regardless of gender identity. However, there is varied consensus on whether or not routine cervical cytology should be continued in FTMs (transmen) who take testosterone therapy (ACOG, 2011).

Any transgender patient who has any type of gender-affirming surgery should be treated like any other postoperative patient with the same risk factors.

CHAPTER REVIEW

Critical Thinking Questions

1. A 60-year-old woman has a weak family history of breast cancer, including two great aunts, both postmenopausal at diagnosis. She would like to pursue *BRCA* testing. How would you address this request? What are the implications of genetic testing? What would you need to know about her history to determine the appropriateness of this test?

2. A 72-year-old woman with comorbidities of obesity and diabetes, who lives alone, is scheduled for a modified radical mastectomy for invasive breast cancer. Discuss the postoperative care of this patient, including discharge planning. How would you modify care if she has a severe hearing impairment? How would you modify care if she has been noncompliant with her medical care in the past? What appropriate resources are available for this patient?

3. When visiting the employee health center to obtain her annual influenza vaccine, a 48-year-old woman with a history of breast cancer and previous mastectomy reports that she has been experiencing vague abdominal discomfort, bloating, flatulence, and increased waist size over the last 6 months. Her next annual physical examination is 6 months from now. What additional information is it important to obtain from her? What recommendations for further follow-up and health care would you provide?

4. A 50-year-old woman is scheduled for a total hysterectomy to treat fibroids. She reports that she anticipates severe symptoms of menopause because her mother and grandmother had severe symptoms. She asks you about medications and herbal substances that can prevent or

minimize menopausal symptoms without increasing her risk of breast cancer or cardiac disease. What is the strength of evidence about medications, including estrogen, and herbal substances to reduce menopausal symptoms? What criteria would you use to determine the strength of that evidence?

NCLEX-Style Review Questions

1. A patient is concerned with developing breast cancer. The nurse recognizes which as the greatest risk factor for developing breast cancer?
   a. Having a first-degree relative who developed breast cancer
   b. Being female and advancing age
   c. Beginning menses before age 12 and never having children
   d. Smoking and obesity

2. A patient asks the nurse when she should be screened for breast cancer. What is the nurse's best response, based on the American Cancer Society's recommendations for breast cancer screening?
   a. Annual screening mammography beginning at age 40, clinical breast examination every 3 years beginning at age 20 and annually beginning at age 40, and practicing breast self-awareness
   b. Annual screening mammography beginning at age 50, annual clinical breast examination beginning at age 50
   c. Screening mammography every other year beginning at age 50, annual clinical breast examination beginning at age 40, monthly breast self-examination

d. Baseline screening mammogram at age 35, annual screening mammography beginning at age 40, breast MRI every 5 years beginning at age 40, annual clinical breast examination beginning at age 20, monthly breast self-examination

3. Which patient would be at highest risk for subsequent development of lymphedema?
   a. A 75-year-old woman with a single focus of biopsy-proven localized ductal carcinoma in situ
   b. A 65-year-old woman with a known benign cyst
   c. A 50-year-old woman with a biopsy-confirmed fibroadenoma
   d. A 62-year-old woman with biopsy-proven invasive ductal carcinoma with palpable axillary lymph nodes and positive node fine-needle aspiration

4. A patient suspects that she may have PMS. The nurse should ask the patient about which symptoms?
   a. Symptoms that occur during the luteal phase of the menstrual cycle
   b. Symptoms that occur during the follicular phase of the menstrual cycle
   c. Symptoms that worsen during menopause
   d. Symptoms that persist throughout the entire menstrual cycle

5. A patient has just been prescribed Lupron for her endometriosis. The nurse should mention which side effects while educating the patient about this drug?
   a. She may experience breakthrough bleeding.
   b. Reversible symptoms of menopause may occur.
   c. The medication will reduce the size of her fibroids.
   d. A form of back-up contraception should be used while taking this drug.

Try these additional resources, available at **http://thepoint.lww.com/Honan2e**, to enhance your learning and understanding of this chapter:
- NCLEX-Style Student Review Questions
- Journal Articles

REFERENCES AND SELECTED READINGS

References and selected readings associated with this chapter can be found on the website that accompanies the book. Visit **http://thepoint.lww.com/Honan2e** to access the references and other additional resources associated with this chapter.

Nursing Management: Patients with Male Reproductive Disorders

Susanne A. Quallich

Learning Objectives

After reading this chapter, you will be able to:

1. Discuss the causes and management of male sexual dysfunction.
2. Compare the types of prostatectomy with regard to advantages and disadvantages.
3. Use the nursing process as a framework for care of the patient undergoing prostatectomy.
4. Describe the various conditions affecting the testes, including pathophysiology, clinical manifestations, and management.
5. Describe the various conditions affecting the penis, including pathophysiology, clinical manifestations, and management.

Disorders of the male reproductive system involve the genitalia and, in some instances, sexuality; as a consequence, the patient may experience anxiety and embarrassment. The effects of trauma, chronic illness, and physical disability on sexual function can be profound. A man's willingness to discuss these issues is influenced directly by his culture, religion, and social community. The nurse must recognize the patient's need for privacy as well as his need for education.

DISORDERS OF MALE SEXUAL FUNCTION

ERECTILE DYSFUNCTION

Erectile dysfunction (ED) is the inability to achieve or maintain an erection sufficient for satisfactory sexual activity. Up to 50% of men 40 years of age and older may report some difficulty with erectile function (Glina, Sharlip, & Hellstrom, 2013).

Pathophysiology

The physiology of erection and ejaculation is complex and involves sympathetic and parasympathetic components. Erection involves the release of nitric oxide into the corpus cavernosum during sexual stimulation; this releases cyclic guanosine monophosphate (cGMP) and causes relaxation of the smooth muscles. This allows flow of blood into the corpus cavernosum, resulting in erection.

ED has both psychogenic and organic causes. Psychogenic causes include anxiety, fatigue, depression, and pressure to perform sexually. Organic causes include occlusive vascular disease, endocrine disease (diabetes, hypogonadism, hyperthyroidism, and hypothyroidism), cirrhosis, chronic kidney failure, postsurgical causes (retroperitoneal surgery), neurologic disorders (neuropathies, parkinsonism, spinal cord injury, and multiple sclerosis), trauma to the pelvic or genital area, alcohol, medications (Box 34-1), and drug abuse.

Clinical Manifestations and Assessment

The diagnosis of ED requires a sexual and medical history; an analysis of presenting symptoms; a physical examination, including a neurologic examination; a detailed assessment of the usage of any medications, alcohol, and drugs; and laboratory studies. Because ED can occur secondary to a variety of disorders and pharmacologic agents, nurses are encouraged to ask the patient questions about erectile function. Numerous tools are available to help nurses introduce the topic of sexual health with their patients. The man may report decreased frequency of erections, inability to achieve a firm erection, or rapid detumescence (subsidence of erection).

Nocturnal penile tumescence tests and Rigiscan® testing are options to evaluate actual erectile function and help to determine whether there is an organic or a psychological cause; these are ordered at the discretion of the provider. Arterial blood flow to the penis can be measured using a Doppler probe. Figure 34-1 describes the evaluation and treatment of ED.

Medical Management

Treatment can be medical, surgical, or both, depending on the cause (Table 34-1). Nonsurgical therapy includes treating

BOX 34-1

Classes of Medications Associated with Erectile Dysfunction

- Antiadrenergics and antihypertensives
- Anticholinergics and phenothiazines
- Antiseizure agents
- Antifungals
- Antiandrogen medications (prostate cancer treatment)
- Antipsychotics
- Antispasmodics
- Anxiolytics, sedative–hypnotics, tranquilizers
- Beta blockers
- Calcium-channel blockers
- Carbonic anhydrase inhibitors
- H_2 antagonists
- Thiazide diuretics
- Tricyclic antidepressants

associated conditions, such as diabetes, and adjusting antihypertensive agents or other medications. Endocrine therapy may reverse the condition. Patients with ED from psychogenic causes are referred to a sex therapist. Patients with ED secondary to organic causes may be candidates for penile implants.

Pharmacologic Therapy

Phosphodiesterase-5 (PDE-5) inhibitors are oral medications that are used to treat ED. Sildenafil citrate (Viagra), the first of these agents, was introduced in 1998 in the United States. Other PDE-5 inhibitors are vardenafil HCl (Levitra), avanafil (Stendra), and tadalafil (Cialis). PDE-5 is an enzyme that destroys cGMP, the nucleotide that causes the cavernosal relaxation necessary for erection to occur. By inhibiting PDE-5, cGMP is allowed to accumulate, thus facilitating relaxation of corporeal smooth muscle in response to sexual stimulation. When these PDE-5 inhibitors are taken about 1 hour before sexual activity, they are effective in producing, with stimulation, an erection that can last 60 to 120 minutes. These medications have side effects and are contraindicated in men who take organic nitrates because together these drugs can cause severe hypotension. Table 34-2 summarizes the dosing and nursing implications of these medications.

Other pharmacologic measures to induce erections include injecting vasoactive agents, such as alprostadil, papaverine, and phentolamine, directly into the penis. Complications include **priapism** (a persistent erection of the penis) and development of fibrotic plaques at the injection sites. Alprostadil also is formulated in a gel pellet that can be inserted into the urethra to promote an erection.

Penile Implants

Penile implants are available in two types: the semirigid rod and inflatable. The semirigid rod results in a permanent semierection, but it is not commonly used. The inflatable

FIGURE 34-1 Evaluation and treatment of men with erectile dysfunction. (From Lue, T. F. (2000). Erectile dysfunction. *New England Journal of Medicine, 342*(24), 1807. © 2000 Massachusetts Medical Society. All rights reserved. Used with permission.)

TABLE 34-1 Treatments for Erectile Dysfunction

Method	Description	Advantages and Disadvantages	Duration
Pharmacologic therapy • Oral medication (sildenafil citrate [Viagra]; vardenafil HCl [Levitra]; avanafil [Stendra]; tadalafil [Cialis]) Oral medication	Smooth muscle relaxant causing blood to flow into penis	Can cause headache and sinus stuffiness Contraindicated for men taking nitrate medications Used with caution in patients with retinopathy or poor exercise tolerance	Taken orally 1 hour before intercourse Stimulation is required to achieve erection.
• Injection (alprostadil, papaverine, phentolamine) Penile injection	Smooth muscle relaxant increasing blood to flow into penis	Firm erections are achievable in more than 50% of cases Pain at injection site; plaque formation, risk of priapism	Injection 20 minutes before intercourse Erection can last up to 1 hour.
• Urethral suppository (alprostadil) Penile suppository	Smooth muscle relaxant increasing blood to flow into penis	May be used twice a day Not recommended with partners who are pregnant or if trying to become pregnant	Inserted 20–30 minutes before intercourse Erection can last up to 1 hour.
Penile implants • Semirigid rod • Inflatable Penile implant	Surgically implanted into corpus cavernosum	Reliable Requires surgery Healing takes up to 3 weeks Semirigid rod results in permanent semierection	Indefinite—must be deflated manually (inflatable device) Inflatable prosthesis: Saline returns from penile receptacle to reservoir.

(continued on page 1042)

TABLE **34-1** Treatments for Erectile Dysfunction (*continued*)

Method	Description	Advantages and Disadvantages	Duration
Negative-pressure (vacuum) devices	Induction of erection with vacuum; maintained with constriction band around base of penis	Few side effects Patients may find it cumbersome to use Vasocongestion of penis can cause pain or numbness	To prevent penile injury, constriction band must not be left in place for longer than 1 hour.

Penile vacuum pump

TABLE **34-2** Pharmacologic Treatment of Erectile Dysfunction

	Sildenafil Citrate (Viagra)	Vardenafil HCl (Levitra)	Avanavil (Stendra)	Tadalafil (Cialis)
Recommended dose	Dosage range is 25–100 mg, based on individual response. Take only once in 24 hours.	Dosage range is 5–20 mg, based on individual response. Take only once in 24 hours.	Dosage range is 50–200 mg, based on individual response. Take only once in 24 hours.	Dosage range is 5–20 mg, based on individual response. Take only once in 24 hours. For patients with decreased liver or kidney function, the maximum dose is 10 mg every 48 hours.
When to take	Take the medication 30 minutes to 4 hours before sexual activity. *There must be sexual stimulation to produce an erection.*	Take the medication 1 hour before sexual activity. The peak action occurs in 30–120 minutes. *There must be sexual stimulation to produce an erection.*	Take the medication at least 15 minutes before sexual activity. The peak action occurs in 30–120 minutes. *There must be sexual stimulation to produce an erection.*	Take the medication before sexual activity. Effect peaks at 2–6 hours; effect may last up to 36 hours. *There must be sexual stimulation to produce an erection.*
Side effects	Side effects include headache, flushing, indigestion, nasal congestion, blue vision.	Side effects include headache, flushing, runny nose, indigestion, sinusitis.	Side effects include headache, flushing, runny nose, back pain.	Tadalafil may cause back pain and muscle aches. Tell your provider if you experience any of these side effects.
Note	Patients must be counseled to seek medical attention for erection lasting longer than 4 hours. Patients must be counseled to seek medical attention in the event of a sudden loss of vision in one or both eyes. Taking more than one of these mediations is not advised; combinations have not been evaluated formally for efficacy or safety. These medications can potentiate the effects of nitrates, alpha blockers, antihypertensives, and alcohol.			
Contraindications	Do not take if you are taking nitrate medications, such as nitroglycerine or isosorbide mononitrate. Do not take if you have high uncontrolled blood pressure, coronary artery disease, or have had a heart attack within the past 6 months. Do not take if you have been diagnosed with a cardiac arrhythmia or kidney or liver dysfunction—discuss with your provider to ensure proper dosing.			
Drug interactions	These medications can react with other medications that you may be taking. Provide your provider with a complete list of all prescribed as well as over-the-counter medications that you are using.			

prosthesis simulates natural erections and natural flaccidity. Complications after implantation include infection and erosion of the prosthesis through the one or both of the corpora cavernosa (see Chapter 32, Fig. 32-7), which may require removal of the implant (Oberlin et al., 2015). Factors to consider in choosing a prosthesis include the expectations of the patient and his partner.

Vacuum Erection Devices

Negative-pressure (vacuum) devices also may be used to induce an erection. A plastic cylinder is placed over the flaccid penis, and negative pressure is applied. When an erection is attained, a constriction band is placed around the base of the penis to maintain the erection.

Nursing Management

Personal satisfaction and the ability to satisfy a partner sexually are common concerns of patients. Men with illnesses and disabilities may need the assistance of a sex therapist to find, implement, and integrate their sexual beliefs and behaviors into a healthy and satisfying lifestyle. The nurse should assess the patient's needs and make appropriate resources available, including information regarding referral to a specialized sex therapist, such as www.aasect.org.

DISORDERS OF EJACULATION

The spectrum of disorders of ejaculation responses ranges from occasional ejaculation through intercourse or self-stimulation to complete inability to ejaculate under any circumstances. For instance, premature ejaculation occurs when a man reaches climax before or shortly after intromission. Treatment modalities depend on the nature and severity of the ejaculation problem. Behavioral therapies may be indicated; these therapies often involve both sexual partners. In some cases, pharmacologic and behavioral therapy together may be effective.

Neurologic disorders (e.g., spinal cord injury, multiple sclerosis, neuropathy secondary to diabetes), surgery (prostatectomy), and medications are the most common causes of inhibited ejaculation. Chemical, vibratory, and electrical methods of stimulation have been used with some success.

CONDITIONS OF THE PROSTATE

PROSTATITIS

Prostatitis is an inflammation of the prostate gland that is caused by infectious agents or other conditions (e.g., urethral stricture, prostatic hyperplasia).

Pathophysiology

Escherichia coli is the organism that is isolated most commonly. Usually microorganisms are carried to the prostate

from the urethra. Prostatitis syndromes are classified as acute bacterial (type I), chronic bacterial (type II), chronic prostatitis/chronic pelvic pain syndrome (CP/CPPS) (type IIIa), inflammatory/chronic prostatitis/chronic pelvic pain syndrome (CP/CPPS) (type IIIb), and noninflammatory and asymptomatic inflammatory prostatitis (type IV) (National Institute of Health; National Institute of Diabetes and Digestive and Kidney Disease [NIH/NIDDK], 2014).

Clinical Manifestations and Assessment

The diagnosis of prostatitis requires a careful history and physical examination. Symptoms of prostatitis may include perineal discomfort, dysuria, urgency, frequency, and pain with or after ejaculation. Prostatodynia (pain in the prostate) is manifested by pain on voiding or perineal pain without evidence of inflammation or bacterial growth in the prostate fluid.

Acute bacterial prostatitis may produce sudden fever and chills as well as pain in the perineum, rectum, or low back. Urinary symptoms, such as dysuria (painful urination), frequency, urgency, and **nocturia** (awakening at night to urinate), may occur. Chronic bacterial prostatitis is a major cause of relapsing urinary tract infection (UTI) in men. Symptoms are usually mild, consisting of frequency, dysuria, and, occasionally, urethral discharge. Complications of prostatitis include swelling of the prostate gland, urinary retention, epididymitis, bacteremia, and pyelonephritis (discussed in Chapter 27).

If the patient does not have acute prostatitis, the provider performs a digital rectal examination (DRE) after collection of a urine sample, which commonly reveals many white blood cells. A DRE should not be performed if acute prostatitis is suspected because of the increased risk of causing bacteremia and septicemia.

Medical Management

The goal of therapy for acute bacterial prostatitis is to avoid the complications of abscess formation and septicemia. A complete blood count (CBC) and blood and urine culture may be ordered. A **prostate-specific antigen** (PSA) test may not be obtained since in many patients the acute inflammatory process causes temporary elevation. However, the PSA test also can provide a means to track the success of treatment as the level should lessen with the use of antibiotics. A broad-spectrum antibiotic, frequently a fluoroquinolone, is administered for 14 to 30 days. Comfort is promoted with analgesic agents, antispasmodic medications, bladder sedatives (to relieve bladder irritability), sitz baths (to relieve pain and spasm), and stool softeners (to prevent pain from straining).

Chronic bacterial prostatitis can be difficult to treat because most antibiotics diffuse poorly from the plasma into the prostatic fluid. Treatment includes alpha-adrenergic blockers to promote relaxation of the bladder and prostate.

Antibiotics, such as trimethoprim-sulfamethoxazole or a fluoroquinolone, may be prescribed.

The treatment of nonbacterial prostatitis is directed toward relief of symptoms.

Nursing Management

A patient experiencing symptoms of acute prostatitis may be hospitalized for IV antibiotic therapy. Nursing management includes administration of prescribed antibiotics and provision of comfort measures, including prescribed analgesic agents and sitz baths. In addition, the patient is cautioned to avoid activities that result in repetitive perineal trauma, such as cycling.

Usually the patient with chronic prostatitis is treated on an outpatient basis and needs to be instructed about the importance of continuing antibiotic therapy. The nurse instructs the patient to complete the prescribed course of antibiotics. Hot sitz baths (10 to 20 minutes) may be taken several times daily. Fluids should be encouraged to keep the urine dilute, and the patient should avoid sitting for long periods to minimize discomfort.

BENIGN PROSTATIC HYPERPLASIA

In approximately one half of men 50 years of age and older, the prostate gland enlarges and obstructs the outflow of urine. This enlargement and obstruction, referred to as benign prostatic hyperplasia (BPH), is evident in 80% of men 80 years of age and older.

Pathophysiology

The hypertrophied lobes of the prostate may obstruct the vesical neck or prostatic urethra, causing incomplete emptying of the bladder and urinary retention. As a result, a gradual dilation of the ureters (hydroureter) and kidneys (hydronephrosis) can occur. UTIs may result from urinary stasis since retained urine serves as a medium for infective organisms.

Risk Factors

The cause of BPH is uncertain. Many African-American men develop BPH at a much younger age (40 years of age) than Caucasian men do, whereas Asian men are unlikely to develop BPH (Sotelo, Azhar, & Morales, 2015). Recent studies have identified smoking (both current and former smoking), heavy alcohol consumption, hypertension, heart disease, and diabetes as risk factors associated with BPH (Moyad, 2014). Other studies suggest that dietary factors may affect prostate growth and BPH (Sotelo et al., 2015).

Clinical Manifestations and Assessment

The obstructive and irritating symptoms associated with BPH include increased frequency of urination, nocturia, urgency, hesitancy in starting urination, abdominal straining with urination, a decrease in the volume and force of the urinary stream, interruption of the urinary stream, dribbling, a sensation of incomplete emptying, possible acute urinary retention, and recurrent UTIs.

DRE may reveal a large, rubbery, and nontender prostate gland, although the size of the prostate correlates poorly with symptom report. Diagnostic studies may be indicated to determine the degree to which the prostate is enlarged, the presence of any changes in the bladder wall, and the efficiency of kidney function. These tests may include urinalysis as well as urodynamic studies to assess urine flow and bladder function. Renal function tests, including serum creatinine levels, may be performed to determine whether renal impairment exists.

Medical Management

The treatment plan depends on the severity of the obstruction and the patient's condition. If the patient is admitted on an emergency basis because of urinary retention, an emergency catheterization is performed. The ordinary catheter may be too soft and pliable to advance through the urethra into the bladder. A Coude catheter (45-degree, semirigid curved tip) is recommended to facilitate passage through the prostatic urethra. If a catheter cannot be placed, an incision is made into the bladder (a suprapubic cystostomy) to provide drainage; however, this is rare. Further details are discussed in Chapter 28 under urinary retention.

Pharmacologic Therapy

Pharmacologic treatment for BPH includes use of alpha-adrenergic blockers and 5-alpha-reductase inhibitors. Alpha-adrenergic blockers relax the smooth muscle of the bladder neck and prostate, improve urine flow, and relieve BPH symptoms. 5-alpha-reductase inhibitors interfere with the conversion of testosterone to dihydrotestosterone (DHT), which is associated with prostate growth. Decreased levels of DHT lead to decreased activity of glandular cells and prostate size. Side effects may include gynecomastia, ED, low volume ejaculate, and flushing.

Saw palmetto is an herbal product some men find helpful in addressing symptoms associated with BPH. In theory, it functions by interfering with the conversion of testosterone to DHT. Research has shown that the efficacy of saw palmetto is similar to that of medications such as finasteride, and the herbal product may be better tolerated and less expensive (Katz & Darves-Bornoz, 2014). The lack of standardization of herbal products should be a source of concern for health care professionals (Katz & Darves-Bornoz, 2014; Porth, 2015), and the nurse should warn men that formulations may be different with each purchase.

Other Therapies

Other treatment options for BPH include surgical options, such as transurethral incision of the prostate (TUIP), balloon dilation, transurethral laser resection, transurethral needle ablation, and microwave thermotherapy (Porth, 2015). Surgical approach of choice depends on the size of the gland, the severity of the obstruction, the age of the patient, any comorbidities, and the function of the bladder, and there are potential postoperative management issues (Box 34-3). Stents (devices made of tubular mesh) may be inserted under local or regional anesthesia to maintain patency of the urethra when patients are a poor risk for prostatic surgery. "Watchful waiting" is another option chosen by many, in which patients are monitored periodically for severity of symptoms, physical findings, and laboratory tests and may undergo diagnostic urologic tests.

CANCER OF THE PROSTATE

Prostate cancer is the most common cancer in men other than nonmelanoma skin cancer. It is the second most common cause of cancer death in American men, exceeded only by lung cancer, and is responsible for 10% of cancer-related deaths in men. Among men diagnosed with prostate cancer, 5-year survival is nearly 100%, 99% survive at least 10 years, and 94% survive 15 years (ACS, 2015a, 2015b).

Risk Factors

Prostate cancer is common in the United States and northwestern Europe but is rare in Asia, Africa, Central America, and South America. The worldwide incidence of prostate cancer is highest in African-American men; possible factors that may explain the increased mortality rate in African-American men include their lower level of engagement in the health care system, disparities in health care, and cultural constraints that define masculinity and health (Tanagho & McAninch, 2012). Other risk factors for prostate cancer include increasing age; more than two thirds of cases occur in men older than 65 years of age (ACS, 2015a). A familial predisposition may occur in men who have a father or brother previously diagnosed with prostate cancer, especially if those relatives were diagnosed at a young age. Data suggest that men who consume a diet containing excessive amounts of red meat or high-fat dairy products are at increased risk for prostate cancer (ACS, 2015b).

Clinical Manifestations and Assessment

Cancer of the prostate in its early stages rarely produces symptoms. If the neoplasm is large enough to encroach on the bladder neck, signs and symptoms of urinary obstruction occur (difficulty and frequency of urination, urinary retention, and decreased size and force of the urinary stream). Hematuria may result if the cancer invades the urethra or bladder, or both.

Prostate cancer can metastasize to bone and lymph nodes. Symptoms related to metastases include backache, hip pain, perineal and rectal discomfort, anemia, weight loss, weakness, nausea, and oliguria (less than 400 mL/day). These symptoms may be the first indications of prostate cancer, although due to contemporary US screening practices, it is uncommon for men to present at this advanced stage.

The American Urological Association (AUA) (2013) recommendation states that "the highest-quality evidence for benefit (lower prostate cancer mortality) was found in men ages 55 to 69 screened at 2- to 4-year intervals," and the organization "does not recommend routine screening in men between ages 40 and 54 years at average risk." The AUA also recommends that men be counseled regarding their potential treatment options prior to screening (AUA, 2013).

In direct contrast, the American Cancer Society (2015) does not support routine PSA screening but recommends that "asymptomatic men who have at least a 10-year life expectancy should have an opportunity to make an informed decision with their health care provider about screening for prostate cancer after receiving information about the uncertainties, risks, and potential benefits associated with screening." These tests are recommended for younger men (40 to 45 years of age) if they are at high risk for prostate cancer; namely, African-American men and men who have a first-degree relative (father, brother, or son) diagnosed with prostate cancer at an early age (under 65 years of age) (ACS, 2015b).

The level of PSA in the blood is proportional to the total prostatic mass and does not necessarily indicate malignancy. There are limitations in the relationship among serum PSA, prostate cancer volume, and higher stages of prostate cancer as measured by the Gleason score, which is the system used most often to grade prostate cancer and to guide the physician in determining the most appropriate treatment (Sher & Eastham, 2015). The combination of DRE and PSA testing appears to be a cost-effective method of detecting prostate cancer. If prostate cancer is detected early, the likelihood of cure is high. This is limited by the methods used to identify prostate cancer from abnormal findings on DRE and serum PSA elevations. Both of those tools have issues related to sensitivity and specificity, adding to the continued lack of consensus regarding "best screening" tools.

Routine repeated rectal palpation of the gland (preferably by the same examiner) is important because early cancer may be detected as a nodule within the substance of the gland. The diagnosis of prostate cancer is confirmed by a histologic examination of tissue. Cancer detected when transurethral resection of the prostate (TURP) is performed for benign prostatic enlargement and lower urinary tract symptoms occurs in about one out of 10 cases (Tanagho & McAninch, 2012).

Needle biopsies of the prostate are guided by transrectal ultrasound (TRUS) and may be indicated for men who have elevated PSA levels and abnormal DRE findings. Other tests that may be used to establish the extent of disease include bone scans to detect metastasis to the bones and computed tomography (CT) scan to identify metastases in the pelvic lymph nodes. Some facilities now offer an MRI/ultrasound fusion biopsy, especially for men with a history of a previous negative ultrasound-guided biopsy and rising PSA. Men who have chosen active surveillance for prostate cancer also may be candidates for this procedure. This new procedure allows the urologist to precisely identify areas of the prostate that should be investigated or biopsied. Patient preparation is the same for a traditional prostate biopsy.

Medical and Nursing Management

Treatment is based on the stage of the disease and the patient's age and symptoms. Review of data from clinical assessment, laboratory and radiology tests, TRUS, and/or biopsy results assists in the treatment decision process.

Surgical Management

Radical prostatectomy is the complete surgical removal of the prostate, seminal vesicles, and, often, the surrounding fat, nerves, lymph nodes, and blood vessels. It is considered the standard first-line treatment for prostate cancer. Although ED commonly follows radical prostatectomy, Da Vinci prostatectomy or robotically assisted laparoscopic radical prostatectomy (RALP) offers advantages of low morbidity and more rapid discharge postprocedure (see below for discussion).

Radiation Therapy

If prostate cancer is detected in its early stage, the treatment may be curative radiation therapy. Two major forms of radiation therapy are used to treat cancer of the prostate: teletherapy (external) and brachytherapy (internal).

Teletherapy (external-beam radiation therapy) involves 6 to 7 weeks of daily (5 days/week) radiation treatments. Current technology sets a dose for the target volume and restricts the dose to adjacent structures. It is thought to be accurate within 1 to 3 mm.

Brachytherapy involves the implantation of interstitial radioactive seeds under anesthesia, via the perineum, into the prostate. Eighty to 100 seeds are placed directly into the prostate, and the patient returns home after the procedure. Exposure of others to radiation is minimal, but the patient should avoid close contact with pregnant women and infants for up to 2 months.

Side effects of teletherapy and brachytherapy include inflammation of the rectum, bowel, and bladder due to their proximity to the prostate and the radiation doses. Men are likely to suffer a decline in erectile function with time. Table 34-3 discusses nursing interventions to minimize side effects. Combination therapy (radiation therapy followed by hormonal therapy) may improve overall survival.

Hormonal Therapy

Hormonal therapy for advanced prostate cancer suppresses androgenic stimuli to the prostate by decreasing the level of circulating plasma testosterone or interrupting the conversion to or binding of DHT. As a result, the prostatic

TABLE 34-3 Management of Radiation-Induced Symptoms

Symptom	Intervention
Cystitis	Maintain hydration. Encourage patient to take prescribed medications (bladder antispasmodics, alpha blockers, analgesics). Avoid known bladder irritants (see Chapter 28).
Diarrhea	Provide low-residue diet. Maintain hydration. Administer antidiarrheals as indicated. Give dietary bulking agents as indicated.
Erectile dysfunction	Assess for level of distress and suggest sexual therapist as appropriate. Provide education regarding appropriate medication.
Proctitis (inflammation of the rectum)	Offer sitz baths. Recommend water-based lubricants. Maintain hydration to avoid constipation. Adjust diet to avoid constipation.

epithelium atrophies. This effect is accomplished either by surgical castration (**orchiectomy**) or by the administration of medications. Orchiectomy is associated with considerable emotional impact. The most appropriate choice, timing, and actual benefits of hormonal therapy are uncertain.

Effective hormonal alternatives to orchiectomy include the nonsteroidal antiandrogen bicalutamide. Newer hormonal therapies include luteinizing hormone–releasing hormone (LHRH) agonists (leuprolide and goserelin) and antiandrogen agents, such as flutamide. LHRH suppresses testicular androgen, while flutamide causes suppression of adrenal androgen. LHRH agonists are used for the following: (1) in the adjuvant and neoadjuvant setting (i.e., before use of hormonal suppressive agents), in combination with radiation therapy; (2) in combination with radical prostatectomy; and (3) in the treatment of recurrence indicated by an elevation in the PSA. Hot flashes can occur with orchiectomy or LHRH-agonist therapy.

Second-Line Medical Treatment

The management of hormone-refractory cancer of the prostate remains somewhat controversial. Administration of second-line hormonal therapy using ketoconazole is an option that lowers testosterone by decreasing both testicular and endocrine production of androgens. There may be benefits in terms of survival with chemotherapy treatment that includes paclitaxel and docetaxel for nonandrogen-dependent prostate cancer.

Other Therapies

Cryosurgery of the prostate is used to ablate prostate cancer in patients who cannot tolerate surgery and in those with recurrent prostate cancer. Transperineal probes are inserted into the prostate under ultrasound guidance to freeze the tissue directly.

Keeping the urethral passage patent may require repeated transurethral (TUR) resections. If this is impractical, catheter drainage is instituted by way of the suprapubic or transurethral route. For men with advanced prostate cancer, palliative measures, such as pain management, complementary and alternative medicine (CAM), and androgen deprivation, can be options. Although cure is unlikely with advanced prostate cancer, many men survive for a long period apparently free of metastatic disease.

Bone lesions resulting from metastasis of prostate cancer can be very painful. Opioid and nonopioid medications are used to control the pain. External-beam radiation therapy can be delivered to skeletal lesions to relieve pain, while radiopharmaceuticals can be injected IV to treat multiple sites of bone metastasis.

More than one third of men with a diagnosis of prostate cancer elect to use some form of CAM. Because of lack of research on many forms of CAM, patients may be forced to rely on anecdotal information or information gained via the Internet to make decisions about its use.

Complications

Each treatment for prostate cancer has some incidence of sexual function issues. With nerve-sparing radical prostatectomy, the likelihood of recovering the ability to have erections is better for men who are younger and in whom both neurovascular bundles (the erectile nerves and blood vessels called neurovascular bundles run along the surface of each side of the prostate) are spared. Hormonal therapy also affects the central nervous system mechanisms that mediate sexual desire and arousability. PDE-5 inhibitors may be effective for treatment of ED in younger men after radical retropubic prostatectomy (discussed shortly), especially if the neurovascular bundles were preserved. They may improve erectile function in men with partial or moderate ED after radiation therapy for localized prostate cancer.

PROSTATE SURGERY

Prostate surgery may be indicated for the patient with BPH or prostate cancer. Prostate surgery should be performed before acute urinary retention develops and damages the upper urinary tract and collecting system or before cancer progresses.

Procedures

Several approaches can be used to remove the hypertrophied portion of the prostate gland: TURP, suprapubic prostatectomy, perineal prostatectomy, retropubic prostatectomy, TUIP, and robotic prostatectomy (Table 34-4). Hyperplastic tissue is removed, leaving behind the capsule of the prostate.

NURSING PROCESS
Patient Undergoing Prostatectomy

ASSESSMENT

The nurse assesses how the underlying disorder (BPH or prostate cancer) has affected the patient's lifestyle. The nurse asks about the patient's family history of cancer and heart or kidney disease, including hypertension. In addition, the nurse observes for weight loss, pallor, ability to get in and out of bed without assistance, and ability to perform activities of daily living (ADL). This information helps determine how soon the patient will be able to return to normal activities after prostatectomy.

DIAGNOSIS

Based on the assessment data, the patient's major nursing diagnoses may include the following:

- Preoperative nursing diagnoses:
  - Anxiety related to surgery and its outcome
  - Acute pain related to bladder distention
  - Deficient knowledge about factors related to the disorder and the treatment protocol
- Postoperative nursing diagnoses:
  - Acute pain related to the surgical incision, catheter placement, and bladder spasms
  - Deficient knowledge about postoperative care and management

Based on the assessment data, the potential complications may include the following:

- Hemorrhage and shock
- Infection
- Deep vein thrombosis (DVT)
- Catheter obstruction
- Sexual dysfunction

PLANNING

The major preoperative goals for the patient may include reduced anxiety and learning about his prostate disorder and the perioperative experience. The major postoperative goals may include maintenance of fluid volume balance, relief of pain and discomfort, ability to perform self-care activities, and absence of complications.

PREOPERATIVE NURSING INTERVENTIONS

REDUCING ANXIETY

The nurse must establish communication with the patient to assess his understanding of the diagnosis and of the planned surgical procedure. The nurse clarifies the nature of the surgery and expected postoperative outcomes, familiarizes the patient with the preoperative and postoperative routines, and initiates

(continued on page 1050)

TABLE **34-4** Surgical Approaches for Treatment of Prostate Disorders

Surgical Approach	Images	Advantages	Disadvantages	Nursing Implications
Transurethral resection of the prostate (TURP) is carried out through endoscopy: the surgical instrument is introduced via the urethra to the prostate, which can then be viewed directly. The gland is removed in small chips with an electrical cutting loop. This procedure may be used for glands of varying size. The procedure is ideal for patients who have small glands and poor surgical risks. Open surgical removal (for prostate cancer; uncommonly used to treat enlarged prostate)	Hypertrophied prostate being cut / Bladder	Avoids abdominal incision Safer for patients with surgical risk Shorter hospitalization and recovery periods Lower morbidity rate Causes less pain	Recurrent obstruction, urethral trauma, and stricture may develop. Delayed bleeding may occur. Retrograde ejaculation due to removal of prostatic tissue at the bladder neck, which causes the seminal fluid to flow backward into the bladder.	Monitor for TUR syndrome. Monitor for hemorrhage. Observe for symptoms of urethral stricture (dysuria, straining, weak urinary stream).
Suprapubic approach Suprapubic prostatectomy is one method of removing the gland through an abdominal incision. An incision is made into the bladder, and the prostate gland is removed from above.	Urethra / Prostate / Bladder	Technically simple Offers wide area of exploration Permits exploration for cancerous lymph nodes Allows more complete removal of obstructing gland Permits treatment of associated bladder lesions	Requires surgical approach through the bladder Difficult to control hemorrhage Urine may leak around the suprapubic tube. Recovery may be prolonged and uncomfortable.	Monitor for indications of hemorrhage and shock. Provide meticulous aseptic care to the area around suprapubic tube.
Perineal approach Perineal prostatectomy involves removal of the gland through an incision in the perineum.	Sound in urethra / Pubis / Testis / Prostate / Bladder / Rectum	Offers direct anatomic approach Permits gravity drainage of catheter Particularly effective for radical cancer therapy Allows hemostasis under direct vision Low mortality rate Low incidence of shock	Higher postoperative incidence of impotence and urinary incontinence Possible damage to rectum and external sphincter Restricted operative field	Avoid using rectal tubes or thermometers and enemas after perineal surgery. Use drainage pads to absorb excess urinary drainage. Possible urinary leakage around the wound after the catheter is removed

Procedure		Advantages	Disadvantages	Nursing considerations
Retropubic approach Retropubic prostatectomy is more common than the suprapubic approach. A low abdominal incision is made, and the prostate gland can be reached between the pubic arch and the bladder without entering the bladder.	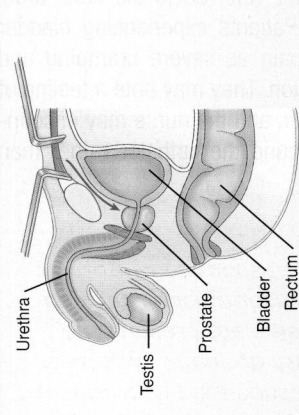	Avoids incision into the bladder Permits surgeon to see and control bleeding Shorter recovery period Less damage to the bladder sphincter	Cannot treat associated bladder disease Increased incidence of hemorrhage from prostatic venous plexus	Monitor for hemorrhage. Anticipate urinary leakage for several days after removing the catheter.
Transurethral incision of the prostate (TUIP) is indicated when the prostate gland is small (30 g or less), and it is an effective treatment for many cases of BPH. An instrument is passed through the urethra. Incisions are made in the prostate and prostate capsule to reduce the prostate's pressure on the urethra and to reduce urethral constriction.	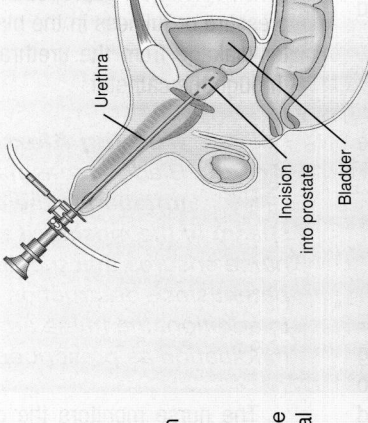	Results comparable to TURP Low incidence of erectile dysfunction and retrograde ejaculation No contracture of the bladder neck Outpatient procedure Low complication rate	Recurrent obstruction and urethral trauma Delayed bleeding	Monitor for hemorrhage.
Robotic prostatectomy (Da Vinci prostatectomy) Laparoscopic prostatectomy provides better visualization of the surgical site and surrounding areas.		Minimally invasive technique Improved patient satisfaction and quality of life Short convalescence More rapid return to normal activity Short indwelling catheter duration Decreased blood loss Improved magnification of operative field	Technically demanding skill set for surgeon Lack of tactile sensation available with open prostatectomy Inability to palpably assess for induration and palpable nodules Inability to delineate the proximity of involvement of the neurovascular bundles due to lack of palpation	Observe for symptoms of urethral stricture (dysuria, straining, weak urinary stream). Monitor for hemorrhage and shock. Provide meticulous aseptic care to the area around the suprapubic tube. Avoid using rectal tubes or thermometers and enemas after perineal surgery. Use drainage pads to absorb excess urinary drainage. Anticipate urinary leakage after the catheter is removed.

Postoperative complications depend on the type of prostatectomy performed and may include hemorrhage, clot formation, catheter obstruction, and sexual dysfunction. All prostatectomies carry a risk of impotence because of potential damage to the pudendal nerves. The anatomic changes in the posterior urethra lead to retrograde ejaculation. For the patient with resulting ED that does not resolve, options are available to produce erections sufficient for sexual intercourse: prosthetic penile implants, vacuum devices, and pharmacologic interventions.

measures to reduce anxiety. Because the patient may be sensitive and embarrassed discussing problems related to the genitalia and sexuality, the nurse provides privacy and establishes a trusting and professional relationship. The patient is encouraged to verbalize his feelings and concerns.

RELIEVING DISCOMFORT

If the patient experiences discomfort before surgery, he is prescribed bed rest, and analgesic agents are administered. If he is hospitalized, the nurse monitors his voiding patterns, watches for bladder distention, and assists with catheterization if indicated. The catheter can help decompress the bladder gradually over several days, especially if the patient is elderly and hypertensive and has diminished kidney function or urinary retention that has existed for many weeks. If the patient cannot tolerate a urinary catheter, he is prepared for a cystostomy (surgical creation of an opening into the bladder, usually with a catheter [e.g., suprapubic tube, see Chapter 28]).

PROVIDING INSTRUCTION

Before surgery, the nurse reviews with the patient the anatomy of the affected structures and their function in relation to the urinary and reproductive systems, using diagrams and other teaching aids if indicated. This instruction often takes place during the preadmission testing visit or in the urologist's office. The nurse explains what will take place as the patient is prepared for surgery (depending on the type of prostatectomy planned). The nurse also describes the type of incision, which varies with the surgery chosen, and informs the patient about the likely type of urinary drainage system and the recovery room procedure. The amount of information given is based on the patient's needs and questions.

PREPARING THE PATIENT

If the patient is scheduled for a prostatectomy, the preoperative preparation described in Chapter 5 is provided.

POSTOPERATIVE NURSING INTERVENTIONS

MAINTAINING FLUID BALANCE

During the postoperative period, the patient is at risk for imbalanced fluid volume due to irrigation of the surgical site during and after surgery. With irrigation of the urinary catheter to prevent its obstruction by blood clots, fluid may be absorbed through the open surgical site and retained, increasing the risk of excessive fluid retention, fluid imbalance, and water intoxication. The patient is observed for signs of fluid volume excess, such as jugular vein distention (JVD), the development of an S_3 gallop, and pulmonary crackles. The urine output and the amount of fluid used for irrigation must be monitored closely to determine whether irrigation fluid is being retained and to ensure adequate urine output. An intake and output record, including the amount of fluid used for irrigation, must be maintained closely. Also the patient is monitored for electrolyte imbalances

(e.g., hyponatremia), increasing blood pressure, confusion, and respiratory distress. Refer to Box 34-2 for details on dilutional hyponatremia after a transurethral prostatectomy (TURP). Additionally, since the prostate is a vascular organ, hemorrhage is an immediate danger postoperatively; thus, the nurse monitors the patient for hypotension, tachycardia, tachypnea, gross hematuria, restlessness, pallor, and decreasing levels of hemoglobin and hematocrit. If deterioration of the patient's condition occurs, the surgeon is notified immediately. The nurse anticipates fluid resuscitation with IV fluids and blood products.

> **Nursing Alert**
> *In assessing urinary output, the nurse anticipates output at a minimum 0.5 mL/kg/hr; thus, if the patient weighs 70 kg, 35 mL of urine is expected hourly. To calculate the actual urine output, the nurse must consider all irrigating fluids instilled against the total drainage of the urine collection bag. If large amounts of irrigating solutions are required postoperatively, the nurse empties the collection bag frequently to prevent overfilling and creating back pressure within the bladder. Meticulous recording of the urinary output is required.*

RELIEVING PAIN

If pain is present, the cause and location are determined, and the severity of pain and discomfort is assessed using a pain scale. The pain may be incisional, referred to the flank area, or caused by bladder spasms. Patients experiencing bladder spasms typically describe the pain as severe cramping and spasmodic in the suprapubic region. They may note a feeling of pressure or fullness in the bladder, and the nurse may encounter leakage from the urethra around the catheter rather than through the catheter.

> **Nursing Alert**
> *Bladder spasms are associated with irritation to the detrusor muscle, causing spasm of the muscle. If spasms are present, the nurse ensures that the urinary drainage system is patent since obstruction is associated with spasms. In addition, the nurse administers antispasmodic medication as prescribed.*

The nurse monitors the drainage tubing and irrigates the system as prescribed to relieve any obstruction that may cause discomfort. Usually, if clots impede urinary drainage, the catheter is irrigated with 50 to 60 mL of irrigating fluid at a time. It is important to make sure that the same amount is recovered in the drainage receptacle. Securing the catheter drainage tubing to the patient's leg or lower abdomen can help decrease tension on the catheter and prevent bladder irritation.

After the patient is ambulatory, he is encouraged to walk but not to sit for prolonged periods because this increases intra-abdominal pressure and the possibility of discomfort and bleeding.

BOX 34-2
Transurethral Resection Syndrome (Symptomatic Dilutional Hyponatremia)

Transurethral resection (TUR) syndrome is a rare (less than 2%) but potentially serious complication of transurethral prostatectomy (TURP). Signs and symptoms are caused by neurologic, cardiovascular, and electrolyte imbalances associated with absorption of the solution used to irrigate the surgical site during the surgical procedure. Hyponatremia, hypo-osmolality, and hypervolemia are dominant findings. Symptoms usually are associated with a serum sodium level of 125 mEq or less (Duke, 2016). The dilutional hyponatremia leads to cerebral edema; thus, the patient exhibits neurologic symptoms, while the volume overload is noted in symptoms of hypertension; arrhythmias; and full, bounding pulse. Patients with poor left ventricular function may develop pulmonary edema. Given the age of many men undergoing TURP and possible comorbidities of cardiac disease, the nurse is aware that fluctuating intravascular volume and myocardial compromise may result in hypotension. Additionally, if the hyponatremia develops rapidly, with the count dropping to less than 120 mEq/L, negative inotropic effects cause hypotension and electrocardiographic changes of widened QRS complexes and ventricular ectopy (Wieder, 2014).

Signs and Symptoms of TUR Syndrome

- Lethargy and confusion
- Hypertension
- Tachycardia
- Nausea and vomiting
- Visual disturbances, such as flashing lights if glycine is used as an irrigant, as it is a neurotransmitter for the retina (Duke, 2016)
- Headache
- Muscle spasms
- Seizures

Interventions

- During the operative procedure, normal saline cannot be used as it conducts electricity. If the patient displays the aforementioned signs and symptoms, the intraoperative irrigating solution of glycine, sorbitol/mannitol, or water is discontinued and replaced with normal saline.
- Administer diuretics as prescribed to facilitate excretion of absorbed fluid.
- Monitor intake and output.
- Monitor the patient's vital signs and level of consciousness.
- Differentiate the lethargy and confusion of TUR syndrome from postoperative disorientation and hyponatremia.
- Maintain patient safety during times of confusion.
- Assess lung and heart sounds for indications of pulmonary edema, heart failure, or both (fluid already present in profound hyponatremia).

MONITORING AND MANAGING POTENTIAL COMPLICATIONS

After prostatectomy, the patient is monitored for major complications, such as hemorrhage, infection, DVT, catheter obstruction, and sexual dysfunction.

Hemorrhage. The immediate dangers after a prostate surgery are bleeding and hemorrhagic shock. This risk is increased with BPH because a hyperplastic prostate gland is very vascular. Bleeding may result in the formation of clots, which then obstruct urine flow. The drainage normally begins as reddish-pink and then clears to a light pink within 24 hours after surgery. Bright red bleeding with increased viscosity and numerous clots usually indicates arterial bleeding and requires surgical intervention. Venous bleeding, which is dark red in color, may be controlled by the provider via "overinflating" the urinary catheter balloon and applying traction to the catheter so that the balloon holding the urinary catheter in place applies pressure to the prostatic fossa. If, after 20 minutes, the bleeding is not controlled, surgical exploration may be considered. Since bleeding is increased when the patient is in the sitting position, which increases bladder and venous pressure, the patient is encouraged to rest in bed with the head of the bed slightly elevated.

Nursing management includes assistance in implementing strategies to stop the bleeding and to prevent or reverse hemorrhagic shock. If hemorrhagic shock occurs, treatments described in Chapter 54 are initiated.

Nursing interventions include closely monitoring vital signs; administering medications, IV fluids, and blood component therapy as prescribed; maintaining an accurate record of intake and output; and carefully monitoring drainage to ensure adequate urine flow and patency of the drainage system.

Infection. After perineal prostatectomy, the surgeon usually changes the dressing on the first postoperative day. Careful aseptic technique is used because the potential for infection is great. Rectal thermometers, rectal tubes, and enemas are avoided because of the risk of injury and bleeding in the prostatic fossa. Sitz baths are used to promote healing.

UTIs and epididymitis (infection of the epididymis, discussed later in the chapter) are possible complications after prostatectomy, and the patient is assessed for their occurrence. Because the risk for infection continues after discharge from the hospital, the patient and family need to be instructed to monitor for signs and symptoms of infection (fever, chills, sweating, myalgia, dysuria, urinary frequency, and urgency).

Deep Vein Thrombosis. Because patients undergoing prostatectomy have a high incidence of DVT and pulmonary embolism, the provider may prescribe prophylactic low-dose heparin therapy. The nurse assesses the patient frequently after surgery for manifestations of DVT and applies elastic compression stockings as needed. Nursing and medical management of DVT and pulmonary embolism are described in Chapters 10 and 18, respectively.

Obstructed Catheter. After any procedure involving the prostate in which a catheter is placed, the catheter must drain well. An obstructed catheter produces distention of the prostatic capsule

(continued on page 1052)

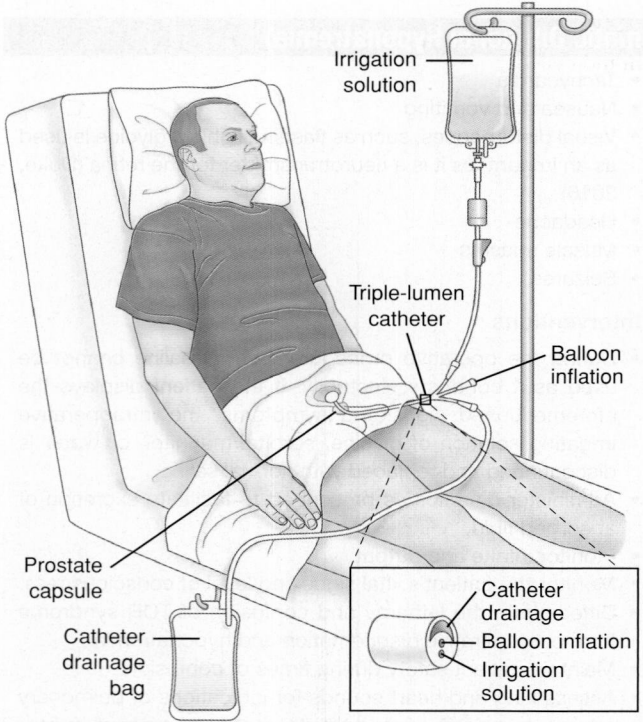

FIGURE 34-2 A three-way system for bladder irrigation.

and resultant hemorrhage. A diuretic may be prescribed to promote urination and initiate postoperative diuresis, thereby helping to keep the catheter patent. The nurse observes the lower abdomen for increasing distention to ensure that the catheter has not become blocked. On percussion of a patient with a blocked catheter, increased dullness will be noted in the suprapubic region.

The drainage bag, dressings, and incisional site are examined for bleeding. The color of the urine is noted and documented; a change in color from pink to amber indicates reduced bleeding. Blood pressure, pulse, and respirations are monitored and compared with baseline preoperative vital signs to detect hypotension. The nurse also observes the patient for restlessness, diaphoresis, pallor, any drop in blood pressure, and an increasing pulse rate.

Drainage of the bladder may be accomplished by gravity through a closed sterile drainage system. A three-way drainage system is useful in irrigating the bladder and preventing clot formation (Fig. 34-2). Continuous bladder irrigation (CBI) may be used after a TURP to maintain the drainage of the urinary catheter, remove blood clots from the bladder that are the result of the procedure, and cleanse the surgical area to promote healing as well as to prevent potentially obstructing clots. The amount of fluid recovered in the drainage bag must equal the amount of fluid infused. Overdistention of the bladder is avoided because it can induce secondary hemorrhage by stretching the coagulated blood vessels in the prostatic capsule.

To prevent traction on the bladder, the drainage tube (not the catheter) is taped to the shaved inner thigh. If a cystostomy catheter is in place, it is taped to the abdomen.

Sexual Dysfunction. The patient may experience sexual dysfunction related to ED, decreased libido, and fatigue. These issues may become a concern to the patient soon after surgery or in the weeks to months of rehabilitation. Options to restore erectile function may include medications, surgically placed implants, or vacuum devices. The patient should be aware that he may experience fatigue during rehabilitation from surgery, which may decrease his libido and alter his enjoyment of usual activities.

Nursing interventions include assessing for the presence of sexual dysfunction after surgery. Providing a private and confidential environment to discuss issues of sexuality is important. The emotional challenges of prostate surgery and its consequences need to be explored carefully with the patient and his partner.

TEACHING PATIENTS SELF-CARE

The patient undergoing prostatectomy may be discharged within several days. The length of the hospital stay depends on the type of prostatectomy performed. The patient and family require instructions about how to manage the urinary drainage system, how to assess for complications, and how to promote recovery. Verbal and written instructions should be provided, and the patient and family need to know about signs and symptoms that should be reported to the physician (e.g., blood in urine, decreased urine output, fever, change in wound drainage, calf tenderness) (Box 34-3).

After the catheter is removed (usually when the urine appears clear), urine may leak out around the wound for several days.

BOX 34-3 **Patient Education**

Self-Care After a Prostatectomy

- Perform Kegel exercises, as they may help with regaining urinary control:
  - Tense the perineal muscles by pressing the buttocks together; hold this position; relax. This exercise can be performed 10–20 times each hour while sitting or standing.
  - Try to interrupt the urinary stream after starting to void; wait a few seconds and then continue to void.
- While the prostatic fossa heals (6–8 weeks), avoid activities that produce Valsalva effects (straining, heavy lifting) as this may increase venous pressure and produce hematuria.
- Avoid long motor trips and strenuous exercise, which increase the tendency to bleed.
- Note that spicy foods, alcohol, and coffee may cause bladder discomfort.
- Maintain fluid intake to avoid dehydration, which increases the tendency for a blood clot to form and obstruct the flow of urine.
- Report signs of complications, such as bleeding, passage of blood clots, a decrease in the urinary stream, urinary retention, or symptoms of UTI, to the urologist.

Some urinary incontinence may occur after catheter removal, and the patient is informed that this is likely to subside over time.

CONTINUING CARE

Referral for home care may be indicated if the patient is elderly or has other health problems, if the patient and family cannot provide care in the home, or if the patient lives alone without available supports. The home care nurse assesses the patient's physical status and provides catheter and wound care. The home care nurse encourages the patient to ambulate and to carry out perineal exercises as prescribed. If the prostatectomy was performed to treat prostate cancer, the patient and family also are instructed about the importance of follow-up and monitoring with the urologist.

EVALUATION

Expected postoperative patient outcomes may include the following:
1. Reports relief of discomfort
2. Exhibits fluid and electrolyte balance:
   a. Irrigation fluid and urinary output are within parameters determined by surgeon
   b. Experiences no signs or symptoms of fluid retention
3. Participates in self-care measures:
   a. Increases activity and ambulation daily
   b. Produces urine output within normal ranges and consistent with intake
   c. Performs perineal exercises and interrupts urinary stream to promote bladder control
   d. Avoids straining and lifting heavy objects
4. Is free of complications:
   a. Maintains vital signs within normal limits
   b. Exhibits wound healing without signs of inflammation or hemorrhage
   c. Maintains acceptable level of urinary elimination
   d. Maintains optimal drainage of catheter and other drainage tubes
   e. Reports understanding of changes in sexual function

CONDITIONS AFFECTING THE TESTES AND ADJACENT STRUCTURES

ORCHITIS AND EPIDIDYMITIS

Orchitis is an inflammation of the testes caused by a variety of factors (bacterial, viral, spirochetal, parasitic, traumatic, chemical, or unknown). Bacterial causes usually spread from an associated epididymitis, which usually descends from an infected prostate or urinary tract. Recommended treatments include rest, elevation of the scrotum, ice packs to reduce scrotal edema, antibiotics, analgesic agents, and anti-inflammatory medications.

Pathophysiology

In men younger than 35 years of age, the major cause of epididymitis or orchitis is *Chlamydia trachomatis*. The infection passes upward through the urethra and the ejaculatory duct and then along the vas deferens to the epididymis, and it can migrate to the testis as well.

Clinical Manifestations and Assessment

The patient complains of unilateral pain and soreness in the inguinal canal along the course of the vas deferens and can develop pain and swelling in the scrotum and the groin. The epididymis becomes swollen and extremely painful. Bacteriuria may be evident, and the patient may experience chills and fever, along with nausea, urinary frequency, urgency, or dysuria. Laboratory assessment includes urinalysis and Gram stain of urethral drainage if there is suspicion of sexually transmitted infection (STI). If the epididymitis is untreated, it can progress to involve the testis.

Medical Management

Treatment of scrotal support, ice, and antibiotic therapy are anticipated on an outpatient basis. If the epididymitis is caused by a chlamydial infection, the patient and his sexual partner must be treated with antibiotics. If no improvement occurs within 2 weeks, an underlying testicular tumor should be considered. An epididymectomy (excision of the epididymis from the testis) may be performed as a last resort for patients who have recurrent, incapacitating episodes of epididymitis or for those with chronic, painful conditions.

Nursing Management

The scrotum is elevated with a scrotal bridge or folded towel to prevent traction on the spermatic cord, to promote venous drainage, and to relieve pain. A folded hand towel is secured under one thigh, allowing the penis and scrotum to be elevated on the midsection of the towel, and then the edge of the towel is secured under opposite thigh. Antimicrobial agents are administered as prescribed until the acute inflammation subsides. Intermittent cold compresses to the scrotum may help ease the pain. Later, local heat or sitz baths may help resolve the inflammation. Analgesic medications are administered for pain relief.

The nurse instructs the patient to avoid straining, lifting, and sexual activity until the infection is resolved. He should continue taking analgesic agents and antibiotics as prescribed and using ice packs if necessary to relieve discomfort. He needs to know that it may take 2 to 3 months for the epididymis to return to normal.

TESTICULAR CANCER

Testicular cancer is the most common cancer in men between 15 and 40 years of age, with the average age at diagnosis of 33 years of age, although it can occur in males of any age. It is a highly treatable and usually curable form of cancer, with a cure rate of greater than 90% for all stages of the disease; in 2015, it was expected that there would be 8,430 cases in the United States (ACS, 2015c).

Classification of Testicular Tumors

The testicles contain several types of cells, each of which may develop into one or more types of cancer. The type of cancer determines the appropriate treatment and affects the prognosis. Testicular cancers are classified as germinal, having their origins within the germ cells of the gonads (testes), or nongerminal (stromal).

Germinal Tumors

More than 90% of all cancers of the testicle are germinal and may be further classified as seminomas or nonseminomas. Seminomas are tumors that develop from the sperm-producing cells of the testes and account for 50% of tumors. Seminomas tend to remain localized, whereas nonseminomatous tumors grow quickly. Nonseminomas tend to develop earlier in life than seminomas, usually occurring in men in their 20s. Many tumors are mixtures of at least two different tumor types.

Nongerminal Tumors

Testicular cancer also may develop in the supportive and hormone-producing tissues, or stroma, of the testicles. The two main types of stromal tumors are Leydig cell tumors and Sertoli cell tumors. These tumors infrequently spread beyond the testicle.

Risk Factors

Risk factors for testicular cancer include undescended testicles (**cryptorchidism**), a family history of testicular cancer, and cancer of one testicle, which increases the risk in the other testicle. Caucasian-American men have a risk that is five times greater than that of African-American men and more than double the risk of Asian-American men (Wieder, 2014).

Clinical Manifestations and Assessment

The symptoms appear gradually, with a mass or lump on the testicle and usually painless enlargement of the testis. The patient may report heaviness in the scrotum, inguinal area, or lower abdomen. Backache (from retroperitoneal node extension), abdominal pain, weight loss, and general weakness may result from metastasis. Enlargement of the testis without pain is a significant diagnostic finding. Testicular tumors tend to metastasize early, spreading from the testis to the lymph nodes in the retroperitoneum and to the lungs. Monthly testicular self-examinations (TSEs) can detect testicular cancer, but recent recommendations argue against this practice in asymptomatic adolescent and adult males (O'Reilly et al., 2016) due to the low incidence of

finding testicular cancer via TSE and the high rate of anxiety associated with self-examination.

Human chorionic gonadotropin (hCG) and alpha-fetoprotein (AFP) are tumor markers that may be elevated. Tumor marker levels in the blood are used for diagnosis, staging, and monitoring the response to treatment. Other diagnostic tests include lactate dehydrogenase (LDH) levels and ultrasound examination to determine the presence and size of the testicular mass.

A CT of the abdomen and pelvis is performed to determine the extent of the disease in the retroperitoneum and pelvis. Also a chest x-ray is performed to assess for lung metastasis. Tissue biopsy is the only definitive way to determine whether cancer is present, and it is performed at the time of surgery rather than as a part of the diagnostic workup, to reduce the risk of promoting spread of the cancer (ACS, 2015c).

Medical Management

Testicular cancer is highly responsive to treatment, with a 5-year survival rate of 95% (National Cancer Institute, 2014). The goals of management are to eradicate the disease and achieve a cure. Treatment selection is based on the cell type and the anatomic extent of the disease. The testis is removed by orchiectomy through an inguinal incision with a high ligation of the spermatic cord. A retroperitoneal lymph node dissection (RPLND) may be performed after orchiectomy if there is evidence of lymph node metastasis. Although libido and climax are usually unimpaired after RPLND, the patient may develop ejaculatory dysfunction. Because men with testicular cancer demonstrate pretreatment subfertility, and treatment of the cancer itself can result in subfertility or infertility, cryopreservation of sperm before treatment should be offered (Yokonishi & Ogawa, 2016).

Seminomatous tumors are more sensitive to radiation therapy, and radiation therapy alone provides excellent results for the majority of patients. Postoperative irradiation of the lymph nodes from the diaphragm to the iliac region is used to treat seminomas. Radiation is delivered only to the affected side; the other testis is shielded from radiation to preserve fertility.

Chemotherapy is reserved for the treatment of stage IIC testicular cancer as well as more advanced stages (ACS, 2015c). Chemotherapy with cisplatin-based regimens results in a high percentage of complete remissions. Even with disseminated testicular cancer, the prognosis is favorable. Follow-up studies may include chest x-rays, hCG levels (a tumor marker with nonseminomatous germ cell tumors), AFP levels (a tumor marker for some men with nonseminomatous germ cell tumors), and LDH levels (an enzyme found in many body tissues, such as heart, skeletal muscle, liver, and kidney, but that also may be elevated in some men with testicular cancer), and serial CT scans to detect recurrent malignancy.

Nursing Management

Nursing management includes assessment of the patient's physical and psychological status and monitoring of the patient for response to and possible effects of surgery, chemotherapy, and radiation therapy (see Chapter 6). Operative care is described in Chapter 5. Because the patient may have difficulty coping with his condition, issues related to body image and sexuality are addressed; he also needs to know that radiation therapy will not necessarily prevent him from fathering children, and unilateral excision of a testis will not necessarily decrease virility.

Banking Sperm

Cryopreserving semen in a sperm bank is an option for men who are about to undergo a procedure or treatment (e.g., radiation therapy to the pelvis, chemotherapy, RPLND) that may affect their fertility. All men undergoing cancer treatment should be offered the opportunity for sperm cryopreservation. This requires visits to the facility, where the sperm is produced by masturbation and collected in a sterile container for storage.

HYDROCELE

A **hydrocele** is a collection of fluid, generally in the tunica vaginalis of the testis, although it also may collect within the spermatic cord. Hydrocele can be differentiated from a hernia by transillumination; the hydrocele will glow red, whereas dense tissue will not illuminate. Acute hydrocele may occur in association with acute infectious disease of the epididymis or as a result of local injury. Chronic hydrocele has no known cause.

Therapy is not required unless the hydrocele becomes tense or if the scrotal mass becomes large, uncomfortable, or embarrassing. In the surgical treatment of hydrocele, an incision is made through the wall of the scrotum down to the distended tunica vaginalis. The sac is resected and is sutured together to collapse the wall. The patient is advised to wear an athletic supporter postoperatively for comfort and support. The major complication is hematoma.

VARICOCELE

A **varicocele** is an abnormal dilation of the veins of the pampiniform venous plexus in the scrotum (the network of veins from the testis and the epididymis that constitute part of the spermatic cord) and is present in 15% to 20% of men (Fig. 34-3). Varicoceles usually occur in the veins on the upper portion of the left testicle in adults because of the angle in which the left spermatic cord inserts into the left

Dilated and tortuous veins

Epididymis

Testis

Scrotal sac

FIGURE 34-3 Varicocele.

renal vein, while the right spermatic cord enters the inferior vena cava. Varicoceles can be associated with infertility in some men. Few symptoms may be produced by the enlarged spermatic vein, and no treatment is required unless fertility is a concern or there is pain. It is corrected microsurgically by ligation of the external spermatic vein. An ice pack may be applied to the scrotum for the first few hours after surgery to relieve edema. Then the patient wears a scrotal supporter.

CONDITIONS AFFECTING THE PENIS

PHIMOSIS AND PARAPHIMOSIS

Phimosis, a condition in which the foreskin is constricted so that it cannot be retracted over the glans, can occur congenitally or as a result of inflammation and edema. If the preputial area is not cleaned, normal secretions accumulate, causing inflammation (balanitis), which can lead to adhesions and fibrosis. It is seen more commonly in adult men with poorly controlled diabetes and obesity. In elderly men, penile carcinoma may develop. Phimosis is corrected by circumcision or dorsal slit.

Paraphimosis is a condition in which the foreskin is retracted behind the glans and, because of narrowness and subsequent edema, cannot be returned to its usual position covering the glans. It is a true urologic emergency, and patients should be directed to the nearest emergency department for treatment. Initial treatment of paraphimosis involves firmly compressing the glans to reduce its size and then pushing the glans back while simultaneously moving the prepuce forward.

Nursing Alert

To catheterize an uncircumcised male, the nurse retracts the foreskin and uses soap and water to clean away the smegma (whitish sebaceous secretion that collects between the glans penis and foreskin) before beginning the sterile procedure. The glans and foreskin are rinsed thoroughly. The nurse follows institutional protocols for male catheterization. Immediately after catheterization, the foreskin is returned to its normal position to prevent an accumulation of fluid within the glans, which may cause paraphimosis (the inability to retract the foreskin to its natural position because of venous and lymphatic congestion caused by constriction by the foreskin). The provider should be notified immediately if the nurse is unable to retract the foreskin.

PRIAPISM

Priapism is a persistent erection that causes the penis to become large, hard, and painful. It results from either neural or vascular causes, including sickle cell thrombosis, leukemic cell infiltration, and tumor invasion of the penis or its vessels. It may occur with use of medications that affect the central nervous system, antihypertensive agents, antidepressant medications, and substances injected into the penis to treat ED.

Priapism is a true urologic emergency. The goal of therapy is to improve venous drainage of the corpora cavernosa to prevent ischemia, fibrosis, and impotence. The corpora may be irrigated with an anticoagulant, which allows stagnant blood to be aspirated. Shunting procedures to divert the blood from the turgid corpora cavernosa to the venous system or into the corpus spongiosum–glans penis compartment may be attempted.

CHAPTER REVIEW

Critical Thinking Exercises

1. A 58-year-old man with type 2 diabetes has undergone TURP. What immediate postoperative assessment is indicated when he arrives from the postanesthetic care unit and for the first 24 hours after surgery? What discharge teaching and preparation are indicated for this patient?

2. One of your patients, a 32-year-old man with a spinal cord injury, tells you that he has seen an advertisement on television for vardenafil HCl (Levitra). He wishes to try this to improve his erectile function. What is the appropriate teaching for this patient?

3. A 21-year-old college athlete who describes his health as excellent comes to the student health clinic because he noticed a painless walnut-size mass in his testicle when showering. What would be your concerns, and what referrals would be warranted for him? What initial laboratory work would be indicated?

NCLEX-Style Review Questions

1. A 45-year-old man complains of a painless swelling in his scrotum. The nurse assesses the patient for which condition?
   a. Prostatitis
   b. Hydronephrosis
   c. Varicocele
   d. Priapism
   e. Hypospadias

2. A 60-year-old patient is complaining of difficulty sustaining his erections. The nurse is aware that he suffered a myocardial infarction approximately 3 months ago. What teaching is relevant to his concern? Select all that apply.
   a. If he increases his physical activity, his function will improve.
   b. Function may improve as his medications are adjusted.
   c. He should avoid the strain with sexual activity.
   d. Men with a heart attack in the preceding 6 months cannot use PDE medications.
   e. His complaint is purely psychological.

3. A 55-year-old man has been diagnosed with prostate cancer. On what factors do his treatment options depend? Select all that apply.
   a. Staging of the tumor
   b. Patient preference
   c. Patient diet
   d. Patient age
   e. Size of his prostate

4. A 50-year-old man is being treated presumptively for acute prostatitis. He asks the nurse why the course of antibiotics is so long. What is the nurse's best response?
   a. His infection is resistant to most antibiotics.
   b. Most antibiotics diffuse poorly from the plasma into the prostatic fluid.
   c. Most of the antibiotic is excreted in the urine, requiring a longer course.
   d. His liver is preventing the antibiotic from working effectively.
   e. Men of his age need a prolonged antibiotic course.

5. A 58-year-old patient has had a prostatectomy. The nurse is preparing him for discharge. What information is important for the nurse to incorporate in the teaching plan?
   a. Do not interrupt the stream after starting to void.
   b. Increased activity is permitted.
   c. Limit fluid intake to prevent hypervolemia.
   d. Note that spicy foods, alcohol, and coffee may cause bladder discomfort.
   e. He should expect immediate return of his erectile function.

Try these additional resources, available at **http://thepoint.lww.com/Honan2e**, to enhance your learning and understanding of this chapter:
• NCLEX-Style Student Review Questions
• Journal Articles

REFERENCES AND SELECTED READINGS

References and selected readings associated with this chapter can be found on the website that accompanies the book. Visit **http://thepoint. lww.com/Honan2e** to access the references and other additional resources associated with this chapter.

Nursing Management: Patients with Sexually Transmitted Infections

Christa Palancia Esposito

Learning Objectives

After reading this chapter, you will be able to:

1. Differentiate between colonization, infection, and disease.
2. Compare the various types of sexually transmitted infections (STIs) and the signs, symptoms, and treatments of each.
3. Use the nursing process as a framework for care of patients with an STI.
4. Develop a teaching plan for the patient with an STI.

A sexually transmitted infection (STI), also known as a sexually transmitted disease (STD), is an infection acquired through sexual contact with an infected person. STIs are the most common infectious diseases in the United States and are epidemic in most parts of the world. To understand the pathophysiology of STIs, it is important to understand the infectious process.

THE INFECTIOUS PROCESS

An infectious disease is any disease caused by the growth of pathogenic microbes in the body. It may or may not be communicable (i.e., contagious). The nurse plays an important role in infection control and prevention. Educating patients can decrease their risk of becoming infected or decrease the sequelae of infection.

The Chain of Infection

A complete chain of events is necessary for infection to occur. The necessary elements for infection to occur are described in Box 35-1.

Colonization, Infection, and Infectious Disease

Relatively few anatomic sites are sterile (e.g., brain, blood, bone, heart, vascular system). Bacteria found throughout the body usually provide beneficial **normal flora** to compete with potential pathogens, to facilitate digestion, or to work in other ways symbiotically with the host.

Colonization

The term *colonization* is used to describe microorganisms present without host interference or interaction. Organisms reported in microbiology test results often reflect colonization rather than infection. *Colony count* represents a visual count of microbes present in a sample. In general, clinicians use a colony count of greater than 100,000/mL or 10^5 bacteria/mL to represent an infection. However, astute clinicians also will consider other local and systemic signs of infection at lower colony counts, such as fever, leukocytosis (elevated white blood cells [WBCs]), erythema (redness), purulent exudate, inflammation, warmth, and the like.

Infection

Infection indicates a host interaction with an organism. A patient colonized with *Staphylococcus aureus* may have staphylococci on the skin without any skin interruption or irritation. However, if the patient had an incision, *S. aureus* could enter the wound, be seen as foreign, and result in an immune system reaction of local inflammation and migration of WBCs to the site. Infection may be suggested based on clinical evidence of erythema, heat, and pain as well as laboratory evidence of WBCs on the wound specimen smear.

Infectious Disease

It is important to recognize the difference between infection and infectious disease. While infection merely indicates interaction between the host and the organism, **infectious disease** is the state in which the infected host displays a decline in

BOX 35-1 Chain of Infection

The chain of infection requires the following elements:
- A causative organism
- A reservoir of available organisms
- A portal or mode of exit from the reservoir
- A mode or route of transmission from reservoir to host
- A susceptible host
- A mode of entry to host

Causative Organism

The types of microorganisms that cause infections are bacteria, rickettsiae (gram-negative bacteria carried by ticks, fleas, and lice), viruses, protozoa, fungi, and helminths (parasitic worms).

Reservoir

Reservoir is the term used for any person, plant, animal, substance, or location that provides nourishment for microorganisms and enables their further dispersal.

Mode of Exit

The organism must have a mode of exit from a reservoir. An infected host must shed organisms to another or to the environment before transmission can occur. Organisms exit through the respiratory tract, the gastrointestinal tract, the genitourinary tract, the skin, or the blood.

Route of Transmission

A route of transmission is necessary and specific to each pathogen in order to connect the infectious source with its new host. Organisms may be transmitted through sexual contact, skin-to-skin contact, percutaneous injection, or through infectious particles carried in the air. A person who carries or transmits an organism but does not have apparent signs and symptoms of infection is called a *carrier*.

Susceptible Host

For infection to occur, the host must be susceptible (not possessing immunity to a particular pathogen). Previous infection or vaccine administration may render the host immune (not susceptible) to further infection with an agent. Although exposure to potentially infectious microorganisms occurs essentially on a constant basis, our elaborate immune systems generally prevent infection from occurring. A person who is immunosuppressed has much greater susceptibility to infection than does a healthy person.

Portal of Entry

A portal of entry is needed for the organism to gain access to the host. For example, airborne *Mycobacterium tuberculosis* does not cause disease when it settles on the skin of an exposed host; the only entry route for *M. tuberculosis* is through the respiratory tract.

---

wellness due to the infection. When the host interacts immunologically with an organism but remains symptom free, the definition of infectious disease has not been met. The microbiology laboratory report is the primary source of bacterial infection identification and should be viewed as a tool to be used along with clinical indicators to determine whether a patient is colonized, infected, or diseased. Microbiology reports from clinical specimens usually show three components: the smear and stain, the culture and organism identification, and the antimicrobial susceptibility (i.e., sensitivity). As a marker for the likelihood of infection, the smear and stain (referred to as *Gram stain*) generally provide the most helpful information because they describe the mix of cells present at the anatomic site at the time of specimen collection and are a guide to the choice of antibiotic pending the culture results. The Gram stain will classify organisms as either gram-positive or gram-negative. The culture will detail the exact organism(s), while the sensitivity will specify antimicrobials most likely to be effective against the organism(s).

SEXUALLY TRANSMITTED INFECTIONS

STIs are acquired through sexual contact with an infected person. Table 35-1 identifies infections that can be classified as STIs and their routes of transmission. Portals of entry of STI-causing microorganisms and sites of infection include the skin and mucosal linings of the urethra, cervix, vagina, rectum, and oropharynx.

Education about prevention of STIs includes information about risk factors and behaviors that can lead to infection. Refer to Box 35-2 for risk factors associated with STIs. The placement of a condom or protective barrier (i.e., dental dam) before any sexual contact is imperative to help prevent the acquisition or transmission of an STI. Refer to Box 35-3

TABLE **35-1** Conditions Classified as Sexually Transmitted Diseases (STDs) and Their Routes of Transmission

Disease	Route(s) of Transmission
Chlamydia	Sexual
Gonorrhea	Sexual
Herpes simplex	Sexual, percutaneous, perinatal
Human papillomavirus (HPV)	Sexual, percutaneous
Syphilis	Sexual, perinatal
Trichomoniasis	Sexual

BOX 35-2

Risk Factors for Sexually Transmitted Infections and Diseases

- Having unprotected sex
- Having multiple partners
- Being under 26 years of age
- Starting sex at an early age
- Using alcohol or illegal drugs
- Using IV drugs
- Having a history of STI
- Participating in prostitution
- Using oral contraceptives as only form of contraception

BOX 35-3

Patient Education

Use of Male Condoms

1. Put on a new condom before any kind of sex.
2. Hold the condom by the tip to squeeze out the air.

3. Unroll the condom all the way over the erect penis.

4. Have sex.
5. Hold the condom so it cannot come off the penis.
6. Pull out.
7. Use a new condom if you want to have sex again or if you want to have sex in a different place (e.g., in the anus and then in the vagina).

Keep condoms cool and dry. Never use skin lotions, baby oil, petroleum jelly, or cold cream with condoms. The oil in these products will cause the condom to break. Products made with water (such as K-Y jelly or glycerin) are safer to use.

for the application of male condom and Figure 35-1 for the application of a female condom.

Nursing Alert
Infection with one STI suggests the possibility of infection with other diseases as well. After one STI is identified, diagnostic evaluation for others should be performed.

SYPHILIS

Pathophysiology

Syphilis is an acute and chronic infectious disease caused by the spirochete *Treponema pallidum.* It is acquired primarily through sexual contact although rarely may be congenital in origin; that is, it is passed from mother to child during pregnancy or childbirth.

Risk Factors

Risk factors include having unprotected sex and being infected with other STIs. The estimated risk of transmission from an individual with primary syphilis to an uninfected individual is 30% per sexual act (Chan & Cu-uvin, 2016).

Clinical Manifestations and Assessment

In the untreated person, the course of syphilis can be divided into three stages: primary, secondary, and tertiary. These stages reflect the time from infection and the clinical manifestations observed in that period and are the basis for treatment decisions.

Primary syphilis occurs 2 to 3 weeks after initial inoculation with the organism. A painless lesion at the site of infection is called a *chancre* (Fig. 35-2). Untreated, these lesions usually resolve spontaneously within about 2 months.

Secondary syphilis occurs when the hematogenous spread of organisms from the original chancre leads to generalized infection. The rash of secondary syphilis occurs about 2 to 8 weeks after the chancre and involves the trunk and the extremities, including the palms of the hands and the soles of the feet. Transmission of the organism can occur through contact with these lesions. Generalized signs of infection may include lymphadenopathy (abnormal enlargement of lymph nodes), arthritis, meningitis (inflammation of the pia mater, arachnoid, and the subarachnoid space), hair loss, fever, malaise, and weight loss. After the secondary stage, there is a period of **latency**, when the infected person has no signs or symptoms of syphilis. Latency can be interrupted by a recurrence of secondary syphilis.

Tertiary syphilis is the final stage in the natural progression of the disease. It is estimated that between 20% and 40% of those infected do not exhibit signs and symptoms in this final stage. Tertiary syphilis has become uncommon in the era of antibiotics and presents as a slowly progressive

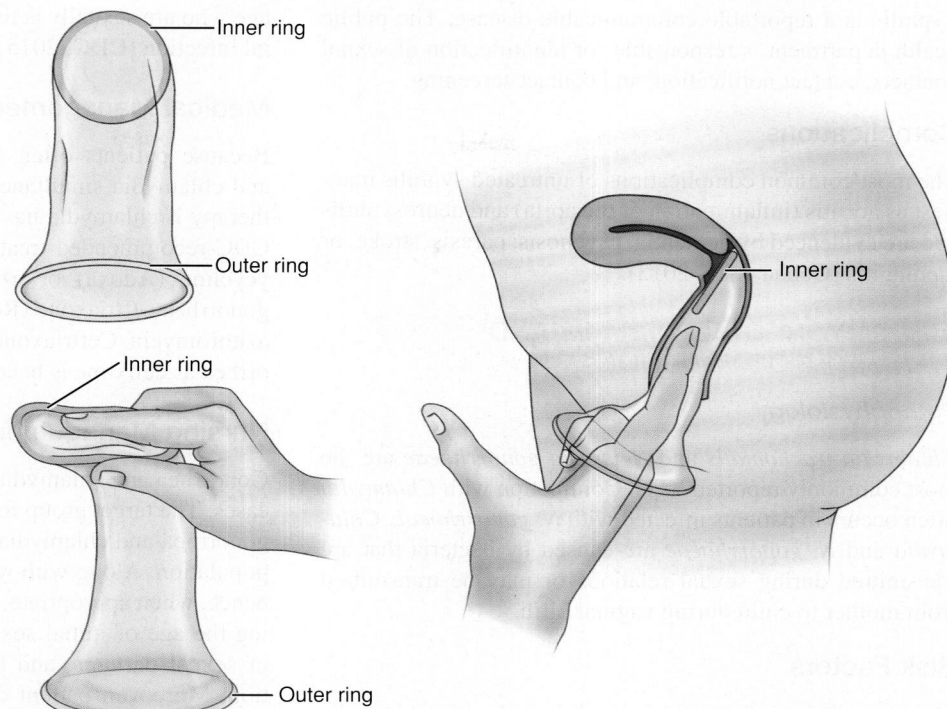

FIGURE 35-1 Female condom. To insert the female condom, hold the inner ring between the thumb and middle finger. Put the index finger on the pouch between the thumb and other fingers and squeeze the ring. Slide the condom into the vagina as far as it will go. The inner ring keeps the condom in place.

inflammatory disease with the potential to affect multiple organs (Cohen, Klausner, Engelman, & Philip, 2013).

The conclusive diagnosis of syphilis can be made by direct identification of the spirochete obtained from the chancre lesions of primary syphilis. Serologic tests used in the diagnosis of secondary and tertiary syphilis require clinical correlation in interpretation. The serologic tests are summarized as follows:

- Nontreponemal or reagin tests, such as the Venereal Disease Research Laboratory (VDRL) or the rapid plasma reagin

FIGURE 35-2 The first stage of a syphilis infection is the appearance of a chancre, a round, usually solitary, painless sore that appears on the glans penis, the shaft of the penis, or may lie within the urethra. If left untreated, it will heal; however, secondary syphilis will develop. (From Goodheart, H. (2003). *Goodheart's photoguide of common skin disorders.* Philadelphia, PA: Lippincott Williams & Wilkins.)

circle card test (RPR-CT), generally are used for screening and diagnosis. After adequate therapy, the test result is expected to decrease quantitatively until it is read as negative, usually about 2 years after therapy is completed.
- Treponemal tests, such as the fluorescent treponemal antibody absorption test (FTA-ABS) and the microhemagglutination assay test (MHA-TP), are used to verify that the screening test did not represent a false-positive result. Positive results usually are positive for life and, therefore, are not appropriate to determine therapeutic effectiveness.

Medical Management

Administration of antibiotics is the treatment of all stages of syphilis. A single dose of penicillin G benzathine intramuscular injection is the medication of choice for early syphilis or early latent syphilis of less than 1 year's duration. Patients with late latent or latent syphilis of unknown duration should receive three injections at 1-week intervals. Usually patients who are allergic to penicillin are treated with doxycycline or tetracycline (Centers for Disease Control and Prevention [CDC], 2015).

Nursing Management

Nursing interventions include administration of the prescribed antibiotics, referral for further STI testing, and education on the pathophysiology and prevention of transmission of syphilis and all STIs. The nurse advises the patient to get retested at 3 and 12 months after treatment.

Syphilis is a reportable communicable disease. The public health department is responsible for identification of sexual contacts, contact notification, and contact screening.

Complications

The most common complications of untreated syphilis manifest as aortitis (inflammation of the aorta) and neurosyphilis and are evidenced by dementia, psychosis, paresis, stroke, or meningitis (Cohen et al., 2013).

CHLAMYDIA TRACHOMATIS AND *NEISSERIA GONORRHOEAE*

Pathophysiology

Chlamydia trachomatis and *Neisseria gonorrhoeae* are the most commonly reported STIs. Coinfection with *Chlamydia* often occurs in patients infected with *N. gonorrhoeae*. *Chlamydia* and *N. gonorrhoeae* are caused by bacteria that are transmitted during sexual relations or may be transmitted from mother to child during vaginal birth.

Risk Factors

Any sexually active person can be infected with *Chlamydia* or *N. gonorrhoeae*, and the risk increases with the number of sexual partners. The group with the greatest risk for *Chlamydia* infection is young women 24 years of age and younger and may be associated with a cervix that has not matured fully (CDC, 2015). The risk for *N. gonorrhoeae* also includes sexually active young women as well as men who have sex with men.

Clinical Manifestations and Assessment

Both *Chlamydia* and *N. gonorrhoeae* infections frequently do not cause symptoms in women and thus are often referred to as "silent" related to clinical presentation. When symptoms are present, the most frequent finding is mucopurulent cervicitis with exudates in the endocervical canal. Women with gonorrhea also can present with symptoms of urinary tract infection (UTI) or vaginitis.

Although men are more likely than women to have symptoms when infected, infection with *N. gonorrhoeae* and/or *Chlamydia* also can be asymptomatic. When symptoms are present in male patients, the symptoms may include burning during urination and penile discharge. Patients with *N. gonorrhoeae* infection also may report painful swollen testicles.

Assessment includes noting fever, discharge (urethral, vaginal, penis, or rectal), and signs of arthritis. Diagnostic methods available include urine testing or swab specimens of the endocervix, urethra, anal canal, and pharynx. **Nucleic acid amplification tests (NAAT)** are most sensitive for the detection of chlamydia. The Gram stain best identifies gonorrhea from the male urethra.

Because many chlamydial infections are asymptomatic, the CDC recommends all women younger than 25 years of age who are sexually active be tested routinely for chlamydial infection (CDC, 2015).

Medical Management

Because patients often are infected with both gonorrhea and chlamydia simultaneously, the CDC recommends dual therapy if chlamydia has not been ruled out by NAAT. The CDC-recommended treatment for chlamydia is either doxycycline (Adoxa) or azithromycin (Zithromax), and for gonorrhea ceftriaxone (Rocephin) or cefixime (Suprax) plus azithromycin. Ceftriaxone is the preferred treatment for gonorrhea as cefixime is becoming less effective (CDC, 2015).

Nursing Management

Gonorrhea and chlamydia are reportable communicable diseases. The target group for preventive patient teaching about gonorrhea and chlamydia is the adolescent and young adult population. Along with reinforcing the importance of abstinence, when appropriate, education should address postponing the age of initial sexual exposure, limiting the number of sexual partners, and use of condoms or barrier protection. Moreover, patient counseling includes abstinence for 1 week after treatment in addition to the completion of the partner's treatment. Test of cure is not recommended unless medication compliance is in question; however, the retesting of females 3 months' posttreatment is recommended due to the possibility of reinfection. Education for males includes that they must inform their female partners of infection, and they must provide literature on STIs and the risk of **pelvic inflammatory disease** (PID) to them.

Complications

In women, PID, **ectopic pregnancy**, endometritis, and infertility are possible complications of either *N. gonorrhoeae* or *Chlamydia* infection. Figure 35-3 demonstrates how microorganisms spread in pelvic infection.

In men, epididymitis, a painful disease that may lead to infertility, may result from infection with either bacterium. In people of either gender, *N. gonorrhoeae* may cause arthritis or bloodstream infection.

HUMAN PAPILLOMAVIRUS

Human papillomavirus (HPV) infection is the most common STI among young, sexually active people. Millions of Americans are infected with HPV, many unaware they carry the virus. Most sexually active men and women acquire genital HPV infection at some point in their lives (CDC, 2015).

Pathophysiology

The virus affects the skin and mucous membranes through sexual contact (i.e., naked rubbing and vaginal/anal intercourse). At least 40 HPV types can infect the genitalia and

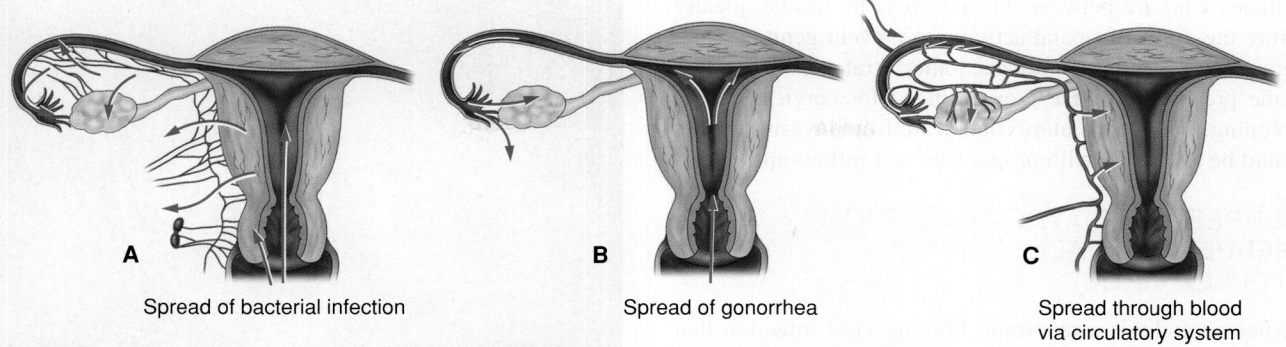

A	B	C
Spread of bacterial infection	Spread of gonorrhea	Spread through blood via circulatory system

FIGURE 35-3 Pathway by which microorganisms spread in pelvic infections. (**A**) Bacterial infection spreads up the vagina, into the uterus, and through the lymphatics. (**B**) Gonorrhea spreads up the vagina, into the uterus, and then to the tubes and ovaries. (**C**) Bacterial infection can reach the reproductive organs through the bloodstream (hematogenous spread).

perineum, including the skin of the penis, vulva, and anus as well as the linings of the vagina, cervix, and rectum. Certain types of HPV can cause the cells of the cervix to become abnormal, contributing to approximately 70% of cervical cancer cases (refer to Chapter 33 for additional details). Other strains of HPV cause genital warts. The virus can be present in the body for a long period of time before detection or symptoms occur (CDC, 2015). Psychologically, the diagnosis of HPV on a pap can be upsetting to patients. This is particularly stressful and difficult to understand for some women after testing negative for years. Explaining the latency of viruses can facilitate understanding. Often HPV is self-limiting due to an effective immune system response; however, smoking has been associated with increased morbidity. Persistent HPV can lead to cervical cancer but with proper management and patient compliance morbidity and mortality are easily minimized. Therefore, best practice pap follow-up is patient specific. Newer guidelines assist providers on making the determination whether to pap yearly or up to every 3 to 5 years depending on risk factors, history, and age.

Risk Factors

Risk factors include being sexually active, having multiple sex partners, and having sex with a partner who has or has had multiple partners.

Clinical Manifestations and Assessment

More than 100 strains of HPV exist, and infection can be latent (asymptomatic and detected only by DNA hybridization tests for HPV), subclinical (visualized only after application of acetic acid followed by inspection under magnification), or clinical (visible warts).

The most common strains of HPV, 6 and 11, usually cause **condylomata** (genital warts) on the female and male genitalia and can be found in the mouth. Often these lesions are visible, flesh-colored, flat, verrucous, or papillary.

Some HPV strains (16, 18, 31, 33, and 45) affect the cervix, resulting in abnormal Papanicolaou (Pap) smears and are strongly associated with cervical cancer (CDC, 2015). Thus, the Pap smear is the detection vehicle identifying HPV DNA. **Colposcopy**-derived biopsies diagnose any cellular changes or dysplasia (changes in cervical cells).

Medical and Nursing Management

Treatment of external genital warts includes topical application of trichloroacetic acid, podophyllin (Podofin), and chemotherapeutic agents as well as injections of interferon administered by a health care provider. Topical agents that can be applied by patients to external lesions include podofilox (Condylox) and imiquimod (Aldara). Electrocautery and laser therapy are alternative therapies that may be indicated for patients with a large number or area of genital warts (CDC, 2015).

Women with HPV should have annual Pap smears because of the potential of HPV to cause dysplasia. Use of condoms can reduce the likelihood of transmission, but transmission also can occur during skin-to-skin contact in areas not covered by condoms.

In many cases, patients are angry about having warts or HPV and do not know who infected them because the incubation period can be long and partners may have no symptoms. Acknowledging the emotional distress that occurs when an STI is diagnosed and providing support and facts are important nursing actions. Likewise, patient education about the likelihood of recurrence in the first 3 months after treatment is encouraged.

Complications

Preventatively, vaccination is recommended for girls and women who are between 11 and 26 years of age, before the onset of sexual activity, against four strains of HPV that account for up to 70% of cervical cancer (CDC, 2015). Also the quadrivalent HPV vaccine should be administered to males who are between 11 and 26 years of age, ideally before the onset of sexual activity, to prevent genital warts. Immunization will not replace other strategies important in the prevention of HPV or the need for cervical cancer screening. Loss of the uterus and death from invasive cancer should be avoidable with proper care and follow-up.

HERPES VIRUS TYPE 2 INFECTION (HERPES GENITALIS, HERPES SIMPLEX VIRUS)

Herpes genitalis is a recurrent, lifelong viral infection that causes herpetic lesions (blisters) on the vulva, vagina, and cervix in females and the penis in males. There are two types of herpes simplex virus (HSV): HSV-1 and HSV-2, which are clinically indistinguishable.

Pathophysiology

HSV-1 is known as the oral type and can be transmitted to the genitalia by oral sex or self-inoculation (i.e., touching a cold sore and then touching the genital area). HSV-2 is always transmitted sexually. Usually the initial infection is very painful and lasts about 1 week, but it also can be asymptomatic. Most HSV infections occur via asymptomatic transmission when neither the carrier nor the recipient manifests lesions (Bernstein et al., 2013).

Recurrences are more common with HSV-2 than HSV-1, are less painful, and usually produce minor itching and burning. Some patients have few or no recurrences, whereas others have frequent bouts. Often recurrences are associated with stress, sunburn, dental work, or inadequate rest or nutrition—all situations that may tax the immune system. When viral replication diminishes, the virus ascends the peripheral sensory nerves and remains inactive in the nerve ganglia. Similar to HPV, HSV can lay dormant without symptoms. Often, HSV is diagnosed through serology testing during STI screening. For many, the diagnosis of HSV comes with emotional distress and sigma necessitating emotional support and reassurance.

Risk Factors

Risk factors include contact with an infected person by the mouth, oropharynx, mucosal surface, vagina, or cervix.

Clinical Manifestations and Assessment

Itching and pain accompany the process as the infected area becomes red and edematous. Primary infection may begin with macules (small flat spots on skin) and papules (small circumscribed elevations) and progress to vesicles (small, serous-filled elevated spots) and ulcers. The vesicular state often appears as a blister, which later coalesces, ulcerates, and encrusts (Fig. 35-4). Influenza-like symptoms may occur 3 or 4 days after the lesions appear. Often inguinal lymphadenopathy (enlarged lymph nodes in the groin),

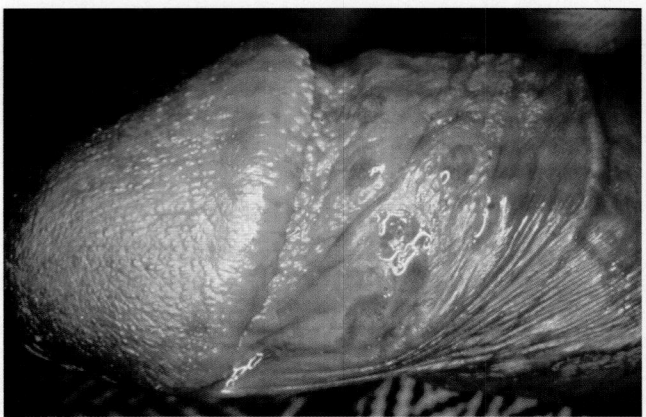

FIGURE 35-4 Herpes simplex may manifest as a painful open ulcer or cluster of superficial vesicles (fluid-filled) with an erythematous base. (From Goodheart, H. (2003). *Goodheart's photoguide of common skin disorders*. Philadelphia, PA: Lippincott Williams & Wilkins.)

minor temperature elevation, malaise, headache, myalgia (aching muscles), and dysuria (pain on urination) are noted. Pain is evident during the first week and then decreases. The lesions subside in about 2 weeks unless secondary infection occurs.

The gold standard for HSV diagnosis is a culture of the lesion. Serology may help determine new versus chronic infection when obtained concurrently with positive culture of a lesion.

Medical Management

There is currently no cure for HSV-2 infection, but treatment is aimed at relieving the symptoms. Antiviral dosing varies, depending on primary, recurrent, or suppressive management. Management goals include preventing the spread of infection, making patients comfortable, decreasing potential health risks, and initiating a counseling and education program. The antiviral agents acyclovir (Zovirax), valacyclovir (Valtrex), and famciclovir (Famvir) are recommended to suppress the viral load and decrease recurrence and shedding (CDC, 2015).

Nursing Management

Patient education is paramount in preventing the transmission of HSV. Counseling regarding suppressive therapy should be offered at the initial diagnosis and has been shown to decrease the risk of recurrence by 70 to 80% (Markle, Conti, & Kad, 2013). The nurse informs patients of their potential to transmit the virus without symptoms or lesions. In addition, patients have a potentially legal and moral obligation to disclose their diagnosis to sexual partners. Moreover, the importance of barrier methods to prevent the transmission is imperative. Often emotional support is needed for the patient who is diagnosed with HSV (CDC, 2015), since herpes can be present without symptoms for years.

Concept Mastery Alert

HSV can be transmitted whether lesions are present or not. A client's consistent use of condoms with sexual activity would be a measure to reduce the risk of transmission and recurrences.

Complications

Rarely, complications may arise from extragenital spread of HSV, such as to the buttocks, upper thighs, or even the eyes as a result of touching lesions and then touching other areas. Patients should be advised to wash their hands after contact with lesions. Other potential problems are aseptic meningitis, neonatal transmission, and severe emotional stress related to the diagnosis.

FEMALE REPRODUCTIVE INFECTIONS ASSOCIATED WITH SEXUAL ACTIVITY

PELVIC INFLAMMATORY DISEASE

PID is an inflammatory condition of the pelvic cavity that may begin with cervicitis (inflammation of the uterine cervix) and may involve the uterus (endometritis), fallopian tubes (salpingitis), ovaries (oophoritis), pelvic peritoneum, or pelvic vascular system. Infection may be acute, subacute, recurrent, or chronic and localized or widespread, and infection usually is caused by bacteria but may be attributed to a virus, fungus, or parasite. Gonorrheal and chlamydial organisms are the most likely causes.

Pathophysiology

PID arises from a polymicrobial infection that ascends upward from the vagina and into the uterus, fallopian tubes, and peritoneal cavity. In bacterial infections that occur after childbirth or abortion, pathogens are disseminated directly through the tissues that support the uterus by way of the lymphatics and blood vessels.

In gonorrheal infections, the gonococci pass through the cervical canal and into the uterus, where the environment, especially during menstruation, allows them to multiply rapidly and spread to the fallopian tubes and into the pelvis (see Fig. 35-3B). Usually the infection is bilateral.

Pelvic infection is caused most commonly by sexual transmission but also can occur with invasive procedures, such as endometrial biopsy, surgical abortion, hysteroscopy, or insertion of an intrauterine device (IUD). Bacterial vaginosis (BV), a vaginal infection, may predispose women to pelvic infection.

Figures 35-3 and 35-5 illustrate the path that organisms can travel from the vagina to the sterile peritoneum, resulting in peritonitis (inflammation of the peritoneum).

Risk Factors

Risk factors for PID include early age at first intercourse, multiple sexual partners, frequent intercourse, intercourse

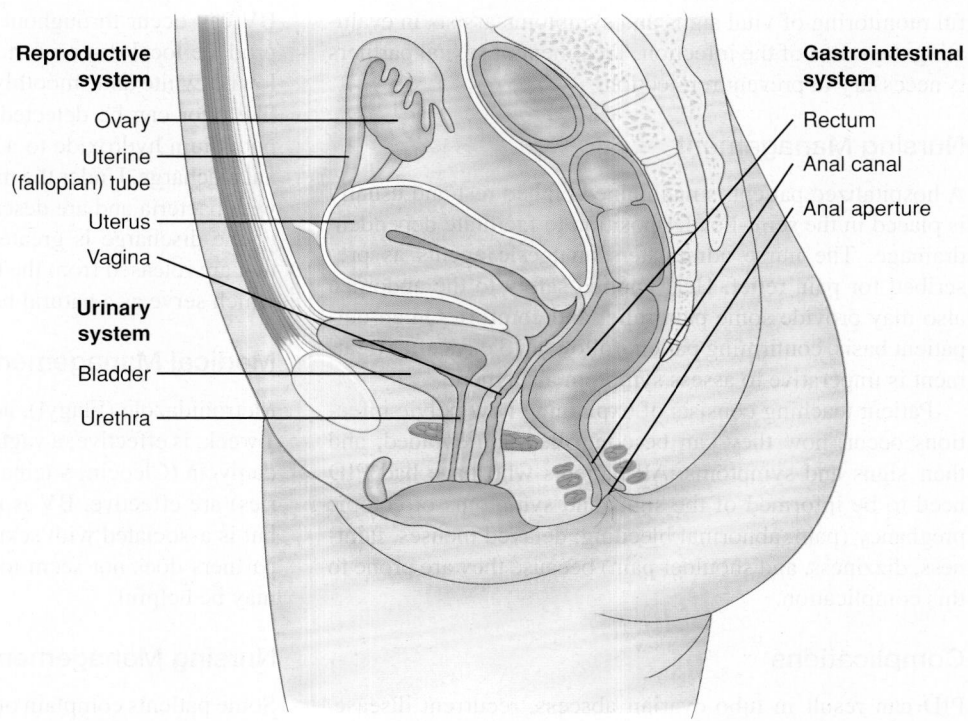

Reproductive system
- Ovary
- Uterine (fallopian) tube
- Uterus
- Vagina

Urinary system
- Bladder
- Urethra

Gastrointestinal system
- Rectum
- Anal canal
- Anal aperture

FIGURE 35-5 Female anatomy. Note the relationship of the reproductive organs to the pelvic peritoneum.

without condoms, intercourse with a partner with an STI, and a history of STIs or previous pelvic infection (CDC, 2015).

Clinical Manifestations and Assessment

Symptoms of pelvic infection usually begin with vaginal discharge, **dyspareunia** (painful sexual intercourse), lower abdominal pelvic pain, and tenderness that occurs after menses. Pain may increase with voiding or with defecation. The minimal criteria for diagnosis and treatment include one, or more, of the following:

• Uterine tenderness,
• Adnexal tenderness (adnexa are the "appendages" of the uterus, namely the ovaries, fallopian tubes, and ligaments that hold the uterus in place), and
• Cervical motion tenderness.

Other symptoms include fever, general malaise, anorexia, nausea, headache, and, possibly, vomiting (CDC, 2015).

Medical Management

Women with mild infections may be treated as outpatients with ceftriaxone IM and doxycycline with or without metronidazole, but hospitalization may be necessary if a patient is nonresponsive to medication, if a surgical emergency (e.g., appendicitis) or abscess formation is suspected, or if the patient is pregnant and salpingitis (inflammation of the fallopian tubes) is suspected (CDC, 2015; Swygard & Cohen, 2016). Intensive therapy includes bed rest, IV fluids, and IV antibiotic therapy. If the patient has abdominal distention or **ileus**, nasogastric intubation and suction are initiated. Careful monitoring of vital signs and symptoms assists in evaluating the status of the infection. Treatment of sexual partners is necessary to prevent reinfection.

Nursing Management

A hospitalized patient is maintained on bed rest and usually is placed in the semi-Fowler position to facilitate dependent drainage. The nurse administers analgesic agents as prescribed for pain relief. Heat applied safely to the abdomen also may provide some pain relief and comfort. On an outpatient basis, confirming patient follow-up 3 days after treatment is imperative to assess symptom abatement.

Patient teaching consists of explaining how pelvic infections occur, how they can be controlled and avoided, and their signs and symptoms. All patients who have had PID need to be informed of the signs and symptoms of ectopic pregnancy (pain, abnormal bleeding, delayed menses, faintness, dizziness, and shoulder pain) because they are prone to this complication.

Complications

PID can result in tubo-ovarian abscess, recurrent disease, pelvic or generalized peritonitis, strictures, fallopian tube obstruction, ectopic pregnancy, and infertility. Adhesions are common and often result in chronic pelvic pain. Other complications include bacteremia with septic shock and thrombophlebitis with possible embolization.

BACTERIAL VAGINOSIS (BV)

The vagina is protected against infection by its normally low pH (3.5 to 4.5), which is maintained in part by *Lactobacillus acidophilus*, the dominant bacteria in a healthy vaginal ecosystem. These bacteria suppress the growth of anaerobes and produce lactic acid, maintaining normal pH. Factors that may initiate or predispose a patient to infections include contact with an infected partner and wearing tight, nonabsorbent, and heat- and moisture-retaining clothing. BV and trichomoniasis are two vulvovaginal infections that are sexually associated.

Pathophysiology

BV is caused by an overgrowth of anaerobic bacteria and *Gardnerella vaginalis* normally found in the vagina and an absence of **lactobacilli**. It is characterized by a fish-like odor that is particularly noticeable after sexual intercourse or during menstruation as a result of an increase in vaginal pH. Usually it is accompanied by a heavier-than-normal discharge.

Risk Factors

Douching after menses, smoking, multiple sex partners, other STIs, and increased sexual activity are risk factors for BV.

Clinical Manifestations and Assessment

BV can occur throughout the menstrual cycle and does not produce local discomfort or pain. Discharge is gray to yellowish white and smoothly coats the vaginal walls. The fish-like odor can be detected before or after adding a drop of potassium hydroxide to a glass slide with a sample of vaginal discharge. Under the microscope, vaginal cells are coated with bacteria and are described as *clue cells*. Usually the pH of the discharge is greater than 4.7 because of the amines that are released from the bacterial overgrowth. Lactobacilli, which serve as a natural host defense, are usually absent.

Medical Management

Metronidazole (Flagyl), administered orally twice a day for 1 week, is effective; a vaginal gel is also available. Also Clindamycin (Cleocin) vaginal cream or ovules (oval suppositories) are effective. BV is not considered an STI exclusively but is associated with sexual activity. Treatment of patients' partners does not seem to be effective, but use of condoms may be helpful.

Nursing Management

Some patients complain of an unpleasant but transient metallic taste when taking metronidazole.

Clindamycin creams are oil-based and will decrease the efficacy of latex condoms. The nurse teaches proper perineal hygiene for prevention (CDC, 2015).

Nursing Alert
Patients taking metronidazole (Flagyl) must be instructed to avoid alcohol during and for 24 hours after treatment to prevent significant gastrointestinal upset (disulfiram-like reaction).

Complications

BV is not considered a serious condition; however, it has been associated with premature labor, endometritis, PID, and recurrent UTI (CDC, 2015).

TRICHOMONIASIS

Pathophysiology

Trichomonas vaginalis (aka "trich") is a flagellated protozoan that causes a common sexually transmitted vaginitis. It may be transmitted by an asymptomatic carrier who harbors the organism in the urogenital tract.

Clinical Manifestations and Assessment

Clinical manifestations include a vaginal discharge that is thin (sometimes frothy), yellow to yellow-green, malodorous, and very irritating. An accompanying vulvitis may result, with vulvovaginal burning and itching. Trich often causes urethritis in men. Diagnosis is made most accurately with NAAT, detecting three to five times more infections than wet mount microscopic analysis (CDC, 2015). Inspection with a speculum often reveals vaginal and cervical erythema (redness) with multiple small petechiae ("strawberry spots"). Testing of a trichomonal discharge demonstrates a pH greater than 4.5.

Medical and Nursing Management

The most effective treatment for trichomoniasis is metronidazole or tinidazole. Both partners receive a one-time loading dose. Test of cure is not needed unless symptoms recur.

Nursing education on abstaining from sexual activity until both partners are treated is imperative.

MALE REPRODUCTIVE INFECTIONS ASSOCIATED WITH SEXUAL ACTIVITY

Several infections affect the male genitourinary tract, including prostatitis (see Chapter 34), epididymitis, and orchitis, often caused by STIs.

Epididymitis usually descends from an infected prostate or urinary tract. The infection passes upward through the urethra, ejaculatory duct, and vas deferens to the epididymis and commonly develops from STIs, such as gonorrhea and

chlamydia. In younger men, the major cause of epididymitis is *C. trachomatis* (Stewart, Ubee, & Davies, 2011).

Orchitis is an inflammation of the testes (testicular congestion) that can be caused by a number of factors: bacterial, viral, spirochetal, parasitic, traumatic, chemical, or unknown. Bacterial causes usually spread from an associated epididymitis in men who are sexually active. Causative organisms include *N. gonorrhoeae, C. trachomatis, Escherichia coli, Klebsiella, Pseudomonas aeruginosa, Staphylococcus* species, and *Streptococcus* species. Additionally, a more common cause of isolated orchitis is mumps. When postpubertal men contract mumps, about one in five develop some form of orchitis 4 to 7 days after the jaw and neck swell, and the testes may show some atrophy. Therefore mumps vaccination is recommended for postpubertal men who have not had mumps or previous mumps vaccination in childhood. Further details related to epididymitis and orchitis may be found in Chapter 34.

NURSING PROCESS
The Patient with a Sexually Transmitted Infection

ASSESSMENT

During the physical examination, the examiner looks for rashes, lesions, drainage, discharge, or swelling. Inguinal nodes are palpated to elicit tenderness and to assess swelling (Fig. 35-6). Women are examined for abdominal or uterine tenderness.

DIAGNOSIS

Appropriate nursing diagnoses of the patient with an STI may include:

• Deficient knowledge about the disease and risk for spread of infection and reinfection

(continued on page 1068)

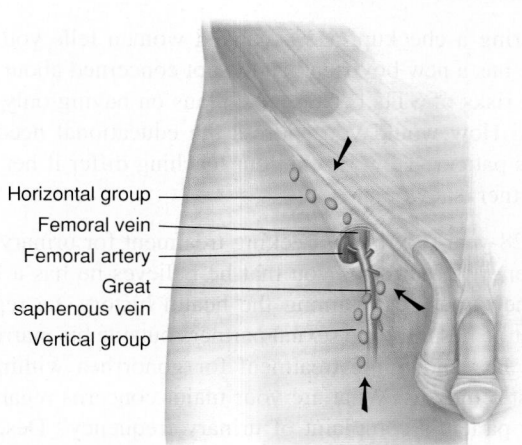

FIGURE 35-6 Superficial inguinal lymph nodes. (Courtesy of Bickley, L. (2013). *Bates' pocket guide to physical examination and history taking*. Philadelphia, PA: Lippincott Wolters Kluwer.)

- Anxiety related to anticipated stigmatization and to prognosis and complications
- Ineffective health maintenance related to high-risk sexual behaviors
- Risk for infection transmission related to lack of measures for STI prevention
- Risk of infection transmission from mother to child during delivery

PLANNING AND GOALS

Major goals are increased patient understanding of the natural history and treatment of the infection, reduced anxiety, increased compliance with therapeutic and preventive goals, and absence of complications.

NURSING INTERVENTIONS

INCREASING KNOWLEDGE AND PREVENTING SPREAD OF DISEASE

Often education about STIs and prevention of the spread to others are accomplished simultaneously. Explanation includes covering the causative organism, the usual course of the infection (including the interval of potential communicability to others), and possible complications. The nurse stresses the importance of following therapy as prescribed and the need to report any side effects or progression of symptoms. The nurse emphasizes that the same behaviors that led to infection with one STI increase the risk for any other STI. Methods used to contact sexual partners should be discussed. The patient should understand that until the partner has been treated, continued sexual exposure to the same person may lead to reinfection. The nurse discusses the relative value of condoms in reducing the risk for infection with STIs.

REDUCING ANXIETY

When appropriate, the nurse encourages the patient to discuss anxieties and fear associated with the diagnosis, treatment, or prognosis. Patients may need help in planning discussion with partners. If the patient is especially apprehensive about this aspect, referral to a social worker or other specialist may be appropriate.

INCREASING COMPLIANCE

In group settings or in a one-to-one setting, open discussion about STI information facilitates patient teaching. Discomfort can be reduced by factual explanation of causes, consequences, treatments, and prevention. Patients can obtain more information by accessing the CDC website (see Resources at the end of the chapter).

EVALUATION

Expected patient outcomes may include the following:
1. Understands infection and treatment:
   a. Verbalizes understanding of infectious process
   b. Demonstrates compliance with medications, barriers, and behaviors
2. Absence of complications, such as ectopic pregnancy, infertility, neurosyphilis, gonococcal meningitis/arthritis, and prostatitis

CHAPTER REVIEW

Critical Thinking Exercises

1. During a checkup, a 23-year-old woman tells you that she has a new boyfriend and is not concerned about sexual risks of STIs because she plans on having only oral sex. How would you address the educational needs of this patient? How would your teaching differ if her new partner is a woman?

2. A 28-year-old man is seeking treatment for urinary frequency. He informs you that he believes he has a UTI. When you are obtaining the health history, he reports that he has multiple sexual partners outside his marriage. He has undergone treatment for gonorrhea within the past 6 months. What are your major concerns regarding the patient's complaint of urinary frequency? Describe important aspects that must be addressed when teaching this patient about safer sex. What community resources should you make available to this patient and his wife?

NCLEX-Style Review Questions

1. A 22-year-old woman presents requesting STI testing after a recent encounter ended with a broken condom. She has cervical cultures but declined having blood work done. Which positive test result would lead the nurse to counsel the patient to seek further blood work related to screening for STIs?
   a. Candida yeast
   b. Group B *Streptococcus*
   c. Trichomoniasis
   d. Gardnerella

2. A 16-year-old girl presents with recurrent painful vulvar lesions. The nurse obtains subsequent test results from her pelvic evaluation and confirms the identification of HSV-2. What counseling is most appropriate for this patient?
   a. HSV-2 is self-limiting and will go away again on its own, no medication needed.

   b. HSV-2 can be transmitted and acquired without obvious symptoms or sores.

   c. A blood test can determine if this is a new infection or subsequent outbreak.

   d. Stress caused the sores; exercise and stress management will prevent them.

3. A 29-year-old woman presents with pelvic pain, fever, and irregular bleeding. She has been trying to get pregnant and fears she is having a miscarriage. Upon examination, the woman yells when her uterus is palpated bimanually and almost jumps off the table with cervical motion tenderness. The pregnancy test is negative. What nursing intervention is most appropriate for this patient?

   a. Administer the antibiotics as prescribed for PID.

   b. Reassure her she is not pregnant.

   c. Refer her to a fertility specialist.

   d. Counsel her on the signs of ectopic pregnancy.

4. A 26-year-old woman recently had a colposcopy that detected cervical dysplasia and HPV types 16 and 18, necessitating the removal of part of her cervix. The patient returns for her postoperative follow-up appointment saying, "I'm glad the cancer thing is over and I don't have to come back again for a long time." Which nursing response is most appropriate?

   a. "You are fortunate the cancer was caught early and you healed fast."

   b. "You still need to return for frequent Pap smears to monitor your cervix."

   c. "Good for you, not smoking helps keep the HPV away for good."

   d. "There will be a problem getting pregnant now after your surgery."

5. A 24-year-old man complains about an ulcer on the shaft of his penis along with complaints of fever and enlarged nodes in the inguinal region. He is diagnosed with syphilis and discharged after receiving one dose of penicillin IM. Which comment made by the patient would alert the nurse of the need to review the management plan with this patient?

   a. I am aware that all my sexual partners will need to be treated.

   b. I know that my blood work (VDRL or RPR titer) may take 12 months to become negative.

   c. This disease cannot be cured, and I will likely develop complications.

   d. I am aware that I must wear a condom every time I have sex.

Try these additional resources, available at **http://thepoint.lww.com/Honan2e,** to enhance your learning and understanding of this chapter:

- NCLEX-Style Student Review Questions
- Journal Articles

REFERENCES AND SELECTED READINGS

References and selected readings associated with this chapter can be found on the website that accompanies the book. Visit **http://thepoint. lww.com/Honan2e** to access the references and other additional resources associated with this chapter.

Problems Related to Immunologic Function

A 45-year-old patient with a history of leukemia has been diagnosed with secondary gout. She is complaining of pain in the wrist and fingers. She recently had a surgical procedure done and believes this is the cause of her current attack.

- What medications would the nurse expect the health care provider to order for this patient?
- Discuss the two phases of medical management.
- What are important components of nursing management for this patient?
- List two possible nursing diagnoses for this patient.

Nursing Assessment: Immune Function

Mary E. Bartlett

Learning Objectives

After reading this chapter, you will be able to:

1. Discuss the body's general immune response.
2. Discuss the stages of the immune response.
3. Differentiate between humoral and cellular immune responses.
4. Complete an assessment on the function of the immune system.

The most basic abilities of the human body to protect itself from disease and illness derive from the various components of the immune system. The term *immunity* refers to the body's specific protective response to an invading foreign agent or organism. The immune system functions as the body's defense mechanism against invasion and allows a rapid response to foreign substances in a specific manner. Responses occur at the genetic and cellular levels.

Immune function is affected by a variety of factors, such as central nervous system integrity, emotional status, medications, and the stress of illness, trauma, or surgery. Dysfunctions involving the immune system occur across the lifespan. When the functions of the immune system are diminished or disturbed, autoimmune and other disorders may develop. Disorders of the immune system may stem from excesses or deficiencies of immunocompetent cells, alterations in the function of these cells, immunologic attack on self-antigens, or inappropriate or exaggerated responses to specific antigens (Table 36-1).

ANATOMIC AND PHYSIOLOGIC OVERVIEW

One of the most effective defense mechanisms is the body's capacity to equip itself rapidly with weapons (antibodies) individually designed to meet each new invader (antigens). Antibodies react with antigens by:

- Coating antigens' surfaces
- Neutralizing the antigens if they are toxins
- Precipitating the antigens out of solution if they are dissolved

Although this system is normally protective, in some cases, the body produces inappropriate or exaggerated responses to specific antigens, and the result is an allergic or hypersensitivity reaction. Before looking at immunity and immune response more closely, it is helpful to understand the basic components of the immune system.

Anatomy of the Immune System

The immune system is composed of an integrated collection of various cell types, each with a designated functional role in defending against infection and invasion by other organisms. Supporting this system are molecules that are responsible for the interactions, modulations, and regulation of the system. These molecules and cells participate in specific interactions with immunogenic **epitopes** or antigenic determinants, which are substances that, when introduced into the body, stimulate the production of an antibody. These epitopes are present on foreign materials and initiate a series of actions in a host, including the inflammatory response, the lysis of microbial agents, and the disposal of foreign toxins. The major components of the immune system include the bone marrow, the white blood cells (WBCs), the lymphoid tissues (including the thymus gland, the spleen, the lymph nodes, and the tonsils and adenoids), and similar tissues in the gastrointestinal (GI), respiratory, and reproductive systems (Fig. 36-1).

Stem cells (undifferentiated cells) in the bone marrow generate lymphocytes (a type of WBC) (Fig. 36-2). There are two types of lymphocytes: **B lymphocytes (B cells)**, which mature in the bone marrow and enter the circulation as precursors to antibody-secreting cells or memory cells, and **T lymphocytes (T cells)**, which move from the bone

TABLE 36-1 Immune System Disorders

Disorder	Description
Autoimmunity	Normal protective immune response paradoxically turns against or attacks the body, leading to tissue damage
Hypersensitivity	Body produces inappropriate or exaggerated responses to specific antigens
Gammopathies	Immunoglobulins are overproduced
Immune Deficiencies	
Primary	Deficiency results from improper development of immune cells or tissues; usually congenital or inherited
Secondary	Deficiency results from some interference with an already developed immune system; usually acquired later in life

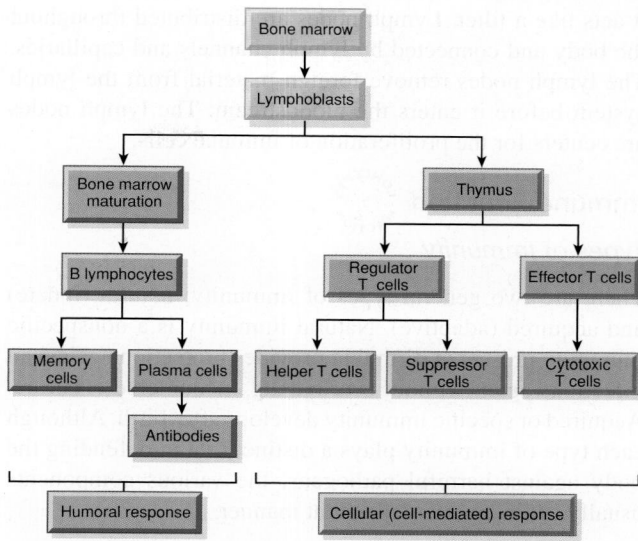

FIGURE 36-2 Development of cells of the immune system.

marrow to the thymus, where they mature into several kinds of cells with different helper functions (Fig. 36-3).

The thymus is a double-lobed organ found in the upper mediastinum. The spleen is located in the left upper quadrant of the abdomen. It is composed of red pulp (where old and injured red blood cells [RBCs] are destroyed) and white pulp (which contains concentrations of lymphocytes), and

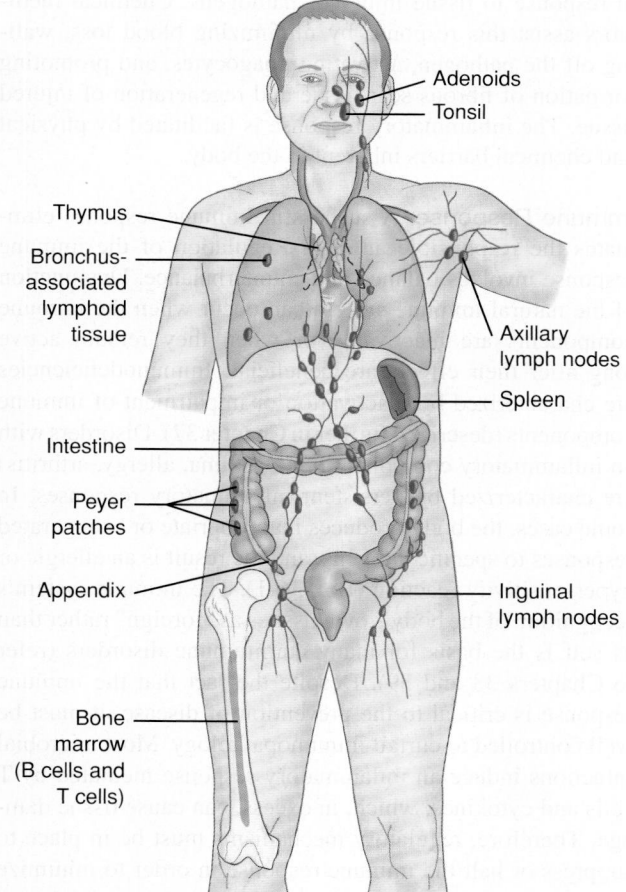

FIGURE 36-1 Central and peripheral lymphoid organs and tissues. (From Grossman, S., Porth, C. M., Conelius, J., Gerard, S. O., Moriber, N., O'Shea, E. R., & Wheeler, K. (2014). *Porth's pathophysiology: Concepts of altered health states*. Philadelphia, PA: Wolters Kluwer Health/Lippincott Williams & Wilkins.)

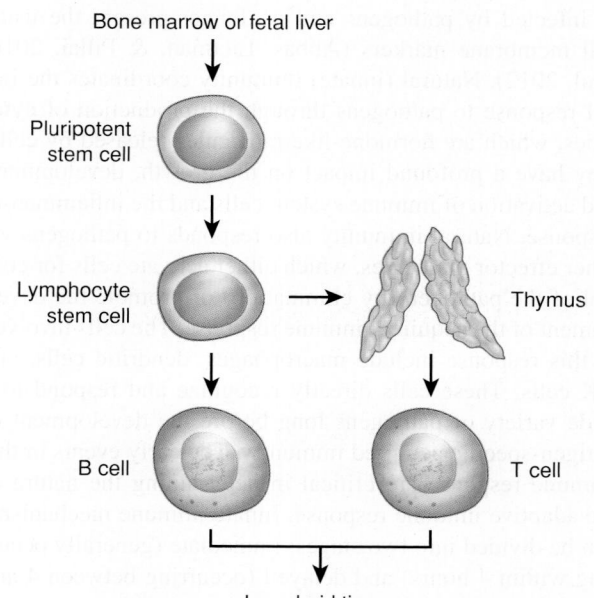

FIGURE 36-3 Lymphocytes originate from stem cells in the bone marrow. B lymphocytes mature in the bone marrow before entering the bloodstream, whereas T lymphocytes mature in the thymus, where they also differentiate into cells with various functions. (From Grossman, S., Porth, C. M., Conelius, J., Gerard, S. O., Moriber, N., O'Shea, E. R., & Wheeler, K. (2014). *Porth's pathophysiology: Concepts of altered health states*. Philadelphia, PA: Wolters Kluwer Health/Lippincott Williams & Wilkins.)

it acts like a filter. Lymph nodes are distributed throughout the body and connected by lymph channels and capillaries. The lymph nodes remove foreign material from the lymph system before it enters the bloodstream. The lymph nodes are centers for the proliferation of immune cells.

Immune Function

Types of Immunity

There are two general types of immunity: natural (innate) and acquired (adaptive). Natural immunity is a nonspecific immunity present at birth that provides protection against an infectious agent without ever having encountered it before. Acquired or specific immunity develops after birth. Although each type of immunity plays a distinct role in defending the body against harmful pathogens, the various components usually act in an interdependent manner.

Natural Immunity
Natural immunity provides a nonspecific response to any foreign pathogen, regardless of the pathogen's composition. Because of its lack of specificity, natural immunity maintains a broad spectrum of defense against and resistance to infection. The basis of this defense mechanism is the ability to distinguish between "self" and "nonself." Recent research in transplantation medicine demonstrates that this is a very simplistic differentiation. **Natural killer** (NK) cells also recognize "missing self" or cells that have been transformed or infected by pathogens and no longer present the usual cell membrane markers (Abbas, Lictman, & Pillai, 2016; Paul, 2012). Natural (innate) immunity coordinates the initial response to pathogens through the production of cytokines, which are hormone-like molecules released by cells; they have a profound impact on the growth, development, and activation of immune system cells and the inflammatory response. Natural immunity also responds to pathogens via other effector molecules, which either activate cells for control of the pathogen (by elimination) or promote the development of the acquired immune response. The cells involved in this response include macrophages, dendritic cells, and NK cells. These cells directly recognize and respond to a wide variety of pathogens long before the development of antigen-specific acquired immunity. The early events in this immune response are critical in determining the nature of the adaptive immune response. Innate immune mechanisms can be divided into two stages: immediate (generally occurring within 4 hours) and delayed (occurring between 4 and 96 hours after exposure).

The development of immunity occurs via physical and chemical barriers, inflammatory response, and immune response.

Physical and Chemical Barriers. Activation of the natural immunity response is enhanced by processes inherent in physical and chemical barriers. The processes prevent or delay the entry into the body of various pathogens before infection can develop. Physical surface barriers include intact skin, mucous membranes, and cilia of the respiratory tract, which prevent pathogens from gaining access to the body. The cilia of the respiratory tract, along with coughing and sneezing responses, filter and clear pathogens from the upper respiratory tract before they can invade the body further. Chemical barriers, such as mucus, acidic gastric secretions, enzymes in tears and saliva, and substances in sebaceous and sweat secretions, act in a nonspecific way to destroy invading bacteria and fungi. For example, in addition to dissolving food, hydrochloric acid in the stomach destroys pathogens present in food or swallowed mucus (Porth, 2015). Viruses are countered by other means, such as interferon (IFN). **Interferon**, one type of biologic response modifier, is a nonspecific viricidal protein that is naturally produced by the body and is capable of activating other components of the immune system.

Inflammatory Response. The inflammatory response is a major function of the natural immune system that is elicited in response to tissue injury or pathogens. Chemical mediators assist this response by minimizing blood loss, walling off the pathogen, activating phagocytes, and promoting formation of fibrous scar tissue and regeneration of injured tissue. The inflammatory response is facilitated by physical and chemical barriers inherent in the body.

Immune Response. A successful immune response eliminates the responsible antigen. Regulation of the immune response involves balance and counterbalance. Dysfunction of the natural immune system can occur when the immune components are inactivated or when they remain active long after their effects are beneficial. Immunodeficiencies are characterized by inactivation or impairment of immune components (described further in Chapter 37). Disorders with an inflammatory component (e.g., asthma, allergy, arthritis) are characterized by persistent inflammatory responses. In some cases, the body produces inappropriate or exaggerated responses to specific antigens, and the result is an allergic or hypersensitivity reaction (Box 36-1). The immune system's recognition of the body's own tissues as "foreign" rather than as self is the basis for many autoimmune disorders (refer to Chapters 38 and 39). Despite the fact that the immune response is critical to the prevention of disease, it must be well controlled to curtail immunopathology. Most microbial infections induce an inflammatory response mediated by T cells and cytokines, which, in excess, can cause tissue damage. Therefore, regulatory mechanisms must be in place to suppress or halt the immune response in order to minimize tissue damage. This is achieved mainly by the production of cytokines and transformation of growth factors that inhibit macrophage activation. In some cases, T-cell activation is so overwhelming that these mechanisms fail, and pathology results. Researchers in gene therapy are attempting to recruit

BOX 36-1
Focus on Pathophysiology

Allergic Reaction

An allergic reaction is a manifestation of tissue injury resulting from interaction between an antigen and an antibody. Allergy is an inappropriate and often harmful response of the immune system to substances that are normally harmless. In this case, the inappropriate substance is termed an *allergen*.

Mast cells located in tissues throughout the body can be activated by a variety of stimuli, causing immediate allergic inflammation. The binding of the antigen and antibodies on the mast cells causes the release of mediators that effect blood vessel, smooth muscle, and glandular secretions. The powerful chemical mediators released from the mast cells cause a sequence of physiologic events, resulting in symptoms of immediate hypersensitivity. There are two types of chemical mediators: primary and secondary. Primary mediators are preformed and are found in mast cells or basophils. Secondary mediators are inactive precursors that are formed or released in response to primary mediators (e.g., leukotrienes, bradykinin, and serotonin).

When in contact with an allergen, the body produces large amounts of IgE, thus causing a hypersensitivity or allergic response (see figure on next page). IgE-producing cells are located in the respiratory and intestinal mucosa. Two or more IgE molecules bind together to an allergen and trigger mast cells or basophils to release chemical mediators, such as histamine and leukotrienes. Maximal intensity of histamine release is reached within about 15 minutes after antigen contact. Effects of histamine release include erythema; localized edema in the form of wheals; pruritus; contraction of bronchial smooth muscle, resulting in wheezing and bronchospasm; dilation of small venules and constriction of larger vessels; and increased secretion of gastric and mucosal cells, resulting in diarrhea. Histamine action results from stimulation of histamine-1 (H_1) and histamine-2 (H_2) receptors found on different types of lymphocytes, particularly T-lymphocyte suppressor cells and basophils. H_1 receptors are found predominantly on bronchiolar and vascular smooth muscle cells; H_2 receptors are found on gastric parietal cells.

Certain medications are categorized by their action at these receptors. Diphenhydramine (Benadryl) is an example of an antihistamine, a medication that displays an affinity for H_1 receptors. Cimetidine (Tagamet) and ranitidine (Zantac) target H_2 receptors to inhibit gastric secretions in cases of peptic ulcer disease.

Leukotrienes, another chemical mediator released by mucosal mast cells, cause smooth muscle contraction, bronchial constriction, mucus secretion in the airways, and the typical wheal-and-flare reaction of the skin. Compared with histamine, leukotrienes are 100 to 1,000 times more potent in causing bronchospasm. Many manifestations of inflammation can be attributed in part to leukotrienes. Medications categorized as leukotriene antagonists or modifiers block the synthesis or action of leukotrienes and prevent the signs and symptoms associated with asthma.

Hypersensitivity

A hypersensitivity reaction is an abnormal, heightened reaction to any type of stimulus. Usually it does not occur with the first exposure to an allergen, but it is a reflection of excessive or atypical immune responses. To promote understanding of the immunopathogenesis of disease, hypersensitivity reactions have been classified into four specific types of reactions: Anaphylactic (type 1) Hypersensitivity, Cytotoxic (type II) Hypersensitivity, Immune Complex (type III) Hypersensitivity, and Delayed-Type (type IV) Hypersensitivity. Most allergies are identified as either type I or type IV hypersensitivity reactions.

Anaphylactic (Type I) Hypersensitivity

The most severe form of hypersensitivity reaction or immune-mediated reaction is **anaphylaxis**. An unanticipated severe allergic reaction that is often explosive in onset, anaphylaxis is characterized by edema in many tissues, including the larynx, and often is accompanied by hypotension, bronchospasm, and cardiovascular collapse in severe cases. Mast cells in any organ system may be involved; however, the primary foci are the cardiovascular, skin, respiratory, and gastrointestinal systems (sites where mast cells are abundant) (Schwartz, 2016). Type I or anaphylactic hypersensitivity is an immediate reaction beginning within minutes of exposure to an antigen. This reaction is mediated by IgE antibodies and typically occurs on re-exposure to a specific antigen. If chemical mediators continue to be released, a delayed reaction may occur up to 24 hours after allergen exposure. Refer to Chapter 38 for more details on anaphylaxis.

Cytotoxic (Type II) Hypersensitivity

Type II, or cytotoxic, hypersensitivity occurs when the system mistakenly identifies a normal constituent of the body as foreign. This reaction may be the result of a cross-reacting antibody, possibly leading to damage to cells and tissues. Several disorders are associated with type II hypersensitivity reactions, including myasthenia gravis, in which the body mistakenly generates antibodies against normal nerve ending receptors; or Goodpasture syndrome, in which antibodies are generated against lung and renal tissue, producing lung damage and kidney failure; or they may be associated with drug-induced immune hemolytic anemia, Rh-hemolytic disease of the newborn, and incompatibility reactions in blood transfusions.

Immune Complex (Type III) Hypersensitivity

Type III, or immune complex, hypersensitivity involves immune complexes that are formed when antigens bind to antibodies. These complexes are cleared from the circulation by phagocytic action. If these type III complexes are deposited in tissues or vascular endothelium, two factors contribute to injury: the increased amount of circulating complexes and the presence of vasoactive amines. As a result, there is an increase in vascular permeability and tissue injury. The joints and kidneys are particularly susceptible to this type of injury. Type III hypersensitivity is associated with systemic lupus erythematosus,

(continued on page 1076)

BOX 36-1 **Focus on Pathophysiology** (*continued*)

rheumatoid arthritis, certain types of nephritis, and some types of bacterial endocarditis.

Delayed-Type (Type IV) Hypersensitivity

Type IV, or delayed-type hypersensitivity, also known as cellular hypersensitivity, occurs 24–72 hours after exposure to an allergen. It is mediated by sensitized T cells and macrophages. An example of this reaction is the effect of an intradermal injection of tuberculin antigen or purified protein derivative (PPD). Sensitized T cells react with the antigen at or near the injection site. Lymphokines are released and attract, activate, and retain macrophages at the site. These macrophages then release lysozymes, causing tissue damage. Edema and fibrin are responsible for the positive tuberculin reaction.

Another example of a type IV hypersensitivity reaction is contact dermatitis resulting from exposure to allergens, such as cosmetics, adhesive tape, topical agents (e.g., povidone-iodine), medication additives, and plant toxins. The most common immune-mediated reaction to local anesthetics is a type IV hypersensitivity reaction. The primary exposure results in sensitization. Re-exposure causes a hypersensitivity reaction with resultant symptoms, such as pruritus, erythema, and raised lesions.

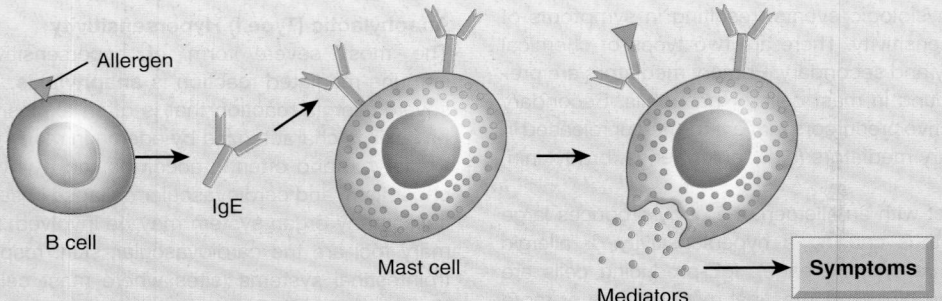

Allergen triggers the B cell to make IgE antibody, which attaches to the mast cell. When that allergen reappears; it binds to the IgE and triggers the mast cell to release its chemicals. (Courtesy of the U.S. Department of Health and Human Services. National Institutes of Health.)

natural components of the immune system to fight cancer through activation of these inhibitory factors (Weiser et al., 2015).

One of the most actively researched areas of immunology involves the inflammatory response and its contribution to chronic conditions, such as diabetes, autoimmune disease, and cancer. Previously, when cells underwent apoptosis (programmed cell death) or phagocytosis (the engulfing of microorganisms or other cells and foreign particles by phagocytes), the death of cells was thought to be a null response that did not contribute to further actions by the immune system. Research into the role of damage-associated molecular pattern molecules (DAMPs) changes this belief and contributes to the evidence that inflammation may be the most important factor of any disease process. DAMPs, also known as alarmins, consist of a wide variety of proteins and other byproducts of cell damage that trigger cascading events in the inflammatory response (Firestein, 2016). As researchers elucidate the contribution of inflammation to chronic disease, further research will determine the role of anti-inflammatory diets and probiotics to counteract these harmful changes.

Acquired Immunity

Acquired immunity—immunologic responses acquired during life but not present at birth—usually develops as a result of exposure to an antigen through immunization (vaccination) or by contracting a disease, both of which generate a protective immune response. Weeks or months after initial exposure to the disease or vaccine, the body produces an immune response that is sufficient to defend against the disease on re-exposure. In contrast to the rapid but nonspecific innate immune response, this form of immunity relies on the recognition of specific foreign antigens. The two components of the immune response are strongly interrelated. Events occurring early in infection dictate the direction of the adaptive response and activate the acquired immune effector mechanisms, which have direct feedback on the cells of the innate (natural) system. The acquired immune response is broadly divided into two mechanisms: the cell-mediated response, involving T-cell activation, and effector mechanisms, involving B-cell maturation and the production of antibodies. With the combination of innate and acquired immune responses, the body is capable of protecting itself immediately as well as against future challenges to its integrity.

The two types of acquired immunity are known as active and passive. In active acquired immunity, the immunologic defenses are developed by the person's own body. This immunity typically lasts many years or even a lifetime. This response is best demonstrated by the response of the body to immunizations. Exposure to attenuated virus, such as the influenza vaccine, prompts the production of antibodies against influenza. Re-exposure to influenza initiates a cascade of immune responses that are more rapid and capable of controlling the virus. Patients either eliminate the virus from their system or have a milder case of influenza. Passive acquired immunity is temporary immunity transmitted from a source outside the body that has developed immunity through previous disease or immunization. For example, immune globulin or antiserum, obtained from the plasma of people with acquired immunity, is used in emergencies to provide temporary immunity to certain diseases, such as hepatitis, immediately after exposure. Immunity resulting from the transfer of antibodies from the mother to an infant in utero or through breastfeeding is another example of passive immunity. Active and passive acquired immunity involve immunologic responses that are both humoral (antibodies produced by B cells) and cellular (cell-mediated T lymphocytes that attack pathogens).

Response to Invasion

When the body is invaded or attacked by bacteria, viruses, or other pathogens, it has three means of defense:

- The phagocytic immune response
- The humoral or antibody immune response
- The cellular immune response

The first line of defense, the **phagocytic immune response**, involves the WBCs (granulocytes and macrophages), which have the ability to ingest foreign particles. These cells move to the point of attack, where they engulf and destroy the invading agents. Phagocytes also remove the body's own dying or dead cells. Dying cells in necrotic tissue release substances that trigger an inflammatory response.

Apoptosis is the body's way of destroying worn-out cells, such as blood or skin cells, or cells that need to be renewed. The cells that have been damaged by infection or genetic change, or cells that are simply in excess of the body's needs, are targeted for removal and destruction by a subgroup of proteases called *caspase*. Once the process of apoptosis begins, generally it is irreversible (Paul, 2012).

Unlike macrophages, eosinophils are only weakly phagocytic. On activation, eosinophils probably kill parasites by releasing specific chemical mediators into the extracellular fluid. Additionally, eosinophils secrete leukotrienes (discussed later in the chapter), prostaglandins, and various cytokines (Paul, 2012; Salmon, 2016).

A second protective response, the **humoral immune response** (sometimes called the **antibody** response), begins with the B lymphocytes, which can transform themselves into plasma cells that manufacture antibodies. These antibodies are highly specific proteins that are transported in the bloodstream and attempt to disable pathogens.

The third mechanism of defense, the **cellular immune response**, involves the T lymphocytes, which can turn into special cytotoxic (or killer) T cells that can attack the pathogens. Table 36-2 summarizes the types of cells involved in immune response.

Basics of Immune Response

The structural part of the invading or attacking organism that is responsible for stimulating antibody production is called an **antigen** (or an immunogen). An antigen can be a small patch of proteins on the outer surface of a microorganism. Some antigens are naturally immunogenic or able to stimulate an immune response directly. Most antigens must be coupled with other molecules to stimulate the immune response. A single bacterium or large molecule, such as a

TABLE **36-2** Lymphocytes Involved in Immune Responses

Type of Immune Response	Cell Type	Function
Humoral	B lymphocyte	Produces antibodies or immunoglobulins (IgA, IgD, IgE, IgG, IgM)
Cellular	T lymphocyte	
	Helper T	Attacks foreign pathogens (antigens) directly
		Initiates and augments inflammatory response
	Helper T$_1$	Increases activated cytotoxic T cells
	Helper T$_2$	Increases B-cell antibody production
	Suppressor T	Suppresses the immune response
	Memory T	Remembers contact with an antigen and on subsequent exposures mounts an immune response
	Cytotoxic T (killer T)	Lyses cells infected with virus; plays a role in graft rejection
Nonspecific	Non-T, non–B lymphocyte (L lymphocytes)	Amplify T cell proliferation
	Null cell	Destroys antigens already coated with antibody
	Natural killer (NK) cell (granular lymphocyte)	Defends against microorganisms and some types of malignant cells; produces cytokines

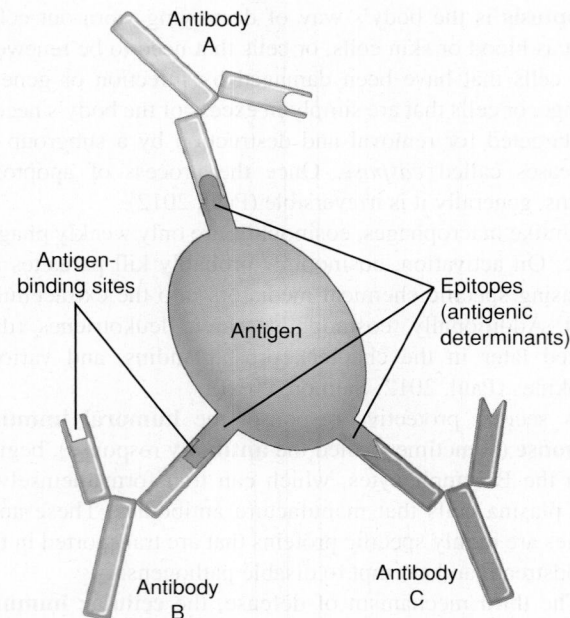

FIGURE 36-4 Complement-mediated immune responses. (From Grossman, S., Porth, C. M., Conelius, J., Gerard, S. O., Moriber, N., O'Shea, E. R., & Wheeler, K. (2014). *Porth's pathophysiology: Concepts of altered health states*. Philadelphia, PA: Wolters Kluwer Health/Lippincott Williams & Wilkins.)

diphtheria or tetanus toxin, may have several antigens, or markers, on its surface, thus inducing the body to produce a number of different antibodies. Once produced, an antibody is released into the bloodstream and carried to the attacking organism. There, it combines with the antigen, binding with it like an interlocking piece of a jigsaw puzzle (Fig. 36-4). There are four well-defined stages in an immune response: recognition, proliferation, response, and effector.

Recognition Stage.
Recognition of antigens as foreign, or nonself, by the immune system is the initiating event in any immune response. The body accomplishes recognition using lymph nodes and lymphocytes for surveillance. Lymph nodes continuously discharge lymphocytes into the bloodstream. These lymphocytes patrol the tissues and vessels that drain the areas served by that node.

The exact way in which circulating lymphocytes recognize antigens on foreign surfaces is through complex rearrangements of genes that produce T-cell antigen receptors (TCR) during cell differentiation and maturation in the thymus. T cells present in primary lymphoid tissue that have not been presented with an antigen are called *naïve* and are capable of responding to a vast array of antigens (Paul, 2012). Macrophages play an important role in helping the circulating lymphocytes process the antigens. Both macrophages and neutrophils have receptors for antibodies and *complement* (a system of proteins found in normal blood plasma that combines with antibodies to destroy pathogens, to be discussed later in this chapter); as a result, they coat microorganisms

with antibodies, complement, or both, enhancing phagocytosis. Then the engulfed microorganisms are subjected to a wide range of toxic intracellular molecules. When foreign materials enter the body, circulating lymphocytes come into physical contact with the surfaces of these materials. Upon contact with the foreign material, naïve lymphocytes, with the help of macrophages, either remove the antigen from the surface or obtain an imprint of its structure, initiating the process of acquired immunity and antigen recognition in preparation for subsequent re-exposure to the antigen (Abbas et al., 2016; Paul, 2012).

Proliferation Stage.
The circulating lymphocyte containing the antigenic message returns to the nearest lymph node. Once in the node, the sensitized lymphocyte stimulates some of the resident dormant T and B lymphocytes to enlarge, divide, and proliferate. T lymphocytes differentiate into cytotoxic (or killer) T cells, whereas B lymphocytes produce and release antibodies. Enlargement of the lymph nodes in the neck in conjunction with a sore throat is one example of the inflammatory response during immune activation.

Response Stage.
In the response stage, the differentiated lymphocytes function in either a humoral or a cellular capacity. The production of antibodies by the B lymphocytes in response to a specific antigen begins the humoral response. *Humoral* refers to the fact that the antibodies are released into the bloodstream and, therefore, reside in the plasma (fluid fraction of the blood).

With the initial cellular response, the returning sensitized lymphocytes migrate to areas of the lymph node other than those areas containing lymphocytes programmed to become plasma cells. Here, they stimulate the residing lymphocytes to become cells that will attack microbes directly, rather than through the action of antibodies. These transformed lymphocytes are known as *cytotoxic (killer) T cells*. The T stands for *thymus*, signifying that, during embryologic development of the immune system, these T lymphocytes spent time in the thymus of the developing fetus. Viral rather than bacterial antigens induce a cellular response. This response is manifested by the increasing number of T lymphocytes (lymphocytosis) seen on the complete blood counts (CBC) of people with viral illnesses, such as infectious mononucleosis (cellular immunity is discussed in further detail later in this chapter).

Most immune responses to antigens involve both humoral and cellular responses, although one usually predominates. For example, during transplant rejection, the cellular response predominates, whereas in cases of bacterial pneumonias and sepsis, the humoral response plays the dominant protective role (Box 36-2).

Effector Stage.
In the effector stage, either the antibody of the humoral response or the cytotoxic (killer) T cell of the cellular response reaches and connects with the antigen on the surface of the foreign pathogen. The connection initiates

BOX 36-2

Examples of Humoral and Cellular Immune Responses

Humoral Responses (B Cells)

- Bacterial phagocytosis and lysis
- Anaphylaxis
- Allergic hay fever and asthma
- Immune complex disease
- Bacterial and some viral infections

Cellular Responses (T Cells)

- Transplant rejection
- Delayed hypersensitivity (tuberculin reaction)
- Graft-versus-host disease
- Tumor surveillance or destruction
- Intracellular infections
- Viral, fungal, and parasitic infections

a series of events that, in most instances, results in the total destruction of the invading microbes or the complete neutralization of the toxin. The events involve interplay of antibodies (humoral immunity), complement, and action by the cytotoxic T cells (cellular immunity). Figure 36-5 summarizes the stages of the immune response.

Humoral Immune Response

The humoral response is characterized by the production of antibodies by B lymphocytes in response to a specific antigen. Although the B lymphocyte is ultimately responsible for the production of antibodies, both the macrophages of natural immunity and the special T-cell lymphocytes of cellular immunity are involved in recognizing the foreign substance and in producing antibodies.

Antigen Recognition. B lymphocytes recognize and respond to invading antigens in more than one way.

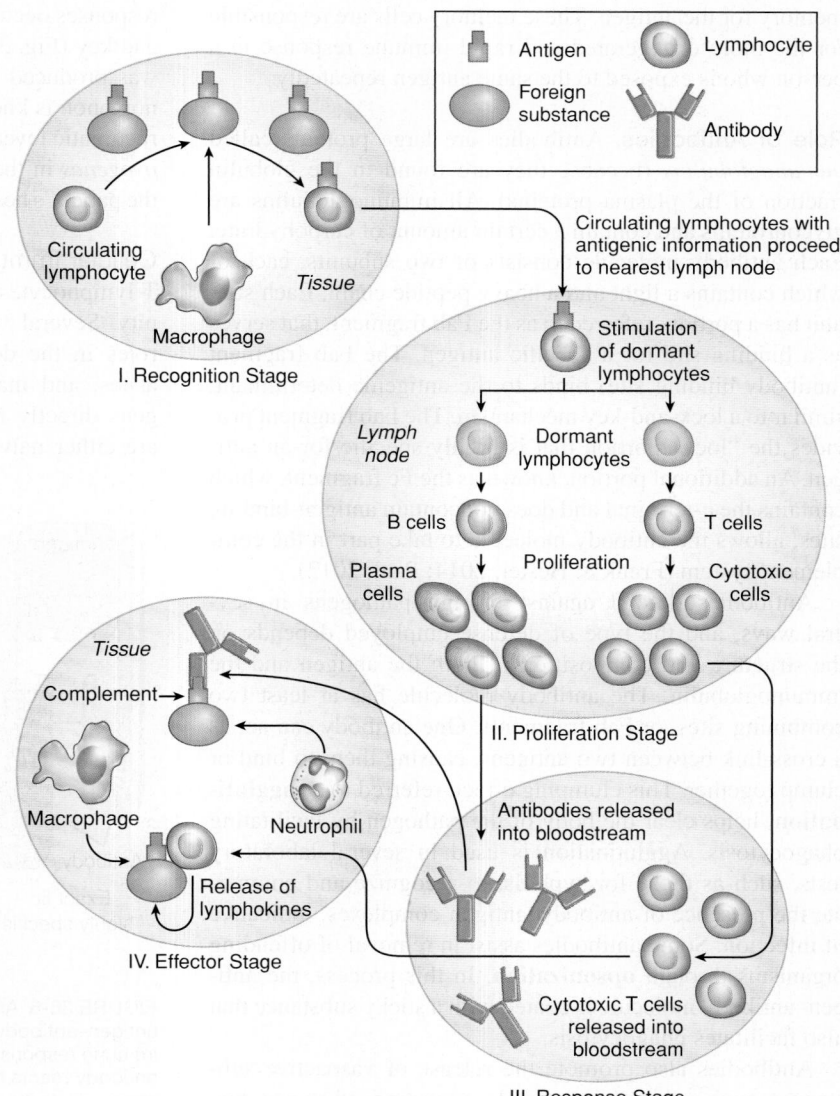

FIGURE 36-5 Stages of the immune response. (I) In the *recognition stage,* antigens are recognized by circulating lymphocytes and macrophages. (II) In the *proliferation stage,* the dormant lymphocytes proliferate and differentiate into cytotoxic (killer) T or B cells responsible for formation and release of antibodies. (III) In the *response stage,* the cytotoxic T cells and the B cells perform cellular and humoral functions, respectively. (IV) In the *effector stage,* antigens are destroyed or neutralized through the action of antibodies, complement, macrophages, and cytotoxic T cells.

The B lymphocytes appear to respond to some antigens by triggering antibody formation directly; however, in response to other antigens, they need the assistance of T cells to trigger antibody formation. The T lymphocytes are part of a surveillance system that is dispersed throughout the body and recycles through the general circulation, tissues, and lymphatic system. With the assistance of macrophages, the T lymphocytes are believed to recognize the antigen of a foreign pathogen. The T lymphocyte picks up the antigenic message, or "blueprint," of the antigen and returns to the nearest lymph node with that message.

B lymphocytes stored in the lymph nodes are subdivided into thousands of clones, each responsive to a single group of antigens having almost identical characteristics. When the antigenic message is carried back to the lymph node, specific clones of the B lymphocyte are stimulated to enlarge, divide, proliferate, and differentiate into plasma cells capable of producing specific antibodies to the antigen. Other B lymphocytes differentiate into B-lymphocyte clones with a memory for the antigen. These memory cells are responsible for the more exaggerated and rapid immune response in a person who is exposed to the same antigen repeatedly.

Role of Antibodies.
Antibodies are large proteins called *immunoglobulins* (because they are found in the globulin fraction of the plasma proteins). All immunoglobulins are glycoproteins and contain a certain amount of carbohydrate. Each antibody molecule consists of two subunits, each of which contains a light and a heavy peptide chain. Each subunit has a portion, referred to as the Fab fragment, that serves as a binding site for a specific antigen. The Fab fragment (antibody-binding site) binds to the antigenic determinant, similar to a lock-and-key mechanism. The Fab fragment provides the "lock" portion that is highly specific for an antigen. An additional portion, known as the Fc fragment, which contains the c-terminal and does not contain antigen-binding sites, allows the antibody molecule to take part in the complement system (Frank & Hester, 2014; Paul, 2012).

Antibodies defend against foreign pathogens in several ways, and the type of defense employed depends on the structure and composition of both the antigen and the immunoglobulin. The antibody molecule has at least two combining sites, or Fab fragments. One antibody can act as a cross-link between two antigens, causing them to bind or clump together. This clumping effect, referred to as **agglutination**, helps clear the body of the pathogen by facilitating phagocytosis. Agglutination is used in several laboratory tests, such as those for syphilis, to recognize and enumerate the presence of antibody–antigen complexes, indicative of infection. Some antibodies assist in removal of offending organisms through **opsonization**. In this process, the antigen–antibody molecule is coated with a sticky substance that also facilitates phagocytosis.

Antibodies also promote the release of vasoactive substances, such as histamine and slow-reacting substance, two of the chemical mediators of the inflammatory response. Antibodies do not function in isolation; rather, they mobilize other components of the immune system to defend against the pathogen. The typical role of antibodies is to focus components of the natural immune system on the pathogen. This includes activation of both the complement system and phagocytosis (Paul, 2012; Salmon, 2016).

The body can produce five different types of immunoglobulins (Ig). Each of the five types, or classes, is identified by a specific letter of the alphabet derived from the name of the heavy chain present on the immunoglobulin: IgA for alpha (α), IgD for delta (δ), IgE for epsilon (ϵ), IgG for gamma (γ), and IgM for mu (μ). Classification is based on the chemical structure and biologic role of the individual immunoglobulin.

Antigen–Antibody Binding.
The portion of the antigen involved in binding with the antibody is referred to as the **antigenic determinant**. The most efficient immunologic responses occur when the antibody and antigen fit like a lock and key (Fig. 36-6). Poor fit can occur with an antibody that was produced in response to a different antigen. This phenomenon is known as *cross-reactivity*. For example, in acute rheumatic fever, the antibody produced against *Streptococcus pyogenes* in the upper respiratory tract may cross-react with the patient's heart tissue, leading to mitral valve abnormalities.

Cellular Immune Response
T lymphocytes are responsible primarily for cellular immunity. Several types of T cells exist, each with designated roles in the defense against bacteria, viruses, fungi, parasites, and malignant cells. T cells attack foreign pathogens directly rather than by producing antibodies. T cells are either naïve—capable of reacting to new antigens—or

FIGURE 36-6 Antigen–antibody binding. (*Left*) A highly specific antigen–antibody complex. (*Middle*) No match and, therefore, no immune response. (*Right*) Poor fit or match with low specificity; antibody reacts to antigen with similar characteristics, producing cross-reactivity.

activated—having the memory of previous antigen exposure (Paul, 2012).

Cellular reactions are initiated by the binding of an antigen to an antigen receptor located on the surface of a naïve T cell. This may occur with or without the assistance of macrophages. The activated T cells then carry the antigenic message, or blueprint, to the lymph nodes, where the production of other T cells is stimulated. Some T cells remain in the lymph nodes and retain a memory for the antigen. Other T cells migrate from the lymph nodes into the general circulatory system and ultimately to the tissues, where they remain until they either come in contact with their respective antigens or die.

Role of T Lymphocytes. T cells include effector T cells, suppressor T cells, and memory T cells. Two major categories of effector T cells exist: helper T cells and cytotoxic T cells. These effector T cells participate in the destruction of foreign organisms. T cells interact closely with B cells, indicating that humoral and cellular immune responses are not separate, unrelated processes but, rather, branches of the immune response that interact.

Helper T cells are activated on recognition of antigens and stimulate the rest of the immune system. When activated, helper T cells secrete **cytokines**, which attract and activate B cells, cytotoxic T cells, NK cells, macrophages, and other cells of the immune system. Separate subpopulations of helper T cells produce different types of cytokines and determine whether the immune response will be the production of antibodies or a cell-mediated immune response. Helper T cells produce **lymphokines**, one category of cytokines. These lymphokines activate other T cells (e.g., interleukin-2 [IL-2]), natural and cytotoxic T cells (e.g., IFN-gamma), and other inflammatory cells (e.g., tumor necrosis factor). Helper T cells produce IL-4 and IL-5, lymphokines that activate B cells to grow and differentiate.

Cytotoxic T cells (killer T cells) attack the antigen directly by altering the cell membrane and causing cell lysis (disintegration) and by releasing cytolytic enzymes and cytokines. Lymphokines can recruit, activate, and regulate other lymphocytes and WBCs. These cells then assist in destroying the pathogen. Delayed-type hypersensitivity is an example of an immune reaction that protects the body from antigens through the production and release of lymphokines (see later discussion).

Another type of cell, the **suppressor T cell**, has the ability to decrease B cell production, thereby keeping the immune response at a level that is compatible with health (e.g., sufficient to fight infection adequately without attacking the body's healthy tissues). **Memory cells** are responsible for recognizing antigens from previous exposure and mounting an immune response.

Roles of Null Lymphocytes and Natural Killer Cells. Null lymphocytes and NK cells are other lymphocytes that assist in combating organisms. These cells are distinct from B and T cells and lack the usual characteristics of those cells. **Null lymphocytes**, a subpopulation of lymphocytes, destroy antigens already coated with antibody. These cells have special Fc receptor sites on their surface that allow them to connect with the Fc end of antibodies; this is known as *antibody-dependent, cell-mediated cytotoxicity*.

NK cells, another subpopulation of lymphocytes, defend against microorganisms and some types of malignant cells (Grossman et al., 2014). NK cells are capable of directly killing pathogens and producing cytokines. The helper T cells contribute to the differentiation of null and NK cells.

Complement System

Circulating plasma proteins, known as **complement**, are made in the liver and other sites and activated when an antibody connects with its antigen. There are more than 35 of these plasma or membrane proteins, and they are an important additional component of the immune system (Paul, 2012). Destruction of an invading or attacking organism or toxin is not achieved merely by the binding of the antibody and antigens; destruction also requires activation of complement, the arrival of killer T cells, or the attraction of macrophages. Complement has three major physiologic functions: defending the body against bacterial infection, bridging natural and acquired immunity, and disposing of immune complexes and the by-products associated with inflammation.

The proteins that comprise complement interact sequentially with one another in a cascading or "falling domino" effect. The complement cascade is important to modifying the effector arm of the immune system. Activation of complement allows for the occurrence of important events, such as removal of infectious agents and initiation of the inflammatory response. These events involve active parts of the pathway that enhance chemotaxis of macrophages and granulocytes, alter blood vessel permeability, change blood vessel diameters, cause cells to lyse, alter blood clotting, and cause other points of modification. These macrophages and granulocytes continue the body's defense by devouring the antibody-coated microbes and by releasing antibacterial products.

Role of Interferons

IFNs are cytokines. They have antiviral and antitumor properties. In addition to responding to viral infection, IFNs are produced by T lymphocytes, B lymphocytes, and macrophages in response to antigens. They modify the immune response by suppressing antibody production and cellular immunity. They also facilitate the cytolytic (cell destruction) role of lymphocytes, macrophages, and NK cells. Research continues on the pathways that IFNs use to transmit signals from cell membranes to the nucleus. IFNs are undergoing extensive testing to evaluate their effectiveness in treating tumors and AIDS (Andzinski et al., 2016).

Advances in Immunology

Genetic Engineering

One of the more remarkable evolving technologies is **genetic engineering**, which uses recombinant DNA technology. Genetic engineering is used in everything from the production of insulin and human growth hormone to the production of experimental mice. One type of genetic engineering permits scientists to combine genes from one type of organism with genes of a second organism. This type of technology allows cells and microorganisms to manufacture proteins, monokines, and lymphokines that can alter and enhance immune system function. This type of technology also produces genetically modified organisms (GMOs) that have been the source of much controversy in the food industry. The second use of recombinant DNA technology involves gene therapy (Grossman et al., 2014). If a particular gene is abnormal or missing, experimental recombinant DNA technology may be capable of restoring normal gene function. For example, a recombinant gene is inserted onto a virus particle. When the virus particle splices its genes, the virus automatically inserts the missing gene, and theoretically corrects the genetic anomaly. Extensive research into recombinant DNA technology and gene therapy is ongoing; successful models of a recombinant DNA vaccine against tumor cells and angiogenesis have been created in mice (Yin et al., 2015).

Stem Cells

Stem cells are potentially immortal cells that are capable of self-renewal and differentiation; they continually replenish the body's entire supply of both RBCs and WBCs. Some stem cells, described as *totipotent cells*, have tremendous capacity to self-renew and differentiate. Embryonic stem cells, described as *pluripotent*, give rise to numerous cell types that are able to form tissues (Grossman et al., 2014). Research and clinical trials have shown that stem cells can restore an immune system that has been destroyed. Stem cell transplantation therapy has been developed for numerous types of conditions, such as severe combined immunodeficiency (SCID), acute myeloid leukemia, periodontal disease, and other types of cancer (Klein & Nör, 2015). Clinical trials using stem cells as therapy are underway in patients with a variety of disorders having an autoimmune component, including systemic lupus erythematosus (SLE), rheumatoid arthritis, scleroderma, multiple sclerosis, and heart disease, specifically in the repair of endothelial cells (Gurtu & Michelakis, 2015).

Gerontologic Considerations

People at the extremes of the lifespan are more likely than middle-aged adults to develop problems related to the functioning of the immune system (Table 36-3). The greatest impact of aging on the immune system is on cell-mediated immunity; age has a lesser but substantial impact on humoral immunity. The frequency and severity of infections are increased in elderly people, possibly due to a decreased ability to respond adequately to pathogens. Both the production and the function of T and B lymphocytes may be impaired. Responses to antigen stimulation may be altered, with increasing proportions of lymphocytes becoming unresponsive with age. An example of this is the recent development of a vaccine for older patients against herpes zoster and postherpetic neuralgia caused by the varicella virus. The antigen present in this vaccine is 14 times the amount of live attenuated virus present in the varicella vaccine for children (Cohen, 2016). The impact of aging on the immune system can best be summarized as *immunosenescence*, a condition thought to be a result of involution of the thymus (Duggal & Lord, 2013).

ASSESSMENT OF THE IMMUNE SYSTEM

Assessment of the immune system involves nearly every organ system of the body.

Health History

Common Complaints

Accurately assessing a patient's immune system can include consideration of nonspecific signs and symptoms, such as fatigue, impaired wound healing, recurrent infections, weight loss, or lymphadenopathy (Fig. 36-7). Or the signs and symptoms may be more specific, such as a butterfly (malar) rash in SLE; joint deformities in rheumatoid arthritis; thrush in HIV; or erythema, hoarseness, and dyspnea with anaphylactic reaction.

FIGURE 36-7 Lymphadenopathy. An enlarged cervical lymph node. (Courtesy of Gehrig, J. S., *Patient assessment tutorials* (3rd ed.). Lippincott, Wolters, Kluwer.)

TABLE 36-3 GERONTOLOGIC CONSIDERATIONS / Age-Related Changes in Immunologic Function

Body System	Structural and Functional Changes	History and Physical Findings
Immune	Impaired function of B and T lymphocytes Failure of lymphocytes to recognize mutant or abnormal cells Decreased antibody production Failure of immune system to differentiate "self" from "non-self" Suppressed phagocytic immune response	Suppressed responses to pathogenic organisms with increased risk for infection Increased incidence of cancers Anergy (lack of response to antigens applied to the skin [PPD, allergens]) Increased incidence of autoimmune diseases Absence of typical signs and symptoms of infection and inflammation Dissemination of organisms usually destroyed or suppressed by phagocytes (e.g., reactivation or spread of tuberculosis)
Gastrointestinal	Decreased gastric secretions and motility Decreased phagocytosis by the liver's Kupffer cells Altered nutritional intake with inadequate protein intake	Proliferation of intestinal organisms, resulting in gastroenteritis and diarrhea Increased incidence and severity of hepatitis B; increased incidence of liver abscesses Suppressed immune response
Urinary	Decreased kidney function and changes in lower urinary tract function (enlargement of prostate gland, neurogenic bladder) Altered flora in the genitourinary tract	Urinary stasis and increased incidence of UTIs
Pulmonary	Impaired ciliary action due to exposure to smoke and environmental toxins	Impaired clearance of pulmonary secretions; increased incidence of respiratory infections
Integumentary	Thinning of skin with less elasticity; loss of adipose tissue	Increased risk of skin injury, breakdown, and infection
Circulatory	Impaired microcirculation	Stasis and pressure ulcers
Neurologic function	Decreased sensation and slowing of reflexes	Increased risk of injury, skin ulcers, abrasions, and burns

Past History

The nurse asks the patient about childhood and adult immunizations and childhood diseases. Known past or present exposure to tuberculosis is assessed, and the dates and results of any tuberculin tests (PPD or tine test) and chest x-rays are obtained. The nurse elicits information related to any recent exposure to any infections and the exposure dates. It is important for the nurse to assess whether the patient has been exposed to any sexually transmitted infections (STIs) or bloodborne pathogens, such as hepatitis A, B, or C viruses and HIV virus. A history of STIs, such as gonorrhea, syphilis, HPV infection, and chlamydia, can alert the nurse that the patient may have been exposed to HIV infection or to hepatitis. However, the Centers for Disease Control and Prevention (CDC) recommend universal HIV testing of all patients over the age of 13 with risk assessment determining the need for repeat testing. The nurse obtains a history of past and present infections and the dates and types of treatments along with a history of any multiple persistent infections, fevers of unknown origin, lesions or sores, or any type of drainage.

Allergy

The nurse asks the patient about any allergies, including types of allergens (e.g., pollens, dust, plants, cosmetics, food, medications, vaccines, latex), the symptoms experienced, and seasonal variations in occurrence or severity in the symptoms. A history of testing and treatments, including prescribed and over-the-counter medications that the patient has taken or is currently taking for these allergies and the effectiveness of the treatments, is obtained. All medication and food allergies are listed on an allergy alert sticker and placed on the front of the patient's health record or chart to alert others. Continued assessment for potential allergic reactions in the patient is vital.

Autoimmune Disorders

Autoimmune disorders affect people of both genders and of all ages, ethnicities, and social classes. The nurse asks the patient about any autoimmune disorders, such as lupus erythematosus, rheumatoid arthritis, or psoriasis. The patient is asked to describe the onset, severity, remissions and exacerbations, functional limitations, treatments that the patient has received or is currently receiving, and the effectiveness of the treatments. Although most specific autoimmune disorders are rare, together they affect approximately 5% of the United States population. The occurrence of different autoimmune diseases within a family strongly suggests a genetic predisposition to more than one autoimmune disease (Paul, 2012).

Neoplastic Disease

If there is a history of cancer in the family, the nurse takes note of the type of cancer, age at onset, and relationship (maternal or paternal) of the patient to the affected family member(s). Dates and results of any cancer screening tests for the patient are obtained. A history of cancer in the patient is also obtained, along with the type of cancer, date of diagnosis, and treatment modalities used. Immunosuppression contributes to the development of cancers; however, cancer itself is immunosuppressive. Hematologic cancers, such as leukemia and lymphoma, are associated with altered production and function of WBCs and lymphocytes (Bierman & Armitage, 2016; Paul, 2012).

The nurse records data about all treatments that the patient has received or is currently receiving, such as radiation or chemotherapy, in the health history. Radiation destroys lymphocytes and decreases the ability to mount an effective immune response. The size and extent of the irradiated area determine the extent of immunosuppression. Whole-body irradiation may leave the patient totally immunosuppressed. Chemotherapy also affects bone marrow function, destroying cells that contribute to an effective immune response and resulting in immunosuppression.

Chronic Illness and Surgery

The nurse notes any history of chronic illness, such as diabetes mellitus, kidney disease, chronic obstructive pulmonary disease (COPD), or fibromyalgia. The onset and severity of illnesses, as well as treatment that the patient is receiving for the illness, are obtained. Chronic illness may contribute to immune system impairments in various ways. Kidney failure is associated with a deficiency in circulating lymphocytes. In addition, immune defenses may be altered by acidosis and uremic toxins. In diabetes, hyperglycemia impairs immune function (decreases the function of WBCs), promotes inflammation, favors the growth of yeast organisms, and is associated with changes in the walls of the blood vessels, resulting in increased risk for infection as well as both microvascular and macrovascular dysfunction. Recurrent respiratory tract infections are associated with COPD as a result of altered inspiratory and expiratory function and ineffective airway clearance.

Special Problems

Conditions such as burns and other forms of injury and infection may contribute to altered immune system function. Major burns cause impaired skin integrity and compromise the body's first line of defense. Loss of large amounts of serum occurs with burn injuries and depletes the body of essential proteins, including immunoglobulins. The physiologic and psychological stressors associated with surgery or injury stimulate cortisol release from the adrenal cortex; increased serum cortisol also contributes to suppression of normal immune responses.

Social History

Poor nutritional status, poor sleep habits, smoking, excessive consumption of alcohol, illicit drug use, STIs, and occupational or residential exposure to environmental radiation and pollutants have been associated with impaired immune function. The nurse needs to assess all of these factors in a detailed patient history.

Nutrition

The importance of optimal nutrition in enhancing immunity is gaining greater recognition. Inadequate intake of vitamins that are essential for synthesis of both DNA and protein may lead to protein–calorie deficiency and, subsequently, to impaired immune function. Vitamins also help in the regulation of cell proliferation and maturation of immune cells. Excess or deficiency of trace elements (i.e., copper, iron, manganese, selenium, or zinc) in the diet generally suppresses immune function.

Fatty acids are the building blocks that make up the structural components of cell membranes. Lipids are precursors of vitamins A, D, E, and K, as well as cholesterol. Both excess and deficiency of fatty acids have been found to suppress immune function.

Depletion of protein reserves results in atrophy of lymphoid tissues, depression of antibody response, reduction in the number of circulating T cells, and impaired phagocytic function. As a result, susceptibility to infection is greatly increased. During periods of infection or serious illness, nutritional requirements may be altered further, potentially contributing to depletion of stores of protein, fatty acid, vitamin, and trace elements and causing even greater risk of impaired immune response and sepsis. Patients whose nutritional status is compromised have a delayed postoperative recovery and often experience more severe infections and delayed wound healing. The nurse must assess the patient's nutritional status and caloric intake. The nurse is responsible for assuming a proactive role in ensuring the best possible nutritional intake for all patients as a vital step in preventing untoward treatment outcomes.

Box 36-3 discusses the role of probiotics.

Medications and Blood Transfusions

The nurse obtains a list of past and present medications that the patient has used or is using. In large doses, antibiotics, corticosteroids, cytotoxic agents, salicylates, nonsteroidal anti-inflammatory drugs (NSAIDs), and anesthetics can cause immune suppression (Table 36-4). The overuse of antibiotics, their effect on the intestinal microbiome, and the use of fecal transplants to restore a depleted microbiome are new areas that the nurse may explore with the patient during an assessment of the immune system.

Nursing Research

Bridging the Gap to Evidence-Based Practice

Probiotics in preventing recurrent urinary tract infections in women: A literature review.

Chisholm, A. H. (2015). Probiotics in preventing recurrent urinary tract infections in women: A literature review. *Urologic Nursing, 35*(1), 18–21, 29.

Increasing antibiotic resistance and increasing resistance to commonly used antibiotics makes treatment and prevention of urinary tract infections (UTIs) difficult. The objective of this study was to evaluate the evidence on probiotics in preventing recurrent UTIs in women.

A literature search was conducted to find research articles about the role of probiotics in preventing UTIs in women. The literature provided low to moderate evidence that probiotics are effective in preventing UTIs in women. Conclusions: Level of Evidence—V; this rating refers to evidence that is obtained from systematic reviews of descriptive and qualitative studies (Polit & Beck, 2012).

Purpose

This study employed a literature review to evaluate the evidence on probiotics in preventing recurrent UTIs in women. Given increasing antibiotic resistance to common medications, alternative methods that can prevent UTIs have become increasingly important.

Design

Using several databases, the researcher gathered articles that illustrated the role of probiotics for the prevention of recurrent UTIs in women.

Findings

The literature demonstrated low to moderate evidence that probiotics are effective in the prevention of recurrent UTIs in women. While more research is needed to strengthen the recommendation, the use of probiotics may be a safe alternative for preventing UTIs in women.

Nursing Implications

Lactobacillus probiotics, taken either orally or vaginally, are likely effective in reducing recurrent UTIs in women. Although more research is needed, probiotics should be considered a useful and safe alternative to antibiotics. The review of the research indicates potential benefits to the use of probiotics for several types of disorders. Patient education focuses on the multitude of strains of probiotics that are commercially available to consumers, from yogurt to nutritional supplements to kombucha and miso. There are no standards developed by the U.S. Food and Drug Administration (FDA) for additions of probiotics to food; nor are there recommended dosages. At this time, the research indicates that probiotics are safe and potentially beneficial for numerous disorders.

The nurse obtains a history of blood transfusions because previous exposure to foreign antigens through transfusion may be associated with the current abnormal immune function. Additionally, although the risk of HIV transmission through blood transfusion is extremely low in patients who received a transfusion after 1985 (the year that testing of blood for HIV was initiated in the United States), a small risk remains. The nurse also assesses for signs or symptoms of hepatitis in patients who have received blood products.

Travel and Occupation

Patients who are immunocompromised should be asked about travel history and occupational history to determine exposure to specific pathogens. For example, patients from the Southwest United States are more likely to be infected with certain types of fungi that are more prevalent in the desert.

Psychoneuroimmunologic Factors

The patient assessment also addresses psychoneuroimmunologic factors. The bidirectional pathway between the brain and immune system is referred to as *psychoneuroimmunology*, a field that has been the focus of research and discussion over the last several decades (Haroon, Raison, & Miller, 2012; Pariante, 2015). It is thought that the immune response is regulated and modulated in part by neuroendocrine influences. Lymphocytes and macrophages have receptors that are capable of responding to neurotransmitters and endocrine hormones. Lymphocytes can produce and secrete adrenocorticotropic hormone and endorphin-like compounds. Cells in the brain, especially in the hypothalamus, can recognize prostaglandins, IFNs, and interleukins as well as histamine and serotonin, which are released during the inflammatory process. Like all other biologic systems functioning in the interest of homeostasis, the immune system is integrated with other psychophysiologic processes and is subject to regulation and modulation by the brain.

Conversely, the immune processes can affect neural and endocrine function, including behavior. Growing evidence indicates that a measurable immune system response can be influenced positively by biobehavioral strategies, such as relaxation and imagery techniques, biofeedback, humor, hypnosis, and conditioning. Therefore, the assessment should address the patient's general psychological status and the patient's use of and response to these strategies.

Physical Assessment

Immune dysfunction may have manifestations in various body systems (Box 36-4). In addition to the assessment

TABLE **36-4** Selected Medications and Effects on the Immune System

Drug Classification (and Examples)	Effects on the Immune System
Antibiotics (in large doses)	**Bone marrow suppression**
ceftriaxone (Rocephin)	Eosinophilia, hemolytic anemia, hypoprothrombinemia, neutropenia, thrombocytopenia
cefuroxime sodium (Ceftin)	Eosinophilia, hemolytic anemia, hypoprothrombinemia, neutropenia, thrombocytopenia
chloramphenicol (Chloromycetin)	Leukopenia, aplastic anemia
dactinomycin (Cosmegen)	Agranulocytosis, neutropenia
fluoroquinolones (Cipro, Levaquin, Tequin)	Hemolytic anemia, methemoglobinemia, eosinophilia, leukopenia, pancytopenia
gentamicin sulfate (Garamycin)	Agranulocytosis, granulocytopenia
macrolides (erythromycin, Zithromax, Biaxin)	Neutropenia, leukopenia
penicillins	Agranulocytosis
streptomycin	Leukopenia, neutropenia, pancytopenia
vancomycin (Vancocin, Vancoled)	Transient leukopenia
Antithyroid drugs	
propylthiouracil (PTU)	Agranulocytosis, leukopenia
Nonsteroidal anti-inflammatory drugs (NSAIDs) (in large doses)	**Inhibit prostaglandin synthesis or release**
aspirin	Agranulocytosis
COX-2 inhibitors (e.g., Celebrex)	Anemia, allergy, no major other adverse effects to the immune system
ibuprofen (Advil, Motrin)	Leukopenia, neutropenia
indomethacin (Indocid, Indocin)	Agranulocytosis, leukopenia
phenylbutazone	Pancytopenia, agranulocytosis, aplastic anemia
Adrenal corticosteroids	**Immunosuppression**
Prednisone	Suppressing or preventing cell-mediated immune reactions reducing leukocyte, monocyte, and eosinophil levels Decreasing immunoglobulin binding to cell surface receptors inhibiting interleukin synthesis
Antineoplastic agents (cytotoxic agents)	**Immunosuppression**
alkylating agents	Leukopenia, bone marrow suppression
cyclophosphamide (Cytoxan)	Leukopenia, neutropenia
mechlorethamine HCl (Mustargen)	Agranulocytosis, neutropenia
cyclosporine	Leukopenia, inhibits T-lymphocyte function
Antimetabolites	**Immunosuppression**
fluorouracil (pyrimidine antagonist)	Leukopenia, eosinophilia
methotrexate (folic acid antagonist)	Leukopenia, aplastic bone marrow
mercaptopurine (6-MP) (purine antagonist)	Leukopenia, pancytopenia

BOX 36-4   Focused Assessment

Immune Dysfunction

Be alert for the following signs and symptoms:

Respiratory System
- Changes in respiratory rate
- Cough (dry or productive)
- Abnormal lung sounds (wheezing, crackles, rhonchi, stridor)
- Rhinitis
- Hyperventilation
- Bronchospasm
- Hypoxemia

Cardiovascular System
- Hypotension
- Tachycardia
- Arrhythmia
- Vasculitis
- Anemia

Gastrointestinal System
- Hepatosplenomegaly
- Colitis
- Vomiting
- Diarrhea

Genitourinary System
- Frequency and burning on urination
- Hematuria
- Discharge

Musculoskeletal System
- Joint mobility, edema, and pain

Skin
- Rashes
- Pruritus
- Lesions
- Dermatitis
- Hematomas or purpura
- Edema, angioedema, or urticaria
- Inflammation
- Flushing
- Discharge

Neurosensory System
- Cognitive dysfunction
- Hearing loss
- Visual changes
- Headaches and migraines
- Ataxia
- Tetany

components described below, the nurse assesses the patient's respiratory, cardiovascular, genitourinary, and neurosensory status for signs and symptoms indicative of immune dysfunction.

Assessment of the Skin

The nurse assesses the skin and mucous membranes for color, lesions, dermatitis, purpura (subcutaneous bleeding), urticaria (hives), inflammation (angioedema [Fig. 36-8]), or any discharge. Purpura may indicate life-threatening infections like meningitis; urticaria indicates an acute or chronic response to allergens, pathogens, or autoimmune disorders.

Assessment of Eyes, Ears, Nose, and Throat

The nurse assesses for injected (redness) of the conjunctivae; periorbital tissues may be swollen and darkened with allergic disorders. The nares may show pale and edematous nasal mucous membranes and swollen turbinates. Assess secretions (typically clear) of the nasal passages or in the posterior pharynx. Thick secretions (yellow or green) may suggest infection. Percussion over the maxillary or frontal sinuses may elicit tenderness in acute sinusitis.

Assessment of the Lungs

The nurse inspects the patient for work of breathing, respiratory rate, use of accessory muscles, presence of retractions of bulging at intercostal space and/or supra- and infraclavicular area, and clubbing; the nurse auscultates the lungs for adventitious sounds. Patients with acute asthma may display

FIGURE 36-8 Angioedema is a diffuse, nonpitting, tense swelling of the dermis and subcutaneous tissue that can develop rapidly. Although usually allergic in nature and sometimes associated with hives, angioedema does not itch. (From Neville, B., Damm, D. D., & White, D. K. (1991). *Color atlas of clinical oral pathology*. Philadelphia, PA: Lea & Febiger. Used with permission.)

tachypnea and auditory wheezes, dyspnea, retractions, and use of accessory muscles of respiration.

Assessment for Signs of Infection

The nurse notes any signs of infection (erythema, warmth, tenderness, drainage). The patient's temperature is recorded, and the patient is observed for chills and sweating. Fever often accompanies infection.

Assessment of the Lymph Nodes

The lymph nodes and thyroid are palpated for enlargement. If palpable nodes are detected, their location, size, consistency, and reports of tenderness on palpation are noted. Lymphadenopathy indicates activation of the immune system against pathogens. Generalized lymphadenopathy, which is manifested by swollen lymph nodes in multiple sites, is often one of the first signs of infection with HIV.

Assessment of the Joints

Joints are assessed for tenderness, swelling, increased warmth, and limited range of motion. These findings indicate inflammation and infiltration by leukocytes, including macrophages and cytokines.

Diagnostic Evaluation

The nurse needs to be aware that patients undergoing evaluation for possible immune system disorders experience not only physical pain and discomfort with certain types of diagnostic procedures but also many psychological reactions. For example, patients may fear test results that demonstrate decreased immune function because the diminished immune system can make them more prone to certain infections, cancers, and other disorders. It is the nurse's role to counsel, educate, and support patients throughout the diagnostic process. Further, many patients may be extremely anxious about the results of diagnostic tests and the possible implications of those results for their employment, insurance, and personal relationships. This is an ideal time for the nurse to provide counseling and education, should these interventions be warranted.

Immune Competence Testing

A series of blood and skin tests and a bone marrow biopsy may be performed to evaluate the patient's immune competence. Specific laboratory and diagnostic tests are discussed in greater detail along with individual disease processes in subsequent chapters in this unit. Selected laboratory and diagnostic tests used to evaluate immune competence are summarized in Box 36-5.

Allergy Testing

Diagnostic evaluation of the patient with allergic disorders commonly includes blood tests, smears of body secretions (nasal, conjunctival, or sputum secretions), skin tests (intradermal injections of solutions at several sites that may provoke an allergic response), and the radioallergosorbent test (RAST). Many health organizations recommend that RAST be phased out in favor of more sensitive tests such as fluorescence enzyme-labeled assays.

Results of laboratory blood studies provide supportive data for various diagnostic possibilities; however, they are not the major criteria for the diagnosis of allergic disease.

> **! Nursing Alert**
> *With allergic condition, the WBC count is usually normal, except with infection. Eosinophils, which are granular leukocytes, normally make up 1% to 3% of the total number of WBCs. A level between 5% and 15% is nonspecific but suggests an allergic reaction. Moderate eosinophilia is defined as 15% to 40% eosinophils and is found in patients with allergic disorders; in patients with malignancy, immunodeficiencies, parasitic infections, or congenital heart disease; and in patients receiving peritoneal dialysis. Severe eosinophilia is defined as 50% to 90% eosinophils and is found in patients with the idiopathic hypereosinophilic syndrome.*

Skin Tests

If a skin test is indicated, there is a reasonable suspicion that a specific allergen is producing symptoms in an allergic patient. However, several precautionary steps must be observed before skin testing with allergens is performed:

- Testing is not performed during periods of bronchospasm.
- Epicutaneous tests (scratch or prick tests) are performed before other testing methods in an effort to minimize the risk of systemic reaction.
- Emergency equipment must be readily available to treat anaphylaxis.

Methods of **skin testing** include prick skin tests, scratch tests, and intradermal skin testing. After negative prick or scratch tests, intradermal skin testing is performed with allergens that are suggested by the patient's history to be problematic. The back is the most suitable area of the body for skin testing because it permits the performance of many tests. The multitest applicator is a commercially available device with multiple test heads that allows simultaneous administration of antigens by multiple punctures at different sites. A negative response on a skin test cannot be interpreted as an absence of sensitivity to an allergen. Such a response may occur with insufficient sensitivity of the test or with use of an inappropriate allergen in testing. Therefore, it is essential to observe the patient undergoing skin testing for an allergic reaction, even if the previous response was negative.

The results of skin tests complement the data obtained from the history. They indicate which of several antigens are most likely to provoke symptoms and provide some clue to

Selected Tests for Evaluating Immunologic Status

Various laboratory tests may be performed to assess activity or dysfunction of the immune system. The studies assess leukocytes and lymphocytes, humoral immunity, cellular immunity, phagocytic cell function, complement activity, hypersensitivity reactions, specific antigen–antibodies, or HIV infection.

Leukocyte and Lymphocyte Tests
- White blood cell count and differential
- Bone marrow biopsy

Humoral (Antibody-Mediated) Immunity Tests
- B-cell quantification with monoclonal antibody
- In vivo immunoglobulin synthesis with T-cell subsets
- Specific antibody response
- Total serum globulins and individual immunoglobulins (by electrophoresis, immunoelectrophoresis, single radial immunodiffusion, nephelometry, isohemagglutinin techniques)

Cellular (Cell-Mediated) Immunity Tests
- Total lymphocyte count
- T-cell and T-cell subset quantification with monoclonal antibody
- Delayed hypersensitivity skin test
- Cytokine production
- Lymphocyte response to mitogens, antigens, and allogenic cells
- Helper and suppressor T-cell functions

Phagocytic Cell Function Tests
- Nitroblue tetrazolium reductase assay

Complement Component Tests
- Total serum hemolytic complement
- Individual complement component titrations
- Radial immunodiffusion
- Electroimmunoassay
- Radioimmunoassay
- Immunonephelometric assay
- Immunoelectrophoresis

Hypersensitivity Tests
- Scratch test
- Patch test
- Intradermal test
- Radioallergosorbent test (RAST)
- Immunofluorescence

Specific Antigen–Antibody Tests
- Radioimmunoassay
- Immunofluorescence
- Agglutination
- Complement fixation test

HIV Infection Tests
- Enzyme-linked immunosorbent assay (ELISA)
- P24 antigen test
- Western blot, replaced by the fourth generation antigen/antibody tests
- CD4 and CD8 cell counts
- Polymerase chain reaction (PCR)

the intensity of the patient's sensitization. Also the dosage of the antigen (allergen) injected is important. Most patients are hypersensitive to more than one allergen. Under testing conditions, they may not react (although they usually do) to the specific allergens that induce their attacks.

Familiarity with and consistent use of a grading system with skin tests are essential. The grading system used should be identified on a skin test sheet for later interpretation. A positive reaction, evidenced by the appearance of an urticarial wheal (round, reddened skin elevation) (Fig. 36-9), localized **erythema** (diffuse redness) in the area of inoculation or contact, or pseudopodia (irregular projection at the end of a wheal) with associated erythema is considered indicative of sensitivity to the corresponding antigen.

False-negative results may occur because of improper technique, outdated allergen solutions, or prior use of medications that suppress skin reactivity. Corticosteroids and antihistamines, including over-the-counter allergy medications, suppress skin test reactivity and usually are withheld for 48 to 96 hours before testing, depending on the duration of their activity. False-positive results may occur because of improper preparation or administration of allergen solutions.

Interpretation of positive or negative skin tests must be based on the history, physical examination, and other laboratory test results. The following guidelines are used for the interpretation of skin test results:

- Skin tests are more reliable for diagnosing atopic sensitivity in patients with allergic rhinoconjunctivitis (nasal congestion, runny nose, postnasal drip, sneezing, red eyes [conjunctivitis], and itching of the nose or eyes) than in patients with asthma.
- Positive skin tests correlate highly with food allergy.
- The use of skin tests to diagnose immediate hypersensitivity to medications is limited because usually metabolites of medications, not the medications themselves, are responsible for causing hypersensitivity.

In cases of doubt about the validity of the skin tests, an RAST or a provocative challenge test may be performed.

Radioallergosorbent Testing
Radioallergosorbent testing (RAST) is a radioimmunoassay that measures allergen-specific IgE in the patient's blood. In addition to detecting an allergen, RAST indicates

FIGURE 36-9 Interpretation of reactions: Negative = wheal soft with minimal erythema. 1+ = wheal present (5 to 8 mm) with associated erythema. 2+ = wheal (7 to 10 mm) with associated erythema. 3+ = wheal (9 to 15 mm) with slight pseudopodia possible with associated erythema. 4+ = wheal (12 mm+) with pseudopodia and diffuse erythema.

Negative wheal

1+ wheal

2+ wheal

3+ wheal

4+ wheal

the quantity of allergen necessary to evoke an allergic reaction. Values are reported on a scale from 0 to 5. Values of 2 or greater are considered significant. The major advantages of RAST over other tests include decreased risk of systemic reaction, stability of antigens, and lack of dependence on skin reactivity modified by medications. The major disadvantages include limited allergen selection and reduced sensitivity compared with intradermal skin tests, lack of immediate results, and higher cost. RAST is being replaced by the more sensitive fluorescence enzyme-labeled assays such as ImmunoCAP, a quantitative test for IgE proteins.

Provocative Testing

Provocative testing involves the direct administration of the suspected allergen to the sensitive tissue, such as the conjunctiva, nasal or bronchial mucosa, or GI tract (by ingestion of the allergen), with observation of target organ response. This type of testing is helpful in identifying clinically significant allergens in patients who have a large number of positive tests. Major disadvantages of this type of testing are the limitation of one antigen per session and the risk of producing severe symptoms, particularly bronchospasm, in patients with asthma.

CHAPTER REVIEW

Critical Thinking Exercises

1. A 36-year-old man was camping and hiking with his partner when he began to run a high temperature and developed a nonproductive cough. He is diagnosed with *Pneumocystis* pneumonia (PCP) and started on antibiotic therapy. He asks why he has developed this problem. How would you respond? What diagnostic tests would you expect to be ordered? Why?

2. A 68-year-old woman is hospitalized for a kidney transplantation, and immunosuppressant medications are prescribed. Describe the parameters you would use to assess her immune function. How would altered immune function affect the care that you provide?

NCLEX-Style Review Questions

1. In which stage of the immune response does the antibody of the humoral response or the cytotoxic (killer) T cell of the cellular response reach and connect with the antigen on the surface of the foreign pathogen?
   a. Recognition stage
   b. Proliferation stage
   c. Response stage
   d. Effector stage

2. A patient is exhibiting anaphylaxis after eating shellfish. What type of reaction is the patient experiencing?
   a. Type I
   b. Type II
   c. Type III
   d. Type IV

3. Disorders of the immune system may stem from excesses or deficiencies of immunocompetent cells, alterations in the functions of these cells, immunologic attack on self-antigens, or inappropriate or exaggerated responses to specific antigens. Which type of immune system disorder is characterized by an overproduction of immunoglobulins?
   a. Autoimmunity
   b. Gammopathies
   c. Hypersensitivity
   d. Secondary immune deficiency

4. A patient is being seen in the dermatology clinic to have allergy testing performed. What statement is accurate regarding this type of testing?
   a. A positive reaction is evidenced by the appearance of an urticarial wheal.
   b. The arms are the most suitable area of the body for skin testing.
   c. A negative response can be interpreted as an absence of sensitivity to an allergen.
   d. There is no risk of a false-negative result.

5. A patient has requested to be tested for an HIV infection. What test might be performed on this patient?
   a. Bone marrow biopsy
   b. Agglutination
   c. Scratch test
   d. ELISA for specific antibodies

Try these additional resources, available at **http://thepoint.lww.com/Honan2e**, to enhance your learning and understanding of this chapter:
- NCLEX-Style Student Review Questions
- Journal Articles

REFERENCES AND SELECTED READINGS

References and selected readings associated with this chapter can be found on the website that accompanies the book. Visit **http://thepoint. lww.com/Honan2e** to access the references and other additional resources associated with this chapter.

Nursing Management: Patients with Immunodeficiency, HIV Infection, and AIDS

Mary E. Bartlett

Learning Objectives

After reading this chapter, you will be able to:

1. Describe the basic aspects of primary immunodeficiency.
2. Describe the essential aspects of secondary immunodeficiency.
3. Summarize the epidemiology of HIV infection and AIDS.
4. Explain the gerontologic considerations of HIV/AIDS in the United States.
5. Describe the pathophysiology, modes of transmission, and prevention of HIV infection.
6. Explain postexposure prophylaxis for health care workers.
7. Explain pre-exposure prophylaxis for patients at high risk.
8. Summarize the clinical manifestations, assessment, and treatment of patients of HIV infection.
9. Use the nursing process as a framework for care of the patient with AIDS.

Nurses have been at the forefront of caring for patients with human immunodeficiency virus (HIV) even before the cause and infectious nature of the virus was known. Today, nurses work as clinicians, researchers, patient advocates, and educators. Certification for registered nurses and advanced practice nurses is offered through the HIV/AIDS Nursing Certification Board (HANCB). Certification is highly valued and provides formal recognition of HIV/AIDS nursing knowledge. Through the concerted effort of policy makers, researchers, and clinicians developing best practices and strategies, nursing is in a unique position to meet the challenges of HIV care. Because the field of HIV nursing and medicine changes rapidly, readers should refer to the most recent guidelines and recommendations at www.iasusa.org.

Immunodeficiency, or the inability for the body's natural defenses to protect itself from outside pathogens, presents in one of its most complicated forms in patients with the infection that causes **acquired immunodeficiency syndrome (AIDS)**.

PRIMARY AND SECONDARY IMMUNODEFICIENCIES

Immunodeficiencies are classified as either primary or secondary and are further classified by the affected components

of the immune system. Primary immunodeficiency diseases are genetic in origin and manifest most commonly in infancy and childhood as abnormally recurrent infections. About 80% of the patients with primary immunodeficiency are less than 20 years of age. Many primary immunodeficiencies may occur alone or as part of a syndrome. More than 250 have been described that affect different components of the immune system. Transmission of these inborn errors is predominantly X-linked; therefore, more than 70% of affected patients are male. Primary immunodeficiencies, classified by the main component of the immune system that is dysregulated, include B lymphocytes (or IgG), T lymphocytes, natural killer (NK) cells, phagocytic cells, or complement proteins. More than 50% of primary immunodeficiency is caused by errors in B lymphocytes, causing decreases in production of immunoglobulin and antibodies. The most common B-cell disorder is selective IgA deficiency (Stiehm, 2014).

In contrast, secondary immunodeficiencies affect the normal immune system of the patient, resulting in increased susceptibility to infection and certain types of cancer. Extrinsic and intrinsic factors, such as nonimmune systemic disorders like HIV infection, immunosuppressive therapy, prolonged illness or hospitalization, and aging, trigger secondary immunodeficiency. These factors cause impaired immune response through loss or destruction of lymphocytes, such as

CD4 cell depletion, or decreased production of lymphocytes, as in the effects of irradiation on bone marrow lymphocyte production (Stiehm, 2014). Patients with immunosuppression from secondary immunodeficiencies are referred to as *immunocompromised hosts*. The most common secondary immunodeficiency is AIDS.

HUMAN IMMUNODEFICIENCY VIRUS AND ACQUIRED IMMUNODEFICIENCY SYNDROME

The Centers for Disease Control and Prevention (CDC) estimate that more than 1.2 million people are living with HIV/AIDS in the United States. The CDC estimates that there were 44,000 new infections in 2014 with a decline of 19% in new diagnoses since 2005. Worldwide, there were 2 million new cases of HIV in 2014. In 2015, UNAIDS/WHO estimated that 36.9 million people are living with HIV/AIDS in the world, and nearly half of those people have access to highly active antiretroviral (ARV) treatment (HAART). While many advances have been made in the treatment and long-term survival of people living with HIV/AIDS, new infections continue. One in eight people infected with HIV is unaware of the diagnosis; these patients are the ones responsible for transmitting most new infections. The recommendation by the CDC is for universal testing for all people between 13 and 64 years of age to lead to early diagnosis and treatment of people infected with HIV and to slow the rate of new infections in the United States (CDC, 2016a).

Epidemiology

The earliest confirmed case of HIV infection was found in blood drawn from an African man in 1959. Most theories about the origin and spread of AIDS point to a mutated simian immunodeficiency virus (SIV) that crossed species to humans, similar to the changes seen with bird and swine influenza viruses today (AVERT, 2016). An analysis of people with a diagnosis of HIV infection by race/ethnicity and risk factor underscores the disproportionate impact of HIV among communities of color and men who have sex with other men (MSM) of all races. In the United States, new infection rates by race/ethnicity show that nearly half of the cases (49%) are African American. Although African Americans make up only 12% of the population of the 34 states surveyed, their rate of HIV infection is 60% higher than that of Caucasians. While the rate of new diagnosis among African-American women fell by 42% since 2005, new diagnosis among African-American men increased by 22% during that same time period. By transmission category, MSM continues to account for the largest number of diagnoses overall, rising to 67% of newly diagnosed cases (CDC, 2014).

Worldwide, AIDS kills more than 1.1 million people every year, and 75% of those deaths occur in sub-Saharan Africa (UNAIDS, 2015). Since the beginning of the epidemic, 15 million children have been orphaned due to AIDS. In sub-Saharan Africa during 2014, there were 190,000 new infections among children. During that same time period, less than 500 children in Europe and the United States were infected; the difference is related directly to a mother's access to ART during pregnancy (UNAIDS, 2015).

New research finds that many patients live longer due to the use of ARV agents but are increasingly susceptible to age-associated non-AIDS diseases. The mechanism suspected is a chronic inflammatory process caused by HIV or the long-term use of ARV medications. In resource-rich countries, such as the United States, the epidemic has changed to one in which patients who are motivated can achieve long-term, if not lifelong, suppression of the virus with safe and tolerable medications. Patients who access and adhere to therapy rarely suffer AIDS-related complications. More likely, these patients will have many non–AIDS-defining cancers, cardiovascular disease, kidney disease, osteopenia/osteoporosis, liver failure, frailty, and neurologic decline. These normal age-related processes occur sooner and more severely in patients infected with HIV (National Institute on Aging [NIA], 2015).

Gerontologic Considerations

Of the 47,000 patients newly diagnosed with HIV infections in 2013, more than 18% of these were over 50 years of age. HIV infection in middle-aged and older populations may be underreported and underdiagnosed because health care professionals erroneously believe that older adults are not at risk for HIV infection. In addition, HIV-related dementia in the older adult may mimic Alzheimer disease and may be misdiagnosed.

In fact, several factors put older adults at risk for HIV infection:

- Older adults recently widowed or divorced are dating again and may not be aware of the risks of HIV infection.
- Many older adults are sexually active but do not use condoms, viewing them only as a means of unneeded birth control.
- Older adults may be IV/injection drug users.
- Older adults may have received HIV-infected blood through transfusions before 1985.
- Normal age-related changes include a reduction in immune system function, which puts the older adult at greater risk for infections, cancers, and autoimmune disorders. Many older adults also experience the loss of loved ones, resulting in depression and bereavement, factors that are associated with depressed immune function.

Physical and mental stress of long-term caregiving and the number of comorbidities are significant predictors of the adequacy of social support in older adults with HIV.

Transmission

HIV is a bloodborne, sexually transmissible virus. **HIV-1** is transmitted in body fluids containing HIV or infected

CD4$^+$ T lymphocytes. These fluids include blood, seminal fluid, vaginal secretions, amniotic fluid, and breast milk. Mother-to-child transmission of HIV-1 may occur in utero or through breastfeeding, but most perinatal infections are thought to occur after exposure during delivery (CDC, 2016a). Inflammation and breaks in the skin or mucosa result in the increased probability of exposure to HIV. HIV is not transmitted through casual contact. Because HIV is harbored within lymphocytes, a type of white blood cell (WBC), any exposure to infected blood results in a significant risk of infection. The amount of virus and infected cells in the body fluid, as well as other host factors, is associated with the risk of new infection after exposure to that fluid.

Transfusion of blood and blood products can transmit HIV to recipients. However, the risk associated with transfusions has been virtually eliminated because of voluntary self-deferral, completion of a detailed health history, extensive testing, heat treatment of clotting factor concentrates, and more effective methods of virus inactivation. Donated blood is tested for antibodies to HIV-1, **HIV-2**, and p24 antigen (an early marker for HIV infection); in addition, since 1999, nucleic acid amplification testing (NAAT) has been performed (CDC, 2015). However, blood donated during the **window period** after infection is highly infectious even though it tests negative for HIV antibodies. The window period is the period between initial infection with HIV and development of a positive antibody test for HIV. Development of a positive HIV antibody test generally occurs within 4 weeks and, with few exceptions, by 6 months (Sax, Cohen, & Kuritzkes, 2014).

Until an effective vaccine is developed, preventing HIV by eliminating or reducing risky behaviors is essential (Box 37-1). Primary prevention efforts through effective educational programs are vital for control and prevention. As noted earlier, HIV is not transmitted by casual contact.

Prevention and Education

To reduce further the incidence of HIV infection, the CDC announced a new initiative, Advancing HIV Prevention (AHP), in 2003. This initiative comprises four strategies: making HIV testing a routine part of medical care, implementing new models for diagnosing HIV infections outside medical settings, preventing new infections by working with HIV-infected people and their partners, and further decreasing perinatal transmission of HIV (CDC, 2007).

BOX 37-1

Risk Behaviors Associated with HIV Infection and AIDS

- Sharing injection drug use equipment (aka "works")
- Having sexual relations with infected individuals (both male and female)
- People who received HIV-infected blood or blood products (especially before blood screening was instituted in 1985)
- Infants born to mothers with HIV infection not taking ART medication

---

BOX 37-2

Health Promotion

Safer Sexual Behaviors

- Encourage patients to be tested for HIV.
- Advise patients to abstain from sharing sexual fluids.
- Advise patients to reduce the number of sexual partners to one.
- Encourage patients to use latex condoms always. If the patient is allergic to latex, polyurethane condoms should be used.
- Advise patients to avoid using cervical caps or diaphragms without using a condom as well.
- Recommend patients always use dental dams for oral–genital or anal stimulation.
- Advise patients to use water-based lubricants to decrease condom breakage.
- Advise patients to avoid anal intercourse because this practice may injure tissues.
- Advise patients to avoid manual–anal intercourse.
- Encourage patients not to ingest urine or semen.
- Educate patients about nonpenetrative sexual activities, such as body massage, social kissing (dry), mutual masturbation, fantasy, and sex films.
- Advise patients to avoid sharing needles, razors, toothbrushes, sex toys, or blood-contaminated articles.
- Encourage patients who are HIV-positive to inform previous, present, and prospective sexual and drug-using partners of their HIV-positive status. If the patient is concerned for his or her safety, advise the patient that many states have anonymous partner notification programs through the public health department to notify people who have been exposed to HIV.
- Advise HIV-positive patients to avoid donating blood, plasma, body organs, or sperm.

Initiation of effective educational programs educates the public regarding safer sexual practices and decreases the risk of transmitting HIV-1 infection to sexual partners (Box 37-2). Other than abstinence, consistent and correct use of condoms is the only method proven to decrease the risk for sexual transmission of HIV infection (see Chapter 35, Box 35-3, Fig. 35-1). Latex condoms should be used during vaginal or anal intercourse. Nonlatex condoms made of natural materials, such as lambskin, are available for people with latex allergy but will not protect against HIV infection. Condoms made from polyurethane provide comparable protection against STDs and HIV to latex condoms (CDC, 2015). A condom should be used for oral contact with the penis, and a dental dam (a piece of latex used by dentists to isolate a tooth for treatment) should be used for oral contact with the vagina or rectum.

The use of a microbicide, nonoxynol-9 (N-9), was widely advocated to reduce the risk of HIV infection until a clinical trial conducted in almost 1,000 female commercial sex workers in African countries revealed that those who used N-9 intravaginally along with condoms were 50% more likely to be infected with HIV than those who did not use the N-9 gel. Based on these results, it is now recommended that intravaginal application of N-9 not be used as a means of HIV prevention. Further research throughout the world continues to investigate the use of other microbicides, especially since the female sex partner controls its use. The challenge lies in developing a microbicide that is antiviral yet not irritating to the genital mucosa.

Other topics important in preventive education include the importance of avoiding sexual practices that might cut or tear the lining of the rectum, penis, or vagina, and avoiding sexual contact with multiple partners or people who are known to be HIV-positive or IV/injection drug users. In addition, people who are HIV-positive or who use injection drugs should be instructed not to donate blood or share drug equipment with others.

Increasingly, needle exchange programs are available so that IV/injection drug users can obtain sterile drug equipment at no cost. Extensive research has demonstrated that needle exchange programs do not promote increased drug use; in fact, they have been found to decrease the incidence of blood-borne infections in people who use IV/injection drugs (Des Jarlais, Kerr, Carrieri, Feelemyer, & Arasteh, 2016). In the absence of needle exchange programs, IV/injection drug users should be instructed on methods to clean their syringes and advised to avoid sharing cotton and other drug use equipment. Drug users interested in treatment programs should be referred to those programs.

Pre-exposure prophylaxis (PrEP), when taken consistently, has been shown in several clinical trials to reduce the rate of transmission of HIV up to 92%. A combination pill of tenofovir and emtricitabine is taken daily to prevent HIV infection among people whose behavior may increase their risk of exposure through sex or injection drug use. This regimen has shown efficacy and safety for people at substantial risk of acquiring HIV infection. However, people on PrEP must commit to medication adherence and regular follow-up with their health care provider (CDC, 2015).

Nursing Alert

Due to the rapidly changing and evolving guidelines for HIV care, it is essential to access reliable Internet resources. As this book is going to press, clinical evidence demonstrates that durable undetectable viral load translates into effectively no risk of transmission of HIV. This is based on years of cohort studies of serodiscordant couples where the HIV positive partner maintains an undetectable viral load, non-adherence to condom use and no infection of the HIV negative partner. Durably undetectable viral load is defined as at least 6 months of undetectable viral loads after starting medications.

Related Reproductive Education

Because HIV infection in women often occurs during the childbearing years, family planning issues need to be addressed. Attempts to achieve pregnancy by couples in which only one partner has HIV, referred to as serodiscordant, exposes the unaffected partner to the virus. Efforts at artificial insemination using processed semen from an HIV-infected partner are underway. At a fertility clinic in Italy, 3,000 successful pregnancies occurred within serodiscordant couples in whom the male partner was HIV-positive through sperm washing. Women who are HIV-positive and considering pregnancy need to have adequate information about the risks for transmitting HIV infection to their partner and their future children and about the benefits of taking ART agents to reduce perinatal HIV transmission. The desire of women who are HIV-positive to bear children is strong, despite health risks to these women, their children, and society in general (Mabileau et al., 2015). Due to effective ARV medications and universal testing of pregnant women and newborns in the United States, mother-to-child transmission rates have dropped dramatically. Women who are HIV-positive should be instructed not to breastfeed their infants because HIV is transmitted through breast milk. The use of medications coupled with women not breastfeeding has allowed the risk of transmission of HIV from mother to child to drop from 25% to less than 1% in the Western world (Mabileau et al., 2015).

Certain contraceptive methods may pose additional health risks for women. The message to women must be that contraception and prevention of HIV or other sexually transmitted infections (STIs) are two separate considerations. Estrogen and progesterone may increase a woman's risk for HIV infection through changes in the cervical mucosa. In addition, women infected with HIV who use estrogen oral contraceptives have shown increased shedding of HIV in vaginal and cervical secretions putting her partner at increased risk for HIV transmission in serodiscordant couples. The female condom (see Chapter 35, Fig. 35-1) is as effective in preventing pregnancy as other barrier methods, such as the diaphragm and the male condom. Unlike the diaphragm, the female condom also is effective in preventing the transmission of HIV infection and STIs. The female condom has the distinction of being the first barrier method that can be controlled by the woman.

Postexposure Prophylaxis

Standard Precautions

In 1996, the CDC and its Hospital Infection Control Practices Advisory Committee (HICPAC) developed guidelines to reduce the risk for exposure of health care workers to HIV through the development of Standard Precautions. Standard Precautions incorporate the major features of Universal Precautions (designed to reduce the risk of transmission of blood-borne pathogens) and Body Substance Isolation (designed to reduce the risk of transmission of pathogens from moist body substances); these standards are applied to all patients in health care facilities regardless of their diagnosis or presumed infectious status (Box 37-3). Standard Precautions apply to blood; all body fluids, secretions,

BOX 37-3 **Standard Precautions**

The following guidelines prevent the transmission of infection during patient care for all patients, regardless of known or unknown infectious status. Barrier protection should be used at all times to prevent contamination of the skin and mucous membrane with blood, body fluids containing visible blood, or other body fluids (cerebrospinal, synovial, pleural, peritoneal, pericardial, and amniotic fluids, as well as semen and vaginal secretions). Barrier protection should be used with *all* tissues. The type of barrier protection used should be appropriate for the type of procedures being performed and the type of exposure anticipated. Examples of barrier protection include disposable laboratory coats, gloves, and eye and face protection. Private rooms and rooms specially equipped with ventilation systems should be used as indicated.

- **Protective body clothing**, such as disposable laboratory coats, should be worn whenever there is a potential for splashing of blood or body fluids:
  - Wear a clean, nonsterile gown to protect the skin and prevent soiling of clothing during procedures and patient care activities that are likely to generate splashes or sprays of blood, body fluids, secretions, or excretions.
  - Remove a soiled gown promptly, avoiding contact with clean clothes, and wash hands/perform hand hygiene to prevent the transfer of microorganisms to other patients or environments.
- Gloves are to be worn when there is a potential for hand or skin contact with blood, other potentially infectious material, or items and surfaces contaminated with these materials.
  - Clean, nonsterile gloves can be used to protect the nurse's hands.
  - Change gloves after contact with materials that may contain a high concentration of microorganisms even when working with the same patient.
  - Remove the gloves promptly after use, and wash hands immediately before touching noncontaminated items and environmental surfaces and before going to another patient.
- Face protection (face shield, mask, and eye protection) should be worn during procedures that are likely to generate droplets of blood or body fluid to prevent exposure to mucous membranes of the mouth, nose, and eyes.
- Environmental control includes the following:
  - Ensure that the hospital has adequate procedures for the routine care, cleaning, and disinfection of environmental surfaces, beds, bed rails, bedside equipment, and other surfaces that are touched frequently.
  - Ensure that procedures are being followed.
  - Advocate for the purchase and correct use of the safest equipment.
- Patient care equipment:
  - Used patient care equipment that is soiled with blood, body fluids, secretions, and excretions should be handled

in a manner that prevents exposure of the skin and mucous membrane, contamination of clothing, and transfer of microorganisms to other patients and the environment.
- Ensure that reusable equipment is not used for the care of another patient until it has been cleaned and reprocessed appropriately.
- Ensure that single-use items are discarded properly.
- Use mouthpieces, resuscitation bags, or other ventilation devices as an alternative to mouth-to-mouth resuscitation methods.
- Used linen that is soiled with blood, body fluids, secretions, and excretions should be handled, transported, and processed in a manner that prevents exposure of the skin and mucous membrane, contamination of clothing, and transfer of microorganisms to other patients and environments.
- **Wash hands** thoroughly and immediately if contaminated with blood, body fluids containing visible blood, or other body fluids to which universal precautions apply:
  - Use soap and water or an antimicrobial agent or waterless antiseptic agent.
  - Wash the hands during procedures for the same patient to prevent cross-contamination of different body sites.
  - Wash the hands and other skin surfaces immediately after gloves are removed.
- **Avoid accidental injuries** that can be caused by needles, scalpel blades, laboratory instruments, and so on when performing procedures, cleaning instruments, handling sharp instruments, disposing of used needles or pipettes, and similar activities. Used needles, disposable syringes, scalpel blades, pipettes, and other sharp items are to be placed in puncture-resistant containers marked with a biohazard symbol for disposal:
  - Use "needleless" systems correctly whenever possible.
  - Never recap used needles or otherwise manipulate them by using both hands or use any technique that involves directing the point of the needle toward any part of the body.
  - Use either a one-handed scoop technique or a mechanical device designed for holding the needle sheath.
  - Do not remove used needles from disposable syringes by hand, and do not bend, break, or otherwise manipulate used needles by hand.
  - Place used disposable syringes and needles, scalpel blades, and other sharp items in appropriate puncture-resistant containers as close as practical to the area in which the items were used.
  - Place reusable syringes and needles in a puncture-resistant container for transport to the reprocessing area.

Adapted from Siegel, J. D., Rhinehart, E., Jackson, M., Chiarello, L., & Health Care Infection Control Practices Advisory Committee. (2007). 2007 Guideline for isolation precautions: Preventing transmission of infectious agents in healthcare settings. *American Journal of Infection Control*, 35(10 Suppl 2), S65–164. Accessed from http://www.cdc.gov/ncidod/dhqp/pdf/guidelines/Isolation2007.pdf

and excretions (except sweat), regardless of whether they contain visible blood; nonintact skin; and mucous membranes (CDC, 2015). The primary purpose of Standard Precautions is to prevent the transmission of nosocomial infection. The first tier, referred to as Standard Precautions, reduces the risk for exposure from all recognized or unrecognized sources of infections in hospitals. New elements, such as Respiratory Hygiene/Cough etiquette, safe injection practices, and the use of masks during catheter placement, effectively address those specific issues centered on patient protection.

Large-scale studies of exposed health care workers continue to be conducted by the CDC and other groups. In November 2000, the Needle-stick Safety and Prevention Act became law, mandating that health care facilities use devices to protect against sharps injuries. A plan of nursing care for a patient with an infectious disease is available online at http://thepoint.lww.com/Honan2e.

Postexposure Prophylaxis for Health Care Providers

Postexposure prophylaxis in response to the exposure of health care personnel to blood or other body fluids reduces the risk for HIV infection. According to the CDC, there have been only 58 confirmed cases of HIV transmission through occupational exposure (CDC, 2014). The CDC recommends that all health care providers who have sustained a significant exposure to HIV be counseled and offered anti-HIV postexposure prophylaxis, if appropriate (Box 37-4). More clinicians are using postexposure prophylaxis for patients exposed to HIV because of high-risk sexual behavior or possible contact through IV/injection drug use. This use of postexposure prophylaxis is controversial because of concern that it may be substituted for safer sex practices and safer IV/injection drug use. Postexposure prophylaxis should not be considered an acceptable method of preventing HIV infection but used for reducing risk after a possible transmission.

The medications recommended for postexposure prophylaxis are those used to treat established HIV infection. Ideally, prophylaxis needs to start immediately after exposure; therapy started more than 72 hours after exposure is thought to offer no benefit due to rapid increases in viral load upon initial infection.

The recommended course of therapy involves taking the prescribed medications for 4 weeks. Those who choose postexposure prophylaxis must be prepared for the side effects of the medications and must be adherent to treatment or face the possible long-term risks due to developing resistance. The cost is also of concern; the average wholesale price of a medication regimen is more than $2,500 (Department of Health and Human Services [DHHS], 2016), in addition to the costs of testing and counseling. Most health care employers and agencies provide access to treatment and medication through Occupational Health Services.

BOX 37-4

Postexposure Prophylaxis for Health Care Providers

If you sustain a puncture injury, such as a needle stick, take the following actions immediately:

- Wash the area thoroughly with soap and water.
- Alert your supervisor/nursing faculty and initiate the injury-reporting system used in the setting.
- Identify the source patient who may need to be tested for HIV, hepatitis B, and hepatitis C. State laws will determine whether written informed consent must be obtained from the source patient before his or her testing. Rapid testing should be used, if possible, if the HIV status of the source patient is unknown because results can be available within 20 minutes.
- Report as quickly as possible to employee health services, the emergency department, or other designated treatment facility. This visit should be documented in the health care worker's confidential medical record.
- Give consent for baseline testing for HIV, hepatitis B, and hepatitis C. Confidential HIV testing can be performed up to 72 hours after the exposure but should be performed as soon as the health care worker can give informed consent for baseline testing.
- Get postexposure prophylaxis for HIV in accordance with CDC guidelines. Start the prophylaxis medications within 2 hours after exposure. Postexposure prophylaxis must be initiated within 72 hours of exposure to be effective. Make sure that you are being monitored for symptoms of toxicity. Practice safer sex until follow-up testing is complete. Continue the HIV medications for 4 weeks.
- Follow up with postexposure testing at 1 month, 3 months, and 6 months.
- Document the exposure in detail for your own records, as well as for the employer.

Pathophysiology

Because HIV infection is an infectious disease, it is important to understand how HIV integrates itself into a person's immune system and how immunity plays a role in the course of infection. This knowledge is also essential for understanding medication therapy and vaccine development.

Viruses are intracellular parasites. HIV belongs to a group of viruses known as **retroviruses**. These viruses carry their genetic material in the form of ribonucleic acid (RNA) rather than deoxyribonucleic acid (DNA). As shown in Figure 37-1, HIV consists of a viral core containing the viral RNA, surrounded by an envelope consisting of protruding glycoproteins (gp). For HIV to enter the targeted cell, the membrane of the viral envelope must be fused with the plasma membrane of the cell, a process mediated by the envelope glycoproteins of HIV and other coreceptors (National Institutes of Health [NIH], 2016).

All viruses target specific cells. Lymphocytes (type of WBC) consist of three major populations: T cells, B cells,

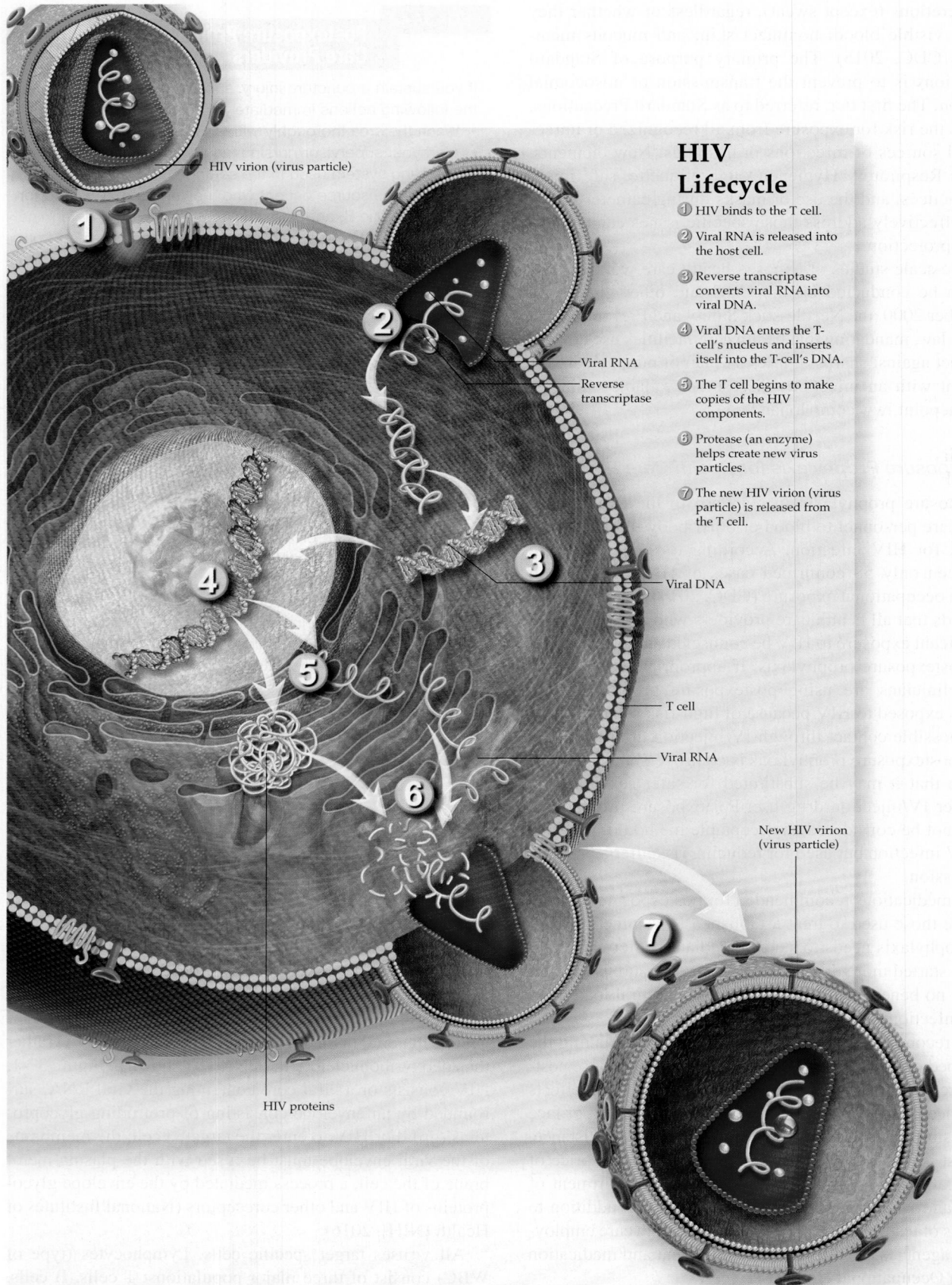

HIV Lifecycle

1. HIV binds to the T cell.

2. Viral RNA is released into the host cell.

3. Reverse transcriptase converts viral RNA into viral DNA.

4. Viral DNA enters the T-cell's nucleus and inserts itself into the T-cell's DNA.

5. The T cell begins to make copies of the HIV components.

6. Protease (an enzyme) helps create new virus particles.

7. The new HIV virion (virus particle) is released from the T cell.

HIV virion (virus particle)

Viral RNA

Reverse transcriptase

Viral DNA

T cell

Viral RNA

HIV proteins

New HIV virion (virus particle)

FIGURE 37-1 HIV life cycle. (Courtesy of Anatomical Chart Company.)

and NK cells. Mature T cells are phenotypically (characteristics of the cells) composed of two major subpopulations, defined by cell surface reciprocal expression of CD4 or CD8. Approximately two thirds of peripheral blood T cells are CD4$^+$, and approximately one third is CD8$^+$. Most people have about 700 to 1,500 CD4$^+$ cells/mm^3, but a count as low as 500 cells/mm^3 can be considered "normal." HIV targets cells with the CD4 glycoprotein expressed on the surface of T lymphocytes, **monocytes**, dendritic cells, and brain microglia. Monocytes and macrophages serve as long-lived reservoirs of HIV. Most primary clinical isolates of HIV use the chemokine coreceptor **CCR5** for cell entry. HIV-1 isolates that appear later in the course of infection often use other chemokine receptors, such as CXCR4, in addition to CCR5 (National Institute of Allergy and Infectious Disease [NIAID], 2016). HIV must attach to both the CD4 and the CCR5 coreceptor binding sites in order to infect CD4$^+$ cells.

A mutation of CCR5 that is common among Caucasians but not other ethnic groups has been identified. About 1% of Caucasians lack functional CCR5 and are highly protected against HIV infection even if exposed (although protection is not absolute); about 18% are not markedly protected against infection but, if infected, demonstrate significantly slower rates of disease progression (Tebas et al., 2014). Reports of a man treated in Berlin, Germany, who received a stem cell transplant for treatment of acute myeloid leukemia from a donor with the Delta 32 mutation at the CCR5 binding site shows promise for further research for HIV treatment. After total intentional destruction of the patient's bone marrow, a procedure with a 30% mortality rate, this patient has had no detectable virus 20 months after transplant and discontinuation of ARV therapy (Symons et al., 2014).

The HIV life cycle is complex (see Fig. 37-1) and consists of the following:

- The HIV gp120 and gp41 attach to the uninfected CD4$^+$ lymphocyte at the CD4 receptor and one of two coreceptors, fusing with the cell membrane.
- The viral core contents are emptied into the host cell, a process known as *uncoating*.
- HIV enzyme **reverse transcriptase** converts the viral genetic material from RNA into double-stranded DNA.
- Double-stranded DNA is spliced into the cellular DNA by the action of integrase, another HIV enzyme.
- During transcription, the integrated DNA or **provirus** makes new viral proteins and viral RNA. Provirus may remain inactive for months to years within the CD4$^+$ cell and other components of the immune system.
- HIV protease cleaves the new proteins (polyproteins).
- The new proteins join the viral RNA into new viral particles.
- New viral particles bud from the cell and start the process all over.

In resting (nondividing) cells, HIV can apparently survive in a latent state as an integrated provirus that produces

TABLE 37-1 Selected Laboratory Tests for Diagnosing and Tracking HIV and Assessing Immune Status

Test	Findings in HIV Infection
Enzyme immunoassay (EIA)	Antibodies are detected, resulting in positive results. May have false-negative results within the window period.
Antigen/antibody	Detects HIV antibodies and p24 antigen; detects early acute infection.
Viral load	Quantifies HIV RNA in the plasma. Monitors efficacy of ART through virologic suppression. Goal is undetectable.
CD4/CD8 ratio	These are markers found on lymphocytes. HIV kills CD4$^+$ cells, which results in a significantly impaired immune system. Used in decision to initiate ART and use of prophylactic medications.

few or no viral particles. These resting CD4$^+$ T cells as well as monocytes and macrophages can be stimulated to produce new particles if something reactivates them. Activation of the infected cell may be achieved by antigens, mitogens, certain cytokines (tumor necrosis factor-α [TNF] or interleukin-1 [IL-1]), or virus gene products of such viruses as **cytomegalovirus** (CMV), Epstein–Barr virus, herpes simplex virus, and hepatitis viruses. Consequently, whenever the infected T cell is activated, HIV replication and budding occur, which often destroys the host cell. Then newly formed HIV is released into the blood plasma and infects other CD4$^+$ cells (see Fig. 37-1). If inadequately suppressed, HIV mutates at a relatively constant rate, enabling it to blunt or completely suppress the effects of HIV medications.

Assessment and Diagnosis

Diagnostic tests are summarized in Table 37-1.

HIV Antibody Tests

Before an HIV antibody test is performed, the meaning of the test and possible test results are explained, and informed consent for the test is obtained from the patient. The CDC recommends universal testing of all patients 13 to 64 years of age through opt-out testing. However, some states still require written informed consent and face-to-face results counseling. Consult state laws about specific requirements related to testing for HIV. When the result of the HIV antibody test is received, it is carefully explained to the patient in private (Box 37-5). All test results are kept confidential. Education and counseling about the test result and about preventing transmission are essential. The

BOX 37-5

HIV Test Results: Implications for Patients

Interpretation of Positive Test Results

- Antibodies to HIV are present in the blood (the patient has been infected with the virus, and the body has produced antibodies).
- HIV is active in the body, and the patient can transmit the virus to others.
- Despite HIV infection, the patient does not necessarily have AIDS.
- The patient is not immune to HIV (the antibodies do not indicate immunity).

Interpretation of Negative Test Results

- Antibodies to HIV are not present in the blood at this time, which can mean that the patient has not been infected with HIV or, if infected, the body has not yet produced antibodies (the patient may be in the window period—usually 4 weeks to 6 months).
- The patient should continue taking precautions. The test result does not mean that the patient is immune to the virus, nor does it mean the patient is not infected; it just means that the body may not have produced antibodies yet. Recommend repeat testing if at high risk for HIV.

patient's psychological response to a seropositive test result may include feelings of panic, depression, and hopelessness. The social and interpersonal consequences of a positive test result can be devastating. The patient may lose his or her sexual partner because of disclosure. The patient may experience discrimination in employment and housing, as well as social ostracism. For these reasons and others, a patient who tests positive may need ongoing counseling, as well as referrals for social, financial, medical, and psychological support services.

Patients whose test results are seronegative may develop a false sense of security, possibly resulting in continued high-risk behaviors or feelings that they are immune to the virus. These patients may need ongoing counseling to help modify high-risk behaviors and to encourage returns for repeated testing. Other patients may experience anxiety regarding the uncertainty of their status.

During initial infection with HIV, the immune system responds by producing antibodies against the virus, usually within 4 to 12 weeks after infection. In 1985, the U.S. Food and Drug Administration (FDA) licensed the first HIV-1 antibody assay that used approximately 5 to 7 mL of blood. The **enzyme immunoassay (EIA)** test, formerly referred to as the enzyme-linked immunosorbent assay (ELISA) test, identifies antibodies directed specifically against HIV. As of 2014, the CDC recommends testing with the newer fourth-generation test for HIV-1 and HIV-2 antibodies and HIV-1 p24 antigen using an immunoassay process. Confirmation testing includes nucleic acid testing (NAT) and no longer utilizes the Western Blot test. This process allows detection of early infections and reduces indeterminate results (CDC, 2014).

Home-based testing for HIV antibodies using a small amount of blood was first proposed in 1985 but was not approved by the FDA until 1995. Although home testing kits are commercially available, they raise concerns because of the lack of counseling and the possibility of inaccurate results, including both false-positive and false-negative results.

Viral Load Tests

Target amplification methods quantify HIV RNA or DNA levels in the plasma and have replaced p24 antigen capture assays. Target amplification methods include reverse transcriptase–**polymerase chain reaction** (RT-PCR) and nucleic acid sequence–based amplification (NASBA). A widely used **viral load test** measures plasma HIV RNA levels. Currently, these tests track viral load and response to treatment of HIV infection. RT-PCR is also used to detect HIV in high-risk seronegative people before antibodies are measurable, to confirm a positive EIA result, and to screen neonates. Viral load is a better predictor of the risk for HIV disease progression than the $CD4^+$ count. The lower the viral load, the longer the time to AIDS diagnosis and the longer the survival time. Increased presence of the virus causes lymphoid dysfunction and other inflammatory responses that affect long-term survival (NIA, 2016).

Stages of HIV Disease

The stage of HIV disease is based on clinical history, physical examination, laboratory evidence of immune dysfunction, signs and symptoms, opportunistic infections, and malignancies. The CDC standard case definition of AIDS categorizes HIV infection and AIDS in adults and adolescents based on clinical conditions associated with HIV infection and $CD4^+$ T-cell counts. The classification system groups clinical conditions into one of three categories, denoted A, B, and C. Each category represents clinical progression of HIV infection in the patient, from asymptomatic (category A) to "full blown" AIDS (category C). Although a patient's health and immune status may improve, the CDC classification of the patient's illness does not change. Universal testing coupled with early diagnosis and treatment attempts to intervene in the natural progression of HIV to maintain as functional an immune system as possible.

Primary Infection (Acute HIV Infection, Acute Retroviral Syndrome)

The period from infection with HIV to the development of antibodies to HIV is known as **primary infection**. This period is characterized by intense viral replication and widespread dissemination of HIV throughout the body. During primary infection, a window period occurs, during which a person with HIV infection tests negative on the HIV antibody blood test. Although antibodies to the HIV envelope glycoproteins typically can be detected in the sera of HIV-infected individuals by 2 to 3 weeks after infection, most of these antibodies lack the ability to inhibit virus infection. By the time neutralizing antibodies can be detected, HIV-1 is firmly established in the host. During this period, there are high levels of viral replication and destruction of $CD4^+$ T cells, resulting in high levels of HIV in the blood and a dramatic drop in $CD4^+$ T-cell counts from the normal range of 500 to 1,500 cells/mm^3 of blood. Detectable levels of virus can occur as early as 72 hours after exposure; this provides the rationale for immediate initiation of prophylaxis.

About 3 weeks into this acute phase, the person may display symptoms similar to mononucleosis, such as fever, enlarged lymph nodes, rash, muscle aches, and headaches. These symptoms resolve within another 1 to 3 weeks as the immune system begins to recuperate. That is, the $CD4^+$ T-cell population responds in ways that cause other immune cells, such as $CD8^+$ lymphocytes, to increase their killing of infected, virus-producing cells. The body produces antibody molecules in an effort to contain the virus; they bind to free HIV particles (outside cells) and assist in their removal. This balance between the amount of HIV in the body and the immune response is referred to as the **viral set point**; it results in a steady state of infection that can last for years.

Primary HIV infection, the time during which the viral burden set point is achieved, includes the acute symptomatic and early infection phases. During this initial stage, viral replication is associated with dissemination in lymphoid tissue (lymph nodes, spleen, tonsils and adenoids, and the thymus) and a distinct immunologic response. The final level of the viral set point is inversely correlated with disease prognosis; that is, the higher the viral set point, the poorer the prognosis. The primary infection stage is part of CDC category A.

HIV Asymptomatic (CDC Category A: More Than 500 CD4$^+$ T Lymphocytes/mm^3)

When a viral set point is reached, a chronic, clinically asymptomatic state begins. Despite its best efforts, the immune system rarely, if ever, fully eliminates the virus. By about 6 months, the rate of viral replication reaches a lower but relatively steady state that is reflected in the maintenance of viral levels at a set point. This set point varies greatly from patient to patient and dictates the subsequent rate of disease progression; on average, 8 to 10 years pass before a major HIV-related complication develops. In this prolonged, chronic stage, patients feel well and have few if any symptoms. Apparent good health continues because $CD4^+$ T-cell levels remain high enough to preserve defensive responses to other pathogens.

HIV Symptomatic (CDC Category B: 200 to 499 CD4$^+$ T Lymphocytes/mm^3)

Over time, the number of $CD4^+$ T cells gradually falls. Category B consists of symptomatic conditions in HIV-infected patients that are not included in the conditions listed in category C. These conditions also must meet one of the following criteria: (1) the condition is due to HIV infection or a defect in cellular immunity, or (2) the condition is considered to have a clinical course or to require management that is complicated by HIV infection.

AIDS (CDC Category C: Fewer Than 200 CD4$^+$ T Lymphocytes/mm^3)

When the $CD4^+$ T-cell level drops below 200 cells/mm^3 of blood, the person has AIDS. As levels decrease to fewer than 100 cells/mm^3, the immune system is significantly impaired. Once a patient has had a category C condition, he or she maintains a permanent diagnosis of AIDS even if the immune system recuperates. This classification has implications for entitlements (i.e., disability benefits, housing, and food stamps) because these programs are often linked to an AIDS diagnosis. Although the revised classification system of the CDC emphasizes $CD4^+$ T-cell counts, it allows for the count of $CD4^+$ T-cells to be expressed as a percentage (percentage of $CD4^+$ T cells compared with total lymphocytes). The $CD4^+$ percentage is less subject to variation on repeated measurements than is the absolute $CD4^+$ T-cell count. A $CD4^+$ percentage of less than 14% of the total lymphocytes is consistent with an AIDS diagnosis. The percentage, as compared with the absolute number of $CD4^+$ T cells, becomes particularly important when the patient has a heightened immune response to infections in addition to HIV.

Clinical Manifestations

During the first stage of HIV infection, the patient may be asymptomatic or may exhibit various signs and symptoms. The patient's health history should alert the health care provider about the need for HIV screening based on the patient's sexual practices, IV/injection drug use, and receipt of blood transfusions. Patients who are in later stages of HIV infection may have a variety of symptoms related to their immunosuppressed state. HIV often causes **opportunistic infections (OIs)**. With widespread availability and improved effectiveness of ARVs, clinical occurrence of OIs has plummeted. OIs and other common manifestations are discussed below.

Respiratory Manifestations

Dyspnea (labored breathing), cough, chest pain, and fever are associated with various OIs, such as those caused by *Pneumocystis jiroveci*, *Mycobacterium avium-intracellulare*, CMV, and *Legionella* species.

Pneumocystic Pneumonia

The most common infection in people with AIDS is *Pneumocystic* pneumonia (PCP). The current guidelines on treatment of OIs (Sax et al., 2014) refer to the causative organism as *P. jiroveci* instead of *P. carinii*, although the infection is still abbreviated as PCP. PCP was one of the first OIs described in association with AIDS, and it is the most common OI resulting in the diagnosis of AIDS. Without prophylactic therapy, 80% of all people infected with HIV will develop PCP.

The clinical presentation of PCP in patients with HIV infection is generally less acute than in people who are immunosuppressed because of other conditions. The time between the onset of symptoms and the actual documentation of disease may be weeks to months. Patients with AIDS initially develop nonspecific signs and symptoms, such as nonproductive cough, fever, chills, dyspnea, and, occasionally, chest pain. PCP may be present despite the absence of crackles. Arterial oxygen concentrations in patients who are breathing room air may be mildly decreased, indicating minimal hypoxemia. Pulse oximetry after exercise, such as walking up and down a flight of stairs is a simple, noninvasive test for outpatient use.

If left untreated, PCP eventually progresses and causes significant pulmonary impairment and respiratory failure. Some patients have a dramatic onset and a fulminating course involving severe hypoxemia, cyanosis, tachypnea, and altered mental status. Respiratory failure can develop within 2 to 3 days after the initial appearance of symptoms.

PCP can be diagnosed definitively by identifying the organism in lung tissue or bronchial secretions. This is accomplished by such procedures as sputum induction, bronchial-alveolar lavage, and transbronchial biopsy (by fiberoptic bronchoscope).

Tuberculosis

Mycobacterium tuberculosis tends to occur in IV/injection drug users and other groups with a pre-existing high prevalence of tuberculosis (TB) infection. TB that occurs late in HIV infection is characterized by the absence of delayed type of hypersensitivity response mediated by T lymphocytes to the tuberculin skin test. This is known as **anergy**, and it occurs because the compromised immune system can no longer respond to the TB antigen. For this reason, TB testing is essential upon initial diagnosis of HIV, with appropriate treatment for patients demonstrating latent TB infection. Nurses administer the Mantoux test to determine infection with TB (refer to Chapter 10 for further discussion). In the later stages of HIV infection, TB may be associated with dissemination to extrapulmonary sites, such as the central nervous system (CNS), bone, pericardium, stomach, peritoneum, and scrotum. Multidrug-resistant strains of the bacillus have emerged and often are associated with a lack of adherence to regimens for antituberculosis medication.

Immune reconstitution syndrome (also known as *paradoxical reactions*) seems to occur more often among patients with TB. Patients can experience high fevers, worsening lymphadenopathy, or transient to severe worsening of pulmonary infiltrates and expanding CNS lesions. Reduction of HIV-1 RNA levels and marked increases in CD4[+] T-lymphocyte counts have been associated with the occurrence of paradoxical

reactions in patients with TB disease or *Mycobacterium avium* complex (MAC). A common mycobacterium, MAC may cause infection in immunosuppressed patients. While affecting the lungs primarily, it can have extrapulmonary impact on the lymph nodes, bones, skin, and other tissues. However, a MAC infection cannot be passed from one person to another. Although the majority of reactions occur within the first few weeks after initiation of ART, some have occurred up to several months after the initiation of TB therapy or ART (Sax et al., 2014).

Gastrointestinal Manifestations

The gastrointestinal (GI) manifestations of AIDS include loss of appetite, nausea, vomiting, oral and esophageal candidiasis, and chronic diarrhea. Diarrhea is a problem in 50% to 90% of all AIDS patients. GI symptoms may be related to the direct effect of HIV on the cells lining the intestines. Some of the enteric pathogens that occur most frequently, identified by stool cultures or intestinal biopsy, are *Cryptosporidium muris, Salmonella* species, *Isospora belli, Giardia lamblia,* CMV, *Clostridium difficile,* and *M. avium-intracellulare.* In patients with AIDS, the effects of diarrhea can be devastating in terms of profound weight loss (more than 10% of body weight), fluid and electrolyte imbalances, perianal skin excoriation, weakness, and inability to perform the usual activities of daily living.

Candidiasis

Candidiasis or *thrush*, a fungal infection, occurs in almost all patients with AIDS and AIDS-related conditions. It commonly precedes other life-threatening infections and is characterized by adherent creamy-white patches in the oral cavity (Fig. 37-2). When left untreated, oral candidiasis progresses to involve the esophagus and stomach. Associated signs and symptoms include difficult, painful swallowing,

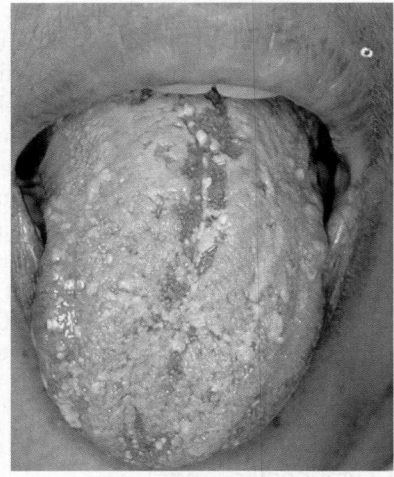

FIGURE 37-2 Oral candidiasis. (From Goodheart, H. P. (2015). Goodheart's photoguide of common skin disorders (4th ed.). Philadelphia, PA: Lippincott Williams & Wilkins.)

and retrosternal pain. Some patients also develop ulcerating oral lesions and are particularly susceptible to dissemination of candidiasis to other body systems.

Wasting Syndrome

Wasting syndrome is part of the category C case definition for AIDS. Diagnostic criteria include profound involuntary weight loss exceeding 10% of baseline body weight and either chronic diarrhea for more than 30 days or chronic weakness and documented intermittent or constant fever in the absence of any concurrent illness that could explain these findings. This protein–energy malnutrition is multifactorial. In some AIDS-associated illnesses, patients experience a hypermetabolic state in which excessive calories are burned and lean body mass is lost. This state is similar to that seen in sepsis or trauma and can lead to organ failure. The distinction between cachexia (wasting) and malnutrition, or between cachexia and simple weight loss, is important because the metabolic derangement seen in wasting syndrome may not be modified by nutritional support alone.

Progressive tissue wasting may occur with only modest GI involvement and without diarrhea. TNF and IL-1 are cytokines that play important roles in AIDS-related wasting syndrome and the inflammatory processes that complicate its course. Both act directly on the hypothalamus to cause anorexia. Cytokine-induced fever accelerates the body's metabolism by 14% for every 1°F increase in temperature. TNF causes inefficient use of lipids by reducing enzymes that are needed for fat metabolism, whereas IL-1 triggers the release of amino acids from muscle tissue. It is believed that infections and sepsis lead to transient increases in TNF, IL-1, and other cell mediators above the chronically elevated levels that often are seen with AIDS (refer to Chapter 54 for discussion of sepsis). These transient increases in TNF and IL-1 trigger muscle wasting. People with AIDS generally experience increased protein metabolism in relation to fat metabolism, which results in significant decreases in lean body mass due to muscle and protein breakdown. Hypertriglyceridemia, seen in people with AIDS and attributed to chronically elevated cytokine levels, can persist for months without tissue wasting and loss of lean body mass. It is also caused by **protease inhibitors** (PIs) and increases the risk for pancreatitis.

Oncologic Manifestations

Patients with AIDS have a higher than usual incidence of cancer, possibly related to HIV stimulation of developing cancer cells or to the immune deficiency that allows cancer-causing substances, such as viruses, to transform susceptible cells into malignant cells. Kaposi sarcoma (KS), certain types of B-cell lymphomas, and invasive cervical carcinoma are included in the CDC classification of AIDS-related malignancies. Carcinomas of the skin, stomach, pancreas, rectum, and bladder also occur more frequently than expected in people with AIDS.

Kaposi Sarcoma

KS, the most common HIV-related malignancy, is a disease that involves the endothelial layer of blood and lymphatic vessels. Since the introduction of ARVs, there has been a significant decrease in the incidence of KS. It is associated with transmission of human herpes virus 8 (HHV-8). Acquired KS occurs in patients who are treated with immunosuppressive agents and commonly in patients who have undergone organ transplantation. In such patients, KS usually resolves once the dose of the immunosuppressive medication is decreased or discontinued. In people with AIDS, epidemic KS is seen most often among male homosexuals and bisexuals. Although the histopathology of all forms of KS is virtually identical, the clinical manifestations differ: AIDS-related KS exhibits a more variable and aggressive course, ranging from localized cutaneous lesions to disseminated disease involving multiple organ systems. Cutaneous signs may be the first manifestation of HIV, appearing in more than 90% of HIV-infected patients as the immune functions deteriorate. These skin signs correlate to low CD4$^+$ counts, usually less than 50. Cutaneous lesions can appear anywhere on the body and are brownish pink to deep purple. They may be flat or raised and surrounded by ecchymoses (hemorrhagic patches) and edema (Fig. 37-3). Rapid development of lesions involving large areas of skin is associated with extensive disfigurement. The location and size of some lesions can lead to venous stasis, lymphedema, and pain. Ulcerative lesions disrupt skin integrity and increase discomfort and susceptibility to infection. The most common sites of visceral involvement are the lymph nodes, GI tract, and lungs. Involvement of internal organs may eventually lead to organ failure, hemorrhage, infection, and death.

Proper identification of these lesions is difficult with darkly pigmented skin; biopsy confirms the diagnosis. Prognosis depends on the extent of the tumor, the presence of other symptoms of HIV infection, and the CD4$^+$ count. Death may result from tumor progression.

FIGURE 37-3 Lesions of AIDS-related Kaposi sarcoma. Whereas some patients may have lesions that remain flat, others experience extensively disseminated, raised lesions with edema.

B-Cell Lymphomas

B-cell lymphomas are the second most common malignancy occurring in people with AIDS. Lymphomas associated with AIDS usually differ from those occurring in the general population. Patients with AIDS are typically much younger than the usual population affected by non-Hodgkin lymphoma. In addition, AIDS-related lymphomas tend to develop outside the lymph nodes, most commonly in the brain, bone marrow, and GI tract. These types of lymphomas are characteristically of a higher grade, indicating aggressive growth and resistance to treatment.

The course of AIDS-related lymphomas includes multiple sites of organ involvement and complications related to OIs. Although aggressive combination chemotherapy is frequently successful in the treatment of non-Hodgkin lymphoma in the patient who is HIV-negative, treatment is less successful in people with AIDS because of severe hematologic toxicity and complications of OIs.

Neurologic Manifestations

An estimated 80% of all patients with AIDS experience some form of neurologic involvement during the course of HIV infection. Many neuropathologic disorders are underreported because patients may have neurologic involvement without overt signs or symptoms. Neurologic complications involve central, peripheral, and autonomic functions. HIV-associated neurocognitive disorders (HAND) can affect memory, attention, language, and executive functioning. Neurologic dysfunction results from direct effects of HIV on nervous system tissue, OIs, primary or metastatic neoplasms, cerebrovascular changes, metabolic encephalopathies, or complications secondary to therapy. Immune system response to HIV infection in the CNS includes inflammation, atrophy, demyelination, degeneration, and necrosis.

HIV Encephalopathy

HIV encephalopathy or HIV-associated dementia (HAD) was formerly referred to as *AIDS dementia complex*. The clinical syndrome is characterized by a progressive decline in cognitive, behavioral, and motor functions. Substantial evidence exists that HIV encephalopathy is a direct result of HIV infection in brain macrophages and microglia. HIV infection is thought to trigger the release of lymphokines and other inflammatory factors that result in cellular dysfunction or interference with neurotransmitter function rather than cellular damage.

Signs and symptoms may be subtle and difficult to distinguish from fatigue, depression, or the adverse effects of treatment for infections and malignancies. Early manifestations include memory deficits, headache, difficulty concentrating, progressive confusion, psychomotor slowing, apathy, and ataxia. Later stages include global cognitive impairments, delay in verbal responses, a vacant stare, spastic paraparesis (a slight weakness or paralysis of both lower extremities), hyperreflexia, psychosis, hallucinations, tremor, incontinence, seizures, mutism, and death.

Confirming the diagnosis of HIV encephalopathy can be difficult. Extensive neurologic evaluation includes a computed tomography (CT) scan, which may indicate diffuse cerebral atrophy and ventricular enlargement. Other tests that may detect abnormalities include magnetic resonance imaging (MRI), analysis of CSF through lumbar puncture, and brain biopsy.

Cytomegalovirus

Retinitis is the most common clinical manifestation of CMV. Before the use of ARVs, 30% of patients experienced CMV retinitis with a high incidence of blindness. The incidence of CMV retinitis has been reduced by 80% with these medications.

Peripheral retinitis might be asymptomatic or present with floaters, scotomata (a loss of vision within the visual field), or reduced visual acuity. CMV retinitis has characteristic fluffy yellow-white retinal lesions with or without intraretinal hemorrhage visualized on funduscopic examination. Blood vessels near the lesions might appear to be sheathed. Patients with CD4+ counts of less than 50 should be examined by an ophthalmologist on a yearly basis (Sax et al., 2014).

Other Neurologic Disorders

Other common infections involving the nervous system include *Toxoplasma gondii, M. tuberculosis*, and syphilis. Additional neurologic manifestations include both central and peripheral neuropathies. Vascular myelopathy is a degenerative disorder that affects the lateral and posterior columns of the spinal cord, resulting in progressive spastic paraparesis, ataxia (inability to coordinate body movements), and incontinence. HIV-related peripheral neuropathy is thought to be a demyelinating disorder. It is associated with pain and numbness in the extremities, weakness, diminished deep tendon reflexes, orthostatic hypotension, and impotence. Peripheral neuropathy is a common adverse effect of many HIV medications.

Depressive Manifestations

The prevalence of depression among people with HIV infection is three times higher than in the HIV-negative population (Mayo, Brouillette, & Fellows, 2016). The causes of depression are multifactorial and may include a history of pre-existing mental illness, neuropsychiatric disturbances, and psychosocial factors. Depression also occurs in people with HIV infection in response to the physical symptoms, including pain and weight loss, as well as isolation. People with HIV/AIDS who are depressed may experience irrational guilt and shame, loss of self-esteem, feelings of helplessness and worthlessness, and suicidal ideation.

Integumentary Manifestations

Cutaneous manifestations are associated with HIV infection and the accompanying OIs and malignancies. KS (described earlier) and OIs, such as herpes zoster and herpes simplex, are associated with painful vesicles that disrupt skin integrity. Molluscum contagiosum is a viral infection characterized by multiple grouped lesions. Seborrheic dermatitis is associated with an indurated, diffuse, scaly rash involving the scalp and face (see Chapter 52). Patients with AIDS also may exhibit a generalized eosinophilic folliculitis associated with dry, flaking skin or atopic dermatitis, such as eczema or psoriasis. Up to 60% of patients treated with trimethoprim-sulfamethoxazole (TMP-SMZ) develop a drug-related rash that is pruritic with pinkish-red macules and papules. Regardless of the origin of these rashes, patients experience discomfort and are at increased risk for additional infection from disrupted skin integrity. See Chapter 51 for how to assess and describe rashes.

Nursing Alert
The viral exanthem associated with acute retroviral syndrome during initial infection with AIDS is one of the few rashes accurately described as maculopapular (flat, erythematous rash on the skin that is covered with small confluent [merging] bumps).

Gynecologic Manifestations

Persistent, recurrent vaginal candidiasis or bacterial vaginosis may be the first sign of HIV infection in women. Past or present genital ulcer disease is a risk factor for the transmission of HIV infection. Women with HIV infection are more susceptible to and have increased rates of incidence and recurrence of genital ulcer disease and venereal warts. Ulcerative STIs, such as chancroid, syphilis, and herpes, are more severe in women with HIV infection. Human papillomavirus (HPV) causes venereal warts and is a risk factor for cervical intraepithelial neoplasia, a cellular change that is frequently a precursor to cervical cancer. Women with HIV are 10 times more likely to develop cervical intraepithelial neoplasia than are those not infected with HIV. HIV-seropositive women with cervical carcinoma present at a more advanced stage of disease and have more persistent and recurrent disease and a shorter interval to recurrence and death than women without HIV infection.

A significant percentage of women who require hospitalization for pelvic inflammatory disease (PID) have HIV infection. Women with HIV are at increased risk for PID, and the associated inflammation may potentiate the transmission of HIV infection (see Chapter 35 for information related to PID). Moreover, women with HIV infection appear to have a higher incidence of menstrual abnormalities, including amenorrhea or bleeding between periods, than do women without HIV infection.

Immunologic Manifestations

Immune reconstitution inflammatory syndromes (IRIS) have been described for mycobacterial infections, including disease caused by MAC and *M. tuberculosis*, PCP, toxoplasmosis, hepatitis B and hepatitis C, CMV infection, varicella-zoster virus infection, cryptococcal infection, and progressive multifocal leukoencephalopathy. Immune reconstitution syndromes are characterized by fever and worsening of the clinical manifestations of the OI, or the appearance of new manifestations developing weeks after the initiation of ART. It is important to determine the absence or reappearance of the underlying OI, new drug toxicity, or a new OI. If the syndrome represents an immune restoration response, adding nonsteroidal anti-inflammatory agents (NSAIDs) or corticosteroids to alleviate the inflammatory reaction is appropriate. The inflammation might take weeks to months to subside (Sax et al., 2014). The nurse should be alert to signs of immune reconstitution syndrome and advise the patient to seek health care if he or she is feeling sicker with no clear explanation.

Medical and Nursing Management
Treatment Regimen

Protocols on treatment of HIV disease change frequently. The U.S. DHHS periodically convenes a team of HIV specialists from across the country to evaluate the latest evidence and make recommendations that are widely disseminated (DHHS, 2016). In general, ARV medications should be offered to all individuals, regardless of CD4 cell count to reduce the morbidity and mortality of HIV infection (DHHS, 2016). In addition, ARV therapy (ART) is recommended to prevent HIV transmission. Even with these overriding recommendations from DHHS, treatment decisions are individualized based on a number of factors, including CD4$^+$ T-cell count, HIV RNA (viral load), severe symptoms of HIV disease or AIDS, and willingness of the patient to adhere to a lifelong treatment regimen. New HIV medications are easier to take, have fewer adverse reactions, and are effective and potent. Monitoring the DHHS website for updates to the recommendations is essential before caring for patients with HIV/AIDS (DHHS, 2016).

ART may be complex, have major side effects, pose difficulties with regard to adherence, and carry serious potential consequences; these include viral resistance resulting from nonadherence to the medication regimen or suboptimal levels of ARV agents. Adherence to ART facilitates long-term success of initial regimens that are easily tolerated and convenient. Poor adherence allows the development of resistance to ART necessitating the use of less tolerable and more complicated regimens. Patient education about adherence continues to be an essential intervention by nurses. The increasing number of ARV agents (Table 37-2) and the rapid evolution of new information have introduced extraordinary complexity into the treatment of HIV infection in the patient with a resistant virus. The goals of treatment include maximal and sustained suppression of viral load, restoration or preservation of immunologic function, improved quality of life, and reduction of HIV-related morbidity and mortality. The DHHS Guidelines recommend viral load testing at the time of diagnosis of HIV

TABLE **37-2** Commonly Used Antiretroviral Agents[a]

Generic Name (Abbreviation) and Trade Names	Food Effect	Adverse Events
Nucleoside Reverse Transcriptase Inhibitors (NRTIs)		
emtricitabine (FTC) Emtriva Truvada (FTC + TDF)	Can be taken without regard to meals	Minimal toxicity; lactic acidosis with hepatic steatosis (rare but potentially life-threatening toxicity with use of NRTIs); combined with tenofovir as part of the PrEP regimen
tenofovir disoproxil fumarate (TDF) Viread Truvada (TDF + FTC)	Can be taken without regard to meals	Asthenia (loss of strength and energy), headache, diarrhea, nausea, vomiting, and flatulence; renal insufficiency; lactic acidosis with hepatic steatosis (rare but potentially life-threatening toxicity with use of NRTIs)
Non-nucleoside Reverse Transcriptase Inhibitors (NNRTIs)		
efavirenz (EFV) Sustiva	High-fat/high-caloric meals increase peak plasma concentrations of capsules by 39% and tablets by 79%; take on an empty stomach.	Rash (rare cases of Stevens–Johnson syndrome have been reported); central nervous system symptoms (dizziness, somnolence, insomnia, abnormal dreams, confusion, abnormal thinking, impaired concentration, amnesia, agitation, depersonalization, hallucinations, and euphoria); increased transaminase levels (ALT/AST or liver enzymes); false-positive cannabinoid test; teratogenic
Protease Inhibitors (PIs)		
atazanavir (ATV) Reyataz	Administration with food increases bioavailability. Should be taken with food; avoid taking with antacids.	Indirect hyperbilirubinemia; prolonged PR interval—some patients experienced asymptomatic first-degree AV block; use with caution in patients with underlying conduction defects or on concomitant medications that can cause PR prolongation; hyperglycemia; fat maldistribution, possible increased bleeding episodes in patients with hemophilia
Fusion Inhibitors		
enfuvirtide (T-20) Fuzeon	Injected subcutaneously	Local injection site reactions—almost 100% of patients (pain, erythema, induration, nodules and cysts, pruritus, ecchymosis); increased rate of bacterial pneumonia; hypersensitivity reaction—symptoms may include rash, fever, nausea, vomiting, chills, rigors, hypotension, or elevated serum liver enzymes
CCR5 Antagonists		
maraviroc (MVC) Selzentry	No food effect; take with or without food.	Abdominal pain; cough; dizziness; musculoskeletal symptoms; pyrexia; rash; upper respiratory infections; hepatotoxicity; orthostatic hypotension
Integrase Inhibitors		
raltegravir (RAL) Isentress	Take with or without food.	Nausea, headache; diarrhea; pyrexia; CPK elevation

[a]Regimens should be individualized based on the advantages and disadvantages of each combination, such as pill burden, dosing frequency, toxicities, drug–drug interaction potential, comorbid conditions, and level of plasma HIV-RNA. Complete listing of medications, adverse effects and patient education available at https://aidsinfo.nih.gov/contentfiles/lvguidelines/adultandadolescentgl.pdf
The nurse is advised to refer to pharmacologic resources for additional information.

disease and every 3 to 4 months thereafter; CD4$^+$ cell counts should be measured at diagnosis and usually every 3 to 6 months thereafter (DHHS, 2016).

Medications
More than 28 approved ARV agents, belonging to 6 classes, are available for the design of combination regimens. Effective regimens contain at least three virologically active medications from at least two classes. The six classes currently approved by the FDA are the

- nucleoside/nucleotide reverse transcriptase inhibitors (NRTIs),
- non-nucleoside reverse transcriptase inhibitors (NNRTIs),
- PIs,

- integrase strand transfer inhibitors (INSTIs),
- CCR5 antagonist, and
- fusion inhibitor (see Table 39-2, [DHHS, 2015]).

Each of these medications attacks HIV at different stages of viral replication in the CD4$^+$ lymphocyte.

As new medications are developed and research is completed, the number and types of recommended drug combinations continue to change (DHHS, 2016). In addition, some pharmaceutical companies have combined two to three agents into one tablet or capsule (such as Kaletra, which is a combination of lopinavir and ritonavir) so that a patient may be taking one tablet or capsule that contains two different medications. With a decrease in the number of tablets or capsules that the patient must take ("pill burden"), the patient is more likely to adhere to prescribed regimens and achieve sustained viral suppression. Efforts are underway to develop additional combinations of ARV medications. The first single tablet for once-a-day use was made available in 2006; Atripla combined Sustiva (efavirenz), Emtriva (emtricitabine), and Viread (tenofovir disoproxil fumarate). Today, there are six of these well-tolerated combination pills available. Simplifying treatment regimens and decreasing the number of medications that must be taken each day increase patients' adherence to therapy (DHHS, 2016).

Adherence

It is difficult to predict which patients will adhere to medication regimens. Adherence rates of 95% minimize the risks of developing a resistant virus. Patients should understand that the first regimen prescribed has the best chance for long-term treatment success with minimal impact on daily functioning and prevention of resistance. Individualized plans of care that take into consideration housing and social support issues, in addition to health indicators, are essential. Adherence to the ART plan involves very complex behavior that can change over the duration of the medication regimen. Self-reported adherence measures can distinguish clinically meaningful patterns of medication-taking behaviors; therefore, nurses should ask patients if they are taking their medications as prescribed. Factors associated with nonadherence include active substance abuse, depression, lack of social support, and treatment fatigue. Gender, race, pregnancy, and history of past substance use have not been associated with nonadherence (DHHS, 2016). Box 37-6 summarizes various strategies that health care providers can use to encourage adherence to the treatment regimen. Every health care encounter should be used as an opportunity to briefly review the treatment regimen and identify any new issues.

Patients who elect to interrupt therapy should be counseled that the HIV viral load would increase, usually to pretreatment levels, resulting in an increased risk for transmission to others during risky behaviors, such as unsafe sex and sharing needles. Because of drug toxicities, drug resistance, quality-of-life issues, and the high cost of medications, some

---

BOX 37-6

Patient Education

Adhering to the Medication Therapy for HIV

With the advent of one daily pill for treatment for most patients, adherence is significantly simplified. To help ensure adherence with more complicated therapy regimens, you need to be able to:

- Correctly identify each medication, preferably by name.
- State the action of each medication.
- State the correct times that medication is to be taken.
- Identify special guidelines to follow when taking medications (e.g., with meals, on an empty stomach, medications that are not to be taken together).
- Demonstrate methods of tracking and storage of the medication regimen and use reminders such as beepers and/or pillboxes.
- Identify specific laboratory tests, such as viral load, that are necessary to monitor the effectiveness of the medication regimen.
- List expected side effects of each medication.
- Identify side effects reportable to health care providers.
- Explain the importance of and necessity for adherence.
- Demonstrate correct administration of intramuscular, subcutaneous, or IV medications.
- Demonstrate correct use and safe disposal of needles, syringes, and other IV equipment.
- Discuss episodes of nonadherence to the medication regimen.

---

patients may choose to take a "drug holiday" or structured treatment interruption. Through an open, honest partnership between the health care provider and the patient, these options can be explored and their effectiveness maximized. Structured intermittent therapy, characterized by alternating short periods on and off medication, appears to be ineffective and may increase mortality.

Evaluation of Therapy

Viral load tests evaluate the results of therapy (DHHS, 2016). Viral load levels should be measured immediately before initiation of ART and again after 2 to 8 weeks. In most patients, adherence to a regimen of potent ARV agents should result in a significant decrease in the viral load by 2 to 8 weeks. The viral load should continue to decline over the following weeks, and, in most individuals, it will drop below detectable levels (currently defined as less than 50 RNA copies/mL) by 16 to 20 weeks. The rate of viral load decline toward undetectable levels is affected by the baseline T-cell count, the initial viral load, the potency of the medication, adherence to the medication regimen, prior exposure to ARV agents, and the presence of any OIs. The confirmed absence of a viral load response in an adherent patient should prompt the health care team to re-evaluate the regimen and check for resistant mutations. The CD4$^+$ count should increase by 100 to 150 cells/mm^3 per year, with an accelerated response in the first 3 months (DHHS, 2016).

FIGURE 37-4 Facial lipoatrophy.

Side Effects

Many of the ARV agents that prolong life may simultaneously cause lipodystrophy syndrome and place the person at risk for early-onset hypercholesterolemia, heart disease, and diabetes. Fat redistribution syndrome, which consists of lipoatrophy (Fig. 37-4), lipohypertrophy, or both in localized areas, is also known as *lipodystrophy syndrome.* This syndrome is one of the most frequent systemic side effects associated with the use of ARV medications, especially PIs, and affects up to 58% of patients (Sax et al., 2014). Many people who have lipodystrophy experience an increase in fat loss in the legs, arms, face, or a buildup of fat around the abdomen and at the base of the neck, or both. Patients also may experience an increase in breast size. All of these adverse effects can have a profound impact on a patient's psychological well-being due to the increased stress of stigmatization.

Facial wasting, characterized as a sinking of the cheeks, eyes, and temples caused by the loss of fat tissue under the skin, may be treated by injectable fillers such as poly-L-lactic acid (Sculptra).

Drug Resistance

Drug resistance can be broadly defined as the ability of pathogens to withstand the effects of medications that are intended to be toxic to them. Resistance develops because of spontaneous genetic mutation of the pathogens or in response to exposure to the medication. Factors associated with the development of drug resistance include serial monotherapy (taking one medication at a time), common during early clinical trials, inadequate suppression of virus replication with suboptimal treatment regimens, difficulty with adherence to complex and toxic regimens, and initiation of therapy late in the course of HIV infection. HIV-1 may find refuge beyond physiologic protective adaptations, such as behind the blood–brain barrier, where diminished drug concentrations in the CNS might induce the development of drug-resistant mutants. HIV-1 persists in lymphoid tissue even in people who appear to have responded well to antiviral therapy, another factor that is limiting discovery of a cure or vaccine for HIV.

Resistance testing has a number of limitations and is more helpful in the elimination of ARV agents rather than in deciding which ones should be used. Deciding whether a medication regimen is effective or ineffective is a complex phenomenon. Some patients demonstrate inconsistent results on virologic, immunologic, and clinical parameters. In general, virologic failure occurs first, followed by immunologic failure, and, finally, by clinical progression. These events may be separated by months to years (DHHS, 2015). Genotypic testing allows detection of amino acid mutations that are either proved or suspected to be associated with phenotypic resistance. Phenotypic testing predicts the susceptibility of resistant virus to inhibition by a particular drug (DHHS, 2016).

In addition to resistance testing, several factors must be considered in choosing medications for a new regimen, once the prior regimen has failed. These factors include the patient's treatment history, viral load, and medication tolerance; the likelihood of the patient's adhering to the medication regimen; and concomitant medical conditions or medications. Resistance testing is of greatest value when it is performed before drugs are discontinued or immediately afterward (within 4 weeks). Most HIV providers perform genotype testing during the initial diagnosis stage as some patients with HIV are infected with a resistant virus. Drug resistance testing is not advised for patients with a viral load of less than 1,000 copies/mL because amplification of the virus is unreliable (DHHS, 2016).

Vaccines

Vaccine research for HIV has two potential areas of application: prevention of new infections and therapy for those already infected with HIV (therapeutic vaccine). Since HIV-1 was discovered, researchers have been working to develop a vaccine. A vaccine is a substance that triggers the production of antibodies to destroy the offending organism. Creation of an HIV vaccine is feasible, but researchers have had difficulty finding an adequate animal model in which to test new vaccines. Because HIV can attack the human immune system as either cell-free or cell-associated virus, a vaccine against HIV must be capable of producing both antibodies and cytotoxic lymphocytes.

Treatment of Opportunistic Infections

Pneumocystis Pneumonia

In the past several years, many advances have been made in the treatment of PCP. TMP-SMZ (Bactrim, Septra), the treatment of choice for PCP in patients with AIDS and in immunocompromised patients without HIV infection, is available in both IV and oral preparations. TMP-SMZ is an antibacterial agent used to treat various organisms causing infection. People with HIV infection who have a T-cell count of less than 200 cells/mm^3 should receive chemoprophylaxis against PCP with TMP-SMZ. PCP prophylaxis can be safely discontinued in patients who are responding to highly active ART (HAART) with a sustained increase in T lymphocytes. TMP-SMZ also confers cross-protection against toxoplasmosis and some common respiratory bacterial infections. Patients with AIDS who are treated with TMP-SMZ experience a high incidence of adverse effects, such as fever, rashes, leukopenia (decreased WBC count), thrombocytopenia (decreased platelet count), and kidney dysfunction. Reintroduction of TMP-SMZ using a gradually increasing dose (desensitization) may be successful in up to 70% of patients (DHHS, 2015).

Pentamidine (Pentacarinat, Pentam 300, NebuPent), an antiprotozoal medication, is used as an alternative agent for combating PCP. Avoid intramuscular administration because of the potential for painful formation of a sterile abscess. In addition, IV pentamidine can cause severe hypotension if it is administered too rapidly. Other adverse effects include impaired glucose metabolism leading to the development of diabetes mellitus from damage to the pancreas, kidney damage, liver dysfunction, and neutropenia. Initially, the success of aerosolized pentamidine led to its use as a treatment for mild to moderate PCP. However, it has proved to be less effective and more costly than TMP-SMZ, and early relapses are common. Because of these limitations, aerosolized pentamidine should not be used (DHHS, 2016).

Mycobacterium Avium Complex

Chemoprophylaxis against disseminated MAC disease is indicated for people infected with HIV whose T-cell count is lower than 50 cells/mm^3. Treatment for MAC infections involves use of either clarithromycin (Biaxin) or azithromycin (Zithromax). Secondary prophylaxis for disseminated MAC may be discontinued in patients who have sustained increases in CD4 counts (at least 100 cells/mm^3) in response to HAART, have completed 12 months of MAC therapy, and have no signs or symptoms attributable to MAC. Primary prophylaxis for disseminated MAC may be discontinued in patients who have responded to HAART with CD4 counts of 100 cells/mm^3 or higher for at least 3 months and may be reintroduced if counts decrease to 50 to 100 cells/mm^3 (DHHS, 2016).

Cytomegalovirus Retinitis

Retinitis caused by CMV is a leading cause of blindness in patients with AIDS. Prophylaxis with oral ganciclovir may be considered for people infected with HIV who have CD4$^+$ T-cell counts of less than 50 cells/mm^3. Two antiviral agents, ganciclovir (DHPG, Cytovene, Vitrasert) and foscarnet (Foscavir), offer effective treatment but not a cure for CMV retinitis. Because ganciclovir and foscarnet do not kill the virus but rather control its growth, they must be taken for

life. Relapse rates associated with the two agents are similar. Discontinuation of the medication is associated with the relapse of retinitis within 1 month.

A common adverse reaction to ganciclovir is severe neutropenia, which limits the concomitant use of zidovudine (AZT, Retrovir). Intravitreal injections of ganciclovir have been effective for patients who cannot tolerate systemic ganciclovir because of severe neutropenia, infection at the venous access site, or the need to take zidovudine. Zidovudine may be given with foscarnet (Foscavir). Common adverse reactions to foscarnet are nephrotoxicity, including acute kidney failure, and electrolyte imbalances, including hypocalcemia, hyperphosphatemia, and hypomagnesemia, which can be life-threatening. Other common adverse effects include seizures, GI disturbances, anemia, phlebitis at the infusion site, and low back pain. Possible bone marrow suppression (producing a decrease in WBC and platelet counts), oral candidiasis, and liver and kidney impairments require close patient monitoring.

Other Infections

Oral acyclovir, famciclovir, or valacyclovir may be used to treat infections caused by herpes simplex or herpes zoster. Patients coinfected with HSV and HIV are more likely to transmit and infect others if not treated for herpes. Esophageal or oral candidiasis is treated topically with clotrimazole (Mycelex) oral troches or nystatin suspension. Chronic refractory candidiasis (thrush) or esophageal involvement is treated with ketoconazole (Nizoral) or fluconazole (Diflucan).

Antidiarrheal Therapy

Although many forms of diarrhea respond to treatment, it is not unusual for this condition to recur and become a chronic problem for the patient with HIV. Therapy with octreotide acetate (Sandostatin), a synthetic analog of somatostatin, has been shown to be effective in managing chronic severe diarrhea. High concentrations of somatostatin receptors have been found in the GI tract and in other tissues. Somatostatin inhibits many physiologic functions, including GI motility and intestinal secretion of water and electrolytes.

Chemotherapy

Kaposi Sarcoma

Usually management of KS is difficult because of the variability of symptoms and the organ systems involved. KS is rarely life-threatening except when there is pulmonary or GI involvement. The treatment goals are to reduce symptoms by decreasing the size of the skin lesions, to reduce discomfort associated with edema and ulcerations, and to control symptoms associated with mucosal or visceral involvement. No one treatment has been shown to increase survival. Localized treatment includes surgical excision of the lesions or application of liquid nitrogen to local skin lesions, and injections of intraoral lesions with dilute vinblastine. Injection of intraoral lesions has been associated with local pain and skin irritation. Radiation therapy is effective as a palliative measure to relieve localized pain due to tumor mass (especially in the legs) and for KS lesions that are in sites such as the oral mucosa, conjunctiva, face, and soles of the feet.

Interferon is known for its antiviral and antitumor effects. Patients with cutaneous KS treated with **alpha-interferon** have experienced tumor regression and improved immune system function. Positive responses have been observed in 30% to 50% of patients, with the best responses seen in those with limited disease and no OIs. Alpha-interferon is administered by the IV, intramuscular, or subcutaneous route. Patients may self-administer interferon at home or receive interferon in an outpatient setting. Rituximab infusions are monoclonal antibodies effective in the treatment of KS and non-Hodgkin lymphoma but may cause a fatal infusion reaction and are administered in the inpatient setting so that the patient can be observed during administration.

Lymphoma

Successful treatment of AIDS-related lymphomas has been limited because of the rapid progression of these malignancies. Combination chemotherapy and radiation therapy regimens may produce an initial response, but it is usually short-lived. Because standard regimens for non-AIDS lymphomas have been ineffective, many clinicians suggest that AIDS-related lymphomas should be studied as a separate group in clinical trials.

Antidepressant Therapy

Treatment for depression in people with HIV infection involves psychotherapy integrated with pharmacotherapy. If depressive symptoms are severe and of sufficient duration, treatment with antidepressants may be initiated. Antidepressants, such as imipramine (Tofranil), desipramine (Norpramin), and fluoxetine (Prozac), may be used because these medications also alleviate the fatigue and lethargy associated with depression. A psychostimulant, such as methylphenidate (Ritalin), may be used in low doses in patients with neuropsychiatric impairment. Electroconvulsive therapy may be an option for patients with severe depression who have not responded to pharmacologic interventions.

Nutrition Therapy

Malnutrition increases the risk for infection and may increase the incidence of OIs. Nutrition therapy should be integrated into the overall management plan and should be tailored to meet the nutritional needs of the patient, whether by oral diet, enteral tube feedings, or parenteral nutritional support, if needed. As with all patients, a healthy diet is essential for the patient with HIV infection. For all patients with AIDS who experience unexplained weight loss, calorie counts should be obtained to evaluate nutritional status and initiate appropriate therapy. The goal is to maintain the ideal weight and, when necessary, to increase weight.

Appetite stimulants have been used successfully in patients with AIDS-related anorexia. Megestrol acetate (Megace), a synthetic oral progesterone preparation used to treat breast cancer, promotes significant weight gain and inhibits cytokine IL-1 synthesis. In patients with HIV infection, it increases body weight primarily by increasing body fat stores. Dronabinol (Marinol), which is a synthetic tetrahydrocannabinol (THC), the active ingredient in marijuana, has been used to relieve nausea and vomiting associated with cancer chemotherapy. Many states now allow the use of medical marijuana for patients who are HIV-positive.

Oral supplements may be used to improve diets that are deficient in calories and protein. Ideally, oral supplements should be lactose-free as many people with HIV infection are lactose intolerant. Parenteral nutrition is the final option because of its prohibitive cost and associated risks, including risk of infections.

Complementary and Alternative Medicine (CAM)

Traditional Western or allopathic medicine focuses on the treatment of disease. These treatments or interventions are taught in medical and nursing schools and are used by health care providers in the care of patients. Complementary and alternative medicine (CAM) is often viewed as consisting of unconventional and unorthodox treatments or interventions. These modalities and therapies stress the need to treat the whole person, recognizing the interaction of the body, mind, and spirit. People with HIV infection report substantial use of CAM for symptom management. The use of CAM in patients with HIV infection and AIDS often results because of disillusionment with standard medical treatment, which to date has provided no cure. Combined with traditional therapies, CAM may improve the patient's overall well-being. However, there can be adverse drug–drug interactions between certain CAM therapies (e.g., St. John wort) and some ARV medications (DHHS, 2016).

CAM can be divided into four categories:

- Spiritual or psychological therapies, which may include humor, hypnosis, faith healing, guided imagery, and positive affirmations.
- Nutritional therapies, which may include vegetarian or macrobiotic diets or supplements of vitamin C or beta-carotene. Also Chinese herbs are used, in addition to compound Q (a Chinese cucumber extract) and *Momordica charantia* (bitter melon).
- Drug and biologic therapies, including medications and other substances not approved by the FDA. Examples are *N*-acetylcysteine, pentoxifylline (Trental), and 1-chloro-2, 4-dinitrobenzene.

- Treatment with physical forces and devices, which may include acupuncture, acupressure, massage therapy, reflexology, therapeutic touch, and yoga.

Although there is insufficient research on the effects of CAM, a growing body of literature reports benefits for modalities involving nutrition, exercise, psychosocial treatment, and Chinese medicine.

Many patients who use these therapies do not report use of CAM to their health care providers. To obtain a complete health history, the nurse should ask about the patient's use of alternative therapies, including all over-the-counter, nutritional supplements and vitamins. Patients may need to be encouraged to report their use of CAM to their primary health care provider. Problems may arise, for example, when patients are using CAM while participating in clinical drug trials; alternative therapies can have significant adverse side effects, making it difficult to assess the effects of the medications in the clinical trial. The nurse needs to become familiar with the potential adverse side effects of these therapies. The nurse who suspects that CAM is causing a side effect needs to discuss this with the patient, the alternative therapy provider, and the primary health care provider. It is important for the nurse to view CAM with an open mind and to try to understand the importance of this treatment to the patient. This approach will improve communication with the patient and reduce conflict.

NURSING PROCESS
The Patient with AIDS

The nursing care of patients with AIDS is challenging because of the potential for any organ system to be the target of infections or cancer. In addition, this disease is complicated by many emotional, social, and ethical issues.

ASSESSMENT

Nursing assessment includes identification of potential risk factors, including a history of risky sexual practices or IV/injection drug use. The nurse assesses the patient's physical and psychological status and should explore all factors affecting the immune system and its function.

NUTRITIONAL STATUS

The nurse assesses nutritional status by obtaining a dietary history and identifying factors that may interfere with oral intake, such as anorexia, nausea, vomiting, oral pain, or difficulty swallowing. In addition, the nurse evaluates the patient's ability to purchase and prepare food. Weight history (i.e., changes over time); anthropometric measurements; and levels of blood urea nitrogen (BUN), serum protein, albumin, and transferrin provide objective measurements of nutritional status.

Nursing Alert
Transferrin, which is synthesized in the liver, is a transport protein that regulates iron absorption by transporting it from the intestines to the bloodstream; therefore, it may be monitored to evaluate iron saturation of the blood. Low levels of transferrin impair hemoglobin production, resulting in anemia. Transferrin levels also decrease with liver disease and poor protein intake, thus this laboratory test may be ordered to assess liver function and nutritional status. High levels of transferrin are associated with immune function and the ability to deal with infection. Normal transferrin levels for adults are 250 to 425 mg/dL or 2.5 to 4.2 g/L. Decreased transferrin levels are seen in microcytic (small red blood cells) anemia, protein calorie malnutrition, chronic infection, acute liver disease, and nephrotic disease (protein loss in urine) (Minchella et al., 2015).

SKIN INTEGRITY

The nurse inspects the skin and mucous membranes daily for evidence of breakdown, ulceration, or infection. Monitoring the oral cavity for redness, ulcerations, and the presence of creamy-white adherent patches detects candidiasis. Assessment of the perianal area for excoriation and infection in patients with profuse diarrhea is important. Cultures of wounds may be indicated and performed by the nurse to identify infectious organisms, especially methicillin-resistant *Staphylococcus aureus* (MRSA).

RESPIRATORY STATUS

The nurse assesses respiratory status by monitoring the patient for cough, sputum production (i.e., amount and color), dyspnea on exertion, orthopnea, tachypnea, and chest pain. Auscultation detects the quality of breath sounds. Other measures of pulmonary function include chest x-ray results, arterial blood gas values, pulse oximetry, and pulmonary function tests.

NEUROLOGIC STATUS

The nurse determines neurologic status by assessing level of consciousness; orientation to person, place, and time; and memory lapses. Assessment of mental status as early as possible during initial care provides a baseline. The nurse assesses the patient for sensory deficits (visual changes, headache, or numbness and tingling in the extremities), motor involvement (altered gait, paresis [slight or partial paralysis], or paralysis), and seizure activity.

FLUID AND ELECTROLYTE BALANCE

Fluid and electrolyte status is determined by examining the skin and mucous membranes for turgor and dryness. Dehydration may be indicated by increased thirst, decreased urine output, postural hypotension, weak and rapid pulse, and urine-specific

(continued on page 1112)

gravity of 1.025 or more. Electrolyte imbalances, such as decreased serum sodium, potassium, calcium, magnesium, and chloride, typically result from profuse diarrhea. The nurse assesses the patient for signs and symptoms of electrolyte deficits, including decreased mental status, muscle twitching, muscle cramps, irregular pulse, nausea, vomiting, and shallow respirations.

KNOWLEDGE LEVEL

The nurse evaluates the patient's level of knowledge about the disease and the modes of disease transmission. In addition, the nurse assesses the level of knowledge of family and friends. The patient's psychological reaction to the diagnosis of HIV infection or AIDS is important to explore. Reactions vary among patients and may include denial, anger, fear, shame, withdrawal from social interactions, and depression. The nurse should identify the patient's resources for support.

DIAGNOSIS

The list of potential nursing diagnoses is extensive because of the complex nature of this disease. However, based on assessment data, major nursing diagnoses for the patient may include the following:

- Impaired skin integrity related to cutaneous manifestations of HIV infection, excoriation, and diarrhea
- Diarrhea related to enteric pathogens, HIV infection, or ARV medications
- Risk for infection related to immunodeficiency
- Activity intolerance related to weakness, fatigue, malnutrition, impaired fluid and electrolyte balance, and hypoxia associated with pulmonary infections
- Disturbed thought processes related to shortened attention span, impaired memory, confusion, and disorientation associated with HIV-related cognitive decline
- Ineffective airway clearance related to PCP, increased bronchial secretions, and decreased ability to cough related to weakness and fatigue
- Pain related to impaired perianal skin integrity secondary to diarrhea, KS, and peripheral neuropathy
- Imbalanced nutrition, less than body requirements, related to decreased oral intake
- Social isolation related to stigma of the disease, withdrawal of support systems, isolation procedures, and fear of infecting others
- Anticipatory grieving related to changes in lifestyle and roles and unfavorable prognosis
- Deficient knowledge related to HIV infection, means of preventing HIV transmission, and self-care

Based on the assessment data, possible complications may include the following:

- OIs
- Impaired breathing or respiratory failure

- Wasting syndrome and fluid and electrolyte imbalance
- Adverse reaction to medications

PLANNING

Goals for the patient may include achievement and maintenance of skin integrity, resumption of usual bowel patterns, absence of infection, improved activity tolerance, improved thought processes, improved airway clearance, increased comfort, improved nutritional status, increased socialization, expression of grief, increased knowledge regarding disease prevention and self-care, and absence of complications.

NURSING INTERVENTIONS

PROMOTING SKIN INTEGRITY

The nurse routinely assesses the skin and oral mucosa for changes in appearance, location and size of lesions, and evidence of infection and breakdown. The nurse assists immobile patients to change position every 1 to 2 hours. Devices such as alternating-pressure mattresses and low-air-loss beds are used to prevent skin breakdown. Patients should avoid scratching; use nonabrasive, nondrying soaps; and apply nonperfumed skin moisturizers to dry skin surfaces. Regular oral care is also encouraged.

The nurse applies medicated lotions, ointments, and dressings to affected skin surfaces as prescribed. Adhesive tape is avoided. Protect patient's skin from friction and rubbing by keeping bed linens free of wrinkles and avoiding tight or restrictive clothing. The nurse advises patients with foot lesions to wear cotton socks and shoes that do not cause the feet to perspire. Antipruritic, antibiotic, and analgesic agents are administered as prescribed.

The nurse assesses the perianal region frequently for impairment of skin integrity and infection. The patient should keep the area as clean as possible. The perianal area should be cleaned after each bowel movement with nonabrasive soap and water to prevent further excoriation and breakdown of the skin. If the area is very painful, soft cloths or cotton sponges may be less irritating than washcloths. In addition, sitz baths or gentle irrigation may facilitate cleaning and promote comfort. It is important to dry the area thoroughly after cleaning. Topical lotions or ointments may be prescribed to promote healing. If infection is suspected, wounds should be cultured to initiate the appropriate antimicrobial treatment. The nurse assists debilitated patients in maintaining hygienic practices.

PROMOTING USUAL BOWEL PATTERNS

The nurse assesses bowel patterns for diarrhea. The nurse monitors the frequency and consistency of stools and the patient's reports of abdominal pain or cramping associated with bowel movements. Factors that exacerbate frequent diarrhea should be avoided. The nurse measures the quantity and volume of liquid stools to document fluid volume losses and obtains stool cultures to identify pathogenic organisms.

The nurse counsels the patient about ways to decrease diarrhea. Recommendations may include restricting oral intake to rest the bowel during periods of acute inflammation associated with severe enteric infections. As the patient's dietary intake is increased, the patient avoids foods that act as bowel irritants, such as raw fruits and vegetables, popcorn, carbonated beverages, and spicy foods. Small, frequent meals help to prevent abdominal distention. The nurse administers prescribed medications, such as anticholinergics, antispasmodics, or opioids, which decrease diarrhea by decreasing intestinal spasms and motility. Administering antidiarrheal agents on a regular schedule may be more beneficial than administering them on an as-needed basis. Also antibiotics and antifungal agents may be prescribed to combat pathogens identified by stool cultures. The nurse also assesses the self-care strategies being used by the patient to control diarrhea, including the use of probiotics.

PREVENTING INFECTION

The nurse instructs the patient and caregivers to monitor for signs and symptoms of infection: fever; chills; night sweats; cough with or without sputum production; shortness of breath; difficulty breathing; oral pain or difficulty swallowing; creamy-white patches in the oral cavity; unexplained weight loss; swollen lymph nodes; nausea; vomiting; persistent diarrhea; frequency, urgency, or pain on urination; headache; visual changes or memory lapses; redness, swelling, or drainage from skin wounds; and vesicular lesions on the face, lips, or perianal area. The nurse monitors laboratory test results that indicate infection, such as the WBC count and differential. Culture specimens of wound drainage, skin lesions, urine, stool, sputum, and blood as well as a culture from the patient's mouth are obtained to identify pathogenic organisms and the most appropriate antimicrobial therapy. The nurse instructs the patient to avoid others with active infections, such as upper respiratory infections.

IMPROVING ACTIVITY TOLERANCE

The nurse assesses activity tolerance by monitoring the patient's ability to ambulate and perform activities of daily living. Patients may be unable to maintain their usual levels of activity because of weakness, fatigue, shortness of breath, dizziness, and neurologic involvement. Assistance in planning daily routines that maintain a balance between activity and rest may be necessary. In addition, patients benefit from instructions about energy conservation techniques, such as sitting while washing or while preparing meals. Personal items that are used frequently should be kept within the patient's reach. Measures, such as relaxation and guided imagery, may be beneficial because they decrease anxiety, which contributes to weakness and fatigue.

Collaboration with other members of the health care team may uncover other factors associated with increasing fatigue and strategies to address them. Physical therapists participate in the plan of care of patients with AIDS at long-term care facilities to increase endurance and tolerance for activities of daily learning. If fatigue is related to anemia, administering epoetin

alfa (Epogen) as prescribed may relieve fatigue and increase activity tolerance.

MAINTAINING THOUGHT PROCESSES

The nurse assesses the patient for alterations in mental status that may be related to neurologic involvement, metabolic abnormalities, infection, side effects of treatment, and coping mechanisms. Manifestations of neurologic impairment may be difficult to distinguish from psychological reactions to HIV infection, such as anger and depression.

If the patient experiences altered mental or cognitive status, the nurse instructs family members to speak to the patient in simple, clear language and give the patient sufficient time to respond to questions. Family members orient the patient to the daily routine by talking about what is taking place during daily activities. They are encouraged to provide the patient with a regular daily schedule for medication administration, grooming, meal times, bedtimes, and awakening times. Posting the schedule in a prominent area (e.g., on the refrigerator), providing nightlights for the bedroom and bathroom, and planning safe leisure activities allow the patient to maintain a regular routine in a safe manner. The nurse encourages activities that the patient previously enjoyed. These should be easy to accomplish and fairly short in duration. Around-the-clock supervision may be necessary, and strategies can be implemented to prevent the patient from engaging in potentially dangerous activities, such as driving or using the stove. The nurse uses strategies for improving or maintaining functional abilities and for providing a safe environment for patients with HIV-related cognitive decline.

IMPROVING AIRWAY CLEARANCE

At least daily, the nurse assesses respiratory status, including rate, rhythm, use of accessory muscles, breath sounds, mental status, and skin color. Any cough and the quantity and characteristics of sputum are documented. The nurse obtains sputum specimens for infectious organism analysis as indicated. Pulmonary therapy (coughing, deep breathing, postural drainage, percussion, and vibration) as often as every 2 hours may be required to prevent stasis of secretions and promote airway clearance. Because of weakness and fatigue, many patients require assistance in attaining a position (such as a semi-Fowler position) that facilitates breathing and airway clearance. The nurse evaluates fluid volume status so that adequate hydration can be maintained. Daily intake is 3 L of fluid unless contraindicated because of renal or cardiac disease. Humidified oxygen may be prescribed, and nasopharyngeal or tracheal suctioning, intubation, and mechanical ventilation may be necessary to maintain adequate ventilation.

RELIEVING PAIN AND DISCOMFORT

The nurse assesses the patient for the quality and severity of pain associated with impaired perianal skin integrity, the lesions of KS, and peripheral neuropathy. In addition, the nurse explores

(continued on page 1114)

the effects of pain on elimination, nutrition, sleep, affect, and communication, along with exacerbating and relieving factors. Cleaning the perianal area, as previously described, can promote comfort. Topical anesthetics or ointments may be prescribed. The nurse increases patient comfort while sitting with the use of soft cushions or foam pads. If necessary, systemic analgesic agents also may be prescribed. Frequently pain from KS is described as a sharp, throbbing pressure and heaviness if lymphedema is present. Pain management may include use of NSAIDs and opioids, plus nonpharmacologic approaches, such as relaxation techniques. When NSAIDs are administered to patients who are receiving zidovudine, the nurse is aware that hepatic and hematologic status is evaluated.

The patient with pain related to peripheral neuropathy frequently describes it as burning, numbness, and "pins and needles." Pain management approaches may include opioids, tricyclic antidepressants, and elastic compression stockings to equalize pressure. Tricyclic antidepressants potentiate the actions of opioids and can be used to relieve pain without increasing the dose of the opioid. Ongoing assessment by the nurse of the use and potential abuse of opioids is part of the collaborative model of pain management.

IMPROVING NUTRITIONAL STATUS

The nurse assesses nutritional status by monitoring weight, dietary intake and output, and levels of serum albumin, BUN, protein, and transferrin. The patient is assessed for factors that interfere with oral intake, such as anorexia, candidal infection, nausea, pain, weakness, fatigue, and lactose intolerance. Based on the results of assessment, the nurse implements specific measures to facilitate oral intake. A dietitian helps to determine the patient's nutritional requirements.

Control of nausea and vomiting with antiemetic medications administered on a regular basis may increase the patient's dietary intake. Inadequate food intake resulting from pain caused by oral lesions or a sore throat may be managed by administering prescribed opioids and viscous lidocaine. Additionally, the nurse encourages the patient to eat foods that are easy to swallow and to avoid rough, spicy, or sticky food items and foods that are excessively hot or cold. The patient should perform oral hygiene before and after meals; in the debilitated patient with AIDS, the nurse will assist in these activities. If fatigue and weakness interfere with intake, the nurse encourages the patient to rest before meals. If the patient is hospitalized, meals should be scheduled so that they do not occur immediately after painful or unpleasant procedures. The nurse advises the patient with diarrhea and abdominal cramping to avoid foods that stimulate intestinal motility and abdominal distention, such as fiber-rich foods or lactose, if the patient is intolerant to lactose. The nurse instructs the patient about ways to enhance the nutritional value of meals. Supplements, such as puddings, powders, milkshakes, and Advera (a nutritional product specifically designed for people with HIV infection or AIDS) also may be useful. Patients who cannot maintain their nutritional status through oral intake may require enteral feedings or parenteral nutrition.

DECREASING THE SENSE OF ISOLATION

People with AIDS are at risk for double stigmatization. Judgments about disease acquisition and lifestyle choices isolate many patients who are HIV-positive. Many people with AIDS are young adults at a developmental stage that is usually associated with establishing intimate relationships, personal goals, and career goals, as well as having and raising children. Their focus changes as they are faced with a disease that threatens their quality of life with no cure. In addition, they may be forced to reveal hidden lifestyles or behaviors to family, friends, coworkers, and health care providers. As a result, people with HIV infection may be overwhelmed with emotions such as anxiety, guilt, shame, and fear. They also may be faced with multiple losses, such as loss of financial security, normal roles and functions, self-esteem, privacy, ability to control bodily functions, ability to interact meaningfully with the environment, and sexual functioning, as well as rejection by sexual partners, family, and friends. Some patients may harbor feelings of guilt because of their lifestyle or because they may have infected others in current or previous relationships. Other patients may feel anger toward sexual partners who transmitted the virus to them. Infection control measures used in the hospital or at home may further contribute to the patient's emotional isolation. Any or all of these stressors may cause the patient with AIDS to withdraw both physically and emotionally from social contact.

Nurses are in a key position to provide an atmosphere of acceptance and understanding for people with AIDS and their families and partners. The nurse assesses the patient's usual level of social interaction as early as possible to provide a baseline for monitoring changes in behaviors that suggest social isolation (e.g., decreased interaction with staff or family, hostility, noncompliance). Patients are encouraged to express feelings of isolation and loneliness with the assurance that these feelings are not unique or abnormal.

Providing information about how to protect themselves and others may help patients avoid social isolation. The nurse reassures patients, family, and friends that AIDS is not spread through casual contact. Patient care conferences that address the psychosocial issues associated with AIDS may help sensitize the health care team to patients' needs.

COPING WITH GRIEF

The nurse helps the patient verbalize feelings and explore and identify resources for support. In addition, the nurse works with the patient to establish mechanisms for coping, especially when the patient is grieving anticipated losses. The patient is encouraged to maintain contact with family, friends, and coworkers and to use local or national AIDS support groups and hotlines. If possible, losses are identified and addressed. The nurse encourages the patient to continue usual activities whenever possible. Consultations with mental health counselors are useful for many patients.

MONITORING AND MANAGING POTENTIAL COMPLICATIONS

Opportunistic Infections. Patients who are immunosuppressed are at risk for OIs. Therefore, anti-infective agents may be prescribed and laboratory tests obtained to monitor their effect. The nurse should report signs and symptoms of OIs, including fever, malaise, difficulty breathing, nausea or vomiting, diarrhea, difficulty swallowing, and any occurrences of swelling or discharge.

Respiratory Failure. Impaired breathing is a major complication that increases the patient's discomfort and anxiety and may lead to respiratory and cardiac failure. The nurse monitors respiratory rate and pattern and auscultates the lungs for abnormal breath sounds. The patient should report shortness of breath and increasing difficulty in carrying out usual activities. The nurse monitors pulse rate and rhythm, blood pressure, and oxygen saturation. Suctioning, if indicated, and oxygen therapy ensure an adequate airway and prevent hypoxia. Mechanical ventilation may be necessary for the patient who cannot maintain adequate ventilation because of pulmonary infection, fluid and electrolyte imbalance, or respiratory muscle weakness. Arterial blood gas values will be obtained to guide ventilator management. Instruct intubated patients in methods to allow communication with the nurse and others. The patient receiving mechanical ventilation should be assessed regarding coping with the stress associated with intubation and ventilator assistance. The possible need for mechanical ventilation in the future should be discussed early in the course of the disease, when the patient is able to make known his or her preferences about treatment. The use of mechanical ventilation should be consistent with the patient's decisions about end-of-life treatment.

Cachexia and Wasting. Wasting syndrome, and fluid and electrolyte disturbances, including dehydration, are common complications of HIV infection and AIDS. The nurse evaluates the patient's nutritional and electrolyte status by monitoring weight gains or losses, skin turgor, ferritin (blood cell protein that contains iron) levels, hemoglobin, hematocrit, and electrolyte levels. Fluid and electrolyte status is monitored on an ongoing basis; fluid intake and output and urine-specific gravity may be monitored daily if the patient is hospitalized with complications. The nurse assesses the skin for dryness and adequate turgor. Vital signs are monitored for decreased systolic blood pressure or increased pulse rate on sitting or standing. The nurse documents and reports signs and symptoms of electrolyte disturbances, such as muscle cramping, weakness, irregular pulse, decreased mental status, nausea, and vomiting to the provider. The nurse also monitors serum electrolyte values and reports abnormalities.

The nurse helps the patient select foods that will replenish electrolytes, such as oranges and bananas (potassium) and cheese and soups (sodium). Fluid intake is 3 L or more per day, unless contraindicated, to replace fluid lost with diarrhea, and measures to control diarrhea are initiated. If fluid and electrolyte imbalances persist, the nurse administers IV fluids and electrolytes as prescribed. The nurse also monitors effects of parenteral therapy.

Side Effects of Medications. Adverse reactions are of concern in patients who receive many medications to treat HIV infection or its complications. Many medications can cause severe toxic effects. The nurse provides information about the purpose of the medications, their correct administration, side effects, and strategies to manage or prevent side effects. Patients and their caregivers need to know which signs and symptoms of side effects should be reported immediately to their primary health care provider (see Table 37-2).

In addition to medications used to treat HIV infection, other medications that may be required include opioids, tricyclic antidepressants, and NSAIDs for pain relief; medications for treatment of OIs; antihistamines (diphenhydramine) for relief of pruritus; acetaminophen or aspirin for management of fever; and antiemetic agents for control of nausea and vomiting. Concurrent use of these medications can cause many drug interactions, resulting in hepatic and hematologic abnormalities. Therefore, careful monitoring of laboratory test results is essential.

During each contact with the patient, it is important for the nurse to ask not only about side effects but also about how well the patient is adhering to the medication regimen.

TEACHING PATIENTS SELF-CARE

The nurse instructs patients, families, and friends about the routes of transmission of HIV. As discussed earlier, the nurse discusses precautions the patient can use to avoid transmitting HIV sexually or through sharing of blood. Patients and their families or caregivers must receive instructions about how to prevent disease transmission, including handwashing techniques and methods for safely handling and disposing of items soiled with body fluids. Clear guidelines about avoiding and controlling infection, maintaining regular health care appointments, managing symptoms, and getting adequate nutrition, rest, and exercise are necessary. Emphasize the importance of personal and environmental hygiene. The nurse teaches caregivers the guidelines (Standard Precautions) described in Box 37-3. Patients and caregivers should clean kitchen and bathroom surfaces regularly with disinfectants to prevent growth of fungi and bacteria. Patients with pets should have another person clean the area soiled by animals, such as birdcages and litter boxes. If this is not possible, patients should use gloves and should wash their hands after they clean the area. Patients should avoid exposure to others who are sick or who have recently received live vaccines. The nurse emphasizes the importance of avoiding smoking, excessive alcohol, and over-the-counter and street drugs. Instruct patients who are HIV-positive or who inject drugs not to donate blood. IV/injection drug users who are unwilling to stop using should avoid sharing drug equipment with others.

The nurse teaches caregivers how to administer medications, including IV preparations, in the home. Often the medication regimens used for patients with HIV infection and AIDS are complex and expensive. If the patient requires enteral or parenteral nutrition, provide instruction to the patient and family about how to administer nutritional therapies at home. Home

(continued on page 1116)

care nurses provide ongoing teaching and support for the patient and family.

PROVIDING CONTINUING CARE

Many people with AIDS remain in their community and continue their usual daily activities, whereas others can no longer work or maintain their independence. Families or caregivers may need assistance in providing supportive care. Many community-based organizations provide a variety of services for people living with HIV infection and AIDS; nurses can help identify these services.

Nurses may refer patients to community programs that offer a range of services for patients, friends, and families, including help with housekeeping, hygiene, and meals; transportation and shopping; individual and group therapy; support for caregivers; telephone networks for the homebound; and legal and financial assistance. These services are typically provided by both professionals and nonprofessional volunteers. A social worker can identify sources of financial support, if needed.

Home care and hospice nurses are called on to provide physical and emotional support to patients and families as patients with AIDS enter the terminal stages of disease. This support takes on special meaning when people with AIDS lose friends and when family members fear the disease or feel anger concerning the patient's lifestyle. The nurse encourages the patient and family to discuss end-of-life decisions and to ensure that care is consistent with those decisions, all comfort measures are employed, and the patient is treated with dignity at all times.

EVALUATION

Expected patient outcomes may include:
1. Maintains skin integrity
2. Resumes usual bowel habits
3. Experiences no OIs
4. Maintains adequate level of activity tolerance
5. Maintains usual level of thought processes
6. Maintains effective airway clearance
7. Experiences increased sense of comfort and less pain
8. Maintains adequate nutritional status
9. Experiences decreased sense of social isolation
10. Progresses through grieving process
11. Reports increased understanding of AIDS and participates in self-care activities
12. Remains free of complications

A plan of nursing care for a patient with AIDS is available online at http://thepoint.lww.com/Honan2e.

Emotional and Ethical Concerns

Nurses in all settings provide care for patients with HIV infection. In doing so, they encounter not only the physical challenges of this epidemic but also emotional and ethical concerns. The concerns raised by health care professionals involve issues such as fear of infection, responsibility for giving care, values clarification, confidentiality, developmental stages of patients and caregivers, and poor prognostic outcomes.

Many patients with HIV infection have engaged in "stigmatized" behaviors. Because these behaviors challenge some traditional religious and moral values, nurses may feel reluctant to care for these patients. In addition, health care providers still may have fear and anxiety about disease transmission despite education concerning infection control and the low incidence of transmission to health care providers. Nurses are encouraged to examine their personal beliefs and to use the process of values clarification to approach controversial issues. The American Nurses Association's Code of Ethics for Nurses also can be used to help resolve ethical dilemmas that might affect the quality of care given to patients with HIV infection and AIDS (refer to Chapter 1).

Nurses are responsible for protecting the patient's right to privacy by safeguarding confidential information. Inadvertent disclosure of confidential patient information may result in personal, financial, and emotional hardships for the patient. The controversy surrounding confidentiality concerns the circumstances in which information may be disclosed to others. Many patients avoid necessary health care appointments due to confidentiality concerns. Health care team members need accurate patient information to conduct assessment, planning, implementation, and evaluation of patient care. Failure to disclose HIV status could compromise the quality of patient care. Sexual partners of patients who are HIV-infected should know about the potential for infection and the need to engage in safer sex practices as well as the possible need for testing and health care. State health departments offer confidential partner notification services. In situations in which a patient cannot or will not inform others, "duty to warn" regulations vary by state. Nurses are advised to discuss concerns about confidentiality with nurse administrators and to consult professional nursing organizations, such as the Association of Nurses in AIDS Care (ANAC), and legal experts in their state to identify the most appropriate course of action.

AIDS has had a high mortality rate, but advances in ARV and multidrug therapy have demonstrated promise in slowing or controlling disease progression. It is not known whether current treatment regimens will remain effective because viral drug resistance has developed with many medications. However, most experts agree that educated, adherent patients can expect to survive for decades living a life that is relatively complication-free. In spite of these advances, many young and middle-aged adults will experience serious illness and may die during the usual course of the disease process. Unlike cancer or other diseases, AIDS is associated with controversies challenging our legal and political systems as well as religious and personal beliefs. Contributing to this stress is personal fears of contagion or disapproval of the patient's lifestyle and behaviors. Nurses who feel stressed and overburdened may experience physical and mental distress in the form of fatigue, headache, changes in appetite and sleep patterns, helplessness, irritability, apathy, negativity, and anger.

Many strategies have been used by nurses to cope with the stress associated with caring for patients with AIDS. Education and provision of up-to-date information help to alleviate apprehension and prepare nurses to deliver safe, high-quality patient care. Interdisciplinary meetings allow participants to support one another and provide comprehensive patient care. Staff support groups give nurses an opportunity to solve problems and explore values and feelings about caring for patients with AIDS and their families; the groups also provide a forum for grieving. Other sources of support include nursing administrators, peers, and spiritual advisors.

CHAPTER REVIEW

Critical Thinking Exercises

1. A 43-year-old man who has been injecting drugs for 20 years says that he is not going to stop his use of drugs but wants to reduce his risk for HIV infection. What would you teach him? What types of community agencies could provide resources to this patient?

2. During a code response in the intensive care unit (ICU), a nursing student was inadvertently stuck with a needle used on a homeless patient who has AIDS. The student states that he is not concerned about contracting any diseases as a result. As his clinical instructor or the nurse manager of the ICU, what actions should you take? What reporting and documentation are needed? What testing, treatment, and counseling are indicated for the student?

3. During a home visit to a family in which two adolescents are HIV-positive, you are instructing the adolescents, their siblings, and their parents about strategies to protect the adolescents from other infections and to protect other family members from HIV transmission. What is the evidence for strategies that you plan to discuss with the adolescents and their family members? What is the strength of that evidence, and what criteria would you use to evaluate the strength of the evidence?

NCLEX-Style Review Questions

1. The patient with a CD4⁺ count of 100 cells/mm³ and not taking any antiretroviral medications is admitted to the hospital after a motor vehicle accident. In addition, the patient has a productive cough, fever, lymphadenopathy, and a history of night sweats. The patient's **purified protein derivative** (PPD) test is negative. What is the nurse's best action?
   a. Use Standard Precautions alone because the patient does not have tuberculosis.
   b. Use Airborne Precautions alone because the patient has not started appropriate therapy for HIV.
   c. Use Standard Precautions and Airborne Precautions because the patient has tuberculosis.
   d. Use Standard and Airborne Precautions until the infectious disease providers verify the patient does not have tuberculosis, and then continue using standard precautions.

2. The patient who just tested HIV-positive has persistent lymphadenopathy. The patient asks, "When will I be capable of transmitting the virus to others?" What is the nurse's best response?
   a. At this stage, you can transmit the virus only through donation of blood or blood products.
   b. If your CD4⁺ T cells drop below 200 cells/mm³ you would be considered infectious.
   c. You cannot transmit the virus as long as you take your prescribed drugs.
   d. The virus can be transmitted at all stages and categories of HIV infection.

3. Which finding in the patient with HIV disease who started HAART 3 months ago indicates that the treatment is effective? Select all that apply.
   a. Increased CD4 cells
   b. Decreased CD4 cells
   c. Decreased viral load
   d. Increased CD8 cells
   e. Decreased HIV antibody levels

4. The nurse suspects a patient has the early signs of an opportunistic infection with CMV. Which one of the early signs that may be present?
   a. Discolorations of the mucous membranes
   b. Cardiac arrhythmias
   c. Hypotension
   d. Visual disturbances

5. Kaposi sarcoma, once a common manifestation of AIDS before HAART was available, is seldom seen. A patient with AIDS wants to know how Kaposi sarcoma presents. What is the nurse's best response?
   a. Thick, white exudate in the mouth
   b. A purple-red lesion on the body
   c. Weight loss
   d. An increase in respiratory secretions

Try these additional resources, available at **http://thepoint.lww.com/Honan2e**, to enhance your learning and understanding of this chapter:

• NCLEX-Style Student Review Questions
• Journal Articles

REFERENCES AND SELECTED READINGS

References and selected readings associated with this chapter can be found on the website that accompanies the book. Visit **http://thepoint. lww.com/Honan2e** to access the references and other additional resources associated with this chapter.

Nursing Management: Patients with Allergic Disorders

Nicole C. Colline

Learning Objectives

After reading this chapter, you will be able to:

1. Describe the management of patients with allergic disorders.
2. Describe measures to prevent and manage anaphylaxis.
3. Discuss the different allergic disorders according to type.

Autoimmune reactions occur when self-antigens are recognized by the body's normal defense mechanisms as foreign. With the presence of these "foreign" antigens, B cells become hyperactive, and increased amounts of immunoglobulin E (IgE) are produced, thus causing a hypersensitivity or allergic response. *Hypersensitivity* is an amplified or inappropriate response to an antigen (on second exposure, see Pathophysiology), leading to inflammation and destruction of healthy tissue. The cause may result from genetic, hormonal, and environmental factors; many times, the etiology is unclear. The reaction time varies and can be within minutes to hours of exposure or may be delayed. Refer to Chapter 36 for details of types of allergic classifications (Table 36-1). Symptoms will vary depending on the classification and may range from a local reaction to the life-threatening systemic response of anaphylaxis. It is important for nurses to recognize signs and symptoms of allergic reactions, understand the risk factors associated with reaction, and become familiar with treatment management.

There are two types of IgE-mediated allergic reactions: atopic (local) and nonatopic disorders. Although the underlying immunologic reactions of the two types of disorders are the same, the predisposing factors and manifestations are different. The atopic disorders are characterized by a hereditary predisposition and production of a local reaction to IgE antibodies, which manifests in one or more of the following three atopic disorders: allergic rhinitis, asthma, and atopic dermatitis/eczema. The nonatopic disorders (e.g., tetanus vaccine, insect venom, airborne allergens) lack the genetic component and organ specificity of the atopic disorders (Porth, 2015). Latex allergy (see pages 1134–1137) may be a type I or type IV **hypersensitivity** reaction, although true latex allergy is considered to be a type I hypersensitivity reaction. Contact dermatitis is considered to be a type IV hypersensitivity reaction (Peng & Novak, 2015).

Unfolding Patient Stories: Jennifer Hoffman • Part 2

Recall from Chapter 11 Jennifer Hoffman, who came to the clinic with continued symptoms of asthma. The nurse confirmed that she was following the asthma action plan; however, Jennifer now returns to the clinic with worsening symptoms. What assessment findings would indicate to the nurse that Jennifer is having a hypersensitivity reaction to an allergen(s)? What questions can assist the nurse in identifying the causative agent(s)? What interventions should be implemented when allergen(s) are identified?

Care for Jennifer and other patients in a realistic virtual environment: *vSim for Nursing* (thepoint.lww.com/vSimMedicalSurgical). Practice documenting these patients' care in (thepoint.lww.com/DocuCareEHR).

ANAPHYLAXIS

Anaphylaxis is defined as a severe allergic reaction that is rapid in onset and can cause various systemic reactions, including death (Ferri, 2016). Anaphylaxis is a clinical response to an immediate (type I hypersensitivity) immunologic reaction between a specific **antigen** and an **antibody**. The reaction results from a rapid release of IgE-mediated chemicals, which can induce a severe, life-threatening allergic reaction.

Pathophysiology

Anaphylaxis occurs when the body's immune system produces specific IgE antibodies toward a substance that is normally nontoxic (e.g., food such as a peanut) (Box 38-1). When the person first ingests the peanut, for example, there are no physical reactions manifested. Instead, antibodies are produced for that specific substance, and then those antibodies are stored in

BOX 38-1

Focus on Pathophysiology

Anaphylaxis

The chain of events for anaphylaxis:

1. Response to antigen. IgM and IgG recognize and bind the antigen.

2. Release of chemical mediators. Activated IgE on basophils promotes release of mediators (histamine, serotonin, and leukotrienes).

3. Intensified response. Mast cells release more histamine and eosinophil chemotactic factor of anaphylaxis (ECF-A), which create venule-weakening lesions.

4. Respiratory distress. In the lungs, histamine causes endothelial cell destruction and fluid leakage into the alveoli.

5. Deterioration. Meanwhile, mediators increase vascular permeability, causing fluid to leak from the vessels.

6. Failure of compensatory mechanisms. Endothelial cell damage causes basophils and mast cells to release heparin and mediator-neutralizing substances. However, anaphylaxis is now irreversible.

Adapted from Lippincott. (2010). *Pathophysiology: An incredibly visual! pocket guide*. Philadelphia, PA: Lippincott Williams & Wilkins.

the immune system for future re-exposure. If the substance is ingested again, the body releases excess amounts of the protein **histamine**. Large amounts of histamine released into the body may cause flushing, urticaria, angioedema, hypotension, and bronchoconstriction (Fig. 38-1). These systemic changes (most commonly in the dermatologic, respiratory, cardiovascular, and gastrointestinal [GI] tracts) characteristically produce clinical manifestations within seconds or minutes after antigen exposure. In severe cases, these symptoms may cause shock. If no medical intervention is sought, death may ensue (Lieberman, 2014).

Box 38-2 lists substances that most commonly cause anaphylaxis.

The diagnosis of anaphylaxis is predominantly based on objective findings during clinical examination, despite potential negative laboratory testing (i.e., serum IgE levels or tryptase levels [a protease of human mast cells that has been implicated as a pathologic mediator of numerous allergic and

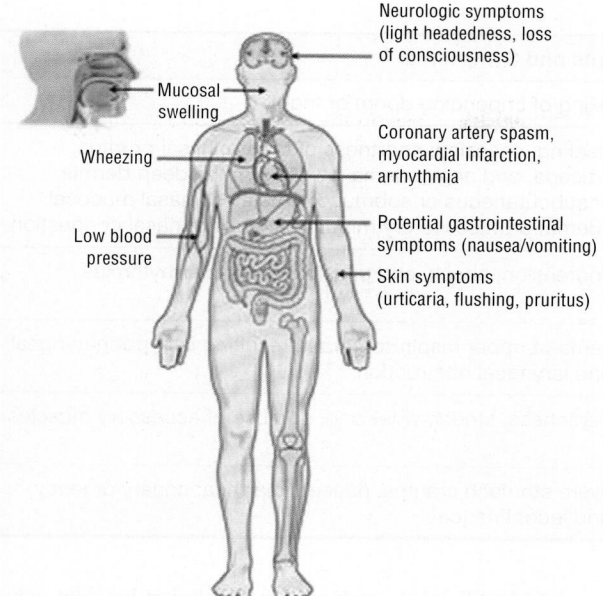

FIGURE 38-1 Anaphylaxis: Systemic symptoms. (Miller, M. D., Chhabra, A. B., Konin, J., & Mistry, D. (2013). *Sports medicine conditions: Return to play: recognition, treatment, planning.* Philadelphia, PA: Lippincott Williams & Wilkins.)

inflammatory conditions]). Some providers continue to utilize prick and intradermal skin testing to assist in diagnosis; however, a positive test result cannot confirm a diagnosis due to asymptomatic sensitization (when the body's cells detect the allergen but re-exposure does not cause physical or immunologic effects). Anaphylaxis continues to be underdiagnosed in the medical community, largely in part from patients not describing all of their symptoms, all the while undermining

---

BOX 38-2
Common Causes of Anaphylaxis

Foods

Peanuts, tree nuts (e.g., walnuts, pecans, cashews, almonds), shellfish (e.g., shrimp, lobster, crab), fish, milk, eggs, soy, wheat

Medications

Antibiotics (especially penicillin and sulfa antibiotics), allopurinol, radiocontrast agents, anesthetic agents (lidocaine, procaine), vaccines, hormones (insulin, vasopressin, adrenocorticotropic hormone [ACTH], aspirin, nonsteroidal antiinflammatory drugs [NSAIDs]).

Other Pharmaceutical/Biologic Agents

Animal serums (tetanus antitoxin, snake venom antitoxin, rabies antitoxin), antigens used in skin testing

Insect Stings

Bees, wasps, hornets, yellow jackets, ants (including fire ants)

Latex

Medical and nonmedical products containing latex

---

their expressed symptoms. Another contributing factor to underdiagnosing an acute anaphylactic episode is that medical providers are not well versed in the complexity of anaphylaxis. As the prevalence of anaphylaxis is rising, proper diagnosis and medical management is imperative to save people's lives.

Clinical Manifestations and Assessment

The severity of previous anaphylactic reactions does not determine the severity of subsequent reactions, which could be the same, more, or less severe. The severity depends on the degree of **allergy** and the dose of **allergen** (Porth, 2015; Simons, 2010).

Anaphylactic reactions consist of three basic patterns: uniphasic, biphasic, and protracted reactions. **Uniphasic** reactions occur as an exclusive incident where the patient develops symptoms within 30 minutes of allergen exposure that resolve spontaneously within 1 to 2 hours, either with or without medical treatment. In **biphasic** responses, the patient will have an initial reaction, followed by subsequent symptoms up to 8 hours after the first reaction. These patients should be managed in the emergency room. Finally, a **protracted** reaction is just that: a reaction that may last for a prolonged period of time, up to 32 hours, and may include cardiogenic or septic shock and respiratory distress despite medical treatment (Lieberman, 2014).

Mild systemic reactions consist of peripheral tingling and a sensation of warmth, possibly accompanied by a sensation of fullness in the mouth and throat. Nasal congestion, periorbital swelling, pruritus, sneezing, and tearing of the eyes also can be expected.

Moderate systemic reactions may include flushing, warmth, anxiety, and itching in addition to any of the milder symptoms. More serious reactions include bronchospasm and edema of the airways or larynx with dyspnea, cough, and wheezing. Both mild and moderate reactions begin within 2 hours of exposure. Severe systemic reactions, however, have an abrupt onset with the same signs and symptoms described previously. These symptoms progress rapidly to bronchospasm, laryngeal edema, severe dyspnea, cyanosis, and hypotension. Dysphagia (difficulty swallowing), abdominal cramping, vomiting, diarrhea, and seizures also can occur. Cardiac arrest and coma may follow. Monitoring the patient with anaphylaxis includes continual assessment of the patient's respiratory rate and pattern, oxygen saturation, assessing for breathing difficulties or abnormal lung sounds, and monitoring for hemodynamic stability (pulse rate and rhythm, and blood pressure). Table 38-1 summarizes the clinical manifestations of various pathophysiologic changes.

Prevention

Strict avoidance of potential allergens is an important preventive measure for the patient at risk for anaphylaxis. For example, patients at risk for anaphylaxis from insect stings should avoid areas populated by insects and should use appropriate clothing, insect repellent, and caution to avoid further stings.

If avoidance of exposure to allergens is impossible, the patient should be instructed to carry and administer epinephrine

TABLE 38-1 Clinical Manifestations of Anaphylaxis

Change	Signs and Symptoms
Activation of IgE and subsequent release of chemical mediators	Feeling of impending doom or fright
Histamine release	Sweating; sneezing; shortness of breath; nasal pruritus, urticaria, and angioedema (swelling of the deep dermis or subcutaneous or submucosal tissues); nasal mucosal edema; profuse watery rhinorrhea; itching; nasal congestion
Increased vascular permeability, subsequent decrease in peripheral resistance and leakage of plasma fluids	Hypotension, shock, and possible cardiac arrhythmias
Increased capillary permeability and mast cell degranulation	Edema of upper respiratory tract, resulting in hypopharyngeal and laryngeal obstruction
Bronchiole smooth muscle contraction and increased mucus production	Hoarseness, stridor, wheezing, and use of accessory muscles
Smooth muscle contraction of intestines and bladder	Severe stomach cramps, nausea, diarrhea; urinary urgency and incontinence

to prevent an anaphylactic reaction in the event of exposure to the allergen. People who are sensitive to insect bites and stings, those who have experienced food or medication reactions, and those who have experienced idiopathic or exercise-induced anaphylactic reactions should always carry an emergency kit that contains epinephrine. The EpiPen from Dey Pharmaceuticals (Napa, CA) is a commercially available first-aid device that delivers premeasured doses of 0.3 mg (EpiPen) or 0.15 mg (EpiPen Jr.) of epinephrine (Fig. 38-2). The autoinjection system requires no preparation, and the self-administration technique is uncomplicated. The patient must be given an opportunity to demonstrate the correct technique for use; an EpiPen training device can be used for teaching correct technique. Verbal and written information about the emergency kit, as well as strategies to avoid exposure to threatening allergens, also must be provided. Failure to administer epinephrine promptly and properly has proven to be fatal in severe anaphylactic reactions.

Screening for allergies before a medication is prescribed or first administered is an important preventive measure. A careful history of any sensitivity to suspected antigens must be obtained before administering any medication, particularly in parenteral form, because this route is associated with the most severe anaphylaxis. Nurses caring for patients in any setting (hospital, home, outpatient diagnostic testing sites, long-term care facilities) must assess patients' risks for anaphylactic reactions. Patients are asked about previous exposure to contrast agents used for diagnostic tests and any allergic reactions as well as reactions to any medications, foods, insect stings, and latex. People who are predisposed to anaphylaxis should wear some

form of identification, such as a medical alert bracelet, which names allergies to medications, food, and other substances.

People who are allergic to insect venom may require venom immunotherapy, which is used as a control measure and not a cure. Immunotherapy administered after an insect sting is very effective in reducing the risk of anaphylaxis from future stings (Schwartz, 2016; Simons, 2010). Insulin-allergic patients with diabetes and those who are allergic to penicillin may require desensitization. Desensitization is based on controlled anaphylaxis, with a gradual release of mediators. Patients who undergo desensitization are cautioned that there should be no lapses in therapy because this may lead to the reappearance of the allergic reaction when the use of the medication is resumed. See further discussion of immunotherapy later in this chapter.

Medical Management

Acute management depends on the severity of the reaction. Initially, respiratory and cardiovascular functions are evaluated. If the patient is in cardiac arrest, cardiopulmonary resuscitation is instituted. Oxygen is provided in high concentrations during cardiopulmonary resuscitation or if the patient is cyanotic, dyspneic, or wheezing. At first response, epinephrine, in a 1:1,000 dilution, is administered subcutaneously in the upper extremity or thigh and may be followed by a continuous IV infusion. Epinephrine is the first-line treatment of anaphylaxis as it is the only medication that may halt cardiac or respiratory arrest, which typically occurs 5 to 30 minutes after exposure to an allergen (Lieberman, 2014). Most adverse events associated with administration of epinephrine (e.g., adrenaline) occur when the dose is excessive or given intravenously. Patients at risk for adverse effects include elderly patients and those with hypertension, arteriopathies (diseases of the arteries), or known ischemic heart disease (Schwartz, 2016; Simons, 2010).

FIGURE 38-2 The EpiPen. Autoinjectors are commercially available first-aid devices that administer premeasured doses of epinephrine. An EpiPen training device is available for patients to practice correct self-injection technique. (Courtesy of Dey L.P., Napa, CA.)

Drug Alert!
To avoid mishaps in dosing, many emergency departments now stock both adult and pediatric EpiPens, which provide the standard adult or pediatric dose (EpiPen, 0.3 mg epinephrine; EpiPen-Jr, 0.15 mg epinephrine) (Schwartz, 2016).

Antihistamines and corticosteroids also may be administered to prevent recurrences of the reaction and to treat urticaria and angioedema, although they are not the first-line treatment. Antihistamines take up to 80 minutes to suppress histamine levels by 50%, and steroids generally work very slowly once administered. IV fluids (e.g., normal saline solution), volume expanders, and vasopressor agents are administered to maintain blood pressure and normal hemodynamic status. In patients with episodes of bronchospasm or a history of bronchial asthma or chronic obstructive pulmonary disease, aminophylline and corticosteroids also may be administered to improve airway patency and function. If hypotension is unresponsive to vasopressors, glucagon may be administered intravenously for its acute inotropic and chronotropic effects (Schwartz, 2016; Simons, 2010). Glucagon stimulates the enzyme adenylate cyclase, and its activation results in the intracellular accumulation of the second messenger cyclic adenosine monophosphate (cAMP). Increased levels of cAMP improve the suppressive actions that epinephrine exerts on the biochemical events responsible for the anaphylactic response.

Patients who have experienced anaphylactic reactions and received epinephrine should be transported to the local emergency department for observation and monitoring because of the risk for a "rebound" reaction usually within 4 to 10 hours after the initial allergic reaction. Patients with severe reactions are monitored closely for 12 to 14 hours in a facility that can provide emergency care, if needed. Because of the potential for recurrence, patients with even mild reactions must be informed about this risk (Lieberman, 2014). Refer to Nursing research brief (Box 38-3) that discusses Emergency Room (ER) management of anaphylaxis.

Nursing Management

If a patient is experiencing an acute allergic response, the nurse's initial action is to assess the patient for signs and symptoms of anaphylaxis. The nurse assesses the airway, breathing pattern, and other vital signs. The patient is observed for signs of increasing edema and respiratory distress. Prompt notification of the provider (or calling 911 if in the community) and preparation for initiation of emergency measures (intubation, administration of emergency medications, insertion of IV lines, fluid administration, oxygen administration) are important to reduce the severity of the reaction and to restore cardiovascular function. The nurse documents the interventions used and the patient's vital signs and response to treatment.

Nursing Alert
In the event of an acute allergic reaction, the nurse recognizes that ET intubation may be difficult or impossible because it can result in increased laryngeal edema, bleeding, and further narrowing of the glottic opening. Fiberoptic ET intubation, needle cricothyrotomy (followed by transtracheal ventilation), or cricothyrotomy may be necessary (Wafer, 2015).

The patient who has recovered from anaphylaxis needs an explanation of what occurred as well as instruction about avoiding future exposure to antigens and how to administer emergency medications to treat anaphylaxis. All patients who have experienced an anaphylactic reaction should receive a prescription for preloaded syringes of epinephrine. The nurse instructs the patient and family in their use and has the patient and family demonstrate correct administration of the medication (Box 38-4).

Long-term preventative measures include proper management of a patients' chronic condition(s), such as asthma, cardiovascular disease, etc., followed by detailed education in regards to treating an acute anaphylactic reaction. All patients are to be informed that anaphylaxis is a potential life-threatening allergy, and immediate treatment can be the difference between life and death.

ALLERGIC RHINITIS

Allergic **rhinitis** (hay fever, seasonal allergic rhinitis), a type I hypersensitivity reaction and the most common form of chronic respiratory allergic disease, remains the fifth most common chronic disease in the United States. It is one of the most common reasons for visits to primary care practitioners. Symptoms are similar to those of viral rhinitis but usually are more persistent and demonstrate seasonal variation; rhinitis is considered to be the allergic form if the symptoms are caused by an allergen-specific IgE-mediated immunologic response. However, a sizable proportion of patients with rhinitis have mixed rhinitis, or coexisting allergic and nonallergic rhinitis (Seidman et al., 2015).

The proportion of patients with the allergic form of rhinitis is greatest among children yet is on the rise among adults. It often occurs with other conditions, such as allergic conjunctivitis, sinusitis, and asthma. If symptoms are severe, allergic rhinitis may interfere with sleep, leisure, and school or work activities. If left untreated, many complications may result, such as allergic asthma, chronic nasal obstruction, chronic otitis media with hearing loss, anosmia (absence of the sense of smell), and, in children, orofacial dental deformities. Early diagnosis and adequate treatment are essential to relieve current symptoms and reduce comorbidities later in life (Rachelefsky & Farrer, 2013).

BOX 38-3 **Nursing Research**

Bridging the Gap to Evidence-Based Practice

Caton, E., & Flynn, M. (2013). Management of anaphylaxis in the ED: A clinical audit, *International Emergency Nursing*, 21(1), 64–70.

Purpose

The purpose of this paper was to review the existing evidence around the effective diagnosis, emergency treatment, and long-term management of anaphylaxis. It then describes a clinical audit that was carried out in the ED of a large University hospital in the United Kingdom.

Design

A retrospective audit design sampled all patients presenting with anaphylaxis in one calendar year; 146 cases were eligible for inclusion. The audit results showed widespread inconsistencies in the diagnosis and treatment of this patient group.

Findings

Of the 507 patients included in the original sample, a total of 29% (n = 146) of the identified cases met all the inclusion criteria for the audit, and the sample was made up of 92 (63%) women and 54 (37%) men. The median age was 34 years, and those under 40 years old accounted for 60% (n = 88) while 14% (n = 21) were over the age of 70 years. Patients in the range between 80 and 89 years of age were the only ones in which the number of men presenting to the ED was greater than the number of women.

In the majority of patients (66%, n = 96) a diagnosis of allergic reaction was documented, with anaphylaxis noted as the reason for presentation in 21% (n = 30) of cases. Angioedema was diagnosed in 8% (n = 12), while allergic rash and drug reactions occurred in a further 4% (n = 6) of cases. One patient self-discharged from the ED prior to being seen by a clinician, and a hypersensitivity reaction was recorded in one other patient.

Adrenaline was administered alone or in combination with antihistamine and or hydrocortisone in 43% (n = 63) of patients. The remaining 57% (n = 83) received hydrocortisone and/or antihistamine without adrenaline. The administration of adrenaline was recorded in 21% (n = 31) of patients where the diagnosis was reported as an allergic reaction. In an additional 5% (n = 7) of patients who had not received adrenaline, a diagnosis of anaphylaxis was recorded. A systolic blood pressure of 90 mm Hg or below was evident in 3% (n = 5) of patients who did not have adrenaline administered, one of whom was discharged with a diagnosis of anaphylaxis. There were only two

diagnoses, allergic rash and hypersensitivity reaction, in which patients did not require adrenaline.

Of the 146 patients included in the audit, 37 (25%) had been diagnosed previously as having asthma, but adrenaline was administered to only half of them (n = 19). A previous anaphylactic episode had occurred in 50% (n = 73) of patients, but an autoinjector of adrenaline was carried by less than half (n = 34). In addition, the discharge diagnosis recorded in 60% (n = 44) of the patients with a known anaphylactic history was documented as an allergic reaction. In 2% (n = 3) of cases, the patient's anaphylaxis history was unknown.

In 54% (n = 79) of cases, patient care and management involved admission to the ED observation ward, while 9% (n = 13) of patients were admitted directly to specialty wards. Discharge directly from the ED accounted for the remaining 37% (n = 54).

Guidelines recommend that all patients treated for anaphylaxis are referred to an allergy specialist, but in this audit no patient was referred to an allergy specialist from the ED. Of the 73 cases with a previous episode of anaphylaxis only 10 had been referred for consultation with an allergy specialist and a further nine patients had appointments pending. However, the majority of patients reporting a history of anaphylaxis (n = 49) had received no specialist referral. Over half (n = 19) of the 34 patients who carried their own adrenaline had not consulted an allergy specialist previously, and only three patients who were known to be asthmatics had been referred previously.

As a result of admission to an inpatient ward from the ED, referral outcomes on eventual hospital discharge were unknown in 14% (n = 20) of cases, and discharge without any follow-up occurred in 28% (n = 41) of cases.

Nursing Implications

The results of this audit are consistent with the published evidence and suggest there is more work to be done to enhance our understanding of the issues surrounding the ED treatment of anaphylaxis, to deliver the best possible patient care. The findings support the notion that the lack of an accepted definition of anaphylaxis generates conflict and confusion for ED practitioners. With no definitive diagnostic criteria, the ED clinicians' subjective interpretation of anaphylactic symptoms can result in a huge divergence among evidence-based guidelines, expert recommendations, and clinical practice.

Because allergic rhinitis is induced by airborne pollens or molds, it is activated by the following seasonal occurrences:

- Early spring: Tree pollen (oak, elm, poplar), mold spores
- Early summer: Rose pollen (rose fever), grass pollen (timothy, red-top)
- Early fall: Weed pollen (ragweed), mold spores

Each year, attacks begin and end at about the same time. Airborne mold spores require warm, damp weather. Although there is no rigid seasonal pattern, these spores appear in early spring, are rampant during the summer, and then taper off and disappear by the first frost.

Clinical Manifestations and Assessment

Typical signs and symptoms of allergic rhinitis include sneezing and nasal congestion; clear, watery nasal discharge; itchy eyes and nose; and lacrimation (Ferri, 2016). Drainage of nasal mucus into the pharynx, otherwise known as *postnasal drip*, results in multiple attempts to clear the throat and results in a dry cough, hoarseness, or scratchy

Patient Education

Self-Administration of Epinephrine

1. After removing the EpiPen autoinjector from its carrying tube, grasp the unit with the black tip (injecting end) pointing downward. Form a fist around the unit with the black tip down; with your other hand, remove the gray safety release cap.

2. Hold the black tip near the outer thigh. Swing and **jab firmly** into the outer thigh until a click is heard with the device perpendicular (90-degree angle) to the thigh.

3. Hold the device firmly against the thigh for approximately 10 seconds.

~10 seconds

4. Remove the unit from the thigh, and massage the injection area for 10 seconds. Call 911, and seek immediate medical attention. Carefully place the used EpiPen, needle-end first, into the device storage tube without bending the needle. Screw on the storage tube completely, and take it with you to the hospital emergency room.

---

throat. Headache, pain over the paranasal sinuses, and epistaxis can accompany allergic rhinitis. The symptoms of this chronic condition depend on environmental exposure and intrinsic host responsiveness. Allergic rhinitis can affect quality of life by also producing fatigue, loss of sleep, poor concentration, and interference with physical activities. Of great concern is the risk of developing persistent asthma and other comorbid conditions (chronic otitis media and sinusitis, obstructive sleep apnea, airway inflammation, etc.) from uncontrolled allergic rhinitis (Seidman et al., 2015).

Diagnosis of seasonal allergic rhinitis is based on history, physical examination, and diagnostic test results. On objective examination, a patient suffering with allergic rhinitis may appear fatigued (the patient may complain of not feeling well-rested after a full night's sleep); the patient may present with any of the following conditions:

- Allergic "shiners" (gray-black discoloration below lower eye lids that some refer to as "raccoon eyes");
- Puffy eyes;

- Clear or cloudy fluid surrounding the tympanic membranes;
- Nasal congestion or rhinorrhea;
- Marked erythema of palpebral conjunctivae associated with increased tearing;
- Enlarged nasal turbinates that are a pale-bluish color and boggy in texture;
- Enlarged anterior cervical lymph nodes;
- Cobblestoned appearance on the posterior pharynx (due to chronic postnasal drip and nasal congestion); and
- Sinus tenderness on palpation (Seidman et al., 2015).

Diagnostic tests include nasal smears, peripheral blood counts, total serum IgE, epicutaneous and intradermal testing, radioallergosorbent test (RAST), food elimination and challenge, and nasal provocation tests. Results indicative of allergy as the cause of rhinitis include increased levels of IgE and eosinophil and positive reactions on allergen testing. False-positive and false-negative responses to these tests, particularly skin testing and provocation tests, may occur, yet they still are considered a highly effective means of identifying agents that are causative of allergic responses (Kim & Mun, 2010; Van Rooyen, 2014).

It is imperative that patients with allergic rhinitis are diagnosed correctly and their treatment is individualized according to the severity of their disease. Then patients must be able to verbalize understanding of their diagnosis and proper treatment modalities.

Medical Management

The goal of therapy is to provide relief from symptoms and encourage adherence to therapeutic regimens. Therapy may include one or all of the following interventions: avoidance therapy, pharmacotherapy, immunotherapy, and homeopathic modalities. Verbal instructions must be reinforced by written information. Knowledge of general concepts regarding assessment and therapy in allergic diseases is important so that the patient can learn to manage certain conditions as well as prevent severe reactions and illnesses.

Avoidance Therapy

In avoidance therapy, every attempt is made to remove the allergens that act as precipitating factors. Often simple measures and environmental controls are effective in decreasing symptoms. Examples include using air cleaners/purifiers, humidifiers, and dehumidifiers; keeping windows closed during periods of high pollen counts and windy conditions; using air conditioning as much as possible in the warmer months; sleeping with windows closed; removing dust-catching furnishings (carpets, stuffed animals, feather bedding, window coverings); removing pets from the home or bedroom; removing cockroaches by professional extermination followed by regular cleaning of the infested area(s); using pillow and mattress covers that are impermeable to dust mites; washing bedding materials biweekly in hot water (55°C); and maintaining a smoke-free environment (Ferri, 2016). Because multiple allergens are often implicated, multiple measures to avoid exposure to allergens are often necessary. High-efficiency particulate air (HEPA) purifiers and vacuum cleaner filters also may be used to reduce allergens in the environment. The patient is instructed to reduce exposure to people with upper respiratory tract infections. If an upper respiratory infection occurs, the patient is encouraged to take deep breaths and to cough frequently to ensure adequate gas exchange and to prevent atelectasis. The patient is instructed to seek medical attention because the presence of allergy symptoms along with an upper respiratory tract infection may compromise adequate lung function (Seidman et al., 2015).

Research has shown that multiple avoidance strategies tailored to a person's risk factors can reduce the severity of symptoms, the number of work or school days missed because of symptoms, and the number of unscheduled health care visits for treatment. In many cases, it is impossible to avoid exposure to all environmental allergens so pharmacologic therapy or immunotherapy is needed.

Pharmacologic Therapy

Although allergen avoidance is clearly the safest and most effective means of treating symptoms associated with allergic rhinitis, some individuals may require pharmacologic therapy to further suppress the effects of histamine on the body.

Antihistamines

Antihistamines, now classified as H_1-receptor antagonists (or H_1-blockers), are used in the management of *mild* allergic disorders. H_1-blockers bind selectively to H_1 receptors, preventing the actions of histamines at these sites. They do not prevent the release of histamine but rather protect the surrounding tissue from the effects of the histamine release.

Oral antihistamines, which are readily absorbed, are most effective when given at the first occurrence of symptoms because they prevent the development of new symptoms. The effectiveness of these medications is limited to certain patients with hay fever, vasomotor rhinitis, **urticaria** (hives), and mild asthma. Examples of antihistamine medications include diphenhydramine (Benadryl), loratadine (Claritin), cetirizine (Zyrtec), levocetirizine (Xyzal), desoloratidine (Clarinex), and fexofenadine (Allegra). Currently, most antihistamines are available over-the-counter in local pharmacies. Refer to Table 38-2 for details.

Patients also need to understand that medications for allergy control should be used only when the allergy is apparent. This is usually on a seasonal basis. Continued use of medications when not required can cause an increased tolerance to the medication, with the result that the medication will not be effective when needed.

Adrenergic Agents

Adrenergic agents, vasoconstrictors of mucosal vessels, are used topically (nasal and ophthalmic formulations) in addition to the oral route. These medications help relieve severity of symptoms by narrowing blood vessels in the nasal passageways, therefore decreasing nasal congestion; however, these medications will not treat the underlying cause of nasal congestion, sinus pressure, etc. The most commonly used oral adrenergic agent is pseudoephedrine hydrochloride (Sudafed). Although considered safe if used as directed, pseudoephedrine hydrochloride has been known to cause some patients to complain of mild shakiness, heart palpitations, and anxiety shortly after ingestion. Pseudoephedrine is to be used cautiously or avoided in patients with underlying cardiac conditions, anxiety disorders, patients who are or plan on becoming pregnant, asthmatics, and those who use herbal supplements on a regular basis. Potential side effects include hypertension, arrhythmias, palpitations, central nervous system stimulation, irritability, tremor, and tachyphylaxis (acceleration of hemodynamic status) (Meltzer, Ratner, & McGraw, 2015).

TABLE **38-2** Selected H₁-Antihistamines

H₁-Antihistamine	Contraindications	Major Side Effects	Nursing Implications and Patient Teaching
First-Generation H₁-Antihistamines (Sedating)			
Diphenhydramine (Benadryl)	Allergy to any antihistamines Third trimester of pregnancy Lactation Use cautiously with narrow-angle glaucoma, asthma, stenosing peptic ulcer, benign prostatic hypertrophy or bladder neck obstruction, elderly patients	Drowsiness, confusion, dizziness, dry mouth, nausea, vomiting, photosensitivity, urinary retention	Administer with food if gastrointestinal upset occurs. Caution patients to avoid alcohol, driving, or engaging in any hazardous activities due to sedative effects of this medication. Suggest sucking on sugarless lozenges or ice chips for relief of dry mouth. Encourage the use of sunscreen and a hat while outdoors. Assess for urinary retention; monitor urinary output.
Chlorpheniramine (Chlor-Trimeton)	Allergy to any antihistamines Third trimester of pregnancy Lactation Use cautiously with narrow-angle glaucoma, asthma, stenosing peptic ulcer, BPH or bladder neck obstruction, elderly patients	Drowsiness, sedation, and dizziness, although less than other sedating agents; confusion, dry mouth, nausea, vomiting, urinary retention, epigastric distress, thickening of bronchial secretions	Caution patients to avoid alcohol, driving, or engaging in any hazardous activities until CNS response to medication is stabilized. Suggest sucking on sugarless lozenges or ice chips for relief of dry mouth. Recommend the use of a humidifier.
Hydroxyzine (Atarax)	Allergy to hydroxyzine or cetirizine (Zyrtec), pregnancy, lactation	Drowsiness, dry mouth, involuntary motor activity, including tremor and seizures	Caution patients to avoid alcohol, driving, or engaging in any hazardous activities until CNS response to medication is stabilized. Suggest sucking on sugarless lozenges or ice chips for relief of dry mouth. Instruct patients to report tremors.
Second-Generation H₁-Antihistamines (Nonsedating)			
Cetirizine (Zyrtec)	Allergy to any antihistamines Narrow-angle glaucoma Asthma Stenosing peptic ulcer BPH or bladder neck obstruction Lactation	Dry nasal mucosa, thickening of bronchial secretions	Can be taken without regard to meals. Instruct patients to use caution if driving or performing tasks that require alertness. Recommend the use of a humidifier.
Desloratadine (Clarinex)	Allergy to loratadine (Alavert, Claritin) Lactation Use cautiously with kidney or liver impairment or with pregnancy	Somnolence, nervousness, dizziness, fatigue, dry mouth	Can be taken without regard to meals. Suggest sucking on sugarless lozenges or ice chips for relief of dry mouth. Recommend the use of a humidifier.
Loratadine (Alavert, Claritin)	Allergy to any antihistamines Narrow-angle glaucoma Asthma Stenosing peptic ulcer BPH or bladder neck obstruction	Headache, nervousness, dizziness, depression, edema, increased appetite	Instruct patients to take on empty stomach (1 hour before or 2 hours after meals or food). Instruct patients to avoid alcohol and to use caution if driving or performing tasks that require alertness. Suggest sucking on sugarless lozenges or ice chips for relief of dry mouth. Recommend the use of a humidifier.

(continued on page 1128)

TABLE **38-2** Selected H$_1$-Antihistamines (*continued*)

H$_1$-Antihistamine	Contraindications	Major Side Effects	Nursing Implications and Patient Teaching
Fexofenadine (Allegra)	Allergy to any antihistamines Pregnancy Lactation Use with caution with liver or kidney impairment and in elderly patients	Fatigue, drowsiness, GI upset	Should not be administered within 15 minutes of ingestion of antacids. Instruct patients to use caution if driving or performing tasks that require alertness. Recommend the use of a humidifier.
Levocetirizine (Xyzal)	Allergy to any antihistamines; Dosage should be selected with caution in geriatric patients (start low dosage range) because of the greater frequency of decreased liver, kidney, and/or cardiac function and of concomitant disease and drug therapy; not recommended in nursing women Contraindicated in children 6 months to 11 years of age with renal impairment.	Somnolence, nasopharyngitis, fatigue, dry mouth, and pharyngitis	Avoid concomitant use with alcohol or other CNS depressants; Maintain fluid intake of 1500–2000 mL/day to decrease viscosity of secretions. May cause false-negative result in allergy skin testing. May cause transient ↑ in serum bilirubin and transaminases.

The topical route (drops and nasal sprays) causes fewer side effects than oral administration; however, the use of drops (e.g., tetrahydrozoline hydrochloride [Visine]) and sprays (e.g., oxymetazoline hydrochloride [Afrin]) should be limited to a few days to avoid rebound congestion. Adrenergic nasal decongestants are applied topically to the nasal mucosa for the relief of nasal congestion. They activate the alpha-adrenergic receptor sites on the smooth muscle of the nasal mucosal blood vessels, reducing local blood flow, fluid exudation, and mucosal edema. Topical ophthalmic drops are used for symptomatic relief of eye irritations caused by allergies. Common ocular complaints warranting use of ophthalmic drops include tearing, scleral and/or conjunctival erythema, and itching.

Mast Cell Stabilizers

Mast cell stabilizers are used prophylactically (before exposure to allergens) to prevent the onset of symptoms and to treat symptoms once they occur. They are also used therapeutically in chronic allergic rhinitis. Intranasal cromolyn sodium (NasalCrom) is a spray that acts by stabilizing the mast cell membrane, thus reducing the release of histamine and other mediators of the allergic response (Ferri, 2016). This spray is as effective as antihistamines but less effective than intranasal corticosteroids in the treatment of seasonal allergic rhinitis. The patient must be informed that the beneficial effects of the medication may take a week or so to manifest.

Corticosteroids

Intranasal **corticosteroids** (INCS) are indicated in more severe cases of acute allergic and perennial rhinitis that cannot be controlled by more conventional medications, such as decongestants, antihistamines, and intranasal cromolyn. Examples of these medications include beclomethasone (Beconase, Vancenase), budesonide (Rhinocort), dexamethasone (Decadron Phosphate Turbinaire), flunisolide (Nasalide), fluticasone (Cutivate, Flonase), and triamcinolone (Nasacort). Studies have proven that INCS are the most effective *maintenance* therapy for chronic allergic rhinitis, regardless of the patient's age, sex, race, or gender. These findings are based on their ability to prevent progression to more severe disease, along with their ability to decrease the likelihood of the evolution of a sleep-related breathing disorder or asthma (Rachelefsky & Farrer, 2013).

Because of their anti-inflammatory actions, these medications are equally effective in preventing or suppressing the major symptoms of allergic rhinitis.

Corticosteroids are administered by metered-spray devices. If the nasal passages are blocked, a topical decongestant may be used to clear the passages before the administration of the INCS. Patients must be aware that full benefit may not be achieved for several days to 2 weeks. Adverse effects of INCS are mild and include drying of the nasal mucosa, potentially causing epistaxis (bloody nose), which is resolved with discontinuing the medication for a few days, as well as burning and itching sensations caused by the vehicle used to administer the medication. Recommended use of this medication is limited to 30 days (Seidman et al., 2015).

Topical nasal medication for moderate to severe seasonal and perennial allergic rhinitis has emerged in the pharmaceutical industry. MP29-02 (Dymista), which consists of azelastine hydrochloride (AZE) and fluticasone propionate (Flonase), has a wider spray angle, lower viscosity, and smaller droplet size. The medicine has a greater ability to retain itself within the nasal cavity mucosa, thus decreasing nasal congestion and allergy symptoms (Rossi et al., 2015).

Immunotherapy

Allergen desensitization (allergen immunotherapy, hyposensitization) is primarily used to treat IgE-mediated diseases by injections of allergen extracts. **Immunotherapy** involves the administration of gradually increasing quantities of specific allergens to the patient until a dose is reached that is effective in reducing disease severity from natural exposure (Schwartz, 2016). Immunotherapy is treatment in the form of vaccine therapy (better known as "allergy shots") and, if available, sublingual medication. This type of therapy provides an adjunct to symptomatic pharmacologic therapy and can be used when avoidance of allergens is not possible. Goals of immunotherapy include reducing the level of circulating IgE, increasing the level of blocking antibody IgG, and reducing the sensitivity of mediator cells. Immunotherapy has been most effective for ragweed pollen; however, treatment also has been effective for grass, tree pollen, cat dander, and house dust mite allergens. Indications and contraindications for immunotherapy are presented in Box 38-5.

Unlike antiallergy medication, allergen immunotherapy has the potential to alter the allergic disease course after 3 to 5 years of therapy. Because it may prevent progression or development of asthma or multiple or additional allergies, it is also considered to be a potential preventive measure. The patient must understand what to expect and the importance of continuing therapy for several years before immunotherapy is accomplished. Subcutaneous immunotherapy (SCIT) treatment consists of injecting extracts of the allergens that cause symptoms in a particular patient. Injections begin with very small amounts and are increased gradually, usually at weekly intervals, until a maximum tolerated dose is attained. Maintenance booster injections are administered at 2- to 4-week intervals, frequently for a period of several years, before maximum benefit is achieved, although some patients will note early improvement in their symptoms. Long-term benefit seems to be related to the cumulative dose of vaccine given over time, lasting 3 or more years after therapy has stopped (Vadlamudi & Shaker, 2015). Immunotherapy should not be initiated during pregnancy; for patients who have been receiving immunotherapy before pregnancy, the dosage should not be increased during pregnancy provided the patient is tolerating and benefiting from the injections.

A newer approach evolving in the treatment of allergies is sublingual immunotherapy (SLIT). The U.S. Food and Drug Administration has recently approved SLIT, yet the treatment has not been utilized much due to lack of treatment options for polysensitized patients. Currently, there are sublingual tablets commercially available for grass and ragweed only. From approximately 8 weeks before the onset of the targeted pollen season continuing through the end of the season, an individual would ingest a pill daily. Benefits of SLIT include self-administration at home, no pain during administration, improvement in comorbid conditions (e.g., asthma, conjunctivitis), and reduced risk of anaphylaxis. Adverse effects include potential bad taste and risk of noncompliance as the patient must adhere to taking the medication daily in order for maximum benefits to be achieved (Lin et al., 2013; Vadlamudi & Shaker, 2015).

 Concept Mastery Alert

Allergy control by immunotherapy usually requires treatment for 3 to 5 years.

Candidates for SLIT therapy are chosen carefully after analyzing the risk/benefit ratio. Although severe systemic reactions occur in fewer than 1% of patients receiving immunotherapy, the risk for systemic and potentially fatal anaphylaxis does exist. It tends to occur most frequently at the induction or "up-dosing" phase. Therefore, the patient must be monitored after administration of immunotherapy. SLIT is to be administered under supervision by the medical provider in the provider's office. The patient remains in the office or clinic for at least 30 minutes after the injection and is observed for possible systemic symptoms. If a large, local swelling develops at the injection site, the next dose should not be increased because this may be a warning sign of a possible systemic reaction (Vadlamudi & Shaker, 2015).

BOX 38-5

Immunotherapy: Indications and Contraindications

Indications

- Allergic rhinitis, conjunctivitis, or allergic asthma
- History of a systemic reaction to *Hymenoptera* and specific IgE antibodies to *Hymenoptera* venom
- Desire to avoid the long-term use, potential adverse effects, or costs of medications
- Lack of control of symptoms by avoidance measures or use of medications

Contraindications

- Use of beta blocker or angiotensin-converting inhibitor therapy, which may mask early signs of anaphylaxis
- Presence of significant pulmonary or cardiac disease or organ failure
- Inability of the patient to recognize or report signs and symptoms of a systemic reaction
- Nonadherence of the patient to other therapeutic regimens and low probability that patient will adhere to immunization schedule (often weekly for an indefinite period)
- Inability to monitor the patient for at least 30 minutes after administration of immunotherapy
- Absence of equipment or adequate personnel to respond to allergic reaction if one occurs

Therapeutic failure is evident when a patient does not experience a decrease of symptoms within 12 to 24 months, fails to develop increased tolerance to known allergens, and cannot decrease the use of medications to reduce symptoms. Potential causes of treatment failure include misdiagnosis of allergies, inadequate doses of allergen, newly developed allergies, and inadequate environmental controls.

Homeopathic Modalities

Anecdotally, the health benefits of traditional Chinese medicine (TCM) which includes herbal therapies, has been reported for years. Studies are evaluating the impact of herbal medications on food allergy responses, such as FAHF-2 which is a formulation of nine Chinese herbs. Preclinical studies report that FAHF-2 blocked peanut-induced anaphylaxis during and after the development peanut hypersensitivity, with effectiveness sustained for up to 6 months after therapy (Slomski, Lack, & Jones, 2014). A phase II clinical trial is in progress. Additionally, probiotic dietary supplements, typically with *Lactobacillus* and *Bifidobacterium* species, has been used in clinical trials to evaluate the preventive impact on atopic disease and the impact on active disease (Slomski et al., 2014).

CONTACT DERMATITIS

Contact dermatitis, a type IV delayed hypersensitivity reaction, is an acute or chronic skin inflammation that results from direct skin contact with chemicals or allergens.

Types

There are four basic types: allergic, irritant, phototoxic, and photoallergic (Table 38-3). Eighty percent of cases are caused by excessive exposure to or additive effects of irritants (e.g., soaps, detergents, plants, organic solvents). Skin sensitivity may develop after brief or prolonged periods of exposure, and the clinical picture may appear hours or weeks after the sensitized skin has been exposed.

Clinical Manifestations and Assessment

Symptoms include itching, burning, **erythema**, skin lesions (vesicles), and edema, followed by weeping, crusting, and, finally, drying and peeling of the skin. In severe responses, hemorrhagic bullae may develop. Repeated reactions may be accompanied by thickening of the skin and pigment changes.

Secondary invasion by bacteria may develop in skin that is abraded by rubbing or scratching. Usually, there are no systemic symptoms unless the eruption is widespread.

The location of the skin eruption and the history of the exposure aid in determining the condition (see Table 38-3). However, in cases of obscure irritants or an unobservant patient, the diagnosis can be extremely difficult, often involving many trial-and-error procedures before the cause is determined. Patch tests on the skin with suspected offending agents may clarify the diagnosis (American Academy of Dermatology, n.d.). Management is discussed in Table 38-3.

ATOPIC DERMATITIS

Atopic dermatitis is a type I immediate hypersensitivity disorder characterized by inflammation and hyperreactivity of the skin, often causing pruritus. Although most commonly seen in children, the prevalence among adults has increased in the past 5 years. Recent studies confirm atopic dermatitis will persist through adulthood in up to 50% of individuals (Mortz et al., 2015). Other terms used to describe this skin disorder include *atopic eczema, atopic dermatitis/eczema,* and *atopic dermatitis/eczema syndrome* (AEDS).

Clinical Manifestations and Assessment

Most patients with atopic dermatitis have significant elevations of serum IgE and peripheral eosinophilia. Pruritus and hyperirritability of the skin (most commonly seen in flexural folds) are the most consistent features of atopic dermatitis and are related to large amounts of histamine in the skin (Fig. 38-3). Excessive dryness of the skin with resultant itching is related to changes in lipid content, sebaceous gland activity, and sweating. In response to stroking of the skin, immediate redness appears on the skin and is followed in 15 to 30 seconds by pallor, which persists for 1 to 3 minutes. Years of chronically irritated skin resulting in excessive itching can cause lichenification, or a leathery hardened appearance to the affected area. Lesions develop secondary to the trauma of scratching and appear in areas of increased sweating and hypervascularity. Atopic dermatitis is chronic, with remissions and exacerbations, reoccurrences often occurring with allergy flare-ups (Mortz, Andersen, Dellgren, Barington, & Bindslev-Jensen, 2015).

It is important to note that atopic dermatitis is often the first step in a process that leads to asthma and allergic rhinitis, otherwise known as the "allergic/atopic triad." It is the result of interactions among susceptibility genes, the environment, defective function of the skin barrier, and immunologic responses. Factors associated with more severe disease states or increased rates of exacerbations include familial history of atopic dermatitis, being the oldest or only child, having a severe case of dermatitis at a very early age, respiratory disease, early onset, and very high serum IgE levels (Seidman et al., 2015).

TABLE **38-3** Types, Testing, and Treatment of Contact Dermatitis

Type	Etiology	Clinical Presentation	Diagnostic Testing	Treatment
Allergic	Results from contact of skin and allergenic substance. Has a sensitization period of 10–14 days.	Vasodilation and perivascular infiltrates on the dermis Intracellular edema Usually seen on dorsal aspects of hand	Patch testing (contraindicated in acute, widespread dermatitis)	Avoidance of offending material Burow solution (aluminum acetate in water) is a drying agent for weeping skin lesions or cool water compress Systemic corticosteroids (prednisone) for 7–10 days Topical corticosteroids for mild cases Oral antihistamines to relieve pruritus
Irritant	Results from contact with a substance that chemically or physically damages the skin on a nonimmunologic basis. Occurs after first exposure to irritant or repeated exposures to milder irritants over an extended time.	Dryness lasting days to months Vesiculation, fissures, cracks Most common on hands and lower arms	Clinical picture Appropriate negative patch tests	Identification and removal of source of irritation Application of hydrophilic cream or petrolatum to soothe and protect Topical corticosteroids and compresses for weeping lesions Antibiotics for infection, and oral antihistamines for pruritus
Phototoxic	Resembles the irritant type but requires sun and a chemical in combination to damage the epidermis.	Similar to irritant dermatitis	Photopatch test	Same as for allergic and irritant dermatitis
Photoallergic	Resembles allergic dermatitis but requires light exposure in addition to allergen contact to produce immunologic reactivity.	Similar to allergic dermatitis	Photopatch test	Same as for allergic and irritant dermatitis

Medical Management

Treatment of patients with atopic dermatitis must be individualized. Guidelines for treatment include decreasing itching and scratching by wearing cotton fabrics; washing with a mild detergent; humidifying dry heat in winter; maintaining room temperature at 20°C to 22.2°C (68°F to 72°F); using antihistamines, such as diphenhydramine (Benadryl); and avoiding animals, dust, sprays, and perfumes. Keeping the skin moisturized with daily baths to hydrate the skin and the use of topical skin emollients is encouraged and remains the main treatment for atopic dermatitis (Ferri, 2016). Topical corticosteroids are used to prevent inflammation, and any infection is treated with antibiotics to eliminate *Staphylococcus aureus* when indicated. Use of immunosuppressive agents, such as cyclosporine (Neoral, Sandimmune), tacrolimus (Prograf, Protopic), and pimecrolimus (Elidel), may be effective in inhibiting T cells and mast cells involved in atopic dermatitis (Moskowitz, 2014).

Nursing Management

Patients who experience atopic dermatitis and their families require assistance and support from the nurse to cope with the disorder. Often the symptoms are disturbing to the patient and disruptive to the family. The appearance of the skin may affect the patient's self-esteem and his or her willingness to interact with others. Instructions and counseling about strategies to incorporate preventive measures and treatments into the lifestyle of the family may be helpful. Instructions include counseling the patient and family on various triggers of atopic dermatitis (e.g., winter months, heat or exercise, emotional stress, hormonal fluxes in women, skin irritants [perfumes], and microorganisms [bacteria, fungi, viruses, and yeast]) that may lead to an exacerbation. The patient and family need to be aware of signs of secondary infection and of the need to seek treatment if infection occurs. The nurse also teaches the patient and family about the side effects of medications used in treatment.

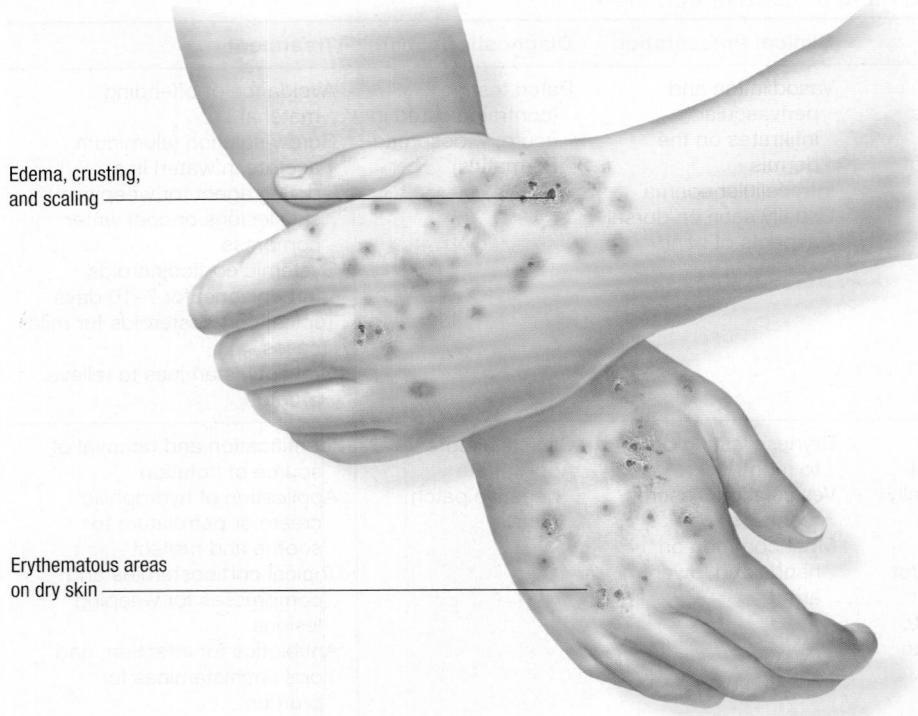

Edema, crusting, and scaling

Erythematous areas on dry skin

FIGURE 38-3 Atopic dermatitis. (Courtesy of Anatomical Chart Company.)

DERMATITIS MEDICAMENTOSA (DRUG REACTIONS)

Dermatitis medicamentosa, a type I hypersensitivity disorder, is the term applied to skin rashes associated with certain medications. Although people react differently to each medication, certain medications tend to induce eruptions of similar types. Rashes are among the most common adverse reactions to medications and occur in approximately 2% to 3% of hospitalized patients.

Clinical Manifestations and Assessment

In general, drug reactions appear suddenly, have a particularly vivid color, manifest with characteristics that are more intense than the somewhat similar eruptions of infectious origin, and, with the exception of bromide and the iodide rashes, disappear rapidly after the medication is withdrawn. Rashes may be accompanied by systemic or generalized symptoms, such as bronchospasm, urticaria, and significant angioedema.

Medical and Nursing Management

Upon discovery of a medication allergy, the causative agent must be discontinued immediately and treatment initiated for any symptoms the patient is experiencing. Once stable, the patient is warned that he or she has a hypersensitivity to a particular medication and is advised not to take it again. Patients should carry information identifying the hypersensitivity, and subsequent reaction experienced, with them at all times.

Skin eruptions related to medication therapy suggest more serious hypersensitivities. Frequent assessment and prompt reporting of the appearance of any eruptions are important so that early treatment can be initiated. Some cutaneous drug reactions may be associated with a clinical complex that involves other organs. These are known as *complex drug reactions.*

URTICARIA AND ANGIONEUROTIC EDEMA

Urticaria (hives) is a type I hypersensitive allergic reaction of the skin characterized by the sudden appearance of pinkish, edematous elevations that vary in size and shape, itch, and cause local discomfort (Fig. 38-4). They may involve any part of the body, including the mucous membranes (especially those of the mouth), the larynx (occasionally with serious respiratory complications), and the GI tract.

Each hive remains for a few minutes to several hours before disappearing. For hours or days, clusters of these lesions may come, go, and return episodically. If this sequence continues for longer than 6 weeks, the condition is called chronic urticaria. Chronic urticaria requires an extensive workup, ruling out numerous autoimmune diseases (e.g., lupus, rheumatoid arthritis, thyroid disease, etc.).

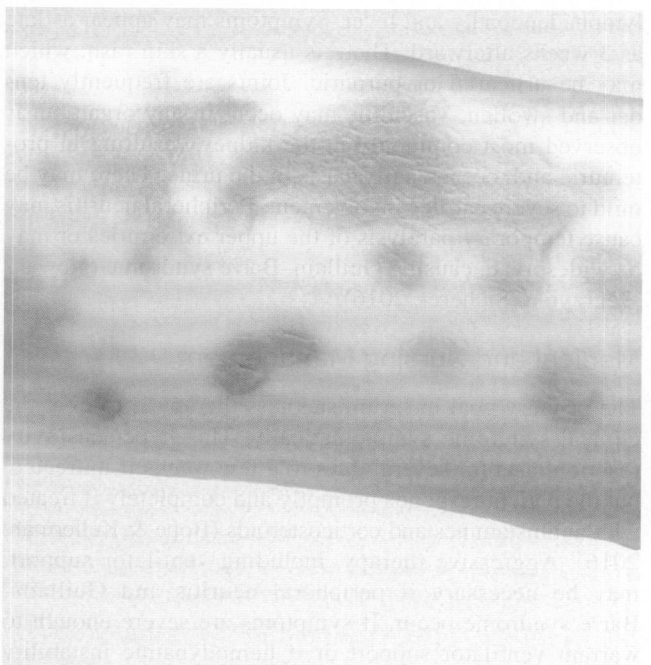

FIGURE 38-4 Hives.

Angioneurotic edema involves the deeper layers of the skin, resulting in more diffuse swelling, rather than the discrete lesions characteristic of hives. On occasion, this reaction covers the entire back. The skin over the reaction may appear normal but often has a reddish hue. The skin does not pit on pressure, as ordinary edema does. The regions most often involved are the lips, eyelids, cheeks, hands, feet, genitalia, and tongue; the mucous membranes of the larynx, the bronchi, and the GI canal also may be affected, particularly in the hereditary type (see discussion in the following section). Swellings may appear suddenly, in a few seconds or minutes, or slowly, in 1 or 2 hours. In the latter case, often their appearance is preceded by itching or burning sensations. Seldom does more than a single swelling appear at one time, although one may develop while another is disappearing. Infrequently, swelling recurs in the same region. Individual lesions usually last 24 to 36 hours. On rare occasions, swelling may recur with remarkable regularity at intervals of 3 to 4 weeks.

FOOD ALLERGY

Pathophysiology

IgE-mediated food allergy, a type I hypersensitivity reaction, occurs in about 2% of the adult population; it is thought to occur in people who have a genetic predisposition combined with exposure to allergens early in life through the GI or respiratory tract or nasal mucosa. Researchers also have identified a second type of food allergy, a non–IgE-mediated food allergy syndrome in which T cells play a major role (Ferri, 2016).

Almost any food can cause allergic symptoms, some even resulting in anaphylaxis. The most common offenders are seafood (lobster, shrimp, crab, clams, fish), legumes (peanuts, peas, beans, licorice), seeds (sesame, cottonseed, caraway, mustard, flaxseed, sunflower seeds), tree nuts, berries, egg white, buckwheat, milk, and chocolate. Peanut and tree nut (e.g., cashew, walnut) allergies are responsible for severe food allergy reactions in children and may result in anaphylactic death. The most common cause of anaphylactic death reported in adults is due to stings from insects, whereas in children, anaphylaxis to food may be more common (Chang, 2010; Schwartz, 2016).

Clinical Manifestations and Assessment

The clinical symptoms are classic allergic symptoms (urticaria, dermatitis, wheezing, cough, laryngeal edema, angioedema) and GI symptoms (itching; swelling of lips, tongue, and palate; abdominal pain; nausea; cramps; vomiting; and diarrhea).

A careful diagnostic workup is required in any patient with a suspected food hypersensitivity. Included are a detailed allergy history, a physical examination, and pertinent diagnostic tests. Skin testing is used to identify the source of symptoms and is useful in identifying specific foods as causative agents.

Medical Management

Therapy for food hypersensitivity includes elimination of the food responsible for the hypersensitivity. Pharmacologic therapy is necessary for patients who cannot avoid exposure to offending foods and for patients with multiple food sensitivities not responsive to avoidance measures. Medication therapy involves the use of H_1-blockers, antihistamines, adrenergic agents, corticosteroids, and cromolyn sodium. An essential aspect of management is teaching patients and family members to recognize symptoms associated with an anaphylactic reaction, when and how to administer life-saving medication (epinephrine), and when to call for emergency help. Many food allergies disappear with time, particularly in children. About one third of proven allergies disappear in 1 to 2 years if the patient carefully avoids the offending food. However, allergies to peanuts, shellfish, fish, and tree nuts have been reported to persist throughout adulthood in 20% of people. Researchers are hopeful that within the next 10 years more studies will have been performed and oral immunotherapy (OIT) will become an effective treatment option for those with certain food allergies (Slomski, 2012; Slomski et al., 2014).

Nursing Management

In addition to participating in management of the allergic reaction, the nurse focuses on preventing future exposure of the patient to the food allergen. If a severe allergic or anaphylactic reaction to food allergens has occurred, the nurse must instruct the patient and family about strategies to prevent its recurrence. The patient is instructed about the importance of carefully assessing foods prepared by others for obvious as well as hidden sources of food allergens and of avoiding locations and facilities where those allergens are likely to be present. This includes careful reading of food labels and monitoring the preparation of food by others to be sure that exposure to even minute amounts of allergenic foods is avoided. One of the dangers of food allergens is that they may be hidden in other foods and not apparent to people who are susceptible to the allergen. For example, often peanuts and peanut butter are used in salad dressings and Asian, African, and Mexican cooking and may result in severe allergic reactions, including anaphylaxis. Previous contamination of equipment with allergens (e.g., peanuts) during preparation of another food product (e.g., chocolate cake) is enough to produce anaphylaxis in people with severe allergy.

The patient and family must be knowledgeable about early signs and symptoms of allergic reactions and must be proficient in emergency administration of epinephrine if a reaction occurs. The nurse also advises the patient to wear a medical alert bracelet or to carry identification and emergency equipment at all times. Patients' food allergies should be noted on their medical records because there may be risk of allergic reactions not only to food but also to some medications containing similar substances.

SERUM SICKNESS

Pathophysiology

Serum sickness is an immune-complex type III hypersensitivity. If these type III complexes are deposited in tissues or vascular endothelium, there is an increase in vascular permeability and tissue injury, resulting in a vasculitis (inflammation of blood vessels). Traditionally serum sickness has resulted from the administration of therapeutic antisera of animal sources for the treatment or prevention of infectious diseases, such as tetanus, pneumonia, rabies, diphtheria, and botulism, as well as the bites of venomous snakes and black widow spiders. With the advent of human antitetanus serum and antibiotics, classic serum sickness is much less common now. However, various medications (primarily penicillin) may cause a serum-sickness–like reaction similar to that caused by foreign sera.

Clinical Manifestations and Assessment

Symptoms are caused by a reaction and immunologic attack on the serum or medication. Antibodies appear to be of the IgE and IgM classes. Early manifestations, beginning 6 to 10 days after administration of the medication, include an inflammatory reaction at the site of injection of the medication, followed by regional and generalized lymphadenopathy and fever. Symptoms may appear as late as 3 weeks afterward. There is usually a skin rash, which may be urticarial or purpuric. Joints are frequently tender and swollen. Vasculitis may occur in any organ but is observed most commonly in the kidney, resulting in proteinuria and, occasionally, casts in the urine. There may be mild to severe cardiac involvement. Peripheral neuritis may cause temporary paralysis of the upper extremities or may be widespread, causing Guillain–Barré syndrome (Nowak-Wegrzyn & Sicherer, 2016).

Medical and Nursing Management

The primary goal in serum sickness therapy is to treat the clinical syndrome symptomatically. This hypersensitivity reaction lasts for several days to a few weeks if untreated, but the patient responds promptly and completely if treated with antihistamines and corticosteroids (Bope & Kellerman, 2016). Aggressive therapy, including ventilator support, may be necessary if peripheral neuritis and Guillain–Barré syndrome occur. If symptoms are severe enough to warrant ventilator support or if hemodynamic instability ensues, the patient is to be admitted to an intensive care unit. See Chapter 46 for nursing management of Guillain–Barré syndrome.

LATEX ALLERGY

Latex allergy, the allergic reaction to natural rubber proteins, has been implicated in rhinitis, conjunctivitis, contact dermatitis, urticaria, asthma, and anaphylaxis. Over the past 80 years, the numbers of individuals affected with this allergy has dropped drastically due to the processing of non-latex materials and nonpowdered latex gloves used in health care settings. Despite numbers and studies confirming this, the severity of illness associated with a latex allergy remains a nursing priority.

Risk Factors

Populations at risk include health care workers, patients with atopic allergies or multiple surgeries, people working in factories that manufacture latex products, and females, as well as patients with spina bifida or spinal cord injuries and congenital abnormalities of the genitourinary tract. Because more food handlers, hairdressers, auto mechanics, and police officers are now wearing latex gloves, they also may be at risk for latex allergy. Latex is the second most common cause of anaphylactic reactions during the intraoperative period (due to repeated latex exposure), preceded only by muscle relaxants (Butterworth, Mackey, & Wasnick, 2013).

Food that has been handled by people wearing latex gloves may stimulate an allergic response in the consumer. Cross-reactions have been reported in people who are allergic

TABLE **38-4** Selected Products Containing Natural Rubber Latex and Latex-Free Alternatives

Products Containing Latex	Examples of Latex-Safe Alternatives[a]
Hospital Environment	
Ace bandage (brown)	Ace bandage, white, all cotton
Adhesive bandages, Band-Aid dressing, Telfa	Cotton pads and plastic or silk tape, Active Strip (3M), Duoderm, Mepilex
Anesthesia equipment	Neoprene anesthesia kit (King)
Blood pressure cuff, tubing, and bladder	Clean Cuff, single-use nylon or vinyl blood pressure cuffs or wrap with stockinette; or apply over clothing
Catheters	All-silicone or vinyl catheters
Catheter leg bag straps	Velcro straps
Crutch axillary pads and hand grips, tips	Cover with cloth, tape
ECG pads	Baxter, Red Dot 3M ECG pads
Elastic compression stockings	Kendall SCD stockings with stockinette
Gloves	Dermaprene, Neoprene, polymer, or vinyl gloves
IV catheters	Jelko, Deseret IV catheters
IV rubber injection ports	Cover Y-sites and ports; do not puncture. Use three-way stopcocks on plastic tubing.
Levin tube	Salem sump tube
Medication vials	Remove rubber stopper
Penrose drains	Jackson-Pratt, Zimmer Hemovac drains
Prepackaged enema kits	Theravac, Fleet Ready-to-use
Pulse oximeters	Nonin oximeters
Resuscitation bags	Laerdal, Puritan Bennett, *certain* Ambu
Stethoscope tubing	PVC tubing; cover with latex-free stockinette
Syringes—single use (Monoject, B & D)	Terumo syringes, Abbott PCA Abboject
Suction tubing	PVC (Davol, Laerdal)
Tapes	Dermicel, Micropore
Thermometer probes	Diatec probe covers
Tourniquets	X-Tourn straps (Avcor)
Thera-Band	New Thera-band Exercisers, plastic tubing
Home Environment	
Balloons	Mylar balloons
Diapers, incontinence pads	Huggies, Always, *some* Attends
Condoms, diaphragms	Polyurethane products, Durex/Avanti and Reality products (female condom)
Feminine hygiene pad	Kimberly-Clark products
Wheelchair cushions	ROHO cushions, Sof Care bed/chair cushions

[a]Confirmation is essential to verify that all items are latex-free before using, especially if risk of latex allergy is present.

TABLE **38-5** **Types of Reactions to Latex**

Type of Reaction	Cause	Signs/Symptoms	Treatment
Irritant contact dermatitis	Damage to skin because of irritation and loss of epidermoid skin layer; not an allergic reaction. Can be caused by excessive use of soaps and cleansers, multiple hand-washings, inadequate hand drying, mechanical irritation (e.g., sweating, rubbing inside powdered gloves), exposure to chemicals added during the manufacturing of gloves, and alkaline pH of powdered gloves. Reaction may occur with first exposure, is usually benign, and is not life-threatening.	Acute: redness, edema, burning, discomfort, itching Chronic: dry, thickened, cracked skin	Referral for diagnostic testing Avoidance of exposure to irritant Thorough washing and drying of hands Use of powder-free gloves with more frequent changes of gloves Changing glove types Use of water- or silicone-based moisturizing creams, lotions, or topical barrier agents Avoidance of oil- or petroleum-based skin agents with latex products because they cause breakdown of the latex product
Allergic contact dermatitis	Delayed hypersensitivity (type IV) reaction. Usually affects only area in contact with latex; reaction is usually to chemical additives used in the manufacturing process rather than to latex itself. Cause of reaction is T cell–mediated sensitization to additives of latex. Reaction is not life-threatening and is far more common than a type I reaction. Slow onset; occurs 18–24 hours after exposure. Resolves within 3–4 days after exposure. More severe reactions may occur with subsequent exposures.	Pruritus, erythema, swelling, crusty thickened skin, blisters, other skin lesions	Referral for diagnosis (patch tests) and treatment Thorough washing and drying of hands Use of water- or silicone-based moisturizing creams, lotions, or topical barrier agents Avoidance of oil- or petroleum-based products unless they are latex-compatible Avoidance of identified causative agent because continued exposure to latex products in the presence of breaks in skin may contribute to latex protein sensitization
Latex allergy	Type I IgE-mediated immediate hypersensitivity to plant proteins in natural rubber latex. In sensitized people, anti-latex IgE antibody stimulates mast cell proliferation and basophil histamine release. Exposure can be through contact with the skin, mucous membranes, or internal tissues, or through inhalation of traces of powder from latex gloves. Severe reactions usually occur shortly after parenteral or mucous membrane exposure. People with any type I reaction to latex are at high risk of anaphylaxis.	Local: swelling, redness, edema, itching Mild systemic: rhinitis, flushing, conjunctivitis Severe systemic: urticaria, laryngeal edema, bronchospasm, asthma, severe vasodilation angioedema, including anaphylaxis, cardiovascular collapse, and death All above reactions can occur within minutes after exposure.	Immediate treatment of reaction with epinephrine, fluids, vasopressors, and corticosteroids, and airway and ventilator support, with close monitoring for recurrence for next 12–14 hours Prompt referral for diagnostic evaluation Treatment and diagnostic evaluation in latex-free environment Strict avoidance of allergy testing and management Assessment of all patients for symptoms of latex allergy Teaching of patients and family members about the disorder and about the importance of preventing future reactions by avoiding latex Encouraging wearing of a medical alert bracelet that identifies latex allergy for emergency situations Warning labels can be attached to car windows to alert police and paramedics about the driver's or passenger's latex allergy in case of a motor vehicle crash. Carrying an EpiPen at all times and being prepared and able to use it

to certain food products, such as kiwis, bananas, pineapples, mangos, passion fruit, avocados, and chestnuts (American Academy of Allergy, Asthma & Immunology, n.d.).

Pathophysiology

Routes of exposure to latex products can be cutaneous, percutaneous, mucosal, parenteral, or aerosol. Allergic reactions are more likely with exposure via the mucous membrane or from the parenteral route but also can occur with cutaneous contact or inhalation. The most frequent source of exposure is cutaneous, which usually involves the wearing of natural latex gloves. The powder used to facilitate putting on latex gloves can become a carrier of latex proteins from the gloves; when the gloves are put on or removed, the particles become airborne and can be inhaled or settle on the skin, mucous membranes, or clothing. Mucosal exposure can occur from the use of latex condoms, catheters, airways, and nipples. Parenteral exposure can occur from IV lines or hemodialysis equipment. In addition to latex-derived medical devices, many household items also contain latex. Examples of medical and household items containing latex and a list of alternative products are found in Table 38-4.

Clinical Manifestations and Assessment

Several different types of reactions to latex are possible: irritant contact dermatitis, allergic dermatitis, and latex allergy. Table 38-5 lists the causes, symptoms, and management of each.

The diagnosis of latex allergy is based on the history and diagnostic test results. Sensitization is detected by skin testing, RAST, or enzyme-linked immunosorbent assay (ELISA). Skin tests should be performed only by clinicians who have expertise in their administration and interpretation and who have the necessary equipment available to treat local or systemic allergic reactions to the reagent.

Medical Management

See Table 38-5 for medical management.

Nursing Management

The nurse can assume a pivotal role in the management of latex allergies in both patients and staff. All patients should be asked about latex allergy, although special attention should be given to those at particularly high risk (e.g., patients with spina bifida, patients who have undergone multiple surgical procedures). Every time an invasive procedure must be performed, the nurse should consider the possibility of latex allergies. Nurses working in operating rooms, intensive care units, short-term procedure units, and emergency departments need to pay particular attention to latex allergy.

Although the type I reaction is the most significant of the reactions to latex, care must be taken in the presence of irritant contact dermatitis and delayed hypersensitivity reaction to avoid further exposure of the person to latex. Patients with latex allergy are advised to notify their health care providers and to wear a medical information bracelet. Patients must become knowledgeable about what products contain latex and what products are safe, nonlatex alternatives. Also, they must become knowledgeable about signs and symptoms of latex allergy as well as emergency treatment and self-injection of epinephrine in case of allergic reaction.

> **Nursing Alert**
> *Chronic exposure to latex and a history of skin atopy increases the risk of sensitization for health care providers. If a patient is exposed to latex through frequent medical procedures utilizing latex products (e.g., repeated urinary catheterization), they, too, should be considered at increased risk for developing a latex allergy.*

Nurses can be instrumental in establishing and participating in multidisciplinary committees to address latex allergy and to promote a latex-free environment. Latex allergy protocols and education of staff about latex allergy and precautions are important strategies to ensure assessment and prompt treatment of affected people.

CHAPTER REVIEW

Critical Thinking Exercises

1. A 17-year-old girl has developed symptoms of asthma thought to be an allergic response to allergens in her environment. Develop an evidence-based plan for avoidance strategies for her while she is living at home and for her move next year to a college dormitory. Describe the strength of the evidence and criteria used to assess its strength. What instructional strategies and outcome measures will you use to educate her about avoidance strategies and to assess the effectiveness of their use?

2. A 72-year-old man is admitted for emergency surgery to treat a strangulated hernia. He reports that he has severe allergies but is unable to be specific about the nature of

his allergies or the allergic reactions that he has experienced in the past. He reports that he has had to use emergency epinephrine on several occasions in the past because of severe allergic reactions. What precautions are needed preoperatively, intraoperatively, and postoperatively for this patient to prevent the occurrence of severe allergic reactions? What interventions and nursing management would be indicated if he developed a severe allergic reaction?

NCLEX-Style Review Questions

1. During a clinical post-conference, the nursing instructor is discussing factors related to the risk of anaphylaxis. Select all statements that properly describe allergic and anaphylactic reactions.
   a. The severity depends on the degree of allergy.
   b. The severity of previous reactions determines the severity of subsequent reactions.
   c. The severity depends on the dose of the allergen.
   d. The severity of previous reactions does not determine the severity of subsequent reactions.

2. Which reaction would be consistent with a mild reaction to an allergen?
   a. Bronchospasm
   b. Warmth
   c. Cough
   d. Tearing of the eyes

3. When reviewing the chart of a patient diagnosed with allergic rhinitis, the nurse understands that this allergic disorder is caused by which type of hypersensitivity reaction?
   a. Type I
   b. Type II
   c. Type III
   d. Type IV

4. A patient is being seen in the dermatology clinic for urticaria. The nurse would expect which medication to be prescribed for the patient?
   a. Pseudoephedrine (Sudafed)
   b. Diphenhydramine (Benadryl)
   c. Dexamethasone (Decadron)
   d. Cromolyn sodium (NasalCrom)

5. What is the most common risk in developing a latex allergy?
   a. Occasional latex condom use
   b. IV line insertions
   c. Use of hemodialysis equipment
   d. Repeated donning of latex gloves

Try these additional resources, available at **http://thepoint.lww.com/Honan2e**, to enhance your learning and understanding of this chapter:
- NCLEX-Style Student Review Questions
- Journal Articles

REFERENCES AND SELECTED READINGS

References and selected readings associated with this chapter can be found on the website that accompanies the book. Visit **http://thepoint. lww.com/Honan2e** to access the references and other additional resources associated with this chapter.

Nursing Management: Patients with Rheumatic Disorders

Linda Alessie Podolak

Learning Objectives

After reading this chapter, you will be able to:

1. Explain the pathophysiology of rheumatic diseases or disorders.
2. Describe the assessment and diagnostic findings seen in patients with a suspected diagnosis of rheumatic disease or disorder.
3. Describe the systemic effects of a connective tissue disease.
4. Discuss the pharmacologic, medical, and nursing management associated with rheumatic disorders.
5. Apply the nursing process as a framework for the care of the patient with a rheumatic disorder.
6. Identify appropriate nursing interventions based on nursing diagnoses that commonly occur with rheumatic disorders.

Rheumatic disorders affect the joints, bones, muscles, and connective tissues. These conditions can be minor illnesses, or they can be life-threatening. Systemic effects caused by rheumatic disorders or diseases result in obvious limitations in mobility and activities of daily living (ADL) as well as more subtle manifestations, such as pain, fatigue, insomnia, and disturbed body image. Organ failure and death may be an end result for some rheumatic disorders. The rheumatic condition may be the patient's primary health problem or a secondary diagnosis. Thorough understanding of rheumatic conditions and their effects on a patient's function and well-being is key to developing an interprofessional plan of care.

OVERVIEW

Commonly called arthritis (inflammation of a joint) and thought of as one condition, the rheumatic diseases are actually more than 100 different types of disorders that primarily affect joints, bones, skeletal muscles, and connective tissues that collectively affect more than 46 million Americans (National Institute of Arthritis and Musculoskeletal and Skin Diseases [NIAMS], 2014a). Some disorders are more likely to occur at a particular time of life or to affect one gender more than the other (see Box 39-1 for Gerontologic Considerations). The symptom that most commonly causes a person to seek medical attention is pain. Other common

symptoms include joint swelling, limited movement, stiffness, weakness, and fatigue. The onset of these conditions may be acute or insidious, with a course possibly marked by periods of remission (a period when disease symptoms are reduced or absent) and exacerbation (a period when symptoms occur or increase).

Assessment includes a complete health history followed by a complete physical examination combined with a functional assessment. Inspection of the patient's general appearance occurs during initial contact. Gait, posture, and general musculoskeletal size and structure are observed. Gross deformities and abnormalities in movement are noted. Also the symmetry, size, and contour of other connective tissues, such as the skin and adipose tissue, are noted and recorded. The functional assessment is a combination of history (what the patient reports that he or she can and cannot do) and examination (observation of activities is made: the patient demonstrates what he or she can and cannot do, such as dressing and getting in and out of a chair). Observation also includes the adaptations and adjustments the patient may have made (sometimes without awareness); for example, with shoulder or elbow involvement, the person may bend over to reach a fork, rather than raising the fork to the mouth.

The history and physical assessment data are supplemented by supportive or confirming diagnostic test findings. Common serum laboratory tests used for patients with rheumatic disorders are described in Table 39-1. Radiologic

Gerontologic Considerations

Although people of all ages may be affected, rheumatic disease is commonly thought of by the patient, family, and society as a whole as an inevitable consequence of aging. Many older people expect and accept the immobility and self-care problems related to the rheumatic disorders and do not seek help, thinking that nothing can be done. Careful diagnosis and appropriate treatment is crucial and can improve the quality of life for older people. An adequate support system for the elderly is also a critical factor in the ability to follow an interdisciplinary plan of care that includes exercise, nutrition, general health maintenance, pharmacotherapy, and non-pharmacologic management. However, the rheumatic disorders do have some special implications for the older adult.

Age alone causes changes in serologic studies (e.g., ESR, ANA), making interpretation of laboratory values more difficult. Decreased vision and altered balance, often present in elderly people, may be problematic if rheumatic disease in the lower extremities affects locomotion. Also, the combination of decreased hearing and visual acuity, memory loss, and depression contributes to failure to follow the treatment regimen in elderly patients.

Pharmacologic treatment of rheumatic disease in older patients is more difficult. Aging brings many physical and metabolic changes that may increase the elderly patient's sensitivity to both the therapeutic and toxic effects of some drugs, making overtreatment or inappropriate treatment possible. If therapeutic medications have an effect on the senses (hearing, cognition), this effect is intensified in the elderly. The cumulative effect of these medications is accentuated because of the physiologic changes of aging. For example, decreased kidney function in the elderly alters the metabolism of certain medications, such as NSAIDs. In addition, elderly patients are more prone to side effects associated with the use of multiple-drug therapy for various disorders (Lehne, 2013; Miller, 2015).

anticoagulated whole blood sample over a specified period of time; it is commonly referred to as a "sed" rate. Often increased "sed" rates are associated with inflammatory states. Normally, the distance an RBC falls in 1 hour is less than 15 mm/hr for men and slightly higher in women. The speed with which the RBC moves is related to the clumping of RBCs. The more clumping, the heavier and higher the speed that an RBC falls. Inflammatory states produce proteins that encourage this clumping, thus high ESR levels are associated with inflammation. The ESR does not diagnose a problem, but it is used to monitor status of a disease and response to therapy (Van Leeuwen & Bladh, 2015).

Treatment can be simple, aimed at localized relief, or it can be complex, directed toward relief of systemic effects. The chronic nature of most of these disorders mandates that the patient understand the disease, have the information necessary to make good self-management decisions, be referred to appropriate community agencies (such as the Arthritis Foundation) for support, and be presented with a therapeutic program that is compatible with his or her lifestyle. The goals and strategies of management of basic rheumatic diseases are outlined in Table 39-2. The trend in management is toward a more aggressive pharmacologic approach earlier in the disease presentation.

Pharmacologic management of rheumatic disorders is used to manage symptoms, control pain and inflammation, and—in some diseases, such as rheumatoid arthritis (RA)—modify the disease course. However, disease typically advances steadily and, as a result, pharmacologic therapy is chronic; thus, success requires motivation and cooperation by the patient. Selection of medication is based on the patient's needs, the stage of disease, and the risk of side effects (Durham, Fowler, Donato, Smith, & Jensen, 2015).

Antiarthritic drugs fall into three major groups: nonsteroidal anti-inflammatory drugs (NSAIDs) including salicylates (e.g., aspirin), disease-modifying antirheumatic drugs (DMARDs), and glucocorticoids (adrenal corticosteroids). These groups differ with reference to time course of effects, toxicity, and ability to slow disease progression. Table 39-3 reviews the medications commonly used in rheumatic disorders, particularly RA.

Nonpharmacologic treatment measures include the use of heat or cold, weight reduction, joint rest and avoidance of joint overuse, orthotic devices (e.g., splints, braces) to support inflamed joints, and an exercise regimen. Occupational and physical therapy can help the patient adopt self-management strategies. Other nonpharmacologic modalities, such as massage, yoga, pulsed electromagnetic fields, transcutaneous electrical nerve stimulation (TENS), and music therapy, have been used in the treatment of arthritis (Berman, Lewith, Manheimer, Bishop, & D'Adamo, 2015; Field, Diego, Delgado, Garcia, & Funk, 2013; Sharma, 2014). In

investigations facilitate early diagnosis, guide treatment, and, ultimately, impact prognosis. Scans, computed tomography (CT), and magnetic resonance imaging (MRI) are not the most cost-effective methods for detection of early disease and are not performed routinely at the time of diagnosis. In some instances, many tests are used to monitor the course of the disease. For example, contrast radiography and MRI play a role in diagnosing advancing systems affected in scleroderma; the erythrocyte sedimentation rate (ESR) reflects inflammatory activity and, indirectly, the progression or remission of disease. Ultimately, the health care provider determines which tests are necessary based on the symptoms, stage of disease, cost, and likely benefit of the test.

Nursing Alert
The ESR is a measure of the rate of sedimentation of red blood cells (RBCs) in an

TABLE **39-1** **Common Serum Laboratory Tests for Rheumatic Diseases**

Test	Normal Value	Implications
Serology		
Erythrocyte Sedimentation Rate (ESR)		
Measures the rate at which red blood cells (RBCs) settle out of unclotted blood in 1 hour	Westergren method *Men,* 0–15 mm/hr, over 50 years of age: 0–20 mm/hr *Women,* 0–20 mm/hr, over 50 years of age: 0–30 mm/hr	Usually increase is seen in inflammatory connective tissue diseases (e.g., RA, SLE, scleroderma), gout, can be seen in elderly An increase indicates rising inflammation; the higher the ESR, the greater the inflammatory activity
Uric Acid		
Measures level of uric acid in serum	*Men,* 3.4–7 mg/dL (202–416 µmol/L) *Women,* 2.4–6 mg/dL (143–357 µmol/L) *Biologic Crystallization Point,* at least 6.8 mg/dL (408 µmol/L)	Increase is seen with gout, where there is an overproduction of uric acids that occurs when there is excessive cell breakdown and catabolism of nucleonic acids
Serum Immunology		
Antinuclear Antibody (ANA)		
Measures antibodies that react with a variety of nuclear antigens Usually the first step, if antibodies are present, further testing determines specific circulating antibodies to extractable nuclear antigens (anti-dsDNA, anti-RNP, anti Ro-SSA).	Screen: negative by ELISA and IFA methods If positive by IFA, specimen is titered. Titer: less than 1:160 Low titers are present in elderly and some healthy adults	Positive test is associated with systemic rheumatic disease, such as mixed connective tissue disease, SLE, RA, scleroderma, CREST syndrome, can be seen in elderly The higher the titer, the greater the inflammation Some negative ANA findings have been found to have positive anti-Ro (SSA)
Anticentromere Antibody Test		
A specific autoantibody, detected by using Hep-2 cells in various stages of cell division, centromere region of the cell chromosomes will stain if positive	Screen: negative by ELISA and IFA methods If positive by IFA, specimen is titered.	Positive test is associated with the CREST syndrome in scleroderma Present in 90% of those with CREST
Anticyclic Citrullinated Peptide (Anti-CCP)		
Disease-specific autoantibody, highly specific diagnostic and prognostic markers for RA Detects patients with early RA at baseline (after 3–6 months of symptoms) Second generation test: CCP2 assay, even higher sensitivity	Negative	Positive in RA Predictive of erosive disease Sensitivity of anti-CCP comparable to rheumatoid factor (RF) but has higher specificity (90–95%) Differentiates other entities that can resemble RA and, at times, be RF positive
Anti–double-stranded DNA (Anti-dsDNA)		
Specific autoantibody to extractable nuclear antigens; differentiates native (i.e., double-stranded) DNA antibodies from other nonnative antibodies; 95% specific for SLE, making it a valuable disease marker	Negative: less than 25 IU by ELISA	DNA-anti-dsDNA immune complexes play a role in SLE pathogenesis, found in 70% of SLE patients Positive: 31–200 IU; strongly positive: over 200 IU Anti-dsDNA concentrations may decrease with successful therapy, may increase with exacerbation of SLE
Autoantibodies, Others		
Specific autoantibodies to extractable nuclear antigens (*anti-RNA, anti-Sm, anti-scl-70*); may reflect disease-specific immune mechanisms but are not pathogenetic by themselves	Negative: less than 20 U/mL by ELISA	Positive: greater than 26 U/mL *Anti-RNA:* mixed connective tissue disease (MCTD), 35–40% of SLE patients *Anti-Sm* (Smith): SLE, MCTD *Anti-scl-70:* Scleroderma

(*continued on page 1142*)

TABLE **39-1** **Common Serum Laboratory Tests for Rheumatic Diseases (***continued***)**

Test	Normal Value	Implications
Complement Levels—C3, C4		
Complement component levels: done if a reduction/consumption of complement component concentration is suspected C3 constitutes 70% of the total protein in the complement system (antigen–antibody complexes)	C3: 75–175 mg/dL (or 0.75–1.75 g/L) C4: 14–40 mg/dL (or 140–400 mg/L)	Decrease may be seen in active SLE, immune complex disease (i.e., RA) Decrease indicates autoimmune activity
C-Reactive Protein Test (CRP)		
Measures the presence of abnormal glycoprotein in response to inflammatory cytokines	Less than 1 mg/dL (less than 10 mg/L)	A positive reading indicates active inflammation Often is positive for RA and SLE More sensitive than ESR test
Immunoglobulin Electrophoresis		
Measures the values of immunoglobulins	IgG: 700–1,500 mg/dL (7.0–15.0 g/L) IgM: 60–300 mg/dL (600–3,000 mg/L)	Increased levels of IgG occurs in RA, autoimmune disorders (i.e., SLE) Increased levels of IgM occurs in RA, SLE
Rheumatoid Factor (RF)		
Measures RFs, antibodies directed against the Fe fragment of IgG Determines the presence of abnormal antibodies seen in connective tissue disease	0–20 U/mL Negative titer	Positive titer greater than 1:80 Present in 80% of those with RA; positive RF also may suggest SLE, MCTD Low titers can be seen in OA The higher the titer (number at right of colon), the greater the inflammation

addition, iontophoresis can be used to deliver medication through the skin using direct electrical current. A combination of methods may be required because different methods often work better at different times.

Common choices of complementary and alternative medicine (CAM) used by patients with rheumatologic disorders include dietary supplements, herbal therapies, mind/body and spiritual practices, manual/manipulative therapies, biostimulation, vagus nerve stimulation, and topical ointments (Cheung, Geisler, & Sunneberg, 2014; Koopman,

Schuurman, Vervoordeldonk, & Tak, 2014; Lu, Hart, Lutgendorf, & Perkhounkova, 2013; Shengelia, Parker, Ballin, George, & Reid, 2013). It is essential that health care providers remain informed on appropriate indications for use, risks, and limitations of such therapies or practices.

Nurses need to understand the classification of rheumatic diseases. One basic system is to classify disease as either monoarticular (affecting a single joint) or polyarticular (affecting multiple joints) and then to further classify it as either inflammatory (e.g., RA) or degenerative,

TABLE **39-2** **Goals and Strategies for Rheumatic Diseases**

Major Goals	Management Strategy
Suppress inflammation and the autoimmune response	Optimize pharmacologic therapy (anti-inflammatory and disease-modifying agents)
Control pain	Protect joints; ease pain with splints/orthoses, thermal modalities, relaxation techniques
Maintain or improve joint mobility	Implement exercise programs for joint motion and muscle strengthening and overall health
Maintain or improve functional status	Make use of adaptive devices and techniques
Increase patient's knowledge of disease process	Provide and reinforce patient teaching
Promote self-management by patient compliance with the therapeutic regimen	Promote social support and encouragement of change-based interventions compatible with therapeutic regimen and lifestyle

TABLE **39-3** Medications Used in Rheumatic Diseases

Medication	Action, Use, and Indication	Nursing Considerations
Nonsteroidal Anti-Inflammatory Drugs (NSAIDs)		
Salicylates		
Acetylated Aspirin *Nonacetylated* Choline salicylate (Arthropan, Trilisate), Salsalate (Disalcid), Sodium salicylate	*Action:* anti-inflammatory, analgesic, antipyretic Acetylated salicylates are platelet aggregation inhibitors Anti-inflammatory doses will produce blood salicylate levels of 20–30 mg/dL	Administer with meals to prevent gastric irritation Assess for tinnitus, gastric intolerance, gastrointestinal (GI) bleeding, and purpuric tendencies Monitor for possible confusion in the elderly
Nonsalicylates		
First-Generation Diclofenac (Voltaren), diflunisal (Dolobid), etodolac (Lodine), flurbiprofen (Ansaid), ibuprofen (Motrin), indomethacin (Indocin), ketoprofen (Orudis, Oruvail), meclofenamate (Meclomen), meloxicam (Mobic), nabumetone (Relafen), naproxen (Naprosyn), oxaprozin (DayPro), piroxicam (Feldene), sulindac (Clinoril), tolmetin sodium (Tolectin)	*Action:* anti-inflammatory, analgesic, antipyretic, inhibition of platelet aggregation, inhibition of prostaglandin synthesis Anti-inflammatory effect occurs 2–4 weeks after initiation NSAIDs are alternative to salicylates for first-line therapy in several rheumatic diseases All NSAIDs are useful for short-term treatment of acute gout attack	Administer NSAIDs with food Monitor for GI, CNS, cardiovascular, renal, hematologic, and dermatologic adverse effects Avoid salicylates; use acetaminophen for additional analgesia Need to be used regularly for maximal effect Watch for possible confusion in the elderly
Second-Generation: COX-2 *Inhibitors* Celecoxib (Celebrex)	*Action*: Selective prostaglandin inhibition, inhibit only cyclooxygenase (COX)-2 enzymes, which are produced during inflammation, and spare COX-1 enzymes, which can be protective to the stomach	Monitoring the same as for other NSAIDs Increased risk of cardiovascular events, including myocardial infarction and stroke Appropriate for the elderly and patients who are at high risk for gastric ulcers
Related Agent Acetaminophen (Tylenol)	*Action*: Inhibits the synthesis of prostaglandins; antipyretic, analgesic, no anti-inflammatory properties	Chronic excessive use of more than 4 g/day may lead to hepatotoxicity or renal or cardiac damage Concurrent use of NSAIDs increases the risk of adverse renal effects
Disease-Modifying Antirheumatic Drugs (DMARDs)		
Nonbiologic DMARDs—Traditional Drugs		
Immunosuppressives Methotrexate (Rheumatrex)	*Action:* Immune suppression, inhibits folic acid reductase, leading to inhibition of DNA synthesis and other cellular effects Acts faster than other DMARDs Methotrexate is gold standard for RA treatment; also useful in SLE	Assess for bone marrow suppression, GI ulcerations, skin rashes, alopecia, bladder toxicity, increased infections Monitor CBC, liver enzymes, creatinine every 2–4 weeks Caution with NSAID use Should be on folic acid Advise patient of contraceptive measures because of teratogenicity
Antimalarials Hydroxychloroquine (Plaquenil), chloroquine (Aralen)	*Action:* Anti-inflammatory, inhibits lysosomal enzymes Slow-acting, onset may take 2–4 months Useful in RA and SLE	Administer concurrently with NSAIDs Assess for visual changes, GI upset, skin rash, headaches, photosensitivity, bleaching of hair Retinopathy may occur; emphasize (every 6–12 months) ophthalmologic examinations

(continued on page 1144)

TABLE **39-3** Medications Used in Rheumatic Diseases (*continued*)

Medication	Action, Use, and Indication	Nursing Considerations
Sulfonamides sulfasalazine (Azulfidine)	*Action:* Anti-inflammatory, reduces lymphocyte response, inhibits angiogenesis Useful in RA, seronegative spondyloarthropathies	Administer concurrently with NSAIDs Do not use in patients with allergy to sulfa medications or salicylates Emphasize adequate fluid intake Assess for GI upset, skin rash, headache, liver abnormalities, anemia
Pyrimidine Synthesis Inhibitor Leflunomide (Arava)	*Action:* Has antiproliferative and anti-inflammatory effects, powerful immunosuppressant Used in moderate to severe RA May be used alone or in combination with other DMARDs (except methotrexate) About as effective as methotrexate but more adverse effects	Long half-life; requires loading dose followed by daily administration Assess for diarrhea, respiratory infection, alopecia, skin rash, mouth sores, nausea Monitor liver function tests Risk for serious infections Contraindicated in patients who are pregnant and breastfeeding Administered orally
Nonbiologic DMARDs—Minor Drugs		
Cyclosporine (Neoral)	*Action:* Immune suppression by inhibiting T lymphocytes Used for severe, progressive RA, unresponsive to other DMARDs Used in combination with methotrexate	Assess slow dose titration upward until response noted or toxicity occurs Assess for toxic effects: bleeding gums, fluid retention, hair growth, tremors Monitor blood pressure and creatinine every 2 weeks until stable
Gold-Containing Compounds Aurothioglucose (Solganol), gold sodium thiomalate (Myochrysine), auranofin (Ridaura)	*Action:* Inhibits T- and B-cell activity, suppresses synovitis during active stage of rheumatoid disease Slow-acting, onset may take 3–6 months IM preparations are given weekly for about 6 months and then every 2–4 weeks	Administer concurrently with NSAIDs Assess for pruritus, stomatitis, diarrhea, dermatitis, proteinuria, hematuria, bone marrow suppression (decreased WBCs and/or platelets), profound hypotension Monitor CBC and urinalysis with every other injection
Penicillamine (Cuprimine, Depen)	*Action:* Anti-inflammatory, inhibits T-cell function, impairs antigen presentation Slow-acting, onset may take 2–3 months Useful in RA and systemic sclerosis	Administer concurrently with NSAIDs Assess for GI irritation, decreased taste, skin rash or itching, bone marrow suppression, proteinuria with CBC, and urinalysis every 2–4 weeks
Minor Immunosuppressants Azathioprine (Imuran), cyclophosphamide (Cytoxan)	*Action:* Immune suppression, affects DNA synthesis and other cellular effects Have teratogenic potential; azathioprine and cyclophosphamide reserved for more aggressive or unresponsive disease	Assess for bone marrow suppression, GI ulcerations, skin rashes, alopecia, bladder toxicity, increased infections Monitor CBC, liver enzymes, creatinine every 2–4 weeks Advise patient of contraceptive measures because of teratogenicity
Biologic DMARDs—Immunomodulators		
Tumor Necrosis Factor (TNF) Inhibitors Adalimumab (Humira), etanercept (Enbrel), infliximab (Remicade), golimumab (Simponi), certolizumab pegol (Cimzia)	*Action:* Biologic response modifier that binds to TNF, a cytokine involved in inflammatory and immune responses Used in moderate to severe RA unresponsive to methotrexate Can be used alone or with methotrexate or other DMARDs Humira is administered every 1–2 weeks, and Enbrel is administered twice a week Simponi is the first treatment that is administered once a month	Patient should be tested for tuberculosis before beginning this medication Teach patient subcutaneous self-injection of adalimumab (Humira) or etanercept (Enbrel) Infliximab (Remicade) is administered by IV over 2 hours or more Medication must be refrigerated Monitor for injection site reactions Educate patient about increased risk for serious infection and to withhold medication if fever occurs Contraindicated in CHF class III/IV, and may pose a risk for new onset of heart failure

Medication	Action, Use, and Indication	Nursing Considerations
T-Cell Activation Inhibitors Abatacept (Orencia)	*Action:* selectively modulates T-cell activation, altering immune response (costimulatory blocker) A cost-effective alternative treatment of moderate to severe RA when conventional DMARDs and TNF inhibitors are inadequate	Contains maltose, may falsely elevate blood glucose High risk for infections Do not give live vaccines
B-Cell Depleting Agents Rituximab (Rituxan)	*Action:* monoclonal antibody directed at the CD20 antigen expressed on mature B and pre-B cells B-cell depletion therapy: a course of two IV infusions, 2 weeks apart with a repeat treatment interval of 6–12 months	Usually patient is premedicated with acetaminophen and diphenhydramine to decrease fever, chills as associated with infusion Caution in patients with cardiac and pulmonary diseases
Interleukin (IL)-1 Receptor Antagonist Anakinra (Kineret)	*Action:* Human IL-1 receptor antagonist; blocks IL-1 receptors, decreasing inflammatory and immunologic responses Used in moderate to severe RA unresponsive to methotrexate Can be used alone or with methotrexate or DMARDs but not with TNF inhibitors	Administered daily by subcutaneous injection Teach patient subcutaneous self-injection to be administered daily Medication must be refrigerated at 36–46°F (2–8°C) and warmed to room temperature for 30 minutes prior to injection Monitor for injection site reactions Educate patient about increased risk for infection and to withhold medication if fever occurs
Interleukin (IL)-6 Receptor Antagonist Tocilizumab (Actemra)	*Action:* Human IL-6 receptor antagonist; blocks IL-6 receptors, decreasing inflammatory and immunologic responses Used in moderate to severe RA unresponsive to a TNF inhibitor Can be used alone or with methotrexate or DMARDs but not with TNF inhibitors	Administered as IV therapy or subcutaneous injection; should be refrigerated at 36–46°F (2–8°C) and warmed to room temperature for 30 minutes prior to injection Risk for serious infections and other serious adverse effects, e.g., liver injury, GI perforation, neutropenia, and thrombocytopenia Can reduce blood levels of other drugs, e.g., oral contraceptives, warfarin, proton pump inhibitors
New Class of DMARDs—Small Molecule Kinase Inhibitors		
Janus Kinase (JAK) Inhibitor Tofacitinib citrate (Xeljanz)	*Action:* JAK inhibitor works deep inside the cell (intracellular) to disrupt activities occurring in signaling pathways that play a role in the inflammation associated with RA Used in moderate to severe RA unresponsive to methotrexate	First oral agent taken p.o. twice a day. Xeljanz should not be given if lymphocyte count, neutrophil count, or red blood cell count is too low or liver tests are too high. Cholesterol levels should be monitored 4–8 weeks after start and as needed after that. High risk for infections Do not give live vaccines
Glucocorticoids		
Adrenal Corticosteroids Prednisone (Deltasone) hydrocortisone sodium succinate (Solu-Cortef) methylprednisolone sodium succinate (Solu-Medrol) methylprednisolone acetate (Depo-Medrol), intra-articular injection	*Action:* Anti-inflammatory Used for shortest duration and at lowest dose possible to minimize adverse effects Useful for unremitting RA, SLE Fast-acting; onset in days Intra-articular injections useful for joints unresponsive to NSAIDs	Assess for toxicity: cataracts, GI irritation, hyperglycemia, hypertension, fractures, avascular necrosis, hirsutism, psychosis Joints most amenable to injections include ankles, knees, hips, shoulders, and hands Repeated injections can cause joint damage

CBC, complete blood count; CNS, central nervous system; RA, rheumatoid arthritis; SLE, systemic lupus erythematosus; WBCs, white blood cells.
Adapted from Lehne, R. A. (2013). *Pharmacology for nursing care* (8th ed.). St. Louis, MO: W. B. Saunders Elsevier.

Focus on Pathophysiology

Rheumatic Disorders

Each **synovial** joint has a given range of motion, and the synovial fluid within a joint has three primary functions: lubrication, nutrient distribution, and shock absorption. Inflammation is manifested in the joints as **synovitis**. Rheumatic disorders always involve damage to the articular cartilages. Because articular cartilages involve some degree of inflammation and degeneration, the rheumatic disorders can be classified as either inflammatory (e.g., RA) or degenerative, noninflammatory (e.g., OA).

In the inflammatory rheumatic disorder classification, the primary process starts with inflammation due to an altered immune function. The inflammatory reaction includes swelling, pain, and loss of function (see Chapter 36 for the inflammatory and immunologic processes). Degeneration then occurs as a secondary process, spreading to the articular surfaces. The cause of degeneration of the articular cartilage is poorly understood but believed to be metabolically active and, therefore, is more accurately called *degradation*.

On the other hand, in the degenerative (noninflammatory) rheumatic disorder classification, inflammation occurs as a secondary process. The resultant secondary synovitis is usually milder, is more likely to be seen in advanced disease, and represents a reactive process. The synovitis is thought to result mainly from degeneration due to mechanical irritation of two bone surfaces. As the articular cartilage becomes damaged, the matrix (noncellular component of tissue) begins to break down; the exposed cartilage changes from a slick, smooth gliding surface to a rough fibrous network of collagen fibers. Later this network may be converted to bone, locking the articulating elements into position. Fixation of a joint, called ankylosis, eliminates the friction but at the drastic cost of immobility.

noninflammatory (e.g., osteoarthritis [OA]). This chapter groups the conditions into those affecting the joints, bones, and muscles and then those affecting the connective tissues.

CONDITIONS AFFECTING THE JOINTS, BONES, AND MUSCLES

Despite the diversity of rheumatic disorders, the joint is the area most commonly affected and involves some degree of inflammation and damage to the articular cartilages, which may occur simultaneously. Understanding normal anatomy and physiology of **articulations**, or joints, is the key to understanding the pathophysiology of the rheumatic disorders (Box 39-2).

Osteoarthritis

Osteoarthritis, also known as degenerative joint disease, is a chronic, noninflammatory (even though inflammation may be present), progressive disorder that causes cartilage deterioration in synovial joints and vertebrae. It particularly affects the weight-bearing joints, knees and hips, and joints of the distal interphalangeal (DIP) and proximal interphalangeal (PIP) joints of the fingers (Shelton, 2013). OA is the most common and most frequently disabling of the joint disorders; it is overdiagnosed and trivialized and frequently over- or undertreated. The functional impact of OA on quality of life, especially for elderly patients, is often ignored.

OA has been classified as both primary (idiopathic), with no prior event or disease related to the OA, and secondary, resulting from previous joint injury or inflammatory disease. The distinction between primary and secondary OA is not always clear, but often the clinical presentation and symptoms are similar.

Risk Factors

Risk factors for OA are summarized in Box 39-3. Age is the risk factor most strongly correlated with OA, while obesity is now well recognized as an important contributing factor (Di Cesare, Haudenschild, Samuels, & Abramson, 2013; Felson & Zhang, 2015).

Risk Factors for Osteoarthritis (OA)

- Aging
- Obesity (mechanical loading from a higher body mass index is associated with an increased risk of knee OA; the link between OA and adipose-derived leptin is now recognized as a metabolically active contributor to inflammatory cascades)
- Genetic predisposition
- Joint location (joint-specific, age-related articular cartilage changes, varying joint responsiveness to cytokines)
- Malalignment of joints (can lead to rapid development of OA; congenital and developmental disorders, e.g., poorly reduced intra-articular fractures, developmental dysplasia of the hip)
- Trauma (also can lead to rapid development of OA; overuse or abuse of joints, as occurs in high-impact sports; previous joint damage; excessive loading or forces, such as that seen in pneumatic drill operators, or frequent squatting position, such as catchers in baseball, where up to 10 times body weight may be transmitted to the knee.)
- Gender (differences in incidence after 50 years of age may be the result of postmenopausal estrogen deficiency; articular chondrocytes possess functional estrogen receptors)

Adapted from Di Cesare, P. E., Haudenschild, D. R., Samuels, J., & Abramson, S. B. (2013). Pathogenesis of osteoarthritis. In G. S. Firestein, R. C. Budd, S. E. Gabriel, I. B. McInnes, & J. R. O'Dell. (Eds.), *Kelley's textbook of rheumatology* (9th ed.). Philadelphia, PA: Saunders Elsevier.

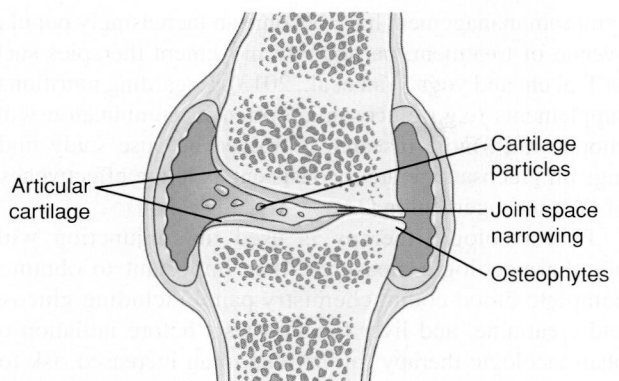

FIGURE 39-1 Osteoarthritic degenerative joint changes: hypertrophy of bone margins resulting in characteristic osteophytes (bone spurs) and narrowing of joint space.

OA generally affects adults 40 years of age and above (American College of Rheumatology [ACR], 2015a; Harris & Crawford, 2015). Prevalence of arthritis in the United States for adults 25 years of age and older having clinical OA of some joint was estimated at nearly 27 million (Nelson & Jordan, 2015). Because of the aging of Western populations and because of the increased prevalence of obesity, a major risk factor, the occurrence of OA is on the rise. In the United States, OA prevalence will increase by 66% to 100% by 2020 (Felson, 2015). Radiologic OA is more prevalent than symptomatic OA. According to the ACR, 70% of people over 70 years of age have x-ray evidence of OA; however, only half ever develop symptoms. OA of the hand, hip, and knee become more frequent with age, and more women are affected than men after 50 years of age (Centers for Disease Control and Prevention [CDC], 2015b).

Pathophysiology

OA may be thought of as the end result of many factors that, when combined, predispose the patient to the disease. In OA, changes in articular cartilage occur first; eventually, changes to secondary soft tissue may occur. OA is characterized by erosion of the articular cartilage combined with hypertrophy of bone at the joint margins, resulting in formation of new bone known as **osteophytes** or bone spurs (Fig. 39-1) and subchondral (the bony plate that supports the articular cartilage) sclerosis. In addition, OA is characterized by a range of biochemical and morphologic alterations of the synovial membrane and joint capsule. In general, a combination of cartilage degradation, bone stiffening, and reactive inflammation of the synovium occurs (Aigner, Schmitz, & Salter, 2015). Understanding of OA has been expanded greatly beyond what previously was thought of as simply "wear and tear" related to aging.

Clinical Manifestations and Assessment

The general clinical manifestations of OA are pain, stiffness, and functional disability (Altman, 2015; Harris & Crawford, 2015). Pain in one or more joints typically is worsened by activities and is alleviated by rest. Although osteoarthritic pain is unusual during the night or at rest, there are exceptions, including in patients with mild OA using joints for several hours, in patients with advanced OA with destructive arthropathy, and in patients with an acute inflammatory flare-up of OA. Stiffness may be defined as a sensation of a gelling or tightening of the involved joint that usually occurs after inactivity, such as in the morning or when rising after sitting for a prolonged period. Morning stiffness usually resolves after less than 10 minutes (no more than 30 minutes' duration), in contrast to prolonged stiffness seen in inflammatory disorders. Functional impairment is reflected in limited range of motion (ROM) and patient report of limited ability to perform day-to-day activities.

The diagnosis of OA is complicated by many contributing factors. The ACR has established clinical classification criteria for OA of specific joints to promote consistency in the diagnosis of OA. Typically OA is diagnosed by an overall clinical impression based on the patient's age and history, location of joint abnormalities, and radiographic findings. Limited passive movement can be the first and only physical sign of symptomatic OA. During joint examination, crepitus, a continuous grating sensation, may be felt or heard as the joint goes through ROM. Physical assessment of the musculoskeletal system reveals joint enlargement, resulting from **joint effusion** or bony swelling or both. This is most easily detected in the patient's knees by the evidence of patellar tap or by the elicitation of a fluid thrill (wave test). Joint deformities reflect advanced disease with joint destruction, which then contributes to misalignment, joint instability (causing a sensation in the knees of "giving way" or "locking"), and limb shortening. Fingers also can be misaligned in the presence of Heberden (enlargements of DIP joints) or Bouchard nodes (enlargements of PIP joints) (Fig. 39-2).

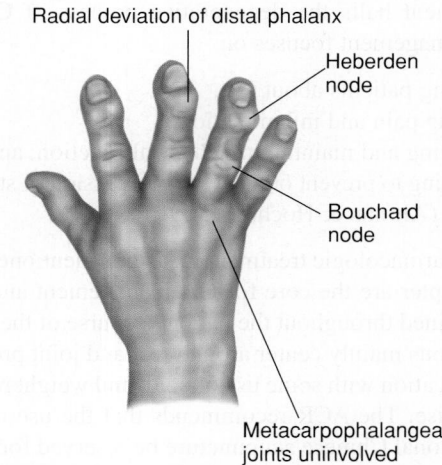

FIGURE 39-2 Heberden and Bouchard nodes. (From Bickley, L. S. (2009). *Bates' guide to physical examination and history taking* (10th ed.). Philadelphia, PA: Lippincott Williams & Wilkins.)

Radiographic assessment has long been considered the gold standard to diagnose OA and to establish severity of joint damage; to monitor disease activity, progression, and response to therapy; and to search for complications of the disorder or the treatment. Standard x-rays of affected joints show osteophytes, the most characteristic feature of OA, and, in more advanced disease, joint space narrowing and sclerosis. One method of classifying the severity of OA (with or without symptoms) is on a plain radiograph using the Kellgren–Lawrence (KL) grading scale. This overall joint scoring system, used extensively in research for more than five decades, grades OA in five levels from 0 (no osteophytes or joint space narrowing) to 4 (severe joint space narrowing with subchondral sclerosis); generally a grade of 2 is considered diagnostic of OA (Nelson & Jordan, 2015). MRI can be used to assess the quantity and function of cartilage, synovium, and bone; however, it is not yet recommended for routine use. Arthroscopy is a more appropriate gold standard in the evaluation of OA, allowing direct visualization of cartilage surface integrity. Routine laboratory testing is rarely required and is primarily used to rule out other conditions, such as metabolic or inflammatory arthropathies. A positive C-reactive protein (CRP) and rheumatoid factors (RFs) can be found in low-grade inflammation in OA. Synovial fluid analysis can be done to differentiate OA from RA. According to the World Health Organization (WHO), biomarkers are an important aspect for clinical diagnosis and treatment for arthritis in general and OA research in particular for drug development. Therefore, molecular biomarkers are currently being explored for clinical utility, such as urinary C-telopeptide fragments of type II collagen (u-CTXII). However, no single marker is yet adequate for predicting or monitoring OA (Altman, 2015; DeGroot, Zuurmond, & Tak, 2013; Nelson & Jordan, 2013).

Medical and Nursing Management

No treatment halts the degenerative process of OA; as a result, management focuses on:

- Educating patients about OA,
- Reducing pain and inflammation,
- Optimizing and maintaining physical function, and
- Attempting to prevent or slow the progression of structural damage (Altman & Hochberg, 2015).

Nonpharmacologic treatment measures mentioned earlier in the chapter are the core for OA management and should be maintained throughout the patient's course of the disease. Interventions mainly center around rest and joint protection, heat application with some use of cold, and weight reduction and exercise. The ACR recommends that the use of TENS and traditional Chinese acupuncture be reserved for patients who are candidates for total joint reconstructive surgery but are either unwilling to undergo the surgery or have medical contraindications to these procedures. CAM therapies for

symptom management have become an increasingly popular avenue of treatment, particularly movement therapies such as T'ai chi and yoga (Yan et al., 2013). Regarding nutritional supplements (e.g., glucosamine often in combination with chondroitin), more research is needed because study findings on glucosamine are inconsistent as to the effectiveness of pain management in OA.

Pharmacologic therapy is used in conjunction with nonpharmacologic measures. It is important to obtain a complete blood count, chemistry panel including glucose and creatinine, and liver function tests before initiation of pharmacologic therapy for OA due to an increased risk for adverse events. In OA, the initial analgesic therapy is acetaminophen with doses recommended by the U.S. Food and Drug Administration (FDA) up to 1,000 mg three times daily (Felson, 2015). The safety profile of acetaminophen has been revisited, in particular when considering a daily dose of 4,000 mg. Study results suggest that high doses (over 3,000 mg) place patients at risk for upper gastrointestinal (GI) complications and hepatic toxicity and has been associated with a prolonged prothrombin time (PT) in patients undergoing Coumadin anticoagulation (Altman & Hochberg, 2015). To promote excretion of the drug, adequate water intake of at least 2,000 mL/day is encouraged.

Nursing Alert *Nurses need to educate patients who are taking acetaminophen to avoid the concomitant use of alcohol and over-the-counter (OTC) products that contain acetaminophen, such as cold preparations and use of combination opioid analgesics such as Tylenol #3 (acetaminophen and codeine). Use of either of these substances simultaneously with acetaminophen can lead to the possibility of hepatic toxicity (Lozada, 2013; Shelton, 2013).*

For the patient who either fails to obtain adequate pain management with acetaminophen or has moderate to severe pain, an NSAID may provide greater relief. If the patient is at risk for or experiences GI complications with an NSAID, supplemental treatment with a protective agent, such as misoprostol (Cytotec), may be indicated. As an alternative to traditional NSAIDs, treatment with the cyclooxygenase (COX)-2 inhibitors celecoxib (Celebrex) or etoricoxib (Arcoxia) may be considered in selected patients. The use of COX-2 inhibitors will be discussed later, in the management of RA.

Other medications that may be considered are the opioids and topical analgesics, such as capsaicin (Capsin, Zostrix) and methyl salicylate. Another therapeutic approach is the intra-articular injection of hyaluronic acid, referred to as *viscosupplementation*. Viscosupplementation is used in patients with OA and is thought to act as a short-term lubricant and provide a biomechanical benefit as well as an analgesic effect by buffering synovial nerve endings directly; it also may have some anti-inflammatory effects, and it may stimulate synovial lining cells to produce hyaluronic acid.

For persistent, moderate to severe OA and erosive RA, reconstructive surgery and corticosteroids are used often. Reconstructive surgery is indicated when pain cannot be relieved by conservative measures and the threat of loss of independence is eminent. Surgical procedures include synovectomy (excision of the synovial membrane), arthrodesis (surgical fusion of the joint), tenorrhaphy (suturing of a tendon), and osteotomy (to alter the distribution of weight within the joint). The procedure used most commonly is **arthroplasty**, a surgical repair and replacement of the joint. Surgery is not performed during disease flare ups.

Tidal irrigation (lavage) and joint debridement of the knee involve the introduction of a large volume of saline into the joint through cannulas and then removal of debris with this fluid. In some cases, this procedure provides pain relief for up to 6 months.

Gout

Gout, one of the most common of the inflammatory arthritides, is a metabolic disorder marked by the deposition of monosodium urate crystals within joints and other tissues. Gout is a heterogeneous group of conditions related to a genetic defect of purine metabolism that results in hyperuricemia (excessive uric acid, a purine end product). The prevalence of gout is reported to be less than 1% to 15.3%, and it appears to be on the rise. It occurs more commonly in males than in females (3–4:1), and the incidence of gout among black men is almost twice that among white men. The general incidence increases with age, body mass index, and increasing levels of serum uric acid (urate) (Burns & Wortmann, 2013; CDC, 2015d; Choi, 2015). While hyperuricemia may indicate an increased risk of gout, the association between hyperuricemia and gout is unclear. Typically, the higher the uric acid level and longer the length of the elevation, the more likely that gout will occur and tophi (deposits of uric acid) will form. On the other hand, some patients with hyperuricemia do not develop gout, and other patients with repeated gout attacks have normal or low levels of serum uric acid (laboratory population–based norm for men is rounded to 8 mg/dL and women is 7 mg/dL) (Van Leeuwen & Bladh, 2015). Therefore, the exact level of uric acid that is considered pathologic is controversial.

Primary gout is characterized by hyperuricemia caused by an overproduction of uric acid or a decreased urate excretion in the kidney. Often primary gout is caused by an inherited disorder in purine metabolism, with a 50% incidence (Keenan, Nowatzky, & Pillinger, 2013; McLean & Dalbeth, 2015). Secondary gout is related to a wide number of diseases or drugs that decrease the kidney's ability to excrete uric acid, increase the production of uric acid, or a combination of both. Conditions associated with secondary gout include diabetic ketoacidosis, severe dieting or starvation, and metabolic syndrome. Disorders, such as multiple myeloma and leukemia, result in increased production of uric acid because of a greater cell turnover and an increase in cell breakdown. Altered renal tubular function, either as a major action or as an unintended side effect of certain pharmacologic agents (e.g., diuretics such as thiazides and furosemide), low-dose salicylates, or ethanol, can contribute to uric acid underexcretion. An excessive intake of foods that are high in purines (shellfish, organ meats) may result in symptoms of gout in susceptible persons.

Pathophysiology

Hyperuricemia denotes an elevated level of uric acid (urate) in the blood, and, in recent years, it has been recognized that the reference ranges are quite wide. The laboratory reference ranges of hyperuricemia often are reported based on population norms, and values vary depending on the population being evaluated. To define individuals with hyperuricemia, current evidence-based reviews recommend that it is more clinically relevant to use the biologic value of 6.8 mg/dL or 408 μmol/L, a level of serum uric acid above the saturation point for crystal formation (Burns & Wortmann, 2013; Edwards, 2015). Asymptomatic hyperuricemia is a laboratory finding, not a disease, but can lead to gout pathogenesis. Attacks of gout appear to be related to sudden increases or decreases of serum uric acid levels. When the uric acid precipitates and then deposits within a joint as urate crystals, an inflammatory response occurs, and an attack of gout begins. With repeated attacks, accumulations of sodium urate crystals, called **tophi**, are deposited in peripheral areas of the body, such as the great toe, the hands, and the ear (lower temperature areas). Renal urate lithiasis (kidney stones), with chronic renal disease secondary to urate deposition, may develop.

Clinical Manifestations and Assessment

Manifestations of the gout syndrome include acute gouty arthritis (recurrent attacks of severe articular and periarticular inflammation), tophi (crystalline deposits accumulating in articular tissue, osseous tissue, soft tissue, and cartilage), gouty nephropathy (renal impairment), and uric acid urinary calculi. Four phases (or stages) of gout can be identified: asymptomatic hyperuricemia, acute gouty arthritis, intercritical or interval gout, and chronic tophaceous gout (acute and intercritical gout together are sometimes noted as one phase). Phase 1, asymptomatic hyperuricemia, is when the serum urate level is high, but gout manifested by arthritis or nephrolithiasis has not yet occurred. People can remain asymptomatic throughout their lifetimes. The subsequent development of gout is directly related to the duration and magnitude of the hyperuricemia. Therefore, the commitment to lifelong pharmacologic treatment of hyperuricemia is deferred until there is an initial attack of gout (phase 2).

Olecranon bursa

Elbow

Wrist
Fingers

Knee

Ankle

Subtalar

1st MTP

Midfoot

FIGURE 39-3 Gout: common sites of involvement. MTP, (metatarsophalangeal) or gout of the knee. (From Stoller, J. K., Nielsen, C., Buccola, J., & Brateanu, A. (2014). *The Cleveland clinic foundation intensive review of internal medicine.* (6th ed.). Philadelphia, PA: Wolters Kluwer Health.)

Acute arthritis is the most common early clinical manifestation of gouty arthritis. The first attack usually occurs between 40 and 60 years of age in men and after 60 years of age in women (Burns & Wortmann, 2013). The patient experiences excruciating pain and inflammation in one or more small joints. The metatarsophalangeal (MTP) joint of the big toe is the joint affected most commonly (up to 90% of patients) and is referred to as **podagra** (Bardin & Desideri, 2013; Edwards, 2015; Roddy, Mallen, & Doherty, 2013). The tarsal area, ankle, or knee also may be affected. Less commonly, the wrists, fingers, and elbows may be affected. Trauma, alcohol ingestion, dieting, medications, surgical stress, or illness may trigger the acute attack (Fig. 39-3). The abrupt onset often occurs at night, awakening the patient with severe pain, redness, swelling, and warmth of the affected joint. Early attacks tend to subside spontaneously over 3 to 10 days even without treatment. The attack is followed by a symptom-free period (the intercritical stage or phase 3) until the next attack, which may not come for months or years. However, with time, attacks tend to occur more frequently, to involve more joints, last longer, and lead to long-term sequelae (phase 4).

In general, tophi are associated with more frequent and severe inflammatory episodes. Higher serum concentrations of uric acid also are associated with more extensive tophus formation. Tophi most commonly occur in the synovium, olecranon bursa, subchondral bone, infrapatellar and Achilles tendons, and subcutaneous tissue on the extensor surface of the forearms and overlying joints. Also they have been found in the aortic walls, heart valves, nasal and ear cartilage, eyelids, cornea, and sclerae. Joint enlargement may cause a loss of joint motion. Uric acid deposits may cause kidney stones and kidney damage.

A definitive diagnosis of gouty arthritis is established by polarized light microscopy of the synovial fluid of the involved joint (ACR, 2015c; Burbage, 2014; Schumacher & Chen, 2015). Uric acid crystals are seen within the polymorphonuclear leukocytes in the fluid. Although the gold standard for diagnosis is correct identification of crystals, clinical impressions are most frequently used.

Medical Management

Treatment of gout is managed in two major phases: management of acute gouty inflammation and long-term management to prevent flare ups and to control hyperuricemia. According to recent ACR guidelines, an acute gout attack should be treated pharmacologically within 24 hours of the onset of symptoms. First-line oral drugs are usually NSAIDs or colchicine. NSAIDs with short half-life are most effective (e.g., indomethacin, naproxen, ibuprofen, and diclofenac). Other agents prescribed to relieve an acute attack of gout are corticosteroids (oral or parenteral) or adrenocorticotropic hormones (ACTH) because of their anti-inflammatory properties and their ability to be used for short periods of time so generally long-term complications can be avoided (Bolzetta, Veronese, Manzato, & Sergi, 2013; Schumacher & Chen, 2015; Stamp & Chapman, 2013; Terkeltaub, 2015).

Drug Alert!
Selection of NSAIDs, colchicine, or corticosteroids is influenced by the patient's comorbid conditions (e.g., renal, cardiac, hepatic, or GI disease). Aging itself is an important risk factor. For instance, age-related decline in kidney function and the use of diuretics in the elderly are common risk factors for NSAID-induced renal injury.

Low-dose colchicine has been used for prophylaxis after resolution of attacks, but it does not prevent accumulation of tophi and urate in joints. Usually management of hyperuricemia, tophi, joint destruction, and kidney disorders is initiated after the acute inflammatory process has subsided. Allopurinol (Zyloprim), a xanthine oxidase inhibitor, is considered the drug of choice for preventing the precipitation of an attack and tophi formation and for promoting the regression of existing tophi. Febuxostat (Uloric) is a nonpurine xanthine oxidase inhibitor that mimics the action of allopurinol and is an effective alternative for patients who experience severe reactions to allopurinol. Uricosuric agents, such as probenecid (Benemid), correct hyperuricemia and stimulate renal urate excretion. Sulfinpyrazone (Anturane) is very similar to probenecid, but it is more potent. Severe blood dyscrasias may occur with use so generally it is reserved for patients with symptoms resistant to other agents. Drugs that metabolize uric acid, such as rasburicase and pegloticase, are called *uricolytic agents*; these new uricases are reserved for refractory tophaceous gout (Bolzetta et al., 2013; Burns & Wortmann, 2013; Harrold, 2013; Mikuls, 2013).

TABLE **39-4** Medications Used to Treat Gout

Medication	Actions and Use	Nursing Implications
Colchicine	Lowers the deposition of uric acid and interferes with leukocyte infiltration, thus reducing inflammation; does not alter serum or urine levels of uric acid; used in acute and chronic management	*Acute management:* Administer when attack begins; dosage increased until pain is relieved or diarrhea develops *Chronic management:* Causes gastrointestinal upset in most patients
Probenecid (Benemid), sulfinpyrazone (Anturane)	Uricosuric agent; inhibits renal reabsorption of urates and increases the urinary excretion of uric acid; prevents tophi formation	Be alert for nausea and rash Risk of uric acid deposition in kidney; patient should ingest large volumes of fluids
Allopurinol (Zyloprim), febuxostat (Uloric)	Inhibits xanthine oxidase; interrupts the breakdown of purines before uric acid is formed; inhibits xanthine oxidase because it blocks uric acid formation	Monitor for side effects, including bone marrow depression, vomiting, and abdominal pain
Pegloticase (Krystexxa)	Recombinant form of uric acid oxidase; Pegloticase is an enzyme that converts uric acid to allantoin, a water-soluble compound that is readily excreted by the kidney	Monitor for infusion reactions, such as urticaria, dyspnea, chest discomfort, erythema, and pruritus

When reduction of the serum urate level is indicated, uricosuric agents are the medications of choice. The recommended target goal of therapy is a serum uric acid level of less than 6 mg/dL, a level below the saturation point of 6.8 mg/dL at which urate crystals precipitate from solution (Burns & Wortmann, 2013; Harrold, 2013). Current practice trends have shown that reducing and maintaining the serum uric acid levels result in crystal dissolution from joints, a reduction in gout attacks (flares), and the prevention or reduction in tophaceous deposits. If the patient has, or is at risk for, renal insufficiency or renal calculi (kidney stones), allopurinol is also effective at a lowered adjusted dose. New therapies for acute gout targeting interleukin-1 β blockage are currently under investigation and show promise for successful gout treatment. Ilaris (canakinumab) was approved by the FDA in 2011 and has shown to extend the time to the next attack and reduce the frequency of subsequent attacks. Although not FDA approved, anakinra (Kineret) may be prescribed by health care providers for very severe attacks of gout (ACR, 2015c; Bardin & Desideri, 2013; Stamp & Chapman, 2013). Corticosteroids may be used in patients who have no response to other therapy. If the patient experiences several acute episodes or there is evidence of tophi formation, prophylactic treatment is considered. Specific treatment is based on the serum uric acid level, 24-hour urinary uric acid excretion, and renal function. Table 39-4 lists the common medications used in treating gout.

Nursing Management

Pain management is the primary concern during the acute phase of an attack. The joint should be rested and elevated, and application of ice, not heat, may help with reducing discomfort. Keeping the bedclothes away from the affected joint using a "bed cage" if available can be of benefit. The management of the intercritical and chronic phases of gout involves teaching self-care measures to decrease the risk of attacks (e.g., avoidance of aspirin [because doses below 2 to 3 g/day impair renal excretion of uric acid retention and higher doses are associated with high renal excretion of uric acids], trauma, stress, alcohol, smoking) and to avoid long-term complications (e.g., importance of medication compliance). During the intercritical period, the patient feels well and may abandon preventive behaviors, which may result in an acute attack. Health care providers recommend that patients restrict consumption of foods high in purines, especially organ meats and shellfish; others believe that limiting protein foods such as red meats, lamb and pork or avoiding trigger foods are sufficient. Patients should be taught to limit alcohol intake, avoid fad starvation diets, and avoid sugary drinks and food that are high in fructose such as fructose corn syrup, sweetened soda, and processed foods. As fructose breaks down in the body, purines are released. The breakdown of purines produces uric acid, the substance that forms painful crystals in the joints and causes gout. Your uric acid levels rise within minutes after you drink high fructose drinks. It is important that patients drink plenty of fluids, at least 2,000 mL daily, to avoid dehydration and lessen renal involvement and the development of urinary stones (ACR, 2015c; Burbage, 2014; Edwards, 2015). Maintenance of normal body weight should be encouraged. Dietary vitamin C supplementation has been shown to reduce the risk of gout. Also, dietary restriction of sodium, fat, and cholesterol can lead to a reduction in gout symptoms and decrease effects associated with coexisting metabolic syndrome. Although research is limited, first acute gout attacks may commonly precede the diagnosis of metabolic abnormalities and associated diseases. Gout studies have shown to be associated with poorer physical health-related quality of life (HRQOL). Both gout-specific features (attack frequency and intensity, intercritical pain and number of joints involved) and comorbid disease were associated with poor HRQOL in all domains. Therefore success of lifelong treatment is dependent on the patient's commitment to treatment. Nurses need to explain lifestyle changes and drug management to the patient as they play a vital role in increasing treatment adherence and, therefore, considerable improvements in patient-centered outcomes (Bardin & Desideri, 2013; CDC, 2015d; Chandratre et al., 2013; Roddy et al., 2013).

Fibromyalgia

Fibromyalgia (FM) is a chronic syndrome characterized by widespread nonarticular musculoskeletal pain or multiple tender points lasting more than 3 months and other general physical symptoms, such as fatigue (NIAMS, 2014b). The pain in FM is not due to tissue damage or inflammation, thus making it fundamentally different from other rheumatic disorders and many other pain conditions. According to the 1990 ACR criteria, which specify 11 or more tender points, FM affects women more frequently than men (10:1 ratio). However, according to alternative ACR criteria for FM, women are only 1.5 times more likely than men to experience chronic widespread pain (CWP) (Clauw, 2015). The newer criteria established in 2010 do not require performing a tender point count, and they are recommended for clinical diagnosis versus the 1990 criteria intended for research. A hallmark of FM is that individuals display diffuse hyperalgesia (increased pain to normally painful stimuli) and/or allodynia (pain to normally nonpainful stimuli). This suggests that these individuals have a fundamental problem with central dysfunction (pain processing mechanisms) that results in central pain sensitization. These findings of centralization of pain have been corroborated by advanced neuroimaging techniques and appear to be due, in part, to imbalances in levels of neurotransmitters that affect pain and sensory transmission (Clauw, 2015; Wolfe & Rasker, 2013). The overall prevalence rate remains at 2% to 5% worldwide (ACR, 2015b; Crofford, 2015).

Clinical Manifestations and Assessment

The core features of CWP and tenderness are almost invariably accompanied by a wide range of symptoms, the most common of which are sleep disturbances, fatigue, morning stiffness, muscle weakness, paresthesias, cognitive dysfunction ("fibro fog"), chronic headaches, mood disturbances, and irritable bowel syndrome (CDC, 2015c; Clauw, 2015; Wolfe & Rasker, 2013). CWP is pain that is typically both above and below the waist on both sides of the body and involves the axial skeleton (neck, back, or chest). The patient complains of a widespread burning pain and often is unable to discriminate if pain occurs in the muscles, joints, or soft tissues. Physical examination typically reveals point

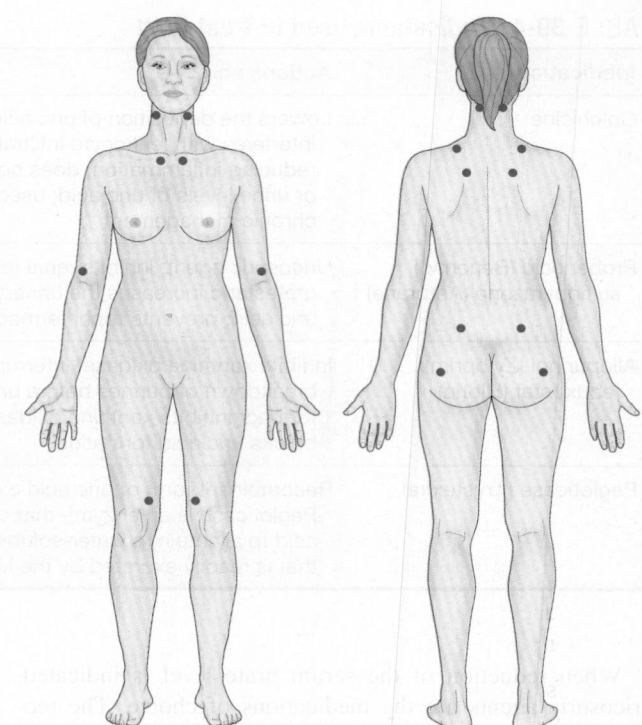

FIGURE 39-4 Fibromyalgia tender points.

tenderness at 11 or more of 18 identified sites characteristically described in ACR 1990 criteria (Fig. 39-4).

Medical Management

It is recommended to use symptom-based pharmacology therapy together with nonpharmacologic therapies. Paying attention to the specific symptoms reported by the patient is important. Patient education, exercise, and cognitive therapy, along with medication, are frequently used.

The pharmacotherapy of FM is mechanism-based; many have been tested to a greater or lesser extent. NSAIDs may be used to treat the diffuse muscle aching and stiffness. Tramadol is the only opiate shown to provide some relief. Many drugs have been used off-label to treat FM. Pregabalin (Lyrica), an analgesic, anxiolytic, and anticonvulsant ($\alpha_{2-\delta}$ receptor ligand agent) is the first to receive FDA approval for FM use. Psychotropic agents have been used to reduce pain centrally, even in the absence of depression: serotonin noradrenaline reuptake inhibitors or SNRIs (duloxetine, milnacipran), least selective serotonin reuptake inhibitors or SSRIs (fluoxetine, paroxetine), dopaminergic agents (pramipexole), and antidepressants, particularly tricyclics (Clauw, 2015; Polston & Wallace, 2013). The two SNRIs, duloxetine (Cymbalta) and milnacipran (Savella), were shown to be effective and are approved by the FDA for symptom relief in FM. Also tricyclic antidepressants in low doses can be used to improve or restore normal sleep patterns. Other drugs acting on the central nervous system also have been used or are under investigation (e.g., gabapentin, cannabinoids). Individualized programs of exercise are used to decrease muscle weakness and discomfort and to improve the general deconditioning that occurs in affected patients. Investigators, Martinez-Amat et al. (2014), found an association of weekly practice of guided physical activity with reduction of falls and symptoms of FM. Nonpharmacologic therapies (e.g., massage, spa treatment, hydrotherapy, acupuncture), including neurostimulation therapies such as peripheral nerve stimulation (PNS), occipital nerve stimulation (ONS), etc. (Dailey et al., 2013), can be extremely helpful and often are underused in clinical practice.

Nursing Management

Typically, patients with FM have endured their symptoms for a long period of time. They may feel as if their symptoms have not been taken seriously. Nurses need to undertake a holistic assessment to identify the influence of any factors on the pain experienced and management strategies. The assessment should include:

1. Beliefs and thoughts about the cause of the condition—talking about how the pain started can lead to shared insight and provide direction for management strategies,
2. Level of functional activity—FM has been associated with lower levels of health-related quality of life and more work productivity loss (CDC, 2015c),
3. Mood status—the nurse should help the patient identify existing psychological stressors that are having an adverse effect on the pain experienced,
4. Sleep patterns—if pain is interfering with the quality of sleep, the patient will often awaken unrefreshed and experience difficulties with cognitive functioning, including concentration, sentence formation, and memory recall, and
5. Patient's role—the nurse should assess if the patient is experiencing emotional or physical difficulties in the workplace or the family setting (Davis, Moder, & Hunder, 2013; Ryan, 2013).

Nurses need to pay special attention to supporting these patients and providing encouragement as they begin their program of therapy. The goal of FM treatment is to improve the physical and mental health of patients and their quality of life. Interventions or strategies should be developed to promote better functioning. Greater education, lower-intensity fatigue, and using aerobic or strength training exercises were predictors of physical functioning (Kaleth, Saha, Jensen, Slaven, & Ang, 2013; Vural et al., 2014). Nurses need to work with the patient to increase independence, avoiding complications of deconditioning, work disability, and the inability to fulfill social roles. FM has been found to be associated with impaired balance and falls (Rutledge, Martinez, Traska, & Rose, 2013). Stretching, aerobic exercise, and strength training should be in every patient's exercise plan.

Nursing Alert
Nurses should focus on patient safety. Nurses caring for people with FM should assess for potential risk factors of falling and offer plans for individualized fall-prevention strategies. One of the Joint Commission (JC) 2015 National Patient Safety Goals aims at reducing falls. The JC recommends a patient evaluation include fall history, review of medications and alcohol consumption, gait and balance screening; assessment of walking aids, assistive technologies, and protective devices; and environmental assessments.

Motivational interviewing (MI) is a client-centered approach that nurses can use to promote behavioral changes (see the Nursing Process section later in the chapter). Meta-analysis of studies using MI when delivered in brief consultations showed efficacy in medical settings for a wide range of behavioral issues, such as exercise, self-management of pain, and medication adherence (Ferguson, Ibrahim, Thomas, & Weinman, 2015; Lundahl et al., 2013). Another meta-analysis supports MI in increasing physical activity in people with chronic health conditions, one of the ten conditions being FM (O'Halloran et al., 2014). Other management approaches include patient support groups and the use of meditation, prayer, and other spiritual practices. Careful listening to patients' descriptions of their concerns and symptoms is essential to help patients make the changes that are necessary to improve their quality of life (Clauw, 2015; Hardcastle et al., 2015; Ryan, 2014b).

DIFFUSE CONNECTIVE TISSUE DISEASES

Rheumatic disorders with diffuse inflammation and degeneration in the connective tissues are referred to as *connective tissue diseases*. These disorders share similar clinical features and may affect some of the same organs. The characteristic clinical course is one of exacerbations and remissions. Although the diffuse connective tissue diseases have unknown causes, they are thought to be the result of immunologic abnormalities in which the immune system loses its ability to tell the difference between foreign invaders and the body's normal cells. The common connective tissue diseases, RA, systemic lupus erythematosus (SLE), and scleroderma, are presented in detail.

Rheumatoid Arthritis

RA is the most common inflammatory arthritic disorder and serves as a prototype for the study of many inflammatory and immune-mediated diseases. RA affects 0.5% to 1% of the general population worldwide, with a female-to-male ratio of between 2:1 and 3:1 using 1987 ACR criteria for the classification of RA (CDC, 2015a; Firestein, 2013; Liao & Karlson, 2015). The most recent 2010 RA criteria identify people with early RA; however, there are no current estimates. Globally, out of 291 conditions studied, RA was ranked as the 42nd highest contributor to global disability (Cross et al., 2014).

Pathophysiology

A variety of predetermined genes (e.g., human leukocyte antigens [HLA]), random events, and environmental (e.g., pathogens, smoking) factors contribute to RA susceptibility and pathogenesis. In RA, numerous cell types are involved, including macrophages, T cells, B cells, fibroblasts, chondrocytes, and dendritic cells. The autoimmune reaction primarily occurs in the synovial tissue. Adaptive and innate immune responses in the synovium have been implicated in the pathogenesis of RA. RF antibodies develop in the synovium against the Immunoglobulin G (IgG) to form immune complexes. The activation of the complement system and release of lysosomal enzymes from leukocytes lead to inflammation. It is unknown why the body produces an antibody (RF) against its own antibody (IgG) and, in consequence, transforms IgG to an antigen or foreign protein that must be destroyed. Phagocytosis produces enzymes (proinflammatory cytokines such as

interleukin [IL]-1, interleukin-6 [IL-6], and tumor necrosis factor [TNF]) within the joint. These cytokines are the primary factors that drive the inflammatory response in RA. The enzymes (especially cytokines) break down collagen, causing edema, proliferation of the synovial membrane, and, ultimately, formation of **pannus** (Fig. 39-5). Pannus, formation of vascular granulation tissue, is a characteristic of RA that differentiates it from other forms of inflammatory arthritis. Pannus has a destructive effect on the adjacent cartilage and bone. If response is not suppressed, the disease progresses and the consequences are loss of articular surfaces and joint motion. Muscle fibers also undergo degenerative changes. Tendon and ligament elasticity and contractile power are lost.

Clinical Manifestations and Assessment

Clinical manifestations of RA vary, usually reflecting the stage and severity of the disease. Physical signs of RA are associated with the pathophysiology of the disease. The manifestations of RA can be categorized as early or late disease and as articular (joint) or extra-articular. Joint pain, swelling, warmth, erythema (redness), and lack of function are classic symptoms. Palpation of the joints reveals spongy or boggy tissue. Often, fluid can be aspirated from the inflamed joint. The hallmark of RA is synovial proliferation and

Right Hand and Wrist

Joint capsule
Pannus
Swelling
Erosion
Joint space narrowing
Pannus

FIGURE 39-5 Joints affected by rheumatoid arthritis.

FIGURE 39-6 Deformity to the hands caused by rheumatoid arthritis.

tenderness in multiple joints, particularly in the small joints of the hands, wrists, and feet. As the disease progresses, the knees, shoulders, hips, elbows, ankles, cervical spine, and temporomandibular joints are affected. In addition to joint pain and swelling, a cardinal sign of inflammatory arthritis that can appear even before pain is morning stiffness, lasting for more than an hour (Brasington, 2015; Shah & Clair, 2015; Sweeney, Harris, & Firestein, 2013).

Deformities of the hands and feet are common in RA (Fig. 39-6). Often the PIP and metacarpophalangeal (MCP) joints of the hands are involved initially. The deformity may be caused by misalignment resulting from swelling, progressive joint destruction, or the subluxation (partial dislocation) that occurs when one bone slips over another and eliminates the joint space.

RA is a systemic disease with multiple extra-articular features. Most common are fever, weight loss, fatigue, anemia, lymph node enlargement, and Raynaud phenomenon (cold- and stress-induced vasospasm causing episodes of digital blanching or cyanosis). Extra-articular disease manifestations occur in about 40% of patients at some time in the course of the disease (Turesson & Matteson, 2015). Rheumatoid nodules may be noted in patients with more advanced RA in about 20% of patients (Brasington, 2015). These nodules are usually nontender and movable in the subcutaneous tissue. They usually appear over bony prominences, most often on extensor surfaces or pressure points, such as the elbow, are varied in size, and can disappear spontaneously. Nodules occur only in people positive for RF. The nodules often are associated with rapidly progressive and destructive disease. Other extra-articular features include arteritis (inflammation of the walls of arteries), neuropathy, scleritis (inflammation of the sclera), pericarditis, splenomegaly, and Sjögren syndrome (dry eyes and dry mucous membranes).

A clinical examination of all synovial joints should be undertaken for evidence of tenderness, swelling, and range of movement. Evidence for synovitis should be seen by a rheumatologist, ideally within 6 weeks after the onset of symptoms to facilitate early diagnosis and clinical management and to achieve optimal outcomes for patients (Beaton, Boers, & Tugwell, 2013; Holers & Deane, 2015; Palmer & El Miedany, 2013; Palmer & El Miedany, 2014; Shah & St. Clair, 2015; Villeneuve, 2013). Presence of deformities, such as hyperextension of PIP joints (swan neck), flexion of PIP joints (Boutonniere), and ulnar deviation, in which fingers point toward the ulna, may be noted on examination. The patient is also assessed for extra-articular changes, such as weight loss, sensory changes, lymph node enlargement, and fatigue.

! Nursing Alert
Patients commonly have the inability to "wring out a wash cloth," need to hold a cup with both hands, and may complain of the sensation of having a "stone in my shoe."

The 2010 RA classification criteria, developed collaboratively by the ACR and the European League Against Rheumatism (EULAR) replaced the 1987 gold standard for disease classification. In addition to active synovitis in at least one joint that cannot be better explained by another diagnosis, additional criteria added include positivity for antibodies to citrullinated proteins (ACPAs or anti-CCP) and abnormal levels of the inflammatory markers, such as the ESR and CRP levels. RF is present in up to 70% to 80% of patients with RA, but its presence alone is not diagnostic of RA. Anticyclic citrullinated peptide (anti-CCP) is a marker that has similar sensitivity but potentially greater specificity to RF (Durham, Fowler, Donato, Smith, & Jensen, 2015; Liao & Karlson, 2015). Some laboratories are currently doing a second generation of the test, called the CCP2 assay. The RBC count and complement C3 and C4 levels are decreased. Complements may be decreased as they are "used up" in some antigen-antibody reactions. Results of antinuclear antibody (ANA), the screening test for autoantibodies (antibodies that form against self), also may be positive. **Arthrocentesis** shows abnormal synovial fluid that is cloudy, milky, or dark yellow and contains numerous inflammatory components, such as leukocytes and complement. The enzyme MMP-3 is increased in the synovial fluid of the patient with RA, and it may be a marker of progressive joint damage. Synovial biopsy can detect inflammatory cells associated with RA. Radiologic studies are not specifically diagnostic in the early stages of RA; however, they do show characteristic bony erosions and narrowed joint spaces occurring later in the disease and help in monitoring the progression of disease and effectiveness of treatment.

Medical and Nursing Management

Drugs remain the cornerstone of RA treatment. Joint inflammation is the main driver of joint damage and is the most important cause of functional disability in the early stages of disease; thus changes in the therapeutic landscape in RA are seen. Today, treatment is more aggressive. The treatment paradigm changed to adopt a "patient-centered" and "treat-to-target" approach aiming at disease remission. Current guidelines recommend starting a course of DMARDs early, within 3 months of RA diagnosis to delay joint degeneration (O'Dell, 2013). NSAIDs provide fast relief of symptoms but do not prevent joint damage nor slow disease progression. Because the effects of DMARDs take weeks or months to develop, whereas the effects of NSAIDs are immediate, an NSAID is given until the DMARD has had time to act.

The use of traditional NSAIDs (salicylates and nonsalicylates) inhibits the production of prostaglandins and provides anti-inflammatory effects as well as analgesia. Effectiveness, side effects, cost, and dosing schedules are considered in the selection of an NSAID. The incidence of adverse reactions (e.g., gastric irritation, kidney damage, changes in liver function) to the NSAIDs increases with age and long-term use. A second-generation NSAID, the COX-2 inhibitor, has been shown to inhibit inflammatory processes, but it does not inhibit the protective prostaglandin synthesis in the GI tract. Therefore, patients who are at increased risk for GI complications, especially GI bleeding, have been managed effectively with COX-2 inhibitors.

Drug Alert!
COX-2 inhibitors must be used with caution because of the associated risk of cardiovascular disease.

The DMARDs can be classified into nonbiologic and biologic DMARDs. The nonbiologic agent, methotrexate (Rheumatrex, Trexall), is one of the first-choice DMARDs and has become the drug of choice due to its potency and time of action (faster than all other DMARDs). Therapeutic effects or improvement may develop in 3 to 6 weeks, compared to other DMARDs, which can take 3 to 4 months to work (Lehne, 2013). A black-box warning exists for unexpected, severe, and sometimes fatal myelosuppression, aplastic anemia, and GI toxicity reported with methotrexate (usually high dose) in combination with some NSAIDs. Additionally, methotrexate is teratogenic (capable of causing birth defects); therefore, a pregnancy test should be performed if a decision is made to begin treatment in a woman of childbearing age.

Nursing Alert
Nurses should alert patients that taking extra doses of methotrexate is dangerous. The drug is administered weekly or twice a week. Nurses need to encourage feedback to ensure that the patient understands the weekly dosing schedule and that the medication should not be used "as needed" for symptom control.
Institute for Safe Medication Practices (ISMP); www.ismp.org

Another preferred nonbiologic DMARD, hydroxychloroquine (Plaquenil), a drug with antimalarial actions, can be initiated early and used with mild symptoms, but as a rule it is used in combination with methotrexate. By itself, hydroxychloroquine does not slow disease progression; however, early use can improve long-term outcomes.

Leflunomide (Arava), a nonbiologic small-molecule DMARD, is a relatively new and powerful immunosuppressant used for patients with RA. Compared with methotrexate, leflunomide is about equally as effective but more dangerous because of the incidence of liver failure; it is reserved for second-line use. Other minor nonbiologic DMARDs, cyclosporine, gold salts, penicillamine, and azathioprine, have been available for many years. These have been used frequently in the past, but their use today is limited. The drugs are generally reserved for patients with severe, progressive RA disease who have failed to respond to safer DMARDs.

Biologic agents (also referred as *immunomodulators*) are expensive, whereas the nonbiologic small-molecule DMARDs cost much less and are easier to manufacture.

Biologic drugs can be categorized based on their mechanism of action and target specific components of the inflammatory process. They can be used to treat patients with moderate to severe disease who have not responded to DMARDs or in combination therapy with an established DMARD, such as methotrexate. Some biologic agents or modifiers interfere with the action of TNF: etanercept (Enbrel), infliximab (Remicade), and adalimumab (Humira). Most recently, golimumab (Simponi) and certolizumab pegol (Cimzia) have been approved for use in RA. The immunosuppressant actions of TNF inhibitors can increase the patient's risk of serious infections, including bacterial sepsis, invasive fungal infection, and tuberculosis. As a result, prior to initiation of TNF inhibitors, patients should be tested for tuberculosis. A different biologic agent, anakinra (Kineret), interferes with IL-1, which modulates immune and inflammatory responses, and thus has efficacy with rheumatic disorders. Like the TNF inhibitors, anakinra poses a risk of serious infections; therefore, anakinra should not be used in combination with TNF inhibitors.

Nursing Alert
Do not give live vaccines to patients on a biologic agent. Nurses need to monitor for signs of infection (e.g., fever, cough, flu-like symptoms, open sores on body). Also nurses should monitor for heart failure in patients on etanercept (Enbrel) or infliximab (Remicade).

The emerging agents show that a new era in treatment has begun, newly targeting B lymphocyte cells, T-cell activation, and IL-6. These constitute new principles for interference with the disease process (Athanasakis, Petrakis, & Kyriopoulos, 2013; Weinblatt et al., 2013). Tofacitinib (Xeljanz), also a type of DMARD, is the first oral medication in a new class of treatments called Janus kinase (JAK) inhibitors and is FDA approved for moderate to severe RA in which methotrexate did not work well. As most biologics fight inflammation from outside the cell, the JAK inhibitor works deep inside the cell to disrupt activities occurring in signaling pathways. These JAK pathways are believed to be involved in the production of cytokines and in the inflammation of RA (Meier & McInnes, 2014; Vollenhoven, 2015).

The third major group of antiarthritic drugs is the glucocorticoids (adrenal corticosteroids). These are powerful anti-inflammatory drugs used in RA especially during exacerbations ("flare ups") of the disease or when needing a "bridging" medication while waiting for the slower DMARDs (e.g., methotrexate) to begin taking effect. Oral glucocorticoids, such as prednisone and prednisolone, are indicated for patients with generalized symptoms. Long-term therapy can cause serious toxicity (e.g., osteoporosis, gastric ulceration, adrenal suppression, diabetes) so glucocorticoids should be limited to patients with RA who have failed to respond adequately to all other treatment options. Intra-articular injections, commonly used in severe RA, may be employed if only one or two joints are affected. Antibiotics, the tetracycline derivatives minocycline (Minocin) and doxycycline (Vibramycin), are given to improve symptoms (morning stiffness, joint pain and tenderness), and enhance ADL in patients with RA. These antibiotics have found to decrease the action of enzymes on cartilage degradation. Usage is seen in patients who have not responded to DMARDs.

The *Prosorba Column*, a blood filtration device used in apheresis, has been approved by the FDA for use in treating patients with more severe and longstanding RA who have had no response to or are intolerant of DMARDs. The device, a protein A immunoadsorption column, is used in 12 weekly 2-hour apheresis treatments to bind IgG (i.e., circulating immune complex). As the patient's blood passes through the column, RF is removed.

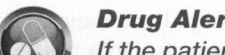 **Drug Alert!**
If the patient is on an angiotensin-converting enzyme (ACE) inhibitor, it should be discontinued prior to treatment using Prosorba Column, as the risk of serious hypotension exists with this treatment.

Through all stages of RA, depression and sleep deprivation may require the short-term use of low-dose antidepressant medications, such as amitriptyline (Elavil), paroxetine (Paxil), or sertraline (Zoloft), to reestablish an adequate sleep pattern and to manage chronic pain. Furthermore, adults with RA are at high risk of falls and fall-related injuries. Strategies to prevent falls should be implemented (Stanmore et al., 2013a, 2013b).

Systemic Lupus Erythematosus

SLE is a chronic inflammatory multisystem autoimmune disease with variable presentations, courses, and prognoses characterized by remissions and exacerbations. National incidence data are difficult to obtain because onset is difficult to determine. The existing estimates of SLE range widely from 1.8 to 7.6 cases per 100,000 in the United States (CDC, 2015e). Occurrence peaks up to 10 to 12 times more frequently in women than in men (predominantly during a woman's childbearing years), and African Americans and Hispanics are affected more frequently than are Caucasians (ACR, 2015d; Lim & Drenkard, 2015; Simard & Costenbader, 2015).

Pathophysiology

SLE is a result of disturbed immune regulation that causes an exaggerated production of autoantibodies and antigens. The immune abnormalities that characterize SLE occur in five phases: susceptibility (genes and environmental factors), abnormal innate and adaptive immune responses, autoantibodies immune complexes, inflammation, and damage. Interactions of predisposing factors (genes, female gender, and environment) result in abnormal immune responses, specifically in B cells and T cells. These responses produce pathogenic autoantibodies and immune complexes that activate complement, form in tissue, and cause inflammation. Inflammation stimulates antigens, which, in turn, stimulate additional antibodies. The cycle repeats and, over time, leads to irreversible organ damage. Some individuals do not progress through all phases (Crow, 2013).

Drug Alert!
Certain medications, such as hydralazine (Apresoline), procainamide (Pronestyl), isoniazid (INH), chlorpromazine (Thorazine), and some antiseizure medications, can trigger an exaggerated immune response and cause a chemical- or drug-induced SLE.

Clinical Manifestations and Assessment

The onset of SLE may be insidious or acute. For this reason, SLE may remain undiagnosed for many years. The most common presenting manifestations are constitutional symptoms (fever, fatigue, and/or weight loss), cutaneous manifestations, and articular manifestations (arthritis and/or arthralgia). Each of these manifestations appears to be present in at least 50% of patients with lupus at the time of diagnosis (Dall'Era & Wofsy, 2013). SLE is an autoimmune systemic disease that can affect any body system. Clinical manifestations can resemble RA and may be mistaken for it, especially early in the course of the disease. Unlike RA, the arthritis is nonerosive and not seen on x-ray.

Several different types of skin manifestations are prevalent in 80% to 90% of patients with SLE. Photosensitivity rashes are most common; however, the most characteristic skin manifestation is an acute cutaneous lesion consisting of a butterfly-shaped rash across the bridge of the nose and

FIGURE 39-7 The characteristic butterfly rash of systemic lupus erythematosus.

cheeks (Dall'Era & Wofsy, 2013; Dvorkina & Ginzler, 2015) (Fig. 39-7). This malar rash manifests as an erythematous, flat or raised lesion, pruritic (itchy) or painful, and can be transient and heal without scarring. In some cases of discoid lupus erythematosus (DLE), only skin involvement occurs. Discoid (coinlike) lesions are scarring and ring-shaped that may result in erythematous, scaling plaques, and alopecia (hair loss). In some patients with SLE, the initial skin involvement is the precursor to more systemic involvement. The lesions often worsen during exacerbations (flares) of the systemic disease and possibly are provoked by sunlight or artificial ultraviolet B light.

Nursing Alert
The nurse should teach patients to avoid sunlight or ultraviolet (UV) exposure and to protect themselves with clothing and sunscreen with at least a sun protection factor (SPF) of 30.

Central nervous system involvement is widespread, encompassing the entire range of neurologic disease (60% prevalence). The varied and frequent neuropsychiatric presentations of SLE are now widely recognized. In general, these are demonstrated by subtle changes in behavior patterns or cognitive ability. Headaches, psychiatric disorders (mood disorder, depression, and psychosis), cognitive dysfunction, and seizures are common (Dvorkina & Ginzler, 2015; Hahn, 2015).

Pericarditis and pleuritis are the most common cardiopulmonary disorders (refer to Chapters 10 and 16). Women who have SLE are also at risk for early atherosclerosis. About

50% of patients with SLE have kidney disease, such as glomerulonephritis. Serum creatinine levels and urinalysis are used in screening for kidney involvement. Early detection allows for prompt treatment so that kidney damage can be prevented. Kidney involvement may lead to hypertension, which also requires careful monitoring and management.

Diagnosis of SLE is based on a complete history, physical examination, and diagnostic tests. SLE has an extreme range of clinical manifestations without classic presentation. Diagnosis is made difficult by the variable manifestations of the disease and relies on the overall clinical picture with the correlation of diagnostic laboratory and imaging studies, possibly including skin biopsy.

The presence of at least four of the criteria established by the ACR is required to make the diagnosis of SLE. Cutaneous manifestations comprise 4 of the 11 diagnostic ACR criteria (malar rash, discoid rash, photosensitivity, and oral ulcers). When performing an assessment, it is critical to inspect skin for erythematous rashes. The nurse asks the patient about the existence of photosensitivity, fatigue, oral ulcers, or pain in joints. Additionally, systemic involvement may encompass several organ systems; therefore, the nurse must review laboratory values or findings that might suggest that the effects of inflammation are targeting organs (e.g., ESR, complete blood count—anemia or thrombocytopenia, creatinine, hematuria).

No single laboratory test confirms SLE. Laboratory features include both hematologic abnormalities (e.g., hemolytic anemia, leukopenia, thrombocytopenia) and immunologic findings indicative of autoimmunity. Most patients with SLE (more than 98%) demonstrate elevated serum levels of ANA, which is another ACR criterion for SLE diagnosis. A small percent of patients will test negative for ANA but will have antibodies to the nuclear antigen anti-Ro (SSA) (Hahn, 2015). Other diagnostic immunologic tests that support SLE diagnosis in the presence of clinical manifestations are CRP, anti–double-stranded DNA (anti-ds DNA), anti-RNA, anti-La (SSB), anti-Sm (Smith) or antiphospholipid antibodies, and high-titer IgG antibodies. The double-stranded DNA test, C3, and C4 indicate whether there is a genetic component that is common in patients with SLE (Dall'Era & Wofsy, 2013).

Medical and Nursing Management

SLE can be life-threatening; however, advances in its treatment have led to improved survival and reduced morbidity. Treatment of SLE includes management of acute and chronic disease. The goals of treatment include preventing progressive loss of organ function, reducing the likelihood of acute disease, minimizing disease-related disabilities, and preventing complications from therapy. Management of SLE involves regular monitoring to assess disease activity and therapeutic effectiveness.

The mainstay of SLE treatment is based on pain management and nonspecific immunosuppression. Therapy includes NSAIDs, DMARDs (including antimalarials) alone or in combination with glucocorticoids, and, in severe SLE cases, immunosuppressive agents (azathioprine, mycophenolate mofetil, methotrexate). Hydroxychloroquine has a central role for long-term treatment. In 2011, the biologic, belimumab (Benlysta) for treatment of mild to moderate SLE became the first FDA-approved drug (ACR, 2015d; Lim & Drenkard, 2015).

Corticosteroids are the single most important medication available for SLE. These drugs are used topically for cutaneous manifestations in low oral doses for minor disease activity and in high doses for major disease activity. IV administration of corticosteroids is an alternative to traditional high-dose oral use (Bertsias, Fanouriakis, & Boumpas, 2013). Important risk factors associated with the use of corticosteroids are osteoporosis and fractures. Corticosteroid toxicity is a major problem, and tapering of the dosage is a primary concern. Treatment of moderate to severe SLE consists of a period of intensive immunosuppressive therapy (induction therapy) followed by a longer period of less intensive maintenance therapy. The main objective of the induction therapy is to stop injury, recover function, and induce remission by managing immunologic activity. The combination of high-dose glucocorticoids with pulses of intravenous cyclophosphamide (CYC), a cyctoxic agent, remains the standard of care for severe SLE with major organ involvement. B-cell–depleting therapies, such as the monoclonal antibodies rituximab (Rituxan) and epratuzumab (humanized anti-CD22 antibody), are the newest form of treatment for SLE and are reserved for patients who have serious forms of SLE that have not responded to conservative therapies.

Nurses also need to be sensitive to the psychological reactions of the patient with SLE. The disease or its treatment may produce dramatic changes in appearance and considerable distress for the patient. The changes and unpredictable course of SLE necessitate expert assessment skills and nursing care.

Scleroderma

Scleroderma ("hard skin") is a relatively rare disease that is poorly understood; the cause is unknown. Potential triggers include exposure to certain environmental and occupational agents (e.g., silica dust, heavy metals, polyvinyl chloride) and drugs (e.g., bleomycin, cocaine, fenfluramine appetite suppressants), infection, and human cytomegalovirus (CMV) and other viruses (Varga & Lafyatis, 2015). Scleroderma is classified into localized and systemic (systemic sclerosis), with subclassifications within each one. Incidence estimates range from 9 to 19 people per million per year (Varga, 2015). Similar to other connective tissue diseases, scleroderma is more frequent in women than men (4.6:1).

Pathophysiology

Like other diffuse connective tissue diseases, scleroderma has a variable course, featuring remissions and exacerbations.

Systemic scleroderma (SSc) is a progressive, chronic, devastating, and debilitating disease with a prognosis not as optimistic as that of SLE. Pathogenesis integrates three cardinal features: vascular injury and damage, activation of innate and adaptive arms of the immune system autoimmunity, and generalized interstitial and vascular fibrosis.

Scleroderma commonly begins with skin involvement. Mononuclear cells cluster on the skin and stimulate lymphokines to stimulate procollagen. Insoluble collagen is formed and accumulates excessively in the tissues. Initially, the inflammatory response causes edema formation, with a resulting skin appearance that is taut, smooth, and shiny. The skin then undergoes fibrotic changes, leading to loss of elasticity and movement. Eventually, the tissue degenerates and becomes nonfunctional. This chain of events, from inflammation to degeneration, also occurs in blood vessels, synovium, skeletal muscles, and internal organ(s) of the heart, lungs, GI tract, and kidneys (Varga, 2013; Varga, 2015).

Clinical Manifestations and Assessment

Scleroderma starts insidiously with Raynaud phenomenon and swelling in the hands. The hallmark of scleroderma is when the skin and the subcutaneous tissues become increasingly hard and rigid and cannot be pinched up from the underlying structures (fibrosis). Wrinkles and lines are obliterated. The skin is dry because sweat secretion over the involved region is suppressed. The extremities stiffen and lose mobility. The condition spreads slowly; for years, these changes may remain localized in the hands and the feet. The face appears masklike, immobile, and expressionless, and the mouth becomes rigid.

The changes within the body, although not visible directly, are vastly more important than the visible changes. The left ventricle of the heart is involved, resulting in heart failure. The esophagus hardens, interfering with swallowing. The lungs become scarred, impeding respiration. Digestive disturbances occur because of hardening (sclerosing) of the intestinal mucosa. Progressive kidney failure may occur.

The patient may manifest a subset of limited cutaneous SSc symptoms referred to as the CREST syndrome (Box 39-4).

BOX 39-4   **Focused Assessment**

Cutaneous Symptoms of Scleroderma

Be alert for the CREST symptoms:
- **C**alcinosis (calcium deposits in the tissues)
- **R**aynaud phenomenon (spasm of blood vessels in response to cold or stress)
- **E**sophageal dysfunction (acid reflux and decrease in mobility of esophagus)
- **S**clerodactyly (thickening and tightening of skin on fingers and hands)
- **T**elangiectasia (capillary dilation that forms vascular red marks on surface of skin)

Assessment focuses on the hallmark sclerotic changes (thickening) in the skin, contractures in the fingers, and color changes or ulcerations in the fingertips due to poor circulation (Boin & Wigley, 2013; Hoogen et al., 2013). Assessment of systemic involvement requires a systems review with special attention to GI, pulmonary, renal, and cardiac symptoms. Limitations in mobility and self-care activities should be assessed along with the impact the disease has had (or will have) on body image.

There is no one conclusive test to diagnose scleroderma, and testing depends on the possibility or extent of organ involvement. A skin biopsy is performed to identify cellular changes specific to scleroderma. Pulmonary studies show ventilation–perfusion abnormalities. Echocardiography evaluates left ventricular function and pulmonary arterial pressure and identifies pericardial effusion (often present with cardiac involvement). Esophageal studies demonstrate reflux esophagitis (early discriminator) and dysmotility in most patients with scleroderma. Autoantibody testing, particularly ANA, is the most useful laboratory test, with a positive result common in more than 95% of patients with scleroderma and antisclerodermal antibody (anti-scl) 70 (Bolster & Silver, 2015; Fett, 2013; Mayes & Assassi, 2015; Varga, 2015). In the presence of CREST syndrome, 90% have a positive anticentromere antibody test. Other autoantibodies demonstrate an association between scleroderma and a specific clinical pattern, such as anti-topoisomerase I antibodies and lung fibrosis or anti-RNA polymerase I/III and scleroderma renal crisis.

Medical and Nursing Management

Management of scleroderma depends on the patient's clinical manifestations and is based on disease comorbidities (Fett, 2013). In scleroderma, treatment includes management of both acute and chronic disease. Acute conditions require interventions directed at controlling increased disease activity or exacerbations that can involve any organ system. Management of the more chronic condition involves periodic monitoring and recognition of meaningful clinical changes requiring adjustments in therapy. Because this is a life-altering disease that has no cure, all patients should receive counseling, during which realistic individual goals may be determined. As in the other rheumatic disorders, support measures include strategies to decrease pain, limit disability, maintain moderate exercise, and prevent joint contractures. No specific medication regimen has proved effective in modifying the disease process in scleroderma, but, along with antiarthritic drugs, various medications are used to treat organ system involvement. Calcium-channel blockers may provide improvement in symptoms of Raynaud phenomenon. ACE inhibitors appear to have improved survival of renal scleroderma crisis, and now there are many therapeutic agents approved for use in pulmonary hypertension (Steen, 2015; Topal & Dhurat, 2013).

In addition to the common problems of rheumatic disorders, nurses need to identify other patient difficulties or needs

related to scleroderma and plan accordingly. For instance, patients with scleroderma have problems associated with impaired skin integrity and imbalanced nutrition that is less than what the body requires. The patient with advanced disease also may have impaired gas exchange, decreased cardiac output, impaired swallowing, and constipation. There has been increased attention on psychosocial issues in SSc, but currently there have been no evidence-based interventions (Malcarne, Fox, Mills, & Gholizadeh, 2013).

Providing meticulous skin care and preventing the effects of Raynaud phenomenon are major nursing challenges. Nurses teach patients to avoid the cold and to protect fingers with mittens. In addition, warm socks and properly fitting shoes are helpful in preventing foot ulcers. Careful, frequent inspection for early ulcers is important, and smoking cessation is critical.

NURSING PROCESS
The Patient with a Rheumatic Disorder

ASSESSMENT

The health history and physical and psychological assessments focus on current and past symptoms, such as fatigue, weakness, pain, stiffness, fever, or anorexia and the effects of these symptoms on the patient's lifestyle and self-image. Also the patient's social support systems are assessed as well as his or her ability to participate in daily activities, comply with the treatment regimen, and manage self-care (Box 39-5). Additional areas assessed include the patient's understanding, motivation, knowledge, coping abilities, past experiences, preconceptions, and fears. The impact of the rheumatic disorder on the patient must be assessed to understand the patient's problems so that a plan of care specific to his or her issues can be developed. The nurse assesses the impact of the condition by asking, "Are there things that you cannot do now that you could do a year ago?" "What is it about your condition that you find most frustrating?" "What do you most enjoy doing?" "What things do you find difficult that you would like to be able to do?" and "How do you manage to get around the tasks that are difficult?" (Woolf, 2015). The nurse's assessment and patient response to these questions may lead to identifying issues and concerns that can be addressed by nursing interventions, and, through collaboration with other interprofessional members, expected patient outcomes can be achieved (Crossland, Field, Ainsworth, Edwards, & Cherry, 2014; Iversen, 2013; Iversen & Sharby, 2015; Kjeken, Dagfinrud, Heiberg, & Kvien, 2015).

DIAGNOSIS

Nursing diagnoses for patients with rheumatic disorders may include, but are not limited to:

- Acute and chronic pain related to inflammation and/or progression of joint deterioration, tissue damage, fatigue, lowered tolerance level, or ineffective pain/comfort measures

Nursing Research

Bridging the Gap to Evidence-Based Practice

What is the Evidence of the Effects of a Self-Care Program in People with Rheumatic Diseases?

Arvidsson, S., Bergman, S., Arvidsson, B., Fridlund, B., & Tingström, P. (2013). Effects of a self-care promoting problem-based learning programme in people with rheumatic diseases: A randomized controlled study. *Journal of Advanced Nursing*, 69(7), 1500–1514.

Purpose

Empowerment is a concept often used in health care. The World Health Organization (WHO) describes empowerment in health promotion work as a process where individuals receive more control over decisions and actions that affect their own life and health. Therefore, the goal of patient education for individuals with RA is that they must participate actively in their own care and have knowledge and skills to manage their self-care in the best way. The purpose of this study was to evaluate the effects of a self-care promoting problem-based learning program for people with rheumatic diseases in terms of health-related quality of life (HRQL), empowerment, and self-care ability.

Design

A randomized controlled design was selected with test at baseline, 1 week, and 6 months postintervention after completing a 1-year program. The participants were assigned randomly to either the experimental group (*n* = 54) or the control group (*n* = 148). The inclusion criteria were that the participants had one or more diagnoses of rheumatic diseases for more than a year, had musculoskeletal pain, and had sleep disturbances

and/or fatigue during the last 3 months. The participants in the experimental group were divided consecutively into seven tutorial groups of seven or eight participants and one tutor. Each tutorial group met for 1½ hours, 10 times in a 1-year period. Starting points in the curriculum were: self-awareness and self-confidence, relationship to others, stress and relaxation, physical activity and rest, medicines and herbal remedies, tobacco and alcohol, and food and drink. The program ran alongside the standard care the participants received at a rheumatology unit.

Findings

The participants in the experimental group had a statistically significant difference demonstrating stronger empowerment after participation in the self-care promoting problem-based learning program compared with the control group, at the 6-month postintervention meeting. Approximately two thirds of the participants in the experimental group stated that they had implemented lifestyle changes due to the program.

Nursing Implications

The results of this study showed that the self-care promoting problem-based learning program enabled people with rheumatic diseases to improve their empowerment compared with the control group. It is important to continue to develop problem-based learning in patient education to find the very best way to use this pedagogical method in the care of patients affected by rheumatologic disorders.

- Fatigue related to inflammatory process and increased disease activity, pain, inadequate sleep/rest, impaired physical and psychosocial functioning (including emotional stress/depression), and inadequate nutrition
- Insomnia related to pain, anxiety/stress, depression, and medications
- Impaired physical mobility related to musculoskeletal impairment, decreased ROM, muscle weakness, pain on movement, limited endurance, lack of or improper use of ambulatory devices
- Self-care deficits (specify) related to limitations secondary to progression of disease, pain, fatigue, contractures, or loss of motion
- Ineffective health self-management (formerly ineffective therapeutic regimen management) related to complexity of chronic health problem and medication compliance, decisional conflicts, economic difficulties, and deficient knowledge regarding disease management
- Disturbed body image related to physical (e.g., joint abnormalities) and psychological (e.g., depression) changes, loss of body function, and dependency imposed by chronic illness
- Ineffective coping related to actual or perceived lifestyle or role changes, chronicity of disease, poor prognosis, and sense of powerlessness

- Risk for injury related to adverse effects of medications, high risk of falls, and potential complications

PLANNING

The major goals for the patient may include relief of pain and discomfort, relief of fatigue, promotion of nutrition and restorative sleep, increased mobility and exercise, maintenance of self-care, motivation and adherence to therapeutic regimen, improved body image, effective coping, absence of complications, and promotion of home care.

NURSING INTERVENTIONS

Pain management and optimal functional ability, including the promotion of a healthy, positive life course adaptation, are major goals of nursing intervention. Patient teaching is an essential nursing intervention in the care of the patient with a rheumatic disorder. Education is the key to successfully enabling the patient to maintain as much independence as possible, to take medications accurately and safely, and to use adaptive devices correctly. Patient teaching focuses on the disorder itself, the possible changes related to the disorder, and the therapeutic regimen prescribed to treat it. Additional teaching is centered on

(continued on page 1162)

the potential side effects of medications, strategies to maintain independence and function, and patient safety.

RELIEVING PAIN AND DISCOMFORT

Pain has quite different effects on different patients. The response to pain and the degree to which it disrupts the patient's life give a more meaningful indication of severity. Does the pain affect their sleep? How has pain affected their mood? What specific functions or activities does it limit? Understanding the problems it causes can guide how best to manage the patient's pain.

The nurse teaches patients to differentiate between joint pain and stiffness. Medications are used on a short-term basis to relieve acute pain. Because the pain may be persistent, non-opioid analgesics, such as acetaminophen, are often used. After administering medications, the nurse needs to reassess pain levels and response to treatment. With persistent pain, assessment findings should be compared with baseline measurements; evaluations of additional measures include exploring coping skills and strategies that have worked in the past.

The nurse teaches the patient about self-administration of pharmacologic agents and the need for safety in doing so. The patient needs to understand the importance of taking medications, such as NSAIDs and DMARDs, exactly as prescribed to achieve maximum benefits. These benefits include relief of pain and anti-inflammatory action as the disease is brought under control. Because disease control and pain relief are delayed, the patient may mistakenly believe the medication is ineffective or may think of the medication as merely "pain pills," taking them only sporadically and failing to achieve control over the disease activity. Alternatively, the patient may not understand the need to continue the medication for its anti-inflammatory actions once pain control has been achieved.

Also heat applications are helpful in relieving pain, stiffness, and muscle spasm. Superficial heat may be applied in the form of warm tub baths or showers and warm, moist compresses. Paraffin baths (dips), which offer concentrated heat, are helpful to patients with wrist and small-joint involvement. Therapeutic exercises can be carried out more comfortably and effectively after heat has been applied. However, in some patients, heat actually may increase pain, muscle spasm, and synovial fluid volume. If the inflammatory process is acute, cold applications in the form of moist packs or an ice bag may be tried. Both heat and cold are analgesic to nerve pain receptors and can relax muscle spasms (Iversen, 2013; Kjeken et al., 2015). The nurse teaches safe use of heat and cold application, in 15- to 20-minute intervals, usually three to four times a day. The nurse checks the temperature of warm soaks and covers cold packs with a towel, particularly for patients with impaired sensation. Further study of the effectiveness of these modalities is needed.

The nurse encourages measures to protect affected joints. There is no clear indication that the use of orthotic devices, such as braces, splints, collars, and shoe modifications, provides pain relief. However, there is preliminary evidence to support the use of extra-depth shoes, with or without semi-rigid insoles, to relieve pain on walking and weight bearing (Kjeken et al., 2015).

Patients should be taught to avoid stooping, bending, or over-reaching and to rest 5 to 10 minutes when trying to complete a task. The nurse educates the patient regarding other strategies for decreasing pain, such as relaxation techniques, imagery, meditation, and distraction.

DECREASING FATIGUE

Fatigue is a common problem for patients with rheumatic disorders (Matcham, Ali, Hotopf, & Chalder, 2015; Rongen-van Dartel et al., 2014). Fatigue related to rheumatic disorders can be both acute (brief and relieved by rest or sleep) and chronic. Chronic fatigue, related to the disease process, is persistent, cumulative, and not eliminated by rest, but it is influenced by biologic, psychological, social, and personal factors. The nurse discusses related causes of fatigue with patients. Disease-related factors that may influence the amount and severity of fatigue include persistent pain, sleep disturbance, impaired physical activity, and disease duration. Pain increases fatigue because additional physical and emotional energy is required to deal with it. Pain also may cause the patient to expend more energy to do tasks in a way that causes less pain. A plan of nursing care for a patient with a rheumatic disorder is available online at http://thepoint.lww.com/Honan2e.

PROMOTING NUTRITION

Dietary intake of high-quality food has declined for most Western cultures. Americans are eating an increased amount of processed animal products and foods (high in trans fatty acids and omega-6 free fatty acids), food additives, preservatives, and high–glycemic-index foods (Berman, Lewith, Manheimer, Bishop, & D'Adamo, 2015; Stamp & Cleland, 2013). These factors directly or indirectly stimulate inflammation by increasing levels of arachidonic acid, a key component of many inflammatory mediators. Evidence has suggested incorporating an anti-inflammatory diet to improve serologic and symptomatic markers of inflammation. Fish oil supplements, and omega-3 or omega-6 fatty acids, can be added to the diet.

An anti-inflammatory diet is a predominantly plant-based diet, avoiding excess and high-glycemic-load calories. There is a strong emphasis on avoidance of foods that may potentially exacerbate the inflammatory response (e.g., trans fats, refined sugars, high saturated fats, alcohol, and caffeine in excess). The majority of the diet should be derived from four areas: whole-grain products, fresh fruits and vegetables, legumes, and seeds and nuts. These sources provide several anti-inflammatory components, such as fiber, isoflavones (e.g., soybeans and soy products), carotenoids, and omega-3 free fatty acids (e.g., flaxseed). Patients can be told to keep a journal to assist in monitoring ongoing diet and symptom changes and not to expect immediate results, allowing at least 12 weeks before reevaluating for any benefits. Consultation with a dietitian is highly recommended for understanding the overall diet and suggestions for meal planning.

Nursing Alert
Some medications (i.e., oral corticosteroids) used in the treatment of rheumatic diseases

stimulate the appetite and, when combined with decreased activity, may lead to weight gain. Therefore, patients may need to be counseled about eating a healthy, calorie-restricted diet.

PROMOTING RESTORATIVE SLEEP

Restful sleep is important in helping the patient to cope with pain, minimize physical fatigue, and deal with the changes necessitated by a chronic disease. In patients with acute disease, sleep time is frequently reduced and fragmented by prolonged awakenings. Also stiffness, depression, and medications may compromise the quality of sleep and increase daytime fatigue. A sleep-inducing routine, medication, and comfort measures may help improve the quality of sleep. The nurse encourages patients to take a warm bath or shower before bedtime to relax muscles; showering first thing in the morning may be beneficial to reduce morning stiffness.

Teaching sleep hygiene strategies may be helpful in promoting restorative sleep. These strategies include establishing a set time to sleep and wake up, creating a quiet sleep environment with a comfortable room temperature, avoiding factors that interfere with sleep (e.g., use of alcohol and caffeine), maintaining proper positioning of joints, using relaxation exercises, and getting out of bed and engaging in another activity (e.g., reading) if unable to fall asleep within 20 to 30 minutes (Taylor, Lillis, Lynn, & LeMone, 2015).

INCREASING MOBILITY

Maintaining some degree of joint mobilization and load on the joints is essential to the preservation of articular cartilage integrity. If the patient is overweight, a weight reduction program is a critical element in relieving stress on painful joints. Proper body positioning is essential to minimize stress on inflamed joints and prevent deformities that limit mobility. All joints should be supported in a position of optimal function. When in bed, the patient should lie flat on a firm mattress, with feet positioned against a footboard and with only one pillow under the head because of the risk of dorsal kyphosis. A pillow should not be placed under the knees, because this promotes flexion contracture. It is best for the patient to lie prone several times daily to prevent hip flexion contracture.

Care must be taken so that splinting for comfort does not restrict mobility later. Regularly removing the splint and exercising the joint through an ROM should be done to prevent joint "freezing." Splint modification may be needed when changes occur in joint structure.

In addition, assistive devices may be necessary for mobility. They should be fitted properly, and the patient should be instructed in their correct and safe use. A cane, long enough to allow for only a slight bend of the elbow, should be held in the hand opposite the affected side. Forearm-trough style crutches (platform crutches) may be needed to protect the upper extremities if the disease also involves the hands and wrists. This is especially important for the patient undergoing rehabilitation after reconstructive surgery on a joint in the lower extremity. Assistive devices can mean the difference between dependence and independence in mobility.

However, keep in mind also that use of assistive devices may alter the patient's body image, which can become a barrier to adherence to the treatment regimen.

ENCOURAGING EXERCISE

The ACR has identified exercise as a fundamental part in the management of rheumatic disorders. Active and active/self-assisted ROM exercises are encouraged because they prevent joint stiffness and increase mobility (Farrokhi, Baker, & Fitzgerald, 2015). Active/self-assisted exercises involve the use of overhead pulleys or wand exercises (shoulder exercises using a wand, stick, or cane). Measures to reinforce proper body posture and increase mobility include walking erect and using chairs with straight backs. When seated, the patient should rest the feet flat on the floor and the shoulders and hips against the back of the chair.

A formal program with occupational and physical therapy should be prescribed to educate the patient about principles of joint protection, pacing activities, work simplification, ROM, and muscle-strengthening exercises. An individualized exercise program is crucial to movement. Exercises appropriate in promoting mobility in patients with rheumatic disorders are summarized in Table 39-5. Appropriate programs of moderate pressure massage therapy and exercise, including T'ai chi, have been shown to decrease pain, improve function, and improve quality of life (Ekelman et al., 2014; Field et al., 2013; Field, Diego, Gonzalez, & Funk, 2014; Iversen, 2013; Sun et al., 2014). The major challenge for the patient and the health care provider is the need to adjust all aspects of treatment according to the activity of the disease. Especially for the patient with an active diffuse connective tissue disease, such as RA or SLE, activity levels may vary from day to day and even within a single day.

FACILITATING SELF-CARE

Self-care includes practices that patients undertake to promote their own health and well-being despite having a chronic illness. Self-care practices must be taught and reinforced so the patient does not develop self-care deficits. The nurse needs to keep in mind that a patient's deformity does not necessarily equate with the severity of limitations or disability. For example, swollen (edematous) hands may be more limiting than deformed hands.

The nurse should assist the patient in identifying any self-care deficit and those factors that interfere with the ability to perform self-care activities. The nurse in a hospital or extended care facility can help preserve the patient's independence by making available adaptive equipment for eating, toileting, bathing, and dressing. In the home, the nurse can encourage use of these devices. Also, the nurse should reemphasize the importance of relief for pain, stiffness, and fatigue and its impact on increasing the patient's ability to perform self-care.

PROMOTING MOTIVATION AND ENHANCING HEALTH MANAGEMENT

Motivating patients to make behavioral changes is an important nursing intervention. MI, proved effective in treating addictions,

(continued on page 1164)

TABLE **39-5** Exercises to Promote Mobility

Type of Exercise	Purpose	Recommended Performance	Precautions
Range of motion	Maintain flexibility and joint motion	Active or active/self-assisted at least daily	Reduce number of repetitions when inflammation is present
Isometric exercise	Improve muscle tone, static endurance, and strength; prepare for dynamic and weight-bearing exercises	Perform at 70% of maximal voluntary contraction daily	Monitor blood pressure; isometric exercises may increase blood pressure and decrease blood flow to muscles
Dynamic exercise	Maintain or increase dynamic strength and endurance; increase muscle power; enhance synovial blood flow; promote strength of bone and cartilage	Start with repetitions against gravity and add progressive resistance; perform 2–3 days per week	May increase biomechanical stress on joints that are unstable or misaligned
Aerobic exercise	Improve cardiovascular fitness and endurance	Perform 3–5 days per week for a maximum of 20–30 minutes of moderate-intensity exercise	Progress slowly as activity tolerance and fitness improve
Aquatic exercise	Water supports or resists movement; warm water may provide muscle relaxation and ease of movement	Provides buoyant medium for performance of dynamic or aerobic exercise	Recommended water temperature (92–94°F); deep water to minimize joint compression; nonslip footwear for safety; receive appropriate instruction in a program designed for people with arthritis

Adapted from Iversen, M. D. (2013). Introduction to physical medicine, physical therapy, and rehabilitation. In G. S. Firestein, R. C. Budd, S. E. Gabriel, I. B. McInnes, & J. R. O'Dell (Eds.), *Kelley's textbook of rheumatology* (9th ed.). Philadelphia, PA: Saunders Elsevier.

has been adapted for managing chronic illnesses. MI is a skillful clinical style for eliciting from patients their own good motivations for making behavior changes in the interest of their health through exploring and resolving ambivalence (Huffman, 2014; Knittle et al., 2014; Westra & Aviram, 2013). MI is an evidence-based counseling approach that can be used by nurses to help patients adhere to health regimens and can be applied in very brief, 10- to 15-minute patient encounters (Droppa & Lee, 2014; Lundahl et al., 2013; Moral et al., 2015). A key to understanding MI is knowing the phenomenon of ambivalence (Miller & Rollnick, 2013). Patients may feel ambivalent about change. Conflicting motivations are normal and common, to simultaneously want and not want. "I want to exercise, but it hurts," "I mean to take my medicine, but I keep forgetting." Nurses need to recognize the telltale sign of ambivalence is the "but" in the middle of their narrative. The nurse's task is to elicit "change talk" rather than resistance from the patient. Resistance is the patient's way of trying to resolve the discomfort created by ambivalence. Resistance is best handled by restating, using a "but" statement. For example, "You say you want to exercise, but it hurts. What things can you do to help ease the pain with activity?" The nurse refrains from persuading and confronting but guides the patient toward an acceptable resolution that triggers change. Patient motivation and readiness to change are dynamic states that can be greatly influenced by interactions between nurse and patient. By guiding the patient on what he or she sees as obstacles (the

"buts"), nurses can play a vital role in motivating the patient toward change (Box 39-6).

As part of standard nursing practice, patient education is the cornerstone to effective health management. Nurses should use therapeutic skills, such as reflective listening and asking open questions, prior to informing (The Advisory Board Company & Nursing Executive Center, 2015). Ask the patient what he or she already knows about the topic before preceding—use the "ask–provide–ask–formula."

Educational topics should include information about the nature and treatment of the disease, pain management strategies, correct posture and body mechanics, correct use of assistive devices, principles of joint protection, energy conservation and pacing techniques, balanced nutrition, weight and stress management, and an individualized exercise program. In the spirit of motivation and enhancement, it is crucial to form a partnership (collaboration) between nurse and patient; the nurse needs to listen and elicit information from the patient, understand the patient's own perspectives (evocation), and recognize that the patient can and does make choices about the course of his or her life (autonomy). In the end, the patient should express confidence in his ability to make treatment decisions and to carry out a health regimen.

IMPROVING BODY IMAGE AND COPING

All aspects of the patient's life, including work role, social life, sexual function, financial status, and perception of self may be

BOX 39-6

Four Guiding Principles of Motivational Interviewing (Acronym RULE)

R: Reflect Resistance

When the nurse suggests change and the patient is resisting and arguing against it, the nurse should "roll with the patient's resistance" (i.e., the nurse acknowledges that resistance to change is expected). The patient is the primary source of arguments and solutions. The nurse should reflect resistance nonjudgmentally.

U: Understand

The nurse expresses empathy and communicates acceptance of the patient's experience, including the patient's ambivalence about change. Be interested in the patient's own concerns, values, and motivations.

L: Listen

By listening to what patients say, the nurse can tell how likely they are to change. Listen for verbs in patient narrative indicating change talk, statements in relation to desire, ability, reasons, need, commitment, and taking action.

E: Empower

Nurses assist patients to explore how they can make a difference in their own health, emphasizing the patient's ability to choose and carry out a plan for change. Outcomes are best when patients take an active role in their own health care.

Adapted from Letourneau, K., & Goodman, J. H. (2014). A patient-centered approach for addressing physical activity in older adults: Motivational interviewing. *Journal of Gerontological Nursing, 40*(11), 26–32; Miller, W. R., & Rollnick, S. (2013). *Motivational interviewing: Helping people change.* (3rd ed.). New York: The Guilford Press.

altered because of the impact and unpredictability of the course of a rheumatoid disorder. Body image changes can lead to social isolation and depression. Hence, the nurse and the family need to understand and be sensitive to the patient's emotional reactions to the disease and provide support and assistance when appropriate.

The nurse should encourage the patient and family to verbalize feelings, perceptions, and fears related to the disease. Additionally, the nurse facilitates communication and aids the patient and family in identifying areas in which they have some control over disease symptoms and treatment. By taking action and involving others, the patient develops or draws on coping skills and possibly community support. The role of the nurse aims at addressing these psychological challenges to optimize the physical and psychological status of each patient (Roberts, 2013; Ryan, 2014a). The nurse also assists the patient to identify past coping mechanisms, as well as use of effective coping strategies, which is a key to positive outcomes.

MONITORING AND MANAGING POTENTIAL COMPLICATIONS

Medications used for treating rheumatic disorders have the potential for serious and adverse effects. Therefore, an important aspect of care is avoiding medication-induced complications. The provider bases the prescribed medication regimen on clinical findings and medical history and then monitors for side effects with periodic clinical assessments and laboratory testing. The nurse plays a major role in working with the primary care provider and pharmacist to help the patient recognize and deal with medication side effects. If side effects occur, the medication may need to be stopped or the dose reduced. The patient may experience an increase in symptoms while the complication is being resolved or a new medication is being initiated. In such cases, the nurse's counseling regarding symptom management may relieve potential anxiety and distress.

PROMOTING HOME CARE

Depending on the severity of the disorder and the patient's resources and supports, referral for home care may or may not be warranted. The patient who is elderly or frail, has a rheumatic disorder that limits function significantly, and lives alone may need a referral for home care. A dietary consultation may be indicated to ensure that the patient is knowledgeable about dietary recommendations given the increased risk of cardiovascular disease. The patient and family should be informed about support services such as Meals on Wheels and local chapters of the Arthritis Foundation.

During home visits, the nurse has the opportunity to assess the home environment and its adequacy for patient safety and management of the disorder. Adherence to the treatment program can be monitored more easily in the home setting, where physical and social barriers to adherence are more readily identified. For example, a patient with diabetes who requires insulin may be unable to fill the syringe accurately or be unable to administer the insulin because of impaired joint mobility. Often appropriate adaptive equipment needed for increased independence is identified more readily when the nurse sees how the patient functions in the home. Any barriers to adherence are identified, and appropriate referrals are made. Referrals to physical and occupational therapists may be made as problems are identified and limitations increase.

Furthermore, with each home visit the nurse assesses the patient's physical and psychological status, adequacy of symptom management, and adherence to the management plan. Previous teaching is reinforced, with emphasis on potential side effects of medications and changes in physical status that indicate disease progression and the need to contact the health care provider for reevaluation. Because of the increased risk of involvement of multiple organ systems, the importance of follow-up appointments is emphasized to the patient and family.

(*continued on page 1166*)

EVALUATION

Expected patient outcomes may include the following:

1. Experiences relief of pain or improved comfort level:
   a. Identifies factors that cause or increase pain
   b. Identifies realistic goals for pain relief
   c. Uses pain management strategies safely and effectively
   d. Reports decreased pain and increased comfort level
2. Experiences reduction in level of fatigue:
   a. Identifies factors that contribute to fatigue
   b. Verbalizes the relationship of fatigue to disease activity
   c. Schedules periodic rest periods, and identifies and uses other measures to prevent or modify fatigue
   d. Reports decreased level of fatigue
   e. Practices energy conservation strategies
   f. Discusses the relationship of the inflammatory process to fatigue and nutrition
3. Improves sleep patterns:
   a. Reports fewer nighttime awakenings
   b. Adheres to sleep-inducing routine
   c. Reports feeling rested on awakening
4. Increases or maintains level of mobility:
   a. Identifies factors that impede mobility
   b. Demonstrates normal or acceptable body alignment and posture
   c. Uses assistive devices appropriately and safely
   d. Participates in activities and exercises that promote or maintain mobility
5. Maintains self-care activities:
   a. Participates in self-care activities within capabilities
   b. Uses adaptive equipment and alternative methods to increase participation in self-care activities
   c. Maintains self-care at highest possible level
6. Enhances motivation and health self-management:
   a. Self-initiates goal-directed behavior
   b. Expresses belief in ability to perform activities
   c. Develops contract for health management with mutually agreeable goals for treatment
   d. Performs self-care and health-related activities consistent with ability
   e. Balances treatment, exercise, work, leisure, rest, and nutrition
7. Experiences improved body image and coping:
   a. Verbalizes concerns about the impact of rheumatic disease on appearance and function
   b. Sets and achieves meaningful goals
   c. States acceptance of self-worth
   d. Adapts to body image changes caused by disease
   e. Identifies and uses effective coping strategies
8. Experiences absence of complications:
   a. Takes medications as prescribed
   b. States potential side effects of medications and names reportable side effects
   c. Verbalizes understanding of rationale for monitoring
   d. Complies with recommendations for monitoring
   e. Identifies strategies to reduce risks of side effects and potential risks for falling

CHAPTER REVIEW

Critical Thinking Exercises

1. A 79-year-old woman with a 10-year history of OA of the right knee complains of pain every day and difficulty walking. Currently, she uses a walker to ambulate but needs to stop and rest every so often because of the pain. What treatment options are available? Develop an evidence-based plan of care for her.

2. A 20-year-old woman complains of alopecia, skin rash, joint pain, weight loss, and fatigue. Her family states that she does not "seem like herself" lately. A diagnosis of SLE is made. What can you explain to her about her diagnosis and her treatment options?

3. You are caring for a patient with a rheumatic disorder. NSAIDs, corticosteroids, and a biologic response modifier have been prescribed. How do the actions, uses, and indications of these medications differ? What instructions and recommendations would you give to the patient to ensure their safe administration?

NCLEX-Style Review Questions

1. When assessing a patient, the nurse knows that which clinical manifestations are shared by rheumatoid arthritis and OA?
   a. Joint space narrowing and a decreased C4 level
   b. Symmetrical knee involvement and joint effusions
   c. Tophi, joint enlargement, and severe pain
   d. Joint swelling, stiffness, and pain

2. The nursing diagnosis identified for a patient with OA is acute pain. Which action by the patient warrants intervention by the visiting nurse?
   a. Acetaminophen (Tylenol) taken PO in doses no more than 3,000 mg/day
   b. Capsaicin (Capsin) applied topically as needed 3 to 4 times a day
   c. Cold application to localized area for 30 minutes 4 to 5 times a day
   d. Paraffin dips providing concentrated heat applied to the wrist before bedtime

3. The nurse has finished the receiving shift report at 7:30 AM. Which patient should the nurse assess first?
   a. The patient with scleroderma who had an episode of dyspnea during the night shift
   b. The patient diagnosed with OA who complains of morning joint stiffness
   c. The patient who needs to receive a scheduled 8 AM IV adrenal corticosteroid
   d. The patient suspected of an acute gout attack who is scheduled for an arthrocentesis

4. A patient with SLE is admitted to the hospital for evaluation and management of acute joint inflammation. Which information obtained in the admission laboratory testing results is of most concern to the nurse?
   a. Elevated blood urea nitrogen (BUN)
   b. Increased C-reactive protein
   c. Positive ANA
   d. Positive RF

5. Which statement indicates the patient requires further teaching regarding the nutritional management of gout?
   a. "I need to limit my alcohol intake."
   b. "I need to avoid fad starvation diets."
   c. "I need to follow a high-protein diet."
   d. "I need to eliminate fructose drinks."

Try these additional resources, available at **http://thepoint.lww.com/Honan2e**, to enhance your learning and understanding of this chapter:
- NCLEX-Style Student Review Questions
- Journal Articles

REFERENCES AND SELECTED READINGS

References and selected readings associated with this chapter can be found on the website that accompanies the book. Visit **http://thepoint. lww.com/Honan2e** to access the references and other additional resources associated with this chapter.

Problems Related to Musculoskeletal Function

A 26-year-old man is being seen in the orthopedic clinic for complaints of low back pain. He is employed as a construction worker. He complains of pain radiating down his left leg. He states that his back pain started after he lifted a steel beam at work.

- Discuss evaluative data that would be important to gather on this patient.
- Describe diagnostic procedures that would lead to a definitive diagnosis.
- Discuss medical and nursing management for this patient.

Nursing Assessment: Musculoskeletal Function

Geriann B. Gallagher

Learning Objectives

After reading this chapter, you will be able to:

1. Describe the basic structure and function of the musculoskeletal system.
2. Discuss the relationship of the health history to the assessment of musculoskeletal health.
3. Describe the significance of physical assessment findings to the diagnosis of musculoskeletal dysfunction.
4. Specify the diagnostic tests used for assessment of musculoskeletal function.

The musculoskeletal system includes the bones, joints, muscles, tendons, ligaments, and bursae of the body. The functions of these components are highly integrated; therefore, disease in or injury to one component adversely affects the others. For instance, an infection in a joint (septic arthritis) causes degeneration of the articular surfaces of the bones within the joint and local muscle atrophy.

Diseases and injuries that involve the musculoskeletal system are commonly implicated in disability and death. In 2006, patients at least 65 years of age had over 2.1 million visits to the emergency department (ED) for injurious falls, which accounts for 10.5% of all ED visits among the elderly. In addition, 29.6% of these visits required hospital admission (Ferri, 2016). Hip fracture is a serious consequence of falls in the elderly; approximately 73% to 90% of hip fractures occur from a fall (Agency for Healthcare Research and Quality [AHRQ], 2015). Fractures increase the risk of mortality and significantly increase the cost of patient care. Musculoskeletal diseases and injuries can significantly affect overall productivity, independence, and quality of life (QOL) in people of all ages. Nurses in all practice areas encounter patients with disruption in musculoskeletal function.

ANATOMIC AND PHYSIOLOGIC OVERVIEW

The health and proper functioning of the musculoskeletal system is interdependent with that of the other body systems. The musculoskeletal system has important functions, including providing protection for vital organs (e.g., brain, heart, liver, kidneys, lungs, spleen) and providing a sturdy framework to support body structures. It also makes mobility possible. Joints hold the bones together and allow the body to move. The muscles attached to the skeleton contract, moving the bones and producing heat that helps maintain body temperature. Movement facilitates the return of deoxygenated blood to the right side of the heart by massaging the venous vasculature. In addition, the musculoskeletal system serves as a reservoir for immature blood cells and essential minerals, including calcium, phosphorus, magnesium, and fluoride. More than 98% of total body calcium is present in the bones. Additionally, the red bone marrow located within bone cavities produces red blood cells (RBCs), white blood cells (WBCs), and platelets through a process referred to as **hematopoiesis**.

Structure and Function of the Skeletal System

The shape and construction of a specific bone are determined by its function and the forces exerted on it.

Bone Types and Tissue

Bones are constructed of two types of bone tissue: **cancellous** (trabecular) or **cortical** (compact). Cancellous bone, or spongy bone, is found in the interior of bones and forms a lattice-like pattern. Red or yellow bone marrow fills the lattice network. Cortical, or compact, bone forms the outer shell of a bone. It has a densely packed, calcified intercellular matrix, making the cortical bone more rigid than cancellous bone (Grossman & Porth, 2014). Varying amounts of both cancellous and cortical bone are found throughout the body in differing proportions depending on the function of the bone.

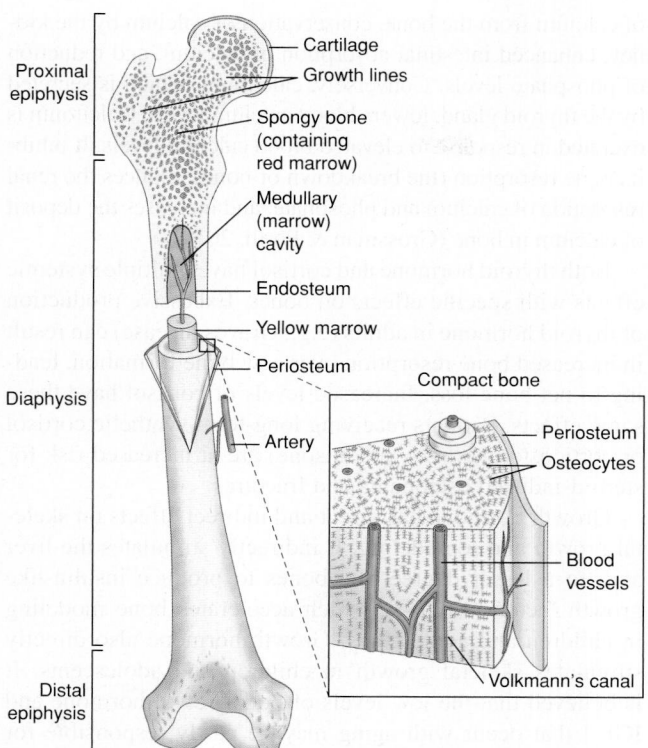

Proximal epiphysis

Cartilage
Growth lines
Spongy bone (containing red marrow)
Medullary (marrow) cavity
Endosteum
Yellow marrow
Periosteum

Diaphysis

Artery

Compact bone
Periosteum
Osteocytes
Blood vessels
Volkmann's canal

Distal epiphysis

FIGURE 40-1 Structure of a long bone; composition of compact bone.

There are 206 bones in the human body, divided into four categories:

- Long bones (e.g., femur)
- Short bones (e.g., metacarpals)
- Flat bones (e.g., sternum)
- Irregular bones (e.g., vertebrae)

Long bones are shaped like rods or shafts with rounded ends (Fig. 40-1). The shaft, known as the **diaphysis**, is primarily cortical bone. The ends of the long bones, called **epiphyses**, are primarily cancellous bone. The epiphyseal plate separates the epiphyses from the diaphysis and is the center for longitudinal growth in children, thus it can be a critical indicator of potential growth problems if fractured in children. It is calcified in adults. The ends of long bones are covered at the joints by articular **cartilage**, which is tough, elastic, avascular tissue. Long bones are designed for weight bearing and movement. Short bones consist of cancellous bone covered by a layer of compact bone. Flat bones are important sites of hematopoiesis and frequently provide protection for vital organs. They are made of cancellous bone layered between compact bone. Irregular bones have unique shapes related to their function. An example of irregular shaped bones is the vertebrae.

Bone is composed of three basic cell types—**osteoblasts**, **osteocytes**, and **osteoclasts**. Osteoblasts function in bone formation by secreting bone matrix. The term *blast* refers to

immature or precursor cell, thus it is foundational for bone formation (Grossman & Porth, 2014). The matrix consists of collagen and ground substances (glycoproteins and proteoglycans) that provide a framework in which inorganic mineral salts are deposited. These minerals are composed primarily of calcium and phosphorus. Osteocytes are mature bone cells involved in bone maintenance. Osteoclasts are multinuclear cells involved in dissolving and resorbing bone. The microscopic functioning unit of mature cortical bone is the **osteon** (Haversian system). The center of the osteon, the Haversian canal, contains blood vessels and nerve supply for the osteon. Around the canal are circles of mineralized bone matrix called **lamellae**. The lamellae follow along the shaft of the long bone to nourish the osteon. Covering the bone is a dense, fibrous membrane known as the **periosteum**. This membranous structure nourishes bone and facilitates its growth. The periosteum contains nerves, blood vessels, and lymphatics. It also provides for the attachment of tendons, which connect muscles to bones, and ligaments, which connect bones to bones. The **endosteum** is a thin, vascular membrane that covers the marrow cavity of long bones and the spaces in cancellous bone.

Bone marrow is a vascular tissue located in the medullary (shaft) cavity of long bones and in flat bones. Red bone marrow, located mainly in the sternum, ilium, vertebrae, and ribs in adults, is responsible for producing RBCs, WBCs, and platelets. In adults, the long bone is filled with fatty, yellow marrow.

Bone tissue is well vascularized. Cancellous bone receives a rich blood supply through metaphyseal and epiphyseal vessels. Periosteal vessels carry blood to compact bone through minute openings called *Volkmann canals*. In addition, nutrient arteries penetrate the periosteum and enter the medullary cavity through foramina (small openings). Nutrient arteries supply blood to the marrow and bone. The venous system may accompany arteries or may exit independently.

Bone Formation

Osteogenesis (bone formation) begins long before birth. **Ossification** is the process by which the bone matrix (collagen fibers and ground substance) is formed and hard mineral crystals composed of calcium and phosphorus (e.g., hydroxyapatite) are bound to the collagen fibers. The mineral components of the bone give it its characteristic strength, whereas the proteinaceous collagen gives bone its resilience.

Bone Maintenance

Bone is a dynamic tissue in a constant state of turnover. During childhood, bones grow and form by a process called *modeling*. By early adulthood (i.e., early 20s), **remodeling** is the primary process that occurs. Remodeling maintains bone structure and function through simultaneous **resorption** (removal/destruction of tissue) and osteogenesis (bone formation). The balance between bone resorption and formation is influenced by physical activity; dietary intake of certain nutrients, especially calcium; and several hormones, including calcitriol (i.e., active vitamin D), parathyroid hormone (PTH), calcitonin, thyroid hormone, cortisol, growth hormone, and the sex hormones estrogen and testosterone. Physical activity, particularly weight-bearing activity, stimulates bone formation and remodeling. Bones subjected to continued weight bearing tend to be thick and strong. Conversely, people who are unable to engage in regular weight-bearing activities, such as those on prolonged bed rest or those with disabilities, have increased bone resorption from calcium loss, and their bones become osteopenic and weak. These weakened bones may fracture easily.

> **Nursing Alert**
>
> *It is important to note that after 30 to 45 years of age, the resorption of bone exceeds bone formation. This imbalance is exaggerated in women after menopause, which increases the risk of osteoporosis-related fractures (Kasper et al., 2015).*

Good dietary habits are integral to bone health. In particular, absorption of daily calcium, approximately 1,200 mg for adults and 1,500 mg for postmenopausal women, is essential to maintaining adult bone mass. This may be achieved through ingesting calcium-rich foods on a daily basis (e.g., through drinking 16 to 24 oz of milk daily) (Box 40-1).

Several hormones are vital in ensuring that calcium is absorbed properly and available for bone mineralization and matrix formation. Biologically active vitamin D (calcitriol) functions to increase the amount of calcium in the blood by promoting absorption of calcium from the gastrointestinal tract. It also facilitates mineralization of osteoid tissue. A deficiency of vitamin D results in bone mineralization deficit, deformity, and fracture.

PTH and calcitonin are the major hormonal regulators of calcium homeostasis. PTH is one of the important regulators of the concentration of calcium and phosphate in the blood. PTH promotes movement of calcium and phosphorus from the bone into the extracellular fluid. In response to low calcium levels in the blood, levels of PTH increase, promoting the mobilization

of calcium from the bone, conservation of calcium by the kidney, enhanced intestinal absorption of calcium, and reduction of phosphate levels. Conversely, calcitonin, which is secreted by the thyroid gland, lowers blood calcium levels. Calcitonin is excreted in response to elevated blood calcium levels. It inhibits bone resorption (the breakdown of bone), reduces the renal resorption of calcium and phosphate, and increases the deposit of calcium in bone (Grossman & Porth, 2014).

Both thyroid hormone and cortisol have multiple systemic effects with specific effects on bones. Excessive production of thyroid hormone in adults (e.g., Graves disease) can result in increased bone resorption over new bone formation, leading to net bone loss. Increased levels of cortisol have these same effects. Patients receiving long-term synthetic cortisol or corticosteroids (i.e., prednisone) are at increased risk for steroid-induced osteopenia and fractures.

Growth hormone has direct and indirect effects on skeletal growth and remodeling. It indirectly stimulates the liver and, to a lesser degree, the bones to produce insulin-like growth factor-1 (IGF-I), which accelerates bone modeling in children and adolescents. Growth hormone also directly stimulates skeletal growth in children and adolescents. It is believed that the low levels of both growth hormone and IGF-I that occur with aging may be partly responsible for decreased bone formation and resultant osteopenia.

The sex hormones testosterone and estrogen have important effects on bone remodeling. Estrogen stimulates osteoblasts and inhibits osteoclasts; therefore, bone formation is enhanced and resorption is inhibited. Low levels of estrogen or increased levels of corticosteroids cause disruption in normal osteoclast and osteoblast homeostasis. Testosterone has both direct and indirect effects on bone growth and formation. It directly causes skeletal growth in adolescence and has continued effects on skeletal muscle growth throughout the lifespan. Increased muscle mass results in greater weight-bearing stress on bones, resulting in increased bone formation. In addition, testosterone converts to estrogen in adipose tissue, providing an additional source of bone-preserving estrogen for aging men.

Blood supply to the bone also affects bone formation. With diminished blood supply or hyperemia (congestion), osteogenesis and bone density decrease. Bone necrosis occurs when the bone is deprived of blood.

Bone Healing

When a bone is fractured, the bone regenerates itself.

Although the exact process of fracture healing is open to controversy, stages of bone healing are identified below (Grossman & Porth, 2014).

1. *Hematoma formation:* The body responds to a fracture by bleeding into the injured tissue and forming a fracture hematoma. The fragmented ends of the fracture become devitalized because of the interrupted blood supply. This hematoma facilitates the formation of fibrin, which will become the framework upon which new bone will

---

BOX 40-1 **Nutrition Alert**

Bone Health

Calcium is important for bone health. Sources of calcium include:

- Milk, yogurt, and cheese
- Rhubarb, cooked collard greens, Chinese cabbage, kale, and broccoli
- Sardines, oysters, clams, canned salmon with bones
- Tofu
- Calcium-fortified fruit juices, fruit drinks, and cereals

grow. The injured area is invaded by macrophages (large phagocytic WBCs), which débride the area. Inflammatory cells that migrate to the injured area release growth factors that stimulate osteoclast and osteoblast activity. Inflammation, swelling, and pain are present. The inflammatory stage lasts several days and resolves with a decrease in pain and swelling.

2. *Inflammatory phase:* New capillaries infiltrate the hematoma, and fibroblasts (cells that produce collagen, the major protein of bone) from the periosteum, endosteum, and bone marrow produce a bridge between the fractured bones. This bridge made of tissue not yet ossified—termed a soft tissue **callus**—establishes a connection between the bone fragment and will, in time, become bone. Under the influence of signaling molecules, cell proliferation and differentiation occur.

3. *Reparative phase:* Chondrocytes (cartilage cells) in the cartilage callus form matrix vesicles, which regulate calcification of the cartilage. Enzymes within these matrix vesicles prepare the cartilage for calcium release and deposit. The calcified cartilage, referred to as *bony callus*, is invaded by blood vessels and becomes resorbed by chondroblasts and osteoclasts. It is replaced by woven bone similar to that of the growth plate.

4. *Remodeling:* Minerals continue to be deposited until the bone is firmly reunited. With major adult long bone fractures, ossification (the making of bone) takes 3 to 4 months. The final stage of fracture repair consists of remodeling the new bone into its former structural arrangement. Remodeling may take months to years, depending on the extent of bone modification needed, the function of the bone, and the functional stresses on the bone. Cancellous bone heals and remodels more rapidly than does compact cortical bone.

Serial x-rays are used to monitor the progress of bone healing. The rate of fracture healing is influenced by the type of bone fractured, the adequacy of blood supply, the surface contact of the fragments, and the age and general health of the person. Adequate immobilization is essential until there is x-ray evidence of bone formation with ossification.

When fractures are treated with open rigid compression plate fixation techniques, the bony fragments can be placed in direct contact. Primary bone healing occurs through cortical bone (Haversian) remodeling. Little or no cartilaginous callus develops. Immature bone develops from the endosteum. There is an intensive regeneration of new osteons, which develop in the fracture line by a process similar to normal bone maintenance. Fracture strength is obtained when the new osteons have become established.

Structure and Function of the Articular System

The junction of two or more bones is called a **joint** (articulation). There are three basic kinds of joints: synarthrosis,

FIGURE 40-2 Hinge joint of the knee.

amphiarthrosis, and diarthrosis joints. Synarthrosis joints are immovable (e.g., the skull sutures). Amphiarthrosis joints (e.g., the vertebral joints and the symphysis pubis) allow limited motion; the bones of amphiarthrosis joints are joined by fibrous cartilage. Diarthrosis joints are freely movable joints.

There are several types of diarthrosis joints:

- *Ball-and-socket* joints (e.g., the hip and the shoulder) permit full freedom of movement.
- *Hinge* joints permit bending in one direction only (e.g., the elbow and the knee) (Fig. 40-2).
- *Saddle* joints allow movement in two planes at right angles to each other. The joint at the base of the thumb is a saddle joint.
- *Pivot* joints are characterized by the articulation between the radius and the ulna. They permit rotation for such activities as turning a doorknob.
- *Gliding* joints allow for limited movement in all directions and are represented by the joints of the carpal bones in the wrist.

The ends of the articulating bones of a typical movable joint are covered with smooth hyaline cartilage. A tough, fibrous sheath called the **joint capsule** surrounds the articulating bones. The capsule is lined with a membrane, the **synovium**, which secretes the lubricating and shock-absorbing synovial fluid into the joint capsule. Therefore, the bone surfaces are not in direct contact. In some synovial joints (e.g., the knee), fibrocartilage disks (e.g., medial meniscus) are located between the articular cartilage surfaces. These disks provide shock absorption.

Ligaments (fibrous connective tissue bands) bind the articulating bones together. Ligaments and muscle tendons, which pass over the joint, provide joint stability. In some joints, intracapsular ligaments (e.g., the cruciate ligaments of the knee) are found within the capsule and add stability to the joint.

A **bursa** is a thin-walled sac lined with synovial fluid that facilitates the movement of tendons and muscles over bony prominences. Bursae are found at the elbow, shoulder, knee, and some other joints.

Structure and Function of the Skeletal Muscle System

Tendons (cords of fibrous connective tissue) or aponeuroses (broad, flat sheets of connective tissue) attach muscles to bones, connective tissue, other muscles, soft tissue, or skin. The muscles of the body are composed of parallel groups of muscle cells (fasciculi) encased in fibrous tissue called **fascia** (or epimysium). The more fasciculi contained in a muscle, the more precise the movements. Muscles vary in shape and size according to the activities for which they are responsible. Skeletal (striated) muscles are involved in body movement, posture, and heat-production functions. Muscles contract to bring the two points of attachment closer together, resulting in movement.

Muscle Tone

The contraction of muscle fibers can result in either isotonic or isometric contraction of the muscle. In **isometric contraction**, the length of the muscles remains constant but the force generated by the muscles is increased; an example of this is pushing against an immovable wall. **Isotonic contraction**, on the other hand, is characterized by shortening of the muscle with no increase in tension within the muscle; an example of this is flexing the forearm. In normal activities, many muscle movements are a combination of isometric and isotonic contraction.

Relaxed muscles demonstrate a state of readiness to respond to contraction stimuli. This state of readiness, known as muscle **tone (tonus)**, is produced by the maintenance of some of the muscle fibers in a contracted state. Muscle spindles, which are sense organs in the muscles, monitor muscle tone. Muscle tone is minimal during sleep and is increased when the person is anxious. A muscle that is limp and without tone is described as **flaccid**; a muscle with greater-than-normal tone is described as **spastic**. In conditions characterized by destruction of lower motor neurons (e.g., polio), denervated muscle becomes **atonic** (soft and flabby) and atrophies.

Muscle Actions

Muscles accomplish movement by contraction. Through the coordination of muscle groups, the body is able to perform a wide variety of movements (Fig. 40-3). The prime mover is the muscle that causes a particular motion. The muscles assisting the prime mover are known as *synergists*. The muscles causing movement opposite to that of the prime mover are known as *antagonists*. An antagonist must relax to allow the prime mover to contract, producing motion. For example, when contraction of the biceps causes flexion of the elbow joint, the biceps are the prime movers, and the triceps are the antagonists. A person with muscle **paralysis** (a loss of movement, possibly from nerve damage) may be able to retrain functioning muscles within the synergistic group to produce the needed movement. Muscles of the synergistic group then become the prime movers.

Exercise, Disuse, and Repair

Muscles need to be exercised to maintain function and strength. When a muscle repeatedly develops maximum or close to maximum tension over a long time, as in regular exercise with weights, the cross-sectional area of the muscle increases. This enlargement, known as **hypertrophy**, results from an increase in the size of individual muscle fibers without an increase in their number. Hypertrophy persists only if the exercise is continued. The opposite phenomenon occurs with disuse of muscle over a long period of time. Age and disuse cause loss of muscular function as fibrotic tissue replaces the contractile muscle tissue. The decrease in the size of a muscle is called **atrophy**. Bed rest and immobility cause loss of muscle mass and strength. When immobility is the result of a treatment modality (e.g., casting, traction), the patient can decrease the effects of immobility by performing isometric exercise of the muscles of the immobilized part.

Gerontologic Considerations

Multiple changes in the musculoskeletal system occur with aging (Table 40-1). Bone mass usually peaks between 18 and 25 years of age (National Osteoporosis Foundation, 2016), after which there is a universal gradual loss of bone. There is also a decrease in muscle mass and strength and an actual loss in the size and number of muscle fibers due to myofibril atrophy with fibrous tissue replacement. Numerous metabolic changes, including menopausal withdrawal of estrogen and decreased activity, contribute to **osteoporosis**. As a result, women lose more bone mass than men and are at higher risk for fractures. In the elderly, the articular cartilage degenerates in weight-bearing areas and heals less readily. Ultimately, ligaments become weak, and this contributes to the development of **osteoarthritis** (degenerative joint disease). Decrease in muscle mass, pain, and decrease in range of motion (ROM) can cause functional impairment in the elderly. Decreased activity, diminished neuron stimulation, and nutritional deficiencies also contribute to loss of muscle strength. In addition, remote musculoskeletal problems for which the patient has compensated may become new problems with age-related changes. For example, people who have had polio and who have been able to function normally by using synergistic muscle groups may discover increasing incapacity because of a reduced compensatory ability. However, many of the effects of aging can be slowed if the body is kept healthy and active through positive lifestyle behaviors.

FIGURE 40-3 Body movements produced by muscle contraction.

TABLE 40-1 GERONTOLOGIC CONSIDERATIONS / Age-Related Changes of the Musculoskeletal System

Musculoskeletal System	Structural Changes	Functional Changes	History and Physical Findings
Bones	Gradual, progressive loss of bone mass after 30 years of age Vertebrae collapse; Decreased osteoblastic activity (reduced production of new bone)	Bones fragile and prone to fracture: vertebrae, hip, wrist	Loss of height Posture changes Kyphosis Loss of flexibility Flexion of hips and knees Back pain Osteoporosis Fracture
Muscles	Increase in collagen and resultant fibrosis Muscles diminish in size (atrophy); wasting Tendons less elastic	Loss of strength and flexibility Weakness Fatigue Stumbling Falls	Loss of strength Diminished agility Decreased endurance Prolonged response time (diminished reaction time) Diminished tone Wide based gait History of falls
Joints	Cartilage shows progressive deterioration Thinning of intervertebral discs	Stiffness, reduced flexibility, and pain interfere with activities of daily living	Diminished range of motion Stiffness Loss of height
Ligaments	Lax ligaments (less than normal strength; weakness)	Postural joint abnormality Weakness	Joint pain on motion; resolves with rest Crepitus Joint swelling/enlargement Osteoarthritis (degenerative joint disease)

ASSESSMENT

The nursing assessment of the patient with musculoskeletal dysfunction includes an evaluation of the effects of the musculoskeletal problem on the patient. The nurse is concerned with assisting patients who have musculoskeletal problems to maintain their general health, accomplish their activities of daily living, and manage their treatment programs. The nurse encourages optimal nutrition and teaches the patient strategies to minimize problems related to mobility. Through an individualized plan of nursing care, the nurse helps the patient achieve maximum health.

Health History

Common Complaints

Common musculoskeletal complaints include pain or tenderness and altered sensations.

Pain

Most patients with diseases and traumatic conditions or disorders of the muscles, bones, and joints experience pain. Bone pain is characteristically described as a dull, deep ache that is "boring" in nature, whereas muscular pain is described as soreness or aching and is referred to as "muscle cramps." Fracture pain is sharp and piercing and is relieved by immobilization. Sharp pain also may result from bone infection, with muscle spasm or pressure on a sensory nerve.

Pain that increases with activity may indicate joint sprain or muscle strain, whereas steadily increasing pain points to the progression of an infectious process (osteomyelitis), degenerative changes, a malignant tumor, or neurovascular complications. Radiating pain occurs in conditions in which pressure is exerted on a nerve root. Pain is variable, and its assessment and nursing management must be individualized. It is important that the patient's pain and discomfort be managed successfully. Not only is pain exhausting, but, if prolonged, it can force the patient to become increasingly preoccupied and dependent (see Chapter 7). The nurse notes body positioning and the influence of appliances, such as casts, traction, and surgical pins, when considering the patient's pain.

Altered Sensations

Frequently sensory disturbances are associated with musculoskeletal problems. The patient may describe **paresthesias**, which are burning, tingling sensations or numbness. Box 40-2 provides assessment questions related to altered sensation. These sensations may be caused by pressure on nerves or by circulatory impairment. Soft tissue swelling or direct trauma can impair function.

Past, Family, and Social History

When taking the history, the nurse assesses for past history pertinent to the musculoskeletal system (e.g., broken bones or any history of musculoskeletal diseases, such as rheumatoid

BOX 40-2
BOX 40-2 Assessing Altered Sensation

Questions that the nurse should ask regarding altered sensations include the following:

- Is the patient experiencing any abnormal sensations or numbness?
- If the abnormal sensation or feeling of numbness involves an extremity, how does this feeling compare to sensation in the unaffected extremity?
- When did the condition begin? Is it getting worse?
- Does the patient also have pain? (If the patient has pain, then the assessment for pain should include questions related to sensation, numbness, onset, duration, location, characteristics, aggravating factors, alleviating factors, etc. Refer to Chapter 7 for aspects of pain assessment.)
- If the affected part is an extremity, the nurse compares the overall appearance in relation to the unaffected extremity, noting size, shape, and symmetry.

- Can the patient move the affected part?
- What is the color of the part distal to the affected area? Is it pale? Dusky? Mottled? Cyanotic?
- Does rapid capillary refill occur? (The nurse can gently squeeze a nail until it blanches, and then release the pressure. The amount of time for the color under the nail to return to normal is noted. Color normally returns within 2 seconds. The return of color is evidence of capillary refill.)
- Is a pulse palpable distal to the affected area? If the affected area is an extremity, how does the pulse compare to that felt in the unaffected extremity?
- Is edema present? If so, is it pitting?
- Is any constrictive device or clothing causing nerve or vascular compression?

---

arthritis). The nurse notes any history of family members who have had limitations that prevented them from performing functional activities. The nurse also assesses the patient's activity level. For example, does the patient do weight-bearing exercises on a regular basis? Is the patient involved in high-risk activities and sports that may put him or her at risk for injury? This may evolve into an opportunity for safety education, such as wearing a helmet when bicycle riding.

Physical Assessment

An examination of the musculoskeletal system ranges from a basic assessment of functional capabilities to sophisticated physical examination maneuvers that facilitate diagnosis of specific bone, muscle, and joint disorders. The extent of assessment depends on the patient's physical complaints, health history, and physical clues that warrant further exploration. The nursing assessment is primarily a functional evaluation, focusing on the patient's ability to perform activities of daily living.

Techniques of inspection and palpation are used to evaluate the patient's posture, gait, bone integrity, joint function, and muscle strength and size. In addition, assessing the skin and neurovascular status is an important part of a complete musculoskeletal assessment. When specific symptoms or physical findings of musculoskeletal dysfunction are apparent, the nurse carefully documents the examination findings and shares the information with the provider, who may decide that a more extensive examination and a diagnostic workup are necessary.

Special precautions must be taken when assessing a patient with a musculoskeletal injury (Box 40-3).

Posture

The normal curvature of the spine is convex through the thoracic portion and concave through the cervical and lumbar portions. Common deformities of the spine include **kyphosis**, an increased forward curvature of the thoracic spine; **lordosis**, an exaggerated curvature of the lumbar spine; and **scoliosis**, a lateral curving deviation of the spine (Fig. 40-4). Frequently kyphosis is seen in elderly patients with osteoporosis and in some patients with neuromuscular diseases. Scoliosis may be congenital, idiopathic (without an identifiable cause), or the result of damage to the paraspinal muscles, as in polio. Frequently lordosis is seen during pregnancy as the woman adjusts her posture in response to changes in her center of gravity.

Gait

Gait is assessed by having the patient walk away from the examiner for a short distance. The nurse observes the

BOX 40-3 The Patient with Musculoskeletal Injury

Special precautions must be taken when assessing a patient who has sustained trauma. If there is injury to an extremity, it is important to assess for soft tissue trauma, deformity, and neurovascular status. If the patient might have a cervical spine injury and is wearing a cervical collar, the collar must not be removed until the absence of spinal cord injury is confirmed by appropriate imaging studies. When the collar is removed, the cervical spine area is assessed gently for swelling, tenderness, deformity, and skin integrity. With pelvic trauma, injuries may occur to abdominal organs. The patient is assessed for abdominal pain, tenderness, hematomas, distention, and the presence or absence of femoral pulses. If blood is present at the urinary meatus, the nurse should suspect bladder and urethral injury, and the patient should not be catheterized. Instead, such findings should be reported immediately to the emergency department physician or the surgeon.

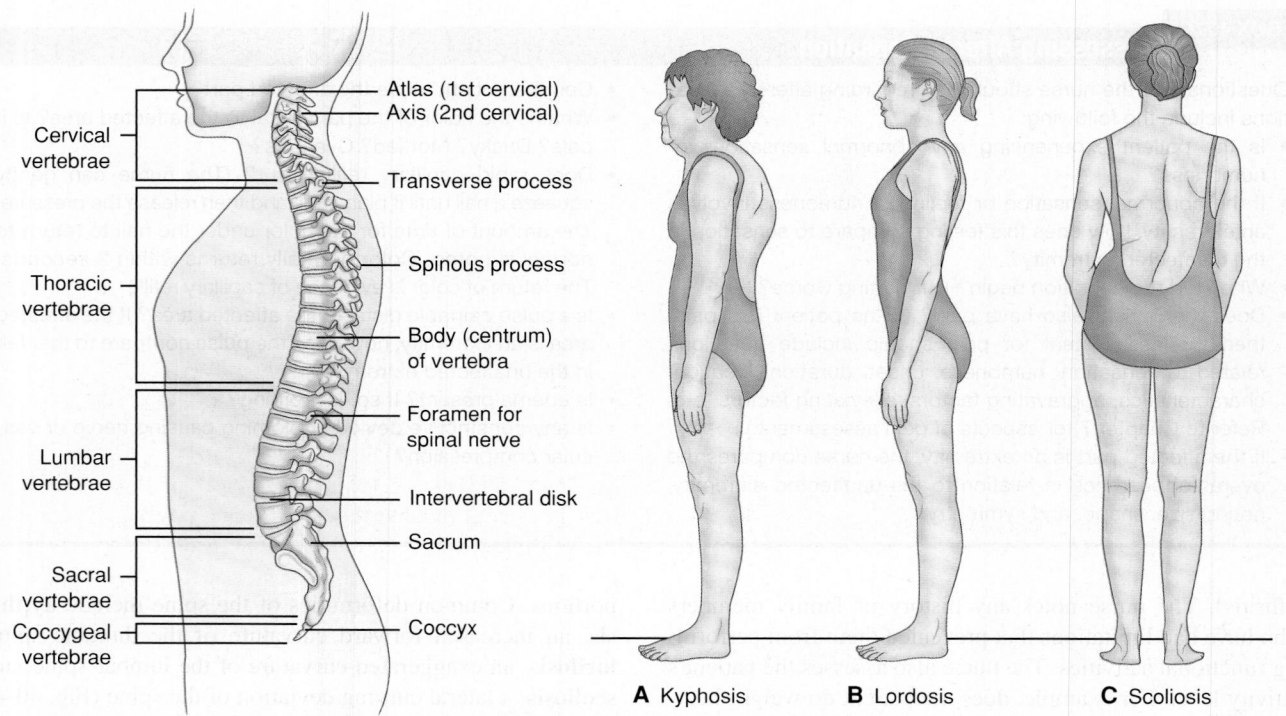

FIGURE 40-4 A normal spine and three abnormalities. **A.** Kyphosis: an increased convexity or roundness of the spine's thoracic curve. **B.** Lordosis: swayback; exaggeration of the curve of the lumbar spine. **C.** Scoliosis: a lateral curvature of the spine.

patient's gait for smoothness and rhythm. Any unsteadiness or irregular movements are considered abnormal. Limited joint motion may affect gait. In addition, a variety of neurologic conditions are associated with abnormal gaits, such as a spastic hemiparesis gait (stroke), steppage gait (lower motor neuron disease), and shuffling gait (Parkinson disease).

Bone Integrity

The bony skeleton is assessed for deformities, alignment, and symmetry. During the examination, body parts are compared from side to side. Shortened extremities, amputations, and body parts that are not in anatomic alignment are noted. Fracture findings may include abnormal angulation of long bones, motion at points other than joints, and crepitus (a grating sound) at the point of abnormal motion. Movement of fracture fragments must be minimized to avoid additional injury.

Joint Function

The articular system is evaluated by noting ROM, deformity, stability, and nodular formation. The tissues surrounding joints are examined for nodule formation, color changes, skin integrity, temperature, and injury. ROM is evaluated both actively (the joint is moved by the muscles surrounding the joint without assistance from the nurse) and passively (the joint is moved by the examiner). The nurse needs to be familiar with the normal ROM of major joints. Limited ROM may be the result of skeletal deformity, joint pathology, or **contracture**

(shortening of surrounding joint structures) of the surrounding muscles, tendons, and joint capsule. With contractures, there is a loss of full movement resulting from a fixed resistance caused either by tonic spasm of muscle (reversible) or by fibrosis of joint structures (permanent). In elderly patients, limitations of ROM associated with osteoarthritis may reduce their ability to perform activities of daily living.

If joint motion is compromised or the joint is painful, the joint is examined for **effusion** (excessive fluid within the capsule), swelling, and increased temperature that may reflect active inflammation. An effusion is suspected if the joint is swollen and the normal bony landmarks are obscured. The most common site for joint effusion is the knee. If inflammation or fluid is suspected in a joint, consultation with a provider is indicated.

Joint deformity may be caused by contracture, dislocation (complete separation of joint surfaces), subluxation (partial separation of articular surfaces), or disruption of structures surrounding the joint. Weakness or disruption of joint-supporting structures may result in a weak joint that requires an external supporting appliance (e.g., brace).

Palpation of the joint while it is moved passively provides information about the integrity of the joint. Normally, the joint moves smoothly. A snap or crack may indicate that a ligament is slipping over a bony prominence. Slightly roughened surfaces, as in arthritic conditions, result in **crepitus** (grating, crackling sound, or sensation) as the irregular joint surfaces move across one another.

FIGURE 40-5 A patient with rheumatoid arthritis with involvement of the metacarpophalangeal joints. Note the severe ulnar drift of the fingers. (From Koopman, W. J., & Moreland, L. W. (2005). *Arthritis and allied conditions: A textbook of rheumatology* (15th ed.). Philadelphia, PA: Lippincott Williams & Wilkins.)

TABLE 40-2 Muscle Strength

Grade	Strength	Physical Findings
0	None	No contraction
1	Trace	Palpable contraction only
2	Poor	Moves joint without gravity
3	Fair	Moves joint against gravity
4	Good	Moves against gravity and resistance
5	Normal	Normal strength

From Staheli, L. T. (2016). *Fundamentals of pediatric orthopedics* (5 ed.). Staheli, Inc.

Nodule formation is associated with rheumatoid arthritis (Fig. 40-5), gout, and osteoarthritis. While the subcutaneous nodules of rheumatoid arthritis are soft and occur within and along tendons, the nodules of gout are hard and lie within and immediately adjacent to the joint capsule itself. Osteoarthritic nodules are hard and painless and represent bony overgrowth that has resulted from destruction of the cartilaginous surface of bone within the joint capsule. They are seen frequently in older adults (refer to Chapter 39 for additional details).

Muscle Strength and Size

The muscular system is assessed by noting muscular strength and coordination, the size of individual muscles, and the patient's ability to change position. Weakness of a group of muscles might indicate a variety of conditions. By palpating the muscle while passively moving the relaxed extremity, the nurse can determine the muscle tone. The nurse assesses muscle strength by having the patient perform certain maneuvers with and without added resistance (Table 40-2). For example, when the biceps are tested, the patient is asked to extend the arm fully and then to flex it against resistance applied by the nurse. A simple handshake may provide an indication of grasp strength.

The nurse may elicit muscle **clonus** (rhythmic contractions of a muscle) in the ankle or wrist by sudden, forceful, sustained dorsiflexion of the foot or extension of the wrist. **Fasciculation** (involuntary twitching of muscle fiber groups) may be observed (Fig. 40-6).

The nurse measures the girth of an extremity to monitor increased size due to exercise, edema, or bleeding into

On stretching the Achilles tendon, the brisk contraction of the agonists initiates a myotatic reflex in the antagonists and so forth, resulting in repetitive contractions

FIGURE 40-6 Clonus. (From Young, P. A., Young, P. H., & Tolbert, D. L. (2015). *Basic clinical neuroscience* (3rd ed.). Philadelphia, PA: Wolters Kluwer.)

the muscle. Girth may decrease due to muscle atrophy. The unaffected extremity is measured and used as the reference standard for the affected extremity. Measurements are taken at the maximum circumference of the extremity. It is important that the measurements be taken at the same location on the extremity, and with the extremity in the same position, with the muscle at rest. Distance from a specific anatomic landmark (e.g., 10 cm below the tibial tuberosity for measurement of the calf muscle) should be indicated in the patient's record so that subsequent measurements can be made at the same point. For ease of serial assessment, the nurse may indicate the point of measurement by marking the skin. Unilateral calf swelling that is more than 3 cm larger than the opposite limb is a clinical variable associated with deep vein thrombosis (DVT) (Kasper et al., 2015).

Skin

In addition to assessing the musculoskeletal system, the nurse inspects the skin for edema, temperature, and color. Palpation of the skin can reveal whether any areas are warmer, suggesting increased perfusion or inflammation, whereas cooler skin suggests decreased perfusion or the presence of edema. Cuts, bruises, skin color, and evidence of decreased circulation or inflammation can influence nursing management of musculoskeletal conditions.

Neurovascular Status

It is important for the nurse to perform frequent neurovascular assessments of patients with musculoskeletal disorders (especially of those with fractures) because of the risk for tissue and nerve damage. Table 40-3 summarizes peripheral vascular assessment. One complication that the nurse needs to be alert for when assessing the patient is *compartment syndrome*, which is described in detail later in this unit. This major neurovascular problem is caused by pressure within a muscle compartment that increases to such an extent that microcirculation diminishes, leading to nerve and muscle anoxia and necrosis. Function can be lost permanently if the anoxic situation continues for longer than 6 hours. Assessment of neurovascular status is frequently referred to as assessment of CSM (circulation, sensation, and movement). Symptoms of neurovascular dysfunction are discussed in Box 40-4.

Diagnostic Evaluation

During the period of assessment, the patient requires support and nursing care, including physical and psychological preparation for examinations and tests. Patient education before the tests (what is to be done; why it is being done; what the patient can expect to experience, including tactile, visual, and auditory sensations; and what patient participation is expected) reduces anxiety and enables the patient to be an active participant in care. The resulting medical

TABLE **40-3** Assessing for Peripheral Nerve Function

Assessment of peripheral nerve function has two key elements: evaluation of sensation and evaluation of motion. The nurse may perform one or all of the following during a musculoskeletal assessment.

Nerve	Test of Sensation	Test of Movement
Peroneal nerve	Stimulate the skin midway between the great and second toe.	Ask the patient to dorsiflex the foot and extend the toes.
Tibial nerve	Stimulate the medial and lateral surface of the sole.	Ask the patient to plantar flex toes and foot.
Radial nerve	Stimulate the skin midway between the thumb and second finger.	Ask the patient to stretch out the thumb, then the wrist, and then the fingers at the metacarpal joints.
Ulnar nerve	Stimulate the distal fat pad of the small finger.	Ask the patient to abduct all fingers.
Median nerve	Stimulate the top or distal surface of the index finger.	Ask the patient to touch the thumb to the little finger. Also observe whether the patient can flex the wrist.

BOX 40-4

Indicators of Peripheral Neurovascular Dysfunction

Circulation

- *Color:* Pale, cyanotic, or mottled
- *Temperature:* Cool
- *Capillary refill:* More than 2 seconds

Motion

- Weakness
- Paralysis

Sensation

- Paresthesia
- Unrelenting pain
- Pain on passive stretch
- Absence of feeling

diagnosis and prescribed treatment regimen affect the nursing management of the patient.

Imaging Procedures

X-Ray Studies

X-ray studies are important in evaluating patients with musculoskeletal disorders. Bone x-rays determine bone density, texture, erosion, and changes in bone relationships. X-ray study of the cortex of the bone reveals any widening, narrowing, or signs of irregularity. Joint x-rays reveal fluid, irregularity, spur formation, narrowing, and changes in the joint structure. Multiple views are needed for full assessment of the structure being examined. Serial x-rays may be indicated to determine if healing of a fractured bone is progressing normally or to determine if a bone affected by disease is stable, deteriorating, or responding to prescribed therapy. After being positioned for the study, the patient must remain still while the x-rays are taken.

Computed Tomography

A computed tomography (CT) scan shows in detail a specific plane of involved bone and can reveal tumors of the soft tissue or injuries to the ligaments or tendons. It is used to identify the location and extent of fractures in areas that are difficult to evaluate (e.g., acetabulum). CT studies, which may be performed with or without the use of contrast agents, can last up to 1 hour. The patient must remain still during the procedure.

Magnetic Resonance Imaging

Magnetic resonance imaging (MRI) is a noninvasive imaging technique that uses magnetic fields, radiowaves, and computers to demonstrate abnormalities (i.e., tumors or narrowing of tissue pathways through bone) of soft tissues, such as muscle, tendon, cartilage, nerve, and fat. Because an electromagnet is used, patients with any metal implants, clips, or pacemakers are not candidates for MRI.

! Nursing Alert

Jewelry, hair clips, hearing aids, credit cards with magnetic strips, and other metal-containing objects must be removed from the patient before the MRI is performed; otherwise they can become dangerous projectile objects or cause burns. Credit cards with magnetic strips may be erased, and nonremovable cochlear devices can become inoperable. Also, transdermal patches that have a thin layer of aluminized backing must be removed before MRI because they can cause burns. The provider should be notified before the patches are removed.

To enhance visualization of anatomic structures, IV contrast agent may be used. During the MRI, the patient needs to lie still for 30 to 60 minutes and hears a rhythmic knocking sound. Patients who experience claustrophobia may be unable to tolerate the confinement of closed MRI equipment without sedation. Open MRI systems are available, but they use lower-intensity magnetic fields that reduce the quality of the imaging; thus, repeated imaging may be required. Advantages of open MRI include increased patient comfort, reduced problems with claustrophobic reactions, and reduced noise.

Arthrography

Arthrography is useful in identifying acute or chronic tears of the joint capsule or supporting ligaments of the knee, shoulder, ankle, hip, or wrist. A radiopaque contrast agent is injected into the joint cavity to outline soft tissue structures and the contour of the joint. The joint is put through its ROM to distribute the contrast agent, and then an MRI is obtained. If a tear is present, the contrast agent leaks out of the joint and is evident on the MRI image.

After an arthrogram, a compression elastic bandage is applied as prescribed and usually the joint is rested for 12 hours. The nurse provides additional comfort measures (mild analgesia, ice) as appropriate. The nurse explains to the patient that it is normal to experience clicking or crackling in the joint for a day or two after the procedure, until the contrast agent or air is absorbed.

! Nursing Alert

If contrast agents will be used for CT scan, MRI, or arthrography, the nurse carefully assesses the patient for possible allergy. This includes previous experience with contrast studies and past reactions. In addition, the nurse is aware that risk factors for adverse reactions include a history of asthma, allergies, diabetes, renal insufficiency, and cardiac disease. Finally, the nurse assesses risk of pregnancy before decisions are made regarding the use of contrast materials.

Bone Densitometry

Bone densitometry is used to estimate bone mineral density (BMD). This can be performed through the use of x-rays or ultrasound. Most commonly, dual-energy x-ray absorptiometry (DEXA) is done. This determines BMD at the wrist, hip, or spine to estimate the extent of osteoporosis and to monitor a patient's response to treatment for osteoporosis. In particular, hip BMD is recommended as an osteoporosis screening for all Caucasian women older than 65 years of age and for other people at increased risk for osteoporosis-related fractures (Grossman & Porth, 2014). See Chapter 41 for a further discussion of osteoporosis risks.

 Concept Mastery Alert

BMD is used in diagnosing osteoporosis. Bone scans are used to detect metastatic and primary bone tumors, osteomyelitis, certain fractures, and aseptic necrosis, but not osteoporosis.

Bone Scan

A bone scan is performed to detect metastatic and primary bone tumors, osteomyelitis, certain fractures, and aseptic necrosis. A bone-seeking radioisotope is injected IV. The scan is performed 1 to 3 hours after the injection. At this point, distribution and concentration of the isotope in the bone are measured. The degree of nuclide uptake is related to the metabolism of the bone. An increased uptake of isotope is seen in primary skeletal disease (osteosarcoma), metastatic bone disease, inflammatory skeletal disease (osteomyelitis), and certain types of fractures.

Before the patient undergoes an imaging study, the nurse assesses for conditions that may require special consideration during the study or that may be contraindications to the study (e.g., pregnancy; claustrophobia; inability to tolerate required positioning due to age, debility, or disability; metal implants). If contrast agents will be used for CT scan, MRI, bone scan, or arthrography, the nurse carefully assesses the patient for possible allergy (see previous Nursing Alert).

Arthroscopy

Arthroscopy is a procedure that allows direct visualization of a joint to diagnose joint disorders. Treatment of tears, defects, and disease processes may be performed through the arthroscope. The procedure is performed in the operating room under sterile conditions; injection of a local anesthetic into the joint or general anesthesia is used. A large-bore needle is inserted, and the joint is distended with saline. The arthroscope is introduced, allowing for visualization of the joint structures, synovium, and articular surfaces. After the procedure, the puncture wound is closed with adhesive strips or sutures and covered with a sterile dressing. Complications are rare but may include infection, hemarthrosis (bleeding into the joint cavity), neurovascular compromise, thrombophlebitis, stiffness, effusion, adhesions, and delayed wound healing.

The joint is wrapped with a compression dressing to control swelling. In addition, ice may be applied to control edema and discomfort. Frequently, the joint is kept extended and elevated to reduce swelling. It is important to monitor neurovascular status. The nurse administers prescribed analgesics to control discomfort. The nurse explains when the patient can resume activity and what weight-bearing limits to follow, as prescribed by the orthopedic surgeon. The nurse also explains to the patient and family the symptoms (e.g., swelling, numbness, cool skin) to observe for in order to determine whether complications are occurring and the importance of notifying the surgeon of these observations. The nurse's verbal instructions are reinforced with written instructions before discharge. Finally, the nurse explains the surgeon's prescription for analgesic medication.

Other Studies

Arthrocentesis

Arthrocentesis (joint aspiration) is carried out to obtain synovial fluid for purposes of examination or to relieve pain due to effusion. Examination of synovial fluid is helpful in the diagnosis of septic arthritis and other inflammatory arthropathies (any joint disease) and reveals the presence of hemarthrosis (bleeding into the joint space), which suggests trauma or a bleeding disorder. Normally, synovial fluid is clear, pale, straw-colored, and scanty in volume. Using aseptic technique, the provider inserts a needle into the joint and aspirates fluid. Anti-inflammatory medications, such as cortisone, may be injected into the joint. A sterile dressing is applied after aspiration. There is a small risk of infection after this procedure.

Electromyography

Electromyography (EMG) provides information about the electrical potential of the muscles and the nerves leading to them. Needle electrodes are inserted into selected muscles, and responses to electrical stimuli are recorded on an oscilloscope. The test is performed to evaluate the electrical potential generated by muscle cells when they are activated. The results can be analyzed to detect medical abnormalities, such as muscle weakness, pain, and disability. The procedure helps to determine any abnormality of function and to differentiate muscle and nerve problems.

Biopsy

Biopsy may be performed to determine the structure and composition of bone marrow, bone, muscle, or synovium to help diagnose specific diseases. The nurse prepares the patient by providing teaching about the procedure and assuring the patient that analgesic agents will be provided. The nurse monitors the biopsy site for edema, bleeding, and infection (fever, erythema, swelling, drainage, and tenderness at site) and asks the patient about their perception of pain. Ice is applied as prescribed to control bleeding and edema. In addition, analgesics are administered as prescribed for comfort.

TABLE **40-4** Blood Chemistry Studies Related to Musculoskeletal Conditions

Blood Chemistry	Musculoskeletal Conditions
Altered serum calcium levels	Osteomalacia, parathyroid dysfunction, Paget disease, metastatic bone tumors, or prolonged immobilization
Serum phosphorus inversely related to calcium levels	Diminished in osteomalacia associated with malabsorption syndrome
Acid phosphatase	Elevated in Paget disease and metastatic cancer
Alkaline phosphatase	Elevated during early fracture healing and in diseases with increased osteoblastic activity (e.g., metastatic bone tumors)
Creatine kinase and aspartate	Elevated with muscle damage
Elevated erythrocyte sedimentation rate (ESR) or C-reactive protein (CRP)	Inflammation, infection, autoimmune disorders, neoplasia, pregnancy, renal insufficiency, advanced age, and hyperlipidemia
Elevated uric acid	Gout, nephrolithiasis
Serum myoglobin	Elevated with muscle trauma
Serum osteocalcin (bone GLA protein)	Indicated rate of bone turnover
Calcitonin levels	Bone metabolism
Parathormone	Bone metabolism
Vitamin D levels	Bone metabolism
Urine calcium levels	Increased with bone destruction (e.g., parathyroid dysfunction, metastatic bone tumors, multiple myeloma)

Laboratory Studies

Examination of the patient's blood and urine can provide information about a primary musculoskeletal problem (e.g., Paget disease), a developing complication (e.g., infection), the baseline for instituting therapy (e.g., anticoagulant therapy), or the response to therapy. The complete blood count includes the hemoglobin level (which is frequently lower after bleeding associated with trauma and surgery) and the WBC count (which is elevated with any inflammatory condition, including acute infections, trauma, acute hemorrhage, and tissue necrosis). Before surgery, coagulation studies are performed to detect bleeding tendencies (because bone is very vascular tissue).

Blood chemistry studies provide data about a wide variety of musculoskeletal conditions; see Table 40-4.

CHAPTER REVIEW

Critical Thinking Exercises

1. A 62-year-old Caucasian woman presents to the family practice clinic where you are the nurse manager for her annual wellness examination. She asks you if she should have "a type of bone scan" because her younger sister recently had a hip fracture. What recommendations might be made for appropriate testing in this patient?

2. You are teaching a class at a senior center on age-associated changes in the musculoskeletal system. What age-related changes do you anticipate finding in this population?

NCLEX-Style Review Questions

1. A 78-year-old woman is complaining of neck and upper back pain. The nurse's assessment reveals an abnormal convex curvature of the cervical and thoracic area. What is the terminology for this finding?
   a. Kyphosis
   b. Lordosis
   c. Kyphoscoliosis
   d. Scoliosis

2. A 12-year-old girl complained to the school nurse about back pain. The nurse's assessment revealed a deviation of the vertebrae to the right, with a raised shoulder and hip. What is the terminology for this finding?
   a. Kyphosis
   b. Lordosis
   c. Osteoporosis
   d. Scoliosis

3. A cast was applied to a patient's fractured leg 4 hours ago. Which finding is associated with neurovascular compromise?
   a. Capillary refill of 5 seconds
   b. Ability to move the toes without limitation
   c. Full sensation
   d. Toes warm to touch

4. What food would the nurse recommend for bone health?
   a. Herbal tea
   b. Yogurt
   c. Liver
   d. Eggs

5. An MRI has been ordered for a patient with low back pain. What should be included in the teaching plan for this patient?
   a. The patient will need to lie still for 3 to 4 hours.
   b. A rhythmic rocking sound will be heard during the procedure.
   c. There is no risk of claustrophobia.
   d. It is an invasive technique.

Try these additional resources, available at **http://thepoint.lww.com/Honan2e**, to enhance your learning and understanding of this chapter:
- NCLEX-Style Student Review Questions
- Journal Articles

REFERENCES AND SELECTED READINGS

References and selected readings associated with this chapter can be found on the website that accompanies the book. Visit **http://thepoint. lww.com/Honan2e** to access the references and other additional resources associated with this chapter.

Nursing Management: Patients with Musculoskeletal Disorders

Geriann B. Gallagher

Learning Objectives

After reading this chapter, you will be able to:

1. Describe the rehabilitation and health education needs of the patient with low back pain.
2. Describe common conditions and nursing care of the upper and lower extremities
3. Explain the pathophysiology, pathogenesis, prevention, and management of osteoporosis.
4. Describe management of the patient with Paget disease.
5. Use the nursing process as a framework for care of the patient with osteomyelitis.
6. Describe medical and nursing management as well as potential complications to be encountered in the patient with a bone tumor.

Musculoskeletal disorders carry a heavy economic and health burden. The financial cost of musculoskeletal disorders in the United States was 7.4% of the nation's gross domestic product when analyzing available data from 2004 to 2006 (McPhail, Schippers, & Marshall, 2014). Adding to this burden is the personal, functional, and psychological limitations imposed on the patient. Musculoskeletal disorders are increased in patients with insufficient physical activity. Negative outcomes associated with a sedentary lifestyle include heart disease, diabetes, and depression. Increasing physical activity, which can vary according to the patient's functional level, can improve cardiovascular and respiratory status, reduce the severity of existing health problems, and reduce the impact of physical decline and falls. Nurses must be aware of the clinical manifestations and management of these disorders.

ACUTE LOW BACK PAIN

Low back pain, one of the most common reasons for a visit to a provider, is primarily caused by one of many musculoskeletal problems, including acute lumbosacral strain, unstable lumbosacral ligaments and weak muscles, osteoarthritis of the spine, spinal stenosis, intervertebral disk problems, and unequal leg length.

Older patients may experience back pain associated with osteoporotic vertebral fractures or bone metastasis. Other causes include kidney disorders, pelvic problems, retroperitoneal tumors, and abdominal aortic aneurysms.

In addition, obesity, stress, and, occasionally, depression may contribute to low back pain. Back pain due to musculoskeletal disorders usually is aggravated by activity, whereas pain due to other conditions is not.

Pathophysiology

The spinal column can be considered an elastic rod constructed of rigid units (vertebrae) and flexible units (intervertebral disks) held together by complex facet joints, multiple ligaments, and paravertebral muscles. Its unique construction allows for flexibility while providing maximum protection for the spinal cord. The abdominal and thoracic muscles help to stabilize the spine and are important in lifting activities, working together to minimize stress on the spinal units. Disuse weakens these supporting muscular structures. Obesity, postural problems, structural problems, and overstretching of the spinal supports may result in back pain.

The intervertebral disks change in character as a person ages. A young person's disks are mainly fibrocartilage with a gelatinous matrix. As a person ages, the fibrocartilage becomes dense and irregularly shaped. Disk degeneration is a common cause of back pain. The lower lumbar disks, L4 to L5 and L5 to S1, are subject to the greatest mechanical stress and the greatest degenerative changes. Disk protrusion (herniated nucleus pulposus) or facet joint changes can cause pressure on nerve roots as they leave the spinal canal, which results in pain that radiates along the nerve.

Clinical Manifestations and Assessment

The initial evaluation of acute low back pain (lasting less than 3 months) includes a focused history and physical examination, including general observation of the patient, back examination, and neurologic testing (reflexes, sensory impairment, straight-leg raising, muscle strength, and assessment of muscle atrophy). Signs and symptoms relate to the corresponding dermatome (see Fig. 43-13) or myotome (the group of muscles served by motor neurons of a spinal cord segment). Pressure on the nerve roots or spinal cord will cause symptoms, such as abnormal or painful sensations (paresthesias or dysesthesias), loss of sensation, weakness, and autonomic dysfunction (most commonly bladder or bowel incontinence) (Barbano, 2016). Pain may be felt directly along the spine itself or may be referred (e.g., aortic aneurysm may present with back pain), or the patient may report pain radiating down the leg, which is known as **radiculopathy** or **sciatica** (pain from irritation of the sciatic nerve, classically felt from the low back to behind the thigh and radiating down below the knee). The presence of this symptom suggests nerve root involvement. The patient's gait, spinal mobility, reflexes, leg length, leg motor strength, and sensory perception may be affected. Careful examination of both sides will cue the nurse into subtle differences. Physical examination may disclose paravertebral muscle spasm (greatly increased muscle tone of the back postural muscles) with a loss of the normal lumbar curve and possible spinal deformity. The findings suggest either nonspecific back symptoms or potentially serious problems, such as sciatica, spine fracture, cancer, infection, or a rapidly progressing neurologic deficit. If the initial examination does not suggest a serious condition, no additional testing is performed during the first 4 weeks of symptoms.

The diagnostic procedures described in Box 41-1 may be indicated for the patient with potentially serious or prolonged low back pain. The nurse prepares the patient for these studies, provides the necessary support during the testing period, and monitors the patient for any adverse responses to the procedures.

Medical and Nursing Management

Management focuses on relief of pain and discomfort, activity modification, use of back-conserving techniques of body mechanics, improved self-esteem, and weight reduction. Most back pain is self-limited and resolves within 4 weeks with analgesics, rest, stress reduction, and relaxation.

Relieving Pain

To relieve pain, the nurse encourages the patient to reduce stress on the back muscles and to change position frequently. The patient is taught to control and modify the perceived pain through behavioral therapies that reduce muscular and psychological tension. Diaphragmatic breathing and relaxation help reduce muscle tension contributing to low back pain. Diverting the patient's attention from the pain to another activity (e.g., reading, conversation, watching television) may be helpful in some instances. Guided imagery, in which the relaxed patient learns to focus on a pleasant event, may be used along with other pain-relief strategies.

If medication is prescribed, the nurse assesses the patient's response to each medication. As the acute pain subsides, medication dosages are reduced as prescribed. Usually nonprescription analgesics are effective in achieving pain relief. At times, a patient may require the addition of muscle relaxants or opioids. Often heat or cold therapy is used and frequently provides temporary relief of symptoms; further study of the effectiveness of heat or cold modalities is needed (Moss et al., 2014). In the absence of symptoms of disease (radiculopathy of the roots of spinal nerves), spinal manipulation performed by a chiropractor or an osteopath may be helpful. Acupuncture, massage, biofeedback, and yoga are other modalities the patient may find to be therapeutic. There is no convincing researched evidence that these modalities are beneficial; however, there is anecdotal evidence that many patients benefit from alternative modalities. Each patient's plan of care should be individualized, and then the nurse evaluates and notes the patient's response to various pain management modalities.

Improving Physical Mobility

Physical mobility is monitored through continuing assessments. The nurse assesses how the patient moves and stands. As the back pain subsides, self-care activities are resumed with minimal strain on the injured structures. Position changes should be made slowly and carried out with assistance as required. The patient should avoid twisting and jarring motions. The nurse encourages the patient to alternate lying, sitting, and walking activities frequently and advises the patient to avoid sitting, standing, or walking for long

---

BOX 41-1

Diagnostic Procedures for Low Back Pain

X-ray of the spine: May demonstrate a fracture, dislocation, infection, osteoarthritis, or scoliosis

Bone scan and blood studies: May disclose infections, tumors, and abnormalities in bone marrow

Computed tomography (CT): Useful in identifying underlying problems, such as obscure soft tissue lesions adjacent to the vertebral column and problems of vertebral disks

Magnetic resonance imaging (MRI): Permits visualization of the nature and location of spinal pathology

Electromyogram (EMG) and nerve conduction studies: Used to evaluate disorders of the spinal nerve root (radiculopathies)

periods. The patient may find that sitting in a chair with arm rests to support some of the body weight and a soft support at the small of the back provides comfort.

With severe pain, the nurse instructs the patient to limit activities for 1 to 2 days (Barbano, 2016). Extended periods of inactivity are not effective and result in deconditioning. An international campaign (the Victorian WorkCover Authority in Australia), called "Back Pain: Don't take it lying down," is an example of stressing the importance of continued mobility in patients with back pain. Lumbar flexion is increased by elevating the head and thorax 30 degrees using pillows or a foam wedge as well as another pillow to allow the patient to flex the knees slightly. Alternatively, the patient can assume a lateral position with knees and hips flexed (curled position) with a pillow between the knees and legs and a pillow supporting the head. A prone position should be avoided because it accentuates lordosis (inward curvature of the spine). The nurse instructs the patient to get out of bed by rolling to one side and placing the legs down while pushing the torso up, keeping the back straight.

As the patient achieves comfort, activities are resumed gradually, and an exercise program is initiated. Initially, low-stress aerobic exercises, such as short walks or swimming, are suggested. After 2 weeks, conditioning exercises for the abdominal and trunk muscles are started. The physical therapist designs an exercise program for the individual patient to reduce lordosis, increase flexibility, and reduce strain on the back. Exercise begins gradually and increases as the patient recovers.

The nurse encourages the patient to adhere to the prescribed exercise program. Erratic exercising is ineffective. Some patients may find it difficult to adhere to a program of prescribed exercises for a long period. These patients are encouraged to improve their posture, use good body mechanics on a regular basis, and engage in regular exercise activities (e.g., walking, swimming) to maintain a healthy back. Activities should not cause excessive lumbar strain, twisting, or discomfort; for example, activities such as horseback riding, basketball, and weight-lifting should be avoided. If there is no improvement within 1 month, additional assessments for physiologic abnormalities are performed. Management is based on findings.

Using Proper Body Mechanics

Good body mechanics and posture are essential to avoid recurrence of back pain. The patient must be taught how to stand, sit, lie, and lift properly. Providing the patient with a list of suggestions helps in making these long-term changes (Box 41-2). If the patient wears high heels, the nurse

---

BOX 41-2 | **Health Promotion**

Activities to Promote a Healthy Back

Standing
Advise the patient to adhere to the following guidelines:
- Avoid prolonged standing and walking.
- When standing for any length of time, rest one foot on a small stool or box to relieve lumbar lordosis.
- Avoid forward flexion work positions.
- Avoid high heels.

Sitting
Discuss the following strategies with the patient:
- Avoid sitting for prolonged periods.
- Sit in a straight-back chair with back well supported and arm rests to support some of the body weight; use a footstool to position knees higher than hips if necessary.
- Eradicate the hollow of the back by sitting with the buttocks "tucked under."
- Maintain back support; use a soft support at the small of the back.
- Avoid knee and hip extension. When driving a car, have the seat pushed forward as far as possible for comfort.
- Guard against extension strains—reaching, pushing, or sitting with legs straight out.
- Alternate periods of sitting with walking.

Lying
Encourage the patient to do the following:
- Rest at intervals; fatigue contributes to spasm of the back muscles.

- Place a firm bed board under the mattress.
- Avoid sleeping in a prone position.
- When lying on the side, place a pillow under the head and one between the legs, with the legs flexed at the hips and knees.
- When supine, use a pillow under the knees to decrease lordosis.

Lifting
Emphasize the importance of the following strategies:
- When lifting, keep the back straight and hold the load as close to the body as possible.
- Lift with the large leg muscles, not the back muscles.
- Use trunk muscles to stabilize the spine.
- Squat while keeping the back straight when it is necessary to pick up something off the floor.
- Avoid twisting the trunk of the body, lifting above waist level, and reaching up for any length of time.

Exercising
Daily exercise is important in the prevention of back problems.
- Walk daily, and gradually increase the distance and pace of walking.
- Perform prescribed back exercises twice daily, increasing exercise gradually.
- Avoid jumping and jarring activities.

encourages changing to low heels with good arch support. The patient who is required to stand for long periods should shift weight frequently and should rest one foot on a low stool, which decreases lumbar lordosis. Patients who stand in place for a long period of time (e.g., cashiers) should stand on a foot cushion made of foam or rubber. The proper posture can be verified by looking in a mirror to see whether the chest is up, the abdomen is tucked in, and the shoulders are down and relaxed (Fig. 41-1). The patient should avoid locking the knees when standing and bending forward for long periods.

When the patient is sitting, the knees and hips should be flexed, and the knees should be level with the hips or higher to minimize lordosis. The feet should be flat on the floor. The back needs to be supported, so the patient should avoid sitting on stools or chairs that do not provide firm back support.

The nurse instructs the patient in the safe and correct way to lift objects—using the strong quadriceps muscles of the

FIGURE 41-2 Proper and improper lifting techniques. (*Left*) Correct position for lifting. This person is using the long and strong muscles of the arms and legs and holding the object so that the line of gravity falls within the base of support. (*Right*) Incorrect position for lifting because pull is exerted on the back muscles and leaning causes the line of gravity to fall outside the base.

thighs, with minimal use of weak back muscles. With feet placed hip-width apart to provide a wide base of support, the patient should bend the knees, tighten the abdominal muscles, and lift the object close to the body with a smooth motion, avoiding twisting and jarring motions (Fig. 41-2). It takes about 6 months for a person to readjust postural habits. Practicing these protective and defensive postures, positions, and body mechanics results in natural strengthening of the back and diminishes the chance that back pain will recur.

Nursing Alert

Nurses, by virtue of their daily work, are a group at high risk for acute back injuries (e.g., transferring patients, repositioning patients in bed, lifting a patient in bed, making an occupied bed). The national problem with obesity (64% of US population is classified as overweight, and 30% classified as obese [McGinley & Bunke, 2008]), only compounds this risk. Use of "lift teams" or lift devices should be available to nursing staff as accompanied by ergonomic instruction on body mechanics principles as described above. Currently, 11 states have enacted "safe patient handling" laws or launched regulations that require health care facilities to provide proper equipment, education, and policies that promote worker health and safety (American Nurses' Association, 2016; Association of Safe Patient Handling Professionals [ASPHP], 2015). The nurse would do well to practice and use the postures described above.

Modifying Nutrition for Weight Reduction

Obesity contributes to back strain by stressing the relatively weak muscles of the back and abdomen. Exercises are less effective and more difficult to perform when the patient is overweight. Weight reduction through diet modification may prevent recurrence of back pain. Weight reduction is based on

FIGURE 41-1 Proper and improper standing postures. (*Left*) Abdominal muscles contracted, giving a feeling of upward pull, and gluteal muscles contracted, giving a downward pull. (*Right*) Slouch position, showing abdominal muscles relaxed and body out of proper alignment.

a sound nutritional plan that includes a change in eating habits to maintain desirable weight. Monitoring weight reduction, noting achievement, and providing encouragement and positive reinforcement facilitate adherence. Frequently, back problems resolve as optimal weight is achieved.

COMMON UPPER EXTREMITY PROBLEMS

The structures in the upper extremities are frequently the sites of painful syndromes. The structures affected most frequently are the shoulder, wrist, and hand.

Bursitis and Tendinitis

Bursitis and **tendinitis** are inflammatory conditions that commonly occur in the shoulder. Bursae are fluid-filled sacs that prevent friction between joint structures during joint activity. When inflamed, they are painful. Tendonitis is inflammation of a tendon. Tendons, which connect muscles to bone, are enclosed in sheaths. At points of friction, the sheath is double layered. The space between the two sheaths is filled with fluid similar to synovial fluid. Overuse of the tendon can result in inflammation and degeneration of the tendon (Grossman & Porth, 2014). Conservative treatment includes rest of the extremity, intermittent ice, heat, ultrasound to the joint, and nonsteroidal anti-inflammatory drugs (NSAIDs) to control the inflammation and pain. Corticosteroid injections may be considered. Stretching and strengthening exercises should be initiated after the acute phase. Further imaging or arthroscopic intervention may be considered if pain and weakness persist.

Impingement Syndrome

Impingement syndrome, or rotator cuff tendinitis, is caused by repeated overhead activity of the shoulder. When the arm is raised overhead, there is decreased space between the humeral head and acromion. The patient may feel a dull achy pain, limited movement, and muscle spasm. Complaints, such as difficulty in dressing oneself and night pain because of difficulty in positioning the shoulders, may be noted. The process may progress to rotator cuff disease (see Chapter 42). Conservative treatment includes rest; application of heat, cold, and ultrasound; NSAIDs; joint injections; and physical therapy (Box 41-3 discusses patient education). Arthroscopic débridement (a minimally invasive surgical procedure that permits evacuation of joint debris) is used for persistent pain. Gentle joint motion is begun after surgery.

Carpal Tunnel Syndrome

Carpal tunnel syndrome is an entrapment neuropathy that occurs when the median nerve at the wrist is compressed by a thickened flexor tendon sheath, skeletal encroachment, edema, or a soft tissue mass. The syndrome is commonly

---

> **BOX 41-3** | **Patient Education**
>
> **Measures to Promote Shoulder Healing of Impingement Syndrome**
>
> - Rest the joint in a position that minimizes stress on the joint structures, to prevent further damage and the development of adhesions.
> - Support the affected arm on pillows while sleeping to keep from turning onto the shoulder.
> - For the first 24–48 hours of the acute phase, apply cold to reduce swelling and discomfort; then, according to the treatment plan, apply heat intermittently to promote circulation and healing.
> - Gradually resume motion and use of the joint. Assistance with dressing and other ADLs may be needed.
> - Avoid working and lifting above shoulder level or pushing an object against a "locked" shoulder.
> - Perform the prescribed daily ROM and strengthening exercises.

---

caused by repetitive hand and wrist movements, but it also may be associated with arthritis, hypothyroidism, or pregnancy. Patients who perform repetitive movements or those whose hands are exposed repeatedly to cold temperatures, vibrations, or extreme direct pressure are at a greater risk for developing carpal tunnel syndrome. The patient experiences pain, numbness, paresthesia, and, possibly, weakness along the median nerve (thumb, index, and middle fingers). Phalen test or Tinel sign may be used to help identify carpal tunnel syndrome (Fig. 41-3). Night pain is common.

Treatment of carpal tunnel syndrome is based on the cause of the condition. Symptoms may be relieved by wrist splints to prevent hyperextension and prolonged flexion of the wrist, avoidance of repetitive flexion of the wrist (e.g., making ergonomic changes at work to reduce wrist strain), use of NSAIDs, and carpal canal cortisone injections. Specific yoga postures, relaxation, and acupuncture may be nontraditional alternatives to relieve carpal tunnel symptoms. In pregnancy, symptoms usually resolve spontaneously weeks after delivery (Ferri, 2016a).

If conservative treatment fails, surgical management options are traditional open nerve release or endoscopic laser surgery. Both of these procedures are performed under local anesthesia and involve making small incisions into the affected wrist and cutting the carpal ligament so that the carpal tunnel is widened. Smaller incisions are made with the endoscopic laser procedure, and there is less scar formation and a shorter recovery time than with the open method. Following either of these procedures, the patient wears a hand splint and limits hand use during healing. The patient may need assistance with personal care and activities of daily living (ADLs). Full recovery of motor and sensory function may take several weeks or months after either type of nerve release surgery.

FIGURE 41-3 There are two ways to assess for carpal tunnel syndrome: Phalen test and Tinel sign. **A.** To perform Phalen test, have the patient hold the position shown for 60 seconds. **B.** To elicit Tinel sign in a patient, percuss lightly over the median nerve, located on the inner aspect of the wrist. If the patient reports tingling, numbness, and pain, the test for Phalen and Tinel sign is considered positive. (From Weber, J. W., & Kelley, J. (2014). *Health assessment in nursing* (5th ed.). Philadelphia, PA: Wolters Kluwer Health, Lippincott Williams & Wilkins.)

Ganglion

A ganglion, a collection of gelatinous material near the tendon sheaths and joints, appears as a round, firm, compressible, cystic swelling, usually on the dorsum of the wrist (60% to 70%). They may be caused by injury or repetitive activity. The ganglion may or may not be locally tender. The pain may be described as aching and can be aggravated by extreme flexion or extension. Ganglion cysts may occur in any age group, but they are found most commonly in people between 20 and 40 years of age. The incidence is greater in females than in males (Meena & Gupta, 2014). Asymptomatic ganglions are monitored, since approximately 50% will resolve without treatment. Other treatments may include aspiration, corticosteroid injection, or surgical excision. After treatment, a compression dressing and immobilization splint are used.

Dupuytren Disease

Dupuytren disease results in a slowly progressive **contracture** of the palmar fascia, called Dupuytren contracture, which causes flexion of the fourth and fifth fingers and, frequently, the middle finger (Fig. 41-4). This renders the

FIGURE 41-4 Dupuytren contracture, a flexion deformity caused by an inherited trait, is a slowly progressive contracture of the palmar fascia, which severely impairs the function of the fourth, fifth, and, sometimes, the middle finger.

fingers more or less useless. It is caused by an inherited autosomal dominant trait and occurs most frequently in men who are older than 50 years of age and who are of northern European descent. While strongly inheritable, it is also associated with drug therapy for epilepsy, diabetes, HIV infection, and alcoholism (Nunn & Schreuder, 2014). It starts as a nodule of the palmar fascia. The nodule may not change, or it may progress so that the fibrous thickening extends to involve the skin in the distal palm and produces a contracture of the fingers. The patient may experience dull aching discomfort, morning numbness, cramping, and stiffness in the affected fingers. The patient often seeks care because contracture of the fingers alters the function of the hand. This condition starts in one hand, but eventually both hands can be affected. Initially, finger-stretching exercises may prevent contractures. With contracture development, patients are referred to a hand specialist. Nonsurgical options of treatment include percutaneous needle fasciotomy (fascia is cut to relieve tension or pressure) and injection of collagenase into the palmer cord. The collagenase breaks down the fibrous thickening, and the patient returns to the surgeon for manipulation of the finger, resulting in increased function. Surgical options include palmar and digital fasciectomies. Finger and hand exercises are begun as prescribed on postoperative day 1 or 2.

Box 41-4 discusses nursing interventions for patients undergoing surgery for upper extremity problems.

COMMON FOOT PROBLEMS

Disorders of the foot are commonly caused by poorly fitting shoes, which distort normal anatomy while inducing deformity and pain.

BOX 41-4

Nursing Interventions for Patient Undergoing Surgery to Treat Upper and Lower Extremity Conditions

Promoting Tissue Perfusion

Neurovascular assessment of the exposed digits every 1–2 hours for the first 24 hours after surgery is essential to monitor the function of the nerves and the perfusion of the tissues. The nurse compares the affected extremity with the unaffected one and the postoperative status with the documented preoperative status. Perfusion is assessed by temperature, color, capillary refill, and grading of peripheral pulses. The nurse asks the patient to describe the sensations in the affected extremity and to demonstrate mobility of the involved area. With tendon repairs and nerve, vascular, or skin grafts, motor function is tested as necessary. Dressings provide support but are not constrictive. If the patient is discharged within several hours after the surgery, the nurse teaches the patient and family how to assess for edema and neurovascular status (circulation, sensation, motion). Compromised neurovascular function can increase the patient's pain.

Relieving Pain

Pain experienced by patients who undergo hand and foot surgery is related to inflammation and edema. Formation of a hematoma may contribute to the discomfort. To control the edema, the extremity should be elevated on several pillows when the patient is sitting or lying. When higher elevation is prescribed for an upper extremity, an elevating sling may be attached to an IV pole or to an overhead frame. If the patient is ambulatory, the affected arm is elevated in a conventional sling with the hand at heart level.

Ice packs applied intermittently to the surgical area during the first 24–48 hours may be prescribed to control edema and provide some pain relief. Dependent positioning of an extremity is uncomfortable, but simply elevating the extremity often relieves the discomfort. Oral analgesics may be used to control the pain. The nurse instructs the patient and family about appropriate use of these medications.

Activity

During the first few days after surgery, the patient may need assistance with ADLs, particularly following surgery of an upper extremity when one hand is bandaged and independent self-care is impaired. The patient may need to arrange for assistance with feeding, bathing and hygiene, dressing, grooming, and toileting. Within a few days, the patient develops skills in one-handed ADLs and is usually able to function with minimal assistance and use of assistive devices. The nurse encourages use of the involved hand, unless contraindicated, within the limits of discomfort. As rehabilitation progresses, the patient resumes use of the injured hand. Physical or occupational therapy–directed exercises may be prescribed. The nurse emphasizes adherence to the therapeutic regimen.

After lower extremity surgery, the patient will have a bulky dressing on the foot, protected by a light cast or a special protective boot. Limits for weight-bearing on the foot will be prescribed by the surgeon. Some patients are allowed to walk on the heel and progress to weight-bearing as tolerated; other patients are restricted to non–weight-bearing activities. Assistive devices (e.g., crutches, walker) may be needed. The choice of the devices depends on the patient's general condition and balance and on the weight-bearing prescription. Safe use of the assistive devices must be ensured through adequate patient education and practice before discharge. Strategies to move around the house safely while using assistive devices are discussed with the patient. As healing progresses, the patient gradually resumes ambulation within prescribed limits. The nurse emphasizes adherence to the therapeutic regimen.

Preventing Infection

Any surgery carries a risk of infection. In addition, percutaneous pins may be used to hold bones in position, and these pins serve as potential sites for infection. Care must be taken to protect the surgical wound from dirt and moisture. When bathing, the patient can secure a plastic bag over the dressing to prevent it from getting wet. Patient instructions concerning aseptic wound care and pin care may be necessary. Refer to Chapter 42 for pin care.

The nurse teaches the patient to monitor for temperature changes and infection. Drainage on the dressing, a foul odor, or increased pain and swelling could indicate infection. The nurse instructs the patient to report any of these findings to the provider promptly. If prophylactic antibiotics are prescribed, the nurse provides instruction about their correct use.

Promoting Home and Community-Based Care

The nurse plans patient teaching for home care, focusing on neurovascular status, pain management, mobility, and wound care.

The nurse instructs the patient to report the following signs and symptoms, which indicate impaired circulation:
- Change in sensation
- Inability to move toes or fingers
- Digits or extremity cool to touch
- Color changes

The nurse also provides instructions for wound care, including:
- Keep the dressing or cast clean and dry.
- Report signs of wound infection (e.g., pain, drainage, fever) immediately.
- Follow the prescribed antibiotic regimen.
- Keep your appointment with the surgeon for the initial dressing change.

Several systemic diseases affect the feet. Patients with diabetes are prone to develop corns and peripheral neuropathies with diminished sensation, leading to ulcers at pressure points of the foot. Patients with peripheral vascular disease and arteriosclerosis can develop ulcers as a result of ischemia. Complaints of burning and itching feet can be seen, resulting in scratching and skin breakdown. Foot deformities may occur with rheumatoid arthritis. Dermatologic problems commonly affect the feet in the form of fungal infections and plantar warts.

The discomforts of foot strain are treated with rest, elevation, physiotherapy, and orthotic devices. The patient must inspect the foot and skin under pads and orthotic devices daily for pressure and skin breakdown. If a "window" is cut into shoes to relieve pressure over a bony deformity, the skin must be monitored daily for breakdown from pressure exerted at the window area. Active foot exercises promote circulation and help strengthen the feet. Walking in properly fitting shoes is considered the ideal exercise.

Plantar Fasciitis

Plantar fasciitis is an inflammation of the foot-supporting fascia. Often, patients experience severe heel pain with the first steps in the morning. The pain is localized to the anterior medial aspect of the heel and diminishes with gentle stretching of the foot and Achilles tendon. Management includes stretching exercises, wearing shoes with support, orthotic devices (e.g., heel cups, arch supports), weight loss for obese patients, and NSAIDs. In approximately 80% of patients, symptoms of plantar fasciitis will resolve in 12 months (Kasper et al., 2015). Unresolved plantar fasciitis may progress to fascial tears at the heel and eventual development of heel spurs.

Hallux Valgus

Hallux valgus (commonly called a bunion) is a deformity in which the great toe deviates laterally (Fig. 41-5A). Associated with this is a marked prominence of the medial aspect of the first metatarsophalangeal joint. There is also osseous enlargement (exostosis) of the medial side of the first metatarsal head, over which a bursa may form (secondary to pressure and inflammation). Acute bursitis symptoms include a reddened area, edema, and tenderness.

Factors contributing to bunion formation may include heredity, ill-fitting shoes, a loss of arch height, and gradual lengthening and widening of the foot associated with aging. Frequently osteoarthritis is associated with hallux valgus. Treatment depends on the patient's age, the degree of deformity, and the severity of symptoms. If a bunion deformity is uncomplicated, wearing a shoe that conforms to the shape of the foot or that is molded to the foot to prevent pressure on the protruding portions may be the only treatment needed. Corticosteroid injections control acute inflammation.

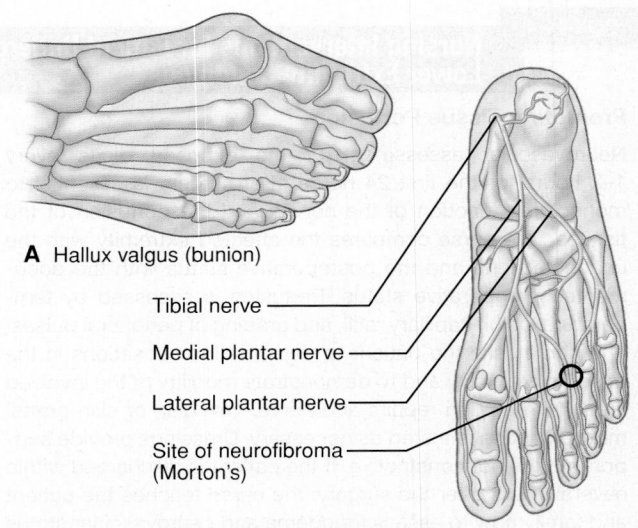

A Hallux valgus (bunion)

Tibial nerve

Medial plantar nerve

Lateral plantar nerve

Site of neurofibroma (Morton's)

B Neurofibroma (Morton neuroma)

FIGURE 41-5 Common foot deformities.

Surgical removal of the bunion (exostosis) and osteotomies to realign the toe may be required to improve function and appearance. Complications related to bunionectomy include limited range of motion (ROM), paresthesias, tendon injury, and recurrence of deformity.

Postoperatively, the patient may have intense throbbing pain at the operative site, requiring liberal doses of analgesic medication. The foot is elevated to the level of the heart to decrease edema and pain. The neurovascular status of the toes is assessed by noting temperature, color, sensation, movement, and capillary refill of the affected toes. The duration of immobility and initiation of ambulation depend on the procedure used. Toe flexion and extension exercises are initiated to facilitate walking. Shoes that fit the shape and size of the foot are recommended.

Morton Neuroma

Morton neuroma (plantar digital neuroma, neurofibroma) is a thickening of the tissues around the third (lateral) branch of the median plantar nerve (see Fig. 41-5B). The third digital nerve, which is located in the third intermetatarsal (web) space, is most commonly involved. Microscopically, digital artery changes cause an ischemia of the nerve.

The result is a throbbing, burning pain in the foot that is usually relieved when the patient rests. Conservative treatment consists of inserting innersoles and metatarsal pads designed to spread the metatarsal heads and balance the foot posture. Local injections of hydrocortisone and a local anesthetic may provide relief. If these fail, surgical excision of the neuroma is necessary. Pain relief and loss of sensation are immediate and permanent.

See Box 41-4 for interventions for patients undergoing surgery for foot problems.

METABOLIC BONE DISORDERS

Osteoporosis

Osteoporosis is a costly disorder, not only in terms of health care dollars but also in terms of human suffering, pain, disability, and death. It is estimated that 10 million Americans had osteoporosis in 2010, and without efforts, by 2030, that number will likely increase to over 13 million (National Osteoporosis Foundation [NOF], 2016). This includes approximately one in two women and two in five men. It is believed to be the underlying cause of 2 million fractures a year (NOF, 2016). Characteristics of osteoporosis include a reduction of bone density and a change in bone structure. The bones become progressively porous, brittle, and fragile; they fracture easily under stresses that would not break normal bone. Osteoporosis frequently results in compression fractures (Fig. 41-6) of the thoracic and lumbar spine, fractures of the neck and intertrochanteric region of the femur, and Colles fractures of the wrist (refer to Chapter 42). These fractures may be the first clinical manifestation of osteoporosis. Fracture risk increases with increasing age and is greatest in Caucasian women.

Pathophysiology

It is thought that 60% to 80% of a person's peak bone mass is genetically determined. Bone mineral density (BMD) in adults is determined by the magnitude of bone acquisition during adolescence and young adulthood coupled with the rate of bone loss that ensues thereafter. By the early to late 20s, peak bone mass is achieved in most people, but differences are seen in timing by skeletal site (e.g., 18 to 20 years of age for proximal femur, 25 to 30 years of age for spine). Typically, peak bone mass is achieved by the third decade, but after this age, rates of bone loss (0.3% to 0.5% per year from the third through fifth decades of life) are seen; the rate of bone resorption (the lysis or breakdown of bone) is greater than the rate of bone formation, resulting in a reduced total bone mass. As individuals age, mismatches in bone remodeling, due to reduced formation, increased resorption, or a combination of both, result in greater rates of bone loss (Weber, 2016).

> ### ⚠ Nursing Alert
> *Nurses are aware that bone density issues in later years are correlated to bone acquisition in younger years. It is important that nurses stress the need for bone health for children and young adults. Early identification of at-risk teenagers and young adults, increased calcium intake, participation in regular weight-bearing exercise, and modification of lifestyle (e.g., reduced use of caffeine, cigarettes, carbonated soft drinks, and alcohol) are interventions that decrease the risk of osteoporosis, fractures, and associated disability later in life.*

FIGURE 41-6 Progressive osteoporotic bone loss and compression fractures. (From Rubin, E., Gorstein, F., Schwarting, R., et al. (2004). *Pathology* (4th ed.). Philadelphia, PA: Lippincott Williams & Wilkins.)

The withdrawal of estrogens at menopause or with oophorectomy causes an accelerated bone resorption that continues during the postmenopausal years. Women develop osteoporosis more frequently and more extensively than men because of lower peak bone mass and the effect of estrogen loss during menopause. Calcium metabolism is illustrated in Figure 41-7.

Secondary osteoporosis is associated with many disease states, nutritional deficiencies, and medications. Coexisting medical conditions, such as gastric bypass, malabsorption syndromes, lactose intolerance, malnutrition, alcohol abuse, kidney failure, liver failure, Cushing syndrome, hyperthyroidism, and hyperparathyroidism, contribute to bone loss and the development of osteoporosis. Medications, including corticosteroids, antiseizure medications, heparin, tetracycline, aluminum-containing antacids, and thyroid supplements, affect the body's use and metabolism of calcium. The degree of osteoporosis is related to the duration of medication therapy. When the therapy is discontinued or the metabolic problem is corrected, the progression of osteoporosis is halted, but restoration of lost bone mass usually does not occur. Specific disease states (e.g., celiac disease, hypogonadism) and medications (e.g., corticosteroids, antiseizure medications) that place patients at risk need to be identified and therapies instituted to reverse the development of osteoporosis.

Risk Factors

Small-framed, nonobese Caucasian women are at greatest risk for osteoporosis. Also, Asian women of slight build

FIGURE 41-7 Calcium metabolism in osteoporosis. Normally, blood absorbs calcium from the digestive system and deposits it into bone. In osteoporosis, blood levels of calcium are reduced. To maintain blood calcium levels, reabsorption of calcium from the bones is increased.

Calcium

Normal absorption of calcium by intestines

Lining of intestine

Calcium stored in bone

Normal bone

Ineffective absorption of calcium by intestines

Increased calcium resorption from bone

Osteoporotic bone

are at risk for low peak bone mineral density (BMD). African-American women, who have a greater bone mass than Caucasian women, are less susceptible to osteoporosis. Men have a greater peak bone mass and do not experience sudden estrogen reduction. As a result, osteoporosis occurs in men at a lower rate and at an older age (about one decade later) (Weber, 2016). It is believed that testosterone and estrogen are important in achieving and maintaining bone mass in men.

Nutritional factors contribute to the development of osteoporosis. A diet that includes adequate calories and nutrients needed to maintain bone, calcium, and vitamin D must be consumed. Vitamin D is necessary for calcium absorption and for normal bone mineralization. Dietary calcium and vitamin D must be adequate to maintain bone remodeling and body functions. While there is some controversy, it is felt that vitamin D deficiency is more prevalent than

previously thought (Kasper et al., 2015) as more than 75% of individuals in the United States are either vitamin D deficient or insufficient (Weber, 2016).

Bone formation is enhanced by the stress of weight and muscle activity. Resistance and impact exercises are most beneficial in developing and maintaining bone mass. Immobility contributes to the development of osteoporosis. Risk factors for osteoporosis are summarized in Figure 41-8.

Gerontologic Considerations

The prevalence of osteoporosis increases with age; although this disorder is not gender specific, there is an increased incidence in women. By the time a woman reaches 80 years of age, the amount of trabecular and cortical bone lost is approximately 40% from the premenopausal peak BMD

FIGURE 41-8 Risk factors for osteoporosis and the effects of these factors on bone.

Nursing Alert

Nurses are aware that corticosteroids are the most frequent cause of medication-related osteoporosis. Often patients with arthritis are prescribed long-term steroids. The combination of the medication and the disease process itself places patients at increased risk for fractures.

Clinical Manifestations and Assessment

Osteoporosis may be undetectable on routine x-rays until there has been 25% to 40% demineralization, resulting in radiolucency of the bones. Frequently, postmenopausal women lose height from vertebral collapse. The gradual collapse of a vertebra may be asymptomatic (1/3 in height loss per year per decade over 50 years of age); it is observed as progressive kyphosis or "dowager's hump" (Fig. 41-9). Multiple compression fractures of the vertebrae result in skeletal deformity. The postural changes result in relaxation of the abdominal muscles and a protruding abdomen. Also the deformity may produce pulmonary insufficiency. Many patients complain of fatigue.

Osteoporosis is diagnosed by dual-energy x-ray absorptiometry (DEXA), which provides information about BMD at the spine and hip. The DEXA scan data are analyzed and reported as T scores (the number of standard deviations [SDs] above or below the average BMD value for a healthy adult at 30 years of age). A normal BMD is less than 1 SD

FIGURE 41-9 Typical loss of height associated with osteoporosis and aging.

(International Osteoporosis Foundation; Szulc & Bouxsein, 2016). Furthermore, elderly people absorb dietary calcium less efficiently and excrete it more readily through their kidneys; therefore, postmenopausal women and the elderly need to consume liberal amounts of calcium. With the aging of the population, the incidence of fractures (more than 2 million osteoporotic fractures per year), pain, and disability associated with osteoporosis is increasing. Most residents of long-term care facilities have a low BMD and are at risk for bone fracture. In addition, restricted sun exposure and a reduced capacity to generate previtamin D in the skin with aging is a consideration.

below the young adult mean value. According to Cosman et al. (2014), BMD is known to correlate with bone strength and is considered an important tool in predicting future fracture risk. It is critical to rule out other conditions associated with low BMD. There is also a fracture risk algorithm (FRAX) developed by the World Health Organization (WHO) to evaluate specific risk factors to assess the 10-year absolute fracture risk for all osteoporotic fractures. The WHO defines osteoporosis as being present when the T score is at least 2.5 SD below the young adult mean value on BMD scan (National Osteoporosis Foundation, 2015). Low bone mass (osteopenia) is diagnosed when the BMD T score is between 1 and 2.5 SD below the young adult mean value. Fracture risk increases progressively as the SD of the T score falls below the mean value.

Quantitative ultrasound studies of the heel and DEXA of the forearm, hip, or spine are used to screen for osteoporosis and to predict the risk of hip and nonvertebral fracture. Current evidence-based guidelines recommend the use of BMD (spine and hip) as the first-line screening test for osteoporosis (Ferri, 2016b; The International Society for Densitometry, 2013) for all postmenopausal women and men over 50 years of age.

BMD studies are useful in identifying low bone mass and osteoporotic bone and in assessing response to therapy. Bone loss and osteoporosis can be reduced through early screening (using both assessment of risk factors and BMD scans), promotion of adequate dietary intake of calcium and vitamin D, encouragement of lifestyle changes, and early institution of preventive medications, resulting in a reduced incidence of fracture.

Other possible medical diagnoses that contribute to bone loss (e.g., multiple myeloma, osteomalacia, hyperparathyroidism, malignancy, celiac disease, hypogonadism in men) can be excluded through the use of x-ray studies or laboratory studies, such as serum calcium, serum phosphate, vitamin D 25OH, bone-specific alkaline phosphatase, urine calcium excretion, testosterone and estrogen studies, hematocrit, and erythrocyte sedimentation rate (ESR).

Medical and Nursing Management

All people should continue to obtain sufficient calcium, vitamin D (Box 41-5), sunshine, and weight-bearing exercise to slow the progression of osteoporosis.

Pharmacologic Therapy

Medications commonly prescribed to treat osteoporosis are classified based on their mechanism of action: anticatabolic (i.e., antiresorptive) and anabolic (i.e., bone building). Anticatabolic medications, or antiresorptives, inhibit osteoclast activity, resulting in reductions in skeletal turnover and bone loss. Bisphosphonates, such as ibandronate, alendronate, and risedronate, reduce spine and hip fractures associated with osteoporosis through inhibition of osteoclast activity, reducing bone resorption and turnover. Adequate calcium and vitamin D intake is needed for maximum effect. Side effects

---

BOX 41-5 | **Nutrition Alert**

Calcium and Vitamin D

A diet rich in calcium and vitamin D throughout life, with an increased calcium intake during adolescence, young adulthood, and the middle years, protects against skeletal demineralization. Such a diet includes three glasses of skim or whole vitamin D–enriched milk (a cup of milk or calcium-fortified orange juice contains about 300 mg of calcium) or other foods high in calcium (e.g., cheese and other dairy products, steamed broccoli, canned salmon with bones) daily. The recommended adequate intake (RAI) level of calcium for the age range of puberty through young adulthood (9–18 years of age) is 1,300 mg/day. The goal of this daily level of calcium is to maximize peak bone mass. The RAI level for adults 19–50 years of age is 1,000 mg/day, and the RAI level for adults 51 years of age and older is 1,200 mg/day.

NOF (2015) recommends an intake of 800–1,000 international units (IU) of vitamin D per day for adults 49 years of age and older. Inadequate intake of calcium or vitamin D over a period of years results in decreased bone mass and the development of osteoporosis.

To ensure adequate calcium intake, a calcium supplement with vitamin D may be prescribed and taken with meals or with a beverage high in vitamin C to promote absorption. The recommended daily dose should be split and not taken as a single dose. Common side effects of calcium supplements are abdominal distention and constipation. Because GI symptoms and abdominal distention are frequent side effects of calcium supplements, the nurse instructs the patient to take the calcium supplements with meals. Also, it is important to teach the patient to drink adequate fluids to reduce the risk of renal calculi.

---

of bisphosphonates include gastrointestinal (GI) symptoms (e.g., dyspepsia, nausea, flatulence, diarrhea, constipation), and some patients may develop esophageal ulcers, esophagitis, gastric ulcers, or osteonecrosis of the jaw related to bisphosphonate use. Patients must take these medications on an empty stomach with a full glass of water upon arising in the morning, and they must sit upright for 30 to 60 minutes after the administration. Other bisphosphonates are administered intravenously.

At natural or surgical menopause, hormone therapy with estrogen and progesterone had been the mainstay of therapy to slow bone loss and reduce the occurrence of fractures. Estrogen replacement decreases bone resorption and increases bone mass, reducing the incidence of osteoporotic fractures. However, studies have demonstrated greater risks, including strokes, venous thromboemboli, and breast cancer, than the benefits of osteoporosis preventive treatment could justify. Although hormone therapy is approved to conserve bone mass and prevent osteoporosis-related fractures, the lowest effective dose for the shortest amount of time is recommended (Cosman et al., 2014).

Selective estrogen receptor modulators (SERMs), such as Raloxifene, reduce the risk of osteoporosis by preserving BMD without estrogenic effects on the uterus. They are indicated for both prevention and treatment of osteoporosis. Raloxifene is the only SERM approved for the treatment of osteoporosis in postmenopausal women as it does not increase the risk of breast or uterine cancer, but it does come with an increased risk of thromboembolism. Duavee®, which is an oral tablet, is a combination of conjugated estrogen and bazedoxifene (another SERM) that is indicated for the prevention of osteoporosis in postmenopausal women. Similarly to raloxifene, bazedoxifene is an estrogen antagonist in the breast and endometrium. The same precautions as with other estrogen products are considered for this drug (e.g., strokes, venous thromboemboli).

Denosumab is approved for the treatment of postmenopausal women with osteoporosis and men who are at high risk for fractures. It is a fully human monoclonal antibody to RANKL, which is a critical determinant of osteoclast activity. Recall osteoclasts dissolve and resorb bone, thus decreasing BMD. Therefore, a RANK-ligand inhibitor is considered a potent inhibitor of osteoclast formation. Denosumab has been shown to increase BMD at the spine, hip, and forearm (Kasper et al., 2015).

Calcitonin directly inhibits osteoclasts, thereby reducing bone loss and may increase osteoblast activity; it also helps to regulate calcium via bone, renal, and GI effects. Calcitonin is administered by nasal spray or by subcutaneous or intramuscular injection. Nasal calcitonin is administered daily, alternating the nares to prevent nasal mucosal dryness. Side effects include nasal irritation, flushing, GI disturbances, and urinary frequency; however, the nasal spray method of delivery has moderate effectiveness. There has been some data to suggest an increase in malignancies, but according to the Food and Drug Administration (FDA, 2015), *"there is no conclusive evidence of a causal relationship between the use of these products and cancer."*

The anticatabolic drugs described previously are effective at slowing bone loss and reducing fracture risk. Another class of medications are anabolic or "bone-building" drugs such as Teriparatide (Forteo), a recombinant human parathyroid hormone. Teriparatide is a medication administered subcutaneously that is given once daily for the treatment of osteoporosis in postmenopausal women and men at risk for fracture. Teriparatide stimulates osteoblasts to build bone matrix and facilitates overall calcium absorption. Teriparatide can reduce the risk of vertebral fractures by about 65% and nonvertebral fragility fractures by about 53% in patients with osteoporosis after an average of 18 months of treatment (Cosman et al., 2014).

Preventing Injury

Physical activity is essential to strengthen muscles, improve balance, prevent disuse atrophy, and slow progressive bone demineralization. Regular weight-bearing exercise promotes bone formation. It is recommended that patients perform 20 to 30 minutes of aerobic exercise (e.g., walking), 3 days or more a week. Weight training stimulates an increase in BMD. In addition, exercise improves balance, reducing the incidence of falls and fractures. Isometric exercises can strengthen trunk muscles. The nurse encourages walking, good body mechanics, and good posture. Daily weight-bearing activity, preferably outdoors in the sunshine to enhance the body's ability to produce vitamin D, is encouraged. Sudden bending, jarring, and strenuous lifting are avoided.

Fracture Management

Fractures of the hip are managed surgically by joint replacement or by closed or open reduction with internal fixation (e.g., hip pinning). Surgery, early ambulation, intensive physical therapy, and adequate nutrition result in decreased morbidity and improved outcomes. In addition, patients need to be evaluated for osteoporosis and treated, if indicated. Refer to Chapter 42 for details on nursing management of patients with a fracture.

One of the most common fractures associated with osteoporosis is vertebral compression fracture. It can affect approximately 25% of postmenopausal women and 200 million individuals worldwide (Zhang et al., 2015). Compression fractures can lead to significant deformity and pain, causing disability and decreased quality of life. Typically osteoporotic compression fractures of the vertebra are managed conservatively with analgesics, external braces, and physical therapy. However, patients with ongoing severe pain may choose vertebral body augmentation, such as kyphoplasty or percutaneous vertebroplasty. Percutaneous vertebroplasty/kyphoplasty includes injection of polymethylmethacrylate bone cement into the fractured vertebra, followed by inflation of a pressurized balloon to restore the shape of the affected vertebra. This procedure can provide rapid relief of acute pain and improve quality of life (QOL). Patients who have not responded to first-line approaches to the treatment of vertebral compression fracture can be considered for the procedure. It is contraindicated in the presence of infection, old fractures, uncorrected coagulopathies, and allergic sensitivity to any of the required components.

Box 41-6 discusses fall prevention. Box 41-7 discusses the impact of nurse practitioners on osteoporosis management.

Paget Disease

Paget disease (osteitis deformans) is a disorder of localized rapid bone turnover, most commonly affecting the skull, femur, tibia, pelvic bones, humerus, scapula, and vertebrae. The disease occurs in about 3% of the population older than 50 years of age and up to 10% in those over 90 years of age (Ferri, 2016c). The incidence is slightly greater in men than in women and increases with aging. A family history has

BOX 41-6 **Gerontologic Considerations**

Fall Prevention

Elderly people fall frequently as a result of environmental hazards, neuromuscular disorders, diminished senses, cardiovascular responses, and responses to medications. The patient and family need to be included in planning for care and preventive management regimens. For example, the home environment should be assessed for safety and elimination of potential hazards (e.g., scatter rugs, cluttered rooms and stairwells, toys on the floor, pets underfoot). Then a safe environment can be created (e.g., well-lighted staircases with secure hand rails, grab bars in the bathroom, properly fitting footwear).

been noted, with siblings often developing the disease. The cause of Paget disease is not known.

Pathophysiology

In Paget disease, there is a primary proliferation of osteoclasts, which produces bone resorption. This is followed by a compensatory increase in osteoblastic activity that replaces the bone. As this chaotic bone turnover continues, a classic mosaic (disorganized) pattern of bone develops. Because the diseased bone is of poor quality, highly vascularized, and structurally weak, pathologic fractures occur. Structural bowing of the legs causes malalignment of the joints of the hip, knee, and ankle, which contributes to the development of arthritis and back and joint pain.

Clinical Manifestations and Assessment

Paget disease is insidious; most patients never experience symptoms but have skeletal deformity. A few patients have symptomatic deformity, and up to 40% of patients who come to medical attention present with bone pain (Ferri, 2016c). The condition is identified most frequently on x-ray studies performed during a routine physical examination or during a workup for another problem. Sclerotic changes, skeletal deformities (e.g., bowing of the femur and tibia, enlargement of the skull, deformity of pelvic bones), and cortical thickening of the long bones occur.

In most patients, skeletal deformity involves the skull or long bones. The skull may thicken, and the patient may report that a hat no longer fits. In some cases, the cranium, but not the face, is enlarged. This gives the patient's face a small, triangular appearance. Most patients with skull involvement have impaired hearing from cranial nerve compression and dysfunction. Other cranial nerves also may be compressed.

The femurs and tibiae tend to bow, producing a waddling gait. The spine is bent forward and is rigid; the chin rests on the chest. The thorax is compressed and immobile on respiration. The trunk is flexed on the legs to maintain balance, and the arms are bent outward and forward and appear long in relation to the shortened trunk. Nerve entrapment may be seen.

Pain, tenderness, and warmth over the bones may be noted. The pain is mild to moderate, deep, and aching; it increases with weight-bearing if the lower extremities are involved. Pain and discomfort may precede skeletal deformities of Paget disease by years and often are wrongly attributed by the patient to old age or arthritis.

BOX 41-7 **Nursing Research**

Bridging the Gap to Evidence-Based Practice

Choi, S.D., & Brings, K., (2016). Work-related musculoskeletal risks associated with nurses and nursing assistants handling overweight and obese patients: A literature review. *Work, 53,* 439–448.

Purpose

Nurses and nursing assistants are susceptible to work-related musculoskeletal disorders and injuries (WMSDs) due to the increase in overweight and obese patients they are handling on a daily basis. This study aimed to review work-related musculoskeletal hazards and risks associated with handling overweight and obese patients as well as summarize the recommended interventions to mitigate musculoskeletal concerns among nurses and nursing assistants.

Design

Approximately 350 publications were screened initially and 22 refereed articles were used for this study on the bases of inclusion/exclusion relevance and strength of evidence on handling overweight or obese patients.

Findings

Evidence suggested that the work-related musculoskeletal risks among nurses and nursing assistants included sprains/

strains; low back pain; and injuries to the wrist, knee, and shoulders. The findings indicated that the risks of WMSD increased when nurses and nursing assistants were moving or lifting patients manually, especially when the patients were overweight or obese. The recommended solutions included the use of lifting/transfer equipment and devices, ergonomic assessments and controls, no-lift policies, and training and education.

Nursing Implications

Nurses should assess their institutional policies on safe lifting, availability of equipment, and available educational programs. To alleviate the risk of musculoskeletal disorders and injuries among nurses and nursing assistants handling overweight or obese patients, additional research and development into what safe patient handling interventions suit this growing population needs to be addressed.

The temperature of the skin overlying the affected bone increases because of increased bone vascularity. Patients with large, highly vascular lesions may develop high-output cardiac failure because of the increased vascular bed and metabolic demands.

Increased osteoblastic activity is reflected by elevated serum ALP concentration or elevated bone-specific alkaline phosphatase (conditions that affect bone growth or cause increased activity of bone cells affect serum ALP) and excretion of urinary N telopeptide. Higher values suggest more active disease. Patients with Paget disease have normal levels of blood calcium.

Concept Mastery Alert

Elevated serum alkaline phosphatase (SAP) levels, but a normal serum calcium level, are indicative of Paget disease.

X-rays confirm the diagnosis of Paget disease. Local areas of demineralization and bone overgrowth produce characteristic mosaic patterns and irregularities. Bone scans demonstrate the extent of the disease. Bone scintigraphy is the most sensitive test to detail the extent and site of pagetic lesions. Bone biopsy may aid in the differential diagnosis.

Medical and Nursing Management

Several medications reduce bone turnover, reverse the course of the disease, relieve pain, and improve mobility. Pain usually responds to NSAIDs. Gait problems from bowing of the legs are managed with walking aids, shoe lifts, and physical therapy. Weight is controlled to reduce stress on weakened bones and malaligned joints. Diets adequate in calcium (up to 1,200 mg per day) and vitamin D (400 to 800 IU) are important as is periodic monitoring to prevent hypocalcemia and secondary hyperparathyroidism during therapy (Kasper et al., 2015).

Medications, such as bisphosphonates and calcitonin, are used to treat Paget disease. They help to suppress further pain and spread of the disease. Bisphosphonates work well for Paget disease; the preferred option is a one-time infusion of Zoldedronate, which has been associated with remission for up to 6 years (Singer et al., 2014). Bisphosphonates produce rapid reduction in bone turnover and relief of pain. They also reduce bone-specific alkaline phosphatase and urinary N telopeptide (a measure of bone turnover) levels. Food inhibits absorption of these medications; therefore, patients ingest the medications on an empty stomach. Calcitonin, a polypeptide hormone, slows bone resorption by decreasing the number and availability of osteoclasts. Calcitonin therapy facilitates remodeling of abnormal bone into normal lamellar bone, relieves bone pain, and helps alleviate neurologic and biochemical signs and symptoms. Calcitonin is administered subcutaneously or by nasal inhalation. Side effects include flushing of the face and nausea. The effect of calcitonin therapy is evident in 3 to 6 months through reduction of bone loss and pain.

Fractures, arthritis, and hearing loss are complications of Paget disease. Fractures are managed according to location. Healing occurs if fracture reduction, immobilization, and stability are adequate. Severe degenerative arthritis may require total joint replacement. Loss of hearing is managed with hearing aids and communication techniques used with people who are hearing-impaired (e.g., speech reading, body language).

Gerontologic Considerations

Because Paget disease tends to affect elderly people, careful assessment of a patient's pain and discomfort is necessary. Patient teaching helps the patient understand the treatment regimen, the need for a diet with adequate calcium and vitamin D, and how to compensate for altered musculoskeletal functioning. The home environment is assessed for safety to prevent falls and to reduce the risk of fracture. Strategies for coping with a chronic health problem and its effect on QOL need to be developed.

MUSCULOSKELETAL INFECTIONS

Osteomyelitis

Osteomyelitis is an infection of the bone; it can be acute or chronic and is usually bacterial in nature. The bone becomes infected in one of three ways:

- Extension of soft tissue infection (e.g., infected pressure or vascular ulcer, incisional infection)
- Direct bone contamination from bone surgery, open fracture, or traumatic injury (e.g., gunshot wound)
- Hematogenous (blood-borne) spread from other sites of infection (e.g., infected tonsils, boils, infected teeth, upper respiratory infections). Osteomyelitis resulting from hematogenous spread typically occurs in a bone in an area of trauma or lowered resistance, possibly from subclinical (nonapparent) trauma. Examples include immunocompromised patients, blood-borne seeding from a distant infection such as a urinary tract infection, pneumonia, and cellulitis.

Patients who are at high risk for osteomyelitis include those who are poorly nourished, elderly, or obese. Other patients at risk include those with impaired immune systems, those who are IV drug users, those with chronic illnesses (e.g., diabetes, rheumatoid arthritis, neuropathy, and arterial insufficiency), and those receiving long-term corticosteroid therapy or immunosuppressive agents.

Postoperative surgical wound infections occur within 30 days after surgery. They are classified as incisional (superficial, located above the deep fascia layer) or deep (involving tissue beneath the deep fascia). If an implant has been used, deep postoperative infections may occur within a year. Deep sepsis after arthroplasty (surgical procedure that replaces damaged joints) may be classified as follows:

- *Stage 1, acute fulminating:* Occurring during the first 3 months after orthopedic surgery; frequently associated with hematoma, drainage, or superficial infection
- *Stage 2, delayed onset:* Occurring between 4 and 24 months after surgery
- *Stage 3, late onset:* Occurring 2 or more years after surgery, usually as a result of hematogenous spread

Bone infections are more difficult to eradicate than are soft tissue infections because the infected bone is mostly avascular (without blood vessels) and not accessible to the body's natural immune response. Also, there is decreased penetration by antibiotics.

Pathophysiology

Between 70% and 80% of bone infections are caused by *Staphylococcus aureus.* Other pathogenic organisms that frequently are found in osteomyelitis include MRSA: methicillin-resistant *S. aureus, Pseudomonas aeruginosa, Escherichia coli, Neisseria gonorrhoeae, Haemophilus influenzae, Fungi,* and *Salmonella* (Grossman & Porth, 2014). There is increasing incidence of infections that are penicillin resistant, nosocomial, gram negative, and anaerobic.

The initial response to infection is inflammation, increased vascularity, and edema. After 2 or 3 days, thrombosis of the blood vessels occurs in the area, resulting in ischemia with bone necrosis. The infection extends into the medullary cavity and under the periosteum and may spread into adjacent soft tissues and joints. Unless the infective process is treated promptly, a bone abscess forms. The resulting abscess cavity contains dead bone tissue (the **sequestrum**), which does not easily liquefy and drain. Therefore, the cavity cannot collapse and heal as it does with abscesses in soft tissue. New bone growth (the **involucrum**) forms and surrounds the sequestrum (Fig. 41-10). Although healing appears to take place, a chronically infected sequestrum remains and produces recurring abscesses throughout the patient's life. This is referred to as chronic osteomyelitis.

FIGURE 41-10 Stages of osteomyelitis.

Clinical Manifestations and Assessment

The hallmark of osteomyelitis is localized pain over the infected bones. When the infection is blood-borne, the onset is usually sudden, occurring often with the clinical and laboratory manifestations of sepsis (e.g., chills, high fever, rapid pulse, and general malaise). The systemic symptoms, such as fever, may overshadow the local signs at first. As the infection extends through the cortex of the bone, it involves the periosteum and the soft tissues. The infected area becomes painful, swollen, and extremely tender. The patient may describe a constant, pulsating pain that intensifies with movement as a result of the pressure of the collecting pus. When osteomyelitis occurs from spread of adjacent infection or from direct contamination, there may be symptoms of sepsis. The area is swollen, warm, painful, and tender to touch.

In acute osteomyelitis, early x-ray findings demonstrate soft tissue swelling. In about 2 weeks, areas of irregular decalcification, bone necrosis, periosteal elevation, and new bone formation are evident. Radioisotope bone scans, particularly the isotope-labeled white blood cell (WBC) scan, and magnetic resonance imaging (MRI) help with early definitive diagnosis. Blood studies reveal leukocytosis (elevated WBCs) and an elevated ESR and C-reactive protein in hematogenous and acute osteomyelitis, but those counts may be normal in chronic contiguous osteomyelitis. Wound and blood culture studies are performed to identify the offending organisms so appropriate antibiotic therapy can be instituted.

With chronic osteomyelitis, large, irregular cavities, raised periosteum, sequestra, or dense bone formations are seen on x-ray. Bone scans may be performed to identify areas of infection. Usually the ESR and the WBC count are normal. Anemia, associated with chronic infection, may be evident. The abscess is cultured to determine the infective organism and appropriate antibiotic therapy. While both acute and chronic osteomyelitis are associated with infections of the bone, they are differentiated by the presence of dead bone in the latter.

Prevention

Prevention of osteomyelitis is the goal. Elective orthopedic surgery should be postponed if the patient has a current infection (e.g., urinary tract infection, sore throat) or a recent history of infection. During orthopedic surgery, careful attention is paid to the surgical environment and to techniques to decrease direct bone contamination. Prophylactic antibiotics, administered to achieve adequate tissue levels at the time of surgery and for 24 hours after surgery, are helpful. Urinary catheters and drains are removed as soon as possible to decrease the incidence of hematogenous spread of infection.

Treatment of focal infections diminishes hematogenous spread. Aseptic postoperative wound care reduces the incidence of superficial infections and osteomyelitis. Prompt management of soft tissue infections reduces extension of infection to the bone. When patients who have had joint replacement surgery undergo dental procedures or other invasive procedures (e.g., cystoscopy), prophylactic antibiotics are recommended frequently. In order to decrease the incidence of osteomyelitis of the foot in patients with diabetes, therapy should be aimed at controlling the blood sugar, decreasing the incidence of peripheral vascular disease.

Medical Management

The initial goal of therapy is to control and halt the infective process. Antibiotic therapy depends on the results of blood and wound cultures. Frequently, the infection is caused by more than one pathogen. General supportive measures (e.g., hydration, a balanced diet, correction of anemia) should be instituted. If necessary, the area affected with osteomyelitis is immobilized to decrease discomfort and to prevent pathologic fracture of the weakened bone.

Pharmacologic Therapy

As soon as the culture specimens are obtained, IV antibiotic therapy begins. The aim is to control the infection before the blood supply to the area diminishes as a result of thrombosis. Around-the-clock dosing is necessary to achieve a sustained high therapeutic blood level of the antibiotic. After results of the culture and sensitivity studies are known, an antibiotic to which the causative organism is sensitive is prescribed. IV antibiotic therapy usually continues for 6 weeks for acute osteomyelitis; chronic osteomyelitis may require a longer course of medication (Ferri, 2016d). After the infection appears to be controlled, the antibiotic may be administered orally for up to 3 months. To enhance absorption of the orally administered medication, antibiotics should not be administered with food.

Surgical Management

If the infection is chronic, surgical débridement may be indicated. The infected bone is surgically exposed, the purulent and necrotic material is removed, and the area is irrigated with sterile saline solution. Antibiotic-impregnated beads may be placed in the wound for direct application of antibiotics for 2 to 4 weeks. IV antibiotic therapy is continued.

In chronic osteomyelitis, antibiotics are adjunctive therapy to surgical débridement. A sequestrectomy (removal of enough involucrum to enable the surgeon to remove the sequestrum) is performed. In many cases, sufficient bone is removed to convert a deep cavity into a shallow saucer (saucerization). All dead, infected bone and cartilage (to the extent possible) must be removed before permanent healing can occur, followed by culture-directed IV antibiotic therapy.

The wound is either closed tightly to obliterate the dead space or packed and closed later by granulation or possibly by grafting. The débrided cavity may be packed with cancellous bone graft to stimulate healing. With a large defect, the cavity may be filled with a vascularized bone transfer or muscle flap (in which a muscle is moved from an adjacent area with blood supply intact). These microsurgery techniques enhance the blood supply. The improved blood supply facilitates bone healing and eradication of the infection. These surgical procedures may be staged over time to ensure healing. A wound-assisted vacuum device may help with closure of the wound. Because surgical débridement weakens the bone, internal fixation or external supportive devices may be needed to stabilize or support the bone to prevent pathologic fracture.

NURSING PROCESS
The Patient with Osteomyelitis

ASSESSMENT

The patient reports an acute onset of signs and symptoms (e.g., localized pain, edema, erythema, abrupt fever with acute osteomyelitis, and persistent low-grade temperature with chronic osteomyelitis); also the patient may describe recurrent drainage of an infected sinus tract with associated pain, edema, and low-grade fever. The nurse assesses the patient for risk factors (e.g., older age, diabetes, long-term corticosteroid therapy, PVD) and for a history of previous injury, infection, or orthopedic surgery. The patient avoids pressure on the area and guards movement. In acute hematogenous osteomyelitis, the patient exhibits generalized weakness due to the systemic reaction to the infection.

Physical examination reveals an inflamed, markedly edematous, warm area that is tender. Purulent drainage may be noted. The patient has an elevated temperature with acute osteomyelitis; whereas with chronic osteomyelitis, the temperature elevation may be low grade, occurring in the afternoon or evening.

Nursing Alert
The nurse recognizes there is a normal in oral temperature in 99% of the population with ranges from 36.0°C (96.8°F) to 37.7°C (99.86°F) with a circadian variation of 1°C or more between the morning nadir and the evening peak (Leggett, 2016).

NURSING DIAGNOSES

Appropriate nursing diagnoses may include:

- Acute pain related to inflammation and edema
- Impaired physical mobility related to pain, use of immobilization devices, and weight-bearing limitations
- Risk for extension of infection: bone abscess formation
- Deficient knowledge related to the treatment regimen

PLANNING

The patient's goals may include relief of pain, improved physical mobility within therapeutic limitations, control and eradication of infection, and knowledge of the treatment regimen.

NURSING INTERVENTIONS

RELIEVING PAIN

The affected part may be immobilized with a splint to decrease pain and muscle spasm. The nurse monitors the neurovascular status of the affected extremity. Frequently the wounds are very painful, and the extremity must be handled with great care and gentleness. Elevation reduces swelling and associated discomfort. Pain is controlled with prescribed analgesics and other pain-reducing techniques.

IMPROVING PHYSICAL MOBILITY

Treatment regimens may consist of activity restriction. The bone is weakened by the infective process and must be protected by immobilization devices and by avoidance of stress on the bone. The patient must understand the rationale for the activity restrictions. The nurse encourages full participation in ADLs within the physical limitations to promote general well-being.

CONTROLLING THE INFECTIOUS PROCESS

The nurse monitors the patient's response to antibiotic therapy and observes the IV access site for evidence of phlebitis, infection, or infiltration. With long-term, intensive antibiotic therapy, the nurse monitors the patient for signs of superinfection (e.g., oral or vaginal candidiasis, loose or foul-smelling stools).

If surgery is necessary, the nurse takes measures to ensure adequate circulation to the affected area (wound suction to prevent fluid accumulation, elevation of the area to promote venous drainage, avoidance of pressure on the grafted area), to maintain needed immobility, and to ensure the patient's adherence to weight-bearing restrictions. The nurse changes dressings using aseptic technique to promote healing and to prevent cross-contamination.

The nurse continues to monitor the general health and nutrition of the patient. A diet high in protein and vitamin C promotes a positive nitrogen balance and healing. The nurse encourages adequate hydration as well.

TEACHING PATIENTS SELF-CARE

The patient and family are taught about the importance of strictly adhering to the therapeutic regimen of antibiotics and preventing falls or other injuries that could result in bone fracture. They need to learn to maintain and manage the IV access and IV administration equipment in the home. Teaching includes medication name, dosage, frequency, administration rate, safe storage and handling, adverse reactions, and necessary laboratory monitoring. In addition, aseptic dressing and warm compress techniques are taught.

The nurse carefully monitors the patient for the development of additional sites that are painful or for sudden increases in body temperature. The nurse instructs the patient and family to observe for and report elevated temperature, drainage, odor, signs of increased inflammation, adverse reactions, and signs of superinfection.

If warranted, the nurse completes a home assessment to determine the patient's and family's abilities regarding continuation of the therapeutic regimen. If the patient's support system is questionable, or if the patient lives alone, a home care nurse may be needed to assist with IV administration of the antibiotics. The nurse monitors the patient for response to the treatment, signs and symptoms of superinfections, and adverse drug reactions. The nurse stresses the importance of follow-up health care appointments and recommends age-appropriate health screening.

EVALUATION

Expected patient outcomes may include:
1. Experiences pain relief:
   a. Reports decreased pain
   b. Experiences no tenderness at site of previous infection
   c. Experiences no discomfort with movement
2. Increases physical mobility:
   a. Participates in self-care activities
   b. Maintains full function of unimpaired extremities
   c. Demonstrates safe use of immobilizing and assistive devices
   d. Modifies environment to promote safety and to avoid falls
3. Shows absence of infection:
   a. Takes antibiotic as prescribed
   b. Reports normal temperature
   c. Exhibits no edema
   d. Reports absence of drainage
   e. Laboratory results indicate normal WBC count and ESR.
   f. Wound cultures are negative.
4. Adheres to therapeutic plan:
   a. Takes medications as prescribed
   b. Protects weakened bones
   c. Demonstrates proper wound care
   d. Reports signs and symptoms of complications promptly
   e. Consumes a diet high in protein and vitamin C
   f. Keeps follow-up health care appointments
   g. Reports increased strength
   h. Reports no elevation of temperature or recurrence of pain, edema, or other symptoms at the site

Septic (Infectious) Arthritis

Septic arthritis refers to infection of a joint by a microorganism. It is an important medical emergency with high morbidity and mortality; inappropriate or delayed treatment can lead to joint damage and a mortality rate of about 10% (Bohler, Dragana, Puchner, Windhager, & Holinka, 2016).

Pathophysiology

Joints can become infected through spread of infection from other parts of the body (hematogenous spread) or directly through trauma or surgical instrumentation. Previous trauma to joints, joint replacement, coexisting arthritis, diabetes mellitus, rheumatoid arthritis, osteoarthritis, alcoholism, cutaneous ulcers, and diminished host resistance contribute to the development of an infected joint. IV drug abusers or those who have intravenous catheters in place to treat other medical conditions are at particular risk for unusual bacterial infection. Patients taking glucocorticosteroids, other immunosuppressive agents, and biologic response modifiers to manage autoimmune diseases, such as rheumatoid arthritis and inflammatory bowel disease, are also at risk. *S. aureus* causes most adult joint infections, followed by *Streptococci*, accounting for 90% of cases of septic arthritis (Matteson & Osmon, 2016). Prompt recognition and treatment of an infected joint are important because accumulating purulent material results in chondrolysis (destruction of hyaline cartilage), which can cause destruction of the surface of the bones.

Clinical Manifestations and Assessment

The patient with acute septic arthritis usually presents with a warm, painful, swollen joint with decreased ROM. The knee is involved in more than 50% of cases (Matteson & Osmon, 2016). Systemic chills, fever, and leukocytosis are present. Elderly patients and patients taking corticosteroids or immunosuppressive medications may not exhibit typical clinical manifestations of infection, and may not have a marked febrile response. Therefore, they require ongoing assessment to detect infection as early as possible in the infectious process. An assessment for the source and cause of infection is performed. Blood cultures, ESR, C-reactive protein, and complete blood count are evaluated. Diagnostic studies include aspiration, examination, and culture of the synovial fluid. Evaluation of the synovial fluid can be critical when choosing the appropriate antibiotic and treatment plan for the patient. Computed tomography (CT) and MRI may reveal inflammation and damage to the joint and may be helpful in assessing osteomyelitis. Radioisotope scanning may be useful in localizing the infectious process.

Medical and Nursing Management

Prompt treatment is essential and may save a joint prosthesis for patients who have one. Broad-spectrum IV antibiotics are started promptly and then changed to organism-specific antibiotics after culture results are available. The IV antibiotics are continued until symptoms disappear. The synovial fluid is monitored for sterility and decrease in WBCs.

In addition to prescribing antibiotics, the provider may aspirate the joint with a needle to remove excessive joint fluid, exudate, and debris. This promotes comfort and decreases joint destruction caused by the action of proteolytic enzymes in the purulent fluid. Occasionally, arthrotomy (incision into a joint) or arthroscopy is used to drain the joint and remove dead tissue.

The inflamed joint is supported and immobilized in a functional position by a splint that increases the patient's comfort. Analgesics may be prescribed to relieve pain. The patient's nutrition and fluid status is monitored. Progressive ROM exercises are prescribed after the infection subsides.

If septic joints are treated promptly, recovery of normal function is expected. The patient is assessed periodically for recurrence. If the articular cartilage was damaged during the inflammatory reaction, joint fibrosis and diminished function may result.

The nurse describes the septic arthritis process to the patient and teaches the patient how to relieve pain using pharmacologic and nonpharmacologic interventions. The nurse also explains the importance of supporting the affected joint, adhering to the prescribed antibiotic regimen, and observing weight-bearing and activity restrictions. In addition, the nurse demonstrates and encourages the patient to practice safe use of ambulatory aids and assistive devices.

The nurse teaches the patient strategies to promote healing through aseptic dressing changes and proper wound care. Then the patient is encouraged to perform ROM exercises after the infection subsides.

BONE TUMORS

Neoplasms of the musculoskeletal system are of various types, including osteogenic, chondrogenic, fibrogenic, muscle (rhabdomyogenic), and marrow (reticulum) cell tumors as well as nerve, vascular, and fatty cell tumors. They may be primary tumors or metastatic tumors from primary cancers elsewhere in the body (e.g., breast, lung, prostate, kidney). Metastatic bone tumors are more common than primary bone tumors.

Benign Bone Tumors

Benign tumors of the bone and soft tissue are more common than malignant primary bone tumors. Benign bone tumors generally are slow growing, well circumscribed, and encapsulated; present few symptoms; and are not a cause of death.

Benign primary neoplasms of the musculoskeletal system include osteochondroma, enchondroma, bone cyst (e.g., aneurysmal bone cyst), osteoid osteoma, rhabdomyoma, and fibroma. Some benign tumors, such as giant cell tumors, have the potential to become malignant.

Osteochondroma is the most common benign bone tumor. It usually occurs as a large projection of bone at the end of the long bones (at the knee or shoulder). It develops during growth and then becomes a static bony mass. In fewer than 1% of patients, the cartilage cap of the osteochondroma may undergo malignant transformation after trauma, and a chondrosarcoma or osteosarcoma may develop.

Enchondroma is a common tumor of the hyaline cartilage that develops in the hand, femur, tibia, or humerus. Usually, the only symptom is a mild ache. Pathologic fractures may occur.

Bone cysts are lesions that expand within the bone. Aneurysmal (widening) bone cysts are seen in young adults, who present with a painful, palpable mass of the long bones, vertebrae, or flat bone. Unicameral (single cavity) bone cysts occur in children and cause mild discomfort and possible pathologic fractures of the upper humerus and femur, which may heal spontaneously.

Osteoid osteoma is a painful tumor that occurs in children and young adults. The neoplastic tissue is surrounded by reactive bone formation that can be identified by x-ray.

Giant cell tumors (osteoclastomas) are benign for long periods but may invade local tissue and cause destruction. They occur in young adults and are soft and hemorrhagic. Eventually, giant cell tumors may undergo malignant transformation and metastasize.

Malignant Bone Tumors

Primary malignant musculoskeletal tumors are relatively rare and arise from connective and supportive tissue cells (sarcomas) or bone marrow elements (multiple myeloma; see Chapter 20). Malignant primary musculoskeletal tumors include osteosarcoma, chondrosarcoma, and Ewing sarcoma. Soft tissue sarcomas include liposarcoma, fibrosarcoma of soft tissue, and rhabdomyosarcoma, which arise in fat cells, fibrous connective tissue, or soft tissue, respectively. Bone tumor metastasis to the lungs is common.

Osteogenic sarcoma (osteosarcoma) is the primary malignant bone tumor that is most common and most often fatal. Prognosis depends on whether the tumor has metastasized to the lungs at the time the patient seeks health care. Osteogenic sarcoma appears most frequently in males between 10 and 25 years of age (in bones that grow rapidly), in older people with Paget disease, and as a result of radiation exposure. Clinical manifestations include pain, edema, limited motion, and weight loss (which is considered an ominous finding). The bony mass may be palpable, tender, and fixed, with an increase in skin temperature over the mass and venous distention. The primary lesion may involve any bone, but the most common sites are the distal femur, the proximal tibia, and the proximal humerus.

Malignant tumors of the hyaline cartilage are called chondrosarcomas. These tumors are the second most common primary malignant bone tumor. They are large, bulky, slow-growing tumors that affect adults. The usual tumor sites include the pelvis, femur, humerus, spine, scapula, and tibia. Metastasis to the lungs occurs in fewer than half of patients. When these tumors are well differentiated, large bloc excision or amputation of the affected extremity results in increased survival rates. These tumors may recur. Refer to a pediatric text for details of the Ewing family of tumors.

Metastatic Bone Disease

Metastatic bone disease (secondary bone tumor) is more common than any primary bone tumor. Tumors arising from tissues elsewhere in the body may invade the bone and produce localized bone destruction (lytic lesions) or bone overgrowth (blastic lesions). The most common primary sites of tumors that metastasize to bone are the kidney, prostate, lung, breast, ovary, and thyroid. Metastatic tumors most frequently attack the skull, spine, pelvis, femur, and humerus, and they often involve more than one bone (polyostotic).

Pathophysiology

A tumor in the bone causes the normal bone tissue to react by osteolytic response (bone destruction) or osteoblastic response (bone formation). Primary tumors cause bone destruction, which weakens the bone, resulting in bone fractures. Adjacent normal bone responds to the tumor by altering its normal pattern of remodeling. The bone's surface changes and the contours enlarge in the tumor area.

Malignant bone tumors invade and destroy adjacent bone tissue. Benign bone tumors, in contrast, have a symmetric, controlled growth pattern and place pressure on adjacent bone tissue. Malignant invading bone tumors weaken the structure of the bone until it can no longer withstand the stress of ordinary use; pathologic fracture commonly results.

Clinical Manifestations and Assessment

Patients with primary malignant and benign bone tumors present with pain, swelling, and, occasionally, pathologic fracture of the involved bone (Doroshow, 2016). Patients with metastatic bone tumor may have a wide range of associated clinical manifestations. They may be symptom free or have pain (mild and occasional to constant and severe), varying degrees of disability, and, at times, obvious bone growth. Weight loss, malaise, and fever may be present. The tumor may be diagnosed only after pathologic fracture has occurred.

With spinal metastasis, spinal cord compression may occur. It can progress rapidly or slowly. Neurologic deficits (e.g., progressive pain, weakness, gait abnormality, paresthesia, paraplegia, urinary retention, loss of bowel or bladder control) must be identified early and treated with decompressive laminectomy to prevent permanent spinal cord injury.

The differential diagnosis is based on the history, physical examination, and diagnostic studies, including CT, bone scans, myelography, arteriography, MRI, biopsy, and biochemical assays of the blood and urine. Frequently serum ALP levels are elevated with osteogenic sarcoma. With metastatic carcinoma of the prostate, serum acid phosphatase levels are elevated. Hypercalcemia is present with bone metastases from breast, lung, or kidney cancer. Symptoms of hypercalcemia include muscle weakness, fatigue, anorexia, nausea, vomiting, polyuria, cardiac arrhythmias, seizures, and coma. Hypercalcemia must be identified and treated promptly. A surgical biopsy is performed for histologic identification. Extreme care is taken during the biopsy to prevent seeding and resultant recurrence after excision of the tumor.

Chest x-rays are performed to determine the presence of lung metastasis. Surgical staging of musculoskeletal tumors is based on tumor grade and site (intracompartmental or extracompartmental) as well as on metastasis. Staging is used for planning treatment.

During the diagnostic period, the nurse explains the diagnostic tests and provides psychological and emotional support to the patient and family. The nurse assesses coping behaviors and encourages use of support systems.

Medical Management

Primary Bone Tumors

The goal of treatment of a primary bone tumor is to destroy or remove the tumor. This may be accomplished by surgical excision (ranging from local excision to amputation and disarticulation), radiation therapy if the tumor is radiosensitive, and chemotherapy (preoperative [neoadjuvant], intraoperative, postoperative, and adjunctive for possible micrometastases). Preoperative imaging studies determine the extent of tumor penetration and impact on adjacent structures. Survival and QOL are important considerations in procedures that attempt to save the involved extremity.

Typically patients are managed with initial neoadjuvant (given before surgery) chemotherapy, delayed resection of the primary tumor, and then further postoperative chemotherapy (Doroshow, 2016). The SAP level, which often is elevated in patients with osteosarcoma, can be used to monitor disease status. Limb-sparing (salvage) procedures are used to remove the tumor and adjacent tissue. A customized prosthesis, total joint arthroplasty, or bone tissue from the patient (autograft) or from a cadaver donor (allograft) replaces the resected tissue. Soft tissue and blood vessels may need grafting because of the extent of the excision. Complications may include infection, loosening or dislocation of the prosthesis, allograft nonunion, fracture, devitalization of the skin and soft tissues, joint fibrosis, and recurrence of the tumor. Function and rehabilitation after limb salvage depend on positive encouragement and reducing the risk of complications.

Surgical removal of the tumor may require amputation of the affected extremity with the amputation extending well above the tumor to achieve local control of the primary lesion (refer to Chapter 42). Because of the danger of metastasis with malignant bone tumors, combined chemotherapy is started before and continued after surgery in an effort to eradicate micrometastatic lesions. The goal of combined chemotherapy is greater therapeutic effect at a lower toxicity rate with reduced resistance to the medications. There is an improved long-term survival rate when a localized osteosarcoma is removed and chemotherapy is initiated. Soft tissue sarcomas are treated with radiation, limb-sparing excision, and adjuvant chemotherapy.

Secondary Bone Tumors

The treatment of metastatic bone cancer is palliative. The therapeutic goal is to relieve the patient's pain and discomfort while promoting QOL.

If metastatic disease weakens the bone, structural support and stabilization are needed to prevent pathologic fracture. At times, large bones with metastatic lesions are strengthened by prophylactic internal fixation. Internal fixation of pathologic fractures, arthroplasty, or methylmethacrylate (bone cement) reconstruction minimizes associated disability and pain. Patients with metastatic disease are at higher risk than other patients for postoperative pulmonary congestion, hypoxemia, deep vein thrombosis, and hemorrhage.

Hypercalcemia results from breakdown of bone. It needs to be recognized promptly. Treatment includes hydration with IV administration of normal saline solution; diuresis; mobilization; and medications such as bisphosphonates, pamidronate, and calcitonin (refer to Chapter 6 for further details on hypercalcemia). Because inactivity leads to loss of bone mass and increased calcium in the blood, the nurse assists the patient to increase activity and ambulation.

Frequently hematopoiesis is disrupted by tumor invasion of the bone marrow or by treatment (chemotherapy or radiation). Blood component therapy restores hematologic factors. Pain can result from multiple factors, including the osseous metastasis, surgery, chemotherapy or radiation side effects, and arthritis. Pain must be assessed accurately and managed with adequate and appropriate opioid, nonopioid, and nonpharmaceutical interventions. In the absence of fracture, external beam radiation may be used for painful metastatic sites. Systemic chemotherapy or endocrine therapy also may be considered for palliation. Patients with multiple bony metastases may achieve pain control with systemically administered "bone-seeking" isotopes (e.g., strontium-89).

Nursing Management

The nursing care of a patient who has undergone excision of a bone tumor is similar in many respects to that of other patients who have had skeletal surgery. Vital signs are monitored; blood loss is assessed; and observations are made to assess for the development of complications, such as deep vein thrombosis, pulmonary emboli, infection, contracture, and disuse atrophy. The affected part is elevated to reduce edema, and the neurovascular status of the extremity is assessed.

Providing Patient Education

Patient and family teaching about the disease process and diagnostic and management regimens is essential. Explanation of diagnostic tests, treatments (e.g., wound care), and expected results (e.g., decreased ROM, numbness, change of body contours) helps the patient deal with the procedures

and changes. Cooperation and adherence to the therapeutic regimen are enhanced through understanding. The nurse can most effectively reinforce and clarify information given by the provider by being present during these discussions.

Relieving Pain

Accurate pain assessment is the foundation for pain management. Pharmacologic and nonpharmacologic pain management techniques are used to relieve pain and increase the patient's comfort level. The nurse works with the patient in designing the most effective pain management regimen, thereby increasing the patient's control over the pain. Prescribed IV or epidural analgesics are used during the early postoperative period. Later, oral or transdermal opioid or nonopioid analgesics are indicated to alleviate pain. In addition to external radiation, systemic radioisotopes may be used to control pain. See Chapter 7 for further discussion of pain management.

Preventing Pathologic Fracture

Bone tumors weaken the bone to a point at which normal activities or even position changes can result in fracture. During nursing care, the affected extremities must be supported and handled gently. External supports (e.g., splints) may be used for additional protection. At times, the patient may elect to have surgery (e.g., open reduction with internal fixation, joint replacement) in an attempt to prevent pathologic fracture. Prescribed weight-bearing restrictions must be followed. The nurse and physical therapist teach the patient how to use assistive devices safely and how to strengthen unaffected extremities.

Promoting Coping Skills

The nurse encourages the patient and family to verbalize their fears, concerns, and feelings. They need to be supported as they deal with the impact of the malignant bone tumor. Feelings of shock, despair, and grief are expected. Referral to a psychiatric advanced practice nurse, psychologist, counselor, or spiritual advisor may be indicated for specific psychological help and emotional support.

Promoting Self-Care

Independence versus dependence is an issue for the patient who has a malignancy. Lifestyle is changed dramatically, at least temporarily. It is important to support the family in working through the adjustments that must be made. The nurse assists the patient in dealing with changes in body image due to surgery and possible amputation. It is helpful to provide realistic reassurance about the future and resumption of role-related activities and to encourage self-care and socialization. The patient participates in planning daily activities. The nurse encourages the patient to be as independent as possible. Involvement of the patient and family throughout treatment encourages confidence, restoration of self-concept, and a sense of being in control of one's life.

Monitoring and Managing Potential Complications

Delayed Wound Healing

Wound healing may be delayed because of tissue trauma from surgery, previous radiation therapy, inadequate nutrition, or infection. The nurse assesses the patient's nutritional status by monitoring weight, percentage of weight loss, and evaluating the serum albumin or prealbumin level. An unintentional weight loss of 10% of usual body weight in 3 months is a risk factor for malnutrition.

Nursing Alert
The nurse monitors and reports laboratory markers related to nutritional status. Serum prealbumin has a shorter half-life (2 days) than albumin (21 days) and is not influenced by fluid balance, making it an excellent marker for malnutrition. A normal prealbumin level is 19 to 38 mg/dL with values of 0 to 5, 5 to 10, and 10 to 15 mg/dL reflecting a severe, moderate, and mild protein depletion, respectively (Fischbach & Dunning, 2014). Interventions that promote homeostasis and wound healing should be initiated as soon as possible. In addition, the nurse considers that the patient's requirements for calories, protein, vitamins, and minerals will be expected to increase in times of stress.

The nurse minimizes pressure on the wound site to promote circulation to the tissues. Repositioning the patient at frequent intervals reduces the incidence of skin breakdown and pressure ulcers. Special therapeutic beds may be needed to prevent skin breakdown and to promote wound healing after extensive surgical reconstruction and skin grafting.

Inadequate Nutrition

Because loss of appetite, nausea, and vomiting are frequent side effects of chemotherapy and radiation therapy, it is necessary to provide adequate nutrition for healing and health promotion. Antiemetics, relaxation techniques, and acupuncture reduce the adverse GI effects of chemotherapy. Stomatitis is controlled with anesthetic or antifungal mouthwash (see Chapter 6). Adequate hydration is essential. Nutritional supplements and enteral or parenteral nutrition may be prescribed to achieve adequate nutrition.

Osteomyelitis and Wound Infections

Prophylactic antibiotics and strict aseptic dressing techniques are used to diminish the occurrence of osteomyelitis and wound infections. During healing, other infections (e.g., upper respiratory infections) need to be prevented so that hematogenous spread does not result in osteomyelitis. If the patient is receiving chemotherapy, it is important to monitor the WBC count and to instruct the patient to avoid contact with people who have colds or other infections.

Hypercalcemia

Hypercalcemia is a dangerous complication of bone cancer. The symptoms must be recognized and treatment initiated promptly. Symptoms include muscular weakness, incoordination, anorexia, nausea and vomiting, constipation, electrocardiographic changes (e.g., shortened QT interval and ST segment, bradycardia, heart blocks), and altered mental states (e.g., confusion, lethargy, psychotic behavior). See Chapter 6, Table 6-6 for a discussion of hypercalcemia and its management.

CHAPTER REVIEW

Critical Thinking Exercises

1. At the general medical clinic where you are a nurse, a 64-year-old woman presents with acute onset of low back pain. You discover that she has a history of long-term alcohol use and has smoked one pack of cigarettes daily for the past 45 years. What musculoskeletal conditions is she at risk of developing? What specific questions would you ask her to determine the status of her bone health? Discuss the strength of the evidence that supports any risk factor reduction strategies you consider implementing.

2. You are a home care nurse who is about to visit a 26-year-old patient with osteomyelitis that occurred after a fracture to the left tibia and fibula sustained in a motorcycle crash. What is the strength of the evidence that identifies factors that affect bone healing? Discuss the significance of these factors in determining your health-teaching strategies for this patient.

3. You are caring for an elderly patient who has advanced cancer. During the afternoon, she complains of muscle weakness, extreme fatigue, anorexia, and nausea. Her urinary output is also elevated. What laboratory value would you assess? What nursing interventions would you implement in light of her new symptoms? What might be the pathophysiology behind these new symptoms?

NCLEX-Style Review Questions

1. A 25-year-old woman experienced an open fracture of the right fibula with major soft tissue damage of her lower leg in a motor vehicle accident. Surgical reduction and fixation of the fibula were performed with débridement of nonviable tissue and drain placement in the damaged soft tissue. Which complication is this patient at risk for?
   a. Osteoporosis
   b. Osteomyelitis
   c. Fat emboli
   d. Compartment syndrome

2. Which assessment finding may indicate to the nurse an acute peripheral neurovascular dysfunction for the patient recovering from surgery of the foot?
   a. Pale skin, atrophy of the limb, with capillary refill of 2 seconds
   b. Absence of feeling, capillary refill of 4 to 5 seconds, and cool skin
   c. Atrophy of limb, increased motion, and thickened toe nails
   d. Pale skin, weakness in motion, and loss of toe hairs

3. Which assessment finding would the nurse expect to find in a patient diagnosed with acute osteomyelitis?
   a. Leukopenia and localized bone pain
   b. Leukocytosis and elevated sedimentation (SED) rate
   c. Leukopenia and elevated fever
   d. Petechiae over the chest and abnormal arterial blood gas (ABG) results

4. A client is diagnosed with osteoporosis. Which statements should the nurse include when teaching the client about the disease? *Select all that apply.*
   a. Osteoporosis is common in females after menopause.
   b. Osteoporosis is a degenerative disease characterized by an increase in bone density.

   c. Osteoporosis can increase the risk for fractures.
   d. The recommended daily calcium dose should be taken as a single dose, and the patient should be instructed not to lie down for 30 minutes.
   e. Weight-bearing exercise should be avoided.
   f. The patient's T score is at least 2.5 SD below the young adult mean value on the BMD scan.

5. What places the patient at risk for impaired wound healing after surgery for a primary bone cancer? *Select all that apply.*
   a. Radiation therapy
   b. Prealbumin level is 28 mg/dL
   c. Weight loss of 18% over the previous 3 months
   d. Anorexia
   e. Satisfactory vitamin C levels

Try these additional resources, available at **http://thepoint.lww.com/Honan2e**, to enhance your learning and understanding of this chapter:
- NCLEX-Style Student Review Questions
- Journal Articles

REFERENCES AND SELECTED READINGS

References and selected readings associated with this chapter can be found on the website that accompanies the book. Visit **http://thepoint. lww.com/Honan2e** to access the references and other additional resources associated with this chapter.

Nursing Management: Patients with Musculoskeletal Trauma

Linda Honan

Learning Objectives

After reading this chapter, you will be able to:

1. Differentiate between contusions, strains, sprains, and dislocations.
2. Specify the clinical manifestations of a fracture and the emergency management of the patient with a fracture.
3. Describe the principles and methods of fracture reduction, fracture immobilization, and management of open fractures.
4. Describe the prevention and management of complications of fractures.
5. Discuss nursing management of the patient with a cast.
6. Discuss nursing management of the patient undergoing joint replacement or amputation.

Injury to any part of the musculoskeletal system necessitates evaluation of the damaged area, along with assessment of the structures and organs that underlie the fracture. For example, if a bone is broken, the adjacent muscles cannot function, blood vessels and nerves may be injured with resultant neurovascular complications, and the organs that lie beneath the fracture may have damage secondary to the trauma.

Treatment of injury to the musculoskeletal system involves providing support to the injured part until healing is complete. Frequently, management includes the use of internal and/or external devices, such as bandages, splints, casts, skin or skeletal traction, artificial joint replacement, pins, or a combination of these. Pharmacologic treatment often includes anti-inflammatory agents, muscle relaxants, and analgesics. They may help diminish edema and relax muscles at risk for spasm that can cause further injury to inflamed muscles or to fractured bones. Pain relief is an important factor to facilitate healing.

Patient education is essential for optimal outcomes. Nursing care is planned to maximize the effectiveness of treatment modalities, prevent potential complications associated with interventions, and observe for the development of untoward signs and symptoms as soon as possible. After the immediate and painful effects of the injury have passed, treatment efforts are focused on preventing fibrosis and atrophy or degeneration of the injured muscles and joint structures, respectively.

COMMON MUSCULOSKELETAL INJURIES

Contusions, Strains, and Sprains

Pathophysiology

A **contusion** is an injury to soft tissue produced by blunt force, such as a blow, kick, or fall, that results in bleeding into soft tissues (ecchymosis, or bruising). A *hematoma* (collection of blood within tissues) develops when the bleeding is sufficient to form an appreciable solid swelling. A muscle **strain**, or a "pulled muscle," is an injury to a musculotendinous unit caused by overuse, overstretching, or excessive stress. It can occur anywhere within the muscle, but it commonly occurs at the distal muscle-tendon junction (Nelson, 2014). Recall, a tendon connects muscle to bone, whereas a ligament connects bone to bone. A **sprain** is an injury to the ligaments and supporting muscle fibers that surround a joint often caused by a trauma, wrenching, or twisting motion. The injury can range from a mild stretching of the ligament to a complete tear. While a history and physical examination are important, diagnostic studies of the affected extremity may be ordered to determine diagnosis.

Risk Factors

The main risk factor for contusions, strains, or sprains is participation in sports and physical fitness activities. Strains and sprains occur after intense activity or are associated with over-use repetitive injuries or trauma, whereas contusions can occur in any soft tissue that suffers blunt trauma. Ankles, knees, and wrists are vulnerable to sprains, while strains frequently occur in the neck, lower back, and hamstring muscle (back of the thigh). Previous injuries are a risk factor for reinjury.

Clinical Manifestations and Assessment

An important question for nurses to ask when assessing for musculoskeletal injury is, "What were you doing at the time of the injury?" For example, many ankle sprains occur because of inversion injury (turning ankle in while walking), while muscle strains occur because of a "pulled muscle" while exercising. The nurse assesses the threes "S's," size, shape, and symmetry, of the involved area in comparison to the opposite region. It is important to note presence of **edema** (swelling), ecchymosis (bruising), tenderness, abnormal joint motion, and pain. Contusions, strains, and sprains can present with similar symptoms of pain, edema, and discoloration from the broken blood vessels. The patient may guard or protect the affected area, and he or she may have difficulty moving the affected area; increased warmth may be noted at the injury site.

With contusions, the nurse notes ecchymosis and edema of the injured area. The patient may complain initially of dull pain at the site that increases as edema develops and subsequent stiffness of the area, usually by the next day. Most contusions resolve in 1 to 2 weeks.

Muscle strains are graded along a continuum based on symptoms and loss of function. A first-degree strain reflects tearing of few muscle fibers and is accompanied by minor edema, tenderness (usually noticed after the activity is over), and mild muscle spasm, without a noticeable loss of function. A second-degree strain involves a tearing of more muscle fibers and is manifested by edema, tenderness, muscle spasm, ecchymosis, and a notable loss of load-bearing strength of the involved extremity. A third-degree strain involves complete disruption of at least one musculotendinous unit that involves separation of muscle from muscle, muscle from tendon, or tendon from bone. Patients present with significant pain, muscle spasm, ecchymosis, a large hematoma, edema, and loss of function. An x-ray should be obtained to rule out bone injury because an avulsion fracture (in which a bone fragment is pulled away from the bone by a tendon) may be associated with a third-degree strain.

Like strains, sprains (ligamentous injuries) are graded to reflect the degree of injury. A mild sprain, termed first-degree sprain (a tear of only a few fibers), may cause minor edema, tenderness, and mild muscle spasm, without a noticeable loss of function. Patients are able to bear weight with minimal pain. A second-degree sprain is an incomplete tear of the ligament (bone-to-bone); as blood vessels rupture, ecchymosis and edema are expected and movement of the joint becomes painful. The degree of disability and pain

---

BOX 42-1 **RICE**

The acronym **RICE**—**R**est, **I**ce, **C**ompression, **E**levation—is helpful for remembering treatment interventions for musculoskeletal injuries.

Rest prevents additional injury and promotes healing. Intermittent application of moist or dry cold packs for 20–30 minutes during the first 24–48 hours after injury produces vasoconstriction, which decreases bleeding, edema, and discomfort. Ensure care to avoid skin and tissue damage from excessive cold. An elastic compression bandage controls bleeding, reduces edema, and provides support for the injured tissues. Elevation controls the swelling.

---

increases during the first 2 to 3 hours after the injury because of the associated swelling and bleeding. There is restricted motion of the affected limb, and weight bearing is painful. A third-degree sprain involves complete ligament tear with resultant complaints of significant pain, muscle spasm, ecchymosis, edema, and loss of function. Patients are unable to bear weight on the affected limb. Tenderness at the distal tibia (inner ankle) or fibula (outer ankle) is associated with an inversion or eversion injury and may indicate a fracture.

Medical and Nursing Management

Treatment of contusions, strains, and sprains consists of resting and elevating the affected part, applying cold, and using a compression bandage (Box 42-1). Immobilization of the affected extremity until definite diagnosis is determined may be appropriate. It is important to monitor the **neurovascular status** of the injured extremity; this is termed **CSM:** Circulation, by way of pulses, color, temperature, and capillary refill; Sensation, by noting awareness of light touch; and Movement, by range of motion (ROM) of the m ost distal digits. The nurse compares the injured limb to the uninjured limb.

After the acute inflammatory stage (e.g., 24 to 48 hours after injury), intermittent heat application (for 15 to 30 minutes, four times a day) relieves muscle spasm and promotes vasodilation, absorption, and repair. Depending on the severity of injury, progressive passive and active exercises may begin in 2 to 5 days. Severe sprains and strains may require 1 to 3 weeks of immobilization before exercises are initiated. Excessive exercise early in the course of treatment delays recovery. Strains and sprains take weeks or months to heal because ligaments and tendons are relatively avascular. Splinting may be used to prevent reinjury.

JOINT DISLOCATIONS

Pathophysiology

With **dislocation** of a joint, the articular surfaces of the bones forming the joint are no longer in anatomic alignment.

The bones are literally "out of joint." Dislocations may be congenital, or present at birth; spontaneous or pathologic; or traumatic, resulting from injury in which the joint is disrupted by force. A **subluxation** is a partial dislocation of the articulating surfaces. Traumatic dislocations are orthopedic emergencies because the associated joint structures, blood supply, and nerves are distorted and severely stressed.

> ### Nursing Alert
> *If the dislocation is not treated promptly, avascular necrosis (AVN), tissue death due to anoxia and diminished blood supply, and nerve palsy may occur. Tenderness at the site, limited ROM, the affected limb being shortened, pain, and asymmetry of limbs is observed. The limb is immobilized and the provider notified.*

Clinical Manifestations and Assessment

Signs and symptoms of a traumatic dislocation include acute pain, change in contour of the joint, change in the length of the extremity (shortening of the affected limb), loss of normal mobility, and change in the axis of the dislocated bones. X-rays confirm the diagnosis and reveal any associated fracture.

Medical and Nursing Management

The affected joint needs to be immobilized while the patient is transported to the hospital. The dislocation is reduced promptly (i.e., displaced parts are brought into normal position) to preserve joint function. Analgesia, muscle relaxants, and, possibly, anesthesia are used to facilitate closed reduction (e.g., noninvasive or nonsurgical reduction). The joint is immobilized by bandages, splints, casts, or traction and is maintained in a stable position. Neurovascular status is monitored (temperature, capillary refill, pulses, color, mobility, sensation). After reduction, if the joint is stable, then gentle, progressive, active, and passive movement is begun to preserve ROM and restore strength. The joint is supported between exercise sessions.

SPECIFIC MUSCULOSKELETAL INJURIES

Common specific musculoskeletal injuries include **rotator cuff** tears, epicondylitis, and injury to the ligaments of the knee. Table 42-1 summarizes key findings and treatment for these common injuries.

FRACTURES

A **fracture** is a break in the continuity of bone caused by direct blows, crushing forces, sudden twisting motions, and extreme muscle contractions. When the bone is broken, adjacent structures also are affected, resulting in soft tissue edema and hemorrhage into the muscles and joints, with potential joint dislocations, ruptured tendons, severed nerves, and damaged blood vessels. Because body organs may be injured by the force that caused the fracture or by fracture fragments, it is important for nurses to have knowledge of the organs that lie beneath the fracture. For example, the nurse is alert for liver injuries with fractures to right ribs 6 through 12 and splenic injuries with fractures to left ribs 9 through 11. In addition to the magnitude of the force on the bone, the nurse needs to consider the strength of the bone, which is related directly to its density. Thus a lower force may create a fracture because of bone weakness (e.g., osteoporosis or bone cysts).

Types of Fractures

Fractures are defined according to the bone involved (e.g., humerus, femur, tibia) and can be categorized in several ways, including the direction of the fracture. A *complete fracture* involves a break across the entire cross-section of the bone and frequently is displaced (removed from its normal position). An *incomplete fracture* (e.g., greenstick fracture) involves a break through only part of the cross-section of the bone. An *oblique fracture* runs across the bone at a diagonal angle of 45 to 60 degrees. A *comminuted* fracture is one that produces several bone fragments, while an *impacted* fracture is one whose ends are driven into each other. A *closed fracture* (simple fracture) is one that does not cause a break in the skin. An *open fracture* (compound or complex fracture) is one in which the wound to the skin or mucous membrane extends to the fractured bone. Some fractures have specific names, for example, a fracture of the distal radius (wrist) is termed a *Colles fracture*. *Stress fractures* occur with repeated bone trauma from athletic activities, most frequently involving the tibia and metatarsals. *Compression fractures* are caused by compression of vertebrae and are associated frequently with osteoporosis. Figure 42-1 depicts types of fractures.

> ### Nursing Alert
> *On x-rays, long bone fractures will be categorized as proximal (closest to or toward the center of the body), middle, or distal (the portion of the bone that is farthest away). The term intra-articular fracture extends into the joint space, whereas fractures not involving the joint are termed extra-articular. In children, fractures are described in relation to the growth plate (physis); thus, if a fracture is seen between the joint and the growth plate, it will be termed an epiphyseal fracture. A diaphysis fracture refers to the shaft of the bone and metaphysis is between the epiphysis and the diaphysis.*

TABLE **42-1** Specific Musculoskeletal Injuries

Injury	Description	Key Assessment Findings	Treatment
Rotator cuff tears	Tear results from an acute injury or from chronic joint stresses; it occurs when there is damage to one or more of the four muscles and their tendons in the shoulder.	• Acromioclavicular joint pain; in many cases, the patient with a rotator cuff tear experiences night pain and cannot sleep on the involved side. • Limited ROM; the patient cannot perform over-the-head activities or activities as simple as putting on a coat. • Muscle weakness	• Rest and modalities such as hot packs, ultrasound, or cold applications, with specific ROM exercises as soon as tolerated. • Nonsteroidal anti-inflammatory drugs (NSAIDs) but most frequent treatment is steroid injection into the shoulder joint or • Arthroscopic débridement (removal of devitalized tissue) • Arthroscopic or open acromioplasty with tendon repair
Epicondylitis (tennis elbow)	Chronic, painful condition that is caused by excessive, repetitive extension and flexion and/ or pronation and supination activities of the forearm. These excessive, repetitious activities result in inflammation (**tendinitis**) and minor tears in the tendons at the origin of the muscles on the medial or lateral epicondyles.	• Pain that usually radiates down the extensor (dorsal) surface of the forearm and generally is relieved with rest and avoidance of the aggravating activity • Weakened grasp	• Application of ice for pain after the activity • NSAIDs for pain • In some instances, immobilization of the arm in a molded splint or cast is necessary. • Local injection of a corticosteroid generally is reserved for patients with severe pain who do not respond to NSAIDs and immobilization because of its degenerative effects on tendons. • After pain subsides, rehabilitation exercises that stretch and strengthen the area (including gentle and gradual increased stretching of the tendons) • Tennis elbow counterforce strap that limits extension of the elbow (may be prescribed when activity is resumed) • Occasionally, surgery to release strictures or to débride the joint
Knee injury	Injury to the anterior cruciate ligament (ACL) or the posterior cruciate ligament (PCL), which stabilize forward and backward motion of the femur and tibia, occurs when the foot is firmly planted and the knee is hyperextended and the person twists the torso and femur. Injury to the lateral or medial collateral ligaments of the knee, which provide stability lateral and medial to the knee, occurs when the foot is firmly planted and the knee is struck either medially or laterally.	• Acute onset of pain • Point tenderness (e.g., tenderness at the site of injury) • Joint instability and inability to walk without assistance • Hemarthrosis (bleeding into the joint) may develop, contributing to the pain.	• Treatment will depend on the severity of the injury, but may include: • RICE • Evaluation of the joint for fracture • Aspiration of joint fluid to relieve pressure • Limited weight bearing • Use of protective elastic bandaging or brace • Surgery; the operation is typically performed as ambulatory arthroscopic surgery, in which the surgeon uses an **arthroscope** to visualize and repair the damage.

Clinical Manifestations and Assessment

The diagnosis of a fracture is based on the patient's symptoms, the physical signs, and the x-ray findings. Usually, the patient reports having sustained an injury to the area. The clinical manifestations of a fracture include pain, loss of function, deformity, shortening, **crepitus** (described shortly),

swelling, and discoloration. These clinical manifestations do not all need to be present in every fracture.

Pain

The pain is immediate, continuous, and increases in severity until the bone fragments are immobilized. The muscle

Avulsion
A fracture in which a fragment of
bone has been pulled away by a
tendon and its attachment

Comminuted
A fracture in which bone has
splintered into several fragments

Compression
A fracture in which bone
has been compressed
(seen in vertebral fractures)

Depressed
A fracture in which fragments
are driven inward (seen frequently
in fractures of skull and facial bones)

Epiphyseal
A fracture through the epiphysis

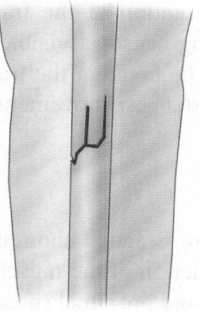

Greenstick
A fracture in which one
side of a bone is broken
and the other side is bent

Impacted
A fracture in which a
bone fragment is driven into
another bone fragment

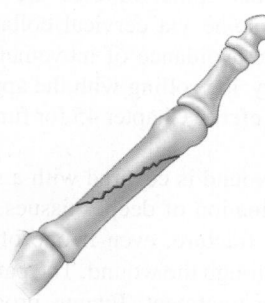

Oblique
A fracture occurring at an
angle across the bone (less
stable than a transverse fracture)

Open
A fracture in which damage also involves
the skin or mucous membranes, also called
a compound fracture

Pathologic
A fracture that occurs through an area of
diseased bone (e.g., osteoporosis, bone cyst,
Paget disease, bony metastasis, tumor); can
occur without trauma or fall

Simple
A fracture that remains contained,
with no disruption of the skin integrity

Spiral
A fracture that twists around
the shaft of the bone

Stress
A fracture that results from repeated
loading of bone and muscle

Transverse
A fracture that is straight
across the bone shaft

FIGURE 42-1 Specific types of fractures.

spasms that accompany a fracture begin shortly after the injury and result in increasing pain intensity and further bony fragmentation or malalignment.

Loss of Function

After a fracture, the extremity cannot function properly because normal function of the muscles depends on the integrity of the bones to which they are attached. Pain contributes to the loss of function. In addition, abnormal movement (false motion) may be present.

Deformity

Displacement, angulation, or rotation of the fragments in a fracture or soft tissue swelling causes a visible or palpable deformity. Movement may be noted at the fracture site, whereas under normal circumstances, movement of bones occurs only at joint.

Shortening

In fractures of long bones, there is actual shortening of the extremity because of the contraction of the muscles that are attached distal (furthest away) and proximal (nearest) to the site of the fracture. The fragments often overlap by as much as 2.5 to 5 cm (1 to 2 in).

Crepitus

Palpation of the extremity reveals a grating sensation, called crepitus, caused by the rubbing of the bone fragments against each other.

Swelling and Discoloration

Localized edema and ecchymosis occur as a result of trauma and bleeding into the tissues.

Fracture Blisters

Fracture blisters are tense blisters or bullae (large blister) associated with high-energy injuries commonly occurring in the ankle, elbow, foot, and/or knee. These sites have less anchoring of epidermal–dermal junction and little subcutaneous fat cushioning than do other areas in the limbs. Nurses should be alert to the potential for compartment syndrome (discussed on page 24) since fracture blisters represent underlying increased pressure. Prompt surgical intervention may reduce the incidence of fracture blister formation (within 4 hours after the acute injury). However, the presence of a fracture blister requires an alteration of the surgical approach or a delay in surgery because of potential increase in infection and skin breakdown (Geiderman & Katz, 2014). If possible, fracture blisters should not be disrupted because of risk of infection with skin flora. An ointment, such as silver sulfadiazine, may be applied to the blister to promote re-epithelialization and to prevent infection (Howe, 2016).

Managing Fractures

Immediately after injury, whenever a fracture is suspected, it is important to immobilize the body part before the patient is moved. If an injured patient must be moved before extremity **splints** can be applied, support the limb distal and proximal to the fracture site to prevent rotation as well as angular motion. It is important to recognize that movement of fracture fragments can cause additional pain, soft tissue damage, and neurovascular damage. Splinting a fracture can include bandaging the legs together, with the unaffected extremity serving as a splint for the injured one. In an upper extremity injury, the arm can be bandaged to the chest, a forearm placed in a **sling**, or a finger can be taped to the adjacent digit. Taping, splinting, or bandaging too tightly may cause impaired distal perfusion and thus is avoided. Immobilization is applied to the joints above and below the fracture. Neurovascular status distal to the injury is assessed before and after splinting to determine the adequacy of peripheral tissue perfusion and nerve function. An assessment of the patient also includes observing for the five warning "P's" associated with acute disruption of arterial flow: **p**ain, **p**oikilothermia (cold limb), **p**allor (paleness), **p**aresthesia (can range from numbness, "pins and needles," burning, itching, and/or tingling), and **p**ulselessness (weak pulses or delayed capillary refill; normal is less than 2 seconds).

If cervical and thoracolumbar spinal injuries are suspected, immobilization of the spine via cervical collar or spinal backboard as well as the avoidance of movement is essential. If moving is necessary, log rolling with the appropriate number of staff is used. Refer to Chapter 45 for further details of spinal fractures.

With an open fracture, the wound is covered with a sterile dressing to prevent contamination of deeper tissues. No attempt is made to reduce the fracture, even if one of the bone fragments is protruding through the wound. The patient is transferred to the hospital for treatment. Tetanus prophylaxis will be administered in the emergency room (ER) if the last known booster was over 5 years ago.

An immediate priority is maintaining hemodynamic stability. Hypovolemic shock, resulting from hemorrhage (both visible and nonvisible blood loss) and from loss of intravascular volume into the interstitial space, may occur in fractures of the extremities, thorax, pelvis, or spine. Because the bone is very vascular, large quantities of blood may be lost as a result of trauma, especially in fractures of the femur and pelvis. A closed fracture of the femur can have an estimated blood loss (EBL) of 1,000 to 1,500 mL, while a closed fracture of the tibia can be 500 to 1,000 mL. A closed humerus fracture can result in the loss of 250 mL, EBL for fracture to the radius and ulna can be 150 to 250 mL, while a pelvic fracture can cause the loss of 3 to 4 L of blood (Geiderman & Katz, 2014). An open fracture results in greater EBL, and increased risk of infection. The nurse is aware that bleeding is a common problem with fractures. The elderly may be

Focused Assessment

Hypovolemic Shock

Be alert for the following signs and symptoms:
- Thirst
- Anxiety, restlessness, altered sensorium
- Elevated heart rate
- Weak pulse (thready)
- Decreased blood pressure
- Cool, clammy skin
- Decreased urine output
- Decreased pulse pressure (difference between the systolic and diastolic pressure)
- Decreased blood pressure; mean arterial pressure (MAP) below 65 mm Hg
- Rapid, shallow respirations
- Delayed capillary refill

at increased risk if vasoconstriction is insufficient to maintain blood pressure. When an acute loss of 15% to 20% of blood volume occurs, a state of inadequate blood volume exists. This has a direct impact on perfusion; as the perfusion decreases, cardiac output falls, and multiple organ failure can occur. Box 42-2 provides focused assessment guidelines for hypovolemic shock. Treatment of shock consists of stabilizing the fracture to prevent further hemorrhage, restoring blood volume and circulation, relieving the patient's pain, providing adequate splinting, and protecting the patient from further injury and other complications.

Surgical Management

Many patients with unstable fractures undergo surgery to correct the condition. Frequent surgical procedures include **open reduction with internal fixation (ORIF)** and closed reduction with internal fixation (the fracture is reduced prior to making a surgical incision for "internal fixation" of the fracture) for fractures; amputation for severe extremity conditions (e.g., massive trauma); **bone graft** for joint stabilization, defect filling, or stimulation of bone healing; and **tendon transfer** for improving motion.

Ongoing Management

Nursing goals include improving function by restoring motion and stability, and relieving pain and disability. The principles of fracture treatment include reduction, immobilization, and regaining of normal function and strength through rehabilitation.

Reduction

Reduction of a fracture ("setting" the bone) refers to restoration of the fracture fragments to anatomic alignment and rotation. Either closed reduction or **open reduction** may be used to reduce a fracture. Before **fracture reduction** and

immobilization, the nurse prepares the patient for the procedure, assures permission for the procedure is obtained, and administers an analgesic as prescribed. The nurse gently handles the injured extremity to avoid additional damage.

Closed Reduction. In most instances, closed reduction is accomplished through manipulation and manual traction. The extremity is held in the desired position while the provider applies a cast, splint, or other device. Reduction under anesthesia with percutaneous pinning may be used. The immobilizing device maintains the reduction and stabilizes the extremity for bone healing. X-rays are obtained to verify that the bone fragments are aligned correctly.

Traction (skin or skeletal) may be used to effect fracture reduction and immobilization. Traction is discussed later in the chapter.

Open Reduction. With an open fracture, surgical intervention is needed to align the bone fragments. **Internal fixation** devices (metallic pins, wires, screws, plates, nails, or rods) are used to hold the bone fragments in position until bone healing occurs (Fig. 42-2). Internal fixation devices ensure firm approximation and fixation of the bony fragments. They

FIGURE 42-2 Techniques of internal fixation. **A.** Plate and six screws for a transverse or short oblique fracture. **B.** Screws for a long oblique or spiral fracture. **C.** Screws for a long butterfly fragment. **D.** Plate and six screws for a short butterfly fragment. **E.** Medullary nail for a segmental fracture.

are not designed to support the body's weight, and they can bend, loosen, or break if stressed. The estimated strength of the bone, the stability of the fracture, reduction and fixation, and the amount of bone healing are important considerations in determining weight-bearing limits. Although the incision may appear healed, the underlying bone requires more time to repair and regain normal strength. Some orthopedic procedures require weight-bearing restrictions. The orthopedic surgeon will prescribe the weight-bearing limits and the use of protective devices (orthoses), if necessary, after surgery.

Management of an Open Fracture

For patients with open fractures, prompt, thorough wound irrigation and **débridement** are necessary to remove foreign bodies, obvious debris, and bacteria. Often this is performed in the operating room. Once the wound is cleaned, the fracture is carefully reduced and stabilized by internal and/or external fixation. All open fractures are considered contaminated and carry risks for osteomyelitis (bone infection), tetanus, and gas gangrene. For this reason, systemic antibiotics are generally ordered and administered within 6 hours after open trauma to reduce the risk of soft tissue infection or osteomyelitis (Sebastin, Chung, & Ono, 2015). The nurse is mindful that fixation of fractures carries a risk of infection. The objectives of management are to prevent infection of the wound, soft tissue, and bone, and to promote healing of soft tissue and bone. Options include sterile dressing changes to allow drainage of wound and edema from heavily contaminated injuries; the use of wound vacuum–assisted closure (VAC) device; or re-exploration of the wound with débridement as necessary to remove infected and devitalized (dead) tissue and increase vascularity in the region. After it has been determined that infection is not present, the wound is closed by grafting of autogenous (patient's own tissue) skin, or a flap, or healing by secondary intention (a full-thickness wound heals from the base upward, by laying down new tissue). The nurse instructs the patient or family to monitor temperature at regular intervals and report signs of infection to their provider (Box 42-3). Infections must be treated promptly. In 4 to 8 weeks, bone grafting may be necessary to bridge bone defects and to stimulate bone healing.

BOX 42-3

Focused Assessment

Infection with an Open Fracture

Be alert for signs and symptoms of infection:
- Elevated temperature
- Tachycardia
- Tachypnea
- Redness, warmth, tenderness, purulent drainage at wound site
- Leukocytosis (elevated WBCs)

Nursing Alert

Do not rely on fever as a marker for infection in the elderly. Consider change in the level of consciousness as an indication of suspicion.

Immobilization

After the fracture has been reduced, the bone fragments must be immobilized, or held in correct position and alignment, until union occurs. Internal fixation, as described above, or external fixation via bandages, casts, and splints are methods used to immobilize fractures. Casts are discussed later in the chapter.

Unfolding Patient Stories: Marilyn Hughes • Part 1

Marilyn Hughes, a 45-year-old female, was brought to the emergency department by her husband after a fall down icy stairs. She is complaining of severe left lower leg pain. She is wearing long pants and boots. What are priority assessments and interventions that the nurse should implement for a suspected lower leg fracture? (Marilyn Hughes' story continues in Chapter 43.)

Care for Marilyn and other patients in a realistic virtual environment: *vSim for Nursing* (thepoint.lww.com/vSimMedicalSurgical). Practice documenting these patients' care in DocuCare (thepoint.lww.com/DocuCareEHR).

Nursing Management

The major goals for the patient with a fracture include knowledge of the treatment regimen, relief of pain, improved physical mobility, achievement of maximum level of self-care, healing of any trauma-associated lacerations and abrasions, maintenance of adequate neurovascular function, and absence of complications.

Teaching Related to Treatment Regimen

Anticipatory guidance is provided to the patient and significant others by explaining the sights, sounds, and sensations (e.g., heat from the hardening reaction of the plaster) associated with application of the internal or external device chosen to treat the fracture. Specific treatment modalities are discussed later in the chapter. Regardless of the treatment modality chosen for the fracture, patient teaching includes self-care, medication information, monitoring for potential complications, and the need for continuing health care supervision. Fracture healing and restoration of full strength and mobility may take many months.

Relieving Pain

The nurse must carefully evaluate pain associated with musculoskeletal conditions, asking the patient to indicate the exact site, character, and intensity of the pain to help determine its cause. Pain associated with the underlying condition (e.g., fracture) is frequently controlled by immobilization. Pain due to edema that is associated with trauma, surgery, or bleeding into the tissues frequently can be controlled by elevation and, if prescribed, intermittent application of cold packs. Ice bags (one third to one half full) or cold application devices are placed on each side of the cast or fixator, if prescribed, making sure not to indent the cast or put undue pressure on external pins. Analgesics are administered as prescribed.

Also pain may be indicative of complications. Unrelenting pain that is unresponsive to usual treatment measures (narcotics, elevation, cold) is associated with compartment syndrome. Severe pain over a bony prominence may warn of an impending pressure ulcer. Discomfort due to pressure on the skin may be relieved by elevation that controls edema or by positioning that alters pressure. However, the affected limb must be elevated no higher than heart level to ensure adequate arterial perfusion. If the fracture is casted, it may be necessary to modify the cast or to apply a new cast.

Nursing Alert

The nurse must never ignore complaints of pain from the patient in a cast because of the possibility of problems such as impaired tissue perfusion or pressure ulcer formation.

Improving Mobility

Every joint and digit that is not immobilized should be exercised and moved through its ROM to maintain function. The nurse encourages the patient to assist in the repositioning, if not contraindicated, by use of the **trapeze** or bed rail. If a patient has a spica cast (a cast that stabilizes the hips and thighs, also known as a body cast), a stabilizing **abduction** bar may be incorporated into the cast to maintain the legs in an abducted position. This bar should never be used as a turning device. If internal fixation is required to stabilize the fracture, the provider determines weight-bearing activity.

Because deep vein thrombosis (DVT) is a significant risk for the immobilized patient, the nurse encourages the patient to do active flexion–extension foot and ankle exercises and isometric contraction of the calf muscles (calf-pumping exercises) every hour while awake to decrease venous stasis in the unaffected limb. In addition, elastic stockings, intermittent compression devices, such as Venodyne boots, and anticoagulant therapy may be prescribed to help prevent thrombus formation. The nurse encourages the patient to move digits and joints distal to the injury hourly when awake to prevent problems related to inactivity (Murr, 2016).

Maintaining Adequate Neurovascular Function

The immobilized extremity's neurovascular status is assessed at least every hour initially, always comparing the affected extremity to the noninjured one. The nurse assesses for the "five P's," as described previously. Edema is a natural response of the tissue to trauma. If the edema is significant, pressure can rise within the area, compromising circulation as well as nerve and motor function. Early recognition of diminished circulation and nerve function, therefore, is essential to prevent loss of function. The affected extremity is adjusted so that it is no higher than heart level to control edema but not impede arterial perfusion. The surgeon is notified at once if signs of compromised neurovascular status are present. The nurse assesses the sensory and motor function of major nerves in the area of injury. Diminished circulation and nerve function must be treated promptly by release of constricting bandages. Refer to Box 42-4 for assessment of peripheral nerves of the upper extremities.

BOX 42-4

GUIDELINES FOR NURSING CARE

Assessing the Radial, Medial, and Ulnar Nerves

Implementation _____

NURSING ACTION	RATIONALE
1. To assess the radial nerve, ask the patient to extend the forefinger against resistance. If you suspect radial nerve damage, check the sensation at the web space between the thumb and index finger by asking the patient to describe the sensation to light touch.	1. Inability to extend finger or lack of sensation suggests radial nerve abnormality.
2. To test for median nerve integrity, ask the patient to make the "OK" sign using the thumb and forefinger to make a ring. Check the strength of the "O" by trying to open it with your fingers. Assess sensation on the distal surface of the index finger.	2. Weakness indicates a median nerve abnormality.
3. To assess the ulnar nerve, ask the patient to spread his fingers as widely as possible. Also check sensation to the little finger and the ulnar half of the ring finger by asking the patient to describe the sensation as you touch the area described.	3. Difficulty spreading fingers or lack of sensation suggests ulnar neuropathy.

Normal findings of the fractured limb include minimal edema and discomfort, pink color, warm to touch, capillary refill less than 2 seconds, normal sensations, and ability to move fingers or toes. Numbness, tingling, and burning may be caused by nerve injury from pressure at the fracture site. The nurse instructs the patient to report any changes in sensation or movement immediately so that they can be evaluated promptly.

Maintaining and Restoring Function

It is important to teach exercises to maintain the health of unaffected muscles and to increase the strength of muscles needed for transferring and for using assistive devices (e.g., crutches, walker, special utensils). The nurse and physical therapist teach patients how to use assistive devices safely. Isometric and muscle-setting exercises (discussed later in the chapter) are encouraged to minimize disuse atrophy and to promote circulation. Participation in activities of daily living (ADLs) is encouraged to promote independent functioning and self-esteem. Gradual resumption of activities is promoted within the therapeutic prescription. With internal fixation, the surgeon determines the amount of movement and weight-bearing stress the extremity can withstand and prescribes the level of activity. Plans are made to help patients modify their home environment as needed and to secure personal assistance if necessary.

Monitoring and Managing Potential Complications

Fat Embolism Syndrome

Emboli are clots that travel. In pelvic or long-bone fractures, in trauma patients, or in orthopedic surgeries, the fat globules released when the bone was fractured may occlude the small blood vessels that supply the lungs, brain, kidneys, and other organs.

At the time of fracture, fat globules may diffuse into the vascular compartment because the marrow pressure is greater than the capillary pressure or because catecholamines elevated by the patient's stress reaction mobilize fatty acids and promote the development of fat globules in the bloodstream (Porth, 2015). The onset of symptoms is rapid, usually within 12 to 72 hours of injury (Newbigin et al., 2016). Risk factors for fat embolism syndrome (FES) include trauma, fracture of long bones or pelvic bones, multiple fractures, crush injuries, or orthopedic surgery (intramedullary nail fixation, fixation of multiple fractures). FES occurs most frequently in young adults (typically in those 20 to 30 years of age) and in elderly adults who experience fractures of the proximal femur (hip fracture). Time to surgery has been implicated as a risk factor for FES; a fivefold decrease in the rate of FES was noted if surgery (intramedullary nail fixation) was performed in the first 24 hours of injury (Newbigin et al., 2016).

Presenting features of FES include a triad of pulmonary, central nervous system (CNS), and skin manifestations, which may include a change in behavior and disorientation combined with respiratory compromise (nearly 90% of symptoms are pulmonary) and a petechial rash (Newbigin et al., 2016). The nurse observes for hypoxia, tachypnea, tachycardia, and pyrexia. The respiratory distress response includes dyspnea, crackles, wheezes, and substernal chest pain. The cerebral disturbances (due to hypoxia and the lodging of fat emboli in the brain) manifest by mental status changes varying from headache and mild agitation to confusion, delirium, and coma. The skin manifestations include petechial rash to the axillary, subconjunctival, or chest (upper anterior torso) region; however, this rash does not appear until 3 to 5 days after the onset of respiratory symptoms and thus is generally not helpful in establishing an early diagnosis (Newbigin et al., 2016).

Occlusion of a large number of small vessels causes the pulmonary pressure to rise. Edema and hemorrhages in the alveoli impair oxygen transport, leading to hypoxia. Arterial blood gas values show the partial pressure of oxygen (PaO_2) to be less than 70 mm Hg, with early respiratory alkalosis (hyperventilation) and later respiratory acidosis (hypoventilation). The chest x-ray reveals a typical "snowstorm" infiltrate; however, this finding is associated with other pathologies, thus a CT of the chest and, in particular, high-resolution CT (HRCT) is the modality of choice to assess for FES (Newbigin et al., 2016). Magnetic resonance imaging (MRI) may be performed to diagnose cerebral fat embolism. Without prompt, definitive treatment, acute pulmonary edema, acute respiratory distress syndrome (ARDS), and heart failure may develop.

With systemic embolization, the patient appears pale. Petechiae, possibly due to a transient thrombocytopenia, are noted in the buccal membranes and conjunctival sacs, on the hard palate, and over the chest and anterior axillary folds. The patient develops a fever greater than 39.5°C (~103°F). Free fat may be found in the urine if emboli are filtered by the renal tubules; however, this is a nonspecific finding in the setting of multitrauma (Newbigin et al., 2016). Acute tubular necrosis and kidney failure may develop.

Immediate immobilization of fractures (including early surgical fixation), minimal fracture manipulation, adequate support for fractured bones during turning and positioning, and maintenance of fluid and electrolyte balance are measures that may reduce the incidence of fat emboli. The nurse monitors high-risk patients (adults between 20 and 30 years of age with long-bone, pelvic, or multiple fractures or crush injuries, and elderly patients with hip fractures, or multiple fixations of fractures) to identify this complication. Prompt initiation of respiratory support is essential to prevent respiratory failure and to correct homeostatic disturbances. Acute pulmonary edema and ARDS are the most common causes of death. Oxygen therapy, mechanical ventilation, and use of positive end-expiratory pressure (PEEP) may be used to maintain arterial oxygenation. Continuous monitoring of oxygen saturation is initiated. Corticosteroids may be administered IV to treat the inflammatory lung reaction and to control cerebral edema in cases of fulminant FES. However, current evidence does not support routine administration in the majority of patients (Newbigin et al., 2016). Vasopressor medications to support cardiovascular function are administered IV to prevent hypotension, shock, and interstitial pulmonary edema. Accurate fluid intake and output records facilitate adequate fluid replacement therapy. In addition, the nurse provides calm reassurance to allay apprehension. FES has a 7% mortality rate; therefore, the nurse must recognize early indications of FES and report them promptly to the provider (Newbigin et al., 2016).

> ### *Nursing Alert*
> *Subtle personality changes, restlessness, irritability, or confusion in a patient who has sustained a fracture are indications for immediate reassessment of the patient (vitals, O$_2$ saturation, physical examination, and laboratory data).*

Delayed Union, Malunion, and Nonunion

When prolonged healing for union of the fracture is noted, it is termed **delayed union**. The fracture eventually does heal. In **malunion**, there is flawed union of fractured bone, whereas **nonunion** results from failure of the ends of a fractured bone to unite in normal alignment. Patient complaints of persistent discomfort and abnormal movement or instability at the fracture site indicate potential delayed union, malunion, or nonunion.

Delayed union may be due to inadequate blood supply, inadequate bone-to bone-contact, infection, or incorrect immobilization of the fracture. It may be associated with a fracture that involved a significant loss of bone, a hematoma at the fracture site, or comorbidity (e.g., diabetes mellitus, autoimmune disease). Malunion is associated with inadequate reduction of the fracture, misalignment of the fracture at the time of immobilization, or infection at the fracture site, and it presents as a deformity at the site visually or on x-ray. In nonunion, fibrocartilage or fibrous tissue exists between the bone fragments; no bone salts have been deposited. Nonunion is associated with infection, inadequate circulation, malignancy, and noncompliance with activity restrictions. Cigarette smoking and poor nutrition place the patient at a higher risk of delayed healing, and higher nonunion rates (Brinker & O'Connor, 2015). Nonunion most commonly occurs with open tibia fractures, scaphoid fractures, fractures of the fifth metatarsal or the hamate (carpal bone in the wrist), and, in elderly people, at the neck of the femur because of their tenuous blood supply. Factors contributing to both nonunion and malunion include interposition of tissue between the bone ends, or manipulation that disrupts callus formation, excessive space between bone fragments (bone gap), limited bone contact, bone or soft tissue loss, and impaired blood supply, resulting in AVN. Finally, a false joint (pseudarthrosis) often develops at the site of the fracture.

> ### *Nursing Alert*
> *Nurses encourage patients with bone fractures to quit smoking since nicotine inhibits vascular ingrowth and early revascularization of bone and diminishes osteoblast activity. Additionally, poor nutrition is a risk factor for impaired fracture healing. A serum albumin level of at least 3.0 g/dL is preferred (Brinker & O'Connor, 2015).*

Nonsteroidal anti-inflammatory drugs (NSAIDs) and older nonselective anti-cyclooxygenase (COX)-2 agents have been implicated in delayed fracture healing, although the magnitude of the effect of these drugs on fracture healing in humans is uncertain, and a causal relationship has not been proven (Solomon, 2015). Cigarette smoking, poor nutrition, excessive alcohol intake, diabetes, and use of steroids place the patient at a higher risk of delayed healing.

Nonunion is treated with internal fixation, bone grafting, electrical bone stimulation (thought to stimulate osteoblasts or bone formation), or a combination of these therapies. Internal fixation stabilizes the bone fragments and ensures bone contact. A bone graft may be an **autograft** (tissue, frequently from the iliac crest, harvested from the patient for his or her own use) or an **allograft** (tissue harvested from a donor for a recipient). The bone graft fills the bone gap, provides a lattice structure for invasion by bone cells, and actively promotes bone growth.

After grafting, immobilization and non–weight-bearing exercises are required while the bone graft becomes incorporated and the fracture or defect heals. Depending on the type of bone grafted, healing may take from 6 to 12 months or longer. Bone grafting problems include wound or graft infection, fracture of the graft, persistent pain, sensory loss, and nonunion (Brinker & O'Connor, 2015).

Venous Thromboemboli

Venous thromboemboli, including DVT and pulmonary emboli (PE), are associated with reduced skeletal muscle contractions and bed rest. Patients with fractures of the lower extremities and pelvis are at high risk for venous thromboemboli. PEs may cause death several days to weeks after injury.

Depending on the size and location of the emboli, symptoms vary. A large PE can cause an increase in pulmonary arterial resistance, which can lead to right heart failure and hypoxemia (DeHart, 2015). Massive emboli can present as shock and loss of consciousness. The most frequent signs are sudden-onset shortness of breath (dyspnea), restlessness, increased respiratory rate, tachycardia, chest pain, cough, and low-grade fever. Pleuritic pain that increases with inspiration is seen with pulmonary infarct. Moderate hypoxemia occurs, without retention of CO$_2$, and a cough that is productive of blood-tinged sputum may be seen. It is important that a high degree of suspicion is maintained for PE since patients may have mild or nonspecific symptoms. Refer to Chapters 18 and 10 for details on DVT and PE.

Disseminated Intravascular Coagulation

Disseminated intravascular coagulation (DIC) is a systemic disorder that results in widespread hemorrhage and microthrombosis with ischemia. Its causes are diverse and can include massive tissue trauma. Early manifestations of DIC include unexpected bleeding after surgery as well as bleeding from the mucous membranes, venipuncture sites, and gastrointestinal and urinary tracts. The treatment of DIC is discussed in Chapter 20.

Avascular Necrosis of Bone

AVN or osteonecrosis occurs when the bone loses its blood supply and dies. The cause of AVN is not well understood but may include vascular occlusion, altered lipid metabolism/fat emboli, intravascular coagulation, mechanical stress, and primary cell death (Qasem, 2016). It may occur after a fracture with disruption of the blood supply (especially of the femoral neck). It is also seen with dislocations, bone transplantation, prolonged high-dose corticosteroid therapy, excessive alcohol intake, cigarette smoking, chronic kidney disease, systemic lupus erythematosus, and other diseases. Use of glucocorticoids and excessive alcohol intake are associated with more than 80% of atraumatic cases of AVN (Jones & Mount, 2014). The devitalized bone may collapse or reabsorb. The patient develops pain and experiences limited movement. X-rays reveal loss of mineralized matrix and structural collapse. Treatment generally consists of attempts to revitalize the bone with bone grafts, prosthetic replacement, or **arthrodesis** (joint fusion).

Reaction to Internal Fixation Devices

Internal fixation devices may be removed after bony union has taken place. However, in most patients, the device is not removed unless it produces symptoms. Common reasons cited for removal include pain, neurologic symptoms, decreased function, or fear of future complications in active individuals (Bessette & Hammert, 2014). Problems may include mechanical failure (inadequate insertion and stabilization); material failure (faulty or damaged device); corrosion of the device, causing local inflammation; allergic response to the metallic alloy used; and osteoporotic remodeling adjacent to the fixation device, in which stress needed for bone strength is transferred to the device, causing a disuse osteoporosis. If the device is removed, the bone needs to be protected from refracture related to osteoporosis, altered bone structure, and trauma. Bone remodeling reestablishes the bone's structural strength.

Reaction to External Fixation Devices

Because the screws or pins are inserted externally (Fig. 42-3), infection is a complication for which nurses must be vigilant. Rates of pin tract infections range from 0.5% to 30% in the literature when looking at external fixation (regardless of site) (Mitchell et al., 2016). Signs of infection include erythema, purulent drainage, warmth, leukocytosis, fever, and loosening pins (pins should be immobile in the bone). It is important to note that in a recent review of international protocols of

FIGURE 42-3 External fixation device. Pins are inserted into bone. The fracture is reduced and aligned and then stabilized by attaching the pins to a rigid portable frame. The device facilitates treatment of soft tissue damaged in complex fractures.

pin-site care where practice varied, no one standard was associated with a 0% infection rate. Currently no consensus exists about which protocol should be applied universally (Lethaby, Temple, & Santy-Tomlinson, 2013; Mitchell et al., 2016). The mainstay of prevention and/or reduction of the incidence of pin-site infections is surgical technique during pin insertion and implementation of one of the existing protocols of pin-site care. Thus, pin care is performed according to hospital and provider protocol (Mitchell et al., 2016, p. 91).

Complex Regional Pain Syndrome

Complex regional pain syndrome (CRPS), formerly called *reflex sympathetic dystrophy* or *RSD*, is a painful sympathetic nervous system problem characterized by constant and intense limb pain associated with vasomotor and neurosensory abnormalities, skin changes, and demineralization of bone (Ferri, 2016a). It occurs in 7% of patients who have limb fractures, limb surgery, or other injuries (burns, stroke) (Bruehl, 2015). When it does occur, it is seen most often in women (60% to 82%); with a mean range of 36 to 46 years of age; whose injury was a fracture (16% to 46%), strain, or sprain (10% to 29%); was acquired postoperatively (3% to 24%); or from a contusion or crush injury (8% to 18%) (Dinakar, 2016). There are two types of CRPS: in *CRPS I* no definable nerve lesion is found, whereas in *CRPS II* definable nerve lesion is seen (Dinakar, 2016).

Clinical manifestations of CRPS include severe burning pain, swelling, hyperesthesia, limited ROM, discoloration, vasomotor skin changes (i.e., fluctuating warm, red, dry and cold, sweaty, cyanotic), and abnormal nail, skin, and hair changes. *Livedo reticularis* is common in CRPS; *Livedo* describes the red, nonblanchable (i.e., does not turn white when pressed) network pattern (reticulated) in the skin. About 60% of patients may report excessive sweating in the affected limbs. Temperature asymmetry between the affected and unaffected sides may exceed 1°C (Dinakar, 2016). The cardinal feature of CRPS is excruciating pain, often described as burning, aching, pricking, or shooting. Also edema of the affected limb frequently is present; initially it may be very mild; however, it may be so severe that a Doppler test is needed to rule out the possibility of a DVT (Dinakar, 2016). This syndrome is frequently chronic, with extension of symptoms to adjacent areas of the body. Disuse muscle atrophy and bone deossification (osteoporosis) occur with persistence of CRPS. Patients may exhibit ineffective individual coping related to the chronic pain. The best treatment is prevention with vitamin C supplementation and early active mobilization, imagery treatment with imagined hand movements and mirror therapy for upper extremity CRPS, and pharmacologic treatment.

Prevention may include elevation of the extremity after injury or surgery and selection of an immobilization device (e.g., external fixator) that allows for the greatest ROM and functional use of the rest of the extremity. Early effective pain relief is the focus of management. Pain may need to be controlled with a variety of agents, including anesthetic nerve blocks, spinal cord stimulation, tricyclic antidepressants, anticonvulsants, NSAIDs, corticosteroids, muscle relaxants, and, for those with severe pain, an opioid. Bisphosphonates also are considered. Physical and occupational therapy (including imagery and mirror therapy), tai chi, and yoga have been recommended (Bruehl, 2015; Jones, Lawson, & Backonja, 2016). With pain relief, the patient can participate in ROM exercises and functional use of the affected area. The nurse needs to help the patient cope with CRPS manifestations and explore multiple ways to control pain (see Chapter 7).

Nursing Alert
Since patients with CRPS feel severe and long-lasting pain to light touch, the nurse avoids using the involved extremity for blood pressure measurements and venipunctures.

Heterotopic Ossification

Heterotopic ossification (myositis ossificans) is the abnormal formation of bone, near bones or in muscle, in response to soft tissue trauma after blunt trauma, fracture, or total joint replacement. It is also commonly seen in patients with traumatic brain injury, spinal cord injury, cerebrovascular accident (CVA), and burns (Harrington, Eliason, & Bockenek, 2015). Heterotopic ossification is both more common and more extensive in patients with severe spasticity, with incidence rates varying from 11% to 75% in patients with severe traumatic brain injury and spinal cord injury (Harrington et al., 2015). The muscle is painful, and normal muscular contraction and movement are limited. Early mobilization may prevent its occurrence. NSAIDs (e.g., ibuprofen [Advil, Motrin]) to decrease inflammation or bone formation and prophylactic low-dose radiation therapy have been shown to help prevent heterotopic ossification after total hip arthroplasty (THA). Usually, the bone lesion resorbs over time, but the abnormal bone eventually may need to be excised if symptoms persist. Exercises to maintain joint ROM are considered the foundation of prevention, and continuous passive motion (CPM) machines are beneficial in increasing ROM after surgical resection.

Fractures of Specific Sites

Injuries to the skeletal structure may vary from a simple linear fracture to a severe crushing injury. The type and location of the fracture and the extent of damage to surrounding structures determine the therapeutic management. Maximum functional recovery is the goal of management.

Clavicle

Fracture of the clavicle (collar bone) is a common injury that results from a fall or a direct blow to the shoulder. These injuries frequently are associated with equestrian sports and cycling, when a rider is thrown forward and lands on the unprotected shoulder. Head or cervical spine injuries may accompany these fractures. They are also seen in the geriatric population after a low-impact fall. When the clavicle is fractured, the patient assumes a protective position, slumping the shoulders and immobilizing the arm to prevent shoulder movements. A deformity of the clavicle may be observed, with obvious local tenderness. The treatment goal is to align the shoulder in its normal position by means of closed reduction and immobilization or, if displaced, an ORIF.

Depending on the site of the clavicular fracture, most minimally displaced or nondisplaced fractures can be treated nonsurgically with a sling or a figure-eight bandage (also called a *clavicular strap* or *broad arm sling*) to pull the shoulders back, reducing and immobilizing the fracture (Fig. 42-4) (Silverstein, Moeller, & Hutchinson, 2016). Each treatment has advantages and disadvantages. When a clavicular strap is used, the axillae are well padded to prevent skin breakdown or a compression injury to the brachial plexus and the axillary artery. In most cases, a simple sling for comfort is adequate over the first few

FIGURE 42-4 Fracture of the clavicle. **A**. Anteroposterior view shows typical displacement in midclavicular fracture. **B**. Immobilization is accomplished with a clavicular strap.

weeks followed by progressive ROM activities (Silverstein et al., 2016). If the clavicle is displaced significantly or if there is significant comminution or excessive shortening (more than 2 cm), referral to an orthopedic surgeon is warranted. When internal fixation is indicated, surgery may be performed with either a plate and screws or an intramedullary device.

The nurse monitors the skin integrity and circulation and nerve function of both arms. An arm sling may be used to support the arm and to relieve pain. A sling may cause the elbow to stiffen so the patient is encouraged to perform elbow ROM exercises to maintain normal function and prevent stiffness. The patient may be permitted to use the arm for light activities within the range of comfort.

With a clavicular fracture, the nurse cautions the patient not to elevate the arm above the shoulder level until the ends of the bone have united (about 6 weeks) but encourages the patient to exercise the elbow, wrist, and fingers as soon as possible. Vigorous activity is limited for 3 months. Complications of clavicular fractures include trauma to the nerves of the brachial plexus, injury to the subclavian vein or artery from a bony fragment, and malunion (faulty union of fractured bone) or nonunion (failure of the ends of a fractured bone to unite in normal alignment). Nonunion occurs more frequently with distal clavicular fractures managed nonsurgically.

Humeral Shaft

Fractures of the shaft of the humerus may injure the nerves and brachial blood vessels in the affected arm; therefore, neurovascular assessment is essential to identify when immediate attention is required. Table 42-2 provides guidelines for neurovascular evaluation. A wrist drop is indicative of radial nerve injury. An inability to oppose the thumb indicates a median nerve lesion, and an inability to spread the fingers indicates an ulnar nerve injury (Acklin & Sommer, 2015). An ORIF of a fracture of the humerus is necessary if the patient has nerve palsy, blood vessel damage, comminuted fracture, or pathologic fracture. There are two distinct populations who are more at-risk for humeral shaft fractures: young adults injured in high-energy motor vehicle accidents, falls from height, or gunshots; and the elderly who falls from a standing height.

If the fracture is uncomplicated, well-padded splints, overwrapped with an elastic bandage, are used to immobilize the upper arm initially and to support the arm in 90 degrees of flexion at the elbow. A sling or collar and cuff support the forearm (Fig. 42-5). The weight of the hanging arm and splints reduces the fracture. Functional bracing is another form of treatment used for these fractures. A contoured thermoplastic sleeve is secured in place with interlocking fabric (Velcro) closures around the upper arm, thus immobilizing the reduced fracture. As swelling decreases, the sleeve is tightened, and uniform pressure and bone stability is maintained. The forearm is supported with a collar and cuff sling. Functional bracing allows active use of muscles, motion in the shoulder and elbow, and good approximation of fracture fragments. After, the first week, pendulum shoulder exercises are performed as prescribed to provide active movement of the shoulder, thereby preventing adhesions of the shoulder joint capsule (Acklin & Sommer, 2015). If an ORIF was required for the humeral fracture, immediate mobilization of the elbow joint and active-assisted shoulder mobilization should be possible (Acklin & Sommer, 2015). Isometric exercises may be prescribed to prevent muscle atrophy. Complications that are seen with humeral shaft fractures include delayed union and nonunion (failure of the ends of a fractured bone to unite).

Elbow

Fractures of the elbow result from motor vehicle crashes, falls on the elbow (in the extended or flexed position), or a direct blow. Radial head fractures are the most common fractures involving the elbow; however, the distal humerus or proximal ulna is also commonly involved. Nondisplaced or minimally displaced fractures can be treated nonoperatively; however, a displaced fracture may require operative treatment. Elbow fractures may result in injury to the median, radial, or ulnar nerves. The patient is evaluated for paresthesia and signs of compromised circulation in the forearm and hand. The most serious complication is *Volkmann contracture* (an acute compartment syndrome [ACS]), which

TABLE **42-2** Neurovascular Assessment and Expected Findings

Assessment Component	Technique	Normal Findings
Skin color	Evaluate the injured area in relation to the noninjured area.	No change is noted compared to other parts of the body.
Skin temperature	Palpate using the dorsum of the hand as it is more sensitive to temperature.	No change is noted compared to other parts of the body.
Pulses	Assess proximal and distal pulses. Grade as 0, absent; 1+, weaker than normal; 2+, normal; or 3+, full and bounding.	No change is noted compared to other extremity.
Capillary refill	Depress the nail bed and note return of color.	Capillary refill is less than 2 seconds.
Sensation	With his eyes closed, evaluate the patient's ability to feel light touch of the affected extremity (e.g., assess on the first web space of foot [between great toe and second toe] for the peroneal nerve, or base of thumb [radial nerve], or little finger [ulnar nerve]). Assess presence of numbness or tingling.	No sensory deficit is noted.
Mobility	Observe the ROM in joints or digits distal to the injury.	Full movement of digits is noted.
	Note edema and tenseness of the injured area.	Minimal edema and ecchymosis are noted.
	Mark and measure circumference if concerned.	In a nontraumatized limb, a difference of 1 cm at the ankles and 2 cm at mid-calf is expected.

results from antecubital swelling or damage to the brachial artery (Fig. 42-6). Contracture of the fingers and wrist occurs as the result of obstructed arterial blood flow to the forearm and hand. The patient is unable to extend the fingers, describes abnormal sensation (e.g., unrelenting pain, pain on passive stretch), and exhibits signs of diminished circulation

to the hand. Although the incidence of Volkmann contracture is low, its devastating complications are preventable if detected early. This serious complication warrants nursing vigilance to minimize limb loss. The nurse needs to monitor the patient regularly for compromised neurovascular status. Refer back to Box 42-4 for focused assessment guidelines for evaluation of the radial, medial, and ulnar nerve in upper extremity fractures. Severe pain at the elbow and increasing tenseness of the forearm are worrisome signs of increasing intracompartmental pressure. Compartment syndrome is discussed on pages 1232–1234.

 Nursing Alert
Absence of a radial pulse is a critical finding that warrants emergency notification of the provider.

FIGURE 42-5 Humeral brace with collar and cuff sling.

FIGURE 42-6 Volkmann contracture.

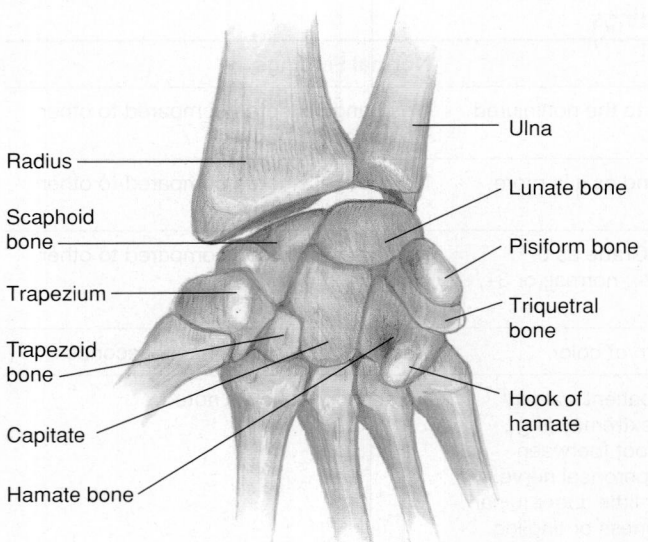

Radius

Scaphoid bone

Trapezium

Trapezoid bone

Capitate

Hamate bone

Ulna

Lunate bone

Pisiform bone

Triquetral bone

Hook of hamate

FIGURE 42-7 Palmar view of Carpal bones. (Courtesy of Anatomical Chart Company.)

Hand

Trauma to the hand often requires extensive reconstructive surgery. The objective of treatment is always to regain maximum function of the hand. Scaphoid fractures (bone on the thumb side of the wrist) are the most common carpal bone fractures, far exceeding all other carpal bone injuries. Fifteen percent of patients with scaphoid displacement exhibit nonunion, and 10% of fractures develop AVN because of disturbances in blood supply (Owens, 2016). Refer to Figure 42-7 for carpel bones details. Patient complaints include radial-sided wrist pain, tenderness in the anatomical snuff box, bruising, and edema (swelling at the base of the thumb). Cast treatment results in healing of the majority of scaphoid fractures. For an undisplaced fracture of the phalanx (finger bone), the finger is splinted for 3 to 4 weeks to relieve pain and to protect the finger from further trauma. Displaced fractures and open fractures may require ORIF, using wires or pins.

Arm

The most frequently broken arm bone is the radius, and the site most commonly affected is the distal radius. Termed a Colles fracture (the broken fragment of the radius tilts upward), the distal radius fracture usually is the result of a fall on an open, dorsiflexed hand. This fracture is frequently seen in elderly women with osteoporotic bones and weak soft tissues that do not dissipate the energy of the fall or in younger people involved in high impact trauma (e.g., falls, sports injuries). The patient presents with a deformed wrist, radial deviation, pain, swelling, weakness, limited finger ROM, and numbness.

Treatment usually consists of closed reduction and immobilization with a short-arm cast if the fracture is nondisplaced or minimally displaced. The extremity may be treated initially in a splint for 5 to 7 days until swelling subsides and then casted in a short-arm cast. For fractures with extensive comminution (bone is broken into a number of pieces) or impaction, ORIF, arthroscopic percutaneous pinning, or external fixation is used to achieve and maintain reduction and to allow for early functional rehabilitation. The wrist and forearm are elevated for 48 hours after reduction to control swelling, and active motion of the fingers and shoulder begins promptly. The nurse monitors for signs of neurovascular compromise comparing findings on the affected limb to the other limb.

Tibia and Fibula

The most common fractures below the knee are tibia and fibula fractures, and these tend to result from a direct blow, falls with the foot in a flexed position, or a violent twisting motion. The patient presents with pain, deformity, obvious hematoma, and considerable edema. Frequently, these fractures are open and involve severe soft tissue damage because there is little subcutaneous tissue in the area.

The peroneal nerve is assessed for damage that may result in foot drop (inability to lift the foot), by checking for sensation of the web between the great and second toes, and for increased sensitivity of the dorsal surfaces of the foot (top). If nerve function is impaired, the patient cannot dorsiflex the great toe and has diminished sensation in the first web space (between first metatarsal and hallux [big toe]). As with all fractures, the patient is observed for signs of neurovascular complications. The development of ACS (see discussion later in this chapter) requires prompt recognition and resolution to prevent permanent functional deficit. Other complications include delayed union, infection, impaired wound edge healing due to limited soft tissue, and loosening of the internal fixation hardware (if ORIF is performed to repair fracture).

Most closed tibial fractures are treated with closed reduction and initial immobilization in a long-leg walking cast or a patellar tendon–bearing cast. Reduction must be relatively accurate in relation to angulation and rotation. Comminuted fractures may be treated with skeletal traction, internal fixation with intramedullary nails or plates and screws, or external fixation. External support may be used with internal fixation.

Pelvis

Numerous classification systems have been used to describe pelvic fractures in relation to pelvic anatomy, stability, and mechanism of injury. Some fractures of the pelvis do not disrupt the pelvic ring; others do—therefore the severity of pelvic fractures varies.

Stable Pelvic Fractures

Stable fractures of the pelvis (Fig. 42-8) heal rapidly because the pelvic bones are mostly cancellous bone, which has a

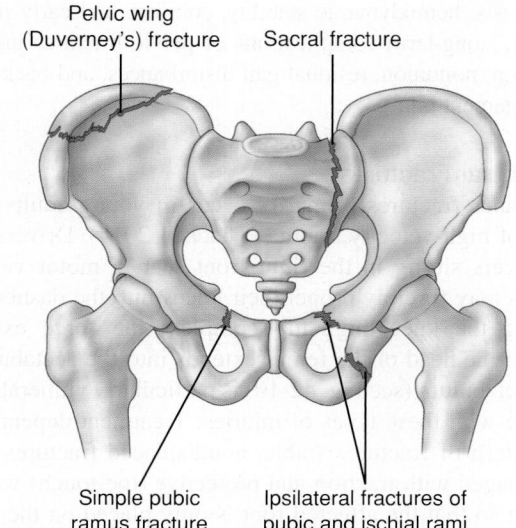

FIGURE 42-8 Stable pelvic fractures.

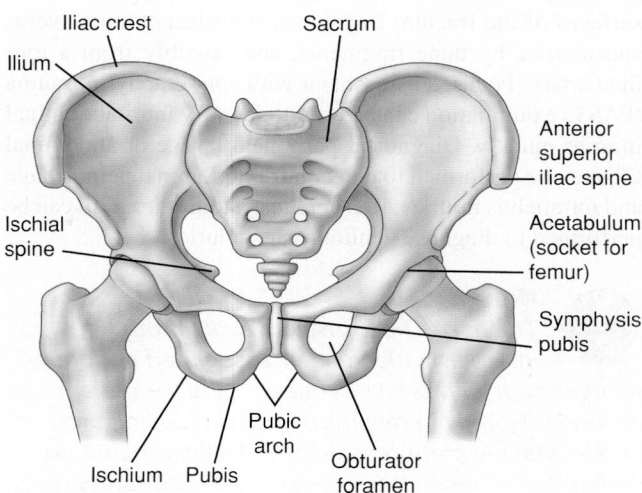

FIGURE 42-10 Pelvic bones.

rich blood supply. The fractures are treated with a few days of bed rest and symptom management until the pain and discomfort are controlled. The patient with a fractured sacrum is at risk for paralytic ileus, and bowel sounds should be monitored.

Unstable Pelvic Fractures

Unstable fractures of the pelvis may result in rotational instability (e.g., the "open book" type, in which a separation occurs at the symphysis pubis with sacral ligament disruption), vertical instability (e.g., the vertical shear type, with superior–inferior displacement), or a combination of both (Fig. 42-9).

Managing Pelvic Fractures

Falls, motor vehicle crashes, and crush injuries can cause pelvic fractures. Pelvic fractures are serious because at least two thirds of affected patients have significant and multiple injuries. Twenty percent of multitrauma patients sustain pelvic fractures

with a mortality rate approaching 15% to 20%, whereas if the pelvic fracture is open, a mortality rate of 25% to 50% is seen (Perkins & Quinnan, 2016). Management of severe, life-threatening pelvic fractures is coordinated with the trauma team. Hemorrhage and thoracic, intra-abdominal, and cranial injuries have priority over treatment of fractures. There is a high mortality rate associated with pelvic fractures related to hemorrhage, pulmonary complications, fat emboli, thromboembolic complications, and infection.

Signs and symptoms of pelvic fracture include ecchymosis; tenderness over the symphysis pubis, anterior iliac spines, iliac crest, sacrum, or coccyx; local edema; numbness or tingling of the pubis, genitals, and proximal thighs; and inability to bear weight without discomfort. Neurovascular assessment of the lower extremities is performed to detect injury to pelvic blood vessels and nerves. Figure 42-10 details the pelvic bones. The peripheral pulses of both lower extremities are palpated; absence of a pulse may indicate a tear in the iliac artery or one of its branches.

Hemorrhage and shock are two of the most serious consequences that may occur. Bleeding arises from the cancellous

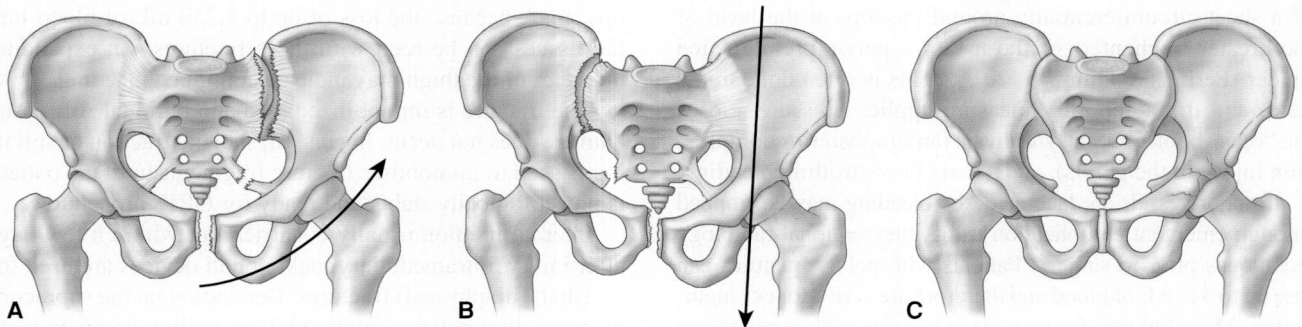

FIGURE 42-9 Unstable pelvic fracture. **A.** Rotationally unstable fracture. The symphysis pubis is separated and the anterior sacroiliac, sacrotuberous, and sacrospinous ligaments are disrupted. **B.** Vertically unstable fracture. The hemipelvis is displaced anteriorly and posteriorly through the symphysis pubis, and the sacroiliac joint ligaments is disrupted. **C.** Undisplaced fracture of the acetabulum.

surfaces of the fracture fragments, from laceration of veins and arteries by bone fragments, and possibly from a torn iliac artery. Focused assessment with sonography in trauma (FAST) examination can be used to identify intra-abdominal injuries quickly. Diagnostic peritoneal lavage or abdominal CT may be performed to detect intra-abdominal hemorrhage and intrapelvis injuries. Retrograde cystourethrogram can be performed to diagnose genitourinary injuries.

> **⚠ Nursing Alert**
> *The risk of hemorrhagic shock from intrapelvic bleeding or associated abdominal injury is high with pelvic fractures, thus the patient is handled gently to minimize further bleeding and shock. Manual compression of the pelvis should be avoided, and, when log rolling the patient, rotation more than 15 degrees is avoided until the patient is stabilized (Perkins & Quinnan, 2016).*

Injuries to the bladder, urethra, rectum, intestines, other abdominal organs, and pelvic vessels and nerves are associated with pelvic fracture. Injuries to the bladder and urethra are seen most commonly (63%) (Perkins & Quinnan, 2016). To assess for urinary tract injury, the patient's urine is examined for blood (hematuria) or blood at the introitus, or if the patient is a male, observed for scrotal hematoma. A urinary drainage catheter should not be inserted until the status of the urethra is known. Ecchymosis of the anterior abdominal wall, flank, or sacral or gluteal region is suggestive of significant internal bleeding. Diffuse and intense abdominal pain, hyperactive or absent bowel sounds, and abdominal rigidity and hyper-resonance (free air) or dullness to percussion (blood) suggest injury to the intestines or abdominal bleeding. Additionally, the nurse is aware that the loss of dullness over the liver (normally percusses a dull sound) indicates the presence of free air and that dullness over regions normally tympanic may indicate the presence of blood or fluid.

Immediate treatment in the emergency department of a patient with an unstable pelvic fracture includes stabilizing the pelvic bones and tamponading or compressing bleeding vessels. A simple method of stabilizing the pelvis is the tying of a sheet circumferentially around the hips at the level of the greater trochanters or the use of a pelvic prefabricated binder (Perkins & Quinnan, 2016). This is often done in the field, and this temporary measure applies pressure, closes the "open-book" pubic symphysis (anteroposterior compression injury to the pelvis), and assists in controlling bleeding.

If major vessels are lacerated, the bleeding may be stopped through emergent embolization using interventional radiology techniques prior to surgery. Patients with pelvic fractures can lose up to 4 to 5 L of blood and therefore are at risk for exsanguination. Mortality rate for patients presenting with hypotension associated with pelvic fractures is approximately 50%. Once the patient is hemodynamically stable, treatment generally involves external fixation or ORIF. These measures promote hemostasis, hemodynamic stability, comfort, and early mobilization. Long-term complications of pelvic fractures include malunion, nonunion, residual gait disturbances, and back pain from ligament injury.

Acetabular Fractures

Acetabular fractures primarily occur in young adults as a result of high-velocity trauma (Thacker, 2014). Drivers and passengers sitting in the right front seat in motor vehicle crashes may forcibly propel their knees into the dashboard, injuring the knee–thigh–hip complex; the force exerted through the head of the femur extends into the acetabulum. The acetabulum (see Fig. 42-10) is particularly vulnerable to fracture with these types of injuries. Treatment depends on the pattern of fracture. Stable, nondisplaced fractures may be managed with traction and protective (toe-touch) weight bearing so that the affected foot is only placed on the floor for balance. Displaced and unstable acetabular fractures are treated with open reduction, joint débridement, and internal fixation or arthroplasty (replacement of all or part of the joint surfaces). Internal fixation permits early non–weight-bearing ambulation and ROM exercise. Complications seen with acetabular fractures include nerve palsy, AVN, heterotopic ossification, and posttraumatic arthritis.

Femoral Shaft

Considerable force is required to break the shaft of the femur in adults since it is the longest and strongest bone in the body. Most femoral fractures are seen in young adults who have been involved in a motor vehicle crash, who have fallen from a high place, or who have received a gunshot wound. Older women with osteoporosis are also at risk for femur shaft fractures after low to moderate level trauma (Gösling & Giannoudis, 2015). Frequently, these patients have associated multiple injuries and significant soft tissue damage.

The nurse assesses for the presence and location of the pain, edema, bruising, deformity, and instability. The patient presents with an enlarged, deformed, painful thigh and cannot move the hip or the knee. The fracture may be transverse, oblique, spiral, or comminuted. Frequently, the patient develops shock because the loss of up to 1,250 mL of blood into the tissues can be seen with these fractures. An expanding diameter of the thigh may indicate continued bleeding.

The fracture is immobilized so that additional soft tissue damage does not occur. In general, skeletal traction or splinting is used to immobilize fracture fragments until the patient is physiologically stable and ready for ORIF procedures.

Internal fixation usually is carried out within a few days after injury. Intramedullary locking nail devices are used for midshaft (diaphyseal) fractures. Depending on the supracondylar fracture pattern, intramedullary nailing or screw plate fixation may be used. Internal fixation permits early mobilization. A thigh cuff orthosis may be used for external support. To preserve muscle strength, the patient is instructed to perform active exercises of the upper and lower extremities on a regular basis. Active muscle movement enhances healing by increasing blood supply and electrical potentials at the fracture site. Prescribed weight-bearing limits are based on the type of fracture. Physical therapy includes ROM and strengthening exercises, safe use of ambulatory aids, and gait training. Functional ambulation stimulates fracture healing. Healing time is 4 to 6 months.

A common complication after fracture of the femoral shaft is restriction of knee motion. Active and passive knee exercises begin as soon as possible, depending on the management approach and the stability of the fracture and knee ligaments.

Femur

Fracture of the proximal femur is termed a *hip fracture* and is classified as either intracapsular or extracapsular. Intracapsular fractures include femoral head and femoral neck fractures, while extracapsular fractures includes trochanteric, intertrochanteric, and subtrochanteric fractures (Fig. 42-11). Fractures of the neck of the femur may damage the vascular system that supplies blood to the head and the neck of the femur, and the bone may become ischemic. For this reason, AVN is common in patients with femoral neck fractures. The elderly are particularly vulnerable to intertrochanteric fractures and generally have a much worse prognosis than do younger patients. It is important for the nurse to be aware that the mortality rate after hip fracture surgical repair is 2% to 3%, and the mortality rate within 1 year in the elderly patients is 25% to 30%. DVT and subsequent PE are well-known complications of patients undergoing hip surgery, with rates of 1.6% within 30 days after surgery. Without prophylaxis, the rate of objectively confirmed DVT occurring within 7 to 14 days after lower extremity orthopedic surgery is around 40% to 60% (Kakkar & Rushton-Smith, 2013, p. 11). Also, older adults have a five- to eightfold increased risk for all-cause mortality during the first 3 months after hip fracture (Ferri, 2016d).

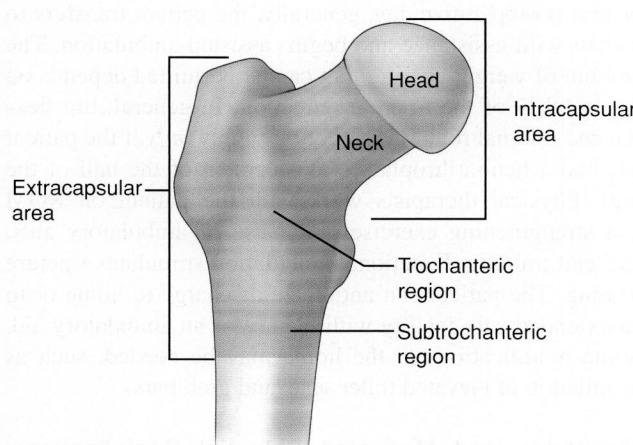

FIGURE 42-11 Regions of the proximal femur.

Head

Neck

Intracapsular area

Extracapsular area

Trochanteric region

Subtrochanteric region

Clinical Manifestations and Assessment

With displaced fractures of the femoral neck, the leg is shortened, abducted, and externally rotated (Murray, 2014). The patient complains of pain in the hip and groin or knee. Nondisplaced fractures (e.g., stress fractures) will not be shortened or externally rotated, but the patient will complain of pain. With most fractures of the femoral neck, the patient cannot move the leg without a significant increase in pain. Impacted intracapsular femoral neck fractures cause moderate discomfort (even with movement), may allow the patient to bear weight, and may not demonstrate obvious shortening or rotational changes. With extracapsular femoral fractures of the trochanteric or subtrochanteric regions, the extremity is significantly shortened, externally rotated to a greater degree than in intracapsular fractures, exhibits muscle spasm that resists positioning of the extremity in a neutral position, and has an associated large hematoma or area of ecchymosis. The diagnosis of fractured hip is confirmed with an x-ray.

Gerontologic Considerations

Elderly people (particularly women) who have brittle bones from osteoporosis and who tend to fall frequently have a high incidence of hip fracture. Weak quadriceps muscles, general frailty due to age, and comorbidities that produce decreased cerebral arterial perfusion (transient ischemic attacks, anemia, emboli, cardiovascular disease, and medication effects) contribute to the incidence of falls.

Often, a fractured hip is a catastrophic event that has a negative impact on the patient's lifestyle and quality of life. Hip fractures are a frequent contributor to death after 75 years of age. Because of the risk of DVT and PE with hip surgery, regional anesthesia is recommended since it reduces the risk for proximal DVT following total hip replacement by two- to threefold and also reduces the overall risk for DVT by at least 20% (Mackenzie & Su, 2016, p. 1832). Additionally, many elderly people hospitalized with hip fractures exhibit delirium as a result of the stress of the trauma, unfamiliar surroundings, sleep deprivation, and medications. An incidence rate of 24% of postoperative delirium following hip fracture repair in elderly patients was seen in a recent systematic review (Yang et al., 2016). Preoperative predictors of postoperative delirium include advanced age, living in an institution, heart failure, multiple comorbidities, THA, and morphine usage. Females were less likely to develop delirium after hip surgery (Yang et al., 2016).

> **Nursing Alert**
> *When a patient presents with a change in the level of consciousness, the nurse recalls the mnemonic DOG: **D**rugs are reviewed to evaluate whether a medication could be associated with the altered sensorium, **O**xygen saturation level is assessed for hypoxemia via pulse oximeter, and a **G**lucose level is obtained to evaluate for hypoglycemia/hyperglycemia via a finger stick since all are associated with altered LOC.*

To prevent complications, the nurse must assess the elderly patient for chronic pre-existing conditions as described above, including polypharmacy. Dehydration and poor nutrition may be present, contributing to hemoconcentration, and this predisposes the patient to the development of venous thromboemboli. Therefore monitoring intake and output in the elderly and assessing for DVT are particularly important.

Muscle weakness and wasting, which may have initially contributed to the fall and fracture, will be further compromised by bed rest and immobility. The nurse encourages the patient to move all joints except the involved hip and knee. Strengthening of the arms and shoulders will facilitate walking with assistive devices. A plan of nursing care for an elderly patient with a fractured hip is available online at http://thepoint.lww.com/Honan2e.

Medical Management

If surgery cannot be performed immediately, the fracture is immobilized so that additional soft tissue damage does not occur. Temporarily, traction can either be applied as skin or skeletal (pins or wires inserted into bones) traction. Each carries risks. Skin traction can put undue pressure on skin for prolonged periods of time, is limited in the amount of weight that can be applied (5 to 7 lb or less), and as a result, has limited use (Gösling & Giannoudis, 2015). Higher weights risk damage to the skin and neurovascular status of the involved extremity.

Skeletal traction is used more frequently to immobilize fracture fragments until the patient is physiologically stable and ready for surgical treatment. However, skeletal traction can increase the risk of infection since sterile pin(s) are drilled or wires are placed into the bone. The weight for skeletal traction is determined by body size and the extent of the injury. With either choice, continued neurovascular monitoring and assessment of the skin is needed.

Additionally, there are several types of traction. *Straight* or *running traction* applies the pulling force in a straight line with the body part resting on the bed. Buck's extension traction is an example of skin traction that is straight traction. It may be used for patients with fractures of the hip as a temporary measure to reduce muscle spasm, immobilize the extremity, and relieve pain. Another type of traction is *balanced suspension traction* (see Fig. 42-14 on page 1237), in which the affected extremity "floats" or is suspended in the traction apparatus by the balanced weights. The line of traction on the extremity remains fairly constant despite patient movement as long as the pull remains constant.

> ### Nursing Alert
> *The nurse must never remove weights from skeletal traction unless an emergency situation occurs. Removal of the weights completely defeats their purpose and may result in injury to the patient.*

The goal of surgical treatment of hip fractures is to obtain a satisfactory fixation so that the patient can be mobilized quickly and avoid secondary medical complications. Surgical intervention is carried out as soon as possible after injury. Surgical treatment consists of one of the following:

- Open or closed reduction of the fracture and internal fixation; a thigh cuff orthosis may be used for external support
- Replacement of the femoral head with a prosthesis (**hemiarthroplasty**). This is usually reserved for fractures that cannot be satisfactorily reduced or securely nailed, or to avoid complications of nonunion and AVN of the head of the femur. It is similar to a total hip replacement but only replaces the ball portion of the hip joint, not the socket (which is replaced in total hip replacement [discussed later in the chapter]).
- Closed reduction with percutaneous stabilization for an intracapsular fracture.

Nursing Management

The immediate postoperative care for a patient with a hip fracture is similar to that for other patients undergoing major surgery.

Encouraging Activity. The patient is encouraged to exercise as much as possible by means of the overbed trapeze. This device helps strengthen the arms and shoulders in preparation for protected ambulation (e.g., toe touch, partial weight bearing). A common complication after fracture of the femoral shaft is restriction of knee motion. In general, active and passive knee exercises begin as soon as possible, depending on the management approach and the stability of the fracture and knee ligaments. To preserve muscle strength, the patient is instructed to exercise the noninjured hip and the lower leg, foot, and toes on a regular basis. The surgeon prescribes the degree of weight bearing and the rate at which the patient can progress to full weight bearing. On the day of surgery or first postoperative day, generally, the patient transfers to a chair with assistance and begins assisted ambulation. The amount of weight bearing that can be permitted depends on the stability of the fracture reduction. In general, hip flexion and internal rotation restrictions apply *only* if the patient has had a hemiarthroplasty (replacement of the ball of the hip). Physical therapists work with the patient on ROM and strengthening exercises, safe use of ambulatory aids, and gait training. Functional ambulation stimulates fracture healing. The patient can anticipate discharge to home or to an extended care facility with the use of an ambulatory aid. Some modifications in the home may be needed, such as installation of elevated toilet seats and grab bars.

Monitoring and Managing Potential Complications. Attention is given to pain management as well as prevention of secondary medical problems, such as hemorrhagic shock, atelectasis, pneumonia, DVT, heart failure, constipation, pressure ulcer development, bladder control problems, and pain. Early mobilization of the patient is important so that independent functioning can be restored. Elderly people with hip fractures are particularly prone to complications that may require more vigorous treatment than the fracture. Frequently, the patient develops shock because the loss of two to three units of blood into the tissues is common with these fractures. Achievement of homeostasis after injury and after surgery is accomplished through careful monitoring of vital signs, wound drainage from dressings and external drains (drains are typically removed 24 to 48 hours after surgery), laboratory results, and physical assessment findings, as well as through collaborative management, including adjustment of therapeutic interventions as indicated. Refer back to Box 42-2 for signs and symptoms of hypovolemic shock.

Neurovascular complications may occur from direct injury to nerves and blood vessels or from increased tissue pressure. Assessment includes checking the neurovascular status of the extremity, especially circulatory perfusion of the lower leg and foot (popliteal, posterior tibial, and pedal pulses; toe capillary refill time; color; temperature; sensation and movement). A Doppler ultrasound device may be needed to assess blood flow. With hip fracture, bleeding into the tissues is expected. Excessive swelling may be observed and may further impair the neurovascular status. Patients may complain of increased pain at the site, and swelling may be noted in the thigh and buttock due to hematoma formation. Ice may be applied to decrease the swelling. The nurse marks the extent of drainage on the dressing by circling the extent and noting initials, date, and time. If excessive, the nurse should notify the provider.

DVT is a common postoperative complication contributing to significant morbidity and mortality in patients undergoing hip fracture surgery. To prevent DVT, the nurse encourages intake of fluids, and ankle and foot exercises. The nurse assesses the patient's legs for signs of DVT, which may include unilateral calf edema, tenderness, warmth, redness, a palpable cord, and Moses sign (pain with calf compression against the tibia) (DeHart, 2015). However, objective evidence is found in fewer than 50% of patients with these classic signs of DVT; therefore, the nurse maintains a high degree of suspicion for this complication (DeHart, 2015). The symptoms are related to inflammatory processes, and, therefore, the nurse also assesses for low-grade fever, malaise, and elevated white blood cell (WBC) count and sedimentation rate (Porth, 2015). The nurse administers the anticoagulant and mechanically based prophylaxis (e.g., elastic compression stockings, sequential compression devices, and prophylactic anticoagulant therapy) as prescribed.

Pulmonary complications, which commonly include atelectasis and pneumonia, are a threat to elderly patients undergoing hip surgery. Deep-breathing exercises, a change

of position at least every 2 hours, and the use of an incentive spirometer hourly help prevent respiratory complications. The nurse assesses breath sounds at least every 4 hours to detect adventitious or diminished sounds. Oxygen saturation should be assessed; supplemental oxygen may be ordered to keep the level above 95%. Pain must be treated with analgesic agents, typically opioids; otherwise, the patient may not be able to readily cough, deep breathe, or engage in prescribed activities. Out-of-bed (OOB) activities will be beneficial for lung function as well as muscle strength.

Heart failure is a frequent cause of mortality in elderly patients with hip fracture. The cumulative effect of trauma, major surgery, and concurrent medical history place the patient at risk for heart failure. The nurse is alert for signs and symptoms associated with left-sided heart failure, including shortness of breath, cough, dyspnea on exertion (DOE), crackles, orthopnea, and paroxysmal nocturnal dyspnea. Right ventricular failure presents with peripheral edema (may be pitting), jugular vein distention, and abdominal distention. Edema will be in dependent areas so the nurse assesses the sacral area as well as extremities. Accurate recording of intake and output (noting decreased urinary output), auscultation of heart (noting presence of S_3) and lung sounds (crackles), and monitoring O_2 saturation and vital signs (noting decreasing blood pressure, tachycardia, and tachypnea) are important nursing responsibilities. The nurse consults with the surgeon if signs and symptoms of excess fluid volume persist or worsen. The nurse expects fluid restriction and administers diuretics as ordered.

Skin breakdown is often seen in elderly patients with hip fracture. Blisters caused by tape are related to the tension of soft tissue edema under the nonelastic tape. An elastic hip spica wrap dressing or elastic tape applied in a vertical fashion may reduce the incidence of tape blisters. In addition, patients with hip fractures tend to remain in one position and may develop pressure ulcers; therefore, the nurse ensures that the patient is changing position at least every 2 hours. Proper skin care, especially on the heels, back, sacrum, and shoulders, as well as turning and frequent repositioning and supporting the legs with pillows and lifting the heels off the mattress all help to relieve pressure. Special mattress may provide protection by distributing pressure evenly.

Reduced GI motility, immobility, and the effects of anesthesia may result in constipation. Accurate assessment of intake and output, assessing bowel sounds, and noting distention of the abdomen are important nursing interventions, as prevention of constipation is the goal. A diet high in fiber and fluids may help stimulate gastric motility and since ambulation improves GI peristalsis, the nurse assists the patient in OOB activities and ambulation as prescribed. If constipation develops, therapeutic measures may include stool softeners, laxatives, suppositories, and enemas. To improve the patient's appetite, the nurse identifies and includes the patient's food preferences, as appropriate, within the prescribed therapeutic diet.

Loss of bladder control (incontinence or retention) may occur. In general, the routine use of an indwelling catheter is avoided because of the high risk for urinary tract infection (UTI). If a catheter is inserted at the time of surgery, it usually is removed on the morning of the first postoperative day. Because urinary retention is common after surgery, the nurse must assess the patient's voiding patterns and amounts, noting bladder distention and voiding of small amounts of urine (less than 100 mL) frequently. To ensure proper urinary tract function, the nurse monitors intake via IV route and/or by mouth if allowed and output. If no pre-existing cardiac disease (e.g., heart failure, coronary artery disease) exists, then liberal intake of fluids is encouraged. The patient is informed to notify the nurse if complaints of bladder fullness or inability to void are noted. A bladder scan can be performed by the nurse to evaluate postvoid residual, which should be less than 100 mL.

Infection is suspected if the patient complains of persistent, moderate discomfort in the hip, experiences chills or malaise, and has an elevated WBC count and erythrocyte sedimentation rate (ESR). The nurse observes the surgical incision for erythema, warmth, and tenderness and notes color, amount, and consistency of wound drainage. In the elderly, symptoms of infection may be nonspecific (e.g., patients may be afebrile without complaints); an important marker is a decline in the patient's functional status and/or the presence of confusion. The closed-wound drainage system is observed for color and amount of drainage and functioning of the drainage device. International research suggests that preoperative serum albumin is a reliable predictor of an infection at the surgical site in patients admitted for elective total joint arthroplasty (Alfargieny, Bodalal, Bendardaf, El-Fadli, & Langhi, 2015).

Delayed complications of hip fractures include malunion, delayed union or nonunion, AVN of the femoral head (particularly with femoral neck fractures), and fixation device problems (e.g., protrusion of the fixation device through the acetabulum, loosening of hardware) (discussed earlier in this chapter). Healing time is 4 to 6 months.

Promoting Health. Osteoporosis screening of patients who have experienced hip fracture is important for prevention of future fractures (Box 42-5). Specific patient education is needed regarding dietary requirements, lifestyle changes, and weight-bearing exercise to promote bone health. Prevention of falls is also important and may be achieved through exercises to improve muscle tone, flexibility, and balance and through the elimination of environmental hazards such as throw rugs. Other environmental considerations are the use of hand rails on the stairs, nonskid surfaces in the bathroom, grab bars in the shower, raised toilet seats, well-fitting shoes with nonskid soles, and adequate home lighting.

BOX 42-5 | **Risk Factors for Osteoporosis**

- Age
- Female
- Caucasian
- Small bone structure
- Postmenopausal
- Sedentary lifestyle
- Chronic obstructive pulmonary disease
- Smoking
- Steroid use
- Family history
- Calcium deficiency
- Poor nutrition
- Excessive alcohol intake
- Excessive caffeine intake
- Malignancy
- Hyperthyroidism
- Rheumatoid arthritis
- Diabetes mellitus
- Cushing disease
- Gastrectomy
- Inflammatory bowel disease
- Malabsorption
- Multiple myeloma

TREATMENT MODALITIES

Cast

A **cast** is a rigid external immobilizing device that is applied for a variety of medical surgical disorders including fractures and deformities. Many injuries that were previously treated with casts may now be treated with other immobilization devices (e.g., immobilizers). In general, casts permit mobilization of the patient while restricting movement of a body part. The cast provides adequate stability to the injured area and does not restrict circulation and nerve supply. Additionally, it must be smooth and free of ridges to prevent pressure on underlying tissue.

Casting Materials

Casts may be made of plaster or nonplaster materials. Refer to Box 42-6 for cast application.

Fiberglass

Nonplaster casts are generally referred to as fiberglass casts. These water-activated polyurethane materials are light in weight, strong, water resistant, and durable. They are made of nonabsorbent fabric impregnated with cool water–activated hardeners that bond and reach full rigid strength in minutes. The material does not soften when wet, which allows for hydrotherapy when appropriate. When wet, the casts are dried with a hair dryer on a cool setting; thorough drying is important to prevent skin breakdown.

BOX 42-6

GUIDELINES FOR NURSING CARE

Assisting with Cast Application

Equipment

Tubular stockinette, casting material as specified by the provider (plaster rolls/plaster splints); sink equipped with plaster trap or bucket of water, gloves, padding, sponge or felt padding (if necessary)

Implementation

NURSING ACTIONS	RATIONALE
1. Support extremity or body part to be casted.	1. Minimizes movement; maintains reduction and alignment; increases comfort
2. Position and maintain body part to be casted in the position indicated by the provider during the casting procedure.	2. Facilitates casting; reduces incidence of complications (e.g., malunion, nonunion, contracture)
3. Drape the patient.	3. Avoids undue exposure; protects other body parts from contact with casting materials
4. Wash and dry the body part to be casted.	4. Reduces incidence of skin breakdown
5. Place knitted material (e.g., stockinette) over the body part to be casted. • Apply the material in a smooth and nonconstrictive manner.	5. Protects skin from casting materials Protects the skin from pressure Folds over edges of cast when finishing application; creates smooth, padded edge; protects skin from abrasion
6. Wrap soft, nonwoven roll padding smoothly and evenly around the body part. Use additional padding around bony prominences to protect superficial nerves (e.g., head of fibula, olecranon process).	6. Protects the skin from pressure of the cast Protects the skin at bony prominences Protects superficial nerves
7. Apply plaster or nonplaster casting material evenly on body part. • Choose appropriate width bandage. • Overlap preceding turn by half the width of the bandage. • Use continuous motion, maintaining constant contact with the body part. • Use additional casting material (splints) at joints and at points of anticipated cast stress.	7. Creates a smooth, solid, well-contoured cast Facilitates smooth application Creates a smooth, solid, immobilizing cast Shapes the cast properly for adequate support Strengthens the cast
8. "Finish" cast: • Smooth the edges. • Trim and reshape with a cast knife or cutter.	8. Protects skin from abrasion Allows full range of motion of adjacent joints
9. Remove particles of casting materials from the skin.	9. Prevents particles from loosening and sliding underneath the cast
10. Support the cast during hardening. • Handle hardening casts with the palms of your hands. • Support the cast on a firm, smooth surface. • Do not rest the cast on hard surfaces or on sharp edges. • Avoid pressure on the cast.	10. Casting materials begin to harden in minutes; maximum hardness of nonplaster cast occurs in minutes; maximum hardness of plaster cast occurs with drying (24–72 hours, depending on environment and thickness of cast) Avoids denting of cast and development of pressure areas
11. Promote drying of cast. • Leave cast uncovered and exposed to air. • Turn patient every 2 hours, supporting the major joints. • Fans may be used to increase air-flow and speed drying.	11. Facilitates drying

Plaster

Traditional casts are made of rolls of plaster bandage that are wet in cool water and applied smoothly to the body. A crystallizing reaction occurs, and heat is given off (an exothermic reaction). The heat given off during this reaction can be uncomfortable, and the patient needs to be informed about the sensation of increasing warmth that generally dissipates after 15 minutes. Additionally, the nurse explains that

the cast needs to be exposed to air (i.e., uncovered) to allow maximum dissipation of the heat and facilitate drying, which can take 24 to 72 hours. Because the plaster cast remains wet and somewhat soft, the cast needs to remain uncovered until it is completely dry. A wet plaster cast appears dull and gray, sounds dull on percussion, feels damp, and smells musty. A dry plaster cast is white and shiny, resonant to percussion, firm, and odorless.

BOX 42-7

Focus on Pathophysiology

Rhabdomyolysis

A wide variety of etiologies are associated with rhabdomyolysis, including seizures, drug reactions (e.g., statins), extreme exercise, soft tissue infections, burns, malignant hyperthermia, extended lithotomy position and lateral decubitus positions, use of pneumatic antishock garments or tourniquet ischemia, compartment syndrome, toxins (alcohol, cocaine, heroin, amphetamines, ecstasy, phencyclidine, snakebite), and electrical and crush injuries. With trauma injuries, the nurse is alert for rhabdomyolysis, in which the crushing injury causes the breakdown of skeletal muscle, resulting in the release of muscle cell contents, including myoglobin (a protein released from muscle when injury occurs), creatine phosphokinase (CPK), phosphate, enzymes, and potassium, into the systemic circulation. Myoglobin, which gives skeletal muscle its color, is released from the damaged muscle and filtered by the kidney, resulting in brown or tea-colored urine. Myoglobinuria does not occur in the absence of rhabdomyolysis; therefore, when present, it is the best marker and diagnostic cornerstone of rhabdomyolysis (Ferri, 2016b). Urine dipstick for blood may be positive because of the cross-reaction with myoglobin; however, microscopic examination of urine may reveal no red blood cells. The myoglobin threatens kidney function due to renal tubular obstruction and direct toxic effects, resulting in acute kidney failure (5–30% of patients develop AKF). The CPK typically peaks 2–5 days after the initial insult and, in general, is in excess of five times the normal serum level. Anion gap metabolic acidosis may be present due to the release of organic acids from damaged muscle (Ferri, 2016b). Goals of management are to prevent acute kidney failure by countering the effects of myoglobin with the use of aggressive fluid resuscitation (reduces the accumulation of toxic intracellular contents), bicarbonate administration (urine that is alkalized lessens myoglobin toxicity), and possibly the administration of mannitol (Osmitrol), an osmotic diuretic to "wash out" the myoglobin. In addition, management of hyperkalemia with insulin/dextrose is expected. The nurse assesses urine output hourly, monitors vital signs, maintains strict intake and output, and assesses for fluid volume deficit (secondary to the trauma) versus fluid volume excess (secondary to overhydration). The nurse monitors for disseminated intravascular coagulation (DIC), which can occur in up to 30% of severe cases and is associated with higher mortality rates (Ferri, 2016c).

Nursing Alert
The nurse ensures that all jewelry is removed from the injured limb that is to be casted since edema is expected in fractures.

Nursing Management

Monitoring and Managing Potential Complications

Compartment Syndrome

There are three types of compartment syndromes: ACS, chronic compartment syndrome, and crush compartment syndrome. *ACS* involves a sudden and severe decrease in blood flow to the tissues distal to an area of injury that results in ischemic necrosis if prompt, decisive intervention does not occur. It is a potentially limb-threatening complication that occurs when increased pressure occurs within a limited space (e.g., cast, muscle compartment) that compresses the blood vessels and nerves within the area. The pressure within the confined space becomes so high that there is massive compromise to circulation and nerve transmission in the affected extremity. Permanent damage develops within a few hours if action is not taken.

Chronic compartment syndrome is characterized by pain, aching, and tightness in a muscle or muscle group that has been subjected to inordinate stress or exercise. In this instance, muscle volume increases by as much as 20% within a short time, resulting in stretching of the fascia and inflammation. *Crush compartment syndrome* is caused by massive external compression or crushing of a compartment; for instance, this may occur when a car jack fails and a car falls on a mechanic. This type of massive injury results in systemic effects that include rhabdomyolysis (Box 42-7) that causes acute kidney failure and that may eventually lead to multiple organ dysfunction syndrome (MODS), further discussed in Chapter 54.

A specific type of compartment syndrome in the arm is Volkmann contracture (discussed on page 1223). It is frequently associated with supracondylar fractures of the humerus (refer to Figure 42-6). The following discussion focuses on ACS.

Fascia is tough connective tissue that surrounds muscle groups, organs, nerves, blood vessels, bones, and internal structures. It does not expand readily. Therefore, if a compartment begins to swell, the pressure in the area rises, leading to venous obstruction, compromising circulation and nerve and motor function to the point at which the limb may need to be amputated (Fig. 42-12).

Risk factors for this complication include trauma from accidents, surgery, or crushing injuries, in which massive edema and bleeding is expected. Casts and tight bandages are also associated with this complication as the external devices increase the pressure within the injured area. In addition, it may be caused by any condition that increases the risk of bleeding or edema in a confined space, including patients with soft tissue injury, without fractures, who are on anticoagulants or have bleeding dyscrasias (e.g., prolonged malposition, burns, electrocutions, snake venom, stressful athletic activity, contusions, and infiltrations from intravenous [IV]

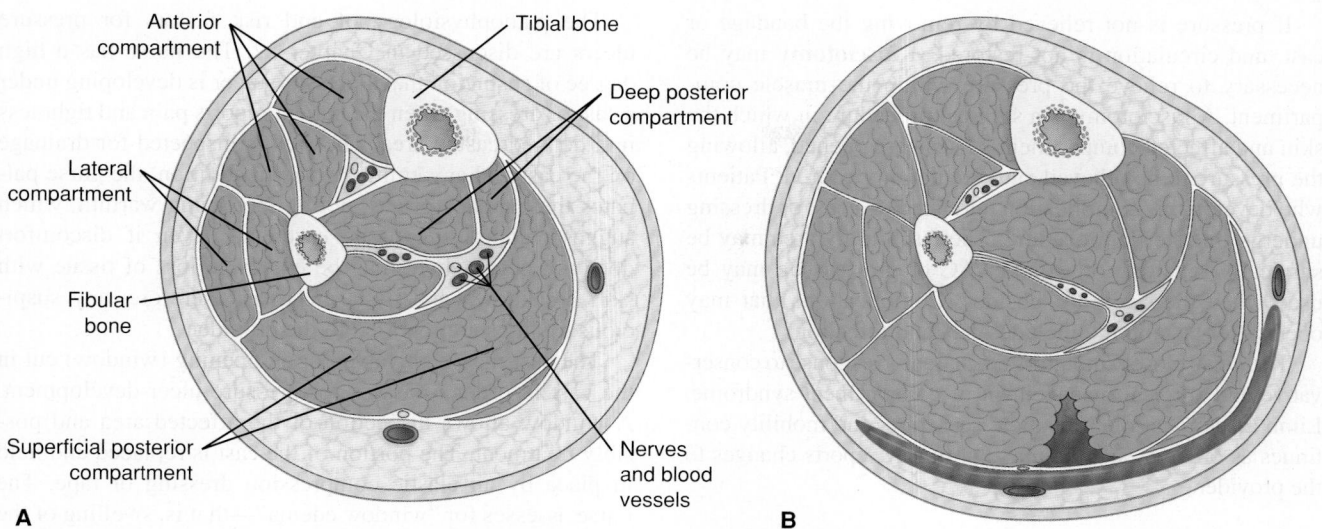

FIGURE 42-12 **A.** Cross-section of normal lower leg with muscle compartments. **B.** Cross-section of lower leg with compartment syndrome. Swelling of muscles causes compression of nerves and blood vessels.

sites). Long bone fractures (open tibial fractures [6% to 9%]; tibial plateau fracture) and multitrauma patients (24%) are implicated in ACS; however, it can occur in other parts, such as the foot, thigh, gluteal region, and abdomen (Ferri, 2016b; Shuler, Roskosky, & Freedman, 2014; Sise, 2016). Further details on ACS of the abdomen are in Chapter 53.

It is essential to detect this complication early. The first clinical finding is loss of light touch sensation in the distribution of the nerve in the compartment (e.g., first web space for lower extremity, see Table 42-2); however, this may be difficult to assess because of altered mentation of patients (unresponsive, uncooperative patient [e.g., ETOH (ethylalcohol and alcohol), overdose], or those with peripheral nerve deficits). Clinical manifestations include paleness of limb, cool skin temperature, delayed capillary refill, weak pulsations, paresthesia (tingling/burning sensation in the involved muscle), decreased sensation and mobility, tight and full muscle, and pain (progressive—not relieved by position changes, ice, or analgesia, or pain that is disproportional to the injury). A hallmark sign is pain that occurs or intensifies with passive ROM. Ominous *late* signs are pallor and loss of pulses. If the nurse is concerned about neurovascular impairment, the provider is notified immediately.

Nursing Alert

It is important to note that late signs *of compartment syndrome are pulselessness and pallor. The presence of a pulse does not rule out compartment syndrome.*

If the complication is secondary to a tight bandage or cast, the nurse anticipates that the bandage would be loosened or removed and the cast bivalved (cut in half longitudinally) to release the constriction. While the surgeon

is bivalving the cast, the nurse assists in maintaining limb alignment (Box 42-8). The affected limb must be elevated no higher than heart level to ensure arterial perfusion. Intracompartmental pressure monitoring may be required to diagnose compartment syndrome. A variety of commercial systems is available for the provider to measure intracompartmental pressure. The intracompartmental pressure of a normal muscle compartment at rest is less than 10 mm Hg (Sise, 2016). A high tissue pressure indicates compartment syndrome. Debate exists on the intracompartmental pressure that mandates fasciotomy, but pressures exceeding 25 mm Hg suggest the need to consider a fasciotomy (Sise, 2016). Another reliable method of assessment for ACS is *perfusion pressure* or ΔP of the limb, which is calculated as

$$\Delta P = \text{diastolic blood pressure} - \text{intracompartmental pressure}$$

A perfusion pressure of less than 30 mm Hg is considered a criterion for fasciotomy (Sise, 2016).

BOX 42-8 **Procedure for Bivalving a Cast**

The following procedure is followed when a cast is bivalved.
1. With a cast cutter, a longitudinal cut is made to divide the cast in half.
2. The under padding is cut with scissors.
3. The cast is spread apart with cast spreaders to relieve pressure and to inspect and treat the skin without interrupting the reduction and alignment of the bone.
4. After the pressure is relieved, the anterior and posterior parts of the cast are secured together with an elastic compression bandage to maintain immobilization.
5. To control swelling and promote circulation, the extremity is elevated (but no higher than heart level) to minimize the effect of gravity on perfusion of the tissues.

If pressure is not relieved by removing the bandage or cast, and circulation is not restored, a **fasciotomy** may be necessary to relieve the pressure within the muscle compartment. A fasciotomy is a surgical procedure in which the skin and affected compartment's fascia are opened, allowing the pressure to be relieved and circulation restored. Patients who develop this complication unrelated to a cast or dressing undergo this sterile procedure. The fasciotomy area may be surgically repaired, or wound VAC or graft tissue may be used when the swelling subsides. Complications that may occur after fasciotomy include AVN and infection.

The nurse closely monitors the patient's response to conservative and surgical management of compartment syndrome. Limb assessment of circulation, sensation, and mobility continues as ordered, and the nurse promptly reports changes to the provider.

> **⚠ Nursing Alert**
> *If ACS is suspected, the injured extremity should not be elevated to decrease edema, as this action will increase the intracompartmental pressure and decrease perfusion to the extremity (Sise, 2016). The extremity should be maintained at heart level (Shuler et al., 2014).*

Pressure Ulcers

Pressure ulcers are breakdowns in the skin caused by prolonged pressure on a body part. Casts or bandages can put pressure on soft tissues, causing tissue anoxia and pressure ulcers. Susceptible sites in the lower extremity include the heel, malleoli, dorsum of the foot, head of the fibula, tibial tuberosity, and anterior surface of the patella (Fig. 42-13). Upper extremity sites are located at the medial and or lateral epicondyle of the humerus, olecranon, and the ulnar styloid.

The pathophysiology of and risk factors for pressure ulcers are discussed in Chapter 52. The nurse has a high degree of suspicion that a pressure ulcer is developing under a cast or dressing when the patient reports pain and tightness in a defined casted area. The area is inspected for drainage on the cast and any emitted odor. In addition, the nurse palpates the bandage or cast noting increasing warmth, which suggests underlying tissue erythema. Even if discomfort does not occur, there may be extensive loss of tissue with skin breakdown and tissue necrosis; therefore, any suspicious findings are reported to the provider.

The cast may be bivalved or an opening (window) cut in the cast in order to assess for pressure ulcer development. A window allows inspection of the affected area and possibly treatment. The portion of the cast is replaced and held in place by an elastic compression dressing or tape. The nurse assesses for "window edema"—that is, swelling of the underlying tissue through the window, which creates pressure areas around the window margins. Patients who have histories of impaired sensation due to neuropathy or neurologic injury are at high risk for ulcer development; thus, removable braces may be used for management of fractures with frequent skin assessments.

Disuse Syndrome

When a muscle is left inactive, it loses its strength and size. Disuse syndrome is the nursing diagnosis defined as muscular deconditioning and atrophy resulting from inactivity or immobilization (Murr, 2016). Depending on the status of the patient and length of time since the initial trauma, strengthening exercises may be ordered. The nurse will teach the patient to tense or contract muscles (isometric muscle contraction) without moving the underlying bone. The internal or external devices stabilize the underlying bone. Isometric activity, such as teaching a patient in an arm

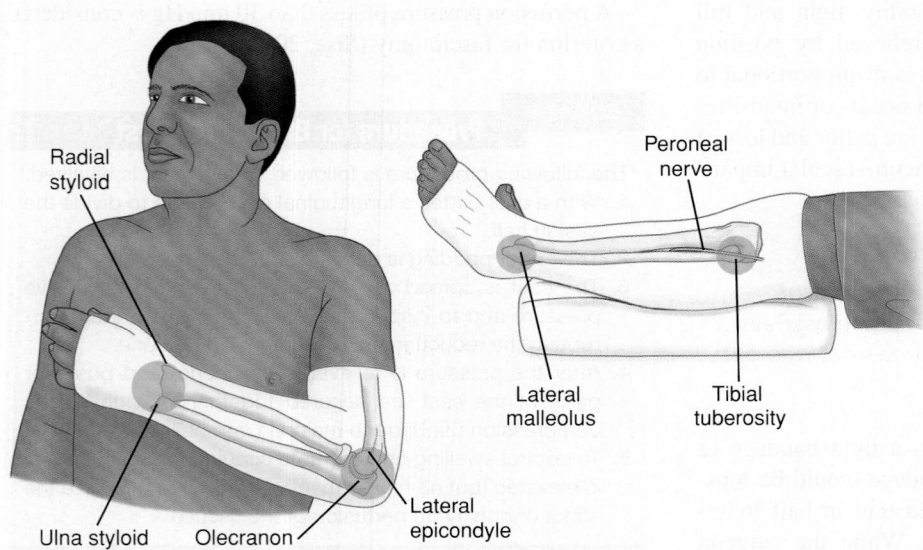

Radial styloid

Ulna styloid   Olecranon   Lateral epicondyle

Peroneal nerve

Lateral malleolus   Tibial tuberosity

FIGURE 42-13 Pressure areas in common types of casts. *Left,* long-arm cast. *Right,* short-leg cast.

Muscle-Setting Exercises

Isometric contractions of the muscle maintain muscle mass and strength and prevent atrophy.

Quadriceps-Setting Exercise
- Position the patient supine with the leg extended.
- Instruct the patient to push his or her knee back onto the mattress by contracting the anterior thigh muscles.
- Encourage the patient to hold the position for 5–10 seconds.
- Let the patient relax.
- Have the patient repeat the exercise 10 times each hour when awake.

Gluteal-Setting Exercise
- Position the patient supine with legs extended, if possible.
- Instruct the patient to contract the muscles of the buttocks.
- Encourage the patient to hold the contraction for 5–10 seconds.
- Let the patient relax.
- Have the patient repeat the exercise 10 times each hour when awake.

cast to "make a fist," helps reduce muscle atrophy and maintain muscle strength. Muscle-setting exercises (e.g., quadriceps-setting and gluteal-setting exercises) are important in maintaining muscles essential for walking (Box 42-9). Isometric exercises should be performed hourly while the patient is awake. Physical therapy can assist in developing an exercise regimen for the patient.

Providing Initial Patient Teaching

The nurse teaches the patient and family that the casted extremity must be uncovered until it is completely dry and supported on pillows to the level of the heart to control swelling; ice packs should be applied as prescribed over the fracture site for 1 or 2 days. The patient is taught to elevate the casted arm or leg when seated to promote venous return and control swelling, unless ACS is suspected, where the extremity is at the level of the heart. The patient needs to understand that the body part will be immobilized after casting.

Positioning

If a body cast is in place, the nurse turns the patient as a unit toward the uninjured side every 2 hours to relieve pressure and to allow the cast to dry. It is important to avoid twisting the patient's body within the cast. Sufficient personnel (depending on the size of the patient and type of cast) are needed when the patient is turned so that the fresh cast can be adequately supported with the palms of the hands at vulnerable points (i.e., body joints) to prevent cracking.

Teaching the Patient Self-Care

Self-care deficits occur when a portion of the body is immobilized. The nurse encourages the patient to participate actively in personal care and to use assistive devices safely. The nurse assists the patient in identifying areas of need and in developing strategies to achieve independence in ADLs. Patient teaching is discussed in Box 42-10.

Providing Continuing Care

The nurse prepares the patient for cast removal or cast changes by explaining that the cast is cut with a cast cutter, which vibrates. The cutter does not penetrate deeply enough to hurt the patient's skin. The cast padding is cut with scissors. Refer to Box 42-11.

The formerly casted body part is weak from disuse, stiff, and may appear atrophied. Therefore, support is needed when the cast is removed. The skin, which is usually dry and

Patient Education

Cast Care
- Move about as normally as possible, but avoid excessive use of the injured extremity, and avoid walking on wet, slippery floors or sidewalks.
- If the cast is on an upper extremity, you may use a sling when you ambulate. To prevent pressure on the cervical spinal nerves, the sling should distribute the supported weight over a large area and not on the back of the neck. Remove the arm from the sling and elevate it frequently.
- Perform prescribed exercises regularly, as prescribed.
- Elevate the casted extremity to heart level frequently to prevent swelling. For example: when lying down, elevate the arm, so that each joint is positioned higher than the preceding proximal joint (e.g., elbow higher than the shoulder, hand higher than the elbow).
- Do not attempt to scratch the skin under the cast. This may cause a break in the skin and result in the formation of a skin ulcer. Cool air from a hair dryer may alleviate an itch. Do not insert objects, such as coat hangers, inside the cast to scratch itching skin. If itching persists, contact your provider.
- Cushion rough edges of the cast with tape.
- Keep the cast dry, but do not cover it with plastic or rubber because this causes condensation, which dampens the cast and skin. Moisture softens a plaster cast (a wet fiberglass cast must be dried thoroughly with a hair dryer on a cool setting to avoid skin burns).
- Report any of the following to the provider: persistent pain; swelling that does not respond to elevation; changes in sensation; decreased ability to move exposed fingers or toes; changes in capillary refill, skin color, and temperature.
- Note odors around the cast, stained areas, warm spots, and pressure areas. Report them to the provider.
- Report a broken cast to the provider; do not attempt to fix it yourself.

BOX 42-11

GUIDELINES FOR NURSING CARE

Removing a Cast

Equipment

Cast scissors, cast saw, and cast spreader (if necessary); eye protection, Ace wraps, splints as indicated, adhesive tape (optional)

Implementation

NURSING ACTIONS	RATIONALE
1. Inform the patient about the procedure.	1. Facilitates cooperation and reduces fear about the procedure
2. Reassure the patient that the electric saw or cast cutter will not cut the skin. (Explain that the blade oscillates to cut the cast and vibrations will be felt.)	2. Reduces anxiety
3. Wear eye protection (patient and operator of the cast cutter).	3. Protects eyes from flying cast particles
4. Bivalve the cast using a series of alternating pressures and linear movements of the blade along the line to be cut.	4. Cuts cast in halves; avoids burning sensation from prolonged contact of oscillating blade with padding
5. Cut the padding with scissors.	5. Releases all of the casting materials
6. Support the body part as it is removed from the cast.	6. Reduces stresses on body part that has been immobilized
7. Gently wash and dry the area that has been immobilized.[a] Apply emollient lotion.	7. Removes dead skin that has accumulated during immobilization; keeps skin supple
8. Teach the patient to avoid rubbing and scratching skin.	8. Prevents skin breakdown
9. Collaborate with the physical therapist to teach the patient to resume active use of the affected body part gradually within the guidelines of the prescribed therapeutic regimen.	9. Protects weakened body part from excessive stress; progressive exercises reduce stiffness and restore muscle strength and function
10. Teach the patient to control swelling by elevating the extremity or using an elastic bandage if prescribed.	10. Facilitates circulation (i.e., venous return) and controls fluid pooling

[a]If a new cast is to be applied, follow guidelines for application of a cast and associated nursing care.

scaly from accumulated dead skin, is vulnerable to injury from scratching. The skin needs to be washed gently and lubricated with an emollient lotion.

The nurse and physical therapist teach the patient to resume activities gradually within the prescribed therapeutic regimen. Exercises prescribed to help the patient regain joint motion are explained and demonstrated. Because the muscles are weak from disuse, the body part that has been casted cannot withstand normal stresses immediately. In addition, the nurse teaches the patient with noticeable swelling of the affected extremity after cast removal to continue to elevate the extremity to control swelling until normal muscle tone and use are reestablished.

SKIN TRACTION

Skin traction is used to control muscle spasms and to immobilize an area before surgery. Skin traction is accomplished by using a weight to pull on traction tape or on a foam boot attached to the skin. The amount of weight applied must not exceed the tolerance of the skin. Adhesive tape and weights greater than 5 to 7 lb (Gösling & Giannoudis, 2015) are avoided as they may cause avulsion of the superficial skin layers.

Buck's Extension Traction

Buck's extension traction (unilateral or bilateral) is skin traction to the lower leg. The pull is exerted in one plane when partial or temporary immobilization is desired. In general, this form of traction is used to immobilize fractures of the proximal femur before surgical fixation or when only a light traction weight is necessary.

Before the traction is applied, the nurse inspects the skin for abrasions and circulatory disturbances. The skin and circulation must be in healthy condition to tolerate the traction. The extremity should be clean and dry before the foam boot or traction tape is applied.

To apply Buck's traction, one nurse elevates and supports the extremity under the patient's heel and knee while another nurse places the foam boot under the leg, with the patient's heel in the heel of the boot. Next, the nurse secures Velcro straps around the leg. Traction tape overwrapped with elastic bandage in a spiral fashion may be used instead of the boot. Excessive pressure is avoided over the malleolus and proximal fibula during application to prevent pressure ulcers and nerve damage. The nurse then passes the rope affixed to the spreader or footplate over a pulley fastened to the end of the bed and attaches the weight—usually 5 lb—to the rope.

Nursing Alert
The nurse must check nonadhesive traction frequently because it tends to slip when the traction weight is applied. Assessment of pressure on the fibula is essential because of the risk of nerve impingement; the peroneal nerve passes around the neck of the fibula just below the knee. Assess for inability to dorsiflex the foot and toes, a foot drop, or sensation in the web between the great toe and second toe.

Skin breakdown, nerve pressure, and circulatory impairment are complications that may develop as a result of skin traction. Skin breakdown results from irritation caused by contact of the skin with the tape or foam and shearing forces. Older adults are at greater risk for this complication because of their sensitive, fragile skin.

Nursing Alert
The nurse must promptly investigate every report of discomfort expressed by the patient in traction.

Circulatory impairment is manifested by cold skin temperature, decreased peripheral pulses, slow capillary refill time, and bluish skin. DVT, a serious circulatory impairment, may be manifested by unilateral calf tenderness, warmth, redness, and swelling (see Chapter 18).

SKELETAL TRACTION

The goals of skeletal traction are to maintain alignment of the injured limb and counteract the shortening of the injured limb from muscle spasm before definitive treatment can occur. Skeletal traction is applied directly to the bone. This method of traction is used occasionally to treat fractures of the femur, the tibia, and the cervical spine. The traction is applied directly to the bone by use of a metal pin or wire (e.g., Steinmann pin or Kirschner wire), which is inserted through the bone distal to the fracture, avoiding nerves, blood vessels, muscles, tendons, and joints. Tongs applied to the head are fixed to the skull to apply traction that immobilizes cervical fractures.

After local anesthesia and skin preparation by the surgeon, using surgical asepsis, a small skin incision is made and sterile pin(s) are drilled or wire is placed through the bone. The patient feels pressure during this procedure and possibly some pain when the periosteum is penetrated.

After insertion, the pin or wire is attached to the traction bow or caliper. The ends of the pin or wire are covered with corks or tape to prevent injury to the patient or caregivers. The weights are attached to the pin or wire bow by a rope-and-pulley system that exerts the appropriate amount and direction of pull for effective traction. Skeletal traction frequently uses 7 to 12 kg (15 to 25 lb) to achieve the therapeutic effect. Usually the weight of 15 to 25 lb of traction is sufficient to restore bone length during the first few days after injury when muscle spasms can be intense. The nurse is aware that the weights applied initially must overcome the spasms of the affected muscles that pull on the fractured bones and shorten the limb.

Often, skeletal traction is balanced traction, which supports the affected extremity, allows for some patient movement, and facilitates patient independence and nursing care while maintaining effective traction. The Thomas splint with a Pearson attachment (Fig. 42-14) is frequently used with skeletal traction for fractures of the femur. Because upward traction is required, an overbed frame is used.

When skeletal traction is discontinued, the extremity is gently supported while the weights are removed. The pin is cut close to the skin and removed by the physician. Then internal fixation, casts, or splints are used to immobilize and support the healing bone.

FIGURE 42-14 Balanced suspension skeletal traction with Thomas leg splint. The patient can move vertically as long as the resultant line of pull is maintained.

External fixators are often used to maintain position of unstable fractures when the use of a cast is prohibited or the patient's condition is unstable and precludes a surgical procedure to stabilize the fracture. They can also be used to manage open fractures with soft tissue damage or severe comminuted (crushed or splintered) fractures while permitting active treatment of damaged soft tissues. Complicated fractures of the humerus, forearm, femur, tibia, and pelvis are often managed with external skeletal fixators. The fracture is reduced, aligned, and immobilized by a series of pins or screws inserted directly into the bone above and below the fracture and secured with the use of a metal frame. Pin position is maintained through attachment to a portable frame. The fixator facilitates patient comfort, early mobility, and active exercise of adjacent uninvolved joints; thus, complications due to disuse and immobility are minimized.

Nursing Alert
The nurse never adjusts the clamps on the external fixator frame. It is the surgeon's responsibility to do so.

Nursing Management

Maintaining Effective Traction

When skeletal traction is used, the nurse checks the traction apparatus at least once per shift to see that the ropes are in the wheel grooves of the pulleys, that the ropes are not frayed, that the weights hang freely, and that the knots in the rope are tied securely. The nurse also evaluates the patient's position because slipping down in bed results in ineffective traction.

Maintaining Positioning

The nurse must maintain alignment of the patient's body in traction as prescribed to promote an effective line of pull. The nurse positions the patient's foot to avoid footdrop (plantar flexion), inward rotation (inversion), and outward rotation (eversion). The patient's foot may be supported in a neutral position by orthopedic devices (e.g., foot supports).

Preventing Skin Breakdown

The patient's elbows frequently become sore, and nerve injury may occur if the patient repositions by pushing on the elbows. In addition, patients frequently push on the heel of the unaffected leg and elbows when they raise themselves in bed. Therefore, the nurse should protect the elbows and heels and inspect them for pressure ulcers. A trapeze should be suspended above the patient, to encourage movement without using the elbows or heels. Areas that are particularly vulnerable to pressure caused by a traction apparatus applied to the lower extremity include the ischial tuberosity, popliteal space, Achilles tendon, and heel. If the patient is not permitted to turn on one side or the other, the nurse must make a special effort to provide back care and to keep the bed

dry and free of crumbs and wrinkles. The patient can assist by holding the overhead trapeze and raising the hips off the bed. If the patient cannot do this, the nurse can push down on the mattress with one hand to relieve pressure on the back and bony prominences and to provide for some shifting of weight. A pressure-relieving air-filled or high-density foam mattress overlay may reduce the risk of pressure ulcer.

For change of bed linens (top to bottom rather than side to side), the patient raises the torso while nurses on both sides of the bed roll down and replace the upper mattress sheet. Then, as the patient raises the buttocks off the mattress, the nurses slide the sheets under the buttocks. Finally, the nurses replace the lower section of the bed linens while the patient rests on the back. Sheets and blankets are placed over the patient in such a way that the traction is not disrupted.

Providing Pin-Site Care

The wound at the pin insertion site requires attention. The goal is to avoid infection and development of **osteomyelitis** (Box 42-12). Osteomyelitis is an acute or chronic inflammation of the bone caused by infection. There is wide variability on pin care, and research on outcomes is scarce, thus further studies are warranted. However, the National Association of Orthopaedic Nurses Guidelines for Orthopaedic Nursing (Smith & Dahlen, 2013) offers specific recommendations for pin care, which are as follows:

- Pins located in areas with considerable soft tissue should be considered at greatest risk for infection.
- At sites with mechanically stable bone–pin interfaces, pin care should be done on a daily or weekly basis (after the first 48 to 72 hours, when drainage may be heavy).

BOX 42-12 | **Focus on Pathophysiology**

Osteomyelitis

Osteomyelitis is an infection in the bone caused by a variety of microorganisms, most commonly *Staphylococcus aureus,* that are introduced during injury, from the bloodstream, through direct inoculation (chronic infection of skin/soft tissue), or during surgery. Once in the bone, the microorganisms proliferate and spread within the bone shaft, causing an inflammatory response that further destroys the bone. Wound cultures identify the organism and antibiotic sensitivity. Difficult to treat, osteomyelitis requires IV therapy, in general, for 6 weeks. Osteomyelitis may be classified as acute (an infection lasting less than 4 weeks) or chronic (more than 4 weeks). Pain over the affected bone is the dominant finding in osteomyelitis. Palpation of the involved bone usually elicits tenderness over the infected area. Increased warmth, erythema, and swelling may be seen at the affected segment but are not always present. The ESR is commonly elevated, and elevated WBC levels may be seen in acute infections (but not always). The WBC count may be normal in chronic osteomyelitis.

- Chlorhexidine 2 mg/mL solution is considered to be the most effective cleansing solution for pin-site care. Saline should be used if chlorhexidine solution is contraindicated such as those with hypersensitivity to Chlorhexidine gluconate or other formula ingredients.
- Strict handwashing should always take place before and after skeletal pin-site care.
- Patients and families should be taught pin care before discharge. They should be required to demonstrate the prescribed care and provided with written instructions that include signs and symptoms of infection.

Note: Follow your facility's specific policy and procedure pertaining to skeletal pin care.

The nurse must inspect the pin sites daily for reaction (i.e., normal changes that occur at the pin site after insertion) and infection. Signs of reaction may include redness, warmth, and serous or slightly sanguinous drainage at the site. These signs are expected to subside after 72 hours. Rates of pin tract infections range from 10% to 15%, with deep infection rates of 3.5% to 8.2% (Mitchell et al., 2016). Signs of infection may mirror those of reaction but also include the presence of edema, purulent drainage, erythema, excessive warmth, tenderness, pin loosening, and odor. In addition, the nurse monitors the patient for fever. The frequency of pin care needs to be increased if mechanical looseness of pins or early signs of infection are present. Minor infections may be readily treated with antibiotics, whereas infections that result in systemic manifestations may additionally warrant pin removal until the infection resolves. When pins are mechanically stable (after 48 to 72 hours), weekly pin site care may be recommended. Crusting may occur at the pin site, and uncertainties currently exist about whether scabs around the pin sites should be removed. Additional research is needed to determine best practice to prevent infection with external fixators. The nurse follows institutional protocol and teaches the patient and family to perform pin-site care prior to discharge from the hospital. Written follow-up instructions that include the signs and symptoms of infection should be provided.

JOINT REPLACEMENT SURGERY

Joint surgery is one of the most frequently performed orthopedic surgeries. Joint disease, disability, or deformity may necessitate surgical intervention to relieve pain, improve stability, and improve function. Conditions contributing to joint degeneration include osteoarthritis (degenerative joint disease), rheumatoid arthritis, trauma, and congenital deformity. As noted previously, some fractures (e.g., femoral neck fracture) may cause disruption of the blood supply and subsequent AVN, and a **joint replacement** may be elected over an ORIF. Joints frequently replaced include the shoulder, hip, or knee (Fig. 42-15), and finger joints. Less frequently, more complex joints (elbow, wrist, or ankle) are replaced.

FIGURE 42-15 Examples of hip and knee replacement.

Timing of these procedures is important to ensure maximum function. Surgery should be performed before surrounding muscles become contracted and atrophied and serious structural abnormalities occur. The surgeon carefully evaluates the patient so that the most appropriate procedure is performed.

Surgical procedures include excision of damaged and diseased tissue, repair of damaged structures (e.g., ruptured tendon), **arthroplasty** (replacement of all or part of the joint surfaces), and **arthrodesis** (immobilizing fusion of a joint).

Most joint replacements consist of metal, ceramic, or polyethylene components. Selection is typically based on the patient's age and activity level as well as the surgeon's preference. Cementless fixation of the femoral and acetabular component has become the standard procedure in the United States. Accurate fitting and the presence of healthy bone with adequate blood supply are important in the use of cementless components. Joint implants may be cemented with a bone-bonding agent, although they usually are reserved for individuals with a life expectancy of 10 years or less (Skinner, Sekiya, Jameel, & McMahon, 2014). Much progress has been made in reducing the prosthesis failure rate through improved techniques, improved materials, and use of bone grafts. The anterior or anterolateral approach for THA (see next section) avoids disruption of the posterior soft tissues and has dislocation rates of less than 1% (McCarthy, McMillan, Busconi, & Pive, 2016). Implant survival rates are 90% to 95% successful at 15 years; however, longevity will vary depending on patient factors, such as weight and activity (Mackenzie & Su, 2016, p. 1830).

With joint replacement, excellent pain relief is obtained in most patients. Return of motion and function depends on preoperative soft tissue condition, soft tissue reactions, and general muscle strength. Early failure of joint replacement is associated with excessive activity and preoperative joint and bone pathology.

Because these are elective procedures, some patients donate their own blood during the weeks preceding their surgery (autologous donation). This blood is used to replace blood lost during surgery. Autologous blood transfusions eliminate many of the risks of transfusion therapy.

TOTAL HIP REPLACEMENT

THA or surgical replacement of the hip joint with an artificial prosthesis, is indicated for idiopathic osteoarthritis, acetabular dysplasia, Paget disease, rheumatoid arthritis, AVN, posttraumatic injury, and other causes.

> **Nursing Alert**
> *Aspirin and NSAIDs should be discontinued at least 1 week prior to surgery because of the risk of perioperative bleeding.*

Preoperative Management

Assessment of the patient and preoperative management are aimed at having the patient in optimal health at the time of surgery. Preoperatively, it is important to evaluate cardiovascular, respiratory, kidney, and liver functions. Additionally, the nurse considers many factors, such as age (over 60 years of age), obesity, preoperative leg edema, a history of any venous thromboemboli, varicose veins, cancer, prolonged immobility, estrogens, and a wide variety of hematologic conditions, as they are indicators of risk for postoperative DVT and PE, the most common causes of postoperative mortality in those undergoing total hip replacement, and every effort is made to prevent them.

Preoperatively, it is important also to assess the neurovascular status of the extremity undergoing joint replacement. Postoperative assessment data are compared with preoperative assessment data to identify changes and deficits. For example, a sensory deficit postoperatively is of concern unless it was also noted preoperatively as nerve palsy can

occur as a result of surgery. A plan of nursing care for a patient with a total hip replacement is available online at http://thepoint.lww.com/Honan2e.

Providing Patient Education

Maintenance of the femoral head component in the acetabular cup is essential. The nurse teaches the patient about positioning the leg in **abduction**, which helps prevent dislocation of the prosthesis. The patient is aware that an abduction splint, a wedge pillow, or pillows will be placed between the knees to keep the hip in abduction if a posterior approach is used. For an anterior approach or anterolateral approach, the patient is instructed to avoid hip extension as well as external rotation beyond neutral. With an anterior THA approach, the hip muscles are left intact, generally leading to a more stable hip, lower complication rates (e.g., lower rate of dislocation, reduced blood loss), earlier restoration of gait, and decreased postoperative restrictions. The nurse should consult with the surgeon regarding the need for specific postoperative hip restrictions. General dislocation precautions include no hip flexion past 90 degrees, avoid hip adduction and internal or external rotation, and do not lie in prone position. In general, hip precautions including raised toilet seats should be employed as they will minimize hip joint flexion in the postoperative period.

> **Nursing Alert**
> *For total hip replacement surgery (posterior approach) the legs should be slightly abducted. Prevent hip flexion beyond 90 degrees, hip adduction, and internal rotation to avoid dislocation of the hip after joint replacement surgery. For an anterior approach, motions that externally rotate the limb as well as hyperextension and flexion of the hip combined with external rotation are avoided.*

Preventing Infection

Preoperative assessment of the patient for infections (including skin, urinary tract, and pulmonary infection) is necessary because of the risk for postoperative infection. Any infection 2 to 4 weeks before planned surgery may result in postponement of surgery. Preoperative skin preparation frequently begins 1 or 2 days before the surgery. Prophylactic antibiotics are given immediately preoperatively (typically less than 2 hours before the surgery) and continued for 24 hours (Mackenzie & Su, 2016).

Intraoperative Management

Blood is conserved during surgery to minimize loss via a pneumatic tourniquet that produces a "bloodless field." Intraoperative blood salvage with reinfusion is used when a large volume of blood loss is anticipated, and this has shown to substantially reduce the need for allogeneic transfusions (transfusion of blood collected from someone other than the patient) (Xie et al., 2015).

Airborne bacteria that contaminate the wound at the time of surgery cause most deep infections. Therefore, as with any surgery, there is strict adherence to aseptic principles, and the operating area is controlled and made as bacteria-free as possible.

Culture of the joint during surgery, before intraoperative antibiotic therapy is begun, may be important in identifying and treating subsequent infections. If osteomyelitis develops, it is difficult to treat. Persistent infection at the site of the prosthesis usually requires removal of the implant and joint revision, which is a complex procedure. Also, it is not always possible to achieve a functional joint when the reconstruction procedure has to be repeated.

Postoperative Management

Repositioning the Patient and Preventing Dislocation

Depending on the surgical approach, the nurse may turn the patient onto the affected or unaffected extremity as prescribed by the surgeon.

Dislocation is more common with the posterolateral approach and is seen when the hip is in full flexion, adducted (legs together), and internally rotated. For this reason, the patient will have either a triangular abduction wedge placed between the legs or pillows placed between the knees prior to positioning, to keep the affected leg in an abducted position and prevent internal rotation. The pillows between the legs are used when in a supine or side-lying position and when turning. The patient's hip is never flexed more than 90 degrees. To prevent hip flexion, the nurse does not elevate the head of the bed more than 60 degrees. Limited flexion is maintained during transfers and when sitting. When the patient is initially assisted out of bed, an abduction splint or pillows are kept between the legs. The nurse encourages the patient to keep the affected hip in extension, instructing the patient to pivot on the unaffected leg with assistance by the nurse, who protects the affected hip from **adduction** (together), flexion, internal or external rotation, and excessive weight-bearing.

When the patient is turned onto his side, proper alignment and supported abduction are maintained with pillows or abduction wedge. The nurse ensures that the straps of the abduction wedge are secured before turning the patient onto his unaffected side and that straps do not cause undue pressure on the peroneal nerve or surrounding skin. If the patient needs to use a bedpan, a fracture bedpan is used; the nurse instructs the patient to flex the unaffected hip and use the trapeze to lift the pelvis onto the pan. The patient is also reminded not to flex the affected hip. In addition, the patient is aware that crossing of legs is prohibited. Elevated toilet seats and chairs are suggested, as well as "reaching devices" that will limit hip flexion to less than 90 degrees. Occupational therapists can provide the patient with devices to assist with dressing below the waist.

High-seat (orthopedic) chairs and semireclining wheelchairs may also be used to minimize hip joint flexion. When sitting, the patient's hips should be higher than the knees. The patient's affected leg should not be elevated when sitting. The patient may flex the knee. A cradle boot may be used to prevent leg rotation and to support the heel off the bed, preventing development of a pressure ulcer. In general, the nurse instructs the patient not to sleep on the operative side without consulting the surgeon. Hip precautions should be enforced for 4 or more months after surgery.

Dislocation may occur with positioning that exceeds the limits of the prosthesis. The nurse must recognize dislocation of the prosthesis. Indicators are as follows:

- Increased pain at the surgical site, swelling, and immobilization
- Acute groin pain in the affected hip or increased discomfort
- Shortening of the leg
- Abnormal external or internal rotation
- Restricted ability or inability to move the leg
- Reported "popping" sensation in the hip

If a prosthesis becomes dislocated, the nurse (or the patient, if at home) immediately notifies the surgeon because the hip must be reduced and stabilized promptly so that the leg does not sustain circulatory and nerve damage. After closed reduction, the hip may be stabilized with Buck's traction or a **brace** to prevent recurrent dislocation. As the muscles and joint capsule heal, the chance of dislocation diminishes. Stresses to the new hip joint should be avoided for the first 3 to 6 months.

Promoting Ambulation

Patients with total hip replacement begin ambulation with a physical therapist, generally within a day after surgery. The nurse and the physical therapist assist the patient in achieving the goal of independent ambulation. At first, the patient may be able to stand for only a brief period because of orthostatic hypotension.

Nursing Alert

Orthostatic hypotension is an abnormal drop in blood pressure on change of position from lying to standing. Approximately 500 to 700 mL of blood momentarily shifts to the lower body when changing position to standing from supine, resulting in decreased venous return and arterial pressure. Complaints of dizziness may be noted. A drop of systolic pressure of 20 mm Hg, a drop in diastolic pressure of 10 mm Hg or more, or an increase in heart rate of 15 bpm within 3 minutes is diagnostic of orthostatic hypotension. It may be related to hypovolemia, dehydration, drug-induced hypotension, or prolonged bed rest. Patients should be encouraged to rise slowly and move their legs prior to rising to facilitate venous return from the extremities.

Patient Education

Avoiding Hip Dislocation After Replacement Surgery

Until the hip prosthesis stabilizes after hip replacement surgery, it is necessary to follow instructions for proper positioning so that the prosthesis remains in place. Dislocation of the hip is a serious complication of surgery that causes pain and loss of function and necessitates reduction under anesthesia to correct the dislocation. Desirable positions include abduction, neutral rotation, and flexion of less than 90 degrees. When you are seated, the knees should be lower than the hip.

Methods for avoiding displacement for posterior hip procedures include the following:
- Keep the knees apart at all times.
- Put two pillows between the legs when sleeping.
- Never cross the legs when seated.
- Avoid bending forward when seated in a chair to pick up an object on the floor.

- Avoid internal rotation of the hip.
- Avoid sitting in a low chair or toilet seat to avoid flexing the hip more than 90 degrees.
- Use a high-seated chair and a raised toilet seat; consider handrails by the toilet.
- Limit sitting to 30 minutes at a time—to minimize hip flexion and the risk of prosthetic dislocation and to prevent hip stiffness and flexion contracture.
- Do not flex the hip to put on clothing such as pants, stockings, socks, or shoes. Consider Occupational therapy devices for dressing and reaching.
- Encourage quadriceps setting and ROM exercises, as directed.
- Positions to avoid after total hip replacement are illustrated below.

Affected leg should not cross the center of the body   Hip should not bend more than 90 degrees   Affected leg should not turn inward

Nettina, S. M. (2014). *Lippincott manual of nursing practice.*

Specific weight-bearing limits on the prosthesis are determined by the surgeon and are based on the patient's condition, the procedure, and the fixation method. Usually, patients with cemented prostheses can proceed to weight bearing as tolerated. If the patient has a press-fit, cementless, ingrowth prosthesis, weight-bearing immediately after surgery may be limited to minimize micromotion of the prosthesis in the bone. As the patient is able to tolerate more activity, the nurse encourages transferring to a chair several times a day for short periods and walking for progressively greater distances. Refer to Box 42-13 for patient education to prevent hip dislocation.

Monitoring for Complications

Complications that may occur include dislocation of the hip prosthesis, excessive wound drainage, thromboembolism, infection, and heel pressure ulcer. Other complications for which the nurse must monitor include those associated with immobility, heterotopic ossification, AVN, and loosening of the prosthesis.

Monitoring Wound Drainage

If extensive blood loss is anticipated after total joint replacement surgery, an autotransfusion drainage system (in which the drained blood is filtered and reinfused into the patient during the immediate postoperative period) may be used to decrease the need for blood transfusions. Because of the risk of contamination, the blood should be administered within 6 hours of initiation of collection. The nurse should follow institutional protocol.

Fluid and blood accumulating at the surgical site may be drained with a portable suction device (PSD). Traditionally PSD was used to prevent accumulation of fluid, which could contribute to discomfort and provide a site for infection. However, recent research reveals that patients with PSD required transfusions and had longer length of stay; in addition, no differences were observed in pain level, wound-related complications, infection, or early functional outcome than in patients managed postoperatively without drains (Fichman, 2016). If drains are used, typically they are removed by 48 hours after surgery.

Preventing Deep Vein Thrombosis

The risk of venous thromboembolism is particularly great after reconstructive hip surgery. Without prophylaxis, the incidence of documented DVT in the patient with total joint arthroplasty is reported in the range of 40% to 60% (Kakkar & Rushton-Smith, 2013). The peak occurrence is 2 to 14 days after surgery (60% of DVTs occur within 2 weeks); however, patients are at risk until 6 months after the operation (Kakkar & Rushton-Smith, 2013). The risk of DVT can be reduced with short intraoperative time, epidural anesthesia, intraoperative heparin administration, elastic stockings, pneumatic devices, foot flexion-extension exercises, and early ambulation. Therefore, the nurse must institute preventive measures and monitor the patient closely for the development of DVT and PE. Signs of DVT include unilateral calf pain, swelling, and tenderness. Measures to promote circulation and decrease venous stasis are priorities for the patient undergoing hip reconstruction. The nurse encourages the patient to consume adequate amounts of fluids, to perform ankle and foot exercises hourly while awake, to use elastic stockings and sequential compression devices as prescribed, and to transfer out of bed and ambulate with assistance beginning on the first postoperative day. There is no consensus on appropriate anticoagulation status post-THA; however, low–molecular-weight heparin (e.g., enoxaparin [Lovenox], dalteparin [Fragmin]) or sometimes unfractionated heparin frequently is prescribed as prophylaxis for DVT after hip replacement surgery. If warfarin is administered, the international normalized ratio (INR) should be maintained between 2.0 and 3.0, typically for 21 days (Mackenzie & Su, 2016; McElroy, Innerfield, Cuccurullo, & Rossi, 2015).

Preventing Infection

Infection, a serious complication of total hip replacement, may necessitate removal of the implant. Patients who are elderly, obese, or poorly nourished, and patients who have diabetes, rheumatoid arthritis, concurrent infections (e.g., UTI, dental abscess), or large hematomas are at high risk for infection.

Because total joint infections are so disastrous, all efforts are made to prevent them. Potential sources of infection are avoided. Typically prophylactic antibiotics are prescribed less than 2 hours before surgery and continued for 24 hours. If indwelling urinary catheters or portable wound suction devices are used, they are removed as soon as possible to avoid infection. Prophylactic antibiotics are prescribed if the patient needs any future surgical or invasive procedures, such as tooth extraction or cystoscopic examination.

BOX 42-14

Risk Factors for Delayed Healing

The nurse is aware that patients who present with the following factors are at risk for delayed healing of fractures:
- Extensive local trauma
- Malnutrition
- Bone loss
- Inadequate immobilization
- Space or tissue between bone fragments
- Infection
- Local malignancy
- Metabolic bone disease (e.g., Paget disease)
- Irradiated bone (radiation necrosis)
- Avascular necrosis (AVN)
- Intra-articular fracture (synovial fluid contains fibrolysins, which lyse the initial clot and restrict clot formation)
- Age (elderly people heal more slowly)
- Corticosteroids (inhibit the repair rate)

Acute infections may occur within 3 months after surgery and are associated with progressive superficial infections or hematomas. Delayed surgical infections may appear 4 to 24 months after surgery and may cause return of discomfort in the hip. Infections occurring more than 2 years after surgery are attributed to the spread of infection through the bloodstream from another site in the body. If an infection occurs, antibiotics are prescribed. Severe infections may require surgical débridement or removal of the prosthesis. Refer to Box 42-14 for risk factors associated with impaired healing.

Teaching the Patient Self-Care

Before the patient prepares to leave the acute care setting, the nurse provides thorough teaching to promote continuity of the therapeutic regimen and active participation in the rehabilitation process. The nurse advises the patient of the importance of the daily exercise program in maintaining the functional motion of the hip joint and strengthening the abductor muscles of the hip, and reminds the patient that it will take time to strengthen and retrain the muscles.

Assistive devices (crutches, walker, or cane) are used for a time. After sufficient muscle tone has developed to permit a normal gait without discomfort, these devices are not necessary. In general, by 3 months, the patient can resume routine ADLs. Frequent walks, swimming, and use of a high rocking chair are excellent for hip exercises. Sexual intercourse can be resumed based upon surgeon recommendation (typically 4 to 6 weeks postoperatively). Sexual positions will depend on surgical approach used for THA and will be individualized based upon the position of the hip that is most unstable.

Assistance in putting on shoes and socks may be needed. The patient should avoid low chairs and maintain restrictions per surgeon's preference. At the present time, weight-bearing restrictions after THA are not standardized and are typically determined by the surgeon's preference. Precautions that minimize hip flexion and risks of prosthetic dislocation, hip stiffness, and flexion **contracture** are reviewed with the patient and significant others. Other activities to avoid typically include tub baths, jogging, lifting heavy loads, and excessive bending and twisting (e.g., lifting, shoveling snow, forceful turning).

 Nursing Alert
The risk of dislocation after THA decreases as time passes without a dislocation. If dislocation occurs, typically it is seen within 6 weeks after surgery and frequently is associated with adhering to postsurgical guidelines.

TOTAL KNEE REPLACEMENT

Total knee replacement surgery is considered for patients who have severe pain and functional disabilities related to destruction of joint surfaces by arthritis (osteoarthritis, AVN, rheumatoid arthritis, posttraumatic arthritis) or bleeding into the joint (e.g., hemarthrosis), such as may result from hemophilia. Metal and acrylic prostheses designed to provide the patient with a functional, painless, stable joint may be used. If the patient's ligaments have weakened, a fully constrained (hinged) or semiconstrained prosthesis may be used to provide joint stability. A nonconstrained prosthesis depends on the patient's ligaments for joint stability.

Postoperative Management

Postoperatively, the knee is dressed with a compression bandage. Ice may be applied to control edema and bleeding. The nurse assesses the neurovascular status of the leg. It is important to encourage active flexion of the foot every hour when the patient is awake. Efforts are directed at preventing complications (thromboembolism, peroneal nerve palsy, infection, limited ROM).

A wound suction drain removes fluid accumulating in the joint. Drainage varies depending on operative event (cement vs. non-cement; use of drains, tourniquets) and patient comorbidities. In general, the surgeon can be expected to remove the drains within 24 hours. If extensive bleeding is anticipated, an autotransfusion drainage system may be used during the immediate postoperative period. The color, type, and amount of drainage are documented, and any excessive drainage or change in characteristics of the drainage is promptly reported to the surgeon.

The use of a CPM device is often dependent on the surgeon's preference. If a CPM machine is used, the patient's leg is placed in the device and ROM movement usually begins on postoperative day 1 at full extension (0 degrees) and 30 degrees of flexion and generally is advanced 5 to 10 degrees per day until 90 degrees of flexion is achieved at approximately 6 weeks postoperatively (McElroy et al., 2015). The physical therapist supervises exercises for strength and ROM, and progression of rehabilitation will be based upon patient tolerance.

The nurse assists the patient to get out of bed on the evening of or the day after surgery. The knee is usually protected with a knee immobilizer (splint, cast, or brace) and is elevated when the patient sits in a chair. The surgeon prescribes weight-bearing limits. Progressive ambulation, using assistive devices and within the prescribed weight-bearing limits, begins on the day after surgery.

After discharge from the hospital, the patient may continue to use the CPM device at home and may undergo physical therapy on an outpatient basis. The overall complication rate of total knee replacement is 8% within the first 6 months postoperatively. Complications include knee stiffness, infection, DVT, poor wound healing, loosening of components, periprosthetic fracture, and nerve injury (McElroy et al., 2015). As with THA, there is no uniform consensus regarding type and duration of anticoagulation therapy after TKA. Medications (warfarin, heparin, aspirin, or enoxaparin) and pneumatic compression devices are often utilized. Patients usually can achieve a pain-free, functional joint and participate more fully in life activities than before the surgery.

AMPUTATION

Amputation is the removal of a body part, usually an extremity. Amputation of a lower extremity is often necessary because of progressive peripheral vascular disease (often a sequela of diabetes mellitus), fulminating gas gangrene, trauma (crushing injuries, burns, frostbite, electrical burns), congenital deformities, chronic osteomyelitis, or malignant tumor. Of all these causes, peripheral vascular disease accounts for 82% of all amputations, with 97% of these in the lower limb (Uustal, 2015). (See Chapter 18 for more information about peripheral vascular disease.) Amputation of an upper extremity occurs less frequently than amputation of a lower extremity and is most often necessary because of either traumatic injury or a malignant tumor. More than 100,000 major amputations occur each year in the United States, and there are currently 1.6 million amputee survivors in the United States, with numbers increasing annually (Uustal, 2015).

Levels of Amputation

Amputation is performed at the most distal point that will heal successfully. The site of amputation is determined by two factors: circulation in the body part and functional usefulness (i.e., meets the requirements for the use of a prosthesis).

The objective of surgery is to conserve as much extremity length as needed to preserve function and possibly to achieve a good prosthetic fit. Preservation of knee and elbow joints is desired. Most amputations involving extremities can be eventually fitted with a prosthesis.

The amputation of toes and portions of the foot causes minor changes in gait and balance. A Syme amputation (modified ankle **disarticulation** amputation) is the most common ankle procedure and is performed frequently for extensive foot trauma; it produces a painless, durable extremity end that can withstand full weight bearing. Below-knee amputation (BKA) is preferred to above-knee amputation (AKA) because of the importance of the knee joint and the energy requirements for walking. Knee disarticulations are most successful with young, active patients who can develop precise control of the prosthesis. When AKAs are performed, all possible length is preserved, muscles are stabilized and shaped, and hip contractures are prevented for maximum ambulatory potential. Most people who have a hip disarticulation amputation must rely on a wheelchair for mobility.

Complications

Complications that may occur with amputation include hemorrhage, infection, skin breakdown, phantom limb pain, and joint contracture. Because major blood vessels have been severed, massive bleeding may occur. Infection is a risk with all surgical procedures. The risk of infection increases with contaminated wounds after traumatic amputation. Skin irritation caused by the prosthesis may result in skin breakdown. **Phantom limb pain** is caused by the severing of peripheral nerves. Joint contracture is caused by positioning and a protective flexion withdrawal pattern associated with pain and muscle imbalance.

The 5-year survival rate for patients with BKA due to vascular disease is 48%, and only 22% for patients with AKA, whereas long-term survival rate for patients with traumatic amputation is near normal life expectancy (Uustal, 2015).

Medical and Nursing Management

Dressings vary according to surgeon preference and may include a closed rigid cast dressing, a removable rigid dressing, or a soft dressing. A closed rigid cast dressing is frequently used to provide uniform compression, support soft tissues, control pain, and prevent joint contractures. Care is taken not to constrict circulation.

For the patient with a lower extremity amputation, the plaster cast may be equipped to attach a temporary prosthetic extension (pylon) and an artificial foot. This rigid dressing technique is used as a means of creating a socket for immediate postoperative prosthetic fitting. The length of the prosthesis is tailored to the individual patient. Early minimal weight bearing on the residual limb with a rigid cast dressing and a pylon attached produces little discomfort. The cast is changed in about 10 to 14 days. Elevated body temperature, severe pain, or a loose-fitting cast may necessitate earlier replacement.

A removable rigid dressing may be placed over a soft dressing to control edema, prevent joint flexion contracture, and protect the residual limb from unintentional trauma during transfer activities. This rigid dressing is removed several days after surgery for wound inspection and is then replaced to control edema. The dressing facilitates residual limb shaping.

A soft dressing with or without compression may be used if there is significant wound drainage, and frequent inspection of the residual limb (stump) is desired. An immobilizing splint may be incorporated in the dressing. Stump (wound) hematomas are controlled with wound drainage devices to minimize infection.

 Nursing Alert
If the cast or elastic dressing inadvertently comes off, the nurse must immediately wrap the residual limb with an elastic compression bandage. If this is not done, excessive edema will develop in a short time, resulting in a delay in rehabilitation. The nurse notifies the surgeon if a cast dressing comes off so that another cast can be applied promptly.

Promoting Rehabilitation

Patients who require amputation because of severe trauma are usually, but not always, young and healthy, heal rapidly, and are physically able to participate in a vigorous rehabilitation program. Because the amputation is the result of an injury, the patient needs psychological support in accepting the sudden change in body image and in dealing with the stresses of hospitalization, long-term rehabilitation, and modification of lifestyle. Patients who undergo amputation need support as they grieve the loss, and they need time to work through their feelings about their permanent loss and change in body image. Their reactions are unpredictable and can include anger, bitterness, and hostility.

The multidisciplinary rehabilitation team (patient, nurse, clinical nurse specialist, physician, social worker, physical therapist, occupational therapist, psychologist, prosthetist, vocational rehabilitation worker) helps the patient achieve the highest possible level of function and participation in life activities. Prosthetic clinics and amputee support groups facilitate this rehabilitation process. Vocational counseling and job retraining may be necessary to help patients return to work.

Psychological issues (e.g., denial, withdrawal) may be influenced by the type of support the patient receives from the rehabilitation team and by how quickly ADLs and use of the prosthesis are learned. Knowing the full options and capabilities available with the various prosthetic devices can give the patient a sense of control over the resulting disability.

Minimizing Altered Sensory Perceptions

A person who has had an amputation may experience phantom limb pain soon after surgery or 2 to 3 months later. It occurs more frequently in patients who have had AKAs. As many as 80% of amputees complain of phantom pain, which is often described as sharp and electric or burning pain of the amputated limb, and highly fluctuant (Andersen, Nanos, Pinzur, & Potter, 2015). The pathogenesis of the phantom limb phenomenon is unknown. When a patient describes phantom pains or sensations, the nurse acknowledges these feelings and helps the patient modify these perceptions. Phantom sensations were thought to diminish over time; however, recent research challenges that notion. Richardson, Crawford, Milnes, Bouch, & Kulkarni, (2015) found that phantom pain was associated with sleep loss and social restrictions, and their results challenge the belief that phantom limb pain reduces over time. Further research is warranted on this complex phenomenon, and a multimodal approach that combines both pharmacologic and nonpharmacologic interventions should be considered. Transcutaneous electrical nerve stimulation (TENS), massage, mirror therapy, ultrasound, acupuncture, hypnosis, hot and cold modalities, or local anesthetics may provide some relief for patients. In addition, beta blockers may relieve dull, burning discomfort; antiseizure medications control stabbing and cramping pain; and tricyclic antidepressants are used to modify pain signals and improve mood and coping ability. Newer treatment modalities include virtual reality in an attempt to extinguish maladaptive memory traces of the amputated limb and extinguish the pain (Sano et al., 2015).

Helping the Patient to Achieve Physical Mobility

Proper positioning prevents the development of hip or knee joint contracture in the patient with a lower extremity amputation. Exercises that preserve essential ROM for hip extension and knee extension also should be part of the therapy program. Abduction, external rotation, and flexion of the lower extremity are avoided. Depending on the surgeon's preference, the residual limb may be placed in an extended position or elevated for a brief period after surgery. Prolonged elevation (after initial 24 hours postoperative) is not recommended as flexion contractions are to be avoided.

 Nursing Alert
The residual limb should not be placed on a pillow because a flexion contracture of the hip may result.

A physical therapist will develop exercises if indicated for muscle strengthening and to prevent abduction and flexion contractures. The nurse encourages the patient to turn from side to side and to assume a prone position, if possible, to stretch the flexor muscles and to prevent flexion contracture of the hip. The nurse discourages sitting for prolonged periods to prevent flexion contracture. The legs should remain close together to prevent an abduction deformity. The nurse encourages the patient to use assistive devices (e.g., reachers) to more readily perform self-care activities and to identify what home modifications should be made to perform these activities in the home environment.

Postoperative ROM exercises are started early because contracture deformities develop rapidly. ROM exercises include hip and knee exercises for BKAs and hip exercises for AKAs. It is important that the patient understand the importance of exercising the residual limb.

The upper extremities, trunk, and abdominal muscles are exercised and strengthened. The extensor muscles in the arm and the depressor muscles in the shoulder play an important part in crutch walking. The major problems that can delay prosthetic fitting during this period are (1) flexion deformities, (2) nonshrinkage of the residual limb, and (3) abduction deformities of the hip. In general, fabrication of the temporary prosthesis begins 3 to 4 weeks after amputation. The wearing time should start with only 1 to 2 hours per day and advance by 1 hour daily if tolerated.

Excessive pressure from the prosthesis can cause skin irritation, pain, skin breakdown, and infection. The nurse observes the operative site for erythema and pain. The introduction of gel liner material improves the ability of the skin to tolerate pressures. However, because of sanitation issues associated with gel liners, daily cleansing of the skin and gel liner is essential to prevent maceration of the skin or development of bacterial and fungal infections (Uustal, 2015). The nurse also assesses for systemic indicators of infection (e.g., elevated temperature, leukocytosis [elevated WBCs] with an increase of at least 10% bands on the differential) and promptly reports indications of infection to the surgeon.

CHAPTER REVIEW

Critical Thinking Exercises

1. You volunteer to provide field first aid for your neighborhood's softball league. Common injuries you expect include sprains, strains, and possibly dislocations and fractures. What specific assessment would you make to differentiate these problems? Describe the standard treatment for any of these common musculoskeletal disorders.

2. A 68-year-old man has had a repair of a fracture of his right tibia. During the evening of his second postoperative day, he complains of increasing pain and slight paresthesias of his right toes. Opioid analgesics have only moderately relieved his pain. The night-shift nurse documents her findings and asks you, as the oncoming day-shift nurse, to report these findings to the orthopedic surgeon when he

makes his rounds. You assess the patient after report and find that he now describes his right lower leg as "feeling tight" and that he has sensations of "pins and needles." His right lower leg has a capillary refill longer than 3 seconds, and his right toes feel much cooler than the left toes. What additional assessments might you make at this time? What is your priority nursing diagnosis and intervention?

3. Mrs. Y, who is postoperative from total hip repair and has a history of ulcers, is complaining of abdominal pain. Her hematocrit this morning is 8/24. One unit of packed cells is administered. One hour after the unit has infused, you are asked to draw a repeat H/H. If Mrs. Y does not have any additional sources of blood loss, what do you expect her H/H to rise by in the repeat laboratory work?

NCLEX-Style Review Questions

1. In the immediate postoperative period, which measure would best prevent a DVT?
   a. Adding a multivitamin to the patient's medication
   b. Early ambulation
   c. Measuring intake and output
   d. Lowering the legs below the level of the heart

2. A 22-year-old man is admitted to the emergency department with a crush injury to both lower legs. He was pinned under a car for 3 hours. On admission, his vital signs are stable; he is alert and oriented and complaining of extreme pain in his legs. Popliteal pulses are strong; pedal and posterior tibial pulses are weak. The ankle and feet appear dusky; the skin is tense, but the skin envelope is not broken. X-rays show no broken bones. Based upon these data, what interventions are most appropriate?
   a. Notify the provider and anticipate that a stat V̇/Q̇ scan will be performed to rule out fat emboli.
   b. Notify the provider and prepare to set up skin traction to decrease the pressure on the calf muscle.

c. Notify the provider and anticipate that the provider will measure the pressure in the compartment and possibly perform a fasciotomy if elevated pressure is noted.
   d. Notify the provider and prepare to give IV antibiotics stat to decrease the risk of osteomyelitis.

3. During assessment of a patient admitted to the emergency room after a motor vehicle collision, he becomes semi-conscious and continues moaning with pain. His blood pressure has now decreased to 100/42, and his pulse has increased to 122. What is the most immediate life-threatening problem for this patient?
   a. Arrhythmias due to hypokalemia
   b. Hypovolemia
   c. Respiratory depression from pain medication
   d. Fat embolus to the lung

4. A 73-year-old patient is placed in skeletal traction prior to surgery for an ORIF of fractured femur. She develops chest pain, tachypnea, and tachycardia the second day in traction. What additional symptom would indicate her symptoms are related to a fat emboli rather than a pulmonary thromboembolic event?
   a. Hypotension
   b. Restlessness
   c. Petechiae of the anterior chest wall
   d. Warm, reddened areas in her leg

5. A 23-year-old patient, experienced an open fracture of the left tibia with major soft tissue damage of his lower leg in a bicycle accident. Surgical reduction and fixation of the tibia were performed with debridement of nonviable tissue and drain placement in the damaged soft tissue. Which finding by the nurse would most likely indicate the development of the osteomyelitis?
   a. Tachycardia
   b. Elevated ESR
   c. Numbness in the left leg and toes
   d. Muscle spasms around the affected bone

REFERENCES AND SELECTED READINGS

References and selected readings associated with this chapter can be found on the website that accompanies the book. Visit **http://thepoint. lww.com/Honan2e** to access the references and other additional resources associated with this chapter.

Problems Related to Neurologic Function

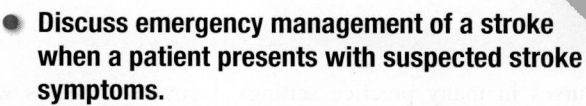

A 65-year-old patient presents to the emergency department by ambulance. The paramedics state that his spouse witnessed the sudden onset of confusion, weakness in his right arm and leg, and difficulty speaking (he could not get the right words out). His symptoms occurred 2 hours prior to arrival at the hospital. He has a history of smoking, hypertension, atrial fibrillation, and prior transient ischemic attacks (TIAs). An initial noncontrast head CT was negative for intracerebral hemorrhage. An acute ischemic stroke in the left hemisphere is suspected.

- Discuss emergency management of a stroke when a patient presents with suspected stroke symptoms.
- What sub-type of ischemic stroke is the patient most likely experiencing?
- Discuss nursing considerations for the patient receiving tPA.
- Describe three of the eight standardized performance measures that are considered for a patient with an ischemic stroke.

Nursing Assessment: Neurologic Function

Dawn K. Beland • **Donna M. Avanecean**

Learning Objectives

After reading this chapter, you will be able to:

1. Describe the structures and functions of the central and peripheral nervous systems.
2. Differentiate between pathologic changes that affect motor control and those that affect sensory pathways.
3. Compare the functioning of the sympathetic and parasympathetic nervous systems.
4. Describe changes in neurologic function associated with aging and their impact on neurologic assessment findings.
5. Describe the significance of physical assessment to the diagnosis of neurologic dysfunction.
6. Describe diagnostic tests used for assessment of suspected neurologic disorders and the related nursing implications.

Nurses in many practice settings encounter patients with altered neurologic function. Disorders of the nervous system can occur at any time during the lifespan and can vary from mild, self-limiting symptoms to devastating, life-threatening disorders. Nurses must be skilled in the assessment of the neurologic system, whether the assessment is generalized or focused on specific areas of function. In either case, assessment requires knowledge of the anatomy and physiology of the nervous system and an understanding of the array of tests and procedures used to diagnose neurologic disorders. Knowledge about the nursing implications and interventions related to assessment and diagnostic testing is also essential.

ANATOMIC AND PHYSIOLOGIC OVERVIEW

The function of the nervous system is control of all motor, sensory, autonomic, cognitive, and behavioral activities. The nervous system consists of two major divisions: the central nervous system (CNS), including the brain and spinal cord; and the peripheral nervous system (PNS), which includes cranial and spinal nerves that lie outside the brain and spinal cord. The PNS can be further divided into the somatic, or voluntary nervous system, and the autonomic, or involuntary nervous system.

Anatomy of the Nervous System

Cells and Neurotransmitters of the Nervous System

Cells of the brain link the motor and sensory pathways, monitor the body's processes, respond to the internal and external environment, maintain homeostasis, and direct all psychological, biologic, and physical activity through complex chemical and electrical messages. The basic functional unit of the brain is the neuron (Fig. 43-1). It is composed of a cell body, a dendrite, and an axon. The **dendrite** is a branch-type structure with synapses (a gap between two neurons, in which impulses jump from one neuron to another) for receiving electrochemical messages. The **axon** is a long projection that carries impulses away from the cell body. Nerve cell bodies occurring in clusters are called *ganglia* or *nuclei*. A cluster of cell bodies with the same function is called a *center* (e.g., the respiratory center).

Neurotransmitters communicate messages from one neuron to another or from a neuron to a specific target tissue and are responsible for all types of brain activity. Each neurotransmitter has an affinity for specific receptors in the postsynaptic bulb. When released, neurotransmitters cross the synaptic cleft and bind to receptors in the postsynaptic cell membrane. The action of a neurotransmitter is to potentiate, terminate, or modulate a specific action, and it can either

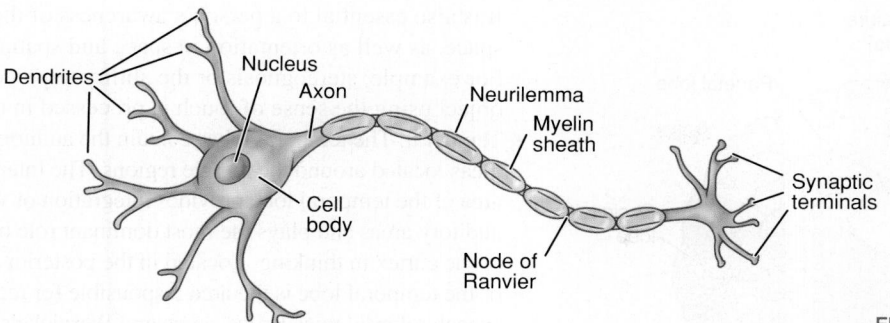

FIGURE 43-1 Neuron.

excite or inhibit the activity of the target cell. Usually, multiple neurotransmitters are at work in the neural synapse. Imbalances or deficiencies of a particular neurotransmitter may cause neurologic dysfunction. Major neurotransmitters are described in Table 43-1.

The Central Nervous System

The Brain

The brain is divided into three major areas: the cerebrum, the brainstem, and the cerebellum. The cerebrum is composed of two hemispheres, the thalamus, the hypothalamus, and the basal ganglia. In addition, connections for the olfactory (cranial nerve I) and optic (cranial nerve II) nerves are found in the cerebrum. The brainstem includes the midbrain, pons, medulla, and connections for cranial nerves III through XII. The cerebellum is located under the cerebrum and behind the brainstem (Fig. 43-2).

Cerebrum. The cerebrum consists of two hemispheres that are incompletely separated by the great longitudinal fissure. This sulcus (a depression or groove) separates the cerebrum into the right and left hemispheres. The two hemispheres are joined at the lower portion of the fissure by the corpus callosum. The outside surface of the hemispheres has many folded layers or convolutions called *gyri*, which increase the surface area of the brain. The external or outer portion of the cerebrum (the cerebral cortex) is made up of gray matter, approximately 2 to 5 mm in depth. White matter makes up the innermost layer and is composed of nerve fibers and neuroglia (support tissue) that form tracts or pathways connecting various parts of the brain. The cerebral hemispheres are divided into pairs of frontal, parietal, temporal, and occipital lobes. The four lobes are as follows (see Fig. 43-2):

• Frontal: The frontal lobe is the largest lobe in the front of the skull. The major functions are concentration, abstract

TABLE 43-1 Major Neurotransmitters

Neurotransmitter	Source	Action	Example of Dysfunction
Acetylcholine (major transmitter of the parasympathetic nervous system)	Many areas of the brain; autonomic nervous system	Usually excitatory; parasympathetic effects sometimes inhibitory (stimulation of heart by vagal nerve)	↓ Leads to Myasthenia gravis
Serotonin	Brainstem, hypothalamus, dorsal horn of the spinal cord	Inhibitory, helps control mood and sleep, inhibits pain pathways	↓ Leads to depression
Dopamine	Substantia nigra and basal ganglia	Usually inhibits, affects behavior (attention, emotions) and fine movement	↓ Leads to Parkinson disease
Norepinephrine (major transmitter of the sympathetic nervous system)	Brainstem, hypothalamus, postganglionic neurons of the sympathetic nervous system	Usually excitatory; affects mood and overall activity	Seen rarely
Gamma-aminobutyric acid (GABA)	Spinal cord, cerebellum, basal ganglia, some cortical areas	Inhibitory	↓ Leads to seizures
Enkephalin, endorphin	Nerve terminals in the spine, brainstem, thalamus and hypothalamus, pituitary gland	Excitatory; pleasurable sensation, inhibits pain transmission	Poor pain control

FIGURE 43-2 View of the external surface of the brain showing lobes, cerebellum, and brainstem.

thought, information storage or memory, and motor function. The motor strip, which lies in the frontal lobe, anterior to the central sulcus, is responsible for muscle movement. Refer to Figure 43-3 for specific locations of control of motor movement. It also contains Broca's area and Wernicke's area (left frontal lobe region in most people), critical for motor control of speech. The frontal lobe is responsible in large part for a person's affect, judgment, personality, emotions, attitudes, and inhibitions, and contributes to the formation of thought processes.

• Parietal: The parietal lobe is the primary sensory cortex, which is located posterior to the motor strip, and is organized topographically similar to the motor strip. This lobe analyzes sensory information such as pressure, vibration, pain, and temperature, and relays the interpretation of this information to the thalamus from the sensory cortex.

FIGURE 43-3 Diagrammatic representation of the cerebrum showing locations for control of motor movement of various parts of the body.

It is also essential to a person's awareness of the body in space, as well as orientation in space and spatial relations. For example, stereognosis or the ability to perceive an object using the sense of touch is processed in this area.

• Temporal: The temporal lobes contain the auditory receptive areas located around the temple regions. The interpretive area of the temporal lobe provides integration of visual and auditory areas and plays the most dominant role of any area of the cortex in thinking. Located in the posterior region of the temporal lobe is the area responsible for receptive speech referred to as Broca's area and Wernicke's area. For most people, whether right- or left-handed, Broca's area and Wernicke's area. is in the left lobe. Long-term memory recall is also associated with this lobe.

• Occipital: The occipital lobe located in the posterior portion of the cerebral hemispheres is known as the primary visual cortex. The occipital lobe also assists in some visual reflexes, as well as allows for some involuntary eye movements.

The corpus callosum (Fig. 43-4) is a thick collection of nerve fibers that connects the two hemispheres of the brain and transmits the information from one side of the brain to the other. Right-handed people and some left-handed people have cerebral dominance on the left side of the brain for verbal, linguistic, arithmetical, calculating, and analytic functions. The nondominant hemisphere is responsible for geometric, spatial, visual, pattern, and musical functions.

The basal ganglia are masses of nuclei located deep in the white matter of the cerebral hemispheres and are responsible for control of fine motor movements. The thalamus lies

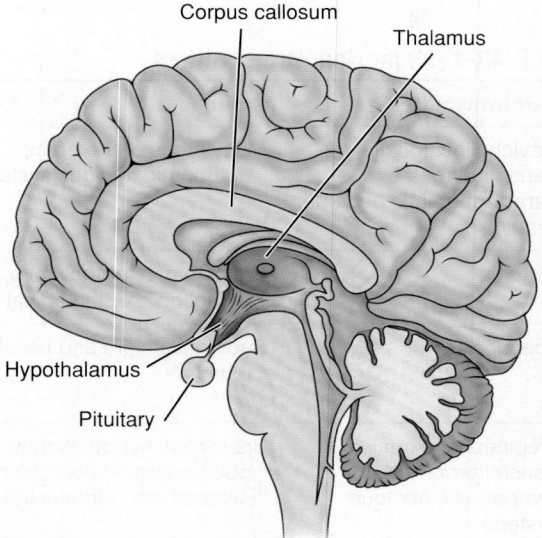

FIGURE 43-4 Medial view of the brain. The brain is divided into the **right and left hemisphere**, and the two halves are connected by the **corpus callosum**. This bundle of nerve tissue contains over 200 million axons (nerve fibers that carry electrical impulses from neurons' cell bodies) by rough estimate. This neural tissue facilitates communication between the two sides of the brain (Healthline, 2015).

on either side of the third ventricle and acts primarily as a relay station for all sensation except smell. All memory also passes through this section of the brain.

The hypothalamus (see Fig. 43-4) is anterior and inferior to the thalamus and lies next to the third ventricle. It includes the optic chiasm (where the two optic tracts cross) and the mammillary bodies (involved in olfactory reflexes and emotional response to odors). The infundibulum of the hypothalamus connects to the posterior pituitary gland. The hypothalamus, important in the endocrine system, regulates the pituitary secretion of hormones influencing metabolism, reproduction, stress response, and urine production. It works with the pituitary to maintain fluid balance (refer to Chapter 29 for further details). In addition, the hypothalamus, the site of the hunger center, is involved in appetite control. It contains centers that regulate the sleep–wake cycle, blood pressure, aggressive and sexual behavior, and emotional responses (i.e., blushing, rage, depression, panic, and fear). The hypothalamus also controls and regulates the autonomic nervous system and maintains temperature regulation by promoting vasoconstriction or vasodilatation.

The pituitary gland is located in the sella turcica at the base of the brain. The pituitary is a common site of brain tumors in adults, which are frequently detected by signs and symptoms traced to the pituitary, such as hormonal imbalance or visual disturbances due to pressure on the optic chiasm (see Chapter 31).

Nerve fibers from the cortex converge in each hemisphere and exit in a tight bundle of nerve fibers known as the *internal capsule*. After entering the pons and medulla, each bundle crosses to the corresponding bundle from the opposite side. Although the various cells in the cerebral cortex are quite similar in appearance, their functions vary widely, depending on location.

Brainstem. The brainstem is responsible for automatic functions such as heart rate, breathing, and swallowing. It consists of the **midbrain, pons,** and **medulla oblongata** and contains motor and sensory pathways (see Fig. 43-2). The midbrain connects the pons and cerebellum with the cerebral hemispheres and serves as the center for auditory and visual reflexes. Cranial nerves III and IV originate in the midbrain. The pons is situated in front of the cerebellum, between the midbrain and the medulla, and acts as a bridge between the cerebrum, the cerebellum, and the medulla. Cranial nerves V through VIII originate in the pons and connect the brain to the pons. Portions of the pons also control the heart rate, respiration, and blood pressure.

The medulla oblongata contains motor fibers from the brain to the spinal cord and sensory fibers from the spinal cord to the brain. Most of these fibers cross, or *decussate* at this level. Cranial nerves IX through XII originate in the medulla and connect the brain to the medulla. The medulla and pons are essential for respiratory function.

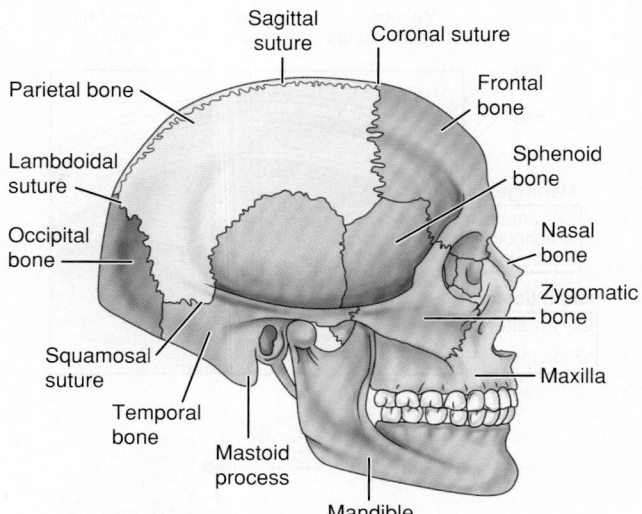

FIGURE 43-5 Bones and sutures of the skull.

Cerebellum. The cerebellum is separated from the cerebral hemispheres by a fold of dura mater, the *tentorium cerebelli.* The cerebellum is largely responsible for coordination of all movement. It also controls fine movement, balance, **position (postural) sense** or proprioception (awareness of where each part of the body is), and integration of sensory input.

Structures Protecting the Brain
Skull. The brain is contained in a rigid skull, protecting it from injury. The major bones of the skull are the frontal, temporal, parietal, and occipital bones (Fig. 43-5). These bones join at suture lines.

Meninges. The meninges (fibrous connective tissues) cover the brain and spinal cord, and provide protection, support, and nourishment. The three layers of the meninges are the **dura, arachnoid, and pia mater** (Fig. 43-6). An easy way to remember the layers is to note that the meninges **"PAD"** the brain (*p*ia, *a*rachnoid, and *d*ura).

The **dura mater**, the outermost layer, covers the brain and the spinal cord. The dura mater is tough, thick, inelastic, fibrous, and gray. There are four extensions of the dura: the **falx cerebri**, which separates the two hemispheres in a longitudinal plane; the **tentorium**, which is an infolding of the dura that forms a tough, membranous shelf between the cerebrum and cerebellum; the **falx cerebelli**, which lies between the two lateral lobes of the cerebellum; and the **diaphragm sellae**, which provides a "roof" for the sella turcica. The tentorium supports the hemispheres and separates them from the lower part of the brain. When excess pressure occurs in the cranial cavity, brain tissue may be compressed against the tentorium or displaced downward, a process called *herniation.*

The epidural space, a *potential space* that has the capacity to expand slightly, lies outside the outermost layer of the

FIGURE 43-6 Meninges and related structures.

dura. In the spinal canal, the dura forms a tubular sheath around the spinal cord. This narrow space between the dura mater and the periosteum (lining of the bones) is where local anesthetic can be injected for pain relief.

The **arachnoid**, the middle membrane, is an extremely thin, delicate membrane resembling a spider web (hence the name arachnoid). It appears white because it has no blood supply. This membrane has unique finger-like projections, **arachnoid villi**, which absorb cerebrospinal fluid (CSF). In the normal adult, approximately 500 mL of CSF is produced each day; all but 125 to 150 mL is absorbed by the villi (Hickey, 2014). When blood enters the system (from trauma or hemorrhagic stroke), the villi become obstructed, and hydrocephalus (increased size of ventricles) may result. The subarachnoid space is between the arachnoid and pia layers and contains CSF.

The pia mater, the innermost membrane, is a thin, transparent layer that hugs the brain closely and extends into every fold of the brain's surface. It is highly vascular.

Cerebrospinal Fluid

CSF, a clear and colorless fluid, is produced in the lateral ventricles by the choroid plexus and is circulated around the brain and spinal cord through the ventricular system. There are four ventricles. The two lateral ventricles, normally containing 25 mL of CSF each, open into the third ventricle at the interventricular foramen or the foramen of Monro. The third and fourth ventricles connect via the aqueduct of Sylvius. The fourth ventricle supplies CSF to the subarachnoid space and down the spinal cord on the dorsal surface. CSF is

returned to the brain and then circulated, where it is absorbed by the arachnoid villi.

The composition of CSF is similar to other extracellular fluids (such as blood plasma), but the concentrations of the various constituents differ. The laboratory report of CSF analysis usually contains information on color, specific gravity, protein count, white blood cell (WBC) count, glucose, and other electrolyte levels. Normal CSF contains a minimal number of WBCs and no red blood cells (RBCs). The intracranial pressure (ICP) within the skull results from a combination of brain tissue, blood flow, and CSF. Normal CSF pressure is approximately 5 to 15 mm Hg (Hickey, 2014), while pressures greater than 20 mm Hg indicate increased ICP.

Nursing Alert

*In the event of a skull fracture, the nurse should be alert for signs of CSF leakage. Suspect rhinorrhea (leakage of CSF via nares) with fractures involving the cribriform plates of the anterior cranial fossa, while otorrhea (leakage of CSF via ear) is suspected with fractures involving the basilar skull. Depending on the site of the fracture, the patient may present with **raccoon eyes** (bruising around the eyes) or **Battle sign** (ecchymosis of the mastoid process of the temporal bone). Leakage of CSF places the patient at risk for meningitis. If a CSF leak is suspected, the nurse is aware that nothing is allowed into the patient's nose or ears (suction or nasogastric catheters, dressings, tissues etc.). See Figure 43-7.*

Cerebral Circulation

The cerebral circulation receives approximately 15% of the cardiac output, or 750 mL per minute. The brain does not store nutrients, has a high metabolic demand, and requires high blood flow. The brain's blood pathway is unique because it flows against gravity; its arteries fill from below, and the veins drain from above. The brain has poor collateral blood flow, which results in irreversible tissue damage when blood flow is occluded for even short time periods.

Arteries. Two internal carotid arteries and two vertebral arteries and their extensive system of branches provide blood supply to the brain (Fig. 43-8). The internal carotids arise from the bifurcation of the common carotid and supply much of the anterior circulation. The vertebral arteries branch from the subclavian arteries, flow back and upward on either side of the cervical vertebrae, and enter the cranium through the foramen magnum. The vertebral arteries join to become the basilar artery at the brainstem; then the basilar artery divides to form the two branches of the posterior cerebral arteries. The vertebrobasilar arteries supply most of the posterior circulation of the brain.

The circle of Willis is formed from the branches of the anterior circulation and posterior circulation connected by one anterior communicating artery and two posterior

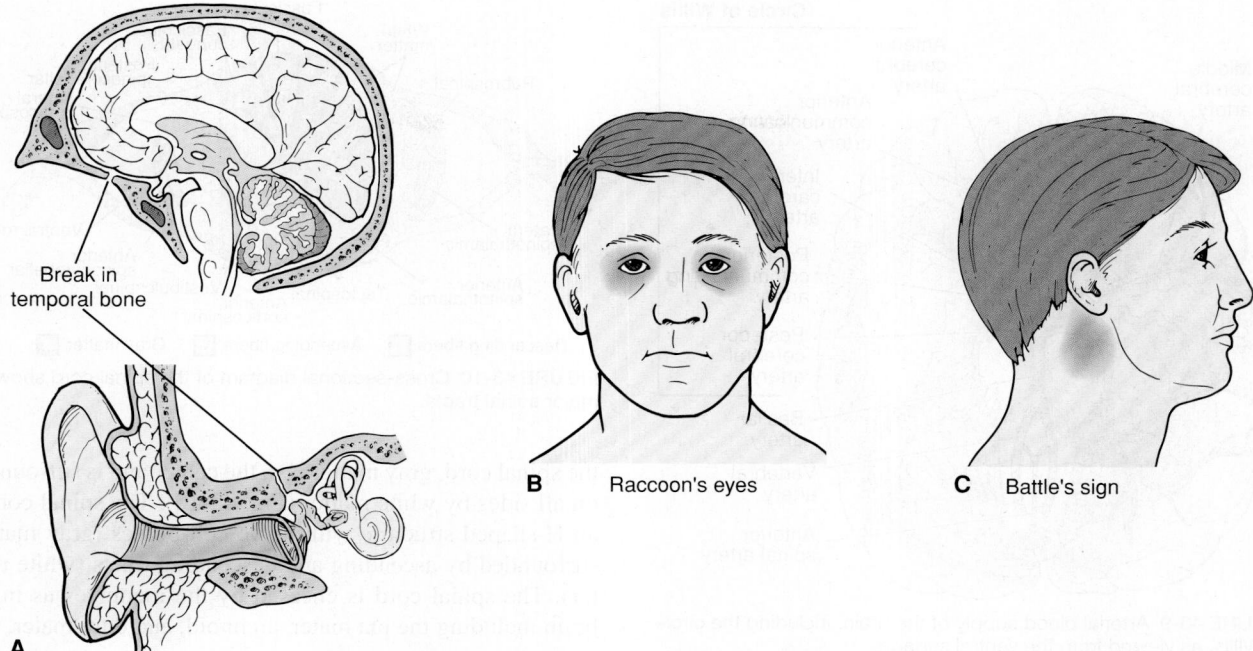

FIGURE 43-7 **A.** Basilar skull fracture in the temporal bone can cause cerebrospinal fluid (CSF) to leak from the nose or ear. **B.** Periorbital ecchymosis, called raccoon's eyes. **C.** Battle sign over the mastoid process. (From Rosdahl, C. B., & Kowalski, M. (2017). *Textbook of basic nursing* (11th ed.). Philadelphia, PA: Wolters Kluwer.)

communicating arteries (Fig. 43-9). The arteries of the circle of Willis can provide collateral circulation if one or more of the four vessels supplying it becomes occluded.

The arterial bifurcations (branches) along the circle of Willis are frequent sites of aneurysm formation. Aneurysms may be congenital or result from changes in the vessel wall associated with atherosclerotic disease. If an artery with an aneurysm bursts, depending on its size and location, catastrophic effects can be seen. Additionally, if a blood vessel becomes constricted by vasospasm, it may lead to diminished

blood flow, causing potential damage to neurons distal to the constriction, leading to cell death. If not aggressively treated, this may result in an ischemic stroke. The effects of the constriction depend on which vessels are involved and the areas these vessels supply.

Veins. Venous drainage for the brain does not follow the arterial circulation, as in other body structures. The veins reach the brain's surface, join larger veins, then cross the subarachnoid space, and empty into the **dural sinuses**, which

The two vertebral arteries (branches of the subclavians) converge to become...

...the basilar artery, which...

...supplies oxygen to the posterior brain.

The common carotids branch into the two internal carotids, which...

...divide further to supply oxygen to the...

...anterior brain and the middle brain.

FIGURE 43-8 Arterial circulation to the brain. (From Lippincott. (2009). *Anatomy and physiology made incredibly visual!* (p. 63). Philadelphia, PA: Lippincott Williams & Wilkins.)

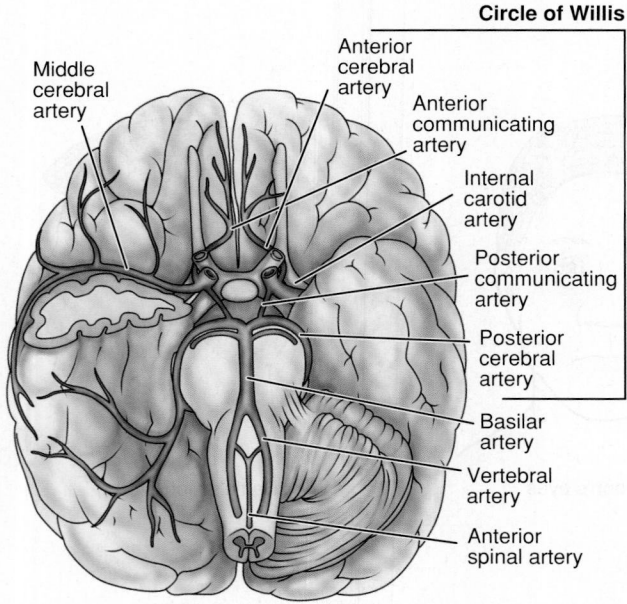

FIGURE 43-9 Arterial blood supply of the brain, including the circle of Willis, as viewed from the ventral surface.

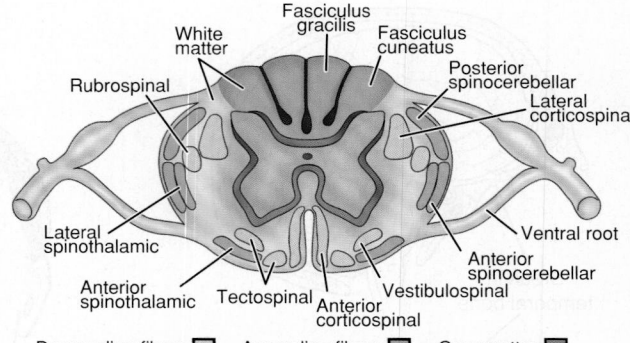

FIGURE 43-10 Cross-sectional diagram of the spinal cord showing major spinal tracts.

are the vascular channels lying within the dura mater (see Fig. 43-6). The network of sinuses empties into the internal jugular vein, returning blood to the heart. Cerebral veins and sinuses are unique because, unlike other veins, they do not have valves to prevent blood from flowing backward and depend on both gravity and blood pressure.

Blood–Brain Barrier

The CNS and its neurons are inaccessible to many substances that circulate in the blood plasma (e.g., dyes, medications, and antibiotics) because of the blood–brain barrier. This barrier is formed by the tight junction of the endothelial cells in the brain's capillaries. All substances entering the CSF must filter through the capillary endothelial cells and astrocytes (Hickey, 2014). The blood–brain barrier has a protective function but can be altered by trauma, cerebral edema, and cerebral hypoxemia; this has implications in the treatment and selection of medication for CNS disorders.

Spinal Cord

The spinal cord and medulla form a continuous structure extending from the cerebral hemispheres and serving as the connection between the brain and the periphery. Approximately 45 cm (18 in) long and about the thickness of a finger, it extends from the foramen magnum at the base of the skull to the lower border of the first lumbar vertebra, where it tapers to a fibrous band called the *conus medullaris*. Continuing below the second lumbar space are the nerve roots that extend beyond the conus, which are called the *cauda equina* because they resemble a horse's tail. Similar to the brain, the spinal cord consists of gray and white matter. Gray matter in the brain is external and white matter is internal; in

the spinal cord, gray matter is in the center and is surrounded on all sides by white matter (Fig. 43-10). The spinal cord is an H-shaped structure with nerve cell bodies (gray matter) surrounded by ascending and descending tracts (white matter). The spinal cord is encased by the meninges as in the brain including the pia mater, archnoid, and dura mater.

Nursing Alert
The nurse understands that the spinal cord extends to L1; therefore, if a lumbar puncture (spinal tap) is to be performed, the site for insertion of the needle will be below L1. Typically the needle is placed in the interspace between L3 and L4 or between L4 and L5, which is a safe distance from the distal spinal cord. The bony landmark for the L4 spinous process is located at the intersection of the line between the top of the iliac crests and the midline of the lumbar spine.

Sensory and Motor Pathways: The Spinal Tracts. The white matter of the cord is composed of **myelinated** and **unmyelinated** nerve fibers. The fast-conducting **myelinated fibers** form bundles that also contain **glial cells**. Fiber bundles with a common function are called *tracts*.

There are six **ascending tracts** (see Fig. 43-10). Two conduct sensation, principally the perception of touch, pressure, vibration, position, and passive motion from the same side of the body. Before reaching the cerebral cortex, these fibers cross to the opposite side in the medulla. The two spinocerebellar tracts conduct sensory impulses from muscle spindles, providing necessary input for coordinated muscle contraction. They ascend essentially uncrossed and terminate in the cerebellum. The last two spinothalamic tracts are responsible for conduction of pain, temperature, proprioception, fine touch, and vibratory sense from the upper body to the brain. They ascend, cross to the opposite side of the brain, and terminate in the thalamus.

There are eight **descending** tracts. The two corticospinal tracts conduct motor impulses to the anterior horn cells from the opposite side of the brain and control voluntary muscle activity. The three vestibulospinal tracts descend uncrossed and are involved in some autonomic functions (sweating, pupil dilation, and circulation) and involuntary muscle control. The corticobulbar tract conducts impulses responsible for voluntary head and facial muscle movement and crosses at the level of the brainstem. The rubrospinal and reticulospinal tracts conduct impulses involved with involuntary muscle movement.

Vertebral Column. The bones of the vertebral column surround and protect the spinal cord and normally consist of seven **cervical**, 12 **thoracic**, and five **lumbar** vertebrae, as well as the **sacrum** (a fused mass of five vertebrae), and terminate in the **coccyx**. Nerve roots exit from the vertebral column through the intervertebral foramina (openings). The vertebrae are separated by disks, except for the first and second cervical, the sacral, and the coccygeal vertebrae. The vertebral body, arch, pedicles, and laminae all encase and protect the spinal cord.

The Peripheral Nervous System

The PNS includes the **cranial nerves**, the **spinal nerves**, and the **autonomic nervous system**.

Cranial Nerves

Twelve pairs of cranial nerves emerge from the lower surface of the brain and pass through the foramina in the skull (Fig. 43-11). Three are entirely sensory (I, II, VIII), five are motor (III, IV, VI, XI, and XII), and four are mixed (V, VII, IX, and X), because they have both sensory and motor functions. Most cranial nerves innervate the head, neck, and special sense structures. Table 43-2 lists the names and primary functions of the cranial nerves.

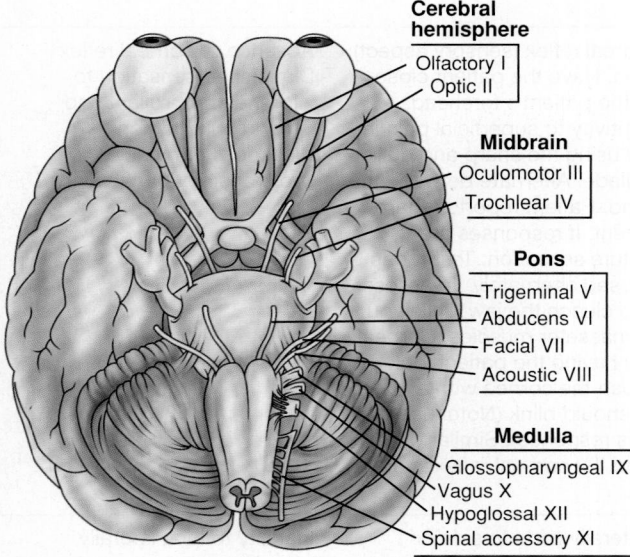

FIGURE 43-11 Diagram of the base of the brain showing entrance or exit of the cranial nerves. The right column shows the anatomic location of the connection of each cranial nerve to the central nervous system.

FIGURE 43-12 Spinal cord and meninges. (From Porth, C. M., & Matfin, G. (2009). *Pathology: Concepts of altered health states* (8th ed.). Philadelphia, PA: Lippincott Williams & Wilkins.)

Spinal Nerves

The spinal cord is composed of **31 pairs of spinal nerves**: eight cervical, 12 thoracic, five lumbar, five sacral, and one coccygeal. Each spinal nerve has a **ventral** and **dorsal** root (Fig. 43-12).

The dorsal roots are sensory and transmit sensory impulses from specific areas of the body known as ***dermatomes*** (Fig. 43-13) to the dorsal ganglia. The sensory fiber may be **somatic**, carrying information about pain, temperature, touch, and position sense (proprioception) from the tendons, joints, and body surfaces; or **visceral**, carrying information from the internal organs.

The ventral roots are motor and transmit impulses from the spinal cord to the body, and these fibers are also either somatic or visceral. The visceral fibers include autonomic fibers that control the cardiac muscles and glandular secretions.

Autonomic Nervous System

The **autonomic nervous system** regulates activities of internal organs, such as the heart, lungs, blood vessels, digestive organs, and glands. Maintenance and restoration of internal homeostasis is largely the responsibility of the autonomic nervous system. There are two major divisions: the **sympathetic nervous system**, with predominantly excitatory responses, most notably the "fight-or-flight" response, and the **parasympathetic nervous system**, which controls mostly visceral functions, known as "rest-and-digest."

The autonomic nervous system is regulated by centers in the spinal cord, brainstem, and hypothalamus. Its regulatory effects are exerted not on individual cells but on large expanses of tissue and on entire organs. The responses elicited do not occur instantaneously but after a lag period. These responses are sustained far longer than other neurogenic responses to

TABLE **43-2** Cranial Nerves

Cranial Nerve (CN)	Type	Assessment	Dysfunction
I (Olfactory)	Sensory	With eyes closed, the patient should be asked to identify two familiar odors (e.g., coffee, tobacco). Each nostril is tested separately. Avoid using strong odors, such as ammonia, as the trigeminal nerve may be stimulated. Testing of this CN is usually deferred.	Inability to identify odor, termed anosmia
II (Optic)	Sensory	Assess visual acuity using a portable eye chart or, if not available, grossly assess vision by having the patient read a card or newspaper from big print to small. Assess visual fields by testing peripheral vision: stand directly in front of the patient. Ask the patient to close one eye and focus on your nose as you assess the patient's ability to see your fingers that are positioned in four visual fields (upper right and left and lower right and left). In combination with CN III, assess the pupils (the light emitted into the pupil begins the process by which constriction is seen; constriction is the function of CN III).	Decreased visual acuity Decreased visual fields
III (Oculomotor)	Motor	CN III controls most extraocular eye movement (EOM), eyelid elevation, and pupillary constriction. To assess EOM, ask the patient to follow your finger through the six cardinal positions (use the letter H as a guide to assess the ability of the eye to move to the left superior, left lateral, left inferior, right superior, right lateral, and right inferior). CN III is responsible for all movements except lateral movement (CN VI) and movement of the eye downward and inward (CN IV). While the patient is looking in the six positions, have him or her hold the position briefly while you assess for nystagmus (rotary oscillation of the eye). Test for pupillary reflexes (constriction of the pupil to light), and inspect the eyelids for ptosis (drooping of the eyelid).	Inability to move the eyes in the visual field described Ptosis of affected eye Nonreactive or dilated pupil
IV (Trochlear)	Motor	This is assessed with EOM as described above. CN IV moves the eye down and in (as if looking toward the nose).	Inability to look down and in
V (Trigeminal)	Mixed	Assess facial sensation, corneal reflex (sensory aspect), and chewing or mastication. Have the patient close the eyes. Touch cotton to the patient's forehead, cheeks, and jaw. Test sensitivity to superficial pain in these same three areas by using the sharp and dull ends of a broken tongue blade. Alternate between the sharp point and the dull end. Patient reports "sharp" or "dull" with each movement. If responses are incorrect, test for temperature sensation. Test tubes of cold and hot water are used alternately. To assess chewing, ask the patient to clench the jaw while you palpate the temporal and masseter muscles. Corneal reflex may be assessed by having the patient look up and away while you brush the cornea with a wisp of cotton; both eyes should blink (Note: use of contact lens decreases this response). Similar to the pupillary reaction (CN II and III), corneal reflexes are a combination CN V and VII.	Absence of corneal reflex Diminished sensation to forehead, maxillary and mandibular region Weakness of muscles responsible for chewing
VI (Abducens)	Motor	Abducens moves the eye laterally (side to side or horizontally) and is assessed with EOMs.	Inability to look laterally, double vision

Cranial Nerve (CN)	Type	Assessment	Dysfunction
VII (Facial)	Mixed	Assess for symmetry of facial movement. Ask the patient to smile, raise the eyebrows, keep eyes and lips closed while you try to open them, and puff out the cheeks. Taste is also a function of this CN, although testing is often deferred. The motor response of closing the eye in response to stimuli is assessed with corneal reflex (combination of CN V and VII).	Facial paralysis Facial asymmetry, droop of mouth Absent nasolabial fold Decreased ability to taste
VIII (Acoustic)	Sensory	Assess hearing by rubbing your fingers, placing a ticking watch, or whispering near each ear. Equilibrium can be assessed with the Romberg test and is usually deferred.	Decreased hearing in affected ear
IX (Glossopharyngeal)	Mixed	This CN's function is primarily innervation of the pharynx and tongue, pharyngeal muscles, and swallowing. Ask the patient to open the mouth and say "Ah." Note symmetrical elevation of the upper palate and uvula in the midline position. Assessing for the gag reflex tests this nerve and CN X, as they travel together. To test gag reflex, use a cotton swab or tongue blade to touch the patient's posterior pharynx; note gag response.	Dysphagia Absence of gag reflex
X (Vagus)	Mixed	This CN is assessed by swallowing and gag reflex as noted above. In addition, the quality of the patient's voice is noted.	Hoarse or nasal quality to voice Slurred speech
XI (Spinal accessory)	Motor	Have the patient shrug the shoulders and turn his or her head from side to side; assess the sternocleidomastoid and trapezius muscles for symmetry.	Inability to shrug shoulders
XII (Hypoglossal)	Motor	Inspect the patient's tongue for atrophy at rest. To assess movement of the tongue, have the patient stick out the tongue and move it internally from cheek to cheek.	Tongue weakness

ensure maximal functional efficiency on the part of receptor organs, such as blood vessels. The autonomic nervous system transmits its impulses by way of nerve pathways, enhanced by chemical mediators.

Sympathetic stimuli are mediated by norepinephrine, and parasympathetic impulses are mediated by acetylcholine. Both divisions produce stimulatory and inhibitory effects. Table 43-3 compares sympathetic and parasympathetic effects on different systems of the body.

Motor and Sensory Functions of the Nervous System

Motor System Function

The motor cortex, a vertical band within each cerebral hemisphere, controls the voluntary movements of the body. The exact locations within the brain at which the voluntary movements of the muscles of the face, thumb, hand, arm, trunk, and leg originate are known (see Fig. 43-3). Stimulation of these cells results in muscle contraction. En route to the pons, the motor fibers converge into a tight bundle

known as the *internal capsule*. A comparatively small injury to the capsule results in paralysis in more muscles than does a much larger injury to the cortex itself.

Within the medulla, the motor axons from the cortex form the **corticospinal** or **pyramidal tracts**. Here, most of the fibers cross (or decussate) to the opposite side. The remaining fibers enter the spinal cord on the same side as the direct pyramidal tract. All of the motor fibers of the spinal nerves represent extensions of the anterior horn cells, with each of these fibers communicating with only one particular muscle fiber. The motor system is complex, and motor function depends on the integrity of the corticospinal tracts, the extrapyramidal system, and cerebellar function.

Upper and Lower Motor Neurons
The voluntary motor system consists of two groups of neurons: **upper motor neurons** and **lower motor neurons**. Upper motor neurons originate in the cerebral cortex, the cerebellum, and the brainstem, where they cross over and descend throughout the corticospinal tract. Their fibers make up the descending motor pathways, are located entirely

FIGURE 43-13 Dermatome distribution.

within the CNS, and modulate the activity of the lower motor neurons. Lower motor neurons are located either in the anterior horn of the spinal cord gray matter or within cranial nerve nuclei in the brainstem. Axons of lower motor neurons in both sites extend through peripheral nerves and terminate in skeletal muscle at the myoneural junction. Lower motor neurons are located in both the CNS and the PNS. The clinical features of lesions of upper and lower motor neurons are discussed in Table 43-4.

Coordination of Movement

The smoothness, accuracy, and strength that characterize muscular movements are attributable to the influence of the cerebellum and the basal ganglia.

The cerebellum (see Fig. 43-2, p. 1252) is responsible for the coordination, balance, and timing of all muscular movements. Through the action of the cerebellum, the contractions of opposing muscle groups are adjusted in relation to each other to maximal mechanical advantage.

The basal ganglia play an important role in planning and coordinating motor movements and posture. Complex neural connections link the basal ganglia with the cerebral cortex. The major effect of these structures is to inhibit unwanted

muscular activity; disorders of the basal ganglia result in exaggerated, uncontrolled movements.

Impaired cerebellar function, which may occur as a result of an intracranial injury, cerebrovascular event, or some type of an expanding mass, results in loss of muscle tone, weakness, and fatigue. Cerebellar signs, such as ataxia and incoordination, as well as CSF obstruction and compression of the brainstem may be seen. Signs of increased ICP, including vomiting, headache, and changes in vital signs and level of consciousness (LOC), are especially common when CSF flow is obstructed.

Destruction or dysfunction of the basal ganglia leads not to paralysis but to muscle rigidity, with disturbances of posture and movement. The patient tends to have involuntary movements. These may take the form of coarse tremors, most often in the upper extremities, particularly in the distal portions; athetosis (movement of a slow, squirming, writhing, twisting type); or chorea (spasmodic, purposeless, irregular, uncoordinated motions of the trunk and the extremities, and facial grimacing). Disorders due to lesions of the basal ganglia include Parkinson disease, Huntington disease, and spasmodic torticollis (a painful condition where neck muscles contract involuntarily, causing the head to twist or turn to one side).

TABLE **43-3** Autonomic Effects of the Nervous System

Structure or Activity	Parasympathetic Effects	Sympathetic Effects
Pupil of the Eye	Constricted	Dilated
Circulatory System		
Rate and force of heartbeat	Decreased	Increased
Blood Vessels		
In heart muscle	Constricted	Dilated
In skeletal muscle	a	Dilated
In abdominal viscera and the skin	a	Constricted
Blood pressure	Decreased	Increased
Respiratory System		
Bronchioles	Constricted	Dilated
Rate of breathing	Decreased	Increased
Digestive System		
Peristaltic movements of digestive tube	Increased	Decreased
Muscular sphincters of digestive tube	Relaxed	Contracted
Secretion of salivary glands	Thin, watery saliva	Thick, viscid saliva
Secretions of stomach, intestine, and pancreas	Increased	a
Conversion of liver glycogen to glucose	a	Increased
Genitourinary System		
Urinary bladder	Contracted	Relaxed
Muscle walls		
Sphincters	Relaxed	Contracted
Muscles of the uterus	Relaxed; variable	Contracted under some conditions; varies with menstrual cycle and pregnancy
Blood vessels of external genitalia	Dilated	a
Integumentary System		
Secretion of sweat	a	Increased
Pilomotor muscles	a	Contracted (gooseflesh)
Adrenal Medulla	a	Secretion of epinephrine and norepinephrine

aNo direct effect.
From Hickey, J. (2014). *Clinical practice of neurological and neurosurgical nursing* (7th ed.). Philadelphia, PA: Lippincott Williams & Wilkins.

TABLE **43-4** **Comparison of Lesions of the Upper Motor Neurons and Lower Motor Neurons**

Upper Motor Neuron Lesions	Lower Motor Neuron Lesions
Loss of voluntary control	Loss of voluntary control
Increased muscle tone	Decreased muscle tone
Muscle spasticity	Flaccid muscle paralysis
No muscle atrophy	Muscle atrophy
Hyperactive and abnormal	Absent or decreased reflexes

Sensory System Function

Integrating Sensory Impulses

The thalamus, a major receiving and transmitting center for the afferent sensory nerves, is a large structure connected to the midbrain (see Fig. 43-4). The thalamus integrates all sensory impulses except olfaction. It plays a role in the conscious awareness of pain and the recognition of variation in temperature and touch. The thalamus is responsible for the sense of movement and position and the ability to recognize the size, shape, and quality of objects.

Receiving Sensory Impulses

Afferent impulses travel from their points of origin to their destinations in the cerebral cortex via the ascending pathways directly, or they may cross at the level of the spinal cord or in the medulla, depending on the type of sensation that is registered. Sensory information may be integrated at the level of the spinal cord or may be relayed to the brain. Knowledge of these pathways is important for neurologic assessment and for understanding symptoms and their relationship to various lesions.

Sensory Losses

Destruction of a sensory nerve results in total loss of sensation in its area of distribution. **Transection** of the spinal cord yields complete anesthesia below the level of injury. Selective destruction or degeneration of the posterior columns of the spinal cord is responsible for a loss of position and vibratory sense in segments distal to the lesion, without loss of touch, pain, or temperature perception. A lesion, such as a cyst, in the center of the spinal cord causes dissociation of sensation—loss of pain at the level of the lesion. This occurs because the fibers carrying pain and temperature cross within the cord immediately on entering; thus, any lesion that divides the cord longitudinally divides these fibers. Other sensory fibers ascend the cord for variable distances, some even to the medulla, before crossing, thereby bypassing the lesion and avoiding destruction.

Lesions affecting the posterior spinal nerve roots may cause impairment of tactile sensation, including intermittent severe pain that is referred to the area of distribution. Tingling of the fingers and the toes can be a prominent symptom of spinal cord disease, presumably due to degenerative changes in the sensory fibers that extend to the thalamus (i.e., belonging to the spinothalamic tract).

Gerontologic Considerations

During the normal aging process, the nervous system undergoes many changes, and it is extremely vulnerable to general systemic illness. Changes throughout the nervous system that occur with age vary in degree. Nerve fibers that connect directly to muscles show little decline in function with age, as do simple neurologic functions that involve a number of connections in the spinal cord. Disease in the elderly often makes it difficult to distinguish normal from abnormal changes. It is important for clinicians not to attribute abnormality or dysfunction to aging without appropriate investigation. Pain in the absence of disease, for example, is not a normal part of aging and should be assessed, diagnosed, and treated. Table 43-5 summarizes structural changes.

Structural Changes

A number of alterations occur with increasing age. Brain weight decreases, as does the number of synapses. A loss of neurons occurs in select regions of the brain. Cerebral blood flow and metabolism are reduced. Temperature regulation becomes less efficient. In the PNS, myelin is lost, resulting

TABLE **43-5** **GERONTOLOGIC CONSIDERATIONS / Age-Related Changes in the Neurologic System**

Structural changes	Brain weight decreases Loss of neurons in the brain Reduced cerebral blood flow Decreased myelin, resulting in decreased nerve conduction in some nerves Decrease in muscle bulk Slowing in deep tendon reflexes Overall slowing of the autonomic and sympathetic nervous system Temperature regulation becomes less efficient Reduced pupillary response
Sensory changes	Atrophy of taste buds Degeneration of olfactory bulb Degeneration of nerve cells in vestibular system of inner ear, cerebellum, and proprioceptive pathways Decreased neural transmission leading to difficulty in discriminating important sounds from background noise; hearing loss becomes more common (Walston, 2016) Stage IV sleep is decreased; sleep apnea becomes more common Presence of cataracts Dulling of tactile sensation

in a decrease in conduction velocity in some nerves. There is an overall reduction in muscle bulk and the electrical activity within muscles. Taste buds atrophy, and nerve cell fibers in the olfactory bulb degenerate. Nerve cells in the vestibular system of the inner ear, cerebellum, and proprioceptive pathways also degenerate. Deep tendon reflexes can be decreased or, in some cases, absent. Hypothalamic function is modified such that stage IV sleep is reduced. There is an overall slowing of autonomic nervous system responses. Pupillary responses are reduced or may not appear at all in the presence of cataracts.

Motor Alterations

Changes in motor function often result in a flexed posture, shuffling gait, and rigidity of movement. These changes create difficulties for the older person in maintaining or recovering balance. Strength and agility are diminished, and reaction time and movement time are decreased. Repetitive movements and mild tremors may be noted during an examination and may be of concern to the person. Observation of gait may reveal a wide-based gait with balance difficulties.

Sensory Alterations

Sensory isolation due to visual and hearing loss can cause confusion, anxiety, disorientation, misinterpretation of the environment, and feelings of inadequacy. Sensory alterations may require modification of the home environment, such as large-print reading materials or sound enhancement for the telephone, as well as extra orientation to new surroundings. Simple explanations of routines, the location of the bathroom, and how to operate the call bell or light are just a few examples of information the elderly patient may need when hospitalized.

Temperature Regulation and Pain Perception

Other manifestations of neurologic changes are related to temperature regulation and pain. The elderly patient may feel cold more readily than heat and may require extra covering when in bed; a room temperature somewhat higher than usual may be desirable. Reaction to painful stimuli may be decreased with age. Because pain is an important warning signal, caution must be used when hot or cold packs are used. The older patient may be burned or suffer frostbite before being aware of any discomfort. Complaints of pain, such as abdominal discomfort or chest pain, may be more serious than the patient's perception might indicate and thus require careful evaluation. Two pain syndromes that are common in the neurologic system in older adults are diabetic neuropathies and postherpetic neuropathies (refer to Chapters 30 and 52 for further information).

Taste and Smell Alterations

The acuity of the taste buds decreases with age; along with an altered olfactory sense, this may cause a decreased appetite and subsequent weight loss. Extra seasoning often increases food intake as long as it does not cause gastric irritation. A decreased sense of smell due to atrophy of olfactory organs may present a safety hazard because elderly people living alone may be unable to detect household gas leaks or fires. Smoke and carbon monoxide detectors, important for all, are critical for the elderly.

Tactile and Visual Alterations

Another neurologic alteration in the elderly patient is the dulling of tactile sensation. There may be difficulty in identifying objects by touch, and because fewer tactile cues are received from the bottom of the feet, the person may become confused about body position and location.

These factors, combined with sensitivity to glare, decreased peripheral vision, and a constricted visual field, may result in disorientation, especially at night when there is little or no light in the room. Because the elderly person takes longer to recover visual sensitivity when moving from a light to dark area, night-lights and a safe and familiar arrangement of furniture are essential.

Mental Status

Mental status is evaluated when obtaining the history. Areas of judgment, intelligence, memory, affect, mood, orientation, speech, and grooming are assessed. Family members who bring the patient to the attention of the health care provider may have noticed changes in the patient's mental status. Drug toxicity should always be suspected as a causative factor when the patient has a change in mental status. **Delirium** (mental confusion, usually with delusions and hallucinations) is seen in elderly patients who have underlying CNS damage or are experiencing an acute condition, such as infection, adverse medication reaction, or dehydration. Many elderly patients admitted to the hospital have delirium, and the cause is often reversible and treatable (e.g., drug toxicity, vitamin B deficiency, thyroid disease). Depression may produce impairment of attention and memory. In elderly patients, delirium, which is an acute change in mental status attributable to a treatable medical problem, must be differentiated from dementia, which is a chronic and irreversible deterioration of cognitive status.

Nursing Implications

Nursing care for patients with age-related changes to the nervous system and for patients with long-term neurologic disability who are aging should include the previously described modifications. In addition, the consequences of any neurologic deficit and its impact on overall function, such as activities of daily living, use of assistive devices, and individual coping, should be assessed and considered in planning patient care.

Patient teaching is also affected because the nurse must understand the altered responses and the changing needs of the elderly patient before beginning to teach. When caring for the elderly patient, the nurse adapts activities, such as preoperative teaching, diet therapy, and instruction about new medications, their timing, and doses, to the patient's needs and capabilities. The nurse considers the presence of decline in fine motor movement and failing vision. When using visual materials for teaching or menu selection, adequate lighting without glare, contrasting colors, and large print are used to offset visual difficulties caused by rigidity and opacity of the lens in the eye and slower pupillary reaction.

Even with hearing loss, the elderly patient often hears adequately if the speaker uses a low-pitched, clear voice; shouting only makes it harder for the patient to understand the speaker. Providing auditory and visual cues aids understanding; if the patient has a significant hearing or visual loss, assistive devices, a signer, or a translator may be needed.

Teaching at an unrushed pace and using reinforcement enhances learning and retention. Material should be short, concise, and concrete. Vocabulary is matched to the patient's ability, and terms are clearly defined. The elderly patient requires adequate time to receive and respond to stimuli, learn, and react. These measures allow comprehension, memory, and formation of association and concepts.

ASSESSMENT

Health History

The history-taking portion of the neurologic assessment is critical and, in many cases of neurologic disease, leads to an accurate diagnosis. The initial interview provides an excellent opportunity to systematically explore the patient's current condition and related events while simultaneously observing overall appearance, mental status, posture, movement, and affect. Depending on the patient's condition, the nurse may need to rely on yes-or-no answers to questions, a review of the medical record, or input from the family or a combination of these.

Common Concerns

An important aspect of the neurologic assessment is the history of the present illness. Neurologic disease may be acute or progressive, characterized by symptom-free periods as well as fluctuations in symptoms. The nurse, therefore, asks about the onset, character, severity, location, duration, and frequency of symptoms and signs; associated complaints; precipitating, aggravating, and relieving factors; progression, remission, and exacerbation; and the presence or absence of similar symptoms among family members.

The clinical manifestations of neurologic disease are as varied as the disease processes themselves. Symptoms may be subtle or intense, fluctuating or permanent, inconvenient or devastating. An introduction to some of the most common

symptoms associated with neurologic disease is given in this chapter. Detailed discussions regarding how specific symptoms relate to a particular disorder are covered in later chapters in this unit.

Pain

Pain is considered an unpleasant sensory perception and emotional experience associated with actual or potential tissue damage or described in terms of such damage. Therefore pain is considered multidimensional and entirely subjective. Pain can be acute or chronic. In general, acute pain lasts for a relatively short period of time and remits as the pathology resolves. In neurologic disease, this type of pain is often associated with spinal disk disease, trigeminal neuralgia, or other neuropathic pathology (e.g., postherpetic neuralgia or painful neuropathies). In contrast, chronic or persistent pain extends for long periods of time and may represent a low level of pathology. This type of pain can occur with many degenerative and chronic neurologic conditions (e.g., cerebral palsy).

Headache and Migraine

Headache, or cephalalgia, is one of the most common of all human physical complaints. Headache is a symptom rather than a disease entity; it may indicate organic disease (neurologic or other disease), a stress response, vasodilation (migraine), skeletal muscle tension (tension headache), or a combination of factors. A **primary headache** is one for which no organic cause can be identified. These types of headache include migraine, tension-type, and cluster headaches. **Migraine headache** is characterized by periodic and recurrent attacks of severe headaches lasting from 4 to 72 hours in adults. The cause of migraine has not been clearly demonstrated, but it is primarily a vascular disturbance that occurs more commonly in women and has a strong familial tendency. The typical time of onset is at puberty, and the highest prevalence in adults occurs between 25 and 55 years of age. Migraine headaches may occur with or without an aura (a sensation that precedes the headache); however, most patients do not exhibit auras. Migraine with aura affects 5% of the adult population, and 90% of auras are visual. Migraine is more prevalent in white people and in those with a lower socioeconomic status or income (Digre, 2016).

A **secondary headache** is a symptom associated with an organic cause, such as a brain tumor or an aneurysm. Although most headaches do not indicate serious disease, persistent headaches require further investigation. Serious disorders related to headache include brain tumors, subarachnoid hemorrhage, stroke, severe hypertension, meningitis, and head injuries.

Temporal arteritis is a cause of headache in the older population, reaching its greatest incidence in those older than 70 years of age. Inflammation of the cranial arteries is characterized by a severe headache localized in the region of the temporal arteries. The inflammation may be generalized (in which case temporal arteritis is part of a vascular disease) or focal (in which case only the cranial arteries are involved) and may be associated with visual loss.

Seizures

Seizures are the result of abnormal paroxysmal discharges in the cerebral cortex, which then manifest as an alteration in sensation, behavior, movement, perception, or consciousness. The alteration may be short, such as a blank stare that lasts only a second, or of longer duration, such as a tonic-clonic seizure that can last several minutes. The type of seizure activity is a direct result of the area of the brain affected. Seizures can occur as isolated events, such as when induced by a high fever, alcohol or drug withdrawal, or hypoglycemia. A seizure may also be the first obvious sign of a brain lesion.

Dizziness and Vertigo

Dizziness is an abnormal sensation of imbalance or movement. It is fairly common in the elderly and one of the most common complaints encountered by health professionals. Dizziness can occur as a result of a variety of medical conditions that include viral syndromes, hypotension, cardiac arrhythmia, hypoglycemia, and middle ear infections, to name a few. One difficulty confronting health care providers when assessing dizziness is the vague and varied terms patients use to describe the sensation.

About 50% of all patients with dizziness have **vertigo**, which is defined as an illusion of movement, usually rotation. Vertigo is usually a manifestation of vestibular dysfunction. It can be so severe as to result in spatial disorientation, light-headedness, loss of equilibrium (staggering), and nausea and vomiting.

Visual Disturbances

Visual defects that cause people to seek health care can range from the decreased visual acuity associated with aging to sudden blindness caused by acute glaucoma. Normal vision depends on functioning visual pathways through the retina and optic chiasm and the radiations into the visual cortex in the occipital lobes. Lesions of the eye itself (e.g., cataract), lesions along the pathway (e.g., tumor), or lesions in the visual cortex (from stroke) interfere with normal visual acuity. Abnormalities of eye movement can also compromise vision by causing **diplopia** or double vision.

Weakness

Weakness, specifically muscle weakness, is a common manifestation of neurologic disease. Weakness frequently coexists with other symptoms of disease and can affect a variety of muscles, causing a wide range of disabilities. Weakness can be sudden and permanent, as in stroke, or progressive, as in many neuromuscular diseases, such as amyotrophic lateral sclerosis (ALS). Any muscle group can be affected.

Abnormal Sensation

Numbness, abnormal sensation, or loss of sensation is a neurologic manifestation of both central and peripheral nerve disease. Altered sensation can affect small or large areas of the body. It is frequently associated with weakness or pain and is potentially disabling. Both numbness and weakness can significantly affect balance and coordination.

History

A review of the medical history, including a system-by-system evaluation, is part of the health history. The nurse should be aware of any history of trauma or falls that may have involved the head or spinal cord.

Family History

The nurse may also use the interview to inquire about any family history of genetic diseases, such as Huntington disease, dystonia, and epilepsy.

Social History

The nurse questions the patient regarding the use of alcohol, medications, and illicit drugs, and assesses for signs and symptoms of withdrawal. Additionally, the nurse is aware that certain agents, such as sedatives, analgesics, or neuromuscular blocking agents, may interfere with an accurate neurologic assessment.

The nurse assesses the impact that any neurologic impairment has on the patient's lifestyle. Issues to consider include the limitations imposed on the patient by any deficit and the patient's role in society, including family and community roles. The plan of care that the nurse develops needs to address and support adaptation to the neurologic deficit and continued function to the extent possible within the patient's support system.

Physical Assessment

The neurologic examination is a systematic process that includes a variety of clinical tests, observations, and assessments designed to evaluate the neurologic status of a complex system. Although the neurologic examination is often limited to a simple screening, the examiner must be able to conduct a thorough neurologic assessment when the patient's history or other physical findings warrant it. An example of a simple screening tool for patients with head injury is the Glasgow Coma Scale (GCS; refer to Box 45-6 in Chapter 45). A GCS score is based on three patient responses: eye opening, motor response, and verbal response. The patient receives a score for his or her best response in each of these areas, and the three scores are added together. The total score will range from 3 to 15; the higher the number, the better. A score of 8 or lower usually indicates coma.

The brain and spinal cord cannot be examined as directly as other systems of the body. Thus, much of the neurologic examination is an indirect evaluation that assesses the function of the specific body part or parts controlled or innervated by the nervous system. A neurologic assessment is divided into five components: cerebral function, cranial nerves, motor system, sensory system, and reflexes. As in other parts of the physical assessment, the neurologic examination follows a logical sequence and progresses from higher levels of cortical function, such as abstract thinking, to lower levels of function, such as the determination of the integrity of peripheral nerves.

Assessing Cerebral Function

Cerebral abnormalities may cause disturbances in mental status, intellectual functioning, and thought content, and in patterns of emotional behavior. There may also be alterations in perception and motor and language abilities, as well as lifestyle.

Interpretation and documentation of neurologic abnormalities, particularly mental status abnormalities, should be specific and nonjudgmental. Lengthy descriptions and the use of terms such as *inappropriate* or *demented* should be avoided. Terms such as these often mean different things to different people and, therefore, are not useful when describing behavior. The examiner records and reports specific observations regarding level of consciousness (LOC), orientation, emotional state, or thought content, all of which permit comparison by others over time. Analysis and the conclusions that may be drawn from these findings usually depend on the examiner's knowledge of neuroanatomy, neurophysiology, and neuropathology.

Level of Consciousness

The first cue to a change in the neurologic function of a patient may be a change in the LOC, which is evaluated clinically as the patient's ability to respond appropriately to stimuli. It involves both wakefulness and cognition. The nurse compares current findings to previous patient baseline and notifies providers when any deterioration is noted. Rather than use terms like *stuporous* or *obtunded*, it is beneficial to describe the behavior in detail rather than use a broad term.

> **Nursing Alert**
> *The major source of energy for the brain is glucose. Neurons of the brain are incapable of creating or storing glucose. Therefore, the brain is dependent on blood flow for brain glucose. When blood glucose drops because of insulin administration, patients exhibit signs of decreased mentation, progressing to unconsciousness. If a patient has a history of diabetes or is receiving insulin treatment for other causes, the nurse should perform a glucose fingerstick to assess blood glucose level when a change in the LOC is noted.*

Mental Status

An assessment of mental status begins by observing the patient's appearance and behavior, noting dress, grooming, and personal hygiene. Posture, gestures, movements, facial expressions, speech, and motor activity often provide important information about the patient.

Assessing orientation to time, place, and person assists in evaluating mental status. Does the patient know what day it is, what year it is, and where he or she is? Is the patient aware of who the examiner is and of his or her purpose for being in the room?

Assessment of mental status also includes both long- and short-term memory, and the ability to concentrate and attend to tasks asked of them as well. A more detailed mental status assessment may also include assessment of an individual's ability to calculate as well as perform abstract reasoning such as "What would you do if you spotted a fire in your kitchen?"

Perception

The examiner may now consider more specific areas of higher cortical function. **Agnosia** is the inability to interpret or recognize objects seen through the special senses. The patient may see a pencil but not know what it is called or what to do with it. The patient may even be able to describe it but not interpret its function. The patient may experience auditory or tactile agnosia as well as visual agnosia. Each of the dysfunctions implicates a different part of the cortex (Table 43-6).

Screening for visual and tactile agnosia provides insight into the patient's cortical interpretation ability. The patient is shown a familiar object and asked to identify it by name. Placing a familiar object (e.g., key, coin) in the patient's hand and having him or her identify it with both eyes closed is an easy way to assess tactile interpretation.

Motor Ability

Nurses assess cortical motor integration by asking the patient to perform a skilled act (comb hair, brush teeth). Successful performance requires the ability to understand the activity desired and normal motor strength. Failure signals cerebral dysfunction.

TABLE **43-6** Types of Agnosia and Corresponding Sites of Lesions

Type of Agnosia	Affected Cerebral Area
Visual	Occipital lobe
Auditory	Temporal lobe (lateral and superior portions)
Tactile	Parietal lobe
Body parts and relationships	Parietal lobe (posteroinferior regions)

TABLE 43-7 Types of Aphasia and Region of Brain Involved

Type of Aphasia	Brain Area Involved
Auditory-receptive	Temporal lobe
Visual-receptive	Parietal-occipital area
Expressive speaking	Inferior posterior frontal areas
Expressive writing	Posterior frontal area

Language Ability

The person with normal neurologic function can understand and communicate in spoken and written language. Does the patient answer questions appropriately? Can he or she read a sentence from a newspaper and explain its meaning? Can the patient write his or her name or copy a simple figure that the examiner has drawn? A deficiency in language function is called *aphasia*. Different types of aphasia result from injury to different parts of the brain (Table 43-7).

Unfolding Patient Stories: Marilyn Hughes • Part 2

Recall from Chapter 42 **Marilyn Hughes**, who came to the hospital after falling on icy stairs. She sustained a left mid shaft tibula-fibula fracture, which requires surgery. Her husband informs the nurse that she also hit her head and did not respond to him for a short time after the fall. Describe the neurologic assessment performed by the nurse. Why should the nurse to report this information promptly to the health care team?

Care for Marilyn and other patients in a realistic virtual environment: ***vSim*** *for Nursing* (thepoint.lww.com/vSimMedicalSurgical). Practice documenting these patients' care in DocuCare (thepoint.lww.com/DocuCareEHR).

Assessing the Cranial Nerves

Refer back to Table 43-2 on page 1258 for assessment of the cranial nerves. Opposite sides of the face and neck are compared throughout the examination. The assessment of multiple cranial nerves may be combined, such as eye movement (CN III, IV, VI) and **dysphagia**, difficulty swallowing (CN IX, X, XII).

Examining the Motor System

A thorough examination of the motor system includes an assessment of muscle size, tone, and strength as well as coordination and balance. The muscles are inspected, and palpated if necessary, for their size and symmetry. Any evidence of atrophy or involuntary movements (tremors, tics) is noted. Muscle **tone** (the tension present in a muscle at rest) is evaluated by palpating various muscle groups at rest and during passive movement.

Resistance to these movements is assessed and documented. Abnormalities in tone include **spasticity** (increased muscle tone), **rigidity** (resistance to passive stretch), and flaccidity.

Strength

Assessing the patient's ability to flex or extend the extremities against resistance tests muscle strength. The function of an individual muscle or group of muscles is evaluated by placing the muscle at a disadvantage. The evaluation of muscle strength compares the sides of the body to each other.

Clinicians use a five-point scale to rate muscle strength:

- 5 indicates full power of contraction against gravity and resistance or normal muscle strength;
- 4 indicates fair but not full strength against gravity and a moderate amount of resistance or slight weakness;
- 3 indicates just sufficient strength to overcome the force of gravity or moderate weakness;
- 2 indicates the ability to move but not to overcome the force of gravity or severe weakness;
- 1 indicates minimal contractile power (weak muscle contraction can be palpated but no movement is noted) or very severe weakness; and
- 0 indicates no movement.

Distal and proximal strength in both upper and lower extremities is recorded.

Nursing Alert

There are occasional situations in which weakness of the upper extremities may be so subtle that the nurse is unsure if weakness is present. In these situations, the pronator drift can help assess for weakness. The patient holds her arms out in front of herself with palms facing the ceiling. The patient is asked to hold the position and close her eyes for approximately 20 seconds. If pronation (turning inward of the palm or the arm) or a downward drift of an arm is noted, the limb is weak. A positive pronator drift is associated with upper motor neurons in the brain and spinal cord that control voluntary movement.

Balance and Coordination

Cerebellar influence on the motor system is reflected in balance control and coordination. Coordination in the upper and lower extremities is tested by having the patient perform rapid, alternating movements and point-to-point testing. Speed, symmetry, and degree of difficulty are noted.

Point-to-point testing for coordination of the upper extremities is accomplished by having the patient touch the examiner's extended finger and then his or her own nose. This is repeated with each arm several times. Coordination in the lower extremities is tested by having the patient run the heel down the anterior surface of the tibia of the other leg. Each leg is tested in turn. **Ataxia** is defined as incoordination of voluntary muscle action, particularly of the muscle groups used in

FIGURE 43-14 Deep tendon reflexes: (**A**) biceps, (**B**) brachioradialis, (**C**) triceps, (**D**) patellar, and (**E**) ankles. (From Rhoads, J. (2006). *Advanced health assessment and diagnostic reasoning*. Philadelphia, PA: Lippincott Williams & Wilkins.)

activities such as walking or reaching for objects. The presence of ataxia or tremors (rhythmic, involuntary movements) during these movements suggests cerebellar disease.

The **Romberg test** is a screening test for balance. The patient stands with feet together and arms at the side, first with eyes open and then with both eyes closed for 20 to 30 seconds. The examiner stands close to reassure the patient of support if he or she begins to fall. Slight swaying is normal, but a loss of balance is abnormal and is considered a positive Romberg test.

Examining the Reflexes

The motor reflexes are involuntary contractions of muscles or muscle groups in response to abrupt stretching near the site of the muscle's insertion. Common reflexes that may be tested include the deep tendon reflexes (biceps, brachioradialis, triceps, patellar, and ankle reflexes, Fig. 43-14) and superficial or cutaneous reflexes (abdominal reflexes and plantar or Babinski reflex).

Deep Tendon Reflexes

The tendon is struck directly with a reflex hammer or indirectly by striking the examiner's digit with the hammer, which is placed firmly against the patient's tendon. Testing these reflexes enables the examiner to assess involuntary reflex arcs that depend on the presence of afferent stretch receptors, spinal synapses, efferent motor fibers, and a variety of modifying influences from higher levels.

Grading. The absence of reflexes is significant, although ankle jerks (Achilles reflex) may be normally absent in older people. Deep tendon reflex responses are often graded on a scale of 0 to 4+. Box 43-1 depicts how to document reflexes using this scale. As stated previously, scale ratings are highly subjective. Findings can be recorded as a fraction, indicating the scale range (e.g., 2/4). Some examiners prefer to use the terms *present*, *absent*, and *diminished* when describing reflexes.

Clonus. When reflexes are very hyperactive, a phenomenon called *clonus* may be elicited. If the foot is abruptly dorsiflexed,

BOX 43-1

Documenting Reflexes

Deep tendon reflexes are graded on a scale of 0 to 4:

0   No response
1+   Diminished (hypoactive)
2+   Normal
3+   Increased (may be interpreted as normal)
4+   Hyperactive (hyperreflexia)

The deep tendon responses and plantar reflexes are commonly recorded on stick figures. The arrow points downward if the plantar response is normal and upward if the response is abnormal.

---

it may continue to "beat" two or three times before it settles into a position of rest. Occasionally, with CNS disease, this activity persists, and the foot does not come to rest while the tendon is being stretched but continues the repetitive activity. The unsustained clonus associated with normal but hyperactive reflexes is not considered pathologic. Sustained clonus always indicates the presence of CNS disease and requires further evaluation.

Superficial Reflexes

The major superficial reflexes include corneal, gag or swallowing, upper/lower abdominal, cremasteric (men only), plantar, and perianal. These reflexes are graded differently than the motor reflexes and are noted to be present (+) or absent (−). Of these, only the corneal, gag, and plantar reflexes are tested commonly.

The corneal reflex is tested carefully using a clean wisp of cotton and lightly touching the outer corner of each eye on the sclera. The reflex is present if the action elicits a blink. Conditions such as a stroke or coma might result in loss of this reflex, either unilaterally or bilaterally. Loss of this reflex indicates the need for eye protection and possible lubrication to prevent corneal damage.

The gag reflex is elicited by gently touching the back of the pharynx with a cotton-tipped applicator; first on one side of the uvula and then the other. Positive response is an equal elevation of the uvula and "gag" with stimulation. Absent response on one or both sides can be seen following a stroke and requires careful evaluation and treatment of the resultant swallowing dysfunction to prevent aspiration of food and fluids.

The plantar reflex, also known as the **Babinski reflex**, is elicited by stroking the lateral side of the foot with a tongue blade or the handle of a reflex hammer. In a person with an intact CNS, if the lateral aspect of the sole of the foot is stroked, the toes contract and draw together. However, in a person who has CNS disease of the motor system, the toes fan out. This is normal in newborns but in adults, the presence of Babinski indicates brain dysfunction (see Fig. 43-15).

Sensory Examination

The sensory system is even more complex than the motor system because sensory modalities are carried in different tracts located in different portions of the spinal cord. The sensory examination is largely subjective and requires the cooperation

FIGURE 43-15 The clinician uses an instrument to stroke the sole of the patient's foot, beginning at the heel and curving upward, causing toe flexion (negative Babinski sign) (**A** and **B**). Toes that fan outward (positive Babinski sign) may indicate injury to the brain or spinal nerves. (From Bickley, L. S., & Szilagyi, P. (2003). *Bates' guide to physical examination and history taking* (8th ed.). Philadelphia, PA: Lippincott Williams & Wilkins.)

of the patient. The examiner should be familiar with dermatomes that represent the distribution of the peripheral nerves that arise from the spinal cord (see Fig. 43-13). Exceptions to this include major destructive lesions of the brain; loss of sensation, which may affect an entire side of the body; and the neuropathies associated with alcoholism, which occur in a glove-and-stocking distribution (i.e., over the entire hand or foot, in areas traditionally covered by a glove or sock).

Assessment of the sensory system involves tests for tactile sensation, superficial pain, vibration, and position sense (proprioception). During the sensory assessment, the patient's eyes are closed. Simple directions and reassurance that the examiner will not hurt or startle the patient encourage cooperation. Comparisons between the left- and right-side findings are documented depending on which modality is found to have a deficit.

Diagnostic Evaluation

Computed Tomography Scanning

Computed tomography (CT) scanning makes use of a narrow x-ray beam to scan the body part in successive layers. The images provide cross-sectional views of the brain, with distinguishing differences in tissue densities of the skull, cortex, subcortical structures, and ventricles. The image is displayed on a monitor and is photographed and stored digitally.

Lesions in the brain are seen as variations in tissue density differing from the surrounding normal brain tissue. Abnormalities of tissue indicate possible tumor masses, brain infarction, displacement of the ventricles, and cortical atrophy. An emergency CT scan is performed in the patient with suspected brain bleed (e.g., subarachnoid hemorrhage) since blood within the basal cisterns is generally evident within the first 24 hours, whereas conventional magnetic resonance imaging (MRI) generally is less sensitive than CT scans for detecting blood (Mayer, 2016).

Procedure

CT scanning is usually performed first without contrast material and then with IV contrast enhancement. The patient lies on an adjustable table with the head held in a fixed position while the scanning system rotates around the head or spine and produces cross-sectional images. The patient must lie perfectly still without talking or moving because motion distorts the image.

CT scanning is noninvasive and painless and has a high degree of sensitivity for detecting lesions. With advances in CT scanning, the number of disorders and injuries that can be diagnosed is increasing.

Nursing Interventions

Essential nursing interventions include preparation for the procedure and patient monitoring. Preparation includes teaching the patient about the need to lie quietly throughout the procedure. A review of relaxation techniques may be helpful for patients with claustrophobia.

Sedation can be used if agitation, restlessness, or confusion will interfere with a successful study. Ongoing patient monitoring during sedation is necessary. If a contrast agent is used, the patient must be assessed before the CT scan for an iodine/shellfish allergy because the contrast agent is iodine-based. An IV line for injection of the contrast agent and a period of fasting (usually 4 hours) are required prior to the study. Patients who receive an IV or inhalation contrast agent are monitored during and after the procedure for allergic reactions, kidney function, and other side effects, including flushing, nausea, and vomiting. Preprocedure hydration, along with the lowest possible dose of contrast for the study, is recommended, since contrast-induced nephropathy is the third most common cause of hospital-acquired kidney failure.

Positron Emission Tomography

Positron emission tomography (PET) is a computer-based nuclear imaging technique that produces images of actual organ functioning.

Procedure

The patient either inhales a radioactive gas or is injected with a radioactive substance that emits positively charged particles. When these positrons combine with negatively charged electrons (normally found in the body's cells), the resultant gamma rays can be detected by a scanning device that produces a series of two-dimensional views at various levels of the brain. This information is integrated by a computer and gives a composite picture of the brain at work.

PET permits the measurement of blood flow, tissue composition, and brain metabolism and thus indirectly evaluates brain function. The brain is one of the most metabolically active organs, consuming 80% of the glucose the body uses. PET measures this activity in specific areas of the brain and can detect changes in glucose use.

In addition, PET is useful in showing metabolic changes in the brain (Alzheimer disease), locating lesions (brain tumor, epileptogenic lesions), identifying blood flow and oxygen metabolism in patients with strokes, evaluating new therapies for brain tumors, and revealing biochemical abnormalities associated with mental illness. The isotopes used have a very short half-life and are expensive to produce, requiring specialized equipment for production.

Nursing Interventions

Key nursing interventions include patient preparation, which involves explaining the test and teaching the patient about inhalation techniques and the sensations (e.g., dizziness, lightheadedness, and headache) that may occur. The IV injection of the radioactive substance produces similar side effects. Relaxation exercises may reduce anxiety during the test.

Single-Photon Emission Computed Tomography

Procedure

Single-photon emission computed tomography (SPECT) is a three-dimensional imaging technique that uses radionuclides and instruments to detect single photons. It is a perfusion study that captures a moment of cerebral blood flow at the time of injection of a radionuclide. Gamma photons are emitted from a radiopharmaceutical agent administered to the patient and are detected by a rotating gamma camera or cameras; the image is sent to a minicomputer. This approach allows areas behind overlying structures or background to be viewed, greatly increasing the contrast between normal and abnormal tissue. It is relatively inexpensive, and the duration is similar to that of a CT scan.

SPECT is useful in detecting the extent and location of abnormally perfused areas of the brain, thus allowing detection, localization, and sizing of stroke (before it is visible by CT scan); localization of seizure foci in epilepsy; detection of tumor progression; and evaluation of perfusion before and after neurosurgical procedures. Pregnancy and breastfeeding are contraindications to SPECT.

Nursing Interventions

The nursing interventions for SPECT primarily include patient preparation and patient monitoring. Teaching about what to expect before the test can allay anxiety and ensure patient cooperation during the test. Premenopausal women are advised to practice effective contraception before and for several days after testing, and the woman who is breastfeeding is instructed to stop nursing for the time period recommended by the nuclear medicine department.

The nurse may need to accompany and monitor the patient during transport to the nuclear medicine department for the scan. Patients are monitored during and after the procedure for allergic reactions to the radiopharmaceutical agent.

Magnetic Resonance Imaging

Procedure

MRI uses a powerful magnetic field to obtain images of different areas of the body. This diagnostic test involves altering hydrogen ions in the body. Placing the patient into a powerful magnetic field causes the hydrogen nuclei (protons) within the body to align like small magnets in a magnetic field. In combination with radiofrequency pulses, the protons emit signals, which are converted to images. There are two magnet strengths available for clinical use; 1.5 T (most common strength) and 3.0 T. An MRI scan can be performed with or without a contrast agent and can identify a cerebral abnormality earlier and more clearly than other diagnostic tests. It can provide information about the chemical changes within cells, allowing the clinician to monitor a tumor's response to treatment. It is particularly useful in the diagnosis of multiple sclerosis and can describe the activity and extent of disease in the brain and spinal cord. MRI does not involve ionizing radiation. At present, MRI is most valuable in the diagnosis of nonacute conditions because the test may take up to an hour to complete.

There are several MRI scanning techniques, including magnetic resonance angiography (MRA), diffusion-weighted imaging (DWI), perfusion-weighted imaging (PWI), and fluid attenuation inversion recovery (FLAIR). The use of MRA allows visualization of the cerebral vasculature without the administration of an arterial contrast agent, but the clarity of the images is enhanced when a contrast agent is used. If an agent is used, kidney function must be assessed.

Nursing Interventions

Patient preparation should include teaching relaxation techniques and informing the patient that he or she will be able to talk to the staff by means of a microphone located inside the scanner. Many MRI suites provide headphones so that patients can listen to the music of their choice during the procedure.

Before the patient enters the room where the MRI is to be performed, all metal objects and credit cards (the magnetic field can erase them) are removed. This includes medication patches that have a metal backing; these can cause burns if not removed. No metal objects may be brought into the room where the MRI is located; this includes oxygen tanks, traditional ventilators, or even stethoscopes. The magnetic field generated by the unit is so strong that any metal-containing items will be strongly attracted and literally can be pulled away with such force that they fly like projectiles toward the magnet. There is a risk of severe injury and death; furthermore, damage to a very expensive piece of equipment may occur. A patient history is obtained to determine the presence of any metal objects (e.g., aneurysm clips, orthopedic hardware, pacemakers, artificial heart valves, intrauterine devices). These objects could malfunction, be dislodged, or heat up as they absorb energy. Cochlear implants will be inactivated by MRI; therefore, other imaging procedures are considered.

The patient lies on a flat platform that is moved into a tube housing the magnet. The scanning process is painless, but the patient hears loud thumping of the magnetic coils as the magnetic field is being pulsed. Because the MRI scanner is a narrow tube, patients may experience claustrophobia; sedation may be prescribed in these circumstances. Newer versions of MRI machines (open MRI) are less claustrophobic than the earlier devices and are available in some locations. However, the images produced on these machines are not optimal, and traditional devices are preferable for accurate diagnosis.

 Nursing Alert
For patient safety, the nurse must make sure no patient care equipment (e.g., portable oxygen tanks) that contains metal or metal parts enters the room where the MRI is located. The patient must be assessed for the presence of medication patches with foil backing (such as nicotine) that may cause a burn.

Cerebral Angiography

Procedure

Cerebral angiography is an x-ray study of the cerebral circulation with a contrast agent injected into a selected artery.

Cerebral angiography is a valuable tool to investigate vascular disease, aneurysms, and arteriovenous malformations and to define their anatomy. It is still considered the gold standard for diagnosing these conditions.

Most cerebral angiograms are performed by threading a catheter through the femoral artery in the groin and up to the desired vessel. After the groin is shaved and prepared, a local anesthetic is administered to prevent pain at the insertion site and to reduce arterial spasm. A catheter is introduced into the femoral artery, flushed with heparinized saline, and filled with contrast agent. Fluoroscopy is used to guide the catheter to the appropriate vessels. During injection of the contrast agent, images are made of the arterial and venous phases of circulation through the brain.

Nursing Interventions

The patient should be well hydrated, and clear liquids are usually permitted up to the time of a regular arteriogram. Before going to the x-ray department, the patient is instructed to void. The locations of the appropriate peripheral pulses are marked with a felt-tip pen. The patient is instructed to remain immobile during the angiogram process and is told to expect a brief feeling of warmth in the face, behind the eyes, or in the jaw, teeth, tongue, and lips, and a metallic taste when the contrast agent is injected.

Nursing care after cerebral angiography includes observation for signs and symptoms of altered cerebral blood flow. In some instances, patients may experience major or minor arterial blockage due to embolism, thrombosis, or hemorrhage, producing a neurologic deficit. Signs of such an occurrence include alterations in the level of responsiveness and consciousness, weakness on one side of the body, motor or sensory deficits, and speech disturbances. Therefore, it is necessary to observe the patient frequently for these signs and to report them immediately if they occur.

The injection site is observed for hematoma formation (a localized collection of blood), and an ice bag may be applied intermittently to the puncture site to relieve swelling and discomfort. Because a hematoma at the puncture site or embolization to a distant artery affects the peripheral pulses, these pulses are monitored frequently. The color and temperature of the involved extremity are assessed to detect possible embolism (the limb would be cool and pale if arterial perfusion is impaired).

Myelography

Procedure

A myelogram is an x-ray of the spinal subarachnoid space taken after the injection of a contrast agent through a lumbar puncture. It outlines the spinal subarachnoid space and shows any distortion of the spinal cord or spinal dural sac caused by tumors, cysts, herniated vertebral disks, or other lesions. Water-based agents have replaced oil-based agents, and their use has reduced side effects and complications; these agents

disperse upward through the CSF. Myelography is performed less frequently today because of the sensitivity of CT and MRI scanning. It is still used occasionally to provide information about the spinal cord and nerve roots (Barbano, 2016).

Nursing Interventions

Because many patients have misconceptions about myelography, the nurse clarifies the explanation given by the provider and answers questions. The patient is informed about what to expect during the procedure and should be aware that changes in position may be made during the procedure. The meal that normally would be eaten before the procedure is omitted. A sedative may be prescribed to help the patient cope with this rather lengthy test. Patient preparation for lumbar puncture is discussed later in this chapter.

After myelography, the patient lies in bed with the head of the bed elevated 30 to 45 degrees. The patient is advised to remain in bed in the recommended position for 3 hours or as prescribed by the provider. The patient is encouraged to drink liberal amounts of fluid for rehydration and replacement of CSF. The blood pressure, pulse, respiratory rate, and temperature are monitored, as well as the patient's ability to void. Untoward signs include headache, fever, stiff neck, **photophobia** (sensitivity to light), seizures, and signs of chemical or bacterial meningitis.

Noninvasive Carotid Flow Studies

Procedure

Noninvasive carotid flow studies use ultrasound imagery and Doppler measurements of arterial blood flow to evaluate carotid and deep orbital circulation. The graph produced indicates blood velocity. Increased blood velocity can indicate stenosis or partial obstruction. These tests are often obtained before arteriography, which carries a higher risk of stroke or death. Carotid Doppler, carotid ultrasonography, oculoplethysmography, and ophthalmodynamometry are four common noninvasive vascular techniques that permit evaluation of arterial blood flow and detection of arterial stenosis, occlusion, and plaques. These vascular studies allow noninvasive imaging of extracranial and intracranial circulation.

Nursing Interventions

When a carotid flow study is scheduled, the procedure is described to the patient. The patient is informed that this is a noninvasive test, that a hand-held transducer will be placed over the neck or orbits of the eyes, and that some type of water-soluble jelly is used on the transducer.

Electroencephalography (EEG)

Procedure

An electroencephalogram (EEG) represents a record of the electrical activity generated in the brain. It is obtained through electrodes applied on the scalp or through microelectrodes placed within the brain tissue. It provides a physiologic assessment of cerebral activity.

The EEG is a useful test for diagnosing and evaluating seizure disorders, coma, or organic brain syndrome. Tumors, brain abscesses, blood clots, and infection may cause abnormal patterns in electrical activity. The EEG is also used in making a determination of brain death.

For a baseline recording, the patient lies quietly with both eyes closed. The patient may be asked to hyperventilate for 3 to 4 minutes and then look at a bright, flashing light for photic stimulation. These activation procedures are performed to evoke abnormal electrical discharges, such as seizure potentials. A sleep EEG may be recorded after sedation because some abnormal brain waves are seen only when the patient is asleep.

Nursing Interventions

To increase the chances of recording seizure activity, it is sometimes recommended that the patient be deprived of sleep on the night before the EEG. Antiseizure agents, tranquilizers, stimulants, and depressants should be withheld 24 to 48 hours before an EEG because these medications can alter the EEG wave patterns or mask the abnormal wave patterns of seizure disorders (Hickey, 2014).

The patient is informed that the standard EEG takes 45 to 60 minutes (12 hours for a sleep EEG). The patient is assured that the procedure does not cause an electric shock and that the EEG is a diagnostic test, not a form of treatment. An EEG requires patient cooperation and ability to lie quietly during the test. Sedation is not advisable because it may lower the seizure threshold in patients with a seizure disorder and it alters brain wave activity in all patients. The nurse needs to check with the physician regarding the administration of antiseizure medication prior to testing.

Routine EEGs use a water-soluble lubricant for electrode contact, which at the conclusion of the study can be wiped off and removed by shampooing. Sleep EEGs involve the use of collodion glue for electrode contact, which requires acetone for removal.

Electromyography (EMG)

Procedure

An electromyogram (EMG) is obtained by inserting needle electrodes into the skeletal muscles to measure changes in the electrical potential of the muscles and the nerves leading to them. The electrical potentials are shown on an oscilloscope and amplified so that both the sound and appearance of the waves can be analyzed and compared simultaneously.

An EMG is useful in determining the presence of neuromuscular disorders and myopathies. It helps distinguish weakness due to neuropathy (functional or pathologic changes in the PNS) from weakness resulting from other causes.

Nursing Interventions

The procedure is explained, and the patient is warned to expect a sensation similar to that of an intramuscular injection as the needle is inserted into the muscle. The muscles examined may ache for a short time after the procedure.

Lumbar Puncture and Examination of Cerebrospinal Fluid

Procedure

A lumbar puncture (spinal tap) is an aseptic procedure carried out by inserting a needle into the lumbar subarachnoid space to withdraw CSF. The test may be performed to obtain CSF for examination, to measure and reduce CSF pressure, to assess for infection, and to determine the presence or absence of blood in the CSF. Antibiotics may be administered intrathecally (into the spinal canal) in certain cases of infection or contrast injected for diagnostic purposes.

The needle is usually inserted into the subarachnoid space between the third and fourth or fourth and fifth lumbar vertebrae. Because the spinal cord divides into a sheaf of nerves at the first lumbar vertebra, insertion of the needle below the level of the third lumbar vertebra prevents puncture of the spinal cord.

A successful lumbar puncture (LP) requires that the patient be relaxed; an anxious patient is tense, and this may increase the pressure reading. CSF pressure with the patient in a lateral recumbent position is normally 70 to 200 mm H_2O. This value is position dependent and will change with a horizontal or sitting position (Fischbach & Dunning, 2014). Pressures of more than 200 mm H_2O are considered abnormal.

An LP may be risky in the presence of an intracranial mass lesion because ICP is decreased by the removal of CSF, and the brain may herniate downward through the tentorium and the foramen magnum. To avoid this complication, a CT scan must be done prior to the procedure for patients with a suspected intracranial mass. Additionally, LPs are avoided in patients on antiplatelet therapy or anticoagulants. See Box 43-2 for nursing guidelines for assisting with a lumbar puncture.

Cerebrospinal Fluid Analysis

The CSF should be clear and colorless. Pink, blood-tinged, or grossly bloody CSF may indicate a subarachnoid hemorrhage. Cloudiness of CSF may be due to increased WBCs or increased protein from microorganisms; whereas xanthochromia (yellow, orange, or brown color) of CNS is usually due to RBC breakdown (Hickey, 2014). Sometimes, with a difficult lumbar puncture, the CSF initially is bloody because of local trauma but then becomes clearer. Usually, specimens are obtained for cell count, culture, and glucose and protein testing. The specimens should be sent to the laboratory immediately because changes will take place and alter the result if the specimens are allowed to stand.

BOX 43-2 Assisting with a Lumbar Puncture

A needle is inserted into the subarachnoid space through the third and fourth or fourth and fifth lumbar interface to withdraw spinal fluid.

Preprocedure

1. Determine whether written consent for the procedure has been obtained.
2. Explain the procedure to the patient and describe sensations that are likely during the procedure (i.e., a sensation of cold as the site is cleansed with solution, a needle prick when local anesthetic is injected).
3. Determine whether the patient has any questions or misconceptions about the procedure; reassure the patient that the needle will not enter the spinal cord or cause paralysis.
4. Instruct the patient to void before the procedure.

Procedure

1. The patient is positioned on one side (knee to chest position) at the edge of the bed or examining table with back toward the provider; the legs are flexed as much as possible to increase the space between the spinous processes of the vertebrae, for easier entry into the subarachnoid space.
2. A small pillow may be placed under the patient's head to maintain the spine in a horizontal position; a pillow may be placed between the legs to prevent the upper leg from rolling forward.
3. The nurse assists the patient to maintain the position to avoid sudden movement, which can produce a traumatic (bloody) tap.
4. The patient is encouraged to relax and is instructed to breathe normally because hyperventilation may lower an elevated pressure.
5. The nurse describes the procedure step by step to the patient as it proceeds.
6. Using an aseptic technique, the provider cleanses the puncture site with an antiseptic solution and drapes the site.
7. The provider injects local anesthetic to numb the puncture site and then inserts a spinal needle into the subarachnoid space through the third and fourth or fourth and fifth lumbar interspace.

8. A specimen of CSF is removed and usually collected in three test tubes, labeled in order of collection. A pressure reading may be obtained. The needle is withdrawn.

Third lumbar vertebra
Dura mater
Subarachnoid space
Cauda equina

9. The provider applies a small dressing to the puncture site.
10. The tubes of CSF are sent to the laboratory immediately.

Postprocedure

Typically patients are instructed to rest in bed for a few hours after a lumbar tap, and fluids are encouraged; however, research reveals no definite differences in the effects of bed rest or hydration of patients. Therefore, the nurse should refer to institutional procedures for postprocedure care.

1. Monitor the patient for complications of lumbar puncture; notify the provider if complications occur:
   a. Common complications: Post–lumbar puncture headache, voiding difficulties, slight elevation of temperature, backache or spasms, stiffness of neck. Typical management of postprocedure headache includes maintaining a supine posture, hydration, and analgesia and/or antiemetics prn; however, the nurse follows institutional procedures until best practices are delineated.
   b. Rare complications: Herniation of intracranial contents, spinal epidural abscess, spinal epidural hematoma, meningitis

Post–Lumbar Puncture Headache

A post–lumbar puncture headache, ranging from mild to severe, may occur a few hours to several days after the procedure. This is the most common complication, occurring in 15% to 30% of patients. It is a throbbing bifrontal or occipital headache, dull and deep in character. It is particularly severe on sitting or standing but lessens or disappears when the patient lies down.

The headache is caused by CSF leakage at the puncture site. The fluid continues to escape into the tissues by way of the needle track from the spinal canal. It is then absorbed promptly by the lymphatic system. As a result of this leak, the supply of CSF in the cranium is depleted to a point at which it is insufficient to maintain proper mechanical stabilization of the brain. This leakage of CSF allows settling of the brain when the patient assumes an upright position, producing tension and stretching the venous sinuses and pain-sensitive structures. Both traction and pain are lessened and the leakage is reduced when the patient lies down for 4 to 8 hours (Fischbach & Dunning, 2014).

Post–lumbar puncture headache may be avoided if a small-gauge needle is used. The postpuncture headache is usually managed by bed rest, analgesic agents, and hydration. However, the Therapeutics and Technology Assessment Subcommittee of the American Academy of Neurology, along with other groups, noted there is no class I or class II evidence to demonstrate that duration of bed rest, position of bed rest (prone or supine), or increased intake influences incidence of LP headache (Afshinmajd et al., 2014). The nurse should follow hospital standards while best practices are being developed. Occasionally, if the headache persists, an epidural blood patch may be used. Blood is withdrawn from the antecubital vein and injected into the epidural space, usually at the site of the previous spinal puncture. The rationale is that the blood acts as a gelatinous plug to seal the hole in the dura, preventing further loss of CSF.

Other Complications of Lumbar Puncture

Herniation of the intracranial contents, spinal epidural abscess, spinal epidural hematoma, and meningitis are rare but serious complications of lumbar puncture. Other complications include temporary voiding problems, slight elevation of temperature, backache or spasms, and stiffness of the neck.

CHAPTER REVIEW

Critical Thinking Exercises

1. A 68-year-old woman presents to your unit with complaints of weakness, headache, and lethargy. After completing the Glasgow Coma Scale, you are asked to perform assessment of her cranial nerves; identify what will be included in this assessment.

2. A 78-year-old patient with a history of chronic pain is admitted to the hospital to rule out an ischemic stroke and is scheduled for an MRI. Explain why the MRI is indicated and what, if any, precautions must be taken because this patient has chronic pain. What nursing observations and assessments are indicated because of the occurrence of these two disorders? What safety precautions are essential in the MRI suite, and why?

3. You are caring for a patient who is scheduled to undergo a lumbar puncture. How can you best assist and support the patient during the procedure? What laboratory studies would you expect to be ordered on the CSF sample? What postprocedure restrictions can you expect and prepare the patient for?

NCLEX-Style Review Questions

1. A patient is undergoing a cerebral angiography to rule out an aneurysm. When preparing the patient for the procedure, what would the nurse include in the instructions?
   a. Expect a metallic taste when the contrast agent is injected.
   b. You will need a full bladder prior to the procedure.
   c. Maintain an NPO status.
   d. General sedation will be given prior to procedure.

2. The nurse is assisting with a lumbar puncture. What is the most common complication for which the nurse should monitor the patient following the procedure?
   a. Post–lumbar puncture headache
   b. Herniation of intracranial contents
   c. Spinal epidural abscess
   d. Meningitis

3. A patient is scheduled for an EEG tomorrow. Which piece of information should the nurse provide to the patient prior to the procedure?
   a. Antiseizure medications need to be taken prior to procedure.
   b. Sedation will be given during the procedure.
   c. There is a slight chance of electric shock.
   d. Maintain a sleep-deprived state the night before the procedure.

4. A patient with Parkinson disease is seen in the neurology clinic for treatment. The nurse identifies this disorder as being caused by a lack of which neurotransmitters?
   a. Acetylcholine
   b. Dopamine
   c. Serotonin
   d. Gamma-aminobutyric acid (GABA)

5. The nurse is testing the cranial nerves of a patient diagnosed with myasthenia gravis. The nurse asks the patient to clench his jaw while she palpates the temporal and masseter muscles. The nurse is correctly testing which cranial nerve?
   a. Abducens
   b. Trigeminal
   c. Acoustic
   d. Hypoglossal

Try these additional resources, available at **http://thepoint.lww.com/Honan2e**, to enhance your learning and understanding of this chapter:

- NCLEX-Style Student Review Questions
- Journal Articles

REFERENCES AND SELECTED READINGS

References and selected readings associated with this chapter can be found on the website that accompanies the book. Visit **http://thepoint. lww.com/Honan2e** to access the references and other additional resources associated with this chapter.

Nursing Management: Patients with Oncologic Disorders of the Brain and Spinal Cord

Jill S. Keller

Learning Objectives

After reading this chapter, you will be able to:

1. Describe the different types of brain tumors, including classification, clinical manifestations, diagnosis, and medical and nursing management.
2. Describe the symptoms and effects of increased intracranial pressure.
3. Differentiate between primary and metastatic brain tumors.
4. Describe the different types of spinal cord tumors, including classification, clinical manifestations, diagnosis, and medical and nursing management.
5. Describe the symptoms and effects of spinal cord compression.

PRIMARY BRAIN TUMORS

Primary brain tumors are localized intracranial lesions that begin in the brain and occupy space within the skull. The tumor is an abnormal growth of cells that forms a mass, but it also can grow diffusely. The effects of neoplasms (tumors or lesions) on the central nervous system (CNS), including seizure activity and focal neurologic signs, are caused by the compression or infiltration of tissue, or both. Tumors may be benign or malignant. Benign tumors are usually slow growing but can occur in a vital area, where they can grow large enough to cause serious effects. Malignant tumors can be rapidly growing in nature, can spread into surrounding tissue, and are considered life-threatening. Primary brain tumors rarely spread to other areas of the body.

Oncologic (cancer) disorders of the brain include several types of neoplasms, each with its own biology, prognosis, and treatment options. Because of the unique anatomy and physiology of the CNS, this collection of neoplasms is challenging to diagnose and treat.

Types of Brain Tumors

There are many different types of brain tumors. They are classified into several groups: those originating within brain tissue (e.g., glioma), those arising from the coverings of the brain (e.g., dural meningioma), those developing in or on the cranial nerves (e.g., acoustic neuroma), and metastatic lesions originating from cancer elsewhere in the body. Tumors of the pituitary and pineal glands and of cerebral blood vessels are also considered types of brain tumors. Relevant clinical considerations when developing a plan of treatment includes the location, size, histologic character of the tumor, and if the tumor can be surgically removed.

Gliomas

Gliomas tumors are a type of intracerebral brain neoplasm. Gliomas are divided into many categories. Box 44-1 lists the classification of these and other brain tumors. Glioblastoma multiforme (GBM) is the most common and aggressive malignant brain tumor (Ray, Bonafede, & Mohile, 2014). In most cases, a tissue biopsy, which can be obtained at the time of surgical removal, is needed to confirm the diagnosis. The grade of the tumor is based on cellular density, cell mitosis, and appearance. Usually, these tumors form in the cerebrum and spread by infiltrating the surrounding neural connective tissue. Treatment for this type of tumor may include surgery, radiation therapy, and/or chemotherapy. Total surgical resection is difficult due to the "finger-like tentacles" the tumor produces. The goal of surgery is to remove as much tumor as possible without causing any neurologic damage. Despite treatment, median life expectancy is 14.6 months (American Brain Tumor Association [ABTA], 2014a).

Classification of Brain Tumors in Adults

I. Intracerebral tumors
  A. Gliomas—infiltrate any portion of the brain:
    1. Astrocytomas (grades I and II)
    2. Glioblastoma multiforme (astrocytoma grades III and IV)
    3. Oligodendrocytoma (low and high grades)
    4. Ependymoma (grades I to IV)
    5. Medulloblastoma
II. Tumors arising from supporting structures
  A. Meningiomas
  B. Neuromas (acoustic neuroma, schwannoma)
  C. Pituitary adenomas
III. Developmental tumors
  A. Angiomas
  B. Dermoid, epidermoid, teratoma, craniopharyngioma
IV. Metastatic lesions

Meningiomas

Meningiomas represent 36.1% of all primary brain tumors and are the most common brain tumors found in adults. Most are characterized as a benign, encapsulated, slow-growing tumor that occurs in people over 60 years of age and found twice as often in women as in men (ABTA, 2014e). These tumors grow on the membrane covering of the brain, called the meninges. Grade I meningiomas are the most common type and can be cured by surgery. Due to the slow-growing nature of this tumor, it is not uncommon that people die unaware they have a meningioma. Grades II and III are less common and grow quickly. They can spread to the brain and spinal cord. These tumors have a poorer prognosis and usually cannot be completely resected. Manifestations depend on the area involved and are the result of compression rather than invasion of brain tissue (National Cancer Institute [NCI], 2015). In some cases this type of tumor can run in families that have the neurofibromatosis syndrome (genetic disorders that cause tumors to grow along various types of nerves and/or non-nervous tissues) that can increase their risk for developing a brain tumor (American Cancer Society [ACS], 2015).

Acoustic Neuromas

An acoustic neuroma (vestibular schwannoma) is a benign tumor of the eighth cranial nerve, the cranial nerve most responsible for hearing and balance. It usually arises within the internal auditory meatus. An acoustic neuroma is a slow-growing tumor and attains considerable size before it is correctly diagnosed. The patient usually experiences loss of hearing, tinnitus, episodes of vertigo, and staggering gait. As the tumor becomes larger, painful sensations of the face may occur on the same side, as a result of the tumor's compression of the fifth cranial nerve (trigeminal nerve) resulting in facial numbness (paresthesia) and pain. Diagnosis is suggested by unilateral sensorineural hearing loss; the Weber and Rinne test may be useful in assessing asymmetric hearing loss (refer to Chapter 48). Most acoustic neuromas can be surgically removed or are suitable for stereotactic radiotherapy. When patients present with small tumors with limited symptomatology, treatment options may include observation over time since some tumors may not progress and may shrink in size.

Pituitary Adenomas

Pituitary tumors represent 12–19% of all primary brain tumors (ABTA, 2017). They are slow growing in nature. A majority of these tumors are benign but, in rare cases, may be malignant. Pituitary tumors are classified as nonfunctioning and functioning. Nonfunctioning tumors do not produce hormones. Functioning tumors can produce one or more hormones, normally by the anterior pituitary. Increase may be seen in prolactin hormone, growth hormone, adrenocorticotropic hormone (ACTH), or thyroid-stimulating hormone. Females are more affected than males, and these tumors are rarely seen in the pediatric population (Lopes, 2013). Endocrine disorders resulting from these tumors are discussed in Chapter 31.

Pressure from a pituitary adenoma may be exerted on the optic nerves, optic chiasm, optic tracts, hypothalamus, or the third ventricle. Headache is a common symptom; there can also be visual dysfunction, hypothalamic disorders (diabetes insipidus, sleep disturbances, and changes in appetite), and increased intracranial pressure (ICP). Advances in transsphenoidal surgery and stereotactic radiotherapy help to normalize hormonal secretion and relieve symptoms and compression on surrounding structures (Melmed & Jameson, 2015).

Angiomas

Brain angiomas (masses composed largely of abnormal blood vessels) are found either in the brain or on its surface. They occur most often in the cerebellum. Some persist throughout life asymptomatically, while others cause symptoms of a brain tumor, such as seizures and headaches. Occasionally, the diagnosis is suggested by the presence of another angioma somewhere in the head or by a bruit (an abnormal sound) that is audible over the skull. Because the walls of the blood vessels in angiomas are thin, affected patients are at risk for hemorrhagic stroke. In fact, cerebral hemorrhage in people younger than 40 years of age should suggest the possibility of an angioma.

Cerebral Metastases

Metastatic disease is the ability for a malignant cell to travel through the circulation and reestablish itself in a second site. Primary sites of cancer that commonly metastasize to the brain include the lung, breast, and gastrointestinal tract as well as melanoma. Primary lung cancer accounts for 50% of all brain metastases (Tse, 2014a).

Risk Factors

The incidence of brain tumors appears to have increased in the past few decades. Epidemiologic data suggest that this is due to more aggressive and more accurate diagnosis rather than to an actual rise in incidence. Better access to care and an increase in the aging population may contribute to the increase in rates. An estimated 68,470 new cases of primary brain (nonmalignant and malignant) and CNS tumors were diagnosed in 2015. Of those tumors, 23,180 will be primary malignant brain tumors. The incidence rate for primary brain and CNS tumors is higher in males than females (Central Brain Tumor Registry of the United States [CBTRUS], 2014).

The cause of most primary brain tumors is unknown. The only known risk factors are exposure to ionizing radiation and cancer-causing chemicals. Additional possible risk factors that require further investigation include non-ionizing consumption of nitrates, cigarette smoking, cell phone use, and exposure to residential power lines (ABTA, 2014a).

There has been some suggestion that there are particular genetic risk factors for certain types of brain tumors. Neurofibromatosis type 1 (NF1), also known as von Recklinghausen disease, is a genetic disorder linked to brain and spinal cord tumors. People with this disorder are at higher risk for schwannomas, meningiomas, and types of gliomas and neurofibromas (benign tumor). Neurofibromatosis type 2 (NF2) is less common and related to acoustic neuromas. People with a condition called tuberous sclerosis are at risk for low-grade astrocytomas (tumors that arise from astrocytes—star-shaped cells that make up the supportive tissue of the brain) and other benign tumors on the body. Li-Fraumeni syndrome increases the risk for developing gliomas, and von Hippel–Lindau disease may cause tumors in the blood vessels of the brain and spinal cord as well as other areas of the body. Other inherited conditions include Gorlin syndrome, Turcot syndrome, and Cowden syndrome (ACS, 2015). However, the cause of the vast majority of brain tumors remains elusive.

Clinical Manifestations

Brain tumors can produce focal (localized) or generalized neurologic symptoms. Symptoms reflect brain invasion, compression by the mass on adjacent structures, or increased ICP. The patient can experience seizures, nausea and vomiting, cognitive impairment, and visual disturbances. Additionally, specific signs and symptoms result from tumors that interfere with functions in specific brain regions. These focal symptoms may also include weakness, sensory loss, aphasia, visual dysfunction, and other manifestations related to

specific neurologic dysfunction because of localized involvement. Figure 44-1 indicates common tumor sites in the brain.

Increased Intracranial Pressure

Symptoms of increased ICP, which is discussed in Chapter 45, result from compression of the brain by the enlarging tumor or edema. Vasogenic (cerebral) edema plays a major role in symptoms related to an increase in mass. Edema can exceed the mass itself, creating increased pressure and disrupting flow of blood or cerebral spinal fluid. Symptoms often include headache, nausea with or without vomiting, papilledema (edema of the optic disk), and visual changes (Gucalp & Dutcher, 2015). Personality changes and a variety of focal deficits, including motor, sensory, and cranial nerve dysfunction, are common. The nurse remains alert for changes in the patient's level of consciousness (LOC) and notifies the primary care provider of any alterations in mental status. Late signs associated with rising ICP related to the vital signs are termed Cushing triad; those signs may include hypertension with a widening pulse pressure (the difference between systolic and diastolic pressure), bradycardia, and respiratory depression.

Headache
Headache, although not always present, is most common in the early morning and improves during the day. Pain is made worse by coughing, straining, or sudden movement. Headache is thought to be caused by the tumor's invading, compressing, or distorting the pain-sensitive structures or by edema that accompanies the tumor. Thus, headaches are related to intracerebral edema and increasing ICP (ABTA, 2014b). Headaches are usually described as deep or expanding or as dull but unrelenting. Location of the headache can correlate to the area of the tumor. Progressive headaches are more common in glioblastoma and secreting pituitary adenomas tumors (Nelson & Taylor, 2014).

> **(!) Nursing Alert**
> *The nurse is aware that headaches in the morning are suggestive of a tumor. When the patient complains of a headache, the nurse assesses the patient's temperature. The nurse knows that fever with headache is associated with an infectious process, such as meningitis or encephalitis, whereas headache without fever may be associated with a tumor or intracerebral bleeding.*

Personality Changes
The location, pressure, and degree of infiltration of the tumor, and edema, if present, influence the changes in personality and mental status. Changes may be subtle with the patient sleeping more, losing interest in activities, and having difficulty with memory. These symptoms may be confused with depression (Wong & Wu, 2016). It is not uncommon for the short-term memory to be affected while still retaining long-term thoughts.

Lateral ventricle
ependymoma
glioblastoma multiforme

3rd ventricle area
ependymoma

Corpus callosum
astrocytoma
oligodendroglioma
lipoma

Cerebrum
astrocytoma
oligodendroglioma
lymphoma
metastatic tumors

Pineal area
pineocytoma
pineoblastoma

Optic chiasm
astrocytoma

Pituitary area
craniopharyngioma
pituitary adenoma
epidermoid cyst

Acoustic nerve
neuroma

Brain stem
astrocytoma
glioblastoma multiforme
metastatic tumors

4th ventricle
ependymoma

Cerebellum
medulloblastoma
astrocytoma
hemangioblastoma
metastatic tumors

FIGURE 44-1 Common brain tumor sites.

Fatigue

Fatigue is a symptom experienced by patients with both malignant and nonmalignant brain tumors. Etiology of fatigue can be multifactorial. The tumor itself, surgery, medications, chemotherapy, and radiation may all contribute to increased fatigue. Patients may complain of a constant feeling of exhaustion, weakness, and lack of energy. It is also important to identify underlying conditions, such as stress, anxiety, and depression, which may play a role in fatigue (ABTA, 2014c).

Vomiting

Vomiting, seldom related to food intake, is usually the result of irritation of the vagal centers in the medulla. Forceful vomiting is described as *projectile vomiting.*

Visual Disturbances

Papilledema is associated with visual disturbances, such as decreased visual acuity, diplopia (double vision), and visual field deficits.

New Onset of Seizures

Seizures are a common symptom among patients with brain tumors due to abnormal electrical activity in the brain. They may present upon initial diagnosis or during the course of

the disease process. Approximately 60% of patients with brain tumors have seizures during their illness (ABTA, 2014d). The type and frequency of seizure vary, related to tumor size, site, and type. Seizures can be characterized as simple partial, complex partial, and secondary generalized seizures (Vecht, Kerkhof, & Duran-Pena, 2014). Figure 44-2 presents an algorithm for initial evaluation of seizures.

Localized Symptoms

Common focal, or localized, symptoms include muscle weakness, sensory loss, aphasia, and visual changes (Wong & Wu, 2016). When specific regions of the brain are affected, additional local signs and symptoms occur, such as motor abnormalities, changes in hearing, alterations in cognition, and language disturbances. The progression of the signs and symptoms is important because it indicates tumor growth and expansion. For example, if a tumor is present in the cerebellar area, the nurse might expect to see changes in balance and coordination. Figure 44-3 reviews specific cerebral structures and function.

Assessment and Diagnostic Findings

The history of the illness as well as the manner and time frame in which the symptoms evolved are key components

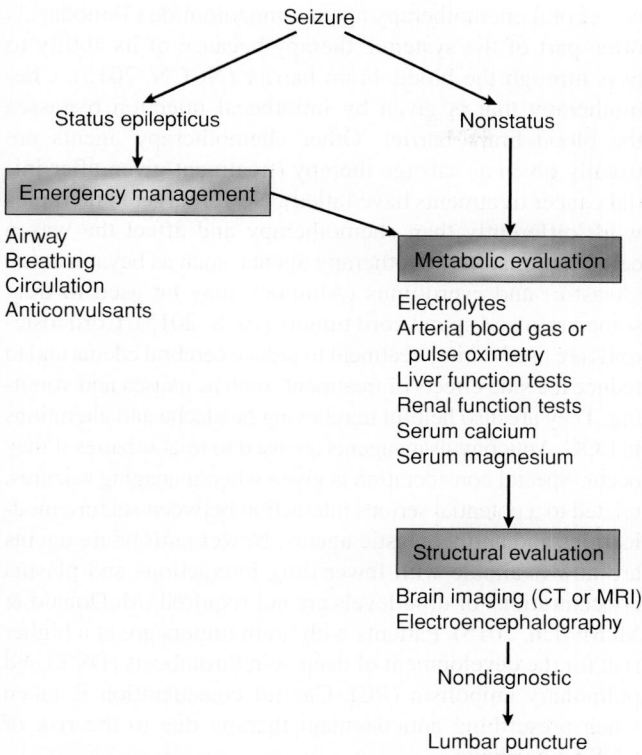

Seizure

Status epilepticus   Nonstatus

Emergency management

Airway
Breathing
Circulation
Anticonvulsants

Metabolic evaluation

Electrolytes
Arterial blood gas or
  pulse oximetry
Liver function tests
Renal function tests
Serum calcium
Serum magnesium

Structural evaluation

Brain imaging (CT or MRI)
Electroencephalography

Nondiagnostic

Lumbar puncture

FIGURE 44-2 Algorithm for initial evaluation of patients with suspected brain tumor based on type of seizure in presenting symptoms. (From Hickey, J. (2015). *The clinical practice of neurological and neurosurgical nursing.* Philadelphia, PA: Lippincott Williams & Wilkins.)

FIGURE 44-4 Low-grade glioma. Magnetic resonance imaging (MRI) of the brain shows an abnormal density in the right temporal lobe. (Courtesy of the Hospital of the University of Pennsylvania, Nuclear Medicine Section, Philadelphia, PA.)

in the diagnosis of a brain tumor. A neurologic examination can be helpful in indicating the areas of the CNS that are involved. To assist in identifying the precise location of the lesion, a battery of tests may need to be performed.

Magnetic resonance imaging (MRI) is the gold standard for detecting brain tumors (McDonald & McMullen, 2015),

particularly smaller lesions, and tumors in the brainstem and pituitary regions, where bone is thick (Fig. 44-4). Computed tomography (CT), enhanced by a contrast agent, can give specific information concerning the number, size, and density of the lesions and the extent of secondary cerebral edema. CT can also provide information about the ventricular system (the communicating network of cavities filled with CSF and located within the brain parenchyma).

FIGURE 44-3 Brain structures and their function. (Adapted with permission from National Brain Tumor Society. (2010). *The essential guide to brain tumors*, p. 9, Retrieved from http://www.braintumor.org/patients-family-friends/about-brain-tumors/publications/essentialguide.pdf.)

Frontal lobe
• movement
• reasoning
• behavior
• memory
• personality
• planning
• decision making
• judgment
• initiative
• inhibition
• mood

Pituitary gland
• hormones
• growth
• fertility

Temporal lobe
• language
  comprehension
• behavior
• memory
• hearing
• emotions

Parietal lobe
• telling right from left
• calculations
• sensations
• reading
• writing

Occipital lobe
• vision

Cerebellum
• balance
• coordination
• fine muscle control

Brainstem
• breathing
• blood pressure
• heartbeat
• swallowing

Positron emission tomography (PET), which measures the brain's activity rather than simply its structure, is useful in differentiating tumor from scar tissue or radiation necrosis. Computer-assisted stereotactic (three-dimensional) biopsy is being used to diagnose deep-seated brain tumors. Cerebral angiography provides visualization of cerebral blood vessels and can localize most cerebral tumors.

Cytologic studies of the CSF may be performed to detect malignant cells because CNS tumors can shed cells into the CSF.

Medical Management of Primary Brain Tumors

A variety of medical treatment modalities, including chemotherapy and external-beam radiation therapy, radiosurgery, or radiotherapy are used alone or in combination with surgical resection (Etame, 2014). Depending on the type and the extent of the tumor, medical treatments may be done for symptom management purposes rather than to cure the patient of a brain tumor. This type of medical management is referred to as *palliative care* and will help improve the patient's quality of life when cure is not possible.

Surgical Management

Surgical intervention provides the best outcome for most brain tumor types. The objective of surgical management is removal of part of or the entire tumor without increasing the neurologic deficit. The surgical approach depends on the type of tumor, its location, and its accessibility. Options include stereotactic biopsy, open biopsy, craniotomy with debulking (surgical removal of part of a malignant tumor that cannot be excised completely), and subtotal or complete resection (National Comprehensive Cancer Network [NCCN], 2015).

Radiation Therapy

Radiation therapy, the cornerstone of treatment for many brain tumors, decreases the incidence of recurrence of incompletely resected tumors. External-beam radiation therapy may be used alone or in combination with surgical resection. Stereotactic radiosurgery may be performed to deep, inaccessible tumors, often in a single session. Precise localization of the tumor is accomplished by the stereotactic approach and by minute measurements and precise positioning of the patient either through the use of Gamma Knife or CyberKnife (McDonald & McMullen, 2015). Gamma Knife is a form of stereotactic radiosurgery, where precise beams of radiation produce a targeted approach of concentrated radiation for the brain, head, and neck, whereas CyberKnife is used to treat cancer anywhere on the body.

Pharmacologic Therapy and Chemotherapy

Chemotherapy may be given intravenously, orally, or intrathecally (injected directly into the subarachnoid space). The newer oral chemotherapy agent temozolomide (Temodar) is often part of the systemic therapy because of its ability to pass through the blood–brain barrier (NCCN, 2015). Chemotherapy that is given by intrathecal injection bypasses the blood–brain barrier. Other chemotherapy agents are usually given as salvage therapy (treatment given after initial cancer treatments have failed). Newer targeted therapies work differently than chemotherapy and affect the way a cell functions. Immunotherapy agents, such as bevacizumab (Avastin) and everolimus (Afinitor), may be used to treat some brain and spinal cord tumors (ACS, 2015). Corticosteroids are used during treatment to reduce cerebral edema and to reduce the side effects of treatment, such as nausea and vomiting. They are also helpful in relieving headache and alterations in LOC. Anticonvulsant agents are used to treat seizures if they occur. Special consideration is given when managing seizures, related to a potential serious interaction between seizure medications and antineoplastic agents. Newer antiseizure agents are now available with fewer drug interactions and plasma concentrations of drug levels are not required (McDonald & McMullen, 2015). Patients with brain tumors are at a higher risk for the development of deep vein thrombosis (DVT) and pulmonary embolism (PE). Careful consideration is taken when prescribing anticoagulant therapy due to the risk of CNS hemorrhage.

Pain is managed by means of a stepped progression with regard to the dosing, delivery method, and type of analgesic agents needed for relief. Headache is often a common complaint of pain in this population of patients. If the patient has severe pain, morphine can be infused into the epidural catheter placed as near as possible to the spinal segment where the pain is projected. Small doses of morphine are administered at prescribed intervals (refer to Chapter 7).

Medical Management of Metastatic Brain Cancer

The treatment of metastatic brain cancer is palliative and involves eliminating or reducing serious symptoms. Even when palliation is the goal, distressing signs and symptoms can be relieved, thereby improving the quality of life for both patient and family. The therapeutic approach includes radiation therapy, surgery (usually for a single intracranial metastasis), and chemotherapy. GammaKnife radiosurgery is considered if three or fewer lesions are present. Survival rates vary, depending on the type and extent of the tumor at the time of diagnosis. The overall prognosis is poor in most cases.

Nursing Management

The effects of increased ICP caused by the tumor mass are reviewed in Chapter 45. The nurse performs neurologic checks, monitors vital signs, maintains a neurologic flow chart, spaces nursing interventions to prevent a rapid increase in ICP, and reorients the patient when necessary to person, time, and place. Patients with changes in cognition

BOX 44-2

Family Caregivers of Patients with a High-Grade Glioma

A Qualitative Study of Their Lived Experience and Needs Related to Professional Care

Coolbrandt, A., Sterckx, W., Clement, P., Borgenon, S., Decruyenaere, M., de Vleeschouwer, S.,...de Casterle, B. D. (2015). Family caregivers of patients with a high-grade glioma: A qualitative study of their lived experience and needs related to professional care. *Cancer Nursing, 38*(5), 406–413.

Purpose
To look at what caregivers of patients with high-grade glioma experienced and their needs for professional help.

Design
The work was based on a qualitative study using the Grounded Theory to help understand how caregivers experience caring for a patient with high-grade gliomas. Caregivers were chosen from a university hospital between February and July 2011 and again between April and November 2012. Caregivers were caring for patients who received chemotherapy and/or radiation therapy or who were in the monitor stage after treatment. Seventeen caregivers participated initially, but one withdrew due to the death of the patient. Semistructured interviews took place at the hospital or in the home. Topics of discussion included diagnosis, symptoms, relationships, support, caregiving tasks, the future, communication, and information. Interviews were audiotaped and transcribed.

Findings
Caregivers reported disbelief and powerlessness. Many reported they felt this way due to the way the diagnosis was communicated to them. Lack of support during diagnosis added to their stress. Life as they knew it was lost. They noted feelings of being socially deprived as they assumed the role of caregiver. At the same time caregivers reported loss of control of their own life as well. Witnessing physical and cognitive decline was painful for the caregiver to watch. Many developed irritation when

they became tired. A sense of loneliness was expressed as the relationship with the patient was no longer the same. Caregivers developed anxiety and uncertainty regarding the future but at the same time tried to remain hopeful. Despite the struggle, caregivers remained completely committed to continuing to give care until the end. They did express that they got little or no professional help on how to care for a patient with a brain tumor and felt they made decisions on their own. They felt that professional help was not available (nights, 24 hours a day). Those who did accept help were fairly positive. Multiple caregivers felt unprepared to care for the patient but stated no one ever questioned the demands on them. When the patient was satisfied, caregivers became more confident, but when the patient could no longer express his or her feelings, once again the caregiver became less confident.

Caregivers did express the need for information on how to care for the patient and side effects of treatment. Follow-up visits were often with a physician in training and did not allow for the opportunity to ask questions. At home caregivers felt that they had no one to turn to. Caregivers wanted professionals to share their goals for the patient in order to provide the best care possible.

Nursing Implications
This study will help nurses caring for patients with brain tumors understand the difficulties the caregivers experience. Nurses are a resource of information to both the patient and the caregivers. Working with home care agencies and asking for social work consultation can provide a benefit in the care of the patient and the caregiver. Nurses need to be aware of the family structure and identify needs for additional assistance.

---

caused by their lesions require frequent reorientation and the use of orienting devices (e.g., personal possessions, photographs, lists, and a clock). Supervision of and assistance with self-care, ongoing monitoring, and interventions for prevention of injury may be required. Patients who have seizures are carefully monitored and protected from injury. Box 44-2 explores the emotional impact of being diagnosed with an aggressive brain tumor.

The nursing process for patients undergoing neurosurgery is discussed in Chapter 45. The patient with a brain tumor may be at increased risk for aspiration due to cranial nerve dysfunction. If the patient is at risk for aspiration, he or she should be placed in a side-lying position with HOB elevated 10 to 30 degrees. The nurse must ensure that suction equipment is at the bedside. Preoperatively, the gag reflex and ability to swallow are evaluated by gently touching each side of the posterior pharyngeal wall with a cotton swab or suction catheter and noting the strength of the gag. The nurse expects to observe a simultaneous elevation of the uvula and "gag" with stimulation of the posterior pharynx. Function

should be reassessed postoperatively because changes can occur because of alterations in cranial nerves IX (glossopharyngeal) and X (vagus) or the pons or medulla. If the gag reflex is impaired, the health care provider is notified and food and fluid are withheld until evaluation of swallowing is determined.

SPINAL CORD TUMORS

Primary spinal tumors are rare. Tumors within the spine are classified according to their anatomic relation to the spinal cord. Intramedullary tumors arise from within the spinal cord. Intradural–extramedullary tumors are within or under the spinal dura but not on the actual spinal cord. Extradural tumors are located outside the dura and often involve the vertebral bodies. These tumors may be either primary or metastatic in nature (Welch, Schiff, & Gerszten, 2015). Spinal tumors causing cord compression are considered a neurologic emergency.

Metastatic Spinal Cord Tumors

Cancer can spread to the spinal cord. The three most common cancers that metastasize to the spinal cord are lung, breast, and those of the gastrointestinal tract. It is the third most common site for metastases behind the lung and liver (Tse, 2014b). Cancer can invade the bone, causing vertebral metastases.

Spinal Cord Compression

Spinal cord compression (SCC) occurs because of tumor extension into the epidural space. The cord can be compressed at any area of the spine, resulting in permanent paralysis if not treated. Patients with myeloma or lymphoma, as well as those with breast, lung, and prostate cancer are at an increased risk for developing SCC.

SCC is considered a medical emergency and requires immediate treatment to prevent permanent neurologic damage. The treatment goal is to relieve cord compression with the use of IV steroids, such as dexamethasone (Decadron), to reduce edema. Additionally, chemotherapy, radiation, or surgery to debulk the tumor is expected to preserve neurologic function. Early intervention is the key to prevent loss of function.

Assessment and Diagnostic Findings

Initial symptoms may present as radicular pain (pain that radiates along the dermatome [sensory distribution] of a nerve), weakness, sphincter dysfunction, and sensory changes. The nurse is alert for early complaints of back pain, which occurs in the region of the tumor. The pain typically increases when the patient is in the prone position. Symmetrical extremity weakness also may be present. Ataxia with back pain should always be a concern for patients with SCC. If left untreated, motor weakness and sensory deficits can progress to paralysis. Neurologic examination and diagnostic studies are used to make the diagnosis. Neurologic examination includes assessment of pain, loss of reflexes above the tumor level, progressive loss of sensation or motor function, and the presence of weakness and paralysis. These changes in neurologic function are related to the mass exerting pressure and compression of the nerve roots or spinal cord. Late symptoms include bladder and bowel dysfunction (urinary incontinence or retention; fecal incontinence or constipation). The patient's ambulatory status is also an important prognostic indicator. MRI is the most commonly used diagnostic tool, detecting epidural SCC and metastases (Schiff, 2015).

Medical Management

Treatment of spinal cord tumors depends on the type, location of the tumor, the presenting symptoms, and physical status of the patient. Surgical intervention, if appropriate, is the primary treatment for most tumors. Other treatment modalities include partial removal of the tumor with decompression of the spinal cord. For metastatic lesions of the spine, radiation therapy can be used to decrease the size of the tumor. Chemotherapy

options are limited due to the blood–brain barrier. Dexamethasone is used temporarily to reduce edema and improve neurologic function until other treatments can take effect.

Tumor removal is desirable but not always possible. The goal is to remove as much tumor as possible while sparing uninvolved portions of the spinal cord to avoid neurologic damage. Microsurgical techniques have improved the prognosis for patients with intramedullary tumors. Prognosis is related to the degree of neurologic impairment at the time of surgery, the speed with which symptoms occurred, and the origin of the tumor. Patients with extensive neurologic deficits before surgery usually do not make significant functional recovery, even after successful tumor removal.

Palliative care may be an option for the medical management of some patients. Relief from symptoms and pain control are the goals of care. Patients may receive palliative treatments, such as radiation, and then transition into hospice care when supportive treatments fail to control tumor growth. Other integrative therapies (complementary/alternative) may be incorporated into part of the patient's treatment plan.

Nursing Management

Providing Preoperative Care

The objectives of preoperative care include recognition of neurologic changes through ongoing assessments, pain control, and the management of altered activities of daily living (ADLs). The nurse assesses for weakness, muscle wasting, spasticity, sensory changes, bowel and bladder dysfunction, and potential respiratory problems, especially if a cervical tumor is present. The patient is also evaluated for coagulation deficiencies. Postoperative pain management strategies are discussed with the patient before surgery.

Assessing the Patient Postoperatively

The patient is monitored for deterioration in neurologic status. A sudden onset of neurologic deficit is an ominous sign and may be due to vertebral collapse associated with spinal cord infarction. Frequent neurologic checks are carried out, with emphasis on movement, strength, and sensation of the upper and lower extremities. Staining of the dressing may indicate leakage of CSF from the surgical site, which may lead to serious infection or to an inflammatory reaction in the surrounding tissues that can cause severe pain in the postoperative period (refer to Chapter 43 for evaluation of CSF leakage).

Managing Pain

The prescribed medication should be administered in adequate amounts and at appropriate intervals to relieve pain and prevent its recurrence. Early symptoms of spinal cord tumors include stiffness and pain that continues to worsen. Pain and bone pain at night is the hallmark of spinal metastasis. Pain may increase in the recumbent position (Welch et al., 2015).

The bed is usually kept flat initially. However the head of the bed position will depend on the specific surgical procedure and the surgeon's preference (Hickey, 2015, p. 312). The nurse turns the patient as a unit, keeping shoulders and hips aligned and the back straight. The side-lying position is usually the most comfortable because this position imposes the least pressure on the surgical site. Placement of a pillow between the knees of the patient in a side-lying position helps to prevent extreme knee flexion.

Promoting Home and Community-Based Care

In preparation for discharge, the patient is assessed for the ability to function independently in the home and for the availability of resources, such as family members, to assist in caregiving. Safety is a key component when arranging for home care. Patients with residual sensory involvement are cautioned about the dangers of extremes in temperature. They should be alerted to the dangers of heating devices (e.g., hot water bottles, heating pads, space heaters). The patient is taught to check skin integrity daily. Patients with impaired motor function related to motor weakness or paralysis may require training in ADLs and safe use of assistive devices, such as a cane, walker, or wheelchair.

The patient and family members are educated about pain management strategies, bowel and bladder management, and assessment for signs and symptoms of neurologic dysfunction, which should be reported promptly.

CHAPTER REVIEW

Critical Thinking Exercises

1. A 48-year-old man is married with two young children and has been newly diagnosed with a metastatic spinal cord tumor. The patient is scheduled to have surgery to debulk the tumor. What nursing assessments should be performed preoperatively? What postoperative nursing assessments should be performed? What assessments would alert the nurse of possible complications? What interventions can the nurse do to provide comfort pre- and postoperatively?

2. A 60-year-old patient with a history of lymphoma who has developed a new onset of low back pain is seen in the clinic. What pertinent questions should the nurse ask the patient that would aid in identifying the cause of the pain? Describe what nursing assessment is the priority. Identify deficits that would indicate that this is an urgent condition and why. What type of medication do you anticipate will be prescribed for this patient?

3. A 50-year-old patient has been recently diagnosed with a glioblastoma brain tumor. He had surgery several weeks ago and is now receiving chemotherapy. He is complaining of feeling exhausted and unable to do his normal work at home. What resources would you use to identify current guidelines for treatment of fatigue? How would this information help you develop a plan to educate your patient in lifestyle changes?

NCLEX-Style Review Questions

1. A patient admitted to the emergency room has a history of a spinal tumor. Which sign and symptom should alert the nurse to the possibility of SCC?
   a. Seizures
   b. Headache
   c. Back pain
   d. Diplopia

2. A patient with a decreased LOC and an absent gag reflex was just admitted to the neurologic unit. In what position should the nurse place the patient?
   a. Prone
   b. Head of bed should be elevated 45 to 90 degrees
   c. Flat
   d. Side lying with head of bed elevated 10 to 30 degrees

3. What is a late sign of rising ICP?
   a. Papilledema
   b. Change in the LOC
   c. Vomiting
   d. Hypertension

4. A patient with a brain tumor is receiving palliative care. What does the nurse understand to be true about palliative care? *Select all that apply.*
   a. Providing comfort care
   b. Early identification of spiritual needs to the patient
   c. Management of symptoms
   d. Does not include pain management
   e. Is not an option with a patient with a brain tumor

5. A patient has just been admitted to the hospital with a diagnosis of brain tumor. She makes a comment that drinking alcohol has caused her brain tumor. What does the nurse understand to be a cause of brain tumor?
   a. Smoking
   b. Ionizing radiation
   c. Diet high in fat
   d. Exposure to the sun

Try these additional resources, available at **http://thepoint.lww.com/Honan2e**, to enhance your learning and understanding of this chapter:

- NCLEX-Style Student Review Questions
- Journal Articles

REFERENCES AND SELECTED READINGS

References and selected readings associated with this chapter can be found on the website that accompanies the book. Visit **http://thepoint.lww.com/Honan2e** to access the references and other additional resources associated with this chapter.

Nursing Management: Patients with Neurologic Trauma

Tara Driesen Jennings

Learning Objectives

After reading this chapter, you will be able to:

1. Differentiate patients with head injuries according to mechanism of injury, clinical signs and symptoms, diagnostic testing, and treatment options.
2. Describe the multiple needs of the patient with altered level of consciousness.
3. Identify the early and late clinical manifestations of increased intracranial pressure (ICP).
4. Describe the management of the patient with increased ICP.
5. Identify the population at risk for spinal cord injury (SCI).
6. Identify common complications and management of complications in patients with SCI.
7. Use the nursing process as a framework for care of patients with SCI.

Trauma involving the central nervous system often can be life-threatening. Even when it is not life-threatening, brain and spinal cord injuries (SCIs) can result in major physical and psychological dysfunction and can alter the patient's life completely. Neurologic trauma affects the patient, the family, the health care system, and society as a whole because of its major sequelae and the costs of acute and long-term care of patients with trauma to the brain and spinal cord.

Ongoing assessment of the patient's neurologic function and health needs, identification of problems, mutual goal setting, development and implementation of care plans (including teaching, counseling, and coordinating activities), and evaluation of the outcomes of care are nursing actions integral to the recovery of the patient with neurologic trauma. The nurse also collaborates with other members of the health care team to provide essential care, offer a variety of solutions to problems, help the patient and family gain control of their lives, and explore the educational and supportive resources available in the community. The goals are to achieve as high a level of function as possible and to enhance the quality of life for the patient with neurologic trauma and his or her family.

HEAD INJURIES

Head injury is a broad classification that includes injury to the scalp, skull, or brain. It is the most common cause of death from trauma in the United States. Approximately 1.4 million people receive treatment for head injuries every year (National Institute of Neurological Disorders and Stroke [NINDS], 2015). Of these, 1.1 million are treated and released by the emergency room, 230,000 are hospitalized, 80,000 have permanent disabilities, 60,000 develop seizure disorders, and 50,000 people die (Dawodu, 2015). Traumatic brain injury (TBI) is the most serious form of head injury. The most common causes of TBI are falls (40.5%), motor vehicle accidents (14.3%), collisions with stationary or moving objects (15.5%), and assaults (10.7%) (CDC, 2015). Males between 15 and 24 years of age are at highest risk for TBI. The very young (children under 5 years of age) and the very old (adults over 75 years of age) are also at increased risk. An estimated 5.3 million Americans today are living with a disability as a result of a TBI (Brain Trauma Foundation, 2007; CDC, 2015). Despite advances in care, only 40% of patients with severe TBI have good outcomes (Seemann, 2014). Patients with TBI often have long-lasting chronic comorbidities, including neuro-endocrine abnormalities, neuropsychiatric disease, insomnia, and chronic pain (Bay & Chartier, 2014). The best approach to head injury is an emphasis on prevention (Box 45-1).

Pathophysiology

Research has shown that not all brain damage occurs at the moment of impact. Damage to the brain from traumatic injury takes two forms: primary injury and secondary injury. Primary injury is the initial damage to the brain that results from the traumatic event. This may include contusions, lacerations, and torn blood vessels due to impact, acceleration/

Health Promotion

Preventing Head and Spinal Cord Injuries

- Advise drivers to obey traffic laws and to avoid speeding or driving when under the influence of drugs or alcohol.
- Advise all drivers and passengers to wear seat belts and shoulder harnesses.
- Caution passengers against riding in the back of pickup trucks.
- Advise motorcyclists, scooter riders, bicyclists, skateboarders, and roller-bladers to wear helmets.
- Promote educational programs that are directed toward prevention of violence and suicide in the community.
- Provide water safety instruction.
- Teach patients steps that can be taken to prevent falls, particularly in the elderly.
- Advise athletes to use protective devices. Recommend that coaches be educated in proper coaching techniques.
- Advise owners of firearms to keep them locked in a secure area where children cannot access them.
- Advise drivers to pay attention to the road and not be a distracted driver; advise against looking away from the road to eat, read, or text while driving.

deceleration, or penetration by a foreign object (Porth & Matfin, 2013). Secondary injury evolves over the ensuing hours and days after the initial injury and can be due to cerebral edema, ischemia, seizures, infection, hyperthermia, hypovolemia, and hypoxia (Loane, Stoica, & Faden, 2015).

An injured brain is different from other injured body areas because of its unique characteristics. It resides within the skull, which is a rigid, closed compartment (Hickey, 2014). Unlike other areas of the body, the confines of the skull do not allow for the expansion of cranial contents. Any bleeding or swelling within the skull increases the volume of contents and therefore can cause increased **intracranial pressure** (ICP). If the increased pressure is high enough, it can cause **herniation** of the brain through or against the rigid structures of the skull. This causes restriction of blood flow to the brain, with resultant ischemia, infarction, irreversible brain damage, and, eventually, **brain death** (Box 45-2).

Skull Fractures

A skull fracture is a break in the continuity of the skull caused by forceful trauma. It may occur with or without damage to the brain. Skull fractures can be classified as simple, comminuted, depressed, or basilar. A simple (linear) fracture is a break in the continuity of the bone. A comminuted skull fracture refers to a splintered fracture line. When bone fragments are embedded into brain tissue, the fracture is depressed. A fracture of the base of the skull is called a basilar or basal skull fracture (Fig. 45-1) (Porth & Matfin, 2013). A fracture may be open, indicating a scalp laceration or tear in the dura, or closed, in which case the dura is intact.

Clinical Manifestations

The symptoms, apart from those of the local injury, depend on the severity and the distribution of the underlying brain injury. Persistent, localized pain suggests that a fracture is present. Fractures of the cranial vault may or may not produce swelling in the region of the fracture.

Fractures of the base of the skull tend to traverse the paranasal sinus of the frontal bone or the middle ear located in the temporal bone. Therefore, they frequently produce hemorrhage from the nose, pharynx, or ears, and blood may appear under the conjunctiva. An area of ecchymosis (bruising) that may be seen over the mastoid (Battle sign), develops 12 to 24 hours after injury (Hickey, 2014). Basilar skull fractures are suspected when cerebrospinal fluid (CSF) escapes from the ears (CSF otorrhea) and the nose (CSF rhinorrhea). A halo sign (a blood stain surrounded by a yellowish stain) may be seen on bed linens or on the head

Focus on Pathophysiology

Traumatic Brain Injury

When the brain is injured, there is no room for swelling within the rigid cranial vault. Any bleeding or swelling causes an increase in the amount of intracranial contents, which, in turn, increases intracranial pressure (ICP). The increased pressure causes vasoconstriction and a decrease in blood flow to the brain. This causes hypoxia and ischemia of brain tissue. If ICP continues to rise, eventually the brain will herniate, causing brain death.

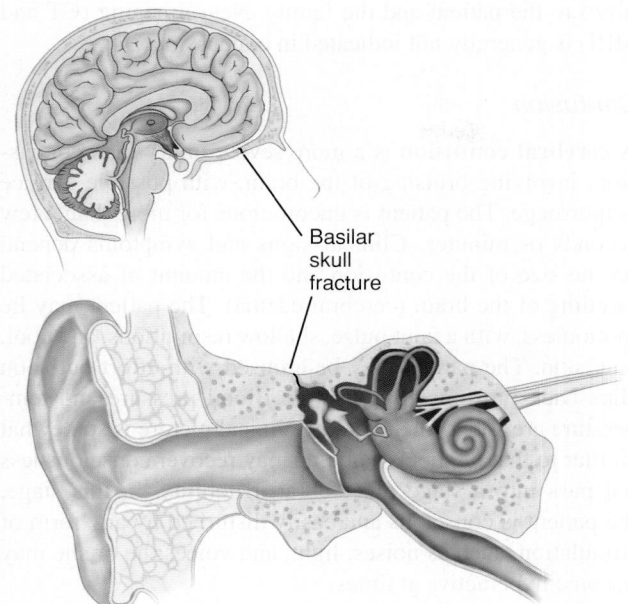

Basilar skull fracture

FIGURE 45-1 Basilar skull fractures allow cerebrospinal fluid to leak from the nose and ears. (Adapted from Hickey, J. V. (2014). *The clinical practice of neurological and neurosurgical nursing* (7th ed.). Philadelphia, PA: Lippincott Williams & Wilkins.)

dressing and is highly suggestive of a CSF leak. Drainage of CSF is a serious problem because meningeal infection, abscess formation, and osteomyelitis can occur if organisms gain access to the cranial contents via the nose, ear, or sinus through a tear in the dura.

Assessment and Diagnostic Findings

Radiologic examination confirms the presence and extent of a skull fracture (Porth & Matfin, 2013). A rapid physical examination and evaluation of neurologic status detects obvious brain injuries, and a computed tomography (CT) scan uses high-speed x-ray scanning to detect less apparent abnormalities.

Magnetic resonance imaging (MRI) is used to evaluate patients with head injury when a more accurate picture of the anatomic nature of the injury is warranted and when the patient is stable enough to undergo this longer diagnostic procedure. See Chapter 43 for further discussion of CT and MRI.

Medical and Nursing Management

Nondepressed skull fractures generally do not require surgical treatment; however, close observation of the patient is essential. Nursing personnel may observe the patient in the hospital, but if no underlying brain injury is present, the patient may be allowed to return home. If the patient is discharged home, specific instructions must be given to the family.

Depressed skull fractures usually require surgery, particularly if contaminated or deformed fractures are present. Large defects can be repaired immediately with bone or artificial grafts; if significant cerebral edema is present, repair of the defect may be delayed for 3 to 6 months. Penetrating wounds require surgical débridement to remove foreign bodies and devitalized brain tissue and to control hemorrhage. IV antibiotic treatment is instituted immediately, particularly with a dural laceration, and blood products are administered if indicated.

As stated previously, fractures of the base of the skull are serious because they are usually open (involving the paranasal sinuses or the middle or external ear). CSF leakage is present in 15% to 20% of patients with skull base fractures (Neville et al., 2014). Clear fluid that is draining from the nose or ears should be collected and tested for glucose. If the drainage is CSF, it will be positive for glucose. Suspicion of a CSF leak should be reported immediately to the provider.

The patient who is conscious is cautioned not to blow his or her nose if there is a CSF leak as this can worsen the leak. The head is elevated 30 degrees to reduce ICP and promote spontaneous closure of the leak (Hickey, 2014). Early detection of a CSF leak may help avoid complications, including meningitis or pneumocephalus (air within the cranial vault). The patient with a basal skull fracture should not have the nose suctioned. If a nasogastric tube is required for patient management, it should be inserted orally. Tears of the dura (protective covering directly on top of the brain) are commonly seen in basal skull fractures. A suction catheter or nasogastric tube is a potential source of infection and may lead to the development of meningitis. Early CSF rhinorrhea (resolving within 3 to 5 days) usually does not require surgery. Late-onset (7 or more days after the initial injury) and persistent CSF rhinorrhea usually requires surgical intervention to prevent development of meningitis. CSF otorrhea typically does not require surgical treatment as 85% of CSF leaks through the ears stop spontaneously (Mateo, Savage, & Jimenez, 2012).

> **! Nursing Alert**
> *Any patient with extensive facial fractures or suspected basilar skull fracture may also have a fracture of the cribriform plate (portion of the ethmoid bone that separates the roof of the nose from the cranial cavity). Attempted intubation with a nasogastric tube or nasotracheal tube or suctioning is prohibited to avoid intracranial penetration of the brain with the tube or catheter.*

BRAIN INJURY

The most important consideration in any head injury is whether or not the brain is injured. Even seemingly minor injury can cause significant brain damage secondary to obstructed blood flow and decreased tissue perfusion. The brain cannot store oxygen or glucose to any significant degree. Because neurons need an uninterrupted blood supply

Traumatic Brain Injury

Be on alert for the following signs and symptoms:

- Altered level of consciousness (LOC)
- Confusion
- Pupillary abnormalities (changes in shape, size, and response to light)
- Sudden onset of neurologic deficits
- Changes in vital signs (altered respiratory pattern, widened pulse pressure, bradycardia, tachycardia, hypothermia, or hyperthermia)
- Vision and hearing impairment
- Sensory dysfunction
- Headache
- Seizures

to obtain these nutrients, irreversible brain damage and cell death occur if the blood supply is interrupted for even a few minutes. Clinical manifestations of **brain injury** (injury to the brain that is severe enough to interfere with normal functioning) are listed in Box 45-3. Closed (blunt) brain injury occurs when the head accelerates and then rapidly decelerates or collides with another object (i.e., a wall, the dashboard of a car) and brain tissue is damaged but there is no opening through the skull and dura. Open brain injury occurs when an object penetrates the skull, enters the brain, and damages the soft brain tissue in its path (penetrating injury), or when blunt trauma to the head is so severe that it opens the scalp, skull, and dura to expose the brain.

Types of Brain Injury

Concussion

A **concussion** (also referred to as a mild TBI) involves an alteration in mental status that results from trauma and may or may not involve loss of consciousness. This typically lasts no longer than 24 hours and may include symptoms such as headache, nausea, vomiting, photophobia (sensitivity to light), amnesia, and blurry vision (McClain, 2015).

Treatment involves observing the patient for symptoms, including headache, dizziness, lethargy, irritability, anxiety, photophobia, phonophobia (fear of sound or of speaking aloud), difficulty concentrating, and memory difficulties. The occurrence of these symptoms after the injury is referred to as *postconcussive syndrome* (Barlow et al., 2014). Giving the patient information, explanations, and encouragement may reduce some of the problems associated with postconcussive syndrome. The patient is advised to resume normal activities slowly; the exact recovery time is not known (McClain, 2015). Once the patient is discharged home, he or she should be closely observed for the next 24 hours and awakened every 2 hours in order to detect any changes in mental status. Box 45-4 provides complete instructions to be

given to the patient and the family. Neuroimaging (CT and MRI) is generally not indicated in concussion.

Contusion

A **cerebral contusion** is a more severe injury than concussion, involving bruising of the brain, with possible surface hemorrhage. The patient is unconscious for more than a few seconds or minutes. Clinical signs and symptoms depend on the size of the contusion and the amount of associated swelling of the brain (cerebral edema). The patient may lie motionless, with a faint pulse, shallow respirations, and cool, pale skin. The patient may be aroused with effort but soon slips back into unconsciousness. Blood pressure and temperature are subnormal, and the clinical picture is somewhat similar to that of shock. Patients may recover consciousness but pass into a stage of cerebral irritability. In this stage, the patient is conscious and easily disturbed by any form of stimulation, such as noises, light, and voices; he or she may become hyperactive at times.

Nursing Alert
When the patient begins to emerge from unconsciousness, every measure that is available and appropriate for calming and quieting the patient should be used. Any form of restraint is likely to be countered with resistance, leading to self-injury or to a dangerous increase in ICP. Therefore, physical restraints should be avoided, if possible.

Gradually, the pulse, respirations, temperature, and other body functions return to normal, but full recovery can be delayed for months. Residual headache and vertigo are common, and impaired mental function or seizures may occur as a result of irreparable cerebral damage.

Teaching Guidelines Following Concussion

Once the patient is discharged home, he or she should be closely observed for the next 24 hours and awakened every 2 hours. The patient and family are instructed to observe for the following signs and symptoms and to notify the provider (or bring the patient to the emergency department) if they occur:

- Difficulty in awakening
- Difficulty speaking
- Confusion
- Seizures
- Severe headache
- Vomiting
- Weakness on one side of the body

The patient should also avoid playing contact sports, driving, drinking alcohol, and using heavy machinery until cleared by a health care provider.

FIGURE 45-2 Abnormal posture response to stimuli. **A.** Decorticate posturing, involving adduction and flexion of the upper extremities, internal rotation of the lower extremities, and plantar flexion of the feet. **B.** Decerebrate posturing, involving extension and outward rotation of upper extremities and plantar flexion of the feet.

Diffuse Axonal Injury

Diffuse axonal injury involves widespread damage to axons in the cerebral hemispheres, corpus callosum, and brainstem. It can be seen with mild, moderate, or severe head trauma. The patient experiences immediate coma, global cerebral edema, decorticate and decerebrate rigidity, or *posturing* (Fig. 45-2). **Decorticate** posturing involves abnormal flexion of the upper extremities and extension of the lower extremities and indicates damage to the upper midbrain; **decerebrate** posturing involves extreme extension of the upper and lower extremities and indicates severe damage to the brain at the lower midbrain and upper pons (Hickey, 2014). Diagnosis of diffuse axonal injury is made by clinical signs in conjunction with a CT or MRI scan. These tests are usually normal; a definitive diagnosis can be made only at autopsy. Recovery depends on the severity of the axonal injury.

Intracranial Hemorrhage (Intracranial Hematoma)

Hematomas (collections of blood) that develop within the cranial vault are the most serious type of brain injury (Hickey, 2014). A hematoma may be epidural (above the dura), subdural (below the dura), or intracerebral (within the brain) (Fig. 45-3). Major symptoms are frequently delayed until the hematoma is large enough to cause distortion of the brain and increased ICP. The signs and symptoms of cerebral ischemia resulting from compression by a hematoma are variable and depend on the speed with which vital areas are affected and the area that is injured (American Association of Neuroscience Nurses [AANN], 2012).

Epidural Hematoma (Extradural Hematoma or Hemorrhage)

After a head injury, blood may collect in the epidural (extradural) space between the skull and the dura. This can result from a skull fracture that causes a rupture or laceration of the middle meningeal artery, the artery that runs between the dura and the skull, inferior to a thin portion of temporal bone. Hemorrhage from this artery causes a rapid increase in pressure on the brain.

Symptoms are caused by the expanding hematoma. Usually a momentary loss of consciousness occurs at the time of injury, followed by an interval of apparent recovery (lucid interval). Although the lucid interval is considered a classic characteristic of an epidural hematoma, no lucid interval

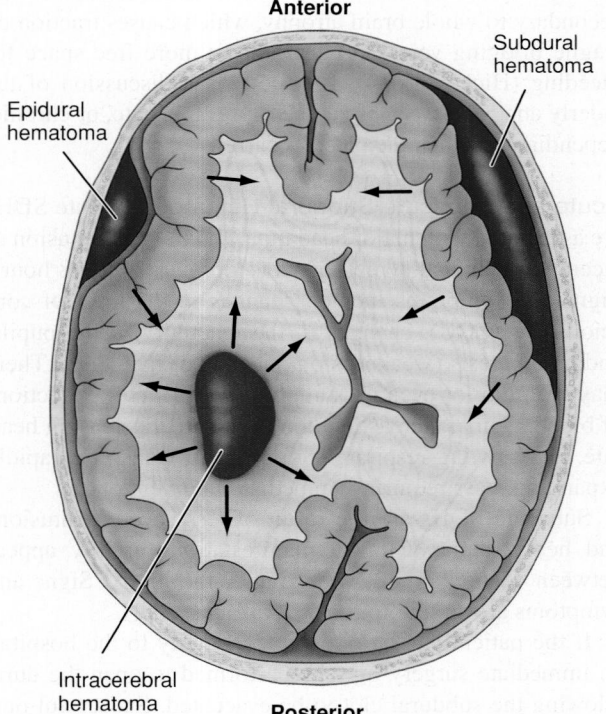

FIGURE 45-3 Location of epidural, subdural, and intracerebral hematomas.

has been reported in many patients with this lesion (Hickey, 2014), and, therefore, it should not be considered a critical defining criterion. During the lucid interval, compensation for the expanding hematoma takes place by rapid absorption of CSF and decreased intravascular volume, both of which help maintain a normal ICP. When these mechanisms can no longer compensate, even a small increase in the volume of the hematoma produces a marked elevation in ICP. Then, often suddenly, signs of compression appear (usually deterioration of consciousness and signs of focal neurologic deficits, such as dilation and fixation of a pupil or paralysis of an extremity), and the patient's condition deteriorates rapidly.

An epidural hematoma is considered an extreme emergency; marked neurologic deficit and respiratory arrest can occur within minutes. Treatment consists of making openings through the skull (burr holes) to decrease ICP emergently, remove the clot, and control the bleeding. A craniotomy (surgical procedure that removes of part of the skull to gain access to the brain) may be required to remove the clot and control the bleeding. A drain may be inserted after creation of burr holes or a craniotomy to prevent reaccumulation of blood.

Subdural Hematoma

A subdural hematoma (SDH) is a collection of blood between the dura and the brain, a space normally occupied by a thin cushion of CSF (see Fig. 45-3). The most common cause of SDH is trauma, but it can also occur as a result of coagulopathies (bleeding disorders) or rupture of an aneurysm. The elderly are at increased risk for subdural hemorrhage secondary to whole brain atrophy, which causes traction on fragile bridging veins and also allows more free space for bleeding (Hickey, 2014). Box 45-5 is a discussion of the elderly and SDHs. SDHs can be acute, subacute, or chronic, depending on when the bleed occurred.

Acute and Subacute Subdural Hematoma.
Acute SDHs are associated with major head injury involving contusion or laceration. Clinical symptoms develop over 24 to 48 hours. Signs and symptoms include changes in the level of consciousness (LOC), changes in the reactivity of the pupils, and hemiparesis (weakness on one side of the body). There may be minor or even no symptoms, with small collections of blood. Coma, increasing blood pressure, decreasing heart rate, and slowing respiratory rate are all signs of a rapidly expanding mass requiring immediate intervention.

Subacute SDHs are the result of less severe contusions and head trauma. Clinical manifestations usually appear between 48 hours and 2 weeks after the injury. Signs and symptoms are similar to those of an acute SDH.

If the patient can be transported rapidly to the hospital, an immediate surgery may be performed to open the dura, allowing the subdural clot to be evacuated. Successful outcome also depends on the control of ICP and careful monitoring of respiratory function. The mortality rate for patients

> **BOX 45-5** **Gerontologic Considerations**
>
> **Subdural Hematomas**
>
> Subdural hematomas (SDHs) are more common in the elderly, occurring most often in patients in their 60s and 70s. SDHs represent a reversible cause of dementia so their detection is vital to accurate diagnosis of dementia in the older adult.
>
> Older adults are more prone to developing SDHs due to cerebral atrophy. This causes fragile bridging veins, which run between the dura and the brain, to tear as the atrophied brain pulls away from the dura. Trauma is the leading cause of SDHs and will often be so trivial that the older adult does not remember it occurring. Alcoholics and patients taking anticoagulation are also at increased risk for developing an SDH.
>
> Common presenting symptoms of SDHs in the older adult are gait disturbance, headache, aphasia (inability to speak), altered mental status, and hemiparesis (weakness on one side of the body). The initial presentation of an SDH is often very subtle, with the patient becoming confused and easily agitated. Diagnosis is made by obtaining a CT scan. Treatment typically consists of surgical evacuation of the hematoma.
>
> When caring for the older adult, it is important to consider the risk for development of an SDH. SDHs represent a common cause of reversible dementia that is easily overlooked due to the subtlety of presenting signs and symptoms.

with acute or subacute SDH is high because of associated brain damage (Hickey, 2014).

Chronic Subdural Hematoma.
Chronic SDHs can develop from seemingly minor head injuries and are seen most frequently in the elderly. The time between injury and onset of symptoms can be lengthy (i.e., 3 weeks to many months) so the actual injury may be forgotten.

The treatment of a chronic SDH typically consists of surgical evacuation of the clot if the patient is symptomatic and the bleed is at least 1 cm in size. Smaller bleeds are monitored until the body has fully reabsorbed the blood (Hickey, 2014).

Intracerebral Hemorrhage and Hematoma

Intracerebral hemorrhage (ICH) is bleeding into the parenchyma of the brain. It is commonly seen in head injuries when force is exerted to the head over a small area (e.g., bullet wounds and stab injuries). These hemorrhages within the brain may also result from:

- Systemic hypertension, which causes degeneration and rupture of a vessel
- Rupture of a saccular aneurysm
- Vascular anomalies
- Intracranial tumors
- Bleeding disorders, such as leukemia, hemophilia, aplastic anemia, and thrombocytopenia
- Complications of anticoagulant therapy

The onset may be insidious, beginning with the development of neurologic deficits followed by headache. Management includes supportive care, control of ICP, and careful administration of fluids, electrolytes, and antihypertensive medications. Surgical intervention by craniotomy permits removal of the blood clot and control of hemorrhage but may not be possible because of the inaccessible location of the bleeding or the lack of a clearly circumscribed area of blood that can be removed. Decompressive craniectomies that are performed up to 24 hours after the initial injury have been shown to improve outcomes. These procedures are performed to allow for swelling of the brain, which decreases ICP. The earlier the craniectomy can be done, the greater benefit it can have for the patient (Takeuchi et al., 2013).

Management of Brain Injuries

Assessment and diagnosis of the extent of injury are accomplished by the initial physical and neurologic examinations. CT and MRI are the primary neuroimaging diagnostic tools of choice and are useful in evaluating the brain structure.

Cervical spine injuries occur in 1.7% to 8% of patients with TBI. Patients at highest risk for cervical spine injury are those involved in motorcycle accidents, those with lower scores on the Glasgow Coma Scale (GCS) (score of 8 or less), and those with skull base fractures (Tomoko, Faul, & Sasser, 2013). The patient is transported from the scene of the injury on a board with the head and neck maintained in alignment with the axis of the body. A hard cervical collar should be applied and maintained until cervical spine x-rays have been obtained and the absence of cervical SCI is documented.

All therapy is directed toward preserving brain homeostasis and preventing secondary brain injury. Common causes of secondary injury include cerebral edema, hypotension, and respiratory depression. Treatments to prevent secondary injury include stabilization of cardiovascular and respiratory function to maintain adequate cerebral perfusion, control of hemorrhage and hypovolemia, and maintenance of optimal blood gas values.

Nursing Alert
Any patient with a head injury is presumed to have a cervical spine injury until such injury is ruled out; therefore, immobilization of the spine via cervical collar, spinal backboard, and the avoidance of movement is essential.

ALTERED LEVEL OF CONSCIOUSNESS AND INCREASED INTRACRANIAL PRESSURE

An **altered level of consciousness** (LOC) is apparent in the patient who is not oriented, does not follow commands, or needs persistent stimuli to achieve a state of alertness.

LOC is gauged on a continuum, with a normal state of alertness and full cognition (consciousness) on one end and coma on the other end. **Coma** is a clinical state of unarousable unresponsiveness in which there are no purposeful responses to internal or external stimuli, although nonpurposeful responses to painful stimuli and brainstem reflexes may be present (Hickey, 2014). The duration of coma is usually limited to 2 to 4 weeks. *Persistent vegetative state* is a condition in which the unresponsive patient resumes sleep–wake cycles after coma but is devoid of cognitive or affective mental function. **Locked-in syndrome** results from a lesion affecting the pons or midbrain and results in **tetraplegia** (formerly called quadriplegia) and inability to speak, but vertical eye movements and lid elevation typically remain intact and are used to indicate responsiveness (Hickey, 2014). The LOC is the most important indicator of the patient's condition.

The volume of the rigid cranial vault is approximately 1,700 mL, containing brain tissue (1,400 mL, or 80%), intravascular blood (150 mL, or 10%), and CSF (150 mL, or 10%). The volume and pressure of these three components are usually in a state of equilibrium, and together they produce the ICP. An alteration in LOC may be the result of increased ICP. Increased ICP is explained by the Monro-Kellie hypothesis. The **Monro-Kellie hypothesis** states that because of the limited space for expansion within the skull, an increase in any one of the components causes a change in the volume of the others. Because brain tissue has limited space to expand, compensation typically is accomplished by increasing absorption or diminishing production of CSF or decreasing cerebral blood volume. Without such changes, ICP will begin to rise. ICP is usually measured in the lateral ventricles, with normal pressure being 5 to 15 mm Hg. Treatment of increased ICP is generally initiated at a pressure of 20 mm Hg (Hickey, 2014).

Pathophysiology

Altered LOC is not a disorder itself; rather, it is the result of multiple pathophysiologic phenomena. The cause may be neurologic (head injury, stroke), toxicologic (drug overdose, alcohol intoxication), or metabolic (liver or kidney failure, diabetic ketoacidosis). Increased ICP affects many patients with acute neurologic conditions. This is because pathologic conditions alter the relationship between intracranial volume and ICP. Elevated ICP is most commonly associated with head injury, although it may also be seen in other neurologic conditions, including brain tumors and subarachnoid hemorrhages. Increased ICP from any cause decreases cerebral perfusion, stimulates further swelling (edema), and may shift brain tissue through openings in the rigid dura, resulting in herniation (Fig. 45-4). The herniated brain tissue exerts pressure on the brain area into which it has shifted, which interferes with the blood supply in that area. Cessation of cerebral blood flow results in cerebral ischemia, infarction,

FIGURE 45-4 Brain with intracranial shifts from supratentorial lesions. (**1**) Herniation of the cingulate gyrus under the falx cerebri. (**2**) Central transtentorial herniation. (**3**) Uncal herniation of the temporal lobe into the tentorial notch. (**4**) Infratentorial herniation of the cerebral tonsils. (Adapted from Porth, C. M., & Matfin, G. (2013). *Pathophysiology: Concepts of altered health states* (9th ed.). Philadelphia, PA: Lippincott Williams & Wilkins.)

and brain death. Herniation is often a dire, and frequently fatal, event (Hickey, 2014).

Increased ICP may significantly reduce cerebral blood flow, resulting in ischemia and cell death. In the early stages of cerebral ischemia, the vasomotor centers are stimulated and the systemic pressure rises to maintain cerebral blood flow. This is typically accompanied by a slow, bounding pulse and respiratory irregularities. These changes in blood pressure, pulse, and respiration are important clinically because they suggest increased ICP.

Cerebral edema is defined as an abnormal accumulation of water or fluid in the intracellular space, extracellular space, or both, and is associated with an increase in the volume of brain tissue. Edema can occur in any part of the brain. As brain tissue swells within the rigid skull, several mechanisms attempt to compensate for the increasing ICP. These compensatory mechanisms include autoregulation and decreased production and flow of CSF. **Autoregulation** refers to the brain's ability to change the diameter of its blood vessels automatically to maintain a constant cerebral blood flow during alterations in systemic blood pressure. This mechanism may be impaired in patients who are experiencing a pathologic and sustained increase in ICP.

A clinical phenomenon known as the **Cushing response** (or Cushing reflex) is seen when cerebral blood flow decreases significantly. When ischemic, the vasomotor center triggers an increase in arterial pressure in an effort to overcome the increased ICP. A sympathetically mediated response causes an increase in the systolic blood pressure,

with a widening of the pulse pressure and cardiac slowing. It is a late sign requiring immediate intervention; however, perfusion may be recoverable if the Cushing response is treated rapidly.

At a certain point, the brain's ability to autoregulate becomes ineffective and decompensation (ischemia and infarction) begins. When this occurs, the patient exhibits significant changes in mental status and vital signs. The bradycardia, hypertension, and bradypnea associated with this deterioration are known as **Cushing triad**, a grave sign. At this point, herniation of the brainstem and occlusion of the cerebral blood flow occur if therapeutic intervention is not initiated immediately.

Clinical Manifestations

Alterations in LOC occur along a continuum, and the clinical manifestations depend on where the patient is along this continuum. As the patient's state of alertness and consciousness decreases, changes will ultimately occur in the pupillary response, eye opening response, verbal response, and motor response. However, initial alterations in LOC may be reflected by subtle behavioral changes, such as restlessness or increased anxiety. The pupils, normally round and briskly reactive to light, become sluggish (response is slower); as the patient becomes comatose, the pupils become fixed (no response to light). The patient in a coma does not open the eyes, respond verbally, or move the extremities in response to a request to do so.

It is important to be familiar with the patient's baseline status as many early signs of increased ICP are subtle; they include sudden onset of restlessness (without apparent cause), confusion, and increasing drowsiness. As ICP increases, the patient becomes stuporous, reacting only to loud or painful stimuli. At this stage, serious impairment of brain circulation is likely taking place, and immediate intervention is required. As neurologic function deteriorates further, the patient becomes comatose and exhibits decorticate and decerebrate posturing or flaccidity (see Fig. 45-2). If the coma is profound, with the patient exhibiting fixed and dilated pupils and impaired or absent respiration, death is usually inevitable.

Assessment and Diagnostic Findings

The patient with an altered LOC is at risk for alterations in every body system. A complete assessment is performed, with particular attention to the neurologic system. The neurologic examination should be as complete as the LOC allows (AANN, 2014a). It includes an evaluation of mental status, cranial nerve function, cerebellar function (balance and coordination), reflexes, and motor and sensory function.

LOC, a sensitive indicator of neurologic function, can be assessed based on the criteria in the GCS, which include eye opening (E), verbal response (V), and motor response (M). The patient's responses are rated on a scale from 3 to 15. Box 45-6

BOX 45-6

Focused Assessment

Glasgow Coma Scale

The Glasgow Coma Scale (GCS) is a tool for assessing a patient's response to stimuli. Scores range from 3 (deep coma) to 15 (normal).

Eye opening response	Spontaneous	4
	To voice	3
	To pain	2
	None	1
Best verbal response	Oriented	5
	Confused	4
	Inappropriate words	3
	Incomprehensible sounds	2
	None	1
Best motor response	Obeys command	6
	Localizes pain	5
	Withdraws	4
	Flexion	3
	Extension	2
	None	1
Total		3 to 15

provides the complete scoring of the GCS. The severity of TBI can be classified based upon the score on the GCS. A score of 13 to 15 is classified as mild TBI, 9 to 12 is moderate TBI, and 3 to 8 is severe TBI (Goldberg, Rojanasarntikul, & Jagoda, 2015; Hickey, 2014). A score of 3 indicates severe impairment of neurologic function, deep coma, brain death, or pharmacologic inhibition of the neurologic response; a score of 8 or less typically indicates an unconscious patient; a score of 15 indicates a fully alert and oriented patient.

The patient's orientation is assessed by asking the patient to identify his or her full name, where he or she is, and the day, month, or season, and what happened to them (person, time, place, and situation). Other questions such as "Who is the president?" may be helpful in determining the patient's processing of information in the environment. Verbal response cannot be evaluated if the patient is intubated or has a tracheostomy; this should be clearly documented.

Alertness is measured by the patient's ability to open the eyes spontaneously or in response to a vocal or noxious stimulus (pressure or pain). Patients with severe neurologic dysfunction cannot do this. The nurse assesses for periorbital edema (swelling around the eyes) or trauma, which may prevent the patient from opening the eyes, and documents any such condition that interferes with eye opening.

Motor response includes spontaneous, purposeful movement (e.g., the awake patient can move all four extremities with equal strength on command), movement only in response to painful stimuli, or abnormal posturing. If the patient is not responding to commands, the motor response is tested by applying a painful stimulus, using the least amount of pressure to elicit a possible response. Suggestions include using central pressure such as a sternal rub or squeezing the muscle masses and tendons. Central stimulation produces an overall body response, compared to peripheral stimulation via nail bed pressure, which can elicit a reflex response, which is not a true indicator of motor activity (Hickey, 2014; Noah, 2004). If the patient attempts to push away or withdraw, the response is recorded as purposeful or appropriate ("patient withdraws to painful stimuli"). This response is considered purposeful if the patient can cross the midline from one side of the body to the other in response to painful stimuli. An inappropriate or nonpurposeful response is random and aimless. Movement of only one side is suggestive of hemiparesis, while withdrawal suggests purposeful behavior. The motor response cannot be elicited if pharmacologic paralyzing agents have been administered to the patient. These must be suspended and time must elapse for the effects to wear off before attempting to elicit a motor response.

In addition to LOC, the nurse monitors parameters such as respiratory status, pupillary response, and vital signs on an ongoing basis. Table 45-1 summarizes the assessment and the clinical significance of the findings. Body functions (circulation, respiration, elimination, fluid and electrolyte balance) are examined in a systematic and ongoing manner.

If the patient is comatose and has localized signs, such as abnormal pupillary and motor responses, it is assumed that neurologic disease is present until proven otherwise. If the patient is comatose but pupillary light reflexes are preserved, a toxic or metabolic disorder is suspected. Common laboratory testing and diagnostic procedures performed on patients with decreased LOC and increased ICP are listed in Table 45-2.

Medical and Nursing Management

The first priority of treatment for the patient with altered LOC is to obtain and maintain a patent airway. The patient may be orally or nasally intubated (unless basilar skull fracture or facial trauma is suspected), or a tracheostomy may be performed. Until the ability of the patient to breathe on his or her own is determined, a mechanical ventilator is used to maintain adequate oxygenation and ventilation. The circulatory status (blood pressure, heart rate) is monitored to ensure adequate perfusion to the body and brain. An IV catheter is inserted to provide access for IV fluids and medications.

Increased ICP is a true emergency and must be treated promptly. Invasive monitoring of ICP is an important component of management. Immediate management to relieve increased ICP requires decreasing cerebral edema, lowering the volume of CSF, and decreasing cerebral blood volume while maintaining cerebral perfusion. These goals are accomplished by administering osmotic diuretics, restricting fluids, draining CSF, controlling fever, maintaining systemic blood pressure and oxygenation, and reducing cellular metabolic demands. Corticosteroids are not recommended in cases of increased ICP resulting from TBI (Hickey, 2014). In patients with severe TBI, there was a significant reduction in mortality when clinicians closely followed the guidelines

TABLE **45-1** **Nursing Assessment of the Unconscious Patient**

Examination	Clinical Assessment	Clinical Significance
Level of responsiveness or consciousness	Eye opening; verbal and motor responses; pupils (size, equality, reaction to light)	Obeying commands is a favorable response and demonstrates a return to consciousness.
Pattern of respiration	Respiratory pattern	Disturbances of respiratory center of brain may result in various respiratory patterns.
	Cheyne–Stokes respiration	Suggests lesions deep in both hemispheres; area of basal ganglia and upper brainstem
	Hyperventilation	Suggests onset of metabolic problem or brainstem damage
	Ataxic respiration with irregularity in depth/rate	Ominous sign of damage to medullary center
Eyes		
Pupils (size, equality, reaction to light)	Equal, normally reactive pupils	Suggests that coma is toxic or metabolic in origin
	Equal or unequal diameter	Helps determine location of lesion
	Progressive dilation	Indicates increasing intracranial pressure
	Fixed dilated pupils	Indicates injury at level of midbrain
Eye movements	Normally, eyes should move from side to side.	Functional and structural integrity of brainstem is assessed by inspection of extraocular movements; usually absent in deep coma
Corneal reflex	When cornea is touched with a wisp of clean cotton, blink response is normal	Tests cranial nerves V and VII; helps determine location of lesion if unilateral; absent in deep coma
Facial symmetry	Asymmetry (sagging, decrease in wrinkles)	Sign of paralysis
Swallowing reflex	Drooling versus spontaneous swallowing	Absent in coma Paralysis of cranial nerves IX, X, and XII
Neck	Stiff neck	Subarachnoid hemorrhage, meningitis
	Absence of spontaneous neck movement	Fracture or dislocation of cervical spine
Response of extremity to noxious stimuli	Firm pressure on a joint of the upper and lower extremity	Asymmetric response in paralysis
	Observe spontaneous movements	Absent in deep coma
Deep tendon reflexes	Tap patellar and biceps tendons.	Brisk response may have localizing value Asymmetric response in paralysis No response in deep coma
Pathologic reflexes	Firm pressure with blunt object on sole of foot, moving along lateral margin and crossing to the ball of foot	Flexion of the toes, especially the great toe, is normal except in newborn Dorsiflexion of toes (especially great toe) indicates contralateral pathology of corticospinal tract (Babinski reflex) Helps determine location of lesion in brain
Abnormal posture	Observation for posturing (spontaneous or in response to noxious stimuli)	Deep extensive brain lesion
	Flaccidity with absence of motor response	Seen with cerebral hemisphere pathology and in metabolic depression of brain function
	Decorticate posture (flexion and internal rotation of forearms and hands)	Decorticate posturing indicates damage to the upper midbrain
	Decerebrate posture (extension and external rotation)	Decerebrate posturing indicates deeper and more severe dysfunction than does decorticate posturing; implies brain pathology; poor prognostic sign

TABLE 45-2 Laboratory and Diagnostic Tests for Patients with Traumatic Brain Injury

Test	Normal Values	Critical Values	Nursing Implications
Complete blood count	WBC: 4.5–10.5 (×1,000/mm³) WBC for Black adults: 3.2–10.0 (×1,000/mm³) HCT: women: 36–48%; men: 42–52%	WBC: >10.5 (×1,000/mm³) HCT: <32%	Assess for any signs or symptoms of infection with increased WBC; assess for any signs or symptoms of occult bleeding with decreased HCT.
Glucose	70–110 mg/dL	>150 mg/dL	Hyperglycemia may worsen outcomes; administer insulin if glucose is elevated.
Serum osmolality	278–300 mOsm/L	≥320 mOsm/L	Osmolality should not exceed 320 mOsm/L to prevent kidney failure in patients receiving mannitol.
Serum sodium	135–145 mEq/L	<130 mEq/L or >145 mEq/L	Hyponatremia may indicate cerebral salt wasting or SIADH. Hypernatremia may indicate diabetes insipidus or be due to mannitol therapy.
Urine specific gravity	1.005–1.015	<1.005 or >1.015	Low specific gravity can mean diabetes insipidus while a high level may mean SIADH.
Chest radiograph	Negative for pneumonia or infiltrate	Presence of pneumonia or infiltrate	Ventilated patients are prone to aspiration and development of pneumonias.
Head CT without contrast	Negative for acute hemorrhage	Positive for epidural, subdural, or intracerebral hemorrhage	Observe for any signs or symptoms of intracranial bleeding.
Serum potassium	3.5–5.0 mEq/L	<3.5 mEq/L	Hypokalemia may be a consequence of mannitol therapy.
Magnesium	1.8–2.6 mg/dL	<1.8 mg/dL	Hypomagnesemia may lower the seizure threshold and cause secondary brain injury; low levels should be corrected.

WBC, white blood cell count; HCT, hematocrit; SIADH, syndrome of inappropriate antidiuretic hormone.
Adapted from Dunning, M., & Fischbach, F. (2015). *Nurses' quick reference to common laboratory and diagnostic tests* (5th ed.). Philadelphia, PA: Lippincott Williams & Wilkins.

from the Brain Trauma Foundation for control of both ICP and cerebral perfusion pressure (CPP) (Gerber, Chiu, Carney, Hartl, & Ghajar, 2013).

Monitoring Intracranial Pressure

Nursing management focuses on detecting early signs of increasing ICP because medical interventions are usually ineffective once later signs develop. Frequent neurologic assessments and documentation and analysis of trends will reveal the subtle changes that may indicate increasing ICP.

Detecting Early Indications of Increasing Intracranial Pressure

The nurse assesses for and immediately reports any of the following early signs or symptoms of increasing ICP:

- Disorientation, restlessness, increased respiratory effort, purposeless movements, and mental confusion; these are early clinical indications of increasing ICP because the

brain cells responsible for cognition are extremely sensitive to decreased oxygenation.
- Pupillary changes and impaired extraocular movements; these occur as the increasing pressure displaces the brain against the oculomotor and optic nerves (cranial nerves II, III, IV, and VI), which arise from the midbrain and brainstem (see Chapter 43).
- Weakness in one extremity or on one side of the body; this occurs as increasing ICP compresses the pyramidal tracts, which control motor function.
- Headache that is constant, increasing in intensity, and aggravated by movement or straining; this occurs as increasing ICP causes pressure and stretching of venous and arterial vessels in the base of the brain.

Nursing Alert
The earliest sign of increasing ICP is a change in LOC. Any changes in LOC should be reported immediately.

Detecting Later Indications of Increasing Intracranial Pressure

As ICP increases, the patient's condition worsens and the following signs and symptoms may be observed:

- LOC continues to deteriorate until the patient is comatose.
- Respiratory rate decreases or becomes erratic, blood pressure and temperature increase. The pulse pressure widens and the pulse fluctuates rapidly, varying from bradycardia to tachycardia.
- Altered respiratory patterns develop, including Cheyne–Stokes breathing (rhythmic waxing and waning of rate and depth of respirations alternating with brief periods of apnea) and ataxic breathing (irregular breathing with a random sequence of deep and shallow breaths).
- Projectile vomiting may occur with increased pressure on the reflex center in the medulla.
- Hemiplegia or decorticate or decerebrate posturing may develop as pressure on the brainstem increases; bilateral flaccidity occurs before death.
- Loss of brainstem reflexes, including pupillary, corneal, gag, and swallowing reflexes, which is an ominous sign of impending death.

Because clinical assessment is not always a reliable guide in recognizing increased ICP, especially in comatose patients, monitoring of ICP is an essential part of management (Hickey, 2014). ICP is monitored closely for continuous elevation or significant increase over baseline. The trend of ICP measurements over time is an important indication of the patient's underlying status. Vital signs are assessed when an increase in ICP is noted.

ICP can be monitored with the use of an intraventricular catheter (ventriculostomy) or a subarachnoid bolt or screw (Fig. 45-5). When a **ventriculostomy** is used for monitoring ICP, a fine-bore catheter is inserted into a lateral ventricle, preferably in the nondominant hemisphere of the brain (Hickey, 2014). The catheter is connected by a fluid-filled system to a transducer, which records the pressure in the form of an electrical impulse. In addition to obtaining continuous ICP recordings, the ventricular catheter allows CSF to drain, particularly during acute increases in pressure. The ventriculostomy can also be used to drain blood from the ventricle. Continuous drainage of CSF under pressure control is an effective method of treating intracranial hypertension. Complications associated with its use include infection, meningitis, ventricular collapse, occlusion of the catheter by brain tissue or blood, and problems with the monitoring system (AANN, 2014a). CSF drainage is frequently performed because the removal of CSF with a ventriculostomy drain can dramatically reduce ICP and restore cerebral perfusion. Caution should be used in draining CSF, however, because excessive drainage may result in collapse of the ventricles and herniation.

The **subarachnoid bolt** or **screw** is a hollow device that is inserted through the skull and dura mater into the cranial subarachnoid space (Hickey, 2014). It has the advantage of

FIGURE 45-5 Intracranial pressure monitoring. A device may be placed in (**A**) the ventricle, (**B**) the subarachnoid space, (**C**) the intraparenchymal space, or (**D**) the subdural space.

not requiring a ventricular puncture. The subarachnoid bolt is attached to a pressure transducer, and the output is recorded on an oscilloscope. This technique also has the advantage of avoiding complications from brain shift and small ventricle size. One disadvantage to using a subarachnoid bolt is the inability to obtain CSF for analysis or drainage purposes. Complications include infection and blockage of the bolt by clot or brain tissue, which leads to a loss of pressure tracing and a decrease in accuracy at high ICP readings.

While ICP monitoring is only performed in an ICU setting, CSF drainage may be carried out in the operating room, emergency room, or intensive care unit. A ventriculostomy without the ICP monitoring catheter is known as an *external ventricular drain* (EVD). Box 45-7 provides guidelines on nursing care of the EVD.

Monitoring and Managing Complications

Potential complications for the patient with altered LOC include respiratory failure, pneumonia, pressure ulcers, and aspiration. Respiratory failure may develop shortly after the patient becomes unconscious. If the patient cannot maintain effective respirations, insertion of an airway and mechanical ventilation is initiated to provide adequate ventilation and to protect the airway. Pneumonia is common in patients receiving mechanical ventilation and in those who cannot maintain and clear the airway. The patient with altered LOC is subject to all the complications associated with immobility, such as pressure ulcers, venous stasis, musculoskeletal deterioration, and disturbed gastrointestinal functioning. Aspiration of gastric contents or feedings may occur, precipitating the development of aspiration pneumonia or airway occlusion.

Endocrine abnormalities, including diabetes insipidus and syndrome of inappropriate antidiuretic hormone (SIADH),

GUIDELINES FOR NURSING CARE

Caring for an External Ventricular Drain (EVD)

Nurses in a variety of acute care settings may receive patients who have an external ventricular drain (EVD) in place to drain off excess CSF. The nurse is responsible for maintaining the EVD while monitoring for any signs or symptoms of infection or CSF leak.

Equipment

- Carpenter's level
- Sterile gloves
- Sterile 4 × 4 gauze pad
- Transparent dressing large enough to cover the gauze (e.g., Tegaderm)

Implementation

NURSING ACTION	RATIONALE
1. Position the head of the bed at 30 degrees with the patient's head and neck in the midline position, taking care to avoid neck flexion.	1. Positioning the head of the bed at 30 degree helps promote venous return, which will assist in keeping ICP within normal limits. Keeping the head and neck in the midline position while avoiding flexion will help prevent any increases in ICP.
2. Using the carpenter's level, set the collection bag even with the external auditory meatus (EAM) of the ear at the level that has been ordered by the physician (measured in centimeters either above or below the EAM).	2. The EAM is level with the foramen of Monro. A level below the EAM will increase drainage of CSF, while a level above the EAM will decrease drainage of CSF.
3. Documentation should include the position of the collection bag, the amount of CSF drainage, and the color and quality of the CSF (clear, cloudy, bloody, etc.).	3. Proper documentation of where the collection bag is placed and the amount of drainage is important for the neurosurgeons to evaluate when to make adjustments to the level and when the EVD is no longer needed. Any change in quality of the CSF may indicate infection or bleeding into the ventricles, which should be reported immediately.
4. If the patient needs to be turned, the head of the bed needs to be adjusted, or when the patient needs to be moved out of bed, the drainage system should be turned off until it can be returned to the ordered position. Once the patient is back in bed and the system has been re-leveled, the drainage system may be opened again.	4. If the drainage system is not turned off and the patient's head is moved, CSF may be forcefully pulled out of the ventricles, potentially causing herniation of the brain.
5. The EVD should always be handled with sterile technique when changing the dressing covering the insertion site. The dressing consists of a sterile 4 × 4 gauze pad that is folded in order to fully cover the insertion site and then covered with a transparent dressing. The insertion site should be monitored for any signs or symptoms of infection and should be kept clean and dry. If the dressing becomes damp, it should be changed and the provider should be notified.	5. The EVD is a closed, sterile system. Risk for infection is high and all precautions should be taken to prevent any infection from entering the brain. The gauze needs to be covered with a clear dressing so that the gauze may be readily inspected for the presence of dampness and blood. If the dressing becomes damp with fluid, the fluid is presumed to be CSF. Presence of a damp dressing may indicate a CSF leak.

EAM, external auditory meatus; EVD, external ventricular drain; ICP, intracranial pressure; CSF, cerebrospinal fluid.

are common complications of TBI. Diabetes insipidus is the result of decreased secretion of antidiuretic hormone (ADH). The patient has excessive urine output, decreased urine osmolality, and serum hyperosmolarity. Therapy consists of administration of fluids, electrolyte replacement, and vasopressin (desmopressin, DDAVP) therapy. SIADH is the result of increased secretion of ADH. The patient becomes volume-overloaded, urine output diminishes, and serum sodium concentration becomes dilute (sodium is less than 134 mEq/L). Treatment of SIADH includes fluid restriction (typically less than 1 L/day with no free water), which is usually sufficient to correct the hyponatremia. Severe cases call for judicious administration of a 3% hypertonic saline solution. If hypertonic saline is administered, usually it is necessary to administer furosemide (Lasix) simultaneously to reduce intravascular volume via diuresis. Hyponatremia presents commonly with a change in mental status ranging from mild confusion to coma; seizures are associated with low sodium levels (less than 115 mEq/L). The more quickly this problem has developed, the more profound the signs and symptoms. Aggressive management may be required to correct hyponatremia as delaying treatment may result in irreversible brain damage. However, overcorrection of the sodium level predisposes the patient to central pontine myelinolysis, a disorder in which the white matter of the pons loses myelin (the protective sheath surrounding nerves); this results in tetraplegia with cranial nerve deficits (Luzzio, 2013). To prevent this complication, the nurse monitors results of sodium levels (initially, these may be ordered hourly) and the patient's response to hypertonic saline treatment. As a general guideline, the plasma sodium concentration should probably be raised by no more than 10 mEq during the first 24 hours.

Because the unconscious patient's protective reflexes are impaired, the quality of nursing care provided literally may mean the difference between life and death. The nurse must assume responsibility for the patient until the basic reflexes (coughing, blinking, and swallowing) return and the patient becomes conscious and oriented. Therefore, the major nursing goal is to compensate for the absence of these protective reflexes.

Potential complications include cerebral edema, high fever, alterations in blood pressure and oxygenation, increased metabolic demand, and seizures. The nurse must maintain oral hygiene, monitor for the presence of pressure ulcers, avoid any complications associated with the eyes (eye care discussed later in this chapter), monitor urinary output and bowel function, and assess nutritional status. The nurse must always remember to be the patient's advocate, as an unconscious patient cannot advocate for him- or herself.

Decreasing Cerebral Edema: Osmotic Diuretics, Fluid Restriction, and Hypothermia

Cerebral edema is the leading cause of secondary brain injury (Kahle, Walcott, & Simard, 2014). Osmotic diuretics, such as mannitol, may be administered to dehydrate the brain tissue and reduce cerebral edema. Osmotic diuretics work by creating a gradient that draws water across intact membranes, thereby reducing the volume of the swollen brain. Secondarily, they reduce blood viscosity and hematocrit and enhance cerebral blood flow (Rickard, Smith, Newell, Bailey, & Mann, 2014). If the patient is receiving osmotic diuretics, serum osmolality should be determined to assess hydration status.

Drug Alert!
Mannitol becomes ineffective when the serum osmolality exceeds 320 mOsm.

Nursing Alert
The serum osmolality is calculated with the following formula:

$2 \times sodium + glucose/18 + Blood\ Urea\ Nitrogen\ (BUN)/2.8$

If a patient's serum sodium is 140 mEq/L, blood sugar is 80 mg/dL, and BUN is 10 mg/dL; then the calculated serum osmolality is

> *280 (sodium) + 4.4 (glucose) + 3.5 (BUN), for a calculated serum osmolality of 288 mOsm/kg.*

Hypertonic saline is another medication that works to reduce cerebral edema. While mannitol is considered the gold standard in reducing increased ICP, hypertonic saline is gaining popularity as an effective osmotic diuretic. Optimal concentration, dosing, timing, and duration of hypertonic saline has yet to be determined (Rickard et al., 2014). The nurse follows institutional policies for hypertonic saline administration.

Another method for decreasing cerebral edema is fluid restriction. Limiting overall fluid intake leads to dehydration and hemoconcentration, which draws fluid across the osmotic gradient and decreases cerebral edema. Fluid needs are met initially by administering the required IV fluids.

Drug Alert!
Hypotonic fluids (e.g., 0.45% NaCl, D$_5$W) should be avoided in patients with TBI as those fluids can cause an increase in cerebral edema.

Researchers have long hypothesized that lowering body temperature decreases cerebral edema by reducing the oxygen and metabolic requirements of the brain, thus protecting the brain from continued ischemia. If body metabolism can be reduced by lowering the body temperature, the collateral circulation in the brain may be able to provide an adequate blood supply to the brain. The effect of hypothermia on ICP requires more study; thus far, induced hypothermia has not consistently been shown to be beneficial for patients with brain injury. Current literature suggests it is beneficial but only when maintained for at least 48 hours. Inducing and maintaining hypothermia is a major clinical treatment that requires knowledge and skilled nursing observation and management (Crossley et al., 2014).

Controlling Fever

High fever in the unconscious patient may be caused by infection of the respiratory or urinary tract, drug reactions, or damage to the hypothalamic temperature-regulating center. Approximately one fifth to one half of fevers are never explained, despite extensive workup. Because of damage to the temperature center in the brain or severe intracranial infection, unconscious patients often develop very high temperatures. Such temperature elevations must be controlled because the increased metabolic demands of the brain can exceed cerebral circulation and oxygenation, resulting in cerebral deterioration (Hickey, 2014). Studies have shown that fever within the first week of injury is associated with poor outcomes and should be treated aggressively (Titus, Furones, Atkins, & Dietrich, 2015). Persistent hyperthermia with no identified clinical source of infection indicates brainstem damage and a poor prognosis.

Strategies for reducing fever include:

- Removing all bedding over the patient (with the possible exception of a light sheet or small drape)
- Administering acetaminophen as prescribed

- Giving cool sponge baths and allowing a fan to blow over the patient to increase surface cooling
- Using a hypothermia blanket

Frequent temperature monitoring is indicated to assess the patient's response to the therapy and to prevent an excessive decrease in temperature and shivering, which increases heat production and cerebral oxygen consumption.

Nursing Alert

If an automatic hyperthermia/hypothermia blanket is used for patient care, the nurse understands that the unit directly and continually monitors the patient's temperature by means of a thermistor probe (e.g., rectal, skin) and alternates heating and cooling cycles as necessary to achieve and maintain the desired body temperature. The nurse inserts the thermistor probe into the patient's rectum or axilla and tapes it in place to prevent accidental dislodgment. If dislodged, the thermistor will be monitoring room temperature rather than the patient's temperature and will warm the patient to the desired temperature. The probe should be checked at frequent intervals to ensure correct placement.

Maintaining Blood Pressure, Oxygenation, and Hyperventilation

Patients with TBI may sustain a secondary insult if they become hypotensive or hypoxic. Due to ethical reasons, no randomized controlled trials have been done to study the effects of hypotension and hypoxia. However, a growing body of evidence shows deleterious effects if the patient experiences either of these conditions. It is recommended that systolic blood pressure be maintained at greater than 90 mm Hg and oxygen saturation be maintained at greater than 90% (Brain Trauma Foundation, 2007; Hickey, 2014).

Hyperventilation, which results in vasoconstriction, was previously used in patients with increased ICP. Research has demonstrated that hyperventilation may not be as beneficial as once thought (Brain Trauma Foundation, 2007). The reduction in partial pressure of carbon dioxide ($PaCO_2$) may result in hypoxia, ischemia, and an increase in cerebral lactate levels (Hickey, 2014). Hyperventilation is an option for patients with ICP who are unresponsive to conventional therapies, but it should be used cautiously and should be avoided for the first 24 hours following the initial injury (Brain Trauma Foundation, 2007).

Pathophysiology Alert

Carbon dioxide (CO_2) is a potent vasodilator or vasoconstrictor. A normal PCO_2 is 35 to 45 mm Hg. As the patient hypoventilates, the PCO_2 rises (hypercarbia), which causes vasodilation. Likewise, as the patient hyperventilates, the PCO_2 decreases (hypocarbia), which causes vasoconstriction. It

seems reasonable that hyperventilation would cause vasoconstriction and, therefore, decrease cerebral blood flow with a resulting decrease in ICP. However, on review, when the PCO_2 was lowered to 25 mm Hg, ischemia of the brain and increased mortality was seen. Therefore, moderate hyperventilation where the target PCO_2 is 30 to 35 mm Hg may be recommended as a temporary measure until definitive treatment is instituted. In general, normocarbia is preferred.

Reducing Metabolic Demands

Cellular metabolic demands may be reduced through the administration of high doses of barbiturates if the patient is unresponsive to conventional treatment. The mechanism by which barbiturates decrease ICP and protect the brain is through inhibition of free radicals, alterations in vascular tone, and suppression of metabolism (Hickey, 2014). Use of high-dose barbiturates should be reserved for patients with refractory increased ICP who do not respond to other medical or surgical treatments. Barbiturates should not be used as prophylaxis to prevent increased ICP (Brain Trauma Foundation, 2007).

Another method of reducing cellular metabolic demand and improving oxygenation is the administration of pharmacologic paralyzing agents, such as pancuronium, vecuronium, and cisatracurium. The patient who receives these agents cannot move; this decreases the metabolic demands and results in a decrease in cerebral oxygen demand. Because the patient cannot respond or report pain, sedation and analgesia must be provided because the paralyzing agents do not provide either.

Patients receiving high doses of barbiturates or pharmacologic paralyzing agents require continuous cardiac monitoring, endotracheal intubation, mechanical ventilation, ICP monitoring, and arterial pressure monitoring.

The ability to perform serial neurologic assessments is lost with the use of barbiturates or paralyzing agents. Therefore, other monitoring tools are needed to assess the patient's status and response to therapy. Important parameters that must be assessed include ICP, blood pressure, heart rate, respiratory rate, and response to ventilator therapy (e.g., "bucking" or "fighting" the ventilator). Refer to Chapters 10 and 55 for ventilator considerations. Potential complications include hypotension due to decreased sympathetic tone and myocardial depression (Hickey, 2014).

Seizure Prophylaxis

Patients with severe TBI are at risk for developing seizures. Seizures that develop after head injury are known as posttraumatic seizures (PTS) and are classified according to when they occur. If they occur within 7 days of injury, they are known as early PTS; if they occur more than 7 days after the injury, they are known as late PTS (Szaflarski, Nazzal, & Dreer, 2014). Box 45-8 lists risk factors for developing PTS. There is evidence to support the use of prophylactic

Risk Factors for Developing Posttraumatic Seizures (PTS)

- Depressed skull fracture
- Penetrating head wound
- Epidural, subdural, or intracerebral hemorrhage
- GCS score below 10
- Cortical contusion

anticonvulsants only for early PTS. It is not recommended that patients be started on seizure prophylaxis more than 1 week after the injury if they have not had any seizures. If the patient develops late PTS, the seizures should be managed in the same way as new-onset seizures (Szaflarski et al., 2014). See Chapter 46 for further discussion on management of seizures.

Providing Mouth Care
To provide care, the mouth is inspected for dryness, inflammation, and crusting. The unconscious patient requires conscientious oral care because there is a risk of parotitis (inflammation of the salivary glands) if the mouth is not kept scrupulously clean (refer to Chapter 22). The mouth is cleansed and rinsed carefully to remove secretions and crusts and to keep the mucous membranes moist. A thin coating of petrolatum on the lips prevents drying, cracking, and encrustations. If the patient has an endotracheal tube, the tube should be moved to the opposite side of the mouth daily to prevent ulceration of the mouth and lips.

Nursing Alert
Oral care in patients at risk for increased ICP has been shown to be safe. However, this should be done with caution in patients who already have elevated ICP as oral interventions may cause modest increases in ICP (McNett & Olson, 2013).

Maintaining Skin and Joint Integrity
Preventing skin breakdown requires continuing nursing assessment and intervention. Special attention is given to unconscious patients because they cannot respond to external stimuli. Assessment includes a regular schedule of turning to avoid pressure, which can cause breakdown and necrosis of the skin. Turning also provides kinesthetic (sensation of movement), proprioceptive (awareness of position), and vestibular (equilibrium) stimulation. After turning, the patient is carefully repositioned to prevent ischemic necrosis over pressure areas.

Preserving Corneal Integrity
Unconscious patients may have their eyes open and have inadequate or absent corneal reflexes. The cornea may become irritated, dried out, or scratched, leading to ulceration. The eyes may be cleansed with cotton balls moistened with sterile normal saline to remove debris and discharge (Hickey, 2014). If artificial tears are prescribed, they may be instilled every 1 to 2 hours. Periorbital edema often occurs after cranial surgery. Cold compresses may be prescribed, and care must be exerted to avoid contact with the cornea. Eye patches should be used cautiously because of the potential for corneal abrasion from contact with the patch.

Managing Nutritional Needs
If the patient does not recover quickly and sufficiently enough to take adequate fluids and calories by mouth, a nasogastric tube or gastrostomy tube is inserted for the administration of enteral feedings. A nutritionist should be involved in the care of the unconscious patient. The nutritionist will determine the patient's caloric needs and will make recommendations for the amount and type of tube feeding that is appropriate. Daily intake and output should be recorded, as well as daily weights to ensure the patient has adequate caloric intake (Hickey, 2014). Box 45-9 gives nutritional considerations of the patient with decreased LOC and increased ICP.

Preventing Urinary Retention
The patient with an altered LOC is often incontinent or has urinary retention. The bladder is palpated or scanned at intervals to determine whether urinary retention is present. If the patient is not voiding, an indwelling urinary catheter is inserted and connected to a closed drainage system. A catheter may also be inserted during the acute phase of illness to monitor urinary output. Because catheters are a major factor in causing urinary tract infection (UTI), the patient is observed for fever, leukocytosis (increased WBCs), and cloudy urine. The urinary catheter is usually removed if the patient has a stable cardiovascular system and if no diuresis, sepsis, or voiding dysfunction existed before the onset of coma. An intermittent catheterization program may be initiated to ensure complete emptying of the bladder at intervals, if indicated.

Nutrition Alert

Nutritional Support Following Traumatic Brain Injury

- Patients with traumatic brain injury (TBI) have increased metabolic expenditure so they have high caloric needs.
- Full nutritional support should be begun no later than 72 hours after the injury to achieve full caloric replacement by postinjury day 7.
- Protein should comprise 15% of total calories.
- When feedings are initiated, glucose levels should be closely monitored as hyperglycemia is associated with worse outcomes.
- Consultation with a dietician is recommended to provide optimal nutritional support.

Promoting Bowel Function

The abdomen is assessed for distention by listening for bowel sounds and measuring the girth of the abdomen with a tape measure. There is a risk for diarrhea from infection, antibiotics, hyperosmolar fluids and enteral feedings.

Immobility and lack of dietary fiber can cause constipation. The nurse monitors the number and consistency of bowel movements and performs a rectal examination for signs of fecal impaction. Stool softeners may be prescribed and can be administered with tube feedings. To facilitate bowel emptying, a glycerin suppository may be indicated. The patient may require an enema every other day to empty the lower colon (Hickey, 2014).

Nursing Alert
The nurse is aware that straining during bowel movement increases intra-abdominal and/or intrathoracic pressure, which impedes venous return and increases ICP. Therefore a bowel program is initiated to prevent constipation.

Protecting the Patient

Care should be taken to prevent injury from invasive lines and equipment, and other potential sources of injury should be identified, such as restraints, tight dressings, environmental irritants, damp bedding or dressings, and tubes and drains.

Protection also includes protecting the patient's dignity during altered LOC. Simple measures, such as providing privacy and speaking to the patient during nursing care activities, preserve the patient's dignity. Not speaking negatively about the patient's condition or prognosis is also important because patients in a light coma may be able to hear. The patient who is comatose has an increased need for advocacy, and the nurse is responsible for seeing that these advocacy needs are met (Hickey, 2014).

New Therapies

Despite many years of extensive research, no new therapies have been shown to improve outcomes after TBI. Research into this area continues to be important as over 5 million Americans currently have some form of disability related to TBI with an estimated annual cost in the United States around $76 billion (Wright et al., 2014). The hormone progesterone initially showed clinical benefit in two phase II randomized controlled trials. However, a large phase III randomized clinical trial did not show any difference between treatment with progesterone and treatment with placebo. The use of progesterone in treatment for TBI is no longer recommended (Skolnick et al., 2014).

Intracranial Surgery

Decompressive craniectomy is a surgical procedure that can be used to help relieve increased ICP. A decompressive craniectomy involves removal of a bone flap from the skull to allow expansion of the brain. The bone flap is then implanted into the abdomen, so the bone remains viable. Once cerebral edema has decreased, the bone flap is replaced back on the skull. No randomized controlled trials have investigated the utility of decompressive craniectomy, although studies have suggested it is helpful (Hickey, 2014).

BRAIN DEATH

When a patient has sustained a severe neurologic injury incompatible with life, the diagnosis of brain death should be considered. Often, it is the nurse who will first notice signs of decompensation and will begin the process of determining if the patient meets criteria for brain death. Approximately 5% to 10% of patients in ICUs who are comatose will be declared brain dead (Hickey, 2014).

Brain death was formally defined by the Ad Hoc Committee at Harvard Medical School in 1968 as an "irreversible coma." In 1981, the President's Commission for the Study of Ethical Problems in Medicine and Biomedical and Behavioral Research published *Guidelines for the Determination of Death.* These guidelines clarified that patients who are considered brain dead must have confirmation of cessation of all brain function resulting from an irreversible cause. Reversible conditions, such as shock, hypothermia, and drug intoxication, must be excluded prior to diagnosis. This study served as the basis for the Uniform Death and Determination Act (UDDA), which is now recognized by all 50 states. The UDDA states that death will be determined with accepted medical standards and that death will indicate irreversible loss of all brain function.

The most recent practice parameters come from the Quality Standards Subcommittee of the American Academy of Neurology (2010) and include three cardinal findings: coma or unresponsiveness, absence of brainstem reflexes, and apnea. The current criteria for brain death are: the condition is irreversible with a known cause; the patient is not under the effects of a CNS depressant or a paralytic; no evidence of electrolyte, severe acid–base, or endocrine abnormality; the patient has apnea; the patient has no brainstem reflexes; the core body temperature is greater than 90°F (36°C); systolic blood pressure is at least 100 mm Hg; and there is neuroimaging evidence of catastrophic CNS damage.

The nurse may assist in the clinical examination for determination of brain death and in the process of organ procurement. Often, there will be a meeting among the attending physician, nurse, social worker, and representative of the organ procurement organization to inform the family of the organ donation process. The family will often look to the nurse for answers about organ donation and an explanation of questions related to the determination of brain death (Jackson, Willmarth-Stec, & Shutter, 2015; Miller, 2015).

SPINAL CORD INJURY

Spinal cord injury (SCI) is a major health problem. An estimated 276,000 people in the United States live each day with a disability from SCI, and an estimated 12,500 new injuries occur each year (National Spinal Cord Injury Statistical Center [NSCISC], 2014). Males account for 79% of SCI in a reported national database (NSCISC, 2014). Young people between 16 and 30 years of age account for more than half of the new SCIs each year. The most common cause of SCI is motor vehicle accidents, which account for 38% of SCI. Violence-related injuries account for 14% of SCIs, with falls causing 30%, and sports-related injuries causing 9% of SCIs (NSCISC, 2014). The frequency of associated injuries and medical complications in SCI is high. The frequency with which these risk factors are associated with SCI serves to emphasize the importance of primary prevention. The same interventions suggested earlier in this chapter for head injury prevention serve to decrease the incidence of SCI as well (see Box 45-1, p. 1288).

Pathophysiology

Damage to the spinal cord ranges from transient concussion (from which the patient fully recovers) to contusion, laceration, and compression of the cord substance (either alone or in combination), to complete **transection** (severing) of the cord (which renders the patient paralyzed below the level of the injury).

SCIs, like head injuries, can be separated into two categories: primary injuries and secondary injuries (Porth & Matfin, 2013). Primary injuries are the result of the initial insult or trauma and are usually permanent. Secondary injuries are usually the result of a contusion or tear injury, in which the nerve fibers begin to swell and disintegrate. A secondary chain of events produces ischemia, hypoxia, edema, and hemorrhagic lesions, which in turn result in destruction of myelin and axons (Hickey, 2014). These secondary reactions, believed to be the principal causes of spinal cord degeneration at the level of injury, are now thought to be reversible during the first 4 to 6 hours after injury. Therefore, if the cord has not suffered irreparable damage, some method of early treatment is needed to prevent partial damage from developing into total and permanent damage (Hickey, 2014) (see later discussion).

The vertebrae most frequently involved in SCI are the fifth, sixth, and seventh cervical (neck) vertebrae (C5 to C7), the twelfth thoracic vertebra (T12), and the first lumbar vertebra (L1). These vertebrae are most susceptible because there is a greater range of mobility in the vertebral column in these areas (Porth & Matfin, 2013).

Clinical Manifestations

Manifestations of SCI depend on the type and level of injury (Box 45-10). **Incomplete spinal cord lesions** (the sensory or motor fibers, or both, are preserved below the lesion) are classified according to the area of spinal cord damage: central, lateral, anterior, or peripheral. The American Spinal Injury Association (ASIA) provides another standard classification of SCI according to the degree of sensory and motor function present after injury (Box 45-11). *Neurologic level* refers to the lowest level at which sensory and motor functions are normal. A motor complete SCI (ASIA Grades A and B) involves no motor function below the neurologic level. ASIA Grade A involves no sensory or motor function all the way down to the sacral segments, S4 and S5. ASIA Grade B involves preserved sensory but not motor function below the neurologic level and includes preservation of the sacral segments S4 and S5. A motor incomplete SCI (ASIA Grades C and D) involves preservation of motor function below the neurologic level. ASIA Grade C involves preserved motor function below the neurologic level with at least half of the key muscles having a grade of less than 3 (see Chapter 43 for discussion of grading muscle strength). ASIA Grade D involves preserved motor function below the neurologic level with at least half of the key muscles having a grade of 3 or greater. A **complete spinal cord lesion** (total loss of sensation and voluntary muscle control below the lesion) can result in **paraplegia** (paralysis of the lower body) or **tetraplegia** (formerly **quadriplegia**—paralysis of all four extremities). Complete SCIs also include loss of all spinal reflexes below the level of the lesion, loss of the ability to perspire below the level of the lesion, dysfunction of the bowel and bladder, and absence of visceral and somatic sensations below the level of the lesion (Hickey, 2014).

If conscious, the patient usually complains of acute pain in the back or neck, which may radiate along the involved nerve. However, absence of pain does not rule out spinal injury, and a careful assessment of the spine should be conducted if the mechanism of injury has involved significant force (i.e., concomitant head injury).

Respiratory dysfunction is related to the level of injury. The muscles contributing to respiration are the abdominals and intercostals (T1 to T11) and the diaphragm (C3 to C5). In high cervical cord injury, acute respiratory failure is the leading cause of death. Functional abilities by level of injury are described in Table 45-3.

Nursing Alert

Ascending edema of the spinal cord in the acute phase of the injury may cause respiratory difficulty that requires immediate intervention. Therefore, the patient's respiratory status must be monitored frequently.

Assessment and Diagnostic Findings

A detailed neurologic examination is performed. Diagnostic x-rays (lateral cervical spine x-rays) and CT are usually performed initially. An MRI may be ordered as further workup if a ligamentous injury is suspected because significant spinal

BOX 45-10 Effects of Spinal Cord Injuries (SCI)

Central Cord Syndrome

- Characteristics: Motor deficits (in the upper extremities compared to the lower extremities; sensory loss varies but is more pronounced in the upper extremities); bowel/bladder dysfunction is variable, or function may be completely preserved.
- Cause: Injury or edema of the central cord, usually of the cervical area. May be caused by hyperextension injuries.

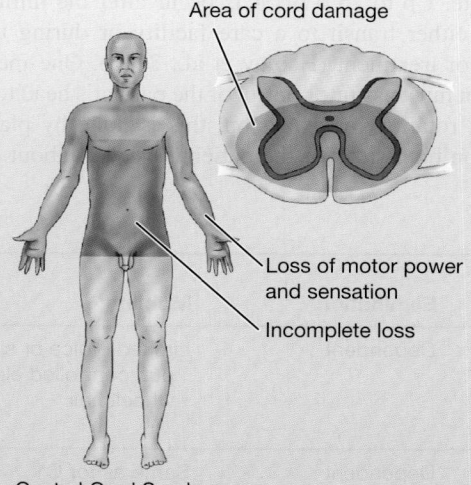

Central Cord Syndrome

Area of cord damage

Loss of motor power and sensation

Incomplete loss

Anterior Cord Syndrome

- Characteristics: Loss of pain, temperature, and motor function are noted below the level of the lesion; light touch, position, and vibration sensations remain intact.
- Cause: The syndrome may be caused by acute disk herniation or hyperflexion injuries associated with fracture-dislocation of vertebra. It also may occur as a result of injury to the anterior spinal artery, which supplies the anterior two thirds of the spinal cord.

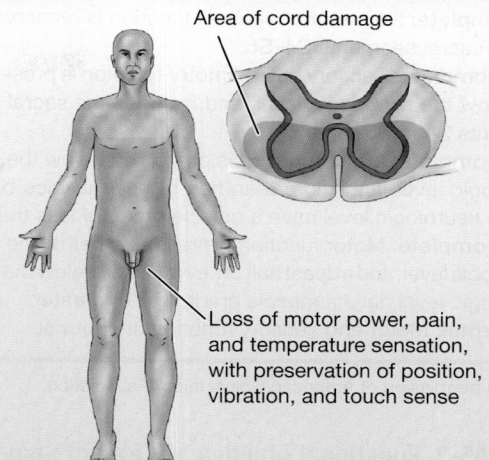

Anterior Cord Syndrome

Area of cord damage

Loss of motor power, pain, and temperature sensation, with preservation of position, vibration, and touch sense

Brown-Séquard Syndrome (Lateral Cord Syndrome)

- Characteristics: Ipsilateral paralysis or paresis is noted, together with ipsilateral loss of touch, pressure, and vibration and contralateral loss of pain and temperature.
- Cause: The lesion is caused by a transverse hemisection of the cord (half of the cord is transected from north to south), usually as a result of a knife or missile injury, fracture-dislocation of a unilateral articular process, or possibly an acute ruptured disk.

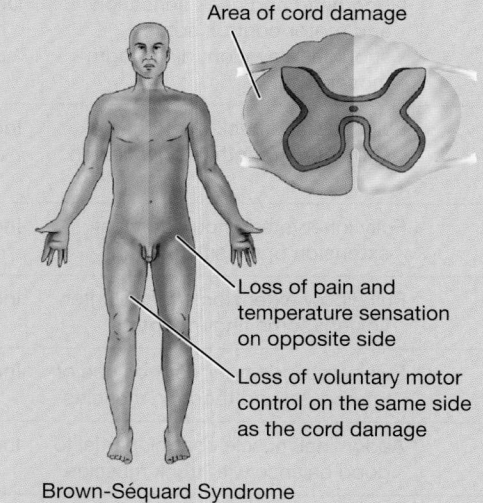

Brown-Séquard Syndrome

Area of cord damage

Loss of pain and temperature sensation on opposite side

Loss of voluntary motor control on the same side as the cord damage

Adapted from Hickey, L. (2014). *The clinical practice of neurological and neurosurgical nursing* (7th ed., pp. 423–425). Philadelphia, PA: Lippincott Williams & Wilkins.

cord damage may exist even in the absence of bony injury. An assessment is made for other injuries because spinal trauma often is accompanied by concomitant injuries, commonly to the head and chest. Continuous cardiac monitoring may be indicated if an SCI is suspected because bradycardia and asystole are common in patients with acute SCIs.

Emergency Management

The immediate management at the scene of the injury is critical because improper handling of the patient can cause further damage and loss of neurologic function. Any patient who is involved in a motor vehicle accident, a diving or contact

ASIA Impairment Scale

A = Complete: No motor or sensory function is preserved in the sacral segments S4–S5.

B = Incomplete: Sensory but not motor function is preserved below the neurologic level, and includes the sacral segments S4 to S5.

C = Incomplete: Motor function is preserved below the neurologic level, and more than half of key muscles below the neurologic level have a muscle grade of less than 3.

D = Incomplete: Motor function is preserved below the neurologic level, and at least half of key muscles below the neurologic level have a muscle grade of 3 or greater.

E = Normal: Motor and sensory function are normal.

Used with permission of American Spinal Injury Association.

sports injury, a fall, or any direct trauma to the head and neck should be considered to have an SCI until such an injury has been ruled out. Initial care should include rapid assessment, immobilization, extrication, stabilization or control of life-threatening injuries, and transportation to the most appropriate medical facility (Ropper, Neal, & Theodore, 2015).

At the scene of the injury, the patient should be immobilized on a spinal (back) board, with head and neck in a neutral position, to prevent an incomplete injury from becoming complete. Up to 25% of SCIs occur after the initial insult, during either transit to a care facility or during the early course of treatment (Hadley et al., 2013). One member of the team must assume control of the patient's head to prevent flexion, rotation, or extension; this is done by placing the hands on both sides of the patient's head at about ear level

TABLE 45-3 Functional Abilities by Level of Spinal Cord Injury

Injury Level	Segmental Sensorimotor Function	Dressing, Eating	Elimination	Mobility[a]
C1	Little or no sensation or control of head and neck; no diaphragm control; requires continuous ventilation	Dependent	Dependent	Limited. Voice or sip-n-puff controlled electric wheelchair
C2–C3	Head and neck sensation; some neck control; independent of mechanical ventilation for short periods	Dependent	Dependent	Same as for C1
C4	Good head and neck sensation and motor control; some shoulder elevation; diaphragm movement	Dependent, may be able to eat with adaptive sling	Dependent	Limited to voice, mouth, head, chin, or shoulder-controlled electric wheelchair
C5	Full head and neck control; shoulder strength; elbow flexion	Independent with assistance	Maximal assistance	Electric or modified manual wheelchair, needs transfer assistance
C6	Fully innervated shoulder; wrist extension or dorsiflexion	Independent or with minimal assistance	Independent or with minimal assistance	Independent in transfers and wheelchair
C7–C8	Full elbow extension; wrist plantar flexion; some finger control	Independent	Independent	Independent; manual wheelchair
T1–T5	Full hand and finger control; use of intercostal and thoracic muscles	Independent	Independent	Independent; manual wheelchair
T6–T10	Abdominal muscle control, partial to good balance with trunk muscles	Independent	Independent	Independent; manual wheelchair
T11–L5	Hip flexors, hip abductors (L1–L3); knee extension (L2–L4); knee flexion and ankle dorsiflexion (L4–L5)	Independent	Independent	Short distance to full ambulation with assistance
S1–S5	Full leg, foot, and ankle control; innervation of perineal muscles for bowel, bladder, and sexual function (S2–S4)	Independent	Normal to impaired bowel and bladder function	Ambulate independently with or without assistance

[a]Assistance refers to adaptive equipment, setup, or physical assistance.
From Porth, C. M., & Matfin, G. (2013). *Pathophysiology: Concepts of altered health states* (9th ed.). Philadelphia, PA: Lippincott Williams & Wilkins.

to limit movement and maintain alignment while a spinal board or cervical immobilizing device is applied. If possible, at least four people should slide the patient carefully onto a board for transfer to the hospital. Any twisting movement may irreversibly damage the spinal cord by causing a bony fragment of the vertebra to cut into, crush, or sever the cord completely (Hickey, 2014). While spine immobilization is necessary, it may lead to worse outcomes in patients with penetrating trauma as immobilization may delay other life-saving treatments (Ropper et al., 2015).

The standard of care is that the patient is referred to a regional spinal injury or trauma center because of the multidisciplinary personnel and support services required to counteract the destructive changes that occur in the first 24 hours after injury. During treatment in the emergency and x-ray departments, the patient is kept on the transfer board. The patient must always be maintained in an extended position. No part of the body should be twisted or turned, nor should the patient be allowed to sit up. Once the extent of the injury has been determined, the patient may be placed on a rotating bed or in a cervical collar. Later, if SCI and bone instability have been ruled out, the patient may be moved to a conventional bed or the collar may be removed without harm. If a rotating bed is needed but not available, the patient should be placed in a hard cervical collar and on a firm mattress.

Medical and Nursing Management

The goals of management are to prevent further SCI and to observe for symptoms of progressive neurologic deficits. Many changes in the treatment of SCI have occurred during the past 20 years. Treatments such as hypothermia, corticosteroids, and naloxone were investigated and used during the 1980s; of these, high-dose corticosteroids had shown the most promise, but their use has become controversial. In the National Acute Spinal Cord Injury Studies (NASCIS) done in 1990 and 1997, the administration of high-dose corticosteroids, specifically methylprednisolone (Solu-Medrol), was found to improve motor and sensory outcomes at 6 weeks, 6 months, and 1 year if given within 8 hours after injury (Hadley et al., 2013). In 2001, The American Association of Neurological Surgeons/Congress of Neurological Surgeons conducted a review of available literature and noted that treatment for either 24 or 48 hours was recommended as an option. They noted, however, that there was more evidence to suggest harmful side effects than there was evidence that suggested clinical benefit (Hadley et al., 2013). Currently, there is no Class I or II evidence to support the benefits of methylprednisolone; and there is Class I, II, and III evidence that use of high-dose steroids is associated with harmful side effects, up to and including death. There also has not been any benefit seen from administration of the biologic agent Syngen (GM-1 ganglioside) and its use is not recommended (Hurlbert et al., 2013).

Biologic agents are currently being investigated for the acute and chronic phases of SCI. Cell-based therapies, including stem cells, have theoretical benefits, but while trials so far have not consistently shown efficacy, they do seem to be relatively safe (Robbins, Kumar, Vaccaro, & Behrend, 2015).

Nonsurgical Management

Treatment of SCI attempts to achieve decompression, stabilization, and realignment of the spinal cord while preserving or improving neurologic function (Hickey, 2014). Cervical fractures are reduced, and the cervical spine is aligned with some form of skeletal traction, such as skeletal tongs or calipers, or with use of the halo device. A variety of skeletal tongs are available, all of which involve fixation in the skull in some manner. The Gardner-Wells tongs require no pre-drilled holes in the skull. Crutchfield and Vinke tongs are inserted through holes made in the skull with a special drill under local anesthesia.

A halo device may be used initially with traction, or may be applied after removal of the tongs. It consists of a stainless-steel halo ring that is fixed to the skull by four pins. The ring is attached to a removable **halo vest**, a device that suspends the weight of the unit circumferentially around the chest. A metal frame connects the ring to the chest. Halo devices provide immobilization of the cervical spine while allowing early ambulation (Fig. 45-6). Refer to Chapter 42 for nursing responsibilities related to pin care.

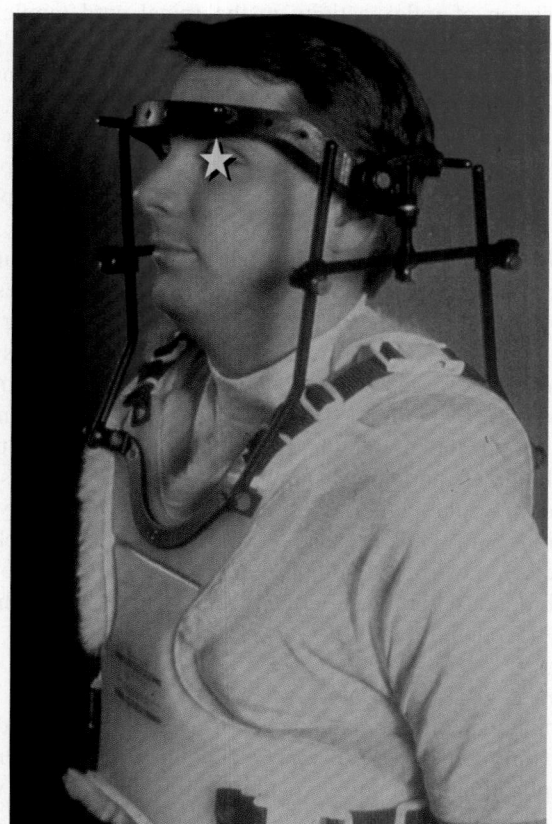

FIGURE 45-6 Halo vest.

Thoracic and lumbar injuries are usually treated with surgical intervention followed by immobilization with a fitted brace. Traction is not indicated either before or after surgery, due to the relative stability of the spine in these regions.

Surgical Management

Surgery is indicated in any of the following instances:

- Compression of the cord
- Fragmented or unstable vertebral body
- Penetrating wound to the spinal cord
- Bone fragments in the spinal canal
- Deterioration of the patient's neurologic status

Surgery is performed to decompress the spinal cord, reduce the spinal fracture or dislocation, or to stabilize the spinal column. Laminectomy is the most common surgical procedure used to decompress or stabilize the spinal column. A **laminectomy** involves excision of the lamina (a portion of the posterior arch) and spinous processes of a vertebra. Various techniques (i.e., fusion or fixation) are used to create a stable spinal column (Hickey, 2014).

Monitoring and Managing Acute Complications of Spinal Cord Injury

Spinal and Neurogenic Shock

The spinal shock associated with SCI reflects a sudden depression of reflex activity in the spinal cord (areflexia) below the level of injury. The muscles innervated by the part of the spinal cord segment below the level of the lesion are without sensation, paralyzed, and flaccid. In particular, the reflexes that initiate bladder and bowel function are affected. Bowel distention and paralytic ileus can be caused by depression of the reflexes and are treated with intestinal decompression by insertion of a nasogastric tube (Hickey, 2014).

Neurogenic shock develops due to the loss of autonomic nervous system function below the level of the lesion (Hickey, 2014). The vital organs are affected, causing the blood pressure and heart rate to decrease. This loss of sympathetic innervation causes a variety of other clinical manifestations, including a decrease in cardiac output, venous pooling in the extremities, and peripheral vasodilation, resulting in mild hypotension, bradycardia, and warm skin. In addition, the patient does not perspire on the paralyzed portions of the body because sympathetic activity is blocked; therefore, close observation is required for early detection of an abrupt onset of fever. Further details on neurogenic shock may be found in Chapter 54.

Deep Vein Thrombosis

Thrombophlebitis, inflammation of a vein related to deep vein thrombosis (DVT), is a relatively common potential complication of immobility and is common in patients with SCI (Chung, Lin, Chang, Sung, & Kao, 2014). DVT occurs in a high percentage of patients with SCI, placing them at risk for pulmonary embolism (PE), which is the third most common cause of death in patients with SCI (Chung et al., 2014). The patient must be assessed for symptoms of both DVT and PE. A low-grade fever may be the first sign of DVT. Manifestations of PE include pleuritic chest pain, anxiety, and shortness of breath.

Thigh and calf measurements should be made daily at consistent sites. The patient is evaluated for the presence of DVT if the circumference of one extremity increases significantly. Diagnostic studies used to detect DVT and PE include Doppler ultrasound, radiocontrast venography, ventilation/perfusion lung scans (Hickey, 2014), a computed tomographic pulmonary angiography (CTPA) (Weitz, 2016), or spiral CT.

Anticoagulation therapy to prevent DVT and PE is initiated once head injury and other systemic injuries have been ruled out and there is low risk for bleeding. There is strong evidence to support the use of low–molecular-weight heparin as well as unfractionated heparin. This may be followed by long-term oral anticoagulation with a vitamin K antagonist (i.e., warfarin) or subcutaneous fractionated heparin injections (Chung et al., 2014). In a review of the literature on treatments for thromboembolism, low–molecular-weight heparin was shown to be more effective at preventing DVT and had fewer bleeding complications than fractionated heparin. However, full-dose enoxaparin should be used with caution as it can lead to compartment syndrome and even limb amputation (Yeung & Formal, 2015). Anticoagulant therapy should be continued for at least 6 to 12 weeks after injury.

Nonpharmacologic measures, including elastic compression stockings or pneumatic compression devices, as well as range-of-motion exercises, are important preventive measures that work to reduce venous pooling and promote venous return. Compression devices should be used for 2 weeks following injury. In some cases, permanent indwelling filters may be placed in the vena cava to prevent emboli (dislodged clots) from migrating to the lungs and causing PE in patients who have developed clots despite receiving anticoagulation (Sarosiek, Crowther, & Sloan, 2013).

Orthostatic Hypotension

For the first 2 weeks following SCI, blood pressure tends to be unstable and quite low. It gradually returns to preinjury levels, but periodic episodes of severe orthostatic hypotension frequently interfere with efforts to mobilize the patient. Orthostatic hypotension is defined as a drop in systolic blood pressure of at least 20 mm Hg or a drop in diastolic pressure of at least 10 mm Hg, regardless of the patient's symptoms (Shen, Huang, Yuan, Zhang, & Li, 2014). Patients with SCI are prone to orthostatic hypotension during position changes due to a loss of reflex vasoconstriction and pooling of blood in the lower extremities and abdominal viscera. This results in decreased venous return to the heart and decreased cardiac output. To compensate, patients develop reflex tachycardia, although this is rarely sufficient to raise blood pressure enough to return to normal levels (Shen et al., 2014). Orthostatic hypotension is a particularly common problem for patients with lesions above T7 and those with tetraplegia (Hickey, 2014).

A number of techniques can be used to reduce the frequency of hypotensive episodes. Close monitoring of vital signs before and during position changes is essential. Vasopressor medication can be used to treat the profound vasodilation. Elastic compression stockings should be applied to improve venous return from the lower extremities. Abdominal binders may also be used to encourage venous return and provide diaphragmatic support when the patient is upright. Activity should be planned in advance, and adequate time should be allowed for a slow progression of position changes from recumbent to sitting and upright.

Autonomic Dysreflexia

Autonomic dysreflexia, also known as autonomic hyperreflexia, sympathetic storming, or autonomic dysfunction syndrome (ADS), is an acute emergency that occurs as a result of exaggerated autonomic responses to stimuli that are harmless in normal people. It only occurs after spinal shock has resolved in patients with cord lesions above T6. This syndrome is characterized by a severe, pounding headache with paroxysmal hypertension, profuse diaphoresis (most often of the forehead), nausea, nasal congestion, and bradycardia (Hickey, 2014). The sudden increase in blood pressure may cause a rupture of one or more cerebral blood vessels or lead to increased ICP. Autonomic dysreflexia is more commonly seen in patients with complete SCIs and in the chronic stages of SCI (Richa, 2014).

A number of stimuli may trigger this reflex: distended bladder (the most common cause); distention or contraction of the visceral organs, especially the bowel (from constipation, impaction); or stimulation of the skin (tactile, pain, thermal stimuli, pressure ulcer). Because this is an emergency situation, the objectives are to remove the triggering stimulus and to avoid the potentially serious complications.

The following measures are carried out:

- The head of the bed is raised, and the patient is placed immediately in a sitting position to lower blood pressure.
- Rapid assessment is performed to identify and alleviate the cause.
- The bladder is emptied immediately via a urinary catheter. If an indwelling catheter is not patent, it is irrigated or replaced with another catheter.
- The rectum is examined for a fecal mass. If one is present, a topical anesthetic such as lidocaine may be inserted 10 to 15 minutes before the mass is removed because visceral distention or contraction can worsen autonomic dysreflexia. The nurse observes for symptoms of flushing, sweating, nasal congestion, and headache while performing a digital examination and ceases the procedure if symptoms appear and assesses blood pressure.
- The skin is examined for any areas of pressure, irritation, or broken skin.

- Any other stimulus that could be the triggering event, such as an object next to the skin or a draft of cold air, must be removed.
- If these measures do not relieve the hypertension and excruciating headache, a ganglionic blocking agent (hydralazine hydrochloride [Apresoline]) is prescribed and administered slowly by the IV route.
- The medical record or chart is labeled with a clearly visible note about the risk for autonomic dysreflexia.
- The patient is instructed about prevention and management measures.
- Any patient with a lesion above the T6 segment is informed that such an episode is possible and may occur even years after the initial injury.

NURSING PROCESS
The Patient with Acute Spinal Cord Injury

ASSESSMENT

The breathing pattern is observed, the strength of the cough is assessed, and the lungs are auscultated because paralysis of abdominal and respiratory muscles diminishes coughing and makes clearing of bronchial and pharyngeal secretions difficult.

The patient is monitored closely for any changes in motor or sensory function and for symptoms of progressive neurologic damage. In the early stages of SCI, determining whether the cord has been severed may be very difficult because signs and symptoms of cord edema are indistinguishable from those of cord transection. Edema of the spinal cord may occur with any severe cord injury and may further compromise spinal cord function.

Motor and sensory functions are assessed through careful neurologic examination. These findings are usually recorded on a flow sheet so that changes in the baseline neurologic status can be monitored closely and accurately. The ASIA classification is commonly used to describe level of function for SCI patients. Box 45-10 gives examples of the effects of altered spinal cord function. At the minimum:

- Motor ability is tested by asking the patient to spread the fingers, squeeze the examiner's hand, and move the toes or turn the feet.
- Sensation is evaluated by gently pinching the skin or touching it lightly with an object such as a tongue blade, starting at shoulder level and working down both sides of the extremities. The patient should have both eyes closed so that the examination reveals true findings, not what the patient hopes to feel. The patient is asked where the sensation is felt.
- Any decrease in neurologic function is reported immediately.

The patient is also assessed for spinal shock, urinary retention, overdistention of the bladder, and paralytic ileus.

(continued on page 1310)

DIAGNOSIS

NURSING DIAGNOSES

Based on the assessment data, the patient's major nursing diagnoses may include the following:

- Ineffective breathing patterns related to weakness or paralysis of abdominal and intercostal muscles and inability to clear secretions
- Ineffective airway clearance related to weakness of intercostal muscles
- Impaired bed and physical mobility related to motor and sensory impairments
- Disturbed sensory perception related to motor and sensory impairment
- Risk for impaired skin integrity related to immobility and sensory loss
- Impaired urinary elimination related to inability to void spontaneously
- Constipation related to presence of atonic bowel as a result of autonomic disruption
- Acute pain and discomfort related to treatment and prolonged immobility

COLLABORATIVE PROBLEMS/POTENTIAL COMPLICATIONS

Potential complications that may develop in patients with SCI include:

- DVT/PE (thrombophlebitis)
- Orthostatic hypotension
- Autonomic dysreflexia

PLANNING AND GOALS

The goals for the patient may include improved breathing pattern and airway clearance, improved mobility, improved sensory and perceptual awareness, maintenance of skin integrity, relief of urinary retention, improved bowel function, promotion of comfort, and absence of complications.

NURSING INTERVENTIONS

PROMOTING ADEQUATE BREATHING AND AIRWAY CLEARANCE

Oxygen is administered to maintain a normal saturation level because hypoxemia can create or worsen a neurologic deficit of the spinal cord. If endotracheal intubation is necessary, extreme care is taken to avoid flexing or extending the patient's neck, which can result in extension of a cervical injury.

Possible impending respiratory failure is detected by observing the patient, noting rate and depth of respirations, assessing lung sounds, accessory muscle use, monitoring oxygen saturation through pulse oximetry, and monitoring arterial blood gas values. Early and vigorous attention to clearing bronchial and pharyngeal secretions can prevent retention of secretions and atelectasis. Suctioning may be indicated, but caution must be

used because this procedure can stimulate the vagus nerve, producing bradycardia, which can result in cardiac arrest.

If the patient cannot cough effectively because of decreased inspiratory volume and inability to generate sufficient expiratory pressure, chest physical therapy and assisted coughing may be indicated.

IMPROVING MOBILITY

Proper body alignment is maintained at all times. The patient is repositioned frequently and is assisted out of bed as soon as the spinal column is stabilized. The feet are prone to footdrop; therefore, various types of splints are used to prevent it. When used, the splints are removed and reapplied every 2 hours. Trochanter rolls, applied from the crest of the ileum to the midthigh of both legs, help prevent external rotation of the hip joints.

Patients with lesions above the midthoracic level have loss of sympathetic control of peripheral vasoconstrictor activity, leading to hypotension. These patients may tolerate changes in position poorly and require monitoring of blood pressure when positions are changed. Usually, the patient is turned every 2 hours by log rolling. Log rolling ensures proper spinal alignment during turning of the patient. The patient should not be turned unless the spine is stable and the provider has indicated that it is safe to do so.

Contractures develop rapidly with immobility and muscle paralysis. A joint that is immobilized too long becomes fixed as a result of contractures of the tendon and joint capsule. Atrophy of the extremities results from disuse. Contractures and other complications may be prevented by range-of-motion exercises that help preserve joint motion and stimulate circulation. Passive range-of-motion exercises should be implemented as soon as possible after injury.

PROMOTING ADAPTATION TO SENSORY AND PERCEPTUAL ALTERATIONS

The nurse assists the patient to compensate for sensory and perceptual alterations that occur with SCI. The intact senses above the level of the injury are stimulated through touch, aromas, flavorful food and beverages, conversation, and music. Additional strategies include the following:

- Providing prism glasses to enable the patient to see from the supine position
- Encouraging use of hearing aids, if indicated, to enable the patient to hear conversations and environmental sounds
- Providing emotional support to the patient
- Teaching the patient strategies to compensate for or cope with these deficits

MAINTAINING SKIN INTEGRITY

Because patients with SCI are immobilized and have loss of sensation below the level of the lesion, they have the highest prevalence of pressure ulcers in the United States. Up to 66% of patients with spinal cord disorders will develop pressure ulcers.

Patients with higher-level SCIs are more likely to develop pressure ulcers than patients with lower-level SCIs (Kruger, Pires, Ngann, Sterling, & Rubayi, 2013). The most common sites for pressure ulcers are over the ischial tuberosity, the greater trochanter, the sacrum, the gluteal region, and the occiput (back of the head). Patients who wear cervical collars for prolonged periods may develop breakdown from the pressure of the collar under the chin, on the shoulders, and at the occiput. The nurse follows institutional policy regarding collar care, which typically may require changing of pads every 24 hours and inspecting and cleaning the skin every shift. In patients with SCI, pressure-relieving cushions (e.g., Roho wheelchair cushions) and bed support surfaces are used to lessen the risk of developing pressure ulcer. The nurse is aware that doughnut-shaped devices are NOT to be used because of the reduced blood flow associated with them.

The patient is repositioned every 2 hours, and careful inspection of the skin is made every time the patient is turned. The skin over pressure points is assessed for redness or breakdown. The patient's skin should be kept clean by washing with a mild soap, rinsing well, and blotting dry. Pressure-sensitive areas should be kept well-lubricated and soft with hand cream or lotion.

MAINTAINING URINARY ELIMINATION

Immediately after SCI, the urinary bladder may become atonic and is unable to contract by reflex activity. Urinary retention typically results. Because the patient has no sensation of bladder distention, overstretching of the bladder and detrusor muscle may occur, delaying the return of bladder function.

Intermittent catheterization is carried out to avoid overdistention of the bladder and UTI. If this is not feasible, an indwelling catheter is inserted temporarily. At an early stage, family members are shown how to carry out intermittent catheterization and are encouraged to participate in this facet of care because they will be involved in long-term follow-up and must be able to recognize complications so that treatment can be instituted.

The patient is taught to record fluid intake, voiding pattern, characteristics of urine, and any unusual sensations that may occur. The management of a neurogenic bladder (bladder dysfunction that results from a disorder or dysfunction of the nervous system) is discussed in detail in Chapter 28.

IMPROVING BOWEL FUNCTION

Immediately after SCI, a paralytic ileus may develop due to neurogenic paralysis of the bowel; therefore, a nasogastric tube is often required to relieve distention and to prevent vomiting and aspiration.

Bowel activity usually returns within the first week following the injury. As soon as bowel sounds are heard on auscultation, the patient is given a high-calorie, high-protein, high-fiber diet, with the amount of food gradually increased. The nurse administers prescribed stool softeners to counteract the effects of immobility and analgesic agents. A bowel regimen is instituted as early as possible. The types of bowel dysfunction most commonly seen in patients with SCI are constipation, fecal incontinence, and fecal impaction. Of these, fecal impaction is the most common and is reported in about 39% of patients (Pan, Liu, Li, Zhang, & Lu, 2014).

PROVIDING COMFORT MEASURES

A patient who has had pins, tongs, or calipers placed for cervical stabilization may have a headache or discomfort for several days after the pins are inserted. Patients initially may be bothered by the rather startling appearance of these devices, but usually they readily adapt to it because the device provides comfort for the unstable neck. The patient may complain of being caged in and of noise created by any object coming in contact with the steel frame of a halo device, but he or she can be reassured that adaptation to this will occur.

The areas around the four pin sites of a halo device are cleaned daily and observed for redness, drainage, and pain. The pins are observed for loosening, which may contribute to infection. If one of the pins becomes detached, the head is stabilized in a neutral position by one person, while another notifies the neurosurgeon. A torque screwdriver should be readily available in case the screws on the frame need tightening.

The skin under the halo vest is inspected for excessive perspiration, redness, and skin blistering, especially on the bony prominences. The vest is opened at the sides to allow the torso to be washed. The liner of the vest should not become wet because dampness causes skin excoriation. The liner should be changed periodically to promote hygiene and good skin care. If the patient is to be discharged with the vest, detailed instructions must be given to the family, with time allowed for them to demonstrate the necessary skills of halo vest care.

PROMOTING HOME AND COMMUNITY-BASED CARE

Teaching Patient Self-Care. In most cases, patients with SCI (i.e., patients with tetraplegia or paraplegia) need long-term rehabilitation. The process begins during hospitalization, as acute symptoms begin to subside or come under better control and the overall deficits and long-term effects of the injury become clear. The goals begin to shift from merely surviving the injury to learning strategies necessary to cope with the alterations that the injury imposes on activities of daily living (ADLs). The emphasis shifts from ensuring that the patient is stable and free of complications to specific assessment and planning designed to meet the patient's rehabilitation needs. Patient teaching may initially focus on the injury and its effects on mobility, dressing, and bowel, bladder, and sexual function. As the patient and family acknowledge the consequences of the injury and the resulting disability, the focus of teaching broadens to address issues necessary for carrying out the tasks of daily living and taking charge of their lives. Teaching begins in the acute phase and continues throughout rehabilitation. Interventions are aimed at increasing function, improving adjustment, increasing social integration, and reducing social stigma (Delparte, Chau, Mills, & Burns, 2014).

(continued on page 1312)

Caring for the patient with SCI at home may at first seem a daunting task to the family. They will require dedicated nursing support to gradually assume full care of the patient. Although maintaining function and preventing complications will remain important, goals regarding self-care and preparation for discharge will assist in a smooth transition to rehabilitation and eventually to the community.

Continuing Care. The ultimate goal of the rehabilitation process is independence. The nurse becomes a support to both the patient and the family, assisting them to assume responsibility for increasing aspects of patient care and management. Care for the patient with SCI involves members of all the health care disciplines, which may include nursing, medicine, rehabilitation, respiratory therapy, physical and occupational therapy, case management, and social services. The nurse often serves as coordinator of the management team and as a liaison with rehabilitation centers and home care agencies (Hickey, 2014). The patient and family often require assistance in dealing with the psychological impact of the injury and its consequences; referral to a psychiatric clinical nurse specialist or other mental health care professional is often helpful. Box 45-12 discusses the higher incidence in depression with SCI and recognition of the importance of assessment of the patient's psychological state early in the rehabilitative process, as early intervention improves long-term patient satisfaction (Hickey, 2014).

As more patients survive acute SCI, they face the changes associated with aging with a disability. Therefore, teaching in the home and community focuses on health promotion and addresses the need to minimize risk factors that increase the risk of mortality. Some risk factors that have been identified include cardiovascular disease, diabetes, psychiatric disorders, and alcohol or substance abuse (Hwang, Zebracki, Chlan, & Vogel, 2014). Home care nurses and others who have contact with patients with SCI are in a position to teach patients about healthy lifestyles, remind them of the need for health screenings, and make referrals as appropriate. Assisting patients to identify accessible health care providers, clinical facilities, and imaging centers may increase the likelihood that they will participate in health screening (van Wyk, Backwell, & Townson, 2015).

EVALUATION

EXPECTED PATIENT OUTCOMES

Expected patient outcomes may include the following:
1. Demonstrates improvement in gas exchange and clearance of secretions, as evidenced by normal breath sounds on auscultation:
   a. Breathes easily without shortness of breath
   b. Performs hourly deep-breathing exercises, coughs effectively, and clears pulmonary secretions
   c. Is free of respiratory infection (i.e., has normal temperature, respiratory rate, and pulse, normal breath sounds, absence of purulent sputum)

BOX 45-12	Nursing Research

Bridging the Gap to Evidence-Based Practice

Williams, R., & Murray, A. (2015). Prevalence of depression after spinal cord injury: A meta-analysis. *Archives of Physical Medicine and Rehabilitation*, 96(1), 133–140.

Purpose
To use meta-analysis to synthesize point prevalence estimates of depressive disorder diagnoses for people who have sustained a spinal cord injury (SCI).

Design
Data Sources searched PsycINFO, PubMed, the Cumulative Index to Nursing and Allied Health Literature (CINAHL), and Dissertation Abstracts International (DAI) for studies examining depression after SCI through 2013. A manual search of the reference sections of included studies was also completed. Nineteen studies, containing 35,676 subjects and 21 effect size estimates, were included in this meta-analysis. All the studies contained people with SCI; used a diagnostic measure of depression (i.e., an unstructured, semi-structured, or structured clinical interview, and/or a clinician diagnosis); and provided a diagnosis of major or minor depressive episodes for the subjects in the study.

Findings
The mean prevalence estimate of depression diagnosis after SCI was 22.2%, with a lower-bound estimate of 18.7% and an upper-bound estimate of 26.3%. Data collection method, *Diagnostic and Statistical Manual of Mental Disorders* version, and diagnostic composition significantly predicted variation in observed effect size estimates, with primary data collection studies having lower estimates compared with secondary data analysis studies; studies using *Diagnostic and Statistical Manual of Mental Disorders*, Fourth Edition; diagnostic criteria having higher estimates compared with studies using *Diagnostic and Statistical Manual of Mental Disorders*, Third Edition; and samples comprising individuals diagnosed only with major depression having lower prevalence estimates.

Nursing Implications
The existing data on depression after SCI indicate that the prevalence of depression after SCI is substantially greater than that in the general medical population. These results underscore the importance of continued research on measuring depression in people with SCI and on treatments for depression after SCI. Since nursing is actively involved in patient care, assessment of the patient's psychological state and referral is crucial as early intervention improves long-term patient satisfaction.

2. Moves within limits of the dysfunction and demonstrates completion of exercises within functional limitations
3. Demonstrates adaptation to sensory and perceptual alterations:
   a. Uses assistive devices (i.e., prism glasses, hearing aids, computers) as indicated
   b. Describes sensory and perceptual alterations as a consequence of injury
4. Demonstrates optimal skin integrity:
   a. Exhibits normal skin turgor; skin is free of reddened areas or breakdown
   b. Participates in skin care and monitoring procedures within functional limitations
5. Regains control of urinary bladder function:
   a. Exhibits no signs of UTI (i.e., has normal temperature; voids clear, dilute urine)
   b. Has adequate fluid intake
   c. Participates in bladder training program within functional limitations

6. Regains control of bowel function:
   a. Reports regular pattern of bowel movement
   b. Consumes adequate dietary fiber and oral fluids
   c. Participates in bowel training program within functional limitations
7. Reports absence of pain and discomfort
8. Is free of complications:
   a. Demonstrates no signs of DVT or PE
   b. Exhibits no manifestations of PE (i.e., no chest pain or shortness of breath; arterial blood gas values are within normal limits)
   c. Maintains blood pressure within normal limits
   d. Reports no lightheadedness with position changes
   e. Exhibits no manifestations of autonomic dysreflexia (i.e., absence of headache, diaphoresis, nasal congestion, or bradycardia)

CHAPTER REVIEW

Critical Thinking Exercises

1. A 70-year-old patient was brought to the emergency department after he fell and hit his head and was unconscious for about 2 minutes. He now seems alert and oriented. What type of injury has he most likely sustained? What discharge instructions are warranted for this patient's family or caregiver? How would you modify your discharge instructions if the patient lives alone?

2. Your 25-year-old patient with a TBI has early signs of increased ICP. Describe the medical management you would anticipate to control the ICP and the nursing measures that are indicated. How would you determine whether your interventions were effective in alleviating the increased ICP? What is the evidence base for these interventions?

3. A 47-year-old man with paraplegia secondary to SCI, diabetes, and obesity is admitted. For what complications is he at risk? What interventions would be appropriate to prevent these complications?

NCLEX-Style Review Questions

1. The nurse assesses the LOC of a patient who suffered a head injury and determines that the patient's GCS score is 15. Which of the following responses did the nurse assess to determine the GCS score? *Select all that apply.*
   a. Spontaneous eye opening
   b. Tachycardia, hypotension, bradycardia
   c. Ability to follow commands
   d. Unequal pupil size
   e. Orientation to person, place, and time

2. A patient sustained a C6 SCI 4 hours ago. What nursing diagnosis is a priority?
   a. Urinary retention
   b. Risk for impaired skin integrity
   c. Ineffective breathing pattern
   d. Powerlessness

3. The nurse notices clear fluid draining from the nose of a patient who sustained a head injury 2 hours ago. This may indicate the presence of what condition?
   a. Cerebral concussion
   b. Basal skull fracture
   c. Brain tumor
   d. Sinus infection

4. A patient is admitted with a closed head injury that was sustained in a motorcycle accident. The patient has been showing an upward trend in ICP measurements. What is the first priority action that the nurse should take with this patient?
   a. Administer 100 mg of IV pentobarbital as ordered
   b. Increase the ventilator settings to a respiratory rate of 20 breaths/min
   c. Administer 20 g of IV mannitol as ordered
   d. Reposition the patient to avoid neck flexion

5. Which interventions should the nurse's plan of care include to help prevent autonomic dysreflexia in a patient with SCI? *Select all that apply.*
a. Check for fecal impactions.
b. Monitor blood pressure for hypotension.
c. Check the urinary drainage system for any obstruction.
d. Monitor bowel movements.
e. Instruct the patient to wear a medic alert bracelet.

Try these additional resources, available at **http://thepoint.lww.com/Honan2e**, to enhance your learning and understanding of this chapter:
• NCLEX-Style Student Review Questions
• Journal Articles

REFERENCES AND SELECTED READINGS

References and selected readings associated with this chapter can be found on the website that accompanies the book. Visit **http://thepoint. lww.com/Honan2e** to access the references and other additional resources associated with this chapter.

Nursing Management: Patients with Neurologic Disorders

Cynthia Bautista

Learning Objectives

After reading this chapter, you will be able to:

1. Identify the various types and causes of seizures.
2. Use the nursing process to develop a plan of care for the patient experiencing seizures.
3. Differentiate among the infectious disorders of the nervous system according to causes, manifestations, medical care, and nursing management.
4. Describe the pathophysiology, clinical manifestations, and medical and nursing management of multiple sclerosis, myasthenia gravis, and Guillain–Barré syndrome.
5. Describe neuromuscular disorders and their manifestations and indicated nursing interventions.
6. Use the nursing process as a framework for care of patients with degenerative neurologic disorders.

SEIZURE DISORDERS

SEIZURES, EPILEPSY, AND STATUS EPILEPTICUS

Seizures are abnormal discharges in the brain for a single event of which results in an abrupt and temporary altered cerebral function state (England & Plueger, 2014). A part or all of the brain may be involved. The term *ictal* refers to an actual seizure or *ictal event*.

Epilepsy is a disease that meets any of the following conditions: (1) at least two unprovoked seizures occurring more than 24 hours apart; (2) one unprovoked seizure and probability of further seizures; (3) diagnosis of an epilepsy syndrome (Fisher et al., 2014). Epileptic syndromes are classified by specific patterns of clinical features, including age at onset, family history, and seizure type.

Status epilepticus is continuous seizure activity for more than 5 minutes or two or more sequential seizures without full recovery of consciousness between seizures (England & Plueger, 2014). Seizures that last longer than 5 to 10 minutes are less likely to stop without intervention. Status epilepticus is a neurologic emergency and can be life-threatening.

> **Nursing Alert**
> *Not all seizures imply epilepsy. Although seizures are the cardinal symptom of epilepsy, seizures also occur as a manifestation of an underlying treatable problem, such as hyponatremia*

or high fever. Once the cause is identified and treated, the seizures cease. Epilepsy is a disease, and refers to recurrent, unpredictable, and unprovoked seizures.

Pathophysiology of Seizures

Messages from the body are carried by the neurons (nerve cells) of the brain by means of discharges of electrochemical energy that sweep along them. These impulses occur in bursts whenever a nerve cell has a task to perform. Sometimes, these cells or groups of cells continue firing after a task is finished. During the period of unwanted discharges, parts of the body controlled by the errant cells may perform erratically. Seizures require three conditions: (1) excitable neurons; (2) increase in excitatory glutaminergic activity (relates to the action of glutamate or to neural or metabolic pathways in which it functions as a transmitter) through recurrent connections to spread the discharge; and (3) reduction in activity of normal inhibitory GABA projection (GABA is an amino acid that is the major inhibitory neurotransmitter in the vertebrate gray matter) (England & Plueger, 2014). When there is an imbalance between inhibition and excitation within the central nervous system (CNS), seizures occur.

> **Nursing Alert**
> *Anyone can have a seizure. Although we all have a unique threshold for seizures, an imbalance in that threshold can provoke a seizure. In fact, 10% of Americans will have a seizure in their*

BOX 46-1 **Classification of Seizures**

Focal Seizures (seizure activity starts in one area of the brain)

- *Focal*—retains awareness: There is no impairment of consciousness, similar to simple partial seizures, may have movement of body parts, may experience an aura.
- *Focal*—altered awareness: There is impairment of consciousness, similar to complex partial seizures, this can spread to both hemispheres of brain.

Partial Seizures

These seizures begin in a part of one hemisphere, generally in the temporal or frontal lobe. The two types of partial seizures, called simple and complex, are based on whether a person remains fully conscious during a seizure.

Simple

Complex

Unknown Seizures (insufficient evidence to classify as focal, generalized, or both)

Generalized Seizures (seizure activity involves both hemispheres of the brain)

Generalized Seizures

These seizures affect both hemispheres of the brain at the same time. Abnormal activity is not focused in one specific area and there generally is no aura at the start.

- *Tonic–clonic seizures:* Generalized seizures that affect the entire brain; they begin with rigidity (tonic phase), followed by repetitive clonic activity of all extremities characterized by stiffening or jerking of the body.
- *Tonic seizures:* Seizures characterized by muscle stiffening, dilation of the pupils, and altered respiratory patterns; the body becomes stiff and the person may fall backward. The seizure usually lasts less than 1 minute, and recovery is rapid.
- *Clonic seizures:* Characterized by jerking movements, which involve muscles on both sides of the body
- *Absence seizures:* Short episodes of staring and loss of awareness
- *Atonic seizures:* Sudden loss of muscle tone, resulting in falls or a "drop" to the ground, with rapid recovery
- *Myoclonic seizure:* Characterized by jerking (myoclonic) movements of a muscle or muscle group, without loss of consciousness

lifetime. It is a matter of imbalance in excitatory activity in the CNS or a reduction in inhibitory activity.

The international classification of seizures differentiates between two main types: focal or partial seizures, which begin in one part of the brain, and generalized seizures, which involve electrical discharges in the whole brain (see Box 46-1). However, it is understood that not all seizures or syndromes fit neatly into these classifications, and patients may have more than one type of seizure.

The specific causes of seizures are varied and can be categorized as idiopathic (genetic, developmental defects) and acquired. Causes of acquired seizures include:

- Cerebrovascular disease
- Hypoxemia of any cause, including vascular insufficiency
- Fever (childhood)
- Head injury
- Hypertension
- CNS infections
- Metabolic and toxic conditions (e.g., kidney failure, hyponatremia, hypocalcemia, hypoglycemia, pesticides)
- Brain tumor
- Drug and alcohol withdrawal; drug toxicity
- Allergies
- Alzheimer disease (see discussion later in this chapter on pp. 1343–1347)

Clinical Manifestations and Assessment

The initial pattern of the seizures indicates the region of the brain in which the seizure originates (see Box 46-1). In focal seizures in which the patient retains awareness, only a finger or hand may shake, or the mouth may jerk uncontrollably. The person may talk unintelligibly, may be dizzy, and may experience unusual or unpleasant sights, sounds, odors, or tastes but without loss of consciousness.

In focal seizures with altered awareness, the person either remains motionless or moves automatically but inappropriately for time and place, or he or she may experience excessive emotions of fear, anger, elation, or irritability. Whatever the manifestations, the person does not remember the episode when it is over.

Generalized seizures involve both hemispheres of the brain, causing both sides of the body to react. Intense rigidity of the entire body may occur, followed by alternating muscle relaxation and contraction (generalized tonic–clonic contraction). The simultaneous contractions of the diaphragm and chest muscles may produce a characteristic epileptic cry. The patient may chew the tongue or bite the inner cheek, and the patient may be incontinent of urine and feces. After 1 or 2 minutes, the convulsive movements begin to subside; the patient relaxes and lies in deep coma, breathing noisily. The respirations at this point are chiefly abdominal. In the postictal (after the seizure) state, the patient is often confused and hard to arouse and may sleep for hours. Many patients report headache, sore muscles, extremity weakness, fatigue, and depression (Bazil & Pedley, 2015).

A medical history is taken, including previous seizure history, alcohol and drug use, medication use, allergy status, and family history. The patient is also questioned about illnesses or head injuries that may have affected the brain. Women should be questioned about their last menstrual period (increase in seizure frequency is noted during menses) and pregnancy status (fetal anomaly is two times higher in women taking antiepileptic medications). The patient is asked about common triggers associated with seizures, which can be olfactory (particular odors), visual (flashing lights), or auditory (certain types of music) in nature, or related to fatigue, sleep deprivation, hypoglycemia, emotional stress, electrical shock, febrile illness, alcohol consumption, certain drugs, drinking too much water, constipation, and hyperventilation (England & Plueger, 2014).

In addition to physical and neurologic evaluations, diagnostic examinations include biochemical, hematologic, and serologic studies. Imaging studies, such as magnetic resonance imaging (MRI), computed tomography (CT) scan, single-photon emission computed tomography (SPECT), and positron emission tomography (PET) may be used to detect lesions, such as focal abnormalities, cerebrovascular abnormalities, and cerebral degenerative changes (Nettina, 2014). The SPECT is useful for identifying the epileptogenic zone so that the area in the brain giving rise to seizures can be removed surgically.

The EEG furnishes diagnostic evidence for a substantial proportion of patients with epilepsy and assists in classifying the type of seizure (Nettina, 2014). Abnormalities in the EEG usually continue between seizures or, if not apparent, may be elicited by hyperventilation or during sleep. Microelectrodes (depth electrodes) can be inserted deep in the brain to probe the action of single brain cells. Some people with clinical seizures have normal EEGs, whereas others who have never had seizures have abnormal EEGs. Telemetry and computerized equipment are used to monitor electrical brain activity while the patient pursues his or her normal activities and to store the readings on computer tapes for analysis. Video recording of seizures taken simultaneously with EEG telemetry is useful in determining the type of seizure as well as its duration and magnitude.

Medical and Nursing Management

The goals of treatment are to stop the seizures as quickly as possible, to ensure adequate cerebral oxygenation, and to maintain the patient in a seizure-free state. In the case of prolonged seizures, as in status epilepticus, the nurse recalls the standard ABCs (airway, breathing, and circulation) of emergency management. An airway and adequate oxygenation are established if the patient shows signs of airway obstruction. Oxygen is administered as ordered via nasal cannula, or intubation may be required, and oxygen is administered via the artificial airway and monitored by pulse oximetry. Suctioning of the airway may also be required. An IV line is established, and IV lorazepam (Ativan), diazepam (Valium), or midazolam (Versed) is administered slowly in an attempt to halt seizures immediately. The IV line is closely monitored because it may become dislodged during seizures. Antiepileptic drugs (AEDs) (levetiracetam, phenytoin, phenobarbital) are administered later to maintain a seizure-free state. In general, a single drug is used to control the seizures. Termed *monotherapy*, the selected drug is determined by the type of seizure, and the dose is increased until symptoms resolve, maximal dose is required, or signs of drug toxicity emerge, at which time alternative therapeutic agents are considered.

Nursing Alert
Phenytoin (Dilantin), if ordered intravenously, must be administered slowly because of its effect on the myocardium and the potential for arrhythmia development. In addition, it is irritating to the vein; thus, the nurse observes for the development of phlebitis. The rate of administration is no faster than 50 mg/min in normal saline solution, since the drug precipitates in D_5W. If the pre-existing solution contained dextrose, the nurse flushes the IV line with normal saline before administering the medication. Many AEDs are highly bound to plasma protein, and the nurse is aware that only the unbound, or "free," serum concentration is available for use by the body. Patients on high-protein tube feedings

(see Chapter 22) may require higher dosages to maintain therapeutic blood levels, while those with hypoalbuminemia because of malnutrition, burns, or liver or kidney disease may require alternative dosing to prevent phenytoin toxicity. Therapeutic range for phenytoin is 10 to 20 mg/L (Lassiter & Henkel, 2014).

Blood samples are obtained to monitor serum electrolytes, glucose, blood cell count, and toxicology/drug screen, and levels of drugs, such as phenobarbital or phenytoin, may be monitored if the patient has been treated with the medication. If the serum concentration of the AED is below therapeutic levels, it suggests that the patient was not taking the medication, the dosage was too low, or factors such as pharmacokinetics of the medication may be involved. EEG monitoring may be useful in determining the nature of the seizure activity. Vital signs and neurologic signs are monitored on a continuing basis. An IV infusion of dextrose is administered if the seizure is caused by hypoglycemia. If initial treatment is unsuccessful, general anesthesia with a short-acting barbiturate may be used. Cardiac involvement or respiratory depression may be life-threatening. The potential for postictal cerebral edema also exists. This varies in clinical presentation and may include deterioration in neurologic signs, ranging from drowsiness to coma, as well as nausea, vomiting, sluggish pupillary response, cardiac arrhythmias, and altered respiratory patterns. The nurse initiates ongoing assessment and monitoring of respiratory and cardiac function because of the risk for delayed depression of respiration and blood pressure secondary to administration of AEDs and sedatives to halt the seizures. Nursing assessment also includes monitoring and documenting the seizure activity and the patient's responsiveness.

A person who has received long-term antiepileptic therapy has a significant risk for fractures resulting from bone disease (osteoporosis, osteomalacia, and hyperparathyroidism), a side effect of therapy. Therefore, during seizures, the patient is protected from injury with the use of seizure precautions, which include placing the bed in a low position, raising the bedside rails, and not letting the patient get up and ambulate without someone's assistance. The patient's room should have suction and oxygen available at the bedside if needed (England & Plueger, 2014). No effort should be made to restrain seizure activity. The patient having seizures can inadvertently injure nearby people, so nurses should protect themselves. Other nursing interventions for the person having seizures are presented in Box 46-2.

During a Seizure

A major responsibility of the nurse is to observe and record the sequence of signs. Before and during a seizure, the patient is assessed and the following items are documented:

- The circumstances before the seizure (visual, auditory, or olfactory stimuli; tactile stimuli; emotional or psychological disturbances; sleep; hyperventilation)

- The occurrence of an aura (a premonitory or warning sensation that can be visual, auditory, gustatory, visceral, or olfactory) that is experienced at the beginning of a seizure and remembered (England & Plueger, 2014)
- The first thing the patient exhibits in the seizure—in what part of the body the movement or stiffness begins, conjugate gaze position (term that denotes both eyes working in unison), and the position of the head at the beginning of the seizure. This information gives clues to the location of the seizure's origin in the brain. (In recording, it is important to state whether the beginning of the seizure was observed).
- The type of movements in the part of the body involved
- The areas of the body involved (turn back bedding to expose patient)
- The size of both pupils and whether the patient's eyes are open
- Whether the patient's eyes or head are/is turned to one side (eyes look away from the side of the seizure)
- The presence or absence of automatisms (involuntary motor activity, such as lip smacking or repeated swallowing)
- Incontinence of urine or stool
- Duration of each phase of the seizure
- Unconsciousness, if present, and its duration
- Any obvious paralysis or weakness of the patient's arms or legs after the seizure
- Inability to speak after the seizure
- Movements at the end of the seizure
- Whether or not the patient sleeps afterward
- Cognitive status (confused or not confused) after the seizure

In addition to providing data about the seizure, nursing care is directed at preventing injury and supporting the patient, not only physically but also psychologically. Steps to prevent or minimize injury are presented in Box 46-2.

After a Seizure

After a patient has a seizure, the nurse's role is to document the events leading to and occurring during and after the seizure and to prevent complications (e.g., aspiration, injury). The patient is at risk for hypoxia, vomiting, and pulmonary aspiration. To prevent complications, the patient is placed in the side-lying position to facilitate drainage of oral secretions, and suctioning is performed, if needed, to maintain a patent airway and prevent aspiration (see Box 46-2). Seizure precautions are maintained, including having available functioning suction equipment with a suction catheter. The bed is placed in a low position with two to three side rails up, if necessary, to prevent injury to the patient. The patient may be drowsy and may wish to sleep after the seizure; he or she may not remember events leading up to the seizure and for a short time thereafter.

Pharmacologic Therapy

Although many medications are available to control seizures, the nurse stresses that the treatment is not curative. The objective is to achieve seizure control with minimal side

BOX 46-2 GUIDELINES FOR NURSING CARE

Nursing Care During a Seizure

- Provide privacy and protect the patient from curious onlookers. (The patient who has an *aura* [warning of an impending seizure] may have time to seek a safe, private place.)
- Ease the patient to the floor, if possible.
- Protect the head with a pad to prevent injury (from striking a hard surface).
- Loosen constrictive clothing, remove eyeglasses.
- Push aside any furniture that may injure the patient during the seizure.
- If the patient is in bed, remove extra pillows and raise the side rails.
- *Do not attempt to pry open the patient's jaws if they are clenched in a spasm or to insert anything.* Broken teeth and injury to the lips and tongue may result from such an action.
- No attempt should be made to restrain the patient during the seizure because muscular contractions are strong and restraint can produce injury.

- If possible, place the patient on one side to facilitate drainage of saliva and mucus. If suction is available, use it if necessary to clear secretions.

Nursing Care After the Seizure

- Keep the patient on one side to prevent aspiration. Make sure the airway is patent.
- There is usually a period of confusion after a tonic–clonic seizure.
- A short apneic period may occur during or immediately after a generalized seizure.
- The patient, on awakening, should be reoriented to the environment.
- If the patient becomes agitated after a seizure (postictal), use calm persuasion.

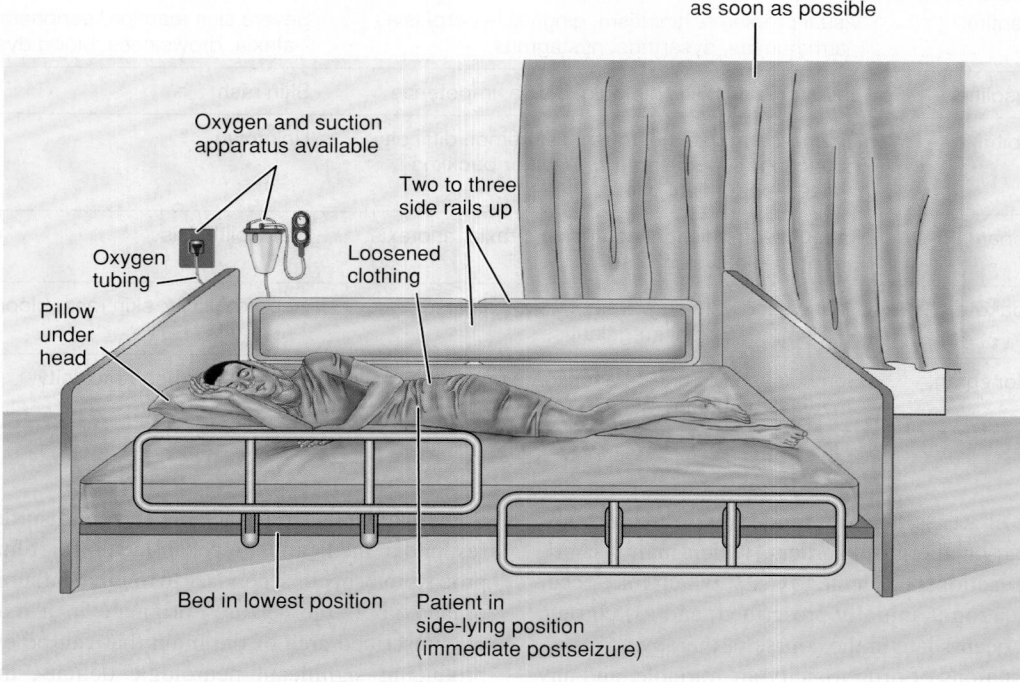

Privacy provided as soon as possible

Oxygen and suction apparatus available

Two to three side rails up

Oxygen tubing

Loosened clothing

Pillow under head

Bed in lowest position

Patient in side-lying position (immediate postseizure)

---

effects. Medications are selected on the basis of the patient's type of seizure and the effectiveness and safety of the medications. If properly prescribed and taken, medications control seizures in 70% to 80% of patients with seizures (Lowenstein, 2014), although approximately 65% of patients with epilepsy are resistant to AEDs (England & Plueger, 2014). In these situations, surgery may reduce seizure frequency or provide complete seizure control.

Treatment usually starts with a single medication. The starting dose and the rate at which the dosage is increased depend on the occurrence of side effects. The medication levels in the blood are monitored because the rate of drug absorption varies among patients. Changing to another medication may be necessary if seizure control is not achieved or if toxicity makes it impossible to increase the dosage. The medication may need to be adjusted because of concurrent illness, weight changes, or increases in stress. Stopping these medications without provider's knowledge can cause seizures to occur with greater frequency or can precipitate the development of status epilepticus (England & Plueger, 2014).

TABLE **46-1** Major Antiseizure Medications

Medication	Dose-Related Side Effects	Toxic Effects
Carbamazepine (Tegretol)	Dizziness, drowsiness, unsteadiness, nausea and vomiting, diplopia, mild leukopenia	Severe skin rash, blood dyscrasias, hepatitis
Clonazepam (Klonopin)	Drowsiness, behavior changes, headache, hirsutism, alopecia, palpitations	Hepatotoxicity, thrombocytopenia, bone marrow failure, ataxia
Ethosuximide (Zarontin)	Nausea and vomiting, headache, gastric distress	Skin rash, blood dyscrasias, hepatitis, systemic lupus erythematosus (SLE)
Gabapentin (Neurotonin)	Dizziness, drowsiness, somnolence, fatigue, ataxia, weight gain, nausea	Leukopenia, hepatotoxicity
Lamotrigine (Lamictal)	Drowsiness, tremor, nausea, ataxia, dizziness, headache, weight gain	Severe rash (Stevens-Johnson syndrome)
Levetiracetam (Keppra)	Somnolence, dizziness, fatigue	Unknown
Oxcarbazepine (Trileptal)	Dizziness, somnolence, double vision, fatigue, nausea, vomiting, loss of coordination, abnormal vision, abdominal pain, tremor, abnormal gait	Hepatotoxicity
Phenobarbital (Luminal)	Sedation, irritability, diplopia, ataxia	Skin rash, anemia
Phenytoin (Dilantin)	Visual problems, hirsutism, gingival hyperplasia, arrhythmias, dysarthria, nystagmus	Severe skin reaction, peripheral neuropathy, ataxia, drowsiness, blood dyscrasias
Primidone (Mysoline)	Lethargy, irritability, diplopia, ataxia, impotence	Skin rash
Tiagabine (Gabitril)	Dizziness, fatigue, nervousness, tremor, difficulty concentrating, dysarthria, weak or buckling knees, abdominal pain	Unknown
Topiramate (Topamax)	Fatigue, somnolence, confusion, ataxia, anorexia, depression, weight loss	Nephrolithiasis
Valproate (Depakote, Depakene)	Nausea and vomiting, weight gain, hair loss, tremor, menstrual irregularities	Hepatotoxicity, skin rash, blood dyscrasias, nephritis
Zonisamide (Zonegran, Excegran)	Somnolence, dizziness, anorexia, headache, nausea, agitation, rash	Leukopenia, hepatotoxicity

Side effects of AEDs may be divided into three groups: (1) idiosyncratic or allergic disorders, which manifest primarily as skin reactions; (2) acute toxicity, which may occur when the medication is initially prescribed; and (3) chronic toxicity, which occurs late in the course of therapy.

The manifestations of drug toxicity are variable, and any organ system may be involved. Gingival hyperplasia (swollen and tender gums) can be associated with long-term use of phenytoin (Dilantin), for example (Lassiter & Henkel, 2014). Periodic physical and dental examinations and laboratory tests are performed for patients receiving medications that are known to have hematopoietic, genitourinary, or hepatic effects. Table 46-1 lists the medications in current use.

Surgical Management

Surgery is indicated for patients whose epilepsy results from intracranial tumors, abscesses, cysts, or vascular anomalies. Some patients have intractable seizure disorders that do not respond to medication. A focal (localized or limited) atrophic process may occur secondary to trauma, inflammation, stroke, or anoxia. If the seizures originate in a reasonably well-circumscribed area of the brain that can be excised without producing significant neurologic deficits, the removal of the area (termed a *lobectomy*) generating the seizures may produce long-term control and improvement (Lowenstein, 2014).

Epilepsy surgery has been aided by several advances, including microsurgical techniques, EEGs with depth electrodes, improved illumination and hemostasis, and the introduction of neuroleptanalgesic agents (droperidol and fentanyl). These techniques, combined with use of local anesthetic agents, enable the neurosurgeon to perform surgery on an alert and cooperative patient. Using special testing devices, electrocortical mapping, and the patient's responses to stimulation, the boundaries of the epileptogenic focus (the abnormal area of the brain) are determined. The abnormal epileptogenic focus is then excised (lobectomy) (England & Plueger, 2014). Resection surgery significantly reduces the incidence of seizures in patients with refractory epilepsy; however, more research is needed to determine the effect of surgery on quality of life, anxiety, and depression, all issues for these patients.

As an adjunct to medication in adolescents and adults with focal seizures, a vagal nerve stimulator may be implanted under the clavicle. The device is connected to the vagus nerve in the cervical area, where it delivers electrical signals to the brain to control and reduce seizure activity (England & Plueger, 2014). An external programming system is used by the physician to change stimulator settings. Patients can turn the stimulator on and off with a magnet. This can be performed as an outpatient surgical procedure.

Gerontologic Considerations

Elderly people (65 years of age and older) have a high incidence of new-onset epilepsy (England & Plueger, 2014). Cerebrovascular disease is the leading cause of seizures in the elderly, but head trauma, dementia, infection, alcoholism, and aging are also associated risk factors (Correll & Bazil, 2014). Treatment depends on the underlying cause. Because many elderly people have chronic health problems, they may be taking other medications that can interact with medications prescribed for seizure control. In addition, the absorption, distribution, metabolism, and excretion of medications are altered in the elderly as a result of age-related changes in kidney and liver function. Therefore, elderly patients must be monitored closely for adverse and toxic effects of AEDs and for osteoporosis. The cost of AEDs can lead to poor adherence to the prescribed regimen in elderly patients on fixed incomes.

NURSING PROCESS
The Patient with Epilepsy and Seizures

ASSESSMENT

The nurse elicits information about the patient's seizure history. The patient is asked about the factors or events that may precipitate the seizures. Alcohol and illicit drug intake is documented. The nurse determines whether the patient has an aura before an epileptic seizure, which may indicate the origin of the seizure (e.g., seeing a flashing light may indicate that the seizure originated in the occipital lobe). Observation and assessment during and after a seizure assist in identifying the type of seizure and its management.

The effects of epilepsy on the patient's lifestyle are assessed. What limitations are imposed by the seizure disorder? Does the patient have a recreational program? Social contacts? Is the

patient working, and is it a positive or stressful experience? What coping mechanisms are used?

DIAGNOSIS

NURSING DIAGNOSES

Based on the assessment data, the patient's major nursing diagnoses may include the following:

- Risk for injury related to seizure activity
- Fear related to the possibility of seizures
- Ineffective individual coping related to stresses imposed by epilepsy
- Deficient knowledge related to epilepsy and its control

COLLABORATIVE PROBLEMS/POTENTIAL COMPLICATIONS

The major potential complications for patients with epilepsy are status epilepticus and medication side effects (toxicity).

PLANNING AND GOALS

Goals for the patient may include prevention of injury, control of seizures, achievement of a satisfactory psychosocial adjustment, acquisition of knowledge and understanding about the condition, and absence of complications.

NURSING INTERVENTIONS

PREVENTING INJURY

Injury prevention for the patient with seizures is a priority. If the type of seizure the patient is having places him or her at risk for injury, the patient should be lowered gently to the floor (if not in bed), and any potentially harmful items nearby (e.g., furniture, eyeglasses) should be removed. The patient should never be restrained or forced into a position, nor should anyone attempt to insert anything into the patient's mouth once a seizure has begun, as protecting the airway is a priority. Place a pillow under the patient's head to cushion it. Patients for whom seizure precautions are instituted should have the bed in the lowest position and side rails raised when in bed.

> **Nursing Alert**
> Since 50% of deaths associated with epilepsy are accidental (drowning, trauma, burns, choking), the nurse reviews safety issues with the patient, such as never swimming alone, taking showers rather than baths, and avoiding activities that could cause harm if the patient were to have a seizure.

REDUCING FEAR OF SEIZURES

Fear that a seizure may occur unexpectedly can be reduced by the patient's adherence to the prescribed treatment regimen. Cooperation of the patient and family and their trust in the prescribed regimen are essential for control of seizures. The nurse emphasizes that the prescribed AED must be taken on a

(continued on page 1322)

continuing basis and that drug dependence or addiction does not occur. Periodic monitoring is necessary to ensure the adequacy of the treatment regimen, to prevent side effects, and to monitor for drug resistance.

In an effort to control seizures, factors that may precipitate them are identified, such as emotional disturbances, new environmental stressors, onset of menstruation in female patients, hypoglycemia, or fever. Online programs, such as SeizureTracker.com and "My seizure event diary," are available for patients to document their seizure activity. The patient is encouraged to follow a regular and moderate routine in lifestyle, diet (avoiding excessive stimulants), exercise, and rest (sleep deprivation may lower the seizure threshold). Moderate activity is therapeutic, but excessive exercise should be avoided. An additional dietary intervention, referred to as the *ketogenic diet,* has been suggested for control of seizures in some patients. This diet is high-fat and protein and low-carbohydrate. Effects of this diet are seen quickly. Because of the high-fat component of this diet and limited replacement of essential nutrients, compliance with this diet is difficult (Klein, Tyrlikova, & Mathews, 2014; Ye, Li, Jiang, Sun, & Liu, 2015).

Photic stimulation (bright flickering lights, television viewing) may precipitate seizures; wearing dark glasses or covering one eye may be preventive. Tension states (anxiety, frustration) induce seizures in some patients. Classes in stress management may be of value. Because seizures are known to occur with alcohol intake, alcoholic beverages should be avoided.

IMPROVING COPING MECHANISMS

The social, psychological, and behavioral problems that frequently accompany epilepsy can be more of a disability than the actual seizures. Epilepsy may be accompanied by feelings of stigmatization, alienation, depression, and uncertainty. The patient must cope with the constant fear of a seizure and the psychological consequences. Adults face potential issues such as the burden of finding employment, restrictions on the ability to drive, concerns about relationships and childbearing, insurance problems, and legal barriers. Alcohol abuse may complicate matters. Family reactions may vary from outright rejection of the person with epilepsy to overprotection. As a result, many people with epilepsy are at risk for psychological and behavioral problems.

> **Nursing Alert**
> *Patients with epilepsy have a depression incidence that is nearly five times higher than that of the general population as well as a higher suicide rate (England & Plueger, 2014). Thus, all patients with epilepsy should be screened for depression.*

Counseling assists the patient and family to understand the condition and the limitations it imposes. Social and recreational opportunities are necessary for good mental health. Nurses can improve the quality of life for patients with epilepsy by teaching them and their families about symptoms and their management.

PROVIDING PATIENT AND FAMILY EDUCATION

Perhaps the most valuable facets of care contributed by the nurse to the person with epilepsy are education and efforts to modify the attitudes of the patient and family toward the disorder. The person who experiences seizures may consider every seizure a potential source of humiliation and shame. This may result in anxiety, depression, hostility, and secrecy on the part of the patient and family. Ongoing education and encouragement should be given to patients to enable them to overcome these reactions. The patient with epilepsy should carry an emergency medical identification card or wear a medical information bracelet. The patient and family need to be educated about medications as well as care during a seizure.

MONITORING AND MANAGING POTENTIAL COMPLICATIONS

Status epilepticus, the major complication, was described previously. Another complication is the toxicity of AEDs. The patient and family are instructed about side effects and are given specific guidelines to assess and report signs and symptoms that indicate medication toxicity. Many AEDs require careful monitoring for therapeutic levels. The patient should plan to have serum drug levels assessed at regular intervals. Many known drug interactions occur with AEDs. A complete pharmacologic profile should be reviewed with the patient to avoid interactions that either potentiate or inhibit the effectiveness of the medications.

EVALUATION

EXPECTED PATIENT OUTCOMES

Expected patient outcomes may include the following:
1. Sustains no injury during seizure activity:
   a. Complies with treatment regimen and identifies the hazards of stopping the medication
   b. Patient and family can identify appropriate care during seizure.
2. Indicates a decrease in fear
3. Displays effective individual coping
4. Exhibits knowledge and understanding of epilepsy:
   a. Identifies the side effects of AEDs
   b. Avoids factors or situations that may precipitate seizures (e.g., flickering lights, hyperventilation, alcohol)
   c. Follows a healthy lifestyle by getting adequate sleep and eating meals at regular times to avoid hypoglycemia
5. Absence of complications

INFECTIOUS NEUROLOGIC DISORDERS

MENINGITIS

Meningitis is an inflammation of the meninges, which are the protective membranes covering the brain and spinal cord. Bacterial or viral infections are the primary causes of meningitis, but it also can be caused by a fungus or parasite. Because of this inflammation close to the brain and spinal cord, meningitis can be life-threatening.

Bacterial Meningitis

Bacterial meningitis is caused by bacteria; commonly, *Streptococcus pneumoniae* and *Neisseria meningitidis* (meningococcus) are infecting organisms. *Haemophilus influenzae* was once a common cause of meningitis in children, but because of vaccination, infection with this organism is now rare in the United States. However, it is still a concern for those not immunized for *H. influenzae*. Outbreaks of *N. meningitidis* infection are most likely to occur in dense community groups, such as college campuses and military installations. Although infections occur year round, incidence of outbreaks is reduced in the summer (VanDemark & Hickey, 2014). Factors that increase the risk for bacterial meningitis include tobacco use and viral upper respiratory infection because they increase the amount of droplet production. Otitis media and mastoiditis increase the risk for bacterial meningitis because the bacteria can cross the epithelial membrane and enter the subarachnoid space. Patients who are immunosuppressed are at risk for the development of bacterial meningitis (organ transplant, diabetes, cancer, asplenia [spleen removed], chronic steroid therapy, HIV infection, malnutrition, etc.), as well as patients who are very young (less than 2 months of age) and the elderly. A study by Fernandes et al. (2014) found that patients admitted with acute bacterial meningitis in the intensive care unit with low Glasgow Coma Scale scores or no signs of fever were at high risk for unfavorable outcomes.

Pathophysiology

The brain is protected by the skull, meninges, and the blood–brain barrier. Any violation to these defenses by a pathogen can result in meningitis. Meningeal infections generally originate in one of two ways: through the bloodstream as a consequence of other infections of the heart, lung, or viscera; or by direct spread, such as might occur after a traumatic injury to the facial bones, infection in the skull or spine, sinusitis, otitis, brain abscess, or secondary to invasive procedures, such as lumbar puncture or ventricular shunting procedures.

> ### ! Nursing Alert
> *Given the risk of bacterial meningitis in patients with traumatic injuries, prophylactic antibiotics are administered to patients who present with cerebrospinal fluid (CSF) escaping from the ears (CSF otorrhea) and the nose (CSF rhinorrhea) as is seen in basal skull fractures, dural tears, and compound skull fractures.*

Once the causative organism enters the bloodstream, it crosses the blood–brain barrier and proliferates in the CSF. The host immune response disrupts the cellular integrity of the microorganism and the breakdown products (cell wall fragments and lipopolysaccharides [LPS]), which enhances the inflammatory response in the involved meninges. Part of this response is the recruitment of neutrophils to the inflammatory site, resulting in thickening (an increase in viscosity) of the CSF. Because the cranial vault contains little room for expansion, the inflammation may cause increased intracranial pressure (ICP). CSF circulates through the subarachnoid space, where inflammatory cellular materials from the affected meningeal tissue enter and accumulate. The thickened CSF can interfere with CSF absorption, resulting in hydrocephalus. CSF studies demonstrate decreased glucose, increased protein levels, and increased white blood cell count (Bloch, 2014).

The prognosis for bacterial meningitis depends on the causative organism, the severity of the infection and illness, and the timeliness of treatment. Acute fulminant presentation may include adrenal damage, circulatory collapse, and widespread hemorrhages (Waterhouse–Friderichsen syndrome). This syndrome is the result of endothelial damage and vascular necrosis caused by the bacteria. Complications include visual impairment, deafness, seizures, paralysis, hydrocephalus, and septic shock.

Clinical Manifestations and Assessment

Headache and fever are frequently the initial symptoms. Fever tends to remain high throughout the course of the illness. An altered level of consciousness (LOC) is frequently seen; however one third of patients present with normal mentation (Bloch, 2014). Meningeal irritation results in a number of other well-recognized signs common to all types of meningitis:

- *Nuchal rigidity (stiff neck):* This is an early sign seen in 30% to 70% of patients (Bloch, 2014). Any attempts at flexion of the head are difficult because of spasms in the muscles of the neck. With the patient in supine position, the head is gently flexed forward and assessed for rigidity.
- *Positive Kernig sign:* When the patient is lying supine with the hip flexed to a 90-degree angle, resistance to passive extension of the knee is a positive Kernig sign (Fig. 46-1A). This pain is caused by inflammation of the meninges and spinal roots.
- *Positive Brudzinski sign:* When the patient's neck is flexed (after ruling out cervical trauma or injury), flexion of the knees and hips is produced; when the lower extremity of one side is passively flexed, a similar movement is seen in the opposite extremity (see Fig. 46-1B). This sign is caused by exudate that is irritating the root of the lumbar region (VanDemark & Hickey, 2014).
- *Photophobia (extreme sensitivity to light):* This finding is common, although the cause is unclear.

FIGURE 46-1 Testing for meningeal irritation. **A.** Kernig sign. **B.** Brudzinski sign.

> **Nursing Alert**
> The classic triad of symptoms of bacterial meningitis is stiff neck/nuchal rigidity, altered LOC, and fever, although all these symptoms are not found routinely. However, 95% of patients with bacterial meningitis suffer from two of the following four symptoms: headache, fever, stiff neck/nuchal rigidity, and altered LOC.

A rash can be a striking feature of *N. meningitidis* infection, occurring in about half of patients with this type of meningitis. Skin lesions develop, ranging from a petechial rash with purpuric lesions to large areas of ecchymosis.

Disorientation and memory impairment are common early in the course of the illness. The changes depend on the severity of the infection, as well as the individual response to the physiologic processes. As the illness progresses, lethargy, unresponsiveness, and coma may develop. Within the first week, seizures occur in 40% to 50% of patients with bacterial meningitis (VanDemark & Hickey, 2014).

ICP increases secondary to the accumulation of purulent exudate and cerebral edema. The initial signs of increased ICP include decreased LOC and focal motor deficits. Vomiting is a frequent finding associated with rising ICP. If ICP is not controlled, the uncus of the temporal lobe may herniate through the tentorium, causing pressure on the brainstem. Brainstem herniation is a life-threatening event that causes cranial nerve dysfunction and depresses the centers of vital functions, such as the medulla. Refer to Chapter 45 to review vital sign changes termed *Cushing's response*. An acute fulminant infection can occur in patients with meningococcal meningitis, producing signs of overwhelming septicemia: an abrupt onset of high fever, extensive purpuric lesions (over the face and extremities), shock, and signs of disseminated intravascular coagulopathy (DIC). Refer to Chapter 20 for details of DIC. Some patients develop hyponatremia or Syndrome of Inappropriate Antidiuretic Hormone (SIADH, refer to Chapter 31). Death may occur within a few hours after onset of the infection.

> **Nursing Alert**
> The nurse recognizes that with fever, tachycardia (increased heart rate) and tachypnea (increased respiratory rate [RR]) are expected. If bradycardia and decreased RR are seen, the nurse should consider ICP as an etiology for the decreased HR and RR.

If the clinical presentation suggests meningitis, diagnostic testing is conducted to identify the causative organism. Bacterial culture and Gram staining of CSF and blood are the "gold standard" for definitive diagnosis. These cultures should be obtained immediately when there is a suspicion of bacterial meningitis (Fischbach & Dunning, 2014). CT scanning is useful for detection of abscesses and lesions that may have provided a route for the bacteria.

Medical and Nursing Management

Successful outcomes depend on the early administration of antibiotics that cross the blood–brain barrier into the subarachnoid space in sufficient concentration to halt the multiplication of bacteria. Penicillin antibiotics (e.g., ampicillin, piperacillin) or one of the cephalosporins (e.g., ceftriaxone sodium, cefotaxime sodium) may be used. Vancomycin hydrochloride alone or in combination with rifampin may be used if resistant strains of bacteria are identified. High doses of the appropriate antibiotic are administered IV.

> **Nursing Alert**
> The nurse understands the difference between empiric antimicrobial therapy versus culture-documented therapy. Empiric therapy refers to selection of an antibiotic based upon the "most likely" suspected organism, while considering variables such as the patient's age, predisposing conditions, geographical region, etc. Empiric therapy is initiated immediately after collecting the culture specimens. Premature initiation of antimicrobial therapy before cultures are obtained can suppress bacterial growth

and impede the diagnosis. While culture-documented therapy will detail this patient's organism and specific sensitivities and/or resistance to certain antibiotics, there is a lapse of 24 to 72 hours before culture results are returned.

The use of dexamethasone as an adjunct therapy in the treatment of acute bacterial meningitis and in pneumococcal meningitis, if administered before the first dose of antibiotic, has been considered. However, recent results of a meta-analysis did not demonstrate significant reduction in death or neurologic disability in patients with steroid use (Brouwer, McIntyre, Prasad, & van de Beek, 2015).

Dehydration and shock are treated with fluid volume expanders. Seizures, which may occur early in the course of the disease, are controlled with phenytoin (Dilantin). Some providers may prophylactically use anticonvulsants and histamine-2-receptor antagonists or proton pump inhibitors (PPI) to prevent GI bleeding. Increased ICP is treated as necessary (see Chapter 45).

The patient with bacterial meningitis is critically ill; therefore, many of the nursing interventions are collaborative with the health care provider, respiratory therapist, and other members of the health care team. The patient's safety and well-being depend on sound nursing judgment.

Neurologic status and vital signs are continually assessed. Pulse oximetry and arterial blood gas (ABG) values are used to quickly identify the need for respiratory support if increasing ICP compromises the patient's LOC. Insertion of a cuffed endotracheal tube (or tracheotomy) and mechanical ventilation may be necessary to maintain adequate tissue oxygenation.

Blood pressure should be monitored to assess for incipient shock, which precedes cardiac or respiratory failure. Rapid IV fluid replacement may be prescribed, but care is taken to prevent fluid overload. Fever also increases the workload of the heart and cerebral metabolism. ICP will increase in response to increased cerebral metabolic demands. Therefore, measures are taken to reduce body temperature as quickly as possible.

Other important components of nursing care include the following measures:

- Protecting the patient from injury secondary to seizure activity or altered LOC
- Monitoring daily body weight; serum electrolytes; and urine volume, specific gravity, and osmolality, especially if SIADH is suspected (refer to Chapter 31).
- Preventing complications associated with immobility, such as pressure ulcers and pneumonia
- Instituting infection control precautions until 24 hours after initiation of antibiotic therapy (oral and nasal discharge is considered infectious)

Any sudden, critical illness can be devastating to the family. Because the patient's condition is often critical and the

prognosis guarded, the family needs to be informed about the patient's condition. Periodic family visits are essential to facilitate coping of the patient and family. An important aspect of the nurse's role is to support the family and assist them in identifying others who can be supportive of them during the crisis.

 Nursing Alert
Since bacterial meningitis is a contagious disease, isolation precautions must be instituted and will depend on the organism and patient status.

Viral Meningitis

Pathophysiology

Viral meningitis, also known as acute aseptic meningitis or acute benign lymphocytic meningitis, is more common than bacterial meningitis. The most common causes are enteroviruses (coxsackievirus, poliovirus, and echovirus). Patients with HIV can present with acute aseptic meningitis. In most cases no specific organism is identified. Children are most often affected, but all age groups can be affected.

Clinical Manifestations and Assessment

Viral meningitis usually starts with a headache, low-grade fever, stiff neck, photophobia, malaise, and symptoms of an upper respiratory viral illness, which are similar to bacterial meningitis. However, altered mental status and seizure activity are not associated with this disorder. Assess patient for a recent systemic viral infection. Patient may receive a CT scan to look for increased ICP. A lumbar puncture should be performed, and the CSF will be clear; results will show increased protein and WBC count as well as normal glucose level but will be free of any bacterial organism.

Medical and Nursing Management

Viral meningitis is managed based on the patient's symptoms and supportive nursing care. Patients may need to be hospitalized because of their discomfort and severe vomiting. Supportive care can include bed rest with head of bed (HOB) elevated 30 degrees and the patient's head in neutral alignment (improves venous drainage), a dark quiet environment, fever management, monitoring fluid intake, and pain management. Recovery should occur within 10 days.

ENCEPHALITIS

Encephalitis is an acute inflammatory process of the brain tissue (cerebral cortex) secondary to viruses, bacteria, fungi, or parasites. Viruses are the most common cause of encephalitis in the United States, and herpes simplex virus (HSV) is the most common of these. There are two HSVs, HSV-1 and HSV-2 (VanDemark & Hickey, 2014). HSV-1 typically affects children and adults. HSV-2 most commonly affects neonates whose mother was infected during pregnancy (Nettina, 2014).

Herpes Simplex Encephalitis

Pathophysiology

HSV-1 causes encephalitis by following a retrograde intraneuronal path to the brain. The olfactory and trigeminal nerves are the paths most commonly involved. A latent virus in brain tissue may reactivate and result in encephalitis. The invading organism causes cerebral edema and petechial hemorrhages of the brain and can directly invade the brain, damaging neurons (VanDemark & Hickey, 2014).

Clinical Manifestations and Assessment

Initial symptoms include fever, headache, stiff neck, and confusion. Focal neurologic symptoms reflect the areas of cerebral inflammation and necrosis and include behavioral changes, focal seizures, dysphasia, hemiparesis, and altered LOC. Patients may also have auditory and visual hallucinations (VanDemark & Hickey, 2014).

Neuroimaging studies, EEG, and CSF examination are used to diagnose HSV encephalitis. The EEG demonstrates periodic high-voltage spikes originating in the temporal lobe, and MRI may reveal temporal lobe edema. Lumbar puncture often reveals a high opening pressure and low-glucose and high-protein levels in CSF samples. Viral cultures are almost always negative. The polymerase chain reaction (PCR) is the standard test for early diagnosis of HSV-1 encephalitis. The validity of PCR is very high between the third and tenth days after symptom onset.

Medical and Nursing Management

Acyclovir (Zovirax), an antiviral agent, is the medication of choice in the treatment of HSV. Studies have indicated that early administration of acyclovir improves the prognosis associated with HSV-1 encephalitis and reduces a mortality rate of 60% to 70% down to 30% if treatment is initiated before the onset of coma (VanDemark & Hickey, 2014). To prevent relapse, treatment should continue for up to 3 weeks. Slow IV administration over at least 1 hour, along with adequate hydration, may prevent crystallization of the medication in the renal tubules, which would be reflected by a rising serum creatinine and blood urea nitrogen (BUN). Assessment of neurologic function is key to monitoring the progression of disease. Comfort measures to reduce headache include dimming the lights, limiting noise, and administering analgesic agents. Opioid analgesic medications may mask neurologic symptoms; therefore, they are used cautiously. Focal seizures and altered LOC require care directed at injury prevention and safety. Nursing care addressing

patient and family anxieties is ongoing throughout the illness. Monitoring of blood chemistry test results and hourly urinary output will alert the nurse to the presence of renal complications related to acyclovir therapy.

Arboviral Encephalitis

Arthropod vectors transmit several types of viruses that cause encephalitis. The primary vector in North America is the mosquito. In cases of West Nile virus, humans are the secondary host; birds are the primary host (refer to Fig. 46-2). Arbovirus infection (transmitted by arthropod vectors) occurs in specific geographic areas during the summer or early fall when the vectors are most active. West Nile virus, the most common type of arboviral encephalitis, was first observed in New York City in 1999 (Jubelt, 2015). The elderly are primarily affected (Jubelt, 2015). The St. Louis arbovirus is seen in the western United States, and the elderly are affected more frequently.

Pathophysiology

Viral replication occurs at the site of the mosquito bite. The host immune response attempts to control viral replication. If the immune response is inadequate, viremia will ensue. The virus gains access to the CNS via the cerebral capillaries, resulting in encephalitis. It spreads from neuron to neuron, predominantly affecting the cortical gray matter, the brainstem, and the thalamus. Meningeal exudates compound

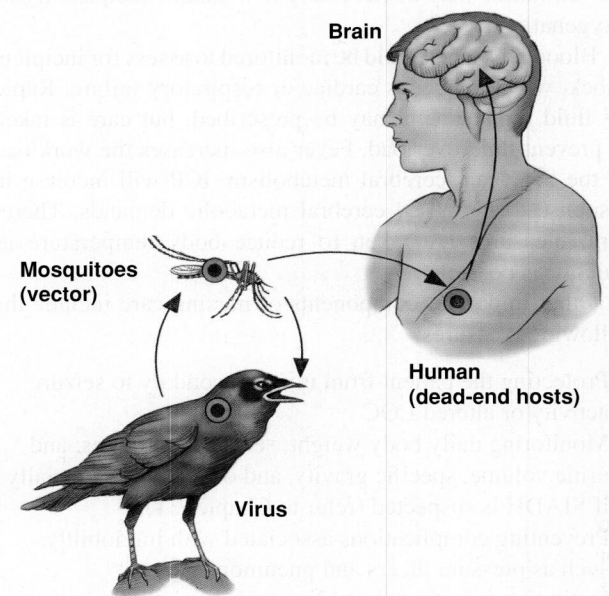

FIGURE 46-2 Transmission routes of West Nile virus. Birds are the reservoir of the West Nile virus, but they are unable to spread it. Mosquitoes serve as the vectors, spreading it from bird to bird and from birds to people. Humans are believed to be "dead-end hosts" because the virus can live and cause illness in humans. (Used with permission from Lippincott's Nursing Advisor.)

the clinical presentation by irritating the meninges and increasing ICP.

Clinical Manifestations and Assessment

An arboviral encephalitis begins with early flu-like symptoms, but specific neurologic manifestations depend on the viral type. After a brief febrile prodrome, neurologic symptoms will reflect the area of the brain that is involved. For example, if meninges are involved, patients can present with nuchal rigidity and headache. A unique clinical feature of St. Louis encephalitis is the development of SIADH with hyponatremia in 25% to 33% of affected patients (Jubelt, 2015). (SIADH is detailed in Chapter 31.) Signs and symptoms specific to West Nile encephalitis include a maculopapular or morbilliform rash (erythematous [red] rash resembling that of measles consisting of macules and papules [or maculopapular]) on the neck, trunk, arms, and legs, and flaccid paralysis. Both West Nile and St. Louis encephalitis can result in parkinsonian-like movements, reflecting inflammation of the basal ganglia.

Neuroimaging and CSF evaluation are useful in the diagnosis of arboviral encephalitis. MRI demonstrates inflammation of the basal ganglia in cases of St. Louis encephalitis and inflammation in the periventricular area in cases of West Nile encephalitis. Immunoglobulin M antibodies to West Nile virus are observed in serum and CSF (Davis & Pirio Richardson, 2015). Serum cultures are not useful because the viremia is brief.

Medical and Nursing Management

No specific medication for arboviral encephalitis exists. Medical management is aimed at controlling the seizures and the increased ICP and supporting respiratory function. If the patient is very ill, hospitalization may be required. The nurse carefully assesses neurologic status and identifies improvement or deterioration in the patient's condition. Injury prevention is key in light of the potential for falls and seizures. Arboviral encephalitis may result in death or lifelong residual health issues, such as neurologic deficits and seizures. The family will need support and teaching to cope with these outcomes.

Public education addressing the prevention of arboviral encephalitis is a key nursing role. Clothing that provides coverage and applying Environmental Protection Agency (EPA)–approved insect repellents containing permethrin or another EPA-registered repellent to clothes will give extra protection. This should be used in high-risk areas to decrease mosquito and tick bites. Avoidance of outdoor activities and control of the mosquito vector are important for control of the disease. Screens should be in good repair in the home, and standing water, such as in birdbaths, should be removed or avoided. Blood donation centers screen all blood for West Nile virus. Cases of West Nile virus are reported to the Centers for Disease Control and Prevention (CDC). People must be warned not to handle a dead bird if found and to call

FIGURE 46-3 Distribution of the facial nerve.

the local health department for instructions on reporting and disposing of the body.

BELL'S PALSY

Bell's palsy (facial paralysis) is caused by unilateral inflammation of the seventh cranial nerve, which results in weakness or paralysis of the facial muscles on the ipsilateral, or same side, of the affected facial nerve (Fig. 46-3).

Pathophysiology

Although the cause is unknown, theories about causes include vascular ischemia, viral disease (herpes simplex, herpes zoster), Lyme disease, autoimmune disease, or a combination of all of these factors. Bell's palsy may be a type of pressure paralysis. The inflamed, edematous nerve becomes compressed to the point of damage, or its blood supply is occluded, producing ischemic necrosis of the nerve.

Clinical Manifestations and Assessment

The face is distorted from paralysis of the facial muscles; there are increased lacrimation (tearing) and painful sensations in the face, behind the ear, and in the eye of the affected side. The ear pain may precede the paralysis by 24 to 48 hours. The patient may experience speech difficulties and may be unable to eat on the affected side because of weakness or paralysis of the facial muscles. A disturbance of taste is a common finding. When asking the patient to show his or her teeth and smile, weakness of the involved nerve will be noted, there will be an absence of wrinkling on the forehead, the affected side will appear mask-like.

Medical and Nursing Management

Corticosteroid therapy (prednisone) may be prescribed to reduce inflammation and edema; this reduces vascular compression and permits restoration of blood circulation to the nerve. Early administration of corticosteroid therapy appears to diminish the severity of the disease, relieve the pain, and prevent or minimize denervation. Prednisone may be combined with Acyclovir to improve facial function (Nettina, 2014).

Facial pain is controlled with analgesic agents. Heat may be applied to the involved side of the face to promote comfort and blood flow through the muscles. Electrical stimulation may be applied to the face to prevent muscle atrophy.

While the paralysis lasts, nursing care involves protection of the eye from injury. Frequently, the eye does not close completely and the blink reflex is diminished, so the eye is vulnerable to injury from dust and foreign particles. Corneal irritation, corneal abrasion, and ulceration may occur. Distortion of the lower lid alters the proper drainage of tears. To prevent injury, the eye may be covered with a protective shield at night. The eye patch may abrade the cornea, however, because there is some difficulty in keeping the partially paralyzed eyelids closed. Eye ointment may be applied at bedtime to promote adherence of the eyelids to prevent injury during sleep. Artificial tears are typically instilled to maintain eye lubrication. The patient can be taught to close the paralyzed eyelid manually before going to sleep. Wraparound sunglasses or goggles may be worn during the day to decrease normal evaporation from the eye.

NEURODEGENERATIVE AND NEUROMUSCULAR DISORDERS

MULTIPLE SCLEROSIS

Multiple sclerosis (MS), the leading cause of nontraumatic disability in young adults, is an immune-mediated, progressive demyelinating disease of the CNS. *Demyelination* refers to the destruction of myelin, the fatty and proteinaceous material that surrounds certain nerve fibers in the brain and spinal cord; it results in impaired transmission of nerve impulses (Fig. 46-4). MS may occur at any age but typically manifests in young adults between the ages of 20 and 40 years; it affects women more frequently than men and rarely affects those over 60 years (Riley & Tullman, 2015).

The etiology of MS is unknown and may result from complex interactions between environmental factors and genetically susceptible individuals that trigger an abnormal immune response that damages the myelin sheath, oligodendrocytes, axons, and neurons (Riley & Tullman, 2015). Evidence for a genetic predisposition is seen in an increased risk for

FIGURE 46-4 The process of demyelination. (**A**) and (**B**) depict a normal nerve cell and axon with myelin. (**C**) and (**D**) show the slow disintegration of myelin, resulting in a disruption in axon function.

Caucasians of northern European ancestry and a decreased risk in others (e.g., Native Americans) (Riley & Tullman, 2015). Researchers found that some environmental exposure (i.e., biomarker of Epstein–Barr virus, infectious mononucleosis, smoking) may play a role in the development of MS (Belbasis, Bellou, Evangelou, Ioannidis, & Tzoulaki, 2015).

Pathophysiology

Sensitized T cells typically cross the blood–brain barrier; their function is to check the CNS for antigens and then leave. B cells and monocytes are also activated; B cells secrete antibodies against myelin. In MS, the sensitized T cells remain in the CNS and promote the infiltration of other agents that damage the immune system. The immune system attack leads to inflammation that damages myelin (which normally insulates the axon and speeds the conduction of impulses along the axon) and the oligodendroglial cells that produce myelin in the CNS.

Demyelination interrupts the flow of nerve impulses and results in a variety of manifestations, depending on the nerves affected. Plaques appear on demyelinated axons, further interrupting the transmission of impulses. Demyelinated axons are scattered irregularly throughout the CNS. The areas most frequently affected are the optic nerves, chiasm, and tracts; the cerebrum; the brainstem and cerebellum; and the spinal cord. Eventually, the axons themselves begin to degenerate, resulting in permanent and irreversible damage (Riley & Tullman, 2015).

Clinical Manifestations and Assessment

The course of MS may assume many different patterns (Fig. 46-5). Between 85% and 90% of patients with MS have a relapsing-remitting (RR) course. With each relapse, recovery is usually complete; however, residual deficits may occur and accumulate over time, contributing to functional decline. Approximately 40% of those with the RR course of MS progress to a secondary progressive course, in which disease progression occurs with or without relapses. About 10% to 15% of patients have a primary progressive course, in which disabling symptoms steadily increase, with rare plateaus and temporary improvement (Riley & Tillman, 2015). Primary progressive MS may result in quadriparesis, cognitive dysfunction, visual loss, and brainstem syndromes. The least common presentation is the progressive relapsing form of MS, which occurs in approximately 5% of patients and is characterized by relapses with continuous disabling progression between exacerbations (Hauser & Goodin, 2014).

The signs and symptoms of MS are varied and multiple, reflecting the location of the lesion (plaque) or combination of lesions. The primary symptoms most commonly reported are unilateral visual loss, typically preceded or accompanied by orbital pain that increases with eye movement (acute optic neuritis), fatigue, depression, weakness, limb (typically legs) numbness, difficulty in coordination, loss of balance, and pain. Visual disturbances due to lesions in the optic nerves or their connections may also include blurring of vision, **diplopia** (double vision), nystagmus (rotary oscillation of the eyes), patchy blindness (scotoma), and total blindness.

Fatigue, defined as a subjective lack of physical or mental energy that interferes with desired activity, is one of the more common symptoms of MS; it is typically worse in the afternoon hours. Depression, heat, anemia, deconditioning, and medication may contribute to fatigue. The etiology of MS-related fatigue is poorly understood; there appears to be no association between fatigue and disease course (Riley & Tillman, 2015).

Like fatigue, pain is a symptom that can contribute to social isolation. Approximately 70% of patients with MS report pain at some point (Riley & Tillman, 2015). Lesions on the sensory pathways cause pain. Lhermitte sign is described as an electrical sensation that is felt down the arms, back, or lower trunk when the patient flexes the neck. It is theorized this acute pain sensation is related to sclerotic plaques on the dorsal nerve roots (Weigel & Hickey, 2014). Many people with MS need daily analgesics. In some cases, pain is managed with opioids, antiseizure medication, or antidepressants. Rarely, surgery may be needed to interrupt pain pathways.

Additional sensory manifestations include paresthesias (abnormal skin sensations, such as tingling, itching, or burning), dysesthesias (unpleasant, abnormal sense of touch), and loss of proprioception (ability to sense the position, location, orientation, and movement of the body and its parts). An objective sensory loss (position, vibration, shape, texture) is noted in 50% of patients with MS (Weigel & Hickey, 2014). Among perimenopausal women, those with MS are more likely to have pain related to osteoporosis. In addition to estrogen loss, immobility and corticosteroid therapy play a role in the development of osteoporosis among women with MS. Bone mineral density (BMD) testing is recommended for this high-risk group (refer to Chapter 40). Diagnosis and treatment of osteoporosis are discussed in Chapter 41.

Spasticity (muscle hypertonicity) of the extremities (usually the legs) and loss of the abdominal reflexes result from involvement of the main motor pathways (pyramidal tracts) of the spinal cord. The spasticity often occurs with painful spasms, which interfere with mobility, sleep, and activities of daily living (ADLs). Gait abnormalities are common and are usually a result of ataxia, weakness, or spasticity. Disruption of the sensory axons may produce sensory dysfunction (paresthesias, pain). Cognitive and psychosocial problems may reflect frontal or parietal lobe involvement. Some degree of cognitive impairment (e.g., memory loss, decreased concentration) occurs in about 65% of patients, but severe cognitive changes with dementia (progressive organic mental disorder) are rare.

Involvement of the cerebellum or basal ganglia can produce **ataxia** (impaired coordination of movements) and

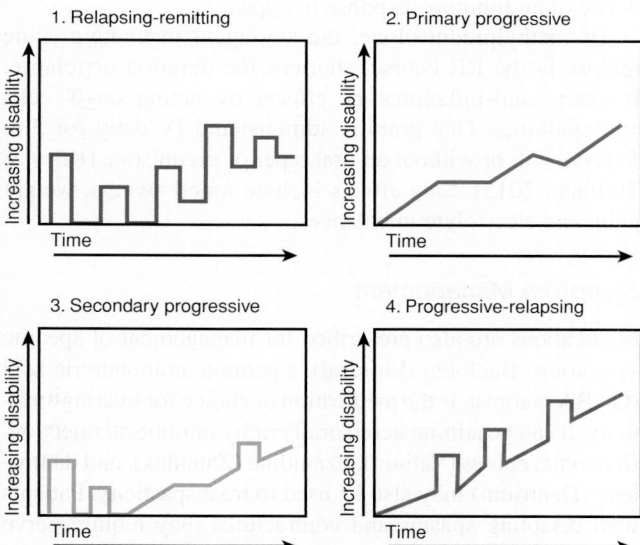

FIGURE 46-5 Types and courses of multiple sclerosis (MS). **1.** Relapsing-remitting (RR) MS is characterized by clearly acute attacks with full recovery or with sequelae and residual deficit upon recovery. Periods between disease relapses are characterized by lack of disease progression. **2.** Primary progressive (PP) MS is characterized by disease showing progression of disability from onset, without plateaus and temporary minor improvements. **3.** Secondary progress (SP) MS begins with an initial RR course, followed by progression of variable rate, which may also include occasional relapses and minor remissions. **4.** Progressive-relapsing (PR) MS shows progression from onset but with clear acute relapses with or without recovery. (From Lublin, F. D., & Reingold, S. C. (1996). Defining the clinical course of multiple sclerosis: Results of an international survey. *Neurology, 46*(64), 907–911. Used with permission from Lippincott Williams & Wilkins.)

tremor. Loss of the control connections between the cortex and the basal ganglia may occur and cause emotional lability and euphoria. Bladder, bowel, and sexual dysfunctions are common. Bladder dysfunction (urinary urgency, frequency, nocturia, and urge incontinence) affects approximately 75% of patients, and in approximately 15% of these, symptoms can be severe enough to socially isolate the patient (Riley & Tillman, 2015).

Secondary complications of MS include urinary tract infections, constipation, pressure ulcers, contracture deformities, dependent pedal edema, pneumonia, reactive depression, and decreased bone density. Emotional, social, marital, economic, and vocational problems may also be a consequence of the disease.

Exacerbations and remissions are characteristic of MS. During exacerbations, new symptoms appear and existing ones worsen; during remissions, symptoms decrease or disappear. Fifteen years after onset, only 20% of patients have no functional limitation (Hauser & Goodin, 2014). Precipitation of symptoms may occur with the following events: periods of emotional and physical stress; cold or humid, hot weather; hot baths; overheating; fever; fatigue; and pregnancy (Weigel & Hickey, 2014). There is no single test for the diagnosis of MS. Diagnosis is established based upon clinical examination, results from MRI ("bright spots" of demyelinated lesions or plaques are easily seen in white matter) and evoked potential studies (EPS), and examination of CSF. Approximately 95% of MS patients' MRI studies reveal abnormalities. Electrophoresis of CSF identifies the presence of oligoclonal banding. EPS can help define the extent of the disease process and monitor changes.

Medical and Nursing Management

No cure exists for MS. The goals of treatment are to treat acute exacerbations, delay the progression of the disease, and manage chronic symptoms. Many patients with MS have a stable disease course and require only intermittent treatment, whereas others experience steady progression of their disease. Symptoms requiring intervention include spasticity, fatigue, bladder dysfunction, and ataxia. Management strategies target the various motor and sensory symptoms and effects of immobility that can occur.

Disease-Modifying Therapies

The disease-modifying medications reduce the frequency of relapse, the duration of relapse, and the number and size of plaques observed on MRI. All of the medications require injection.

Interferon beta-1a (Rebif) and interferon beta-1b (Betaseron) are administered subcutaneously (SQ), and another preparation of interferon beta-1a, Avonex, is administered intramuscularly (IM) once a week. Side effects of all the interferon beta medications include flu-like symptoms, which may be minimized by administration at bedtime, and can be managed with acetaminophen and ibuprofen; these side effects may resolve after a few months. Additional side effects include injection site reaction (seen less frequently with IM preparations), thrombocytopenia, anemia, leukopenia, potential liver damage, fetal abnormalities, and depression. For optimal control of disability, disease-modifying medications should be started early in the course of the disease.

Nursing Alert
MS does not affect fertility or carrying a pregnancy to term. Interestingly women with MS typically do not have relapses during pregnancy; however, there is a relapse incidence of 20% to 40% in the first 3 months after delivery. The relapse does not impact the risk of long-term disability. Research efforts on the effects of hormones and circulating protein on MS may shed light on the course of MS.

Glatiramer acetate (Copaxone) reduces the rate of relapse in the RR course of MS. It decreases the number of plaques noted on MRI and increases the time between relapses. Copaxone is administered SQ daily. It acts by increasing the antigen-specific suppressor T cells. Side effects and injection site reactions are rare. Copaxone is an option for those with an RR course; however, it may take 6 months for evidence of an immune response to appear.

IV methylprednisolone, the key agent in treating acute relapse in the RR course, shortens the duration of relapse. It exerts anti-inflammatory effects by acting on T cells and cytokines. One gram is administered IV daily for 3 to 5 days, with or without an oral taper of prednisone (Riley & Tullman, 2015). Side effects include mood swings, weight gain, and electrolyte imbalances.

Symptom Management

Medications are also prescribed for management of specific symptoms. Baclofen (Lioresal), a gamma-aminobutyric acid (GABA) agonist, is the medication of choice for treating spasticity. It can be administered orally or by intrathecal injection. Benzodiazepines (Valium), tizanidine (Zanaflex), and dantrolene (Dantrium) may also be used to treat spasticity. Patients with disabling spasms and contractures may require nerve blocks or surgical intervention. Fatigue that interferes with ADLs may be treated with amantadine (Symmetrel), pemoline (Cylert), or fluoxetine (Prozac). Ataxia is a chronic problem most resistant to treatment. Medications used to treat ataxia include beta-adrenergic blockers (Inderal), antiseizure agents (Neurontin), and benzodiazepines (Klonopin).

Bladder and bowel problems are often among the most difficult ones for patients, and a variety of medications (anticholinergics, alpha-adrenergic blockers, antispasmodic agents) may be prescribed. Nonpharmacologic strategies also assist in establishing effective bowel and bladder elimination (discussed shortly).

Urinary tract infection is often superimposed on the underlying neurologic dysfunction. Ascorbic acid (vitamin C) may be prescribed to acidify the urine, making bacterial growth less likely. Antibiotics are prescribed when appropriate.

Antidepressants may be prescribed since 25% to 50% of patients with MS are depressed, and the suicide rate is significantly higher than in the general population (Weigel & Hickey, 2014).

An individualized program of physical therapy, rehabilitation, and education is combined with emotional support. An educational plan of care is developed to enable the person with MS to deal with the physiologic, social, and psychological problems that accompany chronic disease.

Promoting Physical Mobility

Relaxation and coordination exercises promote muscle efficiency. Progressive resistive exercises are used to strengthen weak muscles because diminishing muscle strength is often significant in MS.

Exercises. Walking improves the gait and particularly helps with the problem of the loss of the sense of position of the legs and feet. If certain muscle groups are irreversibly affected, other muscles can be trained to compensate. Instruction in the use of assistive devices may be needed to ensure their safe and correct use. Weighted canes, walkers, or limb bracelets may be of value.

Minimizing Spasticity and Contractures. Muscle spasticity is common and, in its later stages, is characterized by severe adductor spasm of the hips, with flexor spasm of the hips and knees. Without relief, fibrous contractures of these joints will occur. Warm packs may be beneficial, but hot baths should be avoided because of risk for burn injury secondary to sensory loss and increasing symptoms that may occur with elevation of the body temperature.

Daily exercises for muscle stretching are prescribed to minimize joint contractures. Special attention is given to the hamstrings, gastrocnemius muscles, hip adductors, biceps, and wrist and finger flexors. Muscle spasticity is common and interferes with normal function. A stretch–hold–relax routine is helpful for relaxing and treating muscle spasticity. Swimming and stationary bicycling are useful, and progressive weight bearing can relieve spasticity in the legs. The patient should not be hurried in any of these activities because this often increases spasticity.

Activity and Rest. The patient is encouraged to work and exercise to a point just short of fatigue. Very strenuous physical exercise is not advisable because it raises the body temperature and may aggravate symptoms. The patient is advised to take frequent short rest periods, preferably lying down. Extreme fatigue may contribute to the exacerbation of symptoms.

Minimizing Effects of Immobility. Because of the decrease in physical activity that often occurs with MS, complications associated with immobility, including pressure ulcers, expiratory muscle weakness, and accumulation of bronchial secretions, need to be considered and steps taken to prevent them. Measures to prevent such complications include assessing and maintaining skin integrity and having the patient perform coughing and deep-breathing exercises.

Preventing Injury

If motor dysfunction causes coordination problems and clumsiness, or if ataxia is apparent, the patient is at risk for falling. To overcome this disability, the patient is taught to walk with feet apart to widen the base of support and to increase walking stability. If the loss of sense of position occurs, the patient is taught to watch the feet while walking. Gait training may require assistive devices (walker, cane, braces, crutches, parallel bars) and instruction about their use by a physical therapist. If the gait remains inefficient, a wheelchair or motorized scooter may be the solution. The occupational therapist is a valuable resource person in suggesting and securing aids to promote independence. The patient is trained in transfer and ADLs.

Because sensory loss may occur in addition to motor loss, pressure ulcers are a continuing threat to skin integrity. The need to use a wheelchair continuously increases the risk. See Chapter 52 for a discussion of the prevention and treatment of pressure ulcers.

Enhancing Bladder and Bowel Control

In general, bladder symptoms fall into the following categories: (1) inability to store urine (hyperreflexic, uninhibited); (2) inability to empty the bladder (hyporeflexic, hypotonic); and (3) a mixture of both types. The patient with urinary frequency, urgency, or incontinence requires special support. The sensation of the need to void must be heeded immediately so the bedpan or urinal should be readily available. A voiding time schedule is set up (every 1.5 to 2 hours initially, with gradual lengthening of the interval). The patient is instructed to drink a measured amount of fluid every 2 hours and then attempt to void 30 minutes after drinking. Use of a timer or wristwatch with an alarm may be helpful for the patient who does not have enough sensation to signal the need to empty the bladder. The nurse encourages the patient to take the prescribed medications to treat bladder spasticity because this allows greater independence. Intermittent self-catheterization has been successful in maintaining bladder control in patients with MS. If a female patient has permanent urinary incontinence, urinary diversion procedures may be considered. The male patient may wear a condom appliance for urine collection.

Bowel problems include constipation, fecal impaction, and incontinence. Adequate fluids, dietary fiber, and a bowel-training program are frequently effective in solving these problems.

Enhancing Communication and Managing Swallowing Difficulties

If the cranial nerves that control the mechanisms of speech and swallowing are affected, dysarthrias (defects of articulation) marked by slurring, low volume of speech, and difficulties in phonation may occur. **Dysphagia** (difficulty swallowing) may also occur. A speech therapist evaluates speech and swallowing and instructs the patient, family, and health team members about strategies to compensate for speech and swallowing problems. The nurse reinforces this instruction and encourages the patient and family to adhere to the plan. Impaired swallowing increases the patient's risk for aspiration; therefore, strategies are needed to reduce that risk. Such strategies include having suction apparatus available, performing careful feeding, and ensuring proper positioning for eating. Refer to Chapters 9 and 10 for information related to aspiration.

Improving Sensory and Cognitive Function

Measures may be taken if visual defects or changes in cognitive status occur.

Vision. The cranial nerves affecting vision may be affected by MS. An eye patch or a covered eyeglass lens may be used to block the visual impulses of one eye if the patient has diplopia (double vision). Prism glasses may be helpful for patients who are confined to bed and have difficulty reading in the supine position. People who are unable to read regular-print materials are eligible for the free "talking book" services of the Library of Congress or may obtain large-print or audio books from local libraries.

Cognition and Emotional Responses. Cognitive impairment and emotional lability occur early in MS in some patients and may impose numerous stresses on the patient and family. Some patients with MS are forgetful and easily distracted.

Patients adapt to illness in a variety of ways, including denial, depression, withdrawal, and hostility. Emotional support assists patients and their families to adapt to the changes and uncertainties associated with MS and to cope with the disruption in their lives. The patient is assisted to set meaningful and realistic goals, to remain as active as possible, and to keep up social interests and activities. Hobbies may help the patient's morale and provide satisfying interests if the disease progresses to the stage at which formerly enjoyed activities can no longer be pursued.

The family should be made aware of the nature and degree of cognitive impairment. The environment is kept structured, and lists and other memory aids are used to help the patient with cognitive changes to maintain a daily routine. The occupational therapist can be helpful in formulating a structured daily routine.

Strengthening Coping Mechanisms. The diagnosis of MS is always distressing to the patient and family. They need to know that no two patients with MS have identical symptoms or courses of illness. Although some patients do experience significant disability early, others have a near-normal lifespan with minimal disability. Some families, however, face overwhelming frustrations and problems. MS affects people who are often in a productive stage of life and concerned about career and family responsibilities. Family conflict, disintegration, separation, and divorce are not uncommon. Often, very young family members assume the responsibility of caring for a parent with MS. Nursing interventions in this area include alleviating stress and making appropriate referrals for counseling and support to minimize the adverse effects of dealing with chronic illness.

The nurse, mindful of these complex problems, initiates home care and coordinates a network of services, including social services, speech therapy, physical therapy, and homemaker services. To strengthen the patient's coping skills, as much information as possible is provided. Patients need an updated list of available assistive devices, services, and resources.

Coping through problem-solving involves helping the patient define the problem and develop alternatives for its management. Careful planning and maintaining flexibility and a hopeful attitude are useful for psychological and physical adaptation.

Improving Home Management

MS can affect every facet of daily living. Certain abilities are often impossible to regain after they are lost. Physical function may vary from day to day. Modifications that allow independence in home management should be implemented (e.g., assistive eating devices, raised toilet seat, bathing aids, telephone modifications, long-handled comb, tongs, modified clothing). Exposure to heat increases fatigue and muscle weakness so air conditioning is recommended in at least one room. Exposure to extreme cold may increase spasticity.

Promoting Sexual Functioning

Patients with MS and their partners face problems that interfere with sexual activity, both as a direct consequence of nerve damage and also from psychological reactions to the disease. Easy fatigability, conflicts arising from dependency and depression, emotional lability and loss of self-esteem compound the problem. Erectile and ejaculatory disorders in men and orgasmic dysfunction and adductor spasms of the thigh muscles in women can make sexual intercourse difficult or impossible. Bladder and bowel incontinence and urinary tract infections add to the difficulties.

An experienced sexual counselor helps bring into focus the patient's or partner's sexual resources and suggests relevant information and supportive therapy. Sharing and communicating feelings, planning for sexual activity (to minimize the effects of fatigue), and exploring alternative methods of sexual expression may open up a wide range of sexual enjoyment and experiences.

MYASTHENIA GRAVIS

Myasthenia gravis (MG), an autoimmune disorder affecting the neuromuscular junction, is characterized by fatigability and degrees of muscle weakness of the voluntary muscles. According to the Myasthenia Gravis Foundation of America, the prevalence of MG in the United States is estimated to be approximately 20 per 100,000 people. MG occurs in both men and women at older ages; however before 40 years of age, the disease is three times more common in women (Penn & Rowland, 2015). A women's average age of onset is 28 years of age whereas the men's average age of onset is 42 years of age (Fowler, Herrington, Koopman, & Ricci, 2013).

Pathophysiology

Normally, a chemical impulse precipitates the release of acetylcholine from vesicles on the nerve terminal at the neuromuscular junction. The acetylcholine attaches to receptor sites on the motor endplate and stimulates muscle contraction. Continuous binding of acetylcholine to the receptor site is required for muscular contraction to be sustained.

In MG, there is a reduction in the number of acetylcholine receptor sites because antibodies directed at the acetylcholine receptor sites impair transmission of impulses across the neuromuscular junction. Therefore, fewer receptors are available for stimulation, resulting in voluntary muscle weakness that escalates with continued activity (Fig. 46-6). Abnormalities of the thymus (located behind the sternum) are found in 80% of patients with MG (Nettina, 2014).

Clinical Manifestations and Assessment

The initial manifestation of MG usually involves the ocular muscles. Diplopia (double vision) and ptosis (drooping of the eyelids) are common. However, the majority of patients also experience weakness of the muscles of the face and throat (bulbar symptoms) and generalized weakness. Weakness of the facial muscles results in a bland facial expression. Laryngeal involvement produces **dysphonia** (voice impairment) and increases the patient's risk for choking and aspiration. Generalized weakness affects all the extremities and the intercostal muscles, resulting in decreasing vital capacity and respiratory failure. MG is purely a motor disorder with no effect on sensation or coordination.

The hallmark of MG is fluctuating muscle weakness, which intensifies with activity, such as exercise, and improves with rest (Koopman & Hickey, 2014).

An acetylcholinesterase test is used to diagnose MG. The acetylcholinesterase inhibitor stops the breakdown of acetylcholine, thereby increasing availability at the neuromuscular junction. The drug used is edrophonium chloride (Tensilon) because it has a rapid onset of 30 seconds and a short duration of 5 minutes (Koopman & Hickey, 2014). Immediate improvement in muscle strength after administration of this agent represents a positive test and usually confirms the diagnosis.

An ice-pack test can help differentiate MG from other causes of ptosis. An ice pack is applied over the patient's closed eyes for 2 minutes. Improvement of the ptosis that is sustained for several minutes is considered a positive ice-pack test and is suggestive of MG. The rationale behind this test is that by cooling the tissues, which include skeletal muscle fibers, the activity of the acetylcholinesterases are inhibited. This test has the advantage of being noninvasive and inexpensive; however, not all patients with MG present with ptosis.

The presence of acetylcholine receptor antibodies is identified in serum. Repetitive nerve stimulation demonstrates a decrease in successive action potentials. The thymus gland may be enlarged in MG, and a CT scan of the mediastinum is performed to detect thymoma or hyperplasia of the thymus.

Medical and Nursing Management

Management of MG is directed at improving function and reducing and removing circulating antibodies. Therapeutic modalities include administration of anticholinesterase medications and immunosuppressive therapy, plasmapheresis, intravenous immunoglobulin, and thymectomy.

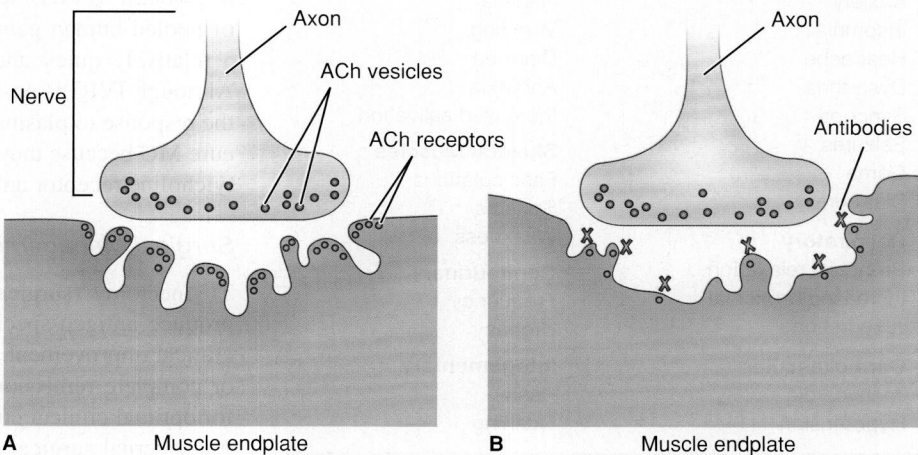

FIGURE 46-6 Myasthenia gravis (MG). **A.** Normal acetylcholine (ACh) receptor site. **B.** ACh receptor site in MG.

Pharmacologic Therapy

Pyridostigmine bromide (Mestinon), an anticholinesterase medication, is the first line of therapy. It provides symptomatic relief by inhibiting the breakdown of acetylcholine and increasing the relative concentration of available acetylcholine at the neuromuscular junction. The dosage is gradually increased to a daily maximum and is administered in divided doses (usually four times a day). The most common adverse effects are gastrointestinal discomfort, increased bronchial and oral secretions, and muscle fasciculations and cramps (Koopman & Hickey, 2014). Pyridostigmine tends to have fewer side effects than other anticholinesterase medications (Box 46-3).

If pyridostigmine bromide does not improve muscle strength and control fatigue, the next agents used are immunosuppressant agents. The goal of immunosuppressive therapy is to reduce production of the antibody. Corticosteroids suppress the patient's immune response, decreasing the amount of antibody production, and this correlates with clinical improvement. An initial dose of prednisone is given daily; as symptoms improve, the medication is tapered and a maintenance alternative-day dosing schedule may be considered. Since long-term steroids carry substantial risks for a variety of dose-dependent side effects (diabetes, osteoporosis, hypertension), this treatment is usually reserved for patients with ocular symptoms. As the corticosteroid dosage is gradually increased, the anticholinesterase dosage is lowered. Cytotoxic medications are used to treat MG if there is inadequate response to steroids. Azathioprine (Imuran), an immunosuppressive drug, inhibits T lymphocytes and reduces acetylcholine receptor antibody levels. Therapeutic effects may not be evident for 3 to 12 months. Leukopenia

and hepatotoxicity are serious adverse effects so monthly evaluation of liver enzymes and white blood cell count is necessary.

> **Nursing Alert**
> *Prophylactic treatment for osteoporosis and careful follow-up for other side effects is mandatory in all patients managed with long-term prednisone.*

A number of medications are contraindicated for patients with MG because they exacerbate the symptoms. The health care provider and the patient should weigh risks and benefits before any new medications are prescribed, including antibiotics, cardiovascular medications, antiseizure and psychotropic medications, morphine, quinine and related agents, beta blockers, and nonprescription medications.

> **Nursing Alert**
> *The patient's dentist should be advised of the diagnosis of MG, and Procaine (Novocain) should be avoided. Since neuromuscular blocking agents may have a very prolonged effect in patients with MG, any anesthetic medication should be evaluated by the primary care provider to ensure it is not capable of exaggerating myasthenic weakness (Fowler et al., 2013).*

Plasmapheresis/Intravenous Immunoglobulin

Plasmapheresis (plasma exchange) is a technique used to treat exacerbations of MG. The patient's plasma and plasma components are removed through a centrally placed large-bore double-lumen catheter. The blood cells and antibody-containing plasma are separated, after which the cells and a plasma substitute are reinfused. Plasma exchange produces a temporary reduction in the level of circulating antibodies. The typical course of plasmapheresis consists of daily or alternate-day treatment, and the number of treatments is determined by the patient's response. IV immunoglobulin (IVIG) treatment involves the administration of pooled human gamma globulin, which usually produces a relatively quick and short-term relief of MG weakness. Although IVIG is easier than plasmapheresis to administer, the response to plasmapheresis is more rapid. No treatments cure MG because they do not stop the production of the acetylcholine receptor antibodies.

Surgical Management

Thymectomy (surgical removal of the thymus gland) can produce antigen-specific immunosuppression and result in clinical improvement. The procedure results in either partial or complete remission. The entire gland must be removed for optimal clinical outcomes; therefore, surgeons prefer the trans-sternal surgical approach. After surgery, the patient is

---

BOX 46-3
Potential Adverse Effects of Anticholinesterase Medications

Central Nervous System
Irritability
Anxiety
Insomnia
Headache
Dysarthria
Syncope
Seizures
Coma
Diaphoresis

Respiratory
Bronchial relaxation
Increased bronchial
  secretions

Cardiovascular
Tachycardia
Hypotension

Gastrointestinal
Abdominal cramps
Nausea
Vomiting
Diarrhea
Anorexia
Increased salivation

Skeletal Muscles
Fasciculations
Spasms
Weakness

Genitourinary
Frequency
Urgency

Integumentary
Rash
Flushing

monitored in an intensive care unit, with special attention to respiratory function. The patient is weaned from mechanical ventilation after thorough respiratory assessment. Thymectomy leads to improvement in almost all patients, but it may take months before the patient sees any benefit from the procedure.

Nursing Management

Because MG is a chronic disease and most patients are seen on an outpatient basis, much of the nursing care focuses on patient and family teaching. Educational topics for outpatient self-care include medication management, energy conservation, strategies to help with ocular manifestations, and prevention and management of complications.

Medication management is a crucial component of ongoing care. Understanding the actions of the medications and taking them on schedule is emphasized, as are the consequences of delaying medication and the signs and symptoms of myasthenic and cholinergic crises. The patient can determine the best times for daily dosing by keeping a diary to determine fluctuation of symptoms and to learn when the medication is wearing off. The medication schedule can then be manipulated to maximize strength throughout the day.

Nursing Alert

Maintenance of stable blood levels of anticholinesterase medications is imperative to stabilize muscle strength. Therefore, the anticholinesterase medications must be administered on time. Any delay in administration of medications may exacerbate muscle weakness and make it impossible for the patient to take medications orally.

To minimize the risk of aspiration, mealtimes should coincide with the peak effects of anticholinesterase medication. In addition, rest before meals is encouraged, to reduce muscle fatigue. The patient is advised to sit upright during meals, with the neck slightly flexed to facilitate swallowing. Soft foods in gravy or sauces can be swallowed more easily; if choking occurs frequently, the nurse can suggest puréed food with a pudding-like consistency. Suction should be available at home, with the patient and family instructed in its use. Supplemental feedings may be necessary in some patients to ensure adequate nutrition.

Impaired vision results from ptosis of one or both eyelids, decreased eye movement, or double vision. To prevent corneal damage when the eyelids do not close completely, many providers may instruct the patient to tape or patch the eyes closed for short intervals and to regularly instill artificial tears. If taping is done, it is important to ensure the lid covers the eye to prevent corneal abrasion from the tape or patch. Patients who wear eyeglasses can have "crutches" attached to help lift the eyelids. Patching of one eye can help with double vision.

The patient is reminded of the importance of maintaining health promotion practices and of following health care screening recommendations. Factors that exacerbate symptoms and potentially cause crisis should be noted and avoided: emotional stress, infections (particularly respiratory infections), vigorous physical activity, some medications, and high environmental temperature.

The patient is also taught strategies to conserve energy. To do this, the nurse helps the patient identify the optimal times for rest throughout the day. If the patient lives in a two-story home, the nurse can suggest that frequently used items (e.g., hygiene products, cleaning products, snacks) be kept on each floor to minimize travel between floors. The patient is encouraged to apply for a handicapped license plate to minimize walking from parking spaces, and to schedule activities to coincide with peak energy and strength levels. Patients are encouraged to wear a medical alert bracelet identifying them as having MG. The Myasthenia Gravis Foundation of America provides support groups, services, and educational materials for patients, families, and health care providers (www.myasthenia.org).

Complications

Cholinergic Crisis

A cholinergic crisis, which is essentially a problem of overmedication, results in severe generalized muscle weakness, respiratory impairment, and excessive pulmonary secretions that may result in respiratory failure. Weak respiratory muscles do not support inhalation. An inadequate cough and an impaired gag reflex, caused by bulbar weakness, result in poor airway clearance and risk of aspiration. Bulbar weakness specifically involves the muscles of the jaw, face, palate, pharynx, larynx, tongue, glossopharyngeal nerve (IX), vagus nerve (X), and hypoglossal nerve (XII). A downward trend of two respiratory function tests, the negative inspiratory force and vital capacity, is the first clinical sign of respiratory compromise.

Nursing Alert

The phrase bulbar weakness *refers to weakness and fatigue in the neck and jaw, and it is named for the nerves that originate from the bulblike part of the brainstem, the medulla. The nurse anticipates the patient will have difficulty talking, chewing, swallowing, and holding the head erect. Patients should be assessed for their ability to communicate, to tolerate oral intake, and to determine their aspiration risk. A marked decrease in oxygen saturation (as measured by pulse oximetry), tachypnea (increased respiration rate), and coughing to a lesser extent after oral intake suggests aspiration. Weakness of the respiratory musculature can lessen the ability to cough.*

Endotracheal intubation and mechanical ventilation may be needed. Cholinesterase inhibitors are stopped when respiratory failure occurs and gradually restarted after the patient demonstrates improvement. Nutritional support may be needed if the patient is intubated for a long period.

Myasthenic Crisis

Myasthenic crisis is a sudden, temporary exacerbation of symptoms of MG. A common precipitating event for myasthenic crisis is an infection. Respiratory distress and varying degrees of dysphagia (difficulty swallowing), dysarthria (difficulty speaking), eyelid ptosis, diplopia, and prominent muscle weakness are symptoms of myasthenic crisis.

Providing ventilatory assistance takes precedence in the immediate management of the patient with myasthenic crisis. Ongoing assessment for respiratory failure is essential. The nurse assesses the respiratory rate and depth, breath sounds, and oxygen saturation and monitors pulmonary function parameters (vital capacity and negative inspiratory force) to detect pulmonary problems before respiratory dysfunction progresses. ABG analysis is performed as needed. Endotracheal intubation and mechanical ventilation may be needed.

If the abdominal, intercostal, and pharyngeal muscles are severely weak, the patient cannot cough, take deep breaths, or clear secretions. Chest physiotherapy, including postural drainage to mobilize secretions and suctioning to remove secretions, may have to be performed frequently. (Postural drainage should not be performed for 30 minutes after feeding.)

Several strategies and supportive measures should be performed during this crisis, including monitoring of laboratory work, input and output, and daily weight, along with vigilant pulmonary assessments. If the patient cannot swallow, nasogastric tube feedings may be prescribed. Sedatives and tranquilizers are avoided because they aggravate hypoxia and hypercapnia and can cause respiratory and cardiac depression.

GUILLAIN–BARRÉ SYNDROME

Guillain–Barré syndrome (GBS) is an autoimmune attack on the peripheral nerve myelin. The result is acute, rapid, segmental demyelination of peripheral nerves and some cranial nerves, producing ascending weakness with **dyskinesia** (inability to execute voluntary movements), hyporeflexia, and **paresthesias** (numbness). An antecedent event (most often a viral infection) precipitates clinical presentation. *Campylobacter jejuni*, cytomegalovirus, Epstein–Barr virus, *Mycoplasma pneumoniae*, *H. influenzae*, and HIV are the most common infectious agents associated with the development of GBS. In a few instances, the patient reports receiving a vaccination prior to the onset of GBS (Hickey, 2014a).

In North America, approximately 1.0 to 2.0 cases of GBS occur for every 100,000 people each year. GBS affects people of all ages and races and females slightly more than men. Given the relationship of GBS to colds and flu-like illnesses, it is expected that GBS would occur more frequently in the fall and winter when these infections are more likely (Hickey, 2014a).

Pathophysiology

Myelin is a complex substance that covers nerves, providing insulation and speeding the conduction of impulses from the cell body to the dendrites. The cell that produces myelin in the peripheral nervous system is the Schwann cell. In GBS, the Schwann cell is spared, allowing for remyelination in the recovery phase of the disease.

GBS is the result of a cell-mediated and humoral immune attack on peripheral nerve myelin proteins that causes inflammatory demyelination. The immune system cannot distinguish between the two proteins and attacks and destroys peripheral nerve myelin. The exact location of the immune attack within the peripheral nervous system is the ganglioside GM1b. With the autoimmune attack, there is an influx of macrophages and other immune-mediated agents that attack myelin, cause inflammation and destruction, and leave the axon unable to support nerve conduction (Fig. 46-7).

Clinical Manifestations and Assessment

GBS typically begins with muscle weakness and diminished reflexes of the lower extremities. Hyporeflexia and weakness may progress to tetraplegia (paralysis of all four limbs). Demyelination of the nerves that innervate the diaphragm and intercostal muscles results in neuromuscular respiratory failure. Sensory symptoms include paresthesias of the hands and feet and pain related to the demyelination of sensory fibers.

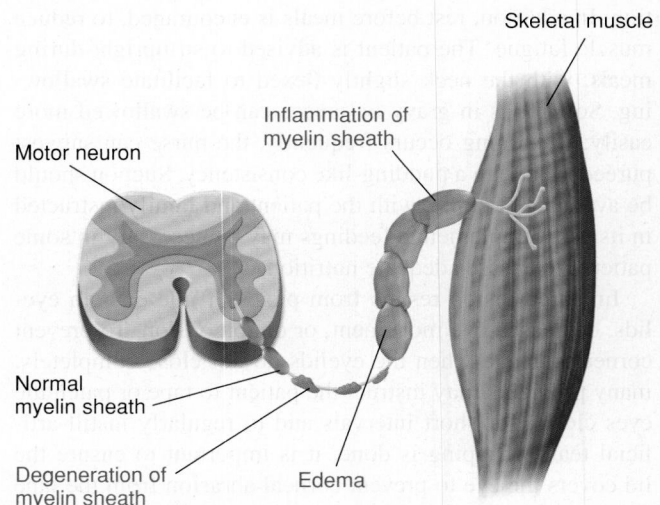

FIGURE 46-7 Peripheral nerve demyelination. (Used with permission from *ACC atlas of pathophysiology*. (2001). Philadelphia, PA: Lippincott Williams & Wilkins.)

The antecedent event usually occurs 2 weeks before symptoms begin. Weakness usually begins in the legs and progresses upward. Maximum weakness, the *plateau,* varies in length but usually includes neuromuscular respiratory failure and bulbar weakness. The duration of the symptoms is variable; complete functional recovery may take up to 2 years (Hickey, 2014a). Any residual symptoms are permanent and reflect axonal damage from demyelination.

Cranial nerve demyelination can result in a variety of clinical manifestations. Optic nerve demyelination may result in blindness. Bulbar muscle weakness related to demyelination of the glossopharyngeal and vagus nerves results in the inability to swallow or clear secretions. Vagus nerve demyelination results in autonomic dysfunction, manifested by instability of the cardiovascular system. The presentation is variable and may include tachycardia, bradycardia, hypertension, or orthostatic hypotension. The symptoms of autonomic dysfunction occur and resolve rapidly. GBS does not affect cognitive function or LOC.

Although the classic clinical features include areflexia and ascending weakness, variation in presentation occurs. There may be a sensory presentation, with progressive sensory symptoms, an atypical axonal destruction, or the Miller–Fisher variant, which includes paralysis of the ocular muscles, ataxia, and areflexia (Hickey, 2014a).

The patient presents with symmetric weakness, diminished reflexes, and upward progression of motor weakness. Changes in vital capacity and negative inspiratory force are assessed to identify impending neuromuscular respiratory failure. Serum laboratory tests are not useful in the diagnosis. However, elevated protein levels are detected in CSF evaluation, without an increase in other cells. EPSs demonstrate a progressive loss of nerve conduction velocity.

Medical and Nursing Management

Because of the possibility of rapid progression and neuromuscular respiratory failure, GBS is a medical emergency, requiring management in an intensive care unit. After baseline values are identified, assessment of changes in muscle strength and respiratory function alert the clinician to the physical and respiratory needs of the patient. Respiratory therapy or mechanical ventilation may be necessary to support pulmonary function and adequate oxygenation. Some clinicians recommend elective intubation before the onset of extreme respiratory muscle fatigue. Mechanical ventilation may be required for an extended period. The patient is weaned from mechanical ventilation after the respiratory muscles can again support spontaneous respiration and maintain adequate tissue oxygenation.

Other interventions are aimed at preventing the complications of immobility. These may include the use of anticoagulant agents and thigh-high elastic compression stockings or sequential compression boots to prevent thrombosis and pulmonary emboli (PE).

Plasmapheresis and IVIG are used to affect directly the peripheral nerve myelin antibody level. Both therapies decrease circulating antibody levels and reduce the amount of time the patient is immobilized and dependent on mechanical ventilation. The cardiovascular risks posed by autonomic dysfunction require continuous electrocardiographic (ECG) monitoring. Tachycardia and hypertension are treated with short-acting medications, such as alpha-adrenergic blocking agents. The use of short-acting agents is important because autonomic dysfunction is very labile. Hypotension is managed by increasing the amount of IV fluid administered.

Maintaining Respiratory Function

Respiratory function can be maximized with incentive spirometry and chest physiotherapy. Monitoring for changes in vital capacity and negative inspiratory force are key to early intervention for neuromuscular respiratory failure. Mechanical ventilation is required if the vital capacity falls, making spontaneous breathing impossible and tissue oxygenation inadequate.

Nursing Alert
To evaluate respiratory muscle strength, maximal inspiratory pressures (MIP) are obtained using a handheld or electronic device that can be attached to an endotracheal tube (if needed), or the patient can place the device around his or her lips. The patient exhales the residual volume and then inhales with maximal force. A normal MIP is usually more negative than –75 cm H$_2$O; when the value is less negative than –20 or –30 cm H$_2$O, weaning from mechanical ventilation may be difficult, and values less positive than 60 cm H$_2$O suggest cough insufficiency (Stoller & Hill, 2016). This simple bedside test also can be used to monitor deterioration or improvement of the strength of the diaphragm and other inspiratory muscles. Respiratory therapy personnel perform this test.

Parameters for determining the appropriate time to begin mechanical ventilation include a vital capacity of less than 15 mL/kg. The potential need for mechanical ventilation should be discussed with the patient and family on admission, to provide time for psychological preparation and decision-making. Intubation and mechanical ventilation will result in less anxiety if it is initiated on a nonemergency basis to a well-informed patient. The patient may require mechanical ventilation for a long period.

Bulbar weakness that impairs the ability to swallow and clear secretions is another factor in the development of respiratory failure in the patient with GBS. Suctioning may be needed to maintain a clear airway.

The nurse assesses the blood pressure and heart rate frequently to identify autonomic dysfunction so that interventions can be initiated quickly if needed. Medications are administered for clinically significant symptoms.

Enhancing Physical Mobility

Nursing interventions to enhance physical mobility and prevent the complications of immobility are key to the function and survival of these patients. The paralyzed extremities are supported in functional positions, and passive range-of-motion (ROM) exercises are performed at least twice daily. Deep venous thrombosis (DVT) and PE are threats to the patient who is paralyzed. Nursing interventions are aimed at preventing DVT. ROM exercises, position changes, anticoagulation, the use of thigh-high elastic compression stockings or sequential compression boots, and adequate hydration decrease the risk for DVT.

Padding may be placed over bony prominences, such as the elbows and heels, to reduce the risk for pressure ulcers. The need for consistent position changes every 2 hours cannot be overemphasized. The nurse evaluates laboratory test results that may indicate malnutrition or dehydration, both of which increase the risk for pressure ulcers. The nurse collaborates with the provider and dietitian to develop a plan to meet the patient's nutritional and hydration needs.

Providing Adequate Nutrition

Paralytic ileus may result from insufficient parasympathetic activity. In this event, the nurse administers IV fluids and parenteral nutrition as prescribed and monitors for the return of bowel sounds and bowel function. If the patient cannot swallow due to **bulbar paralysis** (immobility of muscles), a gastrostomy tube may be placed to administer nutrients. The nurse carefully assesses the return of the gag reflex and bowel sounds before resuming oral nutrition.

Improving Communication

Because of paralysis, the patient cannot talk, laugh, or cry and therefore has no method for communicating needs or expressing emotion. Establishing some form of communication with picture cards or an eye blink system provides a means of communication. Collaboration with the speech therapist may be helpful in developing a communication mechanism that is most effective for a specific patient.

Decreasing Fear and Anxiety

The patient and family are faced with a sudden, potentially life-threatening disease, and anxiety and fear are constant themes for them. The impact of disease on the family depends on the patient's role within the family. Referral to a support group may provide information and support to the patient and family.

The family may feel helpless in caring for the patient. Mechanical ventilation and monitoring devices may frighten and intimidate them. Family members often want to participate in physical care; with instruction and support by the nurse, they should be allowed to do so.

In addition to fear, the patient may experience isolation, loneliness, and lack of control. Nursing interventions that increase the patient's sense of control include providing information about the condition, emphasizing a positive appraisal of coping resources, and teaching relaxation exercises and distraction techniques. The positive attitude and atmosphere of the multidisciplinary team are important to promote a sense of well-being.

Diversional activities are encouraged to decrease loneliness and isolation. Encouraging visitors, engaging visitors or volunteers to read to the patient, listening to music or books on tape, and watching television are ways to alleviate the patient's sense of isolation.

Complications

Thorough assessment of respiratory function at regular and frequent intervals is essential because respiratory insufficiency and subsequent failure due to weakness or paralysis of the intercostal muscles and diaphragm may develop quickly. In addition to the respiratory rate and the quality of respirations, vital capacity is monitored frequently and at regular intervals so that respiratory insufficiency can be anticipated. Decreasing vital capacity associated with weakness of the muscles used in swallowing, which causes difficulty in both coughing and swallowing, indicates impending respiratory failure. Signs and symptoms include breathlessness while speaking, shallow and irregular breathing, use of accessory muscles, tachycardia, and changes in respiratory pattern.

Parameters for determining the onset of respiratory failure are established on admission, allowing intubation and the initiation of mechanical ventilation on a nonemergent basis. This also allows the patient to be prepared for the procedure in a controlled manner, which reduces anxiety and complications.

Other complications include cardiac arrhythmias, which necessitate ECG monitoring; transient hypertension; orthostatic hypotension; DVT; PE; urinary retention; and other threats to any patient who is immobilized and paralyzed. These require monitoring and attention to prevent them and prompt treatment if indicated.

PARKINSON DISEASE

Parkinson disease (PD) is a slowly progressing neurologic movement disorder that eventually leads to disability. The degenerative or idiopathic form is the most common; there is also a secondary form with a known or suspected cause. Although the cause of most cases is unknown, causative factors include genetics, atherosclerosis, excessive accumulation of oxygen-free radicals, viral infections, head trauma, chronic use of antipsychotic medications, and some environmental exposures. Parkinsonian symptoms usually first appear in the fifth decade of life, with diagnosis typically in the sixth and seventh decades of life; however, cases have been diagnosed as early as 30 years of age. It is the second most common **neurodegenerative** disease. PD affects men more frequently than women.

Pathophysiology

PD is associated with decreased levels of dopamine resulting from destruction of pigmented neuronal cells in the substantia nigra in the basal ganglia region of the brain. Fibers or neuronal pathways project from the substantia nigra to the corpus striatum, where neurotransmitters are key to the control of complex body movements. Through the neurotransmitters acetylcholine (excitatory) and dopamine (inhibitory), striatal neurons relay messages to the higher motor centers that control and refine motor movements. The loss of dopamine stores in this area of the brain results in more excitatory neurotransmitters than inhibitory neurotransmitters, leading to an imbalance that affects voluntary movement. Clinical symptoms do not appear until 60% of the pigmented neurons are lost and the striatal dopamine level is decreased by 80%. Cellular degeneration impairs the extrapyramidal tracts that control semiautomatic functions and coordinated movements; motor cells of the motor cortex and the pyramidal tracts are not affected.

Clinical Manifestations and Assessment

PD has a gradual onset, and symptoms progress slowly over a chronic, prolonged course. The cardinal signs are T-R-A-P: **T**remor, **R**igidity of muscles, **A**kinesia/Bradykinesia (without or decreased body movement), and **P**ostural disturbances (gait and balance disorders).

Tremor

The most common reason why individuals seek medical evaluation is the presence of a resting tremor. Resting tremor characteristically disappears with purposeful movement but is evident when the extremities are motionless. The tremor may manifest as a rhythmic, slow-turning motion (pronation–supination) of the forearm and the hand and a motion of the thumb against the fingers as if rolling a pill between the fingers. Tremor is present while the patient is at rest; it increases when the patient is walking, concentrating, or feeling anxious.

Rigidity

Resistance to passive limb movement characterizes muscle rigidity. *Cogwheel rigidity* is characterized by jerky rhythmic tone on passive muscle stretching (Mastrianni, Barton, Shannon, Gilman, & Shakkotai, 2014). Involuntary stiffness of the passive extremity increases when another extremity is engaged in voluntary active movement. Early in the disease, the patient may complain of shoulder pain due to rigidity.

Akinesia/Bradykinesia

Akinesia means a lack of movement, and *bradykinesia* means a slowness of initiation and execution of movement. Patients may take longer to complete activities and have difficulty initiating movement, such as rising from a sitting position or turning in bed.

Postural Disturbances

A loss of postural reflexes occurs, and the patient stands with the head bent forward and walks with a propulsive gait. The posture is caused by the forward flexion of the neck, hips, knees, and elbows. The patient may walk faster and faster, trying to move the feet forward under the body's center of gravity (shuffling gait). Difficulty in pivoting that causes loss of balance (either forward or backward) places the patient at risk for falls.

Other Manifestations

The effect of PD on the basal ganglia often produces autonomic symptoms that include excessive and uncontrolled sweating, paroxysmal flushing, orthostatic hypotension, gastric and urinary retention, constipation, and sexual dysfunction. Cognitive and psychiatric changes are often interrelated and may be predictive of one another. Depression is common; whether it is a reaction to the disorder or is related to a biochemical abnormality is uncertain. Cognitive changes may appear in the form of judgment, reasoning, decision making, and memory deficits, although intellect is not usually affected. A number of psychiatric manifestations (personality changes, psychosis, dementia, and acute confusion) are common in elderly patients with PD.

Patients with PD experience sleep disturbances. This may be related to depression, dementia, or medications. Auditory and visual hallucinations have also been reported in PD and may be associated with depression, dementia, lack of sleep, or adverse effects of medications.

Hypokinesia (abnormally diminished movement) is also common and may appear after the tremor. The *freezing phenomenon* refers to a transient inability to perform active movement and is thought to be an extreme form of bradykinesia. Additionally, the patient tends to shuffle and exhibits a decreased arm swing. As dexterity declines, **micrographia** (small handwriting) develops. The face becomes increasingly mask-like and expressionless, and the frequency of blinking decreases. Dysphonia (soft, low-pitched, and less audible speech) may occur due to weakness of the muscles responsible for speech and paralysis of the soft palate, resulting in a nasal-sounding speech. In many cases, the patient develops dysphagia, begins to drool, and is at risk for choking and aspiration.

Complications associated with PD are common and are typically related to disorders of movement. As the disease progresses, patients are at risk for respiratory and urinary

Stooped posture

Resting tremor

Masklike facial expression

Cogwheel rigidity

Arms flexed at elbows and wrists

Akinesia

Hips and knees slightly flexed

Tremor

Short, shuffling steps

FIGURE 46-8 The clinical features of Parkinson disease: TRAP (Tremor, Rigidity, Akinesia/Bradykinesia, and Postural disturbances). (Adapted from Timby, B. (2010). *Introductory medical-surgical nursing* (10th ed., p. 535). Philadelphia, PA: Lippincott Williams & Wilkins.)

tract infection, skin breakdown, and injury from falls. The adverse effects of medications used to treat the symptoms are associated with numerous complications, such as dyskinesia (impairment of voluntary movements resulting in fragmented or jerky motions) and orthostatic hypotension.

Early diagnosis can be difficult because patients rarely are able to pinpoint when the symptoms started. Often, a family member notices a change, such as stooped posture, a stiff arm, a slight limp, tremor, or slow, small handwriting. The medical history, presenting symptoms, neurologic examination, and response to pharmacologic management are carefully evaluated when making the diagnosis. Currently, the disease is diagnosed clinically from the patient's history and the presence of two of the four cardinal manifestations: tremor, rigidity, akinesia/bradykinesia, and postural disturbances (Fig. 46-8).

Medical and Nursing Management

Treatment is directed at controlling symptoms and maintaining functional independence. Care is individualized for each patient based on presenting symptoms and social, occupational, and emotional needs. Pharmacologic management is the mainstay of treatment, although advances in research have led to increased surgical options. Patients are usually cared for at home and are admitted to the hospital only for complications or to initiate new treatments.

Antiparkinsonian Medications

Levodopa (Larodopa) is the most effective agent and the mainstay of treatment. Levodopa is converted to dopamine in the basal ganglia, producing symptom relief. The beneficial effects of levodopa are most pronounced in the first few years of treatment. Benefits begin to wane and adverse effects become more severe over time. Confusion, hallucinations, depression, and sleep alterations are associated with prolonged use. Levodopa is usually administered in combination with carbidopa (Sinemet), an amino acid decarboxylase inhibitor, which helps to maximize the beneficial effects of levodopa.

Within 5 to 10 years, most patients develop a response to the medication characterized by **dyskinesia** (abnormal involuntary movements), including facial grimacing, rhythmic jerking movements of the hands, head bobbing, chewing and smacking movements, and involuntary movements of the trunk and extremities. The patient may experience an on–off syndrome, in which sudden periods of near-immobility ("off effect") are followed by a sudden return of effectiveness of the medication ("on effect"). Refer to Table 46-2 for additional medical therapies.

Drug Alert!
MAO-B inhibitors may offer some neuroprotective benefits that could postpone the need for levodopa. Since MAO-B is an enzyme that breaks down dopamine, a medication that helps to block the breakdown of dopamine in the brain makes more dopamine available and reduces some of the motor symptoms of PD. When used together with other medications, MAO-B inhibitors may reduce "off" effect and extend "on" effect as described previously. The patient must be educated to avoid an interaction with products containing tyramine (red wine, aged cheese) since sudden and severe hypertension can occur.

Deep Brain Stimulation

Deep brain stimulation is the delivery of high-frequency electrical stimulation to a select targeted area in the brain (Fig. 46-9). A CT scan or MRI determines the target area. Unilateral and/or bilateral deep brain stimulation of the subthalamic nucleus or globus pallidus (the site where most of the degenerative changes of PD occurs) improves the symptoms of PD, and early use (when motor complications are developing) results in significant benefit compared to traditional

TABLE 46-2 Antiparkinsonian Medications

Anticholinergic Therapy Trihexyphenidyl hydrochloride (Artane) Benztropine mesylate (Cogentin)	Used for controlling tremor by counteracting the action of the neurotransmitter acetylcholine; often poorly tolerated in elderly patients. Intraocular pressure must be closely monitored; these medications are contraindicated in patients with narrow-angle glaucoma. Patients with benign prostate hyperplasia (BPH) are monitored for signs of urinary retention.
Antiviral Therapy Amantadine hydrochloride (Symmetrel)	Used for symptoms related to akinesia, as well as tremor. A low incidence of side effects is seen but can include psychiatric disturbances (mood changes, confusion, depression, hallucinations), lower extremity edema, orthostatic hypotension, congestive heart failure, nausea, epigastric distress, urinary retention, headache, and visual impairment.
Dopamine Agonists Bromocriptine mesylate (Parlodel) Pergolide (Permax) Ropinirole hydrochloride (Requip) Pramipexole (Mirapex)	Useful in postponing the initiation of carbidopa or levodopa therapy or added to the medication regimen after carbidopa or levodopa loses effectiveness. Adverse reactions to these medications include nausea, vomiting, diarrhea, lightheadedness, hypotension, impotence, and psychiatric effects. Requip and Mirapex do not have the potentially serious adverse effects of pergolide and bromocriptine mesylate.
Monoamine Oxidase Inhibitors (MAOIs) Selegiline (Eldepryl) Rasagiline (Azilect) Zydis selegiline HCl (Zelapar)	Used in combination with a dopamine agonist to delay the use of carbidopa or levodopa therapy. Adverse effects are similar to those of levodopa.
Catechol-O-Methyltransferase (COMT) Inhibitors Entacapone (Comtan) Tolcapone (Tasmar)	When given in combination with carbidopa or levodopa, they can increase the duration of action. COMT inhibitors block an enzyme that metabolizes levodopa, making more levodopa available for conversion to dopamine in the brain.
Antidepressants	
Tricyclic antidepressants	Used to treat depression; dosing is lower in patients with Parkinson disease, typically one third to one half of the usual dosage.
Amitriptyline hydrochloride (Elavil)	Used for anticholinergic and antidepressant effects
Serotonin reuptake inhibitors (SRIs) Fluoxetine hydrochloride (Prozac)	Effective for treating depression but may aggravate symptoms of Parkinson disease.
Atypical antidepressants Bupropion hydrochloride (Wellbutrin)	Effective for treating depression but may aggravate symptoms of Parkinson disease.

medical treatment (Lang, 2016). In deep brain stimulation, one or more electrodes is placed in specific areas of the brain and connected to a pulse generator that is implanted in a subcutaneous subclavicular or abdominal pouch. The battery-powered pulse generator sends high-frequency electrical impulses through a wire placed under the skin to a lead anchored to the skull. The electrode blocks nerve pathways in the brain that cause tremors. Deep brain stimulation usually results in patients being at their best for longer periods of the day than they were with medication alone.

Improving Mobility

A progressive program of daily exercise will increase muscle strength, improve coordination and dexterity, reduce muscular rigidity, and prevent contractures that occur when muscles are not used. Walking, riding a stationary bicycle, swimming, and gardening are all exercises that help maintain joint mobility. Stretching (stretch–hold–relax) and ROM exercises promote joint flexibility. Postural exercises are important to counter the tendency of the head and neck to be drawn forward and down. A physical therapist may be helpful in developing an individualized exercise program and can provide instruction to the patient and caregiver on exercising safely. Faithful adherence to an exercise and walking program helps to delay the progress of the disease. Warm baths and massage, in addition to passive and active exercises, help relax muscles and relieve painful muscle spasms that accompany rigidity.

Balance may be adversely affected because of the rigidity of the arms (arm swinging is necessary in normal walking). Special walking techniques must be learned to offset the

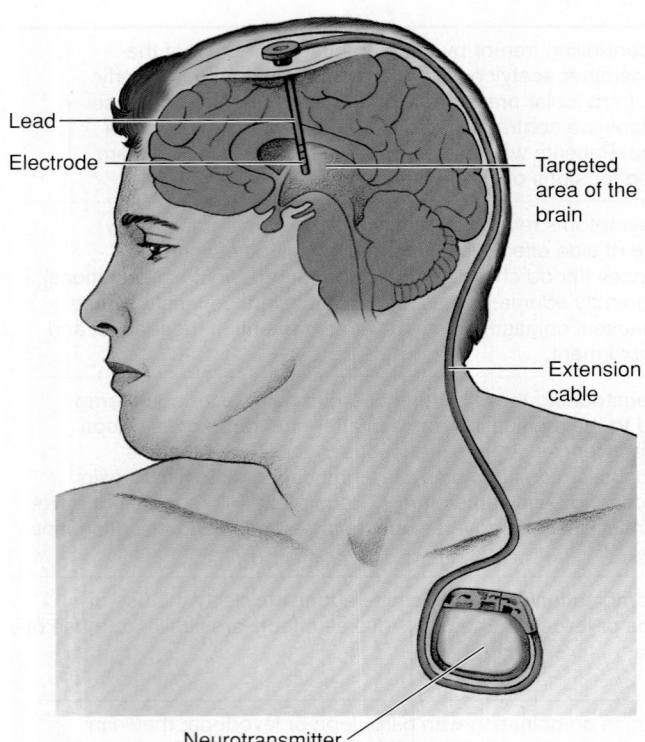

Lead

Electrode

Targeted area of the brain

Extension cable

Neurotransmitter

FIGURE 46-9 Deep brain stimulation. The deep brain stimulation system consists of the stimulating lead (which is implanted to the desired target), the extension cable (which is tunneled under the scalp and soft tissues of the neck to the anterior chest wall), and the pulse generator (which is the programmable source of the electrical impulses). This illustration shows the placement of the stimulator in the patient's body. (Used with permission from Lippincott's Nursing Advisor by Lippincott Williams & Wilkins.)

shuffling gait and the tendency to lean forward. The patient is taught to concentrate on walking erect, to watch the horizon, and to use a wide-based gait (i.e., walking with the feet separated). A conscious effort must be made to swing the arms, raise the feet while walking, and use a heel–toe placement of the feet with long strides. The patient is advised to practice walking to marching music or to the sound of a ticking metronome because this provides sensory reinforcement. Breathing exercises while walking helps to move the rib cage and to aerate parts of the lungs. Frequent rest periods aid in preventing frustration and fatigue.

Enhancing Self-Care Activities

Environmental modifications are necessary to compensate for functional disabilities (removing scatter rugs, installing bathroom handrails, ensuring good lighting, etc.). Patients may have severe mobility problems that make normal activities impossible. Adaptive or assistive devices may be useful. A hospital bed at home with bedside rails, an overbed frame with a trapeze, or a rope tied to the foot of the bed can provide assistance in pulling up without help. An occupational

therapist can evaluate the patient's needs in the home, make recommendations regarding adaptive devices, and teach the patient and caregiver how to improvise.

Improving Bowel Elimination

The patient may have severe problems with constipation. Among the factors causing constipation are weakness of the muscles used in defecation, lack of exercise, inadequate fluid intake, and decreased autonomic nervous system activity. The medications used for the treatment of the disease also inhibit normal intestinal secretions. A regular bowel routine may be established by encouraging the patient to set a specific time of day to sit on the toilet without distractions, consciously increase fluid intake, and eat foods with moderate fiber content. Laxatives should be avoided. A raised toilet seat is useful because the patient has difficulty in moving from a standing to a sitting position.

Improving Nutrition

Patients may have difficulty maintaining their weight. Eating becomes a very slow process, requiring concentration due to a dry mouth from medications and difficulty chewing and swallowing. These patients are at risk for aspiration because of impaired swallowing and the accumulation of saliva. They may be unaware that they are aspirating; subsequently, bronchopneumonia may develop.

Monitoring weight on a weekly basis indicates whether caloric intake is adequate. Supplemental feedings increase caloric intake. As the disease progresses, a nasogastric tube or percutaneous endoscopic gastroscopy may be necessary to maintain adequate nutrition. A dietitian can be consulted regarding nutritional needs.

An electric warming tray keeps food hot and allows the patient to rest during the prolonged time that it may take to eat. Special utensils also assist at mealtime. A plate that is stabilized, a nonspill cup, and eating utensils with built-up handles are useful self-help devices. The occupational therapist can assist in identifying appropriate adaptive devices.

Enhancing Swallowing

Swallowing difficulties are common in PD, and may be associated with poor head control, tongue tremor, hesitancy in initiating swallowing, difficulty in shaping food into a bolus, and disturbances in pharyngeal motility. To offset these problems, the patient should sit in an upright position during mealtime. A semisolid diet with thick liquids is easier to swallow than solids; thin liquids should be avoided. Thinking through the swallowing sequence is helpful. The patient is taught to place the food on the tongue, close the lips and teeth, lift the tongue up and then back, and swallow. The patient is encouraged to chew first on one side of the mouth and then on the other. To control the buildup of saliva, the patient is reminded to hold the head upright and make a conscious effort to swallow.

Improving Communication

Speech disorders are present in most patients with PD. Their low-pitched, monotonous, soft speech requires that they make a conscious effort to speak slowly, with deliberate attention to what they are saying. The patient is reminded to face the listener, exaggerate the pronunciation of words, speak in short sentences, and take a few deep breaths before speaking. A speech therapist may be helpful in designing speech improvement exercises and assisting the family and health care personnel to develop and use a method of communication that meets the patient's needs. A small electronic amplifier is helpful if the patient has difficulty being heard.

Supporting Coping Abilities

Support can be given by encouraging the patient and pointing out that activities will be maintained through active participation. A combination of physiotherapy, psychotherapy, medication therapy, and support group participation may help reduce the depression that often occurs.

Patients often feel embarrassed, apathetic, inadequate, bored, and lonely. These feelings may be due, in part, to physical slowness and the great effort that even small tasks require. The patient is assisted and encouraged to set achievable goals (e.g., improvement of mobility).

Because PD can lead to withdrawal and depression, patients must be active participants in their therapeutic program, including social and recreational events. A planned program of activity throughout the day prevents too much daytime sleeping as well as disinterest and apathy.

Every effort should be made to encourage patients to carry out the tasks involved in meeting their own daily needs and to remain independent. Doing things for the patient merely to save time undermines the basic goal of improving coping abilities and promoting a positive self-concept.

ALZHEIMER DISEASE

Alzheimer disease (AD) is the most common type of dementia. This disease is a progressive, irreversible, degenerative neurologic disease that begins insidiously and is characterized by gradual losses of cognitive function and disturbances in behavior and affect. Although AD can occur in people as young as 40 years of age, it is uncommon before 65 years of age. AD can be classified into two types: familial, or early-onset AD, and sporadic, or late-onset AD. Familial AD is rare, accounting for only 5% to 10% of all cases, and is frequently associated with genetic mutations (four susceptible genes have been identified). It occurs in middle-aged adults. If family members have at least one other relative with AD, then there is a familial component, which nonspecifically includes both environmental triggers and genetic determinants. Sporadic AD generally occurs in people older than 65 years of age, and it has no obvious pattern of inheritance.

Pathophysiology

Specific neuropathologic and biochemical changes are found in patients with AD. These include neurofibrillary tangles (tangled masses of nonfunctioning neurons) and senile or neuritic plaques (deposits of amyloid protein, part of a larger protein called amyloid precursor protein [APP]) in the brain. The neuronal damage occurs primarily in the cerebral cortex and results in brain atrophy. Similar changes are found in the normal brain tissue of older adults, but to a lesser extent. Cells that use the neurotransmitter acetylcholine are those principally affected by AD. Biochemically, the enzyme active in producing acetylcholine, which is specifically involved in memory processing, is decreased.

Clinical Manifestations and Assessment

In the early stages of AD, forgetfulness and subtle memory loss occur. Patients may experience small difficulties in work or social activities but have adequate cognitive function to hide the loss and function independently. Depression may occur. With further progression of AD, the deficits can no longer be concealed. Forgetfulness is manifested in many daily actions; patients may lose their ability to recognize familiar faces, places, and objects, and they may become lost in a familiar environment. They may repeat the same stories because they forget that they have already told them. Trying to reason with people with AD and using reality **orientation** only increases their anxiety without increasing function. Conversation becomes difficult, and word-finding difficulties occur. The ability to formulate concepts and think abstractly disappears; for example, a patient can interpret a proverb only in concrete terms. Patients are often unable to recognize the consequences of their actions and, therefore, will exhibit impulsive behavior. For example, on a hot day, a patient may decide to wade in the city fountain fully clothed. Patients have difficulty with everyday activities, such as operating simple appliances and handling money.

Personality changes are also usually evident. Patients may become depressed, suspicious, paranoid, hostile, and even combative. Progression of the disease intensifies the symptoms: speaking skills deteriorate to nonsense syllables, agitation and physical activity increase, and patients may wander at night. Eventually, assistance is needed for most ADLs, including eating and toileting, because dysphagia and incontinence develop. The late stages, in which patients are usually immobile and require total care, may last months or years. Occasionally, patients may recognize family members or caregivers. Death occurs as a result of complications, such as pneumonia, malnutrition, or dehydration.

A definitive diagnosis of AD is made based on meeting the clinical criteria and histologic evidence based on examination of brain tissue obtained from biopsy or autopsy. The most important goal is to rule out other causes of dementia or reversible causes of confusion, such as other types of dementia, depression, delirium, alcohol or drug abuse, or inappropriate drug dosage or drug toxicity. Refer to Table 46-3 for a summary of differences between AD and delirium.

The health history—including medical history, family history, social and cultural history, and medication history—and the physical examination, including functional and mental health status, are essential to the diagnosis of probable AD. Diagnostic tests, including complete blood count, chemistry profile, and vitamin B_{12} and thyroid hormone levels, as well as screening with EEG, CT, MRI, and examination of the CSF may all refute or support a diagnosis of probable AD.

Depression can closely mimic early-stage AD and coexists in many patients. A depression scale is helpful in screening for underlying depression. Tests of cognitive function, such as the Mini-Mental Status Examination and the clock-drawing test, are useful for screening. CT scans and MRIs of the brain are useful for excluding hematoma, brain tumor, stroke, normal-pressure hydrocephalus, and atrophy but are not reliable in making a definitive diagnosis of AD. Infections, physiologic disturbances such as hypothyroidism, PD, and vitamin B_{12} deficiency can cause cognitive impairment that may be misdiagnosed as AD. Biochemical abnormalities can be excluded through examination of the blood and CSF, but the findings are not sufficiently specific to make the diagnosis. AD is a diagnosis of exclusion, and a diagnosis

TABLE 46-3 Summary of Differences Between Alzheimer Disease and Delirium

	Alzheimer Disease (AD)	Delirium
Etiology	Familial (genetic [chromosomes 1, 14, 21]) Sporadic	Drug toxicity and interactions; acute disease; trauma; chronic disease exacerbation Fluid and electrolyte disorder
Risk factors	Advanced age; genetics (apoE4 gene)	Preexisting cognitive impairment
Occurrence	50–60% of dementias	20% of hospitalized older people
Onset	Slow, progressive	Rapid, acute onset A harbinger of acute medical illness (e.g., pneumonia, urinary tract infection, myocardial infarction, pain)
Age of onset (years)	Early onset AD: 30–65 years of age Late onset AD: 65+ years of age Most commonly: 85+ years of age	Any age but predominantly in older people (over 65 years of age) (Fong, Tulebaev, & Inouye, 2009).
Gender	Males and females equally	Males and females equally
Course	Chronic, irreversible; progressive, regular, downhill	Acute
Duration	2–20 years	Lasts 1 day to 1 month
Symptom progress	Onset insidious. *Early:* Mild and subtle *Middle and late:* Intensified Progression to death (infection or malnutrition)	Symptoms are fully reversible with adequate treatment; can progress to chronicity or death if underlying condition is ignored.
Mood	Early depression (30%)	Variable
Speech/language	Speech remains intact until late in disease *Early:* Mild anomia (cannot name objects); deficits progress until speech lacks meaning; echoes and repeats words and sounds; mutism	Fluctuating; often cannot concentrate long enough to speak
Physical signs	*Early:* No motor deficits *Middle:* Apraxia (70%) (cannot perform purposeful movement) *Late:* Dysarthria (impaired speech) *End stage:* Loss of all voluntary activity; positive neurologic signs	Signs and symptoms of underlying disease
Orientation	Becomes lost in familiar places (topographic disorientation) Has difficulty drawing three-dimensional objects (visual and spatial disorientation) Disorientation to time, place, and person—with disease progression	May fluctuate between lucidity and complete disorientation to time, place, and person

	Alzheimer Disease (AD)	Delirium
Memory	Loss is an early sign of AD; loss of recent memory is soon followed by progressive decline in remote memory as well	Impaired recent and remote memory; may fluctuate between lucidity and confusion
Personality	Apathy, indifference, irritability Early disease—social behavior intact; hides cognitive deficits Advanced disease—disengages from activity and relationships; suspicious; paranoid delusions caused by memory loss; aggressive; catastrophic reactions	Fluctuating; cannot focus attention to converse; alarmed by symptoms (when lucid); hallucinations; paranoid
Functional status, activities of daily living	Poor judgment in everyday activities; has progressive decline in ability to handle money, use telephone, function in home and workplace	Impaired
Attention span	Distractable; short attention span	Highly impaired; cannot maintain or shift attention
Psychomotor activity	Wandering, hyperactivity, pacing, restlessness, agitation	Variable; alternates between high agitation, hyperactivity, restlessness, and lethargy
Sleep–wake cycle	Often impaired; wandering and agitation at nighttime	Takes brief naps throughout day and night

of probable AD is made when the medical history, physical examination, and laboratory tests have excluded all known causes of other dementias.

Medical and Nursing Management

The primary goal in the medical management of AD is to manage the cognitive and behavioral symptoms. There is no cure and no way to slow the progression of the disease. Cholinesterase inhibitors, such as donepezil hydrochloride (Aricept), rivastigmine tartrate (Exelon), and galantamine hydrobromide (Reminyl), enhance acetylcholine uptake in the brain, thus maintaining memory skills for a period of time. The drug memantine (Namenda) is an N-methyl-D-aspartate receptor antagonist that is thought to interfere with glutaminergic overstimulation. Cognitive ability improves within 6 to 12 months of therapy, but cessation of the medications results in cognitive decline commensurate with disease progression.

Behavioral problems, such as agitation and psychosis, can be managed by behavioral and psychosocial therapies. Providing an environment that is controlled and stable can help with behavior problems. Pharmacologic treatment for psychosis in patients with AD can be complicated due to a black box warning by the FDA that both conventional and atypical antipsychotics can increase the risk of death (Madhusoodanan & Ting, 2014). Assessment and diagnosis of depression should occur during the initial evaluation. Associated depression can be treated with antidepressants.

Nursing interventions for AD are aimed at promoting patient function and independence for as long as possible. Other important goals include promoting the patient's physical safety, promoting independence in self-care activities,

reducing anxiety and agitation, improving communication, providing for socialization and intimacy, promoting adequate nutrition, promoting balanced activity and rest, and supporting and educating family caregivers.

Supporting Cognitive Function

Because dementia of any type is degenerative and progressive, patients display a decline in cognitive function over time. In the early phase of AD, minimal cueing and guidance may be all that are needed for the patient to function fairly independently for a number of years. However, as the patient's cognitive ability declines, family members must provide more and more assistance and supervision. A calm, predictable environment helps people with AD interpret their surroundings and activities. Environmental stimuli are limited, and a regular routine is established. A quiet, pleasant manner of speaking, clear and simple explanations, and use of memory aids and cues help minimize confusion and disorientation and give patients a sense of security. Prominently displayed clocks and calendars may enhance orientation to time. Color-coding the doorway may help patients who have difficulty locating their room. Active participation may help patients maintain cognitive, functional, and social interaction abilities for a longer period.

Promoting Physical Safety

A safe home environment allows the patient to move about as freely as possible and relieves the family of constant worry about safety. To prevent falls and other injuries, all obvious hazards are removed and hand rails are installed. A hazard-free environment allows the patient maximum independence and a sense of autonomy. Adequate lighting, especially in halls, stairs, and bathrooms, is necessary. Night lights are helpful, particularly if the patient has increased confusion at night (**sundowning**). Driving is prohibited, and smoking is allowed only with supervision. The patient may have a short attention span and be forgetful. Wandering behavior can often be reduced by gentle persuasion or distraction. Restraints should be avoided because they increase agitation. Doors leading from the house must be secured. Outside the home, all activities must be supervised to protect the patient, and the patient should wear an identification bracelet or neck chain in case he or she becomes separated from the caregiver.

Promoting Independence in Self-Care Activities

Pathophysiologic changes in the brain make it difficult for people with AD to maintain physical independence. Patients should be assisted to remain functionally independent for as long as possible. One way to do this is to simplify daily activities by organizing them into short, achievable steps so that the patient experiences a sense of accomplishment. Frequently, occupational therapists can suggest ways to simplify tasks or recommend adaptive equipment. Direct patient supervision is sometimes necessary, but maintaining personal dignity and autonomy is important for people with AD, who should be encouraged to make choices when appropriate and to participate in self-care activities as much as possible.

Reducing Anxiety and Agitation

Despite profound cognitive losses, patients are sometimes aware of their diminishing abilities. Patients need constant emotional support that reinforces a positive self-image. When losses of skills occur, goals are adjusted to fit the patient's declining ability.

The environment should be kept familiar and noise-free. Excitement and confusion can be upsetting and may precipitate a combative, agitated state known as a *catastrophic reaction* (overreaction to excessive stimulation). The patient may respond by screaming, crying, or becoming abusive (physically or verbally); this may be the person's only way of expressing an inability to cope with the environment. When this occurs, it is important to remain calm and unhurried. Forcing the patient to proceed with the activity only increases the agitation. It is better to postpone the activity until later, even to another day. Frequently, the patient quickly forgets what triggered the reaction. Measures such as moving to a familiar environment, listening to music, stroking, rocking, or distraction may quiet the patient. Structuring activity is also helpful. Becoming familiar with a particular patient's predicted responses to certain stressors helps caregivers avoid similar situations.

Many older people with AD who have progressed to the late stages of the disease typically reside in nursing homes and are predominantly cared for by nurses' aides. Dementia education for caregivers is essential to minimize patient agitation and can be effectively taught by advanced practice nurses.

Improving Communication

To promote the patient's interpretation of messages, the nurse should remain unhurried and reduce noises and distractions. Use of clear, easy-to-understand sentences to convey messages is essential because patients frequently forget the meaning of words or have difficulty organizing and expressing thoughts. In the earlier stages of AD, lists and simple written instructions that serve as reminders may be helpful. In later stages, the patient may be able to point to an object or use nonverbal language to communicate. Tactile stimuli, such as hugs or hand pats, are usually interpreted as signs of affection, concern, and security.

Providing for Socialization and Intimacy Needs

Because socialization with friends can be comforting, visits, letters, and phone calls are encouraged. Visits should be brief and nonstressful; limiting visitors to one or two at a time helps reduce overstimulation. Recreation is important, and people with AD are encouraged to enjoy simple activities. Realistic goals for activities that provide satisfaction are appropriate. Hobbies and activities, such as walking, exercising, and socializing, can improve the quality of life. The nonjudgmental friendliness of a pet may provide stimulation, comfort, and contentment. Care of plants or of a pet can also be satisfying and an outlet for energy.

AD does not eliminate the need for intimacy. Patients and their spouses may continue to enjoy sexual activity. Spouses should be encouraged to talk about any sexual concerns, and sexual counseling may be necessary. Simple expressions of love, such as touching and holding, are often meaningful.

Promoting Adequate Nutrition

Mealtime can be a pleasant social occasion or a time of upset and distress, and it should be kept simple and calm, without confrontations. Patients prefer familiar foods that look appetizing and taste good. To avoid any "playing" with food, one dish is offered at a time. Food is cut into small pieces to prevent choking. Liquids may be easier to swallow if they are converted to gelatin. Hot food and beverages are served warm, and the temperature of the foods should be checked to prevent burns.

When lack of coordination interferes with self-feeding, adaptive equipment is helpful. Some patients may do well eating with a spoon or with their fingers. If this is the case, an apron or a smock, rather than a bib, is used to protect clothing. As deficits progress, it may be necessary to feed the patient. Forgetfulness, disinterest, dental problems, lack of coordination, overstimulation, and choking may all serve as barriers to good nutrition and hydration.

Promoting Balanced Activity and Rest

Many patients with AD exhibit sleep disturbances, wandering, and behaviors that may be considered inappropriate. These behaviors are most likely to occur when there are unmet underlying physical or psychological needs. Caregivers must identify the needs of patients who are exhibiting these behaviors because further health decline may occur if the source of the problem is not corrected. Adequate sleep and physical exercise are essential. If sleep is interrupted or the patient cannot fall asleep, music, warm milk, or a back rub may help the patient to relax. During the day, patients should be encouraged to participate in exercise because a regular pattern of activity and rest enhances nighttime sleep. Long periods of daytime sleeping are discouraged.

Caregiver Burden

The emotional burden on the families of patients with AD is enormous. The physical health of the patient is often very stable, and the mental degeneration is gradual. Family members are faced with numerous difficult decisions (e.g., when the patient should stop driving, when to assume responsibility for the patient's financial affairs). Aggression and hostility exhibited by the patient are often misunderstood by families or caregivers, who feel unappreciated, frustrated, and angry. Feelings of guilt, nervousness, and worry contribute to caregiver fatigue, depression, and family dysfunction.

In some cases, caregivers themselves can become so fatigued as a result of the stress of caregiving that self-neglect or neglect or abuse of the patient can occur. This has been documented in home situations as well as in institutions. Respite care is a commonly provided service in which caregivers can get away from the home for short periods while someone else tends to the needs of the patient.

AMYOTROPHIC LATERAL SCLEROSIS

Amyotrophic lateral sclerosis (ALS) is a degenerative disease characterized by the loss of both upper and lower motor neurons. As motor neuron cells die, the muscle fibers that they supply undergo atrophic changes. Causes of ALS include multiple genetic and environmental factors (Hickey, 2014b). It is estimated that 90% of cases of ALS occur sporadically, but 5% to 10% are familial, usually with an autosomal dominant mode of inheritance (Shaw, 2016).

Clinical Manifestations and Assessment

Clinical manifestations depend on the location of the affected motor neurons because specific neurons activate specific muscle fibers. The chief symptoms are fatigue and limb weakness. There is a gradual onset of asymmetric, progressive weakness. Upper extremity onset causes reduced dexterity, and lower extremity symptoms may be tripping, falling, and changes in gait (Hickey, 2014b). Spasticity usually is present, and the deep tendon stretch reflexes become

brisk and overactive. Usually, the function of the anal and bladder sphincters remains intact because the spinal nerves that control muscles of the rectum and urinary bladder are not affected.

In about 25% of patients, weakness starts in the muscles supplied by the cranial nerves, and difficulty in talking, swallowing, and, ultimately, breathing occurs. When the patient ingests liquids, soft palate and upper esophageal weakness cause the liquid to be regurgitated through the nose. Weakness of the posterior tongue and palate impairs the ability to laugh, cough, or even blow the nose. If bulbar muscles are impaired, speaking and swallowing are progressively difficult, and aspiration becomes a risk. The voice assumes a nasal sound, and articulation becomes so disrupted that speech is unintelligible. Some emotional lability may be present, but intellectual function is not impaired. Eventually, respiratory function is compromised.

The prognosis generally is based on the area of CNS involvement and the speed with which the disease progresses. Death usually occurs as a result of infection, respiratory failure, or aspiration.

ALS is diagnosed on the basis of the signs and symptoms because no clinical or laboratory tests are specific for this disease. An electromyogram (EMG) will demonstrate fibrillations, which are signs of denervation, muscle wasting, and atrophy (Shaw, 2016). An MRI scan may show high signal intensity in the corticospinal tracts; this differentiates ALS from a multifocal motor neuropathy.

Medical and Nursing Management

No specific therapy exists for ALS. The main focus of management is on interventions to maintain or improve function, well-being, and quality of life.

Most patients with ALS are managed at home and in the community, with hospitalization for acute problems. The most common reasons for hospitalization are dehydration and malnutrition, pneumonia, and respiratory failure; recognizing these problems at an early stage in the illness allows for the development of preventive strategies.

Riluzole (Rilutek), a glutamate antagonist, is the only drug approved by the FDA. A dose of 100 mg/day (50 mg BID) provides a modest improvement in the survival rate (additional 3 months of survival) (Shaw, 2016). The action of riluzole is not clear, but its pharmacologic properties suggest that it may have a neuroprotective effect in the early stages of ALS. Liver function tests should be monitored at baseline and monthly.

Symptomatic treatment and rehabilitative measures are employed to support the patient. Baclofen (Lioresal), dantrolene sodium (Dantrium), or diazepam (Valium) may be useful for patients troubled by spasticity, which causes pain and interferes with self-care.

A patient experiencing problems with aspiration and swallowing may require enteral feeding. The American Academy of Neurology practice guidelines suggest the placement of a percutaneous endoscopic gastrostomy tube before the forced vital capacity drops below 50% of the predicted value.

> ### Nursing Alert
> *The nurse observes for paradoxical movement of the abdominal wall during inspiration, SOB, and orthopnea, which may be associated with diaphragmatic weakness. Complaints of interrupted sleep, morning headaches, anorexia, and daytime somnolence may reflect nocturnal retention of carbon dioxide.*

Respiratory management is guided by the results of vital capacity and negative inspiratory force parameters that are measured at regular intervals. The use of noninvasive positive-pressure ventilation (NIPPV) is started as indicated by these measurements. As the disease progresses, the NIPPV will become inadequate, and, if the decision is made to have life prolonged with advanced technology, the patient can proceed to tracheotomy and invasive ventilation (Shaw, 2016).

Decisions about life-support measures are made by the patient and family and should be based on a thorough understanding of the disease, the prognosis, and the implications of initiating such therapy. Patients are encouraged to complete an advance directive or "living will" to preserve their autonomy in decision-making.

DEGENERATIVE DISK DISEASE

Low back pain is a significant public health disorder in the United States, although its prevalence is difficult to quantify. Acute low back pain lasts less than 3 months, whereas chronic or degenerative disease has a duration of 3 months or longer. It is estimated that disk disease, such as protrusion, accounts for only 5% of all low back problems, whereas degenerative changes are commonly associated with low back pain.

Pathophysiology

The intervertebral disk is a cartilaginous plate that forms a cushion between the vertebral bodies (see Fig. 46-10A). This tough, fibrous material is incorporated in a capsule. A ball-like cushion in the center of the disk is called the *nucleus pulposus*. In herniation of the intervertebral disk (ruptured disk), the nucleus of the disk protrudes into the annulus (the fibrous ring around the disk), with subsequent nerve compression. Protrusion or rupture of the nucleus pulposus usually is preceded by degenerative changes that occur with aging. Loss of protein polysaccharides in the disk decreases the water content of the nucleus pulposus. The development of radiating cracks in the annulus weakens resistance to nucleus herniation. After trauma (falls and repeated minor stresses such as lifting incorrectly), the cartilage may be injured.

For most patients, the immediate symptoms of trauma are short-lived, and those resulting from injury to the disk do not appear for months or years. Then, with degeneration in the disk, the capsule pushes back into the spinal canal, or it may rupture and allow the nucleus pulposus to be pushed back against the dural sac or against a spinal nerve as it emerges from the spinal column (see Fig. 46-10B). This sequence produces pain due to **radiculopathy** (pressure in the area of distribution of the involved nerve endings). Continued pressure may produce degenerative changes in the involved nerve, such as changes in sensation and deep tendon reflexes.

Clinical Manifestations and Assessment

Common clinical manifestations are pain, motor and sensory deficits, and alterations of reflexes. A neurologic examination is carried out to determine whether motor, sensory, or reflex impairment from root compression is present and to provide a baseline for future assessment.

MRI has become the diagnostic tool of choice for localizing even small disk protrusions, particularly for lumbar spine disease. If the clinical symptoms are not consistent with the

FIGURE 46-10 **A.** Normal lumbar spine vertebrae, invertebral disks, and spinal nerve root. **B.** Ruptured vertebral disk.

pathology seen on MRI, then CT scanning and myelography are performed. EMG may be used to localize the specific spinal nerve roots involved.

Medical and Nursing Management

Most cases may improve with conservative treatment consisting of 1 to 2 days of bed rest, nonsteroidal anti-inflammatory drugs (NSAIDs), exercise regimens, epidural steroids, and patient education (Strayer & Hickey, 2014).

Surgery is usually indicated if the degenerative disk is causing compression on the spinal cord or if the patient has radiculopathy that fails conservative treatment. The most common procedure is a decompression laminectomy, which is the removal of the laminar portion of the vertebrae to gain access to the spinal cord.

INTERVERTEBRAL DISK HERNIATION

CERVICAL SPINE

The cervical spine is subjected to stresses that result from disk degeneration (due to aging, occupational stresses) and **spondylosis** (degenerative changes occurring in a disk and adjacent vertebral bodies with bulging and, occasionally, herniation). Cervical disk degeneration may lead to lesions that can cause damage to the spinal cord and its roots.

Clinical Manifestations and Assessment

A cervical disk herniation usually occurs at the C5–C6 and C6–C7 interspaces. Pain and stiffness may occur in the neck, the top of the shoulders, and the region of the scapulae. Sometimes patients interpret these signs as symptoms of heart trouble or bursitis. Pain may also occur in the upper extremities and head, accompanied by **paresthesia** (tingling or a "pins and needles" sensation) and numbness of the upper extremities. Cervical MRI usually confirms the diagnosis.

Medical and Nursing Management

The goals of treatment are to rest and immobilize the cervical spine to give the soft tissues time to heal and to reduce inflammation in the supporting tissues and the affected nerve roots in the cervical spine. Bed rest (usually 1 to 2 days) is important because it eliminates the stress of gravity and relieves the cervical spine of the need to support the head. It also reduces inflammation and edema in soft tissues around the disk, relieving pressure on the nerve roots. Proper positioning on a firm mattress may bring dramatic relief from pain.

The cervical spine may be rested and immobilized by a cervical collar. A collar allows maximal opening of the intervertebral foramina and holds the head in a neutral or slightly flexed position. The patient may have to wear the collar 24 hours a day during the acute phase. The skin under the collar is inspected for irritation. After the patient is free of pain, cervical isometric exercises are begun to strengthen the neck muscles.

Analgesic agents are often necessary to manage pain (NSAIDs, acetaminophen). Narcotics are reserved for severe pain (e.g., hydrocodone/tylenol). Sedatives may be administered to control the anxiety that is often associated with cervical disk disease. Muscle relaxants (cyclobenzaprine [Flexeril], methocarbamol [Robaxin], metaxalone [Skelaxin]) are administered to interrupt muscle spasm and to promote comfort. NSAIDs (aspirin, ibuprofen [Motrin, Advil], naproxen [Naprosyn, Anaprox]) or corticosteroids are prescribed to treat the inflammation that usually occurs in the affected nerve roots and supporting tissues. Occasionally, a corticosteroid is injected into the epidural space for relief of radicular (spinal nerve root) pain. Hot, moist compresses (for 10 to 20 minutes) applied to the back of the neck several times daily increase blood flow to the muscles and help relax the patient and reduce muscle spasm.

Surgical excision of the herniated disk may be necessary if there is a significant neurologic deficit, progression of the deficit, evidence of cord compression, or pain that either worsens or fails to improve. A cervical discectomy, with or without fusion, may be performed to alleviate symptoms. An anterior surgical approach may be used through a transverse incision to remove disk material that has herniated into the spinal canal and foramina, or a posterior approach may be used at the appropriate level of the cervical spine. Potential complications with the anterior approach include carotid or vertebral artery injury, recurrent laryngeal nerve dysfunction, esophageal perforation, and airway obstruction. Complications of the posterior approach include damage to the nerve root or the spinal cord due to retraction or contusion of either of these structures, resulting in weakness of muscles supplied by the nerve root or cord.

Microsurgery, such as endoscopic microdiscectomy, may be performed in selected patients through a small incision and using magnification techniques. The patient who undergoes microsurgery usually has less tissue trauma and pain and consequently a shorter hospital stay than after conventional surgical approaches.

> **Nursing Alert**
> *Although NSAIDs are often prescribed for cervical disk herniation, when surgery involving bone fusion is considered, NSAIDs are often discontinued because they can interfere with bone healing. The nurse should collaborate with the health care provider to instruct the patient to avoid these drugs prior to and after surgery.*

LUMBAR SPINE

The most common site of lumbar disk herniation occurs at the L4–L5 or L5–S1 levels (Strayer & Hickey, 2014). A herniated lumbar disk causes low back pain accompanied by varying degrees of motor and sensory impairment.

Clinical Manifestations and Assessment

The patient complains of low back pain with muscle spasms, followed by radiation of the pain into one hip and down into the leg (sciatica). Pain is aggravated by actions that increase intraspinal fluid pressure, such as bending, lifting, or straining (as in sneezing or coughing), and usually is relieved by bed rest. Usually there is some type of postural deformity because pain causes an alteration of the normal spinal mechanics. If the patient lies on the back and attempts to raise a leg in a straight position, pain radiates into the leg; this maneuver, called the *straight leg–raising test*, stretches the sciatic nerve. Additional signs include muscle weakness, alterations in tendon reflexes, and sensory loss.

The diagnosis of lumbar disk disease is based on the history and physical findings and the use of imaging techniques, such as MRI, CT, and myelography. Although MRI has largely replaced myelography (fluoroscopy and an injection of contrast material to evaluate the spinal cord, nerve roots and spinal lining), myelography still may be used occasionally to provide information about the spinal cord and nerve roots.

Medical and Nursing Management

The objectives of treatment are to relieve pain, slow disease progression, and increase the patient's functional ability. Bed rest for patients with severe pain in the lumbar region is limited to a short course (2 days or less), followed by resumption of light activity (Strayer & Hickey, 2014).

Strategies for increasing the patient's functional ability include weight reduction, physical therapy, and biofeedback. Mobilization, walking short distances, is recommended. When symptoms subside, stretching, strengthening, and exercise programs should be initiated.

Because muscle spasm is prominent during the acute phase, muscle relaxants are used. NSAIDs and systemic corticosteroids may be administered to counter the inflammation that usually occurs in the supporting tissues and the affected nerve roots. Moist heat and massage help to relax muscles.

Most patients fear surgery on any part of the spine and therefore need explanations about the surgery and reassurance that it will not weaken the back. When data are being collected for the health history, any reports of pain, paresthesia, or muscle spasm are recorded to provide a baseline for comparison after surgery. Preoperative assessment also includes an evaluation of movement of the extremities, as well as bladder and bowel function. To facilitate the postoperative turning procedure, the patient is taught to turn as a unit (called *logrolling*) as part of the preoperative preparation (Fig. 46-11). Before surgery, the patient is also encouraged to take deep breaths, cough, and perform muscle-setting exercises to maintain muscle tone.

FIGURE 46-11 Before the patient undergoes spinal surgery, the logrolling technique that will be used for turning the patient should be demonstrated. The patient's arms will be crossed and the spine aligned. To avoid twisting the spine, the patient's head, shoulders, knees, and hips are turned at the same time that the patient rolls over like a log. When in a side-lying position, the patient's back, buttocks, and legs are supported with pillows.

In the lumbar region, surgical treatment includes lumbar disk excision through a posterolateral laminotomy and the techniques of microdiscectomy and percutaneous discectomy. In microdiscectomy, an operating microscope is used to visualize the offending disk and compressed nerve roots; it permits a small incision (2.5 cm [1 in]) and minimal blood loss and takes about 30 minutes of operating time. In general, the hospital stay is short, and the patient makes a rapid recovery. Percutaneous discectomy is an alternative treatment for herniated intervertebral disks of the lumbar spine. One approach in current use is through a 2.5-cm (1-in) incision just above the iliac crest. A tube, trocar, or cannula is inserted under x-ray guidance through the retroperitoneal space to the involved disk space. Special instruments are used to remove the disk. The operating time is about 15 minutes. Blood loss and postoperative pain are minimal, and usually the patient is discharged within 2 days after surgery. The disadvantage of this procedure is the possibility of damage to structures in the surgical pathway.

Complications that could occur after surgery include herniation relapse, arachnoiditis (inflammation of the arachnoid), neuritis (inflammation of a nerve), or failed disk syndrome (generalized term to describe continued **pain after surgery**). Herniation relapse may occur at the same level or elsewhere so the patient may become a candidate for another disk procedure. Arachnoiditis may occur after surgery (and after myelography [if used]); it involves an insidious onset of diffuse, frequently burning pain in the lower back, radiating into the buttocks. Disk excision can leave adhesions and scarring around the spinal nerves and dura, which then produce inflammatory changes that create chronic neuritis and neurofibrosis. Disk surgery may relieve pressure on the spinal nerves, but it does not reverse the effects of neural injury and scarring and the pain that results.

Because postoperative neurologic deficits may occur from nerve root injury, the motor strength and sensation of the lower extremities are evaluated at specified intervals, along with the color and temperature of the legs and sensation of the toes. Assessing the patient after surgery, the nurse checks vital signs frequently, and the wound is inspected for hemorrhage because vascular injury is a complication of disk surgery. It is important to assess for urinary retention, another sign of neurologic deterioration.

In discectomy with fusion, the patient has an additional surgical incision if bone fragments were taken from the iliac crest or fibula to serve as wedges in the spine. The recovery period is longer than for those patients who underwent discectomy without spinal fusion because bony union must take place.

To position the patient, a pillow is placed under the head, and the knee rest is elevated slightly to relax the back muscles. When the patient is lying on one side, however, extreme knee flexion must be avoided. The patient is encouraged to move from side to side to relieve pressure and is reassured that no injury will result from moving. When the patient is ready to turn, the bed is placed in a flat position and a pillow is placed between the patient's legs. The patient turns as a unit (logrolls) without twisting the back. To get out of bed, the patient lies on one side while pushing up to a sitting position. At the same time, the nurse or family member eases the patient's legs over the side of the bed. Coming to a sitting or standing posture is accomplished in one long, smooth motion. Most patients walk to the bathroom on the same day as the surgery. Sitting is discouraged except for defecation.

CHAPTER REVIEW

Critical Thinking Exercises

1. Your 40-year-old patient has MG. Her condition has been stable and she has been able to manage without assistance, but she reports increasing weakness and fatigue. What nursing assessments and interventions are warranted for her? What discharge plans are indicated if she is to return home to the care of her family? How would your discharge planning change if she lived alone in an apartment on the third floor of a building without an elevator?

2. Your patient has been admitted to the intensive care unit with a diagnosis of possible Guillain–Barré syndrome. Identify the priorities of assessment for this patient and the nursing and medical interventions that you would anticipate. What medications should you have readily available for this patient?

3. A 50-year-old man newly diagnosed with Parkinson disease asks what type of medication he will be given. What are the possible medications that will be used to treat his disease, and the long-term effects of each? How would your discharge teaching targeted toward medications be modified if the patient lives alone?

NCLEX-Style Review Questions

1. While assessing a client with Parkinson disease, the nurse identifies bradykinesia when the client exhibits which symptom?
   a. Muscle flaccidity
   b. An intention tremor
   c. Paralysis of the limbs
   d. Slow spontaneous movement

2. What is the most common initial symptom that a nurse might expect a client with MS to complain about?
   a. Diarrhea
   b. Headaches
   c. Skin infections
   d. Visual disturbances

3. A client who has GB asks, "Will I ever get better?" Which response would be the most appropriate answer by the nurse?
   a. "You'll notice your strength will improve each day."
   b. "We are doing everything we can to provide the best care."
   c. "You seem concerned about getting better. What do you think?"
   d. "Your chances for recovery are very good, but recovery is slow."

4. What manifestations will the nurse observe in the patient undergoing a tonic–clonic seizure?
   a. Jerking in one extremity that spreads gradually to adjacent areas
   b. Vacant staring and abrupt cessation of all activity
   c. Facial grimaces, patting motions, and lip smacking
   d. Loss of consciousness, body stiffening, and violent muscle contractions

5. The nurse knows that the signs and symptoms of meningeal irritation include which of the following? Select all that apply.
   a. Nuchal rigidity and headache
   b. Kernig and Brudzinski signs
   c. Aphasia and motor weakness
   d. Photophobia
   e. Ptosis

Try these additional resources, available at **http://thepoint.lww.com/Honan2e**, to enhance your learning and understanding of this chapter:

- NCLEX-Style Student Review Questions
- Journal Articles

REFERENCES AND SELECTED READINGS

References and selected readings associated with this chapter can be found on the website that accompanies the book. Visit **http://thepoint. lww.com/Honan2e** to access the references and other additional resources associated with this chapter.

Nursing Management: Patients with Cerebrovascular Disorders

Karin V. Nyström

Learning Objectives

After reading this chapter you will be able to:

1. Describe the incidence and epidemiology of stroke.
2. Identify mechanisms that affect cerebral blood flow.
3. Describe the pathophysiology of ischemic and hemorrhagic stroke, and transient ischemic attack.
4. Identify risk factors and manifestations of stroke syndromes.
5. Describe collaborative care, drug therapy, and nutritional considerations for patients who have had a stroke.
6. Describe the acute care, rehabilitation, and drug and nutritional considerations for patients recovering from stroke.

Cerebrovascular disorder is an umbrella term that refers to abnormalities of the central nervous system (CNS) affecting normal blood supply to the brain and/or spinal cord. There are many vascular abnormalities affecting cerebral blood flow, but the most common cerebrovascular disorder is stroke. The nurse should be well prepared to recognize stroke symptoms be able to care for patients admitted to an acute care facility with a stroke, and identify the common comorbidities that accompany stroke syndromes. The neurologic condition may be the patient's primary health problem or a secondary diagnosis. As such, nurses must be able to develop a care plan for a stroke patient's recovery that considers both neurologic deficits and potential complications associated with those deficits during both acute recovery and rehabilitation. Additionally, the care plan should include important stroke prevention strategies, such as pharmacotherapies and lifestyle changes applicable to patients who have had a stroke and other patient populations at risk for a cerebrovascular event.

STROKE

It was more than 2,000 years ago that Hippocrates recognized stroke and coined the term "apoplexy" (meaning "struck down with violence" in Greek), which characterized sudden body changes that are manifested in patients who have a stroke, such as unilateral paralysis (Nilsen, 2010). It has been only within the last century that clinicians have understood the pathophysiologic mechanisms to describe stroke types and the potential etiologies of these cerebrovascular disorders. Although patients may present with the sudden onset of neurologic symptoms, usually the etiology of this syndrome is related to chronic disease. An organized and expeditious approach to the management of patients during the acute stroke phase becomes key to reducing the leading adult disability in the United States (2016 stroke statistics).

Incidence

Stroke is currently the fifth leading cause of death in the United States, behind heart disease, cancer, chronic respiratory diseases, and accidents (Centers for Disease Control and Prevention [CDC], 2016). Approximately 800,000 people experience a stroke each year in the United States; 600,000 of these are first events, and approximately 200,000 are recurrent strokes. With about 5 million stroke survivors alive today, stroke is the leading cause of serious, long-term adult disability in the United States (Lloyd-Jones, Brown et al., 2010; AHA, 2015). It is estimated that approximately 90% of stroke survivors are left with some residual deficit. The financial impact of stroke is profound, with estimated direct and indirect costs totaling $33 billion (Mozaffarian, 2015). Although strokes can affect people of all ages, older men are more likely to have strokes and older women more frequently tend to die from their stroke. African Americans have a risk for an ischemic stroke that is three times higher than Caucasians; and Asian patients are at higher risk for a hemorrhagic stroke. These patients are in the same category of populations at higher risk for cardiac events and other vascular diseases. There is also a geographic distinction in this country such that Americans living in the southeastern United States have a higher incidence of stroke—thereby nicknaming this region the "stroke belt."

Despite the numerous national campaign efforts (American Heart/Stroke Association [AHA/ASA], 2017; Payne, Fang, Fogle et al., 2010) to increase stroke awareness over the past three decades, several studies have shown that a majority of people cannot name many of the typical stroke symptoms or do not consider calling 911 in the event that they or a family member are experiencing stroke symptoms (Fussman, Rafferty, Lyon-Callo et al., 2012). Delays in recognizing stroke symptom and in activating the Emergency Medical System limit treatment options and lead to worsening long-term recovery outcomes. The AHA/ASA responded to this gap in awareness and adopted the Stroke Chain of Survival (similar to the Heart Chain of Survival established for cardiac care), implementing a prompt pre-hospital and acute care approach to the evaluation of patients with acute stroke symptoms. Also known as the "7 D's," these components highlight key areas in the recognition and evaluation of a patient suspected of having a stroke to reinforce an efficient method for a rapid approach to acute stroke care (Box 47-1).

Strokes continue to be one of the most common neurologic emergencies, and both community hospitals and large tertiary referral medical centers see a high volume of patients admitted with a stroke-related neurologic diagnosis or patients at risk for stroke. Hospitals today are charged with implementing systems of care to treat stroke patients in the acute phase of their illness and to direct patients and their families to the appropriate rehabilitative program to optimize recovery and functional outcome (Schwamm et al. 2013).

Certified Stroke Centers

In 2003, the Joint Commission launched a disease-specific care certification program for medical facilities committed to using evidence-based clinical practice guidelines for best stroke care. The Joint Commission's Primary Stroke Center certification program was developed in collaboration with the ASA and was based on the 2000 Brain Attack Coalition's "Recommendations for the Establishment of Primary Stroke Centers." In 2011, an update to the recommendation for the establishment of Primary Stroke Centers as an approach to acute stroke care was published to improve the medical care of stroke patients and included criteria such as an acute stroke team, a dedicated stroke unit, written care protocols, supporting laboratory and imaging services, and mandatory continuing education related to strokes (Alberts, Latchaw, & Jagoda, 2011). These recommendations followed the 1996 U.S. Food and Drug Administration (FDA) approval of intravenous tissue plasminogen activator (tPA) for the treatment of acute ischemic stroke (NINDS & Stroke rtPA Stroke Study Work Group, 1995). In the past 20 years, intravenous thrombolytic therapy with alteplase (recombinant tissue-type plasminogen activator or rtPA) has shown to improve outcomes in patients with acute ischemic stroke if treated within 3 to 4.5 hours from stroke onset and when additional eligibility criteria (discussed later in the chapter) are met. Certified stroke centers are mandated to collect data on a series of specific practice components, including selected performance measures to monitor and improve the quality of stroke care. These measures apply to patients hospitalized with either an ischemic or hemorrhagic stroke. Currently, eight stroke performance activities have been endorsed by the National Quality Forum and are supported by The Joint Commission. Although not inclusive of all important aspects of acute stroke care, initial data from these metrics support the efforts to improve quality of care and to predict functional outcome (Smith, Saver, & Alexander, 2014). Table 47-1 outlines the specific stroke performance measures and applicable stroke types.

In the last decade, stroke certification options have expanded to include Acute Stroke Ready Hospital (for small facilities equipped to stabilize and treat acute stroke patients prior to transferring to a higher level of care), Thrombectomy-capable Stroke Center (for facilities that meet Primary Stroke Center criteria and have the capability to perform thrombectomy procedures), and Comprehensive Stroke Centers (for facilities capable of managing multiple complex

---

| BOX 47-1 | **Stroke Chain of Survival: The 7 D's** |

1. **Detection of the onset of signs and symptoms of acute stroke.** Early recognition of the hallmark signs and symptoms of acute stroke is critical to improved patient outcomes.
2. **Dispatch of Emergency Medical Services (EMS) by telephoning 911.** This communication activates EMS systems and ensures prompt EMS response.
3. **Delivery of the patient to a medical facility.** Patients should be transported to a stroke hospital or other facility capable of providing acute stroke care, and advanced prehospital notification should be given to the selected medical facility.
4. **Door of the emergency department (ED).** Immediately upon arrival, the patient should undergo general and neurologic assessment in the ED.
5. **Data collection,** including computer tomography (CT) scan and serial neurologic examinations, along with reviews of the patient's file for potential fibrinolytics (tPA) exclusions.
6. **Decision regarding stroke treatment.** If the patient remains a candidate for tissue plasminogen activator (tPA) therapy, review risks and benefits with the patient and family.
7. **Drug administration** as appropriate and postadministration monitoring.

TABLE **47-1** Stroke Performance Measures

Stroke Performance Measures	Stroke Type
Deep venous thrombosis (DVT) prophylaxis: • Nonambulatory patients should start receiving DVT prophylaxis by the end of day 2	Ischemic stroke Hemorrhagic stroke
Discharged on antithrombotic therapy: • Patients prescribed antithrombotic therapy at discharge	Ischemic stroke
Discharged on anticoagulation for patients in atrial fibrillation: • Patients with atrial fibrillation discharged on anticoagulation	Ischemic stroke
Thrombolytic therapy administered: • Patients with acute ischemic stroke who arrive at the hospital within 120 minutes of time last known well and for whom IV tissue plasminogen activator (tPA) was initiated at this hospital within 180 minutes of last known well	Ischemic stroke
Antithrombotic medication by the end of hospital day 2: • Patients received antithrombotic therapy by the end of hospital day 2	Ischemic stroke
Discharged on cholesterol-reducing medication: • Patients with low-density lipoproteins (LDL) above 100 or LDL not measured or on cholesterol-reducer before admission are discharged on cholesterol-reducing drugs	Ischemic stroke
Stroke education: • Patients and caregivers were given education or educational materials prior to discharge to address personal risk factors, stroke warning signs, activation of emergency medical services, need for follow-up after discharge, and medications prescribed	Ischemic stroke Hemorrhagic stroke
Assessed for rehabilitation: • Patients were assessed for rehabilitation	Ischemic stroke Hemorrhagic stroke

stroke patients across the disease trajectory). Certified Comprehensive Stroke Centers are required to report their compliance with the eight Primary Stroke Center measures as well as an additional eight measures (Comprehensive Stroke Center-specific) that reflect care and outcomes for patients who undergo specific treatment interventions. Today, there are nearly 2,000 hospitals certified as Primary Stroke Centers and over 100 hospitals certified as Comprehensive Stroke Centers (Gorelick, 2013). Nursing staff working at a certified stroke center will be familiar with evidence-based stroke protocols and will have specific education requirements to maintain their stroke expertise.

Pathophysiology

Stroke is a heterogeneous syndrome characterized by the onset of one or more focal neurologic deficits (corresponding to the affected area of the brain) caused by reduced cerebral blood flow that leads to brain cell death and functional disability. The two major stroke types that cause an interruption in cerebral blood flow are an occluded artery that deprives blood flow to part of the brain supplied by that blood vessel (called an *ischemic stroke*, Fig. 47-1), or a ruptured artery resulting in bleeding in or around the brain (called a *hemorrhagic stroke*, Fig. 47-2). Hemorrhagic strokes are further subdivided based on the specific intracranial space that is filled with blood: an intraparenchymal hemorrhage (blood within the brain tissue),

and a subarachnoid hemorrhage (SAH) (blood occupying the subarachnoid space). Ischemic strokes account for about 85% of all stroke syndromes. Hemorrhagic strokes account for the remaining 15% (Table 47-2). Regardless of stroke type or mechanism, the concept that "time is brain" has become the mainstay for directing a rapid clinical diagnosis and acute treatment options if patients present within a specific time window from the onset of symptoms.

Although patients suffering from an ischemic or hemorrhagic stroke may present with similar neurologic deficits, initial brain imaging (i.e., noncontrast head CT) will identify the presence of a hemorrhage; any area of ischemia due to an occluded artery typically will be visible only after 4 to 6 hours from symptom onset. Therefore the rapid diagnosis of an acute ischemic stroke is considered a clinical diagnosis and is based on the patient's presenting symptoms and clinical examination. Treatment options and management will vary depending on stroke type.

Ischemic Stroke

Normally, the brain receives approximately 15% of the total cardiac output. Cerebral blood flow is calculated to be 50 to 55 mL of blood per 100 g of brain tissue per minute. For patients who experience an ischemic stroke, disruption of blood flow in or to the brain due to an obstruction of a blood vessel initiates a complex series of circulatory and metabolic

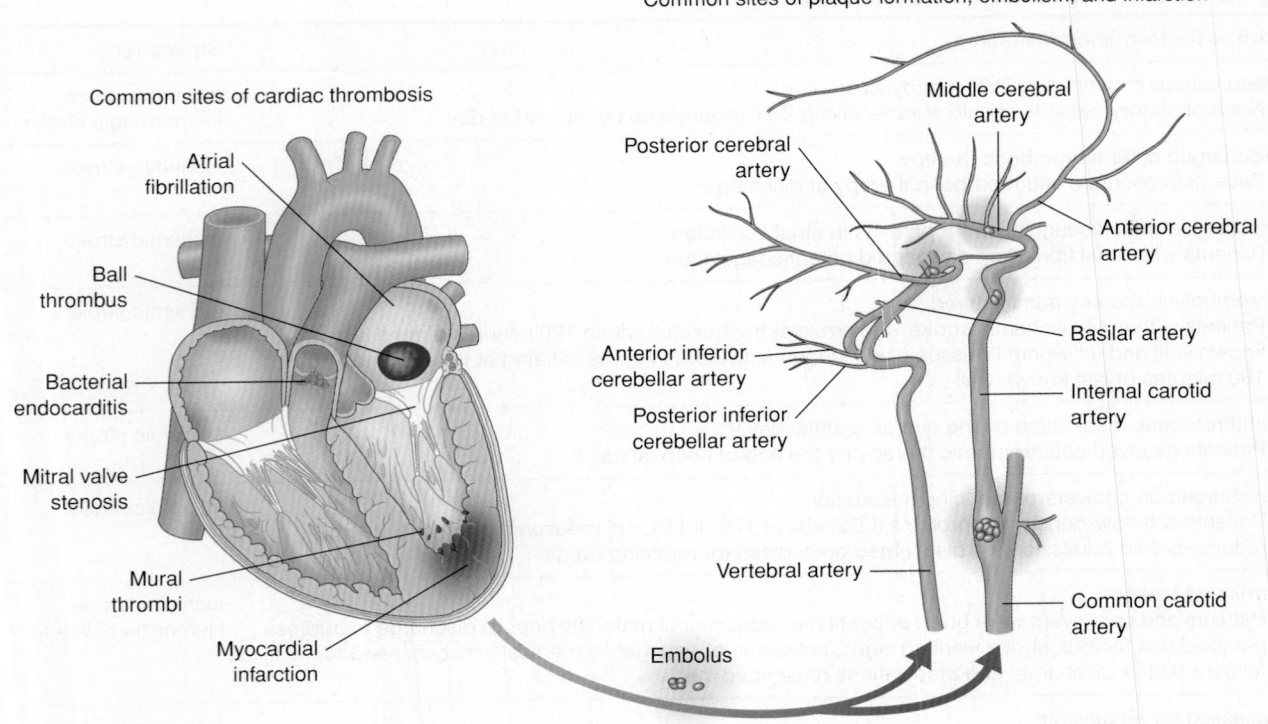

Common sites of cardiac thrombosis

Common sites of plaque formation, embolism, and infarction

FIGURE 47-1 Ischemic stroke.

events referred to as the *ischemic cascade*. The ischemic cascade begins when cerebral blood flow decreases to less than 25 mL/100 g/min. At this point, neurons are no longer able to maintain aerobic respiration. The cell's mitochondria must then switch to anaerobic metabolism, generating large amounts of lactic acid and glutamate, causing a change in pH. This switch to anaerobic metabolism also renders the neuron incapable of producing sufficient quantities of adenosine triphosphate (ATP) to fuel cell depolarization processes. The cell membrane pumps that maintain electrolyte

balances begin to fail, and the cells cease to function (Fig. 47-3). Cell death at the site of occlusion is referred to as the *core infarct*. The surrounding area of affected brain tissue in which blood flow has been reduced is referred to as the *ischemic penumbra*. In selected patients, the penumbra, or stunned brain tissue, is deemed salvageable with early treatment, such as with thrombolysis (*administration of intravenous alteplase or IV tPA*) or with clot retrieval (using a catheter-based intra-arterial approach to extract the clot); see Figure 47-4. Specific inclusion and exclusion criteria for the use of these treatment options assist the clinicians in identifying patients that would have the best outcomes after acute stroke.

Ischemic strokes are further divided into five subtypes according to a mechanism-based classification system: large-artery thrombotic strokes (representing 20% of ischemic strokes); small, penetrating artery thrombotic strokes (25%); cardio embolic strokes (20%); cryptogenic strokes (strokes that cannot be attributable to any specific cause) (30%); and "other" (5%). Each stroke subtype has a characteristic pathophysiologic course, but these types have overlapping clinical features. This subtyping directs both therapeutic interventions and long-term prognosis.

Large-artery thrombotic strokes are caused by atherosclerotic plaques in the large blood vessels of the brain. Thrombus formation and occlusion can occur at the site of the atherosclerosis and result in ischemia and infarction (tissue death).

Common sites of cerebral hemorrhage

FIGURE 47-2 Common sites of cerebral hemorrhage.

TABLE **47-2** Comparison of Major Types of Stroke

Facet	Ischemic	Hemorrhagic
Causes	Large-artery thrombosis Small, penetrating artery thrombosis Cardiogenic embolic Cryptogenic (no known cause) Other	Intracerebral hemorrhage Subarachnoid hemorrhage Cerebral aneurysm Arteriovenous malformation
Main presenting symptoms	Numbness or weakness of the face, arm, or leg, especially on one side of the body	"Exploding headache" Decreased level of consciousness
Additional symptoms	Slurred speech, or difficulty with word finding or comprehension	Nausea/vomiting; visual changes; seizures

Many of these symptoms occur with either stroke type.

Small, penetrating artery thrombotic strokes that affect one or more vessels and cause reduced blood flow are the most common type of ischemic stroke, typically caused by longstanding hypertension, hyperlipidemia, or diabetes. Small artery thrombotic strokes are frequently referred to as *lacunar strokes* or *lacunes* because of the small cavities that are created after the death of infarcted brain tissue.

Cardio embolic strokes are associated with cardiac arrhythmias, such as atrial fibrillation, but can also be associated with valvular heart disease or left ventricular thrombus (as depicted in Fig. 47-1). Emboli originating from the heart that circulate to the cerebral vasculature, most commonly via the left middle cerebral artery, cause ischemia and subsequent infarction.

The last two classifications of ischemic strokes are cryptogenic strokes, which have no identified cause, and strokes-from other-causes, such as illicit drug use (cocaine), coagulopathies, migraine, or spontaneous dissection of the carotid or vertebral arteries. Differentiating

stroke etiologies directs specific treatment and secondary prevention strategies.

Transient Ischemic Attacks

A transient ischemic attack, or TIA (sometimes referred to as a "mini-stroke"), has traditionally been defined as a brief episode of neurologic dysfunction resulting from focal cerebral ischemia not associated with permanent cerebral infarction. A TIA involves the same pathophysiologic mechanism outlined in the ischemic cascade, but symptoms are transient (persisting less than 24 hours) and there is no evidence of cerebral tissue infarction on follow-up brain imaging studies. TIAs have often been referred to as a warning stroke since the causative process is likely to recur (causing cerebral infarction) if no interventions are undertaken. With the advent of better brain imaging techniques, and recognizing that TIAs typically resolve within 60 minutes, a new definition for a TIA was adopted. It has now been operationally defined as a brief episode of neurologic dysfunction caused by focal brain or retinal ischemia, with clinical symptoms typically lasting less than 1 hour, and without evidence of acute infarction (Livesay & Hickey, 2014). The corollary is that persistent clinical signs or characteristic imaging abnormalities change the definition to include ischemic infarction. For the purposes of this chapter, ischemic stroke and TIA are considered one disease process that mandates the same evaluative detail in determining cause, implementing a care plan, and supporting secondary stroke prevention measures (Kernan, Ovbiagele, Black et al., 2014).

Patients diagnosed with a TIA are at a higher risk for a subsequent stroke (Thacker, 2010). Clinicians use a scoring system to determine which TIA patients warrant a more urgent evaluation and possible hospital admission based on selected clinical features. As outlined in Figure 47-5, older patients with elevated blood pressure and multiple symptoms of a longer duration were more likely to have a stroke at the 2-day, 7-day, and 9-day periods, thereby requiring a more urgent evaluation and initiation of secondary stroke prevention therapy.

FIGURE 47-3 Processes contributing to ischemic brain cell injury. Courtesy of the National Stroke Association, Englewood, Colorado.

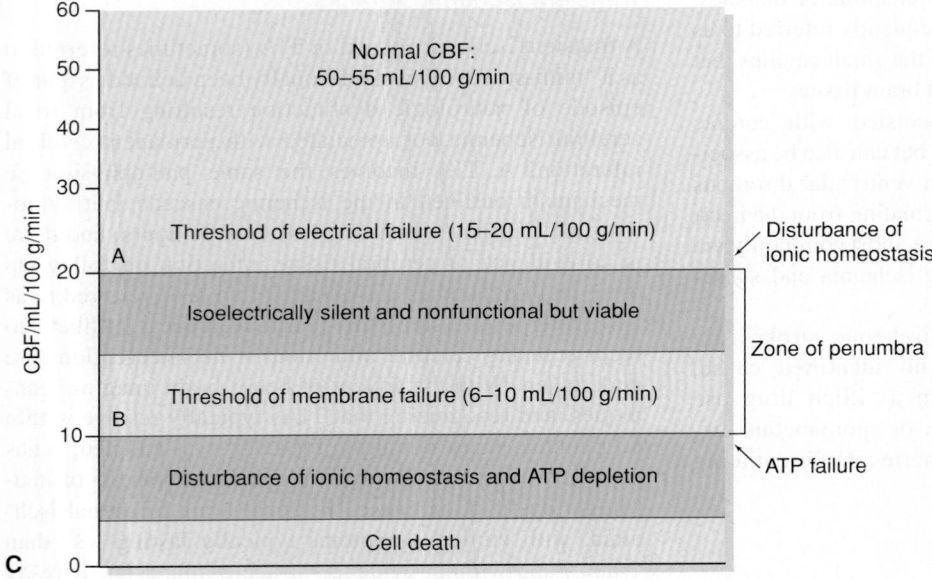

Ischemic Penumbra: Conceptual Basis for Brain Resuscitation
(Prevent or minimize secondary injury by improving
cerebral delivery of oxygen [CDO₂])

FIGURE 47-4 Cerebral blood supply during ischemic events. **A.** See distribution of middle cerebral artery and occlusion of a branch. Note area of infarction and surrounding penumbra with viable but nonfunctional cells. These cells will become either infarcted or recover, depending on treatment. **B.** Ischemic penumbra: normal cerebral blood flow (CBF) = 50 to 55 mL/100 g/min. Variations in CBF are noted. Penumbra is the critical area that may be salvageable with appropriate treatment, or cell death will occur if adequate CBF is not restored. **C.** Ischemic penumbra: conceptual basis for brain resuscitation. ATP, adenosine triphosphate; EEG, electroencephalogram; LOC, level of consciousness. (Adapted from Hickey, J. V. (2014). *The clinical practice of neurological and neurosurgical nursing* (7th ed.). Philadelphia, PA: Lippincott Williams & Wilkins.)

Hemorrhagic Strokes

Hemorrhagic strokes refer to bleeding into the brain tissue (parenchyma), the ventricles, or the subarachnoid space. Normal brain metabolism is disrupted when blood outside the vasculature forms a mass that compresses adjacent brain tissue, causing increased intracranial pressure (ICP), secondary hemorrhage, and further ischemia. In cases where there is significant blood volume in the brain tissue, a condition referred to as *herniation* can occur in which brain tissue is subjected to increased pressure and moves across structures within the skull. If blood extends into the ventricles, it can cause acute hydrocephalus (increase in the amount of cerebral spinal fluid in the brain). These events can impair level of consciousness (LOC) and lead to coma and death.

Hemorrhagic stroke can further be divided into subtypes: intracerebral hemorrhage (ICH) and subarachnoid hemorrhage (SAH). ICH can occur with bleeding into any of the spaces within the cranium, including subarachnoid, epidural, and subdural spaces. Bleeding into the subdural and epidural spaces is primarily associated with trauma. Conversely, SAH, which is bleeding into the subarachnoid space, is associated primarily with hemorrhage due to intracranial aneurysms (commonly in the *vessels that make up* the Circle of Willis), trauma, or arteriovenous malformations (AVMs). An AVM is caused by an abnormality during embryonal development that leads to a tangle of arteries and veins in the brain that lacks a capillary bed. The absence of a capillary bed causes higher pressure within the arterioles to be transmitted directly to the veins. This anomaly leads to dilation of both arteries and veins

Risk Factor	Points	Score
Age ≥ 60 years	1	
Blood pressure Systolic BP ≥ 140 mm Hg *OR* Diastolic BP ≥ 90 mm Hg	1	
Clinical features of TIA *(choose one)* Unilateral weakness with or without speech impairment *OR* Speech impairment without unilateral weakness	2 1	
Duration TIA duration ≥ 60 minutes TIA duration 10–59 minutes	2 1	
Diabetes	1	
Total ABCD^2 score	0–7	

Using the ABCD^2 Score

Higher ABCD^2 scores are associated with greater risk of stroke during the 2, 7, 30, and 90 days after a TIA (Figure). The authors of the ABCD^2 score made the following recommendations for hospital observation[1]:

ABCD^2 Score	2-day Stroke Risk (%)	Comment
0–3	1.0	Hospital observation may be unnecessary without another indication (e.g., new atrial fibrillation)
4–5	4.1	Hospital observation justified in most situations
6–7	8.1	Hospital observation worthwhile

FIGURE 47-5 Transient ischemic attack (TIA): Prognosis and key management considerations. MR, magnetic resonance; TIA, transient ischemic attack. (Used with permission from Johnston, S. C., Rothwell, P. M., Huynh-Huynh, M. N., Giles, M. F., Elkins, J. S., & Sidney, S. (2007). Validation and refinement of scores to predict very early stroke risk after transient ischemic attack. *Lancet, 369,* 283–292; Johnston, S. C., Nguyen-Huynh, M. N., Schwarz, M. E., Fuller, K., Williams, C. E., Joseph-son, S. A.,…Albers, G. W. (2006). National Stroke Association guidelines for the management of transient ischemic attacks. *Annals of Neurology, 60,* 301–313.)

and, if the pressure increases, possible rupture. AVM is a common cause of hemorrhagic stroke in younger patients.

Primary ICH from a spontaneous rupture of small arteries or arterioles accounts for approximately 80% of hemorrhagic strokes and is caused chiefly by uncontrolled hypertension. Blood can accumulate outside the vessels and into the intracranial space over minutes to hours. Symptom presentation can vary from mild deficits to acute loss of consciousness. Because the brain is enclosed in a rigid structure, hemorrhage can dramatically increase ICP, causing shifts in the content volume within the skull and eventual herniation (and

a higher mortality rate) if not acutely treated. ICH occurs most commonly in the cerebral lobes, basal ganglia, thalamus, brainstem (the pons), and cerebellum. Occasionally, bleeding ruptures the wall of the lateral ventricle and causes intraventricular hemorrhage, which is frequently fatal.

ICH can also occur in the setting of an ischemic stroke, when the infarcted tissue becomes susceptible to leaking blood vessels. ICH is also associated with AVMs, intracranial aneurysms, intracranial neoplasms, and with certain medications, such as anticoagulants or abuse of cocaine or amphetamines (Hickey & Livesay, 2014). Cerebral amyloid angiopathy (a condition in which amyloid [fibrous proteins] deposits accumulate inside the walls of arteries in the brain, causing vessel wall breakdown) can predispose patients to cerebral hemorrhage. Amyloid deposits are often seen in conjunction with dementia. Characteristic lobar hemorrhages on magnetic resonance imaging (MRI) may be diagnostic in the absence of a brain tissue biopsy when combined with patient history and clinical presentation (Hickey & Livesay, 2014). An intracranial (cerebral) **aneurysm** is a dilation of the wall of a cerebral artery. These vessel abnormalities may be due to atherosclerosis, which results in vessel wall weakness but also may be due to a congenital defect of the vessel wall, hypertensive vascular disease, head trauma, or advancing age. The cerebral arteries most commonly affected by an aneurysm are the internal carotid artery (ICA), anterior cerebral artery (ACA), anterior communicating artery (ACoA), posterior communicating artery (PCoA), posterior cerebral artery (PCA), and middle cerebral artery (MCA).

Risk Factors

The conditions or risk factors that predispose patients to stroke are diverse and are similar to risk factors for cardiac and peripheral vascular disease. Although some risk factors are applicable to a specific stroke type, most can apply to both ischemic and hemorrhagic strokes. Identifying patient-specific stroke risk factors is part of the patient and family education process during primary stroke prevention and during stroke recovery.

Modifiable Risk Factors

Modifiable risk factors are those that can be altered through lifestyle changes and medical treatment. Common modifiable stroke risk factors include hypertension, smoking and second-hand smoke exposure, diabetes, dyslipidemia, atrial fibrillation, diet (including excessive salt, high alcohol consumption), obesity, sleep apnea, and lack of exercise.

Hypertension is the most important risk factor for both ischemic and hemorrhagic stroke, and, despite the numerous treatment options, it remains underrecognized and undertreated in most communities. In the acute stroke phase, blood pressure is generally liberalized to allow for improved cerebral blood flow, but the general practice in the stroke recovery phase is to achieve normotension, defined as less than 140 mm Hg systolic and less than 90 mm Hg diastolic (JNC 8).

Smoking and second-hand smoke are prevalent among all age groups and pose an increased stroke risk among women who smoke and who are on oral contraceptives. Smoking cessation programs (counseling and nicotine replacement) have been included as part of the post-stroke care plan for all patients identified as current smokers (CDC, 2015).

Diabetes independently increases stroke risk and contributes to the increased prevalence of hypertension and dyslipidemia. Glycemic control alone has not been shown to reduce stroke risk, but in combination with blood pressure and lipid management, patients with diabetes can lower their overall risk (ASA, 2014).

Atrial fibrillation is the most frequently diagnosed arrhythmia in the United States. If left untreated, it puts patients at higher risk for suffering from an ischemic stroke. Approximately 15% to 20% of ischemic strokes can be attributed to atrial fibrillation. Screening for atrial fibrillation in patients over 40 years of age has been recommended since anticoagulation and rate/rhythm control can reduce stroke risk by up to 68% (ACC guidelines for afib-2014).

Obstructive sleep apnea (OSA) is an independent risk factor for stroke, and the mechanism of cause is yet to be elucidated. It has been proposed that intermittent hypoxemia (due to intermittent cessation of breathing) may cause surges in blood pressure with release of vasoconstrictive substances, such as endothelin; additionally increased levels of inflammatory biomarkers are seen in sleep-disordered breathing (Ifergane, Ovanyan, Toledano, et al., 2016). Patients with OSA have a greater functional impairment and higher mortality rates than patients without OSA during an acute stroke. Continuous positive airway pressure (CPAP) treatment is associated with decreased mortality and better functional recovery after stroke (Ifergane, Ovanyan, Toledano, et al., 2016, p. 1207).

Nonmodifiable Risk Factors

Nonmodifiable risk factors are important to highlight from both a primary and secondary stroke prevention standpoint because, while they cannot be changed, stroke risk factors can be identified in a patient's medical profile, and associated modifiable risk factors can be aggressively treated. Having a family history of stroke increases the chance of stroke and can be attributed to genetic influences as well as cultural/environmental influences. Genetic testing is not generally recommended unless there is a suspicion of a rare genetic condition or when other more common causes for stroke cannot be identified. Older age is a risk factor for stroke, and for both ischemic and hemorrhagic strokes the risk doubles every 10 years after 55 years of age. Men tend to have a higher risk for stroke and a higher age-specific stroke incidence rate, but more women tend to die from stroke.

Race and ethnicity impact stroke risk among specific populations. Blacks and Hispanics have a higher incidence of both ischemic and hemorrhagic stroke, and contributing factors may be the higher incidence of diabetes and hypertension in these groups (Livesay & Hickey, 2014).

Clinical Manifestations and Assessment

Common Symptoms

Stroke syndromes produce a wide variety of neurologic deficits, depending on the location in the brain that is affected, the specific blood vessels that are obstructed, the size and area of underperfused brain tissue, and the amount of collateral (secondary or accessory) blood flow to the affected area. The AHA/ASA advises the public to be aware of the symptoms of stroke and to call 911 immediately. The most common symptoms of stroke include:

- Sudden numbness or weakness of the face, arm, or leg, especially on one side of the body
- Sudden trouble speaking or understanding speech
- Sudden visual disturbances
- Difficulty walking, dizziness, or loss of balance or coordination
- Sudden, severe headache

There are additional, less commonly recognized stroke symptoms that also put patients at risk for disabling and devastating outcomes. These include: sudden, unexplained fall; onset of nausea and vomiting; and acute changes in mentation, such as confusion or disorientation. These symptoms have been associated more commonly with strokes that occur in the posterior circulation leading to infarctions in the cerebellum (Arch et al., 2015).

The clinician should be able to correlate commonly presenting neurologic deficits with the location(s) in the brain affected by ischemia or hemorrhage. Box 47-2 compares the symptoms and behaviors seen in patients with right hemispheric strokes with those seen in patients with left hemispheric strokes. Acute neurologic deficits are not stroke-type specific. Patients with a hemorrhagic or ischemic stroke can present with similar neurologic deficits, thus making expedited brain imaging an important aspect of the stroke workup.

Many of the same motor, sensory, cranial nerve, cognitive, and other functions that are disrupted after ischemic stroke are also altered after a hemorrhagic stroke. For patients with cerebral hemorrhages, the most common presenting symptom is a severe headache. Other symptoms that can be observed are vomiting, a slow or sudden change in

LOC, or focal seizures. Patients with a ruptured AVM will typically present with a sudden severe headache and sudden loss of consciousness. There may be posterior neck or spine pain associated with the headache. If there is a slow leakage of blood that leads to formation of a clot at the site of rupture, the patient may show little neurologic deficit. In cases in which severe bleeding occurs, there can be extensive cerebral injury, and the patient may progress to coma and death. Symptoms are described in detail in the following sections.

Motor Loss

The most common motor dysfunction resulting from stroke is hemiparesis, or weakness of one side of the body. Upper and lower motor neurons play a role in mediating muscle and tendon reflex activity. Because the upper motor neurons decussate (cross over from one hemisphere to the other), a disturbance of voluntary motor control on one side of the body may reflect damage to the upper motor neurons on the opposite side of the brain. Motor loss can range from a mild or subtle weakness in an isolated muscle group (such as the muscles controlling wrist flexion) to a dense paresis or plegia in which there are multiple muscle groups affecting multiple limbs rendering a patient unable to sit, stand, or walk.

Communication Loss

Language and communication may also be affected by stroke. While there are several specific areas in the brain responsible for the production and comprehension of speech, a majority of patients have their language center in the left hemisphere. Dysfunctions of language and communication related to cerebral injury include:

- *Dysarthria:* Difficulty in articulating speech, caused by paralysis of the muscles responsible for producing speech; also referring to slurred speech.
- *Dysphasia or aphasia:* Partial or complete impairment of language resulting from brain injury, affecting spoken language and comprehension.
- Aphasias can be further defined as (1) Expressive aphasia, in which the patient has difficulty producing speech and (2) Receptive aphasia, in which the patient has difficulty comprehending speech.
- *Apraxia:* Inability to put sounds and syllables together in the correct order to form words, to produce speech.

Visual Disturbances

Visual-perceptual dysfunctions are caused by disturbances of the primary sensory pathways between the eye and visual cortex. Although there are numerous forms of visual impairment that include diplopia, impaired acuity, and abnormal eye movement, the most common visual impairment after stroke is visual field loss. Homonymous hemianopsia (loss of half of the visual field) may occur from stroke and may be temporary or permanent. Disturbances in visual–spatial relations (perceiving the relationship of two or more objects

---

BOX 47-2

Focused Assessment

Left and Right Hemispheric Strokes

Be alert for the following signs and symptoms:

Left hemispheric stroke:
- Paralysis or weakness on right side of body
- Right visual field deficit
- Aphasia (expressive, receptive, or global)
- Altered intellectual ability
- Slow, cautious behavior

Right hemispheric stroke:
- Paralysis or weakness on left side of body
- Left visual field deficit
- Spatial-perceptual deficits
- Increased distractibility
- Impulsive behavior and poor judgment
- Lack of awareness of deficits

in spatial areas) are frequently seen in patients with right hemispheric damage.

Dysphagia

Dysphagia is one of the most common complications after stroke, leading to problems such as aspiration pneumonia, dehydration, and poor nutrition. It can occur in up to 75% of patients and can prolong hospitalization and overall recovery. Swallowing is a complex process that allows for the transfer of food or fluids from the mouth to the stomach. The swallowing process occurs in four stages using six cranial nerves (trigeminal [CN V], facial [CN VII], glossopharyngeal [CN IIX], vagus [CN X], spinal accessory [CN XI], and hypoglossal [CN XII]). Multiple bedside dysphagia screening tools have been developed to assess patients suspected of having a stroke who are at risk for aspiration prior to administering medications or food. These tools include a clinical assessment of the patient's LOC and ability to swallow (various consistencies, such as thin liquids). Usually these assessments are performed by nurses with a "pass/fail" option for the patient. A patient who fails the assessment is referred to a speech and language pathologist for a formal swallow study, such as videofluoroscopy (VFS) or a fiberoptic endoscopic evaluation of swallowing (FEES).

Sensory Loss

The sensory losses from stroke may range from a slight impairment of touch, to more severe or total loss of sensation, with loss of proprioception (ability to perceive the position and motion of body parts), as well as difficulty in interpreting visual, tactile, and auditory stimuli. *Agnosias* describe the inability to recognize previously familiar objects perceived by one or more of the senses.

Cognitive Impairment and Psychological Effects

If damage has occurred to the frontal lobe, learning capacity, memory, or other higher cortical intellectual functions may be impaired. Such dysfunction may be reflected in a limited attention span, difficulties in comprehension, forgetfulness, and a lack of motivation.

A common sequela is depression, and this may be exaggerated by the patient's natural response to this catastrophic event. Emotional lability, hostility, frustration, resentment, lack of cooperation, and other psychological problems may occur at some point during the recovery period and should be part of a screening process post-stroke.

Acute Stroke Assessment

As a result of the more recent clinical trials in stroke treatment that demonstrated a positive outcome, the concept of defining and performing an acute stroke assessment has now become a standard approach to clinical care in both the pre-hospital field setting as well as the "stroke ready" emergency departments. The Emergency Nurses Association and the American College of Emergency Physicians recommend stroke patients be considered an ESI Level 2 emergency (see Chapter 56 for an explanation of the five-level Emergency Severity Index [ESI]), meaning that the suspected stroke patient "needs immediate assessment," the same as for an unstable trauma patient or a critical-care cardiac patient.

Nurses in the pre-hospital setting or at triage in an emergency department should be familiar with the pre-hospital screening and assessments that are done by members of the EMS team so that they can relay this information to the stroke team prior to arrival. (For a detailed explanation of the pre-hospital care for stroke patients, refer to Interactions within Stroke Systems of Care: A Policy Statement from the American Heart Association/American Stroke Association Expert Panel on Emergency Medical Services Systems and the Stroke Council [Higgashida, Alberts, Alexander, et al., 2013].)

Acute stroke care can be divided into two phases: the hyperacute phase (the first 24 hours of care) and the acute phase (acute care during the hospitalization). Nurses involved in the initial triage process are corresponding with EMS either to confirm a patient suspected of having a stroke is being transported to their facility or to address the immediate needs of a patient who may "walk in" to the emergency department.

Several algorithms have been developed for the hyperacute phase for the initial workup of a patient presenting with acute stroke symptoms as a template to expedite the diagnostic workup (Fig. 47-6). For patients arriving by ambulance (with prenotification by the paramedics that a suspected stroke patient is en route) or by car, the triage nurse will confirm the presenting stroke symptoms and the time the patient was last known to be at his or her baseline. Many of the same motor, sensory, cranial nerve, and cognitive functions are disrupted in both ischemic and hemorrhagic strokes; however, changes in LOC, vomiting, sudden severe headache, and seizure are frequently associated with hemorrhagic strokes.

Specifically, triaging includes eliciting a detailed history and determining time of onset of the patient's symptoms. When the time of symptom onset is not definitive, the time the patient was last known to be at baseline becomes the default time of onset. Determining the time of the onset of symptoms becomes important since drug treatment options and interventional procedures for clot retrieval for an ischemic stroke are time dependent. Vital signs and other key clinical information (e.g., current medications or recent prior surgeries) also will be obtained. This information also may trigger the staff to activate a stroke code at the receiving facility so that the team is prepared to expedite a rapid evaluation.

Figure 47-7 depicts a typical acute stroke protocol.

Diagnostic Evaluation

The diagnosis of an acute stroke is made by history, a precise neurologic examination, and rapid neuroimaging. An initial

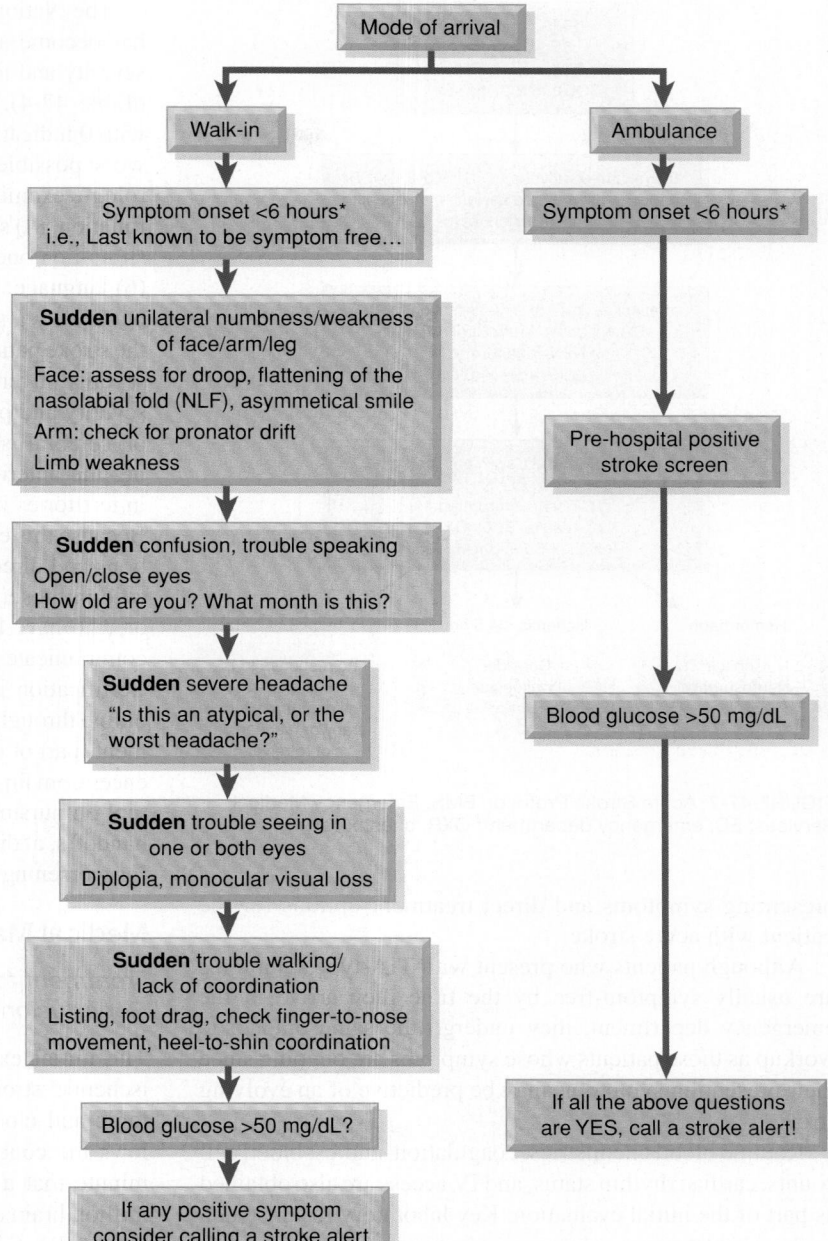

FIGURE 47-6 Triage stroke screen. *While intravenous tPA treatment is administered to eligible patients within 3 to 4.5 hours of symptom onset, patients are frequently evaluated within 6 to 12 hours of symptom onset to determine eligibility for neurointerventional treatment procedures.

noncontrast head CT scan is performed to assess for the presence of intraparenchymal blood. Ischemia will not be readily visible on initial CT scan when it is performed within the first few hours after symptom onset; however, evidence of bleeding (hemorrhage) will almost always be visible. Clinicians will also consider the location of the hematoma, the size and presence of blood in the ventricular system, and evidence of increased ICP. Additional diagnostic testing is done to determine if the hemorrhage is due to a ruptured intracranial aneurysm or AVM.

Although both CT scan and MRI are acceptable initial studies, most facilities have ready access to rapid CT imaging to rule out hemorrhage. Given that "minutes matter" when treatment for brain injury is time dependent, rapid imaging procedures should be part of the evaluation. Both CT and MRI will aid in determining stroke type, size, and location of the infarct or hematoma, any swelling and shift in brain tissue, presence of blood in the ventricles, and presence of hydrocephalus. It is a common practice at most institutions to also acquire intracranial and extracranial vessel imaging (computed tomography angiography [CTA] and magnetic resonance angiography [MRA]) to look for evidence of a significant vessel stenosis, in situ clot, or dissection of a vessel wall that could explain the patient's

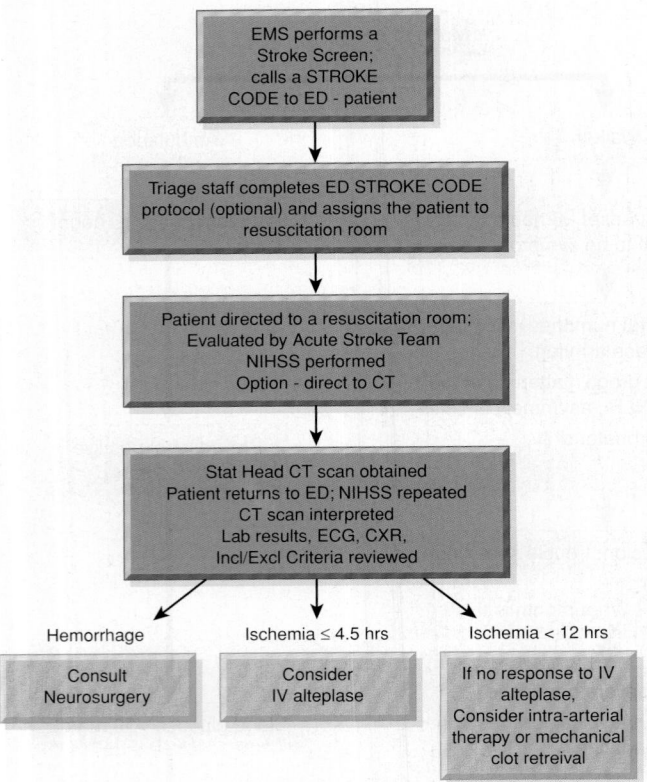

FIGURE 47-7 Acute Stroke Protocol. EMS, Emergency Medical Services; ED, emergency department; CXR, chest x-ray.

presenting symptoms and direct treatment options for the patient with acute stroke.

Although patients who present with TIA-type symptoms are usually symptom-free by the time they arrive in the emergency department, they undergo the same diagnostic workup as those patients whose symptoms are ongoing since their presenting symptoms may be predictive of an evolving stroke.

Routine blood chemistries, coagulation studies, blood cell counts, cardiac rhythm status, and IV access are also obtained as part of the initial evaluation. Key laboratory results (such as the platelet count, glucose, and coagulation profile) will direct decision-making regarding treatment options, such as thrombolysis. Table 47-3 details a variety of diagnostic tests or procedures that are commonly recommended.

The Clinical Examination

The neurologic examination is perceived as a complicated and often poorly performed examination. For clinicians working in acute care (and specifically in the emergency department), a more focused standardized neurologic examination has been a recommended practice in identifying and quantifying the presenting deficits and in facilitating communication among the team members. A standard examination is also an efficient way to assess the patient suspected of having a stroke rapidly during the first minutes after arrival.

The National Institutes of Health Stroke Scale (NIHSS) has become an accepted assessment tool to quantify stroke severity and to assess patient outcome after stroke treatment (Table 47-4). The NIHSS is a 42-point assessment scale, with 0 indicating no neurologic deficits and 42 indicating the worst possible score. It focuses on six major areas of the neurologic examination: (1) LOC, (2) visual function, (3) motor function, (4) sensation and neglect (failure to pay attention to stimuli on one side of the body), (5) cerebellar function, and (6) language. The NIHSS was initially used by stroke teams but is now a standard assessment used by nursing to follow the stroke patient's neurologic deficits and to document stroke severity. It enables the examiner to rapidly determine the severity and possible location of the stroke. While it focuses on cerebral ischemia corresponding to abnormalities affecting the anterior circulation, this scale often misses deficits in territories in the brain dependent on posterior circulation. Because this examination relies heavily on responses to questions and directions, the assessment score becomes less specific in those patients who have a markedly depressed LOC or who have lost language. However, it allows clinicians to communicate findings using a standardized assessment tool. Certification in the use of this assessment tool is available online through the ASA training center and is often a requirement (part of orientation) for nurses working in the neurosciences domain. The NIHSS has become a standard assessment tool on nursing flow sheets for periodic assessments, during handoffs, at discharge, and when there is a neurologic change (or worsening) that warrants an urgent evaluation.

Medical Management

Treatment for Acute Ischemic Stroke: Reperfusion Therapies

The initial expedited diagnostic workup and treatment of ischemic stroke are driven by time-dependent pharmacologic and clot retrieval device treatment options. This follows the concept that "Time is Brain," that says for every minute that a stroke occurs and is not treated, nearly two million brain cells are destroyed. Thrombolysis with recombinant tPA (alteplase) is currently the only FDA-approved drug for acute ischemic stroke within a 3-hour window of symptom onset. Alteplase binds to fibrin and converts plasminogen to plasmin, which is responsible for clot breakdown. Results from the 1995 NINDS trial demonstrated a significant improvement in functional outcome at 3 months post-stroke in those patients who received tPA within 3 hours after symptom onset (NINDS & Stroke rtPA Stroke Study Work Group, 1995).

Results from the 2008 European Cooperative Acute Stroke Study (ECASS 3) demonstrated clinically significant improvement in functional outcome in selected patients who received treatment up to 4.5 hours after symptom onset (Hacke, Kaste, Bluhmi, et al., 2008). Specifically, patients who are under 80 years of age, who have no history of stroke

TABLE **47-3** Diagnostic Procedures for Transient Ischemic Attacks (TIAs) and Stroke

Diagnostic Procedure	Information Provided
Computed tomography (CT) scan without contrast	Important diagnostic test to quickly assess for the presence of blood (hemorrhage), which will preclude treatment with antithrombotics
CT scan with contrast	Useful to rule out lesions that may mimic ischemia, especially when symptoms are related to hemispheric deficits; hypodense areas on CT scan suggest infarction
Magnetic resonance imaging (MRI)	Offers soft tissue contrast discrimination with superior demarcation of mass lesion from surrounding structures, including areas of ischemia and infarction; good visualization of vascular structures; useful for diagnosis of stroke in first 72 hours; a diffusion-weighted MRI can show ischemia in first few hours
Magnetic resonance angiography (MRA)	Less available and higher cost; noninvasive imaging of the carotid, vertebral, basilar, and major intracranial and extracranial arteries to determine occlusion; useful for clot visualization
Carotid ultrasonography	Noninvasive imaging; widely used initial diagnostic in patients with carotid territory symptoms for whom carotid endarterectomy (CEA) is considered
Transcranial Doppler (TCD)	Noninvasive monitoring of blood flow velocities of the major cerebral and carotid arteries to assess degree of stenoses; may be included as part of the stroke workup
Cerebral angiography	Ordered for patients to define precisely the percentage of occlusion and in patients with unusual presentation with aneurysm, vasculitis, and high-grade stenosis
Transthoracic echocardiography (TTE)	Helpful to identify cardioembolic sources; TTE is particularly helpful for diagnosing left ventricular thrombi, left atrial myxomas, and thrombi that protrude into the atrial cavity; they are less reliable for small tumors, laminated thrombi, and thrombi limited to the left or right atrium
Transesophageal echocardiography (TEE)	Benefit of TEE is in greater sensitivity for source of cardioembolic (except ventricular disease); TEE provides better visualization of cardiac structures, especially those at greater depth from chest wall and lesions of the atria (atrial appendage thrombi associated with atrial fibrillation), interatrial septum defects (patent foramen ovale, atrial septal defects), mitral valvular vegetation, and atherosclerotic disease of ascending aortic arch
Electrocardiogram (ECG); 12-lead is recommended initially	12-lead ECG recommended immediately because of the high incidence of heart disease in patients with stroke; ECG also useful when cardiogenic embolic stroke or concurrent coronary artery disease is suspected and to evaluate for atrial fibrillation
Ambulatory ECG monitoring	Reserved for patients who have suspicious palpitations, arrhythmias, or enlarged left atrium
Prothrombotic states	Protein C, protein S, antithrombin III, thrombin time, hemoglobin, electrophoresis, anticardiolipin antibody, lupus anticoagulant, and syphilis serology

From Adams, H. P. Jr., del Zoppo, G., Alberts, M. J., Bhatt, D. L., Brass, L., Furlan, A., . . . Wijdicks, E. F. (2007). Guidelines for the early management of adults with ischemic stroke. *Stroke*, *38*, 1655–1711, reprinted with permission. © 2007 American Heart Association, Inc.

or diabetes, who are not on anticoagulation therapy, and who do not have a severe stroke score of 25 or more are deemed significantly likely to benefit from thrombolysis using this extended time window (Livesay & Hickey, 2014, p. 525). This change in practice has afforded more patients the option for treatment and a better functional outcome after stroke. Stroke centers generally outline their approach to treatment according to the most current ASA guidelines. Once a hemorrhage has been ruled out and the clinical diagnosis of ischemic stroke is made, the acute stroke team must review the eligibility criteria for alteplase administration. For a complete list of inclusion and exclusion criteria for IV thrombolysis, see Figure 47-7.

Nurses are often responsible for administering alteplase, and some facilities expect nurses to mix and prepare the medication for administration. It is a weight-based medication and dosed at 0.9 mg/kg, with a maximum dose of 90 mg. Ten percent of the calculated dose is administered as an IV bolus over 1 minute. The remaining dose (90%) is administered over 1 hour via an infusion pump. Since bleeding is the most common side effect of alteplase, the patient is closely monitored for any suspected bleeding (at IV insertion sites, gums, urine/stools, and intracranially by assessing changes in LOC). Patients are also monitored for angioedema (oral/lingual swelling) and anaphylaxis (allergic reaction) to the medication.

TABLE **47-4** Summary of National Institutes of Health Stroke Scale (NIHSS)

Category	Description	Score
1a. Level of consciousness (LOC)	Alert	0
	Arousable by minor stimulation	1
	Obtunded, strong stimulation to attend	2
	Unresponsive, or reflex responses only	3
1b. LOC questions (month, age)	Answers both correctly	0
	Answers one correctly	1
	Both incorrect	2
1c. LOC, commands (open, close eyes; make fist, let go)	Obeys both correctly	0
	Obeys one correctly	1
	Both incorrect	2
2. Best gaze (eyes open—patient follows examiner's finger or face)	Normal	0
	Partial gaze palsy	1
	Forced deviation	2
3. Visual (introduce visual stimulus/threat to patient's visual field quadrants)	No visual loss	0
	Partial hemianopsia	1
	Complete hemianopsia	2
	Bilateral hemianopsia	3
4. Facial palsy (show teeth, raise eyebrows and squeeze eyes shut)	Normal	0
	Minor loss	1
	Partial loss	2
	Complete loss	3
5a. Motor; arm—left (elevate extremity to 90 degrees for 10 seconds and score drift/movement)	No drift	0
	Drift but maintains in air	1
	Unable to maintain in air	2
	No effort against gravity	3
	No movement	4
	Amputation, joint fusion (explain)	N/A
5b. Motor; arm—right (elevate extremity to 90 degrees for 10 seconds and score drift/movement)	No drift	0
	Drift but maintains in air	1
	Unable to maintain in air	2
	No effort against gravity	3
	No movement	4
	Amputation, joint fusion (explain)	N/A
6a. Motor; leg—left (elevate extremity to 30 degrees for 5 seconds and score drift/movement)	No drift	0
	Drift but maintains in air	1
	Unable to maintain in air	2
	No effort against gravity	3
	No movement	4
	Amputation, joint fusion (explain)	N/A
6b. Motor; leg—right (elevate extremity to 30 degrees for 5 seconds and score drift/movement)	No drift	0
	Drift but maintains in air	1
	Unable to maintain in air	2
	No effort against gravity	3
	No movement	4
	Amputation, joint fusion (explain)	N/A
7. Limb ataxia (finger-to-nose and heel-to-shin testing)	Absent	0
	Present in one limb	1
	Present in two limbs	2
8. Sensory (pin prick to face, arm, trunk, and leg—compare side to side)	Normal	0
	Mild to moderate loss	1
	Severe to total loss	2

Category	Description	Score
9. Best language (name items, describe a picture and read sentences)	No aphasia Mild to moderate aphasia Severe aphasia Mute	0 1 2 3
10. Dysarthria (evaluate speech clarity by having patient repeat words)	Normal Mild to moderate dysarthria Severe dysarthria, mostly unintelligible or worse Intubated or other physical barrier	0 1 2 N/A
11. Extinction and inattention (use information from prior testing to score)	No abnormality Visual, tactile, auditory, or other extinction to bilateral simultaneous stimulation Profound hemi-attention or extinction to more than one modality.	0 1 2
Total score		

Adapted from the version available at the National Institute of Neurological Disorders and Stroke, National Institutes of Health, Bethesda, MD. Retrieved from http://www.ninds.nih.gov/doctors/NIH_Stroke_Scale.pdf. It is recommended that the full scale with all instructions be used.

During the hyperacute phase of a suspected acute stroke, ongoing assessments and meticulous documentation of the patient's neurologic and hemodynamic status are essential, regardless of stroke type and whether or not the patient was a candidate for IV treatment.

Following the publication of several major trials in 2014 and 2015 for treatment of acute ischemic stroke, intra-arterial therapies for acute ischemic stroke were recommended as a standard-of-care option for selected patients with large vessel occlusions. The use of a clot-retrieval device (thrombectomy) with and without intra-arterial alteplase (typically within 6 hours of when patient was last known well) was shown to have a benefit in recanalizing the stenosed or occluded vessel and also demonstrated a statistically significantly improved functional outcome. These procedures have now become an accepted option for patients who present to facilities who support neurointerventional services (Goyal, Menon, & Van Zwam, 2016). Many Primary Stroke Centers, Thrombectomy-capable Stroke Centers, and Comprehensive Stroke Centers have the capability to perform thrombectomies, and patients require postprocedure intensive care monitoring similar to care provided following IV thrombolysis. For a more detailed explanation regarding the management of stroke patients who undergo these procedures, see the Current Treatment Options in Cardiovascular Medicine (2014) article, Intra-arterial Treatment for Acute Ischemic Stroke: the Continued Evolution.

Acute Stroke Recovery Care

Table 47-5 summarizes the nursing care for thrombolysis and nonthrombolysis treatments for patients with acute ischemic stroke. Post-stroke management addresses blood pressure parameters, oxygenation, body temperature, and hyperglycemia. Additionally, there are directives for neurologic assessments, deep vein thrombosis (DVT) prophylaxis, body temperature and oxygen status, cardiac monitoring and screening for impaired swallowing prior to oral intake.

Secondary Stroke Prevention

Once the patient has had a stroke, the patient is at increased risk for a second event. This risk is dependent on the etiology of the index stroke and the steps taken to prevent a recurrent stroke. Once the likely etiology of an ischemic stroke is determined, effective secondary stroke prevention will include the selection of the appropriate antithrombotic medication. The use of antithrombotic agents is a primary focus for secondary stroke prevention.

For patients whose stroke is thought to be cardiogenic embolic (from atrial fibrillation), warfarin or one of the newer anticoagulants is the most effective treatment to reduce stroke risk. For all other ischemic stroke types, antiplatelet treatment is recommended and can comprise one of several medications, including aspirin (at doses of 81 to 325 mg), clopidogrel (75 mg daily), and low-dose aspirin in combination with extended-release dipyridamole (50/200 mg). Additionally, based on the results of several studies, the use of statins for secondary (and primary) stroke prevention is recommended. A lipid profile is reviewed, and the current goal is for the LDL (low-density lipoprotein) to be less than 70 mg/dL. In general, patients are prescribed a high-dose statin (such as atorvastatin) to achieve the goal LDL. Statins also have shown to have an anti-inflammatory effect, which provides further secondary stroke prevention in the first few months after the event.

Acute Hemorrhagic Stroke

During the hyperacute phase, the management of patients with an intracranial hemorrhage focuses on airway, breathing, and circulation (ABCs), with particular attention

TABLE **47-5** Schedule of Neurologic Assessment and Vital Signs and Other Acute Care Assessments in Thrombolysis-Treated and Nonthrombolysis-Treated Patients

Thrombolysis-Treated Patients	Nonthrombolysis-Treated Patients
Neurologic assessment and vital signs (except temperature) every 15 minutes during alteplase infusion, then every 30 minutes for 6 hours, and then every 60 minutes for 16 hours (total of 24 hours) Note: Frequency of blood pressure (BP) assessments may need to be increased if systolic BP stays greater than 180 mm Hg or diastolic BP stays greater than 105 mm Hg during the first 24 hours. Temperature every 4 hours or as required. Treat temperatures > 99.6°F with acetaminophen as ordered.	In intensive care unit (ICU), every hour with neurologic checks or more frequently if necessary. In a non-ICU setting, depending on patient's condition and neurologic assessments; at a minimum check neurologic assessment and vital signs every 4 hours
After 24 hours, call physician if systolic BP greater than 185 or less than 110 mm Hg; diastolic BP greater than 105 or less than 60 mm Hg; pulse less than 50 or greater than 110 per minute; respirations 24 per minute; temperature over 99.6°F; or for worsening of stroke symptoms or other decline in neurologic status	Call physician for further treatment based on physician and institutional preferences/guidelines: Systolic BP above 220 or below 110 mm Hg; diastolic BP above 120 or below 60 mm Hg; pulse below 50 or above 110 per minute; temperature above 99.6°F; respirations 24 per minute; or for worsening of stroke symptoms or other decline in neurologic status
For O_2 saturation below 94%, give O_2 by cannula at 2–3 L/min	For O_2 saturation below 94%, give O_2 by cannula at 2–3 L/min
Monitor for major and minor bleeding complications	N/A
Continuous cardiac monitoring up to 72 hours or more	Continuous cardiac monitoring for 24–48 hours
Measure intake and output	Measure intake and output
Activity – as ordered by the physician	Activity – as ordered by the physician
IV fluids normal saline (NS) at 75–100 mL/hr	IV fluids NS at 75–100 mL/hr
No heparin, warfarin, aspirin, clopidogrel, or aspirin/extended-release dipyridamole for 24 hours, then start antithrombotic as ordered	Antithrombotics should be ordered before the end of hospital day #2
Brain CT or MRI after rtPA therapy	Repeat brain CT scan or MRI may be ordered 24–48 hours after stroke or as needed

Adapted from Summers, D., Leonard, A., Wentworth, D., Saver, J. L., Simpson, J., Spilker, J. A., ... Mitchell, P. H. (2009). Comprehensive overview of nursing and interdisciplinary care of the acute ischemic stroke patient: A scientific statement from the American Heart Association. *Stroke, 40*, 2911–2944. © 2009 American Heart Association, Inc.

paid to the patient's LOC. Immediate complications of a hemorrhage include extension of bleeding causing increased ICP, acute hydrocephalus, potential for herniation, and secondary brain injury. Any evidence of deterioration and ICP (refer to Chapter 45) is reported immediately to the health care team. For patients with a hemorrhage, the Glasgow Coma Scale (GCS) is also used as part of ongoing patient assessment. For patients with a GCS score of 8 or less, immediate intubation is indicated. Monitoring of peripheral oxygenation is expected with a pulse oximeter. Nurses will be directed to elevate the head of bed to 30 degrees, monitor sedation if instituted, and prepare for one or more of the following treatment options: anticoagulation reversal if patient is on anticoagulant, hyperventilation (hypocapnia temporarily causes vascular constriction, resulting in reduced blood flow in vessels not involved with the injury), placement of a ventricular catheter for CSF drainage, administration of mannitol—all to reduce elevated ICP. Because hyperthermia

(temperature above 37.5°C) is associated with a poorer prognosis following acute stroke, the nurse monitors the patient's temperature and is prepared to initiate measures to prevent and control fever collaboratively with the health care team. Additionally, because aspiration is a significant risk, patients should be maintained NPO until they are screened for dysphagia (Livesay & Hickey, 2014).

Clinicians will report an ICH score early in the assessment of a patient with an intracranial hemorrhage to determine prognosis. The scale in Figure 47-8 reviews specific patient-related characteristics to devise a score that is associated with risk for mortality within the first 30 days after hemorrhage. Components of the ICH score include the GCS score, hemorrhage volume, the presence of infratentorial hemorrhage, location of the hemorrhage, and patient age. The higher scores (5 and 6) predict a 100% mortality and, as such, will assist with decisions related to goals of care (Hemphill, Bonovich, Besmertis, et al., 2001).

GCS	
3–4	2 pts
5–12	1 pt
13–15	0 pts

ICH volume	
≥ 30 cm^3	1 pt
< 30 cm^3	0 pts

IVH	
Yes	1 pt
No	0 pts

ICH score	Mortality
0	No mortality
1	13%
2	26%
3	72%
4	97%
5	100%
6	100%

Location	
Infratentorial	1 pt
Supratentorial	0 pts

Age	
≥ 80 yrs	1 pt
< 80 yrs	0 pts

FIGURE 47-8 Determination of the intracerebral hemorrhage (ICH) score and risk of mortality. GCS, Glasgow Coma Scale; ICH, intracerebral hemorrhage; IVH, intraventricular hemorrhage. (Hemphill, J. C., Bonovich, D. C., Besmertis, L., Manley, G. T., & Johnston, S. C. (2001). The ICH score: A simple reliable grading scale for intracerebral hemorrhage. *Stroke, 32,* 891–897.)

 Concept Mastery Alert

For nonthrombolysis-treated patients, antithrombotics should be administered before the end of Day #2.

Surgical evacuation of intracranial bleeding is also considered in selected cases that require immediate intervention and when neurosurgical services are available. Depending on the location and volume of the intracerebral bleed, the degree of neurologic deterioration, and the presence of hydrocephalus and ventricular obstruction, patients may undergo a craniotomy and evacuation of the hematoma. Antihypertensive medications and antiepileptic medications are also mainstays of acute therapy to control bleeding and potential seizures. Blood pressure goals are ordered based on individual patient profiles. Current clinical trials are underway to determine target blood pressure ranges in ischemic stroke; however, generally treatment is avoided unless the systolic BP is greater than 220 mm Hg or diastolic BP is greater than 120 mm Hg (Livesay & Hickey, 2014, p. 525). Pain, fever, and hyperglycemia are addressed in the first 24 hours to reduce further cerebral injury (Livesay & Hickey, 2014).

For patients with a known ruptured aneurysm and subsequent SAH, the 2015 AHA guidelines for SAH describe both surgical clipping and endovascular coiling as beneficial options to reduce the risk of rebleeding. Surgical clipping involves a craniotomy and placement of a clip at the neck of the artery to close the rupture site. Coiling is an endovascular

procedure using a catheter that is accessed from the femoral artery and directed through the vasculature to the location of the aneurysm. Multiple coils are then dispensed through the catheter and packed into the dome of the aneurysm to promote clotting and close the aneurysm. The choice of aneurysm treatment depends on the overall health of the patient, the nature and location of the aneurysm, and the available resources at the hospital. Clinicians also use an assessment scoring tool called the Hunt and Hess Score (Fig. 47-9) to grade patients with SAH to predict surgical mortality. Based on headache quality, focal deficit, and LOC, the patient with a higher score will portend a poor prognosis. Because this score depends on evolving and sometimes fluctuating symptoms, this score can change from what was recorded during the patient's initial admission.

Stroke care in the acute phase is typically designated as the time during which the patient has been admitted to the hospital. The hospital stay can vary from a few days to many weeks, depending on the nature and severity of the stroke, and deficits and complications associated with recovery. In addition to monitoring for potential complications associated with stroke such as deconditioning, aspiration, infection, bowel and bladder dysfunction, and inability to perform self-care, care plans should include an early initiation of rehabilitation to improve functional outcome.

Hunt-Hess Scale

- **Grade 1:**
  Mild headache, normal mental status, no cranial nerve or motor findings – (GCS* score 15, no motor deficits)

- **Grade 2:**
  Severe headache, normal mental status, may have cranial nerve deficit – (GCS score 13–14, no motor deficits)

- **Grade 3:**
  Somnolent, confused, may have cranial nerve or mild motor DEFICIT – (GCS SCORE 13–14, WITH MOTOR DEFICITS)

- **Grade 4:**
  Stupor, moderate to severe motor deficit, may have intermittent reflex posturing – (GCS score 7–12, with or without motor deficits)

- **Grade 5:**
  Coma, reflex posturing or flaccid – (GCS score, 3–6, with or without motor deficits)

FIGURE 47-9 HUNT-HESS scores. (Hunt, W. E., & Hess, R. M. (1968). Surgical risk as related to time of intervention in the repair of intracranial aneurysms. *Journal of Neurosurgery, 28*(1), 14–20.)

Stroke Rehabilitation

The potential for recovery after stroke extends beyond the hospital admission and beyond the time spent in an acute or subacute care facility. Although rehabilitation planning begins on the day of hospital admission, nursing interventions and collaboration with the multidisciplinary rehabilitation team continue throughout the patient's recovery. It is important to understand what the patient was like before the stroke. A history of other illnesses, behavioral characteristics, activities of daily living (ADLs), and neurologic scores (such as the modified Rankin scale) will provide information to develop a realistic plan for recovery. The World Health Organization's International Classification of Functioning (ICF) has been included as one of the five sections outlined in the AHA's Guidelines for Adult Stroke Rehabilitation and Recovery (Winstein, Stein, Arena, et al., 2016). The three components of the model include:

1. The pathophysiologic processes directly related to the stroke and its associated comorbidities
2. The impact this condition has on the individual
3. Contextual variables, such as each survivor's personal and environmental resources

The major goals for the patient (and family) should include all efforts to return the patient to his or her premorbid functioning. Depending on the location of the initial brain injury, patients are assessed for rehabilitative needs to improve mobility, communication, cognition, coordination, balance, and pain relief (from contractures). Potential complications such as aspiration, incontinence, skin breakdown, falls, depression, and disruption of family dynamics are targets for prevention.

Prevention

In a healthy population, risk factors are identified and addressed in a primordial and primary prevention program. *Primordial prevention* refers to strategies designed to decrease the development of disease risk factors (e.g., efforts to decrease the development of obesity, increase exercise, and provide a well-balanced diet). Primordial prevention encompasses the entire population and is not limited to individuals with recognized risk factors for stroke or other cardiovascular diseases (Schwamm, Pancioli, Acker, et al., 2005). *Primary prevention* refers to the treatment of established disease risk factors but for those patients who have not yet had an event. The 2014 Guidelines for the Primary Prevention of Stroke provide a comprehensive overview of established and emerging modifiable and nonmodifiable stroke risk factors (Meschia, Bushnell, Boden-Albala, et al., 2014).

For patients who have had a stroke, risk factor modification is a critical part of the secondary prevention plan. Stroke education for patients and their families addresses the possible causes of stroke, identifies potential stroke risk factors, reinforces compliance with medications, and discusses pertinent lifestyle changes to reduce stroke risk. The 2014 guidelines for the prevention of subsequent stroke after stroke or TIA highlight the following key risk factors: hypertension, diabetes, dyslipidemia, smoking, alcohol consumption, obesity, and sedentary activity. Patient education has become a standard performance measure for practice at certified primary stroke centers.

Optimal medical therapy includes prescribing an antiplatelet medication (such as aspirin, clopidogrel, or aspirin/extended-release dipyridamole), a statin (such as atorvastatin or simvastatin), and an antihypertensive (thiazide diuretic, angiotensin-converting enzyme [ACE] inhibitor or beta blocker). For those patients with paroxysmal or permanent atrial fibrillation, anticoagulation (with warfarin or other anticoagulant) is also recommended (Furie, Kasner, Adams, et al., 2011).

For those patients who have had a hemorrhagic stroke, blood pressure control is critical. The issue of whether to start or resume antithrombotic therapy is highly dependent on the nature and severity of the hemorrhage and the risk for a subsequent thrombotic event (as in the case of a patient with atrial fibrillation or with a mechanical heart valve).

For patients with symptoms of TIA or stroke thought to be caused by significant carotid artery stenosis (70% to 99%), a carotid endarterectomy (CEA) may be recommended. A CEA is the removal of an atherosclerotic plaque or thrombus from the ICA to prevent recurrent stroke. Carotid angioplasty and stenting is an alternative (less invasive) procedure and performed in selected patients when surgery poses a higher risk and the endovascular approach poses a low perioperative complication risk. These procedures are generally recommended once the patient is hemodynamically stable and usually within the first 2 weeks following their event.

In preparation for discharge, teaching patients and families about what to expect within a home or rehabilitation facility will be a focus for nursing, the rehabilitation staff, and the discharge planner. Resources in the community, such as support groups, regional and national heart and stroke associations, and hospital-based social work support should also be part of the discharge materials.

NURSING PROCESS
The Patient with a Stroke

ASSESSMENT

A nursing flow sheet is maintained for the documentation of a complete neurologic assessment.

A systems approach to examining and documenting findings should include a mental status evaluation (orientation, affect, perception, memory, attention span, speech, and language), motor control, swallowing ability, hydration status, fluid output, skin integrity, and activity level. The ongoing nursing assessment continues to focus on alterations in cognition and functional impairment and directs the appropriate nursing diagnoses.

DIAGNOSIS

Appropriate nursing diagnoses may include:

- Altered hemodynamics related to cardiac arrhythmias, hyper-/hypotension, fluid/electrolyte imbalances
- Impaired physical mobility related to hemiparesis, sensory loss, loss of balance or coordination, or visual field deficit
- Impaired verbal communication related to dysarthria, aphasia, altered cognition
- Impaired swallowing/risk for aspiration related to inability to protect airway or altered LOC
- Risk for infection related to smoking history, invasive lines, Foley catheter, nasogastric (NG) tube
- Risk for ineffective peripheral tissue perfusion related to risk for DVT/immobility
- High risk for injury related to visual field, motor, or perception deficits
- Knowledge deficit related to lack of awareness of stroke risk factors, secondary stroke prevention medications, potential lifestyle changes, physical and occupational therapies

PLANNING

Although rehabilitation begins on the day of admission, the process is intensified during convalescence and requires a coordinated team effort. It is helpful for the team to know the patient's baseline function, medical history, mental and emotional state, behavioral characteristics, and ADLs. Additionally, clinicians should be knowledgeable about the relative importance of predictors of stroke outcome (age, comorbidities such as diabetes, and presenting NIHSS score) in order to provide stroke survivors and their families with a realistic recovery trajectory. For example, the NIHSS score is used commonly to communicate the severity of symptoms associated with stroke and is often conducted on admission, at 24 hours and at discharge; other institutions will collect the NIHSS score every shift and use the score to communicate patient status (Livesay & Hickey, 2014). Refer to Table 47-4 for the NIHSS scale.

A commonly used assessment scale for measuring disability as it relates to the patient's dependence with daily activities after stroke is the modified Rankin scale. A 0–6 scale is used to describe the trajectory from "zero" or "no symptoms—able to perform all usual activities" to "five" or "severe disability—bedridden and requiring constant 24-hour care." A score of "six" refers to "death." This tool has been adopted by clinicians, rehabilitation specialists, and researchers to determine pre-stroke capabilities as well as short- and long-term post-stroke degree of disability (Wilson, Hareendran, & Grant, 2002). See Figure 47-10.

The major goals for the patient (and family) may include improved mobility, avoidance of shoulder pain, achievement of self-care, relief of sensory and perceptual deprivation, prevention of aspiration, continence of bowel and bladder, improved

Modified Rankin Scale (MRS)	
0	No symptoms
1	No significant disability, despite symptoms; able to perform all usual duties and activities
2	Slight disability; unable to perform all previous activities but able to look after own affairs without assistance
3	Moderate disability; requires some help, but able to walk without assistance
4	Moderately severe disability; unable to walk without assistance and unable to attend to own bodily needs without assistance
5	Severe disability; bedridden, incontinent, and requires constant nursing care and attention
6	Death

FIGURE 47-10 Modified Rankin scale. (Rankin, J. (1957). Cerebral vascular accidents in patients over the age of 60. *Scottish Medical Journal, 2,* 200–215; Bonita, R., & Beaglehole, R. (1988). Modification of Rankin Scale: Recovery of motor function after stroke. *Stroke, 19*(12), 1497–1500.)

thought processes, optimization of communication, maintaining skin integrity, restored family functioning, improved sexual function, and absence of complications.

NURSING INTERVENTIONS

Nursing care has a significant impact on the patient's recovery. Often, many body systems are impaired as a result of the stroke, and conscientious care and timely interventions can prevent debilitating complications. During and after the acute phase, nursing interventions include a comprehensive approach to physical care and fostering recovery by listening to the patient and asking questions to elicit the meaning of the stroke experience.

IMPROVING MOBILITY AND PREVENTING JOINT DEFORMITIES

When control of the voluntary muscles is lost, the strong flexor muscles exert control over the extensors. The arm tends to adduct (adductor muscles are stronger than abductors) and to rotate internally. The elbow and the wrist tend to flex, the affected leg tends to rotate externally at the hip joint and flex at the knee, and the foot at the ankle joint supinates and tends toward plantar flexion.

Correct positioning is important to prevent contractures; measures are used to relieve pressure, assist in maintaining good body alignment, and prevent compressive neuropathies,

(continued on page 1372)

especially of the ulnar and peroneal nerves. Because flexor muscles are stronger than extensor muscles, a posterior splint applied at night to the affected extremity may prevent flexion and maintain correct positioning during sleep. If splints are in place, the nurse assesses the skin for evidence of impaired circulation, sensation, and/or mobility, as well as any evidence of altered skin integrity.

> **Nursing Alert**
> *Positioning after stroke remains controversial (Hunter et al., 2011; Olavarria et al., 2014). In the acute phase, the goal is to optimize cerebral perfusion and so having the head of bed flat (supine) will enhance blood flow to the brain. The supine position is generally reserved for conscious patients without evidence of dysphagia since they are at low risk for aspiration and can control secretions. The unconscious patient or a patient at risk for aspiration is positioned in side-lying position with the head of the bed elevated 10 to 30 degrees to facilitate the drainage of secretions from the mouth (Livesay & Hickey, 2014). Practices for patient positioning are institution-specific and are outlined in stroke recovery care protocols. In general, most practices include an HOB order of 30 to 45 degrees.*

Preventing Shoulder Adduction. To prevent adduction of the affected shoulder while the patient is in bed, a pillow is placed in the axilla when there is limited external rotation; this keeps the arm away from the chest. A pillow is placed under the arm, and the arm is placed in a neutral (slightly flexed) position, with distal joints positioned higher than the more proximal joints (i.e., the elbow is positioned higher than the shoulder and the wrist higher than the elbow). This helps to prevent edema and the resultant joint fibrosis that will limit range of motion (ROM) if the patient regains control of the arm.

Positioning the Hand and Fingers. The fingers are positioned so that they are barely flexed. The hand is placed in slight supination (palm faces upward), which is its most functional position. If the upper extremity is flaccid, a splint can be used to support the wrist and hand in a functional position. Every effort is made to prevent hand edema.

Spasticity, particularly in the hand, can be a disabling complication after stroke. Researchers have reported that repeated intramuscular injections of botulinum toxin A into wrist and finger muscles significantly reduced upper limb spasticity after stroke and improved upper limb motor function for a period of 3 months; however, the evidence on whether botulinum toxin A injections are useful for improving upper limb capacity is lacking (Kwakkel & Meskers, 2015; Tsuchiya, Morita, & Hara, 2016).

Mirror therapy has also demonstrated improvement in motor functions and ADLs that persisted after 6 months. In this therapy, the patient watches a mirror as movements with the unaffected hand are performed, leaving the impression that his or her affected hand is moving. This therapy is purported to induce neuroplasticity changes in the primary motor cortex that support recovery (Radajewska, 2016).

Establishing an Exercise Program. The affected extremities are exercised passively and put through a full ROM four or five times a day to maintain joint mobility, regain motor control, prevent contractures in the paralyzed extremity, prevent further deterioration of the neuromuscular system, and enhance circulation. Repetition of an activity forms new pathways in the CNS and therefore encourages new patterns of motion. At first, the extremities are usually flaccid. If tightness occurs in any area, the ROM exercises should be performed more frequently. Regularity in exercise is most important. Improvement in muscle strength and maintenance of ROM can be achieved only through daily exercise.

The patient is encouraged and reminded to exercise the unaffected side at intervals throughout the day. It is helpful to develop a written schedule to remind the patient of the exercise activities. The nurse supervises and supports the patient during these activities. The patient can be taught to put the unaffected leg under the affected one to assist in moving it when turning and exercising. Flexibility, strengthening, coordination, endurance, and balancing exercises prepare the patient for ambulation. Quadriceps muscle setting and gluteal setting exercises are started early to improve the muscle strength needed for walking; these are performed at least five times daily for 10 minutes at a time.

Preparing for Ambulation. As soon as possible, the patient is assisted out of bed. Usually, an active rehabilitation program is started as soon as the patient regains consciousness. The patient is first taught to maintain balance while sitting and then to learn to balance while standing. If the patient has difficulty in achieving standing balance, a tilt table, which slowly brings the patient to an upright position, can be used. If orthostatic hypotension is a problem, the nurse can gradually elevate the head of the bed and assess blood pressure, pulse, skin color, and any complaints of dizziness or lightheadedness. If hypotension, tachycardia, paleness, diaphoresis, dizziness, or lightheadedness are noted, the head of the bed may be lowered until the symptoms resolve.

The patient is usually ready to walk as soon as standing balance is achieved. Parallel bars are useful in these first efforts. A chair or wheelchair should be readily available in case the patient suddenly becomes fatigued or feels dizzy.

The training periods for ambulation should be short and frequent. As the patient gains strength and confidence, an adjustable cane can be used for support. In general, a three- or four-pronged cane provides a stable support in the early phases of rehabilitation.

PREVENTING SHOULDER PAIN

As many as 70% of stroke patients suffer pain in the shoulder that prevents them from regaining full ROM, and 88% will have some level of upper extremity dysfunction (Winstein, 2016). Shoulder function is essential in achieving balance and performing transfers and self-care activities. Three problems can occur: painful shoulder, subluxation (partial dislocation) of the shoulder, and shoulder–hand syndrome or reflex sympathetic dystrophy syndrome (RSDS), which features pain (often "burning"); tenderness; vasoconstrictive-related coldness of the affected extremity; trophic changes of hair, nails, skin; and swelling.

A flaccid shoulder joint may be overstretched by the use of excessive force in turning the patient or from overstrenuous arm and shoulder movement. To prevent shoulder pain, the nurse should never lift the patient by the flaccid shoulder or pull on the affected arm or shoulder. If the arm is paralyzed, subluxation at the shoulder can occur as a result of overstretching of the joint capsule and musculature by the force of gravity when the patient sits or stands in the early stages after a stroke. This results in severe pain. Shoulder–hand syndrome (painful shoulder and generalized swelling of the hand) can cause a frozen shoulder and ultimately atrophy of subcutaneous tissues. When a shoulder becomes stiff, it is usually painful.

Many shoulder problems can be prevented by proper patient movement and positioning. The flaccid arm is positioned on a table or with pillows while the patient is seated. Some clinicians advocate the use of a properly worn sling when the patient first becomes ambulatory to prevent the paralyzed upper extremity from dangling without support. ROM exercises are important in preventing painful shoulder. Overly strenuous arm movements are avoided. The patient is instructed to interlace the fingers, place the palms together, and push the clasped hands slowly forward to bring the scapulae forward; he or she then raises both hands above the head. This is repeated throughout the day. The patient is instructed to flex the affected wrist at intervals and move all the joints of the affected fingers. He or she is encouraged to touch, stroke, rub, and look at both hands. Pushing the heel of the hand firmly down on a surface is useful. Elevation of the arm and hand is also important in preventing dependent edema of the hand. When dressing, the sequence of weaker arm, head, followed by stronger arm is followed (Winstein, 2016). Patients with continuing pain after attempted movement and positioning may require the addition of analgesia to their treatment program.

Medications are helpful in the management of post-stroke pain. Opioids are generally prescribed for acute pain but may be considered for patients with chronic pain. If prescribed, the nurse assesses for side effects, tolerance, dependency, and abuse. Adjuvant drugs, such as antidepressants, anticonvulsants, and anxiolytics, may also be considered. Tricyclic antidepressants are often prescribed for neuropathic pain, while anticonvulsants are used for their ability to stabilize neuronal membranes. Gabapentin (Neurontin) is becoming a first-line drug for neuropathic pain (Livesay & Hickey, 2014). The antiseizure medication lamotrigine (Lamictal) has been found to be effective for post-stroke pain. Topical analgesics, such as lidocaine cream or patch, may also be considered.

ENHANCING SELF-CARE

As soon as the patient can sit up, personal hygiene activities are encouraged. The patient is helped to set realistic goals; if feasible, a new task is added daily. The first step is to carry out all self-care activities on the unaffected side. Such activities as combing the hair, brushing the teeth, shaving with an electric razor, bathing, and eating can be carried out with one hand and are suitable for self-care. Although the patient may feel awkward at first, the various motor skills can be learned by repetition, and the unaffected side will become stronger with use. The nurse must be sure that the patient does not neglect the affected side. Assistive devices will help make up for some of the patient's deficits. For example, a small towel is easier to control while drying after bathing, and boxed paper tissues are easier to use than a roll of toilet tissue.

Return of functional ability is important to the patient recovering after a stroke. An early baseline assessment of functional ability with an instrument such as the Functional Independence Measure (FIM™) is important in team planning and goal setting for the patient. The FIM™ is a widely used instrument in stroke rehabilitation and provides valuable information about motor, social, and cognitive function (Livesay & Hickey, 2014). The patient's morale will improve if ambulatory activities are carried out in street clothes. The family is instructed to bring in clothing that is preferably a size larger than that normally worn. Clothing fitted with front or side fasteners or Velcro closures is the most suitable. The patient has better balance if most of the dressing activities are carried out while seated.

Perceptual problems may make it difficult for the patient to dress without assistance because of an inability to match the clothing to the body parts. To assist the patient, the nurse can take steps to keep the environment organized and uncluttered, because the patient with a perceptual problem is easily distracted. The patient has to make many compensatory movements when dressing; these can produce fatigue and painful twisting of the intercostal muscles. Support and encouragement are provided to prevent the patient from becoming overly fatigued and discouraged. Even with intensive training, not all patients can achieve independence in dressing.

MANAGING SENSORY-PERCEPTUAL DIFFICULTIES

Patients with a decreased field of vision should be approached on the side where visual perception is intact. All visual stimuli (e.g., clock, calendar, television) should be placed on this side. The patient can be taught to turn the head in the direction of the defective visual field to compensate for this loss. The nurse should make eye contact with the patient and draw his or her attention to the affected side by encouraging the patient to move the head. The nurse may also want to stand at a position that encourages the patient to move or turn to visualize who is in the room. Increasing the natural or artificial lighting in the room and providing eyeglasses are important aids to increasing vision.

The patient with homonymous hemianopsia (loss of half of the visual field) turns away from the affected side of the body

(continued on page 1374)

and tends to neglect that side and the space on that side; this is called *amorphosynthesis.* In such instances, the patient cannot see food on half of the tray, and only half of the room is visible. It is important for the nurse to constantly remind the patient of the other side of the body, to maintain alignment of the extremities, and, if possible, to place the extremities where the patient can see them.

ASSISTING WITH NUTRITION

Stroke can result in swallowing problems (dysphagia). Patients must be observed for paroxysms of coughing, food dribbling out of or pooling in one side of the mouth, food retained for long periods in the mouth, or nasal regurgitation when swallowing liquids. Swallowing difficulties place the patient at risk for aspiration, pneumonia, dehydration, and malnutrition. A speech therapist will evaluate the patient's gag reflexes and ability to swallow. A validated, nurse-directed dysphagia screening assessment has been recommended as part of post-stroke care to identify a patient's swallowing difficulty. A speech therapist may be consulted for patients who fail an initial screen and require a more formal evaluation. Even if swallowing function is partially impaired, it may return in some patients over time, or the patient may be taught alternative swallowing techniques, advised to take smaller boluses of food, place food on the unaffected side of the patient's mouth, and taught about types of foods that are easier to swallow. The patient may be started on a thick liquid or puréed diet because these foods are easier to swallow than thin liquids. Having the patient sit upright, preferably out of bed in a chair, and instructing him or her to tuck the chin toward the chest as he or she swallows will help prevent aspiration. The diet may be advanced as the patient becomes more proficient at swallowing. If the patient cannot resume oral intake, a gastrointestinal feeding tube will be placed for ongoing tube feedings.

Enteral tubes can be either nasogastric (placed in the stomach) or nasoenteric (placed in the duodenum) to reduce the risk of aspiration. For long-term feedings, a gastrostomy tube is preferred. Refer to Chapter 22 for details on enteral feeding. Nursing responsibilities in feeding include elevating the head of the bed at least 30 degrees to prevent aspiration, checking the position of the tube before feeding, assessing residuals, and ensuring that the cuff of the tracheostomy tube (if in place) is inflated.

ATTAINING BOWEL AND BLADDER CONTROL

After a stroke, the patient may have transient urinary incontinence due to confusion, inability to communicate needs, and inability to use the urinal or bedpan because of impaired motor and postural control. Occasionally, after a stroke, the bladder becomes atonic, with impaired sensation in response to bladder filling. Sometimes control of the external urinary sphincter is lost or diminished. During this period, intermittent catheterization with sterile technique is carried out. After muscle tone increases and deep tendon reflexes return, bladder tone increases and

spasticity of the bladder may develop. Because the patient's sense of awareness is clouded, persistent urinary incontinence or urinary retention may be symptomatic of bilateral brain damage. The voiding pattern is analyzed, and the urinal or bedpan is offered on a pattern or schedule. The upright posture and standing position are helpful for male patients during this aspect of rehabilitation.

Patients may have problems with bowel control, particularly constipation. Unless contraindicated, a high-fiber diet and adequate fluid intake (2 to 3 L/day) should be provided and a regular time (usually after breakfast) should be established for toileting.

IMPROVING THOUGHT PROCESSES

After a stroke, patients may experience changes in cognition and behavior and may exhibit periods of emotional lability. These changes are usually associated with injury to the right hemisphere. Often they are transient and, with aggressive rehabilitation, patients can recover.

Screening for these problems is typically incorporated into the initial rehabilitation assessment and then repeated after discharge. Often a neuropsychologist will be consulted to perform formal neuropsychological testing to make recommendations for the appropriate follow-up treatment. A treatment program for addressing any identified deficit is established in collaboration with the patient's neurologist and primary care provider.

The role of the nurse is supportive. The nurse reviews the results of neuropsychological testing, observes the patient's performance and progress, gives positive feedback, and, most importantly, conveys an attitude of confidence and hope. Interventions capitalize on the patient's strengths and remaining abilities while attempting to improve performance of affected functions. Other interventions are similar to those for improving cognitive functioning after a head injury.

IMPROVING COMMUNICATION

Aphasia, which impairs the patient's ability to express him- or herself and to understand what is being said, may become apparent in various ways. The cortical area that is responsible for integrating the myriad pathways required for the comprehension and formulation of language is called the *Broca area.* It is located in a convolution adjoining the middle cerebral artery. This area is responsible for control of the combinations of muscular movements needed to speak each word. Patients who are paralyzed on the right side (due to damage or injury to the left side of the brain) cannot speak, whereas those paralyzed on the left side are less likely to have speech disturbances. The speech therapist assesses the communication needs of the stroke patient, describes the precise deficit, and suggests the best overall method of communication. Most language intervention strategies can be tailored for the individual patient. The patient is expected to take an active part in establishing goals.

Nursing interventions include strategies to make the atmosphere conducive to communication. This includes being sensitive to the patient's reactions and needs and responding to them in an appropriate manner. A consistent schedule, routines, and repetition help the patient to function despite significant deficits. A written copy of the daily schedule, a folder of personal information (birth date, address, names of relatives), checklists, and an audio-taped list help improve the patient's memory and concentration. The patient may also benefit from a communication board, which has pictures of common needs and phrases. When talking with the patient, it is important for the nurse to gain the patient's attention, speak slowly, and keep the language of instruction consistent. One instruction is given at a time, and time is allowed for the patient to process what has been said. The use of gestures may enhance comprehension. In working with the patient with aphasia, the nurse must remember to talk to the patient during care activities. This provides social contact for the patient.

MAINTAINING SKIN INTEGRITY

The patient who has had a stroke may be at risk for skin and tissue breakdown because of altered sensation and inability to respond to pressure and discomfort by turning and moving. Preventing skin and tissue breakdown requires frequent assessment of the skin, with emphasis on bony areas and dependent parts of the body. During the acute phase, a specialty bed (e.g., low-air-loss bed) may be used until the patient can move independently or assist in moving.

A regular turning schedule (at least every 2 hours) must be adhered to even if pressure-relieving devices are used to prevent tissue and skin breakdown. When the patient is positioned or turned, care must be used to minimize shear and friction forces that may tear the skin and expose the patent to additional sources for infection. The patient's skin must be kept clean and dry; gentle massage of healthy (non-reddened) skin and adequate nutrition are other factors that help to maintain normal skin and tissue integrity.

IMPROVING FAMILY COPING

Family members play an important role in the patient's recovery. Family members are encouraged to participate in counseling and to use support systems that will help with the emotional and physical stress of caring for the patient. Involving others in the patient's care and teaching stress management techniques and methods for maintaining personal health also facilitate family coping.

The family may have difficulty accepting the patient's disability and may be unrealistic in their expectations. They are given information about the expected outcomes and are counseled to avoid doing activities for the patient that he or she can do. They are assured that their love and interest are part of the patient's therapy.

The family needs to be informed that the rehabilitation of the hemiplegic patient requires many months and that progress may be slow. The gains made by the patient in the hospital or rehabilitation unit must be maintained. All caregivers should approach the patient with a supportive and optimistic attitude,

focusing on the patient's remaining abilities. The rehabilitation team, the medical and nursing team, the patient, and the family must all be involved in developing attainable goals for the patient at home.

Most relatives of patients with stroke handle the physical changes better than the emotional aspects of care. The family should be prepared to expect occasional episodes of emotional lability. The patient may laugh or cry easily and may be irritable and demanding or depressed and confused. The nurse can explain to the family that the patient's laughter does not necessarily connote happiness, nor does crying reflect sadness, and that emotional lability usually improves with time.

HELPING THE PATIENT COPE WITH SEXUAL DYSFUNCTION

Sexual functioning can be altered by stroke. Sexual dysfunction after stroke is multifactorial. There may be medical reasons for the dysfunction (neurologic and cognitive deficits, previous diseases, medications), as well as various psychosocial factors. A stroke can potentially be such a catastrophic illness that the patient experiences loss of self-esteem and value as a sexual being. These psychosocial factors play an important role in determining sexual drive, activity, and satisfaction after a stroke.

Nurses in the rehabilitation setting play a crucial role in beginning a dialogue between the patient and his or her partner about sexuality after a stroke. In-depth assessments to determine sexual history before and after the stroke should be followed by appropriate interventions. Interventions for the patient and partner focus on providing relevant information, education, reassurance, adjustment of medications, counseling regarding coping skills, suggestions for alternative sexual positions, and a means of sexual expression and satisfaction.

PROVIDING PATIENT EDUCATION AND PREPARING THE PATIENT FOR THE HOME

Patient and family education is a fundamental component of rehabilitation. The nurse provides teaching about stroke, its causes and prevention, and the rehabilitation process. In both acute care and rehabilitation facilities, the focus is on teaching the patient to resume as much self-care as possible. This may entail using assistive devices or modifying the home environment to help the patient live with a disability. Families are also encouraged to take part in being assessed for their role as caregiver and their readiness to accept the additional responsibilities associated with a family member with both physical and cognitive disabilities.

An occupational therapist may be helpful in assessing the home environment and recommending modifications to help the patient become more independent. For example, a shower is more convenient than a tub for the patient with hemiplegia because most patients do not gain sufficient strength to get up and down from a tub. Sitting on a stool of medium height with rubber suction tips allows the patient to wash with greater ease. A long-handled bath brush with a soap container is helpful to the patient who has only one functional hand. If a shower is not

(continued on page 1376)

available, a stool may be placed in the tub and a portable shower hose attached to the faucet. Handrails may be attached alongside the bathtub and the toilet. Other assistive devices include special utensils for eating, grooming, dressing, and writing.

A program of physical therapy can be beneficial in the home environment. One technique that was shown to result in a reduction in motor impairment concentrates on enhanced exercise of the affected limb. Another technique that showed positive outcomes uses sensorimotor training of the upper limb and the wrist.

Depression is a common and serious problem after stroke. Counseling and antidepressant therapy may help if depression dominates the patient's life. As progress is made in the rehabilitation program, some problems will diminish. The family can help by continuing to support the patient and by giving positive reinforcement for the progress that is being made.

Community-based stroke support groups may allow the patient and family to learn from others with similar problems and to share their experiences. Support groups take the form of in-person meetings as well as web-based support programs. The patient is encouraged to continue hobbies and recreational and leisure interests and to maintain contact with friends to prevent social isolation. Patients should be supported to keep active, adhere to the exercise program, and remain as self-sufficient as possible.

The nurse should recognize the potential effects of caregiving on the family. Not all families have the adaptive coping skills and adequate psychological functioning necessary for the long-term care of another person. The patient's spouse may be elderly, with his or her own health concerns; in some instances, the patient may have been the provider of care to the spouse. Even healthy caregivers may find it difficult to maintain a schedule that includes being available around the clock.

Depressed caregivers are more likely to resort to physical or emotional abuse of the patient and are more likely to place the patient in a nursing home. Respite care (planned short-term care to relieve the family from having to provide continuous 24-hour care) may be available from an adult day care center. Some hospitals also offer weekend respite care that can provide caregivers with needed time for themselves. The nurse encourages the family to arrange for such services and provides information to assist them.

The nurse involved in home and continuing care also needs to remind the patient and family of the need for continuing health promotion and screening practices. Patients who have not been involved in these practices in the past are educated about their importance and are referred to appropriate health care providers, if indicated.

EVALUATION

Expected patient outcomes may include the following:
1. Demonstrates intact neurologic status and normal vital signs and respiratory patterns:
   a. Normal mental status examination, intact cognitive process
   b. Normal speech patterns and language function
   c. Normal/equal strength, movement, and sensation of all four extremities
2. Understands diagnostic procedures and treatment plan:
   a. Review of current and new medications
   b. Proposed physical and occupational therapies
   c. Achieves self-care; uses adaptive equipment
3. Arranges for follow-up appointments with stroke neurologist or primary care provider

CHAPTER REVIEW

Critical Thinking Exercises

1. A 74-year-old man presents to the emergency department with confusion, right-sided weakness, and difficulty getting his words out. He scores an 8 on the NIHSS. His symptoms started 1 hour prior to admission. His head CT scan shows no evidence of a bleed. He weighs 78 kg. What are the inclusion criteria for administering IV alteplase? What is the FDA-approved time-frame for administering alteplase? How is alteplase dosed?

2. An 80-year-old woman is admitted to the hospital with a large SAH and undergoes a coiling procedure for a ruptured aneurysm. What nursing measures should be implemented to prevent rebleeding during her hospital stay?

3. A 48-year-old man with a history of hypertension, dyslipidemia, coronary artery disease, and smoking is admitted to the hospital with a 2-day history of nausea and vertigo. His hospital workup revealed an ischemic stroke in the right cerebellum. What medications might he be sent home with? What risk factor modifications will be recommended? What additional teaching will be important to emphasize his need to seek medical care?

NCLEX-Style Review Questions

1. A patient being cared for on the neurologic unit has a diagnosis of acute ischemic stroke. It has affected the

left hemisphere of the patient's brain. The nurse would expect to assess which deficit in this patient?

a. Left side of body weakness
b. Aphasia
c. Left field visual deficit
d. Lack of awareness of deficits

2. A patient diagnosed with a stroke is experiencing slurred speech. The nurse would accurately document this finding as which clinical manifestation of stroke?

a. Aphasia
b. Dysphasia
c. Dysarthria
d. Apraxia

3. A 73-year-old patient has been diagnosed with ischemic stroke following diagnostic studies. Which medication must be given within a 4.5-hour window of symptom onset to be effective in lysing a clot?

a. Heparin
b. Coumadin
c. Plavix
d. Alteplase

4. What would the nurse expect to document in a patient diagnosed with a right hemispheric stroke?

a. Aphasia
b. Slow, cautious behavior
c. Right visual field deficit
d. Impulsive behavior

5. What initial diagnostic test is recommended to assess for a cerebral bleed?

a. MRI
b. Noncontrast CT
c. CT with contrast
d. Cerebral angiography

Try these additional resources, available at **http://thepoint.lww.com/Honan2e**, to enhance your learning and understanding of this chapter:

• NCLEX-Style Student Review Questions
• Journal Articles

REFERENCES AND SELECTED READINGS

References and selected readings associated with this chapter can be found on the website that accompanies the book. Visit **http://thepoint. lww.com/Honan2e** to access the references and other additional resources associated with this chapter.

Problems Related to Sensorineural Function

A patient with hearing loss in both ears is being seen in the hearing clinic. She sustained the hearing loss in a traumatic accident. The health care provider is giving her information about a cochlear implant.

- What are the criteria that have to be met to receive a cochlear implant?
- What does the surgical procedure involve?
- What does the rehabilitation period consist of?

Nursing Assessment: Sensorineural Function

Linda S. Dune • Lynn S. Bickley • Peter G. Szilagyi

Learning Objectives

After reading this chapter, you will be able to:

1. Identify eye structures and describe their functions.
2. Describe assessment components for the eye.
3. Identify diagnostic tests for assessment of vision and evaluation of visual disabilities.
4. Identify ear structures and describe their functions.
5. Describe assessment components for the ear.
6. Describe methods used to assess hearing and diagnose hearing and balance disorders.

THE EYE

The eye is a sensitive, highly specialized sense organ subject to various disorders, many of which lead to impaired vision. Impaired vision may affect a person's independence in self-care, work and lifestyle choices, sense of self-esteem, safety, ability to interact with society and the environment, and overall quality of life.

Although most people with eye disorders are treated in an ambulatory care setting, many patients receiving health care have an eye disease as a comorbid condition. In addition to understanding the prevention, treatment, and consequences of eye disorders, nurses in all settings assess visual acuity in those at risk, refer patients to eye care specialists as appropriate, implement measures to prevent further visual loss, and help patients adapt to impaired vision.

ANATOMIC AND PHYSIOLOGIC OVERVIEW

Unlike most organs of the body, the eye is available for external examination, and its anatomy is more easily assessed than many other body parts (Fig. 48-1). The eyeball, or globe, sits in a protective bony structure known as the *orbit*. The optic nerve and the ophthalmic artery enter the orbit at its apex through the optic foramen. The eyeball is moved through all fields of gaze by the extraocular muscles. The four rectus muscles and two oblique muscles (Fig. 48-2) are innervated by cranial nerves (CN) III, IV, and VI. Normally, the movements of the two eyes are coordinated, and the brain perceives a single image.

External Eye

The eyelids, composed of thin elastic skin that covers striated and smooth muscles, protect the anterior portion of the eye. The eyelids contain multiple glands, including sebaceous, sweat, and accessory lacrimal glands, and they are lined with conjunctival material. The upper lid normally covers the uppermost portion of the iris and is innervated by the oculomotor nerve (CN III). The lid margins contain meibomian glands, which produce an oil-like substance as a constituent of tears that helps to prevent dry eyes in the inferior and superior puncta, and the eyelashes. The triangular spaces formed by the junction of the eyelids are known as the *inner* or *medial canthus* and the *outer* or *lateral canthus*.

Tears are vital to eye health. They protect the cornea and sclera with lubrication, nutritional support, moisture, and protection from microbes. Tears also contain immunoglobulins that contribute to the increase in tearing during allergic responses. A healthy tear is composed of three layers: lipoid, aqueous, and mucoid. If there is a defect in the composition of any of these layers, the integrity of the cornea may be compromised. Tears are secreted in response to reflex or emotional stimuli. With every blink of the eyes, the lids wash the cornea and conjunctiva with tears.

Nursing Alert
In the absence of the patient's corneal reflex, the nurse must protect the patient's affected

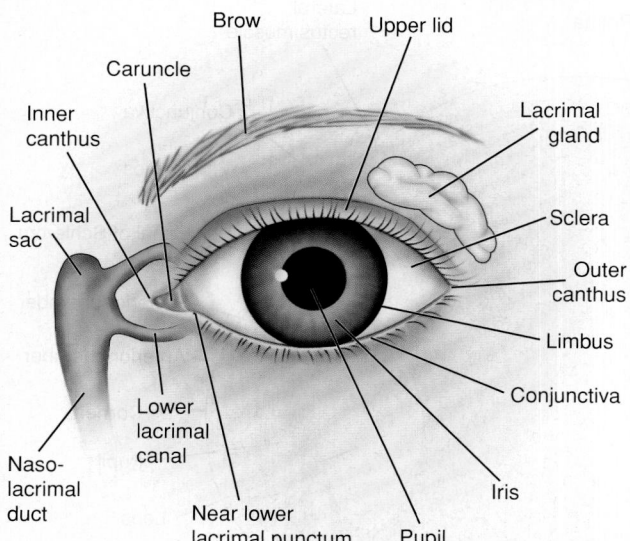

FIGURE 48-1 External structures of the eye and position of the lacrimal structures.

eye from injury by lubricating it with artificial tears to prevent drying.

Nursing Alert

The lacrimal apparatus are located in the eyelid and inner canthus and are essential for tear formation and drainage needed to lubricate the eyes. The lacrimal apparatus, within the inner canthus, contains a tiny fold of mucous membrane that can be blocked by debris when providing eye care (Bickley, 2013). When cleaning the eyes, in order to remove crusting or drainage, the nurse moves from inner to outer canthus. Use only one cotton ball or pledget (small compress) for each eye to remove debris and prevent it from entering the lacrimal duct.

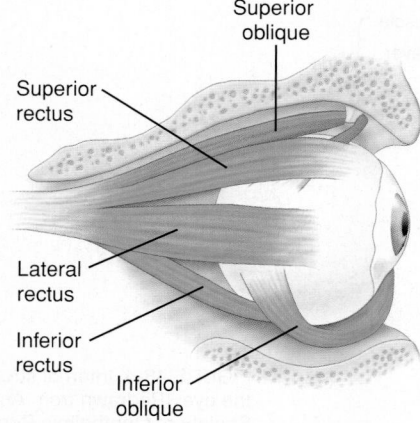

FIGURE 48-2 The extraocular muscles responsible for eye movement. The medial rectus muscle (not shown) is responsible for opposing the movement of the lateral rectus muscle.

Internal Eye

The conjunctiva, a mucous membrane, provides a barrier to the external environment and nourishes the eye. The goblet cells of the conjunctiva secrete lubricating mucus. The bulbar conjunctiva covers the sclera, whereas the palpebral conjunctiva lines the inner surface of the upper and lower eyelids. The junction of the two portions is known as the *fornix.*

The sclera, commonly known as the white of the eye, is a dense, fibrous structure that helps maintain the shape of the eyeball and protects the intraocular contents from trauma (Fig. 48-3). The sclera may have a slightly bluish tinge in young children, a dull white color in adults, a slightly yellowish color in the elderly, or a muddy brown color in African Americans; all are variations of normal. Externally, it is overlaid with conjunctiva, which is a thin, transparent mucous membrane that contains fine blood vessels. The conjunctiva meets the cornea at the **limbus** on the outermost edge of the iris.

The cornea (Fig. 48-4) is a transparent, avascular, dome-like structure that covers the iris, pupil, and anterior chamber. It is the most anterior portion of the eyeball and is the main refracting surface of the eye. The epithelial cells of the cornea are capable of rapid replication and are completely replaced every 7 days. Behind the cornea lies the **anterior chamber**, filled with a continually replenished supply of clear aqueous humor, which nourishes the cornea. The aqueous humor is produced by the ciliary body, and its production is dependent on a normal intraocular pressure (IOP) of 10 to 21 mm Hg.

The uvea consists of the iris, the ciliary body, and the choroid. The iris, or colored part of the eye, is a highly vascularized, pigmented collection of fibers surrounding the pupil. The pupil is a space that dilates and constricts in response to light. Normal pupils are round and constrict symmetrically when exposed to bright, direct light or for accommodation to objects that are near. Dilation and constriction are controlled by the sphincter and dilator pupillae muscles. The dilator muscles are controlled by the sympathetic nervous system, whereas the sphincter muscles are controlled by the parasympathetic nervous system.

Nursing Alert

Approximately 20% of the population may have pupils that are slightly unequal in size but respond equally to light. The term for unequal pupils is physiologic anisocoria, and it can be a benign variant (usually less than 1 mm difference between pupils) or a manifestation of disease, pathologic anisocoria (at least 1 mm difference) (American Association for Pediatric Ophthalmology and Strabismus [AAPOS, 2015]).

Directly behind the pupil and iris lies the lens, a colorless and almost completely transparent biconvex structure. It is

FIGURE 48-3 Three-dimensional cross-section of the eye.

FIGURE 48-4 Internal structures of the eye. (Redrawn from American Society of Ophthalmic Registered Nurses. (2008). *Core curriculum for ophthalmic nursing*. Dubuque, IA: Kendall/Hall Publishing.)

avascular and has no nerve or pain fibers. The lens enables focusing for near vision and refocusing for distance vision. The ability to focus and refocus is called **accommodation**. The lens is suspended behind the iris by zonules (string-like fibers) and is connected to the ciliary body. The ciliary body controls accommodation through the zonular fibers and the ciliary muscles (Fig. 48-4). The aqueous humor is anterior to the lens; posterior to the lens is the vitreous humor. The **posterior chamber** is a small space between the vitreous and the iris. The ciliary body in the posterior chamber produces aqueous fluid. This aqueous fluid flows from the posterior chamber into the anterior chamber, from which it drains through the trabecular meshwork into the canal of Schlemm.

The choroid lies between the retina and the sclera. It is avascular tissue, supplying blood to the portion of the sensory retina closest to it.

The ocular fundus is the largest chamber of the eye and contains the **vitreous humor**, a clear, gelatinous substance, composed mostly of water and encapsulated by a hyaloid membrane. The vitreous humor occupies about two thirds of the eye's volume and helps maintain the shape of the eye. The vitreous humor is in continuous contact with the retina and is attached to the retina by scattered collagenous filaments. The innermost surface of the fundus is the retina. The retina is composed of 10 microscopic layers and has the consistency of wet tissue paper. It is neural tissue, an extension of the optic nerve. Viewed through the pupil, the landmarks of the retina are the optic disc, the retinal vessels, and the macula. The point of entrance of the optic nerve into the retina is the optic disc. The optic disc is pink; it is oval or circular and has sharp margins. In the disc, a physiologic depression or cup is present centrally, with the retinal blood vessels emanating from it. The retinal tissues arise from the optic disc and line the inner surface of the vitreous chamber. The retinal vessels also enter the eye through the optic nerve, branching out through the retina and forming superior and inferior branches. The macula is the area of the retina responsible for central vision. The rest of the retina is responsible for peripheral vision. In the center of the macula is the most sensitive area, the fovea, which is avascular and surrounded by the superior and inferior vascular arcades (arches of blood vessels). Two important layers of the retina are the retinal pigment epithelium (RPE) and the sensory retina. A single layer of cells constitutes the RPE, and these cells have numerous functions, including the absorption of light. The sensory retina contains the photoreceptor cells: **rods** and **cones**. These are long, narrow cells shaped like rods or cones. The rods are mainly responsible for night vision or vision in low light, whereas the cones provide the best vision for bright light, color vision, and fine detail. Cones are distributed throughout the retina, with their greatest concentration in the fovea. Rods are absent in the fovea (Grossman & Porth, 2014).

Vision

Visual acuity depends on a healthy, functioning eyeball and an intact visual pathway (Fig. 48-5). This pathway includes the retina, optic nerve, optic chiasm, optic tracks, lateral

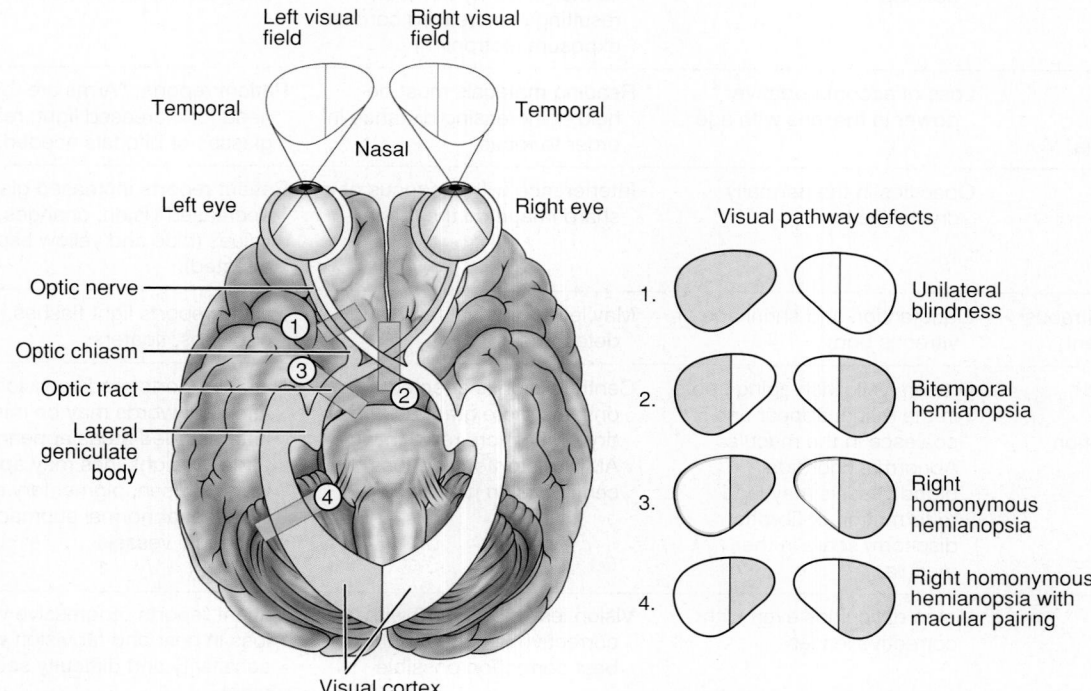

FIGURE 48-5 The visual pathway. (Redrawn from Fuller, J., & Schaller-Ayers, J. (2000). *Health assessment: A nursing approach* (3rd ed.). Philadelphia, PA: Lippincott Williams & Wilkins.)

geniculate bodies, optic radiations, and the visual cortex area of the brain. The pathway is an extension of the central nervous system (CNS). The funduscopic examination allows the only direct visualization of arteries, veins, and the CNS.

The optic nerve is also known as the second cranial nerve (CN II). Its purpose is to transmit impulses from the retina to the occipital lobe of the brain. The optic nerve head, or optic disc, is the physiologic blind spot in each eye. The optic nerve leaves the eye and then meets the optic nerve from the other eye at the **optic chiasm**. The chiasm is the anatomic point at which the nasal fibers from the nasal retina of each eye cross to the opposite side of the brain. The nerve fibers from the temporal retina of each eye remain uncrossed. Fibers from the right half of each eye, which would be the left visual field, carry impulses to the right occipital lobe. Fibers from the left half of each eye, or the right visual field, carry impulses to the left occipital lobe. Beyond the chiasm,

these fibers are known as the *optic tract*. The optic tract continues on to the lateral geniculate body, which leads to the optic radiations and then to the cortex of the occipital lobe of the brain.

Gerontologic Considerations

The eye undergoes many changes as the body ages. All cells formed throughout life are retained by the lens, which makes the cell structure of the lens susceptible to the degenerative effects of aging. The lens continues to grow throughout life, laying down fibers in concentric rings. As the body ages, the gel-like characteristics of the vitreous humor are gradually lost, and various cells and fibers cast shadows that the patient perceives as "floaters." The vitreous humor shrinks and shifts with age. Other age-related changes are summarized in Table 48-1.

TABLE 48-1 GERONTOLOGIC CONSIDERATIONS / Age-Related Changes in the Eye

Component	Structural Change	Functional Change	History and Physical Findings
Dry eye	Dysfunction of meibomian glands	Discomfort and pain with possible vision changes	Patient complains of vision changes, itching, burning, scratching sensation proportional to increased computer screen time.
Eyelids and lacrimal structures	Loss of skin elasticity and orbital fat, decreased muscle tone; wrinkles develop	Lid margins turn in, causing lashes to irritate cornea and conjunctiva (entropion); or lid margins may turn out, resulting in increased corneal exposure (ectropion)	Patient reports burning, foreign-body sensation, increased tearing (epiphora); injection, inflammation, and ulceration may occur.
Refractive changes; presbyopia	Loss of accommodative power in the lens with age	Reading materials must be held at increasing distance in order to focus.	Patient reports, "Arms are too short!;" need for increased light; reading glasses or bifocals needed.
Cataract	Opacities in the normally crystalline lens	Interference with the focus of a sharp image on the retina	Patient reports increased glare, decreased vision, changes in color values (blue and yellow especially affected).
Posterior vitreous detachment	Liquefaction and shrinkage of vitreous body	May lead to retinal tears and detachment	Patient reports light flashes, cobwebs, floaters.
Age-related macular degeneration (AMD)	Drusen (yellowish aging spots in the retina) appear and coalesce in the macula. Abnormal choroidal blood vessels may lead to formation of fibrotic disciform scars in the macula.	Central vision is affected; onset is more gradual in dry AMD, more rapid in wet AMD; distortion and loss of central vision may occur	Patient reports reading vision is affected; words may be missing letters, faded areas appear on the page, straight lines may appear wavy; drusen, pigmentary changes in retina; abnormal submacular choroidal vessels.
Low vision	Vision difficulties even with corrective lenses	Vision less than 20/40 with corrective lenses with the best correction possible	Patient reports progressive vision loss in near and far vision with light sensitivity and difficulty seeing at night.

Chader & Taylor, 2013.

ASSESSMENT

Health History

The nurse, through careful questioning, elicits the necessary information that can lead to the diagnosis of an ophthalmic condition.

Common Complaints

Common symptoms include changes in vision, pain or discomfort, and discharge. For each of the symptoms, the nurse asks:

- Are both eyes affected?
- Is this a recurrence of a previous condition?
- How has the patient self-treated?
- How is the patient affected by the symptom(s)?
- What makes the symptoms improve or worsen?
- What is the duration of the problem?

Changes in Vision

The nurse asks about changes in vision, including diminished visual acuity and blurred, distorted, or double vision. Changes in vision can be associated with problems such as myopia (distant objects appear blurred or nearsightedness), hyperopia (farsightedness), presbyopia (diminished ability to focus on near objects with age, a form of farsightedness), cataracts (opacity of the lens), glaucoma (abnormally high IOP that can damage the optic nerve), aging, diabetes, hypertension, cranial tumors, head trauma, or increased intracranial pressure (ICP).

Pain or Discomfort

The nurse inquires about the type of pain (sharp or dull) and whether it is worse when blinking. Pain while blinking might be present in superficial trauma events, such as corneal abrasions, corneal lacerations, or presence of a foreign body. Discomfort may include itching or a foreign-body sensation. This sensation of the presence of a foreign body is often present in diseases associated with conjunctival irritation. Conjunctival irritation may be found in conditions such as dry eye, bacterial or viral infections (pink eye), and irritation and allergic reactions (Bickley, 2013).

Discharge

It is important to note the color, consistency, and odor of any discharge. Eye discharge commonly results from inflammation or infection of the conjunctiva. Manifestations of other non-eye disorders may have eye discharge, such as erythema multiforme major (Stevens–Johnson syndrome), herpes zoster, and psoriasis vulgaris (refer to Chapter 52).

Past History

The nurse asks if this is a recurrence of a previous condition and notes the presence of any systemic diseases and medications used in their treatment. Medications for medical disorders cause thousands of eye disorders as side effects. For example, if long-term steroids are administered for arthritis, cataracts may develop. The nurse also inquires about concurrent ophthalmic conditions and any history of ophthalmic surgery.

Family History

The nurse asks whether any family members have had the same symptoms or condition, such as glaucoma, refraction disorders, and allergies.

Social History

In ophthalmology, the well-being of the patient physically, emotionally, financially, socially, and spiritually can be at risk when vision is threatened. The patient may equate a decrease in visual acuity with a loss of independence. The loss of a driver's license may force a patient to relocate or give up or change careers.

Major goals should include the preservation of vision and the prevention of further visual loss in patients who have already experienced some degree of loss. Lines of communication must be kept open so that the patient is comfortable exploring all treatment options to promote rehabilitation.

Physical Assessment

Visual Acuity Assessment

Following the health history, the patient's visual acuity is assessed. Most people are familiar with the standard Snellen chart. It is composed of a series of progressively smaller rows of letters and is used to test distance vision. The patient is positioned at the prescribed distance, usually 20 ft, from the chart and is asked to read the smallest line visible. The patient should wear distance correction (eyeglasses or contact lenses) if required, and each eye should be tested separately. A card should be provided to cover one eye to prevent the patient from trying to view the chart between the fingers. The fraction 20/20 is considered the standard of normal vision. The numerator denotes the distance between the patient and the chart, whereas the denominator quantifies the distance at which a normal eye can read the line of letters. A person whose vision is 20/200 can read print from 20 ft away that a person with 20/20 vision can read at 200 ft (Bickley, 2013). Most people can see the letters on the line designated as 20/20 from a distance of 20 ft.

If the patient cannot read the 20/20 line, he or she is given a pinhole occluder and asked to read again using the eye in question. The patient should be encouraged to read every letter possible. Specific visual acuities are then recorded for each eye. If the patient reads all five letters from the 20/20 line with the right eye and three letters of the 20/15 line with the left eye, the examiner records right eye 20/20, left eye 20/15-2. (Note: Medical abbreviations in the past used the terms OD and OS to represent right and left eyes, respectively; however, those abbreviations are no longer recommended because misinterpretation has resulted in harmful medication errors.)

If the patient cannot read the largest letter on the chart (the 20/200 line), the patient should be moved toward the chart or the chart moved toward the patient until the patient can identify the largest letter on the chart. If the patient can recognize only the letter E on the top line at a distance of 10 ft, the visual acuity would be recorded as 10/200. If the patient cannot see the letter E at any distance, the examiner should determine if the patient can count fingers. The examiner holds up a random number of fingers and asks the patient to count the number he or she sees. If the patient correctly identifies the number of fingers at 3 ft, the examiner would record "counts fingers/3 ft."

If the patient cannot count fingers, the examiner raises one hand up and down or moves it side to side and asks in which direction the hand is moving. This level of vision is known as hand motion. A patient who can perceive only light is described as having light perception. The vision of a patient who cannot perceive light is described as no light perception.

Near vision testing is performed to identify the need for reading glasses. **Presbyopia** is the term used for impaired near vision and is often found in middle-aged and older persons. A specially designed handheld card is held 14 in away from the patient's eyes, and the patient is asked to read the chart. Presbyopic people are commonly able to read the chart when it is held farther away.

External Eye Examination

After the visual acuity has been recorded, an external eye examination is performed. While standing directly in front of the patient, the nurse notes the position of the eyelids and alignment of the eyes. Commonly, the upper 2 mm of the iris are covered by the upper lid. The patient is examined for **ptosis** (drooping eyelid) and for lid retraction (too much of the eye exposed). Sometimes, the upper or lower lid turns out, referred to as *ectropion*, affecting closure. Additionally, the eyelid may invert; this is termed *entropion* and causes irritation of the eye. The lid margins and lashes should have no edema, erythema, or lesions. The examiner looks for scaling or crusting, and the sclera is inspected. A normal sclera is opaque and white (except as noted earlier). Lesions on the conjunctiva, discharge, and tearing or blinking are noted.

The pupils are inspected for size, shape, and symmetry. A normal pupil is black in color, round in shape, and symmetrical. Pupil size ranges between 2 and 8 mm depending on extremes of light. In room lighting, usual pupil size is 3 to 5 mm. The room should be darkened so that the pupils can be examined. The nurse checks pupillary response with a penlight to determine if the pupils are equally reactive and regular. The patient is asked to stare at a target; each eye is covered and uncovered quickly while the examiner looks for any shift in gaze. Recall that pupillary inequality of less than 1 mm may be detected in 20% to 40% of normal people (AAPOS, 2015). An artificial eye will have anisocoria. Other notable irregularity may be the result of trauma, previous surgery, or disease.

The pupillary response to light is determined by shining a bright light obliquely into each pupil. Pupils are assessed for *direct reaction*, in which the pupil tested with light constricts, and for *consensual reaction*, in which the pupil of the opposite eye also constricts. The nurse is aware that the pupil of a blind eye will not constrict; however, if a direct light is reflected on the "good eye," a consensual light reaction may be noted in the impaired eye. Obviously, there will be no reaction with a prosthetic eye.

The examiner also observes for **nystagmus** (i.e., oscillating movement of the eyeball). The extraocular movements (EOMs) of the eyes are tested by having the patient follow the examiner's finger, pencil, or a hand light through the six cardinal directions of gaze, a wide H pattern (i.e., up, down, right, left, and both diagonals). Normal EOMs should produce conjugate movements of the eyes in each direction. This is especially important when screening patients for ocular trauma or for neurologic disorders.

Diagnostic Evaluation

Direct Ophthalmoscopy

A direct ophthalmoscope is a handheld instrument enabling magnification of the cornea, lens, and retina. The patient is normally given mydriatic drops to dilate the pupils and assist in the examination of vision. Contraindications to the use of mydriatic drops include head injury or narrow-angle glaucoma. The patient is given a target to gaze at. The examiner holds the ophthalmoscope in the right hand and uses the right eye to examine the patient's right eye. The examiner switches to the left hand and left eye when examining the patient's left eye. During this examination, the room should be darkened, and the examiner should be about 15 in away from the patient and 15 degrees lateral to the patient's line of vision. The patient should be relaxed and able to keep both eyes open and steady.

The examiner shines the light on the patient's pupil to examine the fundus (Fig. 48-6). The fundus of the eye is the interior structure opposite the lens that includes the retina, optic disc, macula, fovea, and posterior pole. A normal orange glow is observed as light is applied to the pupil, known as the **red reflex**. Absence of the red reflex may indicate lens opacity, which is consistent with a cataract, detached retina, or retinoblastoma in children. When the fundus is examined, the vasculature comes into focus first. The examiner focuses on a large vessel and then follows it as it becomes larger in diameter, leading to the optic disc. The central depression in the disc is known as the *cup*. The normal cup is about one third the size of the disc. The size of the physiologic optic

FIGURE 48-6 Normal fundus.

cup should be estimated and the disc margins described as sharp or blurred. The periphery of the retina is examined by having the patient shift his or her gaze. The last area of the fundus to be examined is the macula, because this area is the most sensitive to light.

The healthy fundus should be free of any lesions. The examiner looks for intraretinal hemorrhages, which may appear as red smudges or, if the patient has hypertension, may look somewhat flame-shaped. A yellow lipid may be present in the retina of patients with hypercholesterolemia or diabetes. The examiner looks for microaneurysms, which look like little red dots, and nevi. *Drusen* (small, hyaline, globular growths), commonly found in macular degeneration, appear as yellowish areas with indistinct edges. The examiner should sketch the fundus and document any abnormalities.

Amsler Grid

The Amsler grid is a test often used for patients with macular problems, such as macular degeneration. It consists of a geometric grid of identical squares with a central fixation point. The grid should be viewed by the patient wearing normal reading glasses. Each eye is tested separately. The patient is instructed to stare at the central fixation spot on the grid and report any distortion in the squares of the grid itself. Patients with macular problems typically note that some of the squares may look wavy, blurred, or distorted. Patients with age-related macular degeneration are commonly given these Amsler grids to take home. The patient is encouraged to check them frequently, as often as daily, to detect any early signs of distortion that may indicate the development of a neovascular choroidal membrane, an advanced stage of macular degeneration characterized by the growth of abnormal choroidal vessels.

Tonometry

Tonometry measures IOP by determining the amount of force or pressure necessary to indent or flatten (applanate)

a small anterior area of the globe of the eye. High readings indicate high pressure; low readings indicate low pressure. The procedure is noninvasive and usually painless. A topical anesthetic eye drop is instilled into the lower conjunctival sac, and the tonometer is then used to measure the IOP. Air-puff tonometry may also be done but is not as reliable as a direct contact method (Farhood, 2013).

Two of the most commonly used tonometers are the applanation tonometer and the Tono-Pen. The applanation tonometer is generally used by the more skilled examiner. A drop of fluorescein dye and an anesthetic drop are instilled in the eye. The applanation tip is pressed against the cornea and the examiner, looking through the slit lamp, obtains the IOP reading. The Tono-Pen is a portable, battery-operated, handheld tonometer that is commonly used in many clinical settings. A disposable cover is placed over the tip of the instrument, and it is held against the anesthetized cornea for a few seconds. The tension reading is displayed in a liquid crystal display window.

Perimetry Testing

Perimetry testing evaluates the field of vision. A *visual field* is the area or extent of physical space visible to an eye in a given position. It has a three-dimensional contour representing areas of relative retinal sensitivity; visual acuity is sharpest at the very top of the field and declines progressively toward the periphery. It is most helpful in detecting central **scotomas** (blind areas in the visual field) in macular degeneration and the peripheral field defects in glaucoma and retinitis pigmentosa.

The two methods of perimetric testing are manual and automated perimetry. Manual perimetry involves the use of moving (kinetic) or stationary (static) stimuli or targets. An example of kinetic manual perimetry is the tangent screen. A tangent screen is a black felt material mounted on a wall that has a series of concentric circles bisected by straight lines emanating from the center. It tests the central 30 degrees of the visual field. Automated perimetry uses stationary targets, which are more difficult to detect than moving targets. In this test, a computer projects light randomly in different areas of a hollow dome while the patient looks through a telescopic opening and depresses a button whenever the light stimulus is detected. Automated perimetry is more accurate than manual perimetry.

Slit-Lamp Examination

The slit lamp is a binocular microscope mounted on a table. This instrument enables the user to examine the eye with magnification of 10 to 40 times the actual image. The illumination can be varied from a broad to a narrow beam of light for different parts of the eye. For example, by varying the width and intensity of the light, the anterior chamber can be examined for signs of inflammation. Cataracts may be evaluated by changing the angle of the light. When a handheld lens, such as a three-mirror lens, is used with the slit lamp, the angle of the anterior chamber may be examined, as may the ocular fundus.

Color Vision Testing

The ability to differentiate colors has a dramatic effect on the activities of daily living. For example, the inability to differentiate between red and green can compromise traffic safety. Some careers (e.g., commercial art, color photography, airline pilot, electrician) may be closed to people with significant color deficiencies. Color discrimination allows visualization of a broad spectrum of color. The photoreceptor cells responsible for color vision are the cones, and the greatest area of color sensitivity is in the macula, the area of densest cone concentration. A defect or deficiency in the cones (red, blue, or green) will result in abnormal color vision. There are three basic types of color blindness: red–green, which is the most common deficiency; blue; and total color blindness, also known as *achromatopsia*.

A screening test, such as the polychromatic plates, can be used to establish whether a person's color vision is within normal range. Color vision deficits can be inherited. For example, red–green color deficiencies are inherited in an X-linked manner, affecting approximately 8% of men and 0.5% of women. Acquired color vision losses may be caused by chronic illness (e.g., diabetes, macular degeneration, glaucoma), medications (e.g., digitalis), trauma, industrial toxins, or aging (e.g., cataracts). A simple test, such as asking a patient if the red top on a bottle of eye drops appears redder to one eye than the other, can be an effective tool. A difference in the perception of the intensity of the color red between the two eyes can be a symptom of a neurologic problem and may provide information about the location of the lesion.

Ultrasonography

Lesions in the globe or the orbit may not be directly visible and are evaluated by ultrasonography. Ultrasonography is a very valuable diagnostic technique, especially when the view of the retina is obscured by opaque media, such as cataract or hemorrhage. Ultrasonography can be used to identify orbital tumors, retinal detachment, and changes in tissue composition.

Special techniques can also be used to calculate the power for an intraocular lens implant and to obtain more anatomic information, showing cross-sectional images. Vitreous hemorrhage, retinal detachment, and tumors can be evaluated with minimal discomfort for the patient. Three-dimensional images can be created, and the entire ultrasound examination can be recorded for later use.

Fluorescein Angiography

Fluorescein angiography evaluates clinically significant macular edema, documents macular capillary nonperfusion, and identifies retinal and choroidal neovascularization (growth of abnormal new blood vessels) in age-related macular degeneration. It is an invasive procedure in which fluorescein dye is injected, usually into an antecubital vein. Within 10 to 15 seconds, this dye can be seen coursing through the retinal vessels. Over a 10-minute period, serial black-and-white photographs are taken of the retinal vasculature. The dye may impart a gold tone to the skin of some patients, and urine may turn deep yellow or orange. This discoloration usually disappears in 24 hours.

Nursing Alert
When the nurse administers eye medications, pressure is applied to the inner canthus while placing the medication on the conjunctival sac to prevent systemic absorption.

THE EAR

The ear is a sensory organ with dual functions—hearing and balance. The sense of hearing is essential for normal development and maintenance of speech, as well as for the ability to communicate with others. Balance, or equilibrium, is essential for maintaining body movement, position, and coordination.

ANATOMIC AND PHYSIOLOGIC OVERVIEW

External Ear

The **external ear** includes the auricle (**pinna**) and the **external auditory canal** (Fig. 48-7). The external ear is separated from the middle ear by a disc-like structure called the **tympanic membrane** (eardrum). The auricle, attached to the side of the head by skin, is composed mainly of cartilage, except for the fat and subcutaneous tissue in the earlobe. The auricle collects the sound waves and directs vibrations into the external auditory canal.

The external auditory canal is approximately 2.5 cm long. The external auditory canal ends at the tympanic membrane. The skin of the canal contains hair, sebaceous glands, and ceruminous glands, which secrete a brown, waxlike substance called **cerumen** (earwax). The ear's self-cleaning mechanism moves old skin cells and cerumen to the outer part of the ear.

Middle Ear

The **middle ear**, an air-filled cavity, includes the tympanic membrane laterally and the otic capsule medially. The middle ear is connected by the **eustachian tube** to the nasopharynx and is continuous with air-filled cells in the adjacent mastoid portion of the **temporal bone**. Normally, the eustachian tube

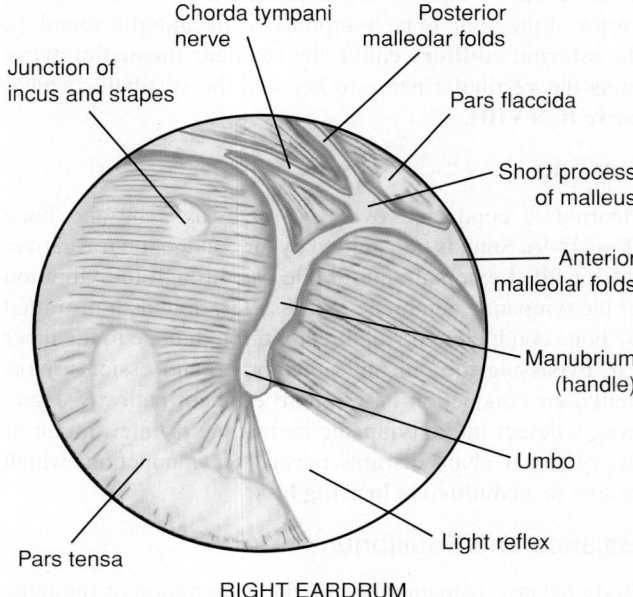

FIGURE 48-7 **A.** Anatomy of the ear. **B.** The inner ear.

is closed, but it opens when the person performs a Valsalva maneuver, yawns, or swallows. It drains normal and abnormal secretions of the middle ear and equalizes pressure in the middle ear with that of the atmosphere.

The tympanic membrane (eardrum), about 1 cm in diameter and very thin, is normally pearly gray and translucent. The tympanic membrane protects the middle ear and conducts sound vibrations from the external canal to the **ossicles**. Figure 48-8 illustrates the distinguishing landmarks of the tympanic membrane.

The middle ear contains the three smallest bones (the ossicles) of the body: the **malleus**, the **incus**, and the **stapes**. The ossicles, which are held in place by joints, muscles, and ligaments, assist in the transmission of sound. Two small fenestrae (oval and round windows), located in the medial wall of the middle ear, separate the middle ear from the inner ear. The footplate of the stapes sits in the **oval window**, secured by a fibrous annulus (ring-shaped structure). The footplate transmits sound to the inner ear. The **round window**, covered by a thin membrane, provides an exit for sound vibrations (see Fig. 48-7).

FIGURE 48-8 The tympanic membrane.

TABLE **48-2** GERONTOLOGIC CONSIDERATIONS / Age-Related Changes in the Ear

Component	Structural Change	Functional Change	History and Physical Findings
Atrophy of the external ears	Pinna loses flexibility	Thinning and drying of ear canal	Pinna longer and thinner with dry cerumen in external ear canal
Hardening of cerumen	Dryer, thicker cerumen	Earwax accumulates	Visible earwax and conductive hearing impairment
Thickening of the eardrum	Stiffness of eardrum	Impaired transmission of sound	Mild hearing impairment
Change in vestibulospinal reflex	Loss of vestibular afferents and neurons	Progressive imbalance and increased falls	Balance and gait tests provoke symptoms of dizziness and postural instability
Degeneration of organ of Corti (presbycusis)	Loss of cochlear pathway neurons, atrophy of vascular cochlear tissue	Loss of ability to discriminate words or comprehend conversations	Decreased ability to hear high frequencies or to interpret consonant sounds

Inner Ear

The **inner ear** is housed deep within the temporal bone. The organs for hearing (**cochlea**) and balance (**semicircular canals**), as well as CN VII (facial nerve) and CN VIII (**vestibulocochlear nerve**), are all part of this complex anatomy (see Fig. 48-7). The three semicircular canals—posterior, superior, and lateral, which lie at 90-degree angles to one another—contain sensory receptor organs, arranged to detect rotational movement. These receptor end organs are stimulated by changes in the rate or direction of a person's movement.

The **organ of Corti**, also called the *end organ for hearing,* transforms mechanical energy into neural activity and separates sounds into different frequencies. This electrochemical impulse travels through the **acoustic** nerve to the temporal cortex of the brain to be interpreted as meaningful sound. In the **internal auditory canal**, the **cochlear (acoustic) nerve** joins the vestibular nerve to become the vestibulocochlear nerve (CN VIII).

Hearing

Hearing is conducted over two pathways: air and bone (Fig. 48-9). Sounds transmitted by air conduction travel over the air-filled external and middle ear through the vibration of the tympanic membrane and ossicles. Sounds transmitted by bone conduction travel directly through bone to the inner ear, bypassing the tympanic membrane and ossicles. Normally, air conduction is the more efficient pathway. However, a defect in the tympanic membrane or interruption of the ossicular chain disrupts normal air conduction, which results in a **conductive hearing loss**.

Balance and Equilibrium

Body balance is maintained by the cooperation of the muscles and joints of the body (proprioceptive system), the eyes (visual system), and the labyrinth (vestibular system). These areas send their information about equilibrium, or balance, to the brain (cerebellar system) for coordination and perception in the cerebral cortex. The vestibular apparatus of the inner ear provides feedback regarding the movements and the position of the head and body in space.

Gerontologic Considerations

Hearing loss is a common finding in the geriatric population, with a full third of those over 60 years of age demonstrating detectable hearing deficits (Fioretti, Poli, Varakliotis, & Eibenstein, 2014). The term *presbycusis* refers to hearing loss associated with degenerative changes. Table 48-2 summarizes age-related changes.

ASSESSMENT

Assessment of the ear includes a health history and physical assessment.

Health History

The nurse should include questions about hearing loss, hearing aids, medications, itching, ear drainage, tinnitus (sensation of noise such as ringing or roaring), vertigo (sensation of motion), ear pain, and environmental exposure to loud or continuous noises in the health history.

Common Complaints

The nurse needs to explore common ear complaints, such as changes in hearing acuity, earache, drainage, and tinnitus. A common complaint of ear pain is associated with a variety of disorders including cerumen impaction, acute external otitis, acute mastoiditis, acute otitis media, and foreign

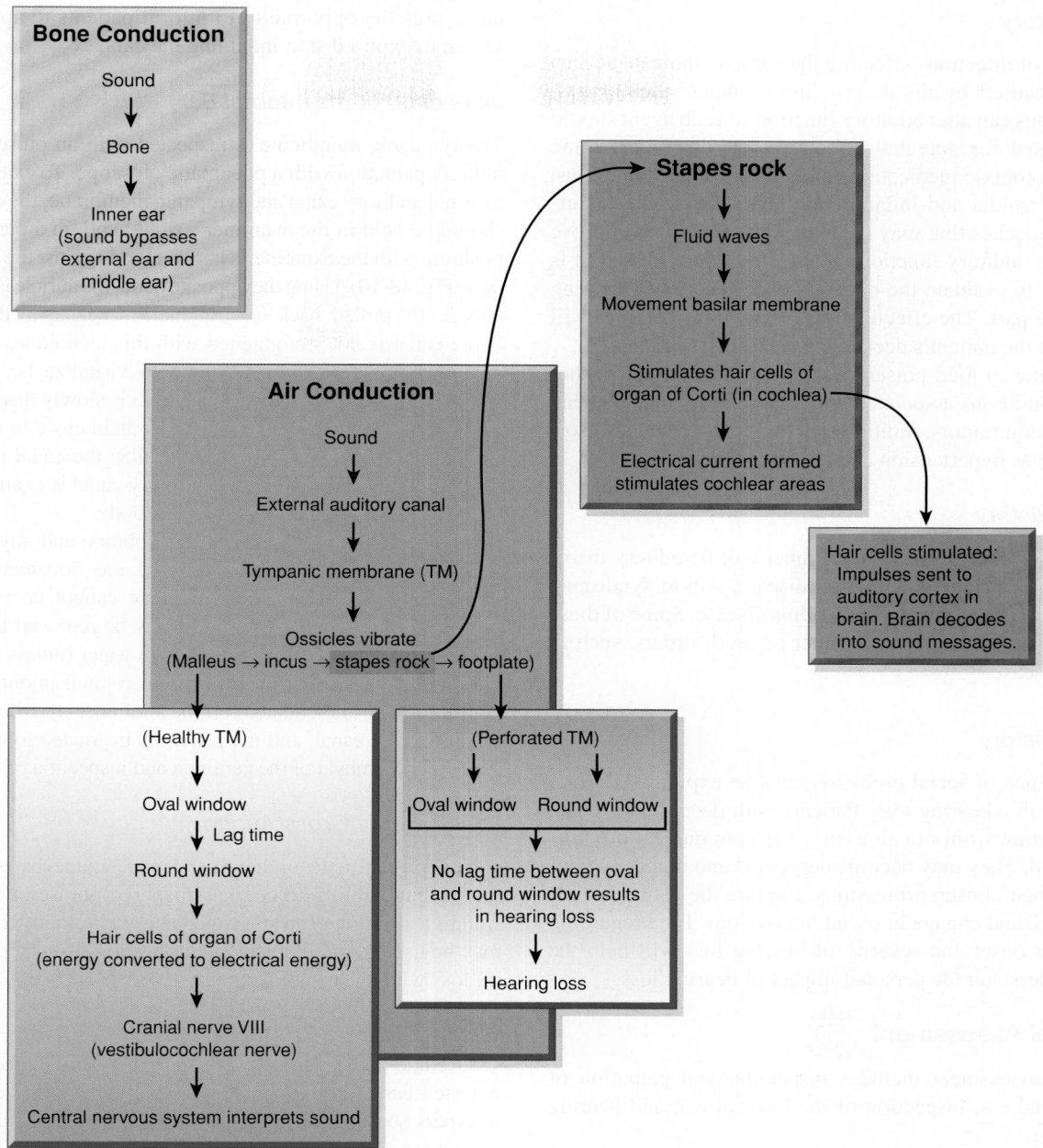

Bone Conduction

Sound
↓
Bone
↓
Inner ear
(sound bypasses
external ear and
middle ear)

Stapes rock
↓
Fluid waves
↓
Movement basilar membrane
↓
Stimulates hair cells of
organ of Corti (in cochlea)
↓
Electrical current formed
stimulates cochlear areas

Hair cells stimulated:
Impulses sent to
auditory cortex in
brain. Brain decodes
into sound messages.

Air Conduction

Sound
↓
External auditory canal
↓
Tympanic membrane (TM)
↓
Ossicles vibrate
(Malleus → incus → stapes rock → footplate)

(Healthy TM)
↓
Oval window
↓ Lag time
Round window
↓
Hair cells of organ of Corti
(energy converted to electrical energy)
↓
Cranial nerve VIII
(vestibulocochlear nerve)
↓
Central nervous system interprets sound

(Perforated TM)
↓   ↓
Oval window   Round window
↓
No lag time between oval
and round window results
in hearing loss
↓
Hearing loss

FIGURE 48-9 Bone conduction compared to air conduction.

bodies. Impaction of cerumen can cause otalgia (a sensation of fullness or pain in the ear), with or without a hearing loss. If, on manipulation of the auricle, the patient complains of pain, the nurse suspects the etiology of the pain is acute external otitis. Tenderness on palpation in the area of the mastoid may indicate acute mastoiditis or inflammation of the posterior auricular node. Acute otitis media, an acute infection of the middle ear, can occur at any age, although it is seen most commonly in children. Symptoms vary with the severity of the infection. In adults, complaints of pain are usually unilateral, and the pain is relieved after

spontaneous perforation or therapeutic incision of the tympanic membrane.

Tinnitus is another common symptom of an underlying disorder of the ear that is associated with hearing impairment and loss, ototoxic substances (see Chapter 50), and a variety of hearing disorders (otosclerosis, Ménière disease, acoustic neuroma) and systemic disorders (thyroid disease, neurologic disorders). Tinnitus may range from mild to severe and is frequently described as a roaring, buzzing, or hissing sound in one or both ears. Refer to Chapter 50 for further details.

Past History

A history of infections affecting the ear may indicate a hearing loss caused by diseases of the tympanic membranes. Medications can alter auditory function so each agent should be evaluated for potential effects on ear disorders. Some common ototoxic medications include antibiotics, diuretics, and nonsteroidal anti-inflammatory agents (NSAIDs). Surgical approaches that may have been performed to improve a patient's auditory function must be explored. If used, it is necessary to evaluate the patient's experience with hearing aids in the past. The effectiveness of previous therapies will determine the patient's decisions on ear interventions.

Exposure to loud noises should also be explored. Other related conditions associated with hearing loss include head trauma, brain tumors, multiple sclerosis, and vascular disorders, such as hypertension and arteriosclerosis.

Family History

Many cases of hearing loss are inherited; hereditary disorders of the ear include Hallgren disease, Alport syndrome, Refsum disease, and Treacher Collins disease. Some of these disorders are associated with other organ disorders, such as kidney disease.

Social History

The presence of social problems must be explored with the patient with a hearing loss. Patients with decreased hearing may withdraw from situations in which communication skills are needed. They may become depressed and unable to continue in their chosen professions. Explore the patient's ability to work and engage in social interactions. Data regarding the age at onset and severity of hearing loss will help the nurse understand the personal impact of hearing loss.

Physical Assessment

Physical assessment includes inspection and palpation of the external ear, inspection of the internal ear, and hearing evaluation.

Inspection and Palpation of the External Ear

Inspection of the external ear is a simple procedure but often overlooked. The external ear is examined by inspection and direct palpation; the auricle and surrounding tissues should be inspected for deformities, lesions, and discharge, as well as size, symmetry, and angle of attachment to the head. If manipulation of the auricle is painful, acute external otitis is suspected. Tenderness on palpation in the area of the mastoid may indicate acute mastoiditis or inflammation of the posterior auricular node. Because the ear is exposed to the sunlight, the nurse should examine the shell of the ear for lesions. Any lesion lasting over 2 weeks should be referred to a skin care specialist for evaluation of skin cancer. The nurse uses the opportunity to inform patients to apply sunscreen to exposed skin including the ears.

Inspection of the Internal Ear

The tympanic membrane is inspected with an otoscope and indirect palpation with a pneumatic otoscope. To examine the external auditory canal and tympanic membrane, the otoscope should be held in the examiner's right hand, in a pencil-hold position, with the examiner's hand braced against the patient's face (Fig. 48-10). Using the opposite hand, the auricle is grasped and gently pulled back to straighten the canal in the adult. If the canal is not straightened with this technique, the tympanic membrane is more difficult to visualize because the canal obstructs the view. The speculum is slowly inserted into the ear canal, with the examiner's eye held close to the magnifying lens of the otoscope to visualize the canal and tympanic membrane. The external auditory canal is examined for discharge, inflammation, or a foreign body.

The position and color of the membrane and any unusual markings or deviations from normal are documented (see Fig. 48-8). If the tympanic membrane cannot be visualized because of cerumen, the cerumen may be removed by gently irrigating the external canal with warm water (unless contraindicated). If adherent cerumen is present, a small amount of mineral oil or over-the-counter cerumen softener may be instilled within the ear canal, and the patient is instructed to return for subsequent removal of the cerumen and inspection of the ear.

Evaluation of Gross Auditory Acuity

A general estimate of hearing can be made by assessing the patient's ability to hear a whispered phrase or a ticking watch, testing one ear at a time. The Weber and Rinne tests may be used to distinguish conductive loss from sensorineural loss when hearing is impaired.

Whisper Test

To exclude one ear from the testing, the examiner covers the untested ear with the palm of the hand. Then the examiner whispers softly from a distance of 1 or 2 ft from the unoccluded ear and out of the patient's sight. The patient with normal hearing acuity can correctly repeat what was whispered.

Weber Test

The Weber test uses bone conduction to test lateralization of sound. A tuning fork (ideally, 512 Hz), set in motion, is placed on the patient's head or forehead (Fig. 48-11). A person with normal hearing hears the sound equally in both ears or describes the sound as centered in the middle of the head. The Weber test is useful for detecting unilateral hearing loss (Table 48-3).

Rinne Test

In the Rinne test, the examiner shifts the stem of a vibrating tuning fork between two positions: against the mastoid bone (for bone conduction), and, when the sound is no longer

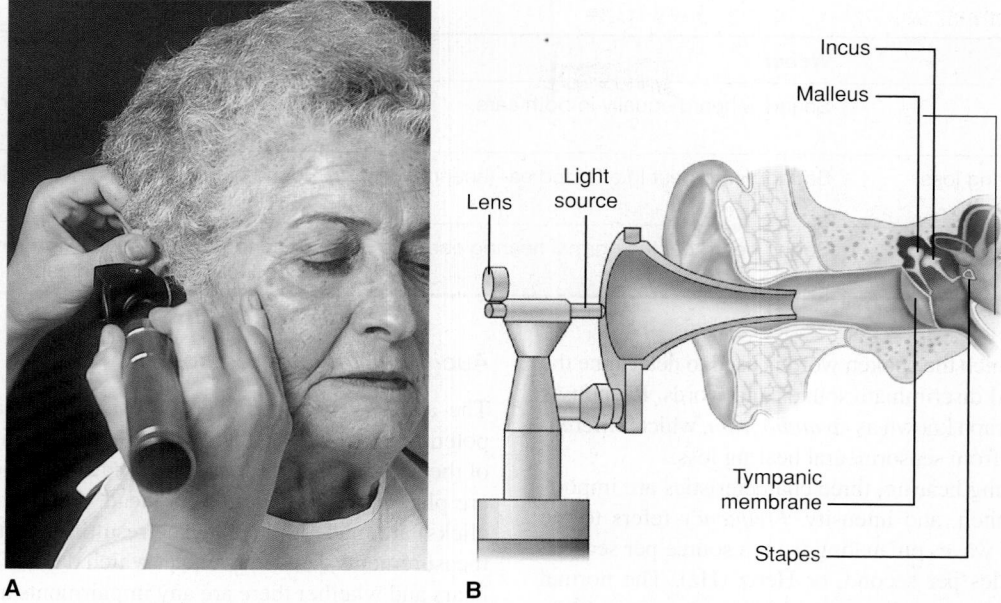

FIGURE 48-10 Proper technique for examining the ear. **A.** Hold the otoscope in the right or left hand, in a "pencil-hold" position. **B.** Steady the hand against the patient's head to avoid inserting the otoscope too far into the external canal.

audible, then the position is shifted 2 in from the opening of the ear canal (for air conduction). As the position changes, the patient is asked to indicate which tone is louder or when the tone is no longer audible. The Rinne test is useful for distinguishing between conductive and **sensorineural hearing loss** (Table 48-3).

Diagnostic Evaluation

Many diagnostic procedures are available to measure the auditory and vestibular systems indirectly. These tests are usually performed by an audiologist whose clinical competence is certified by the American Speech-Language-Hearing Association.

Audiometry

In detecting **hearing loss**, audiometry is the single most important diagnostic instrument. Audiometric testing is of two kinds: *pure-tone audiometry*, in which the sound stimulus consists of a pure or musical tone (the louder the tone before the patient perceives it, the greater the hearing loss), and *speech*

FIGURE 48-11 **A.** The Weber test assesses bone conduction of sound. **B.** The Rinne test assesses both air and bone conduction of sound.

TABLE **48-3** Comparison of Weber and Rinne Tests

Hearing Status	Weber	Rinne
Normal hearing	Sound is heard equally in both ears.	Air conduction is audible longer than bone conduction.
Conductive hearing loss	Sound heard best in affected ear (hearing loss).	Sound heard as long or longer in affected ear (hearing loss).
Sensorineural hearing loss	Sound heard best in normal hearing ear.	Air conduction is audible longer than bone conduction in affected ear.

audiometry, in which the spoken word is used to determine the ability to hear and discriminate sounds and words. Responses are plotted on a graph known as an *audiogram*, which differentiates conductive from sensorineural hearing loss.

When evaluating hearing, three characteristics are important: frequency, pitch, and intensity. *Frequency* refers to the number of sound waves emanating from a source per second, measured as cycles per second, or Hertz (Hz). The normal human ear perceives sounds ranging in frequency from 20 to 20,000 Hz. *Pitch* is the term used to describe frequency; a tone with 100 Hz is considered of low pitch, and a tone of 10,000 Hz is considered of high pitch. The unit for measuring loudness (*intensity* of sound) is the decibel (dB), the pressure exerted by sound. Hearing loss is measured in decibels, a logarithmic function of intensity that is not easily converted into a percentage. The critical level of loudness is approximately 30 dB. The shuffling of papers in quiet surroundings is about 15 dB. Table 48-4 classifies hearing loss based on decibel level.

Tympanogram

A tympanogram or impedance audiometry is used to evaluate the tympanic membrane and status of the middle ear. This test measures middle ear muscle reflex to sound stimulation (movement of the tympanic membrane) and the compliance of the tympanic membrane by changing the air pressure in the sealed ear canal. Compliance is impaired with middle ear disease, such as fluid accumulation in the middle ear or rupture of the tympanic membrane.

TABLE **48-4** Severity of Hearing Loss

Loss in Decibels	Interpretation
0–15	Normal hearing
>15–25	Slight hearing loss
>25–40	Mild hearing loss
>40–55	Moderate hearing loss
>55–70	Moderate to severe hearing loss
>70–90	Severe hearing loss
>90	Profound hearing loss

Auditory Brainstem Response

The auditory brainstem response is a detectable electrical potential from CN VIII and the ascending auditory pathways of the brainstem in response to sound stimulation. Electrodes are placed on the patient's forehead. Acoustic stimuli (e.g., clicks) are made in the ear. The resulting electrophysiologic measurements can determine at which decibel level a patient hears and whether there are any impairments along the nerve pathways (e.g., tumor on CN VIII).

Electronystagmography

Electronystagmography is the measurement and graphic recording of the changes in electrical potentials created by eye movements during spontaneous, positional, or calorically evoked nystagmus. It is also used to assess the oculomotor and vestibular systems and their corresponding interaction. It helps diagnose conditions such as Ménière disease and tumors of the internal auditory canal or posterior fossa. Vestibular suppressants, such as sedatives, tranquilizers, antihistamines, and alcohol, are withheld for 24 hours before testing. Prior to the test, the procedure is explained to the patient.

Platform Posturography

Platform posturography is used to investigate postural control capabilities, such as **vertigo**. It can be used to evaluate if a person's vertigo is becoming worse or to evaluate the person's response to treatment. The integration of visual, vestibular, and proprioceptive cues (i.e., sensory integration) with motor response output and coordination of the lower limbs is tested. The patient stands on a platform, surrounded by a screen, and different conditions, such as a moving platform with a moving screen or a stationary platform with a moving screen, are presented. The responses from the patient on six different conditions are measured and indicate which of the anatomic systems may be impaired. Preparation for the testing is the same as for electronystagmography.

Sinusoidal Harmonic Acceleration

Sinusoidal harmonic acceleration, or a rotary chair, is used to assess the vestibulo-ocular system by analyzing compensatory eye movements in response to the clockwise and counterclockwise rotation of the chair. Although such testing cannot identify the side of the lesion in unilateral disease, it helps identify disease (e.g., Ménière disease and tumors of the auditory canal) and evaluate the course of recovery. The same patient preparation is required as for electronystagmography.

Middle Ear Endoscopy

With endoscopes of very small diameters and acute angles, the ear can be examined by an endoscopist specializing in otolaryngology. Middle ear endoscopy is performed safely and effectively as an office procedure to evaluate suspected perilymphatic fistula, new-onset conductive hearing loss, the anatomy of the round window before transtympanic treatment of Ménière disease, and the tympanic cavity before ear surgery to treat chronic middle ear and mastoid infections.

The tympanic membrane is anesthetized topically for about 10 minutes before the procedure. Then, the external auditory canal is irrigated with sterile normal saline solution. With the aid of a microscope, a tympanotomy is created with a laser beam or a **myringotomy** knife so that the endoscope can be inserted into the middle ear cavity. Video and photo documentation can be accomplished through the scope.

CHAPTER REVIEW

Critical Thinking Exercises

1. An 82-year-old woman who lives at home with her daughter is scheduled for a posturography. She cooks for the family and frequently cooks for and visits older ill friends in the local extended-care facilities. She is very active and walks on her treadmill three times per week. She plans on her usual work at evening church services after her posturography. What should you instruct her regarding preprocedure planning for her examination?

2. A 24-year-old woman was transported to the emergency department after sustaining a corneal irritation from chemical exposure. Following the health history, the patient's visual acuity was assessed. Visual acuity test was to be done by Snellen chart. The patient was positioned 20 ft from the chart and was asked to read the smallest line visible. She was not able to see the chart with the affected eye. She started crying and reported that she used to be able to see perfectly from both eyes. What further assessment is needed at this time? How would you explain this finding to the patient?

NCLEX-Style Review Questions

1. What information from a health history collected from a 70-year-old should be further evaluated as a sign of presbycusis?
   a. "I haven't been going out with friends."
   b. "I am a retired truck driver."
   c. "My hobby is caring for livestock."
   d. "I watch television in the evening with my wife."

2. The nurse assesses a patient who is complaining of an earache. What assessment finding would the nurse expect?
   a. Blue tympanic membrane
   b. Cerumen buildup
   c. Mastoid tenderness
   d. Tympanic retraction

3. A 45-year-old man reports that he is experiencing trouble with close vision that is becoming progressively worse. The nurse explains the reason for the problem. What statement shows that the patient understands the explanation?
   a. "This is a sign that I might have hypertension."
   b. "I might be having early signs of presbyopia."
   c. "So you think I might have had some kind of eye trauma?"
   d. "Which one of my medications caused this?"

4. A patient arrives at a minor emergency center complaining of eye pain after an animal scratch incident. What would the nurse expect to find during the assessment?
   a. An injury to the opposite eye
   b. Pain while blinking
   c. Bleeding from the tear duct
   d. Change in distance vision

5. A patient is being evaluated for conductive versus sensorineural hearing loss. The nurse is performing the Rinne test. What result would the nurse expect to see if the patient has sensorineural hearing loss?
   a. Sound is heard equally in both ears.
   b. Air conduction is equal to bone conduction in the affected ear.
   c. Air conduction is longer than bone conduction in the affected ear.
   d. Air conduction is shorter than bone conduction in the affected ear.

Try these additional resources, available at **http://thepoint.lww.com/Honan2e**, to enhance your learning and understanding of this chapter:

- NCLEX-Style Student Review Questions
- Journal Articles

REFERENCES AND SELECTED READINGS

References and selected readings associated with this chapter can be found on the website that accompanies the book. Visit **http://thepoint.lww.com/Honan2e** to access the references and other additional resources associated with this chapter.

Nursing Management: Patients with Eye and Vision Disorders

Carolynn Spera Bruno

Learning Objectives

After reading this chapter, you will be able to:

1. Define low vision and blindness, and differentiate between functional and visual impairment.
2. List and describe assessment and management strategies for low vision.
3. Demonstrate orientation and mobility techniques for patients with low vision in a hospital setting.
4. Discuss assessment and management of glaucoma.
5. Discuss assessment and management of cataracts.
6. Discuss assessment and management of retinal disorders.
7. Discuss assessment and management of eye trauma.
8. Discuss assessment and management of infectious and inflammatory eye disorders.
9. Demonstrate the instillation of eye drops and ointment.
10. Discuss the postoperative management and discharge instructions of patients undergoing ocular surgery.

Patients admitted to medical surgical units may have acute conditions affecting the eye or comorbidities associated with visual impairment. Many of the leading causes of visual impairment are associated with aging (e.g., cataracts, glaucoma, macular degeneration), and two thirds of the population with impaired vision are older than 65 years of age. Younger people are also at risk for eye disorders, particularly traumatic injuries. Understanding the prevention, treatment, and consequences of eye disorders, nurses in all settings assess visual acuity in those at risk (e.g., patients who are elderly, those with diabetes or AIDS), refer patients to eye care specialists as appropriate, implement measures to prevent further visual loss, and help patients adapt to impaired vision.

IMPAIRED VISION

More than one million Americans are legally blind and 12 million are visually impaired (Centers for Disease Control and Prevention [CDC], 2017). Chief causes of visual impairment or blindness include diabetic retinopathy and age-related eye diseases (i.e., cataracts, macular degeneration, and glaucoma). In 2013, the World Health Organization (WHO) stated in their Global Action Plan 2014–2019 that 80% of all causes of visual impairment can be prevented. Given that the population rates among the aged demographic are increasing dramatically along with the recognition that many eye disorders often are undiagnosed, it is essential for nurses to screen for visual impairment and provide education and appropriate resources to their patients.

Refractive Errors, Low Vision, and Blindness

In refractive errors, vision is impaired because a shortened or elongated eyeball prevents light rays from focusing sharply on the retina. Blurred vision from refractive error can be corrected with eyeglasses or contact lenses. The appropriate eyeglass or contact lens is determined by **refraction**. Ophthalmic refraction consists of placing various types of lenses in front of the patient's eyes to determine which lens best improves the patient's vision.

The depth of the eyeball is important in determining refractive error. Patients for whom the visual image focuses precisely on the macula and who do not need eyeglasses or contact lenses are said to have **emmetropia** (normal vision). People who have **myopia** are said to be nearsighted. They have deeper eyeballs; thus, the distant visual image focuses in front of, or short of, the retina. People who are myopic experience blurred distance vision. When people have a shorter depth to their eyes, the visual image focuses beyond the retina; the eyes are shallower and are called *hyperopic*. People with **hyperopia** are farsighted. These patients experience near vision blurriness, whereas their distance vision is excellent.

Another important cause of refractive error is **astigmatism**, an irregularity in the curve of the cornea. Because astigmatism causes a distortion of the visual image, acuity of both distance and near vision can be decreased. Hard or soft toric contact lenses may be used to correct astigmatic errors, in place of eyeglasses.

Ophthalmology has entered the era of customized vision correction, in its desire to achieve "super-normal vision." A new method of measuring refractive error is called *wavefront technology*. The most promising application for this technology is wavefront-guided refractive surgery.

Low vision is a general term describing visual impairment that requires patients to use devices and strategies in addition to corrective lenses to perform visual tasks. Low vision is defined as a best corrected visual acuity (BCVA) of 20/70 to 20/200.

Blindness is defined as a BCVA that can range from 20/400 to no light perception (NLP). The clinical definition of absolute blindness is the absence of light perception. Legal blindness is a condition of impaired vision in which a person has a BCVA that does not exceed 20/200 in the better eye or whose widest visual field diameter is 20 degrees or less. This definition neither equates with functional ability nor classifies the degrees of visual impairment. Legal blindness ranges from an inability to perceive light to having some vision remaining. A person who meets the criteria for legal blindness may be eligible for government financial assistance, such as social security disability benefits. Nurses may make social service referral for follow-up.

Impaired vision is often accompanied by difficulty in performing functional activities. People with visual acuity of 20/80 to 20/100 and a visual field restriction of 60 degrees to greater than 20 degrees can read at a nearly normal level with optical aids. Their visual orientation is near normal but requires increased scanning of the environment (i.e., systematic use of head and eye movements). In patients with a visual acuity range of 20/200 to 20/400 and a visual field restriction of 20 degrees to greater than 10 degrees, these persons can read slowly with optical aids. In this setting, visual orientation is slow necessitating constant scanning of the environment. People in this category may have the ability to negotiate their environment without auxiliary aids. This ability is termed "travel vision." People with hand motion vision or no vision may benefit from the use of mobility devices (e.g., cane, guide dog) and should be encouraged to learn Braille and to use computer aids.

The most common causes of blindness and visual impairment among adults 40 years of age or older are diabetic retinopathy (refer to Chapter 30), macular degeneration, glaucoma, and cataracts (discussed later in this chapter) (Baloh & Jen, 2016). Macular degeneration is more prevalent among Caucasians, whereas glaucoma is more prevalent among African Americans. Age-related changes in the eye are discussed in Chapter 48.

Clinical Manifestations and Assessment

The assessment of low vision includes a thorough history and the examination of distance and near visual acuity, visual field, contrast sensitivity, glare, color perception, and refraction (see Chapter 48). Specially designed, low-vision visual acuity charts are used to evaluate patients.

During history taking, the underlying cause, course, and duration of the patient's visual impairment are identified. Patients with retinitis pigmentosa, for example, have a genetic abnormality. Patients with diabetic macular edema typically experience fluctuating visual acuity. Deterioration of the central portion of the retina causes macular degeneration and central acuity problems. Risk factors of age-related macular degeneration (AMD) include being 50+ years of age, smoking, and family history, and there is a higher incidence among Caucasians than African Americans or Hispanics/Latinos (National Eye Institute [NEI], 2015). Patients with macular degeneration may experience scotomas (partial or complete visual field cuts surrounded by intact visual fields). Central acuity problems cause difficulty in performing activities that require seeing fine details, such as reading. People with peripheral field defects have more difficulties with mobility. The patient's customary activities of daily living (ADLs), medication regimen, habits (e.g., smoking), acceptance of the physical limitations brought about by the visual impairment, and realistic expectations of low-vision aids must be identified and included in the plan of care, including provision of guidelines for safety and referrals to social services.

Contrast-sensitivity testing measures visual acuity in different degrees of contrast. The initial test may take the form of simply turning on the lights while testing the distance acuity. If the patient can read better with the lights on, the patient can benefit from magnification. Glare testing enables the examiner to obtain a more realistic evaluation of the patient's ability to function in his or her environment. Glare can reduce a person's ability to see, especially in patients with cataracts. Devices that test glare are calibrated to imitate certain objects that create glare, such as a car's headlights at night.

Medical Management

Managing patients with low vision involves magnification and image enhancement through the use of low-vision aids and strategies, and referrals to social services and community agencies serving those with visual impairment. Since macular degeneration is irreversible, goals are to optimize the

TABLE **49-1** Activities Affected by Visual Impairment with Suggestions for Low-Vision Aids

Activity	Optical Aids	Nonoptical Aids
Shopping	Hand magnifier	Lighting, color cues
Fixing a snack	Spectacle magnifier	Color cues, consistent storage plan
Eating out	Hand magnifier	Flashlight, portable lamp
Identifying money	Spectacle, spectacle-mounted or hand magnifier	Arrange paper money in wallet compartments or fold banknotes of different denominations differently
Reading print	Spectacle, spectacle-mounted, dome, hand, or stand magnifier Closed-circuit television	Lighting, high-contrast print, large print, reading slit stand magnifier, electronic books
Writing	Hand magnifier	Lighting, bold-tip pen, black ink
Using a telephone	Telescope hand magnifier	Large print dial or touch tone buttons, hand-printed directory
Crossing streets	Telescope	Cane, ask directions
Finding taxis and bus signs	Telescope	Ask for assistance
Reading medication labels	Hand magnifier	Color codes, large print
Reading stove dials	Hand magnifier	Color codes, raised dots
Adjusting the thermostat	Hand magnifier	Enlarged print model
Using a computer	Spectacle or spectacle-mounted magnifier	High-contrast color, large-print program
Reading signs	Telescope Portable electronic magnifier	Move closer
Watching sporting event	Telescope	Sit in front rows

Adapted from Riordan-Eva, P., & Cunningham, E. (Eds.). (2012). *Vaughan & Asbury's general ophthalmology* (18th ed.). New York: McGraw-Hill Companies.

patient's remaining vision, whether central or peripheral, and assist the patient to perform customary activities. Low-vision aids include optical and nonoptical devices (Table 49-1). The optical devices include convex lens aids, such as magnifiers and spectacles; telescopic devices; antireflective lenses that diminish glare; and electronic reading systems, such as closed-circuit television and computers with large print. Continuing advances in computer software provide very useful products for patients with low vision. Scanners and the appropriate software enable the user to scan printed material and have it read by computer voice or to enlarge the print for reading. Magnifiers can be handheld or attached to a stand with or without illumination. Telescopic devices can be spectacle telescopes or clip-on or handheld loupes.

The Internet continues to expand, and a telephone system has been developed that allows access to the Internet and e-mail using voice commands (Box 49-1).

Referrals to community agencies may be necessary for patients with low vision who live alone and cannot self-administer their medications. Community agencies, such as the Lighthouse National Center for Vision and Aging, offer services to patients with low vision that include training in independent living skills, the provision of occupational and recreational activities, and a wide variety of assistive devices for vision enhancement and orientation and mobility.

BOX 49-1 | **Web Access for the Visually Impaired**

People with impaired vision need not be left behind in the computer age. Various technologies are available. A list of general equipment needs follows:

- *Computer:* Software specifically developed for people with visual impairment
- *Internet service provider* (e.g., AOL, Netscape, Earthlink, Comcast)
- *Screen-reader program:* Converts text on the computer screen to synthesized speech (e.g., JAWS for Windows, Windows Eyes, Slimware Window Bridge, ProTalk 32, Hal Screen Reader, WinVision, outSPOKEN for Windows)
- *Browser program to navigate the World Wide Web* (e.g., Microsoft Internet Explorer, IBM Home Page Reader)

Nursing Management

Coping with blindness involves three types of adaptation: emotional, physical, and social. The emotional adjustment to blindness or severe visual impairment determines the success of the physical and social adjustments of the patient. Successful emotional adjustment means acceptance of blindness or severe visual impairment.

Promoting Coping Efforts

Effective coping may not occur until the patient recognizes the permanence of the blindness. Clinging to false hopes of regaining vision hampers effective adaptation to blindness. A patient who is newly blind and his or her family members (especially those who live with the patient) undergo the various steps of grieving: denial, anger, loss bargaining, depression, and resolution and acceptance (Kübler-Ross, 1969). The ability to accept the changes that must come with visual loss and willingness to adapt to those changes influence the successful rehabilitation of the patient who is blind. Additional aspects to consider are value changes, independence–dependence conflicts, coping with stigma, and learning to function in social settings without visual cues and landmarks.

Promoting Spatial Orientation and Mobility

A person who is blind or severely visually impaired requires strategies for adapting to the environment. ADLs, such as walking to a chair from a bed, require spatial concepts. A patient whose visual impairment results from a chronic progressive eye disorder, such as glaucoma, has better cognitive mapping skills than does the patient who becomes blind suddenly. Patients with progressive eye disorders develop the use of spatial and topographic concepts early and gradually; hence, remembering a room layout is easier for them. Patients who become blind suddenly have more difficulty in adjusting, and emotional and behavioral issues of coping with blindness may hinder their learning. These patients require intensive emotional and physical support.

In the hospital, the bedside table and the call button must always be within reach. The parts of the call button are explained, and the patient is taught to touch and press the buttons or dials until the activity is mastered. The patient must be familiarized with the location of the telephone, water pitcher, and other objects on the bedside table. The food tray's composition is likened to the face of a clock; for example, the main plate may be described as being at 12 o'clock or the coffee cup at 3 o'clock. All articles and furniture must remain in the same positions throughout the patient's hospitalization. Introduction of hospital personnel should be made upon entering and departure from the patient's room.

The nurse should be aware of the importance of techniques in providing physical assistance, encouraging independence, and ensuring safety. Specific guidelines for interacting with the patient with vision loss are presented in Box 49-2. The readiness of the patient and his or her family to learn must be assessed before initiating orientation and mobility training.

Promoting Home and Community-Based Care

The nurse, social worker, family, and others collaborate to assess the patient's home condition and support system. If available, a low-vision specialist or occupational therapist should be consulted, particularly for patients for whom identifying and administering medications pose problems. Contact information for some private and nonprofit services is included in the Internet Resources for this chapter available at http://thepoint.lww.com/Honan2e.

Other interventions that are appropriate for some people with low vision or blindness include Braille and guide dogs. Guide dogs, also known as Seeing-Eye dogs, are dogs that are specially bred and raised and then rigorously trained to assist people who are blind. The guide dog is a constant companion to the person who is blind (also referred to as the animal's handler) and is allowed on airplanes and in restaurants, stores, hotels, and other public places. A guide dog in harness is a working dog and should not be approached without permission of the handler. With the assistance of the guide dog, the person who is blind can be extremely mobile and accomplish normal activities both within and outside of the home and workplace.

Unfolding Patient Stories: Vernon Watkins • Part 2

Recall from Chapter 5 Vernon Watkins, who came to the emergency department with severe abdominal pain and underwent a hemicolectomy for a bowel perforation. During postoperative care the nurse determines that he has poor vision. What measures can the nurse take to maintain a safe environment for a patient with visual impairment? How will the discovery of impaired vision impact the nursing plan of care, discharge planning, and delivery of patient education?

Care for Vernon and other patients in a realistic virtual environment: *vSim for Nursing* (thepoint.lww.com/vSimMedicalSurgical). Practice documenting these patients' care in DocuCare (thepoint.lww.com/DocuCareEHR).

GLAUCOMA

Glaucoma is a group of ocular conditions characterized by optic nerve damage. The optic nerve damage is related to the intraocular pressure (IOP) caused by congestion of aqueous humor in the eye. Ranges of pressures have been considered "normal," but they may be associated with visual loss in some patients. While the average IOP is generally at or below 21 mm Hg, exceptions to this normal value exist. Genetic disposition and central corneal thickness have been

BOX 49-2

Guidelines for Interacting with People Who Are Blind or Have Low Vision

- Remember that the only difference between you and people who are blind or have low vision is that they are not able to see through their eyes what you are able to see through yours.
- Do not be uncomfortable when in the company of a person who is blind or has low vision. Talk with the person as you would talk with any other individual, honestly and without pity; do not be concerned about using words like "see" and "look." There is no need to raise your voice unless the person asks you to do so.
- Identify yourself as you approach the person and before you make physical contact. Tell the person your name and your role. If another person approaches, introduce him or her. When you leave the room, be sure to tell the person that you are leaving and if anyone else remains in the room.
- It is appropriate to touch the person's hand or arm lightly to indicate that you are about to speak.
- When talking, face the person and speak directly to him or her using a normal tone of voice.
- Be specific when communicating direction. Mention a specific distance or use clock cues when possible (e.g., walk left about 2 yards; walk about 20 ft to the right; the telephone is at 2 o'clock). Avoid using phrases such as "over there."
- When you offer to assist someone, allow the person to hold onto your arm just above the elbow and to walk a half-step behind you.

- When offering the person a seat, place the person's hand on the back or the arm of the seat.
- When you are about to go up or down a flight of stairs, tell the person, and place his or her hand on the banister.
- Make sure that the environment is free of obstacles; close doors and cabinets so they are not in the path.
- Offer to read written information, such as a menu.
- If you serve food to the person, use clock cues to specify where everything is on the plate.
- When the person who is blind or who has low vision is a patient in a health care facility:
  - Make sure all objects the person will need are close at hand.
  - Identify the location of objects that the person may need (e.g., "The call light is near your right hand"; "The telephone is on the table on the left side of your bed.")
  - Remove obstacles that may be in the person's pathway and could cause a fall.
  - Place all assistive devices the person uses close at hand; let the person feel the devices so that he or she knows their location.
- Do not distract the service animal unless the owner has given permission.
- Ask the person, "How can I help you?" At some times, the person needs help, but at other times help may not be needed.

This material is adapted from and based in part on *Achieving Physical and Communication Accessibility,* a publication of the National Center for Access Unlimited; *Community Access Facts,* an Adaptive Environments Center publication; and *The Ten Commandments of Interacting with People with Mental Health Disabilities,* a publication of The Ability Center of Greater Toledo.

---

implicated in causing ocular hypertension (OHT), a major precursor to glaucoma (Yanoff & Cameron, 2016). Glaucoma is one of the leading causes of irreversible blindness in the world and is the leading cause of blindness among adults in the United States. There is no cure for glaucoma; research is aimed at identifying risk factors and preventing vision loss and blindness.

Pathophysiology

Aqueous humor flows between the iris and the lens, nourishing the cornea and lens. Most (90%) of the fluid then flows out of the anterior chamber, draining through the spongy trabecular meshwork into the canal of Schlemm and the episcleral veins (Fig. 49-1). About 10% of the aqueous fluid exits through the ciliary body into the suprachoroidal space and then drains into the venous circulation of the ciliary body, choroid, and sclera. Unimpeded outflow of aqueous fluid depends on an intact drainage system and an open angle (about 45 degrees) between the iris and the cornea. A narrower angle places the iris closer to the trabecular meshwork, diminishing the angle. The amount of aqueous humor produced tends to decrease with age, in systemic diseases such as diabetes, and in ocular inflammatory conditions.

IOP is determined by the rate of aqueous production, the resistance encountered by the aqueous humor as it flows out of the passages, and the venous pressure of the episcleral veins that drain into the anterior ciliary vein. When aqueous

FIGURE 49-1. Normal outflow of aqueous humor. **A.** Trabecular meshwork. **B.** Uveoscleral route. (From Kanski, J. J. (2011). *Clinical ophthalmology.* Oxford: Butterworth-Heinemann Ltd.)

Progression of Glaucoma

1. **Initiating events**
   Precipitating factors include illness, emotional stress, congenital narrow angles, long-term use of corticosteroids, and use of mydriatics (i.e., medications causing pupillary dilation).
   ↓
2. **Structural alterations in the aqueous outflow system**
   Tissue and cellular changes caused by factors that affect aqueous humor dynamics lead to structural alterations.
   ↓
3. **Functional alterations**
   Conditions such as increased IOP or impaired blood flow create functional changes.
   ↓
4. **Optic nerve damage**
   Atrophy of the optic nerve is characterized by loss of nerve fibers and blood supply. This fourth stage inevitably progresses to the fifth stage.
   ↓
5. **Visual loss**
   Progressive loss of vision is characterized by visual field defects.

fluid production and drainage are in balance, the IOP is between 10 and 21 mm Hg. When aqueous fluid is inhibited from flowing out, pressure builds up within the eye. Fluctuations in IOP occur with time of day, exertion, diet, and medications. IOP tends to increase with blinking, tight lid squeezing, and upward gazing. Systemic conditions, such as hypertension, and intraocular conditions, such as uveitis and retinal detachment, have been associated with elevated IOP.

There are two accepted theories regarding how increased IOP damages the optic nerve in glaucoma. The direct mechanical theory suggests that high IOP damages the retinal layer as it passes through the optic nerve head. The indirect ischemic theory suggests that high IOP compresses the microcirculation in the optic nerve head, resulting in cell injury and death. Some glaucomas appear as exclusively mechanical, and some are exclusively ischemic types. Typically, most cases are a combination of both. Regardless of the cause of damage, glaucomatous changes typically evolve through clearly discernible stages (Box 49-3).

Classification of Glaucoma

There are several types of glaucoma. Although glaucoma classification is changing as knowledge increases, current clinical forms of glaucoma are identified as open-angle glaucoma, angle-closure glaucoma (also called pupillary block), congenital glaucoma, and glaucoma associated with other conditions, such as developmental anomalies or corticosteroid use. Glaucoma can be primary or secondary, depending on whether associated factors contribute to the rise in IOP. The two common clinical forms of glaucoma encountered in adults are open-angle and angle-closure glaucoma. These are differentiated by mechanisms that cause impaired aqueous outflow. Table 49-2 summarizes the characteristics of the different types of open-angle and angle-closure glaucoma.

Risk Factors

It is estimated that at least 2.7 million Americans have glaucoma (Prevent Blindness in America, 2012). Glaucoma is more prevalent among people older than 40 years of age, and the incidence increases with age. It is also more prevalent among men than women and in African American and Asian populations. Inflammatory processes, such as uveitis, may cause glaucoma in about 10% to 30% of the population (Sarodia, Kulkarni, & Barton, 2016). Uveitic glaucoma (UG) is a secondary glaucoma associated with high IOP and optic nerve damage. There are multiple mechanisms of IOP, which pose significant challenge when treating UG. Glaucoma associated with uveitis results in cellular debris and protein leakage out of the blood vessels into clear, aqueous fluid, blocking drainage. Initially the angle between the iris and cornea may be open. As IOP rises, the iris can bow forward, sticking to the lens, cornea, or sclera, which closes the angle of the anterior chamber. Management often requires both an ophthalmologist specializing in glaucoma in addition to a rheumatologist (Munoz-Negrete, Moreno-Montanes, Hernandez-Martinez, & Rebolleda, 2015) (Box 49-4).

Clinical Manifestations and Assessment

Glaucoma is often called the "silent thief of sight" because most patients are unaware that they have the disease until they have experienced visual changes and vision loss. The patient may not seek health care until he or she experiences blurred vision or "halos" around lights, difficulty focusing, difficulty adjusting eyes in low lighting, loss of peripheral vision, aching or discomfort around the eyes, and headache.

The purpose of a glaucoma workup is to establish the diagnostic category, assess the optic nerve damage, and formulate a treatment plan. The patient's ocular and medical history must be detailed to investigate the history of predisposing factors. Diagnostic examination to detect and manage glaucoma includes the following tests: tonometry to measure the IOP, ophthalmoscopy to inspect the optic nerve, gonioscopy to examine the filtration angle of the anterior chamber, perimetry to assess the visual fields, and pachymetry to measure the thickness of the cornea, which influences IOP readings.

The changes in the optic nerve related to glaucoma are pallor and cupping of the optic nerve disc. The pallor of the optic nerve is caused by a lack of blood supply that results from cellular destruction. Cupping is characterized by exaggerated bending of the blood vessels as they cross the optic disc, resulting in an enlarged optic cup that appears more basin-like compared with a normal cup. The progression of cupping in glaucoma is caused by the gradual loss of retinal

TABLE **49-2** Glaucoma Types, Clinical Manifestation, and Treatment

Types of Glaucoma	Clinical Manifestations	Treatment
Open-Angle Glaucoma		
Usually bilateral, but one eye may be affected more severely than the other. In all three types of open-angle glaucoma, the anterior chamber angle is open and appears normal.		
Chronic open-angle glaucoma (COAG)	Optic nerve damage, visual field defects, IOP >21 mm Hg May have fluctuating IOPs. Usually no symptoms but possible ocular pain, headache, and halos	Decrease IOP 20–50%. Additional topical and oral agents added as necessary. If medical treatment is unsuccessful, laser trabeculoplasty (LT) can decrease IOP by 20%. Glaucoma filtering surgery if continued optic nerve damage despite medication therapy and LT.
Normal tension glaucoma	IOP ≤21 mm Hg; optic nerve damage, visual field defects	Treatment similar to COAG, however, the best management for normal tension glaucoma is yet to be established. Goal is to lower the IOP by at least 30%.
Ocular hypertension	Elevated IOP Possible ocular pain or headache	Decrease IOP by at least 20%
Angle-Closure (Pupillary Block) Glaucoma		
Obstruction in aqueous humor outflow due to the complete or partial closure of the angle from the forward shift of the peripheral iris to the trabecula. The obstruction results in an increased IOP.		
Acute angle-closure glaucoma (AACG)	Rapidly progressive visual impairment, periocular pain, conjunctival hyperemia, and congestion Pain may be associated with nausea, vomiting, bradycardia, and profuse sweating. Reduced central visual acuity, severely elevated IOP, corneal edema Pupil is vertically oval, fixed in a semi-dilated position, and unreactive to light and accommodation	Ocular emergency, requiring administration of hyperosmotics, acetazolamide, and topical ocular hypotensive agents, such as pilocarpine and beta blockers (betaxolol). Possible laser incision in the iris (iridotomy) to release blocked aqueous and reduce IOP Other eye is also treated with pilocarpine eye drops and/or surgical management to avoid a similar spontaneous attack.
Subacute angle-closure glaucoma	Transient blurring of vision, halos around lights; temporal headaches and/or ocular pain; pupil may be semi-dilated	Prophylactic peripheral laser iridotomy Can lead to acute or chronic angle-closure glaucoma if untreated
Chronic angle-closure glaucoma	Progression of glaucomatous cupping and significant visual field loss; IOP may be normal or elevated; ocular pain and headache	Management is similar to that for COAG: includes laser iridotomy and medications.
Other Types of Glaucoma		
Uveitic glaucoma	IOP ≥ 21 mm Hg; optic nerve damage, visual field defects	Decrease IOP; medical treatment or surgery may be necessary

BOX 49-4

Risk Factors for Glaucoma

- Family history of glaucoma
- African American race
- Older age (over 60 years of age)
- Diabetes mellitus
- Cardiovascular disease
- Migraine syndromes
- Nearsightedness (myopia)
- Eye trauma
- Prolonged use of topical or systemic corticosteroids

nerve fibers accompanied by the loss of blood supply, resulting in increased pallor of the optic disc.

As the damage to the optic nerve increases, visual perception in the area is lost. The localized areas of visual loss (i.e., **scotomas**) represent loss of retinal sensitivity and are measured and mapped by perimetry. In patients with glaucoma, there is a distinct pattern that differs from other ocular diseases and is useful in establishing its diagnosis. Figure 49-2 shows the progression of visual field defects caused by glaucoma.

FIGURE 49-2 Progression of glaucomatous visual field defects. A central scotoma at 10 to 20 degrees of fixation near the blind spot is the initial significant finding (**A, B**). As the glaucoma progresses, the scotomas enlarge and deepen, resulting in peripheral vision loss. **C.** Defect within 5 degrees of fixation point nasally. **D.** Peripheral involvement enlarges. **E.** Ringlike scotoma. **F.** Eventually, vision is lost. The resulting "island of vision" becomes the characteristic visual field appearance of glaucoma and correlates with the "tunnel vision," in which peripheral vision is lost. (From Kanski, J. J. (2011). *Clinical ophthalmology.* Oxford: Butterworth-Heinemann Ltd.)

Medical Management

The aim of all glaucoma treatment is prevention of damage to the optic nerve. Lifelong therapy is almost always necessary because glaucoma cannot be cured. Treatment focuses on pharmacologic therapy, laser procedures, surgery, or a combination of these approaches, all of which have potential complications and side effects. The object is to achieve the greatest benefit at the least risk, cost, and inconvenience to the patient. Although treatment cannot reverse damage to the optic nerve, further damage can be controlled. The goal is to maintain an IOP within a range unlikely to cause further damage.

The initial target for IOP among patients with elevated IOP and those with low-tension glaucoma with progressive visual field loss is typically set at 30% lower than the current pressure. The patient is monitored for changes in the appearance of the optic nerve. If there is evidence of progressive damage, the target IOP is lowered again until the optic nerve shows stability.

Medical management of glaucoma relies on systemic and topical ocular medications that lower IOP. Periodic follow-up examinations are essential to monitor IOP, the appearance of the optic nerve, the visual fields, and side effects of medications. Therapy takes into account the patient's health and stage of glaucoma. Comfort, affordability, convenience, lifestyle, and personality are factors to consider in the patient's adherence to the medical regimen.

The patient is usually started on the lowest dose of topical medication and then advanced to increased concentrations until the desired IOP level is reached and maintained. Because of their efficacy, minimal dosing (can be used once each day), and low cost, beta blockers are the preferred initial topical medications. Beta blockers decrease the production of aqueous humor with resultant decrease in IOP. One eye is treated first, with the other eye used as a control in determining the efficacy of the medication; once efficacy has been established, treatment of the other eye is started. If the IOP is elevated in both eyes, both are treated. When results are not satisfactory, a new medication is substituted. The main markers of the efficacy of the medication in glaucoma control are lowering of the IOP to the target pressure, appearance of the optic nerve head, and less deterioration of the visual field.

Surgical management for glaucoma includes several procedures. In laser trabeculoplasty, burns are applied to the inner surface of the trabecular meshwork to open the intratrabecular spaces and widen the canal of Schlemm, thereby promoting outflow of aqueous humor and decreasing IOP. Laser iridotomy, used for pupillary block glaucoma, is an opening made in the iris to eliminate the pupillary block. Laser iridotomy is contraindicated in patients with corneal edema, which interferes with laser targeting and strength.

Filtering procedures for chronic glaucoma are used to create an opening or fistula in the trabecular meshwork to drain aqueous humor from the anterior chamber to the subconjunctival space into a bleb (blister-like fluid collection), thereby bypassing the usual drainage structures. This allows the aqueous humor to flow and exit by different routes (i.e., absorption by the conjunctival vessels or mixing with tears). Trabeculectomy is the standard filtering technique used to remove part of the trabecular meshwork. Complications include hemorrhage, an extremely low (hypotony) or elevated IOP, uveitis, cataracts, bleb failure, bleb leak, and endophthalmitis. Unlike other surgical procedures, the filtering procedure's goal in glaucoma treatment is to achieve incomplete healing of the surgical wound.

Nursing Management

Teaching Patients Self-Care

The medical and surgical management of patients with glaucoma slows the progression of glaucoma but does not cure it. The lifelong therapeutic regimen mandates patient education. The nature of the disease and the importance of strict adherence to the medication regimen must be included in a teaching plan to help ensure compliance. A thorough patient interview is essential to determine systemic conditions, current systemic and ocular medications, family history, and problems with compliance to glaucoma medications. The

BOX 49-5
Patient Education

Managing Glaucoma

- Know your IOP measurement and the desired range.
- Be informed about the extent of your vision loss and optic nerve damage.
- Keep a record of your eye pressure measurements and visual field test results to monitor your own progress.
- Review all your medications (including over-the-counter and herbal medications) with your ophthalmologist, and mention any side effects each time you visit.
- Ask about potential side effects and drug interactions of your eye medications.
- Ask whether generic or less costly forms of your eye medications are available.
- Review the dosing schedule with your ophthalmologist and inform him or her if you have trouble following the schedule.
- Participate in the decision-making process. Let your provider know what dosing schedule works for you and other preferences regarding your eye care.
- Have the nurse observe you instilling eye medication to determine whether you are administering it properly.
- Be aware that glaucoma medications can cause adverse effects if used inappropriately. Eye drops are to be administered as prescribed, not when eyes feel irritated.
- Ask your ophthalmologist to send a report to your provider after each appointment.
- Keep all follow-up appointments.

effects of glaucoma-control medications on vision must also be explained. **Miotics** and sympathomimetics decrease the size of the pupil, facilitating the outflow of aqueous humor and decreasing the IOP, but they may also result in altered focus; therefore, patients need to be cautious in navigating their surroundings.

Nurses in all settings encounter patients with glaucoma. Even patients with longstanding disease and those with glaucoma as a secondary diagnosis should be assessed for knowledge level and compliance with the therapeutic regimen. Box 49-5 contains points to review with patients with glaucoma.

Continuing Care

For the patient with severe glaucoma and impaired function, referral to services that assist the patient in performing ADLs may be needed. The loss of peripheral vision can impact mobility, and patients may benefit from low vision and rehabilitation services. Patients who meet the criteria for legal blindness should be offered referrals to agencies that can assist them in obtaining federal assistance.

Reassurance and emotional support are important aspects of care. A lifelong disease involving possible loss of sight has psychological, physical, social, and vocational ramifications. The family must be integrated into the plan of care, and because the disease has a familial tendency, family members

should be encouraged to undergo examinations at least once every 2 years to detect glaucoma early.

CATARACTS

A cataract is a lens opacity or cloudiness (Fig. 49-3). Cataracts rank behind only arthritis and heart disease as a leading cause of disability in older adults. In fact, cataracts are the most common cause of treatable blindness. It is estimated the prevalence for cataract is 17.2%, with higher rates (77%) appreciated among Caucasian woman over 80 years of age (Klein & Klein, 2013). It is estimated that more than 30 million Americans will develop cataracts by the year 2020 (Ferri, 2016).

Pathophysiology

Cataracts can develop in one or both eyes at any age for a variety of causes (Box 49-6). Visual impairment normally progresses at the same rate in both eyes over many years or in a matter of months. The three most common types of senile (age-related) cataracts are defined by their location in the lens: nuclear, cortical, and posterior subcapsular. The extent of visual impairment depends on their size, density, and location in the lens. More than one type can be present in one eye.

A nuclear cataract is caused by central opacity in the lens and has a substantial genetic component. It is associated with myopia (i.e., nearsightedness), which worsens when the cataract progresses. If dense, the cataract severely blurs vision. Periodic changes in prescription eyeglasses help manage this condition.

A cortical cataract involves the anterior, posterior, or equatorial cortex of the lens. A cataract in the equator or periphery of the cortex does not interfere with the passage of light through the center of the lens and has little effect on vision. Cortical cataracts progress at a highly variable rate. Vision is worse in very bright light.

Posterior subcapsular cataracts occur in front of the posterior capsule. This type typically develops in younger

FIGURE 49-3 A cataract is a cloudy or opaque lens. On visual inspection, the lens appears gray or milky. (From Rubin, E., & Strayer, D. S. (Eds.). (2014). *Rubin's pathology* (7th ed.). Philadelphia, PA: Lippincott Williams & Wilkins.)

Risk Factors for Cataract Formation

Aging:
- Loss of lens transparency
- Clumping or aggregation of lens protein (which leads to light scattering)
- Accumulation of a yellow-brown pigment due to the breakdown of lens protein
- Decreased oxygen uptake
- Increase in sodium and calcium
- Decrease in levels of vitamin C, protein, and glutathione (an antioxidant)

Associated ocular conditions:
- Retinitis pigmentosa
- Myopia
- Retinal detachment and retinal surgery
- Infection (e.g., herpes zoster, uveitis)

Toxic factors:
- Corticosteroids, especially at high doses and in long-term use
- Alkaline chemical eye burns, poisoning

- Cigarette smoking
- Calcium, copper, iron, gold, silver, and mercury, which tend to deposit in the pupillary area of the lens

Nutritional factors:
- Reduced levels of antioxidants
- Poor nutrition
- Obesity

Physical factors:
- Dehydration associated with chronic diarrhea, use of purgatives in anorexia nervosa, and use of hyperbaric oxygenation
- Blunt trauma, perforation of the lens with a sharp object or foreign body, electric shock
- Ultraviolet radiation in sunlight and x-ray

Systemic diseases and syndromes:
- Diabetes mellitus
- Down syndrome
- Disorders related to lipid metabolism
- Kidney disorders
- Musculoskeletal disorders

---

people and, in some cases, is associated with prolonged corticosteroid use, diabetes, or ocular trauma. Near vision is diminished, and the eye is increasingly sensitive to glare from bright light (e.g., sunlight, headlights).

Clinical Manifestations and Assessment

Painless, blurry vision is characteristic of cataracts. The person perceives that surroundings are dimmer, as if his or her glasses need cleaning. Light scattering is common, and the person experiences reduced contrast sensitivity, sensitivity to glare, and reduced visual acuity. Other effects include myopic shift, astigmatism, monocular **diplopia** (double vision), color shift (the aging lens becomes progressively more absorbent at the blue end of the spectrum), brunescens (color values shift to yellow-brown), and reduced light transmission.

Decreased visual acuity is directly proportionate to cataract density. The Snellen visual acuity test, ophthalmoscopy, and slit-lamp biomicroscopic examination are used to establish the degree of cataract formation. The degree of lens opacity does not always correlate with the patient's functional status. Some patients can perform normal activities despite clinically significant cataracts. Others with less lens opacification have a disproportionate decrease in visual acuity; hence, visual acuity is one measure of visual impairment and needs to be considered along with other visual screening techniques and assessments.

Medical Management

Nonsurgical Management

Nonsurgical (medications, eyedrops, eyeglasses) treatment has not been found as curative for people with cataracts nor

does it prevent age-related cataracts. Cigarette smoking, long-term use of corticosteroids, especially at high doses, sunlight and ionizing radiation, diabetes, obesity, and eye injuries can increase the risk for cataracts. In the early stages of cataract development, glasses, contact lenses, strong bifocals, or magnifying lenses may improve vision.

Surgical Management

Surgical management of cataracts is considered when reduced vision interferes with normal activities. In deciding when cataract surgery is to be performed, the patient's functional and visual status should be a primary consideration. Surgery is performed on an outpatient basis and usually takes less than 1 hour. Although complications from cataract surgery are uncommon, they can have significant effects on vision. Restoration of visual function through a safe and minimally invasive procedure is the surgical goal.

When both eyes have cataracts, one eye is treated first, with at least several weeks, preferably months, separating the two procedures. Because cataract surgery is performed to improve visual functioning, the delay for the other eye gives time for the patient and the surgeon to evaluate whether the results from the first surgery are adequate to preclude the need for a second operation.

Intracapsular Cataract Extraction

In intracapsular cataract extraction, the entire lens (i.e., nucleus, cortex, and capsule) is removed and fine sutures are used to close the incision. From the late 1800s until the 1970s, it was the technique of choice for cataract extraction. It is infrequently performed today but is still indicated when there is a need to remove the entire lens, such as with a subluxated cataract (i.e., partially or completely dislocated lens).

Extracapsular Cataract Extraction

The extracapsular cataract extraction technique involves smaller incisional wounds (less trauma to the eye) and maintains the posterior capsule of the lens, thus reducing postoperative complications, particularly aphakic retinal detachment and cystoid macular edema. A portion of the anterior capsule is removed, allowing extraction of the lens nucleus and cortex. The posterior capsule and zonular support are left intact. An intact zonular–capsular diaphragm provides the needed safe anchor for the posterior chamber intraocular lens (IOL). After the pupil has been dilated and the surgeon has made a small incision on the upper edge of the cornea, a viscoelastic substance (clear gel) is injected into the space between the cornea and the lens. This prevents the space from collapsing and facilitates insertion of the IOL.

Phacoemulsification

This method of extracapsular surgery uses an ultrasonic device that liquefies the nucleus and cortex, which are then suctioned out through a tube. The posterior capsule is left intact. Because the incision is even smaller than the standard extracapsular cataract extraction, the wound heals more rapidly, and there is early stabilization of refractive error and less astigmatism. Hardware and software advances in ultrasonic technology—including modern phaco needles that are used to cut and aspirate the cataract—permit safe and efficient removal of nearly all cataracts through a clear cornea incision. With increasing frequency, self-sealing (sutureless) clear corneal incisions (temporal part of the cornea) are performed with phacoemulsification, minimizing postoperative astigmatism and thus decreasing bleeding and subconjunctival hemorrhage and speeding recovery of visual acuity.

Lens Replacement

After removal of the crystalline lens, the patient is considered to have aphakia (i.e., without a lens). The lens, which focuses light on the retina, must be replaced for the patient to see clearly. There are three lens replacement options: aphakic eyeglasses, contact lenses, and IOL implants.

Aphakic glasses, although effective, are rarely used. Objects are magnified by 25%, making them appear closer than they actually are. This magnification creates distortion. Peripheral vision is also limited, and binocular vision (i.e., ability of both eyes to focus on one object and fuse the two images into one) is impossible if the other eye is phakic (normal).

Contact lenses provide patients with almost normal vision, but because contact lenses need to be removed occasionally, the patient also needs a pair of aphakic glasses. Contact lenses are not advised for patients who have difficulty inserting, removing, and cleaning them. Frequent handling and improper disinfection increase the risk for infection.

Insertion of IOLs during cataract surgery is the usual approach to lens replacement. After cataract extraction, or phacoemulsification, the surgeon implants an IOL. Extracapsular cataract extraction and posterior chamber IOLs are associated with a relatively low incidence of complications (e.g., **hyphema** [bleeding into the anterior chamber of the eye], macular edema, secondary glaucoma, damage to the corneal endothelium). IOL implantation is contraindicated in patients with recurrent uveitis, proliferative diabetic retinopathy, neovascular glaucoma, or rubeosis iridis.

The most common IOL is the single-focus lens. Eyeglasses are still needed for distant or close vision because the single-focus lens, unlike the natural lens of the eye, cannot alter its shape to bring objects at different distances into focus. Multifocal IOLs reduce the need for eyeglasses, but patients can experience halos and glare. In the future, aging patients may benefit from a combined surgical approach using customized IOLs and refractive surgery for a customized vision correction.

Toxic Anterior Segment Syndrome

Also known as toxic endothelial cell destruction or sterile endophthalmitis, toxic anterior segment syndrome is a noninfectious inflammation caused by a toxic agent after an uncomplicated and uneventful surgery. This disorder is a complication of anterior chamber surgery that often occurs acutely and is characterized by widespread corneal edema and disseminated breakdown of the blood–aqueous barrier and the presence of fibrin and exudate noted in the anterior chamber (Dotan, Kaiserman, Kremer, Ehrlich, & Bahar, 2014).

Toxic anterior segment syndrome is characterized by corneal edema less than 24 hours after surgery and an accumulation of white cells in the anterior chamber of the eye. Like the classic endophthalmitis, the symptoms include reduction in visual acuity and pain. In the absence of microorganism growth, improvement has occurred with topical steroid treatment alone.

Nursing Management

The patient with cataracts should receive the usual preoperative care for ambulatory surgical patients undergoing eye surgery.

Providing Preoperative Care

It has been common practice to withhold any anticoagulant therapy (e.g., aspirin, warfarin [Coumadin]) to reduce the risk for retrobulbar hemorrhage (after retrobulbar injection) for 5 to 7 days before surgery. Dilating drops are administered every 10 minutes for four doses at least 1 hour before surgery. Additional dilating drops may be administered in the operating room (immediately before surgery) if the affected eye is not fully dilated. Antibiotic, corticosteroid, and anti-inflammatory drops may be administered prophylactically to prevent postoperative infection and inflammation.

Patient Education

Intraocular Lens Implant

- Wear glasses or metal eye shield at all times following surgery, as instructed by the provider.
- Always wash hands before touching or cleaning the postoperative eye.
- Clean the postoperative eye with a clean tissue; wipe the closed eye with a single gesture from the inner canthus outward.
- Bathe or shower; shampoo hair cautiously or seek assistance.
- Avoid lying on the side of the affected eye the night after surgery.
- Keep activity light (e.g., walking, reading, watching television). Resume the following activities only as directed by the surgeon: driving, sexual activity, unusually strenuous activity.
- Remember not to lift, push, or pull objects heavier than 15 lb.
- Avoid bending or stooping for an extended period.
- Be careful when climbing or descending stairs.
- Know when to contact the surgeon.[a]

[a]Contact the surgeon immediately if any of the following problems occur before the next appointment: (1) vision changes; (2) continuous flashing lights appear to the affected eye; (3) redness, swelling, or pain increase in the eye; (4) the amount or type of eye drainage changes; (5) the eye is injured in any way; (6) significant pain is not relieved by acetaminophen.

Providing Postoperative Care

After recovery from anesthesia, the patient receives verbal and written instructions about how to protect the eye, administer medications, recognize signs of complications, and obtain emergency care. Box 49-7 identifies activities to be avoided. The nurse also explains that there should be minimal discomfort after surgery and instructs the patient to take a mild analgesic agent, such as acetaminophen, as needed. Antibiotic, anti-inflammatory, and corticosteroid eye drops or ointments are prescribed postoperatively.

Teaching Patients Self-Care

To prevent accidental rubbing or poking of the eye, the patient wears a protective eye patch for 24 hours after surgery, followed by eyeglasses worn during the day and a metal shield worn at night for 1 to 4 weeks. The nurse instructs the patient and family in applying and caring for the eye shield. Sunglasses should be worn while outdoors during the day because the eye is sensitive to light.

Slight morning discharge, some redness, and a scratchy feeling may be expected for a few days. A clean, damp washcloth may be used to remove slight morning eye discharge. Because cataract surgery increases the risk for retinal detachment, the patient must know to notify the surgeon if new floaters (dots) in vision, flashing lights, decrease in vision, pain, or increase in redness occurs.

Continuing Care

The eye patch is removed after the first follow-up appointment. The patient may experience blurring of vision for several days to weeks. Sutures, if used, are left in the eye but alter the curvature of the cornea, resulting in temporary blurring and some astigmatism. Vision gradually improves as the eye heals. Patients with IOL implants have functional vision on the first day after surgery. Vision is stabilized when the eye is completely healed, usually within 6 to 12 weeks, when final corrective prescription is completed. Visual correction is needed for any remaining nearsightedness or farsightedness (even in patients with IOL implants).

RETINAL DISORDERS

Although the retina is composed of multiple microscopic layers, the two innermost layers, the sensory retina and the retinal pigment epithelium (RPE), are the most susceptible to common retinal disorders. As the film in a camera captures an image, the retina, the neural tissue of the eye, performs the same function. The rods and cones, the photoreceptor cells, are found in the sensory layer of the retina. Beneath the sensory layer lies the RPE, the pigmented layer. When the rods and cones are stimulated by light, an electrical impulse is generated, and the image is transmitted to the brain.

RETINAL DETACHMENT

Retinal detachment refers to the separation of the RPE from the sensory layer. The four types of retinal detachment are rhegmatogenous, traction, a combination of rhegmatogenous and traction, and exudative. Rhegmatogenous detachment is the most common form. In this condition, a hole or tear develops in the sensory retina, allowing some of the liquid vitreous to seep through the sensory retina and detach it from the RPE (Fig. 49-4). People at risk for this type of detachment include those with high myopia or aphakia (absence of lens) after cataract surgery. Trauma may also play a role in rhegmatogenous retinal detachment. Between 5% and 10% of all rhegmatogenous retinal detachments are associated with proliferative retinopathy, a retinopathy associated with diabetic neovascularization (see Chapter 30).

Tension, or a pulling force, is responsible for traction retinal detachment. An ophthalmologist must ascertain all of the areas of retinal break and identify and release the scars or bands of fibrous material providing traction on the retina. In general, patients with this condition have developed fibrous scar tissue from conditions such as diabetic retinopathy, vitreous hemorrhage, or the retinopathy of prematurity. The hemorrhages and fibrous proliferation associated with these conditions exert a pulling force on the delicate retina.

Patients can have both rhegmatogenous and traction retinal detachment. Exudative retinal detachments are the result of the production of a serous fluid under the retina from the

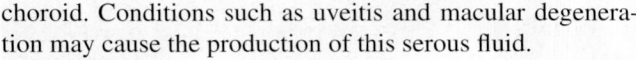

FIGURE 49-4 Rhegmatogenous detachment: the most common form of retinal detachment.

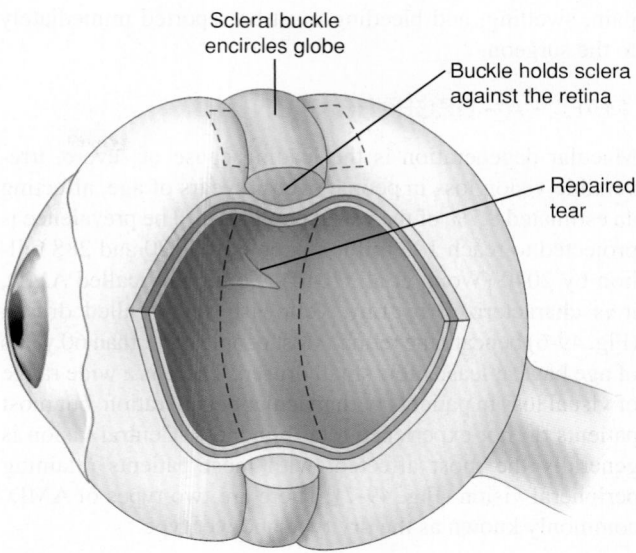

FIGURE 49-5 Scleral buckle.

choroid. Conditions such as uveitis and macular degeneration may cause the production of this serous fluid.

Clinical Manifestations and Assessment

Patients may report the sensation of a shade or curtain coming across the vision of one eye, cobwebs, bright flashing lights, or the sudden onset of a great number of floaters. Patients do not complain of pain.

After visual acuity is determined, the patient must have a dilated **fundus** examination using an indirect ophthalmoscope as well as slit-lamp biomicroscopy. Stereo fundus photography and fluorescein angiography are commonly used during the evaluation.

Increasingly, optical coherence tomography and ultrasound are used for the complete retinal assessment, especially if the view is obscured by a dense cataract or vitreal hemorrhage. All retinal breaks, all fibrous bands that may be causing traction on the retina, and all degenerative changes must be identified.

Medical Management

In rhegmatogenous detachment, an attempt is made to surgically reattach the sensory retina to the RPE. In traction detachment, the source of traction must be removed and the sensory retina reattached. New surgical techniques, as well as advances in instrumentation, have led to an increased rate of success of surgical reattachment and better visual outcomes. The most commonly used surgical interventions are the scleral buckle, the pars plana vitrectomy, and pneumatic retinopexy. The scleral buckle is a procedure in which a piece of silicone plastic or sponge is sewn onto the sclera at the site of the retinal tear. The buckle holds the retina against the sclera until scarring seals the tear (Fig. 49-5).

Nursing Management

For the most part, nursing interventions consist of educating the patient and providing supportive care.

Promoting Comfort

Following surgery, patients will require assistance with meals and walking. While some procedures require a hospital stay, many scleral buckling procedures are performed on an outpatient basis. The nurse should advise patients to avoid heavy lifting or strenuous activity that could increase intraocular pressure. Reading may be restricted until the surgeon gives permission. Patients wear sunglasses during the day and an eye patch at night. Patients often report pain, erythema, and a scratchy sensation after surgery. Ice packs may be applied to counter any edema associated with the conjunctiva. If a vitrectomy was performed with scleral buckling, patients are required to sleep with their head elevated. Air travel must be avoided until the gas bubble, injected during surgery into the vitreous cavity to position the retina, is absorbed. Driving may be restricted until vision stabilizes. Reevaluation of vision and the need for corrective lenses is performed 6 to 8 weeks postoperatively.

Teaching About Complications

Postoperative complications may include increased IOP, endophthalmitis (inflammation of the internal layer of the eye), development of other retinal detachments, development of cataracts, and loss of turgor of the eye. Patients must be taught the signs and symptoms of complications, particularly of increasing IOP and postoperative infection, such as eye pain, sudden change in vision, fever, lid swelling, or conjunctival and/or corneal injection (redness). Excessive pain, swelling, and bleeding must be reported immediately to the surgeon.

MACULAR DEGENERATION

Macular degeneration is the leading cause of severe, irreversible vision loss in people over 60 years of age, affecting an estimated 8.7% of the world population. The prevalence is projected to reach 196 million people by 2020 and 288 million by 2040 (Wong et al., 2014). Commonly called AMD, it is characterized by tiny, yellowish spots called drusen (Fig. 49-6) beneath the retina. Most people older than 60 years of age have at least a few small drusen. There is a wide range of visual loss in patients with macular degeneration, but most patients do not experience total blindness. Central vision is generally the most affected, with most patients retaining peripheral vision (Fig. 49-7). There are two types of AMD, commonly known as the dry type and wet type.

Pathophysiology

Approximately 90% of people with AMD have the dry or nonexudative type, which has an insidious onset and leads to a mild to moderate loss of vision, although peripheral vision is preserved. In dry AMD, the outer layers of the retina slowly break down (Fig. 49-8). With this breakdown comes the appearance of drusen. When the drusen occur outside of the macular area, patients generally have no symptoms. When the drusen occur within the macula, however, there is a gradual blurring of vision that patients may notice when they try to read. There is no known treatment that can cure this type of AMD.

Wet or exudative AMD is characterized by **choroidal neovascularization** (CNV), new growth of blood vessels beneath the retina, which causes severe vision loss in 90% of AMD cases (Normando, Tilley, Guo, & Cordeiro, 2013). Wet AMD may have an abrupt onset. The affected vessels can leak fluid and blood, elevating the retina. Patients report

A Normal Vision

B Age-related Macular Degeneration

FIGURE 49-7 **A.** Normal vision. **B.** Visual loss associated with macular degeneration. (Photos courtesy of the National Eye Institute/National Institutes of Health.)

that straight lines appear crooked and distorted, or that letters in words appear broken. Some patients can be treated with the argon laser to stop the leakage from these vessels. However, this treatment is not ideal because vision may be affected by the laser treatment and abnormal vessels often grow back after treatment.

Medical Management

Visual loss from CNV lesions in AMD is a growing problem. With the growth of these new vessels from the choriocapillary layer, fibrous tissue develops that can, over months, destroy central vision. Laser treatment has been used to close these abnormal vessels, but the very process of photocoagulation carries with it some level of retinal destruction, albeit less than the natural scarring that would occur in the untreated eye.

Photodynamic therapy (PDT) has been developed in an attempt to ameliorate the CNV while causing minimal damage to the retina. Studies have shown that PDT can reduce the risk of visual loss for certain groups of patients who have

FIGURE 49-6 Retina showing drusen and age-related macular degeneration (AMD).

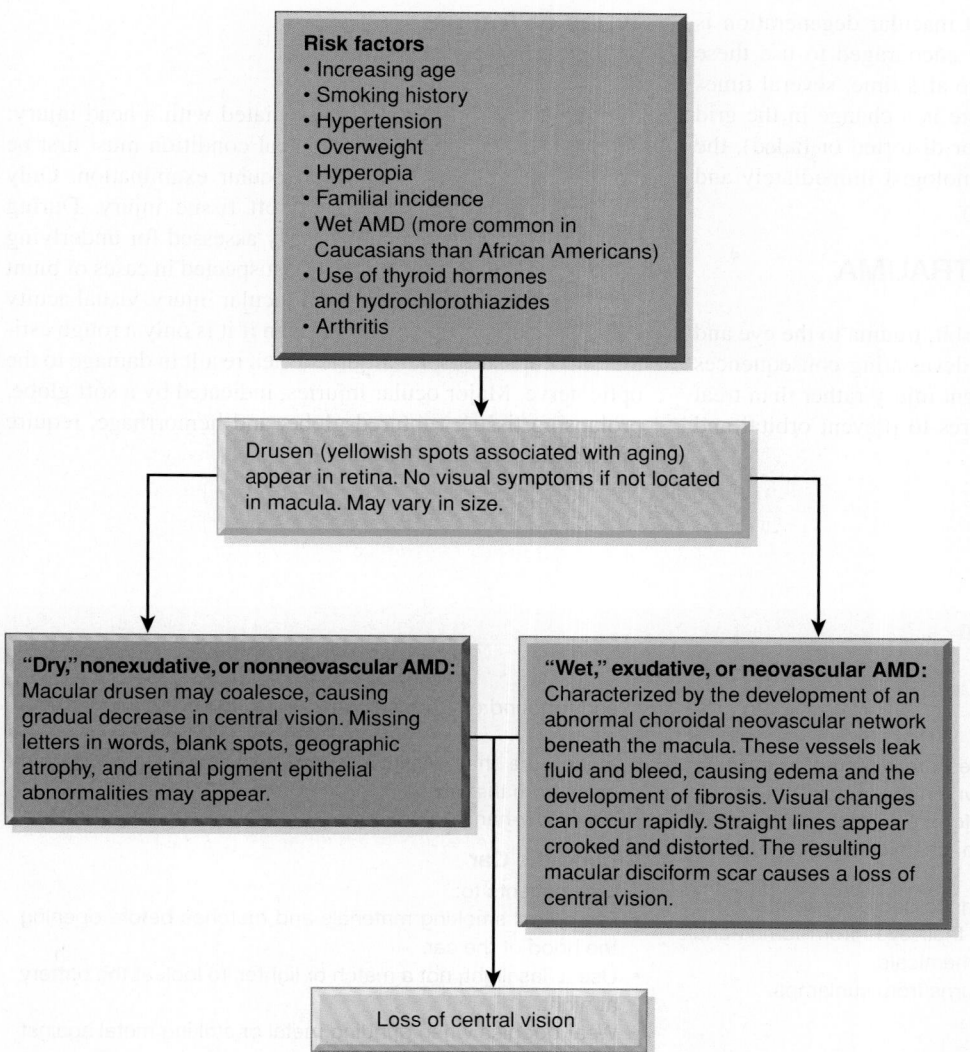

Risk factors
- Increasing age
- Smoking history
- Hypertension
- Overweight
- Hyperopia
- Familial incidence
- Wet AMD (more common in Caucasians than African Americans)
- Use of thyroid hormones and hydrochlorothiazides
- Arthritis

Drusen (yellowish spots associated with aging) appear in retina. No visual symptoms if not located in macula. May vary in size.

"Dry," nonexudative, or nonneovascular AMD: Macular drusen may coalesce, causing gradual decrease in central vision. Missing letters in words, blank spots, geographic atrophy, and retinal pigment epithelial abnormalities may appear.

"Wet," exudative, or neovascular AMD: Characterized by the development of an abnormal choroidal neovascular network beneath the macula. These vessels leak fluid and bleed, causing edema and the development of fibrosis. Visual changes can occur rapidly. Straight lines appear crooked and distorted. The resulting macular disciform scar causes a loss of central vision.

Loss of central vision

FIGURE 49-8 Progression of age-related macular degeneration (AMD): pathways to vision loss.

classic subfoveal CNV due to macular degeneration. PDT is a two-step process. Verteporfin, a photosensitive dye, is infused IV over 10 minutes. Fifteen minutes after the start of the infusion, a diode laser is used to treat the abnormal network of vessels. The dye within the vessels takes up the energy of the diode laser but the surrounding retina does not, thus avoiding damage to adjacent areas. Multiple treatments may be necessary over time.

Verteporfin is a light-activated dye, so patient education is important preoperatively. The dye within the blood vessels near the surface of the skin could become activated with exposure to strong light. This would include bright sunlight, tanning booths, halogen lights, and the bright lights used in dental offices and operating rooms; ordinary indoor light is not a problem. The patient should be instructed to bring dark sunglasses, gloves, a wide-brimmed hat, long-sleeved shirt, and slacks to the setting where PDT will be performed. The patient must be cautioned to avoid exposure to direct sunlight or bright light for 5 days after treatment. Inadvertent

sunlight exposure can lead to severe blistering of the skin and sunburn that may require plastic surgery.

Other treatment options are commonly used in the management of advanced wet AMD; they involve intravitreous injection of vascular endothelial growth factor (VEGF) and inhibitor-like medications. Bleeding risk in intravitreal injections is minimal such that anticoagulation is continued.

Nursing Management

Nursing management is primarily educational. Most patients benefit from the use of bright lighting and magnification devices and from referral to a low-vision center. Some low-vision centers send representatives to the patient's home or place of employment to evaluate the living and working conditions and make recommendations to improve lighting, thereby improving vision and promoting safety.

Amsler grids are given to patients to use in their home to monitor for a sudden onset or distortion of vision. These may provide the earliest sign that macular degeneration is getting worse. Patients should be encouraged to use these grids and to look at them, one eye at a time, several times each week with glasses on. If there is a change in the grid (e.g., if the lines or squares appear distorted or faded), the patient should notify the ophthalmologist immediately and should arrange to be seen promptly.

ORBITAL AND OCULAR TRAUMA

Whether affecting the eye or the orbit, trauma to the eye and surrounding structures may have devastating consequences for vision. It is preferable to prevent injury rather than treat it. Box 49-8 details safety measures to prevent orbital and ocular trauma.

Types of Trauma

Orbital Trauma

Injury to the orbit is usually associated with a head injury; hence, the patient's general medical condition must first be stabilized before conducting an ocular examination. Only then is the globe assessed for soft tissue injury. During inspection, the face is meticulously assessed for underlying fractures, which should always be suspected in cases of blunt trauma. To establish the extent of ocular injury, visual acuity is assessed as soon as possible, even if it is only a rough estimate. Soft tissue orbital injuries often result in damage to the optic nerve. Major ocular injuries, indicated by a soft globe, prolapsing tissue, ruptured globe, and hemorrhage, require immediate surgical attention.

BOX 49-8 | **Health Promotion**

Preventing Eye Injuries

In and Around the House

Advise patients to:

- Make sure that all spray nozzles are directed away from themselves before pressing down on the handle.
- Read instructions carefully before using cleaning fluids, detergents, ammonia, or harsh chemicals, and to wash hands thoroughly after use.
- Use grease shields on frying pans to decrease spattering.
- Wear special goggles to shield their eyes from fumes and splashes when using powerful chemicals.
- Use opaque goggles to avoid burns from sunlamps.

In the Workshop

Advise patients to:

- Protect their eyes from flying fragments, fumes, dust particles, sparks, and splashed chemicals by wearing safety glasses.
- Read instructions thoroughly before using tools and chemicals, and follow precautions for their use.

Around Children

Advise patients to:

- Pay attention to age and maturity level of a child when selecting toys and games, and to avoid projectile toys, such as darts and pellet guns.
- Supervise children when they are playing with toys or games that can be potentially dangerous.
- Teach children the correct way to handle potentially dangerous items, such as scissors and pencils.

In the Garden

Advise patients to:

- Avoid letting anyone stand at the side of or in front of a moving lawn mower.
- Pick up rocks and stones before going over them with the lawn mower (stones can be hurled out of the rotary blades

and rebound off curbs or walls, causing severe injury to the eye).
- Make sure that pesticide spray can nozzles are directed away from the face.
- Avoid low-hanging branches.

Around the Car

Advise patients to:

- Put out all smoking materials and matches before opening the hood of the car.
- Use a flashlight, not a match or lighter, to look at the battery at night.
- Wear goggles when grinding metal or striking metal against metal while performing auto body repair.
- Take standard safety precautions when using jumper cables (wear goggles; make sure the cars are not touching one another; make sure the jumper cable clamps never touch each other; never lean over the battery when attaching cables; and never attach a cable to the negative terminal of a dead battery).

In Sports

Advise patients to:

- Wear protective safety glasses, especially for sports such as racquetball, squash, tennis, baseball, and basketball.
- Wear protective caps, helmets, or face protectors when appropriate, especially for sports such as ice hockey.

Around Fireworks

Advise patients to:

- Wear eye glasses or safety goggles.
- Avoid using explosive fireworks.
- Never allow children to ignite fireworks or stand near others when lighting fireworks.
- Douse firework duds in water instead of attempting to relight them.

Soft Tissue Injury and Hemorrhage

The signs and symptoms of soft tissue injury from blunt or penetrating trauma include tenderness, ecchymosis, lid swelling, **proptosis** (i.e., downward displacement of the eyeball), and hemorrhage. Closed injuries lead to contusions with subconjunctival hemorrhage, commonly known as a *black eye.* Blood accumulates in the tissues of the conjunctiva. Hemorrhage may be caused by a soft tissue injury to the eyelid or by an underlying fracture.

Management of soft tissue hemorrhage that does not threaten vision is usually conservative and consists of thorough inspection, cleansing, and repair of wounds. Cold compresses are used in the early phase, followed by warm compresses. Hematomas that appear as swollen, fluctuating areas may be surgically drained or aspirated; if they are causing significant orbital pressure, they may be surgically evacuated.

Penetrating injuries or a severe blow to the head can result in severe optic nerve damage. Visual loss can be sudden or delayed and progressive. Immediate loss of vision after an ocular injury is usually irreversible. Delayed visual loss has a better prognosis. Corticosteroid therapy is indicated to reduce optic nerve swelling. Surgery, such as optic nerve decompression, may be performed.

Orbital Fractures

Orbital fractures are detected by facial x-rays. Depending on the orbital structures involved, orbital fractures can be classified as blowout, zygomatic or tripod, maxillary, midfacial, orbital apex, and orbital roof fractures. Blowout fractures result from compression of soft tissue and the sudden increase in orbital pressure when the force is transmitted to the orbital floor, the area of least resistance.

The inferior rectus and inferior oblique muscles, with their fat and fascial attachments, or the nerve that courses along the inferior oblique muscle may become entrapped, and the globe may be displaced inward (i.e., enophthalmos). Computed tomography (CT) can identify the muscle and its auxiliary structures that are entrapped. These fractures are usually caused by blunt small objects, such as a fist, knee, elbow, or tennis or golf ball.

Orbital roof fractures are dangerous because of potential complications to the brain. Surgical management of these fractures requires a neurosurgeon and an ophthalmologist. The most common indications for surgical intervention are displacement of bone fragments disfiguring the normal facial contours, interference with normal binocular vision caused by extraocular muscle entrapment, interference with mastication in zygomatic fracture, and obstruction of the nasolacrimal duct. Surgery is usually nonemergent, and a period of 10 to 14 days gives the ophthalmologist time to assess ocular function, especially the extraocular muscles and the nasolacrimal duct. Emergency surgical repair is usually not performed unless the globe is displaced to the maxillary sinus. Surgical repair is primarily directed at freeing the entrapped ocular structures and restoring the integrity of the orbital floor.

Foreign Bodies

Foreign bodies that enter the orbit are usually tolerated, except for copper, iron, and vegetable materials, such as those from plants or trees, which may cause purulent infection. X-rays and CT scans are used to identify the foreign body. A careful history is important, especially if the foreign body has been in the orbit for a period of time and the incident forgotten. It is important to identify metallic foreign bodies because they prohibit the use of magnetic resonance imaging (MRI) as a diagnostic tool.

After the extent of the orbital damage is assessed, the decision to use conservative treatment or surgical removal is made. In general, orbital foreign bodies are removed if they are superficial and anterior in location; have sharp edges that may affect adjacent orbital structures; or are composed of copper, iron, or vegetable material. Surgical intervention is directed at preventing further ocular injury and maintaining the integrity of the affected areas. Cultures are usually obtained, and the patient is placed on prophylactic IV antibiotics that are later changed to oral antibiotics.

Ocular Trauma

Ocular trauma is the leading cause of blindness among children and young adults, especially male trauma victims. The most common circumstances of ocular trauma are occupational injuries (e.g., construction industry), sports (e.g., baseball, basketball, racquet sports, boxing), weapons (e.g., air guns, BB guns), assault, motor vehicle crashes (e.g., broken windshields), and explosions (e.g., blast fragments).

There are two types of ocular trauma in which the first response is critical: chemical burn and foreign object in the eye. With a chemical burn, the eye should be immediately irrigated with tap water or normal saline. With a foreign body, no attempt should be made to remove the foreign object. The object should be protected from jarring or movement to prevent further ocular damage. No pressure or patch should be applied to the affected eye. All traumatic eye injuries should be protected using a metal shield, if available, or a stiff paper cup until medical treatment can be obtained (Fig. 49-9).

A **B**

FIGURE 49-9 Two kinds of eye patches. **A.** Aluminum shield. **B.** Stiff paper cup shield (creative substitute when aluminum shield is unavailable).

Clinical Manifestations and Assessment

The nurse obtains a thorough history, particularly assessing the patient's ocular history, such as preinjury vision in the affected eye or past ocular surgery. Details related to the injury that help in the diagnosis and assessment of need for further tests include the nature of the ocular injury (i.e., blunt or penetrating trauma); the type of activity that caused the injury to determine the nature of the force striking the eye; and whether onset of vision loss was sudden, slow, or progressive. For chemical eye burns, the chemical agent must be identified and tested for pH if the agent is available. The nurse examines the corneal surface for foreign bodies, wounds, and abrasions and then the other external structures of the eye. Pupillary size, shape, and light reaction of the pupil of the affected eye are compared with the other eye. The nurse assesses ocular motility (ability of the eyes to move synchronously up, down, right, and left).

Medical Management

Splash Injuries

Splash injuries are irrigated with normal saline solution before further evaluation occurs. In cases of a ruptured globe, cycloplegic agents (agents that paralyze the ciliary muscle) or topical antibiotics must be deferred because of potential toxicity to exposed intraocular tissues. Further manipulation of the eye must be avoided until the patient is under general anesthesia. Parenteral, broad-spectrum antibiotics are initiated. Tetanus antitoxin is administered, if indicated, as well as analgesics. Tetanus prophylaxis is recommended for full-thickness ocular and skin wounds.

Foreign Bodies and Corneal Abrasions

After removal of a foreign body from the surface of the eye, an antibiotic ointment is applied and the eye is patched. The eye is examined daily for evidence of infection until the wound is completely healed.

Contact lens wear is a common cause of corneal abrasion. The patient experiences severe pain and **photophobia** (ocular pain on exposure to light). Corneal epithelial defects are treated with antibiotic ointment and a pressure patch to immobilize the eyelids. Topical anesthetic eye drops must not be given to the patient to take home for repeated use after corneal injury because their effects mask further damage, delay healing, and can lead to permanent corneal scarring. Corticosteroids are avoided while the epithelial defect exists.

Penetrating Injuries and Contusions of the Eyeball

Sharp penetrating injury or blunt contusion force can rupture the eyeball. When the eye wall, cornea, and sclera rupture, rapid decompression or herniation of the orbital contents into adjacent sinuses can occur. In general, blunt traumatic injuries (with an increased incidence of retinal detachment, intraocular tissue avulsion, and herniation) have a worse prognosis than penetrating injuries. Most penetrating injuries result in marked loss of vision with the following signs: hemorrhagic **chemosis** (edema of the conjunctiva), conjunctival laceration, shallow anterior chamber with or without an eccentrically placed pupil, hyphema (hemorrhage within the anterior chamber), or vitreous hemorrhage.

Hyphema is caused by contusion forces that tear the vessels of the iris and damage the anterior chamber angle. Preventing rebleeding and prolonged increased IOP are the goals of treatment for hyphema. In severe cases, the patient is hospitalized with moderate activity restriction. An eye shield is applied. Topical corticosteroids are prescribed to reduce inflammation. An antifibrinolytic agent, aminocaproic acid (Amicar), stabilizes clot formation at the site of hemorrhage. Aspirin is contraindicated.

A ruptured globe and severe injuries with intraocular hemorrhage require surgical intervention. Vitrectomy, surgical removal of vitreous fluid and stabilization of the retina, is performed for traumatic retinal detachments. Primary **enucleation** (complete removal of the eyeball and part of the optic nerve) is considered only if the globe is irreparable and has NLP. It is a general rule that enucleation is performed within 2 weeks of the initial injury (in an eye that has no useful vision after sustaining penetrating injury) to prevent the risk of **sympathetic ophthalmia** (an inflammation created in the uninjured eye by the affected eye that can result in blindness of the uninjured eye).

Intraocular Foreign Bodies

A patient who complains of blurred vision and discomfort should be questioned carefully about recent injuries and exposures. Patients may be injured in a number of different situations and experience an intraocular foreign body (IOFB). Precipitating circumstances can include working in construction; striking metal against metal; being involved in a motor vehicle crash with facial injury; a gunshot wound; grinding-wheel work; and an explosion.

IOFB is diagnosed and localized by slit-lamp biomicroscopy and indirect ophthalmoscopy, as well as CT or ultrasonography. MRI is contraindicated because most foreign bodies are metallic and magnetic. It is important to determine the composition, size, and location of the IOFB and affected eye structures. Every effort should be made to identify the type of IOFB and whether it is magnetic. Iron, steel, copper, and vegetable matter cause intense inflammatory reactions. The incidence of endophthalmitis is also high. If the cornea is perforated, tetanus prophylaxis and IV antibiotics are administered.

Ocular Burns

Alkali, acid, and other chemically active organic substances, such as Mace and tear gas, cause chemical burns. Alkali burns (e.g., lye, ammonia) result in the most severe injury because they penetrate the ocular tissues rapidly and continue to cause damage long after the initial injury is sustained. They also cause an immediate rise in IOP. Acids (e.g., toilet bowl cleaners, bleach, car battery fluid, refrigerant) generally cause less damage because the precipitated necrotic tissue proteins form a barrier to further penetration and damage. Chemical burns may appear as superficial punctate keratopathy (i.e., spotty damage to the cornea), subconjunctival hemorrhage, or complete marbleizing of the cornea.

In treating chemical burns, every minute counts. Immediate tap-water irrigation should be started on site before transport of the patient to an emergency department. In the Emergency Department, only a brief history and examination are performed, then the corneal surfaces and conjunctival fornices are immediately and copiously irrigated with normal saline or any neutral solution. A local anesthetic is instilled, and a lid speculum is applied to overcome blepharospasm (i.e., spasms of the eyelid muscles that result in closure of the lids). Particulate matter must be removed from the fornices using moistened, cotton-tipped applicators and minimal pressure on the globe. Irrigation continues until the conjunctival pH normalizes (between 7.3 and 7.6). The pH of the corneal surface is checked by placing a pH paper strip in the fornix. Antibiotics are instilled, and the eye is patched.

The goal of intermediate treatment is to prevent tissue ulceration and promote re-epithelialization. Intense lubrication using nonpreserved (i.e., without preservatives to avoid allergic reactions) artificial tears is essential. Re-epithelialization is promoted with patching or therapeutic soft lenses. The patient is usually monitored daily for several days. Prognosis depends on the type of injury and adequacy of the irrigation immediately after exposure. Long-term treatment consists of two phases: restoration of the ocular surface through grafting procedures and surgical restoration of corneal integrity and optical clarity.

Thermal injury is caused by exposure to a hot object (e.g., curling iron, tobacco, ash), whereas photochemical injury results from ultraviolet irradiation or infrared exposure (e.g., exposure to the reflections from snow, sun gazing, viewing an eclipse of the sun without an adequate filter). These injuries can cause corneal epithelial defect, corneal opacity, conjunctival chemosis (edema) and **injection** (congestion of blood vessels), and burns of the eyelids and periocular region. Antibiotics and a pressure patch for 24 hours constitute the treatment of mild injuries. Scarring of the eyelids may require oculoplastic surgery, whereas corneal scarring may require corneal surgery.

INFECTIOUS AND INFLAMMATORY CONDITIONS

Inflammation and infections of eye structures are common. Eye infection is a leading cause of blindness worldwide. Table 49-3 summarizes selected common infections and their treatment. Conjunctivitis and orbital cellulitis are discussed below.

CONJUNCTIVITIS

Conjunctivitis (inflammation of the conjunctiva) is the most common ocular disease worldwide. Its appearance varies from a mildly pink appearance of the conjunctiva (hence the common term *pink eye*) because of subconjunctival blood vessel congestion to copious purulent drainage.

Clinical Manifestations and Assessment

Conjunctivitis may be unilateral or bilateral, but the infection usually starts in one eye and then spreads to the other eye by hand contact.

Clinical features important to evaluate are the type of discharge (watery, mucoid, purulent, or mucopurulent), presence or absence of lymphadenopathy (enlargement of the preauricular and submandibular lymph nodes where the eyelids drain), important symptoms such as a foreign-body sensation, irritation, a scratching or burning sensation, a sensation of fullness around the eyes, crusting of the eyelids, itching, visual blurring, and photophobia (Tu, 2015). Common organisms isolated are *Streptococcus pneumoniae*, *Haemophilus influenzae*, and *Staphylococcus aureus*. Two sexually transmitted agents associated with conjunctivitis are *Chlamydia trachomatis* and *Neisseria gonorrhoeae*. Diagnosis is based on the distinctive characteristics of ocular signs, acute or chronic presentation, and identification of any precipitating events. Positive results of swab smear preparations and cultures confirm the diagnosis.

Types of Conjunctivitis

Conjunctivitis is classified according to its cause. The major causes are microbial infection, allergy, and irritating toxic stimuli. A wide spectrum of organisms can cause conjunctivitis, including bacteria (e.g., *Chlamydia*), viruses, fungi and parasites. Conjunctivitis can also result from an existing ocular infection or can be a manifestation of a systemic disease.

Microbial Conjunctivitis

Bacterial Conjunctivitis
Bacterial conjunctivitis can be acute or chronic. The acute type can develop into a chronic condition. Signs and symptoms can vary from mild to severe. Chronic bacterial conjunctivitis is usually seen in patients with lacrimal duct obstruction, chronic dacryocystitis (infection of the nasolacrimal sac), and chronic blepharitis (eyelid inflammation). The most common causative microorganisms are *S. pneumoniae, H. influenzae,* and *S. aureus.*

Bacterial conjunctivitis manifests with an acute onset of redness, burning, and discharge. There is conjunctival irritation, and injection in the fornices. The exudates are variable

TABLE **49-3** Common Infections and Inflammatory Disorders of Eye Structures

Disorder	Description	Management
Hordeolum (stye)	Acute suppurative infection of the glands of the eyelids caused by *Staphylococcus aureus*. The lid is red and edematous, with a small collection of pus in the form of an abscess. There is considerable discomfort.	Warm compresses are applied directly to the affected lid area three to four times a day for 10–15 minutes. If the condition is not improved after 48 hours, incision and drainage may be indicated. Application of topical antibiotics may be prescribed thereafter.
Chalazion	Sterile inflammatory process involving chronic granulomatous inflammation of the meibomian glands; can appear as a single granuloma or multiple granulomas in the upper or lower eyelids.	Warm compresses applied three to four times a day for 10–15 minutes may resolve the inflammation in the early stages. Most often, however, surgical excision is indicated. Corticosteroid injection to the chalazion lesion may be used for smaller lesions.
Blepharitis	Chronic bilateral inflammation of the eyelid margins. There are two types: staphylococcal and seborrheic. Staphylococcal blepharitis is usually ulcerative and is more serious due to the involvement of the base of hair follicles. Permanent scarring can result.	The seborrheic type is chronic and is usually resistant to treatment, but the milder cases may respond to lid hygiene. Staphylococcal blepharitis requires topical antibiotic treatment. Instructions on lid hygiene (to keep the lid margins clean and free of exudates) are given to the patient.
Bacterial keratitis	Infection of the cornea by *S. aureus*, *Streptococcus pneumoniae*, and *Pseudomonas aeruginosa*	Fortified (high-concentration) antibiotic eyedrops are administered every 60 minutes around the clock for the first 24–48 hours. When a positive response to treatment is demonstrated, antibiotics may be tapered down to every 2–3 hours for 2 weeks. Systemic antibiotics may be administered to fortify topical antibiotics. Cycloplegics are administered to reduce pain caused by ciliary spasm. Corticosteroid therapy and subconjunctival injections of antibiotics are controversial.
Herpes simplex keratitis	Leading cause of corneal blindness in the United States. Symptoms are severe pain, tearing, and photophobia. The dendritic ulcer has a branching, linear pattern with feathery edges and terminal bulbs at its ends. Herpes simplex keratitis can lead to recurrent stromal keratitis and persist to 12 months, with residual corneal scarring.	Many lesions heal without treatment and residual effects. The treatment goal is to minimize the damaging effect of the inflammatory response and eliminate viral replication within the cornea. Penetrating keratoplasty is indicated for corneal scarring and must be performed when the herpetic disease has been inactive for many months.

but are usually present on waking in the morning. The eyes may be difficult to open because of adhesions caused by the exudate. Purulent discharge occurs in severe acute bacterial infections, whereas mucopurulent discharge appears in mild cases. In gonococcal conjunctivitis, the symptoms are more acute and may present with profuse and purulent exudate, lymphadenopathy, and pseudomembranes.

Chlamydial conjunctivitis includes **trachoma** (a bilateral chronic follicular conjunctivitis of childhood that leads to blindness during adulthood if left untreated) and inclusion conjunctivitis. Trachoma is prevalent in areas with hot, dry, and dusty climates, and in areas with poor living conditions. It is spread by direct contact or fomites, and the vectors can be insects such as flies and gnats. Symptoms include red, inflamed eyes, tearing, photophobia, ocular pain, purulent exudates, preauricular lymphadenopathy (anterior to the auricle of the ear), and lid edema. At the middle stage of the disease, an acute inflammation occurs, after which trichiasis

(turning inward of hair follicles) and entropion begin to develop, causing corneal erosion and ulceration. The late stage of the disease is characterized by scarred conjunctiva, subepithelial keratitis (inflammation of the cornea), abnormal vascularization of the cornea (pannus), and residual scars from the follicles. Severe corneal ulceration can lead to perforation and blindness.

Inclusion conjunctivitis affects sexually active people who have genital chlamydial infection. Transmission is by oral–genital sex or hand-to-eye transmission. Indirect transmission can occur in inadequately chlorinated swimming pools. The eye lesions usually appear a week after exposure and may be associated with a nonspecific urethritis or cervicitis.

Viral Conjunctivitis

Viral conjunctivitis can be acute and chronic. The discharge is watery, and follicles are prominent. Severe cases include

FIGURE 49-10 Conjunctival hyperemia in viral conjunctivitis.

pseudomembranes. Pseudomembranes appear as tissue that covers the conjunctiva or sclera but are actually composed of mucus, fibrin, bacteria, or immune system cells. The common causative organisms are adenovirus and herpes simplex virus. Conjunctivitis caused by adenovirus is highly contagious. The condition is usually preceded by symptoms of upper respiratory infection. Corneal involvement causes extreme photophobia. Symptoms include extreme tearing, redness, and foreign-body sensation that can involve one or both eyes. There is lid edema, ptosis, and conjunctival **hyperemia** (dilation of the conjunctival blood vessels) (Fig. 49-10). These signs and symptoms vary from mild to severe and may last for 2 weeks. Viral conjunctivitis, although self-limited, tends to last longer than bacterial conjunctivitis.

 Nursing Alert
The clinical term for hyperemia of the conjunctiva is known as "injected."

Epidemic keratoconjunctivitis (EKC) is a highly contagious viral conjunctivitis that is easily transmitted from one person to another among household members, school children, and health care workers. The outbreak of epidemics is seasonal, especially during the summer, when people use swimming pools. EKC is most often accompanied by preauricular lymphadenopathy and occasionally periorbital pain. EKC can lead to keratopathy (corneal disease).

Allergic Conjunctivitis

Immunologic or allergic conjunctivitis is a hypersensitivity reaction that occurs as part of allergic rhinitis (hay fever), or it can be an independent allergic reaction. Patients often present with a history of atopy, a genetic predisposition toward hypersensitivity reactions. Atopic conditions include allergies (e.g., food and seasonal), asthma, and atopic dermatitis (e.g., eczema). Allergic conjunctivitis is characterized by extreme pruritus, epiphora (i.e., excessive secretion of tears),

injection, and usually severe photophobia. A string-like mucoid discharge is usually associated with rubbing the eyes because of severe pruritus. Vernal conjunctivitis is also known as *seasonal conjunctivitis* because it appears mostly during warm weather.

Toxic Conjunctivitis

Chemical conjunctivitis can be the result of medications; chlorine from swimming pools; exposure to toxic fumes among industrial workers; or exposure to other irritants, such as smoke, hair sprays, acids, and alkalis.

Medical and Nursing Management

The management of conjunctivitis depends on the type (Table 49-4). Most types of mild and viral conjunctivitis are self-limiting, benign conditions that may not require treatment. Box 49-9 includes patient teaching information about viral conjunctivitis. For more severe cases, topical antibiotics, eye drops, or ointments are prescribed. Patients with gonococcal conjunctivitis require urgent antibiotic therapy. If left untreated, this ocular disease can lead to corneal perforation and blindness. The systemic complications can include meningitis and generalized septicemia.

ORBITAL CELLULITIS

Orbital cellulitis is inflammation of the tissues surrounding the eye.

Pathophysiology

Orbital cellulitis may result from bacterial, fungal, or viral inflammatory conditions of contiguous structures, such as the face, oropharynx, dental structures, or intracranial structures. It can also result from foreign bodies and from a pre-existing ocular infection or from generalized septicemia. Infection of the sinuses is the most frequent cause. Infection originating in the sinuses can spread easily to the orbit through the thin bony walls and foramina or by means of the interconnecting venous system of the orbit and sinuses. The most common causative organisms are staphylococci and streptococci in adults and *H. influenzae* in children.

Clinical Manifestations and Assessment

The symptoms include pain, lid swelling, conjunctival edema, **proptosis**, and decreased ocular motility. With such edema, optic nerve compression can occur and IOP may increase.

The severe intraorbital tension caused by abscess formation and the impairment of optic nerve function in orbital cellulitis can result in permanent visual loss. Because of the orbit's proximity to the brain, orbital cellulitis can lead to life-threatening complications, such as intracranial abscess and cavernous sinus thrombosis.

TABLE **49-4** Management of Conjunctivitis

Conjunctivitis	Management
Bacterial Conjunctivitis	Acute bacterial conjunctivitis is almost always self-limiting, lasting 2 weeks if left untreated. If treated with antibiotics, it may last a few days, except for gonococcal conjunctivitis. Gonococcal conjunctivitis ceases within hours of topical antibiotic therapy and may be discontinued 24 hours after treatment. For trachoma, usually broad-spectrum antibiotics are administered topically and systemically. Surgical management includes the correction of trichiasis (eyelashes growing inward toward the conjunctiva and cornea) to prevent conjunctival scarring. Adult inclusion conjunctivitis requires 1 week of antibiotics. Prevention of reinfection is important, and affected individuals and their sexual partners must seek treatment for sexually transmitted disease, if indicated.
Viral Conjunctivitis	Viral conjunctivitis is not responsive to any treatment. Cold compresses may alleviate some symptoms. It is extremely important to remember that viral conjunctivitis, especially epidemic keratoconjunctivitis, is highly contagious. Patient instructions should include an emphasis on hand hygiene and avoiding sharing of hand towels, face cloths, and eye drops. Tissues should be directly discarded into a covered trash can. All forms of tonometry must be avoided unless medically indicated. All multidose medications must be discarded at the end of each day or when contaminated. Infected employees and others must not be allowed to work or attend school until symptoms have resolved, which can take 3–7 days.
Allergic Conjunctivitis	Patients with allergic conjunctivitis, especially recurrent vernal or seasonal conjunctivitis, are usually given corticosteroids in ophthalmic preparations. Depending on the severity of the disease, they may be given oral preparations. Use of vasoconstrictors, such as topical epinephrine solution, cold compresses, ice packs, and cool ventilation usually provide comfort by decreasing swelling.
Toxic Conjunctivitis	For conjunctivitis caused by chemical irritants, the eye must be irrigated immediately and profusely with saline or sterile water.

Medical and Nursing Management

Immediate administration of high-dose, broad-spectrum, systemic antibiotics is indicated. Cultures and Gram-stained smears are obtained. Monitoring changes in visual acuity, degree of proptosis, central nervous system function (e.g., nausea, vomiting, fever, cognitive changes), displacement of the globe, extraocular movements, pupillary signs, and the fundus is extremely important. Consultation with an

---

BOX 49-9 **Patient Education**

Instructions for Patients with Viral Conjunctivitis

Viral conjunctivitis is a highly contagious eye infection. It can easily spread from one person to another. The symptoms can be alarming, but they are not serious. The following information will help you understand this eye condition and how to take care of yourself and/or your family member at home.

- Your eyes will look red and will have watery discharge, and your lids will be swollen for about a week.
- You will experience eye pain, a sandy sensation in your eye, and sensitivity to light.
- Symptoms will resolve after about 1 week.
- You may use light, cold compresses over your eyes for about 10 minutes four to five times a day to soothe the pain.
- You may use artificial tears for the sandy sensation in your eye, and mild pain medications, such as acetaminophen (Tylenol).
- You need to stay at home. Children must not play outside. You may return to work or school after 7 days, when the redness and discharge have cleared. You may obtain a doctor's note to return to work or school.
- Do not share towels, linens, makeup, or toys.
- Wash your hands thoroughly and frequently, using soap and water, including before and after you apply artificial tears or cold compresses.
- Use a new tissue every time you wipe the discharge from each eye. You may dampen the tissue with clean water to clean the outside of the eye.
- You may wash your face and take a shower as you normally do.
- Discard all of your makeup articles. You must not apply makeup until the disease is over.
- You may wear dark glasses if bright lights bother you.
- If the discharge from your eye turns yellowish and pus-like, or you experience changes in your vision, you need to return to the health care provider for an examination.

otolaryngologist is necessary, especially when sinusitis is suspected. In the event of abscess formation or progressive loss of vision, surgical drainage of the abscess or sinus is performed. Sinusotomy and antibiotic irrigation are also performed.

TREATMENT MODALITIES FOR EYE INJURIES AND DISORDERS

Common treatments discussed in this section include surgery and pharmacologic treatment.

SURGICAL PROCEDURES

Orbital Surgeries

Orbital surgeries may be performed to repair fractures, remove a foreign body, or remove benign or malignant growths. The eyeball is lined with muscle, connective, and adipose tissues and is housed in the bony orbit, which is about 4 cm high, wide, and deep. It is shaped roughly like a four-sided pyramid, surrounded on three sides by the sinuses: ethmoid (medially), frontal (superiorly), and maxillary (inferiorly). Surgical procedures involving the orbit and lids affect facial appearance (cosmesis). The goals are to recover and preserve visual function and to maintain the anatomic relationship of the ocular structures to achieve cosmesis. During the repair of orbital fractures, the orbital bones are realigned to follow the anatomic positions of facial structures.

Orbital surgical procedures involve working around delicate structures of the eye, such as the optic nerve, retinal blood vessels, and ocular muscles. Complications of orbital surgical procedures may include blindness as a result of damage to the optic nerve and its blood supply. Sudden pain and loss of vision may indicate intraorbital hemorrhage or compression of the optic nerve. Ptosis and diplopia may result from trauma to the extraocular muscles during the surgical procedure, but these conditions typically resolve after a few weeks.

Prophylaxis with IV antibiotics is the usual postoperative regimen after orbital surgery, especially with repair of orbital fractures and removal of an intraorbital foreign body. IV corticosteroids are used if there is a concern about optic nerve swelling. Topical ocular antibiotics are typically instilled, and antibiotic ointments are applied externally to the skin suture sites.

For the first 24 to 48 hours postoperatively, ice compresses are applied over the periocular area to decrease periorbital swelling, facial swelling, and hematoma. The head of the patient's bed should be elevated to a comfortable position (30 to 45 degrees).

Discharge teaching should include medication instructions for oral antibiotics, instillation of ophthalmic medications, and application of ocular compresses.

Enucleation

Enucleation is the removal of the entire eye and part of the optic nerve. It may be performed for the following conditions:

- Severe injury resulting in prolapse of uveal tissue (iris, ciliary body, and choroid), or loss of light projection (the ability to identify the direction of the light source) or perception
- An irritated, blind, painful, deformed, or disfigured eye, usually caused by glaucoma, retinal detachment, or chronic inflammation
- An eye without useful vision that is producing or has produced sympathetic ophthalmia (inflammation of the eye or conjunctiva) in the other eye
- Intraocular tumors that are untreatable by other means

The procedure for enucleation involves the separation and cutting of each of the ocular muscles, dissection of the Tenon capsule (fibrous membrane covering the sclera), and cutting of the optic nerve from the eyeball. The insertion of an orbital implant typically follows, and the conjunctiva is closed. A large pressure dressing is applied over the area. Box 49-10 discusses ocular prostheses.

Evisceration

Evisceration involves the surgical removal of the intraocular contents through an incision or opening in the cornea or sclera. Evisceration may be performed to treat severe ocular trauma with ruptured globe, severe ocular inflammation, or severe ocular infection. The optic nerve, sclera, extraocular muscles, and sometimes the cornea are left intact. The main advantage of evisceration over enucleation is that the final cosmetic result and motility after fitting the ocular prosthesis are enhanced. This procedure would be more acceptable to a patient whose body image is severely threatened. The main disadvantage is the high risk of sympathetic ophthalmia.

Exenteration

Exenteration is the removal of the eyelids, the eye, and various amounts of orbital contents. It is indicated in malignancies in the orbit that are life-threatening or when more conservative modalities of treatment have failed or are inappropriate. An example is squamous cell carcinoma of the paranasal sinuses, skin, and conjunctiva with deep orbital involvement. In its most extensive form, exenteration may include the removal of all orbital tissues and resection of the orbital bones.

PHARMACOLOGIC TREATMENT

The main objective of ocular medication delivery is to maximize the amount of medication that reaches the ocular site of action in sufficient concentration to produce a beneficial therapeutic effect. This is determined by the dynamics of

BOX 49-10

Ocular Prostheses

Orbital implants and conformers (ocular prostheses usually made of silicone rubber) maintain the shape of the eye after enucleation or evisceration to prevent a contracted, sunken appearance. The temporary conformer is placed over the conjunctival closure after the implantation of an orbital implant. A conformer is placed after the enucleation or evisceration procedure to protect the suture line, maintain the fornices, prevent contracture of the socket in preparation for the ocular prosthesis, and promote the integrity of the eyelids.

All ocular prosthetics have limitations in their motility. There are two designs of eye prostheses (see figure below). The anophthalmic ocular prostheses are used in the absence of the globe. Scleral shells look just like the anophthalmic prosthesis but are thinner and fit over a globe with intact corneal sensation. An eye prosthesis usually lasts about 6 years, depending on the quality of fit, comfort, and cosmetic appearance. When the anophthalmic socket is completely healed, conformers are replaced with prosthetic eyes.

Eye prostheses. (*Left*) Anophthalmic ocular prosthesis. (*Right*) Scleral shell.

An ocularist is a specially trained and skilled professional who makes prosthetic eyes. After the ophthalmologist is satisfied that the anophthalmic socket is completely healed and is ready for prosthetic fitting, the patient is referred to an ocularist. The healing period is usually 6 to 8 weeks. It is advisable for the patient to have a consultation with the ocularist before the fitting. Obtaining accurate information and verbalizing concerns can lessen anxiety about wearing an ocular prosthesis.

Medical Management

Removal of an eye has physical, social, and psychological ramifications for any person. The significance of loss of the eye and vision must be addressed in the plan of care. The patient's preparation should include information about the surgical procedure and placement of orbital implants and conformers and the availability of ocular prosthetics to enhance cosmetic appearance. In some cases, patients may choose to see an ocularist before the surgery to discuss ocular prosthetics.

Nursing Management

Teaching About Postsurgical Care

Patients who undergo eye removal need to know that they will usually have a large ocular pressure dressing, which is

typically removed after a week, and that an ophthalmic topical antibiotic ointment is applied in the socket three times daily. When surgical eye removal is immediate and unexpected, as in the case of ocular trauma, the nurse's role in providing emotional support is crucial.

After the removal of an eye, there is a loss of depth perception. Patients must be advised to take extra caution in their ambulation and movement to avoid miscalculations that may result in injury. It may take some time to adjust to monocular vision. Patients using conformers must be advised that the prosthetic may accidentally fall out of the socket. If this happens, the conformer must be washed, wiped dry, and placed back in the socket.

Teaching Patients Self-Care

Patients need to be taught how to insert, remove, and care for the prosthetic eye. Proper hand hygiene must be observed before inserting and removing an ocular prosthesis. A suction cup may be used if there are problems with manual dexterity. Precautions, such as draping a towel over the sink and closing the sink drain, must be taken to avoid loss of the prosthesis. When instructing patients or family members, a return demonstration is important to assess the level of understanding and ability to perform the procedure.

Before insertion, the inner punctal or outer lateral aspects and the superior and inferior aspects of the prosthesis must be identified by locating the identifying marks, such as a reddish color in the inner punctal area. For people with low vision, other forms of identifying markers, such as dots or notches, are used. The upper lid is raised high enough to create a space. The patient slides the prosthesis up, underneath, and behind the upper eyelid. Meanwhile, the patient pulls the lower eyelid down to help put the prosthesis in place and to have its inferior edge fall back gradually to the lower eyelid. The lower eyelid is checked for correct positioning.

To remove the prosthesis, the patient cups one hand on the cheek to catch the prosthesis, places the forefinger of the free hand against the midportion of the lower eyelid, and gazes upward. Gazing upward brings the inferior edge of the prosthesis nearer the inferior eyelid margin. With the finger pushing inward, downward, and laterally against the lower eyelid, the prosthesis slides out, and the patient's cupped hand acts as the receptacle.

Continuing Care

An eye prosthesis can be worn and left in place for several months. Hygiene and comfort are usually maintained with daily irrigation of the prosthesis in place with normal saline solution, hard contact lens solution, or artificial tears. In the case of dry eye symptoms, the use of ophthalmic ointment lubricants or oil-based drops, such as vitamin E and mineral oil, can be helpful. Removing crusting and mucous discharge that accumulate overnight is performed with the prosthesis in place. Malposition may occur when wiping or rubbing the prosthesis in the socket. The prosthesis can be repositioned with the use of clean fingers. Proper wiping of the prosthesis should be a gentle temporal-to-nasal motion to avoid malpositions.

ocular pharmacokinetics: absorption, distribution, metabolism, and excretion.

Concepts in Ocular Medication Administration

Topical administration of ocular medications results in only a 1% to 7% absorption rate by the ocular tissues. Ocular absorption involves the entry of a medication into the aqueous humor through the different routes of ocular medication administration. The rate and extent of aqueous humor absorption are determined by the characteristics of the medication and the anatomy and physiology of the eye. Natural barriers of absorption that diminish the efficacy of ocular medications include the following:

- *Limited size of the conjunctival sac.* The conjunctival sac can hold only 50 µL, and any excess is wasted. The volume of one eye drop from commercial topical ocular solutions typically ranges from 20 to 35 µL.
- *Corneal membrane barriers.* The epithelial, stromal, and endothelial layers are barriers to absorption.
- *Blood–ocular barriers.* Blood–ocular barriers prevent high ocular tissue concentration of most ophthalmic medications because they separate the bloodstream from the ocular tissues and keep foreign substances from entering the eye, thereby limiting a medication's efficacy.
- *Tearing, blinking, and drainage.* Increased tear production and drainage due to ocular irritation or an ocular condition may dilute or wash out an instilled eye drop; blinking expels an instilled eye drop from the conjunctival sac.

Distribution of an ocular medication into the various ocular tissues varies by tissue type; the various tissues (e.g., conjunctiva, cornea, lens, iris, ciliary body, choroids) absorb medications to varying degrees. Medications penetrate the corneal epithelium by diffusion by passing through the cells (intracellular) or by passing between the cells (intercellular). Water-soluble (hydrophilic) medications diffuse through the intracellular route, and fat-soluble (lipophilic) medications diffuse through the intercellular route. Topical administration usually does not reach the retina in significant concentrations. Because the space between the ciliary process and the lens is small, medication diffusion in the vitreous is slow. When high concentrations of medication in the vitreous are required, intraocular injection is often chosen to bypass the natural ocular anatomic and physiologic barriers.

Aqueous solutions are most commonly used for the eye. They are the least expensive medications and interfere least with vision. However, corneal contact time is brief because tears dilute the medication. Ophthalmic ointments have extended retention time in the conjunctival sac and provide a higher concentration than eye drops. The major disadvantage of ointments is the blurred vision that results after application. In general, eyelids and eyelid margins are best treated with ointments. Contact lenses and collagen shields soaked in antibiotics are alternative delivery methods for treating corneal infections.

Of all these delivery methods, the topical route of administration—instilled eye drops and applied ointments—remains the most common. Topical instillation, which is the least invasive method, permits self-administration of medication and produces fewer side effects.

Preservatives are commonly used in ocular medications. Benzalkonium chloride, for example, prevents the growth of organisms and enhances the corneal permeability of most medications; however, some patients are allergic to this preservative. This may be suspected even if the patient had never before experienced an allergic reaction to systemic use of the medication in question. Eye drops without preservatives can be prepared by pharmacists.

Commonly Used Ocular Medications

Common ocular medications include topical anesthetic, mydriatic, and cycloplegic agents that reduce IOP; anti-infective medications, corticosteroids, nonsteroidal anti-inflammatory drugs (NSAIDs), antiallergy medications, eye irrigants, and lubricants.

Topical Anesthetics

One or two drops of proparacaine hydrochloride (Ophthaine 0.5%) and tetracaine hydrochloride (Pontocaine 0.5%) are instilled before diagnostic procedures such as tonometry. Topical anesthetics are also used for severe eye pain, to allow the patient to open his or her eyes for examination or treatment. The nurse must instruct the patient not to rub his or her eyes while anesthetized because this may result in corneal damage.

Patients with corneal abrasions and erosions experience severe pain and are often tempted to overuse topical anesthetic eye drops. Overuse of these drops results in softening of the cornea. Prolonged use of anesthetic drops can delay wound healing and can lead to permanent corneal opacification and scarring, resulting in visual loss.

Mydriatics and Cycloplegics

Mydriasis, or pupil dilation, is the main objective of the administration of mydriatic and cycloplegic agents (Table 49-5). These two types of medications function differently and are used in combination to achieve the maximal dilation that is needed during surgery and fundus examinations to give the ophthalmologist a better view of the internal eye structures. **Mydriatics** potentiate alpha-adrenergic sympathetic effects that result in the relaxation of the ciliary muscle leading to dilatation of the pupil. The patient may have difficulty reading. The patient is advised to wear sunglasses (most eye clinics provide protective sunglasses). The ability to drive is dependent on the person's age, vision, and comfort level.

TABLE **49-5** Mydriatics and Miotics

Medication	Forms	Indication/Dosages	Action	Duration	Nursing Considerations
Phenylephrine (Dilate, Neofrin)	Solution (0.12%, 2.5%, 10%)	Instill 1 drop per dose and may repeat in 1 hour for: Mydriasis Posterior synechiae and minor eye irritation	Dilates pupil by contracting dilator muscle. Peaks within 10–60 minutes	3–7 hours	Monitor for systemic effects of hypertension if 10% solution is administered.
Atropine (Isopto Atropine)	Ointment (1%) Solution (0.5%–2%)	Instill 1–2 drops for acute iritis, uveitis, or cycloplegic refraction, three to four times daily	Dilates pupil by anticholinergic action. Peaks within 30 minutes–3 hours	7–10 days	Have antidote available, physostigmine salicylate (IM or IV). Watch patient for signs and symptoms of glaucoma.
Scopolamine hydrobromide (Isopto Hyoscine)	Solution (0.25%)	Instill 1–2 drops for acute iritis, uveitis, or cycloplegic refraction, once to four times daily	Same action as atropine Peaks within 15–45 minutes	3–7 days	Observe patient closely for disorientation or delirium. May be given to patients sensitive to atropine.
Pilocarpine hydrochloride (Isopto Carpine)	Gel (4%) Solution (0.25%–1%)	Apply one ribbon of gel into lower conjunctival sac once daily at bedtime. Instill 1–2 drops of solution for open-angle glaucoma, acute angle-closure glaucoma, or mydriasis caused by mydriatic or cycloplegic drugs	Cholinergic effect of pupil constriction (miosis) and deepening of anterior chamber. Peaks within 30–85 minutes	4–8 hours	Monitor vital signs. Monitor drug administration carefully. If taken by mouth, contact poison control center or take patient to ED immediately.

Nursing Alert

Mydriatic and cycloplegic agents affect the central nervous system. Their effects are most prominent in children and elderly patients; these patients must be assessed closely for symptoms, such as increased blood pressure, tachycardia, dizziness, ataxia, confusion, disorientation, incoherent speech, and hallucination. These medications are contraindicated in patients with narrow angles or shallow anterior chambers, and in patients taking monoamine oxidase inhibitors or tricyclic antidepressants.

Antiglaucoma Medications

Therapeutic medications for glaucoma are used to lower IOP by decreasing aqueous production or increasing aqueous outflow. Because glaucoma calls for lifetime therapy, the patient must be instructed regarding both the ocular and systemic side effects of the medications.

Most antiglaucoma medications affect the **accommodation** of the lens and limit light entry through a constricted pupil. Visual acuity and the ability to focus may be affected. Factors to consider in selecting glaucoma medications are efficacy, systemic and ocular side effects, convenience, and cost.

Anti-Infective Medications

Anti-infective medications include antibiotic, antifungal, and antiviral agents. Most are available as drops, ointments, or subconjunctival or intravitreal injections. Antibiotics include penicillin, cephalosporins, aminoglycosides, and fluoroquinolones. The main antifungal agent is amphotericin B (Abelcet). Side effects of amphotericin are serious, and include severe pain, conjunctival necrosis, iritis, and retinal toxicity. Antiviral medications include acyclovir (Zovirax) and ganciclovir (Cytovene). Patients receiving ocular agents are subject to the same side effects and adverse reactions as those receiving anti-infective oral or parenteral medications.

BOX 49-11

GUIDELINES FOR NURSING CARE

Instilling Eye Medications

Equipment

- Medication(s) as ordered
- Cotton balls or gauze
- Optional: Eye dressing

Implementation

ACTION	RATIONALE
1. Ensure adequate lighting.	1. Adequate lighting ensures the procedure will be carried out using appropriate technique.
2. Perform hand hygiene.	2. Hand hygiene and aseptic technique is important to decrease the risk of contamination of supplies and the spread of further infection.
3. Don clean gloves and, if necessary or required, gently clean any crusts or drainage from the eyelid margins, wiping from the inner to the outer canthus and using a fresh gauze pad or cotton ball moistened with warm water for each stroke.	3. Cleaning the eyes promotes patient comfort and promotes absorption of medications. Additionally, debris is removed from the nasolacrimal duct.
4. Prepare medication. Read the label of the eye medication to make sure it is the correct medication. Shake suspensions or "milky" solutions to obtain the desired medication level. Verify which eye is to be treated.	4. Proper checking of medication and which eye is to be treated is an essential right. Mixing of medication in suspension is required.
5. Assume proper position for instillation of eye medications.	5. Positioning of the patient's head in a supine position or, if sitting, hyperextended in a "sniffing position" allows for proper instillation of ophthalmic medication, particularly drops.
6. Do not touch the tip of the medication container to any part of the eye or face. Hold the lower lid down; do not press on the eyeball. Apply gentle pressure to the cheek bone to anchor the finger holding the lid.	6. Maintaining aseptic technique avoids contamination of materials, such as the medication container. Using the cheek bone as a fulcrum to steady the arm allows for improved medication delivery.

7. Apply medication. Instill eye drops before applying ointments.
 	
For eye drops:
 	
Eye drops should be instilled at a distance of approximately 1 in from the eye. Before instilling the eyedrops, instruct the patient to look up and away. The lower lid is gently pulled down to instill the drops in the conjunctival sac. Immediately after instilling eye drops, apply gentle pressure on the inner canthus (punctal occlusion) near the bridge of the nose for 3–5 minutes.
 	
Using a clean tissue, gently pat the skin to absorb excess eyedrops that run onto the patient's cheeks.
 	
For eye ointment:
 	
Apply a ½-in ribbon of ointment to the lower conjunctival sac. Immediately after ointment instillation, ask the patient to roll his or her eyes behind closed lids.
	7. Medication is administered into the conjunctival sac, rather than on the eyeball, which can cause discomfort.
	
	   Gentle pressure on the inner canthus (punctal occlusion) is done to decrease the risk of systemic absorption of the medication.
	
	   Rolling the eye helps to distribute the medication over the surface of the eyeball.

8. Wait 5 minutes before instilling another eye medication.	8. Allow for absorption of one medication to occur prior to applying another one.
9. Perform hand hygiene.	9. Hand hygiene prevents further contamination post instillation.

Corticosteroids and Nonsteroidal Anti-Inflammatory Drugs

The topical preparations of corticosteroids are commonly used in inflammatory conditions of the eyelids, conjunctiva, cornea, anterior chamber, lens, and uvea. Because these topical eye drops are suspensions, the patient is instructed to shake the bottle several times to promote mixture of the medication and maximize its therapeutic effect. The most common ocular side effects of long-term topical corticosteroid administration are glaucoma, cataracts, susceptibility to infection, impaired wound healing, mydriasis, ptosis, and high IOP. To avoid the side effects of corticosteroids, NSAIDs are used as an alternative in controlling inflammatory eye conditions and postoperatively to reduce inflammation.

Antiallergy Medications

Ocular hypersensitivity reactions are extremely common and result primarily from responses to environmental allergens. Most allergens are airborne or carried to the eye by the hand or by other means, although allergic reactions may also be drug-induced. Corticosteroids are commonly used as anti-inflammatory and immunosuppressive agents to control ocular hypersensitivity reactions.

Ocular Irrigants and Lubricants

Irrigating solutions are used to cleanse the external lids to maintain lid hygiene, to irrigate the external corneal surface to regain normal pH (e.g., in chemical burns), to irrigate the corneal surface to eliminate debris, or to inflate the globe intraoperatively. These solutions have various compositions (sodium, potassium, magnesium, calcium, bicarbonate, glucose, and glutathione) that are safe to use with an intact corneal surface; however, the corneal surface should not be irrigated in cases of threatened corneal perforation.

Sterile irrigating solutions, such as Dacriose, for lid hygiene are available. For patients with severe corneal ulcer, specific orders must be obtained regarding whether it is safe to irrigate the corneal surface or just to cleanse the external lids. Although it is good practice to promote hygiene, prevention of complications must be the primary concern.

Lubricants, such as artificial tears, help alleviate corneal irritation, such as dry eye syndrome. Artificial tears are topical preparations of methyl or hydroxypropyl cellulose that are prepared as eye drop solutions, ointments, or ocular inserts (inserted at the lower conjunctival cul-de-sac once each day).

Nursing Management

The objectives in administering ocular medications are to ensure proper administration to maximize the therapeutic effects and to ensure the safety of the patient by monitoring for systemic and local side effects. Absorption of eye drops by the nasolacrimal duct is undesirable because of the potential systemic side effects of ocular medications. To diminish systemic absorption and minimize the side effects, it is important to occlude the puncta (Box 49-11).

Before the administration of ocular medications, the nurse warns the patient that blurred vision, stinging, and a burning sensation are symptoms that ordinarily occur after instillation and are temporary. Risk for interactions of the ocular medication with other ocular and systemic medications must be emphasized; therefore, a careful patient interview regarding the medications being taken must be obtained.

Emphasis must be placed on hand hygiene techniques before and after medication instillation. The tip of the eye drop bottle or the ointment tube must never touch any part of the patient's eye. The medication must be recapped immediately after each use. The patient or the caregiver at home should be asked to demonstrate actual eye drop or ointment instillation and punctal occlusion.

CHAPTER REVIEW

Critical Thinking Exercises

1. You are employed in an eye clinic in which the majority of patients are elderly, and the majority of medications that are prescribed for these patients are topical agents. Develop an evidence-based teaching plan for patients and caregivers that provides instructions in the proper administration of ocular drops and ointments. What evidence supports the medication administration techniques and associated safety precautions that you have included in the teaching plan? What evidence supports the principles of learning that you considered regarding the elderly population that the clinic serves? What is the strength of the evidence? What criteria would you use to determine the strength of the evidence?

2. In the emergency department, you are caring for a man who has been involved in a motor vehicle crash in which there was a broken windshield. He states that he has a headache and a stiff neck, that his vision is "blurry," and that he has a "scratching pain" in his right eye. He requests a cold compress for his eyes. How would you respond to this patient's request? What diagnostic tests do you anticipate would be used to determine the cause for the patient's symptoms of blurred vision and pain in the eye? What information would you communicate to the health care provider?

NCLEX-Style Review Questions

1. When the nurse is gathering a history from a patient newly diagnosed with glaucoma, the patient reports the following statement to the nurse. Which statement would be consistent with the patient's diagnosis?
   a. "I began seeing halos around lights and had dim vision."
   b. "I had a difficult time matching my blue socks."
   c. "My eyes began to tear and itch."
   d. "I could see the street signs better than my hand."

2. Which statement by the patient diagnosed with viral conjunctivitis indicates that more teaching is necessary?
   a. "I will wash my hands frequently."
   b. "I will use a washcloth to clean both my eyes, starting with the infected eye and moving to the uninfected eye."
   c. "I will avoid contact with other people until my symptoms are gone."
   d. "I will discard any leftover eye medication when the infection is gone."

3. The nurse is caring for a baseball player who reports getting hit in the head with a baseball 1 hour prior to admission in the ED. What assessment requires immediate reporting?
   a. Eye pain
   b. Flashing lights in the visual field
   c. Headache, pain intensity rated as 2/10
   d. Superficial head abrasion

4. The patient with significant visual impairment requires assistance with ADLs. The nurse provides support when serving food by performing which action?
   a. Leaving the tray on the patient's bedside table
   b. Serving hot food as quickly as possible
   c. Describing the food on the tray in terms of the face of a clock
   d. Ensuring all food is soft

5. A patient, who is seen in the vision clinic, has been diagnosed with glaucoma. What initial topical medication would the nurse expect to be included in the treatment plan for this patient?
   a. Mydriatic
   b. Antifungal
   c. Beta blocker
   d. Miotic

Try these additional resources, available at **http://thepoint.lww.com/Honan2e**, to enhance your learning and understanding of this chapter:
- NCLEX-Style Student Review Questions
- Journal Articles

REFERENCES AND SELECTED READINGS

References and selected readings associated with this chapter can be found on the website that accompanies the book. Visit **http://thepoint. lww.com/Honan2e** to access the references and other additional resources associated with this chapter.

Nursing Management: Patients with Hearing and Balance Disorders

Carolynn Spera Bruno

Learning Objectives

After reading this chapter, you will be able to:

1. List the manifestations that may be exhibited by a person with a hearing disorder.
2. Identify ways to communicate effectively with a person with a hearing disorder.
3. Differentiate problems of the external ear from those of the middle ear and inner ear.
4. Compare the various types of surgical procedures used for managing middle ear disorders and appropriate nursing care.
5. Describe the different types of inner ear disorders, including the clinical manifestations, diagnosis, and management.

The delicate structure and function of the ear make early detection and accurate diagnosis of disorders necessary for preservation of normal hearing and balance. Medical surgical nurses will care for patients with hearing loss because of a wide variety of reasons. This chapter addresses the assessment and management of hearing and balance disorders common to the adult population.

HEARING LOSS

More than 36 million people in the United States report some form of hearing loss. *Healthy People 2010* initiated a goal to promote the hearing health of the nation through prevention, early detection, treatment, and rehabilitation.

Pathophysiology

Hearing loss may be the result of a conduction problem, a sensorineural loss, mixed, or of a psychogenic issue. Conductive hearing loss usually results from an external ear disorder, such as impacted cerumen, or a middle ear disorder, such as **otitis media** or otosclerosis. In such instances, the efficient transmission of sound by air to the inner ear is interrupted. A sensorineural loss involves damage to the cochlea or vestibulocochlear nerve. Patients with mixed hearing loss have conductive loss and sensorineural loss, resulting from dysfunction of air and bone conduction. A functional (or

psychogenic) hearing loss is nonorganic and unrelated to detectable structural changes in the hearing mechanisms; it is usually a manifestation of an emotional disturbance.

Many environmental factors have an adverse effect on the auditory system and gradually result in permanent **sensorineural hearing loss**. The most common is noise (unwanted and unavoidable sound), which has been identified as one of today's environmental hazards. The volume of noise that surrounds us daily has increased into a potentially dangerous source of physical and psychological damage.

Risk Factors

About 5% of the world population suffers from disabling hearing loss with prevalence increasing with every age decade, and it is higher in men than in women across all age decades (Baloh & Jen, 2016). Box 50-1 summarizes risk factors.

The National Institutes of Deafness and Other Communication Disorders (NIDCD) estimates that approximately 15% (26 million) of Americans between 20 and 69 years of age have high-frequency hearing loss due to exposure to loud sounds or noise at work or in leisure activities. *Noise-induced hearing loss* (NIHL) refers to hearing loss that follows a long period of exposure to loud noise (e.g., heavy machinery, engines, artillery). Occupations such as carpentry, plumbing, and coal mining have the highest risk of noise-induced hearing loss. Recreational activities, such

Risk Factors for Hearing Loss

- Family history of sensorineural impairment
- Congenital malformations of the cranial structure (ear)
- Low birth weight (less than 1,500 g)
- Use of ototoxic medications (e.g., gentamicin, loop diuretics)
- Recurrent ear infections
- Bacterial meningitis
- Chronic exposure to loud noises
- Chronic exposure to loud volume using headphones or earbuds
- Perforation of the tympanic membrane

as listening to loud sounds through earbuds or headphones or exposure to loud concerts, as well as exposure to leaf blowers or lawnmowers can place people at risk for NIHL.

Acoustic trauma refers to hearing loss caused by a single exposure to an extremely intense noise, such as an explosion. Usually, noise-induced hearing loss occurs at a high frequency (about 4,000 Hz). However, with continued noise exposure, the hearing loss can become more severe and include adjacent frequencies. The minimum noise level known to cause NIHL, regardless of duration, is about 85 to 90 dB.

Noise exposure is inherent in many jobs (e.g., mechanics, printers, pilots, musicians) and in hobbies, such as woodworking and hunting. The Occupational Safety and Health Administration requires that workers wear ear protection to prevent noise-induced hearing loss when exposed to noise above the legal limits. Ear protection against noise is the most effective preventive measure available. There are no medications that protect against NIHL; hearing loss is permanent because the hair cells in the organ of Corti are destroyed.

Clinical Manifestations and Assessment

Early manifestations of hearing impairment and loss may include **tinnitus**, increasing inability to hear when in a group, and a need to turn up the volume of the television. Hearing impairment can also trigger changes in attitude, the ability to communicate, the awareness of surroundings, and even the ability to protect oneself, affecting a person's quality of life. In a classroom, a student with impaired hearing may be uninterested, inattentive, and have failing grades. A person at home may feel isolated because of an inability to hear the clock chime, the refrigerator hum, the birds sing, or the traffic pass. A pedestrian who is hearing-impaired may attempt to cross the street and fail to hear an approaching car. People with impaired hearing may miss parts of a conversation. Many people are unaware of their gradual hearing impairment. Often, it is not the person with the hearing loss but the people with whom he or she is communicating who recognize the impairment first (Box 50-2).

For various reasons, some people with hearing loss refuse to seek medical attention or wear a hearing aid. Others feel self-conscious wearing a hearing aid. Insightful people generally ask those with whom they are trying to communicate to let them know whether difficulties in communication exist. These attitudes and behaviors should be taken into account when counseling patients who need hearing assistance. The decision to wear a hearing aid is a personal one that is affected by these attitudes and behaviors.

Focused Assessment

Hearing Loss

Be on the alert for the following signs and symptoms:

- *Speech deterioration:* The person who slurs words or drops word endings, or produces flat-sounding speech, may not be hearing correctly. The ears guide the voice, both in loudness and in pronunciation.
- *Fatigue:* If a person tires easily when listening to conversation or to a speech, fatigue may be the result of straining to hear. Under these circumstances, the person may become irritable very easily.
- *Indifference:* It is easy for the person who cannot hear what others say to become depressed and disinterested in life in general.
- *Social withdrawal:* Not being able to hear what is going on causes a person who is hearing-impaired to withdraw from situations that might prove embarrassing.
- *Insecurity:* Lack of self-confidence and fear of mistakes create a feeling of insecurity in many people who are hearing-impaired. No one likes to say the wrong thing or do anything that might appear foolish.
- *Indecision and procrastination:* Loss of self-confidence makes it increasingly difficult for a person who is hearing-impaired to make decisions.
- *Suspiciousness:* The person who is hearing-impaired, who often hears only part of what is being said, may suspect that others are talking about him or her or that portions of the conversation are deliberately spoken softly so that he or she will not hear them.
- *False pride:* The person who is hearing-impaired wants to conceal the hearing loss and thus often pretends to be hearing when he or she actually is not.
- *Loneliness and unhappiness:* Although everyone wishes for quiet now and then, *enforced* silence can be boring and even somewhat frightening. People with a hearing loss often feel isolated.
- *Tendency to dominate the conversation:* Many people who are hearing-impaired tend to dominate the conversation, knowing that as long as it is centered on them and they can control it, they are not so likely to be embarrassed by some mistake.

Gerontologic Considerations

With aging, changes occur in the ear that may eventually lead to hearing deficits. Although few changes occur in the external ear, cerumen tends to become harder and drier, posing a greater chance of impaction. In the middle ear, the tympanic membrane may atrophy or become sclerotic. In the inner ear, cells at the base of the cochlea degenerate. A familial predisposition to sensorineural hearing loss is also seen, manifested by inability to hear high-frequency sounds, followed in time by the loss of middle and lower frequencies. The term **presbycusis** is used to describe this progressive hearing loss.

In addition to age-related changes, other factors can affect hearing in older adults, such as lifelong exposure to loud noises (e.g., jets, guns, heavy machinery, circular saws). Certain medications, such as aminoglycosides and aspirin, have ototoxic effects when kidney changes (e.g., in the older person) result in delayed medication excretion and increased levels of the medications in the blood. Although the use of quinine for treatment of leg cramps has been banned by the FDA, it was widely used and is found in lower quantities in tonic water. Quinine can cause ringing in the ears or hearing loss. Psychogenic factors and other disease processes (e.g., diabetes) also may be partially responsible for sensorineural hearing loss.

When hearing loss occurs, proper evaluation and treatment are warranted. *Healthy People 2010* identified eight objectives for decreasing the problems caused by hearing loss. One of these objectives for people diagnosed with hearing loss or deafness is to use rehabilitation services and supplemental devices to improve communication with other people. *Healthy People 2020 provide specific target measures for addressing hearing disorder objectives.* Resources are available in workplaces and in schools. The Individuals with Disabilities Education Act (IDEA) was developed to ensure that children and adults, including elderly adults, receive the same opportunities in the educational system as those without hearing impairment.

Care of elderly patients includes recognizing emotional reactions related to hearing loss, such as suspicion of others because of an inability to hear adequately; frustration and anger, with repeated statements such as, "I didn't hear what you said"; and feelings of insecurity because of the inability to hear the telephone or alarms. The Americans with Disabilities Act (ADA) of 1990 required that all emergency services are accessible to people who have text message telephones (TTYs). In addition, in 1998, the Department of Justice mandated that all 911 centers in the United States be accessible to people with Text Telephone (TTYs).

Medical Management

Implanted Hearing Devices

Three types of implanted hearing devices are commercially available: semi-implantable hearing device, fully implantable device, and the cochlear implant, the bone conduction device.

Cochlear implants are for patients with little or no hearing and are discussed below. Bone conduction devices, which transmit sound through the skull to the inner ear, are used in patients with a conductive hearing loss if a hearing aid is contraindicated (e.g., those with chronic infection). The device is implanted postauricularly under the skin into the skull, and an external device—worn above the ear, not in the canal—transmits the sound through the skin. Currently there are two types of implantable hearing aid devices, semi-implantable and fully implantable. Semi-implantable devices consist of a magnetic component that is implanted in the auditory ossicle, a receiver and a sound processor. Whereas, fully implantable middle ear devices consist of a sensor, sound processor along with a driver that is connected to the auditory ossicle.

The bone-anchored hearing aid (BAHA) may be fully or partially implantable. It is surgically implanted behind the ear in the mastoid area. The middle ear implantation (MEI) is implanted in the middle ear cavity and designed to move the bones directly rather than only amplifying sound. The BAHA is used for conductive or mixed hearing loss or unilateral sensorineural hearing loss, while the MEI is used for moderate to severe sensorineural hearing loss.

Cochlear Implant

A cochlear implant is an auditory prosthesis used for people with profound bilateral sensorineural hearing loss who do not benefit from conventional hearing aids. The hearing loss may be congenital or acquired. An implant does not restore normal hearing; rather, it amplifies sound so the person detects medium to loud environmental sounds and conversation. The implant provides stimulation directly to the auditory nerve, bypassing the nonfunctioning hair cells of the inner ear. The microphone and signal processor, worn outside the body, transmit electrical stimuli to the implanted electrodes. The electrical signals stimulate the auditory nerve fibers and then the brain, where they are interpreted.

Candidates for a cochlear implant, who are usually at least 1 year of age, are selected after careful screening by otologic history, physical examination, audiologic testing, x-rays, and psychological testing. Children who receive cochlear implants prior to 18 months of age achieve the greatest hearing, appreciation of sound and music, and development of speech as compared to older children who receive the implants (NIDCD, 2014). Criteria for choosing adults who may benefit from a cochlear implant include the following:

- Profound sensorineural hearing loss in both ears
- Inability to hear and recognize speech well with hearing aids
- No medical contraindication to a cochlear implant or general anesthesia
- Indications that being able to hear would enhance the patient's life (some candidates who are deaf do not view themselves as having a disability that needs to be cured)

FIGURE 50-1 The cochlear implant. The internal coil has a stranded electrode lead. The electrode is inserted through the round window into the scala tympani of the cochlea. The external coil (the transmitter) is held in alignment with the internal coil (the receiver) by a magnet. The microphone receives the sound. The stimulator wire receives the signal after it has been filtered, adjusted, and modified so that the sound is at a comfortable level for the patient. Sound is passed by the external transmitter to the inner coil receiver by magnetic conduction and then is carried by the electrode to the cochlea.

Labels in figure: External coil, Internal coil, Malleus, Incus, Stapes, Acoustic nerve, Cochlea, Active electrode, Ground electrode, Microphone, Earmold, Stimulator wires, External auditory canal, Tympanic membrane, Eustachian tube

 Concept Mastery Alert

Conductive hearing loss is not an indication for cochlear implants. People with profound bilateral sensorineural hearing loss who do not benefit from conventional hearing aids do qualify as candidates for cochlear implants.

The surgery involves implanting a small receiver in the temporal bone through a postauricular incision and placing electrodes into the inner ear (Fig. 50-1). The microphone and transmitter are worn on an external unit. The patient undergoes extensive cochlear rehabilitation with the multidisciplinary team, which includes an audiologist and speech pathologist. Several months may be needed to learn to interpret the sounds heard. Children and adults who lost their hearing before they learned to speak take much longer to acquire speech. There are wide variations of success with cochlear implants, and there is also controversy about their use, especially among the Deaf community. Patients who have had a cochlear implant are cautioned that magnetic resonance imaging (MRI) will inactivate the implant; MRI is to be used only when there is no other diagnostic option.

Aural Rehabilitation

If hearing loss is permanent or cannot be treated by medical or surgical means, or if the patient elects not to undergo surgery, aural rehabilitation may be beneficial. The purpose of aural rehabilitation is to maximize the communication skills of the person with hearing impairment. Aural rehabilitation includes auditory training, speech reading, speech training, and the use of hearing aids and hearing guide dogs.

Auditory training emphasizes listening skills so the person who is hearing-impaired concentrates on the speaker.

Speech reading (formerly known as *lip reading*) can help fill the gaps left by missed or misheard words. The goals of speech training are to conserve, develop, and prevent deterioration of current communication skills.

It is important to identify the type of hearing impairment a person has so that rehabilitative efforts can be directed at his or her particular need. Surgical correction may be all that is necessary to treat and improve a conductive hearing loss by eliminating its cause. With advances in hearing aid technology, amplification for patients with sensorineural hearing loss is more helpful than ever.

Hearing Aids

A hearing aid is a device through which speech and environmental sounds are received by a microphone, converted to electrical signals, amplified, and reconverted to acoustic signals. Many aids available for sensorineural hearing loss depress the low frequencies, or tones, and enhance hearing for the high frequencies. The evolution in technology has led to the availability of many smaller and more effective hearing aids. It is estimated that 98% of all hearing aids sold today are behind-the-ear, in-the-ear, or in-the-canal types (Table 50-1).

A hearing aid should be fitted according to the patient's needs (e.g., type of hearing loss, manual dexterity, and preferences) by a certified audiologist licensed to dispense hearing aids. Many states have consumer protection laws that allow the hearing aid to be returned after a trial use if the patient is not completely satisfied.

A hearing aid makes sounds louder, but it does not improve a patient's ability to discriminate words or understand speech. People who have low discrimination scores (i.e., 20%) on audiograms may derive little benefit from a hearing aid. Hearing aids amplify all sounds, including background

TABLE **50-1** Hearing Aids

Site (and Range of Hearing Loss)	Advantages	Disadvantages
Body, usually on the trunk (mild–profound)	Separation of receiver and microphone prevents acoustic feedback, allowing high amplification. Generally used in a school setting.	Bulky; requires long wire, which may be cosmetically displeasing; some loss of high-frequency response.
Behind the ear (mild–profound)	Economical; powerful, with no long wires; easily used by children—adapts easily as the child grows, with only the ear mold needing replacement.	Large size, are visible.
In the ear (mild–moderately severe)	The in-the-ear (ITE) is custom molded fitting within the outer ear or partially filling the lower outer ear. One-piece custom fit to contour of ear; no tubes or cords; miniature microphone is located in the ear, which is a more natural placement; more cosmetically appealing due to easy concealment.	Smaller size limits output; patients who have arthritis or cannot perform tasks requiring good manual dexterity may have difficulty with the small size of the aid and/or its battery; can require more repair than the behind-the-ear aid.
In the canal (mild–moderately severe)	In-the-canal (ITC) are custom molded to fit partially in the ear canal and are less visible; completely-in-canal (CIC) or the mini CIC is molded to fit inside the ear canal and is the smallest and least visible type, so more cosmetically pleasing.	Smaller aids require good manual dexterity. CICs are prone to earwax building up and dampening the speaker. Small batteries have a short life and are difficult to handle. There is no volume control.

noise, which may be disturbing to the wearer. Box 50-3 identifies additional problems associated with hearing aid use. Computerized hearing aids are available to compensate for background noise or allow amplification at certain programmed frequencies rather than at all frequencies. Occasionally, depending on the type of hearing loss, binaural aids (i.e., one for each ear) may be indicated. Box 50-4 provides tips for hearing aid care.

Hearing Guide Dogs

Specially trained service dogs are available to assist the person with a hearing loss. People who live alone are eligible to apply for a dog trained by, for example, International Hearing Dog, Inc. The dog reacts to the sound of a telephone, a doorbell, an alarm clock, a baby's cry, a knock at the door, a smoke alarm, or an intruder. The dog alerts its handler by physical contact; the dog then runs to the source

---

BOX 50-3 | **Hearing Aid Problems**

Improper Aid Selection

Consumers often find they cannot adjust to the hearing aid, but there are many hearing aids on the market to choose from. One consideration is sound amplification. The amplifier is a transformer that increases the amplitude of the electrical signal sent to the receiver. The receiver takes the sound and transmits it to the ear. A mismatch between receiver and amplifier increases sound distortion and may become intolerable to patients. The open mold provides a full shell or half shell instrument. Aids need to transmit sound well, fit comfortably, and be aesthetically pleasing.

Inadequate Amplification

- Dead batteries
- Cerumen in ear
- Cerumen or other material in mold
- Wires or tubing disconnected from aid

- Aid turned off or volume too low
- Improper mold
- Improper aid for degree of loss

Pain from Mold

- Improperly fitted mold
- Ear skin or cartilage infection
- Middle ear infection
- Ear tumor
- Unrelated conditions of the *temporomandibular* joint, throat, or larynx

Whistling Noise

- Loose ear mold
- Improperly made
- Improperly worn
- Worn out

Patient Education

Tips for Hearing Aid Care
Cleaning
- Behind the ear (BTE) hearing aids may be washed infrequently using soap and water. Ensure that the device is dried thoroughly after cleaning.
- It is recommended to use a soft, cotton cloth to clean and remove dried cerumen for most hearing aid devices, such as in-the-ear hearing aids (ITE).
- Many hearing aid manufacturers advertise online information including cleaning directions.
- Clean the cannula with a small pipe cleaner-like device.
- Prevent complications by proper care of the ear device and keeping the ear canal clean and dry.

Malfunctioning
Inadequate amplification, a whistling noise, or pain from the mold can occur when a hearing aid is not functioning properly.
- Check for malfunctions:
  - Is the switch on properly?
  - Are the batteries charged and positioned correctly?
- If the hearing aid is still not working properly, notify the hearing aid dealer.
- If the unit requires extended time for repair, the dealer may lend you a hearing aid until the repair can be accomplished.

Recognizing Complications
Common medical complications include external otitis media and pressure ulcers in the external auditory canal.
- Be alert for signs and symptoms of these infections, including painful ear, especially when the external ear is touched, canal swelling, redness, difficulty hearing, pain radiating to the jaw area, and fever.
- If any of these symptoms are present, notify your health care provider for evaluation. You may need medication to treat infection, pain, or both.

of the noise. In public, the dog positions itself between the person with hearing impairment and any potential hazard that the person cannot hear, such as an oncoming vehicle or a loud, hostile person. In most states, a certified hearing guide dog is legally permitted access to public transportation, public eating places, and stores, including food markets.

Nursing Management

Communicating Effectively

Nurses who understand the different types of hearing loss are more successful in adopting a communication style to fit the needs and preferences of every patient. Trying to speak in a loud voice to a person who cannot hear high-frequency sounds only makes understanding more difficult. However, strategies such as talking into the less-impaired ear and using gestures and facial expressions can help (Box 50-5).

A major issue for many people who are deaf or hearing-impaired is that they have other health problems that often do not receive attention, in large part because of communication barriers with their health care practitioners and the physical environment. The American Disabilities Act and Section 504 of the 1973 Rehabilitation Act mandates that people with disabilities have access to health care facilities and programs, thereby reducing disparity among individuals who are sensory and physically impaired. To meet the health care needs of patients who are hearing-impaired, practitioners are legally obligated to make accommodations for a patient's inability to hear. Providing interpreters for those who can communicate through sign language is essential in many situations so that the practitioner can effectively communicate with the patient.

During health care and screening procedures, the health care practitioner must be aware that patients who are deaf or hearing-impaired have certain limitations. They are unable to read lips, see a signer, or read written materials in the dark rooms required during some diagnostic tests. The same situation exists if the practitioner is wearing a mask or is not in the direct line of vision. Nurses and other health care practitioners must work with patients who are deaf or hearing-impaired and their families to identify practical and effective means of communication and to ensure accommodations are made. Refer to agency protocols for assistance when communicating with individuals who are hearing-impaired during a health care visit.

Maintaining a Quiet Environment

Loud, persistent noise has been found to cause constriction of peripheral blood vessels, increased blood pressure and heart rate (because of increased secretion of adrenalin), and increased gastrointestinal activity, as well as disturb patterns of sleep. Although research is needed to address the overall effects of noise on the human body, a quiet environment is more conducive to peace of mind (Box 50-6). A person who is ill feels more at ease when noise is kept to a minimum. The World Health Organization set noise guidelines for hospitals since noise negatively affect patient outcomes and staff performance (Berglund, Lindvall, & Schwela, 1999). Infrastructure designs, such as noiseless call bell systems and sound-masking floors and walls, represent attempts to decrease noise in hospitals.

CONDITIONS OF THE EXTERNAL EAR

CERUMEN IMPACTION

Cerumen normally accumulates in the external canal in various amounts and colors. Although wax does not usually need to be removed, impaction occasionally occurs.

BOX 50-5

Communicating with People Who are Hearing-Impaired

For the person who is hearing-impaired whose speech is difficult to understand:

- Consider how the person prefers to communicate with others. Do not assume that writing, gestures, or other means are the best or preferred technique.
- Consider if the person uses sign language. Interpreters are available in person or by video from the American Sign Language Inc., Interpreting Service (ASLI). These specialists provide the best means of communication, and provide accurate, professional services.
- Devote full attention to what the person is saying. Look and listen—do not try to attend to another task while listening.
- Engage the speaker in conversation when it is possible for you to anticipate the replies. This enables you to become accustomed to any peculiarities in speech patterns.
- Try to determine the essential context of what is being said; you can often fill in the details from context.
- Do not try to appear as if you understand if you do not.
- If you cannot understand at all or have serious doubt about your ability to understand what is being said, have the person write the message rather than risk misunderstanding. Having the person repeat the message in speech, after you know its content, also aids you in becoming accustomed to the person's pattern of speech.

- Written communication is an excellent resource. Written material should be written at a third-grade level so that the majority of people can understand it.

For the person who is hearing-impaired who speech reads:

- If you need to get the patient's attention, wave your hand in front of his or her visual field.
- When speaking, always face the person and smile.
- Make sure your face is as clearly visible as possible. Locate yourself so that your face is well lighted; avoid being silhouetted against strong light. Do not obscure the person's view of your mouth in any way; avoid talking with any object held in your mouth.
- Be sure that the patient knows the topic or subject before going ahead with what you plan to say. This enables the person to use contextual clues in speech reading.
- Speak slowly and distinctly, pausing more frequently than you would normally.
- If you question whether some important direction or instruction has been understood, check to be certain that the patient has the full meaning of your message.
- If for any reason your mouth must be covered (as with a mask), and you must direct or instruct the patient, write the message.

Clinical Manifestations and Assessment

Impaction causes **otalgia**, a sensation of fullness or pain in the ear, with or without a hearing loss. Accumulation of cerumen as a cause of hearing loss is especially significant in the older population. Attempts to clear the external auditory canal with cotton-tipped applicators, matches, hairpins, and other implements are dangerous because trauma to the skin, infection, and damage to the tympanic membrane can occur.

Medical and Nursing Management

Cerumen can be removed by irrigation, suction, or instrumentation. Unless the patient has a perforated eardrum or an

BOX 50-6

Nursing Research

Bridging the Gap to Evidence-Based Practice

Darbyshire, J., & Young, J. (2013). An investigation of sound levels on intensive care units with reference to the WHO guidelines. *Darbyshire and Young Critical Care, 17,* R187. Retrieved from http://ccforum.com/content/17/5/R18

Purpose
Patients in intensive care units (ICUs) suffer from sleep deprivation arising from nursing interventions and ambient noise. This may exacerbate confusion and ICU-related delirium. The World Health Organization (WHO) suggests that average hospital sound levels should not exceed 35 dB with a maximum of 40 dB overnight. The authors monitored five ICUs to check compliance with these guidelines.

Design
Sound levels were recorded in five adult ICUs in the United Kingdom. Two sound level monitors recorded concurrently for 24 hours at the ICU central stations and adjacent to patients. Sample values to determine levels generated by equipment and external noise were also recorded in an empty ICU side room.

Findings
Average sound levels always exceeded 45 dBA and, for 50% of the time, exceeded between 52 and 59 dBA in individual ICUs. There was diurnal variation with values decreasing after evening handovers to an overnight average minimum of 51 dBA at 4 am. Peaks above 85 dBA occurred at all sites, up to 16 times per hour overnight and more frequently during the day. WHO guidelines on sound levels could be achieved only in a side room by switching off all equipment.

Nursing Implications
All ICUs had sound levels greater than WHO recommendations, but the WHO recommended levels are so low, they are not achievable in an ICU. Levels adjacent to patients are higher than those recorded at central stations. Unit-wide noise reduction programs or mechanical means of isolating patients from ambient noise, such as earplugs, should be considered.

inflamed external ear (i.e., **otitis externa**), gentle irrigation with tap water usually helps remove impacted cerumen, particularly if it is not tightly packed into the external auditory canal. For successful removal, the water stream must flow behind the obstructing cerumen to move it first laterally and then out of the canal. To prevent injury, the lowest effective pressure should be used. However, if the eardrum behind the impaction is perforated, water can enter the middle ear, producing acute pain, vertigo and infection. If irrigation is unsuccessful, a trained health care provider can perform direct visual, mechanical removal on a cooperative patient.

Instilling a few drops of warmed glycerin, mineral oil, or half-strength hydrogen peroxide into the ear canal for 30 minutes can soften cerumen before its removal. Ceruminolytic agents, such as peroxide in glyceryl (Debrox), are available; however, these compounds may cause an allergic dermatitis reaction. Using any softening solution two or three times a day for several days is generally sufficient. If the cerumen cannot be dislodged by these methods, instruments, such as an ear curette, aural suction, and a binocular microscope for magnification, can be used by a provider with specialized training.

FOREIGN BODIES

Objects may be inserted into the ear canal by children. Occasionally, beads or parts to toys are found in the external ear canal. Some objects are inserted intentionally into the ear by adults who may have been trying to clean the external canal or relieve itching. Insects may also enter the ear canal. In either case, the effects may range from no symptoms to profound pain and decreased hearing.

Removing a foreign body from the external auditory canal can be quite challenging, and in unskilled hands may be dangerous. The object may be pushed completely into the bony portion of the canal, lacerating the skin and perforating the tympanic membrane. The three standard methods for skilled practitioners to remove foreign bodies are the same as those for removing cerumen: irrigation, suction, and instrumentation. The contraindications for irrigation are also the same. Foreign vegetable bodies and insects tend to swell; thus, irrigation is contraindicated. Usually, an insect can be dislodged by instilling mineral oil, which will suffocate the insect and allow it to be removed using alligator forceps or a loop-wired instrument. A referral to a specialist in Ears, Eyes, Nose Throat may be indicated. In some circumstances, the foreign body may have to be extracted in the operating room with the patient under general anesthesia.

CONDITIONS OF THE MIDDLE EAR

TYMPANIC MEMBRANE PERFORATION

Perforation of the tympanic membrane is usually caused by infection or trauma. Sources of trauma include skull fracture, explosive injury, or a severe blow to the ear. Less frequently, perforation is caused by foreign objects (e.g., cotton-tipped applicators, bobby pins, keys) that have been pushed too far into the external auditory canal. In addition to tympanic membrane perforation, injury to the ossicles and even the inner ear may result; thus, attempts by patients to clear the external auditory canal should be discouraged. During infection, the tympanic membrane can rupture if the pressure in the middle ear exceeds the atmospheric pressure in the external auditory canal.

Clinical Manifestations and Assessment

Symptoms of tympanic membrane perforation include whistling sounds upon sneezing and blowing nose, reduced hearing, purulent drainage from ear(s), and/or otalgia.

Medical and Nursing Management

Although most tympanic membrane perforations heal spontaneously within weeks after rupture, some may take several months to heal. Some perforations persist because scar tissue grows over the edges of the perforation, preventing extension of the epithelial cells across the margins and healing. In the case of a head injury or temporal bone fracture, a patient is observed for evidence of cerebrospinal fluid: **otorrhea** or **rhinorrhea**, a clear, watery drainage from the ear or nose, respectively. If present, the nurse is aware that this represents an abnormal communication between the subarachnoid space and the tympanomastoid space, with a risk of a central nervous system (CNS) infection. While healing, the ear must be protected from water.

Perforations that do not heal on their own may require surgery. The decision to perform a **tympanoplasty** (surgical repair of the tympanic membrane) is usually based on the need to prevent potential infection from water entering the ear or the desire to improve the patient's hearing. Performed on an outpatient basis, tympanoplasty may involve a variety of surgical techniques. In all techniques, tissue (commonly from the temporalis fascia) is placed across the perforation to allow healing. Surgery is usually successful in closing the perforation permanently and improving hearing. Postoperative instructions after middle ear surgery are found in Box 50-7.

OTOSCLEROSIS

Otosclerosis involves the stapes and is thought to result from the formation of new, abnormal spongy bone, especially around the oval window, with resulting fixation of the stapes. The efficient transmission of sound is prevented because the stapes cannot vibrate and carry the sound as conducted from the malleus and incus to the inner ear. Otosclerosis is more common in women and frequently hereditary, and pregnancy may worsen it.

Clinical Manifestations and Assessment

Otosclerosis may involve one or both ears and manifests as a progressive conductive or mixed hearing loss. The

BOX 50-7
Patient Education

Self-Care After Middle Ear or Mastoid Surgery

Postoperative instructions for patients who have had middle ear and mastoid surgery may vary among otolaryngologists. General teaching guidelines for the patient may include:

- Take antibiotics and other medications as prescribed.
- Blow the nose gently, one side at a time, for 1 week after surgery.
- Sneeze and cough with the mouth open for a few weeks after surgery.
- Avoid heavy lifting (over 10 lb), straining, and bending over for a few weeks after surgery.
- Popping and crackling sensations in the operative ear are normal for approximately 3–5 weeks after surgery.
- Temporary hearing loss is normal in the operative ear due to fluid, blood, or packing in the ear.
- Report excessive or purulent ear drainage to the surgeon. Some slightly bloody or serosanguineous drainage from the ear is normal after surgery.
- Change the cotton ball in the ear as needed.
- Avoid getting water in the operative ear for 2 weeks after surgery. You may shampoo the hair 2–3 days postoperatively if the ear is protected from water by saturating a cotton ball with petroleum jelly (or some other water-insoluble substance) and loosely placing it in the ear. If the postauricular suture line becomes wet, pat (do not rub) the area and cover it with a thin layer of antibiotic ointment.

patient may or may not complain of tinnitus (ringing in the ear). Otoscopic examination usually reveals a normal tympanic membrane. Bone conduction is better than air conduction on Rinne testing. The audiogram confirms conductive hearing loss or mixed loss, especially in the low frequencies.

Medical and Nursing Management

There is no known nonsurgical treatment for otosclerosis. However, some physicians believe the use of sodium fluoride can mature the abnormal spongy bone growth and prevent the breakdown of the bone tissue. Amplification with a hearing aid also may help.

One of two surgical procedures may be performed, the stapedectomy or the stapedotomy. A stapedectomy involves removing the stapes superstructure and part of the footplate and inserting a tissue graft and a suitable prosthesis (Fig. 50-2). The surgeon drills a small hole into the footplate to hold a prosthesis. The prosthesis bridges the gap between the incus and the inner ear, providing better sound conduction. Stapes surgery is very successful; approximately 95% of patients experience resolution of conductive hearing loss. Balance disturbance or true vertigo, which rarely occurs in other middle ear surgical procedures, may occur during the postoperative period for several days.

MIDDLE EAR MASSES

Other than **cholesteatoma** (middle ear or mastoid tumor), masses in the middle ear are rare. A glomus jugulare tumor is a tumor that arises from the jugular vein and appears as a red blemish on or behind the tympanic membrane upon examination with an otoscope. Glomus jugulare tumors are rarely malignant; however, due to their location, treatment may be necessary to relieve symptoms. The treatment for glomus tumors is surgical excision, except in poor surgical candidates, in whom radiation therapy is used.

A facial nerve neuroma is a tumor on cranial nerve VII, the facial nerve. These types of tumors are usually not visible on otoscopic examination but are suspected when a patient presents with a facial nerve paresis. X-ray evaluation is used to identify the site of the tumor along the facial nerve. The treatment is surgical removal.

CONDITIONS OF THE INNER EAR

Almost 8 million American adults are affected by a chronic problem with balance, and an additional 2.4 million are affected by dizziness alone. Balance or vestibular problems are reported in approximately 9% of the older adult population over 65 years of age. In the United States, there are 1.6 million older adults who are treated for falls in emergency departments each year (NIH, 2015). Disorders of balance are a major cause of falls in the older population. Body balance is maintained by the cooperation of the muscles and joints of the body (proprioceptive system), the eyes (visual system), and the labyrinth (vestibular system). These areas send their information about equilibrium, or balance, to the brain (cerebellar system) for coordination and perception in the cerebral cortex. Since the brain obtains its blood supply from the cardiovascular system, arteriosclerosis can also cause a disturbance in balance. Likewise, impaired vision can have an impact on equilibrium. The vestibular apparatus of the inner ear provides feedback regarding the movements and the position of the head and body in space.

Patients and health care providers frequently use the term *dizziness* to describe any altered sensation of orientation in space. **Vertigo** is defined as the misperception or illusion of motion of the person or the surroundings. Most people with vertigo describe a spinning sensation or say they feel as though objects are moving around them. *Ataxia* is a failure of muscular coordination and may be present in patients with vestibular disease. Syncope, fainting, and loss of consciousness are not forms of vertigo and usually indicate disease in the cardiovascular system.

Nystagmus is an involuntary rhythmic movement of the eyes, and slight oscillation may be a normal variant. However, when nystagmus is pathologic, it is an ocular disorder associated with vestibular dysfunction. Nystagmus can be horizontal, vertical, or rotary and can be caused by a disorder in the central or peripheral nervous system.

FIGURE 50-2 Stapedectomy for otosclerosis. **A.** Normal anatomy. **B.** Arrow points to sclerotic process at the foot of the stapes. **C.** Stapes broken away surgically from its diseased base. The hole in the footplate provides an area where an instrument can grasp the plate. **D.** The footplate is removed from its base. Some otosclerotic tissue may remain, and tissue is placed over it. **E.** Robinson stainless-steel prosthesis in position.

MOTION SICKNESS

Motion sickness is a disturbance of equilibrium caused by constant motion. For example, it can occur aboard a ship, while riding on a merry-go-round or swing, or in the back seat of a car.

Clinical Manifestations and Assessment

Motion sickness manifests itself with diaphoresis, pallor, nausea, and vomiting caused by vestibular overstimulation. These manifestations may persist for several hours after the stimulation stops.

Medical and Nursing Management

Over-the-counter antihistamines, such as dimenhydrinate (Dramamine) or meclizine hydrochloride (Antivert), may provide some relief of nausea and vomiting by blocking the conduction of the vestibular pathway of the inner ear. Anticholinergic medications, such as scopolamine patches, may also be effective because they antagonize the histamine response. These must be replaced every few days. Common side effects, such as dry mouth and drowsiness, may occur. Potentially hazardous activities, such as driving a car or operating heavy machinery, should be avoided.

MÉNIÈRE DISEASE

Ménière disease is a disorder of the inner ear that causes vertigo, tinnitus, a feeling of fullness or pressure in the ear, and fluctuating hearing loss.

Pathophysiology

Ménière disease is believed to be the result of fluctuating pressure within the inner ear or the mixing of inner ear fluids. The membranous labyrinth of the inner ear contains a fluid called *endolymph*. The membranes can become dilated because of malabsorption of the fluid in the endolymphatic sac or a blockage in the drainage of fluid in the endolymphatic duct within the labyrinth. This dilation is termed **endolymphatic hydrops** or a ballooning of the membranous labyrinth, which results in increased pressure in the system or rupture of the inner ear membrane producing symptoms of Ménière disease.

Risk Factors

According to the National Institute on Deafness and Other Communication Disorders (NIDCD), Ménière disease affects approximately 615,000 people in the United States, and 45,500 new cases are diagnosed each year (NIH, 2015). More common in adults, it has an average age of onset in the 40s, with symptoms usually beginning between 20 and 60 years of age. Ménière disease appears to be equally common in both genders and occurs bilaterally in about 20% of patients. About 50% of the patients who have Ménière disease have a positive family history of the disease. Patients who present at greater risk also include those with a recent viral illness or upper respiratory infection, allergy sufferers, smokers, patients with stress or fatigue, alcohol users, and in those who take aspirin.

Clinical Manifestations and Assessment

Symptoms of Ménière disease include fluctuating, progressive sensorineural hearing loss; tinnitus or a roaring sound; a feeling of pressure or fullness in the ear; and episodic, incapacitating vertigo, often accompanied by nausea and vomiting. These symptoms range in severity from a minor nuisance to extreme disability, especially if the attacks of vertigo are severe. At the onset of the disease, perhaps only one or two of the symptoms are manifested.

Some clinicians believe that there are two subsets of the disease, known as atypical Ménière disease: cochlear and vestibular. Cochlear Ménière disease is recognized as a fluctuating, progressive sensorineural hearing loss associated with tinnitus and aural pressure in the absence of vestibular symptoms or findings. Vestibular Ménière disease is characterized as the occurrence of episodic vertigo associated with aural pressure but no cochlear symptoms. Patients may experience either cochlear or vestibular disease symptoms; however, eventually all of these symptoms develop.

Vertigo is usually the most troublesome complaint related to Ménière disease. A careful history is taken to determine the frequency, duration, severity, and character of the patient's vertigo attacks. Vertigo may last minutes to hours, possibly accompanied by nausea or vomiting. Diaphoresis and a persistent feeling of imbalance or disequilibrium may awaken patients at night. Some patients report that these feelings last for days. However, they usually feel well between attacks. Hearing loss may fluctuate, with tinnitus and aural pressure waxing and waning with changes in hearing. These feelings may occur during or before attacks, or they may be constant. Long periods of remission may occur.

Physical examination findings are usually normal, with the exception of those of cranial nerve VIII. Sounds from a tuning fork (Weber test) may lateralize to the unaffected ear. Using a Rinne test, the normal finding of air conduction remaining greater than bone conduction usually is found. An audiogram typically reveals a sensorineural hearing loss in the affected ear. This can be in the form of a "Pike's Peak"

pattern, which looks like a hill or mountain. A sensorineural loss in the low frequencies occurs as the disease progresses. The electronystagmogram may be normal or may show reduced vestibular response. Imaging using magnetic resonance may also prove useful in diagnosis of CNS lesions.

Medical Management

Most patients with Ménière disease can be successfully treated with diet and medication. Many patients can control their symptoms by adhering to a low-sodium (2,000 mg/day) diet, with no caffeine and alcohol. Box 50-8 describes dietary guidelines that may be useful in Ménière disease. The amount of sodium is one of many factors that regulate the balance of fluid within the body. Sodium and fluid retention disrupts the delicate balance between endolymph and perilymph in the inner ear. Medications to control allergies or improve blood circulation of the inner ear prove helpful. Eliminating tobacco use and stress reduction can also decrease the severity of symptoms. Psychological evaluation may be indicated as comorbidity of vertigo and anxiety is well established in the literature. A plan of nursing care for a patient with vertigo is available online at http://thepoint.lww.com/Honan2e.

Pharmacologic Therapy

Pharmacologic therapy for Ménière disease consists of antihistamines, such as meclizine (Antivert), which suppress the vestibular system. Benzodiazepines, such as diazepam

---

BOX 50-8 Nutrition Alert

Dietary Guidelines for Patients with Ménière Disease

Advise patients to:
- Limit foods high in salt or sugar. Be aware of foods with hidden salts and sugars.
- Eat meals and snacks at regular intervals to stay hydrated. Missing meals or snacks may alter the fluid level in the inner ear.
- Eat fresh fruits, vegetables, and whole grains. Limit the amount of canned, frozen, or processed foods with high sodium content.
- Drink plenty of fluids daily. Water, milk, and low-sugar fruit juices are recommended. Limit intake of coffee, tea, and soft drinks. Avoid caffeine because of its diuretic effect.
- Limit alcohol intake. Alcohol may change the volume and concentration of the inner ear fluid and may worsen symptoms.
- Avoid monosodium glutamate (MSG), which may increase symptoms.
- Avoid aspirin and aspirin-containing medications. Aspirin may increase tinnitus and dizziness.

(Valium), may be used in acute instances to help control vertigo. Antiemetics, such as promethazine (Phenergan) suppositories, help control the nausea, vomiting, and vertigo because of their antihistamine effect. Betahistine hydrochloride and diuretic therapy may reduce the severity of symptoms by lowering the pressure in the endolymphatic system. Intake of foods containing potassium (e.g., bananas, cantaloupe, oranges) is necessary if the patient takes a diuretic that causes potassium loss. There is no scientific basis for the use of vasodilators, such as nicotinic acid, papaverine hydrochloride (Pavabid), and methantheline bromide (Banthine), to alleviate the symptoms, but they are often used in conjunction with other therapies. Corticosteroids are useful in reducing edema of the labyrinth and inflammation, in order to improve healing of the inner ear structures.

Surgical Management

Although most patients respond well to conservative therapy, some continue to have disabling attacks of vertigo. If these attacks reduce their quality of life, patients may elect to undergo chemical treatment or surgery for relief. Vestibular rehabilitation can assist to restore function in patients with permanent disorder. Surgical procedures, such as labyrinthectomy, vestibular neurectomy, or endolymphatic sac decompression, may be considered.

Endolymphatic Sac Decompression
Endolymphatic sac decompression, or shunting, theoretically equalizes the pressure in the endolymphatic space. A shunt or drain is inserted in the endolymphatic sac through a postauricular incision. Many otolaryngologists favor this procedure as a first-line surgical approach to treat the vertigo of Ménière disease because it is relatively simple and safe and can be performed on an outpatient basis.

Middle and Inner Ear Perfusion
Ototoxic medications, such as streptomycin or gentamicin, can be administered to patients by infusion into the middle and inner ear. These medications are used to destroy vestibular function and decrease vertigo. The success rate for eliminating vertigo is about 85%, but the risk of significant hearing loss is high. After the procedure, many patients have a period of imbalance that lasts several weeks.

Intraotologic Catheters
In an attempt to deliver medication directly to the inner ear, catheters are being developed to provide a conduit from the outer ear to the inner ear. The route of the catheter is from the external ear canal through or around the tympanic membrane and to the round window niche or membrane. Medicinal fluids can be placed against the round window for a direct route to the inner ear fluids.

Potential uses of these catheters include treatment for sudden hearing loss and various disorders causing intractable vertigo. Future applications may include tinnitus and slowly progressing sensorineural hearing loss. Intratympanic injections of ototoxic medications for round window membrane diffusion can be used to decrease vestibular function. Established surgical techniques can be used for the patient with vertigo who has not responded to medical or physical therapeutic modalities.

Vestibular Nerve Sectioning
Vestibular nerve sectioning provides the greatest success rate (98%) in eliminating the attacks of vertigo. It can be performed by a translabyrinthine approach (i.e., through the hearing mechanism) or in a manner that can conserve hearing (i.e., suboccipital or middle cranial fossa), depending on the degree of hearing loss. Most patients with incapacitating Ménière disease have little or no effective hearing. Cutting the nerve prevents the brain from receiving input from the semicircular canals. This procedure requires a brief hospital stay.

TINNITUS

Tinnitus is a symptom of an underlying disorder of the ear that is associated with hearing loss. This condition affects approximately 10% of the U.S. population between 40 and 70 years of age. The severity of tinnitus may range from mild to severe. Patients describe tinnitus as a roaring, buzzing, or hissing sound in one or both ears. Numerous factors may contribute to the development of tinnitus, including several ototoxic substances (Box 50-9). Underlying disorders that contribute to tinnitus may include thyroid disease, hyperlipidemia, vitamin B_{12} deficiency, psychological disorders (e.g., depression, anxiety), fibromyalgia, otologic disorders (Ménière disease, acoustic neuroma), and neurologic disorders (head injury, multiple sclerosis).

A physical examination should be performed to determine the cause of tinnitus. Diagnostic testing determines if hearing

---

BOX 50-9   Selected Ototoxic Substances

- *Diuretics:* Ethacrynic acid, furosemide, acetazolamide
- *Chemotherapeutic agents:* Cisplatin, nitrogen mustard
- *Antimalarial agents:* Quinine, mefloquine, chloroquine
- *Anti-inflammatory agents:* Salicylates (aspirin), indomethacin
- *Chemicals:* Alcohol, arsenic
- *Aminoglycoside antibiotics:* Amikacin, gentamicin, kanamycin, netilmicin, neomycin, streptomycin, tobramycin
- *Other antibiotics:* Erythromycin, minocycline, polymyxin B, vancomycin
- *ACE inhibitors:* Enalapril, moexipril, ramipril
- *Acetic acids:* Diclofenac, indomethacin, ketorolac
- *Alpha blockers:* Doxazosin
- *Anti-arrhythmics:* Flecainide, propafenone, quinidine, tocainide
- *Calcium-channel blockers:* diltiazem, nifedipine, nisoldipine
- *H_1-blockers:* Cetirizine, fexofenadine
- *Metals:* Gold, mercury, lead

loss is present. An audiograph speech discrimination test or a tympanogram may be used to help determine the cause. Some forms of tinnitus are irreversible; therefore, patients may need teaching and counseling about ways of adjusting to their treatment and dealing with tinnitus in the future.

BENIGN PAROXYSMAL POSITIONAL VERTIGO

Benign paroxysmal positional vertigo (BPPV) is a brief period of incapacitating vertigo that occurs when the position of the patient's head is changed with respect to gravity, typically by placing the head back with the affected ear turned down. The onset is sudden and followed by a predisposition for positional vertigo, usually for hours to weeks but occasionally for months or years. Other symptoms may include lightheadedness, blurred vision, and nausea and vomiting.

Pathophysiology

BPPV is thought to be due to the disruption of debris in the labyrinth, termed **otoconia** (small crystal particles of calcium carbonate that detach and float in the endolymph and cause symptomatology). This is frequently stimulated by head trauma, infection (particularly of the respiratory tract), or other events. Precipitating factors include sneezing or coughing, or the vertigo may be induced by any change in head positioning. Bed rest is recommended for patients with acute symptoms.

Clinical Manifestations and Assessment

Diagnosis of BBPV is performed after an ear examination, audiogram, and test of nerve responses and use of the Dix–Hallpike test, also called the Nylen–Barany test. The test involves making the patient undergo a rapid change from an erect seated position to a supine position with the head hanging over the edge of the examination table to the left, right, or center. Dizziness and peripheral vertigo will be elicited with the affected ear pointing downward. The eyes are examined for a brief period for nystagmus present while the head is maintained in a provoking position, which also commonly accompanies vertigo. Nystagmus and vertigo may be present for less than 30 seconds during maneuvers.

Medical and Nursing Management

Repositioning techniques can be used to treat vertigo, such as the Epley maneuver. The maneuver is designed to reposition the canalith and involves quick movements of the head. The noninvasive procedure is performed by placing the patient in a sitting position and turning the head to a 45-degree angle on the affected side and 30 to 45 degrees backward. Then the patient is quickly moved to the supine position. The procedure is repeated, tilting the head to the opposite side. The patient must not lie flat for 48 to 72 hours after repositioning to prevent the particles from reentering the posterior canal. The procedure is safe, inexpensive, and easy to perform.

Patients with acute vertigo are treated with medications that target vertigo and its related symptoms of nausea, vomiting, and anxiety. Vestibular suppressants that are commonly used originate from classes of anticholinergics (scopolamine), antihistamines (meclizine, dimenhydrinate), and benzodiazepines. Meclizine is often the drug of choice, with patients treated for a 1- to 2- week course of therapy. Antiemetic medications, such as phenothiazines, are used to treat nausea. Meclizine has both vestibular suppressant and antiemetic effects.

Vestibular rehabilitation can be used in the management of vestibular disorders. This strategy promotes active use of the vestibular system through an interdisciplinary team approach, including medical and nursing care, stress management, biofeedback, vocational rehabilitation, and physical therapy. A physical therapist prescribes balance exercises that help the brain compensate for the impairment to the balance system.

OTOTOXICITY

A variety of medications may have adverse effects on the cochlea, vestibular apparatus, or cranial nerve VIII. All but a few, such as aspirin and quinine, cause irreversible hearing loss. At high doses, aspirin toxicity can produce bilateral tinnitus. IV medications, especially the aminoglycosides, are the most common cause of ototoxicity, and they destroy the hair cells in the organ of Corti (see Box 50-9).

To prevent loss of hearing or balance, patients receiving potentially ototoxic medications should be counseled about the side effects of these medications. These medications should be used with caution in patients who are at high risk for complications, such as children, the elderly, pregnant patients, patients with kidney or liver problems, and patients with current hearing disorders. Blood levels of the medications should be monitored, and patients receiving long-term IV antibiotics should be monitored with an audiogram twice each week during therapy.

> **(!) Nursing Alert**
> *Many intravenous medications require careful monitoring of the highest (peak) and lowest (trough) concentration of the drug in the patient's blood to ensure that the dosage is within the therapeutic range and to prevent toxicity. The trough is drawn just before a drug is scheduled to be given whereas the peak is drawn after the drug is administered (typically 30 minutes).*

ACOUSTIC NEUROMA

Acoustic neuromas develop in 1 of every 10,000 people per year. These neuromas account for 5% to 10% of all intracranial tumors and seem to occur with equal frequency in men and women of any age, although most occur during middle age.

Pathophysiology

Acoustic neuromas are slow-growing, benign tumors of cranial nerve VIII, usually arising from the Schwann cells of the vestibular portion of the nerve. Most acoustic tumors arise within the internal auditory canal and extend into the cerebellopontine angle to press on the brainstem, possibly destroying the vestibular nerve.

Clinical Manifestations and Assessment

The most common assessment findings of patients with *acoustic neuromas are unilateral tinnitus and hearing loss with or without vertigo or balance disturbance*. If the tumor is large, the trigeminal nerve may be involved resulting in facial paresthesia, hypesthesia (sensitivity to touch), and discomfort. Facial paresis and disturbance in taste result from facial nerve involvement, which occurs less commonly. It is important to identify asymmetry in audiovestibular test results so that further workup can be performed to rule out an acoustic neuroma. MRI with a paramagnetic contrast agent (i.e., gadolinium or Magnevist) is the imaging study of choice. If the patient is claustrophobic or cannot undergo an MRI for other reasons, or if the scan is unavailable, a computed tomography (CT) scan with contrast dye is performed; however, MRI is more sensitive than CT in delineating a small tumor.

Medical and Nursing Management

Surgical removal of acoustic tumors is the treatment of choice because these tumors do not respond well to radiation or chemotherapy. Because treatment of acoustic tumors crosses several specialties, the interdisciplinary treatment approach involves a neurologist and a neurosurgeon. The objective of the surgery is to remove the tumor while preserving facial nerve function. Most acoustic tumors have damaged the cochlear portion of cranial nerve VIII, and hearing is impaired. In these patients, the surgery is performed using a translabyrinthine approach, and the hearing mechanism is destroyed. If hearing is still good before surgery, a suboccipital or middle cranial fossa approach to removing the tumor may be used. This procedure exposes the lateral third of the internal auditory canal and preserves hearing.

Complications of surgery include facial nerve paralysis, cerebrospinal fluid leakage, meningitis, and cerebral edema. Death from acoustic neuroma surgery is rare.

CHAPTER REVIEW

Critical Thinking Exercises

1. You are visiting an older man for a postoperative home visit following a cholecystectomy. He tells you that he has had severe leg cramps at nighttime and has started drinking tonic daily. He has noticed a significant improvement in the leg cramps. During your assessment, you also learn that he has a significant hearing loss, and his wife tells you that she thinks that his hearing has worsened over the past several months; however, she attributes his hearing loss to advanced age and to anxiety regarding his recent surgery. Devise a teaching plan for this patient and his wife. Provide a rationale for each part of the plan.

2. A 20-year-old man, a member of a college swim team, has recurrent external otitis—his third episode in the past 6 weeks. He is being treated at an ear-nose-throat clinic. Devise an evidence-based teaching plan for this patient including holistic, pharmacologic, and nonpharmacologic measures.

NCLEX-Style Review Questions

1. A 56-year-old patient who is hearing-impaired is scheduled for a colonoscopy. Which nursing action is most appropriate in performing patient education prior to the procedure?
   a. Face the patient directly, smile, and speak slowly.
   b. Continue to administer medications while educating the patient.
   c. Nod to make up for awkward silence, even if you don't know what is being said.
   d. Use only gestures to communicate the highlights of content to be covered.

2. The nurse caring for the patient with Ménière disease restricts the following foods in the dietary plan. Select all that apply.
   a. Coffee
   b. Wine
   c. Baked potato
   d. Cheese
   e. Milk

3. During preoperative teaching, the 25-year-old patient receiving cochlear implants states, "I will be able to fully regain my hearing with the implants." What is the nurse's best response to the patient?
   a. "The implants will assist you to detect medium to loud environmental sound and conversation rather than restoring normal hearing."
   b. "The implant will assist you to restore normal hearing fully."
   c. "The implants will be immediately effective."
   d. "The implant will require minimal rehabilitation in order for you to recognize sounds."

4. How might a patient with tinnitus describe hearing sound to the nurse?
   a. Sputtering
   b. Muffled
   c. Loud
   d. Buzzing

5. A patient taking aspirin for stroke prevention reports the development of hearing disturbances. The appropriate intervention is to decrease the dose in order to prevent which condition?
   a. Ototoxicity
   b. Vertigo
   c. Nystagmus
   d. Otitis externa

Try these additional resources, available at **http://thepoint.lww.com/Honan2e**, to enhance your learning and understanding of this chapter:
- NCLEX-Style Student Review Questions
- Journal Articles

REFERENCES AND SELECTED READINGS

References and selected readings associated with this chapter can be found on the website that accompanies the book. Visit **http://thepoint. lww.com/Honan2e** to access the references and other additional resources associated with this chapter.

Problems Related to Integumentary Function

A 48-year-old electrician has come to the emergency department via ambulance after falling and sustaining a high-voltage electrical burn. He has a full-thickness (third-degree) burn on his abdomen that will need autografting.

- Describe the nursing management of this patient in the emergent phase of burn injury.
- Discuss graft site care and donor site care following an autograft.
- What are the long-term complications for this patient?

Nursing Assessment: Integumentary Function

Commander Patina S. Walton-Battle

Learning Objectives

After reading this chapter, you will be able to:

1. Identify the structures and functions of the skin.
2. Differentiate the composition and function of each skin layer: epidermis, dermis, and subcutaneous tissue.
3. Describe the normal aging process of the skin and skin changes common in elderly patients.
4. List appropriate questions that help elicit information during an assessment of the skin.
5. Describe the components of physical assessment that are most useful when examining the skin, hair, and nails.
6. Identify and describe primary and secondary skin lesions and their pattern and distribution.
7. Discuss common skin tests and procedures used in diagnosing skin and related disorders.

The skin is the largest organ in the body and makes up approximately 12% of body weight. It is responsible for regulation of body temperature, maintenance of normal fluid and electrolyte balance, sensation, and protection from infection and the environment. Nurses care for patients with burns, skin infections, surgical wounds, and secondary skin abnormalities associated with systemic disease; this chapter provides the knowledge necessary to assess, diagnose, and manage skin abnormalities and describes when to seek referrals to the primary care provider or specialist.

ANATOMIC AND PHYSIOLOGIC OVERVIEW

The integumentary system comprises multiple subunits that work simultaneously. The system includes skin and its appendages, such as hair, nails, and sweat or sebaceous glands, which are lined with epidermal cells (Van De Graaff, 2014).

Anatomy of the Skin

The skin is composed of three layers: epidermis (outermost layer), dermis (inner layer), and hypodermis (innermost layer) (Fig. 51-1). Five distinct layers compose the epidermis; from innermost to outermost they are the stratum basale, stratum spinosum, stratum granulosum, stratum lucidum, and stratum corneum (Anderson, 2012). Each layer becomes more differentiated (i.e., mature and with more specific functions) as it rises from the basal stratum germinativum layer to the outermost stratum corneum layer. The stratum lucidum is found only on the skin of the palms and soles (James, Berger, & Elston, 2016a). The epidermis and the dermis are separated by a structure called the basement membrane zone. This zone contains proteins that can target various autoantibodies that can be found in patients with autoimmune blistering diseases (Anderson, 2012). The dermis, which is the thickest layer of skin, is composed principally of collagen, a fibrous protein synthesized primarily by fibroblast cells, which are important in remodeling and repairing skin. This layer is split up into two regions, the papillary dermis and reticular dermis. This connective tissue layer contains nerve endings, sensory receptors, capillaries, and elastic fibers.

Epidermis

The epidermis consists of continuously dividing cells covered on the surface by dead cells that were originally deeper in the dermis but were pushed upward by the newly developing, more differentiated cells underneath. This external layer

FIGURE 51-1 Anatomic structures of the skin.

Labels: Hair, Epidermis, Sebaceous gland, Dermis, Hair follicle, Papilla, Subcutaneous tissue, Sweat pore, Arrector pili muscle, Eccrine sweat gland, Nerve, Arteriole, Venule

is almost completely replaced every 3 to 4 weeks. The dead cells contain large amounts of **keratin**, an insoluble, fibrous protein that forms the outer barrier of the skin and has the capacity to repel pathogens and prevent excessive fluid loss from the body. Keratin is the principal hardening ingredient of the hair and nails.

Melanocytes are the special cells of the epidermis that are primarily involved in producing the pigment **melanin**, which colors the skin and hair. Most of the skin of dark-skinned people and the darker areas of the skin on light-skinned people (e.g., the areola) contain larger amounts of this pigment. Albinism is associated with a lack of melanin and is discussed later in the chapter. Production of melanin is controlled by a hormone secreted from the hypothalamus of the brain called *melanocyte-stimulating hormone.* Melanin provides a natural protection against the harmful effects of ultraviolet light; however, it does not provide complete protection from the sun's damaging rays.

Two other types of cells are common to the epidermis: Merkel and Langerhans cells. **Merkel cells** are receptors that transmit stimuli to the axon through a chemical synapse and therefore are associated with the sense of touch. **Langerhans cells** are accessory cells of the afferent immune system that play a role in cutaneous (skin) immune system reactions. These cells process invading antigens and transport the antigens to the lymph system to activate the T lymphocytes.

The junction of the epidermis (basement membrane zone, BMZ) and dermis is an area of many undulations and furrows called **rete ridges**. This junction anchors the epidermis to the dermis and permits the free exchange of essential nutrients between the two layers. If the BMZ is interrupted,

it must re-form to successfully achieve healing of the tissue (Wysocki, 2016).

Dermis

The dermis makes up the largest portion of the skin, providing strength and structure. It is composed of two layers: papillary and reticular. The papillary dermis lies directly beneath the epidermis and is composed primarily of fibroblast cells capable of producing one form of collagen, a component of connective tissue. The reticular layer lies beneath the papillary layer and also produces collagen and elastic bundles. The dermis is also made up of blood and lymph vessels, nerves, sweat and sebaceous glands, and hair roots. The dermis is often referred to as the "true skin." It is especially thick on the palms and soles, while thin over the eyelids and scrotum; thus, it is not surprising that in conditions of fluid volume excess, patients develop edema in thin skinned areas, resulting in periorbital and scrotal edema. An infection of the dermis that spreads rapidly within the skin and subcutaneous structures is termed *cellulitis.* It is usually caused by staphylococci or streptococci and presents with redness, warmth, swelling, and tenderness, usually of the limbs.

Hypodermis

The subcutaneous tissue, or hypodermis, is the innermost layer of the skin. It is primarily adipose tissue, which provides a cushion between the skin layers, muscles, and bones. It promotes skin mobility, molds body contours, and insulates the body. Fat is deposited and distributed according to the person's gender and in part accounts for the difference in body shape between men and women. Overeating results in increased deposition of fat beneath the skin. The subcutaneous tissues and the amount of fat deposited are important factors in body temperature regulation.

> **Nursing Alert**
> *An area of skin indurated (hardened) from collagen deposits in the cutaneous and subcutaneous tissue as a result of chronic inflammation is termed* sclerosis. *Examples include keloid formation, stasis dermatitis, and scleroderma.*

Anatomy of Hair, Nails, and Glands of the Skin

Hair

An outgrowth of the skin, hair is present over the entire body except for the palms and soles. The hair consists of a root formed in the dermis and a hair shaft that projects beyond the skin. It grows in a cavity called a *hair follicle* (see Fig. 51-1). Proliferation of cells in the bulb of the hair causes the hair to form.

Hair follicles undergo cycles of growth and rest. The rate of growth varies; beard growth is the most rapid, followed by hair on the scalp, axillae, thighs, and eyebrows. The growth or **anagen phase** may last up to 6 years for scalp hair, whereas the telogen or resting phase lasts approximately 4 months. During telogen, hair is shed from the body. The hair follicle recycles into the growing phase spontaneously, or it can be induced by plucking out hairs. Growing and resting hairs can be found side by side on all parts of the body. About 90% of the 100,000 hair follicles on a normal scalp are in the growing phase at any one time, and 50 to 100 scalp hairs are shed each day. In conditions in which inflammation causes damage to the root of the hair, regrowth is possible. However, if inflammation causes damage to the hair follicle, stem cells are destroyed and the hair does not grow.

Hair in different parts of the body serves different functions. The hairs of the eyes (i.e., eyebrows and lashes), nose, and ears filter out dust, microbes, and airborne debris. Hair color is supplied by various amounts of melanin within the hair shaft. Gray or white hair reflects the loss of pigment. Hair quantity and distribution can be affected by endocrine conditions. For example, Cushing syndrome causes **hirsutism**, especially in women; hypothyroidism (i.e., underactive thyroid) causes coarse hair; while hyperthyroidism (i.e., overactive thyroid) is associated with fine hair. In many cases, chemotherapy and radiation therapy cause hair thinning or weakening of the hair shaft, resulting in partial or complete **alopecia** from the scalp and other parts of the body.

Nails

On the dorsal surface of the fingers and toes, a hard, transparent plate of keratin, called the *nail*, overlies the skin. The nail grows from its root, which lies under a thin fold of skin called the *cuticle*. The nail protects the fingers and toes by preserving their highly developed sensory functions, such as for picking up small objects.

Nail growth is continuous throughout life, with an average growth of 0.1 mm daily. Growth is faster in fingernails than toenails and tends to slow with aging. Complete renewal of a fingernail takes about 170 days, whereas toenail renewal takes 12 to 18 months.

Glands of the Skin

There are two types of skin glands: sebaceous glands and sweat glands (see Fig. 51-1). The **sebaceous glands** are associated with hair follicles. The ducts of the sebaceous glands empty **sebum** onto the space between the hair follicle and the hair shaft. For each hair, there is a sebaceous gland, the secretions of which lubricates the hair and renders the skin soft and pliable.

Sweat glands are found in the skin over most of the body surface, but they are heavily concentrated in the palms of the hands and soles of the feet. Only the glans penis, the margins of the lips, the external ear, and the nail bed are devoid of sweat glands. Sweat glands are subclassified into two categories: eccrine and apocrine.

The eccrine sweat glands are found in all areas of the skin. Their ducts open directly onto the skin surface. The thin, watery secretion called *sweat* is produced in the basal, coiled portion of the eccrine gland and is released into its narrow duct.

The apocrine sweat glands are larger than eccrine sweat glands and are located in the axillae, anal region, scrotum, and labia majora. Their ducts generally open onto hair follicles. The apocrine glands become active at puberty. In women, they enlarge and recede with each menstrual cycle. Apocrine glands produce a milky sweat that is sometimes broken down by bacteria to produce the characteristic underarm odor.

Functions of the Skin

Protection

The skin covering most of the body is no more than 1 mm thick, but it provides very effective protection against invasion by aqueous, chemical, and mechanical assault; and bacterial and viral pathogens as well as ultraviolet rays (Wysocki, 2016). The thickened skin of the palms and soles protects against the effects of the constant trauma that occurs in these areas.

The stratum corneum, the outer layer of the epidermis, provides the most effective barrier to epidermal water loss to maintain a homeostatic environment and penetration of environmental factors, such as chemicals, microbes, and insect bites. Various lipids are synthesized in the stratum corneum and are the basis for the barrier function of this layer. These are long-chain lipids that are better suited than phospholipids for water resistance. The presence of these lipids in the stratum corneum creates a relatively impermeable barrier for water egress and for the entry of toxins, microbes, and other substances that come in contact with the surface of the skin.

Some substances do penetrate the skin but meet resistance in trying to move through the channels between the cell layers of the stratum corneum. Microbes and fungi, which are part of the body's normal flora, cannot penetrate unless there is a break in the skin barrier.

Sensation

The receptor endings of nerves in the skin allow the body to constantly monitor the conditions of the immediate environment. The primary functions of the receptors in the skin are to sense temperature, pain, light touch, and pressure (or heavy touch). Different nerve endings respond to each of the different stimuli. Although the nerve endings are distributed over the entire body, they are more concentrated in some areas than in others. For example, the fingertips are more densely innervated than the skin on the back.

Fluid Balance

The stratum corneum, the outermost layer of the epidermis, has the capacity to absorb water, thereby preventing an excessive loss of water and electrolytes from the internal body and retaining moisture in the subcutaneous tissues. When skin is damaged, as occurs with a severe burn, large quantities of fluids and electrolytes may be lost rapidly, possibly leading to circulatory collapse, shock, and death.

The skin is not completely impermeable to water. Small amounts of water continuously evaporate from the skin's surface. This evaporation, called *insensible perspiration*, amounts to approximately 600 mL daily in a normal adult. Insensible water loss varies with the body and ambient temperature. In a person with a fever, the fluid loss increases. If the fever is between 38.3°C (101°F) and 39.4°C (103°F), a loss of 500 mL per 24 hours is anticipated; whereas if the temperature if over 39.4°C (over 103°F), a loss of 1,000 mL at a minimum is expected (Porat & Dinarello, 2015).

Thermoregulation

The body continuously produces heat as a result of the metabolism of food, which produces energy. This heat is dissipated primarily through the skin.

Evaporation from the skin aids heat loss by conduction. Heat is conducted through the skin into water molecules on its surface, causing the water to evaporate. The water on the skin surface may be from insensible perspiration, sweat, or the environment.

Under normal conditions, metabolic heat production is balanced by heat loss, and the internal temperature of the body is maintained constant at approximately 37°C (98.6°F).

The rate of heat loss depends primarily on the surface temperature of the skin, which is a function of the blood flow to the skin. Increased blood flow to the skin results in more heat delivered to the skin and a greater rate of heat loss from the body. In contrast, decreased skin blood flow decreases the skin temperature and helps conserve heat for the body. When the temperature of the body begins to fall, as occurs on a cold day, the blood vessels of the skin constrict, thereby reducing heat loss from the body.

Sweating is another process by which the body can regulate the rate of heat loss. Sweating does not occur until the core body temperature exceeds 37°C (98.6°F), regardless of skin temperature. In extremely hot environments, the rate of sweat production may be as high as 1 L per hour. Under some circumstances (e.g., emotional stress), sweating may occur as a reflex and may be unrelated to the need to lose heat from the body.

Vitamin Synthesis

Skin exposed to ultraviolet light can convert substances necessary for synthesizing vitamin D (cholecalciferol). Vitamin D is essential for preventing osteoporosis and rickets, a condition that causes bone deformities and results from a deficiency of vitamin D, calcium, and phosphorus (Box 51-1).

Immune Response Function

Recent research has confirmed a definite action of **Langerhans cells** (specialized cells in the skin) in facilitating the uptake of IgE-associated allergens. This action plays a pivotal role in the pathogenesis of atopic dermatitis and other allergic diseases, such as asthma and allergic rhinitis (Amin, 2012; James, Berger, & Elston, 2016b). These findings support the concept of a systemic regulatory mechanism as a trigger for allergic diseases and suggest that this trigger can be aggravated by local inflammation (Amin, 2012; James et al., 2016b).

Nursing Alert
Localized opening of the normally tight endothelial junctions leads to interstitial edema in the deep layers of the skin and subcutaneous tissue of the face, tongue, hands, face, and genitalia. Occasionally, the tongue or pharynx can be involved. It may be related to allergy or idiopathic in nature. Histamine that is contained in mast cells is released with a variety or immunologic, nonimmunologic, physical, and/or chemical stimuli. The released histamine causes hyperpermeability of the microvessels, which allows fluid to leak out into affected areas and causes the characteristic appearance. Nurses observe for the tense swelling of the lips that develops rapidly. Angioedema is frequently associated with an allergic reaction and may present with hives. If shortness of breath is

BOX 51-1

Nursing Research

Bridging the Gap to Evidence-Based Practice

Colantonio, S., Bracken, M. B, & Beecker, J. (2014). The association of indoor tanning and melanoma in adults: Systematic review and meta-analysis. *Journal of the American Academy of Dermatology, 70*(5), 847–857.

Purpose

The authors sought to update the evidence of the association of melanoma and indoor tanning, focusing on frequency of use and exposure to newer tanning beds. Databases searched included: Scopus, MEDLINE, and Cumulative Index to Nursing and Allied Health Literature in 2013. All observational studies that included patients with melanoma who had tanned indoors were included. Odds ratios (OR) with 95% confidence intervals (CI) were extracted and combined using generic inverse variance methods assuming a random effects model. In all, 31 studies were included with data available on 14,956 melanoma cases and 233,106 controls.

Findings

Compared with never using, the OR for melanoma associated with ever using indoor tanning beds was 1.16 (95% CI 1.05–1.28).

Similar findings were identified in recent studies with enrollment occurring in the year 2000 onward (OR 1.22, 95% CI 1.03–1.45) and in subjects attending more than 10 tanning sessions (OR 1.34, 95% CI 1.05–1.71). Using tanning beds is associated with a subsequent melanoma diagnosis. Exposure from more than 10 tanning sessions is most strongly associated, and there was no statistically significant difference in this association before and after 2000, suggesting that newer tanning technology is not safer than older models.

Nursing Implications

This study supports the relationship between indoor tanning and melanoma risk and suggests that public education is needed to correct the misunderstanding of the negative effects of indoor tanning. Nurses can play a pivotal role in educational efforts.

also noted, the medical provider must be contacted immediately as severe swelling of the airway and tongue can be life-threatening.

Gerontologic Considerations

The skin undergoes many physiologic changes associated with normal aging. A lifetime of excessive sun exposure, systemic diseases, and poor nutrition can increase the range of skin problems and the rapidity with which they appear. In addition, certain medications (e.g., antihistamines, antibiotics, diuretics) are photosensitizing and increase the damage that results from sun exposure. The outcome is an increasing vulnerability to injury and to certain diseases. Skin problems are common among older people. Refer to Table 51-1 for skin changes in the elderly.

Many skin changes and lesions are part of normal aging. Recognizing these lesions enables the examiner to assist the patient to feel less anxious about changes in skin. Box 51-2 summarizes some changes that are expected to appear as the skin ages. These are normal and require no special attention unless the skin becomes infected or irritated.

ASSESSMENT

Some conditions may subject the patient to a protracted illness, leading to feelings of depression, frustration, self-consciousness, poor self-image, and rejection. Itching and skin irritations, which are features of many skin diseases,

may be a constant annoyance. These discomforts may result in loss of sleep, anxiety, and depression, all of which reinforce the general distress and fatigue that frequently accompany skin disorders.

For patients suffering such physical and psychological discomforts, the nurse needs to provide understanding, explanations of the problem, appropriate instructions related to treatment, nursing support, and encouragement. It is imperative to overcome any aversion that may be felt when caring for patients with unattractive skin disorders. The nurse should show no sign of hesitancy when approaching patients with skin disorders. Such hesitancy only reinforces the psychological trauma of the disorder.

Because patients with skin conditions may be viewed negatively by others, these patients may become distraught and avoid interaction with people. Skin conditions can lead to disfigurement, isolation, job loss, and economic hardship.

Health History

During the health history interview, the nurse asks about any family and personal history of skin allergies; allergic reactions to food, medications, and chemicals; previous skin problems; and skin cancer. The names of cosmetics, soaps, shampoos, and other personal hygiene products are obtained if there have been any recent skin problems noticed with the use of these products. The health history contains specific information about the onset, signs and symptoms, location, and duration of any pain, itching, rash, or other discomfort experienced by the patient. The nurse inquires about tattoos

TABLE 51-1 GERONTOLOGIC CONSIDERATIONS / Age-Related Changes of the Skin

Structural Changes	Associated Physical Findings
Thinning at the junction of the dermis and epidermis result in fewer anchoring sites between the two skin layers, which means that even minor injury or stress to the epidermis can cause it to shear away from the dermis.	Increased vulnerability of aged skin to trauma
The epidermis and dermis thin and flatten.	Wrinkles, sags, and overlapping skin folds
Loss of the subcutaneous tissue substances of elastin, collagen, and fat	Decreased protection and cushioning of underlying tissues and organs, decreased muscle tone, and loss of the insulating properties of fat.
Cellular replacement slows as a result of aging, and there is thinning of the dermal layers.	Skin becomes fragile and transparent.
The blood supply to the skin also changes with age. Vessels, especially the capillary loops, decrease in number and size.	Vascular changes are associated with delayed wound healing.
Sweat and sebaceous glands decrease in number and functional capacity.	Dry and scaly skin
Reduced hormonal levels of androgens	Associated with declining sebaceous gland function
Hair growth gradually diminishes, especially over the lower legs and dorsum of the feet. Thinning is common in the scalp, axilla, and pubic areas.	Decreased hair growth, hair loss
Photoaging (damage from excessive sun exposure)	Profound wrinkling; increased loss of elasticity; mottled, pigmented areas; cutaneous atrophy; and benign or malignant lesions

because they involve the injection of ink into the dermis of the skin and are associated with an increased risk for blood-borne disease, skin infections, and allergic reactions. Box 51-3 lists selected questions useful in obtaining appropriate information.

Benign Changes in Elderly Skin

- Cherry angiomas (bright red "moles")
- Diminished hair, especially on scalp and pubic area
- Dyschromias (color variations):
  - Solar lentigo (liver spots)
  - Melasma (dark discoloration of the skin)
  - Lentigines (freckles)
- Neurodermatitis (itchy spots)
- Seborrheic keratoses (crusty brown "stuck-on" patches)
- Spider angiomas (network of dilated capillaries radiating from a central arteriole)
- Telangiectasias (red marks on skin caused by stretching of the superficial blood vessels)
- Wrinkles (a small fold, ridge, or crease in the skin)
- Xerosis (dryness)
- Xanthelasma (yellowish waxy deposits on upper and lower eyelids)
- Ichthyosis (fish scale appearance of the skin)

Unfolding Patient Stories: Vincent Brody • Part 2

Recall from Chapter 2 Vincent Brody, with chronic obstructive pulmonary disease (COPD), who spends most of the day in a recliner chair smoking and has a poor nutritional intake due to shortness of breath. He is admitted to the hospital with COPD exacerbation. What are the factors related to his diagnosis? What background information can influence skin breakdown? Describe the skin assessment performed by the nurse.

Care for Vincent and other patients in a realistic virtual environment: *vSim for Nursing* (thepoint.lww.com/vSimMedicalSurgical). Practice documenting these patients' care in DocuCare (thepoint.lww.com/DocuCareEHR).

Physical Assessment

Assessment of the skin involves the entire skin area, including the mucous membranes, scalp, hair, and nails. The skin is a reflection of a person's overall health, and alterations commonly correspond to disease in other organ systems. Inspection and palpation are techniques commonly used in examining the skin. The room must be well lighted and

---

BOX 51-3

Health History Related to Skin Disorders

Patient history relevant to skin disorders may be obtained by asking the following questions:

- When did you first notice this skin problem? (Also investigate duration and intensity)
- Has it occurred previously?
- Are there any other symptoms?
- What site was first affected?
- What did the rash or lesion look like when it first appeared?
- Where and how fast did it spread?
- Do you have any itching, burning, tingling, or crawling sensations?
- Is there any loss of sensation?
- Is the problem worse at a particular time or season?
- How do you think it started?
- Do you have a history of hay fever, asthma, hives, eczema, or allergies?
- Who in your family has skin problems or rashes?
- Did the eruptions appear after certain foods were eaten? Which foods?
- When the problem occurred, had you recently consumed alcohol?
- What relation do you think there may be between a specific event and the outbreak of the rash or lesion?
- What medications are you taking?
- What topical medication (ointment, cream, salve) have you put on the lesion (including over-the-counter medications)?
- What skin products or cosmetics do you use?
- What is your occupation?
- What in your immediate environment (plants, animals, chemicals, infections) might be precipitating this disorder? Is there anything new, or are there any changes in the environment?
- Does anything touching your skin cause a rash?
- How has this affected you (or your life)?
- Is there anything else you wish to talk about in regard to this disorder?

---

warm. A penlight may be used to highlight lesions. The patient completely disrobes and is adequately draped. Gloves are worn during skin examination if a rash or lesions are to be palpated.

The general appearance of the skin is assessed by observing color, temperature, moisture or dryness, skin texture (rough or smooth), lesions, vascularity, mobility, and the condition of the hair and nails. Skin turgor, possible edema, and elasticity are assessed by palpation.

Assessing Color

Skin color varies from person to person and ranges from ivory to deep brown to almost pure black. The skin of exposed portions of the body, especially in sunny, warm climates, tends to be more pigmented than the rest of the body.

Almost every process that occurs on the skin causes some color change. For example, **hypopigmentation** may be caused by a fungal infection, eczema, or **vitiligo; hyperpigmentation** can occur after sun injury, as a result of aging, or with disease processes such as Addison because of stimulation of melanocyte-stimulating hormone. The vasodilation that occurs with fever, sunburn, and inflammation produces a pink or reddish hue to the skin. Pallor is an absence of or a decrease in normal skin color and vascularity and is best observed in the conjunctivae or around the mouth. Assessing for pallor in the palms and soles of patients with dark skin may be helpful (Bickley & Szilagyi, 2013).

In people with dark skin, melanin is produced at a faster rate and in larger quantities than in people with light skin. Healthy dark skin has a reddish base or undertone. The buccal mucosa, tongue, lips, and nails normally are pink.

Dark pigment responds with discoloration after injury or inflammation, and patients with dark skin more often experience postinflammatory hyperpigmentation than do those with lighter skin. The hyperpigmentation eventually fades but may require months to a year to do so. Table 51-2 provides an overview of color changes in people who are light-skinned and dark-skinned.

 Concept Mastery Alert

Pallor can best be determined by examining conjunctivae or around the mouth. Nail beds are not necessarily a reliable area when assessing for pallor.

In general, people with dark skin suffer the same skin conditions as those with light skin. They are less likely to have skin cancer but more likely to have keloid or scar formation and disorders resulting from occlusion or blockage of hair follicles.

Erythema

Erythema is redness of the skin caused by the congestion of capillaries. To determine possible inflammation, the skin is palpated for increased warmth and for smoothness (i.e., edema) or hardness (i.e., intracellular infiltration).

Cyanosis

Cyanosis is the bluish discoloration that results from a lack of oxygen in the blood. It appears with shock or with respiratory or circulatory compromise. In people with light skin, cyanosis manifests as a bluish hue to the lips, fingertips, and nail beds (Fig. 51-2). In people who are dark-skinned, the

TABLE **51-2** Color Changes in Light and Dark Skin

Etiology	Light Skin	Dark Skin
Pallor		
Anemia: Decreased hematocrit Shock: Decreased perfusion, vasoconstriction	Generalized pallor	Brown skin appears yellow-brown, dull; black skin appears ashen gray, dull. (Observe areas with least pigmentation: conjunctivae, mucous membranes)
Local arterial insufficiency	Marked localized pallor (lower extremities, especially when elevated)	Ashen gray, dull; cool to palpation
Albinism: Total absence of pigment melanin	Whitish pink	Tan, cream, white
Vitiligo: A condition characterized by destruction of the melanocytes in circumscribed areas of the skin (may be localized or widespread)	Patchy, milky white spots, often symmetric bilaterally	Same
Cyanosis		
Increased amount of unoxygenated hemoglobin:	Dusky blue	Dark but dull, lifeless; only severe cyanosis is apparent in skin. (Observe conjunctivae, oral mucosa, nail beds)
Central: Chronic heart and lung diseases cause arterial desaturation	Bluish discoloration of skin, mucous membranes and nail beds	
Peripheral: Exposure to cold, anxiety	Nail beds dusky	
Erythema		
Hyperemia: Increased blood flow through engorged arterial vessels, as in inflammation, fever, alcohol intake, blushing	Red, bright pink	Purplish tinge, but difficult to see because epidermal melanin may alter disease presentation by masking erythema (Palpate for increased warmth with inflammation, taut skin, and hardening of deep tissues)
Polycythemia: Increased red blood cells, capillary stasis	Ruddy blue in face, oral mucosa, conjunctivae, hands and feet	Well concealed by pigment. (Observe for redness in lips)
Carbon monoxide poisoning	Bright, cherry red in face and upper torso	Cherry red nail beds, lips, and oral mucosa
Stasis dermatitis (venous stasis) is poor venous return in the lower extremities causing hemosiderin staining and cracking of the skin (skin breakdown) that causes stasis ulcers or venous ulcers.	Brown or rusty discoloration of the skin resulting from a buildup of hemosiderin (iron-containing pigment derived from the breakdown of hemoglobin) in the interstitial fluid	More difficult to detect signs of venous insufficiency such as hemosiderin staining (reddish, brown color) (James et al., 2016a; Reddy, Lenzy, Brown, & Gilchrest, 2013)
Venous disease	Edema, hyperpigmentation surrounding the skin (reddish or brown due to hemosiderin), warmth at feet with palpable pulses (exception if no coexisting arterial disease)	Edema, hyperpigmentation surrounding the skin (reddish or brown due to hemosiderin), warmth at feet with palpable pulses (exception if no coexisting arterial disease)

(continued on page 1450)

TABLE 51-2 Color Changes in Light and Dark Skin (*continued*)

Etiology	Light Skin	Dark Skin
Jaundice		
Increased serum bilirubin concentration (>2.5–3 mg/dL) due to liver dysfunction or hemolysis, as after severe burns or some infections	Yellow first in sclerae, hard palate, and mucous membranes; then over skin	Check sclerae for yellow near limbus; do not mistake normal yellowish fatty deposits in the periphery under eyelids for jaundice. (Jaundice is best noted at junction of hard and soft palate, on palms)
Carotenemia: Increased level of serum carotene from ingestion of large amounts of carotene-rich foods	Yellow-orange tinge in forehead, palms and soles, and nasolabial folds, but no yellowing in sclerae or mucous membranes	Yellow-orange tinge in palms and soles
Uremia: Kidney failure causes retained urochrome pigments in the blood	Orange-green or gray overlying pallor of anemia; may also have ecchymoses and purpura	Easily masked. (Rely on laboratory and clinical findings)
Brown-Tan		
Addison disease: Cortisol deficiency stimulates increased melanin production	Bronzed appearance, an "external tan"; most apparent around nipples, perineum, genitalia, and pressure points (inner thighs, buttocks, elbows, axillae)	Easily masked. (Rely on laboratory and clinical findings)
Café-au-lait spots: Caused by increased melanin pigment in basal cell layer	Tan to light brown, irregularly shaped, oval patch with well-defined borders	Often not visible in a person with very dark skin

skin may appear blue and dull or assume a gray hue. The term *central cyanosis* refers to desaturation of oxygen in the blood and this is reflected in the mucous membranes and skin, whereas *peripheral cyanosis* implies increased oxygen extraction from the blood because of sluggish blood flow, or vasoconstriction related to exposure to cold environments, which is reflected in the extremities. The nurse assesses the patient for additional indications of decreased tissue perfusion, including cold, clammy skin; a rapid, thready pulse; and rapid, shallow respirations. The conjunctivae of the eyelids are examined for pallor and **petechiae**.

Nursing Alert
Cyanosis is a late sign and symptom of hypoxemia, as 5 g of hemoglobin (normal level is 15 g/dL) are desaturated before cyanosis is evident. In cases of carbon monoxide poisoning, the level of carboxyhemoglobin does not affect color; therefore, the patient may be profoundly hypoxemic without evidence of cyanosis.

Jaundice
Jaundice, a yellowing of the skin, is directly related to elevations in serum bilirubin and is often first observed in the sclerae and mucous membranes (see Fig. 51-2). The term *icterus* is used to describe yellowing of the sclerae (white of the eyes).

Striae
The nurse assesses for striae (stretch marks), which occurs when the elastic fibers in the reticular dermis rupture. Striae are seen in conditions of weight gain, such as pregnancy and obesity, in muscle building, with prolonged use of oral or topical corticosteroids, or in Cushing syndrome (increased adrenal cortical activity) (see Chapter 31).

Assessing Rash

In instances of pruritus (i.e., itching), the patient is asked to indicate which areas of the body are involved. The skin is then stretched gently to decrease the reddish tone and make the rash more visible. Pointing a penlight laterally across the skin may highlight the rash, making it easier to observe. The differences in skin texture are then assessed by running the

FIGURE 51-2 Examples of skin color changes: the bluish tint of cyanosis (*left*) and the yellow hue of jaundice (*right*).

tips of the fingers lightly over the skin. The borders of the rash may be palpable. The patient's mouth and ears are included in the examination (sometimes rubeola, or measles, causes a red cast to appear on the ears). The patient's temperature is assessed, and the lymph nodes are palpated.

Assessing Skin Lesions

Skin lesions are the most prominent characteristics of dermatologic conditions. They vary in size, shape, and cause and are classified according to their appearance and origin. Skin lesions can be described as primary or secondary. Primary lesions are the initial lesions and are characteristic of the disease itself. Secondary lesions result from external causes, such as scratching, trauma, infections, or changes caused by wound healing. Depending on the stage of development, skin lesions are further categorized according to type and appearance (Table 51-3). The degree of pigmentation of the patient's skin may affect the appearance of a lesion. In patients with darker skin, lesions may be black,

TABLE 51-3 Primary and Secondary Skin Lesions

Lesion	Description	Examples
Primary Lesions		
Macule, patch Macule Patch	Flat, nonpalpable skin color change (color may be brown, white, tan, purple, red) • *Macule:* less than 1 cm, circumscribed border • *Patch:* greater than 1 cm, may have irregular border	Freckles, flat moles, petechia, rubella, vitiligo, port wine stains, ecchymosis
Papule, plaque Papule Plaque	Elevated, palpable, solid mass with a circumscribed border Plaque may be coalesced papules with flat top • *Papule:* less than 0.5 cm • *Plaque:* greater than 0.5 cm	*Papules:* Elevated nevi, warts, lichen planus *Plaques:* Psoriasis, actinic keratosis
Nodule, tumor Tumor	Elevated, palpable, solid mass that extends deeper into the dermis than a papule • *Nodule:* 0.5–2 cm; circumscribed • *Tumor:* greater than 1–2 cm; tumors do not always have sharp borders	*Nodules:* Lipoma, squamous cell carcinoma, poorly absorbed injection, dermatofibroma *Tumors:* Larger lipoma, carcinoma
Vesicle, bulla Bulla Vesicle	Circumscribed, elevated, palpable mass containing serous fluid • *Vesicle:* less than 0.5 cm • *Bulla:* greater than 0.5 cm	*Vesicles:* Herpes simplex/zoster, chickenpox, poison ivy, second-degree burn (blister) *Bulla:* Pemphigus, contact dermatitis, large burn blisters, poison ivy, bullous impetigo
Wheal Wheal	Elevated mass with transient borders; often irregular; size and color vary Caused by movement of serous fluid into the dermis; does not contain free fluid in a cavity (as, for example, a vesicle does)	Urticaria (hives), insect bites

(continued on page 1452)

TABLE 51-3 Primary and Secondary Skin Lesions (*continued*)

Lesion	Description	Examples
Pustule Pustule	Pus-filled vesicle or bulla	Acne, impetigo, furuncles, carbuncles
Cyst Cyst	Encapsulated fluid-filled or semisolid mass in the subcutaneous tissue or dermis	Sebaceous cyst, epidermoid cysts
Secondary Lesions		
Erosion Erosion	Loss of superficial epidermis that does not extend to dermis; depressed, moist area	Ruptured vesicles, scratch marks
Ulcer Ulcer	Skin loss or damage at or extending past the epidermis. May include necrotic tissue development, bleeding or scarring	Stasis ulcer of venous insufficiency, pressure ulcer
Fissure Fissure	Linear crack in the skin that may extend to dermis	Chapped lips or hands, athlete foot
Scales Scales	Flakes secondary to desquamated, dead epithelium that may adhere to skin surface; color varies (silvery, white); texture varies (thick, fine)	Dandruff, psoriasis, dry skin, pityriasis rosea

Lesion	Description	Examples
Crust Crust	Dried residue of serum, blood, or pus on skin surface Large, adherent crust is a scab	Residue left after vesicle rupture: impetigo, herpes, eczema
Scar (cicatrix) Scar	Skin mark left after healing of a wound or lesion; represents replacement by connective tissue of the injured tissue • *Young scars:* red or purple • *Mature scars:* white or glistening	Healed wound or surgical incision
Keloid Keloid	Hypertrophied scar tissue secondary to excessive collagen formation during healing; elevated, irregular, red Greater incidence among African Americans	Keloid of ear piercing or surgical incision
Atrophy Atrophy	Thin, dry, transparent appearance of epidermis; loss of surface markings; secondary to loss of collagen and elastin; underlying vessels may be visible	Aged skin, arterial insufficiency
Lichenification Lichenification	Thickening and roughening of the skin or accentuated skin markings that may be secondary to repeated rubbing, irritation, scratching	Contact dermatitis

maroon, purple, or gray instead of the tan or red seen in patients with light skin.

A preliminary assessment of the eruption or lesion helps identify the type of **dermatosis** and indicates whether the lesion is primary or secondary. At the same time, the anatomic distribution of the eruption should be observed because certain diseases affect certain sites of the body and are distributed in characteristic patterns and shapes (Figs. 51-3 and 51-4). To determine the extent of the regional distribution, the left and right sides of the body should be compared while the color and shape of the lesions are assessed. After observation, the lesions are palpated to determine their texture, shape, and border and to see if they are soft and filled with fluid or hard and fixed to the surrounding tissue.

A disposable metric ruler is used to measure the size of the lesions so that any further extension can be compared with this baseline measurement. Skin lesions are described clearly and in detail on the patient's health record, using precise terminology.

Characteristics of Lesions

After the characteristic distribution of the lesions has been determined, the following information should be obtained and described clearly and in detail:

• Color of the lesion
• Any redness, heat, pain, or swelling
• Size and location of the involved area

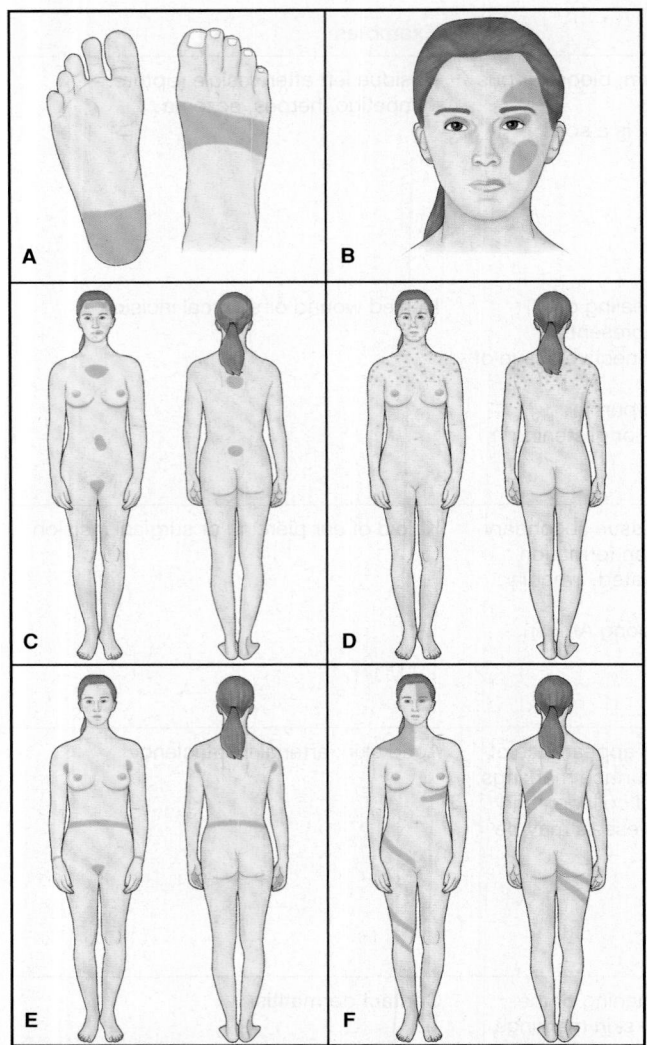

FIGURE 51-3 Anatomic distribution of common skin disorders.
A. Contact dermatitis (shoes). **B.** Contact dermatitis (cosmetics, perfumes, earrings). **C.** Seborrheic dermatitis. **D.** Acne. **E.** Scabies. **F.** Herpes zoster (shingles).

- Pattern of eruption (e.g., macular, papular, scaling, oozing, discrete, confluent)
- Distribution of the lesion (e.g., bilateral, symmetric, linear, circular)

If acute open wounds or lesions are found on inspection of the skin, a comprehensive assessment should be made and documented. This assessment should address the following issues:

- *Wound bed:* Inspect for necrotic, slough, granulation or epithelial tissue, exudate, color, and odor.
- *Wound edges and margins:* Observe for undermining (i.e., extension of the wound under the surface skin) or epibole (rolled edges), and evaluate for condition.
- *Wound size:* Measure in centimeters (cm), as appropriate, to determine diameter and depth of the wound and surrounding erythema.

- *Surrounding skin:* Assess for color, suppleness and moisture, irritation, induration (abnormal firmness of tissue), and scaling.

Assessing Vascularity

After the color of the skin has been evaluated and lesions have been inspected, an assessment of vascular changes in the skin is performed. A description of vascular changes includes location, distribution, color, size, and the presence of pulsations. Common vascular changes include petechiae, ecchymoses, Telangiectasia (spider veins), angiomas, and venous stars. Petechiae are small (less than 2 mm in diameter) lesions that are red or purple in color. They are associated with broken capillaries or indicative of platelet abnormalities, specifically thrombocytopenia (low platelet counts).

Assessing Hydration

Skin moisture, temperature, and texture are assessed primarily by palpation. The turgor (i.e., elasticity) of the skin, which decreases in normal aging, may be a factor in assessing the hydration status of a patient. The forearm, sternum, or forehead is recommended for assessing turgor in the elderly, rather than the hand, owing to the loss of elasticity with aging. The nurse pinches the skin of the sternum with the thumb and index finger, creating a tent of skin. Upon releasing it, normal

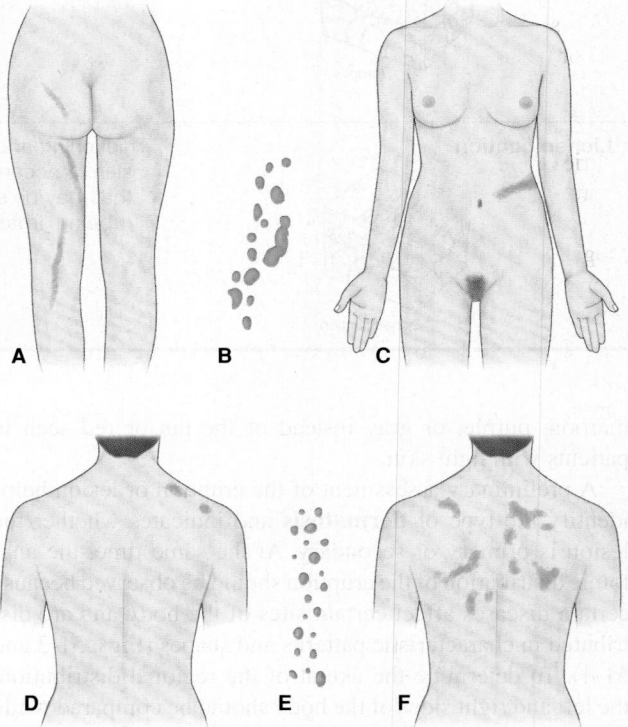

FIGURE 51-4 Skin lesion configurations. **A.** Linear (in a line). **B.** Annular and arciform (circular or arcing). **C.** Zosteriform (linear along a nerve route). **D.** Grouped (clustered). **E.** Discrete (separate and distinct). **F.** Confluent (merged).

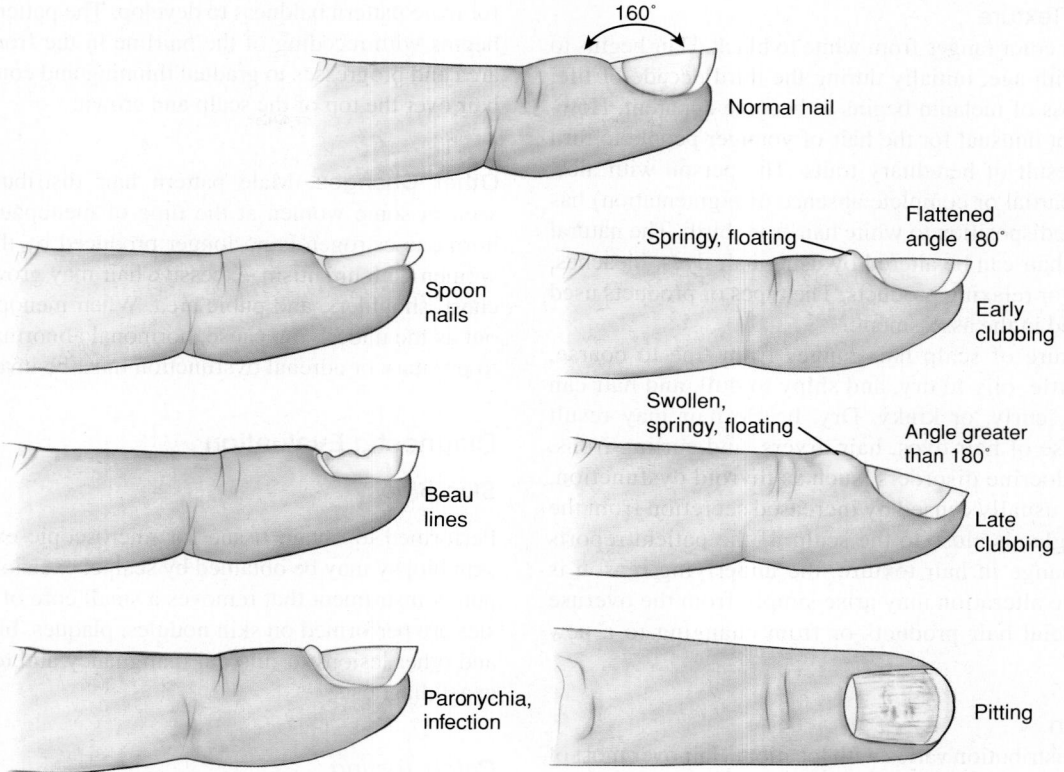

FIGURE 51-5 Common nail disorders.

turgid skin promptly resumes its shape, whereas a persistent fold or tent is associated with fluid volume deficit.

Assessing the Nails

A brief inspection of the nails includes observation of configuration, color, and consistency. Many alterations in the nail or nail bed reflect local or systemic abnormalities in progress or resulting from past events (Fig. 51-5). Transverse depressions known as *Beau lines* in the nails may reflect retarded growth of the nail matrix because of severe illness or, more commonly, local trauma. Ridging, hypertrophy, and other changes may also be visible with local trauma. Paronychia, an inflammation of the skin around the nail, is usually accompanied by tenderness and erythema. The angle between the normal nail and its base is 160 degrees. When palpated, the nail base is usually firm. Clubbing is manifested by a straightening of the normal angle (at least 180 degrees) and softening of the nail base (Box 51-4). The softened area feels sponge-like when palpated.

Assessing the Hair

Hair assessment involves inspection and palpation. Gloves are worn by the examiner, and the examination room should be well lighted. Separating the hair so that the condition of the skin underneath can be easily seen, the nurse assesses color, texture, and distribution. The wooden end of a cotton swab can be used to make small parts in the hair, so that the scalp can be inspected. Any abnormal lesions, evidence of itching, inflammation, scaling, or signs of infestation (i.e., lice or mites) are documented.

BOX 51-4

Assessing for Clubbing

Although the mechanism is unknown for the characteristic changes to the nails, clubbing is frequently associated with hypoxemia. The nail changes are painless and usually found bilaterally. If the underlying cause is removed, clubbing is reversible. To assess for clubbing, have the patient place both forefinger nails together and look between them. If a small diamond space is visible at the nail base then the nails are *not* clubbed (Schamroth sign).

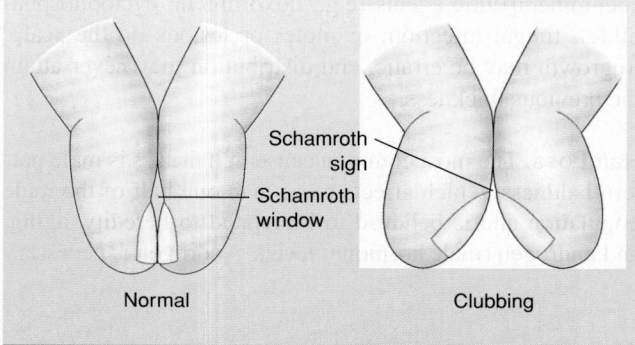

Color and Texture

Natural hair color ranges from white to black. Hair begins to turn gray with age, initially during the third decade of life, when the loss of melanin begins to become apparent. However, it is not unusual for the hair of younger people to turn gray as a result of hereditary traits. The person with albinism (i.e., partial or complete absence of pigmentation) has a genetic predisposition to white hair from birth. The natural state of the hair can be altered by using hair dyes, bleaches, and curling or relaxing products. The types of products used are identified in the assessment.

The texture of scalp hair ranges from fine to coarse, silky to brittle, oily to dry, and shiny to dull, and hair can be straight, curly, or kinky. Dry, brittle hair may result from overuse of hair dyes, hair dryers, and curling irons, or from endocrine disorders, such as thyroid dysfunction. Oily hair is usually caused by increased secretion from the sebaceous glands close to the scalp. If the patient reports a recent change in hair texture, the underlying reason is pursued; the alteration may arise simply from the overuse of commercial hair products or from changing to a new shampoo.

Distribution

Body hair distribution varies with location. Hair over most of the body is fine, except in the axillae and pubic areas, where it is coarse. Pubic hair, which develops at puberty, forms a diamond shape extending up to the umbilicus in boys and men. Female pubic hair resembles an inverted triangle. If the pattern found is more characteristic of the opposite gender, it may indicate an endocrine problem and further investigation is in order. Racial differences in hair are expected, such as straight hair in Asians and curly, coarser hair in people of African descent.

Men tend to have more body and facial hair than do women. Loss of hair, or alopecia, can occur over the entire body or be confined to a specific area. Scalp hair loss may be localized to patchy areas or may range from generalized thinning to total baldness. When assessing scalp hair loss, it is important to investigate the underlying cause with the patient. Patchy hair loss may be from habitual hair pulling or twisting; excessive traction on the hair (e.g., braiding too tightly); excessive use of dyes, straighteners, and oils; chemotherapeutic agents (e.g., doxorubicin, cyclophosphamide); fungal infection; or moles or lesions on the scalp. Regrowth may be erratic, and distribution may never attain the previous thickness.

Hair Loss. The most common cause of hair loss is male pattern baldness, which affects more than one half of the male population and is believed to be related to heredity, aging, and androgen (male hormone) levels. Androgen is necessary for male pattern baldness to develop. The pattern of hair loss begins with receding of the hairline in the frontal-temporal area and progresses to gradual thinning and complete loss of hair over the top of the scalp and crown.

Other Changes. Male pattern hair distribution may be seen in some women at the time of menopause, when the hormone estrogen is no longer produced by the ovaries. In women with hirsutism, excessive hair may grow on the face, chest, shoulders, and pubic area. When menopause is ruled out as the underlying cause, hormonal abnormalities related to pituitary or adrenal dysfunction must be investigated.

Diagnostic Evaluation

Skin Biopsy

Performed to obtain tissue for microscopic examination, a skin biopsy may be obtained by scalpel excision or by a skin punch instrument that removes a small core of tissue. Biopsies are performed on skin nodules, plaques, blisters, ulcers, and other lesions to rule out malignancy and to establish an exact diagnosis.

Patch Testing

Performed to identify substances to which the patient has developed an allergy, patch testing involves applying the suspected allergens to normal skin under occlusive patches. The development of redness, fine elevations, or itching is considered a weak positive reaction; fine blisters, papules, and severe itching indicate a moderately positive reaction; and blisters, pain, and ulceration indicate a strong positive reaction.

Skin Scrapings

Tissue samples are scraped from suspected fungal lesions with a scalpel blade moistened with oil, so that the scraped skin adheres to the blade. The scraped material is transferred to a glass slide, covered with a coverslip, and examined microscopically. The spores and hyphae of dermatophyte infections, as well as infestations such as scabies, can be visualized.

Clinical Photographs

Photographs are taken to document the nature and extent of the skin condition and are used to determine progress or improvement resulting from treatment. They are sometimes used to track the status of moles to document if the characteristics of the mole are changing.

CHAPTER REVIEW

Critical Thinking Exercises

1. You are caring for an elderly African American woman who is hospitalized with a stroke. She has hemiparesis of her right arm and leg and is receiving physical therapy. Because of the patient's age and her limited mobility, what would the patient be at high risk for and what would your assessment include in examining her skin?

2. You are volunteering at the skin cancer screening booth at a community health fair. A middle-aged man approaches you about a skin lesion. He states that he is a landscaper and works long hours all year long. Discuss the possible types of lesions that can be found and how you would describe the lesion after assessing it.

3. An 88-year-old male patient is admitted to the hospital after a visit to his provider's office. Initial nursing assessment reveals that he has a poor skin turgor. What effects will this have on skin integrity?

NCLEX-Style Review Questions

1. A 90-year-old patient with multiple medical problems is admitted to the hospital's geriatric care unit. The nursing assessment reveals weight loss, poor capillary perfusion, and delayed skin turgor. These findings should alert the gerontologic nurse to which condition?
   a. Aspiration
   b. Fluid volume deficit
   c. Pressure ulcers
   d. Contractures

Try these additional resources, available at **http://thepoint.lww.com/Honan2e**, to enhance your learning and understanding of this chapter:
- NCLEX-Style Student Review Questions
- Journal Articles

2. During assessment, what does the nurse recognize as a normal function of the skin?
   a. Thermal regulation
   b. Vitamin E production
   c. Vitamin C production
   d. Releasing of carbon dioxide

3. A patient has returned to the room postoperatively. The nurse examines the patient's nail beds to assess for what condition?
   a. Cyanosis
   b. Respiratory rate
   c. Edema
   d. Cellulitis

4. What does the nurse look for when assessing the characteristics of a lesion? Select all that apply.
   a. Heat
   b. Claudication
   c. Size
   d. Erythema
   e. Pattern

5. What changes in the older adult best describe why aging process increases risk for impairment in skin integrity?
   a. Epidermal cells thicken
   b. Dermal thickness increases
   c. Decreased elastin, collagen, and fat
   d. Maceration

REFERENCES AND SELECTED READINGS

References and selected readings associated with this chapter can be found on the website that accompanies the book. Visit **http://thepoint.lww.com/Honan2e** to access the references and other additional resources associated with this chapter.

Nursing Management: Patients with Dermatologic Problems

Commander Patina S. Walton-Battle

Learning Objectives

After reading this chapter, you will be able to:

1. Describe the general management of the patient with an abnormal skin condition.
2. Describe general principles of wound care
3. Identify stages of pressure ulcers
4. Discuss the general management of a patient with pruritus
5. Describe the health education needs of the patient with infections of the skin and parasitic skin diseases.
6. Discuss care of patients with noninfectious, inflammatory dermatoses, including psoriasis.
7. Describe nursing management of the patient with skin cancer.
8. Describe characteristics of the various types of Kaposi sarcoma.

Regardless of the environment where they work, nurses manage skin care. Additionally, nurses predict patients who will be at risk for skin problems, assess skin changes, and intervene to prevent injury and maintain skin viability. As nurses, it is also important to utilize preventative practices to reduce transmission of infection or further injury, and maintain skin viability.

GENERAL MANAGEMENT OF SKIN DISORDERS

Nursing management of skin disorders includes protecting the skin, preventing infection, reversing inflammation, administering therapeutic baths, and administering medications.

PROVIDING SKIN CARE

Protecting the Skin

Some skin problems are aggravated by bathing. The essence of skin care in bathing a patient with skin problems is as follows:

- A mild, lipid-free soap or soap substitute is used.
- The area is rinsed completely and blotted dry with a soft cloth.
- Deodorant soaps are avoided.

Special care is necessary when changing dressings. Pledgets (small compress of material, usually cotton or gauze) saturated with oil, sterile saline or water, wound cleansers, or another prescribed solution help to loosen crusts, remove exudates, or free an adherent dry dressing.

Preventing Infection

Potentially infectious skin lesions should be regarded strictly as such, and proper precautions should be observed until the diagnosis is established. Most lesions with purulent drainage contain infectious material. The health care provider must adhere to standard contact precautions carried out according to Occupational Safety and Health Administration (OSHA) regulations.

> **Nursing Alert**
> The nurse is aware that, for patients with contact precautions, a gown and gloves should be worn for all interactions that may involve contact with the patient or potentially contaminated areas in the patient's environment. The personal protective equipment (PPE) is donned before room entry and discarded before exiting (Denton, Topping, & Humphreys, 2016).

Reversing Inflammation

The type of skin lesion (e.g., oozing, infected, or dry) usually determines the type of local medication or treatment that is prescribed. As a rule, if the skin is acutely inflamed (i.e., hot), erythematous (red), and edematous (swollen) and draining, it is best to apply wet or specialty dressings and/or soothing lotions. For chronic conditions in which the skin surface is dry and scaly, water-soluble emulsions, creams, ointments, and pastes are used. The therapy is modified as the responses of the skin indicate. The patient and the nurse should note whether the medication or dressings seem to irritate the skin. The success or failure of therapy usually depends on adequate instruction and motivation of the patient and family, and the support of health care personnel promotes adherence to instructions.

Administering Therapeutic Baths (Balneotherapy)

Baths or soaks, known as **balneotherapy**, are useful when large areas of skin are affected. The baths remove crusts, scales, and old medications and relieve the inflammation and pruritus (itching) that accompany acute dermatoses. Additional information about therapeutic baths is given in Box 52-1.

Administering Pharmacologic Therapy

Topical Preparations

Table 52-1 lists some commonly used topical preparations.

BOX 52-1
Therapeutic Baths

Types of Therapeutic Baths

Bath Solution	Effects and Uses
Water	Same effect as wet dressings
Saline	Used for widely disseminated lesions
Colloidal (Aveeno, oatmeal)	Antipruritic, soothing
Sodium bicarbonate (baking soda)	Cooling
Starch	Soothing
Medicated tars	Psoriasis and chronic eczema
Bath oils	Antipruritic and emollient action; acute and subacute generalized eczematous eruptions

Nursing Interventions

- Fill the tub half full.
- Keep the water at a comfortable temperature.
- Do not allow the water to cool excessively.
- Use a bath mat because *medications added to the bath can cause the tub to be slippery.*
- Apply an emollient cream to damp skin after the bath if lubrication is desired.
- Because tars are volatile, the bath area should be well ventilated.
- Maintain a constant room temperature without drafts.
- Encourage the patient to wear light, loose clothing after the bath.

TABLE 52-1 Common Topical Preparations and Medications

Preparation	Product Name
Bath preparations	
With tar	Balnetar, Doak Oil, Lavatar
With colloidal oatmeal	Aveeno Oilated Bath Powder
With oatmeal and mineral oil	Aveeno Bath Oil, Nutra Soothe
With mineral oil	Nutraderm Bath Oil, Lubath, Alpha-Keri Bath Oil
Moisturizer creams	Acid Mantle Cream, Curel Cream, Dermasil, Eucerin, Lubriderm, Noxzema Skin Cream
Moisturizer ointments	Aquaphor Ointment, Eutra Swiss Skin Cream, Vaseline Ointment
Topical anesthetics	Anesthetic drugs such as lidocaine, tetracaine, benzocaine, and prilocaine in a cream, ointment, or gel. EMLA cream (llidocaine 2.5% and prilocaine 2.5%) is an example of one most commonly used.
Topical antibiotics	Bacitracin, Polysporin (bacitracin and polymyxin B), Bactroban ointment or cream (mupirocin 2%), erythromycin 2% (Emgel, Eryderm Solution), clindamycin phosphate 1% (Cleocin cream, gel, solution), gentamicin sulfate 1% (Garamycin cream or ointment), 1% silver sulfadiazine cream (Silvadene)

Lotions

Lotions are used frequently to replenish lost skin oils or to relieve pruritus. They are usually applied directly to the skin, but a dressing soaked in the lotion can be placed on the affected area. Lotions must be applied every 3 or 4 hours for sustained therapeutic effect because if left in place for a long period, they may crust and cake on the skin.

There are two types of lotions: suspensions and liniments. **Suspensions** are medicines that are mixed with a liquid, usually water, in which it cannot dissolve and, therefore, remains intact in the form of small particles. The important thing to remember about suspensions is to shake the medication before giving each dose so that the medicine particles are evenly distributed throughout the liquid. An example is calamine lotion, which provides a rapid cooling and drying effect as it evaporates, leaving a thin, medicinal layer of powder on the affected skin. **Liniments** are lotions with oil added to prevent crusting. An example of a liniment is Ben-Gay for muscle aches.

Powders

Powders usually have a talc, zinc oxide, bentonite, or cornstarch base and are dusted on the skin with a shaker or applied with cotton sponges. Although their therapeutic action is brief, powders act as **hygroscopic** agents that absorb and retain moisture from the air and reduce friction between skin surfaces and clothing or bedding.

Creams and Emulsions

Creams may be suspensions of oil in water or emulsions of water in oil, with additional ingredients to prevent bacterial and fungal growth. Both may cause an allergic reaction, such as contact dermatitis (discussed on page 1473). Oil-in-water creams are easily applied and usually are the most cosmetically acceptable to the patient. Although they can be used on the face, they tend to have a drying effect. Water-in-oil emulsions are greasier and are preferred for drying and flaking dermatoses.

Gels

Gels are semisolid emulsions that become liquid when applied to the skin or scalp. The water-based gels appear to penetrate the skin more effectively, are greaseless and odorless, and cause less stinging on application. They are especially useful for acute dermatitis in which there is weeping exudate (e.g., poison ivy).

Pastes

Pastes are mixtures of powders and ointments and are used in inflammatory blistering conditions. They adhere to the skin and may be difficult to remove without using oil (e.g., olive oil or mineral oil). Pastes are applied with a wooden tongue depressor or gloved hand.

Ointments

Ointments retard water loss and lubricate and protect the skin. Ointments are better moisturizers or hydrators of the skin due to better adherence to the skin and pharmacologic formulations (Kanfer, Tettley-Amialo, Au, & Hughes-Formella, 2016). They are the preferred vehicle for delivering medication to patients with chronic or localized dry skin conditions, such as eczema or psoriasis (e.g., triamcinolone). Other ointments are used to aid in healing and treatment of pressure ulcers, varicose ulcers, and dehiscent wounds (e.g., Xenaderm). Ointments are applied with a wooden tongue depressor or gloved hand and applied up to twice a day.

Sprays and Aerosols

Spray and aerosol preparations may be used on any widespread dermatologic condition (e.g., 3M Cavilon Skin Protectant; Convatec Aloe Vesta Skin Protectant). They evaporate on contact and are used infrequently.

Corticosteroids

Corticosteroids are widely used in treating dermatologic conditions to provide anti-inflammatory, antipruritic, and vasoconstrictive effects. The patient is taught to apply the product sparingly and rub it into the prescribed area

thoroughly. Absorption of topical corticosteroid is enhanced when the skin is hydrated or when the affected area is covered by an occlusive or moisture-retentive dressing. Inappropriate use of topical corticosteroids can result in local and systemic side effects, especially when the medication is absorbed through inflamed and excoriated skin or is used for long periods on sensitive areas. Local side effects may include skin atrophy and thinning, **striae** (bandlike streaks), and telangiectasia (small dilated blood vessels on the surface of the skin). Thinning of the skin results from the ability of corticosteroids to inhibit the synthesis of skin collagen. The thinning process can be reversed by discontinuing the medication, but striae and telangiectasia are permanent. Systemic side effects may include hyperglycemia and symptoms of Cushing syndrome (refer to Chapter 31). Caution is required when applying corticosteroids around the eyes for two reasons: (1) long-term use may cause glaucoma or cataracts, and (2) the anti-inflammatory effect of corticosteroids may mask existing viral or fungal infections.

Concentrated (fluorinated) corticosteroids are never applied on the face or intertriginous areas (i.e., axilla and groin) because these areas have a thinner stratum corneum and absorb the medication much more quickly than do other areas of the body, such as the forearm or legs.

Nursing Alert

It is important for the nurse to consider that penetration of a topical steroid depends on the skin site, which varies based upon the denseness of the stratum corneum, blood supply, and tissue integrity of the involved area. According to Nicol (2016), penetration of topical steroids applied to the eyelids or scrotum is 4 times greater than for the forehead and 36 times greater than the palms and soles. Thus, thinner and less intact skin has a higher absorption and thus poses a higher risk for side effects.

Intralesional Therapy

Intralesional therapy consists of injecting a sterile suspension of medication (usually a corticosteroid) into or just below a lesion. Although this treatment may have an anti-inflammatory effect, local atrophy may result if the medication is injected into subcutaneous fat. Skin lesions treated with intralesional therapy include psoriasis, keloids, and cystic acne.

Systemic Medications

Systemic medications are also prescribed for skin conditions. These include corticosteroids for short-term therapy for contact dermatitis or for long-term treatment of a chronic **dermatosis**, such as pemphigus vulgaris. Other frequently used systemic medications include antibiotics, antifungals, antihistamines, sedatives, tranquilizers, analgesics, and **cytotoxic** (destructive of cells) agents.

CARING FOR WOUNDS

Wound Dressings

There are three types of wound dressings: primary, secondary, and active. Primary dressings have only a protective function and maintain a moist environment for natural healing. They include those that just cover the area (e.g., Duo-DERM, Tegaderm) and may remain in place for several days. Secondary dressings are capable of absorbing wound exudate while (1) maintaining a moist environment in the area of the wound and (2) allowing the surrounding skin to remain dry. They include hydrocolloids, alginates, and hydrogels. Secondary dressings are able to modify the physiology of the wound environment by modulating and stimulating cellular activity and by releasing growth factor (Bryant & Nix, 2016). Active dressings improve the healing process and decrease healing time. They include skin grafts and biologic skin substitutes. Both interactive and active dressings create a moist environment at the interface of the wound with the dressing.

> **Nursing Alert**
> *Primary dressings are usually considered passive and provide protection to the wound, whereas interactive dressings create a moist wound environment and interact with the wound bed components to further enhance wound healing. Interactive dressings may reduce colonization count, reduce the level of exudate, improve wound bed moisture retention, improve wound collagen matrix, remove cellular products, or provide protection for the epithelializing bed (Bryant & Nix, 2016).*

Because so many wound care products are available, it is often difficult to select the most appropriate product for a specific wound. Selection of products should be made carefully because of their expense. Both clinical efficacy and health-related outcomes (e.g., decreased pain, increased mobility) should be used to measure the success of a product for a wound. Even with the availability of a large variety of dressings, an appropriate selection can be made if certain principles are maintained. Table 52-2 is a guide to wound dressing functions and categories.

Occlusive Dressings

Occlusive dressings cover a topical medication that is applied to a skin lesion. The area is kept airtight by using plastic film (e.g., plastic wrap). Plastic film is thin and readily adapts to all sizes, body shapes, and skin surfaces. In general, plastic wrap should be used no more than 12 hours each day.

Transparent Films

Transparent films are thin, transparent, polyurethane, impermeable adhesive films that are used for partial thickness, minimally draining, or closed wounds. They permit visualization of the wound, promote autolysis, reduce friction, and are sometimes used as a secondary dressing. Examples are Op-Site and Tegaderm.

Specialty Absorptive Dressings

These are used for heavily exudating wounds. The dressings absorb copious amounts of drainage. Examples of these are Exudry and ABD pads.

Moisture-Retentive Dressings

Commercially produced moisture-retentive dressing can perform the same functions as wet dressings but are more efficient at removing exudate because of their higher moisture-vapor transmission rate; some have reservoirs that can hold excessive exudate. A number of moisture-retentive dressings are already impregnated with saline solution, petrolatum, zinc-saline solution, hydrogel, or antimicrobial agents, thereby eliminating the need to coat the skin to avoid maceration. Depending on the product used and the type of dermatologic problem encountered, most moisture-retentive dressings may remain in place from 12 to 24 hours; some can remain in place as long as a week.

Hydrogels

Hydrogels are polymers with a water content of 90% to 95%. They are available in impregnated sheets or as gel in a tube. Their high moisture content makes them ideal for autolytic débridement of wounds. They are semitransparent, allowing for wound inspection without dressing removal. They are comfortable and soothing for the painful wound. They require a secondary dressing to keep them in place. Hydrogels are appropriate for superficial wounds with high serous output, such as abrasions, skin graft sites, and draining venous ulcers.

Hydrocolloids

Hydrocolloids are composed of a water-impermeable, polyurethane outer covering separated from the wound by a hydrocolloid material. They are adherent and nonpermeable to water vapor and oxygen. As water evaporates over the wound, it is absorbed into the dressing, which softens and discolors with the increased water content. The dressing can be removed without damage to the wound. As the dressing absorbs water, it produces a foul-smelling, yellowish covering over the wound. This is a normal chemical interaction between the dressing and wound exudate and should not be confused with purulent drainage from the wound. Most can be left in place for as long as 7 days.

Foam Dressings

Foam dressings are nonadherent and require a secondary dressing to keep them in place. Moisture is absorbed into the foam layer, decreasing maceration of surrounding tissue. A moist environment is maintained, and removal of the dressing does not damage the wound. Foams are a good choice

TABLE **52-2** **Quick Guide to Wound Dressing Function and Categories**

Function	Action	Example
Absorption	Absorbs exudate	Alginates, composite dressings, foams, gauze, hydrocolloids, hydrogels
Cleansing	Removes purulent drainage, foreign debris, and devitalized tissue	Wound cleansers
Débridement	*Autolytic*; covers a wound and allows enzymes to self-digest sloughed skin	Absorption beads, pastes, powders; alginates; composite dressings; foams; hydrate gauze; hydrogels; hydrocolloids; transparent films; wound care systems
	Chemical or enzymatic; applied topically to break down devitalized tissue	Enzymatic débridement agents
	Mechanical; removes devitalized tissue with mechanical force	Wound cleansers, gauze (wet to dry), whirlpool
Diathermy	Produces electrical current to promote warmth and new tissue growth	Ultrasound and microwave (diathermy)
Hydration	Adds moisture to a wound	Gauze (saturated with saline solution), hydrogels, wound care systems
Maintain moist environment	Manages moisture levels in a wound and maintains a moist environment	Composites, contact layers, foams, gauze (impregnated or saturated), hydrogels, hydrocolloids, transparent films, wound care systems
Manage high-output wounds	Manages excessive quantities of exudate	Pouching systems
Pack or fill dead space	Prevents premature wound closure or fills shallow areas and provides absorption	Absorbent beads, powders, pastes; alginates, composites, foams, gauze (impregnated and nonimpregnated)
Protect and cover wound	Provides protection from the external environment	Composites, compression bandages/wraps, foams, gauze dressings, hydrogels, hydrocolloids, transparent film dressings
Protect periwound skin	Prevents moisture and mechanical trauma from damaging delicate tissue around the wound	Composites, foams, hydrocolloids, pouching systems, skin sealants, transparent film dressings
Provide therapeutic compression	Provides appropriate levels of support to the lower extremities in venous stasis disease	Compression bandages, wraps, support stockings

for exudative wounds. They are especially helpful over bony prominences because they provide contoured cushioning.

Alginates

Calcium alginates (e.g., AlgiSite M, Kaltostat, Sorbsan, Algicell) are derived from brown seaweed and consist of very absorbent calcium alginate fibers that can absorb 20 times their weight (Bryant & Nix, 2016). They are useful in areas where the tissue is highly irritated or macerated. The alginate dressing forms a moist pocket over the wound while the surrounding skin stays dry. The dressing also reacts with wound fluid and forms a foul-smelling coating. Alginates work well when packed into a deep cavity, wound, or sinus tract with heavy drainage. They are nonadherent and require a secondary dressing.

Antimicrobial Dressings

Antimicrobial dressings are used for partial and full-thickness wounds. They help to control or decrease the bioburden and odor for minimal and heavy exudating wounds. They

are a topical antifungal and antibiotic agent that come in ointments, gels, impregnated gauze, hydrofiber, and pads. Examples are Acticoat 7 and Aquacel Ag (hydrofiber).

Collagen Dressings

These dressings stimulate the wound and accelerate wound healing. Some forms can be left on for up to 7 days. They are used for minimal to moderate exudating wounds that are partial to full thickness. Examples are Promogran and ColActive.

Tissue Engineered Skin

Apligraf and Dermagraft are dressings made up of a bioabsorbable matrix of collagen or suture material that contains living cytokines and fibroblasts. When applied to wounds, these agents stimulate platelet activity and potentially decrease wound-healing time (Bryant & Nix, 2016). Bioengineered skin works by maintaining wound moisture, providing a structure for regeneration of cells, and supplying beneficial cytokines.

Débridement

Débridement is the removal of nonviable tissue from pressure and vascular ulcers, burns, surgical or traumatic wounds, and other types of wounds.

Autolytic Débridement

Autolytic **débridement** is a process that uses the body's own digestive enzymes to break down necrotic tissue. The wound is kept moist with occlusive dressings. Eschar and necrotic debris are softened, liquefied, and separated from the bed of the wound.

Enzymatic Débridement

Several commercially available products contain the same enzymes that the body produces naturally. These are called enzymatic débriding agents; an example is a collagenase (Santyl). Application of these products speeds the rate at which necrotic tissue is removed. This method is slower and no more effective than surgical débridement.

Mechanical Débridement

Wet-to-dry dressings are still used, but not very much. It is considered a nonselective method of débridement, which removes necrotic tissue and absorbs small to large amounts of exudates. This method exposes healthy tissue in the wound and can damage it as well.

Wet dressings (wet compresses applied to the skin) were traditionally used for acute, weeping, inflammatory lesions. They have become almost obsolete because of the many newer products available for wound care (Ramundo, 2016).

Negative Pressure Wound Therapy

In this therapy, an open-cell, reticulated foam, gauze, or specially designed dressing is placed into the wound, sealed with semi-occlusive drape, and exposed to subatmospheric pressure via an evacuation tube connected to a computerized pump. It is used for acute and chronic open wounds. It also can be used on partial to full-thickness wounds, as well as partial-thickness burns.

Hyperbaric Oxygen Therapy

Hyperbaric oxygenation (HBO) is an adjunctive therapy that requires the patient to breathe 100% oxygen while under increased atmospheric pressure in a pressure chamber. It is recommended that hyperbaric therapy be utilized for limb-threatening diabetic wounds of the lower extremities and pressure ulcers. Also, it is used for hypoxic vascular wounds of the lower extremity (Bryant & Nix, 2016). Those who received HBO as part of their wound care regimen healed faster than those who received standard treatment (Ramundo, 2016).

Pharmacologic Therapy

Pain management can be challenging. In managing any patient with acute or chronic wounds, it is important to identify and measure the degree, site, and type of pain. This aids in utilizing the appropriate treatment for pain (Hopt, Shapshak, Junkins, & O'Neil, 2016).

SKIN CONDITIONS

Pruritus

While not a disorder but a manifestation, pruritus (itching) is one of the most common symptoms of patients with dermatologic disorders.

GENERAL PRURITUS

Pathophysiology

Itch receptors are unmyelinated, penicillate (brush-like) nerve endings that are found exclusively in the skin, mucous membranes, and cornea. Although pruritus is usually caused by a primary skin disease with resultant rash or lesions, it may occur without a rash or lesion. This is referred to as *essential pruritus*, which generally has a rapid onset, may be severe, and interferes with normal daily activities.

Pruritus may be the first indication of a systemic internal disease, such as diabetes mellitus, blood disorders, or cancer (occult malignancy of the breast or colon; Hodgkin disease, other lymphomas). It may also accompany kidney, liver, and thyroid diseases (Box 52-2). Some common oral medications, such as aspirin, antibiotics, hormones (i.e., estrogens, testosterone, or oral contraceptives), and opioids (i.e., morphine or cocaine) may cause pruritus directly or by increasing sensitivity to ultraviolet light. Certain soaps

---

BOX 52-2

Systemic Disorders Associated with Generalized Pruritus

- Chronic kidney disease
- Obstructive biliary disease (primary biliary cirrhosis, extrahepatic biliary obstruction, drug-induced cholestasis)
- Endocrine disease (thyrotoxicosis, hypothyroidism, diabetes mellitus)
- Psychiatric disorders (emotional stress, anxiety, neurosis, phobias)
- Malignancies (polycythemia vera, Hodgkin disease, lymphoma, leukemia, multiple myeloma, mycosis fungoides, and cancers of the lung, breast, central nervous system, and GI tract)
- Neurologic disorders (multiple sclerosis, brain abscess, brain tumor)
- Infestations (scabies, lice, other insects)
- Pruritus of pregnancy (pruritic urticarial papules of pregnancy [PUPP], cholestasis of pregnancy, pemphigoid of pregnancy)
- Folliculitis (bacterial, candidiasis, dermatophyte)
- Skin conditions (seborrheic dermatitis, folliculitis, iron deficiency anemia, atopic dermatitis)

and chemicals, radiation therapy, prickly heat (miliaria), and contact with woolen garments are also associated with pruritus. Pruritus may also be caused by psychological factors, such as excessive stress in family or work situations.

Scratching the pruritic area causes the inflamed cells and nerve endings to release histamine, which produces more pruritus, generating a vicious itch–scratch cycle. If the patient responds to an itch by scratching, the integrity of the skin may be altered, and excoriation, erythema, raised areas (i.e., wheals), infection, or changes in pigmentation may result. Pruritus usually is more severe at night and is less frequently reported during waking hours, most likely because the person is distracted by daily activities. At night, when there are few distractions, even the slightest pruritus cannot be ignored easily. Severe itching can be debilitating.

Gerontologic Considerations

Pruritus occurs frequently in elderly people as a result of dry skin. Elderly people are also more likely to have a systemic illness that triggers pruritus, are at higher risk for occult malignancy, and are more likely to be taking multiple medications than younger people. All of these factors increase the incidence of pruritus in elderly people.

Medical and Nursing Management

A thorough history and physical examination usually provide clues to the underlying cause of the pruritus, such as hay fever, allergy, recent administration of a new medication, or a change of cosmetics or soaps. After the causative agent has been identified and removed (if possible), treatment of the condition should relieve the pruritus. Signs of infection and environmental clues, such as warm, dry air or irritating bed linens, should be identified. In general, washing with soap and hot water is avoided. Bath oils containing a surfactant that makes the oil mix with bath water (e.g., Alpha-Keri) may be sufficient for cleaning. A warm bath with a mild soap followed by application of a bland emollient to moist skin can control **xerosis** (dry skin). Applying a cold compress, or cool agents that contain menthol and camphor (which constrict blood vessels) may also help relieve pruritus. If baths have been prescribed, the nurse reminds the patient to use tepid (not hot) water and to shake off the excess water and blot between intertriginous areas (body folds) with a towel. Rubbing vigorously with the towel is avoided because this overstimulates the skin and causes more itching. It also removes water from the stratum corneum (horny layer or outermost layer of the epidermis). Immediately after bathing, the patient should lubricate the skin with an emollient to trap moisture. The nurse instructs patient to avoid situations that cause vasodilation, such as exposure to an overly warm environment and ingestion of alcohol or hot foods and liquids. Activities that result in perspiration should be limited because perspiration may irritate and promote pruritus. If the patient is troubled at night with itching that interferes with

sleep, the nurse can advise wearing cotton clothing next to the skin rather than synthetic materials. The room should be kept cool and humidified. Vigorous scratching should be avoided and nails kept trimmed to prevent skin damage and infection. When the underlying cause of pruritus is unknown and further testing is required, the nurse explains each test and the expected outcome.

Topical corticosteroids may be beneficial as anti-inflammatory agents to decrease itching. Oral antihistamines are even more effective because they can overcome the effects of histamine released from damaged mast cells. An antihistamine, such as diphenhydramine (Benadryl) or hydroxyzine (Atarax), prescribed in a sedative dose at bedtime, may be beneficial in producing a restful and comfortable sleep. Nonsedating antihistamine medications, such as fexofenadine (Allegra), are more appropriate to relieve daytime pruritus. Tricyclic antidepressants may be prescribed for pruritus of neuropsychogenic origin. If pruritus continues, further investigation of a systemic problem is advised.

PERINEAL AND PERIANAL PRURITUS

Pathophysiology

Pruritus of the genital and anal regions may be caused by small particles of fecal material lodged in the perianal crevices or attached to anal hairs. Alternatively, it may result from perianal skin damage caused by scratching, moisture, and decreased skin resistance as a result of corticosteroid or antibiotic therapy. Other possible causes of perianal itching include local irritants such as scabies and lice, local lesions such as hemorrhoids, fungal or yeast infections, and pinworm infestation. Foods associated with anal pruritus include coffee, tea, cola, beer, chocolate, and tomatoes. Occasionally, no cause for genital and anal pruritus can be identified.

Medical and Nursing Management

The nurse instructs the patient to follow proper hygiene measures and to discontinue home and over-the-counter remedies. The perineal or anal area should be rinsed with lukewarm water and blotted dry with cotton balls. Premoistened tissues may be used after defecation. Cornstarch can be applied in the skinfold areas to absorb perspiration.

As part of health teaching, the nurse instructs the patient to avoid bathing in water that is too hot and to avoid using bubble baths, sodium bicarbonate, and detergent soaps, all of which aggravate dryness. To keep the perineal or perianal skin as dry as possible, patients should avoid wearing underwear made of synthetic fabrics. Local anesthetic agents should not be used because of possible allergic effects. The patient should also avoid vasodilating agents or stimulants (e.g., alcohol, caffeine) and mechanical irritants, such as rough or woolen clothing. A diet that includes adequate fiber may help maintain soft stools and prevent minor trauma to the anal mucosa.

ULCERATION

Superficial loss of surface tissue as a result of death of cells is called an ulceration. A simple **ulcer**, such as the kind found in a small, superficial, partial-thickness burn, tends to heal by granulation if kept clean and protected from injury. If exposed to the air, the serum that escapes will dry and form a scab, under which the epithelial cells grow and cover the surface completely. The four most common ulcers noted are arterial, venous, neuropathic/diabetic, and pressure ulcers (Table 52-3).

ARTERIAL ULCERS

Ulcers related to problems with arterial circulation are seen in patients with hypertension, diabetes, cigarette smoking, hypercholesterolemia, obesity, and sedentary lifestyle. Arterial ulcers are caused by lower extremity arterial disease (LEAD), which is inadequate blood flow to the tissue, resulting in severe tissue ischemia, and which can create ulcers that are extremely painful (Doughty & Sparks-Defriese, 2016). This condition is also referred to as peripheral arterial disease (PAD), peripheral vascular disease (PVD), or peripheral arterial occlusive disease (PAOD). In patients with LEAD and

TABLE 52-3 Characteristics of Ulcers

Ulcer Type	Location	Description of Wound Bed	Exudate	Description of Wound Edges
Arterial	Tips of toes, pressure points, areas of trauma	Pale or necrotic	Minimal amount	Well defined
Venous	Commonly located in the lower leg just above the ankle (gaiter region)	Dark red, "ruddy"	Moderate to large amounts	Poorly defined; irregular
Neuropathic	Plantar surface over metatarsal heads	Typically red (unless coexisting ischemia)	Moderate to large amounts	Well defined
Pressure	Any boney prominence	Erythremic or purplish in discoloration due to pressure	Minimal to large amounts	Poorly to well defined

Reprinted with permission from Goodheart, H. P. (2010). *Goodheart's same-site differential diagnosis: A rapid method of diagnosing and treating common skin disorders* (arterial ulcer). Lippincott, Williams, & Wilkins; Nettina, S. M. (2001). *The Lippincott manual of nursing practice* (7th ed.). Lippincott, Williams & Wilkins (venous ulcer); Bickley, L. (2013). *A guide to physical examination and history taking* (11th ed.). Philadelphia, PA: J.B. Lippincott (neuropathic ulcer); and Doughty, D., & McNichol, L. (2015). *Wound, Ostomy and Continence Nurses Society Core Curriculum: Wound management*. Philadelphia, PA: Lippincott, Williams, and Wilkins (pressure ulcer).

ulcers, treatment of the ulcers is concurrent with treatment of the arterial disease. Management includes the use of the dressings and/or tissue perfusion improvement. Perfusion and tissue oxygenation can improve outcomes via surgical options (bypass graft, angioplasty), medications (antiplatelets, vasodilators, hemorheologics [decrease the viscosity of the blood], antilipemics [decrease lipid levels], analgesics), lifestyle changes, and adjunctive therapies (hyperbaric oxygen therapy) (Doughty & Sparks-Defriese, 2016). If these interventions are instituted early in the progression of an ulcer, the condition can often be effectively improved. Surgical amputation of an affected limb is a last resort.

VENOUS ULCERS

Venous ulcers are more common than arterial ulcers. They occur due to impaired return of venous blood from the tissue to the heart, also known as chronic venous insufficiency (CVI) or lower extremity venous disease (LEVD). Risk factors are valvular dysfunction caused by obesity, multiple pregnancies, thrombophlebitis, leg trauma (deep vein thrombosis or fractures), and thrombophilic conditions (increased coagulability of the blood). Other risks factors include arthritis or calf muscle dysfunction, IV drug use involving the affected extremity, sedentary lifestyle, or prolonged standing. Healing can be affected by diabetes, smoking, nutrition, and medications (Carmel & Bryant, 2016). Management includes reduction of edema, prevention of complications, and appropriate topical therapy or specialty dressings (Carmel & Bryant, 2016).

NEUROPATHIC ULCERS

Diabetic foot ulcers are also known as neuropathic ulcers or lower extremity neuropathic disease (LEND). These ulcers occur due to reduced blood supply to the nerves, also known as microvascular damage, which can lead to neuropathy. Neuropathy is classified as loss of sensation. Risk factors include history of amputations or ulcers, long duration of diabetes and/or poor glucose control, limited joint mobility, long history of smoking, obesity, poor vision, poor footwear, vascular insufficiency, structural deformities and callus formation, absence of protective sensation, and autonomic neuropathy, causing decreased sweating and dry feet (Driver, Brentton, Allen, & Park, 2016).

Early prevention can be achieved through comprehensive annual foot examinations, glycemic control, limiting other health complications, and offloading (pressure relief). Wound management may include débridement, treatment of infection if needed, and topical, specialty wound care dressing and/or adjunctive therapies (Driver et al., 2016). For further information related to diabetic neuropathy, refer to Chapter 30.

PRESSURE ULCERS

Pathophysiology

Pressure ulcers involve the breakdown of the skin due to prolonged pressure, friction, and shear forces, and insufficient

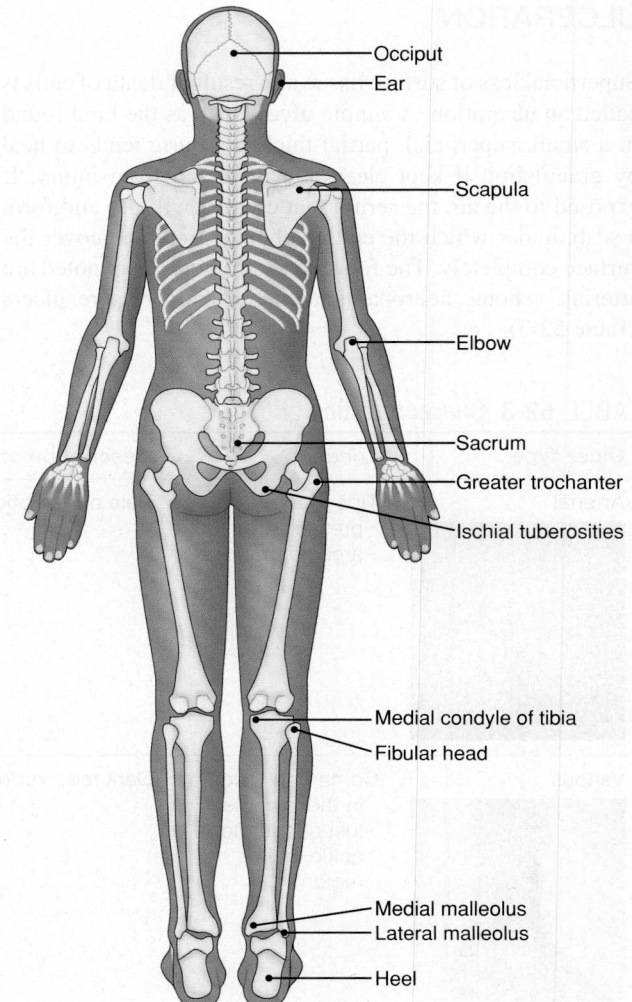

FIGURE 52-1 Areas susceptible to pressure ulcers.

blood supply, usually at bony prominences. Pressure ulcers are localized areas of infarcted soft tissue that occur when pressure applied to the skin over time is greater than normal capillary closure pressure, which is about 32 mm Hg. Weight-bearing bony prominences are most susceptible to pressure ulcer development because they are covered only by skin and small amounts of subcutaneous tissue. Susceptible areas include the sacrum and coccygeal areas, ischial tuberosities (especially in people who sit for prolonged periods), greater trochanter, heel, knee, malleolus, medial condyle of the tibia, fibular head, scapula, and elbow (Fig. 52-1).

Risk Factors

Box 52-3 summarizes risk factors for pressure ulcers.

Clinical Manifestations and Assessment

The initial sign of pressure is erythema (redness of the skin) caused by reactive hyperemia, which normally resolves in less than 1 hour. Unrelieved pressure results in tissue

Risk Factors for Pressure Ulcers

- Immobility, compromised mobility
- Prolonged pressure on tissue
- Altered skin moisture: excessively dry, excessively moist (perspiration, urine, feces, or drainage produces maceration [softening] of the skin)
- Equipment: Casts, traction, restraints
- Impaired sensory perception or cognition
- Decreased tissue perfusion (seen with diabetes, obesity, and edema). Patients who are critically ill have a lower capillary closure pressure and, thus, higher risk.
- Decreased nutritional status (anemia, hypoalbuminemia, vitamin deficiency)
- Friction and shear forces

ischemia or anoxia. The cutaneous tissues become broken or destroyed, leading to progressive destruction and necrosis of underlying soft tissue, and the resulting pressure ulcer is painful and slow to heal. The nurse assesses the patient's mobility, sensory perception, cognitive abilities, tissue perfusion, nutritional status, friction and shear forces, sources of moisture on the skin, age, and skin condition. Scales such as the Braden or Norton scale may be used to facilitate systematic assessment and quantification of a patient's risk for pressure ulcers although the nurse should recognize that the reliability of these scales is not well established for all patient populations. If a pressure area is observed, the nurse notes its size and location and uses a grading system to describe its severity (refer to Box 52-4 for current standards in assessing and staging pressure ulcers). A recent study of

Stages of Pressure Ulcers

Stage I

Description
Ulcer appears as intact skin with nonblanchable erythema of a localized area, usually over a bony prominence. Darkly pigmented skin may not have visible blanching; its color may differ from the surrounding area.

The area may be painful, firm, soft, and warmer or cooler in temperature as compared to adjacent tissue. Stage I may indicate patients who are "at risk" (a heralding sign of risk).

Treatment
To permit healing of Stage I pressure ulcers, the pressure is removed to allow increased tissue perfusion; nutritional status and fluid and electrolyte balance are maintained; friction and shear are reduced; and moisture to the skin is avoided.

stage should not be used to describe skin tears, tape burns, perineal dermatitis, maceration, or excoriation.

Treatment
In addition to measures listed for Stage I pressure ulcers, a moist environment, in which migration of epidermal cells over the ulcer surface occurs more rapidly, should be provided to aid wound healing. The ulcer is gently cleansed with sterile saline solution. Use of a heat lamp to dry the open wound is avoided as is the use of antiseptic solutions that damage healthy tissues and delay wound healing. Semipermeable occlusive dressings, hydrocolloid wafers, or wet saline dressings are helpful in providing a moist environment for healing and in minimizing the loss of fluids and proteins from the body.

Stage III

Description
There is full-thickness tissue loss. Subcutaneous fat may be visible, but bone, tendon, or muscle is not exposed. Slough may be present but does not obscure the depth of tissue loss. The ulcer may include undermining and tunneling.

The depth of a Stage III pressure ulcer varies by anatomical location. The bridge of the nose, ear, occiput and malleolus do not have subcutaneous tissue, and Stage III ulcers here can be

Stage II

Description
Ulcer appears as partial-thickness loss of dermis, presenting as a shallow open ulcer with a red or pink wound bed, without slough. It may also present as an intact or open/ruptured serum-filled blister.

It may be a shiny or dry shallow ulcer without slough or bruising (bruising indicates suspected deep tissue injury). This

(continued on page 1468)

BOX 52-4 **Stages of Pressure Ulcers (*continued*)**

shallow. In contrast, areas of significant adiposity can develop Stage III pressure ulcers that are extremely deep. Bone/tendon is not visible or directly palpable.

Treatment

Stage III and IV pressure ulcers are characterized by extensive tissue damage. In addition to the measures listed for Stage I, these advanced, draining, necrotic pressure ulcers must be cleaned (débrided) to create an area that will heal. Necrotic, devitalized tissue favors bacterial growth, delays granulation, and inhibits healing. Wound cleaning and dressing are uncomfortable; therefore, the nurse must prepare the patient for the procedure by explaining what will occur and administering prescribed analgesia.

Débridement may be accomplished by wet-to-damp dressing changes, mechanical flushing of necrotic and infective exudate, application of prescribed enzyme preparations that dissolve necrotic tissue, or surgical dissection. If an eschar covers the ulcer, it is removed surgically to ensure a clean, vitalized wound. Exudate may be absorbed by dressings or special hydrophilic powders, beads, or gels. Cultures of infected pressure ulcers are obtained to guide the selection of antibiotic therapy.

After the pressure ulcer is clean, a topical treatment is prescribed to promote granulation. New granulation tissue must be protected from reinfection, drying, and damage, and care should be taken to prevent pressure and further trauma to the area. Dressings, solutions, and ointments applied to the ulcer should not disrupt the healing process. Multiple agents and protocols are used to treat pressure ulcers, but consistency is an important key to success. Objective evaluation of the pressure ulcer (e.g., measurement of the size and depth of the pressure ulcer, inspection for granulation tissue) for response to the treatment protocol must be made every 4–6 days. Taking photographs at weekly intervals is a reliable strategy for monitoring the healing process, which may take weeks to months.

Stage IV

Description

There is full-thickness tissue loss with exposed bone, tendon, or muscle. Slough or eschar may be present on some parts of

the wound bed. These ulcers often include undermining and tunneling.

The depth of a Stage IV pressure ulcer varies by anatomical location. The bridge of the nose, ear, occiput, and malleolus do not have subcutaneous tissue, and these ulcers can be shallow. Stage IV ulcers can extend into muscle and/or supporting structures (e.g., fascia, tendon, or joint capsule), making osteomyelitis possible. Exposed bone/tendon is visible or directly palpable.

Treatment

See Stage III treatment. In addition, surgical intervention may be necessary when the ulcer is extensive, when complications (e.g., fistula) exist, and when the ulcer does not respond to treatment. Surgical procedures include débridement, incision and drainage, bone resection, and skin grafting. Osteomyelitis is a common complication of wounds of Stage IV depth. See Chapter 41 for more information on osteomyelitis.

Unstageable

An unstageable lesion shows full-thickness tissue loss in which the base of the ulcer is covered by slough (yellow, tan, gray, green, or brown) and/or eschar (tan, brown or black) in the wound bed.

Until enough slough and/or eschar is removed to expose the base of the wound, the true depth and, therefore, stage cannot be determined. Stable (dry, adherent, intact without erythema or fluctuance) eschar on the heels serves as the body's natural (biologic) cover and should not be removed.

Suspected Deep Tissue Injury (DTI)

Suspected deep tissue injury (DTI) appears as a purple or maroon localized area of discolored intact skin or blood-filled blister due to damage of underlying soft tissue from pressure and/or shear. The area may be preceded by tissue that is painful, firm, mushy, boggy, warmer, or cooler as compared to adjacent tissue.

DTI may be difficult to detect in individuals with dark skin tones. Evolution may include a thin blister over a dark wound bed. The wound may further evolve and become covered by thin eschar. Evolution may be rapid, exposing additional layers of tissue even with optimal treatment.

interrater reliability in identifying classification of pressure ulcers revealed low reliability; therefore, it is imperative that nurses use a consistent scale (Pieper, 2016).

Nursing Alert
Beginning in 2008, Medicare regulations do not reimburse for treatment of pressure ulcers acquired in the hospital, even if the ulcer was present on admission but undocumented. Therefore, it is imperative that accurate recognition and staging of pressure ulcers occurs in all patients.

Medical and Nursing Management

Treatment depends on stage (see Box 52-4). Nursing interventions for prevention and management of pressure ulcers include turning and repositioning the patient every 1 to 2 hours when in bed, and shifting of weight every 15 minutes while in a chair to allow the blood to flow into the ischemic areas to help tissues recover from the effects of pressure. The recumbent position is preferred to the semi-Fowler position because of increased supporting body surface area in this position, with careful attention paid to the repositioning of the patient's ankles, elbows, and shoulders. The nurse inspects the patient's skin at each position change and assesses for temperature elevation. If redness or heat is noted, or if the patient complains of discomfort, pressure on the area must be relieved.

A pillow or commercial heel protector may be used to support the heels off the bed when the patient is supine. Supporting the patient in a 30-degree side-lying position avoids pressure on the trochanter. At times, special equipment and beds may be needed to help relieve the pressure on the skin, such as wheelchair cushions and static support devices (such as high-density foam, air, or liquid mattress overlays). Shear occurs when patients are pulled, allowed to slump, or move by digging heels or elbows into the mattress. Raising the head of the bed by even a few centimeters increases the shearing force over the sacral area; therefore, the semi-reclining position is avoided in patients at risk. The patient is encouraged to remain active and is ambulated whenever possible. Exercise and repositioning improve tissue perfusion. Massage of erythematous areas is avoided because damage to the capillaries and deep tissue may occur.

Strategies to improve cognition and sensory perception may include stimulating the patient to increase awareness of self in the environment, encouraging the patient to participate in self-care, or supporting the patient's efforts toward active compensation for loss of sensation (e.g., a patient with paraplegia lifting up from the sitting position every 15 minutes).

Continuous moisture on the skin must be prevented by meticulous hygiene measures. Perspiration, urine, stool, and drainage must be removed from the skin promptly. The skin may be lubricated with a bland lotion to keep it soft and pliable. Drying agents and powders are avoided. Topical barrier ointments (e.g.,

petroleum jelly) may be helpful in protecting the skin of patients who are incontinent. Absorbent pads that wick moisture away from the body should be used to absorb drainage.

The patient's nutritional status must be adequate, and a positive nitrogen balance must be maintained because pressure ulcers develop more quickly and are more resistant to treatment in patients with nutritional disorders. A high-protein diet with protein supplements may be helpful. Iron preparations may be necessary to raise the hemoglobin concentration so that tissue oxygen levels can be maintained within acceptable limits. Ascorbic acid (vitamin C) is necessary for tissue healing. Other nutrients associated with healthy skin include vitamin A, B vitamins, zinc, and sulfur. See Box 52-5 for a systematic overview of research on preventing pressure ulcers.

Gerontologic Considerations

In older adults, the skin has diminished epidermal thickness, dermal collagen, and tissue elasticity. The skin is drier as a result of diminished activity of the sebaceous and sweat glands. Cardiovascular changes result in decreased tissue perfusion. Muscles atrophy, and bone structures become prominent. Diminished sensory perception and reduced ability to reposition oneself contribute to prolonged pressure on the skin. Therefore, older adults are more susceptible to pressure ulcers, which cause pain and suffering and reduce quality of life.

SEBORRHEIC DERMATITIS

Seborrhea is excessive production of sebum (secretion of sebaceous glands) in areas where sebaceous glands are normally found in large numbers, such as on the face, scalp, eyebrows, eyelids, sides of the nose and upper lip, malar regions (cheeks), ears, axillae, under the breasts, in the groin, and in the gluteal crease of the buttocks. Seborrheic dermatitis is a chronic inflammatory disease of the skin with a predilection for areas that are well supplied with sebaceous glands or lie between skin folds, where the bacteria count is high.

Clinical Manifestations and Assessment

Two forms of seborrheic dermatitis can occur, an oily form and a dry form. Either form may start in childhood and continue throughout life. The oily form appears moist or "greasy." There may be patches of yellowish-red or gray-white, greasy skin, with white dry scaling macules and/or papules, with slight erythema, predominantly on the forehead, nasolabial fold, beard area, scalp, and between adjacent skin surfaces in the regions of the axillae, groin, and breasts (Clark, Pope, & Jaboori, 2015). Small pustules or papulopustules resembling acne may appear on the trunk. The dry form, consisting of flaky desquamation of the scalp with a profuse amount of fine, powdery scales, is commonly called dandruff. The

---

BOX 52-5 Nursing Research

Bridging the Gap to Evidence-Based Practice

Tayyib, N., & Coyer, F. (2016). Effectiveness of pressure ulcer prevention strategies for adult patients in intensive care units: A systematic review. *Worldviews on Evidence-Based Nursing, 13*(6), 432–444.

Purpose

Pressure ulcers are associated with substantial health burden, but could be preventable. Hospital-acquired pressure ulcers (HAPUs) prevention has become a priority for all healthcare settings, as it is considered a sign of quality of care providing. Intensive care unit (ICU) patients are at higher risk for HAPUs development. Despite the availability of published prevention strategies, there is a little evidence about which strategies can be safely integrated into routine standard care and have an impact on HAPUs prevention. The aim was to synthesize the best available evidence regarding the effectiveness of single strategies designed to reduce the incidence and prevalence of HAPUs development in ICUs.

Design

The search strategy was designed to retrieve studies published in English across CINAHL, Medline, Cochrane Central Register of Controlled Trials, Embase, Scopus, and Mednar between 2000 and 2015. All adult ICU participants were aged 18 years or over. This review included randomized controlled trials, quasi-experimental and comparative studies. The studies that were selected for retrieval were assessed by two independent reviewers for methodologic validity prior to inclusion in the review using standardized critical-appraisal instruments.

Findings

The review included 25 studies, and the meta-analysis revealed a statistically significant effect of a silicon foam dressing strategy in reducing HAPUs incidence (effect size = 4.62; 95% CI: 0.05–0.29; p <0.00001, effect size = 4.50; 95% CI: 0.05–0.31; p = 0.00001, respectively) in critically ill patients. Evidence of the effectiveness of nutrition, skin-care regimen, positioning and repositioning schedule, support surfaces, and the role of education in prevention of HAPUs development in the ICU was limited, which precludes strong conclusions.

Nursing Implications

The review provides an evidence-based guide to future priorities for clinical practice. In particular, a silicone foam dressing has positive impact in reducing sacrum and heel HAPUs incidence in the ICU.

---

mild forms of the disease are asymptomatic. When scaling occurs, it is often accompanied by pruritus, which may lead to scratching and secondary infections and excoriation.

Seborrheic dermatitis has a genetic predisposition. Hormones, nutritional status, infection, and emotional stress influence its course. The remissions and exacerbations of this condition should be explained to the patient. If a person has not previously been diagnosed with this condition and suddenly appears with a severe outbreak, a complete history and physical examination should be considered.

Medical and Nursing Management

Because there is no known cure for seborrhea, the objective of therapy is to control the disorder and allow the skin to repair itself. Seborrheic dermatitis of the body and face may respond to a topically applied glucocorticoid cream or low-potency topical steroids (e.g., desonide), which allays the secondary inflammatory response (Clark et al., 2015). However, glucocorticoids should be used with caution near the eyelids, because they can induce glaucoma and cataracts in predisposed patients. Patients with seborrheic dermatitis may develop a secondary candidal (yeast) infection in body creases or folds and may have to use a topical antifungal (e.g., ciclopirox or ketoconazole) (Clark et al., 2015). To avoid this, patients should be advised to ensure maximum aeration of the skin and to clean areas where there are creases or folds in the skin carefully. Patients with persistent candidiasis should

be evaluated for diabetes. Ultraviolet radiation therapy can be beneficial as a form of treatment as well.

The mainstay of dandruff treatment is proper, frequent shampooing (at least three times weekly) with medicated shampoos. Two or three different types of shampoo should be used in rotation to prevent the seborrhea from becoming resistant to a particular shampoo. The shampoo is left on at least 5 to 10 minutes. As the condition of the scalp improves, the treatment can be less frequent. Antiseborrheic shampoos include those containing selenium sulfide suspension, zinc pyrithione, salicylic acid or sulfur compounds, and tar shampoo that contains sulfur or salicylic acid. Instructions for using medicated shampoos are reinforced for people with dandruff who require treatment. Frequent shampooing is contrary to some cultural practices; the nurse should be sensitive to these differences when teaching the patient about home care.

A person with seborrheic dermatitis is advised to avoid external irritants, excessive heat, and perspiration; rubbing and scratching prolong the disorder. To avoid secondary infection, the patient should air the skin and keep skin folds clean and dry.

The patient is cautioned that seborrheic dermatitis is a chronic problem that tends to reappear. The goal is to keep it under control. Patients need to be encouraged to adhere to the treatment program. Those who become discouraged and disheartened by the effect on body image should be treated with sensitivity and encouraged to express their feelings.

VIRAL SKIN INFECTIONS

HERPES ZOSTER

Herpes zoster, also called *shingles*, is an infection caused by the varicella-zoster virus, a member of a group of DNA viruses. The viruses causing chickenpox and herpes zoster are indistinguishable, hence the name varicella-zoster virus. The disease is characterized by a painful vesicular eruption along the area of distribution of the sensory nerves from one or more posterior ganglia.

Pathophysiology

After a case of chickenpox runs its course, the varicella-zoster viruses responsible for the outbreak lie dormant inside nerve cells near the brain and spinal cord. Later, when these latent viruses are reactivated because of declining cellular immunity, they travel by way of the peripheral nerves to the skin, where the viruses multiply and create a red rash of small, fluid-filled vesicles. About 10% of adults get shingles during their lifetimes, usually after 50 years of age. There is an increased frequency of herpes zoster infections among patients with weakened immune systems and cancers (especially leukemias and lymphomas), those on chemotherapy, and in individuals who are HIV infected.

Clinical Manifestations and Assessment

The eruption is usually accompanied or preceded by pain, which may radiate over the entire region supplied by the affected nerves. The pain may be burning, lancinating (tearing or sharply cutting), stabbing, or aching. Some patients have no pain, but itching and tenderness may occur over the area. Sometimes, malaise and gastrointestinal (GI) disturbances precede the eruption. The patches of grouped vesicles appear on the red and swollen skin. The early vesicles, which contain serum, later may become purulent, rupture, and form crusts. The inflammation is usually unilateral, involving the thoracic, cervical, or cranial nerves in a band-like configuration. Usually the blisters are confined to a narrow region of the face or trunk (Fig. 52-2). The clinical course varies from 1 to 3 weeks. If an ophthalmic nerve is involved, the patient may have eye pain. Inflammation and a rash on the trunk may cause pain with the slightest touch. The healing time varies from 7 to 26 days.

Herpes zoster in healthy adults is usually localized and benign. However, in patients who are immunosuppressed, the disease may be severe and disabling.

Medical and Nursing Management

There is evidence that infection is arrested if oral antiviral agents, such as acyclovir (Zovirax), valacyclovir (Valtrex), or famciclovir (Famvir), are administered within 24 hours of the initial eruption. IV acyclovir, if started early, is effective in significantly reducing the pain and halting the progression

FIGURE 52-2 Herpes zoster (shingles).

of the disease. In older patients, the pain from herpes zoster may persist as postherpetic neuralgia (persistent pain of the affected nerve after healing) for months after the skin lesions disappear.

The goals of herpes zoster management are to relieve the pain and to reduce or avoid complications, which include infection, scarring, and postherpetic neuralgia and eye complications. Pain is controlled with analgesics because adequate pain control during the acute phase helps prevent persistent pain patterns. Systemic corticosteroids may be prescribed for patients older than 50 years of age to reduce the incidence and duration of postherpetic neuralgia. Healing usually occurs more quickly in those who have been treated with corticosteroids. Triamcinolone (Aristocort, Kenacort, Kenalog) injected subcutaneously under painful areas is effective as an anti-inflammatory agent.

Ophthalmic herpes zoster occurs when an eye is involved. This is considered an ophthalmic emergency, and the patient should be referred to an ophthalmologist immediately to prevent the possible sequelae of keratitis, uveitis, ulceration, and blindness.

People who have been exposed to varicella by primary infection or by vaccination are not at risk for infection after exposure to patients with herpes zoster.

HERPES SIMPLEX

Herpes simplex is a common skin infection. There are two types of the causative virus, which are identified by viral typing. In general, herpes simplex type 1 occurs on the mouth and type 2 occurs in the genital area, but both viral types can be found in both locations. About 85% of adults worldwide are seropositive for herpes type 1. The prevalence of type 2 is lower; type 2 usually appears at the onset of sexual activity. Herpes simplex type 2 is discussed in detail in Chapter 35.

Serologic testing shows that many more people are infected than have a history of clinical disease.

Herpes simplex infection is classified as a true primary infection, a nonprimary initial episode, or a recurrent episode. True primary infection is the initial exposure to the virus. A nonprimary initial episode is the initial episode of either type 1 or type 2 in a person previously infected with the other type. Recurrent episodes are subsequent episodes of the same viral type.

TINEA

Fungi—tiny members of a subdivision of the plant kingdom that feed on organic matter—are responsible for various common skin infections. In some cases, they affect only the skin and its appendages (hair and nails). In other cases, internal organs are involved, and the diseases may be life-threatening. However, superficial infections rarely cause even temporary disability and usually respond readily to treatment. Secondary infection with bacteria, *Candida*, or both organisms may occur.

The most common fungal skin infection is **tinea** (Fig. 52-3), which is also called *ringworm* because of its characteristic appearance of a ring or rounded tunnel under the skin. Tinea infections affect the head, body, groin, feet, and nails. Table 52-4 summarizes the tinea infections.

To obtain a specimen for diagnosis, the lesion is cleaned and a scalpel or glass slide is used to remove scales from the margin of the lesion. The scales are dropped onto a slide to which potassium hydroxide has been added. The diagnosis is made by examination of the infected scales microscopically for spores and hyphae or by isolating the organism

FIGURE 52-3 Tinea corporis. Tinea is one of several conditions (granuloma annulare, nummular eczema) that produces circular lesions. In tinea, the margin of the lesion contains microvesicles, which are best visualized by peering through the lens of a lighted otoscope, and is raised. The flat central area often shows fine scaling. (Reprinted with permission from Fleisher, G. R., Ludwig, S., & Baskin, M. N. (2004). *Atlas of pediatric emergency medicine.* Philadelphia, PA: Lippincott Williams & Wilkins.)

in culture. Under Wood's light, a specimen of infected hair appears fluorescent; this may be helpful in diagnosing some cases of tinea capitis.

SCABIES

Scabies is an infestation of the skin by the itch mite *Sarcoptes scabiei*. The disease may be found in people living

TABLE 52-4 Tinea (Ringworm) Infections

Type and Location	Clinical Manifestations	Treatment
Tinea corporis (body)	• Begins with red macule, which spreads to a ring of papules or vesicles with central clearing. • Lesions are found in clusters. • Many spread to the hair, scalp, or nails. • Very pruritic. • An infected pet may be the source.	• Mild conditions: topical antifungal creams • Severe conditions: griseofulvin or terbinafine
Tinea cruris (groin area; "jock itch")	• Begins with small, red scaling patches, which spread to form circular elevated plaques. • Very pruritic. • Clusters of pustules may be seen around borders.	• Mild conditions: topical antifungal creams • Severe conditions: griseofulvin or terbinafine
Tinea pedis (foot; "athlete's foot")	• Soles of one or both feet have scaling and mild redness with maceration in the toe webs. • More acute infections may have clusters of clear vesicles on dusky base.	• Soak feet in vinegar and water solution. • Resistant infections: griseofulvin or terbinafine • Terbinafine (Lamisil) daily for 3 months
Tinea unguium (toenails; affects about 50% of adults)	• Nails thicken, crumble easily, and lack luster. • Whole nail may be destroyed.	• Itraconazole (Sporanox) in pulses of 1 week a month for 3 months in cases of terbinafine failure

in substandard hygienic conditions, but it can occur in any-one. Infestations may or may not be associated with sexual activity. The mites frequently involve the fingers, and hand contact may produce infection. In children, overnight stays with friends or the exchange of clothes may be a source of infection.

Clinical Manifestations and Assessment

It takes approximately 4 weeks from the time of contact for the patient's symptoms to appear. The patient complains of severe itching caused by a delayed type of immunologic reaction to the mite or its fecal pellets. During examination, the nurse asks the patient where the pruritus is most severe. A magnifying glass and a penlight are held at an oblique angle to the skin while a search is made for the small, raised burrows created by the mites. The burrows may be multiple, straight or wavy, brown or black, thread-like lesions, most commonly observed between the fingers and on the wrists. Other sites are the extensor surfaces of the elbows, the knees, the edges of the feet, the points of the elbows, around the nipples, in the axillary folds, under pendulous breasts, and in or near the groin or gluteal fold, penis, or scrotum. Red, pruritic eruptions usually appear between adjacent skin areas. However, the burrow is not always visible. Any patient with a rash may have scabies.

One classic sign of scabies is the increased itching that occurs during the overnight hours, perhaps because the increased warmth of the skin has a stimulating effect on the parasite. Hypersensitivity to the organism and its products of excretion also may contribute to the pruritus. If the infection has spread, other members of the family and close friends also complain of pruritus about a month later.

Secondary lesions are quite common and include vesicles, papules, excoriations, and crusts. Bacterial superinfection may result from constant excoriation of the burrows and papules.

The diagnosis is confirmed by recovering *S. scabiei* or the mites' by-products from the skin. A sample of superficial epidermis is scraped from the top of the burrows or papules with a small scalpel blade. The scrapings are placed on a microscope slide and examined through a microscope at low power to demonstrate evidence of the mite (Monsel & Chosidow, 2015).

Gerontologic Considerations

Elderly patients living in long-term care facilities are susceptible to outbreaks of scabies because of close living quarters, poor hygiene due to limited physical ability, and the potential for incidental spread of the organisms by staff members. Although pruritus may be severe in the older patient, the vivid inflammatory reaction seen in younger people seldom occurs. Scabies may not be recognized in the elderly person; the pruritus may be attributed erroneously to the dry skin of old age or to anxiety.

Health care personnel in extended-care facilities should wear gloves when providing hands-on care for a patient

suspected of having scabies until the diagnosis is confirmed and treatment completed. It is advisable to treat all residents, staff, and families of patients at the same time to prevent reinfection. Because geriatric patients may be more sensitive to side effects of the scabicides, they should be observed closely for reactions.

Medical and Nursing Management

The patient is instructed to take a warm, soapy bath or shower to remove the scaling debris from the crusts and then to dry thoroughly and allow the skin to cool. A prescription scabicide, such as lindane (Kwell), crotamiton (Eurax), or 5% permethrin (Elimite), is applied thinly to the entire skin from the neck down, sparing only the face and scalp (which are not affected in scabies). The medication is left on for 12 to 24 hours, after which the patient is instructed to wash thoroughly. One application may be curative, but it is advisable to repeat the treatment in 1 week.

CONTACT DERMATITIS

Contact dermatitis is an inflammatory reaction of the skin to physical, chemical, or biologic agents.

Pathophysiology

The epidermis is damaged by repeated physical and chemical irritations. Contact dermatitis may be of the primary irritant type, in which a nonallergic reaction results from exposure to an irritating substance, or it may be an allergic reaction resulting from exposure of sensitized people to contact allergens. Common causes of irritant dermatitis are soaps, detergents, scouring compounds, and industrial chemicals. Predisposing factors include extremes of heat and cold, frequent contact with soap and water, and a pre-existing skin disease (Box 52-6).

Clinical Manifestations and Assessment

The eruptions begin when the causative agent contacts the skin. The first reactions include pruritus, burning, and erythema, followed closely by edema, papules, vesicles, and oozing or weeping. In the subacute phase, these vesicular changes are less marked, and they alternate with crusting, drying, fissuring, and peeling. If repeated reactions occur or if the patient continually scratches the skin, **lichenification** (thickening of the horny layer of the skin) and pigmentation occur. Secondary bacterial invasion may follow.

Medical and Nursing Management

The objectives of management are to rest the involved skin and protect it from further damage. The distribution pattern of the reaction is identified to differentiate between allergic and irritant contact dermatitis. A detailed history is obtained.

Patient Education

Strategies for Avoiding Contact Dermatitis

The following precautions may help prevent repeated cases of contact dermatitis. Follow these instructions for at least 4 months after your skin appears to be completely healed:

- Study the pattern and location of your dermatitis and think about which things have touched your skin and which things may have caused the problem. Try to avoid contact with these materials.
- Avoid heat, soap, and rubbing, all of which are external irritants.
- Choose bath soaps, laundry detergents, and cosmetics that do not contain fragrance.
- Avoid using a fabric softener dryer sheet (Bounce, Cling Free). Fabric softeners that are added to the washer may be used.
- Avoid topical medications, lotions, or ointments, except those specifically prescribed for your condition.
- Wash your skin thoroughly immediately after exposure to possible irritants.
- When wearing gloves (e.g., for washing dishes or general cleaning), be sure they are cotton-lined. Do not wear them more than 15 or 20 minutes at a time.

If possible, the offending irritant is removed. Local irritation should be avoided, and generally soap is not used until healing occurs.

Many preparations are advocated for relieving dermatitis. In general, a bland, unmedicated lotion is used for small patches of erythema. Cool, wet dressings also are applied over small areas of vesicular dermatitis. Finely cracked ice added to the water often enhances its antipruritic effect.

Wet dressings usually help clear the oozing eczematous lesions. Then a thin layer of cream or ointment containing a corticosteroid may be used. Medicated baths at room temperature are prescribed for larger areas of dermatitis. For severe, widespread conditions, a short course of systemic corticosteroids may be prescribed.

NONINFECTIOUS INFLAMMATORY DERMATOSES

PSORIASIS

Considered one of the most common skin diseases, psoriasis affects approximately 2% of the population, appearing more often in people of European ancestry. It is thought that this chronic, noninfectious, inflammatory disease stems from a hereditary defect that causes overproduction of keratin. Onset may occur at any age, but psoriasis is most common in people between 15 and 35 years of age. Psoriasis has a tendency to improve and then recur periodically throughout life (Augustin & Radtke, 2016).

Pathophysiology

Although the primary cause of psoriasis is unknown, a combination of specific genetic makeup and environmental stimuli may trigger the onset of disease. Current evidence supports an immunologic basis for the disease (Mrowietz & Reich, 2009). Periods of emotional stress and anxiety aggravate the condition, and trauma, infections, and seasonal and hormonal changes also are trigger factors.

Epidermal cells are produced at a rate that is about six to nine times faster than normal. The cells in the basal layer of the skin divide too quickly, and the newly formed cells move so rapidly to the skin surface that they become evident as profuse scales or plaques of epidermal tissue. The psoriatic epidermal cell may travel from the basal cell layer of the epidermis to the stratum corneum and be cast off in 3 to 4 days, which is in sharp contrast to the normal 26 to 28 days. As a result of the increased number of basal cells and rapid cell passage, the normal events of cell maturation and growth cannot take place. This abnormal process does not allow the normal protective layers of the skin to form.

Clinical Manifestations and Assessment

Lesions appear as red, raised patches of skin covered with silvery scales. The scaly patches are formed by the buildup of living and dead skin resulting from the vast increase in the rate of skin cell growth and turnover (Fig. 52-4). If the scales are scraped away, the dark-red base of the lesion is exposed, producing multiple bleeding points. These patches are not moist and may be pruritic. One variation of this condition is called *guttate* (in the shape of a drop) psoriasis because the lesions remain about 1 cm wide and are scattered like raindrops over the body. This variation is believed to be associated with a recent streptococcal throat infection. Psoriasis may range in severity from a cosmetic source of annoyance to a physically disabling and disfiguring disorder.

FIGURE 52-4 Psoriasis. Reprinted with permission from Bickley, L. S. (2013). *Bate's guide to physical examination and history taking*. Philadelphia, PA: Lippincott Williams & Wilkins.

Particular sites of the body tend to be affected most by this condition; they include the scalp, the extensor surface of the elbows and knees, the lower part of the back, and the genitalia. Bilateral symmetry is a feature of psoriasis. In approximately one fourth to one half of patients, the nails are involved, with pitting, discoloration, crumbling beneath the free edges, and separation of the nail plate. When psoriasis occurs on the palms and soles, it can cause pustular lesions called *palmar pustular psoriasis.*

The presence of the classic plaque-type lesions generally confirms the diagnosis of psoriasis. Because the lesions tend to change histologically as they progress from early to chronic plaques, biopsy of the skin is of little diagnostic value. There are no specific blood tests for diagnosing the condition. When in doubt, the health care provider should assess for signs of nail and scalp involvement and for a positive family history.

Complications

Asymmetric rheumatoid factor–negative arthritis of multiple joints occurs in about 5% of people with psoriasis. The arthritic development can occur before or after the skin lesions appear. The relationship between arthritis and psoriasis is not understood, although recent studies suggest there is interplay among genetics, environmental factors, and the immune system (Augustin & Radtke, 2016). Erythrodermic psoriasis, an exfoliative psoriatic state, involves disease progression that affects the total body surface. The patient is acutely ill, with impaired temperature regulation and fluid and protein loss. Erythrodermic psoriasis often appears in people with chronic psoriasis after infections, after exposure to certain medications, or following withdrawal of systemic corticosteroids.

Medical and Nursing Management

The goals of management are to slow the rapid turnover of epidermis, to promote resolution of the psoriatic lesions, and to control the natural cycles of the disease. There is no known cure.

The therapeutic approach should be one that the patient understands; it should be cosmetically acceptable and minimally disruptive to the patient's lifestyle. Treatment involves the commitment of time and effort by the patient and possibly the family. First, any precipitating or aggravating factors are addressed. An assessment is made of lifestyle because psoriasis is significantly affected by stress. The patient is informed that treatment of severe psoriasis can be time-consuming, expensive, and aesthetically unappealing at times.

Removal of Scales

The most important principle of psoriasis treatment is gentle removal of scales. This can be accomplished with baths. Oils (e.g., olive oil, mineral oil, Aveeno Oilated Oatmeal Bath) or coal tar preparations (e.g., Balnetar) can be added to the bath water and a soft brush used to scrub the psoriatic plaques gently. After bathing, the application of emollient creams containing alpha-hydroxy acids (e.g., Lac-Hydrin, Penederm) or salicylic acid continues to soften thick scales. The patient and family should be encouraged to establish a regular skin care routine that can be maintained even when the psoriasis is not in an acute stage.

Pharmacologic Therapy

With the recent addition of biologic medications, four types of therapy are now commonly used: topical, intralesional, oral, and injectable (Table 52-5).

Topical Agents

Topically applied agents are used to slow the overactive epidermis without affecting other tissues. These agents include lotions, ointments, pastes, creams, and shampoos. Topical corticosteroids may be applied for their anti-inflammatory effect. Choosing the correct strength of corticosteroid for the involved site and choosing the most effective vehicle base are important aspects of topical treatment. In general, high-potency topical corticosteroids should not be used on the face and intertriginous areas, and their use on other areas should be limited to a 4-week course of twice-daily applications. A 2-week break should be taken before repeating treatment with the high-potency corticosteroids. For long-term therapy, moderate-potency corticosteroids are used. On the face and intertriginous areas, only low-potency corticosteroids are appropriate for long-term use (see Table 52-6).

Occlusive dressings may be applied to increase the effectiveness of the corticosteroid. Large rolls of tubular plastic can be used to cover the arms and legs. Another option is a vinyl jogging suit. The medication is applied, and the suit is put on over it. The hands can be wrapped in gloves, the feet in plastic bags, and the head in a shower cap. Occlusive dressings should not remain in place longer than 8 hours. The skin should be inspected carefully for the appearance of atrophy, hypopigmentation, striae, and telangiectasias, all side effects of corticosteroids.

When psoriasis involves large areas of the body, topical corticosteroid treatment can be expensive and involve some systemic risk. The more potent corticosteroids, when applied to large areas of the body, have the potential to cause adrenal suppression through percutaneous absorption of the medication. In this event, other treatment modalities (e.g., nonsteroidal topical medications, ultraviolet light) may be used instead or in combination to decrease the need for corticosteroids.

Two topical nonsteroidal treatments introduced within the past few years are calcipotriene (Dovonex) and tazarotene (Tazorac). Treatment with these agents tends to suppress **epidermopoiesis** (i.e., development of epidermal cells) and cause sloughing of the rapidly growing

TABLE **52-5** **Current Pharmacologic Treatment for Psoriasis**

Topical Agents	Use	Selected Agents
Biologicals	Moderate to severe lesions	Cyclosporine (Neoral), alefacept (Amevive), etanercept (Enbrel), infliximab (Remicade)
Topical corticosteroids	Mild to moderate lesions Moderate to severe lesions Severe lesions Lesions on face and groin	Aristocort, Kenalog, Valisone Lidex, Psorcon, Cutivate Temovate, Diprolene, Ultravate Aclovate, DesOwen, Hytone 2.5%
Topical nonsteroidals	Mild to severe lesions	Retinoids, such as tazarotene (Tazorac) Vitamin D_3 derivative calcipotriene (Dovonex)
Coal tar products	Mild to moderate lesions	Coal tar and salicylic acid ointment (Aquatar, Estar gel, Fototar, Zetar); anthralin (AnthraDerm, Dritho-Cream); Neutrogena T-Derm, Psori Gel
Medicated shampoos	Scalp lesions	Neutrogena T-Gel, T-Sal, Zetar, Head & Shoulders, Desenex, Selsun Blue, Bakers P&S (emulsifying agent with phenol, saline solution, and mineral oil)
Intralesional therapy	Thick plaques and nails	Kenalog, Cordran-impregnated tape, Fluoroplex
Systemic therapy	Extensive lesions and nails Psoriatic arthritis	Methotrexate (Folex, Mexate); hydrouria (Hydrea); retinoic acid (Tegison) (not to be used in women of childbearing age) Oral gold (auranofin), etretinate, methotrexate
Photochemotherapy	Moderate to severe lesions	UVA or UVB light with or without topical medications PUVA (combines UVA light with oral psoralens, or topical Trisoralen)

epidermal cells. Calcipotriene 0.05% is a derivative of vitamin D_2. It works by decreasing the mitotic turnover of the psoriatic plaques. Its most common side effect is local irritation. The intertriginous areas and face should be

TABLE **52-6** **Potency: Topical Corticosteroids**

Potency	Topical Corticosteroid
Over-the-counter	0.5–1.0% hydrocortisone
Lowest	Dexamethasone 0.1% (Decaderm) Alclometasone 0.05% (Aclovate) Hydrocortisone 2.5% (Hytone)
Low–Medium	Desonide 0.05% (DesOwen, Tridesilon) Fluocinolone acetonide 0.025% (Synalar) Hydrocortisone valerate 0.2% (Westcort) Betamethasone valerate 0.1% (Valisone) Fluticasone propionate 0.05% (Cutivate)
Medium–High	Triamcinolone acetonide 0.1–0.5% (Aristocort) Fluocinonide 0.05% (Lidex) Desoximetasone 0.05–0.25% (Topicort) Fluocinolone 0.2% (Synalar) Diflorasone diacetate 0.05% (Psorcon)
Very high	Clobetasol propionate 0.05% (Temovate) Betamethasone dipropionate 0.05% (Diprolene) Halobetasol propionate 0.05% (Ultravate)

avoided when using this medication. The patient should be monitored for symptoms of hypercalcemia. Calcipotriene is available as a cream for use on the body and a solution for the scalp. It is not recommended for use by elderly patients because of their more fragile skin or by pregnant or lactating women.

Tazarotene, a retinoid, causes sloughing of the scales covering psoriatic plaques. As with other retinoids, it causes increased sensitivity to sunlight by loss of the outermost layer of skin so the patient should be cautioned to use an effective sunscreen and avoid other photosensitizers (e.g., tetracycline, antihistamines). Tazarotene is listed as a Category X drug in pregnancy; reports indicate evidence of fetal risk, and the risk of use in pregnant women clearly outweighs any possible benefits. A negative result on a pregnancy test should be obtained before initiating this medication in women of childbearing age, and an effective contraceptive should be continued during treatment. Side effects include burning, erythema, or irritation at the site of application and worsening of psoriasis.

Intralesional Agents

Intralesional injections of the corticosteroid triamcinolone acetonide (Aristocort, Kenalog-10, Trymex) can be administered directly into highly visible or isolated patches of psoriasis that are resistant to other forms of therapy. Care must be taken to ensure that the medication is not injected into unaffected skin.

Systemic Agents

Although systemic corticosteroids may cause rapid improvement of psoriasis, their usual risks and the possibility of triggering a severe flare-up on withdrawal limit their use. Systemic cytotoxic preparations, such as methotrexate, have been used in treating extensive psoriasis that fails to respond to other forms of therapy.

Methotrexate appears to inhibit DNA synthesis in epidermal cells, thereby reducing the turnover time of the psoriatic epidermis. However, the medication can be toxic, especially to the liver, kidneys, and bone marrow. Laboratory studies must be monitored to ensure that the hepatic, hematopoietic, and renal systems are functioning adequately. The patient should avoid drinking alcohol while taking methotrexate because alcohol ingestion increases the possibility of liver damage. The medication is teratogenic (produces physical defects in the fetus) and thus should not be administered to pregnant women.

Hydroxyurea (Hydrea) also inhibits cell replication by affecting DNA synthesis. The patient is monitored for signs and symptoms of bone marrow depression.

Cyclosporine A, a cyclic peptide used to prevent rejection of transplanted organs, has shown some success in treating severe, therapy-resistant cases of psoriasis. However, its use is limited by side effects such as hypertension and nephrotoxicity.

Oral retinoids (i.e., synthetic derivatives of vitamin A and its metabolite, vitamin A acid) modulate the growth and differentiation of epithelial tissue. Etretinate is especially useful for severe pustular or erythrodermic psoriasis. Etretinate is a teratogen with a very long half-life; it cannot be used in women with childbearing potential.

Photochemotherapy

One treatment for severely debilitating psoriasis is a psoralen (phototoxic) medication (e.g., methoxsalen) combined with ultraviolet-A (PUVA) light therapy. Ultraviolet light is the portion of the electromagnetic spectrum containing wavelengths ranging from 180 to 400 nm. In this treatment, the patient takes a photosensitizing medication (usually 8-methoxypsoralen) in a standard dose and is subsequently exposed to long-wave ultraviolet light as the medication plasma levels peak. Although the mechanism of action is not completely understood, it is thought that when psoralen-treated skin is exposed to ultraviolet-A light, the psoralen binds with DNA and decreases cellular proliferation. PUVA is not without its hazards; it has been associated with long-term risks of skin cancer, cataracts, and premature aging of the skin (Augustin & Radtke, 2016). The PUVA unit consists of a chamber that contains high-output black-light lamps and an external reflectance system. The exposure time is calibrated according to the specific unit in use and the anticipated tolerance of the patient's skin. The patient is usually treated two or three times each week until the psoriasis clears. An interim period of 48 hours between treatments is necessary; it takes this long for any burns resulting from PUVA therapy to become evident.

After the psoriasis clears, the patient begins a maintenance program. Once little or no disease is active, less potent therapies are used to keep minor flare-ups under control.

Ultraviolet-B (UVB) light therapy is also used to treat generalized plaques. UVB light ranges from 270 to 350 nm, although research has shown that a narrow range, 310 to 312 nm, is the action spectrum. It is used alone or combined with topical coal tar. Side effects are similar to those of PUVA therapy. If access to a light treatment unit is not feasible, the patient can expose himself or herself to sunlight. The risks of all light treatments are similar and include acute sunburn reaction; exacerbation of photosensitive disorders, such as lupus, rosacea, and polymorphic light eruption (a rash related to photosensitivity that can take on many forms); as well as other skin changes, such as increased wrinkles, thickening, and an increased risk for skin cancer.

EXFOLIATIVE DERMATITIS

Exfoliative dermatitis is a serious condition characterized by progressive inflammation in which generalized erythema and shedding of the skin occur. It may be associated with chills, fever, prostration, severe toxicity, and a pruritic scaling of the skin.

Pathophysiology

There is a profound loss of stratum corneum (i.e., outermost layer of the skin), which causes capillary leakage, hypoproteinemia, and negative nitrogen balance. Because of widespread dilation of cutaneous vessels, large amounts of body heat are lost, and exfoliative dermatitis has a marked effect on the entire body.

Exfoliative dermatitis has a variety of causes. It is considered to be a secondary or reactive process to an underlying skin or systemic disease. It may appear as a part of the lymphoma group of diseases and may precede the clinical manifestations of lymphoma.

Clinical Manifestations and Assessment

This condition starts acutely as a patchy or a generalized erythematous eruption accompanied by fever, malaise, and, occasionally, GI symptoms. The skin color changes from pink to dark red. Redness and other color changes are usually not noticed in patients with darker tones. It is recommended that the skin should be compared with the adjacent or opposite area of the body to note skin color changes. The skin should also be assessed for firmness and bogginess when palpated as well as the presence of pain, edema, warmth or cooler temperatures.

After a week, the characteristic exfoliation (i.e., scaling) begins, usually in the form of thin flakes that leave the underlying skin smooth and red, with new scales forming as the older ones come off. Hair loss may accompany this disorder. Relapses are common. The systemic effects include high-output heart failure, intestinal disturbances, breast enlargement, elevated levels of uric acid in the blood (i.e., hyperuricemia), and temperature disturbances.

Medical and Nursing Management

The objectives of management are to maintain fluid and electrolyte balance and to prevent infection. The treatment is individualized and supportive and should be initiated as soon as the condition is diagnosed.

The patient may be hospitalized and placed on bed rest. All medications that may be implicated are discontinued. A comfortable room temperature should be maintained because the patient does not have normal thermoregulatory control as a result of temperature fluctuations caused by vasodilation and evaporative water loss. Fluid and electrolyte balance must be maintained because there is considerable water and protein loss from the skin surface. Administration of plasma volume expanders may be indicated.

BLISTERING DISORDERS

PEMPHIGUS

Pemphigus is a group of serious diseases of the skin characterized by the appearance of bullae (blisters) of various sizes on apparently normal skin (Fig. 52-5) and mucous membranes.

Pathophysiology

Pemphigus is an autoimmune disease involving immunoglobulin G. It is thought that the pemphigus antibody is directed against a specific cell-surface antigen in epidermal cells. A blister forms from the antigen–antibody reaction. The level of serum antibody is predictive of disease severity.

FIGURE 52-5 Vesicles on the chin (in pemphigus). (From Hall, J. C. (2006). *Sauer's manual of skin diseases*. Philadelphia, PA: Lippincott Williams & Wilkins.)

Risk Factors

Genetic factors may also have a role in its development, with the highest incidence among those of Jewish or Mediterranean descent. This disorder usually occurs in men and women in middle and late adulthood. The condition may be associated with the use of penicillins and captopril and with the disorder myasthenia gravis.

Clinical Manifestations and Assessment

Most patients present with oral lesions appearing as irregularly shaped erosions that are painful, bleed easily, and heal slowly. The skin bullae enlarge, rupture, and leave large, painful, eroded areas that are accompanied by crusting and oozing. A characteristic offensive odor emanates from the bullae and the exuding serum. There is blistering or sloughing of uninvolved skin when minimal pressure is applied (Nikolsky sign). The eroded skin heals slowly, and large areas of the body eventually are involved. Bacterial superinfection is common.

Complications

The most common complications arise when the disease process is widespread. Before the advent of corticosteroid and immunosuppressive therapy, patients were very susceptible to secondary bacterial infection. Skin bacteria have relatively easy access to the bullae as they ooze, rupture, and leave denuded (loss of epidermis) areas exposed to the environment. Fluid and electrolyte imbalance results from fluid and protein loss as the bullae rupture. Hypoalbuminemia is common when the disease process includes extensive areas of the body's skin surface and mucous membranes.

Medical and Nursing Management

The goals of therapy are to bring the disease under control as rapidly as possible, to prevent loss of serum and the development of secondary infection, and to promote re-epithelization (i.e., renewal of epithelial tissue).

Corticosteroids are administered in high doses to control the disease and keep the skin free of blisters. The high dosage level is maintained until remission is apparent. In some cases, corticosteroid therapy must be maintained for life. High-dose corticosteroid therapy has serious toxic effects.

Immunosuppressive agents (e.g., azathioprine, cyclophosphamide, gold) may be prescribed to help control the disease and reduce the corticosteroid dose. **Plasmapheresis** temporarily decreases the serum antibody level and has been used with variable success, although it is generally reserved for life-threatening cases.

BULLOUS PEMPHIGOID

Bullous pemphigoid is an acquired disease of flaccid blisters appearing on normal or erythematous skin.

Clinical Manifestations and Assessment

Bullous pemphigoid appears more often on the flexor surfaces of the arms, legs, axilla, and groin. Oral lesions, if present, are usually transient and minimal. When the blisters break, the skin has shallow erosions that heal fairly quickly. Pruritus can be intense, even before the appearance of the blisters. Bullous pemphigoid is common in the elderly, with a peak incidence at about 60 years of age. There is no gender or racial predilection, and the disease can be found in patients throughout the world.

Medical and Nursing Management

Medical treatment includes topical corticosteroids for localized eruptions and systemic corticosteroids for widespread involvement. Systemic corticosteroids (e.g., prednisone) may be continued for months, in alternate-day doses. The patient needs to understand the implications of long-term corticosteroid therapy.

Complications

Infection and Sepsis

The patient is susceptible to infection because the barrier function of the skin is compromised. Bullae are also susceptible to infection, and sepsis may follow. The skin is cleaned to remove debris and dead skin and to prevent infection.

Secondary infection may be accompanied by an unpleasant odor from skin or oral lesions. *Candida albicans* of the mouth (i.e., thrush) commonly affects patients receiving high-dose corticosteroid therapy. The oral cavity is inspected daily, and any changes are reported. Oral lesions are slow to heal.

Infection is the leading cause of death in patients with blistering diseases. Particular attention is given to assessment for signs and symptoms of local and systemic infection. Seemingly trivial complaints or minimal changes are investigated because corticosteroids can mask or alter typical signs and symptoms of infection. The patient's vital signs are monitored, and temperature fluctuations are documented. The patient is observed for chills, and all secretions and excretions are monitored for changes suggesting infection. Results of culture and sensitivity tests are monitored. Antimicrobial agents are administered as prescribed, and response to treatment is assessed. Health care personnel must perform effective hand hygiene and wear gloves.

In hospitalized patients, environmental contamination is reduced as much as possible. Protective isolation measures and standard precautions are warranted.

Fluid and Electrolyte Imbalance

Extensive denudation of the skin leads to fluid and electrolyte imbalance because of significant loss of fluids and sodium chloride from the skin. This sodium chloride loss is responsible for many of the systemic symptoms associated with the disease and is treated by IV administration of saline solution.

A large amount of protein and blood is also lost from the denuded skin areas. Blood component therapy may be prescribed to maintain the blood volume, hemoglobin level, and plasma protein concentration. Serum albumin, protein, hemoglobin, and hematocrit values are monitored.

The patient is encouraged to maintain adequate oral fluid intake. Cool, nonirritating fluids are encouraged to maintain hydration. Small, frequent meals or snacks of high-protein, high-calorie foods (e.g., oral nutritional supplements, eggnog, milkshakes) help maintain nutritional status. Parenteral nutrition is considered if the patient cannot eat an adequate diet.

TOXIC EPIDERMAL NECROLYSIS AND STEVENS–JOHNSON SYNDROME

Toxic epidermal necrolysis (TEN) and Stevens–Johnson syndrome (SJS) are potentially fatal skin disorders and the most severe forms of erythema multiforme.

These diseases are mucocutaneous reactions that constitute a spectrum of reactions, with TEN being the most severe. The mortality rate from TEN is 30% to 35%. TEN and SJS are triggered by a reaction to medications. Antibiotics, especially sulfonamides, antiseizure agents, nonsteroidal anti-inflammatory drugs (NSAIDs), are the medications implicated most frequently (Bryant, 2016).

Risk Factors

These conditions occur in patients of all ages and both genders. The incidence is increased in older people because of their use of many medications. People who are immunosuppressed, including those with HIV infection and AIDS, have a high risk of SJS and TEN. Although the incidence of TEN and SJS in the general population is about 2 to 3 cases per 1 million people in the United States, the risk associated with sulfonamides in HIV-positive individuals may approach 1 case per 1,000 (Bryant, 2016). Most patients with TEN have an abnormal metabolism of the medication; the mechanism leading to TEN seems to be a cell-mediated cytotoxic reaction.

Clinical Manifestations and Assessment

TEN and SJS are characterized initially by conjunctival burning or itching, cutaneous tenderness, fever, cough, sore throat, headache, extreme malaise, and myalgias (i.e., aches and pains). These signs are followed by a rapid onset of erythema involving much of the skin surface and mucous membranes, including the oral mucosa, conjunctiva, and genitalia. In severe cases of mucosal involvement, there may be danger of damage to the larynx, bronchi, and esophagus from ulcerations. Large, flaccid bullae develop in some areas; in other areas, large sheets of epidermis are shed, exposing the underlying dermis. Fingernails, toenails, eyebrows, and eyelashes may be shed along with the surrounding epidermis. The skin is excruciatingly tender, and the loss of skin leaves a weeping surface similar to that of a total-body, partial-thickness burn; hence the condition is also referred to as "scalded skin syndrome."

Histologic studies of frozen skin cells from a fresh lesion and cytodiagnosis of collections of cellular material from a freshly denuded area are conducted. A history of use of medications known to precipitate TEN or SJS may confirm medication reaction as the underlying cause.

Immunofluorescent studies may be performed to detect atypical epidermal autoantibodies. A genetic predisposition to erythema multiforme has been suggested but has not been confirmed in all cases.

Medical and Nursing Management

The goals of treatment include control of fluid and electrolyte balance, prevention of sepsis, and prevention of ophthalmic complications. Supportive care is the mainstay of treatment.

All nonessential medications are discontinued immediately. If possible, the patient is treated in a regional burn center because aggressive treatment similar to that for severe burns is required. Skin loss may approach 100% of the total body surface area. Surgical débridement or hydrotherapy in a Hubbard tank (large steel tub) may be performed to remove involved skin.

Tissue samples from the nasopharynx, eyes, ears, blood, urine, skin, and unruptured blisters are obtained for culture to identify pathogenic organisms. IV fluids are prescribed to maintain fluid and electrolyte balance, especially in the patient who has severe mucosal involvement and who cannot easily take oral nourishment. Because an indwelling IV catheter may be a site of infection, fluid replacement is carried out by nasogastric tube and then orally as soon as possible.

Initial treatment with systemic corticosteroids is controversial. Some experts argue for early high-dose corticosteroid treatment. However, in most cases, the risk of infection, the complication of fluid and electrolyte imbalance, the delay in the healing process, and the difficulty in initiating oral corticosteroids early in the course of the disease outweigh the perceived benefits. In patients with TEN thought to result from a medication reaction, corticosteroids may be administered; however, the patient should be monitored closely for adverse effects.

Protecting the skin with topical agents is crucial. Various topical antibacterial and anesthetic agents are used to prevent wound sepsis and to assist with pain management. Systemic antibiotic therapy is used with extreme caution. Temporary biologic dressings (e.g., pigskin, amniotic membrane) or plastic semi-permeable dressings (e.g., Vigilon) may be used to reduce pain, decrease evaporation, and prevent secondary infection until the epithelium regenerates. Meticulous oropharyngeal and eye care is essential when there is severe involvement of the mucous membranes and the eyes.

As the patient completes the acute inpatient stage of illness, the focus is directed toward rehabilitation and outpatient care or care in a rehabilitation center. Throughout this care, the patient and family members are involved in the care and are instructed in the procedures, such as wound care and dressing changes that will need to be continued at home. The patient and family members are assisted in acquiring dressing supplies that will be needed at home.

The patient and family members are also provided with instructions about pain management, nutrition, measures to increase mobility, and prevention of complications, including prevention of infection. They are taught the signs and symptoms of complications and instructed when to notify the health care provider. When appropriate, instructions are provided in writing to the patient and family so they can refer to these instructions when necessary at later times.

Interdisciplinary follow-up care is imperative to ensure that the patient's progress continues. Some patients will require care in a rehabilitation center before returning home. Others will require outpatient physical and occupational therapy for an extended period. When the patient returns home, the home care nurse coordinates the care provided by the various members of the health care team (e.g., primary care provider, physical therapist, occupational therapist, and dietician). The nurse also monitors the patient's progress, provides ongoing assessment to identify complications, and monitors the patient's adherence to the plan of care. The patient's adaptation to the home care environment and the patient's and family's needs for support and assistance are also assessed. Referrals to community agencies are made as appropriate.

Complications

Sepsis

The major cause of death from TEN is infection, and the most common sites of infection are the skin and mucosal surfaces, lungs, and blood. The organisms involved most often are *Staphylococcus aureus*, *Pseudomonas*, *Klebsiella*, *Escherichia coli*, *Serratia*, and *Candida*. Monitoring vital signs closely and noticing changes in respiratory, renal, and GI function may quickly detect the beginning of an infection. Strict asepsis is always maintained during routine skin care measures. Hand hygiene and wearing sterile gloves when carrying out procedures are essential. When the condition involves a large portion of the body, the patient should be in a private room to prevent possible cross-infection from other patients. Visitors should wear protective garments and wash their hands before and after coming into contact with the patient. People with any infections or infectious disease should not visit the patient until they are no longer a danger to the patient. Refer to Chapter 54 for more details on sepsis.

Conjunctival Retraction, Scars, and Corneal Lesions

The nurse inspects the eyes daily for signs of pruritus, burning, and dryness, which may indicate progression to keratoconjunctivitis, the principal eye complication. Applying a cool, damp cloth over the eyes may relieve burning sensations. The eyes are kept clean and observed for signs of discharge or discomfort, and the progression of symptoms is documented and reported. Administering an eye lubricant, when prescribed, may alleviate dryness and prevent corneal abrasion. Using eye patches or reminding the patient to blink periodically may also counteract dryness. The patient is instructed to avoid rubbing the eyes or putting any medication into the eyes that has not been prescribed or approved by the provider.

BENIGN SKIN TUMORS

Table 52-7 provides descriptions of and treatments for common benign skin lesions.

MALIGNANT SKIN TUMORS

Skin cancer is the most common cancer in the United States. If the incidence continues at the present rate, an estimated one of eight fair-skinned Americans will eventually develop skin cancer, especially basal cell carcinoma. Because the skin is easily inspected, skin cancer is readily seen and detected and is the type of cancer that is treated most successfully.

Exposure to the sun is the leading cause of skin cancer; incidence is related to the total amount of exposure to the sun. Sun damage is cumulative, and harmful effects may be severe by 20 years of age. The increase in skin cancer probably reflects changing lifestyles and the emphasis on sunbathing and related activities in light of changes in the environment, such as holes in the Earth's ozone layer. Changes in the ozone layer from the effects of worldwide industrial air pollutants, such as chlorofluorocarbons, have prompted concern that the incidence of skin cancers, especially malignant melanoma, will increase. The ozone layer, a stratospheric blanket of bluish, explosive gas formed by the sun's ultraviolet radiation, varies in depth with the seasons and is thickest at the North and South Poles and thinnest at the equator. Scientists believe that it helps protect the earth from the effects of solar ultraviolet radiation. Proponents of this theory predict an increase in skin cancers as a consequence of changes in the ozone layer. Other skin cancer risk factors are summarized in Box 52-7. Protective measures should be used throughout life, and nurses should inform patients about risk factors associated with skin cancer.

BASAL CELL AND SQUAMOUS CELL CARCINOMA

The most common types of skin cancer are basal cell carcinoma (BCC) and squamous cell (epidermoid) carcinoma (SCC).

BOX 52-7	**Risk Factors for Skin Cancer**

- Fair-skinned, fair-haired, blue-eyed people, particularly those of Celtic origin, with insufficient skin pigmentation to protect underlying tissues
- People who sustain sunburn and who do not tan
- Chronic sun exposure (certain occupations, such as farming, construction work)
- Exposure to chemical pollutants (industrial workers in arsenic, nitrates, coal, tar and pitch, oils and paraffins)
- Sun-damaged skin (elderly people)
- History of x-ray therapy for acne or benign lesions
- Scars from severe burns
- Chronic skin irritations
- Immunosuppression
- Genetic factors

The third most common type, malignant melanoma, is discussed separately. Skin cancer is diagnosed by biopsy and histologic evaluation.

Clinical Manifestations and Assessment

BCC is the most common type of skin cancer. It generally appears on sun-exposed areas of the body and is more prevalent in regions where the population is subjected to intense and extensive exposure to the sun. The incidence is proportional to the age of the patient (average, 60 years of age) and the total amount of sun exposure, and it is inversely proportional to the amount of melanin in the skin.

BCC usually begins as a small, waxy nodule with rolled, translucent, pearly borders; telangiectatic vessels may be present. As it grows, it undergoes central ulceration and, sometimes, crusting (Fig. 52-6). The tumors appear most frequently on the face. BCC is characterized by invasion and erosion of contiguous (adjoining) tissues. It rarely metastasizes, but recurrence is common. However, a neglected

FIGURE 52-6 Basal cell carcinoma (*left*) and squamous cell carcinoma (*right*). (Reprinted by permission from *New England Journal of Medicine, 326,* 169–170; 1992.)

TABLE **52-7** Benign Skin Lesions

Lesion	Description	Treatment
Cysts	Cysts of the skin are epithelium-lined cavities that contain fluid or solid material.	
	Epidermal cysts (epidermoid cysts) occur frequently and are slow-growing, firm, elevated tumors frequently noted on the face, neck, upper chest, and back.	Removal of the cysts provides a cure.
	Pilar cysts (trichilemmal cysts), formerly called sebaceous cysts, frequently are found on the scalp. They originate from the middle portion of the hair follicle and from the cells of the outer hair root sheath.	Treatment is surgical removal.
Seborrheic and actinic keratoses	**Seborrheic keratoses** are benign, wartlike lesions of various sizes and colors, ranging from light tan to black, that are usually located on the face, shoulders, chest, and back.	Treatment is removal of the tumor tissue by excision, electrodesiccation, and curettage, or application of carbon dioxide or liquid nitrogen.
	Actinic keratoses are premalignant skin lesions that develop in chronically sun-exposed areas of the body. They appear as rough, scaly patches with underlying erythema. A small percentage of these lesions gradually transforms into cutaneous squamous cell carcinoma.	They are usually removed by cryotherapy or shave excision.
Verrucae: Warts	**Warts** are common, benign skin tumors caused by infection with the human papillomavirus, which belongs to the DNA virus group. People of all ages may be affected, but the warts occur most frequently in patients between 12 and 16 years of age.	They may be treated with locally applied laser therapy, liquid nitrogen, salicylic acid plasters, or electrodesiccation.
	Genitalia and perianal warts are known as *condylomata acuminata*. They may be transmitted sexually. Condylomata that affect the uterine cervix predispose the patient to cervical cancer.	They are treated with liquid nitrogen, cryosurgery, electrosurgery, topically applied trichloroacetic acid, and curettage.
Angiomas	**Angiomas** are benign vascular tumors that involve the skin and the subcutaneous tissues. They are present at birth and may occur as flat, violet-red patches (port-wine angiomas) or as raised, bright-red, nodular lesions (strawberry angiomas). The latter tend to involute spontaneously within the first few years of life, but port-wine angiomas usually persist indefinitely.	Most patients use masking cosmetics (i.e., Covermark or Dermablend) to camouflage the lesions. The argon laser is being used on various angiomas with some success. Treatment of strawberry angiomas is more successful if undertaken as soon after birth as possible.
Pigmented nevi: Moles	**Moles** are common skin tumors of various sizes and shades, ranging from yellowish brown to black. They may be flat, macular lesions or elevated papules or nodules that occasionally contain hair. Most pigmented nevi are harmless lesions. However, in rare cases, malignant changes occur, and a melanoma develops at the site of the nevus. Nevi that show a change in color or size, become symptomatic (e.g., itch), or develop irregular borders should be removed to determine if malignant changes have occurred. Moles that occur in unusual places (palms of the hands and soles of the feet) should be examined carefully for any irregularity and for notching of the border and variation in color. Nevi larger than 1 cm should be examined carefully. Excised nevi should be examined histologically.	
Keloids	**Keloids** are benign overgrowths of fibrous tissue at the site of a scar or trauma. They appear to be more common among dark-skinned people. Keloids are asymptomatic but may cause disfigurement and cosmetic concern.	The treatment, which is not always satisfactory, consists of surgical excision, intralesional corticosteroid therapy, and radiation.

lesion can result in the loss of a nose, an ear, or a lip. Other variants of BCC may appear as shiny, flat, gray or yellowish plaques.

SCC is a malignant proliferation arising from the epidermis. Although it usually appears on sun-damaged skin, it may arise from normal skin or from pre-existing skin lesions. It is of greater concern than BCC because it is a truly invasive carcinoma, metastasizing by the blood or lymphatic system.

Metastases account for 75% of deaths from SCC. The lesions may be primary, arising on the skin and mucous membranes, or they may develop from a precancerous condition, such as actinic keratosis (lesions occurring in sun-exposed areas), leukoplakia (premalignant lesion of the mucous membrane), or scarred or ulcerated lesions. SCC appears as a rough, thickened, scaly tumor that may be asymptomatic or may involve bleeding (see Fig. 52-6). The border of an SCC lesion may be wider, more infiltrated, and more inflammatory than that of a BCC lesion. Secondary infection can occur. Exposed areas, especially of the upper extremities and of the face, lower lip, ears, nose, and forehead, are common sites.

The incidence of BCC and SCC is increased in all people who are immunocompromised, including those infected with HIV. Clinically, the tumors have the same appearance as in people who are not HIV-infected; however, in patients with HIV, the tumors may grow more rapidly and recur more frequently. These tumors are managed the same as those for the general population. Frequent follow-up (every 4 to 6 months) is recommended to monitor for recurrence.

Medical Management

The goal of treatment is to eradicate the tumor. The treatment method depends on the tumor location; the cell type, location, and depth; the cosmetic desires of the patient; the history of previous treatment; whether the tumor is invasive; and whether metastatic nodes are present. The management of BCC and SCC includes surgical excision, Mohs' micrographic surgery, electrosurgery, cryosurgery, and radiation therapy.

Surgical Management

The primary goal is to remove the tumor entirely. The best way to maintain cosmetic appearance is to place the incision properly along natural skin tension lines and natural anatomic body lines. In this way, scars are less noticeable. The size of the incision depends on the tumor size and location but usually involves a length-to-width ratio of 3:1.

The adequacy of the surgical excision is verified by microscopic evaluation of sections of the specimen. When the tumor is large, reconstructive surgery with use of a skin flap or skin grafting may be required. The incision is closed in layers to enhance cosmetic effect. A pressure dressing applied over the wound provides support. Infection after a simple excision is uncommon if proper surgical asepsis is maintained.

Mohs' Micrographic Surgery

Mohs' micrographic surgery is the technique that is most accurate and that best conserves normal tissue. The procedure removes the tumor layer by layer. The first layer excised includes all evident tumor and a small margin of normal-appearing tissue. The specimen is frozen and analyzed by section to determine if the entire tumor has been removed. If not, additional layers of tissue are shaved and examined until all tissue margins are tumor-free. In this manner, only the tumor and a safe, normal-tissue margin are removed. Mohs' surgery is the recommended tissue-sparing procedure, with extremely high cure rates for both BCC and SCC. It is the treatment of choice and the most effective for tumors around the eyes, nose, upper lip, and auricular and periauricular areas.

Electrosurgery

Electrosurgery is the destruction or removal of tissue by electrical energy. The current is converted to heat, which then passes to the tissue from a cold electrode. Electrosurgery may be preceded by curettage (excising the skin tumor by scraping its surface with a curette). Then electrodesiccation is implemented to achieve hemostasis and to destroy any viable malignant cells at the base of the wound or along its edges. Electrodesiccation is useful for lesions smaller than 1 to 2 cm (0.4 to 0.8 in) in diameter.

This method takes advantage of the fact that the tumor is softer than surrounding skin and, therefore, can be outlined by a curette, which "feels" the extent of the tumor. The tumor is removed and the base cauterized. The process is repeated twice. Usually, healing occurs within a month.

Cryosurgery

Cryosurgery destroys the tumor by deep-freezing the tissue. A thermocouple needle apparatus is inserted into the skin, and liquid nitrogen is directed to the center of the tumor until the tumor base is −40°C to −60°C. Liquid nitrogen has the lowest boiling point of all cryogens, is inexpensive, and is easy to obtain. The tumor tissue is frozen, allowed to thaw, and then refrozen. The site thaws naturally and then becomes gelatinous and heals spontaneously. Swelling and edema follow the freezing. The appearance of the lesion varies. Normal healing, which may take 4 to 6 weeks, occurs faster in areas with a good blood supply.

Radiation Therapy

Frequently radiation therapy is performed for cancer of the eyelid, the tip of the nose, and areas in or near vital structures (e.g., facial nerve). It is reserved for older patients because x-ray changes may be seen after 5 to 10 years, and malignant changes in scars may be induced by irradiation 15 to 30 years later.

The patient should be informed that the skin may become red and blistered. A bland skin ointment prescribed by the provider may be applied to relieve discomfort. Also the patient should be cautioned to avoid exposure to the sun.

Nursing Management

Because many skin cancers are removed by excision, usually patients are treated in outpatient surgical units. The role of the nurse is to teach the patient about prevention of skin cancer and about self-care after treatment.

Teaching Self-Care

Usually the wound is covered with a dressing to protect the site from physical trauma, external irritants, and contaminants. The nurse instructs the patient about when to report for a dressing change or provides written and verbal information on how to change dressings, including the type of dressing to purchase, how to remove dressings and apply fresh ones, and the importance of hand hygiene before and after the procedure.

The patient watches for excessive bleeding and tight dressings that compromise circulation. If the lesion is in the perioral area, the patient is instructed to drink liquids through a straw and limit talking and facial movement. Dental work should be avoided until the area is completely healed.

After the sutures are removed, an emollient cream may be used to help reduce dryness. Applying a sunscreen over the wound is advised to prevent postoperative hyperpigmentation if the patient spends time outdoors.

Follow-up examinations should be at regular intervals, usually every 3 months for a year, and should include palpation of the adjacent lymph nodes. The nurse instructs the patient to seek treatment for any moles that are subject to repeated friction and irritation, and to watch for indications of potential malignancy in moles as described previously. The importance of life-long follow-up evaluations is emphasized.

Teaching Skin Cancer Prevention

Studies show that regular daily use of a sunscreen with a solar protection factor (SPF) of at least 15 can reduce the recurrence of skin cancer by as much as 40% (Box 52-8). The sunscreen should be applied to head, neck, arms, and hands every morning at least 30 minutes before leaving the house and reapplied every 4 hours if the skin perspires. Intermittent application of sunscreen only when exposure is anticipated has been shown to be less effective than daily use. The longer exposure is believed to contribute to the increasing incidence of melanoma. Although the evidence is insufficient, nurses should discuss the issues with patients who are at high risk of skin cancer.

BOX 52-8

Health Promotion

Preventing Skin Cancer

- Teach patients that sunscreens are rated in strength from 4 (weakest) to 50 (strongest). The solar protection factor, or SPF, indicates how much longer a person can stay in the sun before the skin begins to redden. For example, if the person normally can stay in the sun for 10 minutes before reddening begins, an SPF of 4 will protect the person from reddening for about 40 minutes. A sunscreen with an SPF of 15 or greater is recommended under most conditions and indicates 93% protection; an SPF of 34 indicates 97% protection.
- Remind patients that up to 50% of ultraviolet rays can penetrate loosely woven clothing.
- Remind patients that ultraviolet light can penetrate cloud cover, and sunburn still can occur.
- Teach children to avoid all but modest sun exposure and to use a sunscreen regularly for life-long protection.
- Advise patients to:
  - Avoid tanning if their skin burns easily, never tans, or tans poorly.
  - Avoid unnecessary exposure to the sun, especially during the time of day when ultraviolet radiation (sunlight) is most intense (10 AM to 3 PM).
  - Avoid sunburns.
  - Apply a sunscreen daily to block harmful sun rays.
  - Use a sunscreen with an SPF of 15 or higher that protects against both ultraviolet-A (UVA) and ultraviolet-B (UVB) light.
  - Reapply water-resistant sunscreens after swimming, if heavily sweating, and every 2–3 hours during prolonged periods of sun exposure.
  - Avoid applying oils before or during sun exposure (oils do not protect against sunlight or sun damage).
  - Use a lip balm that contains a sunscreen with an SPF of 15 or higher.
  - Wear protective clothing, such as a broad-brimmed hat and long sleeves.
  - Avoid using sun lamps for indoor tanning, and avoid commercial tanning booths.

Nurses should also encourage skin self-examination (Box 52-9).

MALIGNANT MELANOMA

A malignant melanoma is a cancerous neoplasm in which atypical melanocytes are present in the epidermis and the dermis (and sometimes the subcutaneous cells). It is the most lethal of all the skin cancers and is responsible for about 3% of all cancer deaths (Castiglione et al., 2016). Malignant melanoma can occur in one of several forms: superficial spreading melanoma, lentigo-maligna melanoma, nodular melanoma, and acral-lentiginous melanoma. These types have specific clinical and histologic features as well as different biologic behaviors. Most melanomas arise from

Patient Education

Periodic Self-Examination

Prevention of melanoma/skin cancer is the best weapon against these diseases, but if a melanoma should develop, it is almost always curable if caught in the early stages. Practice periodic self-examination to aid in early recognition of any new or developing lesion. The following is one way of self-examination that will ensure that no area of the body is neglected. To perform your self-examination, you will need a full-length mirror, a hand mirror, and a brightly lit room.

1. Examine the body front and back in the mirror, then the right and left sides, with the arms raised.

2. Bend the elbows, looking carefully at the forearms, back of the upper arms, and palms

3. Next, look at the back of the legs and feet, the spaces between the toes, and the soles of the feet.

4. Examine the back of the neck and the scalp with a hand-held mirror. Part the hair to lift.

5. Finally, check the back and buttocks with a hand mirror.

cutaneous epidermal melanocytes, but some appear in pre-existing nevi (i.e., moles) in the skin or develop in the uveal tract of the eye. Melanomas occasionally appear simultaneously with cancer of other organs.

The worldwide incidence of melanoma doubles every 10 years, an increase that is probably related to increased recreational sun exposure, changes in the ozone layer, and improved methods of early detection. Median age at diagnosis is 50 years of age, although melanoma affects all age groups. The incidence of melanoma is increasing faster than that of almost any other cancer, and the mortality rate is increasing faster than that of any other cancer except lung cancer. In the Unites States, approximately 76,690 new cases of malignant melanoma are diagnosed annually, and 9,480 patients will succumb to this disease, accounting for 1% to 2% of all cancer deaths in the United States (Schuchter, 2016). It is estimated that one of 37 men and one of 56 women will be diagnosed with malignant melanoma (Schuchter, 2016, p. 1373).

Risk Factors

The cause of malignant melanoma is unknown, but ultraviolet rays are strongly suspected based on indirect evidence, such as the increased incidence of melanoma in countries near the equator and in people younger than 30 years of age who have used a tanning bed more than 10 times per year. Ethnicity is a risk factor; in general, 1 in 100 Caucasians acquires melanoma each year. As many as 10% of patients with melanoma are members of a family that is more melanoma-prone. They have multiple changing moles (dysplastic nevi), which are susceptible to malignant transformation. Patients with dysplastic nevus syndrome have been found to have unusual moles, larger and more numerous moles, lesions with irregular outlines, and pigmentation located all over the skin. Microscopic examination of dysplastic moles shows disordered, faulty growth. Box 52-10 lists risk factors for malignant melanoma.

Types

Superficial Spreading Melanoma

Superficial spreading melanoma occurs anywhere on the body and is the most common form of melanoma. It usually affects middle-aged people and occurs most frequently on

BOX 52-10
Risk Factors for Malignant Melanoma

- Fair-skinned or freckled, blue-eyed, light-haired people of Celtic or Scandinavian origin
- People who burn and do not tan or who have a significant history of severe sunburn
- Environmental exposure to intense sunlight (older Americans retiring to the southwestern United States appear to have a higher incidence)
- History of melanoma (personal or family)
- Skin with giant congenital nevi

FIGURE 52-7 Two forms of malignant melanoma: superficial spreading (*left*) and nodular (*right*). (From Bickley, L. S. (2013). *Bates' guide to physical examination and history taking* (10th ed.). Philadelphia, PA: Lippincott Williams & Wilkins.)

the trunk and lower extremities. The lesion tends to be circular, with irregular outer portions. The margins of the lesion may be flat or elevated and palpable (Fig. 52-7). This type of melanoma may appear in a combination of colors, with hues of tan, brown, and black mixed with gray, blue-black, or white. Sometimes a dull pink rose color can be seen in a small area within the lesion.

Lentigo-Maligna Melanoma

Lentigo-maligna melanoma is a slowly evolving, pigmented lesion that occurs on exposed skin areas, especially the dorsum of the hand, the head, and the neck in elderly people. Often, the lesion is present for many years before it is examined by a provider. It first appears as a tan, flat lesion, but in time it undergoes changes in size and color.

Nodular Melanoma

Nodular melanoma is a spherical, blueberry-like nodule with a relatively smooth surface and a relatively uniform, blue-black color (see Fig. 52-7). It may be dome-shaped with a smooth surface. It may have other shadings of red, gray, or purple. Sometimes, nodular melanomas appear as irregularly shaped plaques. The patient may describe this as a blood blister that fails to resolve. A nodular melanoma invades directly into the adjacent dermis (i.e., vertical growth) and, therefore, has a poorer prognosis.

Acral-Lentiginous Melanoma

Acral-lentiginous melanoma occurs in areas not excessively exposed to sunlight and where hair follicles are absent. It is found on the palms of the hands, on the soles, in the nail beds, and in the mucous membranes of people who are dark-skinned. These melanomas appear as irregular, pigmented macules that develop nodules. They may become invasive early.

Clinical Manifestations and Assessment

Biopsy results confirm the diagnosis of melanoma. An excisional biopsy specimen provides information on the type,

level of invasion, and thickness of the lesion. An excisional biopsy specimen that includes a 1-cm margin of normal tissue and a portion of underlying subcutaneous fatty tissue is sufficient for staging a melanoma in situ or an early, noninvasive melanoma. Incisional biopsy should be performed when the suspicious lesion is too large to be removed safely without extensive scarring. Biopsy specimens obtained by shaving, curettage, or needle aspiration are not considered reliable histologic proof of disease.

A thorough history and physical examination should include a meticulous skin examination and palpation of regional lymph nodes that drain the lesional area. Box 52-11 discusses assessing moles. Because melanoma occurs in

---

BOX 52-11 **Assessing the ABCDEs of Moles**

A for Asymmetry

- The lesion does not appear balanced on both sides. If an imaginary line were drawn down the middle, the two halves would not look alike.
- The lesion has an irregular surface with uneven elevations (irregular topography) either palpable or visible. A change in the surface may be noted from smooth to scaly.
- Some nodular melanomas have a smooth surface.

B for Irregular Border

- Angular indentations or multiple notches appear in the border.
- The border is fuzzy or indistinct, as if rubbed with an eraser.

C for Variegated Color

- Normal moles are usually a uniform light to medium brown. Darker coloration indicates that the melanocytes have penetrated to a deeper layer of the dermis.
- Colors that may indicate malignancy if found together within a single lesion are shades of red, white, and blue; shades of blue are ominous.
- White areas within a pigmented lesion are suspicious.
- Some malignant melanomas, however, are not variegated but are uniformly colored (bluish-black, bluish-gray, bluish-red).

D for Diameter

- A diameter exceeding 6 mm (about the size of a pencil eraser) is considered more suspicious, although this finding without other signs is not significant. Many benign skin growths are larger than 6 mm, whereas some early melanomas may be smaller.

E for Elevation, Enlargement, and/or Evolution

- The lesion is raised above the surface, enlarged, and/or has an uneven surface. *Evolution* refers to a lesion that has changed significantly (size, shape, symptoms [e.g., itching, tenderness, crusting, bleeding]) over time.

families, a positive family history of melanoma is investigated so that first-degree relatives, who may be at high risk for melanoma, can be evaluated for atypical lesions. After the diagnosis of melanoma has been confirmed, a chest x-ray, complete blood cell count, liver function tests, and radionuclide or computed tomography scans are usually performed to stage the extent of disease.

Medical and Nursing Management

Treatment depends on the level of invasion and the depth of the lesion. Surgical excision is the treatment of choice for small, superficial lesions. Deeper lesions require wide local excision, after which skin grafting may be necessary. Sentinel node biopsy accurately identifies whether microscopic melanoma cells involve regional lymph nodes. The sentinel lymph node is the first node by which cancer is likely to spread from the primary tumor before spreading to other lymph nodes. This technique is used to sample the nodes nearest the tumor and to spare the patient the long-term sequelae of extensive removal of lymph nodes if the sample nodes are negative. If the sentinel node is positive, then lymph node dissection is performed.

Some investigational therapies include biologic response modifiers (e.g., interferon-alpha, interleukin-2), adaptive immunotherapy (i.e., lymphokine-activated killer cells), and monoclonal antibodies directed at melanoma antigens. Immunotherapy modifies immune function and other biologic responses to cancer. New Immunotherapy approaches for treatment of melanoma and molecularly targeted therapy based upon somatic mutation profile have led to recent FDA approvals that have redefined the standard of care for malignant melanoma. Ipilimumab, which blocks cytotoxic T-lymphocyte antigen (CTLA-4), has shown promise in patients with cases of advanced melanoma (Stage IV), with 3-year survival rate of 21% versus 12% (Schuchter, 2016). Monoclonal antibodies, such as nivolumab, have shown recent success in patients with advanced melanoma. Identification of somatic mutations in the gene encoding the serine-threonine protein kinase B-RAF (*BRAF*) is found in approximately 50% of melanomas (Ferri, 2016). Recently combination targeted therapy with the use of molecularly targeted therapies has shown a response rate of 70% (Schuchter, 2016). Several other studies are attempting to develop and test autologous immunization against specific tumor cells. These studies are in the experimental stage but show promise for future development of a vaccine against melanoma.

Further surgical intervention may be performed to debulk the tumor or to remove part of the organ involved (e.g., lung, liver, or colon). However, the rationale for more extensive surgery is for relief of symptoms, not for cure.

METASTATIC SKIN TUMORS

The skin is an important, although not a common, site of metastatic cancer. All types of cancer may metastasize to the skin, but carcinoma of the breast is the primary source of cutaneous metastases in women. Other sources include cancer of the large intestine, ovaries, and lungs. In men, the most common primary sites are the lungs, large intestine, oral cavity, kidneys, or stomach. Skin metastases from melanomas are found in both genders. The clinical appearance of metastatic skin lesions is not distinctive, except perhaps in some cases of breast cancer in which diffuse, brawny hardening of the skin of the involved breast is seen. In most instances, metastatic lesions occur as multiple cutaneous or subcutaneous nodules of various sizes that may be skin-colored or different shades of red.

KAPOSI SARCOMA

Kaposi sarcoma (KS) is a malignancy of endothelial cells that line the small blood vessels. KS is manifested clinically by lesions of the skin, oral cavity, GI tract, and lungs. The skin lesions consist of reddish-purple to dark-blue macules, plaques, or nodules. KS is subdivided into three categories:

- **Classic KS** occurs predominantly in men of Mediterranean or Jewish ancestry between 40 and 70 years of age. Most patients have nodules or plaques on the lower extremities that rarely metastasize beyond this area. Classic KS is chronic, relatively benign, and rarely fatal.
- **Endemic (African) KS** affects people predominantly in the eastern half of Africa near the equator. Men are affected more often than women, and children can be affected as well. The disease may resemble classic KS, or it may infiltrate and progress to lymphadenopathic forms.
- **Immunosuppression-associated KS** occurs in transplant recipients and people with AIDS. This form of KS is characterized by local skin lesions and disseminated visceral and mucocutaneous diseases. The greater the degree of immunosuppression, the higher the incidence of KS. Immunosuppression-related KS that results from AIDS is an aggressive tumor that involves multiple body organs. Its presentation resembles that of KS associated with immunosuppressive therapy. Most patients are between 20 and 40 years of age. Refer to Chapter 37 for more information about KS and AIDS.

CHAPTER REVIEW

Critical Thinking Exercises

1. You are caring for an elderly woman in her home. She has a long history of peripheral vascular disease and now has developed a venous stasis ulcer on her lower leg just above the ankle. Her health care provider has prescribed a moisture-retentive dressing that is impregnated with hydrogel. The dressing is to be changed every 3 days, and the patient asks you why the dressing is not changed every day. How would you explain to the patient the purpose of the dressing? Identify the evidence that supports the use of moisture-retentive dressings for venous ulcers. Discuss the strength of the evidence regarding their effectiveness in the promotion of wound healing.

2. You are caring for a middle-aged woman who has recently been diagnosed with diabetes mellitus. On preparing for discharge, she tells you that she has had itchy, dry, flaky skin during the winter months for several years and that she bathes every morning and night to try to get rid of the itching and dryness. She also states that it is difficult for her to avoid scratching her itchy skin. What teaching would you provide to this patient? What are this patient's risks of developing more serious skin conditions if the dryness and itching of her skin continue?

3. You are assigned to the emergency department and are caring for a young adult who is being treated for heatstroke following a golf game on a very hot day. As he is awaiting discharge, he tells you that he is concerned about developing skin cancer because he spends so much time in the sun. After providing the patient with information about risk factors for, and prevention of, heatstroke, what other patient education would you provide? What are the risk factors for skin cancer? What health promotion strategies would be encouraged for this patient?

NCLEX-Style Review Questions

1. A patient is seen in the wound clinic for a pressure ulcer on his left leg. There is full-thickness tissue loss with the bone exposed. The nurse would correctly document this wound as being in which stage?
   a. I
   b. II
   c. III
   d. IV

2. The health care provider has ordered Collagenase for a patient with a left leg necrotic ulcer. What does the nurse understands about the use of collagenase?
   a. Removes necrotic tissue and absorbs small to large amounts of exudates
   b. Uses the body's own digestive enzymes to break down necrotic tissue
   c. Speeds the rate at which necrotic tissue is removed
   d. Uses a high moisture-vapor transmission rate to remove exudate

3. A 20-year-old patient is being seen in the dermatology clinic for a basal cell carcinoma on her eye. The nurse would expect the physician to complete which intervention?
   a. Electrosurgery
   b. Mohs' micrographic surgery
   c. Cryosurgery
   d. Radiation

4. Topical corticosteroid therapy has been ordered for a patient with pruritus. What information should be incorporated into the plan of care for this patient?
   a. Apply liberally in the prescribed area.
   b. Absorption is enhanced when skin is dry.
   c. Local side effects may include skin atrophy and thinning.
   d. Absorption is decreased when covered with an occlusive dressing.

5. A 55-year-old patient with leukemia is being seen in the clinic for complaints of burning pain in the back. The patient has been diagnosed with shingles. The nurse would expect which medication classification to be ordered to reduce pain and halt the progression of the disease?
   a. Anti-inflammatory
   b. Antiviral
   c. Antibiotic
   d. Antifungal

Try these additional resources, available at **http://thepoint.lww.com/Honan2e,** to enhance your learning and understanding of this chapter:

- NCLEX-Style Student Review Questions
- Journal Articles

REFERENCES AND SELECTED READINGS

References and selected readings associated with this chapter can be found on the website that accompanies the book. Visit **http://thepoint. lww.com/Honan2e** to access the references and other additional resources associated with this chapter.

Nursing Management: Patients with Burn Injury

Jacqueline Laird

Learning Objectives

After reading this chapter, you will be able to:

1. Discuss the classification system used for burn injuries.
2. Describe the local and systemic effects of a major burn injury.
3. Discuss the potential fluid and electrolyte alterations of the emergent/resuscitative and acute phases of burn management.
4. Describe nursing management of the patient with burn injuries.

In comparison to the larger health care picture, burn patients are few. However, severe burn injuries are catastrophic injuries that often have "long-term consequences regarding physical, psychological, social, vocational, and aesthetic aspects of recovery" (Renneberg et al., 2014). Although overall survival for fire, burn, and smoke inhalation exceeds 96%, approximately 3,400 deaths result annually in the United States (American Burn Association [ABA, 2015], National Burn Repository [ABA, nd]). At the time of injury, at least 50% of the burn fatalities occur because of massive hemorrhaging (Sheridan, 2016).

Burns are categorized as thermal (including electrical burns), radiation, electrical, or chemical. The skin and the mucosa of the upper airways are the sites of tissue destruction. Disruption of the skin can lead to increased fluid loss, infection, hypothermia, compromised immunity, and changes in function, appearance, and body image. The nurse caring for the burn patient requires astute assessment skills and a high level of knowledge about physiologic changes after a major burn injury to detect subtle changes in the patient's condition.

OVERVIEW OF BURN INJURY

Incidence of Burn Injury

The two most common burn etiologies are flame and scald. The home remains the most common place of occurrence, accounting for 65% of burn injuries cared for in burn centers. Scald injuries are the most preventable burn injury in children under 5 years of age (ABA, 2015). A burn can affect any person at any time, in any place. Burns involve people of all ages and socioeconomic groups. Each year, approximately 500,000 people with burn injuries receive medical treatment, and just over 3,000 deaths occur annually from fire and smoke inhalation. Residential fires account for 2,800 of these deaths, with the remaining 300 from motor vehicle accidents (National Hospital Ambulatory Medical Care Survey [NHAMCS], 2011). Approximately 70% of all burn victims are men. Children under 5 years of age represent 19%, and people over 60 years of age represent 13% of burn cases (ABA, 2015). Although prognosis can be influenced by several factors, the most important variables include: severity of the burn, the presence of inhalation injury, associated injuries, the patient's age, and comorbid conditions (DeKoning, 2016).

People who are prone to burn injuries are the elderly, smokers, and people with disabilities, neurologic illness, substance abuse issues, and psychiatric illness.

Gerontologic Considerations

Persons over 60 years of age are likely to live alone and have reduced mobility, changes in vision, and decreased sensation in the feet and hands. These changes place them at risk for suffering a burn. Morbidity and mortality rates associated with burns are greater in the elderly (ABA, 2015) than in the remainder of the population. Thinning and loss of elasticity of the skin predispose them to deep injury from a thermal insult that might cause a less severe burn in a younger person. Furthermore, chronic illnesses decrease the older person's ability to withstand the multisystem stresses imposed by major burn injury. Mortality is nearly 90% in patients who are older than 60 years of age, have a burn that is greater than 40% of the total body surface area (TBSA), and have an inhalation injury (Sheridan, 2016). Successful prevention campaigns have been linked to smoke detectors, carbon monoxide detectors, fire extinguishers, escape plans, sprinkler systems, enforcement of fire codes, and fire safe cigarettes (Pertschuk, Hobart, Paloma, Larkin, & Balbach, 2013).

Classification of Burns

Burn injuries are classified by the depth of the injury and the extent of the TBSA that is burned.

Depth

Burns are classified according to the depth of tissue destruction. Cell damage occurs at temperatures of at least 45°C (113°F). The depth depends on how much of the skin's dermis is affected. Burn depth determines whether spontaneous healing will occur and helps to determine the plan of care.

The following factors are considered in determining the depth of a burn:

- How the injury occurred
- Causative agent, such as flame, scald, chemical, or hot tar
- Temperature of the burning agent
- Duration of contact with the agent
- Thickness of the skin in the burned area

Burns are described as superficial, superficial partial-thickness, deep partial-thickness, or full-thickness injuries (Fig. 53-1; Table 53-1). Formerly referred to as a first-degree burn, a superficial burn damages only the **epidermis** (outer layer of the skin). The area is red and dry, with slight swelling but no blister, and painful, like a sunburn. These burns heal in about 7 days with usually no scarring. In a superficial partial-thickness burn (one of two types of second-degree burns), the epidermis is destroyed and a small portion of the underlying **dermis** (deep, vascular inner portion of skin) is injured. The skin is blistered, the exposed dermis is red and moist, and hair follicles are intact. These burns will heal in 14 to 21 days usually without scarring.

A deep partial-thickness burn (the second of the two types of second-degree burns), extends into the reticular layer of the dermis (dense connective tissue that gives the skin strength and elasticity and houses sweat glands, lymph vessels, and hair follicles) and is hard to distinguish from a full-thickness burn. It is red or white, mottled, and can be moist or fairly dry. The patient is in severe pain. Deep partial burns usually take longer than 3 weeks to heal (3 to 8 weeks) and can heal with permanent scarring (some of these burns tend to have a better appearance when grafted).

A full-thickness burn (formerly called a third- or fourth-degree burn) involves total destruction of the dermis and extends into the subcutaneous fat. It can also involve muscle and bone. It heals by contraction or epithelial migration. Wound color ranges widely from mottled white to red, brown, or black. Skin can appear charred and leathery, and hair follicles and sweat glands are destroyed. These burns are so severe that the patient no longer experiences a pain sensation. Healing does not happen spontaneously; this injury will require surgery, and significant scarring is expected (DeKoning, 2016).

Nursing Alert

It is important for the nurse to acknowledge that even when skin is no longer in contact with the burn source, skin damage can continue. In the case of scald burns, 1 second of contact with hot tap

Epidermis

Dermis

Subcutaneous tissue

Muscle

Superficial burn

Superficial partial-thickness burn

Deep partial-thickness burn

Full-thickness burn

FIGURE 53-1 Depth of burn injury.

TABLE 53-1 Characteristics of Burns According to Depth

Depth of Burn	Causes	Skin Involvement	Symptoms	Wound Appearance	Recuperative Course
Superficial	Thermal injury (heat/cold), electromagnetic energy, solar radiation or topical caustic chemicals	Involves only the epidermis	Erythema and edema of skin	Redness, swelling, does not blister, pain	Three days or less
Superficial partial-thickness (similar to first-degree)	Sunburn Low-intensity flash	Epidermis; possibly a portion of dermis	Tingling Hyperesthesia (supersensitivity) Pain that is soothed by cooling	Reddened; blanches with pressure; dry Minimal or no edema Possible blisters	Complete recovery within 5–10 days; usually no scarring Peeling
Deep partial-thickness (similar to second-degree)	Scalds Flash flame Contact	Epidermis, upper dermis, portion of deeper dermis	Pain Hyperesthesia Sensitive to cold air	Blistered, mottled red base; broken epidermis; weeping surface Edema	Recovery in 3–8 weeks Some scarring and depigmentation contractures Infection may convert it to full thickness
Full-thickness (similar to third-degree)	Flame Prolonged exposure to hot liquids Electric current Chemical Contact	Epidermis, entire dermis, and sometimes subcutaneous tissue; may involve connective tissue, muscle, and bone	Pain free Shock Hematuria (blood in the urine) and possibly hemolysis (blood cell destruction) Possible entrance and exit wounds (electrical burn)	Dry; pale white, leathery, or charred Broken skin with fat exposed Edema	Eschar sloughs Grafting necessary Scarring and loss of contour and function; contractures Loss of digits or extremity possible

water at 68°C (155°F) may result in a burn that destroys both the epidermis and the dermis, causing a full-thickness injury (ABA, 2014a). A deep partial-thickness burn can convert to full-thickness burns within 24 hours of injury, thus immediate assessment and management, which includes the application of cool tap water for a minimum of 5 minutes, is important to decrease the risk of thermal injury (ABA, 2014b). It is imperative that the nurse remove all jewelry, rings, watches, or belts, which are typically made of metal, since they can retain heat, cause thermal injury, and act as a tourniquet with tissue swelling. Burning clothing must be removed immediately, and the wound should be covered with a sterile dressing or clean cloth that is loosely wrapped. If clothing has adhered to the wound, it should not be removed. The use of ice water on large burns can result in hypothermia and increased mortality, whereas tap water is associated with a reduction in pain and may reduce the progression of tissue necrosis and need for skin grafting (Varley, Sarginson, & Young, 2015).

Extent of Body Surface Area Injured

Various methods are used to estimate the TBSA affected by burns; among them are the rule of nines and the Lund and Browder method.

Rule of Nines

The **rule of nines** (Fig. 53-2) is a simple and common way to estimate the extent of burns. The system assigns percentages in multiples of nine to major body surfaces with the perineum forming the remaining 1%. This method must be modified in the pediatric population because of the proportionally larger heads and smaller limbs in children.

Lund and Browder Method

A more precise, age-specific method of estimating the extent of a burn is the Lund and Browder method, which recognizes the percentage of surface area of various anatomic parts, especially the head and legs, in relation to growth. Because of changes in body proportion with growth, the calculated TBSA changes with age as well (Bittner, 2015). By dividing

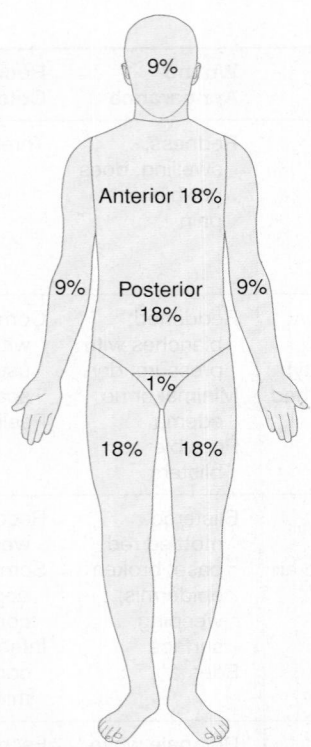

9%

Anterior 18%

9%   Posterior 18%   9%

1%

18%   18%

FIGURE 53-2 The rule of nines: Estimated percentage of total body surface area (TBSA) in the adult is arrived at by sectioning the body surface into areas with a numerical value related to nine. (Note: The anterior and posterior head total 9% of TBSA.)

the body into very small areas and providing an estimate of the proportion of TBSA accounted for by each body part, one can obtain a reliable estimate of TBSA burned.

Severity Grading System

The Severity Grading System (Box 53-1) adopted by the ABA includes: minor, moderate, and major burns.

PATHOPHYSIOLOGY

Burns are a dynamic injury set that result in a cascade of local tissue and systemic inflammatory effects depending on the percentage of TBSA involved. Local effects of burns include the denaturation of protein (which results in the disruption and potential destruction of cells), liberation of vasoactive substances, and the formation of edema. As a result of the cellular injury, the osmotic and hydrostatic pressure gradients are disrupted and intravascular fluid leaks into interstitial spaces. This damage is distributed throughout the injury as some cells die instantly, some are irreversibly damaged, and some—if appropriate interventions occur—will survive. There are three distinct zones that appear in a bull's eye pattern. The zone of coagulation (in the center) is where the tissue is completely destroyed; the zone of stasis surrounds the nonviable tissue and is potentially viable; the

---

BOX 53-1 | **Classification of Extent of Burn Injury**

Minor Burn Injury

- Second-degree burn of less than 15% total body surface area (TBSA) in adults or less than 10% TBSA in children
- Third-degree burn of less than 2% TBSA not involving special care areas (eyes, ears, face, hands, feet, perineum, joints)
- Excludes all patients with electrical injury, inhalation injury, or concurrent trauma and all at-risk patients (i.e., extremes of age, intercurrent disease)

Moderate, Uncomplicated Burn Injury

- Second-degree burns of 15–25% TBSA in adults or 10–20% in children
- Third-degree burns of less than 10% TBSA not involving special care areas
- Excludes all patients with electrical injury, inhalation injury, or concurrent trauma; all at-risk patients (i.e., extremes of age, intercurrent disease)

Major Burn Injury

- Second-degree burns of at least 25% TBSA in adults or at least 20% in children
- All third-degree burns 10% or more TBSA
- All burns involving eyes, ears, face, hands, feet, perineum, joints
- All patients with inhalation injury, electrical injury, or concurrent trauma; all at-risk patients

From Morton, P. G., & Fontaine, D. (2008). *Critical care nursing: A holistic approach* (9th ed.). Philadelphia, PA: Lippincott Williams & Wilkins.

zone of hyperemia has increased blood flow secondary to the natural inflammatory response (Fig. 53-3).

Burns that exceed 20% TBSA may produce a local and a systemic response and are considered major burn injuries. The incidence and significance of pathophysiologic changes are proportional to the extent of burn injury, with a maximal response seen in burns covering 60% or more TBSA (Sheridan, 2016). Additionally, burns of 60% TBSA cause depressed myocardial contractility; this, in combination with the loss of circulating plasma volume, hemoconcentration, and massive edema formation (Latenser, 2015), results in both distributive and hypovolemic shock (see Chapter 54). Fluid volume loss is greatest in the first 6 to 8 hours; capillary integrity returns toward normal by 36 to 48 hours after the burn (Demling, 2015). These patients are best served when transferred to a verified burn center as they are candidates for the occurrence of burn shock.

Burn Shock: Cardiovascular Alterations

Shock occurs when oxygen supply does not meet tissue demand. Burn shock develops from several abnormalities of the circulation. The initial systemic event is hemodynamic

- Zone of coagulation
- Zone of stasis
- Zone of hyperemia

- Skin

- Subcutaneous tissue

FIGURE 53-3 Zones of burn injury. Each burned area has three zones of injury. The inner zone (known as the area of coagulation, in which cellular death occurs) sustains the most damage. The middle area, or zone of stasis, has a compromised blood supply, inflammation, and tissue injury. The outer zone—the zone of hyperemia—sustains the least damage.

instability, which results from loss of capillary integrity and a subsequent shift of fluid, sodium, and protein from the intravascular space into the interstitial spaces. This leaky capillary syndrome increases cell permeability at the burn site, as well as throughout the body. In the major burn, this syndrome far exceeds the useful effect of the inflammatory response. Progressive edema develops in unburned tissue and organs, causing hypoperfusion and hypovolemic shock. As fluid loss continues and vascular volume decreases, the cardiac output (CO) and blood pressure (BP) fall. This is the onset of burn shock. The systemic response is caused by the release of cytokines and other mediators into the systemic circulation. The result is overwhelming; there is an increase in peripheral vascular resistance secondary to the edema formation, a decrease in blood volume, and a decrease in CO (Latenser, 2015). Thus, burn shock is characterized by capillary leak, "third spacing" of fluid, severe hypovolemia, and decreased CO. If the burn patient is not resuscitated adequately, circulatory collapse ensues.

Fluid and Electrolyte Alterations

Prompt fluid resuscitation maintains the BP in the low-normal range and improves CO. In general, the greatest volume of fluid leak occurs in the first 24 to 36 hours after the burn. As the capillaries begin to regain their integrity, burn shock resolves and fluid returns to the vascular compartment. As fluid is reabsorbed from the interstitial tissue into the vascular compartment, blood volume increases. If kidney and cardiac function is adequate, urinary output increases. Lactated Ringer's (LR) solution is the preferred IV fluid for burn

resuscitation because the sodium (130 mEq/L) and potassium (K⁺; 4 mEq/L) concentrations are similar to normal intravascular levels (sodium of 135 to 145 mEq/L and K⁺ of 3.5 to 5 mEq/L). LR also contains lactate (28 mEq/L), which can be converted by the liver to bicarbonate (the blood buffer) to aid in correcting the metabolic acidosis frequently seen in burn shock.

Patients with large burn wounds are at risk for abdominal compartment syndrome, especially if fluid resuscitation is delayed. Fluid shifts into the abdominal cavity, causing increased abdominal distention that interferes with pulmonary ventilation. The volume loss into the peritoneal space results in a decreasing CO, hypotension, and a decreasing urine output. The increased intra-abdominal pressure compresses the inferior vena cava and restricts blood flow and perfusion to abdominal organs, further compromising renal, hepatic, and visceral organ function. The adult patient who is critically ill will have an intra-abdominal pressure that varies with respiration of approximately 5 to 7 mm Hg but may be higher in patients with obesity (Kirkpatrick et al., 2013). Bladder pressures of greater than 25 mm Hg are an indicator of increasing abdominal pressure, resulting in inadequate organ perfusion, and indicate the need for abdominal decompression. Clinical presentation may include a tense, distended abdomen, progressive oliguria (urine output below 400 mL), and increased ventilatory requirements (Sheridan, 2016).

> **Nursing Alert**
> The nurse recognizes that the clinical goal is to administer adequate but not excessive fluid while safeguarding that soft tissues are not rendered ischemic by increasing pressure beneath inelastic eschar or tense muscle compartments (Sheridan, 2016).

> **Nursing Alert**
> Nurses measure intra-bladder pressure (IBP) using a bladder catheter (Foley), a pressure monitor or a manometer, room temperature saline solution, and a 60-mL syringe. A pressure monitor is set up and connected to the catheter drainage bag at the aspiration port via a Luer-lock or needle. Once the bladder is empty, 25 to 50 mL (depending on institutional policy) of saline solution is instilled through the bladder catheter using a 60-mL syringe, and it is clamped. The clamp must be on the drainage tubing below the aspiration port to allow measurement of bladder pressure. Patients must be in a supine position since head of bed elevation can have a significant impact on the reading (Kirkpatrick et al., 2013). The symphysis pubis (at the midaxillary line) is used as the zero reference point for the pressure bag at the midaxillary line. The pressure is recorded, the clamp released, and urine is allowed to flow into the drainage bag. The nurse remembers to subtract

FIGURE 53-4 Measuring intra-bladder pressure. To assess for the development of abdominal compartment syndrome, the intra-bladder pressure may be monitored.

the amount of fluid instilled from the patient's urinary output to maintain an accurate Intake and Output (I&O) record (Fig. 53-4).

Patients with a major burn develop massive systemic edema. As fluid resuscitation proceeds, the edema worsens. As the taut, burned tissue becomes unyielding to the edema underneath its surface, it begins to act like a tourniquet, especially if the burn is circumferential. This complication is similar to a compartment syndrome. The provider may need to perform an **escharotomy**, a surgical incision into the **eschar** (also referred to as "black wound" because of the wounds appearance of thick, dry, black necrotic tissue) to relieve the constricting effect of the burned tissue. Refer to Chapter 42 for details on compartment syndrome.

Burn shock is a physiologic insult combining hypovolemic and distributive shock. Circulating blood volume decreases dramatically during burn shock due to severe capillary leak with variation of serum sodium levels in response to fluid resuscitation. Usually, hyponatremia (sodium depletion) is present. Immediately after burn injury, hyperkalemia (excessive potassium) results from massive cell destruction. The outcome is a dramatic outpouring of fluids, electrolytes, and proteins into the interstitium with rapid equilibrium of intravascular and interstitial compartments. These changes are reflected in loss of circulating plasma volume, hemoconcentration, massive edema formation, decreased urine output, and depressed cardiovascular function (Latenser, 2015). Lactic acidosis is frequently seen in burn shock due to hypovolemia and hypoperfusion; thus, while the lactate in LR IV solution can be converted to base bicarbonate to correct the acidemia, the goal of treatment is aimed at reversing the hypoperfusion. Hypokalemia (potassium depletion) may occur later, with fluid shifts and inadequate potassium replacement. However, plasma lactate levels are significant markers of shock and resuscitation, and appear to be correlated to predict morbidity and outcome. A normal serum lactic acid level in venous blood is 0.5 to 2.2 mEq/L. See discussion of fluid and electrolyte changes in the Emergent/Resuscitative Phase later in the chapter.

Nursing Alert
The nurse is aware that severe lactic acidosis (pH less than 7.2) is associated with a high early mortality. Approximately 17% of patients with a pH below 7.2 are ultimately discharged from the hospital (Seifter, 2016).

Nursing Alert
Ringer's lactate IV solution contains 28 mEq of lactate (28 mmol/L), which is metabolized into bicarbonate by the liver, aiding in correction of metabolic acidosis. However, the nurse is aware that liver function must be assessed to ensure adequate metabolism of this IV solution.

Pulmonary Alterations

Inhalation injury necessitates prolonged hospitalization and remains a major cause of morbidity and mortality. An inhalation injury can occur when a person is trapped inside a burning structure or involved in an explosion that leads to the inhalation of superheated air, steam, and noxious gas. Inhalation injury has a significant impact on a patient's ability to survive (DeKoning, 2016).

Clinical consequences can include upper airway edema, bronchospasm, small airway occlusion, loss of ciliary clearance, increased dead space, intrapulmonary shunting, decreased lung compliance, chest wall compliance, tracheobronchitis, and pneumonia (Sheridan, 2016).

Pulmonary injuries fall into two categories: upper airway injury, and inhalation injury below the glottis, including carbon monoxide poisoning. Upper airway injury results from direct heat and edema. It is manifested by mechanical obstruction of the upper airway as small particles may reach the terminal bronchioles, causing bronchospasms and edema. Direct injury to the upper airway causes airway swelling that typically leads to maximal edema in the first 24 to 48 hours after injury and often requires a short course of endotracheal intubation for airway protection (Friedstat, Endorf, & Gibran, 2014).

Inhalation injury below the glottis results from inhaling noxious gases or steam. The injury results directly from chemical irritation of the pulmonary tissues at the alveolar level. These injuries cause loss of ciliary action, hypersecretion, severe mucosal edema, and possibly bronchospasm. The pulmonary surfactant is reduced, resulting in atelectasis (collapse of alveoli). Expectoration of carbon particles in the sputum is the cardinal sign of this injury.

Carbon monoxide is probably the most common cause of inhalation injury because it is a by-product of the combustion of organic materials and, therefore, is present in smoke. The pathophysiologic effects are caused by tissue hypoxia, a result of carbon monoxide combining with hemoglobin to form **carboxyhemoglobin (COHb or HbCO)**, which competes with oxygen for available hemoglobin-binding sites. The affinity of hemoglobin for carbon monoxide is 250 times greater than that for oxygen. Refer to Table 53-2 for symptoms of CO poisoning. Standard care usually consists of 100% oxygen for 6 hours until the HbCO level is below 10% and the patient is asymptomatic (Ferri, 2016; Sheridan, 2016).

Administering 100% oxygen is essential to accelerate the removal of carbon monoxide from the hemoglobin molecule. Monitor oxygen saturation by pulse oximetry, but be aware that pulse oximetry readings will be falsely elevated in patients with elevated carboxyhemoglobin levels. Simply subtract the measured COHb level from the pulse oximetry value to determine the true oxygen saturation (Drigalla & Gemmill, 2011).

 Nursing Alert
The pulse oximeter contains a light source (light-emitting diode [LED]) and a light detector, the sensor. The light source beams red and infrared light through the skin and blood, and the amount of light received by the detector is measured. The difference of the transmitted light during and between heart beats is calculated and converted to the percent of hemoglobin that is saturated with oxygen, the SpO_2. While the clinical usefulness of pulse oximeter cannot be disputed, there are at least two important limitations that the nurse needs to be aware of:

1. *Unfortunately, pulse oximeters cannot distinguish oxygenated Hb (HbO_2) from carbon monoxide-poisoned hemoglobin, aka carboxyhemoglobin (HbCO). Thus falsely high SpO_2 saturations are seen in CO poisoning despite inadequate oxygenation of Hb. Moreover, the deficit in oxygen delivery to peripheral tissue is exacerbated by the ability of carbon monoxide to impair the release of oxygen that is bound to hemoglobin, often referred to as a decrease in the p50 (oxygen tension at which hemoglobin is 50% saturated).*
2. *While the SpO_2 accurately reflects the percentage of Hb saturation with O_2 under most conditions, it does not measure total O_2 carrying content of the blood. This can be particularly misleading in the anemic patient where the percent of Hb saturation may be normal but total oxygen delivery to tissues is markedly reduced as a consequence of the fall in red blood cell numbers.*

Pulmonary abnormalities are not always immediately apparent. More than half of all patients with burn injuries with pulmonary involvement do not initially demonstrate pulmonary signs and symptoms. Any patient with possible inhalation injury must be observed for at least 24 hours for respiratory complications. Indicators of possible pulmonary damage include the following:

- History indicating that the burn occurred in an enclosed area
- Burns of the face or neck
- Singed nasal hair
- Hoarseness, voice change, dry cough, stridor
- Sooty or bloody sputum
- Labored breathing or tachypnea (rapid breathing) and other signs of reduced oxygen levels (hypoxemia)
- Erythema and blistering of the oral or pharyngeal mucosa

Diagnosis of inhalation injury is an important priority, and nurses should consider assessing if the patient was confined in a closed area, if there are facial burns, were nasal hairs burned, or if there is carbonaceous debris in the mouth or sputum (Sheridan, 2016). Carboxyhemoglobin levels and fiberoptic bronchoscopy are used to assess for inhalation injuries as well. Pulmonary complications secondary to inhalation injuries include acute respiratory failure and acute respiratory distress

TABLE **53-2** **Symptoms of Carbon Monoxide Toxicity**

Blood Carboxyhemoglobin Level (%)	Symptoms
Less than 15–20	Headache, dizziness, occasional confusion
20–40	Disorientation, visual impairment
40–60	Agitation, combativeness, hallucinations, coma, and shock
60	Death

Reprinted with permission from Barash, P., Cullen, B., & Stoelting, R. (2013). *Handbook of clinical anesthesia* (7th ed.). Philadelphia, PA: Lippincott Williams & Wilkins.

syndrome (ARDS). ARDS is common in these patients and can increase mortality to 66%. A 100% mortality was noted where the TBSA was greater than 60% in combination with inhalation injury and ARDS (Friedstat et al., 2014). Refer to Chapter 10 for more information on ARDS.

Renal Alterations

Kidney function may be altered as a result of decreased blood volume. If muscle damage occurs, myoglobin and hemoglobin are released from the muscle cells and excreted by the kidney; this is common in high-voltage injuries or deep thermal burns. The urine will have a pigmented appearance. Adequate fluid volume replacement restores renal blood flow, increasing the glomerular filtration rate and urine volume. Fluids should be titrated to achieve a urine output of 2 mL/kg/hr (Sheridan, 2016). If there is inadequate blood flow through the kidneys, the hemoglobin and myoglobin occlude the renal tubules, resulting in acute tubular necrosis and kidney failure. Blood urea nitrogen (BUN), serum creatinine levels, and urinary output are monitored to evaluate kidney function. Diuretics have no role in this phase of patient management unless fluid overload has occurred (Nemer & Clark, 2016).

Immunologic Alterations

The immunologic defenses of the body are greatly altered by a serious burn injury as it diminishes resistance to infection. The loss of skin integrity is compounded by the release of abnormal inflammatory factors. There is a significant impairment of the production and release of granulocytes and macrophages from bone marrow; the resulting immunosuppression places the patient with burn injury at high risk for sepsis (see Chapter 54 for details on septicemia).

Thermoregulatory Alterations

Loss of skin also results in an inability to regulate body temperature. Therefore patients with burn injuries may exhibit low body temperatures in the early hours after injury. Then, as hypermetabolism resets core temperatures, the patient becomes hyperthermic for much of the post-burn period, even in the absence of infection.

Gastrointestinal Alterations

Two potential gastrointestinal (GI) complications may occur: paralytic ileus (absence of intestinal peristalsis) and Curling ulcer. Decreased peristalsis and bowel sounds are manifestations of paralytic ileus resulting from burn trauma. Gastric distention and nausea may lead to vomiting unless gastric decompression is initiated. Gastric bleeding secondary to massive physiologic stress may be signaled by occult blood in the stool, regurgitation of "coffee ground" material from the stomach, or bloody vomitus. These signs suggest gastric or duodenal erosion (Curling ulcer).

MANAGEMENT OF BURN INJURY

Burn care must be based on burn depth and local response, the extent of the injury, and the presence of a systemic response. Burn care is divided into three phases: emergent/resuscitative phase, acute/intermediate phase, and rehabilitation phase. Although priorities exist for each of the phases, they overlap, and assessment and management of specific problems and complications are not limited to these phases but take place throughout burn care. The three phases and the priorities for care are summarized in Table 53-3. Box 53-2 summarizes emergency care at the burn scene.

Emergent/Resuscitative Phase

Immediate Care

It is important to remember the CABD (circulation, airway, breathing, disability) steps (formerly called ABCs [Airway,

TABLE 53-3 Phases of Burn Care

Phase	Duration	Priorities
Emergent/resuscitative	From onset of injury to completion of fluid resuscitation	• First aid • Prevention of shock • Prevention of respiratory distress • Detection and treatment of concomitant injuries • Wound assessment and initial care
Acute/intermediate	From beginning of diuresis to near completion of wound closure	• Wound care and closure • Prevention or treatment of complications, including infection • Nutritional support
Rehabilitation	From major wound closure to return to patient's optimal level of physical and psychosocial adjustment	• Prevention of scars and contractures • Physical, occupational, and vocational rehabilitation • Functional and cosmetic reconstruction • Psychosocial counseling

BOX 53-2

Emergency Procedures at the Burn Scene

- *Extinguish the flames:* When clothes catch fire, the flames can be extinguished if the person falls to the floor or ground and rolls ("stop, drop, and roll"); anything available to smother the flames, such as a blanket, rug, or coat, may be used. Standing still forces the person to breathe flames and smoke, and running fans the flames. If the burn source is electrical, the electrical source must be disconnected.
- *Cool the burn:* After the flames are extinguished, the burned area and adherent clothing are soaked with *cool* water, briefly, to cool the wound and halt the burning process. Once a burn has been sustained, the application of cool water is the best first-aid measure. Soaking the burn area intermittently in cool water or applying cool towels gives immediate and striking relief from pain and limits local tissue edema and damage. However, *never* apply ice directly to the burn, *never* wrap the person in ice, and *never* use cold soaks or dressings for longer than several minutes; such procedures may worsen the tissue damage and lead to hypothermia in people with large burns.
- *Remove restrictive objects:* If possible, remove clothing immediately. Adherent clothing may be left in place once cooled. Other clothing and all jewelry (especially rings), including all piercings, should be removed to allow for assessment and to prevent constriction secondary to rapidly developing edema.
- *Cover the wound:* The burn should be covered as quickly as possible to minimize bacterial contamination and decrease pain by preventing air from coming into contact with the injured surface. Sterile dressings are best, but any clean, dry cloth can be used as an emergency dressing. Ointments and salves should *not* be used. Other than the dressing, no medication or material should be applied to the burn wound.
- *Irrigate chemical burns:* Chemical burns resulting from contact with a corrosive material are irrigated immediately. Most chemical laboratories have a high-pressure shower for such emergencies. If such an injury occurs at home, brush off the chemical agent, remove clothes immediately, and rinse all areas of the body that have come in contact with the chemical. Rinsing can occur in the shower or any other source of continuous running water. If a chemical gets in or near the eyes, the eyes should be flushed with cool, clean water immediately. Outcomes for the patient with chemical burns are significantly improved by rapid, sustained flushing of the injury at the scene.

Breathing, and Circulation]) of all trauma care during the early post-burn period. Refer to Chapter 56 for further details.

Circulation must be assessed quickly. Apical pulse and BP are monitored frequently. Tachycardia (abnormally rapid heart rate, over 100 bpm) and slight hypotension are expected soon after the burn. A urinary catheter is inserted, and strict intake and output is recorded. Monitoring of hourly urine output and daily weights provides clues about fluid volume status. Any evidence of decreasing urine output or hemodynamic instability requires immediate notification of the provider. A large-bore (16- or 18-gauge) IV catheter should be inserted in a nonburned area for fluid replacement.

It is important to support the *airway* and protect the cervical spine. If edema of the airway develops, endotracheal intubation may be necessary.

The nurse assesses and promotes *breathing*. For mild pulmonary injury, 100% humidified oxygen is administered. Intubation and ventilation may be necessary. The nurse monitors the respiratory rate, lung sounds, and oxygen saturation and notifies the provider if dyspnea, stridor, or changes in respiratory patterns or saturation levels reflect declining ventilation and oxygenation.

! Nursing Alert
Breathing must be assessed and a patent airway established immediately during the initial minutes of emergency care. Immediate therapy is directed toward establishing an airway and administering humidified 100% oxygen. If qualified personnel and equipment are available and the victim has severe respiratory distress or airway edema, the rescuers can insert an endotracheal tube and initiate manual ventilation.

! Nursing Alert
In the event of a high-voltage electrical injury, spinal cord injury can result from the direct effect of electrical current or can occur secondary to trauma associated with blunt injury. Thus, the cervical spine should be immobilized. Additionally, electrical injury interferes with cardiac conduction and can cause direct trauma to cardiac muscle fibers, resulting in a number of arrhythmias, including asystole, ventricular fibrillation, sinus tachycardia, and premature ventricular contractions (PVCs). Because the arrhythmias can present hours after the incident, cardiac monitoring for patients with all electrical injuries for at least 24 hours after cessation of arrhythmia is suggested.

Additionally, related to *disability*, the neurologic status is assessed quickly in the patient with extensive burns. The nurse is aware that restlessness, confusion, difficulty attending to questions, or decreasing level of consciousness may indicate cerebral hypoxia. Often, the patient is awake and alert initially, and vital information can be obtained at that time. A secondary head-to-toe survey of the patient is carried out to identify other potentially life-threatening injuries.

Assessment

Initial priorities in the emergency department remain *CABD*. After adequate circulatory and respiratory functions have been established, and the patient's condition is stable, attention is directed to the burn wound itself.

Information needs to include the time of the burn injury, the source of the burn, how the burn was treated at the scene, and any history of falling with the injury. A history of pre-existing diseases, allergies, medications, and the use of drugs, alcohol, and tobacco is obtained at this point to aid in planning the patient's care. Because poor tissue perfusion accompanies burn injuries, only IV analgesia (usually morphine) is administered, and it should be titrated according to patient need.

If the burn exceeds 20% TBSA, a nasogastric tube should be inserted and connected to low suction. All patients who are intubated should have a nasogastric tube inserted to decompress the abdomen and prevent vomiting.

Assessment of both the TBSA burned and the depth of the burn are completed. Careful attention is paid to keeping the patient warm during wound assessment. Baseline values for height, weight, arterial blood gases, carboxyhemoglobin, hematocrit, electrolyte values, blood alcohol level, drug panel, urinalysis, and baseline electrocardiogram (ECG) are obtained. Because burns are contaminated wounds, tetanus prophylaxis is administered if the patient's immunization status is not current (less than 5 years since last tetanus) or unknown (Advanced Burn Life Support [ABLS], 2012; Ferri, 2016).

Transfer to a Burn Center

The depth and extent of the burn are considered in determining whether the patient should be transferred to a burn center. However, if the patient's prognosis does not support transport to a burn center, nurses may contact burn center nurses via telephone and ask for support in patient management. Examples of criteria for referral to a burn unit can be found at http://ameriburn.org/BurnCenterReferralCriteria.pdf.

Management of Fluid Loss and Shock

Next to managing respiratory difficulties, the most urgent need is preventing irreversible shock by replacing lost fluids and electrolytes (Table 53-4). The total volume and rate of IV fluid replacement are gauged by the patient's response and guided by the resuscitation formula. Numerous fluid resuscitation formulas exist; the nurse needs to be familiar with current institutional protocols. The adequacy of fluid resuscitation is determined primarily by monitoring vital signs and urine output totals, an index of renal perfusion. Urine output totals of 0.5 to 1 mL/kg/hr in adults and 1 mL/kg/hr in children have been used as resuscitation goals (ABLS, 2012). Within the first 24 hours after injury, if the urinary output exceeds 50 mL/hr, the rate of IV fluid administration may be decreased because excessive fluid resuscitation

TABLE 53-4 Fluid and Electrolyte Changes in the Emergent/Resuscitative Phase

Fluid accumulation phase (shock phase)
Plasma → interstitial fluid (edema at burn site)

Observation	Explanation
Generalized dehydration	Plasma leaks through damaged capillaries.
Reduction of blood volume	Secondary to plasma loss, fall of blood pressure, and diminished cardiac output
Decreased urinary output	Secondary to: Fluid loss; Decreased renal blood flow; Sodium and water retention caused by increased adrenocortical activity; Hemolysis of red blood cells, causing hemoglobinuria and myonecrosis or myoglobinuria
Potassium (K^+) excess	Massive cellular trauma causes release of K^+ into extracellular fluid (ordinarily, most K^+ is intracellular).
Sodium (Na^+) deficit	Large amount of Na^+ is lost in trapped edema fluid and exudate and by shift into cells as K^+ is released from cells (ordinarily, most Na^+ is extracellular).
Metabolic acidosis (base–bicarbonate deficit)	Loss of bicarbonate ions accompanies sodium loss.
Hemoconcentration (elevated hematocrit)	Liquid blood component is lost into extravascular space.

may be deleterious for burn patients. Use of advanced technology, such as monitoring with pulmonary artery catheters and esophageal echo-Doppler, to evaluate hemodynamic response in burn-shock resuscitation have utility but carry risks, such as infection and aspiration. Thus, traditional variables of hourly assessment of urinary output and vital signs are used to evaluate the adequacy of fluid replacement therapy. For patients with pre-existing cardiopulmonary disease or kidney disorders, or with patients of extreme age (very young or old), additional hemodynamic parameters may be required to evaluate fluid status (Sheridan, 2016). Factors that are associated with the increased fluid requirements include delayed resuscitation, scald burn injuries, inhalation injuries, high-voltage electrical injuries, hyperglycemia, alcohol intoxication, and chronic diuretic therapy.

The projected fluid requirements for the first 24 hours are calculated by the clinician based on the extent of the burn injury. Formulas have been developed for estimating fluid loss based on the estimated percentage of burned TBSA and the weight of the patient. The length of time since the burn injury occurred is very important in calculating estimated fluid needs. Formulas must be adjusted so that initiation of fluid replacement reflects the time of injury. Resuscitation formulas are approximations only and are individualized to meet the requirements of each patient.

> ### Nursing Alert
> *Intravenous resuscitation formulas are to be used only as guides. The patient's response, evidenced by heart rate, blood pressure, and urine output, is the primary determinant of actual fluid therapy and must be assessed at least hourly.*

The ABA consensus formula provides for the volume of an isotonic solution (e.g., LR) to be administered during the first 24 hours in a range of 2 to 4 mL/kg/% TBSA.

Adults and older children (over 14 years of age, weighing more than 40 kg) receive:

$$2 \text{ mL of LR} \times \text{kg} \times \text{the \% burn}$$

Infants and children (under 14 years of age, weighing less than 40 kg) receive:

$$3 \text{ mL of LR} \times \text{kg} \times \text{the \% burn}$$

Patients with electrical injuries have LR administered:

$$4 \text{ mL} \times \text{kg} \times \text{the \% burn (ABLS, 2012).}$$

For children weighing less than 10 kg, D5LR is typically the solution administered. Half of the calculated total should be given over the first 8 post-burn hours, and the other half should be given over the next 16 hours. The rate and volume of the infusion must be regulated according to the patient's response by changing the hourly infusion rates. Another formula widely used is the Parkland formula, which is 4 mL/kg/% TBSA over 24 hours, using LR. It also administers half of the volume over the first 8 hours post-burn and the remaining half is administered over the next 16 hours. The use of formulas and TBSA methods can improve the accuracy and ease of calculating fluid resuscitation requirements. Again, practitioners should take note that the resuscitation formula serves only as a guideline, and the patient's response to fluid therapy is the best parameter to use.

The following example illustrates use of the consensus formula in a 70-kg (154-lb) patient with a 50% TBSA burn:

1. Consensus formula: 2 to 4 mL/kg/% TBSA
2. $2 \times 70 \times 50 = 7,000$ mL/24 hr
3. Plan to administer: first 8 hours = 3,500 mL, or 437 mL/hr; next 16 hours = 3,500 mL, or 219 mL/hr

Nursing Implications

Nursing assessment in the emergent phase of burn injury focuses on the major priorities for any trauma patient. Vital signs and respiratory status are monitored closely. Circulation, sensation, and mobility (CSM) of burn area is assessed hourly. Refer to Chapter 40 for details on musculoskeletal assessment. Hourly, the nurse will assess warmth, capillary refill, pulses, sensation, and movement of the affected extremity using the unaffected extremity for comparison. A Doppler (ultrasound device) is useful to assess perfusion of the affected extremity. Elevation of burned extremities is crucial to decrease edema. Loss of pulse or sensation must be reported to the provider immediately.

> ### Nursing Alert
> *If a blood pressure cuff is wrapped around a patient's arm, the cuff must be removed from the extremity between readings since it may act as a tourniquet as the extremity swells.*

> ### Nursing Alert
> *Dressings impede circulation if they are wrapped too tightly. The peripheral pulses must be checked frequently and burned extremities elevated on pillows.*

Assessment includes monitoring of fluid intake and output. Urine output is measured hourly. Burgundy-colored/pigmented urine suggests muscle damage. Administering and monitoring IV therapy is a major nursing responsibility.

Body temperature, body weight, current illnesses, and use of medications are assessed. A head-to-toe assessment is performed, focusing on signs and symptoms of concomitant illness, injury, or developing complications. Assessing the extent of the burn wound continues and is facilitated with anatomic diagrams (described previously).

Comorbid conditions coupled with the burn injury contribute to the high mortality rates of patients 60 years of age and older. Decreased function of the cardiovascular, renal, and pulmonary systems increases the need for close observation of elderly patients with even relatively minor burns during the emergent and acute phases. Acute kidney failure is much more common in elderly patients than in those younger than 40 years of age. The margin of difference between hypovolemia and fluid overload is very small. Suppressed immunologic response, a high incidence of malnutrition, and an inability to withstand metabolic stressors further compromise the elderly person's ability to heal. As a result of these issues, close monitoring and prompt treatment of complications are mandatory. A plan of nursing care for a patient during the emergent/resuscitative phase of burn injury is available online at http://thepoint.lww.com/Honan2e.

Acute/Intermediate Phase

The acute or intermediate phase of burn care follows the emergent/resuscitative phase and begins 48 to 72 hours after the burn injury. During this phase, attention is directed

TABLE 53-5 Fluid and Electrolyte Changes in the Acute Phase

Fluid remobilization phase (state of diuresis)
Interstitial fluid → plasma

Observation	Explanation
Hemodilution (decreased hematocrit)	Blood cell concentration is diluted as fluid enters the intravascular compartment; loss of red blood cells destroyed at burn site occurs.
Increased urinary output	Fluid shift into intravascular compartment increases renal blood flow and causes increased urine formation.
Sodium (Na^+) deficit	With diuresis, sodium is lost with water; existing serum sodium is diluted by water influx.
Potassium (K^+) deficit (occurs occasionally in this phase)	Beginning on the fourth or fifth postburn day, K^+ shifts from extracellular fluid into cells.
Metabolic acidosis	Loss of sodium depletes fixed base; relative carbon dioxide content increases.

toward continued assessment and maintenance of respiratory and circulatory status, fluid and electrolyte balance (Table 53-5), and GI function. Infection prevention, burn wound care, pain management, and nutritional support are priorities at this stage.

Maintenance of Circulatory and Respiratory Status

Changes may occur as the effects of resuscitative fluid and the chemical reactions of smoke ingredients with lung tissues become apparent. Pulmonary complications are not unusual.

Pneumonia is the most frequent clinically related complication and occurred in 30% of patients with fire/flame injuries (Sheridan, 2016). The frequency of pneumonia and respiratory failure is much greater in patients with 4 days or more of mechanical ventilation than those with less than 4 days. The incidence of clinically related complications for patients with 0 days of mechanical ventilation increases with age and tops out at nearly 20% for those 80 years of age and over (ABA, 2015). Ideally, the best practice is to remove the endotracheal tube as soon as possible to decrease the risk of infection transmission. The arterial blood gas values and other parameters determine the need for intubation and mechanical ventilation. Humidified oxygen is provided as necessary to maintain adequate oxygen saturation and provide moisture to injured tissues. The nurse assesses breath sounds, and respiratory rate, rhythm, depth, and chest symmetry, and notifies providers with concerns over pulmonary deterioration, such as increasing dyspnea or stridor and

changes in respiratory patterns. As capillaries regain integrity, diuresis begins. If cardiac or renal function is inadequate, fluid overload occurs and symptoms of congestive heart failure may result. Early detection allows for early intervention and carefully calculated fluid intake. Cautious administration of fluids and electrolytes continues during this phase of burn care. Blood components are administered as needed to treat blood loss and anemia.

Infection Prevention

Until recently, a common cause of death in patients with burn wounds was wound sepsis; while early excisions and grafting have made an impact in decreasing its frequency, infection is still a major issue (Sheridan, 2016).

The immunosuppression, absent epithelial barriers, and multiple invasive devices that accompany extensive burn injury place the patient at high risk of sepsis. Despite aseptic precautions and the use of topical antimicrobial agents, the burn wound is an excellent medium for bacterial growth and proliferation. While the wound is healing, it must be protected from infection. A primary source of bacterial infection is the patient's intestinal tract, the source of most microbes. A major secondary source of pathogenic microbes is the environment. Infection control is a major role of the burn team in providing wound care. Gown, mask, and gloves are worn while caring for the patient with open burn wounds. Clean technique is used when caring directly for burn wounds.

Antibiotics are seldom prescribed prophylactically because of the risk of promoting resistant strains of bacteria, and they do not seem to reduce the incidence of septic complications. Systemic antibiotics are administered when there is documentation of positive cultures in, for example, urine, sputum, or blood. Careful attention is paid to antibiotic use because inappropriate use of antibiotics significantly affects the microbial flora present and increases the risk of drug resistance. Fast excisions and grafting are the most effective ways to prevent infection in this population (Sheridan, 2016).

Wound Care

Wound care is the single most time-consuming element of burn care after the emergent phase. The nurse needs to make astute assessments of wound status, use creative approaches to wound dressing, and support the patient and family during the emotionally distressing and very painful experience of wound care.

Various measures are used to clean the burn wound. After the wounds are cleansed, the prescribed method of wound care is performed. Provider preferences, the availability of skilled nursing staff, and resources in terms of number of personnel, supplies, and time must be considered in choosing the best method. The goal is to protect the wound until either spontaneous healing or skin grafting can be achieved. Patient comfort and ability to participate in the prescribed treatment are also important considerations.

Topical Antibacterial Therapy

There is general agreement that some form of antimicrobial therapy applied to the burn wound is the best method of local care. Topical antibacterial therapy does not sterilize the wound; it simply reduces the number of bacteria. For more than 50 years, it has been recognized that silver has bacteriostatic and bacteriocidal properties that make it an excellent treatment agent (Table 53-6).

Criteria for choice of topical agents include the following:

- They are effective against gram-negative organisms and even fungi.
- They are clinically effective.
- They penetrate the eschar but are not systemically toxic.
- They do not lose their effectiveness, allowing another infection to develop.

- They are cost-effective, available, and acceptable to the patient.
- They are easy to apply and remove, minimizing nursing care time.

Wound Débridement

As debris accumulates on the wound surface, it can delay the healing process. **Débridement** has two goals:

- To remove tissue contaminated by bacteria and foreign bodies
- To remove devitalized tissue or burn eschar in preparation for grafting and wound healing

Early surgical excision to remove devitalized tissue along with early burn wound closure is recognized as the most

TABLE 53-6 Overview of Selected Topical Antibacterial Agents Used for Burn Wounds

Agent	Indication	Application	Nursing Implications
Silver sulfadiazine 1% (Silvadene) water-soluble cream	• Most bactericidal agent • Minimal penetration of eschar	Apply 1/16-in layer of cream with a sterile glove 1–3 times daily.	• Watch for leukopenia 2–3 days after initiation of therapy. (Leukopenia usually resolves within 2–3 days.) • Anticipate formation of pseudoeschar (proteinaceous gel), which is removed easily after 72 hours.
Mafenide acetate 5–10% (Sulfamylon) hydrophilic-based cream	• Effective against gram-negative and gram-positive organisms • Diffuses rapidly through eschar • In 10% strength, it is the agent of choice for electrical burns because of its ability to penetrate thick eschar.	Apply thin layer with sterile glove twice a day. Change the dressing every 12 hours as prescribed.	• Monitor arterial blood gas levels and discontinue as prescribed if acidosis occurs. Mafenide acetate is a strong carbonic anhydrase inhibitor that may reduce renal buffering and cause metabolic acidosis. • Premedicate the patient with an analgesic before applying mafenide acetate because this agent causes severe burning pain for up to 20 minutes after application.
Silver nitrate 0.5% aqueous solution	• Bacteriostatic and fungicidal • Does *not* penetrate eschar	Apply solution to gauze dressing and place over wound. Keep the dressing wet but covered with dry gauze and dry blankets to decrease vaporization. Remoisten every 2 hours, and re-dress wound daily as prescribed.	• Monitor serum sodium (Na^+) and potassium (K^+) levels and replace as prescribed. Silver nitrate solution is hypotonic and acts as a wick for sodium and potassium. • Protect bed linen and clothing from contact with silver nitrate, which stains everything it touches black.
Acticoat	• Effective against gram-negative and gram-positive organisms and some yeasts and molds • Delivers a uniform, antimicrobial concentration of silver to the burn wound	Moisten with sterile water only (*never* use normal saline as it will deactivate the silver in the dressing). Apply directly to wound. Cover with absorbent secondary dressing. Remoisten every 3–4 hours with sterile water.	• Do not use oil-based products or topical antimicrobials with Acticoat burn dressing. Keep Acticoat moist, not saturated. May produce a "pseudoeschar" from silver after application. • Can be left in place for 3–5 days. Also available in Acticoat 7, which can be left in place for up to 7 days without the need to change the dressing.

important factor contributing to survival of a patient with a major burn injury.

Wound Coverage

If wounds are full-thickness or extensive, spontaneous healing is not possible, and treatment of the wound is necessary until coverage with a graft of the patient's own skin (**autograft**) is possible. Autografts are the ideal covering for burn wounds because the grafts are the patient's own skin and, therefore, are not rejected by the patient's immune system.

The purposes of wound coverage are to decrease the risk of infection; prevent further loss of protein, fluid, and electrolytes through the wound; and minimize heat loss through evaporation. Once the wound is surgically excised, a wound covering is applied to keep the area moist and promote the granulation process.

Homograft is donor skin from a cadaver. It is a biologic dressing that has several uses. In extensive burns, it save lives by providing temporary wound coverage and protecting the granulation tissue until autografting is possible. Biologic dressings also provide temporary immediate coverage for clean, superficial burns and decrease the wound's evaporative water and protein loss. They decrease pain by protecting nerve endings and are an effective barrier against water loss and entry of bacteria. Biosynthetic and synthetic skin substitutes continue to be used as temporary wound coverings.

In an attempt to develop the ideal burn wound covering product, dermal substitutes have been created. It is believed that skin substitutes enhance the healing process of an open wound when autologous skin is unavailable.

Care of the Graft Site. Occlusive dressings are commonly used initially after grafting to immobilize the graft. Synthetic dressings may be used to protect grafts. The patient is positioned and turned carefully to avoid disturbing the graft or putting pressure on the graft site. If an extremity has been grafted, it is elevated to minimize edema.

Care of the Donor Site. A moist gauze dressing is applied at the time of surgery to maintain pressure and to stop any oozing. With all types of covering, donor sites must remain clean, dry, and free from pressure. Because a donor site is usually a partial-thickness wound, it will heal spontaneously within 7 to 14 days with proper care. Donor sites are painful, and additional pain management must be a part of the patient's care.

Pain Management

Pain is inevitable during recovery from any burn injury. Burn pain has been described as one of the most intense and prolonged types of pain. The pain starts immediately after injury and can last long into the recovery phase. Also the tissue surrounding a thermal burn is usually painful. Hyperalgesia (enhanced intensity of pain sensation) has been known to occur in burn patients; the pain threshold is lowered and pain can last minutes or hours for no apparent reason (Hall, 2012). Pain is related to tissue destruction, as well as to the inflammatory response, which causes the release of histamine, bradykinin, and prostaglandin that are irritating to exposed peripheral nerve endings (Brookman, 2016).

Pain in patients with burn wounds can be divided into four types: (1) Rest pain, constant background, and dull pain; (2) Breakthrough pain, intermittent, short duration, rapid onset (can be excruciating); (3) Procedural, short durations, greatest intensity (wound cleansing, therapy); and (4) Psychogenic pain, anticipatory pain without stimulation (Brookman, 2016). The nurse should be aware that rest pain (background) is best handled by administering regularly scheduled long-acting opioids for continuous coverage; procedural pain requires premedication with analgesic medications before painful procedures (Hall, 2012). Breakthrough pain occurs when blood levels of analgesic agents decrease below the level required to control background pain. Psychogenic pain, which is pain that may be caused by an emotional issue, often fear, depression, stress, or anxiety, may be managed with early psychological evaluation and patient-specific treatment.

Pain changes in time as the wound is covered with new skin, healing takes place, and scars form. Management of the often-severe pain is one of the most difficult challenges facing the burn team. Many factors contribute to the pain experience. These factors include the severity of the pain, the adequacy of the health care provider's assessment of the pain, appropriateness of pharmacologic treatment of pain, multiple procedures involved in burn care, and evaluation of the effectiveness of pain relief measures. Literature suggests that, despite advances in pain management, many burn patients are undertreated for pain. The outstanding features of burn pain are its intensity and long duration; thus, all medical providers should understand that opioid tolerance is not addiction, and pain should be managed when there is a clinical need. Furthermore, necessary wound care carries with it the anticipation of pain and anxiety. Refer to Chapter 7 for discussion of tolerance versus addiction.

In partial-thickness burns, the nerve endings are exposed, resulting in excruciating pain with exposure to air currents. Although nerve endings are destroyed in full-thickness burns, the margins of the burn wound are hypersensitive to pain, and there is pain in adjacent structures. Healing of full-thickness burns creates significant discomfort as regenerating nerve endings become entrapped in scar formation. Most severe burns are a combination of partial-thickness and full-thickness burns.

The patient's pain level must be assessed throughout the day because each type of pain is different, and various management strategies may be needed to address the different types of pain. The nurse uses a pain intensity scale to assess pain level (e.g., 1 to 10), and documents response to the treatment plan consistently. Opioid administration via the IV route, particularly in the emergent and acute phases of burn management, remains the mainstay for pharmacologic management. Titration of analgesic agents to obtain relief while minimizing side effects is crucial. The patient's requirements for analgesia are often high, but fear of addiction on the part of the patient and the health care provider hampers adequate opioid administration. Morphine sulfate remains the analgesic of choice. It is titrated to obtain pain relief based on the patient's self-report of pain. There is increasing evidence that ketamine is a good analgesic in burn pain (Nemer & Clark, 2016).

Fentanyl is another useful opioid, particularly for procedural pain, because it has a rapid onset, high potency, and short duration, all of which make it effective for use with procedures.

Patient-controlled analgesia (PCA) maintains a steady level of opioid for pain relief and enables the patient to administer intermittent doses of medication.

Sustained-release opioids, such as MS Contin or oxycodone (OxyContin), have also been used successfully in the treatment of burn pain. These medications can effectively treat the resting pain that is associated with burn injury. Additional medications must be prescribed with these to cover breakthrough pain.

Also, nursing interventions, such as teaching the patient relaxation techniques, giving the patient some control over wound care and analgesia, and providing frequent reassurance, are helpful and should not be overlooked. Other pain-relieving approaches include distraction through video programs or video games, hypnosis, biofeedback, and behavioral modification.

Anxiety and pain go hand in hand. The entire burn experience can produce severe anxiety, which can, in turn, exacerbate pain. Therefore, the ideal pain management regimen must incorporate the treatment of pain and anxiety and must be individualized for each patient.

It is important for the nurse to differentiate restlessness due to pain from restlessness due to hypoxia; a thorough respiratory assessment can help discriminate the etiology, noting oxygen saturation, lung sounds, chest expansion, and respiratory rate. The nurse also assesses the patient's sleep patterns since lack of sleep and rest interferes with healing, comfort, and restoration of energy. If necessary, sedatives are prescribed.

Nutritional Support

Burn injuries produce profound metabolic abnormalities fueled by the exaggerated stress response to the injury. It is essential to control this response by increasing the anabolic process through adequate nutrition, decreasing heat loss from wounds, and maintaining a warm environment. Controlling secondary stress, such as pain and anxiety, also helps control the stress response.

The most important of these interventions is to provide adequate nutrition and calories. Healing of the burn wound consumes large quantities of energy. Several formulas exist for estimating the daily metabolic expenditure and caloric requirements. The enteral route of feeding is far superior to the parenteral route. Feedings are started as soon as possible. Vitamin and mineral supplements may be prescribed, and the nurse collaborates with the dietitian to plan a protein- and calorie-rich diet that is acceptable to the patient. Other treatment modalities include early excision and skin grafting of the burn wound, aggressive prevention or treatment of infections, and adequate exercise with physical therapy to lessen muscle wasting and increase strength.

Promoting Mobility

An early priority is to prevent complications of immobility. Deep breathing, turning, and proper positioning are essential nursing practices that prevent atelectasis and pneumonia, control edema, and prevent pressure ulcers and contractures. These interventions are modified to meet the patient's needs. Low–air-loss and rotation beds may be useful, and early sitting and ambulation are encouraged. If the lower extremities are burned, elastic pressure bandages should be applied before the patient is placed in an upright position.

Psychological and Emotional Support

Family functioning is disrupted with burn injury. One of the nurse's responsibilities is to support the patient and family. Family members need to be instructed about ways that they can support the patient as adaptation to burn trauma occurs. The burn injury has tremendous psychological, economic, and practical impact on the patient and family. Referrals for social services or psychological counseling should be made as appropriate.

Rehabilitation Phase

Rehabilitation begins immediately after the burn has occurred and often extends for years after injury. In the aftermath of the acute stages of burn injury, the patient increasingly focuses on the alterations in self-image and lifestyle that may occur. Wound healing, psychosocial support, and restoration of maximal functional activity remain priorities so that the patient can have the best quality of life both personally and socially. The body goes through many changes as it heals. As the burn wound becomes a burn scar, the burn survivor may be faced with new complications. Often reconstructive surgery to improve body appearance and function is needed.

Hypertrophic Scarring

The wound is in a dynamic state for 1.5 to 2 years after the burn occurs. If appropriate measures are instituted during this active period, the scar tissue can lose its redness and soften. Healed areas that are prone to hypertrophic scarring require the patient to wear a pressure garment. Pressure needs to be continuous. Gentle superficial massage aids in softening the connective tissue. Patients must be instructed about the need for lubrication and protection of the healing skin and the need to use pressure garments for at least 1 year after the injury. Treatment during rehabilitation is expected to include elastic pressure garments, splints, and exercise under the supervision of an experienced physical and occupational therapy team.

Continuing Care

Follow-up care by an interdisciplinary burn care team is necessary. Patients who receive care in a burn center usually return to the burn clinic for evaluation by the burn team, modification of home care instructions, and planning for reconstructive surgery. Many patients require outpatient physical or occupational therapy. It is often the nurse who is responsible for coordinating all aspects of care and ensuring that the patient's needs are met.

Patients who return home after a severe burn injury need referral for home care. Social services and community nursing services must be contacted to provide optimal care and supervision after hospital discharge. The home care nurse assesses the patient's physical and psychological status, as well as the adequacy of the home setting for safe and adequate care. The nurse monitors the plan of care and notes any problems that interfere with the patient's ability to carry out the care.

Patients who have survived burn injuries frequently suffer profound losses. These include not only a loss of body image due to disfigurement but also losses of personal property, homes, loved ones, and ability to work. The American Burn Association (ABA) has consistently advocated to help uninsured patients with disabling burn injuries receive care through Medicare, and supported the Affordable Healthcare Act (ACA) offering all Americans' the opportunity to secure health care insurance coverage (ABA, n.d.).

The health care team must actively promote a healthy body image and self-concept so that these patients can accept or challenge others' perceptions of those who are disfigured or disabled. Several burn patient support groups and other organizations throughout the United States offer services for burn survivors. They provide caring people (often people who have themselves recovered from burn injuries) who can visit the patient in the hospital or home or telephone the patient and family periodically to provide support and counseling about skin care, cosmetics, and problems related to psychosocial adjustment (www.phoenix-society.org). These organizations, and many regional burn centers, sponsor group meetings and social functions at which outpatients are welcome. Some also provide school-reentry programs and are active in burn prevention activities. If more information is needed regarding burn prevention, the ABA can help locate the nearest burn center and offer current burn prevention tips (www.ameriburn.org).

CHAPTER REVIEW

Critical Thinking Exercises

1. A 75-year-old woman was scalded in the bathtub, where she sustained 25% full-thickness wounds to both lower legs before being found by her niece. It is not known how long the woman was in the tub. She has been independent and living alone for the past 15 years; however, her niece has offered to have her aunt come and live with her family. On admission to the emergency department, the woman's temperature is 94°F (35.5°C) and her weight is 111 lb (50 kg). She has diabetes as well as a history of heart failure and hypertension. What are the priorities in her medical and nursing care during the emergent phase of burn care? What assessment parameters would you monitor closely? Is she a likely candidate for skin grafting?

2. An 18-year-old woman sustained second-degree burns from a tanning bed. Her burns cover her entire chest, abdomen, back, and legs. She has large blisters on her

chest and the backs of her knees. Using the rule of nines, estimate the percent of TBSA burned. Estimate her fluid resuscitation needs. Describe nursing care, including patient teaching that is important for this patient. She is rating her pain level 10 out of 10. What comfort measures can you use to manage her pain?

3. A 50-year-old man who weighs 111 lb (50 kg) was transferred to the emergency department after his truck caught fire. He has circumferential burns on both of his legs, his anterior chest, and his entire right upper extremity. He was unable to extricate himself from the truck and suffered inhalation burns as well. Using the rule of nines chart, estimate the percent of TBSA burned. What are the emergency priorities for this patient? What are the fluid resuscitation requirements for this patient based on his percent of burn and his weight? What assessment parameters would you monitor closely? What pain management strategies would be indicated for this patient?

NCLEX-Style Review Questions

1. The nurse is caring for a 32-year-old with circumferential full-thickness burns to the right arm and trunk. Which nursing intervention has the highest priority in the plan of care?
   a. Assess radial pulses several times a day.
   b. Enforce airborne infection control procedures.
   c. Perform range-of-motion exercises several times per day.
   d. Remove blisters from the burn area.

2. A patient with severe burn injuries to the abdomen and legs becomes combative when it is time to change the dressings. What nursing intervention will be most helpful to this patient?
   a. Allow the patient to determine the time of dressing change.
   b. Premedicate the patient with pain and anxiety medications before dressing change.
   c. Tell the patient it is OK to cry during the dressing change.
   d. Explain the importance of dressing changes.

3. A nurse would suspect an inhalation injury with which of the following findings? Select all that apply.
   a. History of burn occurring in an enclosed space
   b. Carbonaceous sputum
   c. Egophony
   d. Stridor
   e. Singing of nasal hair

4. What is a reasonable option for pain management for a 50-year-old man who has just sustained 20% partial-thickness burns to his right leg and abdomen?
   a. Fentanyl 50 μg intravenously
   b. Morphine sulfate 10 mg IM into the left deltoid
   c. Calm, reassuring words to help relax him
   d. Oxycodone 10 mg PO

5. A patient who was burned at 10:00 AM reports a pre-burn weight of 154 lb (70 kg). The estimated total body surface area (TBSA) burned is 60%. Using the Parkland/Baxter formula, the nurse verifies that the total amount of intravenous lactated Ringer solution to be infused by 6:00 PM on the day of the burn is which of the following?
   a. 5,200 mL
   b. 7,470 mL
   c. 8,400 mL
   d. 16,800 mL

Try these additional resources, available at **http://thepoint.lww.com/Honan2e**, to enhance your learning and understanding of this chapter:
- NCLEX-Style Student Review Questions
- Journal Articles

REFERENCES AND SELECTED READINGS

References and selected readings associated with this chapter can be found on the website that accompanies the book. Visit **http://thepoint. lww.com/Honan2e** to access the references and other additional resources associated with this chapter.

Other Acute Problems

An 80-year-old patient is in acute kidney failure and has been diagnosed with multiple organ dysfunction syndrome (MODS). She underwent a right hip replacement 2 days ago and currently has a temperature of 102.6°F.

- What are treatment measures to reverse MODS?
- What patient populations are at increased risk for developing MODS?
- Discuss nursing care of patients with MODS.

Nursing Management: Shock and Multisystem Failure

Linda Honan • Philip R. Martinez, Jr. • Kelly S. Grimshaw

Learning Objectives

After reading this chapter, you will be able to:

1. Describe shock and its underlying pathophysiology.
2. Compare clinical findings of the preshock, shock, and end-organ damage stages of shock.
3. Describe similarities and differences in hypovolemic, cardiogenic, distributive, and obstructive shock states.
4. Identify medical and nursing management priorities in treating patients in shock.
5. Identify vasoactive medications used in treating shock, and describe nursing implications associated with their use.

Shock is a life-threatening condition with a variety of underlying causes. The progression of shock is neither linear nor predictable. Nurses caring for patients with shock and for those at risk for shock must understand the underlying mechanisms of shock and recognize its subtle as well as more obvious signs. Rapid assessment and response are essential to the patient's recovery.

OVERVIEW

Shock can best be defined as a condition in which tissue perfusion is inadequate to deliver oxygen and nutrients to support vital organs and cellular function. This definition differs from more traditional views of shock because it does **not** depend on absolute criteria for parameters, such as blood pressure (BP).

Nursing Alert

By the time BP drops, damage has already been occurring at the cellular and tissue levels. Therefore, the patient at risk for shock must be assessed and monitored closely before the BP falls.

Adequate blood flow to the tissues and cells requires the following components: adequate cardiac pump, effective vasculature and circulatory system, and sufficient blood volume. If one component is impaired, perfusion to the tissues is threatened or compromised. Without treatment, inadequate blood flow to the tissues results in poor delivery of oxygen and nutrients to the cells, cellular starvation, cell death, organ dysfunction progressing to organ failure, and eventual death.

Shock affects all body systems. It may develop rapidly or slowly, depending on the underlying cause. During shock, the body struggles to survive, utilizing a variety of homeostatic, compensatory mechanisms to restore blood flow. Any insult to the body can create a cascade of events resulting in poor tissue perfusion, which means that nurses should be vigilant about watching for signs of shock in all patients, regardless of their primary problem or diagnosis.

PATHOPHYSIOLOGY

Tissue perfusion is determined by cardiac output (CO) and systemic vascular resistance (SVR). CO is the amount of blood pumped by the heart in liters per minute (usual CO is about 4 to 6 L/min but varies greatly depending on the metabolic needs of the body). CO depends on stroke volume, determined by ventricular preload (volume), and heart rate, which is controlled in large part by the autonomic nervous system. Afterload is related closely to, and often equated with, the aortic pressure. It depends on the contractility of the right or left side of the heart and SVR (the resistance to the flow of blood out from the ventricles and a key determinant of aortic pressure). It is helpful to think of SVR as a vise grip on the aorta. If the vise is tightened, the SVR and aortic

BOX 54-1

Classifications of Shock

- **Hypovolemic shock** occurs when there is a decrease in the intravascular volume. Hypovolemia can be the result of an imbalance of intake and output, such as in patients with **dehydration** or **hemorrhage**.
- **Cardiogenic shock** occurs when the heart has an impaired pumping ability; it may be of coronary or noncoronary event origin.
- **Obstructive shock** occurs when there is decreased oxygen delivery due to an obstructive cause, such as pericardial tamponade, tension pneumothorax, PE, or abdominal compartment syndrome.
- **Distributive shock** is caused by alterations in vascular smooth muscle tone, caused by nervous system injury, inflammatory release causing vasodilation, or complications associated with medications such as epidural anesthesia. **Septic shock** is technically considered a "distributive" type of shock. Sepsis is a complex condition, caused by an infection with profound vasodilation.

pressure rise, and now it requires more work for the ventricle to pump blood out. In contrast, if the vise grip is released from the aorta, there is little resistance to the outflow of blood and the work required of the heart muscle is diminished. Conventionally, the primary underlying pathophysiologic process is used to classify the shock state (Box 54-1 provides classifications). When considering possible causes of shock and potential interventions, nurses should remember that the interplay of these two factors (CO and SVR) is what determines the extent of the course of shock and the prognosis of the patient.

In all types of shock, the cells lack an adequate blood supply and are inadequately oxygenated; therefore, they must produce energy through anaerobic metabolism. This results in an acidotic intracellular environment, along with a host of electrolyte derangements. In stress states such as shock, catecholamines, cortisol, glucagon, and inflammatory cytokines and mediators are released, causing hyperglycemia and insulin resistance in an effort to mobilize glucose for cellular metabolism.

Nursing Alert

Tight glycemic control (blood glucose, 80 to 110 mg/dL) was considered to reduce morbidity and mortality of patients who were acutely ill. While a higher blood glucose concentration has been associated with adverse outcomes in a variety of clinical settings, recent research studies reveal inconsistent results, suggesting that, in patients who are critically ill, a less aggressive glycemic target is appropriate (e.g., a blood sugar of less than or equal to 120 mg/dL was an independent risk factor associated with an increased mortality in patients who were nondiabetic) (Chan et al., 2016). The optimal

strategy for the management of hyperglycemia (also called stress hyperglycemia) in patients who are critically ill with and without diabetes is unknown; however, maintaining the glucose of 140 to 180 mg/dL avoids marked hyperglycemia while minimizing the risk of iatrogenic hypoglycemia (Stapleton & Heyland, 2016).

As the hypoxemia progresses, cellular metabolism becomes anaerobic, which causes the lactic acid level to rise. Excess levels of lactic acid limit the amount of adenosine triphosphate (ATP) produced, and normal cell function cannot be maintained. Recall ATP which is in every cell is responsible for storing and supplying needed energy to the cell. The impaired Na^+/K^+ and ATP membrane pump function results in intracellular accumulation of sodium and loss of K^+. Cellular edema results from the increased intracellular sodium and increased capillary permeability, further decreasing the CO. As the cell membrane becomes more permeable, allowing electrolytes and fluids to seep out of and into the cell, cell structures, primarily the mitochondria, are damaged; and cell death results.

Pathophysiology Alert

Shock often affects the mitochondria within the cell, which normally function at the lowest oxygen tensions in the body (mitochondrial pO_2 is about 5 mm Hg). However, they consume almost all the oxygen used by the body. More than 95% of aerobic chemical energy comes from mitochondrial work (aka oxidative phosphorylation), and the oxygen-dependent combustion of fuel substrates (primarily fats, amino acids, carbohydrates, ketones) into carbon dioxide (CO_2), water, and ATP. Because of this oxygen dependence, the mitochondria of patients in shock can be referred to as "canaries in the coal mine" since often they are affected first during inadequate tissue perfusion. Historically miners would carry canaries into the mine tunnels since the buildup of gases such as carbon monoxide would kill the canary before killing the miners, thus it was a warning to get out! Similarly, without sufficient oxygen, ATP is generated by potential mitochondrial fuels that are anaerobic. Thus lactic acid accumulates in the blood (Jones & Kline, 2014).

STAGES OF SHOCK

Shock is believed to progress along a continuum. One way to understand the physiologic responses and subsequent clinical signs and symptoms is to divide the continuum into separate stages:

- A *nonprogressive stage* (also called the *compensated stage or preshock*)

TABLE **54-1** Clinical Findings in Stages of Shock

Finding	Nonprogressive stage; Compensated stage or Preshock	Progressive stage; Uncompensated Stage or Shock	Irreversible stage or End-Organ Dysfunction
		Stage	
Blood pressure	Near normal	Systolic below 80–90 mm Hg; Mean arterial pressure (MAP) less than 65 mm Hg	Requires mechanical or pharmacologic support
Heart rate	Over 100 bpm	100–150 bpm	Erratic or asystole
Respiratory status	Fewer than 20 breaths/min	Rapid, shallow respirations; crackles	May require assisted ventilation
Skin	Cold, clammy	Mottled, petechiae	Jaundice
Urinary output	Mildly decreased	Severely decreased	Anuric, requires dialysis
Mentation	Confusion	Lethargy	Unresponsive
Acid–base balance	Respiratory alkalosis	Metabolic acidosis	Profound acidosis

- A *progressive stage* (also called the *uncompensated stage or shock*)
- An *irreversible stage* (also called *End-organ dysfunction* which results in irreversible organ damage)

The earlier on this continuum that shock is recognized and interventions are initiated, the greater the patient's chance of survival. Table 54-1 compares clinical findings in the different stages of shock.

NONPROGRESSIVE STAGE (COMPENSATED STAGE OR PRESHOCK)

Pathophysiology

In preshock, or the compensatory stage of shock, the BP often remains within normal limits. Compensatory responses, such as vasoconstriction, increased heart rate, and increased contractility of the heart, contribute to maintaining adequate CO and SVR. This results from stimulation of the sympathetic nervous system and subsequent release of catecholamines (epinephrine and norepinephrine). Patients display the often-described "fight-or-flight" response. Thus, tachycardia or a modest change in systemic blood pressure (increase or decrease) may be the only clinical sign of early shock. Adult patients can often compensate for up to a 10% total volume loss through normal homeostatic mechanisms. Conversely, patients who have other medical problems or who take certain medications (such as beta blockers or calcium channel blockers) may have a diminished ability to compensate.

Clinical Manifestations and Assessment

Despite a near-normal BP, the patient may show other clinical signs indicating inadequate organ perfusion. Tachycardia, peripheral vasoconstriction, and anxiety are common.

Anxiety, along with feelings of doom, are common signs of shock during this early phase and often are not recognized in patients or attributed to something other than developing shock.

Medical and Nursing Management

At this nonprogressive stage, treatment is directed toward identifying the cause of shock, correcting the underlying disorder, and initiating aggressive measures aimed at supporting the body's compensatory mechanisms. Because compensation cannot be maintained indefinitely, measures such as fluid replacement and medication therapy must be initiated early to maintain an adequate BP and reestablish and maintain adequate tissue perfusion. *Early intervention along the continuum of shock is the key to improving the patient's prognosis.* Therefore, the nurse must assess the patient at risk for shock systematically to recognize the subtle clinical signs of the compensatory stage before the patient progresses to uncompensated shock. Box 54-2 highlights considerations for recognizing shock in older patients.

The role of the nurse at this stage is to monitor the patient's hemodynamic status and promptly report deviations to the provider, to assist in identifying and treating the underlying disorder by continuous in-depth assessment of the patient, to administer prescribed fluids and medications, and to promote patient safety. In assessing tissue perfusion, the nurse specifically observes for changes in level of consciousness, vital signs, urinary output, skin, and laboratory values. Constant reassessment is warranted at this stage. Nurses should try to maintain a calm environment for both the patient's and family's sake and also ensure that assessments and interventions are rapid and ongoing. Providing brief explanations about the diagnostic and treatment procedures, supporting the patient during these procedures, and

BOX 54-2

Gerontologic Considerations

Recognizing Shock in Older Patients

The physiologic changes associated with aging, coupled with pathologic and chronic disease states, place older people at increased risk for developing a state of shock and possibly multiple organ dysfunction syndrome (MODS). Elderly people can recover from shock if it is detected and treated early with aggressive and supportive therapies. Nurses play an essential role in assessing and interpreting subtle changes in older patients' responses to illness.

- During hypovolemic states, medications such as beta-blocking agents (metoprolol [Lopressor]) used to treat hypertension may mask tachycardia, a primary compensatory mechanism to increase CO.
- The aging immune system may not mount a truly febrile response (temperature over 40°C or 104°F), but an increasing trend in body temperature should be addressed.
- The heart does not function well in hypoxemic states, and the aging heart may respond to decreased myocardial oxygenation with arrhythmias that may be misinterpreted as a normal part of the aging process.
- Changes in mentation may be inappropriately misinterpreted as dementia. Older people with a sudden change in mentation should be aggressively treated for the presence of infection and organ hypoperfusion.

providing information about their outcomes reduces stress and anxiety and thus promotes the patient's physical and mental well-being. Speaking in a calm, reassuring voice and using gentle touch also help ease the patient's concerns.

> **Nursing Alert**
> *For patients experiencing shock, if perfusion does not improve despite aggressive interventions, the nurse recognizes that the body will shunt blood from organs such as the skin, kidneys, and gastrointestinal (GI) tract to the brain and heart to ensure adequate blood supply to these vital organs. As a result, the skin is cool and clammy, bowel sounds are hypoactive, and urine output decreases.*

PROGRESSIVE STAGE (UNCOMPENSATED STAGE OR SHOCK)

In the progressive stage, the patient loses the ability to compensate for the insult, infection, or injury. It is during this stage that clinical signs become more obvious.

Pathophysiology

The heart and kidneys are among the first organs to show signs of dysfunction. Up until now on the continuum, the myocardium has kept pace by increasing CO, but this can only go on for a limited time. The body's inability to meet

increased oxygen requirements produces ischemia, and biochemical mediators cause myocardial depression. This leads to failure of the cardiac pump, even if the underlying cause of the shock is not of cardiac origin.

The systemic impact of hypotension, and thus hypoperfusion, on the kidneys results in decreased urine output. In addition, the inflammatory response to injury is activated, and proinflammatory and anti-inflammatory cytokines and mediators are released, which, in turn, activate the coagulation system in an effort to reestablish homeostasis. At the same time, acidosis impairs all enzymatic functions, including coagulation. A cascade of progressive organ failure resulting from poor tissue perfusion is illustrated in Figure 54-1. Thus it is common for a systemic inflammatory response, coined SIRS, to occur in patients with shock (see section on Septic Shock, page 1521).

Even if the underlying cause of the shock is reversed, the sequence of compensatory responses to the decrease in tissue perfusion perpetuates the shock state, and a vicious cycle ensues. It is believed that the body's appropriate or inappropriate response in this stage of shock may be the primary factor determining the patient's survival.

Clinical Manifestations and Assessment

Clinical manifestations that may be seen include symptomatic tachycardia, dyspnea, restlessness, diaphoresis, metabolic acidosis, hypotension, prolonged capillary refill (more than 2 seconds), decreasing pulse pressure, and oliguria. The most frequent neurologic finding in patients with shock is alteration in the level of consciousness, ranging from confusion to coma (Rivers, 2016, p. 673). Skin changes will depend on the type of shock and may include cool, clammy skin (related to vasoconstriction) or warm, pink skin (related to peripheral vasodilation of distributive shock).

> **Nursing Alert**
> *Although BP readings alone are unreliable indicators of circulatory status, a single episode of systolic BP of less than 80 mm Hg is associated with an 18% increase in hospital mortality (Rivers, 2016).*

> **Nursing Alert**
> *Pulse pressure is the difference between the systolic and diastolic pressure; for example, for a BP of 120/80, the pulse pressure is 40 mm Hg. Pulse pressure rises when the stroke volume increases and narrows when resistance to outflow decreases (Porth, 2015). The pulse pressure may decrease before the systolic pressure decreases, and in patients with shock pulse pressure is less than 25 mm Hg. Nurses are key to identifying narrowing pulse pressures in patients early in the course of shock and should immediately report a pulse pressure of less*

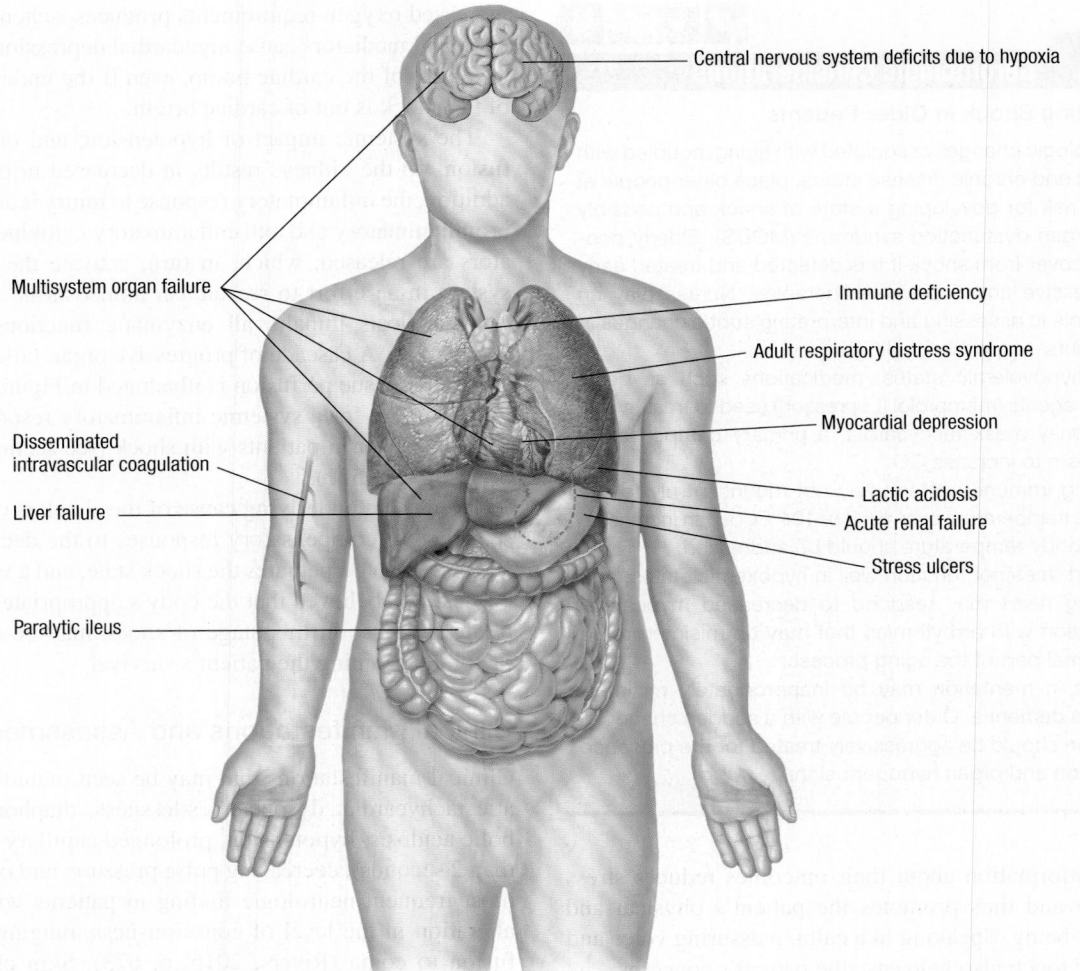

Central nervous system deficits due to hypoxia

Multisystem organ failure

Immune deficiency

Adult respiratory distress syndrome

Myocardial depression

Disseminated intravascular coagulation

Liver failure

Lactic acidosis

Acute renal failure

Stress ulcers

Paralytic ileus

FIGURE 54-1 Multiorgan system effects of shock.

than 25 mm Hg to the provider, even if other signs of shock have not yet manifested.

Medical and Nursing Management

Early and aggressive interventions are essential to the survival of patients in shock; therefore, identifying patients who may be in shock and reporting subtle changes in assessment are imperative. Initially, two large-bore peripheral IVs (at least 16 gauge) are inserted to prepare for fluid administration (Rivers, 2016). Two IV lines allow simultaneous administration of fluid, medications, and blood component therapy if required. Patients in shock are often cared for in the intensive care (ICU) setting in order to

- facilitate close monitoring (hemodynamic monitoring, arterial line insertion, electrocardiographic [ECG] monitoring, arterial blood gases [ABGs], oxygen saturation, serum electrolyte levels, physical and mental status changes);
- allow for rapid and frequent administration of various prescribed medications and fluids;

- provide access for strict measurement of intake and output (Foley catheter may be inserted, and urine output should be measured vigilantly: A urine output of less than 30 mL/hr or 0.5 mL/kg/hr is indicative of renal hypoperfusion and/or hypovolemia); and possibly
- provide interventions with supportive technologies, such as mechanical ventilation, dialysis, extracorporeal membrane oxygenation (ECMO), and intra-aortic balloon pump.

Nursing care of patients in shock requires expertise in assessing and understanding shock and the significance of changes in assessment data.

Specific management of shock depends on the type of shock and its underlying cause, but, in general, care is aimed at achieving the following goals using the acronym ASSESS:

A: Assess frequently the body's response to shock
S: Support the pumping action of the heart
S: Support the respiratory system
E: Encourage patient and family involvement in care, particularly in end-of-life discussions

S: Strengthen the competence of the vascular system
S: Significantly optimize intravascular volume

IRREVERSIBLE STAGE (END-ORGAN DYSFUNCTION)

Pathophysiology

If adequate tissue perfusion is not restored in a timely fashion, irreversible end-organ damage ensues. This represents the point along the shock continuum where end-organ damage is so severe that the patient does not respond to treatment and cannot survive. As the damage increases, acidosis may become so severe that even aggressive therapies such as vasopressor support may not work. For example, kidney and liver failure, compounded by the release of necrotic tissue toxins, will create an overwhelming metabolic acidosis. If the integrity of the gut barrier is compromised, bacteria and their toxins can be translocated into the bloodstream. With severe hypoperfusion of the liver, massive elevations in the enzyme aminotransferase and extensive hepatocellular damage occurs. Anaerobic metabolism contributes to a worsening lactic acidosis. Respiratory system failure prevents adequate oxygenation and ventilation despite mechanical ventilatory support, and the cardiovascular system is ineffective in maintaining an adequate mean arterial pressure (MAP; MAP = $[(2 \times$ diastolic pressure + systolic pressure)/3]) for tissue perfusion. Multiple organ dysfunction progressing to complete organ failure has occurred, and death is imminent. Multiple organ dysfunction can occur as a progression along the shock continuum or as a syndrome unto itself and is described in more detail on page 1528.

> **Nursing Alert**
> *To optimize end-organ perfusion, the nurse monitors the MAP. Although a specific MAP goal has not been established for all shock states, an MAP of at least 60 to 65 mm Hg is a reasonable goal (Rivers, 2016).*

Medical and Nursing Management

Specific therapies in this stage are usually the same as for shock. Although the patient may have progressed from shock to irreversible end-organ damage, the judgment that the shock is irreversible can be made only retrospectively, on the basis of the patient's failure to respond to treatment. As in shock, the nurse focuses on carrying out prescribed treatments, monitoring the patient, preventing complications, protecting the patient from injury, and providing comfort.

Offering brief explanations to the patient about what is happening is essential even if there is no certainty that the patient hears or understands what is being said. Simple comfort measures, including reassuring touches, should continue to be provided despite the patient's nonresponsiveness to verbal stimuli. As it becomes obvious that the patient is unlikely to survive, the family must be informed about the prognosis and likely outcome. Clear, honest communication is imperative as families may not understand what is happening with the patient. Opportunities should be provided, throughout the patient's care, for the family to see, touch, and talk to the patient. Close family friends or spiritual advisors may be of comfort to the family members in dealing with the inevitable death of their loved one. Whenever possible, the patient's family should be approached regarding any living wills, advance directives, or other written or verbal wishes the patient may have shared in the event that he or she became unable to participate in end-of-life decisions. In some cases, ethics committees may assist families and health care teams in making difficult decisions.

GENERAL MANAGEMENT STRATEGIES IN SHOCK

As described previously, and in the discussion of types of shock to follow, management in all types and all phases of shock includes the following:

- Optimization of systemic oxygen delivery to improve tissue oxygenation
- Fluid replacement to restore intravascular volume
- **Vasoactive medications** to restore vasomotor tone and improve cardiac function
- Nutritional support to address the metabolic requirements that are often dramatically increased in shock

Therapies described in this section require collaboration among all members of the health care team to ensure that the manifestations of shock are quickly identified and that adequate and timely treatment is instituted to achieve the best outcome possible (see Fig. 54-2).

Optimize Oxygen Delivery

The first step is to assess oxygenation and provide supplemental oxygen as needed. Oxygen is administered to increase the amount of oxygen carried by available hemoglobin in the blood. A patient who is confused may feel apprehensive with an oxygen mask or cannula in place, and frequent explanations about the need for the mask may reduce some of the patient's fear and anxiety. Frequent assessment of the respiratory status is warranted since many patients with severe shock will require intubation and ventilatory support. Continuous oxygen saturation monitoring is expected. It is important to consider that intubation and mechanical ventilation not only provides for delivery of oxygen and removal of carbon dioxide but also reduces the work of breathing, which, in the patient with hypoperfusion, further exacerbates lactic acidemia (Rivers, 2016). Nurses understand that when patients are "working to breathe," this strenuous use of accessory respiratory muscles can increase

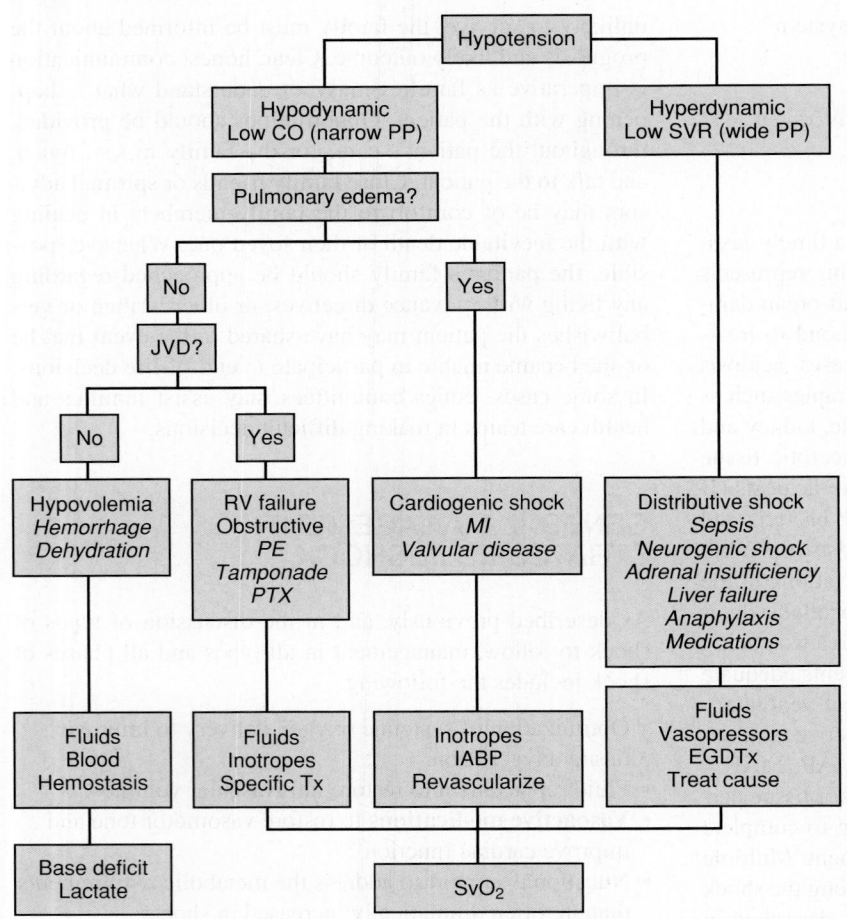

FIGURE 54-2 Shock diagnosis, treatment, and monitoring. CO, cardiac output; PP, pulse pressure; SVR, systemic vascular resistance; JVD, jugular venous distention; PE, pulmonary embolism; PTX, pneumothorax; MI, myocardial infarction; Tx, treatment; IABP, intra-aortic balloon pump; EGDTx, early goal-directed therapy; SvO$_2$, mixed venous oxygen saturation (percent of oxygenated hemoglobin in blood returning to the right heart). (Reprinted with permission from Lawrence, P., Bell, R., Dayton, M., & Hebert, J. (2012). *Essentials of general surgery* (5th ed.). Philadelphia, PA: Lippincott Williams & Wilkins.)

oxygen consumption by 50% to 100% and decrease cerebral blood flow by 50% (Jones & Kline, 2014).

Fluid Replacement

The fluids administered vary but may include **crystalloids** (electrolyte solutions that move freely between intravascular and interstitial spaces), **colloids** (large-molecule IV solutions), and blood components (Table 54-2). The best fluid to treat shock remains controversial. In emergencies, the "best" fluid is often the fluid that is readily available and is dependent on the type of shock and patient presentation. Fluid resuscitation should be initiated early and aggressively in patients with shock to maximize intravascular volume. For example, in patients with septic shock, an intravenous fluid challenge (20 to 30 mL/kg) may be given rapidly of crystalloid IV fluid to improve intravascular volume (Dellinger et al., 2013; Ferri, 2016). A bolus of 500 mL titrated to MAP or measurement of preload is recommended according to Rivers (2016), and repeated based on the absence of pulmonary edema and evidence of improving tissue perfusion. Both crystalloids (e.g., saline and lactated Ringer's [LR] solution) and colloids (e.g., albumin) may be administered to restore intravascular volume. However, IV fluid choice remains

dependent on the type of shock and on the specific patient presentation. For example, in patients with septic shock, crystalloid fluid remains the IV fluid of choice (Dellinger et al., 2013). Conversely, Hespan, a type of colloid fluid, has been shown to cause increased organ damage and mortality in patients who are critically ill, including those with shock (Rivers, 2016). Blood should be given for hypovolemic shock due to trauma and/or hemorrhage, although initially crystalloids may be given to patients to restore intravascular volume while waiting for blood products to transfuse.

Common crystalloid fluids used for resuscitation in hypovolemic shock include 0.9% sodium chloride solution (normal saline) and LR solution. LR is an electrolyte solution containing the lactate ion, which should not be confused with lactic acid. The exogenous lactate is converted to bicarbonate by the liver, thus assisting in treatment of the acidosis. It is important to assess for liver disease when using this solution as the acidosis may worsen when LR is administered to patients with severe liver dysfunction. Additionally, because each liter contains 4 mEq of potassium per liter, it should not be given to patients with severe hyperkalemia. Care also must be taken when administering normal saline rapidly as large volumes result in hyperchloremic metabolic acidosis and coagulopathy (Rivers, 2016). If colloids are administered, the nurse

TABLE 54-2 Fluid Replacement in Shock

Fluids	Advantages	Disadvantages
Crystalloids		
0.9% sodium chloride (normal saline solution)	Widely available, inexpensive	Requires large volume of infusion; can cause hyperchloremic metabolic acidosis, pulmonary edema
Lactated Ringer's (LR)	Lactate ion helps buffer metabolic acidosis	Requires large volume of infusion; can cause pulmonary edema; should not be used in patients with severe hyperkalemia or patients with severe liver dysfunction
Hypertonic saline (3%, 5%, 7.5%)	Small volume needed to restore intravascular volume	Danger of hypernatremia, central pontine myelinolysis, and increased serum osmolality
Colloids		
Albumin (5%, 25%)	Rapidly expands plasma volume	Expensive; requires human donors; limited supply; can cause heart failure
Dextran (40, 70)	Synthetic plasma expander	Interferes with platelet aggregation; not recommended for patients with hemorrhagic shock
Hetastarch	Synthetic; less expensive than albumin; effect lasts up to 36 hours	Prolongs bleeding and clotting times

understands that they expand intravascular volume by exerting oncotic pressure, thereby pulling fluid into the intravascular space. Colloidal solutions have the same effect as hypertonic solutions in increasing intravascular volume, but less volume of fluid is required than with crystalloids. Albumin is a colloid that is commonly ordered to treat hypovolemic shock. The disadvantage of colloids is their high cost, and outcomes of patients with hypovolemic shock are equivalent regardless if they are given crystalloids or albumin (Rivers, 2016). Regardless of the solution administered it is important to avoid "over resuscitation" and thus causing fluid volume excess.

The patient receiving fluid replacement in the context of shock must be monitored frequently for adequate urinary output, changes in mental status, skin perfusion, and changes in vital signs. Lung sounds are auscultated frequently to detect signs of fluid accumulation.

Often, a central venous line is inserted in order to measure central venous pressure (CVP). In addition to physical assessment, the CVP helps in monitoring the patient's response to fluid resuscitation. A normal CVP is 2 to 8 mm Hg. Several readings are obtained to determine a range, and fluid replacement is continued to achieve a CVP of 8 to 12 mm Hg; higher-than-"normal" CVPs readings are desired since ventricles tend to stiffen during shock (Jones & Kline, 2014).

Nursing Alert

The nurse understands that the CVP represents the volume in the right atrium and, therefore, is reflective of the amount of preload to the right ventricle. But in patients with shock, because of the stiffening of the ventricles, the CVP cannot predict what is actually pumped out by the left ventricle; thus the nurse considers parameters such as urinary output (increasing), MAP, and lactate concentrations (decreasing) as measures of improved hemodynamic response to treatment.

With newer technologies, catheters can be placed that allow the monitoring of intravascular pressures and venous oxygen levels. Assessment of mixed venous oxygen saturation (SvO$_2$) or ScvO$_2$ (central venous oxygen saturation) is done with a CVP line or from a special pulmonary artery catheter that has fiber optics capable of calculating the oxygen saturation of hemoglobin. SvO$_2$ reflects the balance between oxygen delivery and oxygen consumption. Knowing the SvO$_2$ in conjunction with pulse oximetry is helpful in evaluating the adequacy of oxygenation; newer technology allows for continuous SvO$_2$/ScvO$_2$ measurements similar to the pulse oximetry. A normal SvO$_2$/ScvO$_2$ is 70% to 80% (i.e., when the blood is returning to the right side of the heart, it has lost only 20% to 30% of its oxygen). An SvO$_2$/ScvO$_2$ of 50% to 70% reveals that more oxygen is being extracted from the RBCs; when the SvO$_2$/ScvO$_2$ is at 30% to 50% the oxygen extraction is becoming exhausted and lactic acidosis begins, and at 25% to 30%, severe lactic acidosis exists. SvO$_2$/ScvO$_2$ below 25% is associated with cellular death (Reyer, 2013). When the SvO$_2$ drops, it reflects the increased consumption of oxygen and the need for intervention.

Knowing the CVP assists in evaluating the intravascular volume. Also the BP, urine output, and base deficit all are suggestive of intravascular volume status. Hemodynamic monitoring with arterial and pulmonary artery lines may be implemented to allow close monitoring of the patient's perfusion and cardiac status, as well as response to therapy. For additional information about hemodynamic monitoring, see Chapter 55.

Vasoactive Medication Therapy

Vasoactive medications can be used in patients with all forms of shock to improve the patient's hemodynamic stability when fluid therapy alone cannot maintain adequate MAP. Different medications work on different aspects of CO, and specific medications are selected depending on the underlying cause (see Chapter 55, Table 55-9). Although most of the medications have several effects, these medications are used to (1) increase the strength of myocardial contractility, (2) regulate the heart rate, (3) reduce myocardial resistance, and (4) initiate vasoconstriction.

Receptors in the sympathetic nervous system are known as alpha-adrenergic and beta-adrenergic receptors. Beta-adrenergic receptors are further classified as beta-1 and beta-2 adrenergic receptors. When alpha-adrenergic receptors are stimulated, blood vessels constrict in the cardiorespiratory and GI systems, skin, and kidneys. When beta-1 adrenergic receptors are stimulated, heart rate and myocardial contraction increase. When beta-2 adrenergic receptors are stimulated, vasodilation occurs in the heart and skeletal muscles, and the bronchioles relax. The medications used in treating shock consist of various combinations of vasoactive medications to maximize tissue perfusion by stimulating or blocking the alpha- and beta-adrenergic receptors.

When vasoactive medications are administered, the nurse must monitor vital signs frequently (at least every 15 minutes until stable, or more often if indicated). Vasoactive medications should be administered through a central venous line because infiltration and extravasation of some vasoactive medications can cause tissue necrosis and sloughing. An IV pump must be used to ensure that the medications are delivered safely and accurately. Often, invasive monitoring using an arterial line is used to titrate medications accurately. Individual medication dosages are usually titrated by the nurse, who adjusts drip rates based on the prescribed dose and the patient's response. Dosages are changed to maintain the MAP at a physiologic level that ensures adequate tissue perfusion (usually above 65 mm Hg). Vasoactive medications should be tapered when possible, and the patient should be weaned from medication with frequent monitoring of BP (at least every 15 minutes).

Nutritional Support

Nutritional support is an important aspect of care for patients with shock. Increased metabolic rates during shock increase energy requirements and, therefore, caloric requirements. The release of catecholamines early in the shock continuum causes depletion of glycogen stores in about 8 to 10 hours. Nutritional energy requirements are then met by breaking down lean body mass. In this catabolic process, skeletal muscle mass is broken down even when the patient has large stores of fat or adipose tissue. Loss of skeletal muscle greatly prolongs the patient's recovery time. Parenteral or enteral nutritional support should be initiated as soon as possible, with some form of enteral nutrition always administered. The integrity of the GI system depends on direct exposure to nutrients. Stress ulcers occur frequently in patients who are acutely ill because of the compromised blood supply to the GI tract. Therefore, antacids (e.g., Carafate), H$_2$ blockers (e.g., famotidine [Pepcid], ranitidine [Zantac]), and/or proton pump inhibitors (e.g., lansoprazole [Prevacid]) are prescribed to prevent ulcer formation by inhibiting gastric acid secretion or increasing gastric pH.

TYPES OF SHOCK

Hypovolemic Shock

Hypovolemic shock, the most common type of shock, is characterized by a decreased intravascular volume. Intracellular fluid accounts for about two thirds of the total body water. The remaining one third of fluid is in the extracellular space that is divided into two compartments: intravascular space (IVS, inside blood vessels) or interstitial space (ISS, surrounding tissues). Approximately three quarters of the extracellular fluid is in the ISS, and the remaining one quarter is in the IVS. Thus, the normal intravascular volume is 4 to 6 L. Hypovolemic shock occurs when there is a reduction in intravascular volume by 15% to 25%, which represents a loss of 750 to 1,500 mL of blood in a 70-kg (154-lb) person.

Pathophysiology

Hypovolemic shock can be caused by sudden fluid losses, such as hemorrhage, or by a gradual deficit in I&O, such as dehydration. See Chapter 56, Table 56-1 for further information on hemorrhagic shock. Figure 54-3 depicts the sequence of events in hypovolemic shock. Box 54-3 discusses risk factors for hypovolemic shock.

Medical Management

Major goals in the treatment of hypovolemic shock are (1) to restore intravascular volume, (2) to reverse the sequence of events leading to inadequate tissue perfusion, and (3) to correct the underlying cause of the fluid loss as quickly as possible. Depending on the severity of shock and the patient's condition, it is likely that efforts will be made to address all three goals simultaneously.

If the patient is hemorrhaging, efforts are made to stop the bleeding. This may involve applying pressure to the bleeding site or a surgery or procedure to stop internal bleeding. If the cause of the hypovolemia is diarrhea or vomiting, medications to treat diarrhea and vomiting are administered while

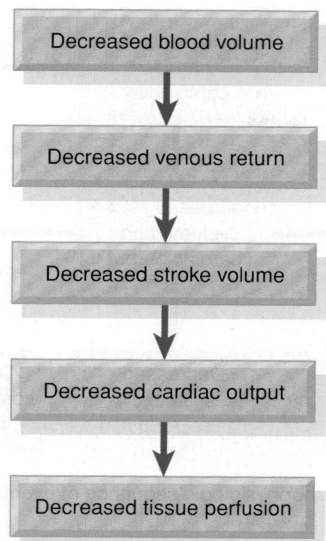

FIGURE 54-3 Pathophysiologic sequence of events in hypovolemic shock.

efforts are made to identify and treat the cause. In elderly patients, dehydration is a common cause of hypovolemia.

If the underlying cause of the hypovolemia is dehydration, medications are also administered to reverse the cause of the dehydration. For example, insulin is administered if dehydration is secondary to hyperglycemia, and desmopressin (DDAVP) is administered for patients with diabetes insipidus.

Beyond reversing the primary cause of the decreased intravascular volume, fluid replacement (also referred to as fluid resuscitation) is of primary concern. At least two large-gauge IV lines are inserted to establish access for fluid administration. Because the goal of the fluid replacement is to restore intravascular volume, it is necessary to administer fluids that will remain in the intravascular compartment, to avoid fluid shifts from the intravascular compartment into

---

BOX 54-3

Risk Factors for Hypovolemic Shock

External: Fluid losses:
- Trauma
- Surgery
- Vomiting
- Diarrhea
- Diuresis
- Diabetes insipidus
- NPO status

Internal: Fluid shifts:
- Hemorrhage
- Burns
- Ascites
- Peritonitis
- Dehydration

---

the intracellular or interstitial compartment. Blood products may need to be administered, particularly if the cause of the hypovolemic shock is hemorrhage. Packed red blood cells are administered to replenish the patient's oxygen-carrying capacity, in conjunction with other fluids that will expand volume. Plasma and platelet transfusions can help with fluid resuscitation and also treat other underlying problems. The need for transfusions is based on the patient's individual perfusion needs, which are determined by vital signs, blood gas values, and clinical appearance rather than an arbitrary laboratory value. An area of active research is the development of synthetic forms of blood (i.e., compounds capable of carrying oxygen in the same way that blood does) as potential alternatives to blood component therapy. Risks inherent to administering blood include the possibility of a transfusion reaction.

Commonly, positioning the patient with his or her head down, known as the *Trendelenburg position*, has been thought to increase blood flow to vital organs by increasing preload. This practice has not been found to be supported by evidence and, in fact, may worsen pulmonary gas exchange and risk of aspiration (Rivers, 2016). An alternative is to elevate the patient's legs slightly to improve cerebral circulation and promote venous return to the heart, but this position is contraindicated for patients with head injuries.

Nursing Management

Primary prevention of shock is an essential focus of nursing care. Hypovolemic shock can be prevented in some instances by closely monitoring patients who are at risk for fluid deficits and assisting with fluid replacement before intravascular volume is depleted. In other circumstances, nursing care focuses on assisting with treatment targeted at the cause of the shock and restoring intravascular volume.

General nursing measures include ensuring safe administration of prescribed fluids and medications and documenting their administration and effects. Another important nursing role is monitoring for signs of complications and side effects of treatment and reporting these signs early in treatment.

Administering blood transfusions safely is a vital nursing role. In emergency situations, it is important to acquire blood specimens quickly, to obtain a baseline complete blood count, and to type and cross-match the blood in anticipation of blood transfusions. A patient who receives a transfusion of blood products must be monitored closely for adverse effects (see Chapter 20).

Fluid replacement complications can occur, often when large volumes are administered rapidly. Therefore, the nurse monitors the patient closely for cardiovascular overload and edema. The risk of these complications is increased in the elderly and in patients with pre-existing cardiac disease. Hemodynamic pressure, vital signs, ABGs, serum lactate levels, hemoglobin and hematocrit levels, and fluid I&O are among the parameters monitored. Temperature should also be monitored closely to ensure that rapid fluid resuscitation does not precipitate hypothermia. IV fluids may need to be warmed during the administration of large volumes. Physical assessment focuses on observing the jugular veins for distention and monitoring CVP. CVP is typically low in hypovolemic shock; it increases with effective treatment, and is significantly increased with fluid overload and heart failure. The nurse must monitor cardiac and respiratory status closely and report to the provider any changes in BP, pulse pressure, heart rate and rhythm, and lung sounds.

CARDIOGENIC SHOCK

Cardiogenic shock occurs when the heart's ability to contract and to pump blood is impaired and the supply of oxygen is inadequate for the heart and tissues. Cardiogenic shock is seen most often in patients with myocardial infarction (MI). Other causes of cardiogenic shock are related to conditions that stress the myocardium (e.g., severe hypoxemia, acidosis, hypoglycemia, and hypocalcemia), as well as in conditions that result in ineffective myocardial function (e.g., cardiomyopathies, valvular damage, and arrhythmias).

Pathophysiology

In cardiogenic shock, CO, which is a function of stroke volume and heart rate, is compromised. When stroke volume and heart rate decrease or become erratic, BP falls (systolic blood pressure is less than 90 mm Hg or there is a decrease from baseline of more than 30 mm Hg for more than 30 minutes), and systemic tissue perfusion is compromised (urine output decreases, skin becomes cool and mottled, mental status changes [sensorium becomes clouded], anxiety is obvious, capillary refill is delayed). Blood supply for the heart muscle itself is inadequate, resulting in further decreases in CO (cardiac index is less than 2.2 L/min/m^2). Additionally, diastolic dysfunction increases left atrial pressure, which leads to pulmonary congestion and hypoxemia that can further exacerbate myocardial ischemia and impair ventricular performance (pulmonary capillary wedge pressure is greater than 18 mm Hg). This can occur rapidly or over a period of days. Patients in cardiogenic shock may experience the pain of angina and develop arrhythmias and hemodynamic instability. Figure 54-4 depicts the pathophysiology of cardiogenic shock.

 Nursing Alert
In the case of heart failure resulting in cardiogenic shock, the nurse assesses for jugular vein distention (JVD), rales, shortness of breath, and S$_3$ gallop.

Medical Management

The goals of management in cardiogenic shock are (1) to limit further myocardial damage and preserve the healthy

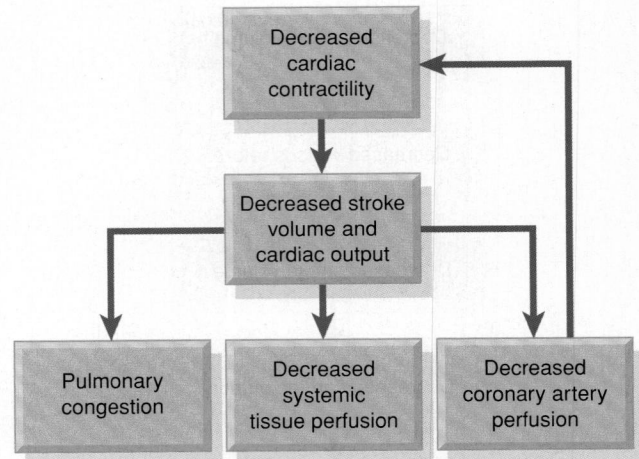

FIGURE 54-4 Pathophysiologic sequence of events in cardiogenic shock.

myocardium and (2) to improve the cardiac function by increasing cardiac contractility, decreasing ventricular afterload, or both. In general, these goals are achieved by increasing oxygen supply to the heart muscle while reducing oxygen demands.

As with all forms of shock, the underlying cause of cardiogenic shock must be corrected. It is necessary first to treat the oxygenation needs of the heart muscle to ensure its continued ability to pump blood to other organs. In the case of cardiogenic shock due to ischemia or infarction, the patient may require thrombolytic therapy, angioplasty, coronary artery bypass graft surgery, intra-aortic balloon pump therapy, ventricular assist device (VAD), or some combination of these treatments. General interventions for cardiogenic shock include supplemental oxygen, controlling chest pain, providing selected fluid support, administering vasoactive medications, controlling heart rate with medication or pacemaker, and using a mechanical assist device if needed. Serial laboratory markers for ventricular dysfunction (e.g., BNP) and cardiac enzyme levels (i.e., troponin-I) are measured, serial 12-lead ECGs are obtained, and frequently an echocardiogram is ordered to assess the degree of myocardial damage or dysfunction.

Pharmacologic Therapy

Oxygen
In the early stages of shock, supplemental oxygen is administered at a rate sufficient to achieve an oxygen saturation exceeding 90%. Monitoring of ABG values and pulse oximetry values helps determine whether the patient requires a more aggressive method of oxygen delivery.

Analgesia
If a patient experiences chest pain, an IV analgesic (commonly morphine sulfate) is administered for pain relief. In addition to relieving pain, morphine dilates the blood

vessels. This reduces the workload of the heart by both decreasing the cardiac filling pressure (preload) and reducing the pressure against which the heart muscle has to eject blood (afterload).

Antiplatelet Agents and Beta Blockers

Antiplatelet agents, such as aspirin, should be given in the case of a patient with acute MI. In addition, a beta blocker is used to decrease workload of the heart and preserve cardiac muscle. The use of these medications in the case of a patient with cardiogenic shock can be complicated since beta blockers will decrease BP. See Chapter 14 for acute treatment of chest pain and MI.

Nursing Alert
During an acute MI, aspirin may be ordered to prevent worsening thrombosis in the coronary arteries. When administering aspirin in this acute situation, the nurse should ask the patient to chew aspirin (162 to 325 mg) rather than swallow a whole enteric-coated aspirin. Chewing aspirin allows for a more rapid absorption rate than does swallowing it whole (Anderson, 2016; Feldman & Cryer, 1999).

Vasoactive Medications

Vasoactive medication therapy consists of multiple pharmacologic strategies to restore and maintain adequate CO. In cardiogenic shock, the aims of vasoactive medication therapy are to improve cardiac contractility, optimize preload and afterload, reduce myocardial oxygen demand, and stabilize heart rate and rhythm. Medications commonly used to treat cardiogenic shock include dobutamine, dopamine, and nitroglycerin. See Table 55-9 for a review of common vasoactive medications.

Nursing Alert
The nurse is vigilant in observing the patient's response to vasoactive agents because of the potential of worsening myocardial ischemia by increasing cardiac work.

Dopamine is a sympathomimetic agent. It acts as an inotrope and a vasopressor (at higher doses). It may be used with dobutamine and nitroglycerin to improve tissue perfusion. Sympathomimetic agents must be used with caution in patients with cardiogenic shock since they increase myocardial oxygen demand and can worsen failure. Also, in patients with severe metabolic acidosis, which occurs in the later stages of shock, the effectiveness of dopamine is diminished. Norepinephrine also may be considered as a first-line agent for hypotension in patients with cardiogenic shock; it is a vasoactive agent that acts primarily as a vasoconstrictor, has a mild inotropic effect, and increases coronary flow while having less of an effect on heart rate in patients with tachycardia (Hollenberg, 2016).

If tissue perfusion remains inadequate, inotropic therapy may be considered with dobutamine, which predominantly affects beta-1 adrenergic receptors (increases the strength of myocardial activity and improves CO). Dobutamine enhances the strength of cardiac contraction, improving stroke volume ejection and overall CO. Because it also has some beta-2 properties, vasodilation occurs (decreased afterload), and the bronchioles relax. The nurse is aware that dobutamine may exacerbate hypotension is some patients (related to vasodilatory effects) and can precipitate tachyarrhythmias (Hollenberg, 2016).

IV nitroglycerin in low doses acts as a venous vasodilator and, therefore, reduces preload. At higher doses, nitroglycerin causes arterial vasodilation and reduces afterload as well. These actions, in combination with dobutamine, increase CO while minimizing cardiac workload. In addition, vasodilation enhances blood flow to the myocardium, improving oxygen delivery to the weakened heart muscle. A combination of medications may be prescribed, depending on the patient's response to treatment. All vasoactive medications have adverse effects, making specific medications more useful than others at different stages of shock.

Nursing Alert
Vasoactive medications should never be stopped abruptly because this could cause severe hemodynamic instability, perpetuating the shock state.

Diuretics

Diuretics such as furosemide (Lasix) may be administered to reduce the workload of the heart by reducing fluid accumulation. Diuretics must be used **cautiously** since they can lead to hypovolemia. In addition, aggressive diuresis can lead to metabolic alkalosis, often referred to as a *contraction alkalosis*. The use of diuretics can also lead to electrolyte abnormalities, the most common of which is hypokalemia.

Antiarrhythmic Medications

Multiple factors, such as hypoxemia, electrolyte imbalances, and acid–base imbalances, contribute to serious cardiac arrhythmias in all patients with shock. In addition, as a compensatory response to decreased CO and BP, the heart rate increases beyond normal limits. This impedes CO further by shortening diastole and thereby decreasing the time for ventricular filling. Consequently, antiarrhythmic medications are required to stabilize the heart rate. For a full discussion of cardiac arrhythmias, as well as commonly prescribed medications, see Chapter 17.

Fluid Status

Appropriate fluid administration is also necessary in the treatment of cardiogenic shock. Administration of fluids must be monitored closely to detect signs of fluid overload. Incremental

IV fluid boluses are cautiously administered to determine optimal filling pressures for improving CO. Nurses should use caution when administering fluids rapidly because rapid fluid administration in patients with cardiac failure may result in acute pulmonary edema. Fluid overload and pulmonary edema are risks because of ineffective cardiac function and accumulation of fluid in the pulmonary tissues.

Mechanical Assistive Devices

If CO does not improve despite supplemental oxygen, vasoactive medications, and fluid boluses, mechanical assistive devices can sometimes be used temporarily to improve the heart's ability to pump. Intra-aortic balloon counterpulsation or left and right ventricular assist devices and total temporary artificial hearts are means of providing temporary circulatory assistance and are reviewed in Chapters 16 and 55.

Nursing Management

Preventing Cardiogenic Shock

In many circumstances, identifying at-risk patients early, promoting adequate perfusion of the heart muscle, and decreasing cardiac workload can prevent cardiogenic shock. Risk factors include advanced age, anterior MI or previous MI, diabetes, hypertension, multivessel CAD, and peripheral vascular and cerebrovascular diseases (Hollenberg, 2016). Patients who have decreased ejection fractions, larger infarctions, and echo results that demonstrate a lack of hyperkinesis in the myocardial remote from the infarction should be considered at risk for cardiogenic shock (Hollenberg, 2016). Minimizing patient risk can be accomplished by conserving the patient's energy, promptly relieving angina, and administering supplemental oxygen, aspirin, and beta blockers. When cardiogenic shock is present, nursing management includes working with other members of the health care team to prevent shock from progressing and to restore adequate cardiac function and tissue perfusion.

Monitoring Hemodynamic Status

A major role of the nurse is monitoring the patient's hemodynamic and cardiac status. Arterial lines and ECG monitoring equipment must be well maintained and functioning properly. The nurse anticipates the medications, IV fluids, and equipment that might be used and is ready to assist in implementing these measures. Changes in hemodynamic, cardiac, pulmonary, and renal status and laboratory values are documented and reported promptly. In addition, adventitious breath sounds, changes in cardiac rhythm, and other abnormal physical assessment findings are reported immediately.

Administering Medications

The nurse documents and records medications and treatments that are administered, as well as the patient's response to treatment.

The nurse must be knowledgeable about the desired effects, as well as the side effects, of medications. For example, it is important to monitor the patient for decreased BP after administering morphine or nitroglycerin. Patients receiving thrombolytic therapy must be monitored for bleeding. Arterial and venous puncture sites must be observed for bleeding, and pressure must be applied at the sites if bleeding occurs. Neurologic assessment is essential after the administration of thrombolytic therapy to assess for the potential complication of cerebral hemorrhage associated with the therapy. IV infusions must be observed closely because tissue necrosis and sloughing may occur if vasopressor medications infiltrate the tissues. Urine output, blood urea nitrogen (BUN), and serum creatinine levels are monitored to detect decreased kidney function secondary to the effects of cardiogenic shock or its treatment.

Enhancing Safety and Comfort

Throughout care, the nurse must take an active role in safeguarding the patient, enhancing comfort, and reducing anxiety. This includes administering medication to relieve chest pain, preventing infection at the multiple arterial and venous line insertion sites, protecting the skin, and monitoring respiratory and kidney function. Proper positioning of the patient promotes effective breathing without decreasing BP and may also increase patient comfort while reducing anxiety.

Brief explanations about procedures that are being performed and the use of comforting touch often provide reassurance to the patient and family. The family is usually anxious and benefits from opportunities to see and talk to the patient. Explanations of treatments and the patient's responses are often comforting to family members.

DISTRIBUTIVE SHOCK

Distributive shock, also sometimes called circulatory shock, occurs when the body's ability to adjust vascular tone is impaired, and thus blood volume is abnormally displaced in the vasculature (e.g., when blood volume pools in peripheral blood vessels). The displacement of blood volume causes a relative hypovolemia because not enough blood returns to the heart, which leads to subsequent inadequate tissue perfusion. The vascular tone is determined both by central regulatory mechanisms, as in BP regulation, and by local regulatory mechanisms, as in tissue demands for oxygen and nutrients. Therefore, distributive shock can be caused either by a loss of sympathetic tone or by release of biochemical mediators from cells.

The varied mechanisms leading to the initial vasodilation in distributive shock further subdivide this classification of shock into three types: (1) **septic shock**, (2) **neurogenic shock,** and (3) **anaphylactic shock**. Other causes of distributive shock are rare but include toxic shock syndrome,

Risk Factors for Distributive Shock

Septic shock:
- Immunosuppression
- Extremes of age (under 1 year of age and over 65 years of age)
- Malnourishment
- Chronic illness
- Invasive procedures

Neurogenic shock:
- Spinal cord injury
- Spinal anesthesia
- Depressant action of medications
- Glucose deficiency

Anaphylactic shock:
- Penicillin sensitivity
- Transfusion reaction
- Bee sting allergy
- Latex sensitivity
- Severe allergy to some foods or medications

drug overdose, neurogenic insults, addisonian crisis, and myxedema coma (Rivers, 2016). In all types of distributive shock, massive arterial and venous dilation allows blood to pool peripherally. The different types of shock cause variations in the pathophysiologic chain of events. Risk factors for distributive shock are summarized in Box 54-4.

SEPTIC SHOCK

Septic shock, the most common type of distributive shock, is caused by widespread, overwhelming infection in combination with a dysregulated host immune response. Because of the increased sophistication of antibiotic therapy and improved recognition of sepsis and initiation of intensive care management, the incidence of septic shock has declined. Approximately 750,000 cases of severe sepsis or septic shock occur annually in the United States, with mortality rates of about 25 to 35%, which is down from rates of 70% in 2010 (Russell, 2016). Finding and aggressively treating the source of infection, as well as providing aggressive cardiopulmonary support, are important determinants of the clinical outcome.

Risk Factors

Nosocomial infections (infections occurring in the hospital) in patients who are critically ill that may progress to septic shock commonly originate in the lungs (pneumonia) and urinary (pyelonephritis) and GI tract (peritonitis, intra-abdominal abscess, cholangitis), although they can originate anywhere in the body (refer to Table 54-3 for common sites related to sepsis). Organisms include gram-positive or negative bacteria, fungi, and, rarely, protozoa or rickettsiae are associated with septic shock; commonly gram-positive bacteria, especially methicillin-resistant *Staphylococcus aureus* (MRSA),

vancomycin-resistant enterococci (VRE), penicillin-resistant *Streptococcus pneumoniae*, and resistant gram-negative bacilli are seen (Russell, 2016). Additional risk factors are age, immunocompromise due to malnutrition, alcoholism, malignancy, diabetes mellitus, and AIDS; invasive procedures and indwelling medical devices; and the increased number of resistant microorganisms. Elderly patients continue to be at particular risk for sepsis because of decreased physiologic reserves and an aging immune system. The incidence of septic shock can be reduced by carrying out infection control practices, including the use of meticulous aseptic technique, properly cleaning and maintaining equipment, and using thorough hand hygiene techniques.

Pathophysiology

When microorganisms invade body tissues, patients exhibit an immune response. This immune response provokes the activation of biochemical cytokines and mediators associated with an inflammatory response and produces a complex cascade of physiologic events that leads to poor tissue perfusion. Widespread endothelial injury leads to increased capillary permeability, which triggers seepage of protein-rich fluid from the capillaries, and vasodilation, which occurs when injured endothelial cells release nitric acid (a potent vasodilator). These two effects interrupt the ability of the body to provide adequate perfusion, oxygen, and nutrients to the tissues and cells. In addition, proinflammatory and anti-inflammatory cytokines released during the inflammatory response activate the coagulation system, which begins to form clots in areas where a clot may or may not be needed, further compromising tissue perfusion. The imbalance of the inflammatory response and the clotting and fibrinolysis cascades are considered critical elements of the devastating physiologic progression that is present in patients with severe sepsis. To illustrate, the increased permeability within the lung is a key component of acute lung injury (ALI), whereas increased permeability in the intestine can lead to translocation of intestinal bacteria.

Clinical Manifestations and Assessment

Sepsis is defined by presence of at least two of the four signs of the systemic inflammatory response syndrome: (1) fever (above 38°C) or hypothermia (below 36°C); (2) tachycardia (more than 90 beats/min); (3) tachypnea (more than 20 breaths/min), hypocapnia (partial pressure of carbon dioxide less than 32 mm Hg), or the need for mechanical ventilatory assistance; and (4) leukocytosis (more than 12,000 cells/μL), leukopenia (fewer than 4,000 cells/μL), or a left shift (more than 0% immature band cells) in the circulating white blood cell differential and suspected or proven infection plus a documented or suspected infection (Russell, 2016, p. 685).

Systemic inflammatory response syndrome (SIRS) presents clinically like sepsis. The only difference between SIRS and sepsis is that an identifiable causative infectious

TABLE **54-3** Common Sites and Diseases Associated with Sepsis/Systemic Inflammatory Response Syndrome (SIRS)

Organ System	Location	Disease
Respiratory	Upper respiratory tract	Sinusitis Mastoiditis
	Lower respiratory tract	Pneumonia Lung abscess Empyema
Gastrointestinal	Mediastinum Hepatobiliary Intra-abdominal	Esophageal rupture/perforation Hepatic abscess Cholangitis Cholecystitis Intestinal infarction/perforation Pancreatitis Intra-abdominal/diverticular abscess
Cardiovascular	Mediastinum Native or prosthetic cardiac valve	Postoperative mediastinitis Endocarditis
Genitourinary	Kidney, ureter, and bladder	Perinephric abscess Pyelonephritis Cystitis
Neurologic	Brain and meninges	Meningitis Intracranial abscess
Dermatologic	Traumatic wound, surgical wound, or burn site	Soft tissue abscess Necrotizing fasciitis Infected decubitus ulcer Full and partial thickness burn
Prosthetic	Central/peripheral venous catheter Arterial catheter Ventriculoperitoneal shunt Dialysis catheter Articular prosthetic device Dialysis graft/shunt	Catheter infection Infected prosthesis
Other	Vascular system	Septic thrombophlebitis

Reprinted with permission from Stenbit, A., & Serio, A. (2010). Sepsis. In R. Irwin & J. Rippe (Eds.), *Manual of intensive care management (Chapter 123)*. Philadelphia, PA: Lippincott Williams & Wilkins.

agent is established in the latter. SIRS/sepsis results in an inflammatory and immunologic response that is overwhelming, thought to be caused in large part by an array of inflammatory cytokines, including but not confined to tumor necrosis factor (TNF). The inflammatory response also leads to increased coagulation, and coagulation triggers inflammation; a positive feedback loop is at play that has the potential to disrupt essential kidney, cardiovascular, and respiratory function (Russell, 2016). Any overwhelming insult can stimulate SIRS and may progress to sepsis; noninfectious disorders include pancreatitis and drug intoxication. Therefore, despite an absence of infection, antibiotic agents still may be administered because of the possibility of unrecognized infection. Additional therapies directed to support patients with SIRS are similar to those for sepsis. If the inflammatory process progresses, septic shock may develop.

Sepsis is an evolving process, without a predictable linear progression. In the past, septic shock has been described as having two phases, a hyperdynamic (warm) and a hypodynamic (cold) phase. Although the division into phases may promote understanding of sepsis, its actual progression into severe sepsis and septic shock is not always easy to recognize clinically. Initially, a hyperdynamic response occurs; it is characterized by a high CO with systemic vasodilation. The BP may remain within normal limits, or the patient may be hypotensive but responsive to fluids. The heart rate increases, progressing to tachycardia. Fever, with warm, flushed skin and bounding pulses, is evident. The respiratory rate is elevated. Urinary output may remain at normal levels or decrease. GI status may be compromised, as evidenced by nausea, vomiting, diarrhea, or decreased bowel sounds. Signs of hypermetabolism include increased serum glucose and insulin resistance. Subtle changes in mental status, such as confusion or agitation, may be present.

As the sepsis progresses, tissues become more underperfused and acidotic, compensation begins to fail, and the

BOX 54-5
Definitions in Sepsis

Bacteremia: The presence of bacteria in the blood

Infection: The presence of microorganisms that trigger an inflammatory response

Systemic inflammatory response syndrome (SIRS): A syndrome resulting from a *severe clinical insult* that initiates an overwhelming inflammatory response by the body; defined as two or more of the following conditions:
- Temperature greater than 38.5°C or less than 35.0°C
- Heart rate of more than 90 bpm
- Respiratory rate of more than 20 breaths/min or $PaCO_2$ of less than 32 mm Hg
- White blood cell count of more than 12,000 cells/mL, less than 4,000 cells/mL, or greater than 10% immature (band) forms

Sepsis: A systemic response to *infection;* may occur after a burn, surgery, or serious illness and is defined as the presence of SIRS, plus the presence of an infectious source (either by documented culture or by visualizing focal infection)

Severe sepsis: Defined as sepsis, plus at least one of the following signs of organ hypoperfusion:

- Areas of mottled skin
- Capillary refill of more than 3 seconds
- Decreased urinary output (less than 0.5 mg/kg for 1 hour) (oliguria)
- Lactate greater than 2 mmol/L (lactic acidosis)
- Abrupt change in mental status (decreased Glasgow Coma Scale)
- Platelet count of less than 100,000 or disseminated intravascular coagulation (DIC) (thrombocytopenia)
- Acute lung injury or acute respiratory distress syndrome (ARDS) (hypoxemia)
- Cardiac dysfunction

Septic shock: Shock associated with sepsis; defined as severe sepsis, plus one of the following:
- Mean arterial pressure (MAP) of less than 60 after fluid resuscitation; systolic blood pressure less than 90 mm Hg or a decrease from baseline that is greater than 40 mm Hg, despite adequate fluid resuscitation.
- Need for vasoactive medication in order to maintain MAP of greater than 60.

Adapted from Annane, D., & Cavaillon, J. M. (2005). Septic shock. *Lancet, 365*(9453), 63–78; Sommers, M. S. (2003). The cellular basis of septic shock. *Critical Care Nursing Clinics of North America, 15*(1), 13–26.

patient becomes more hypodynamic. The cardiovascular system also begins to fail, the BP does not respond to vasoactive agents and fluid resuscitation, and signs of end-organ damage are visible (e.g., kidney failure, pulmonary failure, hepatic failure). As sepsis progresses to septic shock, the BP drops, and the skin becomes cool and pale. Temperature may be normal or below normal. Heart and respiratory rates remain rapid. Urine output decreases, and multiple organ dysfunction syndrome (MODS) develops (discussed on page 1528).

In an effort to promote recognition and earlier treatment of patients with sepsis, the Society of Critical Care Medicine defined a common set of terms and cues for clinicians (Box 54-5).

Medical Management

Current treatment of septic shock involves *identification and elimination of the cause of infection and aggressive cardiopulmonary support* to prevent or limit end-organ damage and death. Specimens of blood, sputum, urine, and wound drainage are collected for culture using aseptic technique. Any potential routes of infection must be eliminated. IV lines may need to be removed and reinserted at other body sites; the patient will require scrupulous sterile techniques for the insertion of catheters, with consideration of the use of antibiotic-impregnated catheters (Russell, 2016). If possible, urinary catheters are removed or replaced. Any abscesses are drained, and necrotic areas are surgically débrided.

Fluid replacement must be instituted to correct the hypovolemia that results from the incompetent vasculature and the inflammatory response. Crystalloids, colloids, and blood products may be administered to increase intravascular volume. IV fluids boluses (in the range of 20 to 40 mL/kg) may be ordered to improve intravascular volume (Rivers, 2016). The CVP, MAP, urinary output, and SvO_2 are used to guide therapy.

Oxygen is administered and guided by the pulse oximeter, SvO_2, and clinical presentation. Many patients will require mechanical ventilation, with a lower tidal volume (typically greater than 6 mL/kg of ideal body weight [IBW]), which has been associated with decreased mortality from ALI and acute respiratory distress syndrome (ARDS). ARDS and ALI are discussed in Chapter 10.

Preventing the progress from sepsis to septic shock necessitates early diagnosis and aggressive resuscitation. The patient's responses to treatment are closely monitored, and resuscitation is continued until CVP is greater than 8, MAP is greater than 65 mm Hg, urine output is 0.5 mL/kg/hr or more, and SvO_2 is greater than 70%. This approach is associated with a decreased mortality and should be considered standard of care in the management of septic shock.

Pharmacologic Therapy

Antibiotics

Before antibiotic therapy is initiated, it is important that all cultures be obtained. However, if obtaining cultures is delayed, the nurse is aware that antimicrobials should be administered within 1 hour of identification of septic shock. The nurse anticipates the need for blood, sputum, urine, and wound cultures, and, depending on the site of the expected infection, additional cultures may be obtained from the cerebrospinal fluid (in the case of suspected meningitis) or pleural space (if empyema is suspected). If the infecting organism is unknown, empiric broad-spectrum antibiotics are started. When culture and sensitivity reports become available, the antibiotic agents can be changed to those that are more specific to the infecting organism and less toxic to the patient.

> **Nursing Alert**
> *It is important for the nurse to consider all possible sources of the infection. Symptoms such as cough, sputum production, adventitious lung sounds and increased work of breathing suggests pneumonia; pleuritic chest pain, decreased fremitus, and a dull, flat sound on percussion suggests empyema; dysuria and costovertebral angle tenderness suggests pyelonephritis; erythema and drainage and warmth from IV lines suggests line sepsis; whereas headache and stiff neck suggest meningitis.*

Vasopressors

Therapy with vasopressors (e.g., norepinephrine, epinephrine) is expected if a mean arterial blood pressure of greater than 65 mm Hg is not achieved by IV hydration alone. The nurse monitors the MAP, the CVP, O_2 saturation, and SvO_2, as well as the hourly urine output (aim is greater than 0.5 mL/kg/hr) to assess evidence of improving perfusion (improved mental status, peripheral perfusion).

Glucocorticoids

Glucocorticoids have been used in the treatment of septic shock with varying effect for decades. The general concept is that, since septic shock represents a significant physiologic stress, dysfunction of the hypothalamic–pituitary–adrenal axis may be one factor that leads to increased mortality. Several studies have attempted to investigate the effect of administering steroids to septic patients. Drawbacks to steroid administration include increased infection rate and increased risk of superinfections, worsening glycemic control, and impaired wound healing. High-dose corticosteroids do not improve outcomes in the full spectrum of patients with sepsis or ARDS, and the evidence supporting the use of low-dose corticosteroids in septic shock remains controversial (Russell, 2016, p. 690). If the patient has not responded to vasopressor support, corticosteroids may be considered.

Nutritional Therapy and Glycemic Control

Aggressive nutritional supplementation is critical in the management of patients with septic shock because malnutrition further impairs the patient's compensatory mechanisms. Nutritional supplementation should be initiated as soon as possible. Enteral feeding, rather than parental nutrition, is associated with improved outcomes, although reasons for this remain unclear. Evidence is particularly strong for enteral nutrition in surgical patients who are critically ill. Regarding glycemic control, intense insulin therapy increases the risk of higher rates of hypoglycemia and perhaps increased mortality and, therefore, is not recommended (Russell, 2016). However, the nurse assesses and alerts the team when the patient's blood glucose level is outside the range of 140 to 180 mg/dL.

Nursing Management

Nurses caring for patients in any setting must keep in mind the risks of sepsis and the high mortality rate associated with sepsis, severe sepsis, and septic shock. All invasive procedures must be carried out with aseptic technique after careful hand hygiene. In addition, IV lines, arterial and venous puncture sites, surgical incisions, traumatic wounds, urinary catheters, and pressure ulcers must be monitored for signs of infection in all patients. Nurses should identify patients who are at particular risk for sepsis and septic shock (i.e., elderly and immunosuppressed patients and those with extensive trauma, burns, or diabetes), keeping in mind that these high-risk patients may not develop typical or classic signs of infection and sepsis. For example, confusion may be the first sign of infection and sepsis in elderly patients.

Monitoring and constant reassessment are primary nursing tasks when caring for a patient with septic shock. Vital signs, hemodynamics (CVP, SvO_2, SVR, CO), urinary output, mental status, and physical assessment findings must be reported accurately and in a timely fashion so that interventions can be instituted. When caring for a patient with septic shock, the nurse collaborates with other members of the health care team to identify the site and source of sepsis and the specific organisms involved. Appropriate specimens for culture and sensitivity are often obtained by the nurse.

Elevated body temperature (hyperthermia) is common in patients with sepsis and raises the patient's metabolic rate and oxygen consumption. Fever is one of the body's natural mechanisms for fighting infections. Therefore, elevated temperatures may not be treated unless they reach dangerous levels (greater than 40°C [104°F]) or unless the patient is uncomfortable. Efforts may be made to reduce the temperature by administering acetaminophen or applying a hypothermia blanket. During these therapies, the nurse monitors the patient closely for shivering, which increases oxygen consumption. Efforts to increase comfort are important if the patient experiences fever, chills, or shivering.

The nurse administers prescribed IV fluids and medications, including antibiotic agents and vasoactive medications, to restore vascular volume. Because of decreased perfusion to the kidneys and liver, serum concentrations of antibiotic agents that are normally cleared by these organs may increase and produce toxic effects. Therefore, the nurse monitors blood levels (antibiotic agent, peak and trough levels of antibiotics (if available), BUN, creatinine, white blood cell count, hemoglobin, hematocrit, platelet levels, coagulation studies) and reports changes to the provider. Daily weights and close monitoring of serum prealbumin levels help determine the patient's protein requirements. Additionally, the nurse expects that deep vein thrombosis (DVT) and stress ulcer prophylaxis will be instituted.

NEUROGENIC SHOCK

Pathophysiology

In neurogenic shock, vasodilation occurs as a result of a loss of balance between parasympathetic and sympathetic stimulation. Sympathetic stimulation causes vascular smooth muscle to constrict, and parasympathetic stimulation causes the vascular smooth muscle to relax or dilate. The patient experiences a predominant parasympathetic stimulation that causes vasodilation lasting for an extended period because of acute interruption of sympathetic function. It is important to understand that the blood volume is adequate, but because the vasculature is dilated, the blood volume is displaced, producing a hypotensive (low BP) state (see Box 54-1, p. 1509). Thus, this is a situation where blood volume is stable, but the drastic dilatation of the vasculature causes a relative hypovolemia. The overriding parasympathetic stimulation that occurs with neurogenic shock causes a severe decrease in the patient's SVR and sometimes bradycardia. Inadequate BP results in the insufficient perfusion of tissues and cells that is common to all shock states.

Nursing Alert
The nurse understands that the preganglionic axons of the SNS have origins in the thoracolumbar region of the spinal cord. Thus, patients with spinal cord injuries in the cervical or upper thoracic spinal cord are at risk for neurogenic shock. Without the tonic sympathetic input to the systemic vasculature, the vagal response of bradycardia and decreased SVR are unopposed and culminate in hypotension. Prompt recognition and treatment is essential to avoid potential organ damage.

Neurogenic shock can be caused by spinal cord injury (commonly above the level of T6), spinal anesthesia, or nervous system damage. It may also result from the depressant action of medications or from lack of glucose (e.g., insulin reaction or shock). Neurogenic shock may have a prolonged course (spinal cord injury) or a short one (syncope or fainting). Normally, during states of stress, the sympathetic stimulation causes the BP and heart rate to increase. In neurogenic shock, the sympathetic system is not able to respond to body stressors.

Clinical Manifestations and Assessment

The clinical characteristics of neurogenic shock are signs of parasympathetic stimulation. It is characterized by **dry,** **warm skin** rather than the cool, moist skin seen in hypovolemic shock. Another characteristic is **hypotension** with **bradycardia**, rather than the tachycardia that characterizes other forms of shock.

Medical Management

Treatment of neurogenic shock involves IV fluid or plasma expanders, vasopressors, and restoring sympathetic tone, either through the stabilization of a spinal cord injury or, in the instance of spinal anesthesia, by positioning the patient properly. Specific treatment depends on cause of the shock. Further discussion of management of patients with a spinal cord injury is presented in Chapter 45. If hypoglycemia (insulin shock) is the cause, glucose is rapidly administered. Hypoglycemia and the insulin reaction are described further in Chapter 30. Current guidelines recommend maintaining an MAP of 85 to 90 mm Hg for 1 week post injury to promote spinal cord perfusion (Hickey, 2014, p. 400).

Nursing Management

In suspected spinal cord injury, neurogenic shock may be prevented by carefully immobilizing the patient to prevent further damage to the spinal cord. The nurse is aware that orthostatic hypotension caused by loss of vasomotor tone below the level of the spinal cord lesion can occur with position changes. Even slightly raising the head of the bed for a new tetraplegic patient can result in a drastic hypotension (Hickey, 2014).

Nursing interventions are directed toward supporting cardiovascular and neurologic function until the usually transient episode of neurogenic shock resolves. Apply sequential compression devices since pooled blood increases the risk for thrombus formation. The nurse must check the patient daily for any lower extremity pain, redness, tenderness, unilateral edema, and warmth of the calves. If the patient complains of pain, and objective assessment of the calf is suspicious, the patient should be evaluated for DVT. Administration of heparin or low–molecular-weight heparin (Lovenox) may prevent thrombus formation. Passive range of motion of the immobile extremities also helps promote circulation.

A patient who has experienced a spinal cord injury may not report pain caused by internal injuries. Therefore, in the immediate postinjury period, the nurse must monitor the patient closely for signs of internal bleeding that could lead to hypovolemic shock. In hemorrhagic shock, the nurse is aware that tachycardia will be present versus bradycardia with neurogenic shock.

ANAPHYLACTIC SHOCK

Anaphylactic shock occurs rapidly and is life-threatening. Annual mortality rates of 1,500 to 2,000 deaths in the United States per year are attributed to systemic anaphylaxis (Schwartz, 2016). Medications (e.g., antibiotics, NSAIDs, contrast media, and blood products) are triggers in 55% of cases, while food (26%) and insect bites (19%) are other frequent causes; combined they are the most common causes of anaphylaxis (Brown & Turner, 2017; Ferri, 2016). Approximately 6% of children and 3% to 4% of adults have food allergy (Brown & Turner, 2017).

Because anaphylactic shock occurs in patients already exposed to an antigen and who have developed antibodies to it, it can sometimes be prevented. Patients with known allergies should understand the consequences of subsequent exposure to the antigen and should wear medical identification that lists their sensitivities. This could prevent inadvertent administration of a medication that would lead to anaphylactic shock. In addition, patients and families need instruction about emergency use of medications for treatment of anaphylaxis.

Nursing Alert

Latex allergies are a risk for health care workers and patients who have multiple mucosal exposures to latex. Nurses should use nonlatex gloves when possible, and patients at risk (patients with spina bifida, spinal cord injuries, and congenital abnormalities of the genitourinary tract) should be catheterized when needed with nonlatex equipment.

Pathophysiology

Anaphylactic shock is caused by a severe allergic reaction when patients who have already produced antibodies to a foreign substance (antigen) develop a systemic antigen–antibody reaction. This reaction provokes mast cells and basophils to release potent vasoactive substances, such as histamine or bradykinin, causing widespread vasodilation, capillary permeability, and potentially catastrophic vascular collapse. Mast cells in any organ system may be involved, depending on the distribution of the instigating stimulus; in general the principal targets include the cardiovascular, cutaneous, respiratory, and GI systems (where mast cells are most abundant) (Schwartz, 2016, p. 1698). An equally important feature of anaphylactic shock is the onset of severe bronchospasm, which causes airway compromise (stridor, wheezing, shortness of breath) and urticaria. A delayed recurrence of the reaction, without re-exposure to the allergen, can sometimes occur. This has been termed a *biphasic reaction* and most commonly occurs 8 to 10 hours after the first symptoms; therefore, patients with severe reactions are generally observed for at least 10 hours.

Clinical Manifestations and Assessment

The clinical manifestations are related to the potent vasoactive and smooth muscle contractile actions due to mast cell release of vasoactive substances. For example, the vasodilatation results in erythema, decreased venous return

to the heart, and subsequent hypotension; activation of multiple inflammatory pathways causes fluid extravasation, seen as angioedema, tissue edema, and hypovolemia; whereas the smooth muscle contraction is associated with bronchospasm and abdominal and pelvic cramps. Thus the nurse observes for generalized hives, pruritus or flushing, angioedema, swelling of the tongue and/or uvula, dyspnea, wheezing, stridor, hypoxemia, and reduced blood pressure. GI symptoms, including nausea, vomiting, abdominal cramps, and diarrhea, may precede the more generalized clinical manifestations described previously after ingestion of an antigen (Haupt & Grandhi, 2017, p. 437). Serum mast cell tryptase (MCT) is the only widely available assay used to confirm the diagnosis of anaphylaxis (Brown & Turner, 2017, p. 354).

Medical Management

Treatment of anaphylactic shock requires removing the causative antigen (e.g., discontinuing an antibiotic agent) and administering medications that restore vascular tone. In addition, the health care team will need to provide emergency airway support, position the patient in supine (see Alert below), administer oxygen, provide ventilation support (endotracheal intubation or tracheotomy may be necessary to establish an airway), perform external chest compressions if cardiac arrest occurs, and prepare for early administration of epinephrine. Epinephrine is usually given intramuscularly in the thigh in a dose of 0.01 mg/kg with a usual dose of 0.2 to 0.5 mg for adults (maximum dose of 0.6 mg), which can be repeated every 5 to 30 minutes if the response is inadequate. Epinephrine is given for its vasoconstrictive action as well its effect of reducing bronchospasm (Brown & Turner, 2017). When epinephrine is given early (before the onset of shock), systemic absorption of IM epinephrine is rapid, with a response seen in minutes. IV epinephrine carries more risks, and incorrect dosing has been associated with serious adverse events (Brown & Turner, 2017). However, in patients with severe anaphylaxis, the nurse considers that decreased perfusion to the muscle may result in slow absorption of epinephrine into the circulation; therefore, IV epinephrine may be necessary. Diphenhydramine (Benadryl), given intramuscularly or intravenously, may be administered to reverse the urticaria and pruritus but is not likely to reduce the hypotension of tissue edema (Schwartz, 2016). Nebulized medications, such as albuterol (Proventil), may also be given to reverse histamine-induced bronchospasm. Glucocorticoids may be considered to prevent a rebound, biphasic reaction, although it is unlikely to be beneficial acutely because of the slow onset of action (Ferri, 2016; Schwartz, 2016). IV lines are inserted to provide access for administering fluids and medications. Aggressive IV fluid resuscitation is expected with hypotension. The patient's cardiac status is monitored, and the electrocardiogram is assessed because anaphylaxis and treatments can be associated with arrhythmias and cardiac ischemia. Pulse oximetry is also expected to monitor oxygenation status and response to treatment. Anaphylaxis and specific chemical mediators are discussed further in Chapter 38.

> ## Nursing Alert
> *It is important to note that Fowler's (upright) or semi-Fowler's (semi recumbent) position has been associated with fatal anaphylaxis. Changing the patient's position to one that is upright reduces venous return to the heart and is proposed to exacerbate the pathophysiologic processes occurring in anaphylaxis; therefore, keeping a patient flat is suggested to improve venous return to the heart, a key aspect of the initial response to anaphylaxis (Brown & Turner, 2017).*

> ## Nursing Alert
> *Nurses understand that epinephrine is typically supplied as 1 mg/mL (1:1,000 dilution). Most authorities recommend that 0.3 to 0.5 mg of the 1:1,000 solution (0.3 to 0.5 mL) be given intramuscularly in the anterolateral aspect of the thigh.*

Nursing Management

The nurse plays an important role in preventing anaphylactic shock. The nurse must assess all patients for allergies or previous reactions to antigens (e.g., medications, blood products, foods, contrast agents, latex) and communicate the existence of these allergies or reactions to others. In addition, the nurse assesses the patient's understanding of previous reactions and the steps taken by the patient and family to prevent further exposure to antigens. When new allergies are identified, the nurse advises the patient to wear or carry identification that names the specific allergen or antigen.

When administering any new medication, the nurse observes all patients for allergic reactions. This is especially important with IV medications. Allergy to penicillin is one of the most common causes of anaphylactic shock. Patients who have a penicillin allergy may also develop an allergy to similar medications. For example, they may react to cefazolin sodium (Ancef) because it has a similar antimicrobial action of attaching to the penicillin-binding proteins found on the walls of infectious organisms. Previous adverse drug reactions increase the risk that the patient will develop an undesirable reaction to a new medication. If the patient reports an allergy to a medication, the nurse must be aware of the risks involved in the administration of similar medications.

In the hospital and outpatient diagnostic testing sites, the nurse must identify patients who are at risk for anaphylactic reactions to the contrast agents (radiopaque, dye-like substances that may contain iodine) that are used for diagnostic tests. These include patients with a known allergy to iodine or fish and those who have had previous allergic reactions to contrast agents. This information must be conveyed to the staff at the diagnostic testing site, including radiology staff. The nurse anticipates that "pre-medication" regimens are likely to be administered in patients with known contrast allergies.

> ## Nursing Alert
> *Pre-medication with steroids and Benadryl may be recommended for patients who have had a previous reaction to contrast agent (gadolinium-based contrast or iodinated contrast) and a similar contrast will be administered (ACR, 2016).*

The nurse must be knowledgeable about the clinical signs of anaphylaxis, must take immediate action if signs and symptoms occur, and must be prepared to begin cardiopulmonary resuscitation if cardiopulmonary arrest occurs. In addition to monitoring the patient's response to treatment, the nurse assists with intubation if needed, monitors the hemodynamic status, ensures IV access for administration of medications, administers prescribed medications and fluids, and documents treatments and their effects.

> ## Nursing Alert
> *If IV epinephrine is required, the nurse carefully titrates the medication to prevent a hypertensive surge. Symptoms of tachycardia, pallor, diaphoresis, and arrhythmias in a patient with normal or raised blood pressure are indicative of epinephrine toxicity. The provider should be notified and the infusion rate reduced (Brown & Turner, 2017). Additionally, the nurse observes carefully the effect of epinephrine in patients with cerebrovascular or coronary artery disease, hypertension, diabetes, hyperthyroidism, cardiomyopathy, or narrow-angle glaucoma, in whom adverse events, such as MI, stroke, or pulmonary edema, can be precipitated (Schwartz, 2016, p. 1702).*

Community health and home care nurses who administer medications, including antibiotic agents, in the patient's home or other settings, must be prepared to administer epinephrine subcutaneously or intramuscularly in the event of an anaphylactic reaction. Prescriptions for prefilled epinephrine syringe (EpiPen or EpiPen Jr.) should be given, and the patient and significant others are instructed on how to administer the EpiPen and that the patient needs to carry it on his or her person at all times. After recovery from anaphylaxis, the patient and family require an explanation of the event. Furthermore, the nurse provides instruction and counseling about avoiding future exposure to antigens and administering emergency medications to treat anaphylaxis.

OBSTRUCTIVE SHOCK

Obstructive shock is caused by a physical obstruction to blood flow, either in the heart or major blood vessels. This causes a decrease in CO and thus a decrease in tissue perfusion. Common causes of obstructive shock include cardiac tamponade, tension pneumothorax, and pulmonary embolism (PE). Obstructive shock is common in the setting of trauma.

Pathophysiology

In the case of tension pneumothorax or hemothorax, air or blood has entered the pleural space and caused a restriction in lung expansion. If enough air is trapped, then eventually pressure builds up and compresses the vessels and myocardium. This compression reduces preload (volume of blood) and increases afterload, in addition to restricting the expansion of the myocardium during filling. Clinical presentation may include JVD, crepitus (with pneumothorax), dyspnea, chest pain, tachycardia and tachypnea, tracheal shifting **away** from the tension pneumothorax, and decreased breath sounds on the affected side. Tension pneumothorax is common in trauma but can also develop spontaneously or as a complication from a procedure such as central line placement. Patients who are mechanically ventilated are at higher risk of developing a clinically significant pneumothorax due to increased ventilatory pressures.

Cardiac tamponade results from excessive blood or fluid inside the pericardium, the sac that surrounds the heart. This can result from a traumatic or infectious cause with a resultant restriction on the pumping ability of the heart. Signs and symptoms of cardiac tamponade include narrowing pulse pressure (difference between the systolic and diastolic pressure; normally 40 mm Hg), chest pain, distant or muffled heart sounds, JVD, hypotension, and tachycardia.

A PE is a clot that gets lodged in the pulmonary vasculature and causes ischemia to the capillary beds. If large enough, the embolism interferes significantly with pulmonary blood flow, which causes blood to back up into the right side of the heart. As the clot increases the pressure in the pulmonary artery, the right heart must beat faster and harder to overcome the pressure. Overall, CO is decreased as the patient goes into right-sided heart failure. Clots that have traveled from the lower extremities cause most PEs. Signs and symptoms of PE include pleuritic chest pain, shortness of breath, tachycardia, and hypoxia (refer to Chapter 10 for more details).

Medical Management

In the case of cardiac tamponade and tension pneumothorax, a procedure done by a qualified clinician should be performed immediately to relieve the obstruction. If the patient is experiencing obstructive shock, then these procedures are done emergently at the bedside. A chest radiograph is often used to diagnose a pneumothorax, although computed tomography (CT) scans and even ultrasound are more sensitive. A chest tube or needle decompression is the primary procedure to relieve tension pneumothorax. Cardiac tamponade is diagnosed similarly, with echocardiography being the most effective. Pericardiocentesis is the treatment for cardiac tamponade and involves inserting a needle into the pericardium to draw off fluid or blood.

The treatment of PE is usually aimed toward preventing clot expansion, although if the patient is experiencing obstructive shock, then other treatment, such as thrombolytic drugs or surgical embolectomy, may be considered. Depending on the severity of the PE, mechanical ventilation and hemodynamic support may be needed to stabilize the patient. PE is usually diagnosed using a CT angiogram, but other imaging and laboratory tests can be used as well.

Nursing Management

Because patients with tension pneumothorax and cardiac tamponade who are experiencing obstructive shock will need an emergent procedure, nurses should focus on facilitating that process. This includes collecting and setting up equipment, communicating effectively with staff, and helping gain consent from the patient and/or family. Careful monitoring of the patient prior to, during, and after the procedure is essential. If a chest tube is placed, then a chest drainage system (e.g., Pleuravac) will need to be set up and connected to suction as ordered. The chest tube setup needs to be monitored to ensure that it is functioning correctly and also to record output. A postprocedure chest radiograph will be ordered, and the results should be followed closely.

Nursing care of a patient with a PE that is causing obstructive shock involves monitoring and initiating ventilatory and hemodynamic support similar to what is done for patients with other types of shock. A primary function of the nurse in this situation is to facilitate diagnostic testing and imaging and then institute treatment in a timely manner. Patients with a PE large enough to cause obstructive shock have a very high mortality and often die within an hour of presentation.

Patients who experience obstructive shock are often quite suddenly acutely ill. This affects the entire health care team as decisions need to be made quickly, and the nurse should work hard to maintain a calm environment. Since obstructive shock usually has a sudden onset, families are quite often surprised when given news about massive PE or other causes of obstructive shock. Having other support personnel in place, such as a social worker or a chaplain, to provide support is advised.

MULTIPLE ORGAN DYSFUNCTION SYNDROME

MODS is altered organ function in patients who are acutely ill that requires medical intervention to support continued organ function. It is another phase in the progression of shock states. The actual incidence of MODS is difficult to determine because it develops with acute illnesses that compromise tissue perfusion. It is defined as severe organ dysfunction of two or more organ systems lasting at least 24 to 48 hours in the setting of sepsis, trauma, burns, or severe inflammatory conditions (Tiesi et al., 2016). It is important to note that the definition includes the number of dysfunctional organs and duration. Mortality rates when two organ systems are involved are 40%; and persistent dysfunction (more than 72 hours) present in three organ systems can result in a mortality risk of 80%.

Nursing Alert
Clinicians may use the SOFA scale to rapidly identify adult patients with organ dysfunction and risk for poor outcomes. The

acronym stands for *Sequential (Sepsis-related) Organ Failure Assessment (SOFA)* and includes parameters such as the PaO_2/FiO_2 ratio (respiratory system), the platelet count (coagulation), bilirubin level (hepatic system), MAP (cardiovascular system), Glasgow Coma Scale (CNS system), and creatinine and urine output (renal system). A higher SOFA score is associated with an increased probability of mortality (Singer et al., 2016).

Pathophysiology

The inflammation, tissue injury, and other sequelae associated with MODS are thought to be caused by an unregulated host response. MODS may result from any form of shock because of inadequate tissue perfusion. As previously described, in patients with shock, all organ systems suffer

Diagnosis	Systemic Blood Pressure	Heart Rate	Central Venous Pressure (CVP)	Pulmonary Artery Pressure	Cardiac Output (CO)	Systemic Vascular Resistance (SVR)
Cardiogenic: Myocardial Infarction (MI), Cardiac Tamponade, Pulmonary Emboli	↓	↑	↑	↑	↓	↑
Hypovolemic: Hemorrhage, Diarrhea, Burns, Dehydration	↓	↑	↓	↓	↓	↑
Septic: Severe Infection	↓	↑	↓	↓	↑↓	↓
Anaphylactic: Type 1 Hypersensitivity Reaction	↓	↑	↓	↓	↓	↓
Neurogenic: Brain Damage, Spinal Cord Injury	↓	↓	↓	↓	↓	↓

FIGURE 54-5 Types of shock. Shock results from (1) an inability of the heart to pump adequately (cardiogenic shock); (2) decreased effective blood volume as a consequence of severely reduced blood or plasma volume (hypovolemic shock); or (3) widespread vasodilation (septic; anaphylactic or neurogenic shock). Increased vascular permeability may complicate vasodilation by contributing to reduced effective blood volume. (Adapted from Lawrence, P., Bell, R., Dayton, M., & Hebert, J. (2012). *Essentials of general surgery* (5th ed.). Philadelphia, PA: Lippincott Williams & Wilkins.)

damage from a lack of adequate perfusion, which can result in organ failure.

Clinical Manifestations and Assessment

Various causes of MODS have been identified, including dead or injured tissue, infection, and perfusion deficits. However, it is not possible as yet to predict which patients will develop MODS, partly because much of the organ damage occurs at the cellular level and, therefore, cannot be directly observed or measured. The most common types of organ dysfunction seen with MODS are acute kidney failure and ARDS. However, organ failure can affect the other body systems:

- Hepatic: jaundice, elevated liver function tests (LFTs), decreased albumin and elevated PT
- Hematologic: decreased platelets, elevated PT/APTT, increased D-dimer
- Central nervous system (CNS): altered level of consciousness (LOC), confusion, psychosis
- Respiratory: tachypnea, hypoxemia, PaO_2/FiO_2 greater than 300 (see Chapter 10)
- Cardiovascular: tachycardia, hypotension, altered CVP and pulmonary artery pressure (PAP) readings

Advanced age, malnutrition, and coexisting diseases appear to increase the risk of MODS in patients who are acutely ill.

Medical Management

Prevention remains the top priority in managing MODS. Elderly patients are at increased risk for MODS because of the lack of physiologic reserve associated with aging and the natural degenerative process, especially immune compromise. Early detection and documentation of initial signs of infection are essential in managing MODS in elderly patients. Subtle changes in mentation and a gradual rise in temperature are early warning signs. Other patients at risk for MODS are those with chronic illness, malnutrition, immunosuppression, or surgical or traumatic wounds.

If preventive measures fail, treatment measures to reverse MODS are aimed at (1) controlling the initiating event, (2) promoting adequate organ perfusion, and (3) providing nutritional support.

Nursing Management

The general plan of nursing care for patients with MODS is the same as that for patients in septic shock. Primary nursing interventions are aimed at early and aggressive hemodynamic support until primary organ insults are halted. Providing information and support to family members is a critical role of the nurse. It is important that the health care team address end-of-life decisions to ensure that supportive therapies are congruent with the patient's wishes (see Chapter 3).

Refer to Figure 54-5 for a review of the various forms of shock.

CHAPTER REVIEW

Critical Thinking Exercises

1. You administer an antibiotic to a patient before he goes to surgery. The patient's chart states that he has no known drug allergies. After 15 minutes, the patient complains of anxiety, shortness of breath, and chest discomfort. He is flushed and visibly uncomfortable. What are your nursing priorities in providing care to this patient? What clinical signs and symptoms would you look for to determine if he is experiencing anaphylactic shock? What nursing interventions and medical treatments would you anticipate?

2. An elderly woman is admitted to the medical floor for a urinary tract infection. You notice that she has become steadily more tachycardic and her urine output has dropped to 15 cc for the last hour. How would you assess this patient for the possibility of sepsis?

3. While working in the emergency department, you see a victim of a motor vehicle accident brought in by ambulance. His pelvis appears deformed, he is pale, diaphoretic, and his heart rate is 124. What type of shock is this patient most likely in? What led you to that conclusion? Name some interventions that would help this patient.

4. You are taking care of a patient in the ICU with a spinal cord injury. His BP has not been responsive to repeated fluid boluses. What type of shock is he mostly likely experiencing? Name some appropriate interventions.

NCLEX-Style Review Questions

1. During a conversation about a patient, a new nurse states to the charge nurse, "His BP is 92/50, so he can't be in shock." Which response by the charge nurse indicates that the new nurse does not completely understand the symptoms of shock?
   a. Patients can have a near-normal BP, yet still have inadequate tissue perfusion.
   b. The cutoff for shock is a systolic pressure of 100 mm Hg.

c. Shock is determined by mean arterial pressure.

d. Shock is determined by a heart rate of over 100.

2. A patient with a GI bleed arrives at the emergency department with the following vital signs: Temperature 37.4°C, HR 112, RR 26, BP 88/44. The nurse recognizes that this patient is most likely experiencing or at risk for which type of shock?

a. Anaphylactic

b. Neurogenic

c. Hypovolemic

d. Septic

3. A patient comes in to the urgent care center complaining of shortness of breath and dizziness after being stung by a bee. The patient loses consciousness in the waiting room. The receptionist has called 911. The nurse anticipates that which medication will be considered first?

a. Diphenhydramine (Benadryl)

b. Phenytoin (Dilantin)

c. Epinephrine IV

d. Epinephrine IM

4. In early goal-directed therapy for shock, the nurse knows that which parameter is the highest priority when evaluating effectiveness of therapy?

a. Heart rate and BP

b. SvO_2 and O_2 saturation

c. Base deficit and hematocrit

d. SvO_2 and CVP

5. A patient develops low BP and tachycardia and is very agitated. The nurse remembers that a central line was placed 3 hours ago. The patient's lung sounds are decreased on one side, and tracheal deviation is present. The nurse realizes that this patient is most likely experiencing which type of shock?

a. Hypovolemic

b. Obstructive

c. Anaphylactic

d. Neurogenic

REFERENCES AND SELECTED READINGS

References and selected readings associated with this chapter can be found on the website that accompanies the book. Visit **http://thepoint.lww.com/Honan2e** to access the references and other additional resources associated with this chapter.

Nursing Management: Critical Care

Kelly S. Grimshaw

Learning Objectives

After reading this chapter, you will be able to:
1. Describe the role of the critical care nurse in health care.
2. Describe nursing management of common problems in the critical care environment.
3. Understand common interventions and equipment used in the critical care environment.

The nurse's priority in caring for patients who are critically ill is to prevent harm and provide physical care, education, and emotional support to patients and families in an effort to return them to the highest possible state of health or to help them toward a peaceful death. Nurses are in the unique position of standing with the patient and family at the center of multisectoral activity. They are at the bedside to act as a care provider and liaison to other health care workers in an effort to coordinate said care. This chapter covers the role of the nurse in critical care and critical care responsibilities and modalities.

THE CRITICAL CARE ENVIRONMENT

Historical tradition dictates the critical care environment to be a separate place or unit within a hospital building. After the Institute of Medicine (IOM) challenge to hospitals to prevent avoidable deaths, over 65% of hospitals in the United States (National Academies of Sciences, Engineering, and Medicine, 2015) have implemented rapid response teams (RRTs). These RRTs usually consist of a doctor, an advanced practice registered nurse (APRN) or physician assistant (PA), a respiratory therapist, and a critical care nurse. These teams were established in hospitals to address the concerns of those patients outside of the intensive care unit (ICU) who were seen as requiring a higher level of care. The RRTs currently in place are able to provide the required higher level of care even when the patient is physically outside of the ICU and awaiting a bed inside the unit, thus making critical care a process and not a place.

NEUROLOGIC ISSUES

A neurologically healthy person is one who is awake, alert, and oriented, with the ability to respond appropriately to his or her environment without sensory or physical limitations.

Whether or not a person is admitted with a specific neurologic or neurosurgical diagnosis, other medical problems or interventions may impact his or her neurologic status.

Altered Level of Consciousness

The causes of altered mental states are numerous and varied but can be remembered using the mnemonic in Table 55-1. Most ICU patients are at risk for mental status changes due to a myriad of potential factors: previously existing mental illness, increased age, severity of illness and comorbidities, sleep deprivation, and/or medications. Assessing changes in level of consciousness (LOC) alerts the nurse to neurologic impairment. A thorough review of possible causes and early intervention can impact a patient's long-term recovery. Refer to Chapter 43 for performing mental status assessment.

Delirium

Delirium is a confused state that has a sudden onset and can last hours to days or weeks; it is characterized by hyperactivity and has the potential to be reversible. For example, the patient who quickly becomes confused and agitated while attempting to pull out IV lines and get out of bed is experiencing delirium. These patients require extensive nursing time and often need someone to be present in the room with them at all times to prevent injury. The consequences of delirium cannot be underestimated. Though probably underdiagnosed, it has been found that delirium leads to a myriad of sequelae including: increased medicinal and restraint interventions, increased length of stay, persistent cognitive impairment with admission to chronic care facilities, and increased mortality (Sangeeta et al., 2015).

Pain and Anxiety

Pain and anxiety are interrelated and should be assessed together. For example, chest pain often produces great anxiety.

TABLE **55-1** Causes of Altered Mental Status

	Cause	Example	Possible Nursing Interventions
A	Alcohol	Intoxication Withdrawal	Institute fall precautions Institute seizure precautions Institute ICU sedation protocol; Clinical Institute Withdrawal Assessment-Alcohol (CIWA-A) scale
E	Epilepsy Endocrine Electrolytes	New onset or low medication level Hypothyroidism Hyper or hyponatremia	Check medication level Check thyroid level IV fluids and serial sodium levels as ordered
I	Insulin	Hypoglycemia	Check glucose level Administer dextrose as ordered
O	Opiates and other drugs	Narcotic overdose	Administer reversal agent as ordered Airway protection with elevated head of bed
U	Uremia	Acute or chronic kidney failure	Follow trends of blood urea nitrogen and creatinine levels Ensure patency of dialysis access shunts and IV lines
T	Trauma Temperature	Hypothermia	Serial temperature measurements Blanket warmer Administer warm IV fluids as ordered
I	Infection	Sepsis	Obtain blood and body fluids for culture as ordered Administer antibiotics as ordered Ensure IV lines and Foley catheters have been changed according to hospital policy
P	Poison	Confusion, seizures, coma	Supportive care until poison is neutralized or removed
S	Shock Stroke Space occupying lesion Subarachnoid hemorrhage	Hypovolemia Thrombolic or hemorrhagic Tumor Trauma or unmonitored anticoagulation use	IV fluids and cardiac pressors to support cerebral blood flow Call for stroke alert if found with acute symptoms Monitor for signs of increased intracranial pressure (ICP) Ensure functioning of ICP monitor or ventricular shunts

Emergency Medicine/Altered Mental Status. (2014). Retrieved on May 13, 2015 from http://en.wikibooks.org/

Pain

Critical care patients can experience pain as a result of their injury or disease as well as its treatment. It is well known that pain elicits a stress response, leading to a catabolic state with increased cardiac workload and an impaired immune response. Care must be taken to ensure that all ICU patients are assessed for any pain, whether or not they are able to communicate their pain level. Prevention and treatment of pain should include both pharmacologic and nonpharmacologic methods in collaboration with the patient (if able) and the medical team. Refer to Chapter 7 for details on pain assessment and management.

Anxiety

Anxiety has been defined as a universal experience with physical side effects and a subjective sense of danger or dread (Silver, Shapiro, & Milrod, 2013). Each hospital also provides scales for objectifying signs and symptoms of anxiety, such as the Richmond Agitation and Sedation Scale (RASS), in order to standardize treatment and minimize its effects (see Fig. 55-1).

Table 55-2 summarizes assessment of anxiety. An ICU stay has inherent stressors of pain, lack of control over one's environment, impaired communication, and possible fears of imminent death, issues that are all causes for severe anxiety. It is estimated that up to 22% of patients admitted to an ICU suffer from posttraumatic stress disorder (PTSD) as a result of their admission, and its prevention is of paramount importance when considering recovery and post discharge quality of life (Rock, 2014).

Dependency and Withdrawal

Use and abuse of illegal and legal drugs is pervasive in the United States, with an estimated incidence of 9.2% of the general population (SAMHSA, 2014) reporting use and abuse.

+4	Combative, violent, of immediate danger to himself and staff
+3	Very agitated, aggressive, pulls or removes tubes or catheters
+2	Agitated frequent nonpurposeful movement, dyssynchronous with the ventilator
+1	Restless, anxious but not aggressive
0	Alert and calm
−1	Drowsy, not fully alert, but has sustained eye-opening/eye contact to *voice* (>10 s)
−2	Light sedation-briefly awakens with eye contact to *voice* (<10 s)
−3	Moderate sedation—moves or opens eyes to *voice* (**but no eye contact**)
−4	Deep sedation. No response to voice. Movement or eye opening to *physical* stimulation
−5	Unarousable. No response to *voice or physical* stimulation

FIGURE 55-1 The Richmond Agitation and Sedation Scale (RASS). (Reprinted with permission from Bigatello, L. M., Alam, H., Allain, R. M., Bittner, E. A., Hess, D., Pino, R. M., & Schmidt, U. (Eds.), *Critical care handbook of the Massachusetts General Hospital*. Philadelphia, PA: Lippincott Williams & Wilkins.)

It is important to realize that people of all ages and from all walks of life may have a chemical dependence issue and that admission to the ICU will not "cure" this problem. It will more likely be that these patients require more pain and sedation medication to achieve desired effects, such as prevention of withdrawal and its sequelae.

Depression

Medical literature is filled with articles and studies demonstrating depression or depressed mood as a component of chronic and critical illness. It is also well known that many of the medications prescribed in the ICU, such as beta blockers, can cause depression. Patients admitted on antidepressive agents should continue them with the shortest interruption possible. Patients exhibiting signs of prolonged or exaggerated mood should be evaluated by a psychiatry provider for adequate diagnosis and treatment in order to facilitate the healing process.

Suicidal ideation, and actions taken with the intent to kill oneself, is another issue requiring assessment in the hospital setting. Suicide ranks as the 10th most common cause of death in the United States and a frequently reported sentinel event in health care institutions (CDC, 2014). The Joint Commission (2015) requires facilities to assess patients for suicidal ideation on admission and throughout their stay as

it poses such a great risk in these institutions. Admission to the ICU during a hospital stay does not diminish the need to assess patients for any suicidal thoughts or actions.

Sensory and Motor Function

Impairment of sensory and motor function (ability to feel and physically react to one's environment) can arise from various sources, including spinal cord injury, peripheral vascular disease, and/or medical restraint devices. Alterations in sensation and motion can be viewed on a negative to positive continuum, ranging from insensate to numbness, normal, tingling, and then pain.

Communication

Communication allows patients and families to interact with health care system professionals in order to satisfy physical, emotional, and spiritual needs. The ICU environment and neurologic status deficits can make communication difficult. It is imperative that critical care nurses work to improve communication in order to satisfy the previously mentioned needs of their patients and families. Suggested methods may include:

- Asking yes or no questions to which the patient may nod his or her head
- Using an electronic tablet for texting

TABLE 55-2 Anxiety Assessment

Assessment	Possible Nursing Interventions
Does my patient have anxiety? If so, at what level?	Presume that all ICU patients are at risk for anxiety! Use appropriate scale to assess level of anxiety, such as the Richmond Agitation and Sedation Scale.
Why is the patient experiencing anxiety?	Provide any information for which the lack of information is the cause of anxiety.
What is the most appropriate medication?	Administer antianxiety medications if ordered.
What is the most appropriate method of delivery?	Assess the patient's ability to tolerate oral medication.
What nonpharmacologic methods of reducing anxiety are available?	Allow for visitation and distraction. Allow pet therapy if available and acceptable to patient.
Is our plan for anxiety relief working?	Reevaluate the patient regularly.
Does my patient have anxiety, and is unable to communicate this?	Observe nonverbal behavior including facial expressions, body language, gaze aversion; advocate for patients.

- Using a board with preprinted phrases to which he or she can point
- Using language and sign language interpreters (from within the hospital or interpreter services)
- Making a paper and pencil available

CARDIOVASCULAR ISSUES

Cardiovascular problems can be broadly categorized as those arising from the heart and vascular system and those affecting the heart and arterial and venous systems (Table 55-3). Patients may be admitted to critical care units for a number of concerns related to the cardiovascular system, including:

- a history of cardiovascular disease requiring careful observation, although not admitted specifically for cardiovascular disease, an active cardiac problem requiring advanced intervention, or
- another active medical problem affecting their cardiovascular status, such as hemorrhage or sepsis.

Monitoring the Patient

Depending upon the individual patient's condition, different levels of monitoring and intervention will be required.

TABLE 55-3 Sources of Cardiac Disease

Sources of Disease	Example
Cardiac	
Myocardial	Left ventricular hypertrophy, congestive heart failure
Ischemic	Coronary artery disease, myocardial infarction
Conductive	Atrial fibrillation, heart blocks
Valvular	Mitral regurgitation, aortic stenosis
Other	
Infection	Pericarditis, sepsis, viral cardiomyopathy
Neurologic system	Spinal shock
Peripheral vascular system	Hypertension, deep vein thrombosis, pulmonary embolism
Respiratory system	Pulmonary hypertension
Renal system	Kidney failure leading to fluid overload
Trauma	Cardiac contusion, cardiac tamponade
Hemorrhage	Circulatory collapse

TABLE 55-4 Monitoring the Cardiac Patient

Conditions and Circumstances	Related Monitoring and Interventions
Patients who are expected to do well, but need additional monitoring in case unexpected complications, such as bleeding, or arrhythmias arise	Vital sign assessment Oxygen saturation Cardiac monitor Peripheral IV access in case of emergency
Patients about to leave the critical care environment and who are awake, hemodynamically stable, and able to eat and drink	All of the above
Patients admitted with singular issues, such as an elective surgery or uncomplicated medical diagnoses, who are expected to recover, but have a cardiac history (such patients may need IV fluids and medications for a limited time period).	All of the above + IV fluids, IV medications, or minimal blood products
Patients who have a medical or surgical issue, in which recovery depends on the medical team's provision of more precise monitoring (such as heart failure)	All of the above + Central venous access and/or arterial line access
Patients who are at risk for complications, or for whom basic monitoring and fluids have failed; patients requiring cardiac pressor support (these patients are often compromised due to sepsis).	All of the above + Vasoactive medications and/or further blood products
Patients who have an unclear cardiac status, have not responded well to lesser interventions, or have undergone cardiac surgery	All of the above + Pulmonary artery catheterization
Cardiac failure due to any cause	All of the above + Counterpulsation via intra-aortic balloon pump
Complete cardiac failure	All of the above + Ventricular assist device

Table 55-4 provides a summary of the different levels of monitoring.

It is important to remember that monitors, invasive lines, and other devices are to assist in confirming or disproving physical examination results and clinical judgments, not replace them.

TABLE **55-5** Effects of Preload and Afterload on the Heart

Factor	Possible Cause	Effects on Heart
Increased preload	Increased fluid volume Vasoconstriction	Increases stroke volume Increases ventricular work Increases myocardial oxygen requirements
Decreased preload	Hypovolemia Vasodilation	Decreases stroke volume Decreases ventricular work Decreases myocardial oxygen requirements
Increased afterload	Hypovolemia Vasoconstriction	Decreases stroke volume Increases ventricular work Increases myocardial oxygen requirements
Decreased afterload	Vasodilation	Increases stroke volume Decreases ventricular work Decreases myocardial oxygen requirements

From Lippincott Williams & Wilkins. (2010). Understanding the cardiac system. In *Hemodynamic monitoring made incredibly visual* (2nd ed., p. 15). Philadelphia, PA: Lippincott Williams & Wilkins.

Intravenous Access in the Cardiac Patient

Peripheral Intravenous Access

At a minimum, peripheral intravenous (IV) access should be obtained on all patients in the critical care environment. Peripheral IVs give the health care team access the vascular system in case of emergency; a potential site for blood sampling; and the ability to provide fluids, medications, and nutrition. Contraindications to specific placements (right vs. left side) will include history of mastectomy, arterial-venous shunt placement, peripherally inserted central catheter (PICC) line placement, thrombus, trauma, and other device placements, such as splints and casts. IV lines in the feet are reserved only for emergencies; they are to be removed as soon as possible and never inserted in the feet of patients with diabetes. Potential complications include bruising, infection, extravasation of fluids and medications, and air embolus.

An arterial line is a peripheral IV in the arterial system used for frequent blood pressure monitoring when a patient requires vasoactive medications (such as nitroprusside) and frequent blood sampling. It is not for administration of fluids or medications. Potential complications include ischemia, thrombosis, infiltration, and exsanguination.

Central Intravenous Lines

Central IV lines (Fig. 55-2) are used for a number of reasons, including:

- Failure to obtain or maintain peripheral access
- Complication of peripheral access
- The patient requires numerous access sites, parenteral nutrition, or hypertonic fluid administration
- Treatment failure with IV fluids necessitates the first level of hemodynamic monitoring for readings of central venous pressure (CVP)
- The patient requires vasoactive medications that place his or her limb at risk if an infiltrate occurs

The triple-lumen catheter is a central line that measures the CVP or the amount of fluid returning to the heart at the level of the right atrium (termed *preload*, see Table 55-5). See Chapter 12 for more information on CVP monitoring.

Pulmonary Artery Catheter

Pulmonary artery catheter (PACs) are used when previous interventions have not yielded the expected outcome (increased urine output with increased IV fluid administration), or when the patient has a complicating factor, such as kidney or heart failure or pulmonary hypertension, that makes clinical judgments difficult without additional information. After decades of its use in practice, there is still no consensus as to whether PACs improve patient outcomes. Without that evidence and because they increase the risk of complications, such as pneumothorax, cardiac arrhythmias, and pulmonary artery rupture, the use of PACs is decreasing. However, they still can be a helpful tool in assisting in the overall evaluation of a patient.

PACs allow the medical and nursing team to monitor, intervene upon, and evaluate:

- Blood volume status
- Blood flow
- Tissue oxygenation

Figure 55-3 illustrates components of the PAC system.

Blood Volume Status

Blood volume status is the amount of blood circulating in the enclosure of the arterial and venous systems. This fluid exerts or creates a pressure that can be monitored to determine preload: The greater the blood volume, the greater the pressure (assuming no confounding variables, such as severe hypertension). Using Starling's Law the volume can be increased to give the heart a greater stretch or potential energy with which to pump blood to the body without

Catheter

Insertion
■ Subclavian vein

Termination
■ Superior vena cava

A

Catheter

Insertion
■ Subclavian vein

Termination
■ Right atrium

B

Catheter

Insertion
■ Internal jugular vein

Termination
■ Superior vena cava

Subclavian vein

C

Catheter

Termination
■ Superior vena cava

Insertion
■ Basilic vein (peripheral)

D

Termination
■ Superior vena cava

Insertion
■ Through a subcutaneous tunnel to the subclavian vein (Antimicrobial cuff helps hold catheter in place)

Subclavian vein

Antimicrobial cuff

Catheter

E

FIGURE 55-2 Central vein catheter pathways showing various insertion and termination sites. Typically, a central vein catheter is inserted in the subclavian or internal jugular vein. (**A**) Subclavian insertion ending in Superior Vena Cava (SVC); (**B**) Subclavian insertion ending in the right atrium; (**C**) Jugular insertion ending in the SVC; (**D**) Peripherally inserted central catheter (PICC) ending in the SVE; (**E**) Hickman Catheter ending in the SVC. (From Lippincott Williams & Wilkins. (2010). *Hemodynamic monitoring made incredibly visual* (2nd ed.). Philadelphia, PA: Lippincott Williams & Wilkins.)

FIGURE 55-3 Components of the pulmonary artery catheter (PAC) monitoring system. (From Lippincott Williams & Wilkins. (2010). *Hemodynamic monitoring made incredibly visual* (2nd ed.). Philadelphia, PA: Lippincott Williams & Wilkins.)

causing overstretch and failure. It can be compared to a sling shot pulled back ever farther to throw a stone farther without stretching the sling to the point of breaking.

A PAC measures and calculates the pressures described in Table 55-6.

It is important to remember that the blood volume measurements describe the total amount of pressure exerted in the vasculature by a particular volume of fluid. They do not describe the components of the blood, such as percentage of red blood cells (RBCs; hematocrit) or plasma. Specific laboratory values, such as the complete blood count (CBC), determine these percentages. The goals of treatment involve restoring and maintaining an adequate blood volume with the right proportions of blood components that best support organ perfusion.

Blood Flow

The right side of the heart pumps blood to the pulmonary system, and the left side pumps blood to itself via the coronary arteries and the rest of the body via the aorta. The PAC

measures how the heart is pumping and how the vasculature is receiving or resisting the flow. Table 55-7 describes PAC blood flow measurements.

It is important to remember that the numbers in the table are general values and that the 98-lb elderly patient will have different requirements than the 200-lb professional defensive lineman. In order to account for differences in body size, index measurements are used (Table 55-8).

Tissue Oxygenation

The ability of tissues to receive and use oxygen depends upon many variables, from physiologic disorders and medical procedures to prescribed medications and their interactions. The health care team is responsible for manipulating these variables to maximize delivery and usage. In general, the following indicate how the patient is doing:

- Arterial pH and partial pressure
- Venous pH and partial pressure
- End organ function, such as urine production

TABLE **55-6** Pulmonary Artery Catheter Pressure Measurements

Measurement	Definition	Formula (If Applicable)	Normal Value (mm Hg)
Mean arterial pressure (MAP)	Average arterial pressure throughout the cardiac cycle	Systolic BP + 2(diastolic BP)/3	70–105
Right atrial pressure (RAP)	Pressure at the level of the right atrium		2–8
Pulmonary artery systolic pressure (PAS)	Pressure in pulmonary artery during systole		20–30
Pulmonary artery diastolic pressure (PAD)	Pressure in the pulmonary artery during diastole		8–15
Mean pulmonary artery pressure (MPAP)	Average pressure in the pulmonary artery throughout the cardiac cycle	PAS + 2(PAD)/3	10–15
Pulmonary artery wedge pressure	The indirect measurement of pressure in the left ventricle at the end of diastole		6–12

TABLE **55-7** Pulmonary Artery Catheter Blood Flow Measurements

Measurement	Definition	Formula (If Applicable)	Normal Value
Heart rate (HR)	The number of beats per minute		60–100 bpm
Stroke volume (SV)	The amount of blood ejected from the left ventricle with each beat	End-diastolic volume – end systolic volume	Patient dependent
Cardiac output	The amount of blood pumped to the body each minute	HR × SV	4–8 L/min
Pulmonary vascular resistance (PVR)		PAM – PAWP/CO × 80	50–150 dynes/sec/cm^{-5}
Systemic vascular resistance (SVR)		MAP – RAP/CO × 80	900–1,200 dynes/sec/cm^{-5}

TABLE **55-8** Pulmonary Artery Catheter Indices

Measurement	Definition	Formula	Normal Value
Stroke volume index	As above accounting for body surface area (BSA)		30–60 mL/beat/m^2
Cardiac index	As above accounting for BSA	CI/BSA	2.4–5 L/min/m^2
Pulmonary vascular resistance index (PVRI)	As above accounting for BSA	PAM – PAWP/CI × 80	200–350 dynes/sec/cm^{-5}
Systemic vascular resistance index (SVRI)	As above accounting for BSA	MAP – RAP/CI × 80	1,800–2,800 dynes/sec/cm^{-5}

- Lactic acid level
- Mixed venous oxygen saturation (MvO_2)

> ### Nursing Alert
> *The lactic acid level represents the end product of anaerobic metabolism used by the body during times of insufficient oxygen supply. Lactic acidosis is generally considered to be present if the plasma lactate concentration is greater than 4 to 5 mEq/L. However, the nurse may see a rise in the lactic acid level as oxygen supplied via blood flow is initially restored. Consider a patient with a vascular blockage to his or her leg during which the leg is not receiving enough oxygen and the extremity is cold and pale without pulses. Lactic acid is building up in the leg, but this lactic acid is not measured because blood flow is blocked. Once vascular flow is restored, marked with a return of warmth and peripheral pulses, there will be an initial rise in lactic acid as the body releases it into the now flowing bloodstream. Thus, the nurse must consider the serum lactic level in conjunction with the patient's clinical situation.*

> ### Nursing Alert
> *As bodies neither make nor store oxygen, humans have evolved and adapted with a safety mechanism to ensure oxygen delivery occurs in times of decreased supply and/or increased demand. The body only uses a portion of the oxygen delivered to the bloodstream during one circuit from the heart and lungs to the rest of the body and back. Consider a person experiencing cardiopulmonary arrest, when 4 to 6 minutes may pass without a heartbeat before brain damage occurs. This is because there is still oxygen in the blood from his last inspiration. The normal value for MvO_2 is 75%. Thus, the body used only 25% of delivered oxygen during the last lap through the body. A decrease in MvO_2 below 75% means the body is not receiving enough oxygen and/or has an increased demand for oxygen.*

The various IV and intra-arterial lines discussed in the previous section are used to monitor cardiac function; they do not change it. To improve a patient's cardiac status, practitioners remove the root cause of the problem and provide support via the use of IV fluids, blood products, vasoactive medications, and medical devices.

Intravenous Fluids and Blood Products

IV fluids are given to obtain and help maintain a euvolemic and isotonic state within the body. The type and amount of fluid will be dependent upon each individual's medical situation. These crystalloid solutions in various concentrations and combinations contain electrolytes and sometimes sugars:

- Saline
- Lactated Ringer's
- 5% dextrose in water

IV solutions with larger molecules designed to expand IV volume with increased oncotic pressures include:

- Albumin
- Hespan™ or Hetastarch™

Blood products can help with hydration and volume expansion, as well as provide additional or replacement oxygen-carrying capacity, clotting factors, and platelets:

- Packed red blood cells (pRBC)
- Fresh-frozen plasma (FFP)
- Pooled platelets
- Cryoprecipitate

McEvoy and Shander (2013) report that up to one third of people admitted to the ICU receive at least one blood product transfusion. Unfortunately, no evidence-based guideline exists to help practitioners determine when the benefits of transfusion outweigh the risks of human error, impaired immune function, and infection that often accompany transfusion.

Vasoactive Medications

Many medications are used to help support cardiovascular function. Vasoactive medications given in the ICU are designed to alter preload, afterload, contractility, and cardiac rhythm, as required by the patient's underlying disease and physiologic condition. These are potent drugs with a myriad of potential adverse effects necessitating close titration and monitoring in an ICU setting. Table 55-9 summarizes those IV medications most commonly used in the ICU.

Medical Devices

Patients in the ICU may require medical devices to assist with cardiac function.

Pacemakers

Pacemakers are medical devices generally used to treat cardiac disease caused by conduction problems. They can be placed temporarily or permanently in order to improve cardiac function with or without adjunct medications. Permanent pacemakers are discussed in Chapter 17.

Temporary pacemakers are used during cardiac surgery and medical emergencies. They can be placed in a variety of ways:

- *External pacemakers:* Involves placement of electrodes on the front and side or back of the chest to deliver repeated shocks

TABLE **55-9** Vasoactive Medications

Medication	Action or Effect	Indications	Dosing Range
Amiodarone	Decreased heart rate	Ventricular Tachycardia Atrial fibrillation	Arrhythmia dependent
Diltiazem	Decreased heart rate and blood pressure	Atrial fibrillation Paroxysmal Supraventricular Tachycardia Hypertension	5–15 mg/hr
Dobutamine	Increased heart contractility Increased blood pressure	Congestive heart failure Low cardiac output	2.5–20 µg/kg/min
Dopamine	Increased heart rate and blood pressure	Bradycardia Hypotension	2–20 µg/kg/min
Epinephrine	Increased heart rate and blood pressure	Anaphylaxis Shock	1–10 µg/min
Esmolol	Decreased heart rate	Tachycardia Hypertension	500 µg/kg load 50–200 µg/kg/min
Nitroglycerin	Decreased blood pressure Arterial vasodilatation	Myocardial ischemia Congestive heart failure Hypertension	10–20 µg/min
Nitroprusside	Decreased blood pressure	Congestive heart failure Hypertensive crisis	3 µg/kg/min—effect
Norepinephrine	Increased blood pressure	Cardiac arrest Hypotension	1–20 µg/min
Phenylephrine	Increased blood pressure	Hypotension	40–200 µg/min
Vasopressin	Increased blood pressure	Diabetes insipidus Gastrointestinal bleed Septic shock	0.02–0.04 units/min

- *Transvenous pacemakers:* Involves placement of a wire into the right ventricle via a central IV catheter
- *Epicardial pacemaker:* Involves surgical placement of wires into the epicardium to prevent and treat postsurgical conduction defects
- *Transthoracic cardiac pacemakers:* Involves introduction of a wire into the right ventricle, which is attached to a generator

Whether temporary or permanent, pacemakers necessitate that care for a patient with a pacemaker includes monitoring of the pacemaker's function and the patient's physical response to the pacing. This will include pain management and sedation for those with external pacers, infection control for newly inserted pacers, and physical assessment of cardiac, pulmonary, renal, and peripheral vascular function. See Chapter 17 for more detailed discussion.

Intra-Aortic Balloon Pump

Patients with temporary or permanent heart muscle damage are unable to adequately perfuse their own heart and other organs. First attempts to improve cardiac muscle function include fluids and medications, but, at times, patients will require additional support in the form of an intra-aortic balloon pump (IABP). A balloon in placed in the descending aorta via a femoral artery. The balloon can be alternately inflated and deflated (Fig. 55-4). It is programmed to inflate during diastole, which pushes blood back toward the cardiac muscle itself, as well as toward the brain. It deflates just before the ejection phase of systole and acts as a vacuum that pulls blood into the aorta with less effort from the left ventricle. An IABP essentially decreases the workload of the heart, allowing the heart muscle to rest and recover while improving organ perfusion. The machine itself can be programmed to assist with every heartbeat or every second, third, or fourth alternate beat, depending upon patient requirements. Care for patients on an IABP includes monitoring cardiac function with the use of a PAC and assessing peripheral circulation to the extremity below its insertion site.

Ventricular Assist Device

A ventricular assist device (VAD) is an implantable device in which cannulas are inserted into the atria or ventricles to

A **B**

FIGURE 55-4 Direction of blood flow when the pump inflates and deflates the balloon. **A.** Balloon inflation: The balloon inflates as the aortic valve closes and diastole begins. Diastole increases perfusion to the coronary arteries. **B.** Balloon deflation: The balloon deflates before ventricular ejection, when the aortic valve opens. This deflation permits ejection of blood from the left ventricle against a lowered resistance. As a result, aortic end-diastolic pressure and afterload decrease and cardiac output rises. (From Lippincott Williams & Wilkins. (2010). *Hemodynamic monitoring made incredibly visual* (2nd ed.). Philadelphia, PA: Lippincott Williams & Wilkins.)

support the right side of the heart, left side of the heart, or both sides by taking over the work of delivering blood to the pulmonary artery and/or aorta (see Fig. 55-5). There are three types of VADs. A right VAD (right ventricular assist device [RVAD]) provides pulmonary support by diverting blood from the right atrium or failing right ventricle to the VAD, which pumps the blood into the pulmonary circulation via the VAD connection to the left pulmonary artery.

With a left VAD (left ventricular assist device [LVAD]), blood flows from the left atrium or ventricle to the VAD, which then pumps blood back to the body via the VAD

connection to the aorta. A RVAD and LVAD combination is referred to as *biventricular* (BiVAD) *support.*

VADs are reserved for patients who cannot be weaned from maximum volume/inotropic support or the IABP, are awaiting cardiac transplantation, or have class IV heart failure but are not candidates for transplantation. This intervention is the last-line treatment for cardiac failure and requires high-intensity nursing care to monitor cardiac function and the myriad of potential adverse effects, which range from infection, bleeding, and neurologic deficits to kidney and device failure. While usually deemed to be a temporary

FIGURE 55-5 Cannulation options. Ventricular assist devices (VADs) divert blood from failing ventricles to a pump that can effectively eject it. This diversion can occur by cannulation of either the atria or the ventricles. LVAD, left VAD; RVAD, right VAD; BiVAD, biventricular support. (From Lippincott Williams & Wilkins. (2010). *Hemodynamic monitoring made incredibly visual* (2nd ed.). Philadelphia, PA: Lippincott Williams & Wilkins.)

measure, VADs are gaining prominence due patients with refractory heart failure who cannot be transplanted who are creating a cohort of patients requiring long-term assistance without definitive cure. Thus VAD support is the destination therapy. These patients are living in communities and should be known to emergency services in case of power outages (refer to Chapter 16 for further details).

RESPIRATORY ISSUES

Respiratory Failure

Respiratory failure and the advent of mechanical ventilation led to the creation of critical care as a specialty service. As times change, so does technology. The use of noninvasive ventilator support (NIV) for respiratory complications is now a first line of treatment for an ever increasing number of patient populations and care settings (Mas & Masip, 2014). The number of patients needing ventilatory support is expected to grow over the next decades. Respiratory failure can generally be divided into two main categories (see Box 55-1).

Oxygen Delivery

In the critical care environment, oxygen is treated as a drug, requiring a providers' order and nursing assessment of the patient's response to this prescription. The need for oxygen therapy and its specific method of delivery varies according to patient condition. Some patients will receive O_2 therapy as a preventative measure. Supplemental oxygen will assist some patients with extra oxygen delivery during acute episodes, such as in cases of myocardial infarction (MI). For the more critically ill, it will serve as an intervention to ensure oxygen delivery when they are unable to maintain their own ventilatory or respiratory function. Oxygen is the most commonly prescribed gas in the critical care environment.

See Chapter 10 for detailed information on oxygen delivery systems and nursing responsibilities.

> ***Nursing Alert***
> *The nurse considers oxygen a drug, which has benefits and risks. The risks associated with oxygen increase as the FiO_2 increases. Healthy lungs may be able to tolerate FiO_2 levels of less than 60%; however, when lungs are damaged, FiO_2 that exceeds 50% may result in a toxic alveolar O_2 concentration (Tokarczyk, Greenberg, & Vender, 2013). Excessive O_2 concentrations have been associated with acute respiratory distress syndrome (ARDS), injury to the lung parenchyma, retinopathy (premature neonates), and resorptive atelectasis (see Chapter 10) (Reardon, Mason, & Clinton, 2014). Although the benefits of oxygen therapy typically outweigh the risks, the nurse is mindful that every intervention employed has to be evaluated for the risk/benefit balance.*

Positive Airway Pressure

As explained by Hess (2013) positive airway pressure machines, whether intermittent or continuous (CPAP), have been used for many years as a method of oxygen delivery in patients requiring assistance with keeping the upper airway open or improving intrathoracic pressure and lung volumes without invasive intubation of the trachea. When initiated for the first time, positive airway pressure is usually started in a highly monitored setting in order to assess for claustrophobia and nausea and vomiting (risk for gastric distention increases with positive pressures above 25 cm H_2O). This therapy requires patient cooperation and spontaneous ventilation, and the patient must also be able to tolerate some periods off the mask in order to eat and drink or perform mouth care and skin assessments. CPAP is most effective when there is a resilient seal around the airway to minimize air leak, but that poses a risk for skin irritation. The nurse assesses pressure areas and provides skin care as needed.

Noninvasive Ventilation

Noninvasive ventilation (NIV) appears similar to the methods of oxygen delivery discussed previously, but it is, in fact, not the same. NIV provides a greater pressure on the inspiratory phase than on expiration, unloading the work of the respiratory muscles and providing complete respiratory support (Hess, 2013).

Intubation and Mechanical Ventilation

Many patients in the ICU will require intubation and mechanical ventilation during their admission. It is hoped that this will be required for only a short time period to assist in supporting the patient's recovery from illness or injury. However, this advanced technology has moved from the

BOX 55-1	**Causes of Respiratory Failure**

Hypoxemic respiratory failure (too little oxygen reaches the tissues):
- Anemia
- Hemorrhage
- Intracardiac shunts
- Acute respiratory distress syndrome (ARDS)

Ventilatory respiratory failure (too little oxygen is exchanged for carbon dioxide):
- Airway obstruction (chronic bronchitis, emphysema, cystic fibrosis)
- Weakness of breathing (acute intoxication, obesity with sleep apnea)
- Muscular weakness (spinal cord injury, muscular dystrophy)
- Lung disease (pneumonia, pulmonary edema)
- Chest wall abnormalities (scoliosis, severe kyphosis)

acute care arena into chronic care facilities and even homes. Intubation and ventilation allow for:

- Airway protection in the event of neurologic deterioration or acute intoxication
- Airway protection during sedation for testing and procedures
- Airway clearance for those unable to manage their own secretions
- Management of respiratory function during surgery
- Rest for the patient with muscular fatigue
- Increased FIO_2 for the arterially hypoxic patient
- Increased flow and pressure to ensure adequate ventilation.

Caring for a patient on mechanical ventilation has become an integral part of nursing care in critical care and progressive care units. Positive patient outcomes depend on an understanding of the indications for and principles of mechanical ventilation, as well as the goals of therapy.

 Nursing Alert
It is important to remember that the right main bronchus is wider, shorter, and more vertical than the left. This physiologic difference may lead to inadvertent intubation of the right lung only. It is essential to listen to both sides of the chest for bilateral breath sounds, mark the correct endotracheal tube (ETT) placement at lip or nares, and monitor for high- and low-pressure alarms.

Types of Ventilators

Today's most commonly used ventilators are programmed to deliver oxygen through positive pressure. The ventilator pushes air into the lungs instead of creating a vacuum or negative pressure to pull air into the lungs when breathing spontaneously. Expiration occurs passively and endotracheal intubation or tracheotomy is necessary. There are three types of positive-pressure ventilators:

- *Time-cycled ventilators:* These terminate inspiration after a preset time. The volume of air the patient receives is regulated by the length of inspiration and the flow rate of the air. These are rarely used in the adult population.
- *Volume-cycled ventilators:* These are the ventilators used most commonly. The volume of air delivered with each inspiration is preset. Once this volume is delivered to the patient, the ventilator cycles off and exhalation occurs passively. The volume of air delivered by the ventilator is relatively constant, ensuring consistent, adequate breaths despite varying airway pressures.
- *Pressure-cycled ventilators:* These deliver a flow of air (inspiration) until it reaches a preset pressure and then cycle off to allow expiration to occur passively. The major limitation is that the volume of air or oxygen can vary as the patient's airway resistance or compliance

changes. The tidal volume delivered may be inconsistent (the amount of air inhaled and exhaled with a normal breath).

Ventilator Modes

Volume-Cycled Ventilators
Controlled Mandatory Ventilation. Controlled mandatory ventilation (CMV) delivers a set tidal volume at a set rate. It is used for the patient who is chemically paralyzed and sedated or whose neurologic status has deteriorated to the point that no drive to breathe exists.

Assist Control. Assist control (AC) also delivers a set tidal volume but allows patients to set their own respiratory rate. When they take a breath, they receive the entire preset tidal volume, thus decreasing their work of breathing. If the rate is set high enough, it is essentially the same as CMV.

Synchronized Intermittent Mandatory Ventilation. Synchronized intermittent mandatory ventilation (SIMV) delivers a number of breaths at a preset tidal volume to ensure a minimum number of breaths with an adequate tidal volume. Patients may breathe spontaneously but will receive only the tidal volume they are able to inspire on their own.

High-Frequency Ventilation. High-frequency ventilation (HFV), or oscillating ventilators, deliver very small tidal volumes from 3 to 6 mL/kg or 50 to 80 mL in a range from 60 to over 200 times a minute. This works on the principle of oxygen diffusion gently pulsating throughout the lungs. Patients on this form of ventilation also require sedation.

Pressure-Cycled Ventilators
Pressure Support Ventilation. Pressure support ventilation (PSV) is a mode of ventilation in which the patient breathes spontaneously but uses additional pressure during inspiration to increase airflow through the ventilator tubing and artificial airway. This decreases the work of breathing caused by a narrowed airway. Patients using pressure support are often in the process of being weaned from the ventilator.

Continuous Positive Airway Pressure. Positive air flow is used via the ETT while the patient is on the ventilator (rather than using a mask, as discussed previously). It is also used as a method of decreasing the work of breathing while weaning the patient from the ventilator.

Airway Pressure Release Ventilation. Airway pressure release ventilation (APRV) is a newer mode of assistance that improves alveolar recruitment using pressure. It is essentially BiPAP on the ventilator using inverse ratio ventilation. It allows patients to breathe with the presence of end expiratory pressure in the alveoli, but this pressure is momentarily released to allow for gas release and ventilation.

Inverse Ratio Ventilation. Inverse ratio ventilation (IRV) changes the normal inspiration to expiration ratios of 1 part inspiration to 2 parts expiration (1:2) to a ratio of 1:1 or more than 1:1 up to 1:4. Prolonging the inspiratory time allows alveolar recruitment (more alveoli used during respiration) at lower pressure levels, thus maintains or improves gas exchange at lower levels of PEEP. This is an uncomfortable way of breathing, and patients may need to be sedated.

Ventilator Settings

The primary provider will order individualized ventilator settings for the patient that will include the following:

Rate
The rate is the number of breaths the machine will give each minute.

Fraction of Inspired Air
Each breath will be given with a specified setting for inspired oxygen level, FIO_2. The goal for the FIO_2 is the lowest possible setting to provide adequate partial pressure of oxygen (PaO_2) in the bloodstream without the side effects of high oxygen percentages, such as nitrogen washout and alveolar collapse.

Tidal Volume
The tidal volume (Tv) is the amount of air given in each breath. This is usually between 5 and 7 mL of air per kilogram of body weight. This allows for air flow without overextending and damaging the alveoli. The Tv multiplied by the rate equals the minute volume (Mv). Patients with ARDS are generally managed with a low tidal volume (6 mL/Kg of ideal body weight).

Positive End Expiratory Pressure
The theory behind positive end expiratory pressure (PEEP) is that it mimics the pressure left in the lungs by closure of the glottis, which is now interrupted by placement of an ETT. PEEP is used to keep alveoli open during exhalation, to allow more time for gas exchange, and to increase *functional residual capacity,* or the amount of air in the lungs at the end of expiration. Levels of PEEP above 5 cm H_2O put the patient at risk for alveolar rupture, pneumothorax, and decreased cardiac output via referred pressure counteracting forward blood flow from the heart. The ventilator-induced damage is termed *barotrauma.*

Nursing Management

Nursing care of the patient who is mechanically ventilated requires expert technical skills.

Care is taken to simultaneously assess, intervene upon, and evaluate both the patient and the technology.

Assessing the Patient
The patient's physiologic response to illness or injury and particular indications for mechanical ventilation will determine the specific ventilator orders. The nurse should continually assess the patient's condition and resulting increase or decrease in ventilatory support required by said condition. For example, a patient with a recent decrease in neurologic function is no longer able to draw spontaneous breaths and will need an increase in the number of breaths provided by the ventilator.

Patients must be able to "allow" the ventilator to perform its function without interference caused by anxiety, biting the ETT, or problems with coughing or increased secretions. If the patient is able to let this happen and coordinate his own breaths with the machine, he is said to have *synchrony* with the ventilator. The nurse must assess the underlying cause of intolerance to mechanical ventilation and remove it in order to promote recovery of respiratory function. Common interventions include sedation, pain control, and adequate suctioning.

Assessing the Equipment
The ventilator needs to be assessed to make sure that it is functioning properly and that the settings are appropriate. While not primarily responsible for the functioning of the ventilator, the nurse is responsible for the patient and, therefore, needs to evaluate how ventilator function affects the patient's overall status.

Ventilator alarms are designed to indicate that the ventilator is unable to deliver what it has been programmed to give the patient or that the patient is unable to tolerate the current settings.

Common problems with the ventilator include:

- Disconnection or kinking of tubing
- Disconnection of tubing from ETT or tracheostomy tube
- Water in the tubing
- Change in air temperature beyond set limits

Common problems with the settings include:

- Limits set too high or too low, especially when exercising or weaning patients

Common problems with the patient include:

- Desynchronized breathing pattern between patient and ventilator
- Biting of the ETT
- Improper placement or inadvertent movement of ETT
- Coughing and/or sputum production interfering with air flow
- Lung or chest cavity fluid and pressure problems, as from congestive heart failure, pulmonary edema, and pneumothorax

Nursing Alert
Pressure limits is one of the ventilator settings with an alarm. Again, either patient

condition or the equipment may be the cause of an alarm. Pressure alarms on the ventilator may indicate a dangerous situation. Low-pressure alarms may indicate disconnection from the machine or displacement of the airway.

A high-pressure alarm usually indicates resistance to or obstruction of airflow from biting on the ETT, a kink in the tubing, or something as severe as bronchospasm or pneumothorax.

Preventing and Managing Adverse Effects of Mechanical Ventilation

As with many medical interventions, mechanical ventilation has the potential to cause complications or undesired secondary effects, and the nurse's priority is patient safety via a focus on preventing problems associated with any treatment modalities.

Ventilator-Associated Pneumonia. Currently, in the critical care world, ventilator-associated pneumonia (VAP) is receiving a lot of attention from patient advocacy groups, health care professionals, and regulatory bodies. It is caused by a patient being placed on a ventilator for a period of at least 48 hours whose oral and nasal secretions pooling above the ETT balloon fall into the lungs upon movement of the pliable balloon. Unfortunately, the mechanical ventilator is both a cause and an assistant in the treatment for pneumonia. The bacterium found in patients with VAP is usually *Pseudomonas*, but any infection not present when a person is placed on a ventilator constitutes VAP.

This infection forces the hospital to develop, implement, and monitor a policy for its prevention. The most important intervention for infection control in the ICU remains handwashing and hand rubbing with alcohol-based solutions. Additional measures include avoiding nasal insertion of endotracheal and gastric tubes, monitoring ETT cuff pressure (above 20 cm H_2O is associated with prevention of bacteria leakage around the cuff into the lower respiratory tract), providing mouth care at a minimum of every 4 hours with an antiseptic such as chlorhexidine to maintain mucosal integrity and prevent pooling of secretions, and keeping the head of the patient's bed elevated to at least 30 degrees (Chastre & Luyt, 2016). Refer to Chapter 10 for more details on VAP.

Increased Intracranial Pressure. Upon receiving air, the positive pressure in the chest decreases venous return and may leave a higher volume of blood in the cranium. This can lead to altered LOC.

Altered Mental Status. Anxiety and discomfort from being placed on a ventilator, the frequent care in the form of suctioning, and persistent ventilator alarms can easily lead to sleep deprivation. Sleep deprivation, in turn, can affect changes in mental status and delay healing, as will be discussed further in this chapter.

Decreased Cardiac Output. The higher pressure in the pulmonary tree makes it difficult for blood to return to the heart from other areas of the body. If there is less blood returning, there is less blood to pump back to the body, causing hypotension and lower cardiac output.

Hypervolemia. The decreased pressure sensed by baroreceptors in the aorta may trick the body into believing hypovolemia exists; it reacts by stimulating production of antidiuretic hormone (ADH). Release of too much hormone may cause an overaccumulation of fluid in the vasculature, necessitating diuretics.

Venous Thromboembolism. Ventilated patients are prone to spending more time in bed due to instability or the practical difficulties of walking around when attached to the ventilator. Pooling of blood in the large veins of the legs (and upper extremities as well) while in bed can lead to clot formation and increase the possibility of pulmonary embolus (PE). With an incidence varying from 10% to 20% among hospitalized patients (Camden & Ludwig, 2014), deep venous thrombosis is an adverse effect with significant morbidity and potential mortality. Prophylaxis in the form of antiembolic stockings, compression boots, range-of-motion (ROM) activity, early mobility, and administration of antiplatelet medications (such as heparin) is advised for all patients who are intubated.

Barotrauma. As the name implies, barotrauma is damage to organs and vessels due to elevated pressures in the thoracic cavity. It is important to remember that this same trauma is possible in the abdominal cavity as well (further details on Abdominal Compartment Syndrome [ACS] are in Chapter 53; Fig. 53-4 details measuring intra-bladder pressure).

Pneumothorax. Pneumothorax is a specific form of barotrauma resulting in the collapse of a lung (it is helpful to compare it to popping an overfilled balloon). Corrective action in the form of a chest tube is often required (Chapter 10 details this complication).

Gastrointestinal Bleeding. It has been found (MacLaren & Campbell, 2014) that most intubated patients develop gastrointestinal damage with up to 5% of these ulcerations causing hemodynamically significant bleeding. Although the reasons remain unclear, it is thought that gut ischemia and reperfusion injury leads to mucosal and/or deep tissue damage in the stomach and duodenum, which leads to ulcers and bleeding. The incidence of GI bleeding has decreased over the last few decades and is largely due to standard administration of proton pump inhibitors (PPIs, such as pantoprazole) or H_2-histamine antagonists (such as ranitidine) in patients with previous or current GI bleeds. Although seen less frequently, the adverse effects of significant bleeding due to stress ulcers cannot be underestimated, and prophylaxis with the medications noted here remains the standard of care. However, recent research reveals that potential harm may be associated with stress ulcer prophylaxis, including increased risk of infectious complications (nosocomial pneumonia and *Clostridium difficile*-associated diarrhea). In addition, for patients with cirrhosis, an increased mortality rate is observed with the use of PPIs (Buendgens, Koch, & Tacke, 2016). Guidelines for intervention are continuously evolving. It is up to the practitioner to keep up with the research findings and to apply the evidence to clinical practice.

Promoting Effective Airway Clearance

The presence of an ETT and continuous positive-pressure ventilation increases the production of secretions, regardless of the patient's underlying condition. Nursing interventions focus on maintaining a clear airway via turning and positioning, meticulous mouth care, and endotracheal/tracheal suctioning as needed.

Promoting Optimal Level of Mobility

The use of a mechanical ventilator limits the patient's mobility. The nurse helps the patient whose condition has become stable to get out of bed and move to a chair as soon as possible. Early mobility and muscle activity are beneficial because they stimulate respirations and improve patient psychological status. If the patient is unable to get out of bed, the nurse encourages performance of active ROM exercises every 6 to 8 hours. If the patient cannot perform these exercises, the nurse performs passive ROM exercises every 8 hours to prevent contractures and venous stasis.

Promoting Optimal Communication

It is important to develop alternative methods of communication for the patient who is receiving mechanical ventilation. The nurse assesses the patient's communication abilities. Once the patient's limitations are known, the nurse offers several appropriate communication approaches: lip reading (use single key words), pad-and-pencil or erasable slate, communication board, electronic tablet, gesturing, sign language, or electric larynx. Use of a "talking" or fenestrated tracheostomy tube may be suggested to the provider; this allows the patient to talk while on the ventilator. The nurse makes sure that the patient's eyeglasses, hearing aid, sign interpreter, and language translator are available if needed to enhance the patient's ability to communicate.

Promoting Coping Ability

Encouraging the family to verbalize their feelings about the ventilator, the patient's condition, and the environment in general is beneficial. Explaining procedures helps reduce anxiety and familiarizes the patient with ventilator procedures. To restore a sense of control, the nurse encourages the patient to participate in decisions about care as appropriate. The patient may become withdrawn or depressed while receiving mechanical ventilation. It is important to provide diversions.

Stress reduction techniques (e.g., a back rub, relaxation measures) help relieve tension and help the patient deal with anxieties and fears about the dependence on the ventilator.

 Concept Mastery Alert

While tidal volume and vital capacity both describe the amount of air inhaled and exhaled, tidal volume is used for a normal breath, and vital capacity is used for the maximum amount of air that can be expelled after a maximum inhalation.

Weaning the Patient from the Ventilator

Mechanical ventilation is not a natural condition, and prolonged intubation carries a number of potentially serious side effects; therefore, every effort is made to make the need for this intervention as short as possible, with weaning from the ventilator initiated at the earliest possible time consistent with patient safety. The goal is to get the patient in the most optimal condition to succeed in weaning from the ventilator. While there are many indicators leading a practitioner to believe a patient is ready to wean, the following have proven the most predictive:

- Vital capacity (the maximum amount of air that can be expelled after a maximum inhalation) should be at least 10 mL per kg of body weight.
- Negative inspiratory force (NIF, the ability to take a deep breath and to generate a cough strong enough to clear secretions; NIF should be at least –20 cm H_2O)
- Tidal volume (amount of air inhaled and exhaled in a normal breath; should be at least 5 mL/kg)
- Minute ventilation (total amount of air inhaled and exhaled in a minute; should be less than 10 L/min)
- Rapid shallow breathing index (RSBI, a ratio determined by the frequency of respirations [breaths per minute] divided by the tidal volume [measured in liters]); an RSBI less than 105 is considered criteria for weaning to extubation, while greater than 120 is considered as predictive of the necessity for ventilator support.

Other criteria to consider include:

- Cardiovascular stability
- Adequate and stable arterial blood gas analysis
- Nutritional support with increasing or normal levels of phosphate, magnesium, and albumin
- Ability to swallow and manage saliva and secretions

ENDOCRINE ISSUES

The endocrine system participates along with the neurologic system to regulate bodily functions, such as growth and development, tissue function, metabolism, and even mood. Disorders of the endocrine system result from the secretion of too much or too little hormone, as well as from too much or too little sensitivity to a particular hormone.

This section covers hormones of particular importance in the critical care environment.

Problems Related to Antidiuretic Hormone

ADH is secreted from the posterior pituitary gland and helps to conserve water in the body. Head trauma and kidney disorders can decrease secretion, while trauma, various cancers, hemorrhage, and infection may lead to excessive secretion of ADH. Decreased secretion leads to diabetes insipidus (DI), while excessive secretion causes syndrome of inappropriate diuretic hormone (SIADH). Recall that DI or SIADH are commonly seen in TBI (see Chapter 45 for further discussion).

Patients at risk for altered ADH secretion should be monitored for neurologic changes as well as volume status via intake and output calculations, serum sodium levels, and serum and urine osmolality. Treatment for increased secretion involves water restriction, saline infusion, and use of demeclocycline, which blocks renal response to ADH. Treatment for decreased secretion is replacement of the hormone via one of the various forms of ADH, more commonly known as *arginine vasopressin*.

Problems Related to Thyroid Hormone

The thyroid gland uses iodine to make thyroxine (T_4) and triiodothyronine (T_3). These hormones are involved in body metabolism, alertness, mood, body temperature, and general energy and oxygen use. Disorders of secretion are viewed in relation to normal function; the trajectory ranges from:

Myxedema coma ↔ Hypothyroidism ↔ Normal function ↔ Hyperthyroidism ↔ Graves disease ↔ Thyroid storm

Critical illnesses, such as cancers and infections, can alter the secretion of these hormones. Metabolism is either adversely increased or decreased at a time when metabolic control is required. Too much hormone results in nervousness, anxiety, hyperthermia, and eventual cardiac failure. Other patients with a history of thyroid disorders or surgery, or those not responding to a range of medical treatments, should have their thyroid hormone levels checked and supplemented, if necessary, to ensure assistance with increased metabolic demands.

Problems Related to Cortisol

Cortisol, secreted by the adrenal glands, is better known as the stress or fight-or-flight hormone. Levels are highest in the morning upon arising, in response to increased activity levels.

Problems related to too little or too much cortisol can be viewed on a continuum from:

Addison disease ↔ Normal function ↔ Cushing disease

At times, the level of this hormone is increased due to factors such as increased and prolonged stress; this leads to impaired cognition, hypertension, decreased thyroid and immune system function, hyperglycemia, and decreased bone density and muscle mass.

More commonly in the ICU, cortisol levels are low due to low perfusion states, infection, or adverse effects of medications. People with low levels of cortisol are unable to mount a physical response to bodily stressors and are likely to have fatigue, lower body temperature, and hypotension. Patients who meet clinical criteria for low cortisol levels are frequently given a cortisol stimulation test to determine if replacement is required to increase the body's metabolic response to illness.

Problems Related to Insulin

The beta cells of the pancreas secrete insulin to help move glucose into the cells to be used as an energy substrate. The majority of people with insulin disorders have type I or type II diabetes mellitus and are at particular risk for acute episodes of hyper- or hypoglycemia with the added stress of a critical illness. Patients with particularly brittle disease may be affected by sugar levels on this continuum:

Hypoglycemia ↔ Normal glucose level ↔ Diabetic ketoacidosis (DKA) or Hyperosmolar hyperglycemic nonketotic syndrome (HHNS), also called hyperglycemic hyperosmolar syndrome (HHS)

Patients with diabetes are frequently admitted to the ICU with complications of their illness, but it is also a disease frequently diagnosed for the first time while hospitalized. All patients admitted to the ICU should have their blood glucose monitored three to four times a day to ensure they are able to maintain their glucose levels below each hospital's prescribed upper limit. For those who are unable to maintain a lower level of glucose, insulin therapy should be initiated according to hospital policy, with frequent monitoring of glucose levels to ensure lower levels without hypoglycemia. The most recent recommendations for insulin therapy target a glucose range of 140 to 180 mg/dL in most patients who are critically ill (Schiffner, 2014).

GASTROINTESTINAL ISSUES

As with oxygen, food and drink becomes a medical prescription in the ICU. It is also regulated by practicalities such as kitchen schedules and nursing time to deliver food to or feed patients.

Nutritional Support

In the critical care unit, nutritional support is required to prevent catabolism of protein stores and provide the necessary elements for healing. The question in the ICU is not whether or not patients should be fed but, rather, when and how. Current trends in feeding lean include early initiation of enteral feedings whenever possible with increases to target energy needs within the first 48 hours of admission (Singer et al., 2014).

Food

Because nature knows best, the optimal method of feeding patients is through oral intake of food and fluids. Specific diets will be altered depending on a patient's diagnoses. These may include altered content (low fat or low salt), altered consistency (soft or pureed), or with altered fluid (fluid restriction). The nurse ensures an environment and physical condition that makes the patient amenable to eating. Prevention of nausea and vomiting, pain relief, and proper positioning in a chair or upright in bed can all increase a person's appetite. At times, smaller more frequent meals consisting of something the patient likes to eat may help increase intake, maintain weight, and provide a diversion from the ICU environment.

Tube Feedings

A percentage of patients have a working GI tract but will not be able to take food orally due to their physiologic condition (dementia with dysphagia) or medical intervention (endotracheal intubation). These patients receive tube feedings. A particular liquid formula is recommended with collaboration of the dietician and medical practitioner. Again, the actual formula will depend upon the patient's diagnosis and current condition. Box 55-2 describes nursing responsibilities for

---

BOX 55-2
Caring for Patients Receiving Tube Feedings

With tube feeding patients, the nurse is responsible for:
- Noting that placement has been verified by the medical team via radiography, which is the gold standard for checking tube placement
- Assess patient's tolerance to medication and feeding administration (noting abdominal distention and complaints of abdominal pain, observing for passage of flatus and stool)
- Double-check placement by measurement of tube length, follow institutional procedures which may include assessing the pH measurement of aspirate (remains an area where further research is warranted); listening for air insufflation over the stomach; this method is common, but its accuracy is controversial
- Preventing accidental dislodgement by patient or staff
- Maintaining patency of the tubes
- Monitoring for intolerance to feeding
- Monitoring for constipation and diarrhea

---

patients receiving tube feedings. Tube feeding pumps deliver the nutrition via a variety of tubes that may include:

- *Nasogastric tube (NGT):* A tube inserted into the nares and ending in the stomach; used for gastric drainage or feeding (may be inserted orally if recommended)
- *Flexible feeding tube:* A synthetic tube of large or small bore (size) inserted into the nares to the stomach; softer, more flexible than the NGT, without the ability to convert to a drainage tube if needed
- *Postpyloric tube:* A longer variety of the flexible feeding tube that reaches past the stomach into the duodenum, in order to use the small bowel when the stomach has the potential to not tolerate feeding or the risk of aspiration is high
- *Percutaneous endoscopic gastrostomy (PEG) tube:* A tube inserted by the physician directly through the abdominal wall into the stomach; removes the discomfort, potential for accidental dislodgement, and potential for sinus infections caused by nasally inserted tubes
- *Gastrojejunostomy (G-J) tube:* A tube that allows for simultaneous feeding of the small bowel and drainage of the stomach

Nursing Alert
Intolerance to feeding is a complicated issue with consequences for deteriorating nutritional status and aspiration pneumonia. Aspiration of GI contents into the lungs leads to increased morbidity and prolonged hospitalization. Risk factors for aspiration may include decreased mental status, placement of the head of the bed at less than 30 degrees, sedatives, vomiting, and high gastric residual volumes.

Parenteral Nutrition

Unfortunately, there are times when a patient is unable to tolerate enteral feeding and nutritional support must be given intravenously. Total parenteral nutrition (TPN) or central parenteral nutrition (CPN) provides amino acids, dextrose, and fat. Because of its high osmolality, it must be given by a central catheter, such as a triple-lumen or Hickman™ catheter, or by a peripheral IV that terminates in a central vein, such as a PICC line. This type of support is used as a method to supplement or completely replace enteral feeding. However, it has numerous potential consequences, including pneumothorax during catheter insertion, catheter infection (due to high concentration of sugar in the solution), and liver failure. The goal is to use this support for as short a time as possible before returning to enteral feeds and eventually to having the patient provide his or her own oral intake. Partial parenteral nutrition (PPN) may be administered via a peripheral IV because of the solution's lower osmolality. A number of metabolic complications are associated with parenteral nutrition, including hyperglycemia, electrolyte abnormalities, and irritation at the IV site.

TABLE **55-10** Immunonutrition

Element	Effects	Comment
Arginine (conditionally nonessential amino acid)	• Stimulation of growth hormone • Precursor in nitric oxide production • Improves immune function • Reduces healing time of injuries (particularly bone) • Increases muscle mass • Improved insulin sensitivity	Its use in septic patients remains controversial as the effects of sepsis on arginine metabolism or of arginine metabolism on sepsis are unclear.
Glutamine (conditionally nonessential amino acid)	• A substrate for DNA synthesis • Major role in protein synthesis • Primary source of fuel for enterocytes • Precursor for rapidly dividing immune cells, thus aiding in immune function • Regulation of acid–base balance in the kidney by producing ammonium • Alternative fuel source for the brain • Blocks cortisol-induced protein catabolism	It remains unclear whether outcomes are improved via enteral or IV administration.
Omega-3 fatty acids	• Reduced Inflammation • Reduced lipid circulation in the bloodstream • Decreased platelet aggregation • Reduced cytokine production • Improved insulin sensitivity	
Copper	• Increased erythrocyte production • Increased absorption of iron • Maintenance of cytochrome p450 cycle • Vitamin C metabolism	
Selenium	• Maintenance of the cytochrome p450 system • DNA repair	
Zinc	• Increased growth hormone • Increased uptake of insulin • Increased cell division and promotion of wound healing • Treatment of diarrhea	

Immunonutrition

A deficit of nutrients can increase infection rates, length of hospital stay, and mortality. These nutrients are additional supplements to the various methods of feeding. Depending on patient diagnosis and condition, the nutrients in Table 55-10 should be considered.

Slow Motility

For a patient to tolerate feedings, the stomach must empty its contents into the small intestine, where nutrients are actually digested. This emptying is partially regulated by cholecystokinin (CCK) and polypeptide YY (PYY) levels that serve to slow gastric emptying. Unfortunately, it has been found that levels of these substances are elevated during critical illness, causing delayed emptying. Diabetes, gastroparesis (delayed gastric emptying), and slowed gut peristalsis due to pain medications are common causes of slow motility. This slow motility of gastric and intestinal contents can lead to

nausea, vomiting, aspiration, and decreased nutritional status, which must be prevented or corrected as soon as possible. Current trends favor the use of promotility drugs, such as metoclopramide and/or erythromycin. It is not yet clear if these medications contribute to improved outcomes, and recommendations may change after future study. Adequate hydration and physical movement also assist in maintaining proper GI function.

If motility cannot be improved, the general consensus dictates movement to small bowel feedings before adding or replacing enteral feeds with parenteral nutrition.

Diarrhea

Diarrhea is frequently seen in the ICU and has been found to be related to enteral therapy, hypoalbuminemia, antibiotic therapy, and sepsis. This makes the issue of diarrhea very difficult as enteral therapy is a treatment for low protein states and antibiotic therapy is required for treatment of overwhelming infections. Once diagnosed, the underlying cause, symptomatology, and potential adverse effects of diarrhea must be addressed and mitigated.

Causes

Enteral Therapy

The use of tube feedings is often required to prevent and treat malnutrition in the ICU. The clinical team needs to evaluate the composition of the prescribed feeding for possible changes required in the fiber or water content or osmolality. Current trends find that continuous feeding via a pump instead of intermittent feeding will decrease the amount of diarrhea. Patient care and testing often require changes of position, transfer, or NPO status, which interrupt feedings because it is considered unsafe to feed a patient while he or she is lying flat during turns and transfers. NPO status for individual medications (Dilantin therapy) or tests also decreases nutritional intake. If possible, nursing needs to plan care in order to limit feeding interruptions. Fewer interruptions in feeding will maintain optimal caloric intake and reduce glucose fluctuations and the risk for diarrhea.

Hypoalbuminemia

Albumin is a protein responsible for maintaining oncotic pressure in the vascular system and, thus, distribution of fluids in the body. Low albumin levels cause water to leave the vasculature and accumulate in other parts of the body, such as the GI tract and tissues.

Antibiotics

The use of antibiotics changes normal gut flora depending upon the sensitivity of bacteria to the prescribed medications. The use of cephalosporins and quinolones is known to place patients at higher risk for overgrowth of *Clostridium difficile*, which forms a covering membrane inside the GI tract. The membrane acts to prevent absorption of fluid and nutrients and causes diarrhea. This particular infection requires yet another antibiotic treatment with metronidazole and vancomycin.

Sepsis

Generalized infections not necessarily specific to the GI tract nonetheless have consequences for this system. Inflammation, cytokine release, and alterations in blood flow and the permeability of GI mucosa have also been found to cause diarrhea.

Symptoms and Adverse Effects

Diarrhea can be uncomfortable, painful, and embarrassing for the patient. It also requires extensive nursing time to keep patients clean and free of complications. The adverse effects of diarrhea are numerous and can impact outcomes. Hemodynamic instability due to fluid and electrolyte losses needs to be corrected with replacement of IV fluids, electrolytes,

and minerals. This prevents cardiac arrhythmias and low perfusion states. Malnutrition due to poor absorption because of diarrhea, at a time when metabolic requirements are elevated, needs intervention with a possible change in feeding formula or supplementation with parenteral nutrition. Fecal contents and even skin cleansers change the normal pH of the skin and can lead to breakdown and the formation of pressure ulcers.

Prevention and Treatment of Diarrhea

The first goal is to prevent diarrhea. The second goal is to stop it as soon as possible if preventative efforts fail. Some of these efforts will be ordered by the provider, with patient response monitored by nursing. Interventions include:

- Change in feeding formula, with higher fiber content or lower osmolality
- Prescription of probiotics, such as *Lactobacillus*, to alter gut flora
- Use of antidiarrheal medications, such as loperamide
- Frequent turning of patient to relieve pressure and enhance evaluation of skin
- Use of skin barrier lotions to prevent contact between skin and fecal contents

Constipation

Patients in the ICU are also at risk for constipation. Incidence varies widely, as do definitions, with levels from 5% to 83% being reported in various studies (Rodrigo & Flávia, 2013). Constipation can be defined as difficulty in or failure to defecate for at least 3 days. Potential causes include decreased fluid intake or hypovolemia, immobility, and side effects of medications such as narcotics. Complications range from mild discomfort and bloating to intolerance to feedings and obstruction and perforation.

Constipation has also been shown to increase bacterial overgrowth and sepsis and is even associated with an increase in the number of days mechanical ventilation is required (Rodrigo & Flávia, 2013). The goal is to prevent constipation via provision of hydration, fiber intake, and the use of pharmacologic agents if prescribed. Various bowel regimens akin to those used in patients with slow motility are employed, including digital extraction of rectal contents, enemas, and suppositories. Once the lower GI tract is cleared, it is possible to provide medication via the upper intestinal tract to clear out fecal contents from areas unreachable by other means.

RENAL ISSUES

Many patients in a critical care unit are either at risk for or have pre-existing renal problems, particularly if they have a history of diabetes or hypertension. Damage to the renal system can be acute, chronic, or acute on chronic. Sources of kidney damage are classified as prerenal, intrarenal, and postrenal (refer to Chapter 27 for further details).

Promotion of Kidney Function

Despite the statistics given previously, many patients admitted to the ICU will have normal kidney function. However, admission to the ICU places patients at risk for kidney dysfunction; therefore, nurses need to monitor urine output and laboratory values such as serum creatinine, blood urea nitrogen, creatinine clearance, and glomerular filtration rates (GFR) in order to ensure continued function or intervene as soon as possible in the event of declining function.

Spontaneous Voiding

The most comfortable method of urinating is to be able to go to the bathroom independently. The ability to do this necessitates functioning kidneys, the mental ability to recognize the need to void, and the physical strength and balance required for mobility. If patients are able to void spontaneously, the nurse should provide them every opportunity to do so. This eliminates the possibility of urinary catheter–related infections. It is important to note, however, that having to go to the bathroom is a very frequent reason for confused patients trying to get out of bed. The practice of toileting patients every few hours prevents the consequences of falls, incontinence, and skin breakdown.

Condom Catheters

Condom catheters are placed on males when they are able to void spontaneously and strict hourly monitoring of urinary output is not required. Additionally, if patients are confused, unable to realize the need to urinate, or lack the ability to use a bathroom or urinal, this provides an alternative to incontinence. Unfortunately, an alternative to condom catheters has not been developed for women.

Urinary Catheters

Urinary catheters are inserted into the bladder by way of the urethra and are used to provide samples of urine for testing, a method of monitoring urine output when concerned with hemodynamic compromise, and as a means for controlling incontinence and skin breakdown. While convenient for staff, urinary catheters are associated with more than 30% of all nosocomial infections in hospitalized patients (Saint, 2014). Standard practice should include aseptic insertion, daily preventative cleaning of the catheter with soap and water, wiping away from the urethra, episodic cleaning after bowel movements as noted previously, maintaining a closed system, ensuring the drainage bag is below the level of the bladder, and proper anchoring of the catheter on the leg to prevent undue strain on it.

According the Centers for Disease Control and Prevention, the most important risk factor for developing a catheter-associated urinary tract infection (CAUTI) is prolonged use of the urinary catheter (2015). Thus the removal of the catheter at the earliest possible time is recommended.

Renal Insufficiency

People with a GFR less than 60 mL/min are said to have renal insufficiency; their ability to filter and excrete metabolic waste products is impaired. Prevention of further deterioration of kidney function is critical. This will include hemodynamic support to maintain blood flow, as the kidneys require up to 20% of the cardiac output. Additionally, the medical team and pharmacists have to evaluate drug dosages because the clearance of medications is impacted by renal excretion. Patients requiring IV contrast for radiographic studies are often prescribed "renal protection" in the form of normal saline and medications, such as acetylcysteine, before their studies. Despite all efforts, some patients will progress from renal insufficiency to kidney failure, so the nurse must remain vigilant to deteriorating function.

Kidney Failure

In patients who are critically ill, the development of acute kidney injury (AKI) is associated with a mortality rate of 50% or greater (Kudlow et al., 2014). Therefore, efforts to mimic normal renal mechanisms are accomplished via renal replacement or dialysis until kidney function resumes. Patients with end-stage renal disease (ESRD), also termed end-stage kidney failure, have the option of complete renal replacement for extended periods of time.

Nursing Alert
Acute tubular necrosis (ATN), commonly related to hypoperfusion and/or nephrotoxic agents, is associated with AKI in patients who are critically ill. Therefore the nurse monitors urinary output hourly in patients who are critically ill, assesses the serum peak and trough levels of nephrotoxic medications, and alerts the provider when urinary output is less than 30 mL/hr (or 0.5 to 1 mL/kg/hr) and/or abnormal peak and trough levels are seen.

Renal Replacement

Renal replacement is accomplished via hemodialysis, peritoneal dialysis, or kidney transplant through either cadaver or living donation. Dialysis can be provided for a short period of time, to allow the kidneys time to recover from an acute injury such as ATN; as a bridge to renal transplantation; or on a permanent basis. Other indications for starting renal replacement therapy include:

- Uremic encephalopathy: Confusion, asterixis, and seizures
- Pericarditis
- Bleeding

- Fluid overload unresponsive to diuretics
- Pleuritis
- Metabolic derangements: Metabolic acidosis, hyperkalemia, hyperphosphatemia, hyper- or hypocalcemia
- Protracted nausea and vomiting
- Weight loss or signs of malnutrition
- Overdose of medications/poisons that are dialyzable

Renal replacement therapies are discussed in detail in Chapter 27.

MUSCULOSKELETAL ISSUES

People admitted to critical care units are usually confined to bed for extended periods of time. Neurologic, cardiovascular, and respiratory instability are reasons why patients are restricted to bed rest in the ICU. Sometimes interventions (ICP monitors, balloon pumps) or the desire to prevent the increased oxygen demands of movement (heart failure, respiratory insufficiency) necessitate bed rest. Other reasons

TABLE **55-11** Effects of Bed Rest

System	Potential Effects
Neurologic	Anxiety Hallucinations
Cardiovascular	Hypovolemia Decreased carotid baroreceptor response Orthostatic hypotension Deep venous thrombosis
Respiratory	Atelectasis Pneumonia Pulmonary Embolus
Gastrointestinal	Ileus Constipation
Genitourinary	Urinary stasis Renal calculi
Endocrine	Insulin resistance Hyperglycemia
Musculoskeletal	Muscular atrophy Bone demineralization Contractures
Skin	Decubitus ulcers
Psychosocial	Depression
Other	Increased catabolism of immunoglobulin G Increased colonization with *Staphylococcus aureus*

From Timmerman, R. A. (2007). A mobility protocol for critically ill adults. *Dimensions of Critical Care Nursing, 26*(5), 175–179; Rubin, M. (1988). The physiology of bed rest. *The American Journal of Nursing, 88*(1), 50–58.

for prolonged bed rest include conflicting priorities in the nursing staff ("Do I spend my time with my patient who is actively hemorrhaging, or with the one who needs to get out of bed?"), or lack of knowledge regarding the importance of physical activity. Being in the recumbent position is not a natural state, and prolonged bed rest has a plethora of adverse effects that are outlined in Table 55-11. Deconditioning is seen in patients after as few as 3 days of bed rest. This leads to a decline in overall ability to function and increases the need for admittance into rehabilitation centers after hospitalization. It is important for nurses to be aware of these potential complications and to create the opportunity for movement and limitation of bed rest activity whenever possible.

ICU-Acquired Weakness

ICU-acquired weakness is an increasingly recognized disorder characterized by the inability of a patient to move against resistance. Witteveena (2015) describes this as a complication associated with increased short- and long-term morbidity and mortality. It encompasses both myopathy and neuropathy with multifactorial causes beyond the scope of this chapter. Patients at risk for this disorder include those with systemic inflammatory response syndrome (SIRS) and sepsis, hyperglycemia, as well as those receiving corticosteroids or neuromuscular blocking agents. Weakness can be difficult to diagnose in the ICU due to confounding issues, such as altered neurologic status, but is often first noticed when patients are unable to be removed from a ventilator. Preventative and rehabilitative measures generally include early identification and treatment of potential causes of multiple organ failure (in particular severe sepsis and septic shock), avoiding unnecessary deep sedation and hyperglycemia, promotion of early mobilization, and thoughtful decisions regarding the risks versus benefits of corticosteroids.

Contractures

Contractures are limitations in ROM of a joint with resultant inability to perform activities of daily living. Dammeyer et al. (2013) note shortening of muscle sarcomeres and the start of contractures begin with just 1 day of bed rest.

Foot drop (Fig. 55-6) is a specific type of contracture defined by the inability to lift the dorsum (anterior surface) of the foot and toes upward (dorsiflexion). It can be caused by neurologic or muscular diseases as well as by inactivity during bed rest. The inability to lift the feet impairs the person's ability to mobilize and improve overall functioning. The use of footboards to maintain dorsiflexion, allowing for some weight bearing by tipping beds forward, and early mobilization in the ICU are recommended nursing interventions.

Nitrogen Wasting

To maintain a healthy state, the body requires equilibrium between the amounts of protein supplied and muscle mass

FIGURE 55-6 Foot drop is a consequence of weakened muscles for dorsiflexion, resulting in permanent plantarflexion. (From Lambert, H. W., & Wineski, L. E. (2010). *Lippincott's illustrated Q&A review of anatomy and embryology* (2nd ed.). Philadelphia, PA: Lippincott Williams & Wilkins.)

breakdown/turnover. Refer to Box 22-2, Establishing Positive Nitrogen Balance, for further details on attaining and maintaining a positive nitrogen balance. Critical illness often leads to increased requirements at a time when protein is either used for healing or lost at a higher rate due to immobility and/or disease processes.

Bone Demineralization

Weight-bearing contributes to calcium uptake by the bones, promoting continued strength and bone formation. When on bed rest, calcium is excreted from the bones at higher levels, while at the same time the patient may be at risk for decreased intake due to anorexia or intolerance to feedings.

Nursing Alert
The variety of ill effects from bed rest demonstrated throughout the literature and in this book should alert every nurse to the need for their patients to move. If out of bed activity is restricted, active/passive ROM should be employed, at a minimum of every shift. It is important to note that while sitting in a chair is helpful, the need to walk is paramount in terms of improving cardiovascular, respiratory, GI, and musculoskeletal status. In short, if allowed, the nurse should encourage and help the patient to get out of bed.

INTEGUMENTARY ISSUES

Admission to the ICU places the patient's skin at risk. Because of decreased mental status or decreased ability to change position, hypoperfusion, fever, immobility, and restraint, a patient may not be able to move in response to discomfort. The state of a patient's skin should be documented

on arrival to the unit, in order to follow changes. This documentation also has financial implications as Medicare is no longer reimbursing hospitals for hospital-acquired alterations in skin integrity, such as pressure ulcers.

Planned Medical Breaks in Skin Integrity

Intravenous Lines

The skin is normally one contiguous unit. The simple act of placing a peripheral IV in a patient disrupts skin continuity and serves as a planned medical break in the skin and a potential source of infection. All IV lines should be monitored for signs of infection (erythema [redness], warmth, and discharge at the IV site or an elevated temperature), and lines should be changed according to hospital policy.

Procedures

Minor procedures, such as pacemaker or PEG placement, are other examples of planned medical interventions that require breaks in the skin. Again, infection control is of paramount importance.

Surgery

Surgical procedures interrupt skin and tissue integrity. Post-surgical infections can arise from deep tissue and organs, but surgical incisions require specific care and attention to prevent infection and poor wound healing.

Unplanned Breaks in Skin Integrity

Skin Tears

A majority of patients in the ICU are elderly and are affected by natural changes in the skin. More specifically, there is a flattening of the dermis and increased movement between the dermis and epidermis. When the two are separated, a skin tear occurs. ICU patients are prone to skin tears due to their age, medication history (chronic steroid use), immobility, and altered mental status. ICU patients are also prone to skin tears due to nursing interventions, such as tape removal, as well as due to friction and shear forces when pulling patients up in bed. Protection of the limbs from skin tears requires vigilance and patience on the part of the nurse. This means asking for enough help to turn or move a large patient.

Pressure Ulcers

A pressure ulcer is a localized injury to the skin and/or underlying tissue, usually over a bony prominence, as a result of pressure alone or pressure in combination with shear and/or friction. These breaks in the skin can progress from the skin to subcutaneous tissue and bone. Because muscle and subcutaneous tissue are more susceptible to pressure-induced injury than skin, pressure ulcers are often worse than their initial appearance. Pressure ulcers are staged to guide clinical

Risk Factors for Pressure Ulcer Development

- Malnutrition
- Hemodynamic instability
- Predisposing diseases, such as diabetes
- Advanced age
- Infection
- Motor/sensory deficits
- Decreased mental status
- Incontinence
- Mobility/activity deficit

Medications, such as sedatives, vasoactive agents, neuro-muscular blocking agents

- Contractures
- Spasms

description of the depth of observable tissue destruction (see Chapter 52). Beinlich and Meehan (2014) state that these wounds cost the Medicare system up to 3.6 billion dollars each year. Box 55-3 provides risk factors for pressure ulcer development.

Unfortunately, many patients in critical care have one or more of these risk factors.

Nursing Alert
Nurses hold the vast majority of responsibility for patient skin assessment, frequent turning, and skin care for pressure ulcer prevention. Early identification of and aggressive treatment for such ulcers is required.

See Chapter 52 for pressure ulcer staging and management.

PSYCHOSOCIAL ISSUES

Entry into an ICU is stressful for patients and for their friends and families. Psychosocial issues can also play a part in the reason for ICU admission. Addiction to legal or illegal drugs, violence, and reckless behavior can all lead to serious accidents and illnesses. Nurses must always consider the possible psychosocial issues and disruptions that patients and families are confronting.

Fear

Every patient and family should be assessed to determine the presence of psychosocial issues. Fear or apprehension, awe, or anxiety due to perceived danger is a frequent entity in critical care. Patients and families can be afraid of death, permanent disability, and the critical care environment itself, where care of oneself or a loved one is entrusted to strangers. Lack of information regarding the plan of care and prognosis, as well as lack of understanding of the information provided,

is also a common cause of fear. Patients who frequently use the call bell or call out for help and family members who are confrontational or demand constant nursing presence in the patient's room provide examples of not coping with the stress of ICU admission. Methods of decreasing fear for patients and families are not complex, yet they require time and patience on the part of nursing staff. Suggestions for allaying fear include:

- Introduction of staff and their roles in caring for the patient
- Explanation of what you are going to do to or with a patient and why
- Allowing family and friends to be present in the room
- Educating patients and families according to needs and desires
- Informing patients and families of progress or failure to progress

Grieving

Grieving is the process of coming to terms with loss: one's impending death, death of a loved one, loss of function and freedom, loss of self-image, and loss of future opportunities. The stages of grief are well defined throughout the literature, and all nurses should be aware of them. People will differ in their coping behaviors, and nurses should help people develop their best coping practices possible. This is a difficult and often time-consuming process. If nurses are unable to spend much time with grieving patients and families, it is imperative to find the patient alternate help: a colleague with more experience with grieving patients, a pastor, a social worker, hospital volunteers, family, or friends.

Violence

Violence in the home and workplace should never be tolerated, but it is a fact that critical care nurses must confront. Patients may have been a victim of past or recent injury. The sad fact is that many nurses can also report being a victim of violence at the hands of their patients. A study by Speroni et al. (2014) found that 76% of nurses experienced violence at the hands of patients and/or visitors. This included intimidation, verbal abuse, threats of physical violence, or actual violence. The nurse's goals are to identify patients at risk for being abused by others in their life, identify patients or families with a potential for violence against hospital staff, and establish a zero-tolerance workplace violence policy across the nation.

Patient Safety

Many people live with violence in their home, either through neglect or outright physical abuse. The elderly requiring significant time and resources from family members may be at increased risk for abuse as others become frustrated with their increasing disabilities. Assessing for a history of past injuries or evidence of current injury with appropriate referrals is warranted.

Patients with suicidal ideation also need to be protected in the acute care setting. This may include:

- A provider's order for one-to-one observation at all times
- A provider's order for chemical or mechanical restraint
- Removal of dangerous objects in the room
- Limit-setting and negotiation with the patient
- Family and/or friend intervention as appropriate

Staff Safety

Patients at risk for harming staff members require specific interventions:

- Notification of security and administration of the potential for violence
- Keeping the patient in view at all times
- Approaching the patient with a calm but firm demeanor only with support from colleagues (and security as required)

END-OF-LIFE ISSUES

The critical care nurse will encounter many patients of various ages who are facing the ends of their lives.

Some of these deaths are unexpected, while others are anticipated. Each critical care nurse needs to be aware of his or her patient's medical prognosis and the patient's and family's response to a poor prognosis. Coping mechanisms will vary widely and range from sitting vigil by the patient to avoidance. An important component of care is providing patients with realistic information about their prognosis and end-of-life care while providing emotional support as they adjust to the idea of death.

Unexpected Death

Society expects that young people will not die. Sadly, accidents, suicides, and illness do claim young lives. This requires nurses to be cognizant of these issues and support patients and families through anger, denial, and the other stages of grief. A number of studies have demonstrated that being with the patient at the end of life is important for many, and those who request it should have someone present whenever they wish—including during resuscitation efforts.

If there is to be any solace in the death of a young or relatively young person, it can be found in the arena of organ and tissue donation. Patients who meet the criteria for past health and current diagnosis of brain death are eligible to donate organs to those on the various transplant lists. This places nurses in a difficult position at times due to their simultaneous obligations to care for a particular patient and their family while informing organ donation services of a potential donor. When the diagnosis of brain death is made, it is usually up to the senior medical staff and organ procurement services to approach the family about the possibility of organ donation.

Expected Death

Patients with a severe chronic illness or those of an advanced age have most likely had a number of experiences with the health care system and may be somewhat more mentally and emotionally prepared for death. ICU nurses need to be aware of their patients' advanced directives and living wills in order to advocate for their wishes during hospital care. These patients may have placed limits on what treatments they will allow in the event they can no longer speak for themselves, and nurses need to support these wishes or changes in those wishes. At this stage of their patient's life, nurses can provide the means to make the patient as comfortable as possible while allowing family and friends to come to terms with the impending loss of a loved one.

OTHER ISSUES

Sleep

Sleep is an essential bodily function, with significant impact on recovery from illness. Critical care patients are known to become sleep deprived due to their illness, ICU admission, pain, medical procedures, and nursing care. No matter the cause, sleep deprivation has been associated with adverse effects in the ICU. A study by Weinhouse (2014) indicated lack of sleep to be a major and memorable stressor for those discharged from an ICU.

Nursing care interferes with patients' ability to move through the stages of sleep toward rapid eye movement (REM), the deepest form of sleep. It requires an average of 90 minutes to reach REM sleep. How often is a patient left comfortable and undisturbed for at least 90 minutes in an ICU? The answer is not often enough.

A number of interventions may assist in promoting sleep:

- Clustering care
- Adequate pain relief
- Ensuring synchrony with the ventilator
- Noise and light reduction
- Day and night routines
- Sleep-promoting medications, such as melatonin
- Relaxation therapy, massage, and white noise
- Alarm limits (set limits appropriate to the individual patient, to minimize nuisance alarms)

Falls

It has been estimated that up to 84% of hospital adverse events are related to patient falls (Aranda-Gallardo et al., 2013). It is also noted that 30% of patient falls lead to injury of which up to 6% lead to serious injury or death (Aranda-Gallardo et al., 2013). Despite the implementation

TABLE **55-12** **Minimizing Falls**

Risk Factors	Nursing Interventions to Decrease Risk for the Individual
History of falls	• Identify the patient as being at risk for falls. • Implement fall protocol.
Fear of falling	• Encourage patient to verbalize feelings. • Institute physical therapy consult to help patient demonstrate their ability to move safely.
Bowel and bladder incontinence	• Implement toileting routine. • Monitor bowel function to prevent diarrhea and constipation.
Cognitive impairment	• Evaluate patient for reversible causes of cognitive impairment/delirium and eliminate causes as possible. • Institute close observation by placing patient in view of nursing staff. • Start one-to-one observation. • Use monitoring devices, such as bed and chair exit alarms.
Mood	• Encourage verbalization of feelings. • Evaluate patient's ability to concentrate and learn new information. • Encourage engagement in daily activities. • Provide diversional activity. • Refer to geriatric psychiatry as appropriate.
Dizziness	• Monitor lying, sitting, and standing blood pressures, and continually evaluate for factors contributing to dizziness. • Set up environment to avoid movements that result in dizziness/vertigo. • If diabetic, monitor blood sugars and facilitate interventions to maintain appropriate blood sugars.
Functional impairment	• Encourage participation in personal care activities at highest level (i.e., if possible, encourage ambulation to bathroom rather than use of bedpan). • Refer to physical and occupational therapy as appropriate.
Medications	• Review medications with medical practitioner and determine need for each medication. • Ascertain that medications are being used at lowest possible dosages to obtain desired results.
Medical problems	• Assure patient that medical problems are not a reason to remain in bed and prevent participation in functional activities.
Environment	• Remove furniture if patient can't sit on it and have his or her feet reach the floor. • Remove clutter. • Make sure furniture and any assistive devices used are in good condition. • Make sure lighting is adequate. • *Avoid* the use of four side rails and other forms of restraint.

From Gray-Micelli, D. (2007). Preventing falls in acute care. In E. Capezuti, D. Zwicker, M. Mezey, & T. Fulmer (Eds.), *Evidence-based geriatric nursing protocols for best practice* (3rd ed.). New York: Springer Publishing Company.

of fall prevention programs, research reveals little impact on decreasing fall rates while a patient is hospitalized. Ideally, the only way to prevent falls is to have a mentally and physically strong enough person be with each patient at all times; something not financially feasible for most hospitals. Realistically, what can be done is to identify risk factors for falling and arrange the care environment as well as possible to reduce the possibility of falls occurring (Table 55-12).

Transport of the ICU Patient

Patients who are critically ill are often safest inside the ICU, where staff and equipment are available for monitoring as

needed. New technology has led to the availability of an ever-increasing number of tests and interventions that are able to be done at the bedside. This includes portable x-rays, endoscopies, and ultrasounds and even minor surgical procedures, such as tracheostomy and PEG tube placement. However, there are a number of times when a patient will require transportation from the ICU to the operating room or, more frequently, to the radiology department. The radiology department may be required for tests such as computed tomography (CT) scan or intervention such as cardiac stent placement. Intra-hospital movement of patients has long been known to be the cause of adverse effects: pain, increased intracranial pressure, hypotension, arrhythmia, hypoxia, VAP, decreased

SBAR (Situation, Background, Assessment, Recommendation)*

NOTE: Pronounced S-BAR and first used by the military to improve the effectiveness of communication between care givers, the SBAR approach is recommended by patient safety experts. SBAR forms vary depending on purpose and setting. Some places use SBAR for giving hand-off situations (when one nurse transfers patient care to another). Some places use SBAR forms like the one below for calling physicians about a problem.

→ Have the chart in hand before you make the phone call, and be sure you can readily communicate all of the following information.

S SITUATION: Have the chart in hand before you make the phone call, and be sure you can readily communicate all the following: Briefly state the issue or problem: what it is, when it happened (or how it started) and how severe it is. Give the signs and symptoms that cause you concern.

B BACKGROUND: Give the date of admission and current medical diagnoses. Determine the pertinent medical history and give a brief synopsis of the treatment to date (eg, medications; oxygen use; nasogastric tube; IVs; code status).

A ASSESSMENT: Give most recent vital signs and any changes in the following:

- ☐ Mental status – neuro signs
- ☐ Respirations
- ☐ Pulse – skin color
- ☐ Comfort – Pain
- ☐ GI status (nausea-vomiting-diarrhea, distention)
- ☐ Urine Output
- ☐ Bleeding-Drainage
- ☐ Other: _____

R RECOMMENDATION: State what you think should be done. For example:

- ☐ Come see the patient now
- ☐ Get a consultation
- ☐ Get additional studies (eg, CXR, ABG, EKG, CBC, other)
- ☐ Transfer the patient to ICU
- ☐ If the patient doesn't improve
- ☐ How frequent do you want vital signs.
- ☐ If there's no improvement, by when do you want us to call you?

*Data from: Haig, K, Sutton, S. and Whittington, J. (2006). SBAR: A Shared Mental Model for Improving Communication Between Clinicians. *Journal of Quality and Patient Safety, 32*(3), 167–175. Available: http://www.jcipatientsafety.org/fpfd/psp/SBAR.pdf

Source: R. Alfaro-LeFevre Handouts © 2007–2013 www.AlfaroTeachSmart.com

FIGURE 55-7 SBAR Tool promotes consistent communication. (From Alfaro-LeFevre, R. (2013). *Applying nursing process*. Philadelphia, PA: Lippincott Williams & Wilkins.)

nutritional intake, hypo- and hyperglycemia, inadvertent disconnection from equipment, and falls.

Patients are placed at risk from transport due to decreased number of staff available to the patient, disruptions in continuity of care, decreased ability to monitor patients in places like the magnetic resonance imaging (MRI) suite, and possible adverse effects of the test itself. With these known risks to patient safety, a number of tools and guidelines have been developed to minimize adverse events associated with transport.

One communication tool, often called a "ticket to ride" using the Situation-Background-Assessment-Recommendation (SBAR; see Fig. 55-7), can be used to exchange information about a patient being transferred to the care of another health care professional. This tool ensures that all pertinent information required is up to date and available on one piece of paper as a reference for the person taking charge of the patient's care (AHRQ, 2015).

Transfer from the ICU

Eventually, all patients with some form of recovery will be discharged from the ICU. This usually occurs after morning provider rounds, when it is decided the patient is well enough to leave the unit for a lower level of care, such as a progressive care/step-down unit or other appropriate nursing unit. However, the need for ICU beds in the United States remains high, and many times, the least ill patient in the ICU is transferred later in the day to make room for someone more critically ill. This frequently happens late in the day or at night, when floor nursing staff levels are lower. It has been found that transfer from the ICU later than 6 PM is associated with readmission to the ICU and increased mortality (Dashiell, 2014). While the decision to transfer a patient is a medical and administrative one, nurses must either advocate for their patients to stay in the ICU or put their patients in the best position to do well outside of the ICU. Doing well outside of the ICU is the goal for all patients.

CHAPTER REVIEW

Critical Thinking Exercises

1. You have received a shift report that your patient, who sustained a femur fracture in a motor vehicle accident, is alert and oriented. Upon your initial assessment, you find the patient agitated and confused. What are some possible causes of this change in mental status?

2. Your patient with congestive heart failure is intubated with a pulmonary artery catheter in place. Your catheter measurements are very different from the measurements taken during the last shift. What are some possible reasons for these differences?

3. Your patient, admitted 14 days ago with respiratory failure, is unable to wean from the ventilator. What are possible causes of his inability to wean from this respiratory support?

NCLEX-Style Review Questions

1. A patient who is an IV drug user has had surgery to fix a broken femur after a motor vehicle accident (MVA). She requests morphine sulfate for pain control every hour, although it is ordered for every 3 hours. What is the nurse's most appropriate response?
   a. Tell her she can only have morphine every 3 hours.
   b. Tell her she is making her addiction stronger.
   c. Give her an extra dose of morphine anyway.
   d. Notify the provider of the patient's request for more frequent pain medication.

2. The nurse is caring for a 72-year-old patient admitted with pneumonia and using a nasal cannula. During the first assessment, the nurse finds the O_2 saturation is 87%. What action will the nurse take first?
   a. Continue the physical assessment.
   b. Increase oxygen by providing an oxygen mask.
   c. Call the provider.
   d. Check to see if the oxygen is actually flowing and the tubing is not kinked.

3. A patient, who underwent a total gastrectomy due to cancer, has just arrived from the operating room. The patient has a Salem sump tube (SST; double-lumen NG tube) in place. Care of this patient and the SST tube include which of the following actions? Select all that apply.
   a. Placing the SST to low continuous wall suction
   b. Frequent and vigorous flushing of the NG tube to ensure patency
   c. Placing a sign at the head of the bed reminding staff not to alter the tube's position
   d. Ensuring the NG tube is securely taped to the patient's nose and noting measurement in the plan of care
   e. Head of bed should be flat to facilitate drainage

4. The nurse knows that the inability to wean from a ventilator is associated with which of the following laboratory or diagnostic studies?
   a. Albumin level of 4.0 g/dL
   b. Tidal volume of 7 mL/kg
   c. Normal sinus rhythm
   d. Negative inspiratory force (NIF) of –15 cm H_2O

5. The nurse knows that complications associated with bed rest include which of the following? Select all that apply.
   a. Hypertension
   b. Constipation
   c. Decubitus ulcer
   d. Kidney stones
   e. Venous stasis

Try these additional resources, available at **http://thepoint.lww.com/Honan2e**, to enhance your learning and understanding of this chapter:
• NCLEX-Style Student Review Questions
• Journal Articles

REFERENCES AND SELECTED READINGS

References and selected readings associated with this chapter can be found on the website that accompanies the book. Visit **http://thepoint. lww.com/Honan2e** to access the references and other additional resources associated with this chapter.

Nursing Management: Emergencies and Disasters

Deborah S. Adelman

Learning Objectives

After reading this chapter, you will be able to:

1. Discuss priority emergency measures instituted for any patient with an urgent condition.
2. Describe primary and secondary survey content and assessment of the emergency patient.
3. Discuss the priorities and assessment of the trauma patient.
4. Describe the fundamental elements of a hospital disaster plan.
5. Discuss how triage in a disaster differs from triage in an emergency.
6. Evaluate the different levels of personal protection and decontamination procedures that may be necessary during an event involving mass casualties or weapons of mass destruction.
7. Identify the effects of chemical and nerve agents, and the decontamination and treatment procedures that are necessary.

The emergency nurse has had specialized education, training, experience, and expertise in assessing and identifying patients' health care problems in crisis situations. The emergency nurse establishes priorities, monitors and continuously assesses patients of all ages who are acutely ill and injured, supports and attends to families, supervises allied health personnel, and teaches patients and families within a time-limited, high-pressured care environment. An additional component of emergency nursing is providing care during disasters, when local resources are overwhelmed.

EMERGENCY NURSING

The nursing process provides a logical framework for problem solving in the emergency department (ED). Patients in the ED have a wide variety of actual or potential problems, and their condition may change constantly. Therefore, nursing assessment must be continuous, and nursing diagnoses must adjust with the patient's condition.

Emergency nursing requires an understanding of triage and assessment and management of common acute disorders and injuries.

FOUNDATIONS OF EMERGENCY NURSING

Triage

Triage is used to sort patients into groups based on the severity of their health problems and the immediacy with which these problems must be treated. All EDs share this characteristic of a hierarchy based on the potential for loss of life. A basic and widely used triage system that was in use for many years consisted of three categories: **emergent**, **urgent**, and **nonurgent** (The ESI Triage Research Team, LLC, 2012; Box 56-1). In this acuity system that was used previously, patients who may have needed many resources yet had a lower acuity need might have been assigned a lower triage level, which did not reflect the care they needed. Additionally, the three-category system did not address issues such as managing patient flow in EDs or issues of overcrowding and wait time, and did not demonstrate consistent reliability and validity.

A more refined comprehensive triage system has been implemented to incorporate the changes in the use of the ED for both emergency and routine health care. The most effective triage systems are simple and require no complex

Traditional Triage Acuity System

Three categories:
- *Emergent:* Patients with the highest priority or life-threatening conditions
- *Urgent:* Patients with serious health problems that are not considered immediately life-threatening
- *Nonurgent:* Patients who do not have life-threatening illnesses

A fourth class was incorporated, termed "fast-track," and includes patients that require simple first aid or basic primary care and may be treated in the emergency department or safely referred to a clinic or health provider's office.

scoring methodology. A four-level system is commonly used in the United States:

1. **Immediate (I—red):** Patients have life-threatening injuries that probably are survivable with immediate treatment. Examples are tension pneumothorax, respiratory distress, major external hemorrhage, and airway injuries. Ideally, with limited resources, the only patients categorized as red will be those who would benefit from immediate short-duration treatment and then could be retriaged as yellow.
2. **Delayed (II—yellow):** Patients require definitive treatment, but no immediate threat to life exists. Patients can wait for treatment without jeopardy. Examples include minor extremity fractures, laceration with hemorrhage controlled, and burns over less than 25% of body surface area.
3. **Minimal (III—green):** Patients have minimal injuries, are ambulatory, and can self-treat or seek alternative medical attention independently. Examples include minor lacerations, contusions, and abrasions.
4. **Expectant (0—black):** Patients have lethal injuries and usually will die despite treatment. Examples include devastating head injuries, major third-degree burns over most of the body, and destruction of vital organs. Retriage of this group may be done as resources become available (Starr, Allen, & Stewart, 2011).

The increased number of triage levels assists the triage nurse to more precisely determine the needs of the patient and the urgency for treatment. There are alternative triage systems that are used in the United States, therefore the nurse should follow institutional policies. For example, the Emergency Severity Index (ESI) has been endorsed by the American College of Emergency Physicians and the Emergency Nurses Association; it is a five-level triage algorithm that considers the patient's clinical presentation, vital signs, and the amount and type of resources (examples include laboratory, IV hydration, radiologic studies, simple or complex procedures, medications, consultation, etc.) needed to treat the patient (The ESI Triage Research

Team, LLC, 2012). Nurses in the triage area collect baseline data: full vital signs including pain assessment, history of the current event and medical history, current medications, brief behavioral/mental status assessment, height, weight, allergies, and system review with a focus on the presenting complaint and clinical presentation. These data are recorded for reference by all health care team members treating the patient. Common assessment data are outlined in Box 56-2.

Primary and Secondary Surveys

A systematic approach to effectively establishing and treating health priorities is the primary survey/secondary survey approach. The primary survey focuses on stabilizing life-threatening conditions. The ED staff work collaboratively and follow the CABD (circulation, airway, breathing, disability) method:

- Evaluate and restore cardiac output by controlling hemorrhage, preventing and treating shock, and maintaining or restoring effective circulation, including the prevention and management of hypothermia.
- Establish a patent airway.
- Provide adequate ventilation, employing resuscitation measures when necessary. Protection of cervical spine in trauma patients is mandatory when ventilating and resuscitation measures are needed.

Data Collected by the Triage Nurse

- Patient's presenting complaint of illness or injury
- Level of pain
- Level of consciousness
- Circumstances, precipitating events, location, and time of the injury or illness
- Treatment of injury or illness prior to arrival in the emergency department (ED)
- Method of arrival to ED
- Physician or health practitioner seen for nonemergent care
- Health status prior to injury or illness
- History of medical illness and previous surgeries
- Previous hospitalizations
- Allergies including medications, eggs, latex, nuts, etc.
- Current medications
- Use of recreational drugs
- Smoking history
- Evaluation of immunizations for currency (tetanus)
- Brief assessment of body systems, including behavioral health screening for depression or suicidal ideation
- Last menstrual period (females of childbearing age)
- Time of last meal or oral intake
- Focused assessment on system involved with presenting complaint
- Special circumstances or requests of patient, especially those related to limitations regarding treatments (i.e., resuscitation status or refusal of blood products)

- Determine neurologic disability by assessing neurologic function using the Glasgow Coma Scale (see Box 45-6 in Chapter 45). Evaluate for spinal cord injury if indicated.

After these priorities have been addressed, the ED team proceeds with the secondary survey. This includes the following:

- A complete health history and head-to-toe assessment
- Diagnostic and laboratory testing
- Insertion or application of monitoring devices, such as electrocardiogram (ECG) electrodes, arterial lines, or urinary catheters
- Splinting of suspected fractures
- Cleansing, closure, and dressing of wounds
- Performance of other necessary interventions based on the patient's condition

Unfolding Patient Stories: Carl Shapiro • Part 2

Recall from Chapter 14 Carl Shapiro, who was diagnosed with hypertension and hyperlipidemia during a routine visit to his primary care provider. He arrives in the ED with a blood pressure of 210/110. The nurse discovers that he stopped his antihypertensive medication due to erectile dysfunction. How does the nurse maintain patient privacy in the ED during discussion of personal issues? What topics should be included in an individualized discharge plan to address his concerns, educational needs, and continuity of care when the nurse receives orders for an ACE inhibitor, captopril (Capoten), and discharge home?

Care for Carl and other patients in a realistic virtual environment: *vSim for Nursing* (thepoint.lww.com/vSimMedicalSurgical). Practice documenting these patients' care in DocuCare (thepoint.lww.com/DocuCareEHR).

CARING FOR LIFE-THREATENING CONDITIONS

Emergency nurses often confront airway obstruction and hemorrhage. These conditions are life-threatening and require immediate intervention to prevent death.

AIRWAY OBSTRUCTION

Acute upper airway obstruction is a life-threatening medical emergency. The airway may be partially or completely occluded. Partial obstruction of the airway can lead to progressive hypoxia, hypercarbia (increased carbon dioxide levels in the blood), and respiratory and cardiac arrest. If the airway is completely obstructed, permanent brain injury or death will occur within 3 to 5 minutes, secondary to hypoxia. Air movement is absent in the presence of complete airway obstruction. Oxygen saturation of the blood decreases rapidly because the obstructed airway prevents entry of air into the lungs. Oxygen deficit occurs in the brain, resulting in unconsciousness, with death following rapidly.

Causes

Upper airway obstruction has a number of causes, including aspiration of foreign bodies, anaphylaxis, viral or bacterial infection, trauma, and inhalation or chemical burns. For elderly patients, especially those in extended-care facilities, sedatives and hypnotic medications, diseases affecting motor coordination (e.g., Parkinson disease), and mental dysfunction (e.g., dementia, mental retardation) are risk factors for asphyxiation by food. In adults, aspiration of a bolus of meat is the most common cause of airway obstruction. In children, small toys, buttons, coins, and other objects are commonly aspirated in addition to food. Peritonsillar abscesses, epiglottitis, and other acute infectious processes of the posterior pharynx can also result in airway obstruction.

> ⚠️ **Nursing Alert**
> *The nurse listens for severe stridor (loud, harsh, vibratory sound of variable pitch); if present and the patient has a persistent pulse, suspicion of aspiration of a foreign body or food should be considered. If this is suspected, a Heimlich maneuver (see Box 56-3) may dislodge the obstructing body.*

Clinical Manifestations and Assessment

Typically, a person with a foreign-body airway obstruction cannot speak, breathe, or cough. The patient may clutch the neck between the thumb and fingers (this is known as the *universal distress signal*). Other common signs and symptoms include choking, apprehensive appearance, inspiratory and expiratory stridor, labored breathing, use of accessory muscles (suprasternal and intercostal retraction), flaring nostrils, increasing anxiety, restlessness, and confusion. Cyanosis and loss of consciousness develop as hypoxia worsens.

Assessment of the patient who has a foreign object occluding the airway may involve simply asking the person whether he or she is choking and requires help. If the person is unconscious, inspection of the oropharynx may reveal the offending object. X-rays, laryngoscopy, or bronchoscopy also may be required.

If the patient can breathe and cough spontaneously, a partial obstruction should be suspected.

Medical and Nursing Management

For partial obstruction, the patient is encouraged to cough forcefully and to persist with spontaneous coughing and breathing efforts as long as adequate air exchange exists. Oxygen saturation should be monitored to evaluate oxygenation. Supplemental oxygen should be administered. There may be some wheezing between coughs. If the patient demonstrates a

Managing a Foreign-Body Airway Obstruction

Heimlich Maneuver (Subdiaphragmatic Abdominal Thrusts)

For conscious patient (sitting or standing):

1. Stand behind the patient and wrap your arms around the patient's waist. If the victim is shorter than the rescuer, the rescuer may kneel behind the victim.
2. Make a fist with one hand.
3. Place the thumb side of the fist against the victim's abdomen, in the midline slightly above the navel and well below the breastbone.
4. Grasp your fist with the other hand and press your fist into the victim's abdomen with a quick upward thrust.
5. Repeat thrusts until the object is expelled from the airway or the victim becomes unresponsive.
6. Give each new thrust with a separate and distinct movement to relieve the obstruction.
   Abdominal thrusts may be performed if the choking victim is responsive and lying down.

Chest Thrusts

For the patient who is conscious and sitting or standing and in advanced stages of pregnancy or markedly obese:

1. Stand behind the patient with your arms under the patient's axillae to encircle the patient's chest.
2. Place the thumb side of your fist on the middle of the patient's sternum, taking care to avoid the xiphoid process and the margins of the rib cage.
3. Grasp your fist with the other hand and perform backward thrusts until the foreign body is expelled or the patient becomes unconscious. Each thrust should be administered with the intent of relieving the obstruction.

Unresponsive Choking, Adult Choking Victim Lying Down

If the choking victim becomes unresponsive, begin the sequence of cardiopulmonary resuscitation (CPR) by calling for support (or activating the emergency response system in a nonhospital setting). When opening the airway to deliver rescue breaths, open the victim's mouth wide, look for any foreign bodies, and remove any objects that can be seen. Be careful not to push any objects deeper into the airway. A blind finger sweep to search for foreign objects is not recommended. If the airway remains obstructed, reposition head and attempt to deliver rescue breaths a second time. Begin compressions and continue with advanced life support measures.

Adapted from American Heart Association (AHA). (2016). *Part 5: Adult basic life support.* Retrieved July 11, 2015 from http://circ.ahajournals.org/content/122/18_suppl_3/S685.full

weak, ineffective cough, a high-pitched noise while inhaling, increased respiratory difficulty, or cyanosis, he should be managed as if there were complete airway obstruction.

After the obstruction is removed, rescue breathing is initiated if the patient has absent or inadequate respiratory effort. If the patient has no pulse, cardiac compressions are instituted. These measures provide oxygen to the brain, heart, and other vital organs until definitive medical treatment can restore and support normal heart and ventilatory activity.

Establishing an Airway

Establishing an airway may be as simple as repositioning the patient's head to prevent the tongue from obstructing the pharynx. Alternatively, other maneuvers, such as abdominal thrusts (also called subdiaphragmatic abdominal thrusts), the head-tilt–chin-lift maneuver, the jaw-thrust maneuver, or insertion of specialized equipment, may be needed to open the airway, remove a foreign body, or maintain the airway. Box 56-3 provides guidelines for performing the Heimlich maneuver and abdominal and chest thrusts. In all maneuvers, the cervical spine must be protected from injury. After these maneuvers are performed, the patient is assessed for breathing by watching for chest movement and listening and feeling for air movement.

The head-tilt–chin-lift maneuver is used only if there is no suspected injury to the cervical spine. It is performed as follows:

- The patient is placed supine on a firm, flat surface.
- If the patient is lying face down, the body is turned as a unit so that the head, shoulders, and torso move simultaneously with no twisting. This requires a minimum of two, preferably three staff members.
- Next, the airway is opened using either the head-tilt–chin-lift maneuver or the jaw-thrust maneuver:
  - In the head-tilt–chin-lift maneuver, one hand is placed on the victim's forehead, and firm backward pressure is applied with the palm to tilt the head back. This will move the tongue forward (away from the back of the throat). The fingers of the other hand are placed under the bony part of the lower jaw (mandible) near the chin, and gently lifted up (Fig. 56-1). The chin and the teeth are lifted so that the teeth are almost brought together.
  - In the jaw-thrust maneuver, after one hand is placed on each side of the patient's jaw, the angles of the patient's lower jaw are grasped and lifted, displacing the mandible forward. This is a safe approach to opening the airway of a patient with suspected neck injury because it can be accomplished without extending the neck.

Oropharyngeal Airway

An oropharyngeal airway is a semicircular tube or tube-like plastic device that is inserted over the back of the tongue into

FIGURE 56-1 The head-tilt–chin-lift maneuver. (LifeART image (© 2010). Lippincott Williams & Wilkins. All rights reserved.)

FIGURE 56-2 Endotracheal intubation in a patient without a cervical spine injury. **A.** The primary glottis landmarks for tracheal intubation as visualized with proper placement of the laryngoscope. **B.** Positioning the endotracheal tube.

the lower posterior pharynx in a patient who is breathing spontaneously but who is unconscious. This type of airway prevents the tongue from falling back against the posterior pharynx and obstructing the airway. It also allows health care providers to suction secretions. It should be reserved for unconscious patients without gag reflex. A nasopharyngeal airway is tolerated better by patients who are not deeply unconscious, but it should be avoided in patients with craniofacial trauma (Carlson & Wang, 2016). (See Box 56-4.)

Intubation

Endotracheal intubation is used to establish and maintain the airway in patients with respiratory insufficiency or hypoxia. Endotracheal intubation is indicated for the following reasons: (1) to establish an airway for a patient who cannot be adequately ventilated with an oropharyngeal airway, (2) to bypass an upper airway obstruction, (3) to prevent aspiration, (4) to permit connection of the patient to a resuscitation bag or mechanical ventilator, and (5) to facilitate the removal of tracheobronchial secretions. Because the procedure requires skill, endotracheal intubation is performed only by those who have had extensive training. However, the emergency nurse is commonly called on to assist with intubation (Fig. 56-2).

If the patient is not hospitalized and cannot be intubated in the field, emergency medical personnel may insert an esophagotracheal airway (The ESI Triage Research Team, LLC, 2012). The tube rapidly provides pharyngeal ventilation and is used in conjunction with a bag-valve mask for ventilation. When the tube is inserted into the trachea, it functions like an endotracheal tube (Fig. 56-3).

FIGURE 56-3 **A.** Combitube in esophageal position. **B.** Combitube in tracheal position. Note: Combitube is one type of esophageal tracheal airway available on the market.

BOX 56-4

GUIDELINES FOR NURSING CARE

Inserting an Oropharyngeal Airway

Equipment

- Oropharyngeal airway
- Nonsterile gloves
- Protective eyewear if secretions are profuse or patient is coughing
- Equipment for suctioning

Implementation

ACTION	RATIONALE
1. Insert only in an unconscious patient who does not have a gag reflex with a risk of airway occlusion and no cervical spine injury, oral trauma, or recent oral surgery.	1. An oropharyngeal airway can prevent the tongue from occluding the airway against the posterior pharynx in an unconscious patient. Patients with known or suspected cervical spine injury may require emergent intubation for airway protection and ventilatory support. It is only used in an unconscious patient since vomiting and laryngospasm may be stimulated by the airway in a conscious or semi-conscious patient. Oral trauma, recent oral surgery may be a contraindication to inserting an oropharyngeal airway.
2. Remove dentures if present before insertion.	2. Remove dentures to prevent them from causing an airway obstruction.
3. Measure the oral airway alongside the head. Correct size of the airway should extend from the corner of the mouth to the tip of the earlobe (Reardon, Mason, & Clinton, 2014).	3. Accurate measurement is needed to ensure the airway is appropriately sized to prevent the tongue from occluding the airway.
4. Extend the patient's head by placing one hand under the bony chin. With the other hand, tilt the head backward by applying pressure to the forehead while simultaneously lifting the chin forward. Open the patient's mouth.	4. When positioning the head for insertion, the head may be tilted back *only* if the patient has had the cervical spine cleared. In the patient with a potential cervical spine injury, use only the jaw-thrust maneuver to aid in positioning the head for airway insertion. Position facilitates insertion.
5. **(A)** Insert the oropharyngeal airway with the tip facing up toward the roof of the mouth until it passes the uvula. **(B)** Rotate the tip 180 degrees so that the tip is pointed down toward the pharynx.	5. This displaces the tongue anteriorly, and the patient then breathes through and around the airway.

| 6. Ensure the distal end of the oropharyngeal airway is in the hypopharynx and the flange is approximately at the patient's lips. Make sure that the tongue has not been pushed into the airway. | 6. An incorrectly placed airway can itself cause airway obstruction by pushing the tongue posteriorly into the hypopharynx. |

The two balloons that surround the tube are inflated after the tube is inserted. One balloon is large (100 mL) and occludes the oropharynx. This permits ventilation by forcing air through the larynx. The smaller balloon is inflated with 15 mL of air and can occlude the trachea if it is inadvertently placed there (Sethi, Desai, Tyagi, & Kumar, 2014). Breath sounds are auscultated after balloon inflation to make sure that the oropharyngeal balloon (or cuff) does not obstruct the glottis. The patient can be ventilated through either one of the two ports (e.g., tracheal or esophageal) of the tube, depending on whether the tube is placed in the trachea or esophagus.

Cricothyroidotomy

Cricothyroidotomy is the opening of the cricothyroid membrane to establish an airway. This procedure is used in emergency situations in which endotracheal intubation is either not possible or contraindicated, as in patients with airway obstruction from extensive maxillofacial trauma, cervical spine injuries, laryngospasm, laryngeal edema (after an allergic reaction or extubation), hemorrhage into neck tissue, or obstruction of the larynx.

Maintaining the Airway

After the airway is determined to be unobstructed, the nurse must ensure that adequate ventilation is maintained. Satisfactory management of ventilations may prevent hypoxia and hypercapnia. The nurse must quickly assess for absent or diminished breath sounds as well as difficulty delivering artificial breaths for the patient. The nurse should monitor pulse oximetry, capnography (monitoring of the amount of exhaled carbon dioxide), and arterial blood gases (ABGs) if the patient requires airway or ventilatory assistance.

The nurse is aware that a tension pneumothorax can mimic hypovolemia, so ventilatory assessment precedes assessment for hemorrhage. A pneumothorax or sucking (open) chest wound is managed with a chest tube; immediate relief of the increasing positive intrapleural pressure (normally, the intrapleural pressure is negative) and maintenance of adequate ventilation should occur (refer to Chapter 10 for information on pneumothorax and chest tube insertion and management).

> **Nursing Alert**
> *Trauma patients are kept on a stretcher to immobilize the spine. A backboard may be used for transporting the patient to the x-ray department, to the operating room, or to the intensive care unit. Cervical spine immobilization is maintained until cervical x-rays have been obtained and cervical spine injury has been ruled out. Ongoing neurologic examinations to assess for spinal cord impairment and change in level of consciousness (LOC) are essential.*

HEMORRHAGE

Stopping bleeding is essential to the care and survival of patients in an emergency or disaster situation. Hemorrhage that results in the reduction of circulating blood volume is a primary cause of shock (see Chapter 54). Minor bleeding, which is usually venous, generally stops spontaneously unless the patient has a bleeding disorder or has been taking anticoagulants.

Clinical Manifestations and Assessment

The patient is assessed for signs and symptoms of shock: cool, moist skin (resulting from poor peripheral perfusion), decreasing blood pressure, decreasing pulse pressure, increasing heart rate, delayed capillary refill, and decreasing urine volume. These criteria are associated with an estimated blood loss of approximately 1,500 to 2,000 mL or 30% to 40% of blood volume; the nurse should assess for the earliest symptom of blood loss: increasing anxiety. Refer to Table 56-1 for estimated fluid and blood losses.

> **Nursing Alert**
> *If the patient is hemorrhaging, the nurse understands that the Trendelenburg position does not improve cardiopulmonary status, and it may predispose the patient to aspiration and worsening pulmonary gas exchange, as well as increasing intracranial pressures. The supine position with passive leg-raising above the level of the heart may be effective. If passive leg-raising results in an increase in blood pressure or cardiac output (CO), then fluid resuscitation is indicated (Nickes & Gaillard, 2016).*

Medical and Nursing Management

The goals of emergency management for patients with blood loss are to control bleeding, maintain adequate circulating blood volume for tissue oxygenation, and prevent shock. Patients who hemorrhage are at risk for cardiac arrest caused by hypovolemia with secondary anoxia; therefore, continuous ECG monitoring is expected. Nursing interventions are carried out collaboratively with other members of the emergency health care team.

Fluid Replacement

Whenever a patient is experiencing hemorrhage—whether external or internal—a loss of circulating blood results in a fluid volume deficit and decreased CO. Therefore, fluid replacement is imperative to maintain circulation. Typically, two large-gauge IV catheters are inserted to provide a means for fluid and blood replacement, and blood samples are obtained for analysis, typing, and cross-matching. Replacement fluids are administered as prescribed, depending on

TABLE **56-1** Classes of Hemorrhagic Shock

Class I Hemorrhage: Loss of up to 15% of Blood Volume (up to 750 mL in 70-kg Adult)	Class II Hemorrhage: Loss of 15–30% of Blood Volume (750–1,500 mL)	Class III Hemorrhage: Loss of 30–40% of Blood Volume (1,500–2,000 mL)	Class IV Hemorrhage: Loss of over 40% of Blood Volume (more than 2,000 mL)
Heart rate (HR) less than 100	HR greater than 100	HR greater than 120	HR greater than 140
Systolic blood pressure (BP) normal	Systolic BP normal	Systolic BP decreased	Systolic BP markedly decreased
Respiratory rate (RR) 14–20	RR 20–30	RR 30–40	RR greater than 35
Increased or normal pulse pressure	Decreased pulse pressure	Decreased pulse pressure	Very narrow pulse pressure
Slight anxiety	Mildly anxious	Significant change in mental status: anxiety or confusion	Depressed mental status: confusion, lethargy, loss of consciousness
30 mL/hr	Small decrease in urine output (20–30 mL/hr)	Marked decrease in urine output (5–15 mL/hr)	Negligible urine output

Adapted from Chan, T. (2014). Hemorrhagic shock. In J. J. Schaider, A. Z. Barkin, R. M. Barkin, R. E. Wolfe, P. Shayne, & S. R. Hayden (Eds.), *Rosen & Barkin's 5-minute emergency medicine consult* (5th ed.). Philadelphia, PA: Lippincott Williams & Wilkins.

clinical estimates of the type and volume of fluid lost. Replacement fluids may include isotonic electrolyte solutions (lactated Ringer's, normal saline), colloids, and blood component therapy.

Packed red blood cells (PRBCs) are infused when there is massive blood loss. In emergencies, if typed and cross-matched blood is not available, then reserve type O-negative blood for females younger than 50 years of age; all others should receive type O-positive. In a situation with a patient requiring resuscitation with massive blood loss, there is no time to type and cross-match or type and screen blood. Type O-negative blood provides safe administration of blood immediately without sensitizing an Rh-negative woman to Rh-positive blood (sensitization can result in neonatal complications during a later pregnancy). Promoting homeostasis and restoring tissue oxygenation is necessary as fast as possible. However, PRBCs will not aid greatly in these processes if plasma and platelets are not also infused.

Once the hemorrhage is controlled, transfusion should cease when the hemoglobin concentration is greater than 10 g/dL (greater than 100 g/L). "Consensus recommendations for transfusion are a hemoglobin concentration between 6 and 7 g/dL (60 to 70 g/L) for those without cardiopulmonary, cerebral, or peripheral vascular disease. [When the hemoglobin is] between 6 and 10 g/dL (60 to 100 g/L), use clinical judgement for transfusion" (Somand & Ward, 2016, para 1). Additional platelets and clotting factors are given when large amounts of blood are needed because transfused PRBCs are deficient in clotting factors. These additional products are given based on the results of coagulation studies that suggest a platelet or clotting deficiency.

Controlling Blood Loss

If a patient is hemorrhaging externally (e.g., from a wound), a rapid physical assessment is performed as the patient's clothing is cut away in an attempt to identify the area of hemorrhage. Direct, firm pressure is applied over the bleeding area or the involved artery at a site that is proximal to (above) the wound (Fig. 56-4). Most bleeding can be stopped or at least controlled by application of direct pressure. Otherwise, unchecked arterial bleeding results in death. A firm pressure dressing is applied, and the injured part is elevated to stop venous and capillary bleeding if possible. If the injured area is an extremity, the extremity is immobilized to control blood loss.

Nursing Alert
In the event of amputated fingers or extremities, the nurse is aware that the body part should be wrapped with a moist, sterile, protective dressing, placed in a waterproof bag, and then placed in a container of ice water for preservation in the event that future reattachment is possible (Singer & Hollander, 2016). It is important to note that the amputated limb should never be placed in ice or water directly as serious cellular damage may occur.

A tourniquet is applied to an extremity only as a *last resort* when the external hemorrhage cannot be controlled in any other way and immediate surgery is not feasible. Care must be taken when applying a tourniquet because of the risk for loss of the extremity. The tourniquet is applied just proximal to the wound and tied tightly enough to control arterial blood flow. Documentation of the application of the

A Temporal   **B** Facial   **C** Carotid

D Subclavian   **E** Brachial

F Radial and ulnar

G Femoral

FIGURE 56-4 Pressure points for control of hemorrhage.

tourniquet is critical so that all providers are aware of the time and placement; suggestions include flow sheet documentation, use of a skin-marking pencil or adhesive tape on the forehead with a "T," labeling the location of the tourniquet and application time. If there is no arterial bleeding, the tourniquet is removed and a pressure dressing is applied. **In general, tourniquets should not be used for more than 30 minutes (Singer & Hollander, 2016).** If the patient has suffered a traumatic amputation with uncontrollable hemorrhage, the tourniquet remains in place until the patient is in the operating room.

If the patient shows no external signs of bleeding but exhibits tachycardia, falling blood pressure, thirst, apprehension, cool and moist skin, or delayed capillary refill, internal hemorrhage is suspected. Typically, PRBCs are administered at a rapid rate, and the patient is prepared for more definitive treatment (e.g., surgery, endoscopy, pharmacologic therapy). In addition, laboratory specimens, including complete blood count (CBC), electrolytes, coagulation studies, type and cross-match, and ABG specimens, are obtained to evaluate pulmonary function and tissue perfusion and to establish baseline hemodynamic parameters, which are then used as an index for determining the amount of fluid replacement the patient can tolerate and the response to therapy. The patient is maintained in the supine position and monitored closely

until hemodynamic or circulatory parameters improve or until he or she is transported for definitive therapy or continued treatment.

Failure to provide adequate fluid resuscitation and definitely control the source of hemorrhage may lead to hypovolemic (hemorrhagic) shock. It is the most common cause of postinjury death and should be suspected in any patient with hypotensive trauma until proven otherwise (Cowell & Moore, 2014). Hypovolemic shock should be anticipated in any emergency situation in which profound blood or fluid (vomiting or diarrhea) loss has occurred. The goals of treatment are to restore and maintain tissue perfusion and to correct physiologic abnormalities. Chapter 54 provides detailed information on the management of hypovolemic shock.

Ongoing nursing surveillance of the *total patient* is maintained. Blood pressure, heart and respiratory rates, skin temperature, color, pulse oximetry, neurologic status, central venous pressure (CVP), ABGs, ECG recordings, hematocrit, hemoglobin, coagulation profile, electrolytes, and urinary output are monitored serially to assess patient response to treatment. Commonly, a flow sheet is used to document these parameters, providing an analysis of trends rather than single values to reveal improvement or deterioration of the patient's condition.

In addition, the body's defense mechanisms are supported. The patient should be reassured and comforted. Sedation may be used judiciously to relieve apprehension. Analgesics are used cautiously to relieve pain. Body temperature is maintained within normal limits to prevent increasing metabolic demands that the body may be unable to meet. Administration of large volumes of IV crystalloids, blood products, or both can result in hypothermia. Hypothermia may be prevented by warming the fluids before they are administered.

CARING FOR TRAUMA

Trauma (an unintentional or intentional wound or injury inflicted on the body from a mechanism against which the body cannot protect itself) is the fourth leading cause of death in the United States (Centers for Disease Control and Prevention [CDC], 2015a). Alcohol and drug abuse are often implicated as factors in both blunt and penetrating trauma.

In assessing and managing any patient with an emergency condition, but especially the patient experiencing trauma, documentation, including descriptions of all wounds, mechanism of injury, and time of events, as well as collection of evidence are essential. In trauma care, the nurse must be exceedingly careful with all potential evidence, handling and documenting it properly.

The basics of care management for patients with traumatic injury include an understanding that trauma in any patient (living or dead) has potential legal or forensic implications if criminal activity is suspected. Hence, proper management

Collection of Forensic Evidence

When clothing is removed from the patient who has experienced trauma, the nurse must be careful not to cut through or disrupt any tears, holes, blood stains, or dirt present on the clothing if criminal activity is suspected. Each piece of clothing should be placed in an individual paper bag. If the clothing is wet, it should be hung to dry. Clothing should not be given to families. Valuables should be placed in the hospital safe or clearly documented as to which family member they were given. If a police officer is present to collect clothing or any other items from the patient, each item is labeled. The transfer of custody to the officer, the officer's name, the date, and the time are documented.

If suicide or homicide is suspected in a trauma patient who is deceased, the medical examiner examines the body on site or has the body moved to the coroner's office for autopsy. All tubes and lines must remain in place. The patient's hands must be covered with paper bags to protect evidence on the hands or under the fingernails. In the patient who survives, tissue specimens may be swabbed from the hands and nails as potential evidence. Photographs of wounds or clothing are essential and should include a reference ruler in one photo and one photo without the ruler.

Documentation should also include any statements made by the patient in the patient's own words and surrounded by quotation marks. A chain of evidence is essential. If the patient's case is adjudicated in the future, clear documentation assists the judicial process and helps to identify the activities that occurred in the emergency department.

from both a medical and forensic perspective is essential. Box 56-5 describes collection of evidence.

Multiple trauma is caused by a single catastrophic event that causes life-threatening injuries to at least two distinct organs or organ systems. Mortality in patients with multiple trauma is related to the severity of the injuries and the number of systems and organs involved. Immediately after injury, the body is hypermetabolic, hypercoagulable, and severely stressed.

Care of the patient with multiple injuries requires a team approach, with one person responsible for coordinating the treatment. The nursing staff assumes responsibility for assessing and monitoring the patient, ensuring airway and IV access, administering prescribed medications, collecting laboratory specimens, and documenting activities and the patient's response.

Gross evidence of trauma may be slight or absent. Patients with multiple traumatic injuries should be assumed to have a spinal cord injury until it is proven otherwise. The injury regarded as the least significant in appearance may be the most lethal. For example, the pelvis fracture not identified until an x-ray is obtained may be the injury from which the patient is exsanguinating into the pelvic cavity. Another example is a tension pneumothorax that is insidiously increasing in size, eventually compressing both the

heart and lungs, while the ED team is focused on repair of external lacerations. An obvious amputation of the arm may have already stopped bleeding from the body's normal response of vasoconstriction, despite being an obvious and devastating injury; meanwhile, the patient may be dying from an internal, less visible, injury.

The goals of treatment are to determine the extent of injuries and to establish priorities of treatment. Any injury interfering with a vital physiologic function (e.g., airway, breathing, circulation) is an immediate threat to life and has the highest priority for immediate treatment. Essential life-saving procedures are performed simultaneously by the emergency team. As soon as the patient is resuscitated, clothes are usually cut off, and a rapid physical assessment is performed. Transfer from field management to the ED must be orderly and controlled, with attention given to the verbal report from emergency medical services (EMS). Treatment in a level I trauma center is appropriate for patients experiencing major trauma.

WOUNDS

Wounds involving injury to soft tissues can vary from minor tears to severe crushing injuries. The primary goal of treatment is to restore the physical integrity and function of the injured tissue while minimizing scarring and preventing infection. Proper documentation of the characteristics of the wound, using precise descriptions and correct terminology, is essential. Such information may be needed in the future for forensic evidence. Photographs are helpful because they provide an accurate, visible depiction of the wound. Photographs also become important for exigent wounds (wounds that will heal and later be unidentifiable). Patients involved in domestic violence or trauma may need the photographs later to visually describe the extent of injury.

Determining *when* and *how* the wound occurred is important because a treatment delay increases infection risk. Using aseptic technique, the clinician inspects the wound to determine the extent of damage to underlying structures. Visible contamination of the wound increases the risk of wound infection. Additionally, the nurse is aware that bite wounds carry significant risk for infection owing to the high bacterial colonization in the mouth. Sensory, motor, and vascular function is evaluated for changes that might indicate complications.

Hair around the wound may be clipped if it is anticipated that the hairs will interfere with wound closure. Shaving should be avoided; it may result in an increased incidence of wound infection since many bacteria reside in hair follicles (Tichter, Carter, & Stone, 2016). Complete removal of eyebrow hairs is avoided as regrowth may not occur; clipping eyebrow hair to 1 to 2 mm above the wound is recommended if hair is interfering with wound care.

If indicated, the area is infiltrated with a local intradermal anesthetic through the wound margins or by regional block. Patients with soft tissue injuries usually have localized pain at the site of injury. The nurse then assists the physician, nurse practitioner, or physician's assistant in cleaning and débriding the wound.

Wound cleaning requires the selection of methods that minimize chemical and mechanical trauma to the wound tissue while removing surface debris and contaminants (Slotts, 2015). Typically, the area around the wound is cleansed with normal saline solution or a polymer agent (e.g., Shur-Clens). Antibacterial agents, such as povidone–iodine (Betadine) or chlorhexidine, can be used to paint the intact skin surrounding the wound but should not be allowed to get into the wound since the solutions are associated with decreasing defense mechanisms and thus increase the risk of wound infection. With the emergence of antibiotic resistance, some researchers call for a reappraisal of the use of antiseptic solutions especially in the management of contaminated and infected wounds (Queirós et al., 2013). At present, a standardized regimen for wound cleaning has yet to be established. Nurses should refer to their facility's protocol.

To decrease the incidence of wound infection, the nurse anticipates both the use of wound irrigation and débridement of dead wound tissue. The wound will be irrigated gently and copiously with sterile isotonic saline solution to remove surface dirt. Approximately 50 to 100 mL of saline irrigation per 1 cm of laceration is considered as a general guideline (Nicks, Ayello, Woo, Nitzki-George, & Sibbald, 2010). The nurse ensures that the **personal protective equipment** (PPE) of face shields is utilized. Devitalized tissue and foreign matter are removed by the physician because they impede healing and may encourage infection. Any small bleeding vessels are clamped or tied. Alternatively, hemostasis of small bleeding vessels is achieved by clamping, tying, or cauterization. After wound treatment, a nonadherent dressing is commonly applied to protect the wound. The dressing may serve as a splint and also as a reminder to the patient that the area is injured.

> **Nursing Alert**
> *The nurse is aware that irrigation may be high pressure or low pressure. High-pressure irrigation is used to clear debris and support reduction of infection. It is defined as approximately 7 psi (50 kPa) or greater and is achieved using any combination of a 30- to 65-mL syringe and a 19-gauge catheter or needle hub, or commercially available splashguard, with forceful depression of the syringe piston. Conversely low-pressure irrigation is defined as approximately 0.5 psi (3.5 kPa) or lower and is achieved with a slow, gentle wash. Low-pressure irrigation may be useful in simple, nonbite, uncontaminated wounds in highly vascular areas, such as the scalp and face (Tichter et al., 2016).*

The decision to suture a wound depends on the nature of the wound, the time since the injury was sustained, the degree of contamination, and the vascularity of tissues. If primary closure is indicated, the wound is sutured or stapled, with the patient receiving either local anesthesia or moderate sedation. Sutures are placed near the wound edge, with the skin edges leveled carefully to promote optimal healing. Instead of sutures, sterile strips of reinforced microporous tape or a bonding agent (skin glue) may be used to close clean, superficial wounds.

Delayed primary closure may be indicated if tissue has been lost or there is a high potential for infection. A thin layer of gauze (to ensure drainage and prevent pooling of exudate), covered by an occlusive dressing, may be used. Other options include split-thickness cadaver allografts or porcine xenografts to simulate the function of epithelium. The wound is splinted in a functional position to prevent motion and decrease the possibility of contracture. Use of antibiotics to prevent infection depends on factors such as how the injury occurred, the age of the wound, the risk of contamination, and the presence of risk factors in the patient's medical history that decrease wound healing (diabetes, steroid use, chemotherapeutic agents, chronic kidney failure, peripheral vascular disease, advanced age, anemia, malnourishment). The site is immobilized and elevated to limit accumulation of fluid in the interstitial spaces of the wound.

Tetanus prophylaxis is administered as prescribed, based on the condition of the wound and the patient's immunization status. If the patient's last tetanus booster was given more than 5 years ago, or if the patient's immunization status is unknown, a tetanus booster must be given. The patient is instructed about signs and symptoms of infection and is instructed to contact the health care provider or clinic if there is sudden or persistent pain, fever or chills, bleeding, rapid swelling, foul odor, drainage, or redness surrounding the wound.

INTRA-ABDOMINAL INJURIES

Intra-abdominal injuries are categorized as penetrating or blunt trauma. Penetrating abdominal trauma (e.g., gunshot wounds, stab wounds) results in a high incidence of injury to hollow organs, particularly the small bowel; thus, they are serious and usually require surgery. The liver is the solid organ that is injured most frequently. In gunshot wounds, the most important factor is the velocity at which the missile (bullet) enters the body. The higher the velocity, the more extensive tissue damage is expected. All abdominal gunshot wounds that cross the peritoneum or are associated with peritoneal signs require surgical exploration. On the other hand, stab wounds may be managed nonoperatively. The nurse accurately documents the location and number of wounds. If abdominal viscera protrude, the area is immediately covered with sterile, moist saline dressings to keep the viscera from drying, and the patient is expected to go directly to the operating room for closure.

Blunt trauma to the abdomen may result from motor vehicle crashes, falls, blows, or explosions. Blunt trauma is commonly associated with extra-abdominal injuries to the chest, head, or extremities. Patients with blunt trauma are a challenge because injuries may be difficult to detect. The incidence of delayed and trauma-related complications is greater than that for penetrating injuries. This is especially true of blunt injuries involving the liver, kidneys, spleen, or blood vessels, which can lead to massive blood loss into the peritoneal cavity.

Clinical Manifestations and Assessment

As the history of the traumatic event is obtained, the abdomen is inspected for obvious signs of injury, including penetrating injuries, bruises, and abrasions. Abdominal assessment continues with auscultation of bowel sounds to provide baseline data from which changes can be noted. Absence of bowel sounds may be an early sign of intraperitoneal involvement. Further abdominal assessment may reveal progressive abdominal distention, involuntary guarding, tenderness, pain, muscular rigidity, or rebound tenderness, along with changes in bowel sounds, all of which are signs of peritoneal irritation (refer to Chapter 21 for further details of gastrointestinal [GI] assessment). Hypotension and signs and symptoms of shock may also be noted. Additionally, the chest and other body systems are assessed for injuries that frequently accompany intra-abdominal injuries.

Studies that aid in assessment include the following:

- Urinalysis to detect hematuria (indicative of a urinary tract injury)
- Ultrasound of abdomen to evaluate fluid collection (Focused Assessment with Sonography in Trauma or *FAST*)
- Peritoneal lavage to evaluate abdominal fluid collection
- Radiology and/or computed tomography (CT) scan to evaluate abdominal organ injury, fluid, foreign particles
- Serial hemoglobin and hematocrit levels to evaluate trends reflecting the presence or absence of bleeding; coagulation studies (prothrombin time [PT]; partial thromboplastin time [PTT]; international normalized ratio [INR]); blood typing
- White blood cell (WBC) count to detect elevation (generally associated with trauma)
- Serum amylase analysis to detect increasing levels, which suggest pancreatic injury or perforation of the GI tract

Hemorrhage frequently accompanies abdominal injury, especially if the liver or spleen has been traumatized. Therefore, the patient is assessed continuously for signs and symptoms of external and internal bleeding. The front of the body, flanks, and back are inspected for bluish discoloration, asymmetry, abrasion, and contusion (see Chapter 21 for descriptions of Cullen and Grey–Turner signs). Abdominal CT scans permit detailed evaluation of abdominal contents and retroperitoneal examination. Abdominal ultrasound studies can rapidly assess hemodynamically unstable patients to detect intraperitoneal bleeding. This is referred to as the Focused Assessment for Sonographic Examination in Trauma (FAST) examination.

The nurse suspects hemoperitoneum and splenic injuries if the patient complains of left shoulder pain. This symptom is termed *Kehr sign* and is referred pain due to diaphragmatic irritation associated with the splenic injury or intra-abdominal hemorrhaging. Pain in the right shoulder can result from laceration of the liver. Referred pain is a significant finding because it suggests intraperitoneal injury. The abdomen is assessed for tenderness, rebound tenderness, guarding, rigidity, spasm, increasing distention, and pain. To determine whether there is intraperitoneal injury and bleeding, the patient is usually prepared for diagnostic procedures, such as abdominal ultrasonography, or abdominal CT scanning. FAST has rapidly replaced **diagnostic peritoneal lavage (DPL)**, owing to its sensitivity (90%), specificity (95%), and accuracy (99%) in determining the presence of intra-abdominal fluid (Jang, 2013; Manthey & Nicks, 2008). Additionally, CT scans, because of their speed and detailed results, have largely replaced DPL in the stable patient. However, peritoneal lavage is useful in assessing hollow organ injury or when serial CT scans cannot be performed, as in patients with severe closed head injury or high spinal cord injury. It involves the instillation of 1 L of warmed lactated Ringer's or normal saline solution into the abdominal cavity. After a minimum of 400 mL has been returned, a fluid specimen is sent to the laboratory for analysis. Positive laboratory findings include a red blood cell count greater than $100,000/mm^3$; a WBC count greater than $500/mm^3$; or the presence of bile, feces, or food.

In patients with stab wounds, the nurse anticipates that a surgeon will assess whether the peritoneal space has been punctured. Fluid resuscitation may be required, and if perforation is confirmed, exploration in the operating room is expected. The need for tetanus booster will be evaluated, and antibiotics administration is anticipated.

Medical and Nursing Management

As indicated by the patient's condition, resuscitation procedures (restoration of circulation, airway, and breathing) are initiated. Circulating blood volume is maintained with IV fluid replacement, including blood component therapy, and the nurse monitors the patient's vital signs, oxygen saturation, urinary output, and mentation to detect stabilization or evidence of deterioration. A patent airway is maintained, and attempts to stabilize the respiratory, circulatory, and nervous systems are made. Bleeding is controlled by application of direct pressure to any external, bleeding wounds and by occlusion of any chest wounds.

Typically, when the patient presents with intra-abdominal injuries, oral fluids are withheld in anticipation of surgery, and a nasogastric tube may be inserted to decompress the stomach and reduce the risk of aspiration. Tetanus prophylaxis and broad-spectrum antibiotics are administered as prescribed.

Throughout the stay in the ED, the patient's condition is continuously monitored for changes. If there is continuing evidence of shock, blood loss, free air under the diaphragm, evisceration, hematuria, severe head injury, or suspected or known abdominal injury, the patient is rapidly transported to surgery. In most cases, blunt injuries to the liver and spleen are managed nonsurgically.

CRUSH INJURIES

Crush injuries occur when a person is caught between opposing forces (e.g., run over by a moving vehicle, compressed by machinery, crushed between two cars, crushed under a collapsed building).

Clinical Manifestations and Assessment

The patient is observed for the following:

- Hypovolemic shock resulting from extravasation of blood and plasma into injured tissues after compression has been released
- Paralysis of a body part
- Erythema and blistering of skin
- Damaged body part (usually an extremity) appearing swollen, tense, and hard
- Kidney dysfunction (prolonged hypotension causes kidney damage and acute renal insufficiency; myoglobinuria secondary to muscle damage can cause acute tubular necrosis and acute kidney failure). See Chapter 42, Box 42-7 for pathophysiology of rhabdomyolysis.

Medical and Nursing Management

In conjunction with maintaining the patient's circulation, airway, and breathing, the patient is observed for acute renal insufficiency. Injury to the back can cause severe kidney damage. Severe muscular damage may cause rhabdomyolysis, a significant release of myoglobin from ischemic skeletal muscle, which can result in acute tubular necrosis. In addition, major soft tissue injuries are splinted early to control bleeding and pain. Fluid resuscitation, as discussed previously, is expected and—in addition to stabilization of vital signs, urine output, and hemodynamic parameters—the serum lactic acid level may be monitored as a parameter of

successful resuscitation. Lactic acid levels are discussed in Chapter 55.

If an extremity is injured, it is elevated to relieve swelling and pressure. To restore neurovascular function, the physician may perform a **fasciotomy** (surgical incision to the level of the fascia). Refer to Chapter 42 for details on compartment syndrome. Medications for pain and anxiety are then administered as prescribed, and the patient is quickly transported to the operating suite for wound débridement and fracture repair. A hyperbaric chamber (if available) may be used for hyperoxygenation of the crushed tissue, if indicated.

GENITOURINARY INJURY

A rectal or vaginal examination is performed by the primary care provider to determine injury to the pelvis, bladder, or intestinal wall. To decompress the bladder and monitor urine output, an indwelling catheter is inserted after a visual examination of the genitourinary area and rectal examination has been completed (not before). In the male patient, a high-riding prostate gland (abnormal position) discovered during a rectal examination indicates a potential urethral injury. Refer to Chapter 28 for details on genitourinary trauma.

ANAPHYLACTIC REACTION

An anaphylactic reaction is an acute systemic hypersensitivity reaction that occurs within seconds or minutes after exposure to certain foreign substances, such as medications, and other agents, such as latex, insect stings, or foods. Repeated administration of parenteral or oral therapeutic agents (e.g., repeated exposures to penicillin) may also precipitate an anaphylactic reaction when initially only a mild allergic response occurred. See Chapter 38 for the pathophysiology and clinical manifestations of anaphylaxis.

With an anaphylactic reaction, establishing a patent airway and ventilation is essential. This is performed while another person administers epinephrine. Early endotracheal intubation is essential to preserve airway patency, and oropharyngeal suction may be necessary to remove excessive secretions. Resuscitative measures are used, especially for patients with stridor and progressive pulmonary edema. If glottal edema occurs, emergent cricothyroidotomy may be necessary to provide an airway.

Simultaneously with airway management, aqueous epinephrine is administered as prescribed to provide rapid relief of the hypersensitivity reaction. Epinephrine may be administered again if necessary and as prescribed. Judgment is used in choosing one of the following routes of administration:

- Subcutaneous injection for mild, generalized symptoms
- IM injection when the reaction is more severe and progressive, and with the knowledge that vascular collapse will delay absorption of the medication
- IV route (aqueous epinephrine diluted in saline solution and administered *slowly*), used in rare instances in which

there is complete loss of consciousness and severe cardiovascular collapse. This method may precipitate cardiac arrhythmias, so ECG monitoring with a readily available defibrillator is necessary. This method is controversial and is not usually recommended because it can lead to more distress than initially present. An IV infusion of saline solution is initiated to provide for emergency access to a vein and to treat hypotension.

Additional treatments may include the following:

- Antihistamines (e.g., diphenhydramine [Benadryl]) to block further histamine binding at target cells
- Aminophylline titrated by IV drip for severe bronchospasm and wheezing refractory to other treatment
- Albuterol (Proventil, Ventolin) inhalers or humidified treatments to decrease bronchoconstriction; crystalloids, colloids, or vasopressors to treat prolonged hypotension
- Isoproterenol (Isuprel) or dopamine (Intropin) for reduced cardiac output; oxygen to enhance tissue perfusion
- IV benzodiazepines (e.g., diazepam [Valium]) for control of seizures, and corticosteroids (e.g., hydrocortisone [Solu-Cortef]) for prolonged reaction with persistent hypotension or bronchospasm

Depending on the severity of the acute symptoms, the patient may be admitted to the hospital for observation. The patient should be informed about ways to prevent anaphylactic reactions in the future.

Drug Alert!
Epinephrine results in α- and β-adrenergic effects, resulting in vasoconstriction and bronchial smooth-muscle relaxation. Epinephrine works rapidly to reduce throat swelling, open up the airways, and maintain blood pressure in patients. Age is not a barrier to epinephrine IM injections in patients with anaphylaxis (Boyce & Austen, 2015; Rowe & Gaeta, 2016).

CARING FOR POISONING

A poison is any substance that, when ingested, inhaled, absorbed, applied to the skin, or produced within the body in relatively small amounts, injures the body by its chemical action. Poisoning from inhalation and ingestion of toxic materials, both intentional and unintentional, constitutes a major health hazard and an emergency situation. Emergency treatment is initiated with the following goals:

- To remove or inactivate the poison before it is absorbed
- To provide supportive care in maintaining vital organ systems
- To administer a specific antidote to neutralize a specific poison

- To implement treatment that hastens the elimination of the absorbed poison

INGESTED (SWALLOWED) POISONS

Swallowed poisons may be corrosive. **Corrosive poisons** include alkaline and acid agents that can cause tissue destruction after coming into contact with mucous membranes. Alkaline products include lye, drain cleaners, toilet bowl cleaners, bleach, nonphosphate detergents, oven cleaners, and button batteries (batteries used to power watches, calculators, or cameras). Acid products include toilet bowl cleaners, pool cleaners, metal cleaners, rust removers, and battery acid.

Medical and Nursing Management

Control of the airway, ventilation, and oxygenation are essential. In the absence of cerebral or renal damage, the patient's prognosis depends largely on successful management of respiration and circulation. Measures are instituted to stabilize cardiovascular and other body functions. ECG, vital signs, and neurologic status are monitored closely for changes. Shock may result from the cardiodepressant action of the substance ingested, from venous pooling in the lower extremities, or from reduced circulating blood volume resulting from increased capillary permeability. An indwelling urinary catheter is inserted to monitor kidney function. Blood specimens are obtained to determine the concentration of drug or poison.

Efforts are made to determine what substance was ingested; the amount of the substance; the time since ingestion; signs and symptoms, such as pain or burning sensations, any evidence of redness or burn in the mouth or throat, pain on swallowing or an inability to swallow, vomiting, or drooling; age and weight of the patient; and pertinent health history.

Measures are instituted to remove the toxin or decrease its absorption. Consultation with a Poison Control Center is strongly recommended for definitive antidote and continued monitoring. The patient who has ingested a corrosive poison is given water or milk to drink for dilution. However, dilution is not attempted if the patient has acute airway edema or obstruction or if there is clinical evidence of esophageal, gastric, or intestinal burn or perforation. The following gastric emptying procedures may be used as prescribed:

- Syrup of ipecac to induce vomiting in the alert patient (*never* use with corrosive poisons)
- Gastric lavage for the obtunded patient. Gastric aspirate is saved and sent to the laboratory for toxicology screens.
- Activated charcoal administration if the poison is one that is absorbed by charcoal
- Cathartic, when appropriate

The specific chemical or physiologic antagonist (antidote) is administered as early as possible to reverse or diminish the effects of the toxin. If this measure is ineffective, procedures may be initiated to remove the ingested substance. These procedures include administration of multiple doses of charcoal, diuresis (for substances excreted by the kidneys), dialysis, or hemoperfusion once admitted to an appropriate inpatient setting. Hemoperfusion involves detoxification of the blood by processing it through an extracorporeal circuit and an adsorbent cartridge containing charcoal or resin, after which the cleansed blood is returned to the patient.

Throughout detoxification, the patient's vital signs, CVP, and fluid and electrolyte balance are monitored closely. Hypotension and cardiac arrhythmias are possible. Seizures are also possible because of central nervous system (CNS) excitement from the poison or from oxygen deprivation. If the patient complains of pain, analgesics are administered cautiously. Severe pain causes vasomotor collapse and reflex inhibition of normal physiologic functions.

Patients presenting with ingested poisoning need to be evaluated for accidental ingestion versus intentional ingestion due to suicide attempt or other psychiatric disturbance. After the patient's condition has stabilized, written material should be given to the patient indicating the signs and symptoms of potential problems related to the poison ingested and signs or symptoms requiring evaluation by the primary care provider.

CARBON MONOXIDE POISONING

Carbon monoxide poisoning may occur as a result of industrial or household incidents or attempted suicide. It is a colorless, odorless gas that is implicated in more deaths than any other toxin except alcohol.

When unintentional carbon monoxide poisoning occurs, the health department should be contacted so that the dwelling or building in question can be inspected. Carbon monoxide exerts its toxic effect by binding to circulating hemoglobin and thereby reducing the oxygen-carrying capacity of the blood.

Clinical Manifestations and Assessment

Because the CNS has a critical need for oxygen, CNS symptoms predominate with carbon monoxide toxicity. A person with carbon monoxide poisoning may appear intoxicated (from cerebral hypoxia). Other signs and symptoms include headache, muscular weakness, palpitation, dizziness, and confusion, which can progress rapidly to coma. Skin color, which can range from pink or cherry-red to cyanotic and pale, is not a reliable sign. Pulse oximetry is also not valid because the hemoglobin is well saturated. It is not saturated with oxygen, but the pulse oximeter only reads whether or not the hemoglobin is saturated; in this case, it is saturated with carbon monoxide rather than oxygen.

Medical and Nursing Management

Exposure to carbon monoxide requires immediate treatment. Goals of management are to reverse cerebral and myocardial

hypoxia and to hasten elimination of carbon monoxide. Whenever a patient inhales a poison, the following general measures apply:

- Carry the patient to fresh air immediately; open all doors and windows.
- Loosen all tight clothing.
- Initiate cardiopulmonary resuscitation if required; administer 100% oxygen.
- Prevent chilling; wrap the patient in blankets.
- Keep the patient as quiet as possible.
- Do not give alcohol in any form or permit the patient to smoke.

In addition, for the patient with carbon monoxide poisoning, **carboxyhemoglobin** levels are analyzed on arrival at the ED and before treatment with oxygen if possible. Oxygen at 100% is administered at atmospheric or preferably hyperbaric pressures to reverse hypoxia and accelerate the elimination of carbon monoxide. Oxygen is administered until the carboxyhemoglobin level is less than 5%. The patient is monitored continuously. Psychoses, spastic paralysis, ataxia, visual disturbances, and deterioration of mental status and behavior may persist after resuscitation and may be symptoms of permanent brain damage.

DISASTER NURSING

The World Health Organization (2015) defines disaster as any man-made or natural event that overwhelms the local community resources. Resources may be required from local, state, and federal agencies. International agency support may be required in cases where extensive intervention is required. Acts of terrorism, warfare, air or rail accidents, pandemic illness, weather-related events, toxic spills, or geologic events such as landslides and earthquakes are examples of some common disaster events that can result in casualties and tax the resources of health care facilities and their communities.

FEDERAL, STATE, AND LOCAL RESPONSES TO EMERGENCIES

When a **mass casualty incident (MCI)** occurs, the initial review and response occurs at the local level. Local emergency response agencies (including volunteer agencies) are typically the first responders. As the magnitude of the MCI is evaluated and scope of services needed is assessed, the progression to enlist aid from state and then federal resources may be made through official channels. Local and state Offices of Emergency Management coordinate interagency efforts. These organizations maintain a corps of emergency management personnel, including responders, planners, and administrative and support staff. A request for federal

TABLE **56-2** Federal Disaster Resources

Federal Disaster Resources	Type of Support Available
Department of Health and Human Services (DHHS)	
Centers for Disease Control and Prevention (CDC)	Collaborates to create the expertise, information, and tools needed to protect the health of the nation and the world
National Disaster Medical System (NDMS)	Has many medical support teams, such as Disaster Medical Assistance Teams (DMATs), Disaster Mortuary Response Teams (DMORTs), Veterinary Medical Assistance Teams (VMATs), and National Medical Response Teams for Weapons of Mass Destruction (NMRTs)
Department of Justice (DOJ)	
Federal Emergency Management Agency (FEMA)	Provides scene control and collection of forensic evidence
Department of Homeland Security	
Federal Bureau of Investigation (FBI)	Can activate teams such as the Urban Search and Rescue Teams (USRTs)

resources generally is made when local resources have become or are expected to become depleted due to the magnitude of the event. Federal resources are available through several departments, although the intent is to support local and state efforts rather than assume responsibility for any disaster response. Table 56-2 lists federal resources.

The Incident Command System (ICS) is the local organization that coordinates personnel, facilities, equipment, and communication in any emergency situation. The ICS has a federal mandate and is an integral part of the National Incident Management System (NIMS). According to the Federal Emergency Management Administration (FEMA, 2015), the ICS can be used at all levels of disaster management to provide a standard management response that organizes and integrates the coordination of response for personnel, facilities, and equipment. It establishes common responses for planning and managing resources at all response levels.

HOSPITAL EMERGENCY PREPAREDNESS PLANS

Health care facilities are required by the Joint Commission to create a plan for emergency preparedness that addresses both internal and external disasters. This plan should be developed with attention to the most likely internal and external disaster potentials. Disaster exercises are required to simulate mass casualty events with participation from multiple agencies.

Components

The Joint Commission has created accreditation standards that cover eight essential areas for disaster operation plans. These emergency management standards include: expectations for plans for managing the consequences of emergencies; development and maintenance of an Emergency Operations Plan; establishing emergency communication strategies; planning for managing resources and assets during emergencies; managing safety and security during emergencies; defining staff roles and responsibilities; establishing strategies for managing utilities during emergencies; and developing strategies for managing patient clinical and support activities during an emergency (Joint Commission, 2012, 2013; McLaughlin, 2014).

Initiating the Disaster Plan

Notification of a disaster situation to a health care facility varies with each situation. In general, the notification to the facility comes from outside sources unless the initial incident occurred at the facility. The disaster activation plan should clearly state how the Emergency Operation Plan (EOP) is to be initiated. If communication is functioning, field incident command will give notice of the approximate number of arriving patients, although the number of self-referring patients will not be known and may impact resource management.

Identifying Patients

Patient tracking is a critical component of casualty management. Disaster tags, which are numbered and include triage priority, name, address, age, location and description of injuries, and treatments or medications given, are used to communicate patient information. The tag should be securely placed on the patient and remain with the patient at all times. The tag number and the patient's name are recorded in a disaster log. The log is used by the command center to track patients, assign beds, and provide families with information.

Triage During Mass Casualty Incidents

In nondisaster situations, health care workers assign a high priority and allocate the most resources to those who are the most critically ill. However, in a disaster, when health care providers are faced with a large number of casualties, the fundamental principle guiding resource allocation is to do the greatest good for the greatest number of people. Decisions are based on the likelihood of survival and consumption of available resources. Therefore, patients with conditions associated with a high mortality rate would be assigned a low triage priority in a disaster situation, even if the person is conscious. Although this may sound uncaring, from an ethical standpoint, the expenditure of limited resources on people with a low chance of survival, and denial of those resources to others with serious but treatable conditions, cannot be justified.

The triage officer rapidly assesses those injured at the disaster scene. Patients are immediately tagged and transported or given life-saving interventions. One person performs the initial triage while other EMS personnel perform life-saving measures (e.g., intubation) and transport patients. Although EMS personnel carry out initial field triage, secondary and continuous triage at all subsequent levels of care is essential.

Staff should control all entrances to the acute care facility so that incoming patients are directed to the triage area first. The triage area may be outside the entry or just at the door of the ED. This allows all patients, including those arriving by medical transport and those who walk in, to be triaged. Some patients already seen in the field may be reclassified in the triage area based on their current presentation.

Triage categories separate patients according to severity of injury. A special color-coded tagging system is used during an MCI so that the triage category is immediately obvious. There are several triage systems in use across the country, and every nurse should be aware of the system used by his or her facility and community. The North Atlantic Treaty Organization (NATO) triage system is one that is widely used and is presented here. It consists of four colors—red, yellow, green, and black (Table 56-3). Each color signifies a different level of priority, with red representing the most significant but potentially survivable injuries through green representing minor injuries. Black designates "expected" death due to nonsurvivable injuries or patients in whom death appears to be imminent.

Communication with Media and Family

Communication is a key component of disaster management. Communication within the vast team of disaster responders is paramount; however, effective, informative communication with the media and worried family members is also crucial and must be addressed in the organization's disaster plan and communicated to staff.

Although the media have an obligation to report the news and can play a significant positive role in communication, the number of reporters and newscasters and their support teams can be overwhelming, possibly compromising

TABLE **56-3** NATO Triage Categories During a Mass Casualty Incident (MCI)

Triage Category	Priority	Color	Typical Conditions
Immediate: Injuries are life-threatening but survivable with minimal intervention. Individuals in this group can progress rapidly to expectant category if treatment is delayed.	1	Red	Sucking chest wound, airway obstruction secondary to mechanical cause, shock, hemothorax, tension pneumothorax, asphyxia, unstable chest and abdominal wounds, incomplete amputations, open fractures of long bones, and second-/third-degree burns of 15–40% total body surface area
Delayed: Injuries are significant and require medical care but can wait hours without threat to life or limb. Individuals in this group receive treatment only after immediate casualties are treated.	2	Yellow	Stable abdominal wounds without evidence of significant hemorrhage; soft tissue injuries; maxillofacial wounds without airway compromise; vascular injuries with adequate collateral circulation; genitourinary tract disruption; fractures requiring open reduction, débridement, and external fixation; most eye and central nervous system injuries
Minimal: Injuries are minor and treatment can be delayed hours to days. Individuals in this group should be moved away from the main triage area.	3	Green	Upper extremity fractures, minor burns, sprains, small lacerations without significant bleeding, behavioral disorders or psychological disturbances
Expectant: Injuries are extensive, and chances of survival are unlikely even with definitive care. Persons in this group should be separated from other casualties but not abandoned. Comfort measures should be provided when possible.	4	Black	Unresponsive patients with penetrating head wounds, high spinal cord injuries, wounds involving multiple anatomical sites and organs, second-/third-degree burns in excess of 60% of body surface area, seizures or vomiting within 24 hours after radiation exposure, profound shock with multiple injuries, agonal respirations; no pulse, no blood pressure, pupils fixed and dilated

operations and patient confidentiality. A clearly defined process for managing media requests that includes a designated spokesperson, a site for the dissemination of information (away from patient care areas), and a regular schedule for providing updates should be part of the disaster plan.

The disaster plan helps prevent the release of contradictory or inaccurate information. Initial statements should focus on current efforts and what is being done to better understand the scope and impact of the situation. Information about casualties should not be released. Security staff should not allow media personnel access to patient care areas.

Friends and family members converging on the scene must be cared for by the facility. They may be feeling intense anxiety, shock, or grief and should be provided with information and updates about their loved ones as soon as possible and regularly thereafter. They should not be in the triage or treatment areas but in a designated area staffed by available social service workers, counselors, therapists, and/or clergy. Access to this area should be controlled to prevent families from being disturbed.

Emotional and behavioral effects vary among affected people. Factors that influence a person's response to disaster include the degree and nature of the exposure to the disaster, loss of friends and loved ones, existing coping strategies, available resources and support, and the personal meaning attached to the event. Other factors, such as loss of home and valued possessions, extended exposure to danger, and exposure to toxic contamination, also influence response and increase the risk for adjustment problems. Those exposed to the dead and injured, those endangered by the event, the elderly, children, emergency first responders, and health care personnel caring for victims are considered to be at higher risk of emotional sequelae.

Nurses can assist victims of disasters and their families through active listening and providing emotional support, giving information, and referring patients to therapists or social workers. Health care workers must refer people to mental health care services because experience has shown that few disaster victims seek these services and early intervention minimizes psychological consequences. Nurses can also discourage victims from subjecting themselves to repeated exposure to the event through media replays and news articles, and encourage them to return to normal activities and social roles when appropriate.

The Nurse's Role in Disaster Response Plans

The role of the nurse during a disaster varies. The nurse may be asked to perform duties outside his or her area of expertise and may take on responsibilities normally held by physicians or advanced practice nurses. Although the exact role of a nurse in disaster management depends on the specific needs of the facility at the time, it should be clear which

nurse or physician is in charge of a given patient care area and which procedures each individual nurse may or may not perform. Assistance can be obtained through the incident command center, and nonmedical personnel can provide services where possible.

New settings and atypical roles for nurses arise during a disaster; for example, the nurse may provide shelter care in a temporary housing area or bereavement support and assistance with identification of deceased loved ones. People may require crisis intervention, or the nurse may participate in counseling other staff members and in critical incident stress management (CISM) (discussed later in this chapter). Special care may be warranted for at-risk populations during a disaster including people who are disabled, elderly, young, pregnant, and members of other vulnerable populations.

Disasters can present a disparity between the resources of the health care agency and the needs of the victims. This generates ethical dilemmas for nurses and other health care providers. Issues include conflicts related to the following:

- Rationing care
- Futile therapy
- Consent
- Duty
- Confidentiality
- Resuscitation

Nurses may find it difficult to not provide medical care to the dying or to withhold information to avoid spreading fear and panic. Clinical scenarios that are unimaginable in normal circumstances confront the nurse in extreme instances. Other ethical dilemmas may arise out of health care providers' instinct for self-protection and protection of their families.

Nurses can plan for the ethical dilemmas they will face during disasters by establishing a framework for evaluating ethical questions before they arise and by identifying and exploring possible responses to difficult clinical situations. They can consider how the fundamental ethical principles of utilitarianism, beneficence, and justice will influence their decisions and care in disaster response. Education and practice of the disaster response plan can assist the nurse in achieving an understanding of the role changes and dilemmas that might impact job performance.

Critical Incident Stress Management

CISM is an approach to preventing and treating the emotional trauma that can affect emergency responders as a consequence of their jobs and that can also occur to anyone involved in a disaster or MCI. CISM is handled by teams trained in the techniques.

Components of CISM plans include defusings, debriefings, demobilization, and follow-up care after the incident. *Defusing* is a process by which the person receives education about recognition of stress reactions and management strategies for handling stress. *Debriefing* is a more complicated intervention; it involves a 2- to 3-hour process during which participants are asked about their emotional reactions to the incident, what symptoms they may be experiencing (e.g., flashbacks, difficulty sleeping, intrusive thoughts), and other psychological ramifications. As an intervention, *demobilization* is usually reserved for large-scale events with large numbers of participants from different disciplines. If separate defusing interventions were attempted for each group, CISM resources might be overwhelmed. Similar to the defusing intervention, responders are presented with information regarding expected stress reactions that they might experience and how to manage them. The responders are also provided an opportunity to rest and eat before returning to their normal, pre-incident routines. In the event of large-scale disasters, it might be appropriate to participate in the demobilization process after each shift of work. In *follow-up*, members of the CISM team contact the participants of a debriefing and schedule a follow-up meeting if necessary. People with ongoing stress reactions are referred to mental health specialists.

PREPAREDNESS AND RESPONSE

As a health care provider, a nurse must be prepared for terrorism and other disasters, which includes awareness of the potential for covert use of weapons of mass destruction (WMD), self-protection, and early detection, containment, or **decontamination** of substances and agents that may affect others by secondary exposure. The strength of many toxins, today's mobile society, and long incubation periods for some organisms and diseases can result in an epidemic that can quickly and silently spread across the entire country. For example, there must be awareness that a formerly healthy person with a rapid onset of flu-like symptoms can have an ominous illness, such as anthrax or severe acute respiratory syndrome (SARS), both of which are discussed in more detail later in the chapter.

Detection

Health care personnel should have a heightened awareness for trends that may suggest deliberate dispersal of toxic or infectious agents. Some general principles should be considered, such as the following:

- Awareness of an unusual increase in the number of people seeking care for fever, respiratory, or GI symptoms.
- Any clusters of patients presenting with the same unusual illness from a single location. Clusters can be from a specific geographic location, such as a city, or from a single sporting or entertainment event.
- Large number of rapidly fatal cases, especially when death occurs within 72 hours after hospital admission.
- Increase in disease incidence in a normally healthy population. These cases should be reported to the state health department and to the CDC, including information about recent travel and contact with others who have been ill or have recently died of a fatal illness.

Suspicions or findings are reported to the appropriate unit in the facility and to proper authorities in the community. Resources for information can include the infection control department, material safety data sheets (MSDS), the state health department, the CDC, the local poison control center, and many Internet sites. Reporting furnishes data elements to those agencies responsible for epidemiology and response. Reporting also allows for sharing of information among facilities and jurisdictions and can help determine the source of infections or exposure and prevent further exposures and even deaths.

Personal Protection

Preparedness and response involves the protection of the health care provider by additional PPE prior to contact with a patient who is contaminated or infected. The purpose of PPE is to shield health care workers from the chemical, physical, biologic, and radiologic hazards that may exist when caring for contaminated patients. The U.S. Environmental Protection Agency (EPA) has divided protective clothing and respiratory protection into four categories, level A through level D (Box 56-6) (U.S. Environmental Protection Agency [EPA], 2015).

BOX 56-6 Environmental Protection Agency Categories of Protective Clothing and Respiratory Protection

- Level A protection is worn when the highest level of protection for the respiratory system, skin, eye, and mucous membrane is required. This includes a self-contained breathing apparatus (SCBA) and a fully encapsulating, vapor-tight, chemical-resistant suit with chemical-resistant gloves and boots.
- Level B protection requires the highest level of respiratory protection but a lesser level of skin and eye protection than with level A situations. This level of protection includes positive-pressure, full face-piece SCBA or positive-pressure supplied air respirator with escape SCBA, inner and outer chemical-resistant gloves, face shield, hooded chemical-resistant clothing, coveralls, and outer chemical-resistant boots.
- Level C protection requires the air-purified respirator, which uses filters or sorbent materials to remove harmful substances from the air. A chemical-resistant coverall with splash hood, chemical-resistant gloves, and boots are included in level C protection.
- Level D protection is the typical work uniform. Level D protective equipment may include gloves, safety glasses, or a face shield.

Decontamination

Decontamination, the process of removing accumulated contaminants, is critical to the health and safety of health care providers by preventing secondary contamination. The decontamination plan should establish procedures and educate employees about decontamination procedures, identify the equipment needed and methods to be used, and establish methods for disposal of contaminated materials.

Effective decontamination must include a minimum of two steps. The first step is removal of the patient's clothing and jewelry and then rinsing the patient with water. Depending on the type of exposure, this step alone can remove a large amount of the contamination and decrease secondary contamination. Ideally, facilities should identify areas where patients can be decontaminated prior to entering the facility, to prevent accidental contamination of the emergency services area, staff, and other hospital areas and personnel. The second step consists of a thorough soap-and-water wash and rinse. When patients arrive at the facility after being assessed and treated by a prehospital provider, it should not be assumed that they have been thoroughly decontaminated.

NATURAL DISASTERS

Natural disasters may result in mass casualties. Natural disasters can occur anywhere at any time and include events such as tornadoes, hurricanes, floods, avalanches, tidal waves (e.g., tsunamis), earthquakes, and volcanic eruptions. In many cases, preparation prior to the natural disaster is the best-laid plan. In the event of a natural disaster, loss of communications, potable water, and electricity are usually the greatest obstacles to a well-coordinated emergency response. Even wireless technology (e.g., mobile or cellular phones, computers, other communication devices) may not be functional.

The majority of the immediate casualties are trauma-related. These mass casualties tax the trauma system to its limits to provide triage, transport of patients (in poor weather and road conditions), and management within the trauma centers. Electrocution is also a common injury and can result in death.

Excessive exposure to the natural elements and the need for food and water (by both patients and emergency responders) are critical issues. Without cover (e.g., buildings may be unsafe or destroyed) or safe water (e.g., water may be either contaminated or unavailable), injuries from exposure to heat, cold, or contaminated food or water can occur. Safety equipment that protects rescue workers from injury, exposure, and potentially dangerous animals must be readily available. Hypothermia can occur rapidly in workers who are exposed to water at temperatures of 75°F or less. As in all disasters, mental health workers and shelters are needed throughout the community. Veterinary assistance is also essential because frequently pets are abandoned and injured. After floods or water disasters, waterborne transmission of agents such as *Escherichia coli*, salmonella, shigella, typhoid, leptospirosis, malaria, and tularemia are common and cause widespread disease.

In some instances, early warning systems have assisted in decreasing the number of deaths from tornadoes and hurricanes. When buildings collapse, rapid response to identify and remove trapped victims is the only means of improving survivability. There is a direct relationship between time trapped and survival as well as the type of building construction and number of stories of the collapsed structure. Larger-scale issues that can cause significant later morbidity and mortality include the absence of water purification, waste removal, removal of human and animal remains, and vector control. Removal or disposal of biologic, chemical, and nuclear agents must also be considered.

BIOLOGIC AGENTS

Biologic weapons are weapons that spread disease among the general population or the military as part of **biologic warfare**. Biologic agents are delivered in either a liquid or dry state, applied to foods or water, or vaporized for inhalation or direct contact. Vaporization may be accomplished through spray or explosives loaded with the agent. Because of increases in business and pleasure travel by people in industrialized nations, an agent could be released in one city and affect people in other cities thousands of miles away. The vector can be an insect, animal, or person, or there may be direct contact with the agent itself.

Anthrax and smallpox are the two of the agents most likely to be used or weaponized. Table 56-4 describes other easily weaponized biologic agents.

 Concept Mastery Alert

Ventilation support of breathing is not recommended for patients exposed to anthrax. Supportive care for clients having direct contact with botulism includes mechanical ventilation.

ANTHRAX

Inhaled anthrax is recognized as the most likely weaponized biologic agent available.

Bacillus anthracis is a naturally occurring gram-positive, encapsulated rod that lives in the soil in the spore state throughout the world. The bacterium is liberated when exposed to air and is infective only in the spore form. Contact with infected animal products (raw meat) or inhalation of the spores results in infection.

Pathophysiology

Animal studies have suggested that small amounts of inhaled anthrax spores (as low as 50 to 98 spores) may be

TABLE **56-4** Examples of Biologic Agents that Can Be Used as Weapons

Agent/ Organism	Contagion	Decontamination and Protective Equipment	Signs and Symptoms	Treatment (Mortality Rate)
Tularemia (*Francisella tularensis*): gram-negative coccobacillus, one of the most infectious bacteria known	Direct contact with infected animals or aerosolized as a bioterror weapon; bites Not contagious through human-to-human contact	Standard barrier precautions Clothing and linens should be laundered under the usual hospital protocol.	*Initial:* Abrupt onset of fever, fatigue, chills, headache, lower backache, malaise, rigor, coryza (acute inflammation of the mucous membrane of the nasal cavities), dry cough, and sore throat without adenopathy. Nausea and vomiting or diarrhea possible. *As disease progresses:* Sweating, fever, progressive weakness, anorexia, and weight loss demonstrate continued illness. *Mortality secondary to:* Pneumonitis (if inhalation is the source) with copious watery or purulent sputum, hemoptysis, respiratory insufficiency, sepsis, and shock.	Streptomycin or gentamicin/ aminoglycoside for 10–14 days. Inhalation tularemia must be treated within 48 hours of onset. In mass casualty situations, doxycycline or ciprofloxacin is recommended. For persons exposed to tularemia, tetracycline or doxycycline is recommended for 14 days. (Mortality rate = 2%)
Botulism (*Clostridium botulinum*): Botulinum blocks acetylcholine-containing vesicles from fusing with the terminal membranes of the motor-neuron end-plate, resulting in a flaccid paralysis.	Direct contact Not contagious through human-to-human contact	Any skin exposure to the botulism toxin can be treated with soap and water or a 0.1% hypochlorite solution. Standard precautions are used when treating patients with botulism.	*Gastrointestinal botulism:* Abdominal cramps, nausea, vomiting, and diarrhea. *Inhalation botulism:* Fever; symmetric descending flaccid paralysis with multiple cranial nerve palsies. Classic signs and symptoms include diplopia, dysphagia, dry mouth, lack of fever, and alert mental status. Other possible symptoms include ptosis of the eyelids, blurred vision, enlarged sluggish pupils, dysarthria, and dysphonia. *Mortality secondary to:* Airway obstruction and inadequate tidal volume.	Supportive ventilatory therapy is necessary if respiratory infection occurs. Aminoglycosides and clindamycin are contraindicated because they exacerbate neuromuscular blockage. Equine antitoxin is used to minimize subsequent nerve damage. There is a 2% rate of anaphylaxis to the antitoxin; therefore, diphenhydramine (Benadryl) and epinephrine must be immediately available for use. Supportive care: Mechanical ventilation, nutrition, fluids, prevention of complications (Mortality rate = 5%)
Plague (*Yersinia pestis*): Nonsporulating gram-negative coccobacillus. The bacterium causes destruction and necrosis of the lymph nodes.	Contagious *Bubonic plague:* transmitted through flea bites with no person-to-person transmission *Pneumonic plague:* transmitted through respiratory droplet contact	Isolation barrier precautions with full face respirators. The patient should wear a mask. Rooms should receive a terminal cleaning. Clothing and linens with body fluids on them should be cleaned with the usual disinfectant. Routine precautions should be used in the case of death.	*Bubonic plague:* Sudden fever and chills, weakness, a swollen and tender lymph node (bubo) in the groin, axilla, or cervical area. The resultant bacteremia progresses to septicemia from the endotoxin and, finally, shock and death. *Primary septicemic plague:* Disseminated intravascular coagulation (DIC), necrosis of small vessels, purpura, and gangrene of the digits and nose (black death). *Pneumonic plague:* Severe bronchospasm, chest pain, dyspnea, cough, and hemoptysis. There is a 100% mortality associated with pneumonic plague if not treated within the first 24 hours.	Streptomycin or gentamicin for 10–14 days. Tetracycline or doxycycline is an acceptable alternative if an aminoglycoside cannot be given. People with close contact exposure (less than 2 m) require prophylaxis with doxycycline for 7 days. (Mortality rate = 50%)

sufficient to cause death in 10% of the exposed human population (Center for Infectious Disease Research and Policy [CIDRAP], 2013). As an aerosol, anthrax is odorless and invisible and can travel a great distance before disseminating; hence, the site of release and the site of infection can be miles apart. Incubation of the inhaled spores can be as long as 7 days.

Clinical Manifestations

Initial symptoms may resemble a common cold. Anthrax does not present as pneumonia. After several days, the symptoms may progress to severe breathing problems and shock.

Medical and Nursing Management

Inhalation anthrax is frequently fatal even with aggressive antibiotic and supportive therapy. Due to the presence of spores, antibiotic treatment is continued for 60 days. Anthrax cannot be spread from person to person, and standard level D universal precautions are sufficient.

SMALLPOX

Pathophysiology

Smallpox (variola) is classified as a DNA virus. It has an incubation period of 10 to 12 days. It is extremely contagious and is spread by direct contact, by contact with clothing or linens, or by inhaled droplets of saliva during contact with an infected person. During the incubation period there are no symptoms. When the virus has multiplied sufficiently to cause the fever and characteristic rash, the affected person not only feels ill but is also at the most infectious period (National Institute of Allergy and Infectious Diseases [NIAID], 2014). Aerosolization of the virus would result in widespread dissemination.

Clinical Manifestations and Assessment

Signs and symptoms of smallpox infection are similar to influenza and include high fever, malaise, headache, backache, and fatigue. After 2 to 3 days, a flat, red, lesioned rash appears, evolving at the same rate, beginning on the face, mouth, pharynx, and forearms. After several days, these lesions become filled with pus (Fig. 56-5) and form crusts in week 2. By week 3, these crusts have become scabs and begin to fall off (NIAID, 2014). There is a large amount of the virus in the saliva and pustules. Smallpox is contagious only after the appearance of the rash. There are two forms of smallpox, variola major and variola minor. Variola major is more common and results in a higher fever and more extensive rash. Variola major has a 30% case-fatality rate. Hemorrhagic smallpox, a subtype of variola major, includes all of the above signs and symptoms plus a dusky erythema and petechiae to frank hemorrhage of the skin and mucous membranes, resulting in death by day 5 or 6.

FIGURE 56-5 Patient with smallpox. (From Knipe, D. M., & Howley, P. M. (Eds.). (2001). *Field's virology* (4th ed.). Philadelphia, PA: Lippincott Williams & Wilkins.)

Medical and Nursing Management

There is no specific treatment for smallpox, and vaccination is preventative. Treatment includes supportive care with antibiotics for any additional infection. The patient must be isolated with the use of transmission precautions. Laundry and biologic wastes should be autoclaved before being washed with hot water and bleach. Standard **decontamination** of the room is effective. All people who have household or face-to-face contact with the patient after the fever begins should be vaccinated within 4 days to prevent the infection or lessen the severity (NIAID, 2014).

SEVERE ACUTE RESPIRATORY SYNDROME

Not all mass casualty biologic events are terrorist-based. The SARS outbreak in 2003 is a prime example of a non–terrorist-based mass casualty biologic event. The disease started as "atypical" pneumonia in China, in February, and had spread to 29 countries throughout the world by July. Air travel and worldwide trade have increased the possibility that any contagious disease process may spread rapidly. The incubation period for SARS is 2 to 10 days.

Clinical Manifestations and Assessment

SARS should be considered in the event of an outbreak of atypical pneumonia with travel to an area with a known SARS outbreak, a health care worker with direct patient contact, or lab worker in a laboratory that contains live SARS-CoV. Early systemic signs are dry cough and shortness of breath with or without other respiratory symptoms. X-ray confirmed pneumonia or acute respiratory distress syndrome (ARDS) is evident at 7 to 10 days, along with fever and respiratory symptoms.

Medical and Nursing Management

Droplet precaution isolation and control of visits to the exposed patient are essential. Treatment is supportive. The overall case fatality rate is 10%, which increases to more than 50% in patients older than 60 years of age, putting frail, elderly people at risk.

> **Nursing Alert**
> *The goal of Droplet Precautions is to prevent the transmission of pathogens spread through close respiratory or mucous membrane contact with respiratory secretions. Because the pathogens do not remain infectious over long distances, special air handling and ventilation are not required to prevent transmission. A single patient room is preferred for patients who require Droplet Precautions; however, if it is not available, consultation with infection control personnel is recommended regarding cohorting of patients. A mask is required for close contact (within 3 ft) with patients who are infectious, which is generally donned upon room entry. If the patient must be transported outside of the room, a mask should be applied (if tolerated), and the patient should be instructed in cough etiquette (cover the mouth/nose when coughing or sneezing, use and dispose of tissues). In addition, hand hygiene should be performed after hands have been in contact with respiratory secretions (CDC, 2015b; Siegel, Rhinehart, Jackson, & Chiarello, 2007).*

CHEMICAL AGENTS

Agents that may be used in **chemical warfare** or terrorism are *overt*, in that the effects are more apparent and occur more quickly than those caused by biologic weapons. Agents are available and well-known, result in major mortality and morbidity, and cause panic and social disruption. There are many agents, including those that affect nerves (sarin, soman), those that affect blood (cyanide), vesicants (lewisite, nitrogen and sulfur mustard, phosgene), heavy metals (arsenic, lead), volatile toxins (benzene, chloroform), pulmonary agents (chlorine), and corrosive acids (nitric acid, sulfuric acid) (refer to Table 56-5).

Chemical agents vary in their absorption and effects. The *volatility* of chemical agents refers to the ability of the agent to become a vapor. Most chemicals are heavier than air, except for hydrogen cyanide, and heavier exposure occurs lower to the ground. *Persistence* of chemical agents means the chemical is less likely to vaporize and disperse. More volatile chemicals do not evaporate quickly and are more commonly used by military and terrorist agents than are industrial chemicals. *Toxicity* of the chemical agent is the ability to cause injury to the body. Toxicity is affected by concentration and length of exposure. *Latency* is the time from absorption to the appearance of symptoms. Sulfur mustards and pulmonary agents have the longest latency, whereas vesicants, nerve agents, and cyanide produce symptoms within seconds.

TABLE 56-5 Common Chemical Agents

Agent	Action	Signs and Symptoms	Decontamination and Treatment
Nerve Agents			
Sarin Soman organophosphates	Inhibition of cholinesterase	Increased secretions, gastrointestinal motility, diarrhea, bronchospasm	Soap and water Supportive care Benzodiazepine Pralidoxime Atropine
Blood Agent			
Cyanide	Inhibition of aerobic metabolism	Inhalation—tachypnea, tachycardia, coma, seizures. Can progress to respiratory arrest, respiratory failure, cardiac arrest, death.	Sodium nitrite Sodium thiocyanate Amyl nitrate Hydroxocobalamin
Vesicant Agents			
Lewisite Sulfur mustard Nitrogen mustard Phosgene	Blistering agents	Superficial to partial-thickness burn with vesicles that coalesce	Soap and water Blot; do not rub dry
Pulmonary Agents			
Phosgene Chlorine	Separation of alveoli from capillary bed	Pulmonary edema, bronchospasm	Airway management Ventilatory support Bronchoscopy

NERVE AGENTS

The most toxic agents in existence are the nerve agents, such as sarin, soman, tabun, VX, and organophosphates (pesticides). They are inexpensive, effective in small quantities, and easily dispersed. In the liquid form, nerve agents evaporate into a colorless, odorless vapor. Organophosphates are similar in nature to the nerve agents used in warfare and are readily available. Nerve agents can be inhaled or absorbed percutaneously or subcutaneously. These agents bond with acetylcholinesterase, so that acetylcholine is not inactivated; the adverse result is continuous stimulation (hyperstimulation) of the nerve endings.

A very small drop of a nerve agent is enough to result in sweating and twitching at the site of exposure. A larger amount results in more systemic symptoms. Effects can begin anywhere from 30 minutes up to 18 hours after exposure. The more common organophosphates and carbamates (e.g., Sevin and malathion) that are used in agriculture result in less severe symptoms than do those used in warfare or in terrorist attacks. In an ordinary situation (e.g., nonwarfare, nonterrorist attack situation), a patient could arrive at the ED having been exposed to organophosphates unintentionally or intentionally, in a suicidal gesture.

Clinical Manifestations and Assessment

Signs and symptoms of nerve gas exposure are those of cholinergic crisis and include bilateral miosis (constriction of the pupil), visual disturbances, increased GI motility, nausea and vomiting, diarrhea, substernal spasm, indigestion, bradycardia and atrioventricular block, bronchoconstriction, laryngeal spasm, weakness, fasciculations (small, localized "twitching"), and incontinence. The patient must be examined in a dark area to truly identify miosis. Neurologic responses include insomnia, forgetfulness, impaired judgment, depression, and irritability. A lethal dose results in loss of consciousness, seizures, copious secretions, fasciculations, flaccid muscles, and apnea.

Medical and Nursing Management

Decontamination with copious amounts of soap and water or saline solution for 8 to 20 minutes is essential. The water is blotted, not wiped, off the skin. A 0.5% hypochlorite solution (bleach) can also be used (Agency for Toxic Substances and Disease Registry [ATSDR], 2014). The airway is maintained, and suctioning is frequently required. Plastic airway equipment will absorb sarin gas, which may result in continued exposure to the agent.

Atropine 2 to 4 mg is administered IV, followed by 2 mg every 3 to 8 minutes for up to 24 hours of treatment. Alternatively, IV atropine 1 to 2 mg/hr may be administered until clear signs of anticholinergic activity have returned (decreased secretions, tachycardia, and decreased GI motility). Another medication that may serve as an antidote is pralidoxime,

which allows cholinesterase to become active against acetylcholine. Pralidoxime 1 to 2 g in 100 to 150 mL of normal saline solution is administered over 15 to 30 minutes. Pralidoxime has no effect on secretions and may have any of the following side effects: hypertension, tachycardia, weakness, dizziness, blurred vision, and diplopia.

Diazepam (Valium) or other benzodiazepines should be administered to control seizures, to decrease fasciculations, and to alleviate apprehension and agitation. Military personnel believed to be at risk for chemical attack are provided with Mark I automatic injectors, which contain 2-mg atropine and 600-mg pralidoxime chloride. Diazepam is administered by a partner.

BLOOD AGENTS

Blood agents, such as hydrogen cyanide and cyanogen chloride, have a direct effect on cellular metabolism, resulting in asphyxiation through alterations in hemoglobin. Cyanide is an agent that has profound systemic effects. It is commonly used in the mining of gold and silver and in the plastics and dye industries.

A cyanide release is often associated with the odor of bitter almonds. In house fires, cyanide is released during the combustion of plastics, rugs, silk, furniture, and other construction materials. There is a significant correlation between blood cyanide and carbon monoxide levels in patients who survive fires, and, in many cases, the cause of death is cyanide poisoning.

Clinical Manifestations and Assessment

Cyanide can be ingested, inhaled, or absorbed through the skin and mucous membranes. Cyanide is protein-bound and inhibits aerobic metabolism, leading to respiratory muscle failure, respiratory arrest, cardiac arrest, and death. Inhalation of cyanide results in flushing, tachypnea, tachycardia, nonspecific neurologic symptoms, stupor, coma, and seizure preceding respiratory arrest.

Medical and Nursing Management

Treatment of patients for cyanide poisoning includes rapid administration of amyl nitrate, sodium nitrite, and sodium thiosulfate, which is essential to the successful management of cyanide exposure. First, the patient is intubated and placed on a ventilator. Next, amyl nitrate pearls are crushed and placed in the ventilator reservoir to induce methemoglobinemia. Cyanide has a 20% to 25% higher affinity for methemoglobin than it does for hemoglobin; it binds with methemoglobin to form either cyanomethemoglobin or sulfmethemoglobin. The cyanomethemoglobin is then detoxified in the liver by the enzyme rhodanese. Next, IV sodium nitrite is administered to induce the rapid formation of methemoglobin. Sodium thiosulfate is then administered by IV; it has a higher affinity for cyanide than methemoglobin does and stimulates the conversion of cyanide to sodium thiocyanate, which can be excreted by the kidneys. Although they may be life-saving, these emergency medications do have side effects: sodium nitrite can result in severe hypotension, and thiocyanate can cause vomiting, psychosis, arthralgia, and myalgia.

The production of methemoglobin is contraindicated in patients suffering from smoke inhalation because they already have decreased oxygen-carrying capacity secondary to the carboxyhemoglobin produced by smoke inhalation. In facilities where a hyperbaric chamber is available, it may be used to provide oxygenation while the previously discussed therapies are initiated. An alternative suggested treatment for cyanide poisoning is hydroxocobalamin (vitamin B_{12a}). Hydroxocobalamin binds cyanide to form cyanocobalamin (vitamin B_{12}). It must be administered IV in large doses. Administration of vitamin B_{12} can result in a transient pink discoloration of mucous membranes, skin, and urine. In high doses, tachycardia and hypertension can occur, but they usually resolve within 48 hours.

CHAPTER REVIEW

Critical Thinking Exercises

1. A young woman arrives at the ED by ambulance after a car crash. She is immobilized on a backboard, with a cervical collar and an oxygen mask in place. There is a bruise across her abdomen where the seatbelt was applied. She complains of nausea and abdominal pain. You note no movement of the left chest wall and an angulated right arm. She has no pulses in her lower extremities and cannot move or feel her legs. How would you prioritize the patient's needs? Develop an assessment strategy, identify diagnostic studies that will benefit the patient, and describe the patient's treatment needs.

2. The following five patients present to the triage desk within minutes of each other. How would you prioritize and categorize each of these patients? Which ones need immediate attention? What initial care would you provide at triage?
   a. A child with medication-controlled asthma presents with rapid, shallow respirations and cyanosis around the lips and is very anxious. He has been this way for about 20 minutes.
   b. A woman who has had a cold for 3 days says she has no primary care physician and must be seen right now because she cannot breathe. Her respirations are normal, pulse oxygenation saturations are 100%, and she has complaints of sinus drainage.
   c. A woman was hit by an automobile while she was riding her bike. Instead of calling 911, a friend drove her to the ED. She is complaining of neck pain and tingling in her upper extremities since the injury. She is beginning to have difficulty taking a deep breath.
   d. A young boy who was riding his skateboard arrives at the ED with an angulated wrist. Pulses are normal, but the wrist is painful.
   e. An elderly woman presents with complaints of 24 hours of vomiting. Her vital signs are normal, but she is diaphoretic and appears weak.

3. You are the triage nurse at the receiving facility for casualties during a hurricane. Five patients arrive at the same time. Together with the surgeon on duty, you must identify the patients' needs. What are the patient needs of the following five patients? How would you classify/tag these patients?
   a. An elderly man with a respiratory rate of 8 breaths/min, color ashen, status unresponsive, with only palpable carotid pulses
   b. A 7-year-old child with a bleeding scalp laceration who needs intubation
   c. The 30-year-old mother of the 7-year-old child, who is crying hysterically and appears to have no pain or visible injuries
   d. A 15-year-old boy who complains of pain in his left leg, with obvious deformity at the calf but good pulses in the foot
   e. A 65-year-old woman who arrives in a police car holding her right wrist, which is cool, ecchymotic, and painful with good pulses

4. Multiple patients begin arriving at the ED complaining of burning eyes and difficulty breathing. All of these people work at the railroad yard, where tanker trucks frequently transport chemical agents. What should you do first? Where do you find information about chemical agents and their treatment?

NCLEX-Style Review Questions

1. When assessing a trauma patient presenting in the ED, what is the most important priority for the nurse?
   a. Controlling hemorrhage
   b. Inserting two large-gauge IV catheters for fluid resuscitation
   c. Obtaining name and phone number of nearest relative to inform them that the patient is in the hospital
   d. Establishing a patent airway

2. A 25-year-old patient is transported by paramedics to the ED following a fall from a second-story balcony during a party. During the primary survey, respirations are noted to be snoring with a heavy alcohol odor to the breath. The patient is receiving 100% O_2 via face mask, and oxygen saturation is 91%. The patient withdraws from painful stimuli but is not speaking or responding appropriately to commands. What are the immediate priorities for care?

   a. Open airway with head tilt-chin lift maneuver and obtain chest x-ray to assess for pneumothorax.

   b. Draw labs for toxicology screen and administer 0.5-mg Ativan to prevent withdrawal seizures.

   c. Perform jaw-thrust maneuver and reassess ventilation effort.

   d. Rapidly transport patient to CT for brain CT to evaluate for neurologic injury.

3. There has been a natural gas explosion in a multistory office building in the city. Initial reports indicate that the ED will be receiving a large number of victims that will overwhelm current resources. What need will the nurse working in the ED anticipate?

   a. Initiate the hospital emergency operation plan.

   b. Call off-duty staff to come in and assist.

   c. Request burn packs from central supply.

   d. Take a meal break quickly before patients arrive.

4. A city has been hit by a tornado, and reports indicate significant numbers of casualties and injuries. The hospital has not been affected, and all systems are operational at this time. As patients arrive, they have been tagged by field responders using the NATO color coding for severity. What does the nurse working in the ED know about this system?

   a. Patients tagged with a green tag require immediate and extensive use of resources for survival.

   b. Patients with a red tag have minor injuries and can wait for care.

   c. Children always receive a red tag.

   d. Patients with a black tag are not a priority for treatment under MCI standards.

5. A 50-year-old patient presents to the ED with complaints of a fever and chills for the past 72 hours, body aches, and appears to be acutely ill. The nurse notes lesions on the patient's arms and face that have appear to be spreading quickly. What are immediate priorities for care?

   a. An assessment of recent travel

   b. Administer an antipyretic to reduce fever and body aches

   c. Isolate from other patients and ensure all staff follow isolation precautions

   d. Assist patient into a hospital gown for an immediate examination and give clothing to family members

---

Try these additional resources, available at **http://thepoint.lww.com/Honan2e**, to enhance your learning and understanding of this chapter:

• NCLEX-Style Student Review Questions
• Journal Articles

REFERENCES AND SELECTED READINGS

References and selected readings associated with this chapter can be found on the website that accompanies the book. Visit **http://thepoint. lww.com/Honan2e** to access the references and other additional resources associated with this chapter.

Appendix A

Major Fluid and Electrolyte Imbalances

Imbalance	Contributing Factors	Signs/Symptoms and Laboratory Findings
Fluid volume deficit (FVD) (hypovolemia)	Loss of water and electrolytes, as in vomiting, diarrhea, fistulas, fever, excess sweating, burns, blood loss, gastrointestinal suction, and third-space fluid shifts; and decreased intake, as in anorexia, nausea, and inability to gain access to fluid Diabetes insipidus and uncontrolled diabetes mellitus also contribute to a depletion of extracellular fluid volume.	Acute weight loss; decreased skin turgor; oliguria; concentrated urine; weak, rapid pulse; prolonged capillary filling time; low CVP; $\downarrow$ blood pressure; orthostatic hypotension; flattened neck veins; dizziness; weakness; thirst and confusion; $\uparrow$ pulse; muscle cramps; sunken eyes *Labs indicate:* $\uparrow$ Hemoglobin and hematocrit, $\uparrow$ serum and urine osmolality and specific gravity, $\uparrow$ BUN out of proportion to serum creatinine
Fluid volume excess (FVE) (hypervolemia)	Compromised regulatory mechanisms, such as kidney failure, heart failure, and cirrhosis; overzealous administration of sodium-containing fluids; and fluid shifts (i.e., treatment of burns). Prolonged corticosteroid therapy, severe stress, and hyperaldosteronism augment fluid volume excess.	Acute weight gain, peripheral edema and ascites, distended jugular veins, crackles, and elevated CVP, shortness of breath, $\uparrow$ blood pressure, bounding pulse and cough, $\uparrow$ respiratory rate *Labs indicate:* $\downarrow$ Hemoglobin and hematocrit, $\downarrow$ serum and urine osmolality, $\downarrow$ urine specific gravity, decreased BUN (due to plasma dilution).
Sodium deficit (hyponatremia) Serum sodium <135 mEq/L	Loss of sodium, as in use of diuretics, loss of GI fluids, kidney disease, and adrenal insufficiency. Gain of water, as in excessive administration of D_5W and water supplements for patients receiving hypotonic tube feedings; disease states associated with SIADH, such as head trauma and oat-cell lung tumor; medications associated with water retention (oxytocin and certain tranquilizers); and psychogenic polydipsia. Patients with congestive heart failure or liver disease may present with hyponatremia despite an excess of total body sodium.	Manifestations of hyponatremia depend on the cause, magnitude, and speed with which the deficit occurs. Symptoms include: Anorexia, nausea and vomiting, headache, lethargy, dizziness, confusion, muscle cramps and weakness, muscular twitching, seizures, papilledema, dry skin, $\uparrow$ pulse, $\downarrow$ BP, weight gain, edema. *Labs indicate:* $\downarrow$ Serum sodium; urine sodium level varies depending on the etiology of the hyponatremia
Sodium excess (hypernatremia) Serum sodium >145 mEq/L	Water deprivation in patients unable to drink at will; hypertonic tube feedings without adequate water supplements; diabetes insipidus; heatstroke; hyperventilation; watery diarrhea; burns; and diaphoresis; excess corticosteroid, sodium bicarbonate, and sodium chloride administration; and salt water near-drowning victims.	Thirst, elevated body temperature, swollen dry tongue and sticky mucous membranes, hallucinations, lethargy, restlessness, irritability, focal or grand mal seizures, pulmonary edema, hyperreflexia, twitching, nausea, vomiting, anorexia, $\uparrow$ pulse, and $\uparrow$ BP *Labs indicate:* $\uparrow$ Serum sodium, increased serum osmolality; $\uparrow$ urine-specific gravity and osmolality (provided the water loss is from a route other than the kidneys); $\downarrow$ CVP

Imbalance	Contributing Factors	Signs/Symptoms and Laboratory Findings
Potassium deficit (hypokalemia) Serum potassium <3.5 mEq/L	Increased output of K^+ (diuretics, diarrhea, vomiting, gastric suction, recent ileostomy, intestinal drains, osmotic diuresis); decreased intake of K^+ (NPO, anorexia, vomiting, alcoholism, fasting diets); or redistribution of K^+ (metabolic alkalosis, insulin administration).	Fatigue, anorexia, nausea and vomiting, muscle weakness, decreased bowel motility, abdominal distention, ileus, ventricular arrhythmias, paresthesias, leg cramps, hypoactive reflexes, increased sensitivity to digitalis *ECG:* Flattened T waves, prominent U waves, ST depression, prolonged PR interval
Potassium excess (hyperkalemia) Serum potassium >5.0 mEq/L	Pseudohyperkalemia, oliguric kidney failure, use of potassium-conserving diuretics in patients with renal insufficiency, metabolic acidosis, Addison disease, crush injury, burns, stored bank blood transfusions, and rapid IV administration of potassium	Vague muscular weakness, tachycardia → bradycardia, arrhythmias, flaccid paralysis, paresthesias, intestinal colic *ECG:* Tall tented T waves, prolonged PR interval and QRS duration, absent P waves, ST depression
Calcium deficit (hypocalcemia) Serum calcium <8.5 mg/dL	Hypoparathyroidism (may follow thyroid surgery or radical neck dissection), malabsorption, pancreatitis, alkalosis, vitamin D deficiency, massive subcutaneous infection, generalized peritonitis, massive transfusion of citrated blood, chronic diarrhea, decreased parathyroid hormone, kidney failure, ↑ PO_4, pancreatic and small bowel fistulas, hypomagnesemia, hypoalbuminemia	Numbness, tingling of fingers, toes, and circumoral region; positive Trousseau sign and Chvostek sign; tetany; seizures, carpopedal spasms, hyperactive deep tendon reflexes, irritability, laryngeal spasm, anxiety. *ECG:* Prolonged QT interval and lengthened ST predisposing to torsades de pointes (form of ventricular tachycardia) *Labs indicate:* Serum calcium concentration is low; ionized serum calcium concentration is also low; ↓ Mg^{++} (inhibits PTH secretion)
Calcium excess (hypercalcemia) Serum calcium >10.5 mg/dL	Hyperparathyroidism, malignant neoplastic disease, prolonged immobilization, overuse of calcium supplements, vitamins A and D excess, oliguric phase of kidney failure, acidosis, thiazide diuretic use	Muscular weakness, confusion, constipation, anorexia, nausea and vomiting, polyuria and polydipsia, dehydration, hypoactive deep tendon reflexes, lethargy, deep bone pain, pathologic fractures, flank pain, and calcium stones. *ECG:* Shortened ST segment and QT interval, bradycardia, heart blocks
Magnesium deficit (hypomagnesemia) Serum magnesium <1.8 mg/dL	Chronic alcoholism, hyperparathyroidism, hyperaldosteronism, diuretic phase of kidney failure, malabsorptive disorders, diabetic ketoacidosis, refeeding after starvation, parenteral nutrition, chronic laxative use, diarrhea, decreased serum K^+ and Ca^{++} and certain pharmacologic agents (such as gentamicin, cisplatin, and cyclosporine)	Neuromuscular irritability, positive Trousseau and Chvostek signs, insomnia, mood changes, anorexia, vomiting, increased tendon reflexes, and potentiation of ventricular and supraventricular arrhythmias. *ECG:* PVCs, flat or inverted T waves, depressed ST segment, prolonged PR interval and widened QRS
Magnesium excess (hypermagnesemia) Serum magnesium >2.7 mg/dL	Renal insufficiency (particularly when magnesium-containing medications are administered IV or excessive ingestion of magnesium-containing antacids or laxatives), adrenal insufficiency	Nausea, vomiting, hypotension, drowsiness, hypoactive reflexes, depressed respirations leading to apnea, bradycardia and hypotension. *ECG:* Prolonged PR interval and QT interval.
Phosphorus deficit (hypophosphatemia) Serum phosphorus <2.5 mg/dL	Refeeding after starvation, alcohol withdrawal, diabetic ketoacidosis, respiratory alkalosis, ↓ magnesium, ↓ potassium, hyperparathyroidism, diarrhea, vitamin D deficiency associated with malabsorptive disorders, burns, acid–base disorders, parenteral nutrition, and diuretic and antacid use	Paresthesias, muscle weakness, bone pain and tenderness, chest pain, confusion, cardiomyopathy, respiratory failure, seizures, tissue hypoxia, and increased susceptibility to infection.

Imbalance	Contributing Factors	Signs/Symptoms and Laboratory Findings
Phosphorus excess (hyperphosphatemia) Serum phosphorus >4.5 mg/dL	Acute and chronic kidney failure, excessive intake of phosphorus, vitamin D excess, respiratory acidosis, hypoparathyroidism, volume depletion, leukemia/lymphoma treated with cytotoxic agents, increased tissue breakdown, rhabdomyolysis	Tetany, signs and symptoms of hypocalcemia; hyperactive reflexes; soft-tissue calcifications in lungs, heart, kidneys, and cornea
Chloride deficit (hypochloremia) Serum chloride <96 mEq/L	GI tube drainage and severe vomiting and diarrhea, laxatives, ileostomy, and fistulas; sodium and potassium deficiency; metabolic alkalosis; loop, osmotic, or thiazide diuretic use; overuse of bicarbonate; rapid removal of ascitic fluid with a high sodium content; intravenous fluids that lack chloride (dextrose and water)	Signs and symptoms of hypochloremia are associated with hyponatremia, hypokalemia, and metabolic alkalosis _Labs indicate:_ ↓ Serum chloride, ↓ serum sodium, ↑ pH, ↑ serum bicarbonate, ↑ total carbon dioxide content, ↓ serum potassium
Chloride excess (hyperchloremia) Serum chloride >108 mEq/L	Excessive sodium chloride infusions with water loss; hypernatremia; kidney failure; corticosteroid use; dehydration; severe diarrhea (loss of bicarbonate); respiratory alkalosis; administration of diuretics; overdose of salicylates; Kayexalate, acetazolamide, phenylbutazone, and ammonium chloride use; hyperparathyroidism; metabolic acidosis	Signs and symptoms of hyperchloremia are typically associated with metabolic acidosis (tachypnea, Kussmaul respirations, lethargy, diminished cognitive ability), and hypernatremia (fluid retention, dyspnea, tachycardia, hypertension) _Labs indicate:_ ↑ Serum chloride, ↑ serum sodium, ↓ serum pH, ↓ serum bicarbonate, normal anion gap

↑ increased; ↓ decreased; BP, blood pressure; BUN, blood urea nitrogen; CVP, central venous pressure; DKA, diabetic ketoacidosis; GI, gastrointestinal; IV, intravenous; PVCs, premature ventricular contractions; SIADH, syndrome of inappropriate secretion of antidiuretic hormone.

Glossary

abduction movement away from the center or median line of the body

ablation purposeful destruction of heart muscle cells, usually in an attempt to control an arrhythmia

abscess localized collection of purulent material surrounded by inflamed tissues, typically associated with signs of infection

absolute neutrophil count (ANC) a mathematical calculation of the actual number of neutrophils in the circulation, derived from the total white blood cells (WBCs) and the percentage of neutrophils counted in a microscope's visual field; provides an estimate of infection risk

absorption phase of the digestive process that occurs when small molecules, vitamins, and minerals pass through the walls of the small and large intestine and into the bloodstream

acanthosis nigricans hyperpigmentation of the skin that typically occurs on the neck, dorsum of hands, axilla, or groin areas

accommodation process by which the eye adjusts for near distance (e.g., reading) by changing the curvature of the lens to focus a clear image on the retina

achalasia absent or ineffective peristalsis (wavelike contraction) of the distal esophagus accompanied by failure of the esophageal sphincter to relax in response to swallowing

achlorhydria lack of hydrochloric acid in digestive secretions of the stomach

acidosis an acid–base imbalance characterized by an increase in H^+ concentration (decreased blood pH); a low arterial pH due to reduced bicarbonate concentration is called metabolic acidosis; a low arterial pH due to increased PCO_2 is respiratory acidosis

acoustic pertaining to sound or the sense of hearing

acromegaly disease process resulting from excessive secretion of somatotropin (growth hormone); causes progressive enlargement of peripheral body parts, commonly the face, head, hands, and feet and enlargement of many body organs

active transport physiologic pump that moves fluid from an area of lower concentration to one of higher concentration; active transport requires adenosine triphosphate (ATP) for energy

acute coronary syndrome (ACS) signs and symptoms that indicate unstable angina or acute myocardial infarction

acute limb ischemia (ACL) sudden decrease in limb arterial perfusion, threatening limb viability

acute lung injury (ALI) an umbrella term for hypoxemic, respiratory failure; ARDS is a severe form of ALI

acute respiratory distress syndrome (ARDS) an inflammatory pulmonary response to a variety of pulmonary and nonpulmonary insults to the lung; characterized by diffuse interstitial infiltrates, alveolar/capillary leak, atelectasis, decreased compliance, refractory hypoxemia and no signs of cardiogenic heart failure

acute tubular necrosis type of acute kidney failure in which there is actual damage to the kidney tubules

addiction a behavioral pattern of substance use characterized by a compulsion to take the substance (drug or alcohol) primarily to experience its psychic effects

Addison disease chronic adrenocortical insufficiency secondary to destruction of the adrenal glands

addisonian crisis acute adrenocortical insufficiency; commonly characterized by shock (acute hypotension, volume depletion), nausea and vomiting; usual laboratory abnormalities include hyponatremia, hyperkalemia, and perhaps hypoglycemia; often precipitated by stress or abrupt withdrawal of therapeutic glucocorticoids

adduction movement toward the center or median line of the body

adherence the process of faithfully following guidelines or directions

adjuvant chemotherapy use of anticancer medications in addition to other treatments such as surgery, radiation to delay or prevent a recurrence of the disease

adnexa the fallopian tubes and ovaries

adrenalectomy surgical removal of one or both adrenal glands

adrenocorticotropic hormone (ACTH) hormone secreted by the anterior pituitary, essential for growth and development; chief function is to stimulate hormones of the adrenal cortex-glucocorticoids (principally cortisol), mineralocorticosteroids (principally aldosterone) and androgens (sex hormones)

adrenogenital syndrome masculinization in women, feminization in men, or premature sexual development in children; result of abnormal secretion of adrenocortical hormones, especially androgens

afterload the amount of resistance to ejection of blood from the ventricle

agglutination clumping effect occurring when an antibody acts as a cross-link between two antigens

agnosia loss of ability to recognize objects through a particular sensory system; may be visual, auditory, or tactile

agonist a substance that when combined with the receptor produces the drug effect or desired effect; endorphins and morphine are agonists on the opioid receptors

AIDS acquired immunodeficiency syndrome; when a person infected with the human immunodeficiency virus (HIV) develops an opportunistic infection or has a CD4$^+$ lymphocyte count below 200

airway pressure release ventilation (APRV) mode of mechanical ventilation that allows unrestricted, spontaneous breaths throughout the ventilatory cycle; on inspiration, patient receives preset level of continuous positive airway pressure, and pressure is periodically released to aid expiration

akathisia restlessness, urgent need to move around, and agitation

alaryngeal communication alternative modes of speaking that do not involve the normal larynx; used by patients whose larynx has been surgically removed

aldosterone hormone synthesized and released by the adrenal cortex; causes the kidneys to reabsorb sodium (and thus water retention) and potassium loss

algogenic causing pain

alkalosis an acid–base imbalance characterized by a reduction in H$^+$ concentration (increased blood pH); a high arterial pH with increased bicarbonate concentration is called metabolic alkalosis; a high arterial pH due to reduced PCO$_2$ is respiratory alkalosis

allergen substance that causes manifestations of allergy

allergy inappropriate and often harmful immune system response to substances that are normally harmless

allograft tissue harvested from a donor for use in another person (*synonym* homograft)

alopecia loss of hair from any cause

alpha$_1$-antitrypsin deficiency a genetic disorder resulting from deficiency of alpha$_1$ antitrypsin, a protective enzyme in the lungs; the deficiency increases the patient's risk for developing emphysema even in the absence of smoking

alpha-interferon protein substance that the body produces in response to infection

altered level of consciousness condition of being less responsive to and aware of environmental stimuli

ambulatory surgery includes outpatient (same-day) surgery that does not require an overnight hospital stay or short stay, with admission to an inpatient hospital setting for less than 24 hours

amenorrhea the absence of menstruation that can be either primary or secondary

amputation the removal of a body part

amylase pancreatic enzyme; aids in the digestion of carbohydrates

anagen phase active phase of hair growth

anaphylactic shock distributive shock state resulting from a severe allergic reaction producing an overwhelming systemic vasodilation and relative hypovolemia in addition to bronchial spasm

anaphylaxis clinical response to an immediate immunologic reaction between a specific antigen and antibody

androgens hormones secreted by the adrenal cortex; stimulate activity of accessory male sex organs and development of male sex characteristics; hormones produced by the ovaries and adrenals that affect many aspects of female health, including follicle development, libido, oiliness of hair and skin, and hair growth

anemia decreased red blood cell (RBC) count

anergy loss or weakening of the body's immunity to an irritating agent or antigen

anesthesia a state of narcosis, analgesia, relaxation, and loss of reflexes

anesthesiologist physician trained to deliver anesthesia and to monitor the patient's condition during surgery

anesthetic the substance, such as a chemical or gas, used to induce anesthesia

anesthetist health care professional, such as a nurse anesthetist, who is trained to deliver anesthesia and to monitor the patient's condition during surgery

aneurysm congenital or acquired localized weakness or dilation of an artery formed at a weak point in the vessel wall

angina pectoris chest pain brought about by myocardial ischemia

angiogenesis formation of new blood vessels, such as in a healing wound or in a malignant tumor

angiography an x-ray picture of a vessel lumen following the injection of a radiopaque contrast material

angioneurotic edema condition characterized by urticaria and diffuse swelling of the deeper layers of the skin

angioplasty an invasive procedure to dilate a stenotic blood vessel

angiotensin-converting enzyme (ACE) inhibitors medications that inhibit the angiotensin-converting enzyme

ankle–brachial index (ABI) ratio of the ankle systolic pressure to the higher of the two brachial systolic pressures; an objective measurement of arterial disease

ankylosis fixation or immobility of a joint

annuloplasty repair of a cardiac valve's outer ring

anovulation lack of ovulation

antagonist a substance that blocks or reverses the effects of the agonist by occupying the receptor site without producing the drug effect; naloxone (Narcan™) is an opi-oid antagonist

anterior chamber space in the eye bordered anteriorly by the cornea and posteriorly by the iris and pupil

antiarrhythmic a medication that suppresses or prevents an arrhythmia

antibody protein substance developed by the body in response to and interacting with a specific antigen

antidiuretic hormone (ADH) hormone secreted by the posterior pituitary gland; causes the kidneys to reabsorb more water; also called *vasopressin*

antigen substance that induces the production of antibodies

antigenic determinant the specific area of an antigen that binds with an antibody combining site and determines the specificity of the antigen–antibody reaction

antihistamine medication that opposes the action of histamine

antireflux valve valve that prevents return or backward flow of fluid

antrectomy removal of the pyloric (antrum) portion of the stomach with anastomosis (surgical connection) to the duodenum (gastroduodenostomy or Billroth I) or anas-tomosis to the jejunum (gastrojejunostomy or Billroth II)

anuria total urine output less than 50 mL in 24 hours

anus last section of the GI tract; outlet for waste products from the system

aortic valve semilunar valve located between the left ven-tricle and the aorta

aphasia impairment of language (including speaking, read-ing, writing, or comprehension) due to an injury of the brain

aphonia impaired ability to use one's voice due to disease or injury to the larynx

apical impulse also called *point of maximum impulse* (PMI); impulse normally palpated at the fifth intercostal space, left midclavicular line (or 7 to 9 cm from the left sternal border); caused by contraction of the left ventricle

aplasia lack of cellular development (e.g., of cells within the bone marrow)

apnea cessation of breathing/airflow for at least 10 seconds

apoptosis programmed cell death

apraxia inability to perform previously learned purposeful motor acts on a voluntary basis

aromatase inhibitors medications that block the produc-tion of estrogens by the adrenal glands

arrhythmia also referred to as *dysrhythmia;* disorder of the formation or conduction (or both) of the electrical impulse within the heart, altering the heart rate, heart rhythm, or both and potentially causing altered perfusion

arterial bypass surgical rerouting of blood around an obstructed artery, using a graft

arteriovenous fistula type of vascular access for dialysis; created by surgically connecting an artery to a vein

arteriovenous graft type of surgically created vascular access for dialysis by which a piece of biologic, semibiologic, or

synthetic graft material connects the patient's artery to a vein

arthrocentesis needle aspiration of synovial fluid

arthrodesis surgical fusion of a joint

arthroplasty the repair of joint problems through the oper-ating arthroscope (an instrument that allows the surgeon to operate within a joint without a large incision) or through open joint surgery

arthroscope surgical instrument used to examine internal joint structures

articulation a joint; the site of close approximation of two or more bones

asbestosis diffuse lung fibrosis resulting from exposure to asbestos fibers

ascites fluid accumulation in the abdominal cavity

aspiration removal of substance by suction; breathing of fluids or foods into the trachea and lungs

assist-control ventilation (A/C) mode of mechanical venti-lation in which the patient's breathing pattern may trigger the ventilator to deliver a preset tidal volume; in the absence of spontaneous breathing, the machine delivers a controlled breath at a preset minimum rate and tidal volume

assisted suicide use of pharmacologic agents to hasten the death of a terminally ill patient; illegal in most states

asterixis involuntary flapping movements of the hands associated with metabolic liver dysfunction

asthma a disease with multiple precipitating mechanisms characterized by the interaction between underlying inflammation, airway hyperresponsiveness, and obstruc-tion to airflow

astigmatism refractive error in which light rays are spread over a diffuse area rather than sharply focused on the ret-ina; a condition caused by differences in the curvature of the cornea and lens

ataxia inability to coordinate muscle movements, resulting in difficulty in walking, talking, and performing self-care activities; irregular, uncoordinated movements

atelectasis collapse or airless condition of the alveoli caused by hypoventilation, obstruction to the airways, or compression

atheroma fibrous cap composed of smooth muscle cells that forms over lipid deposits within arterial vessels and that protrudes into the lumen of the vessel, narrowing the lumen and obstructing blood flow; also called *plaque*

atherosclerosis disease process involving the accumula-tion of lipids, calcium, blood components, carbohydrates, and fibrous tissue on the intimal layer of arteries

atonic without tone; denervated muscle that atrophies

atony lack of normal muscle tone

atopic dermatitis type I hypersensitivity involving inflam-mation of the skin evidenced by itching, redness, and a variety of skin lesions

atrophy shrinkage-like decrease in the size of a muscle

atypical hyperplasia abnormal increase in the number of cells in a specific area within the ductal or lobular areas of the breast; this abnormal proliferation increases the risk for cancer

auscultatory gap a silent interval between systolic and diastolic Korotkoff sounds, causing an underestimation of the systolic pressure

autograft a graft derived from one part of a patient's body and used on another part of that same patient's body

autonomic dysreflexia also called autonomic hyperreflexia; a life-threatening emergency in spinal cord injury patients that causes a hypertensive emergency, occurs in patients with an injury at or above T6

autonomic nervous system division of the nervous system that regulates the involuntary body functions

autonomy self-determination; in the health care context, the right of the individual to make choices about the use and discontinuation of medical treatment

autoregulation ability of cerebral blood vessels to dilate or constrict to maintain stable cerebral blood flow despite changes in systemic arterial blood pressure

avascular necrosis death of tissue due to insufficient blood supply

axon portion of the neuron that conducts impulses away from the cell body

azotemia concentration of urea and other nitrogenous wastes in the blood

Babinski reflex (sign) a reflex action of the toes, indicative of abnormalities in the motor control pathways leading from the cerebral cortex

bacterial vaginosis a vaginal infection caused by an overgrowth of anaerobic bacteria

bacteriuria bacteria in the urine; bacterial count higher than 100,000 colonies/mL

balanced analgesia using more than one form of analgesia concurrently to obtain more pain relief with fewer side effects

balloon angioplasty a technique using a balloon, attached to a catheter, inflated to restore blood flow in blocked arteries

balloon tamponade use of balloons placed within the esophagus and proximal portion of the stomach and inflated to compress bleeding vessels (esophageal and gastric varices)

balneotherapy a bath with therapeutic additives

band cell slightly immature neutrophil

bandemia an excess of immature white blood cells released by the bone marrow into the blood; signifies infection or inflammation

bariatric term that comes from two Greek words meaning "weight" and "treatment"

baroreceptors nerve fibers located in the aortic arch and carotid arteries that are responsible for reflex control of the blood pressure

basal metabolic rate chemical reactions occurring when the body is at rest

basophil type of granulocyte; involved in the inflammatory response

B cells cells that are important for producing a humoral immune response

benign proliferative breast disease various types of atypical, yet noncancerous, breast tissue that increase the risk for breast cancer

benign prostatic hyperplasia (BPH) noncancerous enlargement or hypertrophy of the prostate; BPH is the most common pathologic condition in older men and the second most common cause of surgical intervention in men older than 60 years of age

bereavement period during which mourning for a loss takes place

Biliary tract defined as the organs and ducts that create and store bile and release it into the duodenum (the small intestine)

biologic response modifier (BRM) therapy use of agents or treatment methods that can alter the immunologic relationship between the tumor and the host to provide a therapeutic benefit

biologic warfare use of a biologic agent, such as anthrax, as a weapon of mass destruction

biopsy a diagnostic procedure to remove a small sample of tissue to be examined microscopically to detect malignant cells

blast cell primitive white blood cell

blindness inability to see, usually defined as corrected visual acuity of 20/400 or less, or a visual field of no more than 20 degrees in the better eye

bolus a feeding administered into the stomach in large amounts and at designated intervals

bone graft the placement of bone tissue (autologous or homologous grafts) to promote healing, to stabilize, or to replace diseased bone

borborygmus rumbling noise caused by the movement of gas through the intestines

brace externally applied device to support the body or a body part, control movement, and prevent injury

brachytherapy delivery of radiation therapy through internal implants

bradykinesia very slow voluntary movements and speech

brain death irreversible loss of all brain function, including the brainstem

brain injury an injury to the skull or brain that is severe enough to interfere with normal functioning

BRCA-1 and BRCA-2 genes on chromosome 17 that, when damaged or mutated, place a woman at greater risk for breast cancer and/or ovarian cancer compared with women who do not have the mutation

breakthrough pain a sudden and temporary increase in pain occurring in a patient being managed with opioid analgesia

breast conservation treatment surgery to remove a breast tumor and a margin of tissue around the tumor without removing any other part of the breast; may or may not include lymph node removal and radiation therapy

bronchoscopy direct examination of larynx, trachea, and bronchi using an endoscope

bruit sound produced by turbulent blood flow through an irregular, tortuous, stenotic, or dilated vessel

Budd–Chiari syndrome hepatic vein thrombosis resulting in noncirrhotic portal hypertension

bulbar paralysis immobility of muscles innervated by cranial nerves with their cell bodies in the lower portion of the brainstem

bursa fluid-filled sac found in connective tissue, usually in the area of joints

bursitis inflammation of a fluid-filled sac in a joint

calcitonin hormone secreted by the parafollicular cells of the thyroid gland; participates in calcium regulation (lowers blood calcium and phosphate level)

callus cartilaginous/fibrous tissue at fracture site

cancellous bone lattice-like bone structure; trabecular bone

cancer a disease process whereby cells proliferate abnormally, ignoring growth-regulating signals in the environment surrounding the cells

carboxyhemoglobin hemoglobin that is bound to carbon monoxide and therefore is unable to bind with oxygen, resulting in hypoxemia

carcinogenesis process of transforming normal cells into malignant cells

cardiac output amount of blood pumped by each ventricle in liters per minute; normal cardiac output is 4 to 6 L/min in the resting adult heart

cardiogenic shock shock state resulting from impairment or failure of the myocardium

cardiomyopathy disease of the heart muscle

cardioversion electrical current administered in synchrony with the patient's own QRS complex to stop arrhythmia

cartilage tough, elastic, avascular tissue at ends of bone

cast rigid external immobilizing device molded to contours of body part

CCR5 coreceptor or cell surface molecule needed along with the CD4$^+$ molecule for HIV to infect the host's immune system cells

cellular density the number of living cells in a unit

cellular immune response the immune system's third line of defense, involving the attack of pathogens by T cells

central cyanosis bluish discoloration of the skin or mucous membranes due to hemoglobin carrying reduced amounts of oxygen; often a late sign of hypoxia

central venous access device (CVAD) a device designed and used for long-term administration of medications and fluids into central veins

cerebral contusion bruising of the brain surface

cerebral edema swelling of the brain

cerumen yellow or brown, waxlike secretion found in the external auditory canal

cervical stenosis a narrowing or incomplete opening of the cervical os

cervix bottom (inferior) part of the uterus that is located in the vagina

chemical warfare use of a chemical agent, such as chlorine, as a weapon of mass destruction (WMD)

chemosis edema of the conjunctiva

chemotherapy use of medications to kill tumor cells by interfering with cellular functions and reproduction

chest drainage system use of a chest tube and closed drainage system to reexpand the lung and to remove excess air, fluid, and blood

chest percussion manually cupping over the chest wall to mobilize secretions by mechanically dislodging viscous or adherent secretions in the lungs

chest physiotherapy (CPT) therapy used to remove bronchial secretions, improve ventilation, and increase the efficiency of the respiratory muscles; types include postural drainage, chest percussion, and vibration

cholecystectomy removal of the gallbladder

cholecystitis inflammation of the gallbladder

cholecystokinin-pancreozymin (CCK-PZ) hormone; major stimulus for digestive enzyme secretion; stimulates contraction of the gallbladder

cholelithiasis the presence of calculi in the gallbladder

cholesteatoma tumor of the middle ear or mastoid, or both, that can destroy structures of the temporal bone

cholesterol a lipid that is an integral constituent of cell membranes, transported in the circulatory system bound to low-density and high-density lipoproteins

chordoplasty repair of the tendinous fibers that connect the edges of the atrioventricular valve leaflets to the papillary muscles

choroidal neovascularization new growth of new blood vessels beneath the retina; considered to be abnormal

chronic conditions medical or health problems with associated symptoms or disabilities that require long-term management (3 months or longer)

chronic obstructive bronchitis a disease of the airways defined as the presence of cough and sputum production for at least a combined total of 3 months in each of 2 consecutive years with obstruction to airflow; a category of COPD

chronic obstructive pulmonary disease (COPD) disease state characterized by airflow limitation that is not fully reversible; sometimes referred to as *chronic airway obstruction* or *chronic obstructive lung disease*

chyme mixture of food with saliva, salivary enzymes, and gastric secretions that is produced as the food passes through the mouth, esophagus, and stomach

cilia short hairs that provide a constant whipping motion that serves to propel mucus and foreign substances away from the lung toward the larynx

circulating nurse (or circulator) registered nurse who coordinates and documents patient care in the operating room

cirrhosis a chronic liver disease characterized by fibrotic changes and the formation of dense connective tissue within the liver, subsequent degenerative changes, and loss of functioning cells

clonus abnormal movement marked by alternating contraction and relaxation of a muscle occurring in rapid succession

CMS Center for Medicare Services; the federal agency that administers Medicare, Medicaid, and the Children's Health Insurance programs

cochlea the winding, snail-shaped bony tube that forms a portion of the inner ear and contains the organ of Corti, the transducer for hearing

cochlear (acoustic) nerve the division of the eighth cranial (vestibulocochlear) nerve, which goes to the cochlea

collagen a protein present in skin, tendon, bone, cartilage, and connective tissue

collateral small vessels that may enlarge to carry blood around a blocked vessel

colloids intravenous solutions that contain molecules that are too large to pass through capillary membranes

colonization microorganisms present in or on a host, without host interference or interaction and without eliciting symptoms in the host

colposcopy microscopic examination of the lower genital tract using a magnifying instrument called a colposcope

coma prolonged state of unconsciousness

commissurotomy splitting or separating fused cardiac valve leaflets

community an interacting population of individuals living together within a larger society

compartment syndrome increasing pressure in a muscle compartment causing impaired nerve and blood vessel function

complement series of enzymatic proteins in the serum that, when activated, destroy bacteria and other cells

complete spinal cord lesion a condition that involves total loss of sensation and voluntary muscle control below the lesion in the spinal cord

computed tomographic angiography (CTA) three-dimensional image created by specialized x-ray technique to visualize blood flow

concussion a temporary neurologic dysfunction caused by trauma to the head, classified as mild or classic based on symptoms (mild, without loss of consciousness or memory; classic, includes loss of consciousness and memory)

conduction transmission of electrical impulses from one cell to another

conductive hearing loss loss of hearing in which efficient sound transmission to the inner ear is interrupted by some obstruction or disease process

condyloma external genital warts carrying the human papilloma virus

cones retinal photoreceptor cells essential for visual acuity and color discrimination

congestive heart failure (CHF) a fluid overload condition (congestion) associated with heart failure

consolidation lung tissue that has become more solid in nature due to collapse of alveoli or infectious process (pneumonia)

constructional apraxia inability to draw figures in two or three dimensions

continent urinary diversion (Kock or Charleston pouch) transplantation of the ureters to a segment of bowel with construction of an effective continence mechanism or valve

continuous ambulatory peritoneal dialysis (CAPD) method of peritoneal dialysis whereby a patient performs four or five complete exchanges or cycles throughout the day

continuous cyclic peritoneal dialysis (CCPD) method of peritoneal dialysis in which a peritoneal dialysis machine (cycler) automatically performs exchanges, usually while the patient sleeps

continuous glucose monitoring system (CGMS) a device worn for 72 hours that continuously monitors blood glucose levels; the data are downloaded and analyzed for blood glucose patterns for that time period; presently used diagnostically to elicit patterns and tailor treatment

continuous passive motion (CPM) device a device that promotes range of motion, circulation, and healing

continuous positive airway pressure (CPAP) positive pressure applied throughout the respiratory cycle to a spontaneously breathing patient to promote alveolar and airway stability; may be administered with endotracheal or tracheostomy tube or by mask

continuous renal replacement therapy (CRRT) variety of methods used to replace normal kidney function by circulating the patient's blood through a filter and returning it to the patient

continuous subcutaneous insulin infusion a small device that delivers insulin on a 24-hour basis as basal insulin; it is also programmed by the patient to deliver a bolus dose before eating a meal in an attempt to mimic normal pancreatic function

continuous venovenous hemodialysis (CVVH or CVVHD) form of continuous renal replacement therapy that results in removal of fluid and waste products; venous blood circulates through a hemofilter and returns to the patient

contractility ability of the cardiac muscle to shorten in response to an electrical impulse

contracture abnormal shortening of muscle or joint, or both; fibrosis

control containment of the growth of cancer cells

contusion blunt force injury to soft tissue

cor pulmonale right heart failure due to elevated pulmonary artery pressures or lung disease

coronary artery bypass graft (CABG) a surgical procedure in which a blood vessel from another part of the body is grafted onto the occluded coronary artery below the occlusion in such a way that blood flow bypasses the blockage

corpus luteum site of a follicle that changes after ovulation to produce progesterone

corrosive poison alkaline or acidic agent; causes tissue destruction after contact

cortical bone compact bone

corticosteroids hormones produced by the adrenal cortex or their synthetic equivalents; also referred to as adrenal-cortical hormone and adrenocorticosteroid

crackles soft, high-pitched, discontinuous popping sounds during inspiration caused by delayed reopening of the airways

creatine kinase (CK) an enzyme found in human tissues; one of the three types of CK is specific to heart muscle and may be used as an indicator of heart muscle injury

creatinine endogenous waste product of muscle energy metabolism

crepitus grating or crackling sound or sensation; may occur with movement of ends of a broken bone or irregular joint surface

cricothyroidotomy surgical opening of the cricothyroid membrane to obtain an airway that is maintained with a tracheostomy or endotracheal tube

critical limb ischemia (CLI) chronic severe arterial obstruction with severe pain

cryosurgery of the prostate localized treatment of the prostate by application of freezing temperatures

crystalloids intravenous electrolyte solutions that move freely between the intravascular compartment and interstitial spaces

cure prolonged survival and disappearance of all evidence of disease so that the patient has the same life expectancy as anyone else in his or her age group

Cushing response a compensatory response that attempts to restore blood flow by increasing arterial pressure to overcome the increased intracranial pressure; this includes rising systolic pressure, widening pulse pressure, and bradycardia

Cushing syndrome symptoms resulting from excess free circulating cortisol from the adrenal cortex; characterized by truncal obesity, "moon face," acne, abdominal striae, and hypertension

Cushing triad three classic signs—bradycardia, hypertension, and bradypnea—that represent a loss of compensatory mechanism; a presentation of brainstem dysfunction

cystectomy removal of the urinary bladder

cystitis inflammation of the urinary bladder

cystocele weakness of the anterior vaginal wall that allows the bladder to protrude into the vagina

cytokines hormones produced by leukocytes that are vital to regulation of hematopoiesis, apoptosis, and immune responses; generic term for non-antibody proteins that act as intercellular mediators, as in the generation of immune response

cytologic studies examination of tissue samples (including body fluid) under a microscope, noting the structure, formation, and/or pathology of cells

cytotoxic destructive of cells

cytotoxic T cells lymphocytes that lyse cells infected with virus; also play a role in graft rejection

D-dimer test that measures fibrin breakdown; considered to be more specific than fibrin degradation products in the diagnosis of disseminated intravascular coagulation (DIC)

deafness partial or complete loss of the ability to hear

débridement removal of foreign material and devitalized tissue until surrounding healthy tissue is exposed

debulking surgical removal of all visible tumor in the abdomen

decerebration an abnormal posture associated with severe brain injury, characterized by extreme extension of the upper and lower extremities (extension, adduction and internal rotation of the arm and flexion of the wrist and fingers, extension of the legs, and plantarflexion of the feet)

decompression (intestinal) removal of intestinal contents to prevent gas and fluid from distending the coils of the intestine

decontamination process of removing, or rendering harmless, contaminants that have accumulated on personnel, patients, and equipment

decortication an abnormal posture associated with severe brain injury, characterized by abnormal flexion of the upper extremities (adduction at the shoulder, flexion at the elbow and wrist) and extension of the lower extremities (including hips and knees)

defibrillation electrical current administered to stop an arrhythmia, not synchronized with the patient's QRS complex

dehiscence partial or complete separation of wound edges

delayed union prolongation of expected healing time for a fracture

delirium transient loss of intellectual function, usually due to systemic problems

dementia a progressive organic mental disorder characterized by personality changes, confusion, disorientation, and deterioration of intellect associated with impaired memory and judgment

dendrite portion of the neuron that conducts impulses toward the cell body

dependence occurs when a patient who has been taking opioids experiences a withdrawal syndrome when the opioids are discontinued; often occurs with opioid tolerance and does not indicate an addiction

depolarization electrical stimulation that causes contraction of heart muscle

dermatosis any abnormal skin condition

dermis the second layer of skin containing sweat glands, hair follicles, and nerves

diabetes insipidus condition in which abnormally large volumes of dilute urine are excreted as a result of deficient production of vasopressin (ADH)

diabetes mellitus a group of metabolic diseases characterized by hyperglycemia resulting from defects in insulin secretion, insulin action, or both

diabetic ketoacidosis (DKA) a metabolic derangement in type 1 diabetes that results from a deficiency of insulin; highly acidic ketone bodies are formed, resulting in acidosis; usually requires hospitalization for treatment and is usually caused by nonadherence to the insulin regimen, concurrent illness, or infection

diagnostic peritoneal lavage instillation of lactated Ringer's or normal saline solution into the abdominal cavity to detect red blood cells, white blood cells, bile, bacteria, amylase, or gastrointestinal contents indicative of abdominal injury

dialysate solution that circulates through the dialyzer in hemodialysis and through the peritoneal membrane in peritoneal dialysis

dialyzer "artificial kidney" or dialysis machine; contains a semipermeable membrane through which particles of a certain size can pass

diaphysis shaft of long bone

diastole period of ventricular relaxation resulting in ventricular filling

diastolic heart failure the inability of the heart to pump sufficiently because of an alteration in the ability of the heart to fill; current term used to describe a type of heart failure

differentiation development of functions and characteristics that are different from those of the parent stem cell

diffusion movement of solutes (waste products) from an area of higher concentration to an area of lower concentration *or* exchange of gas molecules from areas of high concentration to areas of low concentration

digestion phase of the digestive process that occurs when digestive enzymes and secretions mix with ingested food and when proteins, fats, and sugars are broken down into their component smaller molecules

dilutional hyponatremia sodium deficiency that develops as a result of fluid retention; associated with excessive antidiuretic hormone secretion in patients with syndrome of inappropriate antidiuretic hormone (SIADH) secretion

diplopia double vision, or the awareness of two images of the same object occurring in one or both eyes

disability restriction or lack of ability to perform an activity in a normal manner; the consequences of impairment in terms of an individual's functional performance and activity; disabilities represent disturbances at the level of the person (e.g., bathing, dressing, communication, walking, grooming)

disarticulation amputation through a joint

dislocation separation of joint surfaces

distributive shock shock state resulting from displacement of blood volume creating a relative hypovolemia and inadequate delivery of oxygen to the cells

diverticulitis inflammation of a diverticulum from obstruction (by fecal matter)

diverticulosis presence of several diverticula in the intestine; common in middle age

dizziness altered sensation of orientation in space

donor site the area from which skin is taken to provide a skin graft for another part of the body

Doppler ultrasonography noninvasive diagnostic procedure to assess blood flow direction, velocity, and turbulence

DRG diagnostic related group; diagnostic categories used by Medicare to classify patients when prospectively paying health care organizations for patient care

dry powder inhaler (DPI) inhalation devices used to deliver medications to the lungs as suspended dry powder

ductal carcinoma in situ (DCIS) cancer cells that start in the ductal system of the breast but have not penetrated the surrounding tissue

dumping syndrome rapid emptying of the stomach contents into the small intestine; characterized by sweating and weakness

duodenum the first part of the small intestine, which connects with the pylorus of the stomach and extends to the jejunum

duplex ultrasound combines grayscale tissue imaging with velocity changes

dysarthria defects of articulation of language (slurred speech)

dyschezia pain with defecation

dyskinesia impaired ability to execute voluntary movements

dyslipidemia abnormal blood lipid levels, including high total, LDL, and triglyceride levels, as well as low HDL levels

dysmenorrhea painful menstruation that is not associated with any type of pathologic process

dyspareunia painful sexual intercourse

dysphagia difficulty swallowing, causing the patient to be at risk for aspiration

dysphonia abnormal voice quality caused by weakness and incoordination of muscles responsible for speech

dysplasia bizarre cell growth resulting in cells that differ in size, shape, or arrangement from other cells of the same type of tissue

dyspnea labored breathing or shortness of breath

dyspnea on exertion (DOE) shortness of breath that occurs with exertion

dysuria painful or difficult urination

ecchymosis bruise

ectopic pregnancy fertilized egg implants anywhere outside of body of the uterus, commonly the fallopian tube

edema soft tissue swelling due to fluid accumulation

effusion excess fluid in joint

EIA (enzyme immunoassay) a blood test that can determine the presence of antibodies to HIV in the blood or saliva; also referred as *enzyme-linked immunosorbent assay* (ELISA); positive results are verified with a Western blot test

ejection fraction percentage of the end-diastolic blood volume ejected from the ventricle with each heartbeat; normal is between 55% and 70%

elimination phase of digestive process that occurs after digestion and absorption, when waste products are evacuated from the body

embolus a piece of thrombus that travels through a vessel and blocks a smaller vessel

emergent triage category signifying potentially life-threatening injuries or illnesses requiring immediate treatment

emmetropia absence of refractive error

emphysema a disease of the airways characterized by destruction of the walls of over distended alveoli; a category of COPD

emptysis the coughing up of blood from the lower respiratory tract

empyema accumulation of purulent material in the pleural space

endocrine secreting internally; hormonal secretion of a ductless gland

endolymphatic hydrops dilation of the endolymphatic space of the inner ear; the pathologic correlate of Ménière disease

endometrial ablation procedure performed through a hysteroscope in which the lining of the uterus is burned away or ablated to treat abnormal uterine bleeding

endometriosis the growth of cells similar to the endometrial lining outside of the uterus causing heavy and painful menses

endometrium lining of the uterus

endorphins, enkephalins, and dynorphins morphine-like substances produced by the body; primarily found in the central nervous system; they have the potential to reduce pain

endoscopic retrograde cholangiopancreatography (ERCP) an endoscopic procedure using fiberoptic technology to visualize the biliary system

endosteum a thin, vascular membrane covering the marrow cavity of long bones and the spaces in cancellous bone

endotracheal intubation insertion of a breathing tube through the nose or mouth into the trachea

end-stage renal disease (ESRD) progressive, irreversible deterioration in renal function that results in retention of uremic waste products

enteroclysis fluoroscopic x-ray of the small intestine; a tube is placed from the nose or mouth through the esophagus and the stomach to the duodenum, a barium-based liquid contrast material is infused through the tube, and x-rays are taken as it travels through the duodenum

enterostomal therapist nurse specially educated in appropriate skin, wound, ostomy, and continence care; often referred to as wound-care specialist or wound–ostomy–continence nurse (WOCN)

enucleation complete removal of the eyeball and part of the optic nerve

eosinophil type of granulocyte; involved in allergic reactions

epidermis the outermost layer of skin

epidermopoiesis development of epidermal cells

epididymitis infection of the epididymis that usually descends from an infected prostate or urinary tract; also may develop as a complication of gonorrhea

epilepsy a group of syndromes characterized by paroxysmal transient disturbances of brain function

epiphysis end of long bone

epistaxis hemorrhage from the nose due to rupture of tiny, distended vessels in the mucous membrane of any area of the nose

epitope any component of an antigen molecule that functions as an antigenetic determinant by permitting the attachment of certain antibodies

erectile dysfunction also called *impotence;* the inability to either achieve or maintain an erection sufficient to accomplish sexual intercourse

erythema redness of the skin caused by congestion of the capillaries

erythrocyte *see* **red blood cell**

erythrocyte sedimentation rate (ESR) laboratory test that measures the rate of settling of red blood cells; elevation is indicative of inflammation; also called the *sed rate*

erythropoiesis process of red blood cell formation

erythropoietin hormone produced primarily by the kidney; necessary for erythropoiesis

eschar devitalized tissue resulting from a burn

escharotomy a linear excision made through eschar to release constriction of underlying tissue

esophagogastroduodenoscopy (EGD) passage of a fiberoptic tube through the mouth and throat into the digestive tract for visualization of the esophagus, stomach, and small intestine; biopsies can be performed

esophagus collapsible tube connecting the mouth to the stomach, through which food passes as it is ingested

estrogen hormone that develops and maintains the female reproductive system

eustachian tube the 3- to 4-cm tube that extends from the middle ear to the nasopharynx

euthanasia Greek for "good death"; has evolved to mean the intentional killing by act or omission of a dependent human being for his or her alleged benefit

euthyroid state of normal thyroid hormone production

evisceration (eye) removal of the intraocular contents through a corneal or scleral incision; the optic nerve, sclera, extraocular muscles, and sometimes, the cornea are left intact

evisceration (wound) protrusion of organs through the surgical incision

excision surgical removal of tissue

exenteration surgical removal of the entire contents of the orbit, including the eyeball and lids

exocrine secreting externally; hormonal secretion from excretory ducts

exophthalmos abnormal protrusion of one or both eyeballs; produces a startled expression; usually due to hyperthyroidism

expressive aphasia difficulty expressing thoughts through speech or written language; inability to express oneself; often associated with damage to the left frontal lobe area (also known as Broca aphasia)

external auditory canal the canal leading from the external auditory meatus to the tympanic membrane; about 2.5 cm in length

external ear the portion of the ear that consists of the auricle and external auditory canal; it is separated from the middle ear by the tympanic membrane

external fixator external metal frame attached to bone fragments to stabilize them

extravasation leakage of medication from the veins into the subcutaneous tissues

fascia (epimysium) fibrous tissue that covers, supports, and separates muscles

fasciculation involuntary twitch of muscle fibers

fasciotomy the incision and diversion of the muscle fascia to relieve muscle constriction, as in compartment syndrome, or to reduce fascia contracture

fasting plasma glucose (FPG) blood glucose determination obtained in the laboratory after fasting for more than 8 hours; although plasma levels are specified in diagnostic criteria, blood glucose levels, which are slightly higher than plasma levels, are more commonly used

feedback the return of information about the results of input given to a person or a system

female-to-male (FTM) a biologic female who is becoming a male

fetor hepaticus sweet, slightly fecal odor to the breath, presumed to be of intestinal origin; prevalent with the extensive collateral portal circulation in chronic liver disease

fibrin filamentous protein; basis of thrombus and blood clot

fibrinogen protein converted into fibrin to form thrombus and clot

fibrinolysis process of breakdown of fibrin clot

fibrinolytic a substance that acts to break up fibrin, the fine filaments of blood clots

fibrocystic breast changes term used to describe certain benign changes in the breast, typically associated with palpable nodularity, lumpiness, swelling, or pain

fibroscopy (gastrointestinal) intubation of a part of the GI system with a flexible, lighted tube to assist in diagnosis and treatment of diseases of that area

fine-needle aspiration insertion of a needle through the chest wall to obtain cells of a mass or tumor; usually performed under fluoroscopy or chest CT guidance

first-intention healing method of healing in which wound edges are surgically approximated and integumentary continuity is restored without granulation

flaccid displaying lack of muscle tone; limp, floppy

follicle-stimulating hormone (FSH) hormone released by the pituitary gland to stimulate estrogen production and ovulation

fornix upper part of the vagina

fraction of inspired oxygen (FiO$_2$) concentration of oxygen delivered (1.0 = 100% oxygen)

fracture a break in the continuity of a bone

fracture reduction restoration of fracture fragments into anatomic alignment and rotation

frequency voiding more frequently than every 3 hours

fulminant hepatic failure sudden, severe onset of acute liver failure that occurs within 8 weeks after the first symptoms of jaundice

functional incontinence physical impairments make it difficult or impossible for the patient to reach the toilet in time for voiding

fundus body of the uterus *or* the interior surface of the eye, opposite the lens, and includes the retina, optic disc, macula and fovea, and posterior pole

gangrene dead tissue

gastric refers to the stomach

gastric outlet obstruction (GOO) any condition that mechanically impedes normal gastric emptying; there is obstruction of the channel of the pylorus and duodenum through which the stomach empties

gastritis inflammation of the stomach

gastroesophageal reflux back-flow of gastric or duodenal contents into the esophagus

gastrostomy surgical creation of an opening into the stomach for the purpose of administering foods and fluids

genetics engineering emerging technology designed to enable replacement of missing or defective genes

gestational diabetes mellitus (GDM) any degree of glucose intolerance with its onset during pregnancy

glomerular filtration rate (GFR) volume of plasma filtered at the glomerulus into the kidney tubules each minute; normal rate is approximately 120 mL/min

glomerulonephritis inflammation of the glomerular capillaries

glomerulus tuft of capillaries forming part of the nephron through which filtration occurs

glucagon a hormone secreted by the alpha cells of the islets of Langerhans of the pancreas that increases the blood glucose by stimulating the liver to convert stored glycogen to glucose

glucocorticoids steroid hormones (i.e., cortisol, cortisone, and corticosterone) secreted by the adrenal cortex in response to ACTH; produces a rise of liver glycogen and blood glucose and counteracts inflammatory responses

glycated hemoglobin (glycosylated hemoglobin, Hgb A$_{1c}$ or A1C) a long-term measure of glucose control that is a result of glucose attaching to hemoglobin for the life of the red blood cell (120 days); the goal of diabetes therapy is a normal to near-normal level of glycolated hemoglobin, the same as in the nondiabetic population

goiter enlargement of the thyroid gland; usually caused by an iodine-deficient diet

graafian follicle ovarian cells that form into a structure on the surface of the ovary that houses the ovum or unfertilized egg

grading identification of the type of tissue from which the tumor originated and the degree to which the tumor cells retain the functional and structural characteristics of the tissue of origin

graft-versus-host disease (GVHD) an immune response initiated by T lymphocytes of donor tissue against the recipient's tissues (skin, gastrointestinal tract, liver); an undesirable response

graft-versus-tumor effect the donor cell response against the malignancy; a desirable response

granulocyte granulated white blood cell (neutrophil, eosinophil, basophil); sometimes used synonymously with neutrophil

granulomas cells surrounded by lymphocytes, which can be found in all layers of the bowel; if present, they strongly suggest Crohn disease

Graves' disease a form of hyperthyroidism; characterized by a diffuse goiter and exophthalmos

grief the personal feelings that accompany an anticipated or actual loss

Hashimoto disease thyroiditis (inflammation of the thyroid gland) characterized by high levels of antimicrosomal antibodies; an autoimmune disorder that is the most common cause of hypothyroidism in the United States

head injury an injury to the scalp, skull, and/or brain

health education a variety of learning experiences designed to promote behaviors that facilitate health

health promotion the art and science of assisting people to change their lifestyle toward a higher state of wellness

hearing loss dysfunction of any component of the auditory system (conductive hearing loss, sensorineural hearing loss, mixed hearing loss)

heart failure (HF) the inability of the heart to pump sufficient blood to meet the needs of the tissues for oxygen and nutrients; signs and symptoms of pulmonary and systemic congestion may or may not be present

Helicobacter pylori a spiral-shaped gram-negative bacterium that colonizes the gastric mucosa; involved in most cases of peptic ulcer disease

helper T cells lymphocytes that attack foreign pathogens (antigens) directly

hematemesis vomiting of blood

hematocrit percentage of total blood volume consisting of red blood cells

hematopoiesis complex process of the formation and maturation of blood cells

hematuria red blood cells in the urine

hemianopsia blindness in half of the field of vision in one or both eyes

hemiarthroplasty the replacement of one of the articular surfaces (e.g., in a hip hemiarthroplasty, the femoral head and neck are replaced with a femoral prosthesis—the acetabulum is not replaced)

hemiplegia/hemiparesis paralysis/weakness on one side of the body, or part or it, due to an injury to the motor areas of the brain

hemodialysis procedure during which a patient's blood is circulated through a dialyzer to remove waste products and excess fluid

hemodynamic monitoring use of devices to measure cardiovascular function

hemoglobin iron-containing protein of red blood cells; delivers oxygen to tissues

hemolysis destruction of red blood cells; can occur within or outside of the vasculature

hemorrhagic stroke a stroke that results from bleeding into the brain tissue itself or into the subarachnoid space or ventricles

hemostasis a dynamic process that involves the cessation of bleeding from an injured vessel, which requires activity of blood vessels, platelets, coagulation, and fibrinolytic systems; intricate balance between clot formation and clot dissolution

hemothorax partial or complete collapse of the lung due to blood accumulating in the pleural space; may occur after surgery or trauma

hepatic encephalopathy central nervous system dysfunction resulting from liver disease; frequently associated with elevated ammonia levels that produce changes in mental status, altered level of consciousness, and coma

hernia protrusion of an organ or part of an organ through the wall of the cavity that normally contains it

herniation abnormal protrusion of tissue through a defect or natural opening

herpes simplex cold sore (cutaneous viral infection with painful vesicles and erosions on the tongue, palate, gingiva, buccal membranes, or lips)

high-density lipoprotein (HDL) a protein-bound lipid that transports cholesterol to the liver for excretion in the bile; composed of a higher proportion of protein to lipid than low-density lipoprotein; exerts a beneficial effect on the arterial wall

hirsutism the condition of having excessive hair growth

histamine substance in the body that causes increased gastric secretion, dilation of capillaries, and constriction of the bronchial smooth muscle

histamine-2 (H₂) receptor antagonist a pharmacologic agent that inhibits histamine action at the H₂ receptors of the stomach, resulting in inhibition of gastric acid secretion

HIV-1 retrovirus isolated and recognized as the etiologic agent of AIDS

HIV-2 virus closely related to HIV-1 that also causes AIDS, predominantly found in West Africa

homeostasis maintenance of a constant internal equilibrium in a biologic system that involves positive and negative feedback mechanisms

hormones chemical transmitter substances produced in one organ or part of the body and carried by the bloodstream to other cells or organs on which they have a specific regulatory effect; produced mainly by endocrine glands (e.g., pituitary, thyroid, gonads)

hospice a coordinated program of interdisciplinary care and services provided primarily in the home to terminally ill patients and their families

humoral immune response the immune system's second line of defense; often termed the *antibody response*

hydrocele a collection of fluid, generally in the tunica vaginalis of the testis, although it also may collect within the spermatic cord

hydrocephalus excessive cerebrospinal fluid (CSF) in the intracranial cavity, commonly due to obstruction of flow in the ventricular system or subarachnoid space

hydrochloric acid acid secreted by the glands in the stomach; mixes with chyme to break it down into absorbable molecules and to aid in the destruction of bacteria

hydrophilic a material that absorbs moisture

hydrostatic pressure the pressure created by the weight of fluid against the wall that contains it; in the body, hydrostatic pressure in blood vessels results from the weight of fluid itself and the force resulting from cardiac contraction

hygroscopic a material that absorbs moisture from the air

hymen tissue that covers the vaginal opening partially or completely before vaginal penetration

hyperemia "red eye" resulting from dilation of the vasculature of the conjunctiva

hyperglycemia elevated blood glucose level; fasting level greater than 110 mg/dL (6.1 mmol/L); 2-hour postprandial level greater than 140 mg/dL (7.8 mmol/L)

hyperglycemic hyperosmolar nonketotic syndrome (HHNS) a metabolic disorder of type 2 diabetes resulting from a relative insulin deficiency initiated by an intercurrent illness that raises the demand for insulin; associated with polyuria and severe dehydration

hyperopia farsightedness; a refractive error in which the focus of light rays from a distant object is behind the retina

hyperpigmentation increase in the melanin of the skin, resulting in an increase in pigmentation

hyperplasia abnormally increased proliferation of normal cells

hypersensitivity abnormal heightened reaction to a stimulus of any kind

hypertension blood pressure of 140/90 mm Hg or greater

hypertensive emergency a situation in which blood pressure is severely elevated and there is evidence of actual or probable target organ damage

hypertensive urgency a situation in which blood pressure is severely elevated but there is no evidence of target organ damage

hypertonic solution a solution with an osmolality higher than that of serum

hypertrophy enlargement; increase in size of muscle

hyphema blood in the anterior chamber

hypochromia pallor within the red blood cell caused by decreased hemoglobin content

hypoglycemia low blood glucose level (<60 mg/dL [<2.7 mmol/L])

hypophysectomy surgical removal of all or part of the pituitary gland

hypopigmentation decrease in the melanin of the skin, resulting in a loss of pigmentation

hyposmia impairment of the sense of smell

hypotension a decrease in blood pressure to less than 90/60 mm Hg

hypotonic solution a solution with an osmolality lower than that of serum

hypovolemic shock shock state resulting from decreased intravascular volume due to fluid loss or deficit; causes include hemorrhage and dehydration

hypoxemia decrease in arterial oxygen tension in the blood

hypoxia decrease in oxygen supply to the tissues and cells

iatrogenic incontinence the involuntary loss of urine due to extrinsic medical factors, predominantly medications

ileal conduit transplantation of the ureters to an isolated section of the terminal ileum, with one end of the ureters brought to the abdominal wall

ileus decreased motility of the GI tract, often the result of irritation of the peritoneum; signs and symptoms include diffuse abdominal discomfort, nausea, vomiting, abdominal distention, hypoactive or absent bowel sounds, absent bowel movement/flatus

immunity the body's specific protective response to an invading foreign agent or organism

immunopathology study of diseases resulting in dysfunctions within the immune system

immunoregulation complex system of checks and balances that regulates or controls immune responses

impaired fasting glucose (IFG), impaired glucose tolerance (IGT) a metabolic stage intermediate between normal glucose homeostasis and diabetes; not clinical entities in their own right but risk factors for future diabetes and cardiovascular disease

impairment loss or abnormality of psychological, physiologic, or anatomic structure or function at the organ level (e.g., dysphagia, hemiparesis); an abnormality of body structure, appearance, and organ or system function resulting from any cause

imperforate hymen membrane at the vaginal opening, or introitus, that is still intact and causing obstruction

implantable cardioverter defibrillator (ICD) a device implanted into the chest to treat arrhythmias

incentive spirometry method of deep breathing that provides visual feedback to help the patient inhale deeply and slowly and achieve maximum lung inflation

incomplete spinal cord lesion a condition where there is preservation of the sensory or motor fibers, or both, below the lesion in the spinal cord

incus the second of the three ossicles in the middle ear; it articulates with the malleus and stapes; the anvil

induration an abnormally hard lesion or reaction, as in a positive tuberculin skin test

infection condition in which the host interacts physiologically and immunologically with a microorganism

infectious disease the consequences that result from invasion of the body by microorganisms that can produce harm to the body and potentially death

informed consent the patient's autonomous decision about whether to undergo a surgical procedure; based on the nature of the condition, the treatment options, and the risks and benefits involved

ingestion phase of the digestive process that occurs when food is taken into the GI tract via the mouth and esophagus

injection congestion of blood vessels

inner ear the portion of the ear that consists of the cochlea, vestibule, and semicircular canals

insulin a hormone secreted by the beta cells of the islets of Langerhans of the pancreas that is necessary for the metabolism of carbohydrates, proteins, and fats

interdisciplinary collaboration communication and cooperation among members of diverse health care disciplines jointly to plan, implement, and evaluate care

interferons proteins formed when cells are exposed to viral or foreign agents; capable of activating other components of the immune system

intermittent claudication a muscular, cramp-like pain in the extremities consistently reproduced with the same degree of exercise or activity and relieved by rest

intermittent mandatory ventilation (IMV) mode of mechanical ventilation that provides a combination of mechanically assisted breaths and spontaneous breaths

internal auditory canal a canal in the petrous portion of the temporal bone that houses the facial and vestibulocochlear nerves (cranial nerves VII and VIII)

internal fixation the stabilization of the reduced fracture by the use of metal screws, plates, wires, nails, and pins

international normalized ratio (INR) a standard method for monitoring prothrombin levels in patients receiving oral anticoagulation (warfarin), eliminating the variation in test results from laboratory to laboratory

interstitial cystitis inflammation of the bladder wall that eventually causes disintegration of the lining and loss of bladder elasticity

interstitial nephritis inflammation within the renal tissue

intracranial pressure pressure exerted by the volume of the intracranial contents within the cranial vault

intraoperative phase period of time from when the patient is transferred to the operating room table to when he or she is admitted to the postanesthesia care unit (PACU)

intrathecal chemotherapy chemotherapeutic agents injected directly into the subarachnoid space

intrinsic factor a gastric secretion that combines with vitamin B_{12} so that the vitamin can be absorbed

introitus perineal opening to the vagina

involucrum new bone growth around a sequestrum

ischemia insufficient tissue oxygenation

ischemic stroke stroke that results from inadequate blood supply to the brain due to partial or complete occlusion of an artery

islet cell transplantation an investigational procedure in which purified islet cells from cadaver donors are injected into the portal vein of the liver, with the goal of having these cells secrete insulin and cure type 1 diabetes

isoelectric line the baseline or flat part of the electrocardiogram (ECG), frequently noted between the T and P waves, or between the P wave and the QRS complex; ST-segment elevation or depression is noted by observing the relationship of the ST-segment to the isoelectric line (above or below)

isometric contraction muscle tension increased, length unchanged, no joint motion

isotonic contraction muscle tension unchanged, muscle shortened, joint moved

isotonic solution a solution with the same osmolality as serum and other body fluids; osmolality falls within normal range for serum (280 to 300 mOsm/kg)

jaundice yellowing discoloration of the skin by abnormally high levels of bilirubin in the blood

jejunum second portion of the small intestine, extending from the duodenum to the ileum

JNC 7 Seventh Joint National Committee on the Prevention, Detection, Evaluation, and Treatment of High Blood Pressure; committee established to study and make recommendations about hypertension in the United States;

findings and recommendations of JNC 7 are contained in an extensive report published in 2003

joint area where bone ends meet; provides for motion and flexibility

joint arthroplasty or replacement the replacement of joint surfaces with metal or synthetic materials

joint capsule fibrous tissue that encloses bone ends and other joint surfaces

joint effusion the escape of fluid from the blood vessels or lymphatics into the joint space

Kegel exercises exercises that contract and relax the pelvic floor muscle, helping to strengthen it

keratin an insoluble, fibrous protein that forms the outer layer of skin

ketone a highly acidic substance formed when the liver breaks down free fatty acids in the absence of insulin

Kock pouch a type of ileostomy in which the surgeon forms an artificial rectum from a section of the ileum

Kussmaul respirations increase in respiration, particularly the tidal volume associated with metabolic acidosis

kyphosis increase in the convex curvature of the spine

lactobacilli vaginal bacteria that limit the growth of other bacteria by producing hydrogen peroxide

lamellae mature compact bone structures that form concentric rings of bone matrix; lamellar bone

laminectomy excision of the posterior arches and spinous processes of a vertebra

Langerhans cells dendritic clear cells in the epidermis that carry surface receptors for immunoglobulin and that are active participants in delayed hypersensitivity of the skin; in addition, these cells are responsible for carrying invading bacteria to lymphocytes in lymph glands where they are neutralized

laparoscopic cholecystectomy removal of gallbladder through endoscopic procedure

large intestine the portion of the GI tract into which waste material from the small intestine passes as absorption continues and elimination begins; consists of several parts—ascending segment, transverse segment, descending segment, sigmoid colon, and rectum

laryngectomy removal of all or part of the larynx and surrounding structures

laryngitis inflammation of the larynx; may be caused by voice abuse, exposure to irritants, or infectious organisms

latency time interval after primary infection when a microorganism lives within the host without producing clinical evidence

lavage flushing of the stomach via the gastric tube with water or other fluids to clear it

leaflet repair repair of a cardiac valve's movable "flaps" (leaflets)

learning the act of gaining knowledge and skill

learning readiness the optimum time for learning to occur; usually corresponds to the learner's perceived need and desire to obtain specific knowledge

leukemia a progressive, malignant disease characterized by uncontrolled proliferation of white blood cells

leukocyte *see* **white blood cell**

leukopenia less than normal amount of white blood cells in circulation

lichenification thickening of the horny layer of the skin

ligament fibrous band connecting bones

limbus junction of the cornea and sclera

liniments lotions with added oil for increased softening of the skin

lipase an enzyme that aids in the digestion of fats

lobular carcinoma in situ (LCIS) atypical change and proliferation of the lobular cells of the breast; previously considered a premalignant condition but now considered a marker of increased risk for invasive breast cancer

locked-in syndrome condition due to a lesion at or below the pons or midbrain, which results in the inability to movement while consciousness is preserved; communication is severely limited

lordosis increase in lumbar curvature of the spine

low-density lipoprotein (LDL) a protein-bound lipid that transports cholesterol to tissues in the body; composed of a lower proportion of protein to lipid than high-density lipoprotein; exerts a harmful effect on the arterial wall

low-profile gastrostomy device (LPGD, G-button) an enteral feeding access device that is flush with the skin and is used for long-term feeding

luteal phase the second half or secretory phase of the menstrual cycle that occurs after ovulation

luteinizing hormone (LH) hormone released by the pituitary gland that stimulates progesterone production

lymphedema chronic swelling of an extremity due to interrupted lymphatic circulation, typically from an axillary lymph node dissection

lymphocyte form of white blood cell involved in immune functions

lymphoid pertaining to lymphocytes

lymphokines substances released by sensitized lymphocytes when they come in contact with specific antigens

lysis destruction of cells

macrophage cells of the reticuloendothelial system (RES) that are capable of phagocytosis

magnetic resonance angiography (MRA) the use of magnetic fields and radio waves to produce two- or three-dimensional images of blood vessels

male-to-female (MTF) a biologic male who is becoming a female

malignant having cells or processes that are characteristic of cancer

malleus the first (most lateral) and largest of the three ossicles in the middle ear; it is connected to the tympanic membrane laterally and articulates with the incus; the hammer

malunion healing of a fractured bone in a malaligned position

mammoplasty surgical procedure to reconstruct or change the size or shape of the breast; can be performed for reduction or augmentation

mass casualty incident (MCI) situation in which the number of casualties exceeds the number of resources

mastalgia breast pain, usually related to hormonal fluctuations or irritation of a nerve

mechanical ventilation a positive- or negative-pressure breathing device that supports ventilation and oxygenation

Medicare Hospice Benefit a Medicare entitlement that provides for comprehensive, interdisciplinary palliative care and services for eligible beneficiaries who have a terminal illness and a life expectancy of less than 6 months

megacolon an acquired or congenital abnormal enlargement of the colon

melanin the substance responsible for melanin

melanocytes cells of the skin that produce coloration of the skin

melena tarry or black stools; indicative of blood in stools

memory cells cells that are responsible for recognizing antigens from previous exposure and mounting an immune response

menarche beginning of menstrual function

Ménière disease condition of the inner ear characterized by a triad of symptoms episodic vertigo, tinnitus, and fluctuating sensorineural hearing loss

meniscectomy the excision of damaged joint fibrocartilage

menopause permanent cessation of menstruation resulting from the loss of ovarian follicular activity

menorrhagia excessive bleeding that occurs in regular cycles

menstruation sloughing and discharge of the lining of the uterus if conception does not take place

Merkel cells cells of the epidermis that play a role in transmission of sensory messages

metabolic syndrome a cluster of metabolic abnormalities including insulin resistance, obesity, dyslipidemia, and hypertension that increase the risk of cardiovascular disease

metaplasia conversion of one type of mature cell into another type of cell

metastasis spread of cancer cells from the primary tumor to distant sites

metered-dose inhaler (MDI) patient-activated medication canister that provides aerosolized medication that the patient inhales into the lungs

metrorrhagia irregular vaginal bleeding that is heavy and prolonged

microcytosis smaller than normal red blood cells

micrographia small and often illegible handwriting

micturition urination or voiding

middle ear the small, air-filled cavity in the temporal bone that contains the three ossicles

migraine headache a severe, unrelenting headache often accompanied by symptoms such as nausea, vomiting, and visual disturbances

mineralocorticoid steroid of the adrenal cortex; primarily aldosterone, which promotes retention of sodium and therefore water and excretion of potassium

minor triage category signifying non–life-threatening injuries or illnesses that can be routinely managed in a clinic or physician's office or that require no medical care

miotics medications that cause pupillary constriction

mitral valve atrioventricular valve located between the left atrium and left ventricle

mittelschmerz midcycle ovulatory pain caused by a ruptured corpus luteum

moderate sedation use of sedation to depress the level of consciousness without altering the patient's ability to maintain a patent airway and to respond to physical stimuli and verbal commands, previously referred to as *conscious sedation*

modified radical mastectomy removal of the breast tissue, nipple–areola complex, and a portion of the axillary lymph nodes

monitored anesthesia care (MAC) moderate sedation administered by an anesthesiologist or anesthetist

monocyte large white blood cell that develop into a macrophage when transported to tissues

Monro–Kellie hypothesis theory that states that due to limited space for expansion within the skull, an increase in volume of any one of the cranial contents—brain tissue, blood, or CSF—must be compensated for by a decrease in volume of another

morbid obesity more than twice ideal body weight, 100 lb or more over ideal body weight, or body mass index (BMI) exceeding 30 kg/m^2

mourning individual, family, group, and cultural expressions of grief and associated behaviors

mouth first portion of the GI tract, through which food is ingested

murmurs sounds created by abnormal, turbulent flow of blood in the heart

mydriatics medications instilled in the eyes that cause pupillary dilation

myeloid pertaining to nonlymphoid blood cells that differentiate into red blood cells, platelets, monocytes and macrophages, neutrophils, eosinophils, basophils, and mast cells

myelopoiesis formation and maturation of cells derived from myeloid stem cell

myelosuppression suppression of the blood cell–producing function of the bone marrow

myocardial infarction (MI) death of heart tissue caused by lack of oxygenated blood flow; if acute, abbreviated as AMI

myocardium muscle layer of the heart responsible for the pumping action of the heart

myoglobinuria iron-containing protein from muscle cells in the urine often following trauma

myomectomy surgical excision of uterine fibroids that preserves fertility

myopia nearsightedness; a refractive error in which the focus of light rays from a distant object is anterior to the retina

myxedema refers to the soft tissue changes in subcutaneous and other interstitial tissues in a person with hypothyroidism

nadir lowest point of white blood cell depression after therapy that has toxic effects on the bone marrow

nasoduodenal tube tube inserted through the nose into the beginning of the small intestine (duodenum)

nasogastric (NG) tube tube inserted through the nose into the stomach

nasojejunal tube tube inserted through the nose into the second portion of the small intestine (jejunum)

natural killer cells (NK cells) lymphocytes that defend against microorganisms and malignant cells

negative feedback regulating mechanism in which an increase or decrease in the level of a substance decreases or increases the function of the organ producing the substance

neoadjuvant chemotherapy preoperative chemotherapy; it is administered preoperatively to shrink a large tumor

neoplasm/tumor/lesion an abnormal mass of tissues, which can be benign or malignant in nature

nephron structural and functional unit of the kidney responsible for urine formation

nephropathy a long-term complication of diabetes in which the kidney cells are damaged; characterized by microalbuminuria in early stages and progressing to end-stage renal disease

nephrosclerosis atherosclerosis of renal arteries causing fibrosis, glomerular damage, ischemia

neurodegenerative a disease, process, or condition that leads to deterioration of normal cells or function of the nervous system

neurogenic bladder bladder dysfunction that results from a disorder or dysfunction of the nervous system; may result in either urinary retention or bladder overactivity, resulting in urinary urgency and urge incontinence

neurogenic shock a type of distributive shock state resulting from loss of sympathetic vascular tone causing low blood pressure

neuropathy a long-term complication of diabetes resulting from damage to the nerve cell

neurovascular status neurologic (motor and sensory components) and circulatory functioning of a body part

neutropenia abnormally low absolute neutrophil count

neutrophil fully mature white blood cell capable of phagocytosis; primary defense against bacterial infection

nociception activation of sensory transduction in nerves by thermal, mechanical, or chemical energy impinging on specialized nerve endings; the nerves involved convey information about tissue damage to the central nervous system

nociceptor a receptor preferentially sensitive to a noxious stimulus

nocturia awakening at night to urinate

nonunion failure of fragments of a fractured bone to heal together

nonurgent triage category signifying episodic or minor injury or illness in which treatment may be delayed several hours or longer without increased morbidity

normal flora persistent nonpathogenic organisms colonizing a host

normal heart sounds referred to as S_1 and S_2, are produced by closure of the atrioventricular (AV) valves (tricuspid, mitral valves) and semilunar valves (pulmonic, aortic valves), respectively

normochromic normal red blood cell color, indicating normal amount of hemoglobin

normocytic normal size of red blood cells

nosocomial pertaining to or originating from a hospitalization; not present at the time of hospital admission

nuchal rigidity stiffness of the neck or inability to bend the neck

nucleated RBC immature form of red blood cell; portion of nucleus remains within the red cell; not normally seen in circulating blood

nucleic acid amplification tests (NAAT) a test that uses nucleic acid to assess for specific pathogens

null lymphocytes lymphocytes that destroy antigens already coated with the antibody

nutrition the science that deals with food and nourishment in humans

nystagmus involuntary oscillation of the eyeball

obstructive shock shock state resulting from the obstruction of the great vessels or heart itself; examples include cardiac tamponade, tension pneumothorax, pulmonary embolism, and abdominal compartment syndrome

odynophagia pain on swallowing

oligomenorrhea infrequent or light menses sometimes occurring at intervals of greater than 35 days

oliguria total urine output less than 400 mL in 24 hours

omentum fold of the peritoneum that surrounds the stomach and other organs of the abdomen

oncology field or study of cancer

oophorectomy surgical removal of the ovaries

open lung biopsy biopsy of lung tissue performed through a limited thoracotomy incision

open reduction the correction and alignment of the fracture after surgical dissection and exposure of the fracture

open reduction with internal fixation (ORIF) open surgical procedure to repair and stabilize a fracture

opioid a morphine-like compound that produces bodily effects including pain relief, sedation, constipation, and respiratory depression; this term is preferred rather than the term *narcotic*

opportunistic infection illness caused by various organisms, some of which usually do not cause disease in persons with normal immune systems

opsonization the coating of antigen–antibody molecules with a sticky substance to facilitate phagocytosis

optic chiasm the area of the brain where optic nerve (CN II) fibers partially cross

orchiectomy surgical removal of one or both of the testes

orchitis inflammation of the testes (testicular congestion) caused by pyogenic, viral, spirochetal, parasitic, traumatic, chemical, or unknown factors

organ of Corti the end organ of hearing, located in the cochlea

orthopnea shortness of breath when lying flat

orthotopic liver transplantation (OLT) grafting of a donor liver into the normal anatomic location, with removal of the diseased native liver

orthotopic transplantation the recipient's heart is removed, and a donor heart is grafted into its normal position in the body of the recipient; the patient has one heart

OSHA Occupational Safety and Health Administration; the federal agency providing oversight to organizations that ensure the safety of employees at work

osmolality the number of osmoles (the standard unit of osmotic pressure) per kilogram of solution, expressed as mOsm/kg; used more often in clinical practice than the term *osmolarity* to evaluate serum and urine; in addition to urea and glucose, sodium contributes the largest number of particles to osmolality

osmolarity the number of osmoles, the standard unit of osmotic pressure per liter of solution, expressed as milliosmoles per liter (mOsm/L); describes the concentration of solutes or dissolved particles

osmosis the process by which fluid moves across a semipermeable membrane from an area of low solute concentration to an area of high solute concentration; the process continues until the solute concentrations are equal on both sides of the membrane

ossicle a small bone; there are three in the middle ear malleus, incus, and stapes

ossification process in which minerals (calcium) are deposited in bone matrix

osteoarthritis degenerative joint disease characterized by destruction of the articular cartilage and overgrowth of bone

osteoblast bone-forming cell

osteoclast bone resorption cell

osteocyte mature bone cell

osteogenesis bone formation

osteoid pertaining to bone matrix tissue; "pre-bone"

osteomyelitis infection of the bone

osteon microscopic functional bone unit

osteophyte a bony outgrowth or protuberance; spur

osteoporosis a disorder in which bones lose density and become porous and fragile

otalgia sensation of fullness or pain in the ear

otitis externa (i.e., external otitis) inflammation of the external auditory canal

otitis media inflammation of the middle ear; may be acute lasting less than 6 weeks or chronic, causing irreversible tissue damage and persistent tympanic membrane perforation

otoconia debris of the inner ear comprised from small, crystalline stones of calcium carbonate

otorrhea drainage from the ear

otosclerosis a condition characterized by abnormal spongy bone formation around the stapes

oval window a fenestra (aperture) between the vestibule of the inner ear and the middle ear, occupied by the base of the stapes

ovaries almond-shaped reproductive organs that produce eggs at ovulation and play a major role in hormone production

overflow incontinence involuntary urine loss associated with overdistention of the bladder due to mechanical or anatomic bladder outlet obstruction

oxyhemoglobin combined form of oxygen and hemoglobin; found in arterial blood

oxytocin hormone secreted by the posterior pituitary; causes myometrial contraction at term and milk release during lactation

P wave the part of an electrocardiogram (ECG) that reflects conduction of an electrical impulse through the atrium; atrial depolarization (contraction)

pain an unpleasant sensory and emotional experience resulting from actual or potential tissue damage

pain threshold the point at which a stimulus is perceived as painful

pain tolerance the maximum intensity or duration of pain that a person is able to endure

palliation relief of symptoms associated with cancer

palliative care comprehensive care for patients whose disease is not responsive to cure; care also extends to patients' families

palliative sedation use of pharmacologic agents, at the request of the terminally ill patient, to induce sedation when symptoms have not responded to other management measures; the purpose is not to hasten the patient's death but to relieve intractable symptoms

pancreaticojejunostomy joining of the pancreatic duct to the jejunum by side-to-side anastomosis; allows drainage of the pancreatic secretions into the jejunum

pancreatitis inflammation of the pancreas; may be acute or chronic

pancytopenia abnormal decrease in white blood cells, red blood cells, and platelets

pannus proliferation of newly formed synovial tissue infiltrated with inflammatory cells

papilledema swelling of the optic disc

paralysis absence of muscle movement suggesting nerve damage

paraplegia paralysis of the lower extremities with dysfunction of the bowel and bladder from a lesion in the thoracic, lumbar, or sacral regions of the spinal cord

parasympathetic nervous system division of the autonomic nervous system active primarily during nonstressful conditions, controlling mostly visceral functions

parenteral nutrition (PN) method of supplying nutrients to the body by an intravenous route

paresthesia abnormal touch sensation (e.g., burning, tingling, numbness)

parotitis inflammation of the parotid gland

paroxysmal an arrhythmia that has a sudden onset and/or termination and is usually of short duration

patient-controlled analgesia (PCA) self-administration of analgesic agents by a patient instructed about the procedure

pelvic inflammatory disease (PID) infection of uterus and fallopian tubes, usually from a sexually transmitted disease

penis male organ for copulation and urination; consists of glans penis, body, and root

penumbra area of ischemic brain tissue surrounding the core infarct that is potentially viable (and therefore an important concept for treatment options for patients with an evolving ischemic stroke)

pepsin a gastric enzyme that is important in protein digestion

percutaneous coronary intervention (PCI) an invasive procedure in which a catheter is placed in a coronary artery, and one of several methods is employed to remove or reduce a blockage within the artery

percutaneous endoscopic gastrostomy (PEG) an endoscopic procedure for inserting a feeding tube into the stomach in order to provide long-term nutritional support

percutaneous thrombectomy endovascular technique to remove thrombus

percutaneous transluminal coronary angioplasty (PTCA) a type of percutaneous coronary intervention in which a balloon is inflated within a coronary artery to break an atheroma and open the vessel lumen, improving coronary artery blood flow

performance status patient activity level; ability to perform activities of daily living (ADLs), work, ambulate; multiple tools exist to measure performance status

pericardiocentesis procedure that involves aspiration of fluid from the pericardial sac

pericardiotomy surgically created opening of the pericardium

perimenopause the period immediately prior to menopause and the first year after menopause

perioperative phase period of time that constitutes the surgical experience; includes the preoperative, intraoperative, and postoperative phases of nursing care

periosteum fibrous connective tissue covering bone

peripheral arterial disease (PAD) process of blood flow reduced to tissue

peripherally inserted central catheter (PICC) a device used for intermediate-term intravenous therapy

peristalsis wavelike movement that occurs involuntarily in the alimentary canal and assists the passage of food through the bowel

peritoneal dialysis procedure that uses the lining of the patient's peritoneal cavity as the semipermeable membrane for exchange of fluid and solutes

peritoneum thin membrane that lines the inside of the wall of the abdomen and covers all the abdominal organs

peritonitis inflammation of the lining of the abdominal cavity, usually as a result of a bacterial infection of an area in the gastrointestinal tract with leakage of contents into the abdominal cavity

personal protective equipment (PPE) equipment beyond standard precautions; may include level A, B, C, and D equipment

pessary a plastic, silicone, rubber, or latex device that is inserted into the vagina

petechiae pinpoint, nonblanchable red spots that appear on the skin as a result of blood leakage into the skin

phagocytic cells cells that engulf, ingest, and destroy foreign bodies or toxins

phagocytic immune response the immune system's first line of defense, involving white blood cells that have the ability to ingest foreign particles

phagocytosis process of ingestion and digestion of bacteria by cells

phantom limb pain pain perceived as being in the amputated limb

pharyngitis inflammation of the throat; usually viral or bacterial in origin

phase I PACU area designated for care of surgical patients immediately after surgery and for patients whose condition warrants close monitoring

phase II PACU area designated for care of surgical patients who have been transferred from a phase I PACU because their condition no longer requires the close monitoring provided in a phase I PACU

phase III PACU setting in which the patient is cared for in the immediate postoperative period and then prepared for discharge from the facility

pheochromocytoma chromaffin cell tumor, usually benign, located in the adrenal medulla; characterized by secretion of catecholamines, resulting in hypertension, severe headache, profuse sweating, visual blurring, anxiety, and nausea

phimosis condition in which the foreskin is constricted so that it cannot be retracted over the glans; can occur congenitally or from inflammation and edema

photophobia ocular pain on exposure to light

physical fitness the condition of being physically healthy as a result of proper exercise and nutrition

pinna the outer part of the external ear, which collects and directs sound waves into the external auditory canal; the auricle

placebo effect analgesia that results from the expectation that a substance will work, not from the actual substance itself

plasma liquid portion of blood

plasmapheresis removal of whole blood from the body, separation of its cellular elements by centrifugation, and reinfusion of them suspended in saline or some other plasma substitute, thereby depleting the body's own plasma without depleting its cells

plasminogen protein that is converted to plasmin to dissolve thrombi and clots

platelet thrombocyte; a cellular component of blood involved in blood coagulation

pleural effusion abnormal accumulation of fluid in the pleural space

pleural space the area between the parietal and visceral pleurae; a potential space

pneumothorax partial or complete collapse of the lung due to positive pressure in the pleural space

podagra gout, especially of the great toe

polycystic ovarian syndrome (PCOS) most common endocrine disorder affecting women of reproductive age that may also cause overproduction of estrogen and testosterone resulting in abnormal thickening of the uterine lining, very heavy and/or irregular periods, as well as acne and facial hair

polycythemia increase in the red blood cell concentration in the blood; in chronic obstructive pulmonary disease (COPD), the body attempts to improve oxygen-carrying capacity by producing increasing amounts of red blood cells

polymenorrhea frequent menstruation occurring 21 days or less

polymerase chain reaction (PCR) a sensitive laboratory technique that can detect and quantify HIV in a person's blood or lymph nodes

polyuria total urine output greater than 3 L in 24 hours

portal hypertension elevated pressure in the portal circulation resulting from obstruction of venous flow into and through the liver

position (postural) sense awareness of position of parts of the body without looking at them; also referred to as *proprioception*

positive end-expiratory pressure (PEEP) positive pressure maintained by the ventilator at the end of exhalation (instead of a normal zero pressure) to increase functional residual capacity and open collapsed alveoli; improves oxygenation with lower FiO_2

postanesthesia care unit (PACU) area where postoperative patients are monitored as they recover from anesthesia; formerly referred to as the *recovery room* or *postanesthesia recovery room*

posterior chamber space between the iris and vitreous

postoperative phase period of time that begins with the admission of the patient to the PACU and ends after a follow-up evaluation in the clinical setting or home

postural drainage positioning the patient to allow drainage from all the lobes of the lungs and airways

postural (orthostatic) hypotension a decrease in systolic blood pressure (SBP) of at least 20 mm Hg or diastolic blood pressure (DBP) of at least 10 mm Hg within 3 minutes of sitting or standing, associated with dizziness, lightheadedness, or syncope

PR interval the part of an electrocardiogram (ECG) that reflects conduction of an electrical impulse from the sinoatrial (SA) node through the atrioventricular (AV) node

preadmission testing (PAT) diagnostic testing performed before admission to the hospital

prediabetes a condition of impaired carbohydrate metabolism that increases the risk of developing diabetes

prehypertension blood pressure 120 to 129/80 to 89 mm Hg

preload degree of stretch of the cardiac muscle fibers at the end of diastole

premenstrual dysphoric disorder (PMDD) a more severe form of PMS that occurs in late luteal phase and recurs cyclically

premenstrual syndrome (PMS) a constellation of symptoms associated with fluctuation of hormones during the luteal phase of the menstrual cycle

preoperative phase period of time from when the decision for surgical intervention is made to when the patient is transferred to the operating room table

presbycusis progressive hearing loss associated with aging

presbyopia describes the condition in which the eye exhibits a progressively diminished ability to focus on near objects with age

pressure support ventilation (PSV) mode of mechanical ventilation in which preset positive pressure is delivered with spontaneous breaths to decrease work of breathing

priapism an uncontrolled, persistent erection of the penis from either neural or vascular causes, including medications, sickle cell thrombosis, leukemic cell infiltration, spinal cord tumors, and tumor invasion of the penis or its vessels

primary amenorrhea the absence of menstruation by age 16 or absence of secondary sex characteristics and menarche by age 14

primary headache a headache for which no specific organic cause can be found

primary hypertension also called essential hypertension; denotes high blood pressure from an unidentified cause

primary infection 4- to 7-week period of rapid viral replication immediately following infection; also known as acute HIV infection

progesterone hormone produced by the corpus luteum

prolapse (of a valve) stretching of an atrioventricular heart valve leaflet into the atrium during systole

prolapse an organ that slips or falls out of place

prophylactic mastectomy removal of the breast to reduce the risk of breast cancer in women considered to be at high risk for development of the disease

proportional assist ventilation (PAV) mode of mechanical ventilation that provides partial ventilatory support in proportion to the patient's inspiratory efforts; decreases the work of breathing

proptosis downward displacement of the eyeball resulting from an inflammatory condition of the orbit or a mass within the orbital cavity

prostaglandins a hormone-like substance that causes rhythmic contraction and relaxation of smooth muscle

prostate gland gland that lies just below the neck of the bladder, surrounds the urethra, and is traversed by the ejaculatory duct, a continuation of the vas deferens; produces a secretion that is chemically and physiologically suitable to the needs of the spermatozoa in their passage from the testes

prostate-specific antigen (PSA) substance that is produced by the prostate gland and measured in a blood specimen; PSA levels are increased with prostate cancer; the PSA test is used in combination with digital rectal examination to detect prostate cancer

prostatitis inflammation of the prostate gland

protease inhibitor medication that inhibits the function of protease, an enzyme needed for HIV replication

proteinuria protein in the urine

proton pump inhibitors pharmacologic agents that block acid secretion by irreversibly binding to and inhibiting the hydrogen–potassium adenosine triphosphatase pump system at the secretory surface of gastric parietal cells; most potent inhibitors of gastric acid secretion

provirus viral genetic material in the form of DNA that has been integrated into the host genome; when it is dormant in human cells, HIV is in a proviral form

ptosis drooping eyelid

pulmonary edema increase in the amount of extravascular fluid in the lung

pulmonary embolism obstruction of the pulmonary vasculature with an embolus; embolus may be due to blood clot, air bubbles, or fat droplets

pulmonary perfusion blood flow through the pulmonary vasculature

pulmonary vascular resistance resistance created by the vasculature of the lungs to the ejection of blood from the right ventricle

pulmonic valve semilunar valve located between the right ventricle and the pulmonary artery

pulseless electrical activity (PEA) condition in which electrical activity is present but there is not an adequate pulse or blood pressure because of ineffective cardiac contraction or circulating blood volume

pulsus paradoxus systolic blood pressure of more than 10 mm Hg higher during exhalation than during inspiration; difference is normally less than 10 mm Hg

purulent consisting of, containing, or discharging pus

pyelonephritis inflammation of the renal pelvis

pyloroplasty surgical procedure to increase the opening of the pyloric orifice

pylorus opening between the stomach and the duodenum

pyrosis heartburn

pyuria white blood cells in the urine

QA/QI quality assurance/quality improvement; a system of continuous monitoring and evaluation of products or services to order to maintain and/or improve quality

QRS complex the part of an electrocardiogram (ECG) that reflects conduction of an electrical impulse through the ventricles; ventricular depolarization (contraction)

QT interval the part of an electrocardiogram (ECG) that reflects the time from ventricular depolarization through repolarization (resting state)

radiation therapy use of ionizing radiation to interrupt the growth of malignant cells

radicular pain pain that radiates along the nerve, caused from irritation or pressure of the nerve root

radiculopathy disease of a nerve root

radioimmunoassay radioisotope-labeled antigen measurement of hormone or other substance

radioisotopes unstable atoms that emit small amounts of energy in the form of gamma rays; used in cardiac nuclear medicine studies

rebound hypertension pressure that is controlled with therapy and that becomes abnormally high with the discontinuation (usually abrupt) of therapy

receptive aphasia difficulty understanding spoken or written language; often associated with damage to the temporal lobe area (Wernicke aphasia)

rectocele weakness of the posterior vaginal wall that allows the rectal cavity to protrude into the submucosa of the vagina

red blood cell (RBC) also *erythrocyte;* a cellular component of blood involved in the transport of oxygen and carbon dioxide

red reflex the reddish-orange reflection from the eye's retina that is observed using an ophthalmoscope under dimly lit or dark conditions

referred pain pain perceived as coming from an area different from that in which the pathology is occurring

reflex an automatic response to stimuli

reflex incontinence involuntary loss of urine due to hyper-reflexia or involuntary urethral relaxation in the absence of normal sensations; usually associated with micturition (voiding)

regurgitation backward flow of blood through a heart valve

reinforcement the process of strengthening a given response or behavior to increase the likelihood that the behavior will continue

remodeling process that ensures bone maintenance through simultaneous bone resorption and formation

renal clearance volume of plasma that the kidneys can clear of a specific solute (e.g., creatinine); expressed in milliliters per minute

renal glycosuria recurring or persistent excretion of glucose in the urine

renal replacement therapy term used to encompass life-supporting treatments for renal failure; includes hemodialysis, peritoneal dialysis, hemofiltration, and renal transplantation

repolarization return of the cell to resting state, caused by reentry of potassium into the cell while sodium exits the cell

residual urine urine that remains in the bladder after voiding

resorption removal/destruction of tissue, such as bone

respiration gas exchange between atmospheric air and the blood, and between the blood and cells of the body

respiratory weaning process of gradual, systematic withdrawal or removal of ventilator, breathing tube, and oxygen

rest pain a persistent pain in the foot at rest that can worsen at night and indicates significant arterial insufficiency

restricted zone area in the operating room where scrub attire and surgical masks are required; includes operating room and sterile core areas

restrictive lung disease disease of the lung that causes a decrease in lung volumes

resuscitation triage category signifying life-threatening injuries or illnesses requiring immediate intervention

rete ridges undulations and furrows that appear at the dermis–epidermis junction and are responsible for cementing together the two layers

reticulocytes slightly immature red blood cells (RBCs), usually only 1% of total circulating RBCs

reticuloendothelial system (RES) complex system of cells throughout body capable of phagocytosis

retinopathy a long-term complication of diabetes in which the microvascular system of the eye is damaged

retrovirus a virus that carries genetic material in RNA instead of DNA and contains reverse transcriptase

reverse transcriptase enzyme that transforms single-stranded RNA into a double-stranded DNA

rhabdomyolysis accumulation of byproducts of skeletal muscle destruction in renal tubule

rhinitis inflammation of the mucous membranes of the nose; may be infectious, allergic, or inflammatory in origin

rhinorrhea drainage of a large amount of fluid from the nose

rhinosinusitis inflammation of the sinuses; may be acute or chronic; may be viral, bacterial, or fungal in origin

RICE acronym for *R*est, *I*ce, *C*ompression, *E*levation

rigidity increase in muscle tone at rest characterized by increased resistance to passive stretch

rods retinal photoreceptor cells essential for bright and dim light

Romberg test test for cerebellar dysfunction requiring the patient to stand with feet together, eyes closed, and arms extended; inability to maintain the position, with either significant stagger or sway, is a positive test

rotator cuff shoulder muscles (supraspinatus, subscapularis, infraspinatus, and teres minor) and their tendons

round window a fenestra between the middle ear and the inner ear at the base of the cochlea, occupied by the round window membrane

rubor reddish blue skin discoloration occurring in skin in dependent position

rule of nines method for calculating body surface area burned by dividing the body into multiples of nine

sciatica inflammation of the sciatic nerve, resulting in pain and tenderness along the nerve through the thigh and leg

sclerotherapy the injection of substances into or around esophagogastric varices to cause constriction, thickening, and hardening of the vessel and thus to stop bleeding

scoliosis lateral curving of the spine

scotomas blind or partially blind areas in the visual field

scrub role registered nurse, licensed practical nurse, or surgical technologist who scrubs and dons sterile surgical attire, prepares instruments and supplies, and hands instruments to the surgeon during the procedure

sebaceous glands glands that exist within the epidermis and secrete sebum to keep the skin soft and pliable

sebum fatty secretion of the sebaceous glands

secondary amenorrhea the absence of menses for 6 or more months after a regular cycle of menstruation has been established

secondary conditions or disorders preventable physical, mental, or social disorders resulting directly or indirectly from an initial disabling condition

secondary headache headache identified as a symptom of another organic disorder (e.g., brain tumor, hypertension)

secondary hypertension high blood pressure from an identified cause, such as renal disease

second-intention healing method of healing in which wound edges are not surgically approximated and integumentary continuity is restored by the process known as granulation

secretin hormone responsible for stimulating secretion of pancreatic juice; also used as an aid in diagnosing pancreatic exocrine disease and in obtaining desquamated pancreatic cells for cytologic examination

seizures paroxysmal transient disturbance of the brain resulting from a discharge of abnormal electrical activity

self-monitoring of blood glucose (SMBG) a method of capillary blood glucose testing in which a drop of blood is applied to a test strip that is read by a meter

self-responsibility personal accountability for one's actions or behavior

semicircular canals the superior, posterior, and lateral bony tubes that form part of the inner ear; contain the receptor organs for balance

semirestricted zone area in the operating room where scrub attire is required; may include areas where surgical instruments are processed

sensitization a heightened response seen after exposure to a noxious stimulus; response to the same stimulus is to feel more pain

sensorineural hearing loss loss of hearing related to damage of the end organ for hearing or cranial nerve VIII, or both

sentinel lymph node first lymph node(s) in the lymphatic basin that receives drainage from the primary tumor in the breast; identified by a radioisotope and/or blue dye

septic shock distributive shock state resulting from combination of infectious trigger and impaired host response, resulting in decreased tissue perfusion

sequestrum dead bone in abscess cavity

serosa thin membrane that forms the outer layer of the stomach

serum portion of blood remaining after coagulation occurs

shock physiologic state in which there is inadequate tissue perfusion

sialadenitis inflammation of the salivary glands

sinoatrial (SA) node primary pacemaker of the heart, located in the right atrium

sinus rhythm electrical activity of the heart initiated by the sinoatrial (SA) node

sling bandage used to support an arm

small intestine longest portion of the GI tract, consisting of three parts—duodenum, jejunum, and ileum—through which food mixed with all secretions and enzymes passes as it continues to be digested and begins to be absorbed into the bloodstream

spacer device a device used to attach to a metered-dose inhaler (MDI) that may improve patients' ability to use their MDI correctly

spastic having greater than normal muscle tone

spasticity sustained increase in tension of a muscle when it is passively lengthened or stretched with exaggeration of the tendon reflexes

spermatogenesis production of sperm in the testes

spinal cord compression tumor extension into the epidural space

spinal cord injury (SCI) an injury to the spinal cord, vertebral column, supporting soft tissue, or intervertebral disks caused by trauma

spirituality personal belief systems that focus on a search for meaning and purpose in life, intangible elements that impart meaning and vitality to life, and a connectedness to a higher or transcendent dimension

spirometry pulmonary function tests that measure specific lung volumes (e.g., FEV_1, forced expired volume in 1 second), capacities (e.g., FVC, forced vital capacity), and flow rates; may be measured before and after bronchodilator administration

splint device designed specifically to support and immobilize a body part in a desired position

spondylosis ankylosis or stiffening of the cervical or lumbar vertebrae

sprain an injury to ligaments and other soft tissues at a joint

ST segment the part of an electrocardiogram (ECG) from the end of the QRS complex to the beginning of the T wave

staging process of determining the size and spread, or metastasis, of a tumor

stapes the third (most medial) ossicle of the middle ear; it articulates with the incus, and its footplate fits into the oval window; the stirrup

status epilepticus episode in which the patient experiences multiple seizure bursts with no recovery time in between

steatorrhea frothy, foul-smelling stools with a high fat content; results from impaired digestion of proteins and fats due to a lack of pancreatic juice in the intestine

stem cell primitive cell, capable of self-replication and differentiation into myeloid or lymphoid stem cell

stenosis narrowing or tightening of an opening or passage in the body

stent a woven mesh that provides structural support to a coronary vessel, preventing its closure

stent-graft tube composed of fabric supported by a metal mesh

stereotactic biopsy computer-guided method of core needle biopsy that is useful when masses in the breast cannot be felt but can be visualized using mammography

stoma artificially created opening between a body cavity (e.g., intestine) and the body surface

stomach distensible pouch into which the food bolus passes to be digested by gastric enzymes

stomatitis inflammation of the oral mucosa

strain a musculotendinous injury

stress incontinence involuntary loss of urine through an intact urethra as a result of a sudden increase in intra-abdominal pressure

stress management behaviors and techniques used to strengthen a person's resources against stress

stress test a test used to evaluate the functioning of the cardiovascular system during a period of increased oxygen demand simulated by walking on a treadmill or medications that mimic the body's physiologic response to exercise

striae band-like streaks on the skin, distinguished by color, texture, depression, or elevation from the tissue in which they are found; usually purplish or white

stroke a syndrome characterized by death of brain cells that occurs when there is a disruption of cerebral blood flow

stroke volume (SV) amount of blood ejected from the ventricle per heartbeat

subarachnoid screw or bolt device placed into the subarachnoid space to measure intracranial pressure

subluxation partial separation or dislocation of joint surfaces

subtotal or supracervical hysterectomy removal of the uterus, fallopian tubes, and ovaries with retention of the cervix

sudden cardiac death immediate cessation of effective heart activity

suppressor T cells lymphocytes that decrease B-cell activity to a level at which the immune system is compatible with life

suprapubic catheter a urinary catheter that is inserted through a suprapubic incision into the bladder

surgical asepsis absence of microorganisms in the surgical environment to reduce the risk for infection

surgical biopsy procedure in which an entire mass or a portion of it is surgically removed for examination under a microscope by a pathologist

suspensions liquid preparations in which powder is suspended, requiring shaking before use

sympathetic nervous system division of the autonomic nervous system with predominantly excitatory responses; the "fight-or-flight" system

sympathetic ophthalmia an inflammatory condition created in the fellow eye by the affected eye (without useful vision); the condition may become chronic and result in blindness (of the fellow eye)

synchronized intermittent mandatory ventilation (SIMV) mode of mechanical ventilation in which the ventilator allows the patient to breathe spontaneously while providing a preset number of breaths to ensure adequate ventilation; ventilated breaths are synchronized with spontaneous breathing

syndrome of inappropriate antidiuretic hormone (SIADH) secretion excessive secretion of antidiuretic hormone (ADH) from the pituitary gland, despite low serum osmolality level, resulting in hyponatremia

synovial pertaining to a complex joint bounded by joint capsule and containing synovial fluid

synovitis inflammation of the synovial membrane

synovium membrane in joint that secretes lubricating fluid

systemic inflammatory response syndrome (SIRS) overwhelming inflammatory response in the absence of known infection causing decreased tissue perfusion

systemic vascular resistance resistance caused by the peripheral circulation to the ejection of blood from the left ventricle

systole period during the cardiac cycle when the ventricles contract, resulting in ejection of blood from the right and left ventricles into the pulmonary artery and aorta

systolic heart failure inability of the heart to pump sufficiently because of an alteration in the ability of the heart to contract; current term used to describe a type of heart failure

T wave the part of an electrocardiogram (ECG) that reflects repolarization of the ventricles

targeted therapies cancer treatments that seek to minimize the negative effects on healthy tissues by disrupting specific cancer cell functions, such as malignant transformation, communication pathways, processes for growth and metastasis, and genetic coding

T cells cells that are important for producing a cellular immune response

teaching the imparting of knowledge

telangiectases spider-like red marks on the skin caused by distention of the superficial blood vessels that blanch on pressure

telemetry ambulatory electrocardiographic monitoring using a battery-operated transmitting device worn by the patient

temporal bone a bone on both sides of the skull at its base; composed of the squamous, mastoid, and petrous portions

temporomandibular disorders a group of conditions that cause pain or dysfunction of the temporomandibular joint (TMJ) and surrounding structures

tendinitis inflammation of a tendon

tendon cord of fibrous tissue connecting muscle to bone

tendon transfer a surgical procedure in which a tendon is incised at its insertion and placed at a site distant from the original insertion site in order to restore or correct the function of a muscle

tenesmus ineffective and sometimes painful straining to eliminate either feces or urine resulting in abscess formation

tension pneumothorax pneumothorax characterized by increasing positive pressure in the pleural space with each breath; this is an emergency situation and the positive pressure needs to be decompressed or released immediately

terminal illness progressive, irreversible illness that despite cure-focused medical treatment will result in the patient's death

testes the ovoid sex glands encased in the scrotum; the testes produce sperm

testicular cancer the most common cancer in men 15 to 35 years of age and the second most common malignancy in those 35 to 39 years of age; its cause is unknown

testosterone male sex hormone secreted by the testes; induces and preserves the male sex characteristics

tetraplegia (formerly quadriplegia) paralysis of both arms and legs, with dysfunction of bowel and bladder from a lesion of the cervical segments of the spinal cord

therapeutic regimen a routine that promotes health and healing

third-intention healing method of healing in which surgical approximation of wound edges is delayed due to contamination and the wound heals initially by second intention (granulation), and later when the wound appears to be clean it is closed surgically

thoracentesis insertion of a needle into the pleural space to remove fluid that has accumulated and decrease pressure on the lung tissue; may also be used diagnostically to identify potential causes of a pleural effusion

thoracotomy surgical opening into the chest cavity

thrombin enzyme necessary to convert fibrinogen into fibrin clot

thrombocyte *see* **platelet**

thrombocytopenia decrease in the number of platelets

thrombocytosis higher than normal platelet count

thrombolysis breakdown of thrombus by pharmacologic means

thrombolytic an agent or process that breaks down blood clots

thyroid storm severe life-threatening form of hyperthyroidism precipitated by stress; usually of abrupt onset; characterized by high fever, extreme tachycardia, and altered mental state

thyroidectomy surgical removal of all or part of the thyroid gland

thyroiditis inflammation of the thyroid gland; may lead to chronic hypothyroidism or may resolve spontaneously

thyroid-stimulating hormone (TSH) released from the pituitary gland; causes stimulation of the thyroid gland, resulting in release of T_3 and T_4

thyrotoxicosis a hypermetabolic response caused by excessive endogenous (T_3 and/or T_4 hormone) or exogenous thyroid hormone

thyroxine (T_4) thyroid hormone; active iodine compound formed and stored in the thyroid; deiodinated in peripheral tissues to form triiodothyronine (T_3); maintains body metabolism in a steady state

tinea a superficial fungal infection on the skin or scalp

tinnitus subjective perception of sound with internal origin; unwanted noises in the head or ear

tolerance occurs when a person who has been taking opioids becomes less sensitive to their analgesic properties (and usually side effects); characterized by the need for increasing doses to maintain the same level of pain relief

tone (tonus) normal tension (resistance to stretch) in resting muscle

tonicity the measurement of the osmotic pressure of a solution; another term for *osmolality*

tophi accumulation of crystalline deposits in articular surfaces, bones, soft tissue, and cartilage

total artificial heart mechanical device used to aid a failing heart, assists both the right and left ventricles

total joint arthroplasty or replacement the replacement of both articular surfaces within a joint with metal or synthetic materials

total mastectomy removal of the breast tissue and nipple–areola complex

total nutrient admixture (TNA) an admixture of lipid emulsions, proteins, carbohydrates, electrolytes, vitamins, trace minerals, and water

trabeculae lattice-like bone structure; cancellous bone

tracheostomy tube indwelling tube inserted directly into the trachea to assist with ventilation

tracheotomy surgical opening into the trachea

trachoma a bilateral chronic follicular conjunctivitis of childhood that leads to blindness during adulthood, if left untreated

traction application of a pulling force to a part of the body

transbronchial through the bronchial wall, as in a transbronchial lung biopsy

transection severing of the spinal cord itself; transection can be complete (all the way through the cord) or incomplete (partially through)

transgender a person who identifies his or her gender with that of the opposite sex

transient ischemic attack (TIA) a brief episode of neurologic dysfunction caused by focal brain or retinal ischemia with clinical symptoms typically lasting less than 1 hour and without evidence of acute infarction

transurethral resection of the prostate (TUR or TURP) resection of the prostate through endoscopy; the surgical and optical instrument is introduced directly through the urethra to the prostate, and the gland is then removed in small chips with an electrical cutting loop

transverse rectus abdominis myocutaneous (TRAM) flap method of breast reconstruction in which a flap of skin, fat, and muscle from the lower abdomen, with its attached blood supply, is rotated to the mastectomy site

trapeze overhead assistive device to promote patient mobility in bed

triage process of assessing patients to determine management priorities

tricuspid valve atrioventricular valve located between the right atrium and right ventricle

triggered in reference to pacemakers, term used to describe the release of an impulse in response to some stimulus

triiodothyronine (T_3) thyroid hormone; formed and stored in the thyroid; released in smaller quantities, biologically more active and with faster onset of action than thyroxine (T_4); widespread effect on cellular metabolism, influences every major organ system

troponin myocardial protein; measurement is used to assess heart muscle injury

trypsin pancreatic enzyme; aids in digestion of proteins

tubular reabsorption movement of a substance from the kidney tubule into the blood in the peritubular capillaries or vasa recta

tubular secretion movement of a substance from the blood in the peritubular capillaries or vasa recta into the kidney tubule

Turner syndrome a female genetic disorder due to a missing or incomplete X chromosome

tympanic membrane the membrane that separates the middle ear from the external auditory canal; also referred to as the *eardrum*

tympanoplasty surgical repair of the tympanic membrane

type 1 diabetes a metabolic disorder characterized by an absence of insulin production and secretion from autoimmune destruction of the beta cells of the islets of Langerhans in the pancreas; formerly called *insulin-dependent* or *juvenile* diabetes

type 2 diabetes a metabolic disorder characterized by the relative deficiency of insulin production and a decreased insulin action and increased insulin resistance; formerly called *non–insulin-dependent* or *adult-onset* diabetes

U wave the part of an electrocardiogram (ECG) that may reflect Purkinje fiber repolarization; usually, it is not seen unless a patient's serum potassium level is low

ulcer an area of tissue erosion or an open sore

ultrafiltration process whereby water is removed from the blood by means of a pressure gradient between the patient's blood and the dialysate

ultrasonography imaging method using high-frequency sound waves to diagnose whether masses are solid or fluid-filled

unrestricted zone area in the operating room that interfaces with other departments; includes patient reception area and holding area

urea nitrogen nitrogenous end product of protein metabolism

uremia the clinical syndrome associated with an excess of urea and other nitrogenous wastes in the blood (fluid and electrolyte, hormonal, and metabolic imbalances)

ureterosigmoidostomy transplantation of the ureters into the sigmoid colon, allowing urine to flow through the colon and out the rectum

ureterovesical or vesicoureteral reflux backward flow of urine from the bladder into one or both ureters

urethritis inflammation of the urethra

urethrovesical reflux backward flow of urine from the urethra into the bladder

urge incontinence involuntary loss of urine associated with urinary urgency due to hypersensory disorders of the bladder, motor instability, or both

urgent triage category signifying serious illness or injury that is not immediately life threatening

urinary casts proteins secreted by damaged kidney tubules

urinary incontinence involuntary or uncontrolled loss of urine from the bladder sufficient to cause a social or hygienic problem

urosepsis sepsis resulting from infected urine, most often a urinary tract infection (UTI)

urticaria hives

uterine prolapse relaxation of pelvic tone that allows the cervix and uterus to descend into the lower vagina

uvulopalatopharyngoplasty (UPPP) surgical removal of the uvula, tonsils, and part of the soft palate to create a larger posterior oropharynx as treatment for obstructive sleep apnea

vagotomy syndrome dumping syndrome; gastrointestinal symptoms, such as diarrhea and abdominal cramping, resulting from rapid gastric emptying

Valsalva maneuver forcible exhalation against a closed glottis followed by a rise in intrathoracic pressure and subsequent possible dramatic rise in arterial pressure; may occur during straining at stool

valve replacement insertion of a prosthetic valve at the site of a malfunctioning heart valve to restore blood flow in one direction through the heart

valvuloplasty repair of a stenosed or regurgitant cardiac valve by commissurotomy, annuloplasty, leaflet repair, or chordoplasty (or a combination of procedures)

variceal banding procedure that involves the endoscopic placement of a rubber band-like device over esophageal varices to ligate the area and stop bleeding

varicocele an abnormal dilation of the veins of the pampiniform venous plexus in the scrotum (the network of veins from the testis and the epididymis, which constitute part of the spermatic cord)

vasculitis inflammation of a blood vessel or lymph vessel

vasoactive medications medications that act on the vessels to either constrict or dilate, resulting in either increased or decreased blood pressure and/or heart rate

vasopressin antidiuretic hormone (ADH) secreted by the posterior pituitary; causes retention of water and raises blood pressure by contraction of smooth muscle, particularly blood vessels

ventilation movement of air in and out of airways

ventilation–perfusion ratio the ratio between ventilation and perfusion in the lung; matching of ventilation to perfusion optimizes gas exchange

ventricular assist device mechanical device used to aid a failing right or left ventricle

ventricular tachycardia (VT) a rapid rhythm that originates in the ventricles

ventriculostomy a catheter placed in one of the lateral ventricles of the brain to measure intracranial pressure and allow for drainage of cerebrospinal fluid (CSF) or blood

vertigo an illusion of movement in which the individual or the surroundings are sensed as moving, usually rotation

vesicant substance that can cause tissue necrosis and damage, particularly when extravasated

vestibulocochlear nerve cranial nerve VIII; contains the cochlear (acoustic) portion and the vestibular portion

vibration a type of massage administered by quickly tapping the chest with the fingertips or alternating the fingers in a rhythmic manner, or by using a mechanical device to assist in mobilizing lung secretions

viral load test measures the quantity of HIV RNA in the blood

viral set point amount of virus present in the blood after the initial burst of viremia and the immune response that follows

vitiligo a localized or widespread condition characterized by destruction of the melanocytes in circumscribed areas of the skin, resulting in white patches

vitreous humor gelatinous material (transparent and colorless) that fills the eyeball behind the lens

volvulus abnormal twisting of the intestines resulting in intestinal obstruction

vulvovaginal candidiasis a vaginal infection caused by fungus or yeast

weapons of mass destruction (WMD) weapons used to cause widespread death and destruction

wellness a condition of good physical and emotional health sustained by a healthy lifestyle

wheezes continuous musical sounds associated with airway narrowing or partial obstruction

white blood cell (WBC) also *leukocytes;* cellular components of blood involved in defense of the body; subtypes include neutrophils, eosinophils, basophils, monocytes, and lymphocytes

window period time from infection with HIV until seroconversion detected on HIV antibody test

wound care specialist a nurse specially educated in appropriate skin, wound, ostomy, and continence care; often referred to as an *enterostomal therapist* or a *wound-ostomy-continence nurse* (WOCN)

xenograft heart valve replacement made of tissue from an animal heart valve (*synonym* heterograft)

xerosis overly dry skin

xerostomia dry oral cavity resulting from decreased function of salivary glands

Zollinger–Ellison tumor hypersecretion of gastric acid that produces peptic ulcers as a result of a non–beta cell tumor of the pancreatic islets

Suggested Answers to Unit Case Studies

UNIT ONE
Basics of Adult Health Nursing

a. Important areas of health education include:
- Adherence to therapeutic regimen
- Willingness to learn
- Health literacy skills
- Learning needs
- Learner readiness

b. Variables that could effect medication compliance include:
- Sensory deficits, such as hearing and visualizing
- Financial constraints
- Inadequate support systems
- Life-time treatment with OTC medications
- Mobility impairments
- Inadequate cognitive, psychomotor, or language skills
- Fear of loss of control in decision making

c. Teaching strategies for this patient include:
- Knowledge of side effects of prescribed medications
- Teaching strategies to accommodate decreased visual and hearing acuity
- Small amounts of material at one time, frequent repetition of information, use of reinforcement techniques
- Minimize distraction

UNIT TWO
Concepts and Challenges in Patient Management

a. Psychosocial aspects of this diagnosis include:
- Body image
- Self-esteem
- Functional and cognitive abilities
- Plan for postoperative rehabilitation
- Prognosis

b. Potential postoperative complications may include:
- Infection
- Bleeding
- Impaired wound healing
- Altered pulmonary or kidney function
- Development of a deep vein thrombosis
- Increased intracranial pressure
- Seizures

c. Special needs of the patient undergoing chemotherapy include:
- Monitoring for nausea, vomiting, fatigue, and depression
- Monitoring white blood cell, hemoglobin, hematocrit, and platelet counts
- Safe administration of chemotherapy
- Monitoring for signs of bone marrow suppression including bleeding, infection, and anemia
- Nutritional status
- Teaching of self-care

UNIT THREE
Problems Related to Gas Exchange and Respiratory Function

a. Potential complications that may arise following a total laryngectomy include:
- Respiratory distress, hypoxia
- Hemorrhage
- Infection
- Wound breakdown
- Aspiration
- Tracheostomal stenosis anxiety and depression

b. Patient teaching areas of self-care include:
- Proper hand hygiene
- Adequate dietary intake
- Safe hygiene, prevention of water entering stoma during a shower
- Signs of infection, indications for notifying provider
- Avoidance of strenuous activities and fatigue
- Carry medical identification
- Performing oral care
- Importance of regular physical examinations
- Tracheostomy suctioning if necessary
- Need for home care

c. Support groups for laryngectomy patients include:
- International Association of Laryngectomees (IAL)
- I Can Cope (American Cancer Society)
- Local area support groups

UNIT FOUR
Problems Related to Cardiovascular and Circulatory Function

a. Current and potential problems related to the patient's nonadherence to medication include:
- Obesity
- Nonadherence with medication regimen
- Smoking
- Congestive heart failure

b. Important areas of teaching to emphasize include:
- Lifestyle changes (smoking cessation, weight loss, regular physical activity)
- Emphasize concept of lifelong blood pressure control rather than cure
- Waist circumference of less than 40 in
- DASH diet
- Limiting alcohol ingestion
- Compliance with medication regimen
- Follow-up appointments

c. Target organs/systems that may be affected by the patient's nonadherence include:
- Heart-Cardiac (MI)
- Kidneys-Renal (kidney failure, elevated BUN, elevated creatinine)
- Brain-Cerebrovascular (TIA or Stroke)

UNIT FIVE
Problems Related to Hematologic Function

a. The only curative treatment for CML is allogeneic stem cell transplantation.
- The efficacy of imatinib is first-line treatment.
- Treatment-related mortality of stem cell transplant limits use of transplant to patients with high risk or relapsed disease, or in those patients who did not respond to therapy with TKI.

b. The three phases of CML include:
- Chronic phase: There is usually adequate numbers of health cells to fight infection; the expected outcome is correction of the chromosomal abnormality.
- Accelerated Phase: Abnormal cells present in higher numbers.
- Blast crisis: The predominant cell type is immature; treatment may resemble induction therapy for acute leukemia, using the same medications as for AML or ALL.
- Most patients are diagnosed in the chronic phase.

c. Nursing considerations of the patient undergoing chemotherapy (Gleevec):
- Monitoring side effects of chemotherapy such as fluid retention.
- Monitoring CBC.
- Monitoring patient for infection; educating patient on signs of infections that would warrant notification of provider.
- Educate patients that antacids and grapefruit juice may limit drug absorption.

UNIT SIX
Problems Related to Digestive, Gastrointestinal, and Metabolic Function

a. Patient selection criteria for bariatric surgery include:
- Table 23-5 Selection Criteria for Bariatric Surgery
- Failure of previous nonsurgical attempts at weight reduction
- Expectation that patient will adhere to postoperative care
- BMI greater than or equal to 35 with obesity-associated comorbidity
- BMI greater than or equal to 40 with no comorbidities

b. Potential lifestyle changes include:
- Box 23-2 Dietary Guidelines for the Patient Who Has Had Bariatric Surgery
- Do not eat and drink at the same time.
- Eat slowly and include two protein snacks per day.
- Patients need extensive counseling before and after the surgery.
- All patients require lifelong monitoring of weight loss, comorbidities, metabolic and nutritional status, and dietary and activity behaviors because they are at risk for developing malnutrition and weight gain.

c. Complications that may be associated with bariatric surgery include:
- Bleeding, blood clots, bowel obstruction, incisional or ventral hernias, and infection
- Peritonitis, stomal obstruction, and stomal ulcers
- Atelectasis and pneumonia
- Nausea, dumping syndrome, diarrhea, and constipation
- Long-term complications are related to nutritional deficiency.

UNIT SEVEN
Problems Related to Urinary Tract Function

a. Areas of teaching for this patient should include:
- Lifestyle changes
- Dietary restrictions
- Encouragement of self-management

- Patient and family teaching regarding the symptoms of worsening renal function; frequent, clear explanations and information
- Dialysis education
- Care of the vascular access; patients with fistulae or grafts are taught to check daily for a thrill over the graft (vibrating or buzzing sensation) and to notify health care provider or dialysis center if absent.

b. Treatment modalities for this patient population include:
- Pharmacologic therapies, which include calcium, phosphorous binders, antihypertensives, antiseizure agents, erythropoietin, and agents to treat metabolic acidosis
- Nutritional therapy and fluid restriction
- Potential blood transfusions

c. Nursing management would include:
- Prevention of infection due to invasive line and catheters
- Meticulous skin care
- Psychosocial care; teaching in brief 10- to 15-minute sessions
- Nutritional and fluid therapy; monitoring fluid and electrolyte balance
- Monitoring weight
- Teaching regarding dietary restrictions
- Monitoring for complications of chronic kidney failure

UNIT EIGHT
Problems Related to Endocrine Function

a. Questions to ask the patient regarding his fluctuating blood sugar levels include:
- What times do you take your blood sugar?
- Have you been sick lately?
- Have you started taking any new medications?
- Do you have all the supplies you need to take your blood sugar?
- Describe a typical meal.
- Tell me what you do for exercise.

b. Areas of teaching with regard to the foot wound for this patient should include:
- Inspect your feet daily; use a mirror to check the bottom of your feet.
- Wash your feet in warm, not hot, water and dry them well.
- Wear shoes and socks at all times; never walk barefoot.
- Put your feet up while sitting.
- Contact your health care provider if you have a cut, sore, blister, or bruise on your foot that does not heal within 3 days or sooner if you see signs of infection.

- Remember that because you have diabetes, it will take longer for you to heal.
- Because you have diabetes, you may experience decreased sensation in your lower legs and feet.
- Maintaining optimal glucose control will aid healing and help to prevent infection.
- Monitor your food intake by using a meal planning guide and by monitoring carbohydrate intake.

c. Aids to assist patient in keeping more accurate records of his blood sugar include:
- Keeping a blood sugar log
- Obtaining blood sugar levels at the same time each day
- Taking blood sugar prior to meals

UNIT NINE
Problems Related to Reproductive Function

a. Risk factors associated with cervical cancer include:
- Lesbian women are at higher risk for cervical cancer due to misinformation, insufficient knowledge and screening.
- The human papillomavirus (HPV) has been implicated.
- Intercourse with an uncircumcised male, high parity, cigarette smoking, multiple sexual partners.
- See also Box 33-11 Risk Factors for Cervical Cancer.

b. Clinical manifestations that the patient may have had prior to the diagnosis include:
- Irregular vaginal bleeding and pelvic pain and pressure
- Malodorous vaginal discharge, which occurs as a result of tumor necrosis
- Dyspareunia and rectal pressure are also common as the tumor increases in size and extent invading surrounding tissue causing other symptoms to develop.

c. The purpose of a colposcopy is:
- To magnify the cervix which has had acetic acid solution applied to it to help differentiate the cervical cells. Biopsies are taken in areas of visible abnormal vascular patterns.
- Approximately 50% of newly diagnosed women with cervical cancer will present with stage I disease.

d. Medical management of cervical cancer includes:
- Cervical conization or cone biopsy
- Cold knife conization and loop electrosurgical excision procedure (LEEP) are other procedures that may be performed to treat high- or low-grade squamous intraepithelial lesions, which are precursors to cervical cancer.
- Cervical conization alone is adequate for those women who want to preserve childbearing ability.
- Patients diagnosed with a stage IB or IIA undergo a radical hysterectomy: removal of the uterus and upper one

third of the vagina, including the cervix, but sparing the ovaries. Pelvic radiation and chemotherapy may follow but depends on the size and extent of the tumor.
- Stage IB carries an increased risk of recurrence.
- Neoadjuvant chemotherapy has demonstrated success in decreasing tumor size and increasing survival when used prior to a radical hysterectomy.

UNIT TEN
Problems Related to Immunologic Function

a. The nurse could expect that the following medications may be ordered for this patient:
- Nonsteroidal anti-inflammatory drugs (indomethacin or ibuprofen) are considered agents of first choice for an acute attack.
- Indomethacin or ibuprofen with colchicines as an alternative or in combination may be considered.
- Low-dose colchicine has been used for prophylaxis after resolution of attacks; not as preventative of accumulation in joints.
- Allopurinol (Zyloprim) is considered the drug of choice for preventing the precipitation of an attack and tophi formation and promoting the regression of existing tophi.
- Uricosuric agents, such as probenecid (Benemid), correct hyperuricemia by inhibiting renal reabsorption and increasing urinary excretion.
- When reduction of the serum urate level is indicated, uricosuric agents are the medications of choice.
- Febuxostat (Uloric) has been approved for the treatment of gout that does not respond to usual treatment. Newer urate-lowering agents, such as uricase, are currently under investigation and show promise for successful gout treatment.
- Corticosteroids are useful for short-term therapy of acute gout and may be used on patients who have no response to other therapy.

b. The two phases of medical management of gout include:
- Management of acute gouty inflammation
- Long-term management to prevent flare-ups and to control hyperuricemia

c. Nursing management of gout includes:
- Pain management is the primary concern during the acute phase of an attack. The joint should be rested and application of ice, not heat, may help with reducing discomfort.
- Patients should be taught to limit alcohol intake and to avoid fad starvation diets, foods high in purines and high in fructose.
- The patient should drink plenty of fluids, at least 2,000 mL daily, to lessen renal involvement and the development of urinary stones.

- Dietary restriction of sodium, fat, and cholesterol can lead to a reduction in gout symptoms and decrease effects associated with coexisting metabolic syndrome.
- Review Table 39-3 Medications Used in Rheumatic Diseases and Table 39-4 Medications Used to Treat Gout

d. Nursing diagnoses for this patient may include:
- Acute and chronic pain related to inflammation and/or progression of joint deterioration.
- Self-care deficits (specify) related to limitations secondary to progression of disease, pain, fatigue, contractures, and loss of motion.
- Risk for injury related to adverse effects of medications and potential complications.
- Insomnia related to pain, anxiety/stress, depression, and medications.

UNIT ELEVEN
Problems Related to Musculoskeletal Function

a. Evaluative data would include:
- A focus on history and physical examination, including general observation of the patient, back examination, and neurologic testing (reflexes, sensory impairment, muscle strength, straight-leg raising, and muscle atrophy).
- The patient may report pain radiating down the leg, which is known as radiculopathy or sciatica.
- The patient's gait, spinal mobility, reflexes, leg length, leg motor strength, and sensory perception may be affected.

b. Diagnostic procedures that could lead to a definitive diagnosis include:
- X-ray of the spine, CT, MRI, EMG
- See Box 41-1 Diagnostic Procedures for Low Back Pain

c. Medical and nursing management of this patient includes:
- Management focuses on relief of pain and discomfort, activity modification, use of back-conserving techniques of body mechanics, improved self-esteem, and weight reduction.
- Most back pain is self-limited and resolves within 4 weeks with analgesics, rest, stress reduction, and relaxation.
- Pain-guided imagery, nonprescription analgesics, diaphragmatic breathing, and relaxation.
- Mobility-position changes should be made slowly and carried out with assistance as required; avoid twisting and jarring movements; alternate lying, sitting, and walking activities frequently; avoid sitting, standing, or walking for long periods.
- As patient achieves comfort, activities are gradually resumed, and an exercise program is initiated (see Box 41-2, p. 1187).

UNIT TWELVE
Problems Related to Neurologic Function

a. Emergency management of stroke includes:
- Acute stroke care can be divided into two phases: hyperacute phase (the first 24 hours of care) and phase 2 (acute care during the hospitalization).
- An algorithm is used in the hyperacute phase for the initial workup of a patient presenting with acute stroke symptoms (see Fig. 47-6, p. 1363).
- The diagnosis is made by history, neurologic examination, and neuroimaging. An initial head CT will determine whether the patient is experiencing a hemorrhagic stroke.
- The National Institutes of Health Stroke Scale (NIHSS) has become an accepted assessment tool to quantify stroke severity and to assess patient outcome after stroke treatment (see Table 47-4, p. 1366).
- Review Table 47-2 Comparison of Major Types of Stroke.
- Review Box 47-1 Stroke Chain of Survival: The 7 D's.

b. The type of stroke that the patient may be experiencing is an ischemic stroke
- In an ischemic stroke, disruption of the cerebral blood flow due to an obstruction of a blood vessel initiates a complex series of metabolic events referred to as the ischemic cascade.

c. Standardized performance measures for ischemic stroke care include:
- Nonambulatory patients should start receiving DVT prophylaxis by the end of day 2.
- Patient is prescribed antithrombotic therapy at discharge.
- Patients with atrial fibrillation are discharged on anticoagulation.
- Patients with acute ischemic stroke who arrive at the hospital within 180 minutes of time last known well may receive tPA.
- Stroke education, cholesterol-lowering medication.
- Review Table 47-1 Stroke Performance Measures.

d. Nursing considerations for the patient receiving t-PA include:
- The penumbra area may be revitalized by administration of tissue plasminogen activator (tPA), which selectively binds fibrin-converting plasminogen to plasmin, causing clot lysis.
- The initial expedited diagnostic workup and treatment of ischemic stroke is driven by time-dependent pharmacologic and clot retrieval device options.
- Thrombolysis with recombinant tissue plasminogen activator (rtPA) is currently the only FDA-approved drug for acute ischemic stroke within a 3-hour window of symptom onset.

- Once a hemorrhage has been ruled out and the clinical diagnosis of ischemic stroke is made, the acute stroke team must review the eligibility criteria for tPA administration
- Review inclusion/exclusion criteria in Figure 47-7 Acute Stroke Protocol.
- Table 47-5 Schedule of Neurologic Assessment and Vital Signs and Other Acute Care Assessments in Thrombolysis-Treated and Nonthrombolysis-Treated Patients summarizes the nursing care for thrombolysis treatment for patients with acute ischemic stroke.

UNIT THIRTEEN
Problems Related to Sensorineural Function

a. Criterion for a cochlear implant includes:
- At least 1 year of age
- Selected after careful screening by otologic history, physical examination, audiologic testing, x-rays, and psychological testing
  Those that benefit from a cochlear implant include:
- Profound sensorineural hearing loss in both ears
- Inability to hear and recognize speech well with hearing aids
- No medical contraindication to a cochlear implant or general anesthesia
- Indications that being able to hear would enhance the patient's life

b. A cochlear implant involves:
- Implantation of a small receiver in the temporal bone through a postauricular incision and placing electrodes into the inner ear
- The microphone and transmitter are worn on the external ear

c. The rehabilitation period includes:
- Extensive cochlear rehabilitation with the multidisciplinary team, which includes an audiologist and speech pathologist.
- Several months may be needed to interpret the sounds heard.
- Children and adults who lost their hearing before they learned to speak take much longer to acquire speech.

UNIT FOURTEEN
Problems Related to Integumentary Function

a. Nursing management for this patient during the emergent phase of burn injury includes:
- ABCs
- In high-voltage electrical injury, spinal cord injury can result; cervical spine immobilization

- Arrhythmias can occur from electrical injury; cardiac monitoring
- Neurologic assessment
- Management of fluid and electrolyte loss and shock (refer to Table 53-4, p. 1498)
- Secondary head-to-toe assessment
- Note time of injury, source of the burn, how the burn was treated at the scene, and any history of falling with the injury
- History of pre-existing disease, allergies, medications, and the use of drugs, alcohol, and tobacco
- IV analgesia
- Assessment of TBSA and depth of injury
- Baseline height, weight, and labs

b. Graft site care includes:
  - Position and turn carefully to avoid disturbing the graft or putting pressure on the graft site.
  - Elevate extremity to minimize edema.
  - Occlusive dressings may be used to immobilize the graft.

  Donor site care includes:
  - A moist gauze dressing is applied at the time of surgery to maintain pressure and to stop any bleeding
  - During healing, site must remain clean, dry, and free of pressure
  - Heals spontaneously within 7 to 14 days
  - Pain management

c. Long-term complications for this patient include:
  - Hypertrophic scarring
  - Immobility
  - Loss of body image due to disfigurement
  - Psychological and economic impact
  - Pain

UNIT FIFTEEN
Other Acute Problems

a. Treatment measures to reverse MODS are aimed at:
  - Controlling the initiating event
  - Promoting adequate organ perfusion
  - Providing nutritional support
  - The nurse is aware that mortality rates are 40% when two organ systems are involved and persistent dysfunction (>72 hours) in three organ systems can result in a mortality risk of 80%. Commonly affected organs are the kidneys (acute kidney failure) and lungs (acute respiratory distress syndrome).

b. Patient populations at increased risk for developing MODS include:
  - Elderly, those with chronic illness, malnutrition, immunosuppression, or surgical or traumatic wounds
  - Early detection and documentation of initial signs of infection are essential in managing MODS in elderly patients. Subtle changes in mentation and a gradual rise in temperature are early warning signs.

c. Nursing management of the patient with MODS includes:
  - The general plan of nursing care for patient with MODS is the same as that for patients in septic shock.
  - Primary nursing interventions are aimed at supporting the patient and monitoring organ perfusion until primary organ insults are halted.
  - Providing information and support to family members is a critical role of the nurse. The health care team needs to address end-of-life decisions to ensure that supportive therapies are congruent with the patient's wishes.

Index

Page numbers followed by b indicate boxes; those followed by f indicate figures; those followed by t indicate tables.

clinical manifestations and assessment, 1317
definition, 1315
in elderly, 1321
medical and nursing management, 1317–1321
nursing care during, 1319b
nursing process, 1321–1322
pathophysiology of, 1315–1316
Neurologic problems. *See also* Critical care
altered level of consciousness, 1532, 1533t
anxiety, 1533, 1534t
communication, 1534–1535
delirium, 1532
dependency and withdrawal, 1533–1534
pain, 1533
sensory and motor function, 1534
Neurologic trauma, 1287–1313. *See also specific disorders*
altered level of consciousness (LOC) and increased ICP, 1293–1303, 1295f, 1296t–1297t
brain death, 1303
brain injury, 1289–1293, 1290b, 1292
head injuries, 1287–1289, 1288b
spinal cord injury (SCI), 1304–1313, 1306t
Neuropathic ulcers, 1466
Neuropathy, 1466
Neurovascular status, evaluation of
contusions, strains, and sprains, 1210
musculoskeletal system, 1180
Neutropenia, 187
assessment in, 567
from chemotherapy, 173
febrile, management, 188
severity, classification of, 566
Neutrophils, 558, 561
Newest Vital Sign tests, literacy skills, 15
Next-generation gene sequencing, 157
Nicotine replacement therapy (NRT), 349, 414
Nicotinic acid, for hyperlipidemia, 425t
Nightingale, Florence, 2
Nilotinib, 176t
Nipple-areola complex (NAC), 1001
Nipple-areolar reconstruction, 1006
Nitrates, for angina, 428
Nitric oxide (NO), exhaled, 364
Nitrogen wash-out, 291
Nitrogen wasting, 1553–1554
Nitroglycerin
in angina, 428
self-administration of, 428b
Nivolumab, 1487
Nizatidine (Axid), 672
for gastritis and peptic ulcer disease, 693t
Nociception, 199

Nociceptors, 199
Nocturia, 848
Nodular melanoma, 1486
Nodule, in rheumatoid arthritis, 1179
Noise exposure, in jobs, 1427
Noise-induced hearing loss (NIHL), 1426
No light perception (NLP), 1398
Nonalcoholic fatty liver disease (NAFLD), 422, 635, 769
Nonallergic rhinitis, 261–262
medical and nursing management, 262–263
signs and symptoms of, 262
Nondepressed skull fractures, 1289
Nondippers, 404
Nonfunctional cysts, 1024
Nongerminal tumors, 1054
Non-Hodgkin lymphoma (NHL), 605–607
clinical manifestations and assessment, 606
high-grade, 606
incidence, 606
low-grade, 606
medical management, 606
nursing management, 606–607
Non-insulin antidiabetic agents
alpha-glucosidase inhibitors, 913t, 915
biguanides, 912, 913t
DPP-4 inhibitors, 912, 914t
GLP-1 agonists, 912, 914t
nonsulfonylurea insulin secretagogues, 914t, 915
sodium glucose co-transporter-2 (SGLT-2) inhibitors, 912, 914t
sulfonylureas, 913t, 914–915
thiazolidinediones, 914t, 915
Noninvasive positive-pressure ventilation (NIPPV), 357, 1348
Noninvasive ventilator support (NIV), 1543
Nonmodifiable risk factors, in stroke, 1360
Nonmyeloablative allogeneic stem cell transplantation, 179
Nonneoplastic polyps, 737–738
clinical manifestations and assessment, 737–738
medical and nursing management, 738
risk factors, 737
Nonpharmacologic pain management
acupuncture, 225
complementary and alternative medicine (CAM), 225–226
cutaneous stimulation and massage, 223–224
distraction, 224
guided imagery, 224–225
hypnosis, 225
meditation, 225
movement therapy, 225
music therapy, 225

relaxation techniques, 224
thermal therapies, 224
transcutaneous electrical nerve stimulation (TENS), 224
Nonprogressive stage
clinical manifestations and assessment, 1510
medical and nursing management, 1510–1511
pathophysiology, 1510
Nonsedating antihistamine medications, 1464
Nonsmall cell lung cancer (NSCLC), 327, 327t. *See also* Lung cancer
Nonsteroidal antiinflammatory drugs (NSAIDs), 214–215, 217t, 1015, 1143t, 1349–1350, 1424
for allergic and nonallergic rhinitis, 262
fracture healing and, 1219, 1221
for gout, 1150, 1151t
OA management, 1148
for pericarditis, 494
for renal stone pain, 865
rheumatic disorder, 1140
for rhinitis, 262
risk of AKI, 817–818, 821
side effects, 215
systemic, 216
tolerance of, 215
topical, 215
use of, 215
Nonthrombolysis-treated patients, 1368
Nontunneled central catheters, 687–688, 688f
Nonunion, 1219
Nonviral hepatitis
alcoholic hepatitis, 766–767
drug-related hepatitis, 767–768
Norepinephrine, 630t, 1519
Normal anion gap acidosis, 85, 87
Normal fremitus, 278
Normal tension glaucoma, 1403t. *See also* Glaucoma
Normochromic, normocytic anemia, 579
Nosebleed. *See* Epistaxis
Nosocomial infections, 1521
Nothing by mouth (NPO status), 671
Nuchal rigidity, 268, 1323
Nuclear cataract, 1405
Nuclear scans, 807
Nucleic acid amplification tests (NAAT), for chlamydia, 1062
Nucleus pulposus, 1348
Null lymphocytes, 1081
Nurse managers, 5
Nurse Practice Act, 3
Nurse practitioners (NPs), 5
Nurse researchers, 5–6